Inborn Errors of Development

OXFORD MONOGRAPHS ON MEDICAL GENETICS

General Editors

ARNO G. MOTULSKY

MARTIN BOBROW

PETER S. HARPER

CHARLES SCRIVER

CHARLES J. EPSTEIN

JUDITH G. HALL

OXFORD MONOGRAPHS ON MEDICAL GENETICS NO. 49

INBORN ERRORS OF DEVELOPMENT

The Molecular Basis of Clinical Disorders of Morphogenesis

Edited by

Charles J. Epstein, M.D.
Robert P. Erickson, M.D.
Anthony Wynshaw-Boris, M.D., Ph.D.

OXFORD
UNIVERSITY PRESS
2004

OXFORD
UNIVERSITY PRESS

Oxford   New York
Auckland   Bangkok   Buenos Aires   Cape Town   Chennai
Dar es Salaam   Delhi   Hong Kong   Istanbul   Karachi   Kolkata
Kuala Lumpur   Madrid   Melbourne   Mexico City   Mumbai
Nairobi   São Paulo   Shanghai   Taipei   Tokyo   Toronto

Copyright © 2004 by Oxford University Press, Inc.

Published by Oxford University Press, Inc.
198 Madison Avenue, New York, New York, 10016
http://www.oup-usa.org

Oxford is a registered trademark of Oxford University Press

Library of Congress Cataloging-in-Publication Data
Inborn errors of development:
the molecular basis of clinical disorders of morphogenesis
(Oxford monographs on medical genetics: no. 49)
/edited by Charles J. Epstein, Robert P. Erickson, Anthony Wynshaw-Boris.
p. ; cm.   Includes bibliographical references and index.
ISBN 0-19-514502-X
1. Genetic disorders.   2. Developmental disabilities—Genetic aspects.
3. Genetic disorders in children.   4. Developmental genetics.
I. Epstein, Charles J. II. Erickson, Robert P., 1939–   III. Wynshaw-Boris, Anthony Joseph.
[DNLM: 1. Abnormalities—genetics.   2. Genetic Diseases, Inborn—genetics.
3. Human Development.
QZ 50 I35 2004]   RB155.5.I536 2004   616′.042—dc21   2003048693

9 8 7 6 5 4 3 2 1
Printed in Hong Kong
on acid-free paper.

To the memory of
    Tracy Lynn Erickson, 1969–1997
                    Robert P. Erickson

To my wife, Diane
                Anthony Wynshaw-Boris

To Lois
    David & Abigail, Jonathan & Teresa,
        Paul & Jennifer, and Joanna
    and most especially
        Jeffrey, Kendra, Jacqueline,
        Genevieve, Violet, and Simon
    who are the hope for the future
                  Charles J. Epstein

Preface

Disorders that affect tissue differentiation, organogenesis, and morphogenesis constitute a significant component of human hereditary disease. These disorders may occur singly or in combination, and their investigation has given rise to the clinical field of dysmorphology. Beginning with David Smith and his seminal work, *Recognizable Patterns of Human Malformations*, dysmorphologists have delineated a large number of multiple malformation syndromes which are often comprised of malformations that affect disparate and seemingly unrelated organs and tissues. Despite a considerable amount of embryological investigation, it has not, however, been possible to begin to understand their causes and pathogenesis until very recently. Two groups of scientific advances have converged to make this new dysmorphology possible. The first is the advances in gene mapping, cloning, and identification which have been fueled by the Human Genome Project. These have greatly facilitated the identification of mutations in human genes that are associated with particular syndromes. They have also permitted comparisons between the human genome and the genomes of other organisms such as mouse and *Drosophila* that have proven to be so valuable both for identifying genes and for understanding what they do. The second group of advances stems from the growing elucidation of the many highly interactive molecular pathways that govern developmental processes. Taken together, these advances are making it possible to discover the genetic bases of an increasing number of human disorders of development and morphogenesis and to establish the links between genotype and phenotype.

It had long been our desire to publish an in-depth analysis of the human syndromes of abnormal morphogenesis for which the responsible genes have been identified, but it was only with the advances just cited that this has become possible. In conceptualizing the approach to be taken in organizing such a volume—indeed, in understanding the entire subject—we were very much influenced by Garrod's concept of inborn errors of metabolism and its profound effect on our understanding of the human biochemical disorders. The relationship between a genetic defect and its ultimate metabolic or biochemical consequences could be understood in terms of the biochemical pathway in which the gene product, usually an enzyme, functioned. Given the fact that the genes involved in development and morphogenesis must also operate within biochemical pathways, although not necessarily enzymatic ones, we and others (see Chapter 1) espoused the notion of inborn errors of development or morphogenesis as a parallel concept to inborn errors of metabolism well before such developmental pathways had actually been elucidated. Although time has proven this approach to be a valid one, it must be acknowledged that the distinction between the two categories of inborn errors has been made more for the sake of organizing thought and presenting information than representing some inherent dichotomy. Ultimately, the pathways that mediate the errors of metabolism and the errors of morphogenesis are components of the overall universe of the expression and interactions of genes and of their products.

PREFACE

The book begins with introductory chapters on congenital malformations and approaches to their understanding, the general principles of differentiation and morphogenesis, model organisms, and the role of the genome project in understanding development. This is followed by a series of 11 chapters on the development of the body plan and of individual tissues and organ systems. The rest of the book is devoted to more than one hundred clinical genetic disorders. These clinical chapters are organized into sections by defined developmental pathways, gene families, or biochemical processes and functions, and almost all of these sections are preceded by a general overview. We adopted the pathway approach described above and grouped the clinical disorders by pathway whenever possible. Thus, sections are devoted to the sonic hedgehog, Wnt (wingless-type), transforming growth factor β, tumor necrosis factor, fibroblast growth factor, glial cell–derived neurotrophic growth factor, endothelin, notch, and sex determination signaling pathways. The many disorders that cannot yet be placed within a specific pathway are grouped according to either the gene families to which the responsible genes belong (homeobox, paired-box, forkhead, T-box) or the processes or functions in which the genes are involved (regulation of chromatin structure and gene expression, transcription factors, posttranslational control and ubiquination, guanine nucleotide–binding proteins, kinases and phosphatases, microtubule motors and cytoskeleton, extracellular matrix, angiogenesis, and transporters).

For each disorder there are descriptions of the disease-causing genes, the role of these genes in development as elucidated in humans and in model organisms, the human mutations that have been identified, and the clinical disorders they cause, along with considerations of therapy and counseling. Each of the clinical chapters concludes with a discussion of the developmental pathogenesis of the condition. It is this discussion, which often proved difficult to write, that tells us how well the link between genotype and phenotype is truly understood.

This book is written for physicians, dentists, genetic counselors, and other health professionals interested in going beyond clinical descriptions of multiple malformation syndromes to gain an understanding of their genetic basis and pathogenesis. It is also intended for basic scientists and students interested in developmental processes and in the human disorders that result from genetic perturbations that affect them.

The good counsel and encouragement of Jeffrey House of Oxford University Press have been much appreciated, as have been the efforts of Leslie Anglin and Ellen Repalda, also of Oxford University Press. We thank Mss. Carole Meyer, Carolyn Henley, Donelle Myers, Debbie Beiley, and Rashaan Lyons for secretarial assistance and Greg Barsh for his advice. Support for the production of this book was received from the Haas Genetics Research Fund.

One of us (R.P.E.) wishes to thank his early mentors in genetics, Tahir Rizki, Leonard and Leonore Herzenberg, and Salome G. Waelsch, for recruiting him to the field, and co-editor Charles J. Epstein and colleague Bryan Hall who guided his education in the clinical aspects of the genetic disorders of development. Above all, he thanks his wife, Sandra, the value of whose support cannot be adequately expressed.

San Francisco, California
Tucson, Arizona
La Jolla, California

C.J.E.
R.P.E.
A.W.-B.

Contents

CONTENTS

Contents

CONTENTS

Part D. Guanine Nucleotide–Binding Proteins

Part E. Kinases and Phosphatases

Part F. Microtubule Motors and Cytoskeleton

Part G. Extracellular Matrix

Contributors

HARUHIKO AKIYAMA, M.D., Ph.D.
Department of Molecular Genetics
The University of Texas
M.D. Anderson Cancer Center
Houston, Texas

KARI ALITALO, M.D., Ph.D.
Molecular/Cancer Biology Laboratory
Haartman Institute and Helsinki
University Central Hospital
University of Helsinki
Helsinki, Finland

MICHAEL J. BAMSHAD, M.D.
Departments of Pediatrics and of Human Genetics
Eccles Institute of Human Genetics
University of Utah
Salt Lake City, Utah

ELENA BELLONI
IFOM (FIRC Institute for Molecular Oncology)
European Institute of Oncology
Milan, Italy

JOHN W. BELMONT, M.D., Ph.D.
Department of Molecular and Human Genetics
Baylor College of Medicine
Houston, Texas

JONATHAN N. BERG, M.D.
Division of Medical and Molecular Genetics
GKT School of Medicine
King's College
London, United Kingdom

FRED B. BERRY, Ph.D.
Departments of Ophthalmology and Medical Genetics
University of Alberta
Edmonton, Alberta, Canada

ETHAN BIER, Ph.D.
Section of Cell and Developmental Biology
Division of Biological Sciences
University of California, San Diego
La Jolla, California

LESLIE G. BIESECKER, M.D.
Genetic Disease Research Branch
Nation Human Genome Research Institute
National Institutes of Health
Bethesda, Maryland

DEBORAH BOURC'HIS, Ph.D.
Institut Jacques Monod
Paris, France

MARTIJN H. BREUNING, M.D., Ph.D.
Department of Clinical Genetics
Leiden University Medical Center
Leiden, The Netherlands

CHRISTOPHER B. BROWN, Ph.D.
Cardiovascular Division
Department of Medicine
University of Pennsylvania Health System
Philadelphia, Pennsylvania

DONALD T. BROWN, D.D.S., M.S.
Covington, Louisiana

RIVKA CARMI, M.D.
Institute of Genetics
Ben Gurion University of the Negav
Negav, Israel

SUZANNE B. CASSIDY, M.D.
Division of Human Genetics
Department of Pediatrics
University of California, Irvine
Orange, California

CONTRIBUTORS

ARAVINDA CHAKRAVARTI, Ph.D.
McKusick-Nathans Institute of Genetic Medicine
Johns Hopkins University School of Medicine
Baltimore, Maryland

M. MICHAEL COHEN, JR., M.D., Ph.D., FCCMG
Department of Pediatrics
Dalhousie University
Halifax, Nova Scotia, Canada

DANIEL H. COHN, Ph.D.
Medical Genetics
Cedars-Sinai Research Institute
Departments of Human Genetics and Pediatrics
David Geffen School of Medicine
University of California, Los Angeles
Los Angeles, California

FRANS P.M. CREMERS, Ph.D.
Department of Human Genetics
University Medical Center Nijmegen
Nijmegen, The Netherlands

COR W.R.J. CREMERS, M.D., Ph.D.
Department of Otorhinolaryngology
University Medical Center Nijmegen
Nijmegen, The Netherlands

MEHUL T. DATTANI, FRCP, M.D.
Biochemistry, Endocrinology, and Metabolism Unit
Institute of Child Health
University College-London
London, England

MICHAEL R. DeBAUN, M.D., M.P.H.
Department of Pediatrics
Washington University School of Medicine
St. Louis Children's Hospital
St. Louis, Missouri

BENOIT DE CROMBRUGGHE, M.D.
Department of Molecular Genetics
The University of Texas
M.D. Anderson Cancer Center
Houston, Texas

JEAN-PIERRE DELAUNOY, Ph.D.
Laboratoire de Diagnostic Génétique
Faculte de Medecine et CHUR
Strasbourg, France

JILL DIXON, M.PHIL., Ph.D.
School of Biological Sciences
University of Manchester
Manchester, United Kingdom

MICHAEL J. DIXON, Ph.D., BDS
Department of Dental Medicine and Surgery
School of Biological Sciences
University of Manchester
Manchester, United Kingdom

OONAGH DOWLING, Ph.D.
Department of Human Genetics
Mount Sinai School of Medicine
New York, New York

MICHAEL R. ECCLES, Ph.D.
Department of Pathology
University of Otago
Dunedin, New Zealand

JAY W. ELLISON, M.D., Ph.D.
Department of Medical Genetics
Mayo Clinic
Rochester, Minnesota

WOLFGANG ENGEL, M.D.
Institute for Human Genetics
University of Göttingen
Göttingen, Germany

CHARLES J. EPSTEIN, M.D.
Department of Pediatrics
University of California, San Francisco
San Francisco, California

ERVIN EPSTEIN, JR., M.D.
Department of Dermatology
University of California, San Francisco
San Francisco, California

JONATHAN A. EPSTEIN, M.D.
Cardiovascular Division
University of Pennsylvania
Philadelphia, Pennsylvania

ROBERT P. ERICKSON, M.D.
Department of Pediatrics
University of Arizona
Tucson, Arizona

VERARAGAVAN P. ESWARAKUMAR, Ph.D.
Department of Pharmacology
Yale University School of Medicine
New Haven, Connecticut

ANDREW P. FEINBERG, M.D., M.P.H.
Department of Medicine, Oncology, and Molecular Biology &
  Genetics
Johns Hopkins University School of Medicine
Baltimore, Maryland

DONNA M. FEKETE, Ph.D.
Department of Biological Sciences
Purdue University
West Lafayette, Indiana

ROBERT E. FERRELL, Ph.D.
Department of Human Genetics
University of Pittsburgh
Pittsburgh, Pennsylvania

DAVID N. FINEGOLD, M.D.
Departments of Pediatrics and Medicine
School of Medicine
University of Pittsburgh
Pittsburgh, Pennsylvania

MARK C. FISHMAN, M.D.
Novartis Institutes for BioMedical Research
Cambridge, Massachusetts

BERTRAND FONTAINE, M.D., Ph.D.
INSERM
Fédération de Neurologie
Faculté de Médecine Pitié-Salpêtrière
Paris, France

JEAN-PIERRE FRYNS, M.D., Ph.D.
Center of Human Genetics
University Hospital Gasthuisberg
Leuven, Belgium

KAZUHITO FUKUOKA, M.D.
Department of Medicine
University of California, San Diego
La Jolla, California

CHERYL E. GARIEPY, M.D.
Department of Pediatrics and Communicable Diseases
University of Michigan
Ann Arbor, Michigan

BRUCE D. GELB, M.D.
Departments of Pediatrics and Human Genetics
Mount Sinai School of Medicine
New York, New York

RICHARD J. GIBBONS, M.D., Ph.D.
MRC Molecular Haematology Unit
Weatherall Institute of Molecular Medicine
University of Oxford
John Radcliffe Hospital
Oxford, United Kingdom

SCOTT F. GILBERT, Ph.D.
Department of Biology
Swarthmore College
Swarthmore, Pennsylvania

RACHEL H. GILES, Ph.D.
Department of Experimental Oncology
University Medical Center
Utrecht, The Netherlands

DAVID GIVOL, Ph.D.
Department of Molecular Cell Biology
Weizmann Institute of Science
Rehovot, Israel

CHRISTOPHER K. GLASS, M.D., Ph.D.
Department of Cellular and Molecular Medicine
University of California, San Diego
La Jolla, California

JOSEPH G. GLEESON, M.D.
Department of Neurosciences
University of California, San Diego
School of Medicine
La Jolla, California

SARAH N. GOLDIN, Ph.D.
Department of Genetics and Development
College of Physicians and Surgeons of Columbia University
New York, New York

FRANCES R. GOODMAN, Ph.D.
Molecular Medicine Unit
Institute of Child Health
London, United Kingdom

JEROME L. GORSKI, M.D.
Department of Pediatrics
University of Michigan School of Medicine
Ann Arbor, Michigan

PETER GRUSS, M.D., Ph.D.
Max-Planck Society
Munich, Germany

DAVID H. GUTMANN, M.D., Ph.D.
Department of Neurology
Washington University School of Medicine
St. Louis, Missouri

JOEL F. HABENER, M.D.
Laboratory of Molecular Endocrinology
Howard Hughes Medical Institute
Massachusetts General Hospital and Harvard Medical School
Boston, Massachusetts

ANDRÉ HANAUER, Ph.D.
Department of Molecular Pathology
Université Louis Pasteur de Strasbourg
Institut de Génétique et de Biologie
Moléculaire et Cellulaire (IGBMC)
Illkirch, France

RAOUL C.M. HENNEKAM, M.D., Ph.D.
Department of Pediatrics
Academic Medical Center
University of Amsterdam
The Netherlands

ELISE HEON, M.D., FRCS(C)
Department of Opthalmology
University of Toronto
Toronto, Canada

OLA HERMANSON, Ph.D.
Department of Cell and Molecular Biology (CMB)
Medical Nobel Institute
Karolinska Institute
Stockholm, Sweden

ROBERT M.W. HOFSTRA, Ph.D.
Department of Medical Genetics
University of Groningen
Groningen, The Netherlands

JEFFREY W. INNIS, M.D., Ph.D.
Departments of Pediatrics and Human Genetics
University of Michigan
School of Medicine
Ann Arbor, Michigan

MIRA IRONS, M.D.
Division of Genetics
Children's Hospital
Harvard Medical School
Boston, Massachusetts

SEIGO IZUMO, M.D.
Department of Medicine
Beth Israel Deaconess Medical Center
Harvard Medical School
Boston, Massachusetts

ETHYLIN WANG JABS, M.D.
Departments of Pediatrics, Medicine, and Plastic Surgery
Johns Hopkins University School of Medicine
Baltimore, Maryland

PETER K. JACKSON, Ph.D.
Department of Pathology
Stanford University School of Medicine
Stanford, California

SYLVIE JACQUOT, Ph.D.
Department of Molecular Pathology
Institut de Génétique et de Biologie
Moléculaire et Cellulaire (IGBMC)
Illkirch, France

LAURA A. JANSEN, M.D., Ph.D.
Department of Neurology
Washington University School of Medicine
St. Louis Children's Hospital
St. Louis, Missouri

PATRICK Y. JAY, M.D., Ph.D.
Department of Cardiology
Children's Hospital
Harvard Medical School
Boston, Massachusetts

KRISTEN JEPSEN, Ph.D.
Department of Medicine
University of California, San Diego
School of Medicine
La Jolla, CA

LYNNE B. JORDE, Ph.D.
Department of Human Genetics
University of Utah
Salt Lake City, Utah

MARIKA J. KARKKAINEN, Ph.D.
Molecular/Cancer Biology Laboratory
Haartman Institute and Helsinki
University Central Hospital
University of Helsinki
Helsinki, Finland

MICHAEL W. KILPATRICK, Ph.D.
Department of Pediatrics
University of Connecticut Health Center
Farmington, Connecticut

SCOTT E. KLEWER, M.D.
Department of Pediatrics
Steele Memorial Children's Research Center
University of Arizona
Tucson, Arizona

JÜRGEN KOHLHASE, M.D.
Institute for Human Genetics
University of Göttingen
Göttingen, Germany

IAN D. KRANTZ, M.D.
Division of Human Genetics and Molecular Biology
Department of Pediatrics
University of Pennsylvania School of Medicine
Philadelphia, Pennsylvania

KENRO KUSUMI, Ph.D.
Division of Human Genetics & Molecular Biology &
*   Orthopaedic Surgery*
Department of Pediatrics
University of Pennsylvania School of Medicine
Philadelphia, Pennsylvania

DAVID J. KWIATKOWSKI, M.D., Ph.D.
Genetics Laboratory, Hematology Division
Brigham and Women's Hospital
Harvard Medical School
Boston, Massachusetts

DEBORAH LANG, Ph.D.
Cardiovascular Division
Department of Medicine
University of Pennsylvania Health System
Philadelphia, Pennsylvania

FRANCOISE LEDEIST, M.D., Ph.D.
Laboratory of Paediatric Ommunology
Necker-Enfants Malades
Paris, France

BRENDAN LEE, M.D., Ph.D.
Howard Hughes Medical Institute
Department of Molecular and Human Genetics
Baylor College of Medicine
Houston, Texas

PETER LONAI, MVD
Department of Molecular Genetics
The Weizmann Institute of Science
Rehovot, Israel

RICHARD L. MAAS, M.D., Ph.D.
Division of Genetics
Department of Medicine
Brigham and Women's Hospital
Harvard Medical School
Boston, Massachusetts

EAMONN R. MAHER, M.D., FRCP
Section of Medical and Molecular Genetics
University of Birmingham Medical School
Birmingham, United Kingdom

SAHAR MANSOUR, BMBS, MRCP
South-West Thames Regional Genetic Service
St. George's Hospital Medical School
London, United Kingdom

DOUGLAS A. MARCHUK, Ph.D.
Department of Genetics
Duke University Medical Center
Durham, North Carolina

JOHN A. MARTIGNETTI, M.D., Ph.D.
Department of Human Genetics
Mount Sinai School of Medicine
New York, New York

RICK A. MARTIN, M.D.
Department of Pediatrics
Washington University School of Medicine
St. Louis Children's Hospital
St. Louis, Missouri

GIUSEPPE MARTUCCIELLO, M.D.
Divisione e Cattedra di Chirugia Pediatrica
Istituto G Gaslini
Genova, Italy

EDWARD R.B. MCCABE, M.D., Ph.D.
Department of Pediatrics
David Geffen School of Medicine
University of California, Los Angeles
Los Angeles, California

ANDREW S. MCCALLION, Ph.D.
McKusick-Nathans Institute of Genetic Medicine
Johns Hopkins University School of Medicine
Baltimore, Maryland

SHAWN E. MCCANDLESS, M.D.
Department of Pediatrics
University of North Carolina School of Medicine
Chapel Hill, North Carolina

WILLIAM MCGINNIS, Ph.D.
Section of Cell and Developmental Biology
Division of Biological Sciences
University of California, San Diego
La Jolla, California

DOUGLAS A. MELTON, Ph.D.
Department of Molecular and Cellular Biology
Howard Hughes Medical Institute
Harvard University
Cambridge, Massachusetts

STANLEY A. MENDOZA, M.D.
Department of Pediatrics
University of California, San Diego
La Jolla, California

NAOYUKI MIURA, M.D., Ph.D.
Department of Biochemistry
Hamamatsu University School of Medicine
Hamamatsu, Japan

ALISON MIYAMOTO, Ph.D.
Department of Biological Chemistry
David Geffen School of Medicine
University of California, Los Angeles
Los Angeles, California

RANDALL T. MOON, Ph.D.
Department of Pharmacology
Center for Developmental Biology
University of Washington
Seattle, Washington

ROY MORELLO, Ph.D.
Department of Molecular and Human Genetics
Baylor College of Medicine
Houston, Texas

DAVID W. MOUNT, Ph.D.
Department of Molecular and Cellular Biology
University of Arizona
Tucson, Arizona

ROBERT T. MOY
Division of Genetics
Department of Medicine
Brigham and Women's Hospital
Harvard Medical School
Boston, Massachusetts

ULRICH MÜLLER, M.D., Ph.D.
Institut für Humangenetik
Justus-Liebig-Universität
Giessen, Germany

SHUNICHI MURAKAMI, M.D., Ph.D.
Department of Molecular Genetics
The University of Texas
M.D. Anderson Cancer Center
Houston, Texas

SARAH E. NEWEY, D.PHIL.
Cold Spring Harbor Laboratory
Cold Spring Harbor, New York

SOPHIE NICOLE, Ph.D.
INSERM
Faculté de Médecine Pitié-Salpêtrière
Paris, France

SANJAY K. NIGAM, M.D.
Departments of Pediatrics, Medicine, and Cellular
* Molecular Medicine*
University of California, San Diego
La Jolla, California

SAHAR NISSIM
Department of Genetics
Harvard Medical School
Boston, Massachusetts

PETER NÜRNBERG, Ph.D.
Gene Mapping Center (GMC)
Max Delbrueck Center for Molecular Medicine
Berlin, Germany

MICHAEL B. O'CONNOR, Ph.D.
Departments of Genetics, Cell Biology, and Development
Howard Hughes Medical Institute
University of Minnesota
Minneapolis, Minnesota

ATSUSHI OHAZAMA, DDS, Ph.D.
Department of Craniofacial Development
Kings College London
Guy's Hospital
London, United Kingdom

MICHAEL OLDRIDGE, DPhil
Weatherall Institute of Molecular Medicine
John Radcliffe Hospital
Oxford, United Kingdom

VIRGINIA E. PAPAIOANNOU, Ph.D.
Department of Genetics and Development
College of Physicians and Surgeons of Columbia University
New York, New York

PRAGNA I. PATEL, Ph.D.
Departments of Neurology, and Molecular and Human Genetics
Baylor College of Medicine
Houston, Texas

ROGER A. PEDERSEN, Ph.D.
Department of Surgery
Addenbrooke's Hospital
University of Cambridge
Cambridge, United Kingdom

FRED PETRIJ, M.D., Ph.D.
Department of Clinical Genetics
Erasmus University Medical Center
Rotterdam, The Netherlands

PETROS PETROU, Ph.D.
Department of Biology
IMBB—University of Crete
Crete, Greece

ANNA PETRYK, M.D.
Department of Pediatrics
University of Minnesota
Minneapolis, Minnesota

JEAN-YVES PICARD, Ph.D.
Developmental Endocrinology
INSERM U493
Clamart, France

ANDREW J. POWELL, M.D.
Department of Cardiology
Children's Hospital
Harvard Medical School
Boston, Massachusetts

LOUIS J. PTÁČEK, M.D.
Department of Neurology
Program in Human Genetics
Howard Hughes Medical Institute
University of California, San Francisco
San Francisco, California

LUIS PUELLES, M.D., Ph.D.
Department of Morphological Sciences
University of Murcia School of Medicine
Murcia, Spain

ALAN RAWLS, Ph.D.
Department of Biology
Arizona State University
Tempe, Arizona

ANDREW READ, Ph.D.
Department of Medical Genetics
St. Mary's Hospital
University of Manchester
Manchester, United Kingdom

LOUIS F. REICHARDT, Ph.D.
Departments of Physiology and Biochemistry and Biophysics
Howard Hughes Medical Institute
University of California, San Francisco
San Francisco, California

DAVID R. RENNER, M.D.
Department of Neurology
University of Utah School of Medicine
Salt Lake City, Utah

JERRY M. RHEE, Ph.D.
Department of Biology
Arizona State University
Tempe, Arizona

MICHAEL G. ROSENFELD, M.D.
Howard Hughes Medical Institute
Department of Medicine
University of California, San Diego
La Jolla, California

WOLFGANG ROTTBAUER, M.D.
Department of Internal Medicine
Cardiovascular Division
University of Heidelberg
Heidelberg, Germany

JOHN L. R. RUBENSTEIN, M.D., Ph.D.
Center for Neurobiology and Psychiatry
Department of Psychiatry
University of California, San Francisco
San Francisco, California

FRANK H. RUDDLE, Ph.D.
Department of Molecular, Cellular, and Developmental Biology
Yale University
New Haven, Connecticut

RAYMOND B. RUNYAN, Ph.D.
Department of Cell Biology and Anatomy
Steele Memorial Children's Research Center
University of Arizona
Tucson, Arizona

RAMSEY A. SALEEM, B.SC.
Departments of Ophthalmology and Medical Genetics
University of Alberta,
Edmonton, Alberta, Canada

MASAHIKO SATODA, M.D.
Departments of Pediatrics and Human Genetics
Mount Sinai School of Medicine
New York, NY

SCOTT SAUNDERS, M.D., Ph.D.
Departments of Pediatrics and Molecular Biology and Pharmacology
Washington University School of Medicine and St. Louis
Children's Hospital
St. Louis, Missouri

PETER J. SCAMBLER, M.D.
Molecular Medicine Unit
Institute of Child Health
London, United Kingdom

STEPHEN SCHERER, Ph.D.
Department of Genetics
Hospital for Sick Children
Toronto, Ontario, Canada

PASCAL SCHNEIDER, Ph.D.
Institute of Biochemistry
University of Lausanne
Epalinges, Switzerland

CONNIE SCHRANDER-STUMPEL, M.D., Ph.D.
Research Institute Growth and Development
Maastricht University
Maastricht, The Netherlands

SCOTT B. SELLECK, M.D., Ph.D.
Departments of Pediatrics and Genetics, Cell Biology
and Development
University of Minnesota
Minneapolis, Minnesota

ELENA V. SEMINA, Ph.D.
Department of Pediatrics and Human and Molecular Genetics Center
Medical College of Wisconsin
Milwaukee, Wisconsin

PAUL T. SHARPE, Ph.D.
Department of Craniofacial Development
Kings College London
Guy's Hospital
London, United Kingdom

VAL C. SHEFFIELD, M.D., Ph.D.
Department of Pediatrics
Division of Medical Genetics
Howard Hughes Medical Institute
University of Iowa College of Medicine
Iowa City, Iowa

LAIRD C. SHELDAHL, Ph.D.
Department of Pharmacology and Center for Development Biology
University of Washington
Seattle, Washington

MICHAEL M. SHEN, Ph.D.
Center for Advanced Biotechnology and Medicine
Department of Pediatrics
UMDNJ-Robert Wood Johnson Medical School
Piscataway, New Jersey

MEGAN C. SHERWOOD, M.D.
Department of Cardiology
Children's Hospital
Harvard Medical School
Boston, Massachusetts

NANCY B. SPINNER, Ph.D.
Division of Human Genetics and Molecular Biology
Department of Pediatrics
University of Pennsylvania School of Medicine
Philadelphia, Pennsylvania

BEN Z. STANGER, M.D., Ph.D.
Department of Molecular and Cellular Biology
Harvard University
Cambridge, Massachusetts

DYLAN STEER, M.D.
Division of Nephrology–Hypertension
Department of Medicine
University of California, San Diego
San Diego, California

EDWIN M. STONE, M.D., Ph.D.
Department of Opthamology and Visual Sciences
University of Iowa College of Medicine
Iowa City, Iowa

SALLY E. STRINGER, Ph.D.
Departments of Pediatrics and Genetics, Cell Biology
  and Development
University of Minnesota
Minneapolis, Minnesota

WAFAA SUWAIRI, M.D.
Department of Pediatrics
Riyadh Armed Forces Hospital
Riyadh, Saudi Arabia

CLIFF TABIN, Ph.D.
Department of Genetics
Harvard Medical School
Boston, Massachusetts

MASAYOSHI TACHIBANA, M.D., Ph.D.
Genome Science Branch
Center for Bioresource-Based Research
Brain Research Institute
Niigata University
Niigata, Japan

TOMOKI TAMAKOSHI, M.AGRI.
Department of Biochemistry
Hamamatsu University School of Medicine
Hamamatsu, Japan

MARCO TARTAGLIA, Ph.D.
Laboratorio di Metabolismo e Biochimica Patologica
Istituto Superiore di Sanità
Rome, Italy

RABI TAWIL, M.D.
Department of Neurology
University of Rochester Medical Center
Rochester, New York

MELISSA K. THOMAS, M.D., Ph.D.
Molecular Endocrinology and Diabetes Units
Massachusetts General Hospital
Harvard Medical School
Boston, Massachusetts

SIGRID TINSCHERT, M.D.
Institute for Medical Genetics
Charite Medical School
Humboldt University
Berlin, Germany

MICHELE TORRE, M.D.
Divisione e Cattedra di Chirurgia Pediatrica
Istituto G Gaslini
Genova, Italy

MARTIN TRISTANI-FIROUZI, M.D.
Department of Pediatrics
University of Utah Health Science Center
Salt Lake City, Utah

PETROS TSIPOURAS, M.D.
Department of Pediatrics
University of Connecticut Health Center
Farmington, Connecticut

PETER D. TURNPENNY, BSc, FRCP, FRCPCH
Department of Clinical Genetics
Royal Devon and Exeter Hospital
Exeter, United Kingdom

LINDA VAN AELST, Ph.D.
Cold Spring Harbor Laboratory
Cold Spring Harbor, New York

MARIE-JOSÉ H. VAN DEN BOOGAARD, M.Sc.
Department of Medical Genetics
Wilhelmina Children's Hospital
University Medical Centre
Utrecht, The Netherlands

VERONICA VAN HEYNINGEN, DPHIL, FRSE, FMEDSCI
MRC Human Genetics Unit
Western General Hospital
Edinburgh, Scotland

JOKE B.G.M. VERHEIJ, M.D.
Department of Medical Genetics
University Hospital Groningen
Groningen, The Netherlands

EVANI VIEGAS-PÉQUIGNOT, M.D.
INSERM
Institut Jacques Monad
Paris, France

MIIKKA VIKKULA, M.D., Ph.D.
Laboratory of Human Molecular Genetics
Christian de Duve Institute and Université catholique de Louvain
Brussels, Belgium

CONTRIBUTORS

ERIC VILAIN, M.D., Ph.D.
Department of Human Genetics
David Geffen School of Medicine
University of California, Los Angeles
Los Angeles, California

TAKAHITO WADA, M.D., Ph.D.
MRC Molecular Haematology Unit
Weatherall Institute of Molecular Medicine
University of Oxford
John Radcliffe Hospital
Oxford, United Kingdom

JOSEPH WAGSTAFF, M.D., Ph.D.
Departments of Pediatrics and Biochemistry &
*   Molecular Genetics*
University of Virginia Health System
Charlottesville, Virginia

CHRISTOPHER A. WALSH, M.D., Ph.D.
Howard Hughes Medical Institute
Department of Neurology
Beth Israel Deaconess Medical Center
Harvard Medical School
Boston, Massachusetts

MICHAEL A. WALTER, Ph.D.
Departments of Ophthalmology and Medical Genetics
University of Alberta
Edmonton, Alberta, Canada

TAO WANG, Ph.D.
Department of Biochemistry
Hamamatsu University School of Medicine
Hamamatsu, Japan

STEPHANIE M. WARE, M.D., Ph.D.
Department of Molecular and Human Genetics
Baylor College of Medicine
Houston, Texas

MATTHEW L. WARMAN, M.D.
Department of Genetics
Case Western Reserve University
School of Medicine
Cleveland, Ohio

GERRY WEINMASTER, Ph.D.
Department of Biological Chemistry
David Geffen School of Medicine
University of California, Los Angeles
Los Angeles, California

LEE S. WEINSTEIN, M.D.
Metabolic Diseases Branch
NIDDK, NIH
Bethesda, Maryland

ANDREW O.M. WILKIE, DM, FRCP
Weatherall Institute of Molecular Medicine
John Radcliffe Hospital
Oxford, United Kingdom

KATHLEEN WILLIAMSON, Ph.D.
MRC Human Genetics Unit
Western General Hospital
Edinburgh, Scotland

MICHAL WITT, M.D., Ph.D.
Institute of Human Genetics
Polish Academy of Sciences
Division of Molecular and Clinical Genetics
Poznań, Poland

KATHRYN WOODS, Ph.D.
Biochemistry, Endocrinology, and Metabolism Unit
Institute of Child Health
London, United Kingdom

ANTHONY WYNSHAW-BORIS, M.D., Ph.D.
Departments of Pediatrics and Medicine
School of Medicine
University of California, San Diego
La Jolla, California

MASASHI YANAGISAWA, M.D., Ph.D.
Department of Molecular Genetics
Howard Hughes Medical Institute
University of Texas Southwestern Medical Center
Dallas, Texas

MARIA ZENIOU, Ph.D.
Department of Molecular Pathology
Institut de Génétique et de Biologie
Moleculaire et Cellulaire (IGBMC)
Illkirch, France

GUANG ZHOU, Ph.D.
Department of Molecular and Human Genetics
Baylor College of Medicine
Houston, Texas

JONATHAN ZONANA, M.D.
Departments of Molecular and Medical Genetics, Pediatrics
Oregon Health Sciences University
Portland, Oregon

I
GENERAL CONCEPTS

1 | Human Malformations and Their Genetic Basis

CHARLES J. EPSTEIN

Of the many problems encountered in the practice of clinical genetics, perhaps the most perplexing, in terms of understanding pathogenesis, have been the conditions characterized by the presence of congenital malformations. Winter (1996) estimated that about 1 in 40 (2.5%) newborns has recognizable congenital abnormalities at birth. These occur singly half the time and half the time as multiple malformations. It has also been estimated that of the more than 1750 inherited human disorders which result in altered morphogenesis, over 1000 are multiple malformation syndromes (Wilson, 1992).

There are several other estimates that place the medical implications of congenital malformations of all etiologies in perspective. Thus, 20%–30% of all infant deaths and 30%–50% of deaths occurring after the neonatal period have been attributed to congenital abnormalities (Berry et al., 1987; Hoekelman and Pless, 1988). The infant death rate for children with a reportable birth defect, which includes chromosomal abnormalities, was 3.9% in Michigan in 1999, a 4.9-fold relative increase over the normal rate (Division for Vital Records and Health Statistics, 2002). Similar increases (4.4- to 4.8-fold) in relative risk were seen for the first 2 and 8 years of life. Incidence rates of the leading categories of structural birth defects have been estimated at 0.87% for heart and circulation, 0.77% for muscles and skeleton, 0.74% for genital and urinary tract, 0.43% for nervous system and eye, 0.14% for club foot, and 0.11% for cleft lip and/or palate (March of Dimes Perinatal Data Center, 2000a). Of the 22.0% of infant deaths attributed to birth defects, 28.2% affected the heart, 12.2% the nervous system, 5.9% the genitourinary tract, and 7.3% the musculoskeletal system (March of Dimes Perinatal Data Center, 2000b). In a survey of admissions to a children's hospital carried out 40 years ago, about 10% were for known genetic conditions of all types and 18% were for congenital defects that were not known to be mendelian or chromosomal in origin (Clow et al., 1973). About 40% of the surgical admissions were for congenital malformations. The latter figure is likely to be too low by current standards, given the large number of surgeries now being performed for congenital heart defects and other previously inoperable conditions.

CLASSIFICATIONS OF MALFORMATIONS

Although both can affect structure, malformations are generally distinguished from dysplasias. *Malformations,* which affect organs or parts of the body, usually large, are considered to result from the abnormal formation of tissues, whereas *dysplasias* are considered to result from the abnormal organization of cells into tissues. In the latter instance, structural abnormalities are the result of aberrant development of a particular tissue type, such as bone or cartilage. Another term, *dyshistogenesis,* is sometimes used in place of *dysplasia,* and Cohen (1997) suggested that it be preferred because of the broad range of senses in which *dysplasia* is often used. Dysplasias (dyshistogeneses) are often apparent at birth but may also change or alter over time as growth proceeds. With regard to skeletal disorders, *osteodysplasias,* which are developmental disorders of chondro-osseous tissues, have been distinguished from *dysostoses,* which are malformations of individual bones or groups of bones (Superti-Furga et al., 2002). However, the distinction is not absolute. Similarly, the distinction between malformations and dysplasias, while useful, is also not absolute; and persons with dysplastic syndromes are often referred to as having malformations.

It is also necessary to discriminate malformations from two other groups of anomalies that can occur in organs and parts of the body, deformations and disruptions. *Deformations* have mechanical causes, such as compression from intrauterine constraint, as of the head in plagiocephaly caused by structural abnormalities of the uterus, or may be the result of abnormal function, as in arthrogryposis, resulting from congenital myopathies. Deformations can also occur secondary to malformations, such as with club feet being caused by spina bifida because of interference with the nerves to the legs. By contrast, *disruptions*, which are associated with tissue damage, result from the breakdown of otherwise normal structures because of factors such as interference with blood supply, anoxia, infection, or mechanical forces. Whereas disruptions may occur during embryonic or fetal life, deformations are usually caused by factors operating later in pregnancy (Cohen, 1997).

Congenital malformations can result from many different types of abnormality of morphogenesis. Cohen (1997) divided these into three categories: incomplete, redundant, and aberrant morphogenesis. In incomplete morphogenesis, there may be absent or hypoplastic development, persistence of an organ or tissue in an early location, or incompleteness of a variety of morphogenetic processes, such as closure or fusion (as in cleft palate), separation (as in syndactyly), recanalization (as in duodenal atresia), septation, migration, rotation, or resolution of an early form. Redundant morphogenesis refers to duplications of structures, such as in polydactyly; and aberrant morphogenesis refers to situations in which organs appear in ectopic locations not accounted for by failures of migration during embryogenesis.

When several malformations are present in the same individual, they can be regarded as being organized into syndromes, sequences, or associations. In a *syndrome*, there is a pattern of multiple abnormalities that are regarded as being pathogenically related or as having a defined genetic or teratological etiology. By contrast, in a *sequence*, the multiple malformations derive from a single initiating event, which could have many different causes. In an *association*, the malformations occur in a nonrandom manner but are not considered to represent either a syndrome or a sequence; in fact, the associations may sometimes be broken down into sequences and/or syndromes (Cohen, 1997). As with some of the other distinctions described above, there is often lack of a clear separation. For example, one of the classical associations, the so-called CHARGE association of *coloboma, heart* defects, choanal *atresia, retarded growth, genital anomalies/hypogonadism, and ear anomalies/deafness, which may have a high concordance in identical twins, has been considered a true syndrome with genetic causes (Tellier et al., 1998). Similarly, the DiGeorge sequence, with abnormalities of the thymus, parathyroids, and heart and great vessels, can have many teratological and genetic causes; but most often it is a component of the velocardiofacial or Shprintzen's syndrome resulting from a deletion of chromosome 22q11.2 (Jones, 1997).

CAUSES OF MALFORMATIONS

Six percent of birth defects are associated with a recognizable chromosomal abnormality, 7.5% are thought to be monogenic in origin, 20% are regarded as multifactorial, and 6%–7% are caused by known environmental factors such as maternal diseases, infections, and teratogens (Winter, 1996). These figures could well change as newer methods for detecting small chromosomal abnormalities and for gene mapping and mutation detection are employed.

The genetic abnormalities underlying the multiple malformation syndromes can be viewed as a continuum, ranging from mutations of individual genes through the deletion of small numbers of adjoining genes (as in the contiguous gene syndromes) to segmental and whole chromosomal aneuploidy. In the latter three instances, the genetic changes involve simultaneous increases or decreases in the dosage of many genes, the genes themselves being structurally and functionally normal. However, in the first instance (single-gene abnormalities that follow mendelian rules of inheritance), the responsible genes can be altered in a variety of ways that affect the level, specificity, and regulation of their expression and of the expression of their gene products.

Single congenital malformations also result from genetic and nongenetic causes. However, they are less likely to result from chromosomal abnormalities and contiguous gene deletions than are multiple malformations. Moreover, there is considerable evidence that many single malformations are multifactorial or complex disorders in which one or more genetic susceptibility factors combine with random developmental (stochastic) events and environmental factors to give rise to the abnormality. For example, two candidate genes, *TGFβ3* and *MSX1*, have been implicated in the genesis of nonsyndromic oral clefts, with *MSX1* perhaps having an interaction with maternal smoking (Beaty et al., 2002). Threshold models have been developed to explain how these factors interact to cause the malformations and why their frequency in near relatives is increased in a predictable manner (Fraser, 1980; Mitchell and Risch, 1992).

Although it is still not known how changes in gene dosage interfere with developmental processes in the chromosomal aneuploidy syndromes (Epstein, 1986), the fact that multiple organs or systems may be involved is not surprising since many different genes are involved. However, for the monogenic conditions and perhaps some of the contiguous gene syndromes, the problem has been how to explain abnormalities in two or more apparently disparate systems or organs being caused by mutations involving single genes. As the following chapters will detail, these explanations are being based on the idea that the genes implicated in these conditions may express in multiple tissues and at different times, may affect cell populations that influence the development of multiple structures, or may be involved in the regulation of more than one developmental pathway.

THE CONCEPT OF INBORN ERRORS OF DEVELOPMENT

One of the great accomplishments of the past century has been the exploitation of human biochemical genetics for the elucidation of many of the intricate details of intermediary metabolism. Starting with a general knowledge of biochemical processes, the analysis of a large number of metabolic defects has led to the discovery and investigation of many previously unsuspected enzymatic pathways. Once this occurred, knowledge of these pathways permitted the explanation of still other biochemical abnormalities. An important aspect of this process is that it is a reciprocal one, in which knowledge of normal biochemical processes and their genetic control has permitted an understanding of the abnormal and, reciprocally, understanding the abnormal has increased our understanding of the normal (Epstein, 1978).

Archibald Garrod is generally regarded as the founder of human biochemical genetics. As early as 1903, and more extensively in his classic *Inborn Errors of Metabolism* published in 1909 (Harris, 1963), he clearly demonstrated this reciprocal process. The success of this approach is certainly attested to by the most recent edition of *The Metabolic and Molecular Bases of Inherited Disease* (Scriver et al., 2001) (formerly *The Metabolic Basis of Inherited Disease*, edited by Stanbury et al.), which details, in four large volumes, the large number of metabolic pathways associated with hereditary disorders.

Garrod was not unaware of the existence of structural malformations. In fact, in describing inborn errors of metabolism, he pointed out that "they are characterized by wide departures from the normal of the species far more conspicuous than individual variations, and one is tempted to regard them as metabolic sports, the *chemical analogues of structural malformation*" (italics mine). In an article discussing developmental abnormalities and a developmental genetics of humans (Epstein, 1978), I suggested that the wording be rearranged somewhat and that we regard hereditary structural malformations as *inborn errors of development*, the structural analogues of Garrod's metabolic sports. Although I did not realize it at the time, Lewis Holmes (1974) had made a similar suggestion a few years earlier in his discussion of "inborn errors of morphogenesis."

Although both Holmes's focus and mine at the time was on single malformations, the existence of inherited multiple malformation syndromes was already well recognized. In his seminal book *Recognizable Patterns of Human Malformation*, David Smith (1970) listed many such syndromes. This book, now in it fifth edition as *Smith's Recognizable Patterns of Human Malformation* (Jones, 1997), serves as the bible for the clinical description of the malformation syndromes. Another very useful compendium is *Syndromes of the Head and Neck* by Gorlin and colleagues (2001). Because of the state of science in the 1970s, there was no conceptual basis for thinking about the genetic mechanisms causing these syndromes. However, with the discovery of the enzymatic basis of conditions such as the mucopolysaccharidoses that cause generalized bony dysplasias (Bach et al., 1973; Neufeld et al., 1975) and of the structural protein defects in osteogenesis imperfecta (Barsh et al., 1982), most thinking turned along the lines of defects in metabolic enzymes and structural proteins such as collagen and fibrillin. In fact, abnormalities of other metabolic enzymes and transporters that cause multiple malformations were eventually recognized, including glutaric aciduria II, which causes facial dysmorphism, enlarged kidneys, abdominal wall muscle defects, and hypospadias (Wilson et al., 1988); vitamin K epoxide reductase deficiency, which causes a form of chondrodysplasia punctata with hypoplasia of the nose, short stature, distal phalangeal hypoplasia, and stippled epiphyses (Pauli et al., 1987); the peroxisomal disorders, which cause Zellweger syndrome and related conditions that have craniofacial dysmorphisms (Brown, 1994; Preuss et al., 2002); and an abnormality of the sulfate transporter, which causes diastrophic dysplasia (Hästbacka et al. 1994).

It was not until 1991, however, with the reports of mutations in the zinc-finger transcription factor gene *GLI3* that result in Greig cephalopolysyndactyly and in the cell adhesion molecule gene *KAL* that result in Kallmann syndrome (with anosmia and hypogonadism), that the first nonmetabolic enzyme, nonstructural protein causes of developmental abnormalities were described. Just 4 years later, a total of 21 genes representing transcription factors, receptors of various types, growth factors, cell adhesion molecules, gap junctions, and G proteins had been shown to cause human birth defects (Epstein, 1995). In several instances, mouse models for the human conditions that were the result of either spontaneous or induced mutations could be identified (Epstein, 1995). As the present volume attests, the number of conditions in which mutations involving developmental processes have been detected is increasing rapidly.

Although I have been making a distinction between metabolic enzymes, structural proteins, and transporters, on the one hand, and transcription factors, receptors, and other molecules more readily identified with developmental processes, on the other, there is certainly no clear line of demarcation between the two. This has already been pointed out with regard to the multiple malformation disorders that result from defects in metabolic enzymes. Another example of a malformation syndrome resulting from a metabolic enzyme defect is the Smith-Lemli-Opitz (SLO) syndrome. In this instance the enzyme is 3-β-hydroxysterol Δ⁷-reductase (7-dehydrocholesterol reductase), the last enzyme in the cholesterol biosynthetic pathway (Porter, 2000). Two other enzyme defects earlier in the pathway also result in dysmorphic syndromes, the CHILD syndrome (congenital *h*emidysplasia with *i*chthyosiform erythroderma and *l*imb *d*efects) and the Conradi-Hünermann syndrome (chondrodysplasia punctata-2) (Kelley and Herman, 2001). A syndrome with craniosynostoses, craniofacial dysmorphisms, and cardiac, renal, genital, and skeletal abnormalities also appears to result from a defect in cholesterol biosynthesis (Kelley et al., 2002).

What makes these syndromes, the SLO syndrome in particular, so interesting is that they provide a compelling example of the overlap

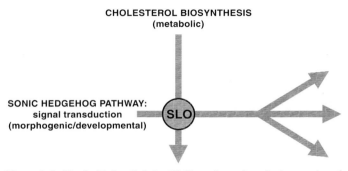

Figure 1–1. The Smith-Lemli-Opitz (SLO) syndrome is at the intersection of the cholesterol biosynthetic (metabolic) and sonic hedgehog signal-transduction morphogenic (developmental) pathways.

between developmental and metabolic pathways, in this case the developmental pathway being the sonic hedgehog (SHH) signal-transduction pathway (Fig. 1–1). This pathway is directly associated with a number of syndromes affecting morphogenesis, including, in addition to SLO, the basal cell nevus (Gorlin) syndrome, Greig cephalopolysyndactyly, Pallister-Hall syndrome, and postaxial poly-dactylies A, IV, and A/II, and indirectly with the Rubinstein-Taybi, Saethre-Chotzen, and Townes-Brock syndromes (Villavicencio et al., 2000). The connection between the cholesterol biosynthetic pathway and the SHH developmental pathways is thought to stem from the role of cholesterol in the action of SHH. Cholesterol is involved in the cleavage of SHH, a secreted ligand, to N-SHH and potentially in the interaction of SHH with its receptor, Patched. The concept, then, is that SLO is simultaneously a disorder of both a metabolic pathway and a developmental pathway that intersect, and understanding its pathogenesis will require understanding the developmental pathway involved. It is not the enzyme defect per se that causes the abnormalities but, rather, the fact that cholesterol is required for normal signal transduction. These issues are discussed in detail in Chapters 16 and 17.

It has been asserted that "metabolic malformation" syndromes such as SLO represent the exceptions rather than the rule (Kelley, 1998). In a strict sense, this may well be the case. However, metabolic pathways and developmental pathways do not sit in exclusively different compartments, and interactions between the two are not only possible but likely. A case in point is provided by the analysis of folate and homocysteine metabolism in mice with a variety of mutations associated with neural tube defects (exencephaly and spina bifida) (Ernest et al., 2002). Mice heterozygous for the mutations *Pax3*^{Sp} *(Splotch)* and *Gli3*^{Xt} *(Extra toes)*, which are also known to cause structural malformations in humans (Waardenburg I and Greig syndromes, respectively), have elevated levels of plasma homocysteine and decreased expression of certain genes related to folate-homocysteine metabolism. The potential significance of the elevated homocysteine concentration is that it itself is known to increase the risk for neural tube defects in humans (Mills et al., 1995).

DEVELOPMENTAL PATHWAYS

In a review several years ago (Epstein, 1995), the only organizational principle that could be used to group the disorders of human morphogenesis was by molecular families, such as *PAX* genes (of which there were three) and genes for zinc finger transcription factors (two) and growth factor receptors (three). However, to understand the developmental mechanisms that were being perturbed, a more satisfactory approach would be to look whenever possible at developmental pathways. This approach is analogous to the organization of metabolic enzyme abnormalities into metabolic pathways composed of series of sequential enzyme reactions. In developmental terms, this might correspond to series of signal-transduction pathways composed of ligands, receptors, enzymes of various types, intracellular mediators, and transcription factors (Downward, 2001; Brivanlou and Darnell, 2002). This has now become possible for several disorders. Even though

many signal-transduction and other developmental pathways are known in some detail, the number of human disorders currently associated with any one of them may be no more than one or perhaps none at all. Because of this, we have used a hybrid type of system to organize the material in the following chapters. For certain conditions, it makes sense to organize the disorders by the pathways that are involved (e.g., SHH, Notch, TGF-β), while in others, where the pathways are not well defined, it seems more appropriate to organize them by classes of genes (e.g., *PAX, HOX, TBX,* G proteins) or by functions of the molecules involved (e.g., extracellular matrix, molecular motors, other transcription factors). Some disorders affect molecules that, for the moment, could be put into neither a group nor a pathway. This organization will undoubtedly change as developmental pathways are better understood and the molecular bases of more human disorders are elucidated.

Although the goal of organizing human developmental disorders on the basis of the developmental pathways involved appears attainable, there will undoubtedly be complexities that will make any such scheme imperfect. As a glance at many of the pathway maps in this book will reveal, developmental pathways are not strictly linear. They are interconnected and have numerous branch points and parallel paths. In fact, there is now a considerable literature that provides evidence for the existence of complex regulatory networks and protein interactions involved in developmental processes (Davidson et al., 2002; Maslov and Sneppen, 2002; Gavin et al., 2002). Further, as Arthur (2002) points out, no developmental pathway exists in isolation from the rest of the developing organism. Therefore, he suggests that terms such as *upstream* and *downstream* be considered relative when used in connection with developmental genes: a gene might be downstream in one pathway and upstream in another. However, this complexity is not greatly different from what is known about intermediary metabolism, and any chart (such as that produced by Boehringer-Mannheim) that summarizes such pathways graphically depicts their interconnectedness and reveals intermediary metabolism to be a complex network. Nevertheless, it has been useful, when trying to understand the human inborn errors of metabolism, to view biochemical pathways as being, for the most part, reasonably linear; and I believe that the same will be true of the inborn errors of development.

ANIMAL MODELS

Although it is not surprising that mouse models of human developmental diseases should exist, it did come as somewhat of a surprise when it was recognized that models also existed in lower organisms, even in invertebrates (see Chapter 3). The prototypic example of this is the *Drosophila* mutation *eyeless (ey)* in a paired-domain/homeobox-containing gene that results in reduction or complete absence of the compound eyes of the fly. The *ey* gene is orthologous to the mouse gene *Pax6*, which in its mutant form, *Pax6*^{Sey}, causes the mouse disorder Small eye. As the name implies, animals heterozygous for this mutation have small eyes, and homozygous animals have no eyes or nose (Glaser et al., 1994). Similarly, *PAX6* mutations in humans result in aniridia in heterozygotes and in anophthalmia, choanal atresia, and brain anomalies in homozygotes (Glaser et al., 1994). Perhaps even more remarkable than these cross-species similarities of genes and disorders is the fact that in targeted gene expression studies the function of the *Drosophila* gene could be reproduced by the mouse gene: targeted expression of mouse *Pax6* could produce an ectopic eye on a fly's leg (Halder et al., 1995). These observations led Halder et al. (1995) to assert that "the genetic control mechanisms for development are much more universal than anticipated," a situation that bodes well for our ability to use model organisms to elucidate the pathogenesis of human developmental disorders. This notion was strengthened by the discovery of the first human disorder resulting from a mutation in a human HOX gene, synpolydactyly, caused by mutations in the *HOXD13* gene (Muragaki et al., 1996), one of a set of vertebrate genes orthologous to the *Drosophila Abd-B* gene (Veraksa et al., 2000). However, in this instance, it is important to keep in mind that developmental genes, or perhaps even the pathways or "cassettes" in which they operate, may, unlike *ey* and *PAX6*, be coopted for different functional roles as development proceeds (Arthur, 2002). Nevertheless, unifying views of developmental gene programs can result from similarities of organ development and function in different species, whereas the differences can provide insight into the evolutionary process that have affected their roles (Thisse and Zon, 2002).

Although our understanding of developmental processes in humans will be informed by an understanding of the functions of orthologous developmental genes in lower organisms, it is not likely that invertebrates will very often provide exact models for human disorders. The principal model organism for human disorders has, of course, been the mouse. Spontaneous mutations and mutations induced by mutagenic agents that affect development have been collected and characterized. As noted earlier, several have been shown to produce developmental abnormalities similar to those found in humans. However, with the introduction of techniques for manipulating the mouse genome, such as transgenesis, and of homologous recombination to produce "knockouts" and "knockins," the modeling of developmental abnormalities has become much more powerful. It is now possible to create models not only for known human mutations but also for developmental pathway mutations that have not yet been recognized in humans. Furthermore, it is possible to dissect specific morphogenetic processes, for example, cardiac morphogenesis, by systematically inducing targeted mutations in the developmental pathways thought to be involved (Srivastava and Olson, 2000).

A large number of mutations, many of which we might regard as being in search of human diseases, have been created in a large number of mouse genes. Descriptions of many of these mutations and their associated phenotypes are contained in a variety of on-line databases: the Jackson Induced Mutant Resource Index of Strains (http://www.jax.org/pub-cgi/imrpub.sh?objtype=stridx); Jackson Strains (http://jaxmice.jax.org/index.shtml); Mouse Genome Informatics (http://www.informatics.jax.org/menus/marker_menu.shtml); Combined Mouse/Human Phenotypes (http://www.informatics.jax.org/searches/noforms_mlc_omim.cgi); ENU Mutagenesis Program (http://www.mgu.har.mrc.ac.uk/mutabase/data/index.html); and Harwell Mutagenesis Project (http://www.mut.har.mrc.ac.uk/servlet/hmp.phenotype.searchforphenotype2).

One of the attractions of using the mouse as a model organism is that it is a mammal and, therefore, presumably quite similar to humans in its development. Nevertheless, many other experimental systems are used for studies on development, and of these, the zebrafish has proven to be very attractive from the genetic point of view. Its transparency in the embryonic stage, rapid generation time, and ease of mutagenesis have made it the subject of several mutagenic screens to search for mutations affecting the organogenesis of numerous organs and systems, including the heart, blood, eye, cartilage, bone, muscle, skin, reproductive system, olfactory system, and gastrointestinal system (Thisse and Zon, 2002; Golling et al., 2002). Some of the mutants that have been obtained provide interesting models for human disorders, including porphyria, hypochromic anemia, thalassemia, polycystic renal disease, the Senior-Loken syndrome (renal-retinal dysplasia), holoprosencephaly, coarctation of the aorta, and hypoplastic right ventricle (Dooley and Zon, 2000; Srivastava and Olson, 2000). An online listing of zebrafish mutations is maintained at the Zebrafish International Resource Center (http://zfin.org/cgi-bin/webdriver?MIval=aa-fishselect.apg&line_type=mutant).

GENETIC MODIFIERS

An important outcome of the study of developmental abnormalities in mice has been the recognition of the importance of genetic modifiers in determining the phenotype of a mutation. Several examples of modifier genes that alter the phenotype of mutant genes affecting development were presented by Nadeau (2001). For example, looking just at morphogenetic abnormalities, unknown strain-specific modifiers affect the penetrance of the mutation disorganization (*Ds*, which causes mirror-image limb duplications, among other abnormalities) (Robin and Nadeau, 2001), the nature of the skeletal abnormalities associated with the mutations undulated (*Pax1^un*) and short-ear (*Bmp5^se*), and the degree of reduction in tail length caused by the mutation *brachy (T)*. However, specific modifier genes have sometimes been identified, for

example, in mice carrying a *Splotch (Pax3^Sp)* mutation, a model for human Waardenburg's syndrome I, which also manifests spina bifida. Whereas the figit mutation (*Fign^fi*) suppresses the occurrence of spina bifida, the gene *curly tail (ct)*, when homozygous, results in more severe spina bifida. The penetrance and expression of the *ct* mutation itself are affected by several other modifier genes (Van Straaten and Copp, 2001). Modifiers have also been identified for many spontaneous mutations affecting other systems in the mouse, and background strain effects presumed to be the result of modifier genes that affect the phenotypes of several targeted mutations in the mouse have also been described (Erickson, 1996; Dipple and McCabe, 2000; Bourdeau et al., 2001; Huang et al., 2001; Nadeau, 2001).

The importance of these findings is twofold. First, they emphasize the care that must be taken in analyzing mouse mutants generated as models for human disorders. Whether the phenotype observed in the mouse model resembles that in humans may depend, in whole or in part, on whether there are modifier genes that can affect the phenotype. As a practical matter, this means that putative mouse models must be bred on a variety of genetic backgrounds, to insure that the desired phenotype is not overlooked. However, of even greater significance is the fact that the penetrance and expression of human developmental mutations are also likely to be influenced by modifier genes of various types. The high degree of variability among individuals carrying the same mutation points to the existence of a variety of factors that could be responsible, chief among which is the genetic background, which is synonymous with genetic modifiers.

Perhaps the best studied human developmental disorder in which there is strong evidence for the existence of modifier genes is Hirschsprung's disease (congenital megacolon). This condition is discussed in detail in Chapter 36, but for the present discussion, I want to make note of the findings in the short-segment type. Following extensive genomewide searches, it has been concluded that, although the essential causative gene is *RET*, there are two independent unidentified polymorphic modifier genes. These modifier genes interact in a multiplicative manner to increase the risk ratio of the short-segment disease for siblings from 0.13% (8.3 times the population risk of 0.016%) when only the *RET* mutation is present to 3% (175 times the population risk) when the two modifier alleles are also present in the genome (Gabriel et al., 2002). The frequencies of the polymorphic alleles were estimated at 4%–5%.

STOCHASTIC FACTORS AND BUFFERING

In addition to modifiers, stochastic and environmental factors may influence the penetrance and expression of developmental phenotypes. Thus, in putting forth an explanation for the fact that atrioventricular septal (endocardial cushion) defects only occur in about half of individuals with trisomy 21, Kurnit et al. (1985) showed how small differences in cell adhesion could, by altering cell migration and division, dramatically affect the fusion of the cushions. Another player in cardiac morphogenesis, the neural crest, may also be subject to stochastic effects since formation of the outflow tracts and valves of the heart depends on the migration of neural crest cells (Chien, 2000) Since many developmental events involve cell migration, adhesion, and division, it is likely that they will be subject to stochastic effects, which may play a significant role in the generation of phenotypic variability.

According to Ozbudak et al. (2002), stochastic mechanisms are ubiquitous to biological systems. They occur not only at the cellular level, as mentioned, but also at the biochemical and molecular levels, where they may give rise to what has been termed *phenotypic noise* because of random fluctuations in gene expression (Ozbudak et al., 2002). Robust buffering mechanisms appear to have evolved to protect against such stochastic variation, as well as against genetic and environmental variation (Rutherford, 2000). Such buffering was termed *canalization* by Waddington (1942; see also McLaren, 1999).

The mechanism of buffering has been extensively explored with regard to metabolic pathways, and it has been concluded, on both theoretical and experimental grounds, that the kinetics of the reactions making up the pathway may have a stabilizing effect. Thus, it has been experimentally shown for many pathways that individual decreases in the activities of constituent enzymes by 50% or more have very little effect on the flux of metabolites through the pathway (Kacser and Burns, 1981). This also appears to be the case for many of the inborn errors of metabolism in which heterozygosity for a null mutation does not have a significant phenotypic effect. However, such buffering does not always work, and there are inborn errors in which 50% of normal enzyme activity, such as in the dominantly inherited porphyrias, do have deleterious consequences (Epstein, 1986).

A similar kinetic mechanism may operate with regard to developmental events. However, developmental pathways may also be buffered by the existence of parallel pathways associated with a redundancy of gene function (Rutherford, 2000). This redundancy, which may be complete or partial, derives from the existence of paralogous genes produced by gene duplication (Wilkins, 1997). In addition, negative feedback control systems can confer great stability on developmental pathways, but positive feedback can, if perturbed, be greatly destabilizing (Freeman, 2000). Furthermore, a "filtering," or buffering, system has been described in *Drosophila* embryos, which insures the precision of morphogenetic gradients necessary for establishment of the anteroposterior axis (Houchmandzadeh et al, 2002).

It has also been suggested that the chaperone heat shock protein 90 (Hsp90) plays an important role in buffering against both genetic and stochastic variation in plants and animals (Rutherford and Linquist, 1998; Queitsch et al., 2002). In experiments with *Drosophila* and *Arabidopsis*, interference with Hsp90 function leads to abnormal morphogenesis, affecting a large number of systems. The protective action of Hsp90 is believed to reside in its ability to chaperone or stabilize metastable proteins, most notably signal transducers such as kinases, transcription factors, and cell cycle regulators, against misfolding. Thus stabilized, these proteins can make the necessary associations with ligands and partner proteins, can be posttranslationally modified, and can be correctly localized (Queitsch et al., 2002).

Despite the presence of several powerful buffering systems, these mechanisms are not always able to prevent abnormalities in development from occurring. This is especially true if other perturbing factors are present, including those that might perturb the buffering systems themselves (e.g., heat in the case of Hsp90). Moreover, there appear to be developmental decisions that are quite sensitive to changes in the concentrations of the reactants in the pathway. Their existence is revealed by the more than 25 developmental disorders that result from haploinsufficiency of transcription factors alone (Hermanns and Lee, 2002; Seidman and Seidman, 2002). Haploinsufficiency results from the presence of one rather than two functional genes at a locus, with a consequent reduction in the level of gene expression by half. Certain classes of transcription factors, such as T-boxes and homeoboxes, show higher proportions of mutations causing haploinsufficiency relative to missense, recessive, or unknown mutations. The sensitivity to haploinsufficiency may be related to the number of independent interactions the factor has with regulatory elements such as proteins and DNA sequences: the greater the number of interactions, the greater the sensitivity (Seidman and Seidman, 2002).

Further evidence for the sensitivity of certain developmental processes to the level of gene expression derives from examples in which decreased and increased expression result in opposite phenotypic effects. This idea, referred to as *type* and *countertype*, was advanced by Jerome Lejeune in his consideration of the phenotypes of duplications and deletions involving the same chromosomes or chromosome segments, and a limited number of examples can be found in the chromosomal abnormality literature (Epstein, 1986). However, with the availability of techniques for manipulating the mouse genome, it is possible to explore the concept further by comparing the phenotypes of spontaneous or engineered gain- and loss-of-function mutations. An interesting example of reciprocal phenotypic effects was described by Clark et al. (2001) for the locus *Lmbr1*, which encodes a multipass transmembrane protein of unknown function. In mice, preaxial polydactyly occurs when there is a gain-of-function mutation and postaxial oligodactyly when there is significant loss of function. Loss of the human orthologues of this gene results in acheiropodia

(acheiropody), with congenital amputations of all limbs and absence of the hands and feet (Ianakiev et al., 2001) (see Chapter 107). The involvement of opposite sides of the limb in the mouse mutants is curious, and a similar example in humans is provided by duplications and deletion of 13q31 → 34, which result, respectively, in postaxial polydactyly and preaxial oligodactyly (Epstein, 1986).

ENVIRONMENTAL FACTORS

When it comes to the role of the environment in the genesis of disorders of development, attention has been principally devoted to two types of factor: teratogenic agents, which cause birth defects, and agents that may prevent them. Teratogenic agents, such as drugs, can certainly act in the absence of known genetic factors, although their effects can be modulated by genetic differences in metabolism. What is perhaps of greater relevance to the present discussion is that teratogenic agents may alter the same developmental pathways that are affected by genetic mutations. A prime example of this comes from the animal literature relating to the teratogenic effects of cyclopamine and jervine, distal inhibitors of cholesterol biosynthesis, which cause holoprosencephaly in exposed lambs (see Chapter 17). This situation is reminiscent of the SLO syndrome, as well as some mutations of the SHH receptor Patched that can sometimes manifest holoprosencephaly (Nowaczyk et al., 2001; Cohen and Shiota, 2002). Investigations of the action of cyclopamine have shown that it inhibits the response of target tissues to signaling through the SHH pathway (Cooper et al., 1998), probably through an action on the Patched or Smoothened protein, downstream of SHH (Taipale et al., 2000).

Another instructive example of the relationship between teratogenic effects and the developmental pathways they may affect is provided by a mouse model for the teratogenicity of valproate, an anticonvulsant in common use. In humans, valproate use during the first trimester has been shown to increase the risk of spina bifida; heart, limb, and craniofacial abnormalities; and cleft palate. In mice, it causes neural tube defects and limb anomalies, the appearance of which is affected by genetic background or modifiers that appear to operate both parentally and embryonically (Faiella et al., 2000). However, what is most interesting is that valproate causes thoracic and lumbar vertebrae to manifest features characteristic of more anterior vertebrae so that, for example, a feature characteristic of T10 and lower does not occur until T11. Such changes, referred to as *anterior homeotic transformations*, have been associated with induced mutations of *Hox* genes; and valproate was shown to cause in vitro changes in *Hox* expression (Faiella et al., 2000).

The protective role of folic acid administration against human neural tube abnormalities is widely known (Wald et al., 2001). However, when it comes to protection against congenital malformations with known genetic causation, the *curly tail* mouse discussed earlier provides an informative system for examining the interaction of environmental and genetic factors. The effect is very dependent on the time of exposure to the agent. Thus, *myo*-inositol, retinoic acid, and several anti-mitogenic agents given at embryonic day 9.5 protect against the development of posterior neural tube abnormalities, whereas retinoic acid, the antimitotics, and hyperthermia at embryonic day 8.5 increase the frequency of exencephaly (Van Straaten and Copp, 2001).

CONCLUSION

Science has finally caught up with human malformations. It is now possible to identify the mutant genes responsible for many multiple malformation syndromes and to study these conditions in animal models. Methods are becoming available for searching for the mutations or polymorphisms that are at the root of many of the more common single malformations. These methods can also be applied to the identification of the genetic modifiers that influence the penetrance and phenotypes of the syndromes that are caused by single-gene mutations. Knowledge of the genetic bases of these conditions will both inform and be informed by an understanding of the developmental pathways that are perturbed. This will, in turn, make it possible to elucidate their pathogenesis and to understand the influence of environmental factors in determining the outcome. Ultimately, the inborn errors of development should be no more mystifying than are the inborn errors of metabolism.

REFERENCES

Arthur W (2002). The emerging conceptual framework of evolutionary developmental biology. *Nature* 415: 757–764.

Bach G, Eisenberg F Jr, Cantz M, Neufeld EF (1973). The defect in the Hunter syndrome: deficiency of sulfoiduronate sulfatase. *Proc Natl Acad Sci USA* 70: 2134–2138.

Barsh GS, David KE, Byers PH (1982). Type I osteogenesis imperfecta: a nonfunctional allele for pro alpha 1 (I) chains of type I procollagen. *Proc Natl Acad Sci USA* 79: 3838–3842.

Beaty T, Hetmanski JB, Zeiger JS, Fan YT, Liang KY, VanderKolk CA, McIntosh I (2002). Testing candidate genes for non-syndromic oral clefts using a case–parent trio design. *Genet Epidemiol* 22: 1–11.

Berry RJ, Buehler JW, Strauss LT, Hogue CJ, Smith JC (1987). Birth weight-specific infant mortality due to congenital anomalies, 1960 and 1980. *Public Health Rep* 102: 171–181.

Bourdeau A, Faughman ME, McDonald M-L, Paterson AD, Wanless IR, Letarte M (2001). Potential role of modifier genes influencing transforming growth factor-β1 levels in the development of vascular defects in endoglin heterozygous mice with hereditary hemorrhagic telangiectasia. *Am J Pathol* 158: 2011–2020.

Brivanlou AH, Darnell JE Jr (2002). Signal transduction and the control of gene expression. *Science* 295: 813–818.

Brown, GK (1994). Metabolic disorders of embryogenesis. *J Inherit Metab Dis* 17: 448–458.

Chien KR (2000). Genomic circuits and the integrative biology of cardiac diseases. *Nature* 407: 227–232.

Clark RM, Marker PC, Roessler E, Dutra A, Schimenti JC, Muenke M, Kingsley DM (2001). Reciprocal mouse and human limb phenotypes caused by gain- and loss-of-function mutations affecting Lmbr1. *Genetics* 159: 715–726.

Clow CL, Fraser FC, Laberge C, Scriver CR (1973). On the application of knowledge to the patient with genetic disease. *Prog Med Genet* 9: 159–213.

Cohen MM Jr (1997). *The Child with Multiple Birth Defects*, 2nd Edition. Oxford University Press, New York.

Cohen MM Jr, Shiota K (2002). Teratogenesis of holoprosencephaly. *Am J Med Genet* 109: 1–15.

Cooper MK, Porter JA, Young KE, Beachy PA (1998). Teratogen-mediated inhibition of target tissue response to Shh signaling. *Science* 280: 1603–1607.

Davidson EH, Rast JP, Oliveri P, Ransick A, Calestani C, et al. (2002). A genomic regulatory network for development. *Science* 295: 1669–1678.

Dipple KM, McCabe ERB (2000). Modifier genes convert "simple" mendelian disorders to complex traits. *Mol Genet Metab* 71: 43–50.

Division for Vital Records and Health Statistics (2002). Birth defects incidence and mortality tables. (http://www.mdmh.state.mi.us/PHA/OSR/BirthDefects/summary.asp)

Dooley K, Zon LI (2000). Zebrafish: a model system for the study of human disease. *Curr Opin Genet Dev* 10: 252–256.

Downward J (2001). The ins and outs of signaling. *Nature* 411: 759–762.

Epstein CJ (1978). Developmental mechanisms and abnormalities: toward a developmental genetics of man. In: *Birth Defects. Proc. 5th International Conference on Birth Defects*. Littlefield JB, deGrouchy J (eds.) Excerpta Medica, Amsterdam, pp. 387–395.

Epstein CJ (1986). *The Consequences of Chromosome Imbalance: Principles, Mechanisms, and Models*. Cambridge University Press, New York.

Epstein CJ (1995). The new dysmorphology: application of insights from basic developmental biology to the understanding of human birth defects. *Proc Natl Acad Sci USA* 92: 8566–8573.

Erickson RP (1996). Mouse models of human genetic disease: which mouse is more like a man? *Bioessays* 18: 993–998.

Ernest S, Christensen B, Gilfix BM, Mamer OA, Hosack A, Rodier M, Colmenares C, McGrath J, Bale A, Balling R, et al. (2002). Genetic and molecular control of folate-homocysteine metabolism in mutant mice. *Mamm Genome* 13: 259–267.

Faiella A, Wernig M, Consalez GG, Hostick U, Hofmann C, Hustert E, Boncinelli E, Balling R, Nadeau JH (2000). A mouse model for valproate teratogenicity: parental effects, homeotic transformations, and altered HOX expression. *Hum Mol Genet* 9: 227–236.

Fraser FC (1980). The William Allan Memorial Award address: evolution of a palatable multifactorial threshold model. *Am J Hum Genet* 32: 796–813.

Freeman M (2000). Feedback control of intercellular signalling in development. *Nature* 408: 313–319.

Gabriel SB, Salomon R, Pelet A, Angrist M, Amiel J, Fornage M, Attie-Bitach T, Olson JM, Hofstra R, Buys C, et al. (2002). Segregation at three loci explains familial and population risk in Hirschsprung disease. *Nat Genet* 31: 89–93.

Gavin A-C, Bösche M, Krause R, Grandl P, Marzioch M, et al. (2002). Functional organization of the yeast proteome by systematic analysis of protein complexes. *Nature* 415: 141–147.

Glaser T, Jepeal L, Edwards JG, Young SR, Favor J, Maas RL (1994). PAX6 gene dosage effect in a family with congenital cataracts, aniridia, anophthalmia and central nervous system defects. *Nat Genet* 7: 464–471.

Golling G, Amsterdam A, Sun Z, Antonelli M, Maldonado E, Chen W, Burgess S, Haldi M, Artzt K, Farrington S, et al. (2002). Insertional mutagenesis in zebrafish rapidly identifies genes essential for early vertebrate development. *Nat Genet* 31: 135–140.

Gorlin RJ, Cohen MM Jr, Hennekam RCM (2001). *Syndromes of the Head and Neck*, 4th Edition. Oxford University Press, New York.

Halder G, Callaerts P, Gehring WJ (1995). Induction of ectopic eyes by targeted expression of the *eyeless* gene in Drosophila. *Science* 267: 1788–1792.

Harris H (1963). *Garrod's Inborn Errors of Metabolism*. Oxford University Press, London.

Hästbacka J, de la Chapelle A, Mahtani MM, Clines G, Reeve-Daly MP, Daly M, Hamilton BA, Kusumi K, Trivedi B, Weaver A, et al. (1994). The diastrophic dysplasia gene encodes a novel sulfate transporter: positional cloning by fine-structure linkage disequilibrium mapping. *Cell* 78: 1073–1087.

Hermanns P, Lee B (2002). Transcriptional dysregulation in skeletal malformation syndromes. *Am J Med Genet* 106: 258–271.

Hoekelman RA, Pless IB (1988). Decline in mortality among young Americans during the 20th century: prospects for reaching national mortality reduction goals for 1990. *Pediatrics* 82: 582–595.

Holmes LB (1974). Inborn errors of morphogenesis. *N Engl J Med* 291: 763–773.

Houchmandzadeh B, Weischaus E, Leibler S (2002). Establishment of developmental precision and proportions in the early Drosophila embryo. *Nature* 415: 798–802.

Huang T-T, Carlson EJ, Kozy HM, Mantha S, Goodman SI, Ursell PC, Epstein CJ (2001) Genetic modification of the development of prenatal lethality and dilated cardiomyopathy in Mn superoxide dismutase mutant mice. *Free Radic Biol Med* 31: 1101–1110.

Ianakiev P, van Baren MJ, Daly MJ, Toledo SP, Cavalcanti MG, Neto JC, Silveira EL, Freire-Maia A, Heutink P, Kilpatrick MW, et al. (2001). Acheiropodia is caused by a genomic deletion in C7orf2, the human orthologue of the *Lmbr1* gene. *Am J Hum Genet* 68: 38–45.

Jones KL (1997). *Smith's Recognizable Patterns of Human Malformation*, 5th Edition. Saunders, Philadelphia.

Kacser H, Burns JA (1981). The molecular basis of dominance. *Genetics* 97: 639–666.

Kelley RI (1998). RSH/Smith-Lemli-Opitz syndrome: mutations and metabolic morphogenesis. *Am J Hum Genet* 63: 322–326.

Kelley RI, Herman GE (2001). Inborn errors of sterol biosynthesis. *Annu Rev Genomics Hum Genet* 2: 299–341.

Kelley RL, Kratz LE, Glaser RL, Netzloff L, Wolf LM, Jabs EW (2002). Abnormal sterol metabolism in a patient with Antley-Bixler syndrome and ambiguous genitalia. *Am J Med Genet* 110: 95–102.

Kurnit DM, Aldridge JF, Matsuoka R, Matthyse S (1985). Increased adhesiveness of trisomy 21 cells and atrioventricular malformations in Down syndrome: a stochastic model. *Am J Med Genet* 20: 385–399.

March of Dimes Perinatal Data Center (2000a). Leading categories of birth defects. (http://www.modimes.org/HealthLibrary2/InfantHealthStatistics/bdtable.htm)

March of Dimes Perinatal Data Center (2000b). Leading causes of infant deaths. United States, 1998. (http://www.modimes.org/HealthLibrary2/InfantHealthStatistics/percent.htm)

Maslov S, Sneppen K (2002). Specificity and stability in topology of protein networks. *Science* 296: 910–913.

McLaren A (1999). Too late for the midwife toad: stress, variability, and Hsp90. *Trends Genet* 15: 169–171.

Mills JL, McPartlin JM, Kirke PN, Lee YJ, Conley MR, et al. (1995). Homocysteine metabolism in pregnancies complicated by neural tube defects. *Lancet* 345: 149–511.

Mitchell LE, Risch N (1992). Mode of inheritance of nonsyndromic cleft lip with or without cleft palate: a reanalysis. *Am J Hum Genet* 51: 323–332.

Muragaki Y, Mundlos S, Upton J, Olsen BR (1996). Altered growth and branching patterns caused by mutations in HOXD13. *Science* 272: 548–551.

Nadeau JH (2001). Modifier genes in mice and humans. *Nat Rev Genet* 2: 165–174.

Neufeld EF, Lim TW, Shapiro LJ (1975). Inherited disorders of lysosomal metabolism. *Annu Rev Biochem* 44: 357–376.

Nowaczyk MJM, Farrell SA, Surkin WA, Velsher L, Krakowiak PA, Waye JS, Porter FD (2001). Smith-Lemli-Opitz (RHS) syndrome: holoprosencephaly and homozygous IVS8-1G → C genotype. *Am J Med Genet* 103: 75–80.

Ozbudak EM, Thattai M, Kurtser I, Grossman AD, van Oudensaarden A (2002) Regulation in the noise in the expression of a single gene. *Nat Genet* 31: 69–73.

Pauli RM, Lian JB, Mosher DF, Suttie JW (1987). Association of congenital deficiency of multiple vitamin K-dependent coagulation factors and the phenotype of the warfarin embryopathy: clues to the mechanism of teratogenicity of coumarin derivatives. *Am J Hum Genet* 41: 566–583.

Porter FD (2000). RSH/Smith-Lemli-Opitz syndrome: a multiple congenital anomaly/mental retardation syndrome due to an inborn error of cholesterol biosynthesis. *Mol Genet Metab* 7: 163–174.

Preuss N, Brosius U, Biermanns M, Muntau AC, Conzelmann E, Gartner J (2002). PEX1 mutations in complementation group 1 of Zellweger spectrum patients correlate with severity of disease. *Pediatr Res* 51: 706–714.

Queitsch C, Sangster TA, Lindquist S (2002). Hsp90 as a capacitor of phenotypic variation. *Nature* 417: 618–624.

Robin NH, Nadeau JH (2001). Disorganization in mice and humans. *Am J Med Genet* 101: 334–338.

Rutherford SL (2000). From genotype to phenotype: buffering mechanisms and the storage of genetic information. *Bioessays* 22: 1095–1105.

Rutherford SL, Linquist S (1998). Hsp90 as a capacitor for morphological evolution. *Nature* 396: 336–342.

Scriver CR, Beaudet AL, Sly WS, Valle D (eds.) (2001). *The Metabolic and Molecular Bases of Inherited Disease*, 8th Edition. McGraw-Hill, New York.

Seidman JG, Seidman C (2002). Transcription factor haploinsufficiency: when half a loaf is not enough. *J Clin Invest* 109: 451–455.

Smith DW (1970). *Recognizable Patterns of Human Malformation. Genetic Embryologic, and Clinical Aspects*. Philadelphia, Saunders.

Srivastava D, Olson EN (2000). A genetic blueprint for cardiac development. *Nature* 407: 221–226.

Superti-Furga A, Bonafé L, Rimoin DL (2002). Molecular-pathogenetic classification of genetic disorders of the skeleton. *Am J Med Genet* 106: 282–293.

Taipale J, Chen JK, Cooper MK, Wang B, Mann RK, Milenkovic L, Scott M, Beachy PA (2000). Effects of oncogenic mutations in *Smoothened* and *Patched* can be reversed by cyclopamine. *Nature* 406: 1005–1009.

Tellier AL, Cormier-Daire V, Abadie V, Amiel J, Sigaudy S, Bonnet D, de Lonlay-Debeney P, Morrisseau-Durand MP, Hubert P, Michel JL, et al. (1998). CHARGE syndrome: report of 47 cases and review. *Am J Med Genet* 76: 402–409.

Thisse C, Zon L (2002). Organogenesis—heart and blood formation from the zebrafish point of view. *Science* 295: 457–462.

Van Straaten HWM, Copp AJ (2001). Curly tail: a 50-year history of the mouse spina bifida model. *Anat Embryol* 203: 225–237.

Veraksa A, Del Campo M, McGinnis W (2000). Developmental patterning genes and their conserved functions: from model organisms to humans. *Mol Genet Metab* 69: 85–100.

Villavicencio EH, Walterhouse DO, Iannacone PM (2000). The Sonic hedgehog-Patched-Gli pathway in human development and disease. *Am J Hum Genet* 67: 1047–1054.

Waddington CH (1942). Canalization of development and the inheritance of acquired characters. *Nature* 150: 563–565.

Wald NJ, Law MR, Morris JK, Wald DS (2001). Quantifying the effect of folic acid. *Lancet* 358: 2069–2073.

Wilkins AS (1997). Canalization: a molecular genetic perspective. *Bioessays* 19: 257–262.

Wilson GN (1992). Genomics of human dysmorphogenesis. *Am J Med Genet* 42: 187–196.

Wilson GN, de Chadarevian J-P, Kaplan P, Loehr JP, Frerman FE, Goodman SI (1988). Glutaric aciduria type II: review of the phenotype and report of an unusual glomerulopathy. *Am J Med Genet* 32: 395–401.

Winter RM (1996). Analysing human developmental abnormalities. *Bioessays* 18: 965–971.

2 | General Principles of Differentiation and Morphogenesis

SCOTT F. GILBERT

Developmental biology is the science connecting genetics with anatomy, and it makes sense out of both. Thus, it is the science that connects the inherited genotype with the observable phenotype and that addresses the mechanisms by which the genome specifies the characteristics of the individual human body. To study human genetics without developmental biology is like studying a culture only by reading its books, and to study anatomy without developmental biology is like visiting a foreign land without knowing its language or history. During the past decade, the basic principles of developmental biology have become known. They cover the following:

- Mechanisms of differential gene expression
- Combinatorial logic of enhancers and promoters
- Signal-transduction pathways linking cell membrane and nucleus
- Mechanisms by which syndromes occur
- Mechanisms producing dominant or recessive traits
- Repertoire of morphogenetic interactions and the molecules causing them
- Role of stochastic variability in morphogenesis

MECHANISMS OF DIFFERENTIAL GENE EXPRESSION

With few exceptions (e.g., lymphocytes and blood cells) every cell nucleus in the body contains the complete genome established in the fertilized egg. In molecular terms, the DNAs of all differentiated cells within an organism are identical. This was vividly demonstrated when entire mammalian organisms were generated from the nuclei of adult cells transplanted into enucleated oocytes (Wilmut et al., 1997; Kato et al., 1998; Wakayama et al., 1998). Thus, the unused genes in differentiated cells are neither destroyed nor mutated, and they retain the potential for being expressed. Only a small percentage of the genome is expressed in each cell, and a portion of the RNA synthesized in the cell is specific for that cell type.

How, then, is the inherited repertoire of genes differentially expressed during development? It appears that this can be accomplished at the four major steps of protein synthesis. Some genes are regulated at different steps in different cells, and certain genes can be regulated at multiple steps in the same cell:

- Differential gene transcription, regulating which of the nuclear genes are transcribed into nuclear (n) RNA
- Selective nRNA processing, regulating which of the transcribed RNAs (or which parts of such an nRNA) enter into the cytoplasm to become messenger (m)RNAs
- Selective mRNA translation, regulating which of the mRNAs in the cytoplasm become translated into proteins
- Differential protein modification, regulating which proteins are allowed to remain or function in the cell

It is estimated (Rockman and Wray, 2002) that the human species has more polymorphism in its regulatory regions than in the amino-acid-encoding exon regions of the genome.

DIFFERENTIAL GENE TRANSCRIPTION

Promoters and Enhancers

Differential gene transcription is by far the best-studied area of developmental gene regulation. To be transcribed, genes have to bind RNA polymerase to their promoters. This is a very tightly regulated task. Promoters of genes that synthesize mRNAs (i.e., genes that encode proteins) are typically located immediately upstream from the site where the RNA polymerase initiates transcription. Most of these promoters contain the sequence TATA, where RNA polymerase will be bound. This site, known as the TATA box, is usually about 30 bp upstream from the site where the first base is transcribed.

Eukaryotic RNA polymerases require additional protein factors to bind efficiently to this promoter sequence. At least six nuclear proteins are necessary for the proper initiation of transcription by RNA polymerase II (Buratowski et al., 1989; Sopta et al., 1989). These proteins are called *basal transcription factors*. The first of these, TFIID, recognizes the TATA box through one of its subunits, TATA-binding protein (TBP). TFIID serves as the foundation of the transcription initiation complex and keeps nucleosomes from forming in this region. Once TFIID is stabilized by TFIIA, it becomes able to bind TFIIB; and once TFIIB is in place, RNA polymerase can bind to this complex. Other transcription factors (TFIIE, -F, and -H) are then used to release RNA polymerase from the complex allowing it to transcribe the gene and to unwind the DNA helix so that the RNA polymerase will have a free template from which to transcribe.

In addition to these basal transcription factors, which are found in each nucleus, there is a set of transcription factors called TBP-associated factors, or TAFs (Buratowski, 1997; Lee and Young, 1998), which can stabilize the TBP. This function is critical for gene transcription, for if the TBP is not stabilized, it can fall off the small TATA sequence. The TAFs are bound by upstream promoter elements on the DNA. These TAFs need not be in every cell of the body, however.

A third set of transcription factors operate in a relatively small subset of cells to activate genes that are specific to these cell types. Cell-limited transcription factors (e.g., the Pax6 and MITF proteins, discussed below) can also activate the gene by stabilizing the transcription initiation complex. They can do so by binding to the TAFs, by binding directly to other factors such as TFIIB, or by destabilizing nucleosomes.

The temporal and spatial regulation of each promoter is controlled by the enhancer region of the gene. An *enhancer* is a DNA sequence that can activate or repress the utilization of a promoter, controlling the efficiency and rate of transcription from that particular promoter. Enhancers can activate only *cis*-linked promoters (i.e., promoters on the same chromosome), but they can do so at great distances (some as great as 50 kb away from the promoter). Moreover, enhancers do not need to be upstream of the gene. They can also be at the 3′ end, in the introns, or even on the complementary DNA strand (Maniatis et al., 1987). The human β-globin gene has an enhancer in its 3′-untranslated region. This sequence is necessary for the temporal and tissue-specific expression of the β-globin gene in adult red blood cell precursors (Trudel and Constantini, 1987). Like promoters, enhancers function by binding transcription factors.

Insulators

Enhancers must be told where to stop. Since enhancers can work at relatively long distances, it is possible for them to activate several nearby promoters. To stop this spreading of the enhancer's power, there are insulator sequences in the DNA (Zhou et al., 1995; Bell et al., 2001). Insulators bind proteins that prevent the enhancer from activating an adjacent promoter. They are often between the enhancer and the promoter. For instance, the chick β-globin enhancers are located in the locus control region (LCR), which is limited by insulators on both sides. On one side is an insulator that prevents the LCR enhancers from activating odorant receptor genes (which are active in the nasal neurons), and on the other side is an insulator preventing the LCR from activating the folate receptor gene.

Transcription Factors

Transcription factors are proteins that bind to enhancer or promoter regions and interact to activate or repress the transcription of a particular gene. Most transcription factors can bind to specific DNA sequences. These proteins can be grouped together into families based on similarities in structure (Table 2–1). The transcription factors within such a family share a framework structure in their DNA-binding sites, and slight differences in the amino acids at the binding site can alter the sequence of the DNA to which the factor binds.

Transcription factors have three major domains. The first is a DNA-binding domain, which recognizes a particular DNA sequence. The second is a *trans*-activating domain, which activates or suppresses the transcription of the gene whose promoter or enhancer it has bound. Usually, the *trans*-activating domain enables the transcription factor to interact with proteins involved in binding RNA polymerase (e.g., TFIIB or TFIIE; see Sauer et al., 1995). In addition, there may be a protein–protein interaction domain, which allows the transcription factor's activity to be modulated by TAFs or other transcription factors.

There are numerous diseases caused by deficiencies of transcription factors. The first identified, "transcription factoropathy," was probably androgen insensitivity syndrome. Here, the testosterone receptor is absent or deficient and, therefore, will not bind to the DNA activating male-specific genes, even in the presence of testosterone (Meyer et al., 1975). One of the first human genetic diseases to be understood from the binding of the ligand to the receptor through the activation of chromatin is Waardenburg's syndrome type II. Here, people heterozygous for the wild-type copy of Microphthalmia (*MITF*) are deaf, have multicolored irises, and have a white forelock in their hair. Activation of this transcription factor through the protein tyrosine kinase cascade enables it to dimerize, to bind to the regulatory regions of particular genes, and to bind a histone acetyltransferase that opens a region of DNA for transcription (Fig. 2–1; see Chapter 77).

Combinatorial Control of Transcription

The binding of a specific transcription factor to the enhancer or promoter does not insure that that gene will be transcribed. Although "master regulatory genes" such as *PAX6* (eye) or *MYOD* (muscles) have been proposed, even they work in concert with other transcription factors to effect cell differentiation. The use of *PAX6* by different organs demonstrates the modular nature of transcriptional regulatory units. The *PAX6* transcription factor is needed for mammalian eye, nervous system, and pancreatic development; and mutations in the human *PAX6* gene cause severe nervous system, pancreatic, and optic abnormalities (Glaser et al., 1994; see Chapters 59, 62). Pax6-binding sequences have been found in the enhancers of vertebrate lens crystallin genes and in the genes expressed in the endocrine cells of the pancreas (insulin, glucagon, and somatostatin).

Transcription factors work in concert with other transcription factors to activate a particular gene. For instance, in the chick δ1 lens crystallin gene, Pax6 works with Sox2, Maf-1, and Sp1. Sp1 is a general transcriptional activator found in all cells. Pax6 is found early in development throughout the head ectoderm. Sox2 is found only in those tissues that will become lens, and it is induced by the presumptive retina when the developing retinal cells contact the outer ectoderm. Thus, only those cells that contain both Sox2 and Pax6 can express the lens crystallin gene. In addition, there is a third site that can bind either an activator (the δEF3 protein) or a repressor (the δEF1 protein) of transcription. It is thought that the repressor may be critical in preventing crystallin expression in the nervous system.

Other regulatory regions that use Pax6 are the enhancers regulating the transcription of the insulin, glucagon, and somatostatin genes of the pancreas. Here, Pax6 cooperates with other transcription factors such as Pdx1 (specific for the pancreatic region of the endoderm) and Pbx1 (Andersen et al., 1999; Hussain and Habener, 1999; Lammert et al., 2001).

Other genes are activated by Pax6 binding, and one of them is the *Pax6* gene itself. Pax6 protein can bind to its own promoter (Plaza et al., 1993). This means that once the *Pax6* gene is turned on, it will continue to be expressed, even if the signal that originally activated it is no longer given.

Thus, three principles can be seen here. The first is that transcription factors function in a combinatorial manner, wherein several work together to promote or inhibit transcription. The second principle is that there are two major routes by which transcription factors become present in the nucleus: the first is through cell lineage, where the presumptive lens tissue acquires its Pax6 by being head ectoderm and the presumptive pancreatic islets acquire Pdx1 through their being endodermal, and the second is through induction, as when the *Sox2* gene becomes expressed when the presumptive retina abuts the presumptive lens. The third principle is that transcription factors can continue to be synthesized after the original signal for their synthesis has ceased. A fourth principle of transcription factors is seen in the example of MITF, mentioned above: the mere presence of transcription factors in the cell is not often sufficient for their binding to DNA and consequently functioning. Often, they have to be activated posttranslationally in order to function. This becomes a major mechanism for the control of differentiation and morphogenesis.

The gene both directs and is directed by protein synthesis. As Angier (1992) wrote:

> A series of new discoveries suggests that DNA is more like a certain type of politician, surrounded by a flock of protein handlers and advisers that must vigorously massage it, twist it and, on occasion, reinvent it before the grand blueprint of the body can make any sense at all.

OTHER MECHANISMS OF DEVELOPMENTAL GENE REGULATION

Regulation of gene expression is not confined to the differential transcription of DNA. Even if a particular RNA transcript is synthesized, there is no guarantee that it will create a functional protein in the cell. To become an active protein, the mRNA must be *(1)* processed into mRNA by the removal of introns, *(2)* translocated from the nucleus to the cytoplasm, and *(3)* translated by the protein-synthesizing apparatus; in some cases, the synthesized protein is not in its mature form

Table 2–1. Transcription Factor Families and Functions

Family	Representative Transcription Factors	Some Functions
Homeodomain		
HOX	HOXA-1, HOXB-2, etc.	Axis formation
POU	PIT1, Unc-86, Oct-2	Pituitary development, neural fate
LIM	Lim-1, Forkhead	Head development
PAX	PAX1, -2, -3, etc.	Neural specification, eye development
Basic helix-loop-helix	MYOD, achaete	Muscle and nerve specification
Basic leucine zipper	C/EBP, AP1	Liver differentiation, fat cell specification
Zinc finger		
Standard	WT1, Krüppel	Kidney, gonad development
Hormone receptors	Estrogen receptor	Secondary sex determination
Sry-Sox	Sry, SOXD, Sox2	Bone, primary sex determination

and *(4)* must be posttranslationally modified to become active. Regulation can occur at any of these steps during development.

Differential Nuclear RNA Processing

In bacteria, differential gene expression can be effected at the levels of transcription, translation, and protein modification. In eukaryotes, however, another possible level of regulation exists: control at the level of RNA processing and transport. There are two major ways in which differential RNA processing can regulate development. The first involves the "censoring" of which nuclear transcripts are processed into cytoplasmic messages. Here, different cells can select different nuclear transcripts to be processed and sent to the cytoplasm as mRNA. The same pool of nuclear transcripts can thereby give rise to different populations of cytoplasmic mRNAs in different cell types. The second mode of differential RNA processing is the splicing of the mRNA precursors into messages for different proteins using different combinations of potential exons. If an mRNA precursor had five potential exons, one cell might use exons 1, 2, 4, and 5; a different cell might utilize exons 1, 2, and 3; and yet another cell type might use a different combination. Thus, one gene can create a family of related proteins by alternative RNA splicing.

This ability to create large numbers of proteins from one gene through differential exon splicing may be extremely important in human development. The average vertebrate nRNA consists of relatively short exons (averaging about 140 bases) separated by introns that are usually much longer. Most mammalian nRNAs contain numerous exons. By splicing together different sets of exons, different cells can make different types of mRNA and, hence, different proteins. Whether a sequence of RNA is recognized as an exon or as an intron is a crucial step in gene regulation. What is an intron in one cell's nucleus may be an exon in another cell's nucleus.

Alternative nRNA splicing is based on determining which sequences can be spliced out as introns. This can occur in several ways. Cells can differ in their ability to recognize the 5′ splice site (at the beginning of the intron) or the 3′ splice site (at the end of the intron), or some cells could fail to recognize a sequence as an intron at all, retaining it within the message. The splicing of nRNA is mediated through a complex called a spliceosome, made up of small nuclear RNAs (snRNA) and proteins, that assembles at a splice site. Whether a spliceosome recognizes the splice sites depends on certain factors in the nucleus that can interact with those sites and compete or cooperate with the proteins that direct spliceosome formation. The 5′ splice site is normally recognized by snRNA U1 and splicing factor 2 (SF2, also known as alternative splicing factor). The choice of alternative 3′ splice sites is often controlled by which splice site can best bind a protein called U2AF. The spliceosome forms when the 5′ and 3′ splice sites are brought together and the intervening RNA is cut out.

Differential RNA processing may be a major source of the human proteome, the number and type of proteins encoded by the genome. Instead of "one gene–one polypeptide," one can have "one gene–one family of proteins." For instance, alternative RNA splicing enables the α-tropomyosin gene to encode brain, liver, skeletal muscle, smooth muscle, and fibroblast forms of this protein (Breitbart et al., 1987). The nRNA for α-tropomyosin contains 11 potential exons, but different sets of exons are used in different cells. Such different proteins encoded by the same gene are called *splicing isoforms* of the protein.

In some instances, alternatively spliced RNAs yield proteins that play similar, yet distinguishable, roles in the same cell. Pax6 has two splicing isoforms, and each is needed for different roles in the body. They cannot compensate for each other, and humans who have a *PAX6* mutation such that they cannot form one of these isoforms have defects in their lenses, corneas, and pupils (Epstein et al., 1994). Similarly, different isoforms of the WT1 protein perform different functions in the development of the gonads and kidneys. The isoform without the extra exon functions as a transcription factor during testis development, while the isoform containing the extra exon appears to be a splicing factor involved in kidney development (Hastie, 2001).

There are some instances where differential splicing may create thousands of different related proteins. *Neurexins* are neuronal cell recognition proteins that appear to be involved in neuron–neuron ad-

hesion and recognition. (The venom of the black widow spider works by binding to neurexins, causing massive neurotransmitter release [Rosenthal and Meldolesi, 1989].) These neurexin genes can be alternatively spliced at several different sites, creating hundreds of proteins from the same gene (Ullrich et al., 1995; Ichtchenko et al., 1995). The champion of making multiple proteins from the same gene is currently the *Drosophila Dscam* gene. This gene is involved in guiding certain axons to their targets during *Drosophila* development. The *Dscam* gene contains 24 exons. Moreover, exons 4, 6, and 9 are each encoded by at least a dozen mutually exclusive alternative sequences (Schmucker et al., 2000). The pre-mRNA of *Drosophila Dscam* is alternatively spliced in different axons and may control the specificity of axon attachments (Celotto and Graveley, 2001). If all the combinations of exons are used, this one gene can produce 38,016 different proteins, and random searches for these combinations indicate that a large fraction of them are actually made. The *Drosophila* genome is thought to contain only 14,000 genes, and here is a gene that potentially encodes three times that number of proteins.

It is estimated that at least 35% of human genes produce alternatively spliced RNAs (Croft et al., 2000). Therefore, even though the human genome may contain only 35,000–50,000 genes, its proteome is probably far more complex. The human homologue of *Drosophila Dscam* was actually discovered prior to its being seen in *Drosophila*. The gene abbreviation stands for "Down syndrome cell adhesion molecule," and it is encoded on the region of chromosome 21 whose trisomies are associated with neurological and coronary symptoms of Down syndrome. Mammalian Dscam is expressed abundantly in the nervous system during development, especially in axonal and dendritic processes within the cerebellum, hippocampus, and olfactory bulb. Dscam is most likely involved in cell–cell interactions during axonal–dendritic development and maintenance of functional neuronal networks. There appear to be several isoforms of this protein, and they are expressed in different subsets of neurons (Yamakawa et al., 1998).

Thus, proper development means not only that genes are transcribed at the appropriate time but also that the nuclear gene products are spliced appropriately. Mutations in the splice sites of genes can therefore prevent certain isoforms from arising, and it is estimated that 15% of all point mutations that result in human genetic disease are those creating splice site abnormalities (Krawzcak et al., 1992; Cooper and Mattox, 1997). For instance, congenital adrenal hypoplasia can be caused by a point mutation in the splice site for the second intron of the *CYP21* gene for 21-hydroxylase. This prevents the intron from being skipped and makes an ineffective protein. Such sequence insertions can also be caused by point mutations that generate new splice sites (Hutchinson et al., 2001). Mutations that interfere with splicing by rendering a splice site inoperative can cause deletion of the exon (Byers et al., 1997). Moreover, mutations may also effect the usage of particular alternative splice sites. Mutations of the 5′ splice site of exon 10 in the gene for FTDP-17 destabilize a potential stem-loop structure that probably regulates the alternative splicing of this exon. This causes a higher percentage of a particular isoform, consistent with the role of this mutant gene in the frontotemporal changes of Pick's disease (Hutton et al., 1998).

There are some proteins and snRNAs that are used throughout the body to effect differential pre-mRNA splicing, and there are some proteins that appear to be cell type-specific and that regulate differential splicing in a manner characteristic for that cell. If the genes encoding these cell set-specific splicing factors are mutated, one could expect several cell-specific isoforms to be aberrant. This appears to be the case in the leading cause of hereditary infant mortality, spinal muscular atrophy. Here, mutations in the gene encoding the SMN (survival of motor neurons) protein prevent the maintenance of motor neurons. This protein is involved in splicing nRNAs in this subset of neurons (Pellizzoni et al., 1999). RNA splicing also appears to be defective in myotonic dystrophy. This abnormality may be caused by binding of the splicing factor CUG-binding protein by the CUG repeats of the mutant DM protein kinase nRNA. Retention of the CUG-binding protein by these CUG repeats may prevent it from its normal functions in alternative splicing of troponin pre-mRNA (Philips et al., 1998).

RNA Translation

Once a message has been transcribed and properly spliced, it can enter the cytoplasm and be translated. However, translation is an intricately regulated mechanism that may also alter phenotypes.

Some genetic diseases are due to mutations that create termination codons. For instance, a complete form of androgen-insensitivity syndrome is caused by a guanine-to-adenine transition at nucleotide 2682, changing codon 717 from tryptophan to a translation stop signal (Sai et al., 1997). Codon 717 is in exon 4, and this truncated receptor thereby lacked most of its androgen-binding domain. Other mutations can alter the longevity of an mRNA. This can greatly affect the number of proteins synthesized from it. For example, hemoglobin α-Constant Spring is a naturally occurring mutation wherein the translation termination codon has been mutated to that of an amino acid codon, and the translation continues for 31 more codons (Wang et al., 1995). This readthrough results in destabilization of the α-globin mRNA, a reduction of greater than 95% of α-globin gene expression from the affected locus, and the resultant clinical disease (α-thalassemia).

In many instances, certain messages are stabilized or brought to the ribosomes by certain proteins. The most prevalent form of inherited mental retardation, fragile X syndrome, may result from translational deficiency of certain neuronal messages. This disease usually results from the expansion and hypermethylation of CGG repeats in the 5'-untranslated region of the *FMR1* gene. This CGG expansion blocks transcription of this gene. This gene encodes an RNA-binding protein, which appears to be critical for the translation of certain messages. Nearly 85% of the FMR1 protein is associated with translating polysomes, while mutants in the RNA-binding domains produce severe forms of the syndrome and are not observed with the cytoplasmic polysomes (Feng et al., 1997a,b). Recent studies (Brown et al., 2001; Darnell et al., 2001) have shown that a particular subset of mouse brain mRNA requires this protein for proper translation. Most of these genes are involved with synapse function or neuronal development. It is probable that FMRP binds to specific mRNAs, either regulating their translation or targeting them to the dendrite, where they might await the signal for translation.

Posttranslational Modification

When a protein is synthesized, the story is still not over. Once a protein is made, it becomes part of a larger level of organization. For instance, it may become part of the structural framework of the cell, or it may become involved in one of the myriad enzymatic pathways for the synthesis or breakdown of cellular metabolites. In any case, the individual protein is now part of a complex "ecosystem," which integrates it into a relationship with numerous other proteins. Thus, several changes can still take place that determine whether or not the protein will be active. Some newly synthesized proteins are inactive without the cleaving away of certain inhibitory sections. This is what happens when insulin is made from its larger protein precursor. Some proteins must be "addressed" to their specific intracellular destinations in order to function. Proteins are often sequestered in certain regions, such as membranes, lysosomes, nuclei, or mitochondria; and specific amino acid sequences are needed either as recognition sequences or as places for such tags. For instance, mucolipidosis II (I-cell disease) is characterized by a deficiency in the mannose-6-phosphate "address tag" put onto enzymes to target them to the lysosome. Here, there is a deficiency in GlcNAc-1-P transferase, which is involved in constructing the mannose-6-phosphate residues (Sly and Fischer, 1982).

Some proteins need to assemble with other proteins to form a functional unit. The hemoglobin protein, the microtubule, and the ribosome are all examples of numerous proteins joining together to form a functional unit. Diseases such as sickle cell anemia and certain types of osteogenesis imperfecta syndrome are caused by the improper assembly of protein subunits. Moreover, some proteins are not active unless they bind an ion such as calcium or are modified by the covalent addition of a phosphate or acetate group. This last type of protein modification will become very important in the next section of this chapter since many important proteins in embryonic cells are just sitting there until some signal activates them.

EMBRYONIC INDUCTION

Induction and Competence

Organs are complex structures composed of numerous types of tissue. In the vertebrate eye, for example, light is transmitted through the transparent corneal tissue and focused by the lens tissue (the diameter of which is controlled by muscle tissue), eventually impinging on the tissue of the neural retina. The precise arrangement of tissues in this organ cannot be disturbed without impairing its function. Such coordination in the construction of organs is accomplished by one group of cells changing the behavior of an adjacent set of cells, thereby causing them to change their shape, mitotic rate, or fate. This kind of interaction at close range between two or more cells or tissues of different history and properties is called *proximate interaction*, or *induction*. There are at least two components to every inductive interaction. The first is the *inducer*, the tissue that produces a signal (or signals) that changes the cellular behavior of the other tissue, and the second is the *responder*, the tissue being induced.

Not all tissues can respond to the signal being produced by the inducer. For instance, if the optic vesicle (presumptive retina) of *Xenopus laevis* is placed in an ectopic location (i.e., in a different place from where it normally forms) underneath the head ectoderm, it will induce that ectoderm to form lens tissue. Only the optic vesicle appears to be able to do this; therefore, it is an inducer. However, if the optic vesicle is placed beneath ectoderm in the flank or abdomen of the same organism, that ectoderm will not be able to respond. Only the head ectoderm is competent to respond to the signals from the optic vesicle by producing a lens (Saha et al., 1989; Grainger, 1992).

This ability to respond to a specific inductive signal is called *competence* (Waddington, 1940). Competence is not a passive state but an actively acquired condition. For example, in the developing chick and mammalian eye, the Pax6 protein appears to be important in making the ectoderm competent to respond to the inductive signal from the optic vesicle. *Pax6* expression is seen in the head ectoderm, which can respond to the optic vesicle by forming lenses; and it is not seen in other regions of the surface ectoderm (Li et al., 1994). Moreover, the importance of Pax6 as a competence factor was demonstrated by recombination experiments using embryonic rat eye tissue (Fujiwara et al., 1994). Pax6 is required for the surface ectoderm to respond to the inductive signal from the optic vesicle. The inducing tissue does not need it. Pax6 is expressed in the anterior ectoderm of the embryo through the interaction of the lateral dorsal head ectoderm with the anterior neural plate (Zygar et al., 1998).

Thus, there is no single inducer of the lens. Studies on amphibians suggest that the first inducers may be the pharyngeal endoderm and heart-forming mesoderm that underlie the lens-forming ectoderm during the early- and mid-gastrula stages (Jacobson, 1966). The anterior neural plate may produce the next signals, including a signal that promotes the synthesis of Pax6 in the anterior ectoderm. Thus, the optic vesicle appears to be *the* inducer, but the anterior ectoderm has already been induced by at least two other factors. (The situation is like that of the player who kicks the "winning goal" of a soccer match.) The optic vesicle appears to secrete two induction factors: one may be BMP4 (Furuta and Hogan, 1998), a protein that induces the transcription of the Sox2 and Sox3 transcription factors, and the other is thought to be FGF8, a signal that induces the appearance of the L-Maf transcription factor (Ogino and Yasuda, 1998; Vogel-Höpker et al., 2000). The combination of Pax6, Sox2, Sox3, and L-Maf ensures the production of the lens.

Cascades of Induction: Reciprocal and Sequential Inductive Events

Another feature of induction is the reciprocal nature of many inductive interactions. Once the lens has begun forming, it can induce other tissues. One of these responding tissues is the optic vesicle itself. Now the inducer becomes the induced. Under the influence of factors secreted by the lens, the optic vesicle becomes the optic cup and the wall of the optic cup differentiates into two layers, the pigmented retina and the neural retina (Cvekl and Piatigorsky, 1996). Such interactions are called *reciprocal inductions*.

At the same time, the developing lens is also inducing the ectoderm above it to become the cornea. Like the lens-forming ectoderm, the cornea-forming ectoderm has achieved a particular competence to respond to inductive signals, in this case the signals from the lens (Meier, 1977). Under the influence of the lens, the corneal ectodermal cells become columnar and secrete multiple layers of collagen. Mesenchymal cells from the neural crest use this collagen matrix to enter the area and secrete a set of proteins (including the enzyme hyaluronidase), which further differentiate the cornea. A third signal, the hormone thyroxine, dehydrates the tissue and makes it transparent (Hay, 1979; Bard, 1990). Thus, there are sequential inductive events and multiple causes for each induction.

Instructive and Permissive Interactions

Howard Holtzer (1968) distinguished two major modes of inductive interaction. In *instructive interaction*, a signal from the inducing cell is necessary for initiating new gene expression in the responding cell. Without the inducing cell, the responding cell would not be capable of differentiating in that particular way. For example, when the optic vesicle is experimentally placed under a new region of the head ectoderm and causes that region of the ectoderm to form a lens, that is an instructive interaction. Wessells (1977) proposed three general principles characteristic of most instructive interactions:

1. In the presence of tissue A, responding tissue B develops in a certain way.
2. In the absence of tissue A, responding tissue B does not develop in that way.
3. In the absence of tissue A but in the presence of tissue C, tissue B does not develop in that way.

The second type of induction is *permissive interaction*. Here, the responding tissue contains all the potentials that are to be expressed and needs only an environment that allows expression of these traits. For instance, many tissues need a solid substrate containing fibronectin or laminin in order to develop. The fibronectin or laminin does not alter the type of cell that is to be produced but only enables what has been determined to be expressed.

Regional Specificity of Induction

Some of the best-studied cases of induction are those involving the interactions of sheets of epithelial cells with adjacent mesenchymal cells. These interactions are called *epithelial–mesenchymal interactions*. Epithelia are sheets or tubes of connected cells; they can originate from any germ layer. Mesenchyme refers to loosely packed, unconnected cells. Mesenchymal cells are derived from the mesoderm or neural crest. All organs consist of an epithelium and an associated mesenchyme, so epithelial–mesenchymal interactions are among the most important phenomena in development. Some examples are listed in Table 2–2.

Using the induction of cutaneous structures as our examples, we will look at the properties of epithelial–mesenchymal interactions. The first of these properties is the regional specificity of induction. Skin is composed of two main tissues: an outer epidermis (an epithelial tissue derived from ectoderm) and a dermis (a mesenchymal tissue derived from mesoderm). The chick epidermis signals the underlying dermal cells to form condensations (probably by secreting Sonic hedgehog and transforming growth factor (TGF)-β2 proteins, which will be discussed below), and the condensed dermal mesenchyme responds by secreting factors that cause the epidermis to form regionally specific cutaneous structures (Nohno et al., 1995; Ting-Berreth and Chuong, 1996). These structures can be the broad feathers of the wing, the narrow feathers of

the thigh, or the scales and claws of the feet. Researchers can separate the embryonic epithelium and mesenchyme from each other and recombine them in different ways (Saunders et al., 1957). These studies demonstrated that the dermal mesenchyme is responsible for the regional specificity of induction in the competent epidermal epithelium. The same type of epithelium develops cutaneous structures according to the region from which the mesenchyme was taken. Here, the mesenchyme plays an instructive role, calling into play different sets of genes in the responding epithelial cells.

Paracrine Factors

How are the signals between inducer and responder transmitted? While studying the mechanisms of induction that produce the kidney tubules and teeth, Grobstein (1956) and others found that some inductive events could occur despite a filter separating the epithelial and mesenchymal cells. Other inductions, however, were blocked by the filter. The researchers therefore concluded that some of the inductive molecules were soluble factors that could pass through the small pores of the filter and that other inductive events required physical contact between the epithelial and mesenchymal cells. When cell membrane proteins on one cell surface interact with receptor proteins on adjacent cell surfaces, these events are called *juxtacrine interactions* (since the cell membranes are juxtaposed). When proteins synthesized by one cell can diffuse over small distances to induce changes in neighboring cells, the event is called a *paracrine interaction*, and the diffusible proteins are called *paracrine factors* or *growth and differentiation factors* (GDFs). We will consider paracrine interactions first and then return to juxtacrine interactions later in the chapter.

Whereas endocrine factors (hormones) travel through the blood to exert their effects, paracrine factors are secreted into the immediate spaces around the cell producing them. These proteins are the "inducing factors" of the classic experimental embryologists. During the past decade, developmental biologists have discovered that the induction of numerous organs is actually effected by a relatively small set of paracrine factors. The embryo inherits a rather compact "toolkit" and uses many of the same proteins to construct the heart, kidneys, teeth, eyes, and other organs. Moreover, the same proteins are utilized throughout the animal kingdom; the factors active in creating the *Drosophila* eye or heart are very similar to those used in generating mammalian organs. Many of these paracrine factors can be grouped into four major families on the basis of their structures: the fibroblast growth factor (FGF) family, the Hedgehog family, the Wingless (Wnt) family, and the TGF-β superfamily.

Fibroblast Growth Factors

Nearly two dozen distinct FGF genes are known in vertebrates, and they can generate hundreds of protein isoforms by varying their RNA splicing or initiation codons in different tissues (see Chapter 32). FGFs can activate a set of receptor tyrosine kinases, the fibroblast growth factor receptors (FGFRs). As we will discuss later in this chapter, receptor tyrosine kinases are proteins that extend through the cell membrane (Fig. 2–1). On the extracellular side is the portion of the protein that binds the paracrine factor. On the intracellular side is a dormant tyrosine kinase (i.e., a protein that can phosphorylate another protein by splitting ATP). When the FGFR binds an FGF (and only when it binds an FGF), the dormant kinase is activated, and it phosphorylates certain proteins within the responding cell. The proteins are now activated and can perform new functions. FGFs are associated with several developmental functions, including angiogenesis (blood vessel formation), mesoderm formation, and axon extension.

Table 2–2. Examples of Organs and Their Epithelial and Mesenchymal Components

Organ	Epithelial Component	Mesenchymal Component
Cutaneous appendages (hair, sweat glands)	Epidermis (ectoderm)	Dermis (mesoderm)
Gut organs	Endodermal epithelium	Mesodermal mesenchyme
Respiratory organs	Endodermal epithelium	Mesodermal mesenchyme
Kidney	Ureteric bud epithelium (mesoderm)	Metanephrogenic (mesodermal) mesenchyme
Tooth	Jaw epithelium (ectoderm)	Neural crest (ectodermal) mesenchyme

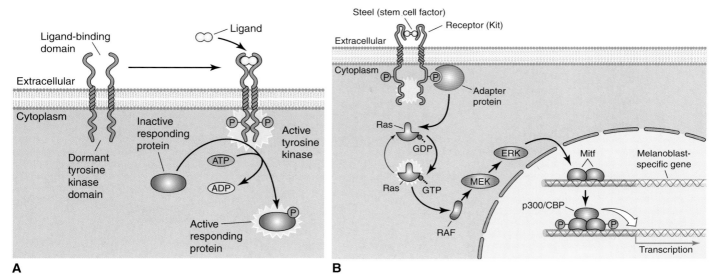

Figure 2–1. Basic pattern of signal transduction. *(A)* The dormant tyrosine kinase is activated by the binding of a ligand by the extracellular portion of the receptor protein. This enzyme activity phosphorylates specific tyrosine residues of certain proteins. These proteins are now activated. They can either enter the nucleus, where they can act as transcription factors, or activate other proteins that will eventually activate transcription factors. *(B)* Activation of the Mitf transcription factor through the binding of stem cell factor by the Kit receptor tyrosine kinase (RTK) protein. The information received at the cell membrane is sent to the nucleus by the RTK signal-transduction pathway. When the Kit protein binds the Steel paracrine factor, Kit dimerizes and becomes phosphorylated. This phosphorylation is used to activate the Ras G protein, which activates the chain of kinases that will phosphorylate the Mitf protein. Once phosphorylated, Mitf can bind the cofactor p300/CBP, acetylate the nucleosome histones, and initiate transcription of the genes for melanocyte development. CBP, cyclic AMP response element binding protein; ERK, extracellular signal–regulated kinase; MEK, mitogen-activated kinase kinase. (After Price et al., 1998; Gilbert, 2003.)

While FGFs can often substitute for one another, their expression patterns give them separate functions. FGF2 is especially important in angiogenesis, and FGF8 is important for the development of the midbrain, eyes, and limbs (Crossley et al., 1996).

Hedgehog Proteins

The Hedgehog proteins constitute a family of paracrine factors that are often used by the embryo to induce particular cell types and to create boundaries between tissues (see Chapter 16). Vertebrates have at least three homologues of the *Drosophila hedgehog* gene: *sonic hedgehog (shh), desert hedgehog (dhh),* and *indian hedgehog (ihh).* Desert hedgehog is expressed in the Sertoli cells of the testes, and mice homozygous for a null allele of *dhh* exhibit defective spermatogenesis. Indian hedgehog is expressed in the gut and cartilage and is important in postnatal bone growth.

Sonic hedgehog is the most widely used of the three vertebrate homologues. Made by the notochord, it is processed so that only the amino-terminal two-thirds of the molecule is secreted. This peptide is responsible for patterning the neural tube such that motor neurons are formed from the ventral neurons and sensory neurons are formed from the dorsal neurons (Yamada et al., 1993). Sonic hedgehog is also responsible for patterning the somites so that the portion of the somite closest to the notochord becomes the cartilage of the spine (Fan and Tessier-Lavigne, 1994; Johnson et al., 1994). Sonic hedgehog mediates the formation of the left–right axis in several vertebrates, initiates the anterior–posterior axis in limbs, induces the regionally specific differentiation of the digestive tube, and induces hair formation. Sonic hedgehog often works with other paracrine factors, such as Wnt and FGF proteins. In the developing tooth, Sonic hedgehog, FGF4, and other paracrine factors are concentrated in the region where cell interactions create the cusps of the teeth (Vaahtokari et al., 1996).

Wnt Family Proteins

The Wnts constitute a family of cysteine-rich glycoproteins. There are at least 15 members of this family in vertebrates (see Chapter 22). Their name comes from fusing the name of the *Drosophila* segment polarity gene *wingless* with the name of one of its vertebrate homologues, *integrated.* While Sonic hedgehog is important in patterning the ventral portion of the somites (causing the cells to become carti-

lage), Wnt1 appears to be active in inducing the dorsal cells of the somites to become muscle (McMahon and Bradley, 1990; Stern et al., 1995). Wnt proteins also are critical in establishing the polarity of insect and vertebrate limbs, and they are used in several steps of urogenital system development.

TGF-β Superfamily Proteins

There are over 30 structurally related members of the TGF-β superfamily, and they regulate some of the most important interactions in development (see Chapter 24). The TGF-β superfamily includes the TGF-β family, the activin family, the bone morphogenetic proteins (BMPs), the Vg1 family, and other proteins, including glia-derived neurotrophic factor (necessary for kidney and enteric neuron differentiation) and müllerian inhibitory factor (which is involved in mammalian sex determination).

TGF-β family members TGF-β1, -2, -3, and -5 are important in regulating the formation of the extracellular matrix between cells and for regulating cell division (both positively and negatively). The members of the BMP family were originally discovered by their ability to induce bone formation; hence, they are the bone morphogenetic proteins. Bone formation, however, is only one of their many functions; they regulate cell division, apoptosis (programmed cell death), cell migration, and differentiation (Hogan, 1996).

Other Paracrine Factors

Although most of the paracrine factors are members of the above-mentioned four families, some have few or no close relatives. Factors such as epidermal growth factor, hepatocyte growth factor, neurotrophins, and stem cell factor are not in the above-mentioned families, but each plays important roles during development. In addition, there are numerous factors involved almost exclusively with developing blood cells: erythropoietin, the cytokines, and the interleukins.

AN INTRODUCTION TO SIGNAL-TRANSDUCTION PATHWAYS

The paracrine factors are inducer proteins. We now turn to the molecules involved in the response to induction. These molecules include the receptors in the membrane of the responding cell, which bind the

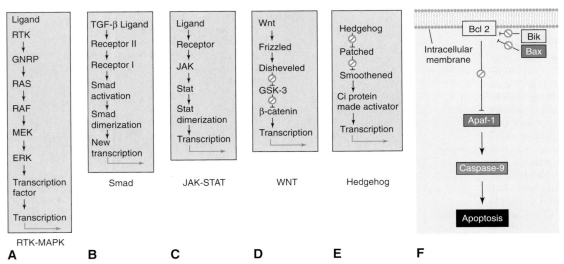

Figure 2–2. Five of the major signal-transduction pathways through which signals on the cell surface are sent into the nucleus. *(A)* The receptor tyrosine kinase–mitogen-activated protein kinase (RTK-MAPK) pathway, *(B)* the Smad pathway used by transforming growth factor β (TGF-β) superfamily proteins, *(C)* the JAK-STAT pathway, *(D)* the Wnt pathway, *(E)* the Hedgehog pathway, and *(F)* one of the apoptosis pathways used by mammalian neurons. ERK, extracellular signal–regulated kinase; MEK, MAPK kinase; JAK, Janus kinase; STAT, signal transducer and activator of transcription; GSK, glycogen synthase kinase; GNRP, guanine nucleotide-releasing protein.

paracrine factor, and the cascade of interacting proteins that transmit a signal through a pathway from the bound receptor to the nucleus. These pathways between the cell membrane and the genome are called *signal-transduction pathways*, and we will outline some of the major ones here. They appear to be variations on a common and rather elegant theme (Fig. 2–1*A*): each receptor spans the cell membrane and has an extracellular region, a transmembrane region, and a cytoplasmic region. When a ligand (the paracrine factor) binds its receptor in the extracellular region, it induces a conformational change in the receptor's structure. This shape change is transmitted through the membrane and changes the shape of the cytoplasmic domains. The conformational change in the cytoplasmic domains gives them enzymatic activity, usually a kinase activity that can use ATP to phosphorylate proteins, including the receptor molecule itself. The active receptor can now catalyze reactions that phosphorylate other proteins, and this phosphorylation activates their latent activities in turn. Eventually, the cascade of phosphorylation activates a dormant transcription factor, which activates (or represses) a particular set of genes. There are numerous modifications of this theme, and some of the most important of these pathways are outlined below (Fig. 2–2).

The Receptor Tyrosine Kinase–Mitogen-Activated Protein Kinase Pathway

The receptor tyrosine kinase (RTK) signal-transduction pathway was one of the first pathways to unite various areas of developmental biology. Researchers studying *Drosophila* eyes, nematode vulvae, and human cancers found that they were all studying homologous genes. The RTK–mitogen-activated protein kinase (MAPK) pathway begins at the cell surface, where an RTK binds its specific ligand. Ligands that bind to RTKs include the FGFs, epidermal growth factors, platelet-derived growth factors, and stem cell factor. Each RTK can bind only one or a small set of these ligands. (Stem cell factor, e.g., will bind to only one RTK, the Kit protein.) The RTK spans the cell membrane, and when it binds its ligand, it undergoes a conformational change that enables it to dimerize with another RTK. This conformational change activates the latent kinase activity of each RTK, and these receptors phosphorylate each other on particular tyrosine residues. Thus, the binding of the ligand to the receptor causes the autophosphorylation of the cytoplasmic domain of the receptor.

The phosphorylated tyrosine on the receptor is then recognized by an adapter protein (Fig. 2–1*B*). The adapter protein serves as a bridge that links the phosphorylated RTK to a powerful intracellular signaling system. While binding to the phosphorylated RTK through one of its cytoplasmic domains, the adapter protein also activates a G pro-

tein (see Chapter 84). Normally, the G protein is in an inactive, GDP-bound state. The activated receptor stimulates the adapter protein to activate the guanine nucleotide-releasing factor. This protein exchanges a phosphate from a GTP to transform the bound GDP into GTP. The GTP-bound G protein is an active form that transmits the signal. After delivering the signal, the GTP on the G protein is hydrolyzed back into GDP. This catalysis is greatly stimulated by the complexing of the Ras protein with the GTPase-activating protein (GAP). In this way, the G protein is returned to its inactive state, where it can await further signaling. Mutations in the genes encoding the small GTP-binding proteins and their regulators can lead to cancers or syndromes such as Aarskog-Scott syndrome, fibrous dysplasia, and neurofibromatosis 1 (see Chapters 85–87).

The active G protein associates with a kinase called Raf. The G protein recruits the inactive Raf protein to the cell membrane, where it becomes active (Leevers et al., 1994; Stokoe et al. 1994). The Raf protein is a kinase that activates the MAPK kinase (MEK) protein by phosphorylating it. MEK is itself a kinase, which activates extracellular signal–regulated kinase (ERK) by phosphorylation, and ERK is a kinase that can enter the nucleus and phosphorylate certain transcription factors. This pathway is critical in numerous developmental processes.

In the migrating neural crest cells of humans and mice, the RTK pathway is important in activating the microphthalmia transcription factor (Mitf) to produce the pigment cells (see Chapter 77). Mitf is transcribed in the pigment-forming melanoblast cells that migrate from the neural crest into the skin and in the melanin-forming cells of the pigmented retina, but this protein is not functional until it receives signals to become active. The clue to these signals lay in two mouse mutants whose phenotypes resemble those of mice homozygous for *microphthalmia* mutations. Like those mice, homozygous *White* mice and homozygous *Steel* mice are white because their pigment cells have failed to migrate. Perhaps all three genes (*Mitf*, *Steel*, and *White*) are on the same developmental pathway. In 1990, several laboratories demonstrated that the *Steel* gene encodes a paracrine protein called stem cell factor (Witte, 1990). Stem cell factor binds to and activates the Kit RTK encoded by the *White* gene (Spritz et al., 1992; Wu et al., 2000). The binding of stem cell factor to the Kit RTK dimerizes the Kit protein, causing it to become phosphorylated. Phosphorylated Kit activates the pathway whereby phosphorylated ERK is able to phosphorylate Mitf (Hsu et al., 1997; Hemesath et al., 1998). Only the phosphor-ylated form of Mitf is able to bind the p300/cyclic AMP response element–binding protein (CBP) coactivator protein, which enables it to activate transcription of the genes encoding tyrosinase and other proteins of the melanin-formation pathway (Price et al. 1998).

The Smad Pathway

Members of the TFG-β superfamily of paracrine factors activate members of the Smad family of transcription factors (Heldin et al., 1997). The TGF-β ligand binds to a type II TGF-β receptor, which allows that receptor to bind to a type I TGF-β receptor. Once the two receptors are in close contact, the type II receptor phosphorylates a serine or threonine on the type I receptor, thereby activating it. The activated type I receptor can now phosphorylate the Smad proteins. (Researchers named the Smad proteins by eliding the names of the first identified members of this family: the *Caenorhabditis elegans* Sma protein and the *Drosophila* Mad protein.) Smads 1 and 5 are activated by the BMP family of TGF-β factors, while the receptors binding activin and the TGF-β family phosphorylate Smads 2 and 3. These phosphorylated Smads bind to Smad 4 and form the transcription factor complex that will enter the nucleus. In vertebrates, the TGF-β superfamily ligand Nodal appears to activate the Smad pathway in those cells responsible for the formation of the mesoderm and for specifying the left–right axis (Nomura and Li, 1998).

The JAK–STAT Pathway

Another important pathway transducing information on the cell membrane to the nucleus is the JAK–STAT pathway. Here, the set of transcription factors consists of the STAT (signal transducers and activators of transcription) proteins (Ihle, 1996). STATs are phosphorylated by certain receptor tyrosine kinases, including FGFRs and the JAK family of tyrosine kinases. The JAK–STAT pathway is extremely important in the differentiation of blood cells and in the activation of the casein gene during milk production. In casein production, for instance, the endocrine factor prolactin binds to the extracellular regions of prolactin receptors, causing them to dimerize. A JAK protein kinase is bound to each of the receptors (in their respective cytoplasmic regions), and these JAK proteins are now brought together, where they can phosphorylate the receptors at several sites. The receptors are now activated and have their own protein kinase activity. Therefore, the JAK proteins convert a receptor into an RTK. The activated receptors can now phosphorylate particular inactive STATs and cause them to dimerize. These dimers are the active form of the STAT transcription factors, and they are translocated into the nucleus, where they bind to specific regions of DNA. In this case, they bind to the upstream promoter elements of the casein gene, causing it to be transcribed.

The STAT pathway is very important in the regulation of human fetal bone growth. Mutations that prematurely activate the STAT pathway have been implicated in some severe forms of dwarfism, such as the lethal thanatophoric dysplasia, wherein the growth plates of the rib and limb bones fail to proliferate. The genetic lesion resides in the gene encoding FGFR3, a receptor expressed in the cartilage precursor cells in the growth plates of the long bones (Rousseau et al., 1994; Shiang et al., 1994). Normally, the FGFR3 protein is activated by an FGF, and it signals the chondrocytes to stop dividing and begin differentiating into cartilage. This signal is mediated by the STAT1 protein, which is phosphorylated by the activated FGFR3 and then translocated into the nucleus. Inside the nucleus, this transcription factor activates the genes encoding a cell cycle inhibitor, the p21 protein (Su et al., 1997). The mutations causing thanatophoric dwarfism result in a gain-of-function phenotype, wherein the mutant FGFR3 is active constitutively, that is, without the need to be activated by an FGF (Deng et al., 1996; Webster and Donoghue, 1996).

The Wnt–β–Catenin Pathway

Members of the Wnt family of paracrine factors interact with transmembrane receptors of the Frizzled family (see Chapter 22). In the classical Wnt pathway, the binding of Wnt by the Frizzled protein causes the Frizzled protein to activate the Disheveled protein. Once the Disheveled protein is activated, it inhibits the activity of the glycogen synthase kinase-3 (GSK-3) enzyme. GSK-3, if it were active, would prevent the dissociation of the β-catenin protein from the APC protein, which targets β-catenin for degradation. However, when the Wnt signal is given and GSK-3 is inhibited, β-catenin can dissociate from the APC protein and enter the nucleus. Once inside the nucleus, it can form a heterodimer with lymphocyte enhancer-binding protein (LEF) or T-cell factor (TCF), becoming a transcription factor. This complex binds to and activates the Wnt-responsive genes (Behrens et al., 1996; Cadigan and Nusse, 1997). This model is undoubtedly an oversimplification (see McEwen and Peifer, 2001). One principle that is readily seen in the Wnt pathway (and evident in the Hedgehog pathway) is that activation is often accomplished by inhibiting an inhibitor. Thus, the GSK-3 protein is an inhibitor that is itself repressed by the Wnt signal.

In addition to sending signals to the nucleus, Wnt can affect the actin and microtubular cytoskeleton. Here, the Disheveled protein interacts with a protein kinase that initiates a cascade that will phosphorylate cytoskeletal proteins and thereby alter cell shape, cell polarity (where the upper and lower portions of the cell differ), or motility (Shulman et al., 1998; Winter et al., 2001).

The Hedgehog Pathway

Members of the Hedgehog protein family function by binding to a receptor called Patched. The Patched protein, however, is not a signal transducer. Rather, it is bound to a signal transducer, the Smoothened protein. The Patched protein prevents the Smoothened protein from functioning. In the absence of Hedgehog binding to Patched, the Smoothened protein is inactive and the Cubitus interruptus (Ci) protein is tethered to the microtubules of the responding cell. While on the microtubules, it is cleaved in such a way that a portion of it enters the nucleus and acts as a transcriptional repressor. This portion of the Ci protein binds to the promoters and enhancers of particular genes and acts as an inhibitor of transcription. When Hedgehog binds to Patched, the Patched protein's shape is altered such that it no longer inhibits Smoothened. The Smoothened protein acts (probably by phosphorylation) to release the Ci protein from the microtubules and to prevent its being cleaved. The intact Ci protein can now enter the nucleus, where it acts as a transcriptional *activator* of the same genes it used to repress (Aza-Blanc et al., 1997).

The Hedgehog pathway is extremely important in limb and neural differentiation in vertebrates (see Chapters 16–20). Here, the homologues of Ci are the GLI proteins. Both the transport of the Hedgehog protein and its reception by the target cell require cholesterol. Therefore, mutations involving cholesterol metabolism and teratogens that block cholesterol synthesis can cause the same spectrum of defects as mutations in sonic hedgehog.

The Notch Pathway: Juxtaposed Ligands and Receptors

While most known regulators of induction are diffusible proteins, some inducing proteins remain bound to the inducing cell surface. In one such pathway, cells expressing the Delta, Jagged, or Serrate protein in their membranes activate neighboring cells that contain the Notch protein in cell membranes (see Chapter 39). Notch extends through the cell membrane, and its external surface contacts Delta, Jagged, or Serrate proteins extending out from an adjacent cell. When complexed to one of these ligands, Notch undergoes a conformational change that enables it to be cut by the presenilin-1 protease. The cleaved portion enters the nucleus and binds to a dormant transcription factor of the CSL *(CBF1, Suppressor of Hairless, Lag-1)* family. When bound to the Notch protein, the CSL transcription factors activate their target genes (Lecourtois and Schweisguth, 1998; Schroeder et al., 1998; Struhl and Adachi, 1998).

Notch proteins are extremely important receptors in the nervous system. In both the vertebrate and *Drosophila* nervous systems, the binding of Delta to Notch tells the receiving cell not to become neural (Chitnis et al., 1995; Wang et al., 1998). In the vertebrate eye, the interactions between Notch and its ligands seem to regulate which cells become optic neurons and which become glial cells (Dorsky et al., 1997; Wang et al., 1998).

THE EXTRACELLULAR MATRIX AS A SOURCE OF CRITICAL DEVELOPMENTAL SIGNALS

Extracellular Matrix Proteins and Functions

The extracellular matrix consists of macromolecules secreted by cells into their immediate environment (see Chapter 95). These macromolecules form a region of noncellular material in the interstices between the cells. The extracellular matrix is a critical region for much of animal development. Cell adhesion, cell migration, and the formation of epithelial sheets and tubes all depend on the ability of cells to form attachments to extracellular matrices. In some cases, as in the formation of epithelia, these attachments have to be extremely strong. In other instances, as when cells migrate, attachments have to be made, broken, and made again. In some cases, the extracellular matrix merely serves as a permissive substrate to which cells can adhere or upon which they can migrate. In other cases, it provides the directions for cell movement or the signal for a developmental event.

Extracellular matrices are made up of collagen, proteoglycans, and a variety of specialized glycoprotein molecules, such as fibronectin and laminin. These large glycoproteins are responsible for organizing the matrix and cells into an ordered structure. Fibronectin plays an important role in cell migration. The "roads" over which certain migrating cells travel are paved with this protein. Fibronectin paths lead germ cells to the gonads and lead heart cells to the midline of the embryo. If chick embryos are injected with antibodies to fibronectin, the heart-forming cells fail to reach the midline and two separate hearts develop (Heasman et al., 1981; Linask and Lash, 1988).

Laminin and type IV collagen are major components of a type of extracellular matrix called the basal lamina. The basal lamina is characteristic of the closely knit sheets that surround epithelial tissue. Adhesion of epithelial cells to laminin (upon which they sit) is much greater than the affinity of mesenchymal cells for fibronectin (to which they must bind and release if they are to migrate). Like fibronectin, laminin plays a role in assembling the extracellular matrix, promoting cell adhesion and growth, changing cell shape, and permitting cell migration (Hakamori et al., 1984).

Bissell and colleagues (1982; Martins-Green and Bissell, 1995) have shown that the extracellular matrix is also capable of inducing specific gene expression in developing tissues, especially those of the liver, testis, and mammary gland, in which the induction of specific transcription factors depends on cell–substrate binding (Liu et al., 1991; Streuli et al., 1991; Notenboom et al., 1996). Often, the presence of bound integrin (the cell membrane receptor for fibronectin and other extracellular matrix molecules) prevents the activation of genes that specify apoptosis (Montgomery et al., 1994; Frisch and Ruoslahti, 1997). The chondrocytes that produce the cartilage of our vertebrae and limbs can survive and differentiate only if they are surrounded by an extracellular matrix and joined to that matrix through their integrins (Hirsch et al., 1997). If chondrocytes from the developing chick sternum are incubated with antibodies that block the binding of integrins to the extracellular matrix, they shrivel up and die.

The extracellular matrix may play especially important roles in mediating the branching of parenchymal organs. Lin and colleagues (2001) showed that murine kidney and lung mesenchymes induce collagen XVIII in different places on the epithelium of murine kidneys and lungs and that this expression is predictive of the branching pattern of the epithelia.

CELL DEATH PATHWAYS

Programmed cell death, or apoptosis, is a normal part of development. In the nematode *C. elegans*, in which we can count the number of cells, exactly 131 cells die according to the normal developmental pattern. All of the cells of this nematode are "programmed" to die unless they are actively told not to undergo apoptosis. In humans, as many as 10^{11} cells die in each adult each day and are replaced by other cells. (Indeed, the mass of cells we lose each year through normal cell death is close to our entire body weight.) Within the uterus, we were constantly making and destroying cells, and we generated about three times as many neurons as we eventually ended up with when we were born.

By the time I was born, more of me had died than survived. It was no wonder I cannot remember; during that time I went through brain after brain for nine months, finally contriving the one model that could be human, equipped for language. (Thomas, 1992)

Apoptosis is necessary not only for the proper spacing and orientation of neurons but also for generating the middle ear space, the vaginal opening, and the spaces between our fingers and toes (Saunders and Fallon, 1966; Rodrigez et al., 1997; Roberts and Miller, 1998). Apoptosis prunes away unneeded structures, controls the number of cells in particular tissues, and sculpts complex organs. Different tissues use different signals for apoptosis. One of the signals often used in vertebrates is BMP4. Some tissues, such as connective tissue, respond to BMP4 by differentiating into bone. Others, such as the surface ectoderm, respond to BMP4 by differentiating into skin. Still others, such as neural crest cells and tooth primordia, respond by degrading their DNA and dying. In the developing tooth, for instance, numerous growth and differentiation factors are secreted by the enamel knot. After the cusp has grown, the enamel knot synthesizes BMP4 and shuts itself down by apoptosis (Vaahtokari et al., 1996).

In several tissues, the cells are programmed to die, and they will remain alive only if some growth or differentiation factor is present to "rescue" them. This happens during the development of mammalian red blood cells. The red blood cell precursors in the mouse liver need the hormone erythropoietin to survive. If they do not receive it, they undergo apoptosis. The erythropoietin receptor works through the JAK–STAT pathway, activating the Stat5 transcription factor (Bittorf et al., 2000; Socolovsky et al., 2001). In this way, the amount of erythropoietin present can determine how many red blood cells enter the circulation.

One of the pathways for apoptosis was largely delineated through genetic studies of *C. elegans*. It was found that the proteins encoded by the *ced-3* and *ced-4* genes were essential for apoptosis but that in the cells that did not undergo apoptosis, those genes were turned off by the product of the *ced-9* gene (Hengartner et al., 1992). The CED-4 protein is a protease activating factor that activates CED-3, a protease that initiates the destruction of the cell. Mutations that inactivate the CED-9 protein cause numerous cells that would normally survive to activate their *ced-3* and *ced-4* genes and die. This leads to the death of the entire embryo. Conversely, gain-of-function mutations of *ced-9* cause the CED-9 protein to be made in cells that would otherwise die. Thus, the *ced-9* gene appears to be a binary switch that regulates the choice between life and death on the cellular level. It is possible that every cell in the nematode embryo is poised to die and that those cells that survive are rescued by activation of the *ced-9* gene.

The CED-3 and CED-4 proteins form the center of the apoptosis pathway that is common to all animals studied. The trigger for apoptosis can be a developmental cue such as a particular molecule (e.g., BMP4 or glucocorticoids) or the loss of adhesion to a matrix. Either type of cue can activate the CED-3 or CED-4 protein or inactivate the CED-9 molecules. In mammals, the homologues of the CED-9 protein are members of the Bcl-2 family of genes. This family includes *Bcl-2*, *Bcl-X*, and similar genes. The functional similarities are so strong that if an active human *BCL-2* gene is placed into *C. elegans* embryos, it prevents normally occurring cell deaths in the nematode embryos (Vaux et al., 1992). In vertebrate red blood cell development (mentioned above), the Stat5 transcription factor activated by erythropoietin functions by binding to the promoter of the *Bcl-X* gene, where it activates the synthesis of that antiapoptosis protein (Socolovsky et al., 1999).

The mammalian homologue of CED-4 is called *Apaf-1* (apoptotic protease activating factor-1), and it participates in the cytochrome c-dependent activation of the mammalian CED-3 homologues caspase-9 and caspase-3 (Shaham and Horvitz, 1996; Cecconi et al., 1998; Yoshida et al., 1998). Activation of the caspases causes autodigestion of the cell. Caspases are strong proteases, and they digest the cell from within. The cellular proteins are cleaved, and the DNA is fragmented.

While apoptosis-deficient nematodes deficient for CED-4 are viable (despite their having 15% more cells than wild-type worms), mice with loss-of-function mutations for either *caspase-3* or *caspase-9* die around birth from massive cell overgrowth in the nervous system (Kuida et al., 1996, 1998; Jacobson et al., 1997). Mice homozygous for targeted deletions of Apaf-1 have severe craniofacial abnormalities, brain overgrowth, and webbing between their toes.

In mammals, there is more than one pathway to apoptosis. Apoptosis of the lymphocytes, for instance, is not affected by deletion of *Apaf-1* or *caspase-9* and works by a separate pathway initiated by the

CD95 protein. Different caspases may function in different cell types to mediate the apoptotic signals (Hakem et al., 1998; Kuida et al., 1998). One of the most interesting involves the "death domain"–containing receptors of the tumor necrosis factor (TNF) family. These receptors can induce apoptosis in several cell systems, and they appear to accomplish this by blocking the antiapoptosis signals sent by other factors. It is likely that the death domain binds a phosphatase that cleaves the phosphates from the RTKs that would be activated by the antiapoptotic signal (Daigle et al., 2002). This prevents their activation and allows apoptosis to commence.

Just as developmental signals (e.g., BMP4) can be used by some cells for apoptosis, so the death domain receptors can, in some instances, be used for nonapoptotic development. One of the developmentally important TNF receptors with a death domain is Edar, a protein required for the development of hair, teeth, and other cutaneous appendages. Mutations of this or of its ligand, Eda, cause hypohidrotic epidermal dysplasia, a syndrome characterized by lack of sweat glands, sparse hair, and poorly formed teeth. An identical syndrome is also produced by a deficiency of the adapter protein that binds the death domain of this receptor. In this instance, instead of producing cell death, activation of the receptor enables continued development (Headon et al., 2001).

THE NATURE OF GENETIC SYNDROMES

Pleiotropy

Research on the expression patterns of transcription factors and paracrine factors has suggested mechanisms that explain some of the genetic syndromes wherein mutations at a single genetic locus can cause numerous different malformations. The production of several conditions by mutations at one locus is called *pleiotropy*. For instance, in humans and mice, heterozygosity for MITF causes a condition that involves iris defects, pigmentation abnormalities, deafness, and inability to produce the normal number of mast cells (see Fig. 2–1B). The skin pigment, the iris of the eye, the inner ear tissue, and the mast cells of the immune system are not related to one another in such a way that the absence of one would produce the absence of the others. Rather, all four parts of the body independently use the MITF protein as a transcription factor. This type of pleiotropy has been called *mosaic pleiotropy* because the relevant organ systems are separately affected by the abnormal gene function.

While the eye pigment, body pigment, and mast cell features of MITF deficiency are separate events, other parts of the syndrome are not. For instance, the failure of MITF expression in the pigmented retina prevents this structure from fully differentiating. This in turn causes a malformation of the choroid fissure of the eye, resulting in drainage of vitreous humor fluid. Without this fluid, the eye fails to enlarge (hence the name *microphthalmia*, which means "small eye"). This phenomenon, in which several developing tissues are affected by the mutation even though they do not express the mutated gene, is called *relational pleiotropy* (see Gruneberg, 1938; 1962).

Genetic Heterogeneity

Another important feature of syndromes is that mutations in different genes can produce the same phenotype. If the genes are part of the same signal-transduction pathway, a mutation in any of them can give a similar result. The phenomenon whereby mutations in different genes produce similar phenotypes is called *genetic heterogeneity*. For example, cyclopia can be produced by mutations in the *Sonic hedgehog* gene or by mutations in cholesterol synthesis genes. Since they are in the same pathway, mutations in one gene generate a phenotype similar or identical to mutations in the other genes. Similarly, as we saw above, mutations in EDA (receptor), EDAR (ligand) or EDARADD (adapter protein) gave the same phenotype of hypohidrotic ectodermal dysplasia (Headon et al., 2001).

Mechanisms of Dominance

Whether a syndrome is dominant or recessive can now be explained at the molecular level. First, many syndromes are referred to as "dominant"

only because the homozygous condition is lethal to the embryo and the fetus never survives. Therefore, the homozygous condition never exists. Second, there are at least four ways of achieving a dominant phenotype.

The first mechanism of dominance is *haploinsufficiency*. This merely means that one copy of the gene (the haploid condition) is not enough to produce the required amount of product for normal development. For example, individuals with Waardenburg's syndrome type II have roughly half the wild-type amount of MITF. This is not enough for full pigment cell proliferation, mast cell differentiation, or inner ear development. Thus, an aberrant phenotype results when only one of the two copies of this gene is absent or nonfunctional.

The second mechanism of dominance is gain-of-function mutations. As mentioned above, thanatophoric dysplasia (as well as milder forms of dwarfism such as achondroplasia) results from a mutation causing the FGFR to be constitutively active. This activity is enough to cause an anomalous phenotype to develop.

The third mechanism of dominance is a dominant negative allele. This situation can occur when the active form of the protein is a multimer, and all proteins of the multimer have to be wild-type for the protein to function. A dominant negative allele is the cause of Marfan syndrome, a disorder of the extracellular matrix. Marfan syndrome is associated with joint and connective tissue anomalies, not all of which are necessarily disadvantageous. Increased height, disproportionately long limbs and digits, and mild to moderate joint laxity are characteristic of this syndrome. However, patients with Marfan syndrome also experience vertebral column deformities, myopia, loose lenses, and (most importantly) aortic problems that may lead to aneurysm (bursting of the aorta) later in life. The mutation is in the gene for fibrillin, a secreted glycoprotein that forms multimeric microfibrils in elastic connective tissue. The presence of even small amounts of mutant fibrillin prohibits the association of wild-type fibrillin into microfibrils. Eldadah and colleagues (1995) have shown that when a mutant human gene for fibrillin is transfected into fibroblast cells that already contain two wild-type genes, incorporation of fibrillin into the matrix is inhibited.

The fourth mechanism of dominance involves subunit interactions wherein the dimer made from the products of two different alleles is superior in function to dimers made exclusively of the product of either allele (Trehan and Gill, 2002).

MODULARITY AND CONTEXTUALITY

During the development of mammals, there are domains set off by the expression of transcription factors. These regions can interact, thereby activating the expression or function of another set of transcription factors. These can further subdivide the domains, or they can initiate the expression of those batteries of genes that cause the differentiated proteins of the particular cell type to emerge. This concept is known as *modularity*. Development occurs through a series of discrete and interacting modules (Riedl, 1978; Gilbert et al., 1996; Raff, 1996; Davidson, 2001). In development, such modules include physical modules (e.g., hair follicles and teeth), morphogenetic fields (e.g., those described for the limb or eye), and physical structures for which there are no adult counterparts (e.g., rhombomeres). Modular units allow certain parts of the body to change without interfering with the functions of other parts.

These fields often provide the genes and proteins with their context. For instance, as we have mentioned above, BMP4 can be a signal for bone development (in somites), apoptosis (in the neural and derivatives), epidermis formation (in the induction of the ectoderm), or lens formation (within the eye). What it does depends on the field in which it is expressed. Unlike the genes for globin or chymotrypsin, the genes expressed early in development are often used for multiple functions. In some instances, these functions can depend on very different properties of the molecule. β-Catenin can play a role on the cell membrane as part of an adhesion complex, or it can play a role in the nucleus as a transcription factor. Similarly, a protein that functions as an enolase or alcohol dehydrogenase enzyme in the liver can function as a structural crystallin protein in the lens (Piatigorsky and Wistow, 1991). Developmental genes work within specific contexts.

These contexts can also determine the effect of a particular gene. It is not uncommon in the context of clinical genetics to identify a mutant allele that produces a mildly abnormal phenotype in one generation and a more abnormal phenotype in another generation. A mutant gene that produces limblessness in one generation can produce only a mild thumb abnormality in the next (Freire-Maia, 1975). Indeed, by following the phenotypes produced in different members of the same family, one can see that the same gene can produce different phenotypes depending on the other genes that are present (Wolf, 1995; Nijhout and Paulsen, 1997). There are even cases where the phenotype depends on whether the mutant allele is passed through the father or the mother (Shore et al., 2002).

MORPHOGENETIC PROCESSES

The Morphogenetic Repertoire

Morphogenesis involves changes in cell behavior. There are two main groups of cells in the embryo: epithelial cells, which are tightly connected to one another in sheets or tubes, and mesenchymal cells, which are unconnected to each other and operate as individual units. Morphogenesis is brought about through a limited repertoire of cellular processes in these two classes of cells: *(1)* the direction and number of cell divisions, *(2)* cell shape changes, *(3)* cell movement, *(4)* cell growth, *(5)* cell death, and *(6)* changes in the composition of the cell membrane and extracellular matrix. How these processes are accomplished can differ between mesenchymal and epithelial cells (Table 2–3; see Larsen, 1997).

Three important morphogenetic events, the orientation of cell division, the orientation of cell polarity, and cell migration, are regulated through the cytoskeleton. The orientation and number of cell divisions are tightly regulated. Given the similarity of facial appearance within a family, it seems that such regulation is under genetic control. The direction of cell divisions is controlled by the orientation of the mitotic spindle. This, in turn, is regulated by the cytoskeleton of the cell, especially by the dynein-rich cortex (O'Connell and Wang, 2000; Dujardin and Vallee, 2002). The positioning of the cytoskeleton can be effected by cell–cell contacts or by paracrine factors such as Wnt proteins (Goldstein, 2000; Le Borgne et al., 2002). Both appear to work by causing changes in the cytoskeleton.

Cell shape changes allow for morphogenesis in several ways.

Many morphogenetic processes, such as neurulation, are caused by changes in the shape of cells. In neurulation, this is especially important for the formation of the neural tube (Smith and Schoenwolf 1997; Zolessi and Arruti, 2001). In mammals, cell shape change is also critical for the formation and polarity of the trophectoderm (Kidder, 2002). Cell shape change is also mediated through the cytoskeleton.

There are several mechanisms that enable cells to migrate from one region of the body to another. These mechanisms involve interactions of the cell surfaces with molecules that give cues as to when to start migrating, where to go, and when to cease migration. Migration is dependent on both the actin cyctoskeleton and the ATPases (e.g., dynein) that drive it. Defects in the regulation of these systems, such as in lissencephaly-1, where the regulation of dynein in certain neuronal precursors is defective (Vallee et al., 2001), result in defective migration. There are two major modes of cell migration, and they are often combined. One mode is to follow a gradient of chemotactic molecules to its source. The other mode is to follow a particular substrate pathway. In addition to attractive signals, repulsive signals can occur.

Chemotaxis is defined as cellular locomotion directed in response to a concentration gradient of a chemical factor in solution. Cells sense the chemical and migrate toward higher concentrations of it until they reach the source secreting it. In the vertebrate lung, brain, and limb, FGFs function as chemotactic proteins (Park et al., 1998; Li and Muneoka, 1999; Kuboto and Ito, 2000). Failure of chemotaxis is found in several systems, especially those affecting the cytoskeleton of neural cells and lymphocytes.

Gradients do not have to be in solution. An adhesive molecule could be present in increasing amounts along an extracellular matrix. A cell that was constantly making and breaking adhesions with such a molecule would move from a region of low concentration to an area where that adhesive molecule was more highly concentrated. Such a phenomenon is called *haptotaxis* (Curtis, 1969). Migration of the pronephric duct cells in salamanders is regulated by haptotaxis (Zackson and Steinberg, 1987; Drawbridge et al., 1995). Moreover, certain human genetic conditions appear to have bases in the haptotactic mode of migration. In Kallmann's syndrome, for instance, the protein anosmin is absent. This protein plays a key role in the migration of gonadotropin-releasing hormone neurons and olfactory nerves to the hypothalamus, and it is thought to be part of the extracellular matrix (Soussi-Yanicostas et al., 1996).

Table 2–3. The Morphogenetic Repertoire

Cell Type	Property	Mechanism	Example
Mesenchyme (and nerves)	Movement	Contact guidance	Amphibian gastrulation
		Haptotaxis	Cell movement in vitro
			Retinal cells mapping to tectum
		Contact inhibition/space	NC invasion of cornea
		Cell repulsion	NC blockage in posterior somite
		Chemotaxis	Neuronal migration in spinal cord
	Apoptosis		Loss of müllerian duct
	Condensation	Migration	Ganglion formation
		Adhesion	Dermal condensations
		Growth	Theoretical
		Traction	Cell aggregation in vitro
		Loss of ECM	Limb precartilage condensations
	Stability		
Epithelia	Polarization		Nephron lumen formation
	Forming folds	Buckling	Ciliary body formation
		Bending of sheet	Neural fold formation
	Forming tubes	Hollowing	Fish neural tube
		Growth	Blood vessels
	Tube branching	Signaling	Trachea
	Cell sorting		*Drosophila* egg chamber formation
	Movement	Passive/growth	Serosal migration in honeybee
			Surface ectoderm
		Rearrangement	Convergent extension
		Cessation	Completion of wound healing
	Tissue integrity		Retinal stability
	Growth		Throughout body

NC, neural cell; ECM, extracellular matrix.
Source: J. Bard, personal communication.

RANDOMNESS AND CHANCE IN MORPHOGENESIS

There are numerous sources of randomness in the human phenotype. In addition to somatic mutation and recombination, the major sources of chance are *(1)* X-chromosome inactivation, *(2)* stochastic interactions, and *(3)* environmental induction.

X-Chromosome Inactivation

In female mammals, including humans, one X chromosome in each cell is inactive, while the other X chromosome is active. Very early in the development of human females, both X chromosomes are active; but as development proceeds, one X chromosome is turned off in each cell. Moreover, this inactivation is random. In some cells, the paternally derived X chromosome is inactivated; in other cells, the maternally derived X chromosome is shut off. This process is irreversible. Once an X chromosome has been inactivated, the same X chromosome is inactivated in all of that cell's progeny. Since X inactivation happens relatively early in development, an entire region of cells derived from a single cell may have the same X chromosome inactivated. Thus, all tissues in female mammals are mosaics of two cell types (see Migeon, 1994).

If one of the X chromosomes contains a mutant allele while the other one does not, the pattern of inactivation can produce different phenotypes. There are several cases of monozygous twins who are heterozygous for an X-linked form of muscular dystrophy. Most heterozygous women do not express any symptoms because the cells expressing the wild-type allele can compensate for the cells expressing the mutant allele. However, if by chance the wild-type allele is on the inactivated X chromosome in a large proportion of her muscle cells, the woman will manifest the disease. There have been several instances where one girl shows the symptoms of the disease while her monmozygous twin sister does not (Pena et al., 1987; Norman and Harper, 1989; Richards et al., 1990; Tremblay et al., 1993). Similarly, there are cases where monozygous female twins are discordant with respect to color blindness or Hunter's syndrome due to X-chromosome inactivation (Jorgensen et al., 1992; Winchester et al., 1992).

Stochastic Variation

Many events in the body are the products of both chance and necessity. The vascularization of the body differs from person to person, as do the intimate details of neural connection. Even in relatively simple animals that are genetically identical and that are given the same homogeneous environment, differences can be seen. The Bristol N2 strain of *C. elegans* has an invariant cell lineage (the cell divisions which occur between the fertilized egg and the adult are largely identical and always produce the same set of tissues), an invariant nervous system whose 302 neurons have reproducible synaptic connectivity, and an invariant genotype. Moreover, this strain of *C. elegans* has a repertoire of behaviors that it performs in a very limited environment, a flat agar surface supplied with a uniform pad of identical bacteria. However, their behavior is not uniform. Jorgensen et al. (1992) isolated mutants wherein most of the mutant worms lie straight in a paralyzed manner. However, a fraction of them consistently take on a quite different "curly" posture. Such differences in a cloned population might be caused by slight differences in neural connectivity, which could be caused by stochastic developmental effects (see Schnabel, 1997). The nervous system seems to encourage such differences by the "winner takes all" mechanisms caused by hebbian rules of neuronal connections.

Stochastic variation may also be important in aging, where oxidative stress and random somatic mutations probably play roles in limiting cell division (Sozou and Kirkwood, 2001).

Perhaps nowhere is chance experience more pronounced than in the development of the human immune system. We respond to external microbes through an immune system based on clonal selection of lymphocytes that recognize specific microbes and their products. Our immune system recognizes a particular microbe, such as a cholera bacterium or a poliovirus, by making lymphocytes, each expressing a different gene product on its cell surface. These genes for immunoglobulin and T-cell receptors form the receptor proteins of the B cells. Each B lymphocyte, for instance, makes one and only one type of antibody, and it places this antibody on the cell surface. One B cell may make an antibody to poliovirus, while its neighboring B cell makes an antibody to diphtheria toxin. When a B cell lymphocyte binds its foreign substance (the antigen), it begins a pathway that causes it to divide repeatedly and to differentiate into an antibody-secreting cell, which secretes the same antibody that originally bound the antigen. Moreover, some of the descendants of that stimulated B cell remain in the body as sentinels against further infection by the same microorganism. When we have a polio vaccine, our body stores B-lymphocyte memory cells, which have receptors to the poliovirus. Thus, identical twins are not identical with respect to their immune systems. Their phenotypes (in this case, both the types of cell in their lymph nodes and their ability to respond against an infectious microorganism) have been altered by the environment.

Environmental Determination of Phenotype

In addition to its role in immunocyte differentiation, the environment plays other significant roles in phenotype production. Obviously, starvation or overeating will change our phenotype, and there are likely to be genes that respond to dietary factors and produce diseases such as diabetes and coronary artery disease. These are diseases where genes interact with environmental conditions to create the pathological states. There are some genetic conditions that can be completely abolished by dietary supplementation. Foremost among these is gulonolactone oxidase deficiency (hypoascorbemia, OMIM 240400), a mutation in the gulonolactone oxidase gene on the short arm of chromosome 8, which causes a syndrome that produces death in childhood due to connective tissue malfunction. Each human being is thought to have this condition. Gulonic acid oxidase is the final enzyme in the pathway leading to ascorbic acid, and while most mammals have this enzyme and can synthesize vitamin C, our genes for this enzyme are mutated and we cannot make this necessary compound. Without this vitamin C replacement therapy from the environment, each of us would die.

Environment can also be extremely important in modulating the effects of mutant alleles. The fetuses most at risk for neural tube defects appear to be those with mutations in genes associated with folate metabolism (Whitehead et al., 1995; De Marco et al., 2000). Folate is a critical substrate for the methylation of homocysteine to methionine, but the mechanisms by which folate deficiency interferes with neural tube closure are not known. Smith-Lemli-Opitz syndrome and phenylketonuria are two other conditions wherein environment interacts with genetics to produce the phenotype. In Smith-Lemli-Opitz syndrome (Chapter 17), dietary cholesterol can offset the mutant alleles that prevent proper cholesterol synthesis. In phenylketonuria, the behavioral and cognitive deficiencies associated with this syndrome can be ameliorated by dietary restriction of phenylalanine.

It is also possible that interactions between the environment and our genome control some of our facial phenotype. Physical stress from the environment is needed to produce bones such as the mammalian patella and the bird fibular crest (Müller and Steicher, 1989; Wu, 1996). Corruccini (1984) and Varrela (1992) have speculated that the reason that nearly a quarter of our population needs orthodontic appliances is that our children's mild-textured diet causes the lower jaw to develop abnormally. Increased chewing causes tension that stimulates mandible bone and muscle growth (Kiliardis et al., 1985; Weijs and Hillen, 1986), and placing young primates on a soft diet will cause malocclusions in their jaws, similar to those in humans (Corruccini and Beecher, 1982, 1984).

The production of phenotype from genotype is regulated at numerous levels. It is regulated at the gene expression levels of gene transcription, mRNA processing, mRNA translation, and posttranslational modification. It is further controlled by cell–cell and cell–substrate interactions and by environmental influences. In all of these levels, the vectors of regulation work both ways. A cell's fate is determined both by the gene expression within it and by the community of cells in which it resides. Even the environment can alter patterns of gene expression, and in the production of the human phenotype, experience is added to endowment (Childs, 1999).

ACKNOWLEDGMENTS

Support for this work came from grants from Swarthmore College and from the National Science Foundation (IBN-0079341).

REFERENCES

Andersen FG, Jensen J, Heller RS, Petersen HV, Larsson L-I, Madsen OD, Serup P (1999). Pax6 and Pdx1 form a functional complex on the rat somatostain gene upstream enhancer. *FEBS Lett* 445: 315–320.

Angier N (1992). A first step in putting genes into action: bend the DNA. *New York Times*, 4 August, pp. C1, C7.

Aza-Blanc P, Ramirez-Weber FA, Laget MP, Kornberg TB (1997). Proteolysis that is inhibited by hedgehog targets Cubitus interruptus protein to the nucleus and converts it to a repressor. *Cell* 89: 1043–1053.

Bard JBL (1990). *Morphogenesis: The Cellular and Molecular Processes of Developmental Anatomy.* Cambridge University Press, Cambridge.

Behrens J, von Kries JP, Kühl M, Bruhn L, Wedlich D, Grosschedl R, Birchmeier W (1996). Functional interaction of β-catenin with the transcription factor LRF-1. *Nature* 382: 638–642.

Bell AC, West AG, Felsenfeld G (2001). Insulators and boundaries: versatile regulatory elements in the eukaryotic genome. *Science* 291: 447–450.

Bissell MJ, Hall HG, Parry G (1982). How does the extracellular matrix direct gene expression? *J Theor Biol* 99: 31–68.

Bittorf T, Seiler J, Ludtke B, Buchse T, Jaster R, Brock J (2000). Activation of STAT5 during EPO-directed suppression of apoptosis. *Cell Signal* 12: 23–30.

Brown V, Jin P, Ceman S, Darnell JC, O'Donnell WT, Tenenbaum SA, Jin X, Feng Y, Wilkinson KD, Keene JD, et al. (2001). Microarray identification of FMRP-associated brain mRNAs and altered mRNA translational profiles in fragile X syndrome. *Cell* 107: 477–487.

Breitbart RA, Andreadis A, Nadal-Ginard B (1987). Alternative splicing: a ubiquitous mechanism for the generation of multiple protein isoforms from single genes. *Annu Rev Biochem* 56: 481–495.

Buratowski S (1997). Multiple TATA-binding factors come back into style. *Cell* 91: 13–15.

Buratowski S, Hahn S, Guarente L, Sharp PA (1989). Five initiation complexes in transcription initiation by RNA polymerase II. *Cell* 56: 549–561.

Byers PH, et al. (1997). Ehler-Danlos syndrome type VIIA and VIIB result from splice-junction mutations or genomic deletions that involve exon 6 in the *COL1A1* and *COL1A2* genes of type I collagen. *Am J Med Genet* 72: 94–105.

Cadigan KM, Nusse R (1997). Wnt signaling: a common theme in animal development. *Genes Dev* 24: 3286–3306.

Cecconi F, Alvarez-Bolado G, Meyer BI, Roth KA, Gruss P (1998). Apaf-1 (CED-4 homologue) regulates programmed cell death in mammalian development. *Cell* 94: 727–737.

Celotto AM, Graveley BR (2001). Alternative splicing of the *Drosophila Dscam* pre-mRNA is both temporally and spatially regulated. *Genetics* 159: 599–608.

Childs B (1999). *Genetic Medicine.* Johns Hopkins University Press, Baltimore.

Chitnis A, Henrique D, Lewis L, Ish-Horowicz D, Kintner C (1995). Primary neurogenesis in *Xenopus* embryos regulated by a homologue of the *Drosophila* gene *Delta*. *Nature* 375: 761–766.

Cooper TA, Mattox W (1997). The regulation of splice-site selection, and its role in human disease. *Am J Hum Genet* 61: 259–266.

Corruccini RS (1984). An epidemiologic transition in dental occlusion in world populations. *Am J Orthod* 86: 419–426.

Corruccini RS, Beecher CL (1982). Occlusal variation related to soft diet in a nonhuman primate. *Science* 218: 74–76.

Corruccini RS, Beecher CL (1984). Occlusofacial morphological integration lowered in baboons raised on soft diet. *J Craniofac Genet Dev Biol* 4: 135–142.

Croft L, Schandorff S, Clark F, Burrage K, Arctander P, Mattick JS (2000). ISIS, the intron information system, reveals the high frequency of alternative splicing in the human genome. *Nat Genet* 24: 340–341.

Crossley PH, Monowada G, MacArthur CA, Martin G (1996). Roles for FGF8 in the induction, initiation, and maintenance of the chick limb development. *Cell* 84: 127–136.

Curtis ASG (1969). The measurement of cell adhesiveness by an absolute method. *J Embryol Exp Morphol* 22: 305–325.

Cvekl A, Piatigorsky J (1996). Lens development and crystallin gene expression: many roles for Pax-6. *Bioessays* 18: 621–630.

Daigle I, Yousefi S, Colonna M, Green DR, Simon HU (2002). Death receptors bind SHP-1 and block cytokine-induced anti-apoptotic signaling in neutrophils. *Nat Med* 8: 61–67.

Darnell JC, Jensen KB, Jin P, Brown V, Warren ST, Darnell RB (2001). Fragile X mental retardation protein targets G quartet mRNAs important for neuronal function. *Cell* 107: 489–499.

Davidson EH (2001). *Genomic Regulatory Systems: Development and Evolution.* Academic Press, New York.

De Marco P, et al. (2000). Folate pathway gene alterations in patients with neural tube defects. *Am J Med Genet* 95: 216–223.

Deng C, Wynshaw-Boris A, Zhou F, Kuo A, Leder P (1996). Fibroblast growth factor receptor-3 is a negative regulator of bone growth. *Cell* 84: 911–921.

Dorsky RI, Chang WS, Rapaport DH, Harris WA (1997). Regulation of neuronal diversity in the *Xenopus* retina by Delta signalling. *Nature* 385: 67–74.

Drawbridge J, Wolfe AE, Delgado YL, Steinberg MS (1995). The epidermis is a source of directional information for the migrating pronephric duct in *Ambystoma mexicanum* embryos. *Dev Biol* 172: 440–451.

Dujardin DL, Vallee RB (2002). Dynein at the cortex. *Curr Opin Cell Biol* 14: 44–49.

Eldadah ZA, Brenn T, Furthmayr H, Dietz HC (1995). Expression of a mutant human fibrillin allele upon a normal human or murine genetic background recapitulates a Marfan cellular phenotype. *J Clin Invest* 95: 874–880.

Epstein JA, Glaser T, Cai J, Jepeal L, Walton DS, Mass RL (1994). Two independent and interactive DNA-binding subdomains of the Pax6 paired domain are regulated by alternative splicing. *Genes Dev* 8: 2022–2034.

Fan CM, Tessier-Lavigne M (1994). Patterning of mammalian somites by surface ectoderm and notochord: evidence for sclerotome induction by a hedgehog homolog. *Cell* 79: 1175–1186.

Feng Y, Absher D, Eberhart DE, Brown V, Malter HE, Warren ST (1997a). FMRP associates with polyribosomes as an mRNP, and the I304N mutation of severe fragile X syndrome abolishes this association. *Mol Cells* 1: 109–118.

Feng Y, Gutekunst CA, Eberhart DE, Yi H, Warren ST, Hersch SM (1997b). Fragile X mental retardation protein: nucleocytoplasmic shuttling and association with somato-dendritic ribosomes. *J Neurosci* 17:1539–1547.

Freire-Maia N (1975). A heterozygote expression of a "recessive" gene. *Hum Hered* 25: 302–304.

Frisch SM, Ruoslahti E (1997). Integrins and anoikis. *Curr Opin Cell Biol* 9: 701–706.

Fujiwara M, Uchida T, Osumi-Yamashita N, Eto K (1994). Uchida rat (rSey): a new mutant rat with craniofacial abnormalities resembling those of the mouse Sey mutant. *Differentiation* 57: 31–38.

Furuta Y, Hogan BLM (1998). BMP4 is essential for lens induction in the mouse embryo. *Genes Dev* 12: 3764–3775.

Gilbert SF (2003). *Developmental Biology*, 7th Edition. Sinauer Associates, Sunderland, MA.

Gilbert SF, Opitz JM, Raff RA (1996). Resynthesizing evolutionary and developmental biology. *Dev Biol* 173: 357–372.

Glaser T, Jepeal L, Edwards JG, Young SR, Favor J, Maas RL (1994). *PAX6* gene dosage effects in a family with congenital cataracts, aniridia, anophthalmia, and central nervous system defects. *Nat Genet* 8: 463–471.

Goldstein B (2000). When cells tell their neighbors which direction to divide. *Dev Dyn* 218: 23–29.

Grainger RM (1992). Embryonic lens induction: shedding light on vertebrate tissue determination. *Trends Genet* 8: 349–356.

Grobstein C (1956). Trans-filter induction of tubules in mouse metanephrogenic mesenchyme. *Exp Cell Res* 10: 424–440.

Grüneberg H (1938). An analysis of the "pleiotropic" effects of a new lethal mutation in the rat (*Mus norwegicus*). *Proc R Soc Lond B* 125: 123–144.

Grüneberg H (1962). *The Pathology of Development.* Blackwell, Oxford.

Hakamori S, Fukuda M, Sekiguchi K, Carter WG (1984). Fibronectin, laminin, and other extracellular glycoproteins. In: *Extracellular Matrix Biochemistry.* Picz KA, Reddi AH (eds.) Elsevier, New York, pp. 229–276.

Hakem R, et al. (1998). Differential requirement for caspase-9 in apoptotic pathways in vivo. *Cell* 94: 339–352.

Hastie ND (2001). Life, sex, and WT1 isoforms—three amino acids can make all the difference. *Cell* 106: 391–394.

Hay ED (1979). Development of the vertebrate cornea. *Int Rev Cytol* 63: 263–322.

Headon DJ, Emmal SA, Ferguson BM, Tucker AS, Justice MJ, Sharpe PT, Zonana J, Overbeek PA (2001). Gene defect in ectodermal dysplasia implicates a death domain adapter in development. *Nature* 414: 913–916.

Heasman J, Hines RD, Swan AP, Thomas V, Wylie CC (1981). Primordial germ cells of *Xenopus* embryos: the role of fibronectin in their adhesion during migration. *Cell* 27: 437–447.

Heldin C-H, Miyazono K, ten Dijke P (1997). TGF-β signaling from cell membrane to nucleus through SMAD proteins. *Nature* 390: 465–471.

Hemesath TJ, Price ER, Takemoto C, Badalian T, Fisher DE (1998). MAP kinase links the transcription factor Microphthalmia to c-Kit signalling in melanocytes. *Nature* 391: 298–301.

Hengartner MO, Ellis RE, Horvitz HR (1992). *Caenorhabditis* elegans gene ced-9 protects from programmed cell death. *Nature* 356: 494–499.

Hirsch MS, Lunsford LE, Trinkaus-Randall V, Svoboda KKH (1997). Chondrocyte survival and differentiation in situ are integrin mediacted. *Dev Dynam* 210: 249–263.

Hogan BLM (1996). Bone morphogenesis proteins: multifunctional regulators of vertebrate development. *Genes Dev* 10: 1580–1594.

Holtzer H (1968). Induction of chondrogenesis: a concept in terms of mechanisms. In: *Epithelial–Mesenchymal Interactions.* Gleischmajer R, Billingham RE (eds.) Williams & Wilkins, Baltimore, pp. 152–164.

Hsu Y-R, et al. (1997). The majority of stem cell factor exists as monomer under physiological conditions. *J Biol Chem* 272: 6406–6416.

Hussain MA, Habener J-F (1999). Glucagon gene transcription activation mediated by synergistic interactions of Pax6 and Cdx2 with the p300 co-activator. *J Biol Chem* 274: 28850–28957.

Hutchinson S, Wordsworth BP, Handford PA (2001). Marfan syndrome caused by a mutation in *FBN1* that gives rise to cryptic splicing and a 33 nucleotide insertion in the coding sequence. *Hum Genet* 109: 416–420.

Hutton M, et al. (1998). Association of missense and 5′-splice-site mutations in tau with the inherited dementia FTDP-17. *Nature* 393: 702–705.

Ihle JN (1996b). STATs: signal transducers and activators of transcription. *Cell* 84: 331–334.

Ichtchenko K, Hata Y, Nguyen T, Ullrich B, Missler M, Moomaw C, Südhof TC (1995). Neuroglian 1: a splice-site specific ligand for β-neurexins. *Cell* 81: 435–443.

Jacobson AG (1966). Inductive processes in embryonic development. *Science* 152: 25–34.

Jacobson MD, Weil M, Raff MC (1997). Programmed cell death in animal development. *Cell* 88: 347–354.

Johnson RL, Riddle RD, Laufer E, Tabin C (1994). Sonic hedgehog: A key mediator of anterior-posterior patterning of the limb and dorso-ventral patterning of axial embryonic structures. *Biochem Soc Trans* 22: 569–574.

Jorgensen AL, Philip J, Raskind WH, Matsushita M, Christensen B, Dreyer V, Motulsky AG (1992). Different pattern of X-inactivation in MZ twins discordant for red–green color-vision deficiency. *Am J Hum Genet* 51: 291–298.

Kato Y, et al. (1998). Eight calves cloned from somatic cells of a single adult. *Science* 282: 2095–2098.

Kidder GM (2002). Trophectoderm development and function: the roles of Na$^+$/K$^+$-ATPase subunit isoforms. *Can J Physiol Pharmacol* 80: 110–115.

Kiliardis S, Engström C, Thilander B (1985). The relationship between masticatory function and craniofacial morphology. *Eur J Orthod* 7: 273–283.

Krawczak M, Reiss J, Cooper DN (1992). The mutational spectrum of single base-pair substitutions in messenger RNA splice junctions of human genes: causes and consequences. *Hum Genet* 90: 41–54.

Kubota Y, Ito K (2000). Chemotactic migration of mesencephalic neural crest cells in the mouse. *Dev Dyn* 217: 170–179.

Kuida K, et al. (1996). Decreased apoptosis in the brain and premature lethality in CPP32-deficient mice. *Nature* 384: 368–372.

Kuida K, et al. (1998). Reduced apoptosis and cytochrome *c*-mediated caspase activation in mice lacking caspase 9. *Cell* 94: 325–337.

Lammert E, Clever O, Melton D (2001). Induction of pancreatic differentiation by signals from blood vessels. *Science* 294: 564–567.

Larsen E (1997). Evolution of development: the shuffling of ancient modules by ubiquitous bureaucracies. In: *Physical Theory in Biology.* Lumsden C, Trainor T, Brandt W (eds.) World Science, Singapore, pp. 431–441.

Le Borgne R, Bellaiche Y, Schweisguth F (2002). *Drosophila* E-cadherin regulates the orientation of asymmetric cell division in the sensory organ lineage. *Curr Biol* 12: 95–104.

Lecourtois M, Schweisguth F (1998). Indirect evidence for Delta-dependent intercellular processing of Notch in *Drosophila* embryos. *Curr Biol* 8: 771–774.

Lee TI, Young RA (1998). Regulation of gene expression by TBP-associated proteins. *Genes Dev* 12: 1398–1408.

Leevers SJ, Paterson HF, Marshall CJ (1994). Requirement for Ras in Raf activation is overcome by targeting Raf to the plasma membrane. *Nature* 369: 411–414.

Li H-S, Yang J-M, Jacobson RD, Pasko D, Sundin O (1994). Pax-6 is first expressed in a region of ectoderm anterior to the early neural plate: implications for stepwise determination of the lens. *Dev Biol* 162: 181–194.

Li S, Muneoka K (1999). Cell migration and chick limb development: chemotactic action of FGF-4 and the AER. *Dev Biol* 211: 335–347.

Lin Y, Shang S, Rehn M, Itäranta P, Tuukkanen J, Heljäsvaara R, Peltoketo H, Pihlajaniemi T, Vainio S (2001). Induced repatterning of type XVIII collagen expression in ureter bud from kidney to lung type: association with sonic hedgehog and ectopic surfactant protein C. *Development* 128: 1573–1585.

Linask KL, Lash JW (1988). A role for fibronectin in the migration of avian precardiac cells. I. Dose-dependent effects of fibronectin antibody. *Dev Biol* 129: 315–323.

Liu J-K, Di Persio MC, Zaret KS (1991). Extracellular signals that regulate liver transcription factors during hepatic differentiation in vitro. *Mol Cell Biol* 11: 773–784.

Maniatis T, Goodbourn S, Fischer JA (1987). Regulation of inducible and tissue-specific gene expression. *Science* 236: 1237–1245.

Martins-Green M, Bissell MJ (1995). Cell-ECM interactions in development. *Semin Dev Biol* 6: 149–159.

McEwen DG, Peifer M (2001). Wnt signaling: the naked truth. *Curr Biol* 11:R524–R526.

McMahon AP, Bradley A (1990). The *Wnt-1* (*int 1*) proto-oncogene is required for the development of a large region of the mouse brain. *Cell* 62: 1073–1086.

Meier S (1977). Initiation of corneal differentiation prior to cornea–lens association. *Cell Tissue Res* 184: 255–267.

Meyer WJ III, Migeon BR, Migeon CJ (1975). Locus on human X chromosome for dihydrotestosterone receptor and androgen insensitivity. *Proc Natl Acad Sci* 72: 1469–1472.

Migeon BR (1994). X-chromosome inactivation: molecular mechanisms and genetic consequences. *Trends Genet* 10:230–235.

Montgomery AMP, Reisfeld RA, Cheresh DA (1994). Integrin $\alpha v \beta 3$ rescues melanoma cells from apoptosis in a three-dimensional dermal collagen. *Proc Natl Acad Sci USA* 91: 8856–8860.

Müller GB, Steicher J (1989). Ontogeny of the syndesmosis tibiofibularis and the evolution of the bird hindlimb: a caenogenetic feature triggers phenotypic novelty. *Anat Embryol* 179: 327–339.

Nijhout HF, Paulsen SM (1997). Developmental models and polygenic characters. *Am Nat* 149: 394–405.

Nohno TW, Kawakami Y, Ohuchi H, Fujiwara A, Yoshioka H, Noji S (1995). Involvement of the sonic hedgehog gene in chick feather formation. *Biochem Biophys Res Commun* 206: 33–39.

Nomura M, Li E (1998). Smad2 role in mesoderm formation, left–right patterning, and craniofacial development. *Nature* 393: 786–790.

Norman A, Harper P (1989). Survey of manifesting carriers of Duchenne and Becker muscular dystrophy in Wales. *Clin Genet* 36: 31–37.

Notenboom RGE, de Poer PAJ, Moorman AFM, Lamers WH (1996). The establishment of the hepatic architecture is a prerequisite for the development of a lobular pattern of gene expression. *Development* 122: 321–332.

O'Connell CB, Wang YL (2000). Mammalian spindle orientation and position respond to changes in cell shape in a dynein-dependent fashion. *Mol Biol Cell* 11: 1765–1774.

Ogino H, Yasuda K (1998). Induction of lens differentiation by activation of a bZIP transcription factor, L-maf. *Science* 280: 115–118.

Park WY, Miranda B, Lebeche D, Hashimoto G, Cardoso WV (1998). FGF-10 is a chemotactic factor for distal epithelial buds during lung development. *Dev Biol* 201: 125–134.

Pellizzoni L, Charroux B, Dreyfuss G (1999). SMN mutants of spinal muscular atrophy patients are defective in binding to snRNP proteins. *Proc Natl Acad Sci USA* 96: 11167–11172.

Pena SDJ, Karpati G, Carpenter S, Fraser FC (1987). The clinical consequences of X-chromosome inactivation: Duchenne muscular dystrophy in one of monozygotic twins. *J Neurol Sci* 79: 337–344.

Philips AV, Timchenko LT, Cooper TA (1998). Disruption of splicing regulated by a CUG-binding protein in myotonic dystrophy. *Science* 280: 737–741.

Piatigorsky J, Wistow G (1991). The recruitment of crystallins: new functions precede gene duplication. *Science* 252: 1078–1079.

Plaza S, Dozier C, Saule S (1993). Quail PAX6 (PAX-QNR) encodes a transcription factor able to bind and transactivate its own promoter. *Cell Growth Differ* 4: 1041–1050.

Price ER, Ding HF, Badalian T, Bhattacharya S, Takemoto C, Yao TP, Hemesath TJ, Fisher DE (1998). Lineage-specific signaling in melanocytes. C-kit stimulation recruits p300/CBP to microphthalmia. *J Biol Chem* 273: 17983–17986.

Raff RA (1996). *The Shape of Life: Genes, Development, and the Evolution of Animal Form.* University of Chicago Press, Chicago.

Richards CS, et al. (1990). Skewed X-inactivation in a female MZ twin results in Duchenne muscular dystrophy. *Am J Hum Genet* 46: 672–681.

Riedl R (1978). *Order in Living Systems: A Systems Analysis of Evolution.* John Wiley & Sons, New York.

Roberts DS, Miller SA (1998). Apoptosis in cavitation of middle ear space. *Anat Rec* 251: 286–289.

Rockman MV, Wray GA (2002). Abundant raw material for cis-regulatory evolution. *Mol Biol Evol* 19:1991–2004.

Rodrigez I, Araki K, Khatib K, Martinou J-C, Vassalli P (1997). Mouse vaginal opening is an apoptosis-dependent process which can be prevented by the overexpression of Bcl2. *Dev Biol* 184: 115–121.

Rosenthal L, Meldolesi J (1989). α-Latrotoxin and related toxins. *Pharm Ther* 42: 115–134.

Rousseau F, et al. (1994). Mutations in the gene encoding fibroblast growth factor receptor-3 in achondroplasia. *Nature* 371: 252–254.

Saha MS, Spann CL, Grainger RM (1989). Embryonic lens induction: more than meets the optic vesicle. *Cell Differ Dev* 28: 153–172.

Sai T, Seino S, Chang C, Trifiro M, Pinsky L, Mhatre A, Kaufman M, Lambert B, Trapman J, Brinkmann AO, et al. (1997). An exonic point mutation of the androgen receptor gene in a family with complete androgen insensitivity. *Am J Hum Genet* 46:1095–1110.

Sato M, Ochi T, Nakase T, Hirota S, Kitamura Y, Nomura S, Yasui N (1999). Mechanical tension-stress induces expression of bone morphogenetic protein BMP-2 and BMP-4, but not BMP-6, BMP-7, and GDF-5 mRNA, during distraction osteogenesis. *J Bone Mineral Res* 14: 1084–1095.

Sauer F, Fondell JD, Ohkuma Y, Roeder RG, Jäckle H (1995). Control of transcription by Krüppel through interactions with TFIIB and TFIIE. *Nature* 375: 162–165.

Saunders JW, Jr., Fallon JF (1966). Cell death and morphogenesis. In: *Major Problems of Developmental Biology.* Locke M (ed.) Academic Press, New York, pp. 289–314.

Schmucker D, Clemens JC, Shu H, Worby CA, Xiao J, Muda M, Dixon JE, Zipursky SL (2000). *Drosophila* Dscam is an axon guidance receptor exhibiting extraordinary molecular diversity. *Cell* 101: 671–684.

Schnabel R (1997). Why does a nematode have an invariant cell lineage? *Semin Cell Dev Biol* 8: 341–349.

Schroeder EH, Kisslinger JA, Kopan R (1998). Notch-1 signalling requires ligand-induced proteolytic release of intracellular domain. *Nature* 393: 382–386.

Shaham S, Horvitz HR (1996). An alternatively spliced *C. elegans* ced-4 RNA encodes a novel cell death inhibitor. *Cell* 86: 201–208.

Shiang R, et al. (1994). Mutations in the transmembrane domain of FGFR3 cause the most common genetic form of dwarfism, achondroplasia. *Cell* 78: 335–342.

Shore EM, Ahn J, Jan de Beur S, Li M, Xu M, Gardner RJ, Zasloff MA, Whyte MP, Levine MA, Kaplan FS (2002). Paternally inherited inactivating mutations of the *GNAS1* gene in progressive osseous heteroplasia. *N Engl J Med* 346: 99–106.

Shulman JM, Perrimon N, Axelrod JD (1998). Frizzled signaling and the developmental control of cell polarity. *Trends Genet* 14: 452–458.

Sly WS, Fischer HD (1982). The phosphomannosyl recognition systems for intracellular and intercellular transport of lysosomal enzymes. *J Cell Biochem* 18: 67–85.

Smith JL, Schoenwolf FC (1997). Neurulation: coming to closure. *Trends Neurosci* 11: 510–517.

Socolovsky M, Fallon AE, Wang S, Brugnara C, Lodish HF (1999). Fetal anemia and apoptosis of red cell progenitors in Stat5a$^{-/-}$5b$^{-/-}$ mice: a direct role for Stat5 in Bcl-X$_L$ induction. *Cell* 98: 181–191.

Socolovsky M, Nam H, Fleming MD, Haase VH, Brugnara C, Lodish HF (2001). Ineffective erythropoiesis in Stat5a$^{-/-}$5b$^{-/-}$ mice due to decreased survival of early erythroblasts. *Blood* 98: 3261–3273.

Sopta M, Burton ZF, Greenblatt J (1989). Structure and associated DNA helicase activity of a general transcription factor that binds to RNA polymerase II. *Nature* 341:410–415.

Soussi-Yanicostas N, Hardelin J-P, del Mar Arroyo-Jimenez M, Ardouin O, Legouis R, Levilliers J, Traincard F, Betton J-M, Cabanie L, Petit C (1996). Initial characterization of anosmin-1, a putative extracellular matrix protein synthesized by definite neuronal cell populations in the central nervous system. *J Cell Sci* 109: 1749–1757.

Sozou P, Kirkwood TB (2001). A stochastic model of cell replicative senescence based on telomere shortening, oxidative stress, and somatic mutations in nuclear and mitochondrial DNA. *J Theor Biol* 213: 573–586.

Spritz RA, Gielbel LB, Holmes SA (1992). Dominant negative and loss-of-function mutations of the c-*kit* (mast/stem cell growth factor receptor) proto-oncogene in human piebaldism. *Am J Hum Genet* 50: 261–269.

Stern HM, Brown AMC, Hauschka SD (1995). Myogenesis in paraxial mesoderm: preferential induction by dorsal neural tube and by cells expressing Wnt-1. *Development* 121: 3675–3686.

Stokoe D, Macdonald SG, Cadwallader K, Symons M, Hancock JF (1994). Activation of Raf as a result of recruitment to the plasma membrane. *Science* 264: 1463–1467.

Streuli CH, Bailey N, Bissell MJ (1991). Control of mammary epithelial differentiation: basement membrane induces tissue specific gene expression in the absence of cell–cell interactions and morphological polarity. *J Cell Biol* 115: 1383–1396.

Struhl G, Adachi A (1998). Nuclear access and action of Notch in vivo. *Cell* 93: 382–386.

Su WC, Kitagawa M, Xue N, Xie B, Garofalo X, Cho J, Deng C, Horton WA, Fu XY (1997). Activation of Stat1 by mutant fibroblast growth-factor receptor in thanatophoric dysplasia type II dwarfism. *Nature* 386: 288–292.

Thomas L (1992). *The Fragile Species.* Macmillan, New York.

Ting-Berreth SA, Chuong C-M (1996). Local delivery of TGFβ-2 can substitute for placode epithelium to induce mesenchymal condensation during skin morphogenesis. *Dev Biol* 179: 347–359.

Trehan KP, Gill KP (2002). Epigenetics of dominance for enzyme activity. *J Biosci* 27: 127–134.

Tremblay JP, et al. (1993). Myoblast transplantation between monozygous twin girl carriers of Duchenne muscular dystrophy. *Neuromuscul Disord* 3: 583–592.

Trudel M, Constantini F (1987). A 3′ enhancer contributes to the stage-specific expression of the human β-globin gene. *Genes Dev* 1: 954–961.

Ullrich B, Uskaryov YA, Südhof TC (1995). Cartography of neurexins: More than 1000 isoforms generated by alternative splicing and expressed in distinct subsets of neurons. *Neuron* 14: 497–507.

Vaahtokari A, Aberg T, Thesleff I (1996). Apoptosis in the developing tooth: association with an embryonic signaling center and suppression by EGF and FGF-4. *Development* 122: 121–129.

Vallee RB, Tai C, Faulkner NE (2001). *LIS1:* cellular function of a disease-causing gene. *Trends Cell Biol* 11: 155–160.

Varrela J (1992). Dimensional variation of craniofacial structures in relation to changing masticatory-functional demands. *Eur J Orthod* 14: 31–36.

Vaux DL, Weissman IL, Kim SK (1992). Prevention of programmed cell death in *Caenorhabditis* elegans by human *bcl-2. Science* 258: 1955–1957.

Vogel-Höpker A, Momose T, Rohrer H, Yasua K, Ishihara L, Rappaport DH (2000). Multiple functions of fibroblast growth factor-8 (FGF-8) in chick eye development. *Mech Dev* 94: 25–36.

Waddington CH (1940). *Organisers and Genes.* Cambridge University Press, Cambridge.

Wakayama T, Perry ACF, Zuccotti M, Johnson KR, Yanagimachi R (1998). Full-term development of mice from enucleated oocytes injected with cumulus cell nuclei. *Nature* 394: 369–374.

Wang S, et al. (1998). Notch receptor activation inhibits oligodendrocyte differentiation. *Neuron* 21: 63–76.

Wang X, Kiledjian M, Weiss IM, Liebhaber SA (1995). Detection and characterization of a 3′ untranslated region ribonucleoprotein complex associated with human α-globin mRNA stability. *Mol Cell Biol* 15:1769–1777.

Webster MK, Donoghue DJ (1996). Constitutive activation of fibroblast growth factor receptor 3 by the transmembrane domain point mutation found in achondroplasia. *EMBO J* 15: 520–527.

Weijs WA, Hillen B (1986). Correlations between the cross-sectional area of the jaw muscles and craniofacial size and shape. *Am J Phys Anthropol* 70: 423–431.

Wessells NK (1977). *Tissue Interaction and Development.* Benjamin Cummings, Menlo Park, CA.

Whitehead AS, et al. (1995). A genetic defect in 5,10-methylenetetrafolate reductase in neural tube defects. *Q J Med* 88: 763–766.

Wilmut I, Schnieke AE, McWhir J, Kind AJ, Campbell KHS (1997). Viable offspring from fetal and adult mammalian cells. *Nature* 385: 810–814.

Winchester B, et al. (1992). Female twin with Hunter disease due to non-random inactivation of the X-chromosome: a consequence of twinning. *Am J Med Genet* 44: 834–838.

Winter CG, Wang B, Ballew A, Royou A, Karess R, Axelrod JD, Luo L (2001). *Drosophila* Rho-associated kinase (Drok) links Frizzled-mediated planar cell polarity signaling to the actin cytoskeleton. *Cell* 105: 81–91.

Witte ON (1990). Steel locus defines new multipotent growth factor. *Cell* 63: 5–6.

Wolf U (1995). Identical mutations and phenotypic variation. *Hum Genet* 100: 305–321.

Wu KC (1996). Entwicklung, Stimulation, und Paralyse der embryonalen Motorick. *Wien Klin Wochenschr* 108: 303–305.

Wu M, et al. (2000). c-Kit triggers dual phosphorylation, which couples activation and degradation of the essential melanocyte factor Mi. *Genes Dev* 14: 301–312.

Yamada T, Pfaff SL, Edlund T, Jessell TM (1993). Control of cell pattern in the neural tube: motor neuron induction by diffusible factors from notochord and floor plate. *Cell* 73: 673–686.

Yamakawa K, Huot YK, Haendelt MA, Hubert R, Chen XN, Lyons GE, Korenberg JR (1998). DSCAM: a novel member of the immunoglobulin superfamily maps in a Down syndrome region and is involved in the development of the nervous system. *Hum Mol Genet* 7: 227–237.

Yoshida H, et al. (1998). Apaf1 is required for mitochondrial pathways of apoptosis and brain development. *Cell* 94: 739–750.

Zackson SL, Steinberg MS (1987). Chemotaxis or adhesion gradient? Pronephric duct elongation does not depend on distant sources of guidance information. *Dev Biol* 124: 418–422.

Zhou K, Hart CM, Laemmli UK (1995). Visualization of chromosomal domains with boundary-element associated factor BEAF-32. *Cell* 81: 879–889.

Zolessi FR, Arruti C (2001). Apical accumulation of MARCKS in neural plate cells during neurulation in the chick embryo. *BMC Dev Biol* 1: 7.

Zygar CA, Cook TL, Jr., Grainger RM (1998). Gene activation during early stages of lens induction in *Xenopus. Development* 125: 3509–3519.

3 | Model Organisms in the Study of Development and Disease

ETHAN BIER AND WILLIAM MCGINNIS

The past two decades have brought major breakthroughs in our understanding of the molecular and genetic circuits that control a myriad of developmental events in vertebrates and invertebrates. These detailed studies have revealed surprisingly deep similarities in the mechanisms underlying developmental processes across a wide range of bilaterally symmetric metazoans (bilateralia). Such phylogenetic comparisons have defined a common core of genetic pathways guiding development and have made it possible to reconstruct many features of the most recent common ancestor of all bilateral animals, which most likely lived 600–800 million years ago (Shubin et al., 1997; Knoll and Carroll, 1999). As flushed out in more detail below and reiterated as a major unifying theme throughout the book, the common metazoan ancestor already had in place many of the genetic pathways that are present in modern-day vertebrates and invertebrates. This ancestor can be imagined as an advanced worm-like or primitive shrimp-like creature which had a few distinct body specializations along the nose-to-tail axis and was subdivided into three distinct germ layers (ectoderm, mesoderm, and endoderm). It also had evolved an inductive signaling system to partition the ectoderm into neural versus nonneural components and is likely to have possessed appendages or outgrowths from its body wall with defined anterior–posterior, dorsal–ventral, and proximo–distal axes, as well as light-sensitive organs, a sensory system for detecting vibrations, a rudimentary heart, a molecular guidance system for initiating axon outgrowth to the midline of the nervous system, ion channels for conducting electrical impulses, synaptic machinery required for neural transmission, trachea, germ cells, and an innate immune system.

The fact that the ancestor of vertebrate and invertebrate model organisms was a highly evolved creature which had already invented complex interacting systems controlling development, physiology, and behavior has profound implications for medical genetics. The central points that we explore in this chapter can be broadly put into two categories: *(1)* the great advantages of model organisms for identifying and understanding genes that are altered in heritable human diseases and *(2)* the functions of many of those genes and the evidence that they were present in the ancestral bilateral organisms and have remained largely intact in both vertebrate and invertebrate lineages during the ensuing course of evolution. In the course of discussing these points, we review the compelling evidence that developmentally important genes have been phylogenetically conserved and the likelihood that developmental disorders in humans will often involve genes controlling similar morphogenetic processes in vertebrates and invertebrates. A systematic analysis of human disease gene homologs in *Drosophila* supports this view since 75% of human disease genes are structurally related to genes present in *Drosophila* and more than a third of these human genes are highly related to their fruit fly counterparts (Bernards and Hariharan, 2001; Reiter et al., 2001; Chien et al., 2002).

Since its inception, the field of human genetics has focused on the identification of genes that, as single entities, can cause disease when mutated. The discovery of such new disease genes has advanced at an accelerating pace in the last decade, and the rate is now over 175 genes per year (Peltonen and McKusick, 2001). This rate is likely to accelerate even further in the near term because of the sequencing of human genome. Most of the 4000–5000 estimated human disease genes should be identified before long. In anticipation of this asymptotic discovery process, the emphasis in human genetics is shifting to understanding the function of these disease genes. An obvious avenue for functional analysis of disease genes is to study them in the closely related mouse using gene knockout techniques to assess the effects of either eliminating the gene's function or inducing specific disease-causing mutations. In some cases, this type of analysis has resulted in excellent mouse models for diseases that have phenotypes very similar to human diseases. In other cases, mouse knockout mutations have been less informative than hoped, either because the greater genetic redundancy in vertebrates masks the effect of mutations in single genes or because the mutations of interest are lethal at an early embryonic stage. Since there are limitations to the mouse system and there are deep ancestrally derived commonalities in the body plan organization and physiology of vertebrate and invertebrate model organisms, particularly flies and nematodes for which there are well-developed and powerful molecular genetic tools, these organisms are likely to play an increasingly important role in the functional analysis of human disease genes. This chapter also compares the strengths and weaknesses of several well-developed model systems, ranging from single-cell eukaryotes to primates, as tools for dissecting the function of human disease genes. We propose that multiple model systems can be employed in cross-genomic analysis of human disease genes to address different kinds of issues, such as basic eukaryotic cellular functions (e.g., yeast and slime molds), assembly of genes into various types of molecular machines and pathways (e.g., flies and nematodes), and accurate models of human disease processes (e.g., vertebrates such as zebrafish and mice).

MODEL ORGANISMS: ADVANTAGES AND LIMITATIONS OF THE VARIOUS SYSTEMS

In this section, we consider the strengths and limitations of several well-studied model organisms with regard to the analysis of human genetic disorders (see Table 3–1). In general, several model systems can be used to analyze the function of a given human disease gene. Unicellular organisms such as yeast (*Saccharomyces*) (Foury, 1997) and the facultatively colonial slime mold (*Dictyostelium*) (Firtel and Chung, 2000; Chung et al., 2001) can be used to analyze phenomena that involve important basic eukaryotic cell functions, such as metabolism, regulation of the cell cycle, membrane targeting and dynamics, protein folding, and DNA repair. Simple invertebrate systems such as *Drosophila* (Bernards and Hariharan, 2001; Reiter et al., 2001; Chien et al., 2002) or *Caenorhabditis elegans* (Aboobaker and Blaxter, 2000; Culetto and Sattelle, 2000) are excellent models for examining the coordinated actions of genes that function as components of a common molecular machine such as a signal-transduction pathway or a complex of physically interacting proteins. These proteins may or may not have highly related sequences in yeast, but if so, the value of the invertebrate system would be most pronounced if the human disease condition involved a tissue-specific requirement for the protein in question (e.g.. metabolic disorders resulting in neurological phenotypes). In contrast, mammalian systems such as the mouse (Benavides and Guenet, 2001), zebrafish (Barut and Zon, 2000; Dooley and Zon, 2000), frog, and chicken and to some extent more complex invertebrates (e.g., echinoderms and primitive chordates) are most likely to provide accurate models for the human disease state, which can be used to assess various strategies for intervening in the disease process.

Table 3–1. Strengths and Limitations of Various Model Organisms

Species	Experimental Advantages	Experimental Limitations

Yeast	Excellent genetics
	    Very powerful second site screening
	Powerful molecular techniques
	    Genes can be easily cloned
	Genome sequence complete
	Possess all basic eukaryotic cell organelles
	Cell cycle control similar to animals
		No distinct tissues

Slime mold	Excellent genetics
	    Very powerful second site screening
	Powerful molecular techniques
	    Genes can be easily cloned
	Genome sequence nearing completion
	Simple cellular behaviors similar to animals
	    Motility
	    Chemotaxis
		Limited cellular diversity

Nematode	Excellent genetics
	    Hermaphrodites, self-fertilization
	    Fast generation time
	    Second site suppressor/enhancer screens
	Powerful molecular techniques
	    Genes can be easily cloned
	        Transposon tagging
	        SNP mapping
	        Rapid cosmid rescue
	        Deletion collections span genome
	    RNAi effective
	Genome sequence complete
	Few cells: 959 cells, 302 neurons
	Morphology fully characterized
	    Serial EM reconstruction
	All cell lineages known
	    Time lapse microscopy of development
	Laser ablation of single identified cells
		Limited external morphology
		Less similar to human than flies (61% of *Drosophila* genes have human counterparts vs. 43% of *C. elegans* genes)
		Detailed direct analysis of gene expression patterns can be difficult
		Some embryological manipulations difficult

Fruit fly	Excellent genetics
	Genome sequence complete
	Targeted gene disruption
	RNAi effective
	Fast generation time
	Second site suppressor/enhancer screens
	Powerful molecular techniques
	Genes can be easily cloned
	    Transposon tagging
	    SNP mapping
	Transgenic animals easily generated
	Targeted misexpression of genes in space and time
	Mosaic analysis: determine where gene acts
		Embryological manipulations difficult
		Targeted gene disruption still difficult, although possible

Zebrafish	Simplest vertebrate with good genetics: nearly saturated for zygotic patterning mutants Genome analysis well under way (good SNP and linkage maps) Easy examination of morphological defects (clear embryos) Embryological manipulations possible Organ systems similar to other vertebrates (e.g., eyes, heart, blood, gastrointestinal tract) Rapid vertebrate development	Not yet trivial to clone genes Cannot easily make transgenic animals No targeted gene disruption
Frog	A vertebrate Ectopic gene expression possible in early embryos, although manipulation of levels difficult Accessibility of embryo (pond no shell) Excellent experimental embryology grafting induction preparations (Keller sandwiches/animal caps, etc.) Injection of RNA into identifiable blastomeres	No genetics, although under development Difficult to create transgenic animals
Chicken	Availability, low cost Accessibility, outside of mother Well suited for embryological manipulation; transplants of limbs, notocord, neural crest Easily transfected by avian retroviruses	Limited genetics Limited genome data at present
Mouse	Mammals; brains similar to human, all homologous areas/cell types "Reverse" genetics: targeted gene knockouts by homologous recombination routine Developmental overview same as for all mammals Large mutant collection Construction of chimeric embryos possible Availability of material at all stages Source of primary cells for culture	Classic "forward" genetics difficult Early-acting mutant phenotypes difficult to study (resorbed by mother) Embryonic manipulations difficult (inside mother) Development and life cycle relatively slow (months)

(Continued)

Table 3–1. *Continued*

Species	Experimental Advantages	Experimental Limitations
Monkey	Very similar to humans	Fetal experiments difficult
	Developmental connections and physiology, postnatal	No genetics
	Anatomy of learning	High cost, for both animals and facilities
	Responses to injury	
Human	Many diseases, self-reporting mutants (>5000 genetically based diseases)	Fetal material difficult
		No experimental access
	Some good family pedigrees	
	Genome sequence complete	
	Detailed behavior/ontogeny	

SNP, single nucleotide polymorphism; RNAi, RNA interference; EM, electrical microscopy.

Unicellular Organisms as Models for Eukaryotic Cell Function

All eukaryotic organisms share an organization of the cell into functionally dedicated, membrane-enclosed compartments such as the nucleus, mitochondria, endoplasmic reticulum/Golgi, and endosomes. In addition, similar mechanisms control the cell cycle, cell division, creation of cell polarity (e.g., bud site selection in yeast or polarity of chemotaxing *Dictyostelium*), and motility (*Dictyostelium*) in unicellular as well as multicellular eukaryotes. Many basic molecular biological processes are also shared by all eukaryotes, including biochemical pathways, DNA replication, DNA repair, transcriptional control, RNA processing, and protein degradation.

The best-studied unicellular eukaryotic systems are yeast (*Saccharomyces cerevisiae*) and slime molds (*Dictyostelium discoideum*). The yeast genome sequence has been completed (http://genome-www.stanford.edu/Saccharomyces/), and several additional genome-scale resources are being developed, such as collections of mutations in every gene and a comprehensive two-hybrid collection defining all two-way interactions between yeast proteins. The *Dictyostelium* genome sequence also is nearly complete (http://glamdring.ucsd.edu/others/dsmith/dictydb.html), and it is possible to knock out specific genes efficiently using the REMI method (Kuspa and Loomis, 1994). Thus, both organisms are excellent molecular systems. In addition, it is possible to carry out genetic selection schemes and screens in these organisms in which greater than a billion progeny can be generated and tested. Genetic schemes of this kind are effective at isolating potential second-site intragenic suppressor loci as well as saturating for second-site mutations which modify the phenotype of a given mutant. These unicellular systems have no equal for establishing the networks of gene action involved in basic cell biological processes.

The chief limitation of unicellular organisms as models for analyzing the function of genes involved in human disease is that pathologies that affect specific tissues, such as the nervous system or organs, or physiological functions that arise from interactions between cells cannot be assessed at the relevant organismal level. This limitation is not restricted to disease genes that do not have obvious homologs in unicellular organisms but also can apply to genes that are present in unicellular organisms but required in a more stringent fashion in certain tissues or expressed as different isoforms in different cell types. For example, defects in enzymes involved in energy metabolism can result in nervous system or muscle-specific defects (Blass et al., 2000; Darras and Friedman, 2000; Guertl et al., 2000; Palau, 2001).

Invertebrate Genetic Systems as Models for Tissue and Organ Function

The most developed invertebrate genetic organisms are fruit flies (*Drosophila melanogaster*, http://flybase.bio.indiana.edu:82/) and nematodes (*C. elegans*, http://www.expasy.ch/cgi-bin/lists?celegans.txt). These model organisms have contributed to many basic biological discoveries, including the organization of genes into independently segregating linear chromosomes, the creation of the first chromosome maps, the one gene–one protein hypothesis, the discovery that X-rays cause increased rates of mutations, the principles of pattern formation and of how genes can act hierarchically in space and time to define distinct positions and cell types, as well as the identification of many genetic pathways that subsequently have been implicated in human disease.

A major strength of these model systems is that they are well suited for second-site modifier screens. These screens can be used to isolate many components in a given genetic pathway once a single gene involved in that process has been identified. The logic of these screens is to partially cripple a process or pathway with a mutation affecting one component and then search for mutations in other genes encoding component functions in the same system. This is accomplished by screening for mutations which critically reduce the function of the pathway in a dominant fashion but only when combined with the first mutation. The cartoon of a simple crank–pulley system designed to hoist a bucket of water illustrates this principle (Fig. 3–1). If one removes any piece entirely, such as either of the gears, the machine is inoperative. If, however, one only files down the teeth on one of the

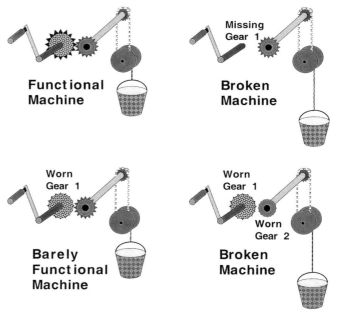

Figure 3–1. Molecular machines and the logic of genetic screens. Several genes typically function in concert as a machine to carry out a particular molecular function. In this diagram, such a "molecular machine" is depicted as a crank and gear assembly that functions to raise a bucket. In this analogy, the various components in the machine can be thought of as genes, which function together to carry out a molecular function such as passing a signal from one cell to another. If one removes either of the two gears, the machine is broken and unable to perform its task. In this complete loss-of-function situation, any further blow to the system has no further consequence. If, on the other hand, one starts out with one of the gears (gear 1) being worn such that the machine barely functions to raise the bucket, then even a small additional insult to another component (e.g., a worn gear 2) will render the machine inoperative. This latter scenario is similar to the genetic conditions one can engineer in a model genetic system wherein a partial loss-of-function mutant in one gene sensitizes the system to even a slight reduction in the function of any other component of that molecular machine. In this way, geneticists can rapidly screen for new mutants that define all the various components of the intact machine.

gears, then it is possible to get a machine that is barely working. If one then damages any other component (e.g., files down another gear), the machine fails. Thus, the barely functioning machine provides a sensitized genetic system that converts an otherwise silent recessive mutation (e.g., 50% reduction in gene dose) into a dominant read-out, which can be easily scored among large numbers of progeny (e.g., 10^5–10^6 individuals).

Because flies and nematodes have closely related counterparts of many human disease genes, identification of new genes functioning as part of a common molecular process in invertebrates will help define new candidate disease genes that are likely also to be involved in the same disease process. An important point regarding the use of invertebrate systems is that it is not necessary that the phenotype resulting from reducing the activity of a pathway in the model system be similar to that of the human disease. The only critical aspect of the invertebrate model is that it faithfully identifies components acting as part of a common molecular machine. A useful example to illustrate this point is the Notch signaling pathway. The Notch pathway controls many different binary cell fate choices during development of *Drosophila* and *C. elegans* (Greenwald, 1998; Simpson, 1998). Two heavily studied phenotypes resulting from mutations in components of this pathway are notching of the wing margin in flies (Irvine, 1999; Wu and Rao, 1999) and defects in vulval development in worms (Greenwald, 1998; Wang and Sternberg, 2001). In the case of the fly, strong reduction in the activities of the ligand Delta, the Notch receptor itself, or the signal transducer Suppressor or Hairless can result in Notched wings. In the case of vertebrates, which have several paralogs of Notch pathway components, reduced function in the Delta-related ligand Delta3 (Kusumi et al., 1998; Bulman et al., 2000) or the Notch homolog Notch1 (Conlon et al., 1995) results in axial skeletal malformations (e.g., spondylocostal dysostosis) as a consequence of somite fusion defects during embryonic development. Mutations in the human *Delta3* gene were originally identified based on previous finding that mutations in mouse *Delta3* gave rise to similar spinal malformations and the fact that the human *Delta3* gene mapped within a genomic interval believed to contain the suspected disease gene. For this reasoning to hold, it was not necessary that the fly phenotype resembled that of the human disease (e.g., humans have no wings and flies do not have bony endoskeletons). The only important facts for this discovery were that mutations in different components of a common signaling pathway in humans led to similar disease phenotypes and that the components of this pathway had been defined by comprehensive saturation screening in model genetic systems.

Vertebrate Genetic Systems as Models for Human Disease

As described above, unicellular and model invertebrate systems can be of great value in defining the molecular components of pathways or processes that depend on the function of several interacting proteins. Once such components have been defined, one can ask whether similar diseases result from defects in more than one of these components in humans. In some cases, the model systems can also serve as models for the disease process itself, as in the polyglutamine repeat neurodegenerative disorders in which there are parallel correlations in *Drosophila* and humans between the length of the polyglutamine repeat and the severity and early onset of neurodegenerative phenotypes (Chan and Bonini, 2000; Fortini and Bonini, 2000). While such examples exist, model invertebrate systems cannot in general be consistently relied on to mimic the human disease state. Rather, the ability to provide an accurate model for the human disease condition is the chief strength of vertebrate systems such as the mouse (*Mus musculus domesticus*, http://www.informatics.jax.org/) and zebrafish (*Danio rerio*, http://www.ncbi.nlm.nih.gov/genome/guide/D_rerio.html).

The great advantage of the mouse system is clearly the ability to make targeted gene knockouts (mutations). The knockout phenotype of a human disease gene counterpart in mice often results in a phenotype resembling that of the human disease. There are notable exceptions to this approach, however, which may result from the significant effect of genetic background on knock-out phenotypes in mice, the genetic variation in human genetic background, or intrinsic differences between the function of mouse and human disease gene homologs. One curious trend is that a corresponding mutation in a given gene in mice and humans often results in a much stronger phenotype in humans. There are even examples in which the heterozygous loss-of-function mutation generates a dominant phenotype in humans comparable to that observed in homozygous null mice knockouts.

Although gene knock-out technology has not yet been developed for zebrafish, systematic genetic screens have been conducted for mutants disrupting various aspects of embryonic development (Driever et al., 1996; Haffter et al., 1996). Among the large number of mutants recovered in these screens, many affected embryonic patterning and formation of organ systems such as the heart (Chen et al., 1996; Stainier et al., 1996; Xu et al., 2002), digestive system (Pack et al., 1996), hematopoetic system (Ransom et al., 1996; Childs et al., 2000), bone and cartilage (Neuhauss et al., 1996; Piotrowski et al., 1996; Schilling et al., 1996), spinal chord/notochord (Odenthal et al., 1996; Stemple et al., 1996), retina (Malicki et al., 1996a; Brockerhoff et al., 1998; Daly and Sandell, 2000), auditory system (Malicki et al., 1996b; Whitfield et al., 1996), and brain (Abdelilah et al., 1996; Brand et al., 1996; Heisenberg et al., 1996; Jiang et al., 1996; Schier et al., 1996; Rodriguez and Driever, 1997). In addition, many mutations were recovered which compromised the pathfinding ability of retinal axons to be guided to their appropriate tectal targets (Baier et al., 1996; Karlstrom et al., 1996; Trowe et al., 1996). High-resolution simple sequence length polymorphisms (SSLPs) and radiation hybrid maps have also been generated for the zebrafish, which greatly aid in the genetic mapping of mutations and cloning of the affected genes (Kelly et al., 2000; Woods et al., 2000; Hukriede et al., 2001).

Nongenetic Model Systems

Although this chapter is focused on model genetic systems for studying genes involved in developmental disorders, there are some significant advantages of nongenetic systems for analyzing certain types of questions. Classic vertebrate embryological systems, for example, *Xenopus* and the chick, offer ease and access to experimental manipulations such as heterotopic transplantation and grafting, which were critical for the identification of organizing centers such as the Spemann organizer, the zone of polarizing activity (ZPA), and the apical ectodermal ridge (AER). Although classic genetic techniques are not available for these systems, some effective experimental alternatives, such as injection of normal or mutant RNAs or virus-mediated gene expression, provide important complementary systems to genetic models.

Higher vertebrate systems, such as birds, cats, ferrets, and primates, also offer advantages with regard to the postnatal development of neural connections. For example, these systems are well suited for analysis of critical periods required for experience-based formation of visual, auditory, sematosensory, and behavioral (e.g., birdsong or language) connections. As many developmental disorders in humans also result in learning or behavioral abnormalities, the more related to humans a species is, the better it can serve as a model for such complex neural functions.

RECONSTRUCTING THE COMMON ANCESTOR OF METAZOANS: OUR DISTANT REFLECTION

The detection of covert similarity in diverse body plans of bilateral animals has resulted from the great advances made in the past 20 years of developmental genetic research. For example, a series of investigations showed that all bilateralia, including humans, possess a common genetic mechanism for patterning the anterior/posterior (A/P) body axis involving the Hox cluster genes (McGinnis and Krumlauf, 1992), the dorsal/ventral (D/V) body axis (Francois and Bier, 1995; DeRobertis and Sasai, 1996), and the three derived axes of the appendages (A/P, D/V, and proximo/distal [P/D]) (Irvine and Vogt, 1997; Panganiban et al., 1997; Shubin et al., 1997). Many of the pathways involved in this discussion are covered in more detail in other sections of the book, but here we use them to illustrate the validity of studying model organisms.

Besides common axial patterning systems, other general architectural features in both vertebrates and invertebrates appear to be controlled by common genetic mechanisms. Humans and insects possess organs of very diverse appearance that serve similar functions, such as eyes for vision (Wawersik and Maas, 2000; Pichaud et al., 2001), and hearts for blood circulation (Bodmer and Venkatesh, 1998; Chen and Fishman, 2000). Traditional views have held that these structures are analogous (i.e., convergently evolved) and therefore likely to be specified by different genetic patterning systems. However, the sum of the evidence discussed below suggests that we now have good reason to call these organs homologous at the level of the genes that control their formation.

Hox Genes Determine Segment Identity along the A/P Axis: From *Drosophila* to Humans

Homeosis was defined by William Bateson (1894) as the phenomenon in which one segment of an organism is transformed in whole or in part to another. The genetic basis for these transformations of the animal body plan was partially revealed by seminal studies on homeotic selector genes (now often referred to as *Hox genes*; see Chapter 46). Mutations in Hox genes often result in homeotic transformations of the body plan in one or a few segments. A systematic collection of homeotic mutations was discovered and studied in *Drosophila* in the labortories of E.B. Lewis, Thomas Kaufman, and others. Two breakthough papers that summarize these studies are Lewis (1978) and Kaufman et al. (1980). The well-known homeotic gene *Ultrabithorax* (*Ubx*) was originally identified by mutations that transform halteres (small club-like balancing organs of flies) into an extra pair of wings. Another classical homeotic phenotype is produced by dominant mutations in the *Antennapedia* (*Antp*) gene, which transform the antenna on the head of a fly into an extra thoracic leg.

Molecular analysis of the genomes of other organisms has revealed that all bilateral animals, including humans, have multiple Hox genes (Fig. 3–2), which carry a common DNA sequence motif called the homeobox (the genesis of the *Hox* acronym). The homeobox motif encodes a similar 60–amino acid motif in Hox proteins, termed the *homeodomain*. Homeodomain proteins such as those of the Hox type are transcription factors and exert their function through activation and repres-

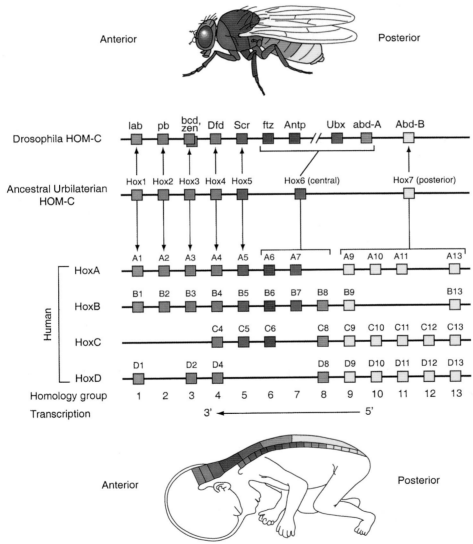

Figure 3–2. Conservation of genomic organization and expression patterns of fly and mammal Hox genes. The lower part of the figure shows the four clusters of Hox genes in mammals and the expression patterns (inferred from mouse expression studies) of the orthologous genes in a diagram of a human embryo. The colored fields in the expression diagram show the anteriormost domains of expression. The posterior extent of many Hox gene expression patterns overlap in more caudal regions. The upper half of the figure shows the *Drosophila* Hox genes aligned with their mammalian orthologs (arrows), with their corresponding expression patterns mapped onto the body plan. The composition of a hypothetical ancestral Hox cluster is shown in the middle. For some of the central and posterior Hox genes, there are no obvious orthology relationships, so groups of genes that are equally related to an ancestral gene are indicated with brackets. *Drosophila bcd, ftz,* and *zen* homeobox genes do not function in the Hox A/P patterning system. They represent insect homeobox genes that have recently diverged from Hox ancestors and now have novel patterning functions.

sion of multiple target genes. Interestingly, the Hox genes are arranged so that the position and order of homologous genes (e.g., *Deformed* [*Dfd*] of *Drosophila* and *HOXD4* of humans) are preserved in the Hox clusters of different animals. The functional significance of the conserved gene order in these clusters is not clearly understood at present. There is, however, evidence that the clustered arrangement has been maintained for more than 500 million years because different genes in the clusters are controlled by the same *cis*-acting DNA regulatory regions. Thus, it can be argued that the clusters function as single, complicated genetic units (Gerard et al., 1996; Gould et al., 1997; Sharpe et al., 1998). In contrast to the unique Hox cluster of *Drosophila* and most other invertebrates, humans and other vertebrates have four clusters of Hox genes (*HOXA, HOXB, HOXC,* and *HOXD*), which apparently evolved by two successive duplications of a primordial cluster.

In addition to conservation of primary sequence and chromosomal organization, Hox gene expression patterns are conserved in diverse animals. Persistent expression of Hox genes in discrete zones on the A/P axis is required to remind embryonic cells of their axial position long after the initial genetic cues are gone. Hox expression zones typically have sharp anterior boundaries, with less well-defined posterior boundaries. The order of anterior boundaries of Hox expression along the A/P axis of the embryo and the timing of activation during development are generally colinear with the order of the genes on the chromosome (Zákány and Duboule, 1999). It is interesting to note that the same Hox gene can have a slightly offset boundary of expression in different tissues, which is especially true for vertebrate embryos (Fig. 3–2). Within the same tissue, however, the relative expression boundaries of different Hox cluster members are almost always preserved.

Conservation of Hox protein sequence and expression patterns suggested that vertebrate Hox genes controlled axial patterning in a manner similar to that in flies. This was confirmed when mouse Hox mutants were obtained and homeotic transformations found in the mutant embryos. For example, in *Hoxc-8* homozygous mutant mice, the most obvious transformations were attachment of the eighth pair of ribs to the sternum and the appearance of a fourteenth pair of ribs on the first lumbar vertebra (Le Mouellic et al., 1992).

Studies in both *Drosophila* and mouse show that Hox loss-of-function mutants generally result in transformations in which more posterior body structures resemble more anterior ones (McGinnis and Krumlauf, 1992). Conversely, many gain-of-function mutations in which a posterior gene is inappropriately expressed in a more anterior region result in the replacement of anterior stuctures with stuctures characteristic of more posterior regions. For example, when *Drosophila* Ubx protein, which is normally confined to the posterior most abdominal region of the fly embryo, is provided ubiquitously under the control of a heat shock promoter, all head and thoracic segments attain a more posterior (abdominal-like) identity. The ability of a more posterior Hox gene to impose its function on more anterior genes is called *posterior prevalence*, or *phenotypic suppression*.

D/V Patterning in *Drosophila*

Establishment of the D/V axis in *Drosophila* is initiated by a cascade of maternally acting genes functioning in both the oocyte and sur-

rounding follicle cells. These genes ultimately create a nuclear gradient of the *rel*-related transcription factor encoded by the *dorsal* gene (Roth et al., 1989; Rushlow et al., 1989; Steward, 1989). The Dorsal nuclear gradient is directly responsible for subdividing the embryo into three primary territories of zygotic gene expression: a ventral zone giving rise to mesoderm, a lateral zone giving rise to neuroectoderm, and a dorsal zone giving rise to dorsal ectoderm and amnioserosa (Fig. 3–3). Dorsal activates expression of genes in ventral and lateral regions of the embryo in a threshold-dependent fashion (reviewed in Rusch and Levine, 1996). High levels of Dorsal are required for activating expression of mesoderm-determining genes such as *snail* (Kosman et al., 1991; Leptin, 1991; Rao et al., 1991; Ray et al., 1991; Thisse et al., 1991; Ip et al., 1992b) and *twist* (Jiang et al., 1991; Kosman et al., 1991; Leptin, 1991; Rao et al., 1991; Ray et al., 1991), whereas lower levels are required to activate genes such as *rhomboid* (*rho*) (Kosman et al., 1991; Leptin, 1991; Rao et al., 1991; Ray et al., 1991; Ip et al., 1992a), *ventral nervous system defective* (*vnd*) (Mellerick and Nirenberg, 1995), *intermediate nervous system defective* (*ind*) (McDonald et al., 1998; Weiss et al., 1998), *short gastrulation* (*sog*) (Francois et al., 1994), and *brinker* (*brk*) (Jazwinska et al., 1999a, 1999b) in the neuroectoderm. The absence of Dorsal defines the dorsal domain since Dorsal represses expression of key genes required for the establishment of dorsal cell fates, such as *decapentaplegic* (*dpp*) (Ray et al., 1991; Jiang et al., 1993; Huang et al., 1993, 1995), *zerknüllt* (*zen*) (Rushlow et al., 1987; Doyle et al., 1989; Ray et al., 1991; Jiang et al., 1992), *tolloid* (*tld*) (Kirov et al., 1994), and *twisted gastrulation* (*tsg*) (Mason et al., 1994).

Mesoderm Specification in *Drosophila*

High levels of Dorsal activate expression of the mesoderm-determining genes *snail* and *twist* (Jiang et al., 1991; Kosman et al., 1991; Leptin, 1991; Rao et al., 1991; Ray et al., 1991; Ip et al., 1992b; see Chapter 34). The *twist* gene encodes a basic helix-loop-helix (bHLH) transcription factor (Thisse et al., 1988), which activates expression of mesoderm-specific target effector genes such as the homeodomain genes *tinman* (Bodmer, 1993; Lee et al., 1997; Yin et al., 1997), *bagpipe* (Azpiazu and Frasch, 1993), and the fibroblast growth factor (FGF) receptor tyrosine kinase *heartless* (Beiman et al., 1996; Gisselbrecht et al., 1996). *snail*, however, encodes Zn^{2+} finger transcription factor (Boulay et al., 1987), which represses expression of neural genes such as *rho* (Kosman et al., 1991; Leptin, 1991; Rao et al., 1991; Ip et al., 1992a), *vnd* (Mellerick and Nirenberg, 1995), and *sog* in ventral cells (Francois et al., 1994). The dual requirement for activation of mesoderm genes and repression of genes specifying alternative fates (e.g., neural genes) is typical of cell fate specification in many settings. This theme of combined activation and repression is echoed in both the neural and non-neural regions of the ectoderm.

Specification of the Lateral Neural Ectoderm in *Drosophila*

Genes required for neural development are expressed in the lateral region of the *Drosophila* embryo. Some of these "neural" genes encode transcription factors that promote neural fates, such as genes of

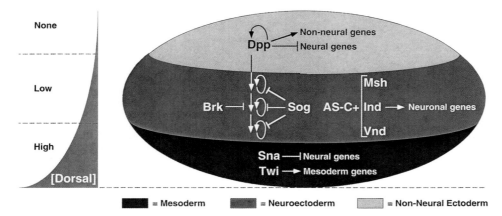

Figure 3–3. Subdivision of the *Drosophila* embryonic dorsal–ventral axis into three primary subdomains. High levels of the maternal morphogen Dorsal specify mesoderm (black ventral domain), intermediate of Dorsal define the neuroectoderm (dark gray lateral domain), and the absence of Dorsal specifies the epidermis (light gray dorsal domain).

the achaete-scute complex (ASC) (Cabrera et al., 1987; Jimenez and Campos-Ortega, 1990; Campuzano and Modolell, 1992; Skeath and Carroll, 1992) and homeodomain protein genes *vnd* (Skeath et al., 1994), *ind* (McDonald et al., 1998; Weiss et al., 1998), and *msh* (D'Alessio and Frasch, 1996). These latter three genes are expressed in three nonoverlapping stripes within the neuroectoderm and are required for the formation of the three primary rows of neuroblasts which derive from those regions. As in the case of the mesoderm, repression also plays an important role in establishing the neural ectoderm since mutations in the repressor *brk* result in ectopic expression of dorsal ectodermal genes, such as *dpp* laterally (Jazwinska et al., 1999b; Rushlow et al., 2001; Zhang et al., 2001).

Sog encodes a secreted antagonist of bone morphogenetic protein (BMP; see Chapter 24) signaling (Francois et al., 1994) and acts in parallel with *brk* to prevent BMP signaling from spreading into the neuroectoderm (Biehs et al., 1996). Sog blocks the activity of the BMP Screw (Scw) (Neul and Ferguson, 1998; Nguyen et al., 1998), which is expressed ubiquitously in the early embryo and acts in concert with Dpp to define peak levels of BMP signaling (Arora et al., 1994). By blocking Scw, Sog interferes with an invasive positive feedback loop of BMP signaling created by Dpp diffusing laterally and activating its own expression in the neuroectoderm (Biehs et al., 1996; Bier, 1997). As discussed further below, this interplay between Sog and Dpp is important for the primary subdivision of the ectoderm into neural versus nonneural domains and has been highly conserved during the course of evolution (Bier, 1997). Thus, as in the case of mesoderm specification, neural genes act by both promoting appropriate neural fates and suppressing the alternative epidermal fate.

Specification of the Dorsal Nonneural Ectoderm

The absence of Dorsal defines the nonneural ectoderm by virtue of Dorsal acting as a repressor of dorsally expressed genes such as *dpp* and *zen* in ventral and lateral cells (Rushlow et al., 1987; Doyle et al., 1989; Ray et al., 1991; Jiang et al., 1992, 1993; Huang et al., 1993, 1995). The key gene involved in development of dorsal cells is *dpp*,

the homolog of vertebrate BMP2/4 (Padgett et al., 1987). To achieve maximal levels of BMP signaling, another BMP family member, Screw (Scw), is also required (Arora et al., 1994). Dpp is essential for BMP signaling in dorsal cells in that the lack of Dpp cannot be compensated for by increasing the levels of Scw. Scw appears to function in more of a helper capacity, however, since elevating Dpp levels can rescue *scw* mutants (Arora et al., 1994). BMP signaling plays two roles in specifying the nonneural ectoderm: it activates expression of genes required for dorsal cell fates, such as *zen* (Ray et al., 1991), and it suppresses expression of neural genes (Skeath et al., 1992; Biehs et al., 1996; von Ohlen and Doe, 2000). One of the genes activated by BMP signaling is *dpp* itself, which results in a positive feedback autoactivation loop (Biehs et al., 1996).

As described in more detail below, a variety of evidence suggests that Dpp acts in a dose-dependent fashion to specify at least two different dorsal cell fates (Ferguson and Anderson, 1992a, b; Wharton et al., 1993; Biehs et al., 1996; Jazwinska et al., 1999b). In this model, peak Dpp activity specifies the dorsalmost cell type (amnioserosa), while lower levels of Dpp signaling specify dorsal nonneural ectoderm.

D/V Patterning in Frogs and Fish

The unfertilized *Xenopus* embryo is visibly subdivided into two hemispheres, a pigmented half known as the vegetal hemisphere and a nonpigmented half known as the animal hemisphere. The A/P and D/V axes are established by a coupled mechanism, which is initiated by the point of sperm entry in *Xenopus* embryos. Fertilization takes place in the animal hemisphere of the egg near the boundary with the vegetal hemisphere and triggers a rotation of the egg cortex away from the point of sperm entry (Fig. 3–4; reviewed in Moon and Kimelman, 1998). The ensuing cortical rotation is believed to result in the activation and displacement of latent dorsalizing factors that previously resided at the vegetal pole of the embryo. A primary response to the cortical activation event is a graded nuclear localization of the Wingless/Wnt pathway (see Chapter 22) signal transducer β-catenin

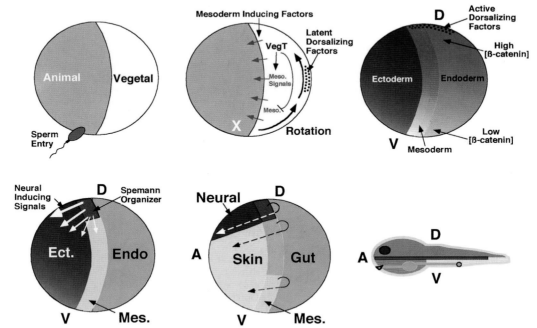

Figure 3–4. Dorsal–ventral patterning of the early *Xenopus* embryo. The point of sperm entry (lower left) defines the future dorsal pole on the opposite side of the embryo by triggering rotation of the cortex and redistribution/activation of putative latent dorsalizing factors. High levels of β-catenin that accumulate in the nuclei of dorsal cells are required for activating expression of genes in dorsal regions. These dorsalizing factors act in concert with mesoderm-inducing factors produced by the vegetal (white domain) hemisphere to induce a band of patterned mesoderm (red domain) within the animal hemisphere (blue domain). The remaining cells of the animal hemisphere will form the ectoderm (purple domain). The transcription factor VegT, which is expressed in vegetal

cells, activates expression of the mesoderm inducing factors but prevents these cells from responding to those factors and directs them instead to become endoderm (green domain). A combination of dorsalizing and mesoderm inducing factors defines a dorsal domain of mesoderm known as the Spemann Organizer, which becomes the source of neural inducing substances such as Chordin and Noggin. The lateral spread of neural inducing substance coupled with their subsequent delivery to overlying cells following involution of the mesoderm (arrows) during gastrulation permits cells to follow their default preference to become neural ectoderm (dorsal purple domain) rather than to give rise to epidermal ectoderm (yellow domain).

(Larabell et al., 1997; Medina et al., 1997), which may occur in a signal (e.g., Wnt) independent fashion (Miller et al., 1999). The maximum point of β-catenin activation defines the dorsal pole of the embryo in much the same fashion that the structurally unrelated Dorsal (and nuclear factor κB [NFκB] family member) initiates patterning along the D/V axis of *Drosophila* embryos (see above). β-Catenin then activates dorsal expression of target genes such as *siamois* (Brannon and Kimelman, 1996; Carnac et al., 1996; Brannon et al., 1997; Fan et al., 1998; Nelson and Gumbiner, 1998), *twin* and *Xnr-3* (Moon and Kimelman, 1998). In addition, the levels of gene expression driven by β-catenin/T-cell transcription factor *siamois* response element are greatest in the dorsalmost cells and diminsh ventrally, suggesting that this enhancer element can sense a β-catenin activity gradient (Brannon et al., 1997). β-Catenin also appears to play a similar role in initiating D/V patterning in early zebrafish embryos (Sumoy et al., 1999).

Establishment of the Marginal Zone and Mesoderm

Following fertilization, a band of equatorial cells, which lie within the animal hemisphere immediately adjacent to the vegetal hemisphere (referred to as marginal cells), are induced to become mesoderm. This inductive event requires the concerted action of FGF (see Chapter 32) and most likely a transforming growth factor-β (TGF-β)/Activin-like signal (see Chapter 24) emanating from the vegetal cells (Fig. 3–4; reviewed in Kimelman and Griffin, 1998, 2000). Vegetal cells cannot themselves respond to these signals by virtue of the fact that they express the transcription factor VegT, which promotes endodermal cell fates, suppresses mesodermal cell fates, and activates expression/activity of secreted TGF-β/Activin/Nodal-related mesodermal inducing factors (Zhang and King, 1996; Zhang et al., 1998; Stennard, 1998; Clements et al., 1999; Xanthos et al., 2001). In response to the nonautonomous induction by vegetal hemisphere–derived signals, marginal cells activate expression of various mesoderm-determining genes such as *brachyury* (Wilkinson et al., 1990; Smith et al., 1991; Conlon et al., 1996; Smith, 2001) and the vertebrate homologs of the *Drosophila twist* (Hopwood et al., 1989; Chen and Behringer, 1995) and *snail* (Nieto et al., 1992; Smith et al., 1992; Essex et al., 1993; Hammerschmidt and Nusslein-Volhard, 1993; Carver et al., 2001; Ciruna and Rossant, 2001) genes. The vertebrate *snail* and *twist* genes may function similarly to the invertebrate counterparts as expression of mesodermal markers is lost in *twist⁻* mice (Chen and Behringer, 1995), while ectopic expression of ectodermal markers but normal mesodermal gene expression is observed in *snail⁻* mice (Carver et al., 2001). Depending on their D/V position, marginal cells give rise to different derivatives, including blood (ventral), muscle (lateral), and notochord (dorsal). The function of *twist* in specifying mesodermal derivatives may be very ancient as a *C. elegans twist* (Harfe et al., 1998) gene is required for the formation of nonstriated muscle (Corsi et al., 2000) and a *twist*-related gene is expressed in mesodermal cells in the jellyfish (Spring et al., 2000). Twist also plays an important developmental role in humans as mutations in this gene lead to dominant inheritance of Saethre-Chotzen syndrome (el Ghouzzi et al., 1997; Howard et al., 1997) and possible recessive inheritance of Baller-Gerold syndrome (Seto et al., 2001). Twist may activate FGF receptor (GFGR) expression in humans as it does in *Drosophila* since mutations in the *FGFR-2* and *FGFR-3* genes also can lead to Saethre-Chotzen syndrome (Lajeunie, 1997; Paznekas et al., 1998).

Establishment of a Dorsal Neural Inducing Center: The Spemann Organizer

As a result of the combined action of mesoderm-inducing factors and transcription factors such as Siamois (Brannon and Kimelman, 1996; Carnac et al., 1996; Brannon et al., 1997; Fan et al., 1998; Nelson and Gumbiner, 1998) and its target gene *goosecoid* (Blum et al., 1992; De Robertis et al., 1992; Steinbeisser and De Robertis, 1993), expressed only in dorsal regions of the embryo, dorsal marginal cells begin to express several secreted neuralizing factors, such as Chordin (Sasai et al., 1994) and Noggin (Smith and Harland, 1992; Lamb et al., 1993; Smith et al., 1993). The first evidence for the existence of such neural inducing substances was provided by the classical embryological transplantation experiments of Spemann and Mangold (1924), who showed that the dorsal mesoderm of amphibian embryos could induce surrounding ventral ectodermal cells to assume neural fates. These neural inducing factors are secreted from the marginal zone and may diffuse in a planar fashion into the neighboring ectoderm and/or may be delivered to overlying dorsal ectodermal cells following invagination of the mesoderm during gastrulation.

Following the landmark work of Spemann and Mangold (1924), a great deal of effort was expended in trying to determine the molecular identity of the neural inducing factor(s). A variety of substances and factors were tested for neural inducing activity, and while many substances could induce second neural axis formation, none of these studies led to isolation of an endogenous neural inducing factor. The first endogenous neural inducer was Noggin, which was identified in a screen for *Xenopus* proteins capable of inducing second neural axes (Smith and Harland, 1992). A subsequent study, based on cloning of genes expressed differentially in the Spemann organizer region of the embryo, identified several other factors with neural inducing activities, including Chordin (Sasai et al., 1994), which is the vertebrate counterpart of *Drosophila sog* (Francois and Bier, 1995).

BMP Signaling Suppresses the Default Ectodermal Fate in Vertebrates and Invertebrates

A variety of evidence indicates that the vertebrate neural inducers Noggin and Chordin and the *Drosophila* counterpart of Chordin (Sog) function by blocking BMP signaling in the neuroectoderm. First, *Drosophila* Dpp and its vertebrate homolog BMP4 are expressed at high levels only in the nonneural ectodermal regions of the embryo (Arendt and Nubler-Jung, 1994), while the neural inducers are expressed in, or adjacent to, neuroectodermal regions of the embryo (Francois and Bier, 1995). Second, Sog and Chd bind to BMPs and prevent these ligands from activating their receptors (Piccolo et al., 1996; Chang et al., 2001; Ross et al., 2001; Scott et al., 2001). Finally, Sog and Chordin function equivalently in cross-species experiments in which Sog can induce a secondary neural axis in *Xenopus* embryos and Chordin can oppose Dpp signaling in *Drosophila* (Holley et al., 1995; Schmidt et al., 1995; Yu et al., 2000).

Although the historical term *neural inducers* connotes a positive action of these factors, they actually function by a double negative mechanism to promote neural fates. Cell dissociation and reaggregation experiments using *Xenopus* ectoderm revealed that BMP4 signaling actively suppresses a default preference of vertebrate ectodermal cells to become neural (Sasai et al., 1995; Wilson and Hemmati-Brivanlou, 1995) and that neural inducers such as Chordin and Noggin function by inhibiting this negative action of BMP4 signaling (reviewed in Hemmati-Brivanlou and Melton, 1997). Likewise, in *Drosophila* embryos, several neural genes, including the critical neural promoting genes of the ASC, are ectopically expressed in *dpp⁻* mutant embryos (Biehs et al., 1996), while ectopic Dpp expression suppresses expression of neural genes in the neuroectoderm. In genetically sensitized *sog⁻* mutant embryos, the autoactivating function of BMP signaling can lead to the spread of *dpp* expression into the neuroectoderm, which then activates expression of Dpp targets and represses expression of neural genes (Biehs et al., 1996). Furthermore, patterning defects in *chordino* mutant zebrafish embryos, which lack function of the *chordin* gene (Schulte-Merker et al., 1997), are strikingly similar to those observed in sensitized *sog⁻* mutant embryos. BMP4 expression autoactivates and expands into the dorsal ectoderm (Hammerschmidt et al., 1996) in *chordino⁻* embryos. The high degree of evolutionary conservation in Dpp/BMP4 and Sog/Chordin function suggests that this patterning system was active in the most recent common ancestor of vertebrates and invertebrates and that the ancestral form of Sog/Chordin protected the neuroectoderm from invasion by Dpp/BMP signaling, permitting cells to follow the default preference of neural development.

Sog and Chordin Also Act as Long-Range Morphogens in the Nonneural Ectoderm

As mentioned above, there is strong evidence that BMP signaling is graded in the dorsal region of the embryo and that different levels of BMP activity define distinct dorsal tissues in a threshold-dependent fashion. Since the level of *dpp* mRNA appears uniform throughout the dorsal zone and *scw* is expressed evenly throughout the embryo (Arora et al., 1994), it has been speculated that a posttranscriptional mechanism is responsible for establishing graded Dpp activity. One mechanism by which this BMP activity gradient might form is long-range diffusion of the antagonist Sog into the dorsal region from the adjacent neuroectodermal domain where it is produced (Francois et al., 1994). Consistent with Sog functioning as a morphogen to define distinct thresholds of BMP signaling in dorsal cells, the gene dose of *sog* determines the width of cells experiencing peak levels of BMP activity (Biehs et al., 1996). This model received additional support when it was found that a metalloprotease known as Tolloid (Shimell et al., 1991), which specifically cleaves and inactivates Sog in vitro (Marques et al., 1997), is expressed in the dorsal region. The combination of Sog expression in the lateral neuroectoderm and Tld degradation of Sog dorsally provides a source and sink configuration, which could create a ventral-to-dorsal concentration gradient of Sog protein in the dorsal region, which in turn generates a reciprocal BMP activity gradient (e.g., highest dorsally and lowest ventrally).

Direct support for the hypothetical Sog gradient in dorsal cells has recently been obtained by histochemical methods (Srinivasan et al., 2002). As predicted, Tolloid proteolysis limits the accumulation of Sog dorsally, which is required to form a stable concentration gradient of Sog. In addition, these studies revealed that Dynamin-mediated endocytosis acts in parallel with Tld-dependent proteolysis to remove active Sog from dorsal cells. Cumulatively, these observations lend strong support to the model that a Sog concentration gradient in dorsal cells creates a reciprocal BMP activity gradient, which partitions the dorsal region into high versus low BMP activity zones. These two domains then give rise, respectively, to an extraembryonic tissue similar to the amnion (amnioserosa) and epidermis proper.

It seems likely that Chordin also acts as a long-range morphogen in vertebrate embryos. First, there are vertebrate homologs of the various *Drosophila* genes involved in sculpting the BMP activity gradient in the nonneural ectoderm, such as the vertebrate counterpart of Tolloid, Xolloid (Piccolo et al., 1997). There is also evidence that BMP signaling plays a role in long-range patterning of the mesoderm and ectoderm in vertebrates. For example, in zebrafish BMP2/4 mutants (e.g., *swirl⁻*), patterning along the entire D/V axis of the embryo is disrupted (Hammerschmidt et al., 1996). Furthermore, as in *Drosophila*, there is no evidence for an asymmetric distribution of BMP2/4 protein or mRNA in the vertebrate nonneural ectoderm and adjacent mesoderm, suggesting that a posttranslational mechanism may also be necessary in vertebrates to establish a gradient of BMP activity, which may be generated by inhibitors such as Chd and Noggin (Jones and Smith, 1998; Blitz et al., 2000). For example, Chordin can block a BMP response far from the site of RNA injection, whereas in control experiments where a truncated dominant negative BMP receptor was injected, a response was elicited only within the progeny of injected cells (Blitz et al., 2000). In addition, cell transplantation experiments indicate that the zebrafish *chordino* gene acts nonautonomously since transplanted wild-type cells restricted to dorsal anterior structures of *chordino* mutants can restore normal patterning along the entire length of the axis (Hammerschmidt et al., 1996).

A Conserved Mechanism for Partitioning the Neuroectoderm into Three Primary Rows?

After being specified by neural inducers, the neuroectoderm is partitioned into three non-overlapping rows of homeobox gene expression, which give rise to the three primary rows of neuroblasts. As in the case of the Hox genes, homologs of these three neuroblast determination genes exist in vertebrates (*Nkx-2, Gsh, Msx*) and invertebrates (*vnd, ind, msh*) and are expressed in the same order relative to the midline of the nervous system (reviewed in Bier, 1997; Arendt and Nubler-Jung, 1999). Although the nervous system forms dorsally in vertebrates and ventrally in invertebrates, the fact that the D/V polarity of the neural plate is inverted during invagination of the neural tube results in the final orientation of the nervous system being similar in both organisms (Fig. 3–5). For example, in both classes of organisms, the outermost row of neuroectodermal cells, which express *msh* or *Msx*, form nearest epidermal cells expressing *dpp* or *BMP4*.

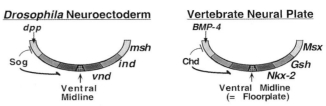

Figure 3–5. Conservation of dorsal–ventral patterning within the neuroectoderm. The *Drosophila* homeobox containing neuroblast determining genes *vnd, ind,* and *msh* are expressed in three adjacent stripes along the dorsal ventral axis of the CNS (left panel). *vnd* (dark gray) is expressed nearest the future ventral midline (hatched) of the CNS and *msh* (light gray) is expressed adjacent to epidermal cells producing Dpp. Vertebrate orthologues of the *Drosophila* neuroblast determining genes (Nkx-2 ⇔ vnd; Gsh ⇔ Ind; Msx ⇔ Msh) are expressed in the same relative position with respect to the future ventral midline of the CNS (= floorplate) and the epidermis (which expresses BPM-4, the vertebrate orthologue of Dpp). In both organisms, neuroectodermal cells contain BMP antagonists (e.g., Sog in *Drosophila* and Chordin in vertebrates).

In *Drosophila*, where the functional interrelationships of these three genes have been well studied, mutants lacking function of any of these genes fail to form neuroblasts derived from the corresponding region. In addition to these genes promoting neuroblast fates appropriate to the three rows of neuroblasts, they engage in cross-regulatory interactions reminiscent of the posterior dominance exhibited by the Hox genes. In this current case, the ventral genes are dominant in the sense that *vnd* represses expression of *ind*, which represses expression of *msh*. Whether a similar cross-regulatory relationship contributes to defining the mutually exclusive patterns of the corresponding vertebrate neuroblast identity genes remains to be determined.

Appendage Outgrowth and Axis Patterning

Appendages typically develop within the context of an already well-organized embryo or larva. The A/P and D/V axes of the appendage therefore derive from the preexisting body axes. Because appendages emerge as outgrowths from the body wall, they have a third direction of polarity, the P/D axis. Although there are significant differences in the structure of appendages forming in vertebrates and invertebrates as well as in the molecular mechanisms underlying their formation, a core set of genetic pathways appears to have defined the primary axes of all appendages (Fig. 3–6).

A/P Axis

Early in appendage development of both vertebrates and invertebrates, A/P axis formation involves creation of a posterior source of the secreted short-range signal Hedgehog (Hh; see Chapter 16). The mechanisms for generating the posterior source of Hh appear to be different in vertebrates and invertebrates, but the effect of Hh is similar, which is to activate expression of a longer-range secondary BMP signal. This posterior source of Hh in vertebrate limbs was identified by classical transplantation experiments (Saunders and Gasseling, 1968) similar to those that defined the Spemann organizer and named the ZPA. The subsequent graded spread of BMPs across the appendage defines positions along the A/P axis, which ultimately leads to the formation of specific structures such as bones in a human hand or veins in a fly wing (reviewed in Pearse and Tabin, 1998; Capdevila and Izpisua Belmonte, 2001).

D/V Axis

Narrow stripes of cells separating the dorsal (e.g., back of the hand) and ventral (e.g., palm) surfaces of limb primordia play critical roles in orchestrating the outgrowth and patterning of vertebrate and invertebrate appendages. These cells arise in response to localized activation of the Notch signaling pathway (see Chapter 39) at the interface between the dorsal and ventral surfaces of the appendage, the AER (reviewed in Capdevila and Izpisua Belmonte, 2001). In both *Drosophila* and vertebrate systems, glycosyl transferases in the Fringe family are required to activate Notch ligands along the margin of the appendage (Irvine, 1999; Wu and Rao, 1999).

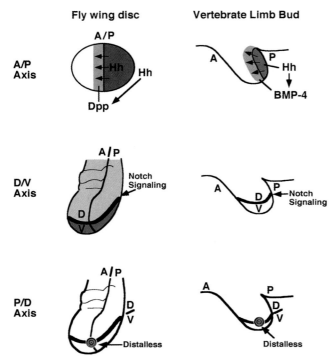

Figure 3–6. Similarities in patterning the primary axes of vertebrate and invertebrate appendages. Anterior–posterior (A/P) axis (top panels): in the primordia of *Drosophila* and vertebrate limbs, posterior cells express the short range signal Hh (dark gray domains), which induces expression of the longer range BMP morphogens (light gray domains). Dorsal–ventral (D/V) axis (middle panels): cells at the interface between dorsal and ventral domains of *Drosophila* and vertebrate limbs are defined by activation of the Notch signaling pathway (black stippled lines). Proximodistal (P/D) axis (bottom panels): Expression of *Distalless* gene (concentric circles), which is activated at the distal tip of *Drosophila* and vertebrate appendages, is required for distal outgrowth of the appendages.

P/D Axis

As appendages grow out from the body wall, they express the homeodomain protein Distalless (Dll) at their distal tips. Dll is also expressed in other tissues of developing animals. In animal systems where function of Dll genes has been determined, it has been found that Dll function is required for appendage outgrowth in many, but not all, cases. The fact that Dll is expressed at the distal tip of all body wall outgrowths, including the tube feet of starfish (Panganiban et al., 1997), suggests that this gene performed a function required to initiate such outgrowth in the bilateral ancestor of vertebrates and invertebrates (Panganiban, 2000; Zerucha and Ekker, 2000).

Early Heart Development

Although the issue of early heart development remains unresolved (see Chapter 9), there are a few examples of genes that are apparently conserved to primarily specify the development of one organ. The term *master control gene* has been coined to denote this class of embryonic patterning genes (Halder et al., 1995). Interestingly, some of these master control proteins also contain homeodomain motifs that are distantly related to the original homeodomain signature found in Hox transcription factors, while others are transcription factors of other types. As seen below, it has been argued that these genes control the development of specific organs, but it is also possible that these genes control regional identities in certain germ layers which just happen to develop functionally similar organs in vertebrates and invertebrates.

One of the so-called master control genes is required for the development of a blood-pumping organ in many animals whose hearts are of diverse shapes and sizes. This work began with the study of a *Drosophila* homeobox gene that was expressed in both dorsal mesoderm and the dorsal vessel (the insect equivalent of the heart). The dor-

sal vessel is a tubular muscle that circulates hemolymph within the open body cavity (Frasch, 1999). The *Drosophila* heart gene was named *tinman*, after the character in *The Wonderful Wizard of Oz* (Baum, 1997), who believes he lacks a heart. Mutations in *tinman* resulted in dead larvae that were missing the dorsal vessel, along with other dorsal mesoderm derivatives (Azpiazu and Frasch, 1993; Bodmer, 1993).

Homology cloning revealed that mice have *tinman*-like genes, one of which is called *Nkx2.5* or *Csx*. The *Nkx2.5/Csx* gene is expressed in the fetal heart primordia (Komuro and Izumo, 1993; Lints et al., 1993), a pattern that is similar to *tinman* gene expression in *Drosophila*. Targeted mutation of *Csx/Nkx2.5* results in embryonic lethality, and embryonic heart development is arrested at the initial stage of heart looping (Lyons et al., 1995). There is also evidence from human genetics that the human *NKX2-5* gene (localized to chromosome 5q35) is required for normal heart morphogenesis. Several cases of familial congenital heart disease with defects in the morphology of the atrial septum and in atrioventricular conduction have been associated with both haploinsufficiency and gain-of-function mutations in the *NKX2-5* gene (Schott et al., 1998). All of this information has led to the proposal that the Csx/NKX2-5/Tinman-like proteins are ancestral determinants of heart and surrounding visceral mesoderm. Ranganayakulu et al. (1998) indicated that the common function of genes in this class may be to specify a positional identity in visceral mesoderm, which in both flies and mice happens to develop into a blood-pumping organ, and that the common ancestor of mammals and insects did not have a blood-pumping organ truly homologous to that in present-day animals.

In addition to heart primordia, the mesodermal layer of the embryo gives rise to muscle, bone, and connective tissues. While the earliest events in specification of the mesoderm vary in different animal groups, one common denominator has been found in the development of skeletal muscle cells: a MADS box gene, *MEF2* (*D-MEF2* in the fly), is an early marker of skeletal muscle lineage in both insects and vertebrates (Lilly et al., 1994, 1995). In vertebrates, MEF2 activates and stabilizes the expression of such well-known muscle-specific genes as the bHLH homologs *Myf5*, *MyoD*, *MRF4*, and *Myogenin* (Brand-Saberi and Christ, 1999). In *Drosophila*, mesoderm fates are initially controlled by Twist and Snail proteins, and Twist directly activates *D-MEF2* (Lilly et al., 1994, 1995; Taylor et al., 1995). D-MEF2 and its vertebrate homologs are required for the completion of myogenesis in all muscles (Baylies et al., 1998; Brand-Saberi and Christ, 1999). Key features of this system have been preserved through millions of years of evolution. Such features include conservation of the MEF2 MADS domain, which mediates sequence-specific DNA binding, and conservation of DNA target sites in regulatory regions of the muscle-specific genes (Lilly et al., 1994, 1995).

Specification of Eye Organ Primordia

Another example of conservation of developmental patterning pathways was shown in a series of experiments that revealed a striking similarity in the mechanisms underlying the formation of eyes and photoreceptor cells in different animals (or the regions of the head that develop those organs, as seen below). As is often the case in genetics, relevant mutations proved crucial for unraveling the molecular pathways underlying eye development. Two such mutations have been known for quite some time: the *Aniridia* defect in humans (Hanson and Van Heyningen, 1995) and the *Small eye* (*Sey*) mutation in mice and rats (Hill et al., 1991; Walther and Gruss, 1991). The human *Aniridia* syndrome is characterized by a reduction in eye size and absence of the iris in heterozygotes. A similar defect is seen in mice that are heterozygous for the *Small eye* mutation. Mice homozygous for *Small eye* completely lack eyes and die in utero.

Molecular analysis revealed that the same gene, *Pax6*, was affected in both the *Aniridia* and the *Small eye* syndromes. Pax6 belongs to a paired box/homeodomain family of transcriptional regulators (see Chapter 59). As expected, the Pax6 protein is abundantly expressed in the eye from the earliest stages until the end of eye morphogenesis: initially in the optic sulcus and subsequently in the eye vesicle, lens, retina, and finally cornea (Hill et al., 1991; Walther and Gruss, 1991). In *Drosophila*, the genes *eyeless* (*ey*) and *twin of eyeless* (*toy*) encode proteins that are homologs of Pax6 (Quiring et al., 1994; Czerny et al.,

1999). Both *ey* and *toy* are expressed at high levels in the cells that will form a photoreceptor field of the *Drosophila* eye, as well as in other regions of the developing nervous system. Weak mutations in *eyeless* lead to the reduction or complete loss of compound eyes, whereas strong mutations are lethal when homozygous (Quiring et al., 1994). Even more striking was the observation that targeted expression of the mouse *Pax6* genes in various fly tissues led to the formation of small ectopic *Drosophila* eyes on the wings, legs, and antennae (Halder et al., 1995). These results demonstrate that the *Pax6* and *eyeless* genes are not only required but sufficient to promote eye development, and they have been called master control genes for eye morphogenesis.

A traditional view, based on the drastic differences observed in eye development and structure in mammals, insects, and mollusks, holds that eye organs evolved independently in different phyla (von Salvini-Plawen and Mayr, 1977). Indeed, this is partly true as the organization of the organ has diverged extensively in different animal lineages. However, the current evidence suggests that a variety of modern animals specify fields of photoreceptor cells using the same *Pax6* controls that triggered the development of the ancestral eye. Recently, *Pax6* homologs have also been identified in other triploblastic animals (e.g., flatworms, nematodes) and even in cnidarians (Callaerts et al., 1999 and references therein). Deep conservation in the visual system is further supported by the fact that all animals use opsins as photoreceptor proteins (Goldsmith, 1990). However, it is also possible that the *Pax6* and *eyeless* genes specify a head regional identity that includes an eye organ in both vertebrate and invertebrate lineages that just happens to include the eye as a specialization of that region. Evidence for this is found in the fact that nematodes, which have no eyes, also conserve a *Pax6*-like gene that is expressed in the head region (Chisholm and Horvitz, 1995); in addition, ablation of *Pax6/eyeless* gene function in *Drosophila* results in headless flies (Jiao et al., 2001).

As described above and in other chapters of this volume, the existence of so many common genetic pathways between distantly related organisms suggests that the ancestor of all bilaterally symmetric animals was a sophisticated creature, with many architectural and organ-specifying genetic systems already in place (De Robertis and Sasai, 1996; Knoll and Carroll, 1999). Figure 3–7 shows a proposed diagram of that ancestral worm-like creature.

Nervous System Wiring

Genes controlling other developmental and physiological functions (see Chapter 71) have also been highly conserved during the evolution of the bilateralia. For example, attractive and repulsive guidance factors directing early outgrowth of axons in the CNS toward or away from the CNS midline have been highly conserved (Kaprielian et al., 2001). A class of factors that act as attractants for most commissural axons, guiding them to the midline, are the netrins (Serafini et al., 1994). In addition, netrins repel a subset of axons from the midline. Analysis of mutants lacking the function of genes encoding the netrins and netrin receptors have revealed a similar requirement for these factors in midline guidance in *C. elegans* (Hedgecock et al., 1990; Ishii

et al., 1992; Leung-Hagesteijn et al., 1992), *Drosophila* (Harris et al., 1996; Kolodziej et al., 1996; Mitchell et al., 1996; Keleman and Dickson, 2001), and mice (Serafini et al., 1996; Fazeli et al., 1997; Leonardo et al., 1997). In all three organisms, loss-of-function *netrin* mutants result in failure of commissural axons to be attracted to the midline as well as failure of a subset of projections to avoid the midline (Hedgecock et al., 1990; Harris et al., 1996; Mitchell et al., 1996; Serafini et al., 1996). Similarly, the attractive and repulsive effects of the Netrins are mediated by two distinct types of Netrin receptor in all three species. Netrin receptors most closely similar in amino acid sequence to the *C. elegans* Unc-40 receptor are required to mediate the attractive component of the Netrins (Hedgecock et al., 1990; Kolodziej et al., 1996; Fazeli et al., 1997) whereas receptors most similar to the *C. elegans* Unc-5 receptor are necessary in the subsets of axons that are repelled by the midline (Hedgecock et al., 1990; Leung-Hagesteijn et al., 1992; Leonardo et al., 1997; Keleman and Dickson, 2001).

Another clear example of a phylogenetically conserved system for midline guidance is axon repulsion mediated by the Slit/Robo signaling system (reviewed in Rusch and Van Vactor, 2000; Guthrie, 2001). Slit is secreted from midline cells (Brose et al., 1999; Kidd et al., 1999; Li et al., 1999) and in a dose-dependent fashion repels Robo-expressing axons from the midline (Kidd et al., 1998a, b). Axons that are most sensitive to the Slit repellent express multiple isoforms of the Robo receptor, while those less sensitive express fewer isoforms (Simpson et al., 2000). Since commissural axons that do cross the midline express Robo, they would be prevented from crossing if it were not for the action of the *commisureless* gene (Tear et al., 1996), which is responsible for down-regulating Robo protein levels in appropriate axons near the midline (Kidd et al., 1998b). This transient down-regulation of Robo allows the attraction mediated by Netrin signaling to overcome the repulsion by low Robo signaling. Once the commissural axons cross the midline, they reexpress Robo on the cell surface and are prevented from recrossing the midline. Since axon fibers expressing differing numbers of Robo isoforms are differentially sensitive to Slit repulsion, they are chased to different distances from the midline and end up following one of three major radially organized axon bundles. In addition to midline repulsion mediated by Slit/Robo activity, a group of Ig domain–containing repellents known as the Semaphorins (Kolodkin et al., 1993) also act in vertebrates and invertebrates to divert axons from the midline (reviewed in Giger and Kolodkin, 2001).

Nervous System Function

Given that the common ancestor of the bilateralia had in place genetic systems for specifying and wiring the nervous system, it is not surprising that it also appears to have evolved the basic molecular processes required for the proper physiological properties of neurons, such as ion channels required for action potential generation and conduction as well as the complex secretory machinery required for release of neurotransmitters.

Ion channels are one of the best studied classes of proteins known. Ever since the mathematical formations of Hodgkin and Huxeley

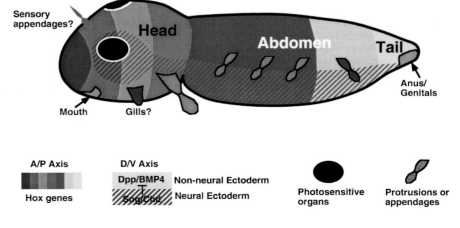

Figure 3–7. Conserved developmental patterning systems. Examples of patterning mechanisms that have been conserved since the divergence of invertebrate and vertebrate lineages include the following: determination of segmental identity along the A/P axis by a series of related Hox genes, subdivision of the ectoderm into neural versus non-neural domains via suppression of BMP signaling in neural domains, speciation of light sensitive primordia by *Eyeless/Pax6*, and patterning the primary axes of protrusions from the body wall (e.g., patterning A/P axis by Hh->BMP signaling, defining border between D/V territories by Notch signaling, and promoting appendage outgrowth by Distalless).

(1952), modeling axons as leaky cables containing voltage gated ion channels, electrophysiological studies have defined detailed in vivo kinetic parameters of ion channels that underlie various electrical phenomena such as the voltage-dependent propagation of action potentials and release of neurotransmitters in presynaptic nerve terminals, the rapid and slow chemical responses of postsynaptic cells to neurotransmitters, and the conduction of electrical impulses in muscle and heart (reviewed in Pallotta and Wagoner, 1992). The similarities in the voltage-dependent properties of action potential propagation in vertebrate in invertebrate axons suggested that similar types of ion channel were involved in defining the electrical behavior of neurons in diverse species. The identification of genes encoding a broad variety of ion channels has confirmed this prediction as there are clear counterparts to vertebrate voltage-gated Na^+, K^+, Ca^+, and Cl^- channels as well as homologs of chemically activated channels such as the acetylcholine, glutamate, GABA, and many peptide transmitters in invertebrates such as *Drosophila* and *C. elegans*. Sequence comparison of these various ion channel proteins reveals that the most recent common ancestor of bilateralia had already evolved specialized prototypes for each of these channel families. Not surpisingly, a variety of neurological disorders in humans have been associated with alterations in ion channel function (reviewed in Cooper and Jan, 1999).

The mechanism by which neurotransmitter-containing vesicles are released following depolarization of axon terminals and Ca^{2+} entry has also been very well studied in both vertebrate and invertebrate systems (Wu and Bellen, 1997; Fernandez-Chacon and Sudhof, 1999; Li and Schwarz, 1999; Lin and Scheller, 2000). Specialized protein complexes have been identified which are required for the vesicle docking (Sec1), fusion (Ca^{2+} activation of the soluble *N*-ethylmaleimide-sensitize factor [NSF] attachment protein [SNAP] receptor [SNARE] complex: Ca^{2+}-bound Synaptotagmin, Synaptobrevin, and SNAP25) of synaptic vesicles at defined release sites in the plasma membrane, followed by ATP-dependent dissociation of the core complex (αSNAP, βSNAP, NSF) and Dynamin-mediated endocytosis of vesicular components. As in the case of ion channels, counterparts of nearly all components identified in vertebrate systems are also present in *Drosophila* and *C. elegans* (Wu and Bellen, 1997; Fernandez-Chacon and Sudhof, 1999; Li and Schwarz, 1999; Lloyd et al., 2000). In a genomewide survey, it was found that *Drosophila* vesicle release proteins on average share approximately 70% amino acid identity with their vertebrate counterparts (Lloyd et al., 2000). The diversity and functional equivalence of homologous ion channel genes and components required for Ca^{2+}-dependent synaptic release strongly suggest that the ancestor of all bilateralia possessed a sophisticated interconnected nervous system and that the basic properties of the nervous system function are shared by all its descendents.

Immune Function

Another striking example of a highly conserved physiological process is the innate immune response, which is mediated by the Toll signaling pathway (reviewed in Wasserman, 2000). The core pathway in both vertebrates and *Drosophila* is initiated by ligand binding to the Toll receptor and assembly of a membrane complex including a conserved kinase, which phosphorylates a cytoplasmic protein in the IκB family (Cactus in *Drosophila*), leading to release and nuclear translocation of a bound transcription factor in the NFκB family (Dif or Dorsal in *Drosophila*). The liberated NFκB-related protein then activates genes that mediate innate immunity (Karin, 1999; Wasserman, 2000). The targets of innate immunity are quite different in vertebrates and flies (e.g., genes mediating cell proliferation, cell–cell signaling, environmental stress, and inflamatory responses in vertebrates [Li et al.,

2001] and bactericidal Cecropins in flies [Ip et al., 1993; Meng et al., 1999; Rutschmann et al., 2000]), but this simple immune system is absolutely required for survival in mammals, whereas loss of the antigen-specific component of the highly specialized vertebrate immune system (e.g., B cell– and T cell–mediated) leads to a less severe and conditionally viable form of immune suppression.

Organism-Specific Thematic Variations

Although we have stressed the similarities of the patterning processes acting in vertebrate and invertebrates in this section, it is also important to note that there are organism-specific variations, which in some cases are quite surprising given the overall conservation of patterning mechanisms. For example, while molecules in the BMP family are expressed in the dorsal region of the developing vertebrate neural tube (where they play a key role in patterning cell fates and suppressing alternative ventral fates) and other regions of the nervous system (e.g., Mowbray et al., 2001), the expression patterns of clear counterparts of these genes can vary significantly between mouse, *Xenopus*, zebrafish, and chicken. Similarly, although the *chordin* and *noggin* genes are expressed in the Spemann organizer equivalent of a chick embryo (Henson's node), these factors do not appear to play as primary a role in establishing neural cell fates by inhibiting BMP signaling in the chick (Connolly et al., 1997; Streit et al., 1998). Other factors/pathways derived from Henson's node may have taken over this primary neural inducing activity (Alvarez et al., 1998; Streit and Stern, 1999; Sasai, 2001). Thus, it is important to bear in mind that even mammalian systems may not always provide accurate models for the role of developmentally important genes in humans.

A BROAD SPECTRUM OF HUMAN DISEASE GENES HAVE INVERTEBRATE COUNTERPARTS

Given the high degree of evolutionary conservation in the genetic circuitry controlling developmental processes in vertebrates and invertebrates, as well as basic physiological processes, a natural question is whether other genes might also be members of conserved molecular machines. Genome-scale gene sequence comparisons indicate that there are many related protein-coding sequences across genomes as diverse as yeast, nematodes, flies, and vertebrates (Table 3–2) (Lander et al., 2001). More focused analyses of genes implicated in genetic forms of human disease indicate that they also have high levels of sequence conservation in model organisms such as fruit flies and nematodes. For example, a systematic analysis of *Drosophila* counterparts of human diseases gene listed in the OMIM database revealed that approximately 74% of all human disease gene entries had matches in flies with expectation values (e values) of $\leq 10^{-10}$. As would be predicted from the greater similarity of the fly versus yeast genome to humans, only 50% of the human disease genes with matches in *Drosophila* (e $\leq 10^{-10}$) also had hits with yeast proteins at comparable stringency. Statistical matches in this probability range typically indicate that matching sequences are nearly certainly related by descent from a common ancestral gene but do not suggest that the genes necessarily carry out equivalent functions. For example, members of large gene families, such as the G protein–coupled receptors, receptor tyrosine kinases, or transcription factor subclasses (e.g., homeobox, helix-loop-helix, and zinc finger), often match other functionally distinct members, with e values in this range. Although e values cannot be used alone to deduce the functional equivalence of two related gene sequences, in general, genes which have been shown to function in cross-phylum experiments have counterparts with e values in the range

Table 3–2. Genome Comparisons of Model Organisms

Organism	Transcriptome Size	Percentage of Genes Similar to a Human Gene	Cellular Complexity	Genetic Screening	Generation Time
Yeast	6,200 genes	46%	1 cell	$>10^9$ progeny	2 hours
Nematode	18,300 genes	43%	959 cells	10^6–10^7 progeny	3 days
Fly	14,400 genes	61%	$>10^6$ cells	10^5–10^6 progeny	10 days
Mouse	30,000–80,000 genes	95%–97%	$>10^9$ cells	10^2–10^3 progeny	6 weeks

Source: Lander et al. (2001). *Nature* 409: 860–921.

Figure 3–8. Percentage of human disease genes with fly counterparts. Black bars show percentage of 1224 human disease genes with match to fly genes; white bars show percentage of 666 fly genes with matches to human disease genes.

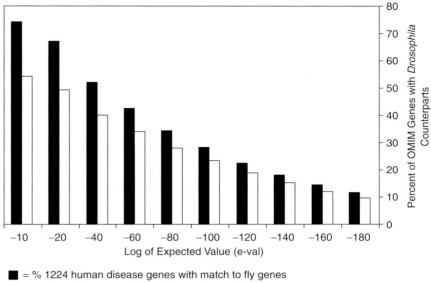

■ = % 1224 human disease genes with match to fly genes
□ = % of 666 fly genes with matches to human disease genes

of $\leq 10^{-100}$. Nearly 30% of human disease genes have matches to genes at this stringent level of sequence similarity (Fig. 3–8). This high degree of cross-species sequence similarity suggests that the *Drosophila* homologs of human disease genes will frequently share important functional characteristics with their human counterparts.

Another important indication that model organisms will be of widespread utility in analyzing the function of conserved molecular machines is that a very broad spectrum of human disease genes have invertebrate counterparts. In the case of *Drosophila*, there are matches to diseases in categories as diverse as cancer, cardiac diseases, neurological diseases, immune dysfunction, metabolic disorders, and, as highlighted in this review, developmental disorders. Furthermore, these human disease genes encode proteins acting in virtually every known biochemical capacity ranging from transcription factors to signaling components to cytoskeletal elements to metabolic enzymes. Thus, it would appear that genes involved in development are likely typical rather than special in being highly conserved functionally during evolution of the bilateralia.

Examples of Human Diseases Caused by Mutations in Developmental Patterning Genes

Disease Phenotypes Associated with Mutations in Hox Genes

Despite the scarcity of available mutations in human and mouse Hox genes, it is possible to make a few generalizations about the observed effects of such genetic lesions. In many cases, mutations involving one or several mammalian Hox genes do result in homeotic transformations, but they are also associated with loss of axial structures and organs and other nonhomeotic malformations (Mark et al., 1997). Part of the reason for the highly complex mutant phenotypes is that Hox genes are involved in an elaborate system of intra-cluster interactions and intercluster redundant functions.

Hox genes are not required solely for the proper development of the rostrocaudal main body axis. In mammals, the posteriormost members of the *HOXC, HOXD,* and *HOXA* clusters (*HOXC9-13, HOXD9-13,* and *HOXA11-13,* respectively) are expressed in developing limb buds (Zákány and Duboule, 1999). Many of the same genes from the *HOXD* and *HOXA* clusters are also expressed in external genitourinary structures (Peterson et al., 1994; Kondo et al., 1997). The limb and genital defects observed in mice and humans that possess mutations in the posterior Hox genes indicate that these expression patterns are crucial for the proper development of the mentioned body parts.

Several groups have reported heterozygous and homozygous synpolydactyly phenotypes that co-segregated with an expansion in a 15-residue polyalanine stretch in exon 1 of the *HOXD13* gene (Akarsu et al., 1996; Muragaki et al., 1996) (Table 3–3). A significant increase of the penetrance and severity of the phenotype correlated with increasing expansion size. Interestingly, the family with the largest expansion included affected males with hypospadias, which is not a fea-

Table 3–3. Mutations in Human HOX Genes and Associated Phenotypes

Disease	Human Gene	Fly Gene	e Value	Component
Heterozygous synpolydactyly: Fingers 3/4 and toes 4/5, with polydactyly in the cutaneous web between digits.	*HOXD13*	*Abd-B*	6×10^{-13}	Transcription factor
Homozygous synpolydactyly: Short hands/feet. Complete soft tissue syndactyly of all four limbs. Preaxial, mesoaxial, and postaxial polydactyly of hands. Loss of tubular shape of carpal, metacarpal, and phalangeal bones.				
Single bone in zeugopod: Radial appearance. Monodactyly with biphalangeal digit and absence of carpal ossification in four limbs. Hypoplastic male external genitalia and cryptorchidism.	*HOXD9-13* deletion	*Abd-B*		
Hand-foot-genital syndrome: Small hands and feet, short great toes, abnormal thumbs. Short first metacarpal and metatarsal, short fifth fingers, carpal and tarsal fusions, small pointed distal phalanx of first toe. Müllerian duct fusion (bicornuate or didelphic uterus). Displaced urethral opening and displaced urethral orifices in bladder wall. Hypospadias.	*HOXA13*	*Abd-B*	4×10^{-12}	Transcription factor
Hand-foot-genital syndrome: Velopharyngeal insufficiency. Persistent ductus botalli.	*HOXA11-13*	*Abd-B*	3×10^{-17}	Transcription factor

ture of classic synpolydactyly but conforms to the genital expression of the gene in mammals.

Two different intragenic *HOXD13* deletions that resulted in premature stop codons have been associated with a phenotype with some features of synpolydactyly and a novel foot malformation (Goodman et al., 1998). Such truncations would eliminate the function of the HOXD13 protein, which suggested that this synpolydactyly phenotypic variant was due to haploinsufficiency for the *HOXD13* gene. Finally, monodactylous limbs and abnormal genitalia were observed in two unrelated patients that were heterozygous for deletions spanning the whole *HOXD* cluster and nearby loci (Del Campo et al., 1999).

Mutations in the posterior genes of the *HOXA* cluster also result in abnormal limb and genital development. The classic hand-foot-genital syndrome is associated with heterozygosity for a nonsense mutation in the homeodomain of HOXA13 (Mortlock et al., 1996) (Table 3–3). This nonsense mutation may generate a truncated protein that would be unable to bind DNA; thus, it is possible that haploinsufficiency for HOXA13 is the mechanism leading to the phenotype. The importance of a diploid dose of the *HOXA* genes is further suggested by the phenotype of a patient with a large deletion spanning the *HOXA* cluster. This patient possessed features of the hand-foot-genital syndrome and other anomalies, possibly caused by deficiency of other members of the cluster (Devriendt et al., 1999).

Conserved Signaling Pathways in Vertebrates and Invertebrates Are Targets for Disease

Systematic genetic analyses of pattern formation in *Drosophila*, *C. elegans,* and *dictyostelium* have uncovered a surprisingly limited number of distinct signaling systems involved in cell fate development. These pathways include the TGF-β-related/BMP, receptor tyrosine kinase (RTK), Notch, Toll, G protein–coupled receptor, Hedgehog (Hh), Wingless (Wg) and Janus kinase/signal transducer and activator of transcription (JAK/STAT) signal-transduction networks. In addition, several signaling systems have been implicated in axonal pathfinding and synapse formation, including by the Netrin, Round About (Robo), Semaphorin, Neuroglian, and BMP-mediated pathways. Disease-causing mutations have been identified in components of nearly all of these major signaling pathway categories (Reiter et al., 2001). Consistent with the high degree of evolutionary conservation between vertebrate and invertebrate genetic systems, many human diseases associated with mutations in signal-transduction pathways lead to developmental disorders, as illustrated by the diseases covered in this volume. Since signaling pathways are also intimately tied to regulation of the cell cycle, another common consequence of disrupting signaling systems is failure of growth control and cancer.

One notable trend among diseases associated with mutations in components of signaling pathways is that defects in extracellular components such as ligands or in ligand-specific receptor subunits often result in limited developmental defects while mutations in more downstream intracellular components, which mediate the action of many ligands, often result in cancer (Reiter et al., 2001). For example, in the BMP pathway, mutations affecting the human BMP2/4 ligand and BMP5/7-specific type I receptor lead to morphological defects such as brachydactyly and hereditary hemoragic telangiectasia, whereas mutations in the shared BMP2 type II receptor or the signal transducer SMAD4 cause cancer (Table 3–4). Similarly, in the case of the RTK pathway, mutations in genes encoding FGFR chain isoforms lead to

restricted conditions such as achondroplasia, while mutations in RAS, the cytoplasmic transducer of all RTKs, lead to cancer (Table 3–5).

CROSS-GENOMIC ANALYSIS OF HUMAN DISEASE GENE FUNCTION USING MODEL SYSTEMS

Model genetic systems have long been appreciated for their value in delineating basic biological mechanisms and uncovering fundamental principles of molecular organization. When work was initiated on such model systems as *Drosophila* and *C. elegans*, the deep genetic homologies between these organisms and humans were not yet evident. The expectations of these studies were largely to provide detailed examples of how various biological processes might be carried out with the hope that these concepts would be helpful in dissecting similar but mechanistically distinct processes in humans. One of the reasons we have gone into such detail in describing the similarities between vertebrate and invertebrate development is that the idea that the common ancestor of bilateral animals was such a highly evolved creature, which had already invented most of the morphogenetic systems in existence today, was initially a great surprise to us all. Prior to these revelations, the images that the field had conjured up of this ancestor were more along the lines of a facultatively colonial organism such as a slime mold.

As the image of our common ancestor has come into clearer focus, it has become increasingly apparent that model systems initially chosen for their experimental advantages might actually be good models for genes involved in human disease. Since the molecular devices which suffer insults causing disease states in humans were likely to have been present in the ancestor of the bilateralia and a high proportion of known human disease genes (e.g., $\approx 30\%$) have extremely good matches ($e \leq 10^{-100}$) to genes present in flies, it seems likely that flies, worms, and humans share many genetic systems involved in the formation and function of these systems. An important challenge now is to find the most effective ways to exploit the deep functional homologies between model genetic systems and humans to help solve defined problems in medical genetics.

"Closing the Loop"

Given that completed genome sequences now exist for nematodes, flies, mice, and humans and given all of the functional homologies described above, the time is now ripe to use cross-genomic approaches to help answer specific questions in medical genetics. Many types of question could in principle benefit from cross-genomics. For example, there are situations in which (1) the function or mechanism of action of the disease genes is unknown, (2) the effector targets of a gene (e.g., a transcription factor or an E-3 ubiquitin ligase) are unknown, and (3) the identity of a human second-site modifier locus is unknown. In addition, only about 20% of the estimated 4000–5000 disease genes have yet been identified.

In this section, we will discuss three examples that illustrate the potential utility of model systems in addressing explicit questions regarding human diseases. In general, the goal is to create mutants in the human disease gene counterpart in the model organism and conduct genetic screens to identify new candidate genes in humans that may play an important role in disease etiology. The final goal in each case is to "close the loop" between the model system and humans by having an explicit test in mind to validate the relevance of candidate

Table 3–4. BMP Pathway Diseases

Disease	Human Gene	Fly Gene	e Value	Component
Fibrodysplasia ossificans progressiva	*BMP2*	*dpp*	6×10^{-76}	Ligand
Fibrodysplasia ossificans progressiva	*BMP4*	*dpp*	2×10^{-76}	Ligand
Brachydactyly type C	*BDC*	*dpp*	3×10^{-36}	Ligand
Acromesomelic dysplasia Hunter-Thompson type	*CDMP1*	*dpp*	3×10^{-36}	Ligand
Hereditary hemorrhagic telangiectasia-2	*ALK1*	*sax*	1×10^{-132}	Specific type I receptor
Persistent müllerian duct syndrome type II	*AMHR*	*wit*	2×10^{-52}	Specific type II receptor
Colorectal cancer, familial nonpolyposis, type 6	*TGFBR2*	*put*	8×10^{-70}	General type II receptor
Polyposis, juvenile intestinal	*JIP*	*med*	1×10^{-10}	Cytoplasmic transducer
Pancreatic cancer	*SMAD4*	*med*	1×10^{-108}	Cytoplasmic transducer

Table 3–5. RTK Pathway Diseases

Disease	Human Gene	Fly Gene	e Value	Signaling Component
Obesity with impaired prohormone processing	PC1	Fur1	1×10^{-165}	Protease: ligand activation?
Crouzon syndrome: achondroplasia, craniosynostosis	FGFR3	htl	1×10^{-129}	Receptor
Pfeiffer syndrome	FGFR1	htl	1×10^{-124}	Receptor
Venous malformations, multiple cutaneous and mucosal	TIE2	htl	6×10^{-63}	Receptor
Apert syndrome: Beare-Stevenson cutis gyrata	FGFR2	htl	1×10^{-131}	Receptor
Mast cell leukemia: mastocytosis, piebaldism	KIT	htl	6×10^{-65}	Receptor
Diabetes mellitus: insulin-resistant, leprechaunism, Rabson-Mendenhall syndrome	INSR	InR	1×10^{-300}	Receptor
Renal cell carcinoma	MET	Alk	6×10^{-53}	Receptor?
Predisposition to myeloid malignancy	CSF1R	CG8222	7×10^{-70}	Receptor?
Elliptocytosis-1	EPB41	cora	1×10^{-130}	Cyoskeletal scaffolding?
Ehlers-Danlos syndrome type X	FN1	Ptp10D	5×10^{-39}	Tyrosine phosphatase
Colon cancer	PTPG1	Ptp99A	4×10^{-46}	Tyrosine phosphatase
Bladder cancer	HRAS	Ras85D	2×10^{-74}	Cytoplasmic transducer
Colorectal adenoma	RASK2	Ras85D	1×10^{-78}	Cytoplasmic transducer
Colorectal cancer	NRAS	Ras85D	6×10^{-73}	Cytoplasmic transducer

genes or allelic variations identified in model systems with respect to a specific question(s) in human medical genetics.

Primary Congenital Glaucoma

Mutations in the human *CYP1B1* gene, which encodes a P-450 protein, cause primary congenital glaucoma (PCG) with high penetrance (Stoilov et al., 1997) as a result of a developmental defect in the formation of the trabecular meshwork, which drains fluid from the eye to maintain intraocular pressure. Curiously, several Saudi Arabian pedigrees have been identified in which some individuals with homozygous or compound heterozygous *CYP1B1* mutant alleles do not develop the glaucoma phenotype (Bejjani et al., 2000). Genetic mapping analysis indicated that unaffected individuals share a modifier locus on the short arm of chromosome 8, which compensates for the loss of *CYP1B1* function. The identity of this second-site suppressor(s) locus remains elusive, however, since the existing inbred pedigrees provide only an approximate map position for this gene(s).

The closing-the-loop goal for PCG is to use a model genetic system to help identify the human PCG suppressor locus. One approach is to make mutations in the single highly related *Drosophila* homolog of CYP1B1 (*cyp18a*) and then conduct genetic screens to identify suppressor loci of *cyp18a* loss-of-function mutants in *Drosophila* that have human counterparts on chromosome 8p. We have generated such loss-of-function mutations (L. Reiter and E. Bier, unpublished) and are collaborating with Dr. Bassem Bejjani (Baylor College of Medicine, Houston, TX) to determine whether this locus or other candidate suppressor loci we identify in *Drosophila* might be homologs of human genes that protect unaffected individuals with mutant copies of the *CYP1B1* gene from developing PCG.

Angelman Syndrome

Angelman syndrome (AS) may hold the best promise for closing the loop between flies and humans. AS causes severe mental retardation and other abnormalities, resulting from inactivation of the human *UBE3A* gene (Matsuura et al., 1997), which encodes an E3 ligase that conjugates ubiquitin to specific protein targets that are to be degraded. We have made mutants in the apparent *Drosophila* structural homolog (*d-as*) of *UBE3A* (L. Reiter, M. Bowers, and E. Bier, unpublished data) and are now screening for second-site modifiers of these loss-of-function *d-as* mutants with the goal of identifying candidate proteins that might be substrates of *UBE3A*-targeted degradation and cause AS phenotypes when over produced. Such candidate *d-as* degradation targets will be analyzed by our collaborator, Dr. A. Beaudet (Baylor College of Medicine), who will test whether levels of the human counterparts of these potential targets are altered in AS patients or mouse models.

Alzheimer Disease

Dr. Jane Wu and colleagues (Washington University, St. Louis, MO) identified two antioxidant proteins (thiol-specific antioxidant and pro- liferation associated gene) that physically interact with the Presenilin (Psn) protein (J. Wu, personal communication). We have coexpressed these proteins with Psn in *Drosophila* using the GAL4/UAS system and found that this results in a strong synergistic reduction in Notch signaling (L. Reiter, M. Wangler, M. McElroy, and E. Bier, unpublished data). We are currently trying to see whether TSA and PAG also interact with mutations in the *Drosophila* homolog of the β-amyloid gene. As a closing-the-loop goal, we will collaborate with various members in the Alzheimer field to determine whether human TSA/PAG-related genes are mutated in any of the five familial forms of Alzheimer disease. We have identified five of the 20 TSA/PAG-related genes in humans which map to intervals harboring new suspected Alzheimer loci (L. Reiter, M. McElroy, and E. Bier, unpublished data).

Multi-tier Cross-genomic Analysis of Human Disease Gene Function

As discussed above, unicellular organisms such as yeast and slime mold can be used to analyze important basic eukaryotic cellular functions such as metabolism, regulation of the cell cycle, membrane targeting and dynamics, protein folding, or DNA repair, while simple invertebrate systems such as flies or nematodes are excellent models for examining the coordinated actions of genes that function as components of a common molecular machine. The primary strength of mammalian systems such as the mouse, zebrafish, frog, and chicken is that they can provide the most accurate models for the human disease state. Given that the different model genetic systems have different strengths and limitations, more than one such system will typically offer advantages for analyzing the function of a given human disease gene. For example, all three levels of genetic systems could make important contributions to the analysis of PCG. As the mutant gene (*CYP1B1*) in PCG is a *P-450* gene, which is a member of a protein class present in yeast, one could attempt to establish assays in yeast that distinguish the function of wild-type versus mutant forms of the gene or to identify endogenous yeast genes that are required for the effect of the human *CYP1B1* gene. Because PCG in humans results from a failure to form the trabecular meshwork, which normally drains fluid from the eye, one would obviously need to turn to a multicellular organism to establish a system in which to analyze the developmental function of *CYP1B1*. Invertebrate models such as the fly (see above) are useful for identifying other genes acting together with the *P-450* gene to carry out its developmental function and to help identify human modifier loci but will not necessarily provide an accurate model for glaucoma (e.g., fly eyes do not have a morphological equivalent of the trabecular meshwork). Finally, the mouse knockout (which exists for the homolog of *CYP1B1*) is best suited for analyzing the primary event responsible for the failure of the trabecular meshwork to develop.

We anticipate that cross-genomic studies will become an integral part of the analysis of human disease gene function. As this field grows, an important goal should be to coordinate studies across the various genetic tiers. For example, in analyzing developmental disorders, one could use model unicellular and invertebrate organisms to identify candidate proteins interacting with the human protein of interest as part of the molecular machines that carry out cellular or developmental functions. The developmental role of these new genes could then be evaluated in a vertebrate model (e.g., by knocking them out alone or in combination in mice) and by asking whether mutations in the human counterparts of these genes result in developmental disorders. One interesting question in this regard would be whether compound heterozygosity for several of these genes in mice could lead to disorders similar to known multigenic disorders in humans. Once new medically relevant target genes have been identified through such a closing-the-loop process, these new genes would become themselves substrates for a second round of cross-genomic analysis. This need not be a purely cyclical process since as the mechanism of disease gene action becomes better defined, it should become increasingly possible to ask more hypothesis-driven questions, which again should in principle be addressed in one or another model system. Such an integrated use of multiple genetic systems should prove far more powerful than reliance on any single system.

Genetic Semantics: Cross-species Translation of Developmental Defects

Bioinformatics is another very important field that will undoubtedly help shape the future of medical genetics. As data sets derived from cross-genomic analyses accumulate, one interesting challenge will be to use bioinformatics tools to make new links between mutant phenotypes in model organisms and human disease phenotypes. This new area of interface between computational and experimental fields could be referred to as "genetic semantics" in that the problem is essentially to translate between the languages of two very different phenotype categories. In the case of model systems, systematic screens typically identify loss-of-function mutations affecting a particular process. One great advantage of such systematic screens is that they can saturate for all genes involved in that process. The famous screen carried out by Nusslein-Volhard and Wieschaus (1980) for developmental patterning mutants in *Drosophila* is a classic example of such a saturating screen. The phenotypes, or lexicon in the linguistic analogy, used to categorize gene function in such screens are often lethal and involve major defects, such as loss of entire sections of the body plan or organs. The equivalent of such homozygous mutations in human counterparts of these genes would typically not be identified as diseases in humans as they would lead to early prenatal lethality.

Because mutations in human genes that completely ablate early crucial developmental functions will not be identified by this phenotype, they tend to be found due to mutations that result in subtle recessive defects or dominant phenotypes resulting from loss of only one gene copy (e.g., haploinsufficiency). Many human disease phenotypes are indeed so subtle that they are known only as a result of the self-reporting tendency of afflicted humans and the remarkable finely honed diagnostic skills of experienced clinicians. The lexicon of this exquisitely subtle language of human disease phenotypes bears little similarity to that of the coarse tongue of loss-of-function genetics in model systems. Because the number of self-reporting mutant humans is significant (e.g., $>10^9$), human genetics is often quasi-saturating in that mutations in many components of various systems have been identified. For example, if one considers inherited cardiac diseases, mutations in nearly all of the known components involved in heart muscle contraction (e.g., actin, myosin, myosin kinase, tropomyosin, and troponin) and electrical conduction (e.g., Na^+, K^+, and Ca^{2+} channels) have been identified. Similarly, if one considers peripheral neuropathies, mutations in several protein components of myelin and peripheral nerve have been assigned to similar but distinct disease subtypes. Signaling pathways provide another example of quasi-saturation in human genetics, as exemplified by the RTK/mitogen-activated protein kinase and BMP pathways (Tables 3–4, 3–5) in which mutations in multiple components have been recovered.

The significant linguistic differences between the genetics of model systems and human disease notwithstanding, any genes which are al-

tered in both humans and model systems will most likely perform the same or very similar molecular functions. How then can one translate between these disparate languages? One way to address this question is to cluster genes into groups using phenotypic similarities in one system and then ask whether the phenotypes associated with mutations in counterparts of these genes in the other system share anything. Text comparing algorithms such as internet search engines could be modified in principle for such purposes, and several commercially available software packages have similar capabilities. As discussed earlier, the Notch pathway illustrates a simple form of this idea. In *Drosophila*, loss-of-function mutations in the Notch pathway lead to a multitude of phenotypes, including hyperplasia of the nervous system at the expense of epidermal cell fates, disruption of D/V patterning of appendages and loss of marginal structures, as well as thickened wing veins. In *C. elegans*, mutants in the Notch (lin12) pathway lead to transformations of cell fates within the vulval cell lineage in which two cells that ordinarily would communicate via Notch signaling to generate two different cell types both develop with the default fate. There are several Notch-related receptors in mice and humans, and mutations in one of these receptors (Notch1) or in one of the Delta-related Notch ligands (Delta3) cause defects in somite segregation, which result in fusion of adjacent somites and subsequent spinal malformations. Given the conservation of signaling pathway organization during evolution, it would be reasonable to ask whether mutations in other components of the Notch pathway might lead to spinal malformations in humans. This seems likely since the mouse knock-out of a gene encoding a glycosyltransferase related to the *Drosophila fringe* gene exhibits spinal malformation phenotypes similar to those observed in Notch1 or Delta3 knockouts. Thus, in this case, one translation of the genetic lexical item Notch is excess neural development in flies, vulval defects in worms, and spinal malformation in humans.

It will not necessarily always be the case that one can identify mutations in all components of a pathway based on there being a shared disease phenotype. For example, as discussed above, a variety of ligands can funnel through a more limited number of receptors whose function may be mediated by only one or a few cytoplasmic transducing molecules. In addition, since humans often have several highly related copies of a gene, which can be expressed in very different patterns, the phenotypes resulting from loss-of-function mutations in various components of a pathway can range from specific developmental conditions (e.g., brachydactyly) to more general loss of cellular growth control (e.g., cancer). Although these factors will complicate phenotypic translation attempts, one can imagine factoring relevant data into clustering programs, such as known gene expression data gathered from the mouse. It is also possible to conduct the analysis in the reverse direction by clustering human diseases based on shared phenotype and then asking whether the counterpart genes in the various model organisms share previously unappreciated similarities. Finally, one can search for patterns of similarity between the phenotypes in mutants of homologous components in more than two organisms (e.g., compare clusters of fly to worm phenotypes and then search carefully for similarities between the disease phenotypes in the human counterparts of this set of genes). Phenotypic homology searches of this kind are likely to uncover hidden genetic relationships that would otherwise remained buried in the vast data fields of the postgenomic era in much the same way that sequence alignment programs such as MIME and Beauty have extracted critical functional information from raw amino acid sequence data (e.g., shared protein motifs).

SUMMARY AND PERSPECTIVES

An important practical consequence of the fact that vertebrates and invertebrates derived from a shared, highly structured, bilateral ancestor is that many types of complex molecular machine which were present in this creature have remained virtually unchanged in both lineages. Given that three-quarters of all known genes which cause disease when mutated in humans have counterparts in model systems such as *Drosophila*, it seems very likely that these genes will often perform similar functions in the context of similar molecular pathways or protein complexes in model organisms and humans. These deep homologies between genetic networks can be exploited to understand the function of genes which can cause disease in humans when altered and should be very useful for identifying new genes in humans involved in disease states.

With the completion of the human genome project and the discovery of many of the most important genes involved in heritable disorders, the primary emphasis in human genetics is shifting to understanding the function of these disease genes. Model organisms ranging from yeast to mice offer distinct advantages for cross-genomic analysis of different aspects of human disease gene function. If unicellular organisms such as yeast and slime molds have closely related sequences to a given human disease gene of interest, these powerful model systems are ideal for conducting systematic screens for new genes that interact with the disease gene as part of a common eukaryotic pathway or cellular process. Since developmental disorders by definition involve interactions between cells in multicellular organisms, there is also a need for model genetic systems such as *Drosophila* and *C. elegans* that can define genes acting at the organismal level. The great advantage offered by these model genetic systems is the ability to design second-site modifier screens to identify new genes involved in a given developmental process or pathway. It is not necessary that these model organism mimic the human disease state as long as the genetic screens are successful in identifying proteins which function as part of a conserved molecular device. Finally, vertebrate model systems such as the mouse or zebrafish are essential for providing accurate models for the human disease state.

As cross-genomic approaches become a routine component in the analysis of human disease function, an interesting and important challenge will be to integrate studies in the various systems into complementary comparative programs. A critical element of this integration will be the use of computational methods to search through large phenotypic and gene expression data sets to extract hidden relationships between individual genes and genetic networks. The next decade should prove to be a very fertile period for forging this new field of comparative functional genomics.

Model Organism Genome Websites

Yeast: http://genome-www.stanford.edu/Saccharomyces/
Slime mold: http://glamdring.ucsd.edu/others/dsmith/dictydb.html
Fly: http://flybase.bio.indiana.edu:82/
Worm: http://www.expasy.ch/cgi-bin/lists?celegans.txt
Zebrafish: http://www.ncbi.nlm.nih.gov/genome/guide/D_rerio.html
Mouse: http://www.informatics.jax.org/
Human disease genes (OMIM): http://www.ncbi.nlm.nih.gov/Omim/

REFERENCES

Abdelilah S, Mountcastle-Shah E, Harvey M, Solnica-Krezel L, Schier AF, Stemple DL, Malicki J, Neuhauss SC, Zwartkruis F, Stainier DY, et al. (1996). Mutations affecting neural survival in the zebrafish *Danio rerio*. *Development* 123: 217–227.

Aboobaker AA, Blaxter ML (2000). Medical significance of *Caenorhabditis elegans*. *Ann Med* 32: 23–30.

Akarsu AN, Stoilov I, Yilmaz E, Sayli BS, Sarfarazi M (1996). Genomic structure of *HOXD13* gene: a nine polyalanine duplication causes synpolydactyly in two unrelated families. *Hum Mol Genet* 5: 945–952.

Alvarez IS, Araujo M, Nieto MA (1998). Neural induction in whole chick embryo cultures by FGF *Dev Biol* 199: 42–54.

Arendt D, Nubler-Jung K (1994). Inversion of dorsoventral axis? *Nature* 371: 26.

Arendt D, Nubler-Jung K (1999). Comparison of early nerve cord development in insects and vertebrates. *Development* 126: 2309–2325.

Arora K, Levine MS, O'Connor MB (1994). The *screw* gene encodes a ubiquitously expressed member of the TGF-beta family required for specification of dorsal cell fates in the *Drosophila* embryo. *Genes Dev* 8: 2588–2601.

Azpiazu N, Frasch M (1993a). *tinman* and *bagpipe*: two homeo box genes that determine cell fates in the dorsal mesoderm of *Drosophila*. *Genes Dev* 7: 1325–1340.

Baier H, Klostermann S, Trowe T, Karlstrom RO, Nusslein-Volhard C, Bonhoeffer F (1996). Genetic dissection of the retinotectal projection. *Development* 123: 415–425.

Barut BA, Zon LI (2000). Realizing the potential of zebrafish as a model for human disease. *Physiol Genomics* 2: 49–51.

Bateson W (1894). *Materials for the Study of Variation*. MacMillan, London.

Baum LF (1900). *The Wonderful Wizard of Oz*. Oxford University Press, Oxford.

Baylies MK, Bate M, Ruiz Gomez M (1998). Myogenesis: a view from *Drosophila*. *Cell* 93: 921–927.

Beiman M, Shilo BZ, Volk T (1996). Heartless, a *Drosophila* FGF receptor homolog, is essential for cell migration and establishment of several mesodermal lineages. *Genes Dev* 10: 2993–3002.

Bejjani BA, Stockton DW, Lewis RA, Tomey KF, Dueker DK, Jabak M, Astle WF, Lup-

ski JR (2000). Multiple *CYP1B1* mutations and incomplete penetrance in an inbred population segregating primary congenital glaucoma suggest frequent de novo events and a dominant modifier locus. *Hum Mol Genet* 9: 367–374.

Benavides F, Guenet JL (2001). Murine models for human diseases. *Medicina* 61: 215–231.

Bernards A, Hariharan IK (2001). Of flies and men—studying human disease in *Drosophila*. *Curr Opin Genet Dev* 11: 274–278.

Biehs B, Francois V, Bier E (1996). The *Drosophila* short gastrulation gene prevents Dpp from autoactivating and suppressing neurogenesis in the neuroectoderm. *Genes Dev* 10: 2922–2934.

Bier E (1997). Anti-neural inhibition: a conserved mechanism for neural induction. *Cell* 89: 681–684.

Blass JP, Sheu RK, Gibson GE (2000). Inherent abnormalities in energy metabolism in Alzheimer disease. Interaction with cerebrovascular compromise. *Ann NY Acad Sci* 903: 204–221.

Blitz IL, Shimmi O, Wunnenberg-Stapleton K, O'Connor MB, Cho KW (2000). Is chordin a long-range- or short-range-acting factor? Roles for BMP1-related metalloproteases in chordin and BMP4 autofeedback loop regulation. *Dev Biol* 223: 120–138.

Blum M, Gaunt SJ, Cho KW, Steinbeisser H, Blumberg B, Bittner D, De Robertis EM (1992). Gastrulation in the mouse: the role of the homeobox gene goosecoid. *Cell* 69: 1097–1106.

Bodmer R (1993a). The gene *tinman* is required for specification of the heart and visceral muscles in *Drosophila*. *Development* 118: 719–729.

Bodmer R, Venkatesh TV (1998). Heart development in *Drosophila* and vertebrates: conservation of molecular mechanisms. *Dev Genet* 22: 181–186.

Boulay JL, Dennefeld C, Alberga A (1987). The *Drosophila* developmental gene *snail* encodes a protein with nucleic acid binding fingers. *Nature* 330: 395–398.

Brand M, Heisenberg CP, Jiang YJ, Beuchle D, Lun K, Furutani-Seiki M, Granato M, Haffter P, Hammerschmidt M, Kane DA, et al. (1996). Mutations in zebrafish genes affecting the formation of the boundary between midbrain and hindbrain. *Development* 123: 179–190.

Brand-Saberi B, Christ B (1999). Genetic and epigenetic control of muscle development in vertebrates. *Cell Tissue Res* 296: 199–212.

Brannon M, Gomperts M, Sumoy L, Moon RT, Kimelman D (1997). A beta-catenin/XTcf-3 complex binds to the siamois promoter to regulate dorsal axis specification in *Xenopus*. *Genes Dev* 11: 2359–2370.

Brannon M, Kimelman D (1996). Activation of Siamois by the Wnt pathway. *Dev Biol* 180: 344–347.

Brockerhoff SE, Dowling JE, Hurley JB (1998). Zebrafish retinal mutants. *Vision Res* 38: 1335–1339.

Brose K, Bland KS, Wang KH, Arnott D, Henzel W, Goodman CS, Tessier-Lavigne M, Kidd T (1999). Slit proteins bind Robo receptors and have an evolutionarily conserved role in repulsive axon guidance. *Cell* 96: 795–806.

Bulman MP, Kusumi K, Frayling TM, McKeown C, Garrett C, Lander ES, Krumlauf R, Hattersley AT, Ellard S, Turnpenny PD (2000). Mutations in the human delta homologue, DLL3, cause axial skeletal defects in spondylocostal dysostosis. *Nat Genet* 24: 438–441.

Cabrera CV, Martinez-Arias A, Bate M (1987). The expression of three members of the *achaete-scute* gene complex correlates with neuroblast segregation in *Drosophila*. *Cell* 50: 425–433.

Callaerts P, Munoz-Marmol AM, Glardon S, Castillo E, Sun H, Li WH, Gehring WJ, Salo E (1999). Isolation and expression of a *Pax-6* gene in the regenerating and intact Planarian Dugesia(G)tigrina. *Proc Natl Acad Sci USA* 96: 558–563.

Campuzano S, Modolell J (1992). Patterning of the *Drosophila* nervous system: the *achaete-scute* gene complex. *Trends Genet* 8: 202–208.

Capdevila J, Izpisua Belmonte JC (2001). Patterning mechanisms controlling vertebrate limb development. *Annu Rev Cell Dev Biol* 17: 87–132.

Carnac G, Kodjabachian L, Gurdon JB, Lemaire P (1996). The homeobox gene *Siamois* is a target of the Wnt dorsalisation pathway and triggers organiser activity in the absence of mesoderm. *Development* 122: 3055–3065.

Carver EA, Jiang R, Lan Y, Oram KF, Gridley T (2001). The mouse snail gene encodes a key regulator of the epithelial–mesenchymal transition. *Mol Cell Biol* 21: 8184–8188.

Chan HY, Bonini NM (2000). *Drosophila* models of human neurodegenerative disease. *Cell Death Differ* 7: 1075–1080.

Chang C, Holtzman DA, Chau S, Chickering T, Woolf EA, Holmgren LM, Bodorova J, Gearing DP, Holmes WE, Brivanlou AH (2001). Twisted gastrulation can function as a BMP antagonist. *Nature* 410: 483–487.

Chen JN, Fishman MC (2000). Genetics of heart development. *Trends Genet* 16: 383–388.

Chen JN, Haffter P, Odenthal J, Vogelsang E, Brand M, van Eeden FJ, Furutani-Seiki M, Granato M, Hammerschmidt M, Heisenberg CP, et al. (1996). Mutations affecting the cardiovascular system and other internal organs in zebrafish. *Development* 123: 293–302.

Chen ZF, Behringer RR (1995). twist is required in head mesenchyme for cranial neural tube morphogenesis. *Genes Dev* 9: 686–699.

Chien S, Reiter LT, Bier E, Gribskov M (2002). Homophila: human disease gene cognates in *Drosophila*. *Nucleic Acids Res* 30: 149–151.

Childs S, Weinstein BM, Mohideen MA, Donohue S, Bonkovsky H, Fishman MC (2000). Zebrafish dracula encodes ferrochelatase and its mutation provides a model for erythropoietic protoporphyria. *Curr Biol* 10: 1001–1004.

Chisholm A, Horvitz R (1995). Patterning of the *Caenorhabditis elegans* head region by the *Pax-6* family member vab-3. *Nature* 377: 52–55.

Chung CY, Funamoto S, Firtel RA (2001). Signaling pathways controlling cell polarity and chemotaxis. *Trends Biochem Sci* 26: 557–566.

Ciruna B, Rossant J (2001). FGF signaling regulates mesoderm cell fate specification and morphogenetic movement at the primitive streak. *Dev Cell* 1: 37–49.

Clements D, Friday RV, Woodland HR (1999). Mode of action of VegT in mesoderm and endoderm formation. *Development* 126: 4903–4911.

Conlon FL, Sedgwick SG, Weston KM, Smith JC (1996). Inhibition of Xbra transcription activation causes defects in mesodermal patterning and reveals autoregulation of Xbra in dorsal mesoderm. *Development* 122: 2427–2435.

Conlon RA, Reaume AG, Rossant J (1995). Notch1 is required for the coordinate segmentation of somites. *Development* 121: 1533–1545.

Connolly DJ, Patel K, Cooke J (1997). Chick noggin is expressed in the organizer and neural plate during axial development, but offers no evidence of involvement in primary axis formation. *Int J Dev Biol* 41: 389–396.

Cooper EC, Jan LY (1999). Ion channel genes and human neurological disease: recent progress, prospects, and challenges. *Proc Natl Acad Sci USA* 96: 4759–4766.

Corsi AK, Kostas SA, Fire A, Krause M (2000). *Caenorhabditis elegans* twist plays an essential role in non-striated muscle development. *Development* 127: 2041–2051.

Culetto E, Sattelle DB (2000). A role for *Caenorhabditis elegans* in understanding the function and interactions of human disease genes. *Hum Mol Genet* 9: 869–877.

Czerny T, Halder G, Kloter U, Souabni A, Gehring WJ, Busslinger M (1999). *twin of eyeless*, a second *Pax-6* gene of *Drosophila*, acts upstream of eyeless in the control of eye development. *Mol Cells* 3: 297–307.

D'Alessio M, Frasch M (1996). msh may play a conserved role in dorsoventral patterning of the neuroectoderm and mesoderm. *Mech Dev* 58: 217–231.

Daly FJ, Sandell JH (2000). Inherited retinal degeneration and apoptosis in mutant zebrafish. *Anat Rec* 258: 145–155.

Darras BT, Friedman NR (2000). Metabolic myopathies: a clinical approach; part I. *Pediatr Neurol* 22: 87–97.

Del Campo M, Jones MC, Veraksa AN, Curry CJ, Jones KL, Mascarello JT, Ali-Kahn-Catts Z, Drumheller T, McGinnis W (1999). Monodactylous limbs and abnormal genitalia are associated with hemizygosity for the human 2q31 region that includes the HOXD cluster. *Am J Hum Genet* 65: 104–110.

De Robertis EM, Sasai Y (1996). A common plan for dorsoventral patterning in Bilateria. *Nature* 380: 37–40.

De Robertis EM, Blum M, Niehrs C, Steinbeisser H (1992). Goosecoid and the organizer. *Dev Suppl* 167–171.

Devriendt K, Jaeken J, Matthijs G, Van Esch H, Debeer P, Gewillig M, Fryns JP (1999). Haploinsufficiency of the *HOXA* gene cluster, in a patient with hand-foot-genital syndrome, velopharyngeal insufficiency, and persistent patent *Ductus botalli*. *Am J Hum Genet* 65: 249–251.

Dooley K, Zon LI (2000). Zebrafish: a model system for the study of human disease. *Curr Opin Genet Dev* 10: 252–256.

Doyle HJ, Kraut R, Levine M (1989). Spatial regulation of *zerknullt*: a dorsal–ventral patterning gene in *Drosophila*. *Genes Dev* 3: 1518–1533.

Driever W, Solnica-Krezel L, Schier AF, Neuhauss SC, Malicki J, Stemple DL, Stainier DY, Zwartkruis F, Abdelilah S, Rangini Z, et al. (1996). A genetic screen for mutations affecting embryogenesis in zebrafish. *Development* 123: 37–46.

el Ghouzzi V, Le Merrer M, Perrin-Schmitt F, Lajeunie E, Benit P, Renier D, Bourgeois P, Bolcato-Bellemin AL, Munnich A, Bonaventure J (1997). Mutations of the *TWIST* gene in the Saethre-Chotzen syndrome. *Nat Genet* 15: 42–46.

Essex LJ, Mayor R, Sargent MG (1993). Expression of *Xenopus* snail in mesoderm and prospective neural fold ectoderm. *Dev Dyn* 198: 108–1122.

Fan MJ, Gruning W, Walz G, Sokol SY (1998). Wnt signaling and transcriptional control of Siamois in *Xenopus* embryos. *Proc Natl Acad Sci USA* 95: 5626–5631.

Fazeli A, Dickinson SL, Hermiston ML, Tighe RV, Steen RG, Small CG, Stoeckli ET, Keino-Masu K, Masu M, Rayburn H, et al. (1997). Phenotype of mice lacking functional Deleted in colorectal cancer (*Dcc*) gene. *Nature* 386: 796–804.

Ferguson EL, Anderson KV (1992a). Decapentaplegic acts as a morphogen to organize dorsal–ventral pattern in the *Drosophila* embryo. *Cell* 71: 451–461.

Ferguson EL, Anderson KV (1992b). Localized enhancement and repression of the activity of the TGF-beta family member, decapentaplegic, is necessary for dorsal–ventral pattern formation in the *Drosophila* embryo. *Development* 114: 583–597.

Fernandez-Chacon R, Sudhof TC (1999). Genetics of synaptic vesicle function: toward the complete functional anatomy of an organelle. *Annu Rev Physiol* 61: 753–776.

Firtel RA, Chung CY (2000). The molecular genetics of chemotaxis: sensing and responding to chemoattractant gradients, Bioessays 22: 603–615.

Fortini ME, Bonini NM (2000). Modeling human neurodegenerative diseases in *Drosophila*: on a wing and a prayer. *Trends Genet* 16: 161–167.

Foury F (1997). Human genetic diseases: a cross-talk between man and yeast. *Gene* 195: 1–10.

Francois V, Bier E (1995). *Xenopus chordin* and *Drosophila short gastrulation* genes encode homologous proteins functioning in dorsal–ventral axis formation. *Cell* 80: 19–20.

Francois V, Solloway M, O'Neill JW, Emery J, Bier E (1994). Dorsal–ventral patterning of the *Drosophila* embryo depends on a putative negative growth factor encoded by the *short gastrulation* gene. *Genes Dev* 8: 2602–2616.

Frasch M (1999). Intersecting signalling and transcriptional pathways in *Drosophila* heart specification. *Semin Cell Dev Biol* 10: 61–71.

Gerard M, Chen JY, Gronemeyer H, Chambon P, Duboule D, Zakany J (1996). In vivo targeted mutagenesis of a regulatory element required for positioning the *Hoxd-11* and *Hoxd-10* expression boundaries. *Genes Dev* 10: 2326–2334.

Giger RJ, Kolodkin AL (2001). Silencing the siren: guidance cue hierarchies at the CNS midline. *Cell* 105: 1–4.

Gisselbrecht S, Skeath JB, Doe CQ, Michelson AM (1996). heartless encodes a fibroblast growth factor receptor (DFR1/DFGF-R2) involved in the directional migration of early mesodermal cells in the *Drosophila* embryo. *Genes Dev* 10: 3003–3017.

Goldsmith TH (1990). Optimization, constraint, and history in the evolution of eyes. *Q Rev Biol* 65: 281–322.

Goodman F, Giovannucci-Uzielli ML, Hall C, Reardon W, Winter R, Scambler P (1998). Deletions in *HOXD13* segregate with an identical, novel foot malformation in two unrelated families. *Am J Hum Genet* 63: 992–1000.

Gould A, Morrison A, Sproat G, White RAH, Krumlauf R (1997). Positive cross-regulation and enhancer sharing: two mechanisms for specifying overlapping Hox expression patterns. *Genes Dev* 11: 900–913.

Greenwald I (1998). LIN-12/Notch signaling: lessons from worms and flies. *Genes Dev* 12: 1751–1762.

Guertl B, Noehammer C, Hoefler G (2000). Metabolic cardiomyopathies. *Int J Exp Pathol* 81: 349–372.

Guthrie S (2001). Axon guidance: Robos make the rules. *Curr Biol* 11: R300–R303.

Haffter P, Granato M, Brand M, Mullins MC, Hammerschmidt M, Kane DA, Odenthal J, van Eeden FJ, Jiang YJ, Heisenberg CP, et al. (1996). The identification of genes with unique and essential functions in the development of the zebrafish. *Danio rerio*. *Development* 123: 1–36.

Halder G, Callaerts P, Gehring WJ (1995). Induction of ectopic eyes by targeted expression of the *eyeless* gene in *Drosophila*. *Science* 267: 1788–1792.

Hammerschmidt M, Nusslein-Volhard C (1993). The expression of a zebrafish gene homologous to *Drosophila snail* suggests a conserved function in invertebrate and vertebrate gastrulation. *Development* 119: 1107–1118.

Hammerschmidt M, Serbedzija GN, McMahon AP (1996). Genetic analysis of dorsoventral pattern formation in the zebrafish: requirement of a BMP-like ventralizing activity and its dorsal repressor. *Genes Dev* 10: 2452–2461.

Hanson I, Van Heyningen V (1995). Pax6: more than meets the eye. *Trends Genet* 11: 268–272.

Harfe BD, Vaz Gomes A, Kenyon C, Liu J, Krause M, Fire A (1998). Analysis of a *Caenorhabditis elegans* Twist homolog identifies conserved and divergent aspects of mesodermal patterning. *Genes Dev* 12: 2623–2635.

Harris R, Sabatelli LM, Seeger MA (1996). Guidance cues at the *Drosophila* CNS midline: identification and characterization of two *Drosophila* Netrin/UNC-6 homologs. *Neuron* 17: 217–228.

Hedgecock EM, Culotti JG, Hall DH (1990). The *unc-5*, *unc-6*, and *unc-40* genes guide circumferential migrations of pioneer axons and mesodermal cells on the epidermis in *C. elegans*. *Neuron* 4: 61–85.

Heisenberg CP, Brand M, Jiang YJ, Warga RM, Beuchle D, van Eeden FJ, Furutani-Seiki M, Granato M, Haffter P, Hammerschmidt M, et al. (1996). Genes involved in forebrain development in the zebrafish. *Danio rerio*. *Development* 123: 191–203.

Hemmati-Brivanlou A, Melton D (1997). Vertebrate embryonic cells will become nerve cells unless told otherwise. *Cell* 88: 13–17.

Hill RE, Favor J, Hogan BL, Ton CC, Saunders GF, Hanson IM, Prosser J, Jordan T, Hastie ND, van Heyningen V (1991). Mouse small eye results from mutations in a paired-like homeobox-containing gene [erratum appears in *Nature* 1992;355:750]. *Nature* 354: 522–525.

Hodgkin AL, Huxley AF (1952). A quantitative description of membrane current and its application to conduction and excitation in nerve. *J Physiol* 108: 37–77.

Holley SA, Jackson PD, Sasai Y, Lu B, De Robertis EM, Hoffmann FM, Ferguson EL (1995). A conserved system for dorsal–ventral patterning in insects and vertebrates involving sog and chordin. *Nature* 376: 249–253.

Hopwood ND, Pluck A, Gurdon JB (1989). A *Xenopus* mRNA related to *Drosophila* twist is expressed in response to induction in the mesoderm and the neural crest. *Cell* 59: 893–903.

Howard TD, Paznekas WA, Green ED, Chiang LC, Ma N, Ortiz de Luna RI, Garcia Delgado C, Gonzalez-Ramos M, Kline AD, Jabs EW (1997). Mutations in *TWIST*, a basic helix-loop-helix transcription factor, in Saethre-Chotzen syndrome. *Nat Genet* 15: 36–41.

Huang JD, Dubnicoff T, Liaw GJ, Bai Y, Valentine SA, Shirokawa JM, Lengyel JA, Courey AJ (1995). Binding sites for transcription factor NTF-1/Elf-1 contribute to the ventral repression of decapentaplegic. *Genes Dev* 9: 3177–3189.

Huang JD, Schwyter DH, Shirokawa JM, Courey AJ (1993). The interplay between multiple enhancer and silencer elements defines the pattern of decapentaplegic expression. *Genes Dev* 7: 694–704.

Hukriede N, Fisher D, Epstein J, Joly L, Tellis P, Zhou Y, Barbazuk B, Cox K, Fenton-Noriega L, Hersey C, et al. (2001). The LN54 radiation hybrid map of zebrafish expressed sequences. *Genome Res* 11: 2127–2132.

Ip YT, Park RE, Kosman D, Bier E, Levine M (1992a). The dorsal gradient morphogen regulates stripes of rhomboid expression in the presumptive neuroectoderm of the *Drosophila* embryo. *Genes Dev* 6: 1728–1739.

Ip YT, Park RE, Kosman D, Yazdanbakhsh K, Levine M (1992b). dorsal–twist interactions establish snail expression in the presumptive mesoderm of the *Drosophila* embryo. *Genes Dev* 6: 1518–1530.

Ip YT, Reach M, Engstrom Y, Kadalayil L, Cai H, Gonzalez-Crespo S, Tatei K, Levine M (1993). *Dif*, a dorsal-related gene that mediates an immune response in *Drosophila*. *Cell* 75: 753–763.

Irvine KD (1999). Fringe, Notch, and making developmental boundaries. *Curr Opin Genet Dev* 9: 434–441.

Irvine KD, Vogt TF (1997). Dorsal–ventral signaling in limb development. *Curr Opin Cell Biol* 9: 867–876.

Ishii N, Wadsworth WG, Stern BD, Culotti JG, Hedgecock EM (1992). UNC-6, a laminin-related protein, guides cell and pioneer axon migrations in *C. elegans*. *Neuron* 9: 873–881.

Jazwinska A, Kirov N, Wieschaus E, Roth S, Rushlow C (1999a). The *Drosophila* gene *brinker* reveals a novel mechanism of *Dpp* target gene regulation. *Cell* 96: 563–573.

Jazwinska A, Rushlow C, Roth S (1999b). The role of *brinker* in mediating the graded response to *Dpp* in early *Drosophila* embryos. *Development* 126: 3323–3334.

Jiang J, Cai H, Zhou Q, Levine M (1993). Conversion of a dorsal-dependent silencer into an enhancer: evidence for dorsal corepressors. *EMBO J* 12: 3201–3209.

Jiang J, Kosman D, Ip YT, Levine M (1991). The dorsal morphogen gradient regulates the mesoderm determinant twist in early *Drosophila* embryos. *Genes Dev* 5: 1881–1891.

Jiang J, Rushlow CA, Zhou Q, Small S, Levine M (1992). Individual dorsal morphogen binding sites mediate activation and repression in the *Drosophila* embryo. *EMBO J* 11: 3147–3154.

Jiang YJ, Brand M, Heisenberg CP, Beuchle D, Furutani-Seiki M, Kelsh RN, Warga RM, Granato M, Haffter P, Hammerschmidt M, et al. (1996). Mutations affecting neurogenesis and brain morphology in the zebrafish, *Danio rerio*. *Development* 123: 205–216.

Jiao R, Daube M, Duan H, Zou Y, Frei E, Noll M (2001). Headless flies generated by developmental pathway interference. Development 128: 3307–3319.

Jimenez F, Campos-Ortega JA (1990). Defective neuroblast commitment in mutants of the achaete-scute complex and adjacent genes of *D. melanogaster. Neuron* 5: 81–89.
Jones CM, Smith JC (1998). Establishment of a BMP-4 morphogen gradient by long-range inhibition. *Dev Biol* 194: 12–17.
Kaprielian Z, Runko E, Imondi R (2001). Axon guidance at the midline choice point. *Dev Dyn* 221: 154–181.
Karin M (1999). The beginning of the end: IkappaB kinase (IKK) and NF-kappaB activation. *J Biol Chem* 274: 27339–27342.
Karlstrom RO, Trowe T, Klostermann S, Baier H, Brand M, Crawford AD, Grunewald B, Haffter P, Hoffmann H, Meyer SU, et al. (1996). Zebrafish mutations affecting retinotectal axon pathfinding. *Development* 123: 427–438.
Kaufman TC, Lewis R, Wakimoto B (1980). Cytogenetic analysis of chromosome 3 in *Drosophila melanogaster*: the homeotic gene complex in polytene chromosome interval 84A-B. *Genetics* 94: 115–133.
Keleman K, Dickson BJ (2001). Short- and long-range repulsion by the *Drosophila* Unc5 netrin receptor. *Neuron* 32: 605–617.
Kelly PD, Chu F, Woods IG, Ngo-Hazelett P, Cardozo T, Huang H, Kimm F, Liao L, Yan YL, Zhou Y, et al. (2000). Genetic linkage mapping of zebrafish genes and ESTs. *Genome Res* 10: 558–567.
Kidd T, Bland KS, Goodman CS (1999). Slit is the midline repellent for the robo receptor in *Drosophila. Cell* 96: 785–794.
Kidd T, Brose K, Mitchell KJ, Fetter RD, Tessier-Lavigne M, Goodman CS, Tear G (1998a). Roundabout controls axon crossing of the CNS midline and defines a novel subfamily of evolutionarily conserved guidance receptors. *Cell* 92: 205–215.
Kidd T, Russell C, Goodman CS, Tear G (1998b). Dosage-sensitive and complementary functions of roundabout and commissureless control axon crossing of the CNS midline. *Neuron* 20: 25–33.
Kimelman D, Griffin KJ (1998). Mesoderm induction: a postmodern view. *Cell* 94: 419–421.
Kimelman D, Griffin KJ (2000). Vertebrate mesendoderm induction and patterning. *Curr Opin Genet Dev* 10: 350–356.
Kirov N, Childs S, O'Connor M, Rushlow C (1994). The *Drosophila* dorsal morphogen represses the *tolloid* gene by interacting with a silencer element. *Mol Cell Biol* 14: 713–722.
Knoll AH, Carroll SB (1999). Early animal evolution: emerging views from comparative biology and geology. *Science* 284: 2129–2137.
Kolodkin AL, Matthes DJ, Goodman CS (1993). The semaphorin genes encode a family of transmembrane and secreted growth cone guidance molecules. *Cell* 75: 1389–1399.
Kolodziej PA, Timpe LC, Mitchell KJ, Fried SR, Goodman CS, Jan LY, Jan YN (1996). frazzled encodes a *Drosophila* member of the DCC immunoglobulin subfamily and is required for CNS and motor axon guidance. *Cell* 87: 197–204.
Komuro I, Izumo S (1993). *Csx*—a murine homeobox-containing gene specifically expressed in the developing heart. *Proc Natl Acad Sci USA* 90: 8145–8149.
Kondo T, Zákány J, Innis JW, Duboule D (1997). Of fingers, toes and penises. *Nature* 390: 29.
Kosman D, Ip YT, Levine M, Arora K (1991). Establishment of the mesoderm-neuroectoderm boundary in the *Drosophila* embryo. *Science* 254: 118–122.
Kuspa A, Loomis WF (1994). REMI-RFLP mapping in the Dictyostelium genome. *Genetics* 138: 665–674.
Kusumi K, Sun ES, Kerrebrock AW, Bronson RT, Chi DC, Bulotsky MS, Spencer JB, Birren BW, Frankel WN, Lander ES (1998). The mouse pudgy mutation disrupts Delta homologue Dll3 and initiation of early somite boundaries. *Nat Genet* 19: 274–278.
Lajeunie E (1997). Genetics of craniofacial malformations. *Ann Chir Plast Esthet* 42: 361–364.
Lamb TM, Knecht AK, Smith WC, Stachel SE, Economides AN, Stahl N, Yancopolous GD, Harland RM (1993). Neural induction by the secreted polypeptide noggin. *Science* 262: 713–718.
Lander ES, Linton LM, Birren B, Nusbaum C, Zody MC, Baldwin J, Devon K, Dewar K, Doyle M, FitzHugh W, et al. (2001). Initial sequencing and analysis of the human genome. *Nature* 409: 860–921.
Larabell CA, Torres M, Rowning BA, Yost C, Miller JR, Wu M, Kimelman D, Moon RT (1997). Establishment of the dorso–ventral axis in *Xenopus* embryos is presaged by early asymmetries in beta-catenin that are modulated by the Wnt signaling pathway. *J Cell Biol* 136: 1123–1136.
Lee YM, Park T, Schulz RA, Kim Y (1997). Twist-mediated activation of the NK-4 homeobox gene in the visceral mesoderm of *Drosophila* requires two distinct clusters of E-box regulatory elements. *J Biol Chem* 272: 17531–17541.
Le Mouellic H, Lallemand Y, Brulet P (1992). Homeosis in the mouse induced by a null mutation in the *Hox-3.1* gene. *Cell* 69: 251–264.
Leonardo ED, Hinck L, Masu M, Keino-Masu K, Ackerman SL, Tessier-Lavigne M (1997). Vertebrate homologues of *C. elegans* UNC-5 are candidate netrin receptors. *Nature* 386: 833–838.
Leptin M (1991). twist and snail as positive and negative regulators during *Drosophila* mesoderm development. *Genes Dev* 5: 1568–1576.
Leung-Hagesteijn C, Spence AM, Stern BD, Zhou Y, Su MW, Hedgecock EM, Culotti JG (1992). UNC-5, a transmembrane protein with immunoglobulin and thrombospondin type 1 domains, guides cell and pioneer axon migrations in *C. elegans. Cell* 71: 289–29.
Lewis EB (1978). A gene complex controlling segmentation in *Drosophila. Nature* 276: 565–570.
Li HS, Chen JH, Wu W, Fagaly T, Zhou L, Yuan W, Dupuis S, Jiang ZH, Nash W, Gick C, et al. (1999). Vertebrate slit, a secreted ligand for the transmembrane protein roundabout, is a repellent for olfactory bulb axons. *Cell* 96: 807–818.
Li J, Schwarz TL (1999). Genetic evidence for an equilibrium between docked and undocked vesicles. *Philos Trans R Soc Lond B Biol Sci* 354: 299–306.
Li J, Peet GW, Balzarano D, Li X, Massa P, Barton RW, Marcu KB (2001). Novel NEMO/IkappaB kinase and NF-kappa B target genes at the pre-B to immature B cell transition. *J Biol Chem* 276: 18579–18590.
Lilly B, Galewsky S, Firulli AB, Schulz RA, Olson EN (1994). D-MEF2: a MADS box transcription factor expressed in differentiating mesoderm and muscle cell lineages during *Drosophila* embryogenesis. *Proc Natl Acad Sci USA* 91: 5662–5666.
Lilly B, Zhao B, Ranganayakulu G, Paterson B, Schulz R, Olson E (1995). Requirement of MADS domain transcription factor D-MEF2 for muscle formation in *Drosophila. Science* 267: 688–693.
Lin RC, Scheller RH (2000). Mechanisms of synaptic vesicle exocytosis. *Annu Rev Cell Dev Biol* 16: 19–49.
Lints TJ, Parsons LM, Hartley L, Lyons I, Harvey RP (1993). *Nkx-2.5*: a novel murine homeobox gene expressed in early heart progenitor cells and their myogenic descendants. *Development* 119: 419–431.
Lloyd TE, Verstreken P, Ostrin EJ, Phillippi A, Lichtarge O, Bellen HJ (2000). A genome-wide search for synaptic vesicle cycle proteins in *Drosophila. Neuron* 26: 45–50.
Lyons I, Parsons L, Hartley L, Li R, Andrews J, Robb L, Harvey R (1995). Myogenic and morphogenetic defects in the heart tubes of murine embryoos lacking the homeo box gene *Nkx2-5. Genes Dev* 9: 1654–1666.
Malicki J, Neuhauss SC, Schier AF, Solnica-Krezel L, Stemple DL, Stainier DY, Abdelilah S, Zwartkruis F, Rangini Z, Driever W (1996a). Mutations affecting development of the zebrafish retina. *Development* 123: 263–273.
Malicki J, Schier AF, Solnica-Krezel L, Stemple DL, Neuhauss SC, Stainier DY, Abdelilah S, Rangini Z, Zwartkruis F, Driever W (1996b). Mutations affecting development of the zebrafish ear. *Development* 123: 275–283.
Mark M, Rijli FM, Chambon P (1997). Homeobox genes in embryogenesis and pathogenesis. *Pediatr Res* 42: 421–429.
Marques G, Musacchio M, Shimell MJ, Wunnenberg-Stapleton K, Cho KW, O'Connor MB (1997). Production of a DPP activity gradient in the early *Drosophila* embryo through the opposing actions of the SOG and TLD proteins. *Cell* 91: 417–426.
Mason ED, Konrad KD, Webb CD, Marsh JL (1994). Dorsal midline fate in *Drosophila* embryos requires twisted gastrulation, a gene encoding a secreted protein related to human connective tissue growth factor. *Genes Dev* 8: 1489–1501.
Matsuura T, Sutcliffe JS, Fang P, Galjaard RJ, Jiang YH, Benton CS, Rommens JM, Beaudet AL (1997). De novo truncating mutations in E6-AP ubiquitin-protein ligase gene (*UBE3A*) in Angelman syndrome. *Nat Genet* 15: 74–77.
McDonald JA, Holbrook S, Isshiki T, Weiss J, Doe CQ, Mellerick DM (1998). Dorsoventral patterning in the *Drosophila* central nervous system: the *vnd* homeobox gene specifies ventral column identity. *Genes Dev* 12: 3603–3612.
McGinnis W, Krumlauf R (1992). Homeobox genes and axial patterning. *Cell* 68: 283–302.
Medina A, Wendler SR, Steinbeisser H (1997). Cortical rotation is required for the correct spatial expression of nr3, sia and gsc in *Xenopus* embryos. *Int J Dev Biol* 41: 741–745.
Mellerick DM, Nirenberg M (1995). Dorsal–ventral patterning genes restrict NK-2 homeobox gene expression to the ventral half of the central nervous system of *Drosophila* embryos. *Dev Biol* 171: 306–316.
Meng X, Khanuja BS, Ip YT (1999). Toll receptor-mediated *Drosophila* immune response requires Dif, an NF-kappaB factor. *Genes Dev* 13: 792–797.
Miller JR, Rowning BA, Larabell CA, Yang-Snyder JA, Bates RL, Moon RT (1999). Establishment of the dorsal–ventral axis in *Xenopus* embryos coincides with the dorsal enrichment of dishevelled that is dependent on cortical rotation. *J Cell Biol* 146: 427–437.
Mitchell KJ, Doyle JL, Serafini T, Kennedy TE, Tessier-Lavigne M, Goodman CS, Dickson BJ (1996). Genetic analysis of netrin genes in *Drosophila*: netrins guide CNS commissural axons and peripheral motor axons. *Neuron* 17: 203–215.
Moon RT, Kimelman D (1998). From cortical rotation to organizer gene expression: toward a molecular explanation of axis specification in *Xenopus. Bioessays* 20: 536–545.
Mortlock DP, Post LC, Innis JW (1996). The molecular basis of hypodactyly (Hd): a deletion in Hoxa 13 leads to arrest of digital arch formation. *Nat Genet* 13: 284–289.
Mowbray C, Hammerschmidt M, Whitfield TT (2001). Expression of BMP signalling pathway members in the developing zebrafish inner ear and lateral line. *Mech Dev* 108: 179–184.
Muragaki Y, Mundlos S, Upton J, Olsen BR (1996). Altered growth and branching patterns in synpolydactyly caused by mutations in *HOXD13. Science* 272: 548–551.
Nelson RW, Gumbiner BM (1998). Beta-catenin directly induces expression of the *Siamois* gene, and can initiate signaling indirectly via a membrane-tethered form. *Ann NY Acad Sci* 857: 86–98.
Neuhauss SC, Solnica-Krezel L, Schier AF, Zwartkruis F, Stemple DL, Malicki J, Abdelilah S, Stainier DY, Driever W (1996). Mutations affecting craniofacial development in zebrafish. *Development* 123: 357–367.
Neul JL, Ferguson EL (1998). Spatially restricted activation of the SAX receptor by SCW modulates DPP/TKV signaling in *Drosophila* dorsal–ventral patterning. *Cell* 95: 483–494.
Nguyen M, Park S, Marques G, Arora K (1998). Interpretation of a BMP activity gradient in *Drosophila* embryos depends on synergistic signaling by two type I receptors, SAX and TKV. *Cell* 95: 495–506.
Nieto MA, Bennett MF, Sargent MG, Wilkinson DG (1992). Cloning and developmental expression of Sna, a murine homologue of the *Drosophila snail* gene. *Development* 116: 227–237.
Nusslein-Volhard C, Wieschaus E (1980). Mutations affecting segment number and polarity in *Drosophila. Nature* 287: 795–801.
Odenthal J, Haffter P, Vogelsang E, Brand M, van Eeden FJ, Furutani-Seiki M, Granato M, Hammerschmidt M, Heisenberg CP, Jiang YJ, et al. (1996). Mutations affecting the formation of the notochord in the zebrafish, Danio rerio. *Development* 123: 103–115.
Pack M, Solnica-Krezel L, Malicki J, Neuhauss SC, Schier AF, Stemple DL, Driever W, Fishman MC (1996). Mutations affecting development of zebrafish digestive organs. *Development* 123: 321–328.
Padgett RW, St Johnston RD, Gelbart WM (1987). A transcript from a *Drosophila* pattern gene predicts a protein homologous to the transforming growth factor-beta family. *Nature* 325: 81–84.
Palau F (2001). Friedreich's ataxia and frataxin: molecular genetics, evolution and pathogenesis. *Int J Mol Med* 7: 581–589.

Pallotta BS, Wagoner PK (1992). Voltage-dependent potassium channels since Hodgkin and Huxley. *Physiol Rev* 72: S49–S67.

Panganiban G (2000). Distal-less function during *Drosophila* appendage and sense organ development. *Dev Dyn* 218: 554–562.

Panganiban G, Irvine SM, Lowe C, Roehl H, Corley LS, Sherbon B, Grenier JK, Fallon JF, Kimble J, Walker M, et al. (1997). The origin and evolution of animal appendages. *Proc Natl Acad Sci USA* 94: 5162–5166.

Paznekas WA, Cunningham ML, Howard TD, Korf BR, Lipson MH, Grix AW, Feingold M, Goldberg R, Borochowitz Z, Aleck K, et al. (1998). Genetic heterogeneity of Saethre-Chotzen syndrome, due to TWIST and FGFR mutations. *Am J Hum Genet* 62: 1370–1380.

Pearse RV 2nd, Tabin CJ (1998). The molecular ZPA. *J Exp Zool* 282: 677–690.

Peltonen L, McKusick VA (2001). Genomics and medicine. Dissecting human disease in the postgenomic era. *Science* 291: 1224–1229.

Peterson RL, Papenbrock T, Davda MM, Awgulewitsch A (1994). The murine Hoxc cluster contains five neighboring AbdB-related *hox* genes that show unique spatially coordinated expression in posterior embryonic subregions. *Mech Dev* 47: 253–260.

Piccolo S, Agius E, Lu B, Goodman S, Dale L, De Robertis EM (1997). Cleavage of Chordin by Xolloid metalloprotease suggests a role for proteolytic processing in the regulation of Spemann organizer activity. *Cell* 91: 407–416.

Piccolo S, Sasai Y, Lu B, De Robertis EM (1996). Dorsoventral patterning in *Xenopus*: inhibition of ventral signals by direct binding of chordin to BMP-4. *Cell* 86: 589–598.

Pichaud F, Treisman J, Desplan C (2001). Reinventing a common strategy for patterning the eye. *Cell* 105: 9–12.

Piotrowski T, Schilling TF, Brand M, Jiang YJ, Heisenberg CP, Beuchle D, Grandel H, van Eeden FJ, Furutani-Seiki M, Granato M, et al. (1996). Jaw and branchial arch mutants in zebrafish II: anterior arches and cartilage differentiation. *Development* 123: 345–356.

Quiring R, Walldorf U, Kloter U, Gehring WJ (1994). Homology of the *eyeless* gene of *Drosophila* to the *small eye* gene in mice and aniridia in humans. *Science* 265: 785–789.

Ranganayakulu G, Elliott DA, Harvey RP, Olson EN (1998). Divergent roles of NK-2 class homeobox genes in cardiogenesis in flies and mice. *Development* 125: 3037–3048.

Ransom DG, Haffter P, Odenthal J, Brownlie A, Vogelsang E, Kelsh RN, Brand M, van Eeden FJ, Furutani-Seiki M, Granato M, et al. (1996). Characterization of zebrafish mutants with defects in embryonic hematopoiesis. *Development* 123: 311–319.

Rao Y, Vaessin H, Jan LY, Jan YN (1991). Neuroectoderm in *Drosophila* embryos is dependent on the mesoderm for positioning but not for formation. *Genes Dev* 5: 1577–1588.

Ray RP, Arora K, Nusslein-Volhard C, Gelbart WM (1991). The control of cell fate along the dorsal–ventral axis of the *Drosophila* embryo. *Development* 113: 35–54.

Reiter LT, Potocki L, Chien S, Gribskov M, Bier E (2001). A systematic analysis of human disease-associated gene sequences in *Drosophila melanogaster*. *Genome Res* 11: 1114–1125.

Rodriguez M, Driever W (1997). Mutations resulting in transient and localized degeneration in the developing zebrafish brain. *Biochem Cell Biol* 75: 579–600.

Ross JJ, Shimmi O, Vilmos P, Petryk A, Kim H, Gaudenz K, Hermanson S, Ekker SC, O'Connor MB, Marsh JL (2001). Twisted gastrulation is a conserved extracellular BMP antagonist. *Nature* 410: 479–483.

Roth S, Stein D, Nusslein-Volhard C (1989). A gradient of nuclear localization of the dorsal protein determines dorsoventral pattern in the *Drosophila* embryo. *Cell* 59: 1189–1202.

Rusch J, Levine M (1996). Threshold responses to the dorsal regulatory gradient and the subdivision of primary tissue territories in the *Drosophila* embryo. *Curr Opin Genet Dev* 6: 416–423.

Rusch J, Van Vactor D (2000). New Roundabouts send axons into the Fas lane. *Neuron* 28: 637–640.

Rushlow C, Colosimo PF, Lin MC, Xu M, Kirov N (2001). Transcriptional regulation of the *Drosophila* gene *zen* by competing Smad and Brinker inputs. *Genes Dev* 15: 340–351.

Rushlow C, Frasch M, Doyle H, Levine M (1987). Maternal regulation of *zerknullt*: a homoeobox gene controlling differentiation of dorsal tissues in *Drosophila*. *Nature* 330: 583–586.

Rushlow CA, Han K, Manley JL, Levine M (1989). The graded distribution of the dorsal morphogen is initiated by selective nuclear transport in *Drosophila*. *Cell* 59: 1165–1177.

Rutschmann S, Jung AC, Zhou R, Silverman N, Hoffmann JA, Ferrandon D (2000). Role of *Drosophila* IKK gamma in a toll-independent antibacterial immune response. *Nat Immunol* 1: 342–347.

Sasai Y (2001). Regulation of neural determination by evolutionarily conserved signals: anti-BMP factors and what next? *Curr Opin Neurobiol* 11: 22–26.

Sasai Y, Lu B, Steinbeisser H, De Robertis EM (1995). Regulation of neural induction by the Chd and Bmp-4 antagonistic patterning signals in *Xenopus*. *Nature* 377: 757.

Sasai Y, Lu B, Steinbeisser H, Geissert D, Gont LK, De Robertis EM (1994). *Xenopus* chordin: a novel dorsalizing factor activated by organizer-specific homeobox genes. *Cell* 79: 779–790.

Saunders JW Jr, Gasseling MT (1968). Ectoderm–mesenchymal interaction in the origin of wing symmetry. In: *Epithelial–mesenchymal interactions*. Fleischmajer R, Billingham RE (eds.) Williams and Wilkins, Baltimore, pp. 159–170.

Schier AF, Neuhauss SC, Harvey M, Malicki J, Solnica-Krezel L, Stainier DY, Zwartkruis F, Abdelilah S, Stemple DL, Rangini Z, et al. (1996). Mutations affecting the development of the embryonic zebrafish brain. *Development* 123: 165–78.

Schilling TF, Piotrowski T, Grandel H, Brand M, Heisenberg CP, Jiang YJ, Beuchle D, Hammerschmidt M, Kane DA, Mullins MC, et al. (1996). Jaw and branchial arch mutants in zebrafish I: branchial arches. *Development* 123: 329–344.

Schmidt J, Francois V, Bier E, Kimelman D (1995). *Drosophila* short gastrulation induces an ectopic axis in *Xenopus*: evidence for conserved mechanisms of dorsal–ventral patterning. *Development* 121: 4319–4328.

Schott JJ, Benson DW, Basson CT, Pease W, Silberbach GM, Moak JP, Maron BJ, Seidman CE, Seidman JG (1998). Congenital heart disease caused by mutations in the transcription factor NKX2-5. *Science* 281: 108–111.

Schulte-Merker S, Lee KJ, McMahon AP, Hammerschmidt M (1997). The zebrafish organizer requires chordino. *Nature* 387: 862–863.

Scott IC, Blitz IL, Pappano WN, Maas SA, Cho KW, Greenspan DS (2001). Homologues of Twisted gastrulation are extracellular cofactors in antagonism of BMP signalling. *Nature* 410: 475–478.

Serafini T, Colamarino SA, Leonardo ED, Wang H, Beddington R, Skarnes WC, Tessier-Lavigne M (1996). Netrin-1 is required for commissural axon guidance in the developing vertebrate nervous system. *Cell* 87: 1001–1014.

Serafini T, Kennedy TE, Galko MJ, Mirzayan C, Jessell TM, Tessier-Lavigne M (1994). The netrins define a family of axon outgrowth-promoting proteins homologous to *C. elegans* UNC-6. *Cell* 78: 409–424.

Seto ML, Lee SJ, Sze RW, Cunningham ML (2001). Another TWIST on Baller-Gerold syndrome. *Am J Med Genet* 104: 323–330.

Sharpe J, Nonchev S, Gould A, Whiting J, Krumlauf R (1998). Selectivity, sharing and competitive interactions in the regulation of *Hoxb* genes. *EMBO J* 17: 1788–1798.

Shimell MJ, Ferguson EL, Childs SR, O'Connor MB (1991). The *Drosophila* dorsal-ventral patterning gene *tolloid* is related to human bone morphogenetic protein 1. *Cell* 67:469–481.

Shubin N, Tabin C, Carroll S (1997). Fossils, genes and the evolution of animal limbs. *Nature* 388: 639–648.

Simpson JH, Bland KS, Fetter RD, Goodman CS (2000). Short-range and long-range guidance by Slit and its Robo receptors: a combinatorial code of Robo receptors controls lateral position. *Cell* 103: 1019–1032.

Simpson P (1998). Introduction: Notch signalling and choice of cell fates in development. *Semin Cell Dev Biol* 9: 581–582.

Skeath JB, Carroll SB (1992). Regulation of proneural gene expression and cell fate during neuroblast segregation in the *Drosophila* embryo. *Development* 114: 939–946.

Skeath JB, Panganiban G, Selegue J, Carroll SB (1992). Gene regulation in two dimensions: the proneural *achaete* and *scute* genes are controlled by combinations of axis-patterning genes through a common intergenic control region. *Genes Dev* 6: 2606–2619.

Skeath JB, Panganiban GF, Carroll SB (1994). The ventral nervous system defective gene controls proneural gene expression at two distinct steps during neuroblast formation in *Drosophila*. *Development* 120: 1517–1524.

Smith DE, Franco del Amo F, Gridley T (1992). Isolation of *Sna*, a mouse gene homologous to the *Drosophila* genes *snail* and *escargot*: its expression pattern suggests multiple roles during postimplantation development. *Development* 116: 1033–1039.

Smith JC (2001). Making mesoderm—upstream and downstream of Xbra. *Int J Dev Biol* 45: 219–224.

Smith JC, Price BM, Green JB, Weigel D, Herrmann BG (1991). Expression of a *Xenopus* homolog of Brachyury (T) is an immediate-early response to mesoderm induction. *Cell* 67: 79–87.

Smith WC, Harland RM (1992). Expression cloning of noggin, a new dorsalizing factor localized to the Spemann organizer in *Xenopus* embryos. *Cell* 70: 829–840.

Smith WC, Knecht AK, Wu M, Harland RM (1993). Secreted noggin protein mimics the Spemann organizer in dorsalizing *Xenopus* mesoderm. *Nature* 361: 547–549.

Spemann H, Mangold H (1924). Uber induction von embryonanlagen durch implantation artfremder organis atoren. *Wilhelm Roux Archiv Fur Entwicklungsmechanik der Organismen* 100: 599–638.

Spring J, Yanze N, Middel AM, Stierwald M, Groger H, Schmid V (2000). The mesoderm specification factor twist in the life cycle of jellyfish. *Dev Biol* 228: 363–375.

Srinivasan S, Rashka KE, Bier E (2002). Creation of a Sog morphogen gradient in the *Drosophila* embryo. *Dev Cell* 2: 91–101.

Stainier DY, Fouquet B, Chen JN, Warren KS, Weinstein BM, Meiler SE, Mohideen MA, Neuhauss SC, Solnica-Krezel L, Schier AF, et al. (1996). Mutations affecting the formation and function of the cardiovascular system in the zebrafish embryo. *Development* 123: 285–292.

Steinbeisser H, De Robertis EM (1993). *Xenopus* goosecoid: a gene expressed in the prechordal plate that has dorsalizing activity. *C R Acad Sci III* 316: 959–971.

Stemple DL, Solnica-Krezel L, Zwartkruis F, Neuhauss SC, Schier AF, Malicki J, Stainier DY, Abdelilah S, Rangini Z, Mountcastle-Shah E, et al. (1996). Mutations affecting development of the notochord in zebrafish. *Development* 123: 117–128.

Stennard F (1998). *Xenopus* differentiation: VegT gets specific. *Curr Biol* 8: R928–R930.

Steward R (1989). Relocalization of the dorsal protein from the cytoplasm to the nucleus correlates with its function. *Cell* 59: 1179–1188.

Stoilov I, Akarsu AN, Sarfarazi M (1997). Identification of three different truncating mutations in cytochrome P4501B1 (CYP1B1) as the principal cause of primary congenital glaucoma (Buphthalmos) in families linked to the GLC3A locus on chromosome 2p21. *Hum Mol Genet* 6: 641–647.

Streit A, Stern CD (1999). Neural induction. A bird's eye view. *Trends Genet* 15: 20–24.

Streit A, Lee KJ, Woo I, Roberts C, Jessell TM, Stern CD (1998). Chordin regulates primitive streak development and the stability of induced neural cells, but is not sufficient for neural induction in the chick embryo. *Development* 125: 507–519.

Sumoy L, Kiefer J, Kimelman D (1999). Conservation of intracellular Wnt signaling components in dorsal–ventral axis formation in zebrafish. *Dev Genes Evol* 209: 48–58.

Taylor MV, Beatty KE, Hunter HK, Baylies MK (1995). *Drosophila* MEF2 is regulated by twist and is expressed in both the primordia and differentiated cells of the embryonic somatic, visceral and heart musculature [erratum appears in *Mech Dev* 1995;51:139–41]. *Mech Dev* 50: 29–41.

Tear G, Harris R, Sutaria S, Kilomanski K, Goodman CS, Seeger MA (1996). Commissureless controls growth cone guidance across the CNS midline in *Drosophila* and encodes a novel membrane protein. *Neuron* 16: 501–514.

Thisse B, Stoetzel C, Gorostiza-Thisse C, Perrin-Schmitt F (1988). Sequence of the *twist* gene and nuclear localization of its protein in endomesodermal cells of early *Drosophila* embryos. *EMBO J* 7: 2175–2183.

Thisse C, Perrin-Schmitt F, Stoetzel C, Thisse B (1991). Sequence-specific transactivation of the *Drosophila twist* gene by the dorsal gene product. *Cell* 65: 1191–1201.

Trowe T, Klostermann S, Baier H, Granato M, Crawford AD, Grunewald B, Hoffmann H, Karlstrom RO, Meyer SU, Muller B, et al. (1996). Mutations disrupting the ordering and topographic mapping of axons in the retinotectal projection of the zebrafish, *Danio rerio*. *Development* 123: 439–450.

von Ohlen T, Doe CQ (2000). Convergence of dorsal, dpp, and egfr signaling pathways subdivides the *Drosophila* neuroectoderm into three dorsal–ventral columns. *Dev Biol* 224: 362–372.

von Salvini-Plawen L, Mayr E (1977). On the evolution of photoreceptors and eyes. *Evol Biol* 10: 207–263.

Walther C, Gruss P (1991). *Pax-6*, a murine paired box gene, is expressed in the developing CNS. *Development* 113: 1435–1449.

Wang M, Sternberg PW (2001). Pattern formation during *C. elegans* vulval induction. *Curr Top Dev Biol* 51: 189–220.

Wasserman SA (2000). Toll signaling: the enigma variations. *Curr Opin Genet Dev* 10: 497–502.

Wawersik S, Maas RL (2000). Vertebrate eye development as modeled in *Drosophila*. *Hum Mol Genet* 9: 917–925.

Weiss JB, Von Ohlen T, Mellerick DM, Dressler G, Doe CQ, Scott MP (1998). Dorsoventral patterning in the *Drosophila* central nervous system: the intermediate neuroblasts defective homeobox gene specifies intermediate column identity. *Genes Dev* 12: 3591–3602.

Wharton KA, Ray RP, Gelbart WM (1993). An activity gradient of decapentaplegic is necessary for the specification of dorsal pattern elements in the *Drosophila* embryo. *Development* 117: 807–822.

Whitfield TT, Granato M, van Eeden FJ, Schach U, Brand M, Furutani-Seiki M, Haffter P, Hammerschmidt M, Heisenberg CP, Jiang YJ, et al. (1996). Mutations affecting development of the zebrafish inner ear and lateral line. *Development* 123: 241–254.

Wilkinson DG, Bhatt S, Herrmann BG (1990). Expression pattern of the mouse T gene and its role in mesoderm formation. *Nature* 343: 657–659.

Wilson PA, Hemmati-Brivanlou A (1995). Induction of epidermis and inhibition of neural fate by Bmp-4. *Nature* 376: 331–333.

Woods IG, Kelly PD, Chu F, Ngo-Hazelett P, Yan YL, Huang H, Postlethwait JH, Talbot WS (2000). A comparative map of the zebrafish genome. *Genome Res* 10: 1903–1914.

Wu JY, Rao Y (1999). Fringe: defining borders by regulating the notch pathway. *Curr Opin Neurobiol* 9: 537–543.

Wu MN, Bellen HJ (1997). Genetic dissection of synaptic transmission in *Drosophila*. *Curr Opin Neurobiol* 7: 624–630.

Xanthos JB, Kofron M, Wylie C, Heasman J (2001). Maternal VegT is the initiator of a molecular network specifying endoderm in *Xenopus laevis*. *Development* 128: 167–180.

Xu X, Meiler SE, Zhong TP, Mohideen M, Crossley DA, Burggren WW, Fishman MC (2002). Cardiomyopathy in zebrafish due to mutation in an alternatively spliced exon of titin. *Nat Genet* 30: 205–209.

Yin Z, Xu XL, Frasch M (1997). Regulation of the *twist* target gene *tinman* by modular *cis*-regulatory elements during early mesoderm development. *Development* 124: 4971–4982.

Yu K, Srinivasan S, Shimmi O, Biehs B, Rashka KE, Kimelman D, O'Connor MB, Bier E (2000). Processing of the *Drosophila* Sog protein creates a novel BMP inhibitory activity. *Development* 127: 2143–2154.

Zákány J, Duboule D (1999). Hox genes in digit development and evolution. *Cell and Tissue Research* 296: 19–25.

Zerucha T, Ekker M (2000). Distal-less-related homeobox genes of vertebrates: evolution, function, and regulation. *Biochem Cell Biol* 78: 593–601.

Zhang H, Levine SE, Ashe HL (2001). Brinker is a sequence-specific transcriptional repressor in the *Drosophila* embryo. *Genes Dev* 15: 261–266.

Zhang J, King ML (1996). *Xenopus* VegT RNA is localized to the vegetal cortex during oogenesis and encodes a novel T-box transcription factor involved in mesodermal patterning. *Development* 122: 4119–4129.

Zhang J, Houston DW, King ML, Payne C, Wylie C, Heasman J (1998). The role of maternal VegT in establishing the primary germ layers in *Xenopus* embryos. *Cell* 94: 515–524.

4 | Consequences of the Genome Project for Understanding Development

DAVID W. MOUNT

The availability of the human and mouse genomes and the genomes of lower organisms has provided developmental biologists with powerful new tools for identifying genes that control development and for analyzing the function, organization, expression, and evolution of these genes. This chapter explains how genomes are analyzed to discover genes that have the same function. Recent experiments in which this information is used in an effort to reconstruct the evolutionary changes that gave rise to species divergence and morphological variation, the "evo-devo" perspective, are then discussed. These analyses are revealing important underlying principles that should help human developmental biologists understand the genetic and evolutionary basis of the diseases they study.

INTRODUCTION TO GENOME PROJECTS

Between the late 1990s and 2002, the complete genome sequences of several eukaryotic organisms, including the human (Lander et al., 2001; Venter et al., 2001), mouse, *Drosophila melanogaster* (Rubin et al., 2000), worm (*Caenorhabditis elegans*) (Chervitz et al., 1998), and budding yeast (*Saccharomyces cerevesiae*), were established. In addition, the genomes of several dozen prokaryotic organisms have been sequenced (see http://www.tigr.org/). Although the precise order of the genes in the human and mouse genomes has not been finally determined, there is enough information to compare gene content and gene order for most of the 30,000–40,000 genes.

Genome sequences are obtained by cloning chromosome fragments into artificial bacterial chromosomes (BACs) and then into smaller fragments of about 500 bp suitable for automatic sequencing. BACs are then assembled into longer units (contigs) by searching for overlapping fragments that have the same sequences. The process is either driven manually, using a map of physical markers (common patterns of restriction enzyme recognition sites), or automatically by having the computer make a comparison of all combinations of fragments to produce a reasonable linear order of the fragments. The former method was used by a consortium of research groups headed by the Whitehead Institute at the Massachusetts Institute of Technology to sequence the human genome (Lander et al., 2001), the latter by Celera, a company originally established by Craig Venter for the purpose of sequencing the human genome (Venter et al., 2001). The presence of repeats makes the gene-ordering process error-prone. Hence, later drafts of the sequence will be prepared as the gene orders are more accurately determined. These sequences also will not be the same for any particular individual.

GENOME SEQUENCE POLYMORPHISMS

Every individual in the human population, except identical twins, has a unique sequence that differs from the sequence of every other individual by one change in every 500–1000 bp. The process of genome sequencing needs to take into account these between-individual, between-population, and between-race polymorphisms, which may influence phenotype. These important variations will affect the level or activity of particular proteins. In humans, some of these differences will be disease-producing variations located within the exons of genes or may lie outside of, and close to, such variant genes. These linked sequence variations are important because they can potentially aid in the identification of both single loci and sets of loci that produce disease. The most common type of variation is the single nucleotide polymorphism (SNP). Great efforts are being expended to collect sequence polymorphisms and to identify those that are correlated with a disease state. Analysis of such data requires an appreciation of the human population structure since the expression of a particular allele may depend on the presence or absence of other genetic variability in the genome. A large number of publicly funded and commercial sources are collecting information on hundreds of thousands of SNPs (e.g., Table 4–1). A far bigger challenge then will arise: to find which of these polymorphisms are associated with disease.

GENE PREDICTION AND VERIFICATION TO GENERATE PROTEIN SEQUENCES

Once sequences approximating the order of genes in the chromosomes have been found, attention is turned to identifying the gene sequences themselves. The problem boils down to trying to predict the location of transcription start and stop signals and intron sequences in the genome sequence. This process of tagging the genome sequence with bits of information is referred to as *annotation*. Following annotation for predicted transcription signals, the exon sequences can be joined to produce a gene model or prediction of the mRNA sequences, which then can be translated into a protein sequence. The total of the predicted protein sequences is known as the *proteome* of the organism. Mathematical models based on the sequence variations that are observed in known genes are used to predict the location of introns of other unidentified genes in the genome sequence. Because introns are generally large and numerous in mammalian genes, this procedure is error-prone and most likely will predict only a portion of the gene correctly.

The only dependable way to obtain the sequence of a gene is to recover its mRNA product from a cell that expresses the gene, produce a cDNA copy of the gene, and sequence that cDNA copy. Since alternative splicing of the mRNA in different tissues or at different stages of development may produce different mRNA sequences or editing of the mRNA may sometimes occur, the laboratory may need to examine the expression of the gene under different conditions. Research groups that are interested in a single gene will identify that cDNA molecule and sequence it. However, many research groups collect very large numbers of partial mRNA sequences at one time (expressed sequence tags) and sequence them without taking the time to isolate a single mRNA molecule. These are partial sequences that generally start at the 3' end of the mRNA from the polyA tail but also go as far as possible toward the 5' end of the mRNA. As done with genomic sequences, these partial sequences may be assembled into contigs, which predict most and perhaps all the mRNA sequence. The contigs may be used to help design further experiments for sequencing the entire mRNA and looking for alternative splicing of mRNAs. Obtaining most gene sequences remains a slow laboratory task. However, the sequences of all expressed genes in human cells will likely become available by 2005. These sequences are needed to provide accurate mRNA sequence information for translation into protein sequences. Until that information is available, it is important to keep in mind that gene predictions provide only an approximate idea of the gene content of human cells. However, this information is sufficient to make comparisons to other genomes and to infer the location and function of all genes in the human genome.

Table 4–1. List of Internet Resources for Exploration of the Human Genome and for Comparison of the Human, Mouse, and Fly Genomes

List of human genome research sites at Oak Ridge National Laboratories
  http://www.ornl.gov/hgmis/research/centers.html
Access to human map linkages
  University of California, Santa Cruz Human Genome Project Working Draft http://genome.ucsc.edu
  e! The ENSEMBL human genome server http://www.ensembl.org/Homo_sapiens
  Locus link at National Center of Biotechnology Information http://www.ncbi.nlm.nih.gov/LocusLink
  Celera http://www.celera.com
Single-nucleotide polymorphisms in the human genome
  The SNP Consortium http://snp.cshl.org/
Mouse and fly comparisons
  Mouse Genome Informatics at Jackson Laboratories http://www.informatics.jax.org/
  Cooperative Human Linkage Center at the National Cancer Institute http://lpg.nci.nih.gov/htmlchlc/ChlcIntegratedMaps.html
  Comparing fly and human genes at the University of California at San Diego http://homophila.sdsc.edu/ (Reiter et al. 2001)
  The gene ontology system for functional classification of genes http://www.geneontology.org/

GENOME COMPARISONS

Related genomes are compared in two ways: the classes of proteins encoded by the genomes and the relative order of the genes that encode these proteins on the genomes. Analysis of all known proteins has revealed three quite startling discoveries (Mount, 2001). The first is that all known proteins have been classified into families based on sequence similarity and into structural fold classes based on structural similarity. Remarkably, proteins are not individual entities. Instead, proteins can be classified into 1000–2000 families based on identity of 50% or more of the amino acids in an alignment of the proteins. These families are believed to arise by repeated gene duplication events in which a new copy of a gene is sometimes replicated adjacent to an existing gene copy (Fig. 4–1). The new sets of genes then can acquire new functions, leaving the earlier sets to provide the original functions. Detailed analyses of gene content in genomes are finding evidence of recent evolutionary duplications in genomes. The duplication can be abortive, leading to production of an unexpressed pseudogene, or productive, leading to a new biological function. Such family expansions by repeated gene duplication events have allowed organisms to develop new biochemical and developmental mechanisms. Many of the gene families in humans are also found in other mammals and, therefore, were developed in an ancestor organism. A second surprise about proteins is that of all the thousands of ways of arranging combinations of secondary structural elements into a three-dimensional configuration, designated a *structural fold*, only 500 have actually been found in an analysis of thousands of structures by experimental methods. This means that many different proteins having entirely different sequences (and, therefore, being in different families) can adopt the same structural fold and that this same fold can provide diverse functions. The relationship of family to fold can be quite complex. Commonly, the same sequence in two families means a similar structural fold. Sometimes, however, two proteins with identical biochemical activities due to a conserved spatial pattern of particular amino acids in an active site have entirely different sequences and folds, thus indicating evolutionary convergence on a single function from two different genetic starting points. The third and final surprise about proteins is that they are comprised of conserved patches of amino acid sequence or sequence building blocks known as *domains*. A given protein may have one or more domains, and protein families tend to have a similar domain composition. Domains are moved around between proteins probably by recombination-like mechanisms, or they are amplified in number within a protein (Fig. 4–2). Domains sometimes correspond to a known structural fold. In

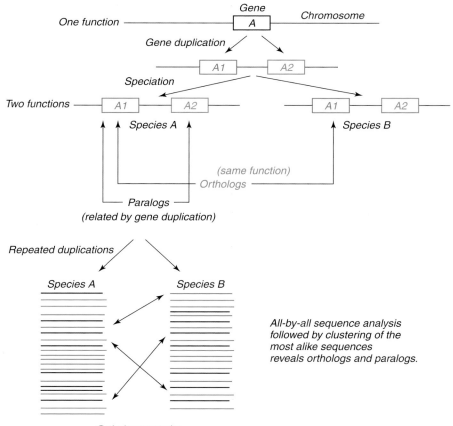

Figure 4–1. Origin of gene families by gene duplication events.

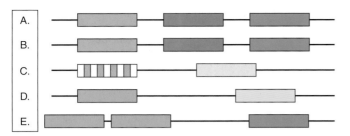

Figure 4–2. Domain structure of hypothetical protein sequences. Proteins are comprised of functional domains defined by conserved amino acid sequences. All five proteins shown have one domain in common, shown in red. The red domain in sequence *C* has evolved somewhat as illustrated by intermittent color, but the remaining residual similarity is sufficient to identify the domain. Of the proteins shown, only *A* and *B* share the same set of sequence domains. If they are from two different organisms and are more alike than any other gene pair between the organisms, they are predicted to be orthologs with the same function. *A* and *B* also include a minor amount of other sequence that is not conserved. These additional sequences may include domains that have not been identified. More complex domain variations are illustrated. *C* and *D* have additional domains (light blue and orange) not present in *A* and *B* and lack two of the conserved domains in *A* and *B*. In sequence *E*, a duplication of the red domain has occurred, probably modifying the associated function of the domain. The green domain present in *A* and *B* is also in *E*, but the blue domain is absent. These sequences share an evolutionary background, but the rearrangements that gave rise to them may be very difficult to reconstruct. If found at adjacent positions on a chromosome, they probably have arisen by gene duplication events, as described in Figure 4–1, a feature of paralogs.

other cases, a relationship has not yet been identified. The best method for identifying known domains in a protein is to search them for sequence variations that are typical of that domain. The interpro resource at http://www.ebi.ac.uk/interpro/ provides a set of domain models that may be used.

Given the above three features of proteins, the proteome of an organism can be analyzed for the presence of proteins that represent known families, a new family represented by orphan genes with no known ancestor, proteins with a particular structural fold, and proteins with a particular domain. The positions of genes on chromosomes sometimes can also provide useful information because closeness implies relatedness dating back to gene duplication events. However, these relationships are often lost due to chromosomal rearrangements taking place over evolutionary time (Mount, 2001).

Comparisons of gene order (*synteny*) in the mouse and human chromosomes have revealed that in localized regions gene order is approximately the same, whereas in larger regions the order is different. Mouse chromosomes can be generated by cutting the human chromosomes and rejoining them in a new order. Repeating this process at least 100 independent times approximately reconstructs the mouse genome. These rearrangements presumably have resulted from a mechanism of random breakage and joining of the human ancestor chromosomes. Attempts have been made to compute mathematically the minimal number of steps that would be required. Based on these types of comparison, it has been proposed that all mammalian chromosomes are rearrangements of approximately the same basic set of genes (O'Brien et al., 1999). Due to the expected origin of genes from gene duplications events, closely linked genes can be predicted to have similar sequences and functions. Therefore, examining localized gene content may be a useful predictive tool for function. However, if clusters of related genes were originally present in an ancestor chromosome, they may have also become disseminated to different locations by chromosomal rearrangements.

GENE-BY-GENE AND PROTEIN-BY-PROTEIN COMPARISONS

There is no simple way to predict the function of a new protein just by examining its sequence. Instead, a search can be made to see if the new sequence can be aligned with a second sequence whose function is known. If the alignment is sufficiently convincing, then the two se-

quences are likely to have the same three-dimensional structure and biochemical activity as well as the same, or a related, biological function. Many human and mouse proteins are comprised of very similar sequences. Protein sequences similar to those of humans and mice may also be encoded by more distantly evolved genomes, such as *Drosophila*, thus revealing that the structure and function of the protein have been conserved over long periods of evolutionary time. However, the genome sequences that specify these proteins are commonly different.

The genome sequence that specifies a particular gene includes the promoter sequence and the introns and the exons within that gene. The genome sequence of the homologous gene in a closely related species (e.g., human vs. mouse) can be quite different due to evolutionary divergence of the genome sequences. The reason is that intron sequences, intron–exon boundaries, use of the genetic code, and other types of evolutionary variation can vary from one genome to the next due to sequence drift during evolution. Hence, a cardinal rule in comparing the gene sequences of two genomes is first to translate them into protein sequences and then to compare the resulting protein sequences. Accordingly, genome-by-genome comparisons generally compare the gene content based on the collective set of predicted proteins, or the proteome.

MODEL ORGANISMS

For the past century, geneticists have used genetic tools to dissect how genes control the metabolism, reproduction, and development of model organisms. At the same time, biochemists and molecular biologists have discovered many of the mechanisms whereby the protein products of these genes regulate biological processes. These model organisms include microbial genomes, the budding yeast *S. cerevisiae*, the worm (nematode) *C. elegans*, the plant *Arabidopsis thaliana*, and the fruit fly *D. melanogaster*. The mouse *Mus musculus* is a genetic model for humans since the two species are so closely related through evolution. As DNA sequencing technology became available, the DNA sequences that encoded the best understood genes became available and were deposited into sequence databases such as GenBank, maintained at the National Center of Biotechnology Information (NCBI), a branch of the U.S. National Library of Medicine (http://www.ncbi.nlm.nih.gov/). The mRNA sequences encoded by the chromosomes could then be quite readily translated to produce the amino acid sequence of the corresponding protein. These protein sequences then became a sequence signature for that particular protein in other organisms. These homologous genes could be found by searching for nucleic acid sequences in these organisms that, when translated, produced a similar protein sequence. The newly identified gene is then predicted to have a similar biological function in the second organism. The NCBI BLAST resource at the above internet address is generally used for this purpose.

As DNA sequencing technology developed further, interest turned toward obtaining the complete genome sequence of model organisms and the human genome and storing these sequences in GenBank so that they could be searched for new genes and the corresponding proteins. A newly identified gene sequence may be compared to the existing database of sequences by aligning the predicted protein sequences. If a gene of unknown function is similar to another of a known function, then the first gene is predicted to have the same function. However, not all gene functions can be identified in this manner. Even in the simplest model organisms, such as *Escherichia coli* and yeast, the functions of only a fraction of the genes are known based on experiment. Hence, different organisms are frequently found to contain the same gene but the function of the gene is not known in either organism. Knowledge of protein domains is helping to alleviate this problem since unknown sequences can be searched for amino acid signatures indicative of structure or biochemical activity. If present, these signatures provide a clue as to function.

If two predicted protein sequences from two genomes are similar enough to produce a convincing alignment of amino acids, then the genes are predicted to have a similar function. Many human genes found to produce disease, for example, are similar to fruit fly genes at the protein sequence level (Rubin et al., 2000). Mutations in the fly gene then provide a biological model for the human disease. In the Homophila project, protein sequences of genes listed in OMIM have been compared to known and predicted *Drosophila* sequences from the *Drosophila* Genome Project, and 714 matching sequences are shown on the web site (Table 4–1) (Reiter et al., 2001). In some cases, a mutation in the functionally homologous gene may not be available. In such cases, disruption of a fly gene by insertion of a transposable element may be used. Similar comparisons may be made between homologous mouse and human genes. A mouse gene inactivated by directed mutagenesis methods (a genetically modified mouse with a knock-out mutation) is now commonly used to examine the effect of mutations in those genes. Table 4–1 lists internet resources that may be utilized for making genome comparisons that can provide the information needed for such experiments. The identification of homologous genes in such different organisms requires an understanding of what constitutes genetic homology.

THE REAL MEANING OF HOMOLOGY

Homology is a term borrowed from evolutionary biology. When a conserved biological function is found between two species, then that function is described as a "homologous" function. There must exist a common ancestor of the two species which had the same function, and these two present species are descendents of this common ancestor. The function is so similar that the chance of it evolving twice by two independent sets of genetic events is extremely small. Thus, because the developmental processes in two organisms are conserved or because two similar organs may exist, they are described as "homologous."

Genes in two organisms are also described as homologous when they are similar at the nucleotide level or when the encoded proteins are so similar at the amino acid sequence level that they almost certainly derived from a common ancestor. Biologists often describe genes as, for example, 40% homologous, meaning that the sequences of the genes or encoded proteins are 40% similar.

Similarity is a measurement made from an optimal sequence alignment of the proteins (Mount, 2001). The alignment includes pairs of aligned amino acids and a few gaps opposite some amino acids that could not be matched with one in the other sequence. The aligned amino acid pairs include identical amino acids, conservative substitutions in which the amino acids are frequently found substituted for each other in related proteins, and mismatched pairs of amino acids which are rarely, if ever, found substituted for each other. The similarity is the fraction of the aligned positions that include identities plus the fraction that includes conservative substitutions. The higher the similarity, the more closely related the proteins and the more likely they are to be homologous.

With the knowledge that proteins are comprised of functional domains, the fraction of each sequence that is included in the alignment of the proteins must also be considered. Figure 4–2 illustrates some possible variations within a hypothetical group of proteins. Although choices should be based on knowledge of specific domains, one criterion may be used. In general, if more than two-thirds of each sequence is included in the alignment, the proteins have a comparable domain structure. Sequences *A* and *B* in Figure 4–2 are examples. However, if only a fraction of each protein sequence is present in the alignment, then the proteins share a domain that can be further analyzed. If the alignment of two sequences within a domain has significant length and sequence similarity, then that domain probably came from a common ancestor domain and represents a homologous relationship. However, the evolutionary history of that domain may be difficult to track since gene rearrangements may have occurred. Sometimes two proteins that have the same conserved amino acid positions in their active sites but are otherwise different at the sequence and secondary structure levels may have two different genetic starting points (Mount, 2001). Thus, two proteins with the same function may have entirely different sequences, indicating that the ancestor genes of these proteins independently converged on the same function.

WHAT GENOME PROJECTS HAVE REVEALED ABOUT GENE FAMILIES

The known and predicted genes of one species may be compared with those of a second organism. In comparing closely related organisms, e.g., mouse and human, in which most genes have been conserved through evolution, these comparisons reveal where homologous genes are located. Some internet sites that allow a visualization of the variations are listed in Table 4–1. From this information, syntenic regions with conserved gene order can be derived, and the types of genome rearrangement that have occurred can be determined.

For more distantly related species that share some developmental processes, e.g., humans and flies, these comparisons provide information as to gene function using the vast amount of genetic and developmental information available for flies. As these comparisons have been extended to other species, genes have been found to occur in families derived from an ancestor gene in a common branch of the evolutionary tree. These genes are *paralogous*, meaning that they originated from repeated gene duplication events followed by evolutionary divergence of the duplicated genes, as illustrated in Figure 4–1. Activities of the resulting proteins may differ slightly or may have acquired a new function by mutation and natural selection. They may also be produced at different stages of development or in different tissues. Sometimes alternative splicing and RNA editing in different tissues may modify the mRNA sequence and the protein sequence so that there is an altered function. If the same gene family is represented in two different species, a cluster analysis may be performed to discover which of the synthesized proteins are most alike and therefore likely to have the same function. The corresponding genes are described as "orthologous." By these types of analysis, much can be learned about the evolution of gene families that influence development.

THE EVO-DEVO PERSPECTIVE OF THE EVOLUTIONARY CONSERVATION OF GENES CONTROLLING DEVELOPMENT

As described above, one commonly used type of genome analysis proceeds by trying to identify those genes in different organisms that serve the same function. Searches are made in the genomes of two organisms for genes whose sequences are sufficiently similar that the two must certainly have the same biological function. Moreover, the two have originated from a common ancestor gene in the evolutionary past. If mutations in one of the genes produce a mutant phenotype, say, a particular developmental defect, then the other gene presumably also has a similar developmental role. This conclusion holds true even though the organisms may have quite different developmental cycles and may be quite unrelated, as in the case of fruit flies and mammals.

Such observations of similar developmental genes have been made sufficiently often that developmental biologists have come to the conclusion that developmentally divergent organisms use the same basic tool kit of genes. They propose that developmental variation is due not so much to variation in the genes that are used for controlling the stages of development as to variation in which genes in this evolutionarily conserved tool kit are used and how they are regulated. This evo-devo view of development (Tautz, 2002) focuses developmental research on identifying the basic set of genes in organisms and then studying how they are regulated in developing cells and tissues. Eric H. Davidson and colleagues (2002) have shown that development of the sea urchin body plan is controlled by large networks of regulatory genes. Analysis of these networks involves a detailed functional identification of specific transcription factors and *cis*-acting binding sites for these factors.

As an extension of this approach, developmental biologists may try to trace the evolutionary and developmental origins of genes that have a possibly related biological feature by searching for them in distantly related organisms. Thus, based on the presence of similar sequences, biologist Walter Gehring (2002) has proposed that eyes evolved only once and may have originated as a light-sensitive body in a microbe that eventually became a chloroplast. However, other evo-devo studies suggest that variations in the genes themselves are also important for evolution and development.

Biologist Claudia Kappen reported that a particular inbred strain of mice can have either a normal or a highly defective skeleton due to the presence of immature cartilage simply by altering the diet (Pennisi, 2002). It appeared that expression of an apparently faulty Hox gene could be suppressed by a substance in the diet. This type of observation has given rise to the notion that accumulated mutations in an important developmental gene may not be expressed until an environmental change occurs (Pennisi, 2002). As in these mice, most of these changes may be deleterious or neutral; but, as with evolution in general, a few of them may be beneficial so that a new developmental scheme appears under the influence of natural selection. The great diversity observed in butterfly wings is also being analyzed from an evolutionary developmental biology perspective and has revealed a link between genetic variation and the phenotypes that are produced. This variation is also considered to be due to the action of natural selection on developmental processes (Beldade and Brakefield, 2002).

CONCLUSION

Comparison of protein sequences encoded by human genes with proteins of other species and similar comparisons among other species have revealed that many genes, including those important for development, have been remarkably conserved through evolutionary time. Fly (*D. melanogaster*) and mouse genes can provide suitable models for human disease. Many genes are members of paralogous families, resulting from repeated gene duplication events. These families share a high degree of sequence similarity. Gene comparisons need to take into account these known family relationships. Care must be taken if the most reliable predictions of orthologous proteins with the same conserved function are to be made. Proteins are also comprised of domains. Proteins that share multiple domains or that align throughout most of their sequence are the most closely related. Other proteins that are only partially similar share domains but are less likely to have a similar biological role.

The availability of genome information, including the location and organization of genes and the above relationships among the encoded proteins, presents the mammalian developmental geneticist with new approaches for learning more about the variations that are observed. One can use not only genetic studies of developmental genes in other organisms as a basis for understanding developmental abnormalities in humans but also information on natural variation in these genes and variation in the way these genes are regulated.

ACKNOWLEDGMENTS

The assistance of Dr. Lisa Nagy in discussing the evo-devo concept is gratefully acknowledged.

REFERENCES

Beldade P, Brakefield PM (2002). The genetics and evo devo of butterfly wing patterns. *Nat Rev Genet* 3: 442–452.

Chervitz SA, Aravind L, Sherlock G, Ball CA, Koonin EV, Dwight SS, Harris MA, Dolinski K, Mohr S, Smith T, et al. (1998). Comparison of the complete protein sets of worm and yeast: orthology and divergence. *Science* 282: 2022–2028.

Davidson EH, Rast JP, Oliveri P, Ransick A, Calestani C, Yuh C, Minokawa T, 1 Amore G, Hinman V, Arenas-Mena C, et al. (2002). A genomic regulatory network for development. *Science* 295: 1669–1678.

Gehring WJ (2002). The genetic control of eye development and its implications for the evolution of the various eye-types. *Int J Dev Biol* 46: 65–73.

Lander ES, Linton LM, Birren B, Nusbaum C, Zody MC, Baldwin J, Devon K, Dewar K, Doyle M, FitzHugh W, et al. (2001). Initial sequencing and analysis of the human genome. *Nature* 409: 860–921.

Mount, DW (2001). *Bioinformatics: Sequence and Genome Analysis*. Cold Spring Harbor Laboratory Press, Cold Spring Harbor, NY.

O'Brien SJ, Menotti-Raymond M, Murphy WJ, Nash WG, Wienberg J, Stanyon R, Copeland NG, Jenkins NA, Womack JE, Marshall Graves JA (1999). The promise of comparative genomics in mammals. *Science* 286:458–462, 479–481.

Pennisi E (2002). Evo-devo devotees eye ocular origins and more. *Science* 296: 1010–1011.

Reiter LT, Potocki L, Chien S, Gribskov M, Bier E (2001). A systematic analysis of human disease-associated gene sequences in *Drosophila melanogaster*. *Genome Res* 11: 1114–1125.

Rubin GM, Yandell MD, Wortman JR, Gabor Miklos GL, Nelson CR, Hariharan IK, Fortini ME, Li PW, Apweiler R, Fleischmann W, et al. (2000). The genome sequence of *Drosophila melanogaster*. *Science* 287: 2204–2215.

Tautz D (2002). Evo-devo graduates to new levels. *Trends Genet* 18: 66–67.

Venter JC, Adams MD, Myers EW, Li PW, Mural RJ, Sutton GG, Smith HO, Yandell M, Evans CA, Holt RA, Gocayne JD, et al. (2001). The sequence of the human genome. *Science* 291: 1304–1351.

II
PATTERNS OF DEVELOPMENT

5 | Developmental Origins of the Mammalian Body Plan

MICHAEL M. SHEN AND ROGER A. PEDERSEN

CONCEPT OF THE BODY PLAN

The concept of the *body plan* refers to the distinguishing features of our bodies as organized three-dimensional structures. Like other vertebrates, mammals are bilaterally symmetrical quadripeds. As such, vertebrates and their close evolutionary relatives are readily distinguished from more distantly related organisms, such as sea anemones with radially symmetrical bodies and starfish with their fivefold symmetry. The vertebrate body plan is marked not only by its bilateral symmetry but also by its polarity, most notably the differences between head and tail features (anterior/posterior [A/P] polarity) and back and front features (dorsal/ventral [D/V] polarity). These asymmetries along two of the major body axes have profound consequences for all aspects of our lives, determining how we eat, move, communicate, and reproduce. Not surprisingly, then, these asymmetrical body axes and their polarity emerge during embryonic development. Moreover, our body's mirror image bilateral symmetry is not absolute but encompasses asymmetries, such as the sidedness of our heart, lungs, stomach, and other organs. This midline symmetry and its exceptions also arise during embryonic development. How the mammalian embryo acquires its body axes with their familiar symmetries and asymmetries is the subject of this chapter.

ORIGINS AND EMERGENCE OF AXIAL ORGANIZATION

The major body axes of a frog or fish embryo become evident within a few hours of fertilization of the egg by a sperm. Identification of the A/P and D/V axes of a frog embryo is aided by the relatively large size of the egg (1–2 mm) and by the reciprocal distribution of pigment and yolk, which also facilitate analysis of how embryonic axes emerge. Conversely, the zygote of eutherian (as distinct from marsupial and monotreme) mammals is small (~0.1 mm diameter), transparent, and virtually featureless, making it difficult to locate landmarks for analysis of any polarity that might be present at the earliest developmental stages. Moreover, mammalian embryos of all eutherian species that have been studied have the remarkable ability of being able to compensate for almost any disturbances in embryonic organization that occur before the embryo's implantation into the uterine wall. Thus, there has been no rush to examine such "preimplantation" stages of mammalian embryos for the emergence of polarity. Instead, the first obvious appearance of A/P polarity at the onset of gastrulation, 1 week after fertilization in the mouse and 2 in the human, was taken as the point of origin for the mammalian body plan (reviewed by Zernicka-Goetz, 2002). However, studies on the development of polarity in mouse embryos point to an earlier origin of embryonic axes in mammalian species and have led to an examination of the organizational role of the precociously differentiating extraembryonic tissues, trophoblast and hypoblast, that were previously thought to have mainly protective and nutritive roles. Finally, the mechanisms responsible for the emergence of the embryo's A/P and D/V axes, which together define the plane of bilateral symmetry (thus, the location of the left and right sides), have been investigated extensively. Surprisingly, the molecular mechanisms responsible for defining the primary embryonic axes also prompt the departures from left/right (L/R) mirror-image symmetry. Thus, we can understand the origins of the mammalian body plan by focusing on genes that are activated during the first fortnight of embryonic life.

MOLECULAR MECHANISMS ESTABLISHING EMBRYONIC POLARITY

As is well known, the major intercellular signaling pathways are used reiteratively during embryogenesis; these are reviewed extensively in later chapters. However, two key signaling pathways figure prominently during the pregastrulation and gastrulation stages of development and are described here.

Nodal Signaling Pathway

The *Nodal* gene was originally identified as being required for formation of the primitive streak and embryonic mesoderm in the mouse embryo (Zhou et al., 1993; Conlon et al., 1994). Subsequently, molecular genetic studies of *Nodal*-related genes in mouse, zebrafish, frog, and chick demonstrated that Nodal signaling is essential for several additional patterning events at the pregastrulation and gastrulation stages of embryogenesis, including A/P axis formation, definitive endoderm formation, and L/R axis specification (reviewed in Schier and Shen, 2000; Whitman, 2001). (Only a single *Nodal* gene has been identified in mouse and chick, but six related genes are known in frog and three in zebrafish.) In addition, Nodal ligands can directly signal over long-range distances in the zebrafish and mouse embryo, thereby acting as classical morphogens (Chen and Schier, 2001; Meno et al., 2001).

Like other ligands of the transforming growth factor-β (TGF-β) family (see Chapter 24), Nodal signals through heteromeric complexes of type I and type II transmembrane receptors with serine-threonine kinase activity (reviewed in Whitman, 2001). In the case of Nodal, the signaling pathway resembles that of Activin in that signaling is mediated by the type I activin receptor ActRIB and the type II receptors ActRIIA (also known as ActRII) and ActRIIB. However, unlike Activin, signaling by Nodal requires the activity of epidermal growth factor–Cripto/FRL1/Cryptic (EGF-CFC) proteins, including mouse Cripto and Cryptic and zebrafish One-eyed Pinhead, extracellular proteins that are attached to the cell surface by a glycosylphosphatidylinositol (GPI) linkage (reviewed in Shen and Schier, 2000) and can act as coreceptors for Nodal (Saijoh et al., 2000; Reissmann et al., 2001; Yeo and Whitman, 2001; Yan et al., 2002). Receptor signaling then leads to phosphorylation and nuclear accumulation of the signal transducer Smad2 (or Smad3) together with the common Smad partner Smad4 (Kumar et al., 2001; Yeo and Whitman, 2001). (Thus, Nodal utilizes the TGF-β/Activin branch of the TGF-β superfamily, as opposed to bone morphogenetic proteins (BMP), which signal through Smads 1, 5, and 8 and form a distinct branch of the TGF-β superfamily.) The activated Smad2/Smad4 complex interacts with nuclear transcription factors that include winged-helix transcription factors of the FoxH (FAST) subfamily (Chen et al., 1996, 1997) as well as the Mixer subfamily of homeodomain proteins (Germain et al., 2000), both of which are essential for many aspects of Nodal signaling (Watanabe and Whitman, 1999; Pogoda et al., 2000; Sirotkin et al., 2000; Hoodless et al., 2001; Yamamoto et al., 2001; Hart et al., 2002). Taken together, these in vivo and biochemical studies indicate that Nodal signaling is mediated by Smad2 and Smad3 in an EGF-CFC- and FoxH1- or Mixer-dependent manner.

Downstream targets of the Nodal pathway include the *Nodal* gene itself, resulting in a positive feedback loop that is required for broad expression of *Nodal* in the epiblast as well as visceral endoderm (Adachi et al., 1999; Norris and Robertson, 1999; Saijoh et al., 2000; Brennan et al., 2001; Norris et al., 2002). Other targets include members of the Lefty subfamily of TGF-β factors, which act as competitive inhibitors of Nodal signaling and may be induced by Nodal in some tissues as part of a negative feedback loop (reviewed in Schier and Shen, 2000). In addition, secreted members of the Cerberus/Dan family can potentially act as trifunctional inhibitors of Nodal, Wnt, and BMP signaling through direct binding interactions (Hsu et al., 1998; Piccolo et al., 1999). Thus, Nodal activity is controlled through regulation of not only ligand production but also ligand propagation as well as receptor interactions at distant cellular targets.

Wnt Signaling Pathway

Originally defined through identification of targets of insertional activation by the mouse mammary tumor virus and through homology with the *Drosophila* segment-polarity gene *wingless,* the *Wnt* gene family of secreted factors has grown to encompass 18 members in humans (reviewed in Wodarz and Nusse, 1998; Peifer and Polakis, 2000; Polakis, 2000; Moon et al., 2002; see also Chapter 22). Members of the Wnt family can signal through at least three distinct intracellular pathways, including the canonical pathway that utilizes β-catenin as well as the noncanonical Janus kinase (JNK)/planar polarity pathway and the less well-characterized Wnt/Ca^{2+} pathway (reviewed in Huelsken and Birchmeier, 2001; Pandur et al., 2002); the noncanonical pathways will not be discussed further here. Following ligand binding to members of the Frizzled family of seven-transmembrane receptors, Wnt signals are transduced intracellularly by members of the Disheveled family, which participate in both canonical and planar polarity pathways. In addition, the low-density lipoprotein (LDL) receptor–related proteins LRP5 and LRP6 act as coreceptors for signaling through the canonical pathway but not for noncanonical Wnt signaling (Pinson et al., 2000; Tamai et al., 2000; Wehrli et al., 2000).

The central component of the canonical pathway is β-catenin, which serves a dual role in cell adhesion as well as Wnt signal transduction (reviewed in Willert and Nusse, 1998). In response to Wnt signaling, steady-state levels of β-catenin protein are stabilized by preventing proteosome-mediated degradation, followed by accumulation in the nucleus. Activated Disheveled blocks phosphorylation and subsequent proteolytic degradation of β-catenin, which is regulated by a two-step phosphorylation involving casein kinase Iα and glycogen-synthase kinase-3 (GSK3) (Liu et al., 2002). The Axin/Conductin proteins together with the adenomatous polyposis coli (APC) tumor-suppressor negatively regulate canonical Wnt signaling by promoting GSK3 activity (Zeng et al., 1997; Behrens et al., 1998). Interestingly, Axin also directly interacts with the intracellular domain of LRP5/6 in response to Wnt signaling, which induces Axin degradation (Mao et al., 2001b). Following accumulation in the nucleus, β-catenin associates with members of the lymphoid enhancer factor/T-cell factor (LEF/TCF) family of transcription factors, which normally recruit co-repressors to repress transcription of target genes but form part of the transcriptional activation complex following binding of β-catenin (reviewed in van Noort and Clevers, 2002).

Extracellular antagonism of Wnt signaling is mediated by several different classes of inhibitors and associated molecular mechanisms. Members of the Frzb class of Wnt inhibitors resemble truncated Frizzled receptors and likely act as competitive inhibitors for receptor binding (reviewed in Jones and Jomary, 2002). In contrast, the novel protein WIF-1 appears structurally unrelated to Frzb proteins and can block Wnt signaling through a direct binding interaction (Hsieh et al., 1999), as is the case for members of the Cerberus/Dan family (Piccolo et al., 1999). The Dickkopf-1 (Dkk1) protein inhibits canonical Wnt signaling by direct binding to the LRP5/6 coreceptors (Bafico et al., 2001; Mao et al., 2001a; Semenov et al., 2001) as well as to members of the Kremen family of transmembrane proteins, which form a complex with LRP5/6 and Dkk1 (Mao et al., 2002). Thus, as is the case for Nodal, canonical Wnt signaling undergoes strict regulation at multiple steps.

PREIMPLANTATION DEVELOPMENT

Polarity within the Oocyte and Zygote

As in other vertebrate species and lower organisms, the mammalian oocyte achieves meiotic maturation as a highly differentiated cell. This large cell has not only specialized cytoplasm capable of programming embryonic development but also an inherent axial organization, manifested in its animal/vegetal polarity. The animal pole is defined by emergence of the first and second polar bodies (products of the meiotic maturation divisions) and is characterized by its lack of microvillar surface features and relative paucity of sperm-binding receptors (Evans et al., 2000). As an apparent consequence of the latter specialization, sperm entry occurs predominantly in the equatorial and vegetal (opposite to animal) regions. The oocyte's animal/vegetal polarity persists to the blastocyst stage, when it is preserved in the position of the polar body (Gardner, 1997) and the localization of blastomeres that descend from either the animal or vegetal region of the cleavage-stage embryo (Ciemerych et al., 2000). Experimental ablation of the oocyte's animal or vegetal pole or deletion or alteration of the embryo's animal/vegetal composition does not prevent development of full-term, fertile offspring (Zernicka-Goetz, 1998; Ciemerych et al., 2000), so it is unlikely that any essential oocyte components are localized to either pole. However, the functional importance of the animal pole was revealed by experiments in which a second animal pole was fused to the vegetal region of mouse oocytes, resulting in arrest at early cleavage stages (Plusa et al., 2002a). The mechanism of this developmental perturbation is unknown but likely involves the effect of the animal pole on cytoskeletal organization and/or function.

The zygote acquires additional polarity as a result of fertilization. This is evident in the relationship between the plane of first cleavage and the boundary between the blastocyst's embryonic region (containing the inner cell mass and polar trophectoderm) and abembryonic region (containing the blastocyst cavity and mural trophectoderm) (Gardner, 2001; Piotrowska et al., 2001) (Fig. 5–1). Moreover, the localization of the sperm entry position in one of the two blastomeres that results from the first cleavage division is associated with the asynchronous (early) division of that blastomere during subsequent cleavages (Piotrowska and Zernicka-Goetz, 2001). This early-dividing two-cell blastomere in turn tends to colonize the embryonic region of the blastocyst. While there is not yet a consensus on the exact relationship between sperm entry position and the first cleavage plane (Davies and Gardner, 2002; Plusa et al., 2002b), the importance of the sperm in orienting the first cleavage plane is apparent from studies on embryos developing in the absence of a sperm. Parthenogenetic mouse embryos and zygotes in which the sperm entry position has been removed microsurgically lose the association between first cleavage plane and the boundary between the embryonic and abembryonic regions that characterizes the unperturbed, fertilized embryo (Piotrowska and Zernicka-Goetz, 2002). Thus, the fertilized mammalian embryo is already highly organized, having two embryonic axes that persist throughout preimplantation development, one arising from the oocyte itself and a second emerging from sperm–egg interaction.

The molecular basis of the polarity that develops in early mammalian embryos is still unknown. By analogy with other vertebrate embryos, it seems that the early embryonic axes are established through cytoskeletal reorganization that accompanies meiotic maturation and sperm entry into the mature oocyte. For example, the sperm entry point establishes the A/P axis of amphibian and worm embryos (see below) through cytoskeleton-based mechanisms. Such a relationship has been difficult to establish in mouse embryos, where the oocyte, rather than sperm, is the source of the microtubule organizing centers that form after fertilization. The role of the cytoskeleton would thus also be clarified in studies of embryos of domestic (e.g., bovine, ovine) or primate (eg., rhesus, human) species, in which a sperm aster dominates cytoskeletal organization after fertilization. Other vertebrate and invertebrate species that acquire their polarity at early embryonic stages may serve as models for such investigations. Where studied, embryos of such species have been shown to accumulate protein and transcripts of genes in asymmetrical patterns that relate to the polarity of the oocyte and play key roles in the subsequent development of the embryonic axes. In *Drosophila* embryos, a number of transcripts, exemplified by the *bicoid* gene, are localized to the oocyte's future anterior pole, while others, exemplified by the *oskar* gene, are localized to its posterior pole, through the action of the RNA-binding protein Staufen, which interacts with microtubule components of the

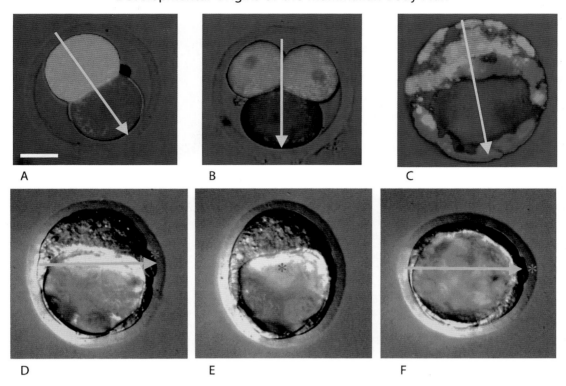

Figure 5–1. Origins of polarity in preimplantation mouse embryos. *A–C:* Origin of embryonic/abembryonic axis in relationship to first cleavage plane and cleavage order. *A:* Two-cell embryo with blastomeres labeled by DiI (red) or DiD (blue). *B:* Three-cell embryo labeled at two-cell stage as in *A*. *C:* Early blastocyst labeled at two-cell stage as in *A*. White arrow indicates orientation and polarity of embryonic/abembryonic axis (arrow points from embryonic region uppermost including inner cell mass toward abembryonic region lower including blastocyst cavity). Note colonization of embryonic region by the cells derived predominantly from the early-dividing two-cell blastomere. *D, E:* Expanding blastocyst seen from three different perspectives to show its animal/vegetal polarity. *D:* Side view of blastocyst focusing on mid-saggital optical section and showing animal pole (polar body asterisk). Yellow arrow indicates orientation and polarity of animal/vegetal axis (arrow points from vegetal pole left toward animal pole, right). *E:* Blastocyst viewed from its animal pole (polar body asterisk). *F:* Blastocyst viewed from its embryonic pole. Yellow arrow oriented as in *D*. Scale bar 25 μm. (Adapted from Piotrowska et al. 2001, and Zernicka-Goetz 2002, with permission of the Company of Biologists Ltd.)

cytoskeleton (reviewed by Lall and Patel, 2001; St Johnston, 2001). The polarized movements of *bicoid* and *oskar* transcripts appear to be mediated, respectively, by the minus end–directed motor protein dynein (Schnorrer et al., 2000) and the plus end–directed microtubule motor protein kinesin 1 (Brendza et al., 2000). In *Caenorhabditis* embryos, sperm entry position initiates the A/P polarity of the embryo through a microtubule-directed process involving the *Par* gene family (Goldstein and Hird, 1996; Wallenfang and Seydoux, 2000). Interestingly, the *Par* genes described in *C. elegans* have homologues with similar developmental roles in *Drosophila* (Riechmann et al., 2002) and similar biochemical functions in vertebrates (Nakaya et al., 2000; reviewed by Bullock and Ish-Horowicz, 2002). In *Xenopus*, embryo transcripts involved in endoderm formation (e.g., *VegT*) accumulate in the vegetal region during oogenesis (King et al., 1999). When the fertilizing sperm enters the amphibian egg, it initiates a reorganization of the cytoskeleton, orienting microtubules in their future A/P polarity (reviewed by De Robertis et al., 2000). This leads to accumulation of proteins (e.g., Disheveled, β-catenin) involved in the dorsalization of the A/P midline of the embryo. Thus, further studies are needed on the roles of mammalian homologues of these and other genes with known functions in establishing embryonic or cellular polarity (Baens and Marynen, 1997; Wickham et al., 1999; Saunders et al., 2000; reviewed by Edwards, 2000, 2001), and of any gene products found to be asymmetrically distributed in oocytes and early embryos, such as Leptin and Stat3 (Antczak and Van Blerkom, 1997) or fibroblast growth factor receptor-2 (FGFR2) (Haffner-Krausz et al., 1999). In this way, it may eventually be possible to understand the mechanistic relationships between mammals and other organisms and, thus, the development of human embryonic polarity in an evolutionary perspective.

Role of the Extraembryonic Lineages

The first cell type to differentiate in embryos of placental (i.e., eutherian) mammals is the trophectoderm, which surrounds the remaining (inner) cells that constitute the pluripotent stem cell progenitors of the entire fetus. Trophectoderm cells similarly constitute the founder population for the chorionic cells of the placenta, which protects the fetus from attack by the maternal immune system and provides it with an organ for exchanging nutrients and oxidative metabolites as necessary for viviparous prenatal life. Accordingly, the trophoblast has typically been understood to be primarily protective and nutritive. The second tissue to differentiate in mammalian embryos is the so-called primitive endoderm, actually a misnomer as it contributes no cells to the fetal gut or endodermal organs but rather populates the absorptive layer of the yolk sac (visceral extraembryonic endoderm) and contributes cells that synthesize the basement membrane utilized by trophoblast cells during implantation. Thus, the primitive endoderm was also regarded as having a primarily nutritive role.

However, studies in mammals and other vertebrate species have shown these extraembryonic tissues in a new light. This is because the extraembryonic tissues have been revealed as the primary candidates for transmitting organizational information from early stages to the stage at which the body plan actually forms (reviewed by Zernicka-Goetz, 2002). In this new perspective, certain cells in the trophectoderm population of the pregastrulation stage mammalian embryo constitute a signaling center that initiates changes leading to gastrulation in the adjacent epiblast cells (Fig. 5–2). Specifically, the distal cells of the extraembryonic ectoderm express BMP4 in a localized manner in mouse embryos; and in the absence of BMP4 gene function, development is blocked at pregastrulation stages (see be-

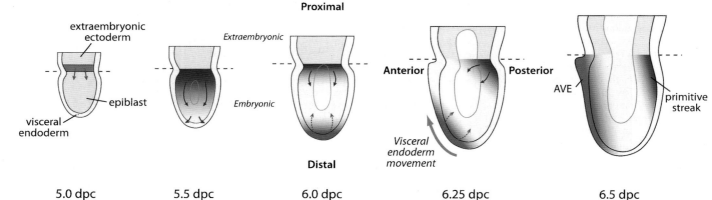

Figure 5–2. Specification of the anterior/posterior axis in mice. Schematic depictions of embryos at early postimplantation stages are shown. A signal(s) from the extraembryonic ectoderm (green arrows) induces *Nodal* expression in the proximal epiblast resulting in propagation of Nodal signaling (blue) throughout the epiblast. Nodal signaling from the epiblast to the visceral en- doderm is required for establishment of the prospective anterior visceral en- doderm (AVE) at the distal end of the egg cylinder which in turn expresses Nodal inhibitors (red) and undergoes movement to the future anterior side. Blue arrows represent Nodal signals while dashed red arrows represent activ- ity of Nodal antagonists.

low). Similarly, the cells of the visceral endoderm (VE) express known morphogenetically active genes in a localized manner, and perturba- tion of the VE function of such genes leads to aberrant development of embryonic polarity during and after gastrulation (reviewed by Bielinska et al., 1999; Lu et al., 2001; Perea-Gomez et al., 2001b). Fi- nally, the pluripotent cells of the epiblast, which serve as the source of all fetal tissues, undergo substantial and continual mixing before and during gastrulation, a cellular behavior that seems incompatible with a role in conveying by itself any localized information from preimplantation stages (Gardner and Cockroft, 1998). By contrast, ex- traembryonic VE in particular develops in a coherent manner so that related descendants tend to remain adjacent to each other during the clonal expansion that occurs with growth in the postimplantation em- bryo (Gardner, 1984; Weber et al., 1999). This pattern of coherent clonal growth is consistent with a role for the VE in localized signal- ing during development of the body plan. Therefore, in addition to the protective, nutritive functions the extraembryonic lineages acquire as fully differentiated tissues, they seem to have a transient early, but crucial, role in establishing the body plan.

Relationship between Early Polarity and the Body Plan

To understand the "peri-implantation" transition between preimplan- tation and postimplantation stages of mammalian development, par- ticularly the role of the extraembryonic tissues in conveying organi- zation between these two phases, it will be helpful to clarify the axial organization at each phase. The two axes recognizable in the preim- plantation embryo are the animal/vegetal (established in the mature oocyte) and the embryonic/abembryonic (established in the fertilized zygote or early cleavage-stage embryo). As the rodent embryo im- plants, it elongates to form a structure known as the "egg cylinder" (Fig. 5–2), which has its own long axis (the proximal/distal [P/D] axis), which was presumed to emerge from embryonic growth along the embryonic/abembryonic axis. However, an investigation of the relation- ship between mouse blastocyst polarity and egg cylinder polarity showed that VE cells arising from the blastocyst animal pole tended to colonize the embryonic (distal) region of the egg cylinder, while VE cells arising from the vegetal pole tended to colonize the ex- traembryonic (proximal) region. Weber et al. (1999) found that VE descendants of labeled inner cell mass (ICM) cells achieved their po- larized distribution through asymmetrical VE movements that precede gastrulation and appear to converge on the future posterior of the em- bryo. This coordinated pregastrulation movement of mouse VE is strikingly similar to a posterior-to-anterior movement known as "polonaise" in the equivalent tissue (hypoblast) of chick embryos (Fo- ley et al., 2000). The embryo's A/P axis, which becomes visible with the onset of gastrulation (see below), is oriented perpendicularly to the egg cylinder's P/D axis. In a landmark study, Thomas and cowork- ers (1998) showed that, shortly before gastrulation, VE cells occupy- ing an initial position at the tip of the egg cylinder moved proximally by about 90 degrees to its future anterior position, thus conveying the P/D axis of the egg cylinder into an A/P one (see below). This ob- servation together with the overall reshaping of VE clones evident in the polonaise movements raised the possibility that the oocyte ani- mal/vegetal axis is transformed initially into the egg cylinder's P/D axis and subsequently into its A/P axis through asymmetrical VE movements (Weber et al., 1999). More generally, finding a relation- ship between polarity of preimplatation and postimplantation embryos raises the question of whether one or more of the body axes (A/P, D/V, L/R) might relate explicitly to the earlier embryonic axes (ani- mal/vegetal, embryonic/abembryonic). While this question remains unresolved, it should be noted that if any axis of the definitive body plan becomes established in the preimplantation embryo, this could also have implications for the other axes. For example, establishment of A/P polarity in response to sperm entry in the *Xenopus* embryo is normally accompanied by early allocation of cells into the left and right halves of the embryo as a result of the first cleavage division (Klein, 1987; Black and Vincent, 1988; reviewed by Yost, 1991). Whether or not such early establishment of the body plan occurs in mammals, it has nevertheless become clear that asymmetrical VE movements together with the unique molecular properties of the par- ticular VE cells that move to an anterior position are responsible for initiating A/P polarity during events preceding gastrulation.

PERI-IMPLANTATION DEVELOPMENT AND ACQUISITION OF THE BODY PLAN

Formation of the A/P Axis

At first glance, the early preimplantation mouse embryo appears rela- tively featureless, to the extent that staging of embryos between im- plantation at 4.5 days postcoitum (dpc) and the onset of gastrulation at 6.5 dpc is difficult. During this time, the egg cylinder superficially ap- pears radially symmetrical, revealing only the overt P/D asymmetry that corresponds to the extraembryonic/embryonic division along the long axis of the egg cylinder. In fact, subtle morphological asymmetries at preimplantation stages have long been noted (Smith, 1980; Gardner, 1997). Moreover, the primary axes of the gastrulating embryo are aligned to the axes of the maternal uterus (Smith, 1980, 1985), sug- gesting that the blastocyst may implant in an oriented fashion to achieve this coordination. As discussed above, fate-mapping studies have sup- ported these early observations by showing that the A/P axis in the postimplantation embryo may be related to preexisting asymmetries within the blastocyst (Weber et al., 1999; Ciemerych et al., 2000).

The A/P axis becomes morphologically apparent at the onset of gas- trulation with the formation of the primitive streak on the posterior side of the egg cylinder. Transplantation and lineage-tracing studies have demonstrated that the anterior (distal) end of the elongating primitive streak corresponds to a classical trunk organizing center (node) (Beddington, 1994; Tam and Steiner, 1999; Kinder et al., 2001). However, a variety of related observations have shown that a second signaling center is located in the extraembryonic anterior visceral endoderm (AVE), which is required for head formation (reviewed in Beddington and Robertson, 1999; also see below). Thus, the early gastrulating mouse embryo contains two distinct signaling centers on opposite ends of the egg cylinder, which together pattern the body plan.

The currently accepted model for A/P axis formation in the mouse was originally proposed by the late Rosa Beddington and colleagues (reviewed in Beddington and Robertson, 1998, 1999). Analysis of the expression pattern of the homeobox gene *Hex* showed that it was expressed at 5.5 dpc in the distal VE and subsequently in the AVE at 6.0 dpc; similarly, expression of *Brachyury* originated in the proximal epiblast adjacent to the extraembryonic boundary and then shifted to the posterior side corresponding to the position of the nascent primitive streak (Thomas et al., 1998). In embryo culture experiments, labeling of cells at the distal end of the VE at 5.5 dpc results in marked cells accumulating in the AVE at 6.5 dpc (Thomas et al., 1998; Weber et al., 1999; Kimura et al., 2000). Based on their findings, Beddington and Robertson (1998, 1999) proposed that the A/P axis is initially generated in a P/D orientation and then undergoes a 90-degree rotation such that the A/P axis becomes aligned orthogonal to its starting position. Thus, distal VE cells migrate to the prospective anterior side, followed by a corresponding shift in gene expression or cell position from the proximal epiblast to the posterior side (Fig. 5–2).

Detailed examination of the premigratory distal VE cells has revealed that they represent a distinct population within the VE, corresponding to a pseudostratified columnar or stratified cuboidal epithelium in histological sections and electron micrographs (Huelsken et al., 2000; Kimura et al., 2000). In principle, the movement of these cells to the anterior side can now be traced in embryo culture using transgenic mice that specifically express green fluorescent protein (GFP) in this cell population (Kimura et al., 2000; Perea-Gomez et al., 2001a; Rodriguez et al., 2001). Such studies should elucidate whether these cell movements occur by an active or passive mechanism and the degree to which they are biased by preexisting asymmetries in the shape of the egg cylinder. Comparable studies of the movement of cells within the epiblast will also be informative as to the nature of A/P patterning at prestreak stages.

Molecular Basis of Pregastrulation Morphogenesis

Until recently, little was known of the molecular pathways that give rise to the asymmetries within the mouse embryo at the onset of gastrulation. However, it is becoming increasingly apparent that many, if not all, of the patterning events at pregastrulation stages can be traced back to existing morphological asymmetries within the early postimplantation embryo and preimplantation blastocyst (reviewed in Lu et al., 2001).

Reciprocal Signaling between the Proximal Epiblast and Extraembryonic Ectoderm

Similar to many other developmental systems, key patterning events in the pregastrulation mouse embryo take place at tissue boundaries. Of particular importance is the boundary between the extraembryonic and embryonic regions of the egg cylinder, which defines the P/D axis of the epiblast. Reciprocal signaling interactions at this boundary appear to be essential for the induction of *Nodal* expression in the proximal epiblast, which is subsequently required for the initial patterning of the A/P axis in the pregastrulation egg cylinder (Brennan et al., 2001).

Analysis of the peri-implantation lethality of *Fgf4* mutant mice and the establishment of trophoblast stem cells has shown that the extraembryonic ectoderm is dependent on FGF4 produced by the epiblast (Feldman et al., 1995; Wilder et al., 1997; Tanaka et al., 1998). Possibly as a consequence, extraembryonic ectoderm is already regionalized at early postimplantation stages, as shown by the restricted expression of *Bmp4* on the extraembryonic side of the extraembry-

onic/embryonic boundary (Lawson et al., 1999). This expression of *Bmp4* is required for formation of a normal node and primitive streak (Fujiwara et al., 2002), as well as generation of primordial germ cells, which are derived from the proximal epiblast (Lawson et al., 1999); similarly, extraembryonic expression of the T-box gene *Eomesodermin* is likely to be required for expression of proximal epiblast markers (Russ et al., 2000). Interestingly, extraembryonic expression of *Bmp4* and *Eomesodermin* is not maintained in *Nodal* mutants, suggesting that Nodal activity is essential for reciprocal signaling from the proximal epiblast to the distal extraembryonic ectoderm (Brennan et al., 2001).

Although the precise mechanisms involved are presently unclear, signaling from the extraembryonic ectoderm is believed to be required for the induction of *Nodal* expression and initial specification of the proximal epiblast (Brennan et al., 2001). Following its initial induction in the proximal epiblast, expression of *Nodal* becomes highly dynamic (Fig. 5–2). The auto-regulation of *Nodal* through its positive feedback loop together with the long-range activity of the Nodal protein result in propagation of *Nodal* expression throughout the epiblast (Varlet et al., 1997; Brennan et al., 2001). Nodal signaling from the epiblast then leads to specification of the distal VE (see below), which in turn expresses Nodal inhibitory activities that downregulate Nodal expression in the distal epiblast, creating a P/D gradient of Nodal expression (Brennan et al., 2001). This proximal epiblast expression of *Nodal* then shifts caudally to the region of the nascent primitive streak prior to the onset of gastrulation (Varlet et al., 1997), concomitant with the overall shift in expression of proximal/posterior markers. Notably, expression of the *EGF-CFC* gene *Cripto* displays a similar pattern to that of *Nodal*, with initial symmetrical expression in the epiblast, followed by a P/D gradient and subsequent shift to the region of the nascent primitive streak (Ding et al., 1998). However, since *Cripto* as well as *Brachyury*, *Fgf8*, and *Wnt3* are not expressed in *Nodal* mutants, expression of each of these proximal/posterior markers appears to be dependent on Nodal activity (Brennan et al., 2001).

Specification of the Distal VE

A second important tissue boundary in the preimplantation mouse embryo occurs between the epiblast and the extraembryonic VE. As mentioned above, Nodal signaling from the epiblast to the extraembryonic VE is required for specification of the distal VE in the pregastrulation egg cylinder (Brennan et al., 2001). Once formed, the distal VE expresses genes encoding Nodal inhibitors, including *Lefty1* and *Cer1* (*Cerberus-like*) (reviewed in Beddington and Robertson, 1999; Lu et al., 2001), which can presumably act on the epiblast in a reciprocal fashion to downregulate Nodal activity in the distal epiblast. As the distal VE initiates movement to the anterior side, its expression of Nodal inhibitors can thereby "clear" Nodal activity in the adjacent proximal/anterior epiblast, setting up the apposition of anterior and posterior signaling centers at the initiation of gastrulation (Fig. 5–2).

Null mutants for *Smad2* also result in failure to express any distal/anterior VE markers, indicating a failure to specify the distal VE (Waldrip et al., 1998; Brennan et al., 2001). In contrast with *Nodal*, however, *Smad2* mutants display widespread expression of proximal/posterior markers throughout the epiblast, including *Nodal* itself, leading to overproduction of extraembryonic mesoderm (Waldrip et al., 1998; Brennan et al., 2001). Based on these findings, Brennan and colleagues (2001) proposed that the initial propagation of *Nodal* signals through the epiblast does not require *Smad2* as its absence can be compensated by *Smad3* but failure to induce distal VE leads to lack of Nodal inhibitory signals that would repress Nodal activity in the distal epiblast.

Anterior Movement of the Distal VE

Several regulatory genes essential for VE movement have been identified. Most strikingly, a specific role of Nodal signaling in A/P axis rotation was originally inferred based on the phenotype of mutants for the *EGF-CFC* gene *Cripto*. In *Cripto* mutants, AVE markers are expressed in the distal VE, while early primitive streak markers are localized in the proximal epiblast; thus, the A/P axis is formed but remains positioned along the P/D axis (Ding et al., 1998). In subsequent work, the phenotype of a hypomorphic *Nodal* mutation as well as of a *FoxH1* null mutation has confirmed the requirement for Nodal signaling in A/P axis rotation (Lowe et al., 2001; Yamamoto et al., 2001).

Additional studies have shown that mutants for *β-catenin* and the homeobox gene *Otx2* also display distal expression of AVE markers, thus implicating these regulatory genes in VE movement (Huelsken et al., 2000; Kimura et al., 2000; Perea-Gomez et al., 2001a). Notably, the role of Wnt signaling in this process remains unclear since no prospective Wnt ligand has been identified that may correspond to this requirement for β-catenin. It is conceivable that this role may be highly redundant among several Wnts or that the requirement of β-catenin in this process may be Wnt-independent. At present, however, how Nodal and Wnt signaling regulate anterior movement of the distal VE is unknown.

EARLY GASTRULATION AND ESTABLISHMENT OF THE BODY PLAN

Cellular Movements and Fate Map of the Gastrulating Embryo

The morphogenetic process of gastrulation converts the embryo into a three-layered structure consisting of mesoderm, endoderm, and ectoderm, the primary germ layers that constitute the "embryo proper," which gives rise to the fetus. Prior to gastrulation, the embryonic region of the mouse egg cylinder is two-layered, with the epiblast layer surrounding the proamniotic cavity and being in turn surrounded by the VE layer. During gastrulation, the VE layer is replaced and displaced from the embryonic region by epiblast-derived definitive endoderm cells, initially at the anterior midline of the primitive streak, then more widely (Lawson et al., 1986; Lawson and Pedersen, 1987). Simultaneously, epiblast precursors of mesoderm converge on the primitive streak, emerging as a new layer between epiblast and endoderm. The primitive streak elongates by progressively incorporating lateral and anterior epiblast regions, which contribute descendants to mesoderm and endoderm populations in an orderly way, enabling the description of a reproducible epiblast fate map (Lawson et al., 1991). Once adjustments are made for the topographic peculiarity of the rodent egg cylinder, the mouse fate map strikingly resembles that of the chick and even the urodele. As in the chick, epiblast is the source of all fetal tissues and of extraembryonic mesoderm. Interestingly, epiblast cells continue to exchange neighbors during gastrulation, rather than develop coherently, and epiblast descendants cross the embryo's midline, which thus does not act as a barrier to clonal spread (Bonnerot and Nicolas, 1993; Bachiller et al., 2000). As development of the mouse fate map has been the subject of several reviews (Tam and Behringer, 1997; Lu et al., 2001; Tam et al., 2001), it will not be covered extensively here.

In amniotes, mesoderm and definitive endoderm formation take place at the primitive streak, with the most anterior region of the mature streak giving rise to the node, which is analogous to the organizer. The anterior derivatives of the streak are fated to form axial mesoderm and definitive endoderm, while successively more posterior derivatives generate paraxial, lateral, and extraembryonic mesoderm. Transplantation studies have revealed the capacity of a small group of cells in the early streak-stage embryo (located where the streak initially forms, near the boundary of the embryonic and extraembryonic regions of the egg cylinder) to induce an ectopic neural axis when they are transplanted as an intact tissue fragment to the late streak-stage embryo (Tam and Behringer, 1997). A population of cells with similar inductive properties has been identified at the anterior end of the streak in mid-streak-stage embryos (Kinder et al., 2001). These studies complement the findings of Beddington (1994), who first demonstrated that the anterior tip of the mouse primitive streak (the node) is capable of inducing a secondary A/P axis. Taken together, these studies show that by the onset of gastrulation the posterior region of the mouse embryo has acquired unique properties involved in induction of the A/P axis. How is this signaling center acquired, and how do its inductive properties become localized?

Molecular Basis for Initial Steps in Mesoderm and Endoderm Differentiation

At the onset of gastrulation, two distinct signaling centers, corresponding to the AVE and the nascent primitive streak, are opposed at the rostral and caudal ends of the mouse egg cylinder. Much work has led to a model in which Nodal and Wnt signals from the nascent streak represent posteriorizing factors in pregastrulation and early gastrulation embryos, while secreted inhibitors of Nodal and Wnt signals produced by the AVE represent anteriorizing factors. This opposition of signaling molecules and secreted antagonists is thought to generate graded levels of Nodal and Wnt activities, which pattern both the nascent mesoderm and the neuroectoderm. This process of axial patterning may primarily arise through the long-range active and/or passive diffusion of signaling factors or inhibitors, thereby generating a graded distribution of signaling activity. This indeed may be the case for the zebrafish Nodal-related protein Squint, which can act as a classical morphogen (Chen and Schier, 2001). Alternatively, graded levels of signaling activity may simply be generated by the rapid displacement of cells that generate such signals as the primitive streak undergoes elongation and as the AVE is displaced by the definitive endoderm.

Formation of the Primitive Streak and Mesoderm Induction

It has become increasingly apparent from molecular genetic studies in several vertebrate systems that the Nodal and Wnt pathways play central roles in the initial events of gastrulation. These Nodal and Wnt signals may act sequentially in the same genetic pathway for mesoderm formation, or they may coordinately regulate common downstream targets; how these two signaling pathways interact to control mesoderm formation is poorly understood at the present time.

Role of Wnt Signaling. A critical role for the canonical Wnt pathway in determining the site of mesoderm formation has long been suggested by studies in fish and frog embryos, demonstrating the essential role of β-catenin in specification of the D/V axis (reviewed in Harland and Gerhart, 1997; De Robertis et al., 2000). In particular, endogenous pathway activity has been shown by the accumulation of nucleus-localized β-catenin on the prospective dorsal side (the site of initial mesoderm formation) in sea urchin, frog, and fish embryos at the blastula stage (Schneider et al., 1996; Larabell et al., 1997; Logan et al., 1999). Indeed, this D/V asymmetry in β-catenin accumulation can be traced in frog embryos back to early cleavage stages and may be generated by the process of cortical rotation that follows fertilization (Larabell et al., 1997). Whether similar asymmetries in β-catenin localization exist in pre- and peri-implantation mouse embryos is currently unknown.

In the mouse embryo, an essential role for Wnt signaling has been demonstrated by analysis of *Wnt3* as well as *β-catenin* null mutants, which lack primitive streak and mesoderm formation (Liu et al., 1999; Huelsken et al., 2000). Conversely, mutations in *Axin*, which negatively regulates Wnt signaling, result in twinned embryos with duplicated primitive streaks (Gluecksohn-Schoenheimer, 1949; Zeng et al., 1997), while overexpression of chick *Wnt8C* results in ectopic streaks in transgenic embryos (Popperl et al., 1997). Notably, in the chick, Wnt8c acts together with the TGF-β factor Vg1 in the posterior marginal zone to induce Nodal expression and consequent streak formation (Skromne and Stern, 2001; Bertocchini and Stern, 2002); thus, in this case, it appears that the requirement for Nodal lies downstream of an initial Wnt signal.

Role of Nodal Signals and Antagonists. As noted above, molecular genetic studies using a variety of experimental approaches in frogs, fish, and mice indicate that Nodal signals play primary roles in mesoderm formation in all vertebrates (reviewed in Schier and Shen, 2000; Whitman, 2001). However, it is likely that other TGF-β factors also play important roles in mesoderm induction, based on studies of *Xenopus Vg1* and *derriere* (Joseph and Melton, 1998; Sun et al., 1999; White et al., 2002). In particular, Derriere may heterodimerize with Nodal-related factors to produce a cooperative interaction between these ligands in mesoderm formation (Eimon and Harland, 2002).

Studies of Nodal inhibitors in frogs, fish, and mice have provided firm evidence for an endogenous gradient of Nodal activity, in which the highest levels of Nodal activity specify definitive endoderm (see below), then axial mesoderm, followed by paraxial and lateral mesoderm, and then extraembryonic mesoderm. Thus, increasing doses of Nodal inhibitors such as *Lefty* or *Cerberus* result in loss of progressively more dorsal mesoderm (Agius et al., 2000; Gritsman et al., 2000; Thisse et al., 2000). Moreover, within the axial mesoderm itself, differential levels of Nodal activity are believed to specify prechordal mesoderm versus notochord (Gritsman et al., 2000). Conversely, the combined deletion of *Lefty1* and *Cerberus-like* in mice results in an overall shift toward axial mesoderm cell fates and depletion of lateral and extraembryonic mesoderm (Perea-Gomez et al., 2002), consistent with the phenotype of a *Nodal* hypomorphic allele (Lowe et al., 2001). These molecular genetic studies are supported by a wealth of older data indicating that the specification of mesoderm subtypes is exquisitely sensitive to the dosage of Nodal signaling (reviewed in Smith, 1995; McDowell and Gurdon, 1999; Gurdon and Bourillot, 2001). (These classical experiments utilized Activin as a mesoderm-inducing factor; however, there is relatively little evidence to support a role for endogenous Activin in mesoderm formation [Schulte-Merker et al., 1994; Matzuk et al., 1995], whereas Nodal signals through an Activin-like pathway.) For example, dissociated cells isolated from *Xenopus* animal caps display sharp thresholds of responses to less than twofold differences in Activin concentrations in culture (Green and Smith, 1990). *In vivo*, these differential responses at the cellular level could be generated through either exposure to graded levels of signal or modulation of the amount of time in which cells receive Nodal signals.

In the mouse embryo, Nodal inhibitors are expressed by the AVE and antagonize the posteriorizing influence of the distal primitive streak (node), which expresses *Nodal*. Evidence for a mutually antagonistic relationship between the AVE and primitive streak in A/P patterning has been generated by genetic studies of *Otx2* mutants and *Otx2;Cripto* and *FoxA2;Lhx1* double mutants (Perea-Gomez et al., 1999; Kimura et al., 2001; Perea-Gomez et al., 2001a) as well as from explant recombination studies (Kimura et al., 2000). The Nodal inhibitors expressed by the AVE correspond, at least in part, to Lefty1 and Cerberus-like, which are required to suppress formation of ectopic primitive streaks and excessive mesoderm (Bertocchini and Stern, 2002; Perea-Gomez et al., 2002). A similar role has been deduced for Nodal inhibitors expressed by the chick hypoblast, which is functionally analogous to the mouse AVE (Bertocchini and Stern, 2002).

Integration of Wnt and Nodal Signals. Subsequent steps in primitive streak elongation and mesoderm differentiation involve the regulatory function of numerous transcription factors and signaling molecules, including homeobox genes such as *Goosecoid* and members of the FGF family, many of which represent targets of Wnt and Nodal signaling (these and other aspects of later stages of gastrulation are reviewed in Tam and Behringer, 1997; De Robertis et al., 2000). Integration of these pathways can take place through direct interactions of TCF/LEF with Smad2/4 complexes on promoter elements, as has been shown for regulation of the *Xenopus twin* homeobox gene, which together with *siamois* is essential for formation of the Spemann organizer (Nishita et al., 2000). Another major target of Wnt and Nodal signaling pathways is the critical T-box transcription factor *Brachyury*, which is essential for caudal primitive streak maintenance and whose promoter contains TCF- and Smad-binding sites that are essential for promoter activity in frogs (Latinkic et al., 1997; Arnold et al., 2000; Vonica and Gumbiner, 2002).

Definitive Endoderm Formation

The Nodal signaling pathway also plays a central role in formation of the definitive endoderm, as has been shown by mutational studies in zebrafish and mice (reviewed in Stainier, 2002). Analysis of a *Nodal* hypomorphic mutant and *Smad2* chimeric mice has provided firm evidence as to the central role of Nodal signaling in endoderm formation (Tremblay et al., 2000; Norris et al., 2002). Nodal signaling in endoderm formation requires the winged-helix transcription factor FoxH1 (Hoodless et al., 2001; Yamamoto et al., 2001). However, the Nodal pathway is also thought to be coupled with the activity of the homeodomain protein encoded by *Mixl1*, which is required for nor-

mal definitive endoderm formation in mice (Hart et al., 2002) and can mediate Smad2/Smad4 binding to downstream targets (Germain et al., 2000). Thus, despite much progress in understanding early steps in endoderm formation, it remains unclear how the definitive endoderm is segregated from the nascent mesoderm.

Targets of Nodal signaling in endoderm formation are likely to include the endoderm-specific *Sox17*, which is required for formation of gut endoderm (Kanai-Azuma et al., 2002). Other Nodal targets are likely to correspond to members of the GATA family, based on the requirement for the zebrafish *gata5 (faust)* gene in endoderm formation (Reiter et al., 1999). Finally, the *FoxA2* gene is required for foregut and midgut formation in mice (Dufort et al., 1998), but it is unclear whether it represents a direct target of Nodal signaling. Interestingly, the differential requirements for *FoxA2* along the A/P axis of the gut endoderm indicate that regional patterning of the endoderm initiates shortly after its formation. Later steps in patterning of the definitive endoderm and formation of its tissue derivatives are described in detail in Chapter 14.

Molecular Basis for Neural Induction

The formation of the nervous system is described in detail in Chapter 7; early steps in neuroectoderm formation are summarized briefly below.

Extensive studies in the frog have led to the "neural default" model, in which the default tendency of ectodermal cells to undergo neural differentiation is blocked by endogenous BMP signaling and BMP inhibitors such as Noggin and Chordin serve as neural inducers (reviewed in Munoz-Sanjuan and Brivanlou, 2002). However, the phenotype of *Noggin; Chordin* double mutants in mice demonstrates that extensive neural differentiation and patterning take place in the absence of these BMP inhibitors (Bachiller et al., 2000), indicating that other factors are necessary. Indeed, studies of embryonic stem cell differentiation have suggested the existence of an as yet unidentified factor (stromal cell–derived inducing activity) that is responsible for facilitating neural differentiation in culture (Kawasaki et al., 2000). In addition, an alternative mechanism for inhibition of BMP activity may occur through heterodimerization with Nodal and related TGF-β factors (Yeo and Whitman, 2001), which may account for the extensive neural differentiation found in *Cripto* and *oep* mutants (Schier et al., 1997; Ding et al., 1998). Finally, work in the chick embryo has indicated important roles for Wnt and FGF signaling in pre-gastrulation steps of neural induction (reviewed in Wilson and Edlund, 2001; Stern, 2002).

Although the sources of neural inducing signals were historically considered to emanate from mesoderm, it is now apparent from molecular genetic analyses in mice, fish, and frogs that neuroectoderm formation and considerable patterning can take place in the absence of mesoderm (Ding et al., 1998; Gritsman et al., 1999; Klingensmith et al., 1999; Agius et al., 2000; Wessely et al., 2001). In the mouse, the likely source of neural inducing signals is the AVE since its surgical removal results in loss of forebrain markers such as *Hesx1* (Thomas and Beddington, 1996). However, although the AVE expresses several secreted molecules that can act as Nodal, BMP, and/or Wnt inhibitors, such as Dickkopf-1, targeted deletion of *Dickkopf-1* results in forebrain defects through its loss in anterior mesendoderm, not the AVE (Mukhopadhyay et al., 2001). In contrast, transcription factors such as Otx2 and Lim1 are required for head formation and have been shown by chimera analysis to be required in the VE for early steps in head induction (Rhinn et al., 1998; Shawlot et al., 1999).

Once acquired, the maintenance of anterior neural fate requires signals from three adjacent territories: the axial mesoderm (prechordal mesoderm), the anterior definitive endoderm, and the anterior neural ridge. Maintenance of the neuroectoderm and its regional specification along the A/P axis are described in detail in Chapter 7.

DEVELOPMENT OF L/R ASYMMETRY

Embryonic Origins of Bilateral Asymmetry

Of the three major body axes, the L/R axis has generally been thought to be the last to be determined during vertebrate embryogenesis. Most of the known molecular events involved in initial specification of the L/R axis occur at late stages of gastrulation, prior to the earliest appearance of asymmetrical gene expression, which occurs during early somite formation in the mouse. While in principle the L/R axis is already specified as being orthogonal to the other preexisting axes, the correct determination of the left and right sides of the body has long been recognized as representing a profound problem in development (Brown and Wolpert, 1990).

Although the initial molecular events that specify the L/R axis occur prior to somite formation, most of the tissue-specific manifestations of morphological asymmetry become apparent much later in development, throughout organogenesis into the late fetal period (reviewed in Burdine and Schier, 2000; Capdevila et al., 2000; Mercola and Levin, 2001; Hamada et al., 2002). The first morphological appearance of L/R asymmetry in all vertebrates occurs during early somitogenesis, with an initial rightward bending of the linear heart tube that presages the direction of cardiac looping. In the mouse, another early sign of laterality is the counterclockwise direction of embryonic turning that inverts the three primary germ layers of the embryo. However, most morphological L/R asymmetry arises at significantly later stages of organogenesis, when unilateral tissues such as the stomach are positioned on one side or when bilateral paired tissues such as the lung form asymmetrically. At late fetal stages, L/R laterality decisions occur within the vasculature, when an initially symmetrical system partially regresses on one side or the other (Kaufman and Bard, 1999).

Mutations that lead to defects in L/R patterning can lead to several distinct phenotypic outcomes. While the term *situs solitus* refers to the wild-type pattern of L/R laterality, *situs inversus* corresponds to complete reversal of L/R polarity and is observed at high frequencies in mouse mutants for *inversion of embryonic turning (inv)*, which encodes a novel intracellular protein (Yokoyama et al., 1993; Mochizuki et al., 1998; Morgan et al., 1998). A far more common outcome, however, is *heterotaxia*, in which each tissue can adopt its own L/R patterning independently of other tissues. In such circumstances, the pat-

terning of individual tissues can become *randomized*, as would be observed with the placement of the stomach on the left or right side, or *isomerized*, as in the case of bilateral paired tissues such as the lung, which normally has four lobes on the right side and one lobe on the left in the mouse. Classical mouse mutations that lead to heterotaxia include *inversus viscerum (iv)* and *left/right dynein (lrd)*, which encodes a novel dynein (Supp et al., 1997, 1999).

Molecular Basis for L/R Asymmetries

The present flowering of molecular studies on L/R specification has been largely inspired by the seminal work from the Tabin laboratory on L/R asymmetrical gene expression and function in the chick embryo (Levin et al., 1995). Since this initial publication, molecular genetic studies performed in chick, frog, zebrafish, and mouse systems have led to a conceptual pathway for L/R axis determination in vertebrates (Fig. 5–3). In this proposed pathway, an initial event that breaks L/R symmetry is believed to occur in or around the embryonic node and the resulting L/R positional information is transferred outward to the lateral plate mesoderm, where it is interpreted to generate the *situs* of individual tissues (reviewed in Burdine and Schier, 2000; Capdevila et al., 2000; Mercola and Levin, 2001; Hamada et al., 2002).

Most of the known genes implicated in L/R patterning have been identified on the basis of their transient L/R asymmetrical expression, particularly in the chick embryo, and/or on the basis of mutational phenotypes in the mouse. Accordingly, the ordering of regulatory relationships has largely derived from gain-of-function ectopic expression experiments in the chick and from analysis of expression patterns in mouse loss-of-function mutants. For example, the *iv* and *inv* genes are believed to reside at or near the beginning of the L/R pathway since the corresponding mutants affect the expression patterns of all known asymmetrically expressed mouse genes (Collignon et al., 1996; Lowe et al., 1996; Meno et al., 1996; Piedra et al., 1998; Ryan et al., 1998; Campione et al., 1999).

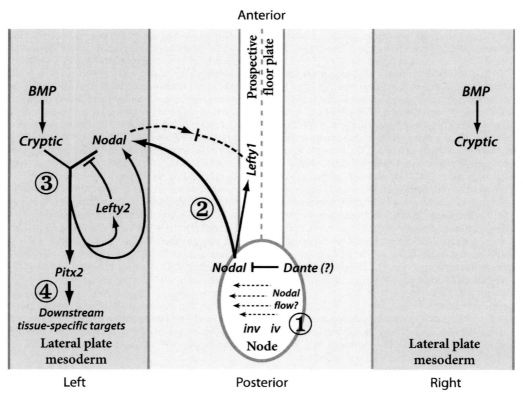

Figure 5–3. Specification of the left/right axis in mice. The embryo is depicted schematically in flattened form viewed from above. Stages of left/right specification shown correspond to *(1)* initial events taking place in and around the node, *(2)* propagation of left/right patterning information to the lateral plate mesoderm, *(3)* maintenance of specification in the left lateral plate, and *(4)* generation of tissue-specific laterality. Details of the molecular pathways are described in the text. BMP, bone morphogenetic protein.

At a conceptual level, the molecular pathway for L/R patterning can be divided into four distinct stages: *(1)* initial breaking of L/R symmetry, *(2)* propagation and establishment of L/R asymmetry, *(3)* maintenance of L/R asymmetrical gene expression, and *(4)* generation of tissue-specific laterality. These stages correspond to a flow of L/R patterning information from the center of the embryo (the node) to the periphery (lateral plate mesoderm), which is responsible for generation of most of the asymmetrical tissues in the body. Interestingly, as discussed below, L/R defects in human patients have been traced to mutations in each of these stages.

Initial Breaking of L/R Symmetry

Although much work on initial events in L/R specification has focused on late gastrulation stages, recent evidence suggests that the L/R asymmetries may exist at early cleavage stages in some vertebrate species. In particular, asymmetrical H^+/K^+-ATPase expression has been shown to occur at early cleavage stages in *Xenopus* embryos, while pharmacological inhibition of H^+/K^+-ATPase results in heterotaxia in frog and chick embryos (Levin et al., 2002), perhaps consistent with the requirement of intact gap junctional communication for correct L/R patterning (Levin and Mercola, 1998, 1999). Thus, the mammalian L/R axis could conceivably also be established at preimplantation stages through mechanisms similar to those responsible for establishing the embryonic/abembryonic and P/D axes.

However, most previous studies have presumed that an initial L/R symmetry is "broken" at the molecular level at mid- to late gastrulation. Indeed, elegant transplantation experiments in the chick embryo have suggested that early events in the generation of L/R asymmetry occur in the vicinity of the node (Pagan-Westphal and Tabin, 1998). Within the mouse node, the ventral cells in the pit of the node are monociliated, each with a single cilium containing a 9+0 microtubule arrangement (reviewed in Hamada et al., 2002). Several lines of evidence have provided strong evidence that these node monocilia play an essential role at an early step in L/R patterning. Mutations in *lrd*, *polaris*, *KIF3B*, and other genes involved in ciliary function result in absence or severe disruption of node monocilia, as well as L/R laterality defects (Nonaka et al., 1998; Supp et al., 1999; Murcia et al., 2000). Moreover, similar monocilia can be found in embryonic structures associated with L/R patterning in chick, zebrafish, and frog, implying a conserved function in this process (Essner et al., 2002).

An elegant model for the role of node monocilia in L/R patterning has been proposed (Nonaka et al., 1998; reviewed in Hamada et al., 2002). In wild-type mouse embryos, the node monocilia rotate unidirectionally *in vivo* and are capable of propelling small particles toward the left side of the node; in contrast, the node monocilia in *lrd* mutants are immotile (Nonaka et al., 1998; Okada et al., 1999; Supp et al., 1999). On this basis, Nonaka and colleagues (1998) proposed that the unidirectional rotation of node monocilia is reponsible for the "flow" of a diffusible signaling factor to the left side of the node, thereby generating an asymmetry in protein distribution that can be amplified into differences in gene expression. Cultured mouse embryos can be subjected to an artificial "nodal flow" that can rescue the phenotype of *lrd* mutants and induce defective L/R patterning in wild-type embryos (Nonaka et al., 2002).

Somewhat confusingly, one of the primary candidate molecules for the signaling molecule propelled by nodal flow is Nodal itself. In the mouse, *Nodal* is expressed in cells at the edges of the node (crown cells) in a symmetrical pattern at presomite stages but later becomes expressed at higher levels on the left side at early somite stages (Collignon et al., 1996; Lowe et al., 1996). This upregulation of *Nodal* expression on the left side of the node requires activation of the *Nodal* autoregulatory enhancer (Norris et al., 2002), suggesting that asymmetrical distribution of Nodal activity around the node is responsible for asymmetrical *Nodal* expression.

Despite these observations, there are several inconsistencies with the "nodal flow" hypothesis, including the diversity of patterning outcomes that arise from seemingly similar disruptions to node monocilia in various mouse mutants (Wagner and Yost, 2000), as well as the failure to observe reversed directionality of nodal flow in *inv* mutants, which instead have slower rates of nodal flow (Okada et al., 1999).

Other functions of node monocilia include potential mechanosensory or chemosensory roles, based on analogous roles for monocilia in other systems. The ability of mechanosensory cilia to induce intracellular calcium fluxes may correlate with the observations that the *pkd-2* (*polycystin-2*) gene encodes a calcium channel and is required for L/R patterning (Pennekamp et al., 2002). Consistent with this idea, Inversin (*inv* gene product) function requires a protein domain that can associate with calmodulin (Yasuhiko et al., 2001; Morgan et al., 2002).

Several regulatory genes for L/R patterning are thought to act in the vicinity of the node, perhaps immediately downstream of the initial symmetry break, though the exact roles of each remain unclear. For example, the *EGF-CFC* gene *Cryptic* is expressed in both the node and lateral plate mesoderm and is required for left-sided specification (Yan et al., 1999); thus, *Cryptic* may function in the node to mediate Nodal signaling, but such a role has not yet been established. In addition, canonical Wnt signaling mediated by *Wnt8c* is required for up-regulation of left-sided *Nodal* expression in the chick node, even though it is expressed only on the right side of the node (Rodriguez-Esteban et al., 2001). Finally, the TGF-β family member Gdf1 is required for left-sided specification in the mouse (Rankin et al., 2000). Notably, mammalian *Gdf1* is most closely related to *Xenopus Vg1*, which has also been implicated in L/R patterning (Hyatt and Yost, 1998).

Another gene that has been implicated in early stages of L/R specification is *Sonic hedgehog*, which was initially implicated as a master regulator of L/R patterning upstream of asymmetrical midline *Nodal* expression in the chick (Levin et al., 1995; Pagan-Westphal and Tabin, 1998). Although *Sonic hedgehog* mutant mice display a left isomerism phenotype (Izraeli et al., 1999; Meyers and Martin, 1999; Tsukui et al., 1999), this laterality defect could be explained as a secondary consequence of a midline defect due to the absence of floor plate and *Lefty1* expression (discussed further below). However, double mutants for *Sonic hedgehog* and *Indian hedgehog*, as well as *Smoothened*, mutants, all of which lack Hedgehog signaling, completely lack left-sided patterning (Zhang et al., 2001), consistent with the idea that Hedgehog signaling plays an essential role in L/R patterning. Interestingly, *Smoothened* mutants lack expression of *Cryptic* and *Gdf1* in the node, suggesting that the role of Hedgehog signaling in L/R patterning is to upregulate these genes in the axial midline (Zhang et al., 2001).

Propagation and Establishment of Asymmetry in the Lateral Plate Mesoderm

At the heart of the pathway for L/R specification is a highly conserved cassette of genes that are asymmetrically expressed in the left lateral plate mesoderm. The core of this cassette is *Nodal*, which was originally implicated in L/R axis specification based on its transiently asymmetrical expression in the left lateral plate mesoderm and on gain-of-function studies in the chick, frog, and fish (reviewed in Burdine and Schier, 2000; Capdevila et al., 2000). Signaling by Nodal in the left lateral plate mesoderm leads to upregulation of *Lefty2*, which maintains left-sided specification by inhibiting excess Nodal signals, and of the homeobox gene *Pitx2*, which is a primary regulator of tissue-specific laterality (discussed below).

Once the initial L/R symmetry break has occurred in or around the node, this positional information needs to be propagated to the left lateral plate mesoderm. Such a propagative role was proposed in the chick for *Caronte*, a member of the Cerberus family that is expressed in the paraxial and lateral plate mesoderm and upregulated on the left side by Sonic hedgehog (Rodriguez Esteban et al., 1999; Yokouchi et al., 1999; Zhu et al., 1999). *Caronte* was thought to function by inhibiting BMP function in the lateral plate mesoderm, thereby leading to upregulation of *Nodal* expression. However, BMP activation (rather than inhibition) is required for upregulation of *Nodal* expression in the lateral plate mesoderm, most likely in an indirect manner through bilateral upregulation of *Cryptic* expression (Fischer et al., 2002; Fujiwara et al., 2002; Piedra and Ros, 2002; Schlange et al., 2002). Instead, given the ability of Nodal to signal over a long range, it is plausible that asymmetrical activity of Nodal in crown cells of the node may directly induce *Nodal* expression in the left lateral plate mesoderm. This model is supported by studies demonstrating a requirement for node-derived Nodal in establishing asymmetrical expression of *Nodal* in the left lateral plate mesoderm (Brennan et al., 2002). In such a scenario, the lack of induced *Nodal* expression in the intervening paraxial mesoderm could simply be attributed to the absence of *Cryptic* expression in this region.

Nodal signaling has long been considered to function primarily in the lateral plate mesoderm to effect L/R patterning, although it is now evident that the Nodal pathway also functions in the node and axial midline (Brennan et al., 2002). Strong support for a central requirement of *Nodal* in L/R patterning has been provided by analysis of *Nodal* hypomorphic mutations (Lowe et al., 2001; Norris et al., 2002) and by targeted disruption of components of the Nodal signaling pathway, including the *EGF-CFC* gene *Cryptic* (Gaio et al., 1999; Yan et al., 1999), *ActRIIB* (Oh and Li, 1997), and *Smad2* (Heyer et al., 1999). In each of these cases, however, the requirements for Nodal signaling in the axial midline versus lateral plate mesoderm have not been clearly distinguished.

As would be expected for a central pathway in left-sided specification, defects in Nodal signaling consistently lead to a right-sided phenotype, typified by right pulmonary isomerism. However, such mutant mice also display a complex mixture of heterotaxia and randomizations of organ *situs,* as well as cardiac defects that are not obviously related to L/R patterning. For example, *Cryptic* null mutants display defects in all known L/R visceral asymmetries, with phenotypes including randomized abdominal *situs,* pulmonary right isomerism, vascular heterotaxia, transposition of the great arteries, and cardiac atrial and septal defects (Gaio et al., 1999; Yan et al., 1999). In *Cryptic* mutant embryos, expression of *Nodal, Lefty2,* and *Pitx2* is abolished in the lateral plate mesoderm, indicating that Nodal signaling is essential for all aspects of L/R patterning.

Maintenance of L/R Specification in the Lateral Plate Mesoderm

Once asymmetrical left-sided expression of *Nodal* is established around the node and in the lateral plate mesoderm, it needs to be maintained on the left side. The requirement for an intact axial midline (prechordal mesoderm, notochord, and floor plate) for maintenance of L/R patterning has been demonstrated by surgical manipulations in frog and mouse embryos (Danos and Yost, 1996; Davidson et al., 1999). These experiments have demonstrated a requirement for a physical midline barrier to maintain left-sided specification; in its absence, the outcome is bilateral expression of *Nodal* and its downstream targets in the lateral plate mesoderm. Notably, numerous mouse mutations that result in defective midline patterning are also associated with L/R patterning defects (*e.g.,* Melloy et al., 1998; Izraeli et al., 1999), but this does not imply that the corresponding genes have any direct role in L/R specification.

In principle, an intact axial midline is required to prevent accidental diffusion of Nodal (or other) signals from the left side to the right or *vice versa.* Such a midline barrier may simply have a physical role in blocking transport of extracellular signals, as is the case for gap junctional communication (Levin and Mercola, 1999). Alternatively, a midline requirement may reflect the midline expression of a "molecular barrier," which has been suggested for the function of *Lefty1* (reviewed in Hamada et al., 2002). Consistent with this model, *Lefty1* is expressed in the left prospective floor plate, and deletion of *Lefty1* results in bilateral expression of *Nodal, Lefty2,* and *Pitx2* in the lateral plate mesoderm (Meno et al., 1996, 1997, 1998). Expression of GFP-tagged proteins in chick embryos suggests that Lefty proteins can diffuse faster than Nodal; thus, midline expression of Lefty proteins can potentially block Nodal activation on the right side through competitive inhibition of Nodal receptors (Sakuma et al., 2002).

Similar findings have been reported for *Lefty2* mutants that lack the Nodal-responsive enhancer that is responsible for *Lefty2* expression in the left lateral plate mesoderm (Meno et al., 2001). In the absence of *Lefty2,* there is prolonged *Nodal* expression that is still restricted to the left lateral plate mesoderm, but the unrestricted diffusion of excess Nodal leads to bilateral expression of *Pitx2* and subsequent left isomerism. Thus, tight regulation of Nodal signaling in the left lateral plate mesoderm is required in addition to a midline barrier to prevent "spillover" of Nodal activity to the right side.

At present, it is unclear whether there is a distinct pathway for right-sided specification that operates in conjunction with the left-sided Nodal signaling pathway or whether right-sided activities merely exist to prevent ectopic Nodal signaling. For example, asymmetrical expression of the Cerberus-related gene *Dante* at higher levels on the right side of the node has been proposed to antagonize left-sided Nodal activity (Pearce et al., 1999). In addition, repression of Nodal activity on the right side of the node may involve N-cadherin, which could antagonize canonical Wnt signaling by Wnt8c through β-catenin (Garcia-Castro et al., 2000; Rodriguez-Esteban et al., 2001). Finally, the Snail-related zinc finger transcription factor encoded by *cSnR* is expressed in the right lateral plate mesoderm of the chick embryo and is believed to repress Nodal target genes in the absence of Nodal signaling (Isaac et al., 1997; Sefton et al., 1998; Patel et al., 1999).

Generation of Tissue-Specific Laterality

Following the generation of L/R asymmetry throughout the embryo, this positional information must be interpreted on a tissue-by-tissue basis. However, the mechanisms by which downstream components of the L/R pathway generate tissue-specific differences in L/R laterality are poorly understood. The *Pitx2* homeobox gene represents a primary regulator of these tissue-specific laterality decisions since it is expressed on the left side of many tissues and required for left-sided patterning of these tissues (Logan et al., 1998; Piedra et al., 1998; Ryan et al., 1998; Yoshioka et al., 1998; Campione et al., 1999). Analysis of the *Pitx2* promoter in transgenic mice has shown that expression of the left side-specific *Pitx2c* isoform is initially dependent on a Nodal-responsive element and subsequently can be maintained by a distinct pathway utilizing tissue-specific transcription factors of the Nkx2 homeodomain family (Shiratori et al., 2001).

The mechanism by which *Pitx2* expression confers left-sided patterning upon multiple individual tissues remains obscure. Since tissue lateralities are randomized rather than abolished in the absence of *Pitx2* expression (e.g., in *Cryptic* mutants), *Pitx2* is likely to function in "biasing" tissue laterality toward a left-sided fate, instead of directly specifying left-sided differentiation. Consistent with this view, analyses of mouse hypomorphic mutants indicate that levels of *Pitx2* activity are critical in determining the *situs* of individual tissues on a tissue-by-tissue basis (Liu et al., 2001). However, the normal cardiac looping and stomach positioning observed in *Pitx2* null mutants indicates that other downstream genes in the L/R pathway remain to be identified (Gage et al., 1999; Kitamura et al., 1999; Lin et al., 1999; Lu et al., 1999).

The interaction between *Pitx2* expression and tissue-specific specification of laterality is perhaps best understood in the case of cardiac patterning (reviewed in Kathiriya and Srivastava, 2000). Despite their normal cardiac looping, *Pitx2* mutants display cardiac phenotypes that indicate a requirement during cardiac morphogenesis (Gage et al., 1999; Kitamura et al., 1999; Lin et al., 1999; Lu et al., 1999). Detailed examination and lineage-tracing analysis have shown that the complex pattern of *Pitx2* expression in the developing heart tube corresponds to left-sided regions of the prospective cardiac chambers (Campione et al., 2001). Moreover, analysis of *iv* mutant mice shows that atrial and ventricular left-sided *Pitx2* expression patterns are independent of each other as well as the direction of cardiac looping, while abnormal expansion of *Pitx2* expression is correlated with formation of double outlet right ventricle (Campione et al., 2001). However, the basis for numerous other cardiac patterning defects that occur as a consequence of defective L/R specification remains to be elucidated.

Differences between Vertebrate Systems

The molecular pathway for L/R patterning is generally well conserved among vertebrate species, but several surprising differences do exist, in addition to those mentioned above. For example, many genes that display transient asymmetry of expression around Hensen's node in the chick embryo are not asymmetrically expressed in the mouse (or fish or frog), including *activin-βB, activin receptor IIA,* and *Sonic hedgehog* (reviewed in Ramsdell and Yost, 1998; Beddington and Robertson, 1999). However, these asymmetries in gene expression may simply reflect a transient morphological asymmetry that exists in Hensen's node but not in the organizer of other vertebrates (Dathe et al., 2002). More interestingly, *Fgf8* has been implicated in right-sided patterning in the chick and rabbit but in left-sided patterning in the mouse, suggesting a fundamental reversal in the role of FGF8 signaling (Boettger et al., 1999; Meyers and Martin, 1999; Fischer et al., 2002). Similarly, the homeobox gene *Nkx3.2* appears to be regulated by FGF8 signaling and is asymmetrically expressed on opposite sides in chick and mouse (Schneider et al., 1999). Thus, some of the regulatory details of the L/R pathway have evolved differently in diverse vertebrate species, possibly including humans.

CONCLUSIONS

Early Developmental Arrest as a Disease Entity

The high rate of spontaneous human embryonic wastage, with an estimated two-thirds of oocytes exposed to sperm either failing to fertilize or dying during subsequent gestation (Leridon, 1987), could have a combination of physiological and environmental etiologies. However, the abundance of embryolethal phenotypes generated in mouse knockouts suggests that genetic abnormalities could play a significant role in spontaneous early human embryonic demise. The potential role of oocyte proteins and transcripts in the establishment of early mammalian polarity introduces the possibility of embryonic defects arising through maternal inheritance. If the embryo's natural regulative ability could not compensate for an abnormality, the most likely outcome would be pre- or peri-implantation embryo death. In addition, there are numerous examples of mouse mutations that manifest their homozygous phenotype during the early postimplantation period (Cross et al., 1994; Copp, 1995; Ihle, 2000). Many of the known embryolethal phenotypes arise because of defects in the interactions between the early tissue lineages (as described in this chapter), while others represent deficiencies in the initial steps of embryonic–maternal interactions. If their human counterparts had similar phenotypes, the affected embryos would in most cases die before or soon after the recognition of pregnancy. Humans carrying such genotypes would likely be diagnosed as infertile or subfertile. This emphasizes the need for further research into the molecular mechanisms of early embryogenesis, including the development of novel models for human embryogenesis based on embryonic stem cells (Xu et al., 2002).

Implications for Human Disease

The genetic complexity of early development implies that the major signaling pathways that have early functions in extraembryonic or embryonic tissues of the conceptus will generally have critical roles at later stages of development. Moreover, due to extensive partial genetic redundancy for components of these pathways, many single-gene mutations will result in relatively mild perturbations of signaling pathways, which will become phenotypically manifest as congenital patterning defects or disease syndromes.

It is already apparent that major classes of human genetic disorders can arise through defective patterning of the major body axes at early stages of embryogenesis. For instance, holoprosencephaly can arise through defects in the formation or maintenance of the axial mesoderm or anterior definitive endoderm (reviewed in Muenke and Beachy, 2000; Roessler and Muenke, 2001); this is covered in detail in Chapter 18. As another example, perturbations of L/R patterning can be evident in human patients with laterality defects (Chapter 26), but subtle laterality defects may underlie many cases of major congenital cardiac abnormalities such as transposition of the great arteries (Goldmuntz et al., 2002). Thus, understanding early embryological processes at the molecular level has provided numerous critical insights into the genetic basis of human disease, which is the subject of the remainder of this volume.

REFERENCES

Adachi H, Saijoh Y, Mochida K, Ohishi S, Hashiguchi H, Hirao A, Hamada H (1999). Determination of left/right asymmetric expression of *nodal* by a left side-specific enhancer with sequence similarity to a *lefty-2* enhancer. *Genes Dev* 13: 1589–1600.

Agius E, Oelgeschlager M, Wessely O, Kemp C, De Robertis EM (2000). Endodermal Nodal-related signals and mesoderm induction in *Xenopus*. *Development* 127: 1173–1183.

Antczak M, Van Blerkom J (1997). Oocyte influences on early development: the regulatory proteins leptin and STAT3 are polarized in mouse and human oocytes and differentially distributed within the cells of the preimplantation stage embryo. *Mol Hum Reprod* 3: 1067–1086.

Arnold SJ, Stappert J, Bauer A, Kispert A, Herrmann BG, Kemler R (2000). *Brachyury* is a target gene of the Wnt/β-catenin signaling pathway. *Mech Dev* 91: 249–258.

Bachiller D, Klingensmith J, Kemp C, Belo JA, Anderson RM, May SR, McMahon JA, McMahon AP, Harland RM, Rossant J, et al. (2000). The organizer factors Chordin and Noggin are required for mouse forebrain development. *Nature* 403: 658–661.

Baens M, Marynen P (1997). A human homologue (*BICD1*) of the *Drosophila bicaudal-D* gene. *Genomics* 45: 601–606.

Bafico A, Liu G, Yaniv A, Gazit A, Aaronson SA (2001). Novel mechanism of Wnt signalling inhibition mediated by Dickkopf-1 interaction with LRP6/Arrow. *Nat Cell Biol* 3: 683–686.

Beddington RS (1994). Induction of a second neural axis by the mouse node. *Development* 120: 613–620.

Beddington RSP, Robertson EJ (1998). Anterior patterning in mouse. *Trends Genet* 14: 277–284.

Beddington RSP, Robertson EJ (1999). Axis development and early asymmetry in mammals. *Cell* 96: 195–209.

Behrens J, Jerchow BA, Wurtele M, Grimm J, Asbrand C, Wirtz R, Kuhl M, Wedlich D, Birchmeier W (1998). Functional interaction of an Axin homolog, Conductin, with β-catenin, APC, and GSK3β. *Science* 280: 596–599.

Bertocchini F, Stern CD (2002). The hypoblast of the chick embryo positions the primitive streak by antagonizing nodal signaling. *Dev Cell* 3: 735–744.

Bielinska M, Narita N, Wilson DB (1999). Distinct roles for visceral endoderm during embryonic mouse development. *Int J Dev Biol* 43: 183–205.

Black SD, Vincent JP (1988). The first cleavage plane and the embryonic axis are determined by separate mechanisms in *Xenopus laevis*. II. Experimental dissociation by lateral compression of the egg. *Dev Biol* 128: 65–71.

Boettger T, Wittler L, Kessel M (1999). FGF8 functions in the specification of the right body side of the chick. *Curr Biol* 9: 277–280.

Bonnerot C, Nicolas JF (1993). Clonal analysis in the intact mouse embryo by intragenic homologous recombination. *C R Acad Sci III* 316: 1207–1217.

Brendza RP, Serbus LR, Duffy JB, Saxton WM (2000). A function for kinesin I in the posterior transport of *oskar* mRNA and Staufen protein. *Science* 289: 2120–2122.

Brennan J, Lu CC, Norris DP, Rodriguez TA, Beddington RS, Robertson EJ (2001). Nodal signalling in the epiblast patterns the early mouse embryo. *Nature* 411: 965–969.

Brennan J, Norris DP, Robertson EJ (2002). Nodal activity in the node governs left-right asymmetry. *Genes Dev* 16: 2339–2344.

Brown NA, Wolpert L (1990). The development of handedness in left/right asymmetry. *Development* 109: 1–9.

Bullock SL, Ish-Horowicz D (2002). Cell polarity: Oskar seeks PARtner for a stable relationship. *Nat Cell Biol* 4: E117–E118.

Burdine RD, Schier AF (2000). Conserved and divergent mechanisms in left-right axis formation. *Genes Dev* 14: 763–776.

Campione M, Steinbeisser H, Schweickert A, Deissler K, van Bebber F, Lowe LA, Nowotschin S, Viebahn C, Haffter P, Kuehn MR, Blum M (1999). The homeobox gene *Pitx2*: mediator of asymmetric left-right signaling in vertebrate heart and gut looping. *Development* 126: 1225–1234.

Campione M, Ros MA, Icardo JM, Piedra E, Christoffels VM, Schweickert A, Blum M, Franco D, Moorman AF (2001). *Pitx2* expression defines a left cardiac lineage of cells: evidence for atrial and ventricular molecular isomerism in the *iv/iv* mice. *Dev Biol* 231: 252–264.

Capdevila J, Vogan KJ, Tabin CJ, Izpisua Belmonte JC (2000). Mechanisms of left-right determination in vertebrates. *Cell* 101: 9–21.

Chen Y, Schier AF (2001). The zebrafish Nodal signal Squint functions as a morphogen. *Nature* 411: 607–610.

Chen X, Rubock MJ, Whitman M (1996). A transcriptional partner for MAD proteins in TGF-β signalling. *Nature* 383: 691–696.

Chen X, Weisberg E, Fridmacher V, Watanabe M, Naco G, Whitman M (1997). Smad4 and FAST-1 in the assembly of activin-responsive factor. *Nature* 389: 85–89.

Ciemerych MA, Mesnard D, Zernicka-Goetz M (2000). Animal and vegetal poles of the mouse egg predict the polarity of the embryonic axis, yet are nonessential for development. *Development* 127: 3467–3474.

Collignon J, Varlet I, Robertson E J (1996). Relationship between asymmetric *nodal* expression and the direction of embryonic turning. *Nature* 381: 155–158.

Conlon FL, Lyons KM, Takaesu N, Barth KS, Kispert A, Herrmann B, Robertson EJ (1994). A primary requirement for *nodal* in the formation and maintenance of the primitive streak in the mouse. *Development* 120: 1919–1928.

Copp AJ (1995). Death before birth: clues from gene knockouts and mutations. *Trends Genet* 11: 87–93.

Cross JC, Werb Z, Fisher SJ (1994). Implantation and the placenta: key pieces of the development puzzle. *Science* 266: 1508–1518.

Danos MC, Yost HJ (1996). Role of notochord in specification of cardiac left-right orientation in zebrafish and *Xenopus*. *Dev Biol* 177: 96–103.

Dathe V, Gamel A, Manner J, Brand-Saberi B, Christ B (2002). Morphological left-right asymmetry of Hensen's node precedes the asymmetric expression of *Shh* and *Fgf8* in the chick embryo. *Anat Embryol (Berl)* 205: 343–354.

Davidson BP, Kinder SJ, Steiner K, Schoenwolf GC, Tam PP (1999). Impact of node ablation on the morphogenesis of the body axis and the lateral asymmetry of the mouse embryo during early organogenesis. *Dev Biol* 211: 11–26.

Davies TJ, Gardner RL (2002). The plane of first cleavage is not related to the distribution of sperm components in the mouse. *Hum Reprod* 17: 2368–2379.

De Robertis EM, Larrain J, Oelgeschlager M, Wessely O (2000). The establishment of Spemann's organizer and patterning of the vertebrate embryo. *Nat Rev Genet* 1: 171–181.

Ding J, Yang L, Yan YT, Chen A, Desai N, Wynshaw-Boris A, Shen MM (1998). *Cripto* is required for correct orientation of the anterior–posterior axis in the mouse embryo. *Nature* 395: 702–707.

Dufort D, Schwartz L, Harpal K, Rossant J (1998). The transcription factor HNF3β is required in visceral endoderm for normal primitive streak morphogenesis. *Development* 125: 3015–3025.

Edwards RG (2000). The role of embryonic polarities in preimplantation growth and implantation of mammalian embryos. *Hum Reprod* 15(Suppl 6): 1–8.

Edwards RG (2001). Regulatory systems in early mammalian development, with especial reference to polarity and totipotency. *Ital J Anat Embryol* 106: 85–100.

Eimon PM, Harland RM (2002). Effects of heterodimerization and proteolytic processing on Derriere and Nodal activity: implications for mesoderm induction in *Xenopus*. *Development* 129: 3089–3103.

Essner JJ, Vogan KJ, Wagner MK, Tabin CJ, Yost HJ, Brueckner M (2002). Left–right development: conserved function for embryonic nodal cilia. *Nature* 418: 37–38.

Evans JP, Foster JA, McAvey BA, Gerton GL, Kopf GS, Schultz RM (2000). Effects of perturbation of cell polarity on molecular markers of sperm–egg binding sites on mouse eggs. *Biol Reprod* 62: 76–84.

Feldman B, Poueymirou W, Papaioannou VE, DeChiara TM, Goldfarb M (1995). Requirement of FGF-4 for postimplantation mouse development. *Science* 267: 246–249.

Fischer A, Viebahn C, Blum M (2002). FGF8 acts as a right determinant during establishment of the left–right axis in the rabbit. *Curr Biol* 12: 1807–1816.

Foley AC, Skromne I, Stern CD (2000). Reconciling different models of forebrain induction and patterning: a dual role for the hypoblast. *Development* 127: 3839–3854.

Fujiwara T, Dehart DB, Sulik KK, Hogan BL (2002). Distinct requirements for extra-embryonic and embryonic bone morphogenetic protein 4 in the formation of the node and primitive streak and coordination of left–right asymmetry in the mouse. *Development* 129: 4685–4696.

Gage PJ, Suh H, Camper SA (1999). Dosage requirement of *Pitx2* for development of multiple organs. *Development* 126: 4643–4651.

Gaio U, Schweickert A, Fischer AN, Muller T, Ozcelik C, Lankes W, Strehle M, Britsch S, Blum M, Birchmeier C (1999). A role of the *cryptic* gene in the correct establishment of the left–right axis. *Curr Biol* 9: 1339–1342.

Garcia-Castro MI, Vielmetter E, Bronner-Fraser M (2000). N-Cadherin, a cell adhesion molecule involved in establishment of embryonic left–right asymmetry. *Science* 288: 1047–1051.

Gardner RL (1984). An in situ cell marker for clonal analysis of development of the extraembryonic endoderm in the mouse. *J Embryol Exp Morphol* 80: 251–288.

Gardner RL (1997). The early blastocyst is bilaterally symmetrical and its axis of symmetry is aligned with the animal–vegetal axis of the zygote in the mouse. *Development* 124: 289–301.

Gardner RL (2001). Specification of embryonic axes begins before cleavage in normal mouse development. *Development* 128: 839–847.

Gardner RL, Cockroft DL (1998). Complete dissipation of coherent clonal growth occurs before gastrulation in mouse epiblast. *Development* 125: 2397–2402.

Germain S, Howell M, Esslemont GM, Hill CS (2000). Homeodomain and winged-helix transcription factors recruit activated Smads to distinct promoter elements via a common Smad interaction motif. *Genes Dev* 14: 435–451.

Gluecksohn-Schoenheimer S (1949). The effects of a lethal mutation responsible for duplication and twinning in mouse embryos. *J Exp Zool* 110: 47–76.

Goldmuntz E, Bamford R, Karkera JD, de la Cruz J, Roessler E, Muenke M (2002). *CFC1* mutations in patients with transposition of the great arteries and double-outlet right ventricle. *Am J Hum Genet* 70: 776–780.

Goldstein B, Hird SN (1996). Specification of the anteroposterior axis in *Caenorhabditis elegans*. *Development* 122: 1467–1474.

Green JB, Smith JC (1990). Graded changes in dose of a *Xenopus* activin A homologue elicit stepwise transitions in embryonic cell fate. *Nature* 347: 391–394.

Gritsman K, Zhang J, Cheng S, Heckscher E, Talbot WS, Schier AF (1999). The EGF-CFC protein one-eyed pinhead is essential for nodal signaling. *Cell* 97: 121–132.

Gritsman K, Talbot WS, Schier AF (2000). Nodal signaling patterns the organizer. *Development* 127: 921–932.

Gurdon JB, Bourillot PY (2001). Morphogen gradient interpretation. *Nature* 413: 797–803.

Haffner-Krausz R, Gorivodsky M, Chen Y, Lonai P (1999). Expression of *Fgfr2* in the early mouse embryo indicates its involvement in preimplantation development. *Mech Dev* 85: 167–172.

Hamada H, Meno C, Watanabe D, Saijoh Y (2002). Establishment of vertebrate left–right asymmetry. *Nat Rev Genet* 3: 103–113.

Harland R, Gerhart J (1997). Formation and function of Spemann's organizer. *Annu Rev Cell Dev Biol* 13: 611–667.

Hart AH, Hartley L, Sourris K, Stadler ES, Li R, Stanley EG, Tam PP, Elefanty AG, Robb L (2002a). *Mixl1* is required for axial mesendoderm morphogenesis and patterning in the murine embryo. *Development* 129: 3597–3608.

Heyer J, Escalante-Alcalde D, Lia M, Boettinger E, Edelmann W, Stewart CL, Kucherlapati R (1999). Postgastrulation *Smad2*-deficient embryos show defects in embryo turning and anterior morphogenesis. *Proc Natl Acad Sci USA* 96: 12595–12600.

Hoodless PA, Pye M, Chazaud C, Labbe E, Attisano L, Rossant J, Wrana JL (2001). *FoxH1 (Fast)* functions to specify the anterior primitive streak in the mouse. *Genes Dev* 15: 1257–1271.

Hsieh JC, Kodjabachian L, Rebbert ML, Rattner A, Smallwood PM, Samos CH, Nusse R, Dawid IB, Nathans J (1999). A new secreted protein that binds to Wnt proteins and inhibits their activities. *Nature* 398: 431–436.

Hsu DR, Economides AN, Wang X, Eimon PM, Harland RM (1998). The *Xenopus* dorsalizing factor Gremlin identifies a novel family of secreted proteins that antagonize BMP activities. *Mol Cell* 1: 673–683.

Huelsken J, Birchmeier W (2001). New aspects of Wnt signaling pathways in higher vertebrates. *Curr Opin Genet Dev* 11: 547–553.

Huelsken J, Vogel R, Brinkmann V, Erdmann B, Birchmeier C, Birchmeier W (2000). Requirement for β-catenin in anterior–posterior axis formation in mice. *J Cell Biol* 148: 567–578.

Hyatt BA, Yost HJ (1998). The left–right coordinator: the role of Vg1 in organizing left–right axis formation. *Cell* 93: 37–46.

Ihle JN (2000). The challenges of translating knockout phenotypes into gene function. *Cell* 102: 131–134.

Isaac A, Sargent MG, Cooke J (1997). Control of vertebrate left–right asymmetry by a snail-related zinc finger gene. *Science* 275: 1301–1304.

Izraeli S, Lowe LA, Bertness VL, Good DJ, Dorward DW, Kirsch IR, Kuehn MR (1999). The *SIL* gene is required for mouse embryonic axial development and left–right specification. *Nature* 399: 691–694.

Jones SE, Jomary C (2002). Secreted Frizzled-related proteins: searching for relationships and patterns. *Bioessays* 24: 811–820.

Joseph EM, Melton DA (1998). Mutant Vg1 ligands disrupt endoderm and mesoderm formation in *Xenopus* embryos. *Development* 125: 2677–2685.

Kanai-Azuma M, Kanai Y, Gad JM, Tajima Y, Taya C, Kurohmaru M, Sanai Y, Yonekawa H, Yazaki K, Tam PP, et al. (2002). Depletion of definitive gut endoderm in *Sox17*-null mutant mice. *Development* 129: 2367–2379.

Kathiriya IS, Srivastava D (2000). Left–right asymmetry and cardiac looping: implications for cardiac development and congenital heart disease. *Am J Med Genet* 97: 271–279.

Kaufman MH, Bard JBL (1999). *The Anatomical Basis of Mouse Development*. Academic Press, San Diego.

Kawasaki H, Mizuseki K, Nishikawa S, Kaneko S, Kuwana Y, Nakanishi S, Nishikawa SI, Sasai Y (2000). Induction of midbrain dopaminergic neurons from ES cells by stromal cell-derived inducing activity. *Neuron* 28: 31–40.

Kimura C, Yoshinaga K, Tian E, Suzuki M, Aizawa S, Matsuo I (2000). Visceral endoderm mediates forebrain development by suppressing posteriorizing signals. *Dev Biol* 225: 304–321.

Kimura C, Shen MM, Takeda N, Aizawa S, Matsuo I (2001). Complementary functions of *Otx2* and *Cripto* in initial patterning of mouse epiblast. *Dev Biol* 235: 12–32.

Kinder SJ, Tsang TE, Wakamiya M, Sasaki H, Behringer RR, Nagy A, Tam P P (2001). The organizer of the mouse gastrula is composed of a dynamic population of progenitor cells for the axial mesoderm. *Development* 128: 3623–3634.

King ML, Zhou Y, Bubunenko M (1999). Polarizing genetic information in the egg: RNA localization in the frog oocyte. *Bioessays* 21: 546–557.

Kitamura K, Miura H, Miyagawa-Tomita S, Yanazawa M, Katoh-Fukui Y, Suzuki R, Ohuchi H, Suehiro A, Motegi Y, Nakahara Y, et al. (1999). Mouse *Pitx2* deficiency leads to anomalies of the ventral body wall, heart, extra- and periocular mesoderm and right pulmonary isomerism. *Development* 126: 5749–5758.

Klein SL (1987). The first cleavage furrow demarcates the dorsal–ventral axis in *Xenopus* embryos. *Dev Biol* 120: 299–304.

Klingensmith J, Ang SL, Bachiller D, Rossant J (1999). Neural induction and patterning in the mouse in the absence of the node and its derivatives. *Dev Biol* 216: 535–549.

Kumar A, Novoselov V, Celeste AJ, Wolfman NM, ten Dijke P, Kuehn MR (2001). Nodal signaling uses activin and transforming growth factor-β receptor-regulated Smads. *J Biol Chem* 276: 656–661.

Lall S, Patel NH (2001). Conservation and divergence in molecular mechanisms of axis formation. *Annu Rev Genet* 35: 407–437.

Larabell CA, Torres M, Rowning BA, Yost C, Miller JR, Wu M, Kimelman D, Moon RT (1997). Establishment of the dorso-ventral axis in *Xenopus* embryos is presaged by early asymmetries in β-catenin that are modulated by the Wnt signaling pathway. *J Cell Biol* 136: 1123–1136.

Latinkic BV, Umbhauer M, Neal KA, Lerchner W, Smith JC, Cunliffe V (1997). The *Xenopus Brachyury* promoter is activated by FGF and low concentrations of activin and suppressed by high concentrations of activin and by paired-type homeodomain proteins. *Genes Dev* 11: 3265–3276.

Lawson KA, Pedersen RA (1987). Cell fate, morphogenetic movement and population kinetics of embryonic endoderm at the time of germ layer formation in the mouse. *Development* 101: 627–652.

Lawson KA, Meneses JJ, Pedersen RA (1986). Cell fate and cell lineage in the endoderm of the presomite mouse embryo, studied with an intracellular tracer. *Dev Biol* 115: 325–339.

Lawson KA, Meneses JJ, Pedersen RA (1991). Clonal analysis of epiblast fate during germ layer formation in the mouse embryo. *Development* 113: 891–911.

Lawson KA, Dunn NR, Roelen BA, Zeinstra LM, Davis AM, Wright CV, Korving JP, Hogan BL (1999). *Bmp4* is required for the generation of primordial germ cells in the mouse embryo. *Genes Dev* 13: 424–436.

Leridon H (1987). Spontaneous fetal mortality. Role of maternal age, parity and previous abortions. *J Gynecol Obstet Biol Reprod (Paris)* 16: 425–431.

Levin M, Mercola M (1998). Gap junctions are involved in the early generation of left-right asymmetry. *Dev Biol* 203: 90–105.

Levin M, Mercola M (1999). Gap junction–mediated transfer of left-right patterning signals in the early chick blastoderm is upstream of *Shh* asymmetry in the node. *Development* 126: 4703–4714.

Levin M, Johnson RL, Stern CD, Kuehn M, Tabin C (1995). A molecular pathway determining left-right asymmetry in chick embryogenesis. *Cell* 82: 803–814.

Levin M, Thorlin T, Robinson K, Nogi T, Mercola M (2002). Asymmetries in H^+/K^+-ATPase and cell membrane potentials comprise a very early step in left–right patterning. *Cell* 111: 77–89.

Lin CR, Kioussi C, O'Connell S, Briata P, Szeto D, Liu F, Izpisua-Belmonte JC, and Rosenfeld MG (1999). Pitx2 regulates lung asymmetry, cardiac positioning and pituitary and tooth morphogenesis. *Nature* 401: 279–282.

Liu P, Wakamiya M, Shea MJ, Albrecht U, Behringer RR, Bradley A (1999). Requirement for *Wnt3* in vertebrate axis formation. *Nat Genet* 22: 361–365.

Liu C, Liu W, Lu MF, Brown NA, Martin JF (2001). Regulation of left-right asymmetry by thresholds of *Pitx2c* activity. *Development* 128: 2039–2048.

Liu C, Li Y, Semenov M, Han C, Baeg GH, Tan Y, Zhang Z, Lin X, He X (2002). Control of β-catenin phosphorylation/degradation by a dual-kinase mechanism. *Cell* 108: 837–847.

Logan M, Pagan-Westphal SM, Smith DM, Paganessi L, Tabin CJ (1998). The tran-

scription factor Pitx2 mediates situs-specific morphogenesis in response to left-right asymmetric signals. *Cell* 94: 307–317.
Logan CY, Miller JR, Ferkowicz MJ, McClay DR (1999). Nuclear β-catenin is required to specify vegetal cell fates in the sea urchin embryo. *Development* 126: 345–357.
Lowe LA, Supp DM, Sampath K, Yokoyama T, Wright CV, Potter SS, Overbeek P, Kuehn MR (1996). Conserved left–right asymmetry of *nodal* expression and alterations in murine situs inversus. *Nature* 381: 158–161.
Lowe LA, Yamada S, Kuehn MR (2001). Genetic dissection of *nodal* function in patterning the mouse embryo. *Development* 128: 1831–1843.
Lu MF, Pressman C, Dyer R, Johnson RL, Martin JF (1999). Function of Rieger syndrome gene in left–right asymmetry and craniofacial development. *Nature* 401: 276–278.
Lu CC, Brennan J, Robertson EJ (2001). From fertilization to gastrulation: axis formation in the mouse embryo. *Curr Opin Genet Dev* 11: 384–392.
Mao B, Wu W, Li Y, Hoppe D, Stannek P, Glinka A, Niehrs C (2001a). LDL-receptor-related protein 6 is a receptor for Dickkopf proteins. *Nature* 411: 321–325.
Mao J, Wang J, Liu B, Pan W, Farr GH, 3rd Flynn C, Yuan H, Takada S, Kimelman D, Li L, et al. (2001b). Low-density lipoprotein receptor-related protein-5 binds to Axin and regulates the canonical Wnt signaling pathway. *Mol Cell* 7: 801–809.
Mao B, Wu W, Davidson G, Marhold J, Li M, Mechler BM, Delius H, Hoppe D, Stannek P, Walter C, et al. (2002). Kremen proteins are Dickkopf receptors that regulate Wnt/β-catenin signalling. *Nature* 417: 664–667.
Matzuk MM, Kumar TR, Bradley A (1995). Different phenotypes for mice deficient in either activins or activin receptor type II. *Nature* 374: 356–360.
McDowell N, Gurdon JB (1999). Activin as a morphogen in *Xenopus* mesoderm induction. *Semin Cell Dev Biol* 10: 311–317.
Melloy PG, Ewart JL, Cohen MF, Desmond ME, Kuehn MR, Lo CW (1998). *No turning*, a mouse mutation causing left–right and axial patterning defects. *Dev Biol* 193: 77–89.
Meno C, Saijoh Y, Fujii H, Ikeda M, Yokoyama T, Yokoyama M, Toyoda Y, Hamada H (1996). Left–right asymmetric expression of the TGF beta-family member lefty in mouse embryos. *Nature* 381: 151–155.
Meno C, Ito Y, Saijoh Y, Matsuda Y, Tashiro K, Kuhara S, Hamada H (1997). Two closely-related left–right asymmetrically expressed genes, *lefty-1* and *lefty-2*: their distinct expression domains, chromosomal linkage and direct neuralizing activity in *Xenopus* embryos. *Genes Cells* 2: 513–524.
Meno C, Shimono A, Saijoh Y, Yashiro K, Mochida K, Ohishi S, Noji S, Kondoh H, Hamada H (1998). lefty-1 is required for left-right determination as a regulator of *lefty-2* and *nodal*. *Cell* 94: 287–297.
Meno C, Takeuchi J, Sakuma R, Koshiba-Takeuchi K, Ohishi S, Saijoh Y, Miyazaki J, ten Dijke P, Ogura T, Hamada H (2001). Diffusion of nodal signaling activity in the absence of the feedback inhibitor Lefty2. *Dev Cell* 1: 127–138.
Mercola M, Levin M (2001). Left–right asymmetry determination in vertebrates. *Annu Rev Cell Dev Biol* 17: 779–805.
Meyers EN, Martin GR (1999). Differences in left-right axis pathways in mouse and chick: functions of FGF8 and SHH. *Science* 285: 403–406.
Mochizuki T, Saijoh Y, Tsuchiya K, Shirayoshi Y, Takai S, Taya C, Yonekawa H, Yamada K, Nihei H, Nakatsuji N, et al. (1998). Cloning of inv, a gene that controls left/right asymmetry and kidney development. *Nature* 395: 177–181.
Moon RT, Bowerman B, Boutros M, Perrimon N (2002). The promise and perils of Wnt signaling through β-catenin. *Science* 296: 1644–1646.
Morgan D, Turnpenny L, Goodship J, Dai W, Majumder K, Matthews L, Gardner A, Schuster G, Vien L, Harrison W, et al. (1998). *Inversin*, a novel gene in the vertebrate left-right axis pathway, is partially deleted in the *inv* mouse. *Nat Genet* 20: 149–156.
Morgan D, Goodship J, Essner JJ, Vogan KJ, Turnpenny L, Yost J, Tabin CJ, Strachan T (2002). The left-right determinant inversin has highly conserved ankyrin repeat and IQ domains and interacts with calmodulin. *Hum Genet* 110: 377–384.
Muenke M, Beachy PA (2000). Genetics of ventral forebrain development and holoprosencephaly. *Curr Opin Genet Dev* 10: 262–269.
Mukhopadhyay M, Shtrom S, Rodriguez-Esteban C, Chen L, Tsukui T, Gomer L, Dorward DW, Glinka A, Grinberg A, Huang SP, et al. (2001). *Dickkopf1* is required for embryonic head induction and limb morphogenesis in the mouse. *Dev Cell* 1: 423–434.
Munoz-Sanjuan I, Brivanlou AH (2002). Neural induction, the default model and embryonic stem cells. *Nat Rev Neurosci* 3: 271–280.
Murcia NS, Richards WG, Yoder BK, Mucenski ML, Dunlap JR, Woychik RP (2000). The *Oak Ridge Polycystic Kidney (orpk)* disease gene is required for left–right axis determination. *Development* 127: 2347–2355.
Nakaya M, Fukui A, Izumi Y, Akimoto K, Asashima M, Ohno S (2000). Meiotic maturation induces animal–vegetal asymmetric distribution of aPKC and ASIP/PAR-3 in *Xenopus* oocytes. *Development* 127: 5021–5031.
Nishita M, Hashimoto MK, Ogata S, Laurent MN, Ueno N, Shibuya H, Cho KW (2000). Interaction between Wnt and TGF-β signalling pathways during formation of Spemann's organizer. *Nature* 403: 781–785.
Nonaka S, Tanaka Y, Okada Y, Takeda S, Harada A, Kanai Y, Kido M, Hirokawa N (1998). Randomization of left–right asymmetry due to loss of nodal cilia generating leftward flow of extraembryonic fluid in mice lacking KIF3B motor protein. *Cell* 95: 829–837.
Nonaka S, Shiratori H, Saijoh Y, Hamada H (2002). Determination of left–right patterning of the mouse embryo by artificial nodal flow. *Nature* 418: 96–99.
Norris DP, Robertson EJ (1999). Asymmetric and node-specific nodal expression patterns are controlled by two distinct *cis*-acting regulatory elements. *Genes Dev* 13: 1575–1588.
Norris DP, Brennan J, Bikoff EK, Robertson EJ (2002). The FoxH1-dependent autoregulatory enhancer controls the level of Nodal signals in the mouse embryo. *Development* 129: 3455–3468.
Oh SP, Li E (1997). The signaling pathway mediated by the type IIB activin receptor controls axial patterning and lateral asymmetry in the mouse. *Genes Dev* 11: 1812–1826.
Okada Y, Nonaka S, Tanaka Y, Saijoh Y, Hamada H, Hirokawa N (1999). Abnormal nodal flow precedes situs inversus in *iv* and *inv* mice. *Mol Cell* 4: 459–468.
Pagan-Westphal SM, Tabin CJ (1998). The transfer of left–right positional information during chick embryogenesis. *Cell* 93: 25–35.
Pandur P, Maurus D, Kuhl M (2002). Increasingly complex: new players enter the Wnt signaling network. *Bioessays* 24: 881–884.
Patel K, Isaac A, Cooke J (1999). Nodal signalling and the roles of the transcription factors SnR and Pitx2 in vertebrate left–right asymmetry. *Curr Biol* 9: 609–612.
Pearce JJ, Penny G, Rossant J (1999). A mouse Cerberus/Dan-related gene family. *Dev Biol* 209: 98–110.
Peifer M, Polakis P (2000). Wnt signaling in oncogenesis and embryogenesis—a look outside the nucleus. *Science* 287: 1606–1609.
Pennekamp P, Karcher C, Fischer A, Schweickert A, Skryabin B, Horst J, Blum M, Dworniczak B (2002). The ion channel polycystin-2 is required for left-right axis determination in mice. *Curr Biol* 12: 938–943.
Perea-Gomez A, Shawlot W, Sasaki H, Behringer RR, Ang S (1999). HNF3β and *Lim1* interact in the visceral endoderm to regulate primitive streak formation and anterior–posterior polarity in the mouse embryo. *Development* 126: 4499–4511.
Perea-Gomez A, Lawson KA, Rhinn M, Zakin L, Brulet P, Mazan S, Ang SL (2001a). Otx2 is required for visceral endoderm movement and for the restriction of posterior signals in the epiblast of the mouse embryo. *Development* 128: 753–765.
Perea-Gomez A, Rhinn M, Ang SL (2001b). Role of the anterior visceral endoderm in restricting posterior signals in the mouse embryo. *Int J Dev Biol* 45(1): 311–320.
Perea-Gomez A, Vella FD, Shawlot W, Oulad-Abdelghani M, Chazaud C, Meno C, Pfister V, Chen L, Robertson E, Hamada H, et al. (2002). Nodal antagonists in the anterior visceral endoderm prevent the formation of multiple primitive streaks. *Dev Cell* 3: 745–756.
Piccolo S, Agius E, Leyns L, Bhattacharyya S, Grunz H, Bouwmeester T, De Robertis EM (1999). The head inducer Cerberus is a multifunctional antagonist of Nodal, BMP and Wnt signals. *Nature* 397: 707–710.
Piedra ME, Ros MA (2002). BMP signaling positively regulates Nodal expression during left/right specification in the chick embryo. *Development* 129: 3431–3440.
Piedra ME, Icardo JM, Albajar M, Rodriguez-Rey JC, Ros MA (1998). Pitx2 participates in the late phase of the pathway controlling left/right asymmetry. *Cell* 94: 319–324.
Pinson KI, Brennan J, Monkley S, Avery BJ, Skarnes WC (2000). An LDL-receptor-related protein mediates Wnt signalling in mice. *Nature* 407: 535–538.
Piotrowska K, Zernicka-Goetz M (2001). Role for sperm in spatial patterning of the early mouse embryo. *Nature* 409: 517–521.
Piotrowska K, Zernicka-Goetz M (2002). Early patterning of the mouse embryo—contributions of sperm and egg. *Development* 129: 5803–5813.
Piotrowska K, Wianny F, Pedersen RA, Zernicka-Goetz M (2001). Blastomeres arising from the first cleavage division have distinguishable fates in normal mouse development. *Development* 128: 3739–3748.
Plusa B, Grabarek JB, Piotrowska K, Glover DM, Zernicka-Goetz M (2002a). Site of the previous meiotic division defines cleavage orientation in the mouse embryo. *Nat Cell Biol* 4: 811–815.
Plusa B, Piotrowska K, Zernicka-Goetz M (2002b). Sperm entry position provides a surface marker for the first cleavage plane of the mouse zygote. *Genesis* 32: 193–198.
Pogoda HM, Solnica-Krezel L, Driever W, Meyer D (2000). The zebrafish forkhead transcription factor FoxH1/Fast1 is a modulator of nodal signaling required for organizer formation. *Curr Biol* 10: 1041–1049.
Polakis P (2000). Wnt signaling and cancer. *Genes Dev* 14: 1837–1851.
Popperl H, Schmidt C, Wilson V, Hume CR, Dodd J, Krumlauf R, Beddington RS (1997). Misexpression of *Cwnt8C* in the mouse induces an ectopic embryonic axis and causes a truncation of the anterior neuroectoderm. *Development* 124: 2997–3005.
Ramsdell AF, Yost HJ (1998). Molecular mechanisms of vertebrate left-right development. *Trends Genet* 14: 459–465.
Rankin CT, Bunton T, Lawler AM, Lee SJ (2000). Regulation of left-right patterning in mice by growth/differentiation factor-1. *Nat Genet* 24: 262–265.
Reissmann E, Jornvall H, Blokzijl A, Andersson O, Chang C, Minchiotti G, Persico MG, Ibanez CF, Brivanlou AH (2001). The orphan receptor ALK7 and the Activin receptor ALK4 mediate signaling by Nodal proteins during vertebrate development. *Genes Dev* 15: 2010–2022.
Reiter JF, Alexander J, Rodaway A, Yelon D, Patient R, Holder N, Stainier DY (1999). Gata5 is required for the development of the heart and endoderm in zebrafish. *Genes Dev* 13: 2983–2995.
Rhinn M, Dierich A, Shawlot W, Behringer RR, Le Meur M, Ang SL (1998). Sequential roles for *Otx2* in visceral endoderm and neuroectoderm for forebrain and midbrain induction and specification. *Development* 125: 845–856.
Riechmann V, Gutierrez GJ, Filardo P, Nebreda AR, Ephrussi A (2002). Par-1 regulates stability of the posterior determinant Oskar by phosphorylation. *Nat Cell Biol* 4: 337–342.
Rodriguez TA, Casey ES, Harland RM, Smith JC, Beddington RS (2001). Distinct enhancer elements control *Hex* expression during gastrulation and early organogenesis. *Dev Biol* 234: 304–316.
Rodriguez Esteban C, Capdevila J, Economides AN, Pascual J, Ortiz A, Izpisua Belmonte JC (1999). The novel Cer-like protein Caronte mediates the establishment of embryonic left–right asymmetry. *Nature* 401: 243–251.
Rodriguez-Esteban C, Capdevila J, Kawakami Y, Izpisua Belmonte J C (2001). Wnt signaling and PKA control *Nodal* expression and left–right determination in the chick embryo. *Development* 128: 3189–3195.
Roessler E, Muenke M (2001). Midline and laterality defects: left and right meet in the middle. *Bioessays* 23: 888–900.
Russ AP, Wattler S, Colledge WH, Aparicio SA, Carlton MB, Pearce JJ, Barton SC, Surani MA, Ryan K, Nehls MC, et al. (2000). *Eomesodermin* is required for mouse trophoblast development and mesoderm formation. *Nature* 404: 95–99.
Ryan AK, Blumberg B, Rodriguez-Esteban C, Yonei-Tamura S, Tamura K, Tsukui T, de la Pena J, Sabbagh W, Greenwald J, Choe S, et al. (1998). Pitx2 determines left–right asymmetry of internal organs in vertebrates. *Nature* 394: 545–551.
Saijoh Y, Adachi H, Sakuma R, Yeo CY, Yashiro K, Watanabe M, Hashiguchi H, Mochida K, Ohishi S, Kawabata M, et al. (2000). Left-right asymmetric expression of *lefty2* and *nodal* is induced by a signaling pathway that includes the transcription factor FAST2. *Mol Cell* 5: 35–47.
Sakuma R, Ohnishi Yi Y, Meno C, Fujii H, Juan H, Takeuchi J, Ogura T, Li E, Miya-

zono K, Hamada H (2002). Inhibition of Nodal signalling by Lefty mediated through interaction with common receptors and efficient diffusion. *Genes Cells* 7: 401–412.

Saunders PT, Pathirana S, Maguire SM, Doyle M, Wood T, Bownes M (2000). Mouse staufen genes are expressed in germ cells during oogenesis and spermatogenesis. *Mol Hum Reprod* 6: 983–991.

Schier AF, Shen MM (2000). Nodal signalling in vertebrate development. *Nature* 403: 385–389.

Schier AF, Neuhauss SCF, Helde KA, Talbot WS, Driever W (1997). The *one-eyed pinhead* gene functions in mesoderm and endoderm formation in zebrafish and interacts with *no tail*. *Development* 124: 327–342.

Schlange T, Arnold HH, Brand T (2002). BMP2 is a positive regulator of Nodal signaling during left–right axis formation in the chicken embryo. *Development* 129: 3421–3429.

Schneider S, Steinbeisser H, Warga RM, Hausen P (1996). β-catenin translocation into nuclei demarcates the dorsalizing centers in frog and fish embryos. *Mech Dev* 57: 191–198.

Schneider A, Mijalski T, Schlange T, Dai W, Overbeek P, Arnold HH, Brand T (1999). The homeobox gene *NKX3.2* is a target of left–right signalling and is expressed on opposite sides in chick and mouse embryos. *Curr Biol* 9: 911–914.

Schnorrer F, Bohmann K, Nusslein-Volhard C (2000). The molecular motor dynein is involved in targeting *swallow* and *bicoid* RNA to the anterior pole of *Drosophila* oocytes. *Nat Cell Biol* 2: 185–190.

Schulte-Merker S, Smith JC, Dale L (1994). Effects of truncated activin and FGF receptors and of follistatin on the inducing activities of BVg1 and activin: does activin play a role in mesoderm induction? *EMBO J* 13: 3533–3541.

Sefton M, Sanchez S, Nieto MA (1998). Conserved and divergent roles for members of the Snail family of transcription factors in the chick and mouse embryo. *Development* 125: 3111–3121.

Semenov MV, Tamai K, Brott BK, Kuhl M, Sokol S, He X (2001). Head inducer Dickkopf-1 is a ligand for Wnt coreceptor LRP6. *Curr Biol* 11: 951–961.

Shawlot W, Wakamiya M, Kwan KM, Kania A, Jessell TM, Behringer RR (1999). *Lim1* is required in both primitive streak-derived tissues and visceral endoderm for head formation in the mouse. *Development* 126: 4925–4932.

Shen MM, Schier AF (2000). The *EGF-CFC* gene family in vertebrate development. *Trends Genet* 16: 303–309.

Shiratori H, Sakuma R, Watanabe M, Hashiguchi H, Mochida K, Sakai Y, Nishino J, Saijoh Y, Whitman M, Hamada H (2001). Two-step regulation of left-right asymmetric expression of *Pitx2*: initiation by nodal signaling and maintenance by Nkx2. *Mol Cell* 7: 137–149.

Sirotkin HI, Gates MA, Kelly PD, Schier AF, Talbot WS (2000). *Fast1* is required for the development of dorsal axial structures in zebrafish. *Curr Biol* 10: 1051–1054.

Skromne I, Stern CD (2001). Interactions between Wnt and Vg1 signalling pathways initiate primitive streak formation in the chick embryo. *Development* 128: 2915–2927.

Smith LJ (1980). Embryonic axis orientation in the mouse and its correlation with blastocyst relationships to the uterus. Part 1. Relationships between 82 hours and 4 1/4 days. *J Embryol Exp Morphol* 55: 257–277.

Smith LJ (1985). Embryonic axis orientation in the mouse and its correlation with blastocyst relationships to the uterus. II. Relationships from 4 1/4 to 9 1/2 days. *J Embryol Exp Morphol* 89: 15–35.

Smith JC (1995). Mesoderm-inducing factors and mesodermal patterning. *Curr Opin Cell Biol* 7: 856–861.

Stern CD (2002). Induction and initial patterning of the nervous system—the chick embryo enters the scene. *Curr Opin Genet Dev* 12: 447–451.

St Johnston D (2001). The beginning of the end. *EMBO J* 20: 6169–6179.

Stainier DY (2002). A glimpse into the molecular entrails of endoderm formation. *Genes Dev* 16: 893–907.

Sun BI, Bush SM, Collins-Racie LA, LaVallie ER, DiBlasio-Smith EA, Wolfman NM, McCoy JM, Sive HL (1999). derriere: a TGF-β family member required for posterior development in *Xenopus*. *Development* 126: 1467–1482.

Supp DM, Witte DP, Potter SS, Brueckner M (1997). Mutation of an axonemal dynein affects left–right asymmetry in *inversus viscerum* mice. *Nature* 389: 963–966.

Supp DM, Brueckner M, Kuehn MR, Witte DP, Lowe LA, McGrath J, Corrales J, Potter SS (1999). Targeted deletion of the ATP binding domain of left-right dynein confirms its role in specifying development of left–right asymmetries. *Development* 126: 5495–5504.

Tam PP, Behringer RR (1997). Mouse gastrulation: the formation of a mammalian body plan. *Mech Dev* 68: 3–25.

Tam PP, Steiner KA (1999). Anterior patterning by synergistic activity of the early gastrula organizer and the anterior germ layer tissues of the mouse embryo. *Development* 126: 5171–5179.

Tam PP, Gad JM, Kinder SJ, Tsang TE, Behringer RR (2001). Morphogenetic tissue movement and the establishment of body plan during development from blastocyst to gastrula in the mouse. *Bioessays* 23: 508–517.

Tamai K, Semenov M, Kato Y, Spokony R, Liu C, Katsuyama Y, Hess F, Saint-Jeannet JP, He X (2000). LDL-receptor-related proteins in Wnt signal transduction. *Nature* 407: 530–535.

Tanaka S, Kunath T, Hadjantonakis AK, Nagy A, Rossant J (1998). Promotion of trophoblast stem cell proliferation by FGF4. *Science* 282: 2072–2075.

Thisse B, Wright CV, Thisse C (2000). Activin- and Nodal-related factors control antero-posterior patterning of the zebrafish embryo. *Nature* 403: 425–428.

Thomas P, Beddington R (1996). Anterior primitive endoderm may be responsible for patterning the anterior neural plate in the mouse embryo. *Curr Biol* 6: 1487–1496.

Thomas PQ, Brown A, Beddington RSP (1998). *Hex*: a homeobox gene revealing peri-implantation asymmetry in the mouse embryo and an early transient marker of endothelial cell precursors. *Development* 125: 85–94.

Tremblay KD, Hoodless PA, Bikoff EK, Robertson EJ (2000). Formation of the definitive endoderm in mouse is a Smad2-dependent process. *Development* 127: 3079–3090.

Tsukui T, Capdevila J, Tamura K, Ruiz-Lozano P, Rodriguez-Esteban C, Yonei-Tamura S, Magallon J, Chandraratna R A, Chien K, Blumberg B, et al. (1999). Multiple left–right asymmetry defects in *Shh*$^{-/-}$ mutant mice unveil a convergence of the shh and retinoic acid pathways in the control of *Lefty-1*. *Proc Natl Acad Sci USA* 96: 11376–11381.

van Noort M, Clevers H (2002). TCF transcription factors, mediators of Wnt-signaling in development and cancer. *Dev Biol* 244: 1–8.

Varlet I, Collignon J, Robertson EJ (1997). *nodal* expression in the primitive endoderm is required for specification of the anterior axis during mouse gastrulation. *Development* 124: 1033–1044.

Vonica A, Gumbiner B (2002). Zygotic Wnt activity is required for *Brachyury* expression in the early *Xenopus laevis* embryo. *Dev Biol* 250: 112.

Wagner MK, Yost HJ (2000). Left–right development: the roles of nodal cilia. *Curr Biol* 10: R149–R151.

Waldrip WR, Bikoff EK, Hoodless PA, Wrana JL, Robertson EJ (1998). Smad2 signaling in extraembryonic tissues determines anterior–posterior polarity of the early mouse embryo. *Cell* 92: 797–808.

Wallenfang MR, Seydoux G (2000). Polarization of the anterior–posterior axis of *C. elegans* is a microtubule-directed process. *Nature* 408: 89–92.

Watanabe M, Whitman M (1999). FAST-1 is a key maternal effector of mesoderm inducers in the early *Xenopus* embryo. *Development* 126: 5621–5634.

Weber RJ, Pedersen RA, Wianny F, Evans MJ, Zernicka-Goetz M (1999). Polarity of the mouse embryo is anticipated before implantation. *Development* 126: 5591–5598.

Wehrli M, Dougan ST, Caldwell K, O'Keefe L, Schwartz S, Vaizel-Ohayon D, Schejter E, Tomlinson A, DiNardo S (2000). arrow encodes an LDL-receptor-related protein essential for Wingless signalling. *Nature* 407: 527–530.

Wessely O, Agius E, Oelgeschlager M, Pera EM, De Robertis EM (2001). Neural induction in the absence of mesoderm: β-catenin-dependent expression of secreted BMP antagonists at the blastula stage in *Xenopus*. *Dev Biol* 234: 161–173.

White RJ, Sun BI, Sive HL, Smith JC (2002). Direct and indirect regulation of *derriere*, a *Xenopus* mesoderm-inducing factor, by VegT. *Development* 129: 4867–4876.

Whitman M (2001). Nodal signaling in early vertebrate embryos. Themes and variations. *Dev Cell* 1: 605–617.

Wickham L, Duchaine T, Luo M, Nabi IR, DesGroseillers L (1999). Mammalian staufen is a double-stranded-RNA- and tubulin-binding protein which localizes to the rough endoplasmic reticulum. *Mol Cell Biol* 19: 2220–2230.

Wilder PJ, Kelly D, Brigman K, Peterson CL, Nowling T, Gao QS, McComb RD, Capecchi MR, Rizzino A (1997). Inactivation of the *FGF-4* gene in embryonic stem cells alters the growth and/or the survival of their early differentiated progeny. *Dev Biol* 192: 614–629.

Willert K, Nusse R (1998). Beta-catenin: a key mediator of Wnt signaling. *Curr Opin Genet Dev* 8: 95–102.

Wilson SI, Edlund T (2001). Neural induction: toward a unifying mechanism. *Nat Neurosci* 4(Suppl): 1161–1168.

Wodarz A, Nusse R (1998). Mechanisms of Wnt signaling in development. *Annu Rev Cell Dev Biol* 14: 59–88.

Xu RH, Chen X, Li DS, Li R, Addicks GC, Glennon C, Zwaka TP, Thomson JA (2002). BMP4 initiates human embryonic stem cell differentiation to trophoblast. *Nat Biotechnol* 20: 1261–1264.

Yamamoto M, Meno C, Sakai Y, Shiratori H, Mochida K, Ikawa Y, Saijoh Y, Hamada H (2001). The transcription factor FoxH1 (FAST) mediates Nodal signaling during anterior–posterior patterning and node formation in the mouse. *Genes Dev* 15: 1242–1256.

Yan Y-T, Gritsman K, Ding J, Burdine RD, Corrales JD, Price SM, Talbot WS, Schier AF, Shen MM (1999). Conserved requirement for *EGF-CFC* genes in vertebrate left–right axis formation. *Genes Dev* 13: 2527–2537.

Yan YT, Liu JJ, Luo Y, E C, Haltiwanger RS, Abate-Shen C, Shen MM (2002). Dual roles of Cripto as a ligand and coreceptor in the Nodal signaling pathway. *Mol Cell Biol* 22: 4439–4449.

Yasuhiko Y, Imai F, Ookubo K, Takakuwa Y, Shiokawa K, Yokoyama T (2001). Calmodulin binds to inv protein: implication for the regulation of inv function. *Dev Growth Differ* 43: 671–681.

Yeo C, Whitman M (2001). Nodal signals to Smads through Cripto-dependent and Cripto-independent mechanisms. *Mol Cell* 7: 949–957.

Yokouchi Y, Vogan KJ, Pearse RV 2nd, Tabin, CJ (1999). Antagonistic signaling by *Caronte*, a novel *Cerberus*-related gene, establishes left–right asymmetric gene expression. *Cell* 98: 573–583.

Yokoyama T, Copeland NG, Jenkins NA, Montgomery CA, Elder FFB, Overbeek PA (1993). Reversal of left–right asymmetry: a situs inversus mutation. *Science* 260: 679–682.

Yoshioka H, Meno C, Koshiba K, Sugihara M, Itoh H, Ishimaru Y, Inoue T, Ohuchi H, Semina EV, Murray JC, et al. (1998). *Pitx2*, a bicoid-type homeobox gene, is involved in a lefty-signaling pathway in determination of left–right asymmetry. *Cell* 94: 299–305.

Yost HJ (1991). *Development* of the left–right axis in amphibians. *Ciba Found Symp* 162: 165–181.

Zeng L, Fagotto F, Zhang T, Hsu W, Vasicek TJ, Perry WLI, Lee JJ, Tilghman SM, Gumbiner BM, Constantini F (1997). The mouse *Fused* locus encodes axin, an inhibitor of the Wnt signaling pathway that regulates embryonic axis formation. *Cell* 90: 181–192.

Zernicka-Goetz M (1998). Fertile offspring derived from mammalian eggs lacking either animal or vegetal poles. *Development* 125: 4803–4808.

Zernicka-Goetz M (2002). Patterning of the embryo: the first spatial decisions in the life of a mouse. *Development* 129: 815–829.

Zhang XM, Ramalho-Santos M, McMahon AP (2001). Smoothened mutants reveal redundant roles for Shh and Ihh signaling including regulation of L/R symmetry by the mouse node. *Cell* 106: 781–792.

Zhou X, Sasaki H, Lowe L, Hogan BL, Kuehn MR (1993). Nodal is a novel TGF-β-like gene expressed in the mouse node during gastrulation. *Nature* 361: 543–547.

Zhu L, Marvin MJ, Gardiner A, Lassar AB, Mercola M, Stern CD, Levin M (1999). Cerberus regulates left-right asymmetry of the embryonic head and heart. *Curr Biol* 9: 931–938.

6 | Neural Crest Formation and Craniofacial Development

DEBORAH LANG, CHRISTOPHER B. BROWN, AND JONATHAN A. EPSTEIN

The neural crest is an intriguing population of cells that gives rise to multiple cell types throughout the body and is associated with a large variety of human developmental disorders. A thorough discussion of the molecular pathways involved in neural crest development is relevant to the discussion of the genetic basis of human disease. Several chapters in this book focus on specific aspects of neural crest maturation and associated diseases. This chapter will serve as an overview of neural crest-related developmental biology and genetics so that the reader may place specific defects in perspective. Several recent reviews and authoritative books summarize the classic studies that have elucidated the cell biology of the neural crest in the context of developmental biology, and the reader is referred to these texts for details (Hall and Hörstadius, 1988; Hall, 1999; Le Douarin and Kalcheim, 1999). Only the relevant highlights will be summarized here, with special attention to the genetic and molecular mechanisms that have emerged from recent studies. The number of specific genes associated with neural crest–related defects in animal models and in humans continues to grow at a remarkable pace, and it is not our intention to provide an exhaustive list. Specific examples of gene defects associated with instructive developmental disorders will be highlighted here and in later chapters.

DISCOVERY OF THE NEURAL CREST

Wilhelm His, a Swiss anatomist, is credited with first identifying a discrete collection of cells residing between the neural tube and the presumptive embryonic ectoderm that gives rise to spinal and cranial ganglia. In 1868, he called this layer of cells the "intermediate cord," identifying a population of cells renamed "neural crest" by Arthur Milnes Marshal in 1879 (Hall, 1999). The origin and developmental potential of the neural crest were the subject of controversy for many years. Dramatic advances became possible in the 1960s and 1970s, when investigators turned to avian embryos as an experimental model and quail-chick chimera studies pioneered by Nicole Le Douarin resolved many of the conflicts. These studies allowed for the fate mapping of neural crest populations and demonstrated the pluripotency and plasticity of neural crest populations (Le Douarin and Kalcheim, 1999).

Brian Hall (2000) has presented convincing arguments that the neural crest qualifies as a fourth germ layer which has arisen in craniates. Ectoderm and endoderm, the primary germ layers, are present at early stages of development. Inductive interactions between ectoderm and endoderm give rise to a secondary germ layer, mesoderm, early during embryogenesis. In a similar fashion, inductive interactions between neural and epidermal ectoderm (perhaps with contributions from neighboring mesoderm) produce the neural crest. Hence, the neural crest can be considered a secondary germ layer. Like other germ layers, the neural crest is capable of giving rise to numerous cell types and to multiple organs and tissues (Table 6–1).

Neural crest cells are characteristic of craniates and vertebrates and are not evident in most invertebrates. While evolutionary ancestors of vertebrate neural crest cells may exist in cephalochordates and urochordates (Hall, 1999), this migratory cell population appears to have arisen relatively late in evolution, allowing craniates to develop complex head structures and peripheral tissues, including the peripheral nervous system. This important evolutionary step required three critical and coordinated activities: induction of neural crest, migration of determined neural crest cells to specific locations in the developing embryo, and differentiation of precursor cells into mature derivatives. Human genetic mutations that result in neural crest defects can affect each of these processes, as described in subsequent chapters. Our current understanding of the general mechanisms and molecular factors regulating these events will be discussed below.

INDUCTION OF THE NEURAL CREST

Classic studies have focused on the specific tissue–tissue interactions required for induction of the neural crest (LaBonne and Bronner-Fraser, 1998, 1999; Hall, 1999; Le Douarin and Kalcheim, 1999). Neural ectoderm and epidermal ectoderm are required for neural crest induction at the neural plate border (Fig. 6–1), and neural crest markers are induced when these tissues are juxtaposed in vitro (LaBonne and Bronner-Fraser, 1999). Nonaxial mesoderm may provide critical inductive signals as well (Bang et al., 1997; Bonstein et al., 1998; Marchant et al., 1998; LaBonne and Bronner-Fraser, 1999). Extensive investigations have focused on the timing and specific spatial requirements that define the competence of presumptive neural crest. The reader is referred elsewhere for these details (Le Douarin and Kalcheim, 1999), while emerging regulatory pathways that control neural crest development will be discussed below. Molecular signals involved in neural crest induction have been identified, though many details remain to be elucidated.

Members of the bone morphogenetic protein (BMP) family of secreted factors may contribute to the specification of the neural plate border region (Liem et al., 1995; Selleck et al., 1998). BMP4 is expressed by both the dorsal neural tube and the presumptive embryonic ectoderm, and BMP7 is transiently expressed in the nonneural ectoderm (Dudley and Robertson, 1997; Dick et al., 2000). BMP expression precedes that of the neural crest marker *Slug* (LaBonne and Bronner-Fraser, 1999), and BMP inhibitors can prevent neural crest induction (Selleck et al., 1998). The precise timing and level of BMP signaling may be critical since conflicting results have been reported by investigators using different concentrations of BMPs and studying different organisms. For example, inhibition of BMP signaling augments neural crest induction in *Xenopus*, while it blocks induction in chick assays (LaBonne and Bronner-Fraser, 1999). These differences may reflect true species variations but more likely reflect significant differences in assay conditions and timing. The timing and tissue source of the required BMP signal remain to be conclusively demonstrated.

Fibroblast growth factor (FGF) signaling has also been implicated in neural crest induction (see Chapter 32). Studies in *Xenopus* embryos have demonstrated that dominant-negative FGF receptor 1 can prevent the expression of some neural crest-specific genes (Mayor et al., 1997) but not others (Kroll and Amaya, 1996). FGF signals may act in concert with BMP-mediated signals, as has been suggested in other developmental systems such as tooth bud formation (Bei and Maas, 1998). Wnt signaling has also been strongly implicated in neural crest induction. Ectopic mis-expression of Wnt factors can induce ectopic expression of neural crest markers (Saint-Jeannet et al., 1997; LaBonne and Bronner-Fraser, 1998). Multiple members of the Wnt family are expressed in appropriate locations to affect neural crest induction, and the specific family members may vary between organisms. For instance, avian explants can induce neural crest markers un-

Table 6–1. Tissue and Cell Derivatives of Neural Crest Precursors

Pigment cells	Melanoblasts, melanocytes, pigment cells
Peripheral nervous system	Sympathoadrenal precursor cells, sympathetic ganglia including the enteric nervous system, parasympathetic ganglia, dorsal root ganglia, sensory neurons, Schwann cells, glial cells, Rohon-Beard cells
Skeletal system and connective tissues	Odontoblasts, osteoblasts, osteocytes, chondroblasts, chondrocytes, fibroblasts, mesenchymal cells, adipocytes
Circulatory system	Angioblasts, fibroblasts, smooth myoblasts, cardiac mesenchyme
Endocrine glands	Calcitonin-producing C cells, parafollicular cells, adrenal medulla, connective tissue of thyroid, parathyroid, thymus, pituitary, lacrimal glands

der conditions in which Wnt-1 and Wnt-3a cannot be detected (Dickinson et al., 1995), while murine embryos lacking Wnt-1 and Wnt-3a display a gross deficiency of neural crest derivatives (Ikeya et al., 1997). This discrepancy could be explained if Wnts are required for persistence or survival of neural crest cells shortly after induction.

Several transcription factors are expressed by neural crest cells dur-

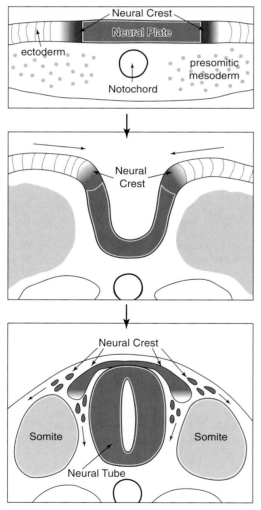

Figure 6–1. Schematic representation of neural crest induction and development. *(Top)* area of neural crest induction at the neural plate border in early presomitic embryo. *(Middle)* specified neural crest cells located at the dorsal region of closing neural folds. *(Bottom)* subsequently, neural crest cells migrate along multiple pathways throughout the body prior to differentiation into numerous cell types

ing and after induction. In *Xenopus* embryos, *Slug* and *Snail* are among the earliest markers of specified neural crest cells (Nieto et al., 1994; LaBonne and Bronner-Fraser, 1998, 2000; Carl et al., 1999). *Slug* and *Snail* are related to the *Drosophila Snail* gene, which encodes a zinc finger transcriptional repressor. In avian embryos, *Slug* is expressed by early neural crest, while in murine embryos, *Snail* is expressed in a similar domain (Jiang et al., 1998; Carl et al., 1999). *Slug/Snail* may play a role in neural crest specification since overexpression expands the neural crest–forming regions (LaBonne and Bronner-Fraser, 1998). However, inactivation of the murine *Slug* gene does not produce obvious neural crest defects (Jiang et al., 1998).

Pax3 is a member of the paired box family of transcription factors and is expressed in the dorsal neural tube and neural crest in all vertebrates (Goulding et al., 1991). Mouse embryos lacking functional Pax3 have neural tube defects and severe neural crest deficiencies (Auerbach, 1954). These include cardiac defects, which can be prevented by replacing Pax3 function in premigratory neural crest using transgenic approaches, thus confirming the critical role of Pax3 in cardiac neural crest in mammals (Li et al., 1999). A closely related family member, Pax7, is also expressed by some populations of neural crest and may be partially redundant with Pax3 in these cells (Jostes et al., 1990). Mice lacking *Pax7* have defects of cranial neural crest (Mansouri et al., 1996). Humans with *PAX3* mutations have Waardenburg-syndrome, which is characterized by multiple neural crest–related defects including facial dysmorphology, pigmentation abnormalities, and deafness resulting from a deficiency of neural crest melanocytes contributing to the inner ear (Hoth et al., 1993; Tassabehji et al., 1993; see Chapters 78 and 80).

FoxD3 is another transcription factor gene that has been implicated in the induction of neural crest. Interestingly, FoxD3 is thought to act as a transcriptional repressor, suggesting that it may promote neural crest fate by repressing alternate pathways (Dottori et al., 2001). FoxD3 is expressed by premigratory and migrating neural crest and functions downstream of Pax3 (Dottori et al., 2001; Kos et al., 2001). In chick and *Xenopus,* FoxD3 overexpression induces neural crest markers (Dottori et al., 2001; Kos et al., 2001; Sasai et al., 2001). Molecular pathways involving FoxD3, Pax3, Slug/Snail, and growth factors such as Wnts, FGFs, and BMPs have yet to be elucidated in detail.

MIGRATION OF THE NEURAL CREST

One of the hallmark features of the neural crest is the ability to migrate to distant locations throughout the developing embryo. While cell migration during embryogenesis is not restricted to neural crest descendents, it is a function absolutely critical to neural crest lineages. The process of migration requires several steps, including delamination from the neuroepithelium, degradation of the extracellular matrix, cytoskeletal reorganization and locomotion, pathfinding, and the ability to determine when the final location has been reached.

Classic studies performed during the last half-century have documented precise pathways followed by various subpopulations of neural crest cells (Le Douarin, 1984; Le Douarin and Kalcheim, 1999). For instance, melanocyte precursors follow a relatively superficial path just below the epidermal ectoderm, while a distinct population travels medially between the neural tube and the somites. Some neural crest cells migrate through the somitic mesoderm, but even here the migratory pathways are exquisitely prescribed; neural crest cells migrate along the dermatome–myotome boundary and are restricted to the rostral half of each somite (Gilbert, 2000).

Transplantation studies have underscored the fact that important migratory cues emanate from the mesenchyme, through which neural crest migrates (Le Douarin and Kalcheim, 1999). Cells transplanted from alternate locations will generally follow the migratory path of the cells that they have replaced, rather than trying to seek their original routes, indicating that migratory fate is not determined prior to transplantation (Le Douarin and Ziller, 1993). These studies have also emphasized the plasticity of neural crest progenitors since derivatives of transplanted tissues can adopt fates not normally found in descendants of the transplant. Likewise, ablation of a specific region of the neural crest can be partially or completely compensated for by adjacent neural crest populations.

To a large extent, factors that initiate neural crest migration remain unknown. Transforming growth factor-β (TGF-β) signaling has been implicated in early stages of neural crest migration (Delannet and Duband, 1992; see Chapter 24). Hepatocyte growth factor/scatter factor (HGF) is capable of triggering migratory behavior in multiple cell types expressing the appropriate receptor: c-Met. Expression of both ligand and receptor has been demonstrated in neural crest, but inactivation of these genes does not result in a neural crest-deficient phenotype (Bladt et al., 1995). Hence, the roles and importance of these pathways remain unknown. At the onset of migration, neural crest cells alter intrinsic gene expression characteristics. They express tenascin and cadherin-7, while they downregulate neural cell adhesion molecule (Duband et al., 1985; Balak et al., 1987). These changes undoubtedly alter cell–cell and cell–matrix interactions such that migration is potentiated. RhoB is also upregulated (Liu and Jessel, 1998). RhoB is a member of the Rho family of GTP-binding proteins and plays an important role in cytoskeletal reorganization, a process critical to motility and cell shape change that accompanies migration. Chemical inhibition of RhoB function during development results in neural crest (and other) defects (Wei et al., 2002).

The ephrin family of signaling molecules has been extensively studied in the context of neural growth cone pathfinding and repellant signaling. Class A ephrin ligands are tethered to the cell surface through glycosylphosphatidylinositol linkages, while B subclass ephrins are transmembrane molecules. The ephrin receptors constitute a large and highly conserved group of transmembrane tyrosine kinases. Receptor complexity is further increased by insertions, deletions, and substitutions, including potential dominant-negative soluble receptor forms that arise by alternative splicing and differential polyadenylation (Zisch and Pasquale, 1997). Ephrin receptors are subclassified as Eph-A or Eph-B based on their binding preference for ephrin A or ephrin B ligand, respectively. Many ephrin ligand–receptor pairs are expressed in reciprocal domains. This complementarity of expression is in accord with the observed repulsive nature of ephrin signaling in the CNS. Subdomains within the CNS can be permissive or restrictive to Ephrin expressing growth cones based on the unique set of local ephrin ligands expressed and the unique set of Ephrin receptors present on the growth cone. In the case of Ephrin-B ligands, the complementarity of receptor and ligand expression can apparently be augmented by two-way signaling. Following receptor binding, B-class ligands can be phosphorylated on their intracellular tails, presumably supplying information to the ligand-expressing cell (Holland et al., 1996; Bruckner et al., 1997).

The ephrin family of growth factors and receptors has been implicated in neural crest pathfinding during migration (see Chapter 101). Rat Ephrin-B2 and chicken Ephrin-B1 are expressed in the caudal half of somites, restricting migration of Ephrin-B2-expressing neural crest cells to the rostral somite (Krull et al., 1997; Wang and Anderson, 1997). In mice, removal of the intracellular tail from the ligand Ephrin-B2 perturbs vascular patterning but does not interfere with cranial neural crest migration. This observation supports the concept of bidirectional signaling between receptor- and ligand-expressing cells and argues that cell populations can obtain different information from the same ligand–receptor pair (Adams et al., 2001). Like many signaling systems, the use of several ephrin–receptor pairs in the same cell population appears to result in functional redundancy. Homozygous null *EphB2(Nuk)* mice display defects in pathfinding in anterior commissure axons. Mice homozygous null for another Eph-B receptor, *EphB3(Sek4)* have defects in corpus callosum formation. Mice homozygous null for both *EphB2* and *EphB3* exhibit much more severe defects in the two axon tracts and die due to complications of cleft secondary palate (Orioli et al., 1996). The receptor tyrosine kinase-like protein Ryk is a mediator of the crosstalk between Eph-B2 and Eph-B3. Mice homozygous null for *Ryk* display the cleft palate of the Eph-B2/Eph-B3 double null along with other craniofacial defects (Halford et al., 2000). Thus, members of the Eph-B class of receptors are important in neural crest-dependant craniofacial morphogenesis. The exact role of individual ephrins and their receptors in neural crest mi-

gration is an area of ongoing study. These studies will be facilitated by the establishment of multiple gene knock-outs and knock-outs in common signaling pathway members such as Ryk.

For migration to proceed, alterations in the extracellular matrix must occur. Neural crest cells produce secreted proteases and plasminogen activators that modify extracellular components to permit migration (Valinsky and Le Douarin, 1985; Menoud et al., 1989; Cai et al., 1998). Alternate components of the extracellular matrix are sufficient to either promote or inhibit neural crest migration and can therefore account, at least partially, for the specificity of the migration route. For instance, neural crest will migrate along adhesive surfaces containing fibronectin or hyaluronan but will avoid surfaces covered with chondroitin sulfate (Landolt et al., 1995; Kubota et al., 1999; Perissinotto et al., 2000).

Emerging data indicate a series of reciprocal signaling pathways that mediate communication between neural crest and surrounding tissues during migration. In some cases, these pathways mimic similar interactions that govern axon guidance in the CNS, an observation consistent with the idea that the neural crest represents an evolutionary extension of the CNS into the periphery.

The Semaphorin family of membrane-bound and secreted proteins is defined by the presence of a semaphorin domain (Yu and Kolodkin, 1999; Tamagnone and Comoglio, 2000). Members of this family are found in species as divergent as flies and humans. They were first identified by their ability to mediate repellent axon guidance in the CNS. Addition of Semaphorin 3A (Sema3A) to extending axons causes growth cone collapse (Luo et al., 1993). Sema3A secreted by neighboring cells is sensed by axons through its binding to heterodimeric receptors composed of neuropilin and plexin subunits (Kolodkin et al., 1997; Winberg et al., 1998). It remains unclear how plexin/neuropilin receptor complexes signal intracellularly; they do not possess intrinsic tyrosine kinase activity.

Several members of the semaphorin family and putative receptors are expressed by neural crest cells, and Sema3A affects migration of dorsal root ganglia axons (Tanelian et al., 1997; Brown et al., 2001; Feiner et al., 2001). Nonneural components of migrating neural crest are also affected by Semaphorin activities. Inactivation of *Sema3C* in the mouse leads to developmental cardiac defects similar to those produced by ablation of premigratory neural crest (Feiner et al., 2001). Sema3C is expressed by mesenchymal cells surrounding the migration route of cardiac neural crest, and a putative receptor component for Sema3C, PlexinA2, is expressed by migrating cardiac neural crest (Brown et al., 2001). It remains unclear if Sema3C regulates cardiac neural crest migration via repellent guidance cues or whether it affects other vital functions, such as survival or differentiation. Nevertheless, it is clear that Semaphorin signaling is one mechanism by which neural crest cells interact with the environment and neighboring cells in a manner that is critical for subsequent development and function.

A similar system of crosstalk between neural crest and local tissues takes place utilizing another secreted ligand–receptor system. The endothelin family of secreted factors consists of three members, each produced as a precursor molecule that is modified by a converting enzyme prior to secretion. Endothelin receptors are composed of dimers consisting of two A subunits, two B subunits, or an A and a B subunit (Baynash et al., 1994; Clouthier et al., 1998; Yanagisawa et al., 1998). Endothelins are produced by endothelial cells, mediate potent vasoconstriction, and are secreted by mesenchymal cells broadly in the developing embryo. Endothelin receptors are expressed by migrating neural crest cells. Inactivation of either the ligands, the converting enzyme, or the receptors leads to neural crest developmental defects, including those affecting the heart and enteric ganglia. In humans, endothelin receptor B mutations are found in some patients with Hirschsprung disease (toxic megacolon) and Waardenburg syndrome (Puffenberger et al., 1994; Edery et al., 1996; Hofstra et al., 1996; see Chapters 37 and 38).

The importance of understanding the complex relationship between migrating neural crest and the environment through which the cells migrate is underscored by recent results relevant to the pathogenesis of the DiGeorge syndrome. This neural crest–related syndrome results in congenital heart defects; thymus, thyroid, and parathyroid abnormalities; and learning disorders. It is often associated with deletions on human chromosome 22q11, which is the most common chromosomal deletion syndrome in humans. While many investigators have sought intrinsic abnormalities in neural crest cells in affected patients or in animal models, some recent results suggest that a critical defect may lie in neighboring cells. Animal studies, described in detail in Chapter 68, have implicated *TBX1* as a key gene in the 22q11 region that is responsible for the cardiovascular, thymic, and parathyroid defects seen in DiGeorge syndrome (Lindsay et al., 1999, 2001; Merscher et al., 2001). *TBX1* appears not to be expressed by neural crest cells but, rather, to be expressed throughout the pharyngeal mesenchyme and in regions of pharyngeal endoderm. *TBX1* encodes a transcription factor and presumably affects the expression of a secreted or cell surface molecule that indirectly affects neural crest–derived structures. Further elucidation of this pathway is likely to enhance our understanding of noncell autonomous mechanisms of neural crest development.

DIFFERENTIATION OF THE NEURAL CREST

One of the most fascinating aspects of neural crest biology is the multiple cell types that are produced from neural crest precursors. The mechanisms that regulate tissue-specific differentiation of neural crest cells remain largely unknown, and fundamental questions remain unanswered. For instance, it is not clear if there is a single common neural crest "stem cell" that has the ability to differentiate into all possible neural crest derivatives given the correct environmental cues. It is possible that several classes of stem cells exist that are capable of adopting some fates and not others. It is also unclear at what stages during development restriction of cell fate occurs.

The position along the anterior–posterior axis of the embryo is important for determining some aspects of neural crest cell fate, though in some cases this may have more to do with the local environment than with intrinsic differences in neural crest progenitors. The cranial crest gives rise to bones and cartilage of the face, the vagal crest gives rise to parasympathetic neurons, and the trunk crest gives rise to sympathetic sensory and autonomic ganglia (Le Douarin and Kalcheim, 1999). Cell transplantation experiments have emphasized the plasticity of different crest populations, indicating that the position rather than intrinsic differences account for this segmentation. However, the trunk crest is generally unable to form cartilage when transplanted to cranial regions (though it can form teeth in some experiments), indicating that some intrinsic differences do exist (Noden, 1983, 1986; Le Douarin and Kalcheim, 1999).

Expression of clustered Hox genes may account, at least in part, for some of the differences in the ability of crest populations to differentiate into facial bones. The most anterior (cranial) crest cells do not express Hox genes and are capable of responding to an unknown signal derived from foregut endoderm that is important for patterning the forming facial skeleton (Couly et al., 2002). Transplantation experiments indicate that Hox-expressing neural crest cells cannot respond to the endoderm-derived signal. Intriguingly, the relative orientation of an endoderm explant can determine the orientation of the forming bone, suggesting that patterning of the facial skeleton relative to the embryonic body axis is determined by endodermal orientation and signaling (Couly et al., 2002).

At any given level along the body axis, neural crest cells emerge from the neural tube and adopt a wide variety of cell fates. The factors that influence these cell fate decisions remain generally unknown. Significant advances in elucidating these factors have come from the laboratories of David Anderson and others, who have identified conditions, growth factors, and transcription factors that affect cell fate decisions during differentiation of sympathetic and autonomic neurons. Although it remains unclear if one pluripotent neural crest precursor cell can give rise to all components of the peripheral nervous system, one type of progenitor cell, the sympathoadrenal cell, can be induced to differentiate into either neurons or chromaffin cells. Nerve growth factor (NGF) promotes a sympathetic neuron phenotype, while glucocorticoids induce chromaffin cell-like differentiation (Anderson and Axel, 1986; Anderson et al., 1991; Carnahan and Patterson, 1991).

In addition, cells that display chromaffin cell morphology can transdifferentiate into sympathetic neurons when treated with NGF (Aloe and Levi-Montalcini, 1979; Doupe et al., 1985).

In *Drosophila*, *achaete-scute* genes play a pivotal role in the development of the CNS as well as sensory organs in the peripheral nervous system (Jimenez and Campos-Ortega, 1990). There are two mammalian homologues to these basic helix-loop-helix transcription factors in the mouse (Johnson et al., 1990). One of these, *mammalian achaete-scute homologue 1 (MASH1)*, is transiently expressed by precursors of the sympathetic and enteric neurons but not by the sensory neuron population (Lo et al., 1991, 1998). *MASH1* expression in neural crest cells is downregulated during neuronal differentiation. Targeted mutation of *MASH1* severely affects the development of sympathetic, parasympathetic, and olfactory epithelium and is thought to be a key factor in cell fate determination (Guillemot et al., 1993).

Several growth factors regulate *MASH1* gene expression, including members of the BMP family, which are also involved in initial neural crest specification (see above). BMP2 is expressed in the dorsal aorta proximal to the area where the sympathetic neurons form (Lyons et al., 1995). BMP2 can induce expression of MASH1 and neurogenesis in a neural crest cell population (Shah et al., 1996). Paradoxically, in other neural populations, BMPs inhibit the induction of neurogenesis and promote apoptosis (Graham et al., 1994). Several BMPs, including BMP2, promote degradation of olfactory receptor neurons (Shou et al., 1999). These data suggest an exquisite dosage sensitivity to BMPs during neural crest differentiation.

A downstream target of *MASH1* is Phox2a, a paired homeodomain transcription factor. In *MASH1*-deficient mice, Phox2a expression is significantly reduced (Hirsch et al., 1998; Lo et al., 1998). Constitutive expression of MASH1 induces expression of both Phox2a and the tyrosine kinase receptor c-RET and promotes neuronal differentiation. Overexpression of Phox2a induces expression of c-RET but is insufficient to promote neuronal differentiation, suggesting that other downstream effectors of MASH1 function are required in addition to Phox2a for induction of a neuronal cell fate (Lo et al., 1998).

Several genes in addition to *MASH1* and *Phox2a* have been implicated in the development of sympathoadrenal cells. These include *neurogenin 1* and *2*, *Phox2b*, *eHAND* and *dHAND*, and *GATA2* and *3*. Several growth factors and receptors have also been implicated, including the BMPs, NGFs, and neurotrophins (NT3) and their receptors $p75^{ntr}$ and the Trks, glia derived neurotrophic factor and its receptor c-RET, and endothelin 3 and its receptor endothelin receptor B.

Hindbrain Segmentation and Cranial Neural Crest

Although the plasticity of premigratory neural crest has been emphasized, there is evidence that some cranial crest progenitors are prepatterned prior to emigration from the neural folds. When cranial crest is transplanted to thoracic regions, it retains the capacity to differentiate into cartilage (Noden, 1983) despite the fact that endogenous crest in the thoracic region cannot. Likewise, transplantation of cells from the mesencephalon, which normally contribute to the lower jaw, to the hindbrain region produces evidence of ectopic lower jaw tissues (Noden, 1983). This result suggests that the transplanted cells are "programmed" to adopt a lower jaw fate prior to excision and are not patterned by the environment through which they migrated or by the target tissue.

The molecular mechanisms by which cephalic neural crest cells are prepatterned include pathways regulated by *Hox* genes and related transcription factors that are expressed in precise domains along the anterior–posterior axis during development (Trainor and Krumlauf, 2001). *Hox* genes were first identified in *Drosophila* as the genetic mutations responsible for homeotic transformations in which one body part was replaced by another. For instance, mutant flies in which a leg segment replaced the normal antenna were found have mutations in a *Hox* gene that was named *antennapedia*. All *Hox* genes contain a relatively conserved 60–amino acid DNA-binding domain called a "homeobox." In flies and higher organisms, including mammals, important groups of related *Hox* genes are clustered within the genome and ordered on the chromosome in the sequence in which they are expressed during development and in which they appear along the anterior–posterior axis. In mammals, four sets of clustered *Hox* genes replace the single set of homologous genes in the fly. The retained genomic clustered organization is likely to be due to complex regulatory mechanisms that control entire clusters in an interdependent fashion (reviewed in Duboule, 1994; see Chapter 46).

Dramatic experiments over the past decade have bolstered the hypothesis that a "*Hox* code" governs positional identity along the neuraxis (Krumlauf, 1994). This model states that positional information and, to some degree, cell fate determination along the anterior–posterior axis are specified by the overlapping expression of clustered *Hox* genes. Deletion or mutation of a single *Hox* gene (or set of homologous/redundant *Hox* genes) results in homeotic transformation in mice. For example, inactivation of *HoxA2* by homologous recombination in embryonic stem cells results in mice with a duplication of the lower jaw (Barrow and Capecchi, 1999). Hence, the final fate adopted by cranial neural crest cells is significantly affected by the homeotic gene expression pattern prior to emigration from the neural folds. This result helps to explain the transplantation results of Noden summarized above. Dietary, environmental, and genetic perturbations that affect *Hox* gene expression patterns at early stages may be associated with craniofacial defects. Likewise, alterations of the expression of genes normally regulated by relative *Hox* gene expression can also be implicated.

The pattern of *Hox* gene expression along the neural axis is paralleled by morphologically apparent segmentation of the cranial neural tube, which appears as a series of constrictions dividing the neural tube into "neuromeres." In the hindbrain, vertebrates have eight distinct segments, called "rhombomeres," that are numbered r1–r8 (cranial to caudal) (Gilbert, 2000). Neural crest cells emerge from these segments and maintain their relative anterior–posterior identity as they populate the branchial arches. Cells emerging from r1–r2 populate branchial arch 1 (the maxillomandibular arch); cells from r4 populate the second branchial arch (the hyoid arch), and cells from r6 enter branchial arch 3. Significant numbers of neural crest cells do not apparently migrate laterally from r3 or r5 (Kulesa et al., 2000; Kulesa and Fraser, 2000). This may be due to two distinct mechanisms. First, migrating neural crest cells from r3 and r5 travel longitudinally to adjacent rhombomeres prior to migrating laterally. Second, neural crest cells from r3 and r5 undergo apoptotic cell death (Graham et al., 1994) with timing that corresponds to enhanced expression of *BMP4* (a TGF-*β* family member) and *Msx2* (a homeobox gene).

Krox20 is a zinc finger transcription factor that is expressed specifically in r3 and r5. Inactivation of *Krox20* in the mouse leads to failure of normal hindbrain segmentation and altered expression of clustered *Hox* genes (Maconochie et al., 2001). In the absence of Krox20, cells normally fated to r3 or r5 adopt the fate of adjacent even-numbered rhombomeres (Voiculescu et al., 2001). Thus, Krox20 is an early regulator of hindbrain segmentation and aspects of cranial neural crest specification.

NEURAL CREST AND CRANIOFACIAL DEVELOPMENT

In vertebrates, many components of the head derive from cranial neural crest, including mesenchymal tissues such as connective tissue, muscle, and bone (Le Douarin and Kalcheim, 1999). This observation originally caused significant controversy since it violated existing dogma that mesenchyme always originated from mesoderm according to von Baer's 1828 germ layer theory. However, a number of cell lineage tracing experiments in a variety of organisms have now clearly established that neural crest of ectodermal origin differentiates into mesenchymal cell types in the head. This tissue is collectively termed *ectomesenchyme* or *mesectoderm*.

Throughout the body, most of the dermis derives from somitic mesoderm. However, in the head, most (Noden, 1978a, b) or all dermis derives from the neural crest (Le Lievre and Le Douarin, 1975). The neural crest also composes the connective tissue of the face, intermingling with muscle of mesodermal origin. Neural crest cells contribute to the tunica media of the arterial vessels in the head, differentiating into connective tissue and smooth muscle. Hence, large

portions of the face and head are of neural crest origin, and gene mutations that affect subclasses of cranial crest can be predicted to result in craniofacial developmental defects.

Some bones of the head, including those that compose the base of the skull, the occipital bone, and components of the otic capsule, derive from somitic and cephalic paraxial mesoderm (mesodermal cells that originate adjacent to the neural tube). These cells mature into bony derivatives after passing through a cartilaginous stage. However, large portions of the facial skeleton, including the frontal bone, the maxilla, the parietal bone, and portions of the otic capsule, derive from neural crest that differentiates into bone without first displaying characteristics of cartilage. Other bony neural crest derivatives in the head, namely Meckel's cartilage, the nasal capsule, and the hyoid bone, are considered cartilaginous bones. Hence, ossification of neural crest can proceed along multiple developmental pathways consistent with the plasticity of neural crest progenitors.

Traditionally, the skull has been described as consisting of two components (Sadler and Langman, 2000): the neurocranium comprises the bones that encase the brain, and the viscerocranium comprises the jaw and facial skeleton. The flat bones of the neurocranium arise by membranous ossification of neural crest–derived mesenchyme. The individual bones of the neurocranium are separated by sutures of neural crest–derived connective tissue known as fontanelles. Neurocranial defects range from complete absence of the cranial vault (cranioschisis) with associated anencephaly to premature fusion of cranial sutures. The viscerocranium is derived predominantly from neural crest remodeling of pharyngeal arches 1 and 2. Neural crest in the first arch gives rise to the maxilla, zygomatic bone, and parts of the temporal bone in the dorsal region and the mandibular process in the ventral region. Neural crest–derived mesenchyme surrounding Meckel's cartilage, in the mandibular process, undergoes membranous ossification to form the mandible. Within the oral cavity, neural crest is also critically involved in the formation and proper fusion of the palate. Craniofacial malformations in humans can occur in isolation or in association with more extensive "neurocristopathy" syndromes affecting multiple organ systems.

While craniofacial abnormalities are common in humans, the vast majority of these defects represent what could be considered small perturbations in neural crest function, such as cleft palate and malformed or misaligned bones of the face and skull. Particularly severe malformations, such as complete absence of the cranial vault (cranioschisis), mandibular agenesis (agnathia), and cyclopia, are quite rare as severe perturbations probably result in disruption of numerous developmental systems and embryonic lethality. Experimental embryology and gene knock-out technology in the mouse are beginning to uncover the molecular pathways which regulate craniofacial development.

Members of the Wnt family of secreted signaling molecules have been implicated in the formation of neural crest, as discussed above (Ikeya et al., 1997; Dorsky et al., 1998; Christiansen et al., 2000; Patapoutian and Reichardt, 2000). At least seven Wnt family members are expressed in the brain and spinal cord. Expression of Wnt proteins by neural crest precursors has been elegantly demonstrated using a transgenic mouse line in which Cre recombinase is expressed under the control of the Wnt-1 enhancers. When these mice are bred to a second line in which *β*-galactosidase is activated in the presence of Cre recombinase, all cells derived from Wnt-1-expressing precursors are permanently labeled (Chai et al., 2000; Jiang et al., 2000). These cells include craniofacial neural crest derivatives. The role of Wnts in neural crest formation and development has been difficult to ascertain, however, due to issues of overlapping ligand expression and functional redundancy. Recent experiments have taken advantage of the *Wnt-1 Cre* transgenic mouse line to remove a critical transcriptional mediator of Wnt signaling, the transcription factor *β*-catenin, specifically in neural crest cells. Neural crest-specific ablation of Wnt signaling results in complete loss of neural crest–derived craniofacial bones (Brault et al., 2001).

Orofacial clefting syndromes represent some of the most commonly observed craniofacial anomalies in humans (Slavkin, 1984; Vekemans and Biddle, 1984; Poswillo, 1988). Facial clefts are highly variable in presentation, ranging from cleft upper lip over a spectrum of isolated and paired clefting of the hard and soft palates to severe bilateral cleft-ing of the face and palate (Ferguson, 1988; Gorlin et al., 2001). Combined cleft lip and palate is most common. Facial clefts can be directly linked to specific errors in palatogenesis. By the fourth week in human development the embryonic face consists of a large frontal prominence. The nasal placodes arise as bilateral ectodermal swellings on the ventrolateral aspects of the frontal prominence. Rapid proliferation of neural crest–derived ectomesenchyme results in nasal swellings surrounding the nasal placodes. This primary structure is actively remodeled by selective apoptosis and proliferation, resulting in extension of the developing olfactory pits into the developing oral cavity. Ectomesenchymal proliferation during the fifth and sixth weeks results in significant mediolateral expansion of the bilateral nasal prominences, and midline fusion of the bilateral structures occurs between the sixth and seventh weeks. Concomitant expansion of crest ectomesenenchyme occurs in the maxillary swellings in the first pharyngeal arch, extending the maxillary processes toward the developing nasal prominences. Fusion of the lateral aspect of the maxillary swellings with fused nasal prominence occurs between the sixth and seventh weeks. The upper lip is therefore composed centrally of the fused medial aspects of the nasal prominences and laterally of the maxillary swellings.

The primary palate is the wedge of tissue created by fusion of the paired nasal prominences, the intermaxillary segment (Ferguson, 1988). The primary palate comprises the philtrum (the central indented area of the upper lip) and a triangle of palatal bone including the four maxillary incisors. Clefts of the lip and palate occur along the lines of fusion both centrally between the paired nasal prominences (very rare central cleft) and laterally between the nasal prominence and one or both of the maxillary swellings. While fusion of the nasal prominence and maxillary swellings forms the upper lip and palate medially, the dorsolateral edges of the nasal prominences simultaneously expand toward the developing eyes. The nasolacrimal groove is the deep furrow separating the lateral aspects of the nasal prominences and the maxillary swellings dorsolaterally. Rather than simple cleft lip and palate, failure of fusion along this line results in more severe oblique facial clefts, which can extend from the upper lip and palate to the corner of the eye, usually exposing the nasolacrimal duct.

The secondary palate comprises the remainder of the tissues of the hard and soft palates. While fusion of the ventrolateral maxillary swellings with the nasal prominence encloses the lateral aspects of the upper jaw, formation of the hard and soft palates medially is more complex. Structures called palatal shelves arise on the medial surfaces of the maxillary swellings. The palatal shelves extend down and medially into the oral cavity. Expansion and elevation of the shelves are most vigorous near the primary palate. Expansion begins around week 7, and the process continues until complete fusion occurs around week 10. Fusion requires specific thinning by apoptosis of the epithelium on the leading shelf edges. This loss of epithelium allows direct fusion of the palatine mesenchymal cores. Neural crest–derived ectomesenchyme comprises the mesenchymal cores of the palatal shelves and is responsible for shelf elevation. What role crest derived cells may play in de-epithelialization of the shelves and subsequent fusion is unclear.

Several growth factors and transcription factors have been implicated in palatogenesis. One such factor is TGF-β3 (Heldin et al., 1997). TGF-β family members are homodimers that are secreted in inactive forms and activated at the site of action (see Chapter 24). TGF-β ligands signal through a complex of type I and type II serine/threonine kinase receptors (Massague, 1992, 1996). The canonical signaling pathway requires cross-phosphorylation of the type I receptor by the type II receptor kinase following ligand binding. The type I receptor phosphorylates receptor-associated Smad proteins. The receptor-associated Smads then associate with Smad4 and translocate to the nucleus, where they regulate transcription of target genes (Derynck et al., 1998; Wrana, 2000). All three mammalian TGF-β ligands (TGF-β1, TGF-β2, and TGF-β3) signal through similar receptor complexes. Mice homozygous null for TGF-β3 but not TGF-β1 or TGF-β2 exhibit cleft secondary palate with 100% penetrance (Proetzel et al., 1995). TGF-β3 is expressed by the palatal epithelium and not by the

ectomesenchyme. Therefore, the defect in these mice is not a primary one of the neural crest–derived ectomesenchyme. In these mice, the palatal shelves form and elevate normally but fail to fuse at the midline. This defect has been interpreted as a failure of the palatal shelves to adhere to one another and a concomitant failure in thinning of the epithelium covering the palatal shelves that allows direct fusion of the shelf ectomesenchyme.

Msx1 is a homeobox transcription factor expressed in vertebrates in many locations, including the developing mandible and teeth. Mice homozygous null for *Msx1* exhibit cleft secondary palate with 100% penetrance (Satokata and Maas, 1994). Null mice also exhibit deficient alveolar mandible and maxilla; abnormalities of the nasal, frontal, and parietal bones; and failure of tooth development. The palatal shelves form and elevate normally in *Msx1* nulls but are greatly reduced in size and not fused at the time of birth, apparently due to a developmental delay. Msx1 is expressed both in the cephalic neural crest at the time of emergence from the neural tube as well as in the differentiating ectomesenchyme of the pharyngeal arches. Msx1 is expressed in mesenchymal cells at numerous locations where epithelial–mesenchymal interactions are utilized during development. It has therefore been suggested that Msx1 may be involved in the integration of epithelial signals that regulate growth, differentiation, or apoptosis in the target mesenchyme (Satokata and Maas, 1994). A recent study identified both *TGF-β3* and *MSX1* as candidate genes for nonsyndromic facial clefting in humans (Beaty et al., 2002).

Another transcription factor, the *Lim* homeobox gene *Lhx8*, is similarly expressed in the palatal mesenchyme (Zhao et al., 1999). Homozygous null *Lhx8* mice exhibit cleft secondary palate with incomplete penetrance. Unlike *Msx1* mutants, all other craniofacial structures appear unaffected in *Lhx8* nulls. The exact mechanism of Msx1 and Lhx8 function and whether or not they interact to regulate palatogenesis remain unclear.

A member of the T-box transcription factor family, *TBX22*, was shown to be the gene mutated in X-linked cleft palate and ankyloglossia syndrome in humans (Braybrook et al., 2001).

Although a growing list of growth factors and transcription factors have been demonstrated to affect craniofacial development, few signaling pathways have been elucidated. One important exception is the endothelin pathway. Endothelin signaling regulates the development of several neural crest lineages, as described above (Baynash et al., 1994; Puffenberger et al., 1994; Clouthier et al., 1998; Yanagisawa et al., 1998). The endothelin-A receptor is expressed in the neural crest–derived ectomesenchyme, while the ligand endothelin-1 (ET-1) is expressed in the pharyngeal arch epithelium and in the mesodermally derived arch core (Clouthier et al., 2000). Expression of the basic helix-loop-helix transcription factor *dHAND* is down-regulated in the pharyngeal arches of ET-1 mutants (Thomas et al., 1998). This down-regulation is the result of loss of Dlx6, a member of the distal-less family of homeodomain transcription factors (Charite et al., 2001). Interestingly, mutations in *Dlx1* and *Dlx2* (Qiu et al., 1997) result in cleft palate associated with other craniofacial malformations. These results represent examples of emerging molecular pathways that regulate craniofacial development deduced from a synthesis of studies involving animal models and human genetics.

In summary, both classic transplantation studies and modern molecular genetic approaches have enhanced our understanding of the signaling processes required for development and function of neural crest cells. Examples of the prominent pathways involved in induction, migration, and differentiation of the neural crest have been reviewed; and several subsequent chapters will examine the effects of individual gene mutations in greater detail. The plasticity of neural crest cells and the complex mechanisms of cell–cell interactions required for patterning and subsequent development have fascinated developmental biologists for over a century and will continue to do so in the future.

REFERENCES

Adams RH, Diella F, Hennig S, Helmbacher F, Deutsch U, Klein R (2001). The cytoplasmic domain of the ligand ephrinB2 is required for vascular morphogenesis but not cranial neural crest migration. *Cell* 104: 57–69.
Aloe L, Levi-Montalcini R (1979). Nerve growth factor–induced transformation of im-

mature chromaffin cells in vivo into sympathetic neurons: effect of antiserum to nerve growth factor. *Proc Natl Acad Sci USA* 76: 1246–1250.

Anderson DJ, Axel R (1986). A bipotential neuroendocrine precursor whose choice of cell fate is determined by NGF and glucocorticoids. *Cell* 47: 1079–1090.

Anderson DJ, Carnahan JF, Michelsohn A, Patterson PH (1991). Antibody markers identify a common progenitor to sympathetic neurons and chromaffin cells in vivo and reveal the timing of commitment to neuronal differentiation in the sympathoadrenal lineage. *J Neurosci* 11: 3507–3519.

Auerbach R (1954). Analysis of the developmental effects of a lethal mutation in the house mouse. *J Exp Zool* 127: 305–329.

Balak K, Jacobson M, Sunshine J, Rutishauser U (1987). Neural cell adhesion molecule expression in *Xenopus* embryos. *Dev Biol* 119: 540–550.

Bang AG, Papalopulu N, Kintner C, Goulding MD (1997). Expression of Pax-3 is initiated in the early neural plate by posteriorizing signals produced by the organizer and by posterior non-axial mesoderm. *Development* 124: 2075–2085.

Barrow JR, Capecchi MR (1999). Compensatory defects associated with mutations in Hoxa1 restore normal palatogenesis to Hoxa2 mutants. *Development* 126: 5011–5026.

Baynash AG, Hosoda K, Giaid A, Richardson JA, Emoto N, Hammer RE, Yanagisawa M (1994). Interaction of endothelin-3 with endothelin-B receptor is essential for development of epidermal melanocytes and enteric neurons. *Cell* 79: 1277–1285.

Beaty TH, Hetmanski JB, Zeiger JS, Fan YT, Liang KY, VanderKolk CA, McIntosh I (2002). Testing candidate genes for non-syndromic oral clefts using a case–parent trio design. *Genet Epidemiol* 22: 1–11.

Bei M, Maas R (1998). FGFs and BMP4 induce both Msx-1-independent and Msx-1-dependent signaling pathways in early tooth development. *Development* 125: 4325–4333.

Bladt F, Riethmacher D, Isenmann S, Aguzzi A, Birchmeier C (1995). Essential role for the c-met receptor in migration of myogenic precursor cells into the limb bud. *Nature* 376: 768–771.

Bonstein L, Elias S, Frank D (1998). Paraxial-fated mesoderm is required for neural crest induction in *Xenopus* embryos. *Dev Biol* 193: 156–168.

Brault V, Moore R, Kutsch S, Ishibashi M, Rowitch DH, McMahon AP, Sommer L, Boussadia O, Kemler R (2001). Inactivation of the beta-catenin gene by Wnt1-Cre-mediated deletion results in dramatic brain malformation and failure of craniofacial development. *Development* 128: 1253–1264.

Braybrook C, Doudney K, Marcano AC, Arnason A, Bjornsson A, Patton MA, Goodfellow PJ, Moore GE, Stanier P (2001). The T-box transcription factor gene *TBX22* is mutated in X-linked cleft palate and ankyloglossia. *Nat Genet* 29: 179–183.

Brown CB, Feiner L, Lu MM, Li J, Ma X, Webber AL, Jia L, Raper JA, Epstein JA (2001). PlexinA2 and semaphorin signaling during cardiac neural crest development. *Development* 128: 3071–3080.

Bruckner K, Pasquale EB, Klein R (1997). Tyrosine phosphorylation of transmembrane ligands for Eph receptors. *Science* 275: 1640–1643.

Cai H, Kratzschmar J, Alfandari D, Hunnicutt G, Blobel CP (1998). Neural crest-specific and general expression of distinct metalloprotease-disintegrins in early *Xenopus laevis* development. *Dev Biol* 204: 508–524.

Carl TF, Dufton C, Hanken J, Klymkowsky MW (1999). Inhibition of neural crest migration in *Xenopus* using antisense slug RNA. *Dev Biol* 213: 101–115.

Carnahan JF, Patterson PH (1991). Isolation of the progenitor cells of the sympathoadrenal lineage from embryonic sympathetic ganglia with the SA monoclonal antibodies. *J Neurosci* 11: 3520–3530.

Chai Y, Jiang X, Ito Y, Bringas P Jr, Han J, Rowitch DH, Soriano P, McMahon AP, Sucov HM (2000). Fate of the mammalian cranial neural crest during tooth and mandibular morphogenesis. *Development* 127: 1671–1679.

Charite J, McFadden DG, Merlo G, Levi G, Clouthier DE, Yanagisawa M, Richardson JA, Olson EN (2001). Role of Dlx6 in regulation of an endothelin-1-dependent, dHAND branchial arch enhancer. *Genes Dev* 15: 3039–3049.

Christiansen JH, Coles EG, Wilkinson DG (2000). Molecular control of neural crest formation, migration and differentiation. *Curr Opin Cell Biol* 12: 719–724.

Clouthier DE, Hosoda K, Richardson JA, Williams SC, Yanagisawa H, Kuwaki T, Kumada M, Hammer RE, Yanagisawa M (1998). Cranial and cardiac neural crest defects in endothelin-A receptor-deficient mice. *Development* 125: 813–824.

Clouthier DE, Williams SC, Yanagisawa H, Wieduwilt M, Richardson JA, Yanagisawa M (2000). Signaling pathways crucial for craniofacial development revealed by endothelin-A receptor-deficient mice. *Dev Biol* 217: 10–24.

Couly G, Creuzet S, Bennaceur S, Vincent C, Le Douarin NM (2002). Interactions between Hox-negative cephalic neural crest cells and the foregut endoderm in patterning the facial skeleton in the vertebrate head. *Development* 129: 1061–1073.

Delannet M, Duband JL (1992). Transforming growth factor-beta control of cell-substratum adhesion during aviation neural crest cell emigration in vitro. *Development* 116: 275–287.

Derynck R, Zhang Y, Feng XH (1998). Smads: transcriptional activators of TGF-beta responses. *Cell* 95: 737–740.

Dick A, Hild M, Bauer H, Imai Y, Maifeld H, Schier AF, Talbot WS, Bouwmeester T, Hammerschmidt M (2000). Essential role of Bmp7 (snailhouse) and its prodomain in dorsoventral patterning of the zebrafish embryo. *Development* 127: 343–354.

Dickinson ME, Selleck MA, McMahon AP, Bronner-Fraser M (1995). Dorsalization of the neural tube by the non-neural ectoderm. *Development* 121: 2099–2106.

Dorsky RI, Moon RT, Raible DW (1998). Control of neural crest cell fate by the Wnt signalling pathway. *Nature* 396: 370–373.

Dottori M, Gross MK, Labosky P, Goulding M (2001). The winged-helix transcription factor Foxd3 suppresses interneuron differentiation and promotes neural crest cell fate. *Development* 128: 4127–4138.

Doupe AJ, Landis SC, Patterson PH (1985). Environmental influences in the development of neural crest derivatives: glucocorticoids, growth factors, and chromaffin cell plasticity. *J Neurosci* 5: 2119–2142.

Duband JL, Tucker GC, Poole TJ, Vincent M, Aoyama H, Thiery JP (1985). How do the migratory and adhesive properties of the neural crest govern ganglia formation in the avian peripheral nervous system? *J Cell Biochem* 27: 189–203.

Duboule D (1994). *Guidebook to the Homeobox Genes*. Oxford University Press, Oxford.

Dudley AT, Robertson EJ (1997). Overlapping expression domains of bone morphogenetic protein family members potentially account for limited tissue defects in BMP7 deficient embryos. *Dev Dyn* 208: 349–362.

Edery P, Attie T, Amiel J, Pelet A, Eng C, Hofstra RM, Martelli H, Bidaud C, Munnich A, Lyonnet S (1996). Mutation of the endothelin-3 gene in the Waardenburg-Hirschsprung disease (Shah-Waardenburg syndrome). *Nat Genet* 12: 442–444.

Feiner L, Webber AL, Brown CB, Lu MM, Jia L, Feinstein P, Mombaerts P, Epstein JA, Raper JA (2001). Targeted disruption of semaphorin 3C leads to persistent truncus arteriosus and aortic arch interruption. *Development* 128: 3061–3070.

Ferguson MW (1988). Palate development. *Development* 103: 41–60.

Gilbert SF (2000). Developmental biology. Sunderland, Mass., Sinauer Associates.

Gorlin RJ, Cohen MM, Hennekam RCM (2001). *Syndromes of the Head and Neck*. Oxford University Press, Oxford.

Goulding MD, Chalepakis G, Deutsch U, Erselius JR, Gruss P (1991). Pax-3, a novel murine DNA binding protein expressed during early neurogenesis. *EMBO J* 10: 1135–1147.

Graham A, Francis-West P, Brickell P, Lumsden A (1994). The signalling molecule BMP4 mediates apoptosis in the rhombencephalic neural crest. *Nature* 372: 684–686.

Guillemot F, Lo LC, Johnson JE, Auerbach A, Anderson DJ, Joyner AL (1993). Mammalian achaete-scute homolog 1 is required for the early development of olfactory and autonomic neurons. *Cell* 75: 463–476.

Halford MM, Armes J, Buchert M, Meskenaite V, Grail D, Hibbs ML, Wilks AF, Farlie PG, Newgreen DF, Hovens CM, et al. (2000). Ryk-deficient mice exhibit craniofacial defects associated with perturbed Eph receptor crosstalk. *Nat Genet* 25: 414–418.

Hall BK (1999). *The Neural Crest in Development and Evolution*. Springer, New York.

Hall BK (2000). The neural crest as a fourth germ layer and vertebrates as quadroblastic not triploblastic. *Evol Dev* 2: 3–5.

Hall BK, Hörstadius S (1988). *The Neural Crest: Including a Facsimile Reprint of The Neural Crest by Sven Hörstadius*. Oxford University Press, New York.

Heldin CH, Miyazono K, ten Dijke P (1997). TGF-beta signalling from cell membrane to nucleus through SMAD proteins. *Nature* 390: 465–471.

Hirsch MR, Tiveron MC, Guillemot F, Brunet JF, Goridis C (1998). Control of noradrenergic differentiation and Phox2a expression by MASH1 in the central and peripheral nervous system. *Development* 125: 599–608.

Hofstra RM, Osinga J, Tan-Sindhunata G, Wu Y, Kamsteeg EJ, Stulp RP, van Ravenswaaij-Arts C, Majoor-Krakauer D, Angrist M, Chakravarti A, et al. (1996). A homozygous mutation in the endothelin-3 gene associated with a combined Waardenburg type 2 and Hirschsprung phenotype (Shah-Waardenburg syndrome). *Nat Genet* 12: 445–447.

Holland SJ, Gale NW, Mbamalu G, Yancopoulos GD, Henkemeyer M, Pawson T (1996). Bidirectional signalling through the EPH-family receptor Nuk and its transmembrane ligands. *Nature* 383: 722–725.

Hoth CF, Milunsky A, Lipsky N, Sheffer R, Clarren SK, Baldwin CT (1993). Mutations in the paired domain of the human *PAX3* gene cause Klein-Waardenburg syndrome (WS-III) as well as Waardenburg syndrome type I (WS-I). *Am J Hum Genet* 52: 455–462.

Ikeya M, Lee SM, Johnson JE, McMahon AP, Takada S (1997). Wnt signalling required for expansion of neural crest and CNS progenitors. *Nature* 389: 966–970.

Jiang R, Lan Y, Norton CR, Sundberg JP, Gridley T (1998). The *Slug* gene is not essential for mesoderm or neural crest development in mice. *Dev Biol* 198: 277–285.

Jiang X, Rowitch DH, Soriano P, McMahon AP, Sucov HM (2000). Fate of the mammalian cardiac neural crest. *Development* 127: 1607–1616.

Jimenez F, Campos-Ortega JA (1990). Defective neuroblast commitment in mutants of the achaete-scute complex and adjacent genes of *D. melanogaster*. *Neuron* 5: 81–89.

Johnson JE, Birren SJ, Anderson DJ (1990). Two rat homologues of *Drosophila* achaete-scute specifically expressed in neuronal precursors. *Nature* 346: 858–861.

Jostes B, Walther C, Gruss P (1990). The murine paired box gene, *Pax7*, is expressed specifically during the development of the nervous and muscular system. *Mech Dev* 33: 27–37.

Kolodkin AL, Levengood DV, Rowe EG, Tai YT, Giger RJ, Ginty DD (1997). Neuropilin is a semaphorin III receptor. *Cell* 90: 753–762.

Kos R, Reedy MV, Johnson RL, Erickson CA (2001). The winged-helix transcription factor FoxD3 is important for establishing the neural crest lineage and repressing melanogenesis in avian embryos. *Development* 128: 1467–1479.

Kroll KL, Amaya E (1996). Transgenic Xenopus embryos from sperm nuclear transplanations reveal FGF signaling requirements during gastrulation. *Development* 122: 3173–3183.

Krull CE, Lansford R, Gale NW, Collazo A, Marcelle C, Yancopoulos GD, Fraser SE, Bronner-Fraser M (1997). Interactions of Eph-related receptors and ligands confer rostrocaudal pattern to trunk neural crest migration. *Curr Biol* 7: 571–580.

Krumlauf R (1994). Hox genes in vertebrate development. *Cell* 78: 191–201.

Kubota Y, Morita T, Kusakabe M, Sakakura T, Ito K (1999). Spatial and temporal changes in chondroitin sulfate distribution in the sclerotome play an essential role in the formation of migration patterns of mouse neural crest cells. *Dev Dyn* 214: 55–65.

Kulesa P, Bronner-Fraser M, Fraser S (2000). In ovo time-lapse analysis after dorsal neural tube ablation shows rerouting of chick hindbrain neural crest. *Development* 127: 2843–2852.

Kulesa PM, Fraser SE (2000). In ovo time-lapse analysis of chick hindbrain neural crest cell migration shows cell interactions during migration to the branchial arches. *Development* 127: 1161–1172.

LaBonne C, Bronner-Fraser M (1998). Neural crest induction in *Xenopus*: evidence for a two-signal model. *Development* 125: 2403–2414.

LaBonne C, Bronner-Fraser M (1999). Molecular mechanisms of neural crest formation. *Annu Rev Cell Dev Biol* 15: 81–112.

LaBonne C, Bronner-Fraser M (2000). Snail-related transcriptional repressors are required in *Xenopus* for both the induction of the neural crest and its subsequent migration. *Dev Biol* 221: 195–205.

Landolt RM, Vaughan L, Winterhalter KH, Zimmermann DR (1995). Versican is selectively expressed in embryonic tissues that act as barriers to neural crest cell migration and axon outgrowth. *Development* 121: 2303–2312.

Le Douarin N, Kalcheim C (1999). *The Neural Crest*. Cambridge University Press, Cambridge.

Le Douarin NM (1984). Cell migrations in embryos. *Cell* 38: 353–360.

Le Douarin NM, Ziller C (1993). Plasticity in neural crest cell differentiation. *Curr Opin Cell Biol* 5: 1036–1043.

Le Lievre CS, Le Douarin NM (1975). Mesenchymal derivatives of the neural crest: analysis of chimaeric quail and chick embryos. *J Embryol Exp Morphol* 34: 125–154.

Li J, Liu K, Jin F, Epstein JA (1999). Transgenic rescue of congenital heart disease and spina bifida in Splotch mice. *Development* 126: 2495–2503.

Liem KF Jr, Tremml G, Roelink H, Jessell TM (1995). Dorsal differentiation of neural plate cells induced by BMP-mediated signals from epidermal ectoderm. *Cell* 82: 969–979.

Lindsay EA, Botta A, Jurecic V, Carattini-Rivera S, Cheah YC, Rosenblatt HM, Bradley A, Baldini A (1999). Congenital heart disease in mice deficient for the DiGeorge syndrome region. *Nature* 401: 379–383.

Lindsay EA, Vitelli F, Su H, Morishima M, Huynh T, Pramparo T, Jurecic V, Ogunrinu G, Sutherland HF, Scambler PJ, et al. (2001). Tbx1 haploinsufficieny in the DiGeorge syndrome region causes aortic arch defects in mice. *Nature* 410: 97–101.

Liu JP, Jessell TM (1998). A role for rhoB in the delamination of neural crest cells from the dorsal neural tube. *Development* 125: 5055–5067.

Lo L, Tiveron MC, Anderson DJ (1998). MASH1 activates expression of the paired homeodomain transcription factor Phox2a, and couples pan-neuronal and subtype-specific components of autonomic neuronal identity. *Development* 125: 609–620.

Lo LC, Johnson JE, Wuenschell CW, Saito T, Anderson D J (1991). Mammalian achaete-scute homolog 1 is transiently expressed by spatially restricted subsets of early neuroepithelial and neural crest cells. *Genes Dev* 5: 1524–1537.

Luo Y, Raible D, Raper JA (1993). Collapsin: a protein in brain that induces the collapse and paralysis of neuronal growth cones. *Cell* 75: 217–227.

Lyons KM, Hogan BL, Robertson EJ (1995). Colocalization of BMP 7 and BMP 2 RNAs suggests that these factors cooperatively mediate tissue interactions during murine development. *Mech Dev* 50: 71–83.

Maconochie MK, Nonchev S, Manzanares M, Marshall H, Krumlauf R (2001). Differences in Krox20-dependent regulation of Hoxa2 and Hoxb2 during hindbrain development. *Dev Biol* 233: 468–481.

Mansouri A, Stoykova A, Torres M, Gruss P (1996). Dysgenesis of cephalic neural crest derivatives in Pax7−/− mutant mice. *Development* 122: 831–838.

Marchant L, Linker C, Ruiz P, Guerrero N, Mayor R (1998). The inductive properties of mesoderm suggest that the neural crest cells are specified by a BMP gradient. *Dev Biol* 198: 319–329.

Massague J (1992). Receptors for the TGF-beta family. *Cell* 69: 1067–1070.

Massague J (1996). TGFbeta signaling: receptors, transducers, and Mad proteins. *Cell* 85: 947–950.

Mayor R, Guerrero N, Martinez C (1997). Role of FGF and noggin in neural crest induction. *Dev Biol* 189: 1–12.

Menoud PA, Debrot S, Schowing J (1989). Mouse neural crest cells secrete both urokinase-type and tissue-type plasminogen activators in vitro. *Development* 106: 685–690.

Merscher S, Funke B, Epstein JA, Heyer J, Puech A, Lu MM, Xavier RJ, Demay MB, Russell RG, Factor S, et al. (2001). TBX1 is responsible for cardiovascular defects in velo-cardio-facial/DiGeorge syndrome. *Cell* 104: 619–629.

Nieto MA, Sargent MG, Wilkinson DG, Cooke J (1994). Control of cell behavior during vertebrate development by *Slug*, a zinc finger gene. *Science* 264: 835–839.

Noden DM (1978a). The control of avian cephalic neural crest cytodifferentiation. I. Skeletal and connective tissues. *Dev Biol* 67: 296–312.

Noden DM (1978b). The control of avian cephalic neural crest cytodifferentiation. II. Neural tissues. *Dev Biol* 67: 313–329.

Noden DM (1983). The role of the neural crest in patterning of avian cranial skeletal, connective, and muscle tissues. *Dev Biol* 96: 144–165.

Noden DM (1986). Patterning of avian craniofacial muscles. *Dev Biol* 116: 347–356.

Orioli D, Henkemeyer M, Lemke G, Klein R, Pawson T (1996). Sek4 and Nuk receptors cooperate in guidance of commissural axons and in palate formation. *EMBO J* 15: 6035–6049.

Patapoutian A, Reichardt LF (2000). Roles of Wnt proteins in neural development and maintenance. *Curr Opin Neurobiol* 10: 392–399.

Perissinotto D, Iacopetti P, Bellina I, Doliana R, Colombatti A, Pettway Z, Bronner-Fraser M, Shinomura T, Kimata K, Morgelin M, et al. (2000). Avian neural crest cell migration is diversely regulated by the two major hyaluronan-binding proteoglycans PG-M/versican and aggrecan. *Development* 127: 2823–2842.

Poswillo D (1988). The aetiology and pathogenesis of craniofacial deformity. *Development* 103: 207–212.

Proetzel G, Pawlowski SA, Wiles MV, Yin M, Boivin GP, Howles PN, Ding J, Ferguson MW, Doetschman T (1995). Transforming growth factor-beta 3 is required for secondary palate fusion. *Nat Genet* 11: 409–414.

Puffenberger EG, Hosoda K, Washington SS, Nakao K, deWit D, Yanagisawa M, Chakravart A (1994). A missense mutation of the endothelin-B receptor gene in multigenic Hirschsprung's disease. *Cell* 79: 1257–1266.

Qiu M, Bulfone A, Ghattas I, Meneses JJ, Christensen L, Sharpe PT, Presley R, Pedersen RA, Rubenstein JL (1997). Role of the Dlx homeobox genes in proximodistal patterning of the branchial arches: mutations of *Dlx-1*, *Dlx-2*, and *Dlx-1* and *-2* alter morphogenesis of proximal skeletal and soft tissue structures derived from the first and second arches. *Dev Biol* 185: 165–184.

Sadler TW, Langman J (2000). *Langman's Medical Embryology*. Lippincott Williams & Wilkins, Philadelphia.

Saint-Jeannet JP, He X, Varmus HE, Dawid IB (1997). Regulation of dorsal fate in the neuraxis by Wnt-1 and Wnt-3a. *Proc Natl Acad Sci USA* 94: 13713–13718.

Sasai N, Mizuseki K, Sasai Y (2001). Requirement of FoxD3-class signaling for neural crest determination in *Xenopus*. *Development* 128: 2525–2536.

Satokata I, Maas R (1994). Msx1 deficient mice exhibit cleft palate and abnormalities of craniofacial and tooth development. *Nat Genet* 6: 348–356.

Selleck MA, Garcia-Castro MI, Artinger KB, Bronner-Fraser M (1998). Effects of Shh and Noggin on neural crest formation demonstrate that BMP is required in the neural tube but not ectoderm. *Development* 125: 4919–4930.

Shah NM, Groves AK, Anderson DJ (1996). Alternative neural crest cell fates are instructively promoted by TGFbeta superfamily members. *Cell* 85: 331–343.

Shou J, Rim PC, Calof AL (1999). BMPs inhibit neurogenesis by a mechanism involving degradation of a transcription factor. *Nat Neurosci* 2: 339–345.

Slavkin HC (1984). Morphogenesis of a complex organ: vertebrate palate development. *Curr Top Dev Biol* 19: 1–16.

Tamagnone L, Comoglio PM (2000). Signalling by semaphorin receptors: cell guidance and beyond. *Trends Cell Biol* 10: 377–383.

Tanelian DL, Barry MA, Johnston SA, Le T, Smith GM (1997). Semaphorin III can repulse and inhibit adult sensory afferents in vivo. *Nat Med* 3: 1398–1401.

Tassabehji M, Read AP, Newton VE, Patton M, Gruss P, Harris R, Strachan T (1993). Mutations in the *PAX3* gene causing Waardenburg syndrome type 1 and type 2. *Nat Genet* 3: 26–30.

Thomas T, Kurihara H, Yamagishi H, Kurihara Y, Yazaki Y, Olson EN, Srivastava D (1998). A signaling cascade involving endothelin-1, dHAND and msx1 regulates development of neural-crest-derived branchial arch mesenchyme. *Development* 125: 3005–3014.

Trainor PA, Krumlauf R (2001). Hox genes, neural crest cells and branchial arch patterning. *Curr Opin Cell Biol* 13: 698–705.

Valinsky JE, Le Douarin NM (1985). Production of plasminogen activator by migrating cephalic neural crest cells. *EMBO J* 4: 1403–1406.

Vekemans MJ, Biddle FG (1984). Genetics of palate development. *Curr Top Dev Biol* 19: 165–192.

Voiculescu O, Taillebourg E, Pujades C, Kress C, Buart S, Charnay P, Schneider-Maunoury S (2001). Hindbrain patterning: Krox20 couples segmentation and specification of regional identity. *Development* 128: 4967–4978.

Wang HU, Anderson DJ (1997). Eph family transmembrane ligands can mediate repulsive guidance of trunk neural crest migration and motor axon outgrowth. *Neuron* 18: 383–396.

Wei L, Imanaka-Yoshida K, Wang L, Zhan S, Schneider MD, DeMayo FJ, Schwartz RJ (2002). Inhibition of Rho family GTPases by Rho GDP dissociation inhibitor disrupts cardiac morphogenesis and inhibits cardiomyocyte proliferation. *Development* 129: 1705–1714.

Winberg ML, Noordermeer JN, Tamagnone L, Comoglio PM, Spriggs MK, Tessier-Lavigne M, Goodman CS (1998). Plexin A is a neuronal semaphorin receptor that controls axon guidance. *Cell* 95: 903–916.

Wrana JL (2000). Regulation of Smad activity. *Cell* 100: 189–192.

Yanagisawa H, Hammer RE, Richardson JA, Williams SC, Clouthier DE, Yanagisawa M (1998). Role of Endothelin-1/Endothelin-A receptor-mediated signaling pathway in the aortic arch patterning in mice. *J Clin Invest* 102: 22–33.

Yu HH, Kolodkin AL (1999). Semaphorin signaling: a little less per-plexin. *Neuron* 22: 11–14.

Zhao Y, Guo YJ, Tomac AC, Taylor NR, Grinberg A, Lee EJ, Huang S, Westphal H (1999). Isolated cleft palate in mice with a targeted mutation of the LIM homeobox gene *lhx8*. *Proc Natl Acad Sci USA* 96: 15002–15006.

Zisch AH, Pasquale EB (1997). The Eph family: a multitude of receptors that mediate cell recognition signals. *Cell Tissue Res* 290: 217–226.

7 | Development of the Nervous System

JOHN L.R. RUBENSTEIN AND LUIS PUELLES

ORGANIZATION OF THE NERVOUS SYSTEM

The nervous system has peripheral and central parts. The peripheral nervous system (PNS) is derived from subsets of neural crest cells (see Chapter 6) and from ectodermal placodes (e.g., olfactory and otic). PNS structures are organized as ganglia (e.g., sympathetic, parasympathetic, dorsal root, and enteric) or sensory epithelia (e.g., olfactory and otic; see Chapter 8). The CNS is derived from the neural plate. CNS structures are categorized according to their location within the neural tube. This chapter focuses on a description of major steps that control development of the CNS and how these steps can be derailed to cause birth defects. We will begin with a morphological description of CNS development (reviewed in Rubenstein et al., 1998; Puelles, 2001).

Induction of the neural plate takes place around the onset of gastrulation and specifies a large region of the embryonic ectoderm to develop into the CNS and PNS. The neural plate can be considered to have several parts, which are characterized by their morphology, position, and molecular constitution (Fig. 7–1). The lateral edges of the neural plate are continuous with the adjacent nonneural ectoderm and generally have a ridge-like shape; this region has the progenitors of the neural crest. During *neurulation* (closure of the neural tube, see below), neural crest cells delaminate into the adjacent mesenchyme and then migrate to distinct locations, where subsets of these cells form the ganglia of the PNS (sensory, motor, and enteric). Other subsets differentiate into dermal melanocytes, craniofacial skeletal elements, and additional organ systems (see Chapters 6, 9, and 15).

As the neural plate folds into the neural tube (neurulation), the fusion of the lateral edges creates the roof plate (dorsal midline) of the neural tube and separates the CNS from the surface ectoderm (Fig. 7–1) (Colas and Schoenwolf, 2001). The fusion occurs at loci in the midbrain and hindbrain; a zippering process in rostral and caudal directions closes the neural tube. The last regions to close are the rostral and caudal neuropores (transient open portions of the tube). Disruption of this process leads to open neural tube defects such as exencephaly (open brain) and spina bifida (open spinal cord). Defects in neurulation can be caused by mutations in genes that are expressed in the neural ridge, such as *Dlx5* (Depew et al., 1999), or by mutations in genes, such as *Apaf1* (Honarpour et al., 2001), that have general effects on neural tube proliferation/survival.

At the rostral limit of the neural plate is a structure called the anterior neural ridge (ANR) (Fig. 7–1). There is little or no neural crest produced in this region; the rostralmost neural crest forms at the prospective thalamic level (Couly et al., 1998). The ANR contains much of the prospective telencephalic primordium (Cobos-Sillero et al., 2001).

There is a groove in the midline of the neural plate that overlies the axial mesendoderm (prechordal plate and notochord); this groove stops short of the ANR. Following neurulation, the deepest part of this groove will give rise to the floor plate and the adjacent region will become the basal plate (i.e., the motor-related part of the mature CNS) (Fig. 7–1). The region between the prospective basal and roof plates represents the anlage of the alar plate (the sensory-related part of the mature CNS). The roof, alar, basal, and floor plates are the principal longitudinal, or dorsoventral, subdivisions of the CNS (Shimamura et al., 1995); the left and right parts of the longitudinal domains are continuous across the rostral and caudal midlines, in the forebrain and

tailbud, respectively. Abnormalities in the induction of these subdivisions in the forebrain cause dysmorphologies, such as holoprosencephaly (see Chapter 18).

By neurulation, the CNS is subdivided into its major transverse parts: the prosencephalon (forebrain), mesencephalon (midbrain), rhombencephalon (hindbrain), and spinal cord (Figs. 7–2, 7–3). Smaller transverse subdivisions, called "neuromeres," are apparent in the rhombencephalon and the caudal part of the prosencephalon (this region becomes the caudal diencephalon) (Lumsden and Krumlauf, 1996; Rubenstein et al., 1998). Additional neuromeres in the rostral part of the prosencephalon (secondary prosencephalon) have been postulated (Rubenstein et al., 1998; Puelles, 2001). During this period, the morphology of the brain is further complicated due to the formation of cervical, rhombic, and cephalic flexures.

During and after neurulation, distinct vesicles evaginate from the prosencephalon (Figs. 7–1, 7–2). The largest are the paired telencephalic and optic vesicles; these expand from the walls of the secondary prosencephalon. Smaller unpaired outpouchings form in the dorsal prosencephalic midline (pineal gland and subfornical organ) and in the ventral midline (posterior pituitary). Thus, the prosencephalon consists of the diencephalon, optic vesicles, and telencephalic vesicles. The caudal limit of the diencephalon contacts the mesencephalon, establishing continuity of the forebrain/midbrain basal and alar plates (Figs. 7–2, 7–3).

The alar diencephalon consists of the pretectum, the epithalamus (habenula), the caudal thalamus (formerly dorsal thalamus), the rostral thalamus (formerly ventral thalamus: reticular nucleus, zona incerta, and ventral lateral geniculate nucleus), and the alar hypothalamus (includes the preoptic, anterior hypothalamic, and supraoptoparaventricular areas) (Figs. 7–2, 7–3). The caudal and rostral parts of the thalamus are separated by a cell-poor boundary region known as the zona limitans intrathalamica (ZLI) (Rubenstein et al., 1998) (Figs. 7–2, 7–3). The ZLI becomes progressively thinner over time (Larsen et al., 2001) and separates predominantly inhibitory cell populations in the rostral thalamus from the caudal thalamus, characterized by thalamocortical excitatory neurons.

The basal diencephalon caudal to the ZLI contains prerubral (basal) and ventral tegmental (paramedian floor) domains analogous to the midbrain tegmentum and includes dopaminergic cells related to the substantia nigra and ventral tegmental area, justifying the newly coined term *nigral tegmentum* (Figs. 7–2, 7–3) (Puelles and Verney, 1998). The basal diencephalon rostral to the ZLI includes the basal prethalamus (includes classical posterior hypothalamic and retro[supra]mammillary areas) and the basal hypothalamus (includes mammillary and infundibular hypothalamus: dorsomedial, ventromedial, and arcuate areas and the neurohypophysis).

The telencephalon is connected to the rostral alar diencephalon through a stalk region (peduncle); the peduncle contains, rostrally, the preoptic area and anterior entopeduncular area and, caudally, the eminentia thalami (a transitional area placed dorsal to the rostral thalamus) (Figs. 7–2, 7–3). The rostral part of the stalk is continuous with the telencephalic subpallium (basal ganglia), and the caudal part is continuous with the pallium (cortex and claustroamygdaloid nuclei). The subpallium is primarily constituted by the primordia of the striatum and the globus pallidus (Figs. 7–2, 7–3). The pallium can be considered to have the following principal subdivisions: the medial, dorsal, and lateral/ventral pallium (Puelles et al., 2000). These parts

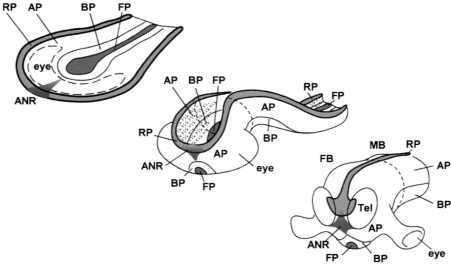

Figure 7–1. Graphic schematic representation of the neurulation process viewed from the rostrolateral end of the brain. Nonneural structures of the head primordium are not shown. As the borders of the neural plate approach each other and fuse at the dorsal midline, the eye vesicles evaginate and the forebrain and midbrain (MB, delimited by a transverse dashed line) gradually acquire their characteristic shape. The schema ends when the telencephalic vesicles (Tel) start to evaginate and the rostral neuropore closes. The fundamental four-tiered longitudinal structure of the CNS has its simplest form at initial neural plate stages. These display the topology of the prospective floor plate (FP, red), basal plate (BP), alar plate (AP), and roof plate (RP, violet) longitudinal domains, which are continuous from left to right across the midline at

the front of the neural plate. The initial eye field, which is conceived to lie within the AP, also bridges the rostral midline. The anterior neural ridge (ANR), postulated to be a secondary organizer for the forebrain, is shown in blue. We base the blue area on the early expression of the *Hesx1* and *Six3* genes. As neurulation proceeds, the mutual topologic relationships of these domains are not altered. The rostral end of the FP will form choroidal tissue at the roof of ventricle III and the medial wall of the lateral ventricles (Tel). The ANR (blue) persists at the telencephalic commissural plate (median septum), the lamina terminalis, and the prospective optic chiasm. The rostralmost FP area is where neurohypophysis will develop.

correspond to the hippocampus, the isocortex (neocortex), and the olfactory cortex/claustral/endopiriform complex, respectively (Figs. 7–2, 7–4). Each region is further subdivided. For example, the isocortex is composed of multiple motor and sensory areas. The septum and amygdalar areas are composed of both pallial and subpallial parts.

The functional organization of structures caudal to the forebrain

tends to have sensory processing structures in the dorsal part (alar plate) and motor processing/output structures in the ventral aspect (basal plate) (Fig. 7–3). For instance, the midbrain consists of dorsal (tectal) and ventral (tegmental) parts. The tectum (superior and inferior colliculi) processes visual and auditory information, whereas the tegmentum participates in motor functions through the substan-

Figure 7–2. *(A)* Axial flexures produced during early morphogenesis of the neural tube and other associated shape changes (evagination of the telencephalon and protrusion of the cerebellum, Cb), with characteristic sectioned appearance at multiple locations *(B–F)*. *(A)* The axial dimension is represented jointly by three lines: *(1)* the floor plate (FP, darkly spotted), which ends at the median eminence and neurohypophysis (HP), overlying the prechordal plate axial mesoderm (PP); *(2)* the plate/alar basal plate boundary (BP/AP, large dashes), which crosses the midline under the optic stalks (eye, also see Fig. 7–1); and *(3)* the roof plate (RP, thick black line), which stops rostrally at the anterior commissure (not shown). All three are parallel to each other and reveal that the neuraxis is sharply bent ventrally under the pretectum (PT) and the midbrain (M), as well as under the caudal hindbrain (medulla). There is a dorsal concavity at the hindbrain level, emphasized by cerebellar overgrowth. The hindbrain, composed of an isthmic domain (Is), rhombomeres r1–r6, and pseudorhombomeres 7–11, overlies the notochord (NC). The isthmomesencephalic boundary, a secondary organizer domain, is indicated by a thick transverse black line. The diencephalic zona limitans intrathalamica (zli), another presumptive secondary organizer, also appears as a thick black line. Other transverse (interneuromeric) boundaries are represented as thin black lines. The thalamic region of the forebrain AP is divided by the zli into a caudal thalamus (classically known as "dorsal thalamus," DT) and a rostral thalamus (classically known as "ventral thalamus," VT). The reinterpreted view favored here is consistent with the axial landmarks defined above (FP, AP, BP, RP). The caudal thalamus is capped dorsally by the epithalamus or habenular region (Hab) and epiphysis (EP), whereas the rostral thalamus is similarly capped by the eminentia thalami at the caudal part of the hemispheric stalk (EMT, it forms a bridge into the telencephalic pallium). Rostral to the thalamus, the large hypothalamic region can be roughly divided in two portions (caudal and rostral; both connect with the telencephalic subpallium, lateral ganglionic eminence [LGE] and medial ganglionic eminence [MGE] dorsalward). The caudal part of the hypothalamus contains the locus of the paraventricular (PV) and supraoptic nuclei, the posterior hypothalamus (PH), the subthalamic nucleus, and the mammillary complex (Mam). The rostral part of the hypothalamus contains

dorsally the preoptic area (PO, which can also be conceived as a telencephalon [Tel] impar portion) and the anterior (AH), suprachiasmatic, retrochiasmatic, and infundibular (IH) hypothalamic domains, including the neurohypophysis and median eminence. The optic vesicles evaginate from the AP of this rostral hypothalamic region. H, horizontal section plane; T, transversal section plane; Tel, telencephalon. *(B)* Topologically transverse section at the front of the forebrain intersects the telencephalon and the rostral hypothalamus (i.e., extends from RP to FP, note also the BP/AP boundary). The telencephalon appears divided into four pallial subregions (medial, dorsal, lateral, and ventral, separated by thin lines) and two subpallial domains (LGE and MGE, the primordia for the striatum and pallidum, respectively). The pallial domains form largely cortex (Cx, isocortex and allocortex) as well as claustral/endopiriform and amygdaloid nuclei (basolateral complex). Arrows represent some of the radial migratory routes of immature neurons as they move from the progenitor zone (hatched territory adjacent to the ventricle) to the overlying mantle zone. *(C)* Cross-section at early stages through the optic stalk, which is topologically horizontal to the axial landmarks and therefore shows periodic outward bulges of the wall separated by ventricular ridges. Most of the section traverses AP domains of successive transverse elements of the neural tube (compare with A). A more caudal section, i.e., across the IH and Mam, would intersect a series of BP sectors. This is the sort of morphological evidence that has been adduced for forebrain prosomeres. A number of gene expression domains respect such boundaries. *(D)* Cross-section through the posterior commissure and pretectum, which is topologically transverse. Note the relatively greater extent of the AP relative to the other longitudinal domains. *(E)* Cross-section through the caudal midbrain (inferior colliculus), which is topologically horizontal to the rostral hindbrain and thus again shows a number of bulging areas separated by constrictions, corresponding to hindbrain rhombomeres. Most of the section traverses AP domains of successive transverse elements of the neural tube (compare with A). *(F)* Cross-section through the rostral medulla (rhombomere 6), which is again topologically transverse; it illustrates the expanded choroidal RP of the hindbrain.

tia nigra, the red nucleus, and the oculomotor nucleus. Similarly, the dorsal hindbrain processes craniofacial or global sensory information (cranial nerve sensory columns and cerebellum), whereas the ventral hindbrain contains cranial nerve motor nuclei and related parts of the reticular formation. Likewise, the dorsal spinal cord (dorsal horn) processes sensory information of the body, whereas the ventral spinal cord contains motor nuclei and integrative local circuits for body musculature and autonomic ganglia control. Neurons located in an intermediate dorsoventral position in the midbrain/hindbrain reticular formation and in the spinal cord tend to be interneurons that regulate sensorimotor circuitry (i.e., postural reflexes and locomotion) and coordinate basic physiological processes such as respiration.

Dorsal (alar) and ventral (basal) parts of the diencephalon proper and the secondary prosencephalon are hierarchically upstream relative to brain-stem components. Dorsal diencephalic elements send sensory signals to the telencephalon (caudal thalamus) or analyze them for suprasegmental reflex actions (pretectum and rostral thalamus). Basal plate elements in the underlying tegmentum integrate complex premotor signals (i.e., for vertical gaze control). The classic hypothalamus in the secondary prosencephalon embodies a diversity of high-level systemic homeostatic servomechanisms, distributed across its

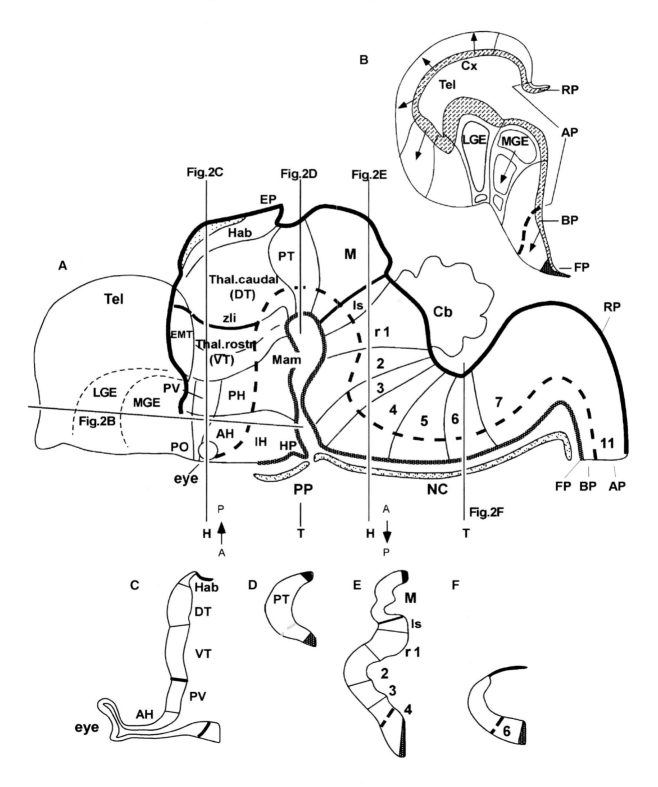

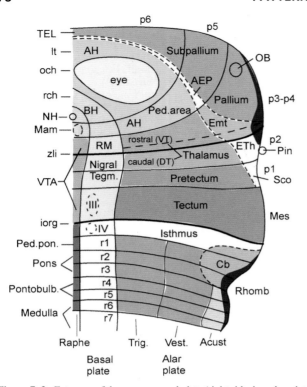

Figure 7–3. Fate map of the mouse neural plate (right side, based on data from Inoue et al. [2000] and extrapolating some chicken data from Fernandez-Garre et al., 2002; Cobos-Sillero et al., 2001; Marín and Puelles, 1995). Fate map appears divided in longitudinal domains, corresponding to the early floor, basal, alar, and roof plates (choroidal roof plate in dark gray; see Fig. 7–1), as well as transverse domains (rhombomeres, isthmus, midbrain, prosomeres. Floor region is divided into a prechordal part (neurohypophysis [NH] and mammillary complex [Mam]) attached to the basal hypothalamus (BH), and an epichordal part. The latter decomposes into two plurisegmental domains: the ventral tegmental area (VTA, underlying the nigral tegmentum in the basal plate) and the hindbrain raphe domain. These two domains are characterized by the formation of dopaminergic and serotoninergic neurons, respectively. The midbrain and isthmic basal plate areas contain the oculomotor and trochlear nuclei (III, IV). The main prospective areas derived from the alar plate are indicated. The alar hypothalamus (AH) surrounds the eye domain and includes caudally the peduncular area (which contains the paraventricular nucleus). Rostral to the midbrain, a series of dorsal specialized territories, such as the subcommissural organ (Sco, under the posterior commissure) and the epithalamus and pineal gland (ETh, Pin), are continuous rostrally with the eminentia thalami (Emt) and anterior entopeduncular area (AEP), which form the so-called hemispheric stalk domains. The Emt borders upon the pallial telencephalon (which includes the olfactory bulb [OB]), whereas the AEP borders upon the subpallial telencephalon. The neural plate rim rostral to the choroidal roof contains the prospective septal domain. The topological arrangement of pallium and subpallium in the neural plate shows that the pallium is primarily caudal to the subpallium. Acust, cochlear column; Cb, cerebellum; DT, dorsal thalamus; iorg, isthmic organizer; lt, lamina terminalis; Mes, mesencephalon; Nigral Tegm, nigral tegmentum; och, optic chiasma; p1–p6, prosomeres 1–6; Ped.area, peduncular area; Ped.pon., pedunculopontine region; Pontobulb, pontobulbar region; r1–r6, rhombomeres; r7, pseudorhombomere 7; rch, retrochiasmatic area; Rhomb., rhombencephalon; RM, retromammillary area; TEL, telencephalon; Trig., trigeminal column; Vest, vestibular column; VT, ventral thalamus; Zli, zona limitans intrathalamica.

alar and basal portions, and is also a site for direct neurohumoral efferent action (through the median eminence and posterior pituitary).

Neurons that use monoamine-type neurotransmitters tend to be clustered within the brain-stem reticular formation as sets of nuclei that send widely ramified axons. These nuclei serve as neuromodulators of various motor and behavioral states. Dopaminergic neurons occupy the basal plate of the posterior diencephalon and midbrain (substantia nigra and ventral tegmental areas, see Fig. 7–3); serotonergic neurons appear largely in the paramedian basal plate of the hindbrain (raphe nuclei; Fig. 7–3), and most noradrenergic neurons lie in the

alar plate of the hindbrain (the locus caeruleus formed in rhombomere 1 is the largest aggregate of such cells).

The topography of the CNS can be imagined using a three-dimensional model. Anteroposterior and dorsoventral patterning of the neural plate generates a two-dimensional grid of spatial coordinates that subdivides the early CNS primordium into an array of differently specified progenitor domains (Fig. 7–3). However, the primordia of regions that form as secondary fields, such as the telencephalon, appear not to be organized according to a rectilinear grid, or this is grossly deformed during the evagination of the hemisphere (Cobos-Sillero et al., 2001). Each of these progenitor domains is programmed to produce a given set of neurons and glia, which migrate away from the progenitor zone to form the laminae and nuclei that constitute the third dimension of the CNS wall (Fig. 7–4). While this model may be oversimplified, it is a useful framework when confronting the daunting task of understanding neuroanatomy.

MOLECULAR GENETICS OF BRAIN DEVELOPMENT

In the last 10 years, huge advances have been made in elucidating the mechanisms underlying the principal steps in brain development. Here, we highlight examples that illustrate major principles.

Induction and Anteroposterior Regionalization of the Neural Plate

Neural induction, the process of converting embryonic ectoderm to a neural fate, is regulated by the secretion of proteins from organizer tissues. This process involves both activation of receptor tyrosine kinases, perhaps through fibroblast growth factors (FGFs) and/or insulin-like growth factors (Streit et al., 2000; Wilson et al., 2000; Pera et al., 2001), and inhibition of transforming growth factor-β (TGF-β) signaling through the noggin and chordin proteins, which bind to bone morphogenetic proteins (BMPs) (Harland, 2000; De Robertis et al., 2000; Wilson and Edlund, 2001; see Chapters 24 and 32 for details about TGF-β and FGF signaling). Furthermore, wingless (WNT) signaling appears to inhibit neural induction in chickens (Wilson et al., 2001; see Chapter 22 for a description of WNT signaling).

Early neural induction generates anterior neural plate structures; anterior specification depends upon the action of the secreted proteins described above in combination with proteins that inhibit signaling through WNT receptors and activin-type TGF-β receptors. Molecules such as Cerberus (which binds BMPs, WNTs, and nodal-type TGF-β proteins) and Dickkopf (which inhibits WNT coreceptors) are implicated in anterior specification (Beddington and Robertson, 1999; Kiecker and Niehrs, 2001). These molecules are secreted by patterning centers adjacent to the anterior neural plate, such as the anterior visceral endoderm and the prechordal mesendoderm. Anterior specification is mediated through homeobox transcription factors such as Otx2, Lim1, and Hesx1 (Cheah et al., 2000; Acampora et al., 2001; Thomas et al., 2001).

Later neural induction generates posterior neural tissues. The mechanisms that specify posterior fate are less well characterized but do not seem to require inhibition of WNT signaling and appear to involve retinoids and FGFs (Lamb and Harland, 1995; Blumberg et al., 1997; Gavalas and Krumlauf, 2000). Posterior fate is regulated by the Hox family of homeobox genes, which are expressed in overlapping patterns along the anteroposterior axis of the CNS (Trainor and Krumlauf, 2000; Barrow et al., 2000; Liu et al., 2001; see Chapter 46).

As the anterior and posterior halves of the CNS are formed, two new patterning centers are generated within the developing brain: one is the ANR, and the other is at the transition between the midbrain and hindbrain (isthmus). The latter is formed through repressive interactions between the *Otx2* and *Gbx2* genes (Simeone, 2000; Li and Joyner, 2001) and the positive action of Pax2 (Ye et al., 2001). These centers express FGF8 and are implicated in specifying anteroposterior position within adjacent areas of the brain (Wilson and Rubenstein, 2000; Nakamura, 2001). They function in part through repressing Otx2 and Emx2 and inducing En1 (Martinez et al., 1999; Crossley et al., 2001). The isthmus is essential for the formation and patterning of the cerebellum and the midbrain, whereas the ANR plays a similar role in patterning the telencephalon (Shanmugalingam et al., 2000; Storm

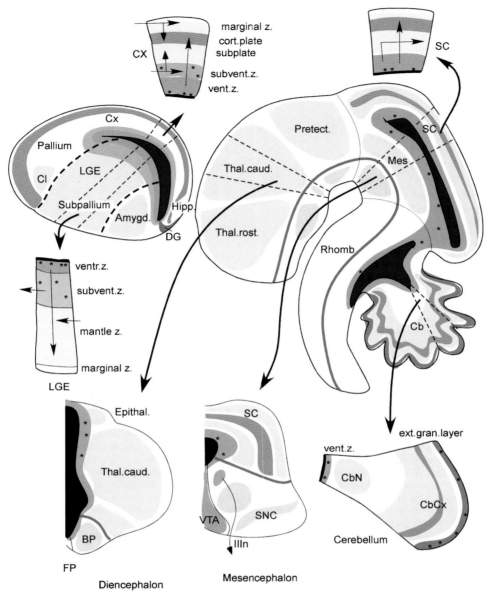

Figure 7–4. Schema of a lateral parasagittal section through the embryonic mammalian brain, to illustrate the variations in the arrangement and location of the proliferative compartments (ventricular zone, subventricular zone, subpial proliferative zones) and the differentiation compartment (mantle zone, cortical or nuclear). Large arrows point to details of sections at different positions. The most extensive proliferation compartment is the radially organized ventricular zone. This zone, which is derived from the neural tube neuroepithelium, is found throughout the CNS, covering all fluid-filled ventricular spaces (ventricular zone represented as blue areas, small asterisks within indicate ventricularly attached mitoses). Proliferation in the ventricular zone ends earlier in the basal plate than in the alar plate, thus explaining the latter's larger relative growth (red line represents the alar/basal boundary). There is a second stratum of proliferating and migrating cells, the subventricular zone; this lacks an epithelial organization (i.e., no radial elements) and contains extraventricular mitoses (subventricular zone as green areas in the schema, asterisks within these areas represent extraventricular mitoses). The subventricular zone is particularly prominent in the telencephalon, where it is thicker in the subpallium than in the pallium. In most places of the brain, postmitotic neurons and various sorts of glia cell migrate out of the deep proliferative compartments and accumulate after some radial or tangential migration into the mantle zone (yellow). Sometimes the mantle zone becomes structured as nuclei, and other times it develops cortical primordia (red areas parallel to brain surface). In that case, a dense cortical plate forms initially, which later differentiates into a number of sublayers. Finally, in some brain regions, superficial (subpial) proliferative zones are established from the migration of ventricular zone progenitors. These cell sources often produce neurons postnatally, even throughout the lifetime of the animal. Examples of such late subpial proliferative zones are the telencephalic source of dentate gyrus elements and the cerebellar external granular layer (both mauve-colored). Amygd., amygdala; BP, basal plate; Cb, cerebellum; CbCx, cerebellar cortex; CbN, cerebellar nucleus; Cl, claustrum; Cx, cortex; DG, dentate gyrus; Epithal., epithalamus; ext.gran.layer, external granular layer; Hipp, hippocampus; IIIn, oculomotor nerve; LGE, lateral ganglionic eminence; mantle z., mantle zone; marginal z., marginal zone; Mes, mesencephalon; Pretect., pretectum; Rhomb, rhombencephalon; SC, superior colliculus; SNC, substantia nigra compacta; subvent.z., subventricular zone; Thal.caud., caudal thalamus; Thal.rost., rostral thalamus; vent.z., ventricular zone; VTA, ventral tegmental area.

et al., 2003). Later expression of Fgf8 in the rostral midline of the telencephalon is implicated in patterning of the cerebral cortex (Fukuchi-Shimogori and Grove, 2001; Garel et al., 2003).

An additional transverse patterning center forms between the rostral and caudal diencephalon. The ZLI may function as a boundary to restrict the action of patterning signals and later, through expression of sonic hedgehog and other signals, may pattern adjacent tissues (Shimamura and Rubenstein, 1997; Zeltser et al., 2001).

As development proceeds, anteroposterior specification of the CNS becomes further refined, as reflected by the formation of transverse subdivisions, or neuromeres (Figs. 7–2, 7–3). In the hindbrain, the rhombomeres have segment-like properties (Lumsden and Krumlauf, 1996; Lumsden, 1999). Cell mixing between adjacent rhombomeres appears to be restricted through repulsive actions of Eph/Ephrin molecules (Mellitzer et al., 1999). In the forebrain, prosomeres of the caudal diencephalon have similarities and differences with the rhombomeres, perhaps reflecting some distinct development mechanisms (Puelles and Rubenstein, 1993; Figdor and Stern, 1993; Puelles, 1995, 2001; Larsen et al., 2001).

During regionalization, neural crest progenitors delaminate from the neural ridge of the spinal cord, hindbrain, midbrain, and posterior diencephalon (see Chapter 6). Therefore, the processes that control regional specification of the CNS also have an important role in regulating the properties of the neural crest (Trainor and Krumlauf, 2000).

Dorsoventral Specification of Longitudinal CNS Subdivisions and Specification of Neuronal Cell Types

Shortly after neural induction and anteroposterior specification have begun, involution of the axial mesendoderm under the medial neural plate initiates ventral specification. Prior to the effects of the axial mesendoderm, the neural plate probably has dorsal molecular properties due to the influence of BMPs produced in the neural ridge and adjacent ectoderm (Barth et al., 1999). Then, through the action of substances produced by the prechordal plate and notochord (anterior and posterior parts of the axial mesendoderm), the medial neural plate expresses transcription factors that confer ventral CNS identity. Sonic hedgehog (SHH) is the best-characterized substance produced by the axial mesendoderm that regulates ventral identity (see Chapters 16 and 18). SHH esterification with cholesterol is critical for its function. Disruption of SHH signaling results in loss of ventral CNS tissues, thereby causing CNS disorders such as holoprosencephaly and cyclopia (see Chapters 17 and 18).

SHH may function as a concentration-dependent inducer of cell fate in the ventral CNS. Decreasing concentrations of SHH may induce six major types of neural progenitor in the ventral spinal cord: FP, V3, Mn, V2, V1, and V0 (Briscoe et al., 2000; Marquardt and Pfaff, 2001). Floor plate progenitors are the ventralmost and lie adjacent to the notochord. V3–V0 progenitors produce distinct types of interneuron, whereas Mn progenitors produce motor neurons. The formation of sharp domains of transcription factor expression is mediated by mutual repression between SHH-induced transcription factors (e.g., the Nkx2 and Nkx6 genes) and transcription factors that are not regulated directly by SHH (Pax6 and Irx) (Briscoe et al., 2000). The repression is controlled in part by interactions between the homeodomain proteins with groucho proteins (Muhr et al., 2001).

SHH is not the only substance that generates ventral CNS patterning as much of this can be formed in mice that lack both SHH and the transcription factor Gli3 (Litingtung and Chiang, 2000; see Chapter 20). Gli3 antagonizes SHH signaling; relieving this repression reveals an underlying pattern that must be generated by a yet unknown mechanism. Nodal-type TGF-β proteins are required for ventral patterning of the zebrafish forebrain (Wilson and Rubenstein, 2000) and are presently being investigated for a similar role in mammals.

Thus, SHH-mediated ventral specification of the floor and basal plates generates a set of ventral progenitor zones that extend along the CNS (there are some differences in these longitudinal zones at different anteroposterior positions). Moreover, BMP-mediated patterning of the roof and alar plates appears to participate in generating an analogous set of dorsal progenitor zones (Lee and Jessell, 1999). Defects in the patterning of dorsal structures through mutations in Zic2 and transforming-growth factor-β-induced factor (TGIF) cause dysmorphic syndromes, such as lobar holoprosencephaly (Wallis and Muenke, 2000; see Chapter 18).

WNT signaling is largely active in the same regions where BMP signaling occurs. For instance, mutations that reduce WNT signaling in the dorsal telencephalon lead to deletion of dorsal telencephalic structures (e.g., the hippocampus) (Galceran et al., 2000; Lee et al., 2000). WNT signaling is also essential at the isthmus for generation of the cerebellum, where WNT and FGF functions are closely linked (Liu and Joyner, 2001).

Generation of these dorsal and ventral progenitors is the first step in the specification of different types of neuron and glia. For instance, in the hindbrain, V3 progenitors generate V3 interneurons and serotonin neurons, whereas Mn progenitors generate motor neurons (Briscoe et al., 1999, 2000). Thus, specification of dorsoventral progenitor identity is linked to specification of neuronal identity. A similar process takes place in the telencephalon, where Nkx genes specify ventral progenitors and cell types (cholinergic neurons), Gsh genes specify intermediate cell types (GABAergic neurons), and genes such as Gli3 are required to specify dorsal cell types (glutamatergic neurons) (reviewed in Wilson and Rubenstein, 2000). However, this analogy is an oversimplification as fate maps show that "ventral" parts of the telencephalon are topologically anterior, while "dorsal" parts are posterior (Cobos-Sillero et al., 2001). During evagination of the telencephalon, topologically anterior parts of the telencephalon secondarily obtain "ventral" molecular properties (Crossley et al., 2001).

The early expression of patterning genes in the ventral CNS may change with time. At early stages of spinal cord development, Nkx2.2 expression is restricted to the V3 domain; at later stages, it expands dorsally (Marquardt and Pfaff, 2001). Nkx2.2 coexpression with the Olig2 basic helix-loop-helix (bHLH) transcription factor is required for the production of oligodendrocytes (Qi et al., 2001; Sun et al., 2001; Zhou et al., 2001).

Neural Progenitor Cells

Progenitor (neuroepithelial) cells in the developing CNS are organized as a pseudostratified epithelium that lines the ventricular surface of the neural tube. This is known as the ventricular zone (Fig. 7–4). At early neural tube stages, the apical surface of neuroepithelial cells maintains contact with the ventricular lumen and the cells extend a basal process toward the outer or pial surface. The cell nuclei move away from the lumen during the S phase of the cell cycle and then move toward it as they proceed through mitosis, or M phase (Caviness et al., 1995).

It is likely that rapid symmetrical mitoses lead to surface growth of the neural tube and particularly to expansion of the optic and telencephalic vesicles. The mitogenic mechanisms underlying this process are poorly understood, although there is evidence that receptor tyrosine kinase signaling through FGF and epidermal growth factor ligands participate in regulating mitosis in the embryonic CNS (Martens et al., 2000; Korada et al., 2002).

Once neurogenesis has begun, asymmetrical mitoses generate one progenitor and one immature neuron. The mechanisms underlying the role of asymmetrical cell division in controlling neural cell fate are best understood in Drosophila, where a number of proteins, including Numb, have key roles (Jan and Jan, 1998). Neural progenitors have basal processes that extend to the pial surface. For a number of reasons, including the fact that they express some markers found in astrocytes, some neuroepithelial cells have been named "radial glia." Now, it is recognized that radial glia in the cerebral cortex can produce both neurons and glia (Noctor et al., 2001; Hartfuss et al., 2001). Radial progenitor cells initially produce neurons and then at later developmental stages astrocytes.

As development proceeds, secondary progenitor zones are generated in specific areas of the neural tube. These include the telencephalic subventricular zone, which is composed of proliferating progenitors not arranged as an epithelium (Fig. 7–4). The subventricular zone is superficial to the ventricular zone and deep to the differentiating cortical or basal ganglia primordial. Subventricular zones produce neurons at early stages (Anderson et al., 1997) and appear to become primarily gliogenic later (Katika and Goldman, 1999).

In the cerebellum, a subpial progenitor zone is formed (the external granule cell layer) that transiently generates granule cells pre- and postnatally (Fig. 7–4). SHH produced by cerebellar Purkinje cells serves as a mitogen for granule cell precursors in the external granule cell layer (Wechsler-Reya and Scott, 2001).

The only parts of the adult mammalian brain certain to have active progenitor cells are the subventricular zone of the rostral telencephalon and the dentate gyrus of the hippocampus (Fig.7–4) (Luskin, 1998; Palmer et al., 2000; Alvarez-Buylla et al., 2001; Gritti et al., 2002). In the adult CNS, ependymal cells line the ventricle. These cells serve primarily a role as an epithelial barrier, although it is unclear whether they may also have neural progenitor properties (Alvarez-Buylla et al., 2001; Cassidy and Frisen, 2001).

Differentiation

Neurodifferentiation involves progressive changes in gene expression that define new cell biological states. As described above, these processes occur in progenitor cells to generate cells that are programmed to produce different types of neuron (e.g., depending on the dorsoventral position), to generate progenitors with different mitotic behavior (e.g., cell cycle rate, symmetrical or asymmetrical divisions), or to generate secondary progenitor zones.

A major step in neurodifferentiation is when progenitor cells are programmed to produce neurons. Neurons do not have the capacity to reenter the cell cycle (Caviness et al., 1995). The mechanisms that underlie the arrest of neurons at the G_0 stage of the cell cycle are poorly understood. Once a neuron is born, it usually migrates away from the progenitor zone toward the mantle zone, forming at the basal aspect of the neuroepithelium. Neurons mature in the mantle zone (Fig. 7–4). Generally, newborn neurons move to the mantle directly overlying the progenitor zone where they were born. This is called *radial migration*. Radial migration can involve either the translocation of the soma within a preexistent radial cytoplasmic process or free migration of the whole cell, guided by the process of an adjacent radial glial cell (*gliophilic migration*) (Puelles and Bendala, 1978; Hatten, 1999; Gleeson and Walsh, 2000). Alternatively, some neurons migrate long distances tangentially (i.e., orthogonally to the radial dimension of the neuroepithelium) to populate other regions of the CNS (*neurophilic migration*, see below).

Molecular mechanisms that control the timing of differentiation in the vertebrate nervous system appear to function in part through lateral inhibition effects mediated by Notch signaling (see Chapters 39–41) (Chitnis, 1995; Henrique et al., 1997). Notch is a cell surface receptor that is activated by DSL ligands (Delta, Serrate, Lag-2). Mammals have four Notch genes (*Notch 1–4*) and five DSL ligand genes (*Delta1, -3,* and *-4, Jagged1,* and *-2*) (Lindsell et al., 1996). Ligand-induced Notch signaling involves proteolytic cleavage of Notch, which releases its intracellular domain (Notch-IC) and allows its translocation to the nucleus. Notch-IC directly modulates the function of a transcription factor known as CSL (CBF1, Suppressor of Hairless [SuH], Lag-1). Notch activation of CSL induces expression of WRPW-bHLH transcription factors, which inhibit neuronal differentiation (e.g., *HES* genes), and represses the expression of proneural bHLH transcription factors (e.g., Mash1) (Robey, 1997; Artavanis-Tsakonas et al., 1999). An increase in Notch signaling biases progenitor cells not to differentiate, whereas a decrease in Notch signaling facilitates their maturation.

There are several classes of proneural bHLH genes expressed in the mammalian telencephalon, including *Mash1* and *Olig2* (primarily in the subpallium) and *Neurogenin 1* and *2* (restricted to the pallium) (Fode et al., 2000; Lu et al., 2000).

Mash1 is required for the expression of Delta; in its absence, early-born subpallial cells are not formed and the subventricular zone prematurely differentiates (Casarosa et al., 1999; Horton et al., 1999; K. Yun et al., 2002). The *Dlx1* and *Dlx2* homeobox genes are required for late differentiation in the subpallium (Anderson et al., 1997). In the absence of both *Dlx1* and *Dlx2*, immature neurons have elevated levels of *Hes* expression, which is indicative of increased Notch signaling (K. Yun et al., 2002). Thus, both bHLH and homeobox transcription factors participate in mediating the effects of Notch signaling to regulate the differentiation of progenitor cells.

As immature neurons migrate and settle into their final positions, their differentiation is regulated by autonomous and non-autonomous mechanisms. For instance, in the subpallium, while Dlx1 and Dlx2 are expressed primarily in progenitor cells, Dlx5 and Dlx6 are also expressed in postmitotic neurons (Anderson et al., 1997). Dlx1/2 expression is required for the proper induction of Dlx5/6 expression (Anderson et al., 1997). In the spinal cord, secretion of retinoids by early-born motor neurons is implicated in controlling the development of later-born adjacent motor neurons (Sockanathan and Jessell, 1998).

The molecular mechanisms that regulate motor neuron development provide the best example of how transcription factors define progressively more defined states of differentiation (Jessell, 2000; Lee and Pfaff, 2001). Specification of motor neuron progenitors is regulated by Nkx6.1 and Olig2 (Sander et al., 2000; Mizuguchi et al., 2001; Novitch et al., 2001). These progenitors are then specified to become either somatic or visceral motor neurons through the action of the *MNR2, HB9,* and *Phox2* genes (Tanabe et al., 1998; Arber et al., 1999). Somatic motor neurons are subdivided into different columns (e.g., medial and lateral), which innervate muscles in different regions of the body (e.g., body wall or limbs) through the action of Lim-homeodomain proteins (Kania et al., 2000). These genes control the projection pathways that motor neuron axons follow. Within the different columns, ETS transcription factors define motor neuron pools that regulate the branching of motor neuron axons and thereby control the innervation of different groups of muscles within a region (Arber et al., 2000). Subpools of motor neurons that innervate different types of muscle (e.g., fast, slow, extrafusal, and intrafusal) are defined by yet unknown transcription factors. It is anticipated that similar cascades of transcription factors will be discovered to control neuronal subtypes in all regions of the CNS.

CELL MIGRATION

Neurons and glia move away from the progenitor zones where they are produced via either radial or tangential trajectories (Figs. 7–4, 7–5). As noted above, there are two modes of radial migration. At early stages in development, when the width of the neural tube is relatively small, immature neurons extend a process to the pial surface; the cell body then follows by translocation (Puelles and Bendala, 1978; Nadarajah et al., 2001). At later stages, radially migrating detached neurons use the processes of radial glia as a guidance substrate (Puelles and Bendala, 1978; Gleeson and Walsh, 2000). Tangentially migrating cells follow unknown (but cell type- and locus-specific) guidance cues as they move from the primordium where they are generated to their target tissues; finally, in some cases, they migrate again radially into their final location (Hatten, 1999; Marin and Rubenstein, 2001). It is thought that, in general, telencephalic projection neurons follow radial migratory pathways, whereas local circuit neurons tend to follow tangential migrations (Marin and Rubenstein, 2001).

The mouse pallium (cortex) exemplifies the differential development of projection and local circuit neurons. Pallial projection neurons, which are glutamatergic, are generated by the pallial progenitor zone, whereas most of the eventual pallial local circuit neurons, which are GABAergic, are generated from subpallial progenitors (Marin and Rubenstein, 2001). The radial migration of projection neurons maintains the positional information to which their progenitors were exposed; this could be important for the generation of topographic connectivity maps (Rakic, 2000). It is unclear why the glutamatergic and GABAergic neurons of the pallium are produced by different progenitor zones, but it may be due to the coupling of regional and cell type specification processes described above. Thus, pallial progenitors may be genetically predisposed to generate specifically glutamatergic cells, whereas subpallial progenitors can generate only GABAergic cells. Therefore, it might have been functionally advantageous during telencephalic phylogeny for subpallial GABAergic cells to evolve tangential migration into the pallium, to enable these cells to participate in pallial circuitry.

The molecular mechanisms that regulate neuronal migration are a subject of intense investigation. Most of the studies have focused on radial migration in the neocortex in mice and humans. The neocortex is a hexalaminar structure that contains projection neurons with related properties in given layers (McConnell, 1995). The first neurons that reach the cortical mantle are called the primordial cortex or "pre-

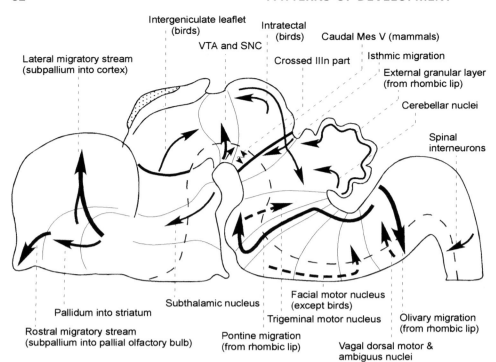

Lateral migratory stream
(subpallium into cortex)

Intergeniculate leaflet
(birds)

VTA and SNC

Intratectal
(birds)

Caudal Mes V (mammals)

Crossed IIIn part

Isthmic migration

External granular layer
(from rhombic lip)

Cerebellar nuclei

Spinal
interneurons

Pallidum into striatum

Subthalamic nucleus

Facial motor nucleus
(except birds)

Trigeminal motor nucleus

Olivary migration
(from rhombic lip)

Rostral migratory stream
(subpallium into pallial olfactory bulb)

Pontine migration
(from rhombic lip)

Vagal dorsal motor &
ambiguus nuclei

Figure 7–5. Schema illustrating the location, extent, and topological relationships of the major known cases of tangential neuronal migration in the brain. This schema is based on Figure 7–2 as regards brain subdivisions and labels the diverse migratory routes. The crossed oculomotor migration occurs across the ventral midline of the midbrain. It is remarkable that all of these migrations are oriented in three-dimensional space, suggesting that the migratory cells utilize positional information along their trajectory to reach their destination analogous to that used by axons (see Fig. 7–6). SNC, substantia nigra compacta; VTA, ventral tegmental area.

plate." Subsequently arriving neurons form the "cortical plate," which splits the preplate into a superficial layer called the marginal zone (layer 1) and a transient deep layer called the "subplate" (Marín-Padilla, 1983; Allendorfer and Shatz, 1994). As new neurons arrive, they progressively stack inside-out on top of the older cells, building cortical layers 2–6; thus, layer 6 neurons are born before layer 2 neurons.

Migration defects of neocortical projection neurons can be classified on the basis of the stage in which radial migration is affected (reviewed in Gleeson and Walsh, 2000; Rice and Curran, 2001; see Chapters 90, 92, and 93). The onset of migration is disrupted by mutations in the X-linked *filamin* gene. Filamin is an actin-binding protein; defects in its expression lead to ectopic collections of neurons near the ventricle (Gleeson and Walsh, 2000). Mutations in the *doublecortin* and *lis* genes disrupt migration and cortical lamination by altering microtubule function (Gleeson and Walsh, 2000; see Chapter 92). In humans, they cause lissencephalies, or smooth brain syndromes. Mutations in genes in the reelin pathway lead to an inversion and disorganization of cortical layers (see Chapter 93). Reelin is a secreted protein produced by Cajal-Retzius cells in the marginal zone. The lipoprotein receptors VLDLR and APOER2 appear to be reelin receptors; they signal through the DAB adaptor and the CDK5, p35, and p39 proteins. Reelin expression is controlled by TBR1 and EMX2; these transcription factors regulate differentiation of Cajal-Retzius cells (Mallamaci et al., 2000; Hevner et al., 2001). The BRN1 and BRN2 transcription factors control p35 and p39 expression (McEvilly et al., 2002). Mutations in presenilin and α6 integrin lead to neurons migrating out of the brain into the meninges; these mutants phenocopy type II lissencephalies such as Fukuyama syndrome.

The mechanisms that control tangential migrations appear to be extremely diverse (reviewed in Marin and Rubenstein, 2001). Because these cells travel over long distances and follow trajectories similar to major axon tracts, it is possible that they use mechanisms related to axonal pathfinding (Fig. 7–5). For instance, semaphorin/neuropilin signaling has been implicated in regulating the sorting of tangentially migrating subpallial cells to distinct telencephalic targets (Marin et al., 2001). Likewise Slit/Robo and Ephrin/Eph signaling are implicated in the tangential migration of precursors for olfactory bulb interneurons (Conover et al., 2000; Wong et al., 2001). The tangential migration of neurons of the inferior olivary nucleus is regulated by netrin/DCC signaling (Yee et al., 1999).

FORMATION AND GROWTH OF DENDRITES

Each type of neuron has a characteristic dendritic arbor and axonal trajectory. Axons are designed to conduct an axon potential and release neurotransmitters from their terminal, whereas dendrites are designed to receive neurotransmitter signals. Dendrites can have an extremely complex and stereotyped architecture. Here, we review some of the salient features of axonal and dendritic development and illustrate a few of the mechanisms that control these processes.

As a neuron differentiates, it produces multiple thin protrusions called neurites, one of which will become the axon; the others will form dendrites (reviewed in Jan and Jan, 2001). Semaphorins can orient the growth of axons and dendrites in the cerebral cortex. Semaphorin3a is an attractant for the apical dendrite and a repellent for the axon (Polleux et al., 2000). Several mechanisms can regulate the growth and branching of neurites and dendrites. For instance, Notch signaling inhibits neurite outgrowth (Sestan et al., 1999). Branching of dendrites is regulated by intrinsic factors that change the organization of the cytoskeleton, such as members of the Rho family of small GTPases (Luo, 2000) and the Plakin cytoskeletal anchor proteins (Gao et al., 1999), and by putative transcription factors (e.g., Sequoia) that may orchestrate the program of dendritic morphogenesis (Brenman et al., 2001).

Extrinsic mechanisms also regulate dendritic outgrowth and branching, such as Sema3a, BMP7, CPG15, and neurotrophins (reviewed in Jan and Jan, 2001). Dendritic growth is slowed by increases in neuronal activity, which may be mediated through cell adhesion molecule kinase II (CAMKII) (reviewed in Cline, 2001). Dendritic morphogenesis is sensitive to the position of other structures in the environment that arrest the growth of the dendritic tree (the "tiling" process). For instance, mutation of the *Drosophila* Flamingo seven-pass membrane protein, which resembles G-protein receptors, blocks dendritic tiling (Gao et al., 2000).

Dendrites are occasionally covered with small protrusions called "spines," where some specific synapses form. Spine formation is affected by mutations in *Spinophilin*, which encodes an anchor protein for actin and protein phosphatase (Feng et al., 2000a), and the *Fragile X* gene *(FMR1)*, which is important in mediating dendritic protein synthesis in response to activity (Comery et al., 1997). Neurotransmitter receptors mediate spine function. The sequence of appearance of ionotropic glutamate receptors during development is similar to that in which they appear in response to events that change synaptic strength (synaptic plasticity) (reviewed in Jan and Jan, 2001).

AXONAL PATHFINDING

Axons grow across considerable distances, follow complex trajectories, and send branches to several target areas, where they synapse upon discrete sets of cells (Fig. 7–6). To accomplish these tasks, growing axons react to an ordered set of cues provided by their environment, which is regulated by multiple mechanisms (see reviews by Tessier-Lavigne and Goodman, 1996; O'Leary and Wilkinson, 1999; Brose and Tessier-Lavigne, 2000; Benson et al., 2001; Jacob et al., 2001).

Tessier-Lavigne and Goodman (1996) describe four general mechanisms that guide axons: "attractive and repulsive cues, which can either be short-range or long-range." The molecular bases for these guidance forces are rapidly being elucidated. However, generalizations about the roles of specific molecules are precarious. For instance, the attractant Netrin1 can be converted into a repellant by Laminin1 (Hopker et al., 1999). These guidance forces regulate processes such as growth along the dorsoventral or anteroposterior axis, sprouting of collateral axons, fasciculation with pioneer axons, channeling into narrow passages, crossing midline structures, and choosing synaptic targets.

Many of the choices that an axon makes are generated by the growth cone. The growth cone is at the distal end of immature axons; it integrates environmental signals and generates corresponding modifications of the cytoskeleton that promote either elongation, turning, growth arrest, or retraction of the axon. Once it reaches its target, the growth cone and the targeted cell develop into pre- and postsynaptic structures, respectively. At the beginning of this section, we distill some of the central principles about axonal pathfinding and synapse formation by describing the development of axons that grow from retinal ganglion cells and extend to their various targets in the diencephalon and mesencephalon. At the end of this section, we discuss additional mechanisms that are also used for axonal pathfinding.

Retinal ganglion cells are the projection neurons of the eye. They send axons that variously synapse on specific target neurons in the hypothalamus (e.g., suprachiasmatic nucleus), in the thalamus (e.g., ventral and dorsal lateral geniculate nuclei), the pretectum (e.g., the pupillary reflex center or olivary pretectal nucleus), and the midbrain (superior colliculus) (Fig. 7–6).

Within the eye, retinal ganglion cell axons (RGCAs) grow in topographical order toward the optic disc, where they enter the optic stalk to form the optic nerve. Netrin, EphB2/B3, and immunoglobulin-related cell adhesion molecules (IgCAMs) are implicated in regulating the growth toward the optic disc (Birgbauer et al., 2001). The EphB2 and EphB3 receptor tyrosine kinases appear to function as inhibitory cues that prevent dorsal RGCAs from growing into the ventral retina. Mutations in either netrin or DCC (one of its receptors) lead to RGCA pathfinding errors at the optic disc (Deiner and Sretavan, 1999).

Within the embryonic optic stalk, RGCAs interact with astroglia. Mutation of either the *Vax1* or *Pax2* transcription factor gene, expressed in these glia, disrupts their interactions with the RGCAs (Torres et al., 1996; Bertuzzi et al., 1999).

After RGCAs leave the optic stalk, they reach the chiasmatic plate, where the majority grow across the midline and form the contralateral optic tract (Marcus et al., 1999); a minority of the axons form the ipsilateral optic tract. RGCAs fail to enter the chiasmatic plate in Vax1 mutants and, thus, do not form the optic chiasm (Bertuzzi et al., 1999). In these mutants, expression of Netrin1 and EphB3 is reduced in the area of the chiasmatic plate. EphB2/B3, Netrin, and Vax1 also affect the development of other brain commissures, such as the corpus callosum (Serafini et al., 1996; Henkemeyer et al., 1996; Bertuzzi et al., 1999).

These and other studies (Mason and Sretavan, 1997) provide evidence that glial cells have a prominent role in regulating axonal pathfinding, particularly at commissures. Slit1, a secreted molecule that binds to the Robo receptors, also plays a prominent role in regulating axon crossing at multiple commissures (Erskine et al., 2000; Bagri et al., 2002; Plump et al., 2002).

The mechanisms that sort ipsilateral and contralateral RGCAs at the optic chiasm remain a mystery. It is likely that positional information present in the retinal ganglion cells participates in this process because a neuron's location along the nasotemporal axis of the retina determines whether its axon will cross at the optic chiasm.

Once the RGCAs reach the optic tract, they grow posteriorly through the alar plate (Fig. 7–6). Little is known about the mechanisms that control the anteroposterior growth of axons. However, signals that instruct an axon about its dorsoventral position are more clearly elucidated. There is evidence that Slit/Robo and Netrin/DCC signaling are important in dorsoventral patterning of growing axons and of axon tracts. For instance, in Slit2, Slit1/2, and Nkx2.1 mutants (which have reduced Slit2 expression), corticofugal fibers are displaced ventrally into the hypothalamic region, which normally has Slit2 expression (Bagri et al., 2002; Marin et al., 2002). A similar defect is seen in the optic tract (Plump et al., 2002). Netrin and DCC mutants also affect the position of the optic tract (Deiner and Sretavan, 1999).

RGCAs grow along the marginal zone of the neural tube. Little is known about the mechanisms that prevent them from inappropriately invading the underlying mantle zone. At specified locations, some RGCAs sprout branches that grow collaterals into the mantle zone of targets, such as the lateral geniculate nucleus of the thalamus. It has been suggested that shared expression of specific cadherin proteins in RGCAs and their target neurons, as well as in other neural systems, may guide synaptic selectivity (Wöhrn et al., 1998; Redies, 2000; Redies and Puelles, 2001).

The mechanisms that regulate sprouting of axonal branches are poorly understood, but there is evidence that Slit2 can regulate sprouting into the spinal cord from the central axonal projections of dorsal root ganglion neurons (Wang et al., 1999). Furthermore, once RGCAs reach the superior colliculus, the growth cones frequently overshoot their target zones; however, axonal branches then form at the topographically correct positions (Yates et al., 2001).

The formation of topographic synaptic maps in target tissues is regulated by the Eph receptors and their ligands, the Ephrins (Flanagan and Vanderhaeghen, 1998). To date, EphB and EphrinB proteins are implicated primarily in axonal pathfinding in the retina and at the optic chiasm, whereas EphA and EphrinA proteins are important in the formation of the nasotemporal retinal map in the midbrain. RGCAs from the nasal side of the retina project to the caudal part of the superior colliculus, whereas RGCAs from the temporal side of the retina project to the rostral part. RGCAs from different positions of the dorsoventral axis of the retina project along the lateromedial axis of the superior colliculus. EphrinA2 and -A5 are expressed in a low-rostral to high-caudal gradient in the superior colliculus, whereas EphA5 and -A6 are expressed in a low-nasal to high-temporal gradient in the retinal ganglion cells. Because Ephrin activation of Eph signaling repels axons, it is hypothetized that Eph/Ephrin interactions contribute to the formation of retinocollicular topographic maps. Indeed, mice that have either decreased or increased levels of EphrinA expression in their retinal ganglion cells show alterations in the topography of RGCA projections in the superior colliculus (Feldheim et al., 2000; Brown et al., 2000).

While development of the retinal projections provides an instructive vignette into axonal pathfinding and target selection, additional mechanisms that participate in axonal guidance are important to describe: semaphorin signaling, integrin signaling, interactions via cadherins and IgCAMs, and the effects of cyclic nucleotide second messengers.

Semaphorins generally repel axons that express either Neuropilins or Plexins (Yu and Kolodkin, 1999). This process is illustrated by examining the development of commissural axons in the spinal cord. Commissural neurons are sensory processing cells located in the dorsal horns of the spinal cord; they extend axons ventrally that cross the ventral midline (floor plate); on reaching the contralateral side, they coalesce to form a rostral-growing ventral tract that extends to the hindbrain reticular formation. Expression of Semaphorins, as well as

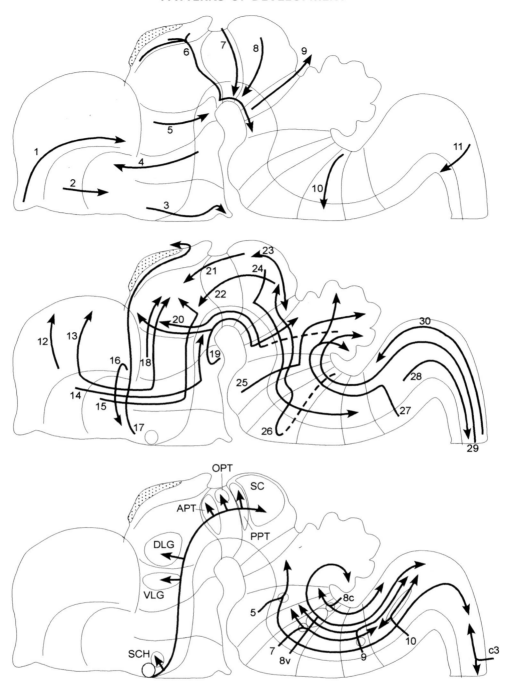

Slits, in the floor plate and adjacent parts of the ventral spinal cord is implicated in preventing these axons from recrossing the floor plate. Furthermore, these proteins are thought to participate in preventing the axons from entering the neuron-rich mantle zone and thereby "squeezing" them into a tract (Zou et al., 2000).

Transduction of extracellular signals into changes in axon growth and trajectory is mediated in part through cyclic nucleotide second messengers. Growth cone responses to semaphorins, neurotrophin-3, and netrin can be modulated by the levels of cAMP or cGMP (Song et al., 1998). For instance, semaphorin-induced repulsion can be converted to attraction by activation of the cGMP signaling pathways (Song et al., 1998).

Integrins are cell surface receptors that coordinate the interaction of growing axons and migrating cells with extracellular matrix molecules such as the laminins and fibronectin (Reichardt et al., 1992). Laminins are multisubunit proteins, parts of which resemble netrins,

which regulate diverse processes, including axon growth and synapse formation (Sanes and Lichtman, 2001).

Molecular homophilic interactions are important in mediating mutual adhesion between axons, forming axon fascicles (fasciculation), and forming synapses (Van Vactor, 1998; Kamiguchi et al., 1998; Redies, 2000). These interactions are mediated via the cadherin and IgCAM families. These proteins can affect mitogen-activated protein kinase (MAPK) signaling, perhaps through FGF receptors, which leads to increasing axon growth (Doherty et al., 2000). Cadherins are calcium-dependent homophilic adhesion proteins. Based on their expression patterns, they are implicated in coordinating the modularity and connectivity of brain circuitry (Takeichi et al., 1997; Redies, 2000; Yoon et al., 2000; Redies and Puelles, 2001). IgCAMs are also involved in heterophilic interactions (De Angelis et al., 1999).

Axonal interactions have been implicated in coordinating reciprocal connections, such as the development of connections between spe-

Figure 7–6. This triple schema illustrates the topological relationships of a number of fiber tracts with the longitudinal and transverse subdivisions of the brain wall. The tracts shown are by no means a complete set and were selected merely for coverage of different parts of the brain and variety of navigational course. In principle, all brain tracts allow an analogous representation. The general principle illustrated is that, as in the case of tangential migration, axonal navigation tends to respect the primary internal boundaries in the wall so that the course selected at given decision points results in a trajectory that is either parallel or orthogonal to neighboring boundaries. The courses of all of these fibers reflect the overall bending of the neural tube axis. Note that several early fiber tracts are elaborated before or during neural tube axial bending, while many others are formed afterward (revealing that the fibers follow intrinsic topological cues, which do not change because of morphogenetic deformations). *Upper schema* displays tracts (or connections) using mainly a transverse course in different parts of the brain (see list below for identifications). *Middle schema* shows tracts disposed longitudinally or with mixed longitudinal and transverse sectors in their course (contralateral parts of courses appear dashed, see list below for identification). *Lower schema* concentrates on two systems of axons. Rostrally it shows the optic pathway in the forebrain and midbrain, illustrating its overall longitudinal course within the alar plate and a set of retinorecipient fields at different transverse parts of the brain wall. This schema does not imply that each ganglion cell axon from the retina gives collaterals to all retinorecipient nuclei since there is evidence of some target selectivity. The retinotopic projection maps produced along this pathway after synaptogenesis are also aligned with the orthogonal grid of primary brain boundaries. Lower schema shows caudally the characteristic topology in the hindbrain alar plate of the primary sensory afferents from the cranial nerves (and of a cervical spinal nerve). Trigeminal and cervical somatosensory fibers

(5, C3); facial, glossopharyngeal, and vagal viscerosensory fibers (7, 9, 10); and vestibular and cochlear sensorial fibers (8v, 8c) are represented. In all of these cases, again, the primary fibers adopt longitudinal courses along the corresponding plurisegmental sensory column (see Fig. 7–3) and will give out collaterals at different transverse levels (again with some target selectivity, as in the retinal fields; details not shown). Note that some nerves contain fibers of different functional modalities (i.e., somatosensory and viscerosensory components in 7, 9, and 10), which will each enter into the appropriate column (not shown). The entrance points of the afferents are indicated by circles or ovals. List of tracts: 1, lateral olfactory tract; 2, striopallidal projection; 3, preoptohypophysary tract; 4, subthalamopallidal projection; 5, tegmental projection from ventral thalamus; 6, habenulointerpeduncular (retroflex) tract; 7, posterior commissure; 8, crossed tectotegmental tract; 9, trochlear nerve; 10, cochleo-olivary tract; 11, dorsal horn into ventral horn projection; 12, claustrocortical projection; 13, bidirectional thalamocortical connection; 14, strionigral tract; 15, pallidothalamic (ansa lenticularis) tract; 16, stria terminalis; 17, stria medullaris; 18, reticular nucleus into dorsal thalamus; 19, mammillotegmental and mammillothalamic tracts; 20, dentatothalamic tract; 21, tectothalamic connection (brachium of superior colliculus); 22, brachium of inferior colliculus; 23, tectoparabigeminal projection; 24, tectoreticular tract; 25, pontocerebellar tract (brachium pontis); 26, trapezoid body and lateral lemniscus; 27, olivocerebellar (climbing) fibers; 28, reticulospinal tracts; 29, dorsal spinocerebellar tract; 30, dorsal column tract. List of structures: SCH, suprachiasmatic nucleus; VLG, ventral lateral geniculate nucleus; DLG, dorsal lateral geniculate nucleus; APT, anterior pretectal nucleus; OPT, olivary pretectal nucleus; PPT, posterior pretectal nucleus; SC, superior colliculus; 5, 7, 8v, 8c, 9, 10, trigeminus, facial, vestibular, cochlear, glossopharyngeal, and vagal cranial nerves; c3, third cervical.

cific thalamic nuclei and distinct areas of the neocortex. There is growing evidence that interactions between corticothalamic and thalamocortical axons have a central role in this process (Ghosh and Shatz, 1993; Molnar et al., 1998; Hevner et al., 2001). Furthermore, there is evidence that the environment through which these axons grow is important for maintaining the topography of their early projections within their target zones (Garel et al., 2002).

Once axons reach their general target area, they search for their specific targets. For instance, thalamocortical fibers from the lateral geniculate nucleus (LGN) grow to the visual area of the neocortex. There, they preferentially form stable synapses with the neurons in layer 4 (Sanes and Yamagata, 1999). Within layer 4, a given axon forms synapses with multiple neurons. Activity-dependent competition between the synapses of several axons results in the mature circuitry. For instance, different layers of the LGN process information from either the left or the right eye or from either X or Y ganglion cell types. Axonal projections from these LGN layers initially overlap within layer 4 of the visual cortex; activity-dependent competition results in the production of alternating stripes of left or right eye innervation within layer 4 (the ocular dominance columns) (Crair et al., 1998; Crowley and Katz, 2000) and a stratification of X versus Y inputs. Thus, the mechanisms underlying synaptic formation, transmission efficiency, and stabilization (known generically as "synaptic plasticity") are essential for later stages of neural histogenesis.

The molecular mechanisms that are implicated in regulating how an axon chooses its synaptic partners (e.g., other neurons or muscle cells) include many of the same molecules that control axonal pathfinding, such as the cadherins, protocadherins, and ephrins (Redies, 2000; Feng et al., 2000b; Lee et al., 2001; Benson et al., 2001; Sanes and Lichtman, 2001). In the CNS, initiation of synapse formation appears to be coordinated by interactions between the growth cone and the filipodia of dendrites (Benson et al., 2001) and may be mediated by the neurexin and neuroligin membrane proteins (Scheiffele et al., 2000).

The complexity of the molecular mechanisms that control the specificity of synapse formation between different targets still evades systematic analysis. In the olfactory bulb, olfactory receptor proteins decorating the afferent axons participate in regulating the specificity of synapse choice (Buck, 2000). In mammals, there are over 1000 olfactory receptor genes (Mombaerts, 1999); thus, in this case, a large number of distinct molecules control the specificity of synapse formation. It remains to be seen whether other complex mechanisms sim-

ilarly regulate the specificity of synapse formation in other regions of the brain.

Synapse formation is also regulated by adjacent astrocytic glial cells. There is evidence that astrocytes increase synapse formation by secreting cholesterol-containing lipoproteins (Mauch et al., 2001). This is an intriguing result because these lipoproteins, or their receptors, are implicated in Alzheimer's disease, as well as in Reelin-signal transduction and synaptic plasticity (Barres and Smith, 2001).

MYELINATION

Many axons in the CNS and PNS are ensheathed by myelinating glial cells, called "oligodendrocytes" and "Schwann cells," respectively (Mirsky and Jessen, 1996). Production of oligodendrocytes is restricted to specific loci in the CNS ventricular zone, from where they colonize diverse axon tracts (Pérez-Villegas et al., 1999; Olivier et al., 2001; Spassky et al., 2001, 2002). Myelination increases the speed at which action potentials are conducted along the axon and appears to modulate synaptic function (Ullian and Barres, 1998). Myelination is a protracted process that continues postnatally and is regulated both by an intrinsic genetic program (Wegner, 2000) and extrinsic factors that include interactions with the axon (Barres and Raff, 1999) and with thyroid hormone and retinoic acid (Barres et al., 1994).

SURVIVAL

Neurogenesis and synaptogenesis produce more neurons and synapses than can be assimilated adaptively in the mature brain. Thus, elimination of neurons and synapses is important in sculpting the nervous system (Raff et al., 1993). There are several mechanisms that regulate these processes. In general, elimination of neurons is controlled by inducing apoptosis (Kuan et al., 2000), which is controlled by a cascade of proteases called "caspases" (Oppenheim et al., 2001). There are multiple pathways that activate caspases in the developing brain. These include the Janus kinase (JNK) protein kinases (Kuan et al., 1999) and signals mediated through neurotrophin receptors (Huang and Reichardt, 2001; Sofroniew et al., 2001). Neurons that succeed in forming synapses obtain from the postsynaptic cells trophic substances that promote their survival. For instance, secretion of neurotrophins by postsynaptic cells (e.g., nerve growth factor, brain-derived neurotrophic factor, neurotrophin-3) promotes the survival of neurons that have made a synapse upon them; neurons that fail to form synapses die (Huang and Reichardt, 2001). Neurotrophins signal through receptor tyrosine kinases via the MAPK and Akt pathways and through the p75 receptor via the JNK, p53, and nuclear factor-κB pathways (Kaplan and Miller, 2000). Neurotrophins and other trophic signals tend to have functions that extend beyond survival as they have roles in the differentiation and morphogenesis of neurons and glia.

REFERENCES

Acampora D, Gulisano M, Broccoli V, Simeone A (2001). Otx genes in brain morphogenesis. *Prog Neurobiol* 64: 69–95.

Allendoerfer KL, Shatz CJ (1994). The subplate, a transient neocortical structure: its role in the development of connections between thalamus and cortex. *Annu Rev Neurosci* 17: 185–218.

Alvarez-Buylla A, Garcia-Verdugo JM, Tramontin AD (2001). A unified hypothesis on the lineage of neural stem cells. *Nat Rev Neurosci* 2: 287–293.

Anderson SA, Qiu M, Bulfone A, Eisenstat DD, Meneses J, Pedersen R, Rubenstein JLR (1997). Mutations of the homeobox genes *Dlx-1* and *Dlx-2* disrupt the striatal subventricular zone and differentiation of late born striatal neurons. *Neuron* 19: 27–37.

Arber S, Han B, Mendelsohn M, Smith M, Jessell TM, Sockananthan S (1999). Requirement for the homeobox gene *Hb9* in the consolidation of motor neuron identity. *Neuron* 23: 659–674.

Arber S, Ladle DR, Lin JH, Frank E, Jessell TM (2000). ETS gene *Er81* controls the formation of functional connections between group Ia sensory afferents and motor neurons. *Cell* 101: 485–498.

Artavanis-Tsakonas S, Rand MD, Lake RJ (1999). Notch signaling: cell fate control and signal integration in development. *Science* 284: 770–776.

Bagri A, Marin O, Plump AS, Mak J, Pleasure SJ, Rubenstein JL, Tessier-Lavigne M (2002). Slit proteins prevent midline crossing and determine the dorsoventral position of major axonal pathways in the mammalian forebrain. *Neuron* 33: 233–248.

Barres BA, Raff MC (1999). Axonal control of oligodendrocyte development. *J Cell Biol* 147: 1123–1128.

Barres BA, Smith SJ (2001). Neurobiology. Cholesterol—making or breaking the synapse. *Science* 294: 1296–1297.

Barres BA, Lazar MA, Raff MC (1994). A novel role for thyroid hormone, glucocorticoids and retinoic acid in timing oligodendrocyte development. *Development* 120: 1097–1108.

Barrow JR, Stadler HS, Capecchi MR (2000). Roles of Hoxa1 and Hoxa2 in patterning the early hindbrain of the mouse. *Development* 127: 933–944.

Barth KA, Kishimoto Y, Rohr K, Seydler C, Schulte-Merker S, Wilson SW (1999). Bmp activity establishes a gradient of positional information throughout the entire neural plate. *Development* 126: 4977–4987.

Beddington RS, Robertson EJ (1999). Axis development and early asymmetry in mammals. *Cell* 96: 195–209.

Benson DL, Colman DR, Huntley GW (2001). Molecules, maps and synapse specificity. *Nat Rev Neurosci* 2: 899–909.

Bertuzzi S, Hindges R, Mui SH, O'Leary DD, Lemke G (1999). The homeodomain protein vax1 is required for axon guidance and major tract formation in the developing forebrain. *Genes Dev* 13(23): 3092–3105.

Birgbauer E, Oster SF, Severin CG, Sretavan DW (2001). Retinal axon growth cones respond to EphB extracellular domains as inhibitory axon guidance cues. *Development* 128: 3041–3048.

Blumberg B, Bolado J Jr, Moreno TA, Kintner C, Evans RM, Papalopulu N (1997). An essential role for retinoid signaling in anteroposterior neural patterning. *Development* 124: 373–379.

Brenman JE, Gao FB, Jan LY, Jan YN (2001). Sequoia, a tramtrack-related zinc finger protein, functions as a pan-neural regulator for dendrite and axon morphogenesis in *Drosophila*. *Dev Cell* 1: 667–677.

Briscoe J, Sussel L, Serup P, Hartigan-O'Connor D, Jessell TM, Rubenstein JL, Ericson J (1999). Homeobox gene *Nkx2.2* and specification of neuronal identity by graded Sonic hedgehog signalling. *Nature* 398: 622–627.

Briscoe J, Pierani A, Jessell TM, Ericson J (2000). A homeodomain protein code specifies progenitor cell identity and neuronal fate in the ventral neural tube. *Cell* 101: 435–445.

Brose K, Tessier-Lavigne M (2000). Slit proteins: key regulators of axon guidance, axonal branching, and cell migration. *Curr Opin Neurobiol* 10: 95–102.

Brown A, Yates PA, Burrola P, Ortuno D, Vaidya A, Jessell TM, Pfaff SL, O'Leary DD, Lemke G (2000). Topographic mapping from the retina to the midbrain is controlled by relative but not absolute levels of EphA receptor signaling. *Cell* 102: 77–88.

Buck LB (2000). The molecular architecture of odor and pheromone sensing in mammals. *Cell* 100: 611–618.

Casarosa S, Fode C, Guillemot F (1999). Mash1 regulates neurogenesis in the ventral telencephalon. *Development* 126: 525–534.

Cassidy R, Frisen J (2001). Neurobiology. Stem cells on the brain. *Nature* 412: 690–691.

Caviness VS Jr, Takahashi T, Nowakowski RS (1995). Numbers, time and neocortical neuronogenesis: a general developmental and evolutionary model. *Trends Neurosci* 18: 379–383.

Cheah SS, Kwan KM, Behringer RR (2000). Requirement of LIM domains for LIM1 function in mouse head development. *Genesis* 27: 12–21.

Chitnis AB (1995). The role of Notch in lateral inhibition and cell fate specification. *Mol Cell Neurosci* 6: 311–321.

Cline HT (2001). Dendritic arbor development and synaptogenesis. *Curr Opin Neurobiol* 11: 118–126.

Cobos-Sillero I, Shimamura K, Rubenstein JLR, Martinez S, Puelles L (2001). Fate map of the avian forebrain at stage 8 with quail-chick chimeras. *Dev Biol* 239: 46–67.

Colas JF, Schoenwolf GC (2001). Towards a cellular and molecular understanding of neurulation. *Dev Dyn* 221: 117–145.

Comery TA, Harris JB, Willems PJ, Oostra BA, Irwin SA, Weiler IJ, Greenough WT (1997). Abnormal dendritic spines in fragile X knockout mice: maturation and pruning deficits. *Proc Natl Acad Sci USA* 94: 5401–5404.

Conover JC, Doetsch F, Garcia-Verdugo JM, Gale NW, Yancopoulos GD, Alvarez-Buylla A (2000). Disruption of Eph/ephrin signaling affects migration and proliferation in the adult subventricular zone. *Nat Neurosci* 3: 1091–1097.

Couly G, Grapin-Botton A, Coltey P, Ruhin B, Le Douarin NM (1998). Determination of the identity of the derivatives of the cephalic neural crest: incompatibility between Hox gene expression and lower jaw development. *Development* 125: 3445–3459.

Crair MC, Gillespie DC, Stryker MP (1998). The role of visual experience in the development of columns in cat visual cortex. *Science* 279: 566–570.

Crossley PH, Martinez S, Ohkubo Y, Rubenstein JL (2001). Coordinate expression of Fgf8, Otx2, Bmp4, and Shh in the rostral prosencephalon during development of the telencephalic and optic vesicles. *Neuroscience* 108: 183–206.

Crowley JC, Katz LC (2000). Early development of ocular dominance columns. *Science* 290: 1321–1324.

De Angelis E, MacFarlane J, Du JS, Yeo G, Hicks R, Rathjen FG, Kenwrick S, Brummendorf T (1999). Pathological missense mutations of neural cell adhesion molecule L1 affect homophilic and heterophilic binding activities. *EMBO J* 18: 4744–4753.

Deiner MS, Sretavan DW (1999). Altered midline axon pathways and ectopic neurons in the developing hypothalamus of netrin-1- and DCC-deficient mice. *J Neurosci* 19: 9900–9912.

Depew MJ, Liu JK, Long JE, Presley R, Meneses JJ, Pedersen RA, Rubenstein JLR (1999). Dlx5 regulates regional development of the branchial arches and sensory capsules. *Development* 126: 3831–3846.

De Robertis EM, Larrain J, Oelgeschlager M, Wessely O (2000). The establishment of Spemann's organizer and patterning of the vertebrate embryo. *Nat Rev Genet* 1: 171–181.

Doherty P, Williams G, Williams EJ (2000). CAMs and axonal growth: a critical evaluation of the role of calcium and the MAPK cascade. *Mol Cell Neurosci* 16: 283–295.

Erskine L, Williams SE, Brose K, Kidd T, Rachel RA, Goodman CS, Tessier-Lavigne M, Mason CA (2000). Retinal ganglion cell axon guidance in the mouse optic chiasm: expression and function of robos and slits. *J Neurosci* 20: 4975–4982.

Feldheim DA, Kim YI, Bergemann AD, Frisen J, Barbacid M, Flanagan JG (2000). Genetic analysis of ephrin-A2 and ephrin-A5 shows their requirement in multiple aspects of retinocollicular mapping. *Neuron* 25: 563–574.

Feng G, Laskowski MB, Feldheim DA, Wang H, Lewis R, Frisen J, Flanagan JG, Sanes JR (2000a). Roles for ephrins in positionally selective synaptogenesis between motor neurons and muscle fibers. *Neuron* 25: 295–306.

Feng J, Yan Z, Ferreira A, Tomizawa K, Liauw JA, Zhuo M, Allen PB, Ouimet CC, Greengard P (2000b). Spinophilin regulates the formation and function of dendritic spines. *Proc Natl Acad Sci USA* 97: 9287–9292.

Fernández-Garre P, Rodríguez-Gallardo L, Gallego-Díaz V, Alvarez I, Puelles L (2002). Fate map of the chicken neural plate at stage 4. *Development* 129: 2807–2822.

Figdor MC, Stern CD (1993). Segmental organization of embryonic diencephalon. *Nature* 363: 630–634.

Flanagan JG, Vanderhaeghen P (1998). The ephrins and Eph receptors in neural development. *Annu Rev Neurosci* 21: 309–345.

Fode C, Ma Q, Casarosa S, Ang SL, Anderson DJ, Guillemot F (2000). A role for neural determination genes in specifying the dorsoventral identity of telencephalic neurons. *Genes Dev* 14: 67–80.

Fukuchi-Shimogori T, Grove EA (2001). Neocortex patterning by the secreted signaling molecule FGF8. *Science* 294: 1071–1074.

Galceran J, Miyashita-Lin EM, Devaney E, Rubenstein JL, Grosschedl R (2000). Hippocampus development and generation of dentate gyrus granule cells is regulated by LEF1. *Development* 127: 469–482.

Garel S, Yun K, Grosschedl R, Rubenstein JLR (2002). Topography of connections between the neocortex and thalamus is regulated by intermediate structures. *Development* 129: 5621–5634.

Gao FB, Brenman JE, Jan LY, Jan YN (1999). Genes regulating dendritic outgrowth, branching, and routing in *Drosophila*. *Genes Dev* 13: 2549–2561.

Gao FB, Kohwi M, Brenman JE, Jan LY, Jan YN (2000). Control of dendritic field formation in *Drosophila*: the roles of flamingo and competition between homologous neurons. *Neuron* 28: 91–101.

Garel S, Huffman KJ, Rubenstein JLR (2003). A caudal shift in neocortical patterning in a *Fgf8* hypomorphic mouse mutant. *Development* 130: 1903–1914.

Gavalas A, Krumlauf R (2000). Retinoid signaling and hindbrain patterning. *Curr Opin Genet Dev* 10: 380–386.

Gavalas A, Trainor P, Ariza-McNaughton L, Krumlauf R (2001). Synergy between Hoxa1 and Hoxb1: the relationship between arch patterning and the generation of cranial neural crest. *Development* 128: 3017–3027.

Ghosh A, Shatz CJ (1993). A role for subplate neurons in the patterning of connections from thalamus to neocortex. *Development* 117: 1031–1047.

Gleeson JG, Walsh CA (2000). Neuronal migration disorders: from genetic diseases to developmental mechanisms. *Trends Neurosci* 23: 352–359.

Gritti A, Bonfanti L, Doetsch F, Caille I, Alvarez-Buylla A, Lim DA, Galli R, Verdugo JM, Herrera DG, Vescovi AL (2002). Multipotent neural stem cells reside into the rostral extension and olfactory bulb of adult rodents. *J Neurosci* 22: 437–445.

Harland R (2000). Neural induction. *Curr Opin Genet Dev* 10: 357–362.

Hartfuss E, Galli R, Heins N, Götz M (2001). Characterization of CNS precursor subtypes and radial glia. *Dev Biol* 229: 15–30.

Hatten ME (1999). Central nervous system neuronal migration. *Annu Rev Neurosci* 22: 511–539.

Henkemeyer M, Orioli D, Henderson JT, Saxton TM, Roder J, Pawson T, Klein R (1996). Nuk controls pathfinding of commissural axons in the mammalian central nervous system. *Cell* 86: 35–46.

Henrique D, Hirsinger E, Adam J, Le Roux I, Pourquie O, Ish-Horowicz D, Lewis J (1997). Maintenance of neuroepithelial progenitor cells by Delta-Notch signalling in the embryonic chick retina. *Curr Biol* 7: 661–670.

Hevner RF, Shi L, Justice N, Hsueh Y, Sheng M, Smiga S, Bulfone A, Goffinet AM, Campagnoni AT, Rubenstein JL (2001). Tbr1 regulates differentiation of the preplate and layer 6. *Neuron* 29: 353–366.

Honarpour N, Gilbert SL, Lahn BT, Wang X, Herz J (2001). Apaf-1 deficiency and neural tube closure defects are found in fog mice. *Proc Natl Acad Sci USA* 98: 9683–9687.

Hopker VH, Shewan D, Tessier-Lavigne M, Poo M, Holt C (1999). Growth-cone attraction to netrin-1 is converted to repulsion by laminin-1. *Nature* 401: 69–73.

Horton S, Meredith A, Richardson JA, Johnson JE (1999). Correct coordination of neuronal differentiation events in ventral forebrain requires the bHLH factor MASH1. *Mol Cell Neurosci* 14: 355–369.

Huang EJ, Reichardt LF (2001). Neurotrophins: roles in neuronal development and function. *Annu Rev Neurosci* 24: 677–736.

Jacob J, Hacker A, Guthrie S (2001). Mechanisms and molecules in motor neuron specification and axon pathfinding. *Bioessays* 23: 582–595.

Jan YN, Jan LY (1998). Asymmetric cell division. *Nature* 392: 775–778.

Jan YN, Jan LY (2001). Dendrites. *Genes Dev* 15: 2627–2641.

Jessell TM (2000). Neuronal specification in the spinal cord: inductive signals and transcriptional codes. *Nat Rev Genet* 1: 20–29.

Kakita A, Goldman JE (1999). Patterns and dynamics of SVZ cell migration in the postnatal forebrain: monitoring living progenitors in slice preparations. *Neuron* 23: 461–472.

Kamiguchi H, Hlavin ML, Yamasaki M, Lemmon V (1998). Adhesion molecules and inherited diseases of the human nervous system. *Annu Rev Neurosci* 21: 97–125.

Kania A, Johnson RL, Jessell TM (2000). Coordinate roles for LIM homeobox genes in directing the dorsoventral trajectory of motor axons in the vertebrate limb. *Cell* 102: 161–173.

Kaplan DR, Miller FD (2000). Neurotrophin signal transduction in the nervous system. *Curr Opin Neurobiol* 10: 381–391.

Kiecker C, Niehrs C (2001). The role of prechordal mesendoderm in neural patterning. *Curr Opin Neurobiol* 11: 27–33.

Korada S, Zheng W, Basilico C, Schwartz ML, Vaccarino FM (2002). Fibroblast growth factor 2 is necessary for the growth of glutamate projection neurons in the anterior neocortex. *J Neurosci* 22: 863–875.

Kuan CY, Yang DD, Samanta Roy DR, Davis RJ, Rakic P, Flavell RA (1999). The Jnk1 and Jnk2 protein kinases are required for regional specific apoptosis during early brain development. *Neuron* 22: 667–676.

Kuan CY, Roth KA, Flavell RA, Rakic P (2000). Mechanisms of programmed cell death in the developing brain. *Trends Neurosci* 23: 291–297.

Lamb TM, Harland RM (1995). Fibroblast growth factor is a direct neural inducer, which combined with noggin generates anterior–posterior neural pattern. *Development* 121: 3627–3636.

Larsen CW, Zeltser LM, Lumsden A (2001). Boundary formation and compartition in the avian diencephalon. *J Neurosci* 21: 4699–4711.

Lee CH, Herman T, Clandinin TR, Lee R, Zipursky SL (2001). N-Cadherin regulates target specificity in the *Drosophila* visual system. *Neuron* 30: 437–450.

Lee KJ, Jessell TM (1999). The specification of dorsal cell fates in the vertebrate central nervous system. *Annu Rev Neurosci* 22: 261–294.

Lee SK, Pfaff SL (2001). Transcriptional networks regulating neuronal identity in the developing spinal cord. *Nat Neurosci* 4(Suppl): 1183–1191.

Lee SM, Tole S, Grove E, McMahon AP (2000). A local Wnt-3a signal is required for development of the mammalian hippocampus. *Development* 127: 457–467.

Li JY, Joyner AL (2001). Otx2 and Gbx2 are required for refinement and not induction of mid-hindbrain gene expression. *Development* 128: 4979–4991.

Lindsell CE, Boulter J, diSibio G, Gossler A, Weinmaster G (1996). Expression patterns of *Jagged, Delta1, Notch1, Notch2,* and *Notch3* genes identify ligand–receptor pairs that may function in neural development. *Mol Cell Neurosci* 8: 14–27.

Litingtung Y, Chiang C (2000). Specification of ventral neuron types is mediated by an antagonistic interaction between Shh and Gli3. *Nat Neurosci* 3: 979–985.

Liu A, Joyner AL (2001). Early anterior/posterior patterning of the midbrain and cerebellum. *Annu Rev Neurosci* 24: 869–896.

Liu JP, Laufer E, Jessell TM (2001). Assigning the positional identity of spinal motor neurons. Rostrocaudal patterning of Hox-c expression by FGFs, Gdf11, and retinoids *Neuron* 32: 997–1012.

Lu QR, Yuk D, Alberta JA, Zhu Z, Pawlitzky I, Chan J, McMahon AP, Stiles CD, Rowitch DH (2000). Sonic hedgehog–regulated oligodendrocyte lineage genes encoding bHLH proteins in the mammalian central nervous system. *Neuron* 25: 317–329.

Lumsden A (1999). Closing in on rhombomere boundaries. *Nat Cell Biol* 1: E83–85.

Lumsden A, Krumlauf R (1996). Patterning the vertebrate neuraxis. *Science* 274: 1109–1115.

Luo L (2000). Rho GTPases in neuronal morphogenesis. *Nat Rev Neurosci* 1: 173–180.

Luskin MB (1998). Neuroblasts of the postnatal mammalian forebrain: their phenotype and fate. *J Neurobiol* 36: 221–233.

Mallamaci A, Mercurio S, Muzio L, Cecchi C, Pardini CL, Gruss P, Boncinelli E (2000). The lack of Emx2 causes impairment of Reelin signaling and defects of neuronal migration in the developing cerebral cortex. *J Neurosci* 20: 1109–1118.

Marcus RC, Shimamura K, Srevatan D, Lai E, Rubenstein JLR, Mason CA (1999). Domains of regulatory gene expression and the developing optic chiasm: correspondence with retinal axon paths and candidate signaling cells. *J Comp Neurol* 403: 346–358.

Marin F, Puelles L (1995). Morphological fate of rhombomeres in quail/chick chimeras: a segmental analysis of hindbrain nuclei. *Eur J Neurosci* 7: 1714–1738.

Marin O, Rubenstein JL (2001). A long, remarkable journey: tangential migration in the telencephalon. *Nat Rev Neurosci* 2: 780–790.

Marin O, Yaron A, Bagri A, Tessier-Lavigne M, Rubenstein JL (2001). Sorting of striatal and cortical interneurons regulated by semaphorin-neuropilin interactions. *Science* 293: 872–875.

Marin O, Baker J, Puelles L, Rubenstein JL (2002). Patterning of the basal telencephalon and hypothalamus is essential for guidance of cortical projections. *Development* 129: 761–773.

Marín-Padilla M (1983). Structural organization of the human cerebral cortex prior to the appearance of the cortical plate. *Anat Embryol* 168: 21–40.

Marquardt T, Pfaff SL (2001). Cracking the transcriptional code for cell specification in the neural tube. *Cell* 106: 651–654.

Martens DJ, Tropepe V, van Der Kooy D (2000). Separate proliferation kinetics of fibroblast growth factor-responsive and epidermal growth factor-responsive neural stem cells within the embryonic forebrain germinal zone. *J Neurosci* 20: 1085–1095.

Martinez S, Crossley PH, Cobos I, Rubenstein JL, Martin GR (1999). FGF8 induces formation of an ectopic isthmic organizer and isthmocerebellar development via a repressive effect on Otx2 expression. *Development* 126: 1189–1200.

Mason CA, Sretavan DW (1997). Glia, neurons, and axon pathfinding during optic chiasm development. *Curr Opin Neurobiol* 7: 647–653.

Mauch DH, Nagler K, Schumacher S, Goritz C, Muller EC, Otto A, Pfrieger FW (2001). CNS synaptogenesis promoted by glia-derived cholesterol. *Science* 294: 1354–357.

McConnell SK (1995). Constructing the cerebral cortex: neurogenesis and fate determination. *Neuron* 15: 761–768.

McEvilly RJ, de Diaz MO, Schonemann MD, Hooshmand F, Rosenfeld MG (2002). Transcriptional regulation of cortical neuron migration by POU domain factors. *Science* 295: 1528–1532.

Mellitzer G, Xu Q, Wilkinson DG (1999). Eph receptors and ephrins restrict cell intermingling and communication. *Nature* 400: 77–81.

Mirsky R, Jessen KR (1996). Schwann cell development, differentiation and myelination. *Curr Opin Neurobiol* 6: 89–96.

Mizuguchi R, Sugimori M, Takebayashi H, Kosako H, Nagao M, Yoshida S, Nabeshima Y, Shimamura K, Nakafuku M (2001). Combinatorial roles of olig2 and neurogenin2 in the coordinated induction of pan-neuronal and subtype-specific properties of motoneurons. *Neuron* 3: 757–771.

Molnar Z, Adams R, Blakemore C (1998). Mechanisms underlying the early establishment of thalamocortical connections in the rat. *J Neurosci* 18: 5723–5745.

Mombaerts P (1999). Seven-transmembrane proteins as odorant and chemosensory receptors. *Science* 286: 707–711.

Muhr J, Andersson E, Persson M, Jessell TM, Ericson J (2001). Groucho-mediated transcriptional repression establishes progenitor cell pattern and neuronal fate in the ventral neural tube. *Cell* 104: 861–873.

Nadarajah B, Brunstrom JE, Grutzendler J, Wong RO, Pearlman AL (2001). Two modes of radial migration in early development of the cerebral cortex. *Nat Neurosci* 4: 143–150.

Nakamura H (2001). Regionalisation and acquisition of polarity in the optic tectum. *Prog Neurobiol* 65: 473–488.

Noctor SC, Flint AC, Weissman TA, Dammerman RS, Kriegstein AR. (2001). Neurons derived from radial glial cells establish radial units in neocortex. *Nature* 409: 714–720.

Novitch BG, Chen AI, Jessell TM (2001). Coordinate regulation of motor neuron subtype identity and pan-neuronal properties by the bHLH repressor Olig2. *Neuron* 31: 773–789.

O'Leary DD, Wilkinson DG (1999). Eph receptors and ephrins in neural development. *Curr Opin Neurobiol* 9: 65–73.

Olivier C, Cobos I, Perez Villegas EM, Spassky N, Zalc B, Martinez S, Thomas JL (2001). Monofocal origin of telencephalic oligodendrocytes in the anterior entopeduncular area of the chick embryo. *Development* 128: 1757–1769.

Oppenheim RW, Flavell RA, Vinsant S, Prevette D, Kuan CY, Rakic P (2001). Programmed cell death of developing mammalian neurons after genetic deletion of caspases. *J Neurosci* 21: 4752–4760.

Palmer TD, Willhoite AR, Gage FH (2000). Vascular niche for adult hippocampal neurogenesis. *J Comp Neurol* 425: 479–494.

Pera EM, Wessely O, Li SY, De Robertis EM (2001). Neural and head induction by insulin-like growth factor signals. *Dev Cell* 1: 655–665.

Perez Villegas EM, Olivier C, Spassky N, Poncet C, Cochard P, Zalc B, Thomas JL, Martinez S (1999). Early specification of oligodendrocytes in the chick embryonic brain. *Dev Biol* 216: 98–113.

Plump A, Erskine L, Sabatier C, Brose K, Epstein CJ, Goodman CS, Mason CA, Tessier-Lavigne M. (2002). Slit1 and Slit2 cooperate to prevent premature midline crossing of retinal axons in the mouse visual system. *Neuron* 33: 219–232.

Polleux F, Morrow T, Ghosh A (2000). Semaphorin 3A is a chemoattractant for cortical apical dendrites. *Nature* 404: 567–573.

Puelles L (1995). A segmental morphological paradigm for understanding vertebrate forebrains. *Brain Behav Evol* 46: 319–337.

Puelles L (2001). Brain segmentation and forebrain development in amniotes. *Brain Res Bull* 55: 695–710.

Puelles L, Bendala MC (1978). Differentiation of neuroblasts in the chick optic tectum up to the eight day of incubation: a Golgi study. *Neuroscience* 3: 207–325.

Puelles L, Rubenstein JLR (1993). Expression patterns of homeobox and other putative regulatory genes in the embryonic mouse forebrain suggest a neuromeric organization. *Trends Neurosci* 16: 472–479.

Puelles L, Verney C (1998). Early neuromeric distribution of tyrosine-hydroxylase and dopamine-β-hydroxylase immunoreactive neurons in human embryos. *J Comp Neurol* 394: 283–308.

Qi Y, Cai J, Wu Y, Wu R, Lee J, Fu H, Rao M, Sussel L, Rubenstein J, Qiu M (2001). Control of oligodendrocyte differentiation by the Nkx2.2 homeodomain transcription factor. *Development* 128: 2723–2733.

Raff MC, Barres BA, Burne JF, Coles HS, Ishizaki Y, Jacobson MD (1993). Programmed cell death and the control of cell survival: lessons from the nervous system. *Science* 262: 695–700.

Rakic P (2000). Radial unit hypothesis of neocortical expansion. Novartis Found Symp 228: 30–52.

Redies C (2000). Cadherins in the central nervous system. *Prog Neurobiol* 61: 611–648.

Redies C, Puelles L (2001). Modularity in CNS development. *Bioessays* 23: 1100–1111.

Reichardt LF, Bossy B, de Curtis I, Neugebauer KM, Venstrom K, Sretavan D (1992). Adhesive interactions that regulate development of the retina and primary visual projection. *Cold Spring Harb Symp Quant Biol* 57: 419–429.

Rice DS, Curran T (2001). Role of the reelin signaling pathway in central nervous system development. *Annu Rev Neurosci* 24: 1005–1039.

Robey E (1997). Notch in vertebrates. *Curr Opin Genet Dev* 7: 551–557.

Rubenstein JLR, Shimamura K, Martinez S, Puelles L (1998). Regionalization of the prosencephalic neural plate. *Annu Rev Neurosci* 21: 445–478.

Sander M, Paydar S, Ericson J, Briscoe J, Berber E, German M, Jessell TM, Rubenstein JL (2000). Ventral neural patterning by Nkx homeobox genes: *Nkx6.1* controls somatic motor neuron and ventral interneuron fates. *Genes Dev* 14: 2134–2139.

Sanes JR, Lichtman JW (2001). Development induction, assembly, maturation and maintenance of a postsynaptic apparatus. *Nat Rev Neurosci* 2: 791–805.

Sanes JR, Yamagata M (1999). Formation of lamina-specific synaptic connections. *Curr Opin Neurobiol* 9: 79–87.

Scheiffele P, Fan J, Choih J, Fetter R, Serafini T (2000). Neuroligin expressed in non-neuronal cells triggers presynaptic development in contacting axons. *Cell* 101: 657–669.

Serafini T, Colamarino SA, Leonardo ED, Wang H, Beddington R, Skarnes WC, Tessier-Lavigne M (1996). Netrin-1 is required for commissural axon guidance in the developing vertebrate nervous system. *Cell* 87: 1001–1014.

Sestan N, Artavanis-Tsakonas S, Rakic P (1999). Contact-dependent inhibition of cortical neurite growth mediated by notch signaling. *Science* 286: 741–746.

Shanmugalingam S, Houart C, Picker A, Reifers F, Macdonald R, Barth A, Griffin K, Brand M, Wilson SW (2000). Ace/Fgf8 is required for forebrain commissure formation and patterning of the telencephalon. *Development* 127: 2549–2561.

Shimamura K, Rubenstein JLR (1997). Inductive interactions direct early regionalization of the mouse forebrain. *Development* 124: 2709–2718.

Shimamura K, Hartigan DJ, Martinez S, Puelles L. and Rubenstein JLR (1995). Longitudinal organization of the anterior neural plate and neural tube. *Development* 121: 3923–3933.

Simeone A (2000). Positioning the isthmic organizer where Otx2 and Gbx2 meet. *Trends Genet* 16: 237–240.

Sockanathan S, Jessell TM (1998). Motor neuron-derived retinoid signaling specifies the subtype identity of spinal motor neurons. *Cell* 94: 503–514.

Sofroniew MV, Howe CL, Mobley WC (2001). Nerve growth factor signaling, neuroprotection, and neural repair. *Annu Rev Neurosci* 24: 1217–1281.

Song H, Ming G, He Z, Lehmann M, McKerracher L, Tessier-Lavigne M, Poo M (1998). Conversion of neuronal growth cone responses from repulsion to attraction by cyclic nucleotides. *Science* 281: 1515–1518.

Spassky N, Olivier C, Cobos I, LeBras B, Goujet-Zalc C, Martinez S, Zalc B, Thomas JL (2001). The early steps of oligodendrogenesis: insights from the study of the plp lineage in the brain of chicks and rodents. *Dev Neurosci* 23: 318–326.

Spassky N, de Castro F, Le Bras B, Heydon K, Queraud-LeSaux F, Bloch-Gallego E, Chedotal A, Zalc B, Thomas JL (2002). Directional guidance of oligodendroglial migration by class 3 semaphorins and netrin-1. *J Neurosci* 22: 5992–6004.

Storm E, Rubenstein JLR, Martin GR (2003). Dosage of Fgf8 determines whether cell survival is positively or negatively regulated in the developing forebrain. *Proc Natl Acad Sci USA* 100: 1757–1762.

Streit A, Berliner AJ, Papanayotou C, Sirulnik A, Stern CD (2000). Initiation of neural induction by FGF signalling before gastrulation. *Nature* 406: 74–78.

Sun T, Echelard Y, Lu R, Yuk DI, Kaing S, Stiles CD, Rowitch DH (2001). Olig bHLH proteins interact with homeodomain proteins to regulate cell fate acquisition in progenitors of the ventral neural tube. *Curr Biol* 11: 1413–1420.

Takeichi M, Uemura T, Iwai Y, Uchida N, Inoue T, Tanaka T, Suzuki SC (1997). Cadherins in brain patterning and neural network formation. *Cold Spring Harb Symp Quant Biol* 62: 505–510.

Tanabe Y, William C, Jessell TM (1998). Specification of motor neuron identity by the MNR2 homeodomain protein. *Cell* 95: 67–80.

Tessier-Lavigne M, Goodman CS (1996). The molecular biology of axon guidance. *Science* 274: 1123–1133.

Thomas PQ, Dattani MT, Brickman JM, McNay D, Warne G, Zacharin M, Cameron F,

Hurst J, Woods K, Dunger D, et al. (2001). Heterozygous *HESX1* mutations associated with isolated congenital pituitary hypoplasia and septo-optic dysplasia. *Hum Mol Genet* 10: 39–45.

Torres M, Gomez-Pardo E, Gruss P (1996). Pax2 contributes to inner ear patterning and optic nerve trajectory. *Development* 122: 3381–3391.

Trainor PA, Krumlauf R (2000). Patterning the cranial neural crest: hindbrain segmentation and Hox gene plasticity. *Nat Rev Neurosci* 1: 116–124.

Ullian EM, Barres BA (1998). The Schwann song of the glia-less synapse. *Neuron* 21: 651–652.

Van Vactor D (1998). Adhesion and signaling in axonal fasciculation. *Curr Opin Neurobiol* 8: 80–86.

Wallis D, Muenke M (2000). Mutations in holoprosencephaly. *Hum Mutat* 16: 99–108.

Wang KH, Brose K, Arnott D, Kidd T, Goodman CS, Henzel W, Tessier-Lavigne M (1999). Biochemical purification of a mammalian slit protein as a positive regulator of sensory axon elongation and branching. *Cell* 96: 771–784.

Wechsler-Reya R, Scott MP (2001). The developmental biology of brain tumors. *Annu Rev Neurosci* 24: 385–428.

Wegner M (2000). Transcriptional control in myelinating glia: flavors and spices. *Glia* 31: 1–14.

Wilson SI, Edlund T (2001). Neural induction: toward a unifying mechanism. *Nat Neurosci* (Suppl): 1161–1168.

Wilson SI, Graziano E, Harland R, Jessell TM, Edlund T (2000). An early requirement for FGF signalling in the acquisition of neural cell fate in the chick embryo. *Curr Biol* 10: 421–429.

Wilson SI, Rydstrom A, Trimborn T, Willert K, Nusse R, Jessell TM, Edlund T (2001). The status of Wnt signalling regulates neural and epidermal fates in the chick embryo. *Nature* 411: 325–330.

Wilson SW, Rubenstein JL (2000). Induction and dorsoventral patterning of the telencephalon. *Neuron* 28: 641–651.

Wöhrn J-CP, Puelles L, Nagakawa S, Takeichi M, Redies C (1998). Cadherin expression in the retina and retinofugal pathways of the chicken embryo. *J Comp Neurol* 396: 20–38.

Wong K, Ren XR, Huang YZ, Xie Y, Liu G, Tang H, Wen L, Brady-Kalnay SM, Mei L, et al. (2001). Signal transduction in neuronal migration. roles of gtpase activating proteins and the small gtpase cdc42 in the slit-robo pathway. *Cell* 107: 209–221.

Yates PA, Roskies AL, McLaughlin T, O'Leary DD (2001). Topographic-specific axon branching controlled by ephrin-as is the critical event in retinotectal map development. *J Neurosci* 21: 8548–8563.

Ye W, Bouchard M, Stone D, Liu X, Vella F, Lee J, Nakamura H, Ang SL, Busslinger M, Rosenthal A (2001). Distinct regulators control the expression of the mid-hindbrain organizer signal FGF8. *Nat Neurosci* 4: 1175–1181.

Yee KT, Simon HH, Tessier-Lavigne M, O'Leary DM (1999). Extension of long leading processes and neuronal migration in the mammalian brain directed by the chemoattractant netrin-1. *Neuron* 24: 607–622.

Yoon MS, Puelles L, Redies C (2000). Formation of cadherin-expressing brain nuclei in diencephalic alar plate divisions. *J Comp Neurol* 427: 461–480.

Yu HH, Kolodkin AL (1999). Semaphorin signaling: a little less per-plexin. *Neuron* 22: 11–14.

Yun K, Fischman S, Johnson J, Hrabe de Angelis M, Weinmaster G, Rubenstein JLR (2002). Modulation of the notch signaling by Mash1 and Dlx1/2 regulates sequential specification and differentiation of progenitor cell types in the subcortical telencephalon. *Development* 129: 5029–5040.

Zeltser LM, Larsen CW, Lumsden A (2001). A new developmental compartment in the forebrain regulated by Lunatic fringe. *Nat Neurosci* 4: 683–684.

Zhou Q, Choi G, Anderson DJ (2001). The bHLH transcription factor Olig2 promotes oligodendrocyte differentiation in collaboration with Nkx2.2. *Neuron* 31: 791–807.

Zou Y, Stoeckli E, Chen H, Tessier-Lavigne M (2000). Squeezing axons out of the gray matter: a role for slit and semaphorin proteins from midline and ventral spinal cord. *Cell* 102: 363–375.

8 | Development of the Ear

DONNA M. FEKETE

The inner ear subserves two distinct sensory systems: hearing and balance. The outer and middle ear are integral parts of hearing and must also be considered. Constructing the vertebrate ear poses special challenges because it is so anatomically complex and there are multiple embryonic origins of the cells and tissues that comprise it. Coordination of these disparate cell populations necessarily involves inductive interactions and probably includes orchestrated feedback loops.

Virtually all of the tissue types in the body are represented in the three parts of the ear, including squamous, cuboidal, pseudostratified, and secretory epithelium as well as nerve, vasculature, dermis, muscle, tendon, cartilage, and bone. Cells originate from the otic placode, craniofacial neural crest, ectoderm, mesoderm, or endoderm. As a functional part of the nervous system, neurons of the inner ear must project to the CNS and form appropriate synaptic contacts with it. Thus, it should not be surprising to learn that more than 400 types of human hereditary hearing loss with syndromal associations have been categorized (Gorlin et al., 1995). These authors grouped syndromal forms of deafness by involvement of the external ear (7%), the eye (10%), the musculoskeletal system (21%), the kidney (6%), the CNS (16%), endocrine and metabolic conditions (13%), the skin (14%), and the mouth and teeth (2%). Remaining syndromes were associated with chromosomal disorders (3%) or miscellaneous tissue disorders (9%). Discovery of the genetic basis of the many forms of hereditary hearing loss and balance disorder will therefore be aided by exploring many organ systems in addition to the ear. To date, more than 100 loci responsible for syndromic deafness in humans have been mapped, and the gene responsible has been identified for over 60 of these (Griffith and Friedman, 2002). The Hereditary Hearing Loss Website is an excellent resource, which posts the latest advances in identifying human deafness genes (Van Camp and Smith, 2002).

Hundreds of genes are suspected to play a role in ear development because they are expressed at key stages in the developing ear of different vertebrate species (Holme et al., 2002). Many of these are especially provocative in the context of syndromal birth defects because they belong to gene families that are known to play a role in the morphogenesis of other developing organ systems. This chapter is focused on a subset of these genes for which there are experimental data supporting a role in development of the outer, middle, or inner ear.

TIMETABLE OF OUTER, MIDDLE, AND INNER EAR DEVELOPMENT

The inner ear derives from a cranial placode, which is a transient, focal thickening of the head ectoderm. Cranial placodes have evolved in concert with the specialization of peripheral sensory structures of the head, including cranial ganglion neurons, the lens of the eye, the olfactory mucosa, and the inner ear. The otic placode originates on either side of the hindbrain, at its dorsolateral margin, late in the third week of gestation in humans (Larsen, 2001). The ectoderm thickens and begins to invaginate into the otic cup (Fig. 8–1). The cup deepens and eventually pinches off entirely, severing itself from the overlying ectoderm through focal programmed cell death of the connecting stalk cells at the end of the fourth week (Represa et al., 1990). The resulting fluid-filled ball of cells, now called the "otic vesicle," will undergo complex morphogenesis and growth over the next 4 weeks (Fig. 8–2). It will give rise to the sensory organs of hearing and balance; their associated canals, vestibules, and ducts; and the sensory

neurons of the statoacoustic ganglion, which innervate the organs and project into the brain.

Early on, three distinct regions of the otic vesicle can be recognized: a dorsal endolymphatic appendage (pars endolymphaticus), an expanded middle region (pars superior) that will generate the utricle and the three semicircular canals, and an elongating ventral protrusion (pars inferior) that will give rise to the saccule and the cochlear duct. At the same time, the initial stages of middle ear development begin as condensations of the lateral mesoderm, which will eventually become the middle ear ossicles.

During the fifth week, the semicircular canal pouches become visible and the cochlear duct begins its characteristic coil. The fifth week also coincides with the beginning of outer ear development, which progresses slowly over several months to generate the auricle (pinna), the external auditory meatus (ear canal), and the outer layer of the tympanic membrane (eardrum). These structures arise from cells of the first and second pharyngeal arches. Overt morphogenesis of the semicircular canals and their ampullary enlargements, where the sensory cristae are housed, occurs during the seventh week. Two weeks later, the surrounding mesenchymal cells begin to coordinate with the inner ear, eventually generating a cartilaginous otic capsule.

The region between the otic capsule and the membranous labyrinth, called the "perilymphatic cavity," arises through vacuolization of the cartilage during the third to fifth months. This space will be filled with perilymphatic fluid and become contiguous with the subarachnoid space (Fig. 8–1). It remains completely separated from the specialized fluid bathing the sensory cells of the inner ear, called "endolymph." Endolymph is unusually high in potassium and essential for mechanotransduction. The cartilage of the otic capsule is replaced by bone between 16 and 23 weeks. A schematic diagram compares the timing of human ear development with that of the mouse, a valuable mammalian model system (Fig. 8–1).

THE INNER EAR

Otic Placode Induction

The tissue interactions that underlie otic placode induction have been studied since the early 20th century, although a molecular understanding is only beginning to be realized (reviewed by Baker and Bronner-Fraser, 2001; Normaly and Grainger, 2002). Classical experiments focused on two basic questions: Which tissues have otic inducing properties? Which tissues can respond to otic inducers, thereby demonstrating competence? Modern experimenters tend to search for mutants or genetic manipulations that reduce or eliminate the otic field. So far, there are no examples where a single genetic manipulation causes a catastrophic failure of otic induction in an otherwise normal embryo. This may indicate that there is no "master ear gene," or it may reflect the need for a combination of factors acting synergistically. At present, the best candidates for bona fide otic inducers include members of the fibroblast growth factor (Fgf) family, perhaps acting in concert with one or more members of the Wingless (Wnt) family, as detailed below. The hindbrain and mesoderm are likely sources of these otic inducers. With respect to otic competence, much and perhaps all ectoderm appears to possess it during gastrulation, with a gradual restriction down to the endogenous region as development proceeds (Groves and Bronner-Fraser, 2000).

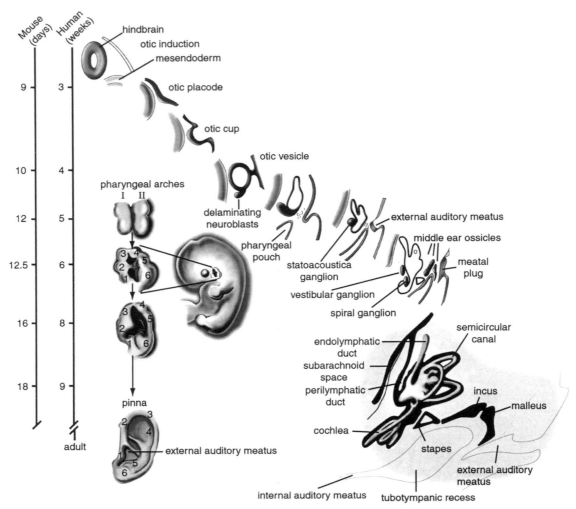

Figure 8–1. Timetable of ear development. Inner ear induction begins just prior to the third week of pregnancy in humans. The major morphogenetic changes in the ectodermal components of the inner ear occur over the following 5–6 weeks. Interactions with and remodeling of the surrounding periotic mesenchyme continue for several months. Meanwhile, beginning at about the fifth week of gestation, development of the middle and outer ear ensues. These two parts of the ear interact to form the tympanic membrane between the external auditory meatus and the tubotympanic recess of the middle ear cavity. The external auditory meatus originates at the cleft between the first and second pharyngeal arches, whose hillocks will morph into the pinna. The approximate ages at which these major events are observed in the mouse are indicated on the far left. (Modified with permission from Larsen, 2001.)

Early Otic Markers (*Sox, Six, Eya, Dlx, Pax,* and *Clnd* Genes)

Before discussing the results, it is helpful to consider the assays. The classical criterion to confirm otic induction was the presence of a hollow epithelial sphere, a relatively late event. Modern studies score for otic tissue more specifically and at much earlier stages using the expression of molecular markers as a defining criterion. In this way, tissue that never makes it to the vesicle stage, perhaps due to defective morphogenesis, can nevertheless be recognized as having assumed an otic identity.

Some markers of the otic placode are initially expressed in a broad U-shaped domain that flanks the anterior neural plate. This region is presumed to be a general "preplacodal field" that gives rise to all placodes, including the olfactory, lens, otic, cranial ganglia, and/or epibranchial (Torres and Giraldez, 1998; Baker and Bronner-Fraser, 2001). Figure 8–3A shows a rough fate map of the preplacodal field for the chicken embryo. With time, the broad expression of marker genes shrinks down to foci representing one or more of the individual placodal types (reviewed in Baker and Bronner-Fraser, 2001). In several species, transcription factors of the *Sox, Six, Eya,* and/or *Dlx* gene families are expressed early in the preplacodal field and later in presumptive otic placode. While they are likely to play important and as yet unknown roles in determining the otic placode, their lack of specificity means that other markers are more valuable to unambiguously detect otic induction.

The most rigorous criterion for an otic placode marker would be one that labels a unique subdomain within the preplacodal field that gives rise exclusively to the otic placode by fate-mapping. In this context, the best fate mapping data are from the zebrafish (Kozlowski et al., 1997; reviewed by Whitfield et al., 2002). *Pax* genes are early markers of presumptive otic tissue in zebrafish (Pfeffer et al., 1998) (see Chapter 59). *Pax8* expression begins prior to overt placode formation, i.e., before there is a focal thickening of the ectoderm, when gastrulation is about 85% complete. At the anterior end, where *Pax8* is first expressed in the prospective otic ectoderm, the mesoderm (a potential inducing tissue) has already moved into position beneath it. *Pax8* is also expressed in the otic placode at similar stages in *Xenopus* (Heller and Brandli, 1999) and mouse (Pfeffer et al., 1998). The onset of *Pax8* expression is followed shortly by *Pax2* genes. *Pax2* is also a well-known early marker of otic tissue in chickens, followed by *Lmx1* (Giraldez, 1998; Groves and Bronner-Fraser, 2000) and then several members of the Fgf, bone morphogenetic protein (Bmp), Wnt, and Notch signaling systems (Baker and Bronner-Fraser, 2001) (Fig. 8–3C).

Another early marker of the otic placode in zebrafish is *claudin-a* (*cldna*) mRNA, which encodes a membrane protein (Kollmar et al., 2001). *Cldna* has been touted as "the only completely ear-specific marker so far described, being expressed exclusively in the otic pre-placode, placode, and vesicle from the end of gastrulation until at

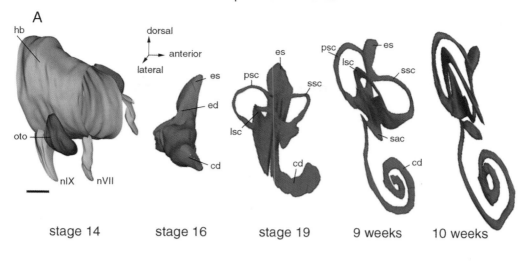

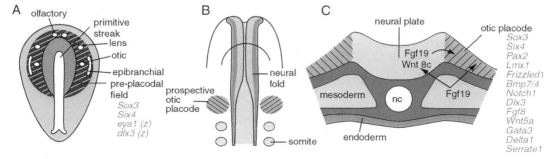

Figure 8–2. Serial reconstructions through the developing inner ear of the human embryo. *(A)* Lateral views of the right ear. At stage 14, the surrounding hindbrain and nerve roots for the seventh and ninth cranial nerves are indicated. *(B)* The same ears are shown from the posterior perspective, now drawn to scale so that the tremendous growth of the membranous labyrinth can be appreciated. (Images kindly provided by Wolfgang H. Arnold, modified from Arnold and Lang, 2001.) cd, cochlear duct; ed, endolymphatic duct; es, endolymphatic sac; hb, hindbrain; lsc, lateral semicircular canal; nIX, ninth cranial nerve; nVII, seventh cranial nerve; oto, otocyst; psc, posterior semicircular canal; sac, saccule; ssc, superior semicircular canal.

least 2 days" (Whitfield et al., 2002). It will be important to study the function of this gene further, not only in zebrafish but also in other vertebrates.

In summary, members of the *Pax* gene family have become standard early indicators of otic identity in studies of otic induction and competence. Another potentially valuable marker may be *Tbx2*, which is expressed slightly later than *Pax8* in presumptive otic placode of zebrafish and *Xenopus* (Baker and Bronner-Fraser, 2001).

Inducing Tissues and Molecules (Fgfs, Wnts)

I first address the question of which tissues have otic-inducing properties. The obvious candidates are the tissues located in close proximity to the presumptive otic ectoderm. The simplest manipulation is to remove each of these tissues at various stages and determine whether otic ectoderm has formed. Extirpation experiments have focused on the hindbrain, which lies adjacent to the otic placode, and the paraxial cranial mesoderm (or mesendoderm), which is located beneath the otic placode. Both tissues have otic-inducing activity, and in some assays they appear to function synergistically and are required over a relatively prolonged period (Baker and Bronner-Fraser, 2001).

There is confusion in the literature about the function of Fgfs in otic induction, due in part to variable onset and location of expression across species and possible redundancy among family members (see discussion by Normaly and Grainger, 2002 and Chapter 32). Fgf19 and Fgf4 are candidates for the mesodermal factor in the chick because they are expressed in a band of mesoderm beneath the pre-

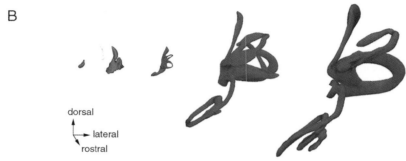

Figure 8–3. Origin and induction of the otic placode. *(A)* Approximate fate map of the cranial placodes at the primitive streak stage of embryonic development in a chicken. Genes expressed in the preplacodal field are shown. Those identified in zebrafish (z) are indicated. *(B)* At the neural fold stage, the prospective otic placode is located just anterior to the first somites in the chicken. *(C)* A model of the tissue interactions and secreted molecules potentially involved in induction or specification of the otic placode in the chicken. Genes are shown in the approximate sequence of their appearance. (Figure based on Baker and Bronner-Fraser, 2001, and Ladher et al., 2000.)

sumptive otic placode (Shamim and Mason, 1999; Ladher et al., 2000). Fgf19 can substitute for the mesoderm in otic induction assays of chicken ear. A second factor, Wnt8c, enhances the ability of Fgf19 to induce otic markers in naive ectoderm (Ladher et al., 2000). *Wnt8c* is expressed in the hindbrain at the level of the prospective otic placode. The working model is that Fgf19 in the mesoderm (and subsequently in the hindbrain) leads to upregulation of Wnt8c in the hindbrain. Together, the two secreted factors act synergistically on the nearby ectoderm to induce otic placode (Fig. 8–3C). These studies do not rule out that other factors may be present in hindbrain and/or mesendoderm that could also contribute to otic induction in the normal embryo.

The possibility that Fgf3 is an endogenous otic inducer has been controversial. In the chick, *Fgf3* is expressed in the hindbrain and can induce competent ectoderm to initiate otic formation following virus-mediated overexpression (Vendrell et al., 2000). Beads soaked in Fgf3 (or Fgf2) can induce ectopic otic vesicles in the frog (Lombardo et al., 1998; Lombardo and Slack, 1998). Although reduction of Fgf3 (by antibodies or antisense oligos) blocks otic vesicle formation in the chick (Represa et al., 1990), *Fgf3* gene knockout in the mouse does not (Mansour et al., 1993). Likewise, elimination of the gene encoding one Fgf receptor isoform, Fgfr2(IIIb) that binds Fgf3 (or Fgf10), does not eliminate the mouse otic vesicle, although it is severely hypomorphic (De Moerlooze et al., 2000; Pirvola et al., 2000). Furthermore, *Fgf3* is not expressed in the hindbrain of *kreisler* mutant mice, yet the otocyst still forms, although it fails to thrive (McKay et al., 1996). Finally, depletion of the gene in zebrafish (by *Fgf3* morpholino injection) does not completely block the appearance of otocyst, although it is reduced in size (Phillips et al., 2001; Whitfield et al., 2002). One interpretation is that the chick is especially dependent on hindbrain-derived Fgf3, while in other vertebrates Fgf3 activity is redundant with other Fgfs for otic induction. An alternative interpretation, based on the stages at which the chicken *Fgf3* gain-of-function experiments were performed, is that the requirement for Fgf3 is rather late, with the responding tissue having already been rendered competent to respond to it by other otic inducers.

In both zebrafish and mouse, other Fgfs may enhance or complement possible inductive activity of Fgf3. In fish, knockdowns of *Fgf8* function, either in the *acerebellar* mutant or by morpholino injection, yield small, abnormal otic vesicles (Whitfield et al., 1996; Phillips et al., 2001). In a double knockdown of both *Fgf3* and *Fgf8*, the effects are additive and the otic tissue is nearly or completely absent (Raible and Brand, 2001). Likewise, a double knockout of *Fgf3* and *Fgf10* in the mouse is associated with total or near total absence of the inner ear (Wright and Mansour, 2002).

In summary, otic induction appears to require one or more members the Fgf family of secreted proteins, particularly Fgf19, Fgf8, Fgf10, and/or Fgf3. The source of these molecules includes the mesendoderm and/or the hindbrain. The inductive activity of the Fgfs may be augmented by secretion of Wnt8c from the hindbrain, at least in the chick. Finally, while the ear program can sometimes be initiated by ectopic expression of a single Fgf, it usually aborts at an early stage in the absence of other factors, including Fgf3.

Competent Tissues

The question of which tissues are competent to respond to otic inducers has been most actively explored in embryos which are readily accessible to tissue transplantation, including zebrafish, newts, axolotls, and chickens (Fritzsch et al., 1998; reviewed by Baker and Bronner-Fraser, 2001; Kiernan et al., 2002; Whitfield et al., 2002). In amphibians, ventral ectoderm from neurula stages is competent to form the otic vesicle (Gallagher et al., 1996). In chicken, anterior epiblast (preotic ectoderm fated to give rise to the extraembryonic ectoderm) from late gastrula/early neurula stages is also competent: when transplanted into the otic region, it will express *Pax2* (Groves and Bronner-Fraser, 2000).

Trunk ectoderm loses competence to form otic vesicles by the midneural fold stages in *Xenopus* and chicken. However, if assayed by *Pax2* expression rather than otic vesicle formation, the competence of transplanted trunk and preotic ectoderm persists for several additional stages (Groves and Bronner-Fraser, 2000). When otic competence is tested by exposure to Fgf3, a strip of dorsolateral ectoderm extending from the rostral hindbrain to the level of the sixth somite retains competence up to the 15-somite stage (day 2) in chicks (Vendrell et al., 2000). Curiously, chick limb ectoderm retains competence in transplantation assays for a surprisingly long time (stage 28, day 6 [Kaan, 1926]). In summary, otic competence is relatively broadly distributed in the embryonic ectoderm, with different regions losing competence at different stages.

Early Ear Development and Patterning

Hindbrain Influences

It has long been appreciated that morphogenesis of the inner ear is strongly influenced by the adjacent hindbrain. This has become even more evident in recent years, with so much attention being placed on the genetic control of hindbrain segmentation and the acquisition of segment identity. The hindbrain, through its associated neural crest derivatives, makes only a minor cellular contribution to the inner ear in the form of melanocytes of the stria vascularis, satellite cells of the statoacoustic ganglion, and possibly a subset of vestibular neurons in the chicken (D'Amico-Martel and Noden, 1983). Because the direct cellular contribution from hindbrain is so sparse, hindbrain influence is primarily indirect. It is probable that the hindbrain secretes factors that generate axial polarity or otherwise influences regional specification of the ear. At the moment, relatively little is known about the molecular nature of such secreted signals, with the possible exception of Fgf3 (detailed below).

In birds and mammals, the otocyst arises adjacent to hindbrain segments (rhombomeres) 5 and 6. Rhombomere 4 (r4) and r5 give rise to neural crest cells, which stream past the otocyst anteriorly to colonize the second pharyngeal arch. Arch II neural crest derivatives give rise to the stapes, which presumably must interact with the inner ear to coordinate placement of the stapes footplate within the oval window of the inner ear. Motor neurons located in r4 and r5 will generate the facial (VII) cranial nerve, which serves cells of the second arch. Later, a branch of this nerve will innervate one of the middle ear muscles. Crest cells that pass posterior to the otocyst arise from r5 and r6 and settle in the third pharyngeal arch. Both arches I and II may contribute to periotic mesenchyme, which probably interacts with otic ectoderm from relatively early stages.

Genetic defects leading to changes in hindbrain segmentation or segment identity, in particular r5, appear to be most influential on ear patterning (Fig. 8–4). Examples include several transcription factors (*Hoxa1*, *Hoxb1*, *Krm1*, and *Krox20*) as well as at least two diffusible signaling systems, Fgf and retinoic acid. Ear defects resulting from mutant *Hox* genes, whether direct or mediated through retinoic acid signaling, have been reviewed (Fritzsch et al., 1998; Fekete, 1999; Kiernan et al., 2002; see Chapter 46). Because *Krox20*, *Krm1*, and the *Hox* genes are transcription factors expressed in hindbrain but not otic vesicle, they must exert their influence indirectly, presumably through secreted factors. Direct versus indirect effects of several other genes are harder to distinguish because both the hindbrain and the otocyst express them: this includes *Lmx1* and genes regulating retinoid and Fgf signaling.

bZIP Genes (*Krm1, kreisler*). The mouse mutant *kreisler* has defects in both hindbrain segmentation and ear development (Deol, 1964). The otocyst is small and laterally displaced away from the hindbrain and fails to undergo morphogenesis (Frohman et al., 1993; McKay et al., 1994). Instead, it becomes enlarged and cystic. One of the earliest signs of ear morphogenesis, outgrowth of the endolymphatic duct, fails (Fig. 8–4). Some vestibular sensory tissue eventually differentiates. Deol (1964) suggested that the ear defects were probably an indirect result of the hindbrain perturbations. It was another 30 years before this was verified molecularly. *Kreisler* was cloned and its expression localized to r5 and r6 but not the ear. The gene proved to be a transcription factor of the bZIP *Maf* family and was called *Krm1* (Cordes and Barsh, 1994). Subsequent analysis of mutant hindbrains showed that only r5 was definitively missing, while

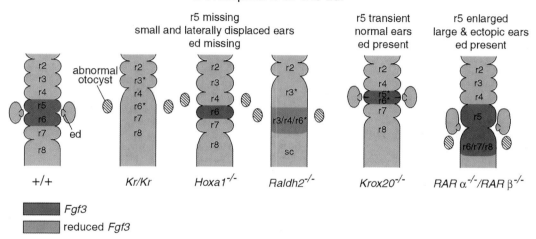

Figure 8–4. Defects in hindbrain segmentation lead to alterations in early ear morphogenesis in mouse. See text (Hindbrain Influences) for details. r, rhom-bomere; ed, endolymphatic duct. (Figure modified with permission from Kiernan et al., 2001.)

r3 and r6 were abnormal (Manzanares et al., 1999). This mutant points squarely at r5 (and possibly r6) as being especially crucial to otic vesicle placement near the hindbrain. Whether the subsequent developmental defects are due to the reduced size of the otocyst or to the fact that it forms too far from the hindbrain to receive inductive signals (from the other rhombomeres) remains open.

Homeobox Genes (*Hoxa1*, *Hoxb1*, *Lmx1a*, and *Pax3*). Knock-out of the *Hoxa1* gene leads to disruptions in rhombomere identity that are different from the *kreisler* mutant, although the effects on the ear are remarkably similar (Lufkin et al., 1991; Chisaka et al., 1992). In the *Hoxa1* knockout, r3 is expanded, r4 is reduced, and r5 is missing (Carpenter et al., 1993; Mark et al., 1993). Once again, the otocyst forms abnormally far from the hindbrain and the endolymphatic duct is missing (Fig. 8–4). In the most penetrant phenotypes, the otocyst is cystic and morphogenesis fails, although some vestibular sensory tissue does differentiate. Double knockouts of *Hoxa1* and *Hoxb1* show even more profound defects in r3 (enlarged further) and r4 (reduced or absent) and increased penetrance of the ear phenotypes (Gavalas et al., 1998; Rossel and Capecchi, 1999) (see Chapter 46).

As a counterexample to the knockouts of *Krm1* and *Hoxa1*, consider the knockout of *Krox20*. This gene is expressed in r3 and r5 even before the constrictions separating rhombomeres are evident. In the absence of *Krox20*, neither r3 nor r5 differentiates (Schneider-Maunoury et al., 1993; Swiatek and Gridley, 1993). However, paradoxically, ear development is remarkably normal (Fig. 8–4). How is it that r5 now has so little influence? Careful molecular analysis revealed that r5 may make a transient appearance in the *Krox20* null mutant at embryonic day (E) 9.5 (Schneider-Maunoury et al., 1997) before disappearing entirely a day later. Perhaps there is a short critical period of r5 requirement, after which the ear develops autonomously. Alternatively, because the otocyst develops close to the hindbrain (compared to the *Hoxa1* knockout), it may be in a better position to receive morphogenetic signals, either transiently from the disappearing r5 or sustained from r4 and/or r6.

Lmx1a is a LIM homeodomain transcription factor that is expressed in both the hindbrain and the dorsal and lateral parts of the otic cup and vesicle (Giraldez, 1998). A spontaneous mouse mutant, *Dreher*, has defective development of the hindbrain roofplate and abnormal ear morphogenesis (Manzanares et al., 2000; Millonig et al., 2000). The endolymphatic apparatus is unusually large and distended, and there are defects in both vestibular and cochlear components of the ear. Correct expression of *Lmx1* in the ear requires signals from the hindbrain: ablations of the ventral hindbrain lead to upregulation of the gene in the adjacent parts of the otic vesicle (Giraldez, 1998). Based on its expression pattern, *Lmx1* appears to be especially important in dorsal/ventral (D/V) patterning of the hindbrain and early ear.

Pax3 may also be involved in D/V patterning. It is expressed in the dorsal part of the neural tube but not apparently in the early ear (Ep-

stein et al., 1991; Goulding et al., 1991). The mouse mutant *Splotch* has a mutated *Pax3* gene that leads to defects in both neural tube and ear (Deol, 1966; Goulding et al., 1991).

Retinoid Signaling. Retinoids regulate *Hox* genes and thereby influence hindbrain development, but there is also evidence that they directly affect the developing ear in chickens (Choo et al., 1998). Nonetheless, in several recent knockouts that alter retinoid levels, there is a familiar confluence of defective hindbrain segmentation and ear abnormalities. It is likely that at least some components of the ear phenotypes are secondary to the hindbrain defects. Knockout of the retinaldehyde dehydrogenase-2 gene (*Raldh2*) blocks the synthesis of retinoic acid. All rhombomeres posterior to r2 are abnormal, with no clear segmentation (Niederreither et al., 2000). Gene expression analysis suggests that the r3–r6 territory is partially divided into two domains: one that may be an enlarged r3 and another that is an abnormal r3/r4/r6 territory expressing reduced levels of Fgf3. There is no clear evidence that r5 is present, based on the absence of the r5 marker *Krox20*. The otocyst arises at approximately its normal anterior/posterior (A/P) level of the abnormal r6 but is abnormally displaced away from the hindbrain (Fig. 8–4). Once again, in the absence of r5, the endolymphatic duct fails to form. While the embryo dies too early (E10.5) to assess the ear for further defects in morphogenesis, it clearly has patterning problems: based on gene expression, it appears to be entirely lateralized (Neidderreither et al., 2000).

The *Raldh2* null phenotype contrasts with that seen with a double knockout of the genes encoding two retinoic acid receptors, RARα and RARβ, which leads to an enlarged r5: the ear field is expanded (Dupe et al., 1999). The otic pit can be elongated in the A/P dimension, sometimes breaking apart into a second additional otic pit or vesicle (Fig. 8–4). With time, the ear field seems to regulate back to a normal size, the ectopic vesicles disappear, and eventually a normal inner ear forms. Once again, the importance of r5 is apparent.

There seems to be a correlation across all of these hindbrain mutants with regard to outgrowth of the endolymphatic duct: it always fails in the absence of r5 or of an r5/r6 boundary and/or when the ear arises adjacent to a rhombomere expressing little or no *Fgf3* (Fig. 8–4).

Fgf Signaling (Fgf3). Both gain-of-function and loss-of-function experiments appear to confirm that Fgf3 is especially important in the formation or outgrowth of the endolymphatic duct. The *Fgf3* knockout fails to form an endolymphatic duct (Mansour et al., 1993). In its absence, the ear develops hydrops, presumably because the endolymphatic fluid is unable to drain into the fourth ventricle of the brain as it would normally. Despite this problem, the ear does show some evidence of morphogenetic development of the cochlea and canals, and some sensory patches differentiate. Significantly, there is no initial lateral displacement of the otic vesicle in this mutant. The endolymphatic duct also fails to form with a knockout of a specific isoform of the

Fgf receptor, Fgfr2(IIIb), which should bind Fgf3 and is expressed by the ear ectoderm (De Moerlooze et al., 2000; Pirvola et al., 2000). In a reciprocal manipulation, overexpression of *Fgf3* in chicken embryos using virus-mediated gene transfer leads to elongation of the endolymphatic duct (Vendrell et al., 2000).

A detailed understanding of the precise function of Fgf3 in ear development is complicated by the fact that it is expressed not only in r5 and r6 but also in the otic placode (in some species), then in the neurogenic region of the developing otocyst, and even later in the sensory patches (Wilkinson et al., 1989; McKay et al., 1996). The picture might be clarified with more in-depth analysis of *Fgf3* and *Fgfr2(IIIb)* knockouts, mapping gene expression domains in the ear (is the ear also lateralized?) and hindbrain (what happens to rhombomere identities?). Even more illuminating would be generation of a conditional knockout of *Fgf3* restricted to either the ear or the hindbrain but not both.

Early Ear Morphogenesis

Pax/Six/Eya/Dach. It has been proposed that a conserved genetic regulatory network involving the *Pax*, *Six*, *Eya*, and *Dach* gene families may be active in all cranial sensory placodes (Baker and Bronner-Fraser, 2001). This network was first identified in the developing fly eye, and subsequent work has shown that it also functions in the specification of the vertebrate eye and myogenesis in the chick. Specificity across systems, including the cranial placodes, is thought to depend on which family members of each gene are expressed. In the ear ectoderm, one can find expression of at least one member of each of these gene families if data are combined from zebrafish, *Xenopus*, chick, and mouse. This includes *Six1* or *-4*; *Pax2*, *-5*, and/or *-8*; *Eya1* or *-4*; and *Dach1* (references in Baker and Bronner-Fraser, 2001). Of these, knockout of *Eya1* has proven especially devastating to ear development. This transcriptional coactivator is related to the fly gene *eyes absent*. Knockout mice have rudimentary inner ears that lack all evidence of cytodifferentiation or vestibulocochlear ganglion cells (Xu et al., 1999). The outer and middle ear are also defective in the *Eya1* knockout mouse, as described later. A zebrafish mutant, *dog-eared*, has been mapped to the *eya1* gene, and it also has widespread defects in ear development (Kozlowski et al., unpublished, cited by Whitfield et al., 2002). Both *Eya1* and *Pax2* are induced by overexpression of *Sox3* in the medaka fish, leading to formation of ectopic otic vesicles and/or absence of endogenous ears (Koster et al., 2000). The absolute levels of Sox3 may be important to the specification of ear tissue from within the general preplacodal field and to the subsequent control of the Pax/Six/Eya/Dach regulatory network. Together these data suggest that Eya1, and perhaps the entire regulatory pathway, functions shortly after otic induction to initiate ear morphogenesis. Both hypomorphic alleles of *Eya1* as well as the *Pax2* knockout affect primarily the cochlea and will be discussed later.

Gata3. Like *Eya1*, knockout of the zinc finger transcriptional regulator *Gata3* leads to severe dysgenesis of the inner ear (Karis et al., 2001). The ear is present but rudimentary. The gene is normally expressed throughout the otic cup and then in a broad lateral region of the otic epithelium. This is followed by a complex and changing expression pattern in sensory and nonsensory tissues as development progresses (Lawoko-Kerali et al., 2002). However, *Gata3* is also expressed in the hindbrain and periotic mesenchyme (Nardelli et al., 1999), suggesting that multiple interactions could be perturbed in the mutant.

Axial Polarity

A major unresolved issue in ear development is an understanding of the rules governing axial polarity, pattern formation, and cell fate specification of the otic vesicle during its morphogenesis into the complex labyrinth of the inner ear (see Chapter 5). We do not know whether the epithelium is organized into separate compartments that can instruct cells as to their identity, whether gradients of patterning molecules provide positional or axial information to the cells, or whether both mechanisms are present. Otic polarity and patterning are established and/or maintained by signals from the surrounding tissue, although the molecular nature of these signals is unclear.

With respect to axial polarity, gene expression patterns can provide clues and are especially informative during the early stages. Shortly after otic induction, several otic markers are broadly expressed throughout the otic field, including *Pax2* and others. Some of these recede into more restricted domains even before otic vesicle closure is complete. This begins as the otic cup invaginates in birds and mammals or as the bolus of otic ectoderm cavitates in zebrafish and continues into the otic vesicle stages. Asymmetry in gene expression is the earliest indicator that cells are acquiring information for A/P, medial/lateral (M/L), and D/V axial polarity.

During this early phase of changing gene expression, it is difficult to detect obvious boundaries of gene expression. Instead, the intensity of expression can gradually fade away at the limits of the domains. This suggests that gradients of gene expression, perhaps reflecting focal sources of one or more morphogens or other signaling molecules, may be the predominant means of inducing axial polarity in the inner ear. However, most of the known asymmetric markers expressed within the otocyst proper are actually transcription factors rather than secreted factors, so the search continues for morphogen-like signaling molecules. A notable exception is *Bmp4*, which becomes focused at the anterior and posterior poles of the otic vesicle in mouse, chicken and frog (Oh et al., 1996; Morsli et al., 1998; Kil and Collazo, 2001). *Bmp4* expression is thought to reflect the initial stages of sensory organ specification at the poles of the vesicle rather than a symmetry-breaking secreted factor (see The Sensory Patches, below).

In zebrafish and chicks, one can find examples of genes that are regionally or focally restricted even prior to otic vesicle formation, showing that axis specification has been initiated (Kiernan et al., 1997; Haddon et al., 1998; Smithers et al., 2000). However, fixation of the axes does not occur until much later, at least in the chick (Wu et al., 1998). Rotation of the otic ectoderm has shown that the axes are gradually specified and/or fixed in the following order: A/P, M/L, and then D/V. In the chicken, the D/V axis remains plastic at least up to stages 18–20 on E3.

A Compartment-Boundary Model

Once the otic vesicle begins to assume a tear-dropped shape in the chicken, some gene expression domains begin to sharpen (Kiernan et al., 1997). By the time the endolymphatic duct begins its outgrowth near the dorsal pole of the vesicle, an identifiable gene expression boundary is present next to the duct. It is defined by the juxtaposition of Pax2 protein, which has become confined to the medial and ventral vesicle, and by several genes, including *Gata3* and two *Hmx* genes that are expressed in the lateral vesicle (Brigande et al., 2000b; Lawoko-Kerali et al., 2002). Fate mapping at the otic cup stage revealed that cells do not move across this M/L boundary, suggesting that it also represents a lineage boundary (Brigande et al., 2000a). A second putative lineage boundary that bisects the dorsomedial otocyst into anterior and posterior halves was also discovered by fate mapping. Remarkably, this A/P boundary within the endolymphatic duct is aligned almost precisely with the r5/r6 boundary of the hindbrain. Recall that the r5/r6 boundary, combined with normal levels of *Fgf3* in r5 and r6, was correlated with successful endolymphatic duct outgrowth (Fig. 8–4).

Orthogonal to these two putative boundaries would be a D/V boundary. Its existence is suggested by a broad ventral swath of the vesicle that expresses *Lunatic-fringe* (*Lfng*) and *Serrate1* (*Ser1*) in the chick (Cole et al., 2000). These and other gene expression data from mouse and chicken suggest that the otic vesicle may become segregated into developmental compartments (Fekete, 1996; Fekete and Wu, 2002). This is shown schematically in Figure 8–5.

Such an arrangement of lineage-restricted compartments could facilitate the subsequent differentiation of the ear into its component parts. A relatively limited set of broad, partially overlapping gene expression domains could specify smaller compartments if a combinatorial code were used. Furthermore, compartment boundaries could provide restricted sources of secreted factors to induce development of more focal structures, including the sensory organs (Fekete, 1996; Kiernan et al., 1997; Brigande et al., 2000b; Fekete and Wu, 2002).

Figure 8–5. A compartment-boundary model of inner ear morphogenesis. Ears are viewed from the anterior pole. *(a)* The otic vesicle may be divided into regions that function as compartments of lineage restriction. Signaling can occur across boundaries to specify cell fates (e.g., sensory patch formation) or morphogenetic events (e.g., outgrowth of the endolymphatic duct). *(b)* Genes with partially overlapping expression domains may help to define the compartments. *(c)* One possible fate map, showing where the compartment-boundaries may be located as the ear develops. Note that sensory organs may arise adjacent to compartments but may also straddle a boundary. *(d)* A suggestion for how each of the sensory patches may be related to the otic vesicle compartments. The precise location of the saccular macula and cochlea with respect to the boundaries is unknown. A, anterior; AC, anterior crista; ADL, anterior-dorsal-lateral; ADM, anterior-dorsal-medial; AVL, anterior-ventral-medial; AVM, anterior-ventral-medial; BP, basilar papilla (birds); D, dorsal; L, lateral; LC, lateral crista; M, medial; oC, organ of Corti (mammals); P, posterior; PC, posterior crista; PDL, posterior-dorsal-lateral; PDM, posterior-dorsal-medial; PVL, posterior-ventral-lateral; PVM, posterior-ventral-medial; SM, saccular macula; UM, utricular macula; V, ventral. (Modified with permission from Fekete and Wu, 2002; see original paper for a color version of the figure.)

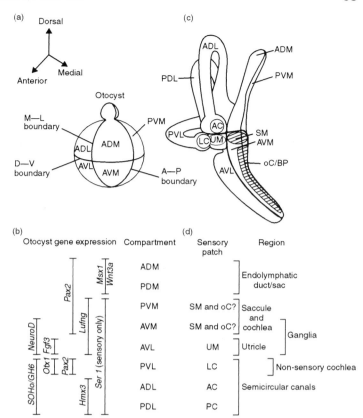

It is clear that sensory patches often arise near the boundary of a broad gene expression domain, as predicted (Kiernan et al., 1997; Brigande et al., 2000b). It may be that the boundaries are involved in establishing the limit of a sensory patch (the sensory/nonsensory border) rather than, or in addition to, specifying sensory identity via a secreted factor arising at the boundary.

While still largely theoretical, the model nevertheless provides a framework to begin to analyze the myriad gene expression patterns and phenotypes displayed when ear genes are mutated. Only a few genes that are expressed in subdomains of the otocyst have yielded relatively specific defects in the inner ear following their functional inactivation, which might be interpreted as the loss of a developmen-

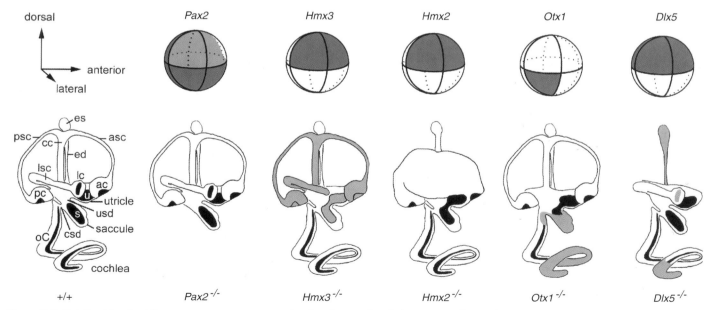

Figure 8–6. Relationship of putative compartments, gene expression domains *(top)*, and loss of different structural parts of the ear following gene knockout in the mouse *(bottom)*. Ears are viewed from the lateral side. When a particular defect is only partially penetrant or not consistent between several independent knockout lines, the affected region is shaded gray. See text for further descriptions. ac, anterior canal; asc, anterior semicircular canal; csd, cochleo-saccular duct; ed, endolymphatic duct; es, endolymphatic sac; lc, lateral crista; lsc, lateral semicircular canal; oC, organ of Corti; pc, posterior crista; psc, posterior semicircular canal; s, saccular macula; u, utricular macula. (After Brigande et al., 2000b.)

tal compartment or the sensory patch that arises within it. Several such mutants are shown schematically in Figure 8–6. While these may be important in trying to identify compartments, they are discussed more descriptively below (see Morphogenesis).

Fate Mapping

The compartment-boundary model could be readily disproved if there were convincing fate-mapping data showing that the borders of gene expression domains do not correspond to regions of lineage restriction. Lineage restriction is believed to be an important component that keeps groups of cells segregated to create boundaries, such as the parasegment interface in the developing fly for focal release of morphogens (Lawrence and Struhl, 1996). However, it is important to point out that compartment boundaries can be transient. Once the appropriate signaling has taken place across the boundary to regulate gene expression and effect cell fate specification, the boundaries can be violated by migrating cells. This has been observed in the vertebrate hindbrain (Birgbauer and Fraser, 1994). In the search for lineage boundaries in the developing ear, we must be careful to include a range of survival times so that transient lineage boundaries will not be overlooked.

To date, surprisingly few studies have been aimed at fate mapping the otic cup or vesicle (reviewed by Kil and Collazo, 2002). The zebrafish holds great promise since a high-resolution fate-mapping method is already available. This involves injecting embryos at the one or two cell stage with caged fluorochromes. The molecules are subsequently uncaged in one or a few cells using focal laser illumination, rendering the cells fluorescent and therefore traceable (Kozlowski and Weinberg, 2000b). Preliminary fate mapping at the otic vesicle stage suggests that clonally related cells do not disperse widely throughout the zebrafish ear as morphogenesis progresses (Kozlowski and Weinberg, 2000a).

The zebrafish data are generally consistent with lineage analysis and fate-mapping studies performed in a higher vertebrate, the chicken. My colleagues and I used retrovirus-mediated lineage analysis to map the distribution of labeled clones. Our data showed that viral infection at the otic vesicle stage yielded small, focal clones 2 weeks later (Lang and Fekete, 2001). That is, clonally related cells did not disperse widely even as the ear enlarged massively and completed its morphogenesis. This result might be expected if each major part of the ear represents a different developmental compartment. However, the clone sizes were sufficiently small that the chance of a clone abutting a boundary was limited.

Fate mapping the rim of the chicken otic cup has been accomplished by targeted injections of fluorochromes. Again, labeled cells tended to remain cohesive, forming linear streaks as the ear expanded dorsally over 2 days of development (Brigande et al., 2000a). Survival times were not long enough to map the sensory patches.

The lack of information about the origin of sensory cells in the chicken is notable in view of surprising results from the frog (Kil and Collazo, 2001). The *Xenopus* otic cup and vesicle were fate-mapped using injections of lipophilic dyes that labeled fewer than 100 cells or up to nearly an entire quadrant of the vesicle. Results showed that progeny derived from a labeled cluster could end up in any of the four quadrants of the ear. For example, cells labeled by a posterior injection could colonize both posterior and anterior sensory patches. While a complete fate map was not attempted, these data certainly raise questions about the presence of lineage boundaries in this species. It will be important to extend these studies to include smaller injections, clonal analysis if possible, and a fate map that includes both sensory and nonsensory parts of the ear.

Fate mapping the mouse by a direct labeling method will be difficult since the relevant stages of development occur in utero. To circumvent this problem, Li and colleagues (1978) used organ culture to perform what is actually called a "specification" assay. They removed the otocyst, cultured it in a neutral environment, and determined whether the tissue had already acquired positional information. The otic vesicle was bisected through one of three orthogonal planes, and each half (D vs. V, M vs. L, or A vs. P) was cultured separately. It was possible to judge by gross morphogenesis which of the various

parts of the ear (e.g., endolympatic duct, semicircular canals, cochlea) and their associated sensory organs arose from each hemi-ear. These data provided evidence that regional specification of the otic vesicle was already under way by E11.0 in the mouse.

Morphogenesis

The Cochlea and Saccule

The cochlea and saccule comprise the *pars inferior* of the mammalian ear. It is not known whether the two chambers and their sensory organs arise from common developmental compartments, as indicated schematically in Figure 8–5. They become obviously separated by a cochleosaccular duct as development progresses. The genetic regulation of cochlear morphogenesis has been reviewed (Cantos et al., 2000, and references therein). Likewise, references for the gene knockouts and expression patterns described in this section can be found elsewhere (Torres and Giraldez, 1998; Fekete, 1999; Brigande et al., 2000b; Holme et al., 2002).

Paired Homeobox (Pax2). The *Pax2* knockout made a big splash in the hearing research field when it was first reported in 1996. For the first time, there was a gene that was shown to be specifically required to make a cochlea. Two different groups described complete agenesis of the cochlea and its associated spiral ganglion in *Pax2* mutant mice (Torres et al., 1996; Favor et al., 1996). The mutant mice were deaf and had other associated defects in brain, eye, and kidney, leading to the conclusion that a mouse model of renal-coloboma syndrome had been identified. *Pax2* is expressed in a broad medial domain in the otocyst that includes more that just the region fated to become cochlea (Lawoko-Kerali et al., 2002): it includes a presumptive saccule and endolymphatic duct (Fig. 8–6). Expression remains high in the cochlea and the saccule as late as E17.5 in the mouse fetus. It is unclear why only the cochlea is so sensitive to the absence of *Pax2*.

Eya1. A hypomorphic allele of *Eya1*, Eya^{bor}, shows a far less severe phenotype in ear morphogenesis compared with a complete knockout of the gene (described earlier). With the *bor* allele, the cochlear duct is severely truncated and the associated auditory ganglion cells are missing (Johnson et al., 1999). Although in normal mouse embryos *Eya1* is initially expressed throughout the entire otic placode, it becomes confined to the ventromedial wall of the otocyst (where the organ of Corti arises) and the statoacoustic ganglion (Kalatzis et al., 1998). This later expression correlates with the structures altered in the Eya^{bor} mutant. The phenotype also mimics that seen in branchio-oto-renal (BOR) and BO syndromes of humans, which are caused by allelic defects of *EYA1* (Abdelhak et al., 1997; Vincent et al., 1997).

Other Genes: *Otx1/2*, *Dlx5*, *Ngn1*, *Brn4*. Several gene knockouts display alterations in the length, shape, and/or smoothness of cochlear duct coiling (reviewed by Cantos et al., 2000). Some of these, like the orthodenticle homologs *Otx1* and *Otx2*, are expressed in the ventral part of the otocyst, which will give rise to the cochlear duct (Fig. 8–6). In these two genes, total gene dosage is important: a combination of $Otx1^{-/-}, Otx2^{+/-}$ shows more severe defects in cochlear length and shape than the *Otx1* null alone. A similar dosage effect was also described for effects on the shape and size of the saccule. Absence of the *atonal* homolog *neurogenin1* (*Ngn1*) leads to absence of inner ear ganglion cells (see below), for which it is best known. In addition, though, the *Ngn1* knockout shows a reduction in the length of the cochlear duct and fusion of the saccule and utricle (Ma et al., 2000). The cochlea and saccule probably arise from an area that partially overlaps with the neurogenic region (see Fig. 8–5), which may explain the constellation of defects. Knockout of *Dlx5* also leads to a reduction in the length of the cochlea, although this result is puzzling since this gene is primarily expressed more dorsally in the otocyst. Another mutation leading to a shortened cochlear duct is absence of the POU transcription factor *Pou3f4*, also called *Brn4*. This gene is expressed in periotic mesenchyme but not in the otic ectoderm, so its requirement in cochlear morphogenesis must be mediated indirectly from the mesenchyme.

The Utricle and Semicircular Canals

The *pars superior* of the inner ear consists of the utricle and the three orthogonal semicircular canals (Fig. 8–6). The utricle houses a vestibular sensory organ, the utricular macula, and connects to the endolymphatic duct medially and to the saccule ventrally through narrow ducts. Each of the three semicircular canals emerges from the utricle at the point of the enlarged ampullary chambers within which the cristae of the canals are located. The canals loop around and reconnect to the utricle either alone (the horizontal or lateral canal) or through a joint attachment duct called the "common crus" (the anterior and posterior canals).

Development of the semicircular canals involves complex reorganization of the dorsal otic epithelium (Fig. 8–7). The anterior and posterior canals arise from a common superior pouch, while the lateral arises from a horizontally directed pouch. For each canal, the epithelial sheets on each side of the pouch approach each other, eventually fusing in the center while leaving the outer rim open. This central region is called a "fusion plate." After the fusion plate cells disappear, the toroidal duct of each semicircular canal is left behind. In some vertebrates, including chickens and *Xenopus*, disappearance of the fusion plate is accompanied by extensive programmed cell death. In others, such as the mouse and zebrafish, there is little or no cell death in the fusion plates and its cells are presumed to become resorbed into the enlarging rim of the canal (Fekete et al., 1997; Bever and Fekete, 1999). The continued outgrowth of the canals is accompanied by cell proliferation confined mostly to the outer rim of the ducts in the chicken (Lang et al., 2000). The outer rim preferentially expresses the two chicken *Hmx* genes (Kiernan et al., 1997), whereas the inner rim preferentially expresses the guidance molecule *netrin1* (Salminen et al., 2000). The molecular control of the vestibular parts of the ear has been reviewed in detail (Chang et al., 2002).

Hmx (Nkx) Genes. Two related homeobox genes, *Hmx2* and *Hmx3*, are closely linked in the mouse genome, and each is required for morphogenesis of the semicircular canals (see Wang et al., 2001, and references therein). Two different groups reported knocking out *Hmx3*, a gene that is normally expressed in the dorsolateral otocyst

(Hadrys et al., 1998; Wang et al., 1998). The less severe of these lost the ampulla of the lateral canal, including its associated sensory organ (Fig. 8–6). Constriction between the saccule and utricle failed to form, leading to fusion of the two sensory maculae of these two compartments. A more severe phenotype was reported by a second group: the entire lateral canal failed to form. Furthermore, the anterior and posterior canals were sometimes hypomorphic (Hadrys et al., 1998). Perhaps the genetic background explains the different degrees of penetrance in the two *Hmx3* null lines. Alternatively, the more severe phenotype may be caused by partial loss of function of the adjacent *Hmx2* in addition to *Hmx3*. When *Hmx2* alone was knocked out, all three canals were hypomorphic (Wang et al., 2001). Like *Hmx3*, the utricular and saccular maculae were fused, with significant reductions in the size of the utricular macula. The *Hmx2* gene comes on later than *Hmx3* but in roughly the same territory, although it eventually is present throughout the entire *par superior* and in part of the cochlea. Within this expression domain, no apparent defects in the endolymphatic duct or cochlea were evident in the knockout.

Dlx Genes. The *distalless* homolog *Dlx5* is required in the two vertical canals in the mouse (Fig. 8–6). Absence of *Dlx5* causes a striking phenotype: complete loss of both vertical canals with virtually normal development of the remainder of the inner ear (Acampora et al., 1999; Depew et al., 1999). This mutant supports the idea that the ear may be subdivided into developmental compartments, with *Dlx5* acting as a "selector" gene for those that will generate the two vertical canals. Several other members of the *Dlx* gene family are expressed in the early ear, including *Dlx6* in mouse and *Dlx3* and *Dlx7* in zebrafish (Ekker et al., 1992; Akimenko et al., 1994; Quint et al., 2000). Their function in ear morphogenesis has not been reported, but their expression in the preplacodal field during gastrulation suggests that they act extremely early in ear specification.

Otx Genes. While *Dlx5* may control development of the vertical canals, *Otx1* is especially important for development of the lateral canal in mice (Fig. 8–6). The entire canal is missing in the *Otx1* knock-

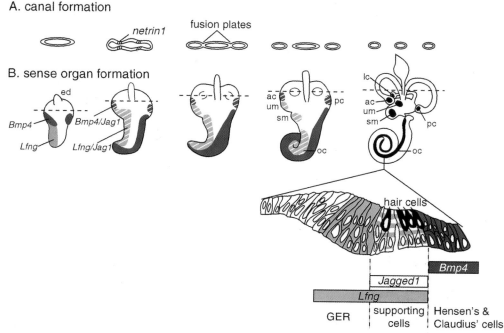

Figure 8–7. Morphogenesis and sensory cell fate specification of the inner ear. *(A)* Representations of cross-sections through the otocyst (dashed lines in *B*) at various stages to show the fusion of epithelial surfaces that takes place to hollow out the center of each canal. Formation of the anterior and posterior canals (ac, pc) are indicated. *(B)* Spatial and temporal map of the expression domains of several genes that mark the incipient sensory patches or adjacent cells. Medial view. Anterior is to the left and dorsal is up. Details of the de-

veloping organ of Corti (oc) are shown for the last stage, emphasizing how the region is segregated into a variety of cell types. Hair cells, shown in black, would express Jagged-2 at this perinatal stage. Most cells in the greater epithelial ridge (GER) will die during early postnatal development in the mouse. sm, saccular macula; um, utricular macula; lc, lateral crista. (Modified from Kiernan et al., 2002, and Chang et al., 2002.)

out. Neither the human *OTX2* gene nor the fly homolog, *Otd*, can substitute for *Otx1* in this capacity, even when they are put under the control of the *Otx1* promoter by knocking them into the *Otx1* locus. This was notable in view of the fact that either gene could rescue the *Otx1* null phenotype in all other parts of the embryo and ear except for the lateral canal (Morsli et al., 1999).

Prx Genes. The lateral canal is the last to develop in the mouse inner ear, and it seems especially prone to disappear in various knockouts. Simultaneous loss of two related genes, *Prx1* and *Prx2*, will lead to absence of the lateral canal (ten Berge et al., 1998). Additionally, the vertical canals are thickened and there is a reduced otic capsule. Both genes are expressed in the lateral periotic mesenchyme, while only *Prx2* is expressed in the dorsolateral otocyst. The canal defects may therefore be due to a combined effect on both the epithelium and the mesenchyme.

Gli3. A mouse mutant, *Extratoes*, is associated with reduction in *Gli3*, and is missing the lateral canal. The anterior canal is also truncated (Johnson, 1967; Hui et al., 1994). The gene is expressed in periotic mesenchyme, suggesting a mesenchymal-to-epithelial interaction for proper canal formation.

Pou Domain Gene. *Brn4* (*Pou3f4*) was already mentioned as a periotic transcription factor that can influence cochlear development. Absence of the gene also affects canal morphogenesis: the anterior semicircular canal is narrower than normal (Minowa et al., 1999; Phippard et al., 1999). The canal defect may underlie balance problems seen in the knockout mice or in the mouse mutant *sex-linked fidget*, which has a chromosomal inversion that eliminates *Brn4* expression in the ear but not the neural tube (Phippard et al., 2000).

Netrin1. Fusion of the canal plates requires intact *Netrin1* (*Ntn1*), whose expression arises in the walls of the canal pouches prior to their approach to generate a fusion plate (Salminen et al., 2000). This localization and its role in canal morphogenesis, were surprising since the protein had earned its reputation as an axon guidance molecule. It has been suggested that Ntn1 protein may indirectly contribute to the approach of the fusion plates by causing a local increase in cell proliferation in the mesenchyme, which may literally "push" together the apposing apical surfaces.

BMP Signaling. Inhibition of BMP signaling can cause severe truncations of the canals. This was seen following periotic implantation of beads soaked in the BMP inhibitor noggin as well as following misexpression of *noggin* using retroviral gene transfer (Chang et al., 1999; Gerlach et al., 2000). There is evidence for an effect on canal pouch formation if the beads are implanted early or for continued maintenance of canal structure if the beads are implanted later in chicken embryos (Chang et al., 2002).

Retinoid Signaling. Manipulating levels of retinoic acid can also affect canal outgrowth. Beads soaked in retinoic acid cause a dose-dependent loss of the canals but not, surprisingly, the common crus in the chicken (Choo et al., 1998).

The Endolymphatic Duct
The endolymphatic duct arises at the dorsal pole of the otocyst, expanding at its distal tip to form the endolymphatic sac. The function of the duct and sac is crucial to fluid homeostasis in the ear: the structures channel endolymph out of the ear to drain into the cerebrospinal fluid at the fourth ventricle. The duct arises early and acquires a unique identity based on the expression of several different marker genes.

Homeobox Genes. *Msx1*, *Dlx5*, and *Pax2* have expression domains that include the endolymphatic duct. *Msx1* is confined to the duct itself, while the other genes include lateral (*Dlx5*) or medial (*Pax2*) structures. The *Dlx5* knockout mouse lacks the endolymphatic duct with variable penetrance, while the anterior and posterior canals are always missing (Acampora et al., 1999; Depew et al., 1999).

Fgf3 Signaling. Formation of the endolymphatic duct is sensitive to the levels of *Fgf3* expressed in the fifth and sixth rhombomeres of the adjacent hindbrain, as discussed earlier (Fig. 8–4). The *Fgf3* knockout mouse lacks the endolymphatic duct (Mansour et al., 1993). The resulting expansion into a cystic ear probably results from failure to drain endolymphatic fluid appropriately, and subsequent endolymphatic hydrops ensues.

Wnt Signaling. Two *Wnt* and several *Frizzled* genes encoding receptors for Wnts are expressed in the early otocyst near where the endolymphatic duct arises (Hollyday et al., 1995; Jasoni et al., 1999; Stark et al., 2000). The role of this pathway is only beginning to be explored experimentally. Our preliminary data show that ectopic activation of Wnt signaling causes dysmorphogenesis of the ear, but the endolymphatic duct arises at its normal location (Stevens and Fekete, unpublished observations).

Cell Fate Specification
The plethora of cell types in the inner ear ensures that the genetic control of cell fate specification will be exceedingly complex. An example of the sequence and type of binary decisions that might be encountered as certain cell types are determined is shown in Figure 8–8. We find that several successive decisions depend on Notch signaling, with the basic helix-loop-helix (bHLH) factors also involved in the implementation of neuronal and sensory fates, the two most thoroughly understood to date.

The Neurons
The neurogenic region of the otic vesicle is located on its anteroventral wall (Fig. 8–5). Here, a subset of otic epithelial cells leave the vesicle and move medially to coalesce as the statoacoustic, or eighth cranial ganglion. Shortly after emigrating, the cells begin to express neuronal markers even as they continue to divide. Generation of a neurogenic population appears to involve Notch signaling as well as bHLH neurogenic genes related to the fly gene *atonal*. Ganglionogenesis also relies on several early otic transcription factors and Fgf signaling. Subsequent survival of the statoacoustic neurons requires two neurotrophins secreted from the sensory organs.

Notch Signaling. Expression of several components of Notch signaling within the neurogenic region implicates this pathway in the specification of neural fate (see Fekete and Wu, 2002, for summary and references). Included among these are *Notch1*, *Delta1*, *Ser1* (called *Jagged1* in the mouse), and *Lufng*. Within the otic placode and vesicle, *Notch* is widely expressed. The Notch ligand *Delta1* is expressed by isolated cells in the neurogenic region; these are presumed to be nascent neuroblasts preparing to emigrate. *Delta1* is not coexpressed with neuronal markers until the cells leave the vesicle.

Notch signaling is often used in the context of lateral inhibition to allow an equipotential cell population to choose between two fates. In this case, the likely choice is between a neuronal fate and an otic epithelial fate. In the simple case of lateral inhibition in other model systems, the cell receiving the Notch signal is the one inhibited. The most parsimonious explanation is that the Delta-expressing neuroblasts inhibit their neighbors from assuming the same fate, perhaps as a way of controlling the total numbers of neurons generated. This interpretation is supported by the zebrafish *mind bomb* mutant, where a block in Notch signaling leads to generation of an excessive number of otic ganglion neurons.

The Notch-expressing cells remaining behind in the neurogenic region of the otocyst continue to express Ser1/Jag1 and *Lufng* and presumably go on to generate at least some sensory patches, including the saccule, cochlea, and utricle (see Fig. 8–5). This additional role for Notch signaling will be discussed later.

bHLH Genes (*Ngn1* and *Neurod1*). Two neurogenic genes, *Neurogenin1* (*Ngn1*, also called *Neurod3*) and *Neurod1*, are required in the ear for neuronal specification and delamination, respectively. Both are distant relatives of the fly proneural gene *atonal*, which is required for development of the chordotonal organ, a mechanoreceptive sensory patch and associated neuron. The evolutionary and

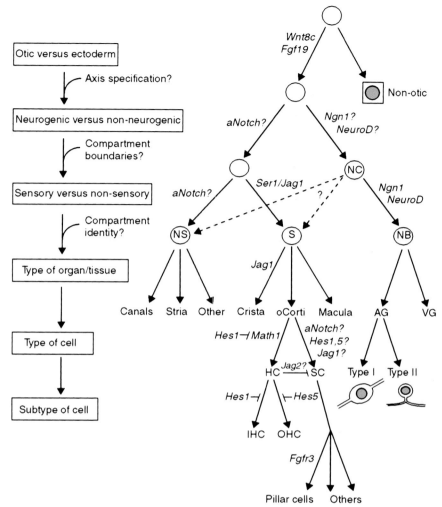

Figure 8–8. Possible cell fate decisions in the developing inner ear and some of the molecular determinants that influence these decisions. AG, auditory ganglion neuron; aNotch, activated Notch; HC, hair cell; IHC, inner hair cell; NB, neuroblast; NC, neural competent progenitor; NS, non-sensory progenitor; S, sensory progenitor; OHC, outer hair cell; SC, supporting cell; VG, vestibular ganglion neuron. (Reproduced with permission from Fekete and Wu, 2002.)

molecular conservation between invertebrate and vertebrate mechano-sensors has not escaped notice by investigators in this field (Eddison et al., 2000; Fritzsch et al., 2000). In the *Ngn1* knockout, neuroblasts are completely missing (Ma et al., 2000). In contrast, neuroblasts are transiently present in the *Neurod1* knockout but fail to emigrate from the vesicle and then die (Liu et al., 2000; Kim et al., 2001).

Pou Domain Gene (*Brn3a*). *Brn3a* (*Brn3.0*) is the next gene required during otic ganglion cell development. It is expressed in the otic neuroblasts shortly after they delaminate, and in its absence the neurons fail to differentiate properly (Huang et al., 2001).

Other Genes: *Gata3, Eya1, Fgfs, Pax2,* and *Hmx2*. Genes that regulate early morphogenesis of the ear usually show an associated absence of the ganglion neurons in the knockout. These include *Gata3, Eya1,* and *Fgfr2(IIIb)*, which were discussed earlier. The zebrafish *ace* mutant implicates *Fgf8* in both ear and ganglion development: a mutation in the gene causes significant loss of neurons in conjunction with a tiny, abnormal otic vesicle (reviewed by Whitfield et al., 2002). *Fgf8* is transiently expressed in the neurogenic part of the otocyst, and Fgf8- or Fgf2-soaked beads implanted near this region appear to induce excess numbers of ganglion cells (Adamska et al., 2001).

How the neuronal population differentiates into auditory vs. vestibular subsets is unknown. Preferential loss of these two major classes of ganglion neurons seems to correlate with the presence or absence of

the part of the ear that it innervates. So, for example, auditory, but not vestibular, neurons are missing in mutants that lead to gross cochlear hypomorphism, such as *Pax2* (Torres et al., 1996) and *Eya*bor (Xu et al., 1999). However, reduced numbers of vestibular neurons are seen in the *Hmx2* knockout, which is missing the canals (Wang et al., 2001). Mutants that selectively disrupt the specification of vestibular ganglion neurons (as opposed to their survival) have not been reported. The glial cells of the eighth cranial ganglion originate not from the otic vesicle but from the cranial neural crest (D'Amico-Martel and Noden, 1983). Their development will not be covered in this chapter.

Neurotrophins and Neuronal Survival. Auditory and vestibular ganglion neurons have different requirements for neurotrophic survival factors (Fritzsch et al., 1997, 1999). In brief, developing neurons express one or more receptors for brain-derived neurotrophic factor (BDNF), neurotrophin3 (NT3), or nerve growth factor. The former two are survival factors for the otic neurons. Secretion of these factors from the sensory epithelium or their reception by the appropriate TrkC or TrkB receptors have been shown by knockouts to be required for the survival of different subtypes of neuron in the inner ear. Neurons innervating the cristae have a specific requirement for BDNF, which is the neurotrophin expressed there. The cochlea expresses *Bdnf* and *Nt3* mRNA in spatially and temporally complex and mostly nonoverlapping patterns, which explains the differential loss of neurons projecting to the basal vs. the apical hearing organ.

The Sensory Patches

There are at least three general features of sensory organ specification that need to be considered. The first is the specification of each cell or, more likely, a group of cells as sensory (Figs. 8–7, 8–8). The second is the choice of sensory organ type: macula, crista, or organ of Corti. The third is the specification of different cell types within each sensory patch (Fekete, 1996; Fekete and Wu, 2002). Most inner ear sensory organs contain only two major cell types, hair cells and supporting cells. Most organs also have at least two distinct types of hair cells, which can vary in morphology, connectivity with afferents and efferents, and physiological properties. The mammalian organ of Corti has additional complexity in the myriad different types of supporting cells found there.

Specification of both the sensory patches and the cell types within them appears to be influenced by Notch signaling. *Bmps* are expressed at the onset of sensory organ specification of the cristae in all vertebrates, and expression persists in different cell types during sensory organ development. Additional transcription factors of the *Pax*, *Eya*, *Otx*, and *Msx* families may be associated with the specification of sensory organ type and/or differentiation, perhaps reflecting their more general role in specification of the larger part (or compartment) of the ear in which each sensory organ arises (see section on Morphogenesis above). Finally, many kinds of molecule can influence proliferation, programmed cell death, and differentiation of the sensory patches. Foremost among these are bHLH and Pou domain transcription factors, which control hair cell fate and differentiation, respectively. Other molecules important in cell fate specification or differentiation include the Fgf signaling pathways, cytoskeletal and motor proteins, membrane proteins, extracellular matrices, and cell cycle inhibitors.

Notch Signaling. The transmembrane receptor *Notch1* is expressed widely in the developing otocyst. Notch ligands are among the earliest markers of the sensory patches in mouse, chicken, and zebrafish. *Ser1/Jag1* are initially expressed throughout the sensory patches before becoming confined to supporting cells in chicken and mice (Adam et al., 1998; Morrison et al., 1999). In the chicken, *Ser1*, together with *Lufng*, has been proposed to mark a broad domain in the ventromedial otocyst that has sensory competence (Cole et al., 2000). However, there is little in the way of a working model for how this might be accomplished. The situation is complicated by the fact that the same region presumed to have sensory competence also gives rise to neuroblasts that leave the otocyst to form the ganglion, at least in the anterior part of the domain. This makes it difficult to distinguish between Notch involvement in neurogenesis vs. its later involvement in sensory organ specification.

Several lines of evidence suggest that changes in the level of Notch signaling can affect the size of sensory patches. In the zebrafish *mind bomb*, which is blocked in Notch signaling, sensory hair cells develop prematurely, apparently in a broader region than normal (Haddon et al., 1998). In the mouse, the *Jag2* knockout makes extra rows of hair cells in the cochlea (Langford et al., 1999; Zheng et al., 2000). A similar phenotype is seen in two mouse mutants with missense mutations in *Jag1* (Kiernan et al., 2001; Tsai et al., 2001). These effects can be mimicked in culture using antisense oligos to block Notch signaling (Zine et al., 2000). Because both *Jag1* and *Notch1* are highly expressed in the prospective sensory patches, one possibility is that Notch activation is at high levels throughout the patch, with *Jag1* serving to block the premature differentiation of prosensory cells into hair cells.

A later role for Notch signaling occurs during specification of hair cells vs. supporting cells. The spatial arrangement of the two cell types as a mosaic pattern, with every hair cell surrounded by supporting cells, suggests that lateral inhibition could be operating (Lewis, 1998). The idea is that the whole prosensory region begins as an equivalence group, with every cell possessing equal potential to become either a hair cell or a supporting cell. The initial, default fate is to become a hair cell; but as a small number of cells begin to assume this fate, they inhibit the cells in their immediate vicinity from acquiring the same fate. The neighbors become the secondary fate, which is to be a supporting cell.

With a Notch lateral inhibition model, the primary (hair cell) fate should be associated with gradual upregulation of the ligand and down-regulation of Notch, while the secondary (supporting cell) fate should be associated with the opposite regulation of ligand and receptor. In fact, the gene expression pattern supports this to some extent. As differentiation progresses, hair cells begin to express the ligands *Delta1* and *Jag2*, while supporting cells continue to express *Notch1* (Figs. 8–7, 8–8). However, the supporting cells also continue to express a different Notch ligand, Jag1/Ser1, leading to the suggestion that Notch signaling may be involved in lateral induction between supporting cells (see discussion by Eddison et al., 2000).

Lateral inhibition among a field of equivalent cells necessarily rules out a role for lineage whereby separate progenitors are set aside for each cell type. As predicted, hair cells and supporting cells indeed arise from a common progenitor in the inner ear, often as a pair of sister cells (Fekete et al., 1998; Lang and Fekete, 2001). These data from the chick have been confirmed by preliminary studies in the mouse cochlea and saccule (Brigande and Fekete, unpublished observations).

A lateral inhibitory model of cell specification in the ear predicts that inhibition of Notch signaling should result in the generation of hair cells at the expense of supporting cells. The model received dramatic support from the sensory organ phenotype displayed by *mind bomb*. With the block of Notch signaling (by an unknown mechanism), all cells in the sensory patches differentiate as hair cells, presumably due to the lack of lateral inhibition (Haddon et al., 1998). The hair cells are unable to survive without the supporting cells to tether them to the epithelium and are extruded from the epithelium within a few days. A similar, albeit less pronounced, effect is seen in zebrafish mutants carrying a dominant-negative *DeltaA* allele, which also gives rise to excess hair cells at the expense of supporting cells (Riley et al., 1999).

This extreme phenotype has not been observed in mouse models where Notch signaling is perturbed due to loss of either Notch itself or its ligands. Eliminating *Jag2* leads to extra hair cell rows in the cochlea, but it appears that both hair cells and supporting cells are overproduced (Langford et al., 1999). Perhaps there is genetic redundancy with *Delta1*, also expressed in hair cells, that limits the severity of the phenotype.

Many kinds of manipulation lead to the generation of excess rows of hair cells. Even normal rat cochleas show this effect when placed in culture (Abdouh et al., 1994). The tendency is enhanced with the addition of retinoic acid (Kelley et al., 1993); downregulation of Notch signaling (Zine et al., 2000) or its putative downstream targets, such as the *Hes* genes (Zheng et al., 2000); or following a knockout of the cyclin inhibitor *p27^{kip1}* (Chen and Segil, 1999). These manipulations can lead to supernumerary inner hair cells, outer hair cells, and/or supporting cells. It is worth considering that lateral spread of sensory cells may reflect a prior perturbation in the choice between sensory and nonsensory cell fates. In this organ, at least, the task appears to require a delicate balance in the levels of several different factors, each of which contributes to the final spatial arrangement. Interestingly, this fate switch from nonsensory to sensory can be induced in cells that are clearly postmitotic.

bHLH Genes (*Math1*, *Hes1*, and *Hes5*). Sensory patches contain receptor cells that make synaptic connections with primary sensory neurons, so sensory organs are generally considered to be specialized neuronal tissues. It is therefore not surprising that the molecular pathways involved in neuronal specification are active in sensory organ or sensory cell fate specification in the ear. Most notable is a requirement for the neurogenic gene *Math1*, the murine homolog to *Drosophila atonal*. *Math1* is absolutely required for hair cell fate specification in mice (Bermingham et al., 1999). Furthermore, a transient cell population adjacent to the cochlea, the greater epithelial ridge cells, can form hair cells if transfected with *Math1* in the cultured cochlea of the neonatal rat (Zheng and Gao, 2000). Curiously, in the absence of detectable *Math1* expression, immortalized cell lines derived from the immature cochlea will turn on many hair cell markers when raised to a temperature permissive for differentiation (Rivolta et al., 2002). How these phenotypic hair cells have managed to bypass the requirement for *Math1* remains to be discovered.

While *Math1* appears to promote a hair cell fate, several *Hes* genes may inhibit hair cell fate acquisition in the surrounding supporting cells. In fact, promotion of a hair cell fate by *Math1* transfection into greater epithelial cells can be blocked by co-transfection of *Hes1* (Zheng et al., 2000). Knockout of *Hes1* or *Hes5* revealed upregulation in the production of cells on the inner or outer hair cell side of the organ of Corti, respectively (Zine et al., 2001). It remains to be determined whether the *Hes* genes are absolutely essential for supporting cell fate specification, as might be predicted if the hair cell and supporting cell fates are simply acquired through up- or downregulation of *Math1* via the *Hes* transcriptional suppressors (Fig. 8–8).

Pou Genes. Following *Math1* expression, there is an essential requirement for *Pou4f3* (*Brn3.1*) in hair cell differentiation. Although hair cells never actually differentiate in the *Pou4f3* knockout, some early markers suggest that they do arise but that their development is quickly aborted and the cells die (Erkman et al., 1996; Xiang et al., 1997, 1998).

Transforming Growth Factor-β (Tgf-β)–Related Signaling (see Chapter 24). In all vertebrate ears, expression of the TGF-β family member *Bmp4* is associated with the development of the cristae (Wu and Oh, 1996; Morsli et al., 1998; Kil and Collazo, 2001; Mowbray et al., 2001). In the chicken and frog, the gene is also expressed in all other sensory patches of the developing ear. It has been difficult to ascertain whether the role of this signaling molecule is cell-autonomous in sensory patches or whether it acts on the surrounding tissues because the knockout animal is an embryonic lethal. In the mammalian cochlea, *Bmp4* is restricted to nonsensory parts of the duct (Fig. 8–7) (Morsli et al., 1998).

The linear arrangement of hair cells into four rows in the mammalian cochlea poses more complex patterning problems than those of the other sensory patches. Its geometry suggests that there may be a linear source of a secreted molecule that initiates the pattern. This could be an inductive influence from the inner hair cell side since this is the first row to differentiate or an inhibitory influence from the opposite side, beyond the outer hair cells. In this context, it is interesting that *Bmp4*, a molecule that blocks neuronal differentiation in early development, is expressed immediately beyond the third row of outer hair cells during cochlear differentiation (Fig. 8–7). Further studies aimed at reducing *Bmp4* signaling exclusively in the ear will be of great interest, given that it is one of the earliest markers associated with incipient sensory patches.

Fgf Signaling (see Chapter 32). It has been difficult to assess the precise role of Fgfs in cell fate specification in the ear because gene knockouts of the *Fgfs* or their receptors have such profound effects on early ear morphogenesis, as described earlier. Nonetheless, expression of *Fgf3* or Fgf receptor in the cells of the sensory patches suggests that Fgfs will also be involved in these later events (Wilkinson et al., 1988; Peters et al., 1993). One example is the requirement for *Fgfr3* in the specification of the pillar cells that create the tunnel of Corti and separate inner and outer hair cells (Colvin et al., 1996).

Wnt Signaling (see Chapter 22). Preliminary data have indicated that the Wnt pathway may be active at stages corresponding to the specification of sensory patches. Messages for several different Wnt receptors, the *Frizzleds*, are expressed in or around the incipient sensory patches in the chick (Stevens et al., in press). The nuclear localization of β-catenin follows Wnt activation, leading to transcription regulation in concert with the transcription factors T-cell-specific transcription factor and lymphoid enhancer binding factor. An activated form of β-catenin that constitutively moves to the nucleus can bypass the need for Wnt ligand. We used retroviral gene transfer of activated β-catenin to effect such a gain of function in the otocyst prior to sensory organ specification. Two striking phenotypes were observed: the presence of ectopic patches on hair cells in nonsensory regions and conversion of auditory into vestibular sensory patches (Stevens et al., in press). The conversion included the hair cells, supporting cells, and the overlying extracellular matrix. This is the first

indication of a molecular manipulation that can influence the important cell fate decision between auditory and vestibular sensory identity.

The Stria Vascularis and Fluid Homeostatis

Mechanotransduction is exquisitely sensitive to the ionic composition of the endolymphatic fluid that bathes the apical surfaces of hair cells. Endolymph is high in potassium and low in sodium ions. It is responsible for a high positive resting potential (approximately 100 mV) across the surface of the cochlear epithelium, called the "endocochlear potential." The endocochlear potential is the driving force needed to send potassium ions down their electrochemical gradient into hair cells when the mechanically gated channels are opened by deflection of the stereociliary bundles. Endolymph is secreted by a specialized tissue on the wall of the cochlea called the "stria vascularis." The stria is composed of cells derived from different embryonic origins. The luminal layer of marginal cells is derived from the otic ectoderm. Beneath it lies a layer of intermediate cells that includes a type of melanocyte derived from the neural crest. These make strong gap-junctional connections with the deepest layer of basal cells. The stria is highly vascularized, perhaps due to the high metabolic requirements of the strial ion pumps. The ionic regulatory function of the stria may be the reason defects of the inner ear often share syndromal associations with defects of the kidney.

Potassium Channels and Transporters. Potassium ion recycling through a series of cells connected by gap junctions is proposed to be essential for maintaining fluid and ionic homeostatis in the ear (Kikuchi et al., 1995; Spicer and Schulte, 1996). The hypothesis is as follows. Cations are secreted from the strial marginal cells, flow into the hair cells during transduction, and then are shuttled laterally from the organ of Corti through the various layers of supporting cells to return to the stria for another round of secretion. Components that are involved in either potassium ion secretion, transport, uptake, or recycling are important; and perturbations in this process cause hearing and balance disorders in humans. Examples include two potassium channels, *Kcnq1* (*Kvlqt1*) and *KCNE1*, that are expressed by the marginal cells (Vetter et al., 1996; Neyroud et al., 1997; Schulze-Bahr et al., 1997; Lee et al., 2000; Casimiro et al., 2001). A K-Na-Cl cotransporter, *Slc12a2*, is expressed in cells of the stria vascularis and other parts of the cochlear duct. Mutant alleles of this gene are found in three different mouse models of deafness and vestibular dysfunction (Delpire et al., 1999; Dixon et al., 1999).

Junctional Proteins. Several gap-junctional proteins create a continuous intracellular pathway for ion movement. Gap junctions are composed of connexin proteins assembled at the interface of two communicating cells. Mutations in four different *connexins* (*connexins 26, 30, 31* and *43*) have been linked with nonsyndromal hearing loss in humans (Van Camp and Smith, 2002). Another human deafness gene encodes the tight junctional protein, *claudin14*. Such a protein could be involved in the maintenance of an ion-impermeable barrier lining the endolymph, which is necessary to maintain the endocochlear potential (Wilcox et al., 2001).

Pendrin. Pendred syndrome and nonsyndromic deafness in humans have been traced to a gene, *pendrin*, expressed in the endolymphatic duct and sac (Everett et al., 1997; Li et al., 1998). It has been suggested that *pendrin* may encode an anion transporter (Everett et al., 2001). This protein may be important in fluid homeostasis in the ear, although its wider expression in a variety of ear tissues suggests that it may have additional functions (Everett et al., 1999). Knockout mice have evidence of endolymphatic hydrops and eventual loss of sensory cells.

Pou Domain. A correlation of hearing loss and defective development of some of the cell types through which the ions are presumed to flow provides further support for the hypothesis that potassium recycling and a healthy endocochlear potential are both essential for hearing. The *Pou3f4* knockout has abnormalities in the fibrous cells underlying the stria vascularis, which is part of the putative potassium ion-recycling system (Phippard et al., 1999). *Pou3f4* mutations are associated with hearing loss in mice and humans.

Genes Regulating Neural Crest–Derived Melanocytes (*Sox10, Kit, Mgf, Mitf, End3,* and *Ednrb*).

Developmentally, absence of the neural crest contribution to the melanocyte population of the stria vascularis has been implicated in deafness in mice. Genes required in the neural crest for proper migration of this population to the inner ear include *Sox10, Kit, Mgf, Mitf, End3,* and *Ednrb* (reviewed by Steel et al., 2002). Although the exact role of melanocytes in hearing is unknown, these mutants provide strong evidence that melanocytes are a crucial functional component in the development of the endocochlear potential and ionic balance in the endolymph.

The Extracellular Matrix (Tectorins, Collagens)

The ear is a complex organ with several important extracellular matrices specialized for coupling fluid movement or pressure changes with deflection of the bundles on top of the hair cells (Goodyear and Richardson, 2002). Cupular membranes are located above the cristae of the semicircular canals and provide a mass that bends the stereocilia projecting into them when the head turns. The tectorial membrane lies over the organ of Corti, and it contains two major extracellular matrix proteins, the tectorins, that have been associated with nonsyndromal hearing loss in humans (Verhoeven et al., 1998; Van Camp and Smith, 2002). A different matrix, the otoconial membrane, lies above the macular sense organs and surrounds the calcarean crystals (otoliths) that typify these organs. Ear extracellular matrices also contain collagens. Defects in several different collagen molecules have been associated with at least two types of syndromal deafness in humans (Van Camp and Smith, 2002). It is not known whether the primary defects are in the membranes overlying the sensory organs or in other parts of the inner ear.

THE OUTER AND MIDDLE EAR

Origin and Morphogenesis

The pinna and the external auditory meatus of the outer ear funnel sound onto the flexible tympanic membrane. These structures arise from the first and second pharyngeal arches, with the pinna derived from the pharyngeal bulges and the groove between them deepening into the auditory meatus and terminating as the outer layer of the tympanic membrane. Functionally and structurally, the middle ear forms a bridge between the sound waves impinging on the surface of the tympanic membrane and pressure changes in the fluid-filled ducts of the inner ear that will cause deflection of the stereociliary bundles on the hair cells. Middle ear components include the inner two layers of the tympanic membrane and the bony tympanic ring that supports it during development, the air-filled middle ear cavity, the middle ear ossicles, two small muscles that attach to the ossicles, and associated nerves and blood vessels (Fig. 8–9). Because of its location, the development of the middle ear requires a coordinated interplay between tissues derived from pharyngeal arch ectoderm, pharyngeal arch mesoderm (of both neural crest and paraxial mesoderm origin), and pharyngeal endoderm. For this reason, defects in outer or middle ear morphogenesis can occur in the context of other defects in craniofacial development, skeletogenesis, and organogenesis elsewhere in the body.

An understanding of the molecular genetics of middle ear development has benefited from analyses of mouse mutants, especially those generated by gene knockout. An excellent review of the field by Mallo (2001) forms the basis of the overview presented here, including the diagrams shown in Figure 8–9. The reader is directed to Mallo's treatise for a full set of literature citations. So far, the genes involved include those encoding secreted factors that have been implicated in epithelial–mesenchymal interactions and transcription factors involved primarily in patterning the cranial neural crest and its derivatives. Of major importance are the signaling molecules endothelin1 and Fgf8, the steroid retinoic acid, and transcription factors of the *Eya, Paired-box* (*Prx*), *Hox, Dlx,* and *Goosecoid* (*Gsc*) gene families.

The Middle Ear Ossicles

The middle ear bones are first evident as local condensations of mesenchymal cells in the proximal part of the first and second pharyngeal (branchial) arches. The maxillary part of the first arch is the origin of the incus (dark blue, Fig. 8–9). The malleus arises from the mandibular part of the first arch (red, Fig. 8–9), and the stapes comes from the second arch (pale blue, Fig. 8–9). In addition to the malleus, the tympanic ring arises from arch I, but it then elongates in a circular path around the pharyngeal cleft to encroach into arch II territory. The tympanic ring is usually present only during embryogenesis in mammals; it eventually merges with the temporal bone in adults. Its primary role may be to coordinate formation of the tympanic membrane (see below).

Transcription Factors: *Dlx, Prx, Hoxa2,* and *Gsc* Genes

One or more of the four skeletal elements (the three ossicles and the tympanic ring) are defective in knockouts of *Dlx1, Dlx2, Prx1, Hoxa2,* and *Gsc,* as shown in Figure 8–9. Most commonly, the affected elements are malformed or hypomorphic. The *Hoxa2* knockout is an interesting exception, showing apparent mirror-image duplications of the first arch elements in addition to absence of the second arch-derived stapes. This phenotype suggests that the second branchial arch may have undergone a homeotic transformation to the first arch.

One can ask whether there is a correlation between the structures affected by a knockout and the normal gene expression domain. It appears that the correlation is often direct but may also be influenced by other factors. Consider the *Dlx* genes as an example. *Dlx1* expression is confined to arch II, the origin of the stapes. The stapes is the only middle ear ossicle altered in the *Dlx1* null, where it is severely hypomorphic (Qiu et al., 1997). *Dlx2* is expressed in the migratory neural crest, which gives rise to the derivatives of both the incus and stapes, both affected by its absence. However, its effects on the two bones are quite different. In the *Dlx2* null (Qiu et al., 1995), the stapes is reduced in size while the incus may be duplicated (Fig. 8–9). Since the gene is also expressed in arch ectoderm, it may be that at least some of its effects on ossicular development are indirect.

Signaling Molecules: Fgf8, Endothelin, Retinoids

Fgf8, endothelin1, and retinoic acid play important roles in pharyngeal arch morphogenesis (Francis-West et al., 1998). This helps to explain their critical role in development of the middle ear (reviewed by Mallo, 2001). Catastrophic defects in middle ear ossicles were found with knockouts of the genes for endothelin1, endothelinA receptor, endothelin converting enzyme-1, and the dHAND transcription factor regulated by this signaling pathway (reviewed by Fekete, 1999). All three ossicles are missing or severely malformed. When *Fgf8* was selectively reduced in arch I ectoderm (in *Fgf8;Nes-cre* mice), the malleus and incus were missing or hypomorphic but not the stapes (Trumpp et al., 1999). The latter may also have a requirement for *Fgf8,* but proof will require an appropriate way to reduce *Fgf8* in arch II. Complementary defects were found when retinoic acid signaling was reduced: defects were severe for the stapes but mild (incus) or absent (malleus) for the arch I derivates.

The Tympanic Membrane, External Auditory Meatus and Outer Ear

At the same time that the mesenchyme is condensing to form the ossicles, two epithelial sheets approach the area: one externally from the pharyngeal cleft and the other internally from the pharyngeal pouch (Figure 8–9). The two sheets meet and stretch around an extension of the malleus, the manubrium. Captured between the two membranous sheets are a small number of fibrous mesenchymal cells. In this way, the cellular components of the tympanic membrane include derivatives from all three germ layers: ectoderm, mesoderm, and endoderm.

Transcription Factors: *Gsc, Prx1, Hoxa1,* and *Hoxb1*

The earliest evidence of specification in the middle ear anlage is expression of the transcription factors *Gsc* and *Prx1* in some mes-

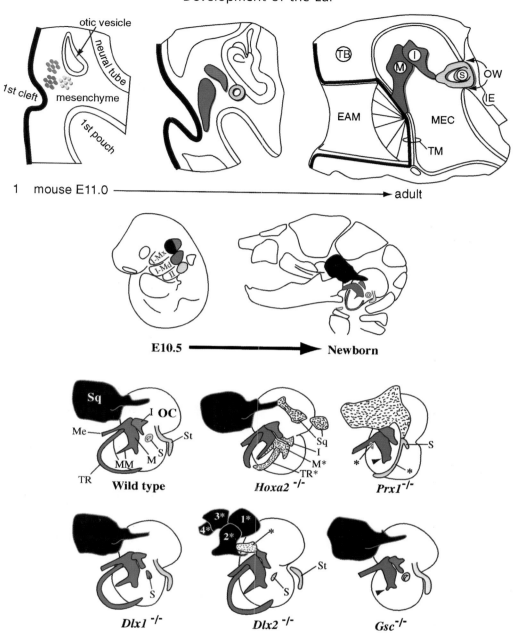

Figure 8–9. Development and malformations of the mouse middle ear. *(Top)* Schematic showing condensation of mesenchyme to form the middle ear ossicles between the first pharyngeal cleft and pouch. The latter two epithelial sheets deepen and eventually meet to form the tympanic membrane. The groove made by the pharyngeal cleft becomes the external auditory meatus. The involution of the pharyngeal pouch forms the tubotympanic recess of the middle ear cavity. *(Middle)* Derivation of the middle ear bones from the first and second pharyngeal arch mesenchyme. *(Bottom)* Defects resulting from knockouts of *Hoxa2*, *Prx1*, *Dlx1*, *Dlx2*, and *Gsc*. EAM, external auditory meatus; I-Mx, maxillary arch I; I-Md, mandibular arch I; II, arch II; I, incus; IE, inner ear; M, malleus; Me, Meckel's cartilage; MEC, middle ear cavity; MM, manubrium of the malleus; OC, otic capsule; OW, oval window; S, stapes; Sq, squamous; St, styloid process; TB, temporal bone; TM, tympanic membrane; TR, tympanic ring; *, extra structures. (Figure modified with permission from Mallo, 2001.)

enchymal cells. These transcription factors will eventually be localized to the tympanic ring, which fails to develop in their absence (Fig. 8–9). Expression of *Gsc* and *Prx1* requires signaling from Fgf8 and endothelin1. Chimeric analysis suggests that *Gsc* has two roles: it acts non-cell-autonomously to recruit mesenchymal cells into a condensing mass and cell-autonomously to induce osteogenesis in the mass (Rivera-Perez et al., 1999). The first role presumably involves transcriptional regulation of unknown secreted factors that can act at a distance. The molecular role of *Prx1* in tympanic ring formation is uncertain. A small piece of the tympanic ring seems to be present in the *Prx1* null mouse. Perhaps the initiation of mesenchymal condensation in the proximal part of the first arch can occur but not the subsequent growth of the anlage around the cleft and into the second arch.

Hoxa1 and *Hoxb1* are required for ring formation, but their expression in second, but not first, arch mesenchyme implies an inductive effect. It is not known whether such induction, if present, is direct from the arch II mesenchyme or mediated through the cleft ectoderm (see discussion by Mallo, 2001).

Knockout mutations in *Gsc* and the two *Hox* genes also alter pinna development in the mouse, emphasizing the importance of the arch mesenchyme in addition to the cleft that forms between these two hillocks.

Signaling Molecules: Endothelin, Fgfs, and Retinoids

Based on the sequence of anatomical events in the normal embryo, in vitro tissue recombination assays, and results of mutant phenotypes, Mallo (2001) has proposed that a series of epithelial–mesenchymal interactions lead to induction of the tympanic ring, the tympanic membrane, and the external auditory meatus. First, there is an epithelial-to-mesenchymal signal: the pharyngeal ectoderm secretes Fgf8 and endothelin1, which diffuse into the underlying mesoderm to induce expression of Gsc and Prx1 in tympanic ring precursors. Second, there is a mesenchymal-to-epithelial signal: the incipient tympanic ring tissue signals back to the overlying ectoderm, causing it to invaginate to form the external auditory meatus. The molecular nature of this putative mesenchymal signal is currently unknown. Third, there is a new epithelial-to-mesenchymal signal: the invaginating ectoderm of the forming meatus induces a cartilaginous condensation of the mesenchyme that will become the manubrium of the malleus. Fourth, there is yet another mesenchymal-to-epithelial signal, this time recruiting the endoderm of the middle ear cavity onto the medial side of the tympanic membrane. Again, the putative signaling molecule is unknown.

The signaling that induces formation of the external canal may also be required for the overt development of the pinna. Defects in the outer ear are found with knockouts of various components of endothelin1 signaling (Fekete, 1999).

SUMMARY AND FUTURE DIRECTIONS

Research in the field of vertebrate ear development is progressing at a furious pace. This chapter describes a subset of more than 400 genes already identified as being expressed in the ear during its development and differentiation (Holme et al., 2002). Emphasis has been placed on genes for which there is experimental evidence for a developmental function, usually by analysis of functional knockdowns or knockouts in animal models. The identification of human birth defects that are proven to be correlates of these animal models, while lagging behind somewhat, has also been accelerating due to rapid progress in sequencing of the human genome.

Animal models will continue to play a key role in understanding congenital human hearing loss, including syndromic deafness. At one end of the spectrum, there are genes whose mutant phenotypes cause embryonic lethality; these animal model systems can be valuable in understanding ear formation, but they may be of less interest clinically. At the other end of the spectrum, certain genes specific to the specialized cell types or physiological nuances of the ear usually have far fewer global consequences. For these, the frequent involvement of the vestibular system can be advantageous for spotting mutations. In the course of genetic screens in mice and fish or simply through spontaneous mutations, animals suffering from congenital sensorineural deafness are often first noticed because their vestibular defects cause them to spin in circles or manifest other peculiar balance behaviors. In this way, a handful of genes specific to inner ear development, cell differentiation, or cell physiology have been identified, although there are certain to be many others.

In contrast, defects involving the conductive portions of the ear, such as the ear canal or middle ear components, may not be associated with imbalance and might generate only moderate hearing loss, although they often manifest additional, syndromic defects in craniofacial development. Genes with a unique or specialized function in development of the sound conduction apparatus are most likely to be identified in genetic screens that specifically include hearing tests. Such screens are currently in progress in Europe and the United States for both mice and zebrafish.

As more genes involved in ear development are identified through expression analysis, genetic screens, microarray technology, or other approaches, their functional roles can be further explored using animal models. The future promises continued progress in understanding exactly how each of these genes contributes to building one of the most anatomically complex sensory systems in the human body.

REFERENCES

Abdelhak S, Kalatzis V, Heilig R, Compain S, Samson D, Vincent C, Weil D, Cruaud C, Sahly I, Leibovici M, et al. (1997). A human homologue of the *Drosophila* eyes absent gene underlies branchio-oto-renal (BOR) syndrome and identifies a novel gene family. *Nat Genet* 15: 157–164.

Abdouh A, Despres G, Romand R (1994). Histochemical and scanning electron microscopic studies of supernumerary hair cells in embryonic rat cochlea in vitro. *Brain Res* 660: 181–191.

Acampora D, Merlo GR, Paleari L, Zerega B, Postiglione MP, Mantero S, Bober E, Barbieri O, Simeone A, Levi G (1999). Craniofacial, vestibular and bone defects in mice lacking the Distal-less-related gene *Dlx5*. *Development* 126: 3795–3809.

Adam J, Myat A, Le Roux I, Eddison M, Henrique D, Ish-Horowicz D, Lewis J (1998). Cell fate choices and the expression of Notch, Delta and Serrate homologues in the chick inner ear: parallels with *Drosophila* sense-organ development. *Development* 125: 4645–4654.

Adamska M, Herbrand H, Adamski M, Kruger M, Braun T, Bober E (2001). FGFs control the patterning of the inner ear but are not able to induce the full ear program. *Mech Dev* 109: 303–313.

Akimenko MA, Ekker M, Wegner J, Lin W, Westerfield M (1994). Combinatorial expression of three zebrafish genes related to *distal-less*: part of a homeobox gene code for the head. *J Neurosci* 14(6): 3475–3486.

Arnold WH, Lang T (2001). Development of the membranous labyrinth of human embryos and fetuses using computer aided 3D-reconstruction. *Ann Anat* 183: 61–66.

Baker CV, Bronner-Fraser M (2001). Vertebrate cranial placodes I. Embryonic induction. *Dev Biol* 232: 1–61.

Bermingham NA, Hassan BA, Price SD, Vollrath MA, Ben-Arie N, Eatock RA, Bellen HJ, Lysakowski A, Zoghbi HY (1999). *Math1*: an essential gene for the generation of inner ear hair cells. *Science* 284: 1837–1841.

Bever MM, Fekete DM (1999). Ventromedial focus of cell death is absent during development of Xenopus and zebrafish inner ears. *J Neurocytol* 28: 781–793.

Birgbauer E, Fraser SE (1994). Violation of cell lineage restriction compartments in the chick hindbrain. *Development* 120: 1347–1356.

Brigande JV, Iten LE, Fekete DM (2000a). A fate map of chick otic cup closure reveals lineage boundaries in the dorsal otocyst. *Dev Biol* 227: 256–270.

Brigande JV, Kiernan AE, Gao X, Iten LE, Fekete DM (2000b). Molecular genetics of pattern formation in the inner ear: do compartment boundaries play a role? *Proc Natl Acad Sci USA* 97: 11700–11706.

Cantos R, Cole LK, Acampora D, Simeone A, Wu DK (2000). Patterning of the mammalian cochlea. *Proc Natl Acad Sci USA* 97: 11707–11713.

Carpenter EM, Goddard JM, Osamu C, Manley NR, Capecchi MR (1993). Loss of HoxA1 (Hox1.6) function results in the reorganization of the murine hindbrain. *Development* 118: 1063–1075.

Casimiro MC, Knollmann BC, Ebert SN, Vary JC Jr, Greene AE, Franz MR, Grinberg A, Huang SP, Pfeifer K (2001). Targeted disruption of the *Kcnq1* gene produces a mouse model of Jervell and Lange-Nielsen syndrome. *Proc Natl Acad Sci USA* 98: 2526–2531.

Chang W, Nunes FD, De Jesus-Escobar JM, Harland R, Wu DK (1999). Ectopic noggin blocks sensory and nonsensory organ morphogenesis in the chicken inner ear. *Dev Biol* 216: 369–381.

Chang W, Cole L, Cantos R, Wu DK (2002). Molecular genetics of vestibular organ development. In: *Anatomy and Physiology of the Central and Peripheral Vestibular System*. Highstein SM, Fay RR, Popper, AN (eds.) Springer, New York (in press).

Chen P, Segil N (1999). p27(Kip1) links cell proliferation to morphogenesis in the developing organ of Corti. *Development* 126: 1581–1590.

Chisaka O, Musci TS, Capecchi MR (1992). Developmental defects of the ear, cranial nerves and hindbrain resulting from targeted disruption of the mouse homeobox gene *Hox-1.6*. *Nature* 355: 516–520.

Choo D, Sanne JL, Wu DK (1998). The differential sensitivities of inner ear structures to retinoic acid during development. *Dev Biol* 204: 136–150.

Cole LK, Le Roux I, Nunes F, Laufer E, Lewis J, Wu DK (2000). Sensory organ generation in the chicken inner ear: contributions of bone morphogenetic protein 4, serrate1, and lunatic fringe. *J Comp Neurol* 424: 509–520.

Colvin JS, Bohne BA, Harding GW, McEwen DG, Ornitz DM (1996). Skeletal overgrowth and deafness in mice lacking fibroblast growth factor receptor 3. *Nat Genet* 12: 390–397.

Cordes SP, Barsh GS (1994). The mouse segmentation gene *kr* encodes a novel basic domain-leucine zipper transcription factor. *Cell* 79: 1025–1034.

D'Amico-Martel A, Noden DM (1983). Contributions of placodal and neural crest cells to avian cranial peripheral ganglia. *Am J Anat* 166: 445–468.

Delpire E, Lu J, England R, Dull C, Thorne T (1999). Deafness and imbalance associated with inactivation of the secretory Na-K-2Cl co-transporter. *Nat Genet* 22: 192–195.

De Moerlooze L, Spencer-Dene B, Revest J, Hajihosseini M, Rosewell I, Dickson C (2000). An important role for the IIIb isoform of fibroblast growth factor receptor 2 (FGFR2) in mesenchymal–epithelial signalling during mouse organogenesis. *Development* 127:483–492.

Deol MS (1964). The abnormalities of the inner ear in *kr* mice. *J Embryol Exp Morphol* 12:475–490.

Deol MS (1966). Influence of the neural tube on the differentiation of the inner ear in the mammalian embryo. *Nature* 209: 219–220.

Depew MJ, Liu JK, Long JE, Presley R, Meneses JJ, Pedersen RA, Rubenstein JL (1999). Dlx5 regulates regional development of the branchial arches and sensory capsules. *Development* 126:3831–3846.

Dixon MJ, Gazzard J, Chaudhry SS, Sampson N, Schulte BA, and Steel KP (1999). Mutation of the Na-K-Cl co-transporter gene *Slc12a2* results in deafness in mice. *Hum Mol Genet* 8: 1579–1584.

Dupe V, Ghyselinck NB, Wendling O, Chambon P, Mark M (1999). Key roles of retinoic acid receptors alpha and beta in the patterning of the caudal hindbrain, pharyngeal arches and otocyst in the mouse. *Development* 126: 5051–5059.

Eddison M, Le Roux I, Lewis J (2000). Notch signaling in the development of the inner ear: lessons from *Drosophila*. *Proc Natl Acad Sci USA* 97:11692-11699.

Ekker M, Akimenko MA, Bremiller R, Westerfield M (1992). Regional expression of three homeobox transcripts in the inner ear of zebrafish embryos. *Neuron* 9: 27–35.

Epstein DJ, Vekemans M, Gros P (1991). Splotch (Sp²H), a mutation affecting development of the mouse neural tube, shows a deletion within the paired homeodomain of Pax-3. *Cell* 67: 767–774.

Erkman L, McEvilly RJ, Luo L, Ryan AK, Farideh H, O'Connell SM, Keithley EM, Rapaport DH, Ryan AF, Rosenfeld MG (1996). Role of transcription factors Brn-3.1 and Brn-3.2 in auditory and visual system development. *Nature* 381: 603–606.

Everett LA, Glaser B, Beck JC, Idol JR, Buchs A, Heyman M, Adawi F, Hazani E, Nassir E, Baxevanis AD, et al. (1997). Pendred syndrome is caused by mutations in a putative sulphate transporter gene (*PDS*). *Nat Genet* 17: 411–422.

Everett LA, Morsli H, Wu DK, Green ED (1999). Expression pattern of the mouse ortholog of the Pendred's syndrome gene (*Pds*) suggests a key role for pendrin in the inner ear. *Proc Natl Acad Sci USA* 96: 9727–9732.

Everett LA, Belyantseva IA, Noben-Trauth K, Cantos R, Chen A, Thakkar SI, Hoogstraten-Miller SL, Kachar B, Wu DK, Green ED (2001). Targeted disruption of mouse Pds provides insight about the inner-ear defects encountered in Pendred syndrome. *Hum Mol Genet* 10: 153–161.

Favor J, Sandulache R, Neuhauser-Klaus A, Pretsch W, Chatterjee B, Senft E, Wurst W, Blanquet V, Grimes P, Sporle R, Schughart K (1996). The mouse Pax2 (1Neu) mutation is identical to a human PAX2 mutation in a family with renal-coloboma syndrome and results in developmental defects of the brain, ear, eye and kidney. *Proc Natl Acad Sci USA* 93: 13870–13875.

Fekete DM (1996). Cell fate specification in the inner ear. *Curr Opin Neurobiol* 6: 533–541.

Fekete DM (1999). Development of the vertebrate ear: insights from knockouts and mutants. *Trends Neurosci* 22: 263–269.

Fekete DM, Wu DK (2002). Revisiting cell fate specification in the inner ear. *Curr Opin Neurobiol* 12:35–42.

Fekete DM, Homburger SA, Waring MT, Riedl AE, Garcia LF (1997). Involvement of programmed cell death in morphogenesis of the vertebrate inner ear. *Development* 124: 2451–2461.

Fekete DM, Muthukumar S, Karagogeos D (1998). Hair cells and supporting cells share a common progenitor in the avian inner ear. *J Neurosci* 18: 7811–7821.

Francis-West P, Ladher R, Barlow A, Graveson A (1998). Signalling interactions during facial development. *Mech Dev* 75: 3–28.

Fritzsch B, Silos-Santiago I, Bianchi LM, Farinas I (1997). Effects of neurotrophin and neurotrophin receptor disruption on the afferent inner ear innervation. *Semin Cell Dev Biol* 8: 277–284.

Fritzsch B, Barald KF, Lomax MI (1998). Early embryology of the vertebrate ear. In: *Development of the Auditory System.* Rubel EW, Popper AN, Fay RR (eds.) Springer-Verlag, New York, pp. 80–145.

Fritzsch B, Pirvola U, Ylikoski J (1999). Making and breaking the innervation of the ear: neurotrophic support during ear development and its clinical implications. *Cell Tissue Res* 295: 369–382.

Fritzsch B, Beisel KW, Bermingham NA (2000). Developmental evolutionary biology of the vertebrate ear: conserving mechanoelectric transduction and developmental pathways in diverging morphologies. *Neuroreport* 11: R35–R44.

Frohman MA, Martin GR, Cordes SP, Halamek LP, Barsh G (1993). Altered rhombomere-specific gene expression and hyoid bone differentiation in the mouse segmentation mutant, *kreisler (kr)*. *Development* 117: 925–936.

Gallagher BC, Henry JJ, Grainger RM (1996). Inductive processes leading to inner ear formation during *Xenopus* development. *Dev Biol* 175:95–107.

Gavalas A, Studer M, Lumsden A, Rijli FM, Krumlauf R, Chambon P (1998). Hoxa1 and Hoxb1 synergize in patterning the hindbrain, cranial nerves and second pharyngeal arch. *Development* 125:1123–1136.

Gerlach LM, Hutson MR, Germiller JA, Nguyen-Luu D, Victor JC, Barald KF (2000). Addition of the BMP4 antagonist, noggin, disrupts avian inner ear development. *Development* 127: 45–54.

Giraldez F (1998). Regionalized organizing activity of the neural tube revealed by the regulation of lmx1 in the otic vesicle. *Dev Biol* 203: 189–200.

Goodyear RJ, Richardson GP (2002). Extracellular matrices associated with the apical surfaces of sensory epithelia in the inner ear: molecular and structural diversity. *J Neurobiol* (in press).

Gorlin RJ, Toriello HV, Cohen JMM (1995). *Hereditary Hearing Loss and Its Syndromes.* Oxford University Press, New York.

Goulding MD, Chalepakis G, Deutsch U, Erselius J, Gruss P (1991). Pax-3, a novel murine DNA binding protein expressed during early neurogenesis. *EMBO J* 32767: 1135–1147.

Griffith AJ, Friedman TB (2002). Autosomal and X-linked auditory disorders. In: *Genetics and Auditory Disorders.* Keats BJB, Popper AN, Fay RR (eds.) Springer, New York.

Groves AK, Bronner-Fraser M (2000). Competence, specification, and commitment in otic placode induction. *Development* 127: 3489–3499.

Haddon C, Jiang YJ, Smithers L, Lewis J (1998). Delta-Notch signalling and the patterning of sensory cell differentiation in the zebrafish ear: evidence from the mind bomb mutant. *Development* 125: 4637–4644.

Hadrys T, Braun T, Rinkwitz-Brandt , Arnold HH, Bober E (1998). Nkx5-1 controls semicircular canal formation in the mouse inner ear. *Development* 125: 33–39.

Heller N, Brandli AW (1999). *Xenopus Pax-2/5/8* orthologues: novel insights into *Pax* gene evolution and identification of *Pax-8* as the earliest marker for otic and pronephric cell lineages. *Dev Genet* 24: 208–219.

Hollyday M, McMahon JA, McMahon AP (1995). *Wnt* expression patterns in chick embryo nervous system. *Mech Dev* 52: 9–25.

Holme RH, Bussoli TJ, Steel KP (2002). Table of gene expression in the developing ear. (http://www.ihr.mrc.ac.uk/Hereditary/genetable/index.shtml)

Huang EJ, Liu W, Fritzsch B, Bianchi LM, Reichardt LF, Xiang M (2001). Brn3a is a transcriptional regulator of soma size, target field innervation and axon pathfinding of inner ear sensory neurons. *Development* 128:2421–2432.

Hui CC, Slusarski D, Platt KA, Holmgren R, Joyner AL (1994). Expression of three mouse homologs of the *Drosophila* segment polarity gene cubitus interruptus, *Gli, Gli-2,* and *Gli-3* in ectoderm- and mesoderm-derived tissues suggests multiple roles during postimplantation development. *Dev Biol* 162:402–413.

Jasoni C, Hendrickson A, Roelink H (1999). Analysis of chicken Wnt-13 expression demonstrates coincidence with cell division in the developing eye and is consistent with a role in induction. *Dev Dyn* 215: 215–224.

Johnson DR (1967). Extra-toes: a new mutant gene causing multiple abnormalities in the mouse. *J Embryol Exp Morphol* 17: 543–581.

Johnson KR, Cook SA, Erway LC, Matthews AN, Sanford LP, Paradies NE, Friedman RA (1999). Inner ear and kidney anomalies caused by IAP insertion in an intron of the *Eya1* gene in a mouse model of BOR syndrome. *Hum Mol Genet* 8:645–653.

Kaan HW (1926). Experiments on the development of the ear of *Amblystoma punctatum. J Exp Zool* 46: 13–61.

Kalatzis V, Sahly I, El-Amraoui A, Petit C (1998). Eya1 expression in the developing ear and kidney: towards the understanding of the pathogenesis of branchio-oto-renal (BOR) syndrome. *Dev Dyn* 213: 486–499.

Karis A, Pata I, van Doorninck JH, Grosveld F, de Zeeuw CI, de Caprona D, Fritzsch B (2001). Transcription factor GATA-3 alters pathway selection of olivocochlear neurons and affects morphogenesis of the ear. *J Comp Neurol* 429: 615–630.

Kelley MW, Xu XM, Wagner MA, Warchol ME, Corwin JT (1993). The developing organ of Corti contains retinoic acid and forms supernumerary hair cells in response to exogenous retinoic acid in culture. *Development* 119: 1041–1053.

Kiernan AE, Nunes F, Wu DK, Fekete DM (1997). The expression domain of two related homeobox genes defines a compartment in the chicken inner ear that may be involved in semicircular canal formation. *Dev Biol* 191: 215–229.

Kiernan AE, Ahituv N, Fuchs H, Balling R, Avraham KB, Steel KP, Hrabe de Angelis M (2001). The Notch ligand Jagged1 is required for inner ear sensory development. *Proc Natl Acad Sci USA* 98: 3873–3878.

Kiernan AE, Steel KP, Fekete DM (2002). Development of the mouse inner ear. In: *Mouse Development: Patterning, Morphogenesis and Organogenesis.* Rossant J, Tam PPL (eds.) Academic Press, San Diego, pp. 539–566.

Kikuchi T, Kimura RS, Paul DL, Adams JC (1995). Gap junctions in the rat cochlea: immunohistochemical and ultrastructural analysis. *Anat Embryol (Berl)* 191: 101–118.

Kil SH, Collazo A (2001). Origins of inner ear sensory organs revealed by fate map and time-lapse analyses. *Dev Biol* 233: 365–379.

Kil SH, Collazo A (2002). A review of inner ear fate maps and cell lineage studies. *J Neurobiol* (in press).

Kim WY, Fritzsch B, Serls A, Bakel LA, Huang EJ, Reichardt LF, Barth DS, Lee JE (2001). NeuroD-null mice are deaf due to a severe loss of the inner ear sensory neurons during development. *Development* 128: 417–426.

Kollmar R, Nakamura SK, Kappler JA, Hudspeth AJ (2001). Expression and phylogeny of claudins in vertebrate primordia. *Proc Natl Acad Sci USA* 98: 10196–10201.

Koster RW, Kuhnlein RP, Wittbrodt J (2000). Ectopic Sox3 activity elicits sensory placode formation. *Mech Dev* 95: 175–187.

Kozlowski D, Weinberg E (2000a). High resolution analysis of otic vesicle cell fates in wild-type and mutant zebrafish embryos by fate mapping with caged-fluorescein dextran. *Assoc Res Otolaryngol Abs* Abstract.

Kozlowski DJ, Weinberg ES (2000b). Photoactivatable (caged) fluorescein as a cell tracer for fate mapping in the zebrafish embryo. *Methods Mol Biol* 135: 349–355.

Kozlowski DJ, Murakami T, Ho RK, Weinberg ES (1997). Regional cell movement and tissue patterning in the zebrafish embryo revealed by fate mapping with caged fluorescein. *Biochem Cell Biol* 75: 551–562.

Ladher RK, Anakwe KU, Gurney AL, Schoenwolf GC, Francis-West PH (2000). Identification of synergistic signals initiating inner ear development. *Science* 290: 1965–1968.

Lang H, Fekete DM (2001). Lineage analysis in the chicken inner ear shows differences in clonal dispersion for epithelial, neuronal, and mesenchymal cells. *Dev Biol* 234: 120–137.

Lang H, Bever MM, Fekete DM (2000). Cell proliferation and cell death in the developing chick inner ear: spatial and temporal patterns. *J Comp Neurol* 417: 205–220.

Langford PJ, Lan Y, Jiang R, Lindsell C, Weinmaster G, Gridley T, Kelley MW (1999). Notch signalling pathway mediates hair cell development in mammalian cochlea. *Nat Genet* 21: 289–292.

Larsen WJ (2001). Human Embryology. Churchill Livingstone, New York.

Lawoko-Kerali G, Rivolta MN, Holley M (2002). Expression of the transcription factors GATA3 and Pax2 during development of the mammalian inner ear. *J Comp Neurol* 442: 378–391.

Lawrence PA, Struhl G (1996). Morphogens, compartments, and pattern: lessons from *Drosophila*? *Cell* 85: 951–961.

Lee MP, Ravenel JD, Hu RJ, Lustig LR, Tomaselli G, Berger RD, Brandenburg SA, Litzi TJ, Bunton TE, Limb C, et al. (2000). Targeted disruption of the *Kvlqt1* gene causes deafness and gastric hyperplasia in mice. *J Clin Invest* 106: 1447–1455.

Lewis J (1998). Notch signalling and the control of cell fate choices in vertebrates. *Semin Cell Dev Biol* 9: 583–589.

Li CW, Van De Water TR, Ruben RJ (1978). The fate mapping of the eleventh and twelth day mouse otocyst: an in vitro study of the sites of origin of the embryonic inner ear sensory structures. *J Embryol Exp Morphol* 157: 249–268.

Li XC, Everett LA, Lalwani AK, Desmukh D, Friedman TB, Green ED, Wilcox ER (1998). A mutation in PDS causes non-syndromic recessive deafness. *Nat Genet* 18: 215–217.

Liu M, Pereira FA, Price SD, Chu M, Shope C, Himes D, Eatock RA, Brownell WE, Lysakowski A, Tsai MJ (2000). Essential role of BETA2/NeuroD1 in development of the vestibular and auditory systems. *Genes Dev* 14: 2839–2854.

Lombardo A, Slack JM (1998). Postgastrulation effects of fibroblast growth factor on *Xenopus* development. *Dev Dyn* 212: 75–85.

Lombardo A, Isaacs HV, Slack JM (1998). Expression and functions of FGF-3 in *Xenopus* development. *Int J Dev Biol* 42: 1101–1107.

Lufkin T, Dierich A, LeMeur M, Mark M, Chambon P (1991). Disruption of the *Hox-1.6* homeobox gene results in defects in a region corresponding to its rostral domain of expression. *Cell* 66: 1105–1119.

Ma Q, Anderson DJ, Fritzsch B (2000). Neurogenin 1 null mutant ears develop fewer, morphologically normal hair cells in smaller sensory epithelia devoid of innervation. *J Assoc Res Otolaryngol* 1: 129–143.

Mallo M (2001). Formation of the middle ear: recent progress on the developmental and molecular mechanisms. *Dev Biol* 231: 410–419.

Mansour SL, Goddard JM, Capecchi MR (1993). Mice homozygous for a targeted disruption of the proto-oncogene *int-2* have developmental defects in the tail and inner ear. *Development* 117: 13–28.

Manzanares M, Trainor PA, Nonchev S, Ariza-McNaughton L, Brodie J, Gould A, Marshall H, Morrison A, Kwan CT, Sham MH, et al. (1999). The role of kreisler in segmentation during hindbrain development. *Dev Biol* 211: 220–237.

Manzanares M, Trainor PA, Ariza-McNaughton L, Nonchev S, Krumlauf R (2000). Dorsal patterning defects in the hindbrain, roof plate and skeleton in the dreher (dr[J]) mouse mutant. *Mech Dev* 94: 147–156.

Mark M, Lufkin T, Vonesch JL, Ruberte E, Olivo JC, Dolle P, Gorry P, Lumsden A, Chambon P (1993). Two rhombomeres are altered in Hoxa-1 mutant mice. *Development* 119: 319–338.

McKay IJ, Muchamore I, Krumlauf R, Maden M, Lumsden A, Lewis J (1994). The *kreisler* mouse: a hindbrain segmentation mutant that lacks two rhombomeres. *Development* 120: 2199–2211.

McKay IJ, Lewis J, Lumsden A (1996). The role of FGF-3 in early inner ear development: an analysis in normal and *kreisler* mutant mice. *Developmental Biology* 174: 370–378.

Millonig JH, Millen KJ, Hatten ME (2000). The mouse Dreher gene *Lmx1a* controls formation of the roof plate in the vertebrate CNS. *Nature* 403: 764–769.

Minowa O, Ikeda K, Sugitani Y, Oshima T, Nakai S, Katori Y, Suzuki M, Furukawa M, Kawase T, Zheng Y, et al. (1999). Altered cochlear fibrocytes in a mouse model of DFN3 nonsyndromic deafness. *Science* 285: 1408–1411.

Morrison A, Hodgetts C, Gossler A, Hrabe de Angelis M, Lewis J (1999). Expression of Delta1 and Serrate1 (Jagged1) in the mouse inner ear. *Mech Dev* 84: 169–172.

Morsli H, Choo D, Ryan A, Johnson R, Wu DK (1998). Development of the mouse inner ear and origin of its sensory organs. *J Neurosci* 18: 3327–3335.

Morsli H, Tuorto F, Choo D, Postiglione MP, Simeone A, Wu DK (1999). Otx1 and Otx2 activities are required for the normal development of the mouse inner ear. *Development* 126: 2335–2343.

Mowbray C, Hammerschmidt M, Whitfield TT (2001). Expression of BMP signalling pathway members in the developing zebrafish inner ear and lateral line. *Mech Dev* 108: 179–184.

Nardelli J, Thiesson D, Fujiwara Y, Tsai FY, Orkin SH (1999). Expression and genetic interaction of transcription factors GATA-2 and GATA-3 during development of the mouse central nervous system. *Dev Biol* 210: 305–321.

Neyroud N, Tesson F, Denjoy I, Leibovici M, Donger C, Barhanin J, Faure S, Gary F, Coumel P, Petit C, et al. (1997). A novel mutation in the potassium channel gene *KVLQT1* causes the Jervell and Lange-Nielsen cardioauditory syndrome. *Nat Genet* 15: 186–189.

Niederreither K, Vermot J, Schuhbaur B, Chambon P, Dolle P (2000). Retinoic acid synthesis and hindbrain patterning in the mouse embryo. *Development* 127: 75–85.

Normaly S, Grainger RM (2002). Determination of the embryonic inner ear. *J Neurobiol* 53: 100–128.

Oh SH, Johnson R, Wu DK (1996). Differential expression of bone morphogenetic proteins in the developing vestibular and auditory sensory organs. *J Neurosci* 16: 6463–6475.

Peters K, Ornitz D, Werner S, Williams L (1993). Unique expression pattern of the FGF receptor 3 gene during mouse organogenesis. *Dev Biol* 155: 423–430.

Pfeffer PL, Gerster T, Lun K, Brand M, Busslinger M (1998). Characterization of three novel members of the zebrafish Pax2/5/8 family: dependency of Pax5 and Pax8 expression on the Pax2.1 (noi) function. *Development* 125: 3063–3074.

Phillips BT, Bolding K, Riley BB (2001). Zebrafish fgf3 and fgf8 encode redundant functions required for otic placode induction. *Dev Biol* 235: 351–365.

Phippard D, Lu L, Lee D, Saunders JC, Crenshaw EB 3rd (1999). Targeted mutagenesis of the POU-domain gene *Brn4/Pou3f4* causes developmental defects in the inner ear. *J Neurosci* 19: 5980–5989.

Phippard D, Boyd Y, Reed V, Fisher G, Masson WK, Evans EP, Saunders JC, Crenshaw EB 3rd (2000). The sex-linked fidget mutation abolishes *Brn4/Pou3f4* gene expression in the embryonic inner ear. *Hum Mol Genet* 9: 79–85.

Pirvola U, Spencer-Dene B, Xing-Qun L, Kettunen P, Thesleff I, Fritzsch B, Dickson C, Ylikoski J (2000). FGF/FGFR-2(IIIb) signaling is essential for inner ear morphogenesis. *J Neurosci* 20: 6125–6134.

Qiu M, Bulfone A, Martinez S, Meneses JJ, Shimamura K, Pedersen RA, Rubenstein JL (1995). Null mutation of Dlx2 results in abnormal morphogenesis of proximal first and second branchial arch derivatives and abnormal differentiation in the forebrain. *Genes Dev* 9: 2523–2538.

Qiu M, Bulfone A, Ghattas I, Meneses JJ, Christensen L, Sharpe PT, Presley R, Pedersen RA, Rubenstein JLR (1997). Role of the Dlx homeobox genes in proximodistal patterning of the branchial arches: mutations of *Dlx-1, Dlx-2,* and *Dlx-1* and *-2* alter morphogenesis of proximal skeletal and soft tissue structures derived from the first and second arches. *Dev Biol* 185: 165–184.

Quint E, Zerucha T, Ekker M (2000). Differential expression of orthologous Dlx genes in zebrafish and mice: implications for the evolution of the Dlx homeobox gene family. *J Exp Zool* 288: 235–241.

Raible F, Brand M (2001). Tight transcriptional control of the ETS domain factors Erm and Pea3 by Fgf signaling during early zebrafish development. *Mech Dev* 107: 105–117.

Represa JJ, Moro JA, Pastor F, Gato A, Barbosa E (1990). Patterns of epithelial cell death during early development of the human inner ear. *Ann Otol Rhinol Laryngol* 99: 482–488.

Riley BB, Chiang M, Farmer L, Heck R (1999). The *deltaA* gene of zebrafish mediates lateral inhibition of hair cells in the inner ear and is regulated by pax2.1. *Development* 126: 5669–5678.

Rivera-Perez JA, Wakamiya M, Behringer RR (1999). Goosecoid acts cell autonomously in mesenchyme-derived tissues during craniofacial development. *Development* 126: 3811–3821.

Rivolta MN, Halsall A, Johnson CM, Tones MA, Holley M (2002). UB/OC-1 is a GER-derived cell line with the potential to differentiate into hair cells without the need of Math1. *Assoc Res Otolaryngol Abs*

Rossel M, Capecchi MR (1999). Mice mutant for both Hoxa1 and Hoxb1 show extensive remodeling of the hindbrain and defects in craniofacial development. *Development* 126: 5027–5040.

Salminen M, Meyer BI, Bober E, Gruss P (2000). Netrin 1 is required for semicircular canal formation in the mouse inner ear. *Development* 127: 13–22.

Schneider-Maunoury S, Topilko P, Seitandou T, Levi G, Cohen-Tannoudji M, Pournin S, Babinet C, Charnay P (1993). Disruption of Krox-20 results in alteration of rhombomeres 3 and 5 in the developing hindbrain. *Cell* 75: 1199–1214.

Schneider-Maunoury S, Seitanidou T, Charnay P, Lumsden A (1997). Segmental and neuronal architecture of the hindbrain of Krox-20 mouse mutants. *Development* 124: 1215–1226.

Schulze-Bahr E, Wang Q, Wedekind H, Haverkamp W, Chen Q, Sun Y, Rubie C, Hordt M, Towbin JA, Borggrefe M, et al. (1997). KCNE1 mutations cause jervell and Lange-Nielsen syndrome. *Nat Genet* 17: 267–268.

Shamim H, Mason I (1999). Expression of Fgf4 during early development of the chick embryo. *Mech Dev* 85: 189–192.

Smithers L, Haddon C, Jiang Y, Lewis J (2000). Sequence and embryonic expression of deltaC in the zebrafish. *Mech Dev* 90: 119–123.

Spicer SS, Schulte BA (1996). The fine structure of spiral ligament cells relates to ion return to the stria and varies with place-frequency. *Hear Res* 100: 80–100.

Stark MR, Biggs JJ, Schoenwolf GC, Rao MS (2000). Characterization of avian frizzled genes in cranial placode development. *Mech Dev* 93: 195–200.

Steel KP, Erven A, Kiernan AE (2002). Mice as models for human hereditary deafness. In: *Genetics and Auditory Disorders.* Keats BJB, Fay RR, Popper AN (eds.) Springer, New York.

Stevens CB, Davies AL, Battista S, Lewis JH, Fekete DM (2003). Forced activation of Wnt signaling alters morphogenesis and sensory organ identity in the chicken inner ear. *Dev Biol* (in press).

Swiatek PJ, Gridley T (1993). Perinatal lethality and defects in hindbrain development in mice homozygous for a targeted mutation of the zinc finger gene *Krox20. Genes Dev* 7: 2071–2084.

ten Berge D, Brouwer A, Korving J, Martin JF, Meijlink F (1998). Prx1 and Prx2 in skeletogenesis: roles in the craniofacial region, inner ear and limbs. *Development* 125: 3831-3842.

Torres M, Giraldez F (1998). The development of the vertebrate inner ear. *Mech Dev* 71: 5–21.

Torres M, Gomez-Pardo E, Gruss P (1996). *Pax2* contributes to inner ear patterning and optic nerve trajectory. *Development* 122: 3381–3391.

Trumpp A, Depew MJ, Rubenstein JL, Bishop JM, Martin GR (1999). Cre-mediated gene inactivation demonstrates that FGF8 is required for cell survival and patterning of the first branchial arch. *Genes Dev* 13: 3136–3148.

Tsai H, Hardisty RE, Rhodes C, Kiernan AE, Roby P, Tymowska-Lalanne Z, Mburu P, Rastan S, Hunter AJ, Brown SD (2001). The mouse slalom mutant demonstrates a role for Jagged1 in neuroepithelial patterning in the organ of Corti. *Hum Mol Genet* 10: 507–512.

Van Camp G, Smith RJH (2002). Hereditary Hearing Loss Homepage. (http://dnalab-www.uia.ac.be/dnalab/hhh/)

Vendrell V, Carnicero E, Giraldez F, Alonso MT, Schimmang T (2000). Induction of inner ear fate by FGF3. *Development* 127: 2011–2019.

Verhoeven K, Van Lear L, Kirschhofer K, Legan PK, Hughes DC, Schatteman I, Verstreken M, VanHauwe P, Coucke P, Chen A, et al. (1998). Mutations in the human alpha-tectorin gene cause autosomal dominant non-syndromic hearing impairment. *Nat Genet* 19: 60–62.

Vetter DE, Mann JR, Wangemann P, Liu J, McLaughlin KJ, Lesage F, Marcus DC, Lazdunski M, Heinemann SF, Barhanin J (1996). Inner ear defects induced by null mutation of the *isk* gene. *Neuron* 17: 1251–1264.

Vincent C, Kalatzis V, Abdelhak S, Chaib H, Compain S, Helias J, Vaneecloo FM, Petit C (1997). BOR and BO syndromes are allelic defects of EYA1. *Eur J Hum Genet* 5: 242–246.

Wang W, Vand De Water T, Lufkin T (1998). Inner ear and maternal reproductive defects in mice lacking the Hmx3 homeobox gene. *Development* 125: 621–634.

Wang W, Chan EK, Baron S, Van de Water T, Lufkin T (2001). Hmx2 homeobox gene control of murine vestibular morphogenesis. *Development* 128: 5017–5029.

Whitfield TT, Granato M, van Eeden FJM, Schach U, Brand M, Furutani-Seiki M, Haffter P, Hammerschmidt M, Heisenberg C-P, Jiang Y-J, et al. (1996). Mutations affecting development of the zebrafish inner ear and lateral line. *Development* 123: 241–254.

Whitfield TT, Riley BB, Chiang M-Y, Phillips B (2002). Development of the zebrafish inner ear. *Dev Dyn* 223: 427–458.

Wilcox ER, Burton QL, Naz S, Riazuddin S, Smith TN, Ploplis B, Belyantseva I, Ben-Yosef T, Liburd NA, Morell RJ, et al. (2001). Mutations in the gene encoding tight junction claudin-14 cause autosomal recessive deafness DFNB29. *Cell* 104: 165–172.

Wilkinson DG, Peters G, Dickson C, McMahon AP (1988). Expression of the FGF-related proto-oncogene *int-2* during gastrulation and neurulation in the mouse. *EMBO J* 7: 691–695.

Wilkinson DG, Bhatt S, McMahon AP (1989). Expression pattern of the FGF-related proto-oncogene *int-2* suggests multiple roles in fetal development. *Development* 105: 131–136.

Wright TJ, Mansour SL (2002). Fgf-3 and Fgf-10 in mouse inner ear development. *Assoc Res Otolaryngol Abs* 190.

Wu DK, Oh S-H (1996). Sensory organ generation in the chick inner ear. *J Neurosci* 16: 6454–6462.

Wu DK, Nunes FD, Choo D (1998). Axial specification for sensory organs versus nonsensory structures of the chicken inner ear. *Development* 125: 11–20.

Xiang M, Gan L, Li D, Chen ZY, Zhou L, O'Malley BWJ, Klein W, Nathans J (1997). Essential role of POU-domain factor Brn-3c in auditory and vestibular hair cell development. *Proc Natl Acad Sci USA* 94: 9445–9450.

Xiang M, Gao W-Q, Hasson T, Shin JJ (1998). Requirement for Brn-3c in maturation, migration and survival, but not in fate determination of inner ear hair cells. *Development* 125(20): 3935–3946.

Xu PX, Adams J, Peters H, Brown MC, Heaney S, Maas R (1999). Eya1-deficient mice lack ears and kidneys and show abnormal apoptosis of organ primordia. *Nat Genet* 23: 113–117.

Zheng JL, Gao WQ (2000). Overexpression of Math1 induces robust production of extra hair cells in postnatal rat inner ears. *Nat Neurosci* 3: 580–586.

Zheng JL, Shou J, Guillemot F, Kageyama R, Gao WQ (2000). Hes1 is a negative regulator of inner ear hair cell differentiation. *Development* 127: 4551–4560.

Zine A, Van De Water TR, de Ribaupierre F (2000). Notch signaling regulates the pattern of auditory hair cell differentiation in mammals. *Development* 127: 3373–3383.

Zine A, Aubert A, Qiu J, Therianos S, Guillemot F, Kageyama R, de Ribaupierre F (2001). Hes1 and Hes5 activities are required for the normal development of the hair cells in the mammalian inner ear. *J Neurosci* 21: 4712–4720.

9 | Development of the Heart and Vasculogenesis

WOLFGANG ROTTBAUER AND MARK C. FISHMAN

Genetic dissection helped to define the unitary logic underlying body plan development in *Drosophila* (Nusslein-Volhard and Wieschaus, 1980). Recent work indicates that vertebrate heart and vessel development is similarly amenable to genetic dissection. The genes that drive heart-cell differentiation in vertebrates and *Drosophila* are similar, even though the *Drosophila* "heart" is a simple tube and the vertebrate heart is a complex, multichambered organ. Mutational analyses in mice and zebrafish have revealed additional genes required for fashioning new organotypic "modules" with evolution of the vertebrate heart, including new chambers and the endothelial lining of the heart and vessels (Chen and Fishman, 2000).

In this chapter, we will review the known molecular players essential for heart development and vasculogenesis. However, it is not possible to review all of the many mutations that affect heart development and vasculogenesis and certainly not the breadth of embryology and development, for which there are other sources (Fishman and Chien, 1997; Fishman and Olson, 1997; Harvey and Rosenthal, 1998; Frasch, 1999; Schwartz and Olson, 1999; Roman and Weinstein, 2000).

DEVELOPMENT OF THE HEART

Specification of Cardiomyocyte Lineage

In all metazoan animals with a circulatory system, the heart (or its homologue) is a mesodermal organ. Despite the profound differences between different vertebrate species in embryonic morphology and the mechanisms of gastrulation (Tam and Quinlan, 1996), all show a common origin for cardiac progenitors. In vertebrate embryos, aggregates of cardiomyocyte progenitor cells are distinguished from the mesodermal population at or shortly after gastrulation (Fig. 9–1). These clusters of cells are initially bilaterally organized and migrate together to the midline, forming a single linear heart tube comprised of an inner layer, the endocardium, surrounded by an outer layer of myocardium. These two layers are separated by a space containing an extracellular matrix material known as "cardiac jelly." The endocardium becomes continuous with the endothelium of the peripheral vasculature.

The contractile dorsal vessel of *Drosophila* functions in a manner analogous to the vertebrate heart but pumps hemolymph through the interstices of tissues rather than through a vascular system. The *Drosophila* heart is located along the dorsal midline, in contrast to the ventral position of the vertebrate heart, consistent with an overall inversion of embryonic dorsal/ventral orientation between *Drosophila* and vertebrates (Lacalli, 1995; Ferguson, 1996). The *Drosophila* heart lacks an endocardial layer. However, the myogenic cells of the *Drosophila* heart are similar to vertebrate cardiomyocytes at the ultrastructural level and in the protein components of the contractile apparatus. In addition, at the molecular level, the regulatory programs responsible for allocation of cells into the cardiogenic lineage are conserved between flies and vertebrates.

Cardiac precursor cells are fated very early in development to become either endocardial or myocardial cells, atrial or ventricular myocardial cells, or cells of the cardiac conduction system. In the mouse embryo, myocardial and endocardial precursors have been mapped to the same regions of the mouse epiblast (Tam et al., 1997). Retroviral labeling studies in chick (Cohen-Gould and Mikawa, 1996) and cell-lineage tracing in zebrafish embryos (Lee et al., 1994) also indicate that myocardial and endocardial lineages are distinct prior to gastrulation. In embryos of the zebrafish mutant *cloche*, the endocardial layer of the heart and anterior endothelial tissue are absent and initial myocardial differentiation is unaffected (Stainier et al., 1995). The clonal cell line QCE-6, which is derived from the cardiogenic mesoderm of quail embryos, behaves like a lineage precursor of both cell types and differentiates into a mixed population of endocardial and myocardial cells (Eisenberg and Bader, 1995, 1996; Eisenberg et al., 1997). Within the chick embryo myocardial precursors, distinct populations giving rise to atrial and ventricular myocytes have also been distinguished (Yutzey et al., 1995; Yutzey and Bader, 1995). These correspond to posterior and anterior regions of the cardiac mesoderm in the early gastrula, respectively. There is also evidence for the early divergence of atrial and ventricular myocyte lineages in zebrafish (Stainier and Fishman, 1992). Genetic screens for early developmental mutants in zebrafish have identified mutations in which the ventricle is either selectively reduced or absent (Chen et al., 1996; Stainier et al., 1996). Studies of the chick have even identified a further lineage division that separates precursors of the Purkinje fibers from ventricular myocytes (Mikawa and Fischman, 1996).

Early Cardiogenic Signals in *Drosophila*

At the molecular level, the regulatory programs responsible for allocation of cells into the cardiogenic lineage are mostly conserved between flies and vertebrates.

The form of the dorsal vessel in *Drosophila* depends on signals, both stimulatory and inhibitory, from adjacent tissues and germ layers. The *Drosophila* embryo is composed of repeated units. Many of the segmentation genes that determine the periodic subdivision of the ectoderm, such as *wingless* (see Chapter 22) and *hedgehog* (see Chapter 16), are also involved in the subdivision of mesoderm. After gastrulation, the heart precursors form sequentially repeated clusters before coming together to form the heart tube. These clusters are adjacent to the *wingless* expression domain in the ectoderm. Heart progenitors are missing in Drosophila embryos mutant in *wingless* (Wu et al., 1995) and in genes encoding components of the Wingless signaling pathway (*dishevelled, zeste-white3, armadillo,* and *pangolin*) (reviewed in Frasch, 1999). The impact of *hedgehog* on heart formation is less clear, but it appears to inhibit late steps in cardiomyocyte generation (Jagla et al., 1997).

In *Drosophila* embryos, the gene *decapentaplegic* (*dpp*) (see Chapter 24) is required for allocation of mesodermal cells to the cardiac lineage (Frasch, 1995). The bone morphogenetic protein (BMP)-like protein DPP is expressed in ectodermal cells immediately adjacent to the heart-forming region in the dorsal mesoderm, and expansion of the DPP-expressing region in transgenic embryos results in a corresponding expansion of the heart (Frasch, 1995). Within the cardiac lineage, *dpp* promotes the expression of *tinman* (Frasch, 1995), a transcription factor of the NK homeobox protein family. Expression of *tinman* in wild-type *Drosophila* embryos is restricted to the heart and some adjacent musculature, and mutations of *tinman* prevent the formation of these structures (Bodmer, 1993). Maintenance of mesodermal *tinman* expression depends on expression of *dpp* in the adjacent ectoderm (Frasch, 1995) and on expression of the *dpp* receptor *thick-vein* and the *smad4* homologue *medea* in the mesoderm (Xu et al., 1998b).

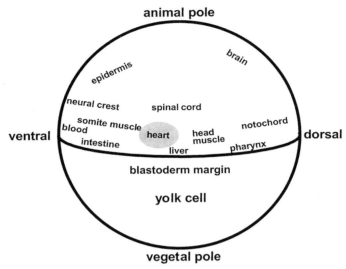

Figure 9–1. Fate map of the zebrafish blastomere; the deep cell layer at gastrula onset of the zebrafish embryo. Ectodermal fates map nearest the animal pole, and mesoderm maps in a broad marginal ring. Heart progenitors (highlighted in gray) arise from the mesodermal blastomere margin.

Tinman directly activates transcription of the *mef2* gene, which encodes a transcription factor that controls myocyte differentiation (Gajewski et al., 1997). Tinman cooperates with zinc-finger transcription factors of the GATA family to activate cardiac gene expression (Durocher et al., 1997); these two classes of cardiac transcription factors also regulate each others' expression (Schwartz and Olson, 1999).

Mutation of the gene *heartless* (Beiman et al., 1996; Gisselbrecht et al., 1996; Shishido et al., 1997), which encodes a fibroblast growth factor (FGF) receptor, leads to a phenotype very similar to that seen in the absence of *tinman*, suggesting that both BMP-type signaling and FGF-type signaling are required for allocation of cells into the *Drosophila* cardiac lineage (Wu et al., 1995).

Alone, *tinman* is not sufficient to drive complete cardiogenesis (Frasch, 1995). Other factors are needed. One of the three known *Drosophila* GATA genes, *pannier*, coregulates heart formation with *tinman*. When either *tinman* or *pannier* is ectopically expressed in the mesoderm, each induces ectopic cardiac gene expression but only to a modest level and in restricted domains. However, when the two genes are co-expressed, the ectopic cardiac gene expression is much stronger and the ectopic expression domains expand to the entire cephalic region and throughout the dorsal and ventral trunk mesoderm (Gajewski et al., 1999).

Early Cardiogenic Signals in Vertebrates

Although similar families of genes are used in *Drosophila* and vertebrates, distinctive mechanisms for fashioning of the heart reflect the accommodation of this organ to very different body forms. The borders of the heart field in vertebrates do not appear to reflect segmental patterns of gene expression. Rather, the posterior border of the heart field can be determined, in part, by inhibitory influences from the anterior end of the notochord. Posterior expansion of Nkx2.5 expression is evident in zebrafish *no tail* mutant embryos, in which the notochord is undifferentiated, and in notochord-ablated zebrafish embryos (Goldstein and Fishman, 1998). Laser ablation studies in the zebrafish show that mesodermal cells anterior to the heart progenitor domain can switch to a cardiac fate after the removal of heart progenitors (Serbedzija et al., 1998). Therefore, in vertebrates, in contrast to *Drosophila*, the neural tube and adjacent notochord are especially potent sources of signals that repress cardiogenesis in neighboring mesoderm (Fig. 9–2). Surgical removal of the anterior neural tube leads to heart formation in head mesenchyme. Coculture of neural tube and notochord with anterior mesodermal explants suppresses the heart-inducing activity of anterior endoderm (Tzahor and Lassar, 2001). Inclusion of

adjacent neural plate and notochord in culture blocks terminal cardiac differentiation, although early markers of cardiac fate are still activated (Climent et al., 1995). The heart-inhibitory factors that emanate from the neural tube appear to be members of the Wnt family (Marvin et al., 2001; Schneider and Mercola, 2001; Tzahor and Lassar, 2001). There are numerous *wnt* genes in vertebrates, many of which are highly expressed in the neural tube (reviewed in Polakis, 2000). Among these, *wnt-3a* and *wnt-8* block cardiogenesis when misexpressed in the anterior heart-forming regions of chick and frog embryos (Schneider and Mercola, 2001; Tzahor and Lassar, 2001).

Wnts (see Chapter 22) bind to the Frizzled family of transmembrane cell surface receptors, activating an intracellular signal-transduction cascade that represses glycogen synthase kinase-3 (GSK-3) (Polakis, 2000). In the absence of Wnt signaling, GSK-3 is active and phosphorylates the cytoplasmic protein β-catenin, resulting in its degradation by ubiquitin-mediated proteolysis. Activation of Wnt signaling inhibits GSK-3, thereby preventing phosphorylation of β-catenin, which is then able to move to the nucleus, where it associates with members of the lymphoid enhancer factor-1/T-cell factor (LEF-1/TCF) family of transcription factors and activates transcription of Wnt target genes. Consistent with the notion that Wnt signaling blocks cardiogenesis, overexpression of GSK-3 in posterior mesoderm activates heart formation in inappropriate sites (Schneider and Mercola, 2001).

The Wnt signaling pathway is blocked by a family of secreted proteins that share homology with the extracellular ligand–binding domain of the Wnt receptor (Schneider and Mercola, 2001). One such antagonist, *crescent*, is expressed in the anterior endoderm. Overexpression of *crescent* in posterior mesoderm represses blood-cell formation and induces formation of beating cardiac muscle cells (Marvin et al., 2001; Schneider and Mercola, 2001). Another secreted Wnt antagonist, *dickkopf*, is expressed in a pattern overlapping that of *crescent* and also suffices for induction of heart formation in posterior mesoderm (Marvin et al., 2001; Schneider and Mercola, 2001).

In the vertebrate embryo, Wnt and BMP (see Chapter 24) signaling pathways influence antagonistically the decision of early mesodermal cells to become heart (Fig. 9–2). Similar to *Drosophila*, BMP signaling plays a permissive role in heart formation. Precardiac mesoderm is in contact with BMP-expressing tissue during the period when

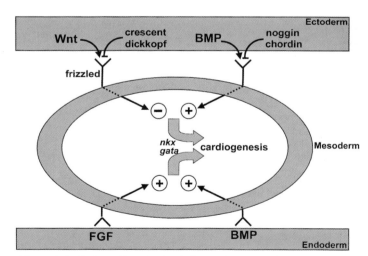

Figure 9–2. Early cardiogenic signals in vertebrates. Cardiogenesis depends on signals, both stimulatory (+) and inhibitory (−), from adjacent tissues and germ layers. Signals from the ectoderm and the endoderm drive anterior mesoderm cells toward a cardiac fate by regulating expression of the transcription factors nkx and gata. Wnt signaling through the frizzled receptor suppresses cardiogenesis in mesodermal tissue. Signals from the endoderm, like crescent and dickkopf, can block Wnt signaling and induce cardiogenesis. Bone morphogenetic protein (BMP) signals from the ectodermal and endodermal germ layers play a permissive role in heart formation, while anterior endoderm-derived fibroblast growth factor (FGF)-signaling has an instructive role in specifying cardiac fate.

it becomes specified to a cardiac fate. Ectoderm overlying the pre-cardiac mesoderm expresses BMP-4 and BMP-7. BMP-2 is expressed in the endoderm, which underlies the precardiac mesoderm (Schultheiss et al., 1997). Differentiation of specified cardiac mesendoderm in explant culture is blocked by exposure to the BMP antagonist noggin.

In addition to its permissive role, endoderm adjacent to the cardiac precursors is a source of instructive signaling capable of respecifying noncardiac mesoderm to a cardiac fate (Nascone and Mercola, 1995; Schultheiss et al., 1995). The heart does not form if anterior endoderm is extirpated from embryos. Explant assays in chick indicate that the anterior endoderm secretes factors that initiate the cardiogenic program in the adjacent mesoderm (Sugi and Lough, 1994; Nascone and Mercola, 1995; Schultheiss et al., 1995). In the explant assay, FGF-4 can substitute for anterior endoderm in maintaining cardiogenesis in isolated anterior mesoderm. However, FGF-4 does not convert posterior mesoderm, which is normally not cardiogenic, to a cardiac fate. Similarly, BMP-2 is incapable of inducing cardiac differentiation in posterior mesoderm. A combination of BMP-2 and FGF-4, however, can convert posterior mesoderm to the cardiac lineage (Lough et al., 1996). These results are consistent with a model in which BMP-2 allocates unspecified mesodermal cells to the cardiac lineage, and FGF-4 promotes the proliferation and survival of these already specified cells (Lough et al., 1996). This model is consistent with the paradigm from *Drosophila*, where both transforming growth factor-β (TGF-β) and FGF signaling pathways (i.e., *decapentaplegic* and *heartless*) are involved in the specification of the cardiomyocyte lineage.

Mutations in the mouse *bmp-2* gene cause mostly early death from defects in the amnion (Zhang and Bradley, 1996). The few mutant embryos that survive this stage display defects in heart morphogenesis: the heart tube forms, but in the exocoelomic space rather than within the pericardial cavity. Mutation of the mouse *bmp-4* (Winnier et al., 1995) or *fgf-4* (see Chapter 32) (Feldman et al., 1995) gene also causes early embryonic lethality. In the zebrafish, mutations in *bmp-2* (*swirl*) abolish *nkx2.5* and *nkx2.7* expression (Kishimoto et al., 1997), and expression of *nkx2.5* and *gata-4* is downregulated in zebrafish embryos with mutant *fgf-8* (*acerebellar*, or *ace*) (Reifers et al., 2000). Introduction of *fgf-8* to *ace* mutant embryos can restore *nkx2.5* and *gata-4* expression (Reifers et al., 2000). In the chick, BMP-2 can induce both *nkx2.5* and *gata-4* expression in the anterior mesoderm (Schultheiss et al., 1997).

Transcription factors of the NKX and GATA families are also essential for vertebrate heart formation. However, no single gene mutation has been described to abrogate selectively and totally the cardiomyogenic fate in vertebrates. This is probably due to a redundancy of several elements in the pathways generating heart cells. For example, five *tinman*-related genes (*nkx2.3*, *nkx2.5*, *nkx2.6*, *nkx2.7*, and *nkx2.8*) are expressed in cardiomyogenic cells (reviewed in Tanaka et al., 1998). Targeted mutation of *nkx2.5* perturbs only late heart maturation (Lints et al., 1993), whereas, at least in frogs, dominant inhibition of several members of this family prevents the appearance of cardiomyogenic cells (Fu et al., 1998; Grow and Krieg, 1998). In *Xenopus* embryos, ectopic expression of *nkx2.5* causes a general increase in heart size (Cleaver et al., 1996). A similar increase in heart size has been reported in zebrafish embryos, which occasionally also show ectopic myosin heavy chain (MHC)-positive cells (Chen and Fishman, 1996).

So far, four zebrafish mutations, *swirl* (*swr*), *one-eyed pinhead* (*oep*), *faust* (*fau*), and *acerebellar* (*ace*), have been reported to affect *nkx2.5* expression in myocardial precursors. These genes encode, respectively, *bmp-2b* (Kishimoto et al., 1997); *oep*, a member of the epidermal growth factor–Cripto/FRL1/Cryptic (EGF-CFC) family that is essential for Nodal signaling (Gritsman et al., 1999); the zinc-finger transcription factor *gata-5* (Reiter et al., 1999); and *fgf-8* (Reifers et al., 2000). Gain-of-function experiments with *gata-5* and *fgf-8* indicate that *gata-5* is required for the initiation of *nkx2.5* expression, whereas *fgf-8* is required for its maintenance (Reiter et al., 1999; Reifers et al., 2000).

There are three *gata* genes in mice that are expressed in precardiac mesoderm and implicated as regulators of cardiogenic differentiation (Jiang et al., 1999). *gata-4*, *gata-5*, and *gata-6* are expressed in distinct, overlapping domains that include the cardiac mesoderm prior to heart tube formation. In later development, their expression becomes restricted to heart, gut, and visceral endoderm, respectively (Laverriere et al., 1994; Jiang and Evans, 1996; Gove et al., 1997; Morrisey et al., 1997). Functional GATA-binding sites have been identified in the promoters of several cardiac-specific genes, including atrial natriuretic peptide (ANP), brain natriuretic peptide (BNP), and MHC. Targeted disruption of the mouse *gata-4* gene does not prevent cardiac differentiation. Rather, mouse embryos mutant in *gata-4* have bilateral heart tubes and a diminished number of cardiomyocytes (Kuo et al., 1997; Molkentin et al., 1997). Differentiated cardiomyocytes form in homozygous mutant embryos, and markers of terminal cardiac differentiation are expressed normally. This likely reflects functional redundancy among the GATA factors, which is supported by increased levels of *gata-6* transcripts in *gata-4* mutant embryos. *gata-4* mutant embryonic stem cells can differentiate into beating myocytes (Narita et al., 1997), indicating that the defect in cardiomyocytes is not autonomous to these cells. Specific depletion of *gata-4* by antisense oligonucleotides blocks dimethyl sulfoxide–induced cardiac differentiation in the mouse embryonic stem cell line P19 (Grepin et al., 1997). Overexpression of *gata-4* in the same cells increases the number of terminally differentiated cells, as well as molecular markers such as Nkx2.5. *gata-5* mutant mouse embryos are viable (Molkentin et al., 1997), and *gata-6* mutant embryos die soon after implantation (Morrisey et al., 1998; Koutsourakis et al., 1999). Overexpression of *gata-6* in *Xenopus* embryos, however, inhibits terminal differentiation within the myocardium (Gove et al., 1997). The zebrafish *gata-5* mutation *faust* demonstrates cardia bifida and diminished cardiac mesoderm (Reiter et al., 1999). Cardia bifida is also noted in two additional zebrafish mutants that lack endodermal tissues, *casanova* (see below) and *one-eye-pinhead* (Alexander and Stainier, 1999). Thus, notochord- and endoderm-derived signals, by coordinating migration and differentiation of cardiac progenitors, are crucial to fashioning of the heart field.

In vertebrates, several genes are expressed throughout the cardiomyocyte population prior to fusion of the linear heart tube (i.e., shortly after allocation of mesodermal cells into the cardiac lineage) and remain expressed thereafter. These genes include *nkx2.5* (a vertebrate homologue of *Drosophila tinman*), *mef-2C* (encoding a transcription factor), *cardiac actin*, and *desmin*, among others (Lyons, 1994). Thus, well before the assembly of sarcomeres, these cells express cardiomyocyte markers and are specified to a cardiogenic fate.

Studies of the *nkx2.5* mutant phenotype have identified several genes that lie downstream of Nkx2.5 in the cardiogenic program. In the mouse, the basic helix-loop-helix (bHLH) transcription factor *ehand* is expressed in a strongly left-dominant fashion within the myocardium as part of a complex embryonic expression pattern (Biben and Harvey, 1997). In the *nkx2.5* mutant, asymmetrical expression of *ehand* is disrupted (Biben and Harvey, 1997), suggesting that *ehand* expression in the myocardium is regulated, either directly or indirectly, by Nkx2.5. In chick embryos, antisense depletion of both *ehand* and *dhand* transcripts, but not either alone, causes arrest of cardiac development immediately prior to looping (Srivastava et al., 1995). In *dhand* knockout mice, heart looping is incomplete and the right ventricle fails to form (Srivastava et al., 1997). Transcript levels for the *gata-4* transcription factor are significantly reduced in the heart but normal in other regions of the embryo. However, several markers of cardiac muscle differentiation appear to be expressed normally in *nkx2.5* mutant mouse embryos. One notable exception is the ventricle-specific myosin light chain gene (*mlc-2v*), expression of which is severely reduced. A short motif in the proximal promoter is necessary for tissue- and stage-specific expression of an *mlc-2v* transgene (Ross et al., 1996). This motif binds cardia-specific ankyrin repeat protein (CARP) (Zou et al., 1997). Expression of CARP is itself abolished in the *nkx2.5* mutant.

Generation and Looping of the Heart Tube

Bilateral cardiogenic precursors move medially to form a single heart tube (Fig. 9–3). The precise mechanism appears to involve cell migration and embryonic folding but with variable contributions de-

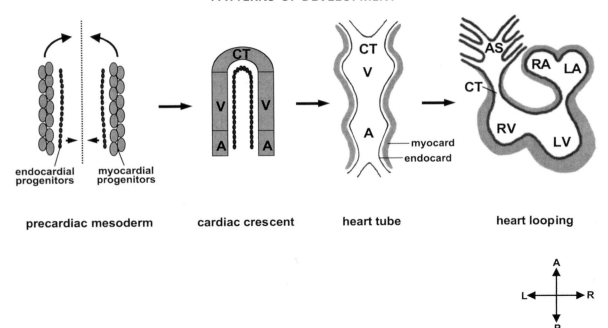

Figure 9–3. From precardiac mesoderm to the four-chamber heart. Aggregates of cardiomyocyte progenitor cells are initially bilaterally organized in the precardiac mesoderm and migrate together to the midline, forming the cardiac crescent, which is already specified to form specific segments (A, atrium; V, ventricle; CT, conotruncus) of the linear heart tube. The single linear heart tube is comprised of an inner layer, the endocardium, surrounded by an outer layer of myocardium. The endocardium becomes continuous with the endothelium of the peripheral vasculature. Each cardiac chamber balloons out from the outer curvature of the looped heart tube in a segmental fashion. AS, aortic sac; CT, conotruncus; RV, right ventricle; LV, left ventricle; RA, right atrium; LA, left atrium.

pending on species. The genes critical to this process are conserved among vertebrates.

The heart tube is organized from the time of its formation, with the rostral end fated to become the outflow region of the mature heart and the caudal end fated to become the inflow region. The early heart tube is demarcated into (from rostral to caudal) the aortic sac, the bulbus cordis (the future cono-truncus and right ventricle), the future left ventricular chamber, the future atrial chamber(s), and the sinus venosus. The aortic sac connects the early heart to the aortic arch arteries, which in turn connect to the dorsal aortae and peripheral circulation. The sinus venosus collects blood from the umbilical, cardinal, and vitelline veins. Therefore, an important step in generation of the primitive chambers of the primitive heart tube, after generation of proper cell fates, is proper anterior/posterior (A/P) placement of the two nascent chambers. This decision is perturbed in the zebrafish *heart and soul* (*has*) mutation. *has* is protein kinase C (PKC) λ, an atypical PKC required for proper A/P polarity during early embryogenesis of *Caenorhabditis elegans* and for epithelial polarity in several vertebrate tissues (Horne-Badovinac et al., 2001; Peterson et al., 2001). As its first evident cardiac effect, the *has* mutation appears to perturb the proper zippering of cardiocytes at the midline along the A/P axis. The consequence is an unusual phenotype, in which a pumping ventricle forms within the atrium (Stainier et al., 1996).

Generation of a single tube requires normal endoderm. In part, this may reflect the need for physical approximation of a substrate for migration. Incision of endoderm in the chick prevents fusion and causes formation of a left and a right heart tube. The endoderm also provides an appropriate matrix for migration. Fibronectin is an important component of this matrix (George et al., 1993, 1997). Fibronectin and MesP1 (a bHLH factor) mutations (Saga et al., 1999) affect the migration of the heart cells but not their early differentiation. Mouse embryos lacking the transcription factor *gata-4* (Kuo et al., 1997; Molkentin et al., 1997) also form laterally paired heart tubes containing differentiated cardiomyocytes. *gata-4* is therefore not necessary for cardiomyocyte specification but, rather, has a role in morphogenic processes that promote the assembly of cardiomyocytes into the heart tube at the ventral midline. In zebrafish, the genes for several cardia

bifida mutations have been isolated (reviewed in Stainier, 2001) and can be separated into distinct classes. As established above, signals derived from the mesoderm play crucial roles in guiding the migration and differentiation of cardiac precursors. Hence, the zebrafish *faust* gene (see above) controls the differentiation of both the endodermal and myocardial cells (Reiter et al., 1999). Mutations such as *casanova*, which encodes a sox-related gene (Alexander et al., 1999; Dickmeis et al., 2001; Kikuchi et al., 2001), or *bonnie-and-clyde*, which encodes a mix-type homedomain protein (Kikuchi et al., 2000), control endoderm formation. These endoderm-interruption mutants result in cardia bifida by abrogation of signals necessary for migration of the precursors to the midline or their differentiation once they have arrived. Zebrafish *miles apart* (Kupperman et al., 2000) encodes a G protein–coupled receptor that binds lysosphingolipids and seems to control migration of the myocardial cells (but not their differentiation); thus, unable to migrate to their central position, the cardiac precursors continue to develop in their lateral positions. The zebrafish mutant *hands off*, which encodes the bHLH transcription factor *hand-2* and is expressed in the migrating myocardial cells (Yelon et al., 2000), controls myocardial, but not endodermal, differentiation. Thus, the logic of these modules is parsed by genetic dissection.

After midline fusion of the endocardial tubes in the higher vertebrates, the single cardiac tube loops to the right (Fig. 9–3). Looping bends the tube such that the future left and right ventricles now assume adjacent left/right positions. Looping requires, but does not appear to be a consequence of, growth per se and, rather, is an active morphogenic process intrinsic to the embryonic heart (Taber et al., 1995).

The direction of cardiac looping is determined by an asymmetrical axial signaling system, which also affects the position of the lungs, liver, spleen, and gut (Capdevila et al., 2000; reviewed in Bisgrove and Yost, 2001). Before organ formation begins, this signaling cascade directs the asymmetrical expression of Sonic hedgehog and Nodal, a member of the TGF family, in the lateral mesoderm. Interpretation of left/right signals is mediated in part by the transcription factor *pitx-2*, which is expressed along the left side of developing organs, including the early heart tube. Mouse models of left/right defects demonstrate absent, bilaterally symmetrical, or reversed *nodal* and *pitx-2* expression.

The bHLH transcription factors *dhand* and *ehand* are expressed in a compartment-specific manner in the early mouse heart (Srivastava et al., 1997). Both genes are expressed throughout the early linear heart tube and remain coexpressed in the conotruncus in later embryos. These two genes represent the earliest markers of chamber-specific regionalization within the heart tube. At the time of looping, *dhand* expression becomes downregulated in the future left ventricle and *ehand* expression is extinguished in the future right ventricle. The ventricular expression patterns of *dhand* and *ehand* are therefore complementary.

In *dhand* mutant mice, heart looping is incomplete and the right ventricle fails to form (Srivastava et al., 1997). The *dhand* gene therefore is required for specification of the future right ventricle. However, it is unclear if the cells that would normally be right ventricular cardiomyocytes are mis-specified in mutant embryos and incorporated into the left ventricle, or if these cells fail to survive. *ehand* has been implicated in left ventricular development. However, early placental defects of *ehand* mutant mice have precluded detailed analysis of its role in the heart (Firulli et al., 1998; Riley et al., 1998).

Interestingly, the chick homologues of *dhand* and *ehand* are expressed in an overlapping pattern, without left/right regionalization. Only suppression of the expression of both genes together generates in chick embryos a phenotype (Srivastava et al., 1995) analogous to the *dhand* mutant phenotype in mice, indicating that left/right specificity may be generated through different regulatory mechanisms in different species.

In zebrafish, embryos mutant in *dhand/hand-2* (*hands off*) have cardiac precursors that express *nkx2.5* but fail to differentiate into myocardial tissue and lack nearly all ventricular tissue. Furthermore, as already outlined above, a null allele of *hands off* blocks the fusion of bilateral heart primordia and results in cardia bifida. This suggests that *dhand* might play a role in heart morphogenesis as well as generation of cardiac cell fate (Yelon et al., 2000).

The MEF-2 class of transcription factors is required for the expression of a number of terminal cardiomyocyte genes, such as *desmin*, *mlc-2v*, and *myosin heavy chain β*. The *Drosophila* analogue DMEF-2 is a direct target for *tinman* (Gajewski et al., 1997). DMEF-2 encodes a MADS (MCM1, Agamous Deficiens, Serum Responsive factor) transcription factor necessary for cardiac and somatic muscle differentiation. By mutational analysis (Bour et al., 1995), *dmef-2* is not required for initial specification of cardiac cells but, rather, for terminal differentiation.

In vertebrates, there are four *MEF-2* genes (identified by the suffixes A–D). *MEF-2C* is the first to be expressed in the heart tube, prior to formation of the linear heart tube, and the other *MEF* genes become active in a spatially overlapping pattern shortly thereafter (Edmondson et al., 1994). In mice, targeted disruption of the *mef-2C* gene interferes with embryonic heart formation (Lin et al., 1997). A linear heart tube still forms in these embryos but subsequently fails to undergo looping and appears to lack the right ventricle. This phenotype is very similar to the *dhand* mutation. Interestingly, *dhand* expression is substantially reduced in *mef-2C* mutants. Therefore, both MEF-2C and dHAND may be required for right ventricular fate. Alternatively, the *mef-2C* mutation could affect an independent aspect of ventricular development, with the reduction of *dhand* expression simply reflecting the absence of right ventricular tissue. Expression of *mef-2B* is highly upregulated in the hearts of *mef-2C* mutant mice, raising the possibility that functional redundancy between MEF-2 family members ameliorates the severity of the *mef-2C* mutant phenotype. The *mef-2B* gene has been mutated in the mouse without cardiovascular consequences (Lin et al., 1997).

Segmentation and Growth of Cardiac Chambers

The structural innovations of the vertebrate heart deliver blood through an oxygenating interface (gills or lungs) and then deliver it at sufficiently high pressure to perfuse the tissues of larger animals. All vertebrates accomplish this task by driving blood in a closed circuit within a distinctive vascular system. At least three elements are essential to

ensure this unidirectional blood flow: the ventricle, a thick-walled high pressure–generating chamber; valves, which prevent backflow of blood; and a pacemaking/conducting system, which coordinates cardiac contraction. Genetic screens in zebrafish and targeted mutations in mice have begun to reveal the genes that generate and pattern these "new" elements of form and function.

Each cardiac chamber differs in its morphological and contractile properties and its patterns of gene expression. Morphological differences between the cardiac chambers are first apparent after the linear heart tube forms and starts to beat, although the underlying molecular events clearly begin much earlier. Embryological studies in chick and zebrafish have implicated retinoic acid (RA) in chamber formation, and genetic studies in mouse have given further support to this model (Xavier-Neto et al., 1999, 2000). Endogenous RA signaling seems to promote atrial development at the expense of ventricular development. Genetic analysis in zebrafish has revealed that the ventricle, the main pumping chamber of the heart, seems to be particularly sensitive to genetic lesions, possibly indicating that atrial fate is more of a default state and that additional molecular events are required to form a ventricle. Specifically, mutations such as *oep*, *faust/gata-5*, *ace/fgf-8*, *hands-off/hand-2*, and *pandora* seem preferentially to affect formation of the ventricle (Reiter et al., 1999; Reifers et al., 2000; Yelon et al., 2000; Keegan et al., 2002).

Chamber Specification and Maturation

Ventricles. In all vertebrates, the early embryonic heart consists of two chambers (Fig. 9–3): an atrium, which remains thin-walled and receives venous return at low pressures; and a ventricle, the myogenic layer which thickens during development by both hyperplasia and hypertrophy. There already are distinctions between atrial and ventricular tissues prior to chamber formation. Atrial and ventricular pathways are genetically separable in the zebrafish. *dHAND* mutation dramatically reduces ventricular size, suggesting more uniform dependence for ventricular formation on this single *dHAND* gene in teleosts than in mammals (Yelon et al., 2000). Zebrafish *pandora* and *lonely atrium* selectively ablate the ventricle (Chen et al., 1996; Stainier et al., 1996; Keegan et al., 2002). *pandora* encodes the elongation factor SPT-6, which promotes transcription in the zebrafish embryo (Keegan et al., 2002). bHLH genes also play an important role in cardiac chamber formation. As discussed above, *dhand/hand-2* is expressed in and responsible for formation of the primitive right ventricle, whereas *ehand/hand-1* is expressed predominantly in the primitive left ventricular segment in mice (Srivastava et al., 1995, 1997), although early placental defects of *ehand* mutant mice precluded detailed analysis of its role in the heart (Firulli et al., 1998; Riley et al., 1998).

Maturation of the ventricular chambers requires several developmental processes: growth and thickening of the outer ventricular chamber wall; elaboration of the trabecular layer within the ventricular lumen; and, in species with two ventricles, growth of the interventricular septum.

Concentric thickening of the ventricle appears to be very sensitive to genetic perturbation in the mouse (reviewed in Fishman and Chien, 1997). A surprising number of mutations in mice give rise to an underdeveloped hypoplastic ventricular chamber, with embryonic lethality. These include the genes that encode the transcription factors N-MYC (Moens et al., 1993), RXR (Moens et al., 1993; Kastner et al., 1994), WT-1 (Kreidberg et al., 1993), and TEF-1 (Chen et al., 1994); the cell surface receptor gp130 (Yoshida et al., 1996); and the G protein–coupled receptor kinase βARK-1 (Jaber et al., 1996). The common phenotype seen in these mutants generally involves failure to expand the compact zone of the ventricular chamber wall, with a corresponding deficiency in the ventricular septum. Usually, both ventricles are affected, although in some there is a trend toward a greater deficiency in one or the other chamber. Even though the hypoplastic phenotype is manifest in the cardiomyocyte population, not all of these genes may function autonomously in the cardiomyocytes.

Heart growth parallels embryonic growth (Gould, 1966). As the embryo size doubles, so does that of the heart. This allometric relationship is critical for most vertebrate embryos, given dependence on blood flow once tissue thickness exceeds 1 mm. Heart mass in the early embryo increases principally by addition of new cells. This process is at least partially regulated by the DNA-stimulated ATPases Reptin and Pontin via the β-catenin pathway (Rottbauer et al., 2002). It is clear late in life, when growth is by hypertrophy, that the work of the heart is an important regulator of growth. In part, this is assayed by calcium-dependent pathways. Early embryonic heart growth may also be calcium-dependent. Loss-of-function mutations in the cardiac L-type calcium channel α-1 subunit in zebrafish *island beat* mutant embryos reduce by half the number of ventricular cells (Rottbauer et al., 2001).

Soon after the ventricular myocardium thickens, the inner wall of the ventricle becomes corrugated. Genetic evidence suggests that the generation of this irregular thickening, termed *trabeculation*, involves signals from the endocardium to the myocardium. Neuregulin growth factors, secreted from the endocardium, and their myocardial receptors Erb-B2 and Erb-B4 are required for the development of trabeculae (Lee et al., 1995). In mice, mutation of the *neuregulin* gene or the genes that encode the neuregulin receptors *erb-B2* and *erb-B4* causes failure to elaborate the trabecular layer and embryonic lethality (Gassmann et al., 1995; Lee et al., 1995; Meyer and Birchmeier, 1995). Lethality might be a direct consequence of the lack of trabecular outgrowth, given the importance of the trabecular layer to cardiac contraction (Sedmera and Thomas, 1996).

Mouse mutants of the *sos-1* gene evidence trabecular disorganization (Wang et al., 1997). The SOS protein is involved in mediating signal transduction between cell surface receptors and RAS and interacts genetically with the EGF receptor in epithelium (Wang et al., 1997). The EGF receptor mutation does not appear to affect the heart. Therefore, it is conceivable that the *sos-1* trabecular phenotype results from an impairment of neuregulin signaling in the myocardium (Threadgill et al., 1995). Defects in ventricular trabeculation have also been observed in mice lacking angiogenic factors, such as vascular endothelial growth factor (Carmeliet et al., 1996) and angiopoietin-1 (Suri et al., 1996), which are expressed in the endocardium. In zebrafish embryos, the *cloche* gene is required for allocation of the endocardial lineage (Stainier et al., 1995). Embryos lacking the *cloche* gene have no endocardium and less ventricular myocyte growth, compatible with an important role for the endocardium in directing myocardial growth.

Atria. There is an atrial-specific program of transcriptional regulation, and several genes (i.e., *ANP*, myosin light chains-1A [*MLC-1A*], *MLC-2A*) are expressed in an atria-specific pattern. However, little is known about the genetics of atrial development. Zebrafish genetic screens have identified loci that are involved in normal atrial chamber maturation (Chen et al., 1996; Stainier et al., 1996), although the molecular nature of these loci has not been determined.

The most clinically relevant aspect of atrial chamber maturation in mammals is the formation of two sequential septae that together form the atrial septum. In the embryo, the atrial septum initially remains open to ensure that oxygenated blood is shunted from the right to the left atrial chamber, where it is then passed to the left ventricle and pumped into the peripheral circulation. The interatrial opening (foramen ovale) normally closes after birth, when the pulmonary system exchanges gases and returns oxygen-rich blood directly to the left atrium.

The orphan nuclear receptor COUP-TFII is expressed in atrial precursors and required for atrial, but not ventricular, growth (Pereira et al., 1999). Retinoid signaling has also been implicated in atrial specification and in regulation of the atrioventricular border along the A/P axis of the heart tube (Dyson et al., 1995).

Some patients heterozygous for mutations in *nkx2.5* have atrial septal defects (Schott et al., 1998), and those heterozygous for mutations in *tbx-5* (Holt–Oram syndrome) have both atrial and ventricular septal defects (Basson et al., 1997; Li et al., 1997).

Atrioventricular Canal and Valve Formation. Appropriate placement and function of cardiac valves is essential for division of the chambers and to ensure the unidirectional flow of blood through the heart. Early in development, septation of the cardiac tube into distinct chambers is achieved through regional swellings of extracellular matrix, known as cardiac cushions, which form the *anlage* of the atrioventricular and ventriculoarterial valves.

Heart valve formation depends on site-specific interactions between endocardium and myocardium. Endocardial cells in both the atrioventricular canal and the outflow tract migrate away from the endocardial surface and form mesenchymal components of the prevalvular structures (cushions) (Brown et al., 1999). These mesenchymal cells differentiate into the fibrous tissue of the valves. The endocardial–mesenchymal transformation seems to be under the influence of myocardia-derived signals, including TGF-1 and TGF-3 (Potts and Runyan, 1989; Potts et al., 1991). Although both *tgf-1* and *tgf-2* are expressed in the mouse heart, only *tgf-2* null embryos have defects in valves and the outflow tract septum (Sanford et al., 1997).

Gene targeting in mice has also revealed important roles for the NF-ATc and Smad6 transcription factors in the formation of cardiac valves. Targeted gene disruption of murine *NF-ATc*, a transcription factor activated and transported to the nucleus by calcineurin-induced dephosphorylation, prevents formation of pulmonary and aortic valves, reflecting a potential role for calcineurin in transduction of signals for valvulogenesis (de la Pompa et al., 1998; Ranger et al., 1998). Smad6, which is implicated in the activation of gene expression in response to TGF signaling, also is expressed in cardiac valve precursors. Disruption of *smad6* leads to abnormally thickened, gelatinous valves in mice (Galvin et al., 2000). In addition, several other mouse mutations affect valve formation, including mutations in the genes that encode versican, hyaluronic acid synthase-2 and vinculin (Mjaatvedt et al., 1998; Xu et al., 1998a; Camenisch et al., 2000).

In the zebrafish, two mutations, *jekyll* and *cloche*, disturb the formation of cardiac cushions and valves (Stainier et al., 1995, 1996; Walsh and Stainier, 2001). For example, *jekyll* mutants are deficient in the initiation of heart valve formation. The *jekyll* mutation disrupts a homologue of Drosophila Sugarless, a uridine 5′-diphosphate-glucose dehydrogenase required for heparan sulfate, chondroitin sulfate, and hyaluronic acid production. The atrioventricular border cells do not differentiate from their neighbors in *jekyll* mutants, suggesting that *jekyll* is required in cell-signaling events that establish a boundary between the atrium and ventricle.

Septation and Remodeling of the Outflow Tract

The advent of air breathing during evolution brought a need for a separate pulmonary circulation and separation of oxygenated from deoxygenated blood. Fish have no septa dividing atria or ventricles. Amphibians have an atrial septum and rely upon streaming of blood within the ventricle to keep oxygenated blood separated from deoxygenated blood. Reptiles, birds, and mammals have both atrial and ventricular septae. The septum of the outflow tract in these species, which separates pulmonary artery from aorta (deoxygenated from oxygenated blood, respectively) is neural crest–derived.

Ventricular and atrial septae are generated by growth from the adjacent myocardial walls. Thus, gene mutations that perturb myocardial wall growth, for example, of *vcam1* and *rxr*, cause septal defects (reviewed in Fishman and Chien, 1997). The BMP1-related gene *tolloid-like 1* (*tll-1*), appears to have a primary role in ventricular septation. In *tll-1* mutant embryos, there is incomplete formation of the muscular inter-ventricular septum while the remainder of the myocardium appears unaffected (Clark et al., 1999). Genes required for development of the atrial septum (*nkx2.5*, *tbx-5*) have been discussed above.

Cardiac neural crest cells migrate from the neural folds into the pharyngeal arches and heart (Fig. 9–3), where they have essential roles in septation of the single outflow of the heart (the truncus arteriosus) into the aorta and pulmonary artery, in the formation of the conotruncal portion of the ventricular septum, and in the formation of cholinergic cardiac ganglia of the parasympathetic plexus (Kirby et al., 1983; Kirby and Waldo, 1995). Removel of these prior to migration causes several defects (Kirby and Waldo, 1990), including persistent truncus arteriosus (PTA), double outlet right ventricle (DORV), tetralogy of Fallot with an overriding aorta, ventricular septal defect, and variable regression of the great arteries. These phenotypes are collectively referred to as the "neural crest ablation model" of defective heart development (for review, see Creazzo et al., 1998). In addition to cardiac outflow tract defects, disturbed development of the neural crest is associated with craniofacial skeletal defects, abnormalities of pharyngeal derivatives (thymus, thyroid, and parathyroids), sensorineural deafness, pigmentation disturbances, and aganglionic bowel (Hirschsprung's disease) (reviewed in Leatherbury and Kirby, 1996).

The most striking functional abnormality of neural crest–ablated chick embryos is decreased ventricular contractility (Tomita et al., 1991; Leatherbury and Kirby, 1996). In addition, these embryos often exhibit incomplete looping of the cardiac tube, altered conotruncal shape, and dilated ventricles. These features exist 48 hours before neural crest cells have migrated into the outflow tract (Waldo et al., 1998). Therefore, there must be a neural crest–related factor, either diffusible or passed from cell to cell, that influences myocardial development. One possible source is pharyngeal endoderm. Migration of the neural crest into the pharyngeal arches might alter signaling in a manner that would facilitate myocardial maturation. In the absence of cardiac neural crest, signaling would be prolonged, to the detriment of the myocardium. It appears that the FGF family is involved in this signaling (Farrell et al., 2001).

Mutations that perturb the cardiac neural crest cause anomalies of the outflow tract (Fig. 9–4; reviewed in Creazzo et al., 1998). Mutations of the genes encoding the signaling peptide *endothelin-1* (ET-1) (Kurihara et al., 1995) and the transcription factor *pax-3* (*Splotch*) (Franz, 1989) result in PTA and/or abnormalities of the aortic arch artery. *ET-1* is expressed in the endothelium of the aortic sac and may be a signal that is interpreted by the arriving neural crest. Mice lacking *et-1* or its G protein–coupled receptor, *ETA*, have post-migratory cardiac neural crest defects, cleft palate, and other craniofacial anomalies reminiscent of 22q11 deletion syndrome in humans (Kurihara et al., 1995; Clouthier et al., 1998). dHAND and eHAND, normally expressed in the neural crest–derived pharyngeal and aortic arches, are downregulated in these structures in mice deficient in *et-1* or *ETA*, suggesting that the HAND proteins are regulated by ET-1 signaling

(Thomas et al., 1998b). Consistent with this notion, *dhand* null mice also exhibit a severe defect in survival of pharyngeal and aortic arch mesenchyme (Srivastava et al., 1997; Thomas et al., 1998b). Neuropilin-1 is downregulated in *dhand* mutants, and targeted mutation of *neuropilin-1* results in a phenotype similar to that of *et-1* mutants. This suggests that ET-1, dHAND, and neuropilin-1 may function in a common pathway regulating neural crest development (Kawasaki et al., 1999; Yamagishi et al., 2000). The *splotch* (Sp2H) mouse mutant manifests a phenotype remarkably similar to cardiac neural crest ablation in the chick embryo. *Splotch* mutation disrupts neural crest development. The *splotch* mutant mouse contains a 32 bp deletion of the DNA-binding transcription factor *pax3* (Goulding et al., 1993). *Pax-3* (see Chapters 59, 61) is a transcription factor that is broadly expressed in the neural tube and in the initial population of migratory neural crest. In the *pax-3* mutant background, initial migration of neural crest cells occurs normally but secondary migration into the aortic sac fails (Conway et al., 1997).

Mutation of the *neurofibromatosis-1 (NF-1)* gene in mice causes DORV (Brannan et al., 1994; Jacks et al., 1994). NF-1 is a negative regulator of cytoplasmic signal transduction through the RAS pathway, suggesting that an external inductive signal is received and transduced through the RA signaling pathway during the course of conotruncal morphogenesis.

Perturbation of the RA signal-transduction pathway causes several types of outflow tract defect. Excess RA during embryonic development causes a spectrum of conotruncal malformations (Shenefelt, 1972; Lammer et al., 1985). Mutation of several of the RA receptor genes (Kastner et al., 1995; Lee et al., 1997) or dietary deficiency of vitamin A (Wilson and Warkany, 1949) results in a similar spectrum of malformations. Mutation of RA receptor genes causes PTA but without a significant degree of thymic, thyroid, or parathyroid hypoplasia (Mendelsohn et al., 1994; Lee et al., 1997). The RA receptor gene mutations may affect secondary migration of crest cells

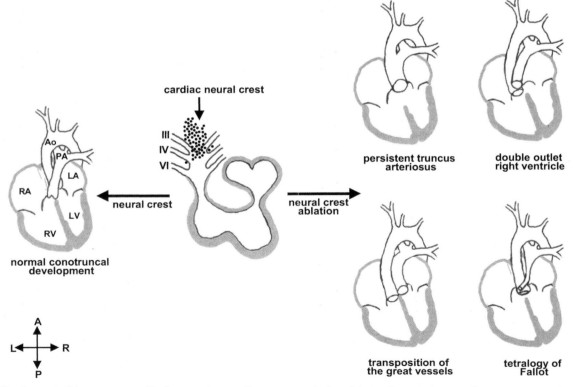

Figure 9–4. Development of the conotruncus. Cardiac neural crest cells populate the bilaterally symmetrical aortic arch arteries (III, IV, and VI) and aortic sac, where they have essential roles in septation of the single outflow of the heart (the truncus arteriosus) into the aorta (Ao) and pulmonary artery (PA) and in the formation of the conotruncal portion of the ventricular septum. Perturbation of the cardiac neural crest pathway causes several outflow tract defects, including persistent truncus arteriosus, double outlet right ventricle, transposition of the great vessels, and tetralogy of Fallot. RA, right atrium; LA, left atrium; RV, right ventricle; LV, left ventricle.

specifically into the aortic sac or their terminal differentiation once there. This is consistent with the temporal requirement for vitamin A during the period when neural crest cells are already resident within the aortic sac (Wilson et al., 1953). Mice lacking combinations of RA receptors (RAR/RXR) also have a variety of outflow tract and aortic arch defects (Gruber et al., 1996).

Endocardium

In the heart, the endocardial layer provides the trabeculation signals and a component of the valves. The first endothelial tubes, including endocardium, are assembled by vasculogenesis, the coalescence of scattered mesodermal angioblasts. At least some of these angioblasts are believed to share a lineage with the first intraembryonic blood cells, both deriving from a common precursor, termed the *hemangioblast* (Choi et al., 1998). Mutation of the *cloche* gene in zebrafish prevents formation of blood and of endothelium, including endocardium (Stainier et al., 1995). The *cloche* mutation appears to affect an early step in formation of the endothelial cell lineage as expression of the endothelia-specific receptor tyrosine kinase genes *flk-1* and *tie* is also affected (Liao et al., 1997).

Epicardium

The epicardium is the outermost layer of the heart. It originates as a population of cells from near the sinus venosus that migrate to cover the developing heart and provide precursors to the coronary arteries. Absence of the cell adhesion molecules α4-integrin (Yang et al., 1995) and VCAM-1 (Gurtner et al., 1995; Kwee et al., 1995) results in failure of the epicardium to adhere to the myocardium and thus the disintegration of the epicardium. VCAM-1 is expressed by the myocardium, and α4-integrin is expressed in the epicardium. VCAM-1 protein physically interacts with α4-integrin. Physical adherence of the epicardium to the myocardium depends on the integrity of the α4-integrin–VCAM-1 interaction. In addition, the myocardium in either mutant background is hypoplastic, suggesting compromised maturation of the compact zone. This may be due to absence of coronary vessels or to lack of trophic signals from epicardium to myocardium.

Conduction System and Pacemaking

The primitive chordate heart contracts in a peristaltic fashion and alternates the primary pacemaker site between its ends. Vertebrate hearts have developed a means to ensure that all parts of a single chamber contract nearly simultaneously. Guarantees of unidirectional flow include use of a single pacemaker site in the atrium, a slowly conducting node at the atrioventricular junction to delay onset of the ventricular beat, rapidly conducting specialized tissue to ensure that all myocytes of each chamber contract in relative synchrony, and valves between the chambers. It appears that the cells of the distal conduction system originate from a subset of ventricular cardiomyocytes that surround the developing coronary arteries and differentiate in response to arterial ET-1 signaling (Hyer et al., 1999).

The development of micro-electrophysiological tools have permitted recording of rhythmicity in developing mice in vivo and revealed the role of several genes in instituting pacemaking and conduction. For instance, mice that lack *Cx40* have first-degree atrio-ventricular block with associated bundle branch block (Simon et al., 1998).

In zebrafish, rhythmicity mutants have been discovered by direct inspection of the developing embryo. Zebrafish *slow mo* causes sinus bradycardia by perturbation of the fast component of I_h, the pacemaker potential (Baker et al., 1997); *reggae* prevents impulse exit from the sinus venosus to the atrium (Stainier et al., 1996); *breakdance* and *hip hop* interfere with conduction between the chambers, so the atrium beats several times before the ventricle does (Chen et al., 1996); *polka* and *tremblor* perturb conduction between cells (Chen et al., 1996; Stainier et al., 1996); and *island beat* causes atrial fibrillation by abolishing the L-type calcium current (Rottbauer et al., 2001). The phenotypes of the zebrafish mutations are evident before there is a fully formed specialized conduction system, so it is likely that they perturb ion channels or gap junctions responsible for generating and transmitting the action potential at the level of the myocytes rather than by affecting the specialized conduction system.

In humans, mutations in the genes for the *kvlqt1*, *minK*, and *herg* potassium channels or the *scn5A* sodium channels cause the long QT syndrome, marked by a propensity to ventricular arrhythmia (reviewed in Vincent, 1998).

VASCULOGENESIS

Vasculogenesis refers to the initial events in vascular growth in which endothelial cell precursors migrate to defined locations, differentiate in situ, and assemble into tubes or solid endothelial cords. The subsequent branching and remodeling of these primitive vessels into a mature vascular network is referred to as *angiogenesis*. We focus here on the molecular pathways involved in vasculogenesis.

Hemangioblast

In vertebrates, the development of the endothelial lineage occurs in very close association with that of the hematopoietic lineage. In the yolk sac mesoderm, blood islands, consisting of an internal core of hematopoietic precursors and an external ring of endothelial precursors, give rise to primitive erythrocytes and the yolk sac vasculature (Risau and Flamme, 1995). Additionally, in the embryo proper, hematopoietic cells first appear as intra-aortic cell clusters at the ventral wall of the dorsal aorta (Jaffredo et al., 1998). These observations implicate a common precursor cell for both the endothelial and hematopoietic lineages, termed the *hemangioblast*. Angiogenic and hematopoietic precursors express common molecular markers. Embryonic stem cells, which express the receptor tyrosine kinase vascular endothelial growth factor receptor-2 (*vegfr-2*, also known as *flk-1*) have the potential to give rise to hematopoietic progenitors, committed angioblasts, or both cell types (Jaffredo et al., 1998). *Vegfr-2* mutant mice lack yolk sac blood islands, do not build organized blood vessels, and show a severe reduction in hematopoietic progenitors (Shalaby et al., 1995). Furthermore, both hematopoietic and endothelial cell precursors express the bHLH transcription factor *scl* (also known as *tal-1*). Scl is required for the development of the blood lineage and for remodeling of the yolk sac vascular plexus (Porcher et al., 1996; Robb et al., 1996; Visvader et al., 1998).

Studies of the *cloche* mutant in zebrafish further support the existence of the hemangioblast (Stainier et al., 1995; Liao et al., 1997). In the zebrafish embryo, blood and trunk endothelial precursors arise from the posterior ventrolateral mesoderm, migrate toward the midline, and form the intermediate cell mass (ICM) between the notochord and endoderm (Roman and Weinstein, 2000). In zebrafish *cloche* mutants, no blood vessels form and markers specific for primitive endothelial cells and hematopoietic cells, including *vegfr-2*, are absent (Liao et al., 1997). Both the endothelial and hematopoietic lesions in *cloche* are cell-autonomous, as revealed by cell-transplantation studies (Stainier et al., 1995; Parker and Stainier, 1999). Overexpression of *scl* in *cloche* mutants partially rescues endothelial and hematopoietic cell defects (Liao et al., 1997). Overexpression of *scl* in wild-type embryos increases both endothelial cell and red blood cell number, indicating that *scl* can drive mesodermal cells toward vascular and hematopoietic fates (Gering et al., 1998).

Angioblast Specification and Tubule Formation

Vasculogenic angioblasts arise from cephalic and trunk paraxial mesoderm and from lateral splanchnopleural mesoderm (Coffin and Poole, 1988; Noden, 1988; Couly et al., 1995; Fouquet et al., 1997; Cleaver and Krieg, 1998). Patterning of the embryonic vasculature depends on extrinsic signals that direct angioblast migration and tube formation (Pardanaud et al., 1987; Noden, 1989; Poole and Coffin, 1989). Angioblasts differentiate in response to FGF signaling (Smith et al., 1989). VEGFR-2 also plays a crucial role in differentiation of mesoderm to endothelial and hematopoietic lineages (Dumont et al., 1995). Targeted disruption of the *vegfr-2* gene in mice results in the development of immature angioblasts, which are incapable of aggregating and forming tubular networks (Shalaby et al., 1995). Furthermore, *vegfr-2*-deficient cells are unable to contribute to the vascular network when placed in wild-type hosts, indicating that *vegfr-2* is required for reception of a signal that directs angioblasts to their proper positions

(Shalaby et al., 1997). The related receptor VEGFR-1 (also known as *flt-1*) is also expressed exclusively in endothelial cells. However, in contrast to *vegfr-2* mutant mice, *vegfr-1* mutants have increased numbers of differentiated angioblasts (Fong et al., 1995, 1999), implicating unique roles for these receptors in vasculogenesis.

Early steps in vasculogenesis are also likely to be controlled by several transcription factors. *Fli* and *ets-1,* members of the Ets-domain family of transcription factors, are expressed early in mesodermal regions that give rise to angioblasts and later transiently in all nascent endothelial cells, indicating a role in transducing an extrinsic signal, which might promote migration and maturation of the endothelial lineage (Vandenbunder et al., 1989; Pardanaud and Dieterlen-Lievre, 1993; Meyer et al., 1995, 1997). *Hex*, a homeobox-containing transcription factor, is transiently expressed in the nascent blood islands of the visceral yolk sac and later in embryonic angioblasts and endocardium (Thomas et al., 1998a). However, in contrast to *fli* and *ets-1, hex* is not expressed until isolated migratory angioblasts reach their final destinations (Newman et al., 1997). Overexpression of *hex* increases the number of endothelial cells that participate in vessel formation but finally leads to vascular disorganization, implicating a role in endothelial cell differentiation, proliferation, and tubule formation (Newman et al., 1997). Early hemangioblast differentiation also requires *vezf, a* zinc-finger transcription factor, expression of which correlates temporally and spatially with the early differentiation of angioblasts into the endothelial cell lineage and the proliferation of endothelial cells (Xiong et al., 1999), *Hox* genes (Boudreau et al., 1997; Belotti et al., 1998), members of the GATA family, and bHLH factors (Elefanty et al., 1997; Robertson et al., 2000). The earliest markers common to endothelial and hematopoietic precursors so far identified are CD31, CD34, and VEGFR-2 (Yamaguchi et al., 1993).

Endoderm and Midline Signaling in Vasculogenesis

Angioblasts arise specifically from endoderm-associated, but not ectoderm-associated, lateral mesoderm (Coffin and Poole, 1988; Noden, 1988). Therefore, primitive endoderm signals might guide mesodermal cells toward an endothelial cell fate. In the mouse, *vegf* is expressed in both embryonic and extraembryonic endoderm (Dumont et al., 1995). In frogs, *vegf* is also expressed in pharyngeal endoderm, which underlies cardiogenic mesoderm, and in the hypochord, a midline structure of endodermal origin (Cleaver et al., 1997, 2000). The hypochord-derived *vegf* transcript encodes a freely diffusible molecule in the form of a homodimer (Houck et al., 1992), indicating that a hypochord-derived VEGF gradient is responsible for patterning the frog dorsal aorta (Cleaver and Krieg, 1998).

An essential role of midline signaling in vasculogenesis is also revealed by several zebrafish mutants. Zebrafish normally form a single midline dorsal aorta just below the notochord. However, mutants that fail to form the notochord do not build the aorta (Fouquet et al., 1997; Sumoy et al., 1997). Dorsal aorta formation can be rescued by clones of wild-type notochord cells (Fouquet et al., 1997). Evidence for an additional midline signal comes from zebrafish mutants with U-shaped somites (van Eeden et al., 1996). The genes responsible for two of these mutations, *you too* (*syu*) and *you too* (*yot*), have been identified as sonic hedgehog (*shh*) and *gli-2*, a hedgehog response gene (Schauerte et al., 1998; Karlstrom et al., 1999). Although *syu* and *yot* form a normal notochord, they fail to form the midline aorta (van Eeden et al., 1996), suggesting that SHH, which is produced by the notochord and floorplate, plays an essential role in patterning the dorsal aorta. Interestingly, VEGF is expressed in the ventromedial part of the somites of frogs, zebrafish, mice, and birds (Cleaver et al., 1997; Aitkenhead et al., 1998; Liang et al., 1998; Miquerol et al., 1999), raising the possibility that somite-derived VEGF might relay a midline SHH signal to angioblasts (Roman and Weinstein, 2000).

Angiogenic Remodeling and Sprouting

Once the basic pattern of major vessels and plexuses is formed by vasculogenesis, further maturation of the vascular network occurs by angiogenic sprouting of new vessels from preexisting vessels and by angiogenic remodeling of the plexuses into mature networks of large and small vessels (reviewed in Flamme et al., 1997; Roman and Weinstein, 2000).

As in vasculogenesis, VEGF and VEGFR-2 are also important in angiogenesis. VEGF and VEGFR-2 are expressed at sites of active angiogenesis during embryogenesis and adulthood (reviewed in Achen and Stacker, 1998). VEGF induces endothelial cell proliferation and capillary sprouting. VEGF can bind to Neuropilin-1, a receptor for the collapsin/semaphorin family of secreted proteins (He and Tessier-Lavigne, 1997). Binding of VEGF to Neuropilin-1 potentiates its binding to VEGFR-2 (Soker et al., 1998). Overexpression of *neuropilin-1* increases blood vessel formation (Kitsukawa et al., 1995). By contrast, targeted inactivation of *neuropilin-1* results in insufficient vascularization of the neural tube and disorganization of the yolk sac vascular plexus (Kawasaki et al., 1999). In addition, targeted inactivation of *vegfr-3*, also known as *flt-4*, impairs remodeling of the yolk sac and perineural vascular plexuses in mouse embryos (Dumont et al., 1998), indicating a role for VEGFR-3 in angiogenic remodeling.

Angioblasts and endothelial cells also express two members of another class of receptor tyrosin kinases, *tie-1* and *tie-2* (Dumont et al., 1995). Targeted disruption of the *tie* genes in mice, either singly (Dumont et al., 1994; Puri et al., 1995; Sato et al., 1995) or in combination (Puri et al., 1999), revealed that neither is required for assembly of the primitive vascular network. However, *tie-2* seems to be required for endocardial morphogenesis and angiogenic remodeling (Sato et al., 1995), whereas *tie-1* seems to play a role in maintenance of the structural integrity of the microvasculature (Puri et al., 1995; Sato et al., 1995). Several angiopoeitins are known ligands for TIE-2: angiopoietin (ANG)-1 and ANG-4, which promote receptor autophosphorylation, and ANG-2 and ANG-3, which antagonize the effects of ANG-1 and ANG-4 (Davis et al., 1996; Maisonpierre et al., 1997; Valenzuela et al., 1999). Targeted inactivation of *ang-1* results in defects similar to those seen in *tie-2*-deficient embryos, including endocardial malformations and impaired remodeling of the yolk sac and of perineural vascular plexuses (Suri et al., 1996).

A third family of receptor tyrosine kinases and their ligands, the Eph-B receptors and ephrin-B ligands, also seems to play an important role in embryonic angiogenesis (Daniel et al., 1996). Targeted inactivation of ephrin-B2 or Eph-B4 results in failure of remodeling of both the perineural and yolk sac vascular plexuses (Wang et al., 1998; Gerety et al., 1999). A similar phenotype is observed in mice mutant in both Eph-B2 and Eph-B3 (Adams et al., 1999).

Arterial versus Venous Identity

Until recently, it was assumed that acquisition of arterial or venous identity is a relatively late event in embryonic vessel formation and is largely determined by blood flow. However, accumulating evidence suggests that arterial and venous endothelial cells have distinct molecular identities prior to patent vessel formation. Lineage tracking in zebrafish embryos shows that angioblast precursors for the trunk artery and vein are spatially mixed in the lateral posterior mesoderm. Progeny of each angioblast, however, are restricted to one of the vessels (Zhong et al., 2001).

Within the vasculature, prior to the onset of circulation, ephrin-B2 is expressed solely by arterial cells and Eph-B4 is expressed almost exclusively by venous cells (Wang et al., 1998; Gerety et al., 1999). Targeted inactivation of ephrin-B2 inhibits remodeling of both the arterial and venous components of the perineural and yolk sac vascular plexuses and disrupts formation of vessels, which connect the intersomitic arteries to the intersomitic veins (Wang et al., 1998). Eph-B4 mutant mice show essentially the same phenotype as ephrin-B2 mutant mice (Gerety et al., 1999). These results suggest that reciprocal signaling between ephrin-B2 and Eph-B4 is required for angiogenic remodeling at sites of arterial–venous connections. Interestingly, ephrin-B2 mutant mice retain appropriate arterial expression of a knocked-in transgene, so ephrin-B2–Eph-B4 interaction cannot be proximally responsible for determining arterial or venous identity.

In zebrafish, components in the Notch signaling pathway (see Chapter 39) specifically identify arterial endothelial cells before blood circulation is established (Lawson et al., 2001). DeltaC, a ligand for the Notch family of receptors that controls binary cell fate decisions (reviewed in Artavanis-Tsakonas et al., 1999), is expressed in endothelial cells that contribute to the rudiment of the dorsal aorta but not

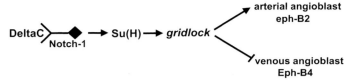

Figure 9–5. The notch-gridlock pathway regulates vasculogenesis by adjudicating an arterial versus venous cell fate decision. DeltaC, a ligand for the Notch family of receptors, activates suppressor of hairless (Su[H]), an intermediary in the Notch signaling pathway. Su(H) activates transcription of gridlock, a member of the Hairy/Enhancer-of-split related family of basic helix-loop-helix proteins, which act as transcriptional repressors. Gridlock drives preangioblast toward an arterial fate and suppresses venous angioblast development.

the posterior cardinal vein prior to the onset of blood flow (Smithers et al., 2000). Therefore, lateral inhibition mediated by Notch ligand–Notch interactions may play an early role in defining arterial endothelial cells. *notch-1*, *notch-4*, and *jagged-1*, another Notch ligand, also known as *serrate-1*, are also expressed in endothelial cells of chick and mouse, although expression restricted to either arterial or venous cells was not observed (Reaume et al., 1992; Myat et al., 1996; Uyttendaele et al., 1996). Further support for the role of the Notch pathway in the definition of arterial and venous populations comes from studies of the *gridlock* mutant in zebrafish (Fig. 9–5). *gridlock* mutant embryos show a localized tissue defect at the junction between the paired lateral dorsal aortae and the single medial dorsal aorta (Weinstein et al., 1995). Positional cloning of the *gridlock* gene revealed it to be a member of the Hairy/Enhancer-of-split-related family of bHLH proteins (Zhong et al., 2000), transcriptional repressors that are downstream effectors of Notch signaling (Kokubo et al., 1999). Three related genes, *hrt1–3*, have been identified in mouse (Nakagawa et al., 1999). *gridlock* is expressed as early as the 10-somite stage in bilateral mesodermal stripes that give rise to angioblasts. *gridlock*-positive cells then migrate medially, contributing only to the dorsal aorta and not the posterior cardinal vein (Zhong et al., 2000). Therefore, similar to ephrin-B2 and deltaC, *gridlock* expression distinguishes arterial from venous endothelial cells prior to the onset of circulation. In zebrafish, graded reduction of *gridlock* expression, by mutation or morpholino antisense oligonucleotides, progressively ablates regions of the dorsal artery and expands contiguous regions of the vein, preceded by an increase in expression of the venous marker EphB-4 receptor and diminution of expression of the arterial marker ephrin-B2.

Interference with *notch* signaling, by blocking *suppressor of hairless*, similarly reduces the artery and increases the vein in zebrafish, indicating that *gridlock* acts downstream of Notch signaling. Conversely, ectopic activation of Notch signaling leads to repression of venous cell fate (Lawson et al., 2001). Thus, a *notch–gridlock* pathway controls assembly of the first embryonic artery, apparently by adjudicating an arterial versus venous cell fate decision (Zhong et al., 2001).

REFERENCES

Achen MG, Stacker SA (1998). The vascular endothelial growth factor family; proteins which guide the development of the vasculature. *Int J Exp Pathol* 79: 255–265.

Adams RH, Wilkinson GA, Weiss C, Diella F, Gale NW, Deutsch U, Risau W, Klein R (1999). Roles of ephrinB ligands and EphB receptors in cardiovascular development: demarcation of arterial/venous domains, vascular morphogenesis, and sprouting angiogenesis. *Genes Dev* 13: 295–306.

Aitkenhead M, Christ B, Eichmann A, Feucht M, Wilson DJ, Wilting J (1998). Paracrine and autocrine regulation of vascular endothelial growth factor during tissue differentiation in the quail. *Dev Dyn* 212: 1–13.

Alexander J, Stainier DY (1999). A molecular pathway leading to endoderm formation in zebrafish. *Curr Biol* 9: 1147–1157.

Alexander J, Rothenberg M, Henry GL, Stainier DY (1999). Casanova plays an early and essential role in endoderm formation in zebrafish. *Dev Biol* 215: 343–357.

Artavanis-Tsakonas S, Rand MD, Lake RJ (1999). Notch signaling: cell fate control and signal integration in development. *Science* 284: 770–776.

Baker K, Warren KS, Yellen G, Fishman MC (1997). Defective "pacemaker" current (Ih) in a zebrafish mutant with a slow heart rate. *Proc Natl Acad Sci USA* 94: 4554–4559.

Basson CT, Bachinsky DR, Lin RC, Levi T, Elkins JA, Soults J, Grayzel D, Kroumpouzou E, Traill TA, Leblanc-Straceski J, et al. (1997). Mutations in human TBX5 [corrected] cause limb and cardiac malformation in Holt-Oram syndrome. *Nat Genet* 15: 30–35.

Beiman M, Shilo BZ, Volk T (1996). Heartless, a *Drosophila* FGF receptor homolog, is essential for cell migration and establishment of several mesodermal lineages. *Genes Dev* 10: 2993–3002.

Belotti D, Clausse N, Flagiello D, Alami Y, Daukandt M, Deroanne C, Malfoy B, Boncinelli E, Faiella A, Castronovo V (1998). Expression and modulation of homeobox genes from cluster B in endothelial cells. *Lab Invest* 78: 1291–1299.

Biben C, Harvey RP (1997). Homeodomain factor Nkx2-5 controls left/right asymmetric expression of bHLH gene *eHand* during murine heart development. *Genes Dev* 11: 1357–1369.

Bisgrove BW, Yost HJ (2001). Classification of left–right patterning defects in zebrafish, mice, and humans. *Am J Med Genet* 101: 315–323.

Bodmer R (1993). The gene *tinman* is required for specification of the heart and visceral muscles in *Drosophila*. *Development* 118: 719–729.

Boudreau N, Andrews C, Srebrow A, Ravanpay A, Cheresh DA (1997). Induction of the angiogenic phenotype by HoxD3. *J Cell Biol* 139: 257–264.

Bour BA, O'Brien MA, Lockwood WL, Goldstein ES, Bodmer R, Taghert PH, Abmayr SM, Nguyen HT (1995). *Drosophila* MEF2, a transcription factor that is essential for myogenesis. *Genes Dev* 9: 730–741.

Brannan CI, Perkins AS, Vogel KS, Ratner N, Nordlund ML, Reid SW, Buchberg AM, Jenkins NA, Parada LF, Copeland NG (1994). Targeted disruption of the neurofibromatosis type-1 gene leads to developmental abnormalities in heart and various neural crest–derived tissues. *Genes Dev* 8: 1019–1029.

Brown CB, Boyer AS, Runyan RB, Barnett JV (1999). Requirement of type III TGF-beta receptor for endocardial cell transformation in the heart. *Science* 283: 2080–2082.

Camenisch TD, Spicer AP, Brehm-Gibson T, Biesterfeldt J, Augustine ML, Calabro A Jr, Kubalak S, Klewer SE, McDonald JA (2000). Disruption of hyaluronan synthase-2 abrogates normal cardiac morphogenesis and hyaluronan-mediated transformation of epithelium to mesenchyme. *J Clin Invest* 106: 349–360.

Capdevila J, Vogan KJ, Tabin CJ, Izpisua Belmonte JC (2000). Mechanisms of left–right determination in vertebrates. *Cell* 101: 9–21.

Carmeliet P, Ferreira V, Breier G, Pollefeyt S, Kieckens L, Gertsenstein M, Fahrig M, Vandenhoeck A, Harpal K, Eberhardt C, et al. (1996). Abnormal blood vessel development and lethality in embryos lacking a single VEGF allele. *Nature* 380: 435–439.

Chen JN, Fishman MC (1996). Zebrafish tinman homolog demarcates the heart field and initiates myocardial differentiation. *Development* 122: 3809–3816.

Chen JN, Fishman MC (2000). Genetics of heart development. *Trends Genet* 16: 383–388.

Chen Z, Friedrich GA, Soriano P (1994). Transcriptional enhancer factor 1 disruption by a retroviral gene trap leads to heart defects and embryonic lethality in mice. *Genes Dev* 8: 2293–2301.

Chen JN, Haffter P, Odenthal J, Vogelsang E, Brand M, van Eeden FJ, Furutani-Seiki M, Granato M, Hammerschmidt M, Heisenberg CP, et al. (1996). Mutations affecting the cardiovascular system and other internal organs in zebrafish. *Development* 123: 293–302.

Choi K, Kennedy M, Kazarov A, Papadimitriou JC, Keller G (1998). A common precursor for hematopoietic and endothelial cells. *Development* 125: 725–732.

Clark TG, Conway SJ, Scott IC, Labosky PA, Winnier G, Bundy J, Hogan BL, Greenspan DS (1999). The mammalian Tolloid-like 1 gene, *Tll1*, is necessary for normal septation and positioning of the heart. *Development* 126: 2631–2642.

Cleaver O, Krieg PA (1998). VEGF mediates angioblast migration during development of the dorsal aorta in *Xenopus*. *Development* 125: 3905–3914.

Cleaver OB, Patterson KD, Krieg PA (1996). Overexpression of the tinman-related genes *XNkx-2.5* and *XNkx-2.3* in *Xenopus* embryos results in myocardial hyperplasia. *Development* 122: 3549–3556.

Cleaver O, Tonissen KF, Saha MS, Krieg PA (1997). Neovascularization of the *Xenopus* embryo. *Dev Dyn* 210: 66–77.

Cleaver O, Seufert DW, Krieg PA (2000). Endoderm patterning by the notochord: development of the hypochord in *Xenopus*. *Development* 127: 869–879.

Climent S, Sarasa M, Villar JM, Murillo-Ferrol NL (1995). Neurogenic cells inhibit the differentiation of cardiogenic cells. *Dev Biol* 171: 130–148.

Clouthier DE, Hosoda K, Richardson JA, Williams SC, Yanagisawa H, Kuwaki T, Kumada M, Hammer RE, Yanagisawa M (1998). Cranial and cardiac neural crest defects in endothelin-A receptor-deficient mice. *Development* 125: 813–824.

Coffin JD, Poole TJ (1988). Embryonic vascular development: immunohistochemical identification of the origin and subsequent morphogenesis of the major vessel primordia in quail embryos. *Development* 102: 735–748.

Cohen-Gould L, Mikawa T (1996). The fate diversity of mesodermal cells within the heart field during chicken early embryogenesis. *Dev Biol* 177: 265–273.

Conway SJ, Henderson DJ, Copp AJ (1997). Pax3 is required for cardiac neural crest migration in the mouse: evidence from the splotch (Sp2H) mutant. *Development* 124: 505–514.

Couly G, Coltey P, Eichmann A, Le Douarin NM (1995). The angiogenic potentials of the cephalic mesoderm and the origin of brain and head blood vessels. *Mech Dev* 53: 97–112.

Creazzo TL, Godt RE, Leatherbury L, Conway SJ, Kirby ML (1998). Role of cardiac neural crest cells in cardiovascular development. *Annu Rev Physiol* 60: 267–286.

Daniel TO, Stein E, Cerretti DP, St John PL, Robert B, Abrahamson DR (1996). ELK and LERK-2 in developing kidney and microvascular endothelial assembly. *Kidney Int Suppl* 57: S73–S81.

Davis S, Aldrich TH, Jones PF, Acheson A, Compton DL, Jain V, Ryan TE, Bruno J, Radziejewski C, Maisonpierre PC, et al. (1996). Isolation of angiopoietin-1, a ligand for the TIE2 receptor, by secretion-trap expression cloning. *Cell* 87: 1161–1169.

de la Pompa JL, Timmerman LA, Takimoto H, Yoshida H, Elia AJ, Samper E, Potter J, Wakeham A, Marengere L, Langille BL, et al. (1998). Role of the NF-ATc transcription factor in morphogenesis of cardiac valves and septum. *Nature* 392: 182–186.

Dickmeis T, Mourrain P, Saint-Etienne L, Fischer N, Aanstad P, Clark M, Strahle U, Rosa F (2001). A crucial component of the endoderm formation pathway, CASANOVA, is encoded by a novel sox-related gene. *Genes Dev* 15: 1487–1492.

Dumont DJ, Gradwohl G, Fong GH, Puri MC, Gertsenstein M, Auerbach A, Breitman

ML (1994). Dominant-negative and targeted null mutations in the endothelial receptor tyrosine kinase, tek, reveal a critical role in vasculogenesis of the embryo. *Genes Dev* 8: 1897–1909.

Dumont DJ, Fong GH, Puri MC, Gradwohl G, Alitalo K, Breitman ML (1995). Vascularization of the mouse embryo: a study of flk-1, tek, tie, and vascular endothelial growth factor expression during development. *Dev Dyn* 203: 80–92.

Dumont DJ, Jussila L, Taipale J, Lymboussaki A, Mustonen T, Pajusola K, Breitman M, Alitalo K (1998). Cardiovascular failure in mouse embryos deficient in VEGF receptor-3. *Science* 282: 946–949.

Durocher D, Charron F, Warren R, Schwartz RJ, Nemer M (1997). The cardiac transcription factors Nkx2-5 and GATA-4 are mutual cofactors. *EMBO J* 16: 5687–5696.

Dyson E, Sucov HM, Kubalak SW, Schmid-Schonbein GW, DeLano FA, Evans RM, Ross J Jr, Chien KR (1995). Atrial-like phenotype is associated with embryonic ventricular failure in retinoid X receptor alpha$^{-/-}$ mice. *Proc Natl Acad Sci USA* 92: 7386–7390.

Edmondson DG, Lyons GE, Martin JF, Olson EN (1994). *Mef2* gene expression marks the cardiac and skeletal muscle lineages during mouse embryogenesis. *Development* 120: 1251–1263.

Eisenberg CA, Bader D (1995). QCE-6: a clonal cell line with cardiac myogenic and endothelial cell potentials. *Dev Biol* 167: 469–481.

Eisenberg CA, Bader DM (1996). Establishment of the mesodermal cell line QCE-6. A model system for cardiac cell differentiation. *Circ Res* 78: 205–216.

Eisenberg CA, Gourdie RG, Eisenberg LM (1997). Wnt-11 is expressed in early avian mesoderm and required for the differentiation of the quail mesoderm cell line QCE-6. *Development* 124: 525–536.

Elefanty AG, Robb L, Birner R, Begley CG (1997). Hematopoietic-specific genes are not induced during in vitro differentiation of scl-null embryonic stem cells. *Blood* 90: 1435–1447.

Farrell MJ, Burch JL, Wallis K, Rowley L, Kumiski D, Stadt H, Godt RE, Creazzo TL, Kirby ML (2001). FGF-8 in the ventral pharynx alters development of myocardial calcium transients after neural crest ablation. *J Clin Invest* 107: 1509–1517.

Feldman B, Poueymirou W, Papaioannou VE, DeChiara TM, Goldfarb M (1995). Requirement of FGF-4 for postimplantation mouse development. *Science* 267: 246–249.

Ferguson EL (1996). Conservation of dorsal–ventral patterning in arthropods and chordates. *Curr Opin Genet Dev* 6: 424–431.

Firulli AB, McFadden DG, Lin Q, Srivastava D, Olson EN (1998). Heart and extra-embryonic mesodermal defects in mouse embryos lacking the bHLH transcription factor Hand1. *Nat Genet* 18: 266–270.

Fishman MC, Chien KR (1997). Fashioning the vertebrate heart: earliest embryonic decisions. *Development* 124: 2099–2117.

Fishman MC, Olson EN (1997). Parsing the heart: genetic modules for organ assembly. *Cell* 91: 153–156.

Flamme I, Frolich T, Risau W (1997). Molecular mechanisms of vasculogenesis and embryonic angiogenesis. *J Cell Physiol* 173: 206–210.

Fong GH, Rossant J, Gertsenstein M, Breitman ML (1995). Role of the Flt-1 receptor tyrosine kinase in regulating the assembly of vascular endothelium. *Nature* 376: 66–70.

Fong GH, Zhang L, Bryce DM, Peng J (1999). Increased hemangioblast commitment, not vascular disorganization, is the primary defect in flt-1 knock-out mice. *Development* 126: 3015–3025.

Fouquet B, Weinstein BM, Serluca FC, Fishman MC (1997). Vessel patterning in the embryo of the zebrafish: guidance by notochord. *Dev Biol* 183: 37–48.

Franz T (1989). Persistent truncus arteriosus in the Splotch mutant mouse. *Anat Embryol* 180: 457–464.

Frasch M (1995). Induction of visceral and cardiac mesoderm by ectodermal Dpp in the early *Drosophila* embryo. *Nature* 374: 464–467.

Frasch M (1999). Intersecting signalling and transcriptional pathways in *Drosophila* heart specification. *Semin Cell Dev Biol* 10: 61–71.

Fu Y, Yan W, Mohun TJ, Evans SM (1998). Vertebrate tinman homologues XNkx2-3 and XNkx2-5 are required for heart formation in a functionally redundant manner. *Development* 125: 4439–4449.

Gajewski K, Kim Y, Lee YM, Olson EN, Schulz RA (1997). D-mef2 is a target for Tinman activation during *Drosophila* heart development. *EMBO J* 16: 515–522.

Gajewski K, Fossett N, Molkentin JD, Schulz RA (1999). The zinc finger proteins Pannier and GATA4 function as cardiogenic factors in *Drosophila*. *Development* 126: 5679–5688.

Galvin KM, Donovan MJ, Lynch CA, Meyer RI, Paul RJ, Lorenz JN, Fairchild-Huntress V, Dixon KL, Dunmore JH, Gimbrone MA Jr, Falb D, Huszar D (2000). A role for smad6 in development and homeostasis of the cardiovascular system. *Nat Genet* 24: 171–174.

Gassmann M, Casagranda F, Orioli D, Simon H, Lai C, Klein R, Lemke G (1995). Aberrant neural and cardiac development in mice lacking the ErbB4 neuregulin receptor. *Nature* 378: 390–394.

George EL, Georges-Labouesse EN, Patel-King RS, Rayburn H, Hynes RO (1993). Defects in mesoderm, neural tube and vascular development in mouse embryos lacking fibronectin. *Development* 119: 1079–1091.

George EL, Baldwin HS, Hynes RO (1997). Fibronectins are essential for heart and blood vessel morphogenesis but are dispensable for initial specification of precursor cells. *Blood* 90: 3073–3081.

Gerety SS, Wang HU, Chen ZF, Anderson DJ (1999). Symmetrical mutant phenotypes of the receptor EphB4 and its specific transmembrane ligand ephrin-B2 in cardiovascular development. *Mol Cell* 4: 403–414.

Gering M, Rodaway AR, Gottgens B, Patient RK, Green AR (1998). The *SCL* gene specifies haemangioblast development from early mesoderm. *EMBO J* 17: 4029–4045.

Gisselbrecht S, Skeath JB, Doe CQ, Michelson AM (1996). heartless encodes a fibroblast growth factor receptor (DFR1/DFGF-R2) involved in the directional migration of early mesodermal cells in the *Drosophila* embryo. *Genes Dev* 10: 3003–3017.

Goldstein AM, Fishman MC (1998). Notochord regulates cardiac lineage in zebrafish embryos. *Dev Biol* 201: 247–252.

Gould SJ (1966). Allometry and size in ontogeny and phylogeny. *Biol Rev Camb Philos Soc* 41: 587–640.

Goulding M, Sterrer S, Fleming J, Balling R, Nadeau J, Moore KJ, Brown SD, Steel KP, Gruss P (1993). Analysis of the *Pax-3* gene in the mouse mutant splotch. *Genomics* 17: 355–363.

Gove C, Walmsley M, Nijjar S, Bertwistle D, Guille M, Partington G, Bomford A, Patient R (1997). Over-expression of GATA-6 in *Xenopus* embryos blocks differentiation of heart precursors. *EMBO J* 16: 355–368.

Grepin C, Nemer G, Nemer M (1997). Enhanced cardiogenesis in embryonic stem cells overexpressing the GATA-4 transcription factor. *Development* 124: 2387–2395.

Gritsman K, Zhang J, Cheng S, Heckscher E, Talbot WS, Schier AF (1999). The EGF-CFC protein one-eyed pinhead is essential for nodal signaling. *Cell* 97: 121–132.

Grow MW, Krieg PA (1998). Tinman function is essential for vertebrate heart development: elimination of cardiac differentiation by dominant inhibitory mutants of the tinman-related genes, *XNkx2-3* and *XNkx2-5*. *Dev Biol* 204: 187–196.

Gruber PJ, Kubalak SW, Pexieder T, Sucov HM, Evans RM, Chien KR (1996). RXR alpha deficiency confers genetic susceptibility for aortic sac, conotruncal, atrioventricular cushion, and ventricular muscle defects in mice. *J Clin Invest* 98: 1332–1343.

Gurtner GC, Davis V, Li H, McCoy MJ, Sharpe A, Cybulsky MI (1995). Targeted disruption of the murine *VCAM1* gene: essential role of VCAM-1 in chorioallantoic fusion and placentation. *Genes Dev* 9: 1–14.

Harvey RP, Rosenthal N (1998). *Heart Development*. Academic Press, San Diego.

He Z, Tessier-Lavigne M (1997). Neuropilin is a receptor for the axonal chemorepellent Semaphorin III. *Cell* 90: 739–751.

Horne-Badovinac S, Lin D, Waldron S, Schwarz M, Mbamalu G, Pawson T, Jan Y, Stainier DY, Abdelilah-Seyfried S (2001). Positional cloning of heart and soul reveals multiple roles for PKC lambda in zebrafish organogenesis. *Curr Biol* 11: 1492–1502.

Houck KA, Leung DW, Rowland AM, Winer J, Ferrara N (1992). Dual regulation of vascular endothelial growth factor bioavailability by genetic and proteolytic mechanisms. *J Biol Chem* 267: 26031–26037.

Hyer J, Johansen M, Prasad A, Wessels A, Kirby ML, Gourdie RG, Mikawa T (1999). Induction of Purkinje fiber differentiation by coronary arterialization. *Proc Natl Acad Sci USA* 96: 13214–13218.

Jaber M, Koch WJ, Rockman H, Smith B, Bond RA, Sulik KK, Ross J Jr, Lefkowitz RJ, Caron MG, Giros B (1996). Essential role of beta-adrenergic receptor kinase 1 in cardiac development and function. *Proc Natl Acad Sci USA* 93: 12974–12979.

Jacks T, Shih TS, Schmitt EM, Bronson RT, Bernards A, Weinberg RA (1994). Tumour predisposition in mice heterozygous for a targeted mutation in Nf1. *Nat Genet* 7: 353–361.

Jaffredo T, Gautier R, Eichmann A, Dieterlen-Lievre F (1998). Intraaortic hemopoietic cells are derived from endothelial cells during ontogeny. *Development* 125: 4575–4583.

Jagla K, Frasch M, Jagla T, Dretzen G, Bellard F, Bellard M (1997). ladybird, a new component of the cardiogenic pathway in *Drosophila* required for diversification of heart precursors. *Development* 124: 3471–3479.

Jiang Y, Evans T (1996). The *Xenopus GATA-4/5/6* genes are associated with cardiac specification and can regulate cardiac-specific transcription during embryogenesis. *Dev Biol* 174: 258–270.

Jiang Y, Drysdale TA, Evans T (1999). A role for GATA-4/5/6 in the regulation of Nkx2.5 expression with implications for patterning of the precardiac field. *Dev Biol* 216: 57–71.

Karlstrom RO, Talbot WS, Schier AF (1999). Comparative synteny cloning of zebrafish you-too: mutations in the Hedgehog target gli2 affect ventral forebrain patterning. *Genes Dev* 13: 388–393.

Kastner P, Grondona JM, Mark M, Gansmuller A, LeMeur M, Decimo D, Vonesch JL, Dolle P, Chambon P (1994). Genetic analysis of RXR alpha developmental function: convergence of RXR and RAR signaling pathways in heart and eye morphogenesis. *Cell* 78: 987–1003.

Kastner P, Mark M, Chambon P (1995). Nonsteroid nuclear receptors: what are genetic studies telling us about their role in real life? Cell 83: 859–869.

Kawasaki T, Kitsukawa T, Bekku Y, Matsuda Y, Sanbo M, Yagi T, Fujisawa H (1999). A requirement for neuropilin-1 in embryonic vessel formation. *Development* 126: 4895–4902.

Keegan BR, Feldman JL, Lee DH, Koos DS, Ho RK, Stainier DY, Yelon D (2002). The elongation factors Pandora/Spt6 and Foggy/Spt5 promote transcription in the zebrafish embryo. *Development* 129: 1623–1632.

Kikuchi Y, Trinh LA, Reiter JF, Alexander J, Yelon D, Stainier DY (2000). The zebrafish *bonnie and clyde* gene encodes a Mix family homeodomain protein that regulates the generation of endodermal precursors. *Genes Dev* 14: 1279–1289.

Kikuchi Y, Agathon A, Alexander J, Thisse C, Waldron S, Yelon D, Thisse B, Stainier DY (2001). casanova encodes a novel Sox-related protein necessary and sufficient for early endoderm formation in zebrafish. *Genes Dev* 15: 1493–1505.

Kirby ML, Waldo KL (1990). Role of neural crest in congenital heart disease. *Circulation* 82: 332–340.

Kirby ML, Waldo KL (1995). Neural crest and cardiovascular patterning. *Circ Res* 77: 211–215.

Kirby ML, Gale TF, Stewart DE (1983). Neural crest cells contribute to normal aorticopulmonary septation. *Science* 220: 1059–1061.

Kishimoto Y, Lee KH, Zon L, Hammerschmidt M, Schulte-Merker S (1997). The molecular nature of zebrafish swirl: BMP2 function is essential during early dorsoventral patterning. *Development* 124: 4457–4466.

Kitsukawa T, Shimono A, Kawakami A, Kondoh H, Fujisawa H (1995). Overexpression of a membrane protein, neuropilin, in chimeric mice causes anomalies in the cardiovascular system, nervous system and limbs. *Development* 121: 4309–4318.

Kokubo H, Lun Y, Johnson RL (1999). Identification and expression of a novel family of bHLH cDNAs related to *Drosophila* hairy and enhancer of split. *Biochem Biophys Res Commun* 260: 459–465.

Koutsourakis M, Langeveld A, Patient R, Beddington R, Grosveld F (1999). The transcription factor GATA6 is essential for early extraembryonic development. *Development* 126: 723–732.

Kreidberg JA, Sariola H, Loring JM, Maeda M, Pelletier J, Housman D, Jaenisch R (1993). WT-1 is required for early kidney development. *Cell* 74: 679–691.

Kuo CT, Morrisey EE, Anandappa R, Sigrist K, Lu MM, Parmacek MS, Soudais C, Leiden JM (1997). GATA4 transcription factor is required for ventral morphogenesis and heart tube formation. *Genes Dev* 11: 1048–1060.

Kupperman E, An S, Osborne N, Waldron S, Stainier DY (2000). A sphingosine-1-phosphate receptor regulates cell migration during vertebrate heart development. *Nature* 406: 192–125.

Kurihara Y, Kurihara H, Oda H, Maemura K, Nagai R, Ishikawa T, Yazaki Y (1995). Aortic arch malformations and ventricular septal defect in mice deficient in endothelin-1. *J Clin Invest* 96: 293–300.

Kwee L, Baldwin HS, Shen HM, Stewart CL, Buck C, Buck CA, Labow MA (1995). Defective development of the embryonic and extraembryonic circulatory systems in vascular cell adhesion molecule (VCAM-1) deficient mice. *Development* 121: 489–503.

Lacalli TC (1995). Dorsoventral axis inversion. *Nature* 373: 110–111.

Lammer EJ, Chen DT, Hoar RM, Agnish ND, Benke PJ, Braun JT, Curry CJ, Fernhoff PM, Grix AW, Jr Lott IT, et al. (1985). Retinoic acid embryopathy. *N Engl J Med* 313: 837–841.

Laverriere AC, MacNeill C, Mueller C, Poelmann RE, Burch JB, Evans T (1994). GATA-4/5/6, a subfamily of three transcription factors transcribed in developing heart and gut. *J Biol Chem* 269: 23177–23184.

Lawson ND, Scheer N, Pham VN, Kim CH, Chitnis AB, Campos-Ortega JA, Weinstein BM (2001). Notch signaling is required for arterial-venous differentiation during embryonic vascular development. *Development* 128: 3675–3683.

Leatherbury L, Kirby ML (1996). Cardiac development and perinatal care of infants with neural crest–associated conotruncal defects. *Semin Perinatol* 20: 473–481.

Lee RK, Stainier DY, Weinstein BM, Fishman MC (1994). Cardiovascular development in the zebrafish. II. Endocardial progenitors are sequestered within the heart field. *Development* 120: 3361–3366.

Lee KF, Simon H, Chen H, Bates B, Hung MC, Hauser C (1995). Requirement for neuregulin receptor erbB2 in neural and cardiac development. *Nature* 378: 394–398.

Lee RY, Luo J, Evans RM, Giguere V, Sucov HM (1997). Compartment-selective sensitivity of cardiovascular morphogenesis to combinations of retinoic acid receptor gene mutations. *Circ Res* 80: 757–764.

Li QY, Newbury-Ecob RA, Terrett JA, Wilson DI, Curtis AR, Yi CH, Gebuhr T, Bullen PJ, Robson SC, Strachan T, et al. (1997). Holt-Oram syndrome is caused by mutations in *TBX5*, a member of the *Brachyury (T)* gene family. *Nat Genet* 15: 21–29.

Liang D, Xu X, Chin AJ, Balasubramaniyan NV, Teo MA, Lam TJ, Weinberg ES, Ge R (1998). Cloning and characterization of vascular endothelial growth factor (VEGF) from zebrafish, *Danio rerio*. *Biochim Biophys Acta* 1397: 14–20.

Liao W, Bisgrove BW, Sawyer H, Hug B, Bell B, Peters K, Grunwald DJ, Stainier DY (1997). The zebrafish gene *cloche* acts upstream of a flk-1 homologue to regulate endothelial cell differentiation. *Development* 124: 381–389.

Lin Q, Schwarz J, Bucana C, Olson EN (1997). Control of mouse cardiac morphogenesis and myogenesis by transcription factor MEF2C. *Science* 276: 1404–1407.

Lints TJ, Parsons LM, Hartley L, Lyons I, Harvey RP (1993). Nkx-2.5: a novel murine homeobox gene expressed in early heart progenitor cells and their myogenic descendants. *Development* 119: 419–431.

Lough J, Barron M, Brogley M, Sugi Y, Bolender DL, Zhu X (1996). Combined BMP-2 and FGF-4, but neither factor alone, induces cardiogenesis in non-precardiac embryonic mesoderm. *Dev Biol* 178: 198–202.

Lyons GE (1994). In situ analysis of the cardiac muscle gene program during embryogenesis. *Trends Cardiovasc Med* 4: 70–77.

Maisonpierre PC, Suri C, Jones PF, Bartunkova S, Wiegand SJ, Radziejewski C, Compton D, McClain J, Aldrich TH, Papadopoulos N, et al. (1997). Angiopoietin-2, a natural antagonist for Tie2 that disrupts in vivo angiogenesis. *Science* 277: 55–60.

Marvin MJ, Di Rocco, G, Gardiner A, Bush SM, Lassar AB (2001). Inhibition of Wnt activity induces heart formation from posterior mesoderm. *Genes Dev* 15: 316–327.

Mendelsohn C, Lohnes D, Decimo D, Lufkin T, LeMeur M, Chambon P, Mark M (1994). Function of the retinoic acid receptors (RARs) during development (II). Multiple abnormalities at various stages of organogenesis in RAR double mutants. *Development* 120: 2749–2771.

Meyer D, Birchmeier C (1995). Multiple essential functions of neuregulin in development. *Nature* 378: 386–390.

Meyer D, Stiegler P, Hindelang C, Mager AM, Remy P (1995). Whole-mount in situ hybridization reveals the expression of the *Xl-Fli* gene in several lineages of migrating cells in *Xenopus* embryos. *Int J Dev Biol* 39: 909–919.

Meyer D, Durliat M, Senan F, Wolff M, Andre M, Hourdry J, Remy P (1997). Ets-1 and Ets-2 proto-oncogenes exhibit differential and restricted expression patterns during *Xenopus laevis* oogenesis and embryogenesis. *Int J Dev Biol* 41: 607–620.

Mikawa T, Fischman DA (1996). The polyclonal origin of myocyte lineages. *Annu Rev Physiol* 58: 509–521.

Miquerol L, Gertsenstein M, Harpal K, Rossant J, Nagy A (1999). Multiple developmental roles of VEGF suggested by a LacZ-tagged allele. *Dev Biol* 212: 307–322.

Mjaatvedt CH, Yamamura H, Capehart AA, Turner D, Markwald RR (1998). The *Cspg2* gene, disrupted in the hdf mutant, is required for right cardiac chamber and endocardial cushion formation. *Dev Biol* 202: 56–66.

Moens CB, Stanton BR, Parada LF, Rossant J (1993). Defects in heart and lung development in compound heterozygotes for two different targeted mutations at the N-myc locus. *Development* 119: 485–499.

Molkentin JD, Lin Q, Duncan SA, Olson EN (1997). Requirement of the transcription factor GATA4 for heart tube formation and ventral morphogenesis. *Genes Dev* 11: 1061–1072.

Morrisey EE, Ip HS, Tang Z, Lu MM, Parmacek MS (1997). GATA-5: a transcriptional activator expressed in a novel temporally and spatially-restricted pattern during embryonic development. *Dev Biol* 183: 21–36.

Morrisey EE, Tang Z, Sigrist K, Lu MM, Jiang F, Ip HS, Parmacek MS (1998). GATA6

regulates HNF4 and is required for differentiation of visceral endoderm in the mouse embryo. *Genes Dev* 12: 3579–3590.

Myat A, Henrique D, Ish-Horowicz D, Lewis J (1996). A chick homologue of Serrate and its relationship with Notch and Delta homologues during central neurogenesis. *Dev Biol* 174: 233–247.

Nakagawa O, Nakagawa M, Richardson JA, Olson EN, Srivastava D (1999). HRT1, HRT2, and HRT3: a new subclass of bHLH transcription factors marking specific cardiac, somitic, and pharyngeal arch segments. *Dev Biol* 216: 72–84.

Narita N, Bielinska M, Wilson DB (1997). Cardiomyocyte differentiation by GATA-4-deficient embryonic stem cells. *Development* 124: 3755–3764.

Nascone N, Mercola M (1995). An inductive role for the endoderm in *Xenopus* cardiogenesis. *Development* 121: 515–523.

Newman CS, Chia F, Krieg PA (1997). The *XHex* homeobox gene is expressed during development of the vascular endothelium: overexpression leads to an increase in vascular endothelial cell number. *Mech Dev* 66: 83–93.

Noden DM (1988). Interactions and fates of avian craniofacial mesenchyme. *Development* 103: 121–140.

Noden DM (1989). Embryonic origins and assembly of blood vessels. *Am Rev Respir Dis* 140: 1097–1103.

Nusslein-Volhard C, Wieschaus E (1980). Mutations affecting segment number and polarity in *Drosophila*. *Nature* 287: 795–801.

Pardanaud L, Dieterlen-Lievre F (1993). Emergence of endothelial and hemopoietic cells in the avian embryo. *Anat Embryol (Berl)* 187: 107–114.

Pardanaud L, Altmann C, Kitos P, Dieterlen-Lievre F, Buck CA (1987). Vasculogenesis in the early quail blastodisc as studied with a monoclonal antibody recognizing endothelial cells. *Development* 100: 339–349.

Parker L, Stainier DY (1999). Cell-autonomous and non-autonomous requirements for the zebrafish gene *cloche* in hematopoiesis. *Development* 126: 2643–2651.

Pereira FA, Qiu Y, Zhou G, Tsai MJ, Tsai SY (1999). The orphan nuclear receptor COUP-TFII is required for angiogenesis and heart development. *Genes Dev* 13: 1037–1049.

Peterson RT, Mably JD, Chen JN, Fishman MC (2001). Convergence of distinct pathways to heart patterning revealed by the small molecule concentramide and the mutation heart-and-soul. *Curr Biol* 11: 1481–1491.

Polakis P (2000). Wnt signaling and cancer. *Genes Dev* 14: 1837–1851.

Poole TJ, Coffin JD (1989). Vasculogenesis and angiogenesis: two distinct morphogenetic mechanisms establish embryonic vascular pattern. *J Exp Zool* 251: 224–231.

Porcher C, Swat W, Rockwell K, Fujiwara Y, Alt FW, Orkin SH (1996). The T cell leukemia oncoprotein SCL/tal-1 is essential for development of all hematopoietic lineages. *Cell* 86: 47–57.

Potts JD, Runyan RB (1989). Epithelial-mesenchymal cell transformation in the embryonic heart can be mediated, in part, by transforming growth factor beta. *Dev Biol* 134: 392–401.

Potts JD, Dagle JM, Walder JA, Weeks DL, Runyan RB (1991). Epithelial–mesenchymal transformation of embryonic cardiac endothelial cells is inhibited by a modified antisense oligodeoxynucleotide to transforming growth factor beta 3. *Proc Natl Acad Sci USA* 88: 1516–1520.

Puri MC, Rossant J, Alitalo K, Bernstein A, Partanen J (1995). The receptor tyrosine kinase TIE is required for integrity and survival of vascular endothelial cells. *EMBO J* 14: 5884–5891.

Puri MC, Partanen J, Rossant J, Bernstein A (1999). Interaction of the TEK and TIE receptor tyrosine kinases during cardiovascular development. *Development* 126: 4569–4580.

Ranger AM, Grusby MJ, Hodge MR, Gravallese EM, de la Brousse FC, Hoey T, Mickanin C, Baldwin HS, Glimcher LH (1998). The transcription factor NF-ATc is essential for cardiac valve formation. *Nature* 392: 186–190.

Reaume AG, Conlon RA, Zirngibl R, Yamaguchi TP, Rossant J (1992). Expression analysis of a Notch homologue in the mouse embryo. *Dev Biol* 154: 377–387.

Reifers F, Walsh EC, Leger S, Stainier DY, Brand M (2000). Induction and differentiation of the zebrafish heart requires fibroblast growth factor 8 (fgf8/acerebellar). *Development* 127: 225–235.

Reiter JF, Alexander J, Rodaway A, Yelon D, Patient R, Holder N, Stainier DY (1999). Gata5 is required for the development of the heart and endoderm in zebrafish. *Genes Dev* 13: 2983–2995.

Riley P, Anson-Cartwright L, Cross JC (1998). The Hand1 bHLH transcription factor is essential for placentation and cardiac morphogenesis. *Nat Genet* 18: 271–275.

Risau W, Flamme I (1995). Vasculogenesis. *Annu Rev Cell Dev Biol* 11: 73–91.

Robb L, Elwood NJ, Elefanty AG, Kontgen F, Li R, Barnett LD, Begley CG (1996). The *scl* gene product is required for the generation of all hematopoietic lineages in the adult mouse. *EMBO J* 15: 4123–4129.

Robertson SM, Kennedy M, Shannon JM, Keller G (2000). A transitional stage in the commitment of mesoderm to hematopoiesis requiring the transcription factor SCL/tal-1. *Development* 127: 2447–2459.

Roman BL, Weinstein BM (2000). Building the vertebrate vasculature: research is going swimmingly. *Bioessays* 22: 882–893.

Ross RS, Navankasattusas S, Harvey RP, Chien KR (1996). An HF-1a/HF-1b/MEF-2 combinatorial element confers cardiac ventricular specificity and established an anterior–posterior gradient of expression. *Development* 122: 1799–1809.

Rottbauer W, Baker K, Wo ZG, Mohideen MA, Cantiello HF, Fishman MC (2001). Growth and function of the embryonic heart depend upon the cardiac-specific L-type calcium channel alpha1 subunit. *Dev Cell* 1: 265–275.

Rottbauer W, Saurin AJ, Lickert H, Shen X, Burns CG, Wo ZG, Kemler R, Kingston R, Wu C, Fishman MC (2002). Reptin and Pontin antagonistically regulate heart growth in zebrafish embryos. *Cell* 111: 661–672.

Saga Y, Miyagawa-Tomita S, Takagi A, Kitajima S, Miyazaki J, Inoue T (1999). MesP1 is expressed in the heart precursor cells and required for the formation of a single heart tube. *Development* 126: 3437–3447.

Sanford LP, Ormsby I, Gittenberger-de Groot AC, Sariola H, Friedman R, Boivin GP,

Cardell EL, Doetschman T (1997). TGFbeta2 knockout mice have multiple developmental defects that are non-overlapping with other TGFbeta knockout phenotypes. *Development* 124: 2659–2670.
Sato TN, Tozawa Y, Deutsch U, Wolburg-Buchholz K, Fujiwara Y, Gendron-Maguire M, Gridley T, Wolburg H, Risau W, Qin Y (1995). Distinct roles of the receptor tyrosine kinases Tie-1 and Tie-2 in blood vessel formation. *Nature* 376: 70–74.
Schauerte HE, van Eeden FJ, Fricke C, Odenthal J, Strahle U, Haffter P (1998). Sonic hedgehog is not required for the induction of medial floor plate cells in the zebrafish. *Development* 125: 2983–2993.
Schneider VA, Mercola M (2001). Wnt antagonism initiates cardiogenesis in *Xenopus laevis*. *Genes Dev* 15: 304–315.
Schott JJ, Benson DW, Basson CT, Pease W, Silberbach GM, Moak JP, Maron BJ, Seidman CE, Seidman JG (1998). Congenital heart disease caused by mutations in the transcription factor NKX2-5. *Science* 281: 108–111.
Schultheiss TM, Xydas S, Lassar AB (1995). Induction of avian cardiac myogenesis by anterior endoderm. *Development* 121: 4203–4214.
Schultheiss TM, Burch JB, Lassar AB (1997). A role for bone morphogenetic proteins in the induction of cardiac myogenesis. *Genes Dev* 11: 451–462.
Schwartz RJ, Olson EN (1999). Building the heart piece by piece: modularity of *cis*-elements regulating Nkx2-5 transcription. *Development* 126: 4187–4192.
Sedmera D, Thomas PS (1996). Trabeculation in the embryonic heart. *Bioessays* 18: 607.
Serbedzija GN, Chen JN, Fishman MC (1998). Regulation in the heart field of zebrafish. *Development* 125: 1095–1101.
Shalaby F, Rossant J, Yamaguchi TP, Gertsenstein M, Wu XF, Breitman ML, Schuh AC (1995). Failure of blood-island formation and vasculogenesis in Flk-1-deficient mice. *Nature* 376: 62–66.
Shalaby F, Ho J, Stanford WL, Fischer KD, Schuh AC, Schwartz L, Bernstein A, Rossant J (1997). A requirement for Flk1 in primitive and definitive hematopoiesis and vasculogenesis. *Cell* 89: 981–990.
Shenefelt RE (1972). Morphogenesis of malformations in hamsters caused by retinoic acid: relation to dose and stage at treatment. *Teratology* 5: 103–118.
Shishido E, Ono N, Kojima T, Saigo K (1997). Requirements of DFR1/Heartless, a mesoderm-specific *Drosophila* FGF-receptor, for the formation of heart, visceral and somatic muscles, and ensheathing of longitudinal axon tracts in CNS. *Development* 124: 2119–2128.
Simon AM, Goodenough DA, Paul DL (1998). Mice lacking connexin40 have cardiac conduction abnormalities characteristic of atrioventricular block and bundle branch block. *Curr Biol* 8: 295–298.
Smith JC, Cooke J, Green JB, Howes G, Symes K (1989). Inducing factors and the control of mesodermal pattern in *Xenopus laevis*. *Development* 107: 149–159.
Smithers L, Haddon C, Jiang Y, Lewis J (2000). Sequence and embryonic expression of deltaC in the zebrafish. *Mech Dev* 90: 119–123.
Soker S, Takashima S, Miao HQ, Neufeld G, Klagsbrun M (1998). Neuropilin-1 is expressed by endothelial and tumor cells as an isoform-specific receptor for vascular endothelial growth factor. *Cell* 92: 735–745.
Srivastava D, Cserjesi P, Olson EN (1995). A subclass of bHLH proteins required for cardiac morphogenesis. *Science* 270: 1995–1999.
Srivastava D, Thomas T, Lin Q, Kirby ML, Brown D, Olson EN (1997). Regulation of cardiac mesodermal and neural crest development by the bHLH transcription factor, dHAND. *Nat Genet* 16: 154–160.
Stainier DY (2001). Zebrafish genetics and vertebrate heart formation. *Nat Rev Genet* 2: 39–48.
Stainier DY, Fishman MC (1992). Patterning the zebrafish heart tube: acquisition of anteroposterior polarity. *Dev Biol* 153: 91–101.
Stainier DY, Weinstein BM, Detrich HW, 3rd Zon, LI, Fishman MC (1995). *Cloche*, an early acting zebrafish gene, is required by both the endothelial and hematopoietic lineages. *Development* 121: 3141–3150.
Stainier DY, Fouquet B, Chen JN, Warren KS, Weinstein BM, Meiler SE, Mohideen MA, Neuhauss SC, Solnica-Krezel L, Schier AF, et al. (1996). Mutations affecting the formation and function of the cardiovascular system in the zebrafish embryo. *Development* 123: 285–292.
Sugi Y, Lough J (1994). Anterior endoderm is a specific effector of terminal cardiac myocyte differentiation of cells from the embryonic heart forming region. *Dev Dyn* 200: 155–162.
Sumoy, L, Keasey JB, Dittman TD, Kimelman D (1997). A role for notochord in axial vascular development revealed by analysis of phenotype and the expression of VEGR-2 in zebrafish flh and ntl mutant embryos. *Mech Dev* 63: 15–27.
Suri C, Jones PF, Patan S, Bartunkova S, Maisonpierre PC, Davis S, Sato TN, Yancopoulos GD (1996). Requisite role of angiopoietin-1, a ligand for the TIE2 receptor, during embryonic angiogenesis. *Cell* 87: 1171–1180.
Taber LA, Lin IE, Clark EB (1995). Mechanics of cardiac looping. *Dev Dyn* 203: 42–50.
Tam PP, Quinlan GA (1996). Mapping vertebrate embryos. *Curr Biol* 6: 104–106.
Tam PP, Parameswaran M, Kinder SJ, Weinberger RP (1997). The allocation of epiblast cells to the embryonic heart and other mesodermal lineages: the role of ingression and tissue movement during gastrulation. *Development* 124: 1631–1642.
Tanaka M, Kasahara H, Bartunkova S, Schinke M, Komuro I, Inagaki H, Lee Y, Lyons GE, Izumo S (1998). Vertebrate homologs of tinman and bagpipe: roles of the homeobox genes in cardiovascular development. *Dev Genet* 22: 239–249.
Thomas PQ, Brown A, Beddington RS (1998a). *Hex*: a homeobox gene revealing periimplantation asymmetry in the mouse embryo and an early transient marker of endothelial cell precursors. *Development* 125: 85–94.
Thomas T, Kurihara H, Yamagishi H, Kurihara Y, Yazaki Y, Olson EN, Srivastava D (1998b). A signaling cascade involving endothelin-1, dHAND and msx1 regulates development of neural-crest-derived branchial arch mesenchyme. *Development* 125: 3005–3014.
Threadgill DW, Dlugosz AA, Hansen LA, Tennenbaum T, Lichti U, Yee D, LaMantia C, Mourton T, Herrup K, Harris RC, et al. (1995). Targeted disruption of mouse EGF receptor: effect of genetic background on mutant phenotype. *Science* 269: 230–234.
Tomita H, Connuck DM, Leatherbury L, Kirby ML (1991). Relation of early hemodynamic changes to final cardiac phenotype and survival after neural crest ablation in chick embryos. *Circulation* 84: 1289–1295.
Tzahor E, Lassar AB (2001). Wnt signals from the neural tube block ectopic cardiogenesis. *Genes Dev* 15: 255–260.
Uyttendaele H, Marazzi G, Wu G, Yan Q, Sassoon D, Kitajewski J (1996). *Notch4/int-3*, a mammary proto-oncogene, is an endothelial cell-specific mammalian *Notch* gene. *Development* 122: 2251–2259.
Valenzuela DM, Griffiths JA, Rojas J, Aldrich TH, Jones PF, Zhou H, McClain J, Copeland NG, Gilbert DJ, Jenkins NA, et al. (1999). Angiopoietins 3 and 4: diverging gene counterparts in mice and humans. *Proc Natl Acad Sci USA* 96: 1904–1909.
Vandenbunder B, Pardanaud L, Jaffredo T, Mirabel MA, Stehelin D (1989). Complementary patterns of expression of c-ets 1, c-myb and c-myc in the blood-forming system of the chick embryo. *Development* 107: 265–274.
van Eeden FJ, Granato M, Schach U, Brand M, Furutani-Seiki M, Haffter P, Hammerschmidt M, Heisenberg CP, Jiang YJ, Kane DA, et al. (1996). Mutations affecting somite formation and patterning in the zebrafish, *Danio rerio*. *Development* 123: 153–164.
Vincent GM (1998). The molecular genetics of the long QT syndrome: genes causing fainting and sudden death. *Annu Rev Med* 49: 263–274.
Visvader JE, Fujiwara Y, Orkin SH (1998). Unsuspected role for the T-cell leukemia protein SCL/tal-1 in vascular development. *Genes Dev* 12: 473–479.
Waldo K, Miyagawa-Tomita S, Kumiski D, Kirby ML (1998). Cardiac neural crest cells provide new insight into septation of the cardiac outflow tract: aortic sac to ventricular septal closure. *Dev Biol* 196: 129–144.
Walsh EC, Stainier DY (2001). UDP-glucose dehydrogenase required for cardiac valve formation in zebrafish. *Science* 293: 1670–1673.
Wang DZ, Hammond VE, Abud HE, Bertoncello I, McAvoy JW, Bowtell DD (1997). Mutation in Sos1 dominantly enhances a weak allele of the EGFR, demonstrating a requirement for Sos1 in EGFR signaling and development. *Genes Dev* 11: 309–320.
Wang HU, Chen ZF, Anderson DJ (1998). Molecular distinction and angiogenic interaction between embryonic arteries and veins revealed by ephrin-B2 and its receptor Eph-B4. *Cell* 93: 741–753.
Weinstein BM, Stemple DL, Driever W, Fishman MC (1995). Gridlock, a localized heritable vascular patterning defect in the zebrafish. *Nat Med* 1: 1143–1147.
Wilson JG, Warkany J (1949). Aortic arch and cardiac anomalies in the offspring of vitamin A deficient rats. *Am J Anat* 85: 113–155.
Wilson JG, Roth CB, Warkany J (1953). An analysis of the syndrome of malformations induced by maternal vitamin A deficiency. Effects of restoration of vitamin A at various times during gestation. *Am J Anat* 92: 189–217.
Winnier G, Blessing M, Labosky PA, Hogan BL (1995). Bone morphogenetic protein-4 is required for mesoderm formation and patterning in the mouse. *Genes Dev* 9: 2105–2116.
Wu X, Golden K, Bodmer R (1995). Heart development in *Drosophila* requires the segment polarity gene wingless. *Dev Biol* 169: 619–628.
Xavier-Neto, J Neville, CM Shapiro, MD Houghton, L Wang, GF Nikovits, W Jr, Stockdale FE, Rosenthal N (1999). A retinoic acid-inducible transgenic marker of sino-atrial development in the mouse heart. *Development* 126: 2677–2687.
Xavier-Neto J, Shapiro MD, Houghton L, Rosenthal N (2000). Sequential programs of retinoic acid synthesis in the myocardial and epicardial layers of the developing avian heart. *Dev Biol* 219: 129–141.
Xiong JW, Leahy A, Lee HH, Stuhlmann H (1999). Vezf1: a Zn finger transcription factor restricted to endothelial cells and their precursors. *Dev Biol* 206: 123–141.
Xu W, Baribault H, Adamson ED (1998a). Vinculin knockout results in heart and brain defects during embryonic development. *Development* 125: 327–337.
Xu X, Yin Z, Hudson JB, Ferguson EL, Frasch M (1998b). Smad proteins act in combination with synergistic and antagonistic regulators to target Dpp responses to the *Drosophila* mesoderm. *Genes Dev* 12: 2354–2370.
Yamagishi H, Olson EN, Srivastava D (2000). The basic helix-loop-helix transcription factor, dHAND, is required for vascular development. *J Clin Invest* 105: 261–270.
Yamaguchi TP, Dumont DJ, Conlon RA, Breitman ML, Rossant J (1993). flk-1, an flt-related receptor tyrosine kinase is an early marker for endothelial cell precursors. *Development* 118: 489–498.
Yang JT, Rayburn H, Hynes RO (1995). Cell adhesion events mediated by alpha 4 integrins are essential in placental and cardiac development. *Development* 121: 549–560.
Yelon D, Ticho B, Halpern ME, Ruvinsky I, Ho RK, Silver LM, Stainier DY (2000). The bHLH transcription factor hand2 plays parallel roles in zebrafish heart and pectoral fin development. *Development* 127: 2573–2582.
Yoshida K, Taga T, Saito M, Suematsu S, Kumanogoh A, Tanaka T, Fujiwara H, Hirata M, Yamagami T, Nakahata T, et al. (1996). Targeted disruption of gp130, a common signal transducer for the interleukin 6 family of cytokines, leads to myocardial and hematological disorders. *Proc Natl Acad Sci USA* 93: 407–411.
Yutzey KE, Bader D (1995). Diversification of cardiomyogenic cell lineages during early heart development. *Circ Res* 77: 216–219.
Yutzey K, Gannon M, Bader D (1995). Diversification of cardiomyogenic cell lineages in vitro. *Dev Biol* 170: 531–541.
Zhang H, Bradley A (1996). Mice deficient for BMP2 are nonviable and have defects in amnion/chorion and cardiac development. *Development* 122: 2977–2986.
Zhong TP, Rosenberg M, Mohideen MA, Weinstein B, Fishman MC (2000). *gridlock*, an HLH gene required for assembly of the aorta in zebrafish. *Science* 287: 1820–1824.
Zhong TP, Childs S, Leu JP, Fishman MC (2001). Gridlock signalling pathway fashions the first embryonic artery. *Nature* 414: 216–220.
Zou Y, Evans S, Chen J, Kuo HC, Harvey RP, Chien KR (1997). CARP, a cardiac ankyrin repeat protein, is downstream in the *Nkx2-5* homeobox gene pathway. *Development* 124: 793–804.

10 | Development of Muscle and Somites

ALAN RAWLS AND JERRY M. RHEE

Vertebrate skeletal muscle is derived from paraxial and head mesoderm that appears on either side of the neural tube during gastrulation. A fundamental understanding of the cellular events associated with myogenesis has been gained from classic embryological studies. The first appearance of myogenic cells is within individual somites derived from paraxial mesoderm. During embryonic development, these cells must undergo rapid expansion, migration, differentiation, and remodeling to generate the morphologically and functionally diverse perinatal muscle groups. Myogenic cells must also respond to spatial and temporal cues that lead to differences in cell fate along the anterior/posterior (A/P) and dorsal/ventral (D/V) axes. In addition, development of the skeletal muscle must be coordinated with the development of the bone and peripheral nerves. During the past 15 years, gain-of-function and loss-of-function approaches have been used to reveal the complex genetic network that integrates these processes. In this chapter, we will discuss our current understanding of the genetic regulation of somitogenesis and skeletal muscle development.

SOMITOGENESIS

Somites arise from the paraxial mesoderm, which involutes through the anterior region of the late primitive streak and migrates to form two discrete bands flanking the notochord and prospective neural plate (reviewed by Christ and Ordhal, 1995). The primitive streak continues to supply the cells of the paraxial mesoderm for the formation of the trunk somites until secondary axis formation begins around 10 days postcoitum (*dpc*) in mice (~30 somites) (Wilson and Beddington, 1996). Afterward, a population of proliferating mesenchymal stem cells located in the tail bud becomes the source of the cells of the paraxial mesoderm until axis elongation ceases at 13.25 dpc (65 somites) (Tam and Tan, 1992). These cells undergo an increase in cell number, density, and expression of extracellular matrix proteins (Keynes and Stern, 1988; for review, see Tam and Trainor, 1994). This results in the transient transition of mesenchymal cells of the presomitic mesoderm into an epithelial ball.

In response to signals emanating from the surrounding axial structures, the somite matures into three morphologically distinct compartments: sclerotome, myotome, and dermomyotome (Fig. 10–1). First, cells in the ventral/medial quadrant of the somite reacquire a mesenchymal phenotype in response to factors secreted from the notochord and floor plate of the neural tube. These cells combine with cells in the somitocoel to create the sclerotome, which is the anlagen for the ribs and vertebrae (Christ and Wilting, 1992). The rest of the somite remains epithelial and is referred to as the "dermomyotome." Cells from the dorsal/medial and ventral/lateral lips of the dermomyotome delaminate and migrate subjacently to form the myotome, which is fated to form embryonic skeletal muscle (Kaehn et al., 1988). At the cervical and limb levels, a small number of cells delaminate from the ventral/lateral lip of the dermomyotome and migrate into the limbs, hypoglossal cords, and septum transversum. These cells will give rise to the appendicular muscles, the tongue, and the diaphragm. The remaining cells of the dermomyotome eventually disperse and migrate under the developing ectoderm to form the dermis.

Specification to the Paraxial Mesoderm Lineage

Epiblast cells fated to become the paraxial mesoderm are located in the anterior primitive streak, adjacent to the node. Specification of these cells during gastrulation is dependent on instructive signals from members of the Wingless (Wnt) and fibroblast growth factor (FGF) family of secreted factors (Fig. 10–2). The Wnt family is comprised of cysteine-rich secreted glycoproteins that play roles in axis formation, morphogenesis, and tissue patterning (Wodarz and Nusse, 1998). Wnts stimulates an intracellular cascade by binding cell surface receptors, *Frizzled1* and *-2*. Activation of Frizzled1 results in the release of β-catenin from a large protein complex that includes Dishevelled, Casein kinase I-α, glycogen synthase kinase-3β (GSK-3β), Axin, and APC. Free β-catenin is then able to move to the nucleus, where it interacts with T-cell factor (TCF) or lymphoid enhancer factor (LEF) to activate transcription of proliferation and determination-specific genes (reviewed in Wodarz and Nusse, 1998)(see Chapter 22). In late-streak gastrula, *Wnt-3a* transcripts are present in the epiblast but not in the migrating mesodermal cells. Targeted disruption of *Wnt-3a* results in loss of paraxial mesoderm posterior to the first six somites (Yoshikawa et al., 1997). The paraxial mesoderm was replaced by neural structures in these mutants, demonstrating a role for Wnt-3a in its specification. Further, compound null mutations in two downstream target genes of Wnt-3a, *Lef1* and *Tcf1*, resulted in similar phenotypes (Galceran et al., 1999).

Respecification of paraxial mesoderm to a neural ectodermal fate has also been observed in embryos where the FGF signaling pathway has been disrupted. FGF is a large family of secreted signaling molecules (18 members in mammals) that activate one of four receptor-tyrosine kinase receptors (FGFRs) (see Chapter 32). One receptor in particular is important in specifying the paraxial mesoderm, FGFR1. FGFR1 regulates the migration of cells through the primitive streak, presumably by controlling the epithelial–mesenchymal transition of ectodermal cells in the epiblast (Ciruna et al., 1997). *Fgf8* has been proposed as the likely ligand for FGFR1 since it is expressed in the primitive streak and *Fgf8⁻/⁻* embryos fail to form paraxial mesoderm (Sun et al., 1999). The creation of a chimeric embryo possessing cells null for *FGFR1* in a wild-type background resulted in the replacement of paraxial mesodermal derivatives with neural ectoderm, demonstrating that a second function for FGFR1 is specification of the paraxial mesoderm (Ciruna et al., 1997). Due to the early block in development in these mutants, it is not clear whether FGF8 also directs cell specification through FGFR1.

Possible downstream targets of Wnt-3a and FGF8 signaling include *Brachyury* (*T*) and *Tbx-6*, two members of the T box–containing family of homeobox transcription factors (see Chapter 67). These genes are coexpressed with Wnt-3a during gastrulation, and mice deficient in either *T* or *Tbx-6* have a similar phenotype. Furthermore, T expression was lost from epiblast cells fated to form paraxial mesoderm in *Wnt-3a⁻/⁻* embryos, while *Tbx-6* was mildly downregulated (Yamaguchi et al., 1999). *T* and *Tbx-6* expression was altered in the *fgf8⁻/⁻* embryos as well. These results led to a model whereby FGF and Wnt signaling interact through the T-box transcription factors to specify paraxial mesoderm (Pourquie, 2001).

Additional regulatory genes have been identified that are associated with the specification of paraxial mesoderm (Fig. 10–2). These genes are expressed in the paraxial mesoderm but not the epiblast, suggesting that they lie downstream of FGF8 and Wnt-3a signaling. *PMesogenin1*, a basic helix-loop-helix (bHLH) transcription factor, is transcribed in an overlapping pattern with *T* and *Tbx-6* in the posterior two-thirds of the presomitic mesoderm (PSM) (Yoon et al., 2000).

Figure 10–1. A schematic of the maturation of somites into lineage-specific cellular compartments.

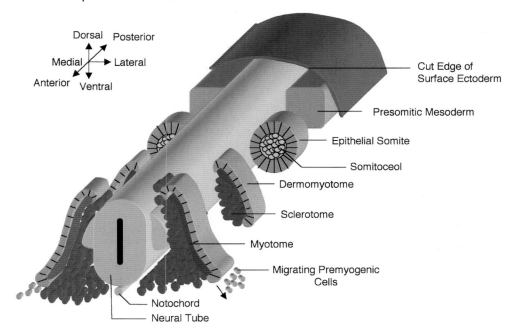

Further, ectopic expression of pMesogenin1 in cap experiments with *Xenopus* embryos led to expression of the *T-box* genes, establishing a regulatory link between these genes. The role of *pMesogenin1* in the specification of paraxial mesoderm is further supported by the fact that *pMesogenin*-deficient embryos fail to form the paraxial mesoderm that is fated to give rise to trunk and tail muscle and skeleton (Yoon and Wold, 2000). Two members of the forkhead class of transcription

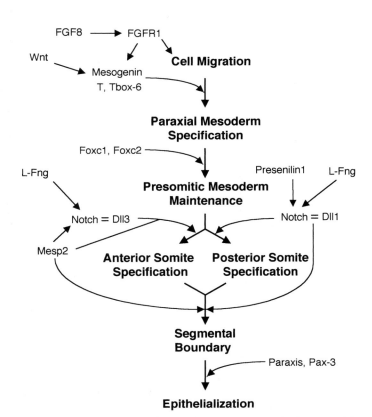

Figure 10–2. Flow diagram of genes that regulate events in the presomitic mesoderm and are critical for somitogenesis. The morphological events that begin with gastrulation and end at somitogenesis have been divided into discrete, demonstrable steps (bold type). Genes that regulate these steps are noted by arrows. Protein–protein interactions are denoted by two horizontal lines.

factors, *Foxc1* and *Foxc2*, are also expressed in the early paraxial mesoderm (Winnier et al., 1997; Kume et al., 2001) (see Chapter 64). Individual targeted null mutations demonstrate a role for these genes in the proliferation of sclerotomal cells and permissivity toward a cartilaginous fate (Kume et al., 2001). However, compound null mutants failed to form somites or express anterior PSM-specific genes. In contrast, posterior PSM gene markers were unaffected, suggesting that these genes have overlapping roles in the specification or maintenance of the paraxial mesoderm. Considering that the posterior PSM was specified normally in these embryos, *Foxc1* and *Foxc2* likely function downstream of pMesogenin and the T-box genes.

Segmentation Is Regulated through an Intrinsic Clock

Somites are generated in register across the neural tube at a rate of approximately one somite every 120 minutes in mice. To explain the connection between the spatial and temporal periodicity of forming somites, various developmental models have been developed (Stern and Vasiliauskas, 2000). Among these, the "clock and wavefront" model proposed by Cooke and Zeeman (1976) has the most experimental support. In this model, a cell-autonomous clock controls the oscillation of cells within a field between different functional states. Arresting the oscillation, and thus determining the proper amplitude of somite boundary formation, is accomplished by a signaling wavefront. Thus, segments will form only when the permissive cells in an oscillating field collide with the wavefront.

Genetic evidence for the existence of an oscillating clock has come from transcriptional analysis of members of the Notch signaling pathway in the PSM (see Chapter 39). In the mouse, there are four Notch homologs, *Notch 1–4* (Del Amo et al., 1992; Weinmaster et al., 1992; Lardelli and Lendahl, 1993; Lardelli et al., 1994; Uyttendaele et al., 1996), two of which (Notch 1+2) are expressed in the paraxial mesoderm. Notch receptors are heterodimeric transmembrane proteins (Weinmaster et al., 1991; Roehl et al., 1996; Kurooka et al., 1998; Artavanis-Tsakonas et al., 1999; Hamada et al., 1999) that interact with the membrane-bound ligands *Delta-like1 (Dll1)* (Bettenhausen et al., 1995), *Dll3* (Dunwoodie et al., 1997), *Jagged1 (Jag1)*, and *Jag2* (Lendahl, 1998; Lindsell et al., 1995; Shawber et al., 1996a). Ligand binding leads to a proteolytic cleavage of the Notch intracellular domain (NICD) that is mediated by a γ–secretase, presenilin. The NICD is transported to the nucleus (Artavanis-Tsakonas et al., 1995, 1999; Greenwald, 1998; Saxena et al., 2001), where it interacts with the transcription factor CBF1/recombination signal binding protein (RBP)-Jκ to regulate the transcription of genes involved in cell fate specification (Bailey and Posakony, 1995; Schroeter et al., 1998; Struhl and Adachi, 1998). In response to Notch activation, mammalian homologs of the *Drosophila enhancer of split complex* (E[spl]), *hairy enhancer of split-1 (HES-1)*, *HES-5*, *HES-7*, and the HES-related genes *HESR* and *HEY* are upregulated (Sasai et al., 1992; Jarriault et al., 1995; de la Pompa et al., 1997; Lee et al., 1999; Ohtsuka et al., 1999). In the PSM, *Lunatic Fringe (L-Fng)* and members of the *HES* and *HEY* families are expressed in an oscillating pattern that moves in a posterior to anterior direction (Palmeirim et al., 1997; McGrew et al., 1998; Aulehla and Johnson, 1999; Leimeister et al., 1999; Jouve et al., 2000). Associated with this wave of expression is a second band at presumptive somite −2 that condenses to the width of a half-somite during the length of the oscillation. Embryos with null mutations in genes of the Notch signaling pathway have disrupted oscillatory gene expression within the presomitic mesoderm. The most severe effects are seen in *Dll1* and *RBP-Jκ* mutants, while milder expression perturbations have been reported for *Notch1* and the *Dll3^pu* (pudgy) mutant allele (Kusumi et al., 1998; Barrantes et al., 1999; Jouve et al., 2000; Leimeister et al., 2000). This suggests that Notch signaling is essential for the propagation of the oscillation. It remains to be determined whether Notch works through a positive feedback loop (de Celis and Bray, 1997; Huppert et al., 1997; Kimble and Simpson, 1997) or maintains the oscillation by synchronizing neighboring cells (Jiang et al., 2000).

The temporal oscillation of gene expression is translated into spatial periodicity based on the influence of *L-fng* on the Notch signaling pathway at the anterior end of the presomitic mesoderm (Evrard et al., 1998; McGrew et al., 1998; Zhang and Gridley, 1998; Barrantes et al., 1999). The involvement of Notch signaling in somitogenesis is further supported by the phenotype of targeted null mutations in several components of the Notch pathway, including *Notch1* (Swiatek et al., 1994 ; Conlon et al., 1995), *Dll1* (Hrabe de Angelis et al., 1997), *Dll3* (Kusumi et al., 1998), *Presenilin1* (Shen et al., 1997; Wong et al., 1997), and *RBP-Jκ* (Oka et al., 1995; de la Pompa et al., 1997). In all of the Notch pathway gene mutant embryos, formation of somitic boundaries is delayed and out of register across the neural tube. In all of these mutations, the severity of the disruption in somitogenesis is increased in the sacral somites derived solely from the tail bud, indicating a difference in the regulatory requirement of Notch signaling. Further, the fact that segmental boundaries do eventually form between the cervical, thoracic, and lumbar somites suggests that other regulatory factors are sufficient to direct segmentation.

Support for the existence of the wavefront has come from experiments using the chick model. In an elegant paper, Dubrulle et al. (2001) argued that the anterior border of *FGF8* expression in the PSM defines a "determination front," which maintains cells of the posterior PSM in an undetermined state. This front recedes posteriorly at a constant rate, which is determined by the elongation of the embryo along the A/P axis. Simultaneously, the inherent clock drives expression of the cycling genes in the posterior segmental plate such that the amplitude occurs just anterior to the determination front. Placement of FGF8-soaked heparin beads along the undetermined area forced an extra oscillation in the cells within the field so that segment borders formed anterior to the normal position. Therefore, the field posterior to the front essentially serves as a block to the wavefront of maturation, as described by Cooke and Zeeman (1976).

Regulation of the segmentation also depends on other genes (Fig. 10–2). For example, *Mesp1* and *-2* in mouse (Saga et al., 1997), *cMeso1* in chicken (Buchburger et al., 1998), *thylacine1* in *Xenopus* (Sparrow et al., 1998), and *Mesp-a* and *-b* in zebrafish (Sawada et al., 2000) make up a family of highly related bHLH transcription factors that are transcribed in the region of the anterior PSM that demarcates presumptive somite −2. A targeted null mutation in mouse *Mesp2* disrupts normal segmentation without altering epithelialization of the tissue (Saga et al., 1997). *Mesp2* appears to form a complex feedback loop with *Notch1* and *Dll1*. *Notch1* and *Dll1* transcription is reduced in the absence of *Mesp2*, while mutations in either *Notch1* or *Dll1* result in a reduction of *Mesp2* transcription (Saga et al., 1997; Barrantes et al., 1999).

Regulation of Somite Epithelialization

At the time of somite formation, the mesenchymal cells in the PSM condense into an epithelial ball with a mesenchymal lumen. This process is associated with an increase in the expression of Ca^{2+}-dependent cell adhesion molecules such as N-cadherin, cadherin-11, nerve cell adhesion molecule (NCAM), and extracellular matrix proteins, including laminin and fibronectin (Tam and Trainor, 1994). It had long been believed that the process of epithelialization was the driving force behind segmentation. However, recent mutations in the bHLH transcription factor *paraxis* and the paired homeobox gene *Pax-3* have revealed that the two processes are separable. Paraxis is expressed exclusively in the presomitic mesoderm and the developing somite and when inactivated results in presomitic tissue that forms intersomitic boundaries but fails to epithelialize (Burgess et al., 1995, 1996). The mutant somites still adopt all three cell lineages at the appropriate time, indicating that specification occurs independently of the epithelial state of the cells. Natural mutations in *Pax-3*, a paired domain-containing homeobox transcription factor that is expressed in an overlapping pattern with *paraxis,* exhibit a similar loss of somite epithelialization (Schubert et al., 2001) (see Chapter 59).

Downstream targets of *paraxis* and *Pax-3* that mediate epithelialization have not been identified. In the case of *Pax-3*, a chimeric analysis using *Splotch* embryonic stem (ES) cells in a wild-type background revealed a decrease in cell adhesion of the mutant cells (Mansouri et al., 2001). Similarly, Ca^{2+}-dependent cell adhesion activity was reduced in the *paraxis^{−/−}* somites (J. Rhee and A. Rawls, personal communication). Interestingly, inactivation of several of the candidate cell adhesion molecules, alone or in combination, did not produce an epithelial defect as severe as that observed in the *paraxis* or *Pax-3* mutants (Radice et al., 1997; Horikawa et al., 1999). This would argue that paraxis and Pax-3 regulate an intracellular pathway that is common to all cell adhesion molecules, such as cytoskeletal remodeling.

A/P Polarity of Newly Formed Somites

At the time of formation, each somite possesses distinct anterior and posterior halves, which are required for the segmental patterning of the peripheral nerves and the resegmentation of the sclerotome during vertebrae formation. Polarity along the A/P axis is manifested by the differential expression of genes that regulate patterning of the vertebrae and peripheral nerves, including *Unc4.1, Pax-1, Pax-9,* and *ephinB2* (reviewed in Rawls et al., 2000). As the somite matures, the posterior half of the sclerotome adopts a more compact morphology. Neural crest cells migrate selectively from the dorsal neural tube to the anterior half of the sclerotome, thus imposing a segmental pattern on the dorsal root ganglia (DRG). Formation of individual vertebrae is associated with resegmentation of the sclerotome such that the anterior half of one somite associates with the posterior half of the adjacent somite. By this process, the vertebrae are offset from the muscle by half a segment, which is important for the attachment of the deep back muscles to the intervertebral discs (reviewed by Dockter, 2000). Thus, establishing A/P polarity is critical to the proper segmentation of the vertebral column and its spatial relationship to the developing muscle.

Specification of somitic cells to an anterior or posterior fate is established in the presomitic mesoderm prior to overt somitogenesis (Aoyama and Asamoto, 1988). At the genetic level, specification of A/P polarity is linked to segmentation (Fig. 10–2). Null mutations in the Notch signaling pathway, including the ligands *Dll1* and *Dll3*, resulted in a disruption in anterior- and posterior-specific gene expression, fusion of the vertebrae, and failure of the peripheral nerves to set up in a segmental pattern (Swiatek et al., 1994; Conlon et al., 1995; Oka et al, 1995; de la Pompa et al., 1997; Hrabe de Angelis et al., 1997; Barrantes et al., 1999; Dunwoodie et al., 2002). The role of Notch in this process is predicted by the expression pattern of three of its ligands. *Dll1* and *Jag1* are coexpressed in the posterior half of somite I and the forming somite (−I), while *Dll3* is expressed in the anterior halves of both (Dunwoodie et al., 1997; Mitsiadis et al., 1997; Zhang and Gridley, 1998; Barrantes et al., 1999). This suggests that the juxtaposition of *Dll1/Jag1* and *Dll3* across the forming somite boundary as well as within the forming somite directs differential responses of Notch in the two domains (Fig. 10–2). Consistent with this, *Presenilin1* is selectively required for Notch-dependent transcription in the posterior half of the forming somites (Koizumi et al., 2001).

Specification of the anterior half of the somite is also dependent on the activity of *Mesp2* (Saga et al., 1997; Takahashi et al., 2000). *Mesp2* is transcribed in a broad domain that encompasses presumptive somite −2 and becomes restricted to the anterior half of the presumptive somite prior to the formation of the newest somite. A null mutation in Mesp2 results in loss of anterior-specific transcription in the PSM and somites (Saga et al., 1997; Takahashi et al., 2000). The restriction of the *Mesp2* pattern is dependent on Notch signaling since the band of transcription remains broad in the *Presenilin1*-null, where posterior specification is lost (Koizumi et al., 2001). This also suggests that downregulation of Mesp2 in the posterior half is essential for specification of cells to a posterior fate (Fig. 10–3). Interestingly, replacement of *Mesp2* with an activated form of membrane-tethered intracellular Notch (*Mesp2^{N/N}*) resulted in partial recovery of the *Mesp2^{−/−}* phenotype (Takahashi et al., 2000). This would argue that Notch lies upstream of specification of both halves of the somite. Further studies will be required to sort out this complex regulatory network.

Paraxis and *Pax-3*, which are associated with the regulation of somite epithelialization, have also been implicated in the A/P polarity of somites. *Paraxis* appears to be required downstream of the spatial specification of the two halves of the somite in the PSM (Johnson et al., 2001). In *paraxis^{−/−}* embryos, transcription of *Mesp2* and components of the Notch signaling pathway are unaltered in the PSM.

In contrast, posterior-specific genes in the newly formed somite are broadly transcribed across the mutant somite. These observations are consistent with a failure to maintain the existing polarity. It has been proposed that paraxis participates in a cell adhesion-dependent mechanism of maintaining a boundary between the two halves of the somite after specification (Johnson et al., 2001).

MUSCLE DEVELOPMENT

Skeletal muscle is one of the most intensely studied tissues in vertebrate embryo development. A combination of *in vivo* and *in vitro* genetic approaches has led to a complex circuitry of regulatory factors controlling discrete events during embryonic myogenesis (Fig. 10–3). At the center of the circuitry are the MyoD family of myogenic bHLH transcription factors, which are crucial for almost every aspect of muscle development. In this section, we will discuss how discrete components of the regulatory circuitry direct *(1)* specification of premyogenic cells to the myogenic lineage, *(2)* proliferation and migration of premyogenic cells, *(3)* differentiation of mononucleated myoblasts into multinucleated contractile myofibers, *(4)* expansion of the muscle mass through hyperplastic and hypertrophic growth of the myofibers, and *(5)* establishment of individual muscle groups through remodeling of muscle masses.

Cellular Events during Myotome Formation

To understand the genetic basis for myogenesis, it is important to first describe the cellular events involved. In response to ventral signals from the notochord and dorsal signals from the surface ectoderm, the newly formed epithelial somite divides into a ventral/medial mes-

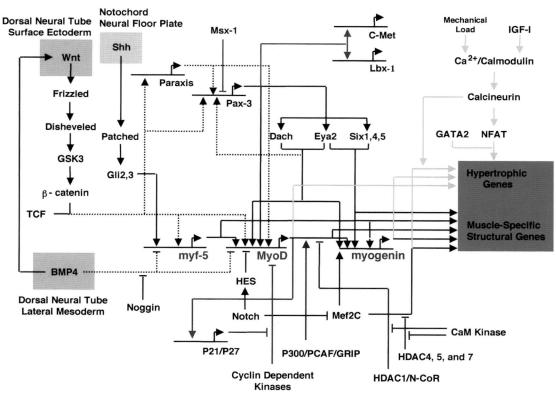

Figure 10–3. The genetic circuitry of genes that regulate muscle differentiation. The genes that regulate distinct events during myogenesis have been incorporated into a single complex circuit. The myogenic basic helix-loop-helix factors that are common regulators to all of these processes are central in the circuit. Red lines indicate inductive and inhibitory events associated with cell cycle regulation. Green lines indicate regulatory relationships between genes that regulate nucleosome remodeling. Yellow lines indicate regulatory relationships among genes involved in regulating fiber type-specific gene expression and hypertrophy. Blue lines indicate the regulatory relationship between genes that regulate the migration of premyogenic cells into the limb. Solid lines represent direct regulation. Dotted lines indicate that it is not known if the regulation is direct. Flat lines indicate that the gene acts as a repressor. Shh, sonic hedgehog; GSK, glycogen synthase kinase; TCF, T-cell factor; BMP, bone morphogenetic protein; CaM kinase, calcium/calmodulin-dependent protein kinase; HES, hairy enhancer of split; HDAC, histone deacetylase; Mef, myocyte enhancer factor; PCAF, p300/CBP-associated factor; N-COR, nuclear reeptor corepressor; NFAT, nuclear factor of activated cell; GRIP, glucocorticoid receptor interactive protein.

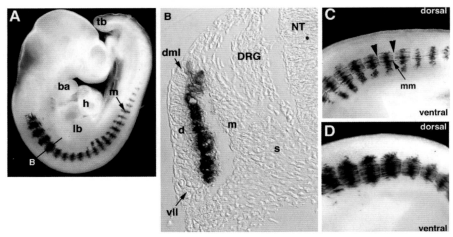

Figure 10–4. Expression of *β-Galactosidase* from the myogenin promoter in mouse 9.5 days postconception (*dpc*). The formation of the myotome can be visualized by staining embryos carrying a muscle-specific *β-Galactosidase* transgene for LacZ enzymatic activity. *(A)* Lateral view of a 9.5 dpc transgenic mouse. The differences in the degree of myotome formation along the anterior/posterior axis can be visualized. ba, branchial arch; lb, limb bud; h, heart; tb, tailbud; m, myotome. *(B)* Transverse section through the thoracic somite. The myotome (m) forms between the sclerotome (s) and the dermomyotome (d) through the migration of cells from the dorsal medial (dml) and ventral lat- eral (vll) lips of the dermomyotome. DRG, dorsal root ganglia; NT, neural tube. *(C)* Lateral view of the lower thoracic somites. Myoblasts have differentiated into mononuclear myotubes (mm), which span the width of the myotome. Myotubes are arranged in a parallel manner, with the nuclei aligned at the midline. The hypaxial (ventral) myotome has begun to form at this stage, though many of the cells have not yet adopted the morphology of the myotubes in the epaxial myotome. Arrows demarcate somite boundaries. *(D)* Lateral view of more mature cervical somites, in which the increase in density of the myotubes associated with a second wave of migration can be seen.

enchymal compartment (sclerotome) and an epithelial sheet (dermomyotome). The origins of skeletal muscle lie within two highly mitogenic, premyogenic cell populations located at the dorsal/medial and ventral/lateral margins of the epithelial dermomyotome (Fig. 10–4B). The first evidence of myogenesis occurs around 8.0 *dpc*, when cells from the dorsal/medial lip of the dermomyotome migrate subjacently, creating a third cellular compartment, the myotome (Fig. 10–4B) (Ordahl and Le Douarin, 1992; Denetclaw et al., 1997). These cells become postmitotic and differentiate into mononucleated myofibers, which are arrayed in a side-by-side manner (Fig. 10–4A, C) (Holtzer et al., 1975). Subsequent expansion of the myotome dorsally and along the medial/lateral axis occurs through successive waves of myofiber migration from the dorsal/medial lip and the anterior and posterior lips of the dermomyotome (Fig. 10–4D) (Denetclaw et al., 1997; Kahane et al., 1998; Denetclaw and Ordahl, 2000; Ordahl et al., 2001). Fusion of mononucleated myofibers into the multinucleated muscle fibers that resemble the epaxial (deep back) muscles begins around 11.5 *dpc* in the dorsal domain of the myotome (Venters et al., 1999).

A second round of myotome expansion begins around 10.0 *dpc* with the migration of cells from the ventral/lateral lip of the dermomyotome (Fig. 10–4B). The lateral myotome then expands ventrally, penetrating the somatopleure of the lateral mesoderm to give rise to the hypaxial muscles of the body wall, including the segmented intercostal muscles, the abdominal wall muscle (internal and external obliques and transverse abdominis), and the rectus abdominis at the ventral midline. In the occipital and cervical somites, myogenic progenitor cells from the dorsolateral lip of the dermomyotome will also migrate to populate the muscle primordia of the hypoglossal muscles of the tongue (Noden, 1983) and the diaphragm (Bladt et al., 1995) and into the limb bud to form the girdle and appendicular muscles (Christ and Ordahl, 1995).

Muscle Differentiation

The genetic basis of muscle differentiation has been an area of intense study. Cell culture systems have been developed in which muscle differentiation can be induced in mononucleated myoblasts or fibroblasts. These studies led to the identification of the MyoD family of bHLH transcription factors (MyoD, myf-5, myogenin, and muscle regulatory factor 4 [MRF4]). These factors auto- and cross-regulate their expression and collaborate with members of the myocyte enhancer factor 2 (MEF2) family of MADS box MCMI, agamous, deficiens, and SRF transcription factors to directly activate the transcription of

muscle-specific genes (Fig. 10–3) (reviewed in Molkentin and Olson, 1996; Yun and Wold, 1996; Black and Olson, 1998; Arnold and Braun, 2000). Recently, the genetic pathway has been revealed to be more complex with the identification of additional cofactors that control cell cycle progression and chromatin remodeling.

During embryonic development, the myogenic bHLH genes are expressed in an overlapping pattern in the myotome. *Myf-5* mRNA transcripts are first detected in cells at the medial edge of the myotome at 8.0 *dpc* (Ott et al., 1991), and expression spreads ventrolaterally with the expansion of the myotome. *Myogenin* is transcribed next in the myotome at 8.5 *dpc* in mice, followed by transient expression of *MRF4* (9.0 and 11.5 *dpc*) (Sassoon et al., 1989; Hinterberger et al., 1991; Bober et al., 1991). *MyoD* is expressed last at 10.0 *dpc*. In the somites of the trunk, the pattern of *MyoD* expression is distinct from that of the other bHLH factors in that it is highest in the myoblasts at the lateral edge of the myotome. The sequential transcription of the myogenic bHLH factors is recapitulated in the developing muscle of the limb buds. The first gene to be transcribed is *myf-5* at 10.0 *dpc*, followed by *MyoD* and *myogenin* (Montarras et al., 1991).

The overlapping but unique expression patterns of the myogenic bHLH factors suggested that each gene played a distinct role during embryonic muscle development. However, gene knockout experiments revealed that *myf-5* and *MyoD* possess redundant functions and are required for the specification of cells to the myogenic lineage (Braun et al., 1992; Rudnicki et al., 1992, 1993). Mice deficient for either *myf-5* or *MyoD* have the normal array of muscles, while mice lacking both genes are devoid of cells expressing muscle-specific genes. A difference in the spatial expression of *myf-5* and *MyoD* and a difference in their role in the onset of epaxial and hypaxial muscle differentiation suggest that the genes represent two distinct entry points into myogenesis (Braun et al., 1994; Braun and Arnold, 1996; Kablar et al., 1997). Differentiation of muscle is dependent on the expression of *myogenin*, *MRF4*, and *MyoD* downstream of specification as muscle. *Myogenin* is required for the differentiation of the majority of embryonic muscle. In targeted *myogenin-null* mutants, the muscle mass is populated with a few muscle fibers and mononucleated myoblasts (Hasty et al., 1993; Nabeshima et al., 1993). The role of *MRF4* is less clear since deletion of the gene results in an increase in *myogenin* levels and normal muscle development (Zhang et al., 1995). However, compound mutant mice deficient for *MyoD* and *MRF4* failed to express myogenin and showed a deficiency similar to the *myogenin-null*, suggesting that these genes lie upstream in the regulation of *myogenin* (Rawls et al., 1998). Mice deficient for *MyoD, myogenin,* and *MRF4* fail to form any muscle fibers, indicating that *myf-5* is not sufficient to direct the muscle differentiation program (Valdez et al., 2000).

The phenotypes of individual and compound null mutants of the myogenic bHLH genes suggest that these factors can be split into a specification subclass (*myf-5* and *MyoD*) and a differentiation subclass (*myogenin* and *MRF4*). This is supported by the observation that *myogenin* is not sufficient to promote myogenesis when knocked into the *myf-5* locus (Wang and Jaenisch, 1997). Similarly, *MyoD* is unable to initiate muscle differentiation in the place of *myogenin* in ES cells (Myer et al., 2001). Differences in the activity of the two subclasses have also been observed in vitro. MyoD and myf-5 have a greater intrinsic ability to regulate the cell cycle, synergize with MEF2C, activate transcriptionally silent endogenous genes, and induce chromatin remodeling (Gerber et al., 1997; Black et al., 1998; de la Serna et al., 2001; Kitzmann and Fernandez, 2001).

A key component of muscle differentiation is the balance between cell proliferation and differentiation. A mitotically active population of cells that is specified to the myogenic lineage must be maintained in order to supply cells to the differentiating postmitotic muscle. Recent studies have implicated MyoD and myf-5 in regulating the cell cycle of dividing myoblasts. MyoD is degraded at G_1/S by a phosphorylation-dependent pathway mediated by cyclin-dependent kinases (cdks). Stabilization of MyoD by inhibition of G_1/S cdks by cdk inhibitors and interaction with retinoblastoma protein (pRb) results in exit from the cell cycle and onset of muscle differentiation (Reynaud et al., 2000; Porrello et al., 2000; Kitzmann and Fernandez, 2001). Myf-5, which is normally degraded at mitosis, can disrupt the cell cycle if present at high enough levels (Lindon et al., 2000). Though there is no direct evidence that these mechanisms are critical during the in vivo regulation of the cell cycle, the cdk inhibitor p21 is regulated by MyoD in the developing embryo and a p21/p57 compound null mutant displays severe muscle defects (Parker et al., 1995; Zhang et al., 1999).

Role of Nucleosome Remodeling in Regulating Myogenesis

Chromatin structure and the acetylation state of histones play an important role in the regulation of gene expression. In the deacetylated state, DNA is packaged around histones in repeating units of condensed chromatin, called "nucleosomes" (reviewed in Strahl and Allis, 2000). Acetylation of the histones weakens the interaction between the positively charged residues on the histone tail and the negatively charged phosphates in the backbone of the DNA, resulting in relaxation of the nucleosome. Two families of antagonistic enzymes, histone acetyltransferases (HATs) and histone deacetylases (HDACs), catalyze these events and thereby act as transcriptional activators and repressors, respectively. Regulation of histone acetylation has been demonstrated to control the muscle differentiation program by activating or repressing muscle-specific transcription (McKinsey et al., 2001). The transcriptional switch appears to occur through the association of the myogenic bHLH and MEF2 proteins with HATs and HDACs. This link between cell type-specific transcription factors and ubiquitous chromatin remodeling factors provides a model for the activation or repression of transcriptional programs.

MyoD forms a complex with p300 and p300/cAMP response element binding protein (CBP)–associated factor (PCAF), a transcriptional co-activator that possesses intrinsic HAT activity (Eckner et al., 1996). When MyoD binds to the E box in the enhancers of the muscle-specific genes, this targets the HAT enzymes to the appropriate nucleosomes (Fig. 10–3). A second function of p300 binding is acetylation of MyoD, which increases the affinity of the transcription factor for muscle-specific promoters (Sartorelli et al., 1997; Polesskaya et al., 2000). Disruption of this complex with an anti-p300 antibody resulted in repression of MyoD-dependent muscle-specific transcription (Yuan et al., 1996; Puri et al., 1997a; Sartorelli et al., 1997). Interestingly, deletion of the HAT domain in p300 does not disrupt MyoD-dependent transcription. In contrast, PCAF HAT activity is critical to MyoD-dependent transcription and muscle differentiation (Puri et al., 1997b). This suggests that the role of p300 may be to act as a

bridge between MyoD and PCAF. Recruitment of p300 and PCAF to transcriptional complexes requires the steroid receptor coactivator glucocorticoid receptor interacting protein (GRIP). Consistent with this, disruption of GRIP using antisense RNA blocks muscle differentiation in C2 muscle cell lines, indicating that it is required for muscle-specific transcription (Chen et al., 2000).

Members of the HDAC family are potent inhibitors of muscle-specific transcription and differentiation. The inhibitory activity of HDAC4, HDAC5, and HDAC7 is mediated through an interaction with MEF2 (Sparrow et al., 1999; Miska et al., 1999; Wang et al., 1999; Lu et al., 2000a; Lemercier et al., 2000). In contrast, HDAC1 inhibits muscle-specific transcription by binding to MyoD as part of a complex with the nuclear receptor corepressor (N-CoR) (Bailey et al., 1999; Mal et al., 2001). Regulation of myogenesis by HDAC4 and HDAC5 appears to be related to the subcellular localization of the proteins (Fig. 10–3). HDACs are exported from the nucleus in response to the phosphorylation of two conserved serine residues by calcium/calmodulin-dependent kinase (Lu et al., 2000b; McKinsey et al., 2000a). The phosphorylation releases MEF2, and HDAC is transported out of the nucleus in a complex with 14-3-3, the intracellular chaperone protein (Grozinger and Schreiber, 2000; McKinsey et al., 2000b; Wang et al., 2000). MEF2 is subsequently available to participate in muscle-specific transcription.

Initiation of Myogenesis

Initiation of the genetic program that leads to muscle specification and ultimately differentiation is the result of a combination of signals originating from the surrounding dorsal and ventral tissues (Munsterberg et al., 1995; Pownall et al., 1996; Marcelle et al., 1999). Opposing gradients of dorsal and ventral signals appear to act synergistically at the dorsal medial lip of the dermomyotome to induce myogenic specification. Interestingly, these same signaling gradients act antagonistically in the specification of dorsal and ventral structures of the somite (Pourquié et al., 1993; Johnson et al., 1997), underscoring the subtle balance of factor concentrations and activity required for proper muscle development. Candidate factors include members of the Wnt family of signaling molecules expressed in the dorsal neural tube and surface ectoderm and Sonic Hedgehog (Shh) produced by the notochord and floor plate of the neural tube (see Chapter 16).

Components of the Wnt signaling pathway, including *Frizzled1, -2,* and *-7* receptors, are expressed broadly in the epithelial somite (Cauthen et al., 2001). Transcription of *Frizzled1* becomes restricted first to the dermomyotome and then the myotome. This is consistent with a role in regulating the induction of muscle-specific transcription (Schmidt et al., 2000). Ectopic expression of Wnt-1, -3a, and -4 in avian somites is sufficient to activate the transcription of *Pax-3, paraxis,* and *MyoD* (Wagner et al., 2000). Since Pax-3 and paraxis are able to direct the transcription of *MyoD* in the hypaxial myotome, it is not clear whether the induction of *MyoD* by Wnts is direct or indirect. The myogenic activity of Wnt-1 and -3a can be recapitulated by overexpression of β-catenin in avian somites and P19 cells (Capdevila et al., 1998; Petropoulos and Skerjanc, 2002). Wnt activation of the myogenic pathway is spatially restricted to the dorsal/medial lip of the dermomyotome. This appears to be due in part to the expression of Frzb and Srfp2 in the ventral half of the somite (Ladher et al., 2000; Terry et al., 2000). These are secreted forms of the Frizzled receptor that inhibit Wnt signaling.

During somitogenesis, the Shh signaling pathway was initially identified for its role in specifying cells in the ventral somite to the sclerotome lineage (reviewed in Hammerschmidt et al., 1997). Shh binding to Patched on the cell surface activates a family of zinc finger transcription factors, *Gli1, -2,* and *-3.* Shh is able to regulate the specification of the epaxial muscles by inducing *myf-5* transcription in premyogenic cells in the dorsal/medial lip (Borycki et al., 1999; Gustafsson et al., 2002). Expression of *Pax-3* and *MyoD* was affected by Shh, suggesting that it does not have the same role during hypaxial muscle development from the ventral/lateral dermomyotome (Marcelle et al., 1999). However, local Shh signals in the limb appear to be required for the survival and proliferation of myogenic hypaxial cells after migration (Krüger et al., 2001).

Proper specification of the myotome and sclerotome are dependent on crosstalk between the Wnt and Shh signaling pathways. Transcription of *Gli2* and *Gli3* in the dermomyotome and myotome require Wnt-1 and Wnt-4, produced by the dorsal neural tube. Since Wnt activity can be recapitulated by expression of β-catenin (Borycki et al., 2000), inductive activity of Shh is dependent on Wnt signaling. Conversely, Shh is able to induce expression of the Wnt inhibitor *Srfp2* in the ventral somite (Lee et al., 2000). It is presumed that this will limit the dorsalizing activity of Wnts in the region of the somite fated to form the sclerotome.

Bone morphogenetic factor 4 (BMP4), a member of the transforming growth factor β (TGF-β) superfamily of signaling molecules, is also important for the spatial regulation of myogenesis (Pourquié et al., 1996) (see Chapter 24). Both inhibitory and inductive activities have been reported for BMP4. Exposure of somitic cells to BMP4 expressed from the lateral mesoderm or dorsal neural tube results in inhibition of myogenesis. In contrast, BMP4 acting on cells in the neural tube induces expression of Wnt-1 and -3a, which in turn promotes myogenesis (Marcelle et al., 1999). The inhibitory activity of BMP4 can be antagonized by Noggin and follistatin, which are secreted proteins that bind with high affinity to members of the TGF-β family. Both Noggin and follistatin are expressed in the dorsal/medial lip of the dermomyotome. Inactivation of *Noggin* results in loss of the myotome, supporting a role for this gene in neutralizing BMP4 activity (McMahon et al., 1998).

In cell culture, it has been demonstrated that Notch signaling can also prevent muscle cell differentiation (Kato et al., 1997; Kopan et al., 1994; Lindsell et al., 1995; Shawber et al., 1996b). This is mediated through upregulation of *HES-1*, which is able to block MyoD-induced myogenesis (Jarriault et al., 1995). Inhibition also occurs by the direct binding of activated Notch to MEF2C, which disrupts its ability to synergize with MyoD (Wilson-Rawls *et al.*, 1999b). Notch may inhibit myogenesis by antagonizing Wnt signaling. This may occur by Wnt binding to the Notch receptor or through an interaction between intracellular components of the two pathways (reviewed in Strooper and Annaert, 2001). In chick somites, the *Notch1* receptor is expressed in postmitotic cells of the myotome while *Dll1* and *Serrate2* transcripts are detected in subsets of differentiating myogenic cells (Delfini et al., 2000; Hirsinger et al., 2001). Misexpression of Dll1 in the early myotome or muscle mass of the limbs results in the specific downregulation of *MyoD* in postmitotic cells. In contrast, *myf-5* and *Pax-3* transcription is unaffected, suggesting that the Notch pathway regulates myogenesis downstream of specification.

Six-Eya-Dach Pathway

The *Six* genes are a family of homeobox-containing transcription factors that have recently been identified as important regulators of muscle differentiation (see Chapter 46). The first member of the family, *sine ocutis* (*so*), was identified in *Drosophila*. This gene is a component of a regulatory network that includes *eyeless* (*ey*), *eye absent* (*eya*), and *dachsund* (*dach*), which are required for compound eye development (Cheyette et al., 1994; Serikaku and O'Tousa, 1994). In vertebrates, three members of the Six family have been identified that are expressed in an embryonic pattern consistent with a role in regulating muscle development. *Six1* and *Six4* are expressed in somites and adult skeletal muscle, while *Six5* is expressed only in skeletal muscle (Oliver et al., 1994; Kawakami et al., 1996; Boucher et al., 1996; Heath et al., 1997; Ohto et al., 1998). All three of these factors are able to bind in a sequence-specific manner to the MEF3 regulatory element (consensus sequence TCAGGTT), which is found in the promoter of *myogenin* and other muscle-specific genes, such as *aldolase A* and *muscle creatine kinase* (Cheng et al., 1993; Yee and Rigby, 1993; Hidaka et al., 1993; Salminen et al., 1996; Spitz et al., 1998). In cell culture, *Six4* is able to activate transcription of *myogenin* in an MEF3-dependent manner, alone or synergistically with *Eya* (Ohto et al., 1999). The Six genes are also able to induce myogenesis *in vivo*. Overexpression of avian *Six1* and *Eya2* in somite explants was sufficient to induce transcription of *MyoD*, *myogenin*, and *Myosin Heavy Chain* (*MHC*) (Heanue et al., 1999). Further, *Six5* in humans is located immediately downstream of the CTG trinucleotide repeats whose

expansion causes myotonic dystrophy (Boucher et al., 1995). Transcription of *Six5* is reduced in myotonic dystrophy patients, suggesting a potential role in the developmental difficulties associated with the disease (Klesert et al., 1997; Winchester et al., 1999). However, a targeted null mutation in *Six4* did not result in a defect in skeletal muscle development (Ozaki et al., 2001). Considering the overlapping expression patterns and binding activity, it is possible that *Six1* or *Six5* is able to compensate for the absence of *Six4*.

The observation that *Eya* genes can act synergistically with *Six1* and *Six4* to activate muscle-specific transcription suggests that a regulatory network initially described for *Drosophila* eye development is required for vertebrate muscle development. Interestingly, there are significant similarities in both regulatory systems. Genetic studies in *Drosophila* have demonstrated that compound eye development is dependent on *ey*, the *Drosophila* homolog of the vertebrate *Pax-6*. Ey activates the transcription of *so*, *eya*, and *dach* (Chen et al., 1997). Physical interactions between *so* and *eya* and between *eya* and *dach* lead to synergistic activation of eye-specific genes as well as a positive feedback loop with *ey* (Pignoni et al., 1997; Halder et al., 1998; Chen et al., 1997; Shen and Mardon, 1997). In addition to *Six* genes, *Eya1*, *Eya2*, *Eya4*, and *Dach2* are expressed in the epithelial somite before becoming restricted to the dorsal/medial and ventral/lateral lips of the dermomyotome (Heanue et al., 1999). Subsequently, they appear in the muscle precursors of the myotome and limbs (Xu et al., 1997; Mishima and Tomarev, 1998; Borsani et al., 1999; Heanue et al., 1999). Similar to their function in the eye, eya2 and dach2 interact in somitic cells and synergistically induce transcription of the myogenic factors *MyoD* and *myogenin* and differentiation-specific genes such as *MHC* (Heanue et al., 1999). Little is known about how *Dach* genes direct transcription. Based on sequence similarities with the transcription factors Ski and Sno, it has been proposed that Dach dimerizes through its DD2 domain and binds to transcriptional complexes in a DNA-independent manner (Nomura et al., 1999; Heanue et al., 1999).

In contrast to eye development, *Pax-6* is not expressed in the epithelial somite. However, the closely related genes *Pax-3* and *Pax-7* are transcribed in an overlapping pattern with genes in the *Six-Eya-Dach* pathway. *Pax-3* participates in a positive feedback loop with *Dach2* and *Eya2* in somitic tissue (Heanue et al., 1999). These observations suggest that the regulatory pathway is recruited to function downstream of different members of the Pax gene family, depending on the developmental context. This is supported by the activation of *Eya1*, *Six1*, and *Six2* by *Pax-2* during otic and kidney development (Xu et al., 1999). The combination of *Eya* and *Six* genes expressed varies with the developing tissue. For example, *Eya2*, *Six1*, *Six4*, and *Six5* are expressed in muscle, while *Eya1* and *Six2* are expressed in the kidney. Therefore, tissue specificity may be induced by the combination of genes activated by the *Pax* genes.

Regulation of Myogenesis in the Migratory Muscles

The hypaxial muscles that are derived from the ventral/lateral lip of the dermomyotome can adopt one of two fates. These cells can migrate into the myotome, where they will contribute to the intercostal and abdominal muscles of the body wall. Alternatively, they can migrate away from the somites to populate the regions of the embryo that will give rise to muscles of the pectoral and pelvic girdles, appendages, septum transversum, and hypoglossal chord. The migratory muscles are able to delay the expression of the myogenic factors and remain proliferative, which is important for establishing a myogenic stem cell population at remote sites. Regulation of the migratory myogenic cells follows a pathway similar to that of the nonmigratory muscles in that the cells must become specified to the myogenic lineage, proliferate, and differentiate. However, these cells must also maintain the premyogenic state away from the dermomyotome and migrate to the correct target site.

The origins of the nonmigratory premyogenic cell population in the dermomyotome are unclear. A series of spontaneous mutations in *Pax-3* (*Splotch* alleles) resulted in failure of muscles to develop in the limbs, tongue, and diaphragm, identifying *Pax-3* as an important regulator of the migratory hypaxial muscle (Bober et al., 1994) (see Chapter 61). *Pax-3* is transcribed throughout the epithelial somite before becoming restricted to the dorsal/medial and ventral/lateral lips of the dermomyotome. As premyogenic cells migrate into the periphery, *Pax-3* transcripiton is maintained in the cells until the time of differentiation. *Pax-3^Splotch/Splotch* embryos have an increase in apoptosis of premyogenic cells in the ventral/lateral dermomyotome and a reduction in the number of cells that migrate away from the dermomyotome (Daston et al., 1996; Tremblay et al., 1998). This predicts that Pax-3 plays an important early role in maintaining the mitogenically active cell population in the dermomyotome. *Pax-3* is expressed exclusively in mitogenically active premyogenic cells in the developing limb muscle mass, suggesting that Pax-3 performs the same function in the limb (Goulding et al., 1998; Amthor et al., 1999). It is not clear whether Pax-3 is directly involved in regulating cell migration. The transcription of other genes believed to participate in migration, such as *c-met* and *Lbx1*, is reduced in the *Pax-3^Splotch/Splotch* embryo, raising the possibility that Pax-3 is indirectly involved in this process (Mennerich et al., 1998; Dietrich et al., 1999).

The role of *Pax-3* in myogenesis is not restricted to the migratory premyogenic cells in the dermomyotome. Ectopic expression of *Pax-3* in avian embryos results in the induction of *MyoD* transcription, indicating that the gene is also involved in initiating muscle differentiation (Maroto et al., 1997). This is supported by the generation of compound null mice between *Pax-3* and *Myf-5*, which fail to develop skeletal muscle in the trunk and limbs (Tajbakhsh et al., 1997). Since *Myf-5* is required for the specification of hypaxial muscles, it was concluded that *Pax-3* is integral for establishing all of the hypaxial muscles. Therefore, two contrasting activities, differentiation and maintenance in a premyogenic state, have been ascribed to Pax-3 in the ventral/lateral dermomyotome. It has been proposed that the differentiation-specific activity of Pax-3 is inhibited in the migratory population until the appropriate time. A likely candidate for inhibition is *Msx-1*, a homeobox transcription factor that can interfere with the DNA-binding activity of Pax-3 *in vivo* and *in vitro* (Woloshin et al., 1995; Bendall et al., 1999; Houzelstein et al., 1999). *Msx-1* is coexpressed with *Pax-3* in migrating premyogenic cells and downregulated at the onset of differentiation (see Chapter 51).

Similar to somite epithelialization, *paraxis* appears to be linked to *Pax-3* in the regulation of the hypaxial premyogenic cell population. *Paraxis* is transcribed in a broader pattern than *Pax-3* in the maturing somite that temporarily includes the sclerotome (Burgess et al., 1995). In the absence of *paraxis*, cell proliferation is dramatically reduced in premyogenic cells (Wilson-Rawls et al., 1999a). *Pax-3* transcription is absent in the newly formed somites of 9.5 *dpc* mutant embryos and reappears at the lateral edge of the dermomyotome. Further, compound *paraxis/myf-5* null mutants experience a reduction in migratory hypaxial muscles and loss of epaxial and nonmigratory hypaxial muscles. This suggests that the activity of paraxis distinguishes between the migratory and nonmigratory myogenic precursor cells.

Migration of myogenic precursor cells is dependent on the delamination of cells from the epithelial sheet of the dermomyotome. Delamination requires an interaction between hepatocyte growth factor (HGF) and its tyrosine kinase receptor, c-Met (Bladt et al., 1995; Maina et al., 1996). *c-met* is expressed in the lateral dermomyotome and medial lip of all somites. In contrast, *HGF* is expressed in the lateral mesenchyme of the limbs and branchial arches adjacent to the somites (Bladt et al., 1995; Takayama et al., 1996; Yang et al., 1996; Dietrich et al., 1999). Therefore, the spatial restriction of the ligand along the A/P axis leads to selective activation of the c-Met receptor in the somites, which will give rise to the migratory cells. Though constant exposure of c-Met-expressing cells to HGF would seem to be a likely mechanism to direct cell migration, addition of ectopic HGF in the interlimb region of chick embryos directs delamination but not migration (Brand-Saberi et al., 1996; Heymann et al., 1996). However, continued activation of c-Met is important for maintaining the migratory cells in a proliferative state, as required for the establishment of a remote premyogenic cell population (Scaal et al., 1999).

The migration of premyogenic cells to specific domains of the developing limb bud is dependent on the homeobox-containing transcription factor (Jagla et al., 1995) *Lbx1* and an interaction between the receptor tyrosine kinase receptor EphA4 and its ligand ephrinA5. *Lbx1* is expressed in premyogenic cells fated to the migratory lineage prior to delamination and maintained in the migrating cells until differentiation (Mennerich et al., 1998; Dietrich et al., 1998, 1999). In the limb, cells migrate to either the proximal/ventral or proximal/dorsal region and will give rise to the extensor and flexor muscles, respectively. In the *Lbx1*-null, the majority of cells that would normally migrate to the proximal/ventral domain aberrantly migrate into the ventral body wall (Schäfer and Braun, 1999; Brohmann et al., 2000; Gross et al., 2000). *EphA4* is also expressed in premyogenic cells in the ventral/lateral lip of the dermomyotome and maintained throughout the migration process (Swartz et al., 2001). Its ligand, ephrinA5, is expressed in the lateral mesoderm of the limb bud, except in the regions of the ventral and dorsal muscle masses. Interaction of Eph receptors with their ligands, ephrins, influences axon guidance, cell migration, and the formation of cellular boundaries in the developing nervous system (Krull et al., 1997; Wang and Anderson, 1997; Smith et al., 1997; Mellitzer et al., 1999; Kullander et al., 2001; Wilkinson, 2001). In the case of axon guidance, ephrin binding to Eph receptor results in a inhibitory response by collapsing the growth cone. This occurs due to remodeling of cytoskeletal actin via the Rho family of GTPases in the Eph-expressing cell (Wahl et al., 2000). The migratory path of EphA4 expressing premyogenic cells in the limb can be altered by ephrinA5 (Swartz et al., 2001). It is unlikely that EphA4 is the sole regulator of cell migration since *EphA4^−/−* mice do not exhibit limb muscle defects.

Differentiation of migratory cells follows a regulatory pathway similar to that of nonmigratory myoblasts of the myotome. Entry into the myogenic lineage begins with transcription of either *myf-5* or *MyoD*. Along with *Mef2*, *myf-5* and *MyoD* direct the transcription of *myogenin* and the structural genes involved in muscle differentiation. The novel requirement of regulating muscle differentiation in the limb is to maintain a subpopulation of cells in a proliferative, nondifferentiated state. A balance between proliferation and differentiation is important for maintaining the local premyogenic cell population required for muscle growth (Amthor et al., 1999; Bendall et al., 1999). Pax-3 is implicated in regulating the onset of myogenic differentiation by inducing *MyoD* transcription (Maroto et al., 1997), and overexpression of Pax-3 in the chick limb can lead to premature differentiation. The action of Pax-3 is antagonized by the homeobox factor Msx1, which is expressed in the migratory cells up until the time of differentiation (Woloshin et al., 1995; Houzelstein et al., 1999; Bendall et al., 1999). Paraxis is also expressed in the migratory cells and downregulated at the time of differentiation (Delfini and Duprez, 2000). It is possible that paraxis is required for the maintenance of a MyoD-dependent subpopulation within the limb bud. This is supported by the observation of reduced limb muscle in *paraxis^−/−/myf-5^−/−*, but not in *myf-5^−/−* or *paraxis^−/−*, embryos (Wilson-Rawls et al., 1999a).

Maturation of Individual Muscle Groups

Formation of individual muscle groups from the paraxial mesoderm requires the coordination of differentiation with local morphogenic processes. Once committed to the myogenic lineage, cells migrate to the site of myogenesis, align, and fuse. In mice, myogenesis occurs in two distinct waves (reviewed in Miller et al., 1999). The primary wave consists of myotubes that establish the muscle organization and act as a scaffold for additional myotubes that are generated in a secondary wave. Additional growth occurs through the fusion of mononucleated cells to the existing fibers (Harris et al., 1989; Wigmore et al., 1992; Zhang and McLennan, 1995). At the time of primary myotube formation, muscle groups exhibit heterogeneity in their contractility and fatigue properties, which is based largely on the expression of metabolic enzymes and fast- or slow-twitch isoforms of MHC. The second wave of myogenesis is associated with muscle-specific changes in the composition of fast- and slow-twitch myotubes. The emergence of adult muscles is associated with a change from embryonic to adult MHC isoforms. Maturation of muscles is influenced by innervation, hormonal factors, and the functional demands on individual muscles (Gardahaut et al., 1992; Lefeuvre et al., 1996; Bruekner and Porter, 1997; Washabaugh et al., 1998).

The embryonic origins of fiber-type heterogeneity remain unclear. In avian models, distinct lineages of slow and fast myoblasts have been identified. Myoblasts that will give rise to slow muscles in the limb migrate away from the ventral/lateral edge of the dermomyotme before the fast muscle myoblasts (Van Swearingen and Lance-Jones, 1995). Further, clonal myoblast lines derived from chicken embryos remained committed to either the fast or slow fiber type (Miller and Stockdale, 1986a,b; Miller et al., 1993). Thus, these cells become committed to a specific fiber type prior to muscle differentiation. Interestingly, the commitment of cells to a single fiber type has not been observed in mice. Murine clonal lines are able to express fast and slow MHC (Robson and Hughes, 1997). Reconciliation between the murine and avian systems likely lies in the extent to which local environmental cues affect the predisposition of myoblasts to a specific fate. In the mouse, local environmental cues likely play a larger role in influencing fiber type gene expression.

Insight into the genetic control of slow and fast fiber types has come from the study of the calcineurin-activated, Ca^{2+}-dependent pathway (reviewed by Olson and Williams, 2000). Calcineurin is a calcium/calmodulin-dependent serine/threonine phosphatase that links intracellular Ca^{2+} concentrations with differentiation-specific muscle transcription. Calcineurin-dependent signals are transduced to target genes by the dephosphorylation of members of the nuclear factor of activated T-cell (NFAT), which allows for transport to the nucleus. (Chin et al., 1998). The importance of this pathway is underscored by the block in the transcription of differentiation-specific genes in cells treated with the calcineurin inhibitor cyclosporin A (CsA) (Abbott et al., 1998). In addtion, dephosphorylated NFAT is actively transported to the nucleus of differentiating myoblasts. Others have reported that calcineurin does not act exclusively through NFAT but is also able to activate MEF2 through dephosphorylation (H. Wu et al., 2000, 2001).

Activation of calcineurin appears to be the intermediate step between motor nerve stimulation and the regulation of fiber type-specific gene expression. Nerve stimulation leads to the release of acetylcholine, which stimulates the release of intracellular Ca^{2+} stored in the sarcoplasmic reticulum. Fast fibers are characterized by sporadic excitation, which leads to large but transient oscillations in intracellular concentrations of Ca^{2+}. In contrast, slow fibers produce sustained excitation, which leads to sustained high Ca^{2+} concentrations. Cross-innervation or electrical pacing experiments that alter the rate or pattern of neuromuscular activation result in changes in the expression pattern of fiber type-specific genes (reviewed by Pette, 2001). Several lines of evidence point to innervation working through the calcineurin pathway. Muscle-specific enhancers for slow fiber subtypes of *myoglobin* and *troponin I* contain NFAT and MEF2 binding sites that are responsive to calcineurin activation (Chin et al., 1998; Calvo et al., 1999; H. Wu et al., 2000, 2001). Further, an increase in the proportion of slow fiber types seen in chronically stimulated muscles can be recapitulated by the ectopic expression of constitutively active *calcineurin* under the control of the *muscle creatine kinase* enhancer (Naya et al., 2000). However, transcription of slow isoforms of *Troponin I* and fast alkali *myosin light chain 1f/3f* is directed by enhancer elements that do not contain binding sites for NFAT, MEF2, or the myogenic factors (Rao et al., 1996; Calvo et al., 1999, 2001). This suggests that a calcineurin-independent mechanism is also at work in regulating fiber type diversity.

Another important aspect of muscle remodeling is growth, or muscle hypertrophy, which also acts through the calcineurin pathway. Insulin-like growth factors (IGFs), inducers of muscle hypertrophy, increase the Ca^{2+} concentration by stimulation of L-type Ca^{2+} channels and expression of calcineurin (Bruton et al., 1999; Musaro et al., 1999; Semsarian et al., 1999; Wang et al., 1999). Treatment of cells with CsA is sufficient to block IGF-induced hypertrophy, indicating that calcineurin is a critical component of the pathway. In addition to stimulation of the calcineurin pathway, IGF stimulates expression of GATA2, which is able to interact with the nonphosphorylated form of NFAT to stimulate transcription (Musaro et al., 1999). An alternative pathway for muscle hypertrophy is through chronic overload associated with exercise. The increase in the mechanical load on the muscles is also associated with an increase in the intracellular con-

centration of Ca^{2+}, implicating the calcineurin pathway in this type of hypertrophy. In support of this hypothesis, treatment of rats with CsA blocks hypertrophy stimulated by mechanical overload (Dunn et al., 1999).

FUTURE DIRECTIONS

The intense study of myogenesis has resulted in insight into the complex genetic circuitry that regulates distinct events such as specification, proliferation, differentiation, and remodeling. This information can be used to explain most aspects of the development of theoretically fast and slow fiber type muscles. The next challenge is to integrate this information into the regulatory network that establishes the complex muscle groups found in the organism. Certainly, this network will include some well-established regulatory elements such as the *Hox* genes as well as poorly understood local signals that refine the morphology of individual muscles.

REFERENCES

Abbott KL, Friday BB, Thaloor D, Murphy TJ, Pavlath GK (1998). Activation and cellular localization of the cyclosporine A-sensitive transcription factor NF-AT in skeletal muscle cells. *Mol Biol Cell* 9: 2905–2916.

Amthor H, Christ B, Patel K (1999). A molecular mechanism enabling continuous embryonic muscle growth—a balance between proliferation and differentiation. *Development* 126: 1041–1053.

Aoyama H, Asamoto K (1988). Determination of somite cells: independence of cell differentiation and morphogenesis. *Development* 104: 15–28.

Arnold HH, Braun T (2000). Genetics of muscle determination and development. *Curr Top Dev Biol* 48: 129–164.

Artavanis-Tsakonas S, Matsuno K, Fortini ME (1995). Notch signaling. *Science* 268: 225–232.

Artavanis-Tsakonas S, Rand MD, Lake RJ (1999). Notch signaling: cell fate control and signal integration in development. *Science* 284: 770–776.

Aulehla A, Johnson RL (1999). Dynamic expression of *lunatic fringe* suggests a link between *notch* signaling and an autonomous cellular driving somite segmentation. *Dev Biol* 207: 49–61.

Bailey AM, Posakony JW (1995). Suppressor of hairless directly activates transcription of enhancer of split complex genes in response to Notch receptor activity. *Genes Dev* 9: 2609–2622.

Bailey P, Downes M, Lau P, Harris J, Chen SL, Hamamori Y, Sartorelli V, Muscat GE (1999). The nuclear receptor corepressor N-CoR regulates differentiation: N-CoR directly interacts with MyoD. *Mol Endocrinol* 13: 1155–1168.

Barrantes I, Elia AJ, Wunsch K, Hrabe De Angelis M, Mak TW, Rossant J, Conlon RA, Gossler A, de la Pompa JL. (1999). Interaction between Notch signalling and Lunatic fringe during somite boundary formation in the mouse. *Curr Biol* 9: 470–480.

Bendall AJ, Ding J, Hu G, Shen MM, Abate-Shen C (1999). Msx1 antagonizes the myogenic activity of Pax3 in migrating limb muscle precursors. *Development* 126: 4965–4976.

Bettenhausen B, Hrabe de Angelis M, Simon D, Guenet JL, Gossler A (1995). Transient and restricted expression during mouse embryogenesis of *Dll1*, a murine gene closely related to *Drosophila* Delta. *Development* 121: 2407–2418.

Black BL, Olson EN (1998). Transcriptional control of muscle development by myocyte enhancer factor-2 (MEF2) proteins. *Annu Rev Cell Dev Biol* 14: 167–196.

Black BL, Molkentin JD, Olson EN (1998). Multiple roles for the MyoD basic region in transmission of transcriptional activation signals and interaction with MEF2. *Mol Cell Biol* 18: 69–77.

Bladt F, Riethmacher D, Isenmann S, Aguzzi A, Birchmeier C (1995). Essential role for the c-met receptor in the migration of myogenic precursor cells into the limb bud. *Nature* 376: 768–771.

Bober E, Lyons GE, Braun T, Cossu G, Buckingham M, Arnold HH (1991). The muscle regulatory gene, Myf-6, has a biphasic pattern of expression during early mouse development. *J Cell Biol* 113: 1255–1265.

Bober E, Franz T, Arnold HH, Gruss P, Tremblay P (1994). Pax-3 is required for the development of limb muscles: a possible role for the migration of dermomyotomal muscle progenitor cells. *Development* 120: 603–612.

Borsani G, DeGrandi A, Ballabio A, Bulfone A, Bernard L, Banfi S, Gattuso C, Mariani M, Dixon M, Donnai D, et al. (1999). *EYA4*, a novel vertebrate gene related to *Drosophila* eyes absent. *Hum Mol Genet* 8: 11–23.

Borycki AG, Brunk B, Tajbakhsh S, Buckingham M, and Emerson CP Jr. (1999). Sonic hedgehog controls epaxial muscle determination through Myf5 activation. *Development* 126:4053-4063.

Borycki AG, Brown AMC, Emerson CP Jr (2000). Shh and Wnt signaling pathways converge to control *Gli* gene activation in avian somites. *Development* 127: 2075–2087.

Boucher CA, King SK, Carey N, Krahe R, Winchester CL, Rahman S, Creavin T, Meghji P, Bailey ME, Chartier FL, et al. (1995). A novel homeodomain-encoding gene is associated with a large CpG island interrupted by the myotonic dystrophy unstable $(CTG)_n$ repeat. *Hum Mol Genet* 4: 1919–1925.

Boucher CA, Carey N, Edwards YH, Siciliano MJ, Johnson KJ (1996). Cloning of the human *SIX1* gene and its assignment to chromosome 14. *Genomics* 33: 140–142.

Brand-Saberi B, Muller TS, Wilting J, Christ B, Birchmeier C (1996). Scatter factor/hepatocyte growth factor (SF/HGF) induces emigration of myogenic cells at interlimb level. *Dev Biol* 179: 303–308.

Braun T, Arnold HH (1996) *Myf-5* and *myoD* genes are activated in distinct mesenchymal stem cells and determine different skeletal muscle cell lineages. *EMBO J* 15: 310–318.

Braun T, Rudnicki MA, Arnold HH, Jaenisch R (1992). Targeted inactivation of the muscle regulatory gene *Myf-5* results in abnormal rib development and perinatal death. *Cell* 71: 369–382.

Braun T, Bober E, Rudnicki MA, Jaenisch R, Arnold HH (1994). MyoD expression marks the onset of skeletal myogenesis in myf-5 mutant mice. *Development* 120: 3083–3092.

Brohmann H, Jagla K, Birchmeier C (2000). The role of Lbx1 in migration of muscle precursor cells. *Development* 127: 437–445.

Brueckner JK, Porter J (1997). Modulation of extraocular muscle maturation by the developing visuomotor system. *J Muscle Res Cell Motil* 18: 203.

Bruton JD, Katz A, Westerblad H (1999). Insulin increases near-membrane but not global Ca^{2+} in isolated skeletal muscle. *Proc Natl Acad Sci USA* 96: 3281–3286.

Buchberger A, Seidl K, Klein C, Eberhardt H, Arnold HH (1998). cMeso-1, a novel bHLH transcription factor, is involved in somite formation in chicken embryos. *Dev Biol* 199: 201–215.

Burgess R, Cserjesi P, Ligon KL, Olson EN (1995). *Paraxis*: a basic helix-loop-helix protein expressed in paraxial mesoderm and developing somites. *Dev Biol* 168: 296–306.

Burgess R, Rawls A, Brown D, Bradley A, Olson EN (1996). Requirement of the *paraxis* gene for somite formation and musculoskeletal patterning. *Nature* 384: 570–573.

Calvo S, Venepally P, Cheng J, Buonanno A (1999). Fiber-type-specific transcription of the troponin I slow gene is regulated by multiple elements. *Mol Cell Biol* 19: 515–525.

Calvo S, Vullhorst D, Venepally P, Cheng J, Karavanova I, Buonanno A (2001). Molecular dissection of DNA sequences and factors involved in slow muscle-specific transcription. *Mol Cell Biol* 21: 8490–8503.

Capdevila J, Tabin C, Johnson RL (1998). Control of dorsoventral somite patterning by Wnt-1 and beta-catenin. *Dev Biol* 193: 182–194.

Cauthen CA, Berdougo E, Sandler J, Burrus LW (2001). Comparative analysis of the expression patterns of Wnts and Frizzleds during early myogenesis in chick embryos. *Mech Dev* 104: 133–138.

Chen R, Amoui M, Zhang Z, Mardon G (1997). Dachshund and eyes absent proteins form a complex and function synergistically to induce ectopic eye development in *Drosophila*. *Cell* 91: 893–903.

Chen SL, Dowhan DH, Hosking BM, Muscat GE (2000). The steroid receptor coactivator, GRIP-1, is necessary for MEF-2C-dependent gene expression and skeletal muscle differentiation. *Genes Dev* 14: 1209–1228.

Cheng TC, Wallace MC, Merlie JP, Olson EN (1993). Separable regulatory elements governing myogenin transcription in mouse embryogenesis. *Science* 261: 215–218.

Cheyette BNR, Green PK, Martin K, Garren H, Hartenstein V, Zipursky SL (1994). The *Drosophila sine oculis* locus encodes a homeodomain-containing protein required for the development of the entire visual system. *Neuron* 12: 977–996.

Chin ER, Olson EN, Richardson JA, Yang Q, Humphries C, Shelton JM, Wu H, Zhu W, Bassel-Duby R, Williams RS (1998). A calcineurin-dependent transcriptional pathway controls skeletal muscle fiber type. *Genes Dev* 12: 2499–2509.

Christ B, Ordahl CP (1995). Early stages of chick somite development. *Anat Embryol (Berl)* 191: 381–396.

Christ B, Wilting J (1992). From somites to vertebral column. *Ann Anat* 174: 23–32.

Ciruna BG, Schwartz L, Harpal K, Yamaguchi TP, Rossant J (1997). Chimeric analysis of *fibroblast growth factor receptor-1 (Fgfr1)* function: a role for FGFR1 in morphogenetic movement through the primitive streak. *Development* 124: 2829–2841.

Conlon RA, Reaume AG, Rossant J (1995). *Notch1* is required for the coordinate segmentation of somites. *Development* 121: 1533–1545.

Cooke J, Zeeman EC (1976). A clock and wavefront model for control of the number of repeated structures during animal morphogenesis. *J Theor Biol* 58: 455–476.

Daston G, Lamar E, Olivier M, Goulding M (1996). Pax-3 is necessary for migration but not differentiation of limb muscle precursors in the mouse. *Development* 122: 1017–1027.

de Celis JF, Bray S (1997). Feed-back mechanisms affecting Notch activation at the dorsoventral boundary in the *Drosophila* wing. *Development* 124: 3241–3251.

Del Amo FF, Smith DE, Swiatek PJ, Gendron-Maguire M, Greenspan RJ, McMahon AP, Gridley T (1992). Expression pattern of Motch, a mouse homolog of *Drosophila* Notch, suggests an important role in early postimplantation mouse development. *Development* 115: 737–744.

de la Pompa JL, Wakeham A, Correia KM, Samper E, Brown S, Aguilera RJ, Nakano T, Honjo T, Mak TW, Rossant J, et al. (1997). Conservation of the Notch signalling pathway in mammalian neurogenesis. *Development* 124: 1139–1148.

de la Serna IL, Carlson KA, Imbalzano AN (2001). Mammalian SWI/SNF complexes promote MyoD-mediated muscle differentiation. *Nat Genet* 27: 187–190.

Delfini MC, Duprez D (2000). Paraxis is expressed in myoblasts during their migration and proliferation in the chick limb bud. *Mech Dev* 96: 247–51.

Delfini M, Hirsinger E, Pourquie O, Duprez D (2000). Delta 1-activated notch inhibits muscle differentiation without affecting Myf5 and Pax3 expression in chick limb myogenesis. *Development* 127: 5213–5224.

Denetclaw WF, Ordahl CP (2000). The growth of the dermomyotome and formation of early myotome lineages in thoracolumbar somites of chicken embryos. *Development* 127: 893–905.

Denetclaw WF Jr, Christ B, Ordahl CP (1997). Location and growth of epaxial myotome precursor cells. *Development* 124: 1601–1610.

Dietrich S, Schubert FR, Healy C, Sharpe PT, Lumsden A (1998). Specification of the hypaxial musculature. *Development* 125: 2235–2249.

Dietrich S, Abou-Rebyeh F, Brohmann H, Bladt F, Sonnenberg-Riethmacher E, Yamaai T, Lumsden A, Brand-Saberi B, Birchmeier C (1999). The role of SF/HGF and c-Met in the development of skeletal muscle. *Development* 126: 1621–1629.

Dockter JL (2000). Sclerotome induction and differentiation. *Curr Top Dev Biol* 48: 77–127.

Dubrulle J, McGrew MM, Pourquie O (2001). FGF signaling controls somite boundary position and regulates segmentation clock control of spatiotemporal Hox gene activation. *Cell* 106: 219–232.

Dunn SE, Bums JL, Michel RN (1999). Calcineurin is required for skeletal muscle hypertrophy. *J Biol Chem* 274: 21908–21912.

Dunwoodie SL, Henrique D, Harrison SM, Beddington RSP (1997). Mouse *Dll3*: a novel divergent *Delta* gene which may complement the function of other Delta homologues during early pattern formation in the mouse embryo. *Development* 124: 3065–3076.

Dunwoodie SL, Clements M, Sparrow DB, Sa X, Conlon RA, Beddington RSP (2002). Axial skeletal defects caused by mutation in the spondylocostal dysplasia/pudgy gene *Dll3* are associated with disruption of the segmentation clock within the presomitic mesoderm. *Development* 129: 1795–1806.

Eckner R, Yao TP, Oldread E, Livingston DM (1996) Interaction and functional collaboration of p300/CBP and bHLH proteins in muscle and B-cell differentiation. *Genes Dev* 10: 2478–2490.

Evrard YA, Lun Y, Aulehla A, Gan L, Johnson RL (1998). Lunatic fringe is an essential mediator of somite segmentation and patterning. *Nature* 394: 377–381.

Galceran J, Farinas I, Depew MM, Clevers H, Grosschedl R (1999). *Wnt3a*$^{-/-}$-like phenotype and limb deficiency in *Lef1*$^{-/-}$Tcf1$^{-/-}$ mice. *Genes Dev* 13: 709–717.

Gardahaut MF, Fontaine-Perus J, Rouaud R, Bandman E, Ferrand R (1992). Developmental modulation of myosin expression by thyroid hormone in avian skeletal muscle. *Development* 115: 1121–1131.

Gerber AN, Klesert TR, Bergstrom DA, Tapscott SJ (1997). Two domains of MyoD mediate transcriptional activation of genes in repressive chromatin: a mechanism for lineage determination in myogenesis. *Genes Dev* 11: 436–450.

Goulding M, Lumsden A, Paquette AJ (1998). Regulation of Pax-3 expression in the dermomyotome and its role in muscle development. *Development* 120: 957–971.

Greenwald I (1998). LIN-12/Notch signaling: lessons from worms and flies. *Genes Dev* 12: 1751–1762.

Gross MK, Moran-Rivard L, Velasquez T, Nakatsu MN, Jagla K, Goulding M (2000). Lbx1 is required for muscle precursor migration along a lateral pathway into the limb. *Development* 127: 413–424.

Grozinger CM, Schreiber SL (2000). Regulation of histone deacetylase 4 and 5 and transcriptional activity by 14-3-3-dependent cellular localization. *Proc Natl Acad Sci USA* 97: 7835–7840.

Gustafsson MK, Pan H, Pinney DF, Liu Y, Lewandowski A, Epstein DJ, Emerson CP Jr. (2002). Myf5 is a direct target of long-range Shh signaling and Gli regulation for muscle specification. *Genes Dev* 16: 114–126.

Halder G, Callaerts P, Flister S, Walldorf U, Kloter U, Gehring WJ (1998). Eyeless initiates the expression of both *sine oculis* and *eyes absent* during *Drosophila* compound eye development. *Development* 125: 2181–2191.

Hamada Y, Kadokawa Y, Okabe M, Ikawa M, Coleman JR, Tsujimoto Y (1999). Mutation in ankyrin repeats of the mouse *Notch2* gene induces early embryonic lethality. *Development* 126: 3415–3424.

Hammerschmidt M, Brook A, McMahon AP (1997). The world according to hedgehog. *Trends Genet* 13: 14–21.

Harris AJ, Duxson MJ, Fitzsimons RB, Rieger F (1989). Myonuclear birthdates distinguish the origins of primary and secondary myotubes in embryonic mammalian skeletal muscles. *Development* 107: 771–784.

Hasty P, Bradley A, Morris JH, Edmondson DE, Venuti JM, Olson EN, Klein WH (1993). Muscle deficiency and neonatal death in mice with a targeted mutation in the *myogenin* gene. *Nature* 364: 501–506.

Heanue TA, Reshef R, Davis RJ, Mardon G, Oliver G, Tomarev S, Lassar AB, Tabin CJ (1999). Synergistic regulation of vertebrate muscle development by *Dach2, Eya2,* and *Six1,* homologs of genes required for *Drosophila* eye formation. *Genes Dev* 13: 3231–3243.

Heath SK, Carne S, Hoyle C, Johnson KJ, Wells DJ (1997). Characterisation of expression of *mDMAHP*, a homeodomain-encoding gene at the murine DM locus. *Hum Mol Genet* 6: 651–657.

Heymann S, Koudrova M, Arnold HH, Koster M, Braun T (1996). Regulation and function of SF/HGF during migration of limb muscle precursor cells in chicken. *Dev Biol* 180: 566–578.

Hinterberger TJ, Sassoon DA, Rhodes SJ, Konieczny SF (1991) Expression of the muscle regulatory factor MRF4 during somite and skeletal myofiber development. *Dev Biol* 147: 144–156.

Hirsinger E, Malapert P, Dubrulle J, Delfini MC, Duprez D, Henrique D, Ish-Horowicz D, Pourquie O (2001). Notch signalling acts in postmitotic avian myogenic cells to control MyoD activation. *Development* 128: 107–116.

Holtzer H, Strahs K, Biehl J, Somlyo AP, Ishikawa H (1975). Thick and thin filaments in postmitotic, mononucleated myoblasts. *Science* 188: 943–945.

Horikawa K, Radice G, Takeichi M, Chisaka O (1999). Adhesive subdivisions intrinsic to the epithelial somites. *Dev Biol* 215: 182–189.

Houzelstein D, Auda-Boucher G, Cheraud Y, Rouaud T, Blanc I, Tajbakhsh S, Buckingham ME, Fontaine-Perus J, Robert B (1999). The homeobox gene *Msx1* is expressed in a subset of somites, and in muscle progenitor cells migrating into the forelimb. *Development* 126: 2689–2701.

Hrabe de Angelis M, McIntyre J II, Gossler A (1997). Maintenance of somite borders in mice requires the Delta homologue Dll1. *Nature* 386: 717–721.

Huppert SS, Jacobsen TL, Muskavitch MA (1997). Feedback regulation is central to Delta–Notch signalling required for *Drosophila* wing vein morphogenesis. *Development* 124: 3283–3291.

Jagla K, Dolle P, Mattei MG, Jagla T, Schuhbaur B, Dretzen G, Bellard F, Bellard M (1995). Mouse Lbx1 and human LBX1 define a novel mammalian homeobox gene family related to the *Drosophila* ladybird genes. *Mech Dev* 53: 345–356.

Jarriault S, Brou C, Logeat F, Schroeter EH, Kopan R, Israel A (1995). Signalling downstream of activated mammalian Notch. *Nature* 377: 355–358.

Jarriault S, Hirsinger E, Pourquié O, Logeat F, Strong CF, Brou C, Seidah N, Israel A (1998). Delta-1 activation of Notch1 signalling results in HES-1 trans-activation. *Mol Cell Biol* 18: 7423–7431.

Jiang Y-J, Aerne BL, Smithers L, Haddon C, Ish-Horowicz D, Lewis J (2000). Notch signalling and the synchronization of the somite segmentation clock. *Nature* 408: 475–479.

Johnson J, Rhee J, Parsons SM, Brown D, Olson EN, Rawls A (2001). The anterior/posterior polarity of somites is disrupted in paraxis-deficient mice. *Dev Biol* 229: 176–187.

Johnson RL, Laufer E, Riddle RD, Tabin C (1997). Ectopic expression of sonic hedgehog alters dorsal–ventral patterning of somites. *Cell* 79: 1165–1173.

Jouve C, Palmeirim I, Henrique D, Beckers J, Gossler A, Ish-Horowicz D, Pourquie O (2000). Notch signalling is required for cyclic expression of the hairy-like gene *HES1* in the presomitic mesoderm. *Development* 127: 1421–1429.

Kablar B, Krastel K, Ying C, Asakura A, Tapscott SJ, Rudnicki MA (1997). MyoD and Myf-5 differentially regulate the development of limb versus trunk skeletal muscle. *Development* 124: 4729–4738.

Kaehn K, Jacob H, Christ B, Hinrichsen K, Poelmann RE (1988). The onset of myotome formation in the chick. *Anat Embryol* 177: 191–201.

Kahane N, Cinnamon Y, Kalcheim C (1998). The cellular mechanism by which the dermomyotome contributes to the second wave of myotome development. *Development* 125: 4259–4271.

Kato H, Taniguchi Y, Kurooka H, Minoguchi S, Sakai T, Nomura-Okazaki S, Tamura K, Honjo T (1997). Involvement of RBP-J in biological functions of mouse Notch1 and its derivatives. *Development* 124: 4133–4141.

Kawakami K, Ohto H, Ikeda K, Roeder RG (1996). Structure, function and expression of a murine homeobox protein AREC3, a homologue of Drosophila sine oculis gene product, and implication in development. *Nucleic Acids Res* 24: 303–310.

Keynes RJ, Stern CD (1988). Mechanisms of vertebrate segmentation. *Development* 103: 413–429.

Kimble J, Simpson P (1997). The LIN-12/Notch signaling pathway and its regulation. *Annu Rev Cell Dev Biol* 13: 333–361.

Kitzmann M, Fernandez A (2001). Crosstalk between cell cycle regulators and the myogenic factor MyoD in skeletal myoblasts. *Cell Mol Life Sci* 58: 571–579.

Klesert TR, Otten AD, Bird TD, Tapscott SJ (1997). Trinucleotide repeat expansion at the myotonic dystrophy locus reduces expression of DMAHP. *Nat Genet* 16: 402–406.

Koizumi K, Mitsunari N, Yuasa S, Saga Y, Sakai T, Kuriyama T, Shirasawa T, Koseki H (2001). The role of presenilin 1 during somite segmentation. *Development* 128: 1391–1402.

Kopan R, Nye JS, Weintraub H (1994). The intracellular domain of mouse Notch: a constitutively activated repressor of myogenesis directed at the basic helix-loop-helix region of MyoD. *Development* 120: 2385–2396.

Krüger M, Mennerich D, Fees S, Schäfer R, Mundlos S, Braun T (2001). Sonic hedgehog is a survival factor for hypaxial muscles during mouse development. *Development* 128: 743–752.

Krull CE, Lansford R, Gale NW, Collazo A, Marcelle C, Yancopoulos GD, Fraser SE, Bronner-Fraser M (1997). Interactions of Eph-related receptors and ligands confer rostrocaudal pattern to trunk neural crest migration. *Curr Biol* 7: 571–580.

Kullander K, Mather NK, Diella F, Dottori M, Boyd AW, Klein R (2001). Kinase-dependent and kinase-independent functions of EphA4 receptors in major axon tract formation in vivo. *Neuron* 29: 73–84.

Kume T, Jiang H, Topczewska JM, Hogan BL (2001). The murine winged helix transcription factors, Foxc1 and Foxc2, are both required for cardiovascular development and somitogenesis. *Genes Dev* 15: 2470–2482.

Kurooka H, Kuroda K, Honjo T (1998). Roles of the ankyrin repeats and C-terminal region of the mouse notch1 intracellular region [erratum appears in *Nucleic Acids Res* 1999;27(5):1407]. *Nucleic Acids Res* 26: 5448–5455.

Kusumi K, Sun ES, Kerrebrock AW, Bronson RT, Chi DC, Bulotsky MS, Spencer JB, Birren BW, Frankel WN, Lander ES (1998). The mouse pudgy mutation disrupts *Delta* homologue *Dll3* and initiation of early somite boundaries. *Nat Genet* 3: 274–278.

Ladher RK, Church VL, Allen S, Robson L, Abdelfattah A, Brown NA, Hattersley G, Rosen V, Luyten FP, Dale L, et al. (2000). Cloning and expression of the Wnt antagonists Sfrp2 and Frzb during chick development. *Dev Biol* 218: 183–198.

Lardelli M, Lendahl U (1993). Motch A and motch B—two mouse Notch homologues coexpressed in a wide variety of tissues. *Exp Cell Res* 204: 364–372.

Lardelli M, Dahlstrand J, Lendahl U (1994). The novel Notch homologue mouse Notch 3 lacks specific epidermal growth factor-repeats and is expressed in proliferating neuroepithelium. *Mech Dev* 46: 123–136.

Lee CS, Buttitta LA, May NR, Kispert A, Fan CM (2000). SHH-N upregulates Sfrp2 to mediate its competitive interaction with WNT1 and WNT4 in the somitic mesoderm. *Development* 127: 109–118.

Lee JS, Ishimoto A, Honjo T, Yanagawa S (1999). Murine leukemia provirus-mediated activation of the *Notch1* gene leads to induction of HES-1 in a mouse T lymphoma cell line, DL-3. *FEBS Lett* 455: 276–280.

Lefeuvre B, Crossin F, Fontaine-Perus J, Bandman E, Gardahaut MF (1996). Innervation regulates myosin heavy chain isoform expression in developing skeletal muscle fibers. *Mech Dev* 58: 115–127.

Leimeister C, Externbrink A, Klamt B, Gessler M (1999). *Hey* genes: a novel subfamily of hairy- and Enhancer of split related genes specifically expressed during mouse embryogenesis. *Mech Dev* 85: 173–177.

Leimeister C, Dale K, Fischer A, Klamt B, Hrabe de Angelis M, Radtke R, McGrew MJ, Pourquie O, Gessler M (2000). Oscillating expression of c-hey2 in the presomitic mesoderm suggests that the segmentation clock may use combinatorial signaling through multiple interacting bHLH factors. *Dev Biol* 227: 91–103.

Lemercier C, Verdel A, Galloo B, Curtet S, Brocard MP, Khochbin S (2000). mHDA1/HDAC5 histone deacetylase interacts with and represses MEF2A transcriptional activity. *J Biol Chem* 275: 15594–15599.

Lendahl U. (1998). A growing family of Notch ligands. *Bioessays* 20: 103–107.

Lindon C, Albagli O, Domeyne P, Montarras D, Pinset C (2000). Constitutive instability of muscle regulatory factor Myf-5 is distinct from its mitosis-specific disappearance, which requires a D-box-like motif overlapping the basic domain. *Mol Cell Biol* 20: 8923–8932.

Lindsell CE, Shawber CJ, Boulter J, Weinmaster G (1995). Jagged: a mammalian ligand that activates Notch1. *Cell* 80: 909–917.

Lu J, McKinsey TA, Nicol RL, Olson EN (2000a). Signal-dependent activation of the MEF2 transcription factor by dissociation from histone deacetylases. *Proc Natl Acad Sci USA* 97: 4070–4075.

Lu J, McKinsey TA, Zhang CL, Olson EN (2000b). Regulation of skeletal myogenesis by association of the MEF2 transcription factor with class II histone deacetylases. *Mol Cell* 6: 233–244.

Maina F, Casagranda F, Audero E, Simeone A, Comoglio PM, Klein R, Ponzetto C (1996). Uncoupling of Grb2 from the Met receptor reveals complex roles in muscle development. *Cell* 87: 531–542.

Mal A, Sturniolo M, Schiltz RL, Ghosh MK, Harter ML (2001). A role for histone deacetylase HDAC1 in modulating the transcriptional activity of MyoD: inhibition of the myogenic program. *EMBO J* 20: 1739–1753.

Mansouri A, Pla P, Larue L, Gruss P (2001). Pax3 acts cell autonomously in the neural tube and somites by controlling cell surface properties. *Development* 128: 1995–2005.

Marcelle C, Algren S, Bronner-Fraser M (1999). In vivo regulation of somite differentiation and proliferation by Sonic Hedgehog. *Dev Biol* 214: 277–287.

Maroto M, Reshef R, Münsterberg AE, Koester S, Goulding M, Lassar AB (1997). Ectopic Pax-3 activates MyoD and Myf-5 expression in embryonic mesoderm and neural tissue. *Cell* 89: 139–148.

McGrew MJ, Dale JK, Fraboulet S, Pourquie O (1998). The lunatic fringe gene is a target of the molecular clock linked to somite segmentation in avian embryos. *Curr Biol* 8: 979–982.

McKinsey TA, Zhang CL, Lu J, Olson EN (2000a). Signal-dependent nuclear export of a histone deacetylase regulates muscle differentiation. *Nature* 408: 106–111.

McKinsey TA, Zhang CL, Olson EN (2000b). Activation of the myocyte enhancer factor-2 transcription factor by calcium/calmodulin-dependent protein kinase–stimulated binding of 14-3-3 to histone deacetylase 5. *Proc Natl Acad Sci USA* 97: 14400–14405.

McKinsey TA, Zhang CL, Olson EN (2001). Control of muscle development by dueling HATs and HDACs. *Curr Opin Genet Dev* 11: 497–504.

McMahon JA, Takada S, Zimmerman LB, Fan CM, Harland RM, McMahon AP (1998). Noggin-mediated antagonism of BMP signaling is required for growth and patterning of the neural tube and somite. *Genes Dev* 12: 1438–1452.

Mellitzer G, Xu Q, Wilkinson DG (1999). Eph receptors and ephrins restrict cell intermingling and communication. *Nature* 400: 77–81.

Mennerich D, Schäfer K, Braun T (1998). Pax-3 is necessary but not sufficient for lbx1 expression in myogenic precursor cells of the limb. *Mech Dev* 73: 147–158.

Miller JB, Stockdale FE (1986a). Developmental origins of skeletal muscle fibers: clonal analysis of myogenic cell lineages based on fast and slow myosin heavy chain expression. *Proc Natl Acad Sci USA* 83: 3860–3864.

Miller JB, Stockdale FE (1986b). Developmental regulation of the multiple myogenic cell lineages of the avian embryo. *J Cell Biol* 103: 2197–2208.

Miller JB, Everitt EA, Smith TH, Block NE, Dominov JA (1993). Cellular and molecular diversity in skeletal muscle development: news from in vitro and in vivo. *Bioessays* 15: 191–196.

Miller JB, Schaefer L, Dominov JA (1999). Seeking muscle stem cells. *Curr Top Dev Biol* 43: 191–219.

Mishima N, Tomarev S (1998). Chicken Eyes absent 2 gene: isolation and expression pattern during development. *Int J Dev Biol* 42: 1109–1115.

Miska EA, Karlsson C, Langley E, Nielsen SJ, Pines J, Kouzarides T (1999). HDAC4 deacetylase associates with and represses the MEF2 transcription factor. *EMBO J* 18: 5099–5107.

Mitsiadis TA, Henrique D, Thesleff I, Lendahl U (1997). Mouse Serrate-1 (Jagged-1): expression in the developing tooth is regulated by epithelial-mesenchymal interactions and fibroblast growth factor-4. *Development* 124: 1473–1483.

Molkentin JD, Olson EN (1996). Defining the regulatory networkds for muscle development. *Curr Opin Genet Dev* 6: 445–453.

Montarras D, Chelly J, Bober E, Arnold H, Ott MO, Gros F, Pinset C (1991). Developmental patterns in the expression of Myf5, MyoD, myogenin, and MRF4 during myogenesis. *New Biol* 3: 592–600.

Munsterberg A, Kitajewski J, Bumcrot D, McMahon A, Lassar A (1995). Combinatorial signaling by Sonic hedgehog and Wnt family members induces myogenic bHLH gene-expression in the somite. *Genes Dev* 9: 2911–2922.

Musaro A, McCullagh KJ, Naya FJ, Olson EN, Rosenthal N (1999). IGF-1 induces skeletal myocyte hypertrophy through calcineurin in association with GATA-2 and NF-ATcl. *Nature* 400: 581–585.

Myer A, Olson EN, Klein WH (2001). MyoD cannot compensate for the absence of myogenin during skeletal muscle differentiation in murine embryonic stem cells. *Dev Biol* 229: 340–350.

Nabeshima YK, Hanaoka K, Hayasaka H, Esumi S, Li S, Nonaka I (1993). *Myogenin* gene disruption results in perinatal lethality because of severe muscle defect. *Nature* 364: 532–535.

Naya FJ, Mercer B, Shelton J, Richardson JA, Williams RS, Olson EN (2000). Stimulation of slow skeletal muscle fiber gene expression by calcineurin in vivo. *J Biol Chem* 275: 4545–4548.

Noden DM (1983). The embryonic origins of avian cephalic and cervical muscles and associated connective tissues. *Am J Anat* 168: 257–276.

Nomura T, Khan MM, Kaul SC, Dong HD, Wadhwa R, Colmenares C, Kohno I, Ishii S (1999). Ski is a component of the histone deacetylase complex required for transcriptional repression by Mad and thyroid hormone receptor. *Genes Dev* 13: 412–423.

Ohto H, Takizawa T, Saito T, Kobayashi M, Ikeda K, Kawakami K (1998). Tissue and developmental distribution of *Six* family gene products. *Int J Dev Biol* 42: 141–148.

Ohto H, Kamada S, Tago K, Tominaga S, Ozaki H, Sato S, Kawakami K (1999). Cooperation of Six and Eya in activation of their target genes through nuclear translocation of Eya. *Mol Cell Biol* 19: 6815–6824.

Ohtsuka T, Ishibashi M, Gradwohl G, Nakanishi S, Guillemot F, Kageyama R (1999). Hes1 and Hes5 as notch effectors in mammalian neuronal differentiation. *EMBO J* 18: 2196–2207.

Oka C, Nakano T, Wakeham A, de la Pompa JL, Mori C, Sakai T, Okazaki S, Kawaichi M, Shiota K, Mak TW, et al. (1995). Disruption of the mouse *RBP-J kappa* gene results in early embryonic death. *Development* 121: 3291–3301.

Oliver G, Wehr R, Jenkins NA, Copeland NG, Cheyette BN, Hartenstein V, Zipursky SL, Gruss P (1994). Homeobox genes and connective tissue patterning. *Development* 121: 693–705.

Olson EN, Williams RS (2000). Calcineurin signaling and muscle remodeling. *Cell* 101: 689–692.

Ordahl CP, Le Douarin NM (1992). Two myogenic lineages within the developing somite. *Development* 114: 339–353.

Ordahl CP, Berdougo E, Venters SJ, Denetclaw WF Jr (2001). The dermomyotome dorsomedial lip drives growth and morphogenesis of both the primary myotome and dermomyotome epithelium. *Development* 128: 1731–1744.

Ott M-O, Bober E, Lyons G, Arnold HH, Buckingham M (1991). Early expression of the myogenic regulatory gene, *myf-5*, in precursor cells of skeletal muscle in the mouse embryo. *Development* 111: 1097–1107.

Ozaki H, Watanabe Y, Katsumasa T, Kitamura K, Tanaka A, Urase K, Momoi T, Sudo K, Sakagami J, Asano M, et al. (2001). *Six4*, a putative *myogenin* gene regulator, is not essential for mouse embryonal development. *Mol Cell Biol* 21: 3343–3350.

Palmeirim I, Henrique D, Ish-Horowicz D, Pourquie O (1997). Avian *hairy* gene expression identifies a molecular clock linked to vertebrate segmentation and somitogenesis. *Cell* 91: 639–648.

Parker SB, Eichele G, Zhang P, Rawls A, Sands AT, Bradley A, Olson EN, Harper JW, Elledge SJ (1995). P53-independent expression of p21cip1 in muscle and other terminally differentiating cells. *Science* 267: 1024–1027.

Petropoulos H, Skerjanc IS (2002). Beta-catenin is essential and sufficient for skeletal myogenesis in p19 cells. *J Biol Chem* 277: 15393–15399.

Pette D (2001). Historical perspectives: plasticity of mammalian skeletal muscle. *J Appl Physiol* 90: 1119–1124.

Pignoni F, Hu B, Zavitz KH, Xiao J, Garrity PA, Zipursky SL (1997). The eye-specification proteins So and Eya form a complex and regulate multiple steps in *Drosophila* eye development [erratum appears in *Cell* 1998;92(4):585]. *Cell* 91: 881–891.

Polesskaya A, Duquet A, Naguibneva I, Weise C, Vervisch A, Bengal E, Hucho F, Robin P, Harel-Bellan A (2000). CREB-binding protein/p300 activates MyoD by acetylation. *J Biol Chem* 275: 34359–34364.

Porrello A, Cerone MA, Coen S, Gurtner A, Fontmaggi G, Cimino L, Piaggio G, Sacchi A, Soddu S (2000). p53 regualtes myogenesis by triggering the differentiation activity of pRb. *J Cell Biol* 151: 1295–1303.

Pourquie O (2001). Vertebrate somitogenesis. *Annu Rev Cell Dev Biol* 17: 311–350.

Pourquié O, Coltey M, Teillet MA, Ordahl C, Le Douarin N (1993). Control of dorsoventral patterning of somitic derivatives by notochord and floor plate. *Proc Natl Acad Sci USA* 90: 5242–5246.

Pourquié O, Fan C, Coltey M, Hirsinger E, Watanabe Y, Bréant C, Francis-West P, Brickell P, Tessier-Lavigne M, Le Douarin N (1996). Lateral and axial signals involved in avian somite patterning: a role for BMP4. *Cell* 84: 461–471.

Pownall M, Strunk K, Emerson C (1996). Notochord signals control the transcriptional cascade of myogenic bHLH genes in somites of quail embryos. *Development* 122: 1475–1488.

Puri PL, Avantaggiati ML, Balsano C, Sang N, Graessmann A, Giordano A, Levrero M (1997a). p300 is required for MyoD-dependent cell cycle arrest and muscle-specific gene transcription. *EMBO J* 16: 369–383.

Puri PL, Sartorelli V, Yang XJ, Hamamori Y, Ogryzko VV, Howard BH, Kedes L, Wang JY, Graessmann A, Nakatani Y, et al. (1997b). Differential roles of p300 and PCAF acetyltransferases in muscle differentiation. *Mol Cell* 1: 35–45.

Radice GL, Rayburn H, Matsunami H, Knudsen KA, Takeichi M, Hynes RO (1997). Developmental defects in mouse embryos lacking N-cadherin. *Dev Biol* 181: 64–78.

Rao MV, Donoghue MJ, Merlie JP, Sanes JR (1996). Distinct regulatory elements control muscle-specific, fiber-type-selective, and axially graded expression of a myosin light-chain gene in transgenic mice. *Mol Cell Biol* 16: 3909–3922.

Rawls A, Valdez MR, Zhang W, Richardson J, Klein WH, Olson EN (1998). Overlapping functions of the myogenic bHLH genes *MRF4* and *MyoD* revealed in double mutant mice. *Development* 125: 2349–2358.

Rawls A, Wilson-Rawls J, Olson EN (2000). Genetic regulation of somite formation. *Curr Top Dev Biol* 47: 131–154.

Reynaud EG, Leibovitch MP, Tintignac LAJ, Pelpel K, Guillier M, Leibovitch SA (2000). Stabilization of MyoD by direct binding to $p57^{kip2}$. *J Biol Chem* 275: 18767–18776.

Robson LG, Hughes SM (1999). Local signals in the chick limb bud can override myoblast lineage commitment: induction of slow myosin heavy chain in fast myoblasts. *Mech Dev* 85: 59–71.

Roehl H, Bosenberg M, Blelloch R, Kimble J (1996). Roles of the RAM and ANK domains in signaling by the *C. elegans* GLP-1 receptor. *EMBO J* 15: 7002–7012.

Rudnicki MA, Braun T, Hinuma S, Jaenisch R (1992). Inactivation of MyoD in mice leads to up-regulation of the myogenic HLH gene *Myf-5* and results in apparently normal muscle development. *Cell* 71: 383–390.

Rudnicki MA, Schnegelsberg PN, Stead RH, Braun T, Arnold HH, Jaenisch R (1993). MyoD or Myf-5 is required for the formation of skeletal muscle. *Cell* 75: 1351–1359.

Saga Y (1998). Genetic rescue of segmentation defect in MesP2-deficient mice by *MesP1* gene replacement. *Mech Dev* 75: 53–66.

Saga Y, Hata N, Koseki H, Taketo MM (1997). *Mesp2*: a novel mouse gene expressed in the presegmented mesoderm and essential for semgentation initiation. *Genes Development* 11: 1827–1839.

Salminen M, Lopez S, Maire P, Kahn A, Daegelen D (1996). Fast-muscle-specific DNA-protein interactions occurring in vivo at the human aldolase A M promoter are necessary for correct promoter activity in transgenic mice. *Mol Cell Biol* 16: 76–85.

Sartorelli V, Huang J, Hamamori Y, Kedes L (1997). Molecular mechanisms of myogenic coactivation by p300: direct interaction with the activation domain of MyoD and with the MADS box of MEF2C. *Mol Cell Biol* 17: 1010–1026.

Sasai Y, Kageyama R, Tagawa Y, Shigemoto R, Nakanishi S (1992). Two mammalian helix-loop-helix factors structurally related to *Drosophila* hairy and Enhancer of split. *Genes Dev* 6: 2620–2634.

Sassoon D, Lyons G, Wright WE, Lin V, Lassar A, Weintraub H, Buckingham M (1989). Expression of two myogenic regulatory factors myogenin and MyoD1 during mouse embryogenesis. *Nature* 341: 303–307.

Sawada A, Fritz A, Jiang Y, Yamamoto A, Yamasu K, Kuroiwa A, Saga Y, Takeda H (2000). Zebrafish *Mesp* family genes, *mesp-a* and *mesp-b* are segmentally expressed in the presomitic mesoderm, and *Mesp-b* confers the anterior identity to the developing somites. *Development* 127: 1691–1702.

Saxena MT, Schroeter EH, Mumm JS, Kopan R (2001). Murine Notch homologs (N1-4) undergo presenilin-dependent proteolysis. *J Biol Chem* 276: 40268–40273.

Scaal M, Bonafede A, Dathe V, Sachs M, Cann G, Christ B, Brand-Saberi B (1999). SF/HGF is a mediator between limb patterning and muscle development. *Development* 126: 4885–4893.

Schäfer K, Braun T (1999). Early specification of limb muscle precursor cells by the homeobox gene *Lbx1h*. *Nat Genet* 23: 213–216.

Schmidt M, Tanaka M, Münsterberg A (2000). Expression of β-catenin in the developing chick myotome is regulated by myogenic signals. *Development* 127: 4105–4113.

Schroeter EH, Kisslinger JA, Kopan R (1998). Notch-1 signalling requires ligand-induced proteolytic release of intracellular domain. *Nature* 393: 382–386.

Schubert FR, Tremblay P, Mansouri A, Faisst AM, Kammandel B, Lumsden A, Gruss P, Dietrich S (2001). Early mesodermal phenotypes in splotch suggest a role for Pax3 in the formation of epithelial somites. *Dev Dyn* 222: 506–521.

Semsarian C, Wu MJ, Ju YK, Marciniec T, Yeoh T, Allen DG, Harvey RP, Graham RM (1999). Skeletal muscle hypertrophy is mediated by a Ca^{2+} dependent calcineurin signaling pathway. *Nature* 400: 576–581.

Serikaku MA, O'Tousa JE (1994). *Sine oculis* is a homeobox gene required for *Drosophila* visual system development. *Genetics* 138: 1137–1150.

Shawber C, Boulter J, Lindsell CE, Weinmaster G. (1996a). *Jagged2:* a serrate-like gene expressed during rat embryogenesis. *Dev Biol* 180: 370–376.

Shawber C, Nofziger D, Hsieh JD, Lindsell C, Bögler O, Hayward D, Weinmaster G (1996b). Notch signaling inhibits muscle cell differentiation through a CBF1-independant pathway. *Development* 122: 3765–3773.

Shen J, Bronson RT, Chen DF, Xia W, Selkoe DJ, Tonegawa S (1997). Skeletal and CNS defects in Presenilin-1-deficient mice. *Cell* 89: 629–639.

Shen W, Mardon G (1997). Ectopic eye development in *Drosophila* induced by directed dachshund expression. *Development* 124: 45–52.

Smith A, Robinson V, Patel K, Wilkinson DG (1997). The EphA4 and Eph B1 receptor tyrosine kinases and ephrin-B2 ligand regulate the targeted migration of branchial neural crest cells. *Curr Biol* 7: 561–570.

Sparrow DB, Jen WC, Kotecha S, Towers N, Kintner C, Mohun TJ (1998). Thylacine 1 is expressed segmentally within the paraxial mesoderm of the *Xenopus* embryo and interacts with the Notch pathway. *Development* 125: 2041-2051.

Sparrow DB, Miska EA, Langley E, Reynaud-Deonauth S, Kotecha S, Towers N, Spohr G, Kouzarides T, Mohun TJ (1999). MEF-2 function is modified by a novel co-repressor, MITR. *EMBO J* 18: 5085–5098.

Spitz F, Demignon J, Porteu A, Axel K, Concordet JP, Daegelen D, Maire P (1998). Expression of myogenin during embryogenesis is controlled by Six/*sine oculis* homeoproteins through a conserved MEF3 binding site. *Proc Natl Acad Sci USA* 95: 14220–14225.

Stern CD, Vasiliauskas D (2000). Segmentation: a view from the border. Somitogenesis *Curr Top Dev Biol* 47: 107–129.

Strahl BD, Allis CD (2000). The language of covalent histone modifications. *Nature* 403: 41–45.

Strooper B, Anneart W (2001). Where Notc and wnt signaling meet: the presenilin hub. *J Cell Biol* 152: F17–F19.

Struhl G, Adachi A (1998). Nuclear access and action of notch in vivo. *Cell* 93: 649–660.

Sun X, Meyers EN, Lewandoski M, Martin GR (1999). Targeted disruption of *Fgf8* causes failure of cell migration in the gastrulating mouse embryo. *Genes Dev* 13: 1834–1846.

Swartz ME, Eberhart J, Pasquale EB, Krull CE (2001). EphA4/ephrin-A5 interactions in muscle precursor cell migration in the avian forelimb. *Development* 128: 4669–4680.

Swiatek PJ, Lindsell CE, del Amo FF, Weinmaster G, Gridley T (1994) Notch1 is essential for postimplantation development in mice. *Genes Dev* 8: 707–719.

Tajbakhsh S, Rocancourt D, Cossu G, Buckingham M (1997). Redefining the genetic hierarchies controlling skeletal myogenesis: Pax-3 and Myf-5 act upstream of MyoD. *Cell* 89: 127–138.

Takahashi Y, Koizumi K, Takagi A, Kitajima S, Inoue T, Koseki H, Saga Y (2000). Mesp2 initiates somite segmentation through the Notch signalling pathway. *Nat Genet* 25: 390–396.

Takayama H, La Rochelle WJ, Anver M, Bockman DE, Merlino G (1996). Scatter factor/ hepatocyte growth factor as a regulator of skeletal muscle and neural crest development. *Proc Natl Acad Sci USA* 93: 5866–5871.

Tam PP, Tan SS (1992). The somitogenetic potential of cells in the primitive streak and the tail bud of the organogenesis-stage mouse embryo. *Development* 115: 703–715.

Tam PP, Trainor PA (1994). Specification and segmentation of the paraxial mesoderm. *Anat Embryol (Berl)* 189: 275–305.

Terry K, Magan H, Baranski M, Burrus LW (2000). Sfrp-1 and sfrp-2 are expressed in overlapping and distinct domains during chick development. *Mech Dev* 97: 177–182.

Tremblay P, Dietrich S, Mericskay M, Schubert FR, Li Z, Paulin D (1998). A crucial role for Pax3 in the development of the hypaxial musculature and the long-range migration of muscle precursors. *Dev Biol* 203: 49–61.

Uyttendaele H, Marazzi G, Wu G, Yan Q, Sassoon D, Kitajewski J (1996). Notch4/int-3, a mammary proto-oncogene, is an endothelial cell-specific mammalian *Notch* gene. *Development* 122: 2251–2259.

Valdez R, Richardson JA, Klein WH, Olson EN (2000). Failure of myf5 to support myogenic differentiation without myogenin, MyoD, and MRF4. *Dev Biol* 219: 287–298.

Van Swearingen J, Lance-Jones C (1995). Slow and fast muscle fibers are preferentially derived from myoblasts migrating into the chick limb bud at different developmental times. *Dev Biol* 170: 321–337.

Venters SJ, Thorsteinsdottir S, Duxson MJ (1999). Early development of the myotome in the mouse. *Dev Dyn* 216: 219–232.

Wagner J, Schmidt C, Nikowits W Jr, Christ B (2000). Compartmentalization of the somite and myogenesis in chick embryos are influenced by Wnt expression. *Dev Biol* 228: 86–94.

Wahl S, Barth H, Ciossek T, Aktories K, Mueller BK (2000). Ephrin-A5 induces collapse of growth cones by activating Rho and Rho kinase. *J Cell Biol* 49: 263–270.

Wang AH, Bertos NR, Vezmar M, Pelletier N, Crosato M, Heng HH, Th'ng J, Ha J, Yang XJ (1999). HDAC4, a human histone deacetylase related to yeast HDA1, is a transcriptional corepressor. *Mol Cell Biol* 19: 7816–7827.

Wang AH, Kruhlak MJ, Wu J, Bertos NR, Vezmar M, Posner BI, Bazett Jones DP, Yang XJ (2000). Regulation of histone deacetylase 4 by binding of 14-3-3 proteins. *Mol Cell Biol* 20: 6904–6912.

Wang H, Anderson DJ (1997). Eph family of transmembrane ligands can mediate repulsive guidance of trunk neural crest cell migration and motor axon outgrowth. *Neuron* 18: 383–396.

Wang Y, Jaenisch R (1997). Myogenin can substitute for Myf5 in promoting myogenesis but less efficiently. *Development* 124: 2507–2513.

Wang Z-M, Messi ML, Renganathan M, Delbono O. (1999). Insulin-like growth factor-1 enhances rat skeletal muscle charge movement and L-type Ca^{2+} channel gene expression. *J Physiol (Lond)* 516: 331–341.

Washabaugh CH, Ontell MP, Shan Z, Hoffman EP, Ontell M (1998). Role of the nerve in determining fetal skeletal muscle phenotype. *Dev Dyn* 211: 177–190.

Weinmaster G, Roberts VJ, Lemke G (1991). A homolog of *Drosophila* Notch expressed during mammalian development. *Development* 113: 199–205.

Weinmaster G, Roberts VJ, Lemk G. (1992). *Notch2*: a second mammalian *Notch* gene. *Development* 116: 931–941.

Wigmore PM, Baillie HS, Morrison EH, Khan M, Mayhew TM (1992). Nuclear number during muscle development. *Muscle Nerve* 15: 1301–1302.

Wilkinson DG (2001). Multiple roles of EPH receptors and ephrins in neural development. *Nat Rev Neurosci* 2: 155–164.

Wilson V, Beddington RSP (1996). Cell fate and morphogenetic movement in the late mouse primitive streak. *Mech Dev* 55: 79–89.

Wilson-Rawls J, Hurt CR, Parsons SM, Rawls A (1999a). Differential regulation of epaxial and hypaxial muscle development by paraxis. *Development* 126: 5217–5229.

Wilson-Rawls J, Molkentin J, Black B, Olson EN (1999b). Activated Notch inhibits myogenic activity of the MADS-Box transcription factor myocyte enhancer factor 2C. *Mol Cell Biol* 19: 2853–2862.

Winchester CL, Ferrier RK, Sermoni A, Clark BJ, Johnson KJ (1999). Characterization of the expression of DMPK and SIX5 in the human eye and implications for pathogenesis in myotonic dystrophy. *Hum Mol Genet* 8: 481–492.

Winnier GE, Hargett L, Hogan BL (1997). The winged helix transcription factor MFH1 is required for proliferation and patterning of paraxial mesoderm in the mouse embryo. *Genes Dev* 11: 926–940.

Wodarz A, Nusse R (1998). Mechanisms of Wnt signaling in development. *Annu Rev Cell Dev Biol* 14: 59–88.

Woloshin P, Song K, Degnin C, Killary AM, Goldhamer DJ, Sassoon D, Thayer MJ (1995). MSX1 inhibits myoD expression in fibroblast × 10T1/2 cell hybrids. *Cell* 82: 611–620.

Wong PC, Zheng H, Chen H, Becher MW, Sirinathsinghji DJ, Trumbauer ME, Chen HY, Price DL, Van der Ploeg LH, Sisodia SS (1997). Presenilin 1 is required for Notch1 and DII1 expression in the paraxial mesoderm. *Nature* 387: 288–292.

Wu H, Naya FJ, McKinsey TA, Mercer B, Shelton JM, Chin ER, Simard AR, Michel RN, Bassel-Duby R, Olson EN, et al. (2000). MEF2 responds to multiple calcium-regulated signals in the control of skeletal muscle fiber type. *EMBO J.* 19: 1963–1973.

Wu H, Rothermel B, Kanatous S, Rosenberg P, Naya FJ, Shelton JM, Hutcheson KA, DiMaio JM, Olson EN, Bassel-Duby R, et al. (2001a). Activation of MEF2 by muscle activity is mediated through a calcineurin-dependent pathway. *EMBO J* 20: 6414–6423.

Wu XY, Li H, Park EJ, Chen JD (2001b). SMRTe inhibits MEF2C transcriptional activation by targeting HDAC4 and 5 to nuclear domains. *J Biol Chem* 276: 24177–24185.

Xu PX, Woo I, Her H, Beier DR, Maas RL (1997). Mouse Eya homologues of the *Drosophila eyes absent* gene require Pax6 for expression in lens and nasal placode. *Development* 124: 219–231.

Xu PX, Adams J, Peters H, Brown MC, Heaney S, Maas R (1999). Eya1-deficient mice lack ears and kidneys and show abnormal apoptosis of organ primordia. *Nat Genet* 23: 113–117.

Yamaguchi TP, Takada S, Yoshikawa Y, Wu N, McMahon AP (1999). *T* (Brachyury) is a direct target of Wnt3a during paraxial mesoderm specification. *Genes Dev* 13: 3185–3190.

Yang XM, Vogan K, Gros P, Park M (1996). Expression of the met receptor tyrosine kinase in muscle progenitor cells in somites and limbs is absent in Splotch mice. *Development* 122: 2163–2171.

Yee SP, Rigby PW (1993). The regulation of myogenin gene expression during the embryonic development of the mouse. *Genes Dev* 7: 1277–1289.

Yoon JK, Wold B (2000). The bHLH regulator pMesogenin1 is required for maturation and segmentation of paraxial mesoderm. *Development* 14: 3204–3214.

Yoon JK, Moon RT, Wold B (2000). The bHLH class protein pMesogenin1 can specify paraxial mesoderm phenotypes. *Dev Biol* 222: 376–391.

Yoshikawa Y, Fujimori T, McMahon AP, Takada S (1997). Evidence that absence of *Wnt-3a* signaling promotes nuralization instead of paraxial mesoderm development in the mouse. *Dev Biol* 183: 234–242.

Yuan W, Condorelli G, Caruso M, Felsani A, Giordano A (1996). Human p300 protein is a coactivator for the transcription factor MyoD. *J Biol Chem* 271: 9009–9013.

Yun KS, Wold BJ (1996). Skeletal muscle determination and differentiation: story of a core regulatory network and its context. *Curr Opin Cell Biol* 8: 877–889.

Zhang M, McLennan IS (1995). During secondary myotube formation, primary myotubes preferentially absorb new nuclei at their ends. *Dev Dyn* 204: 168–177.

Zhang N, Gridley T (1998). Defects in somite formation in lunatic fringe-deficient mice. *Nature* 394: 374–377.

Zhang P, Wong C, Liu D, Finegold M, Harper JW, Elledge S (1999). p21^{CIP1} and p57^{KIP2} control muscle differentiation at the myogenin step. *Genes Dev* 13: 213–224.

Zhang W, Behringer RR, Olson EN (1995). Inactivation of the myogenic bHLH gene *MRF4* results in up-regulation of *myogenin* and rib anomalies. *Genes Dev* 9: 1388–1399.

11 | Development of Bone and Cartilage

SHUNICHI MURAKAMI, HARUHIKO AKIYAMA, AND BENOIT DE CROMBRUGGHE

The formation of bones occurs through two distinct mechanisms. More than 95% of the skeleton is formed by the complex process of endochondral ossification, which involves a cartilage intermediate. The other bones, namely some craniofacial bones, are formed directly from condensations of mesenchymal cells without cartilage intermediates, a process described as intramembranous ossification. Bones contain both bone-forming osteoblasts, which arise from mesenchymal cells, and bone-resorbing osteoclasts, which arise from macrophage/ monocytic cells. The coexistence of the two cell types insures bone homeostasis, which is the result of a functional steady state characterized by an equilibrium between bone synthesis and bone resorption. In cartilage, a single cell lineage, represented by different subpopulations of chondrocytes, constitutes the only cell type of this tissue. Cartilage in articular surfaces, which line the extremities of many bones, and cartilage in the nose, ears, and throat are never replaced by bone and persist as permanent cartilage. It is not clearly understood why chondrocytes in such cartilage do not develop into bone.

As in the formation of other organs, two broad classes of regulatory factors are involved in the formation of the skeleton: (1) patterning factors, which control the shape, size, and number of the primordia of the different skeletal elements, and (2) differentiation factors, which control the differentiation of the constituent cells of the skeletal elements and the maintenance of their phenotype. An initial step in the formation of both endochondral and membranous skeletal elements is provided by patterning signals outlining the three-dimensional coordinates that determine the shape of the cell condensations into which mesenchymal cells are recruited (Tickle, 1995; Johnson and Tabin, 1997).

These mesenchymal precursor cells differentiate in two possible directions. In mesenchymal condensations of membranous skeletal elements, cells differentiate into osteoblasts, whereas in endochondral skeletal elements, cells in condensations differentiate into chondrocytes to form the cartilages that will later be replaced by bones. The molecules that pattern skeletal elements include both signaling polypeptides and transcription factors. To the first group belong a small number of families of signaling molecules that are not unique to skeletal development because they also have key roles in the overall body plan and in the formation of other organs. They include members of the bone morphogenetic protein (BMP) family, other members of the transforming growth factor-β (TGF-β) superfamily, members of the Wingless (Wnt) family, the Hedgehog family, fibroblast growth factors (FGFs), and others (Erlebacher et al., 1995; DeLise et al., 2000). The transcription factors that have a patterning role in the skeleton include members of the Pax, Hox, homeodomain-containing, basic-helix-loop-helix (bHLH), and forkhead families, as well as others (Karsenty, 1999; Olsen et al., 2000). This chapter will not discuss the role of patterning molecules that control shape, size, and numbers of skeletal elements but will focus instead on factors that have key roles in the differentiation of the major constituent cells of the skeleton.

During endochondral bone development, cells in chondrogenic mesenchymal condensations differentiate into chondrocytes and synthesize abundant amounts of cartilage-specific extracellular matrix (ECM) proteins, which include types II, IX, and XI collagen; aggrecan; link protein; epiphycan; and many others (Fig. 11–1). These cells then sustain a series of additional changes as they form the growth plate of endochondral bones (Erlebacher et al., 1995). Chondrocytes first flatten and undergo unidirectional proliferation, resulting in parallel stacks of dividing cells, a process that is largely responsible for the longitudinal growth of bones. Cells at the bottom of these stacks of proliferating cells then exit the cell cycle and, in successive steps, change their genetic programs to become prehypertrophic and then hypertrophic. The ECM around the most advanced hypertrophic chondrocytes becomes mineralized before these cells undergo apoptosis and are replaced by bone cells. It is this characteristic cellular organization that gives the growth plate its unique aspect (Mundlos and Olsen, 1997). When the growth plate is being established, cells surrounding cartilage form the perichondrium, a specialized structure consisting of thin layers of mesenchymal cells. In the centers of skeletal elements, where the perichondrium surrounds the zone of hypertrophic chondrocytes, perichondrial cells begin to differentiate into osteoblasts. Together with blood vessels and osteoclasts or a subpopulation of these cells called chondroclasts (Vu et al., 1998), these cells invade the mineralized cartilage matrix. Osteoclasts degrade the mineralized cartilage matrix, the remnants of which constitute a scaffold for the deposition of a bone-specific matrix by osteoblasts. At the same time, osteoblasts in the perichondrium produce a similar matrix to form bone collars.

Although intramembranous ossification appears to be very different from endochondral ossification, the phenotype of osteoblasts in the membranous skeleton is indistinguishable from that of osteoblasts in the endochondral skeleton, suggesting that common factors control the differentiation of osteoblasts in the two modes of bone formation.

Several levels of control regulate the pathways of differentiation of chondrocytes, osteoblasts, and osteoclasts, the three cell types that will be discussed in this chapter. One essential level of control is provided by specific transcription factors that are required for the differentiation of these cells. Another crucial level of control is provided by signaling molecules that control discrete steps in these pathways. Because the major physiological properties of both cartilage and bone are imparted by the nature of the ECM synthesized by either chondrocytes or osteoblasts, the integrity of the ECM is needed to maintain the overall function of cartilage and bone. In addition, in the endochondral skeleton the ECM is needed for the proper cellular organization of the growth plate. Thus, the role of each of these three different classes of molecules will be discussed. Much recent information on the function of specific molecules in cartilage and bone formation has come from understanding the consequences of mutations in the genes for these polypeptides in both humans and mice.

CHONDROCYTE DIFFERENTIATION AND CARTILAGE FORMATION

Transcription Factors

Sox9

Campomelic dysplasia (CD), a rare human genetic disease, is caused by heterozygous mutations in and around the Sox9 gene (Foster et al., 1994; Wagner et al., 1994; Meyer et al., 1997; see Chapter 43). It is a generalized disease characterized by hypoplasia of most endochondral skeletal elements. In addition, CD is associated with nonskeletal symptoms that include XY sex reversal and, more rarely, heart and kidney anomalies. The disease is severe, and most patients die in the perinatal period from pulmonary complications. The underlying cause of the disease is haploinsufficiency of Sox9, i.e., 50% of the normal levels of Sox9 being insufficient to fulfill its functions. In agreement

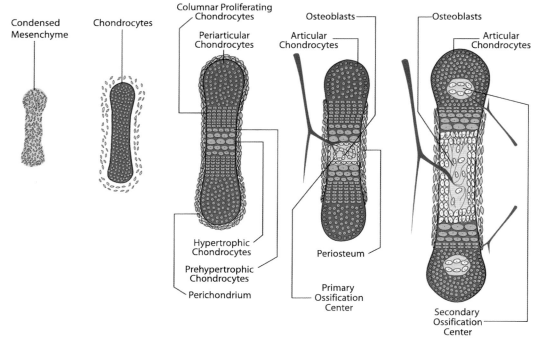

Figure 11–1. Schematic representation of the steps involved in endochondral bone formation.

with the skeletal symptoms of CD, in mouse embryos, *Sox9* is expressed in all chondroprogenitor cells and chondrocytes (Fig. 11–2), but its expression is completely abolished in hypertrophic chondrocytes. Also consistent with the nonskeletal symptoms found in some infants with CD, *Sox9* is expressed in the Sertoli cells of the male gonad and in heart and kidney. *Sox9* is also expressed in neural crest cells and pancreas (Wright et al., 1995; Ng et al., 1997; Zhao et al., 1997). Thus, although *Sox9* expression is not restricted to cells of the chondrocyte lineage, both the skeletal anomalies of CD and the pattern of expression of *Sox9* during chondrogenesis in mouse embryos suggested that Sox9 had a major role in chondrocyte differentiation.

Members of the Sox family of transcription factors contain a high-mobility-group (HMG) box DNA-binding domain whose sequence displays at least 50% identity with that of the sex-determining factor SRY. Based on sequence identities both within and outside the HMG box domain (Wegner, 1999), the Sox family is divided into several subgroups. Like other Sox proteins, Sox9 binds to a specific sequence in the minor groove of DNA. Sox9 also contains a potent transcription activation domain located at its carboxy end. Further support for the hypothesis that *Sox9* has a role in chondrocyte differentiation came from observations that Sox9 bound to and activated several chondrocyte-specific promoters and enhancers, such as those in the *Col2a1*, *Col11a2,* and *CD-RAP* genes, in vitro and activated the *Col2a1* gene in vivo (Bell et al., 1997; Lefebvre et al., 1997; Bridgewater et al., 1998; Xie et al., 1999).

The creation of a null allele of *Sox9* in embryonic stem (ES) cells led to the generation of heterozygous *Sox9* mouse mutants. These mouse mutants faithfully reproduced the skeletal anomalies of CD, including perinatal death, hypoplasia of endochondral bones, bending and angulation of long bones, and cleft palate (Bi et al., 2001). Characterization of the abnormal phenotypes of these mutants during embryonic development indicated that Sox9 haploinsufficiency affects two processes in the pathway of chondrocyte differentiation. One is mesenchymal condensation: smaller and delayed condensations produced the hypoplasia of endochondral bones characteristic of CD. The second is chondrocyte hypertrophy: the enlarged zones of hypertrophic chondrocytes in the mutant and the premature mineralization that occurred in a number of bones indicate that Sox9 has a distinct role in regulating the rate of chondrocyte transition into hypertrophy. Thus, a normal second function of Sox9 would be to maintain the chondrocyte phenotype by inhibiting hypertrophic chondrocyte differentiation. Normal inhibition of hypertrophic chondrocyte differentiation would require a level of Sox9 activity that is not reached in the prehypertrophic chondrocytes of Sox9 heterozygous mutants.

Because heterozygous Sox9 mutant mice die at birth, no homozygous *Sox9*-null mutants could be generated by the conventional method of mating heterozygous mutants with each other. To examine the consequences of a complete absence of Sox9 on chondrogenesis in vivo, mouse chimeras were generated by injecting *Sox9* homozygous mutant ES cells into wild-type blastocysts. Both wild-type and mutant cells con-

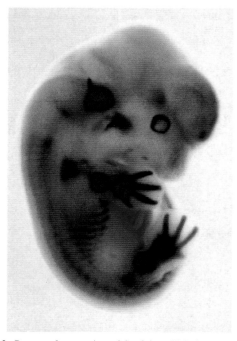

Figure 11–2. Pattern of expression of Sox9 in a 12.5-day postcoitus mouse embryo. A *lacZ* gene was inserted in the *Sox9* gene by homologous recombination in mouse embryonic stem cells. X-gal staining reveals expression of *lacZ*, which reproduces expression of *Sox9*, in all cartilages and cartilage progenitors.

tribute to the cellular composition of these chimeras, but the mutant cells are easily identified because the *lacZ* gene, which had been knocked-in at the *Sox9* locus, is expressed in a *Sox9*-specific pattern. Before chondrogenic mesenchymal condensations occur, the *Sox9*-null mutants were intermingled with wild-type cells in the chondrogenic fields of these chimeras. In contrast, the *Sox9* mutant cells were excluded from all chondrogenic mesenchymal condensations and later from all cartilages (Bi et al., 1999). In addition, the *Col2a1, Col9a2, Col11a2,* and *aggrecan* genes, which are normally first expressed in mesenchymal condensations, were not expressed at all in mutant cells.

These experiments indicated that Sox9 is needed for formation of chondrogenic mesenchymal condensations. How Sox9 controls mesenchymal condensation is not yet understood, but one possible mechanism is that Sox9 may control genes encoding cell-surface proteins that are needed for mesenchymal condensation. Thus, Sox9 is completely required at an early step in the pathway of chondrocyte differentiation, the step of mesenchymal condensations. In addition, the extension of the zone of hypertrophic chondrocytes in heterozygous *Sox9* mutants suggests an inhibitory role for Sox9 in a late step, the transition of chondrocytes to hypertrophic chondrocytes. It is not known, however, what factors induce expression of Sox9 in mesenchymal precursor cells. BMPs increase *Sox9* expression (Murtaugh et al., 1999; Zehentner et al., 1999; Semba et al., 2000), and a similar role can be attributed to Sonic Hedgehog (Murtaugh et al., 1999); however, it is unclear whether the signaling pathways triggered by these molecules act directly on the *Sox9* gene. In vitro experiments suggest that several genes for cartilage ECM components are direct downstream targets of Sox9 and, hence, that Sox9 has a role in the overt differentiation of mesenchymal cells into chondrocytes. Experiments using a conditional allele of Sox9 will help to clarify this question. In addition, because Sox9 has a role and is expressed in several nonchondrogenic tissues, other transcription factors are needed to increase its specificity in chondrocytes.

L-Sox5 and Sox6

Two other Sox family members, L-Sox5, a larger isoform of Sox5, and Sox6, have essential roles in chondrocyte differentiation. Their genes are coexpressed with *Sox9* during chondrogenesis (Lefebvre et al., 1998), and like *Sox9*, the *Sox5* and *Sox6* genes are completely turned off in hypertrophic chondrocytes. Both genes are also expressed in several other nonchondrogenic tissues. L-Sox5 and Sox6 have a high degree of sequence identity, particularly in their HMG box DNA-binding domain and in a coiled domain through which they form homodimers and heterodimers with each other. These dimers bind much more efficiently to pairs of HMG box-binding sites than to single DNA-binding sites. In contrast, Sox9 binds as efficiently to a single HMG box as to double sites. L-Sox5 and Sox6 belong to a different subgroup of Sox proteins than Sox9 and have no sequence homology with Sox9 except in the HMG box. Unlike Sox9, L-Sox5 and Sox6 have no transcriptional activation domain; but in DNA transfection experiments, they cooperate with Sox9 to activate the endogenous *Col2a1* and a*ggrecan* genes (Lefebvre et al., 1998). L-Sox5 and Sox6 may be architectural proteins that organize the DNA and/or chromatin in target genes to help recruit other transcription factors.

The coexpression of *Sox5* and *Sox6* during chondrogenesis and the high degree of sequence identity of the proteins suggested that they might have redundant functions. This hypothesis was confirmed by genetic experiments. Indeed, whereas individual *Sox5*-null mutant mice and *Sox6*-null mutant mice are born with relatively mild skeletal anomalies, double *Sox5, Sox6*-null fetuses die in utero with very severe defects in cartilage formation (Smits et al., 2001). In these double mutants, normal chondrogenic mesenchymal condensations occur, but there is no overt chondrocyte differentiation, normally characterized by the abundant synthesis of cartilage ECM components. Indeed, expression of genes for cartilage ECM components, such as *Col2a1, Col9a2, Col11a2, aggrecan,* and *link protein,* is severely reduced and marker genes preferentially expressed in proliferating chondrocytes, such as *matrilin, comp,* and *epiphycan,* show practically no expression. In addition, the typical cellular organization of the cartilage growth plate is virtually absent in the double mutants. Levels of *Sox9*

RNA in the double mutants are, however, comparable to those observed in wild-type cartilages. Hence, expression of *Sox9* does not require L-Sox5 and Sox6.

After an abnormally long delay, cells in the mesenchymal condensations of the double *Sox5, Sox6*-null mutants begin to proliferate but only after they have accumulated a modest amount of ECM. Perhaps the ECM is needed for the signaling molecules that stimulate proliferation in the cartilage growth plate. Delayed activation of typical markers of prehypertrophic and hypertrophic chondrocytes occurs in $Sox5^{-/-}$, $Sox6^{-/-}$ cells despite their inability to undergo overt chondrocyte differentiation, but morphological hypertrophy is very limited. This late maturation also results in induction of bone collar formation (Smits et al., 2001). Because analogous growth plate and bone formation defects were described in mice lacking one of the main cartilage matrix components (collagen type II, aggrecan, link protein) (Watanabe et al., 1994; Li et al., 1995; Watanabe and Yamada, 1999), it is likely that the severe matrix deficiency of *Sox5, Sox6*-double-null cartilages contributes greatly to these late defects. DNA-binding sites for L-Sox5- and Sox6-containing pairs of HMG-like sites have been identified in the chondrocyte-specific enhancers of the *Col2a1* and *Col11a2* genes (Bridgewater et al., 1998; Lefebvre et al., 1998). These and presumably many other genes that are preferentially or specifically expressed in chondrocytes are, therefore, likely direct targets for L-Sox5 and Sox6.

In summary, Sox9, L-Sox5, and Sox6 have essential functions in cartilage formation and control distinct steps in the chondrocyte differentiation pathway (Fig. 11–3). Sox9 is needed for chondrogenic mesenchymal condensations, whereas L-Sox5 and Sox6 are not. L-Sox5 and Sox6 are required after mesenchymal condensations, when high levels of expression of chondrocyte marker genes such as *Col2a1, aggrecan,* and others are needed.

Runx2

Runx2 is a transcription factor that is required for osteoblast differentiation (see below, Osteoblast Differentiation and Bone Formation). In addition, Runx2 is expressed in hypertrophic chondrocytes and stimulates hypertrophic chondrocyte differentiation. Indeed, a *Runx2*-null mutation not only blocks osteoblast differentiation in mice but also inhibits the maturation of chondrocytes into hypertrophic chondrocytes in many, but not all, skeletal elements; mineralization of the distal hypertrophic zone of the endochondral skeleton is also significantly reduced (Komori et al., 1997; Inada et al., 1999; see also Chapter 29). To distinguish between the roles of *Runx2* in osteoblast differentiation and in hypertrophic chondrocyte maturation, transgenic mice were generated that overexpressed Runx2 in chondrocytes. In these mice, endochondral ossification was accelerated (Takeda et al., 2001; Ueta et al., 2001). When *Runx2* is overexpressed in chondrocytes of *Runx2*-null embryos, partial rescue of the phenotype of *Runx2*-deficient embryos is seen; that is, in the rescued animals, the defects in hypertrophic chondrocyte differentiation are corrected but the arrest of osteoblast differentiation persists (Takeda et al., 2001).

Other Transcription Factors

Several other transcription factors have important roles in chondrocyte differentiation. These include ATF-2, Pbx1, P105, and P130. The role of the first two will be briefly described here.

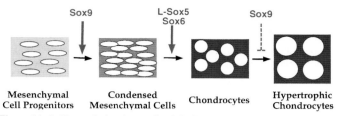

Figure 11–3. Transcription factors Sox9, L-Sox5, and Sox6 are needed in sequential steps of chondrocyte differentiation. Sox9 is needed for chondrogenic mesenchymal condensations; L-Sox5 and Sox6 are needed for overt chondrocyte differentiation. Evidence also favors a role of Sox9 in inhibiting the maturation of chondrocytes into hypertrophic chondrocytes.

ATF-2. Activating transcription factor-2 (ATF-2) is a basic region leucine zipper protein whose DNA target sequence is the widely distributed cAMP response element. Homozygous ATF-2 mutant mice show reduced proliferation of chondrocytes and dwarfism (Reimold et al., 1996). Levels of cyclin D1 protein are greatly reduced in chondrocytes isolated from *ATF-2*-deficient mice (Beier et al., 1999). Growth plates from *cyclin D1*-deficient mice also display a smaller zone of proliferating chondrocytes (Beier et al., 2001). These observations strongly suggest that ATF-2 is a regulator of chondrocyte proliferation in the growth plate and that this is mediated by cyclin D1.

Pbx1. Pbxl is a homeodomain protein originally identified as the product of an oncogene in a subset of childhood leukemias. *Pbx1*-null mutant mice die at embryonic day 15/16 with widespread patterning defects of the axial and appendicular skeleton (Selleri et al., 2001). In affected domains of limbs and ribs, Pbxl deficiency results in reduced proliferation of chondrocytes, acceleration of hypertrophic chondrocytes, and premature cartilage mineralization, indicating that Pbxl regulates chondrocyte proliferation and hypertrophic chondrocyte differentiation. No major changes in the overall patterns of expression of *fibroblast growth factor receptor3 (Fgfr3), Sox9, indian hedgehog (Ihh), parathyroid hormone–related peptide (PTHrP),* and *PTH/PTHrP receptor (PPR)* were detected in rib cartilages, indicating that Pbxl is not an upstream regulator of these genes.

Signaling Molecules

Both the unidirectional proliferation of chondrocytes, which results in parallel stacks of dividing cells, and the rate of transition of chondrocytes into hypertrophic chondrocytes are crucial in endochondral bone formation. Several signaling molecules have critical roles in these processes (Fig. 11–4, Table 11–1).

Fibroblast Growth Factors

FGFs and FGFR3 have major roles in endochondral bone formation (see Chapters 32 and 33). FGFR3 is expressed in proliferating and prehypertrophic chondrocytes in the developing bones (Peters et al., 1993; Delezoide et al., 1998; Naski et al., 1998; Ohbayashi et al., 2002). Activating mutations in FGFR3 cause achondroplasia, hypochondroplasia, and thanatophoric dysplasia, the most common forms of dwarfism in humans (Shiang et al., 1994; Rousseau et al., 1994, 1995; Bellus et al., 1995; Tavormina et al., 1995). Expression of activated *FGFR3* mutants in mice, which reproduces the dwarfism phenotype of these diseases, causes a marked decrease in the proliferation rate of the columnar proliferating chondrocytes and a decrease in size of the zone of hypertrophic chondrocytes (Naski et al., 1998;

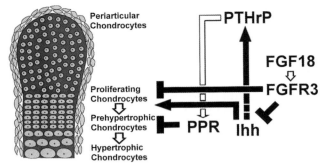

Figure 11–4. Signaling pathways that control proliferation and hypertrophic differentiation of chondrocytes in the growth plate. Fibroblast growth factor 18 (FGF18) is expressed in the perichondrium. FGF18 binds to FGF receptor 3 (FGFR3) expressed in chondrocytes. Signaling from FGFR3 inhibits chondrocyte proliferation, while Indian hedgehog (Ihh) expressed in prehypertrophic chondrocytes promotes chondrocyte proliferation. FGFR3 signaling inhibits *Ihh* expression. Ihh also induces parathyroid hormone–related peptide (*PTHrP*) expression in periarticular chondrocytes. PTHrP binds to the PTH/PTHrP receptor (PPR) and inhibits hypertrophic chondrocyte differentiation.

Wang et al., 1999; Li et al., 1999; Segev et al., 2000; Iwata et al., 2000, 2001; Chen et al., 2001). Interestingly, in these mice, there is also a reduction in expression of *Ihh* and *patched (Ptc),* a downstream target gene of Ihh. In contrast, lack of FGFR3 in mice causes skeletal overgrowth, indicating that a normal function of FGFR3 is to inhibit endochondral bone growth (Colvin et al., 1996; Deng et al., 1996).

Several signaling pathways are activated by FGF, including the signal transducer and activator of transcription Stat1 (Su et al., 1997; Sahni et al., 1999). In chondrocytes in culture, FGF treatment induces the phosphorylation of Stat1 and its translocation to the nucleus of the cell as well as increased expression of the cell cycle inhibitor p21. Nuclear localization of Stat1 and increased levels of p21 expression are observed in chondrocytes of human thanatophoric dysplasia. Although Stat1 mutants do not show a major skeletal phenotype, Stat1 deficiency rescues the chondrodysplasia phenotype of transgenic mice that show systemic expression of FGF2 under the control of a general promoter (Sahni et al., 2001). These observations strongly suggested that Stat1 activation could be involved in the dwarf phenotype of achondroplasia, hypochondroplasia, and thanatophoric dysplasias. Among various FGF ligands expressed in the developing bones, *Fgf18* is expressed in the perichondrium, and mice homozygous for a tar-

Table 11–1. Signaling Molecules that Control Chondrocyte Differentiation

	Sites of Expression	Function
FGF2	Proliferating chondrocytes, hypertrophic chondrocytes	
FGF18	Perichondrium, developing joints	Inhibits chondrocyte proliferation, inhibits Ihh expression, promotes osteogenesis
Ihh	Prehypertrophic chondrocytes	Promotes chondrocyte proliferation, specifies the location of bone collar formation, induces PTHrP expression in periarticular chondrocytes
PTHrP	Periarticular chondrocytes	Inhibits hypertrophic differentiation of chondrocytes
BMP2	Perichondrium, hypertrophic chondrocytes, developing joints	
BMP3	Perichondrium	
BMP4	Perichondrium	Rib cage, digit development
BMP5	Perichondrium	Sternal development
BMP6	Hypertrophic chondrocytes, developing joints	
BMP7	Perichondrium	Rib cage, digit development
GDF5	Developing joints	Specifies presumptive joint positions, segmentation of mesenchymal condensation, sternal development
GDF6	Developing joints	
TGF-β	Mesenchymal condensation, hypertrophic chondrocytes	Inhibits hypertrophic differentiation of chondrocytes, maintains articular cartilage
CNP	Proliferating and prehypertrophic chondrocytes	Promotes chondrocyte proliferation
VEGF	Hypertrophic chondrocytes	Recruits endothelial cells and osteoclasts
Wnt4	Developing joints	Accelerates maturation of chondrocytes, accelerates onset of bone collar formation
Wnt5a	Perichondrium	Delays maturation of chondrocytes, delays onset of bone collar formation
Wnt5b	Prehypertrophic chondrocytes, outer layer of perichondrium	
Wnt14	Developing joints	Induces GDF5 expression

FGF, Fibroblast growth factor; Ihh, Indian hedgehog; PTHrP, parathyroid hormone–related peptide; BMP, bone morphogenetic protein; GDF, growth and differentiation factor; TGF, transforming growth factor; CNP, C-type natriuretic peptide; VEGF, vascular endothelial growth factor; Wnt, Wingless.

geted disruption of *Fgf18* exhibit a growth plate phenotype similar to that observed in mice lacking *Fgfr3*. These data suggest that FGF18 may act as a physiological ligand for FGFR3 (Liu et al., 2002; Ohbayashi et al., 2002).

In recent experiments, expression of *Sox9* was increased by FGFs in chondrocytes in culture. Upregulation of *Sox9* by FGFs in these cells was mediated by the mitogen-activated protein kinase (MAPK) pathway (Murakami et al., 2000). A functional assay for the transcriptional activity of Sox9 was used to show that the activity of Sox9 was also increased by activating mutations of FGFR3 that cause the human dwarfisms. It is thus possible that an increase in the activity of the MAPK pathway and an increase in expression of *Sox9* could have a role, possibly in collaboration with Stat1, in the inhibition of chondrocyte proliferation in the growth plate and the development of dwarfism caused by activating mutations in FGFR3. The inhibition of chondrocyte proliferation could be due to the combined enhancement of Stat1 activity and increased activity of the MAPK pathway.

Indian Hedgehog

Ihh has multiple roles during skeletogenesis, in both the chondrocyte and the osteoblast differentiation pathways (see Chapter 16). *Ihh* is first expressed in skeletal elements in cells that overtly differentiate into chondrocytes right after mesenchymal condensations. Its expression is then downregulated in the central cells of these cartilages, which become hypertrophic; and later, its expression is restricted to the prehypertrophic zone of growth plates (St-Jacques et al., 1999). Ihh, like the other members of the hedgehog family, signals through a complex cellular signaling pathway that includes Ptc and smoothened (Smo) receptors and downstream Gli transcription factors (McMahon, 2000). *Ptc* expression is strongly stimulated by Hedgehog family members so that the extent of Ptc expression in skeletal primordia can be regarded as the domain of active signaling by Ihh. In chick embryos, overexpression of *Ihh* increased the expression of *PTHrP* in periarticular chondrocytes, markedly delaying both hypertrophic chondrocyte maturation and bone formation (Vortkamp et al., 1996). Whether this activation of *PTHrP* expression by Ihh in the growth plate is a direct effect or is mediated by a relay signal is not clear. Loss of Ihh function in mice illustrated the multiple roles of Ihh (St-Jacques et al., 1999). First, these null mice showed severe dwarfism of endochondral skeletal elements, but the absence of Ihh had no effect on intramembranous ossification. In mutant mice, chondrocyte proliferation was markedly reduced and the typical stacks of proliferating chondrocytes were missing, indicating that Ihh is required for normal chondrocyte proliferation. The ability of Ihh to stimulate cell proliferation is also a property of another member of the hedgehog family, sonic hedgehog (Shh). Indeed, Shh increases cell proliferation in a variety of tissues during mouse development. In addition, mutations that cause constitutive activation of the Hedgehog signaling pathway are associated with several specific human tumors, including basal cell carcinoma of the skin and glioblastoma (Gailani et al., 1996; Hahn et al., 1996; Johnson et al., 1996; Raffel et al., 1997).

The severely reduced chondrocyte proliferation rate in *Ihh*-null mutants is not due to lack of PTHrP signaling. Indeed, overexpression of constitutively active PPR in chondrocytes of *Ihh*-null mutants did not rescue the short-limbed dwarfism and decreased proliferation rate of chondrocytes of these mice (Karp et al., 2000). However, another abnormal characteristic of *Ihh*-null embryos, namely the presence of ectopic hypertrophic chondrocytes in close proximity to the articular surface, where no hypertrophic chondrocytes are seen in wild-type embryos, could be corrected by PTHrP signaling in chondrocytes. In addition, in *Ihh*-null mice, there was a complete absence of cortical and trabecular bone formation in the endochondral skeleton, indicating that Ihh is required for osteoblast differentiation in endochondral bones. Ihh signaling could function in the maturation of the layer of osteogenic cells of the periosteum that are precursors of osteoblasts in the endochondral skeleton. In agreement with this hypothesis, no expression of *Runx2* was seen in the perichondrium of *Ihh*-null embryos. Furthermore, results of experiments in mouse chimeras were consistent with the notion that Ihh signals the location in the perichondrium where mesenchymal cells differentiate into osteoblasts to

form cortical bone and invade the mineralized matrix of hypertrophic chondrocytes.

Thus, Ihh controls at least three different critical steps in the endochondral growth plate: *(1)* normal proliferation of chondrocytes and establishment of characteristic columns of proliferating chondrocytes in the cartilage growth plate, a critical process for the growth of endochondral bones; *(2) PTHrP* expression by periarticular chondrocytes) (PTHrP then inhibits the conversion of proliferating and prehypertrophic chondrocytes into hypertrophic chondrocytes and maintains an appropriate pool of proliferating chondrocytes), and *(3)* differentiation of osteoblast precursors in the perichondrium flanking the zone of hypertrophic chondrocytes. Hence, several essential steps in endochondral bone formation that are part of the chondrocyte differentiation pathway and the osteoblast pathway are coordinated by Ihh signaling. The role of Ihh in osteoblast differentiation is a unique feature of endochondral bone formation. Indeed, membranous ossification is not affected in *Ihh*-null embryos.

Heterozygous missense mutations in human IHH have been associated with brachydactyly type A-1, a skeletal syndrome characterized by shortening or missing middle phalanges (Gao et al., 2001). In humans haploinsufficiency of Ihh may be the cause of this syndrome.

PTHrP

PTHrP is an 84–amino acid polypeptide, so named because the sequence of the N-terminal 34 amino acids presents a high degree of identity with that of PTH. In the cartilage growth plate, PTHrP regulates the rate at which proliferative chondrocytes exit the cell cycle and are converted into postproliferative hypertrophic chondrocytes (Kronenberg and Chung, 2001).

This major checkpoint has a key role in regulating longitudinal bone growth during endochondral bone formation. In the developing skeleton, PTHrP is expressed mainly in periarticular chondrocytes, whereas transcripts for its receptor, PPR, which is also the receptor for PTH, are found at low levels in proliferating chondrocytes and at much higher levels in prehypertrophic chondrocytes. *PPR* is also expressed in osteoblasts of skeletal elements. In *PTHrP*-null mice as well as in *PPR*-null mice, proliferation of chondrocytes stops prematurely and the columns of proliferating chondrocytes in the growth plate are short and irregular (Karaplis et al., 1994; Lanske et al., 1996). Humans who harbor null mutations in PPR have similar anomalies (Jobert et al., 1998; Karperien et al., 1999). In contrast, overexpression of *PTHrP* in chondrocytes lengthens the columns of proliferating chondrocytes in the growth plate, delays the conversion of these cells into hypertrophic chondrocytes, and causes retardation of bone formation (Weir et al., 1996; Schipani et al., 1997). As indicated earlier in this chapter, *PTHrP* expression in chondrocytes requires Ihh, a secreted polypeptide of the hedgehog family. PPR is a seven-transmembrane receptor coupled to two different G proteins, one linked to the pathway that activates protein kinase A (PKA), the other linked to activation of phospholipase C (Lanske and Kronenberg, 1998). Upon binding to PPR, PTHrP triggers activation of adenylyl cyclase and, through an increase in the intracellular concentrations of cAMP, activates the cAMP-dependent PKA. Such activation presumably results in the phosphorylation of a number of target proteins, which include transcription factors.

Sox9 harbors two consensus PKA phosphorylation sites and can be phosphorylated by PKA both in a cell-free sytem and in transfection experiments (Huang et al., 2000). This phosphorylation increases the DNA-binding activity and the transcriptional activity of Sox9. Furthermore, in DNA transfection experiments, PTHrP treatment causes phosphorylation of Sox9, detected by a phosphospecific antibody directed against one of the two consensus PKA sites of Sox9, and increased transcriptional activity of Sox9 (Huang et al., 2001). This PTHrP-dependent increase in transcriptional activity is mediated by PKA as it was inhibited by a PKA-specific inhibitor. Thus, Sox9 is likely to be a target of PTHrP signaling and could mediate at least some of the effects of PTHrP in the growth plate. The PTHrP-mediated increase in transcriptional activity of Sox9, probably together with that of other transcription factors, would help maintain the chondrocyte phenotype of cells in the prehypertrophic zone and inhibit their maturation to hypertrophic chondrocytes. Hence, a link exists between PTHrP, a hormone known to control an important checkpoint in the pathway of chondrogenesis, and Sox9, a key transcription factor required for chondrocyte differentiation.

PKA phosphorylation of the ubiquitous transcription factor cAMP-responsive element binding protein (CREB) increases its transcriptional activity. This is the best-studied example illustrating the cAMP-mediated transcriptional stimulation of gene expression. Surprisingly, in *PTHrP*-null mutants, there was no difference in the number of chondrocytes in which CREB was phosphorylated at Ser^{133}, the site that is phosphorylated by PKA (Long et al., 2001). Similarly, phosphorylation at a conserved PKA consensus site in the related transcription factors cAMP-responsive element modulator (CREM) and ATF-1 was unchanged in *PTHrP*-null embryos. Thus, other signaling pathways could control the phosphorylation and activity of CREB family members in the growth plate. However, it is clear that these CREB family members have an important role in the growth plate because chondrocyte expression in transgenic mice of a dominant-negative CREB that decreased the activity of all three family members caused dwarfism associated with inhibition of chondrocyte proliferation and of Ihh signaling. The function of CREB phosphorylation at Ser^{133} in chondrocytes may be to increase expression of Ihh.

BMPs

BMPs were originally identified as proteins capable of inducing ectopic endochondral bone formation in subcutaneous implants. Subsequent molecular cloning revealed that the BMP family consists of a number of related molecules that belong to the TGF-β superfamily (see Chapter 24). Based on sequence homology, most of the growth and differentiation factors (GDFs) have been added to this family. Among the BMP family members, *Bmp2, Bmp3, Bmp4, Bmp5,* and *Bmp7* are expressed in the perichondrium; *Bmp2* and *Bmp6* are expressed in hypertrophic chondrocytes; and *Bmp2, Bmp6, Gdf5,* and *Gdf6* are expressed in developing joints (Storm and Kingsley, 1996; Naski et al., 1998; Solloway et al., 1998; St-Jacques et al., 1999; Minina et al., 2001).

Despite their dramatic bone-inducing activity and potent modulation of differentiation in cell culture, the physiological roles of BMPs in chondrocyte differentiation remain elusive. Analysis of the skeletal phenotypes caused by genetic inactivation of individual Bmps and their receptors along with the study of their expression patterns suggest functional redundancy among these molecules. This view is confirmed by the more severe phenotypes displayed by several double mutants compared with those of individual mutants. For instance, mutations in the *Bmp5* gene result in reduced size of the ear, body size, and number of ribs and deformities in or absence of the xiphoid appendix. Mutations in Gdf5 in the brachypodism (bp) mouse mutant cause reduction in the length of several long bones and segmentation defects of the phalangeal skeletal elements (Storm et al., 1994). Mutations in CDMP1, the human Gdf5 homolog, are associated with Hunter-Thompson chondrodysplasia, chondrodysplasia Grebe type, and brachydactyly type C (Thomas et al., 1996, 1997; Polinkovsky et al., 1997; see Chapter 27).

Despite the widespread expression of *BmprIB* throughout the developing skeleton, defects in *BmprIB*$^{-/-}$ mice are largely restricted to the appendicular skeleton (Yi et al., 2000). Proliferation of prechondrogenic cells and chondrocyte differentiation in the phalangeal region are markedly reduced in *BmprIB* mutant mice. *Bmp5/6* double mutant mice display an exacerbation of the sternal defects observed in *Bmp5* mutants (Solloway et al., 1998). *Gdf5/Bmp5* double mutants also show sternal defects that are not seen in any of the single mutants (Storm and Kingsley, 1996). *Bmp4/7* double heterozygotes have a higher frequency of rib cage and digit abnormalities than single heterozygotes (Katagiri et al., 1998). *BmprIB/Bmp7* double mutants exhibit severe appendicular skeletal defects, suggesting that *BmprIB* and *Bmp7* act in distinct but overlapping pathways (Yi et al., 2000). Mice carrying a *Gdf5*-null mutation and a deletion in *cis*-regulatory sequences for limb expression of *BmprIB* show synergistic malformations in the carpal and tarsal bones (Baur et al., 2000).

In addition to the distinct expression patterns of each of the BMP ligands and receptors, the activity of BMP is regulated by interaction with Noggin and Chordin, antagonists that bind and inactivate BMP. In mice lacking Noggin, cartilage condensations initiate normally but hyperplasia develops, suggesting that excess BMP enhances the recruitment of cells into cartilage (Brunet et al., 1998).

Thus, although the exact role of BMPs during chondrogenesis is not entirely clear, they certainly have important roles, probably in different steps of the chondrocyte differentiation pathway.

TGF-β

Members of the TGF-β superfamily are secreted growth factors that regulate many aspects of development (see Chapter 24). *TGF-β1–3* mRNAs are expressed in condensing mesenchyme during the early stages of chondrocyte differentiation (Pelton et al., 1991). TGF-β mRNAs were not detected in hypertrophic chondrocytes, but TGF-β immunoreactivity was observed in the matrix surrounding these cells. In vitro, TGF-β inhibits the transition of chondrocytes into hypertrophic chondrocytes (Kato et al., 1988; Ballock et al., 1993; Dieudonne et al., 1994), and in transgenic mice, expression of a cytoplasmically truncated, functionally inactive, dominant-negative TGF-β type II receptor in the growth plate and articular chondrocytes produced increased immunostaining of type X collagen in the growth plate and hypertrophic differentiation of articular chondrocytes (Serra et al., 1997). In addition, mutant mice homozygous for a targeted disruption of Smad3, a signaling molecule downstream of TGF-β, show abnormal hypertrophic differentiation of articular chondrocytes, leading to progressive loss of articular cartilage (Yang et al., 2001). These observations indicate that TGF-β signaling inhibits hypertrophic differentiation of chondrocytes and plays a role in maintaining articular cartilage.

Natriuretic Peptides

The natriuretic peptide family consists of three structurally related ligands, atrial, brain, and C-type natriuretic peptides (ANP, BNP, and CNP) (Levin et al., 1998). Two guanylyl cyclase (GC)–coupled receptors, GC-A and GC-B, mediate the biological functions of these ligands; and the biologically silent natriuretic peptide receptor (NPR)-C is thought to act as a clearance or decoy receptor. The natriuretic peptides that bind to NPR-C are internalized and enzymatically degraded. CNP and its receptor GC-B are expressed in proliferating and prehypertrophic chondrocytes in the growth plate (Chusho et al., 2001). *CNP*-deficient mice show severe achondroplasia-like dwarfism, characterized by reduced proliferation of growth plate chondrocytes. The reduced proliferation is, however, independent of *Ihh* expression. By contrast, mice homozygous for null mutations in NPR-C and transgenic mice with elevated plasma BNP levels show skeletal overgrowth (Suda et al., 1998; Matsukawa et al., 1999). These observations indicate that natriuretic peptide signaling positively regulates chondrocyte proliferation in the growth plate.

Vascular Endothelial Growth Factor

During endochondral ossification, the avascular cartilage matrix is invaded by blood vessels and subsequently replaced by bone. Vascular endothelial growth factor (VEGF), a dimeric glycoprotein that stimulates endothelial cells and induces angiogenesis, plays an important role in coordinating the process of vascular invasion, cartilage resorption and bone formation. VEGF is initially expressed in the perichondrium and surrounding tissue of cartilage templates of future bones (Zelzer et al., 2002). This peripheral expression is lost by the time high levels of VEGF expression appear in hypertrophic chondrocytes in the growth plate (Gerber et al., 1999; Horner et al., 1999; Colnot and Helms, 2001). VEGF is a chemoattractant for both endothelial cells and osteoclasts (Engsig et al., 2000). When a soluble chimeric VEGF receptor, which sequesters the VEGF polypeptide, was injected into 24-day-old mice, blood vessels failed to penetrate the hypertrophic cartilage matrix and there was a deep reduction in the number of tartrate-resistant acid phosphatase (TRAP)-positive osteoclasts/chondroclasts that express matrix metalloproteinase-9 (MMP-9) at cartilage–bone junctions (Gerber et al., 1999). In these mice, the zone of hypertrophic chondrocytes was considerably expanded. In contrast, chondrocyte proliferation and maturation of hypertrophic chondrocytes were normal. Deletion of a single *VEGF-A* allele in chondrocytes using the Cre-loxP system also resulted in an expanded hypertrophic zone and reduced vascular invasion (Haigh et al., 2000). These observations indicate that VEGF produced by hypertrophic chondrocytes plays a critical role in regulating vascular invasion of cartilaginous matrix and bone formation. Interestingly, mice deficient in MMP-9 display a growth plate phenotype similar to mice in which VEGF signaling is disrupted (Vu et al., 1998), that is, a considerable expansion of the hypertrophic zone and a delay in vascular invasion and osteoclast recruitment. MMP-9 is highly expressed in cells of the osteoclast lineage (Reponen et al., 1994; Tezuka et al., 1994; Wucherpfennig et al., 1994; Okada et al., 1995). MMP-9 degrades components of the ECM with high specific activity for denatured collagens (gelatin) and releases matrix-bound VEGF in culture (Bergers et al., 2000). These observations indicate that MMP-9 expressed in osteoclasts and VEGF expressed in hypertrophic chondrocytes coordinately regulate vascular invasion and osteoclast recruitment during endochondral ossification.

Wnts

Wnt proteins form a family of highly conserved secreted signaling molecules that play crucial roles during embryonic development (see Chapter 22). During chick limb development, the *Wnt-5a*, *Wnt-5b*, *Wnt-4*, and *Wnt-14* genes are expressed in skeletal elements: *Wnt-5a* is expressed in the perichondrium, *Wnt-5b* is expressed in a subpopulation of prehypertrophic chondrocytes and in the outermost cell layer of the perichondrium, and *Wnt-4* and *Wnt-14* are expressed in cells of the joint region (Kawakami et al., 1999; Hartmann and Tabin, 2000, 2001). Misexpression experiments using a retrovirus vector have indicated distinct roles for these Wnt proteins. While Wnt-4 misexpression accelerates maturation of chondrocytes and the onset of bone collar formation, Wnt5a misexpression delays these processes (Hartman and Tabin, 2000). Wnt-14 misexpression induces morphological and molecular signs of joint formation (Hartman and Tabin, 2001). Wnt ligands bind to receptors of the Frizzled family of proteins and transduce signals to β-catenin, which then enters the nucleus and forms a complex with T-cell factor to activate transcription of target genes. Misexpression of a constitutively active form of β-catenin resulted in accelerated chondrocyte maturation, similar to Wnt-4 misexpression (Hartmann and Tabin, 2000). Misexpression of dominant-negative forms of Frizzled-1 and Frizzled-7 delayed chondrocyte maturation, indicating a role for endogenous Wnt proteins in regulating chondrocyte differentiation (Hartman and Tabin, 2000). Thus, Wnt proteins and their downstream target molecules regulate several steps of chondrocyte differentiation. Identification of physiological receptors for each of the Wnt ligands and of their downstream target molecules should further clarify the diverse effects of Wnt proteins on skeletal development.

ECM Molecules

Cartilage is a specialized connective tissue consisting of chondrocytes, which produce large amounts of ECM components that are characteristic of cartilage (see Chapter 95). Among the major components are fibril-forming collagens and aggrecan. Aggrecan is the most predominant proteoglycan in cartilage. It forms macromolecular complexes with hyaluronic acid and link protein in the ECM. Chondrocytes also produce various other matrix molecules. Defects in these matrix components lead to associated skeletal abnormalities in humans. In mice harboring mutations in each of these matrix molecules, ECM molecules not only serve as structural components but also play critical roles in maintaining the normal cellular organization that is characteristic of growth plate cartilages and in regulating chondrocyte differentiation.

During endochondral ossification, chondrocytes synthesize a particular set of collagen types depending on the stage of differentiation. Chondrocytes in the resting and proliferating zones synthesize collagen types II (the most abundant collagen of cartilage), IX, and XI. Hypertrophic chondrocytes are characterized by the synthesis of type X collagen. Various mutations in the genes for collagens have been identified in human skeletal dysplasia syndromes. Mutations in the collagen type II gene (*COL2A1*) have been associated with either lethal or severe chondrodysplasias, primary generalized osteoarthritis, and Stickler syndrome, an autosomal dominant disorder that affects the eye and joints. In mouse homozygous mutants for *Col2a1*, which show a complete lack of extracellular fibrils discernible by electron microscopy, there was no endochondral bone or epiphyseal growth plate in long bones, although cortical bone formation in these skeletal elements was less affected. Similarly, the cartilage of mutant vertebrae was completely disorganized, and the notochord persisted until birth. The vertebral chondrocytes in *Col2a1*-null embryos undergo a normal sequence of differentiation, producing cartilage lineage-specific matrix components, such as collagen types IX, XI, and X. These data show that collagen type II is not essential for chondrocyte differentiation and hypertrophy, but it plays a crucial role in organizing the growth plate in long bones and the normal structures of vertebrae (Li et al., 1995; Aszódi et al., 1998).

Cartilage matrix deficiency (cmd) is a well-characterized genetic disorder of mouse aggrecan (Rittenhouse et al., 1978; Kimata et al., 1981; Brown and Harne, 1982; Brennan et al., 1983). The cmd phenotype is caused by a 7 bp deletion in *aggrecan* exon 5, resulting in a premature stop codon, a truncated aggrecan core protein, and no mature aggrecan product in the matrix (Watanabe et al., 1994). Mice homozygous for the mutation exhibit cleft palate; short limbs, snout, and tail; and perinatal lethality (Houghton et al., 1989). Growth plates of homozygous *cmd* mutant mice are characterized by disorganization of chondrocytes with no columnar structures and a marked reduction of hypertrophic chondrocytes. These mice show an altered expression pattern of other matrix genes in the growth plate. These include *Link protein*, *Syndecan 3*, *Col10a1*, *Col11a2*, and the alternative transcripts *Col2a1 type IIA* and *Col9a1* (Wai et al., 1998). These results indicate that a deficiency in one matrix component can affect expression of other matrix molecules.

Link protein stabilizes the interaction of aggrecan with hyaluronic acid. Homozygous mutant mice show defects in cartilage development and delayed bone formation with short limbs and craniofacial anomalies (Watanabe and Yamada, 1999). The cartilage contains significantly reduced aggrecan depositions in the hypertrophic zone and decreased numbers of prehypertrophic and hypertrophic chondrocytes, indicating that Link protein is important for the formation of proteoglycan aggregates and normal organization of growth plates. Interestingly, expression of *Ihh* and *PPR* was reduced in these mice (Watanabe and Yamada, 1999). These results indicate that normal expression of local regulators of chondrocyte proliferation and differentiation is dependent on the integrity of the cartilage matrix. It is possible, therefore, that the overall phenotype of mice deficient in one of the matrix components could result from compound effects of matrix deficiency and altered expression or availability of cytokines.

Perlecan is a large heparan sulfate proteoglycan present in basement membrane and in some other tissues such as cartilage. The molecule interacts with FGF family members in vitro (Aviezer et al., 1994). Mice that are homozygous mutants for perlecan exhibit severe disorganization of the columnar structures of chondrocytes and defective endochondral ossification (Arikawa-Hirasawa et al., 1999). Proliferation of chondrocytes is reduced and the size of the prehypertrophic zone in the growth plate is diminished. Cartilage of homozygous null mice contain reduced and disorganized collagen fibrils, suggesting that perlecan has an important role in the overall organization of the ECM. Some of the characteristics of these mutants are similar to those of human thanatophoric dysplasia, a dwarfism syndrome caused by activating mutations in FGFR3, and to those of *Fgfr3* gain-of-function mice, suggesting that the physiological role of perlecan in cartilage might be to bind FGFs and sequester their activity. ECM molecules might thus provide mechanisms to regulate cytokine activity, affecting the entire process of chondrocyte proliferation and maturation in the growth plate. Anomalies of cartilage in mice with null mutations in individual ECM components such as type II Collagen, aggrecan, Link protein, and perlecan are severe and present several common defects, including marked disorganization of the growth plate, particularly of the regular columns of proliferating chondrocytes. Furthermore, the severe anomalies of these mutants have similarities with those of *Sox5*, *Sox6*-double-null mutants, which are characterized by a severe reduction in the expression of numerous cartilage ECM components.

JOINT FORMATION

Joint formation is one of the most remarkable aspects of skeletal development. Cartilage differentiation initially takes place as a continuous rod-like structure, which is subsequently separated into individual elements. During this process, cells at the presumptive joint space first increase in density, flatten, and then downregulate some of the chondrocyte markers such as *Col2a1* (Craig et al., 1987; Hartmann and Tabin, 2001; Wang et al., 2001). They subsequently undergo apoptosis, leading to formation of the joint cavity (Mori et al., 1995; Nalin et al., 1995; Kimura and Shiota, 1996). *Gdf5*, *Gdf6*, and *Wnt-14* are early markers that are known to be expressed in the presumptive joint positions, suggesting crucial roles for these molecules in joint development (Storm et al., 1994; Hartmann and Tabin, 2001). The characterization of both mouse and human mutations in Gdf5 indicate that this BMP family member has a critical role in joint formation. Indeed, Gdf5 is mutated in the brachypodism (bp) mouse mutant (Storm et al., 1994), which is characterized by a segmentation defect and lack of joint formation of the phalangeal skeletal elements (Grüneberg and Lee, 1973; Storm and Kingsley, 1996).

Mutations of CDMP-1, the human ortholog of Gdf5, cause acromesomelic chondrodysplasias (Hunter-Thompson type and Grebe type), which are characterized by short limbs, especially the distal part of the limbs, and by the absence of several phalangeal joints (Thomas et al., 1996, 1997; see Chapter 27). Autosomal dominant brachydactyly type C is also caused by mutation in the *CDMP-1* gene (Polinkovsky et al., 1997). Joint formation is also regulated by Noggin, a secreted polypeptide that binds and antagonizes BMP family members (see Chapter 25). Indeed, in *noggin*-null mice, joints fail to develop in both the axial and appendicular skeletons (Brunet et al., 1998). This loss of joint formation correlates with loss of Gdf5 expression in the presumptive joint regions. In addition, dominant mutations in human Noggin have been identified in proximal symphalangism (SYM1, OMIM 185800) and multiple synostosis syndrome (SYNS1, OMIM 186500); both syndromes are characterized by multiple joint fusions (Gong et al., 1999).

Wnt-14, a member of the *Wnt* gene family, is expressed in joint-forming regions in a pattern similar to Gdf5 (Hartmann and Tabin, 2001). If Wnt-14 is misexpressed in the developing chick limb using a recombinant retrovirus, morphological changes consistent with joint formation appear, and *Gdf5* is expressed in infected chondrogenic regions, strongly suggesting that Wnt-14 plays a critical role in initiating synovial joint formation and is generally upstream of Gdf5.

In humans, joint fusion has also been associated with Apert, Pfeiffer, and Jackson-Weiss syndromes. These syndromes are caused by activating mutations of FGFR2 (Jabs et al., 1994; Rutland et al., 1995; Wilkie et al., 1995; see Chapter 33).

OSTEOBLAST DIFFERENTIATION AND BONE FORMATION

Recent gene-targeting experiments have provided evidence that two transcription factors play essential roles in sequential steps of this cellular pathway. Osteoblasts produce an ECM that is composed of type I collagen and noncollagenous proteins and mineralizes the bone matrix. Bone is constantly regenerated throughout life, and total bone mass is controlled by a precisely balanced process involving bone resorption by osteoclasts and bone formation by osteoblasts. The function of osteoblasts is controlled by both transcription factors and signaling molecules that act either locally or systemically (Fig. 11–5).

Transcription Factors

Runx2

Runx2 is a member of the Runt-domain family of transcription factors, which in mammals contains two additional members, AML1/

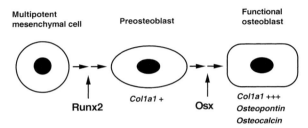

Figure 11–5. Pathway of osteoblast differentiation. Multipotential mesenchymal cells first differentiate into preosteoblasts, a process for which Runx2 is needed. Preosteoblasts do not express osteoblast marker genes, except low levels of *Col1a1*. Preosteoblasts then differentiate into functional osteoblasts expressing high levels of osteoblast marker genes, including *Col1a1, Osteopontin*, and *Osteocalcin*. This process requires Osx.

Runx1, a critical regulator of hematopoiesis, and AML2/Runx3 (Ito, 1999). Runx polypeptides form heterodimers with a single ubiquitous polypeptide called PEBP2β, which does not bind to DNA by itself but increases the efficiency of DNA binding of the heterodimers. In addition to the Runx DNA-binding domain, Runx2 contains an active transcription activation domain rich in glutamine and alanine residues. Expression of *Runx2* in mouse embryos begins as early as embryonic day (E) 9.5 in the notochord; it is expressed later in prechondrogenic mesenchymal condensations and in chondrocytes (Otto et al., 1997). Around E13.5, when both the perichondrium and the organization of the different cellular layers of the cartilage growth plate begin, expression of *Runx2* is observed in the perichondrium/periosteum and soon thereafter in hypertrophic chondrocytes. Later, *Runx2* is expressed in osteoblasts of all endochondral and membranous bones (Ducy et al., 1997). In tissue culture cells, forced expression of *Runx2* activates the osteocalcin and some other osteoblast marker genes.

The human genetic disease cleidocranial dysplasia, which is characterized by hypoplastic clavicles, large open spaces between frontal and parietal bones of the skull, and other skeletal dysplasias, is caused by heterozygous mutations in the *Runx2* gene (Mundlos and Olsen, 1997; see Chapter 29). The disease is due to haploinsufficiency of Runx2. *Runx2*-null mice are characterized by a block in osteoblast differentiation and the absence of both endochondral and intramembranous bone formation (Komori et al., 1997; Otto et al., 1997). Thus, Runx2 has an essential function in osteoblast differentiation. In null embryos, no degradation of the cartilage matrix of hypertrophic chondrocytes occurs because no invasion of this matrix by cells of the periosteum/perichondrium takes place; further, no osteoclasts/chondroclasts appear in this matrix. The lack of matrix invasion by cells of the periosteum is likely due to the defects in hypertrophic chondrocyte differentiation in these mutants. Indeed, Runx2 has two distinct functions in bone formation. First, it has an essential role in the differentiation of mesenchymal progenitors into osteoblasts both in the endochondral and in the intramembranous skeleton. The second function of Runx2, described earlier in this chapter, is to stimulate hypertrophic chondrocyte differentiation. The signals, including VEGF, that stimulate the invasion of the cartilage matrix by blood vessels and osteoclast and osteoblast precursors originate in the hypertrophic zone. Therefore, by stimulating hypertrophic chondrocyte differentiation, Runx2 has a role in priming the replacement of cartilage by bone during endochondral bone formation.

Osterix

Recently, a second transcription factor required for osteoblast differentiation was identified. This transcription factor, called Osterix (Osx), is specifically expressed in osteoblasts of all endochondral and membranous bones (Nakashima et al., 2002). Osx contains a DNA-binding domain consisting of three C2H2-type zinc fingers at its C terminus that share a high degree of sequence identity with similar motifs in Sp1, Sp3, and Sp4. In addition, it contains a proline- and serine-rich transcription activation domain that bears no clear similarities to any other polypeptides except that it is rich in proline residues. When overexpressed in C2C12 cells in culture, Osx activates expression of the *osteocalcin* and *type I collagen* genes. In *Osx*-null mutant mice, no endochondral and no intramembranous bone formation occurs. Mesenchymal cells in *Osx*-null mutant mice do not deposit bone matrix, and cells in the periosteum and the condensed mesenchyme of membranous skeletal elements cannot differentiate into osteoblasts, although these cells express normal levels of *Runx2*. In contrast to what is seen in *Runx2*-null mice, mesenchymal cells of the periosteum in *Osx*-null mutants invade the zone of hypertrophic chondrocytes together with blood vessels and osteoclasts. Arrest in osteoblast differentiation occurs at a later step than in *Runx2*-null mice. Indeed, expression of *Osx* requires Runx2, indicating that Osx acts downstream of Runx2. These studies strongly support the model that osteoblast progenitors in mesenchymal condensations of both endochondral and membranous skeletal elements first differentiate through one or several steps into preosteoblasts and that Runx2 has an essential role in this process. The *Runx2*-expressing preosteoblasts then differentiate in one or more steps into mature osteoblasts and express characteristic osteoblast marker genes, a process that requires Osx. Thus, Osx could be the main effector of the osteoblast program and activate a series of osteoblast-specific genes. It is also possible that Runx2 and Osx cooperate with each other in the activation of downstream genes.

Interestingly, in preosteoblasts of *Osx*-null mice, chondrocyte-specific markers, including *Sox9*, *Sox5*, and *Col2a1*, are expressed, suggesting the hypothesis that preosteoblasts are bipotential cells, having the potential to differentiate into both osteoblasts and chondrocytes.

Other Transcription Factors

Several transcription factors either directly or indirectly control Runx2 expression. Msx1 and Msx2 are homeodomain-containing transcription factors that have important roles in skeletal development (Satokata and Maas, 1994; Satokata et al., 2000). Missense mutations of MSX2 (P148H) cause Boston-type craniosynostosis in humans (see Chapter 52). *Msx2*-null mice show defects in bones of the skull due to defective proliferation of osteoprogenitor cells during morphogenesis of calvaria (Satokata et al., 2000). These mice also display defective endochondral ossification and a postnatal decrease in Runx2. Interestingly, in *Msx1* $^{-/-}$, *Msx2* $^{-/-}$-double-null mutants, the defects of *Msx2*-null mutants are considerably exacerbated (Satokata et al., 2000). This is illustrated by the lack of ossification of membranous bones in the head of double mutants. Thus, Msx1 and Msx2 have partially redundant functions in bone formation. They appear to be required for membranous bone formation, and it is likely that they act upstream of Runx2.

Dlx5 and Dlx6 are members of the distalless homeodomain-containing family of transcription factors expressed in developing bones (Simeone et al., 1994; Chen et al., 1996). *Dlx5* $^{-/-}$ mutant mice show complex craniofacial anomalies affecting derivatives of the branchial arches and a decrease of the thickness of the periosteum in long bones (Acampora et al., 1999; Depew et al., 1999). Expression *Runx2* is not affected in *Dlx5* $^{-/-}$ mutants. It is likely that Dlx5 and Dlx6, which are coexpressed in many tissues, including skeletal elements, have redundant functions during osteogenesis. A recent genetic study reported that *Dlx5* $^{-/-}$, *Dlx6* $^{-/-}$-double-null mutants had severe cartilage and bone defects caused by disruption of craniofacial development, endochondral ossification, and limb bud development, resulting in a phenocopy model of the human autosomal dominant form of the split-hand/split-foot malformation (Robledo et al., 2002). Thus, Dlx5 and Dlx6 are essential for craniofacial, axial, and appendicular skeletal development.

In vitro studies show that Msx2 is able to inhibit the transcriptional activity of Runx2 by interacting with it. Furthermore, Dlx5 interferes with the ability of Msx2 to interact with Runx2 and to repress its transcriptional activity (Newberry et al., 1998; Shirakabe et al., 2001). Indeed, Dlx5 promotes activation of the *Osteocalcin* gene by forming heterodimers with Msx2, which antagonizes the Msx2-mediated repression of Osteocalcin. These results suggest that regulation of the activity of Runx2 by Msx2 and Dlx5 plays an important role in osteoblast development.

Signaling Molecules

Ihh

The essential role of Ihh in osteoblast differentiation of endochondral bones was discussed earlier in this chapter. In contrast, in membranous bones, Ihh appears to have no role and is completely dispensable for the differentiation of osteoblasts (St-Jacques et al., 1999).

FGF18

Recent genetic studies demonstrate that FGF18 is another essential growth factor for osteoblast differentiation. As noted earlier *FGF18*-deficient mice exhibit a growth plate phenotype similar to that observed in *Fgfr3*-deficient mice, but they also display delayed ossification in the developing long bones and delayed suture closure in the skull (Liu et al., 2002; Ohbayashi et al., 2002). These data suggest that FGF18 positively regulates osteoblast proliferation and differentiation.

BMPs

When BMPs are implanted into subcutaneous or muscular tissues of rodents, they induce ectopic bone formation through the sequential processes of endochondral ossification (Wozney et al., 1988). Although a number of in vitro studies suggest that BMPs promote osteoblast differentiation (Katagiri et al., 1990; Takuwa et al., 1991), gene deletion studies of BMPs in vivo have not clarified their proposed stimulatory actions on osteoblast differentiation (Dudley et al., 1995; Winnier et al., 1995; Luo et al., 1995; Zhang and Bradley, 1996; Solloway et al., 1998). Because BMPs have prominent roles during embryonic development in the establishment of the body plan and in organogenesis, inactivation of several BMP genes, their receptors, and their intracellular signaling molecules often leads to early embryonic lethality. In other cases, redundancy of some of the signaling molecules might mask their precise function. The study of Tob, an antiproliferative protein, provides indirect evidence that BMP signaling controls osteoblast differentiation in vivo (Yoshida et al., 2000). BMPs bind to BMP type I and type II serine/threonine kinase receptors and transduce signals via Smad proteins. Tob is an intracellular negative regulator of BMP/Smad signaling in osteoblasts. Indeed, overproduction of Tob represses BMP2-induced, Smad-mediated transcriptional activation, and Tob-deficient mice have a greater bone mass resulting from an increased numbers of osteoblasts. Another finding suggesting involvement of BMPs in osteogenesis is that BMPs upregulate the expression of Runx2 and Osx in mesenchymal cells in cultures (Bae et al., 2001; Nakashima et al., 2002).

TGF-β

TGF-β is one of the components present in bone matrix. Accumulating evidence shows that TGF-β plays an important role in osteoblast differentiation and acts during bone growth and remodeling (Bonewald and Mundy, 1990; Bonewald and Dallas, 1994). For example, in vivo administration of TGF-β induces callus formation in normal bones (Noda and Camilliere, 1989) and increases bone formation during fracture repair (Joyce et al., 1990). Osteoblast-specific overexpression of TGF-β2 from the osteocalcin promoter results in progressive bone loss associated with both an increase in osteoblastic matrix deposition and osteoclastic bone resorption (Erlebacher and Derynck, 1996), suggesting that TGF-β2 functions as a local positive regulator of bone remodeling. Furthermore, in transgenic mice that express a cytoplasmically truncated type II TGF-β receptor in osteoblasts, trabecular bone mass increases with age, due to decreased bone resorption by osteoclasts, probably via both the induction of osteoblastic secretion of macrophage colony-stimulating factor (M-CSF) and a modification of the osteoprotegerin/receptor activator of nuclear factor (RANK)/RANK ligand κβ (RANKL) system described below (Takai et al., 1998; Sells Galvin et al., 1999; Thirunavukkarasu et al., 2001). These experiments suggest that TGF-β functions as a physiological regulator of osteoblast differentiation and acts as a component of the mechanism that couples bone formation and resorption during bone remodeling.

PTH

PTH is essential for the maintenance of calcium homeostasis through direct actions on bone and kidney and indirect actions on the gastrointestinal tract (Fitzpatrick and Bilezikian, 1996). PTH promotes calcium release from bone and increases the extracellular calcium level. In vitro studies showed that PTH increases collagenase synthesis, decreases type I collagen synthesis, and reduces alkaline phosphatase activity in osteoblasts (Bringhurst and Potts, 1981; Heath et al., 1984; Hall and Dickson, 1985; Simon et al., 1988; Partridge et al., 1989). Primary hyperparathyroidism results from excess production of PTH, mostly due to single parathyroid adenomas (Black and Utley, 1968; Spiegel, 1991; Khan and Bilezikian, 2000). It causes osteitis fibrosa, characterized by thinning and weakening of the bones and fractures of the femoral neck. However, intermittent administration of a small dose of PTH increases osteoblast numbers and trabecular bone formation enough to prevent the weakening and fractures (Tam et al., 1982; Hock and Gera, 1992). PTHrP was originally identified as a factor responsible for the hypercalcemia associated with malignancy. Clinical evidence shows that its role in malignancy is as a mediator of bone resorption associated with osteolytic metastasis. Both PTH and PTHrP bind to a common receptor (PPR) with equal affinity and activate intracellular signaling pathways with the same efficacy (Jüppner et al., 1991; Karaplis et al., 1994). The bones in *PPR*-deficient mice exhibit a striking increase in osteoblast number and matrix accumulation in the bone collar (Lanske et al., 1999). However, these mice show a dramatic decrease in trabecular bone formation in the primary spongiosa, due to a decrease in osteoblasts. Thus, PTH/PTHrP receptor signaling regulates osteoblast differentiation and bone formation differently in primary spongiosa and in bone collars.

Leptin

Leptin is a hormone secreted by adipocytes that controls body weight through the hypothalamus, where a leptin-specific receptor is expressed (Spiegelman and Flier, 1996; Friedman and Halaas, 1998). Interestingly, both *leptin*-deficient (*ob/ob*) and *leptin receptor*-deficient (*db/db*) mice show increased bone formation, despite their hypogonadic and hypercortisolic states, which by themselves cause decreased bone formation (Ducy et al., 2000). In addition, intracerebroventricular infusion of leptin causes bone loss in *leptin*-deficient and wild-type mice. These in vivo studies of the role of leptin during bone remodeling have shown that total bone mass is modulated through the hypothalamus.

Signaling Through Low-Density Lipoprotein Receptor–Related Protein

The autosomal recessive disorder osteoporosis-pseudoglioma syndrome dramatically lowers bone mass and produces fractures and deformity of bones (Gong et al., 2001). This congenital disease is caused by mutations in the *low-density lipoprotein* (LDL) *receptor–related protein 5* (*Lrp5*) gene. This protein is expressed in osteoblasts and is involved in Wnt signal transduction, suggesting that Wnt-mediated signaling via Lrp5 plays important roles in osteoblast differentiation and in the establishment of bone mass. An in vivo study showed that *Lrp5*-deficient mice develop a low bone mass phenotype postnatally, secondary to decreased osteoblast proliferation and bone formation, even though *Runx2* expression is not altered (Kato et al., 2002). In vitro studies show that Lrp5 acts as a co-receptor for Wnt proteins and that it can directly bind Wnt proteins (Tamai et al., 2000; Wehrli et al., 2000), thus suggesting that Wnt proteins could be involved in the postnatal control of bone formation in a Runx2-independent manner.

ECM Molecules

Type I collagen is the most abundant fibrillar collagenous extracellular protein of bones and determines the strength of bones. It consists of a long continuous triple helix, which assembles into highly organized fibrils (Rossert and de Crombrugghe, 1996). These fibrils have a very high tensile strength and play a key role in providing a structural frame for bones. Each molecule of type I collagen is typically composed of two $\alpha 1$ chains and one $\alpha 2$ chain coiled around each other in a characteristic triple helix. Mutations within *COL1A1* or *COL1A2*

cause a heritable disorder, osteogenesis imperfecta (OI), characterized by bony deformities, excessive fragility with fracturing, and short stature, as well as connective-tissue abnormalities which may involve the eyes (blue sclerae), ears, teeth, joints, and skin (Sillence et al., 1979; Beighton et al., 1988). Many mutations are heterozygous with a dominant-negative effect; they disrupt formation of the triple helical structure of the collagen or the higher-order assembly of collagen fibrils. Histological analysis of OI bones shows that the osteoblast population increases and osteoclast activity is raised, leading to a high bone turnover rate. The major reason for bone fragility in OI is the failure of osteoblasts to synthesize normal type I collagen (Cole, 1994). Transgenic mice harboring a minigene version of human *COL1A1*, which lacks a large part of the central triple helical region, had a lethal variant of OI (Khillan et al., 1991). The shortened pro-$\alpha 1$ (I) chains synthesized from the minigene in the mutant mice become disulfide-linked to pro-$\alpha 1$ (I) chains synthesized from the endogenous mouse gene, resulting in a phenotype that includes extensive fractures of the ribs and long bones, much like the fractures seen in lethal variants of human OI.

Osteocalcin is the most abundant osteoblast-specific noncollagenous protein. *Osteocalcin*-deficient mice develop a phenotype marked by higher bone mass due to an increase in bone formation but without impairment of bone resorption (Ducy et al., 1996).

Osteopontin is another abundant noncollagenous protein in bone matrix. *Osteopontin*-deficient mice exhibit normal skeletal size and normal skeletal patterning (Liaw et al., 1998; Rittling et al., 1998). Interestingly, however, these mice are resistant to ovariectomy-induced bone resorption, suggesting that osteopontin may be needed for the development of postmenopausal osteoporosis (Yoshitake et al., 1999).

Osteonectin is abundant in bone and is also expressed in tissues that undergo consistent turnover at sites of injury and disease (Bradshaw and Sage, 2001). In vitro studies indicate that osteonectin can bind collagen and regulate angiogenesis, metalloproteinase expression, cell proliferation, and cell–matrix interactions. *Osteonectin*-deficient mice have decreased bone formation and decreased osteoblast and osteoclast surface and number, leading to decreased bone remodeling with a negative bone balance that causes profound osteopenia (Gilmour et al., 1998; Delany et al., 2000). These data indicate that osteonectin supports bone remodeling and the maintenance of bone mass.

OSTEOCLAST DIFFERENTIATION

Osteoclasts are giant multinucleated cells derived from hematopoietic precursors of the monocyte-macrophage lineage. These cells have the unique capacity to resorb mineralized tissues, control total bone mass, and maintain calcium homeostasis. This occurs through a controlled balance of bone resorption by osteoclasts and bone formation by osteoblasts, a process called "bone remodeling." Disruption of the balance of bone remodeling results in the development of osteoporosis, a disorder in which there is a relative increase of bone resorption over bone formation. In addition, defects in the normal functioning of osteoclasts lead to osteopetrosis, a group of congenital diseases that prevent formation of bone marrow and increase bone mass. Recent studies of osteoclast biology using in vitro culture systems as well as mouse genetics have unraveled much of the molecular mechanisms underlying osteoclast differentiation. In this process, several transcription factors and signaling molecules have been assigned essential roles (Fig. 11–6).

Transcription Factors

Pu.1

Pu.1 is an ETS domain–containing transcription factor specifically expressed in the myeloid and B-lymphoid lineages (Klemsz et al., 1990). Pu.1-deficient mice lack both osteoclasts and macrophages in their bone marrow and develop severe osteopetrosis (Scott et al., 1994; McKercher et al., 1996; Tondravi et al., 1997). The osteopetrotic phenotype of *Pu.1*-deficient mice is rescued by bone marrow transplantation, with complete restoration of osteoclast and macrophage differentiation, verifying that the Pu.1 lesion is intrinsic to hematopoietic

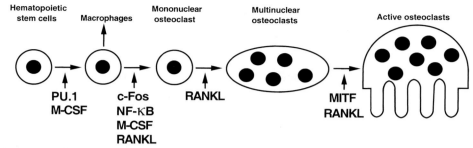

Figure 11–6. Pathway of osteoclast differentiation. Osteoclasts are derived from hematopoietic stem cells. Hematopoietic stem cells differentiate into cells of the monocyte/macrophage lineage, which can form both osteoclasts and monocyte-macrophages. This process requires PU.1 and macrophage colony-stimulating factor (M-CSF). These bipotential cells proliferate and differenti- ate to become mononuclear osteoclasts, a process for which c-Fos, nuclear fac- tor κB (NF-κB), M-CSF, and receptor activator of NF-κB ligand (RANKL) are needed. Mononuclear osteoclasts fuse to form multinuclear osteoclasts, and these multinuclear osteoclasts are activated to resorb bones. Microphthalmia (MITF), RANKL, and a variety of signaling molecules regulate these processes.

cells. These results suggest that Pu.1 regulates the initial stage of myeloid differentiation and further support the notion that osteoclasts are derived from cells of the monocyte-macrophage lineage.

c-Fos

Another transcription factor, the protooncogene c-fos, is also required for osteoclast differentiation. c-fos-deficient mice develop osteopet- rosis due to an early differentiation block in the osteoclast lineage (Johnson et al., 1992; Wang et al., 1992; Grigoriadis et al., 1994); this osteopetrosis too is rescued by bone marrow transplantation. In addi- tion, the observation that c-fos-deficient mice have increased numbers of macrophages indicates that c-Fos acts downstream of Pu.1 and reg- ulates differentiation of hematopoietic precursor cells at the branch point between monocyte-macrophages and osteoclasts.

Nuclear Factor κB

Nuclear factor κB (NF-κB), a dimeric transcription factor, is another important molecule involved in osteoclast differentiation. The subunits of NF-κB are p50, p52, p65, c-Rel, and RelB (Verma et al., 1995). NF- κB plays a regulatory role in the expression of several cytokines, and the genes for NF-κB subunits are themselves also targets of cytokines involved in osteoclast differentiation. Indeed, p50, p52 double knock- out mice develop severe osteopetrosis caused by an arrest of osteoclast differentiation (Franzoso et al., 1997; Iotsova et al., 1997).

Microphthalmia Transcription Factor

The microphthalmia transcription factor (MITF), a bHLH zipper fac- tor, regulates distinct target genes in several cell types, including os- teoclasts. Mitf-deficient mice develop severe osteopetrosis caused by a failure to resorb bones, although the formation of multinucleated osteoclasts occurs normally (Hodgkinson et al., 1993). A possible mechanism of MITF in osteoclast differentiation is that it activates osteoclast-specific marker genes through direct interaction with Pu.1 (Sato et al., 1999; Luchin et al., 2001).

Signaling Molecules

M-CSF

M-CSF is one of the factors essential for the differentiation of osteo- clasts and monocytes-macrophages. A mutation within the M-CSF gene present in the mouse mutant strain op/op causes osteopetrosis with a severe deficiency of osteoclasts, monocytes, and peritoneal macrophages (Marks et al., 1984; Yoshida et al., 1990). Administra- tion of recombinant M-CSF restored impaired bone resorption in op/op mice. Osteoblast/stromal cells produce M-CSF, and osteoclasts ex- press c-fmc, the gene encoding the receptor for M-CSF. These find- ings support the notion that osteoblast/stromal cells are crucially in- volved in osteoclast development.

Osteoprotegerin, RANK, RANKL

Accumulating in vitro evidence shows that cell-to-cell contact between osteoblast/stromal cells and hematopoietic cells is required for the in- duction of osteoclast differentiation (Martin and Ng, 1994; Suda et al., 1996; Martin et al., 1998). Recently, a group of secreted mole- cules regulating osteoclast differentiation has been identified. Osteo- protegerin (OPG) belongs to the tumor necrosis factor (TNF) recep- tor superfamily but contains no transmembrane-spanning sequences, indicating that it is secreted as a soluble receptor (Simonet et al., 1997; Tsuda et al., 1997). OPG is expressed in a variety of tissues, includ- ing lung, heart, kidney, liver, and bone. Several lines of evidence in- dicate that OPG inhibits osteoclast differentiation. First, overexpres- sion of OPG in transgenic mice results in profound osteopetrosis, coincident with a decrease in later stages of osteoclast differentiation. Second, the same effects are observed upon administration of recom- binant OPG into normal mice. Finally, OPG-deficient mice develop early-onset osteoporosis with significant trabecular bone loss, which is caused by an increased number of osteoclasts (Bucay et al., 1998; Mizuno et al., 1998).

The molecular mechanism of OPG function was revealed by the identification of its ligand. RANKL is a membrane-bound, TNF-re- lated cytokine expressed in osteoblast/stromal cells (Darnay et al., 1998; Lacey et al., 1998). RANKL binds to OPG and to hemato- poietic progenitor cells that are committed to the osteoclast lineage. Systemic administration of RANKL into normal adult mice leads to increased bone resorption through osteoclast activation. RANKL- deficient mice show severe osteopetrosis and completely lack osteo- clasts as a result of an inability of osteoblasts to support osteoclast differentiation (Kong et al., 1999).

RANK, a member of the TNF receptor superfamily, binds to RANKL and is expressed in osteoclasts and osteoclast precursor cells (Anderson et al., 1997; Dougall et al., 1999; Hsu et al., 1999). RANK binds RANKL and induces osteoclast differentiation, suggesting that RANKL, which resides on the surface of osteoblast/stromal cells, in- duces osteoclast differentiation by binding to the RANK receptor on the surface of osteoclast precursor cells. Indeed, polyclonal antibody against the RANK extracellular domain promotes osteoclastogenesis in bone marrow culture; transgenic mice expressing a soluble RANK- Fc fusion protein have severe osteopetrosis because of a reduction in osteoclasts; similar to OPG transgenic mice, and RANK-deficient mice have profound osteopetrosis due to a lack of osteoclasts.

A number of other cytokines and systemic hormones, including PTH, 1,25-dihydroxyvitamin D_3, IL-11, and prostaglandin E_2, exert their effects on osteoclast differentiation, in part by regulating the ex- pression of OPG, RANKL, and M-CSF in osteoblast/stromal cells (Roodman, 1999; Suda et al., 1999).

In summary, M-CSF and RANKL expressed in osteoblast/stromal cells induce osteoclast differentiation by binding to their receptors, c-Fms and RANK, respectively, on osteoclasts and osteoclast pre- cursors. OPG blocks the stimulatory effects of RANKL on osteoclast differentiation.

Despite the recent major molecular and genetic advances that re- sulted in identifying and characterizing the molecules that have criti- cal roles in the differentiation of chondrocytes, osteoblasts, and os- teoclasts, a number of important questions remain. One unresolved question is how Sox9 controls the condensation of chondrogenic mesenchymal cells, an initial step in the pathway of chondrocyte differentiation. Another question is the precise mechanisms by which the major transcription factors, which have essential roles in the differentiation of either chondrocytes, osteoblasts, and osteoclasts, control the complex repertoires of their target genes. It is also critical to examine the mechanisms by which Sox9 cooperates with L-Sox5 and Sox6 and how Runx2 might cooperate with Osterix and other factors. Still another question is which signaling pathways affect the expression and activities of these key transcription factors. Equally important is to better understand how the differentiation of chondrocytes and osteoblasts is coordinated and how the replacement of cartilage by bone during endochondral ossification is orchestrated. Finally, it is important to comprehend how the physiological balance of bone formation and bone resorption is achieved. Answers to these questions and many more should also provide further insights for the design of potential therapeutic approaches for some of the major chronic diseases of the skeleton.

ACKNOWLEDGMENTS

Shunichi Murakami and Harukiko Akiyama contributed equally to this chapter. Work in the laboratory of the authors was supported by National Institutes of Health grants PO-AR42919, RO1-HL41264, and RO1-AR49072, a grant of the G. Harold and Leila Y. Mathers Charitable Foundation to Benoit de Crombrugghe, and an Arthritis Investigator Award of the Arthritis Foundation to Shunichi Murakami. We thank Karen Clayton and Janie Finch for editorial assistance and Francisco Vergaray for the drawings.

REFERENCES

Acampora D, Merlo GR, Paleari L, Zerega B, Postiglione MP, Mantero S, Bober E, Barbieri O, Simeone A, Levi G (1999). Craniofacial, vestibular and bone defects in mice lacking the Distal-less-related gene Dlx5. *Development* 126: 3795–3809.

Anderson DM, Maraskovsky E, Billingsley WL, Dougall WC, Tometsko ME, Roux ER, Teepe MC, DuBose RF, Cosman D, Galibert L (1997). A homologue of the TNF receptor and its ligand enhance T-cell growth and dendritic-cell function. *Nature* 390: 175–179.

Arikawa-Hirasawa E, Watanabe H, Takami H, Hassell JR, Yamada Y (1999). Perlecan is essential for cartilage and cephalic development. *Nat Genet* 23: 354–358.

Aszódi A, Chan D, Hunziker E, Bateman JF, Fässler R (1998). Collagen II is essential for the removal of the notochord and the formation of intervertebral discs. *J Cell Biol* 143: 1399–1412.

Aviezer D, Hecht D, Safran M, Eisinger M, David G, Yayon A (1994). Perlecan, basal lamina proteoglycan, promotes basic fibroblast growth factor-receptor binding, mitogenesis, and angiogenesis. *Cell* 79: 1005–1013.

Bae SC, Lee KS, Zhang YW, Ito Y (2001). Intimate relationship between TGF-beta/BMP signaling and runt domain transcription factor, PEBP2/CBF. *J Bone Joint Surg Am* 83(Suppl 1): S48–S55.

Ballock RT, Heydemann A, Wakefield LM, Flanders KC, Roberts AB, Sporn MB (1993). TGF-beta 1 prevents hypertrophy of epiphyseal chondrocytes: regulation of gene expression for cartilage matrix proteins and metalloproteases. *Dev Biol* 158: 414–429.

Baur ST, Mai JJ, Dymecki SM (2000). Combinatorial signaling through BMP receptor IB and GDF5: shaping of the distal mouse limb and the genetics of distal limb diversity. *Development* 127: 605–619.

Beier F, Lee RJ, Taylor AC, Pestell RG, LuValle P (1999). Identification of the cyclin D1 gene as a target of activating transcription factor 2 in chondrocytes. *Proc Natl Acad Sci USA* 96: 1433–1438.

Beier F, Ali Z, Mok D, Taylor AC, Leask T, Albanese C, Pestell RG, LuValle P (2001). TGFbeta and PTHrP control chondrocyte proliferation by activating cyclin D1 expression. *Mol Biol Cell* 12: 3852–3863.

Beighton P, de Paepe A, Danks D, Finidori G, Gedde-Dahl T, Goodman R, Hall JG, Hollister DW, Horton W, McKusick VA, et al. (1988). International nosology of heritable disorders of connective tissue, Berlin, 1986. *Am J Med Genet* 29: 581–594.

Bell DM, Leung KK, Wheatley SC, Ng LJ, Zhou S, Ling KW, Sham MH, Koopman P, Tam PP, Cheah KS (1997). SOX9 directly regulates the type-II collagen gene. *Nat Genet* 16: 174–178.

Bellus GA, McIntosh I, Smith EA, Aylsworth AS, Kaitila I, Horton WA, Greenhaw GA, Hecht JT, Francomano CA (1995). A recurrent mutation in the tyrosine kinase domain of fibroblast growth factor receptor 3 causes hypochondroplasia. *Nat Genet* 10: 357–359.

Bergers G, Brekken R, McMahon G, Vu TH, Itoh T, Tamaki K, Tanzawa K, Thorpe P, Itohara S, Werb Z, et al. (2000). Matrix metalloproteinase-9 triggers the angiogenic switch during carcinogenesis. *Nat Cell Biol* 2: 737–744.

Bi W, Deng JM, Zhang Z, Behringer RR, de Crombrugghe B. (1999). Sox9 is required for cartilage formation. *Nat Genet* 22: 85–89.

Bi W, Huang W, Whitworth DJ, Deng JM, Zhang Z, Behringer RR, de Crombrugghe B (2001). Haploinsufficiency of Sox9 results in defective cartilage primordia and premature skeletal mineralization. *Proc Natl Acad Sci USA* 98: 6698–6703.

Black WC, Utley JR (1968). The differential diagnosis of parathroid adenoma and chief cell hyperplasia. *Am J Clin Pathol* 49: 761–775.

Bonewald LF, Dallas SL (1994). Role of active and latent transforming growth factor beta in bone formation. *J Cell Biochem* 55: 350–357.

Bonewald LF, Mundy GR (1990). Role of transforming growth factor-beta in bone remodeling. *Clin Orthop* 250: 261–276.

Bradshaw AD, Sage EH (2001). SPARC, a matricellular protein that functions in cellular differentiation and tissue response to injury. *J Clin Invest* 107: 1049–1054.

Brennan MJ, Oldberg A, Ruoslahti E, Brown K, Schwartz N (1983). Immunological evidence for two distinct chondroitin sulfate proteoglycan core proteins: differential expression in cartilage matrix deficient mice. *Dev Biol* 98: 139–147.

Bridgewater LC, Lefebvre V, de Crombrugghe B (1998). Chondrocyte-specific enhancer elements in the *Col11a2* gene resemble the Col2a1 tissue-specific enhancer. *J Biol Chem* 273: 14998–15006.

Bringhurst FR, Potts JT Jr (1981). Bone collagen synthesis in vitro: structure/activity relations among parathyroid hormone fragments and analogs. *Endocrinology* 108: 103–108.

Brown KS, Harne L (1982). Brachymorphic (bmm/bmm) cartilage matrix deficiency (cmd/cmd) and disproportionate micromelia (Dmm/Dmm); three inborn errors of cartilage biosynthesis in mice. *Prog Clin Biol Res* 94: 245–249.

Brunet LJ, McMahon JA, McMahon AP, Harland RM (1998). Noggin, cartilage morphogenesis, and joint formation in the mammalian skeleton. *Science* 280: 1455–1457.

Bucay N, Sarosi I, Dunstan CR, Morony S, Tarpley J, Capparelli C, Scully S, Tan HL, Xu W, Lacey DL, et al. (1998). Osteoprotegerin-deficient mice develop early onset osteoporosis and arterial calcification. *Genes Dev* 12: 1260–1268.

Chen L, Li C, Qiao W, Xu X, Deng C (2001). A Ser(365) → Cys mutation of fibroblast growth factor receptor 3 in mouse downregulates Ihh/PTHrP signals and causes severe achondroplasia. *Hum Mol Genet* 10: 457–465.

Chen X, Li X, Wang W, Lufkin T (1996). Dlx5 and Dlx6: an evolutionary conserved pair of murine homeobox genes expressed in the embryonic skeleton. *Ann NY Acad Sci* 785: 38–47.

Chusho H, Tamura N, Ogawa Y, Yasoda A, Suda M, Miyazawa T, Nakamura K, Nakao K, Kurihara T, Komatsu Y, et al. (2001). Dwarfism and early death in mice lacking C-type natriuretic peptide. *Proc Natl Acad Sci USA* 98: 4016–4021.

Cole W (1994). Osteogenesis imperfecta as a consequence of naturally occurring and induced mutations of type I collagen. In: Bone and Mineral Research, Volume 8. Heersche JKJ (ed.) Elsevier, New York, pp. 67–204.

Colnot CI, Helms JA (2001). A molecular analysis of matrix remodeling and angiogenesis during long bone development. *Mech Dev* 100: 245–250.

Colvin JS, Bohne BA, Harding GW, McEwen DG, Ornitz DM (1996). Skeletal overgrowth and deafness in mice lacking fibroblast growth factor receptor 3. *Nat Genet* 12: 390–397.

Craig FM, Bentley G, Archer CW (1987). The spatial and temporal pattern of collagens I and II and keratan sulphate in the developing chick metatarsophalangeal joint. *Development* 99: 383–391.

Darnay BG, Haridas V, Ni J, Moore PA, Aggarwal BB (1998). Characterization of the intracellular domain of receptor activator of NF-kappaB (RANK). Interaction with tumor necrosis factor receptor–associated factors and activation of NF-kappab and c-Jun N-terminal kinase. *J Biol Chem* 273: 20551–20555.

Delany AM, Amling M, Priemel M, Howe C, Baron R, Canalis E (2000). Osteopenia and decreased bone formation in osteonectin-deficient mice. *J Clin Invest* 105: 915–923.

Delezoide AL, Benoist-Lasselin C, Legeai-Mallet L, Le Merrer M, Munnich A, Vekemans M, Bonaventure J (1998). Spatio-temporal expression of FGFR 1, 2 and 3 genes during human embryo-fetal ossification. *Mech Dev* 77: 19–30.

DeLise AM, Fischer L, Tuan RS (2000). Cellular interactions and signaling in cartilage development. *Osteoarthritis Cartilage* 8: 309–334.

Deng C, Wynshaw-Boris A, Zhou F, Kuo A, Leder P (1996). Fibroblast growth factor receptor 3 is a negative regulator of bone growth. *Cell* 84: 911–921.

Depew MJ, Liu JK, Long JE, Presley R, Meneses JJ, Pedersen RA, Rubenstein JL (1999). Dlx5 regulates regional development of the branchial arches and sensory capsules. *Development* 126: 3831–3846.

Dieudonne SC, Semeins CM, Goei SW, Vukicevic S, Nulend JK, Sampath TK, Helder M, Burger EH (1994). Opposite effects of osteogenic protein and transforming growth factor beta on chondrogenesis in cultured long bone rudiments. *J Bone Miner Res* 9: 771–780.

Dougall WC, Glaccum M, Charrier K, Rohrbach K, Brasel K, De Smedt T, Daro E, Smith J, Tometsko ME, Maliszewski CR, et al. (1999). RANK is essential for osteoclast and lymph node development. *Genes Dev* 13: 2412–2424.

Ducy P, Desbois C, Boyce B, Pinero G, Story B, Dunstan C, Smith E, Bonadio J, Goldstein S, Gundberg C, et al. (1996). Increased bone formation in osteocalcin-deficient mice. *Nature* 382: 448–452.

Ducy P, Zhang R, Geoffroy V, Ridall AL, Karsenty G (1997). Osf2/Cbfa1: a transcriptional activator of osteoblast differentiation. *Cell* 89: 747–754.

Ducy P, Amling M, Takeda S, Priemel M, Schilling AF, Beil FT, Shen J, Vinson C, Rueger JM, Karsenty G (2000). Leptin inhibits bone formation through a hypothalamic relay: a central control of bone mass. *Cell* 100: 197–207.

Dudley AT, Lyons KM, Robertson EJ (1995). A requirement for bone morphogenetic protein-7 during development of the mammalian kidney and eye. *Genes Dev* 9: 2795–2807.

Engsig MT, Chen QJ, Vu TH, Pedersen AC, Therkidsen B, Lund LR, Henriksen K, Lenhard T, Foged NT, Werb Z, et al. (2000). Matrix metalloproteinase 9 and vascular endothelial growth factor are essential for osteoclast recruitment into developing long bones. *J Cell Biol* 151: 879–889.

Erlebacher A, Derynck R (1996). Increased expression of TGF-beta 2 in osteoblasts results in an osteoporosis-like phenotype. *J Cell Biol* 132: 195–210.

Erlebacher A, Filvaroff EH, Gitelman SE, Derynck R (1995). Toward a molecular understanding of skeletal development. *Cell* 80: 371–378.

Fitzpatrick LA, Bilezikian JP (1996). Actions of parathyroid hormone. In: Principles of Bone Biology. Bilezikian JP, Raisz LG, Rodan, G (eds.) Academic Press, San Diego, pp. 339–346.

Foster JW, Dominguez-Steglich MA, Guioli S, Kowk G, Weller PA, Stevanovic M, Weissenbach J, Mansour S, Young ID, Goodfellow PN, et al. (1994). Campomelic dysplasia and autosomal sex reversal caused by mutations in an *SRY*-related gene. *Nature* 372: 525–530.

Franzoso G, Carlson L, Xing L, Poljak L, Shores EW, Brown KD, Leonardi A, Tran T,

Boyce BF, Siebenlist U (1997). Requirement for NF-kappaB in osteoclast and B-cell development. *Genes Dev* 11: 3482–3496.

Friedman JM, Halaas JL (1998). Leptin and the regulation of body weight in mammals. *Nature* 395: 763–770.

Gailani MR, Stahle-Backdahl M, Leffell DJ, Glynn M, Zaphiropoulos PG, Pressman C, Unden AB, Dean M, Brash DE, Bale AE, et al. (1996). The role of the human homologue of *Drosophila* patched in sporadic basal cell carcinomas. *Nat Genet* 14: 78–81.

Gao B, Guo J, She C, Shu A, Yang M, Tan Z, Yang X, Guo S, Feng G, He L (2001). Mutations in IHH, encoding Indian hedgehog, cause brachydactyly type A-1. *Nat Genet* 28: 386–388.

Gerber HP, Vu TH, Ryan AM, Kowalski J, Werb Z, Ferrara N (1999). VEGF couples hypertrophic cartilage remodeling, ossification and angiogenesis during endochondral bone formation. *Nat Med* 5: 623–628.

Gilmour DT, Lyon GJ, Carlton MB, Sanes JR, Cunningham JM, Anderson JR, Hogan BL, Evans MJ, Colledge WH (1998). Mice deficient for the secreted glycoprotein SPARC/osteonectin/BM40 develop normally but show severe age-onset cataract formation and disruption of the lens. *EMBO J* 17: 1860–1870.

Gong Y, Krakow D, Marcelino J, Wilkin D, Chitayat D, Babul-Hirji R, Hudgins L, Cremers CW, Cremers FP, Brunner HG, et al. (1999). Heterozygous mutations in the gene encoding noggin affect human joint morphogenesis. *Nat Genet* 21: 302–304.

Gong Y, Slee RB, Fukai N, Rawadi G, Roman-Roman S, Reginato AM, Wang H, Cundy T, Glorieux FH, Lev D, et al. (2001). LDL receptor–related protein 5 (LRP5) affects bone accrual and eye development. *Cell* 107: 513–523.

Grigoriadis AE, Wang ZQ, Cecchini MG, Hofstetter W, Felix R, Fleisch HA, Wagner EF (1994). c-Fos: a key regulator of osteoclast-macrophage lineage determination and bone remodeling. *Science* 266: 443–448.

Grüneberg H, Lee AJ (1973). The anatomy and development of brachypodism in the mouse. *J Embryol Exp Morphol* 30: 119–141.

Hahn H, Wicking C, Zaphiropoulous PG, Gailani MR, Shanley S, Chidambaram A, Vorechovsky I, Holmberg E, Unden A B, Gillies S, et al. (1996). Mutations of the human homolog of *Drosophila* patched in the nevoid basal cell carcinoma syndrome. *Cell* 85: 841–851.

Haigh JJ, Gerber HP, Ferrara N, Wagner EF (2000). Conditional inactivation of VEGF-A in areas of collagen2a1 expression results in embryonic lethality in the heterozygous state. *Development* 127: 1445–1453.

Hall AK, Dickson IR (1985). The effects of parathyroid hormone on osteoblast-like cells from embryonic chick calvaria. *Acta Endocrinol (Copenh)* 108: 217–223.

Hartmann C, Tabin CJ (2000). Dual roles of Wnt signaling during chondrogenesis in the chicken limb. *Development* 127: 3141–3159.

Hartmann C, Tabin CJ (2001). Wnt-14 plays a pivotal role in inducing synovial joint formation in the developing appendicular skeleton. *Cell* 104: 341–351.

Heath JK, Atkinson SJ, Meikle MC, Reynolds JJ (1984). Mouse osteoblasts synthesize collagenase in response to bone resorbing agents. *Biochim Biophys Acta* 802: 151–154.

Hock JM, Gera I (1992). Effects of continuous and intermittent administration and inhibition of resorption on the anabolic response of bone to parathyroid hormone. *J Bone Miner Res* 7: 65–72.

Hodgkinson CA, Moore KJ, Nakayama A, Steingrimsson E, Copeland NG, Jenkins NA, Arnheiter H (1993). Mutations at the mouse microphthalmia locus are associated with defects in a gene encoding a novel basic-helix-loop-helix-zipper protein. *Cell* 74: 395–404.

Horner A, Bishop NJ, Bord S, Beeton C, Kelsall AW, Coleman N, Compston JE (1999). Immunolocalisation of vascular endothelial growth factor (VEGF) in human neonatal growth plate cartilage. *J Anat* 194(4): 519–524.

Houghton MJ, Carey JC, Seegmiller RE (1989). Pulmonary hypoplasia in mice homozygous for the cartilage matrix deficiency (*cmd*) gene: a model for human congenital disorder. *Pediatr Pathol* 9: 501–512.

Hsu H, Lacey DL, Dunstan CR, Solovyev I, Colombero A, Timms E, Tan HL, Elliott G, Kelley MJ, Sarosi I, et al. (1999). Tumor necrosis factor receptor family member RANK mediates osteoclast differentiation and activation induced by osteoprotegerin ligand. *Proc Natl Acad Sci USA* 96: 3540–3545.

Huang W, Zhou X, Lefebvre V, de Crombrugghe B (2000). Phosphorylation of SOX9 by cyclic AMP-dependent protein kinase A enhances SOX9's ability to transactivate a Col2a1 chondrocyte-specific enhancer. *Mol Cell Biol* 20: 4149–4158.

Huang W, Chung UI, Kronenberg HM, de Crombrugghe B (2001). The chondrogenic transcription factor Sox9 is a target of signaling by the parathyroid hormone–related peptide in the growth plate of endochondral bones. *Proc Natl Acad Sci USA* 98: 160–165.

Inada M, Yasui T, Nomura S, Miyake S, Deguchi K, Himeno M, Sato M, Yamagiwa H, Kimura T, Yasui N, et al. (1999). Maturational disturbance of chondrocytes in Cbfa1-deficient mice. *Dev Dyn* 214: 279–290.

Iotsova V, Caamano J, Loy J, Yang Y, Lewin A, Bravo R (1997). Osteopetrosis in mice lacking NF-kappaB1 and NF-kappaB2. *Nat Med* 3: 1285–1289.

Ito Y (1999). Molecular basis of tissue-specific gene expression mediated by the runt domain transcription factor PEBP2/CBF. *Genes Cells* 4: 685–696.

Iwata T, Chen L, Li C, Ovchinnikov DA, Behringer RR, Francomano CA, Deng CX (2000). A neonatal lethal mutation in FGFR3 uncouples proliferation and differentiation of growth plate chondrocytes in embryos. *Hum Mol Genet* 9: 1603–1613.

Iwata T, Li CL, Deng CX, Francomano CA (2001). Highly activated Fgfr3 with the K644M mutation causes prolonged survival in severe dwarf mice. *Hum Mol Genet* 10: 1255–1264.

Jabs EW, Li X , Scott AF, Meyers G, Chen W, Eccles M, Mao JI, Charnas LR, Jackson CE, Jaye M (1994). Jackson-Weiss and Crouzon syndromes are allelic with mutations in fibroblast growth factor receptor 2. *Nat Genet* 8: 275–279.

Jobert AS, Zhang P, Couvineau A, Bonaventure J, Roume J, Le Merrer M, Silve C (1998). Absence of functional receptors for parathyroid hormone and parathyroid hormone-related peptide in Blomstrand chondrodysplasia. *J Clin Invest* 102: 34–40.

Johnson RL, Tabin CJ (1997). Molecular models for vertebrate limb development. *Cell* 90: 979–990.

Johnson RL, Rothman AL, Xie J, Goodrich LV, Bare JW, Bonifas JM, Quinn AG, Myers RM, Cox DR, Epstein EH Jr, et al. (1996). Human homolog of patched, a candidate gene for the basal cell nevus syndrome. *Science* 272: 1668–1671.

Johnson RS, Spiegelman BM, Papaioannou V (1992). Pleiotropic effects of a null mutation in the *c-fos* proto-oncogene. *Cell* 71: 577–586.

Joyce ME, Jingushi S, Bolander ME (1990). Transforming growth factor-beta in the regulation of fracture repair. *Orthop Clin North Am* 21: 199–209.

Jüppner H, Abou-Samra AB, Freeman M, Kong XF, Schipani E, Richards J, Kolakowski LF Jr, Hock J, Potts JT Jr, Kronenberg HM (1991). A G protein–linked receptor for parathyroid hormone and parathyroid hormone–related peptide. *Science* 254: 1024–1026.

Karaplis AC, Luz A, Glowacki J, Bronson RT, Tybulewicz VL, Kronenberg HM, Mulligan RC (1994). Lethal skeletal dysplasia from targeted disruption of the parathyroid hormone-related peptide gene. *Genes Dev* 8: 277–289.

Karp SJ, Schipani E, St-Jacques B, Hunzelman J, Kronenberg H, McMahon AP (2000). Indian hedgehog coordinates endochondral bone growth and morphogenesis via parathyroid hormone–related protein-dependent and -independent pathways. *Development* 127: 543–548.

Karperien M, van der Harten HJ, van Schooten R, Farih-Sips H, den Hollander NS, Kneppers SLJ, Nijweide P, Papapoulos SE, Löwik CWGM (1999). A frame-shift mutation in the type I parathyroid hormone (PTH)/PTH-related peptide receptor causing Blomstrand lethal osteochondrodysplasia. *J Clin Endocrinol Metab* 84: 3713–3720.

Karsenty G (1999). The genetic transformation of bone biology. *Genes Dev* 13: 3037–3051.

Katagiri T, Yamaguchi A, Ikeda T, Yoshiki S, Wozney JM, Rosen V, Wang EA, Tanaka H, Omura S, Suda T (1990). The non-osteogenic mouse pluripotent cell line, C3H10T1/2, is induced to differentiate into osteoblastic cells by recombinant human bone morphogenetic protein-2. *Biochem Biophys Res Commun* 172: 295–299.

Katagiri T, Boorla S, Frendo JL, Hogan BL, Karsenty G (1998). Skeletal abnormalities in doubly heterozygous Bmp4 and Bmp7 mice. *Dev Genet* 22: 340–348.

Kato M, Patel MS, Levasseur R, Lobov I, Chang BH, Glass DA 2nd, Hartmann C, Li L, Hwang TH, Brayton CF, et al. (2002). Cbfa1-independent decrease in osteoblast proliferation, osteopenia, and persistent embryonic eye vascularization in mice deficient in Lrp5, a Wnt coreceptor. *J Cell Biol* 157: 303–314.

Kato Y, Iwamoto M, Koike T, Suzuki F, Takano Y (1988). Terminal differentiation and calcification in rabbit chondrocyte cultures grown in centrifuge tubes: regulation by transforming growth factor beta and serum factors. *Proc Natl Acad Sci USA* 85: 9552–9556.

Kawakami Y, Wada N, Nishimatsu SI, Ishikawa T, Noji S, Nohno T (1999). Involvement of Wnt-5a in chondrogenic pattern formation in the chick limb bud. *Dev Growth Differ* 41: 29–40.

Khan A, Bilezikian J (2000). Primary hyperparathyroidism: pathophysiology and impact on bone. *CMAJ* 163: 184–187.

Khillan JS, Olsen AS, Kontusaari S, Sokolov B, Prockop DJ (1991). Transgenic mice that express a mini-gene version of the human gene for type I procollagen (*COL1A1*) develop a phenotype resembling a lethal form of osteogenesis imperfecta. *J Biol Chem* 266: 23373–23379.

Kimata K, Barrach HJ, Brown KS, Pennypacker JP (1981). Absence of proteoglycan core protein in cartilage from the cmd/cmd (cartilage matrix deficiency) mouse. *J Biol Chem* 256: 6961–6968.

Kimura S, Shiota K (1996). Sequential changes of programmed cell death in developing fetal mouse limbs and its possible roles in limb morphogenesis. *J Morphol* 229: 337–346.

Klemsz MJ, McKercher SR, Celada A, Van Beveren C, Maki RA (1990). The macrophage and B cell-specific transcription factor PU.1 is related to the ets oncogene. *Cell* 61: 113–124.

Komori T, Yagi H, Nomura S, Yamaguchi A, Sasaki K, Deguchi K, Shimizu Y, Bronson RT, Gao YH, Inada M, et al. (1997). Targeted disruption of Cbfa1 results in a complete lack of bone formation owing to maturational arrest of osteoblasts. *Cell* 89: 755–764.

Kong YY, Yoshida H, Sarosi I, Tan HL, Timms E, Capparelli C, Morony S, Oliveira-dos-Santos AJ, Van G, Itie A, et al. (1999). OPGL is a key regulator of osteoclastogenesis, lymphocyte development and lymph-node organogenesis. *Nature* 397: 315–323.

Kronenberg HM, Chung U (2001). The parathyroid hormone–related protein and Indian hedgehog feedback loop in the growth plate. *Novartis Found Symp* 232: 144–157.

Lacey DL, Timms E, Tan HL, Kelley MJ, Dunstan CR, Burgess T, Elliott R, Colombero A, Elliott G, Scully S, et al. (1998). Osteoprotegerin ligand is a cytokine that regulates osteoclast differentiation and activation. *Cell* 93: 165–176.

Lanske B, Kronenberg HM (1998). Parathyroid hormone-related peptide (PTHrP) and parathyroid hormone (PTH)/PTHrP receptor. *Crit Rev Eukaryot Gene Expr* 8: 297–320.

Lanske B, Karaplis AC, Lee K, Luz A, Vortkamp A, Pirro A, Karperien M, Defize LH, Ho C, Mulligan RC, et al. (1996). PTH/PTHrP receptor in early development and Indian hedgehog–regulated bone growth. *Science* 273: 663–666.

Lanske B, Amling M, Neff L, Guiducci J, Baron R, Kronenberg HM (1999). Ablation of the PTHrP gene or the PTH/PTHrP receptor gene leads to distinct abnormalities in bone development. *J Clin Invest* 104: 399–407.

Lefebvre V, Huang W, Harley VR, Goodfellow PN, de Crombrugghe B (1997). SOX9 is a potent activator of the chondrocyte-specific enhancer of the pro alpha1(II) collagen gene. *Mol Cell Biol* 17: 2336–2346.

Lefebvre V, Li P, de Crombrugghe B (1998). A new long form of Sox5 (L-Sox5), Sox6 and Sox9 are coexpressed in chondrogenesis and cooperatively activate the type II collagen gene. *EMBO J* 17: 5718–5733.

Levin ER, Gardner DG, Samson WK (1998). Natriuretic peptides. *N Engl J Med* 339: 321–328.

Li C, Chen L, Iwata T, Kitagawa M, Fu XY, Deng CX (1999). A Lys644Glu substitution in fibroblast growth factor receptor 3 (FGFR3) causes dwarfism in mice by activation of STATs and ink4 cell cycle inhibitors. *Hum Mol Genet* 8: 35–44.

Li SW, Prockop DJ, Helminen H, Fässler R, Lapveteläinen T, Kiraly K, Peltarri A, Arokoski J, Lui H, Arita M, et al. (1995). Transgenic mice with targeted inactivation of the *Col2a1* gene for collagen II develop a skeleton with membranous and periosteal bone but no endochondral bone. *Genes Dev* 9: 2821–2830.

Liaw L, Birk DE, Ballas CB, Whitsitt JS, Davidson JM, Hogan BL (1998). Altered wound healing in mice lacking a functional osteopontin gene (spp1). *J Clin Invest* 101: 1468–1478.

Liu Z, Xu J, Colvin JS, Ornitz DM (2002). Coordination of chondrogenesis and osteogenesis by fibroblast growth factor 18. *Genes Dev* 16: 859–869.

Long F, Schipani E, Asahara H, Kronenberg H, Montminy M (2001). The CREB family of activators is required for endochondral bone development. *Development* 128: 541–550.

Luchin A, Suchting S, Merson T, Rosol TJ, Hume D A, Cassady AI, Ostrowski MC (2001). Genetic and physical interactions between Microphthalmia transcription factor and PU.1 are necessary for osteoclast gene expression and differentiation. *J Biol Chem* 276: 36703–36710.

Luo G, Hofmann C, Bronckers AL, Sohocki M, Bradley A, Karsenty G (1995). BMP-7 is an inducer of nephrogenesis, and is also required for eye development and skeletal patterning. *Genes Dev* 9: 2808–2820.

Marks SC Jr, Seifert MF, McGuire JL (1984). Congenitally osteopetrotic (oplop) mice are not cured by transplants of spleen or bone marrow cells from normal littermates. *Metab Bone Dis Relat Res* 5: 183–186.

Martin TJ, Ng KW (1994). Mechanisms by which cells of the osteoblast lineage control osteoclast formation and activity. *J Cell Biochem* 56: 357–366.

Martin TJ, Romas E, Gillespie MT (1998). Interleukins in the control of osteoclast differentiation. *Crit Rev Eukaryot Gene Expr* 8: 107–123.

Matsukawa N, Grzesik WJ, Takahashi N, Pandey KN, Pang S, Yamauchi M, Smithies O (1999). The natriuretic peptide clearance receptor locally modulates the physiological effects of the natriuretic peptide system. *Proc Natl Acad Sci USA* 96: 7403–7408.

McKercher SR, Torbett BE, Anderson KL, Henkel GW, Vestal DJ, Baribault H, Klemsz M, Feeney AJ, Wu GE, Paige CJ, et al. (1996). Targeted disruption of the *PU.1* gene results in multiple hematopoietic abnormalities. *EMBO J* 15: 5647–5658.

McMahon AP (2000). More surprises in the Hedgehog signaling pathway. *Cell* 100: 185–188.

Meyer J, Südbeck P, Held M, Wagner T, Schmitz ML, Bricarelli FD, Eggermont E, Friedrich U, Haas O A, Kobelt A, et al. (1997). Mutational analysis of the *SOX9* gene in campomelic dysplasia and autosomal sex reversal: lack of genotype/phenotype correlations. *Hum Mol Genet* 6: 91–98.

Minina E, Wenzel HM, Kreschel C, Karp S, Gaffield W, McMahon AP, Vortkamp A (2001). BMP and Ihh/PTHrP signaling interact to coordinate chondrocyte proliferation and differentiation. *Development* 128: 4523–4534.

Mizuno A, Amizuka N, Irie K, Murakami A, Fujise N, Kanno T, Sato Y, Nakagawa N, Yasuda H, Mochizuki S, et al. (1998). Severe osteoporosis in mice lacking osteoclastogenesis inhibitory factor/osteoprotegerin. *Biochem Biophys Res Commun* 247: 610–615.

Mori C, Nakamura N, Kimura S, Irie H, Takigawa T, Shiota K (1995). Programmed cell death in the interdigital tissue of the fetal mouse limb is apoptosis with DNA fragmentation. *Anat Rec* 242: 103–110.

Mundlos S, Olsen BR (1997). Heritable diseases of the skeleton. Part II: Molecular insights into skeletal development-matrix components and their homeostasis. *FASEB J* 11: 227–233.

Murakami S, Kan M, McKeehan WL, de Crombrugghe B (2000). Up-regulation of the chondrogenic Sox9 gene by fibroblast growth factors is mediated by the mitogen-activated protein kinase pathway. *Proc Natl Acad Sci USA* 97: 1113–1118.

Murtaugh LC, Chyung JH, Lassar AB (1999). Sonic hedgehog promotes somitic chondrogenesis by altering the cellular response to BMP signaling. *Genes Dev* 13: 225–237.

Nakashima K, Zhou X, Kunkel G, Zhang Z, Deng JM, Behringer RR, de Crombrugghe B (2002). The novel zinc finger–containing transcription factor osterix is required for osteoblast differentiation and bone formation. *Cell* 108: 17–29.

Nalin AM, Greenlee TK Jr, Sandell LJ (1995). Collagen gene expression during development of avian synovial joints: transient expression of types II and XI collagen genes in the joint capsule. *Dev Dyn* 203: 352–362.

Naski MC, Colvin JS, Coffin JD, Ornitz DM (1998). Repression of hedgehog signaling and BMP4 expression in growth plate cartilage by fibroblast growth factor receptor 3. *Development* 125: 4977–4988.

Newberry EP, Latifi T, Towler DA (1998). Reciprocal regulation of osteocalcin transcription by the homeodomain proteins Msx2 and Dlx5. *Biochemistry* 37: 16360–16368.

Ng LJ, Wheatley S, Muscat GE, Conway-Campbell J, Bowles J, Wright E, Bell DM, Tam PP, Cheah KS, Koopman P (1997). SOX9 binds DNA, activates transcription, and coexpresses with type II collagen during chondrogenesis in the mouse. *Dev Biol* 183: 108–121.

Noda M, Camilliere JJ (1989). In vivo stimulation of bone formation by transforming growth factor-beta. *Endocrinology* 124: 2991–2994.

Ohbayashi N, Shibayama M, Kurotaki Y, Imanishi M, Fujimori T, Itoh N, Takada S (2002). FGF18 is required for normal cell proliferation and differentiation during osteogenesis and chondrogenesis. *Genes Dev* 16: 870–879.

Okada Y, Naka K, Kawamura K, Matsumoto T, Nakanishi I, Fujimoto N, Sato H, Seiki M (1995). Localization of matrix metalloproteinase 9 (92-kilodalton gelatinase/type IV collagenase = gelatinase B) in osteoclasts: implications for bone resorption. *Lab Invest* 72: 311–322.

Olsen BR, Reginato AM, Wang W (2000). Bone development. *Annu Rev Cell Dev Biol* 16: 191–220.

Otto F, Thornell AP, Crompton T, Denzel A, Gilmour KC, Rosewell IR, Stamp GW, Beddington RS, Mundlos S, Olsen BR, et al. (1997). *Cbfa1*, a candidate gene for cleidocranial dysplasia syndrome, is essential for osteoblast differentiation and bone development. *Cell* 89: 765–771.

Partridge NC, Dickson CA, Kopp K, Teitelbaum SL, Crouch EC, Kahn AJ (1989). Parathyroid hormone inhibits collagen synthesis at both ribonucleic acid and protein levels in rat osteogenic sarcoma cells. *Mol Endocrinol* 3: 232–239.

Pelton RW, Saxena B, Jones M, Moses HL, Gold LI (1991). Immunohistochemical localization of TGF beta 1, TGF beta 2, and TGF beta 3 in the mouse embryo: expression patterns suggest multiple roles during embryonic development. *J Cell Biol* 115: 1091–1105.

Peters K, Ornitz D, Werner S, Williams L (1993). Unique expression pattern of the FGF receptor 3 gene during mouse organogenesis. *Dev Biol* 155: 423–430.

Polinkovsky A, Robin NH, Thomas JT, Irons M, Lynn A, Goodman FR, Reardon W, Kant SG, Brunner HG, van der Burgt I, et al. (1997). Mutations in CDMP1 cause autosomal dominant brachydactyly type C. *Nat Genet* 17: 18–19.

Raffel C, Jenkins RB, Frederick L, Hebrink D, Alderete B, Fults DW, James CD (1997). Sporadic medulloblastomas contain PTCH mutations. *Cancer Res* 57: 842–845.

Reimold AM, Grusby MJ, Kosaras B, Fries JW, Mori R, Maniwa S, Clauss IM, Collins T, Sidman RL, Glimcher MJ, et al. (1996). Chondrodysplasia and neurological abnormalities in ATF-2-deficient mice. *Nature* 379: 262–265.

Reponen P, Sahlberg C, Munaut C, Thesleff I, Tryggvason K (1994). High expression of 92-kD type IV collagenase (gelatinase B) in the osteoclast lineage during mouse development. *J Cell Biol* 124: 1091–1102.

Rittenhouse E, Dunn LC, Cookingham J, Calo C, Spiegelman M, Dooher GB, Bennett D (1978). Cartilage matrix deficiency (cmd): a new autosomal recessive lethal mutation in the mouse. *J Embryol Exp Morphol* 43: 71–84.

Rittling SR, Matsumoto HN, McKee MD, Nanci A, An XR, Novick KE, Kowalski AJ, Noda M, Denhardt DT (1998). Mice lacking osteopontin show normal development and bone structure but display altered osteoclast formation in vitro. *J Bone Miner Res* 13: 1101–1111.

Robledo RF, Rajan L, Li X, Lufkin T (2002). The *Dlx5* and *Dlx6* homeobox genes are essential for craniofacial, axial, and appendicular skeletal development. *Genes Dev* 16: 1089–1101.

Roodman GD (1999). Cell biology of the osteoclast. *Exp Hematol* 27: 1229–1241.

Rossert J, de Crombrugghe B (1996). Type I collagen: structure, synthesis, and regulation. In: Principles of Bone Biology. Bilezikian JP, Raisz LG, Rodan G (eds.) Academic Press, San Diego, pp. 127–142.

Rousseau F, Bonaventure J, Legeai-Mallet L, Pelet A, Rozet JM, Maroteaux P, Le Merrer M, Munnich A (1994). Mutations in the gene encoding fibroblast growth factor receptor-3 in achondroplasia. *Nature* 371: 252–254.

Rousseau F, Saugier P, Le Merrer M, Munnich A, Delezoide AL, Maroteaux P, Bonaventure J, Narcy F, Sanak M (1995). Stop codon FGFR3 mutations in thanatophoric dwarfism type 1. *Nat Genet* 10: 11–12.

Rutland P, Pulleyn LJ, Reardon W, Baraitser M, Hayward R, Jones B, Malcolm S, Winter RM, Oldridge M, Slaney SF, et al. (1995). Identical mutations in the *FGFR2* gene cause both Pfeiffer and Crouzon syndrome phenotypes. *Nat Genet* 9: 173–176.

Sahni M, Ambrosetti DC, Mansukhani A, Gertner R, Levy D, Basilico C (1999). FGF signaling inhibits chondrocyte proliferation and regulates bone development through the STAT-1 pathway. *Genes Dev* 13: 1361–1366.

Sahni M, Raz R, Coffin JD, Levy D, Basilico C (2001). STAT1 mediates the increased apoptosis and reduced chondrocyte proliferation in mice overexpressing FGF2. *Development* 128: 2119–2129.

Sato M, Morii E, Takebayashi-Suzuki K, Yasui N, Ochi T, Kitamura Y, Nomura S (1999). Microphthalmia-associated transcription factor interacts with PU.1 and c-Fos: determination of their subcellular localization. *Biochem Biophys Res Commun* 254: 384–387.

Satokata I, Maas R (1994). Msx1 deficient mice exhibit cleft palate and abnormalities of craniofacial and tooth development. *Nat Genet* 6: 348–356.

Satokata I, Ma L, Ohshima H, Bei M, Woo I, Nishizawa K, Maeda T, Takano Y, Uchiyama M, Heaney S, et al. (2000). Msx2 deficiency in mice causes pleiotropic defects in bone growth and ectodermal organ formation. *Nat Genet* 24: 391–395.

Schipani E, Lanske B, Hunzelman J, Luz A, Kovacs CS, Lee K, Pirro A, Kronenberg HM, Jüppner H (1997). Targeted expression of constitutively active receptors for parathyroid hormone and parathyroid hormone-related peptide delays endochondral bone formation and rescues mice that lack parathyroid hormone-related peptide. *Proc Natl Acad Sci USA* 94: 13689–13694.

Scott EW, Simon MC, Anastasi J, Singh H (1994). Requirement of transcription factor PU.1 in the development of multiple hematopoietic lineages. *Science* 265: 1573–1577.

Segev O, Chumakov I, Nevo Z, Givol D, Madar-Shapiro L, Sheinin Y, Weinreb M, Yayon A (2000). Restrained chondrocyte proliferation and maturation with abnormal growth plate vascularization and ossification in human FGFR-3(G380R) transgenic mice. *Hum Mol Genet* 9: 249–258.

Selleri L, Depew MJ, Jacobs Y, Chanda SK, Tsang KY, Cheah KS, Rubenstein JL, O'-Gorman S, Cleary ML (2001). Requirement for Pbx1 in skeletal patterning and programming chondrocyte proliferation and differentiation. *Development* 128: 3543–3557.

Sells Galvin RJ, Gatlin CL, Horn JW, Fuson TR (1999). TGF-beta enhances osteoclast differentiation in hematopoietic cell cultures stimulated with RANKL and M-CSF. *Biochem Biophys Res Commun* 265: 233–239.

Semba I, Nonaka K, Takahashi I, Takahashi K, Dashner R, Shum L, Nuckolls GH, Slavkin HC (2000). Positionally-dependent chondrogenesis induced by BMP4 is co-regulated by Sox9 and Msx2. *Dev Dyn* 217: 401–414.

Serra R, Johnson M, Filvaroff EH, LaBorde J, Sheehan DM, Derynck R, Moses HL (1997). Expression of a truncated, kinase-defective TGF-beta type II receptor in mouse skeletal tissue promotes terminal chondrocyte differentiation and osteoarthritis. *J Cell Biol* 139: 541–552.

Shiang R, Thompson LM, Zhu YZ, Church DM, Fielder TJ, Bocian M, Winokur ST, Wasmuth JJ (1994). Mutations in the transmembrane domain of FGFR3 cause the most common genetic form of dwarfism, achondroplasia. *Cell* 78: 335–342.

Shirakabe K, Terasawa K, Miyama K, Shibuya H, Nishida E (2001). Regulation of the activity of the transcription factor Runx2 by two homeobox proteins, Msx2 and Dlx5. *Genes Cells* 6: 851–856.

Sillence DO, Senn A, Danks DM (1979). Genetic heterogeneity in osteogenesis imperfecta. *J Med Genet* 16: 101–116.

Simeone A, Acampora D, Pannese M, D'Esposito M, Stornaiuolo A, Gulisano M, Mallamaci A, Kastury K, Druck T, Huebner K, et al. (1994). Cloning and characterization of two members of the vertebrate *Dlx* gene family. *Proc Natl Acad Sci USA* 91: 2250–2254.

Simon LS, Slovik DM, Neer RM, Krane SM (1988). Changes in serum levels of type I and III procollagen extension peptides during infusion of human parathyroid hormone fragment (1–34). *J Bone Miner Res* 3: 241–246.

Simonet WS, Lacey DL, Dunstan CR, Kelley M, Chang MS, Lüthy R, Nguyen HQ, Wooden S, Bennett L, Boone T, et al. (1997). Osteoprotegerin: a novel secreted protein involved in the regulation of bone density. *Cell* 89: 309–319.

Smits P, Li P, Mandel J, Zhang Z, Deng JM, Behringer RR, de Croumbrugghe B, Lefebvre V (2001). The transcription factors L-Sox5 and Sox6 are essential for cartilage formation. *Dev Cell* 1: 277–290.

Solloway MJ, Dudley AT, Bikoff EK, Lyons KM, Hogan BL, Robertson EJ (1998). Mice lacking Bmp6 function. *Dev Genet* 22: 321–339.

Spiegel AM (1991). Pathophysiology of primary hyperparathyroidism. *J Bone Miner Res* 6(Suppl 2):S15–S17, S31–S32.

Spiegelman BM, Flier JS (1996). Adipogenesis and obesity: rounding out the big picture. *Cell* 87: 377–389.

St-Jacques B, Hammerschmidt M, McMahon AP (1999). Indian hedgehog signaling regulates proliferation and differentiation of chondrocytes and is essential for bone formation. *Genes Dev* 13: 2072–2086.

Storm EE, Kingsley DM (1996). Joint patterning defects caused by single and double mutations in members of the bone morphogenetic protein (BMP) family. *Development* 122: 3969–3979.

Storm EE, Huynh TV, Copeland NG, Jenkins NA, Kingsley DM, Lee SJ (1994). Limb alterations in brachypodism mice due to mutations in a new member of the TGF beta-superfamily. *Nature* 368: 639–643.

Su WC, Kitagawa M, Xue N, Xie B, Garofalo S, Cho J, Deng C, Horton WA, Fu XY (1997). Activation of Stat1 by mutant fibroblast growth-factor receptor in thanatophoric dysplasia type II dwarfism. *Nature* 386: 288–292.

Suda M, Ogawa Y, Tanaka K, Tamura N, Yasoda A, Takigawa T, Uehira M, Nishimoto H, Itoh H, Saito Y, et al. (1998). Skeletal overgrowth in transgenic mice that overexpress brain natriuretic peptide. *Proc Natl Acad Sci USA* 95: 2337–2342.

Suda T, Udagawa N, Takahashi N (1996). Cells of bone: osteoclast generation. In: Principles of Bone Biology. Bilezikian JP, Raisz LG, Rodan G (eds.) Academic Press, San Diego, pp. 87–102.

Suda T, Takahashi N, Udagawa N, Jimi E, Gillespie MT, Martin TJ (1999). Modulation of osteoclast differentiation and function by the new members of the tumor necrosis factor receptor and ligand families. *Endocr Rev* 20: 345–357.

Takai H, Kanematsu M, Yano K, Tsuda E, Higashio K, Ikeda K, Watanabe K, Yamada Y (1998). Transforming growth factor-beta stimulates the production of osteoprotegerin/osteoclastogenesis inhibitory factor by bone marrow stromal cells. *J Biol Chem* 273: 27091–27096.

Takeda S, Bonnamy JP, Owen MJ, Ducy P, Karsenty G (2001). Continuous expression of Cbfa1 in nonhypertrophic chondrocytes uncovers its ability to induce hypertrophic chondrocyte differentiation and partially rescues Cbfa1-deficient mice. *Genes Dev* 15: 467–481.

Takuwa Y, Ohse C, Wang EA, Wozney JM, Yamashita K (1991). Bone morphogenetic protein-2 stimulates alkaline phosphatase activity and collagen synthesis in cultured osteoblastic cells, MC3T3-E1. *Biochem Biophys Res Commun* 174: 96–101.

Tam CS, Heersche JNM, Murray TM, Parsons JA (1982). Parathyroid hormone stimulates the bone apposition rate independently of its resorptive action: differential effects of intermittent and continuous administration. *Endocrinology* 110: 506–512.

Tamai K, Semenov M, Kato Y, Spokony R, Liu C, Katsuyama Y, Hess F, Saint-Jeannet JP, He X (2000). LDL-receptor-related proteins in Wnt signal transduction. *Nature* 407: 530–535.

Tavormina PL, Shiang R, Thompson LM, Zhu YZ, Wilkin DJ, Lachman RS, Wilcox WR, Rimoin DL, Cohn DH, Wasmuth JJ (1995). Thanatophoric dysplasia (types I and II) caused by distinct mutations in fibroblast growth factor receptor 3. *Nat Genet* 9: 321–328.

Tezuka K, Nemoto K, Tezuka Y, Sato T, Ikeda Y, Kobori M, Kawashima H, Eguchi H, Hakeda Y, Kumegawa M (1994). Identification of matrix metalloproteinase 9 in rabbit osteoclasts. *J Biol Chem* 269: 15006–15009.

Thirunavukkarasu K, Miles RR, Halladay DL, Yang X, Galvin RJ, Chandrasekhar S, Martin TJ, Onyia JE (2001). Stimulation of osteoprotegerin (OPG) gene expression by transforming growth factor-beta (TGF-beta). Mapping of the OPG promoter region that mediates TGF-beta effects. *J Biol Chem* 276: 36241–36250.

Thomas JT, Lin K, Nandedkar M, Camargo M, Cervenka J, Luyten FP (1996). A human chondrodysplasia due to a mutation in a TGF-beta superfamily member. *Nat Genet* 12: 315–317.

Thomas JT, Kilpatrick MW, Lin K, Erlacher L, Lembessis P, Costa T, Tsipouras P, Luyten FP (1997). Disruption of human limb morphogenesis by a dominant negative mutation in CDMP1. *Nat Genet* 17: 58–64.

Tickle C (1995). Vertebrate limb development. *Curr Opin Genet Dev* 5: 478–484.

Tondravi MM, McKercher SR, Anderson K, Erdmann JM, Quiroz M, Maki R, Teitelbaum SL (1997). Osteopetrosis in mice lacking haematopoietic transcription factor PU.1. *Nature* 386: 81–84.

Tsuda E, Goto M, Mochizuki S, Yano K, Kobayashi F, Morinaga T, Higashio K (1997). Isolation of a novel cytokine from human fibroblasts that specifically inhibits osteoclastogenesis. *Biochem Biophys Res Commun* 234: 137–142.

Ueta C, Iwamoto M, Kanatani N, Yoshida C, Liu Y, Enomoto-Iwamoto M, Ohmori T, Enomoto H, Nakata K, Takada K, et al. (2001). Skeletal malformations caused by overexpression of Cbfa1 or its dominant negative form in chondrocytes. *J Cell Biol* 153: 87–100.

Verma IM, Stevenson JK, Schwarz EM, Van Antwerp D, Miyamoto S (1995). Rel/NF-kappaB/IkappaB family: intimate tales of association and dissociation. *Genes Dev* 9: 2723–2735.

Vortkamp A, Lee K, Lanske B, Segre GV, Kronenberg HM, Tabin CJ (1996). Regulation of rate of cartilage differentiation by Indian hedgehog and PTH-related protein. *Science* 273: 613–622.

Vu TH, Shipley JM, Bergers G, Berger JE, Helms JA, Hanahan D, Shapiro SD, Senior RM, Werb Z (1998). MMP-9/gelatinase B is a key regulator of growth plate angiogenesis and apoptosis of hypertrophic chondrocytes. *Cell* 93: 411–422.

Wagner T, Wirth J, Meyer J, Zabel B, Held M, Zimmer J, Pasantes J, Bricarelli F D, Keutel J, Hustert E (1994). Autosomal sex reversal and campomelic dysplasia are caused by mutations in and around the *SRY*-related gene *SOX9*. *Cell* 79: 1111–1120.

Wai AW, Ng LJ, Watanabe H, Yamada Y, Tam PP, Cheah KS (1998). Disrupted expression of matrix genes in the growth plate of the mouse cartilage matrix deficiency (cmd) mutant. *Dev Genet* 22: 349–358.

Wang Q, Green RP, Zhao G, Ornitz DM (2001). Differential regulation of endochondral bone growth and joint development by FGFR1 and FGFR3 tyrosine kinase domains. *Development* 128: 3867–3876.

Wang Y, Spatz MK, Kannan K, Hayk H, Avivi A, Gorivodsky M, Pines M, Yayon A, Lonai P, Givol D (1999). A mouse model for achondroplasia produced by targeting fibroblast growth factor receptor 3. *Proc Natl Acad Sci USA* 96: 4455–4460.

Wang ZQ, Ovitt C, Grigoriadis AE, Mohle-Steinlein U, Ruther U, Wagner EF (1992). Bone and haematopoietic defects in mice lacking c-fos. *Nature* 360: 741–745.

Watanabe H, Yamada Y (1999). Mice lacking link protein develop dwarfism and craniofacial abnormalities. *Nat Genet* 21: 225–229.

Watanabe H, Kimata K, Line S, Strong D, Gao LY, Kozak CA, Yamada Y (1994). Mouse cartilage matrix deficiency (cmd) caused by a 7 bp deletion in the aggrecan gene. *Nat Genet* 7: 154–157.

Wegner M (1999). From head to toes: the multiple facets of Sox proteins. *Nucleic Acids Res* 27: 1409–1420.

Wehrli M, Dougan ST, Caldwell K, O'Keefe L, Schwartz S, Vaizel-Ohayon D, Schejter E, Tomlinson A, DiNardo S (2000). Arrow encodes an LDL-receptor-related protein essential for Wingless signalling. *Nature* 407: 527–530.

Weir EC, Philbrick WM, Amling M, Neff LA, Baron R, Broadus AE (1996). Targeted overexpression of parathyroid hormone–related peptide in chondrocytes causes chondrodysplasia and delayed endochondral bone formation. *Proc Natl Acad Sci USA* 93: 10240–10245.

Wilkie AOM, Slaney SF, Oldridge M, Poole MD, Ashworth GJ, Hockley AD, Hayward RD, David DJ, Pulleyn LJ, Rutland P, et al. (1995). Apert syndrome results from localized mutations of *FGFR2* and is allelic with Crouzon syndrome. *Nat Genet* 9: 165–172.

Winnier G, Blessing M, Labosky PA, Hogan BL (1995). Bone morphogenetic protein-4 is required for mesoderm formation and patterning in the mouse. *Genes Dev* 9: 2105–2116.

Wozney JM, Rosen V, Celeste AJ, Mitsock LM, Whitters MJ, Kriz RW, Hewick RM, Wang EA (1988). Novel regulators of bone formation: molecular clones and activities. *Science* 242: 1528–1534.

Wright E, Hargrave MR, Christiansen J, Cooper L, Kun J, Evans T, Gangadharan U, Greenfield A, Koopman P (1995). The *Sry*-related gene *Sox9* is expressed during chondrogenesis in mouse embryos. *Nat Genet* 9: 15–20.

Wucherpfennig AL, Li YP, Stetler-Stevenson WG, Rosenberg AE, Stashenko P (1994). Expression of 92 kD type IV collagenase/gelatinase B in human osteoclasts. *J Bone Miner Res* 9: 549–556.

Xie WF, Zhang X, Sakano S, Lefebvre V, Sandell LJ (1999). Trans-activation of the mouse cartilage-derived retinoic acid-sensitive protein gene by Sox9. *J Bone Miner Res* 14: 757–763.

Yang X, Chen L, Xu X, Li C, Huang C, Deng CX (2001). TGF-beta/Smad3 signals repress chondrocyte hypertrophic differentiation and are required for maintaining articular cartilage. *J Cell Biol* 153: 35–46.

Yi SE, Daluiski A, Pederson R, Rosen V, Lyons KM (2000). The type I BMP receptor BMPRIB is required for chondrogenesis in the mouse limb. *Development* 127: 621–630.

Yoshida H, Hayashi S, Kunisada T, Ogawa M, Nishikawa S, Okamura H, Sudo T, Shultz LD (1990). The murine mutation osteopetrosis is in the coding region of the macrophage colony stimulating factor gene. *Nature* 345: 442–444.

Yoshida Y, Tanaka S, Umemori H, Minowa O, Usui M, Ikematsu N, Hosoda E, Imamura T, Kuno J, Yamashita T, et al. (2000). Negative regulation of BMP/Smad signaling by Tob in osteoblasts. *Cell* 103: 1085–1097.

Yoshitake H, Rittling SR, Denhardt DT, Noda M (1999). Osteopontin-deficient mice are resistant to ovariectomy-induced bone resorption. *Proc Natl Acad Sci USA* 96: 8156–8160.

Zehentner BK, Dony C, Burtscher H (1999). The transcription factor Sox9 is involved in BMP-2 signaling. *J Bone Miner Res* 14: 1734–1741.

Zelzer E, McLean W, Ng YS, Fukai N, Reginato AM, Lovejoy S, D'Amore PA, Olsen BR (2002). Skeletal defects in VEGF(120/120) mice reveal multiple roles for VEGF in skeletogenesis. *Development* 129: 1893–1904.

Zhang H, Bradley A (1996). Mice deficient for BMP2 are nonviable and have defects in amnion/chorion and cardiac development. *Development* 122: 2977–2986.

Zhao Q, Eberspaecher H, Lefebvre V, de Crombrugghe B (1997). Parallel expression of Sox9 and Col2a1 in cells undergoing chondrogenesis. *Dev Dyn* 209: 377–386.

12 | Development of the Limbs

SAHAR NISSIM AND CLIFF TABIN

Morphological development of a limb begins with a relatively simple outgrowth of cells, which acquires increasing complexity and detail over time. This phenomenon can be viewed as a collaboration of several processes, including changes in cell number, differentiation of cell types, and elaboration of patterning. How these processes are orchestrated in a consistent and orderly way to allow a bird to fly, a mouse to run, and a human to write is astounding.

The human limbs first appear as small buds of cells that emerge from the body wall during week 4 of gestation. By week 8, these buds have formed much of the mature limb structures from the upper arm to the digits, including a cartilage primordium of the entire limb skeleton, the muscle masses, innervation, and vasculature. In approximately 2 of every 1000 births, this carefully regulated process goes awry, leading to major limb malformations (Moore and Persaud, 1998). Most of these defects arise from genetic causes, though environmental causes such as maternal use of thalidomide and intrauterine mechanical influences have also been implicated. Research in limb development has made tremendous advances in identifying and understanding the function of genes responsible for congenital limb defects. Furthermore, many of the genetic pathways that regulate limb development are important in other organ systems as well. The developing limb has therefore been a valuable model for gaining insight into general mechanisms of embryonic development.

Much of the progress in understanding limb development comes from studies in chick and mouse embryos. Though limbs of these species differ greatly from human limbs in structure and function, their basic layout is very similar (each has an upper arm, a lower arm, a wrist, and digits), and the molecular and cellular processes behind their development are remarkably well conserved. The developing chick limb has been thoroughly studied because it is easily accessible for both surgical manipulation and gene manipulation via viral vectors through a window created in the egg. The developing mouse limb has been studied because of the powerful transgenic and knock-out technology available. Moreover, natural and experimentally induced limb malformations are readily characterized in both organisms. Most of the research on these two model organisms falls into four general approaches. First, "classical" experiments relied greatly on surgical manipulations in the chick limb bud. Second, cell-labeling studies have documented where cells move and which cells comprise various limb structures. Third, techniques for visualizing spatial and temporal patterns of gene expression are routine and indispensable. Fourth, the function of genes can be tested by targeted disruption and misexpression. Over several decades, these approaches have offered a vast amount of information and an increasingly detailed view of how limbs develop.

This chapter will review our current understanding of how the limb develops as gathered from experiments in chick and mouse embryos. Emphasis will be given to the genes and molecular pathways that pattern the limb. In the first section, an anatomical and histological overview of limb development will be presented, introducing key structures and the three major axes of the developing limb. The rest of the chapter is organized around some of the most basic questions that have driven limb developmental biology. What determines where limb buds form? How does limb bud formation begin? How is the limb bud patterned along its three axes of asymmetry? How is positional information interpreted in the limb bud? What specifies a forelimb versus a hindlimb? These questions will be addressed, high-

lighting the principle genes and molecular pathways involved. Descriptions of limb malformations caused by genetic mutations are organized according to gene families in subsequent chapters.

ANATOMICAL AND HISTOLOGICAL OVERVIEW OF LIMB DEVELOPMENT

The first visible sign of a limb developing is a small protrusion that arises from the body wall of the embryo (Fig. 12–1A). In human embryos, the forelimb buds appear by day 27 of gestation and the hindlimb buds appear by day 28. The limb bud forms from proliferation of lateral plate mesoderm cells in a region of the flank called the "limb field" (Fig. 12–2). Prior to limb bud formation, proliferation in the body flank is uniform. However, emergence of the limb bud is associated with continued cell proliferation in the limb field in contrast to diminished cell proliferation in nonlimb regions (Searls and Janners, 1971).

The emerging bud of proliferating mesenchymal cells is covered by an epithelial sheet of ectodermal cells. Soon after the limb bud emerges, a specialized epithelial structure called the apical ectodermal ridge (AER) forms at the distal tip. The AER is a tight ridge of pseudostratified (in the chick) or stratified (in the mouse) epithelial cells, which are separated from underlying mesenchymal cells by a basement membrane (Kelley and Fallon, 1976). At the distal tip of the limb bud, the AER runs from anterior to posterior along the boundary between the dorsal and ventral ectoderm (Fig. 12–1). Signals from underlying mesoderm induce formation of the AER in the ectoderm, and it is positioned by signals in the ectoderm. The AER is critical for outgrowth of the limb bud. If it is removed, limb bud outgrowth is drastically reduced and the mature limb is truncated.

As the limb bud continues to grow out, mesenchymal cells directly under the AER remain undifferentiated, whereas mesenchymal cells that are distanced from the AER begin to condense and undergo chondrogenesis. This process forms the cartilage primordium of the limb skeleton in a proximal-to-distal sequence. Thus, in the forelimb, the humerus primordium appears first, followed by the radius and ulna, and then the wrist and digits. The distal end of the limb bud acquires a flattened paddle shape, called the hand or foot plate. In humans, this occurs by day 32 in the forelimb and day 36 in the hindlimb. Mesenchyme in the hand or foot plate begins condensing to form a chondrogenic ray that represents the forming digits. By this time, the AER regresses. Initially, a webbing of mesenchyme exists between the digital rays, but this intervening mesenchyme subsequently breaks down through apoptosis to form separated digits. This occurs by day 46 in the hand and day 49 in the foot of human embryos. By week 8 of human development, a cartilage primordium of all the limb bones has formed and ossification begins.

The limb bud mesenchyme contributes to most of the mature limb structures, including bone, cartilage, tendons, ligaments, and dermis. Muscles, nerves, and blood vessels are derived from tissue originating outside the limb. Muscle forms by the migration of myogenic precursors from the somites into the limbs (Fig. 12–2). These precursors proliferate to form a dorsal and ventral muscle mass in the early limb bud, and these masses then further divide to form individual muscles. This process coincides with innervation. The pattern of muscles is established by the connective tissue surrounding the muscle masses.

Thus, in the span of 4 weeks in human development, a limb bud

Figure 12–1. The axes of limb development. *(A)* A day 30 human embryo. The forelimb and hindlimb buds are visible. *(B)* Schematic of the forelimb, illustrating the proximal/distal and anterior/posterior axes. The apical ectodermal ridge (AER) lies at the distal tip of the limb bud, and the zone of polarizing activity (ZPA) is functionally mapped to a posterior region of the limb bud. *(C)* Cross-section of the limb bud illustrates the dorsal/ventral axis. The AER lies at the juncture of the dorsal and ventral ectoderm. *(D)* Skeletal derivatives of the stylopod, zeugopod, and autopod segments of the developing limb.

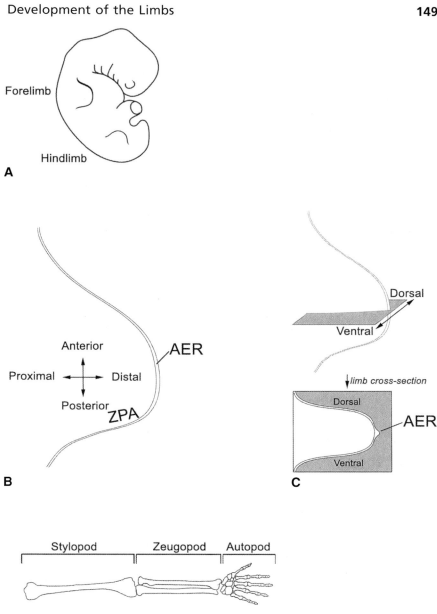

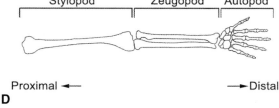

emerges, grows out, and acquires a mature morphology, a full cartilage primordium, musculature, and innervation. This entire process happens in only a few days in the chick and mouse embryo.

THE MAJOR AXES OF LIMB DEVELOPMENT

Patterning of the limb bud can be viewed along three axes of asymmetry: the proximal/distal (P/D) axis, the anterior/posterior (A/P) axis, and the dorsal/ventral (D/V) axis (Fig. 12–1). The limb bud begins as a relatively round and symmetrical mass of cells. However, asymmetry is an essential property of the mature limb, and much research has focused on how mesenchymal cells in the limb bud are patterned along these axes to develop asymmetrical structures. The P/D axis runs from the shoulder to the digits. Three segments along the P/D axis are typical of all tetrapod vertebrate limbs: the stylopod (humerus/femur), the zeugopod (radius, ulna/tibia, and fibula), and the autopod (carpal/tarsal elements and digits). The A/P axis runs from the thumb to the little finger in the hand. A small region of mesenchyme at the posterior margin, called the "zone of polarizing activity" (ZPA), instructs asymmetry along the A/P axis. Finally, the D/V axis runs from the back of

the hand to the palm. Information for D/V patterning is mediated by signaling between the limb ectoderm and mesoderm. Together, asymmetrical patterning along these axes sculpts the three-dimensional structure of the limb. The tissues and molecular mechanisms that perform this patterning and the coordination between these axes will be described in more detail here.

STARTING LIMB FORMATION: WHERE AND HOW

Hox Genes Specify Where Limbs Grow

Outgrowth of the limb begins as a bud projecting from the body flank. The bud arises by proliferation of mesenchymal cells in the lateral plate mesoderm (Fig. 12–2). The forelimb buds always develop at a level adjacent to the cervical–thoracic transition of the vertebral column, and the hindlimb buds always develop at the level of the lumbar–sacral transition. This is true in a variety of vertebrates, even though these species vary in number of axial segments (Burke et al., 1995). How then is the position of limb bud outgrowth determined along the A/P axis of the body?

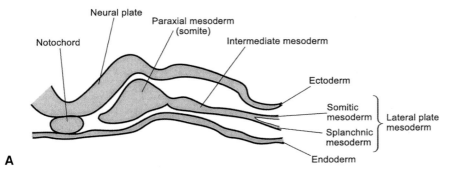

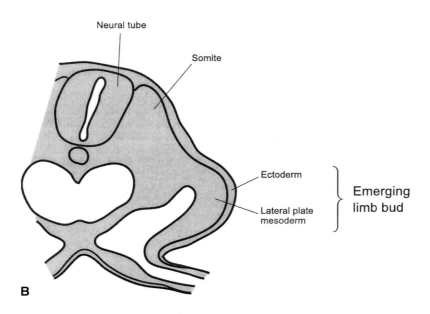

Figure 12–2. Origins of the limb bud. *(A)* Cross-section through a day 20 human embryo. *(B)* Cross-section through a day 24 human embryo. Proliferation of cells in the lateral plate mesoderm results in emergence of a limb bud. Myogenic progenitors migrate from the somites into the limb bud.

One attractive model posits that *Hox* genes determine where the outgrowth occurs (see Chapter 46 for general discussion of *Hox* genes). The *Hox* genes are expressed in a variety of tissues during development, including the neural tube, somitic mesoderm, intermediate mesoderm, and lateral plate mesoderm. Expression of these genes is patterned in a nested fashion along the A/P (rostral–caudal) axis; the particular combination of *Hox* genes expressed at any A/P level are thought to set up a "Hox code," which defines regional identity along the A/P axis (Kessel and Gruss, 1990). This function of *Hox* genes has been demonstrated by both loss of function and misexpression along the A/P axis. For example, an anterior shift in *Hox* gene expression results in a corresponding shift in the axial specification of vertebral structures such that normally cervical vertebrae instead have a thoracic morphology (Kessel and Gruss, 1991). This role has been well established in the neural tube and somitic mesoderm. Hence, *Hox* genes might play a similar role in the intermediate mesoderm and lateral plate mesoderm to define the axial level at which a limb can form.

Support for this model comes from several observations. First, comparison of different animals reveals that the same *Hox* genes are expressed at the level where limbs form in all species examined, potentially representing a *Hox* code for the limb field (Burke et al., 1995). For example, transposition of the forelimbs from somite level 17–18 in the chick to somite level 10–11 in the mouse correlates with changes in the level of *Hoxc-5* expression, suggesting that *Hoxc-5* may influence the position of the forelimb (Burke et al., 1995). This model predicts that changes in the *Hox* code should either eliminate formation of limbs or cause shifts in the location where they form. By and large, this has not been the case, perhaps because of redundancy requiring alteration of several *Hox* genes in concert to produce such an effect.

However, in at least one case, mice defective in *Hoxb-5* do exhibit an anterior shift in the attachment of the forelimb to the shoulder girdle (Rancourt et al., 1995).

Second, as will be discussed below, signals initiating the formation of the limb bud appear to originate, at least in part, from the intermediate mesoderm. Indeed, barriers placed between the intermediate and lateral plate mesoderm abrogate limb formation (Stephens and McNulty, 1981). Thus, *Hox* genes in the intermediate mesoderm may be the key to specifying the limb field. A *Hox* code for the limb field seems to be a consistent feature of the lateral plate mesoderm as well. However, the *Hox* code in this tissue would appear to be secondary to induction of the limb bud: when limbs are ectopically induced in the flank of chick embryos, *Hox* gene expression changes from the normal lateral plate pattern to the pattern found at the wing or leg level, and whether a wing or leg forms correlates with the change in *Hox* gene expression (Cohn et al., 1997).

A Cascade of Wingless and Fibroblast Growth Factor Signals Initiates Limb Outgrowth

While *Hox* genes in the intermediate mesoderm may position the axial level of limb outgrowth, the limb buds form from the lateral plate mesoderm. Therefore, signals downstream of the *Hox* genes in the intermediate mesoderm must be required to initiate the proliferation of cells in the lateral plate limb field, leading to limb outgrowth. The first clue that the intermediate mesoderm is the source of such inductive signals came from foil barrier and extirpation studies (Stephens and McNulty, 1981; Strecker and Stephens, 1983; Geduspan and Solursh, 1992). If a barrier is placed between the intermediate and lateral plate mesoderm, limbs will not form. Similarly, surgical removal of the intermediate mesoderm leads to loss of adjacent limb tissue.

These observations suggest that signals from the intermediate mesoderm are necessary to induce proliferation of the lateral plate mesoderm during limb outgrowth. However, the lateral plate mesoderm subsequently produces its own signals, which are sufficient to promote limb outgrowth. The presence of these signals can be shown by the ability to induce an ectopic limb in the flank of an embryo (Saunders and Reuss, 1974). For example, grafting a piece of presumptive limb lateral plate mesoderm to an ectopic location results in formation of an ectopic fifth limb. In contrast, grafts of presumptive limb ectoderm or lateral plate mesoderm from outside the limb fields do not have this effect. Put together, these classical manipulations suggest that at the level of the limb field signals from the intermediate mesoderm are required to initiate limb formation, after which signals from the lateral plate mesoderm are sufficient for limb outgrowth. What are these signals?

A number of secreted signals have been identified as being expressed in either the intermediate mesoderm or the lateral plate mesoderm at a time consistent with their playing a role in limb bud initiation. In particular, secreted proteins of the fibroblast growth factor (FGF) and Wingless (WNT) families have been implicated (see Chapters 22 and 32). *Fgf-8* is transiently expressed in the intermediate mesoderm and specifically expressed adjacent to the limb-forming regions at times when barrier experiments suggest the intermediate mesoderm plays its inductive role (Crossley et al., 1996; Vogel et al., 1996). At approximately the same time, *Wnt-2b* is also expressed in the intermediate mesoderm and lateral plate mesoderm of the forelimb (Kawakami et al., 2001). In the hindlimb, *Wnt-8c* is expressed in the lateral plate mesoderm, although its timing of expression is less well correlated with limb bud initiation (Kawakami et al., 2001). Shortly after *Fgf-8* expression in the intermediate mesoderm, *Fgf-10* is broadly expressed in the lateral plate mesoderm and becomes restricted to the level of the forelimbs and hindlimbs just before limb bud outgrowth (Ohuchi et al., 1997; Xu et al., 1998). These FGF and WNT factors are therefore good candidates for the endogenous signals that induce limb outgrowth.

To test the functional significance of these gene-expression patterns, beads soaked in these factors or cells expressing them have been implanted into the chick flank. In this assay, several members of the FGF family, including FGF-8 and FGF-10 (Cohn et al., 1995; Crossley et al., 1996; Vogel et al., 1996; Ohuchi et al., 1997), as well as WNT-2b and WNT-8c (Kawakami et al., 2001) can induce the formation of an ectopic limb in the flank. The necessity of these factors in limb induction has also been examined. The requirement of endogenous FGF-8 from the intermediate mesoderm for limb induction has been difficult to address because loss-of-function mutants have an early embryonic lethality and an appropriate conditional mutant has not been made. However, mouse mutant embryos that do not produce *Fgf-10* fail to form limbs (Min et al., 1998; Sekine et al., 1999). Furthermore, mice missing the FGF receptor FGFR-2, isoforms of which are expressed in both the ectoderm and mesoderm of the limb, also fail to form limbs, demonstrating the absolute requirement of these factors for limb bud initiation. Genetic experiments have not been carried out to assess the endogenous roles of *Wnt-2b* and *Wnt-8c*. However, overexpression of Axin, which blocks the β-catenin pathway of WNT signaling, completely abrogates forelimb and hindlimb outgrowth (Kawakami et al., 2001). Put together, these experiments demonstrate that FGF and WNT signals are both sufficient and necessary for induction of limb outgrowth.

How do these FGF and WNT signals interact in limb induction? When WNT activity is blocked by overexpression of Axin, *Fgf-10* is not expressed (Kawakami et al., 2001). This observation puts WNT activity upstream of FGF-10 in the cascade of limb induction. As their relative expression patterns would indicate, *Fgf-8* also appears to act upstream of *Fgf-10* in this process. Indeed, when a bead soaked in FGF-8 is implanted in the flank, *Fgf-10* transcripts appear in the mesoderm around the bead, followed by induction of limb-specific transcripts in the overlying ectoderm. In contrast, when a bead soaked in FGF-10 is implanted in the flank, gene-expression changes are directly induced in the overlying ectoderm (Ohuchi et al., 1997). Thus, while the relationship between *Wnt-2b* and *Fgf-8* has yet to be established,

these two medial signals in the forelimb field induce *Fgf-10* in the lateral plate mesoderm, which in turn affects gene expression in the overlying ectoderm. A similar cascade might operate in the hindlimb, where *Wnt-8c* and *Fgf-8* may induce *Fgf-10* to affect gene expression in the overlying ectoderm.

As indicated above, the cascade of WNT and FGF signals in the limb field mesoderm results in gene-expression changes in the overlying ectoderm. The first limb-specific ectodermal gene to be expressed is another member of the WNT family, *Wnt-3a* (Kengaku et al., 1998). Subsequently, *Fgf-8* is expressed in an overlapping domain (Crossley et al., 1996; Kengaku et al., 1998). This order is recapitulated in response to FGF-10 application to the limb, activating *Wnt-3a* in the ectoderm, followed by *Fgf-8* a few hours later (Kawakami et al., 2001). The functional significance of this temporal order is shown by the ability of ectopic *Wnt-3a* to induce ectopic *Fgf-8* in the ectoderm; conversely, expression of a dominant-negative form of *Lef-1*, which interferes with β-catenin signaling of the WNT pathway, blocks *Fgf-8* expression in the ectoderm (Kengaku et al., 1998). Thus, initiation of forelimb outgrowth is characterized by a cascade of alternating WNT and FGF signals from medial tissue out to the ectoderm: FGF-8 and WNT-2b in the intermediate mesoderm induce FGF-10 in the lateral plate mesoderm, activating WNT-3a in the overlying ectoderm, which in turn induces FGF-8 in the ectoderm.

Fgf-8 expression in the limb ectoderm is localized to a specialized structure, the AER. As will be discussed below, this *Fgf-8* expression is critical for limb bud outgrowth and for induction of a number of genes in the underlying mesenchyme. Among these important roles is maintenance of *Fgf-10* after the limb-initiating signals are no longer present from medial tissues. If the AER, which expresses *Fgf-8*, is removed from a limb bud, *Fgf-10* expression is rapidly lost from the mesenchyme; but it can be rescued by FGF-8 application (Ohuchi et al., 1997). Moreover, if a bead soaked in FGF-10 is applied to the flank, *Fgf-8* is induced in the overlying ectoderm, after which *Fgf-10* is induced in the mesenchyme. This observation has led to a model of an FGF signaling loop that mediates limb outgrowth. It is thought that FGF-10 in the lateral plate mesoderm induces FGF-8 via WNT-3a in the overlying ectoderm and that FGF-8 then reciprocates by inducing FGF-10 in the underlying mesoderm. This feedback interaction between the limb epithelium and limb mesenchyme is thought to persist through limb outgrowth. This allows FGF-10 to be maintained and cell proliferation to continue in the mesoderm of the growing limb bud.

The receptors that mediate this reciprocal loop are two isoforms of FGFR-2 that differ in the third Ig loop, FGFR-2IIIb and FGFR-2IIIc. FGFR-2IIIb is localized to the surface ectoderm and is specific for FGF-10, whereas FGFR-2IIIc is localized to the underlying mesoderm and is specific for FGF-8 (Orr-Urtreger et al., 1993; Xu et al., 1999; see also Chapter 33). This differential localization and specificity of FGFRs is consistent with the notion of a paracrine loop: FGF-10 acts through FGFR-2IIIb in the ectoderm to induce FGF-8, and FGF-8 acts through FGFR-2IIIc in the underlying mesoderm to maintain FGF-10. In further support for this model, mouse embryos mutant in both FGFR-2 isoforms fail to turn on *Fgf-8* in the limb ectoderm and gradually lose *Fgf-10* expression in the underlying mesoderm (Xu et al., 1998).

In addition, a specific splice variant of the transmembrane glycoprotein CD44 may be necessary to present FGF signals from the AER to the underlying mesenchyme (Sherman et al., 1998). This CD44 splice variant is expressed in the AER and binds and presents FGF-8 to mesenchymal cells in vitro. When CD44 is blocked, limb outgrowth ceases, suggesting that this presentation mechanism is necessary.

To summarize, the proliferation of lateral plate mesoderm that forms the emerging limb bud is initiated by a relay of WNT and FGF signals (Fig. 12–3). At the forelimb level, WNT-2b and FGF-8 induce *Fgf-10* in the lateral plate mesoderm. FGF-10 in turn acts through *Wnt-3a* to activate *Fgf-8* in the overlying ectoderm and future AER. FGF-8 then acts back on the underlying mesoderm to maintain *Fgf-10* levels and cell proliferation. If *Hox* genes in the lateral plate mesoderm do in fact specify where limbs grow, it remains to be seen how these transcription factors act in relation to the secreted signals that initiate limb bud outgrowth.

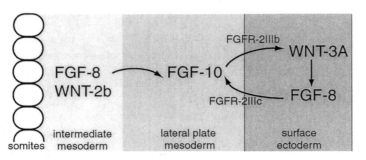

Figure 12–3. Initiation of limb development. A cascade of fibroblast growth factor (FGF) and Wingless (WNT) signals initiates limb bud formation. At the forelimb level, FGF-8 and WNT-2b induce FGF-10 in the lateral plate mesoderm. FGF-10 in turn acts via FGFR-2IIIb to activate WNT-3a and FGF-8 in overlying ectoderm and the future apical ectodermal ridge. FGF-8 reciprocally maintains FGF-10 in the lateral plate mesoderm via the FGFR-2IIIc receptor. This relay initiates proliferation of lateral plate mesoderm cells and emergence of the limb bud.

The AER

The relay of WNT and FGF signals culminates in the emergence of a limb bud. Soon after a bud is visible, the AER forms at the distal tip of the bud. This structure is necessary for maintaining proliferation, preventing cell death in underlying cells, and hence continued outgrowth of the limb. This section summarizes evidence that the function of the AER is mediated by FGFs and describes the mechanisms for positioning and forming the AER.

The Function of the AER Is Mediated by FGFs

Numerous classical manipulations demonstrate that the AER is a critical signaling center in limb outgrowth. If the AER is cut off of a limb bud, growth of the limb bud is interrupted such that the adult limb will have truncations in distal skeletal elements (Saunders, 1948; Summerbell, 1974). Thus, the AER is thought to be the source of signals that keep underlying cells in a proliferating and undifferentiated state, allowing the limb bud to grow. As will be described below, signals from the AER are also thought to coordinate limb outgrowth with A/P patterning of the limb. What are these signals?

Once again, FGF proteins are thought to be critical. Several *Fgf* genes are expressed in the AER, including *Fgf-4* (Niswander et al., 1994), *Fgf-8* (Ohuchi et al., 1994; Crossley et al., 1996; Vogel et al., 1996), *Fgf-9* (Colvin et al., 1999), and *Fgf-17* (Sun et al., 2000) in all species studied, as well as *Fgf-2* in the chick (Fallon et al., 1994). While other genes have been detected in the AER, only FGF proteins can completely substitute for the function of the AER in maintaining limb outgrowth. Thus, in chick embryos, a bead soaked in FGF-2 (Fallon et al., 1994), FGF-4 (Niswander et al., 1994), or FGF-8 (Vogel et al., 1996; Tanaka et al., 1997) is capable of rescuing a limb from truncation after the AER is surgically removed. Each of these AER factors is entirely sufficient to replace the AER, even though none can induce an AER once it has been extirpated.

The necessity of these *Fgf* genes in limb formation has therefore been assessed genetically in mice. Interestingly, normal limbs develop in mice that have a loss of function in *Fgf-2* (Ortega et al., 1998), *Fgf-4* (Moon et al., 2000; Sun et al., 2000), *Fgf-9* (Colvin et al., 2001), or *Fgf-17* (Xu et al., 2000). Only loss of function of *Fgf-8* leads to limb defects. In mice with a conditional disruption of *Fgf-8* in the limb bud, hypoplasia or aplasia occurs in specific skeletal elements throughout the limb, revealing a role for *Fgf-8* in proper limb outgrowth and formation of the stylopod, zeugopod, and autopod (Lewandoski et al., 2000; Moon et al., 2000). This phenotype is similar but not identical to the truncations that result when the AER is resected from chick limbs. The disparity may be due to functional redundancy of *Fgf* genes in the AER. For example, in one type of conditional *Fgf-8* mutant, posterior limb structures are less severely affected or normal, possibly because *Fgf-4* is expressed and can compensate in the posterior region of the AER (Moon et al., 2000). Indeed, when both *Fgf-8* and *Fgf-4* are conditionally removed, the forelimb skeletal phenotype is more severe and hindlimb skeletal elements are completely absent (Sun et al., 2002). Similarly, it is likely that the other *Fgf* genes fail to exhibit mutant phenotypes in the limb because of functional redundancy in the AER.

Altogether, these data demonstrate that FGFs are critical mediators of AER function. The specific roles of these FGF signals as mitogens and cell-survival factors will be discussed below. There is also evidence that FGF signals may act as chemotactic agents to regulate migration of mesenchymal cells (Li and Muneoka, 1999).

Dorsal and Ventral Ectodermal Genes Position the AER

While mesodermal signals induce limb bud outgrowth and formation of an AER, additional factors must be involved in positioning the AER. The simple fact that the AER always appears to form at the boundary between the dorsal and ventral territories of an embryo attests to these additional factors (Fig. 12–1C). Furthermore, ectopic limbs induced by implanting FGF beads in the chick flank will invariably form at the D/V boundary (Cohn et al., 1995; Crossley et al., 1996; Vogel et al., 1996). More rigorous demonstration that the AER forms at this boundary comes from cell lineage studies. In chick embryos, DiI-labeling or quail-chick chimera experiments reveal that the limb ectoderm is divided into dorsal and ventral compartments (Michaud et al., 1997; Altabef et al., 1997). Precursors to the AER are initially spread over a broad domain of ectoderm and gradually consolidate to form a mature AER, which lies right at the boundary between the dorsal and ventral compartments. Similarly, in mouse embryos, use of retroviral labeling *in utero* shows restriction of cell lineage to a dorsal or ventral compartment (Kimmel et al., 2000). Again, the boundary between the dorsal and ventral compartments runs through the AER. This overlap is more than simply coincidence. When pieces of dorsal or ventral limb ectoderm are inserted into the opposite limb domain, ectopic AERs form at the borders of the inserted piece (Tanaka et al., 1997). These observations link specification of dorsal and ventral ectoderm with positioning of the AER. What is the molecular basis for this link?

Clues came from investigation of genes that are differentially expressed along the D/V axis (Fig. 12–4A). Such genes have several possible functions: (1) they may establish dorsal or ventral compartments in the ectoderm, restricting cell lineage to one compartment or the other; (2) they may confer dorsal or ventral identity to the ectoderm, including the ability to instruct underlying mesodermal fate to become dorsal or ventral adult structures; or (3) they may be involved in forming and positioning the AER along the D/V axis. Two genes have been implicated in the last function. The secreted factor *Radical fringe* is expressed in the dorsal ectoderm and through the AER in the chick (Laufer et al., 1997; Rodriguez-Esteban et al., 1997) and weakly in the mouse (Moran et al., 1999). The transcription factor *Engrailed-1* is expressed in ventral ectoderm and the ventral half of the AER in the chick (Davis et al., 1991; Gardner and Barald, 1992; Logan et al., 1997) and the mouse (Wurst et al., 1994).

A focus on *Radical fringe* stemmed from molecular parallels between AER formation in the vertebrate limb and margin formation in the *Drosophila* wing (Laufer et al., 1997; Rodriguez-Esteban et al., 1997). In *Drosophila*, *fringe* is expressed in the dorsal compartment of the wing disc (Irvine and Wieschaus, 1994). The juxtaposition of cells expressing *fringe* in the dorsal compartment and cells not expressing *fringe* in the ventral compartment induces formation of a margin and wing outgrowth. Remarkably, the same role has been demonstrated for the vertebrate homolog *Radical fringe* in chick embryos. The AER forms at the boundary between *Radical fringe*–expressing cells in the dorsal ectoderm and nonexpressing cells in the ventral ectoderm (Laufer et al., 1997; Rodriguez-Esteban et al., 1997). Moreover, ectopic misexpression of *Radical fringe* leads to matching ec-

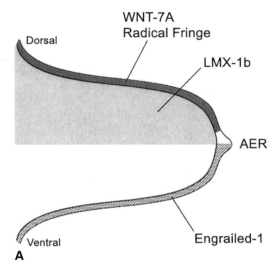

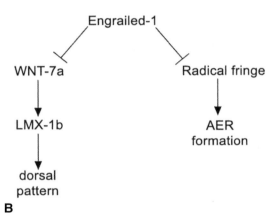

Figure 12–4. Dorsal/ventral patterning of the limb. *(A)* Cross-section of the limb illustrates the restriction of several genes in dorsal or ventral ectoderm. *Engrailed-1* is expressed in the ventral ectoderm and ventral half of the apical ectodermal ridge (AER). *WNT-7a* and *Radical fringe* are expressed in the dorsal ectoderm, and *LMX-1b* is expressed in the dorsal mesenchyme. *(B)* In the chick embryo, *Engrailed-1* links dorsal/ventral patterning with the positioning of the AER. *WNT-7a* instructs dorsal patterning by inducing *LMX-1b* in the dorsal mesenchyme. *Engrailed-1* inhibits *WNT-7a* from the ventral ectoderm, allowing ventral patterning. *Engrailed-1* also inhibits *Radical fringe* from ventral ectoderm. The AER, which forms at a boundary between *Radical fringe*–expressing and nonexpressing ectoderm, is therefore positioned between the dorsal and ventral ectoderm.

topic AER formation, presumably by creating new boundaries of expressing and nonexpressing cells; indeed, the ectopic AERs form only in the ventral ectoderm and not in the dorsal ectoderm, where *Radical fringe* is widely expressed. Because its normal expression is in the dorsal ectoderm, *Radical fringe* creates a boundary at the D/V border, where the AER will consistently form.

The *Engrailed-1* transcription factor is thought to position this border of *Radical fringe*–expressing and nonexpressing cells. When *Engrailed-1* is ectopically misexpressed in chick limb ectoderm, the AER is disrupted and/or ectopic AERs form, depending on the pattern of misexpression (Laufer et al., 1997; Logan et al., 1997). The ectopic AERs form only on the dorsal side. This is the opposite of the ventral ectopic AERs that form following *Radical fringe* misexpression. Furthermore, the disrupted AERs match a disrupted expression of *Radical fringe* following misexpression of *Engrailed-1*. These observations support the idea that *Engrailed-1* represses *Radical fringe*. Normally expressed in the ventral ectoderm, *Engrailed-1* would therefore

restrict *Radical fringe* to the dorsal ectoderm, creating a sharp boundary at which the AER will form. This model draws greatly from experiments in the chick. A mouse *Radical fringe* gene has been reported in the dorsal ectoderm and AER, but loss of function of this gene does not seem to result in any limb abnormalities (Moran et al., 1999). While it is possible that other Fringe genes have redundant function in the limb, it remains to be seen if the role of *Radical fringe* in positioning the AER is conserved in mammals.

The data summarized here implicate the ectodermal genes *Radical fringe* and *Engrailed-1* in positioning the AER (function *3* above), but *Engrailed-1* has also been established as a key signal for informing D/V mesodermal identity (function *2* above). Mice mutants of *Engrailed-1* develop bidorsal paws (Loomis et al., 1996). While the mechanism for D/V mesodermal specification will be described below, the important point here is that *Engrailed-1* may serve two functions in the ventral ectoderm: it restricts *Radical fringe* to appropriately position the AER, and it instructs the D/V identity of underlying mesoderm (Fig. 12–4*B*). Thus, *Engrailed-1* links the position of the AER with D/V specification, ensuring that the AER consistently forms at the border between dorsal and ventral limb domains.

As will be discussed below, *Engrailed-1* represses *Wnt-7a* in the ventral ectoderm. Altering this pathway downstream of *Engrailed-1* does not affect the location at which the AER forms but does affect D/V patterning. Mice mutants of the ectodermally expressed gene *Wnt-7a* develop biventral limbs but have an AER at the correct location (Parr and McMahon, 1995). Conversely, chick limbs that have developed bidorsally due to misexpression of the gene *Wnt-7a* or its mesenchymal target *Lmx-1* have a normal AER (Riddle et al., 1995; Vogel et al., 1995). Thus, the process that positions the AER (function *3* above) can be separated from the process that informs mesoderm D/V identity (function *2* above). It is unclear how the D/V restriction of *Engrailed-1* and *Radical fringe* expression relates to the cellular compartments identified in cell lineage experiments. For example, *Engrailed-1* misexpression in mice and chick limbs can disrupt AER position but will not disrupt cell lineage restriction into dorsal and ventral compartments (Altabef et al., 1997; Kimmel et al., 2000). Thus, the process that positions the AER can also be separated from the process that defines compartment borders between the dorsal and ventral limb ectoderm (function *2* above).

The ectodermal signals described in this section help position the AER at the D/V midline of the limb. Of course, this process must act in conjunction with the mesodermal signals that induce AER formation. The WNT and FGF cascade in the mesoderm triggers morphogenesis of the distal limb ectoderm into an AER, while Engrailed-1 and Radical fringe in the ectoderm ensure that this process happens in the correct place.

The *Notch* Pathway May Be Required Downstream of *Radical fringe* for Proper AER Formation

The ventral expression of *Engrailed-1* helps position a boundary of *Radical fringe*–expressing and nonexpressing cells in the limb ectoderm. The AER will form at this boundary. How then does a boundary of *Radical fringe* lead to formation of the AER? Evidence suggests that a *Radical fringe* boundary triggers signaling through the Notch pathway (see Chapter 39) to induce the AER. It has been demonstrated that the biochemical role of Fringe is to modulate the Notch receptor, making cells less responsive to one Notch ligand, Serrate, but more responsive to another Notch ligand, Delta (Panin et al., 1997; Fleming et al., 1997). The developmental use of this modulation can be seen in wing margin formation in *Drosophila*, where signaling through the Notch receptor is critical for proper margin formation at the D/V border. The dorsal cells of the wing disc express *fringe* as well as the *Serrate* ligand for Notch (Speicher et al., 1994). The Notch ligand encoded by *Delta* is initially expressed throughout the wing (Doherty et al., 1996). Because *fringe* modulates the responsiveness of Notch in dorsal cells, Serrate more potently signals from dorsal to ventral cells and Delta more potently signals from ventral to dorsal cells. Moreover, the Serrate signal upregulates Delta and the Delta signal upregulates Serrate (de Celis and Bray, 1997). The upshot of this positive feedback loop is that expression of the Notch ligands Serrate and Delta becomes focused at the D/V border, and this leads to formation of the wing margin.

Do these parallels extend to vertebrates? *Serrate-2* and *Notch-1* are expressed in the AER of chick and mouse embryos (Swiatek et al., 1994; Myat et al., 1996; Shawber et al., 1996; Laufer et al., 1997). Moreover, mice with a targeted deletion in *Serrate-2* exhibit a hyperplastic AER that encroaches on the underlying mesenchyme. This abnormal regulation of the AER ultimately leads to forelimb and hindlimb syndactyly in adult mice (Sidow et al., 1997; Jiang et al., 1998). Thus, Notch signaling potentially modulated by a *Radical fringe* border may be involved in proper formation of the AER. More data are necessary to elucidate how Notch signaling participates in forming or regulating the AER.

Proper Formation of the AER Requires Distinct Dorsal and Ventral AER Compartments

A number of questions remain about how the AER is formed and positioned. One area of growing interest is the function of genes that subdivide the AER. Classically, the AER has been considered a single entity, a uniform signaling center that promotes the proliferation of underlying mesenchyme; however, expression of *Engrailed-1* through the ventral half of the AER suggests that this classical understanding may be too simplistic (Fig. 12–4*B*). What is the significance of this expression through half the AER?

This question has been assessed by ectopically expressing *Engrailed-1* in the dorsal AER using an AER-specific promoter (Kimmel et al., 2000). In mice hemizygous for the transgene, the AER appears severely fragmented and adult forelimbs and hindlimbs are missing elements of the autopod. In mice homozygous for the transgene, the AER forms but quickly regresses and adults have severe truncations of the forelimbs and almost no hindlimbs. This demonstrates that differences in the dorsal and ventral halves of the AER are critical for its proper formation and maintenance.

This conclusion is upheld by loss-of-function studies. In mice lacking *Engrailed-1* function, the AER is flattened and extends into the ventral ectoderm (Loomis et al., 1996). While the dorsal end of the AER appears to compact normally, the ventral end fails to compact at the midline and occasionally forms a secondary AER. Another gene, *Wnt-7a*, appears to have a role in this formation of rare ectopic AERs. Normally a marker of dorsal ectoderm, *Wnt-7a* ectopically appears in the ventral ectoderm of *Engrailed-1$^{-/-}$* mice and seems to border any secondary AER that forms. However, in *Engrailed-1$^{-/-}$Wnt-7a$^{-/-}$* double-mutant mice, the AER is surprisingly normal and no secondary AER forms (Loomis et al., 1998). Thus, *Wnt-7a* seems to have a role in the failure of the AER to compact in *Engrailed-1* mutant mice. One explanation may be that, normally, *Wnt-7a* confers on dorsal AER the ability to draw AER precursors into a compact ridge (Loomis et al., 1998). In *Engrailed-1$^{-/-}$* mice, ectopic *Wnt-7a* in the ventral ectoderm could then confer the same properties on the ventral AER as well, causing the AER to compact both dorsally and ventrally and resulting in a secondary AER.

While more evidence is needed to prove these models, it is clear that delineating dorsal and ventral compartments in the AER is necessary for its formation, maintenance, and possibly function. It will therefore be interesting to identify and characterize other genes that are patterned within the AER.

p63 May Be Required for Proper AER Formation

In mice carrying mutations in the gene *p63*, the AER fails to form (Yang et al., 1999). Instead, weak *Fgf-8* expression can be detected in the ventral pre-AER ectoderm. The *p63* gene is a homolog of the *p53* tumor-suppressor and is found in basal or progenitor layers of epithelial tissues. In the limb bud, *p63* is expressed in the AER and surrounding ectoderm. It is thought that *p63* is necessary for the pre-AER ectoderm to stratify at the D/V boundary. Therefore, mice lacking *p63* function lack a proper AER and consequently exhibit severe limb truncations.

D/V Patterning

Adult limbs have a D/V polarity to them. In the hand, the formation of hair and nails on the dorsal side and a palm on the ventral side ex-

emplifies this asymmetry. The internal musculoskeletal, vascular, and neural architecture in the limb is also patterned along the D/V axis. In the embryonic limb, this asymmetry is even more intuitive as it is demarcated by the AER. This section describes the molecular mechanisms that inform this D/V asymmetry.

Ectodermal *Wnt-7a* and *Engrailed-1* Control D/V Patterning

Thus far, a signaling interaction between the limb ectoderm and mesoderm has been highlighted in AER induction and limb outgrowth. Another aspect of limb development in which epithelial–mesenchymal crosstalk plays a central role is D/V patterning. The first clues regarding the regulation of D/V patterning came from classical surgical experiments in chick embryos. When chick limb bud ectoderm is removed from the mesoderm, rotated 180 degrees, and fixed back on the limb bud, the polarity of the distal limb structures that develop is likewise inverted about the D/V axis, particularly in distal structures (MacCabe et al., 1974). This finding indicates that D/V polarity is a stable property of the ectoderm at the time the rotations are done and, moreover, that signals from the limb ectoderm instruct the dorsal or ventral fate of underlying mesoderm. What are these signals?

Logical candidates for such signals are genes expressed differentially along the D/V axis (Fig. 12–4*A*). The secreted factor encoded by *Wnt-7a* is expressed in the dorsal but not ventral ectoderm (Dealy et al., 1993; Parr et al., 1993). Misexpression experiments in chick and targeted gene-disruption experiments in mouse demonstrate that this ectodermal factor has a pivotal role in assigning a dorsal fate. When *Wnt-7a* is ectopically expressed on the ventral side of chick limbs, the underlying limb bud mesoderm exhibits bidorsal expression of genes normally restricted to the dorsal mesoderm (Riddle et al., 1995). Conversely, mice defective in *Wnt-7a* develop limbs that are biventral in the distal region, with sole pads on both surfaces of the paws (Parr and McMahon, 1995). Thus, ectodermal *Wnt-7a* provides a dorsalizing signal, in the absense of which limbs become biventral.

As noted above, *Engrailed-1*, a transcription factor expressed in the ventral ectoderm, is also involved in D/V patterning (Fig. 12–4). Ectopic expression of *Engrailed-1* in the dorsal ectoderm of chick limbs represses *Wnt-7a* (Logan et al., 1997). Moreover, in *Engrailed-1* mutant mice, *Wnt-7a* becomes ectopically expressed in the ventral ectoderm (Loomis et al., 1996). As a result, *Engrailed-1$^{-/-}$* mice develop limbs that are bidorsal distally. These observations suggest that *Engrailed-1* functions as a ventralizing factor by restricting *Wnt-7a* to the dorsal ectoderm.

How does *Wnt-7a* in the dorsal ectoderm instruct underlying mesoderm to become dorsal? A key target in the underlying mesenchyme appears to be the LIM-homeodomain protein Lmx-1b, which is expressed specifically in dorsal mesoderm (Fig. 12–4). Interestingly, a related LIM-homeodomain protein, apterous, is similarly expressed in the dorsal domain of the *Drosophila* wing disc, where it is involved in dorsal patterning of the wing (Diaz-Benjumea and Cohen, 1993). Mice carrying a targeted mutation in *Lmx-1b* develop limbs which are morphologically biventral (Chen et al., 1998). Conversely, when *Lmx-1b* is ectopically expressed in the ventral mesoderm of chick limbs, the distal limbs develop a bidorsal phenotype, showing that this gene is sufficient for dorsalizing mesoderm (Vogel et al., 1995; Riddle et al., 1995). When *Wnt-7a* is ectopically expressed in the ventral ectoderm, it induces *Lmx-1b* ectopically in underlying ventral mesoderm, showing that *Wnt-7a* is sufficient to induce expression of this dorsalizing factor (Vogel et al., 1995; Riddle et al., 1995). Consistent with this observation, the ectopic ventral expression of *Wnt-7a* seen in *Engrailed-1* mutant mice is accompanied by ectopic expression of *Lmx-1b* in the ventral mesenchyme, and the resulting limbs are bidorsal distally (Loomis et al., 1998). This ectopic *Lmx-1b* depends on ectopic ventral *Wnt-7a* as it does not occur in *Engrailed-1$^{-/-}$ Wnt-7a$^{-/-}$* double-mutant mice. All of these findings support the conclusion that ectodermal *Wnt-7a* promotes dorsal patterning by inducing *Lmx-1b* in the dorsal mesoderm.

The current model therefore implicates ectodermal genes in D/V specification of the distal limb. Ectodermal *Wnt-7a* is a dorsalizing factor that is restricted from the ventral ectoderm by *Engrailed-1* and acts by inducing *Lmx-1b* in the dorsal mesoderm. The genetic evidence is consistent with the notion that a ventral fate occurs by default in the distal limb and that this state is altered by *Wnt-7a* in the dorsal limb.

While this model accurately predicts the results of several genetic alterations, some questions remain. First, manipulation of these genes appears to influence only the most distal limb structures. Indeed, in the proximal regions of the limb bud, expression and dorsal restriction of *Lmx-1b* are surprisingly normal in *Engrailed-1* and *Wnt-7a* mutants (Loomis et al., 1998). Thus, additional mechanisms may govern the D/V specification of more proximal limb regions. Second, the mechanisms upstream that pattern *Wnt-7a* and *Engrailed-1* in the limb ectoderm remain to be identified. Evidence suggests that D/V information is transferred to the ectoderm from underlying mesodermal structures before the limb bud forms. Grafting and barrier experiments in chick embryos prior to limb bud formation suggest that somites provide a dorsalizing signal and that lateral somatopleure provides a ventralizing signal (Michaud et al., 1997). The molecular details and the relative contribution of ectoderm and mesoderm in establishing D/V patterning upstream of *Wnt-7a* and *Engrailed-1* remain to be characterized. Finally, genes acting downstream of *Lmx-1b* presumably govern the dorsal patterning of muscles, tendons, epithelium, and other limb structures. These genes remain to be discovered.

A/P Patterning

Asymmetry in adult limbs is apparent along the A/P axis. In the hand, differences in length and shape between the thumb on the anterior end and the other four digits have obvious functional importance. This section will describe the molecular mechanisms that have been uncovered for establishing A/P patterning in the limb. Classical tissue manipulations show that the ZPA of the posterior limb bud polarizes the limb along the A/P axis. Thus, three questions will be addressed here. First, what is the molecular nature of this polarizing activity? Second, how do signals from the ZPA act on limb mesenchyme? Third, how is the ZPA correctly positioned in the limb bud?

Sonic hedgehog Mediates Effects of the ZPA

Major progress in understanding A/P patterning was made through manipulations of the chick limb bud. The chick wing is a useful system for addressing this problem because it has three clearly distinct digits, designated 2-3-4 from anterior to posterior. The pattern of the digits can therefore serve as a read-out of A/P positional information. When small pieces of distal posterior mesenchyme are grafted into an ectopic anterior position in the limb bud, a remarkable outcome is seen: mirror-image duplications of the autopod are induced, such that a 4-3-2-2-3-4 digit pattern develops instead of 2-3-4 (Saunders and Gasseling, 1968). Importantly, grafts of quail mesenchyme into chick prove that the additional digits are from the host and not the graft. Thus, the graft both increases proliferation of anterior mesenchyme and changes the fate of this mesenchyme to mirror posterior mesenchyme. The area of posterior mesenchyme capable of this effect is the ZPA (Fig. 12–1*B*).

Several observations have led to the hypothesis that a morphogen mediates the effects of the ZPA. First, to polarize the entire presumptive autopod, the ZPA apparently must influence digit patterning at a distance. Indeed, the ZPA has effects over a distance of 150–200 μm, or 10–20 cell diameters (Honig, 1981). Second, the ZPA seems to influence digit identity in a graded fashion. Indeed, dose dependence can be demonstrated by varying the number of ZPA cells grafted into the anterior limb bud (Tickle, 1981). Grafting a saturating number of cells gives rise to the full 4-3-2-2-3-4 digit duplication, whereas fewer grafted cells result in 3-2-2-3-4 and 2-2-3-4 digit duplications. The hypothesis that a morphogen mediates ZPA effects prompted a search for diffusible signals emanating from the ZPA that are necessary and sufficient for its polarizing activity.

The expression domain of the gene *Sonic hedgehog* (see Chapter 16) was discovered to match that of the operationally defined ZPA in mice and chicks (Fig. 12–5) (Echelard et al., 1993; Riddle et al., 1993). *Sonic hedgehog* was cloned as a putative secreted signal by virtue of

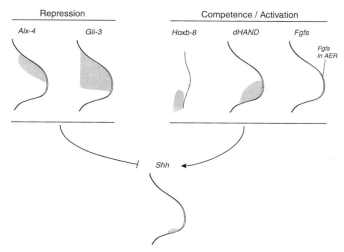

Figure 12–5. Regulation of *Sonic hedgehog (Shh)* expression. Several modes of regulation control the spatial and temporal expression of *Sonic hedgehog*. The genes *Alx-4* and *Gli-3* actively repress *Sonic hedgehog*, confining its expression in the posterior limb mesenchyme. Expression of *Hoxb-8* and *dHAND* correlates with competence to express *Sonic hedgehog*. A positive signal from the apical ectodermal ridge (AER), most likely a fibroblast growth factor (FGF), is required for *Sonic hedgehog* expression.

its homology to the *Drosophila* segment polarity gene *hedgehog*. When chick fibroblasts transfected to express *Sonic hedgehog* are grafted into anterior mesenchyme, they produce the same mirror-image limb as do transplants of the ZPA (Riddle et al., 1993). Recombinant *Sonic hedgehog* protein also produces such ZPA effects (Lopez-Martinez et al., 1995). Additional findings corroborate the conclusion that *Sonic hedgehog* mediates ZPA effects. First, various methods for mimicking the ZPA seem to operate via expression or induction of *Sonic hedgehog*. For example, application of retinoic acid causes mirror duplications (Tickle et al., 1982) and induces *Sonic hedgehog* (Riddle et al., 1993). As another example, grafting pieces of the notochord or floor plate of the neural tube can recapitulate ZPA effects (Wagner et al., 1990), and all of these tissues express *Sonic hedgehog* (Riddle et al., 1993; Echelard et al., 1993; Krauss et al., 1993). Conversely, posterior limb mesenchyme harvested from mice defective in *Sonic hedgehog* exhibits no ZPA activity when grafted into chick limb buds (Chiang et al., 2001). These data convincingly show that *Sonic hedgehog* mediates the effects of the ZPA.

To mediate the effects of the ZPA, *Sonic hedgehog* may act directly as a morphogen or indirectly by inducing secondary signals with polarizing activity. If it acts directly as a morphogen, sonic hedgehog (SHH) must function over a long range and must specify different skeletal elements at different concentration thresholds. This is certainly possible since immunohistochemistry detects SHH protein in a gradient at distances over 200 μm (about 20 cell diameters) anterior from the *Sonic hedgehog* expression domain in the posterior limb bud (Lewis et al., 2001; Zeng et al., 2001). Downstream target genes such as *Patched-1*, the gene encoding the SHH receptor, are also expressed in a similar gradient long distances from the *Sonic hedgehog* expression domain (Goodrich et al., 1996; Marigo et al., 1996). Whether SHH acts directly as a morphogen has been further tested by varying the range or level of its activity. These experiments were performed in mice and lend strong support to the idea that SHH acts as a morphogen. First, the range of SHH activity has been varied by altering its processing. The active form of SHH is produced by autocatalytic cleavage. This process generates an active N-terminal fragment of SHH, which is covalently linked to cholesterol (Porter et al., 1996). Mice have been designed to express the active N-terminal fragment of SHH such that none of the SHH protein undergoes cholesterol modification (Lewis et al., 2001). The range of SHH protein in these mutant mice, as indicated by SHH protein levels and activation of target genes, is sharply curtailed to the posterior limb bud. As a result, a 1-4-5 digit pattern develops instead of the normal mouse 1-2-3-4-5 digit pattern, from anterior to posterior. This suggests that long-range activity of SHH in more anterior regions of the autopod is necessary for digits 2 and 3 to form. In contrast, when the level of SHH activity is reduced using a conditional knockout, a 1-2-3/4 digit pattern results (Lewis et al., 2001). Presumably, the low levels of SHH activity in these latter mice are sufficient for anterior digits to form, but highest levels of SHH activity are required for posterior digits to form. Thus, these two experiments suggest that SHH is required over a long range and that the SHH gradient that exists in the autopod patterns different digits at distinct levels of activity.

It remains possible that, in addition to its direct action, *Sonic hedgehog* acts indirectly by activating a cascade of secondary signals. These secondary signals could contribute to a polarizing gradient across the autopod. One possible secondary signal is *Bone morphogenetic protein-2 (Bmp-2)*, which is expressed in the posterior mesenchyme in an area broader than *Sonic hedgehog* (Francis et al., 1994). *Bmp-2* can be induced by ectopic *Sonic hedgehog* and is drastically reduced in the absence of *Sonic hedgehog* (Laufer et al., 1994; Kawakami et al., 1996; Chiang et al., 2001). However, when *Bmp-2* is ectopically expressed in the anterior mesenchyme, it can at most duplicate digit 2 to yield a 2-2-3-4 pattern, showing that *Bmp-2* has only weak polarizing activity (Duprez et al., 1996). Noggin (see Chapter 25), an antagonist of BMPs, appears to interfere with ZPA effects when added after *Sonic hedgehog*; in such limbs, multiple digits form in response to anterior *Sonic hedgehog*, but these digits often are of the same identity, yielding a 3-3-3-4 pattern (Drossopoulou et al., 2000). Still, misexpression of *Noggin* in the posterior of developing chick limb buds has no effect on A/P patterning and hence does not provide support for the idea that BMP-2 is an important component of polarizing activity (Capdevila and Johnson, 1998). More data are necessary to clarify the role, if any, of *Bmp-2* in polarization activity. Interestingly, observations of *Sonic hedgehog* mutant mice are consistent with a model that BMP-2 can act independently of SHH to specify the anteriormost digit in the mouse autopod (Lewis et al., 2001). Indeed, in the absence of SHH, the hindlimbs retain a digital element that resembles digit 1. Furthermore, when the range of SHH is restricted to the posterior by abrogating cholesterol modification, digits 2 and 3 are lost from the anterior autopod but digit 1 still forms. In both of these *Sonic hedgehog* mutants, expression of *Bmp-2* is reduced but not eliminated. Thus, it remains a possibility that BMP-2 specifies the anteriormost digit 1 in mice. Again, more data are necessary to clarify this possible role of *Bmp-2*.

Though manipulations of the ZPA implicate *Sonic hedgehog* in A/P patterning of the autopod, the proximal extent of its influence is not obvious from these experiments. A mouse mutant in *Sonic hedgehog* reveals that this gene is required for normal formation of the autopod and zeugopod but not the stylopod (Chiang et al., 2001). The humerus and femur form normally in mutant mice. In contrast, the mutant forelimb exhibits only a single zeugopod element and a single autopod element, and the mutant hindlimb exhibits severely truncated zeugopod elements and a single digit in the autopod. The elements that do form in these limbs are not simple cylinders but have A/P morphological asymmetries. Moreover, polar gene expression is still observed in early limb buds of mutant mice, suggesting that additional mechanisms encode A/P information independently of *Sonic hedgehog*. Indeed, the early limb bud must already have A/P information to attain the proper localized expression of *Sonic hedgehog*, as will be discussed below. Nonetheless, *Sonic hedgehog* is the molecule assayed in ZPA transplants which causes digit duplicates and appears to play a key role in establishing a normal A/P pattern.

Sonic hedgehog May Influence A/P Digit Identity by Modulating Signals in the Interdigital Mesenchyme

Sonic hedgehog establishes a gradient of polarizing activity in the early limb bud. Since *Sonic hedgehog* is no longer expressed by the time digits actually form, other factors must provide a molecular memory of A/P positional information. It had been assumed that such information was carried in the cells of the future digit cartilage, but it now appears that the memory is carried in the interdigital mesenchyme. This idea emerged from experimental manipulations of the chick foot.

In the chick foot, the four digits can be easily distinguished because each has a different number of phalanges and the phalanges have different morphology such that the digit identity can be assessed by studying of the bones. Assuming that the number of phalanges indicates digit identity, changes in the number of phalanges can be interpreted as a transformation of digit identity. *Sonic hedgehog* expression ceases in the autopod when a cartilage primordium of the digits begins to appear but before the digits have developed morphological differences. If digit primordia are bisected in this time window, the posterior half develops as it would prior to bisection, but the anterior half appears to undergo a homeotic transformation, taking on the digit identity of the next anterior digit. This observation implied that digit identity was not a fixed property of the digit primordium and could be altered even after *Sonic hedgehog* expression disappears.

Further manipulations supported the idea that A/P identity was instructed by the interdigital mesoderm (Dahn and Fallon, 2000). The interdigital mesoderm is an area of mesenchyme between the condensing cartilage of the digits, and it ultimately regresses by apoptosis to generate the free digits of adults. If the interdigital mesoderm between the primordia of digit 2 and digit 3 is removed, digit 2 transforms into a digit 1, but digit 3 develops normally. If the interdigital mesoderm between primordia of digit 3 and digit 4 is removed, digit 3 transforms into a digit 2, but digit 4 develops normally. These observations are consistent with a model that interdigital mesoderm determines digit identity. The positional information is graded: more posterior interdigital mesoderm specifies more posterior digit identities, and digit identity is governed by the most posterior cues it receives.

The nature of the interdigital cues is unclear. One hypothesis is that BMP activity encodes this A/P positional information, with higher levels of BMP specifying more posterior digit fates. Indeed, BMP-2, BMP-4, and BMP-7 are expressed in a graded fashion in the interdigital mesenchyme. To test this idea, beads soaked in N-Sonic hedgehog were placed in interdigital mesoderm as a way of upregulating *Bmp-2*, *Bmp-4*, and *Bmp-7* (Dahn and Fallon, 2000). Indeed, N-Sonic hedgehog caused flanking digits to develop with an additional phalanx, interpreted as a posterior transformation. However, it is unclear whether the extra phalanx was due to BMPs or to the maintenance of FGFs in the AER by prolonged exposure to Sonic hedgehog (see below). Coadministration of Noggin, a BMP antagonist, blocked the ability of N-Sonic hedgehog to posteriorize digit identity, potentially arguing that BMPs are responsible for the extra phalanx. However, a definitive interpretation of these data cannot be made without considering the role of BMPs in cartilage formation. BMPs are critical for prechondrogenic condensation and chondrocyte differentiation, and Noggin is known to block these process (Capdevila and Johnson, 1998; Pizette and Niswander, 2000). Thus, the effects of applying interdigital Noggin and Sonic hedgehog are difficult to interpret. Finally, direct application of beads soaked in BMP-2 or BMP-4 into interdigital mesoderm fails to posteriorize digits; instead, cartilage and joint abnormalities result, arguing against a role for BMPs in informing digit identity (Dahn and Fallon, 2000). Nonetheless, it is clear that the interdigital mesenchyme has a memory of early polarizing activity in the limb and plays a key role in directing digit patterning. The molecular nature of this memory remains to be clarified.

Sonic hedgehog Regulates *HoxD* Gene Expression

Though it is still not completely clear how the ZPA mediates A/P patterning, it is known the ZPA can modulate genes that pattern elements along the P/D axis. In particular, *Sonic hedgehog* can influence expression of the 5' *HoxD* genes. The genes *Hoxd-13, Hoxd-12, Hoxd-11, Hoxd-10,* and *Hoxd-9* are expressed in the posterior limb mesenchyme, raising the possibility that they are regulated by the ZPA (Dolle and Duboule, 1989). Indeed, when the ZPA is grafted to the anterior mesenchyme, ectopic and mirror-image *HoxD* expression occurs (Nohno et al., 1991; Izpisua-Belmonte et al., 1991; Riddle et al., 1993).

The patterns of *HoxD* ectopic expression induced by *Sonic hedgehog* change over time, indicating that the way limb mesenchyme interprets *Sonic hedgehog* can change. Three phases of *HoxD* gene expression have been reported, and these will be described in more detail later (Nelson et al., 1996). Here, suffice it to say that when *HoxD* genes are expressed in the presumptive stylopod, their expression is independent of *Sonic hedgehog*. However, when *HoxD* expression occurs in the presumptive zeugopod, it follows a posteriorly nested pattern, with *Hoxd-13* closest to the ZPA and *Hoxd-12*, *Hoxd-11*, *Hoxd-10*, and *Hoxd-9* more broad and anterior. In this phase, application of *Sonic hedgehog* to the anterior mesenchyme will activate these *HoxD* genes in a similar, mirror-image, nested pattern (Nelson et al., 1996). In the next phase, *HoxD* expression appears to pattern the presumptive autopod. At this time, *HoxD* expression follows an opposite posteriorly nested pattern, with *Hoxd-9* closest to the ZPA and *Hoxd-10*, *Hoxd-11*, *Hoxd-12*, and *Hoxd-13* more broad and anterior. When *Sonic hedgehog* is ectopically applied in this phase, *Hox* genes are again induced but the mirror-image *HoxD* gene expression is opposite from that induced in the previous phase. Thus, the way limb mesenchyme interprets *Sonic hedgehog* changes over time, and this change corresponds to differential patterning along the P/D axis.

Interestingly, while *Sonic hedgehog* is sufficient to induce ectopic *HoxD* expression in an appropriately nested pattern, observations of mice lacking *Sonic hedgehog* support the idea that the earliest phase of *Hox* gene expression is patterned independently of *Sonic hedgehog*. In mice mutant for *Sonic hedgehog*, expression of *HoxD* genes is greatly reduced; nonetheless, these genes can still be detected in an asymmetrical expression pattern (Chiang et al., 2001). Thus, additional mechanisms likely induce and regulate the expression of *HoxD* genes. Once these genes are induced, *Sonic hedgehog* may be required to amplify or maintain them in correct patterns as well as to regulate their expression in subsequent phases.

Proper Positioning of *Sonic hedgehog* Requires Competence, Activation, and Repression

Given its potency in patterning the limb, the spatial and temporal control of *Sonic hedgehog* must be tightly regulated. Studies on the control of the ZPA have uncovered three modes of regulating precisely where and when *Sonic hedgehog* is expressed. First, intrinsic cues may confer competence for expression of *Sonic hedgehog*. Second, extrinsic cues are necessary for induction of *Sonic hedgehog*. Third, intrinsic cues can prohibit the expression of *Sonic hedgehog*. These three modes of regulation will be described here.

One observation that informed the regulation of *Sonic hedgehog* is that a broad area of tissue can express *Sonic hedgehog* if grafted into the anterior limb mesenchyme. For example, before the discovery of *Sonic hedgehog*, studies mapping polarizing activity discovered a high level of polarizing activity in the flank mesoderm of the presumptive wing field just prior to wing bud outgrowth (Hornbruch and Wolpert, 1991). However, *Sonic hedgehog* is not normally expressed in this region before limb outgrowth (Echelard et al., 1993; Riddle et al., 1993). In fact, only when grafted into the anterior mesenchyme does this tissue express *Sonic hedgehog* and exhibit ZPA effects (Yonei et al., 1995). These experiments manifest two aspects of *Sonic hedgehog* regulation: cells must be competent to express *Sonic hedgehog*, and they can do so only in a permissive environment.

What defines the competence of cells to express *Sonic hedgehog*? Two genes have been implicated in this role: *Hoxb-8* and *dHAND* (Fig. 12–5). The expression domain of the gene *Hoxb-8* overlaps the area of the lateral plate mesoderm capable of polarizing activity, making it a good candidate for this competence factor (Lu et al., 1997). In the chick, *Hoxb-8* is upregulated in the lateral plate mesoderm and its anterior limit coincides with the anterior border of the wing field; at the time of *Sonic hedgehog* induction, *Hoxb-8* is expressed through the posterior half of the forelimb mesenchyme. Transgenic mice have been made expressing *Hoxb-8* under the control of a promoter that drives ectopic expression of *Hoxb-8* in the anterior mesenchyme. These transgenic mice exhibit ectopic *Sonic hedgehog* expression in the anterior mesenchyme with ensuing mirror-image duplications of the forelimb (Charite et al., 1994). Thus, *Hoxb-8* may define the competence of cells for expressing *Sonic hedgehog*. While this intrinsic cue may be sufficient for competence, these experiments do not prove it is necessary for cells to express *Sonic hedgehog*. In fact, mice lacking *Hoxb-8* have normal limbs, demonstrating that *Hoxb-8* is not re-

quired for A/P patterning of the forelimb, perhaps due to functional redundancy (van den Akker et al., 1999).

A second gene that may define the competence of cells to express *Sonic hedgehog* is the basic helix-loop-helix transcription factor *dHAND*, which was isolated for its role in cardiac morphogenesis (Srivastava et al., 1995). Prior to limb bud formation, *dHAND* is expressed throughout the lateral plate mesoderm, but it subsequently becomes restricted to the posterior end of the emerging limb bud in both chick (Fernandez-Teran et al., 2000) and mouse (Charite et al., 2000). This expression domain precedes and encompasses the domain of *Sonic hedgehog*. When *dHAND* is ectopically expressed in the anterior chick limb bud, digit duplications occur that resemble the effects of moderate polarizing activity in the anterior limb bud (Fernandez-Teran et al., 2000). Similarly, transgenic mice designed to express *dHAND* throughout the limb exhibit dramatic mirror duplications of autopod and zeugopod posterior elements (Charite et al., 2000). In both chick and mouse, these phenotypes are paralleled by ectopic gene expression of *Sonic hedgehog* and its response gene *Hoxd-11*, as expected. Conversely, mice defective in *dHAND* have small, underdeveloped limbs that fail to express *Sonic hedgehog* (Charite et al., 2000). Thus, dHAND is both sufficient and necessary for initiating *Sonic hedgehog* expression and polarizing activity in the posterior limb bud. In both chick and mouse, *Sonic hedgehog* appears to positively regulate *dHAND* expression, suggesting a feedback loop between the two genes. However, polar expression of *dHAND* does not require *Sonic hedgehog* since *dHAND* retains a posterior, though greatly reduced, expression domain in *Sonic hedgehog* null mice (Charite et al., 2000). This observation reiterates that some A/P information must exist independently of *Sonic hedgehog*.

While the *Hoxb-8* and *dHAND* expression domains may delineate tissue capable of polarizing activity, not all of this tissue will express *Sonic hedgehog*. Additional factors must be required to activate *Sonic hedgehog* in competent cells. Indeed, in the limb, *Sonic hedgehog* is specifically activated in the posterior mesenchyme adjacent to the AER or in tissue grafted adjacent to the AER in anterior mesenchyme. Furthermore, removal of the AER results in loss of polarizing activity and *Sonic hedgehog* expression (Vogel and Tickle, 1993; Laufer et al., 1994; Niswander et al., 1994). This suggests that an extrinsic cue from the AER is necessary for *Sonic hedgehog* expression. Indeed, *Sonic hedgehog* expression is maintained if an FGF-soaked bead is applied to a limb bud concomitantly with AER removal, suggesting that an FGF is the required extrinsic cue (Fig. 12–5).

If *Hoxb-8* and *dHAND* indeed define tissue competent to express *Sonic hedgehog*, what controls *Hoxb-8* and *dHAND* expression? There is evidence that retinoic acid plays a role in inducing these genes and ultimately the ZPA. Prior to the discovery of *Sonic hedgehog*, it was shown that ectopic retinoic acid applied to the anterior limb bud can cause ZPA-like duplications (Tickle et al., 1982). When retinoic acid is applied to the anterior mesenchyme, *Hoxb-8* expression is stimulated first, followed by *dHAND* expression and then *Sonic hedgehog* expression, leading to digit duplications (Riddle et al., 1993; Lu et al., 1997; Fernandez-Teran et al., 2000). Conversely, when retinoid synthesis is blocked or retinoic acid receptor antagonists are applied to the limb field, *Hoxb-8* expression is downregulated and *Sonic hedgehog* activation is blocked (Stratford et al., 1996; Helms et al., 1996; Lu et al., 1997). These results indicate that retinoic acid has a critical role in forming the ZPA.

A naturally occurring manifestation of aberrant ZPA regulation is pre-axial (anterior) polydactyly. Numerous mouse mutants exhibiting preaxial polydactyly have ectopic anterior expression of *Sonic hedgehog* (Chan et al., 1995; Masuya et al., 1995, 1997). Thus, while a posteriorization of digits is not obvious (because the posterior four digits all have similar morphology), these phenotypes are considered to be related to the digit duplications observed following ectopic ZPA grafts in chick. Ectopic anterior expression of *Sonic hedgehog* in these mutants suggests that active repression may be an additional mechanism for regulating the ZPA in normal limbs.

Characterization of a few polydactylous mutants concurs with this idea. The mutant *Strong's luxoid (lst)* exhibits preaxial polydactyly, and mutations map to the gene *Alx-4* (Qu et al., 1998; Takahashi et al., 1998). The *Alx-4* gene encodes a transcription factor that contains a paired-type homeodomain. During development, *Alx-4* is expressed in various mesenchymal tissues, including the anterior limb mesenchyme, in a pattern opposite the distribution of polarizing activity (Fig. 12–5) (Hornbruch and Wolpert, 1991; Qu et al., 1997; Takahashi et al., 1998). Both *lst* mice and mice with a targeted mutation in *Alx-4* exhibit preaxial polydactyly, and this is preceded embryonically by ectopic anterior *Sonic hedgehog* expression, (Qu et al., 1997, 1998). These observations put forth the model that *Alx-4* suppresses *Sonic hedgehog* from expression in the anterior limb mesenchyme.

Another polydactylous mouse that has been characterized is the *Extra Toes* (*Xt*) mutant. Again, preaxial polydactyly in *Xt* mice is preceded by ectopic anterior *Sonic hedgehog* expression (Masuya et al., 1995). This phenotype results from a mutation in the gene *Gli-3* (Hui and Joyner, 1993; Schimmang et al., 1993; see also Chapter 20). Heterozygous *Xt/+* mice exhibit preaxial polydactyly of the hindlimbs, while homozygous *Xt/Xt* mice exhibit severe polydactyly of up to nine digits in both the forelimb and hindlimb. The heteroyzgous *Xt/+* is thought to mimic the Greig cephalopolysyndactyly disorder in humans, which also maps to *GLI-3* (Vortkamp et al., 1991). The *Gli-3* gene encodes a zinc-finger transcription factor (Ruppert et al., 1990). Its expression in the limb bud begins throughout the A/P axis but is restricted to the anterior mesenchyme as *Sonic hedgehog* initiates expression (Fig. 12–5) (Marigo et al., 1996). The ectopic appearance of *Sonic hedgehog* when *Gli-3* is lost from anterior mesenchyme suggests that *Gli-3* functions to repress *Sonic hedgehog*. This is quite similar to the role of *Cubitus interruptus*, the *Drosophila Gli* homolog; *Cubitus interruptus* is expressed in anterior cells of the wing disc, where it confines Hedgehog secretion to posterior cells (Dominguez et al., 1996). Thus, *Gli-3* may assist patterning of *Sonic hedgehog* by confining it to the posterior limb mesenchyme.

While loss of function of the two putative repressors, *Alx-4* and *Gli-3*, leads to ectopic anterior *Sonic hedgehog* expression, it is not clear how these two pathways interact in regulating the ZPA. Interestingly, in *Alx-4* mutant mice, *Gli-3* is not lost from the anterior mesenchyme and therefore coincides with ectopic anterior *Sonic hedgehog* expression (Qu et al., 1997; Milenkovic et al., 1999). This suggests that these and other regulators of *Sonic hedgehog* expression may act independently. Also, this emphasizes that misexpression experiments with putative regulators need to be performed to assess their exact role in modulating *Sonic hedgehog* expression.

To summarize, several modes of regulation have been elucidated for controlling the spatial and temporal expression of *Sonic hedgehog* (Fig. 12–5). Expression of *Hoxb-8* and *dHAND* correlates with competence to express *Sonic hedgehog*. However, cells also require a positive signal from the AER, most likely an FGF. Finally, preaxial polydactyly mutants suggest that *Sonic hedgehog* is confined to the posterior limb mesenchyme by active repression from the anterior mesenchyme. These prodigious modes of regulation collaborate to ensure that the ZPA forms in the correct place.

P/D Patterning

Perhaps the most obvious asymmetry in adult limbs is along the P/D axis. Differences in the structure of skeletal elements from the proximal humerus to the distal phalanges have obvious importance in the functionality of the limb. However, of all the asymmetrical axes of limb development, patterning along the P/D axis is least understood in molecular terms. This section will discuss models for how different structures are patterned along the P/D axis as the limb develops. A classical hypothesis, the progress zone model, will first be described. Then, evidence challenging the progress zone model will be presented and alternative models for patterning along the P/D axis will be discussed.

The Progress Zone Model: Time in the Progress Zone Specifies P/D Fate

Most ideas about how P/D patterning occurs have come from classical tissue manipulations. A central experiment involves surgical removal of the AER. The AER is required for outgrowth of the limb, during which proximal structures form first and distal structures form last. When the AER is removed, limb outgrowth is drastically reduced, resulting in distal truncations of the adult limb. Importantly, the extent of the truncations depends on the time in limb development at which the AER is removed. Early removal of the AER results in truncations of both distal and proximal structures (e.g., loss of the zeugopod and autopod), whereas later removal of the AER results in more distal truncations (e.g., loss of only the autopod). That limb outgrowth is reduced following removal is not surprising since the AER is a source of FGF signals that are thought to promote the proliferation of cells in underlying mesenchyme. However, it is not obvious why the level of truncation due to AER removal changes over time.

One explanation might be that the AER presents different signals over time to the underlying mesenchyme such that early signals specify proximal structures and late signals specify distal structures. However, this hypothesis would predict that transplanting an old AER onto young limb mesoderm would lead to loss of proximal structures and formation of distal structures. In fact, complete limbs form in these heterochronic transplants (Rubin and Saunders, 1972). Definitive evidence against the notion that AER signals change over time is that a bead soaked in a single FGF can entirely replace the AER in forming a complete limb with normal P/D patterning (Niswander et al., 1993; Fallon et al., 1994; Vogel et al., 1996). Though signals from the AER may change over time, these changes are not necessary for P/D patterning.

A longstanding model for P/D patterning is the progress zone model (Fig. 12–6) (Summerbell et al., 1973). The progress zone is a label for the region of distal mesenchyme about 200 μm that lies immediately under the AER. The progress zone model argues that limb mesenchymal cells have an autonomous "clock" that progressively changes the specification of cells to more distal fates. Thus, cells are said to be progressively distalized. The clock remains active under the influence of the AER, allowing cells in the progress zone that are in proximity to the AER to be progressively distalized. Once the cells exit the progress zone, however, they are out of range of the influence of the AER, so their distalization clock shuts off and their P/D specification becomes fixed. Thus, the longer cells spend in the progress zone under the influence of the AER, the more distal their specification will be. Cells that leave the progress zone early will develop into proximal structures, whereas cells that leave the progress zone later will develop into distal structures. This model nicely explains why truncations would vary with the time of AER removal. When the AER is removed, the distalization clock is shut off and cells have not been in the progress zone long enough to assume distal fates; thus, distal structures are missing. The earlier the AER is removed, the less time cells spend in the progress zone and the more proximal the truncation. An additional observation that is explained by the progress zone model is the effect of irradiation on limbs (Wolpert et al., 1979). X-Irradiation of early limbs reduces the rate at which cells leave the progress zone, hence increasing the time cells spend there. As a result, proximal structures are lost. Increasing the dose of irradiation leads to greater loss of proximal structures, but distal structures remain intact. This observation is interpreted as a sign that slowing the exit from the progress zone forces cells to be specified more distally, therefore leading to loss of proximal structures.

The progress zone model sets several criteria. First, cells in the progress zone must be capable of progressive respecification from more proximal to more distal fates. In regard to D/V and A/P specification, classical experiments suggest that cells in the progress zone do remain uncommitted. For example, manipulations that alter D/V specification, such as ectodermal reversals, or that alter A/P specification, such as ZPA grafts, are interpreted to suggest that cells in the progress zone remain uncommitted to these axes (MacCabe et al., 1974; Summerbell and Lewis, 1975). In regard to the P/D axis, however, lineage experiments suggest that cells are committed to a P/D fate early in limb development and progressive respecification does not occur (Dudley and Tabin, unpublished data). These data, contrary to the progress zone model, will be described below.

Second, an autonomous clock must register the time cells spend in the progress zone and encode that time into P/D positional identity. An obvious way to register time in the progress zone is by number of

Figure 12–6. Models for proximal/distal (P/D) patterning. The progress zone model is compared to the progenitor expansion model in a time course of limb development. According to the progress zone model, cells in the limb mesenchyme have an autonomous "clock" that progressively changes the specification of cells to more distal fates. The clock remains active in cells in the progress zone (PZ), so these cells are progressively distalized. Once cells exit the PZ, the clock shuts off and their proximal/distal specification becomes fixed. Thus, cells that leave the PZ early will develop into proximal structures, whereas cells that leave the PZ later will develop into distal structures. In contrast, the progenitor expansion model states that distal mesenchyme of the early limb is already stratified into stylopod, zeugopod, and autopod progenitor populations. These progenitor populations expand to attain a threshold number of cells necessary to form a skeletal element. These skeletal elements form as progenitors move proximally and begin to differentiate. AER, apical ectodermal ridge.

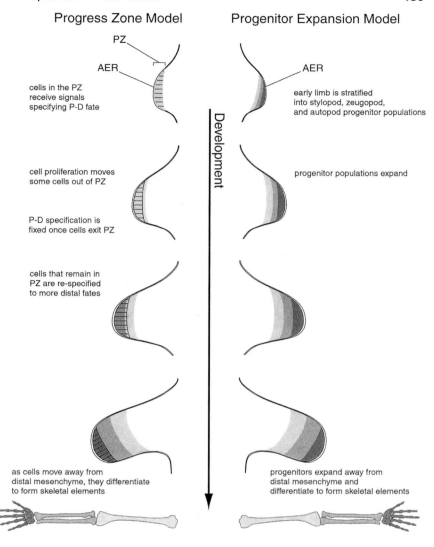

cell cycles. However, the proliferation rate of cells does not change as cells exit the progress zone (Dudley and Tabin, unpublished data), so this parameter must cease to influence specification once cells exit the progress zone. This possibility has not been demonstrated.

Third, the progress zone model predicts a permissive signal from the AER that allows the specification clock to operate in progress zone cells. Given that FGFs can entirely replace the AER, this permissive signal would likely be an FGF. As described below, this prediction has been challenged by studies of mice in which FGF activity has been eliminated. Another possibility is that the AER is the source of an instructive signal and duration of exposure to this signal influences cell specification. However, this model further requires that an FGF signal has a cumulative influence on cell fate in addition to a mitogenic role. None of these criteria has been demonstrated.

Alternative Models for P/D Patterning

Any model for AER function must take into account that beads soaked in FGF can entirely substitute the AER to form a normal limb. The progress zone model argues that signals from the AER are necessary to allow cells in the progress zone to be progressively distalized. Removal of the AER stops the distalization, leading to loss of distal structures; but the presence of FGF, as with FGF-soaked beads, can prevent these distal truncations. This suggests that an FGF is the AER signal that allows progressive distalization of cells in the progress zone. One way to test this prediction is to eliminate FGF activity in the AER. To this end, mice have been generated with a conditional double knock-out of *Fgf-4* and *Fgf-8* in the AER (Sun et al., 2002).

The promoter driving the conditional knockout in these mice is expressed after *Fgf-4* and *Fgf-8* expression initiates in the forelimbs, so *Fgf-4* and *Fgf-8* are transiently expressed but then inactivated in the forelimbs. According to the progress zone model, loss of FGF activity in the AER should curtail the distalization of cells and hence cause preferential loss of distal structures. However, the forelimbs of double knockout mice develop skeletal structures along the full extent of the P/D axis, and abnormalities are observed in all levels of this axis. This result demonstrates that these FGF proteins are not necessary to distalize cells and, thus, does not support the progress zone model.

Another prediction of the progress zone model is that an absence of FGF at early stages followed by restoration of FGF at late stages of limb outgrowth should delay distalization and thereby cause preferential loss of distal structures. In fact, the opposite occurs. This experiment has been performed in mice lacking only *Fgf-8* in the AER. Since *Fgf-8* precedes expression of other *Fgf* genes in the AER, these mutant mice lack any FGF signals from the AER at the earliest stages of limb outgrowth; but in later stages, other *Fgf* genes, such as *Fgf-4*, appear. Thus, in the AER of these mutant mice, FGF is absent at early stages but present at later stages; but rather than losing distal structures preferentially, mutant hindlimbs exhibit *phocomelia*, a preferential loss of proximal structures. The femur is almost entirely absent, whereas the tibia and fibula are only mildly hypoplastic and only one digit is missing. This result is contrary to the progress zone model.

A third prediction of the progress zone model is that the P/D specification of cells inside the progress zone is not fixed and is distalized over time. This changing specification becomes fixed once cells leave the progress zone. This tenet of the progress zone model has been examined by cell lineage studies in chick limbs (Dudley et al., 2002). Cells in the early wing bud can be labeled with dye or retroviral infection, and the progeny of labeled cells can be mapped as the wing develops. Consistent with the progress zone model, all of the progeny of cells labeled outside the putative progress zone are restricted to a particular segment along the P/D axis. In contrast, one might expect that as cells in the progress zone proliferate, the progeny of a single cell would acquire different P/D fates as they exit the progress zone at different times. As a result, labeled progeny might appear in different limb segments along the P/D axis. This anticipated result never occurs. Instead, all of the progeny of cells labeled inside the putative progress zone are restricted to a particular segment along the P/D axis. Cells just under the AER give rise to the developing autopod, whereas cells farther away give rise to either the zeugopod or the stylopod. This counters the notion of a progress zone in the distal mesenchyme in which P/D cell fates are constantly changing. Instead, the distal mesenchyme may be stratified into domains of cells corresponding to different segments along the P/D axis, and the fate of cells is specified very early in limb outgrowth.

The chick lineage analyses are consistent with a new view of P/D patterning in limb outgrowth (Dudley et al., 2002). When the limb bud emerges, it appears that the distal mesenchyme is stratified into stylopod, zeugopod, and autopod progenitor populations. These progenitor populations expand to attain a threshold number of cells necessary to form a skeletal element. The most distal cells receive signals preventing differentiation. More proximal cells no longer receive these signals and initiate differentiation. Thus, a wave of differentiation and condensation occurs from proximal to distal, forming the stylopod first and the autopod last.

Analyses of FGF mouse mutants that challenge the progress zone model are in accord with this new view (Sun et al., 2002). In the forelimbs of *Fgf-4* and *Fgf-8* double knockout mice, loss of FGF throughout much of limb outgrowth diminishes the expansion of progenitors of all limb segments, so skeletal elements of all segments are reduced in size. Furthermore, the phocomelia observed in the hindlimbs of *Fgf-8* knockout mice can also be explained. As described above, FGF is absent at early stages but present at later stages in the hindlimbs of these mice. Because the stylopod progenitor population condenses first, it cannot expand to a necessary threshold size before it condenses. In contrast, the zeugopod and autopod progenitor populations condense later, so the FGF signals that appear later are sufficient to expand these populations before they condense. Thus, the stylopod is almost entirely absent, whereas the zeugopod and autopod are only mildly affected.

The new view of P/D patterning argues that cell positional identity is already specified in the early limb bud (Fig. 12–6). Proper formation of skeletal elements requires the expansion of specified cells to a threshold size. For this model to be correct, it must also account for the classical experimental data previously viewed as evidence for the progress zone model. The first classical observation is that earlier removal of the AER leads to more proximal truncations. The original interpretation of this result assumed that removal of the AER would allow remaining mesenchyme to differentiate as specified, so removal of the AER at different time points could be a way to generate a temporal specification map (Summerbell, 1974). However, this interpretation does not consider the effects of AER removal on cell death and proliferation in underlying mesenchyme. Indeed, analyses in chick limbs have revealed that significant cell death and decreased proliferation occur following removal of the AER (Dudley et al., 2002). Removal of the AER at different times results in a domain of cell death of approximately 200 μm in the distal mesenchyme. By corresponding this domain of cell death with detailed fate maps of the progenitors giving rise to each skeletal element, it becomes clear that cell death in earlier limb buds will eliminate progenitors of more skeletal elements, leading to more proximal truncations. Thus, the cell death and loss of proliferation that result from AER removal can entirely explain the limb truncations that ensue. Moreover, the occurrence of cell death and decreased proliferation following AER removal puts into question the temporal specification map that argued for the progress zone model.

The second classical observation supporting the progress zone model is that X-irradiation can lead to preferential loss of proximal skeletal elements. It was initially interpreted that X-irradiation slows the exit of cells from the progress zone, thereby causing greater distalization and loss of proximal structures. However, an alternative interpretation takes into consideration the distal mesenchyme where progenitor populations are maintained in an undifferentiated and proliferative state. After X-irradiation, these distal progenitor populations would be able to restore their numbers before they differentiate. In contrast, more proximal progenitor populations have begun to differentiate and undergo limited proliferation, and these populations would be less able to recover from X-irradiation. Given the stratified organization of skeletal element progenitors, progenitors of proximal skeletal elements would thus be more susceptible to X-irradiation than the progenitors of distal skeletal elements.

To summarize, several mouse *Fgf* mutants and chick lineage experiments counter the progress zone model and support a new view of P/D patterning in the limb (Fig. 12–6). This view posits that distal limb mesenchyme is stratified into stylopod, zeugopod, and autopod progenitor populations. These progenitor populations expand to attain a threshold number of cells necessary to form a skeletal element, and these skeletal elements form as progenitors move away from the distal mesenchyme and begin to differentiate. This model not only explains the recent mouse *Fgf* mutants and chick lineage experiments but also is consistent with classical experimental observations previously thought to support the progress zone model. The molecular basis for progenitor specification, expansion, and differentiation remains to be elucidated.

COORDINATING THREE AXES OF PATTERNING

The mechanisms described above for patterning along the D/V, A/P, and P/D axes must be synchronized in time and space for a normal limb to form. How are these mechanisms coordinated? This section will describe evidence that the distinct signals involved in patterning the three axes are in fact interdependent such that interfering with signals important for one axis will compromise patterning or growth along all three axes. Evidence for a positive feedback loop between the AER and ZPA will be presented, followed by data that couple D/V patterning and the ZPA.

A Positive Feedback Loop between *Sonic hedgehog* and *Fgf-4* Integrates A/P Patterning and Limb Outgrowth

Throughout limb outgrowth, the operationally defined ZPA and the expression domain of *Sonic hedgehog* are found proximal to the posterior AER (Maccabe et al., 1973; Riddle et al., 1993). Both disappear at the time the AER regresses. These observations suggest that the AER may play a role in maintaining the ZPA during limb outgrowth. To test this, the posterior AER was surgically removed. Within 24 hours after this manipulation, *Sonic hedgehog* expression and polarizing activity disappear (Vogel and Tickle, 1993; Laufer et al., 1994). Thus, signals from the posterior AER are necessary to maintain the ZPA (Fig. 12–7). *Fgf-4* is expressed in the posterior AER (Niswander and Martin, 1992) and, hence, is a good candidate for mediating this signal. Indeed, a bead soaked in FGF-4 is sufficient to maintain operationally defined polarizing activity and *Sonic hedgehog* expression after removal of the posterior AER (Vogel and Tickle, 1993; Niswander et al., 1993; Laufer et al., 1994). However, in *Fgf-4* mutant mice, *Sonic hedgehog* expression appears normal, indicating that *Fgf-4* is not alone necessary to maintain the ZPA (Sun et al., 2000; Moon et al., 2000). Two other genes, *Fgf-9* and *Fgf-17*, are also expressed in the posterior AER. Like *Fgf-4*, loss of *Fgf-17* does not disrupt *Sonic hedgehog* maintenance or normal limb development (Sun et al., 2000; Xu et al., 2000). However, though it has not been shown, it is likely that these FGFs act in a redundant manner to mediate signaling from the AER to the ZPA.

Just as signals from the AER maintain the ZPA, there is evidence that signals from the ZPA polarize and maintain the AER. Misexpression of *Sonic hedgehog* in the anterior limb mesenchyme is suf-

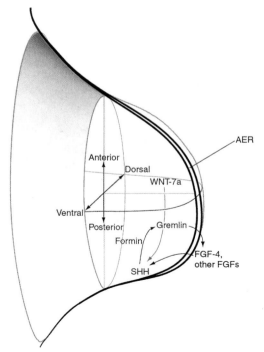

Figure 12–7. Coordinating the axes of limb development. A three-dimensional diagram of a left limb. A positive feedback loop between *Sonic hedgehog* (SHH) in the zone of polarizing activity and fibroblast growth factor 4 (*Fgf-4*) in the apical ectodermal ridge (AER) integrates anterior-posterior patterning and limb outgrowth. *Sonic hedgehog* induces the bone morphogenetic protein antagonist *Gremlin* in posterior mesenchyme through a process that requires *formin*, and *Gremlin* in turn induces *Fgf-4* in the posterior AER. FGF signals are in turn required to maintain *Sonic hedgehog* expression. In addition, *Wnt-7a* in the dorsal ectoderm is required for proper expression of *Sonic hedgehog* in the posterior mesenchyme. This interaction couples dorsal/ventral patterning with anterior/posterior patterning.

ficient to ectopically induce *Fgf-4* in the anterior AER (Laufer et al., 1994; Niswander et al., 1994). Thus, *Sonic hedgehog* may be responsible for maintaining the polar expression of *Fgf-4* in the posterior AER. Indeed, *Fgf-4* is gradually lost from the posterior AER in mice that lack *Sonic hedgehog* (Zuniga et al., 1999). Signals from the ZPA are also thought to be important in maintaining the integrity of the AER throughout limb outgrowth. When a barrier is placed through the middle of the AER and separating the anterior limb mesenchyme from the ZPA, the anterior ridge regresses (Zwilling, 1961; reviewed in Tabin, 1991). This classical observation led to the notion of an AER maintenance factor in the posterior mesenchyme. Consistent with this, experiments in which the ZPA was removed surgically or *Sonic hedgehog* gene expression was blocked pharmacologically demonstrated truncations along the P/D as well as A/P axes, suggesting that loss of *Sonic hedgehog* can compromise the normal function of the AER in outgrowth (Pagan et al., 1996; Bell et al., 1999). A similar result has been obtained in mice with a targeted disruption of the *Sonic hedgehog* gene. In these mice, the AER forms normally, but it becomes disorganized and gradually loses expression of *Fgf-4* in the posterior and *Fgf-8* throughout (Zuniga et al., 1999; Kraus et al., 2001; Chiang et al., 2001). These effects correlate with truncations observed in the zeugopod and autopod structures of these mice. Thus, *Sonic hedgehog* is required to maintain the integrity of the AER and its normal expression of *Fgf* genes during limb outgrowth.

As described above, the reciprocal interactions between the ZPA and AER appear to be mediated in part by a positive feedback loop between *Sonic hedgehog* and *Fgf-4* (Fig. 12–7). *Sonic hedgehog* upregulates *Fgf-4* and other *Fgf* genes in the posterior AER, and these FGFs in turn can maintain the expression of *Sonic hedgehog* in the posterior mesenchyme. Signals that relay the pathway from *Sonic hedgehog* in the posterior mesenchyme to *Fgf-4* in the posterior AER

have been uncovered by analysis of the *limb deformity* (*ld*) mouse mutant (Chan et al., 1995; Haramis et al., 1995). The *ld* mouse mutant has a homozygous mutation in the *formin* gene, leading to oligodactyly and syndactyly of autopod skeletal elements as well as fusion of zeugopod skeletal elements (Woychik et al., 1985). These defects ensue from an incomplete and poorly differentiated AER. Molecular analysis of *ld* mutant limbs reveals that *Fgf-4* fails to be activated in the posterior AER, whereas *Fgf-8* is expressed. Anterior grafts of *Sonic hegdehog*–expressing cells can induce ectopic *Fgf-4* in the AER of wild-type limbs, but they fail to induce *Fgf-4* in the AER of *ld* mutant limbs, even though mesenchymal targets of *Sonic hedgehog* are induced by these grafts (Zuniga et al., 1999). Thus, the *formin* gene appears to be a necessary signal for *Sonic hedgehog* to activate *Fgf-4* in the AER. *Formin* is thought to function in cytokinesis or cell polarization, but how it mediates signaling from the ZPA to the AER is unknown (Zeller et al., 1999). Another player in this pathway may be the secreted BMP antagonist *Gremlin* (Zuniga et al., 1999; Capdevila et al., 1999). When *Gremlin*-expressing cells are implanted into *ld* mutant limbs, *Fgf-4* is activated in the AER. *Noggin*, another BMP antagonist, can mimic this effect, indicating that *Gremlin* does indeed act by interfering with BMP signaling to induce *Fgf-4*. Normally, *Gremlin* is expressed in a domain broader than and overlapping that of *Sonic hedgehog*. Furthermore, *Gremlin* can be activated in the mesenchyme by ectopic *Sonic hedgehog*. In contrast, this response does not occur in *ld* mutant limbs. Thus, it seems that *Sonic hedgehog* induces *Gremlin* in posterior mesenchyme through a process that requires *formin*, and *Gremlin* in turn induces *Fgf-4* in the posterior AER (Fig. 12–7). In the absence of *formin*, *ld* mutants cannot induce *Gremlin*, so *Fgf-4* is never activated in the AER. The precision of this pathway is demonstrated when the range of *Sonic hedgehog* is reduced by precluding its cholesterol modification (Lewis et al., 2001). With a smaller range of *Sonic hedgehog* activity in the posterior mesenchyme, the *Gremlin* expression domain is reduced; hence, the *Fgf-4* expression domain is reduced. More data are necessary to elucidate this role of BMP antagonism in the differentiation and *Fgf* gene expression of the AER.

A feedback loop between the ZPA and AER allows the two signaling centers to be coordinately regulated, thereby integrating A/P patterning with limb outgrowth. Another mechanism that integrates patterning with outgrowth is the requirement of both *Fgf-4* and *Sonic hedgehog* in the activation of mesodermal genes (Laufer et al., 1994). The genes *Hoxd-13* and *Bmp-2* are expressed in response to *Sonic hedgehog* in the posterior mesenchyme, and ectopic expression can be induced anteriorly by ectopic *Sonic hedgehog*. However, *Sonic hedgehog* can induce this ectopic expression only when introduced close to the AER, suggesting that signals from the AER are also required. Indeed, when the anterior AER is removed, ectopic *Sonic hedgehog* fails to induce ectopic *Hoxd-13* or *Bmp-2* in the anterior mesenchyme; but when a bead soaked in FGF-4 is administered after the anterior AER is removed, ectopic *Sonic hedgehog* induces these mesodermal genes. This experiment indicates that both *Sonic hedgehog* in the posterior mesenchyme and *Fgf-4* in the posterior AER are necessary for activation of mesodermal genes *Hoxd-13* and *Bmp-2* (Laufer et al., 1994). Thus, signals from the ZPA and AER are required together for proper patterning.

Regulation of *Sonic hedgehog* by *Wnt-7a* Integrates A/P Patterning with D/V Patterning

In addition to the interaction between the AER and ZPA, there is evidence for an interaction between the dorsal limb ectoderm and the ZPA. When the dorsal ectoderm is removed from developing chick limbs, the level of *Sonic hedgehog* expression decreases, resulting in loss of posterior skeletal elements (Yang and Niswander, 1995). This indicates that signals from the dorsal ectoderm regulate expression of *Sonic hedgehog*. A good candidate for these signals is *Wnt-7a*, which is specifically expressed in the dorsal ectoderm. Indeed, viral expression of *Wnt-7a* following removal of the dorsal ectoderm is sufficient to restore normal levels of *Sonic hedgehog* expression and posterior skeletal elements. Thus, even though *Wnt-7a* is expressed uniformly throughout the dorsal ectoderm, it appears to regulate the expression of *Sonic hedgehog* in the posterior mesenchyme (Fig. 12–7). This conclusion is corroborated by parallel observations in the mouse *Wnt-7a* null mutant (Parr and McMahon, 1995). In mice lacking *Wnt-7a*, expression of *Sonic hedgehog* is reduced and the most posterior skeletal elements fail to be specified. The most posterior digit 5 and the ulna are often missing or abnormal, and the frequency of digit abnormalities increases from anterior to posterior. Thus, *Wnt-7a* is necessary for proper expression of *Sonic hedgehog*. Notably, expression of *Fgf-4* in the posterior AER is also curtailed in *Wnt-7a* mutant mice; but it is not clear if this reflects direct regulation of *Fgf-4* by *Wnt-7a* or indirect regulation via *Sonic hedgehog* since a feedback loop exists between *Sonic hedgehog* and *Fgf-4*, as described above.

These results demonstrate an interaction between the dorsal ectoderm and ZPA. As detailed earlier, signals from the dorsal ectoderm instruct the dorsal fate of underlying limb mesenchyme. *Wnt-7a* in the dorsal ectoderm is necessary for dorsal pattern specification. Thus, an interaction between *Wnt-7a* and *Sonic hedgehog* coordinates D/V patterning with A/P patterning.

Put together, these experiments reveal an interaction between the ZPA, AER, and dorsal ectoderm. This interaction ensures the coordinated regulation of growth and patterning along all three axes of limb development.

INTERPRETING POSITIONAL INFORMATION: *Hox* GENES AND MORPHOGENESIS

The mechanisms described to this point instruct the asymmetry of three axes in limb development. Together, these coordinated patterning mechanisms collaborate to confer positional information on mesenchymal cells throughout the emerging limb bud. How is this positional information interpreted and translated into stereotypical patterns of cell proliferation, movement, differentiation, and death? Though much progress has been made in understanding the initial mechanisms that pattern the limb, very little is known about this question. One family of genes that likely has an important role in executing positional information is the *Hox* gene family. This section will review the most salient themes in the role of *Hox* genes in limb morphogenesis.

Hox Genes Exhibit Complex Expression Patterns in Developing Limbs

Much insight about how *Hox* genes are patterned and act in embryogenesis comes from studies in *Drosophila* (see Chapter 46). Homeotic genes in *Drosophila* are regulatory transcription factors that bind DNA via a homeodomain (Gehring et al., 1990). These genes have successive expression domains along the A/P axis of the *Drosophila* embryo, and this pattern is important for their role in specifying segment identity (Gehring, 1987). The expression pattern of these genes exhibits a property called *spatial colinearity*: the genes are clustered in the genome, and their order on the chromosome is related to their spatial expression (Lewis, 1978). This property of spatial colinearity has been conserved in vertebrate *Hox* genes. There are four clusters of *Hox* genes in the mammalian genome (*HoxA, HoxB, HoxC, HoxD*), and genes within these clusters exhibit spatial colinearity such that 3′ genes are expressed in more anterior positions while 5′ genes are progressively more posterior (Duboule and Dolle, 1989; Graham et al., 1989). This is especially obvious in the CNS and prevertebrae along the primary body axis, but it is also true in secondary axes such as the limb buds, the digestive tract, and the genital ridge. Spatial colinearity may be related to the sequential activation of *Hox* genes beginning at the 3′ end, also called *temporal colinearity*. Similar to *Drosophila*, there is evidence that this successive patterning of *Hox* genes specifies the A/P level along the primary body axis; for example, *Hox* genes may specify the identity of vertebrae along the A/P axis and may determine the level where limbs form, as described earlier. Then, what is the extent of colinearity in the limbs, and does it have significance for *Hox* gene function?

Studies in chick and mouse have demonstrated that colinearity is a property of some *Hox* genes in the limb (Dolle and Duboule, 1989; Nelson et al., 1996). Particular attention has been given to gene members of the *HoxA* and *HoxD* complexes that are structurally related to the *Drosophila* gene *AbdominalB*. These genes are *Hoxa-9* to *Hoxa-13* and *Hoxd-9* to *Hoxd-13*, and they are sequentially expressed in a 3′ to 5′ fashion such that paralogs 9 appear first and paralogs 13 appear last. This temporal colinearity is thought to reflect a progressive 3′ to 5′ opening of chromatin, which allows stepwise accessibility of *Hox* genes for transcription (van der Hoeven et al., 1996). Generally, the domains of expression are nested, such that paralogs 9 are most broad and proximal, whereas paralogs 13 are most restricted and distal. However, these successive domains of *Hox* expression are in fact a composite of three independently regulated phases of expression. Careful study of the changes in *Hox* expression during limb outgrowth reveals a discrete contribution of each phase to the overall limb expression pattern. The first phase begins at the time of initial limb outgrowth and is characterized by uniform expression of *Hoxd-9* and *Hoxd-10* throughout the limb mesenchyme. In the second phase, *Hox* expression follows spatial and temporal colinearity. *Hoxd-9* through *Hoxd-13* are sequentially activated in a nested pattern, with *Hoxd-13* restricted to the most distal and posterior location. In the third phase, *Hox* expression seems to be the reverse of phase II and opposite the 3′ to 5′ spatial and temporal colinearity rule. *Hoxd-13* through *Hoxd-10* are sequentially activated, with *Hoxd-10* restricted to the most distal and posterior location. These three phases are regulated independently but overlap. The patterns of *HoxA* genes can similarly be viewed as overlapping phases of nested expression domains (Nelson et al., 1996). The sum contribution of these phases gives a complex pattern of *Hox* gene expression throughout the emerging limb bud. As a result, cells at different positions of the limb mesenchyme express different combinations of *Hox* genes.

Exceptions to *Hox* gene colinearity have been found in the limb (Nelson et al., 1996). For example, the *HoxC* genes are differently expressed in the forelimb and hindlimb. Though the more 3′ *HoxC* genes are expressed in the forelimb and the more 5′ *HoxC* genes are expressed in the hindlimb, there is no spatial colinearity within each limb bud. In general, the *HoxB* and *HoxC* genes do not exhibit colinearity and are often expressed in the forelimb or hindlimb but not both. Their differential expression in the fore- or hindlimb and their potential redundant function with *HoxA* or *HoxD* genes may explain why some mutants of *HoxA* or *HoxD* genes exhibit phenotypes mostly in one or the other pair of limbs.

Hox Genes Influence the Growth of Cartilaginous Elements According to Where They Are Expressed and "Posterior Prevalence"

The intricate sum of *Hox* gene expression in the limb generates different combinations of *Hox* genes in different positions. *Hox* genes may therefore encode positional information along the A/P and P/D axes of limb development. According to this model, the particular combination of *Hox* genes expressed in any given cell dictates the proliferation or differentiation of that cell. Furthermore, the genes that pattern the A/P and P/D axes instruct which *Hox* genes are expressed where, thereby creating patterns of proliferation or differentiation across the limb bud. If this is true, experimental alterations in genes that pattern these axes should lead to corresponding alterations in *Hox* gene expression preceding the ultimate alterations in skeletal elements. Indeed, when *Sonic hedgehog* is ectopically misexpressed in the anterior limb bud, the mirror-image duplications that occur in skeletal elements are preceded by mirror-image duplications of *Hox* gene expression (Riddle et al., 1993). This result suggests that *Hox* genes may act downstream of patterning cues in the formation of skeletal elements.

To elucidate the role of *Hox* genes, mice have been generated lacking function of specific *Hox* genes or combinations of *Hox* genes. The resulting mutants have complex malformations. Representative limb defects are highlighted below:

- *Hoxa-9* and *Hoxd-9* mutant mice have defects in the humerus (Fromental-Ramain et al., 1996).
- *Hoxa-10* mutant mice have defects in the femur and sesamoid bones of the knee (Favier et al., 1996).
- *Hoxa-11* mutant mice have defects in the ulna, radius, and carpal bones of the forelimb and in the distal tibia and fibula (Small and Potter, 1993; Davis et al., 1995).

- *Hoxd-11* mutant mice have minor shortening of the radius and ulna, fusions of some carpals, and shortened metacarpals and phalanges (Davis and Capecchi, 1994).
- *Hoxd-12* mutant mice have shortened metacarpals and phalanges and an abnormal carpal bone (Davis and Capecchi, 1996).
- *Hoxd-13* mutant mice have severe truncations or absence of metacarpals, metatarsals, and some phalanges (Dolle et al., 1993; see also Chapter 47).

These mutants do not simply lack a particular skeletal element or have a transformation of one skeletal element into another. Rather, they exhibit complex defects in size and shape of many skeletal elements and in different segments of the limb. This observation indicates that Hox genes do not simply specify particular skeletal structures. Instead, they are thought to influence several steps in the growth of cartilage elements.

While the *Hox* mutant limb defects are complex, they do reveal a correlation between the paralog of the disrupted gene and the P/D level affected. As can be seen in the mutants described above, the 3′ genes (*Hoxa-9*, *Hoxd-9*) are important for morphogenesis of more proximal structures, whereas the 5′ genes (*Hoxa-13*, *Hoxd-13*) are important for more distal structures. If *Hox* genes do not specify particular skeletal structures, how does this correlation arise? Two properties accurately predict which limb structures are affected in these various *Hox* mutants. First, which skeletal elements are affected in the mutants corresponds to where the disrupted gene is normally expressed. Second, "posterior prevalence" describes the observation that when two or more *Hox* genes are coexpressed in the same cell, the most 5′ gene of the *Hox* cluster dominates (e.g., *Hoxd-13* dominates over *Hoxd-9*). Posterior prevalence is thought to be a consequence of functional antagonism without transcriptional repression, for example, by competition for target sites or titration of cofactors (Duboule and Morata, 1994). These two properties together explain the correlation between the paralog of the disrupted gene and the P/D level affected. Thus, in *Hoxa-9* and *Hoxd-9* mutants, the stylopod is most severely affected because paralog 9 genes are expressed in the limb mesenchyme during phase I, when the stylopod begins to form while more 5′ genes are not broadly expressed. The zeugopod is most severely affected in *Hoxa-11* and *Hoxd-11* mutants because these genes are widely expressed during phase II, when the zeugopod begins to form; in this phase, paralog 11 genes dominate over more 3′ genes and more 5′ genes are restricted to the extreme posterior margin. Lastly, the autopod is most severely affected in *Hoxa-13* and *Hoxd-13* mutants because these genes are expressed in the distal limb at the time the autopod is being formed and because these genes exert a prevalent effect over more 3′ *Hox* genes expressed there. Altogether, the complex *Hox* expression patterns combined with the property of posterior prevalence result in a correlation between the paralog of a gene and the level of its mutant phenotype.

The single *Hox* gene mutants above suggest that *Hox* genes influence the growth of cartilage elements in different positions of the limb bud but are not involved in the initial specification of cartilage elements. This conclusion is supported by the dramatic phenotype of *Hoxa-11/Hoxd-11* double-mutant mice (Davis et al., 1995). Mutants of either *Hoxa-11* or *Hoxd-11* genes exhibit minor defects or shortening of the radius and ulna. However, *Hoxa-11/Hoxd-11* double mutants exhibit drastic reduction of the radius and the ulna, as well as homeotic transformations of the axial skeleton and kidney defects. It is likely that the zeugopod is severely affected in these double mutants because no other genes of paralog 11 are available: there is no *Hoxb-11*, and *Hoxc-11* is expressed only in the hindlimb. Nevertheless, formation and bifurcation of the radius and ulna anlage occur, and vestiges of the radius and ulna are still detectable, even though subsequent growth of these elements fails to occur. Thus, *Hox* genes are not involved in initial specification of these cartilage elements but, rather, influence their growth.

The phenotype of the *Hoxa-11/Hoxd-11* double mutant is remarkably similar to the phenotype of another mouse mutant, *Ulnaless*. Much like the double mutant mice, *Ulnaless* mice have a severe reduction in the size of the radius and ulna. The *Ulnaless* mutation was generated by X-ray irradiation (Morris, 1967) and is thought to disrupt a *cis*-acting enhancer 5′ of the *HoxD* cluster (Herault et al., 1997;

Peichel et al., 1997). As a result of this mutation, the *HoxD* genes are deregulated in the limb such that *Hoxd-13* and *Hoxd-12* are ectopically expressed in the presumptive zeugopod during phase II. As predicted by posterior prevalence, ectopic expression of *Hoxd-13* and *Hoxd-12* antagonizes *Hoxd-11* and *Hoxd-10* in the presumptive zeugopod. In this way, misexpression of *Hoxd-13* and *Hoxd-12* in the *Ulnaless* mouse yields a phenocopy of the loss of paralog 11 genes in the *Hoxa-11/Hoxd-11* double mutant.

In this section, *Hox* gene expression data in chick and mouse and knockout data in mouse have been summarized. These data demonstrate that several phases of *Hox* gene expression occur in the limb bud with varying degrees of colinearity. As a result, different combinations of *Hox* genes are expressed at different positions of the limb bud. This complex pattern of *Hox* genes influences the growth of cartilage elements in the developing limb.

Hox Genes Exhibit Functional Redundancy and Dosage Effects

A significant degree of overlap is evident in the limb expression domains of *Hox* genes. This raises the possibility that *Hox* genes interact. This idea has been explored by crossing different mouse mutants together. The results of these breedings reveal several important properties of *Hox* gene function, which will be described here.

Two related properties of *Hox* gene function are redundancy and dosage. While *Hox* genes of different paralogs seem to be necessary for different P/D levels of the limb, genes of the same paralog are often functionally redundant. This is indicated when a double-mutant phenotype is worse than the sum of either single-mutant phenotype since loss of redundancy in the double mutant can lead to novel effects. For example, *Hoxa-13* and *Hoxd-13* single homozygous mutants exhibit different defects of the autopod (Dolle et al., 1993; Fromental-Ramain et al., 1996). However, when combined, double homozygous mutant mice are missing almost all elements of the autopod. This is a novel phenotype that suggests a loss of redundancy. Moreover, results of varying the number of copies of wild-type *Hoxa-13* or *Hoxd-13* alleles suggest that the combined dose of the two genes rather than relative levels influences phenotype. For example, though each heterozygote is nearly normal, the compound heterozygote *Hoxa-13*$^{+/-}$*Hoxd-13*$^{+/-}$ phenotype more closely resembles the homozygous mutant phenotype of either gene. This suggests that some of the mutant effects result from a reduction in the total amount of Hoxa-13 and Hoxd-13 proteins. This redundancy and dosage effect is not such a surprise if the proteins share some target binding sites. By the same token, the fact that the combined heterozygote is not identical to either single homozygous mutant indicates that some effects do depend on the loss of Hoxa-13 or of Hoxd-13. A corroborating example of redundancy is with *Hoxa-11* and *Hoxd-11*. Though each single mutant has relatively minor effects on the radius and ulna, the double mutant exhibits almost complete loss of the radius and ulna (Davis et al., 1995). Partial loss of the radius and ulna is seen in a dose-dependent manner as more copies of paralog 11 genes are removed. These examples demonstrate that *Hox* genes of the same paralog are at least partially redundant in function.

Interestingly, functional redundancy can also occur among *Hox* genes of different paralogs. For example, various combinations of mice heterozygous for *Hoxd-11*, *Hoxd-12*, and *Hoxd-13* exhibit phenotypes more severe than the added phenotypes of single heterozygotes (Davis and Capecchi, 1996). The severity of the combined heterozygotes again resembles that of single homozygous mutants. Similarly, *Hoxa-10* and *Hoxd-11* double-mutant mice show synergistic mutant effects, indicating some functional redundancy (Favier et al., 1996). Thus, the function of different paralogs is also partially redundant. Again, this is not so surprising given the overlapping expression and the possibility that different HOX proteins share the same binding sites.

Hox Genes May Influence Adhesiveness of Limb Mesenchyme

How is the positional information encoded by *Hox* genes translated into morphogenesis of limb skeletal elements? Very little is known about the downstream molecular mediators of *Hox* genes. The phenotypic effects of *Hox* gene mutations on skeletal elements has led to speculation that *Hox* genes regulate chondrogenesis, proliferation of chondrocytes, segmentation of skeletal elements, and/or rate of ossification.

Another interesting possibility is that *Hox* genes modulate the adhesiveness of prechondrogenic mesenchyme, thereby shaping the condensation of cartilage elements. Evidence for this idea comes from a misexpression experiment and *in vitro* analysis (Yokouchi et al., 1995). When *Hoxa-13* is transfected into a chick limb and the limb mesenchyme is subsequently dissociated and cultured, the *Hoxa-13*-expressing cells sort themselves out from nonexpressing cells. This indicates that *Hoxa-13* expression alters the homophilic cell-adhesive properties of these cells.

How critical this function is for cartilage patterning is not established. However, this finding nicely complements the observation that limb mesenchyme can self-organize after disaggregation (Zwilling, 1964). The limb mesoderm can be removed from the overlying ectoderm, dissociated, and reaggregated. This procedure randomly disperses any patterned cells or organizing centers such as the ZPA. However, when reconstructed with ectoderm and implanted back onto a chick embryo, these disorganized limbs develop normal distal cartilage elements, indicating that signaling centers such as the ZPA can self-organize. This self-organization could be explained if differential adhesive properties are patterned by *Hox* genes in the limb mesenchyme. For example, the cell-adhesion molecule cadherin-11 is expressed in a P/D gradient in the developing limb and seems to be involved in the sorting of limb mesenchymal cells *in vitro* (Simonneau et al., 1995; Kimura et al., 1995). *Hox* genes may be involved in patterning the expression of such adhesion molecules.

FORELIMB VS. HINDLIMB SPECIFICATION

Though the forelimb buds emerge shortly before the hindlimb buds, all four outgrowths initially appear quite similar. As growth and patterning proceed, the stereotypical differences that distinguish the forelimbs from hindlimbs become more pronounced. Evolutionarily, the limbs are considered serially homologous structures (Ruvinsky and Gibson-Brown, 2000). Consistent with this view, many of the molecular pathways that pattern the two pairs are the same. Indeed, almost all of the gene expression domains and patterning mechanisms described in this chapter are pertinent to both pairs; but while morphological parallels are obvious, the functional importance of differences between forelimbs and hindlimbs is also obvious. What molecular cues lead to these differences? This section will describe mechanisms thought to be involved in specifying forelimb and hindlimb fates.

Tbx-5, *Tbx-4*, and *Pitx-1* Specify Forelimb vs. Hindlimb Identity

Classical manipulations in chick embryos offered some clues on how limb identity is determined. In particular, recombinant limbs have been constructed in which the ectoderm and mesoderm of forelimbs and hindlimbs are interchanged (Zwilling, 1955). These experiments demonstrate that information specifying limb identity (hindlimb or forelimb morphology) resides in the mesoderm. Furthermore, transplantation of lateral plate mesoderm of the limb field revealed that this information exists even prior to limb bud outgrowth. Elucidating how limb identity is specified could therefore be approached by a search for genes that are differentially expressed in the lateral plate tissue that will become the forelimb and hindlimb mesoderm.

Two members of the T-box gene family, *Tbx-4* and *Tbx-5*, were discovered to be specifically expressed in the hindlimb and forelimb buds, respectively (Gibson-Brown et al., 1996). These genes belong to a family of transcription factors that share a conserved DNA-binding T domain with the mouse *Brachyury (T)* gene (Bollag et al., 1994; see also Chapters 67 and 69). Another gene, *Pitx-1*, which encodes a transcription factor of the Otx-related subclass of paired-type homeodomain proteins, is also expressed specifically in the hindlimb bud (Lamonerie et al., 1996; Szeto et al., 1996). In line with the classical manipulations, *Tbx-4*, *Tbx-5*, and *Pitx-1* are expressed in the respec-

tive limb fields prior to limb bud outgrowth (Logan et al., 1998). Furthermore, this expression is retained in recombinant limbs in which mesoderm and ectoderm have been interchanged, as predicted by classical experiments (Gibson-Brown et al., 1998; Isaac et al., 1998). Lastly, when ectopic limbs are induced by placement of an FGF-soaked bead in the interlimb flank, expression of these genes in the induced limb correlates with the axial level and the ultimate limb identity: beads placed more rostrally induce *Tbx-5* expression and form wings, whereas beads placed more caudally induce *Tbx-4* and *Pitx-1* expression and form legs (Isaac et al., 1998; Logan et al., 1998). The differential expression and behavior of *Tbx-5* in the forelimb and *Tbx-4* and *Pitx-1* in the hindlimb make these genes good candidates for the determinants of limb identity. The related genes *Tbx-2* and *Tbx-3* are also expressed during limb development in the anterior and posterior margins of the limb buds, but these are similar in forelimbs and hindlimbs.

Misexpression experiments in chick and genetic manipulations in mouse support the role of these genes in specifying limb identity. Misexpression of *Tbx-4* and *Pitx-1* can induce leg-like features in the wing, and misexpression of *Tbx-5* can induce wing-like features in the leg (Rodriguez-Esteban et al., 1999; Takeuchi et al., 1999; Logan and Tabin, 1999). Moreover, these experiments elucidate interactions among these genes: *Tbx-5* appears to downregulate *Tbx-4*, whereas *Pitx-1* appears to upregulate *Tbx-4*. Finally, a mouse deficient in *Pitx-1* exhibits abnormal morphogenesis of the hindlimbs, with some structural features that resemble the forelimbs (Szeto et al., 1999).

These data are consistent with the model that *Tbx-5* functions in the determination of the forelimb and *Tbx-4* and *Pitx-1* play a role in the determination of the hindlimb, although the transformants observed in these experiments are incomplete enough that parallel pathways may also be involved. Definitive proof will come with more loss-of-function experiments and by completely reversing the expression of these genes. The mechanisms that cause the differential expression of these genes are unknown. If *Hox* genes play a role in specifying the A/P level of limb formation, they may also influence which limb identity genes are expressed. Lastly, how differential expression of these genes is translated into patterning and morphological differences in the limbs remains to be determined.

CLOSING

Our understanding of limb development represents a convergence of many different fields, including classical embryology, evolutionary biology, clinical medicine, and genetics. We have explored our initial knowledge of limb histology and signaling centers to greater and greater resolution so that we now can explain much of the underlying molecular and cellular biology. This chapter has reviewed the major genetic pathways involved in limb development, with attention to how these pathways interact and how they are regulated. Because these same pathways recur in a variety of developmental contexts, advances in the genetics of limb development can offer insight into how other organ systems are patterned. Moreover, this information has improved our understanding of congenital limb defects and ultimately may help guide the treatment of these defects. Finally, this information may one day be harnessed for the healing, repair, and regeneration of adult limb structures.

REFERENCES

Altabef M, Clarke JD, Tickle C (1997). Dorso-ventral ectodermal compartments and origin of apical ectodermal ridge in developing chick limb. *Development* 124: 4547–4556.

Bell SM, Schreiner CM, Scott WJ (1999). Disrupting the establishment of polarizing activity by teratogen exposure. *Mech Dev* 88: 147–157.

Bollag RJ, Siegfried Z, Cebra-Thomas JA, Garvey N, Davison EM, Silver LM (1994). An ancient family of embryonically expressed mouse genes sharing a conserved protein motif with the T locus. *Nat Genet* 7: 383–389.

Burke AC, Nelson CE, Morgan BA, Tabin C (1995). Hox genes and the evolution of vertebrate axial morphology. *Development* 121: 333–346.

Capdevila J, Johnson RL (1998). Endogenous and ectopic expression of noggin suggests a conserved mechanism for regulation of BMP function during limb and somite patterning. *Dev Biol* 197: 205–217.

Capdevila J, Tsukui T, Rodriquez Esteban C, Zappavigna V, Izpisua Belmonte JC (1999). Control of vertebrate limb outgrowth by the proximal factor Meis2 and distal antagonism of BMPs by Gremlin. *Mol Cells* 4: 839–849.

Chan DC, Laufer E, Tabin C, Leder P (1995). Polydactylous limbs in Strong's Luxoid mice result from ectopic polarizing activity. *Development* 121: 1971–1978.

Charite J, de Graaff W, Shen S, Deschamps J (1994). Ectopic expression of Hoxb-8 causes duplication of the ZPA in the forelimb and homeotic transformation of axial structures. *Cell* 78: 589–601.

Charite J, McFadden DG, Olson EN (2000). The bHLH transcription factor dHAND controls Sonic hedgehog expression and establishment of the zone of polarizing activity during limb development. *Development* 127: 2461–2470.

Chen H, Lun Y, Ovchinnikov D, Kokubo H, Oberg KC, Pepicelli CV, Gan L, Lee B, Johnson RL (1998). Limb and kidney defects in Lmx1b mutant mice suggest an involvement of LMX1B in human nail patella syndrome. *Nat Genet* 19: 51–55.

Chiang C, Litingtung Y, Harris MP, Simandl BK, Li Y, Beachy PA, Fallon JF (2001). Manifestation of the limb prepattern: limb development in the absence of sonic hedgehog function. *Dev Biol* 236: 421–435.

Cohn MJ, Izpisua-Belmonte JC, Abud H, Heath JK, Tickle C (1995). Fibroblast growth factors induce additional limb development from the flank of chick embryos. *Cell* 80: 739–746.

Cohn MJ, Patel K, Krumlauf R, Wilkinson DG, Clarke JD, Tickle C (1997). Hox9 genes and vertebrate limb specification. *Nature* 387: 97–101.

Colvin JS, Feldman B, Nadeau JH, Goldfarb M, Ornitz DM (1999). Genomic organization and embryonic expression of the mouse fibroblast growth factor 9 gene. *Dev Dyn* 216: 72–88.

Colvin JS, White AC, Pratt SJ, Ornitz DM (2001). Lung hypoplasia and neonatal death in Fgf9-null mice identify this gene as an essential regulator of lung mesenchyme. *Development* 128: 2095–2106.

Crossley PH, Minowada G, MacArthur CA, Martin GR (1996). Roles for FGF8 in the induction, initiation, and maintenance of chick limb development. *Cell* 84: 127–136.

Dahn RD, Fallon JF (2000). Interdigital regulation of digit identity and homeotic transformation by modulated BMP signaling. *Science* 289: 438–441.

Davis AP, Capecchi MR (1994). Axial homeosis and appendicular skeleton defects in mice with a targeted disruption of hoxd-11. *Development* 120: 2187–2198.

Davis AP, Capecchi MR (1996). A mutational analysis of the 5′ *HoxD* genes: dissection of genetic interactions during limb development in the mouse. *Development* 122: 1175–1185.

Davis AP, Witte DP, Hsieh-Li HM, Potter SS, Capecchi MR (1995). Absence of radius and ulna in mice lacking hoxa-11 and hoxd-11. *Nature* 375: 791–795.

Davis CA, Holmyard DP, Millen KJ, Joyner AL (1991). Examining pattern formation in mouse, chicken and frog embryos with an En-specific antiserum. *Development* 111: 287–298.

Dealy CN, Roth A, Ferrari D, Brown AM, Kosher RA (1993). Wnt-5a and Wnt-7a are expressed in the developing chick limb bud in a manner suggesting roles in pattern formation along the proximodistal and dorsoventral axes. *Mech Dev* 43: 175–186.

de Celis JF, Bray S (1997). Feed-back mechanisms affecting Notch activation at the dorsoventral boundary in the Drosophila wing. *Development* 124: 3241–3251.

Diaz-Benjumea FJ, Cohen SM (1993). Interaction between dorsal and ventral cells in the imaginal disc directs wing development in Drosophila. *Cell* 75: 741–752.

Doherty D, Feger G, Younger-Shepherd S, Jan LY, Jan YN (1996). Delta is a ventral to dorsal signal complementary to Serrate, another Notch ligand, in *Drosophila* wing formation. *Genes Dev* 10: 421–434.

Dolle P, Duboule D (1989). Two gene members of the murine HOX-5 complex show regional and cell-type specific expression in developing limbs and gonads. *EMBO J* 8: 1507–1515.

Dolle P, Izpisua-Belmonte JC, Brown J, Tickle C, Duboule D (1993). Hox genes and the morphogenesis of the vertebrate limb. *Prog Clin Biol Res* 383A: 11–20.

Dominguez M, Brunner M, Hafen E, Basler K (1996). Sending and receiving the hedgehog signal: control by the *Drosophila* Gli protein Cubitus interruptus. *Science* 272: 1621–1625.

Drossopoulou G, Lewis KE, Sanz-Ezquerro JJ, Nikbakht N, McMahon AP, Hofmann C, Tickle C (2000). A model for anteroposterior patterning of the vertebrate limb based on sequential long- and short-range Shh signalling and Bmp signalling. *Development* 127: 1337–1348.

Duboule D, Dolle P (1989). The structural and functional organization of the murine HOX gene family resembles that of *Drosophila* homeotic genes. *EMBO J* 8: 1497–1505.

Duboule D, Morata G (1994). Colinearity and functional hierarchy among genes of the homeotic complexes. *Trends Genet* 10: 358–364.

Dudley AT, Ros MA, Tabin CJ (2002). A re-examination of proximodistal patterning during vertebrate limb development. *Nature* 418: 539–544.

Duprez DM, Kostakopoulou K, Francis-West PH, Tickle C, Brickell PM (1996). Activation of *Fgf-4* and *HoxD* gene expression by BMP-2 expressing cells in the developing chick limb. *Development* 122: 1821–1828.

Echelard Y, Epstein DJ, St-Jacques B, Shen L, Mohler J, McMahon JA, McMahon AP (1993). Sonic hedgehog, a member of a family of putative signaling molecules, is implicated in the regulation of CNS polarity. *Cell* 75: 1417–1430.

Fallon JF, Lopez A, Ros MA, Savage MP, Olwin BB, Simandl BK (1994). FGF-2: apical ectodermal ridge growth signal for chick limb development. *Science* 264: 104–107.

Favier B, Rijli FM, Fromental-Ramain C, Fraulob V, Chambon P, Dolle P (1996). Functional cooperation between the non-paralogous genes *Hoxa-10* and *Hoxd-11* in the developing forelimb and axial skeleton. *Development* 122: 449–460.

Fernandez-Teran M, Piedra ME, Kathiriya IS, Srivastava D, Rodriguez-Rey JC, Ros MA (2000). Role of dHAND in the anterior–posterior polarization of the limb bud: implications for the Sonic hedgehog pathway. *Development* 127: 2133–2142.

Fleming RJ, Gu Y, Hukriede NA (1997). Serrate-mediated activation of Notch is specifically blocked by the product of the gene *fringe* in the dorsal compartment of the *Drosophila* wing imaginal disc. *Development* 124: 2973–2981.

Francis PH, Richardson MK, Brickell PM, Tickle C (1994). Bone morphogenetic proteins and a signalling pathway that controls patterning in the developing chick limb. *Development* 120: 209–218.

Fromental-Ramain C, Warot X, Lakkaraju S, Favier B, Haack H, Birling C, Dierich A, Doll EP, Chambon P (1996). Specific and redundant functions of the paralogous *Hoxa-9* and *Hoxd-9* genes in forelimb and axial skeleton patterning. *Development* 122: 461–472.

Gardner CA, Barald KF (1992). Expression patterns of engrailed-like proteins in the chick embryo. *Dev Dyn* 193: 370–388.

Geduspan JS, Solursh M (1992). A growth-promoting influence from the mesonephros during limb outgrowth. *Dev Biol* 151: 242–250.

Gehring WJ (1987). Homeo boxes in the study of development. *Science* 236: 1245–1252.

Gehring WJ, Muller M, Affolter M, Percival-Smith A, Billeter M, Qian YQ, Otting G, Wuthrich K (1990). The structure of the homeodomain and its functional implications. *Trends Genet* 6: 323–329.

Gibson-Brown JJ, Agulnik SI, Chapman DL, Alexiou M, Garvey N, Silver LM, Papaioannou VE (1996). Evidence of a role for T-box genes in the evolution of limb morphogenesis and the specification of forelimb/hindlimb identity. *Mech Dev* 56: 93–101.

Gibson-Brown JJ, Agulnik SI, Silver LM, Niswander L, Papaioannou VE (1998). Involvement of T-box genes *Tbx2–Tbx5* in vertebrate limb specification and development. *Development* 125: 2499–2509.

Goodrich LV, Johnson RL, Milenkovic L, McMahon JA, Scott MP (1996). Conservation of the hedgehog/patched signaling pathway from flies to mice: induction of a mouse *patched* gene by Hedgehog. *Genes Dev* 10: 301–312.

Graham A, Papalopulu N, Krumlauf R (1989). The murine and *Drosophila* homeobox gene complexes have common features of organization and expression. *Cell* 57: 367–378.

Haramis AG, Brown JM, Zeller R (1995). The limb deformity mutation disrupts the SHH/FGF-4 feedback loop and regulation of 5′ *HoxD* genes during limb pattern formation. *Development* 121: 4237–4245.

Helms JA, Kim CH, Eichele G, Thaller C (1996). Retinoic acid signaling is required during early chick limb development. *Development* 122: 1385–1394.

Herault Y, Fraudeau N, Zakany J, Duboule D (1997). Ulnaless (Ul), a regulatory mutation inducing both loss-of-function and gain-of-function of posterior *Hoxd* genes. *Development* 124: 3493–3500.

Honig LS (1981). Positional signal transmission in the developing chick limb. *Nature* 291: 72–73.

Hornbruch A, Wolpert L (1991). The spatial and temporal distribution of polarizing activity in the flank of the pre-limb-bud stages in the chick embryo. *Development* 111: 725–731.

Hui CC, Joyner AL (1993). A mouse model of Greig cephalopolysyndactyly syndrome: the extra-toes mutation contains an intragenic deletion of the *Gli3* gene. *Nat Genet* 3: 241–246.

Irvine KD, Wieschaus E (1994). fringe, a Boundary-specific signaling molecule, mediates interactions between dorsal and ventral cells during *Drosophila* wing development. *Cell* 79: 595–606.

Isaac A, Rodriguez-Esteban C, Ryan A, Altabef M, Tsukui T, Patel K, Tickle C, Izpisua-Belmonte JC (1998). *Tbx* genes and limb identity in chick embryo development. *Development* 125: 1867–1875.

Izpisua-Belmonte JC, Tickle C, Dolle P, Wolpert L, Duboule D (1991). Expression of the homeobox *Hox-4* genes and the specification of position in chick wing development. *Nature* 350: 585–589.

Jiang R, Lan Y, Chapman HD, Shawber C, Norton CR, Serreze DV, Weinmaster G, Gridley T (1998). Defects in limb, craniofacial, and thymic development in Jagged2 mutant mice. *Genes Dev* 12: 1046–1057.

Kawakami Y, Ishikawa T, Shimabara M, Tanda N, Enomoto-Iwamoto M, Iwamoto M, Kuwana T, Ueki A, Noji S, Nohno T (1996). BMP signaling during bone pattern determination in the developing limb. *Development* 122: 3557–3566.

Kawakami Y, Capdevila J, Buscher D, Itoh T, Rodriguez Esteban C, Izpisua Belmonte JC (2001). WNT signals control FGF-dependent limb initiation and AER induction in the chick embryo. *Cell* 104: 891–900.

Kelley RO, Fallon JF (1976). Ultrastructural analysis of the apical ectodermal ridge during vertebrate limb morphogenesis. 1. The human forelimb with special reference to gap junctions. *Dev Biol* 51: 241–256.

Kengaku M, Capdevila J, Rodriguez-Esteban C, De La Pena J, Johnson RL, Belmonte JC, Tabin CJ (1998). Distinct WNT pathways regulating AER formation and dorsoventral polarity in the chick limb bud. *Science* 280: 1274–1277.

Kessel M, Gruss P (1990). Murine developmental control genes. *Science* 249: 374–379.

Kessel M, Gruss P (1991). Homeotic transformations of murine vertebrae and concomitant alteration of Hox codes induced by retinoic acid. *Cell* 67: 89–104.

Kimmel RA, Turnbull DH, Blanquet V, Wurst W, Loomis CA, Joyner AL (2000). Two lineage boundaries coordinate vertebrate apical ectodermal ridge formation. *Genes Dev* 14: 1377–1389.

Kimura Y, Matsunami H, Inoue T, Shimamura K, Uchida N, Ueno T, Miyazaki T, Takeichi M (1995). Cadherin-11 expressed in association with mesenchymal morphogenesis in the head, somite, and limb bud of early mouse embryos. *Dev Biol* 169: 347–358.

Kraus P, Fraidenraich D, Loomis CA (2001). Some distal limb structures develop in mice lacking Sonic hedgehog signaling. *Mech Dev* 100: 45–58.

Krauss S, Concordet JP, Ingham PW (1993). A functionally conserved homolog of the *Drosophila* segment polarity gene *hh* is expressed in tissues with polarizing activity in zebrafish embryos. *Cell* 75: 1431–1444.

Lamonerie T, Tremblay JJ, Lanctot C, Therrien M, Gauthier Y, Drouin J (1996). Ptx1, a bicoid-related homeo box transcription factor involved in transcription of the pro-opiomelanocortin gene. *Genes Dev* 10: 1284–1295.

Laufer E, Nelson CE, Johnson RL, Morgan BA, Tabin C (1994). Sonic hedgehog and Fgf-4 act through a signaling cascade and feedback loop to integrate growth and patterning of the developing limb bud. *Cell* 79: 993–1003.

Laufer E, Dahn R, Orozco OE, Yeo CY, Pisenti J, Henrique D, Abbott UK, Fallon JF, Tabin C (1997). Expression of Radical fringe in limb-bud ectoderm regulates apical ectodermal ridge formation. *Nature* 386: 366–373.

Lewandoski M, Sun X, Martin GR (2000). Fgf8 signalling from the AER is essential for normal limb development. *Nat Genet* 26: 460–463.

Lewis EB (1978). A gene complex controlling segmentation in *Drosophila*. *Nature* 276: 565–570.

Lewis PM, Dunn MP, McMahon JA, Logan M, Martin JF, St-Jacques B, McMahon AP (2001). Cholesterol modification of sonic hedgehog is required for long-range signaling activity and effective modulation of signaling by Ptc1. *Cell* 105: 599–612.

Li S, Muneoka K (1999). Cell migration and chick limb development: chemotactic action of FGF-4 and the AER. *Dev Biol* 211: 335–347.

Logan C, Hornbruch A, Campbell I, Lumsden A (1997). The role of Engrailed in establishing the dorsoventral axis of the chick limb. *Development* 124: 2317–2324.

Logan M, Tabin CJ (1999). Role of Pitx1 upstream of Tbx4 in specification of hindlimb identity. *Science* 283: 1736–1739.

Logan M, Simon HG, Tabin C (1998). Differential regulation of T-box and homeobox transcription factors suggests roles in controlling chick limb-type identity. *Development* 125: 2825–2835.

Loomis CA, Harris E, Michaud J, Wurst W, Hanks M, Joyner AL (1996). The mouse Engrailed-1 gene and ventral limb patterning. *Nature* 382: 360–363.

Loomis CA, Kimmel RA, Tong CX, Michaud J, Joyner AL (1998). Analysis of the genetic pathway leading to formation of ectopic apical ectodermal ridges in mouse Engrailed-1 mutant limbs. *Development* 125: 1137–1148.

Lopez-Martinez A, Chang DT, Chiang C, Porter JA, Ros MA, Simandl BK, Beachy PA, Fallon J F (1995). Limb-patterning activity and restricted posterior localization of the amino-terminal product of Sonic hedgehog cleavage. *Curr Biol* 5: 791–796.

Lu HC, Revelli JP, Goering L, Thaller C, Eichele G (1997). Retinoid signaling is required for the establishment of a ZPA and for the expression of Hoxb-8, a mediator of ZPA formation. *Development* 124: 1643–1651.

Maccabe AB, Gasseling MT, Saunders JW Jr (1973). Spatiotemporal distribution of mechanisms that control outgrowth and anteroposterior polarization of the limb bud in the chick embryo. *Mech Ageing Dev* 2: 1–12.

MacCabe JA, Errick J, Saunders JW Jr (1974). Ectodermal control of the dorsoventral axis in the leg bud of the chick embryo. *Dev Biol* 39: 69–82.

Marigo V, Scott MP, Johnson RL, Goodrich LV, Tabin CJ (1996). Conservation in hedgehog signaling: induction of a chicken patched homolog by Sonic hedgehog in the developing limb. *Development* 122: 1225–1233.

Masuya H, Sagai T, Wakana S, Moriwaki K, Shiroishi T (1995). A duplicated zone of polarizing activity in polydactylous mouse mutants. *Genes Dev* 9: 1645–1653.

Masuya H, Sagai T, Moriwaki K, Shiroishi T (1997). Multigenic control of the localization of the zone of polarizing activity in limb morphogenesis in the mouse. *Dev Biol* 182: 42–51.

Michaud JL, Lapointe F, Le Douarin NM (1997). The dorsoventral polarity of the presumptive limb is determined by signals produced by the somites and by the lateral somatopleure. *Development* 124: 1453–1463.

Milenkovic L, Goodrich LV, Higgins KM, Scott MP (1999). Mouse patched1 controls body size determination and limb patterning. *Development* 126: 4431–4440.

Min H, Danilenko DM, Scully SA, Bolon B, Ring BD, Tarpley JE, DeRose M, Simonet WS (1998). Fgf-10 is required for both limb and lung development and exhibits striking functional similarity to *Drosophila* branchless. *Genes Dev* 12: 3156–3161.

Moon AM, Boulet AM, Capecchi MR (2000). Normal limb development in conditional mutants of Fgf4. *Development* 127: 989–996.

Moore KL, Persaud TVN (1998). The Developing Human: Clinically Oriented Embryology, 6th edition. Saunders, Philadelphia.

Moran JL, Levorse JM, Vogt TF (1999). Limbs move beyond the radical fringe. *Nature* 399: 742–743.

Morris T (1967). New mutants. *Mouse News Lett* 36: 34.

Myat A, Henrique D, Ish-Horowicz D, Lewis J (1996). A chick homologue of Serrate and its relationship with Notch and Delta homologues during central neurogenesis. *Dev Biol* 174: 233–247.

Nelson CE, Morgan BA, Burke AC, Laufer E, DiMambro E, Murtaugh LC, Gonzales E, Tessarollo L, Parada LF, Tabin C (1996). Analysis of Hox gene expression in the chick limb bud. *Development* 122: 1449–1466.

Niswander L, Martin GR (1992). Fgf-4 expression during gastrulation, myogenesis, limb and tooth development in the mouse. *Development* 114: 755–768.

Niswander L, Tickle C, Vogel A, Booth I, Martin GR (1993). FGF-4 replaces the apical ectodermal ridge and directs outgrowth and patterning of the limb. *Cell* 75: 579–587.

Niswander L, Tickle C, Vogel A, Martin G (1994). Function of FGF-4 in limb development. *Mol Reprod Dev* 39: 83–89.

Nohno T, Noji S, Koyama E, Ohyama K, Myokai F, Kuroiwa A, Saito T, Taniguchi S (1991). Involvement of the Chox-4 chicken homeobox genes in determination of anteroposterior axial polarity during limb development. *Cell* 64: 1197–1205.

Ohuchi H, Yoshioka H, Tanaka A, Kawakami Y, Nohno T, Noji S (1994). Involvement of androgen-induced growth factor (FGF-8) gene in mouse embryogenesis and morphogenesis. *Biochem Biophys Res Commun* 204: 882–888.

Ohuchi H, Nakagawa T, Yamamoto A, Araga A, Ohata T, Ishimaru Y, Yoshioka H, Kuwana T, Nohno T, Yamasaki M, et al. (1997). The mesenchymal factor, FGF10, initiates and maintains the outgrowth of the chick limb bud through interaction with FGF8, an apical ectodermal factor. *Development* 124: 2235–2244.

Orr-Urtreger A, Bedford MT, Burakova T, Arman E, Zimmer Y, Yayon A, Givol D, Lonai P (1993). Developmental localization of the splicing alternatives of fibroblast growth factor receptor-2 (FGFR2). *Dev Biol* 158: 475–486.

Ortega S, Ittmann M, Tsang SH, Ehrlich M, Basilico C (1998). Neuronal defects and delayed wound healing in mice lacking fibroblast growth factor 2. *Proc Natl Acad Sci USA* 95: 5672–5677.

Pagan SM, Ros MA, Tabin C, Fallon JF (1996). Surgical removal of limb bud Sonic hedgehog results in posterior skeletal defects. *Dev Biol* 180: 35–40.

Panin VM, Papayannopoulos V, Wilson R, Irvine KD (1997). Fringe modulates Notch–ligand interactions. *Nature* 387: 908–912.

Parr BA, McMahon AP (1995). Dorsalizing signal Wnt-7a required for normal polarity of D–V and A–P axes of mouse limb. *Nature* 374: 350–353.

Parr BA, Shea MJ, Vassileva G, McMahon AP (1993). Mouse Wnt genes exhibit discrete domains of expression in the early embryonic CNS and limb buds. *Development* 119: 247–261.

Peichel CL, Prabhakaran B, Vogt TF (1997). The mouse Ulnaless mutation deregulates posterior *HoxD* gene expression and alters appendicular patterning. *Development* 124: 3481–3492.

Pizette S, Niswander L (2000). BMPs are required at two steps of limb chondrogenesis: formation of prechondrogenic condensations and their differentiation into chondrocytes. *Dev Biol* 219: 237–249.

Porter JA, Young KE, Beachy PA (1996). Cholesterol modification of hedgehog signaling proteins in animal development. *Science* 274: 255–259.

Qu S, Niswender KD, Ji Q, van der Meer R, Keeney D, Magnuson MA, Wisdom R (1997). Polydactyly and ectopic ZPA formation in Alx-4 mutant mice. *Development* 124: 3999–4008.

Qu S, Tucker SC, Ehrlich JS, Levorse JM, Flaherty LA, Wisdom R, Vogt TF (1998). Mutations in mouse Aristaless-like4 cause Strong's luxoid polydactyly. *Development* 125: 2711–2721.

Rancourt DE, Tsuzuki T, Capecchi MR (1995). Genetic interaction between *hoxb-5* and *hoxb-6* is revealed by nonallelic noncomplementation. *Genes Dev* 9: 108–122.

Riddle RD, Johnson RL, Laufer E, Tabin C (1993). Sonic hedgehog mediates the polarizing activity of the ZPA. *Cell* 75: 1401–1416.

Riddle RD, Ensini M, Nelson C, Tsuchida T, Jessell TM, Tabin C (1995). Induction of the LIM homeobox gene Lmx1 by WNT7a establishes dorsoventral pattern in the vertebrate limb. *Cell* 83: 631–640.

Rodriguez-Esteban C, Schwabe JW, De La Pena J, Foys B, Eshelman B, Belmonte JC (1997). Radical fringe positions the apical ectodermal ridge at the dorsoventral boundary of the vertebrate limb. *Nature* 386: 360–366.

Rodriguez-Esteban C, Tsukui T, Yonei S, Magallon J, Tamura K, Izpisua Belmonte JC (1999). The T-box genes *Tbx4* and *Tbx5* regulate limb outgrowth and identity. *Nature* 398: 814–818.

Rubin L, Saunders JW Jr (1972). Ectodermal–mesodermal interactions in the growth of limb buds in the chick embryo: constancy and temporal limits of the ectodermal induction. *Dev Biol* 28: 94–112.

Ruppert JM, Vogelstein B, Arheden K, Kinzler KW (1990). GLI3 encodes a 190-kilodalton protein with multiple regions of GLI similarity. *Mol Cell Biol* 10: 5408–5415.

Ruvinsky I, Gibson-Brown JJ (2000). Genetic and developmental bases of serial homology in vertebrate limb evolution. *Development* 127: 5233–5244.

Saunders JW Jr (1948). The proximo-distal sequence of origin of the parts of the chick wing and the role of the ectoderm. *J Exp Zool* 108: 363–403.

Saunders JW, Gasseling MT (1968). Ectodermal and mesenchymal interactions in the origin of limb symmetry. In: *Epithelial Mesenchymal Interactions*. Fleischmajer R, Billingham RE (eds). William and Wilkins, Baltimore, pp. 78–97.

Saunders JW Jr, Reuss C (1974). Inductive and axial properties of prospective wing-bud mesoderm in the chick embryo. *Dev Biol* 38: 41–50.

Schimmang T, van der Hoeven F, Ruther U (1993). Gli3 expression is affected in the morphogenetic mouse mutants add and Xt. *Prog Clin Biol Res* 383A: 153–161.

Searls RL, Janners MY (1971). The initiation of limb bud outgrowth in the embryonic chick. *Dev Biol* 24: 198–213.

Sekine K, Ohuchi H, Fujiwara M, Yamasaki M, Yoshizawa T, Sato T, Yagishita N, Matsui D, Koga Y, Itoh N, et al. (1999). Fgf10 is essential for limb and lung formation. *Nat Genet* 21: 138–141.

Shawber C, Boulter J, Lindsell CE, Weinmaster G (1996). *Jagged2*: a serrate-like gene expressed during rat embryogenesis. *Dev Biol* 180: 370–376.

Sherman L, Wainwright D, Ponta H, Herrlich P (1998). A splice variant of CD44 expressed in the apical ectodermal ridge presents fibroblast growth factors to limb mesenchyme and is required for limb outgrowth. *Genes Dev* 12: 1058–1071.

Sidow A, Bulotsky MS, Kerrebrock AW, Bronson RT, Daly MJ, Reeve MP, Hawkins TL, Birren BW, Jaenisch R, Lander ES (1997). Serrate2 is disrupted in the mouse limb-development mutant syndactylism. *Nature* 389: 722–725.

Simonneau L, Kitagawa M, Suzuki S, Thiery JP (1995). Cadherin 11 expression marks the mesenchymal phenotype: towards new functions for cadherins? *Cell Adhes Commun* 3: 115–130.

Small KM, Potter SS (1993). Homeotic transformations and limb defects in Hox A11 mutant mice. *Genes Dev* 7: 2318–2328.

Speicher SA, Thomas U, Hinz U, Knust E (1994). The Serrate locus of *Drosophila* and its role in morphogenesis of the wing imaginal discs: control of cell proliferation. *Development* 120: 535–544.

Srivastava D, Cserjesi P, Olson EN (1995). A subclass of bHLH proteins required for cardiac morphogenesis. *Science* 270: 1995–1999.

Stephens TD, McNulty TR (1981). Evidence for a metameric pattern in the development of the chick humerus. *J Embryol Exp Morphol* 61: 191–205.

Stratford T, Horton C, Maden M (1996). Retinoic acid is required for the initiation of outgrowth in the chick limb bud. *Curr Biol* 6: 1124–1133.

Strecker TR, Stephens TD (1983). Peripheral nerves do not play a trophic role in limb skeletal morphogenesis. *Teratology* 27: 159–167.

Summerbell D (1974). A quantitative analysis of the effect of excision of the AER from the chick limb-bud. *J Embryol Exp Morphol* 32: 651–660.

Summerbell D, Lewis JH (1975). Time, place and positional value in the chick limb-bud. *J Embryol Exp Morphol* 33: 621–643.

Summerbell D, Lewis JH, Wolpert L (1973). Positional information in chick limb morphogenesis. *Nature* 244: 492–496.

Sun X, Lewandoski M, Meyers EN, Liu YH, Maxson RE Jr, Martin GR (2000). Conditional inactivation of Fgf4 reveals complexity of signalling during limb bud development. *Nat Genet* 25: 83–86.

Sun X, Mariani FV, Martin GR (2002). Functions of FGF signalling from the apical ectodermal ridge in limb development. *Nature* 418: 501–508.

Swiatek PJ, Lindsell CE, del Amo FF, Weinmaster G, Gridley T (1994). Notch1 is essential for postimplantation development in mice. *Genes Dev* 8: 707–719.

Szeto DP, Ryan AK, O'Connell SM, Rosenfeld MG (1996). P-OTX: a PIT-1-interacting homeodomain factor expressed during anterior pituitary gland development. *Proc Natl Acad Sci USA* 93: 7706–7710.

Szeto DP, Rodriguez-Esteban C, Ryan AK, O'Connell SM, Liu F, Kioussi C, Gleiberman AS, Izpisua-Belmonte JC, Rosenfeld MG (1999). Role of the Bicoid-related homeodomain factor Pitx1 in specifying hindlimb morphogenesis and pituitary development. *Genes Dev* 13: 484–494.

Tabin CJ (1991). Retinoids, homeoboxes, and growth factors: toward molecular models for limb development. *Cell* 66: 199–217.

Takahashi M, Tamura K, Buscher D, Masuya H, Yonei-Tamura S, Matsumoto K, Naitoh-Matsuo M, Takeuchi J, Ogura K, Shiroishi T, et al. (1998). The role of Alx-4 in the establishment of anteroposterior polarity during vertebrate limb development. *Development* 125: 4417–4425.

Takeuchi JK, Koshiba-Takeuchi K, Matsumoto K, Vogel-Hopker A, Naitoh-Matsuo M, Ogura K, Takahashi N, Yasuda K, Ogura T (1999). *Tbx5* and *Tbx4* genes determine the wing/leg identity of limb buds. *Nature* 398: 810–814.

Tanaka M, Tamura K, Noji S, Nohno T, Ide H (1997). Induction of additional limb at the dorsal–ventral boundary of a chick embryo. *Dev Biol* 182: 191–203.

Tickle C (1981). The number of polarizing region cells required to specify additional digits in the developing chick wing. *Nature* 289: 295–298.

Tickle C, Alberts B, Wolpert L, Lee J (1982). Local application of retinoic acid to the limb bud mimics the action of the polarizing region. *Nature* 296: 564–566.

van den Akker E, Reijnen M, Korving J, Brouwer A, Meijlink F, Deschamps J (1999). Targeted inactivation of Hoxb8 affects survival of a spinal ganglion and causes aberrant limb reflexes. *Mech Dev* 89: 103–114.

van der Hoeven F, Zakany J, Duboule D (1996). Gene transpositions in the HoxD complex reveal a hierarchy of regulatory controls. *Cell* 85: 1025–1035.

Vogel A, Tickle C (1993). FGF-4 maintains polarizing activity of posterior limb bud cells in vivo and in vitro. *Development* 119: 199–206.

Vogel A, Rodriguez C, Warnken W, Izpisua Belmonte JC (1995). Dorsal cell fate specified by chick Lmx1 during vertebrate limb development. *Nature* 378: 716–720.

Vogel A, Rodriguez C, Izpisua-Belmonte JC (1996). Involvement of FGF-8 in initiation, outgrowth and patterning of the vertebrate limb. *Development* 122: 1737–1750.

Vortkamp A, Gessler M, Grzeschik KH (1991). GLI3 zinc-finger gene interrupted by translocations in Greig syndrome families. *Nature* 352: 539–540.

Wagner M, Thaller C, Jessell T, Eichele G (1990). Polarizing activity and retinoid synthesis in the floor plate of the neural tube. *Nature* 345: 819–822.

Wolpert L, Tickle C, Sampford M (1979). The effect of cell killing by x-irradiation on pattern formation in the chick limb. *J Embryol Exp Morphol* 50: 175–193.

Woychik RP, Stewart TA, Davis LG, D'Eustachio P, Leder P (1985). An inherited l imb deformity created by insertional mutagenesis in a transgenic mouse. *Nature* 318: 36–40.

Wurst W, Auerbach AB, Joyner AL (1994). Multiple developmental defects in Engrailed-1 mutant mice: an early mid-hindbrain deletion and patterning defects in forelimbs and sternum. *Development* 120: 2065–2075.

Xu J, Liu Z, Ornitz DM (2000). Temporal and spatial gradients of Fgf8 and Fgf17 regulate proliferation and differentiation of midline cerebellar structures. *Development* 127: 1833–1843.

Xu X, Weinstein M, Li C, Naski M, Cohen RI, Ornitz DM, Leder P, Deng C (1998). Fibroblast growth factor receptor 2 (FGFR2)–mediated reciprocal regulation loop between FGF8 and FGF10 is essential for limb induction. *Development* 125: 753–765.

Xu X, Weinstein M, Li C, Deng C (1999). Fibroblast growth factor receptors (FGFRs) and their roles in limb development. *Cell Tissue Res* 296: 33–43.

Yang A, Schweitzer R, Sun D, Kaghad M, Walker N, Bronson RT, Tabin C, Sharpe A, Caput D, Crum C, et al. (1999). p63 is essential for regenerative proliferation in limb, craniofacial and epithelial development. *Nature* 398: 714–718.

Yang Y, Niswander L (1995). Interaction between the signaling molecules WNT7a and SHH during vertebrate limb development: dorsal signals regulate anteroposterior patterning. *Cell* 80: 939–947.

Yokouchi Y, Nakazato S, Yamamoto M, Goto Y, Kameda T, Iba H, Kuroiwa A (1995). Misexpression of Hoxa-13 induces cartilage homeotic transformation and changes cell adhesiveness in chick limb buds. *Genes Dev* 9: 2509–2522.

Yonei S, Tamura K, Ohsugi K, Ide H (1995). MRC-5 cells induce the AER prior to the duplicated pattern formation in chick limb bud. *Dev Biol* 170: 542–552.

Zeller R, Haramis AG, Zuniga A, McGuigan C, Dono R, Davidson G, Chabanis S, Gibson T (1999). Formin defines a large family of morphoregulatory genes and functions in establishment of the polarising region. *Cell Tissue Res* 296: 85–93.

Zeng X, Goetz JA, Suber LM, Scott WJ Jr, Schreiner CM, Robbins DJ (2001). A freely diffusible form of Sonic hedgehog mediates long-range signalling. *Nature* 411: 716–720.

Zuniga A, Haramis AP, McMahon AP, Zeller R (1999). Signal relay by BMP antagonism controls the SHH/FGF4 feedback loop in vertebrate limb buds. *Nature* 401: 598–602.

Zwilling E (1955). Ectoderm–mesoderm relationship in the development of the chick embryo limb bud. *J Exp Zool* 128: 423–442.

Zwilling E (1961). Limb morphogenesis. *Adv Morphogen* 1: 301–330.

Zwilling E (1964). Development of fragmented and dissociated limb bud mesoderm. *Dev Biol* 9: 20–37.

13 | Development of the Genitourinary System

DYLAN STEER, KAZUHITO FUKUOKA, STANLEY A. MENDOZA, AND SANJAY K. NIGAM

The morphogenetic processes that govern embryonic genitourinary development have important implications for human disease. Renal abnormalities attributable to inborn errors of development account for the majority of pediatric chronic renal failure. Moreover, complex adult phenotypes, such as hypertension, may have their origins in subtle defects in more than one developmental pathway. As a model of organ development, kidney organogenesis can shed light on a variety of fundamental developmental patterns, pathways, and programs applicable to different areas of developmental biology. Specifically, kidney development involves complex mesenchymal–epithelial interactions whereby the epithelium transforms from a simple outbudding of the Wolffian duct into an arborized collecting system and the surrounding mesenchyme is rescued from an apoptotic fate to undergo epithelialization, forming the tubular nephron. Furthermore, the nascent renal tubule interacts with the developing vasculature both by de novo vasculogenic mechanisms and by recruitment of extrinsic blood vessels to form the glomerulus. This elaborate program involves initiators (e.g., growth factors and receptors), intracellular mediators (e.g., transcription factors), and extracellular effectors (e.g., matrix proteases and proteoglycans) that affect fundamental developmental processes such as cell differentiation, proliferation, apoptosis, adhesion, and migration. Significant developmental abnormalities have been ascribed to aberrations in many of the processes central to this inductive program.

Experimentation into the processes that govern genitourinary development dates at least to 1927, when Boyden surgically obliterated the Wolffian duct in chickens and consequently inhibited metanephric development. In the 1940s and 1950s, Grobstein (1953, 1955, 1956) developed an in vitro culture system to investigate the cellular mechanisms that govern renal organogenesis and described the induction of the mesenchyme by a variety of embryonic tissues. At approximately the same time, transplantation of embryonic gonadal primordia was used to examine the mechanisms of gonadal sex determination (Jost, 1953; Jost et al., 1973). These initial experiments of the premolecular era provide the foundation for the molecular and genetic progress achieved thus far. The remarkable advances in technology and molecular biology of the past several decades have led to elaboration of the basic morphologic and cellular principles proposed by these pioneers. The description of the events of urogenital development in cellular and molecular terms has led to an improved understanding of the pathogenesis of diseases attributable to defects in genitourinary development. In many ways, understanding the underpinnings of developmental disease has furthered our understanding of normal development.

This chapter provides a context for the fundamental genetic and molecular events that initiate, propagate, and maintain urinary and genital tract development. The development of these two systems is closely intertwined as they arise from common progenital structures and shared early genetic events help to shape the destinies of both. The details of the significant pathways and molecules are provided in subsequent chapters.

OVERVIEW OF KIDNEY DEVELOPMENT

Fundamentally, the normal kidney is charged with several missions. It filters blood via diffusive and convective forces across a complex basement membrane, it regulates plasma volume and chemical composition by selective tubular reabsorption and secretion, and it has endocrine functions critical to blood and calcium/phosphorus homeosta-

sis. To perform these functions, the kidneys receive approximately 20% of the cardiac output. The kidney contains roughly one million nephrons, each of which is a highly specialized functional unit. The prototypical nephron consists of a glomerulus, tubule, and collecting system. The glomerulus contains an elaborate capillary network lined internally by a fenestrated endothelium and surrounded by unique epithelial cells, called *podocytes*, which extend interdigitated "foot processes" that help to regulate the composition of fluid filtered into the urinary space. The capillary stalks are held together by the glomerular mesangium, a matrix secreted by mesangial cells. The urinary ultrafiltrate is collected within Bowman's capsule and enters the long tubular nephron. Each segment of the tubule (proximal convoluted, loop of Henle, distal convoluted, and collecting duct) has unique transport properties, which tightly regulate the volume and composition of the filtrate. The nephron takes a circuitous course, originating in the cortex and extending deep into the kidney medulla. As the tubular fluid returns from the medulla, it passes by its parent glomerulus and then courses through the terminal portions of the tubule and into the collecting duct. The ducts funnel the filtrate into the ureter, and the urine then empties into the bladder. These structures and their subsequent functions arise from a tightly regulated sequence of development.

The urinary system has its developmental origins in the intermediate mesoderm between the paraxial and lateral plates. Proceeding in a spatiotemporally regulated, craniocaudal fashion, three successive nephric systems develop in mammals and birds: the pronephros, mesonephros, and metanephros. In certain ways, the more complex nephric systems seem to recapitulate basic mechanisms involved in the development of earlier urinary systems. In humans, the vestigial pronephros degenerates completely, and until recently there has been little interest in the molecular mechanisms of pronephric development. Developments in the molecular biology of transparent zebrafish and *Xenopus* have renewed interest in understanding pronephric development as a model of subsequent metanephric development. The mesonephros forms as the second nephric structure and is transiently functional in human embryonic development. Mammalian mesonephric structures associate with structures derived from the cloaca to form the genital system. The mammalian kidney is derived from the metanephros, and the majority of experimental investigation has been done in the field of metanephric development.

Pronephros

The pronephros arises at human embryonic day 22 (day 8 in mice) from cells located in the cervical intermediate mesoderm. This primordial system foreshadows the future metanephric kidney as it consists of three prototypical structures: the glomerulus, tubule, and pronephric duct. The pronephros is functional in fish and amphibian larvae. There appear to be contiguous, bounded, prepatterned regions within these cervical nephrotomes that contribute to the individual structures of the pronephros. In zebrafish, these spatially restricted domains exhibit unique combinations of transcription factor gene expression. For example, pretubular cells express *Wt1* and *Pax2.1* but not *Sim1*, whereas cells destined to form the pronephric glomerulus express only *Wt1* (Serluca and Fishman, 2001). *Pax8* may also have a role in pronephric development (Carroll and Vize, 1999). The pronephric duct then elongates by recruiting a subset of cells from the intermediate mesoderm and inducing their epithelialization. In *Xenopus*, *Xlim1* is expressed early in pronephric development. Transfection with a dominant-negative mutant of *Xlim1* inhibits growth and elongation of the pronephric rudiment, which suggests that the LIM class of homeobox genes is important in normal pronephric development (Chan et al., 2000). In mammals, the pronephros undergoes apoptosis and degenerates (Pole et al., 2002), and the human glomerular and tubular aspects of the pronephros degenerate by day 25. The cranial portion of the pronephric duct also degenerates, while the caudal pronephric duct remains functional, becoming the mesonephric or Wolffian duct.

Mesonephros

Paired swellings of intermediate mesoderm begin to condense in a craniocaudal distribution along the mesonephric duct, beginning at approximately human embryonic day 24. These mesonephric segments give rise to 30–40 tubules, which connect to the mesonephric duct from the upper thoracic to mid-lumbar level. This sequence of events is morphologically similar to later metanephric development; however, the molecular signals that initiate mesonephric development are not well defined. As with the pronephros, mesonephric duct development appears to require expression of the transcription factors *Lim1* and *Pax2*, and *Lim1* appears to be required for mesodermal differentiation (Tsang et al., 2000). *Lim1* continues to be expressed during mesonephric development and then maintains its expression in the metanephric ureteric bud (UB) and in structures derived from the metanephric mesenchyme (Fujii et al., 1994). Although most mice with homozygous mutations of *Lim1* die prior to metanephric development, a few surviving embryos do not have either kidneys or mesodermally derived gonads (Shawlot and Behringer, 1995). As noted above, Pax2 continues to be expressed in the mesonephros. In mice with perturbation of normal Pax2 expression, structures derived from the intermediate mesoderm and the caudal portion of the mesonephric duct are missing. Mesonephric tubules, metanephric kidneys, and genital tracts do not form (Torres et al., 1995).

There appear to be differences within mammalian species regarding the functionality of the mesonephros, but the significance of this finding is unknown. The mesonephros is functional in humans and produces small amounts of urine between the sixth and tenth weeks, whereas in the mouse the mesonephros does not appear to possess an excretory function. As detailed below, the Wolffian ducts in females ultimately undergo complete apoptosis and Wolffian duct derivatives in males develop into the vas deferens, seminal vesicles, and tubules of the epididymis.

Metanephros

The metanephric kidney (Fig. 13–1) develops through spatially restricted, reciprocal inductive events between a loose collection of un-

differentiated mesenchyme and an invading epithelium (Saxen, 1987). The epithelial structure that originates from the Wolffian duct is termed the ureteric bud (UB), which undergoes multiple iterations of branching and elongation and is destined to form the collecting system of the kidney and the ureter. The mesenchyme, a product of the intermediate mesoderm, initially condenses around the branching tips of the UB and then ultimately undergoes mesenchymal to epithelial transformation (MET). Tissue derived from the metanephric mesenchyme (MM) forms the glomerulus and the tubular nephron (i.e., proximal tubule, loop of Henle, and distal tubule). The genetic programs that lead to metanephric development are discussed in detail below.

The first step in definitive metanephric development is induction of the UB by the mesenchyme (Fig. 13–2a), which typically occurs at day 10.5 days postconception (dpc) in mice, day 13.5 dpc in rats, and day 28 dpc in humans. Factors expressed by the metanephric mes-

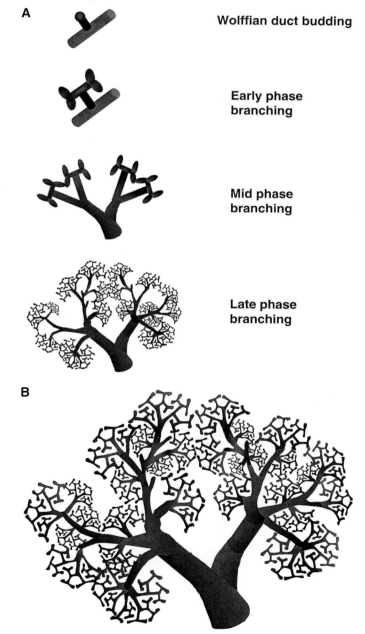

Figure 13–2. Schematic representation of ureteric bud branching morphogenesis. *A*: From top to bottom represents the initial budding of the ureteric bud, followed by early-, mid-, and late-phase branching. *B*: A schematic of the final ureteric "tree."

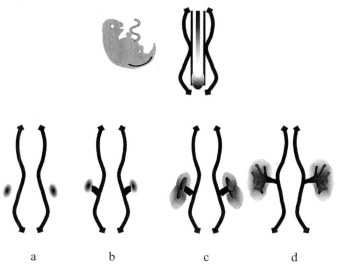

Figure 13–1. Schematic representation of metanephrogenesis. *a*: Wolffian ducts with the undifferentiated metanephric mesenchyme nearby. *b*: The ureteric bud is induced and invades the metanephric mesenchyme. *c*: The ureteric bud undergoes branching, and mesenchymal to epithelial transformation begins. *d*: Kidney formation is nearly complete.

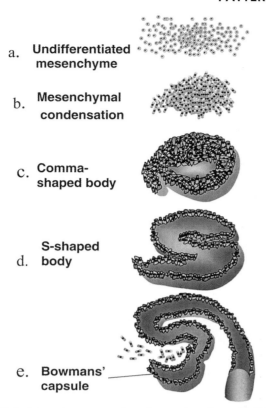

a. **Undifferentiated mesenchyme**

b. **Mesenchymal condensation**

c. **Comma-shaped body**

d. **S-shaped body**

e. **Bowmans' capsule**

Figure 13–3. Schematic representation of mesenchymal to epithelial transformation with the formation of the glomerulus and the renal tubule. *a*: The mesenchyme is initially undifferentiated. *b*: The mesenchyme condenses at the tip of the ureteric bud. *c–e*: The mesenchyme forms a comma-shaped body, which then elongates into an S-shaped body that develops further into Bowman's capsule.

undergo MET (Fig. 13–3). These two processes appear to be independent of cell–cell contact as they can be reproduced *in vitro* using soluble growth factors (Barasch et al., 1999b; Qiao et al., 1999a; Plisov et al., 2001). Mesenchymal transformation into a polarized epithelial tissue is a highly regulated event with distinct morphologic stages. Initially, the loose collection of metanephric mesenchyme condenses into a cap-like aggregated focus of tissue at the tips of the branching UB. There appear to be two distinct portions of this aggregate: the cap, which overlies the majority of each UB branch tip, and the pretubular aggregate, which lies at the lateral edge of tips. This aggregate undergoes dramatic proliferation and is destined to form the nephron (Fig. 13–4) (Bard et al., 2001; Sariola, 2002). A specific cell population within the mesenchyme, termed the *stroma*, may have significant modulatory roles in both mesenchymal and ureteric induction. In addition to losing markers of mesenchymal tissues and gaining markers of epithelial cells, the condensed pretubular mesenchyme forms tight junctions and becomes polarized columnar epithelia, forming a structure termed the *renal vesicle*. Morphologically, this vesicle initially takes on a "comma"-shaped appearance, then elongates into an S-shaped body as it develops. The UB fuses with the most distal limb of the S-shaped body, and the resultant metanephric tubule is now connected to a collecting system. The more proximal elements form each segment of the renal tubule (proximal tubule, loop of Henle, and distal convoluted tubule), and structures derived from the UB form the collecting system and ureter.

Glomerulogenesis requires coordinated development of epithelial podocyte, mesangial, and endothelial vascular elements. This process begins relatively rapidly in the developing kidney and continues throughout nephric development. Although the 11 dpc mouse embryo has begun collecting system development and nephron formation, the kidney remains avascular. Between 12 and 13 dpc, the mouse metanephros acquires rudimentary capillary networks located between the branching UB and the developing tubular structures. As the S-shaped body folds in on itself, the outer cells become the glomerular (Bowman's) capsule, the inner cells become the epithelial podocytes of the glomerulus, and endothelial cells begin to populate the region between the maturing podocytes and tubular cells in the clefts of the S-shaped primordial nephrons. The upper cleft of the S-shaped body appears to recruit these vascular precursors. The embryonic kidney contains endogenous angioblasts and, thus, appears to have the capability for in situ vasculogenesis; however, recruitment of extra-kidney endothelial cell precursors may play a significant role. Finally, by 14 dpc, the deepest cortical nephrons develop glomerular loops and mesangial cells. Between the sixth and ninth weeks of human development, the kidneys ascend from their lumbar location along a path close to the aorta. During this cranial migration, the ascending

enchyme cause focal proliferation and sprouting of the UB from a discrete portion of the Wolffian duct. The UB then invades the surrounding mesenchyme. Without a signal(s) provided by this invading UB, the mesenchyme undergoes rapid apoptosis. The next step in metanephric development is a remarkable sequence of reciprocal inductive events between the UB and MM. The MM induces the UB to undergo a series of repetitive branching and elongating events, termed *branching morphogenesis*, and the UB induces the mesenchyme to

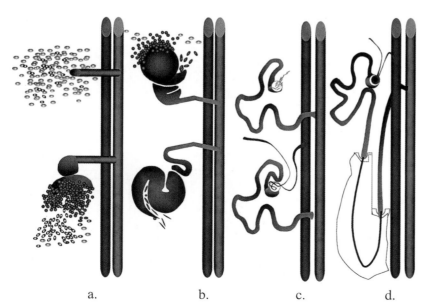

a.   b.   c.   d.

Figure 13–4. Schematic representation of nephron formation. *a*: The ureteric bud grows toward the undifferentiated mesenchyme (*top*), which the condenses around the tip of the bud (*bottom*). *b*: As the ureteric bud branches, the mesenchyme forms a comma-shaped body (*top*) and then an S-shaped body (*bottom*). *c*: Bowman's capsule is formed (*top*), and arterioles grow in forming the glomerular loops and mesangial cells (*bottom*). *d*: The tubule elongates, forming the proximal tubule, the loop of Henle, and the distal convoluted tubule of the mature nephron.

kidney appears to be progressively vascularized by arteries arising from the aorta. These immature arteries do not elongate with the ascending kidney, and as the kidney ascends, the inferior immature renal arteries regress and new, more cranial arteries are recruited. Nephrogenesis occurs in the nephrogenic zone of the outer renal cortex throughout embryogenesis and even into early postnatal life in some mammalian species.

OVERVIEW OF GONADAL DEVELOPMENT

The gonadal primordium arises from the urogenital ridge, which consists of a thickening of the ventrolateral surface of the mesonephros, and initially forms a bipotent or indifferent gonad. The genital tracts are formed from the Wolffian ducts in males and the mullerian ducts in females. The mullerian (paramesonephric) ducts initially develop as an invagination of the coelomic cavity within the mesonephros. Extraembryonic primordial germ cells actively migrate from allantoic mesoderm, through the hindgut and mesonephros, and into the urogenital ridge (Ginsburg et al., 1990). Sex determination, however, does not appear to require primordial germ cell migration. The indifferent gonad undergoes testicular development as a result of expression of *Sry*, which apparently is the only gene on the Y chromosome necessary to trigger Sertoli cell differentiation (Swain and Lovell-Badge, 1999). Ovarian development seems to occur as a result of the absence of *Sry* expression and expression of other "antitestis" factors.

SPECIFIC MODELS FOR STUDYING THE MOLECULAR DEVELOPMENT OF THE GENITOURINARY SYSTEM

The initial classical work in kidney development was typically done in ex vivo organ culture models whereby the kidney is cultured on a porous filter (Fig. 13–5). These models, for example, allowed for the identification of nonspecific inducers of mesenchyme, such as embryonic spinal cord, and continue to remain valid to examine kidney development. Several other models and molecular techniques deserve specific mention as they have been used to develop recent molecular data.

Knockout and Transgenic Techniques

The ability to target specific genes for deletion via homologous recombination or overexpression via transgenic techniques has provided an extremely powerful in vivo tool, providing insight into the functional molecular mechanisms of development. Much of our current understanding of urogenital development derives from these targeted mutations. A discussion of the specific advantages and drawbacks of gene knockout, transgenic, and conditional expression techniques is found in other chapters; but there are several issues specific to studies of renal development. First, functional mutations of genes involved in pro- and mesonephric developmental programs may lead to meta-nephric and sex phenotypes by interrupting these earlier processes. This could lead to the incorrect conclusion that these genes are required for metanephrogenesis or sex determination per se. Second, there appears to be a great degree of redundancy in morphogenetic programs. Several regulatory factors, which appear to be necessary in ex vivo and/or cell culture models of renal development, do not have expected kidney phenotypes when functionally deleted. Finally, since the metanephric kidney develops through reciprocal induction of the UB and the MM, disturbances of one could result from an abnormality in the development of either.

Organ Culture Systems

While whole embryonic kidney organ culture can identify modulators of renal development, the specific effects on mesenchyme or UB cannot be determined. Recent assays have been developed to examine the effects of factors on mesenchyme and UB. The isolated UB (i.e., free of surrounding mesenchyme) has been induced to branch in vitro in a cell-free extracellular matrix in the presence of factors found in medium that has been conditioned by immortalized metanephric mesenchymal cells and supplemented with glial cell line–derived neurotrophic factor (GDNF) (Qiao et al., 1999a). As discussed below, this

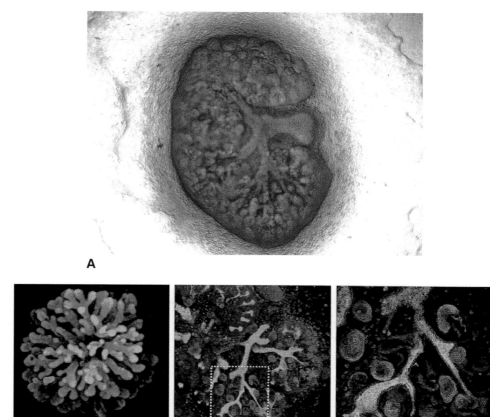

Figure 13–5. *A*: The kidney of a fetal rat grown in organ culture. The fetal kidney was removed at day 13 postconception and the kidney grown in culture for an additional 6 days. The ureteric bud with its main branches can be seen. In addition, there has been significant differentiation of the metanephric mesenchyme. (Figure provided by Dr. Rosemary Sampogna.) *B*: In this experiment, ureteric buds were isolated and grown in culture for 7–10 days (*left*). The cultured bud was then removed from the extracellular matrix in which it was grown and combined with mesenteric mesenchyme freshly isolated from embryonic day 13 fetal kidneys. The recombined bud and mesenchyme were then cultured for an additional 5 days. After culture, the sample was double-stained with Dolichos biflorus lectin, which is specific for ureteric bud–derived structures (green stain) and with peanut agglutinin lectin, which is specific for mesenchyme-derived structures (red stain). This is shown at low power (*center*). The boxed area is enlarged (*right*) and indicates that ureteric buds cultured in vitro can induce nephrogenesis. (Figure from Qiao et al., 1999a, *Proc Natl Acad Sci USA* 96: 7330–7335.)

modified organ culture technique has led to the identification of factors secreted by the mesenchyme that appear to influence UB growth and elongation. In a similar fashion, the MM can be cultured ex vivo on a filter and induced to undergo rudimentary nephrogenesis when exposed to soluble factors that have been isolated from medium conditioned by cultured UB cells (Barasch et al., 1999b; Plisov et al., 2001). These model systems suggest that soluble factors are sufficient for branching morphogenesis and MET to occur, and cell–cell contact is not necessary.

Cell Culture Models of Kidney Development

There are several cell culture–based model systems used to study kidney development. Immortalized embryonic cells derived from the UB, when cultured as a single-cell suspension in an appropriate matrix, can be stimulated by growth factors to proliferate, migrate, and form rudimentary tubules (Sakurai et al., 1997a). In a similar fashion but under different conditions, immortalized cells derived from the adult murine inner medullary collecting duct (mIMCD) can also be stimulated to form multicellular branching structures (Cantley et al., 1994; Sakurai and Nigam, 1997). Other cell culture models of tubulogenesis have utilized adult Madin-Darby canine kidney (MDCK) cells and have helped to elucidate some of the morphologic events critical to tubule lumen formation (Pollack et al., 1998). However, several growth factors that stimulate tubulogenesis in this model, such as hepatocyte growth factor (HGF) and epidermal growth factor (EGF) receptor ligands, fail to do so in culture models utilizing embryonic cells or in the isolated UB culture system.

Gene Array Technology

The development of high-density genetic arrays has allowed surveys of gene expression during kidney development (Stuart et al., 2001). Whole rat kidneys isolated during embryonic metanephric and neonatal development as well as adult kidneys have been surveyed for expressed genes. From these studies, several unique patterns of global gene expression emerged: early in fetal kidney development, the majority of expressed genes appeared to be involved with anatomical developmental processes (e.g., cell division, differentiation, etc.), whereas during later stages of development, the majority of genes assumed functional tasks, such as transport and metabolism. Unexpectedly, during the interval immediately surrounding birth, a large number of retrotransposons were expressed. The functional significance of this finding is unknown. This new technology is currently being focused on individual developmental programs, including branching morphogenesis of the isolated UB and mesenchymal induction and epithelialization.

MORPHOGENETIC DEVELOPMENT OF THE METANEPHRIC KIDNEY

As detailed above, the metanephric kidney undergoes several distinct stages of development, beginning with the initiation of UB outgrowth from the Wolffian duct and continuing with mesenchymal induction of ureteric branching morphogenesis and ureteric induction of mesenchymal condensation and differentiation. The stages have been reviewed in detail (Kuure et al., 2000; Sariola, 2002), and a new classification of developmental disorders of the kidney has been proposed based on their effects on various stages of development (Pohl et al., 2002). The individual steps or stages involved in kidney development do not necessarily occur in temporal series; indeed, several of these processes, including the reciprocal induction of metanephric mesenchyme and epithelial UB, occur simultaneously. Many of the molecules essential to one process of development also have roles in later downstream events. Although a large number of molecules are involved in these steps, the remainder of this chapter will focus on key control genes involved in each of these stages, including transcription factors, growth factors, and matrix components, among others.

Transcription Factors

As noted earlier, the transcription factors *Lim1* and *Pax2* (see Chapters 59–63) are required for the Wolffian duct to form. In the absence of either of these genes, UB outgrowth does not occur and renal agenesis ensues. Heterozygous mutations in the *Pax2* gene lead to kidney hypoplasia in mice and humans. Both of these transcription factors have roles during later stages of metanephric development as well. *Pax2* expression is normally downregulated in later stages of tubular development; however, prolonging its expression produces a phenotype reminiscent of congenital nephrotic syndrome. Interestingly, although mesenchymal expression of *Pax2* occurs in cells of both the cap and pretubular aggregate, *Lim1* is found only in the mesenchymal cells of the pre-tubular aggregate. *Lim1* is also expressed in cells at the tip of the UB (Fujii et al., 1994).

A transcription factor encoded by the Wilms' tumor-suppressor gene (*Wt1*) is expressed in the mesenchyme surrounding the Wolffian duct at the site of UB induction (Buckler et al., 1991; Armstrong et al., 1993). *Wt1* expression increases in induced mesenchyme, reaching its highest level in the early glomerular cells (Ryan et al., 1995). Wt1 is required for initial UB induction. The *Wt1* knockout mouse has a normal Wolffian duct, but the UB does not form and there is apoptosis of the mesenchyme, resulting in renal agenesis (Kreidberg et al., 1993). Furthermore, *Wt1* appears to be necessary for MM responsiveness to inductive signals as nonspecific inducers of the MM, such as spinal cord, were unable to induce nephrogenesis in *Wt1* null embryos (Kreidberg et al., 1993). Normal Wt1 is also required during later stages of development as mice heterozygous for a *Wt1* mutation that causes truncation of Wt1 in one of its zinc fingers develop mesangial sclerosis and male genital defects (Patek et al., 1999). This phenotype is similar to the Denys-Drash and Fraser's syndromes in humans, and humans with these syndromes also have mutations in the *WT1* gene (Little and Wells, 1997).

EYA1 (see Chapter 55) is the human ortholog of the *Drosophila eyes absent* gene and encodes a transcription factor that is expressed in the mesenchyme surrounding initial UB outgrowth. In homozygous null mice, the UB fails to develop from the Wolffian duct and subsequent renal development is absent (Xu et al., 1999). These mice express *Pax2*, but not *Gdnf* or *Six*, suggesting that *Eya1* acts as a mediator of a mesenchymal signal cascade that leads to UB induction. The *Pax-Eya-Six* signal cascade may be an evolutionarily conserved pathway. Significantly, the human branchio-oto-renal syndrome, characterized by deafness and a variety of severe renal malformations, is due to mutations in or near a highly conserved region of *EYA1* (Abdelhak et al., 1997).

The genes for three forkhead/winged transcription factors, *Foxc1* (*Mf1*), *Mf2*, and *Foxc2* (*Mfh1*), affect ureteral development by modulating UB induction and branching. These factors are expressed in the MM surrounding the Wolffian duct and branching UB. One strain of mice with homozygous null mutations for *Foxc1* has renal duplication, multiple ureters, and hydroureter/hydronephrosis (Kume et al., 2000b). This phenotype was uncommon in a second strain with the same mutation, illustrating the importance of the genetic background when interpreting results of gene-knockout experiments. Similar developmental abnormalities were seen in 20%–40% of mice homozygous for null mutations of *Mf2* (Kume et al., 2000a). While *Foxc1* and *Foxc2* heterozygotes do not display a renal phenotype, the compound heterozygote has hypoplastic kidneys and hydroureter.

Several homeobox (*Hox*) genes (see Chapter 46) are expressed in both the mesonephros and metanephros and may be important in patterning of the nephric structures. *Hoxb7* is expressed in tissues derived from the Wolffian duct, including the ureter, UB, and collecting ducts; and its promoter is sufficient to drive reporter gene expression specifically to UB-derived structures (Argao et al., 1995). *Hoxa11* and *-d11* are functionally redundant and expressed in metanephric mesenchyme (Davis et al., 1995). The double-mutant mouse, but not the respective single mutant, has a renal phenotype that includes agenesis or severe hypoplasia, and there appears to be modification of an anterior/posterior renal axis. The double-mutant mouse expresses neither *Gdnf* nor *Bf2*, indicating failure of mesenchymal development, perhaps at the level of the stromal cell (Patterson et al., 2001).

Emx2 (see Chapter 49), a homeobox transcription factor involved in cerebral neurite growth and possibly area patterning, is also expressed in the epithelial UB. In *Emx2* mutant mice, the UB invades the metanephric mesenchyme but the bud does not branch and the mesenchyme undergoes apoptosis. Initially, *Pax2* and *Ret* (coding for a GDNF receptor) expression is normal in the Wolffian duct, as is *Wt1* and *Gdnf* in the mesenchyme. However, the mutant mouse fails to sustain *Pax2*, *Ret*, and *Lim1* expression in the UB and expression of *Gdnf* and *Wnt4* in the mesenchyme is markedly reduced (Miyamoto et al., 1997). Furthermore, mutant animals completely lack urogenital organs. The defect is likely to be a primary one in the UB as the mesenchyme from mutant animals could be normally induced ex vivo by spinal cord but not by UB.

Gata3, a transcription factor expressed during ureteric development as well as during myeloerythropoiesis, appears to be involved in both UB branching and MM differentiation. Homozygous null mice die at day 11.5 dpc, and display little metanephric differentiation (Pandolfi et al., 1995), and haploinsufficiency of Gata3 causes the human hypoparathyroidism, deafness, and renal anomalies syndrome (Van Esch et al., 2000).

A mammalian ortholog of the *Drosophila* circadian clock gene *Timeless* is differentially expressed in UB cells undergoing tubulogenesis in a cell culture model of branching morphogenesis. *Timeless* is expressed in areas of mesenchymal condensation and ureteric branching. Perturbation of *Timeless* using antisense oligonucleotides decreases ureteric branching in both whole organ culture and isolated UB culture (Li et al., 2000). This suggests that clock-related genes, such as *Timeless*, may have a role in regulating the degree or extent of branching of the ureteric tree.

Stromal cells play a significant role in normal kidney development. This cell population is derived from the intermediate mesoderm and may modulate the dialogue between mesenchymal and epithelial cells. The winged-helix transcription factor *Bf2* displays restricted stromal cell expression. Mice with *Bf2* null mutations display normal UB and mesenchymal induction but thereafter show decreased rates of MET as well as decreased UB branching (Hatini et al., 1996). The mechanisms of this *Bf2* involvement are unclear, but they may be related to other stromal functions such as regulation of the GDNF axis, as discussed below.

Pod1 codes for a basic helix-loop-helix transcription factor expressed in embryonic and adult tissues of mesodermal origin. In embryonic mice, *Pod1* is expressed in the kidney, lung, intestine, and pancreas at sites of epithelial-mesenchymal interaction (Quaggin et al., 1998). Homozygous null mice display delayed condensation of mesenchyme around the UB tips and further delayed transformation of this mesenchyme into epithelial tubules (Quaggin et al., 1999). UB branching is also markedly inhibited. Finally, inhibition of *Pod1* in whole-kidney explants using antisense oligonucleotides results in both decreased mesenchymal condensation and decreased ureteric branching (Quaggin et al., 1998). Although the primary mechanism of inhibition of metanephric development is unclear, *Pod1* appears to act downstream of *Pax2* and *Wnt4*, and markers of stromal cell involvement, such as *Bf2* and *Gdnf*, are normal in *Pod1* mutant animals. In addition to its role in ureteric and mesenchymal development, *Pod1* is expressed in epithelial podocytes of the developing glomerulus and *Pod1* null mice display a block in glomerular differentiation.

Growth Factors

GDNF (see Chapter 35), a soluble growth factor belonging to the transforming growth factor-β (TGF-β) superfamily, is secreted by the metanephric mesenchyme (Pepicelli et al., 1997). In whole-organ culture, GDNF-soaked beads placed near the Wolffian duct induce sprouting of ectopic UBs from the duct (Sainio et al., 1997). In the isolated UB model of branching morphogenesis, GDNF is required for survival of explanted UB and initiation of branching morphogenesis, and the nascent UB dies in the absence of GDNF (Qiao et al., 1999a). Ret is a receptor tyrosine kinase encoded by the c-*ret* oncogene, which binds GDNF and is expressed in the UB concurrent with and adjacent to GDNF expression in the mesenchyme. Perturbation of either GDNF or Ret function leads to renal agenesis due to defective ureteric branching (Schuchardt et al., 1994, 1996; Pichel et al., 1996). Mice with heterozygous mutations in *Gdnf* display a variety of renal abnormalities, ranging from unilateral agenesis to hypoplasia to normal; in one

strain, for example, mice display 30% fewer nephrons but have otherwise normal-appearing kidneys (Cullen-McEwen et al., 2001). The GDNF signaling mechanism also includes a glycosylphosphatidylinositol (GPI)-linked coreceptor, GDNFRα, and homozygous null mice for this receptor display a phenotype similar to that of the GDNF and *Ret* deletions whereby the majority of mice display agenesis or severe hypoplasia (Tomac et al., 2000).

Deletion of retinoic acid receptors (RARs) RARα and RARβ2, which are typically expressed in the stromal mesenchyme, leads to downregulation of Ret in the developing UB and impaired ureteric branching (Mendelsohn et al., 1999). This is consistent with the renal malformation phenotype seen with gestational vitamin A (retinoic acid) deficiency. Forced ureteric expression of Ret in RAR double-mutant mice restored both UB growth and stromal cell patterning (Batourina et al., 2001). Interestingly, in a slightly different transgenic line, nonrestricted overexpression of the *Ret* promoter throughout the ureter, under the control of the *HoxB7* promoter, led to the development of small, dysplastic, cystic kidneys (Srinivas et al., 1999). This seems to support the concept that spatially restricted high concentrations of growth factors or their cognate receptors, rather than diffuse nonspecific expression, helps to regulate branching. Furthermore, it appears that stromal cells, whose origins are mesenchymal but which can be distinguished from other components of the metanephric mesenchyme, can modulate the classic epithelial–mesenchymal inductive interactions.

Several members of the TGF-β superfamily (see Chapter 24) can regulate metanephric development. In cell culture models utilizing both embryonic and adult cells, TGF-β appears to decrease the degree of branching tubulogenesis and instead induces the formation of elongated, nonbranching tubules (Santos and Nigam, 1993; Sakurai et al., 1997a). As discussed below, this finding may reflect altered expression of matrix metalloproteases.

The bone morphogenic proteins (BMPs) (see Chapter 24), which are also members of the TGF-β superfamily, have significant roles in the maintenance and modeling of the metanephric mesenchyme as well as coordinating outgrowth, elongation, and branching of the UB. In early organogenesis, *Bmp4* is expressed in the mesenchymal cells that surround the Wolffian duct and in the mesenchyme that surrounds the initial ureteric stalk. Mice that are homozygous null for *Bmp4* have early embryonic lethality, prior to renal organogenesis (Winnier et al., 1995); but heterozygotes display a variety of malformations of both the kidney and urinary tract, including renal hypoplasia, uretero-vesical junction obstruction with hydronephrosis, and duplex kidneys with bifid ureters (Miyazaki et al., 2000). Remarkably, this range of malformations is seen within an individual litter of heterozygous animals. Two BMP type I receptor genes, which can bind BMP4, are expressed either ubiquitously (*ALK3/BMPR-IA*) or exclusively in the duct and branching ureteric epithelium (*ALK6/BMPR-IB*). These two receptors may have functions in patterning sites of UB outgrowth and branching. Depending on the presence of sulfated glycosaminoglycans, BMP4 in conjunction with its receptors prevents aberrant budding of the UB from the Wolffian duct and promotes elongation of the "proper" bud (Miyazaki et al., 2000). BMP4 furthermore appears to have a role in rescuing metanephric mesenchyme from apoptotic signals, thereby modeling the mesenchyme.

During organogenesis, *Bmp7* is expressed by the Wolffian duct and in the metanephric mesenchyme. *Bmp7*-deficient mice have normal-appearing UB induction from the Wolffian duct but display diminished mesenchymal condensation around UB tips, with the mesenchyme undergoing dramatic apoptosis and degeneration (Dudley et al., 1995; Luo et al., 1995a). Mesenchymal expression of *Pax2*, *Wt1*, and *Wnt4* is reduced; and no nephrons are formed. Exogenous BMP7 inhibits apoptosis of cultured isolated mesenchyme and, in combination with FGF2, can potentiate tubulogenesis in *ex vivo* mesenchyme cocultured with spinal cord (Dudley et al., 1999). BMP7 may also play a role in UB branching morphogenesis. In an IMCD cell culture model, BMP7 exhibits dose-dependent stimulatory or inhibitory effects on cell survival, apoptosis, and subsequent branching morphogenesis (Godin et al., 1998). These effects appear to be mediated by glypican3, a cell-surface proteoglycan, and by Smad1, an intracellular messenger involved in TGF-β signaling (Grisaru et al., 2001; Piscione et al., 2001). It may be that BMP7 induces mesenchymal cells to form the stromal component of the mesenchyme, rather than the tubular portion, thereby mediating its effects on both UB branching and mesenchymal differentiation.

Several fibroblast growth factors (FGFs) (see Chapter 32) have roles in the development of a branching ureteric tree. In the isolated UB model of branching, some FGFs have the ability to induce a "branching and elongation" morphology (FGF1 and FGF10) or a hyperproliferative morphology characterized by branching but no elongation (FGF7 and FGF2) (Qiao et al., 2001). In particular, supplementation of mesenchyme-conditioned medium with FGF1 in this model induces the development of a complicated, arborized structure from the nascent bud. FGF2 has potential roles in both mesenchymal differentiation (discussed below) and ureteric development. In UB cells, FGF2 can induce cells to undergo rudimentary branching morphogenesis (Sakurai et al., 1997a). FGF1 and FGF2 single and double knockouts, however, do not have a kidney phenotype. FGF7 is expressed in the MM and in the stromal cells surrounding the developing ureteric tree (Qiao et al., 1999b), and its receptor, FGFR2-IIIb, is expressed by the UB (Qiao et al., 2001). Animals with homozygous mutations for FGF7 have decreased ureteric branching and approximately 30% fewer nephrons. In the isolated UB culture model of branching morphogenesis, addition of either blocking antibodies to FGF7 or soluble (and nontransducing) FGFR2-IIIb decreased the degree of branching morphogenesis but did not abolish it completely (Qiao et al., 2001). Furthermore, addition of exogenous FGF7 appeared to induce proliferation but not selective branching or elongation of the UB. Taken together, it appears that one or more FGFs play important modulatory roles in the patterning of the developing ureteric tree by modulating branch growth, elongation, and differentiation.

Pleiotrophin, an 18 kDa protein involved in neurite outgrowth and expressed in a number of developing organs that involve epithelial–mesenchymal interactions, is expressed in the condensed mesenchyme surrounding the UB. It has been identified in media conditioned by cultured immortalized embryonic MM and promotes impressive UB branching morphogenesis in modified organ culture of the isolated UB (with GDNF) and cell culture of UB-derived cells (Sakurai et al., 2001). These effects are enhanced by, but do not require, FGF, further suggesting that the FGFs listed above play modulatory roles in branching morphogenesis. The pleiotrophin receptor is currently unknown.

Other receptor tyrosine kinase ligands may be involved in ureteric development. HGF is expressed in the MM, and its receptor, Met, is expressed in the UB. Knockouts for either of these do not display a kidney phenotype and die in utero due to liver malformation. Nevertheless, ex vivo organ and cell culture data suggest that HGF induces branching morphogenesis of the UB and inhibits apoptosis of mesenchyme (Santos et al., 1994). Ligands for the EGF receptor, such as EGF and TGF-α, can induce branching structures in some cell culture models of branching morphogenesis (Barros et al., 1995; Sakurai et al., 1997b). Depending on the genetic background, homozygous null EGF receptor mice initially display normal branching but subsequently deformed collecting systems (Sibilia and Wagner, 1995; Threadgill et al., 1995).

Reciprocal induction of epithelia and mesenchyme implies that, in addition to mesenchymal secretion of growth factors essential for branching morphogenesis of the UB, the UB also secretes factors that induce mesenchymal differentiation and tubule formation. Leukemia inhibitory factor (LIF), a member of the TGF-β superfamily, is secreted into media conditioned by cultured embryonic UB cells and induces mesenchymal differentiation and tubule formation when combined with FGF2 and TGF-α (Barasch et al., 1999b). It is likely that the combination of FGF2 and TGF-α prevents mesenchymal apoptosis and stimulates proliferation but does not directly induce tubulogenesis. LIF alone only weakly induces explanted mesenchyme. TGF-β2 is also found in UB conditioned media and, in combination with FGF2, can induce delayed mesenchymal differentiation. The synergistic combination of LIF, TGF-β2, and FGF2 induces robust differentiation after 72 hours of coculture (Plisov et al., 2001). The contribution of LIF and FGF2/TGF-β2 to mesenchymal induction and differentiation appears to be Wnt-dependent (see Chapter 22) as administration of exogenous secreted frizzled related protein-1 (sfrp1), which antagonizes Wnt4 activity, inhibited mesenchymal induction.

The origins of the glomerular endothelial cells of the kidney are currently debated. Endothelial cells may differentiate in situ from precursor cells via a process termed vasculogenesis; alternatively, they may derive from sprouting and ingrowth of extrarenal vessels, termed angiogenesis. Support for the latter theory derives from observations that explanted metanephroi grown in culture develop avascular glomerular structures, although this may be secondary to normoxic culture conditions. Further evidence supporting the extrarenal origin of the renal vasculature principally derives from interspecies transplantation experiments. For example, when mouse metanephroi are transplanted onto avian chorioallantoic membranes, donor glomeruli contain host (avian) endothelial cells (Sariola et al., 1983). Finally, when metanephroi were cocultured with extrinsically labeled endothelial cells, the extrinsic endothelial cells invaded the metanephroi and formed capillary structures. There is evidence, however, for in situ vasculogenesis. Angioblasts have been identified in the MM prior to the formation of capillary networks (Robert et al., 1996; Tufro-McReddie et al., 1997), and exposure of these avascular metanephroi to increased levels of vascular endothelial growth factor (VEGF) induced formation of capillary networks (Tufro et al., 1999). Finally, endothelial cells can derive from the MM depending on the site of transplantation (Abrahamson et al., 1998)

Several growth factors play a significant role in glomerulogenesis, including VEGF (see Chapter 101) and its receptor tyrosine kinases Flk1 and Flt1 as well as the angiopoietin/TIE signaling pathway. In metanephric development, VEGF is initially expressed in the S-shaped body and then by the developing glomerular epithelium as well as tubular cells (Breier et al., 1992; Simon et al., 1995; Tufro et al., 1999). Concurrent with VEGF expression in the epithelium, Flk1 and Flt2 are expressed in the glomerular and capillary endothelial cells. In fact, Flk1 and Flt1 expression can be observed in mesenchymal endothelial precursor cells prior to capillary development. Knockouts of Vegf, Flk1, or Flt1 die prior to renal development. When exogenous VEGF is added to cultures of explanted mesenchymal cells, the population of Flk1-containing cells proliferates and rudimentary capillaries with lumens are seen (Tufro et al., 1999). Under normoxic culture conditions, VEGF expression is decreased (Tufro-McReddie et al., 1997). This is consistent with other models of inducible VEGF expression, whereby ARNT/HIF-1a heterodimerization is uncoupled by normoxia and VEGF expression is subsequently downregulated. Furthermore, Flk1 expression is also decreased under normoxic culture conditions. However, when explanted kidneys are engrafted onto the anterior eye chamber, Flk1 expression increases and there is formation of an extensive microvasculature (Robert et al., 1998). When organ culture is carried out under hypoxic conditions, VEGF and Flk1 expression are increased and microvessels develop. Antibodies to VEGF abrogate this response. Finally, under coculture conditions, mouse glomerular endothelial cells invade the avascular embryonic day 14 rat metanephroi and form rudimentary capillary-like structures. As expected, this response is increased under hypoxic conditions and inhibited by anti-VEGF antibodies (Tufro, 2000). The inducers of VEGF/Flk-1 expression during renal vascular and glomerular development remain undefined. It is likely that regulated expression of these factors, in a manner similar to the regulated expression of factors involved in collecting system and nephron formation, is critical to proper glomerular and vascular formation.

Angiopoietin (ANG) family ligands bind the TIE family of receptors and may modulate renal vascular development. ANG1 binds TIE2 and induces receptor phosphorylation and signal transduction. ANG2 also binds TIE2 but does not induce intracellular signaling and, thus, acts as an inhibitor of ANG1/TIE2-mediated signal transduction. Ang1 and Tie2 knockout mice display abnormal vascular networks (Sato et al., 1995; Suri et al., 1996) and die prior to renal development. This phenotype is replicated with Ang2 transgenic overexpression (Maisonpierre et al., 1997). In vivo, Ang1, Ang2, and Tie2 are expressed during metanephric development (Yuan et al., 1999); and addition of exogenous ANG1 to whole-organ culture increases the number of vascularized glomeruli (Kolatsi-Joannou et al., 2001).

The complex mechanisms guiding the final architecture of both the intra- and extra-glomerular blood vessels likely depend on factors in addition to the VEGF- and angiopoeitin-mediated signaling cascades. One attractive candidate for this patterning is the Eph/ephrin family of receptor ligands, which are involved in extrarenal aspects of vascular definition as well as directional targeting of growth. Descriptions of the expression of ephrin-B1 and ephrin-B2 and their receptors, EphB1 and EphB4, respectively, during glomerular development suggest roles for this system in targeting of glomerular endothelial and mesangial progenitors (Abrahamson et al., 1998; Takahashi et al., 2001).

Development of the glomerular mesangium is also critical for proper glomerulogenesis. Platelet-derived growth factor B (PDGF-b) and its receptor, PDGFR-b, are essential for the appearance of the mesangial cell in the glomerulus. Knockout mice deficient for PDGF-b or its receptor display no mesangial cellularity, and the glomeruli that form have one large irregular capillary loop (Leveen et al., 1994; Soriano, 1994). PDGF-b is initially expressed in vascular endothelial cells and PDGFR-b in the perivascular mesenchyme (Lindahl et al., 1998). In later glomerular development, PDGFR-b-containing cells are found in the mesangium, suggesting that at least some mesangial cells are derived from the perivascular mesenchyme. After birth, mesangial cells appear to originate in part from extrarenal sources. In chimeric mice with transgenic bone marrow–expressing green fluorescent protein (GFP), cells originating in the bone marrow repopulate the mesangium during renal repair after injury (Imasawa et al., 2001). Furthermore, in lethally irradiated mice given bone marrow stem cells from syngenic mice transgenic for GFP, 60% of isolated mesangial cells are GFP-positive after 24 weeks. It is unknown if bone marrow–derived stem cells have a role during embryonic organogenesis and mesangial development.

Congenital perturbation of podocyte function can result in a variety of renal phenotypes. Mutations of nephrin, a protein encoded by the gene *NPHS1* and involved in the podocyte slit diaphragm, and CD2-associated protein (*CD2-AP*), which interacts with nephrin, cause congenital nephrosis (Kestila et al., 1998; Shih et al., 1999). Mutations in *NPHS2*, the gene coding for the production of podocin, another protein exclusively expressed by podocytes, are also seen in patients with early nephrosis (Fuchshuber et al., 1995; Boute et al., 2000; Roselli et al., 2002). It appears that nephrin and podocin form a structure that can stimulate intracellular signaling and support the ultrastructure and function of the podocyte (Huber et al., 2001). Mice lacking laminin-β2 also display congenital nephrosis due to malformation of the glomerular basement membrane (Noakes et al., 1995). Finally, one cause of familial, autosomal-dominant focal and segmental glomerulosclerosis is a mutation in the gene encoding α-actinin-4 (*ACTN4*) (Kaplan et al., 2000). Mutated α-actinin-4 more avidly binds filamentous actin than does wild-type α-actinin-4, and disordered regulation of the actin cytoskeleton in podocytes may account for the development of this form of focal and segmental glomerulosclerosis.

Genes Affecting the Basement Membrane and Extracellular Matrix

Interactions with local basement membrane appear to be important in regulating initial UB outgrowth, elongation, and branching as well as MET. The integrin subunit α8 is expressed by the mesenchyme surrounding the Wolffian duct and upregulated in mesenchymal condensates (but not mesenchyme that has begun to undergo MET) during UB outgrowth. The integrin α8 knockout mouse displays delayed initial UB outgrowth. Furthermore, branching morphogenesis and MET are impaired. This leads to renal agenesis or severely hypoplastic kidneys (Muller et al., 1997). In mice with integrin α3 deletion, the number of medullary collecting ducts is diminished but the total number of nephrons is unchanged, suggesting a defect in early branching events of the UB (Kreidberg et al., 1996). In addition, there are a variety of abnormalities in the structure of both renal tubules and glomeruli. Although the integrin α6 knockout does not have a renal phenotype (Georges-Labouesse et al., 1996), the kidneys in the double integrin α3/α6 knockout do not have proper ureters and the renal

parenchyma appears similar to the α3 knockout (De Arcangelis et al., 1999). In the isolated UB model, blocking antibodies to integrin subunits α3 or α6 markedly decrease branching morphogenesis, and this effect is exaggerated when blocking antibodies to both α3 and α6 are added (Zent et al., 2001). Blocking the function of integrin subunit β1 and laminin-5, which is a ligand of integrin α6β4 and α3β1, also decreased branching morphogenesis. Integrin-mediated interactions with the basement membrane thus appear to play roles in regulating both ureteric branching morphogenesis and tubular structure.

The developing kidney actively remodels the extracellular matrix via the activity of matrix metalloproteinases (MMPs; see Chapter 95). MMP2 and MMP9 can degrade various components of the basement membrane, including collagen types IV and V, aggrecan, and elastin. MMP9 and MMP2 are inhibited by tissue inhibitor of metalloproteinase-1 (TIMP-1) and TIMP-2, respectively, although MMP9 requires TIMP-2 binding for activation (Gomez et al., 1997). The expression of metalloproteases and their inhibitors appears to be tightly regulated during kidney development (Reponen et al., 1992; Tanney et al., 1998; Barasch et al., 1999a). MMP9 and MMP2 as well as their respective TIMPs are predominantly expressed in the mesenchyme of early developing kidneys (Legallicier et al., 2001). MT1-MMP, a membrane-associated MMP that can bind to and activate MMP2, is expressed in the UB (Ota et al., 1998). The knockout of MMP2 does not result in an abnormal renal phenotype, but the mice appear to grow slower (Itoh et al., 1997). Inhibition of the MMP2/MT1-MMP/TIMP2 axis in organ culture leads to disparate results, with no significant perturbation in development of explants of mouse embryonic day 11 kidneys but significant perturbations in explants of mouse embryonic day 13 metanephroi (Kanwar et al., 1999). Addition of either TIMP2 or ilomostat, a chemical inhibitor of MMP function, markedly decreases branching in both the UB cell culture model and the isolated UB organ culture model of branching morphogenesis (Pohl et al., 2000a). Finally, addition of TGF-β to the IMCD cell culture model, which selectively inhibits normal in vitro branching, alters the ratio of MMPs and TIMPs, which suggests that MMP activity can help define branching patterns of tubulogenesis (Sakurai and Nigam, 1997).

Inhibition of MMP9 with blocking antibodies or with exogenous TIMP-1 impairs branching morphogenesis of the UB in whole-kidney organ culture (Lelongt et al., 1997). Targeted deletion of MMP9 also does not appear to result in an obvious renal phenotype, but there may be a subtle defect in the degree of branching morphogenesis as these kidneys displayed a slight reduction in overall nephron number (Vu et al., 1998; Lelongt et al., 2001). When bound by the hyaluronic acid receptor CD44, MMP9 can degrade TGF-β and may thus modulate UB growth via a primary effect on growth factor signaling in addition to its effects on matrix degradation (Yu and Stamenkovic, 2000). Furthermore, inhibition of CD44 blocked UB cell branching morphogenesis in a cell culture model of renal development (Pohl et al., 2000b). CD44 expression in this model system was restricted to the tips of the branching ureteric structures, and the interaction between CD44 and hyaluronic acid appeared to regulate the survival and branching of UB-derived cells.

Heparan sulfate proteoglycans (HSPGs) appear to have central roles in modulating UB branching morphogenesis. HSPGs bind a number of critical growth factors, leading to altered local concentrations of growth factors and modulated presentation to their cognate receptors. These large molecules consist of long, sulfated sugar side chains linked to a protein core. Perturbation of either the core protein or the side chains dramatically affects branching morphogenesis. Embryonic mice that are homozygous for a gene-trap mutation of the heparan sulfate 2-sulfotransferase gene (*HS2ST*) display UBs that invade the MM but fail to divide and are typically stillborn (Bullock et al., 1998). The abnormal HS in these animals displays a decreased affinity for both FGF1 and FGF2, but the downstream FGF signaling cascade is otherwise intact (Merry et al., 2001). In whole embryonic kidney organ culture, perturbations of sulfation of HS moieties lead to decreased ureteric branching (Davies et al., 1995). Disruption of HSPG sulfation or synthesis, but not of chondroitin sulfate proteoglycan, inhibits branching morphogenesis in the isolated UB culture system (D. L. Steer et al., unpublished data).

Knockout of glypican-3, a GPI-linked cell surface HSPG, leads to increased ureteric proliferation and branching and to increased mesenchymal apoptosis in mutant mice (Cano-Gauci et al., 1999). The phenotype results in disorganized tubules and medullary cysts. As mentioned above, glypican-3 also has a role in modulating BMP signals, and it may be that in these mice disordered BMP signaling secondary to lack of glypican-3 leads to the observed phenotype (Grisaru et al., 2001). In humans, a defect in glypican-3 is the cause of the Simpson-Golabi-Behmel syndrome (see Chapter 96).

Endostatin (ES), which is found in the extracellular matrix as a cleavage product of collagen XVIII, has roles in both endothelial and epithelial cell biology. ES can induce endothelial cell apoptosis and prevent de novo angiogenesis (O'Reilly et al., 1997; Dhanabal et al., 1999). Collagen XVIII is expressed during renal development initially throughout the epithelial ureteric bud but then becomes restricted to the ureteric stalk and loses expression at the bud tips (Lin et al., 2001). In renal epithelial cell culture, administration of ES prevents branching morphogenesis (Karihaloo et al., 2001). This inhibition is dependent on glypican-3 as cells from the glypican-3 null mouse are not similarly inhibited by ES and in vitro transfection of the glypican-3 null cells with glypican-1 reconstitutes the ES-induced inhibition. Finally, ES inhibits branching morphogenesis of the isolated UB culture, and a neutralizing antibody to ES increases the extent of branching.

Other Gene Products Involved in Metanephrogenesis

In addition to transcription factors, growth factors and genes affecting the basement membrane and the extracellular matrix, a number of other genes play an important role in nephrogenesis. In addition to limb deformities, the limb-deformity (ld) mutation can cause a variety of renal developmental abnormalities, ranging from renal agenesis (usually unilateral) to normal kidneys (Maas et al., 1994). UB outgrowth from the Wolffian duct is markedly delayed in homozygous mutant animals, and extension into the surrounding MM is incomplete. Since nonspecific inducers, such as spinal cord, can induce the MM in animals with homozygous ld mutations, the phenotype likely arises as a primary defect in UB outgrowth. The ld locus codes for four differentially spliced genes, which code for proteins called formins that are expressed in the UB. Specific targeted disruption of formin IV leads to renal abnormalities in the absence of limb deformities (Wynshaw-Boris et al., 1997). In a cell culture model of tubulogenesis, formin IV is translocated from submembrane and perinuclear compartments to the cytosol and nucleus in a mitogen-activated protein kinase–dependent fashion (O'Rourke et al., 2000).

The Wnt superfamily (see Chapter 22) of secreted glycoproteins plays central roles in the development of a variety of tissues, including kidney and genitalia. Wnts bind to members of the Frizzled family of cell surface receptors and can stimulate T-cell factor (TCF)–dependent gene transcription. There are differential patterns of expression of individual Wnts during development of the UB and the MM (Kispert et al., 1996, 1998). Wnt4 is expressed in the condensed mesenchyme at the tips of the branching UB. In animals that are homozygous null for Wnt4, initial UB branching appears normal, Wt1 and Pax2 are normally expressed, and the MM condenses at the UB tips (Stark et al., 1994). Pretubular aggregates, however, fail to form, and expression of Pax8, which is normally confined to pretubular cell aggregates in the kidney (Plachov et al., 1990), is lost. There is failure of further mesenchymal induction; hence, no nephrons are formed. Addition of exogenous Wnt4 induces mesenchymal differentiation in these mutant animals, and spinal cord, which expresses a variety of Wnt family members, can induce mesenchymal induction in both Wnt4 null and normal mesenchyme. Interestingly, spinal cord from Wnt4 null mice can also induce mesenchyme from Wnt4 null mice, suggesting that Wnt signaling may be redundant (Kispert et al., 1998; Vainio and Uusitalo, 2000). Wnt11 expression, which is normally confined to UB tips, is not sufficient to initiate tubulogenesis in isolated MM but may have autoregulatory functions at the UB tip (Kispert et al., 1996).

Wnt signaling is regulated by HSPGs and by secreted proteins. Both sugarless and sulfateless, Drosophila genes involved in HSPG biosynthesis, as well as dally, a Drosophila ortholog of the human HSPG glypican, mediate Wingless/Wnt signal transduction (Hacker et al., 1997; Lin et al., 1999; Tsuda et al., 1999). Furthermore, perturbation of proteoglycan sulfation inhibits Wnt4-mediated tubulogenesis. It thus appears that proteoglycans may restrict or organize Wnt signaling.

Wnt signaling is mediated by the Frizzled class of receptors (Chan et al., 1992; Wang et al., 1996). Secreted frizzled-related protein (sfrp), which contains the Wnt-binding domain of the Frizzled receptors but lacks the transmembrane domains, is normally expressed in mesenchymal condensate and subsequent epithelial tubules and can further modulate Wnt signaling (Leimeister et al., 1998; Yoshino et al., 2001). Addition of sfrp-1 to mesenchyme culture inhibits epithelial transformation in response to normally inductive media. In a complex fashion, sfrp-1, which is secreted by the developing tubule, antagonizes Wnt4-mediated mesenchymal differentiation. Coadministration of sfrp-2, which is normally expressed by the stroma and upregulated during Wnt4 expression, can rescue mesenchymal differentiation and thus appears to modulate sfrp-1-mediated inhibition (Lescher et al., 1998; Yoshino et al., 2001). In summary, it appears that by modulating Wnt activity the sfrps likely establish a boundary of focal Wnt activity and restrict epithelialization of the mesenchyme to a specific subset of cells.

Summary of Metanephric Development

Normal metanephrogenesis results from the coordinated action of a large number of gene products. In some cases, there are apparently redundant processes that allow for the kidneys to form normally in spite of the absence of an important gene. Fundamentally, the genetic programs must allow for regulated cell proliferation, apoptosis, migration, and differentiation. The coordinated and often reciprocal expression of a variety of transcription factors, growth factors, and matrix proteins underlies metanephric development. Furthermore, there is increasing support for the concept of regulated initiation and termination signals in organizing the vectorial branching and elongating pattern of branching morphogenesis. Certain stimulatory or inhibitory factors appear to display both spatially and temporally restricted patterns of activity and expression. The focus of activity, whether it is a UB-branching event or mesenchymal condensation, may result from the concerted activities of a number of factors distributed in gradients across an "active" zone (Santos and Nigam, 1993; Nigam, 1995; Pohl et al., 2000b).

Prior to UB development, the MM derives from the mesoderm by the coordinated action of genes, including Pax2, Lim1, Wt1, Eya1, and genes coding for several forkhead/winged transcription factors. This mesenchyme then induces the UB to sprout from the Wolffian duct, which appears to be dependent on the expression of GDNF by the mesenchyme and its appropriate receptors in the epithelial bud. A distinct cell population within the mesenchyme, the stroma, may modulate this signaling. Emx2, timeless, and perhaps formin IV appear to be epithelial genes required for initial competence of the branching program. Other factors, such as pleiotrophin, FGF1, FGF7, BMP7, and perhaps Wnt2b, as well as HSPGs, specific integrins, and matrix proteases, are also critically involved in establishing an arborized ureteric tree derived from the initial bud. In turn, the UB rescues the mesenchyme from an apoptotic fate and initiates MET by secreting factors such as LIF, TGF-β, and FGF2. Other factors, such as Wnt4, which is secreted by the induced mesenchyme, may further carry nephron formation in an autocrine fashion. Regulators of Wnt activity, such as the sfrps and proteoglycans, may limit Wnt activity to induced cells. Glomerular development appears to involve both de novo vasculogenesis and extrinsic angiogenesis, under the regulation of both VEGF and angiopoietin signaling pathways. Other specialized cells of the glomerulus, such as mesangial cells and glomerular podocytes, require specific factors for their proper development as well.

SEXUAL DEVELOPMENT

Sexual development shares origins with renal development. Gonadal development arises from perimesonephric structures, and several genes critical for kidney development also play roles in sexual development. The initial step in sexual development consists of the development of the indifferent (or bipotent) gonads. This is followed by sexual determination, which is defined as the commitment of the bipotent gonad to either testicular or ovarian development. Sexual determination is ultimately a function of genetic sex. Finally, sexual differentiation, which is the development of the male or female phenotype, occurs and is predominantly determined by hormonal expression patterns. The classical surgical experiments of Jost (1953), whereby rabbit embryos were castrated *in utero* prior to sexual differentiation and developed as phenotypic females, demonstrated that both sexes contained the genetic information required to develop as females. Furthermore, transplantation of fetal testis into an XX embryo led to male phenotypic development. In general, sexual development has been thought to occur such that the basal pathway of development appears to be female and several pro- or antitesticular factors determine testicular development with consequential male phenotypic development. Recent evidence supports a more complicated mechanism of female sexual development, whereby ovarian and female genital tract development occurs via a regulated, rather than a default, pathway.

The precise mechanisms underlying the genetic control of events in early gonadal development can be difficult to determine as genes involved in kidney development also have significant roles in genital development and there are many potential pathways that could be disrupted by perturbations of one gene. *WT1*, a complex gene that can encode multiple different regulatory proteins, is expressed throughout the intermediate mesoderm beginning just prior to urogenital development. Perturbations of *Wt1* in mutant rodents and *WT1* mutations in humans lead to defects in both meso- and metanephric development as well as gonadal development. XY patients with Denys-Drash syndrome, wherein a heterozygous missense *WT1* mutation in a DNA-binding domain likely acts in a dominant-negative fashion, often display an ambiguous or female phenotype (Pelletier et al., 1991). Furthermore, XY patients with Frasier's syndrome, which is characterized by loss of the +KTS isoform of *WT1* that is thought to be involved in RNA processing, also develop as phenotypic females (Barbaux et al., 1997). Finally, mice with homozygous mutations of the +KTS Wt1 isoform have markedly decreased expression of Sry (see below) and subsequent XY female sex reversal, and it appears that Wt1 may thus regulate gonadal fate (Hammes et al., 2001).

Steroidogenic factor 1 (SF1), an orphan nuclear receptor, is a zinc-finger DNA-binding transcription factor which activates genes involved in steroid biosynthesis (Lala et al., 1992; Morohashi et al., 1993). During development, the gonads, adrenals, pituitary, and hypothalamus express SF1. Antibodies to Sf1 identify a single group of cells in the mesoderm that are destined to form the gonads and cortical cells of the adrenals, and homozygous knockout of *Sf1* leads to mice that lack both gonads and adrenal glands (Ikeda et al., 1994; Ingraham et al., 1994; Luo et al., 1994, 1995b; Hatano et al., 1996). In these mice, the genital ridges form normally and primordial germ cells migrate in via the hindgut; however, the gonadal primordia arrest development at 11–11.5 dpc (after 24–36 hours of development) and then undergo apoptosis. Thus, SF1 may have a direct role in maintenance or growth of the indifferent gonad and may induce expression of either prosurvival or antiapoptotic factors.

Not surprisingly, other genes involved in mesonephric development also have roles in gonadal development. As noted above, mice with homozygous knockout of *Lim1* do not develop either mesonephric or metanephric derivatives, including kidneys and gonads (Shawlot and Behringer, 1995). Homozygous deletion of *Pax2*, which is normally in pro-, meso-, and metanephric mesenchyme, results in loss of kidneys and genital structures derived from the Wolffian and Mullerian ducts; but the gonads of both sexes are spared. Finally, *Emx2*, a homeobox-containing transcription factor, is also involved in urogenital development. As discussed above, *Emx2* is expressed in the Wolffian duct, genital ridge, and mesonephric tubules and acts downstream of Wt1. In addition to disrupted invasion of the mesenchyme by the UB, homozygous null mice display impaired gonadal development. They have apparently normal adrenal glands, and the defect therefore is unlikely to involve Sf1-mediated pathways.

SEXUAL DETERMINATION

Although genetic sex is established at fertilization, sexual determination occurs during gonadal development. The cells of the bipotent gonad can become either the Sertoli and Leydig cells of the testis or the follicular and thecal cells of the ovary. In mammals, the Y chromosome acts dominantly to direct testicular development through expression of Sry (see Chapter 42). Sry triggers the differentiation of Sertoli cells in the testis, and the Sertoli cell then likely directs further testicular development. In individuals with primary sex reversal, that is, when chromosomal sex and phenotypic sex are not matched, the majority of XX patients with male phenotype have aberrant expression of *Sry* and a group of XY patients with female phenotypes display mutations in the *Sry* gene (Hawkins et al., 1992). XX mice with transgenic expression of *Sry* developed as males (Koopman et al., 1991).

Sry is transiently expressed in the male genital ridge at approximately 10.5–11 dpc in an anterior-to-posterior fashion (Hacker et al., 1995; Jeske et al., 1995). On the molecular level, Sry has a high-mobility group (HMG) box DNA-binding motif, which is highly conserved across mammalian species. In cases of human XY female sex reversal, almost all mutations involving Sry cluster in the HMG box domain (Harley et al., 1992). Sry, like other proteins containing HMG box domains, can bind to DNA in its minor groove and induce an acute bend in the double helix (Ferrari et al., 1992). This architectural distortion can exert major influences on other nearby DNA–protein interactions and can, for example, change the efficiency of local promoter regions, thereby exerting its transcriptional control.

Signals downstream from Sry that are also involved in Sertoli cell (and testis) determination include the *Sox* genes, which share homology with the *Sry* HMG box gene. In addition to their HMG box, these conserved genes have strong transactivating domains. Although *Sry* is expressed only in mammals, *Sox9* is expressed in all vertebrates and appears to be a conserved sex-determining factor (Morais da Silva et al., 1996; Spotila et al., 1998). *Sox9* has low-level expression in the indifferent gonad but, immediately after Sry expression, is markedly upregulated in the male (and turned off in the female). By day 12.5, Sox9 shows restricted Sertoli-cell expression (Kent et al., 1996; Morais da Silva et al., 1996). XY female sex-reversed humans often display mutations in one Sox9 allele (Foster et al., 1994; Kent et al., 1996). These haplo-insufficient humans have mutations that can include various portions of the gene, including the HMG box and transactivating domains (Kwok et al., 1995; Meyer et al., 1997). Most mutations in the campomelic dysplasia/sex reversal syndrome are in the transactivating domain of Sox9 (Sudbeck et al., 1996).

Sf1 plays a role in sex determination as well as in earlier gonadal development. Following *Sry* expression, *Sf1* expression in the testis increases in both Leydig cells (as would be expected for steroidogenesis to occur) as well as Sertoli cells. *Dax1*, an X-linked member of the nuclear hormone receptor family, can inhibit *Sf1* activity, thereby acting as an "antitestis" (or pro-ovarian) factor. Expression of *Dax1* is colocalized but slightly lagging that of *Sf1* in the adrenal, gonads, hypothalamic, and pituitary structures (Ikeda et al., 1996). As opposed to the restricted expression of *Sry*, *Dax1* is expressed in the genital ridges of both males and females (Swain et al., 1996). After *Sry* expression ceases in the testis and coincident with *Sox9* testicular expression, *Dax1* expression is downregulated in the testis but persists in the nascent ovary. Transgenic expression of *Dax1* causes XY female sex reversal in mice (Swain et al., 1998), and duplications of the *Dax1* containing portion of the X chromosome have been found in human XY female sex reversal (Muscatelli et al., 1994; Zanaria et al., 1994). Finally, inactivation of Dax1 does not appear to affect testicular development. In sum, *Sf1*, *Sox9*, and *Dax1* appear to act in concert to define gonadal development. The exact sequence of and crosstalk between these regulatory mechanisms is currently being defined. These data indicate that a key function of mammalian sex development is Sertoli-cell determination in the testis. This event appears to be initiated by *Sry* in mammals and maintained by *Sox9* and *SF1*. In nonmammalian organisms, *Sox9* expression is upregulated by other inducers of sex determination, such as temperature.

Once pre-Sertoli cells are determined, they express antimullerian hormone (AMH), which induces regression of the Mullerian ducts, thereby directing genital tract development from the Wolffian duct. It is likely that AMH expression is regulated by elements downstream of Sry, namely, Sf1 and Sox9. The *Amh* promoter contains a consensus site for binding of Sf1 as well as for binding of proteins containing HMG box domains, such as Sry and Sox9 (De Santa Barbara et al., 1998); *Amh* is expressed only by Sox9-expressing cells. The AMH receptor is expressed in the mesenchyme surrounding the Mullerian duct and upregulated by Sf1 (Baarends et al., 1994; Barbara et al., 1998). In some nonmammalian vertebrates, Amh expression precedes that of Sox9 (Western et al., 1999). Wt1 can also regulate Amh expression by acting in concert with Sf1, perhaps as a coactivator (Nachtigal et al., 1998). Furthermore, Dax1 can repress the synergistic action of Wt1 on Sf1-mediated Amh. Thus, it appears that several factors acting in a coordinated fashion restrict Amh expression.

The restricted expression of the Amh receptor to the mesenchyme surrounding the epithelial Mullerian duct implies that Mullerian duct regression is a consequence of mesenchymal–epithelial interactions (Roberts et al., 1999). The Amh receptor is a member of the TGF-β superfamily of receptors, and Amh appears to use a BMP7-like signaling cascade, involving Alk2 and Smad6, in inducing Mullerian duct regression. (Gouedard et al., 2000; Clarke et al., 2001; Visser et al., 2001). As in kidney development, members of the Wnt family appear to have central roles in mediating paracrine mesenchymal–epithelial interactions in gonadal development. During normal development, Wnt4 expression is initially expressed in the genital ridge but then downregulated in the testis and maintained in the ovary. Female mice with homozygous Wnt4 mutations demonstrated loss of Mullerian ducts and masculinization of the Wolffian duct; male mice developed normally (Vainio et al., 1999). Mesenchymal Wnt4 expression, then, appears to support Mullerian duct survival, but it is unclear if the knockout phenotype is mediated by loss of repression of testosterone biosynthesis or direct apoptosis of the Mullerian duct. Wnt7a is normally expressed in Mullerian duct epithelia, and knockout of Wnt7a leads to persistent Mullerian ducts in males due to loss of expression of Amh receptor in the mesenchyme (Parr and McMahon, 1998). Finally, in association with lymphoid enhancer factor-1, β-catenin, which is involved in Wnt signaling, appears to mediate Amh-induced Mullerian duct apoptosis (Allard et al., 2000). One downstream effector target gene of Amh signaling appears to be MMP2, which is upregulated in the Mullerian mesenchyme in response to Amh (Roberts et al., 2002).

In addition to Amh expression, Sertoli cells are thought to direct formation of the remainder of the testis. Although the molecular mechanisms are less clear, Sertoli cells likely secrete factors or act via cell–cell interactions to direct the further differentiation of the testis. In organ culture, mesonephric cells migrate into the gonad to give rise to the endothelial and peritubular myoid cells of the testis but not of the ovary, which suggest dependence of the formation of testicular cords on a Sertoli cell–derived signal (Martineau et al., 1997).

Other factors that regulate ovarian determination are currently unknown, and it is likely that there are pro-ovarian factors in addition to the antiovarian factors discussed above. The remainder of sexual development is predominantly determined by the action of testicular and ovarian hormones on the Wolffian and Mullerian ducts, respectively. The process of sexual differentiation is covered in other chapters.

Summary of Sex Determination

There are several general principles involved in the molecular determination of the gonad. First, the development of the indifferent gonad is dependent on a number of transcription factors that are also involved in mesonephric development, including Pax2, SF1, Lim1, and WT1. Second, development of the testes from the indifferent gonads depends on transient Sry expression in mammals. Sry sets in motion a cascade of events, including Sox9 expression, that direct Sertoli-cell development. In the absence of Sry and Sox9, the gonad becomes an ovary. There may be inhibitors of testicular development, such as Dax1, that help direct ovarian differentiation. Furthermore, some downstream effectors of sexual phenotype, such as AMH and Wnt4,

are dependent on both the integration of crosstalk between these early transcription factors and critical mesenchymal–epithelial interactions.

REFERENCES

Abdelhak S, Kalatzis V, Heilig R, Compain S, Samson D, Vincent C, Weil D, Cruaud C, Sahly I, Leibovici M, et al. (1997). A human homologue of the *Drosophila eyes absent* gene underlies Branchio-Oto-Renal (BOR) syndrome and identifies a novel gene family. *Nat Genet* 15: 157–164.

Abrahamson DR, Robert B, Hyink DP, St John PL, Daniel TO (1998). Origins and formation of microvasculature in the developing kidney. *Kidney Int Suppl* 67: S7–S11.

Allard S, Adin P, Gouedard L, di Clemente N, Josso N, Orgebin-Crist MC, Picard JY, Xavier F (2000). Molecular mechanisms of hormone-mediated mullerian duct regression: involvement of beta-catenin. *Development* 127: 3349–3360.

Argao EA, Kern MJ, Branford WW, Scott WJ Jr, Potter SS (1995). Malformations of the heart, kidney, palate, and skeleton in alpha-MHC-Hoxb-7 transgenic mice. *Mech Dev* 52: 291–303.

Armstrong JF, Pritchard-Jones K, Bickmore WA, Hastie ND, Bard JB (1993). The expression of the Wilms' tumour gene, *WT1*, in the developing mammalian embryo. *Mech Dev* 40: 85–97.

Baarends WM, van Helmond MJ, Post M, van der Schoot PJ, Hoogerbrugge JW, de Winter JP, Uilenbroek JT, Karels B, Wilming LG, Meijers JH, et al. (1994). A novel member of the transmembrane serine/threonine kinase receptor family is specifically expressed in the gonads and in mesenchymal cells adjacent to the mullerian duct. *Development* 120: 189–197.

Barasch J, Yang J, Qiao J, Tempst P, Erdjument-Bromage H, Leung W, Oliver JA (1999a). Tissue inhibitor of metalloproteinase-2 stimulates mesenchymal growth and regulates epithelial branching during morphogenesis of the rat metanephros. *J Clin Invest* 103: 1299–1307.

Barasch J, Yang J, Ware CB, Taga T, Yoshida K, Erdjument-Bromage H, Tempst P, Parravicini E, Malach S, Aranoff T, et al. (1999b). Mesenchymal to epithelial conversion in rat metanephros is induced by LIF. *Cell* 99: 377–386.

Barbara PS, Moniot B, Poulat F, Boizet B, Berta P (1998). Steroidogenic factor-1 regulates transcription of the human anti-mullerian hormone receptor. *J Biol Chem* 273: 29654–29660.

Barbaux S, Niaudet P, Gubler MC, Grunfeld JP, Jaubert F, Kuttenn F, Fekete CN, Souleyreau-Therville N, Thibaud E, Fellous M, et al. (1997). Donor splice-site mutations in WT1 are responsible for Frasier syndrome. *Nat Genet* 17: 467–470.

Bard JB, Gordon A, Sharp L, Sellers WI (2001). Early nephron formation in the developing mouse kidney. *J Anat* 199: 385–392.

Barros EJ, Santos OF, Matsumoto K, Nakamura T, Nigam SK (1995). Differential tubulogenic and branching morphogenetic activities of growth factors: implications for epithelial tissue development. *Proc Natl Acad Sci USA* 92: 4412–4416.

Batourina E, Gim S, Bello N, Shy M, Clagett-Dame M, Srinivas S, Costantini F, Mendelsohn C (2001). Vitamin A controls epithelial/mesenchymal interactions through Ret expression. *Nat Genet* 27: 74–78.

Boute N, Gribouval O, Roselli S, Benessy F, Lee H, Fuchshuber A, Dahan K, Gubler MC, Niaudet P, Antignac C (2000). NPHS2, encoding the glomerular protein podocin, is mutated in autosomal recessive steroid-resistant nephrotic syndrome. *Nat Genet* 24: 349–354.

Boyden E (1927). Experimental obstruction of the mesonephric ducts. *Proc Soc Exp Biol Med* 24: 572–576.

Breier G, Albrecht U, Sterrer S, Risau W (1992). Expression of vascular endothelial growth factor during embryonic angiogenesis and endothelial cell differentiation. *Development* 114: 521–532.

Buckler AJ, Pelletier J, Haber DA, Glaser T, Housman DE (1991). Isolation, characterization, and expression of the murine Wilms' tumor gene (*WT1*) during kidney development. *Mol Cell Biol* 11: 1707–1712.

Bullock SL, Fletcher JM, Beddington RS, Wilson VA (1998). Renal agenesis in mice homozygous for a gene trap mutation in the gene encoding heparan sulfate 2-sulfotransferase. *Genes Dev* 12: 1894–1906.

Cano-Gauci DF, Song HH, Yang H, McKerlie C, Choo B, Shi W, Pullano R, Piscione TD, Grisaru S, Soon S, et al. (1999). Glypican-3-deficient mice exhibit developmental absent overgrowth and some of the abnormalities typical of Simpson-Golabi-Behmel syndrome. *J Cell Biol* 146: 255–264.

Cantley LG, Barros EJG, Gandhi M, Rauchman MI, Nigam SK (1994). Regulation of mitogenesis, motogenesis and morphogenesis by hepatocyte growth factor in inner medullary collecting duct cells. *Am J Physiol* 267: F271–F280.

Carroll TJ, Vize PD (1999). Synergism between Pax-8 and lim-1 in embryonic kidney development. *Dev Biol* 214: 46–59.

Chan SD, Karpf DB, Fowlkes ME, Hooks M, Bradley MS, Vuong V, Bambino T, Liu MY, Arnaud CD, Strewler GJ, et al. (1992). Two homologs of the *Drosophila* polarity gene *frizzled* (*fz*) are widely expressed in mammalian tissues. *J Biol Chem* 267: 25202–25207.

Chan TC, Takahashi S, Asashima M (2000). A role for Xlim-1 in pronephros development in *Xenopus laevis*. *Dev Biol* 228: 256–269.

Clarke TR, Hoshiya Y, Yi SE, Liu X, Lyons KM, Donahoe PK (2001). Mullerian inhibiting substance signaling uses a bone morphogenetic protein (BMP)-like pathway mediated by ALK2 and induces SMAD6 expression. *Mol Endocrinol* 15: 946–959.

Cullen-McEwen LA, Drago J, Bertram JF (2001). Nephron endowment in glial cell line-derived neurotrophic factor (GDNF) heterozygous mice. *Kidney Int* 60: 31–36.

Davies J, Lyon M, Gallagher J, Garrod D (1995). Sulphated proteoglycan is required for collecting duct growth and branching but not nephron formation during kidney development. *Development* 121: 1507–1517.

Davis AP, Witte DP, Hsieh-Li HM, Potter SS, Capecchi MR (1995). Absence of radius and ulna in mice lacking hoxa-11 and hoxd-11. *Nature* 375: 791–795.

De Arcangelis A, Mark M, Kreidberg J, Sorokin L, Georges-Labouesse E (1999). Synergistic activities of alpha3 and alpha6 integrins are required during apical ectodermal ridge formation and organogenesis in the mouse. *Development* 126: 3957–3968.

De Santa Barbara P, Bonneaud N, Boizet B, Desclozeaux M, Moniot B, Sudbeck P, Scherer G, Poulat F, Berta P (1998). Direct interaction of SRY-related protein SOX9 and steroidogenic factor 1 regulates transcription of the human anti-mullerian hormone gene. *Mol Cell Biol* 18: 6653–6665.

Dhanabal M, Ramchandran R, Waterman MJ, Lu H, Knebelmann B, Segal M, Sukhatme VP (1999). Endostatin induces endothelial cell apoptosis. *J Biol Chem* 274: 11721–11726.

Dudley AT, Lyons KM, Robertson EJ (1995). A requirement for bone morphogenetic protein-7 during development of the mammalian kidney and eye. *Genes Dev* 9: 2795–2807.

Dudley AT, Godin RE, Robertson EJ (1999). Interaction between FGF and BMP signaling pathways regulates development of metanephric mesenchyme. *Genes Dev* 13: 1601–1613.

Ferrari S, Harley VR, Pontiggia A, Goodfellow PN, Lovell-Badge R, Bianchi ME (1992). SRY, like HMG1, recognizes sharp angles in DNA. *EMBO J* 11: 4497–4506.

Foster JW, Dominguez-Steglich MA, Guioli S, Kowk G, Weller PA, Stevanovic M, Weissenbach J, Mansour S, Young ID, Goodfellow PN, et al. (1994). Campomelic dysplasia and autosomal sex reversal caused by mutations in an SRY-related gene. *Nature* 372: 525–530.

Fuchshuber A, Jean G, Gribouval O, Gubler MC, Broyer M, Beckmann JS, Niaudet P, Antignac C (1995). Mapping a gene (*SRN1*) to chromosome 1q25-q31 in idiopathic nephrotic syndrome confirms a distinct entity of autosomal recessive nephrosis. *Hum Mol Genet* 4: 2155–2158.

Fujii T, Pichel JG, Taira M, Toyama R, Dawid IB, Westphal H (1994). Expression patterns of the murine LIM class homeobox gene *lim1* in the developing brain and excretory system. *Dev Dyn* 199: 73–83.

Georges-Labouesse E, Messaddeq N, Yehia G, Cadalbert L, Dierich A, Le Meur M (1996). Absence of integrin alpha 6 leads to epidermolysis bullosa and neonatal death in mice. *Nat Genet* 13: 370–373.

Ginsburg M, Snow MH, McLaren A (1990). Primordial germ cells in the mouse embryo during gastrulation. *Development* 110: 521–528.

Godin RE, Takaesu NT, Robertson EJ, Dudley AT (1998). Regulation of BMP7 expression during kidney development. *Development* 125: 3473–3482.

Gomez DE, Alonso DF, Yoshiji H, Thorgeirsson UP (1997). Tissue inhibitors of metalloproteinases: structure, regulation and biological functions. *Eur J Cell Biol* 74: 111–122.

Gouedard L, Chen YG, Thevenet L, Racine C, Borie S, Lamarre I, Josso N, Massague J, di Clemente N (2000). Engagement of bone morphogenetic protein type IB receptor and Smad1 signaling by anti-mullerian hormone and its type II receptor. *J Biol Chem* 275: 27973–27978.

Grisaru S, Cano-Gauci D, Tee J, Filmus J, Rosenblum ND (2001). Glypican-3 modulates BMP- and FGF-mediated effects during renal branching morphogenesis. *Dev Biol* 231: 31–46.

Grobstein C (1953). Morphogenetic interaction between embryonic mouse tissues separated by a membrane filter. *Nature* 172: 869–871.

Grobstein C (1955). Inductive interaction in the development of the mouse metanephros. *J Exp Zool* 130: 319–340.

Grobstein C (1956). Trans-filter induction of tubules in mouse metanephrogenic mesenchyme. *Exp Cell Res* 10: 424–440.

Hacker A, Capel B, Goodfellow P, Lovell-Badge R (1995). Expression of *Sry*, the mouse sex determining gene. *Development* 121: 1603–1614.

Hacker U, Lin X, Perrimon N (1997). The *Drosophila sugarless* gene modulates Wingless signaling and encodes an enzyme involved in polysaccharide biosynthesis. *Development* 124: 3565–3573.

Hammes A, Guo JK, Lutsch G, Leheste JR, Landrock D, Ziegler U, Gubler MC, Schedl A (2001). Two splice variants of the Wilms' tumor 1 gene have distinct functions during sex determination and nephron formation. *Cell* 106: 319–329.

Harley VR, Jackson DI, Hextall PJ, Hawkins JR, Berkovitz GD, Sockanathan S, Lovell-Badge R, Goodfellow PN (1992). DNA binding activity of recombinant SRY from normal males and XY females. *Science* 255: 453–456.

Hatano O, Takakusu A, Nomura M, Morohashi K (1996). Identical origin of adrenal cortex and gonad revealed by expression profiles of Ad4BP/SF-1. *Genes Cells* 1: 663–671.

Hatini V, Huh SO, Herzlinger D, Soares VC, Lai E (1996). Essential role of stromal mesenchyme in kidney morphogenesis revealed by targeted disruption of Winged helix transcription factor BF-2. *Genes Dev* 10: 1467–1478.

Hawkins JR, Taylor A, Goodfellow PN, Migeon CJ, Smith KD, Berkovitz GD (1992). Evidence for increased prevalence of SRY mutations in XY females with complete rather than partial gonadal dysgenesis. *Am J Hum Genet* 51: 979–984.

Huber TB, Kottgen M, Schilling B, Walz G, Benzing T (2001). Interaction with podocin facilitates nephrin signaling. *J Biol Chem* 276: 41543–41546.

Ikeda Y, Shen WH, Ingraham HA, Parker KL (1994). Developmental expression of mouse steroidogenic factor-1, an essential regulator of the steroid hydroxylases. *Mol Endocrinol* 8: 654–662.

Ikeda Y, Swain A, Weber TJ, Hentges KE, Zanaria E, Lalli E, Tamai KT, Sassone-Corsi P, Lovell-Badge R, Camerino G, et al. (1996). Steroidogenic factor 1 and Dax-1 colocalize in multiple cell lineages: potential links in endocrine development. *Mol Endocrinol* 10: 1261–1272.

Imasawa T, Utsunomiya Y, Kawamura T, Zhong Y, Nagasawa R, Okabe M, Maruyama N, Hosoya T, Ohno T (2001). The potential of bone marrow-derived cells to differentiate to glomerular mesangial cells. *J Am Soc Nephrol* 12: 1401–1409.

Ingraham HA, Lala DS, Ikeda Y, Luo X, Shen WH, Nachtigal MW, Abbud R, Nilson JH, Parker KL (1994). The nuclear receptor steroidogenic factor 1 acts at multiple levels of the reproductive axis. *Genes Dev* 8: 2302–2312.

Itoh T, Ikeda T, Gomi H, Nakao S, Suzuki T, Itohara S (1997). Unaltered secretion of beta-amyloid precursor protein in gelatinase A (matrix metalloproteinase 2)-deficient mice. *J Biol Chem* 272: 22389–22392.

Jeske YW, Bowles J, Greenfield A, Koopman P (1995). Expression of a linear Sry transcript in the mouse genital ridge. *Nat Genet* 10: 480–482.

Jost A (1953). Studies on sex differentiation in mammals. *Recent Prog Horm Res* 8: 379–418.

Jost A, Vigier B, Prepin J, Perchellet J (1973). Studies on sex differentiation in mammals. *Recent Prog Horm Res* 29: 1–41.

Kanwar YS, Ota K, Yang Q, Wada J, Kashihara N, Tian Y, Wallner EI (1999). Role of membrane-type matrix metalloproteinase 1 (MT-1-MMP), MMP-2, and its inhibitor in nephrogenesis. *Am J Physiol* 277: F934–F947.

Kaplan JM, Kim SH, North KN, Rennke H, Correia LA, Tong HQ, Mathis BJ, Rodriguez-Perez JC, Allen PG, Beggs AH, et al. (2000). Mutations in ACTN4, encoding alpha-actinin-4, cause familial focal segmental glomerulosclerosis. *Nat Genet* 24: 251–256.

Karihaloo A, Karumanchi SA, Barasch J, Jha V, Nickel CH, Yang J, Grisaru S, Bush KT, Nigam S, Rosenblum ND, et al. (2001). Endostatin regulates branching morphogenesis of renal epithelial cells and ureteric bud. *Proc Natl Acad Sci USA* 98: 12509–12514.

Kent J, Wheatley SC, Andrews JE, Sinclair AH, Koopman P (1996). A male-specific role for SOX9 in vertebrate sex determination. *Development* 122: 2813–2822.

Kestila M, Lenkkeri U, Mannikko M, Lamerdin J, McCready P, Putaala H, Ruotsalainen V, Morita T, Nissinen M, Herva R, et al. (1998). Positionally cloned gene for a novel glomerular protein—nephrin—is mutated in congenital nephrotic syndrome. *Mol Cell* 1: 575–582.

Kispert A, Vainio S, Shen L, Rowitch DH, McMahon AP (1996). Proteoglycans are required for maintenance of Wnt-11 expression in the ureter tips. *Development* 122: 3627–3637.

Kispert A, Vainio S, McMahon AP (1998). Wnt-4 is a mesenchymal signal for epithelial transformation of metanephric mesenchyme in the developing kidney. *Development* 125: 4225–4234.

Kolatsi-Joannou M, Li XZ, Suda T, Yuan HT, Woolf AS (2001). Expression and potential role of angiopoietins and Tie-2 in early development of the mouse metanephros. *Dev Dyn* 222: 120–126.

Koopman P, Gubbay J, Vivian N, Goodfellow P, Lovell-Badge R (1991). Male development of chromosomally female mice transgenic for Sry. *Nature* 351: 117–121.

Kreidberg JA, Sariola H, Loring JM, Maeda M, Pelletier J, Housman D, Jaenisch R (1993). WT-1 is required for early kidney development. *Cell* 74: 679–691.

Kreidberg JA, Donovan MJ, Goldstein SL, Rennke H, Shepherd K, Jones RC, Jaenisch R (1996). Alpha 3 beta 1 integrin has a crucial role in kidney and lung organogenesis. *Development* 122: 3537–3547.

Kume T, Deng K, Hogan BLM (2000a). Minimal phenotype of mice homozygous for a null mutation in the forkhead/winged helix gene, *Mf2*. *Mol Cell Biol* 20: 1419–1425.

Kume T, Deng K, Hogan BLM (2000b). Murine forkhead/winged helix genes *Foxc1* (*Mf1*) and *Foxc2* (*Mfh1*) are required for the early organogenesis of the kidney and urinary tract. *Development* 127: 1387–1395.

Kuure S, Vuolteenaho R, Vainio S (2000). Kidney morphogenesis: cellular and molecular regulation. *Mech Dev* 92: 31–45.

Kwok C, Weller PA, Guioli S, Foster JW, Mansour S, Zuffardi O, Punnett HH, Dominguez-Steglich MA, Brook JD, Young ID, et al. (1995). Mutations in SOX9, the gene responsible for campomelic dysplasia and autosomal sex reversal. *Am J Hum Genet* 57: 1028–1036.

Lala DS, Rice DA, Parker KL (1992). Steroidogenic factor I, a key regulator of steroidogenic enzyme expression, is the mouse homolog of fushi tarazu-factor I. *Mol Endocrinol* 6: 1249–1258.

Legallicier B, Trugnan G, Murphy G, Lelongt B, Ronco P (2001). Expression of the type IV collagenase system during mouse kidney development and tubule segmentation. *J Am Soc Nephrol* 12: 2358–2369.

Leimeister C, Bach A, Gessler M (1998). Developmental expression patterns of mouse *sFRP* genes encoding members of the secreted frizzled related protein family. *Mech Dev* 75: 29–42.

Lelongt B, Trugnan G, Murphy G, Ronco PM (1997). Matrix metalloproteinases MMP2 and MMP9 are produced in early stages of kidney morphogenesis but only MMP9 is required for renal organogenesis in vitro. *J Cell Biol* 136: 1363–1373.

Lelongt B, Legallicier B, Piedagnel R, Ronco PM (2001). Do matrix metalloproteinases MMP-2 and MMP-9 (gelatinases) play a role in renal development, physiology and glomerular diseases? *Curr Opin Nephrol Hypertens* 10: 7–12.

Lescher B, Haenig B, Kispert A (1998). sFRP-2 is a target of the Wnt-4 signaling pathway in the developing metanephric kidney. *Dev Dyn* 213: 440–451.

Leveen P, Pekny M, Gebre-Medhin S, Swolin B, Larsson E, Betsholtz C (1994). Mice deficient for PDGF B show renal, cardiovascular, and hematological abnormalities. *Genes Dev* 8: 1875–1887.

Li Z, Stuart RO, Qiao J, Pavlova A, Bush KT, Pohl M, Sakurai H, Nigam SK (2000). A role for Timeless in epithelial morphogenesis during kidney development. *Proc Natl Acad Sci USA* 97: 10038–10043.

Lin X, Buff EM, Perrimon N, Michelson AM (1999). Heparan sulfate proteoglycans are essential for FGF receptor signaling during Drosophila embryonic development. *Development* 126: 3715–3723.

Lin Y, Zhang S, Rehn M, Itaranta P, Tuukkanen J, Heljasvaara R, Peltoketo H, Pihlajaniemi T, Vainio S (2001). Induced repatterning of type XVIII collagen expression in ureter bud from kidney to lung type: association with sonic hedgehog and ectopic surfactant protein C. *Development* 128: 1573–1585.

Lindahl P, Hellstrom M, Kalen M, Karlsson L, Pekny M, Pekna M, Soriano P, Betsholtz C (1998). Paracrine PDGF-B/PDGF-Rbeta signaling controls mesangial cell development in kidney glomeruli. *Development* 125: 3313–3322.

Little M, Wells C (1997). A clinical overview of *WT1* gene mutations. *Hum Mutat* 9: 209–225.

Luo X, Ikeda Y, Parker KL (1994). A cell-specific nuclear receptor is essential for adrenal and gonadal development and sexual differentiation. *Cell* 77: 481–490.

Luo G, Hofmann C, Bronckers ALJJ, Sohocki M, Bradley A, Karsenty G (1995a). BMP-7 is an inducer of nephrogenesis, and is also required for eye development and skeletal patterning. *Genes Dev* 9: 2808–2820.

Luo X, Ikeda Y, Lala DS, Baity LA, Meade JC, Parker KL (1995b). A cell-specific nu-

clear receptor plays essential roles in adrenal and gonadal development. *Endocr Res* 21: 517–524.
Maas R, Elfering S, Glaser T, Jepeal L (1994). Deficient outgrowth of the ureteric bud underlies the renal agenesis phenotype in mice manifesting the limb deformity (ld) mutation. *Dev Dyn* 199: 214–228.
Maisonpierre PC, Suri C, Jones PF, Bartunkova S, Wiegand SJ, Radziejewski C, Compton D, McClain J, Aldrich TH, Papadopoulos N, et al. (1997). Angiopoietin-2, a natural antagonist for Tie2 that disrupts in vivo angiogenesis. *Science* 277: 55–60.
Martineau J, Nordqvist K, Tilmann C, Lovell-Badge R, Capel B (1997). Male-specific cell migration into the developing gonad. *Curr Biol* 7: 958–968.
Mendelsohn C, Batourina E, Fung S, Gilbert T, Dodd J (1999). Stromal cells mediate retinoid-dependent functions essential for renal development. *Development* 126: 1139–1148.
Merry CL, Bullock SL, Swan DC, Backen AC, Lyon M, Beddington RS, Wilson VA, Gallagher JT (2001). The molecular phenotype of heparan sulfate in the Hs2st$^{-/-}$ mutant mouse. *J Biol Chem* 276: 35429–35434.
Meyer J, Sudbeck P, Held M, Wagner T, Schmitz ML, Bricarelli FD, Eggermont E, Friedrich U, Haas OA, Kobelt A, et al. (1997). Mutational analysis of the *SOX9* gene in campomelic dysplasia and autosomal sex reversal: lack of genotype/phenotype correlations. *Hum Mol Genet* 6: 91–98.
Miyamoto N, Yoshida M, Kuratani S, Matsuo I, Aizawa S (1997). Defects of urogenital development in mice lacking Emx2. *Development* 124: 1653–1664.
Miyazaki Y, Oshima K, Fogo A, Hogan BL, Ichikawa I (2000). Bone morphogenetic protein 4 regulates the budding site and elongation of the mouse ureter. *J Clin Invest* 105: 863–873.
Morais da Silva S, Hacker A, Harley V, Goodfellow P, Swain A, Lovell-Badge R (1996). Sox9 expression during gonadal development implies a conserved role for the gene in testis differentiation in mammals and birds. *Nat Genet* 14: 62–68.
Morohashi K, Zanger UM, Honda S, Hara M, Waterman MR, Omura T (1993). Activation of *CYP11A* and *CYP11B* gene promoters by the steroidogenic cell-specific transcription factor, Ad4BP. *Mol Endocrinol* 7: 1196–1204.
Muller U, Wang D, Denda S, Meneses JJ, Pedersen RA, Reichardt LF (1997). Integrin alpha8beta1 is critically important for epithelial–mesenchymal interactions during kidney morphogenesis. *Cell* 88: 603–613.
Muscatelli F, Strom TM, Walker AP, Zanaria E, Recan D, Meindl A, Bardoni B, Guioli S, Zehetner G, Rabl W, et al. (1994). Mutations in the *DAX-1* gene give rise to both X-linked adrenal hypoplasia congenita and hypogonadotropic hypogonadism. *Nature* 372: 672–676.
Nachtigal MW, Hirokawa Y, Enyeart-VanHouten DL, Flanagan JN, Hammer GD, Ingraham HA (1998). Wilms' tumor 1 and Dax-1 modulate the orphan nuclear receptor SF-1 in sex-specific gene expression. *Cell* 93: 445–454.
Nigam SK (1995). Determinants of branching tubulogenesis. *Curr Opin Nephrol Hypertension* 4: 209–214.
Noakes PG, Miner JH, Gautam M, Cunningham JM, Sanes JR, Merlie JP (1995). The renal glomerulus of mice lacking s-laminin/laminin beta 2: nephrosis despite molecular compensation by laminin beta 1. *Nat Genet* 10: 400–406.
O'Reilly MS, Boehm T, Shing Y, Fukai N, Vasios G, Lane WS, Flynn E, Birkhead JR, Olsen BR, Folkman J (1997). Endostatin: an endogenous inhibitor of angiogenesis and tumor growth. *Cell* 88: 277–285.
O'Rourke DA, Liu ZX, Sellin L, Spokes K, Zeller R, Cantley LG (2000). Hepatocyte growth factor induces MAPK-dependent formin IV translocation in renal epithelial cells. *J Am Soc Nephrol* 11: 2212–2221.
Ota K, Stetler-Stevenson WG, Yang Q, Kumar A, Wada J, Kashihara N, Wallner EI, Kanwar YS (1998). Cloning of murine membrane-type-1-matrix metalloproteinase (MT-1-MMP) and its metanephric developmental regulation with respect to MMP-2 and its inhibitor. *Kidney Int* 54: 131–142.
Pandolfi PP, Roth ME, Karis A, Leonard MW, Dzierzak E, Grosveld FG, Engel JD, Lindenbaum MH (1995). Targeted disruption of the *GATA3* gene causes severe abnormalities in the nervous system and in fetal liver haematopoiesis. *Nat Genet* 11: 40–44.
Parr BA, McMahon AP (1998). Sexually dimorphic development of the mammalian reproductive tract requires Wnt-7a. *Nature* 395: 707–710.
Patek CE, Little MH, Fleming S, Miles C, Charlieu JP, Clarke AR, Miyagawa K, Christie S, Doig J, Harrison DJ, et al. (1999). A zinc finger truncation of murine WT1 results in the characteristic urogenital abnormalities of Denys-Drash syndrome. *Proc Natl Acad Sci USA* 96: 2931–2936.
Patterson LT, Pembaur M, Potter SS (2001). Hoxa11 and Hoxd11 regulate branching morphogenesis of the ureteric bud in the developing kidney. *Development* 128: 2153–2161.
Pelletier J, Bruening W, Kashtan CE, Mauer SM, Manivel JC, Striegel JE, Houghton DC, Junien C, Habib R, Fouser L, et al. (1991). Germline mutations in the Wilms' tumor suppressor gene are associated with abnormal urogenital development in Denys-Drash syndrome. *Cell* 67: 437–447.
Pepicelli CV, Kispert A, Rowitch DH, McMahon AP (1997). GDNF induces branching and increased cell proliferation in the ureter of the mouse. *Dev Biol* 192: 193–198.
Pichel JG, Shen L, Sheng HZ, Granholm AC, Drago J, Grinberg A, Lee EJ, Huang SP, Saarma M, Hoffer BJ, et al. (1996). Defects in enteric innervation and kidney development in mice lacking GDNF. *Nature* 382: 73–76.
Piscione TD, Phan T, Rosenblum ND (2001). BMP7 controls collecting tubule cell proliferation and apoptosis via Smad1-dependent and -independent pathways. *Am J Physiol* 280: F19–F33.
Plachov D, Chowdhury K, Walther C, Simon D, Guenet JL, Gruss P (1990). *Pax8*, a murine paired box gene expressed in the developing excretory system and thyroid gland. *Development* 110: 643–651.
Plisov SY, Yoshino K, Dove LF, Higinbotham KG, Rubin JS, Perantoni AO (2001). TGF-beta2, LIF and FGF2 cooperate to induce nephrogenesis. *Development* 128: 1045–1057.
Pohl M, Sakurai H, Bush KT, Nigam SK (2000a). Matrix metalloproteinases and their inhibitors regulate in vitro ureteric bud branching morphogenesis. *Am J Physiol* 279: F891–F900.
Pohl M Stuart RO, Sakurai H, Nigam SK (2000b). Branching morphogenesis during kidney development. *Annu Rev Physiol* 62: 595–620.
Pohl M, Sakurai H, Stuart RO, Nigam SK (2000c). Role of hyaluronan and CD44 in in vitro branching morphogenesis of ureteric bud cells. *Dev Biol* 224: 312–325.
Pohl M, Bhatnagar V, Mendoza SA, Nigam SK (2002). Toward an etiological classification of developmental disorders of the kidney and upper urinary tract. *Kidney Int* 61: 10–19.
Pole RJ, Qi BQ, Beasley SW (2002). Patterns of apoptosis during degeneration of the pronephros and mesonephros. *J Urol* 167: 269–271.
Pollack AL, Runyan RB, Mostov KE (1998). Morphogenetic mechanisms of epithelial tubulogenesis: MDCK cell polarity is transiently rearranged without loss of cell–cell contact during scatter factor/hepatocyte growth factor–induced tubulogenesis. *Dev Biol* 204: 64–79.
Qiao J, Sakurai H, Nigam SK (1999a). Branching morphogenesis independent of mesenchymal–epithelial contact in the developing kidney. *Proc Natl Acad Sci USA* 96: 7330–7335.
Qiao J, Uzzo R, Obara-Ishihara T, Degenstein L, Fuchs E, Herzlinger D (1999b). FGF-7 modulates ureteric bud growth and nephron number in the developing kidney. *Development* 126: 547–554.
Qiao J, Bush KT, Steer DL, Stuart RO, Sakurai H, Wachsman W, Nigam SK (2001). Multiple fibroblast growth factors support growth of the ureteric bud but have different effects on branching morphogenesis. *Mech Dev* 109: 123–135.
Quaggin SE, Vanden Heuvel GB, Igarashi P (1998). Pod-1, a mesoderm-specific basic-helix-loop-helix protein expressed in mesenchymal and glomerular epithelial cells in the developing kidney. *Mech Dev* 71: 37–48.
Quaggin SE, Schwartz L, Cui S, Igarashi P, Deimling J, Post M, Rossant J (1999). The basic-helix-loop-helix protein Pod1 is critically important for kidney and lung organogenesis. *Development* 126: 5771–5783.
Reponen P, Sahlberg C, Huhtala P, Hurskainen T, Thesleff I, Tryggvason K (1992). Molecular cloning of murine 72-kDa type IV collagenase and its expression during mouse development. *J Biol Chem* 267: 7856–7862.
Robert B, St John PL, Hyink DP, Abrahamson DR (1996). Evidence that embryonic kidney cells expressing flk-1 are intrinsic, vasculogenic angioblasts. *Am J Physiol* 271: F744–F753.
Robert B, St John PL, Abrahamson DR (1998). Direct visualization of renal vascular morphogenesis in Flk1 heterozygous mutant mice. *Am J Physiol* 275: F164–F172.
Roberts LM, Hirokawa Y, Nachtigal MW, Ingraham HA (1999). Paracrine-mediated apoptosis in reproductive tract development. *Dev Biol* 208: 110–122.
Roberts LM, Visser JA, Ingraham HA (2002). Involvement of a matrix metalloproteinase in MIS-induced cell death during urogenital development. *Development* 129: 1487–1496.
Roselli S, Gribouval O, Boute N, Sich M, Benessy F, Attie T, Gubler MC, Antignac C (2002). Podocin localizes in the kidney to the slit diaphragm area. *Am J Pathol* 160: 131–139.
Ryan G, Steele-Perkins V, Morris JF, Rauscher FJ 3rd, Dressler GR (1995). Repression of Pax-2 by WT1 during normal kidney development. *Development* 121: 867–875.
Sainio K, Suvanto P, Davies J, Wartiovaara J, Wartiovaara K, Saarma M, Arumae U, Meng X, Lindahl M, Pachnis V, et al. (1997). Glial-cell-line-derived neurotrophic factor is required for bud initiation from ureteric epithelium. *Development* 124: 4077–4087.
Sakurai H, Nigam SK (1997). Transforming growth factor-beta selectively inhibits branching morphogenesis but not tubulogenesis. *Am J Physiol* 272: F139–F146.
Sakurai H, Barros EJ, Tsukamoto T, Barasch J, Nigam SK (1997a). An in vitro tubulogenesis system using cell lines derived from the embryonic kidney shows dependence on multiple soluble growth factors. *Proc Natl Acad Sci USA* 94: 6279–6284.
Sakurai H, Tsukamoto T, Kjelsberg CA, Cantley LG, Nigam SK (1997b). EGF receptor ligands are a large fraction of in vitro branching morphogens secreted by embryonic kidney. *Am J Physiol* 273: F463–F472.
Sakurai H, Bush KT, Nigam SK (2001). Identification of pleiotrophin as a mesenchymal factor involved in ureteric bud branching morphogenesis. *Development* 128: 3283–3293.
Santos OF, Nigam SK (1993). HGF-induced tubulogenesis and branching of epithelial cells is modulated by extracellular matrix and TGF-beta. *Dev Biol* 160: 293–302.
Santos OF, Barros EJ, Yang XM, Matsumoto K, Nakamura T, Park M, Nigam SK (1994). Involvement of hepatocyte growth factor in kidney development. *Dev Biol* 163: 525–529.
Sariola H (2002). Nephron induction revisited: from caps to condensates. *Curr Opin Nephrol Hypertens* 11: 17–21.
Sariola H, Ekblom P, Lehtonen E, Saxen L (1983). Differentiation and vascularization of the metanephric kidney grafted on the chorioallantoic membrane. *Dev Biol* 96: 427–435.
Sato TN, Tozawa Y, Deutsch U, Wolburg-Buchholz K, Fujiwara Y, Gendron-Maguire M, Gridley T, Wolburg H, Risau W, Qin Y (1995). Distinct roles of the receptor tyrosine kinases Tie-1 and Tie-2 in blood vessel formation. *Nature* 376: 70–74.
Saxen L (1987). *Organogenesis of the Kidney.* Barlow P, Green P, White C (eds.) Cambridge University Press, Cambridge.
Schuchardt A, D'Agati V, Larsson-Blomberg L, Costantini F, Pachnis V (1994). Defects in the kidney and enteric nervous system of mice lacking the tyrosine kinase receptor Ret. *Nature* 367: 380–383.
Schuchardt A, D'Agati V, Pachnis V, Costantini F (1996). Renal agenesis and hypodysplasia in ret-k-mutant mice result from defects in ureteric bud development. *Development* 122: 1919–1929.
Serluca FC, Fishman MC (2001). Pre-pattern in the pronephric kidney field of zebrafish. *Development* 128: 2233–2241.
Shawlot W, Behringer RR (1995). Requirement for Lim1 in head-organizer function. *Nature* 374: 425–430.
Shih NY, Li J, Karpitskii V, Nguyen A, Dustin ML, Kanagawa O, Miner JH, Shaw AS (1999). Congenital nephrotic syndrome in mice lacking CD2-associated protein. *Science* 286: 312–315.
Sibilia M, Wagner EF (1995). Strain-dependent epithelial defects in mice lacking the EGF receptor. *Science* 269: 234–238.
Simon M, Grone HJ, Johren O, Kullmer J, Plate KH, Risau W, Fuchs E (1995). Expres-

sion of vascular endothelial growth factor and its receptors in human renal ontogenesis and in adult kidney. *Am J Physiol* 268: F240–F250.

Soriano P (1994). Abnormal kidney development and hematological disorders in PDGF beta-receptor mutant mice. *Genes Dev* 8: 1888–1896.

Spotila LD, Spotila JR, Hall SE (1998). Sequence and expression analysis of WT1 and Sox9 in the red-eared slider turtle, *Trachemys scripta*. *J Exp Zool* 281: 417–427.

Srinivas S, Wu Z, Chen CM, D'Agati V, Costantini F (1999). Dominant effects of RET receptor misexpression and ligand-independent RET signaling on ureteric bud development. *Development* 126: 1375–1386.

Stark K, Vainio S, Vassileva G, McMahon AP (1994). Epithelial transformation of metanephric mesenchyme in the developing kidney regulated by Wnt-4. *Nature* 372: 679–683.

Stuart RO, Bush KT, Nigam SK (2001). Changes in global gene expression patterns during development and maturation of the rat kidney. *Proc Natl Acad Sci USA* 98: 5649–5654.

Sudbeck P, Schmitz ML, Baeuerle PA, Scherer G (1996). Sex reversal by loss of the C-terminal transactivation domain of human SOX9. *Nat Genet* 13: 230–232.

Suri C, Jones PF, Patan S, Bartunkova S, Maisonpierre PC, Davis S, Sato TN, Yancopoulos GD (1996). Requisite role of angiopoietin-1, a ligand for the TIE2 receptor, during embryonic angiogenesis. *Cell* 87: 1171–1180.

Swain A, Lovell-Badge R (1999). Mammalian sex determination: a molecular drama. *Genes Dev* 13: 755–767.

Swain A, Zanaria E, Hacker A, Lovell-Badge R, Camerino G (1996). Mouse Dax1 expression is consistent with a role in sex determination as well as in adrenal and hypothalamus function. *Nat Genet* 12: 404–409.

Swain A, Narvaez V, Burgoyne P, Camerino G, Lovell-Badge R (1998). Dax1 antagonizes Sry action in mammalian sex determination. *Nature* 391: 761–767.

Takahashi T, Takahashi K, Gerety S, Wang H, Anderson DJ, Daniel TO (2001). Temporally compartmentalized expression of ephrin-B2 during renal glomerular development. *J Am Soc Nephrol* 12: 2673–2682.

Tanney DC, Feng L, Pollock AS, Lovett DH (1998). Regulated expression of matrix metalloproteinases and TIMP in nephrogenesis. *Dev Dyn* 213: 121–129.

Threadgill DW, Dlugosz AA, Hansen LA, Tennenbaum T, Lichti U, Yee D, LaMantia C, Mourton T, Herrup K, Harris RC, et al. (1995). Targeted disruption of mouse EGF receptor: effect of genetic background on mutant phenotype. *Science* 269: 230–234.

Tomac AC, Grinberg A, Huang SP, Nosrat C, Wang Y, Borlongan C, Lin SZ, Chiang YH, Olson L, Westphal H, et al. (2000). Glial cell line–derived neurotrophic factor receptor alpha1 availability regulates glial cell line–derived neurotrophic factor signaling: evidence from mice carrying one or two mutated alleles. *Neuroscience* 95: 1011–1023.

Torres M, Gomez-Pardo E, Dressler GR, Gruss P (1995). Pax-2 controls multiple steps of urogenital development. *Development* 121: 4057–4065.

Tsang TE, Shawlot W, Kinder SJ, Kobayashi A, Kwan KM, Schughart K, Kania A, Jessell TM, Behringer RR, Tam PP (2000). Lim1 activity is required for intermediate mesoderm differentiation in the mouse embryo. *Dev Biol* 223: 77–90.

Tsuda M, Kamimura K, Nakato H, Archer M, Staatz W, Fox B, Humphrey M, Olson S, Futch T, Kaluza V, et al. (1999). The cell-surface proteoglycan Dally regulates Wingless signalling in *Drosophila*. *Nature* 400: 276–280.

Tufro A (2000). VEGF spatially directs angiogenesis during metanephric development in vitro. *Dev Biol* 227: 558–566.

Tufro A, Norwood VF, Carey RM, Gomez RA (1999). Vascular endothelial growth factor induces nephrogenesis and vasculogenesis. *J Am Soc Nephrol* 10: 2125–2134.

Tufro-McReddie A, Norwood VF, Aylor KW, Botkin SJ, Carey RM, Gomez RA (1997). Oxygen regulates vascular endothelial growth factor–mediated vasculogenesis and tubulogenesis. *Dev Biol* 183: 139–149.

Vainio SJ, Uusitalo MS (2000). A road to kidney tubules via the Wnt pathway. *Pediatr Nephrol* 15: 151–156.

Vainio S, Heikkila M, Kispert A, Chin N, McMahon AP (1999). Female development in mammals is regulated by Wnt-4 signalling. *Nature* 397: 405–409.

Van Esch H, Groenen P, Nesbit MA, Schuffenhauer S, Lichtner P, Vanderlinden G, Harding B, Beetz R, Bilous RW, Holdaway I, et al. (2000). GATA3 haplo-insufficiency causes human HDR syndrome. *Nature* 406: 419–422.

Visser JA, Olaso R, Verhoef-Post M, Kramer P, Themmen AP, Ingraham HA (2001). The serine/threonine transmembrane receptor ALK2 mediates mullerian inhibiting substance signaling. *Mol Endocrinol* 15: 936–945.

Vu TH, Shipley JM, Bergers G, Berger JE, Helms JA, Hanahan D, Shapiro SD, Senior RM, Werb Z (1998). MMP-9/gelatinase B is a key regulator of growth plate angiogenesis and apoptosis of hypertrophic chondrocytes. *Cell* 93: 411–422.

Wang Y, Macke JP, Abella BS, Andreasson K, Worley P, Gilbert DJ, Copeland NG, Jenkins NA, Nathans J (1996). A large family of putative transmembrane receptors homologous to the product of the *Drosophila* tissue polarity gene frizzled. *J Biol Chem* 271: 4468–4476.

Western PS, Harry JL, Graves JA, Sinclair AH (1999). Temperature-dependent sex determination in the American alligator: AMH precedes SOX9 expression. *Dev Dyn* 216: 411–419.

Winnier G, Blessing M, Labosky PA, Hogan BL (1995). Bone morphogenetic protein-4 is required for mesoderm formation and patterning in the mouse. *Genes Dev* 9: 2105–2116.

Wynshaw-Boris A, Ryan G, Deng CX, Chan DC, Jackson-Grusby L, Larson D, Dunmore JH, Leder P (1997). The role of a single formin isoform in the limb and renal phenotypes of limb deformity. *Mol Med* 3: 372–384.

Xu PX, Adams J, Peters H, Brown MC, Heaney S, Maas R (1999). Eya1-deficient mice lack ears and kidneys and show abnormal apoptosis of organ primordia. *Nat Genet* 23: 113–117.

Yoshino K, Rubin JS, Higinbotham KG, Uren A, Anest V, Plisov SY, Perantoni AO (2001). Secreted Frizzled-related proteins can regulate metanephric development. *Mech Dev* 102: 45–55.

Yu Q, Stamenkovic I (2000). Cell surface–localized matrix metalloproteinase-9 proteolytically activates TGF-beta and promotes tumor invasion and angiogenesis. *Genes Dev* 14: 163–176.

Yuan HT, Suri C, Yancopoulos GD, Woolf AS (1999). Expression of angiopoietin-1, angiopoietin-2, and the Tie-2 receptor tyrosine kinase during mouse kidney maturation. *J Am Soc Nephrol* 10: 1722–1736.

Zanaria E, Muscatelli F, Bardoni B, Strom TM, Guioli S, Guo W, Lalli E, Moser C, Walker AP, McCabe ER, et al. (1994). An unusual member of the nuclear hormone receptor superfamily responsible for X-linked adrenal hypoplasia congenita. *Nature* 372: 635–641.

Zent R, Bush KT, Pohl ML, Quaranta V, Koshikawa N, Wang Z, Kreidberg JA, Sakurai H, Stuart RO, Nigam SK (2001). Involvement of laminin binding integrins and laminin-5 in branching morphogenesis of the ureteric bud during kidney development. *Dev Biol* 238: 289–302.

14 | Development of Endodermal Derivatives in the Lung, Liver, Pancreas, and Gut

BEN Z. STANGER AND DOUGLAS A. MELTON

The derivatives of endoderm display an extraordinary diversity of function, including gas exchange, digestion, nutrient absorption, detoxification, and endocrine regulation. A wide range of developmental disorders are attributable to abnormalities of endoderm function. The spectrum of these disorders is a reflection of the developmental steps that must normally occur, including (*1*) endoderm formation (*gastrulation*) and spatial specification (*patterning*), (*2*) physical formation of the primitive organ anlagen (*budding*), (*3*) shaping of tissue architecture (*morphogenesis*), and (*4*) creation of specific functional cell types within the organ (*differentiation*). This chapter reviews the development of the lung, liver, pancreas, and gut, focusing on the molecular determinants of each of these processes.

OVERVIEW OF ENDODERMAL DEVELOPMENT

Although the lung, liver, pancreas, and gut contain tissue derived from the mesoderm and ectoderm (smooth muscle, blood vessels, nerves, etc.), the specialized epithelial (parenchymal) tissue of these organs is directly descended from the endoderm layer. Endoderm forms through the process of gastrulation, during which certain cells from the epiblast layer migrate through the primitive streak to give rise to the mesodermal and endodermal cell layers. With the formation of the primitive streak and gastrulation, all the axes of the embryo are established: the anterior/posterior (A/P) axis is defined by the primitive streak, which is located at the posterior end of the embryo; the dorsal/ventral (D/V) axis is defined by the ectodermal (dorsal) and endodermal (ventral) germ layers; and the right/left (medial/lateral) axis is defined by the previous two (Fig. 14–1A). Even in the gastrula-stage embryo, cells of the endoderm already have an A/P identity. However, this identity does not render the cells irreversibly determined to develop into the given organ that position alone would suggest. Thus, cells at this stage are not committed to particular fates; rather, they exhibit *plasticity*.

At the conclusion of gastrulation, the three-layered mammalian embryo is a disc resting on the convex surface of the egg cylinder, which contains both embryonic and extraembryonic tissues (Fig. 14–1A). The endoderm lies on the outermost surface of this cylinder. Subsequently, the endoderm becomes internalized through the process of *turning*, whereby the curvature of the embryonic disc is inverted so that the endoderm lines the innermost layer of the now concave surface (Fig. 14–1B). In parallel, the anteriormost segment of endoderm folds over itself to form a blind-end loop known as the anterior intestinal portal (AIP). A similar fold forms posteriorly (caudally) a bit later to give rise to the caudal intestinal portal (CIP). These loops become tubes through the lateral and ventral growth of the endoderm and grow toward each other until they meet at the yolk stalk (Fig. 14–1B). During this time, additional signals derived from adjacent tissues further commit endoderm cells to their ultimate fates. Shortly thereafter, small buds can be detected along the gut tube, and changes in epithelial cell morphology along the tube are seen (Fig. 14–1C).

Finally, buds expand into recognizable organs through a combination of tissue expansion (proliferation) and regulated movements (morphogenesis). Distinctive cell types differentiate from progenitor cells in the expanding buds. Gross anatomical changes, including elongation, rotation, and duct fusion, take place. Vasculogenesis, innervation, and development of the mucosal immune system complete the final stages of organ development.

Remarkably, a small number of regulatory programs seem to be used repeatedly in the development of the endoderm and its derivatives. The molecules involved include cell-cell signals such as fibroblast growth factors (FGFs), hedgehog (HH) proteins, Notch, and transforming growth factors (TGFs), including the subset of TGFs known as bone morphogenic proteins (BMPs). These signals are interpreted in context-dependent ways, allowing them to have specific effects at different times and places during development. All of these developmental pathways are described in detail below (see Principles of Endodermal Patterning).

ESTABLISHMENT OF THE ENDODERMAL CELL LAYER

Gastrulation

Following implantation, the embryonic structures known as the node and the primitive streak appear in the posterior half of the undifferentiated epiblast layer (Fig. 14–1A). Cells migrate posteriorly toward and down through the primitive streak, giving rise to embryonic mesoderm and embryonic endoderm. With the formation of these distinct germ layers at the conclusion of gastrulation, the endoderm has begun to adopt features of competence and restriction. *Competence* (or potential) refers to the ability of cells within the endoderm layer to form the normal derivatives of endoderm, a property not generally shared by the cells within the mesoderm or ectoderm layers. Conversely, *restriction* refers to the inability of endoderm cells to form mesodermal or ectodermal derivatives. Thus, the complete potential of cells within the early embryo to become any cell type (*totipotency*) becomes reduced to a limited set of possibilities whose range is dictated by the germ layer in which the cells reside. Some recent studies have suggested that certain adult stem cells have the potential to generate progeny that cross germ layer restrictions. While these findings may challenge classically held notions of gastrulation and competence, the restrictions imposed by gastrulation appear to hold for the majority of cells.

Fate maps, in which individual cells are marked at one point in time and then traced during development, illustrate patterns of cell destination. Fate maps of the epiblast demonstrate that gastrulation proceeds in a stereotyped way (Rosenquist, 1971; Lawson et al., 1991). In particular, the endoderm is derived from the epiblast cells that surround the anterior primitive streak; more anterior epiblast cells give rise to more anterior endoderm. Although these morphogenetic movements are coordinated, the epiblast fate map has large regions of overlap; thus, predicting the fate of a single epiblast cell is probabilistic rather than exact. It should be noted that prior to gastrulation, the tissue layer below the epiblast is referred to as either the "hypoblast" or the "visceral endoderm." Confusion arises because this visceral endoderm is displaced by definitive endoderm during gastrulation and does not contribute to the embryo proper (Fig. 14–1A).

Several signals have been identified that are required for proper gastrulation and endodermal formation. Notably, not all of these signals are derived from embryonic tissue. For example, some signals are required in the extraembryonic visceral endoderm to "pattern" the epiblast; these include TGFβ; see Chapter 24 signals (Conlon et al., 1994; Waldrip et al., 1998) and hepatocyte nuclear factor-3β (HNF-3β) (Dufort et al., 1998). Other signals are needed in the gastrulating epiblast cells themselves, most notably the FGFs; see Chapter 32 (Feldman et al., 1995; Ciruna et al., 1997).

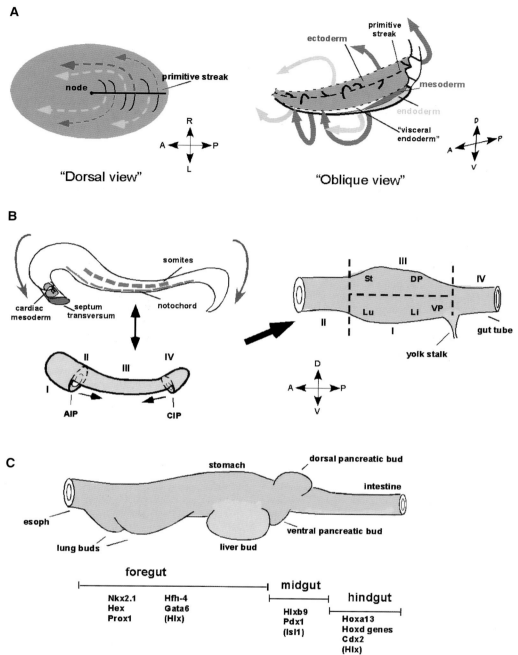

Figure 14–1. Overview of endodermal development. (*A*) Gastrulation (embryonic day [e] 6–7.5 of mouse gestation). (*Left*) shows the epiblast (blue) viewed from above. Epiblast cells (solid black) migrate through the primitive streak and arise as mesoderm (dashed red) or endoderm (dashed yellow) cells. (*Right*) shows an oblique view of cell movements. Note that the newly formed mesoderm (red) and endoderm (yellow) cell layers are displacing the visceral endoderm anteriorly. (*B*) Tube formation and patterning (e7.5–9 of mouse gestation). (*Left*) the ectoderm and mesoderm have been peeled away to reveal the endoderm below. At this stage, the anterior endoderm is in contact with the cardiac mesoderm and septum transversum, while portions of the dorsal endoderm are in contact with the notochord. The anterior intestinal portal (AIP) and caudal intestinal portal (CIP) have formed and are extending toward the midline to form the gut tube. Blue arrows indicate the process of turning, following which the embryo will conform to a concave shape with the endoderm "inside." Roman numerals show the regions corresponding to the fate map of the late streak embryo. (Adapted from Wells and Melton, 1999.) (*Right*) the gut tube has completely formed. Organ domains have been specified, and their position relative to the initial endoderm sheet can be seen. Lu, lung; Li, liver; St, stomach; DP, dorsal pancreatic bud; VP, ventral pancreatic bud. (*C*) Budding and morphogenesis (e9.5 of mouse gestation to birth). The mesoderm and ectoderm have been completely removed to show the position of early organ buds. Several transcription factors required for organogenesis are grouped according to the endodermal domain in which they are required. Transcription factors in parentheses are required in the mesoderm (see text for details).

Some steps in early development may not be governed by absolute requirements for gene products but, rather, through a more subtle relative signal integration. An example of this can be seen in the analysis of "chimeric" embryos containing both wild-type and FGF receptor 1 (*Fgfr1*)-deficient cells. Mutant cells fail to traverse the primitive streak and pile up at the streak, where they differentiate into ectopic ectoderm (neural) derivatives (Ciruna et al., 1997). One is tempted to interpret this result as a requirement for FGFR1 in either migration of epiblast cells or differentiation of endoderm and mesoderm, but in contrast to these results is the phenotype of embryos in which *every* cell bears a targeted mutation in *Fgfr1*. These mutants die over a 2-day period around gastrulation (embryonic day [e] 7.5–9.5), yet many of these embryos do, in fact, gastrulate and develop mesoderm (Yamiguchi et al., 1994; Deng et al., 1994), suggesting that FGFR1 is not absolutely required for either migration or differentiation. The fact that *Fgfr1*-deficient cells fail to gastrulate in a chimeric environment when they are given a choice, but not when all cells share the same disadvantage, suggests that relative preferences may guide cell movements and differentiation decisions. These experiments also demonstrate one potential pitfall in interpreting null mutant phenotypes.

It is unclear when and how the cells that migrate through the primitive streak become mesoderm or endoderm. It is possible that signals are provided before, during, or after gastrulation; and a variety of factors that could influence cell decisions during gastrulation are expressed in the primitive streak and other gastrulation-stage structures (reviewed in Wells and Melton, 1999). Significantly, several transcription factors have been identified in frogs and zebrafish, including *Sox17*, *Mixer*, and *Casanova*, that can induce pluripotent embryonic cells to become endoderm (Hudson et al., 1997; Henry and Melton 1998; Kikuchi et al., 2001). It remains unclear whether similar endoderm "master regulatory pathways" exist in higher vertebrates.

Tube Formation

Following gastrulation, two ventral invaginations form at the anterior and posterior ends of the embryo. The first, at the anterior end, is the AIP, followed shortly by a posterior invagination, the CIP. These invaginations, which incorporate both endoderm and mesoderm, continue toward the midline such that endoderm from the anterior end of the embryo folds back on itself and ends up at the yolk stalk, the umbilical position from which the yolk sac emanates. This means that derivatives of the ventral endoderm closest to the future umbilicus (the liver and ventral pancreas) are descended from what was once the anteriormost endoderm (Fig. 14–1B). The sides of the tube are formed by a lateral-to-ventral movement of endoderm. The splanchnic mesoderm surrounding this tube differentiates into submucosal tissue and smooth muscle, and the endoderm itself is prepared to undergo further changes associated with organogenesis. The molecular signals leading to AIP and CIP formation are unknown, but it does not appear that the ectoderm or mesoderm are needed to initiate the process (reviewed in Roberts, 2000). Nevertheless, several genes have been identified that are necessary for tube formation to proceed.

One of these genes encodes GATA-4 (Table 14–1), a transcription factor containing a zinc finger DNA-binding motif. *Gata-4* mutant mice develop endoderm but have severe problems with folding and formation of ventral structures; they do not develop a foregut as a result of faulty AIP formation (Molkentin et al., 1997; Kuo et al., 1997). *Gata-4* is expressed in the AIP (Molkentin et al., 1997), and chimeric analysis has demonstrated that *Gata-4* acts within the endoderm to allow normal folding and formation of ventral structures (Narita et al.,

1997), although it is not clear whether this activity is provided by visceral endoderm or definitive endoderm. This role in gut development appears to be evolutionarily conserved in organisms as distantly related to humans as flies (Rehorn et al., 1996).

The *Hnf-3β* transcription factor (which bears a "winged helix" DNA-binding motif) is required in visceral endoderm for proper morphogenesis of the node and notochord (Table 14–1); mutant animals form definitive endoderm, which is incapable of invaginating to form a gut tube (Ang and Rossant, 1994; Weinstein et al., 1994). *Hnf-3β* chimeric embryos that progress beyond this block demonstrate that *Hnf-3β* has another separate role in the formation of foregut and midgut, but not hindgut, endoderm (Dufort et al., 1998). Finally, TGF-β signals also appear to be involved in tube formation. Mice with mutations in the gene encoding the Furin protease also fail to undergo ventral closure, possibly as a result of defective processing of TGF-β family signals (Roebroek et al., 1998). One TGF-β signal, BMP4, is required for closure of the ventral mesoderm (Winnier et al., 1995).

Although the mechanism by which these mutations interfere with tube formation is unclear, a requirement for HNF and GATA persists through multiple stages of endodermal development. Development appears to occur through a hierarchy of competence, in which cells become progressively competent to respond to subsequent signals. Dissection of the liver-specific albumin gene enhancer has provided a molecular model for endodermal competence (and restriction), in which the regulated binding of GATA and HNF transcription factors to critical elements in DNA sequentially confers competence for further endodermal differentiation (Bossard and Zaret, 1998).

The albumin enhancer region contains binding sites for both GATA and HNF-3. In vivo footprint analysis has demonstrated that the enhancer exists in three tissue-specific states: (*1*) in neural tube cells, which lack GATA and HNF3, the enhancer is empty; (*2*) in dorsal gut endoderm, which does not transcribe albumin, the enhancer is bound by GATA and HNF-3; and (*3*) in nascent liver bud cells, the enhancer is bound by GATA, HNF-3, and several other transcription factors that confer full transcriptional activity of the enhancer. There is evidence that HNF-3 and/or GATA may be capable of altering chromatin structure through direct effects on histones. Thus, competence may be achieved by the partial occupancy of critical enhancers, imparting a "ready and waiting" status to precursor cells (Zaret, 1999). At present, it is unclear whether these changes are primary determinants of competence or secondary effects, but such observations nevertheless provide a useful framework.

Conclusions

Prior to gastrulation, certain cells in the epiblast have received cues that predispose them to become endoderm cells. A series of morpho-

Table 14–1. Transcription Factors Involved in Endodermal Development

Gene Class	Role
GATA genes	
Gata factors (*Gata4*)	Broad requirement in the early endoderm, endodermal competence
Gata6	Required for lung endodermal development
HNF genes	
Hnf factors (*Hnf-3β*)	Broad requirement in the early endoderm, endodermal competence
Hnf-4α	Hepatocyte differentiation
bHLH genes	
Hes1	Negatively regulates endocrine; secretory fates in pancreas, gut, lung
ngn3, NeuroD	Downstream of (and repressed by) Hes1, "proendocrine" genes
p48	Pancreatic exocrine differentiation
Homeobox genes	
Hex, Prox1	Hepatoblast migration into septum transversum mesenchyme
Hlx	Expression in septum transversum mesenchyme promotes liver development, required for gut elongation and looping
Hlxb9	Dorsal pancreatic bud formation
Isl1	Dorsal pancreatic bud formation and endocrine cell development
Nkx2.1	Tracheoesophageal septation
Nkx2.2	Pancreatic alpha-, beta-, and PP-cell differentiation
Nkx6.1	Pancreatic beta-cell differentiation
Pax4	Pancreatic beta- and delta-cell differentiation
Pax6	Pancreatic alpha-cell differentiation
Pdx1	Dorsal and ventral pancreatic buds, insulin expression

HNF, hepatocyte nuclear factor; bHLH, basic helix-loop-helix; PP, pancreatic polypeptide.

genetic events result in formation of the endoderm germ layer, which then folds on itself to become a tube. The molecular mechanisms controlling endoderm specification are not well understood, but some genes have been identified which are important in the early formation and competence of the endoderm, most notably those encoding HNF and GATA.

PRINCIPLES OF ENDODERMAL PATTERNING

Patterning refers to the stereotyped commitment or specification of cells to certain fates. In the endoderm, patterning results in a series of domains within the primitive gut tube that are predetermined to become the different organs, ensuring that the lung is always anterior to the liver. For early endoderm, the A/P axis is critical as it determines which fate the cells will ultimately adopt.

How is the A/P pattern established? There are two possibilities. Cells may already have an intrinsic (cell-autonomous) identity and know their position by virtue of some genetic identifier. Alternatively, cells may receive signals from adjacent structures (notochord, node, primitive streak) or germ layers (mesoderm, ectoderm) that induce their fate. The details of A/P patterning are not fully understood, but it appears that both mechanisms, intrinsic and inductive, contribute to regionalized identity.

The expression of many genes is regionally restricted along the A/P axis of the endoderm at the end of gastrulation (e.g., *Cerberus*, *Otx1*, and *IFABP*; reviewed in Wells, 1999). Similarly, the endoderm itself has different inductive properties along the A/P axis, as exemplified by the ability of anterior (but not posterior) endoderm to induce cardiac myogenesis (Schultheiss et al., 1995). However, if gastrulation-stage endoderm is recombined with heterologous tissue, the endoderm can be induced to adopt new fates, demonstrating that the endoderm remains plastic to outside influence despite extant functional differences. Thus, the early endoderm can be said to be specified but not committed. This plasticity is short-lived and diminishes soon after gastrulation.

Genetic Control of the Body Plan: *Hox* Genes

The spatial organization of endoderm is precisely regulated. Organs must be correctly oriented relative not only to each other (along the A/P axis) but also to the derivatives of other germ layers, resulting in a coordinated body plan. Theoretically, several mechanisms could regulate the identity and patterning of endoderm cells: (*1*) identity could be "hardwired" (i.e., conferred directly to the endoderm) according to some (genetic) body-plan code; (*2*) identity could be instructed by adjacent tissues (which are themselves prepatterned by a code); or (*3*) it may be achieved through a combination of the two, with reenforcing or modulating crosstalk between adjacent cell layers. Such later signaling interactions between adjacent tissues might ensure that the correct spatial relationships between germ layers have been achieved.

In *Drosophila*, where the genetic mechanism of regionalization is better understood, the endoderm clearly relies on interactions with the mesoderm for patterning. Critical for these interactions are a group of transcription factors containing a homeobox DNA-binding motif encoded by the *Hox* genes (see Chapter 46). In vertebrates, homeobox genes are categorized by their genomic organization. They are divided into four *Hox* clusters (a through d) of up to 13 paralogous genes (e.g., *Hoxa1*, *Hoxb1*, *Hoxd1*, etc.), as well as the so-called dispersed homeobox genes, including those of the ParaHox cluster, consisting of *Pdx1*, *Cdx2*, and *Gsh1*.

In the mesoderm and ectoderm, expression of a subset of these genes confers positional identity. Mis-expression of certain mouse *Hox* genes causes anterior or posterior transformation of axial skeleton and neural tissue, so-called homeotic transformation. *Hox* genes may represent the mechanism by which A/P identity is established in the endoderm as well. This could occur through either direct action of *Hox* genes in endoderm cells or their action in the mesoderm, which in turn could instruct the endoderm (the mechanism apparently used in the developing *Drosophila* gut). Since vertebrate *Hox* genes are expressed in both endoderm and mesoderm, it is impossible to distinguish *a priori* between these models.

Other signals may confer A/P positional identity upon the endoderm, either independent of or through their effects on *Hox* gene expression. The vitamin A derivative retinoic acid (RA) may be such a signal. RA is necessary for patterning in the hindbrain, where it regulates the expression of a number of *Hox* genes (reviewed in Gavalas and Krumlauf, 2000). Although there is no evidence that RA has a role in endoderm patterning, its involvement in ectoderm and mesoderm patterning makes this an area deserving of future study.

What evidence suggests a role for homeobox genes in regionalization of the vertebrate gut? There is widespread and "colinear" expression (i.e., expression which mirrors the genomic organization) of homeobox genes in the developing gut (Yokouchi et al., 1995). In both the endoderm and mesoderm, *Hox* genes (as well as the related paired box [*Pax*] and ParaHox cluster genes) are expressed in overlapping but restricted domains that typically correlate with organ boundaries (Grapin-Botton and Melton, 2000; Beck et al., 2000). Mutations in a number of *Hox* genes result in defective endodermal development, including phenotypes in thyroid (*Hoxa3*) (Manley and Capecchi 1995), lung (*Hoxa5*) (Aubin et al., 1997), esophagus (*Hoxc4*) (Boulet and Capecchi, 1996), and hindgut (*Hoxa13* and *Hoxd4-13*) (Kondo et al., 1996; Warot et al., 1997; Zakany and Duboule, 1999). Furthermore, mutations in a number of "dispersed" homeobox-containing genes, including *Pdx1*, *Nkx2.1*, *Hlx*, and *Hex*, have profound effects on the organogenesis of endoderm derivatives, apparently through their activity in the endoderm (discussed in detail below). For example, mice lacking one copy of the homeobox gene *Cdx2*, which is expressed in the posterior endoderm, develop polyp-like lesions in the colon. These lesions have lost the normal *Cdx2* allele and resemble stomach and small intestinal epithelium, suggesting that *Cdx2* normally directs endoderm to adopt a posterior fate (Beck et al., 1999).

The existence of a homeotic transformation in the endoderm would be the best evidence for a critical role of *Hox* genes in endodermal patterning. However, most attempts to observe such phenotypes have failed, presumably because of the high degree of redundancy between these genes and the difficulty in distinguishing such transformations across large areas of seemingly homogenous gut. Moreover, if a *Hox* prepattern exists within the mesoderm, which is then solely responsible for patterning the endoderm, then *Hox* misexpression might be expected to have no effect unless it is ectopically expressed in the mesoderm.

Such transformations have been seen following *Hox* misexpression in the mesoderm. For example, the misexpression of a posteriorly expressed *Hox* gene (*Hoxd13*) in the embryonic midgut mesoderm causes partial conversion of the underlying endoderm to a hindgut phenotype (Roberts et al., 1998). It has been proposed that the signaling molecule Sonic Hedgehog (*Shh*; see Chapter 16) may mediate this effect as it is expressed in the endoderm and is able to induce expression of certain *Hox* genes in the adjacent mesoderm (Roberts et al., 1995). However, *Shh* is widely expressed in embryonic endoderm, and it is thus not clear how it could regulate *Hox* gene expression in a region-specific manner. A recent study in which a dominant-negative approach was used to inhibit endodermal *Hoxa13* resulted in posterior gut malformations, suggesting that epithelial *Hox* expression is indeed critical (de Santa Barbara and Roberts, 2002).

Conclusions

The spatial regulation of homeobox-containing genes is likely to establish the A/P pattern of the endoderm. *Hox* gene expression may be regulated by other soluble signals, like RA. Positional information may be contained within the endoderm itself, provided by adjacent mesoderm, or both. The formula by which a certain combination of homeobox genes confers positional information and the mechanism by which their expression is regionally restricted remain unknown.

STRUCTURES INVOLVED IN PATTERNING

Whatever organizational role homeobox-containing genes may play in patterning, the process itself is not static. Multiple signals, in particular those received from neighboring cells, are needed to progressively refine developmental progression. Such external signals can be divided into two classes: *permissive* signals, which allow a tissue to progress to a fate that has already been established, and *instructive* signals, which divert a tissue to a new path that would not otherwise have been followed. Historically, such signals have been identified through transplantation studies, in which endoderm is placed adjacent to various embryonic structures and the resulting cell type is determined. Investigators have begun to identify candidates for the active components of these signals.

Complicating these efforts, some signals appear to be *reciprocal*; for example, some endoderm-derived signals act on underlying mesodermal cells, which in turn make signals that affect the endoderm. Moreover, the ability of endoderm to respond to a signal (*competence*) is time-dependent. Thus, signals that may have no effect on a 7.5-day-old embryo (*gastrulation stage*) may be able to induce organ differentiation in its competent counterpart a day later (*somite stage*). Finally, the ability to conclude that a given fate has been established depends on how cell fate is defined: tissue differentiation can be evaluated by looking for markers of cytodifferentiation (by mRNA identification or immunohistochemistry) or by characteristic morphogenetic changes. This is significant because experimental manipulations may result in cytodifferentiation that is not always in agreement with the expected morphogenetic change.

Signals from Other Germ Layers

It has long been appreciated that patterning is normally influenced by interactions between mesoderm derivatives (mesenchyme) and endoderm (Le Douarin, 1975; Haffen et al., 1989). Nevertheless, there are cases in which the endodermal differentiation program does not appear to be under mesodermal control (Hayashi et al., 1988; Duluc et al., 1994). Both instructive and permissive signals contribute to patterning. Among the earliest instructive signals appear to come from adjacent germ layers. For example, culture of gastrulation-stage anterior endoderm with posterior mesoderm/ectoderm can induce posterior endoderm markers; conversely, anterior mesoderm/ectoderm grafts induce posterior endoderm markers (Wells and Melton, 2000). Although there is evidence for an early prepattern in both endoderm and mesoderm, it is clear that the two layers slide relative to each other during growth of the gut tube, causing loss of contact between tissues that were initially adjacent to each other (Rawdon, 2001). Thus, the mechanism of epithelial–mesenchymal interactions that induces or refines endoderm fate must take into account the dynamic nature of the relationship between these two layers, and experiments that identify inductive signals between germ layers must be interpreted in this context.

The epithelial–mesenchymal interactions in the developing chick stomach represent one of the best-studied examples of induction. The stomach consists of the anterior proventriculus and the posterior gizzard. The proventriculus has a predominantly chemical digestive role and is characterized by a glandular epithelium that secretes pepsinogen. The gizzard is involved in crushing and separating food and is consequently surrounded by a thick muscular layer. Conventional recombination experiments have assessed the ability of heterologous mesoderm to induce endoderm fates along the A/P axis. These studies have revealed that anterior endoderm can express pepsinogen when recombined with proventricular mesenchyme (Takiguchi et al., 1986). Similarly, coculture of gizzard endoderm with small intestine mesoderm causes the endoderm to become small intestine-like (reviewed in Rawdon, 2001).

Thus, in many instances, endoderm fate is determined by the identity of the mesenchyme. However, there are caveats. First, the inductive activity of mesenchyme is under spatial regulation. In contrast to its activity on anterior endoderm, proventriculus mesenchyme cannot induce pepsinogen when recombined with posterior (small intestine or allantois) endoderm (Hayashi et al., 1988). This suggests that anterior endoderm retains its competence to respond to mesodermal cues longer than posterior endoderm. Second, the observation that the endodermal and mesodermal cell layers move dramatically relative to each other during development makes the interpretation of recombination studies more complicated. Finally, the results of such recombination studies can vary depending on whether cytodifferentiation or morphogenesis is being assayed.

Signals from Adjacent Structures

Development of the postgastrulation embryo is dynamic; thus, mesoderm that appears homogenous on day 7 of mouse embryogenesis has begun to differentiate or condense into distinct structures a day or two later (see Chapter 5). These structures include somites, cardiac mesoderm, septum transversum mesoderm, notochord, and blood vessels. Signals continue to be released and received after these primitive morphological changes have taken place, allowing better definition of the regional origins of these signals. While many of these mesodermal derivatives influence adjacent endoderm, the signals in most cases appear to be permissive, allowing implementation of a pattern that has already been established. The absence of these permissive signals can lead to profound disruption of the endodermal pattern.

Cardiac Mesoderm

As the AIP forms, the ventral anterior endoderm begins to fold back on itself in an anterior-to-posterior direction (Fig. 14–1*B*). Adjacent to this ventral foregut endoderm is the newly formed cardiac mesoderm (see Chapter 9), which plays a role in the specification of the underlying endoderm into liver. Studies performed over two decades ago showed that somite-stage ventral endoderm transplanted into posterior mesenchyme fails to stain for liver glycogen unless it is grafted along with cardiac mesoderm (LeDouarin, 1975). Other grafting studies demonstrated the dynamic nature of endodermal competence and commitment. For example, while early (4–6 somites) somite-stage ventral endoderm exhibits plasticity with respect to signals from cardiac mesoderm, the endoderm becomes committed to its fate a short time (less than a day) later (7–8 somites) (LeDouarin, 1964, cited in Gualdi et al., 1996).

Although these classic experiments defined the space and time during which liver specification occurs, recent experiments have called into question the basic assumption that liver specification is wholly dependent on signals from the cardiac mesoderm. Relying on an in vitro coculture system and a reverse transcription PCR assay for albumin (as a marker for liver specification), Gualdi et al. (1996) showed that cardiac mesoderm promotes liver fate through a nondiffusible factor. Surprisingly, and in contrast to previous transplantation studies, *dorsal* endoderm was capable of turning on albumin simply when removed from its surrounding mesenchyme. The discrepancy of these results with older experiments may stem from the greater sensitivity of PCR for albumin mRNA compared to staining histological sections for glycogen (highlighting again how the differentiation assay may influence the experimental interpretation). Caution must be exercised in accepting this interpretation, however, since glycogen may represent a more specific and reliable marker of liver differentiation than albumin.

If the detection of albumin truly represents liver induction, the results raise the possibility that a substantial portion of endoderm has hepatic potential and that signals from adjacent mesenchyme are capable of *either* restricting (in the case of dorsal mesoderm) or permitting (in the case of cardiac mesoderm) this competence. More generally, mesenchyme may instruct cell fate by repressing "default" states within the endoderm.

Further studies of the interaction between cardiac mesoderm and ventral endoderm have led to other surprising conclusions. The prehepatic endoderm in contact with the cardiac mesoderm is adjacent to the "leading edge" of the AIP; this leading edge forms a lip of endoderm that is fated to become the ventral pancreas. Deutsch et al. (2001) hypothesized that these adjacent regions of endoderm share the potential to become liver or pancreas and that it is only because this lip fails to contact the cardiac mesoderm that it adopts a pancreatic fate. Supporting this model, ventral endoderm isolated from early somite-stage embryos expresses a number of pancreatic markers, while coculture of this endoderm with cardiac mesoderm results in reduction or elimination of the expression of pancreatic markers. By contrast, isolated anterior dorsal endoderm does not express pancreatic markers but does express albumin when its adjacent mesenchyme is removed (as discussed above).

Taken together, these studies support a model in which different segments of the endoderm have intrinsic fates that are reprogrammed by mesenchyme. According to this model, such defaults (a pancreatic fate for ventral endoderm and a hepatic fate for dorsal endoderm) are imposed early in patterning (by *Hox* gene regulation or other unknown signals). The role of the mesenchyme is then to respecify the endoderm to the "appropriate" fate. Thus, ventral endoderm may be reprogrammed by cardiac mesoderm to become liver, while dorsal endoderm may be reprogrammed by dorsal mesenchyme to become gut. Although this model does not account for the specification of all endoderm derivatives, such mesodermal repressive activity could be the mechanism by which intestinal fate is specified. In particular, dorsal mesoderm can exert a repressive effect on prehepatic ventral endoderm, preventing ventral endoderm/cardiac mesoderm cocultures from expressing albumin (Bossard and Zaret, 2000). Thus, a repressive mechanism may be used to ensure that nonintestinal fates are limited to particular domains of the endoderm and that an intestinal default program results in all other regions. This model does not, of course, explain how the pattern is established in the first place.

Notochord

Three pieces of evidence suggest that the notochord could be involved in endoderm patterning. First, the notochord forms during gastrulation in close approximation with the endoderm, a contact that persists well into the mid-somite-stage embryo (e8 in mice). Second, there is a wealth of evidence that the notochord contributes to D/V patterning in the neural tube and medial/lateral patterning of the somites, making it an obvious candidate source of endodermal patterning signals as well. Third, patients with apparent notochord developmental defects exhibit not only vertebral abnormalities but also gastrointestinal malformations (Elliott et al., 1970).

The pancreas has both ventral and dorsal components, which arise from well-separated regions of the endoderm (Fig. 14–1C). Accumulated evidence, including the apparent differences described in the previous section, makes it likely that the dorsal and ventral pancreatic lobes are specified by different mechanisms. Specification of the dorsal pancreas in mouse occurs prior to the 13-somite stage, a period when the prepancreatic endoderm is in close contact with the notochord (Wessels and Cohen, 1967). Significantly, a series of in vivo dissection and in vitro reassociation experiments demonstrated that signals from the notochord are necessary and sufficient for prepancreatic endoderm to express pancreatic genes (Kim et al., 1997). Notochord cannot induce nonpancreatic endoderm to express pancreatic genes; thus, the notochord signals that specify pancreas are permissive rather than instructive. However, regionalized expression of a number of genes along the A/P axis of the notochord raises the possibility that the notochord itself participates in A/P patterning of the endoderm. Such genes include members of the *Tgf* and *Bmp* families as well as segmental expression of *Hox* genes (reviewed in Cleaver and Krieg, 2001).

Blood Vessels

Shortly before the first signs of pancreatic budding, the notochord becomes separated from the early dorsal endoderm by the medial movement and fusion of the dorsal aortae into a single midline structure (~e8.5–9 in mouse). Other blood vessels begin to form elsewhere in the embryo shortly before organ morphogenesis begins. Two recent studies suggest that blood vessels (see Chapter 9) have a role in endodermal patterning.

Lammert et al. (2001) studied the role of blood vessels (and their endothelial cell constituents) in pancreatic specification and growth. Blood vessels are found in contact with prepancreatic endoderm just prior to budding (e9 in the mouse), adjacent to the aorta dorsally and to the vitelline veins ventrally. When dorsal endoderm is cocultured in vitro with aorta (or other endothelium-containing tissues), the resulting endoderm expands and gives rise to cells expressing the pancreas-specific gene insulin. Conversely, careful dissection of aortic precursor cells in vivo results in loss of cells expressing pancreatic markers, with no effect on other structures, including gut, notochord, and neural tube. The creation of extra blood vessels outside of the pancreatic domain induced by ectopic expression of vascular endothelial growth factor results in the formation of ectopic insulin-producing cells.

Matsumoto et al. (2001) used *flk-1* mutant mice, which are incapable of forming mature endothelial cells or blood vessels, to address the role of blood vessels in hepatogenesis. Although there are no large blood vessels in contact with the prehepatic endoderm, the adjacent septum transversum mesenchyme is rich with endothelial cells when budding begins (e9–9.5 in the mouse). In *flk-1* mutant animals, a number of liver markers (albumin, *Hex*) are expressed where the hepatic bud would normally form, but the endoderm fails to expand into a nascent liver.

Thus, endothelial cells and blood vessels appear to have at least two activities in endodermal development. In the pancreas, blood vessels are required for endoderm to become pancreas; without an aorta, pancreas is not specified, while ectopic blood vessels can induce pancreas formation. In the liver, by contrast, hepatic specification occurs in the absence of mature endothelial cells, but outgrowth and expansion of the endoderm into the liver is defective.

Conclusions

Signals from mesoderm-derived tissues (mesenchyme) influence endodermal fate along the A/P axis as early as gastrulation. As development proceeds, mesenchymal condensation results in defined structures that specify the domains that will give rise to organs. These mesenchymal effects may be inductive, permissive, or restrictive. The most important of these mesenchymal structures involved in the specification of the liver and pancreas are the cardiac mesoderm, notochord, and blood vessels/endothelial cells. Little is known about the specification of the prepulmonary endoderm.

THE MOLECULAR BASIS OF PATTERNING

Molecules Involved in Patterning

Fibroblast Growth Factors

There are 22 members of the FGF family (see Chapter 32) and four FGF receptors. FGFs and their receptors are subject to tissue-specific regulation of splicing; thus, the number of functionally important FGF variants may be much higher (Ornitz and Itoh, 2001). Different receptors have different signaling properties, and ligand-binding specificity is conferred by several factors, including splice variation and interactions with heparin sulfate proteoglycans (Ornitz et al., 1996). Thus, the repertoire of potential FGF signaling combinations is complex, with the prospect of substantial tissue and temporal-specific regulation.

The earliest role postulated for an FGF is that of FGF4, which is expressed in the primitive streak and required for postimplantation development of the embryo (Feldman et al., 1995). FGF4 is one of a small number of FGFs known to be expressed in the gastrulation-stage embryo. It is unique in its ability to induce isolated streak-stage endoderm to express posterior markers in a concentration-dependent manner, suggesting that it is one of the signals that instructs posterior endoderm (Wells and Melton, 2000).

There is evidence that FGFs constitute at least part of the cardiac mesoderm signal that specifies anterior ventral endoderm as liver. Several FGFs are expressed in the cardiac mesoderm of the mouse when endodermal specification occurs, including FGFs1, 2, and 8. Addition of FGFs1, 2, or 8b to isolated ventral endoderm in vitro induces albumin, suggesting that one or all of these FGFs contribute to hepatic specification and that they may be the active factors by which cardiac mesoderm specifies liver. Consistent with this possibility, addition of soluble (inhibitory) FGF receptors can partially block the normal induction of liver markers that occurs when ventral endoderm is cocultured with cardiac mesoderm (Jung et al., 1999).

Consistent with a "bipotential" model of ventral endodermal fate, ventral endodermal explants, which would normally express the pancreatic marker *Pdx1* in the absence of mesenchyme, turn off *Pdx1* and express albumin in the presence of FGF2 (Deutsch et al., 2001). By contrast, dorsal endoderm cocultured with FGF2 expresses pancreatic markers (*Pdx1* and insulin), highlighting the regional differences that constitute the competence of endoderm (Hebrok et al., 1998). More recent studies suggest that BMPs expressed by the septum transversum mesenchyme act in concert with cardiac mesoderm FGFs in hepatic specification (Rossi et al., 2001; discussed in more detail below).

While FGF signals may mediate some of the hepatic/pancreatic specification program, a detailed understanding of FGF function is lacking. Determining which particular ligands and receptors are active in vivo will be difficult. Each of the FGFs mentioned in this section can bind multiple receptor isoforms, and FGF expression in the embryo has been only partially characterized. Only a few of the *Fgf* genes knocked out so far are absolutely required for development prior to organogenesis (*Fgf4*, *Fgf8*, and *Fgf15*) (Ornitz and Itoh, 2001). The role of other FGFs in pancreatic and lung organogenesis, which is better understood, will be discussed in greater detail below.

Sonic Hedgehog

The HHs are a family of extracellular signaling molecules (see Chapter 16) that mediate patterning in a variety of embryonic contexts. There are three mammalian HHs, Indian, Sonic, and Desert, all of which bind to the receptor Patched 1 (PTC1). *Shh* represents a good candidate mediator of endodermal patterning because it is expressed during the initial formation of the gut, specifically in the endoderm of the AIP and CIP. Studies now suggest that *Shh* is involved in at least two processes in endodermal patterning: specification of the pancreas and regionalization of the gut.

Shh is expressed widely in the endoderm, with the striking exception of the prepancreatic regions (both dorsal and ventral), where it is specifically excluded. Notochord signals are required for specification of the dorsal pancreas, and it was hypothesized that notochord signals are responsible for regulating *Shh* expression and pancreatic induction. Indeed, dissection of the notochord away from the dorsal (prepancreatic) endoderm allows *Shh* expression, while grafting of the notochord to ventral endoderm results in downregulation of *Shh* at this ectopic site, demonstrating that the notochord directly regulates *Shh* expression (Hebrok et al., 1998). Grafting of other mesodermal structures (e.g., somites) has no effect on *Shh* expression. Two signaling molecules expressed by the notochord, FGF2 and activin-βB (a member of the TGF-β family), are each able to produce the downregulation of *Shh* when cultured with isolated dorsal endoderm. By contrast, coculture of ventral endoderm with FGF2 induces *Shh* and the subsequent expression of hepatic markers (Deutsch et al., 2001), implying that FGF2 is not the only signal to specify pancreas.

SHH activity can be inhibited with blocking antibodies or cyclopamine, a steroid alkaloid. Treatment of prepancreatic endoderm with blocking antibodies against SHH results in the expression of *Pdx1* and insulin to the same extent as coculture with notochord (Hebrok et al., 1998), and treatment of embryos with cyclopamine results in ectopic pancreas formation (Kim and Melton, 1998). These results suggest that inhibition of dorsal endoderm *Shh* is sufficient for pancreatic differentiation. Evidence that such down-regulation is also necessary comes from studies in which addition of recombinant SHH to ventral endoderm results in the absence of the expected pancreatic fate (Deutsch et al., 2001).

Downregulation of *Shh* appears to be a critical step in the formation of both the dorsal and ventral pancreas. While the notochord mediates this effect dorsally, the source of the *Shh*-repression signal in the ventral endoderm is unknown. Also unknown are the signals that become active or inactive as a result of *Shh* repression. The *Ptc1* receptor is expressed in both the endoderm and mesenchyme of the pancreatic anlagen (Hebrok et al., 1998); and while disruption of the *Shh* gene has no effect on pancreas specification, disruption of *Ptc1* results in loss of pancreatic markers (Hebrok et al., 2000). The intriguing possibility that SHH activity must be suppressed in the endoderm, rather than the mesenchyme, was suggested by the finding that isolated endoderm can express *Pdx1* when incubated with anti-SHH blocking antibodies (Hebrok et al., 1998).

Finally, there is the possibility that *Shh* contributes more generally to patterning of the endoderm. Ectopic expression of *Shh* in the hindgut induces *Hoxd13* expression (Roberts et al., 1995), and ectopic expression of *Hoxd13* in midgut mesoderm results in a partial transformation of the midgut endoderm to a hindgut phenotype (Roberts et

al., 1998). It is therefore tempting to speculate that *Shh* normally acts on the hindgut mesoderm to induce *Hoxd13*. However, *Shh* expression eventually spreads to include the entire endoderm, and it is therefore not clear how such induction would be regionalized. Moreover, *Shh* mutants appear to have normal regional expression of some of the posterior *Hox* genes, including *Hoxd13* (Ramalho-Santos et al., 2000).

Bone Morphogenetic Proteins

The BMPs are members of the TGF-β family of secreted proteins (see Chapter 24). Their potential relevance to *Shh* and gut development was first suggested by parallels to *Drosophila*, in which the BMP ortholog *decapentaplegic* (*dpp*) lies downstream of *hh* and is necessary for midgut patterning.

At least three BMPs are expressed in the developing mouse gut mesenchyme: BMPs2, 4, and 7. Inactivation of *Bmp2* results in death prior to e10.5, with associated amnion/chorion and heart malformation; mutants have not been extensively examined for gut defects (Zhang and Bradley, 1996). *Bmp4* is required for early mesodermal differentiation and closure of the ventral mesoderm; null mutants die between e6.5 and e9.5 of mouse development (Winnier et al., 1995). *Bmp7* is required for kidney and eye development (Luo et al., 1995; Dudley et al., 1995).

Recent studies provide strong evidence that BMPs are critical for specification and development of the liver. We have already seen that FGFs secreted by the cardiac mesoderm help specify anterior ventral endoderm to become liver. If, however, anterior endoderm/cardiac mesoderm explants are exposed to the BMP inhibitor Noggin, induction of liver markers is blocked, suggesting that BMP signals are also necessary for liver specification (Rossi et al., 2001). *Bmp4* is expressed in the septum transversum; and through careful examination of ventral endoderm isolates, "contaminating" levels of *Bmp4* could be detected. Thus, in retrospect, it appears that septum transversum cells, which are difficult to remove from endoderm explants, were likely still present in previous studies of cardiac mesoderm and hepatic specification. These observations raise general questions about the interpretation of ex vivo recombination studies of induction. Despite these cautionary implications, the study of Rossi et al. (2001) provides evidence that BMPs (expressed by the septum transversum) act together with FGFs (expressed by the cardiac mesoderm) to specify hepatic fate.

BMP/SHH Crosstalk.
There is further evidence for the involvement of BMPs in the regional specification of the gut, a process that occurs somewhat later than specification of the lung, liver, and pancreas. The chick stomach, consisting of its glandular proventriculus and muscular gizzard, has already been described as a paradigm of epithelial–mesenchymal signaling; and some studies suggest that BMP signals may control specification in the chick stomach.

Bmp2 is expressed exclusively in the proventriculus mesenchyme of the glandular proventriculus. Inhibition of BMP signals with Noggin abrogates gland formation (Narita et al., 2000), suggesting that mesenchymal BMPs are necessary to specify proventriculus. Overexpression studies have shown that ectopically expressed *Bmp2* enhances gland formation in the proventriculus, while ectopically expressed *Bmp4* in the gizzard causes smooth muscle thinning (Roberts et al., 1998; Smith et al., 2000). Taken together, these studies suggest that BMPs have two proventriculus-promoting activities: enhancement of gland formation and inhibition of muscle growth. The observation that *Bmp2* is incapable of causing gland formation in the gizzard (Narita et al., 2000) suggests that regionalization of the chick stomach may be achieved through spatially restricted responsiveness to BMP signals.

It has been proposed that *Shh* regulates the spatial expression of *Bmp* family members. *Shh* is expressed in the leading edges of AIP and CIP endoderm during gut tube formation and induces *Bmp4*. However, *Shh* cannot induce *Bmp4* in the gizzard, which may permit this part of the gut to develop its thick muscular layer (Roberts et al., 1995, 1998). Such a simple model of gut specification is likely to be incomplete, however, as *Shh* mutant mice have thinning of intestinal smooth muscle, the opposite of what would be expected if an *Shh* → *Bmp4* signal acts to negatively regulate gut smooth muscle (Ramalho-Santos et al., 2000).

Sphincters

Sphincters demarcate different regions of the gut and regulate passage of intestinal contents. Homeodomain-containing genes are involved in sphincter formation; for example, mutant mice in which both the *Hoxa13* and *Hoxd13* genes have been inactivated develop defective anal sphincters (Warot et al., 1997). Similarly, mutant mice with a deletion of *Hoxd4-d13* are unable to form an ileocecal valve, the sphincter-like structure found at the border of small and large intestine (Zakany and Duboule, 1999). Might spatial regulation of BMP signals participate in the formation of sphincters, just as they appear to regulate the formation of the proventriculus–gizzard boundary?

Shh is incapable of inducing *Bmp4* at the junction of the small intestine and stomach, a boundary that corresponds to the pyloric sphincter in the adult. The homeobox gene *Nkx2.5* is a specific marker of the pyloric sphincter and is both necessary and sufficient to induce endoderm to become pyloric epithelium (Smith et al., 2000). Ectopic expression of *Bmp4* in the gizzard induces *Nkx2.5* and conversion to a pyloric sphincter-like endoderm, while inhibition of BMP signaling with Noggin leads to downregulation of *Nkx2.5* (Smith and Tabin, 1999). Thus, BMP signaling seems important for pyloric sphincter specification. Other homeobox genes may be involved in the organization of sphincter boundaries. For example, inactivation of the mouse *Pdx1* gene, which is required for pancreatic development and expressed in a region including the distal stomach and proximal duodenum, results in a shrunken and misshapen pyloric sphincter (Offield et al., 1996).

Conclusions

The identification of the mesenchymal structures that participate in endodermal regionalization has made it possible to ask what specific signals mediate such specification. Crosstalk between a number of signaling molecules (FGFs, BMPs, and HH) contributes to the correct organization of gut structures through epithelial–mesenchymal interactions and regulation of homeobox gene expression. While some of the most important signaling molecules have been identified, a comprehensive model of signal integration during endodermal development is currently lacking. Further characterization of the spatial regulation of soluble signals, and their crosstalk, may make it possible in the future to apply a "network approach" to endodermal regionalization.

ORGANOGENESIS AND MORPHOGENESIS

Following establishment of an A/P axis and midline tube, specific portions of the endoderm form buds and expand into the surrounding mesenchyme, giving rise to the anlagen of lung, liver, and pancreas. This process of organogenesis can be thought of as having two components: (*1*) disruption of the two-dimensional epithelial plane (bud initiation) and (*2*) subsequent growth and movement of epithelium and mesenchyme (morphogenesis). The same molecular pathways are used

repeatedly in different contexts to achieve a particular pattern. Factors from the same families we have already discussed (homeobox-containing genes, FGFs, BMPs, and Shh) play roles in the organogenesis of all of the endoderm-derived organs. What distinguishes these pathways in different organs is the exact identity of each involved family member and its spatial and temporal expression (Table 14–2).

Lung

The molecular specification of prepulmonary endoderm is poorly understood. By contrast, the subsequent outgrowth of lung epithelium (so-called branching morphogenesis) has been better studied. The first lung buds form at approximately e9.5 of mouse development, after the liver and around the same time as the pancreas. Two coordinated activities participate in the formation of the primitive lung. In one step, a newly formed septum divides the foregut into two tubes, the dorsal esophagus and the ventral trachea. In parallel, two small primary buds arise from the ventrolateral wall of the tracheal primordium and give rise to the main bronchi. Different molecular mechanisms regulate formation of the tracheoesophageal septum and initiation of budding. Genes involved in both of these processes have been identified.

Clues about the genetic control of mammalian lung bud formation came from studies of the *Drosophila* respiratory system, demonstrating a central role for FGF signals (reviewed in Metzger and Krasnow, 1999). Initially, two basic helix-loop-helix (bHLH) proteins, *trachealess* and *tango*, drive the formation of small bud-like "sacs." The vertebrate counterparts of these genes, if they exist, are unknown. Subsequently, an FGF receptor ortholog (*breathless*) is expressed in the sac epithelium and receives precisely regulated signals from an FGF-like protein (*branchless*) that result in outgrowth of the primary branches. Additional genes modulate the Branchless–Breathless signal by restricting the area over which the ligand is active.

Trachea Formation

In mouse lung development, foregut septation and trachea formation require the homeobox-containing gene *Nkx2.1* (also called *TTF-1* or *T/ebp*). *Nkx2.1* expression in the anterior endoderm is limited to the small number of anterior foregut cells that will give rise to the trachea, and mutant mice lacking *Nkx2.1* fail to form a septum and, hence, have no trachea (Minoo et al., 1999). Despite the absence of a trachea, lung development (budding and branching) proceeds in mutant mice, although the lungs are hypoplastic and morphologically disorganized.

Septation also requires signals from endodermally derived *Shh* as embryos with homozygous mutations in *Shh* fail to form the septum between esophagus and trachea (Litingtung et al., 1998; Pepicelli et al., 1998). The trachea also fails to form in mice with mutations in the *Shh* target genes *Gli2* and *Gli3*. As will be discussed below, *Shh* assumes additional roles during primary bud formation and subsequent branching morphogenesis.

Primary Bud Induction

Mammalian regulation of lung bud induction resembles that of *Drosophila*; most notably, initiation of lung budding involves FGF fam-

Table 14–2. Soluble Signals Involved in Endodermal Development, Grouped by Organ

Tissue	Signals	Comments
Lung	*Fgf10*	Outgrowth of expanding lung buds
	Shh	Modulates responsiveness to *Fgf10* during branching morphogenesis (along with *Bmp4*, TGF-β1, *Sprouty*)
	Bmp4	Proximal-distal differentiation of the lung
	Notch	Pulmonary neuroendocrine cell differentiation
Liver	*Fgfs*	Cardiac mesoderm FGFs (1, 2, and/or 8) specify prehepatic endoderm, promote liver bud outgrowth
	Bmps	Septum transversum BMPs act with FGFs to specify prehepatic endoderm, also promote outgrowth
	Hgf/c-Met	Promote hepatoblast growth, inhibit apoptosis (may also involve *Sek1*, c-*Jun*, N-*myc*, and TNF)
Pancreas	*Shh*	Repression required to specify prepancreatic endoderm, maintenance of repression required for morphogenesis
	Fgf10	Outgrowth of pancreatic epithelium
	Notch	Exocrine/endocrine cell fate decisions
	TGF-β	Exocrine/endocrine cell fate decisions
Gut	*Shh*, *Bmps*	Crosstalk involved in intestinal patterning, *Shh* regulates gut radial axis

FGF, fibroblast growth factor; Shh, sonic hedgehog; BMP, bone morphogenetic protein; TNF, tumor necrosis factor; TGF, transforming growth factor.

ily members. FGF10 is the most important of these signals so far identified; it is locally expressed in the mesenchyme at the sites where primary lung buds will form, and its predominant receptor (*Fgfr2*) is expressed in the adjacent endoderm. Mice with mutations in *Fgf10* have a block in lung development prior to budding, although formation of the trachea proceeds normally (Min et al., 1998). A similar phenotype is seen when the *Fgfr2* receptor is disrupted through gene targeting or overexpression of a dominant-negative receptor, demonstrating that FGF10–FGFR2 signals are necessary for budding. Such signals are likely to mediate primary bud formation as well as subsequent secondary and tertiary bud formation during branching morphogenesis.

The question of whether *Fgf10* is sufficient to induce primary buds is more complicated. When distal lung endoderm is cultured with FGF10 in the absence of adjacent mesoderm, the outgrowth of bud-like structures is observed (Bellusci et al., 1997b). However, the placement of FGF10-coated beads adjacent to tracheal or proximal lung explants (containing endoderm in association with its underlying mesenchyme) does not result in ectopic budding (Park et al., 1998). These results imply that responsiveness to FGF10 is spatially and temporally regulated in the lung and that proximal lung mesenchyme may contain signals that inhibit FGF10-induced budding. Thus, while *Fgf10* is both necessary and sufficient for lung bud initiation *in vitro*, its activity *in vivo* is subject to more complex regulation.

HH signals are involved in all steps of lung development, including primary lung bud induction. The *Gli2* and *Gli3* zinc finger transcription factors, which lie downstream of *Shh*, are necessary for early lung development. Mice missing both copies of *Gli2* have foregut abnormalities, while superimposed mutations in *Gli3* result in profound (dose-dependent) lung defects. Specifically, *Gli2* null mutants lacking one copy of *Gli3* ($Gli2^{-/-}\ Gli3^{+/-}$ animals) have delayed lung budding and additional foregut defects (including esophageal atresia and tracheoesophageal fistula), while double-null mutants ($Gli2^{-/-}$, $Gli3^{-/-}$) fail to form any recognizable lung, trachea, or esophagus (Motoyama et al., 1998).

Branching Morphogenesis

Following trachea formation and primary bud initiation, the bud epithelium expands and branches into a tree-like structure. The position of secondary branch points is tightly regulated by pulmonary mesenchyme. It is believed that FGF10 is the major signal for all branching, and two models have emerged which explain how the formation of secondary and tertiary buds might be spatially regulated (Hogan, 1999). The first model proposes that *Fgf10* is expressed by mesenchymal cells whose location along the primary bud axis has been genetically "hardwired." The second model proposes that inhibitory signals generated by the epithelial cells at the distal tip of an advancing bud might inhibit *Fgf10*. The expanding distal tip would be halted by these inhibitors; thus, budding and outgrowth would shift to more proximal sites along the bud (Fig. 14–2).

These models are not mutually exclusive. A genetically determined signal might control the site of primary bud initiation, while a more dynamic interaction between mesenchymal and epithelial factors might control the position of secondary and tertiary buds (Hogan, 1999). Such an inductive–inhibitory network is utilized by *Drosophila*, in which the genes *pointed* and *sprouty* induce or inhibit secondary branching. Several vertebrate inhibitory factors have been identified that could modulate *Fgf10* activity in an analogous way.

One apparent branching regulator is *Shh*. The protein is expressed at highest levels in distal tip cells, where it appears to restrict mesenchymal expression of *Fgf10*. Transgenic mice overexpressing *Shh* in the lungs have an expanded mesenchymal component and a reduction of *Fgf10* expression (Bellusci et al., 1997a,b). Conversely, the normally restricted expression pattern of *Fgf10* is dramatically expanded in *Shh* null mutant mice (Pepicelli et al., 1998). Although *Shh* appears to regulate FGF10 levels, FGF10 does not regulate *Shh*; thus, some other factor(s) must induce *Shh* in the distal tips.

Other candidate regulators of *Fgf10* include the TGF-β family members *Bmp4* and *TGF-β1* itself. *Bmp4* is one of three *Bmp* genes expressed in the embryonic lung, and mice lacking *Bmp4* die prior to lung organogenesis (Winnier et al., 1995). In contrast to other endo-

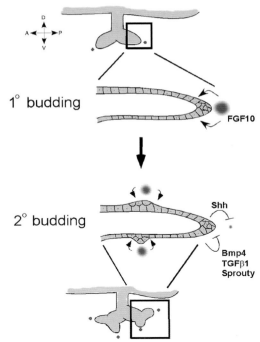

Figure 14–2. Epithelial–mesenchymal signals during branching morphogenesis in the lung. (*Top*) Primary lung buds sprouting from the endoderm (yellow) at the sites of mesenchymal FGF10 expression (red). After a period of growth, signals are induced that have a negative effect on the mitogenic activity of FGF10; these signals include SHH, BMP4, TGF-β1, and Sprouty. Negative regulators arrest growth of the distal tip, and new foci of FGF10 expression emerge and induce secondary budding (*bottom*). FGF, Fibroblast growth factor; Shh, sonic hedgehog; Bmp, bone morphogenetic protein; TGF, transforming growth factor.

derm derivatives, lung expression of *Bmp4* is predominantly epithelial. *Bmp4* is induced in distal tip cells by *Fgf10*. Its expression follows budding; thus, it does not appear to be required for bud formation (Weaver et al., 2000). Transgenic misexpression of *Bmp4* in mice causes lungs to be smaller, with fewer terminal buds and an expanded mesenchyme (Bellusci et al., 1996). Moreover, addition of purified BMP4 to lung endoderm cultures inhibits FGF10-induced budding, while addition of the BMP inhibitor Noggin enhances budding (Weaver et al., 2000). These studies suggest that BMP4 is induced by FGF10, resulting in arrest of the expansion of the distal tip and selection of other sites for budding and outgrowth. *TGF-β1* has similar inhibitory activities, but it is expressed in the mesenchyme. Overexpression of a dominant-negative TGF-β receptor in organ cultures stimulates branching, while addition of recombinant TGF-β1 to similar cultures inhibits branching (reviewed in Cardoso, 2001).

In *Drosophila*, the membrane-associated Sprouty protein is a major regulator of branching. It is induced by Breathless (the FGF receptor ortholog) and limits the number of branches formed. Four mouse (and three human) orthologs of *sprouty* have been identified. Mouse *Sprouty2* expression is regulated by FGF10, and it is found in an expression pattern similar to that of *Shh* and *Bmp4*, with highest levels in the distal epithelial buds. Misexpression of *Sprouty2* results in reduced branching (Mailleux et al., 2001), while inhibition using antisense oligonucleotides stimulates branching in culture (Tefft et al., 1999). Two other *sprouty* orthologs, 1 and 4, are also expressed in pulmonary endoderm (Zhang et al., 2001), but their role in branching morphogenesis has yet to be studied. Thus, a regulatory loop in which an FGF binding to its receptor simultaneously induces both branching and inhibitors of branching is conserved from flies to mice.

It is not clear how the inductive activity of the pulmonary mesenchyme (i.e., *Fgf10*) is regulated. One candidate regulatory gene is *Hoxa5*, which is expressed exclusively in the mesenchyme. *Hoxa5* mutant mice have reduced and disorganized branching, presumably as a result of defective mesenchyme (Aubin et al., 1997). Other evidence supports a role for RA receptors. Specifically, RA signals are down-regulated during branching morphogenesis, and treatment of lung explants with exogenous RA disrupts the budding pattern and alters the expression of *Fgf10* and *Bmp4*, suggesting that inhibition of RA signals is required before distal budding can occur (Malpel et al., 2000).

While FGF10 appears to be the major family member to regulate budding, it is possible that other distinct FGFs are induced by FGF10 in the epithelium. These epithelial FGFs could then relay a feedback signal to the mesenchyme, as occurs during limb development (Martin, 1998). Genetic evidence for such a regulatory loop comes from studies of *Fgf9*, which is expressed early in lung epithelium. Targeted inactivation of *Fgf9* causes reduced pulmonary mesenchyme and decreased branching (Colvin et al., 2001). Thus, reciprocal signaling between FGFs in the mesenchyme (FGF10) and epithelium (FGF9) may regulate lung size and branching.

Additional Pathways

Other genes required for the initial stages of lung development include those that control left–right asymmetry. Vertebrates have more lobes in the right lung than in the left, and many of the genes known to specify left–right asymmetry in the embryo are expressed prior to the initiation of lung budding. One of these, the winged-helix *hfh-4* gene, regulates not only left–right asymmetry but also the development of ciliated cells, possibly through the regulation of dynein genes (Chen et al., 1998).

Finally, early lung development requires GATA-6, a transcription factor necessary in the pre-implantation embryo. *Gata-6* expression is found in primitive pulmonary endoderm, and *Gata-6⁻/⁻* embryonic stem cells are unable to contribute to the pulmonary epithelium of chimeric mice (Morrisey et al. 1998). Further chimeric analysis has demonstrated that *Gata-6* activity is required within epithelial cells and that GATA-6 function is necessary for branching (Keijzer et al., 2001).

Liver

Liver budding and outgrowth require signals similar to those used during lung development: homeobox genes, FGFs, and BMPs. Liver budding begins with the thickening of endodermal cells adjacent to the cardiac mesoderm, which together with septum transversum mesenchyme specifies the hepatic fate (discussed above). As the cardiac mesoderm moves anteriorly, cells of the nascent liver bud grow into the underlying septum transversum mesenchyme (Fig. 14–1*B*), giving rise to a complex network of endoderm-derived hepatocytes and mesenchyme-derived sinusoids. Shortly thereafter, the fetal liver becomes the major site of embryonic hematopoiesis.

As in the lung, a mesenchymally expressed FGF seems to be one of the first factors to induce hepatic morphogenesis. This activity is in addition to the requirement of FGFs in hepatic specification described above. Although *Fgf* expression by the septum transversum has not been well characterized, explants of ventral foregut endoderm express two types of FGF receptors, *Fgfr2* and *Fgfr4*. Such explants exhibit robust outgrowth when cultured with cardiac mesoderm. This outgrowth can be blocked with a soluble fusion protein consisting of the FGFR4 extracellular domain and the IgG heavy chain (Jung et al., 1999). Further studies have demonstrated that *Fgf8* (which along with *Fgf1* and *Fgf2* is expressed in the cardiac mesoderm) is permissive for outgrowth (Jung et al., 1999). These experiments show that FGF signals are necessary but not sufficient for liver bud outgrowth.

Further analysis suggests that BMPs are also necessary. In contrast to the lung, where epithelial *Bmp4* negatively regulates growth to mold the branching pattern, *Bmp4* expressed by the septum transversum appears to have a positive effect on prehepatocyte (hepatoblast) growth. Two experiments reported by Rossi et al. (2001) support an *in vivo* role for BMPs in liver morphogenesis. First, *Bmp4* null mutants have delayed liver budding. Second, the BMP inhibitor Noggin blocks the normal outgrowth of ventral foregut endoderm from *Bmp4* mutant, but not wild-type, embryos (Rossi et al., 2001) This observation suggests that the nascent liver endoderm can discern exquisitely low levels of BMPs.

Liver outgrowth into the septum transversum requires at least three homeobox-containing genes: *Hex*, *Hlx*, and *Prox1*. *Hex* (Table 14–1) is expressed in the anterior visceral endoderm prior to formation of the primitive streak, making it the first marker of A/P asymmetry in the embryo (Thomas et al., 1998). It is expressed later in the first cells of definitive endoderm to exit the streak, which in turn become the anterior endoderm cells that ultimately give rise to the liver. Mice with null mutations in *Hex* form a small hepatic diverticulum (Martinez Barbera et al., 2000; Keng et al., 2000), but hepatoblasts are unable to migrate into the septum transversum mesenchyme.

The *Prox1* gene is also required for the migration of hepatoblasts into the septum transversum; in *Prox1* mutant mice, hepatoblasts that would normally invade the septum transversum remain clustered around the hepatic diverticulum (Sosa-Pineda et al., 2000). Despite the paucity of migrating hepatocytes, a liver that is 30% of the normal size does form in *Prox1* null mutant. The livers of these mutants have an expanded mesenchymal component, suggesting that the mesenchyme contains much of the morphogenetic information needed for organ formation.

Mice with an inactivation of the *Hlx* gene have an even earlier arrest in liver outgrowth. A day and a half after wild-type mouse embryos display the first signs of liver budding, *Hlx* mutant mice still have no bud (Hentsch et al., 1996). At later stages, a small diverticulum does form, giving rise to a liver that contains 3% of the normal number of cells, with no increase in apoptosis or decrease in cell viability (Hentsch et al., 1996). *Hlx* is normally expressed in the septum transversum mesenchyme, and it is thus likely required in the mesenchymal support of liver bud formation and outgrowth. The possibility that *Hlx* might regulate *Bmp4* has not been explored.

The liver undergoes tremendous growth in the period following budding, a process that again depends on both epithelial and mesenchymal signals. One of the mesenchymal signals is hepatocyte growth factor (HGF), which is expressed by cells of the septum transversum mesenchyme and binds to the c-Met receptor on hepatoblasts. Inactivation of either c-*met* or *Hgf* results in marked hepatocyte apoptosis, without apparent effect on the sinusoids (Schmidt et al., 1995; Bladt et al., 1995), although this phenotype has not been observed in all analyses of *Hgf* mutant mice (Uehara et al., 1995). Hepatocyte apoptosis is also seen following inactivation of the N-*myc* (Giroux and Charron, 1998) or c-*jun* transcription factors (Hilberg et al., 1993) or the stress-responsive kinase *Sek1* (Nishina et al., 1999). As *Sek1* is an activator of c-*jun* and c-*jun* is known to also be downstream of c-*met*, it is possible that a c-*met*/Sek1/c-*jun* signaling pathway mediates hepatoblast growth and survival during development, although direct evidence for such a cascade is lacking. The absence of increased apoptosis in *Hlx* mutants suggests that *Hlx* does not induce the *Hgf* pathway.

These phenotypes demonstrate that hepatocyte apoptosis is a critically important and developmentally regulated process. Other studies have suggested that hepatocyte apoptosis is also regulated by the tumor necrosis factor (TNF)–nuclear factor κB (NF-κB) signaling pathway. Increased liver cell apoptosis follows inactivation of genes involved in NF-κB signaling (*Ikkb*, *Ikkg*, *RelA*), while double mutant mice lacking both the TNF receptor 1 and either *Ikkβ* or *RelA* have no liver apoptosis (Li et al., 1999b; Doi et al., 1999; Rosenfeld et al., 2000). These studies suggest that a TNF signal present in the embryonic liver is prevented from inducing apoptosis through the action of NF-κB. How the NF-κB and HGF apoptotic pathways might interact is unclear.

Pancreas

The pancreatic buds emerge from the dorsal and ventral surfaces of endoderm. These buds will become approximated and fuse with later rotation of the gut. Budding is first apparent at e9.5, with the development of the ventral bud lagging slightly behind that of the dorsal bud. During morphogenesis of the pancreas, the expanding epithelial tree gives rise to differentiated endocrine cells, which detach from the epithelial layer and migrate into the mesenchyme, coalescing into the islets of Langerhans, the endocrine compartment of the pancreas.

As in lung and liver, homeobox genes, FGFs, and mesenchymal factors play a critical role in the morphogenesis of the pancreas. We have already seen how the dorsal and ventral components utilize different mechanisms to downregulate *Shh*, an early signal in pancreatic specification. This manner of organization (the use of different mesenchymal signals for dorsal and ventral specification) apparently also permits or requires the use of different developmental pathways later during organogenesis as a number genes differ in their activity in the two lobes.

Inactivation of the homeobox-containing *Hlxb9* gene (Table 14–1), which is expressed in both lobes, results in failure of only the dorsal bud to form. Strikingly, the ventral bud forms and is grossly normal, although defects in the structure of the pancreatic islets of Langerhans are observed (Li et al., 1999a; Harrison et al., 1999). *Hlxb9* mutant animals do not exhibit ectopic *Shh* expression; thus, a failure to down-regulate *Shh* in *Hlxb9* mutants is not the mechanistic basis for the failure of dorsal budding (Li et al., 1999a). Interestingly, *Hlxb9* expression must be transient as transgenic mice with enforced expression beyond e10 have multiple defects in pancreatic morphology and differentiation (Li and Edlund, 2001).

Another gene that reflects differences in dorsal and ventral pancreatic development is the LIM homeodomain gene *Isl1* (Table 14–1). In the embryonic pancreas, *Isl1* is expressed in the epithelial layer of both pancreatic compartments but exclusively in the mesenchyme of the dorsal pancreas. Moreover, *Isl1* is expressed in all mature islet cells in the adult. Mice with an inactivated *Isl1* gene have a loss of dorsal mesenchyme and subsequently fail to form a dorsal pancreas or any endocrine cells (Ahlgren et al., 1997). This suggests two separate requirements for *Isl1*: expression in dorsal pancreatic mesenchyme is required for growth of the mesenchyme, which in turn is required for development of the dorsal pancreas. Expression in the epithelium is required for the development of endocrine cells. Although *Isl1* and *Hlxb9* mutant animals share the phenotype of dorsal pancreas agenesis, *Isl1* does not appear to be downstream of *Hlxb9*; although *Hlxb9* mutant animals have a loss of epithelial *Isl1* expression, mesenchymal *Isl1* expression is preserved (Li et al., 1999a; Harrison et al., 1999). The possibility that *Isl1* could regulate *Hlxb9* has not been explored.

Repression of *Shh* in both dorsal and ventral buds of the pancreas is a necessary step for pancreatic specification during patterning. While signals from the notochord mediate the effect in dorsal endoderm, the signals or structures causing ventral repression are not known. Furthermore, it appears that subsequent maintenance of *Shh* repression throughout development is also required for pancreatic morphogenesis. Late overexpression of *Shh* in the pancreatic endoderm of transgenic mice (under the control of the *Pdx1* promoter) results in the normal cytodifferentiation of cells within the pancreatic epithelium but conversion of epithelial and mesenchymal components toward a small intestine-like morphology (Apelqvist et al., 1997).

The *Shh* signal constitutes part of a reciprocal signaling loop, in which one kind of mesenchyme (i.e., notochord) signals endoderm to become pancreatic and this endoderm in turn signals the adjacent mesenchyme to become pancreatic mesenchyme. What is striking about this reciprocal loop is that the *absence* of *Shh* serves as the signal to the mesenchyme, suggesting that pancreas may represent a default fate for mesenchyme. Different *HH* family members may have different roles in the regulation of pancreatic morphogenesis. For example, the *Indian hedgehog (Ihh)* gene is expressed in the pancreas, unlike its relative *Shh*. Increased numbers of pancreatic endocrine cells and malformations resembling the human condition annular pancreas are observed in mice with inactivation of either *Ihh* or *Shh* (Hebrok et al., 2000; Ramalho-Santos et al., 2000).

How is the *Shh* expression domain regulated? Several secreted molecules can mimic the effect of notochord on the expression of *Shh* and pancreatic markers in isolated endoderm (Hebrok et al., 1998). One of these is activin-βB, a member of the TGF-β family. Activin receptors are expressed broadly in foregut organ primordia, and compound mutants lacking one or both alleles of type IIA and IIB activin receptors develop a variety of abnormalities in the size, shape, and boundaries of multiple foregut organs (Kim et al., 2000). These mutants have an expanded *Shh* expression domain, accounting in part for the observed reduction in pancreas size and suggesting that signals through activin receptors restrict the expression of *Shh*.

The homeobox gene *Pdx1* is expressed in a domain that includes the stomach, duodenum, and pancreas (Table 14–1); in adults, *Pdx1* is expressed in islet cells, where it is a major transcriptional regulator of insulin (Ohlsson et al., 1993). Inactivation of *Pdx1* causes the absence of both dorsal and ventral components of the pancreas (Jonsson et al., 1994), the result of an intrinsic defect in epithelial cell growth and differentiation (Offield et al., 1996; Ahlgren et al., 1996). There is also evidence that *Pdx1* is itself sufficient to promote a pancreatic program. Specifically, ectopic expression of *Pdx1* in the chick gut causes cells to bud from the epithelium and initiate the first steps in a pancreatic transcriptional program, turning on *Hlxb9* and turning off *Shh* (Grapin-Botton et al., 2001). While *Pdx1* is required for morphogenesis and differentiation of all epithelial derivatives (the endocrine and exocrine cells of the pancreas), signals from the post-budding pancreatic epithelium are not necessary for growth of the mesenchyme as pancreatic mesenchyme forms normally in *Pdx1* mutant animals (Ahlgren et al., 1996).

Early pancreatic budding occurs in mouse embryos lacking *Pdx1* or chick embryonic cultures lacking a notochord, although all subsequent development is arrested (Offield et al., 1996; Ahlgren et al., 1996; Kim et al., 1997). These results, taken together with the more severe phenotype observed upon inactivation of *Isl1*, suggest that epithelial–mesenchymal interactions in the embryonic pancreas occur in two phases: an early phase of pancreatic budding (which requires *Isl1*) and a later phase of outgrowth, branching, and differentiation (which requires *Pdx1*). Such a possibility was first raised by Wessels and Cohen (1967), who observed that heterologous mesenchyme could substitute for pancreatic mesenchyme in supporting the late stages of pancreatic development but not the early stages, which required pancreatic mesenchyme. The morphogenic signals from "mesenchymal factors," which are required for outgrowth, branching, and differentiation of the pancreatic epithelium, have been the focus of much interest over the past 30 years (Slack, 1995).

FGF10 has been identified as one of these mesenchymal factors. *Fgf10* is transiently expressed in the pancreatic mesenchyme, and mice with a targeted inactivation of *Fgf10* have arrested pancreatic development at the bud stage. FGF10 appears to act as a mitogen for progenitor cells as mutant animals have a depletion of cells that are positive for both PDX1 and bromodeoxyuridine (Bhushan et al., 2001). FGFR2b is thought to mediate all of the effects of FGF10, and a role for FGF10 had earlier been inferred by the ability of antisense oligonucleotides or a soluble form of *Fgfr2b* to inhibit the growth of pancreatic explants (Miralles et al., 1999). However, transgenic mice in which a dominant-negative form of *Fgfr2b* is expressed under the control of the *Pdx1* promoter have no overt pancreatic abnormalities (Hart et al., 2000), apparently in conflict with the observations of *Fgf10* mutant mice. It is possible that only a small amount of FGF10–FRFR2b signal is needed and that expression of the dominant-negative transgene is inadequate or too late to eliminate all remaining FGF10. Alternatively, FGF10 may be able to signal through other receptors under certain circumstances.

Morphogenesis of the distinctive endocrine islets of Langerhans occurs separately from the growth and branching of the pancreatic ductal system. Islet formation is an active process, in which endocrine precursors bud from expanding duct-like structures, migrate, and combine into the islets of Langerhans. Extrication and migration of these precursors requires their interaction with each other and with the extracellular matrix, a process involving matrix metalloproteinases and cell adhesion molecules (reviewed in Kim and Hebrok, 2001). One adhesion molecule in particular, E-cadherin, is necessary for the insulin-producing beta cells to aggregate (Dahl et al., 1996). Chimeric analysis has demonstrated that islets are not clonal but rather derived from multiple precursor cells (Deltour et al., 1991).

Gut

Comparatively little is known about the molecular control of gut morphogenesis, which involves both large-scale and microscopic movements. The intestines undergo dramatic elongation during embryogenesis, growing approximately 1000-fold in size between the fifth and fortieth weeks of human development (Menard, 1989). The gut also undergoes gross rotational changes, including a transient stage of physiological umbilical herniation, during which portions of the intestine extend beyond the abdominal wall. One gene that promotes the growth and looping of the gut is *Hlx*, which has already been discussed in the context of liver organogenesis. *Hlx* is also expressed in midgut and hindgut mesenchyme and has a sharp border of expression within the duodenum. Targeted inactivation of this gene results in a shortened, single-loop gut that undergoes apparently normal differentiation (Hentsch et al., 1996). The *Pdx1* gene is also required for gross morphogenesis as mice with inactivation of *Pdx1* have severe malformations of the stomach and duodenum. Nevertheless, these phenotypes give little mechanistic insight. Since errors in rotation and position constitute important diseases of the newborn, a better understanding of the factors that control gut looping and rotation is needed.

The morphology of lumenal gut derivatives follows a relatively simple pattern, varying mainly in the shape of the epithelium (i.e., the relative size of villi and crypts) and composition of the underlying mesenchyme. The arrangement of cells within the gut tube has been referred to as the *radial axis*, the normal circumferential distribution of innermost epithelium, lamina propria, muscularis mucosae, submucosa, and outer muscular layers. Variation in the lumenal diameter and shape of mucosal folds constitutes another set of morphologically distinct features along the A/P axis of the gut. There is minimal migration or branching during development of the lumenal gut organs, and it is thus possible that the same signals that specify the identity of the epithelial component may also specify the epithelial–mesenchymal morphology.

We have already examined how epithelial–mesenchymal interactions contribute to the organization of the chick stomach, a process that appears to involve a regulated interplay between *Shh* and *Bmp* genes. *Bmp* expression affects not only patterning but also the degree of muscularity of the adjacent mesenchyme, suggesting that it may participate in determining radial gut morphology (Roberts et al., 1998). Other experiments suggest that *Shh* regulates the radial axis. Based on gut explant studies, Sukegawa et al. (2000) put forward a model in which gut mesenchymal cells have an intrinsic tendency to differentiate into smooth muscle and *Shh* expressed by the lumenal epithelial cells prevents mesenchymal cells from adopting this fate. Thus, epithelial *Shh* may promote the differentiation of inner mesenchyme to lamina propria or submucosa, while the outer mesenchyme, farther from the *Shh* signal, would adopt a smooth muscle fate. Consistent with this model, treatment of explants with cyclopamine (which blocks the *Shh* signal) causes smooth muscle differentiation throughout a thinned mesenchymal layer. *Shh* may also have effects on epithelial morphology, as treatment of mouse embryos with blocking anti-Shh monoclonal antibodies causes severe abnormalities in crypt-villous structure (Wang et al., 2002).

Conclusions

Organogenesis begins with the budding of cells from the patterned endodermal layer within regions that are characterized by expression of certain homeobox genes: *Nkx2.1* (lung), *Hex* (liver), *Hlxb9*, and *Pdx1* (pancreas). The observation that buds still form in the absence of some of these genes implies that they are not required for initial patterning. Rather, these homeobox genes may be used during organogenesis to ensure that other signals used during organogenesis (FGFs, BMPs, and SHH) are interpreted in a tissue-specific manner. This may help explain how these same signaling molecules could have such dramatically different functions in endodermal patterning and organ morphogenesis.

The outgrowth and morphogenesis of lung, liver, and pancreatic epithelia are critically dependent on interactions with mesenchyme. The model that has emerged for the dynamic regulation of branching morphogenesis in the lung begins with expression by the mesenchyme of *Fgf10*. Subsequently, *Bmp4*, *Sprouty,* and other negative regulators are induced in the adjacent epithelium. These, in turn, inhibit proliferation of the tip cells, while *Shh* extinguishes *Fgf10* expression in the

adjacent mesenchyme. Other foci of FGF10 expression then form more proximally, and the process is iterated (Lebeche et al., 1999).

The pancreas also requires signals from the mesenchyme for growth and morphogenesis. In particular, expression of *Isl1* and the absence of *Shh* are necessary for mesenchymal support of pancreatic development. As in the lung, FGF10 may act as a mitogen for pancreatic progenitor cells. Other FGFs and BMPs appear to be required for the first steps of liver bud expansion into the septum transversum. Later in liver development, other growth factors and antiapoptotic factors stimulate hepatocyte growth.

DIFFERENTIATION WITHIN ORGANS

Each of the endoderm-derived organs contains multiple differentiated cell types. A review of the signals that regulate the formation of each of these cell types is well beyond the scope of this chapter. Instead, a few examples will be chosen that give insight into the general mechanism of differentiation. These examples are meant to shed light on the key question of differentiation during organogenesis: how are cells chosen from an apparently uniform pool of progenitors to become one type of specialized cell versus another?

A commonly used mechanism for controlling such cell fate decisions is the Notch pathway (see Chapter 39). The *Notch* genes encode a highly conserved family of membrane receptors that participate in cell fate decisions in most multicellular organisms; it has been suggested that in *Drosophila Notch* signals are involved in the formation of virtually every tissue (Artavanis-Tsakonas et al., 1999). *Notch* functions include the generation of tissue borders (e.g., somite formation), cell fate determination, patterning, and maintenance of a population of stem cells within developing tissues. Vertebrates have four *Notch* ligands (Delta 1 and 2, Jagged 1 and 2) and four receptors (Notch 1–4). Upon ligand binding, a cytoplasmic fragment of the Notch receptor migrates into the nucleus, where it regulates transcription by activating a cascade of bHLH proteins.

Cell–cell signaling through *Notch* commonly involves a process known as "lateral inhibition." During lateral inhibition, the cell that has secreted ligand and the cell that has bound ligand receive distinct cell-autonomous reenforcing signals that irreversibly establish different developmental paths for the two types of cell. The pleiotropic activities of *Notch* are thought to result from context-dependent modulation of a basic signaling pathway. Thus, in the context of lymphoid development, Notch signals may promote T cells at the expense of B cells (Robson MacDonald et al., 2001), while in the context of the heart, Notch signals may promote mesocardium and pericardium at the expense of myocardium (Rones et al., 2000). There is strong evidence that Notch signals play a role in pancreatic cell fate decisions and growing evidence for a role in lung, liver, and gut.

Another feature of organogenesis is that genes (most notably, transcription factors) involved in the early development of an organ are also important in the regulation of terminal differentiation genes within that organ. For example, *Pdx1* is required for morphogenesis early in pancreatic development and again as a major transcription regulator of insulin in pancreatic beta cells (Ohlsson et al., 1993). For example, *Isl1* participates in both pancreatic development and islet cell transcription. HNF and GATA are necessary for both foregut (liver) development and albumin expression, and p48 mediates the development of exocrine pancreatic tissue as well as the transcription of exocrine-specific genes. These observations suggests some parsimony of evolutionary design, in which the commitment of cells to a particular tissue type is modulated using the same molecules involved in the transcriptional control of terminally differentiated cells.

Studies of differentiation rely on assumptions about the lineage relationship between progenitor cells and their progeny. For example, pancreatic islet cells were believed to come from neural crest cells until more careful analyses revealed an endodermal origin. It is clearly more difficult to study the signals that mediate islet differentiation without first understanding something about the origin of islets. Investigation of cell fate determination likewise requires some sense of what other fates were available to a progenitor cell (i.e., its *competence*). While some lineage analyses have been performed in the pancreas and the gut, to a great extent the lineage relationships of cells in the endoderm are inferred rather than proven.

Pancreas

The adult pancreas can be divided into two functional units: the exocrine pancreas, which is composed of enzyme-secreting acinar cells and ducts that modify and carry the digestive juice to the small intestine, and the endocrine pancreas, which secretes hormones that regulate the organism's response to feeding. The endocrine pancreas is itself subdivided into at least four types of cell, which are categorized according to the hormones they make. Alpha and beta cells, which secrete glucagon and insulin, respectively, maintain glucose homeostasis. Delta cells, which secrete somatostatin, downregulate a number of other gastrointestinal regulatory peptides, resulting in suppression of gastric acid secretion. PP cells, which secrete pancreatic polypeptide, appear to regulate the activity of the exocrine pancreas and gallbladder.

A number of approaches have been taken to understand pancreatic lineage relationships, including *in vitro* culture of rudiments, ablation studies, and quail chick chimeric analysis (reviewed in Slack, 1995). Genetic tools, including use of the Cre recombinase, have recently made it possible to irreversibly tag progenitor cells and their progeny. Such an analysis shows that all mature pancreatic cells (exocrine cells, islet cells, and duct cells) are derived from progenitor cells that expressed *Pdx1* during the early bud stage (Gu et al., 2002). Histologically, the expanding pancreatic bud contains multiple branched duct-like structures from which endocrine progenitor cells sprout and coalesce into islets.

It is likely that pancreatic progenitor cells are directed down an exocrine or endocrine differentiation pathway by the presence or absence of a Notch signal. To review this evidence, we must describe in slightly more detail the early response to a Notch signal. Following ligand binding, the intracellular portion of Notch migrates to the nucleus, where it interacts with the product of the *Suppressor of hairless* gene (called RBP-Jκ in vertebrates), leading to transcription of the bHLH gene *Hes1*. *Hes1* in turn downregulates a number of "proneural" (or "proendocrine") genes, among them the bHLH genes *Ngn3* and *NeuroD*. Notch signals appear to maintain cells in an undifferentiated state, and the *removal* of a Notch signal promotes differentiation. If this model applies to the pancreas, then mutations that interfere with Notch signaling at any step along this signal-transduction pathway, from ligand to transcriptional mediator, should promote endocrine cell differentiation at the expense of exocrine cell differentiation.

Analysis of multiple mutant lines is consistent with this model. Specifically, mice with mutations that abrogate Notch signaling (inactivation of the Notch ligand (*Delta*), RBP-Jκ, or *Hes1*) have pancreatic hypoplasia and precocious development of endocrine cells (Apelqvist et al., 1999; Jensen et al., 2000). Conversely, mice with inactivation of *Ngn3* have no endocrine cells whatsoever (Gradwohl et al., 2000), while mice with inactivation of *NeuroD* have a more selective depletion of pancreatic beta cells (Naya et al., 1997). Similarly, early overexpression of *Ngn3* in the pancreas leads to precocious differentiation of glucagon-expressing endocrine cells (Apelqvist et al., 1999; Schwitzgebel et al., 2000), while ectopic expression of *Ngn3* in the gut is also capable of inducing glucagon-positive cells (Grapin-Botton et al., 2001).

It is unclear whether the Notch ligands (*Delta* or *Jagged*) lie at the apex of the fate decision tree or whether other factors control the activation of these ligands. It is also unclear how this model would account for exocrine development: does prolonged Notch signaling beyond an endocrine "window" of competence result in an exocrine fate, or are other genes activated by Notch that somehow compete with proendocrine signals? One clue about how Notch might regulate exocrine fate comes from another bHLH gene, *p48* (Table 14–1). The *p48* gene encodes the DNA-binding subunit of a transcription factor complex called PTF1, which specifically binds to multiple exocrine-specific enhancer regions (Krapp et al., 1996). Inactivation of *p48* results in the selective absence of exocrine tissue (Krapp et al., 1996),

and recent studies have shown that p48 binds to the Notch signaling mediator RBP-Jκ (Obata et al., 2001).

Signals from the TGF-β family (see Chapter 24) also appear to be involved in the endocrine versus exocrine fate decision. Addition of TGF-β1 to pancreatic bud explants results in an increase in the proportion of endocrine cells that arise in the culture (Sanvito et al., 1994). Treatment of pancreatic bud explants with Follistatin, which binds and inhibits ligands of the TGF-β superfamily, results in an increase in the number of exocrine (amylase-positive) cells with a concomitant decrease in the number of insulin-positive cells (Miralles et al., 1998). Moreover, mice with mutations in the receptor for activin, a TGF-β family member, have a dramatic reduction in endocrine cell number. These results are consistent with a model in which TGF-β signals promote endocrine differentiation at the expense of exocrine differentiation. How such regulation might be integrated with Notch signals is unclear; it has been suggested that integration occurs through the action of TGF-β signals on the Notch pathway (Kim and Hebrok, 2001).

Within the endocrine compartment, additional genes control the differentiation of different classes of endocrine cells. These genes include homeodomain transcription factors belonging to the *Pax* and *Nkx* families (Table 14–1). *Pax6* is necessary selectively for the development of alpha cells (St.-Onge et al., 1997; Sander et al., 1997), while *Pax4* is required for the development of beta and delta cells (Sosa-Pineda et al., 1997). Disruption of the *Nkx2.2* gene results in the absence of mature beta cells and a reduction in the number of alpha and PP cells (Sussel et al., 1998). This phenotype appears to represent a block in differentiation rather than specification as mutant animals still generate abundant endocrine-like cells; however, these cells lack markers of terminal differentiation, including insulin. *Nkx6.1* is also required for beta-cell development, and genetic epistasis analysis suggests that the *Nkx6.1* gene lies downstream of *Nkx2.2* (Sander et al., 2000).

The molecular signals that regulate pancreatic duct cell formation are poorly understood. Tubular duct-like structures are widespread in the developing pancreas, but it is not clear whether mature duct cells are derived from these primitive structures. Recent lineage analysis demonstrates that duct cells are derived from progenitors that express *Pdx1* (but not *Ngn3*) at approximately e10.5 of mouse embryogenesis (Gu et al., 2002). Other factors likely govern ductal differentiation, and exposure of pancreatic explants to epidermal growth factor increases the proportion of duct cells (Sanvito et al., 1994).

Gut

The gut derivatives of endoderm differ dramatically along the A/P axis. Sections of the elongating gut tube are specified to become distinct tubular structures that in mammals comprise several distinct "lumenal" organs: the esophagus, stomach, small intestine, and large intestine. Each of these organs contains an array of differentiated cell types, and a detailed discussion of these cells is well beyond the scope of this chapter.

Esophagus and Stomach

The adult esophagus consists of a stratified squamous epithelium with interspersed mucus-secreting glands. The mechanism by which esophageal epithelial composition is determined is poorly understood. The common condition of Barrett's metaplasia, in which the normal squamous epithelium is converted into intestine- or stomach-like columnar epithelium, demonstrates the ease with which epithelial cell types may be interconverted under the appropriate circumstances.

The mammalian stomach has a complex microanatomy and is divisible into histologically distinct regions. The mature stomach is composed of mucus-producing neck cells, acid-producing parietal cells, pepsinogen-producing chief cells, and enteroendocrine cells (which make gastrin, somatostatin, or histamine). These cells are organized within the "gastric pit," the structural unit of the stomach.

Ablation studies have implicated parietal cells as "organizers" of the gastric pit; selective removal of parietal cells results in defects in other lineages and an apparent increase in progenitor cell number (Li et al., 1996). As in the pancreas, the Notch pathway plays an important role in gastric enteroendocrine cell differentiation (Jensen et al.,

2000). *Shh* is required for development of the gastric epithelium (Ra-malho-Santos et al., 2000) and regulates the proliferation of gastric epithelial precursors in the adult (van den Brink et al., 2001); we have already discussed the role of *Shh* in the formation of different cell types in the avian stomach.

Small and Large Intestine

The intestinal epithelium is composed of absorptive enterocytes, crypt cells (including Paneth cells, goblet cells, and stem cells), and several types of endocrine cell. Unlike enterocytes, whose function is mainly absorptive, Paneth, goblet, and endocrine cells are considered secretory because they secrete small peptides, mucus, and hormones, respectively. The timing of the appearance of each of these intestinal cell types has been described elsewhere (Menard, 1989). Similar to the pancreas, in which Notch signals determine whether cells will adopt an exocrine or endocrine fate, Notch signals appear to control whether gut cells become enterocytes or secretory cells.

Several mutant studies support the notion that release of cells from Notch signaling is sufficient to induce a secretory fate. Inactivation of *Hes1*, the most proximal target of Notch signaling, results in increased numbers of intestinal enteroendocrine and goblet cells, analogous to its activity as a negative regulator of endocrine fate in the pancreas (Jensen et al., 2000). Among the genes that *Hes1* negatively regulates is the bHLH gene *Math1*. Inactivation of the *Math1* gene causes depletion of all secretory lineages but has no effect on enterocyte number (Yang et al., 2001). Thus, progenitor cells that express *Math1* may be directed to secretory cell fates, while cells that express *Hes1*, and therefore turn off *Math1*, adopt an enterocyte fate.

Other signals may further modulate cell fate within the secretory lineage once this initial decision is made. For example, lineage ablation studies have demonstrated that multiple enteroendocrine lineages (i.e., cells expressing cholecystokinin, peptideYY/glucagon, or secretin) are descended from a secretin-expressing progenitor (Rindi et al., 1999). *NeuroD*, a bHLH gene that is also negatively regulated by *Hes1*, is expressed in all endocrine cells. Its inactivation in mice results in the selective depletion of secretin- and cholecystokinin-expressing cells, with no effect on other endocrine cell types (Naya et al., 1997). Likewise, the differentiation of some intestinal cell types depends on the *Rac1* GTPase; overexpression of constitutively active or dominant-negative forms of *Rac1* changes the relative abundance of Paneth cells, goblet cells, and enterocytes (Stappenbeck and Gordon, 2000).

Lung

The highly branched epithelium of the adult lung changes in character as one moves from larger (proximal) to smaller (distal) airways. The proximal epithelium is columnar, containing ciliated and secretory cells, which help to clear secretions. Mucus-secreting submucosal glands are found in the largest airways. The distal airways terminate in the squamous air sacs and alveoli, which are composed of thin type I pneumocytes, across which gas exchange occurs, and type II pneumocytes, which secrete surfactant protein. Rare pulmonary neuroendocrine cells (PNECs), which may be involved in sensing oxygen, are dispersed throughout the lung. PNECs are the first cells to differentiate within the lung, while the differentiation of distal pneumocytes occurs late in embryonic development or after birth. The process of lung differentiation can be clearly dissociated from morphogenesis as a number of mutations affecting morphogenesis (e.g., *Shh*, *Fgf9*) have no effect on the differentiation of these specialized cells.

BMP signals, in addition to their apparent role in lung morphogenesis (discussed above), appear to regulate proximal–distal cell fate decisions. The surfactant protein promoter/enhancer has been used to over-express BMP inhibitors (Noggin or a dominant-negative BMP receptor) in the distal airways. Inhibition of BMP function by these methods results in a shift from a distal to a proximal phenotype (Weaver et al., 1999). *Bmp4* expression is greatest at the distal tips of expanding lung bud epithelium (Bellusci et al., 1996), consistent with a model in which expression of *Bmp4* at the bud tips causes a distal fate while absence of *Bmp4* signals elsewhere in the epithelial tree results in a proximal fate. It is not clear how *Bmp* signals are themselves

regulated or whether other signals are required for proximal differentiation. Nevertheless, it is enticing to imagine that a single signaling mechanism, involving an "apical signaling center" at the lung bud tips, regulates both branching morphogenesis and proximal–distal differentiation (Weaver et al., 1999).

Mesenchymal cues influence whether distal cells become type I or II pneumocytes. Coculture of distal lung bud mesenchyme with tracheal epithelium results in induction of branching and differentiation of type II alveolar cells (Shannon, 1994). Further explant studies showed that type II cell induction by mesenchyme could be replaced by a partially defined medium. The successive removal of components from this defined medium showed that either FGF1 or FGF7 must be present for type II differentiation to occur, although neither growth factor was able to induce differentiation on its own (Shannon et al., 1999).

Mirroring the pattern seen in all other endoderm derivatives, endocrine differentiation in the lung is associated with a release from Notch signals. PNECs are absent in mice lacking *Mash1*, a bHLH gene that is negatively regulated by Notch and *Hes1* (Borges et al., 1997). By contrast, mice with inactivation of *Hes1*, which lies directly downstream of Notch, have increased numbers of PNECs (Ito et al., 2000).

Liver

Mature adult hepatocytes are intercalated between two complex networks: the vascular network (consisting of portal venules and hepatic arterioles) and the intrahepatic bile duct (IHBD) network. Cells that are in contact with branches of the future portal vein adopt duct-like characteristics, forming a sleeve of cells known as the "ductal plate." The ductal plate is remodeled during the second half of gestation, giving rise to the cholangiocytes that line the complex IHBD system. The mechanism of ductal plate cell differentiation is unknown but appears to involve portal vein branches in particular as ductal plates do not form around hepatic vein branches (Desmet, 1998).

Hepatocytes and cholangiocytes make up the vast majority of cells within the liver parenchyma. Both types of cell appear to be endodermally derived and to be derived from a common progenitor, the hepatoblast. It is not known how hepatoblast fate is determined. The finding that Alagille syndrome, in which there is a paucity of bile ducts, is caused by mutations in the Notch ligand *Jagged1* (Li et al., 1997; Oda et al., 1997) suggests that *Notch* signals are central to this cell fate decision.

Hepatocytes carry out multiple homeostatic functions, including biosynthesis of serum proteins, cholesterol metabolism, and detoxification. Many transcription factors regulate the expression of genes involved in these processes. One of these, the HNF-4a transcription factor, is found in the earliest stages of liver bud formation. HNF-4α is required in the visceral endoderm early in embryogenesis, and embryos with inactivation of HNF-4α fail to gastrulate (Chen et al., 1994). The technique of tetraploid embryo aggregation, whereby chimeric mice have normal extraembryonic tissues but lack HNF-4α, has been used to show that HNF-4α has a distinct role in hepatocyte differentiation. Specifically, mutant heptocytes fail to express a number of liver-specific genes, despite having normal liver specification and morphology (Li et al., 2000). Thus, the "full" differentiation of hepatocytes requires genes like *Hnf-4a* to activate the transcription of hepatocyte-specific genes. This may be analogous to the pancreatic phenotype of *Nkx6.1* and *Nkx2.2* mutant mice, which undergo partial but incomplete islet differentiation.

Other types of cell residing within the liver parenchyma include Kuppfer, Ito, stellate, and oval cells. The lineage relationship between these other cell types has not been well characterized; thus, there are no definitive data on which cell types are epithelially derived and which are mesenchymally derived. The ability to genetically mark progenitor cells should make it possible to address these questions in the future.

Conclusions

Within each endoderm derivative, specialized cell types differentiate from a multipotent progenitor pool. Notch signals are a common mechanism through which cell fate decisions are made, controlling the dif-

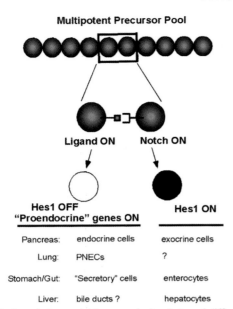

Multipotent Precursor Pool

Ligand ON   Notch ON

Hes1 OFF
"Proendocrine" genes ON   Hes1 ON

Pancreas:	endocrine cells	exocrine cells
Lung:	PNECs	?
Stomach/Gut:	"Secretory" cells	enterocytes
Liver:	bile ducts ?	hepatocytes

Figure 14–3. Speculative model for control of endodermal differentiation by Notch. From a pool of multipotent precursor cells, certain cells acquire greater expression of Notch ligand (Delta or Jagged) compared to their neighbors. This difference leads to a state where Notch signals are present in one cell (Notch ON) and absent in its neighbor (Ligand ON). These states are reenforced, and the cells acquire distinct fates. Cellular context determines the outcome of having a Notch signal present or absent. Likely cell fates associated with removal of Notch signals are shown on the left. Cell fates that may result from persistence of Notch signals are shown on the right. (See text for detailed discussion of this model.) PNEC, pulmonary neuroendocrine cell.

ferentiation of endocrine cells within the pancreas and lung and the secretory lineages within the gut (Fig. 14–3). Signals from TGF-β family members, including TGF-β and activin in the pancreas and BMP4 in the lung, are also involved in the regulation of cell fate. Following these early instructive signals, other genes, such as *Nkx* and *Pax* transcription factors, seem to be involved in guiding subsequent cell fate decisions. Although some studies suggest that differentiation signals come from the mesenchyme, the evidence for epithelial–mesenchymal interactions in guiding differentiation decisions is weaker than for other stages of endodermal development.

FUTURE DIRECTIONS

A detailed understanding of the mechanisms underlying patterning and cell fate decisions remains elusive. In particular, how does an organism encode its body plan and ensure that its varied cell types are present in appropriate abundance? Similarly, how does the organism regulate organ size to ensure proportionality? Also, while progenitor cells play a central role during development, to what extent do similar cells exist in adult tissues as "stem cells," which can be called upon if necessary for tissue regeneration?

The study of stem cells may inform our understanding of development. For example, Suzuki et al. (2002) have described the isolation of embryonic liver stem cells which have the capacity to self-renew and differentiate into both hepatocytes and cholangiocytes. Such stem cells can also differentiate into a variety of intestinal and pancreatic cells in vitro, suggesting lineage relationships that may not have been suspected previously. These studies provide an experimental framework for studying the signals involved in cell fate decisions. They also carry great clinical implications since the ability to purify and manipulate progenitors may lead to future cell-based therapies, in which normal developmental processes may be recapitulated in an adult to rescue failing organs.

REFERENCES

Ahlgren U, Jonsson J, Edlund H (1996). The morphogenesis of the pancreatic mesenchyme is uncoupled from that of the pancreatic epithelium in IPF1/PDX1-deficient mice. *Development* 122: 1409–1416.

Ahlgren U, Pfaff S, Jessell T, Edlund T, Edlund H (1997). Independent requirement for ISL1 in formation of pancreatic mesenchyme and islet cells. *Nature* 385: 257–260.

Ang SL, Rossant J (1994). HNF-3 beta is essential for node and notochord formation in mouse development. *Cell* 78: 561–574.

Apelqvist A, Ahlgren U, Edlund H (1997). Sonic hedgehog directs specialised mesoderm differentiation in the intestine and pancreas. *Curr Biol* 7: 801–804.

Apelqvist A, Li H, Sommer L, Beatus P, Anderson D, Honjo T, Hrabe de Angelis M, Lendahl U, Edlund H (1999). Notch signaling controls pancreatic cell differentiation. *Nature* 400: 877–881.

Artavanis-Tsakonas S, Rand MD, Lake RJ (1999). Notch signaling: cell fate control and signal integration in development. *Science* 284: 770–776.

Aubin J, Lemieux M, Tremblay M, Berard J, Jeannotte L (1997). Early postnatal lethality in *Hoxa-5* mutant mice is attributable to respiratory tract defects. *Dev Biol* 192: 432–445.

Beck F, Chawengsaksophak K, Waring P, Playford R, Furness J (1999). Reprogramming of intestinal differentiation and intercalary regeneration in *Cdx2* mutant mice. *Proc Natl Acad Sci USA* 96: 7318–7323.

Beck F, Tata F, Chawengsaksophak K (2000). Homeobox genes and gut development. *Bioessays* 22: 431–441.

Bellusci S, Henderson R, Winnier G, Oikawa T, Hogan B (1996). Evidence from normal expression and targeted misexpression that *bone morphogenetic protein-4 (Bmp-4)* plays a role in mouse embryonic lung morphogenesis. *Development* 122: 1693–1702.

Bellusci S, Furuta Y, Rush M, Henderson R, Winnier G, Hogan B (1997a). Involvement of Sonic hedgehog (*Shh*) in mouse embryonic lung growth and morphogenesis. *Development* 124: 53–63.

Bellusci S, Grindley J, Emoto H, Itoh N, Hogan B (1997b). Fibroblast growth factor 10 (FGF10) and branching morphogenesis in the embryonic mouse lung. *Development* 124: 4867–4878.

Bhushan A, Itoh N, Kato S, Thiery J, Czernichow P, Bellusci S, Scharfmann R (2001). *Fgf10* is essential for maintaining the proliferative capacity of epithelial progenitor cells during early pancreatic organogenesis. *Development* 128: 5109–5117.

Bladt F, Riethmacher D, Isenmann S, Aguzzi A, Birchmeier C (1995). Essential role for the *c-met* receptor in the migration of myogenic precursor cells into the limb bud. *Nature* 376: 768–771.

Borges M, Linnoila RI, van de Velde HJ, Chen H, Nelkin BD, Mabry M, Baylin SB, Ball DW (1997). An achaete-scute homologue essential for neuroendocrine differentiation in the lung. *Nature* 386: 852–855.

Bossard P, Zaret K (1998). GATA transcription factors as potentiators of gut endoderm differentiation. *Development* 125: 4909–4917.

Bossard P, Zaret K (2000). Repressive and restrictive mesodermal interactions with gut endoderm: possible relation to Meckel's diverticulum. *Development* 127: 4915–4923.

Boulet AM, Capecchi MR (1996). Targeted disruption of hoxc-4 causes esophageal defects and vertebral transformations. *Dev Biol* 177: 232–249.

Cardoso WV (2001). Molecular regulation of lung development. *Annu Rev Physiol* 63: 471–494.

Chen J, Knowles HJ, Hebert JL, Hackett BP (1998). Mutation of the mouse hepatocyte nuclear factor/forkhead homologue 4 gene results in an absence of cilia and random left–right asymmetry. *J Clin Invest* 102: 1077–1082.

Chen WS, Manova K, Weinstein DC, Duncan SA, Plump AS, Prezioso VR, Bachvarova RF, Darnell JE, Jr. (1994). Disruption of the HNF-4 gene, expressed in visceral endoderm, leads to cell death in embryonic ectoderm and impaired gastrulation of mouse embryos. *Genes Dev* 8: 2466–2477.

Ciruna B, Schwartz L, Harpal K, Yamaguchi T, Rossant J (1997). Chimeric analysis of *fibroblast growth factor receptor-1 (Fgfr1)* function: a role for FGFR1 in morphogenetic movement through the primitive streak. *Development* 124: 2829–2841.

Cleaver O, Krieg P (2001). Notochord patterning of the endoderm. *Dev Biol* 234: 1–12.

Colvin J, White A, Pratt S, Ornitz D (2001). Lung hypoplasia and neonatal death in *Fgf9*-null mice identify this gene as an essential regulator of lung mesenchyme. *Development* 128: 2095–2106.

Conlon FL, Lyons KM, Takaesu N, Barth KS, Kispert A, Herrmann B, Robertson EJ (1994). A primary requirement for nodal in the formation and maintenance of the primitive streak in the mouse. *Development* 120: 1919–1928.

Dahl U, Sjodin A, Semb H (1996). Cadherins regulate aggregation of pancreatic β-cells in vivo. *Development* 122: 2895–2902.

Deltour L, Leduque P, Paldi A, Ripoche MA, Dubois P, Jami J (1991). Polyclonal origin of pancreatic islets in aggregation mouse chimaeras. *Development* 112: 1115–1121.

Deng C, Wynshaw-Boris A, Shen M, Daugherty C, Ornitz D, Leder P (1994). Murine FGFR-1 is required for early postimplantation growth and axial organization. *Genes Dev* 8: 3045–3057.

de Santa Barbara P, Roberts DJ (2002). Tail gut endoderm and gut/genitourinary/tail development: a new tissue-specific role for Hoxa13. *Development* 129: 551–561.

Desmet VJ (1998). Ludwig symposium on biliary disorders—part I. Pathogenesis of ductal plate abnormalities. *Mayo Clin Proc* 73: 80–89.

Deutsch G, Jung J, Zheng M, Lora J, Zaret K (2001). A bipotential precursor population for pancreas and liver within the embryonic endoderm. *Development* 128: 871–881.

Doi T, Marino M, Takahashi T, Yoshida T, Sakakura T, Old L, Obata Y (1999). Absence of tumor necrosis factor rescues RelA-deficient mice from embryonic lethality. *Proc Natl Acad Sci USA* 96: 2994–2999.

Dudley AT, Lyons KM, Robertson EJ (1995). A requirement for bone morphogenetic protein-7 during development of the mammalian kidney and eye. *Genes Dev* 9: 2795–2807.

Dufort D, Schwartz L, Harpal K, Rossant J (1998). The transcription factor HNF3β is required in visceral endoderm for normal primitive streak morphogenesis. *Development* 125: 3015–3025.

Duluc I, Freund J-N, Leberquier C, Kedinger M (1994). Fetal endoderm primarily holds the temporal and positional information required for mammalian intestinal development. *J Cell Biol* 126: 211–221.

Elliott GB, Tredwell SJ, Elliott KA (1970). The notochord as an abnormal organizer in

production of congenital intestinal defect. *Am J Roentgenol Radium Ther Nucl Med* 110: 628–634.
Feldman B, Poueymirou W, Papaioannou V, DeChiara T, Goldfarb M (1995). Requirement of FGF-4 for postimplantation mouse development. *Science* 267: 246–249.
Gavalas A, Krumlauf R (2000). Retinoid signalling and hindbrain patterning. *Curr Opin Genet Dev* 10: 380–386.
Giroux S, Charron J (1998). Defective development of the embryonic liver in *N-myc*-deficient mice. *Dev Biol* 195: 16–28.
Gradwohl G, Dierich A, LeMeur M, Guillemot F (2000). *neurogenin3* is required for the development of the four endocrine cell lineages of the pancreas. *Proc Natl Acad Sci U S A* 97: 1607–1611.
Grapin-Botton A, Melton DA (2000). Endoderm development: from patterning to organogenesis. *Trends Genet* 16: 124–130.
Grapin-Botton A, Majithia AR, Melton DA (2001). Key events of pancreas formation are triggered in gut endoderm by ectopic expression of pancreatic regulatory genes. *Genes Dev* 15: 444–454.
Gu G, Dubauskaite J, Melton D (2002). Direct evidence for the pancreatic lineage: NGN3+ cells are islet progenitors and are distinct from duct progenitors. *Development* 127: 2317–2322.
Gualdi R, Bossard P, Zheng M, Hamada Y, Coleman J, Zaret K (1996). Hepatic specification of the gut endoderm in vitro: cell signaling and transcriptional control. *Genes Dev* 10: 1670–1682.
Haffen K, Kedinger M, Simon-Assmann P (1989). Cell contact dependent regulation of enterocytic differentiation. In: *Human Gastrointestinal Development.* Lebenthal E (ed.) Raven Press, New York.
Harrison K, Thaler J, Pfaff S, Gu H, Kehrl J (1999). Pancreas dorsal lobe agenesis and abnormal islets of Langerhans in *Hlxb9*-deficient mice. *Nat Genet* 23: 71–75.
Hart A, Baeza N, Apelqvist A, Edlund H (2000). Attenuation of FGF signalling in mouse β-cells leads to diabetes. *Nature* 408: 864–868.
Hayashi K, Yasugi S, Mizuno T (1988). Pepsinogen gene transcription induced in heterologous epithelial–mesenchymal recombinations of chicken endoderms and glandular stomach mesenchyme. *Development* 103: 725–731.
Hebrok M, Kim S, Melton D (1998). Notochord repression of endodermal Sonic hedgehog permits pancreas development. *Genes Dev* 12: 1705–1713.
Hebrok M, Kim S, St-Jacques B, McMahon A, Melton D (2000). Regulation of pancreas development by hedgehog signaling. *Development* 127: 4905–4913.
Henry G, Melton D (1998). *Mixer*, a homeobox gene required for endoderm development. *Science* 281: 91–96.
Hentsch B, Li R, Hartley L, Lints T, Adams J, Harvey R (1996). *Hlx* homeo box gene is essential for an inductive tissue interaction that drives expansion of embryonic liver and gut. *Genes Dev* 10: 70–79.
Hilberg F, Aguzzi A, Howells N, Wagner E (1993). c-Jun is essential for normal mouse development and hepatogenesis. *Nature* 365: 179–181.
Hogan B (1999). Morphogenesis. *Cell* 96: 225–233.
Hudson C, Clements D, Friday RV, Stott D, Woodland HR (1997). Xsox17alpha and -beta mediate endoderm formation in *Xenopus*. *Cell* 91: 397–405.
Ito T, Udaka N, Yazawa T, Okudela K, Hayashi H, Sudo T, Guillemot F, Kageyama R, Kitamura H (2000). Basic helix-loop-helix transcription factors regulate the neuroendocrine differentiation of fetal mouse pulmonary epithelium. *Development* 127: 3913–3921.
Jensen J, Pedersen EE, Galante P, Hald J, Heller RS, Ishibashi M, Kageyama R, Guillemot F, Serup P, Madsen OD (2000). Control of endodermal endocrine development by Hes-1. *Nat Genet* 24: 36–44.
Jonsson J, Carlsson L, Edlund T, Edlund H (1994). Insulin-promoter-factor 1 is required for pancreas development in mice. *Nature* 371: 606–609.
Jung J, Zheng M, Goldfarb M, Zaret K (1999). Initiation of mammalian liver development from endoderm by fibroblast growth factors. *Science* 284: 1998–2003.
Keijzer R, van Tuyl M, Meijers C, Post M, Tibboel D, Grosveld F, Koutsourakis M (2001). The transcription factor GATA6 is essential for branching morphogenesis and epithelial cell differentiation during fetal pulmonary development. *Development* 128: 503–511.
Keng V, Yagi H, Ikawa M, Nagano T, Myint Z, Yamada K, Tanaka T, Sato A, Muramatsu I, Okabe M, et al. (2000). Homeobox gene *Hex* is essential for onset of mouse embryonic liver development and differentiation of the monocyte lineage. *Biochem Biophys Res Commun* 276: 1155–1161.
Kikuchi Y, Agathon A, Alexander J, Thisse C, Waldron S, Yelon D, Thisse B, Stainier D (2001). *casanova* encodes a novel Sox-related protein necessary and sufficient for early endoderm formation in zebrafish. *Genes Dev* 15: 1493–1505.
Kim S, Hebrok M (2001). Intercellular signals regulating pancreas development and function. *Genes Dev* 15: 111–127.
Kim S, Hebrok M, Melton D (1997). Notochord to endoderm signaling is required for pancreas development. *Development* 124: 4243–4252.
Kim SK, Melton DA (1998). Pancreas development is promoted by cyclopamine, a hedgehog signaling inhibitor. *Proc Natl Acad Sci USA* 95: 13036–13041.
Kim SK, Hebrok M, Li E, Oh SP, Schrewe H, Harmon EB, Lee JS, Melton DA (2000). Activin receptor patterning of foregut organogenesis. *Genes Dev* 14: 1866–1871.
Kondo T, Dolle P, Zakany J, Duboule D (1996). Function of posterior *HoxD* genes in the morphogenesis of the anal sphincter. *Development* 122: 2651–2659.
Krapp A, Knofler M, Frutiger S, Hughes GJ, Hagenbuchle O, Wellauer PK (1996). The p48 DNA-binding subunit of transcription factor PTF1 is a new exocrine pancreas-specific basic helix-loop-helix protein. *EMBO J* 15: 4317–4329.
Kuo C, Morrisey E, Anandappa R, Sigrist K, Lu M, Parmacek M, Soudais C, Leiden J (1997). GATA4 transcription factor is required for ventral morphogenesis and heart tube formation. *Genes Dev* 11: 1048–1060.
Lammert E, Cleaver O, Melton D (2001). Induction of pancreatic differentiation by signals from blood vessels. *Science* 294: 564–567.
Lawson KA, Meneses JJ, Pedersen RA (1991). Clonal analysis of epiblast fate during germ layer formation in the mouse. *Development* 113: 891–911.
Lebeche D, Malpel S, Cardoso WV (1999). Fibroblast growth factor interactions in the developing lung. *Mech Dev* 86: 125–136.
Le Douarin (1975). An experimental analysis of liver development. *Med Biol* 53: 427–455.
Li Q, Karam SM, Gordon JI (1996). Diphtheria toxin-mediated ablation of parietal cells in the stomach of transgenic mice. *J Biol Chem* 271: 3671–3676.
Li L, Krantz ID, Deng Y, Genin A, Banta AB, Collins CC, Qi M, Trask BJ, Kuo WL, Cochran J, et al. (1997). Alagille syndrome is caused by mutations in human Jagged1, which encodes a ligand for Notch1. *Nat Genet* 16: 243–251.
Li H, Arber S, Jessell T, Edlund H (1999a). Selective agenesis of the dorsal pancreas in mice lacking homeobox gene *Hlxb9*. *Nat Genet* 23: 67–71.
Li Q, van Antwerp D, Mercurio F, Lee K-F, Verma I (1999b). Severe liver degeneration in mice lacking the IκB kinase 2 gene. *Science* 284: 321–325.
Li J, Ning G, Duncan SA (2000). Mammalian hepatocyte differentiation requires the transcription factor HNF-4alpha. *Genes Dev* 14: 464–474.
Li H, Edlund H (2001). Persistent expression of *Hlxb9* in the pancreatic epithelium impairs pancreatic development. *Dev Biol* 240: 247–253.
Litingtung Y, Lei L, Westphal H, Chiang C (1998). Sonic hedgehog is essential to foregut development. *Nat Genet* 20: 58–61.
Luo G, Hofmann C, Bronckers AL, Sohocki M, Bradley A, Karsenty G (1995). BMP-7 is an inducer of nephrogenesis, and is also required for eye development and skeletal patterning. *Genes Dev* 9: 2808–2820.
Mailleux AA, Tefft D, Ndiaye D, Itoh N, Thiery JP, Warburton D, Bellusci S (2001). Evidence that SPROUTY2 functions as an inhibitor of mouse embryonic lung growth and morphogenesis. *Mech Dev* 102: 81–94.
Malpel S, Meldelsohn C, Cardoso W (2000). Regulation of retinoic acid signaling during lung morphogenesis. *Development* 127: 3057–3067.
Manley NR, Capecchi MR (1995). The role of Hoxa-3 in mouse thymus and thyroid development. *Development* 121: 1989–2003.
Martin G (1998). The roles of FGFs in the early development of vertebrate limbs. *Genes Dev* 12: 1571–1586.
Martinez Barbera J, Clements M, Thomas P, Rodriguez T, Meloy D, Kioussis D, Beddington R (2000). The homeobox gene *Hex* is required in definitive endodermal tissues for normal forebrain, liver and thyroid formation. *Development* 127: 2433–2445.
Matsumoto K, Yoshitomi H, Rossant J, Zaret KS (2001). Liver organogenesis promoted by endothelial cells prior to vascular function. *Science* 294: 559–563.
Menard D (1989). Growth-promoting factors and the development of the human gut. In: *Human Gastrointestinal Development.* Lebenthal E (ed.) Raven Press, New York.
Metzger RJ, Krasnow MA (1999). Genetic control of branching morphogenesis. *Science* 284: 1635–1639.
Min H, Danilenko DM, Scully SA, Bolon B, Ring BD, Tarpley JE, DeRose M, Simonet WS (1998). Fgf-10 is required for both limb and lung development and exhibits striking functional similarity to *Drosophila* branchless. *Genes Dev* 12: 3156–3161.
Minoo P, Su G, Drum H, Bringas P, Kimura S (1999). Defects in tracheoesophageal and lung morphogenesis in Nkx2.1(−/−) mouse embryos. *Dev Biol* 209: 60–71.
Miralles F, Czernichow P, Scharfmann R (1998). Follistatin regulates the relative proportions of endocrine versus exocrine tissue during pancreatic development. *Development* 125: 1017–1024.
Miralles F, Czernichow P, Ozaki K, Itoh N, Scharfmann R (1999). Signaling through fibroblast growth factor receptor 2b plays a key role in the development of the exocrine pancreas. *Proc Natl Acad Sci USA* 96: 6267–6272.
Molkentin J, Lin Q, Duncan S, Olson E (1997). Requirement of the transcription factor GATA4 for heart tube formation and ventral morphogenesis. *Genes Dev* 11: 1061–1072.
Morrisey EE, Tang Z, Sigrist K, Lu MM, Jiang F, Ip HS, Parmacek MS (1998). GATA6 regulates HNF4 and is required for differentiation of visceral endoderm in the mouse embryo. *Genes Dev* 12: 3579–3590.
Motoyama J, Liu J, Mo R, Ding Q, Post M, Hui CC (1998). Essential function of *Gli2* and *Gli3* in the formation of lung, trachea and oesophagus. *Nat Genet* 20: 54–57.
Narita N, Bielinska M, Wilson D (1997). Wild-type endoderm abrogates the ventral developmental defects associated with GATA-4 deficiency in the mouse. *Dev Biol* 189: 270–274.
Narita T, Saitoh K, Kameda T, Kuroiwa A, Mizutani M, Koike C, Iba H, Yasugi S (2000). BMPs are necessary for stomach gland formation in the chicken embryo: a study using virally induced BMP-2 and Noggin expression. *Development* 127: 981–988.
Naya FJ, Huang HP, Qiu Y, Mutoh H, DeMayo FJ, Leiter AB, Tsai MJ (1997). Diabetes, defective pancreatic morphogenesis, and abnormal enteroendocrine differentiation in *BETA2/neuroD*-deficient mice. *Genes Dev* 11: 2323–2334.
Nishina H, Vaz C, Billia P, Nghiem M, Sasaki T, De la Pompa J, Furlonger K, Paige C, Hui C-c, Fischer K-D, et al. (1999). Defective liver formation and liver cell apoptosis in mice lacking the stress signaling kinase SEK1/MKK4. *Development* 126: 505–516.
Obata J, Yano M, Mimura H, Goto T, Nakayama R, Mibu Y, Oka C, Kawaichi M (2001). p48 subunit of mouse PTF1 binds to RBP-Jkappa/CBF-1, the intracellular mediator of Notch signalling, and is expressed in the neural tube of early stage embryos. *Genes Cells* 6: 345–360.
Oda T, Elkahloun AG, Pike BL, Okajima K, Krantz ID, Genin A, Piccoli DA, Meltzer PS, Spinner NB, Collins FS, et al. (1997). Mutations in the human *Jagged1* gene are responsible for Alagille syndrome. *Nat Genet* 16: 235–242.
Offield MF, Jetton TL, Labosky PA, Ray M, Stein RW, Magnuson MA, Hogan BL, Wright CV (1996). PDX-1 is required for pancreatic outgrowth and differentiation of the rostral duodenum. *Development* 122: 983–995.
Ohlsson H, Karlsson K, Edlund T (1993). IPF1, a homeodomain-containing transactivator of the insulin gene. *EMBO J* 12: 4251–4259.
Ornitz D, Itoh N (2001). Fibroblast growth factors. *Genome Biol* 2: 3001–3012.
Ornitz D, Xu J, Colvin J, McEwen D, MacArthur C, Coulier F, Gao G, Goldfarb M (1996). Receptor specificity of the fibroblast growth factor family. *J Biol Chem* 271: 15292–15297.
Park W, Miranda B, Lebeche D, Hashimoto G, Cardoso W (1998). FGF-10 is a chemotactic factor for distal epithelial buds during lung development. *Dev Biol* 201: 125–134.

Pepicelli CV, Lewis PM, McMahon AP (1998). Sonic hedgehog regulates branching morphogenesis in the mammalian lung. *Curr Biol* 8: 1083–1086.

Ramalho-Santos M, Melton DA, McMahon AP (2000). Hedgehog signals regulate multiple aspects of gastrointestinal development. *Development* 127: 2763–2772.

Rawdon B (2001). Morphogenesis of gut and distribution of the progenitors of gut endocrine cells at cranial somite level of the chick embryo. *Dev Dyn* 222: 153–164.

Rehorn K-P, Thelen H, Michelson A, Reuter R (1996). A molecular aspect of hematopoiesis and endoderm development common to vertebrates and *Drosophila*. *Development* 122: 4023–4031.

Rindi G, Ratineau C, Ronco A, Candusso ME, Tsai M, Leiter AB (1999). Targeted ablation of secretin-producing cells in transgenic mice reveals a common differentiation pathway with multiple enteroendocrine cell lineages in the small intestine. *Development* 126: 4149–4156.

Roberts D (2000). Molecular mechanisms of development of the gastrointestinal tract. *Dev Dyn* 219: 109–120.

Roberts D, Johnson R, Burke A, Nelson C, Morgan B, Tabin C (1995). Sonic hedgehog is an endodermal signal inducing *Bmp-4* and *Hox* genes during induction and regionalization of the chick hindgut. *Development* 12: 3163–3174.

Roberts D, Smith D, Goff D, Tabin C (1998). Epithelial–mesenchymal signaling during the regionalization of the chick gut. *Development* 125: 2791–2801.

Robson MacDonald H, Wilson A, Radtke F (2001). Notch1 and T-cell development: insights from conditional knockout mice. *Trends Immunol* 22: 155–160.

Roebroek A, Umans L, Pauli I, Robertson E, van Leuven F, Van de Ven W, Constam D (1998). Failure of ventral closure and axial rotation in embryos lacking the proprotein convertase Furin. *Development* 125: 4863–4876.

Rones MS, McLaughlin KA, Raffin M, Mercola M (2000). Serrate and Notch specify cell fates in the heart field by suppressing cardiomyogenesis. *Development* 127: 3865–3876.

Rosenfeld M, Pritchard L, Shiojiri N, Fauso N (2000). Prevention of hepatic apoptosis and embryonic lethality in RelA/TNFR-1 double knockout mice. *Am J Pathol* 156: 997–1007.

Rosenquist G (1971). The location of the pregut endoderm in the chick embryo at the primitive streak stage as determined by radioautographic mapping. *Dev Biol* 26: 323–335.

Rossi J, Dunn N, Hogan B, Zaret K (2001). Distinct mesodermal signals, including BMPs from the septum transversum mesenchyme, are required in combination for hepatogenesis from the endoderm. *Genes Dev* 15: 1998–2009.

Sander M, Neubuser A, Kalamaras J, Ee HC, Martin GR, German MS (1997). Genetic analysis reveals that PAX6 is required for normal transcription of pancreatic hormone genes and islet development. *Genes Dev* 11: 1662–1673.

Sander M, Sussel L, Conners J, Scheel D, Kalamaras J, Dela Cruz F, Schwitzgebel V, Hayes-Jordan A, German M (2000). Homeobox gene *Nkx6.1* lies downstream of *Nkx2.2* in the major pathway of beta-cell formation in the pancreas. *Development* 127: 5533–5540.

Sanvito F, Herrera PL, Huarte J, Nichols A, Montesano R, Orci L, Vassalli JD (1994). TGF-beta 1 influences the relative development of the exocrine and endocrine pancreas in vitro. *Development* 120: 3451–3462.

Schmidt C, Bladt F, Goedecke S, Brinkmann V, Zschiesche W, Sharpe M, Gherardi E, Birchmeier C (1995). Scatter factor/hepatocyte growth factor is essential for liver development. *Nature* 373: 699–702.

Schultheiss T, Xydas S, Lassar A (1995). Induction of avian cardiac myogenesis by anterior endoderm. *Development* 121: 4203–4214.

Schwitzgebel VM, Scheel DW, Conners JR, Kalamaras J, Lee JE, Anderson DJ, Sussel L, Johnson JD, German MS (2000). Expression of neurogenin3 reveals an islet cell precursor population in the pancreas. *Development* 127: 3533–3542.

Shannon JM (1994). Induction of alveolar type II cell differentiation in fetal tracheal epithelium by grafted distal lung mesenchyme. *Dev Biol* 166: 600–614.

Shannon JM, Gebb SA, Nielsen LD (1999). Induction of alveolar type II cell differentiation in embryonic tracheal epithelium in mesenchyme-free culture. *Development* 126: 1675–1688.

Slack J (1995). Developmental biology of the pancreas. *Development* 121: 1569–1580.

Smith D, Tabin C (1999). BMP signalling specifies the pyloric sphincter. *Nature* 402: 748–749.

Smith D, Nielsen C, Tabin C, Roberts D (2000). Roles of BMP signaling and NKX2.5 in patterning at the chick midgut–foregut boundary. *Development* 127: 3671–3681.

Sosa-Pineda B, Chowdhury K, Torres M, Oliver G, Gruss P (1997). The *Pax4* gene is essential for differentiation of insulin-producing beta cells in the mammalian pancreas. *Nature* 386: 399–402.

Sosa-Pineda B, Wigle J, Oliver G (2000). Hepatocyte migration during liver development requires *Prox1*. *Nat Genet* 25: 254–255.

Stappenbeck TS, Gordon JI (2000). *Rac1* mutations produce aberrant epithelial differentiation in the developing and adult mouse small intestine. *Development* 127: 2629–2642.

St-Onge L, Sosa-Pineda B, Chowdhury K, Mansouri A, Gruss P (1997). *Pax6* is required for differentiation of glucagon-producing alpha-cells in mouse pancreas. *Nature* 387: 406–409.

Sukegawa A, Narita T, Kameda T, Saitoh K, Nohno T, Iba H, Yasugi S, Fukuda K (2000). The concentric structure of the developing gut is regulated by Sonic hedgehog derived from endodermal epithelium. *Development* 127: 1971–1980.

Sussel L, Kalamaras J, Hartigan-O'Connor DJ, Meneses JJ, Pedersen RA, Rubenstein JL, German MS (1998). Mice lacking the homeodomain transcription factor Nkx2.2 have diabetes due to arrested differentiation of pancreatic beta cells. *Development* 125: 2213–2221.

Suzuki A, Zheng Y, Kaneko S, Onodera M, Fukao K, Nakauchi H, Taniguchi H (2002). Clonal identification and characterization of self-renewing pluripotent stem cells in the developing liver. *J Cell Biol* 156: 173–184.

Takiguchi K, Yasugi S, Mizuno T (1986). Gizzard epithelium of chick embryos can express embryonic pepsinogen antigen, a marker protein of proventriculus. *Roux Arch Dev Biol* 195: 475–483.

Tefft J, Lee M, Smith S, Leinwand M, Zhao J, Bringas P Jr, Crowe D, Warburton D (1999). Conserved function of *mSpry-2*, a murine homology of *Drosophila sprouty*, which negatively modulates respiratory organogenesis. *Curr Biol* 9: 219–222.

Thomas P, Brown A, Beddington R (1998). *Hex*: a homeobox gene revealing peri-implantation asymmetry in the mouse embryo and an early transient marker of endothelial cell precursors. *Development* 125: 85–94.

Uehara Y, Minowa O, Mori C, Shiota K, Kuno J, Noda T, Kitamura N (1995). Placental defect and embryonic lethality in mice lacking hepatocyte growth factor/scatter factor. *Nature* 373: 702–705.

van den Brink GR, Hardwick JC, Tytgat GN, Brink MA, Ten Kate FJ, Van Deventer SJ, Peppelenbosch MP (2001). Sonic hedgehog regulates gastric gland morphogenesis in man and mouse. *Gastroenterology* 121: 317–328.

Waldrip W, Bikoff E, Hoodless P, Wrana J, Robertson E (1998). Smad2 signaling in extraembryonic tissues determines anterior–posterior polarity of the early mouse embryo. *Cell* 92: 797–808.

Wang LC, Nassir F, Liu ZY, Ling L, Kuo F, Crowell T, Olson D, Davidson NO, Burkly LC (2002). Disruption of hedgehog signaling reveals a novel role in intestinal morphogenesis and intestinal-specific lipid metabolism in mice. *Gastroenterology* 122: 469–482.

Warot X, Fromental-Ramain C, Fraulob V, Chambon P, Dolle P (1997). Gene dosage-dependent effects of the *Hoxa-13* and *Hoxd-13* mutations on morphogenesis of the terminal parts of the digestive and urogenital tracts. *Development* 124: 4781–4791.

Weaver M, Yingling JM, Dunn NR, Bellusci S, Hogan BL (1999). Bmp signaling regulates proximal-distal differentiation of endoderm in mouse lung development. *Development* 126: 4005–4015.

Weaver M, Dunn N, Hogan B (2000). Bmp4 and Fgf10 play opposing roles during lung bud morphogenesis. *Development* 127: 2695–2704.

Weinstein DC, Ruiz i Altaba A, Chen WS, Hoodless P, Prezioso VR, Jessell TM, Darnell JE Jr (1994). The winged-helix transcription factor HNF-3 beta is required for notochord development in the mouse embryo. *Cell* 78: 575–588.

Wells J, Melton D (1999). Vertebrate endoderm development. *Annu Rev Cell Dev Biol* 15: 393–410.

Wells J, Melton D (2000). Early mouse endoderm is patterned by soluble factor from adjacent germ layers. *Development* 127: 1563–1572.

Wessells N, Cohen J (1967). Early pancreas organogenesis: morphogenesis, tissue interactions, and mass effects. *Dev Biol* 15: 237–270.

Winnier G, Blessing M, Labosky P, Hogan B (1995). Bone morphogenetic protein-4 is required for mesoderm formation and patterning in the mouse. *Genes Dev* 9: 2105–2116.

Yamiguchi T, Harpal K, Henkemeyer M, Rossant J (1994). *fgfr-1* is required for embryonic growth and mesodermal patterning during mouse gastrulation. *Genes Dev* 8: 3032–3044.

Yang Q, Bermingham NA, Finegold MJ, Zoghbi HY (2001). Requirement of Math1 for secretory cell lineage commitment in the mouse intestine. *Science* 294: 2155–2158.

Yokouchi Y, Sakiyama J-I, Kuroiwa A (1995). Coordinated expression of *Abd-B* subfamily genes of the *HoxA* cluster in the developing digestive tract of chick embryos. *Dev Biol* 169: 76–89.

Zakany J, Duboule D (1999). Hox genes and the making of sphincters. *Nature* 401: 761–762.

Zaret K (1999). Developmental competence of the gut endoderm: genetic potentiation by GATA and HNF3/fork head proteins. *Dev Biol* 209: 1–10.

Zhang H, Bradley A (1996). Mice deficient for BMP2 are nonviable and have defects in amnion/chorion and cardiac development. *Development* 122: 2977–2986.

Zhang S, Lin Y, Itaranta P, Yagi A, Vainio S (2001). Expression of Sprouty genes 1, 2 and 4 during mouse organogenesis. *Mech Dev* 109: 367–370.

15 | Development of Epidermal Appendages: Teeth and Hair

ATSUSHI OHAZAMA AND PAUL T. SHARPE

Skin serves several functions, including thermoregulation, protection from the external environment, maintaining internal tissue fluid from evaporation, reduction of friction in water, sensation, defense against predation and infection, and supporting the hair and feathers. The distribution of pigment in skin and odors from the skin are also important for social interaction and defense. To fulfill these multiple functions, skin develops many structures as epidermal appendages (e.g., scales, feathers, hair, horns, nails, claws, sweat glands, sebaceous glands, and mammary glands). In addition, other epidermal appendages, most notably teeth, develop from the same ectoderm as skin in the oral cavity.

Vertebrate skin is composed of two distinct tissues: an outer epidermis (presumptive epithelium) derived from ectoderm and a dermis (presumptive mesenchyme) derived from mesoderm. All skin appendages develop from these two tissues. The typical skin appendage organ contains cells from both tissues. Part of the dermis of the head and the ventral tissue of the neck contain cells derived from neural crest. Cranial neural crest cells migrate into the frontonasal, maxillary, and mandibular processes from the midbrain, hindbrain, and forebrain regions of the neural tube. The mesenchyme from neural crest cells is called "ectomesenchyme" since neural crest cells are derived from neuroectoderm. Neural crest cells form the mesenchymal component of several ectodermal appendages, such as teeth and whiskers. Neural crest cells also make an important contribution to hair development, namely as melanocytes.

Although diverse structural phenotypes of appendages occur, they share common morphological features in the early stages of development. During the early development of skin appendages, epithelial components usually originate as thickenings that subsequently form buds around which the underlying mesenchymal cells condense. Interactions between the epithelial and mesenchymal tissues play central roles in regulating the morphogenesis of the appendages. When cultured alone, neither the epithelial nor mesenchymal components of these structures can differentiate into specific cells. It is also known that epithelial-mesenchymal interactions are sequential and reciprocal; i.e., there is a chain of interactive events that govern advancing development occurring in both directions between the epithelial and mesenchymal tissues (Sengel, 1986; for review, see Thesleff et al., 1995; Thesleff and Sharpe, 1997).

Experimental evidence for the role of specific genes in ectodermal appendage development has come from *in vivo* experiments using targeted mutagenesis and *in vitro* experiments with explant cultures of early skin appendage primordia. The past decade has seen remarkable advances in our understanding of the genetic control of organ development, in particular that of teeth and hair, which show many similarities in their early development.

There are many similarities (i.e., expression pattern of several genes, signaling cascades, etc.) between feathers and hair development in the early stages of development. Data on the development of feathers in chick have proven useful in understanding hair development and will be included here.

TOOTH DEVELOPMENT

Initiation

The first morphological sign of tooth development is a narrow band of thickened epithelium (primary epithelial band) on the developing jaw primodia. The buds form at discrete locations in these bands by secondary thickening of the epithelium and invagination into the underlying mesenchyme (Fig. 15–1). Narrow bands in the jaws specify the area of epithelium from which teeth can form. These bands occur in four zones, one in each quadrant of the developing mandible and maxilla. Initiation involves the mechanisms which control where a tooth will form on the developing mandibular and maxillary processes. Classical tissue recombination experiments (between tooth epithelium or mesenchyme and epithelium or mesenchyme from other parts of body), with proteolytic enzymes separating the epithelium from the mesenchyme, have been used to determine which cells carry the instructive information for the developing teeth. These classic studies (Kollar and Baird, 1969) demonstrated that the dental mesenchyme could instruct the overlying ectoderm to differentiate. When tooth mesenchyme was recombined with another source of ectoderm, such as plantar (foot) or limb ectoderm, the mesenchyme induced the ectoderm to differentiate into an enamel organ. However, any other mesenchyme, such as limb, when combined with jaw ectoderm, resulted only in keratinized cells characteristic of skin. Conversely, other evidence showed that the oral epithelium is able to induce tooth development in nonoral mesenchyme as long as the mesenchyme is neural crest derived. For example, second branchial arch and oral mesenchyme are unable to induce tooth development when recombined with any epithelium apart from the oral epithelium. Teeth formed in combinations of cranial neural crest with mandibular arch epithelium but not in combinations of cranial neural crest with limb bud epithelium (Mina and Kollar, 1987; Lumsden, 1988). Utilizing the pattern of expression of tooth specific homeobox genes such as *Msx-1* and *Barx-1* in mesenchyme, new data have resolved these inconsistencies. In the mandibular primordia of mouse, removal of epithelium at embryonic day (E) 9.5 and E10.5 (the *E* designation will be used exclusively for mouse studies) results in loss of *Msx-1* and *Barx-1* expression in the mesenchyme. When epithelium is removed from explants at E11.5, the mesenchyme retains correct spatial expression of these genes. Taken together, these results suggest that prior to E10 all ectomesenchyme cells in the mandibular arch are equally responsive to epithelial signals, indicating that there is no pre-specification of the cells into different populations and suggesting that tooth development is instructed by the epithelium. At E11, expression in mesenchyme becomes independent of epithelial signals such that removal of the epithelium does not affect spatial ectomesenchymal gene expression (Ferguson et al., 2000). From the bud stage, the direction of communication is then reversed and signals pass from the condensing mesenchyme to the epithelium.

Initiation begins before the organ anlagen is morphologically visible. Bone morphogenetic proteins (Bmps), fibroblast growth factors (Fgfs), wingless (Wnts), sonic hedgehog (Shh), and lymphoid enhancer factor-1 (Lef-1) genes are expressed in the presumptive tooth epithelium before thickening.

Sonic Hedgehog

Hedgehog proteins (see Chapter 16) constitute a family of signaling molecules involved in the development of invertebrates and vertebrates (reviewed by Hammerschmidt et al., 1997). Hedgehog gene products are secreted and interact with cell receptor ligands; they have been described as growth-modulating factors. Shh is present during feather, hair, and tooth development (Iseki et al., 1996; St-Jacques et

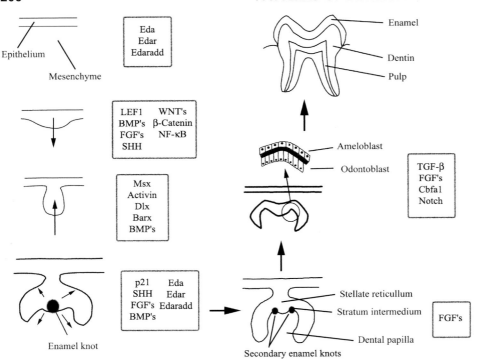

Figure 15–1. Shematic diagram showing the morphology of tooth development and the signals and transcription factors mediating the signaling as tooth development advances. The signals and transcription factors are framed and shown at right, and the corresponding morphological stages are shown at left. Signals and transcription factors form pathways and networks regulating development of the tooth from initiation through bud, cap, and bell stages. NF-κB, nuclear factor-κB; BMP, bone morphogenetic protein; FGF, fibroblast growth factor; WNT, Wingless; SHH, sonic hedgehog; TGF, transforming growth factor; LEF, lymphoid enhancer factor.

al., 1998; Chiang et al., 1999). In tooth development, *Shh* is expressed in dental epithelium at several stages, starting in the early epithelial thickenings, then reappearing in the enamel knot (see below) and subsequently in ameloblast cells (Vaahtokari et al., 1996; Iseki et al., 1996). During the initiation of mammalian tooth development, boundaries that distinguish oral from dental ectoderm must be formed to correctly position the sites of tooth formation. Interactions between the Wnts (see Chapter 22) and hedgehog signaling pathways play a role in establishing boundaries between ectodermal cells in *Drosophila* segmentation. In tooth development, *Wnt-7b* is expressed throughout the oral ectoderm except for presumptive dental ectoderm, which expresses *Shh*. *Wnt-7b* represses *Shh* expression in oral ectoderm, thus maintaining the boundaries between oral and dental ectodermal cells (Sarkar et al., 2000). Furthermore, in the developing mandible, expression of *Ptc* (see Chapter 19) and *Gli-1* are rapidly lost following removal of the epithelium, the source of Shh ligands. This is followed by ectopic expression of *Ptc* and *Gli-1* in diastema mesenchyme, which occupies the region between the sites of incisor and molar tooth formation (Sharpe et al., unpublished). Transplanting diastema epithelium onto intact incisor tooth explants results in loss of *Ptc* and *Shh* expression. It is conceivable that the diastema epithelium produces an Shh protein inhibitory factor and control of the positions of tooth inhibition thus involves a combination of specific expression of Shh at sites where teeth are required and inhibition of Shh signaling at sites where teeth are not required.

BMPs

BMPs are members of the transforming growth factor-β (TGF-β) superfamily and constitute one of the signal families that has widespread signaling functions throughout the animal kingdom (Hogan, 1996) (see Chapter 24). The best-characterized member is the *Drosophila* morphogen decapentaplegic (Dpp), which is homologous with vertebrate BMP-2 and BMP-4. During early tooth development, *Bmp-4* transcripts are present in the thickened presumptive dental epithelium. BMP-4 protein in the epithelium induces tooth-specific *Msx-1* (see Chapter 51) expression in the underlying mesenchyme (Vainio et al., 1993; ten Berge et al., 1998; Tucker et al., 1998). Expression of *Bmp-4* then shifts from the epithelium to the condensing dental mesenchyme around the tooth bud. This shift corresponds to the transfer of the potential to induce tooth formation from epithelium to mesenchyme (Neubüser et al., 1997).

Lef-1 and Wnts

Lef-1 is a transcription factor which is a member of the high-mobility group (HMG) box family of DNA-binding proteins (see Chapter 22). Interestingly, *Lef-1* was shown to be a necessary regulatory molecule for both tooth and hair development since teeth, vibrissae, and mammary glands are missing in *Lef-1* knockout mice (van Genderen et al., 1994). *Lef-1* is expressed in dental epithelial thickenings and in condensing mesenchyme of the tooth buds. Tooth development is arrested at the bud stage in *Lef-1* mutant mice (van Genderen et al., 1994). Recombination experiments using *Lef-1* mutant and wild-type tissues have revealed that *Lef-1* is required in the early thickened epithelium for tooth development (Kratochwil et al., 1996). *Lef-1* interacts with β-catenin in the cell cytoplasm, resulting in transport of the Lef-1 protein into the nucleus. β-Catenin is a component of the cell adhesion molecule E-cadherin, expression of which is localized to tooth epithelial thickenings (Kemler, 1993; Behrens et al., 1996; Huber et al., 1996). *β-Catenin* is downstream of *Wnt* signaling in *Xenopus*. Since some *Wnt* genes co-localize with *Lef-1* and *E-cadherin* in tooth epithelial thickenings, a pathway involving *Wnt* regulation of *Lef-1* expression, resulting in activation of *E-cadherin* with β-catenin as an intermediate, may be important in early tooth development (Dassule and McMahon, 1998; Sharpe, 2000). *Wnt* genes encode small proteins that are secreted from cells and interact with cell surface receptors from the *Frizzled* family. Wnt protein binding to *Frizzled* and arrow receptors activate a cascade of events within the cell that leads to signal transduction of *β-catenin* and ultimate transcription of *Wnt* gene targets. *Mouse Frizzled6* (*Mfz-6*) and Wnt agonists/antagonists *Mfrzb1*, *Wnt-10a*, and *Wnt-10b* have been identified in developing tooth primordia (Sarkar and Sharpe, 1999, 2000).

Bud Formation

As mentioned above, gene expression in mesenchyme at E11 in mice becomes independent of epithelial signals such that removal of the epithelium does not affect spatial ectomesenchymal gene expression (Ferguson et al., 2000). Following the initial signal from the thickened epithelium to the underlying mesenchyme, the direction of communication is then reversed and signals pass from the condensing mesenchyme to the epithelium (Fig. 15–1). The odontogenic mesenchyme gains the ability to instruct nondental epithelium to form tooth-specific structures, which synthesize enamel proteins (Mina and Kollar, 1987; Lumsden, 1988). This shift occurs during budding of tooth epithelium. The tooth bud can first be seen as an outgrowth of the dental lamina, which subsequently grows and undergoes organ-specific morphogenesis. Budding of the lamina marks the shifting of inductive potential from the tooth epithelium to the mesenchyme.

Msx

Msx-1-deficient mice have cleft palate, and their teeth do not develop beyond the bud stage (Satokata and Maas, 1994). *Msx-1* is expressed only in mesenchyme throughout tooth development, whereas *Msx-2* (see Chapters 51 and 52) shows spatially restricted expression in presumptive tooth epithelia and mesenchyme. *Msx-1* mutants have teeth which arrest at the bud stage, whereas *Msx-1/Msx-2* double mutants have tooth anomalies which arrest earlier than the tooth bud stage (Maas et al., 1996; Bei and Maas, 1998). In contrast, *Msx-2* mutant teeth develop normally throughout the lamina, bud, and cap stages. Necrosis of ameloblast and hypoplasia of enamel due to abnormal stratum intermedium and stellate reticulum are observed in *Msx-2* mutants (Satokata et al., 2000).

Many other genes are expressed in condensing tooth bud mesenchyme such as *Bmp-4* and *Activin-βA* (Åberg et al., 1997; Ferguson et al., 1998; see Chapter 24). The level of *Bmp-4* expression is reduced in tooth bud mesenchyme of *Msx-1* mutants, and this reduction can be rescued by addition of beads coated in BMP-4. *Msx-1* thus regulates *Bmp-4* in condensing mesenchyme during the bud stage (Chen et al., 1996). Expression of *Shh* and *Bmp-2* is downregulated in the dental epithelium of *Msx-1* mutant tooth buds, where *Bmp-4* is significantly reduced in the dental mesenchyme. Beads soaked with BMP-4 protein restore the expression of both *Shh* and *Bmp-2* in the *Msx-1* mutant epithelium. BMP-4 is also required for the maintenance of Shh and Bmp-2 expression in the dental epithelium (Zhang et al., 2000). Thus, mesenchymal BMP-4 may represent a component of a feedback signal for further tooth epithelial development beyond the bud stage (Chen and Maas, 1998).

Arrest of tooth development in *Msx-1* mutants is also associated with downregulation of *Fgf-3*, *Lef-1*, *Dlx-2*, and *Syndecan-1* in the molar mesenchyme of the tooth buds (Chen et al., 1996; Bei and Maas, 1998; Zhang et al., 1999). Addition of beads coated in BMP-4 to the *Msx-1* mutant tooth germ could partly rescue the tooth phenotype and induce *Lef-1* and *Dlx-2* expression in the absence of *Msx-1* (Chen et al., 1996; Bei and Maas, 1998). Ectopic expression of a *Bmp-4* transgene driven by the mouse Msx-1 promoter in the dental mesenchyme also restored expression of *Lef-1* and *Dlx-2* (Zhao et al., 2000). Downregulation of Bmp-4 in the molar mesenchyme may also account for the downregulation of *Lef-1* and *Dlx-2*. Fgf-3 is expressed in the dental mesenchyme from the bud stage in wild-type (Thesleff and Vaahtokari, 1992), and ectopic expression of the *Bmp-4* transgene cannot restore *Fgf-3* and *Syndecan-1* in the Msx-1 mutant molar tooth germ (Zhao et al., 2000). Expression of *Fgf-8* in dental epithelium can induce *Fgf-3* expression in the dental mesenchyme via an Msx-1-dependent mechanism distinct from that by which epithelial BMP-4 induces its own gene expression in dental mesenchyme (Bei and Maas, 1998). Downregulation of *Fgf-3* may be responsible for the downregulation of *Syndecan-1* in the Msx-1 mutant since FGFs induce *Syndecan-1* expression in dental mesenchyme (Chen et al., 1996).

Patterning

Teeth have characteristic shapes at each position in the jaws. The shape and position are specific for an animal's diet, and dentitions have diversified for particular specialized feeding functions. Incisors are conical or chisel-shaped and located at the front of the jaws, where they are used not only for obtaining and cutting food but also for grooming and defense functions. Molars are triangular, rectangular, or multicuspid in shape and located toward the back of the jaws; they are for processing food, by either cutting, grinding, or crushing. Our understanding of the formation of different shapes of teeth at their correct positions in the jaws has advanced gradually in recent years.

Classical tissue recombination experiments between presumptive incisor and molar tissues have been used to determine which cells (epithelium or ectomesenchyme) carry the instructive information to determine tooth type. These experiments indicate that tooth type is de-

termined by the epithelium (Millar, 1969; Lumsden, 1988). However, other evidence has suggested that it is the cranial neural crest–derived ectomesenchymal cells that determine tooth type (Kollar and Baird, 1969; Noden, 1983). Following observations that several homeobox genes show highly restricted expression patterns in ectomesenchyme along the proximodistal axis of the mandibular and maxillary processes, a model for tooth patterning was proposed whereby expression of these genes determines tooth type (Sharpe, 1995; Thomas and Sharpe, 1998; Thomas et al., 1998). *Dlx-2* and *Barx-1* are expressed in mesencyhmal cells that will contribute to the development of molar teeth, and *Msx-1* and *Msx-2* are expressed in mesenchymal cells that will form incisors. Expression overlaps, for example, between *Msx* and *Dlx* genes, may code for the canine and premolars of other mammals. Spatially restricted gene expression is also observed in oral epithelium, where *Bmp-4* is expressed in distal epithelium (presumptive incisor region) and *Fgf-8* expression is restricted to proximal epithelium (presumptive molar region). As previously mentioned, prior to E11.5 in mice, tooth mesenchyme is dependent on signals from the epithelium but, from E11.5, expression is independent of epithelium (Ferguson et al., 2000). *Bmp-4* expressed in the incisor epithelium induces mesenchymal expression of *Msx-1* and other homeobox genes in this region (ten Berge et al., 1998; Tucker et al., 1998). BMP-4 also inhibits FGF-8-induced expression of *Barx-1* and thereby restricts expression of this gene to presumptive molar mesenchyme. Inhibition of BMP signaling in the distal cells of E10 mandibular primordia using Noggin resulted in a transformation of tooth type from incisor to molar (Tucker et al., 1998). This transformation was probably mediated by a combination of loss of BMP-inducible distal ectomesenchymal gene expression such as *Msx-1* and ectopic expression of the proximal gene *Barx-1*, which is repressed by *Bmp-4*. Thus, tooth identity is determined by spatially restricted homeobox genes in the ectomesenchyme, but these domains are generated by positional signals from the epithelium.

Mice with targeted null mutations of both *Dlx-1* and *Dlx-2* homeobox genes have a tooth patterning phenotype where development of maxillary molar teeth is inhibited but development of all other teeth is normal (Thomas et al., 1997). Mice lacking either *Dlx-1* or *Dlx-2* (single knockouts) have normal development of all teeth. *Dlx-5* and *Dlx-6* are expressed in proximal regions of the developing mandible but not the maxilla, whereas *Dlx-1* and *Dlx-2* are coexpressed at the molar region of maxilla and mandibule. Development of mandibular molars in these mice is believed to result from the expression of *Dlx-5* and *Dlx-6*, which are functionally redundant for *Dlx-1* and *Dlx-2*. Reciprocal cell transplantations between molar regions of mandibular and maxillary arch ectomesenchymal cells show that the donor cells retain their characteristic gene expression. For example, when mandibular cells are transplanted into the maxilla, they continue to express *Dlx-5* and *-6* in an environment where they are surrounded by non-*Dlx-5*- and *-6*- expressing cells. These experiments reveal intrinsic differences between these populations of cranial neural crest–derived cells. This suggests that the cranial neural crest cells that populate these two primodia are different from each other but that, within each individual population, all cells are uncommitted with respect to hard tissue morphogenesis (Ferguson et al., 2000).

Targeted mutants in *Activin-βA*, a member of the TGF-β superfamily, develop no incisor teeth and no mandibular molars but normal maxillary molars (Ferguson et al., 1998). This phenotype is thus the reciprocal of the *Dlx-1/Dlx-2* double mutant mouse; but unlike the phenotype that can be explained by functional redundancy with other *Dlx* genes expressed in the proximal mandible, the *Activin-βA* mutant phenotype cannnot be explained by redundancy since *Activin-βA/-βB* double mutants have the same tooth phenotype as *Activin-βA* single mutants. *Activin-βA* is expressed in the mesenchyme of all developing teeth from E11 (epithelial thickening stage) in wild-type mice. Expression of Follistatin, a protein that can bind to Activin, is lost in the maxillary molar tooth germs in *Activin-βA* mutants. In addition, compound heterozygous mutants of Activin receptors can show the same tooth phenotype as *Activin-βA*, suggesting that activin receptors are not required for maxillary molar development (Heikinheimo et al., 1997; Ferguson et al., 1998, 2000). Thus, Activin signaling is required for incisor and mandibular molar development but not maxillary molar development. The molecular basis of this phenotype has yet be explained.

Origins of Epithelium Patterning

In mutants of *Ikkα*, a gene involved in the nuclear factor κB (NF-κB) pathway, incisor tooth germ epithelium does not invaginate into the underlying mesenchyme but, rather, evaginates outward into the developing oral cavity. The same phenomenon is observed in the mutant hair primordia. In these mutants, anomalies are found only in ectodermal appendages that develop through ectodermal epithelial–mesenchymal interactions (e.g., skin and whiskers) and not organs that develop through endodermal epithelial–mesenchymal interactions (e.g., lung, liver, etc.) or ectodermal placode organs (e.g., eyes, ears, and nose). Surprisingly, the anomalies are not observed in mutant molar teeth, which are thought to develop through ectodermal epithelial–mesenchymal interactions. It is thus possible that the epithelium of molar teeth is not derived from ectoderm (Sharpe et al., unpublished data).

Mineralized tooth-like structures are observed in the endodermal pharynx of some species of fish such as the zebrafish, *Danio rerio*. There is in vitro evidence that endoderm is required along with ectoderm and neural crest–derived mesenchyme for tooth development in amphibians (Cassin and Capuron, 1979; Barlow and Northcutt, 1995; Graveson et al., 1997). Elegant lineage tracing methods have also shown that even in mammals endodermal cells may contribute to the epithelial components of teeth (Imai et al., 1998). The expression pattern of the early endoderm marker gene *Claudin-6* extends into the oral cavity, into what has been considered to be ectoderm. Thus, presumptive molar epithelium that expresses *Fgf-8* also expresses *Claudin-6*, whereas presumptive incisor epithelium that expresses *Bmp-4* does not express *Claudin-6*.

This suggests that embryonic oral epithelium in the region where teeth develop is a composite of ectoderm and endoderm, with incisors being derived from ectoderm and molars from endoderm (Sharpe et al., unpublished).

Morphogenesis

Once spatial information is provided to specify development of a tooth germ into an incisor or molar, genes that control the shaping process must be activated, to produce cusps.

The patterning mechanisms outlined above are responsible for directing tooth germ cells down particular cuspal pathways of morphogenesis. A significant gap in our current understanding of patterning of the dentition is the nature of the molecules (e.g., mesenchymal genes *Dlx*, *Barx-1*, etc.) that direct the temporal and spatial folding of the internal enamel epithelium to generate cusps. Some clues have emerged from the discovery of the enamel knot as a specialized group of epithelial cells in tooth germs that act as a signaling center (Vaahtokari et al., 1996; Tucker and Sharpe, 1999). Although there is no direct evidence for an organizing capacity of the enamel knot, many of the same signals are expressed in well-known signaling or organizing centers in the embryo, such as apical ectodermal ridge in limb buds (Niswander and Martin, 1992; Riddle et al., 1993; Francis et al., 1994; Parr and McMahon, 1995; Tickle, 1995; Yang and Niswander, 1995; Crossley et al., 1996a,b). The enamel knot is a transient population of cells in the center of the invaginating dental epithelium originally identified in histological sections of cap-stage tooth germs. The cells of the enamel knot are distinct in that they are non-proliferative compared to the surrounding epithelium and mesenchyme, which have high proliferation (Vaahtokari et al., 1996). Expression of *p21*, which has a role in apoptosis, is observed in enamel knot cells. The enamel knot is transient and disappears by the late cap stage (E15 in mice). In the molars, however, secondary enamel knots develop, which are clearly visible by the use of molecular markers such as *Fgf-4* at the bell stage (E18). The only evidence for the role of enamel knots in cusp formation comes from analysis of molar development in mouse mutants with hypohidrotic (anhidrotic) ectodermal dysplasia, which are characterized by congenital defects in several organs, including hair, teeth, and some exocrine glands, in particular sweat glands. The spontaneous mouse mutation *Tabby* has an ectodermal dysplasia phenotype, and the *Tabby* gene is analogous to the gene ectodysplasin-A (Eda), a type II membrane protein of the tumor necrosis factor (TNF) ligand family (see Chapter 30) containing an internal collagen-like domain that is responsible for X-linked hypohidrotic (anhidrotic) ectodermal dysplasia in humans (Kere et al., 1996). Another spontaneous mouse mutation, *Downless*, encodes Edar, a novel member of the TNF receptor family containing the characteristic extracellular cysteine-rich fold, a single transmembrane region, and a death homology domain (Headon and Overbeek, 1999). The Tabby and Downless phenotypes are indistinguishable in adult animals. *Tabby* and *Downless* mutant mice have abnormally shaped or absent teeth (Grüneberg 1965), missing sweat glands, and absence of some hair types (Sundberg, 1994). In *Tabby* mutants, there is a recognizable but small enamel knot, whereas in *Downless* mutants the enamel knot is elongated (Pispa et al., 1999; Tucker et al., 2000). *Crinkled*, another mutant with the same phenotype, encodes Edaradd, a protein with an intracellular domain of Edar (Falconer et al., 1951; Headon et al., 2001). *Downless* and *Crinkled* are coexpressed in epithelial cells during hair follicle and tooth formation (Headon et al., 2001). As mentioned above, the *Tabby* gene encodes Eda, which is a ligand for Edar, the product of the *Downless* gene. Thus, there is a pathway in which Edar is activated by Eda and uses Edaradd as an adapter to build an intracellular signal-transducing complex. Death receptors are capable of activating NF-κB, and Edar also activates NF-κB (Yan et al., 2000; Kumar et al., 2001; Döffinger et al., 2001). Edaradd overexpression activates the NF-κB receptor gene (Headon et al., 2001).

TNFs can activate the NF-κB pathway, and NF-κB transcription factors are essential not only for inflammation and immune responses but also for bone morphogenesis, skin proliferation, and differentiation. Mice with supressed NF-κB activity, as demonstrated by ubiquitous expression of an NF-κB super-repressor, revealed defective early morphogenesis of hair follicles, exocrine glands, and teeth, identical to *Tabby* and *Downless* mutant mice. NF-κB may acts as a survival factor downstream of TNF receptor family members (Schmidt-Ullrich et al., 2001). Moreover, an NF-κB essential modulator, Ikkγ (NEMO), encoded by an X-linked gene in mice and humans, is required for NF-κB activation and resistance to TNF-induced apoptosis. Female mice heterozygous for *Ikkγ/NEMO* deficiency develop a very similar phenotype to the human genetic disorder incontinental pigmenti, which is characterized by abnormal skin pigmentation, absence of hair, and abnormal teeth (Makris et al., 2000; Schmidt-Supprian et al., 2000; Zonana et al., 2000; Döffinger et al., 2001).

Cytodifferentiation

From the cap stage onward, tooth development is characterized by cytodifferentiation of inner enamel epithelial cells into ameloblasts and dental papilla mesenchymal cells into odontoblasts. Dental mesenchyme cells will also form the tooth supporting tissue (dental follicle) and pulp (dental papilla). Ameloblasts progress through three main developmental stages: (*1*) presecretory, (*2*) secretory, and (*3*) maturation. Differentiation of odontoblasts comprises a sequence of cytological and functional changes, such as withdrawal from the cell cycle, cytoplasmic polarization, and finally, secretion and mineralization of predentin.

During dentinogenesis and amelogenesis, several tissue-specific extracellular matrix molecules are secreted, such as amelogenin and enamelin in enamel and dentin phosphoprotein (DPP) and dentin sialoprotein (DSP) in dentin. It is believed that the extracellular matrix associated with dentin or enamel plays a crucial role in controlling the mineralization process. DSP and DPP are encoded by the same gene, *dentin sialophosphoprotein (DSPP)* (Ritchie et al., 1997; MacDougall et al., 1997), which is expressed not only by differentiating and mature odontoblasts but also by a specific population of ameloblast precursors present in the inner dental epithelium (D'Souza et al., 1997; Ritchie et al., 1997; Bègue-Kirn et al., 1998). Amelogenin is also detected in both epithelial and mesenchymal cells and tissues at early stages of development, prior to the onset of dentin mineralization (Bronckers et al., 1993). Here, in common with morphogenesis, cytodifferentiation is also regulated by epithelial–mesenchymal interactions.

The specific localization patterns of growth factors during cytodifferentiation of the ameloblast lineage and/or odontoblast lineage indicate that they might play a role in their cytodifferentiation. FGF-1 might contribute to the mineralization process of the dentin matrix, and FGF-2 might be involved in the control of polarization and differentiation of odontoblasts and/or ameloblasts (Cam et al., 1992). Insulin-like growth factor (IGF)-I is also involved in dentinogenesis and amelogenesis (Joseph et al., 1993, 1994), and TGF-β1 induces odontoblast differentiation (Ruch et al., 1995).

Cbfa-1 is a transcription factor that is a key determinant of the osteoblast lineage. Evidence to support the role of Cbfa-1 as crucial for differentiation of osteoblasts was provided by genetic studies in Cbfa-1 mutant mice, which completely lack bone (Otto et al., 1997; Komori et al., 1997). Cbfa-1 is also involved in tooth crown morphogenesis and cytodifferentiation of odontoblasts and ameloblasts (D'Souza et al., 1999; Bronckers et al., 2001).

It is well established that the Notch signaling pathway (see Chapter 39) enables neighboring cells to adopt different fates (Artavanis-Tsakonas et al., 1999). Moreover, Notch is involved in the formation of boundaries that direct organ growth and patterning (Fanto and Mlodzik, 1999; Micchelli and Blair, 1999; Rauskolb et al., 1999). Notch and its ligands are also expressed in tooth development, where they are linked with the determination of rotation of incisor epithelial growth through which they acquire their characteristic shape (Mucchielli and Mitsiadis, 2000; Pouyet and Mitsiadis, 2000). In addition to these early stages of tooth development, Notch signaling correlates with ameloblast and odontoblast differentiation and is regulated by BMPs and TGF-β1 (Mitsiadis et al., 1998). Surprisingly, Notch signaling is still involved in ameloblast differentiation in adults. Mouse incisors erupt continuously throughout the life of the animal. In adult incisor teeth, stem cells reside in the cervical loop epithelium and give rise to transient amplifying progeny, which differentiate into ameloblasts. FGF signaling from the mesenchyme regulates the Notch pathway in dental epithelial stem cells (Harada et al., 1999).

HAIR DEVELOPMENT

Initiation and Bud Formation

Hair, wool, and quills are produced by follicles, which are cylindrical ingrowths of epidermis enclosing a papilla of mesodermal cells in their bases. The first recognizable structure of the site of the future hair is a placode. Placodes consist of a clump of mesenchymal cells beneath a small symmetric invagination of the epidermis (Fig. 15–2). The hair bud soon becomes club-shaped, forming a hair bulb. The epithelial cells of the hair bulb constitute the germinal matrix, which later produces the hair. The hair bulb becomes invaginated from below by a condensation of mesoderm called the "dermal papilla." The peripheral cells of the developing hair follicle form the epithelial root sheath, and the surrounding mesenchymal cells differentiate into the dermal root sheath. Proliferation of the hair bulb cells continues, thereby pushing the hair shaft upward until it emerges on the skin surface. Meanwhile, melanoblasts from the neural crest migrate into the hair bulbs and differentiate into melanocytes. The melanin produced by these cells is transferred to the hair-forming cells in the germinal matrix. By this means, the hair becomes pigmented. Arrector pili muscles, small bundles of smooth muscle fibers, differentiate from the mesenchyme surrounding the hair follicle and attach to the dermal root sheath of the hair follicles and the papillary layer of the dermis. Constrictions of the arrector pili muscles depress the skin over their attachment and elevate the skin around the hair shafts, forming tiny "goose bumps" on the surface of the skin. In the region of the neck of the hair follicles, a series of flask-shaped outgrowths from the inner coat form the sebaceous glands. In mice, the first hairs to appear on the skin surface are of fine texture and known as "lanugo." Later, these are cast off at about the time of birth and replaced by coarser hairs.

As previously mentioned, the data obtained for development of feathers in chick have proven useful for understanding hair development; thus, relevant data on feather development will be briefly described here. In feather development, the first visible sign of an individual feather rudiment is a white spot on the surface of the body; this is an epidermal placode, a localized thickening in the epidermis which then becomes underlain by a condensation of cells in the dermis, also seen in development. Each dermal papilla and the ectoderm above it proliferate, and the entire structure becomes extended into an elevated epidermal cylinder with a dermal core, the feather bud. The two sides grow unequally so that the apex moves posteriorly, and the entire structure lies almost flat on the surface of the skin (Bellairs and Osmond, 1997).

The distribution of hair over the body is relatively sparse in humans, although in mice, footpads are the only area entirely devoid of hair. The distribution of hair follicles is established during development since no additional hair follicles form after birth. Experiments with chick and mouse embryo skin, in which epidermis and meso-

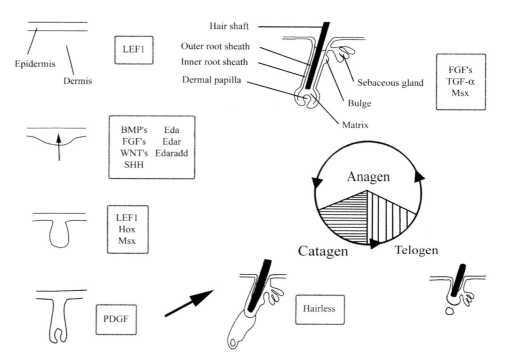

Figure 15–2. Shematic diagram showing the morphology of hair development and postnatal cycling. Signals and transcription factors mediating the signaling during advancing hair development. Signals and transcription factors are framed and shown at right, and the corresponding morphological stages are shown at left. Signals and transcription factors are involved in epithelial–mesenchymal interaction. The pie chart shows the proportion of the time the hair follicle spends in each stage. PDGF, platelet-derived growth factor; BMP, bone morphogenetic protein; FGF, fibroblast growth factor; WNT, Wingless; SHH, sonic hedgehog; TGF, transforming growth factor; LEF, lymphocytic enhancer factor.

derm are recombined and transplanted, have demonstrated that the site on the body from which the mesoderm originates plays a crucial role in the spacing of hair and feathers. When dermis is recombined with epidermis in the chick, the type of cutaneous structure made by the ectoderm is determined by the original location of the dermis (Saunders et al., 1957). These and many subsequent experiments suggest that embryonic dermis instructs overlying ectoderm to initiate placode formation. The placode transmits a signal generating a dermal condensation with hair follicle–inductive properties, and the condensation in turn sends a signal to nascent follicle keratinocytes, stimulating their proliferation, downgrowth into the developing dermis, and reorganization to form the mature follicle (Fig. 15–2) (reviewed in Sengel, 1986; Hardy, 1992; Oro and Scott, 1998).

In common with tooth development, BMP (see Chapter 24), FGF (see Chapter 32), WNT (see Chapter 22), SHH (see Chapter 16), and LEF-1 genes are expressed in the presumptive hair epithelium before thickening.

Sonic Hedgehog

At early stages of hair development, *Shh* is expressed in distinct regions of the epidermis where future hair follicles will develop. *Shh* mutant mice have anomalies of hair follicles, which are arrested after the initial stage of development. *Shh* mutants have normally spaced hair follicle placodes (Chiang et al., 1999), suggesting that *Shh* is unlikely to have an essential role in hair placode spacing in mouse embryos (St-Jacques et al., 1998; Chiang et al., 1999). No evidence has been reported of any hair anomalies in *Gli* mutants (Mo et al., 1997), although *Gli* expression is observed in hair primordia. Thus, the Shh pathway in hair development may be independent of *Gli* and/or *Ptc*. However, *Shh* is expressed in the posterior–distal feather bud epithelium and *Wnt-7a* is restricted to the posterior–proximal placode epithelium (Chuong et al., 1996). *Shh* mediates the anterior–posterior patterning of limb buds (Riddle et al., 1993), and *Wnt-7a* is involved in the dorsal–ventral patterning of limb buds (Parr and McMahon, 1995). These results suggest that these genes may also be involved in the determination of feather orientation. When Shh was ectopically expressed by a retroviral vector, feather buds with abnormal orientation were produced (Ting-Berreth and Chuong, 1996).

FGFs and BMPs

Time course studies using a synchronized epithelium–mesenchyme recombinant of chick skin showed that FGF-4, BMP-2, and BMP-4 are expressed earlier than Shh in feather primordia (Chuong et al., 1996). Feather placode formation is controlled by competition between FGF-4 and BMP-2 or BMP-4 (Oro and Scott, 1998). Transcription of all three of these genes is induced in the epithelium by the underlying dermis early in hair and feather placode formation (Oro and Scott, 1998). FGF-4-soaked beads in unpatterned epithelium induce ectopic feather buds, whereas viruses driving BMP-2 or BMP-4 production dramatically inhibit placode formation. FGF-4 also induces *Shh* in feather development. In addition, the BMP antagonist Noggin can promote feather bud formation (Jung and Chuong, 1998; Noramly and Morgan, 1998). During hair follicle development, Noggin is expressed in the follicular mesenchyme, and *Noggin* knockout mice show significant retardation of hair follicle induction. Hair placodes are induced by FGF-2 and surrounded by cells prevented from adopting a placode fate by inhibitors such as BMP-2 and BMP-4. Although these studies show that BMPs inhibit placode formation, *Bmp-4* mutant mice show retardation in the development of whisker hair follicles (Blessing et al., 1993). The precise role of BMP in the hair follicle–inductive signaling cascade may thus be more complicated (Botchkarev et al., 1999).

Notch Signaling Pathway

FGF-2-soaked beads can restore the permissive properties of scaleless epidermis and induce *Delta-1* expression and feather bud formation at the same time (Viallet et al., 1998). The positioning of *Delta-1* may be under the control of FGF-2. In hair development, Delta-1 is produced in the early placodes and inhibits surrounding cells from forming placodes (Crowe et al., 1998). Once established by FGF/BMP

competition for initial placode formation, the early placode may be further refined by the Notch signaling pathway. Favier et al. (2000) speculated, from the expression pattern of Notch-related genes in hair development, that *Delta-1*, *Notch-2*, and *Lunatic Fringe* may play a predominant role in the segregation of mesenchymal cells forming the dermal condensation.

Lef-1 and Wnts

Lef-1 expression appears in epithelium and mesenchymal components as early as the ectodermal placode stage (Zhou et al., 1995). *Lef-1* mutants lack whisker placodes and have abnormalities in body hair growth and differentiation. Tissue recombination studies show that *Lef-1* function is required in the dermis early in whisker development and later in the epidermis of the differentiating body hair (Kratochwil et al., 1996). Transgenic mice overexpressing *Lef-1* activated β-*catenin* in the ectoderm (Zhou et al., 1995; Gat et al., 1998). *Wnt-11* and *Wnt-7a* have been associated with feather development (Tanda et al., 1995; Chuong et al., 1996; Widelitz et al., 1999), and *Wnt-10b* has been confirmed in developing vibrissa follicles (Wang and Shackleford, 1996). In common with tooth development, the *Lef-1* pathway also implicates β-*catenin* and *Wnt* signaling in hair development (Gat et al., 1998). It is also possible that these signaling pathways interact with *Bmp* and *Shh* signaling pathways in hair development. In fact, a mesenchymal signal that stimulates hair follicle induction, *Noggin*, operates through antagonistic interaction with BMP-4, which results in upregulation of *Lef-1* transcription (Botchkarev et al., 1999). *Bmp-2* and -4 and *Shh* expression is lost in β-*catenin* mutant mice (Huelsken et al., 2001), and β-*catenin* overexpression in the chick results in ectopic expression of *Bmp-4* and *Shh* (Noramly et al., 1999), revealing that *Bmp-4* and *Shh* are genetically located downstream of β-*catenin*.

TNF Signaling

The Tabby (Eda, TNF ligand), Downless (Edar, TNF receptor), and Crinkled (Edaradd, intracellular domain of Downless) gene products (Fig. 15–3) are responsible for ectodermal dysplasia, which displays a phenotype in three kinds of ectodermal organ: teeth, hair, and some glands. In *Tabby* mice, hair follicle composition is abnormal because of the four different hair types normally found in mice (mice-zigzags, guard hairs, auchenes, and awls); only hairs resembling abnormal awls are found. The tooth phenotype is characterized by missing incisors and third molars, albeit with a variable penetrance, and the cusps of the first and second molars are reduced in size and number (Grüneberg, 1965). The timing of follicle development is also abnormal since development starts later than in wild-type mice (Kindred, 1967; Clax-

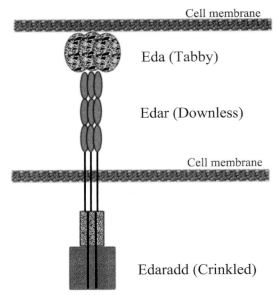

Figure 15–3. Shematic diagram showing the interaction between Eda (Tabby), Edar (Downless), and Edaradd (Crinkled).

ton, 1967). A link between *Tabby* and epidermal growth factor (EGF) signaling (Isaacs et al., 1998) has been proposed since injection of EGF can rescue the sweat gland phenotype (Blecher et al., 1990) and promote epidermal thickening and inhibition of hair fiber growth (Moore et al., 1985). Furthermore, dermal fibroblasts from *Tabby* mice have a lower amount of EGF receptor (EGFR) protein (Vargas et al., 1996). *Egf-R* mouse mutants have hair defects (Isaacs et al., 1998). *Shh* is not expressed in complementary clusters of epidermal cell in *Tabby* mutant skin at the sites of placode initiation (Headon and Overbeek, 1999). TNF signaling may be involved in hair development through the *Shh* pathway and *Egf* pathway. It has also been suggested that the *Downless* pathway is upstream of BMP expression due to the complete absence of patterned BMP expression seen in *Downless* mice. The TNF signaling pathway seems to regulate a wide variety of pathways in hair development (Headon and Overbeek, 1999).

Activin

Activin-βA null mice show normal vibrissa pad development but do not produce hair fibers (Jhaveri et al., 1998). Mouse mutants deficient in the Activin antagonist *Follistatin* show significant whisker anomalies (Matzuk et al., 1995). However, the precise role of *Activin* and *Follistatin* in hair development is not clear.

Platelet-Derived Growth Factors

Platelet-derived growth factor (PDGF) is produced by many cell types, including endothelial cells, keratinocytes, and fibroblasts; and PDGF is a known chemoattractant for fibroblasts (Seppa et al., 1982). PDGF-A and -B and their receptors, PDGF-Rα and PDGF-Rβ, have been confirmed as being present during hair follicle development. PDGF-A and -B are observed in the hair germ, while the respective receptors are expressed in the dermal papillae (Orr-Urtreger and Lona, 1992; Akiyama et al., 1996; Karlsson et al., 1999), suggesting that PDGFs may be important for epithelium–mesenchyme communication. Blocking PDGF-Rα with monoclonal antibodies during neonatal development stops the maturation of hair follicles, further supporting a role for PDGF during hair follicle differentiation (Takakura et al., 1996). Mice with a null mutation for postnatal *Pdgf-A* develop abnormal hair follicles with small dermal papillae and abnormal dermal sheaths (Karlsson et al., 1999). PDGF-A has a role in stimulating the proliferation of dermal mesenchymeal cells, which may contribute to the formation of dental papillae, mesenchymal sheaths, and dermal fibroblasts. PDGFs may be involved in hair development by regulating dermal papillae and dermal sheath development. The mutation in *Patch* that was identified as a deletion of the PDGF-Rα gene demonstrates first branchial arch deformities due to deletion of cranial neural crest–derived ectomesenchymal cells. Thus, this phenotype may result from a defect in PDGF-A ligand-mediated signal transduction using PDGF-Rα. In tooth development, PDGF-A and PDGF-Rα regulate the size and stage of tooth development via an autocrine mechanism (Chai et al., 1998).

Hox

Hox genes encode a set of evolutionarily conserved transcription factors. In mice and humans, there are 39 *Hox* genes arranged in four linkage groups (HoxA–D) on separate chromosomes (see Chapter 46). In general, the position of a gene within each complex determines the anterior limits of its expression. The 3′ genes have the most anterior limits of expression, and the anterior expression boundaries of more 5′ genes are progressively more posterior. This colinearity of expression boundaries and the position in the complex are conserved between mouse and fly. *Hoxc-13* is expressed in vibrissae, the filiform papillae of the tongue, and hair follicles throughout the body, a pattern that apparently violates spatial colinearity. Mice with mutations for *Hoxc-13* have defects in hair, vibrissa, nail, and filiform papillae development as well as in caudal vertebrae (Duboule, 1998; Godwin and Capecchi, 1998).

Skin appendage development can be divided into two stages. First, there is a decision to make a skin appendage; second, there is determination of the phenotypes (Hardy, 1968; Dhouailly, 1973; Dhouailly and Sengel 1973). Chuong et al. (1996) suggested that *Hox* genes and

neural cell adhesion molecule (NCAM) are involved in determination of the phenotypes of skin appendages mediating mesenchymal condensation. They postulated that FGFs, BMPs, and other peptide growth factors may first interact to establish a skin appendage domain. The decision made in the mesenchyme is then transmitted to the epithelium. The epithelium responds by forming placodes and expressing Shh, Wnt-7a, and Msx in the placode. Several experiments show that perturbation with reagents such as retinoic acid transforms hair into glands (Hardy, 1968), scales into feathery scales (Dhouailly et al., 1980), and feathers into scale-like structures (Chuong et al., 1992).

Patterning and Morphogenesis

Different types of hair may be produced by different kinds of follicle, and the type of hair produced in any particular follicle can change with age or under the influence of hormones. The duration of activity of follicles, or anagen, varies greatly in any species from region to region. In the rat, the dorsal hair is fully formed in 3 weeks and the shorter ventral hair in only 12 days (Johnson, 1958). Animals characteristically have both an overcoat of stiff guard hairs and an undercoat of fine hairs, but many kinds of follicle and fiber have been described. Many species also have large vibrissae or sinus hairs, which are sensory and produced from special follicles containing erectile tissue. The arrector pili muscles are poorly developed in the hairs of the axilla and in certain parts of the face, although the eyebrows and the cilia forming the eyelashes have no arrector pili muscles. Differentiation of the facial integument begins at E11.5 in the mouse, whereas body skin differentiation does not occur before E14.5. Recombination experiments have shown that regional specificity of hair is linked mainly to the origin of the dermis (Dhouaillly, 1977). It is conceivable that not all hair follicles behave identically and different types of hair may use different mechanisms of induction (Headon and Overbeek, 1999). *Lef-1* knockout mice lack whisker placodes and have abnormalities in body hair growth and differentiation but a hairy tail (van Genderen et al., 1994). *Downless* mice lack a hairy tail but have only a mild reduction in the number of whiskers (Headon and Overbeek, 1999). These data suggest that the Wnt/β-catenin/Lef-1 pathway and the *Downless* pathway may be capable of independent parallel action in whiskers and tail hairs but are likely to cooperate in a serial manner in the development of most body hairs (Barsh, 1999). *Activin* signaling also seems to be involved in the development of different types of hair since *Activin-βA* mutants show a body hair anomaly with normal whiskers (Jhaveri et al., 1998) and *Follistatin* mutants show a reciprocal phenotype (Matzuk et al., 1995).

Cycling

Unlike other organs in the adult, the hair follicle is remarkably dynamic and continuously cycles through periods of active growth (*anagen*), followed by regression (*catagen*), and inactivity (*telogen*) (Fig.15–2). The morphogenetic program that accompanies the transition from telogen to anagen bears similarities to follicle development during embryogenesis. Rapidly proliferating matrix cells in the hair bulb produce the hair shaft, whose bulk (cortex) is composed of hair-specific intermediate filaments and associated proteins. Pigment in the hair shaft is produced by melanocytes interspersed among the matrix cells. As the matrix cells differentiate and move upward, they are compressed and funneled into their final shape by the rigid inner root sheath, whose dimensions and curvature largely determine the shape of the hair. The dermal papilla, which is composed of specilized fibroblasts located at the base of the follicle, is thought to control the number of matrix cells and, thus, the size of the hair. At the onset of each new follicular cycle in adults, the dermal papillae interact with secondary germ cells in the hair follicle bulge to regenerate the low follicle. The bulge consists of a cluster of biochemically distinct cells in the outer root sheath, which are located near the insertion of the arrector pili muscle. These cells have the characteristic properties of epithelial multipotent stem sells: they are the slowest cycling and longest living epithelial cells within the hair follicle (Oshima et al., 2001). The stem cells develop into epidermis cells or sebaceous gland cells in the absence of β-catenin, whereas stem cells develop into hair follicles in the presence of β-catenin (Huelsken et al., 2001).

Msx

Msx-1 (see Chapter 51) and *Msx-2* (see Chapter 52) are also expressed during feather and hair placode development. Although mostly overlapping, there are differences between the expression of the two *Msx* genes, *Msx-1* being expressed more toward the anterior feather bud and *Msx-2* more toward the distal feather bud (Noveen et al., 1995). This may reveal that *Msx-1* and *Msx-2* also are involved in the determination of feather orientation as well as *Shh* and *Wnt-7a*. *Msx-1* and *-2* are likely to be involved in the early stages of hair development since their expression is observed from an early stage. In the skin of *Msx-1* and *-2* double mutants, the number of hair follicles is reduced to one-third that in wild-type animals, indicating the requirement of *Msx-1* and *-2* for early hair follicle induction when both genes are co-expressed in follicular mesenchyme (Reginelli et al., 1995). However, *Msx-2* is dispensable for hair initiation but essential for hair maintainance. In *Msx-2* mutant mice, hair loss is temporally associated with premature entry into the catagen phase of the hair growth cycle. Upon catagen onset, *Msx-1* is downregulated, whereas *Msx-2* expression expands to the inner root sheath, although *Msx-1* and *Msx-2* are co-expressed during the initial anagen phase (Satokata et al., 2000). This may reveal that there is functional redundancy between *Msx-1* and *Msx-2* at early stages of hair development.

TGF-β

Overexpression of *Tgf-β1* (see Chapter 24) restricted to the epidermis in transgenic mice results in suppression of epithelial cell proliferation, reduced hair follicle development, and severely curtailed life span (Sellheyer et al., 1993). *Tgf-β1* mutant mice show only a slightly reduced number of hair follicles (Foitzik et al., 1999). *Tgf-β2* mutant mice have a reduced density of hair follicles in pelage skin (Foitzik et al., 1999).

FGF-5

FGFs (see Chapter 32) can influence the growth and differentiation of cells from both the ectoderm and mesoderm. Only cursory research has been conducted on the presence and significance of FGF family members and their receptors in the hair follicle. The spontaneous mouse mutation *Angora* involves a sequence deletion in the *Fgf-5* gene. *Angora* mice have very long pelage hair due to a prolonged anagen growth phase (Sundberg et al., 1997). In addition, widely scattered hair follicles produce structurally defective shafts that twist within the follicle, presumably causing secondary hyperplasia of the outer root sheath and epidermis adjacent to the follicle. These may reveal that the length and size of hair are adjusted by regulating the hair cycle via *Fgf-5*.

Vascular Endothelial Growth Factor

Vascular endothelial growth factor (VEGF; see Chapter 101) is a tumor cell–derived factor that induces vascular hyperpermeability in response to plasma protein. VEGF plays an important role in mediating angiogenesis during development, as well as in a number of inflammatory and neoplastic diseases associated with neovascularization (Senger et al., 1983). Overexpression of *Vegf* increases the thickness of hair, whereas inhibition of *Vegf* using VEGF antibodies decreases hair number and thickness (Detmar et al., 1998; Yano et al., 2001). VEGF may be important in hair follicle embryogenesis and development of appropriate capillary blood supply for the dermal papilla.

TGF-α

TGF-α is an EGF family member. TGF-α overexpression in the epidermis of transgenic mice leads to stunted dystrophic hair growth (Vassar and Fuchs, 1991; Luetteke et al., 1993). Mice with a null mutation of *Tgf-α* have dystrophic hair follicles, producing a pelage of wavy hair equivalent to the spontaneous *Waved-1* mouse mutation (Mann et al., 1993). *Tgf-α* is expressed in epidermis, inner and outer root sheath, and the bulge region during anagen. This means that *Tgf-α* in anagen is involved in determining hair shape. Although the precise role of TGF-α in waved hair development is not clear, *Tgf-α* may affect hair development through *Downless* and *Tabby* since EGF signaling seems to be linked with TNF signaling, as previously mentioned.

Winged-Helix Nude

Nude mice have tiny hair, and their hair is easily shed after anagen phase, making them appear to completely lack hair. Nude mice are often used for transplantation because of their low immune activity. They lack T cells due to a defect of the thymus. Mutation in the winged-helix nude (*Whn*) gene results in the nude mouse and rat phenotype. The pleiotropic nude phenotype, which affects the hair, skin, and thymus, suggests that *Whn* plays a pivotal role in the development and/or maintenance of these organs (Brissette et al., 1996; Schlake et al., 1997). Some evidence shows that *Whn* is a key regulatory factor involved in maintaining the balance between keratinocyte growth and differentiation. Although *Whn* is likely to affect the cycling of hair, its precise role is not clear.

Hairless

The first hairs that appear (lanugo hairs) are fine, soft, and lightly pigmented. Lanugo hairs help to hold the vernix caseosa on the skin. These hairs are replaced during the perinatal period by coarser hairs. The *hairless* gene encodes a putative transcription factor with restricted expression in the skin and brain. Mutation in *hairless* results in progressive shedding of the lanugo hairs and lack of coarser hairs. Colocalization of *hairless* with the site of the morphological defects in mutant skin may implicate *hairless* as a key factor in regulating basic cellular processes during catagen, including club hair formation, maintainance of dermal papilla epithelial integrity, formation of an inner root sheath, and keratinocyte apoptosis in the hair follicle matrix (Panteleyev et al., 2000). However, the precise role of *hairless* in the hair cycle is not clear.

More than 100 mutations affecting mouse skin or hair have been described (Sundberg et al., 1995). The *lanceolate hair* mouse is characterized by a generalized form of alopecia associated with the breakage of abnormally formed hair shafts (Montagutelli et al., 1996). Hair shafts are short with a pronounced enlargement at their tips resembling a lance head. The *balding* mutation of the mouse causes autosomal recessive alopecia and waves of hair shedding. The hair lesions include separation of the inner and outer root sheath in anagen follicles, resulting in the hair fiber being plucked easily from the follicle (Koch et al., 1997; Montagutelli et al., 1997).

SUMMARY

Teeth and hair develop as ectodermal appendages. Although diverse in their structural phenotypes, they share morphological features and are formed by epithelial–mesenchymal interactions in the early stages of development. *Fgfs* act as inductive signals in both hair and tooth development. *Lef-1* signaling through *β-catenin* and *Wnts* is likely to similarly influence development of both tissues. *Shh* and *Activin-βA* signaling is conserved in both tissues. Redundancy between Msx-1 and −2 is observed in both tooth and hair development. The relationship between *Shh* and *Wnts* is conserved in both organs for controlling their positional expression. The *TNF* signaling pathway, involving Eda, Edar, and Edaradd, is required for normal development of teeth and hair but probably plays slightly different roles in each. *Bmps* act as inductive signals in tooth development, whereas they may act as inhibitors in hair development. *Barx-1*, *Dlx-1*, and *Dlx-2* are involved in tooth development but not in hair development. *Hoxc-13*, *Hairless*, and *Whn* are involved in hair development but not in tooth development. Each organ develops using conserved pathways for development as an ectodermal appendage and other organ-specific pathways for acquiring individual phenotypes.

ACKNOWLEDGMENTS

Work in the authors' laboratory is supported by the Medical Research Council, the Wellcome Trust, and the Biotechnology and Biological Science Research Council. A.O. is supported by Showa University (Tokyo, Japan) and Odontis, Ltd. We thank Dr. Chris Healy for critical reading of the manuscript.

REFERENCES

Åberg T, Wozney J, Thesleff I (1997). Expression patterns of bone morphogenetic proteins (Bmps) in the developing mouse tooth suggest roles in morphogenesis and cell differentiation. *Dev Dyn* 210: 383–396.

Akiyama M, Smith LT, Holbrook KA (1996). Growth factor and growth factor receptor localization in the hair follicle bulge and associated tissue in human fetus. *J Invest Dermatol* 106: 391–396.

Artavanis-Tsakonas S, Rand MD, Lake RJ (1999). Notch signaling: cell fate control and signal integration in development. *Science* 284: 770–776.

Barlow LA, Northcutt RG (1995). Embryonic origin of amphibian taste buds. *Dev Biol* 169: 273–285.

Barsh G (1999). Of ancient tales and hairless tails. *Nat Genet* 22: 315–316.

Bégue-Kirn C, Ruch JV, Ridall AL, Butler WT (1998). Comparative analysis of mouse DSP and DPP expression in odontoblasts, preameloblasts, and experimentally induced odontoblast-like cells. *Eur J Oral Sci* 106 (Suppl): 254–259.

Behrens J, von Kries JP, Kuhl M, Bruhn L, Wedlich D, Grosschedl R, Birchmeier W (1996). Functional interaction of beta-catenin with the transcription factor LEF-1. *Nature* 382: 638–642.

Bei M, Maas R (1998). FGFs and BMP4 induce both Msx1-independent and Msx1-dependent signaling pathways in early tooth development. *Development* 125: 4325–4333.

Bellains R, Osmond M (1997). Integument. In: *The Atlas of Chick Development*. Bellains R, Osmond M (eds.) Academic Press, London, UK pp. 69–72.

Blecher SR, Kapalanga J, Lalonde D (1990). Induction of sweat glands by epidermal growth factor in murine X-linked anhidrotic ectodermal dysplasia. *Nature* 345: 542–544.

Blessing M, Nanney LB, King LE, Jones CM, Hogan BL (1993). Transgenic mice as a model to study the role of TGF-beta-related molecules in hair follicles. *Genes Dev* 7: 204–215.

Botchkarev VA, Botchkareva NV, Roth W, Nakamura M, Chen LH, Herzog W, Lindner G, McMahon JA, Peters C, Lauster R, et al. (1999). Noggin is a mesenchymally derived stimulator of hair-follicle induction. *Nat Cell Biol* 1: 158–164.

Brissette JL, Li J, Kamimura J, Lee D, Dotto GP (1996). The product of the mouse nude locus, Whn, regulates the balance between epithelial cell growth and differentiation. *Genes Dev* 10: 2212–2221.

Bronckers AL, D'Souza RN, Butler WT, Lyaruu DM, van Dijk S, Gay S, Woltgens JH (1993). Dentin sialoprotein: biosynthesis and developmental appearance in rat tooth germs in comparison with amelogenins, osteocalcin and collagen type-I. *Cell Tissue Res* 272: 237–247.

Bronckers AL, Engelse MA, Cavender A, Gaikwad J, D'Souza RN (2001). Cell-specific patterns of Cbfa1 mRNA and protein expression in postnatal murine dental tissues. *Mech Dev* 101: 255–258.

Cam Y, Neumann MR, Oliver L, Raulais D, Janet T, Ruch JV (1992). Immunolocalization of acidic and basic fibroblast growth factors during mouse odontogenesis. *Int J Dev Biol* 36: 381–389.

Cassin C, Capuron A (1979). Buccal organogenesis in pleurodeles waltlii michah (urodele amphibian). Study by intrablastocelic transplantation and in vitro culture. *J Biol Buccale* 7: 61–76.

Chai Y, Bringas P Jr, Mogharei A, Shuler CF, Slavkin HC (1998). PDGF-A and PDGFR-alpha regulate tooth formation via autocrine mechanism during mandibular morphogenesis in vitro. *Dev Dyn* 213: 500–511.

Chen Y, Bei M, Woo I, Satokata I, Maas R (1996). Msx1 controls inductive signaling in mammalian tooth morphogenesis. *Development* 122: 3035–3044.

Chen YP, Maas, R (1998). Signaling loops in the reciprocal epithelial mesenchymal interaction of mammlian tooth development. In: *Molecular Basis of Epidermal Appendage Morphogenesis*. Chuong C-M (ed.) R.G. Landes, Austin, TX, pp. 265–282.

Chiang C, Swan RZ, Grachtchouk M, Bolinger M, Litingtung Y, Robertson EK, Cooper MK, Gaffield W, Westphal H, Beachy PA, et al. (1999). Essential role for Sonic hedgehog during hair follicle morphogenesis. *Dev Biol* 205: 1–9.

Chuong CM, Ting SA, Widelitz RB, Lee YS (1992). Mechanism of skin morphogenesis. II. Retinoic acid modulates axis orientation and phenotypes of skin appendages. *Development* 115: 839–852.

Chuong CM, Widelitz RB, Ting-Berreth S, Jiang TX (1996). Early events during avian skin appendage regeneration: dependence on epithelial–mesenchymal interaction and order of molecular reappearance. *J Invest Dermatol* 107: 639–646.

Claxton JH (1967). The initiation and development of the hair follicle population in tabby mice. *Genet Res* 10: 161–171.

Crossley PH, Martine S, Martin GR (1996a). Midbrain development induced by FGF8 in the chick embryo. *Nature* 380: 66–68.

Crossley PH, Minowada G, MacArthur CA, Martin GR (1996b). Roles for FGF8 in the induction, initiation, and maintainance of chick limb development. *Cell* 84: 127–136.

Crowe R, Henrique D, Ish-Horowicz D, Niswander L (1998). A new role for Notch and Delta in cell fate decisions: patterning the feather array. *Development* 125: 767–775.

Dassule HR, McMahon AP (1998). Analysis of epithelial–mesenchymal interactions in the initial morphogenesis of the mammalian tooth. *Dev Biol* 202: 215–227.

Detmar M, Brown LF, Schon MP, Elicker BM, Velasco P, Richard L, Fukumura D, Monsky W, Claffey KP, Jain RK (1998). Increased microvascular density and enhanced leukocyte rolling and adhesion in the skin of VEGF transgenic mice. *J Invest Dermatol* 111: 1–6.

Dhouailly D (1973). Dermo–epidermal interactions between birds and mammals: differentiation of cutaneous appendages. *J Embryol Exp Morphol* 30: 587–603.

Dhouailly D (1977). Regional specification of cutaneous appendages in mammal. *Roux Arch Dev Biol* 181: 3–10.

Dhouailly D, Sengel P (1973). Morphogenic interactions between reptilian epidermis and birds or mammalian dermis. *C R Acad Sci Hebd Seances Acad Sci D* 277: 1221–1224.

Dhouailly D, Hardy MH, Sengel P (1980). Formation of feathers on chick foot scales: a stage-dependent morphogenetic response to retinoic acid. *J Embryol Exp Morphol* 58: 63–78.

Döffinger R, Smahi A, Bessia C, Geissmann F, Feinberg J, Durandy A, Bodemer C, Kenwrick S, Dupuis-Girod S, Blanche S, et al. (2001). X-linked anhidrotic ectodermal dysplasia with immunodeficiency is caused by impaired NF-kappaB signaling. *Nat Genet* 27: 277–285.

D'Souza RN, Cavender A, Sunavala G, Alvarez J, Ohshima T, Kulkarni AB, MacDougall M (1997). Gene expression patterns of murine dentin matrix protein 1 (Dmp1) and dentin sialophosphoprotein (DSPP) suggest distinct developmental functions in vivo. *J Bone Miner Res* 12: 2040–2049.

D'Souza RN, Aberg T, Gaikwad J, Cavender A, Owen M, Karsenty G, Thesleff I (1999). Cbfa1 is required for epithelial–mesenchymal interactions regulating tooth development in mice. *Development* 126: 2911–2920.

Duboule D (1998). Hox is in the hair: a break in colinearity? *Genes Dev* 12: 1–4.

Falconer DS, Fraser AS, King JWB (1951). The genetics and development of "crinkled" a new mutant in the mouse. *J Genet* 50: 324–344.

Fanto M, Mlodzik M (1999). Asymmetric Notch activation specifies photoreceptors R3 and R4 and planar polarity in the *Drosophila* eye. *Nature* 397: 523–526.

Favier B, Fliniaux I, Thelu J, Viallet JP, Demarchez M, Jahoda CA, Dhouailly D (2000). Localisation of members of the notch system and the differentiation of vibrissa hair follicles: receptors, ligands, and fringe modulators. *Dev Dyn* 218: 426–437.

Ferguson CA, Tucker AS, Christensen L, Lau AL, Matzuk MM, Sharpe PT (1998). Activin is an essential early mesenchymal signal in tooth development that is required for patterning of the murine dentition. *Genes Dev* 12: 2636–2649.

Ferguson CA, Tucker AS, Sharpe PT (2000). Temporospatial cell interactions regulating mandibular and maxillary arch patterning. *Development* 127: 403–412.

Foitzik K, Paus R, Doetschman T, Dotto GP (1999). The TGF-beta2 isoform is both a required and sufficient inducer of murine hair follicle morphogenesis. *Dev Biol* 212: 278–289.

Francis PH, Richardson MK, Brickell PM, Tickle C (1994). Bone morphogenetic proteins and a signalling pathway that controls patterning in the developing chick limb. *Development* 120: 209–218.

Gat U, DasGupta R, Degenstein L, Fuchs E (1998). De novo hair follicle morphogenesis and hair tumors in mice expressing a truncated beta-catenin in skin. *Cell* 95: 605–614.

Godwin AR, Capecchi MR (1998). Hoxc13 mutant mice lack external hair. *Genes Dev* 12: 11–20.

Graveson AC, Smith MM, Hall BK (1997). Neural crest potential for tooth development in a urodele amphibian: developmental and evolutionary significance. *Dev Biol* 188: 34–42.

Grüneberg H (1965). Genes and genotypes affecting the teeth of the mouse. *J Embryol Exp Morphol* 14: 137–159.

Hammerschmidt M, Brook A, McMahon AP (1997). The world according to hedgehog. *Trends Genet* 13: 14–21.

Harada H, Kettunen P, Jung HS, Mustonen T, Wang YA, Thesleff I (1999). Localization of putative stem cells in dental epithelium and their association with Notch and FGF signaling. *J Cell Biol* 147: 105–120.

Hardy MH (1968). Glandular metaplasia of hair follicles and other responses to vitamin A excess in cultures of rodent skin. *J Embryol Exp Morphol* 19: 157–180.

Hardy MH (1992). The secret life of the hair follicle. *Trends Genet* 8: 55–61.

Headon DJ, Overbeek PA (1999). Involvement of a novel Tnf receptor homologue in hair follicle induction. *Nat Genet* 22: 370–374.

Headon DJ, Emmal SA, Ferguson BM, Tucker AS, Justice MJ, Zonana J, Overbeek PA (2001). Gene defect in ectodermal dysplasia implicates a novel death domain adaptor in development. *Nature* 414: 913–916.

Heikinheimo K, Begue-Kirn C, Ritvos O, Tuuri T, Ruch JV (1997). The activin-binding protein follistatin is expressed in developing murine molar and induces odontoblast-like cell differentiation in vitro. *J Dent Res* 76: 1625–1636.

Hogan BL (1996). Bone morphogenetic proteins in development. *Curr Opin Genet Dev* 6: 432–438.

Huber O, Korn R, McLaughlin J, Ohsugi M, Herrmann BG, Kemler R (1996). Nuclear localization of beta-catenin by interaction with transcription factor LEF-1. *Mech Dev* 59: 3–10.

Huelsken J, Vogel R, Erdmann B, Cotsarelis G, Birchmeier W (2001). Beta-catenin controls hair follicle morphogenesis and stem cell differentiation in the skin. *Cell* 105: 533–545.

Imai H, Osumi N, Eto K (1998). Contribution of foregut endoderm to tooth initiation of mandibular incisor in rat embryos. *Eur J Oral Sci* 106(Suppl l): 19–23.

Isaacs K, Brown G, Moore GP (1998). Interactions between epidermal growth factor and the Tabby mutation in skin. *Exp Dermatol* 7: 273–280.

Iseki S, Araga A, Ohuchi H, Nohno T, Yoshioka H, Hayashi F, Noji S (1996). Sonic hedgehog is expressed in epithelial cells during development of whisker, hair, and tooth. *Biochem Biophys Res Commun* 218: 688–693.

Jhaveri S, Erzurumlu RS, Chiaia N, Kumar TR, Matzuk MM (1998). Defective whisker follicles and altered brainstem patterns in activin and follistatin knockout mice. *Mol Cell Neurosci* 12: 206–219.

Johnson E (1958). Quantitative studies of hair growth in the albino rat. I. Normal males and females. *J Endcrinol* 16: 337–350.

Joseph BK, Savage NW, Young WG, Gupta GS, Breier BH, Waters MJ (1993). Expression and regulation of insulin-like growth factor-I in the rat incisor. *Growth Factors* 8: 267–275.

Joseph BK, Savage NW, Young WG, Waters MJ (1994). Insulin-like growth factor-I receptor in the cell biology of the ameloblast: an immunohistochemical study on the rat incisor. *Epithelial Cell Biol* 3: 47–53.

Jung HS, Chuong CM (1998). Periodic pattern formation of the feathers. In: *Molecular Basis of Epithelial Appendage Morphogenesis*. Chuong CM (ed.) R.G. Landes, Austin, TX, pp. 359–370.

Karlsson L, Bondjers C, Betsholtz C (1999). Roles for PDGF-A and sonic hedgehog in development of mesenchymal components of the hair follicle. *Development* 126: 2611–2621.

Kemler R (1993). From cadherins to catenins: cytoplasmic protein interactions and regulation of cell adhesion. *Trends Genet* 9: 317–321.

Kere J, Srivastava AK, Montonen O, Zonana J, Thomas N, Ferguson B, Munoz F, Morgan D, Clarke A, Baybayan P, et al. (1996). X-linked anhidrotic (hypohidrotic) ectodermal dysplasia is caused by mutation in a novel transmembrane protein. *Nat Genet* 13: 409–416.

Kindred B (1967). Some observations on the skin and hair of tabby mice. *J Hered* 58: 197–199.
Koch PJ, Mahoney MG, Ishikawa H, Pulkkinen L, Uitto J, Shultz L, Murphy GF, Whitaker-Menezes D, Stanley JR (1997). Targeted disruption of the pemphigus vulgaris antigen (desmoglein 3) gene in mice causes loss of keratinocyte cell adhesion with a phenotype similar to pemphigus vulgaris. *J Cell Biol* 137: 1091–1102.
Kollar EJ, Baird GR (1969). The influence of the dental papilla on the development of tooth shape in embryonic mouse tooth germs. *J Embryol Exp Morphol* 21: 131–148.
Komori T, Yagi H, Nomura S, Yamaguchi A, Sasaki K, Deguchi K, Shimizu Y, Bronson RT, Gao YH, Inada M, et al. (1997). Targeted disruption of Cbfa1 results in a complete lack of bone formation owing to maturational arrest of osteoblasts. *Cell* 89: 755–764.
Kratochwil K, Dull M, Farinas I, Galceran J, Grosschedl R (1996). Lef1 expression is activated by BMP-4 and regulates inductive tissue interactions in tooth and hair development. *Genes Dev* 10: 1382–1394.
Kumar A, Eby MT, Sinha S, Jasmin A, Chaudhary PM (2001). The ectodermal dysplasia receptor activates the nuclear factor-kappaB, JNK, and cell death pathways and binds to ectodysplasin A. *J Biol Chem* 276: 2668–2677.
Luetteke NC, Qiu TH, Peiffer RL, Oliver P, Smithies O, Lee DC (1993). TGF alpha deficiency results in hair follicle and eye abnormalities in targeted and waved-1 mice. *Cell* 73: 263–278.
Lumsden AG (1988). Spatial organization of the epithelium and the role of neural crest cells in the initiation of the mammalian tooth germ. *Development* 103(Suppl): 155–169.
Maas R, Chen YP, Bei M, Woo I, Satokata I (1996). The role of *Msx* genes in mammalian development. *Ann NY Acad Sci* 785: 171–181.
MacDougall M, Simmons D, Luan X, Nydegger J, Feng J, Gu TT (1997). Dentin phosphoprotein and dentin sialoprotein are cleavage products expressed from a single transcript coded by a gene on human chromosome 4. Dentin phosphoprotein DNA sequence determination. *J Biol Chem* 272: 835–842.
Makris C, Godfrey VL, Krahn-Senftleben G, Takahashi T, Roberts JL, Schwarz T, Feng L, Johnson RS, Karin M (2000). Female mice heterozygous for IKK gamma/NEMO deficiencies develop a dermatopathy similar to the human X-linked disorder incontinentia pigmenti. *Mol Cells* 5: 969–979.
Mann GB, Fowler KJ, Gabriel A, Nice EC, Williams RL, Dunn AR (1993). Mice with a null mutation of the TGF alpha gene have abnormal skin architecture, wavy hair, and curly whiskers and often develop corneal inflammation. *Cell* 73: 249–261.
Matzuk MM, Lu N, Vogel H, Sellheyer K, Roop DR, Bradley A (1995). Multiple defects and perinatal death in mice deficient in follistatin. *Nature* 374: 360–363.
Micchelli CA, Blair SS (1999). Dorsoventral lineage restriction in wing imaginal discs requires Notch. *Nature* 401: 473–476.
Millar WA (1969). Inductive changes in early tooth development. I. A study of mouse tooth development on the chick choriallantois. *J Dent Res* 48: 719–725.
Mina M, Kollar EJ (1987). The induction of odontogenesis in non-dental mesenchyme combined with early murine mandibular arch epithelium. *Arch Oral Biol* 32: 123–127.
Mitsiadis TA, Hirsinger E, Lendahl U, Goridis C (1998). Delta-notch signaling in odontogenesis: correlation with cytodifferentiation and evidence for feedback regulation. *Dev Biol* 204: 420–431.
Mo R, Freer AM, Zinyk DL, Crackower MA, Michaud J, Heng HH, Chik KW, Shi XM, Tsui LC, Cheng SH, et al. (1997). Specific and redundant functions of Gli2 and Gli3 zinc finger genes in skeletal patterning and development. *Development* 124: 113–123.
Montagutelli X, Hogan ME, Aubin G, Lalouette A, Guenet JL, King LE Jr, Sundberg JP (1996). Lanceolate hair (lah): a recessive mouse mutation with alopecia and abnormal hair. *J Invest Dermatol* 107: 20–25.
Montagutelli X, Lalouette A, Boulouis HJ, Guenet JL, Sundberg JP (1997). Vesicle formation and follicular root sheath separation in mice homozygous for deleterious alleles at the balding (bal) locus. *J Invest Dermatol* 109: 324–328.
Moore GP, Panaretto BA, Carter NB (1985). Epidermal hyperplasia and wool follicle regression in sheep infused with epidermal growth factor. *J Invest Dermatol* 84: 172–175.
Mucchielli ML, Mitsiadis TA (2000). Correlation of asymmetric Notch2 expression and mouse incisor rotation. *Mech Dev* 91: 379–382.
Neubüser A, Peters H, Balling R, Martin GR (1997). Antagonistic interactions between FGF and BMP signaling pathways: a mechanism for positioning the sites of tooth formation. *Cell* 90: 247–255.
Niswander L, Martin GR (1992). Fgf-4 expression during gastrulation, myogenesis, limb and tooth development in the mouse. *Development* 114: 755–768.
Noden DM (1983). The role of the neural crest in patterning of avian cranial skeletal, connective, and muscle tissues. *Dev Biol* 96: 144–165.
Noramly S, Morgan BA (1998). BMPs mediate lateral inhibition at successive stages in feather tract development. *Development* 125: 3775–3787.
Noramly S, Freeman A, Morgan BA (1999). Beta-catenin signaling can initiate feather bud development. *Development* 126: 3509–3521.
Noveen A, Jiang TX, Ting-Berreth SA, Chuong CM (1995). Homeobox genes *Msx-1* and *Msx-2* are associated with induction and growth of skin appendages. *J Invest Dermatol* 104: 711–719.
Oro AE, Scott MP (1998). Splitting hairs: dissecting roles of signaling systems in epidermal development. *Cell* 95: 575–588.
Orr-Urtreger A, Lonai P (1992). Platelet-derived growth factor-A and its receptor are expressed in separate, but adjacent cell layers of the mouse embryo. *Development* 115: 1045–1058.
Oshima H, Rochat A, Kedzia C, Kobayashi K, Barrandon Y (2001). Morphogenesis and renewal of hair follicles from adult multipotent stem cells. *Cell* 104: 233–245.
Otto F, Thornell AP, Crompton T, Denzel A, Gilmour KC, Rosewell IR, Stamp GW, Beddington RS, Mundlos S, Olsen BR, et al. (1997). Cbfa1, a candidate gene for cleidocranial dysplasia syndrome, is essential for osteoblast differentiation and bone development. *Cell* 89: 765–771.
Panteleyev AA, Paus R, Christiano AM (2000). Patterns of hairless (hr) gene expression in mouse hair follicle morphogenesis and cycling. *Am J Pathol* 157: 1071–1079.
Parr BA, McMahon AP (1995). Dorsalizing signal Wnt-7a required for normal polarity of D–V and A–P axes of mouse limb. *Nature* 374: 350–353.
Pispa J, Jung HS, Jernvall J, Kettunen P, Mustonen T, Tabata MJ, Kere J, Thesleff I (1999). Cusp patterning defect in Tabby mouse teeth and its partial rescue by FGF. *Dev Biol* 216: 521–534.
Pouyet L, Mitsiadis TA (2000). Dynamic Lunatic fringe expression is correlated with boundaries formation in developing mouse teeth. *Mech Dev* 91: 399–402.
Rauskolb C, Correia T, Irvine KD (1999). Fringe-dependent separation of dorsal and ventral cells in the *Drosophila* wing. *Nature* 401: 476–480.
Reginelli AD, Wang YQ, Sassoon D, Muneoka K (1995). Digit tip regeneration correlates with regions of Msx1 (Hox 7) expression in fetal and newborn mice. *Development* 121: 1065–1076.
Riddle RD, Johnson RL, Laufer E, Tabin C (1993). Sonic hedgehog mediates the polarizing activity of the ZPA. *Cell* 75: 1401–1416.
Ritchie HH, Berry JE, Somerman MJ, Hanks CT, Bronckers AL, Hotton D, Papagerakis P, Berdal A, Butler WT (1997). Dentin sialoprotein (DSP) transcripts: developmentally-sustained expression in odontoblasts and transient expression in pre-ameloblasts. *Eur J Oral Sci* 105: 405–413.
Ruch JV, Lesot H, Begue-Kirn C (1995). Odontoblast differentiation. *Int J Dev Biol* 39: 51–68.
Sarkar L, Sharpe PT (1999). Expression of Wnt signalling pathway genes during tooth development. *Mech Dev* 85: 197–200.
Sarkar L, Sharpe PT (2000). Inhibition of Wnt signaling by exogenous Mfrzb1 protein affects molar tooth size. *J Dent Res* 79: 920–925.
Sarkar L, Cobourne M, Naylor S, Smalley M, Dale T, Sharpe PT (2000). Wnt/Shh interactions regulate ectodermal boundary formation during mammalian tooth development. *Proc Natl Acad Sci USA* 97: 4520–4524.
Satokata I, Maas R (1994). Msx1 deficient mice exhibit cleft palate and abnormalities of craniofacial and tooth development. *Nat Genet* 6: 348–356.
Satokata I, Ma L, Ohshima H, Bei M, Woo I, Nishizawa K, Maeda T, Takano Y, Uchiyama M, Heaney S, et al. (2000). Msx2 deficiency in mice causes pleiotropic defects in bone growth and ectodermal organ formation. *Nat Genet* 24: 391–395.
Saunders JW Jr, Cairns JM, Gasseling MT (1957). The role of the apical ectodermal ridge of ectoderm in the differentiation of the morphological structure of and inductive specificity of limb parts of the chick. *J Morphol* 101: 57–88.
Schlake T, Schorpp M, Nehls M, Boehm T (1997). The nude gene encodes a sequence-specific DNA binding protein with homologs in organisms that lack an anticipatory immune system. *Proc Natl Acad Sci USA* 94: 3842–3847.
Schmidt-Supprian M, Bloch W, Courtois G, Addicks K, Israel A, Rajewsky K, Pasparakis M (2000). NEMO/IKK gamma-deficient mice model incontinentia pigmenti. *Mol Cell* 5: 981–992.
Schmidt-Ullrich R, Aebischer T, Hulsken J, Birchmeier W, Klemm U, Scheidereit C (2001). Requirement of NF-kappaB/Rel for the development of hair follicles and other epidermal appendices. *Development* 128: 3843–3853.
Sellheyer K, Bickenbach JR, Rothnagel JA, Bundman D, Longley MA, Krieg T, Roche NS, Roberts AB, Roop DR (1993). Inhibition of skin development by overexpression of transforming growth factor beta 1 in the epidermis of transgenic mice. *Proc Natl Acad Sci USA* 90: 5237–5241.
Sengel P (1986). Epidermal–dermal interaction. In: *Biology of the Integument 2. Vertebrates*. Bereiter-Hahn J, Matoltsy AG, Richards KS (eds.) Springer-Verlag, Berlin, pp. 374–408.
Senger DR, Galli SJ, Dvorak AM, Perruzzi CA, Harvey VS, Dvorak HF (1983). Tumor cells secrete a vascular permeability factor that promotes accumulation of ascites fluid. *Science* 219: 983–985.
Seppa H, Grotendorst G, Seppa S, Schiffmann E, Martin GR (1982). Platelet-derived growth factor in chemotactic for fibroblasts. *J Cell Biol* 92: 584–588.
Sharpe PT (1995). Homeobox genes and orofacial development. *Connect Tissue Res* 32: 17–25.
Sharpe PT (2000). Homeobox genes in initiation and shape of teeth during development in mammalian embryos. In: *Development, Function and Evolution of Teeth*. Teaford MF, Smith MM, Fergason MWJ (eds.) Oxford University Press, Oxford, pp. 133–151.
St-Jacques B, Dassule HR, Karavanova I, Botchkarev VA, Li J, Danielian PS, McMahon JA, Lewis PM, Paus R, McMahon AP (1998). Sonic hedgehog signaling is essential for hair development. *Curr Biol* 8: 1058–1068.
Sundberg JP (1994). The downless (dl) and Sleek (Dl^{seek}) mutations, chromosome 10. In: *Handbook of Mouse Mutations with Skin and Hair Abnormalities*. Maibach HI (ed.) CRC Press, Boca Raton, FL, pp. 241–229.
Sundberg JP, Oliver RF, McElwee KJ, King LE Jr (1995). Alopecia areata in humans and other mammalian species. *J Invest Dermatol* 104: 32S–33S.
Sundberg JP, Rourk MH, Boggess D, Hogan ME, Sundberg BA, Bertolino AP (1997). Angora mouse mutation: altered hair cycle, follicular dystrophy, phenotypic maintenance of skin grafts, and changes in keratin expression. *Vet Pathol* 34: 171–179.
Takakura N, Yoshida H, Kunisada T, Nishikawa S, Nishikawa SI (1996). Involvement of platelet-derived growth factor receptor-alpha in hair canal formation. *J Invest Dermatol* 107: 770–777.
Tanda N, Ohuchi H, Yoshioka H, Noji S, Nohno T (1995). A chicken *Wnt* gene, *Wnt-11*, is involved in dermal development. *Biochem Biophys Res Commun* 211: 123–129.
ten Berge D, Brouwer A, el Bahi S, Guenet JL, Robert B, Meijlink F (1998). Mouse *Alx3*: an aristaless-like homeobox gene expressed during embryogenesis in ectomesenchyme and lateral plate mesoderm. *Dev Biol* 199: 11–25.
Thesleff I, Sharpe P (1997). Signalling networks regulating dental development. *Mech Dev* 67: 111–123.
Thesleff I, Vaahtokari A (1992). The role of growth factors in determination and differentiation of the odontoblastic cell lineage. *Proc Finn Dent Soc* 88(Suppl 1): 357–368.
Thesleff I, Vaahtokari A, Partanen AM (1995). Regulation of organogenesis. Common molecular mechanisms regulating the development of teeth and other organs. *Int J Dev Biol* 39: 35–50.
Thomas BL, Sharpe PT (1998). Patterning of the murine dentition by homeobox genes. *Eur J Oral Sci* 106(Suppl 1): 48–54.

Thomas BL, Tucker AS, Qui M, Ferguson CA, Hardcastle Z, Rubenstein JL, Sharpe PT (1997). Role of *Dlx-1* and *Dlx-2* genes in patterning of the murine dentition. *Development* 124: 4811–4818.

Thomas BL, Tucker AS, Ferguson C, Qui M, Rubenstein JL, Sharpe PT (1998). Molecular control of odontogenic patterning: positional dependent initiation and morphogenesis. *Eur J Oral Sci* 106(Suppl 1): 44–47.

Tickle C (1995). Verterate limb development. *Curr Opin Genet Dev* 5: 478–484.

Ting-Berreth SA, Chuong CM (1996). Sonic hedgehog in feather morphogenesis: induction of mesenchymal condensation and association with cell death. *Dev Dyn* 207: 157–170.

Tucker AS, Sharpe PT (1999). Molecular genetics of tooth morphogenesis and patterning: the right shape in the right place. *J Dent Res* 78: 826–834.

Tucker AS, Matthews KL, Sharpe PT (1998). Transformation of tooth type induced by inhibition of BMP signaling. *Science* 282: 1136–1138.

Tucker AS, Headon DJ, Schneider P, Ferguson BM, Overbeek P, Tschopp J, Sharpe PT (2000). Edar/Eda interactions regulate enamel knot formation in tooth morphogenesis. *Development* 127: 4691–4700.

Vaahtokari A, Aberg T, Jernvall J, Keranen S, Thesleff I (1996). The enamel knot as a signaling center in the developing mouse tooth. *Mech Dev* 54: 39–43.

Vainio S, Karavanova I, Jowett A, Thesleff I (1993). Identification of BMP-4 as a signal mediating secondary induction between epithelial and mesenchymal tissues during early tooth development. *Cell* 75: 45–58.

van Genderen C, Okamura RM, Farinas I, Quo RG, Parslow TG, Bruhn L, Grosschedl R (1994). Development of several organs that require inductive epithelial–mesenchymal interactions is impaired in LEF-1-deficient mice. *Genes Dev* 8: 2691–2703.

Vargas GA, Fantino E, George-Nascimento C, Gargus JJ, Haigler HT (1996). Reduced epidermal growth factor receptor expression in hypohidrotic ectodermal dysplasia and Tabby mice. *J Clin Invest* 97: 2426–2432.

Vassar R, Fuchs E (1991). Transgenic mice provide new insights into the role of TGF-alpha during epidermal development and differentiation. *Genes Dev* 5: 714–727.

Viallet JP, Prin F, Olivera-Martinez I, Hirsinger E, Pourquie O, Dhouailly D (1998). Chick *Delta-1* gene expression and the formation of the feather primordia. *Mech Dev* 72: 159–168.

Wang J, Shackleford GM (1996). Murine Wnt10a and Wnt10b: cloning and expression in developing limbs, face and skin of embryos and in adults. *Oncogene* 13: 1537–1544.

Widelitz RB, Jiang TX, Chen CW, Stott NS, Chuong CM (1999). Wnt-7a in feather morphogenesis: involvement of anterior–posterior asymmetry and proximal–distal elongation demonstrated with an in vitro reconstitution model. *Development* 126: 2577–2587.

Yan M, Wang LC, Hymowitz SG, Schilbach S, Lee J, Goddard A, de Vos AM, Gao WQ, Dixit VM (2000). Two-amino acid molecular switch in an epithelial morphogen that regulates binding to two distinct receptors. *Science* 290: 523–527.

Yang Y, Niswander L (1995). Interaction between the signalling molecules WNT7a and SHH during vertebrate limb development: dorsal signals regulate anteroposterior patterning. *Cell* 80: 939–947.

Yano K, Brown LF, Detmar M (2001). Control of hair growth and follicle size by VEGF-mediated angiogenesis. *J Clin Invest* 107: 409–417.

Zhang Y, Zhao X, Hu Y, St Amand T, Zhang M, Ramamurthy R, Qiu M, Chen Y (1999). Msx1 is required for the induction of Patched by Sonic hedgehog in the mammalian tooth germ. *Dev Dyn* 215: 45–53.

Zhang Y, Zhang Z, Zhao X, Yu X, Hu Y, Geronimo B, Fromm SH, Chen YP (2000). A new function of BMP4: dual role for BMP4 in regulation of Sonic hedgehog expression in the mouse tooth germ. *Development* 127: 1431–1443.

Zhao X, Zhang Z, Song Y, Zhang X, Zhang Y, Hu Y, Fromm SH, Chen Y (2000). Transgenically ectopic expression of Bmp4 to the Msx1 mutant dental mesenchyme restores downstream gene expression but represses Shh and Bmp2 in the enamel knot of wild type tooth germ. *Mech Dev* 99: 29–38.

Zhou P, Byrne C, Jacobs J, Fuchs E (1995). Lymphoid enhancer factor 1 directs hair follicle patterning and epithelial cell fate. *Genes Dev* 9: 700–713.

Zonana J, Elder ME, Schneider LC, Orlow SJ, Moss C, Golabi M, Shapira SK, Farndon PA, Wara DW, Emmal SA, et al. (2000). A novel X-linked disorder of immune deficiency and hypohidrotic ectodermal dysplasia is allelic to incontinentia pigmenti and due to mutations in IKK-gamma (NEMO). *Am J Hum Genet* 67: 1555–1562.

III

DEFINED PATHWAYS

Part A.
The Sonic Hedgehog Signaling Pathway

16 | An Introduction to Sonic Hedgehog Signaling

M. MICHAEL COHEN, JR.

Members of the hedgehog family of secreted proteins act on intercellular signals in a host of different processes. Hedgehog (*Hh*; human homologues including *Sonic Hedgehog* or *SHH*) genes play a key role in embryonic patterning. Nüsslein-Volhard and Wieschaus (1980), in screening for mutations that disrupt the *Drosophila* larval body plan, identified several that resulted in duplication of the bristles; their projection from the larval cuticle suggested the spines of a hedgehog to the authors.

The term "hedgehog signaling pathway" is most commonly used. However, the "pathway" is so complex, and such strikingly different phenotypes can result from various types of mutations (Table 16–1), the term "hedgehog signaling network" seems more appropriate. Phenotypes include, among others, holoprosencephaly, nevoid basal cell carcinoma syndrome, Greig cephalopolysyndactyly, Pallister-Hall syndrome, Rubinstein-Taybi syndrome, isolated basal cell carcinoma, and medulloblastoma (Cohen, 1999). Additional phenotypes possibly include multiple exostoses and VACTERL. One target gene upregulates a pathway involved in adenomatous polyposis coli (*APC*).

The hedgehog signaling network has been reviewed by Hahn et al. (1999), Ingham and McMahon (2001), Bale (2002), Ho and Scott (2002), Mullor et al. (2002), Nybakken and Perrimon (2002), Ruiz i Altaba et al. (2002), Cohen (2003b), and Roessler and Muenke (2003). This chapter is based on Cohen (2003b).

The hedgehog signaling network is illustrated in Figures 16–1, 16–2 (*Drosophila* genes; human homologues in parentheses), and 16–3.

Table 16–2 lists some human genes in the network, their chromosome map locations, and their expression patterns.

A general description of the signaling network is presented first. An analysis of each component follows. The last section deals with mutations, gene overexpression, and teratogens that involve the hedgehog signaling network and cholesterol biosynthesis in animals.

GENERAL DESCRIPTION OF THE SIGNALING NETWORK

Although great progress has been made in understanding the hedgehog signaling network, many uncertainties remain to be elucidated in the future. A speculative model of interactions within and between signaling and responding cells is shown in Figure 16–2.

Four features of the hedgehog signaling network are highly unusual. First, autoprocessing generates an active Hedgehog ligand with a C-terminal cholesterol moiety. Then palmitoylation results in an N-terminal palmitate. Thus, the active Hedgehog ligand becomes double lipid-modified (Fig. 16–4).

Second, most membrane-bound receptors activate downstream signaling on ligand binding. In contrast, patched is *repressed* by its Hedgehog ligand, freeing Smoothened for downstream signaling (Fig. 16–1).

Third, Patched (Ptch) (Fig. 16–5) and Smoothened (Smo) may shuttle oppositely between the plasma membrane and endocytic vesicles

Table 16–1. Genetic Disorders in the Sonic Hedgehog Signaling Network

Condition	Mutation Reported in	References
Holoprosencephaly	SHH	Belloni et al. (1996)
		Roessler et al. (1996)
		Roessler et al. (1997)
		Nanni et al. (1999)
	PTCH	Ming et al. (2002)
	GLI2	Roessler et al. (2002)
Nevoid basal cell carcinoma syndrome	PTCH	Hahn et al. (1996)
		Johnson et al. (1996)
		Lench et al. (1997)
		Wicking et al. (1997)
	PTCH2?[a]	Smyth et al. (1999)
	SHH?[a]	Oro et al. (1997)
	SMO?[a]	Reifenberger et al. (1998)
		Xie et al. (1998)
	GLI1?[a]	Dahmane et al. (1997)
Greig cephalopolysyndactyly	GLI3	Biesecker et al. (1997)
		Wild et al. (1997)
Pallister-Hall syndrome	GLI3	Biesecker et al. (1997)
		Kang et al. (1997)
Rubinstein-Taybi syndrome	CBP[b]	Petrij et al. (1995)
		Blough et al. (2000)
Basal cell carcinoma	PTCH	Gailani et al. (1996)
		Johnson et al. (1996)
		Wolter et al. (1997)
		Reifenberger et al. (1998)
		Lam et al. (1997)
	PTCH2	Smyth et al. (1999)
	SHH[a]	Oro et al. (1997)
	SMO	Xie et al. (1998)
		Reifenberger et al. (1998)
		Lam et al. (1999)
Medulloblastoma	PTCH[c]	Raffel et al. (1997)
		Wolter et al. (1997)
	PTCH2	Smyth et al. (1999)
	SMO	Reifenberger et al. (1998)
	SUFU	Taylor et al. (2002)
	GLI3	Erez et al. (2001)
	SHH	Oro et al. (1997)
Meningioma	PTCH[d]	Xie et al. (1997)
Primitive neuroectodermal tumor	PTCH	Wolter et al. (1997)
		Vorechovsky et al. (1997a)
Breast cancer	SHH	Oro et al. (1997)
	PTCH	Xie et al. (1997)
Squamous cell carcinoma	PTCH	Ahmadian et al. (1998)
		Ping et al. (2001)
Trichoepithelioma	PTCH	Vorechovsky et al. (1997b)
Esophageal carcinoma	PTCH	Maesawa et al. (1998)
Fetal rhabdomyoma	PTCH[e]	Klijanienko et al. (1988)
		DiSanto et al. (1992)
Rhabdomyosarcoma	PTCH[e]	Beddis et al. (1983)

[a]To date, the nevoid basal cell carcinoma syndrome has not been reported with mutations in PTCH2, SHH, SMO, or GLI1, but there are reasons for believing that such mutations might rarely be possible in the syndrome (see Cohen, 1999).

PTCH2 has been reported with a mutation in a medulloblastoma by Smyth et al. (1999). Medulloblastoma is a feature of the nevoid basal cell carcinoma in about 3%–5% of cases.

A mutation in SHH has been found in one isolated basal cell carcinoma (Oro et al., 1997), although this association has been questioned (Wicking et al., 1998). However, Oro et al. (1997) showed that basal cell carcinomas and skeletal malformations were found in hypersonic transgenic mice.

Mutations in SMO have been reported in isolated basal cell carcinomas (Reifenberger et al., 1998; Xie et al., 1998).

Dahmane et al. (1997) found unambiguous expression of GLI1 in almost all isolated basal cell carcinomas studied.

[b]Mutations in CBP have been found in Rubinstein-Taybi syndrome by Petrij et al. (1995) and Blough et al. (2000). CBP enhances transcription mediated by many other transcription factors. However, Akimaru et al. (1997) have shown that Drosophila CBP (dCBP) functions as a co-activator of cubitus interruptus, which is part of the hedgehog network.

[c]Goodrich et al. (1997) found that mice lacking a functional copy of the Ptch gene developed medulloblastomas frequently.

[d]Most reported meningiomas in the nevoid basal cell carcinoma syndrome are secondary to radiation treatment for medulloblastomas. However, a few examples of true meningioma have been observed. Xie et al. (1997) noted an isolated meningioma with a PTCH mutation.

[e]These tumors are rare in the nevoid basal cell carcinoma syndrome and no syndrome case to date with a PTCH mutation has been recorded with them. However, in the Ptch mouse model of the syndrome, rhabdomyosarcomas have been reported (Hahn et al., 1998).

in response to Hedgehog ligand (Fig. 16–2). They may not interact physically, with Patched acting catalytically rather than stoichiometrically (Denef et al., 2000; Ingham et al., 2000; Taipale et al., 2002). In contrast, Incardona et al. (2002) suggested that Patched and Smoothened colocalize in the absence of Hedgehog and that both proteins endocytose on ligand binding after which Smoothened subsequently segregates from the Patched/Hedgehog complex.

Fourth, the network has a bifunctional transcription regulator, Cubitus interruptus (Ci) (Fig. 16–6). In the absence of Hedgehog ligand, a truncated transcriptional repressor is generated that binds target genes and blocks their transcription (Fig. 16–3). In the presence of Hedgehog ligand, a full-length transcriptional activator binds target genes and upregulates their transcription (Fig. 16–3).

Hedgehog is capable of both short- and long-range signaling. It is

HEDGEHOG ABSENT   HEDGEHOG PRESENT

Figure 16–1. Classical model for regulation of Smo activity by Ptch and Hh. Both Ptch and Smo are membrane bound. Ptch inhibits Smo when Hedgehog is absent. Hedgehog modified by palmitate (PAL) and cholesterol (CHOL) binds to Ptch, inducing a conformational change, freeing Smo for downstream signaling. Hh-N, autoprocessed N-terminal signaling domain. (From Cohen, 2003b.)

highly regulated at many levels. Cholesterol-modified Hedgehog, which should be tethered to the cell membrane, can be further modified at the lipid rafts where it multimerizes and becomes soluble and diffusable (Zeng et al., 2001).

Dispatched (Disp) functions to release multimeric Hedgehog, making it available for long-range signaling (Burke et al., 1999) (Fig. 16–2).

The movement of multimeric Hedgehog is also regulated by Toutvelu (Ttv)-dependent synthesis of heparan sulfate proteoglycan (HSPG) (Bellaiche et al., 1998). One possibility is that HSPG pre-

sents multimeric Hedgehog to its Patched receptor in a fashion similar to HSPG in fibroblast growth factor (FGF) signaling. Perhaps it targets multimeric Hedgehog specifically to endocytic vesicles. Another possibility is that HSPG allows Hedgehog to move from cell to cell (Fig. 16–2).

Besides Patched, Megalin can also bind Hedgehog with high affinity (McCarthy et al., 2002). Perhaps Megalin-mediated endocytosis of multimeric Hedgehog may regulate its availability to Patched by competing with Patched to limit the levels of multimeric Hedgehog. Al-

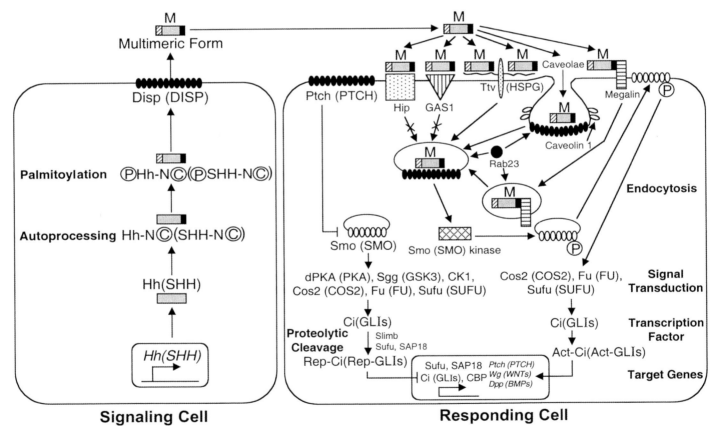

Figure 16–2. Hedgehog signaling network; a speculative model of interactions within and between signaling and responding cells. *Drosophila* genes are shown with human homologues in parentheses. Signaling cell: Autoprocessing generates an N-terminal signaling domain Hh-N with a C-terminal cholesterol moiety (Hh-N©). Then palmitoylation results in an N-terminal palmitate (℗Hh-N©). Cholesterol-modified Hedgehog can be further modified at the lipid rafts where it multimerizes and becomes soluble and diffusible. Disp functions to release multimeric Hedgehog (M), making it available for long range signaling. Responding cell: The movement of multimeric Hedgehog is regulated by Ttv-dependent synthesis of HSPG. One possibility is that HSPG presents multimeric Hedgehog to Ptch. Besides Ptch, Megalin can also bind multimeric Hedgehog. Without Hedgehog ligand binding, Ptch inhibits Smo from downstream signaling. Ptch and Smo shuttle oppositely between the plasma membrane and endocytic vesicles in response to Hedgehog binding to Ptch. Ptch and Smo do not interact physically. Ptch acts catalytically rather than stoichiometrically. Ci is a bifunctional transcription regulator. In the absence of Hedgehog ligand, a truncated transcriptional repressor (Rep-Ci) is generated that binds target genes (*Ptch, Wg, Dpp*) and blocks their transcription. In the presence of Hedgehog ligand, a full length transcriptional activator (Act-Ci) binds target genes and upregulates their transcription. For further details about Ci's role as a transcriptional regulator, see Figure 16–3. For details about Megalin, Hip, GAS1, Rab23, Slimb, and SAP18, see text. In this diagram, the N-terminal signaling portion of Hedgehog is not truncated because it would be too small for use in the diagram. See Figure 16–4 for autoprocessing and palmitoylation of SHH. (From Cohen, 2003b.)

Figure 16–3. *Left:* In downstream signaling, Ci, Cos2, Fu, and Sufu form a tetrameric complex that results in the nuclear transcription and activity of Ci. In the absence of Hedgehog stimulation, the complex is tethered to the microtubules by Cos2. Both Cos2 and Sufu retain Ci in the cytoplasm, the former being bound to Ci's CORD domain and the latter being bound to its Sufu domain. Cos2 promotes proteolysis of Ci, generating the truncated 75-kDa repressor form of Ci (Rep-Ci). The process requires phosphorylation of Ci by dPKA, CK1, and Sgg, and also the activities of Slimb, Sufu, and SAP18. Translocation of Rep-Ci to the nucleus prevents transcription of target genes *Ptch*, *Wg*, and *Dpp*. *Right:* With intermediate levels of Hedgehog stimulation, the Ci, Cos2, Fu, Sufu complex dissociates from the microtubules, inhibiting the cleavage of Ci, possibly through dephosphorylation of Ci. The full-length 155-kDa activator form of Ci (Act-Ci) binds to Sufu, an interaction that restricts its nuclear translocation. Sufu attenuates its transcriptional activity. Higher levels of Hedgehog stimulation promote dissociation of Sufu from Act-Ci, which together with cofactor dCBP upregulates target genes *Ptch*, *Wg*, and *Dpp*. (From Cohen, 2003b.)

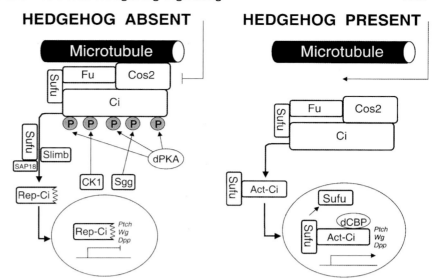

ternatively, Megalin may deliver multimeric Hedgehog to vesicular pools of Patched (Fig. 16–2).

Hedgehog interacting protein (Hip) and growth arrest specific 1 (GAS1) may both attenuate Hedgehog signaling (Chuang and McMahon, 1999, Lee et al., 2001a) (see Fig. 16–2).

Table 16–2. Some Genes of the Hedgehog Signaling Network Together with Their Chromosome Map Locations and Expression Patterns

Gene	Chromosome Map Location	Expression Pattern[a]
SHH	7q36	Node, head process, notochord, floorplate, ventrolateral midbrain, ventral forebrain, branchial arches, cardiac morphogenesis, limb bud and anterior-posterior patterning of limb skeleton, regulation of right/left asymmetry
IHH	2q35-q36	Stimulates endothelial cell production in yolk sac, activation of hematopoiesis, coordination of proliferation/differentiation in endochondral bone formation
DHH	12q13	Peritubular cell development, maturation of testes, Sertoli-Leydig cell interactions, male germ line development, masculization, formation of peripheral nerve sheaths
PTCH	9q22.3	Mesenchymal condensations surrounding epidermal ingrowth, epithelial cells adjacent to SHH-expressing cells
PTCH2	1p32-p34	Co-expressed in epithelium with SHH
DISP	1q42	Ubiquitous early embryonic expression with some tissue-specific variations in level
SMO	7q31-q32	Early neural folds, neural tube, presomitic mesoderm and somites, developing limb bud, gut, eye
SUFU	10q24.3	Multiple embryonic and adult tissues
GLI1	12q13	Widespread mesodermal expression, ventral neural tube
GLI2	2q14	Widespread mesodermal expression, posterior neural tube, overlapping expression with *Gli3*
GLI3	7p13	Widespread mesodermal expression, posterior neural tube, overlapping expression with *Gli2*
CBP	16p13.3	Nucleus

Source: Data from Ruppert et al. (1990), Hui et al. (1994), Alcedo et al. (1996), Hahn et al. (1996), Johnson et al. (1996), Matsumoto et al. (1996), Reifenberger et al. (1996), Stone et al. (1996), Hammerschmidt et al. (1997), Motoyama et al. (1998), Smyth et al. (1999), Stone et al., 1999, Blough et al. (2000), Ingham and McMahon (2001), Ma et al. (2002), and Taylor et al. (2002).

[a]Only some expression patterns are provided in this table. For more complete coverage, see Hui et al. (1994), Hammerschmidt et al. (1997), and Ingham and McMahon (2001).

Multimeric Hedgehog and Patched colocalize in subcellular vesicles (Incardona et al., 2000b) (Fig. 16–2). Whether Patched eventually separates from Hedgehog with Hedgehog being directed to lysosomes for degradation and with the Patched returning to the cell surface is unclear at present.

Patched is also a target gene in the hedgehog signaling network (Fig. 16–2). The upregulation of Patched expression, resulting in Patched protein at the cell membrane, sequesters Hedgehog and limits its spread beyond the cells in which it is produced (Chen and Struhl, 1996). Thus, a balance is created by the antagonism of Hedgehog and Patched, whose relative concentrations alternate with respect to each other (Cohen, 1999).

ANALYSIS OF COMPONENTS

Hedgehog Genes

Unlike one Hedgehog gene found in *Drosophilia* (*Hh*), three Hedgehog genes, first identified in the mouse, are found in vertebrates. These include *Desert hedgehog* (*Dhh*), *Indian hedgehog* (*Ihh*), and *Sonic*

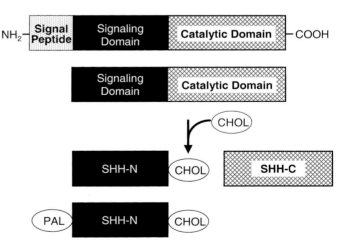

Figure 16–4. *Sonic Hedgehog* (*SHH*) has an N-terminal signaling domain (SHH-N) and a C-terminal catalytic domain (SHH-C) that causes autocleavage of the protein, resulting in an ester-linked cholesterol moiety (CHOL) at the C-terminal end of the signaling portion; the catalytic portion diffuses away. An amide-linked N-terminal palmitate (PAL) is critical for signaling activity. Following the addition of the C-terminal cholesterol adduct, palmitoylation requires the action of Skinny hedgehog (Ski) acyltransferase. (Modified from Cohen, 1999 and Cohen and Shiota, 2002.)

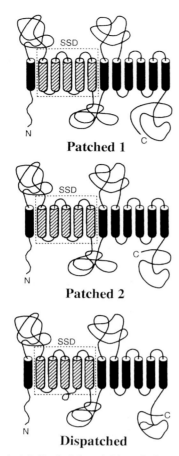

Figure 16–5. Patched 1, Patched 2, and Dispatched are 12-pass transmembrane proteins. The N- and C-terminal domains of Patched 2 are different from Patched 1, including the absence of 150 amino acid residues in the C-terminal domain of Patched 2. Two large extracellular loops are for Hedgehog ligand binding. Dispatched functions to release cholesterol modified Hedgehog from its tether to the plasma membrane, making it available for long range signaling. The sterol-sensing domain (SSD) is shown with hatched cylinders enclosed within a rectangle formed with dashed lines. (From Cohen, 2003b.)

hedgehog (*Shh*).[1] *Dhh* is most closely related to *Hh*; *Ihh* and *Shh* are more closely related to each other and represent a more recent gene duplication. Further duplications within the Ihh and Shh classes have occurred in teleost fishes (Ingham and McMahon, 2001). Phylogenetic relationships in the vertebrate Hedgehog gene family (Zardoya et al., 1996) are shown in Figure 16–7. Human hedgehog genes (*SHH*, *IHH*, and *DHH*), their chromosome map locations, and their expression patterns are summarized in Table 16–2.

Sonic Hedgehog (Shh)

Sonic hedgehog (*Shh*) gene expression has been demonstrated in the floorplate of the neural tube. Targeted gene disruption in the mouse produces cyclopia with absence of ventral neural tube cells. The *Shh* mutation is recessive, resulting in a severe phenotype (Chiang et al., 1996). In contrast to the mouse, human *SHH* mutations are heterozygous, and the holoprosencephalic phenotype is more variable (Belloni et al., 1996; Roessler et al., 1996, 1997; Nanni et al., 1999).

Autoprocessing Reaction

SHH has an N-terminal signaling domain (SHH-N), and a C-terminal catalytic domain (SHH-C) that causes autocleavage of the protein,

[1]The term is named after "Sonic, the Hedgehog," a computer game played by children. Sonic has two closely-set eyes with a common scleral rim, suggesting holoprosencephaly. The murine null mutation (*Shh*[−/−]) demonstrates holoprosencephaly.

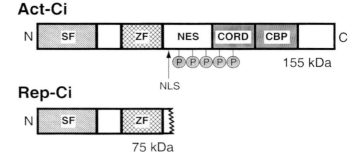

Figure 16–6. Act-Ci, a 155-kDa target activator. Rep-Ci, a 75-kDa target repressor. Motifs include a Suppression of Fused-binding domain (SF), zinc finger DNA-binding domain (ZF), nuclear localization signal (NLS), cleavage site (↑), nuclear export signal (NES), protein kinase A (PKA), phosphorylation sites (P), costal 2-binding domain (CORD), and CREB-binding protein (CPB). (From Cohen, 2003b.)

producing an ester-linked cholesterol moiety at the C-terminal end of SHH-N. The autocleavage of SHH proceeds via a thioester intermediate that undergoes a nucleophilic attack by cholesterol, resulting in a covalently linked cholesterol adduct and activation of the SHH-N signaling portion. The SHH-C catalytic portion diffuses away (Porter et al., 1996) (Fig. 16–4).

Palmitoylation

Following the autoprocessing reaction, palmitoylation of the most N-terminal cysteine of the SHH-N signaling portion takes place, requiring the action of Skinny hedgehog (Ski) acyltransferase (Pepinsky et al., 1998, Chamoun et al., 2001)[2] (Fig. 16–4).

Mutations in Sonic Hedgehog Signaling Network and Linked Pathways

Known human mutations for holoprosencephaly are summarized in Table 16–3 (see Chapter 18). Because various pathways are linked to the sonic hedgehog signaling network, the mutations are interrelated (Muenke and Beachy, 2001) (Fig. 16–8). *SHH* (Belloni et al., 1996; Roessler et al., 1996, 1997; Nanni et al., 1999), *PTCH* (Ming et al., 2002), and *GLI2* (Roessler et al., 2002) are within the sonic hedgehog signaling network itself. *DHCR7* (Wassif et al., 1998; Witsch-Baumgartner et al., 2000; Yu et al., 2000) involves 7-dehydrocholesterol reductase in cholesterol biosynthesis. *ZIC2* (Brown et al., 1998, 2001) and *GLI2* are related; Gli proteins are translocated to cell nuclei by coexpressed Zic proteins (Brewster et al., 1998; Koyabu et al., 2001). *TDGF1* (de la Cruz et al., 2002), *TGIF* (Gripp et al., 2000), and *FAST1* (Ouspenskaia et al., 2002) involve *Nodal/TGFβ* signaling. *SIX3* (Wallis et al., 1999) has not been linked to any of these interrelated pathways to date.

Mechanisms of Hedgehog Protein Transport

The ester-linked cholesterol moiety and the amide-linked palmitate should tether the Shh signaling portion to the plasma membrane of the producing cell. However, transport to responding cells can occur through three mechanisms: (1) formation of multimeric Hedgehog (Zeng et al., 2001); (2) function of Dispatched (Disp) in releasing the lipid-anchored protein (Burke et al., 1999; Ma et al., 2002); and (3) diffusion of the protein by Ttv (Bellaiche et al., 1998; The et al., 1999) (Fig. 16–2).

Multimeric Hedgehog (M-Hh-N, M-Shh-N)

Zeng et al. (2001) demonstrated a soluble and diffusable form of double lipid-modified Shh that is multimeric and biologically potent. They suggested that modified Shh might be formed at the lipid rafts where it multimerizes with its lipid attachments sequestered in the interior of the multimer. This soluble form could then diffuse from its pro-

[2]Besides Skinny hedgehog (Ski), other terms for the same acyltransferase are known, such as rasp, sightless (sit), and central missing (cmn) (Amanai et al., 2001; Lee and Treisman, 2001).

Figure 16–7. Phylogenetic relationships among members of the vertebrate *Hedgehog* gene family. Sequences can be classified into three orthology groups: *Sonic Hedgehog, Indian Hedgehog,* and *Desert Hedgehog* (three vertical black bars). A 50% majority-rule neighbor-joining bootstrap tree is based on aligned amino acid Hedgehog (Hh) sequences (328 characters). Numbers above the branches indicate the percentage of neighbor-joining bootstrap values (1000 replications). Numbers below the branches indicate the maximum percentage of parsimony bootstrap values (1000 replications). (From Zardoya et al., 1996.)

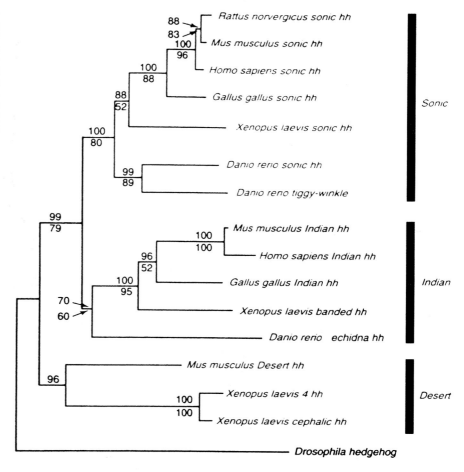

ducing cell, making it available for long-range signaling (Fig. 16–2). In this chapter, the multimeric form of Hedgehog is abbreviated as either M-Hh-N or M-Shh-N.

Dispatched (Disp)

Burke et al. (1999) identified a 12-pass transmembrane protein, Dispatched (Disp), with sequence similarity to *Drosophila* and vertebrate Ptch. Disp has ubiquitous early embryonic expression with some tissue-specific variations in level. Human DISP maps to 1q42 (Ma et al., 2002). Although both Disp and Ptch have sterol sensing domains, they play opposite roles (Fig. 16–5). Disp functions to release cholesterol-modified Hh from its tether to the plasma membrane, making it available for long-range signaling (Fig. 16–2). However, the precise mechanism by which this is accomplished remains unknown to date (Burke

et al., 1999). Zeng et al. (2001) speculated that Disp might be involved in packaging multimeric and soluble Shh protein or targeting it to the lipid rafts.

Ma et al. (2002) noted that Disp showed sequence similarity to the prokaryotic RND permease superfamily. These superfamily proteins are known to function as proton-driven anteporters. They have a conserved GxxxD motif in the middle of TM4 and an aspartic acid residue within this motif, which is important as a proton-binding site. Disp has three aspartic acid residues, suggesting the possibility that Disp and bacterial proteins might act by a similar mechanism.

Tout-velu (Ttv)

Bellaiche et al. (1998) characterized a 760–amino acid protein that mediates movement of M-Hh-N across responding cells. They iden-

Table 16–3. Known Mutated Genes in Holoprosencephaly[a]

Mutated Gene	Chromosome Map Location	Holoprosencephalic Phenotype	Frequency among All Cases of Holoprosencephaly
SHH	7q36	Great variability (severe to mild)	17% of familial cases; 3.7% of sporadic cases
ZIC2	13q32	Severe brain defect; normal or mildly dysmorphic face	3%–4%
SIX3	2p21	Variable	1.3%
TGIF	18p11.3	Variable	1.5%
PTCH	9q22.3	Variable	Rare (4 cases); *PTCH* mutations common in nevoid basal cell carcinoma syndrome and in isolated basal cell carcinomas
GLI2	2q14	Variable	1.8%
FAST1	8q24.3	Variable	20 missense variants in 100 holoprosencephaly cases and in 350 patients with congenital heart defects; 3 mutations were found in both holoprosencephaly and in cardiac defects
TDGF1	3p21-p23	Variable	0.5%
DHCR7	11q12-q13	Holoprosencephalic faces	2%–4% of Smith-Lemli-Opitz syndrome cases

[a]See text for references.

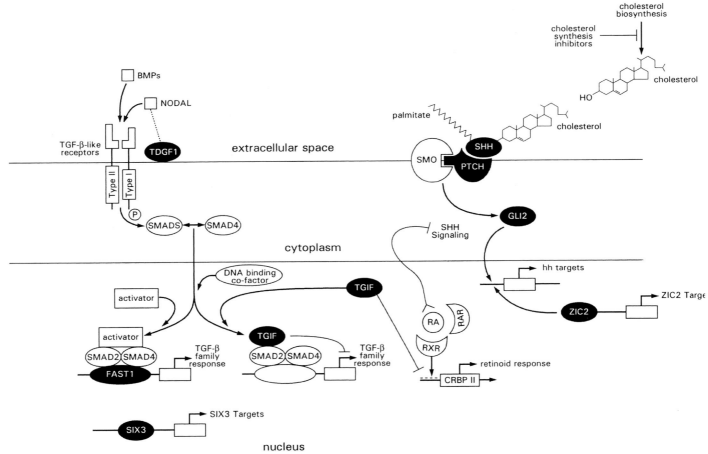

Figure 16–8. Mutations for holoprosencephaly in black: *SHH, PTCH, GLI2, ZIC2, TGIF, TDGF1, FAST1,* and *SIX3*. Another mutation *DHCR7*, involving 7-dehydrocholesterol reductase deficiency, is one of the cholesterol synthesis inhibitors (upper right). Because various pathways are linked to the sonic hedgehog signaling network, the mutations are interrelated: *SHH, PTCH,* and *GLI2* are within the network itself. *ZIC2* and *GLI2* are related: GLI proteins are translocated to cell nuclei by coexpressed ZIC proteins. *TDGF1, TGIF,* and *FAST1* involve Nodal/TGFβ signaling. *SIX3* has not been linked to any of these interrelated pathways to date. (From Muenke and Beachy, 2001. Modified and updated through the courtesy of M. Muenke, Bethesda, MD.)

tified mutants in the gene which they called *Tout-velu* (*Ttv*), meaning "all hair" because of their "hairy" appearance.

Ttv is closely related to the *EXT* gene family involved in human multiple exostoses. It is more homologous to *EXT2* with 44% protein identity than to *EXT1* with 26% protein identity (The et al., 1999).[3] EXT proteins are implicated in HSPG biosynthesis. EXT1 and EXT2 are glycosyltransferases required for the biosynthesis of heparan sulfate (Lind et al., 1998; McCormick et al., 1998). For example, in EXT2, a GalNAc transferase determines a heparan sulfate chain (instead of a chondroitin sulfate chain) attached to the linker region of HSPG (Kitagawa et al., 1999; Simmons et al., 1999).

The movement of M-Hh-N is regulated by Ttv-dependent synthesis of HSPG. One possibility is that HSPG may present M-Hh-N to its receptor Ptch in a fashion similar to HSPG in FGF signaling; perhaps it targets M-Hh-N specifically to endocytotic vesicles (Fig. 16–2). Another possibility is that HSPG allows M-Hh-N to move from cell to cell.

Patched (Ptch, Ptch1)

The symbols for *Patched* are *Ptc* and *PTC*. Recently, *Ptch* and *PTCH* have been used by some authors, and there are compelling reasons for continuing this trend. The ability to taste phenylthiocarbamide is genetically controlled, and numerous articles, beginning as early as 1931, refer to this as PTC (OMIM 171200; Kim et al., 2003); the genetic term PTC for this has been well known to human geneticists for years.

Patched (*Ptch*) encodes a transmembrane protein that acts as a neg-

ative regulator of *hedgehog* (*Hh*) signaling (see Chapter 18). The 1500-amino-acid glycoprotein has 12 hydrophobic membrane-spanning domains, intracellular N- and C-terminal regions, and two large hydrophilic extracellular loops where Hh ligand binding occurs (Hooper and Scott, 1989; Marigo et al., 1996) (Fig. 16–5).

Ptch has dual roles in sequestering and transducing Hh (Chen and Struhl, 1996). When the second large extracellular loop, essential for ligand binding, is deleted by a *Ptch* mutation, Hh binding to Ptch cannot occur, but Ptch's repression of Smo is unaffected (Briscoe et al., 2001). When a C-terminal truncation is caused by a *Ptch* mutation, Ptch can no longer repress Smo, but Hh binding to Ptch is unaffected (Johnson et al., 2000).

Helms et al. (1997) demonstrated that retinoic acid inhibited both Shh and Ptch expressions in the craniofacial primorida of chick embryos; the polarizing activity in these tissues was abolished. These findings are of particular interest because human mutations in both *SHH* (Roessler et al., 1996, 1997, Nanni et al., 1999) and *PTCH* (Ming et al., 2002) have been shown to cause holoprosencephaly.

Human *PTCH*, a tumor suppressor gene, maps to 9q22.3. Mutations in *PTCH* have been identified in patients with nevoid basal cell carcinoma syndrome, isolated basal cell carcinoma, medulloblastoma, meningioma, neuroectodermal tumor, breast carcinoma, esophageal carcinoma, squamous cell carcinoma, and trichoepithelioma (Cohen, 1999) (Table 16–1). Most mutations have resulted in protein truncation. However, four rare *PTCH* missense mutations have resulted in holoprosencephaly—two in the extracellular loops required for SHH binding and two in intracellular loops that may be involved in PTCH–SMO interaction (Ming et al., 2002).

---

[3]In an earlier report by this group (Bellaiche et al., 1998), Ttv is said to be 56% identical to EXT1 and 25% identical to EXT2.

Patched 2 (Ptch2)

A second gene, *Ptch2*, has been detected in the adult mouse eye. In humans, *PTCH2* maps to 1p32-p34 and encodes a 1204-amino-acid protein. PTCH2 has a 54% overall identity to PTCH and a 90% identity to Ptch2 in mice (Carpenter et al., 1998). The Ptch2 protein also contains 12 transmembrane domains and two large extracellular loops. However, both N- and C-terminal regions are different from *Ptch* (*Ptch1*), including the absence of 150-amino-acid residues in the C-terminal domain (Fig. 16–5). Ptch and Ptch2 are differentially expressed during development of the epidermis, suggesting that the two proteins may have different functions (Motoyama et al., 1998; Smyth et al., 1999), although the function of Ptch2 remains unclear to date (see Table 16–2 for expression patterns of PTCH and PTCH2). Rare *PTCH2* mutations have been reported in medulloblastoma and basal cell carcinoma (Smyth et al., 1999).

Translocation in Renal Cell Carcinoma 8 (TRC8)

Translocation in Renal Cell Carcinoma 8 (TRC8) is a 664-amino-acid 10-pass transmembrane protein with some similarities to *PTCH*; it maps to 8q24. In a series of sporadic renal cell carcinomas, a *TRC8* mutation was identified and Gemmill et al. (1998) suggested that *TRC8* may define an additional pathway of mutations resulting in renal and thyroid carcinomas.

Amino acids 344 to 443 in TRC8 have a 60% identity to amino acids 883 to 979 in PTCH, which corresponds to the second large extracellular loop of PTCH involved in SHH binding. Another similarity, a sterol-sensing domain (SSD) between amino acids 22 and 179 in TRC8, has a 63% identity to the SSD between amino acids 440 and 600 in PTCH. TRC8 transcripts are expressed in many tissues, including the testis, placenta, adrenal, kidney, and thyroid (Gemmill et al., 1998).

Sterol Sensing Domain (SSD)

Ptch, Ptch2, and Disp each have a SSD consisting of approximately 180 amino acids that make up five membrane-spanning domains (Fig. 16–5). SSD-containing proteins, such as HMGCR, SCAP, NPC1, and 7DHCR, play key roles in different aspects of cholesterol homeostasis or cholesterol-linked signaling. They share common properties such as rapid trafficking between organelles, cargo transport, and modification of their activity by sterol and/or lipoprotein concentrations (Kuwabara and Labouesse, 2002).

The SSD of Ptch is essential for its activity, but its role remains unclear to date. The hypothesis that the SSD of Ptch plays a role in targeting cholesterol-modified Hh is not supported because absence of the cholesterol adduct does not alter the affinity of Ptch for Hh (Pepinsky et al., 1998). Mutations in the SSD of Ptch in *Drosophila* do not interfere with Hh binding (Martin et al., 2001; Strutt et al., 2001), but cholesterol does affect the potency and range of Hh movement, and the same is true for Shh movement in vertebrates (Chen and Struhl, 1996; Marigo et al., 1996; Stone et al., 1996; Lewis et al., 2001). In *Drosophila*, Ptch cannot effectively sequester Hh without the cholesterol adduct, which results in an *extended* range of Hh signaling (Chen and Struhl, 1996; Burke et al., 1999). In contrast, when Shh without a cholesterol adduct in mice is used, signaling activity is *reduced* (Lewis et al., 2001). Such differences have not been easy to explain to date (Kuwabara and Labouesse, 2002).

Ptch, like NPC1, shuttles between the plasma membrane and endosomes by a dynamin-driven process (Martin et al., 2001; Strutt et al., 2001). Experiments using neural tube explants in chicks demonstrate that Ptch mediates the endocytosis of Shh (Incardona et al., 2000b). Because Ptch, like NPC1, shares sequence similarities to RND permeases, the question can be raised whether Ptch also has transport activity (Kuwabara and Labouesse, 2002).

A dominant-negative mutation in the SSD of Ptch—the same one that makes SCAP resistant to high levels of cholesterol—releases Smo from inhibition and increases its activity; the mutant retains the ability to sequester and endocytose Hh (Chen and Struhl, 1996; Martin et al., 2001; Strutt et al., 2001).

The genome of *C. elegans* contains 24 predicted proteins that have sequence similarities to Ptch (*Caenorhabditis elegans* Sequencing Consortium, 1998; Kuwabara et al., 2000). Deletion of the *Ce-ptch1* gene disrupts cytokinesis, suggesting that Ptch must have other functions besides inhibiting Smo and sequestering Hh (Kuwabara et al., 2000).

Smoothened (Smo)

The symbols for *Smoothened* are *Smo* and *SMO*. Some authors have used slightly different symbols (*Smoh, SMOH*) (Reifenberger et al., 1998).

Smo encodes a 1024-amino-acid transmembrane protein that acts as a transducer of the hedgehog (Hh) signal. Smo protein has 7 hydrophobic membrane-spanning domains, an extracellular N-terminal region, and an intracellular C-terminal region. Smo bears some similarity to G protein–coupled receptors and is most homologous to the Frizzled (Fz) family of serpentine proteins (Alcedo et al., 1996; van den Heuvel and Ingham, 1996).

In humans, *SMO* maps to 7q31-q32. In the absence of Hh, Ptch prevents Smo from signaling. When M-Hh-N binds to Ptch, however, Smo is free to upregulate downstream genes in the network. Activating mutations in *SMO* have been identified in sporadic basal cell carcinomas (Reifenberger et al., 1998, Xie et al., 1998).

Relationship Between Patched (Ptch) and Smoothened (Smo)

The classical interpretation of the relationship between Ptch and Smo transmembrane proteins indicates that Ptch suppresses Smo from downstream signaling. Hedgehog binding to Ptch alleviates Ptch-mediated repression of Smo by a conformational change that frees Smo for downstream signaling (Stone et al., 1996; Alcedo and Noll, 1997; Chen and Struhl, 1998; Murone et al., 1999) (Fig. 16–1).

For more recent interpretation, see the reviews of Denef et al. (2000), Ingham et al. (2000), Kalderon (2000), Ingham and McMahon (2001), Ho and Scott (2002), Incardona et al. (2002), Mullor et al. (2002), Nybakken and Perrimon (2002), Taipale et al. (2002), and Cohen (2003b). Kalderon (2000) reviewed four models for the regulation of Smo by Ptch and Hh. The first model, the classical one, has already been discussed above. A second model postulates that Hh activates Smo by causing dissociation of the Ptch/Smo complex. In a third model, Ptch inhibits Smo through a diffusible intermediate and Hh binding to Ptch alters the activity of the intermediate, allowing Smo to become activated. In a fourth model, Ptch acts catalytically via a small molecule to suppress Smo, and on Hh binding to Ptch, Smo is activated by becoming dissociated from Ptch and the small molecule.

Intracellular localization of Ptch was demonstrated by Capdevila et al. (1994), who induced a mutation in *Shibire* that affects endocytosis. Incardona et al. (2000), noting that M-Shh-N and Ptch colocalize in subcellular vesicles, suggested that internalization of M-Shh-N is mediated by Ptch.[4] Denef et al. (2000) suggested that Ptch and Smo shuttle oppositely between the plasma membrane and cytoplasmic vesicles in response to M-Hh-N ligand.

In the absence of M-Hh-N binding, Ptch may be found principally at the cell membrane. At the same time, Smo may occupy intracellular vesicles. The binding of M-Hh-N to Ptch triggers a dynamin-mediated internalization into endosomes (Capdevila et al., 1994; Incardona et al., 2000b; Martin et al., 2001; Strutt et al., 2001), and this results, indirectly, in the migration of vesicular Smo to the cell membrane (Fig. 16–2).

Caveolae and caveolin-1 protein, which coats calveolae, may play a role in M-Hh-N uptake by Ptch. Karpen et al. (2001) demonstrated both Ptch and Smo in caveolin-1 enriched lipid rafts. However, only Ptch interacts specifically with caveolin-1 while Smo does not (Fig. 16–2).

Ptch mediates the post-translational modification of the C-terminal domain of Smo (Ingham et al., 2000). Modification may include potential

---

[4]Whether Ptch eventually separates from M-Shh-N with M-Shh-N being directed to lysosomes for degradation and with Ptch returning to the cell surface is unclear at present.

enzymatic candidates such as a phosphatase, protein kinase A, or cyclin B1 that alter the phosphorylation status of Smo, affecting its stability, activity, and subcellular localization (Alcedo et al., 2000; Denef et al., 2000; Barnes et al., 2001). When Smo moves to the cell surface, hyperphosphorylation takes place—a putative Smo kinase increasing its activity (Denef et al., 2000; Kalderon, 2000) (Fig. 16–2). How closely linked phosphorylation of Smo is to its transport to the cell surface is not known at present (Nybakken and Perrimon, 2002). Unstimulated Ptch may promote dephosphorylation of Smo, a putative Smo phosphorylase decreasing Smo's activity (Denef et al., 2000, Kalderon, 2000).

Denef et al. (2000) provided some evidence that Ptch and Smo do not interact physically in transducing M-Hh-N signals. They suggested that the regulatory interaction between Ptch and Smo need not be stoichiometric. Taipale et al. (2002) indicated that Ptch acts catalytically rather than stoichiometrically. They found that Ptch and Smo are not significantly associated together within responding cells (Fig. 16–2). They demonstrated that Ptch, unbounded by M-Hh-N, acts substoichiometrically to suppress the activity of Smo. Extremely low levels of Ptch were sufficient to reduce the activity of Smo substantially. For example, a Ptch/Smo ratio of 1:45 suppressed nearly 80% of Smo activity. Taipale et al. (2002) suggested that in the absence of M-Hh-N, Ptch may translocate a small molecule across the lipid bilayer that regulates the activity state of Smo.

In contrast, Incardona et al. (2002) provided some evidence that supported a model in which colocalization of Ptch and Smo occurs in the absence of M-Shh-N. On M-Shh-N binding to Ptch, both Ptch and Smo may undergo simultaneous transport into the endocytic pathway where Smo is subsequently segregated from the Ptch/M-Shh-N complex, which is destined for lysosomal degradation. Possibly, late endosomal sorting may control the generation of active Smo.

Megalin

Megalin (also known as gp330) is a multiligand receptor belonging to the low-density lipoprotein (LDL) receptor family. It mediates endocytosis of ligands and targets them for lysosomal degradation or transcytosis (McCarthy et al., 2002). A null mutation in megalin produces holoprosencephaly in mice (Willnow et al., 1996).

McCarthy et al. (2002) showed that M-Shh-N binds to megalin with high affinity. Direct signal transduction by megalin seems unlikely. Perhaps megalin-mediated endocytosis of M-Shh-N may regulate its availability to Ptch by competing with Ptch for limiting the levels of M-Shh-N. Alternatively, megalin may deliver M-Shh-N to vesicular pools of Ptch (Fig. 16–2).

The mechanism by which megalin ligands bypass lysosomal degradation is not known. Based on considerations of pH, McCarthy et al. (2002) suggested that M-Shh-N may traffic in complex with megalin and thus be recycled and/or transcytosed.

Ras-like in Rat Brain 23 (Rab23)

The *Shh* and *Opb* (*Open brain*) genes have opposite roles in neural patterning, *Shh* being required for ventral cell types and *Opb* being required for dorsal cell types. *Shh* mutants are holoprosencephalic (Chiang et al., 1996), and *Opb* mutants are exencephalic (Günther et al., 1994).

Eggenschwiler et al. (2001) cloned *Opb* and found that it encodes Rab23. Rab proteins make up the largest branch of the Ras superfamily of GTPases. The term Rab stands for "*Ra*s-like in rat *b*rain (Martinez and Goud, 1998). Rabs cycle between GDP-bound and GTP-bound conformation. They regulate specific transport steps along the biosynthetic/secretory and endocytic pathways (Chavrier and Goud, 1999).

The activity of Rab23 is downstream of Shh and upstream of Shh target genes. It could affect Shh signaling by regulating endocytosis of Shh/Ptch from the cell surface or by regulating endocytotic vesicles containing Shh/Ptch or Shh/megalin (Eggenschwiler et al., 2001, Nybakken and Perrimon, 2002) (Fig. 16–2).

Hedgehog-Interacting Protein (Hip)

Chuang and McMahon (1999) isolated Hedgehog-interacting protein (*Hip*), which is found in vertebrates but not in *Drosophila*. Hip encodes a membrane-bound glycoprotein that binds to Shh, Ihh, and Dhh. Hip attenuates M-Shh-N signaling (Fig. 16–2), thus reducing its effective range.

Growth Arrest Specific 1 (GAS1)

Growth arrest specific 1 (GAS1) is a 45-kDa glycophosphatydlinositol (GPI)-linked protein originally identified for arresting the cell cycle when overexpressed (Del Sal et al., 1992, 1994, 1995; Stebel et al., 2000). Lee et al. (2001) suggested that GAS1 attenuated M-Shh-N signaling (Fig. 16–2), thus reducing its effective range.

Downstream Signaling

Many factors are involved in downstream signaling. Costal 2 (Cos2), Fused (Fu), and Suppressor of fused (Sufu)[5] regulate the nuclear transcription and activity of Cubitus interruptus (Ci) (Fig. 16–3). Other factors include protein kinase A (dPKA), glycogen synthase kinase 3 (GSK3), casein kinase 1 (CK1), Supernumerary limbs (Slimb), SAP18, and CREB-bound protein (dCBP) (Fig. 16–3). The three target genes are *Patched* (*Ptch*), *Wingless* (*Wg*), and *Decapentaplegic* (*Dpp*). Separate sections on these factors appear below, followed by a discussion about their interactions.

Cubitus interruptus (*Ci*) and *Gli* Gene Family

The segment polarity gene *Cubitus interruptus* (*Ci*), a zinc-finger gene in *Drosophila*, is the ortholog of the *Gli* gene family in vertebrates. The sequence similarity is striking with a 54.3% identity in a 278-amino-acid overlap beginning 13 amino acids before the first zinc finger and extending approximately 100 amino acids beyond the last zinc finger. Between the twelfth amino acid residue of the second repeat and after the end of the fifth repeat, there are 108 amino acids with a 93% identity (Orenic et al., 1990).

Ci is a 155-kDa protein that contains five zinc fingers. It appears as a truncated 75-kDa target repressor or a full-length 155-kDa target activator (Orenic et al., 1990; Aza-Blanc et al., 1997; Ruiz i Altaba et al., 1997; Tabin and McMahon, 1997; Chen et al., 1999a). A diagram of Ci appears in Figure 16–6. Motifs include a suppressor of fused (Sufu)-binding domain (SF), zinc finger (ZF) DNA-binding domain, nuclear localization signal (NLS), cleavage site (↑), nuclear export signal (NES), protein kinase A (PKA) phosphorylation sites (P), Costal 2 (Cos2)-binding domain (CORD), and CREB-binding protein (CBP) domain (Wang et al., 2000b).

The *Gli* gene family was identified originally by the amplification of human GLI1 in glioblastoma (Kinzler et al., 1987, 1988, 1990). GLI1, GLI2, and GLI3 share five highly conserved tandem C2H2 zinc fingers and a conservative histidine-cysteine linker sequence between zinc fingers (Ruppert et al., 1988). In humans, GLI1 has two isoforms, GLI2 has three alternatively spliced exons, and GLI3 has only one isoform. GLI, encoding a 1106-amino-acid protein, maps to 12q13; GLI2, encoding 812, 829, 1241, or 1258 amino acids, maps to 2q14; and GLI3, encoding 1595 amino acids, maps to 7p13[6] (Ruppert et al., 1988, 1990; Matsumoto et al., 1996; Reifenberger et al., 1996; Villavicencio et al., 2000).

Less is known about Gli family function in vertebrates than is known about Ci function in *Drosophila* (see Chapter 20). Gli1 is an activator of hedgehog target genes, but it does not appear to require CBP as a coactivator. Apparently, Gli1 does not undergo proteolytic cleavage and does not function as a repressor. Gli2 has both activator and repressor forms (Ingham and McMahon, 2001).

Gli3 can undergo proteolytic cleavage, resulting in a truncated 83-kDa repressor form (Wang et al., 2000a). Although evidence for a

---

[5]*Suppressor of fused* has been commonly abbreviated as *Su(fu)*. However, in discussing human mutations for medulloblastoma caused by *Suppressor of Fused*, Taylor et al. (2002) set the precedent of simplifying the term; they used *SUFU* rather than *SU(FU)*.

[6]Unfortunately, *Human Krüppel-Related Gene 4* (*HKR4*), which maps to 8q24.3, has been misclassified as a member of the *GLI* gene family and was called *GLI4* by Kas et al. (1996). Also, in *Drosophila*, the *Gli* gene is not an ortholog of *Gli*; it is an unrelated gene in which *Gli* stands for *Gliotactin* (Ruppert et al., 1988).

Gli3 activator form is weak, some studies have suggested this possibility. Dai et al. (1999), in tissue culture, showed that Gli3 activates a Gli1 promoter in an Shh-dependent manner and is further potentiated by CBP. Gli3 has also been shown to interact with vertebrate Sufu and with human FU (Pearse et al., 1999; Murone et al., 2000), which might be expected if Shh resulted in a Gli3 activator form that was translocated to the nucleus.

Ruiz i Altaba et al. (2002) showed that in mice Shh can induce Gli1 and Gli2 but Shh-Gli1 seems to have a mutually repressive interaction with Gli3. GLi2 may also induce Gli1. Fgf2 was found to induce the expression of Gli2 and Gli3. Target genes of Gli1, Gli2, and Gli3 include Wnt, Igf2, and Pdgfrα.

Three distinct Gli proteins in vertebrates instead of one Ci ortholog in *Drosophila* allow more complex responses within target fields. Thus, cellular response to hedgehog signaling might not simply depend on the level of ligand exposure but also on the particular *Gli* genes expressed (Ingham and McMahon, 2001). Vertebrate *Gli* genes may be tissue specific; may have unevenly partitioned activator and repressor functions; may be coexpressed, possibly being competitive or working synergistically; or may be partially redundant (Ruiz i Altiba, 1997, 1999; Aza-Blanc et al., 2000).

GLI1 is commonly expressed in almost all isolated basal cell carcinomas (Dahmane et al., 1997). Nilsson et al. (2000) overexpressed Gli1 in transgenic mice, inducing basal cell carcinomas and trichoepitheliomas. *GLI2* mutations in humans have been reported with holoprosencephaly (Roessler et al., 2002).

GLI3 mutations cause Greig cephalopolysyndactyly (Biesecker et al., 1997; Wild et al., 1997) and Pallister-Hall syndrome (Biesecker et al., 1997; Kang et al., 1997). Biesecker (1997) indicated that the syndromes do not overlap clinically to any significant extent. He further indicated that in Greig cephalopolysyndactyly, *GLI3* mutations are of the translocation, deletion, missense, splicing, and frameshift types, whereas in Pallister-Hall syndrome, only frameshift mutations occur. Biesecker (see Chapter 20) hypothesized that syndrome differences could be explained by the effects that the two groups of mutations have on the balance of activator and repressor forms of GLI3.

Isolated medulloblastoma is found rarely, if ever, with *GLI3* mutations, although two patients with Greig cephalopolysyndactyly and medulloblastoma have been reported with *GLI3* mutations (Erez et al., 2002).

Mice with a null mutation for Gli2 or for Gli2 plus a heterozygous mutation in Gli3 mimic VACTERL association including vertebral, anal, cardiac, tracheoesophageal, renal, and limb anomalies (Kim et al., 2001). Pallister-Hall syndrome and VACTERL association share in common anal atresia, cardiac anomalies, renal abnormalities, and limb defects. Perhaps patients with VACTERL association might be worked up for digenic heterozygous mutations in Gli2 plus Gli3.

Phosphorylation of Ci, PKA, GSK3, and CK1

The proteolysis of Ci from the 155-kDa form to the repressive 75-kDa form requires phosphorylation of Ci (Figs. 16–3 and 16–6). Chen et al. (1999b) found that PKA phosphorylates four consensus sites on Ci; three involve serine (Ser838, Ser856, and Ser892) and one involves threonine (Thr1006). The three phosphoserines are essential for Ci proteolysis and transcriptional activity. Phosphothreonine does not affect Ci function; Prorok and Lawrence (1989) demonstrated that phosphothreonine is a poor substrate for PKA activity.

Following PKA-primed phosphorylation of Ci, GSK3[7] and CK1 further phosphorylate Ci on serines near PKA phosphorylation sites (Fig. 16–3). This is essential for proteolytic processing because alteration of GSK3 or CK1 sites *prevents* proteolysis (Jia et al., 2002; Price and Kalderon, 2002).

Hedgehog signaling, resulting in the active 155-kDa form, probably reduces the Ci phosphorylation level by the action of a phosphatase (Aza-Blanc et al., 1997; Chen et al., 1999a; Wang and Holmgren, 1999).

[7]Shaggy (Sgg), also known as Zest-white 3 (Zw3), is the *Drosophila* ortholog of vertebrate GSK3 (Jia et al., 2002).

Costal 2 (Cos2)

Costal 2 (Cos2) is a microtubule-associated kinesin-like protein. Kinesins are motor proteins defined by their motor domain of approximately 320 amino acid residues that bind and hydrolyse ATP and bind to microtubules. The motor domain is commonly coupled to additional structural or regulatory domains that can attach to other cofactors, adaptor proteins, or interaction modules (Kamal and Goldstein, 2002; Mandelkow and Mandelkow, 2002). Woehlke et al. (1997) located the microtubule-binding site in three loops that cluster on the motor surface. The core of the microtubule-binding interface resides in a highly conserved loop and helix (L12/α5). Critical residues are positively charged while microtubules are negatively charged.

Fused (*vide infra*) is known to phosphorylate Cos2 at two positions—one in the region between the motor domain and the heptad repeats at serine 572 and, to a lesser extent, in the C-terminal domain at serine 931 (Nybakken et al., 2002). Cos2 binds to the microtubules, to the CORD domain of Ci, and to the C-terminal domain of Fused (Wang et al., 2000b, Ascano et al., 2002) (Figs. 16–3 and 16–6). Monnier et al. (2002) found, in contrast to Wang et al. (2000b), that Cos2 can bind closer to the N terminus of Ci between the Sufu binding domain and the zinc finger domain (Fig. 16–6).

Fused (Fu)

Fused (*Fu*), a segment polarity gene, is a serine/threonine kinase. In *Drosophila*, the original weak *Fu* mutation has a maternal effect; females have tumorous ovaries (Préat et al., 1990). Phosphorylation of Fu occurs in response to hedgehog signaling and involves an activation loop for Fu transcription (Fukumoto et al., 2001). The C-terminal domain then binds to Cos2 and phosphorylates it (Ascano et al., 2002; Nybakken et al., 2002). Thérond et al. (1999) demonstrated that Fu is required to maintain Ptch and Wingless (Wg) expression (Fig. 16–3).

Suppressor of Fused (Sufu)

Suppressor of fused (*Sufu*)[5] has been identified in *Drosophila* (Préat, 1992), chicks, mice (Pearse et al., 1999), and humans (*SUFU*)[5] (Stone et al., 1999). Human SUFU exhibits a 37% sequence identity with *Drosophila* Sufu and a 97% sequence identity with mouse Sufu. Two alternately spliced protein isoforms include a 433-amino-acid 48-kDa form and a 484-amino-acid 54-kDa form. The protein differs only by the inclusion or exclusion of 52 amino acids at the C terminus (Stone et al., 1999).

Human SUFU contains a PEST domain (Stone et al., 1999). A PEST motif is an amino acid sequence rich in proline (P), glutamic acid (E), serine (S), and threonine (T). It is often found in proteins that undergo rapid degradation. Serine/threonine residues are phosphorylated as part of or all of the signal to degrade the protein (Rechsteiner and Rogers, 1996).

In *Drosophila*, Sufu binds to the Sufu domain of Ci near the N terminus and also binds to Fu. However, transcription of activator 155-kDa Ci is attenuated in the nucleus by Sufu, which stabilizes the latent form of Ci. With high levels of hedgehog signaling, Ci is converted into a labile and active form, possibly by dissociating it from Sufu (Wang et al., 2000b) (Fig. 16–3).

Stone et al. (1999) found that human SUFU interacts with GLI1, GLI2, GLI3, and Slimb, indicating that SUFU is a negative regulator of the hedgehog signaling network. They suggested that SUFU can inhibit GLI-mediated transactivation and also serve as an adaptor protein that links GLI to the Slimb-dependent proteasomal degradation pathway. Cheng and Bishop (2002) found that Sufu represses Gli-mediated transcription by recruiting SAP18, a component of the histone deacetylase complex Sin3.

Human SUFU is widely expressed in fetal and adult tissues. Its presence in adult tissues suggests a functional hedgehog signaling network in which SUFU suppresses GLI activity. *SUFU* maps to 10q24-q25, a region that is deleted in glioblastoma, prostate cancer, malignant melanoma, and endometrial cancer (Gray et al., 1995; Rasheed et al., 1995; Albarosa et al., 1996; Pfeiffer-Schneider et al., 1998; Stone et al., 1999). Taylor et al. (2002) reported a subset of children with medulloblastoma and SUFU mutations, both germline and somatic, accompanied by loss of heterozygosity of the wild-type allele.

Supernumerary Limbs (Slimb)

Supernumerary limbs (Slimb) is an F-box/WD40-repeat protein functioning in the ubiquitin-proteasome pathway (Jiang and Struhl, 1998; Patton et al., 1998; Kipreos and Pagano, 2000) (Fig. 16–3). Slimb is the *Drosophila* ortholog of vertebrate βTrCP. Slimb is required for Ci proteolysis to the 75-kDa repressor form, although it remains unclear how Slimb recognizes phosphorylated Ci. Slimb (βTrCP) can recognize paired GSK3 phosphorylation sites on β-catenin; however, the sites occur in a specific consensus sequence DS(P)XXS(P) and the sites on Ci do not conform to this sequence. Perhaps Slimb recognizes more epitopes than are currently known or perhaps multiple weak binding sites on Ci collectively allow it to associate with Slimb (Price and Kalderon, 2002). It is also possible that phosphorylation underlies the known isoforms of Slimb (Spenser et al., 1999). Ko et al. (2002) suggested that the phosphorylation status of Slimb (βTrCP) might modulate its ability to interact with target proteins.

Other Factors (Sil, COUP-TFII, Dyrk1, Twist)

Sil (*SCL interrupting locus*) encodes a 150-kDa cytosolic protein of unknown function. It is highly conserved in vertebrates but has no homologous regions to any known protein. Sil is an essential component of the sonic hedgehog signaling network acting downstream to Ptch. Mouse null mutants $Sil^{-/-}$ are characterized by neural tube defects, left/right axis abnormalities, holoprosencephaly-like features, and early lethality. $Sil^{+/-}$ heterozgotes are normal (Izreali et al., 2001).

Human *SIL*, mapping to 1p32, encodes a protein of 1287 amino acid residues beginning at the third exon. Human SIL and murine Sil have a 73% overall identity. No human mutations for holoprosencephaly have been found (Karkera et al., 2002).

Krishnan et al. (1997) identified an Shh response element in *chicken ovalbumin upstream promoter-transcription factor II* (COUP-TFII). They suggested that Shh signaling may result in dephosphorylation of a target factor required for activating COUP-TFII, Islet-1, and Gli response element–dependent gene expression.

Mao et al. (2002) investigated the cellular role of dual specificity Yak1-related kinase 1 (Dyrk1), finding that it enhanced Gli1-dependent gene transcription. However, Shh failed to stimulate Dyrk1 activity, suggesting the possibility of a separate pathway mediated by Dyrk1 that may functionally interact with the sonic hedgehog signaling network.

Villavicencio et al. (2000) suggested that murine Twist protein can activate human GLI1 at the transcriptional level by interacting with E-boxes in the first intron. However, no published study to date has demonstrated this.

Cyclic AMP Response Element-Binding Protein (CPB)

The cAMP-regulated enhancer (CRE) binds many transcription factors, including CRE-binding (CREB) protein (CPB), which is activated as a result of phosphorylation by PKA. CPB is a 2441-amino-acid 265-kDa nuclear protein that is a coactivator for a number of transcription factors, including 155-kDa activator Ci (Chrivia et al., 1993; Akimaru et al., 1997) (Fig. 16–3). In humans, CBP maps to 16p13.3. Microdeletions resulting in haploinsufficiency of CBP cause Rubinstein-Taybi syndrome (Petrij et al., 1995; Blough et al., 2000).

Interactions of Ci, Cos2, Fu, and Sufu

In downstream signaling, Ci, Cos2, Fu, and Sufu form a tetrameric complex that results in the nuclear transcription and activity of Ci (Fig. 16–3). In the absence of hedgehog stimulation, the complex is tethered to the microtubules by Cos2. Both Cos2 and Sufu retain Ci in the cytoplasm, the former being bound to Ci's CORD domain and the latter being bound to its Sufu domain (SF) (Fig. 16–6). Cos2 promotes proteolysis of Ci, generating the truncated 75-kDa repressor form of Ci (Rep-Ci). The process requires phosphorylation of Ci by dPKA, CK1, and Sgg, and also the activities of Slimb, Sufu, and SAP18. Translocation of Rep-Ci to the nucleus prevents transcription of target genes *Ptch*, *Wg*, and *Dpp* (Robbins et al., 1997; Ruiz i Altaba, 1997; Tabin and McMahon, 1997; Monnier et al., 1998; Wang et al., 2000b; Ingham and McMahon, 2001; Mullor et al., 2002; Nybakken and Perrimon, 2002).

With intermediate levels of hedgehog stimulation, the Ci, Cos2, Fu, Sufu complex dissociates from the microtubules, inhibiting the cleavage of Ci (Fig. 16–3), possibly through dephosphorylation of Ci. The full-length 155-kDa activator form of Ci (Act-Ci) binds to Sufu, an interaction that restricts its nuclear translocation. Sufu attenuates its transcriptional activity. Higher levels of hedgehog stimulation promote dissociation of Sufu from Act-Ci, which together with cofactor dCBP upregulate target genes *Ptch*, *Wg*, and *Dpp* (Robbins et al., 1997; Ruiz i Altaba, 1997; Tabin and McMahon, 1997; Monnier et al., 1998; Wang et al., 2000b; Ingham and McMahon, 2001; Mullor et al., 2002; Nybakken and Perrimon, 2002).

Target Genes

Target genes in *Drosophila* include *Ptch*, *wingless* (*Wg*), and *decapentaplegic* (*Dpp*). These are the orthologs of the vertebrate target genes: *Ptch* (PTCH), the *Wnt* (WNT) family, and the *bone morphogenetic proteins* (BMPs) of the TGFβ superfamily; they are essential for normal embryonic development and differentiation of many adult tissues.

The upregulation of Ptch expression, resulting in Ptch protein at the cell membrane, sequesters hedgehog and limits its spread beyond the cells in which it is produced (Chen and Struhl, 1996). Thus, a balance is created by the antagonism of Hedgehog and Ptch, whose relative concentrations alternate with respect to each other (Cohen, 1999). A detailed discussion of Ptch appears in Cohen (2003b) (also *vide supra*).

Wnt genes encode a family of secreted glycoproteins that share overall sequence identity and a conserved pattern of 23-24 cysteine residues (see Chapter 22). The original ones defined were *Drosophila Wingless* (*Wg*) and murine *Wnt1*. *Drosophila* possesses 4 and the mouse at least 18 *Wnt* genes. They have been implicated in many developmental processes such as cell differentiation, cell polarity, cell migration, and cell proliferation. Misregulation of Wnt signaling is implicated in developmental defects and oncogenesis (Moon et al., 1997; Miller et al., 1999; Kühl et al., 2000; Taipale and Beachy, 2001).

There are two Wnt signaling pathways: Wnt/β-catenin and Wnt/Ca^{2+}. Members of the Frizzled (Fz) family of 7-pass transmembrane proteins serve as receptors of Wnt signaling. They have an extracellular cysteine-rich domain (CRD) at the N terminus that binds Wnt. An LDL-receptor-related protein is a coreceptor for Wnt and binds to a Fz CRD in a Wnt-dependent manner. Sulfated glycosaminoglycans are also required for optimal Wg activity (Cumberledge and Reichsman, 1997; Miller et al., 1999; Kühl et al., 2000; Dann et al., 2001). Dubois et al. (2001) demonstrated that regulated endocytic routing modulates Wg signaling in *Drosophila* embryos.

In the canonical Wnt/β-catenin signaling pathway, a Frizzled receptor with a Wnt ligand increases cytoplasmic β-catenin, which translocates to the nucleus and, together with LEF/TCF, upregulates target genes. Some components of the pathway—Wnt, Fz, and Armadillo (Arm)—are positive, activated during signaling. Other components—GSK3 and TCF-Groucho-CBP—are negative, inhibited during signaling. Mutations in β-catenin have been identified in many human cancers, including, among others, colorectal cancer, endometrial cancer, hepatocellular carcinoma, ovarian cancer, uterine cancer, prostate cancer, melanoma, and pilomatrixoma. In *APC*, a tumor suppressor gene that is part of the Wnt/β-catenin pathway, mutations are known to cause colorectal polyposis and adenocarcinoma (Miller et al., 1999, Nusse et al., 1999, Kühl et al., 2000).

Activation of the Wnt/Ca^{2+} pathway results in intracellular Ca^{2+} release and activation of Ca^{2+}-sensitive enzymes: Ca^{2+}-calmodulin–dependent protein kinase II (CamKII) and protein kinase C (PKC) (Miller et al., 1999; Kühl et al., 2000).

Dpp, most closely related to BMP2 and BMP4 (Massagué et al., 1994), acts at short range to provide dorsal-ventral positional information to the embryonic ectoderm. Dpp positional information in multiple target fields requires synergistic signaling between two different BMP receptor–ligand pairs (Podos and Ferguson, 1999). The heteromeric receptor complex consists of two types of serine-threonine kinases (Cohen, 2002, 2003a). On Dpp ligand binding, the type II receptor (*Punt*, *Put*) phosphorylates the type I receptor (*Thick veins*, *Tkv*), which activates Mad and Med followed by transcription of target genes. A second type I receptor (*Saxaphone*, *Sax*) and its ligand (either *Screw*, *Scw*, or *Glassbottom boat*, *Gbb*) are also essential for normal patterning in each tissue (Podos and Ferguson, 1999).

Entchev et al. (2000) demonstrated that long-range Dpp movement involves intracellular trafficking by dynamin-mediated endocytosis of Dpp and its type I receptor (Tkv). They suggested that a balance between recycling and degradation of Dpp ligand determines the shape of the gradient.

MUTATIONS, GENE OVEREXPRESSION, AND TERATOGENS IN ANIMALS

Table 16–4 summarizes mutations, gene overexpression, and teratogens involving the hedgehog signaling network and cholesterol biosynthesis in animals. The null mutation $Shh^{-/-}$ in mice produces a severe phenotype: holoprosencephaly and distal anteroposterior limb deficiences (Chiang et al., 1996, 2001). Overexpression of *Shh* (*Shh* ↑↑) in mice results in basal cell carcinomas and skeletal anomalies (Oro et al., 1997).

Two teratogens, AY9944[8] and BM15.766,[8] block sterol Δ^7-reductase, resulting in the accumulation of 7-dehydrocholesterol and reduced serum cholesterol with the production of holoprosencephaly in rats (Barbu et al., 1984; Kolf-Clauw et al., 1996, 1997; Gofflot et al., 1999). Lanoue et al. (1997) studied mice with a targeted modification of the *alipoprotein B* (*apoB*) gene; when treated with BM15.766, sterol Δ^7-reductase was blocked, resulting in reduced serum cholesterol and the accumulation of 7-dehydrocholesterol. Phenotypic findings were similar to those found in Smith-Lemli-Opitz syndrome and included holoprosencephaly together with limb and genital defects (see Chapter 17, "Cholesterol Deficiency: Smith-Lemli-Opitz and Cyclopamine Teratogens"). The specific block in cholesterol biosynthesis found in Smith-Lemli-Opitz syndrome is identical to that produced by the two teratogens, AY9944 and BM15.766, which results in holoprosencephaly in experimental animals (Fig. 16–9).

Triparanol[8] is a sterol Δ^{24}-reductase inhibitor that results in an accumulation of desmosterol and reduced serum cholesterol (Fig. 16–9). Triparanol has been used experimentally in rats to produce a wide range of malformations, including holoprosencephaly (Roux, 1964). In contrast to triparanol-treated rats with holoprosencephaly, no instances of frank holoprosencephaly have been reported in human desmosterolosis to date, although one instance of a hypoplastic corpus callosum has been noted. Other blocks in cholesterol biosynthesis are known that also do not result in holoprosencephaly (Kelley, 2000).

Cooper et al. (1998) found that when AY9944, triparanol, cyclopamine, or jervine were added to cells with a stably integrated construct for expressing Shh, the autoprocessed Shh-N was detected with the same mobility as cholesterol-modified Shh-N. The cholesterol adduct was efficiently replaced by 7-dehydrocholesterol in AY9944-treated cells and desmosterol in triparanol-treated cells. It is possible that other 27-carbon cholesterol precursors might also be able to serve as sterol adducts in the Shh autoprocessing reaction. However, neither cyclopamine nor jervine replace the sterol adduct (Cooper et al., 1998).

To examine the possibility that AY9944, triparanol, cyclopamine, and jervine caused their effects on target tissues, Cooper et al. (1998) used a neural plate explant, a target tissue that does not contain Shh but has the ability to respond to it. They found that these teratogens inhibited the response of target tissues to Shh-N. Thus, teratogens such as AY9944 and triparanol still permit Shh autoprocessing by using cholesterol precursors as sterol adducts of Shh-N, and even though Shh-N is active, the target tissues still fail to respond to Shh-N signaling.

Incardona et al. (1998) studied the effects of AY944 and cyclopamine on neural plate explants, also finding that both teratogens blocked the response of target tissues to Shh-N. When exogenous cholesterol supplementation was added to the explants, the response to Shh-N was restored in AY9944-treated explants but not in cyclopamine-treated explants, suggesting that cyclopamine-induced teratogenesis may produce a more direct antagonism to Shh signaling transduction.[9]

Cooper et al. (1998) suggested that defects in intracellular cholesterol transport and homeostasis are the common basis for the induction of holoprosencephaly by cyclopamine and 7-dehydrocholesterol inhibitor AY9944. The study of Incardona et al. (2001a) did not support the hypothesis of Cooper et al. (1998); they found that cyclopamine inhibition of sonic hedgehog signaling transduction is not mediated through effects on cholesterol transport.

Megalin is a receptor for apoB-containing lipoproteins and is expressed in the yolk sac endoderm and the embryonic neuroectoderm (Farese and Herz, 1998). McCarthy et al. (2002) demonstrated that M-Shh-N binds to megalin with high affinity. With megalin deficiency, holoprosencephaly is observed in mouse embryos, suggesting a perturbation of the Shh signaling network (Willnow et al., 1996).

Holoprosencephaly in newborn lambs has been traced to the ingestion of the range plant *Veratrum californicum* by pregnant ewes (Binns et al., 1963), Keeler and Binns (1968) identified steroidal alkaloids in the plant as the cause of holoprosencephaly; two of the isolated compounds were cyclopamine and jervine (Table 16–4), which have some similarities to cholesterol (Fig. 16–10). Beachy et al. (1997) tested jervine-treated cells and found reduced levels of cholesterol and an apparent increase in the cholesterol precursor zymosterol.

Chick embryos treated with ethanol show loss of Shh and other transcripts involving the sonic hedgehog signaling network (Ahlgren et al., 2002).

In the mouse null mutation for *Ihh*, hypertrophic chondrocytes predominate in the growth plate (Lanske et al., 1996; Vortkamp et al., 1996). In humans, heterozygous missense mutations in *IHH* (Glu95Lys, Asp100Glu, and Glu131Lys) cause brachydactyly type A-1 (Gao et al., 2001). Homozygous *IHH* mutations cause acrocapitofemoral dyplasia (Hellemans et al., 2003). The mouse null mutation for *Dhh* results in male infertility with absence of mature sperm (Bitgood et al., 1996).

A mouse null mutation $mDispA^{-/-}$ was found to produce a neural plate defect in the prospective forebrain consistent with later developing holoprosencephaly. However, further embryonic development permitting full-blown holoprosencephaly was precluded by concomitant cardiac defects (Ma et al., 2002).

The mouse $Ptch^{+/-}$ mutation is characterized by skeletal defects and tumors, suggestive of some nevoid basal cell carcinoma syndrome–like features. They include neural tube defects, generalized overgrowth, syndactyly or extra digits uncommonly, cerebellar medulloblastomas, rhabdomyosarcomas, and other tumors (Goodrich et al., 1997; Hahn et al., 1998, 1999) (Table 16–4). The null mutation ($Ptch^{-/-}$) is lethal with an open and overgrown neural tube (Goodrich et al., 1997).

In *Drosophila*, $Ptch^{1130X}$ causes a C-terminal truncation that abolishes repression of Smo but does not affect Hh binding (Johnson et al., 2000). In chick embryos, $Ptch^{\Delta loop2}$ produces loss of the second large extracellular loop so that Shh binding cannot take place (Briscoe et al., 2001).

Several *Ptch* sterol sensor mutations have been induced in *Drosophila* (Gly477Arg, Asp584Asn, Tyr442Cys) and in mice (Tyr438Cys, Asp585Asn) (Strutt et al., 2001; Johnson et al., 2002). *Drosophila* mutations Gly477Arg and Asp584Asn abolish repression of Smo but do not affect Hh ligand binding (Strutt et al., 2001). Johnson et al. (2002) found that Tyr438Cys and Asp585Asn had no effect in mice. They also found that Tyr442Cys in *Drosophila* had no effect, whereas Asp584Asn had dominant negative activity. However, both mutations confer resistance to the sterol regulator in SCAP, indicating that mutations in sterol sensor motifs function differently between sterol sensor family members.

---

[8]Experimental animal teratogens AY9944, BM15.766, and triparanol can affect multipostsqualene enzymes, although AY9944 and BM15.766 primarily block sterol Δ^7-reductase and triparanol blocks primarily sterol Δ^{24}-reductase.

[9]Presumably, the same would be true for the closely-related compound jervine (Fig. 16–10), although this possibility was not tested by Incardona et al. (1998).

Table 16–4. Mutations, Gene Overexpression, and Teratogens Involving the Hedgehog Signaling Network and Cholesterol Biosynthesis in Animals

Mutated Gene, Overexpressed Gene, or Teratogen	Species	Phenotype	Comment	Reference
$Shh^{-/-}$	Mouse	Cyclopia, limb anomalies	Mutation is recessive, resulting in severe phenotype; holoprosencephaly and severe distal anteroposterior limb deficiencies	Chiang et al. (1996, 2001)
$Shh \uparrow\uparrow$	Mouse	Tumors and malformations	Overexpression results in basal cell carcinomas and skeletal malformations	Oro et al. (1997)
AY9944[a]	Rat	Holoprosencephaly	Teratogen blocking sterol Δ^7-reductase. Results in reduced serum cholesterol and accumulation of 7-dehydro-cholesterol	Barbu et al. (1984), Kolf-Clauw et al. (1996), Gofflot et al. (1999)
BM15.766[b]	Rat	Holoprosencephaly	Teratogen blocking sterol Δ^7-reductase. Results in reduced serum cholesterol and accumulation of 7-dehydro-cholesterol	Kolf-Clauw et al. (1997), Dehart et al. (1995)
Hypomorphic apoB + BM15.766[b]	Mouse	Holoprosencephaly	Mice with targeted modification of the alipoprotein B (apoB) gene. When treated with teratogen BM15.766, sterol Δ^7-reductase is blocked resulting in reduced serum cholesterol and accumulation of 7-dehydrocholesterol. Phenotype includes holoprosencephaly, limb defects, and genital anomalies	Lanoue et al. (1997)
Triparanol[c]	Rat	Holoprosencephaly	Teratogen blocking sterol Δ^{24}-reductase. Results in reduced serum cholesterol and accumulation of desmosterol	Roux (1964)[d]
Megalin$^{-/-}$	Mouse	Holoprosencephaly	Holoprosencephaly is found in mouse embryos deficient in megalin, a member of the low-density lipoprotein (LDL) receptor family that is expressed in embryonic neuroectoderm and binds and internalizes LDL.	Willnow et al. (1996)
Cyclopamine	Sheep	Cyclopia	Steroid isolated from desert plant *Veratrum californicum*	Binns et al. (1963, 1965), Keeler and Binns (1966)
	Rat	Cyclopia		Keeler (1975)
	Mouse			Keeler (1975)
	Hamster			Keeler (1975), Coventry et al. (1998)
	Rabbit	Cyclopia		Keeler (1970)
	Chick	Holoprosencephaly		Bryden et al. (1973), Incardona et al. (1998)
Cyclopamine	Chick	Inhibition of Shh signal transduction	Not mediated through effects on cholesterol transport	Incardona et al. (2001a)
Jervine	Rat, mouse, hamster	Holoprosencephaly	Steroid isolated from desert plant *Veratrum californicum*	Keeler (1975)
	Treated COS7 cultured cells		Reduced levels of cholesterol and abnormal accumulation of zymosterol	Beachy et al. (1997)
Ethanol	Chick embryos	Loss of Shh and other transcripts involving the sonic hedgehog signaling network	Cranial neural crest cell death	Ahlgren et al. (2002)
$Ihh^{-/-}$	Mouse	Growth palate defect	Hypertrophic chondrocytes predominate in growth plate; absent PTHrP in growth plate	St-Jacques et al. (1999)
$Ihh \uparrow\uparrow$	Chick	Growth plate defect	Hypertrophic chondrocytes delayed in growth plate	Lanske et al. (1996), Vortkamp et al. (1996)
$IHH^{BDA-1/+}$	Human	Brachydactyly type A-1	Heterozygous missense mutations	Gao et al. (2001)
$IHH^{ACF/ACF}$	Human	Acrocapitofemoral dysplasia	Autosomal recessive disorders of cone-shaped epiphyses in hands and hips	Hellemans et al. (2003)
$Dhh^{-/-}$	Mouse	Male infertility	Absence of mature sperm; Dhh regulates Sertoli-Leydig cell interactions and spermatogenesis	Bitgood et al. (1996)
$mDispA^{-/-}$	Mouse	Neural plate defect in region of prospective forebrain	Findings consistent with holoprosencephaly, but cardiac defects preclude further embryonic development; other anomalies noted	Ma et al. (2002)
$Ptch^{+/-}$	Mouse	Skeletal defects and tumors	Some nevoid basal cell carcinoma syndrome–like features: skeletal abnormalities, neural tube defects, generalized overgrowth, syndactyly or extra digits uncommonly, cerebellar medulloblastomas, rhabdomyosarcomas,	Goodrich et al. (1997), Hahn et al. (1998, 1999)

(continued)

Table 16–4. *Continued*

Mutated Gene, Overexpressed Gene, or Teratogen	Species	Phenotype	Comment	Reference
			intestinal adenocarcinoma, cystadenoma, endometrial stromal sarcoma, and primitive neuroectodermal-like tumor	
$Ptch^{-/-}$	Mouse	Lethal with neural tube defect	Lethal; open and overgrown neural tube	Goodrich et al. (1997)
$Ptch^{1130X}$	*Drosophila*		Mutation causes C-terminal truncation; abolishes Smo repression but does not affect Hh ligand binding	Johnson et al. (2000)
$Ptch^{\Delta loop2}$	Chick embryo	Loss of second large extra-cellular loop; mouse $Ptch^{\Delta loop2}$ used in chick embryo	Cannot bind Shh ligand	Briscoe et al. (2001)
Ptch sterol sensor mutations (Gly477Arg, Asp584Asn)	*Drosophila*		Mutations abolish Smo repression but do not affect Hh ligand binding	Strutt et al. (2001)
Ptch sterol sensor mutations (Tyr442Cys, Asp584Asn)	*Drosophila*		Tyr442Cys has no effect; Asp584Asn has dominant negative activity	Johnson et al. (2002)
Ptch sterol sensor mutations (Tyr438Cys, Asp585Asn)	Mouse		Neither mutation has an effect; in contrast, analogous mutations confer resistance to the sterol regulator in SCAP	Johnson et al. (2002)
$Ptch^{+/-}$ + cyclopamine	Mouse	Tumor inhibition	Medulloblastoma growth inhibition by hedge-hog network blockade	Berman et al. (2002)
$Ptch^{-/-}$ + cyclopamine $Smo \uparrow\uparrow$ + cyclopamine	Mouse	Reversal of oncogenic mutations	In humans, haploinsufficient *PTCH* mutations and activating *SMO* mutations cause basal cell carcinoma	Taipale et al. (2000)
$Smo^{-/-}$	Mouse	Neural plate defect in region of prospective forebrain	Findings consistent with holoprosencephaly, but cardiac defects preclude further embryonic development; other anomalies noted	Ma et al. (2002)
$Gli1^{zfd/zfd e}$	Mouse	Normal	No phenotypic abnormalities	Park et al. (2000)
$Gli1 \uparrow\uparrow$	Frog	Tumors	Skin tumors in tadpoles	Dahmane et al. (1997)
$Gli1 \uparrow\uparrow$	Mouse	Basal cell carcinomas and trichoepitheliomas		Nilsson et al. (2000)
$Gli2^{zfd/+}$	Mouse	Normal	No discernable abnormalities	Mo et al. (1997)
$Gli2^{zfd/zfd}$	Mouse	Multiple anomalies	Cleft palate, tooth defects, vertebral anomalies, short limbs; floorplate throughout midbrain, hindbrain and spinal cord fails to form; notochord does not regress as in normal embryo	Mo et al. (1997), Matise et al. (1998)
$Gli2^{zfd/zfd}$ $Gli2^{zfd/zfd} + Gli3^{zfd/+}$	Mouse	VACTERL-like association	Mimics human VACTERL (vertebral anal, cardiac, tracheoesophageal, renal, and limb defects	Kim et al. (2001)
$Gli1^{zfd/zfd} + Gli2^{zfd/zfd}$	Mouse	Spinal cord abnormality	Failure of spinal cord formation similar to $Gli2^{zfd/zfd}$	Matise et al. (1998)
$Gli3^{XtJ/+ e}$	Mouse	Limb defects and other anomalies	Anterior and posterior digit duplication suggestive of duplicated digits in Greig cephalopolysyndactyly; white belly spot; interfrontal bone (abnormal in mice); increased frequency of hydrocephalus	Johnson (1967, 1969), Pohl et al. (1990), Hui and Joyner (1993), Schimmang et al. (1994), Mo et al. (1997), Maynard et al. (2002)
$Gli3^{XtJ/XtJ}$	Mouse	Limb defects and multiple anomalies	Frequently stillborn; abnormal limbs with severe syndactyly; partial exencephaly; abnormal skull ossification; abnormal olfactory nerves; microphthalmia; absent lateral semicircular canals; abnormal sternum; fused neural arches	Johnson (1967, 1969), Pohl et al. (1990), Hui and Joyner (1993), Schimmang et al. (1994), Mo et al. (1997), Maynard et al. (2002)
$Gli2^{zfd/+} + Gli3^{XtJ/XtJ}$	Mouse	Severe phenotype	More severe phenotype than $Gli3^{XtJ/XtJ}$, indicating some redundancy of *Gli2* and *Gli3*	Mo et al. (1997)
$Shh^{-/-} + Gli3^{XtJ/XtJ}$	Mouse	Severe phenotype	Limb phenotype indistinguishable from $Gli3^{XtJ/XtJ}$. Shh has no effect on skeletal patterning in absence of *Gli3*. Thus, *Gli3* is implicated as an obligate component of the zone of polarizing activity function required in responding cells for Shh to exert polarizing activity.	Liftingtung et al. (2002)
$CBP^{+/-}$	Mouse	Phenotype with some Rubinstein-Taybi syndrome–like features	Insertional mutation resulting in CBP-deficient mice	Oike et al. (1999)

[a]*trans*-1,4-bis (2-chlorobenzyl-amino-methyl)cyclohexine dihydrochloride.
[b]4-(2-[1-(4-chlorocinnamyl) piperazin-4-yl]ethyl)-benzoic acid.
[c]triparanol also induces microphthalmia, cervical block fusion, craniorachischisis, and urogenital anomalies (Roux, 1964).
[d]See also the photograph of triparanol-induced ethmocephaly in Figure 9 of the article by Kolf-Clauw et al. (1997).
[e]A "zinc-finger deletion" is symbolized as zfd, for example, $Gli2^{zfd/+}$ (Mo et al., 1997). Several abnormal alleles in *Gli3* are subsumed under the category "extra toes," for example, $Gli3^{Xt/+}$ (Johnson, 1967). The original Xt allele contains a 5′ deletion (Schimmang et al., 1992). The XtJ allele, for example $Gli3^{XtJ}$, contains an 81-kb deletion (Maynard et al., 2002). Both homozygotes ($Gli3^{Xt/Xt}$ and $Gli3^{XtJ/XtJ}$) lack Gli3 expression, indicating that heterozygous dominant phenotypes in mice are due to haploinsufficiency.

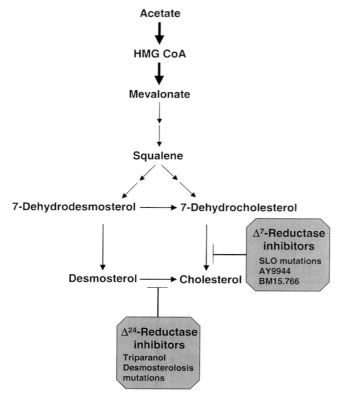

Figure 16–9. Partial, simplified cholesterol biosynthesis pathway. Double arrows indicate multiple steps missing. Note sterol Δ^7-reductase inhibitors: Smith-Lemli-Opitz (SLO) mutations (*DHCR7*[-1-]) and teratogens AY9944 and BM15.766. They result in a reduced serum cholesterol and an accumulation of 7-dehydrocholesterol. Holoprosencephaly occurs in about 4% of Smith-Lemli-Opitz syndrome cases. AY9944 and BM15.766 induce holoprosencephaly in rats. BM15.766 and hypomorphic apoB cause holoprosencephaly in mice. Note the sterol Δ^{24}-reductase inhibitors: teratogen triparanol and mutations in human desmosterolosis. Triparanol is associated with various malformations in rats, and holoprosencephaly has been described. The clinical phenotype of human desmosterolosis has not included holoprosencephaly to date, although a hypoplastic corpus callosum has been noted in one case. (From Cohen and Shiota, 2002.)

Berman et al. (2002) demonstrated that a *Ptch*[+/-] mutation in mice that induces medulloblastomas could be inhibited from growing by blocking the hedgehog signaling network with cyclopamine. In humans, *PTCH*[-/-] and activating mutations in *SMO* result in basal cell carcinomas. Taipale et al. (2000) showed that when cyclopamine was given to mice with *Ptch*[-/-] or *Smo* ↑↑, the oncogenic mutational effects could be reversed.

In contrast, Ma et al. (2002) induced a null mutation in *Smo*, finding a neural plate defect in the region of the prospective forebrain consistent with later developing holoprosencephaly. However, further embryonic development permitting full-blown holoprosencephaly was precluded by concomitant cardiac defects.

Many mutations have been induced in *Gli1*, *Gli2*, and *Gli3*. In mice, several abnormal alleles in *Gli3* are subsumed under the category "extra toes" (*Gli3*[Xt]) (Johnson, 1967). The original Xt allele contains a 5′ deletion (Schimmang et al., 1992). The *XtJ* allele contains a 51.5-kb deletion (Maynard et al., 2002). Both homozgotes (*Gli3*[Xt/Xt] and

Gli3[XtJ/XtJ]) lack Gli3 expression, indicating that heterozygous dominant phenotypes in mice are due to haploinsufficiency. A zinc-finger deletion is symbolized as zfd, for example, *Gli2*[zfd/+] (Mo et al., 1997).

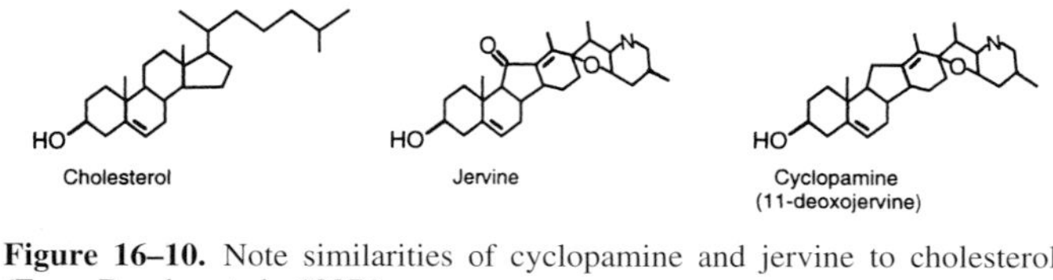

The null mutation *Gli1*[zfd/zfd] in mice has a surprisingly normal phenotype (Park et al., 2000). Overexpression of Gli1 (Gli1 ↑↑) in frogs produces skin tumors in tadpoles (Dahmane et al., 1997). Overexpression of Gli1 (Gli1 ↑↑) in mice produces basal cell carcinomas and trichoepitheliomas (Nilsson et al., 2000).

In the mouse, a *Gli2* heterozygote (*Gli2*[zfd/+]) has no detectable abnormalities, but in the null mutation (*Gli2*[zfd/zfd]), multiple anomalies are found: cleft palate, tooth defects, vertebral anomalies, short limbs, CNS floorplate abnormalities, and failure of notochordal regression (Mo et al., 1997; Matise et al., 1998). In double null *Gli1*[zfd/zfd]; *Gli2*[zfd/zfd], failure of spinal cord formation is similar to that observed with *Gli2*[zfd/zfd] (Matise et al., 1998).

Kim et al. (2001) found that the null mutation *Gli2*[zfd/zfd] in mice mimics human VACTERL association with vertebral, anal, cardiac, tracheoesophageal, and limb defects. They found that *Gli2*[zfd/zfd]; *Gli3*[zfd/+] also caused a VACTERL-like association with renal anomalies in addition.

In mice with heterozygous *Gli3*[XtJ/+], the phenotype consists of limb defects and other anomalies: anterior and posterior digit duplications similar to those found in human Greig cephalopolysyndactyly, white belly spot, interfrontal bone (abnormal in mice), and an increased frequency of hydrocephalus (Johnson, 1967, 1969; Hui and Joyner, 1993; Schimmang et al., 1994; Mo et al., 1997; Maynard et al., 2002). In the null mutation *Gli3*[XtJ/XtJ], abnormalities include frequent stillborns, abnormal limbs with severe syndactyly, partial exencephaly, abnormal skull ossification, abnormal olfactory nerves, microphthalmia, absent semicircular canals, abnormal sternum, and fused neural arches (Johnson, 1967, 1969; Pohl et al., 1990; Hui and Joyner, 1993; Schimmang et al., 1994; Mo et al., 1997; Maynard et al., 2002). In the double mutant *Gli2*[zfd/+]; *Gli3*[XtJ/XtJ], the phenotype is more severe than with *Gli3*[XtJ/XtJ], indicating some redundancy of *Gli2* and *Gli3* (Mo et al., 1997).

In the double null mutant *Shh*[-/-]; *Gli3*[XtJ/XtJ], the limb phenotype is indistinguishable from that of *Gli3*[XtJ/XtJ]. Shh has no effect on skeletal patterning in the absence of Gli3. Thus, Gli3 is implicated as an obligate component of the zone of polarizing activity function required in responding cells for Shh to exert polarizing activity (Liftingtung et al., 2002).

An insertional mutation in *CBP*, resulting in CBP-deficient (*CBP*[+/-]) mice, produces a phenotype with some Rubinstein-Taybi syndrome–like features (Oike et al., 1999).

REFERENCES

Ahlgren SC, Thakur V, Bronner-Fraser M (2002). Sonic Hedgehog rescues cranial neural crest from cell death induced by ethanol exposure. *Proc Natl Acad Sci USA* 99: 10476–10481.

Ahmadian A, Ren ZP, Williams C, Ponten F, Odeberg J, Ponten J, Uhlen M, Lundeberg J (1998). Genetic instability in the 9q22.3 region is a late event in the development of squamous cell carcinoma. *Oncogene* 17: 1837–1843.

Akimaru H, Chen Y, Dai P, Hou DX, Nonaka M, Smolik SM, Armstrong S, Goodman RH, Ishii S (1997). *Drosophila* CMP is a co-activator of cubitus interruptus in hedgehog signaling. *Nature* 386: 735–738.

Albarosa R, Colombo BM, Roz L, Magnani I, Pollo B, Cirenei N, Giani C, Conti AM, DiDonato S, Finocchiaro G (1996). Deletion mapping of gliomas suggests the presence of two small regions for candiate tumor-suppressor genes in a 17-cM interval on chromosome 10q. *Am J Hum Genet* 58: 1260–1267.

Alcedo J, Zou Y, Noll M (2000). Posttranscriptional regulation of smoothened is part of a self-correcting mechanism in the Hedgehog signaling system. *Mol Cell* 6: 457–465.

Alcedo J, Ayzenzon M, Von Ohlen T, Noll M, Hooper JE (1996). The *Drosophila smoothened* gene encodes a seven-pass membrane protein, a putative receptor for the hedgehog signal. *Cell* 86: 221–232.

Amanai K, Jiang J (2001). Distinct roles of Central missing and Dispatched in sending the Hedgehog signal. *Development* 128: 5119–5127.

Ascano M Jr, Nybakken KE, Sosinski J, Stegman MA, Robbins DJ (2002). The carboxyl-terminal domain of the protein kinase fused can function as a dominant inhibitor of hedgehog signaling. *Mol Cell Biol* 22: 1555–1566.

Aza-Blanc P, Lin HY, Ruiz i Altaba A, Kornberg TB (2000). Expression of the vertebrate Gli proteins in *Drosophila* reveals a distribution of activator and repressor activities. *Development* 127: 4293–4301.

Aza-Blanc P, Ramirez-Weber F-A, Laget M-P, Schwartz C, Kornberg TB (1997). Proteolysis that is inhibited by hedgehog targets Cubitus Interruptus protein to the nucleus and converts it to a repressor. *Cell* 89: 1043–1053.

Bale AE (2002). Hedgehog signaling and human disease. *Annu Rev Genomics Hum Genet* 3: 47–65.

Figure 16–10. Note similarities of cyclopamine and jervine to cholesterol. (From Beachy et al., 1997.)

Barbu V, Roux C, Dupuis R, Gardette J, Maziere JC (1984). Teratogenic effect of AY9944 in rats: importance of the day of administration and maternal plasma cholesterol level. *Proc Soc Exp Biol Med* 176: 54–59.

Barnes EA, Kong M, Ollendorff V, Donoghue DJ (2001). Patched1 interacts with cyclin B1 to regulate cell cycle progression. *EMBO J* 20: 2214–2223.

Beachy PA, Cooper MK, Young KE, von Kessler DP, Park W-J, Tanaka Hall TM, Leahy DJ, Porter JA (1997). Multiple roles of cholesterol in hedgehog protein biogenesis and signaling. *Cold Spring Harb Symp Quant Biol* LXII: 191–204.

Beddis IR, Mott MG, Bullimore J (1983). Case report: nasopharyngeal rhabdomyosarcoma and Gorlin's naevoid basal cell carcinoma syndrome. *Med Pediatr Oncol* 11: 178–179.

Bellaiche Y, The I, Perrimon N (1998). *Tout-velu* is a *Drosophila* homologue of the putative tumor suppressor *EXT-1* and is needed for Hh diffusion. *Nature* 394: 85–88.

Belloni E, Muenke M, Roessler E (1996). Identification of Sonic Hedgehog as a candidate gene responsible for holoprosencephaly. *Nat Genet* 14: 353–356.

Berman DM, Karhadkar SS, Hallahan AR, Pritchard JI, Eberhart CG, Watkins DN, Chen JK, Cooper MK, Taipale J, Olson JM, Beachy PA (2002). Medulloblastoma growth inhibition by Hedgehog pathway blockade. *Science* 297: 1559–1561.

Biesecker LG (1997). Strike three for *GLI3*. *Nat Genet* 17: 259–260.

Binns W, James LF, Shupe JL, Everett G (1963). A congenital cyclopian-type malformation in lambs induced by maternal ingestion of a range plant, *Veratrum californicum*. *Am J Vet Res* 24: 1164–1175.

Binns W, Shupe JL, Keeler RF, James LF (1965). Chronologic evaluation of teratogenicity in sheep fed *Veratrum californicum*. *J Am Vet Med Assoc* 147: 839–842.

Bitgood MJ, Shen L, McMahon AP (1996). Sertoli cell signaling by Desert hedgehog regulates the male germline. *Curr Biol* 1: 6(3): 298–304.

Blough RI, Petrij F, Dauwerse JG, Milatovich-Cherry A, Weiss L, Saal HM, Rubinstein JH (2000). Variation in microdeletions of the cyclic AMP-responsive element-binding protein gene at chromosome band 16p13.3 in the Rubinstein-Taybi syndrome. *Am J Med Genet* 90: 29–34.

Brewster R, Lee J, Ruiz i Altaba A (1998). Gli/Zic factors pattern the neural plate by defining domains of cell differentiation. *Nature* 393: 579–583.

Briscoe J, Chen Y, Jessell TM, Struhl G (2001). A Hedgehog-insensitive form of Patched provides evidence for direct long-range morphogen activity of Sonic Hedgehog in the neural tube. *Mol Cell* 7: 1279–1291.

Brown LY, Odent S, David V, Blayau M, Dubourg C, Apacik C, Delgado MA, Hall BD, Reynolds JF, Sommer A, et al. (2001). Holoprosencephaly due to mutations in *ZIC2*. Alanine tract expansion mutations may be caused by parental somatic recombination. *Hum Mol Genet* 10: 791–796.

Brown SA, Warburton D, Brown LY, Yu C-Y, Roeder ER, Stengel-Rutkowski S, Hennekam RCM, Muenke M (1998). Holoprosencephaly due to mutations in *ZIC2*, a homologue of *Drosophila odd-paired*. *Nat Genet* 20: 180–183.

Bryden MM, Perry C, Keeler RF (1973). Effects of alkaloids of *Veratrum californicum* on chick embryos. *Teratology* 8: 19–28.

Burke R, Mellen D, Bellotto M, Hafen E, Senti K-A, Dickson BJ, Basler K (1999). Dispatched, a novel sterol-sensing domain protein dedicated to the release of cholesterol-modified hedgehog from signaling cells. *Cell* 99: 803–815.

Caenorrhabditis elegans Sequencing Consortium (1998). Genome sequence of the nematode *C. elegans*: a platform for investigating biology. *Science* 282: 2012–2018.

Capdevila J, Pariente F, Sampedro J, Alonso JL, Guerrero I (1994). Subcellular localization of the segment polarity protein patched suggests an interaction with the wingless reception complex in *Drosophila* embryos. *Development* 120: 987–998.

Carpenter D, Stone DM, Brush J, Ryan A, Armanini M, Frantz G, Rosenthal A, De Sauvage FJ (1998). Characterization of two patched receptors for the vertebrate hedgehog protein family. *Proc Natl Acad Sci USA* 95: 13630–13634.

Chamoun Z, Mann RK, Nellen D, von Kessler DP, Bellotto M, Beachy PA, Basler K (2001). Skinny hedgehog, an acyltransferase required for palmitoylation and activity of the hedgehog signal. *Science* 293: 2080–2084.

Chavrier P, Goud B (1999). The role of ARF and Rab GTPases in membrane transport. *Curr Opin Cell Biol* 11: 466–475.

Chen C-H, von Kessler DP, Park W, Wang B, Ma Y, Beachy PA (1999a). Nuclear trafficking of Cubitus interruptus in the transcriptional regulation of Hedgehog target gene expression. *Cell* 98: 305–316.

Chen SY, Bishop JM (2002). Suppressor of Fused represses Gli-mediated transcription by recruiting the SAP18-mSin3 corepressor complex. *Proc Natl Acad Sci USA* 99: 5442–5447.

Chen Y, Struhl G (1996). Dual roles for Patched in sequestering and transducing Hedgehog. *Cell* 87: 553–563.

Chen Y, Struhl G (1998). In vivo evidence that Patched and Smoothened constitute distinct binding and transducing components of a Hedgehog receptor complex. *Development* 125: 4943–4948.

Chen Y, Cardinaux J-R, Goodman RH, Smolik SM (1999b). Mutants of *cubitus interruptus* that are independent of PKA regulation are independent of *hedgehog* signaling. *Development* 126: 3607–3616.

Chiang C, Litingtung Y, Harris MP, Simandl BK, Li Y, Beachy PA, Fallon JF (2001). Manifestation of the limb prepattern: limb development in the absence of Sonic hedgehog function. *Dev Biol* 235: 421–433.

Chiang C, Litingung Y, Lee E, Young KE, Corden JE, Westphal H, Beachy PA (1996). Cyclopia and defective axial patterning in mice lacking sonic hedgehog gene function. *Nature* 383: 407–413.

Chrivia JC, Kwok RPS, Lamb N, Hagiwara M, Montming MR, Goodman RH (1993). Phosphorylated CREB binds specifically to the nuclear protein CBP. *Nature* 365: 855–859.

Chuang P-T, McMahon AP (1999). Vertebrate Hedgehog signalling modulated by induction of a Hedgehog-binding protein. *Nature* 397: 617–621.

Cohen MM Jr (1999). Nevoid basal cell carcinoma syndrome: molecular biology and new hypotheses. *Int J Oral Maxillofac Surg* 28: 216–223.

Cohen MM Jr (2002). Bone morphogenetic proteins with some comments on fibrodysplasia ossificans progressiva and NOGGIN. *Am J Med Genet* 109: 87–92.

Cohen MM Jr (2003a). TGFβ/Smad signaling system and its pathologic correlates. *Am J Med Genet* 116A: 1–10.

Cohen MM Jr (2003b). The hedgehog signaling network. *Am J Med Genet* In press.

Cohen MM Jr, Shiota K (2002). Teratogenesis of holoprosencephaly. *Am J Med Genet* 109: 1–15.

Cooper MK, Porter JA, Young KE, Beachy PA (1998). Teratogen-mediated inhibition of target tissue response to *Shh* signaling. *Science* 290: 1603–1607.

Coventry S, Kapur RP, Siebert JR (1998). Cyclopamine-induced holoprosencephaly and associated craniofacial malformations in the Golden hamster: anatomic and molecular events. *Pediatr Dev Pathol* 1: 29–41.

Cumberledge S, Reichsman F (1997). Glycosaminoglycans and WNTs: just a spoonful of sugar helps the signal go down. *Trends Genet* 13: 421–423.

Dahmane N, Lee J, Robins P, Heller P, Ruiz i Altaba A (1997). Activation of the transcription factor Gli1 and the Sonic hedgehog signalling pathway in skin tumors. *Nature* 389: 876–881.

Dai P, Akimaru H, Tanaka Y, Maekawa T, Nakafuku M, Ishii S (1999). Sonic Hedgehog-induced activation of the Gli1 promoter is mediated by GLI3. *J Biol Chem* 274: 8143–8152.

Dann CE, Hsieh J-C, Rattner A, Sharma D, Nathans J, Leahy DJ (2001). Insights into Wnt binding and signalling from the structures of two Frizzled cysteine-rich domains. *Nature* 412: 86–90.

Dehart DB, Lanoue L, Tint GS, Sulik KK (1995). Altered cholesterol biosynthesis in rats: a model for Smith-Lemli-Opitz syndrome. *Teratology* 51: 165.

de la Cruz JM, Bamford RN, Burdine RD, Roessler E, Barkovich AJ, Donnai D, Schier AF, Muenke M (2002). A loss-of-function mutation in the CFC domain of *TDGF1* is associated with human forebrain defects. *Hum Genet* 110: 422–428.

Del Sal G, Ruaro ME, Philipson L, Schneider C (1992). The growth arrest-specific gene, *gas1*, is involved in growth suppression. Cell 70: 595–607.

Del Sal G, Collavin L, Ruaro ME, Edomi P, Saccone S, Valle GD, Schneider C (1994). Structure, function, and chromosome mapping of the growth-suppressing human homologue of the murine gas1 gene. *Proc Natl Acad Sci USA* 91: 1846–1852.

Del Sal G, Ruaro EM, Utrera R, Cole CN, Levine AJ, Schneider C (1995). Gas1-induced growth suppression requires a transactivation-indepedent p53 function. *Mol Cell Biol* 15: 7152–7160.

Denef N, Neubuser D, Perez L, Cohen SM (2000). Hedgehog induces opposite changes in turnover and subcellular localization of patched and smoothened. *Cell* 102: 521–531.

DiSanto S, Abt AB, Boal DK, Krummel TM (1992). Fetal rhabdomyoma and nevoid basal cell carcinoma syndrome. *Pediatr Pathol Lab Med* 12: 441–447.

Dubois L, Lecourtois M, Alexandre C, Hirst E, Vincent J-P (2001). Regulated endocytic routing modulates *wingless* signaling in *Drosophila* embryos. *Cell* 105: 61–624.

Eggenschwiler JT, Espinoza E, Anderson KV (2001). Rab23 is an essential negative regulator of the mouse Sonic hedgehog signalling pathway. *Nature* 412: 194–198.

Entchev EV, Schwabedissen A, González-Gaitán M (2000). Gradient formation of the TGFβ-homolog Dpp. *Cell* 103: 981–991.

Erez A, Ilan T, Amariglio N, Muler I, Brok-Simoni F, Rechavi G, Izraeli S (2002). Gli3 is not mutated commonly in sporadic medulloblastomas. *Cancer* 95: 28–31.

Farese RV Jr, Herz J (1998). Cholesterol metabolism and embryogenesis. *Trends Genet* 14: 115–120.

Fukumoto T, Watanabe-Fukunaga R, Fujisawa K, Nagata S, Fukunaga R (2001). The fused protein kinase regulates hedgehog-stimulated transcriptional activation in *Drosophila* Schneider 2 cells. *J Biol Chem* 276: 38441–38448.

Gailani MR, Stahle-Backdahl M, Leffell DJ (1996). The role of the human homologue of Drosophila Patched in sporadic basal cell carcinomas. *Nat Genet* 14: 78–81.

Gao B, Guo J, She C, Shu A, Yang M, Tan Z, Yang X, Guo S, Feng G, He L (2001). Mutations in *IHH*, encoding Indian hedgehog, cause brachydactyly type A-1. *Nat Genet* 28: 386–388.

Gemmill RM, West JD, Boldog F, Tanaka N, Robinson LJ, Smith DI, Li F, Drabkin HA (1998). The hereditary renal cell carcinoma 3;8 translocation fuses *FHIT* to a *patched*-related gene, *TRC8*. *Proc Natl Acad Sci USA* 95: 9572–9577.

Gofflot F, Kolf-Clauw M, Clotman F, Ropux C, Picard JJ (1999). Absence of ventral cell populations in the developing brain in a rat model of the Smith-Lemli-Opitz syndrome. *Am J Med Genet* 87: 207–216.

Goodrich LV, Milenkovic L, Higgins KM, Scott MP (1997). Altered neural cell fates and medulloblastoma in mouse *patched* mutants. *Science* 277: 1109–1113.

Grachtchouk M, Mo R, Yu S, Zhang X, Sasaki H, Hui CC, Dlugosz AA (2000). Basal cell carcinoma in mice overexpressing Gli2 in skin. *Nat Genet* 24: 216–217.

Gray IC, Phillips SM, Lee SJ, Neoptolemos JP, Weissenbach J, Spurr NK (1995). Loss of the chromosomal region 10q23-25 in prostate cancer. *Cancer Res* 55: 4800–4803.

Gripp KW, Wolton D, Edwards MC, Roessler E, Adès L, Meinecke P, Richieri-Costa A, Zackai EH, Massagué J, Muenke M (2000). Mutations in *TGIF* cause holoprosencephaly and link NODAL signalling to human neural axis determination. *Nat Genet* 25: 205–208.

Günther T, Struwe M, Aguzzi A, Schughart K (1994). *Open brain*, a new mouse mutant with severe neural tube defects, shows altered gene expression patterns in the developing spinal cord. *Development* 120: 3119–3130.

Hahn H, Christiansen J, Wicking C, Zaphiropoulos P, Chidambaram A, Gerrard B, Vorechovsky I, Bale A, Toftgard R, Dean M, Wainwright B (1996). A mammalian patched homolog is expressed in target tissues of sonic hedgehog and maps to a region associated with developmental abnormalities. *J Biol Chem* 271: 12125–12128.

Hahn H, Wicking C, Zaphiropoulos PG (1996). Mutations of the human homolog of *Drosophila Patched* in the nevoid basal cell carcinoma syndrome. *Cell* 85: 841–851.

Hahn H, Wojnowski L, Zimmer AM, Hall J, Miller G, Zimmer A (1998). Rhabdomyosarcomas and radiation hypersensitivity in a mouse model of Gorlin syndrome. *Nat Med* 4: 619–622.

Hahn H, Wojnowski L, Miller G, Zimmer A (1999). The patched signaling pathway in tumorigenesis and development: lessons from animal models. *J Mol Med* 77: 459–468.

Hammerschmidt M (1997). The world according to *Hedgehog*. *Trends Genet* 13: 14–21.

Hellemans J, Coucke PJ, Giedion A, De Paepe A, Kramer P, Beemer F, Mortier GR (2003). Homozygous mutations in *IHH* cause acrocapitofemoral dysplasia, an autosoaml recessive disorder with cone-shaped epiphyses in hands and hips. *Am J Hum Genet* 72: 1040–1046.

Helms JA, Kim CH, Hu D, Minkoff R, Thaller C, Eichele G (1997). Sonic hedgehog participates in craniofacial morphogenesis and is downregulated by teratogenic doses of retinoic acid. *Dev Biol* 187: 25–35.

Ho KS, Scott MP (2002). Sonic Hedgehog in the nervous system: functions, modifications and mechanisms. *Curr Opin Neurobiol* 12: 57–63.

Hooper JE, Scott MP (1989). The *Drosophila patched* gene encodes a putative membrane protein required for segmental patterning. *Cell* 59: 751–765.

Hui C-C, Joyner AL (1993). A mouse model of Greig cephalopolysyndactyly syndrome: the *extra-toes* mutation contains an intragenic deletion of the *Gli3* gene. *Nature Genet* 3: 241–246.

Hui C-C, Slusarski D, Platt KA, Holmgren R, Joyner A (1994). Expression of three mouse homologs of the *Drosophila* segment polarity gene *cubitus interruptus*, GLI-1, GLI-2, and GLI-3, in ectoderm- and mesoderm-derived tissue suggest multiple roles during postimplantation development. *Dev Biol* 162: 402–413.

Incardona JP, Gaffield W, Kapur RP, Roelink H (1998). The teratogenic *Veratrum* alkaloid cyclopamine inhibits sonic hedgehog signal transduction. *Development* 125: 3553–3562.

Incardona JP, Gaffield W, Lange Y, Cooney A, Pentchev PG, liu S, Watson JA, Kapur RP, Roelink H (2000a). Cyclopamine inhibition of sonic hedgehog signal transduction is not mediated through effects on cholesterol transport. *Dev Biol* 234: 440–452.

Incardona JP, Lee JH, Robertson CP, Enga K, Kapur RP, Roelink H (2000b). Receptor-mediated endocytosis of soluble and membrane-tethered Sonic hedgehog by Patched-1. *Proc Natl Acad Sci USA* 971: 12044–12049.

Incardona JP, Gruenberg J, Roelink H (2002). Sonic hedgehog induces the segregation of patched and smoothened in endosomes. *Curr Biol* 12: 983–995.

Ingham PW, McMahon AP (2001). Hedgehog signaling in animal development: paradigms and principles. *Genes Dev* 15: 3059–3087.

Ingham PW, Nystedt S, Nakano Y, Brown W, Stark D, van den Heuvel M, Taylor AM (2000). Patched represses the Hedgehog signalling pathway by promoting modification of the Smoothened protein. *Curr Biol* 10: 1315–1318.

Izraeli S, Lowe LA, Bertness VL, Campaner S, Hahn H, Kirsch IR, Kuehn MR (2001). Genetic evidence that Sil is required for the sonic hedgehog response pathway. *Genesis* 31: 72–77.

Jia J, Amanai K, Wang G, Tang J, Wang B, Jiang J (2002). Shaggy/GSK3 antagonizes hedgehog signalling by regulating Cubitus interruptus. *Nature* 416: 548–552.

Jiang J, Struhl G (1998). Regulation of the Hedgehog and Wingless pathways by the F-box/WD-repeat protein Slimb. *Nature* 391: 493–496.

Johnson DR (1967). Extra-toes: a new mutant gene causing multiple abnormalities in the mouse. *J Embrol Exp Morphol* 17: 543–581.

Johnson DR (1969). Brachyphalangy, an allele of extra-toes in the mouse. *Genet Res* 13: 275–280.

Johnson RL, Rothman AL, Xie J, Goodrich LV, Bare JW, Bonifas JM, Quinn AG, Myers RM, Cox DR, Epstein EH Jr, Scott MP (1996). Human homolog of *patched*, a candidate gene for the basal cell nevus syndrome. *Science* 272: 1668–1671.

Johnson RL, Milenkovic L, Scott MP (2000). In vivo functions of the patched protein: requirement of the C terminus for target gene inactivation but not Hedgehog sequestration. *Mol Cell* 6: 467–478.

Johnson RL, Zhou L, Bailey EC (2002). Distinct consequences of sterol sensor mutations in *Drosophila* and mouse *patched* homologs. *Dev Biol* 242: 224–235.

Kalderon D (2000). Transducing the Hedgehog signal. *Cell* 103: 371–374.

Kamal A, Goldstein LS (2002). Principles of cargo attachment to cytoplasmic motor proteins. *Curr Opin Cell Biol* 14: 63–68.

Kang S, Graham JM Jr, Olney AH, Biesecker LG (1997). *GLI3* frameshift mutations cause autosomal dominant Pallister-Hall syndrome. *Nat Genet* 15: 266–268.

Karkera JD, Izraeli S, Roessler E, Dutra A, Kirsch L, Muenke M (2002). The genomic structure, chromosomal localization, and analysis of *SIL* as a candidate gene for holoprosencephaly. *Cytogenet Genome Res* 97: 62–67.

Karpen HE, Bukowski JT, Hughes T, Gratton J-P, Sessa WC, Gaillani MR (2001). The Sonic hedgehog receptor Patched associates with Caveolin-1 in cholesterol-rich microdomains of the plasma membrane. *J Biol Chem* 276: 19503–19511.

Kas K, Wlodarska I, Meyen E, Van den Berghe H, Van de Ven WJ (1996). Assignment of the gene encoding human Krüppel-related zinc finger protein 4 (GLI4) to 8q24.3 by fluorescent in situ hybridization. *Cytogenet Cell Genet* 72: 297–298.

Keeler RF (1970). Teratogenic compounds of *Veratrum californicum* (Durand) X. Cyclopia in rabbits produced by cyclopamine. *Teratology* 3: 175–180.

Keeler RF (1975). Teratogenic effects of cyclopamine and jervine in rats, mice, and hamsters. *Proc Soc Exp Biol Med* 149: 302–306.

Keeler RF, Binns W (1966). Teratogenic compounds of *Veratrum californicum*. II. Production of ovine fetal cyclopia by fractions and alkaloid preparations. *Can J Biochem* 44: 829–838.

Keeler RF, Binns W (1968). Teratogenic compounds of *Veratrum californicum* (Durand). V. Comparison of cyclopian effects of steroidal alkaloids from the plant and structurally related compounds from other sources. *Teratology* 1: 5–10.

Kelley RI (2000). Inborn errors of cholesterol biosynthesis. *Adv Pediatr* 47: 1–53.

Kim PCW, Mo R, Hui C-c (2001). Murine models of VACTERL syndrome: role of Sonic Hedgehog signaling pathway. *J Pediatr Surg* 36: 381–384.

Kim U-k, Jorgenson E, Coon H, Leppert M, Risch N, Drayna D (2003). Positional cloning of the human quantitative trait locus underlying taste sensitivity to phenylthiocarbamide. *Science* 299: 1221–1225.

Kinzler KW, Bigner SH, Bigner DD, Trent JM, Law ML, O'Brien SJ, Wong AJ, Vogelstein B (1987). Identification of an amplified, highly expressed gene in a human glioma. *Science* 236: 70–73.

Kinzler KW, Ruppert JM, Bigner SH, Vogelstein B (1988): The *GLI* gene is a member of the Krüppel family of zinc finger proteins. *Nature* 332: 371–374.

Kinzler KW, Vogelstein B (1990). The *GLI* gene encodes a nuclear protein which binds specific sequences in the human genome. *Mol Cell Biol* 10: 634–642.

Kipreos ET, Pagano M (2000). The F-box protein family. *Genome Biol* 1: 30021–30027.

Kitagawa H, Shimakawa H, Sugahara K (1999). The tumor suppressor *EXT*-like gene *EXTL2* encodes an α1,4-N-acetylhexosaminyltransferase that transfers N-acetylgalactosamine and N-acetylglucosamine to the common glycosaminoglycan-protein linkage region. The key enzyme for the chain initiation of heparan sulfate. *J Biol Chem* 274: 13933–13937.

Klijanienko J, Çaillaud JM, Micheau C, Flamant F, Schwaab G, Avril MF, Ponzio-Prion A (1988). Basal-cell nevomatosis associated with multifocal fetal rhabdomyoma. A case. *Presse Méd* 17: 2247–2250.

Ko HW, Jiang J, Edery I (2002). Role for Slimb in the degradation of *Drosophila* Period protein phosphorylated by Doubletime. *Nature* 420: 673–678.

Kolf-Clauw M, Chevy F, Wolf C, Siliart B, Citadelle D, Roux C (1996). Inhibition of 7-dehydrocholesterol reductase by the teratogen AY9944: a rat model for Smith-Lemli-Opitz syndrome. *Teratology* 54: 115–125.

Kolf-Clauw M, Chevy F, Siliart B, Wolf C, Mulliez N, Roux C (1997). Cholesterol biosynthesis inhibited by BM15.766 induces holoprosencephaly in the rat. *Teratology* 56: 188–200.

Koyabu Y, Nakata K, Mizugishi K, Aruga J, Mikoshiba K (2001). Physical and functional interactions between Zic and Gli proteins. *J Biol Chem* 276: 6889–6892.

Krishnan V, Pereira FA, Qiu Y, Chen C-H, Beachy PA, Tsai SY, Tsai M-J (1997). Mediation of Sonic Hedgehog-induced expression of COUP-TFII by a protein phosphatase. *Science* 278: 1947–1950.

Kühl M, Sheldahl LC, Park M, Miller JR, Moon RT (2000). The Wnt/Ca^{2+} pathway: a new vertebrate Wnt signaling pathway takes shape. *Trends Genet* 16: 279–283.

Kuwabara PE, Lee M-H, Schedl T, Jefferis GSXE (2000). A *C. elegans* patched gene, *ptc-1* functions in germ-line cytokinesis. *Genes Dev* 14: 1933–1944.

Kuwabara PE, Labouesse M (2002). The sterol-sensing domain: multiple families, a unique role? *Trends Genet* 18: 193–201.

Lam CW, Xie J, To KF, Ng HK, Lee KC, Yuen NW, Lim PL, Chan LY, Tong SF, McCormick F (1999). A frequent activated *smoothened* mutation in sporadic basal cell carcinomas. *Oncogene* 18: 833–836.

Lanoue L, Dehart DB, Hinsdale ME, Maeda N, Tint GS, Sulik KK (1997). Limb, genital, CNS, and facial malformations result from gene/environment-induced cholesterol deficiency: further evidence for a link with sonic hedgehog. *Am J Med Genet* 73: 24–31.

Lanske B, Karaplis AC, Lee K, Luz A, Vortkamp A, Pirro A, Karpenien M, Defize LHK, Ho C, Mulligan RC, et al. (1996). PTH/PTHrP receptor in early development and Indian hedgehog regulated bone growth. *Science* 273: 663–666.

Lee CS, Buttitta L, Fan CM (2001). Evidence that the WNT-inducible growth arrest-specific gene 1 encodes an antagonist of sonic hedgehog signaling in the somite. *Proc Natl Acad Sci USA* 98: 11347–11352.

Lee JD, Treisman JE (2001). Sightless has homology to transmembrane acyltransferases and is required to generate active Hedgehog protein. *Curr Biol* 11: 1147–1152.

Lench NJ, Telford EAR, High AS (1997). Characterisation of human *Patched* germ line mutations in nevoid basal cell carcinoma syndrome. *Hum Genet* 100: 497–502.

Lewis PM, Dunn MP, McMahon JA, Logan M, Martin JF, St-Jacques B, McMahon AP (2001). Cholesterol modification of Sonic hedgehog is required for long-range signaling activity and effective modulation of signaling for Ptc1. *Cell* 105: 599–612.

Lind T, Tufaro F, McCormick C, Lindahl U, Lidholt K (1998). The putative tumor suppressors *EXT1* and *EXT2* are glycosyltransferases required for the biosynthesis of heparan sulfate. *J Biol Chem* 273: 26265–26268.

Litingtung Y, Dahn RD, Li Y, Fallon JF, Chiang C (2002). *Shh* and *Gli3* are dispensable for limb skeleton formation but regulate digit number and identity. *Nature* 418: 979–983.

Ma Y, Erkner A, Gong R, Yao S, Taipale J, Basler K, Beachy PA (2002). Hedgehog-mediated patterning of the mammalian embryo requires transporter-like function of dispatched. *Cell* 111: 63–75.

Maesawa C, Tamura G, Iwaya T (1998). Mutations in the human homologue of the *Drosophila Patched* gene in esophageal squamous cell carcinoma. *Genes Chromosomes Cancer* 21: 276–279.

Mandelkow E, Mandelkow E-M (2002). Kinesin motors and disease. *Trends Cell Biol* 12: 585–591.

Mao J, Maye P, Kogerman P, Tejedor FJ, Toftgård R, Xie W, Wu G, Wu D (2002). Regulation of Gli1 transcriptional activity in the nucleus by Dyrk1. *J Biol Chem* 277: 35156–35161.

Marigo V, Davey RA, Zuo Y, Cunningham JM, Tabin CJ (1996). Biochemical evidence that Patched is the Hedgehog receptor. *Nature* 384: 176–179.

Martin V, Carrillo G, Torroja C, Guerrero I (2001). The sterol-sensing domain of Patched protein seems to control Smoothened activity through Patched vesicular trafficking. *Curr Biol* 11: 601–607.

Martinez O, Goud B (1998). Rab proteins. *Biochim Biophys Acta* 1404: 101–112.

Massagué J, Attisano L, Wrana JL (1994). The TGF-β family and its composite receptors. *Trends Cell Biol* 4: 172–178.

Matise MP, Epstein DJ, Park HL, Platt KA, Joyner AL (1998). *Gli2* is required for induction of floor plate and adjacent cells, but not most ventral neurons in the mouse central nervous system. *Development* 125: 2759–2770.

Matsumoto N, Fujimoto M, Kato R, Niikawa N (1996). Assignment of the human *Gli2* gene to 2q14 by fluorescence in situ hybridization. *Genomics* 36: 220–221.

Maynard T, Jain M, Balmer C, LaMantia A (2002). High-resolution mapping of *Gli3* mutation Extra-toesJ reveals a 51.5 kb deletion. *Mamm Genome* 13: 58–61.

McCarthy RA, Barth JL, Chintalapudi MR, Knaak C, Argraves WS (2002). Megalin functions as an endocytic Sonic hedgehog receptor. *J Biol Chem* 277: 25660–25667.

McCormick C, Leduc Y, Martindale D, Mattison K, Esford LE, Dyer AP, Tufaro F (1998). The putative tumour suppressor *EXT1* alters the expression of cell-surface heparan sulfate. *Nat Genet* 19: 158–161.

Micchelli CA, The I, Selva E, Mogita V, Perrimon N (2002). *Rasp*, a putative transmembrane acyltransferase, is required for Hedgehog signaling. *Development* 129: 843–851.
Miller JR, Hocking AM, Brown JD, Moon RT (1999). Mechanism and function of signal transduction by the Wnt/β-catenin and Wnt/Ca^{2+} pathways. *Oncogene* 18: 7860–7872.
Ming JE, Kaupas ME, Roessler E, Brunner HG, Golabi M, Stratton RF, Sujansky E, Bale SJ, Muenke M (2002). Mutations in *Patched*-1, the receptor for Sonic Hedgehog, are associated with holoprosencephaly. *Hum Genet* 110: 297–301.
Mo R, Freer AM, Zinyk DL, Crackower MA, Michaud J, Heng HH, Chik KW, Shi XM, Tsui LC, Cheng SH, et al. (1997). Specific and redundant functions of Gli2 and Gli3 zinc finger genes in skeletal patterning and development. *Development* 124: 113–123.
Monnier V, Dussillol F, Alves G, Lamour-Isnard C, Plessis A (1998). Suppressor of fused links Fused and Cubitus interruptus on the Hedgehog signalling pathway. *Curr Biol* 8: 583–586.
Monnier V, Ho KS, Sanial M, Scott MP, Plessis A (2002). Hedgehog signal transduction proteins: contacts of the Fused kinase and Ci transcription factor with the Kinesin-related protein Costal2. *BMC Dev Biol* 2: 4.
Moon RT, Brown JD, Torres M (1997). WNTs modulate cell fate and behavior during vertebrate development. *Trends Genet* 13: 157–162.
Motoyama J, Takabatake T, Takeshima K, Hui C-C (1998). *Ptch2*, a second mouse Patched gene is co-expressed with Sonic hedgehog. *Nat Genet* 18: 1094–106.
Muenke M, Beachy PA (2001). Holoprosencephaly. In: *The Metabolic and Molecular Bases of Inherited Disease*, Eighth Edition. Scriver CR, Beaudet AL, Sly WS, Valle D, Childs B, Kinzler KW, Vogelstein B (eds.) McGraw-Hill Inc., New York, pp. 6203–6230.
Mullor JL, Sánchez P, Ruiz i Altaba A (2002). Pathways and consequences: Hedgehog signaling in human disease. *Trends Cell Biol* 12: 562–569.
Murone M, Luoh SM, Stone D, Li W, Gurney A, Armanini M, Grey C, Rosenthal A, de Sauvage FJ (2000). Gli regulation by the opposing activities of fused and suppressor of fused. *Nat Cell Biol* 2: 310–312.
Nanni L, Ming JE, Bocian M, Steinhaus K, Bianchi DW, Die-Smulders C, Giannotti A, Imaizumi K, Jones KL, Campo MD, et al. (1999). The mutational spectrum of the *Sonic Hedgehog* gene in holoprosencephaly: *SHH* mutations cause a significant proportion of autosomal dominant holoprosencephaly. *Hum Mol Genet* 8: 2479–2488.
Nilsson M, Unden AB, Krause D, Malmqwist U, Raza K, Zaphiropoulos PG, Toftgård R (2000). Induction of basal cell carcinomas and trichoepitheliomas in mice overexpressing GLI-1. *Proc Natl Acad Sci USA* 97: 3438–3443.
Nusse R (1999). WNT targets: repression and activation. *Trends Genet* 15: 1–3.
Nüsslein-Volhard C, Wieschaus E (1980). Mutations affecting segment number and polarity in Drosophila. *Nature* 287: 795–801.
Nybakken K, Perrimon N (2002). Hedgehog signal transduction: recent findings. *Curr Opin Genet Dev* 12: 503–511.
Nybakken KE, Turck CW, Robbins DJ, Bishop JM (2002). Hedgehog-stimulated phosphorylation of the kinesin-related protein costal2 is mediated by the serine/threonine kinase fused. *J Biol Chem* 277: 24638–24647.
Oike Y, Hata A, Mamiya T, Kaname T, Noda Y, Suzuki M, Yasue H, Nabeshima T, Araki K, Yamumura K-i (1999). Truncated CBP protein leads to classical Rubinstein-Taybi syndrome phenotype in mice: implications for a dominant-negative mechanism. *Hum Mol Genet* 8: 387–396.
Orenic, TV, Slusarski DC, Kroll KL, Holmgren RA (1990). Cloning and characterization of the segment polarity gene *cubitus interruptus Dominant* of *Drosophila*. *Genes Dev* 4: 1053–1067.
Oro AE, Higgins KM, Hu Z (1997). Basal cell carcinomas in mice overexpressing Sonic Hedgehog. *Science* 276: 817–821.
Ouspenskaia MV, Karkera JD, Roessler E, Shen MM, Goldmunts E, Bowers P, Towbin J, Belmont J, Muenke M (2002). Role of *FAST1* gene in the development of holoprosencephaly (HPE) and congenital cardiac malformations in humans. 52nd Annual Meeting of the American Society of Human Genetics, October 15–19, Baltimore, MD, abstract 822, p. 313.
Park HL, Bai C, Platt KA, Matise MP, Beeghly A, Hui CC, Nakashima N, Joyner AL (2000). Mouse *Gli1* mutants are viable but have defects in SHH signaling in combination with a *Gli2* mutation. *Development* 127: 1593–1605.
Patton EE, Willems AR, Tyers M (1998). Combinatorial control in ubiquitin-dependent proteolysis: don't Skp the F-box hypothesis. *Trends Genet* 14: 236–243.
Pearse RV II, Collier LS, Scott MP, Tabin CJ (1999). Vertebrate homologs of *Drosophila suppressor of fused* interact with the Gli family of transcriptional regulators. *Dev Biol* 212: 323–336.
Peiffer-Schneider S, Noonan FC, Mutch DG, Simpkins SB, Herzog T, Rader J, Elbendary A, Gersell KC, Goodfellow PJ (1998). Mapping an endometrial cancer tumor suppressor gene at 10q25 and development of a bacterial clone contig for the consensus deletion interval. *Genomics* 52: 9–16.
Pepinsky RB, Zeng C, Wen D, Rayhorn P, Baker DP, Williams KP, Bixler SA, Ambrose CM, Garber EA, Miatkowski K, et al. (1998). Identification of a palmitic acid-modified form of Human Sonic hedgehog. *J Biol Chem* 273: 14037–14045.
Petrij F, Giles RH, Dauwerse HG, Saris JJ, Hennekam RC, Masuno M, Tommerup N, van Ommen GJ, Goodman RH, Peters DJ, et al. (1995). Rubinstein-Taybi syndrome caused by mutations in the transcriptional co-activator *CBP*. *Nature* 376: 348–351.
Ping XL, Ratner D, Zhang H, Wu XL, Zhang MJ, Chen FF, Silvers DN, Peacock M, Tsou HC (2001). *PTCH* mutations in squamous cell carcinoma of the skin. *J Invest Dermatol* 116: 614–616.
Podos SD, Ferguson EL (1999). Morphogen gradients: new insights from DPP. *Trends Genet* 15: 396–402.
Pohl TP, Mattei M-G, Rüther U (1990). Evidence for allelism of the recessive insertional mutation *add* and the dominant mouse mutation *extra toes* (*Xt*). *Development* 110: 1153–1157.
Porter JA, Ekken SC, Park W-J, von Kessler DP, Young KE, Chen C-H, Ma Y, Woods AS, Cotten RJ, Koonin EV, et al. (1996). Hedgehog patterning activity: role of a lipophilic modification mediated by the carboxy-terminal autoprocessing domain. *Cell* 86: 21–34.
Préat T (1992). Characterization of *Suppressor of fused*, a complete suppressor of the *fused* segment polarity gene of *Drosophila melanogaster*. *Genetics* 132: 725–736.
Préat T, Thérond P, Lamour-Isnard C, Limbourg-Boucher B, Tricoire H, Erk I, Mariol M-C, Busson D (1990). A putative serine/threonine protein kinase encoded by the segment polarity fused gene of *Drosophila*. Nature 347: 85–89.
Price MA, Kalderon D (2002). Proteolysis of the Hedgehog signaling effector Cubitus interruptus requires phosphorylation by glycogen synthase kinase 3 and casein kinase 1. *Cell* 108: 823–835.
Prorok M, Lawrence DS (1989). Intrasubstrate steric interaction in the active site control the specificity of the cAMP-dependent protein kinase. *Biochem Biophys Res Commun* 158: 136–140.
Raffel C, Jenkins RB, Frederick L, Hebrink D, Alderete B, Fults DW, James CD (1997). Sporadic medulloblastomas contain *PTCH* mutations. *Cancer Res* 57: 842–845.
Rasheed BK, McLendon RE, Friedman HS, Friedman AH, Fuchs HE, Bigner DD, Bigner SH (1995). Chromosome 10 deletion mapping in human gliomas: a common deletion region in 10q25. *Oncogene* 10: 2243–2246.
Rechsteiner M, Rogers SW (1996). PEST sequences and regulation by proteolysis. *Trends Biochem Sci* 21: 267–271.
Reifenberger G, Ichimura K, Reifenberger J, Elkahloun AG, Meltzer PS, Collins VP (1996). Refined mapping of 12q13-q15 amplicons in human malignant gliomas suggests CDK4/SAS and MDM2 as independent amplification targets. *Cancer Res* 56: 5141–5145.
Reifenberger J, Wolter M, Weber RG, Megahed M, Ruzicka T, Lichter P, Reifenberger G (1998). Missense mutations in *SMOH* in sporadic basal cell carcinomas of the skin and primitive neuroectodermal tumors of the central nervous system. *Cancer Res* 58: 1798–1803.
Robbins DJ, Nybakken KE, Kobayashi R, Sisson JC, Bishop JM, Thérond PP (1997). Hedgehog elicits signal transduction by means of a large complex containing the kinesin-related protein costal2. *Cell* 90: 225–234.
Roessler E, Muenke M (2003). How a Hedgehog might see HPE. *Hum Mol Genet* In press.
Roessler E, Belloni E, Gaudenz K, Vargas F, Scherer SW, Tsui L-C, Muenke M (1997). Mutations in the C-terminal domain of *Sonic Hedgehog* cause holoprosencephaly. *Hum Mol Genet* 6: 1847–1853.
Roessler E, Belloni E, Gaudenz K, Jay P, Berta P, Scherer SW, Tsui L-C, Muenke M (1996). Mutations in the human *Sonic Hedgehog* gene cause holoprosencephaly. *Nat Genet* 14: 357–360.
Roessler E, Du Y, Mullor JL, Casas E, Allen WP, Ellis I, Gillessen-Kaesbach G, Roeder E, Ming JE, Ruiz i Altaba A, et al. (2002). Loss-of-function mutations in the human *GLI2* gene cause holoprosencephaly and familial pan-hypopituitarism. 52nd Annual Meeting of the American Society of Human Genetics, October 15–19, Baltimore, MD, abstract No. 132, p. 190.
Roux C (1964). Action teratogenie du triparanol chez l'animal. *Arch Franç Pédiatr* 21: 451–464.
Ruiz i Altaba A (1997). Catching a Gli-mpse of Hedgehog (1997). *Cell* 90: 193–196.
Ruiz i Altaba A (1999). *Gli* proteins and Hedgehog signaling. *Trends Genet* 15: 418–425.
Ruiz i Altaba A, Sanchez P, Dahmane N (2002). *Gli* and hedgehog in cancer: tumors, embryos and stem cells. *Nat Rev Cancer* 2: 361–372.
Ruppert JM, Kinzler KW, Wong AJ, Bigner SH, Kao F-T, Law ML, Seuanez HN, O'Brien SJ, Vogelstein B (1988). The *GLI-Krüppel* family of human genes. *Mol Cell Biol* 8: 3104–3113.
Ruppert JM, Vogelstein B, Arheden K, Kinzler KW (1990). *GLI3* encodes a 190-kilodalton protein with multiple regions of GLI similarity. *Mol Cell Biol* 10: 5408–5415.
Schimmang T, Oda SI, Rüther U (1994). The mouse mutant polydactyly Nagoya (Pdn) defines a novel allele of the zinc finger gene *Gli3*. *Mamm Genome* 5L384–386.
Simmons AD, Musy MM, Lopes CS, Hwang L-Y, Yang Y-P, Lovett M (1999). A direct interaction between EXT proteins and glycosyltransferases is defective in hereditary multiple exostoses. *Hum Mol Genet* 8: 2155–2164.
Smyth I, Narang MA, Evans T, Heimann C, Nakamura Y, Chenevix-Trench G, Pietsch T, Wicking C, Wainwright BJ (1999). Isolation and characterization of human *Patched 2* (*PTCH2*), a putative tumour suppressor gene in basal cell carcinoma and medulloblastoma on chromosome 1p32. *Hum Mol Genet* 8: 291–297.
Spenser E, Jiang J, Chen Z (1999). Signal-induced ubiquination of $\kappa\beta\alpha$ by the F-box protein Slimb/β-TrCP. *Genes Dev* 13: 284–294.
Stebel M, Vatta P, Ruaro ME, Del Sal G, Parton RG, Schneider C (2000). The growth suppressing gas1 product is a GPI-linked protein. *FEBS Lett* 481: 152–158.
St-Jacques B, Hammerschmidt M, McMahon AP (1999). Indian hedgehog signaling regulates proliferation and differentation of chondrocytes and is essential for bone formation. *Genes Dev* 13: 2072–2086.
Stone DM, Hynes M, Armanini M, Swanson TA, Gu Q, Johnson RL, Scott MP, Pennica D, Goddard A, Phillips H, et al. (1996). The tumor-suppressor gene patched encodes a candidate receptor for Sonic hedgehog. *Nature* 384: 129–134.
Stone DM, Murone M, Luoh S-M, Ye W, Armanini MP, Gurney A, Phillips H, Brush J, Goddard A, de Sauvage FJ, Rosenthal A (1999). Characterization of the human Suppressor of fused, a negative regulator of the zinc-finger transcription factor Gli. *J Cell Sci* 112: 4437–4448.
Strutt H, Thomas C, Nakano Y, Stark D, Neave B, Taylor AM, Ingham PW (2001). Mutations in the sterol-sensing domain of *Patched* suggest a role for vesicular trafficking in Smoothened regulation. *Curr Biol* 11: 608–613.
Tabin CJ, McMahon AP (1997). Recent advances in Hedgehog signalling. *Trends Cell Biol* 7: 442–446.
Taipale J, Beachy P (2001). The Hedgehog and Wnt signalling pathways in cancer. *Nature* 411: 349–354.
Taipale J, Cooper MK, Maiti T, Beachy PA (2002). *Patched* acts catalytically to suppress the activity of Smoothened. *Nature* 418: 892–896.
Taipale J, Chen JK, Cooper MK, Wang B, Mann RK, Milenkovic L, Scott MP, Beachy PA (2000). Effects of oncogenic mutations in *Smoothened* and *Patched* can be reversed by cyclopamine. *Nature* 406: 1005–1009.

Taylor MD, Liu L, Raffel C, Hui C-c, Mainprize TG, Zhang X, Agatep R, Chiappa S, Gao L, Lowrance A, et al. (2002). Mutations in *SUFU* predispose to medulloblastoma. *Nat Genet* 31: 306–310.

The I, Bellaiche Y, Perrimon N (1999). Hedgehog movement is regulated through *tout velu*-dependent synthesis of a heparan sulfate proteoglycan. *Mol Cell* 4: 633–639.

Thérond PP, Limbourg-Bouchon B, Gallet A, Dussilol F, Pietri T, van den Heuvel M, Tricoire H (1999). Differential requirements of the Fused kinase for Hedgehog signaling in the *Drosophila* embryo. *Development* 126: 4039–4051.

van den Heuvel M, Ingham PW (1996). *Smoothened* encodes a receptor-like serpentine protein required for *Hedgehog* signalling. *Nature* 382: 547–551.

Villavicencio EH, Walterhouse DO, Iannaccone PM (2000). The Sonic Hedgehog-Patched-Gli pathway in human development and disease. *Am J Hum Genet* 67: 1047–1054.

Vorechovsky I, Tingby O, Hartman M, Stromberg B, Nister M, Collins VP, Toftgard R (1997a). Somatic mutations in the human homologue of *Drosophila patched* in primitive neuroectodermal tumours. *Oncogene* 15: 361–366.

Vorechovsky I, Unden AB, Sandstedt B (1997b). Trichoepitheliomas contain somatic mutations in the overexpressed *PTC* gene: support for a gatekeeper mechanism in skin tumorigenesis. *Cancer Res* 57: 4677–4681.

Vortkamp A, Lee K, Lanske B, Segre GV, Kronenberg M, Tabin CJ (1996). Regulation of rate of cartilage differentiation by Indian hedgehog and PTH related protein. *Science* 273: 613–622.

Wallis DE, Roessler E, Hehr U, Nanni L, Wiltshire T, Richieri-Costa A, Gillessen-Kaesbach G, Zackai EH, Romens J, Muenke M (1999). Mutations in the homeodomain of the human *SIX3* gene cause holoprosencephaly. *Nat Genet* 22: 196–198.

Wang B, Fallon JF, Beachy PA (2000a). Hedgehog-related processing of Gli3 produces anterior/posterior repressor gradient in the developing vertebrate limb. *Cell* 100: 423–434.

Wang G, Amanai K, Wang B, Jiang J (2000b). Interactions with Costal2 and Suppressor of fused regulate nuclear translocation and activity of cubitus interruptus. *Genes Dev* 14: 2893–2905.

Wang QT, Holmgren RA (1999). The subcellular localization and activity of *Drosophila* cubitus interruptus are regulated at multiple levels. *Development* 126: 5097–5106.

Wassif CA, Maslen C, Kachilele-Linjewile S, Lin D, Linck TM, Connor WE, Steiner RD, Porter FD (1998). Mutations in the human *sterol Δ7-reductase* gene at 11q12-13 cause Smith-Lemli-Opitz syndrome. *Am J Hum Genet* 63: 53–62.

Wicking C, Shanley S, Smyth I, Gillies S, Negus K, Graham S, Suthers G, Haites N, Edwards M, Wainwright B, et al. (1997). Most germ-line mutations in the nevoid basal cell carcinoma syndrome lead to a premature termination of the PATCHED protein, and no genotype-phenotype correlations are evident. *Am J Hum Genet* 60: 21–26.

Wicking C, Evans T, Henk B (1998). No evidence for the HI33Y mutation in *Sonic Hedgehog* in a collection of common tumour types. *Oncogene* 16: 1091–1093.

Wild A, Kalft-Suske M, Vortkamp A (1997). Point mutations in human *GLI3* cause Greig syndrome. *Hum Mol Genet* 6: 1979–1984.

Willnow TE, Hilpert J, Armstrong SA, Rohlmann A, Hammer RE, Burns DK, Herz J (1996). Defective forebrain development in mice lacking gp330/megalin. *Proc Natl Acad Sci USA* 93: 8460–8464.

Witsch-Baumgartner M, Fitzky BU, Ogorelkova M, Kraft HG, Moebius FF, Glossmann H, Seedorf U, Gillessen-Kaesbach G, Hoffmann GF, Clayon P, et al. (2000). Mutational spectrum in the *Δ7-sterol reductase* gene and genotype-phenotype correlation in 84 patients with Smith-Lemli-Opitz syndrome. *Am J Hum Genet* 66: 402–412.

Woehlke G, Ruby AK, Hart CL, Ly B, Hom-Booher N, Vale RD (1997). Microtubule interaction site of the kinesin motor. *Cell* 90: 207–216.

Wolter M, Reifenberger J, Sommer C, Ruzicka T, Reifenberger G (1997). Mutations in the human homologue of *Drosophila* segment polarity gene *patched (PTCH)* in sporadic basal cell carcinomas of the skin and primitive neuroectodermal tumors of the central nervous system. *Cancer Res* 57: 2581–2585.

Xie J, Johnson RL, Zhang X (1997). Mutations of the *Patched* gene in several types of sporadic extracutaneous tumors. *Cancer Res* 57: 2369–2372.

Xie J, Murone M, Luch S, Ryan A, Gu Z, Zhang C, Bonifas JM, Rosenthal A, Epstein EH Jr, de Sauvage FG (1998). Activating *SMOOTHENED* mutations in sporadic basal-cell carcinoma. *Nature* 391: 90–92.

Yu H, Lee M-H, Starck L, Elias ER, Irons M, Salen G, Patel SB, Tint GS (2000). Spectrum of *Δ7-dehydrocholesterol reductase* mutations in patients with the Smith-Lemli-Opitz (RSH) syndrome. *Hum Mol Genet* 9: 1385–1391.

Zardoya R, Abouheif E, Meyer A (1996). Evolution and orthology of *hedgehog genes*. *Trends Genet* 12: 496–497.

Zeng X, Goetz JA, Suber LM, Scott WJ Jr, Schreiner CM, Robbins DJ (2001). A freely diffusible form of Sonic hedgehog mediates long-range signalling. *Nature* 411: 716–720.

17 | *DHCR7* and the Smith-Lemli-Opitz (RSH) Syndrome and Cyclopamine Teratogenesis

MIRA IRONS

LOCUS AND DEVELOPMENTAL PATHWAY

The importance of cholesterol metabolism in humans has been recognized for decades. Cholesterol is a major structural component of cell membranes and of myelin. It is also a precursor of bile acids and steroid hormones. While the role of cholesterol in these important biochemical processes has been known for some time, the essential role of cholesterol and the cholesterol metabolic pathway in human development has only been more recently appreciated with the identification of inborn errors of cholesterol metabolism that result in human phenotypes, which include structural malformations as well as growth and mental retardation.

While cholesterol is the important end product of the pathway, the cholesterol biosynthetic pathway itself is a complex multistep process (Fig. 17–1) that begins with the two-carbon acetyl coenzyme A (CoA) and through a series of enzymatic reactions forms the five-carbon isopentenyl-PP (pyrophosphate). This is the basic C_5 isoprene unit that is the building block of all subsequent isoprenoids, which are composed of one or more C_5 isoprene units and function in many different cellular processes (Goldstein and Brown, 1990; Waterham and Wanders, 2000). Isopentenyl-PP is a precursor of isopentenyl-tRNA, which is involved in protein translation. The C_{10} isoprenoid, geranyl-PP, and the C_{15} isoprenoid, farnesyl-PP, are involved in protein prenylation, which is important in cell signaling and differentiation. Farnesyl-PP is also a precursor of dolichol, heme A, and the ubiquinones, which have roles in protein glycosylation and in the mitochondrial electron transport and respiratory chain (Nwokoro et al., 2001). The C_{30} molecule squalene, made up of six isoprene units, is the first intermediate in the production of the sterol isoprenoids that ultimately leads to the biosynthesis of cholesterol. The enzyme 3-hydroxy-3-methylglutaryl CoA reductase (HMG-CoA reductase), which catalyzes the formation of mevalonate, is the rate-limiting enzyme of the pathway (Brown and Goldstein, 1980). The gene encoding HMG-CoA reductase contains the sterol regulatory element 1 (SRE-1) within its promoter region, which responds to the level of cholesterol. A low level of cholesterol leads to activation of transcription of HMG-CoA reductase and is mediated by SRE-1 binding protein and, ultimately, SRE-1 (Goldstein and Brown, 1990; Honda et al., 2000). It is within this complex biochemical pathway whose intermediates have roles in a myriad of important biologic functions that 7-dehydrocholesterol reductase (DHCR7) and the Smith-Lemli-Opitz syndrome (SLOS) reside.

SLOS was first described in 1964 (Smith et al., 1964) as a multiple malformation syndrome that results in a characteristic physical phenotype consisting of dysmorphic facial characteristics, major structural anomalies, and growth and mental retardation. The etiology of SLOS was not known until 1993, when it was noted that several patients with SLOS had a biochemical phenotype characterized by low cholesterol levels and elevation of the cholesterol precursors 7- and 8-dehydrocholesterol (7-DHC and 8-DHC) (Irons et al., 1993; Tint et al., 1994). This biochemical pattern raised the possibility that there was deficiency of the microsomal enzyme DHCR7 (3β-hydroxysterol-Δ7-reductase), which catalyzes the conversion of 7-DHC to cholesterol. Shortly thereafter, defective conversion of 7-DHC to cholesterol was demonstrated in cultured fibroblasts from affected patients (Honda et al., 1995) and deficiency of DHCR7 activity was confirmed in liver microsomes from SLOS homozygotes (Shefer et al., 1995).

In 1998, the cDNA for the human *DHCR7* gene was cloned (Moebius et al., 1998) and the gene was localized to chromosome 11q13 (Fitzky et al., 1998). Mutations in the *DHCR7* gene in patients with SLOS were independently reported that same year by three groups (Fitzky et al., 1998; Wassif et al., 1998; Waterham et al., 1998), confirming the molecular defect of SLOS.

While the biochemical and molecular defects that cause SLOS have only recently been identified, it is still unclear what causes the clinical features seen in this condition. Deficiency of cholesterol needed for cell membrane and steroid hormone synthesis during embryogenesis may be an important factor. Lack of cholesterol, necessary for cell membrane stability and myelin production both pre- and postnatally, may explain the growth and mental retardation. Toxicity of the cholesterol precursors 7- and 8-DHC may also play a role. Finally, the role of cholesterol in the function of the hedgehog class of embryonic signaling proteins may hold the answer.

CLINICAL FEATURES

Since its first description in 1964 in a report of three affected infants (Smith et al., 1964), over 100 affected individuals have been reported. Before the biochemical defect was discovered, the diagnosis was made by clinical recognition of the syndrome, most often based on the characteristic facial appearance in the presence of growth and mental retardation. The presence of genital malformations more easily appreciated in males (hypospadias, ambiguous genitalia) than females (labial hypoplasia) most likely explains the reported male predominance.

The classic description of the syndrome included a characteristic facial appearance (Fig. 17–2), the presence of usually non-life-threatening structural malformations, and growth and mental retardation. Failure to thrive and hypotonia were commonly seen in affected patients. A more severe form of the condition which included multiple visceral malformations, sex reversal of XY males, and a high rate of either fetal demise or early neonatal death, called SLOS type II, was reported by Donnai et al. (1986) and Curry et al. (1987). Initially, it was unclear whether SLOS type I and SLOS type II were the same condition with varying degrees of expressivity or separate genetic conditions. We now know that SLOS types I and II both result from deficiency of DHCR7, with type II patients having a more severe defect of cholesterol biosynthesis (Tint et al., 1995a).

The array of clinical findings seen in SLOS is quite broad and ranges from severely growth-retarded, dysmorphic infants with multiple visceral malformations, cholestatic liver disease, and a high incidence of death either in the fetal/newborn period or first year of life to very mildly affected patients with subtle facial characteristics of the condition, mild hypotonia, often 2-3 syndactyly of the toes (Fig. 17–3), and mild developmental and/or learning problems. Therefore, an appreciation of the spectrum of clinical findings seen in SLOS is important in the evaluation of children with congenital malformations, dysmorphic features, failure to thrive, hypotonia, and developmental delay/mental retardation.

Since the biochemical basis for this condition was identified, attempts have been made to determine if there is a correlation between clinical severity and either cholesterol or precursor (7-DHC and/or 8-DHC) levels. Infants with severe growth retardation and multiple visceral anomalies often have the lowest cholesterol levels (<15–20 mg/dl) and the

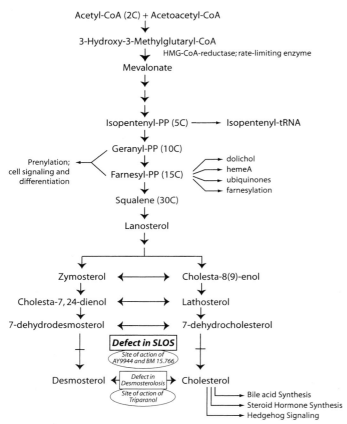

Acetyl-CoA (2C) + Acetoacetyl-CoA
↓
3-Hydroxy-3-Methylglutaryl-CoA
↓   HMG-CoA-reductase; rate-limiting enzyme
Mevalonate
↓
↓
Isopentenyl-PP (5C) ⟶ Isopentenyl-tRNA
↓
Geranyl-PP (10C)   ⟶ dolichol
Prenylation;   ⟶ hemeA
cell signaling and   Farnesyl-PP (15C)   ⟶ ubiquinones
differentiation   ⟶ farnesylation
↓
Squalene (30C)
↓
Lanosterol
↓
Zymosterol ⟷ Cholesta-8(9)-enol
↓   ↓
Cholesta-7,24-dienol ⟷ Lathosterol
↓   ↓
7-dehydrodesmosterol ⟷ 7-dehydrocholesterol
↓   ↓
Defect in SLOS
Site of action of
AY9944 and BM 15.766
↓   ↓
Desmosterol ⟷ *Defect in* Cholesterol
Desmosterolosis
Site of action of
Triparanol
⟶ Bile acid Synthesis
⟶ Steroid Hormone Synthesis
⟶ Hedgehog Signaling

Figure 17–1. Outline of the cholesterol biosynthetic pathway. Sites of action of the chemical inhibitors AY 9944, BM 15.776, and triparanol as well as enzyme deficiencies in Smith-Lemli-Opitz syndrome (SLOS) and desmosterolosis shown.

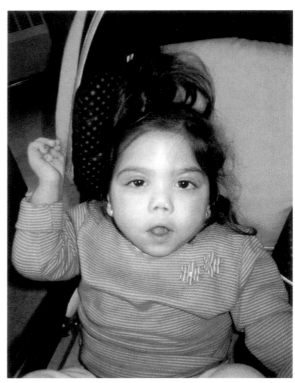

Figure 17–2. Facial phenotype of a child with Smith-Lemli-Opitz syndrome.

ent in the newborn period, when the face tends to be rounder and the anteverted nares, ptosis, and micrognathia not as apparent; thus, the diagnosis is often not thought of in the newborn period. However, by 2–3 months of age, elongation of the face, together with ptosis being more easily appreciated when the eyes are more often open and the nose beginning to take on the characteristic anteverted appearance, often leads to the classic dysmorphic features that raise this diagnostic possibility.

highest precursor levels, while those with hypotonia and mild cognitive delay may have normal levels of cholesterol and only mild elevations of 7- and 8-DHC (Irons, unpublished observation). Normal cognitive development has been reported in three patients with minor dysmorphic features, 2-3 toe syndactyly, normal cholesterol levels, and slightly elevated levels of 7- and 8-DHC (Langius et al., 2000). Between these two extremes are patients with the characteristic facial features, non-life-threatening anomalies, and moderate mental retardation who present with cholesterol levels generally in the 30–70 mg/dl range and 7- and 8-DHC levels in the moderately elevated range (Irons, unpublished observation). Tint et al. (1995a) reported that survival was most compromised in infants with the lowest cholesterol levels, and Cunniff et al. (1997) found a distinct inverse correlation between clinical severity and plasma cholesterol level for all ages and a slight correlation between clinical severity and plasma level of 7-DHC for older patients (>2 years of age). Witsch-Baumgartner et al. (2000) found a significant correlation between severity score and the DHC fraction. Children with variant presentations of SLOS have also shown mild physical and developmental abnormalities and a phenotype consistent with that seen in SLOS but biochemical sterol abnormalities that are different from those seen in classical SLOS. These children are postulated to have a novel disorder that may affect intracellular sterol transport (Anderson et al., 1998).

As previously noted, the clinical findings in SLOS are quite variable and will be discussed below. Detailed reviews of the clinical spectrum of findings seen in SLOS are available for more information (Gorlin et al., 1990; Cunniff et al., 1997; Ryan et al., 1998; Krajewska-Walasek et al., 1999; Kelley and Hennekam, 2000; Kelley, 2000; Nowaczyk and Waye, 2001).

Craniofacial Features

Most children with SLOS have a characteristic facial appearance that is easily recognizable. However, the facial phenotype is often not pres-

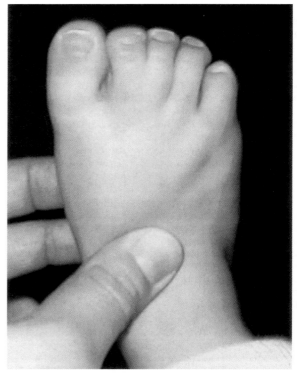

Figure 17–3. Typical 2-3 toe syndactyly seen in Smith-Lemli-Opitz syndrome.

Characteristic craniofacial features include microcephaly, bitemporal narrowing, epicanthal folds, ptosis (unilateral or bilateral), a broad nasal bridge and short nasal root, anteverted nares, micrognathia, and often low-set and/or posteriorly rotated ears (Fig. 17–2). Abnormalities of the palate include a high narrow palate, cleft of the soft or hard palate, submucous cleft palate, or bifid uvula. Broad maxillary alveolar ridges are commonly seen. The tongue is often small. Cataracts can also be seen in the severely affected neonate or can appear later in life. Strabismus can also be seen, although vision is generally not severely affected. The neck is often short, with redundant skin at the nape.

Central Nervous System

A wide range of developmental abnormalities of the CNS can be seen, which range from a normal-appearing, microcephalic (80%–84% of patients) brain (Ryan et al., 1998; Kelley and Hennekam, 2000) to holoprosencephaly (5%) (Kelley and Hennekam, 2000). Other CNS findings include hypo- or delayed myelination, abnormalities of the corpus callosum or cerebellum, ventricular dilatation, or Dandy-Walker malformation or its variants.

Cardiopulmonary Features

Incomplete lobation of the lungs or pulmonary hypoplasia has been seen in more severely affected patients. Anomalies of the laryngeal and tracheal anatomy or cartilages can occur. Cardiovascular anomalies are seen in up to 50% of patients. The most common cardiovascular anomalies include atrial septal defect, ventricular septal defect, posterior descending artery, and atrioventricular canal defects and total anomalous pulmonary venous return (Lin et al., 1997).

Abdominal Features

Renal anomalies are seen in approximately 29%–40% of patients and include renal agenesis or hypoplasia, cystic and/or dysplastic kidneys, or ureteral abnormalities (Ryan et al., 1998; Kelley and Hennekam, 2000). Gastrointestinal (GI) anomalies include pyloric stenosis or Hirschsprung's disease. Large adrenals and pancreatic islet cell "giant cell" hyperplasia have been reported (Gorlin et al., 1990). Genital abnormalities include hypospadias or ambiguous genitalia due to failure of masculinization in males and labial hypoplasia in females.

Skeletal Features

Syndactyly 2-3 of the toes (Fig. 17–3) is seen in approximately 85%–95% of patients (Cunniff et al., 1997; Ryan et al., 1998; Kelley and Hennekam, 2000), and 2-3 syndactyly of the fingers can also rarely be seen. Either unilateral or bilateral postaxial polydactyly of the hands and/or feet is common. The fingers are often long, and the thumb is often proximally placed and short with a narrow proximal portion resulting in a so-called swan's neck appearance. Other findings include short halluces, valgus or varus deformities of the foot, clubfoot deformity, and dislocation of the hip, either congenital or secondary to hypertonia later in life.

Natural History and Other Medical Problems

The problems experienced by infants and children with SLOS are generally secondary to the severity of the biochemical defect and the structural malformations present. More severely affected patients can have multiple medical problems and require the care of many different specialists, while more mildly affected children do not require significant medical care.

In the newborn period, infants with SLOS frequently have feeding problems due to a combination of hypotonia, oral–motor incoordination, and numerous GI problems including dysmotility/hypomotility and intolerance to usual infant formulas. Infants with lower cholesterol levels tend to have more of these problems than those with cholesterol levels in the moderately or mildly decreased ranges. The feeding problems seen in the more severely affected infants lead to placement of gastrostomy tubes, often in the newborn period. Formula intolerance is common, and many severely affected infants require a hypoallergenic, elemental formula. Many of these infants are often too hypotonic to take adequate amounts of breastmilk or formula orally,

while other infants have problems with oral feeding due to structural anomalies of the palate and jaw.

Gastroesophageal reflux and vomiting are common problems and require careful evaluation and treatment. Elemental formulas are more easily tolerated, and often several are tried before finding one that the infant tolerates well. Pyloric stenosis can also be seen with increased frequency in the early weeks of life, although there is some suggestion that the frequency of this is decreased in infants treated with cholesterol supplementation from birth (Kelley and Hennekam, 2000). Constipation is a frequent finding secondary to GI hypomotility and must be distinguished from that due to Hirschsprung's disease. Cholestatic liver disease manifested by elevated transaminases and bilirubin can be seen in more severely affected infants and often resolves with cholesterol and/or bile acid therapy.

Cardiorespiratory problems can occur, usually secondary to structural malformations of the heart and/or respiratory tract. Structural malformations of the larynx or trachea can lead to obstructive apnea (Kelley and Hennekam, 2000). Infants can also develop obstructive sleep apnea due to a combination of their anatomy and hypotonia, which leads to collapse of the airway while sleeping, necessitating either nasal continuous positive airway pressure at night or tracheostomy (Irons, unpublished observation).

Adrenal insufficiency and other endocrine problems have been reported in children with SLOS, which is not surprising given the fact that cholesterol is a precursor of steroid hormones, including cortisol, aldosterone, and testosterone. Sudden death, electrolyte disturbances (hyponatremia and hyperkalemia), hypoglycemia, and/or hypertension during intercurrent illness or stress are most likely due to cortisol and/or aldosterone deficiency secondary to lack of available cholesterol precursor required during periods of increased demand for adrenal hormones (Andersson et al., 1999; Nowaczyk et al., 2001d). Treatment with stress steroids in doses customarily used for children with congenital adrenal hyperplasia is recommended during periods of illness, stress, or prolonged decrease in oral intake. Other abnormalities of endocrine function include an unusual pattern of steroid sulfates in newborns (Chasalow et al., 1985), decreased testosterone levels in male infants (Chasalow et al., 1985; Irons, unpublished), and an exaggerated 17-hydroxyprogesterone response to ACTH in obligate heterozygotes (Chasalow et al., 1985).

Other endocrine problems include failure of masculinization of male genitalia secondary to decreased testosterone levels that requires hormonal and surgical therapy. Precocious puberty on a central basis has also been seen in two girls with SLOS (Starck et al., 1999; Irons, unpublished). A rapid advancement through puberty has been reported in a girl with SLOS with very low initial cholesterol levels after exogenous cholesterol treatment was begun (Elias et al., 1997).

Ophthalmologic problems include cataracts, strabismus, and ptosis, which may require surgical repair if it is severe enough to affect vision. Other ophthalmologic findings include optic atrophy and optic nerve hypoplasia (Atchaneeyasakul et al., 1998). Electroretinographic abnormalities, indicative of some effect of abnormal sterols on the retinal membrane, have been noted, although their clinical consequence is as yet unknown (Elias et al., 2000).

Orthopedic problems include syndactyly of the hands and/or feet and polydactyly. The early hypotonia and late hypertonia seen in many patients also require orthopedic management, including the need for ankle-foot orthosis and other orthotics for stability of the feet/legs and treatment of dislocations of the hips in severely affected patients who develop hypertonia later in life.

Photosensitivity is commonly seen (57% in one series; Ryan et al., 1998) and can be quite severe. Brief exposure to sunlight can result in significant sunburn, so many children need to avoid anything but brief sun exposure. Others experience increased photosensitivity but can tolerate varying periods of sun exposure if properly clothed and protected with a sunscreen with UVA and UVB protection. There is no correlation between levels of 7-DHC and severity of photosensitivity, suggesting that it is not due to a direct toxic effect mediated by 7-DHC (Anstey et al., 1999). The photosensitivity seen in this condition has a distinct phenotype with onset of a sunburn-like erythema within minutes of sun exposure, which persists up to 24–48 hours before fading and appears to be UVA-mediated (Charman et al., 1998; Anstey et al., 1999; Anstey and Taylor, 1999). Photosensitivity testing has revealed an immediate and persistent reaction to low-dose UVA at 350 nm and an abnormal erythemal response to visible light at 400 nm (Charman et al., 1998).

Other medical problems include increased frequency of upper and/or lower respiratory infections, recurrent otitis media necessitating placement of tympanostomy tubes, splenomegaly, and hearing loss, which can be either conductive, sensorineural, or mixed. Higher red blood cell deformability at lower shear stress has been reported in a patient with SLOS, which may be due to a more pliable cell membrane (Hardeman and Ince, 1999), an interesting observation given that patients with SLOS often have abnormalities of red cell appearance on peripheral blood smears (Elias and Irons, unpublished observations).

Almost all affected infants have some degree of hypotonia that interferes with feeding and acquisition of motor milestones. Physical therapy is helpful and can lead to some functional improvement. Seizures can occur but are not particularly common.

A multitude of behavioral and neuropsychologic problems are seen in SLOS. Cognitive abilities range from borderline intellectual function to severe mental retardation, but occasionally normal cognitive function can be seen in those with a mild variant. Tierney et al. (2000, 2001) reported a behavioral phenotype which includes sensory hyperreactivity, irritability, language impairment, sleep cycle disturbance, self-injurious behavior (hand biting and/or head banging), autism spectrum behaviors (46%–53% of patients), opisthokinesis defined as throwing the body backward in a characteristic upper body movement (50%), stereotypic stretching motion of the upper body accompanied by hand flicking, temperament dysregulation, and social and communication deficits. Sleep disturbance, self-abusive behavior, aggressiveness, and difficulty of control are commonly seen in older, untreated patients. Many of these patients require very little sleep, often only several hours/night, which causes problems in the home, especially if the children are ambulatory (Ryan et al., 1998; Irons, unpublished). Depression and other psychiatric problems have also been reported in older patients. Treatment with haloperidol, which has a high affinity for the DHCR7 substrate binding site, should be avoided as it can further inhibit DHCR7 and exacerbate the biochemical sterol abnormalities (Kelley and Hennekam, 2000). It is likely that other

drugs of this class will also cause increased levels of 7-DHC through inhibition of DHCR7.

MOLECULAR GENETICS OF DHCR7 DEFICIENCY

In 1998, the cDNA for the human *DHCR7* gene was cloned (Moebius et al., 1998) and the gene localized to chromosome 11q13 (Fitzky et al., 1998). Mutations in the *DHCR7* gene in patients with SLOS were independently reported that same year by three groups (Fitzky et al., 1998; Wassif et al., 1998; Waterham et al., 1998), confirming the molecular defect of SLOS.

The *DHCR7* gene contains nine exons and eight introns and spans approximately 14 kb; the DHCR7 protein is encoded by exons 3–9 (Witsch-Baumgartner et al., 2001). The gene has an open reading frame of 1425 nucleotides and encodes a 475–amino acid polypeptide with a predicted molecular weight of 54.5 kDa (Fitzky et al., 1998; Wassif et al., 1998; Waterham et al., 1998; Porter, 2000).

Modeling of the peptide predicts an integral membrane protein with nine α-helix transmembrane-spanning domains; the large fourth cytoplasmic loop is believed to contain the active site of the enzyme and the binding site for NADPH, with the C terminus predicted to be located within the endoplasmic reticulum (Fitzky et al., 1998, 1999; Porter, 2000; Witsch-Baumgartner et al., 2001). DHCR7 is 35% identical and 60% similar to the *Arabidopsis thalania* sterol Δ^7–reductase and has strong homology to other sterol reductases, including the sterol Δ^{14}- and Δ^{24}-reductases and the transmembrane domain of the lamin B receptor, which facilitates the attachment of chromatin to the nuclear membrane (Porter, 2000).

Over 70 different mutations have been identified in over 200 patients with SLOS (Fitzky et al., 1998; Wassif et al., 1998; Waterham et al., 1998; De Die-Smulders et al., 1999; De Brasi et al., 1999; Witsch-Baumgartner et al., 2000; Yu et al., 2000a,b; Kozak et al., 2000; Krakowiak et al., 2000; Patrono et al., 2000; Loffler et al., 2000; Porter, 2000; Jira et al., 2001). The most recent data regarding mutant alleles and their frequency are shown in Figure 17–4. Most patients with SLOS have been found to be compound heterozygotes for two different mutant alleles, with an overall mutation detection rate in one large series of 133 patients of 96% (Witsch-Baumgartner et al., 2001). The most frequently found mutant allele (32%) is IVS8-1G → C, a splice site acceptor mutation in the last base of intron 8 that leads to an alternative

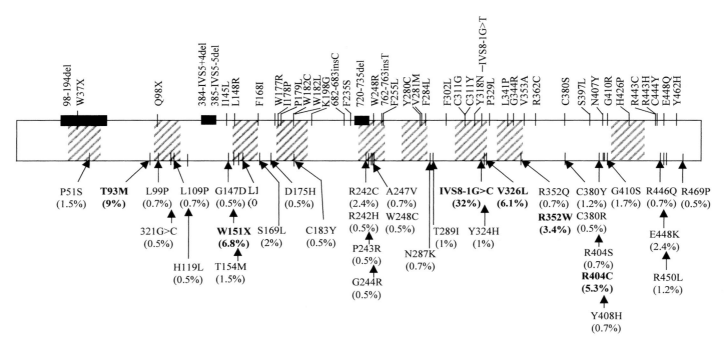

Figure 17–4. Schematic diagram of the DHCR7 protein and mutations identified in Smith-Lemli-Opitz syndrome, with shaded areas representing predicted transmembrane domains. Common mutations are shown in bold type, and the frequency of mutations found more than once is given in parentheses (diagram courtesy of Dr. Forbes D. Porter).

upstream cryptic splice acceptor site. This results in the insertion of 134 bp of intronic sequence into the *DHCR7* mRNA, which shifts the reading frame and leads to a premature stop codon. Other common mutant alleles include T93M, W151X, V26L, R404C, and R352W, which together with IVS8-1G → C account for 62% of the mutant alleles seen in SLOS. Over 90% of mutations are missense mutations scattered over all coding exons, in addition to a relatively few nonsense and frameshift mutations that presumably result in loss of enzymatic activity and represent functional null alleles (Witsch-Baumgartner et al., 2001). Simple PCR-based assays have been developed for detection of the IVS8-1G → C mutation (Battaile et al., 1999) and for several of the other common DHCR7 mutations (Krakowiak et al., 2000).

It has been difficult to establish any clear genotype–phenotype correlations since most patients are compound heterozygotes for different mutant alleles. Patients homozygous for the two functional null alleles, IVS8-1G → C and W151X, or the missense R404C allele were found to have a severe phenotype (Witsch-Baumgartner et al., 2000; Loffler et al., 2000). High severity scores were also found in patients who were compound heterozygotes for these mutations in combination or compound heterozygotes for another mutation and either the IVS8-1G → C or the W151X mutation.

While the mutations seen in affected patients are scattered over all coding exons without any apparent hot spots, most mutations were localized in a spatial pattern at the protein level. Witsch-Baumgartner et al. (2000, 2001) found that approximately two-thirds of mutations were located in the transmembrane domain (TM) or nearby with most of the remaining mutations divided between the fourth cytoplasmic loop (4L) and within the carboxy terminus tail (CT) of the protein. No mutations were identified in the presumed cytosolic amino terminus, in any of the other three cytoplasmic loops, or in the large loop that is believed to be located in the lumen of the endoplasmic reticulum. They classified mutations into four types, including 0 (null), TM, 4L, and CT, to analyze whether a relationship existed between location of the mutation(s) and severity score, and found that the severity score increased from mild to severe in the following order of genotypes: TM/CT → TM/TM → 0/TM → , 4L/TM → 0/4L → 4L/4L → 0/0 (Witsch-Baumgartner et al., 2000, 2001). The frequency of the 0 and 4L alleles was higher in the most severely affected patients. Milder phenotypes may result from combination of a more mild mutation along with a null mutation depending on where the non-null mutation resides. Of interest is the identification of two patients with a severe phenotype who were homozygous for the missense mutation R404C, which resides in the fourth cytoplasmic loop, indicating that its location within 4L is important to the structure or function of the protein. There is also preliminary evidence to suggest that factors in addition to genotype may affect the phenotype. Porter (2000) found a clear bimodal distribution of severity scores in 14 patients with the T93M/null phenotype. However, although there appears to be some correlation with grade of severity and site of mutation(s), prediction of phenotype from a known genotype is not possible, other than perhaps for patients with two null mutations.

INCIDENCE AND DIAGNOSIS

The incidence of SLOS is not known but has variably been estimated to range from 1 in 10,000 to 1 in 60,000 in those of northern or central European ancestry (Porter, 2000); it is less common in those of Asian or African ancestry. Opitz (1998) reported a birth prevalence of 1 in 9000 in middle Bohemia in 1958–1982, and Holmes (1994) estimated a prevalence of 1 in 30,000 in New England. These estimates are based on identification of the clinical phenotype. Since the advent of biochemical testing, newer estimates are now available. Bzduch (2000b) reported an incidence of 1 in 15,000 to 1 in 20,000 in Slovakia, and Nowaczyk et al. (2001c) reported an incidence of at least 1 in 22,700 in Ontario, although pooling data from the two laboratories in the United States that did most of the testing between 1995 and 1998 gives an estimated incidence of less than 1 in 60,000 births (Kelley and Hennekam, 2000). Newborn screening for SLOS will provide more information regarding the true incidence in live births once instituted.

While the incidence of SLOS is not known, most clinical geneticists do not feel that it is a common condition and would most likely agree with an observed incidence figure of approximately 1 in 40,000 to 1 in 60,000 based on their own experience. However, recent evidence obtained by testing for the common IVS8-1G → C mutation in several populations suggests otherwise. Battaile et al. (2001) identified 16 carriers in 1503 anonymous newborn filter paper–dried blood spots, which translates to a carrier frequency for all mutations of approximately 1 in 30. This is turn would predict a disease incidence of 1 in 1590 to 1 in 13,500. Likewise, Nowaczyk et al. (2001c) found 24 heterozygotes for the same mutation in an anonymous group of DNA samples from unrelated individuals from Ontario, Canada, also predicting that the carrier rate may be as high as 1 in 30 and suggesting a disease incidence of 1 in 1700 to 1 in 13,400. Clearly, these incidence figures are higher than what is observed. One explanation may be that many children are not diagnosed either because of a severe phenotype that results in intrauterine fetal demise or early neonatal death prior to evaluation by a geneticist or because of a mild phenotype that is not associated with dysmorphic features and does not prompt referral to a geneticist.

Postnatal Diagnosis

The diagnosis of SLOS is often first raised on the basis of the characteristic phenotype. Confirmation of the diagnosis requires analysis of sterols in blood, tissue, amniotic fluid, or chorionic villus with subsequent identification of the characteristic sterol profile, which includes elevation of the cholesterol precursors 7-DHC and 8-DHC, usually in the presence of decreased levels of cholesterol (Tint et al., 1994, 1995b; Kelley, 1995).

Most patients will have decreased cholesterol levels in blood or other body tissues; however, there have been patients with mild or variant forms of the condition who have normal cholesterol levels but elevation of 7-DHC and 8-DHC. Therefore, measurement of sterols by gas-chromatography (GC) or by GC/mass spectrometry (MS), which can separate the sterols and measure each independently, is necessary for a proper diagnostic evaluation as it is the elevation of 7- and 8-DHC that confirms the diagnosis of SLOS. Measurement of cholesterol by the method employed in most hospital laboratories will not identify all patients as this measures total cholesterol (cholesterol plus the precursors), which can result in cholesterol levels in the normal range. Patients with variant forms of SLOS have also presented with normal sterol profiles in blood but accumulation of sterol precursors in fibroblasts or lymphoblasts (Anderson et al., 1998).

In cases where blood is not available, tissue can be sent for sterol analysis. Sterols from tissue from stored pathologic specimens, either frozen tissue or tissue blocks, can also be extracted for diagnostic testing.

Other laboratory testing should include analysis of electrolytes, glucose, and indices of liver function to evaluate for the presence of cholestasis or coagulopathy in a severely affected newborn and endocrine hormonal testing for cortisol deficiency or abnormal male steroid hormones.

Newborn screening for SLOS has not been possible as an easily implemented, reproducible technique for identification of 7-DHC or 8-DHC from filter paper–dried blood spots has not been established. However, time-of-flight secondary ion MS to measure the cholesterol/dehydrocholesterol ratio (Zimmerman et al., 1997), measurement of 7-DHC and 8-DHC by GC/MS (Starck and Lovgren, 2000), and measurement of the 7-DHC/cholesterol ratio by electrospray ionization tandem MS (Johnson et al., 2001), all from dried blood spots, are promising techniques for future use.

Carrier Testing

Carrier detection by biochemical analysis is more problematic. Obligate carriers do not have significantly lower cholesterol levels or significantly higher levels of 7-DHC or 8-DHC than noncarriers (Irons, unpublished; Nowaczyk et al., 2000a), eliminating sterol analysis of plasma as a potential test for carrier detection. Carrier detection is possible either by measurement of DHCR7 activity (Shefer et al., 1997) or by measurement of the rate of reduction of the ergosterol C-7 double bond (Honda et al., 1998) in cultured skin fibroblasts, although neither technique is readily available and both may potentially miss some carriers due to overlap of activity into the normal range. Molecular analysis of *DHCR7* gene mutations will provide the easiest and most reliable method of carrier detection.

Prenatal Diagnosis

Prenatal diagnosis of SLOS is indicated for pregnancies at risk because of previously affected children or pregnancies where abnormal ultrasound findings or low maternal estriol levels have raised the possibility of SLOS (Irons and Tint, 1998). While there have been reports of abnormal prenatal ultrasound findings in fetuses subsequently confirmed to have SLOS, there is no pathognomonic ultrasound pattern associated with this condition. Intrauterine growth retardation; major malformations of the heart, kidneys, or limbs; and ambiguous genitalia, especially female-appearing genitalia or severe hypospadias in an XY fetus, can be seen. Other nonspecific findings include persistently increased nuchal translucency, polydactyly, cystic hygroma, and nonimmune hydrops. However, the majority of SLOS fetuses most likely have normal ultrasound examinations.

Low or undetectable unconjugated estriol (uE3) levels in maternal serum and amniotic fluid have also been reported (Canick et al., 1997). Since cholesterol is a precursor in the feto-placental biosynthesis of estriol, low levels of uE3 are a manifestation of fetal cholesterol deficiency. There may also be a characteristic pattern of low maternal α-fetoprotein, uE3, and human chorionic gonadotropin in affected pregnancies, with uE3 levels generally being lowest (Bradley et al., 1999). Since fetal demise or steroid sulfatase deficiency can also result in very low or undetectable maternal serum uE3 levels, ultrasound and testing for steroid sulfatase deficiency should be performed. While maternal serum uE3 levels can be significantly decreased in pregnancies affected with SLOS, they are often normal, so a normal maternal serum screen does not rule out an affected fetus.

Prenatal diagnosis of SLOS is possible by measurement of sterols and identification of elevated levels of 7-DHC in amniotic fluid obtained generally after 15 weeks of gestation. Unlike what is seen in plasma or other tissues, cholesterol levels are often normal in amniotic fluid in pregnancies where the fetus is affected, so the diagnosis relies on demonstration of elevated levels of 7-DHC. This method is very reliable; and since testing is done in amniotic fluid and does not require cultured amniocytes, results are available within days (Abuelo et al., 1995; Kelley, 1995; Tint et al., 1998). Enzyme deficiency can also be demonstrated in cultured amniocytes (Honda et al., 1995), and amniocyte culture may be required when there is a family history of a variant or very mild form of SLOS.

Prenatal diagnosis is also available in tissue obtained by chorionic villus sampling. Elevated levels of 7-DHC have been reported as early as 7 weeks' gestation in both direct and cultured chorionic villi (Mills et al., 1996; Sharp et al., 1997). Enzyme deficiency can also be demonstrated in cultured chorionic villus cells (Wanders et al., 1997; Linck et al., 2000b). Caution must be exercised when there is a family history of a mild or variant form of SLOS as diagnostic abnormalities in the 7DHC/sterol ratio may not be seen and prenatal testing later in gestation by amniotic fluid analysis may provide more accurate information (Nowaczyk et al., 2000).

In cases where both mutations in the family are known, prenatal testing can be performed by molecular analysis of chorionic villus in the first trimester (Bzduch et al., 2000a; Nowaczyk et al., 2001b). However, for couples who plan to choose amniocentesis rather than chorionic villus sampling, results of sterol analysis of amniotic fluid will often be available before molecular testing can be completed.

There is also potential for prenatal diagnosis of SLOS by analysis of the dehydrosteroids dehydroestriol and dehydropregnanetriol in maternal urine during pregnancy as a non-invasive means (Shackleton et al., 1999a,b, 2001).

TREATMENT

When developing a treatment strategy for any given condition, it is important to know what the underlying cause of the problem is so that the treatment can be focused on that problem. In most inborn errors of metabolism, the clinical phenotype is caused by the biochemical abnormality present; either accumulation of a toxic metabolite or deficiency of a product that is not made in adequate amounts. Developing a treatment strategy for SLOS has been difficult because it is still unclear whether the clinical phenotype of SLOS is secondary to a deficiency of cholesterol, a "toxic" or other effect from accumulation of 7-DHC and/or 8-DHC, an abnormality in lipid transfer from mother to fetus, other as yet unknown metabolites that may be secondarily increased or decreased due to the primary deficiency of DHCR7, or a combination of factors. While cholesterol levels are low in SLOS, there are other inborn errors of metabolism that also result in hypocholesterolemia, which are not associated with the clinical problems seen in SLOS. In addition, there are individuals who do not have a known metabolic disorder and have no neurologic or cognitive problems but have levels of cholesterol in the 90–110 mg/dl range, which are seen in some patients with mild or variant forms of SLOS who do have neurodevelopemental problems. Therefore, it appears that all of the neurodevelopmental problems cannot be explained by hypocholesterolemia alone.

It is possible that not all features of the clinical phenotype are caused by the same biochemical abnormality. For example, the structural anomalies may be due to a deficiency of cholesterol during embryonic development and the neurodevelopmental problems and growth retardation may be due to either the cholesterol deficiency or a toxic effect of 7- or 8-DHC replacing cholesterol in myelin or in other cell membranes. Both 7-DHC and 8-DHC differ only in having an extra double bond from cholesterol and are therefore structurally very similar to cholesterol and can easily take the place of cholesterol in cell membranes or as substrate for some enzyme systems that can accept them (Jira et al., 2000).

Some of the neurodevelopmental problems seen in SLOS are due to fixed developmental problems caused by abnormalities in embryonic brain development, limiting the ability to provide a neurodevelopmental "cure." However, as cholesterol is an important component of myelin and as myelination continues into the first few years of life, attempts to raise cholesterol levels may prove to be beneficial in maximizing ultimate neurodevelopmental outcome. Cholesterol is also a precursor of bile acids and steroid hormones, so GI, endocrine, and some behavioral problems may be responsive to cholesterol therapy.

Treatment strategies to date have focused on supplying exogenous cholesterol in an attempt to increase cholesterol levels and to secondarily decrease levels of the precursors 7-DHC and 8-DHC by feedback inhibition of HMG-CoA reductase, the rate-limiting enzyme in cholesterol biosynthesis. This strategy was tested in a pharmacologic rat model given the DHCR7 inhibitor BM 15.766, which developed the biochemical pattern of sterols seen in SLOS. The rats were then fed a diet high in cholesterol, which led to increased levels of cholesterol and decreased levels of 7-DHC and 8-DHC, indicating that there was some merit to this strategy (Xu et al., 1995). However, while most treatment protocols have focused on supplying exogenous cholesterol to affected patients, the specific form of cholesterol (food-derived vs. purified crystalline) and dose have not been determined.

Human treatment protocols have utilized exogenous cholesterol supplied in the form of a suspension of purified crystalline cholesterol in oil (soy, corn, grapeseed), crystalline cholesterol in an aqueous pharmaceutical suspending agent (Ora-Plus), or egg yolk (either hardboiled or powdered). Doses of cholesterol have varied with the degree of cholesterol deficiency or age of the child in the various reports. Some authors have titrated the cholesterol dose to the plasma cholesterol level, while others have utilized one or two specific doses for all patients regardless of the initial cholesterol level.

A suspension of crystalline cholesterol in soy oil, used with or without the bile acids ursodeoxycholic acid and chenodeoxycholic acid, was first used in 1994. Cholesterol doses range from 40–275 mg/kg daily depending on the patients' initial cholesterol levels. The suspension is well-tolerated and has shown no toxicity after 8 years of use. Biochemical indices monitored include levels of plasma cholesterol, 7-DHC, and 8-DHC. The ratio of cholesterol to total sterols is also monitored as the primary biochemical goal of therapy is to increase cholesterol and decrease precursor levels, thereby increasing this ratio. This therapy has resulted in statistically significant increases in cholesterol levels, decreased levels of 7-DHC and 8-DHC, and an increase in the ratio of cholesterol to total sterols (Irons et al., 1994, 1997, 2001a; Elias et al., 1997). Other investigators have also used crystalline cholesterol, either as a powder directly added to food, as a suspension in oil, or as an aqueous pharmaceutical suspending agent, and have reported increased cholesterol levels with variable changes in precursors (Nwokoro and Mulvihill, 1997; Starck et al., 1999).

Others have focused their treatment strategies on supplying cholesterol from food sources such as egg yolk. Linck et al. (2000a) reported increased plasma cholesterol levels and decreased levels of 7-DHC after long-term treatment with egg yolk in four patients whose initial cholesterol levels ranged from 38 to 76 mg/dl (Linck, 2000). Other investigators have also reported variable improvement in sterol levels using egg yolk or other food sources of cholesterol (Pauli et al., 1997; Starck et al., 1999). These results are promising and indicate that egg yolk, which is easily obtained and administered, can be used in patients with SLOS who have mild to moderate cholesterol deficiency. It is also possible that cholesterol from egg yolk may be more easily or efficiently absorbed compared with crystalline cholesterol since it is a natural food source. However, it is unclear whether enough cholesterol can be supplied in this form easily to children with severe cholesterol deficiency as higher doses of cholesterol can more easily be administered using crystalline cholesterol. This may be especially important during times of illness, when cholesterol levels fall and children are often unable to tolerate oral feedings and, thus, would not be able to ingest adequate amounts of cholesterol when it is most needed.

Cholesterol can also be supplied in the form of fresh frozen plasma (which contains low-density lipoprotein (LDL) cholesterol) to acutely ill children or to those who cannot take oral forms of cholesterol. This has been shown to be helpful in treating infants with acute infections or enhancing wound healing in postsurgical patients (Kelley, 2000; Irons, unpublished data). Monitoring of blood pressure is important during the administration of fresh frozen plasma as mild hypertension that resolved spontaneously has been noted in several infants following this form of therapy (Irons, unpublished data).

Prenatal therapy of a fetus identified with SLOS in the third trimester has also been reported (Irons et al., 1999). Transfusion of fresh frozen plasma to the fetus through the umbilical vein and into the fetal peritoneum was associated with increased fetal cholesterol levels and increased fetal mean corpuscular volume.

Initial treatment protocols have also used bile acids in conjunction with exogenous cholesterol. The bile acids included ursodeoxycholic acid, chenodeoxycholic acid, cholic acid, and sodium taurocholate (Irons et al., 1994, 1997; Elias et al., 1997; Nwokoro and Mulvihill, 1997; Starck et al., 1999; Behulova et al., 2000). The rationale for the inclusion of bile acids recognizes the facts that cholesterol is a precursor of bile acids and that bile acids are necessary for cholesterol absorption. Supplying bile acids would not only increase bile acid levels but also aid with absorption of the exogenous cholesterol that was being supplied. The bile acids were tolerated well but did not add any benefit over therapy with cholesterol alone. In addition, there was evidence to suggest that treatment with ursodexoycholic acid might actually interfere with cholesterol absorption and result in lower levels of plasma cholesterol (Irons et al., 1997). It has also been shown that bile acid synthesis in patients with SLOS who are mildly to moderately affected is normal, indicating that addition of bile acids to treatment strategies may not be necessary (Steiner et al., 2000). Bile acid therapy may be indicated in an infant with severe SLOS and cholestatic liver disease or in the early stages of therapy of an infant with a severe form of SLOS with significant cholesterol deficiency who would need some bile acid supplementation to be able to absorb the cholesterol provided. This treatment would continue until the infant's cholesterol levels were high enough to allow for endogenous bile acid synthesis.

While treatment with exogenous cholesterol has resulted in improvement in plasma sterol profiles, it is unclear whether this form of therapy will cause any change in sterol levels in the brain. Most evidence suggests that cholesterol in the human brain is made locally and that cholesterol does not cross the blood–brain barrier (Edmond et al.,

1991). However, it is unknown whether the blood–brain barrier is normal in patients with SLOS and whether some of the exogenous cholesterol can cross in areas that do not have an intact blood–brain barrier. Preliminary data utilizing magnetic resonance spectroscopy technology did show changes in brain lipid peaks in two patients who were studied prior to therapy and then on therapy, indicating that exogenous cholesterol may lead to change in brain lipids (Irons et al., 2001b). Measurement of cerebrospinal fluid (CSF) sterol levels in one patient treated with dietary cholesterol supplementation revealed no change in CSF cholesterol levels after 4 months of treatment, although there was a mild decrease in CSF 7-DHC and 8-DHC levels (van Rooij et al., 1997). To address this issue, Jira et al. (2000) studied the use of simvastatin, both without and with cholesterol supplementation, in two patients with SLOS. The rationale for using simvastatin involves the fact that the statins are HMG-CoA reductase inhibitors and can thereby directly affect cholesterol precursor levels both in the plasma and in the brain as simvastatin has lipophilic properties and can cross the blood–brain barrier. The two patients initially had several exchange transfusions that resulted in improvement in plasma sterol levels lasting only 3 days. Simvastatin therapy for several months resulted in improvement in the precursor/cholesterol ratio in the plasma, erythrocyte membrane, and CSF and improvement in anthropometric parameters. No toxicity was noted. The long-term risks and benefits of statin therapy in patients with SLOS are not known. The two patients had moderate DHCR7 deficiency; therefore, the risk of statin therapy in patients with a severe form of SLOS who have little or no residual DHCR7 activity is unclear.

While treatment with exogenous cholesterol leads to improvement in plasma sterol profiles, the clinical effects of therapy are striking in some areas and more variable in others (Irons et al., 1994, 1997: Elias et al., 1997; Nwokoro and Mulvihill, 1997; Pauli et al., 1997; Linck, 2000a). Clinical improvement has been noted in weight, height, head circumferance, and feeding behavior. Patients have fewer infections and recover from illness in shorter time periods. Improvement in GI symptoms, including feeding intolerance, dysmotility, and recurrent GI bleeding, has been reported (Elias et al., 1997). Two patients with delayed puberty rapidly progressed through several pubertal stages once cholesterol that could be used as substrate for steroid hormones was supplied (Elias et al., 1997). Improvement in symptoms of peripheral neuropathy as verified by improved nerve conduction velocities (Starck et al., 1999), hearing (Irons et al., 1997), and cholestatic liver disease (Irons, unpublished data), have been seen. Significant improvements in photosensitivity have also been noted (Elias et al., 1997; Azurdia et al., 2001).

The most striking gains have been noted in behavioral and other "neurodevelopmental" characteristics that are more difficult to objectively quantify. Significant improvements in behavior that begin fairly soon after institution of cholesterol therapy and result in a better quality of life have been reported (Irons et al., 1997; Elias et al., 1997; Pauli et al., 1997; Nwokoro and Mulvihill, 1997; Martin et al., 2001). Patients are described as being happier, more alert, more sociable, and "stronger." One patient began to walk independently after beginning therapy at the age of 14 years (Irons et al., 1997). A decrease in irritability, angry outbursts, and self-abusive behavior is seen, along with improvement in sleep duration (Kelley, 2000). Caretakers describe patients as happier, more calm, and easier to care for while on cholesterol.

While it seems clear that cholesterol therapy leads to improvement in mood and behavior, the effect of therapy on cognitive function is not known. The ability to answer this question has been hampered by many problems, including the fact that double-blinded, placebo-controlled studies have not been possible because the wide range of severity seen in patients and the varying ages at which patients have been identified for treatment make it difficult to find age-matched, severity-matched controls. It would also be difficult to have an untreated group since cholesterol is available in food and, therefore, even untreated patients would be "treated" if they were fed foods that contained cholesterol. In addition, many, if not the majority of, children with SLOS have developmental abnormalities of the brain that will result in cognitive problems that are fixed and not amenable to change. In these children, the goal of therapy would be to enhance whatever developmental potential was possible. Adequate testing tools have also not been available to document the gains made by patients on therapy since many gains are in the areas of attention and behavior and many developmental tests utilized in early infancy and childhood rely heavily on muscle tone, strength, and motor function, which are more significantly affected and do not respond as readily to therapy.

The results of preliminary studies of development in children with SLOS on therapy are somewhat mixed. Elias et al. (1997) reported an improved rate of developmental progress as well as improvement in language and cognitive skills in several patients, while others have not observed similar improvement in cognitive skills (Ullrich et al., 1996; Ruggiero et al., 2000). Therefore, while many beneficial effects of cholesterol therapy have been reported and no toxicity has been documented from the therapy, whether this therapy can improve cognition is unclear. Perhaps the most improvement can be expected from children with more mild or variant forms of SLOS who do not have developmental abnormalities of the brain itself and who are started on therapy early in life.

MUTATIONS IN ORTHOLOGOUS GENES AND ANIMAL MODELS

The nearly simultaneous discoveries of a cholesterol biosynthetic defect as the cause of SLOS, a multiple malformation syndrome, in 1993 and the role of cholesterol in Sonic Hedgehog processing in 1995 (Porter et al., 1995, 1996) generated renewed scientific interest in the role of cholesterol and sterols in morphogenesis. However, while there is much evidence to suggest that abnormal cholesterol metabolism may be causally related to abnormal morphogenesis, the exact nature of the interaction is not known.

Clear evidence of the teratogenic potential of inhibitors of distal cholesterol synthesis was first shown in the 1960s in a series of elegant studies by Roux and colleagues (1964, 1966). Treatment of rat embryos during the first days of gestation with triparanol, a chemical that inhibits Δ^{24}-dehydrocholesterol reductase (Fig. 17–1), was found to cause holoprosecephaly and abnormalities of the vertebrae and limbs (Roux, 1964). Human deficiency of this enzyme was found to cause the condition desmosterolosis, first identified in an infant with macrocephy, visceral anomalies, dysmorphic features, shortened limbs, and abnormalities of bone (Fitzpatrick et al., 1998). Use of the chemicals AY 9944 and BM 15.766, each an inhibitor of Δ^7-dehydrocholesterol reductase (Fig. 17–1), also resulted in CNS anomalies in the holoprosencephaly spectrum as well as craniofacial, limb, and genital anomalies similar to those seen in SLOS (Roux and Aubry, 1966; Kolf-Clauw et al., 1997; Lanoue et al., 1997). Since all three substances resulted in hypocholesterolemia, these findings suggested that a deficiency of cholesterol during embryonic development was an important etiologic factor in the development of fetal malformations. This appears to have been borne out by recent work demonstrating that in a rat model treated with AY 9944, embryonic development was normal as long as cholesterol supplementation was concurrently given (Gaoua et al., 2000; Roux et al., 2000). Additional work demonstrated that while cholesterol supplementation could restore the growth of embryos exposed to AY 9944, 7-DHC did not restore growth and further impaired the beneficial effects of cholesterol added simultaneously, as well as exerting an additional embryotoxic effect which the authors postulated might occur via oxidized by-products (Gaoua et al., 1999), indicating that the antenatal growth retardation in SLOS might be secondary to accumulation of 7-DHC and not to deficiency of cholesterol.

Additional evidence suggesting that normal cholesterol metabolism is important in embryonic development has also come from several different areas, beginning with studies of the corn lily Veratrum californicum, which produces two steroidal alkaloids, cyclopamine and jervine, that are structurally similar to cholesterol. An epidemic of cyclopia in sheep and lambs who ingested this lily in the 1950s led to research that proved that these compounds were teratogenic and caused cyclopia, cebocephaly, anophthalmia, or microphthalmia (Keeler, 1978).

Mutation of other genes involved in cholesterol metabolism has also been shown to cause fetal CNS anomalies. Mutation of the gene for gp330/megalin in a knockout mouse model resulted in holoprosencephalic-spectrum anomalies (Willnow et al., 1996). Megalin is believed to function as an endocytic receptor that mediates the cellular uptake of essential nutrients, possibly LDL cholesterol, from the amniotic fluid into the embryonic neuroepithelium (Willnow et al., 1996).

Apolipoprotein B (apoB) is a key structural component of several lipoproteins, which transport cholesterol, lipids, and vitamin E in the circulation. apoB is also believed to have a role in the transport of lipid nutrients to the embryo via the yolk sac during gestation (Farese et al., 1996). Targeted modification of the apoB gene results in a high incidence of exencephaly and hydrocephaly in homozygous animals and a low but significant incidence of hydrocephaly in heterozygous individuals (Homanics et al., 1995), as well as embryonic lethality and reduced concentrations of cholesterol and α-tocopherol in tissues of $apoB^{-/-}$ embryos (Farese et al., 1996).

Mutations of genes involved in hedgehog signaling have also resulted in anomalies similar to those seen in SLOS. The hedgehog genes encode intracellular signaling molecules that play important roles in embryonic patterning in both vertebrates and invertebrates (these are covered in more detail in Chapter 16. Sonic hedgehog (Shh) begins as a precursor protein that consists of an N-terminal signaling domain and a C-terminal catalytic domain. Autocatalytic cleavage of the molecule occurs; and during this process, cholesterol is covalently attached to the N-terminal signaling portion, which then attaches to the cell surface (Porter et al., 1995, 1996). Palmitate is also bound to this domain; some believe that the lipids linked to Shh are involved in tissue and spatial distribution of the protein and short-range/long-range signaling (Woollett, 2001). The Shh signaling network also contains two other proteins, PATCHED (PTC) and SMOOTHENED (SMO) (Tabin and McMahon, 1997). PTC, which has a sterol sensing domain, functions as a negative regulator of Shh signaling by inhibiting SMO. When the active signaling portion of Shh bound to cholesterol attaches to the cell surface and to PTC, the inhibition of SMO is released and it is free to signal, activating target gene transcription, such as the Gli/Ci family of DNA-binding proteins (Woollett, 2001). Homozygous mutations of Shh in the mouse result in cyclopia (Chiang et al., 1996), while heterogyous mutations of Shh and PTC in humans cause holoprosecephaly as well as nevoid basal cell carcinoma syndrome (Roessler et al., 1996; Ming and Muenke, 1998; Cohen, 1999). The PTC mutations that cause holoprosencephaly are located where Shh binding occurs (Cohen and Shiota, 2002). Total absence of SMO results in a phenotype similar to that produced by loss of Hh (Tabin and McMahon, 1997). Indian hedgehog mutations result in short-limbed dwarfism and other abnormalities of the skeleton, much like those seen in desmosterolosis (Karp et al., 2000).

Two $Dhcr7^{-/-}$ mouse models were created in 2001. Wassif et al. (2001) disrupted the Dhcr7 gene to produce a null mutation and created a mouse model with no detectable Dhcr7 activity and sterol profiles in tissue and serum samples that were similar to those found in humans with SLOS. The $Dhcr7^{-/-}$ animals had retention of the nasal plug, intrauterine growth retardation, and cleft palate (9%). Marked neurologic abnormalities were noted, including decreased movement and inability to suck, which were reminiscent of problems seen in infants with SLOS. Further neurophysiologic investigation revealed that while frontal cortex neurons responded normally to GABA, their response to glutamate was impaired, which may play a role in the pathogenesis of the neurologic problems seen in SLOS.

Fitzky et al. (2001) reported a second murine $Dhcr7^{-/-}$ animal model, also with a null mutation, that was easily identified by its small size, respiratory difficulty, blue coloration, lack of movement, and absence of suckling. The pups died shortly after birth. Isolated cleft palate and distended urinary bladders were found in 12% and 90% of the $Dhcr7^{-/-}$ pups, respectively, but not in any of the $Dhcr7^{+/-}$ or $Dhcr7^{+/+}$ littermates.

While both animal models had cleft palate, other major malformations were found in $Dhcr7^{-/-}$ pups. Fitzky et al. (2001) found that the cholesterol/7-DHC ratios in the liver of pups were considerably higher than those in severely affected children with SLOS. Both groups (Wassif et al., 2001; Fitzky et al., 2001) suggested that one explanation for this might be that since the fetal mouse receives a greater amount of cholesterol from the mother than does the human fetus, elevated transfer of cholesterol from mother to fetus in early gestation protected the fetus from development of the craniofacial and limb anomalies seen in the human. This theory correlates well with earlier animal studies using the DHCR7 inhibitor AY 9944, which led to maternal cholesterol deficit and craniofacial and CNS anomalies and intrauterine growth retardation in the embryos (Gaoua et al., 2000). Feeding the mothers cholesterol prevented the teratogenic effects.

Fitzky et al. (2001) also used their model to study sterol metabolism and found that, while mRNA levels for HMG-CoA reductase were normal, protein levels and activity of HMG-CoA reductase were reduced. Further study revealed that 7-DHC accelerated the proteolysis of HMG-CoA reductase and that, therefore, the accumulated 7-DHC suppressed sterol biosynthesis post-translationally, which they postulated could exacerbate fetal cholesterol deficiency (Fitzky et al., 2001).

DEVELOPMENTAL PATHOGENESIS

Deficiency of DHCR7 results in a clinical phenotype that consists of structural malformations, dysmorphic facial features, intrauterine and postnatal growth retardation, cognitive deficits, and other symptoms of abnormal neurologic, GI, and endocrine function. Affected patients have a characteristic sterol profile of decreased cholesterol and elevation of the cholesterol precursors 7-DHC and 8-DHC in plasma and other body organs and tissues. Cholesterol is not only an important component of cell membranes and myelin but also a precursor of bile acids and steroid hormones. Therefore, the pathogenesis of the clinical features of SLOS will necessarily be due to multiple processes and will not be easily explained by a single mechanism.

The importance of cholesterol in cell membrane structure and cell–cell interactions may help to explain the postnatal growth retardation and GI problems seen in this condition. The fact that cholesterol makes up 25% of myelin could also account for some of the neurodevelopmental problems seen, such as mental retardation or developmental delay, hearing deficit, or peripheral neuropathy. Other as yet unidentified factors, such as the abnormal response of frontal neurons to glutamate documented in the *Dhcr7* $^{-/-}$ mouse model (Wassif et al., 2001), may also help to explain the abnormal neurologic problems in this condition.

GI symptoms, such as dysmotility and cholestasis, may be attributable to a deficiency of bile acids in patients with severe SLOS who do not have adequate amounts of cholesterol to make bile acids. The lack of cholesterol for steroid hormone synthesis will lead to adrenal insufficiency, especially in the severely affected patient or during acute stress or illness, when cholesterol levels fall and there is no substrate for cortisol and mineralocorticoid synthesis, as well as failure of masculinization and delayed puberty due to inadequate substrate for pubertal steroid hormone synthesis. While elevated levels of 7-DHC might predispose to the photosensitivity seen in this condition, there appears to be no relation to 7-DHC levels, although cholesterol therapy is beneficial. The cause of the behavioral abnormalities seen in this condition is also not yet known, although they appear to be responsive to cholesterol supplementation very soon after supplementation is started, which is intriguing given that exogenously supplied cholesterol is not believed to cross the blood–brain barrier and exert any influence centrally. Therefore, while we might attribute many of the clinical problems noted in this condition to deficiency of cholesterol and to the role of cholesterol in numerous physiologic systems, the exact cause of these problems is not known.

Much emphasis has been placed on the etiology of the structural malformations seen in SLOS and how disordered cholesterol synthesis interacts with Shh to produce structural anomalies. Data from studies reviewed in the previous section appear to indicate that cholesterol deficiency, and not accumulation of cholesterol precursors, during crucial periods of development plays the most important role in the etiology of the malformations in SLOS. Since maternal transport of cholesterol to the fetus in humans makes up at most 20% of the cholesterol that reaches the fetus (Carr and Simpson, 1982), the human fetus relies primarily on de novo cholesterol synthesis and deficiency of

DHCR7 would necessarily limit the available amount of cholesterol during important periods of embryogenesis. Possible sites of action include the Shh pathway or the cell membrane itself, which is important in cell–cell interactions and embryonic differentiation (Roux et al., 2000).

The exact role of cholesterol in Shh function and where cholesterol deficiency might affect Shh signaling are not yet known. Cholesterol is important for the autocatalytic processing of Shh and its binding to cholesterol-rich membrane rafts on the cell surface and to PTC. However other sterols, such as 7-DHC, function in Shh autocatalytic processing, so the prime site of action of cholesterol deficiency or the presence of cholesterol precursors is not believed to be in the biogenesis of Shh. What is not known is whether Shh bound to a sterol other than cholesterol would have the same signaling activity or whether attachment to different sterols would affect association with membrane rafts (Incardona and Roelink, 2000). While deficiency of cholesterol may not affect Shh biogenesis, it appears that the site of action of cholesterol deficiency is in Shh signal transduction within target cells, although the exact site is unknown. Current areas of investigation involve PTC since it contains a sterol sensing domain and has similarity to the Niemann-Pick C1 protein, which is involved in the vesicular trafficking of cholesterol (Incardona and Roelink, 2000).

In addition, other modifying genes or factors may play a role in the pathogenesis of SLOS. The phenotypic heterogeneity of SLOS even within families raises the possibility of other modifying genes in the pathogenesis of this disorder. One suggestion involves the possibility that different levels of expression of ApoB, which is required for the transfer of cholesterol from the mother to the embryo and for the packaging of lipids in the yolk sac endoderm, may explain some of the phenotypic heterogeneity seen in this condition (Roux et al., 2000).

Further study of all of these areas will be needed before we have a full understanding of the developmental pathogenesis of SLOS. In addition, information from the study of DHCR7 deficiency will educate us not only about the pathogenesis of SLOS but also about the pathogenesis of structural malformations in humans.

REFERENCES

Abuelo DM, Tint GS, Kelley R, Batta AK, Shefer S, Salen G (1995). Prenatal detection of the cholesterol synthetic defect in the Smith-Lemli-Opitz syndrome by the analysis of the amniotic fluid sterols. *Am J Med Genet* 56: 281–285.

Anderson AJ, Stephan MJ, Walker WO, Kelley RI (1998). Variant RSH/Smith-Lemli-Opitz syndrome with atypical sterol metabolism. *Am J Med Genet* 78: 413–418.

Andersson HC, Frentz J, Martinez JE, Tuck-Muller CM, Bellizaire J (1999). Adrenal insufficiency in Smith-Lemli-Opitz syndrome. *Am J Med Genet* 82: 382–384.

Anstey AV, Taylor CR (1999). Photosensitivity in the Smith-Lemli-Opitz syndrome: The US experience of a new congenital photosensitivity syndrome. *J Am Acad Dermatol* 41: 121–123.

Anstey AV, Ryan A, Rhodes LE, Charman ER, Arlett CF, Tyrrell RM, Taylor CR, Pearse AD (1999). Characterization of photosensitivity in the Smith-Lemli-Opitz syndrome: a new congenital photosensitivity syndrome. *Br J Dermatol* 141: 406–414.

Atchaneeyasakul L-O, Linck LM, Connor WE, Weleber RG, Steiner RD (1998). Eye findings in 8 children an a spontaneously aborted fetus with RSH/Smith-Lemli-Opitz syndrome. *Am J Med Genet* 80: 501–505.

Azurdia RM, Anstey AV, Rhodes LE (2001). Cholesterol supplementation objectively reduces photosensitivity in the Smith-Lemli-Opitz syndrome. *Br J Dermatol* 144: 143–147.

Battaile KP, Steiner RD (2000). Smith-Lemli-Opitz syndrome: The first malformation syndrome associated with defective cholesterol synthesis. *Mol Genet Metab* 71:154–162.

Battaile KP, Maslen CL, Wassif CA, Krakowiak P, Porter FD, Steiner RD (1999). A simple PCR-based assay allows detection of a common mutation, IVS8-1G>C, in DHCR7 in Smith-Lemli-Opitz syndrome. *Genet Test* 3:361–363.

Battaile KP, Battaile BC, Merkens LS, Maslen CL, Steiner RD (2001). Carrier frequency of the common mutation IVS8-1G>C in DHCR7 and estimate of the expected incidence of Smith-Lemli-Opitz syndrome. *Mol Genet Metab* 72: 67–71.

Behulova D, Bzduch V, Skodova J, Dello Russo A, Corso G, Ponec J, Barosova J, Nebesonakova E (2000). Effect of cholesterol supplementation on serum lipid and apolipoprotein levels in children with Smith-Lemli-Opitz syndrome. *J Inherit Metab Dis* 23: Suppl. 1, 197.

Bradley IA, Palomaki GE, Knight GJ, Haddow JE, Opitz JM, Irons M, Kelley RI, Tint GS (1999). Levels of unconjugated estriol and other maternal serum markers in pregnancies with Smith-Lemli-Opitz (RSH) syndrome fetuses. *Am J Med Genet* 82: 355–358.

Brown MS, Goldstein JL (1980). Multivalent feedback regulation of HMG CoA reductase, a control mechanism coordinating isoprenoid synthesis and cell growth. *J Lipid Res* 21: 505–516.

Bzduch V, Kozak L, Francova H, Behulova D (2000a). Prenatal diagnosis of Smith-Lemli-Opitz syndrome by mutation analysis. *Am J Med Genet* 95: 85.

Bzduch V, Behulova D, Skodova J (2000b). Incidence of Smith-Lemli-Opitz syndrome in Slovakia. *Am J Med Genet* 90: 260.

Canick JA, Abuelo DN, Bradley LA, Tint GS (1997). Maternal serum marker levels in two pregnancies affected with Smith-Lemli-Opitz syndrome. *Prenat Diagn* 17: 187–189.

Carr BR, Simpson ER (1982). Cholesterol synthesis in human fetal tissues. *J Clin Endocrinol Metab* 55: 447–452.

Charman CR, Ryan A, Tyrrell RM, Pearse AD, Arlett CF, Kurwa HA, Shortland G, Ansley A (1998). Photosensitivity associated with the Smith-Lemli-Opitz syndrome. *Br J Dermatol* 138: 855–863.

Chasalow FI, Blethan SL, Taysi K (1985). Possible abnormalities of steroid secretion in children with Smith-Lemli-Opitz syndrome and their parents. *Steroids* 46: 827–843.

Chiang C, Litingtung Y, Lee E, Young KE, Corden JL, Westphal H, Beachy PA (1996). Cyclopia and defective axial patterning in mice lacing Sonic hedgehog gene function. *Nature* 383: 407–413.

Cohen MM (1999). Nevoid basal cell carcinoma syndrome: molecular biology and new hypotheses. *Int J Oral Maxillofac Surg* 28: 216–223.

Cohen MM, Shiota K (2002). Teratogenesis of holoprosencephaly. *Am J Med Genet* 109: 1–15.

Cuniff C, Kratz LE, Moser A, Natowicz MR, Kelley RI (1997). Clinical and biochemical spectrum of patients with RSH/Smith-Lemli-Opitz syndrome and abnormal cholesterol metabolism. *Am J Med Genet* 68: 263–269.

Curry CJ, Carey J, Holland JS, Chopra D, Fineman R, Golabi M, Sherman S, Pagon RA, Allanson J, Shulman S (1987). Smith-Lemli-Opitz syndrome-type II: multiple congenital anomalies with male pseudohermaphroditism and frequent early lethality. *Am J Med Genet* 26: 45–57.

De Brasi D, Esposito T, Rossi M, Parenti G, Sperandeo MP, Zuppaldi A, Bardaro T, Ambruzzi MA, Zelante L, Ciccodicola A, et al. (1999). Smith-Lemli-Opitz syndrome: evidence of T93M as a common mutation of Δ7-sterol reductase in Italy and report of three novel mutations. *Eur J Hum Genet* 7: 937–940.

De Die-Smulders CEM, Waterham HR, Fryns JP (1999). Unexpected molecular findings in 2 previously described brothers with Smith-Lemli-Opitz syndrome. *Genet Couns* 10: 403.

Donnai D, Young ID, Owne WG, Clark SA, Miller PF, Knox WF (1986). The lethal multiple congenital anomaly syndrome of polydactyly, sex reversal, renal hypoplasia, and unilobar lungs. *J Med Genet* 23: 64–71.

Edmond JRA, Korsak JW, Morrow G, Torok-Both G, Catlin DH (1991). Dietary cholesterol and the origin of cholesterol in the brain of developing rats. *J Nutr* 121: 1323–1330.

Elias ER, Irons MB, Hurley AD, Tint GS, Salen G (1997). Clinical effects of cholesterol supplementation in six patients with the Smith-Lemli-Opitz syndrome (SLOS). *Am J Med Genet* 68: 305–310.

Elias ER, Fulton AL, Mayer DL, Hansen RM (2000). Retinal dysfunction in patients with the Smith-Lemli-Opitz syndrome (SLOS). *Am J Hum Genet* 67(Suppl 2): 36.

Farese RV, Cases S, Ruland SL, Kayden HJ, Wong JS, Young SG, Hamilton RL (1996). A novel function for apolipoprotein B: lipoprotein synthesis in the yolk sac is critical for maternal–fetal lipid transport in mice. *J Lipid Res* 37: 347–360.

Fitzky BU, Witsch-Baumgartner M, Erdel M, Lee JN, Paik Y-K, Glossmann H, Utermann G, Moebius FF (1998). Mutations in the Δ7-sterol reductase gene in patients with the Smith-Lemli-Opitz syndrome. *Proc Natl Acad Sci USA* 95: 8181–8186.

Fitzky BU, Glossmann H, Utermann G, Moebius FF (1999). Molecular genetics of the Smith-Lemli-Opitz syndrome and postsqualene sterol metabolism. *Curr Opin Lipidol* 10: 123–131.

Fitzky BU, Moebius FF, Asaoka H, Waage-Baudet H, Xu L, Xu G, Mobuyo M, Kluckman K, Hiller S, Yu H, et al. (2001). 7-Dehydrocholesterol-dependent proteolysis of HMG-CoA reductase suppresses sterol biosynthesis in a mouse model of Smith-Lemli-Opitz/RSH syndrome. *J Clin Invest* 108: 905–915.

Fitzpatrick DR, Keeling JW, Evans MJ, Kan AE, Bell JE, Porteous ME, Mills K, Winter RM, Clayton PT (1998). Clinical phenotype of desmosterolosis. *Am J Med Genet* 75: 145–152.

Gaoua W, Chevy F, Roux C, Wolf C (1999). Oxidized derivatives of 7-dehydrocholesterol induce growth retardation in cultured rat embryos: a model for antenatal growth retardation in the Smith-Lemli-Opitz syndrome. *J Lipid Res* 40: 456–463.

Gaoua W, Wolf C, Chevy F, Ilien F, Roux C (2000). Cholesterol deficit but not accumuation of aberrant sterols is the major cause of the teratogenic activity in the Smith-Lemli-Opitz syndrome animal model. *J Lipid Res* 41: 637–646.

Goldstein JL, Brown MS (1990). Regulation of the mevalonate pathway. *Nature* 343: 425–430.

Gorlin RJ, Cohen MM, Levin LS (1990). Smith-Lemli-Opitz syndromes. In: *Syndromes of the Head and Neck,* 3rd Edition. Oxford University Press, New York, pp. 890–894.

Hardeman MR, Ince C (1999). Clinical potential of *in vitro* measured red cell deformability, a myth? *Clin Hemorheol Microcirc* 21: 277–284.

Holmes L (1994). Prevalence of Smith-Lemli-Opitz syndrome (SLO). *Am J Med Genet* 50: 334.

Homanics GE, Maeda N, Traver MG, Kayden HJ, Dehart DB, Sulik KK (1995). Exencephaly and hydrocephaly in mice with targeted modification of the apolipoprotein B (*Apob*) gene. *Teratology* 51: 1–10.

Honda A, Tint GS, Salen G, Batta AK, Chen TS, Shefer S (1995). Defective conversion of 7-dehydrocholesterol to cholesterol in cultured skin fibroblasts from Smith-Lemli-Opitz homozygotes. *J Lipid Res* 36: 1595–1601.

Honda M, Tint GS, Shefer S, Honda A, Batta AK, Xu G, Chen TS, Salen G (1998). Accurate detection of Smith-Lemli-Opitz syndrome carriers by measurement of the rate of redution of the ergosterol C-7 double bond in cultured skin fibroblasts. *J Inherit Metab Dis* 21: 761–768.

Honda M, Tint GS, Honda A, Salen G, Shefer S, Batta AK, Matsuzaki Y, Tanaka N (2000). Regulation of cholesterol biosynthetic pathway in patients with the Smith-Lemli-Opitz syndrome. *J Inherit Metab Dis* 23: 464–474.

Incardona JP, Roelink H (2000). The role of cholesterol in Shh signaling and teratogen-induced holoprosencephaly. *Cell Mol Life Sci* 57: 1709–1719.

Irons MB, Tint GS (1998). Prenatal diagnosis of Smith-Lemli-Opitz syndrome. *Prenat Diagn* 18: 369–372.

Irons M, ELias ER, Salen G, Tint GS (1993). Defective cholesterol biosynthesis in Smith-Lemli-Opitz syndrome. *Lancet* 341: 1414.

Irons MB, Elias ER, Tint GS, Salen G, Frieden R, Buie TM, Ampola M (1994). Abnormal cholesterol metabolism in Smith-Lemli-Opitz syndrome: report of clinical and biochemical findings in four patients and treatment in one patient. *Am J Med Genet* 50: 347–352.

Irons M, Elias ER, Abuelo D, Bull MJ, Greene CL, Johnson VP, Keppen L, Schanen C, Tint GS, Salen G (1997). Treatment of Smith-Lemli-Opitz syndrome: results of a multicenter trial. *Am J Med Genet* 68: 311–314.

Irons MB, Nores J, Stewart TL, Craigo SD, Bianchi DW, D'Alton ME, Tint GS, Salen G, Bradley LA (1999). Antenatal therapy of Smith-Lemli-Opitz syndrome. *Fetal Diagn Ther* 14: 133–137.

Irons M, Elias ER, Bay C, Pober B, Tint GS, Salen G (2001a). Improvement in sterol levels with cholesterol therapy in Smith-Lemli-Opitz syndrome (SLOS). *Am J Hum Genet* 69(Suppl): 679.

Irons M, Elias ER, Poussaint TY, Caruso P, Tzika A (2001b). MR and MRS findings in Smith-Lemli-Opitz syndrome. *Genet Med* 3:239.

Jira PE, Wevers RA, De Jong J, Rubio-Gozalbo E, Janssen-Zijlstra SM, Van Heyst AFJ, Sengers RCA, Smeitink JAM (2000). Simvastatin: a new therapeutic approach for Smith-Lemli-Opitz syndrome. *J Lipid Res* 41: 1339– 1346.

Jira PE, Wanders RJA, Smeitink JAM, De Jong J, Wevers RA, Oostheim W, Tuerlings HAM, Hennekam RCM, Sengers RCA, Waterham HR (2001). Novel mutations in the 7-dehydrocholesterol reductase gene of 13 patients with Smith-Lemli-Opitz syndrome. *Ann Hum Genet* 65: 229–236.

Johnson DW, Ten Brink JH, Jakobs C (2001). A rapid screening procedure for cholesterol and dehydrocholesterol by electrospray ionization tandem mass spectrometry. *J Lipid Res* 42: 1699–1705.

Karp SJ, Schipani E, St-Jacques B, Hunzelman J, Kronenberg H, McMahon AP (2000). Indian hedgehog coordinates endochondral bone growth and morphogenesis via parathyroid hormone–related protein–dependent and –independent pathways. *Dev Suppl* 127: 543–548.

Keeler RF (1978). Cyclopamine and related steroidal alkaloid teratogens: Their occurrence, structural relationship, and biologic effects. *Lipids* 13: 708–715.

Kelley RI (1995). Diagnosis of Smith-Lemli-Opitz syndrome by gas chromatography/mass spectrometry of 7-dehyrocholesterol in plasma, amniotic fluid and cultured skin fibroblasts. *Clin Chim Acta* 236: 45–58.

Kelley RI (2000). Inborn errors of cholesterol biosynthesis. *Adv Pediatr* 47: 1–53.

Kelley RI, Hennekam RCM (2000). The Smith-Lemli-Opitz syndrome. *J Med Genet* 37:321–335.

Kolf-Clauw M, Chevy F, Siliart B, Wolf C, Mulliez N, Roux C (1997). Cholesterol biosynthesis inhibited by BM15.766 induces holoprosencephaly in the rat. *Teratology* 56: 188–200.

Kozak L, Francova H, Hrabincova E, Prochazkova D, Juttneroba V, Bzduch V, Simek P (2000). Smith-Lemli-Opitz syndrome: molecular-genetic analysis of ten families. *J Inherit Metab Dis* 23: 409–412.

Krajewska-Walasek M, Gradowska W, Ryzko J, Socha P, Chmielik J, Szaplyko W, Kasprzyk J, Gorska B, Szreter M, Wolski J, et al. (1999). Further delineation of the classical Smith-Lemli-Opitz syndrome phenotype at different patient ages: clinical and biochemical studies. *Clin Dysmorphol* 8: 29–40.

Krakowiak PA, Nwokoro NA, Wassif CA, Battaile KP, Nowaczyk MJM, Connor WE, Maslen C, Steiner RD, Porter FD (2000). Mutation analysis and description of sixteen RSH/Smith-Lemli-Optiz syndrome patients: polymerase chain reaction–based assays to simplify genotyping. *Am J Med Genet* 94: 214–227.

Langius FAA, Waterham HR, Koster J, Dorland L, Duran M, De Koning TJ, Beemer FA, Wanders RJA, Poll The B-T (2000). Smith-Lemli-Opitz syndrome: the mild end of the clinical and biochemical spectrum. *J Inherit Metab Dis* 23(Suppl 1): 196.

Lanoue L, Dehart DB, Hinsdale ME, Maeda N, Tint GS, Sulik KK (1997). Limb, genital, CNS, and facial malformations result from gene/environment-induced cholesterol deficiency: further evidence for a link to Sonic Hedgehog. *Am J Med Genet* 73: 24–31.

Lin AE, Ardinger HH, Ardinger RH, Cunniff C, Kelley RI (1997). Cardiovascular malformations in Smith-Lemli-Opitz syndrome. *Am J Med Genet* 68: 270–278.

Linck LM, Lin DS, Flavell D, Connor WE, Steiner RD (2000a). Cholesterol supplementation with egg yolk increases plasma cholesterol and decreases plasma 7-dehydrocholesterol in Smith-Lemli-Opitz syndrome. *Am J Med Genet* 93: 360–365.

Linck LM, Hayflick SJ, Lin DS, Battaile KP, Ginat S, Burlingame T, Gibson KM, Honda M, Honda A, Salen G, et al. (2000b). Fetal demise with Smith-Lemli-Opitz syndrome confirmed by tissue sterol analysis and the absence of measureable 7-dehydrocholesterol Δ7-reductase activity in chorionic villi. *Prenat Diagn* 20: 238–240.

Loffler J, Trojovsky A, Casati B, Kroisel PM, Utermann G (2000). Homozygosity for the W151X stop mutation in the Δ7-sterol reductase gene (DHCR7) causing a lethal form of Smith-Lemli-Opitz syndrome: retrospective molecular diagnosis. *Am J Med Genet* 95: 174–177.

Martin A, Koenig K, Scahill L, Tierney E, Porter FD, Nwokoro NA (2001). Smith-Lemli-Opitz syndrome. *J Am Acad Child Adolesc Psychiatry* 40: 506–507.

Mills K, Mandel H, Montemagno R, Soothill P, Gershoni-Baruch R, Clayton PT (1996). First trimester prenatal diagnosis of Smith-Lemli-Opitz syndrome (7-dehydrocholesterol reductase deficiency). *Pediatr Res* 39: 816–819.

Ming JE, Muenke M (1998). Holoprosencephaly: from Homer to hedgehog. *Clin Genet* 53: 155–163.

Moebius FF, Fitzky BU, Lee JNO, Paik Y-K, Glossman H (1998). Molecular cloning and expression of the human Δ7-sterol reductase. *Proc Natl Acad Sci USA* 95: 1899–1902.

Nowaczyk MJM (2000). Plasma measurement of 7-dehydrocholesterol to detect carriers of Smith-Lemli-Opitz syndrome. *Prenat Diagn* 20: 168–170.

Nowaczyk MJM, Waye JS (2001). The Smith-Lemli-Opitz syndrome: a novel metabolic way of understanding developmental biology, embryogenesis, and dysmorphology. *Clin Genet* 59: 375–391.

Nowaczyk MJM, Heshka T, Kratz LE, Kelley RE (2000). Difficult prenatal diagnosis in mild Smith-Lemli-Opitz syndrome. *Am J Med Genet* 95: 396–398.

Nowaczyk MJM, Nakamura LM, Eng B, Porter FD, Waye JS (2001a). Frequency and ethnic distribution of the common DHCR7 mutation in Smith-Lemli-Opitz syndrome. *Am J Med Genet* 102: 383–386.

Nowaczyk MJM, Garcia DM, Eng B, Waye JS (2001b). Rapid molecular prenatal diagnosis of Smith-Lemli-Opitz syndrome. *Am J Med Genet* 102: 387–388.

Nowaczyk MJM, McCaughey D, Whelan DT, Porter FD (2001c). Incidence of Smith-Lemli-Opitz syndrome in Ontario, Canada. *Am J Med Genet* 102: 18–20.

Nowaczyk MJM, Siu VM, Krakowiak PA, Porter FD (2001d). Adrenal insufficiency and hypertension in a newborn infant with Smith-Lemli-Opitz syndrome. *Am J Med Genet* 103: 223–225.

Nwokoro NA, Mulvihill JJ (1997). Cholesterol and bile acid replacement therapy in children and adults with Smith-Lemli-Opitz (SLO/RSH) syndrome. *Am J Med Genet* 68: 315–321.

Nwokoro NA, Wassif CA, Porter FD (2001). Genetic disorders of cholesterol biosynthesis in mice and humans. *Mol Genet Metab* 74: 105–119.

Opitz JM (1998). The RSH syndrome: paradigmatic metabolic malformation syndrome. In: *Diagnosis and Treatment of the Unborn Child.* New MI (ed.) Idelson-Gnocchi, Naples, Italy, pp. 43–55.

Patrono C, Rizzo C, Tessa A, Giannotti A, Borrelli P, Carrozzo R, Piemonte F, Bertini E, Dionisi-Vici A, Santorelli FM (2000). Novel 7-DHCR mutation in a child with Smith-Lemli-Opitz syndrome. *Am J Med Genet* 91: 138–140.

Pauli RM, Williams MS, Josephson KD, Tint GS (1997). Smith-Lemli-Opitz syndrome: thirty-year follow-up of "S" of "RSH" syndrome. *Am J Med Genet* 68: 260–262.

Porter FD (2000). RSH/Smith-Lemli-Opitz syndrome: a multiple congenital anomaly/mental retardation syndrome due to an inborn error of cholesterol biosynthesis. *Mol Genet Metab* 71: 163–174.

Porter JA, Von Kessler DP, Ekker SC, Young KE, Lee JJ, Moses K, Beachy PA (1995). The product of hedgehog autoproteolytic cleavage active in local and long-range signaling. *Nature* 374: 363–366.

Porter JA, Young KE, Beachy PA (1996). Cholesterol modification of Hedgehog signaling proteins in animal development. *Science* 274: 255–259.

Roessler E, Belloni E, Gaudenz K, Jay P, Berta P, Scherer SW, Tsui L-C, Muenke M (1996). Mutations in the human Sonic Hedgehog gene cause holoprosencephaly. *Nat Genet* 14: 357–360.

Roux C (1964): Action teratogene du triparanol chez l'animal. *Arch Pediatr* 21: 451–464.

Roux C, Aubry A (1966). Action teratogene chez le rat d'un inhibiteur de la synthese du cholesterol, le AY9944. *C R Soc Biol* 160: 1353–1357.

Roux C, Wolf C, Mulliez N, Gaoua W, Cormier V, Chevy F, Citadelle D (2000). Role of cholesterol in embryonic development. *Am J Clin Nutr* 71(Suppl): 1270S–1279S.

Ruggiero M, Pettit-Kekel K, Sikora D, Linck L, Connor WE, Steiner RD (2000). Cholesterol supplementation does not alter developmental progress in Smith-Lemli-Opitz syndrome. *J Inherit Metab Dis* 23(Suppl 1): 196.

Ryan AK, Bartlett K, Clayton P, Eaton S, Mills L, Donnai D, Winter RM, Burn J (1998). Smith-Lemli-Opitz syndrome: a variable clinical and biochemical phenotype. *J Med Genet* 35: 558–565.

Shackleton CHL, Roitman E, Kratz LE, Kelley RI (1999a). Equine type estrogens produced by a pregnant woman carrying a Smith-Lemli-Opitz syndrome fetus. *J Clin Endocrinol Metab* 84: 1157–1159.

Shackelton CHL, Roitman E, Kratz LE, Kelley RI (1999b). Midgestational maternal urine steroid markers of fetal Smith-Lemli-Opitz (SLO) syndrome (7-dehydrocholesterol 7-reductase deficiency). *Steroids* 64: 446–452.

Shackleton CHL, Roitman E, Kratz L, Kelley R (2001). Dehydro-oestriol and dehydropregnanetriol are candidate analytes for prenatal diagnosis of Smith-Lemli-Opitz syndrome. *Prenat Diagn* 21: 207–212.

Sharp P, Haan E, Fletcher JM, Khong TY, Carey WF (1997). First-trimester diagnosis of Smith-Lemli-Opitz syndrome. *Prenat Diagn* 17: 355–361.

Shefer S, Salen G, Batta AK, Honda A, Tint GS, Irons M, Elias ER, Chen TC, Holick MF (1995). Markedly inhibited 7-dehydrocholesterol-Δ7-reductase activity in liver microsomes from Smith-Lemli-Opitz homozygotes. *J Clin Invest* 96: 1779–1785.

Shefer S, Salen G, Honda A, Batta A, Hauser S, Tint GS, Honda M, Chen T, Holick MF, Nguyen LB (1997). Rapid identification of Smith-Lemli-Opitz syndrome homozygotes and heterozygotes (carriers) by measurement of deficient 7-dehydrocholesterol-Δ7-reductase activity in fibroblasts. *Metabolism* 46: 844–850.

Smith DW, Lemli L, Opitz JM (1964). A newly recognized syndrome of multiple congenital anomalies. *J Pediatr* 64: 210–217.

Starck L, Lovgren A (2000). Diagnosis of Smith-Lemli-Opitz syndrome from stored filter paper blood specimens. *Arch Dis Child* 82: 490–492.

Starck L, Bjorkhem I, Ritzen EM, Nilsson BY, Von Dobeln U (1999). Beneficial effects of dietary supplementation in a disorder with defective synthesis of cholesterol. A case report of a girl with Smith-Lemli-Opitz syndrome, polyneuropathy and precocious puberty. *Acta Paediatr* 88: 729–733.

Steiner RD, Linck LM, Flavell DP, Lin DS, Connor WE (2000). Sterol balance in the Smith-Lemli-Opitz syndrome. Reduction in whole body cholesterol synthesis and normal bile acid production. *J Lipid Res* 41: 1437–1447.

Tabin CJ, McMahon AP (1997). Recent advances in Hedgehog signaling. *Trends Cell Biol* 7: 442–446.

Tierney E, Nwokoro NA, Kelley RI (2000). Behavioral phenotype of RSH/Smith-Lemli-Opitz syndrome. *Ment Retard Dev Disabil Res Rev* 6: 131–134.

Tierney E, Nwokoro NA, Porter FD, Freund LS, Ghuman JK, Kelley RI (2001). Behavior phenotype in the RSH/Smith-Lemli-Opitz syndrome. *Am J Med Genet* 98: 191–200.

Tint GS, Irons M, Elias ER, Batta AK, Frieden R, Chen TS, Salen G (1994). Defective cholesterol biosynthesis associated with the Smith-Lemli-Opitz syndrome. *N Engl J Med* 330: 107–113.

Tint GS, Salen G, Batta AK, Shefer S, Irons M, Elias ER, Abuelo DN, Johnson VP, Lambert M, Lutz R (1995a). Correlation of severity and outcome with plasma sterol levels in variants of the Smith-Lemli-Opitz syndrome. *J Pediatr* 127: 82–87.

Tint GS, Saller M, Hughes-Benzie R, Batta AK, Shefer S, Genest D, Irons M, Elias E, Salen G (1995b). Markedly increased tissue concentrations of 7-dehydrocholesterol combined with low levels of cholesterol are characteristic of the Smith-Lemli-Opitz syndrome. *J Lipid Res* 36: 89–95.

Tint GS, Abuelo D, Till M, Cordier MP, Batta AK, Shefer S, Honda A, Honda M, Xu G, Irons M, et al. (1998). Fetal Smith-Lemli-Opitz syndrome can be detected accurately and reliably by measuring amniotic fluid dehydrocholesterols. *Prenat Diagn* 18: 651–658.

Ullrich K, Koch H-G, Meschede D, Flotmann U, Seedorf U (1996). Smith-Lemli-Opitz syndrome: treatment with cholesterol and bile acids. *Neuropediatrics* 27: 111–112.

Van Rooij A, Nijenhuis AA, Wijburg FA, Schutgens RBH (1997). Highly increased CSF concentrations of cholesterol precursors in Smith-Lemli-Opitz syndrome. *J Inherit Metab Dis* 20: 578–580.

Wanders RJA, Romeijn GJ, Wijburg F, Hennekam RCM, De Jong J, Wevers RA, Dacremont G (1997). Smith-Lemli-Opitz syndrome: deficient 7-reductase activity in cultured skin fibroblasts and chorionic villus fibroblasts and its application to pre- and postnatal detection. *J Inherit Metab Dis* 20: 432–436.

Wassif CA, Maslen C, Kachilele-Linjewile S, Lin D, Linck LM, Connor WE, Steiner RD, Porter FD (1998). Mutations in the human sterol Δ7-reductase gene at 11q12-13 cause Smith-Lemli-Opitz sydrome. *Am J Hum Genet* 63: 55–62.

Wassif CA, Zhu P, Kratz L, Krakowiak PA, Battaile KP, Weight FF, Grinberg A, Steiner RD, Nwokoro NA, Kelley RI, et al. (2001). Biochemical, phenotype and neurophysiological characterization of a genetic mouse model of RSH/Smith-Lemli-Opitz syndrome. *Hum Mol Genet* 10: 555–564.

Waterham HR, Wanders RJA (2000). Biochemical and genetic aspects of 7-dehydrocholesterol reductase and Smith-Lemli-Opitz syndrome. *Biochim Biophys Acta* 1529: 340–356.

Waterham HR, Wijburg FA, Hennekam RCM, Vreken P, Poll-The BE, Dorland L, Duran M, Jura PE, Smeitink JAM, Wevers RA, et al. (1998). Smith-Lemli-Opitz syndrome is caused by mutations in the 7-dehydrocholesterol reductase gene. *Am J Hum Genet* 63: 329–338.

Willnow TE, Hilpert J, Armstrong SA, Rohlmann A, Hammer PE, Burns DK, Herz J (1996). Defective forebrain development in mice lacking gp330/megalin. *Proc Natl Acad Sci USA* 93: 8460–8464.

Witsch-Baumgartner M, Fitzky BU, Ogorelkova M, Kraft HG, Moebius FF, Glossmann H, Seedorf U, Gillessen-Kaesbach G, Hoffmann GF, Clayton P, et al. (2000). Mutational spectrum in the Δ7-sterol reductase gene and genotype–phenotype correlation in 84 patients with Smith-Lemli-Opitz syndrome. *Am J Med Genet* 66: 401–412.

Witsch-Baumgarner M, Loffler J, Utermann G (2001). Mutations in the human *DHCR7* gene. *Hum Mutat* 17: 172–182.

Woollett LA (2001). Fetal lipid metabolism. *Front Bio* 6: 536–545.

Xu G, Salen G, Shefer S, Ness GC, Thomas S, Zhao Z, Tint GS (1995). Reproducing abnormal cholesterol biosynthesis as seen in the Smith-Lemli-Opitz syndrome by inhibiting the conversion of 7-dehydrocholesterol to cholesterol in rats. *J Clin Invest* 95: 76–81.

Yu H, Tint GS, Salen G, Patel SB (2000a). Detection of a common mutation in the RSH or Smith-Lemli-Opitz syndrome by a PCR-RFLP assay: IVS8-1G>C is found in over sixty percent of US propositi. *Am J Med Genet* 90: 347–350.

Yu H, Lee M-H, Starck L, Elias ER, Irons M, Salen G, Patel SB, Tint GS (2000b). Spectrum of Δ7-dehydrocholesterol reductase mutations in patients with the Smith-Lemli-Opitz (RSH) syndrome. *Hum Mol Genet* 9:1385–1391.

Zimmerman PA, Hercules DM, Naylor EW (1997). Direct analysis of filter paper blood specimens for identification of Smith-Lemli-Opitz syndrome using time-of-flight secondary ion mass spectrometry. *Am J Med Genet* 68: 300–304.

| *SHH* and Holoprosencephaly

M. MICHAEL COHEN, JR.

Topics covered in this chapter are organized under the following headings: clinical description (definition, central nervous system, and face); epidemiology; etiology; molecular biology (mutations in *SHH*, *ZIC2*, *SIX3*, *TGIF*, *PTCH*, *GLI2*, *FAST1*, *TDGF1*, and *DHCR7*); establishing the diagnosis (diagnosis and recurrence risk, prenatal diagnosis); management; and perspectives: past, present, and future.

CLINICAL DESCRIPTION

Definition

Holoprosencephaly is a developmental field defect of impaired midline cleavage of the embryonic forebrain. In alobar holoprosencephaly, the prosencephalon fails to cleave* sagittally into cerebral hemispheres, transversely into telencephalon and diencephalon, and horizontally into olfactory tracts and bulbs. Although the classic definition is unambiguous, problems are encountered at the less severe end of the phenotypic spectrum. The classic anatomic definition of holoprosencephaly and the variable definitions used in genetics are both valid and depend on the context in which they are used (Cohen, 2001).

Central Nervous System

In *alobar holoprosencephaly*, a small monoventricular cerebrum lacking interhemispheric division is present (Fig. 18–1). The thalami and the corpora striata are undivided across the midline. Olfactory tracts and bulbs are always absent, as is the corpus callosum, although a few commissural fibers may cross the midline (DeMyer, 1977). DeMyer (1977) further subdivided alobar holoprosencephaly, depending on the degree to which the dorsal lip of the holotelencephalon rolls over to cover the membranous ventricular roof. The three common external configurations of alobar holoprosencephaly are the pancake type, the cup type, and the ball type.

In *semilobar holoprosencephaly*, rudimentary cerebral lobes are present and, although the interhemispheric fissure is never complete, it may be present posteriorly. Commonly, the olfactory tracts and bulbs are absent, but in some instances, they may be hypoplastic. The corpora striata are continuous across the midline. The corpus callosum is not a distinct bundle, although some commissural fibers may cross the midline (DeMyer, 1977).

In *lobar holoprosencephaly*, the brain has well-formed lobes, which may be of normal size. Although a distinct interhemispheric fissure is present, there may be some midline continuity of the cingulate gyrus. The olfactory tracts and bulbs may be absent or hypoplastic and the corpus callosum may be absent, hypoplastic, or normal. Midline cleavage of the thalami and the corpora striata may be incomplete (DeMyer, 1977).

At the mild end of the holoprosencephalic spectrum are malformations such as absence of the corpus callosum and *arhinencephaly* (absence of the olfactory tracts and bulbs) (DeMyer, 1977). Defects of the corpus callosum result from a variety of different mechanisms (DeMyer, 1977; Cohen and Sulik, 1992). In some instances, absence of the corpus callosum clearly represents the holoprosencephalic spectrum. In other instances, isolated absence of the corpus callosum is

*Although *cleave* is the commonly used term, no splitting actually occurs. In the sagittal plane, budding of the telencephalic vesicles takes place. In the transverse plane, "cleavage" is an arbitrary designation given to regions. In the horizontal plane, budding of the olfactory tracts takes place (Cohen, 2001).

not related to the holoprosencephalic spectrum (DeMyer, 1977; Cohen, 1989b, 2001; Cohen and Sulik, 1992).

In alobar holoprosencephaly, electroencephalography shows various abnormal waves, ranging from asynchrony between the right and left sides of the head to synchronous and asynchronous spikes. In lobar holoprosencephaly, multifocal spikes are common (DeMyer, 1977).

Patients with alobar holoprosencephaly may be completely amented. However, evidence of vision, hearing, and social smiling has been observed in some cases with median cleft lip, lateral cleft lip, or less severe facial dysmorphism. Length of survival is correlated with facial type. With cyclopia, ethmocephaly, and cebocephaly, 50% may survive for 1–2 days. With median cleft lip, 50% survive for 4–5 months. For infants with less severely malformed or normal faces, 50% may survive as long as 12–18 months. In general, patients with semilobar or lobar holoprosencephaly tend to have better survival rates than patients with alobar holoprosencephaly (Barr and Cohen, 1999). At the less severe end of the holoprosencephalic spectrum, patients may have mild or moderate mental retardation and may have sufficient intelligence to live freely in society (DeMyer, 1977).

Face

In a classic article, DeMyer et al. (1963) discussed a graded series of facial anomalies that occur with holoprosencephaly (Fig. 18–2, Table 18–1). The face predicts the brain approximately 80% of the time. The other 20% of the time, the facial features are nondiagnostic (DeMyer, 1977; Cohen, 1989b). In cyclopia, the most extreme variant, a single median eye with varying degrees of doubling of the intrinsic ocular structures is associated with arhinia and usually with proboscis formation. In ethmocephaly, two separate hypoteloric eyes are associated with arhinia and usually with proboscis formation. In cebocephaly, hypotelorism is associated with a blind-ended, single-nostril nose. With median cleft lip, hypotelorism is associated with a flat nose and a median cleft because of agenesis of the primary palate. Less severe facial dysmorphism may include hypotelorism or hypertelorism, lateral cleft lip, and/or iris coloboma (Cohen and Sulik, 1992). Barr and Cohen (2002) reported essentially normal faces in some autosomal-recessive cases of alobar holoprosencephaly.

A number of minor anomalies have been found with holoprosencephaly (Berry et al., 1984; Cohen and Sulik, 1992; Gurrieri et al., 1993; Aylsworth et al., 1994; Martin et al., 1996; Lo et al., 1998; Martin and Jones, 1998). Single maxillary central incisor (Berry et al., 1984; Cohen, 1989b) and, much less commonly, absence of nasal septal cartilage (Hennekam et al., 1991) can be useful markers in autosomal dominant holoprosencephaly. Other identified defects have included stenosis of the pyriform aperture (Aylsworth et al., 1994; Lo et al., 1998), absence of the labial frenum (Martin and Jones, 1998), and absence of the philtral ridges (Martin et al., 1996).

EPIDEMIOLOGY

Croen and colleagues (1996) found a birth prevalence of 1.2 per 10,000 (*n* = 121). Of all cases, 41% had a chromosomal defect, most commonly trisomy 13. Rasmussen et al. (1996) found an overall birth prevalence of 0.86 per 10,000 (*n* = 63). The rate increased from 0.58 per 10,000 in 1968–1972 to 1.2 per 10,000 in 1988–1992. The frequency of holoprosencephalic abortuses is high, being approximately 40 per 10,000 (Matsunaga and Shiota, 1977). Birth weights tend to be

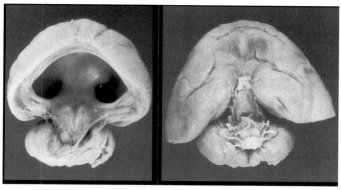

Figure 18–1. Alobar holoprosencephaly resulting from failure of "cleavage" of the embryonic forebrain. (From Pettersen, 1976.)

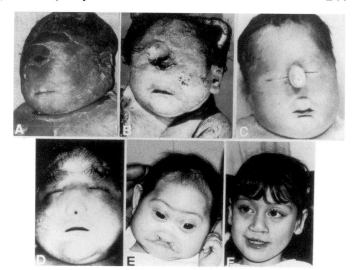

Figure 18–2. Spectrum of dysmorphic faces associated with variable degrees of holoprosencephaly. *A*: Cyclopia without proboscis formation. Note single central eye. *B*: Cyclopia with proboscis. *C*: Ethmocephaly. Ocular hypotelorism with proboscis located between the eyes. *D*: Cebocephaly. Ocular hypotelorism with single-nostril nose. *E*: Median cleft lip, flat nose, and ocular hypotelorism. *F*: Ocular hypotelorism and surgically repaired cleft lip. (*A–D, F* from Cohen et al., 1971, and Cohen, 1982; *E* from DeMyer et al., 1963.)

low, except in holoprosencephalic infants of diabetic mothers. The sex ratio in alobar holoprosencephaly has a 3:1 female predilection. In contrast, the sex ratio is 1:1 in lobar holoprosencephaly. Major facial dysmorphism occurs more frequently in females than in males, particularly with cyclopia (Cohen, 1989a).

ETIOLOGY

Human holoprosencephaly is etiologically heterogeneous and pathogenetically variable. The condition has been reviewed extensively elsewhere (DeMyer et al., 1963, 1964; DeMyer, 1977; Matsunaga and Shiota, 1977; Cohen, 1989a,b; Siebert et al., 1990; Cohen and Sulik, 1992; Croen et al., 1996; Rasmussen et al., 1996; Ming and Muenke, 1998; Roessler and Muenke, 1998; Barr and Cohen, 1999; Wallis and Muenke, 1999; Muenke and Cohen, 2000; Muenke and Beachy, 2001; Cohen, 2002). Identifiable genetic causes in humans account for about 15%–20% of all cases of holoprosencephaly. These are monogenic and chromosomal (Table 18–2). Molecularly defined holoprosencephaly accounts for only a very small percentage of all cases.

Monogenic inheritance of nonsyndromic holoprosencephaly includes autosomal dominant transmission with wide expressivity and incomplete penetrance (Benke and Cohen, 1983; Cohen, 1989a), autosomal recessive transmission (Cohen and Gorlin, 1969; Cohen et al., 1971), and X-linked transmission (Morse et al., 1987; Hockey et al., 1988). Mutations for human holoprosencephaly have been found in a number of genes: *Sonic Hedgehog* (*SHH*) (Roessler et al., 1996, 1997; Nanni et al., 1999), *TGIF* (Gripp et al., 2000), *ZIC2* (Brown et al., 1998, 2001), *SIX3* (Wallis et al., 1999), *Patched* (*PTCH*) (Ming and Muenke, 1998), *GLI2* (Roessler et al., 2002), *TDGF1* (de la Cruz et al., 2002), *FAST1* (Ouspenskaia et al., 2002), and *DHCR7* (Kelley et al., 1996). Known mutated genes, their chromosomal map locations, holoprosencephalic phenotypes, and the frequencies with which they occur are summarized in Table 18–3.

SONIC HEDGEHOG SIGNALING NETWORK AND ORTHOLOGOUS GENES

For a discussion of the sonic hedgehog signaling network and orthologous genes, see Chapter 16.

MOLECULAR BIOLOGY

SHH Mutations

Shh gene expression has been demonstrated in the floorplate of the neural tube. Targeted gene disruption in the mouse produces cyclopia with absence of ventral neural tube cells. The *Shh* mutation is recessive, resulting in a severe phenotype (Chiang et al., 1996). In humans, *SHH* maps to 7q36. In contrast to the mouse, *SHH* mutations are heterozygous and the holoprosencephalic phenotype is more variable (Roessler et al., 1996, 1997; Nanni et al., 1999).

SHH has an N-terminal signaling domain (SHH-N) and a C-terminal catalytic domain (SHH-C) that causes autocleavage of the protein, resulting in an ester-linked cholesterol moiety at the C-terminal end of SHH-N. The autocleavage of SHH proceeds via a thioester intermediate, which undergoes a nucleophilic attack by cholesterol, resulting in a covalently linked cholesterol adduct and activation of the

Table 18–1. Holoprosencephalic Faces

Facial Type*	Main Facial Features	Brain
Cyclopia	Median monophthalmia, synophthalmia, or anophthalmia. Proboscis may be single or absent. Hypognathism in some cases.	Alobar holoprosencephaly
Ethmocephaly	Ocular hypotelorism with proboscis.	Alobar holoprosencephaly
Cebocephaly	Ocular hypotelorism and blind-ended, single-nostril nose.	Usually alobar holoprosencephaly
Median cleft lip	Ocular hypotelorism, flat nose, and median cleft lip.	Usually alobar holoprosencephaly
Less severe facial dysmorphism	Variable features including ocular hypotelorism or hypertelorism, flat nose, unilateral or bilateral cleft lip, iris coloboma, or other anomalies. Minimal facial dysmorphism in some cases.†	Semilobar or lobar holoprosencephaly

*Transitional facial forms are known to occur.
†Autosomal recessive alobar holoprosencephaly with an essentially normal face has been reported (Barr and Cohen, 2002).
Source: Modified after DeMyer et al. (1964).

Table 18–2. Syndromes and Associations with Holoprosencephaly

Chromosomal	Hydrolethalus syndrome
Trisomy 13	Kallmann syndrome
del(13q)	CHARGE syndrome (AD, AR)
Trisomy 18	Hartsfield syndrome
Triploidy	Brachial amelia-facial clefts
dup(3p)	Agnathia-holoprosencephaly (AR?)
Many uncommon types	Agnathia-holoprosencephaly-situs inversus
Monogenic or presumed monogenic	Agnathia-holoprosencephaly (sporadic, 42 cases)
Meckel syndrome (AR)	Teratogenic
Pseudotrisomy 13 syndrome (AR)	Maternal insulin-dependent diabetes mellitus
XK aprosencephaly syndrome (AR)	Alcohol abuse during pregnancy
Aprosencephaly (sporadic)	Retinoic acid embryopathy
Heterotaxy and holoprosencephaly (AR)	Other
Holoprosencephaly-fetal hypokinesia syndrome (XR)	del (22q11) syndrome
Genoa syndrome (AR)	Holoprosencephaly ectopia cordis, and embryonal neoplasms
Martin syndrome (AD)	Associations
Grote syndrome (AR?)	Neural tube defect association
Steinfeld syndrome (AD?)	Frontonasal dysplasia association
Lambotte syndrome (AR)	Caudal dysgenesis association
Pallister-Hall syndrome (AD)	DiGeorge association
Rubinstein-Taybi syndrome	Branchial arch syndrome association

Source: Modified from Cohen (1989a) and Cohen and Sulik (1992).

SHH-N signaling portion. The SHH-C catalytic portion diffuses away (Porter et al., 1996) (Fig. 18–3).

Following the autoprocessing reaction, palmitoylation of the most amino-terminal cysteine of the SHH-N signaling portion takes place, requiring the action of Skinny hedgehog (Ski) acyltransferase (Pepinsky et al., 1998; Chamoun et al., 2001) (Fig. 18–3). The ester-linked cholesterol moiety and the amide-linked palmitate might be expected to anchor the SHH signaling portion to the membranes of the producing cells. However, signaling extends many cells beyond its source, and long-range action of SHH depends on Dispatched (DISP), which releases SHH from the cell membranes (Burke et al., 1999; Ingham and McMahon, 2001; Ma et al., 2002).

SHH mutations of the missense, nonsense, deletion, and frameshift types have been identified in exons 1, 2, and 3 (Nanni et al., 1999; Muenke and Beachy, 2001) (Table 18–4). Nonsense, deletion, and frameshift mutations may truncate SHH-N, altering biological activity or interfering with the autoprocessing reaction by affecting SHH-C (Fig. 18–3). Thus, haploinsufficiency results in holoprosencephaly. Great variability in expression characterizes autosomal dominant *SHH* families, some being minimally affected with holoprosencephalic microforms (*vide supra*) and others being severely affected. No

genotype–phenotype correlations have been found (Nanni et al., 1999; Muenke and Beachy, 2001).

Numerous missense mutations occur throughout the entire coding region of *SHH* (Table 18–4), and their functional significance is more difficult to interpret. If *SHH* mutations involve haploinsufficiency, holoprosencephaly results; but whether missense mutations alone are sufficient to cause holoprosencephaly has been questioned. Roessler et al. (1996) identified two missense mutations in exon 2, involving an invariant amino acid, Trp117 (Table 18–4), that immediately follows the crucial α-helix-1 motif; they suggested that mutations in Trp117 might destabilize SHH-N. It is also possible that other genes in the Shh signaling network or in other developmental pathways might work synergistically with *SHH* missense mutations. At least three patients have been reported with *SHH* mutations together with additional gene mutations: one with a *ZIC2* mutation (*vide infra*) and two with deletions involving *TGIF* (*vide infra*) (Nanni et al., 1999; Gripp et al., 2000).

In mice, double heterozygotes result in holoprosencephaly, whereas single heterozygotes do not (Ming and Muenke, 2002). Animal models of digenic inheritance of holoprosencephaly have been discussed by several authors (Varlet et al., 1997; Nomura and Li, 1998; Song et

Table 18–3. Known Mutated Genes in Holoprosencephaly*

Mutated Genes	Chromosome Map Locations	Holoprosencephalic Phenotypes	Frequencies
SHH	7q36	Great variability (severe to mild)	17% of familial cases, 3.7% of sporadic cases
ZIC2	13q32	Severe brain defect, normal or mildly dysmorphic face	3%–4%
SIX3	2p21	Variable	1.3%
TGIF	18p11.3	Variable	1.5%
PTCH	9q22.3	Variable	Rare (4 cases), *PTCH* mutations common in nevoid basal cell carcinoma syndrome and in isolated basal cell carcinomas
GLI2	2q14	Variable	1.8%
FAST1	8q24.3	Variable	20 missense variants in 100 holoprosencephaly cases and 350 patients with congenital heart defects; 3 mutations were found in both holoprosencephaly and in cardiac defects
TDGF1	3p21-p23	Variable	0.5%
DHCR7	11q12-q13	Holoprosencephalic faces	2%–4% of Smith-Lemli-Opitz syndrome cases

*See text for references.

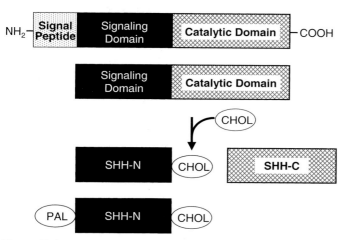

Figure 18–3. *Sonic Hedgehog (SHH)* has an N-terminal signaling domain (SHH-N) and a C-terminal catalytic domain (SHH-C), which causes auto-cleavage of the protein, resulting in an ester-linked cholesterol moiety (CHOL) at the carboxy-terminal end of the signaling portion; the catalytic portion diffuses away. An amide-linked amino-terminal palmitate (PAL) is critical for signaling activity. Following the addition of the carboxy-terminal cholesterol adduct, palmitoylation requires the action of Skinny hedgehog acyltransferase. (From Cohen, 1999, and Cohen and Shiota, 2002.)

al., 1999; Bachiller et al., 2000; Jin et al., 2001; Klingensmith et al., 2001) (Table 18–5).

Some unusual phenotypes have been reported with *SHH* alterations. Nanni et al. (2001) reported an autosomal dominant family with a single maxillary central incisor only, and a novel *SHH* mutation, Ile111Phe, not found in the holoprosencephaly population. Schimmenti et al. (2003) noted a proband and his mother with iris and uve-oretinal colobomas without optic nerve involvement; a novel 24 bp deletion in *SHH* was identified. Watkins et al. (2003) found extensive *SHH* signaling in the respiratory epithelium of a subset of small-cell lung carcinomas.

Table 18–4. *Sonic Hedgehog (SHH)* **Mutations in Holoprosencephaly**

	Nucleotide Change	Amino Acid Change
Exon 1		
	160_161insGCTG	3-4ins
	189_196del	13-15del (frameshift)
	GCG → AGG	Gly31Arg
	GAT → GTT	Asp88Val
	CAG → TAG	Gln100Stop
	CAG → CAC	Gln100His
Exon 2		
	AAG → TAG	Lys105Stop
	AAC → AAA	Asn115Lys
	TGG → GGG	Trp117Gly
	TGG → CGG	Trp117Arg
	TAC → TAG	Tyr158Stop
Exon 3		
	GAG → CAG	Glu188Gln
	CAG → TAG	Gln209Stop
	GAC → AAC	Asp222Asn
	GTG → GAG	Val224Glu
	GCG → ACG	Ala226Thr
	AGC → AGA	Ser236Arg
	GAG → TAG	Glu256Stop
	939_959del	263-269del
	GAG → TAG	Glu284Stop
	GGC → GAC	Gly290Asp
	1283_1291del	378-380del
	GCG → ACG	Ala284Thr
	1361_1375del	404-408del
	CCG → GCG	Pro424Ala
	TCG → TTG	Ser436Leu

Source: Adapted from Nanni et al. (1999).

Table 18–5. **Animal Models of Digenic Inheritance of Holoprosencephaly**

Nodal$^{+/-}$ + *HNF3b$^{+/-}$*
Otx2$^{+/-}$ + *HNF3b$^{+/-}$*
Smad2$^{+/-}$ + *Nodal$^{+/-}$*
ActRIIA$^{-/-}$ + *Nodal$^{+/-}$*
Noggin$^{+/-}$ + *Chordin$^{-/-}$*
Noggin$^{-/-}$ + *Chordin$^{-/-}$*

Source: Adapted from Varlet et al. (1997), Nomura and Li (1998), Song et al. (1999), Bachiller et al. (2000), Jin et al. (2001), Klingensmith et al. (2001).

ZIC2 Mutations

ZIC2, which maps to 13q32, is a homologue of the *Drosophila odd-paired (opa)* gene (Aruga et al., 1996) and the zebrafish *odd-paired-like (opl)* gene. The *Zic* gene family consists of zinc finger proteins bearing some similarity to the Gli proteins (Grinblat et al., 1998). Zic2 is expressed in the neuroepithelium (Foley et al., 1997). Muenke et al. (2002) reported the clinical and neuroradiological findings and suggested that ZIC2 is expressed in the dorsal neural tube, in contrast to SHH, which is expressed in the ventral neural tube.

In humans, heterozygous *ZIC2* mutations cause holoprosencephaly either (*1*) by small insertions or deletions, leading to frameshifts and premature stop codons, thus truncating the protein, or (*2*) by alanine tract expansion (Brown et al., 1998, 2001; Muenke et al., 2002; Dubourg et al., 2002). Brown et al. (2002a) observed that many mutations occurred in the carboxy terminus outside the DNA-binding domain, including some patients with identical expansions of a carboxy-terminal alanine tract. In these instances, DNA-binding is normal, suggesting that the transactivating function of the ZIC2 protein is interrupted and that protein–protein interactions are critical for normal activity.

Most patients have alobar or semilobar holoprosencephaly, but lobar holoprosencephaly and syntelencephaly have been noted on occasion (Brown et al., 2001; Muenke et al., 2002). Before *ZIC2* was identified and mapped to 13q32, Cohen (1982) observed that when patients with holoprosencephaly had del(13q), facial dysmorphism was mild. Brown et al. (2001) and Muenke et al. (2002) studied 28 patients with *ZIC2* mutations and found no instance of cyclopia, ethmocephaly, cebocephaly, or median cleft lip but, rather, a normal or mildly dysmorphic face. Children with *ZIC2* mutations live longer than children with *SHH* mutations, who also have the same severe holoprosencephaly but often with severe facial dysmorphism (Muenke et al., 2002).

Muenke et al. (2002) found that two of 19 families with *ZIC2* mutations had three pregnancies resulting in anencephaly. Targeted *Zic2* mutations in mice can produce neural tube defects as well as holoprosencephaly (Nagai et al., 2000). Brown et al. (2002b) found no *ZIC2* mutations in human neural tube defects but suggested a possible association with a polyhistidine tract polymorphism in the *ZIC2* gene.

SIX3 Mutations

The *so/SIX* family of transcription factors consists of a distantly related group of homeobox-containing genes characterized by the presence of a SIX domain (contiguous homology domain), which is thought to participate in transcriptional activation (Kawakami et al., 1996). *Six3* genes participate in midline forebrain development and in formation of the eye in several species (Oliver et al., 1996, 1999; Kobayashi et al., 1998; Loosli et al., 1999). Human *SIX3* maps to 2p21 (Schell et al., 1996; Wallis et al., 1999).

Wallis et al. (1999) identified four heterozygous mutations in the homeodomain of *SIX3*, including three missense mutations and one 9 bp deletion. Dubourg et al. (2002) reported five mutations.

TGIF Mutations

TG-Interacting Factor (TGIF), which maps to 18p11.3, modulates TGFβ components that cause holoprosencephaly in animals. TGIF is an atypical homeodomain protein that is localized in the nucleus (Wallis and Muenke, 1999; Muenke and Cohen, 2000; Muenke and Beachy, 2001). TGIF acts as a corepressor of SMAD2 by forming a complex with SMAD2/SMAD4 and recruiting histone deacetylases to the complex (Wotton et al., 1999). TGIF can also bind to the RXR binding site of the cellular retinol-binding protein II promotor (CRBPII RXRE) (Bertolino et al., 1995), but TGIF and RXR compete for binding to the promotor element (Bertolino et al., 1996). Thus, TGIF can repress retinoic acid–regulated gene transcription. *TGIF* mutations may produce loss of function as a repressor, resulting in overactivity of retinoic acid–regulated genes, simulating the effect of excessive retinoic acid exposure in humans (Lammer et al., 1985) and in mice (Webster et al., 1986; Sulik et al., 1988, 1995). Helms et al. (1994, 1997) demonstrated an interrelationship between the Shh and retinoic acid pathways in the chick.

To date, at least six heterozygous missense mutations in *TGIF* have been identified in human holoprosencephaly (Gripp et al., 2000; Dubourg et al., 2002; Herbergs et al., 2002). The mutation reported by Herbergs et al. (2002) was also found in one parent who had hypotelorism and microcephaly.

PTCH Mutations

Ptch is part of the Shh signaling network. Helms et al. (1997) demonstrated that retinoic acid inhibited Shh and Ptch expression in the craniofacial primordia of chick embryos; the polarizing activity in these tissues was abolished. These findings are of particular interest because human mutations in both *SHH* (Roessler et al., 1996, 1997; Nanni et al., 1999) and *PTCH* (Ming et al., 1998) have been shown to cause holoprosencephaly.

PTCH, which maps to 9q22.3, is a 12-pass transmembrane protein for which SHH is the ligand. Mutations in *PTCH* have been identified in patients with nevoid basal cell carcinoma syndrome, isolated basal cell carcinoma, medulloblastoma, meningioma, neuroectodermal tumor, breast carcinoma, esophageal squamous cell carcinoma, and trichoepithelioma (Cohen, 1999). Most mutations have resulted in protein truncation. However, four rare *PTCH* missense mutations have resulted in holoprosencephaly, two in extracellular loops that may be required for SHH binding and two in intracellular loops that may be involved in PTCH-SMO interaction (Ming et al., 2002).

GLI2 Mutations

GLI2, which maps to 2q14 (Matsumoto et al., 1996), is part of the Shh signaling network. Transgenic mice overexpressing Gli2 in cutaneous keratinocytes develop multiple basal cell carcinomas (Grachtchouk et al., 2000). Roessler et al. (2002) studied 390 familial and sporadic cases of holoprosencephaly. They identified seven sequence variations in *GLI2*. Functional studies showed four mutations with loss of function. Two mutations truncated the zinc finger domain. Another mutation was in the invariant splice donor consensus sequence. A frameshift mutation was found segregating in a large pedigree associated with panhypopituitarism.

FAST1 Mutations

The *FAST1* (*Forkhead Activin Signal Transducer 1*) gene, which maps to 8q24.3 (Zhou et al., 1998), encodes a transcription factor that complexes with SMAD2 and SMAD4, mediating the TGFβ, Activin, and Nodal pathways. Ouspenskaia et al. (2002) screened 100 patients with familial holoprosencephaly and 350 patients with congenital heart defects. They identified missense mutations, two deletions, and one 13 bp insertion. Several mutations were found with holoprosencephaly and with congenital heart defects. Thus, *FAST1* is the first human gene with mutations causing both midline defects (holoprosencephaly) and lateral defects (anomalies of cardiac looping) (Ouspenskaia et al., 2002).

TDGF1 Mutations

TDGF1 (*Teratocarcinoma-Derived Growth Factor 1*) (*CRIPTO*), an EGF-CFC family member, maps to 3p21-p23 (Ciccodicola et al., 1989; Saccone et al., 1995). In mice, Tdgf1 is essential for germ layer formation, positioning of the anterior-posterior axis, and neural patterning (Shen and Schier, 2000). EGF-CFC proteins are cofactors in Nodal signaling. They are membrane-associated, glycosylated, and have a characteristic epidermal growth factor (EGF)-like motif and a cysteine-rich (CFC) domain (Shen and Schier, 2000). de la Cruz et al. (2002) screened 83 familial and 327 sporadic cases of holoprosencephaly. They identified two loss-of-function mutations in the CFC domain of *TDGF1*. One patient had semilobar holoprosencephaly and median orofacial clefting; the other had a dysplastic forebrain, hypoplastic corpus callosum, and absent septum pellucidum.

DHCR7 Mutations

Holoprosencephaly can be caused by perturbations in cholesterol biosynthesis, including human *DHCR7* (sterol Δ^7-reductase) mutations and animal teratogens AY9944, BM15.766, and triparanol. Theoretically, perturbations in cholesterol homeostasis may result from a defect in normal Shh cholesterol autoprocessing or from interference with the ability of target tissues to sense or transduce the Shh signal. Experimental evidence supports the latter hypothesis (Beachy et al., 1997; Cooper et al., 1998).

In the autosomal recessively inherited Smith-Lemli-Opitz syndrome, *DHCR7* maps to 11q12-q13 (Moebius et al., 1998) and various mutations have been identified (Wassif et al., 1998; Yu et al., 2000; Witsch-Baumgartner et al., 2000; Waterham et al., 2001). These result in accumulation of 7-dehydrocholesterol and reduced serum and tissue cholesterol. Although increased 7-dehydrocholesterol levels enable definitive diagnosis of Smith-Lemli-Opitz syndrome, the clinical severity best correlates inversely with the level of cholesterol or with the level of cholesterol as a fraction of total sterols (Cunniff et al., 1997). About 2%–4% of Smith-Lemli-Opitz syndrome cases are associated with holoprosencephaly (Kelley et al., 1996). Incomplete penetrance of holoprosencephaly may possibly be explained by supplementation via placental exchange from heterozygous mothers with essentially normal sterol metabolism (Muenke and Beachy, 2001).

ESTABLISHING THE DIAGNOSIS

Diagnosis and Recurrence Risk

Diagnosis is based on the overall pattern of anomalies, chromosome analysis, molecular studies in selected cases, and family history. Careful examination of the proband's family for microforms of holoprosencephaly is essential, especially for anosmia or hyposmia, mild hypotelorism, microcephaly, or single maxillary central incisor (Cohen and Sulik, 1992). A family history of short stature, endocrinopathy (particularly hypopituitarism and diabetes mellitus), or CNS anomalies other than holoprosencephaly may be significant (Cohen, 1989b; Cohen and Sulik, 1992).

For nonsyndromic cases, if the findings are consistent with autosomal dominant holoprosencephaly and the family is negative for *SHH* mutations, the risk for an obligate carrier is on the order of 16%–21%; the risk for an incomplete form or microform is on the order of 13%–14%; and the overall effect for some risk, either mild or severe, is on the order of 29%–35% (Cohen, 1989a). Affected sibs in the absence of familial microforms in more than one generation are consistent with autosomal recessive inheritance (Cohen, 1989a). A sporadic case with negative family history except for consanguinity certainly suggests that the recurrence risk may be as high as 25% (Cohen, 1989a). For sporadic, nonchromosomal, nonsyndromic holoprosencephaly, a recurrence risk of approximately 6% may be given. This risk is based on the genetic study of Roach et al. (1975) of 30 families with holoprosencephalic probands; only two of their pedigrees represented examples of familial holoprosencephaly. Mutations in several genes have been identified as causative of holoprosencephaly (*vide supra*). The best known of these is *SHH* (Roessler et al., 1996, 1997; Nanni et al., 1999). Mutations occur in 17% of familial cases and 3.7% of sporadic cases. *ZIC2* mutations occur in 3%–4% of all cases of holoprosencephaly. The frequencies of other genes causing holoprosencephaly are summarized in Table 18–3; they may occur sporadically, but familial instances have been noted.

The causes of most cases of holoprosencephaly remain unknown. Most instances are not associated with chromosomal aberrations and do not represent monogenic syndromes. For diagnostic purposes, severe facial dysmorphism accompanying holoprosencephaly is obvious. However, in some instances, involvement may be mild. MRI characteristics of holoprosencephaly are summarized in Table 18–6. Since holoprosencephaly with facial dysmorphism is frequently part of a broader pattern of anomalies, a careful search for extracephalic and internal anomalies should be done. Because 41% of all sporadic cases are associated with chromosomal anomalies, high-resolution banding should be routine.

Table 18–6. MRI Characteristics of Holoprosencephaly

Alobar type
  Complete absence of interhemispheric fissure and falx cerebri
  Holoprosencephalon (often shield-shaped)
  Absence of corpus callosum
  Horseshoe-shaped supratentorial monoventricle
  Absence of third ventricle
  Absence of superior sagittal, inferior sagittal, and straight sinuses; absent internal cerebral veins
  Increased frequency of azygous anterior cerebral arteries with hypoplastic middle cerebral arteries
Semilobar type
  Partial formation of posterior interhemispheric fissure, falx cerebri, and associated dural sinuses
  Absent or rudimentary corpus callosum
  Partial differentiation of ventricle into temporo-occipital horns
  Rudimentary third ventricle
  Variable, minimal development of deep veins
Lobar type
  Nearly complete interhemispheric fissure; falx cerebri may be shallow anteriorly
  Partial fusion of frontal lobes with direct continuity of gray and white matter across midline
  Well-formed occipital and temporal horns with narrow bodies of lateral ventricles
  Squared-off, fused frontal horns with absent septum pellucidum

Source: Naidich and Zimmerman (1987).

When holoprosencephaly occurs with severe facial dysmorphism and associated anomalies, the condition is likely to be chromosomal. The only known monogenic syndrome with severe facial dysmorphism together with associated anomalies is the Meckel syndrome (Fig. 18–4). When face–brain dysmorphism is relatively mild, the condition is likely to be monogenic, except for del(13q) syndrome (Cohen and Sulik, 1992). With *ZIC2* mutations (13q32), the facial phenotype is normal or mildly dysmorphic, despite alobar holoprosencephaly (Brown et al., 2001).

Prenatal Diagnosis

Prenatal diagnosis is possible in families with *SHH* and familial instances of other mutated genes (Table 18–3). Molecularly undefined monogenic forms of holoprosencephaly, both nonsyndromic and syndromic (Table 18–2), may permit prenatal diagnosis. Ultrasonic detection of holoprosencephaly is based on measurable parameters, including microcephaly, occasional hydrocephalus, absent midline echo at the level of the cerebral hemispheres due to absence of the falx cerebri and interhemispheric fissure, and orbital hypotelorism. Absence of midline echo is not pathognomonic for holoprosencephaly and may also occur with hydranencephaly or a large porencephalic cyst. For proper prenatal identification of holoprosencephaly, both or-

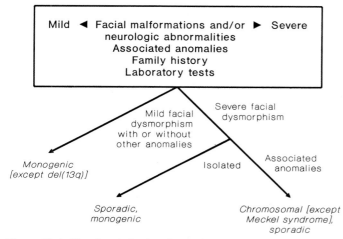

Figure 18–4. Flowchart indicating diagnostic considerations in holoprosencephaly. (From Cohen and Sulik, 1992.)

bital hypotelorism and absence of midline echo must be observed. It should also be recognized that some diagnoses will be missed even with such strict criteria because autosomal recessive alobar holoprosencephaly is found on occasion with an essentially normal face. Furthermore, pathologic changes in lobar and semilobar holoprosencephaly may be too subtle to detect by prenatal ultrasound (Chervenak et al., 1984; Cohen and Sulik, 1992).

If holoprosencephaly is detected by prenatal ultrasound examination, an amniocentesis should be carried out to determine the fetal karyotype; 41% of infants with holoprosencephaly have chromosomal anomalies.

MANAGEMENT

It has been stated repeatedly that holoprosencephaly is lethal and that affected infants will die soon after birth. *This is not always true, and families should be properly counseled. For those who survive, management becomes very important* (Table 18–7).

Virtually all newborns with cyclopia, ethmocephaly, and cebocephaly die within a week of birth. Those with alobar holoprosencephaly and median cleft lip, unilateral cleft lip, bilateral cleft lip, or a more normal face may die before the age of 4–5 months. However, 20%–30% will live for at least 1 year, and survival to at least 8 years

Table 18–7. Survival, Performance, and Management

Neurological
  Seizures (anticonvulsant medications); hypertonicity; unlike some other disorders, there is not a strong tendency to develop joint contractures; when hydrocephalus is markedly excessive, shunting may be necessary
Fluid balance
  Diabetes insipidis (hormone replacement therapy)
Behavioral
  Fluctuations between calmness and irritability (holding, cuddling); day–night confusion (TV or radio as background noise day and night; does not interfere with child's sleep and allows parents to sleep)
Feeding
  Major problems with choking spells, gagging, spitting up, or vomiting (gastrostomy); may have gastroesophageal reflux with risk of aspiration pneumonia (fundoplication accompanying gastrostomy); with clefting of the lip, surgical repair may make feeding easier
Intestinal gas
  Excessive swallowing (careful burping during feeding; gentle stomach massage; medications to decrease peristalsis and/or promote stomach emptying)
Elimination
  Constipation is common, particularly in those with spasticity (altered diet; rectal suppositories; sometimes more rigorous bowel emptying programs)
Growth
  Delay is common even with optimal feeding
Hearing
  Reaction to noise and voices in predictable ways
Vision
  If the eyes are not involved by malformation, children can see, focus on nearby objects, track moving objects, and respond to facial expression
Memory
  Can learn and remember; can anticipate games that involve touching and tickling and can recognize familiar voices and sounds
Language
  May use particular sounds to indicate particular reactions or needs
Voice
  High-pitched; less often hoarse or "barking"
Motor skills
  Minimal
Respiration
  Irregular breathing with alternating rapid and slow breathing; respiratory infection may be life-threatening
Heart rate
  Often irregular; marked and persistent irregularity may presage impending death
Temperature
  Often erratic; elevated temperatures may occur in the absence of infection (when infection has been excluded, no treatment is necessary)

Source: Adapted from Barr and Cohen (1997, 1999).

has been reported. For children with less severe forms of holoprosencephaly, survival is generally longer and life well into adulthood is not uncommon (Barr and Cohen, 1997, 1999) (Table 18–7).

PERSPECTIVES: PAST, PRESENT, AND FUTURE

Chromosomal anomalies associated with holoprosencephaly have been reviewed by Cohen and Sulik (1992), and there are many. The more common ones include trisomy 13 and del(13q). Less commonly associated are trisomy 18 and triploidy (Table 18–2). Some chromosomal deletions, such as del(2q), del(3p), del(7q), del(8q), del(9q), del(13q32), and del(18p), are now known to harbor specific genes for holoprosencephaly (Table 18–3). Cohen and Sulik (1992) noted other chromosomal anomalies associated with holoprosencephaly on occasion, involving chromosomes 1, 5, 6, 14, 20, and 21. Roessler and Muenke (1998) reviewed holoprosencephaly loci and suggested some candidate genes, including 21q22.3 (*Lanosterol Synthase*?) (Muenke et al., 1995), 14q13 (*Thyroid Transcription Factor1*?) (*TTF1*?) (Chen et al., 1997), and 20p13 (*SNAP-25*?) (Roessler and Muenke, 1998). Ma et al. (2002) suggested *DISPA,* which maps to 1q42-qter, as a candidate gene for holoprosencephaly; *DispA*$^{-/-}$ is known to cause holoprosencephaly in mice. No candidate genes have been suggested for 5p or 6q26-qter (Norman et al., 1995).

Translocation breakpoints in 7q36 do not disrupt the *SHH* gene but occur outside the coding region (Belloni et al., 1996; Roessler et al., 1997). Also, balanced translocations and inversions involving 2p21 do not disrupt the *SIX3* gene but occur outside the coding region (Schell et al., 1996; Muenke and Beachy, 2001). These may affect the regulatory elements acting in *cis* on the expression of the gene such as the promoter or enhancer/silencer, or they may affect the local heterochromatin configuration or locus control regions, thus altering expression (Ming and Muenke, 1998; Muenke and Beachy, 2001). Such position effects have been reported for other genes in human disorders, including, among others, *SOX9* (Foster et al., 1994), *PAX6* (Fantes et al., 1995), *TBX5* (Li et al., 1997), and *GLI3* (Vortkamp et al., 1991).

Many animal models for holoprosencephaly are known, and these have been reviewed by Muenke and Beachy (2001) and Cohen and Shiota (2002). Candidate genes are based on important factors in the developing forebrain and in the dorsal-ventral patterning of the forebrain. These genes include, among others, *Dickkopf-1* (*dkk-1*), *HFN3β*, *cerberus* (*cer*), *floating head* (*flh*), *masterblind* (*mbl*), *bozozok* (*boz*), and genes involved in cholesterol biosynthesis (Muenke and Beachy, 2001).

In conclusion, candidate genes for holoprosencephaly should exhibit one or more of the following criteria: (*1*) genes that map to minimal critical regions of chromosomes associated with holoprosencephaly; (*2*) altered genes that cause holoprosencephaly in animals; (*3*) genes in the signaling pathways of SHH, retinoic acid, and Nodal/TGFβ; (*4*) components involved in the transcriptional regulation of opa/ZIC2, so/SIX3, and others; (*5*) genes involved in cholesterol biosynthesis; and (*6*) factors of importance in dorsal-ventral patterning of the forebrain (Muenke and Beachy, 2001).

REFERENCES

Aruga J, Nagai T, Tokuyama T, Hayashizaki Y, Okazaki Y, Chapman VM, Mikoshiba K (1996). The mouse zic gene family. Homologues of the *Drosophila* pair-rule gene *odd-paired*. *J Biol Chem* 271: 1043–1047.

Aylsworth AS, Hicks RPB, Drake AF (1994). Support for the hypothesis that congenital nasal pyriform aperture stenosis (CNPAS) is a phenotype at the mild end of the holoprosencephaly spectrum. 15th David W. Smith Workshop of Malformations and Morphogenesis, Tampa, FL, August 4–9.

Bachiller D, Klingensmith J, Kemp C, Belo JA, Anderson RM, May SR, McMahon JA, McMahon AP, Harland RM, Rossant J, De Robertis EM (2000). The organizer factors Chordin and Noggin are required for mouse forebrain development. *Nature* 403: 658–661.

Barr M Jr, Cohen MM Jr (1997). Holoprosencephaly—Information for Parents, Unpublished Brochure.

Barr M Jr, Cohen MM Jr (1999). Holoprosencephaly survival and performance. *Am J Med Genet* 89: 116–120.

Barr M Jr, Cohen MM Jr (2002). Autosomal recessive alobar holoprosencephaly with essentially normal faces. *Am J Med Genet* 112: 28–30.

Beachy PA, Cooper MK, Young KE, von Kessler DP, Park W-J, Tanaka Hall TM, Leahy DJ, Porter JA (1997). Multiple roles of cholesterol in hedgehog protein biogenesis and signaling. *Cold Spring Harb Symp Quant Biol* LXII: 191–204.

Belloni E, Muenke M, Roessler E, Traverso G, Siegel-Bartelt J, Frumkin A, Mitchell HF (1996). Identification of *Sonic Hedgehog* as a candidate gene responsible for holoprosencephaly. *Nat Genet* 14: 353.

Benke PJ, Cohen MM Jr (1983). Recurrence of holoprosencephaly in families with a positive history. *Clin Genet* 24: 324–328.

Berry SA, Pierpont ME, Gorlin RJ (1984). Single central incisor in familial holoprosencephaly. *J Pediatr* 104: 877–880.

Bertolino E, Reimund B, Wildt-Perinic D, Clerc RG (1995). A novel homeobox protein which recognizes a TGT core and functionally interferes with a retinoid-responsive motif. *J Biol Chem* 270: 31178–31188.

Bertolino E, Wildt S, Richards G, Clerc RG (1996). Expression of a novel murine homeobox gene in the developing cerebellar granular layer during its proliferation. *Dev Dyn* 205: 410–420.

Brown SA, Warburton D, Brown LY, Yu C-Y, Roeder ER, Stengel-Rutkowski S, Hennekam RCM, Muenke M (1998). Holoprosencephaly due to mutations in *ZIC2*, a homologue of *Drosophila odd-paired*. *Nat Genet* 20: 180–183.

Brown LY, Odent S, David V, Blayau M, Dubourg C, Apacik C, Delgado MA, Hall BD, Reynolds JF, Sommer A, et al. (2001). Holoprosencephaly due to mutations in *ZIC2*: alanine tract expansion mutations may be caused by parental somatic recombination. *Hum Mol Genet* 10: 791–796.

Brown SA, Abiginia M, Brown LY (2002a). In-vitro analysis of *Zic2* mutations indicates that holoprosencephaly results from a loss of transactivating function. American Society of Human Genetics 52nd Annual Meeting, Baltimore, MD, October 15–19, p. 166. Abstract nr. 15.

Brown LY, Hodge SE, Johnson WG, Guy SG, Nye JS, Brown S (2002b). Possible association of NTDs with a polyhistidine tract polymorphism in the *ZIC2* gene. *Am J Med Genet* 108: 128–131.

Burke R, Nellen D, Bellotto M, Hafen E, Senti K-A, Dickson BJ, Basler K (1999). Dispatched, a novel sterol-sensing domain protein dedicated to the release of cholesterol-modified hedgehog from signaling cells. *Cell* 99: 803–815.

Chamoun Z, Mann RK, Nellen D, von Kessler DP, Bellotto M, Beachy PA, Basler K (2001). Skinny hedgehog, an acetyltransferase required for palmitoylation and activity of hedgehog signal. *Science* 293: 2080–2084.

Chen C-P, Lee C-C, Chuang C-Y, Jan S-W (1997). Prenatal diagnosis of de novo proximal interstitial deletion of 14q associated with cebocephaly. *J Med Genet* 34: 777–778.

Chervenak FA, Isaacson G, Mahoney JF, Tortora M, Mesologites T, Hobbins JC (1984). The obstetric significance of holoprosencephaly. *Obstet Gynecol* 63: 115–121.

Chiang C, Litingung Y, Lee E, Young KE, Corden JE, Westphal H, Beachy PA (1996). Cyclopia and defective axial patterning in mice lacking *sonic hedgehog* gene function. *Nature* 383: 407–413.

Ciccodicola A, Dono R, Obici S, Simeone A, Zollo M, Persico MG (1989). Molecular characterization of a gene of the "EGF family" expressed in undifferentiated human NTERA2 teratocarcinoma cells. *EMBO J* 8: 1987–1991.

Cohen MM Jr (1982). *The Child with Multiple Birth Defects*. Raven Press, New York.

Cohen MM Jr (1982). An update on the holoprosencephalic disorders. *J Pediatr* 101: 865–869.

Cohen MM Jr (1989a). Perspectives on holoprosencephaly. Part I. Epidemiology, genetics, and syndromology. *Teratology* 40: 211–235.

Cohen MM Jr (1989b). Perspectives on holoprosencephaly. Part III. Spectra, distinctions, continuities, and discontinuities. *Am J Med Genet* 34: 271–288.

Cohen MM Jr (1999). Nevoid basal cell carcinoma syndrome: molecular biology and new hypothesis. *Int J Oral Maxillofac Surg* 28: 216–223.

Cohen MM Jr (2001). On the definition of holoprosencephaly. *Am J Med Genet* 103: 183–187.

Cohen MM Jr (2002). Craniofacial disorders. In: *Emery and Rimoin's Principles and Practice of Medical Genetics, 4th Edition*, Volume 3. Rimoin DL, Connor JM, Pyeritz RE, Korf BR (eds.) Churchill Livingstone, London, pp. 3689–3727.

Cohen MM Jr, Gorlin RJ (1969). Genetic considerations in a sibship of cyclopia and clefts. *Birth Defects* 5(2): 113–118.

Cohen MM Jr, Shiota K (2002). Teratogenesis of holoprosencephaly. *Am J Med Genet* 109: 1–15.

Cohen MM Jr, Sulik KK (1992). Perspectives on holoprosencephaly. Part II. Central nervous system, craniofacial anatomy, syndrome commentary, diagnostic approach, and experimental studies. *J Craniofac Genet Dev Biol* 12: 196–244.

Cohen MM Jr, Jirásek JE, Guzman RT, Gorlin RJ, Peterson MQ (1971). Holoprosencephaly and facial dysmorphia: nosology, etiology and pathogenesis. *Birth Defects* 7(7): 125–135.

Cooper MK, Porter JA, Young KE, Beachy PA (1998). Teratogen-mediated inhibition of target tissue responses to Shh signaling. *Science* 280: 1603–1607.

Croen LA, Shaw GM, Lammer EJ (1996). Holoprosencephaly: epidemiologic and clinical characteristics of a California population. *Am J Med Genet* 64: 465–472.

Cunniff C, Kratz LE, Moser A, Natowicz MR, Kelley RI (1997). Clinical and biochemical spectrum of patients with RSH/Smith-Lemli-Opitz syndrome and abnormal cholesterol metabolism. *Am J Med Genet* 68: 263–269.

de la Cruz JM, Bamford RN, Burdine RD, Roessler E, Barkovich AJ, Donnai D, Schier AF, Muenke M (2002). A loss-of-function mutation in the CFC domain of *TDGF1* is associated with human forebrain defects. *Hum Genet* 110: 422–428.

DeMyer WE (1977). Holoprosencephaly (cyclopia-arhinencephaly). In: *Handbook of Clinical Neurology*. Vinken PJ, Bruyn GW, (eds.) North-Holland Publishing Company, North-Holland, Amsterdam, pp. 431–478.

DeMyer WE, Zeman W, Palmer CG (1963). Familial holoprosencephaly (arhinencephaly) with median cleft lip palate. *Neurology* 13: 913–918.

DeMyer WE, Zeman W, Palmer CG (1964). The face predicts the brain: diagnostic significance of median facial anomalies for holoprosencephaly (arhinencephaly). *Pediatrics* 34: 256–263.

Dubourg C, Pasquier L, Blayau M, Lazaro L, Durou MR, Aguilella C, Odent S, David V

(2002). Holoprosencephaly: mutational screening and functional analysis of human *SHH* missense variants. *American Society of Human Genetics 52nd Annual Meeting*, Baltimore, MD, October 15–19, p. 516. Abstract Nr. 2020.

Fantes J, Redecker B, Breen M, Boyle S, Brown J, Fletcher J, Jones S, Bickmore W, Fukushima Y, Mannens M, et al. (1995). Aniridia-associated cytogenetic rearrangements suggest that a position effect may cause the mutant phenotype. *Hum Mol Genet* 4: 415–422.

Foley AC, Storey KG, Stern CD (1997). The prechordal region lacks neural inducing ability, but can confer anterior character to more posterior neuroepithelium. *Development* 124: 2983.

Foster JW, Dominguez-Steglich MA, Guioli S, Kwok C, Weller PA, Stevanovic M, Weissenbach J, Mansour S, Young ID, Goodfellow PN, et al. (1994). Campomelic dysplasia and autosomal sex reversal caused by mutations in an *SRY*-related gene. *Nature* 372: 525–530.

Grachtchouk M, Mo R, Yu S, Zhang X, Sasaki H, Hui C, Dlugosz AA (2000). Basal cell carcinomas in mice overexpressing Gli2 in skin. *Nat Genet* 24: 216–217.

Grinblat Y, Gamse J, Patel M, Sive H (1998). Determination of the zebrafish forebrain: induction and patterning. *Development* 125: 4403.

Gripp KW, Wotton D, Edwards MC, Roessler E, Adès L, Meinecke P, Richieri-Costa A, Zackai EH, Massagué J, Muenke M (2000). Mutations in *TGIF* cause holoprosencephaly and link NODAL signalling to human neural axis determination. *Nat Genet* 25: 205–208.

Gurrieri F, Trask BJ, van den Engh G (1993). Physical mapping of the holoprosencephaly critical region on chromosome 7q36. *Nat Genet* 3: 247–251.

Helms JA, Thaller C, Eichele G (1994). Relationship between retinoic acid and sonic hedgehog, two polarizing signals in the chick wing bud. *Development* 120: 3267–3274.

Helms JA, Kim CH, Hu D (1997). Sonic hedgehog participates in craniofacial morphogenesis and is down-regulated by teratogenic doses of retinoic acid. *Dev Biol* 187: 25–35.

Hennekam RCM, Van Noort G, de la Fuente FA (1991). Agenesis of the nasal septal cartilage: another sign in autosomal dominant holoprosencephaly. *Am J Med Genet* 39: 121–122.

Herbergs J, Moerland HW, Van der Smagt JJ, Mancini GMS, Van Haelst M, Smeets HJM (2002). Mutations in the *TGIF* gene and *SIX3* gene in patients with holoprosencephaly. *American Society of Human Genetics 52nd Annual Meeting*, Baltimore, MD, October 15–19, p. 518. Abstract Nr. 2040.

Hockey A, Crowhurst J, Cullity G (1988). Microcephaly, holoprosencephaly, hypokinesia—second report of a new syndrome. *Prenat Diagn* 8: 683–686.

Ingham PW, McMahon AP (2001). Hedgehog signaling in animal development: paradigms and principles. *Genes Dev* 15: 3059–3087.

Jin O, Harpal K, Ang SL, Rossant J (2001). Otx2 and HNF3β genetically interact in anterior patterning. *Int J Dev Biol* 45: 357–365.

Kawakami K, Ohto H, Takizawa T, Saito T (1996). Identification and expression of *Six* family genes in mouse retina. *FEBS Lett* 393: 259.

Kelley RI, Roessler E, Hennekam RCM, Feldman GL, Kosaki K, Jones MC, Palumbos JC, Muenke M (1996). Holoprosencephaly in RSH/Smith-Lemli-Opitz syndrome: does abnormal cholesterol metabolism effect the function of *Sonic Hedgehog*? *Am J Med Genet* 66: 478–484.

Klingensmith J, Stottmann R, Nordgren A, Anderson R (2001). The mouse organizer and its secreted factors Chordin and Noggin are unnecessary for anterior-posterior axis formation but are required for head development. *Dev Biol* 235: 283.

Kobayashi M, Toyama R, Takada H, Dawid IB, Kawakami K (1998). Overexpression of the forebrain-specific homeobox gene *Six3* induces rostral forebrain enlargement in zebrafish. *Development* 125: 2973.

Lammer E, Chen D, Hoar R, Agnish N, Benke P, Braun J, Curry C, Fernhoff P, Grix A, Lott I, et al. (1985). Retinoic acid embryopathy. *N Engl J Med* 313: 837–841.

Li Q-Y, Newbury-Ecob RA, Terett JA, Wilson DI, Curtis ARJ, Yi C-H, Gebuhr T, Bullen PI, Robson SC, Strachan T, et al. (1997). Holt-Oram syndrome is caused by mutations in *TBX5*, a member of the *Brachyury (T)* gene family. *Nat Genet* 15: 21–29.

Lo FS, Lee YJ, Lin SP, Shen EY, Huang JK, Lee KS (1998). Solitary maxillary central incisor and congenital nasal pyriform aperture stenosis. *Eur J Pediatr* 157: 39.

Loosli F, Winkler S, Wittbrodt J (1999). Six3 overexpression initiates the formation of ectopic retina. *Genes Dev* 13: 649.

Ma Y, Erkner A, Gong R, Yao S, Taipale J, Basler K, Beachy PA (2002). Hedgehog-mediated patterning of the mammalian embryo requires transporter-like function of Dispatched. *Cell* 111: 63–75.

Martin RA, Jones KL (1998). Absence of the superior labial frenulum in holoprosencephaly: a new diagnostic sign. *J Pediatr* 133: 150–153.

Martin RA, Jones KL, Benirshke K (1996). Absence of the lateral philtral ridges: a clue to the structural basis of the philtrum. *Am J Med Genet* 65: 117–123.

Matsumoto N, Fujimoto M, Kato R, Niikawa N (1996). Assignment of the human *GLI2* gene to 2q14 by fluorescence in situ hybridization. *Genomics* 36: 220–221.

Matsunaga E, Shiota K (1977). Holoprosencephaly in human embryos: epidemiologic studies of 150 cases. *Teratology* 16: 261–272.

Ming JE, Muenke M (1998). Holoprosencephaly: from Homer to hedgehog. *Clin Genet* 53: 155–163.

Ming JE, Muenke M (2002). Multiple hits during early embryonic development: digenic diseases and holoprosencephaly. *Am J Hum Genet* 71: 1017–1032.

Ming JE, Kaupas ME, Roessler E, Brunner HG, Golabi M, Stratton RF, Sujansky E, Bale SJ, Muenke M (2002). Mutations in Patched-1, the receptor for Sonic Hedgehog, are associated with holoprosencephaly. *Hum Genet* 110: 297–301.

Moebius FF, Fitzky BU, Lee JN, Paik YK, Glossmann H (1998). Molecular cloning and expression of the human delta 7-sterol reductase. *Proc Natl Acad Sci USA* 95: 1899–1902.

Morse RP, Rawnsley E, Sargent SK, Graham JM Jr (1987). Prenatal diagnosis of a new syndrome: holoprosencephaly with hypokinesia. *Prenat Diagn* 7: 631–638.

Muenke M, Beachy PA (2001). Holoprosencephaly. In: Scriver CR, Beaudet AL, Sly WS, Valle D, Childs B, Kinzler KW, Vogelstein B (eds). *The Metabolic and Molecular Basis of Inherited Disease, 8th Edition*, Volume 4. McGraw-Hill, New York, pp. 6203–6230.

Muenke M, Cohen MM Jr (2000). Genetic approaches to understanding brain development: holoprosencephaly as a model. *Ment Retard Dev Disabil* 6: 15–21.

Muenke M, Bone LJ, Mitchell HF, Hart I, Walton K, Hall-Johnson K, Ippel EF, Dietz-Band J, Kvaløy K, Fan C-M, et al. (1995). Physical mapping of the holoprosencephaly critical region in 21q22.3, exclusion of *SIM2* as a candidate gene for holoprosencephaly, and mapping of *SIM2* to a region of chromosome 21 important for Down syndrome. *Am J Hum Genet* 57: 1074–1079.

Muenke M, Slavotinek A, Odent S, David V, Brown S, Carter Center for Holoprosencephaly and Related Brain Malformations (2002). Holoprosencephaly due to *ZIC2* mutations: clinical, neuroradiological, and molecular studies. *American Society of Human Genetics 52nd Annual Meeting*, Baltimore, MD, October 15–19, p. 196. Abstract Nr. 26.

Nagai T, Aruga J, Minowa O, Sugimoto T, Ohno Y, Noda T, Mikoshiba K (2000). Zic2 regulates the kinetics of neurulation. *Proc Natl Acad Sci USA* 97: 1618–1623.

Naidich TP, Zimmerman RA (1987). Common congenital malformations of the brain. In: *Magnetic Resonance Imaging*. Brant-Zawadski M, Normal D (eds): Raven Press, New York, pp. 131–141.

Nanni L, Ming JE, Bocian M, Steinhaus K, Bianchi DW, Die-Smulders C, Giannotti A, Imaizumi K, Jones KL, Campo MD, et al. (1999). The mutational spectrum of the *Sonic Hedgehog* gene in holoprosencephaly: *SHH* mutations cause a significant proportion of autosomal dominant holoprosencephaly. *Hum Mol Genet* 8: 2479–2488.

Nanni L, Ming JE, Du Y, Hall RK, Aldred M, Bankier A, Muenke M (2001). *SHH* mutation is associated with solitary median maxillary central incisor: a study of 13 patients and review of the literature. *Am J Med Genet* 102: 1–10.

Nomura M, Li E (1998). Smad2 role in mesoderm formation, left–right patterning and craniofacial development. *Nature* 393: 786–790.

Norman MG, McGillivrary B, Kalousek DK, Hill A, Poskitt J (1995). Holoprosencephaly: defects of the mediobasal prosencephalon. In: *Congenital Malformations of the Brain: Pathological, Embryological, Clinical, Radiological and Genetic Aspects*. Oxford University Press, New York, pp. 187–221.

Oliver G, Loosli F, Koster R, Wittbrodt J, Gruss P (1996). Ectopic lens induction in fish in response to the murine homeobox gene *Six3*. *Mech Dev* 60: 233.

Oliver G, Marihos A, Wehr R, Copeland NG, Jenkins NA, Gruss P (1999). *Six3*, a murine homolog of the *sine oculus* gene, demarcates the most anterior border of the developing neural plate and is expressed during eye development. *Development* 121: 4045.

Ouspenskaia MV, Karkera JD, Roessler E, Shen MM, Goldmunts E, Bowers P, Towbin J, Belmont J, Muenke M (2002). Role of *FAST1* gene in the development of holoprosencephaly (HPE) and congenital cardiac malformations in humans. *American Society of Human Genetics 52nd Annual Meeting*, Baltimore, MD, October 15–19, p. 313. Abstract Nr. 822.

Pepinsky RB, Zeng C, Wen D, Rayhorn P, Baker DP, Williams KP, Bixler SA, Ambrose CM, Garber EA, Miatkowski K, et al. (1998). Identification of a palmitic acid–modified form of human sonic hedgehog. *J Biol Chem* 273: 14037–14045.

Pettersen JC (1976). An anatomical study of the two cases of cebocephaly. In: *Development of the Basicranium*, Bosma JR Jr (ed.): US Department of Health Education and Welfare Publication (NIH) 76-989, Bethesda, MD, pp. 240–265.

Porter JA, Young KE, Beachy PA (1996). Cholesterol modification of hedgehog signaling proteins in animal development. *Science* 274: 255–259.

Rasmussen SA, Moore CA, Khoury MJ, Cordero JF (1996). Descriptive epidemiology of holoprosencephaly and arhinencephaly in metropolitan Atlanta, 1968–1992. *Am J Med Genet* 66: 320–353.

Roach E, DeMyer W, Palmer K, Connelly M, Merritt A (1975). Holoprosencephaly: birth data, genetic and demographic analysis of 30 families. *Birth Defects* 11(2): 294–313.

Roessler E, Muenke M (1998). Holoprosencephaly: a paradigm for the complex genetics of brain development. *J Inherit Metab Dis* 21: 481–497.

Roessler E, Belloni E, Gaudenz K, Jay P, Berta P, Scherer SW, Tsui L-C, Muenke M (1996). Mutations in the human *Sonic Hedgehog* gene cause holoprosencephaly. *Nat Genet* 14: 357–360.

Roessler E, Belloni E, Gaudenz K, Vargas F, Scherer SW, Tsui L-C, Muenke M (1997). Mutations in the C-terminal domain of *Sonic Hedgehog* cause holoprosencephaly. *Hum Mol Genet* 6: 1847–1853.

Roessler E, Du Y, Mullor JL, Casas E, Allen WP, Ellis I, Gillessen-Kaesbach G, Roeder E, Ming JE, Ruiz A, et al. (2002). Loss-of-function mutations in the human *GLI2* gene cause holoprosencephaly and familial panhypopituitarism. *American Society of Human Genetics 52nd Annual Meeting*, Baltimore, MD, October 15–19, p. 190. Abstract Nr.132.

Saccone S, Rapisarda A, Motta S, Dono R, Persico GM, Della Valle G (1995). Regional localization of the human EGF-like growth factor *CRIPTO* gene (*TDGF-1*) to chromosome 3p21. *Hum Genet* 95: 229–230.

Schell U, Weinberg J, Kohler A, Bray-Ward P, Ward DE, Wilson WG, Allen WP, Lebel RR, Sawyer JR, Campbell PL, et al. (1996). Molecular characterization of breakpoints in patients with holoprosencephaly and definition of the HPE2 critical region 2p21. *Hum Mol Genet* 5: 223–229.

Schimmenti LA, de la Cruz J, Lewis RA, Karkera JD, Manligas GS, Roessler E, Muenke M (2003). Novel mutation in *Sonic Hedgehog* in non-syndromic colobomatous microphthalmia. *Am J Med Genet* 116A: 215–221.

Shen MM, Schier AF (2000). The *EGF-CFC* gene family in vertebrate development. *Trends Genet* 16: 303–309.

Siebert JR, Cohen MM Jr, Sulik KK, Shaw C-M, Lemire RJ (1990). *Holoprosencephaly: An Overview and Atlas of Cases*. Wiley-Liss, New York.

Song J, Oh SP, Schrewe H, Nomura M, Lei H, Okano M, Gridley T, Li E (1999). The type II activin receptors are essential for egg cylinder growth, gastrulation, and rostral head development in mice. *Dev Biol* 213: 157–169.

Sulik KK, Cook CS, Webster WS (1988). Teratogens and craniofacial malformations: relationships to cell death. *Development* 103: 213–232.

Sulik KK, Dehart DB, Rogers JM (1995). Teratogenicity of low doses of all-trans retinoic acid in presomite mouse embryos. *Teratology* 51: 398–403.

Varlet I, Collignon J, Norris DP, Robertson EJ (1997). Nodal signaling and axis formation in the mouse. *Cold Spring Harb Symp Quant Biol* 62: 105–113.

Vortkamp A, Gessler M, Grzeschik KH (1991). *GLI3* zinc finger gene interrupted by translocations in Greig syndrome families. *Nature* 352: 539–540.

Wallis DE, Muenke M (1999). Molecular mechanisms of holoprosencephaly. *Mol Genet Metab* 68: 126–138.

Wallis DE, Roessler E, Hehr U, Nanni L, Wiltshire T, Richieri-Costa A, Gillessen-Kaesbach G, Zackai EH, Romens J, Muenke M (1999). Mutations in the homeodomain of the human *SIX3* gene cause holoprosencephaly. *Nat Genet* 22: 196–198.

Wassif CA, Maslen C, Kachilele-Linjewile S, Lin D, Linck TM, Connor WE, Steiner RD, Porter FD (1998). Mutations in the human *sterol Δ^7-reductase* gene at 11q12-13 cause Smith-Lemli-Opitz syndrome. *Am J Hum Genet* 63: 53–62.

Waterham HR, Koster J, Romeijn GJ, Hennekam RCM, Vreken P, Andersson HC, Fitz-Patrick DR, Kelley RI, Wanders RJA (2001). Mutations in the *3-β-hydroxysterol Δ^{24}-reductase* gene cause desmosterolosis, an autosomal recessive disorder of cholesterol biosynthesis. *Am J Hum Genet* 69: 685–694.

Watkins DN, Berman DM, Burkholder SG, Wang B, Beachy PA, Baylin SB (2003). Hedgehog signalling within airway epithelial progenitors and in small-cell lung cancer. *Nature* 422: 313–317.

Webster WS, Johnston MC, Lammer EJ (1986). Isotretinoin embryopathy and the cranial neural crest: an in vivo and in vitro study. *J Craniofac Genet* 6: 211–222.

Witsch-Baumgartner M, Fitzky BU, Ogorelkova M, Kraft HG, Moebius FF, Glossmann H, Seedorf U, Gillessen-Kaesbach G, Hoffmann GF, Clayon P, et al. (2000). Mutational spectrum in the *Δ^7-sterol reductase* gene and genotype–phenotype correlation in 84 patients with Smith-Lemli-Opitz syndrome. *Am J Hum Genet* 66: 402–412.

Wotton D, Lo RS, Lee S (1999). A Smad transcriptional corepressor. *Cell* 97: 29–39.

Yu H, Lee M-H, Starck L, Elias ER, Irons M, Salen G, Patel SB, Tint GS (2000). Spectrum of *Δ7-dehydrocholesterol reductase* mutations in patients with the Smith-Lemli-Opitz (BSH) syndrome. *Hum Mol Genet* 9: 1385–1391.

Zhou S, Zawel L, Lengauer C, Kinzler KW, Vogelstein R (1998). Characterization of human FAST-1, a TGF beta and activin signal transducer. *Mol Cell* 2: 121–127.

19 | *PTCH* and the Basal Cell Nevus (Gorlin) Syndrome

ERVIN EPSTEIN, JR.

The basal cell nevus syndrome (BCNS) is a rare affliction that is inherited as an autosomal dominant trait and characterized by a wide panoply of clinical manifestations, especially the development of large numbers of cutaneous basal cell carcinomas (BCCs). Causative mutations occur in the *PATCHED1* (*PTCH1*) gene, which encodes an inhibitor of hedgehog signaling. This identification has led to the novel finding that sporadic BCCs, the commonest human cancer, are driven by pivotal mutations in genes encoding proteins that are components of the hedgehog signaling pathway. In addition to postnatal tumors of the skin and, less commonly, of other tissues, BCNS patients have malformations (e.g., of the ribs and skull) and overgrowth that are explicable on the basis of abnormal PATCHED1 function during embryogenesis.

MUTANT LOCUS

PTCH1, the site of the causative mutations, is the human homologue of the *Drosphila* gene *ptc*. Its major known function is to suppress the hedgehog signaling pathway, and the clinical manifestations of BCNS appear to be due to dysregulated hedgehog signaling, both during development and postnatally.

CLINICAL DESCRIPTION

BCNS (nevoid BCC syndrome, Gorlin syndrome) is named for its most prominent clinical feature, a propensity to develop large numbers of BCCs of the skin. However, patients may also have a variety of extracutaneous abnormalities, some of which are developmental (Table 19–1). Although several patients with BCNS were reported earlier in the 20th century, wider awareness in the general medical community followed a report emphasizing extracutaneous manifestations in 1960 by the dentist Robert Gorlin and the dermatologist Robert Goltz (Binkley and Johnson, 1951; Howell and Caro, 1959; Gorlin and Goltz, 1960; McKelvey et al., 1960; Howell, 1980). Since then, numerous case reports and review series have identified dozens of clinical abnormalities to which these patients are prone, and clinical criteria for diagnosis have been proposed (Gorlin, 1987; Evans et al., 1993; Shanley et al., 1994; Kimonis et al., 1997; Lo Muzio et al., 1999). None of the clinical abnormalities occurs in 100% of affected persons. Therefore, the diagnosis depends on the presence of a sufficient number of findings, all of which are non-diagnostic and most of which are unusual in non-BCNS persons. The identification in 1996 of causative mutations in *PTCH1* (Hahn et al., 1996b; Johnson et al., 1996) followed a decade of positional cloning efforts, which were spurred by the hope that success would identify a new tumor-suppressor gene, which, like the *Rb* and *APC* genes, would be instructive about the molecular abnormalities in the sporadic tumors (Knudson, 1971). The identification of the mutant gene as one known to be crucial in development has focused further interest not only on the developmental abnormalities in these patients but also on the role of ptc in developmental processes and in control of hedgehog signaling.

The inheritance of BCNS clearly is autosomal dominant, but many patients have no known affected relatives. Since in large families the penetrance of BCNS approaches 100%, the large number of patients without known affected relatives argues for a high rate of new mutations, as is expected for autosomal dominant traits. Nonetheless, there is no reduced fecundity in BCNS patients, and for most patients, life span does not appear to be reduced significantly, if at all. The incidence is estimated at approximately 1:100,000.

Clinical manifestations of BCNS can be divided for heuristic purposes into those that arise postnatally and those that arise prenatally, although it is not known whether abnormal gene function in those clinically manifest postnatally is limited to postnatal life or whether the "seeds" of these abnormalities arise earlier.

POSTNATAL PERIOD

BCCs

Patients most commonly are diagnosed with BCNS when they develop large numbers of BCCs, sometimes starting as early as age 5 or even, rarely, at birth (Meyvisch et al., 1993) but more commonly postpuberty. The appearance of the tumors may vary from tiny (e.g., 1–2 mm, sometimes visible only by careful examination using side lighting) translucent papules, with or without pigmentation, located especially on the trunk, to more typical, invasive, larger (e.g., 4 mm in diameter) papules located especially on the face (Fig. 19–1). The appearance of the larger BCCs is identical to that of sporadic BCCs; smaller BCCs may be confused with nevocellular nevi ("moles") thus giving the syndrome the name *basal cell nevus* to indicate that the papules may resemble nevi but on biopsy are found to have the histology of BCCs. As the patient ages, the BCCs tend to become more numerous. Like sporadic BCCs, some may invade locally and impair skin function (e.g., of the eyelids) and may cause death through aggressive local invasion or even through distant metastases (Southwick and Schwartz, 1979; Winkler and Guyron, 1987; Berardi et al., 1991; Lo et al., 1991). However, BCC metastasis (whether in the sporadic case or as part of the BCNS) is very rare, a fortunate feature of this by far most common of human cancers (approximately 750,000/year in the United States alone [Miller and Weinstock, 1994]). More typically, the clinically significant problem caused by the BCCs is the need for repeated painful and disruptive surgeries with consequent significant scarring, especially of the face.

BCNS patients develop large numbers of papulonodular BCCs on the face and (usually) superficial BCCs on the trunk and limbs. Superficial BCCs of the lower extremities are common in BCNS patients but quite rare in sporadic patients. Although most BCCs in BCNS patients occur on the face, the relative ratio of lesions of the trunk/limbs to those of the face is higher in BCNS patients (38%) than in sporadic cases (13%), suggesting that sunlight may have less of a role in BCC formation in BCNS patients than in sporadic patients (Goldstein et al., 1993). Irrespective of the exact etiologic role of sunlight, it is clear that BCNS is one of the few known human abnormalities in which patients have a well-documented predisposition to ionizing radiation–induced carcinogenesis. Thus, patients may develop sheets of BCCs in portals of ionizing radiation therapy used to treat medulloblastomas; and in one family whose business was a shoe store, repeated demonstrations by affected teenagers of fluoroscopy of the feet (used to help determine the proper shoe size of young customers) produced BCCs of the feet.

The histology of BCCs is varied, ranging from the common small nests of dark staining cells palisaded along the periphery to superficially spreading cells. In some patients, microscopically controlled removal (Mohs' surgery) is frustrating because even random biop-

Table 19–1. Diagnostic Findings in Adults with Basal Cell Nevus Syndrome

Developmental	Hyper/Neoplastic
FREQUENCY ≤ 50%	
Enlarged occipitofrontal circumference (macrocephaly, frontoparietal bossing, in index cases only?)	Multiple basal cell carcinomas
High-arched palate	
Palmar or plantar pits	Odontogenic keratocysts of
Rib anomalies (e.g., splayed, fused, partially missing, bifid)	jaws
Spina bifida occulta of cervical or thoracic vertebrae	Epidermal cysts of skin
Calcified falx cerebri	
Calcified diaphragma sellae (bridged sella, fused clinoids)	
Hyperpeumatization of paranasal sinuses	
FREQUENCY 15%–49%	
Calcification of tentorium cerebelli and petroclinoid ligament	Calcified ovarian fibromas
Short fourth metacarpals	Pseudocystic lytic lesion of
Kyphoscoliosis or other vertebral anomalies	bones (hamartomas)
Lumbarization of sacrum	
Narrow sloping shoulders	
Prognathism	
Pectus excavatum or carinatum	
Strabismus (exotropia)	
FREQUENCY < 14% BUT NOT RANDOM	
Inguinal hernia (?)	Medulloblastoma
True ocular hypertelorism	Meningioma
Ovarian fibrosarcoma	Lymphomesenteric cyst
Marfanoid build	Cardiac fibroma
Anosmia	Fetal rhabdomyoma
Agenesis of corpus callosum	
Cyst of septum pellucidum	
Cleft lip and/or palate	
Low-pitched female voice	
Polydactyly, postaxial in hands or feet	
Sprengel deformity of scapula	
Syndactyly	
Congenital cataract, glaucome, coloboma of iris, retina, optic nerve, medullated retinal nerve fibers	
Subcutaneous calcifications of skin (possibly underestimated frequency)	
Minor kidney malformations	
Hypogonadisms in male subjects	
Mental retardation	

Source: Adapted from Gorlin (1987), with permission.

Figure 19–1. Basal cell carcinomas (BCCs) on the skin of patients with basal cell nevus syndrome. *A:* Small translucent shiny papule. *B:* Flat, irregularly pigmented BCC with tiny translucent papules. *C, D:* Scarring of face and upper body due to invasion by and treatment of previous BCCs; active BCCs outlined in ink. *E:* Lower back with scarring and active flat, pink superficial BCCs. *F:* Lower leg with outlined superficial BCCs.

Pits

Pits are small (e.g., 1–3 mm) sharply localized defects in the stratum corneum of the palms and the soles (Fig. 19–2). They may be easier to see before bathing: dirt may become lodged in and thus highlight the pits. Although a few patients have dozens of pits, more commonly patients have only a few. These are unusual to rare in persons without BCNS, so their presence, if in large numbers, is fairly diagnostic of BCNS. They must be differentiated clinically from *keratoses*, elevated accumulations of excess stratum corneum (the exact opposite of these holes in the stratum corneum), which may be manifestations of chronic arsenic exposure. This differentiation can be of importance since chronic arsenic poisoning also produces multiple cutaneous BCCs. Although there are reports of BCCs arising at the base of a pit, this is uncommon, and usually pits themselves are not of clinical importance and do not require biopsy.

Extracutaneous Tumors

A variety of non-BCC tumors have been reported in BCNS patients. Most of these occur in a small minority of BCNS patients, and so for at least some of them it is difficult to know whether the report is of a chance occurrence or an unusual yet pathogenetically related manifestation. Some of these tumors, however, are so rare in the population that their report in even a handful of BCNS patients is strong evidence of an actual causal relationship.

Clearly, medulloblastomas occur more commonly in BCNS patients than in persons without the syndrome. One estimate is that approximately 3%–5% of BCNS patients develop medulloblastomas and approximately 1%–2% of patients with medulloblastomas have BCNS (Evans et al., 1991, 1993) As expected, medulloblastomas, like BCCs and odontogenic keratocysts, tend to occur at a younger age in BCNS patients than in sporadic cases (Cowan et al., 1997).

Meningiomas are less common in BCNS patients than medulloblastomas, but multiple patients with meningiomas have been reported, probably with an incidence higher than that in the normal population (Albrecht et al., 1994). Rhabdomyosarcomas and cardiac fibromas are tumors sufficiently rare that the several case reports of each occurring in BCNS patients indicate an actual relationship (Jones et al., 1986; Cotton et al., 1991; Herman et al., 1991; DiSanto et al., 1992). Calcified ovarian fibromas have occurred in several BCNS patients, in some at a very early age, as have mesenteric lymphatic cysts, which may reach very large sizes (Scully et al., 1976; Johnson et al., 1986). Cysts of the skin appear to be more common in BCNS patients than in others, but again, they are not in themselves distinguishable from those in sporadic cases. Fibrosarcoma of the jaw has been reported, likely due to ionizing radiation therapy of facial BCCs (Binkley and Johnson, 1951; Tamoney, 1969). However, this tumor has not been reported in the skull following ionizing radiation treatment of medulloblastomas.

Calcification

Although calcification of the falx is very common in healthy adults, the presence of lamellar calcification of the falx in younger persons, e.g., those of 20 years of age, is almost diagnostic of BCNS (Ratcliffe et al., 1995a). Calcification of other parts of the brain and loss of calcification in areas of the skull in BCNS are common in BCNS patients and may strongly suggest an incorrect diagnosis of cancer, as may sclerotic lesions of other bone (Yee et al., 1993). The bone loss appears to be due to replacement of bone by hamartomas, which may be multiple and radiologically worrisome but clinically banal (Miller and Cooper, 1972). X-ray films of the hands may identify flame-shaped lucencies of the phalanges, which also have been reported to be diagnostic of BCNS (Dunnick et al., 1978).

sies of clinically normal skin have budding from the bottom of the epidermis, what appear to be incipient tumors, making the achievement of a tumor-free margin impossible. In addition to the same histology as BCCs in sporadic patients, the skin tumors may resemble cells of the hair, thus fueling the controversy as to whether BCCs themselves arise from follicles as opposed to interfollicular epidermis.

Odontogenic Keratocysts

Odontogenic keratocysts often are the initially diagnosed manifestation of BCNS, arising by the end of the first decade of life. They may occur in either the upper or lower jaw, may be asymptomatic and identified only by X-ray, or may erode enough bone to cause pain and loss of teeth; untreated, they may even invade the sinus (Friedlander et al., 1988). They tend to be more aggressive in BCNS patients than in sporadic cases, and they more often recur after surgical removal (Forssell et al., 1988). Like BCCs, an individual jaw keratocyst in a BCNS patient cannot be differentiated from one arising sporadically.

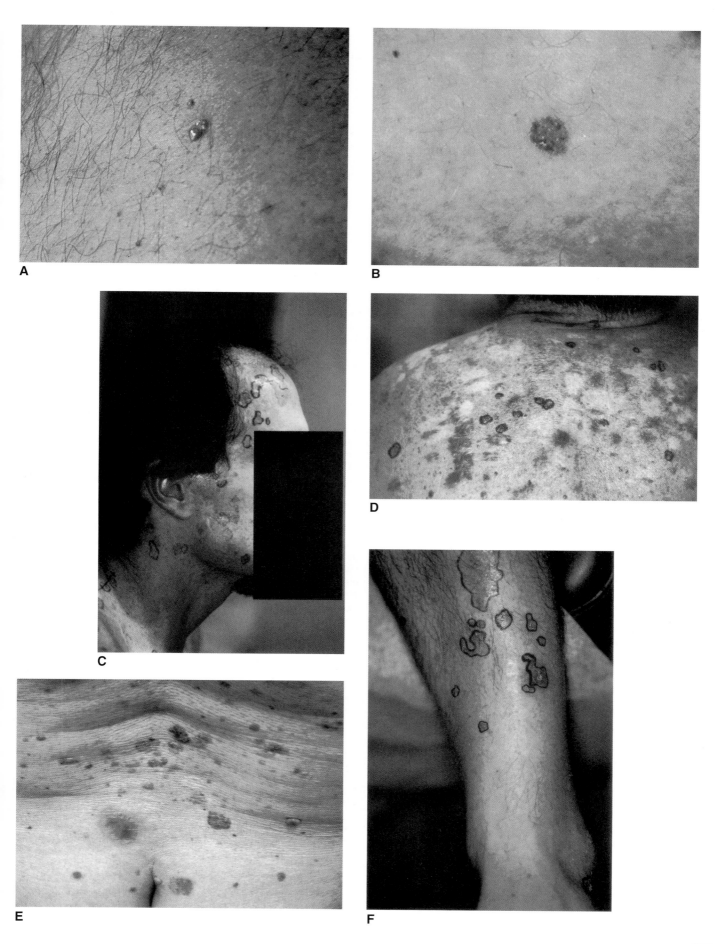

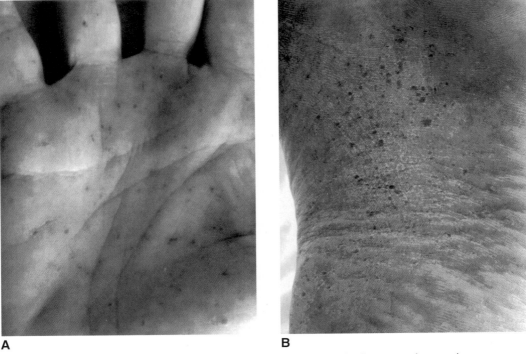

Figure 19–2. Usually florid pits of palm (*A*) and sole (*B*) in basal cell nevus syndrome patients.

PRENATAL PERIOD

Developmental Aspects

Patients with BCNS tend to be larger (taller and heavier) than expected on the basis of the size of their parents and siblings. Sometimes the exaggerated length of the limbs suggests the diagnosis of Marfan syndrome. They tend to have large, overhanging foreheads (large calvaria with frontal and bitemporal bossing) (Dahl et al., 1976), although one study argued that the occipitofrontal head circumference exceeded normal only in probands and not in their affected relatives (Bale et al., 1991). Their enlarged head size may lead to an incorrect diagnosis of hydrocephalus during infancy, but congenital hydrocephalus has been reported (Meyvisch et al., 1993). The ribs, as detected radiologically, may be duplicated, fused, splayed, or otherwise misshapen; and spina bifida occulta occurs commonly (Ratcliffe et al., 1995b). The presence of spinal fusion problems in mice with hedgehog signaling abnormalities suggests that the spina bifida occulta in human BCNS patients is a genuine part of the syndrome (vide infra).

Molecular Genetics

The first successful effort in the positional cloning of the BCNS mutant gene was the identification in 1992 in sporadic BCCs of a region of frequent allelic loss on chromosome 9q and the identification in BCNS families of linkage of the inheritance of the syndrome with inheritance of the same chromosomal region (Gailani et al., 1992). Subsequently, no family with BCNS has been reported in which linkage analysis has excluded this region as the site of the causative mutation. The 1996 identification of *PTCH1* as the chromosome 9q gene harboring mutations causing BCNS and its frequent mutation in sporadic BCCs has been amply confirmed subsequently, although *PTCH1* mutations can be identified in only approximately 50% of patients with typical clinical manifestations of BCNS (Gailani et al., 1996; Unden et al., 1996; Aszterbaum et al., 1998; Bodak et al., 1999; D'Errico et al., 2000). Described mutations (www.cybergene.se/PTCH/) are scattered throughout the gene; many are predicted to encode premature truncations. The high incidence of loss of sequences encoding *PTCH1* in BCCs (as high as 85% of BCCs have *PTCH1* coding region losses [Ling et al., 2001]) as well as the high incidence of mutations predicted to encode truncated proteins (and which, because of nonsense-

mediated RNA decay, may produce unstable mRNA) argue that the mechanism of disease is through loss of gene function rather than through the production of abnormal proteins that acquire new deleterious functions. (This conclusion is muddied a bit, however, by the lack of good studies of the protein products of mutant alleles.) This idea is consistent with the general impression by clinicians that the clinical manifestations of the disease vary as much within a single kindred as they do among different kindreds, suggesting that, irrespective of the exact site and type of mutation, the primary abnormality is a pure loss of *PTCH1* function, that the clinical variability is due to allelic variation at non-*PTCH1* genes and to differences in environment, and that genotype–phenotype correlation is not to be expected (Wicking et al., 1997). As an easily explained but nonetheless dramatic example of varying expression being due to variability at non-*PTCH1* loci, BCNS patients of African descent with dark pigmentation and, hence, good protection of the DNA of their epidermal cells from the sun have few to no BCCs but may have the usual extracutaneous BCNS abnormalities (Goldstein et al., 1994). As an example of the clinical variability caused by environmental differences, BCNS patients in Australia have more BCCs at an earlier age than do those in northern Europe or the United States. Furthermore, there is no clear correlation reported between morphologic abnormalities (e.g., body size, coarse features, etc.) and numbers of tumors, either BCCs or those of a non-BCC type.

Diagnosis

Since no single clinical abnormality is entirely diagnostic of BCNS and since *PTCH1* mutations can be identified in only approximately 50% of patients with clinically typical BCNS, diagnosis (at least in the 50% with undetectable mutations) must depend on a constellation of clinical findings. Criteria for diagnosis have been formulated (Table 19–2) but have not been tested against the "gold standard" of diagnosis by *PTCH1* mutation. Examination for diagnostic purposes should include a careful examination of the total skin surface, with biopsy of several even slightly suspicious lesions since BCCs in BCNS may appear as banal moles resembling nevocellular nevi. Pits of the palms and soles should be looked for specifically. X-ray examination of the jaws (Panorex films), skull, chest, and hands is useful for detection of cysts, early-onset lamellar calcification of the falx (in some instances, early enough in childhood to be present at the same time

Table 19–2. BCNS Diagnostic Criteria

Major Criteria	Minor Criteria
1. More than two basal cell carcinomas or one under the age of 20 years	1. Macrocephaly determined after adjustment for height
2. Odontogenic keratocysts of the jaw proven by histology	2. Congenital malformations: cleft lip or palate, frontal bossing, "coarse face," moderate or severe hypertelorism
3. Three or more palmar and/or plantar pits	3. Skeletal abnormalities: Sprengel deformity, marked pectus deformity, or marked syndactyly of the digits
4. Bilamellar calcification of the falx cerebri (if less than 20 years old)	4. Radiological abnormalities: bridging of the sella turcica, rib anomalies such as bifid or splayed ribs, vertebral anomalies such as hemivertebrae, fusion or elongation of the vertebral bodies, modeling defects of the hands and feet, or flame shaped lucencies of the hands or feet
5. Fused, bifid, or markedly splayed ribs.	5. Ovarian fibroma
6. First-degree relative with basal cell nevus syndrome	6. Medulloblastoma
7. *PTC* gene mutation in normal tissue	

Source: Modified from Kimonis et al. (1997).

as a medulloblastoma), abnormal ribs, spina bifida occulta, and flame-shaped lucencies. Mutations can be detected at several academic centers (e.g., Allen Bale at Yale University: bale@biomed.med.yale.edu) and commercially at GeneDx, Inc. (www.genedx.com). One report describes several children with medulloblastomas with skull changes similar to those in patients with BCNS in which the causative mutation was not in *PTCH1* but rather in the *SUFU* gene, which encodes a more downstream inhibitor of hedgehog signaling (Taylor et al., 2002).

Management

Genetic counseling regarding the uniformly autosomal dominant inheritance of BCNS is highly useful for families in which an affected member is known, and prenatal diagnosis is available by standard DNA-based techniques. If the prospective parent is the only affected individual in the family and if the *PTCH1* mutation cannot be identified, it may be possible to determine which chromosome carries the mutant allele by studying allelic deletion in multiple BCCs in the affected person. This should be possible because such somatic allelic deletion, as expected by the two-hit hypothesis, uniformly deletes the wild-type allele (Bonifas et al., 1994).

Prophylaxis against the clinical manifestations currently is limited to efforts to reduce mutagenesis of the skin and consequent BCC development, by avoidance of sun exposure and of ionizing radiation exposure. Patients should be counseled seriously to avoid outdoor activities in midday, to wear hats and other protective clothing, and to use higher-SPF sunscreens frequently and in thick applications. The most likely source of ionizing radiation is its therapeutic use vs. tumors, especially BCCs and medulloblastomas. For BCCs, other therapeutic options are nearly always available; for medulloblastomas, radiotherapy may be needed, despite the likely subsequent development of large numbers of BCCs of the skin through which the tumors are treated. Oral retinoids clearly can reduce the development of new BCCs, but often the side effects at the high dose needed for preventive efficacy outweigh the therapeutic benefits (Peck et al., 1982; Cristofolini et al., 1984; Hodak et al., 1987; Goldberg et al., 1989; Sanchez-Conejo-Mir and Camacho, 1989). No careful study of the long-term effects of topical retinoids on the skin of BCNS patients has been published. The benefits of a low-fat diet on BCC development in non-BCNS patients (Black et al., 1995) make dietary counseling of BCNS patients attractive, but no study of the actual effects of diet on BCNS has been published.

Therefore, the touchstone of current management is frequent and careful application of standard medical diagnosis and treatment to re-

duce the magnitude of interventions that are needed. Thus, depending on the "activity" of the skin, patients may require dermatologic care as often as monthly, at each visit BCCs being removed by techniques likely to leave as little scarring as possible, e.g., freezing. Topical 5-fluorouracil, imiquomid, retinoids (e.g., tazarotene), photodynamic therapy, and physical (e.g., laser) removal of the epidermis may reduce the rate of development of new BCCs in treated areas (Strange and Lang, 1992; Peris et al., 1999; Kagy and Amonette, 2000). Similarly, patients may need jaw films yearly or even more often, depending on the frequency with which they develop cysts. It is important that patients become knowledgable about the multiple manifestations of the disease since most physicians have little to no knowledge of this rare syndrome.

ANIMAL MODELS

PTCH1 is the human homologue of the *Drosophila ptc* gene. The abnormal developmental phenotype produced by the fly *ptc* mutation was described in the initial report of the Nusslein-Volhard/Wieschaus screen for developmental mutations (Nusslein-Volhard and Wieschaus, 1980). The *Drosophila ptc* gene was cloned in 1989 (Hooper and Scott, 1989; Nakano et al., 1989), and the mouse *ptc1* gene was identified in 1996 (Goodrich et al., 1996; Hahn et al., 1996a). Like $ptc^{-/-}$ flies, $ptc^{-/-}$ mice die early during embryonic development. $Ptc^{+/-}$ mice, like BCNS patients with the $PTCH1^{+/-}$ genotype, are viable, fertile, and relatively normal at birth (Corcoran and Scott, 2001). A small percentage of them have hindlimb syndactyly or extra digits (Goodrich et al., 1997). They tend to be larger than their normal littermates and, perhaps dependent on their background strain, may develop spontaneous tumors, most prominent among which are medulloblastomas and rhabdomyosarcomas. Since similar phenotypes have been described for knockouts at either exons 1 or 2 (Goodrich et al., 1997) or at exon 6 (Hahn et al., 1998), it is likely that these abnormalities indeed are related to loss of ptc1 function. The $ptc^{+/-}$ mice are hypersensitive in utero to ionizing radiation-induced teratogenesis (Hahn et al., 1998). The medulloblastomas generally arise within the first few months of life, and they may retain one normal allele of *ptc*. They appear to arise in the setting of hemizygosity for a functioning *ptc* allele rather than only after loss of the wild-type allele (Wetmore et al., 2000; Zurawel et al., 2000).

The skin of $ptc^{+/-}$ mice appears normal at birth, and unperturbed, the only abnormality detectable is the presence of tiny, microscopically detectable clusters of basaloid cells in the superficial dermis at, e.g., 1 year of age. However, if treated either with repeated doses of UV radiation or with a single dose of ionizing radiation, $ptc^{+/-}$ mice develop BCCs and other closely related tumors whose histology resembles more that of cells of various regions of the hair follicle (Aszterbaum et al., 1999). When 3 times/week UV radiation is begun at 6 weeks of age, the microscopic lesions are easily seen by 6 months of age and occur eventually in 100% of treated $ptc^{+/-}$ mice. After 9–12 months of UV treatment, $ptc^{+/-}$ mice develop grossly visible skin tumors of the irradiated areas. Of these, approximately one-fourth are BCCs, one-fourth are squamous cell carcinomas (SCCs), and one-half are fibrosarcomas. Because deletion of *ptc* exons 1 and 2 was accompanied by insertion of the lacZ gene, areas of upregulated *ptc* expression will stain for β-galactosidase enzyme. The BCCs and fibrosarcomas, like the medulloblastomas and rhabdomyosarcomas, stain blue (positive for β-galactosidase); the SCCs do not. Consistent with this staining pattern, loss of the wild-type *ptc* allele occurs frequently in both BCCs and fibrosarcomas, but such loss did not occur in the SCCs studied (Aszterbaum et al., 1999). Fibrosarcomas occur in UV-treated mice of normal *ptc1* genotype, and it is unclear whether they arise from dermal cells or from epidermal cells that undergo an epithelial to mesenchymal transition (Morison et al., 1986). However, treatment with UV of $ptc^{+/+}$ mice that are littermates of the $ptc^{+/-}$ mice thus far has not produced grossly visible tumors of any type. Thus, the grossly visible fibrosarcomas and SCCs are inconsistent with the human BCNS phenotype and suggest that the $ptc^{+/-}$ mice have a currently unexplained tendency to skin tumorigenesis beyond BCC formation. Consistent with the hypersensitivity to ionizing radiation–induced BCCs of BCNS patients, mice treated with Cs[137] ionizing radiation also develop microscopically detectable and then eventually grossly visible tumors of the BCC lineage, and tumorigensis is dose-dependent (Aszterbaum et al., 1999). In the skin, ionizing radiation induces only BCCs, not the fibrosarcomas and SCCs seen after UV radiation. The cause of this difference is not clear. One possibility is that the broader spectrum of tumor types in $ptc^{+/-}$ mice after UV radiation is due to the immunosuppressive effects of UV radiation (Nishigori et al., 1996). Of interest, ionizing radiation does not appear to induce large numbers of extracutaneous tumors in $ptc^{+/-}$ mice. This is consistent both with the general lack of induction of tumors other than BCCs in patients treated with ionizing radiation, e.g., for medulloblastomas (some bone sarcomas have been reported in BCNS patients subjected to large doses of ionizing radiotherapy of BCCs, but these reports are quite rare), and with the general lack of upregulation of hedgehog target genes in sporadic human cancers other than BCCs and medulloblastomas (Hu et al., 2003). Thus, the hypersensitivity to ionizing radiation–induced carcinogenesis seems in large part to be limited to the skin keratinocytes in both humans and mice, one reported exception being the hypersensitivity of $ptc^{+/-}$ mice to teratogenesis following in utero exposure to ionizing radiation (Hahn et al., 1998).

The mesenchymal dysplasia (mes) mouse mutation arose spontaneously and is due to a 32 bp deletion in the ptc1 gene (Makino et al., 2001). This deletion is predicted to disrupt the C-terminal cytoplasmic tail of ptc1. $mes^{+/-}$ mice have no visible abnormalities; $mes^{-/-}$ mice have several abnormalities, including overgrowth of some tissues, polydactyly, skeletal defects, and abnormal facies (Sweet et al., 1996). The mes allele partially rescues the early embryonic lethality of the $ptc^{-/-}$ mouse; ptc^-/ptc mes mice survive to near the end of gestation, suggesting that an intact C-terminal tail is not essential to some of the developmental functions of ptc protein.

DEVELOPMENTAL PATHOGENESIS

As expected from the growing knowledge of the multiple essential roles of hedgehog signaling during development, homozygous deletion of ptc1 is lethal in flies and mice. Patients or mice with the $PTCH1^{+/-}$ genotype, however, in the overwhelming number of instances, are developmentally nearly normal. Each of the many reported developmental abnormalities, for the most part, affects only a minority of BCNS individuals. Replication of some of these in the $ptc1^{+/-}$ mouse confirms that they truly are caused by the abnormal genotype and are not just a random occurrence of two rare abnormalities in a single BCNS patient. In parallel, identification of phenotypic abnormalities in $ptc1^{+/-}$ mice, e.g., reduced pancreas size and abnormal glucose tolerance (Hebrok et al., 2000) or abnormalities in mammary gland development (Lewis et al., 1999), may inform a search for phenotypic abnormalities not previously appreciated to be of greater than background incidence in BCNS patients

Perhaps most prominent among these developmental abnormalities is the oft-recognized but unquantitated increased body size of BCNS patients compared to others in their family. $ptc1^{+/-}$ mice also are approximately 15% heavier than their $ptc^{+/+}$ littermates, and abnormally increased ptc expression causes decreased size (Goodrich et al., 1997; Milenkovic et al., 1999). Furthermore, BCNS patients may have a marfanoid habitus, with relatively long limbs and a short trunk. One postulated non-cell-autonomous mechanism by which hedgehog signaling might enhance growth has come from evidence that Igf2 is a hedgehog target gene, is upregulated in medulloblastomas and rhabdomyosarcomas, and appears to be necessary for the development of these tumors (Hahn et al., 1998, 2000). Mice with loss of Igf2 are dwarfed; mice with enhanced Igf2 expression are large. However, experimental mice with hedgehog-mediated overgrowth do not have increased levels of Igf2.

Most explanations, however, have focused on the effects on cells that themselves receive the hedgehog signal; hedgehog tends to enhance cell proliferation and to inhibit cell differentiation. There is evidence that hedgehog overexpression increases ovarian stem cells in flies (Zhang and Kalderon, 2001). Several mammalian model systems

have been studied relatively extensively. One of these is the formation of endochondral bone, which appears to have direct relevance to the long-limbed phenotype of BCNS patients. Indian hedgehog (Ihh) directly enhances chondrocyte proliferation. Thus, loss of Ihh or smoothened (smo) inhibits and overexpression of Ihh or the presence of a constitutively activated smo promotes chondrocyte proliferation during mouse bone development; and levels of cyclin D1 change in parallel with changes in hedgehog signaling (Long et al., 2001).

Another model system is the action of hedgehog on the precursors of the neurons of the cerebellum. During development, these granular cell precursors are at the surface of the cerebellum, the external germinal layer, and are targets of the release of hedgehog from underlying Purkinje cells, which maintains their proliferation and inhibits their differentiation (Wechsler-Reya and Scott, 1999; Dahmane and Ruiz-i-Altaba, 1999). Experimental manipulation of hedgehog signaling causes congruent changes in external germinal layer cellularity: enhanced signaling increases cellularity, and decreased signaling decreases cellularity. Part of this effect also may be mediated by upregulation of cyclin D1 expression, although this upregulation appears to occur via intermediate steps since the mRNA induction is cycloheximide-sensitive (Kenney and Rowitch, 2000).

A third studied system is the epidermal keratinocyte. In culture, sonic hedgehog (Shh) opposes normal calcium-induced differentiation with resultant continued cell proliferation and augments the replicative capacity even at low calcium concentrations (Fan and Khavari, 1999). These effects on cultured keratinocytes are consistent with suggestions that BCCs resemble epidermal stem cells (Bonifas et al., 2001; Taipale and Beachy, 2001; Zhang and Kalderon, 2001).

The mechanism for development of tumors is, at first approximation, consistent with the classic two-hit model for inactivation of tumor-suppressor genes: somatic loss of function of the second allele of PTCH1 in BCNS patients causes the cell to become tumorous. In BCCs, this likely is accurate, for half of BCCs arising in BCNS patients have loss of one allele of PTCH1, and the allele lost invariably is the wild-type allele (Bonifas et al., 1994). Furthermore, sporadic BCCs, in as high as 85% of cases, lose one copy of PTCH1 (Ling et al., 2001), and PTCH1 single-base mutations also frequently can be detected in BCCs. Similarly, PTCH1 loss of heterozygosity has been detected in odontogenic keratocysts (Matsumura et al., 2000; Barreto et al., 2000). These findings are consistent with the idea that loss of PTCH1 produces abnormalities via dysregulated hedgehog signaling: all BCCs have increased expression of hedgehog target genes (e.g., GLI1, HIP, and PTCH1 itself); some BCCs and medulloblastomas have mutant SMO alleles, which appear to make the encoded protein resistant to inhibition by PTCH1; and mice engineered to overexpress shh, mutant SMO, gli1, or gli2 develop tumors strongly resembling human BCCs (Dahmane et al., 1997; Fan et al., 1997; Xie et al., 1998; Reifenberger et al., 1998; Lam et al., 1999; Grachtchouk et al, 2000; Nilsson et al., 2000; Bonifas et al., 2001).

Therefore, it is somewhat surprising that several investigators have identified retention of one normal allele of PTCH1 in mouse medulloblastomas (Zurawel et al., 2000; Wetmore et al., 2000), despite the oft-reported upregulation of hedgehog target gene expression and of PTCH1 or SMO mutations in many of these tumors, as in BCCs, in mice and in humans arising in BCNS patients or sporadically (Pietsch et al., 1997; Raffel et al., 1997; Vorechovsky et al., 1997; Wolter et al., 1997; Reifenberger et al., 1998; Dong et al., 2000). One possibility is that the role of hedgehog signaling in medulloblastomas is to increase the precursor cell population and therefore expand the possible targets for other tumorigenic mutations. However, marked upregulation of hedgehog target gene expression in medulloblastomas has been reported repeatedly, a finding not reported in normal cells of $ptc^{+/-}$ mice or of $PTCH1^{+/-}$ humans (Hahn et al., 1998; Aszterbaum et al., 1999; Pomeroy et al., 2002). The mechanism whereby the medulloblastoma cell escapes the expected inhibition of hedgehog target gene expression by the apparently normal overexpressed PTCH1 allele is unknown and suggests that our understanding of hedgehog regulation by PTCH1 may be less complete than we would like.

Since the mechanisms by which PTCH1 loss produces tumors may differ among tumor types, it seems likely that the mechanisms by which the *PTCH1*$^{+/-}$ genotype causes the *developmental* abnormalities also may differ according to the type of abnormality. Thus, several authors have made the appealing suggestion that developmental abnormalities which occur frequently and are symmetric (e.g., both legs are equally long in BCNS patients with marfanoid changes) are likely to be due to haploinsufficiency of *PTCH1* (Bale, 1997; Hahn et al., 1998). By contrast, those developmental abnormalities that occur more sporadically and in a haphazard distribution seem more likely to be due to loss of the normal *PTCH1* allele in some cell critically important to some developmental process. In the former category of symmetric abnormalities would be overgrowth, marfanoid habitus, and characteristic skull shape changes such as frontal bossing and hypertelorism. The degree of these abnormalities can vary markedly within a single family, all members of which carry the same *PTCH1* mutation. It seems likely that they are subject to modification by background genes and perhaps by environmental factors of unknown nature. The influence of such background genes is suggested by a differing incidence of rhabdomyosarcomas in mice of different inbred strains carrying the same *ptc1* mutation (Hahn et al., 1998). In the latter category of asymmetric abnormalities are polydactyly and rib abnormalities. The identification of somatic loss of the normal *PTCH1* allele in perhaps a single, nonproliferative cell that fails to function properly at a critical time in development and thereby causes splitting or fusing of a rib presents a significant challenge indeed. However, it remains possible that differences in non-hedgehog signaling pathway gene expression that occur very locally and perhaps transiently also can affect these phenotypes. Thus, excess or deficient hedgehog signaling in mice of normal *ptc1* genotype can cause changes in rib splitting or fusion that are inconsistent among the limbs of an individual mouse.

REFERENCES

Albrecht S, Goodman J, Rajagopalan S, Levy M, Cech D, Cooley L (1994). Malignant meningioma in Gorlin's syndrome: cytogenetic and *p53* gene analysis. *J Neurosurg* 81: 466–71.

Aszterbaum M, Rothman A, Johnson RL, Fisher M, Xie J, Bonifas JM, Zhang X, Scott MP, Epstein EH Jr (1998). Identification of mutations in the human *PATCHED* gene in sporadic basal cell carcinomas and in patients with basal cell nevus syndrome. *J Invest Dermatol* 110: 885–888.

Aszterbaum M, Epstein J, Oro A, Douglas V, LeBoit PE, Scott MP, Epstein EH Jr (1999). Ultraviolet and ionizing radiation enhance the growth of BCCs and trichoblastomas in patched heterozygous knockout mice. *Nat Med* 5: 1285–1291.

Bale A (1997). Variable expressivity of patched mutations in flies and humans. *Am J Hum Genet* 60: 10–12.

Bale SJ, Amos CI, Parry DM, Bale AE (1991). Relationship between head circumference and height in normal adults and in the nevoid basal cell carcinoma syndrome and neurofibromatosis type I. *Am J Med Genet* 40: 206–210.

Barreto DC, Gomez RS, Bale AE, Boson WL, De Marco L (2000). *PTCH* gene mutations in odontogenic keratocysts. *J Dent Res* 79: 1418–1422.

Berardi R, Korba J, Melton J, Chen H (1991). Pulmonary metastasis in nevoid basal cell carcinoma syndrome. *Int Surg* 76: 64–66.

Binkley GW, Johnson HHJ (1951). Epithelioma adenoides cysticum: basal cell nevi, agenesis of the corpus callosum and dental cysts. *Arch Dermatol Syph* 63: 73–84.

Black HS, Thornby JI, Wolf JE Jr, Goldberg LH, Herd A, Rosen T, Bruce S, Tschen JA, Scott LW, Jaax S, et al. (1995). Evidence that a low-fat diet reduces the occurence of non-melanoma skin cancer. *Int J Cancer* 62: 165–169.

Bodak N, Queille S, Avril MF, Bouadjar B, Drougard C, Sarasin A, Daya-Grosjean L (1999). High levels of patched gene mutations in basal-cell carcinomas from patients with xeroderma pigmentosum. *Proc Natl Acad Sci USA* 96: 5117–5122.

Bonifas JM, Bare JW, Kerschmann RL, Master SP, Epstein EH Jr (1994). Parental origin of chromosome 9q22.3-q31 lost in basal cell carcinomas from basal cell nevus syndrome patients. *Hum Mol Genet* 3: 447–448.

Bonifas JM, Pennypacker S, Chuang PT, McMahon AP, Williams M, Rosenthal A, DeSauvage FJ, Epstein EH Jr (2001). Activation of expression of hedgehog target genes in basal cell carcinomas. *J Invest Dermatol* 116: 739–742.

Corcoran R, Scott M (2001). A mouse model for medulloblastoma and basal cell nevus syndrome. *J Neurooncol* 53: 307–318.

Cotton JL, Kavey R-EW, Palmier CE, Tunnessen WW Jr (1991). Cardiac tumors and the nevoid basal cell carcinoma syndrome. *Pediatrics* 87: 725–727.

Cowan R, Hoban P, Kelsey A, Birch J, Gattamaneni R, Evans D (1997). The gene for the naevoid basal cell carcinoma syndrome acts as a tumour-suppressor gene in medulloblastoma. *Br J Cancer* 76: 141–145.

Cristofolini M, Zumiani G, Scappini P, Piscioli F (1984). Aromatic retinoid in the chemoprevention of the progression of nevoid basal-cell carcinoma syndrome. *J Dermatol Surg Oncol* 10: 778–781.

Dahl E, Kreiborg S, Jensen B (1976). Craniofacial morphology in the nevoid basal cell carcinoma syndrome. *Int J Oral Surg* 5: 300–310.

Dahmane N, Ruiz-i-Altaba A (1999). Sonic hedgehog regulates the growth and patterning of the cerebellum. *Development* 126: 3089–3100.

Dahmane N, Lee J, Robins P, Heller P, Ruiz i Altaba, A (1997). Activation of the tran-

scription factor Gli1 and the Sonic hedgehog signalling pathway in skin tumors. *Nature* 389: 876–881.

D'Errico M, Calcagnile A, Canzona F, Didona B, Posteraro P, Cavalieri R, Corona R, Vorechovsky I, Nardo T, Stefanini M, et al. (2000). UV mutation signature in tumor suppressor genes involved in skin carcinogenesis in xeroderma pigmentosum patients. *Oncogene* 19: 463–467.

DiSanto S, Abt A, Boal D, Krummel T (1992). Fetal rhabdomyoma and nevoid basal cell carcinoma syndrome. *Pediatr Pathol* 12: 441–447.

Dong J, Gailani MR, Pomeroy SL, Reardon D, Bale AE (2000). Identification of PATCHED mutations in medulloblastomas by direct sequencing. *Hum Mutat* 16: 89–90.

Dunnick NR, Head GL, Peck GL, Yoder FW (1978). Nevoid basal cell carcinoma syndrome: radiographic manifestations including cystlike lesions of the phalanges. *Radiology* 127: 331–334.

Evans DG, Ladusans EJ, Rimmer S, Burnell LD, Thakker N, Farndon PA (1993). Complications of the naevoid basal cell carcinoma syndrome: results of a population based study. *J Med Genet* 30: 460–464.

Evans DGR, Farndon PA, Burnell LD, Gattamaneni HR, Birch JM (1991). The incidence of Gorlin syndrome in 173 consecutive cases of medulloblastoma. *Br J Cancer* 64: 959–961.

Fan H, Khavari PA (1999). Sonic hedgehog opposes epithelial cell cycle arrest. *J Cell Biol* 147: 71–76.

Fan H, Oro A, Scott M, Khavari P (1997). Induction of basal cell carcinoma features in transgenic human skin expressing Sonic Hedgehog. *Nat Med* 3: 788–792.

Forssell K, Forssell H, Kahnberg K-E (1988). Recurrence of keratocysts: a long-term follow-up study. *Int J Oral Maxillofac Surg* 17: 25–28.

Friedlander AH, Herbosa EG, Peoples JR (1988). Ocular hypertelorism, facial basal cell carcinomas, and multiple odontogenic keratocysts of the jaws. *J Am Dent Assoc* 116: 887–889.

Gailani MR, Bale SJ, Leffell DJ, DiGiovanna JJ, Peck GL, Poliak S, Drum MA, Pastakia B, McBride OW, Kase R, et al. (1992). Developmental defects in Gorlin syndrome related to a putative tumor suppressor gene on chromosome 9. *Cell* 69: 111–117.

Gailani MR, Stahle-Backdahl M, Leffell DJ, Glynn M, Zaphiropoulos PG, Pressman C, Unden AB, Dean M, Brash DE, Bale AE, et al. (1996). The role of the human homologue of *Drosophila* patched in sporadic basal cell carcinomas. *Nat Genet* 14: 78–81.

Goldberg LH, Hsu SH, Alcalay J (1989). Effectiveness of isotretinoin in preventing the appearance of basal cell carcinomas in basal cell nevus syndrome. *J Am Acad Dermatol* 21: 144–145.

Goldstein AM, Bale SJ, Peck GL, DiGiovanna JJ (1993). Sun exposure and basal cell carcinomas in the nevoid basal cell carcinoma syndrome. *J Am Acad Dermatol* 29: 34–41.

Goldstein AM, Pastakia B, DiGiovanna JJ, Poliak S, Santucci S, Kase R, Bale AE (1994). Clinical findings in two African-American families with the nevoid basal cell carcinoma syndrome (NBCC). *Am J Med Genet* 50: 272–281.

Goodrich LV, Johnson RL, Milenkovic L, McMahon JA, Scott MP (1996). Conservation of the hedgehog/patched signaling pathway from flies to mice: induction of a mouse patched gene by Hedgehog. *Genes Dev* 10: 301–312.

Goodrich LV, Milenkovic L, Higgins KM, Scott MP (1997). Altered neural cell fates and medulloblastoma in mouse *patched* mutants. *Science* 277: 1109–1113.

Gorlin RJ (1987). Nevoid basal cell carcinoma syndrome. *Medicine* 66: 98–109.

Gorlin RJ, Goltz RW (1960). Multiple nevoid basal-cell epithelioma, jaw cysts and bifid ribs: a syndrome. *N Engl J Med* 262: 908–912.

Grachtchouk M, Mo R, Yu S, Zhang X, Sasaki H, Hui CC, Dlugosz AA (2000). Basal cell carcinomas in mice overexpressing Gli2 in skin. *Nat Genet* 24: 216–217.

Hahn H, Christiansen J, Wicking C, Zaphiropoulos P, Chidambaram A, Gerrard B, Vorechovsky I, Bale A, Toftgard R, Dean M, et al. (1996a). A mammalian patched homolog is expressed in target tissues of sonic hedgehog and maps to a region associated with developmental abnormalities. *J Biol Chem* 271: 12125–12128.

Hahn H, Wicking C, Zaphiropoulos PG, Gailani MR, Shanley S, Chidambaram A, Vorechovsky I, Holmberg E, Unden AB, Gillies S, et al. Mutations of the human homologue of *Drosophila* patched in the nevoid basal cell carcinoma syndrome. *Cell* 85: 841–851.

Hahn H, Wojnowski L, Zimmer AM, Hall J, Miller G, Zimmer A (1998). Rhabdomyosarcomas and radiation hypersensitivity in a mouse model of Gorlin syndrome. *Nat Med* 4: 619–622.

Hahn H, Wojnowski L, Specht K, Kappler R, Calzada-Wack J, Potter D, Zimmer A, Mullerl U, Samson E, Quintanilla-Martinez L, et al (2000). Patched target Igf2 is indispensable for the formation of medulloblastoma and rhabdomyosarcoma. *J Biol Chem* 15: 28341–28344.

Hebrok M, Kim S, St Jacques B, McMahon A, Melton D (2000). Regulation of pancreas development by hedgehog signaling. *Development* 127: 4905–4913.

Herman TE, Siegel MJ, McAlister, WH (1991). Cardiac tumor in Gorlin syndrome. *Pediatr Radiol* 21: 234–235.

Hodak E, Ginzburg A, David M, Sandbank M (1987). Etretinate treatment of the nevoid basal cell carcinoma syndrome. *Int J Dermatol* 26: 606–609.

Hooper JE, Scott, MP (1989). The *Drosophila* patched gene encodes a putative membrane protein required for segmental patterning. *Cell* 59: 751–765.

Howell J (1980). The roots of the naevoid basal cell carcinoma syndrome. *Clin Exp Dermatol* 5: 339–348.

Howell JB, Caro MR (1959). Basal cell nevus: its relationship to multiple cutaneous cancers and associated anomalies of development. *Arch Dermatol* 79: 67–80.

Hu Z, Bonifas JM, Aragon G, Kopelovich L, Liang Y, Ohta S, Israel MA, Bickers DR, Aszterbaum M, Epstein EH Jr (2003). Evidence for lack of enhanced hedgehog target gene expression in common extracutaneous tumors. *Cancer Res* 63: 923–928.

Johnson AD, Hebert AA, Esterly NB (1986). Nevoid basal cell carcinoma syndrome: bilateral ovarian fibromas in a 3 1/2-year-old girl. *J Am Acad Dermatol* 14: 371–374.

Johnson RL, Rothman AL, Xie J, Goodrich LV, Bare JW, Bonifas JM, Quinn AG, Myers RM, Cox DR, Epstein EH Jr, et al. (1996). Human homolog of *patched* a candidate gene for the basal cell nevus syndrome. *Science* 272: 1668–1671.

Jones K, Wolf P, Jensen P, Dittrich H, Benirschke K, Bloor C (1986). The Gorlin syndrome: a genetically determined disorder associated with cardiac tumor. *Am Heart J* 111: 1013–1015.

Kagy MK, Amonette R (2000). The use of imiquimod 5% cream for the treatment of superficial basal cell carcinomas in a basal cell nevus syndrome patient. *Dermatol Surg* 26: 577–578.

Kenney A, Rowitch D (2000). Sonic hedgehog promotes G(1) cyclin expression and sustained cell cycle progression in mammalian neuronal precursors. *Mol Cell Biol* 20: 9055–9067.

Kimonis VE, Goldstein AM, Pastakia B, Yang ML, Kase R, DiGiovanna JJ, Bale AE, Bale SJ (1997). Clinical manifestations in 105 persons with nevoid basal cell carcinoma syndrome. *Am J Med Genet* 69: 299–308.

Knudson A (1971). Mutation and cancer: statistical study of retinoblastoma. *Proc Natl Acad Sci USA* 68: 820–823.

Lam CW, Xie J, To KF, Ng HK, Lee KC, Yuen NW, Lim PL, Chan LY, Tong SF, McCormick F (1999). A frequent activated smoothened mutation in sporadic basal cell carcinomas. *Oncogene* 18: 833–836.

Lewis MT, Ross S, Strickland PA, Sugnet CW, Jimenez E, Scott MP, Daniel CW (1999). Defects in mouse mammary gland development caused by conditional haploinsufficiency of Patched-1. *Development* 126: 5181–5193.

Ling G, Ahmadian A, Persson A, Unden A, Afink G, Williams C, Uhlen M, Toftgard R, Lundeberg J, Ponten F (2001). *PATCHED* and *p53* gene alterations in sporadic and hereditary basal cell cancer. *Oncogene* 20: 7770–7778.

Lo JS, Snow SN, Reizner GT, Mohs FE, Larson PO, Hruza GJ (1991). Metastatic basal cell carcinoma: report of twelve cases with a review of the literature. *J Am Acad Dermatol* 24: 715–719.

Lo Muzio L, Nocini P, Savoia A, Consolo U, Procaccini M, Zelante L, Pannone G, Bucci P, Dolci M, Bambini F, et al. (1999). Nevoid basal cell carcinoma syndrome. Clinical findings in 37 Italian affected individuals. *Clin Genet* 55: 34–40.

Long F, Zhang X, Karp S, Yang Y, McMahon A (2001). Genetic manipulation of hedgehog signaling in the endochondral skeleton reveals a direct role in the regulation of chondrocyte proliferation. *Development* 128: 5099–5108.

Makino S, Masuya H, Ishijima J, Yada J, Shiroishi T (2001). A spontaneous mouse mutation, mesenchymal dysplasia (mes), is caused by a deletion of the most C-terminal cytoplasmic domain of patched (ptc). *Dev Biol* 239: 95–106.

Matsumura Y, Nishigori C, Murakami K, Miyachi Y (2000). Allelic loss at the *PTCH* gene locus in jaw cysts but not in palmar pits in patients with basal cell nevus syndrome. *Arch Dermatol Res* 292: 475–476.

McKelvey L, Albright C, Prazak G (1960). Multiple hereditary familiar epithelial cysts of the jaws with the associated anomaly of trichoepithelioma. *Oral Surg Oral Med Oral Pathol* 13: 111–116.

Meyvisch K, Andre J, Song M, Ledoux M (1993). Basal cell nevus syndrome and congenital hydrocephaly. *Dermatology* 186: 311–312.

Milenkovic L, Goodrich L, Higgins K, Scott M (1999). Mouse patched1 controls body size determination and limb patterning. *Development* 126: 4431–4440.

Miller DL, Weinstock MA (1994). Non-melanoma skin cancer in the United States: incidence. *J Am Acad Dermatol* 30: 774–778.

Miller R, Cooper R (1972). Nevoid basal cell carcinoma syndrome. Case report: histopathology of skeletal lesions. *Clin Orthop* 89: 246–252.

Morison W, Jerdan M, Hoover T, Farmer E (1986). UV radiation-induced tumors in haired mice: identification as squamous cell carcinomas. *J Natl Cancer Inst* 77: 1155–1162.

Nakano Y, Guerrero A, Hidalgo A, Taylor A, Whittle JRS, Ingham PW (1989). A protein with several possible membrane-spanning domains encoded by the *Drosophila* segment polarity gene patched. *Nature* 341: 5078–5018.

Nilsson M, Unden AB, Krause D, Malmqwist U, Raza K, Zaphiropoulos PG, Toftgard R (2000). Induction of basal cell carcinomas and trichoepitheliomas in mice overexpressing GLI-1. *Proc Natl Acad Sci USA* 97: 3438–3443.

Nishigori C, Yarosh D, Donawho C, Kripke M (1996). The immune system in ultraviolet carcinogenesis. *J Investig Dermatol Symp Proc* 1: 143–146.

Nusslein-Volhard C, Wieschaus E (1980). Mutations affecting segment number and polarity in Drosophila. *Nature* 287: 795–801.

Peck G, Gross E, Butkus D, DiGiovanna J (1982). Chemoprevention of basal cell carcinoma with isotretinoin. *J Am Acad Dermatol* 6: 815–823.

Peris K, Fargnoli M, Chimenti S (1999). Preliminary observations on the use of topical tazarotene to treat basal-cell carcinoma. *N Engl J Med* 341: 1767–1768.

Pietsch T, Waha A, Koch A, Kraus J, Albrecht S, Tonn J, Sorensen N, Berthold F, Henk B, Schmandt N, et al. (1997). Medulloblastomas of the desmoplastic variant carry mutations of the human homologue of *Drosophila* patched. *Cancer Res* 57: 2085–2088.

Pomeroy S, Tamayo P, Gaasenbeek M, Sturla L, Angelo M, McLaughlin M, Kim J, Goumnerova L, Black P, Lau C, et al. (2002). Prediction of central nervous system embryonal tumour outcome based on gene expression. *Nature* 415: 436–442.

Raffel C, Jenkins RB, Frederick L, Hebrink D, Alderete B, Fults DW, James CD (1997). Sporadic medulloblastomas contain PTCH mutaions. *Cancer Res* 57: 842–845.

Ratcliffe JF, Shanley S, Ferguson J, Chenevix-Trench G (1995a). The diagnostic implication of falcine calcification on plain skull radiographs of patients with basal cell naevus syndrome and the incidence of falcine calcification in their relatives and two control groups. *Br J Radiol* 68: 361–368.

Ratcliffe JF, Shanley S, Chenevix-Trench G (1995b). The prevalence of cervical and thoracic congenital skeletal abnormalities in basal cell naevus syndrome; a review of cervical and chest radiographs in 80 patients with BCNS. *Br J Radiol* 68: 596–599.

Reifenberger J, Wolter M, Weber RG, Megahed M, Ruzicka T, Lichter P, Reifenberger G (1998). Missense mutations in SMOH in sporadic basal cell carcinomas of the skin and primitive neuroectodermal tumors of the central nervous system. *Cancer Res* 58: 1798–1803.

Sanchez-Conejo-Mir J, Camacho F (1989). Nevoid basal cell carcinoma syndrome: combined etretinate and surgical treatment. *J Dermatol Surg Oncol* 15: 868–871.

Scully R, Galdabini J, McNeely B (1976). Case records of the Massachusetts General Hospital. Weekly clinicopathological exercises. Case 14-1976. *N Engl J Med* 294: 772–777.

Shanley S, Ratcliffe J, Hockey A, Haan E, Oley C, Ravine D, Martin N, Wicking C, Chenevix-Trench G (1994). Nevoid basal cell carcinoma syndrome: review of 118 affected individuals. *Am J Med Genet* 50: 282–290.

Southwick GJ, Schwartz RA (1979). The basal cell nevus syndrome: disasters occurring among a series of 36 patients. *Cancer* 44: 2294–2305.

Strange PR, Lang PG (1992). Long-term management of basal cell nevus syndrome with topical tretinoin and 5-fluorouracil. *J Am Acad Dermatol* 27: 842–845.

Sweet H, Bronson R, Donahue L, Davisson M (1996). Mesenchymal dysplasia: a recessive mutation on chromosome 13 of the mouse. *J Hered* 87: 87–95.

Taipale J, Beachy P (2001). The Hedgehog and Wnt signalling pathways in cancer. *Nature* 411: 349–354.

Tamoney HJ (1969). Basal cell nevoid syndrome. *Am Surg* 35: 279–283.

Taylor MD, Liu L, Raffel C, Hui C, Mainprize T, Zhang X, Agatep R, Chiappa S, Gao L, Lowrance A, et al. (2002). Mutations in SUFU predispose to medulloblastoma. *Nat Genet* 31: 306–310.

Unden A, Holmberg E, Lundh-Rozell, Stahle-Backdahle M, Zaphiropolous P, Toftgard R, Vorechovsky I (1996). Mutations in the human homolog of *Drosophila* patched (PTCH) in basal cell carcinomas and the Gorlin syndrome: different in vivo mechanisms of PTCH inactivation. *Cancer Res* 56: 4562–4565.

Vorechovsky I, Tingby O, Hartman M, Stromberg B, Nister M, Collins VP, Toftgard R (1997). Somatic mutations in the human homologue of *Drosophila* patched in primitive neuroectodermal tumours. *Oncogene* 15: 361–366.

Wechsler-Reya R, Scott M (1999). Control of neuronal precursor proliferation in the cerebellum by Sonic Hedgehog. *Neuron* 22: 103–114.

Wetmore C, Eberhart DE, Curran T (2000). The normal patched allele is expressed in medulloblastomas from mice with heterozygous germ-line mutation of patched. *Cancer Res* 60: 2239–2246.

Wicking C, Shanley S, Smyth I, Gillies S, Negus K, Graham S, Suthers G, Haites N, Edwards M, Wainwright B, et al. (1997). Most germ-line mutations in the naevoid basal cell carcinoma syndrome lead to a premature termination of the PATCHED protein, and no genotype–phenotype correlations are evident. *Am J Hum Genet* 60: 21–26.

Winkler PA, Guyuron B (1987). Multiple metastases from basal cell naevus syndrome. *Br J Plast Surg* 40: 528–531.

Wolter M, Reifenberger J, Sommer C, Ruzicka T, Reifenberger G (1997). Mutations in the human homologue of *Drosophila* segment polarity gene patched (PTCH) in sporadic basal cell carcinomas of the skin and primitive neuroectodermal tumors of the central nervous system. *Cancer Res* 57: 2581–2585.

Xie J, Murone M, Luoh S, Ryan A, Gu Q, Zhang C, Bonifas JM, Rosenthal A, Epstein EH Jr, de Sauvage FJ (1998). Activating SMOOTHENED mutations in sporadic basal-cell carcinoma. *Nature* 391: 90–92.

Yee KC, Tan CY, Bhatt KB, Davies AM (1993). Case report: sclerotic bone lesions in Gorlin's syndrome. *Br J Radiol* 66: 77–80.

Zhang Y, Kalderon D (2001). Hedgehog acts as a somatic stem cell factor in the *Drosophila* ovary. *Nature* 410: 599–604.

Zurawel RH, Allen C, Wechsler-Reya R, Scott MP, Raffel C (2000). Evidence that haploinsufficiency of Ptch leads to medulloblastoma in mice. *Genes Chromosomes Cancer* 28: 77–81.

20 | *GLI3* and the Pallister-Hall and Greig Cephalopolysyndactyly Syndromes

LESLIE G. BIESECKER

Pallister-Hall syndrome (PHS) and Greig cephalopolysyndactyly syndrome (GCPS) are distinct, pleiotropic developmental anomaly syndromes that are caused by mutations in *GLI3* and inherited in an autosomal dominant pattern. The major anomalies in PHS include hypothalamic hamartoma, central or postaxial polydactyly, and airway anomalies. The major anomalies of GCPS include macrocephaly with hypertelorism and pre- or postaxial polydactyly. Both disorders have a wide spectrum of severity but are clinically distinct. The *GLI3* gene encodes a C2H2-type zinc finger transcription factor that is downstream in the sonic hedgehog signaling pathway. The mutational spectrum of *GLI3* mutations in patients with GCPS is broad, including translocations, gross and molecular deletions, amino acid substitutions, and frameshift and nonsense mutations. The mutational spectrum of PHS is narrow, including only frameshift mutations that preserve the zinc finger binding domain. A hypothesis has been proposed to explain the correlation of these two phenotypes and the associated mutations.

LOCUS AND DEVELOPMENTAL PATHWAY

GLI3 is a paralog of the *GLI* gene family, which also includes *GLI1* and *GLI2* (Kinzler et al., 1988; Ruppert et al., 1988, 1990). These genes encode zinc finger transcription factor proteins, the single largest cluster of orthologous genes in the human genome. The human *GLI1* locus is on chromosome 12q13 (Reifenberger et al., 1996), *GLI2* is on chromosome 2q14 (Matsumoto et al., 1996), and *GLI3* is on chromosome 7p13 (Ruppert et al., 1990). These three gene products share six domains of conserved sequence in addition to the zinc finger DNA-binding domain, which conforms to the C2H2 subtype. The genomic structures of the three genes are distinct. Although *GLI1* and *GLI3* are similarly organized (11 or 13 small exons, followed by a terminal exon that encodes about half of the protein), *GLI1* occupies only about 12–13 kb of genomic DNA, whereas *GLI3* is spread over nearly 300 kb. *GLI2* has 12 exons spread over nearly 200 kb of genomic DNA, but the large exon is exon 10, with two smaller exons, 11 and 12. Furthermore, *GLI2* has three exons that can be alternatively spliced to yield four mRNA isoforms, whereas *GLI1* has two putative isoforms (Wang and Rothnagel, 2001) and *GLI3* only a single known isoform. The GLI proteins are orthologs of the *Drosophila cubitus interruptus* (*ci*) gene (Ruppert et al., 1988) (note that the Drosophila *Gli* gene is gliotactin and is not an ortholog of vertebrate *Gli*).

The *GLI1* cDNA open reading frame encodes a predicted protein of 1106 amino acids; *GLI2* is predicted to encode 812, 829, 1241, or 1258 amino acids; and *GLI3* is predicted to encode 1595 amino acids. A total of 16 GLI proteins are identified in the GenBank database. These include three each for human, mouse, *Xenopus*, and zebrafish. In addition, one or two GLI homologs have been identified in rat, quail, and chicken. The chicken *GLI2* gene product designated in some early studies was actually *GLI3*. There are several higher numbered GLI paralogs in human, mouse, and *Xenopus*; however, these may be better classified as human krüppel-related (HKR) proteins instead of GLIs. Other closely related proteins include YY1 and the ZIC protein family. Like *Drosophila*, *Caenorhabditis elegans* has a single GLI homolog, *tra-1*. The zinc finger binding domains of these proteins are extremely well conserved.

Studies of the developmental expression pattern of *GLI* family genes have been performed in mice and chickens. The murine data will be summarized here (Hui et al., 1994). Transcription of all *Gli* transcripts is first detected at 7.5 to 8.5 days postconception. Mesodermal expression of all three paralogs was widespread, but no significant expression was detected in the ectoderm. Ectodermal expression showed interesting differences. *Gli1* expression is mostly limited to the ventral neural tube, whereas *Gli2* and *Gli3* expression was more widespread throughout the ectoderm. As development progressed, it became clear that *Gli2* and *Gli3* were expressed more in the posterior neural tube. At organogenesis, expression of all three genes faded, becoming undetectable when fetuses had completed organogenesis. There is a definite overlap in the expression patterns of *Gli2* and *Gli3*, both of which are distinct from the pattern of *Gli1* expression. This similarity will arise again in the discussion of the murine mutants below. However, it is critical to keep in mind that expression of *Gli* transcripts may not directly correlate with Gli protein effector functions as at least some of the Gli proteins have complex posttranslational regulation (see below, Developmental Pathogenesis).

The functions of these genes have been studied in mice and chickens through natural mutants, knockout experiments, and experimental manipulation of gene expression. Surprisingly, no phenotypic abnormalities have been detected in animals that are null for *Gli1*. The gene expression pattern clearly suggests a role for *Gli1* in dorsal-ventral polarization of the developing neural tube (Lee et al., 1997). Nevertheless, there is no functional or histologic evidence of spinal cord abnormalities in these animals. *Gli2* knockouts have a significant phenotype that includes cleft palate, tooth defects, vertebral anomalies, and short limbs but no polydactyly (Mo et al., 1997). GLI2 is also reported to have a role in tax-associated retroviral replication. The evidence for the developmental importance of *GLI3* derives from a series of mutant animals, including several alleles grouped as extra toes (*Gli3^{Xt}*) (Johnson, 1967), anterior digit deformity (Pohl et al., 1990), polydactyly Nagoya (Schimmang et al., 1994), and brachyphalangy (Johnson, 1969). The best studied of these is *Gli3^{XtJ}*, which is caused by a deletion that includes exons 10–14 and 51,530 bp of sequence (Maynard et al., 2002). Exquisitely detailed studies with drawings of the anomalies were performed by Johnson (1967). These studies showed the anterior and posterior digit duplications, which are remarkably consistent with those seen in humans with GCPS. Other abnormalities seen in heterozygotes include a white belly spot, the presence of an interfrontal bone (an abnormal finding in mice), and an elevated incidence of hydrocephalus. Homozygotes showed additional severe malformations and were often stillborn. These malformations include parietal exencephaly with numerous other brain abnormalities. Other than ectopic adrenal glands, there were few visceral abnormalities. Other abnormalities included abnormal olfactory nerves, microphthalmia, absent lateral semicircular canals, abnormal skull ossification, fused neural arches of vertebra, abnormal sternum, and severe limb anomalies. The limb anomalies include high-order polydactyly (as many as nine digits per limb), abnormal metacarpals, phalangeal hypoplasia or aplasia, radial hypo- or aplasia, and short and thick proximal limbs. Closure of the neural tube was delayed. Crosses of *Gli2* knockout and *Gli3^{XtJ}* animals showed that animals with three alleles had a more severe presentation, especially in *Gli2^{KO}/+*, *Gli3^{XtJ}/Gli3^{XtJ}* animals, demonstrating a degree of redundancy of *Gli2* and *Gli3* (Mo et al., 1997). These studies of murine *Gli2* and *Gli3* mutants demonstrate a range of anomalies that show both distinct anomalies and a significant degree of overlap with the human disorders PHS and GCPS.

CLINICAL FEATURES

GCPS

The story of these allelic disorders is best developed in the historical order of their development. The phenotypic descriptor *Greig cephalopolysyndactyly syndrome* is now used to describe a syndrome of macrocephaly with broad and prominent forehead, hypertelorism (Fig. 20–1), and polysyndactyly (Gorlin et al., 1990). The eponym was coined to credit the clinical descriptions of David Middleton Greig,* a surgeon from Edinburgh, Scotland (Greig, 1926). Initially, the term *Greig's syndrome* (absent the word *cephalopolysyndactyly*) was used to describe the dyad of macrocephaly with hypertelorism. However, this latter descriptor is neither specific nor useful, and its use is discouraged. The limb anomalies of GCPS are markedly variable. While it is classically considered to include preaxial polydactyly (Fig. 20–2), postaxial polydactyly may be more common, at least in the hands. Thus, the combination of postaxial duplication in the hands and preaxial duplication in the feet is most common (sometimes termed *crossed polydactyly*). The duplications are not often complete and may instead define a spectrum of great toe or thumb widening, which can be mild or severe. The postaxial polydactyly may also be subtle, comprising a nubbin or vestigial digit along the lateral aspect of the limb. The syndactyly is also markedly variable: some patients have nearly complete cutaneous syndactyly, and some patients have none. Other anomalies seen in GCPS are fairly low in frequency: mental retardation or learning disabilities, agenesis of the corpus callosum, and inguinal or abdominal hernias.

As there are no clear diagnostic criteria for GCPS, the boundaries of the syndrome are undefined. At the severe end, there is substantial

*This surname is pronounced 'greg,' not 'greeg.' The latter is the pronunciation of the Norwegian composer (Grieg).

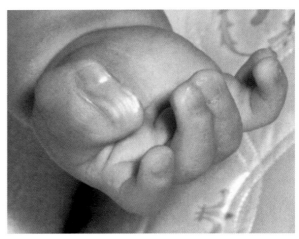

Figure 20–2. Polysyndactyly of Greig cephalopolysyndactyly syndrome. This patient has partial duplication of the thumb with cutaneous syndactyly of digits 3 and 4. (Photo courtesy of R.N. Schimke.)

overlap with the acrocallosal syndrome (ACLS) (Schinzel, 1982; Schinzel and Kaufmann, 1986). In addition to macrocephaly, hypertelorism, and polysyndactyly, patients with ACLS are thought to have mental retardation, seizures, hydrocephalus, inguinal and umbilical hernias, and absence of the corpus callosum. The distinction of ACLS from GCPS is problematic in several ways. Schinzel (1982) coined the *ACLS* designation on the basis of several affected individuals who were born in nearby cantons of Switzerland with this syndrome. A number of subsequent cases were identified, including affected siblings with normal parents. Taken together, these data strongly suggested the existence of a syndrome distinct form GCPS and inherited in an autosomal recessive pattern. However, prior to that report and subsequently, a number of sporadic patients have been described; but by definition, the inheritance pattern cannot be determined in these cases. Most often, the physician presumes that when a child is born with sporadic macrocephaly, hypertelorism, and polysyndactyly, the most appropriate diagnosis is ACLS if the child has other anomalies, mental retardation, and seizures and GCPS if these features are absent. This leads to circular reasoning: patients are diagnosed with ACLS if severe and GCPS if mild, and it is then concluded that the diagnosis correlates with the severity of the manifestations. Although it is very likely that ACLS is a distinct disorder, it is not clear that the current phenotypic classification of patients in the medical literature is valid.

At the other end of the severity spectrum from ACLS is the issue of patients with preaxial polysyndactyly or crossed polydactyly with normal craniofacial manifestations or mild craniofacial alterations insufficient to warrant a diagnosis of GCPS. Most practitioners would code these patients as preaxial polydactyly type 4, crossed polydactyly, or nonsyndromic polysyndactyly. Again, as in the ACLS/GCPS problem denoted above, the boundaries are not defined and there are precious little data that include detailed clinical characterizations with mutation studies. There may be a tendency to discount craniofacial features such as macrocephaly or hypertelorism when they are mild and unassociated with functional consequences.[†] Because of these issues, GCPS should be provisionally considered as a spectrum of anomalies that ranges from isolated preaxial polydactyly through more severe polysyndactyly into typical GCPS with polydactyly, craniofacial alterations, and normal intelligence and finally to a severe picture of limb and craniofacial anomalies with mental retardation and other anomalies that is difficult to distinguish from ACLS. It is hoped that careful genotype–phenotype studies will resolve these questions; but at this time, there are a number of good clinical surveys and a number of elegant

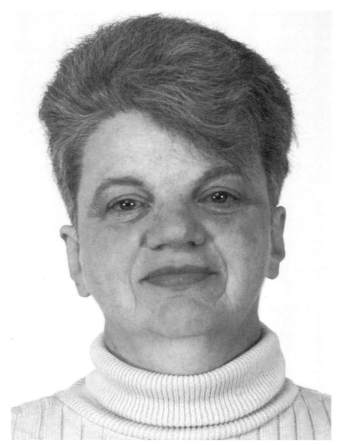

Figure 20–1. Craniofacial features of Greig cephalopolysyndactyly syndrome. This patient has a high, broad, and prominent forehead; hypertelorism; and a widened nasal bridge.

[†]It is worth noting that many persons consider mild to moderate hypertelorism as a positive attribute. A number of models and actors have apparent hypertelorism. This may lead families and physicians to ignore this finding and classify mild GCPS patients as non-syndromic polydactyly.

molecular biology papers, but none includes both. These issues will be revisited below following the discussion of the molecular etiology.

PHS‡

The syndrome of hypothalamic hamartoma (Fig. 20–3), polydactyly (Fig. 20–4), imperforate anus, and epiglottic, laryngeal, or other airway anomalies (Fig. 20–5) was described in the modern medical literature by Philip Pallister, Judith Hall, and colleagues (Hall et al., 1980). In 1980, they reported on a series of six infants, all of whom were sporadic and died in the neonatal period. The cause of death was believed to be a combination of intractable aspiration from the airway anomalies and panhypopituitarism secondary to the hypothalamic hamartoma. PHS was determined to be familial in 1993 and 1994, when a number of families were reported with autosomal dominant inheritance (Sills et al., 1993; Topf et al., 1993; Penman Splitt et al., 1994; Sama et al., 1994). The manifestations of PHS are remarkably variable (Bonnemann et al., 1995; Biesecker and Graham, 1996; Haskins-Olney, 1996). The disorder displays the common pattern for dominantly inherited traits where larger families are typically mildly affected and sporadic cases are more often severe. Of course, founders can also be mildly affected, but these children may not be diagnosed with PHS due to widespread misunderstanding of the range of variability of the disorder.

Hypothalamic hamartoma§ is a rare lesion that has a high but not perfect diagnostic specificity. It can occur as an isolated anomaly. In such cases, it is commonly associated with either endocrine or neuro-

‡Synonyms include congenital hamartomablastoma syndrome, Hall-Pallister syndrome, cerebroacroviseral early lethality syndrome.
§Some authors use the term *hamartoblastoma*. This is due to the immature appearance of the histological specimens taken from infants. Biopsies of older persons are described as "hamartomas." It is believed that the difference is due to maturation with the ageing of the patient, not to histological heterogeneity.

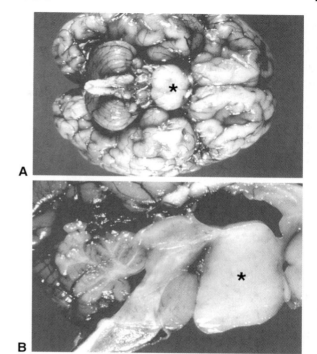

Figure 20–3. Gross anatomy of the hypothalamic hamartoma in a patient with Pallister-Hall syndrome. (*A*) View of the inferior surface of the brain showing the position of the hamartoma (*) anterior (right) to the brain stem. (*B*) Midline sagittal brain view showing the position of the hamartoma (*) in the anterior floor of the third ventricle anterior to the brain stem. (Photo courtesy of J.M. Graham, Jr.)

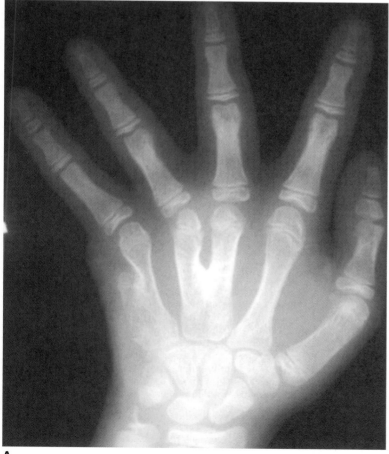

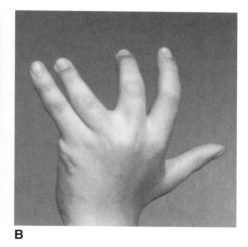

Figure 20–4. The hand in Pallister-Hall syndrome (PHS). (*A*) This radiograph shows the residual osseous malformations in a young adult with PHS. The third and fourth metacarpals (counting from the thumb or radial side) appear fused at their bases. In addition, there is a partial duplication of the fifth metacarpal. This patient had a well-formed digit articulating with the partial sixth metacarpal that was removed when he was young. (*B*) The same hand, illustrating the splaying of the third and fourth fingers due to deviation of the metacarpal heads.

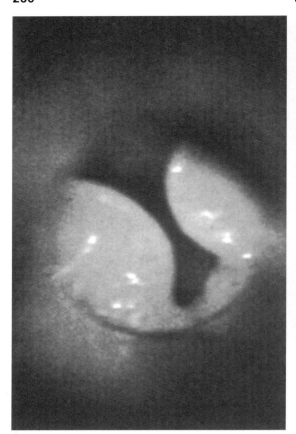

A

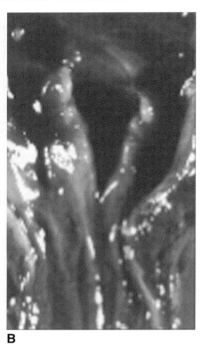

B

Figure 20–5. Airway malformations are common in Pallister-Hall syndrome. (*A*) Endoscopic photograph of a bifid epiglottis. These lesions are nearly always asymptomatic. (*B*) Photograph from an autopsy case showing a cleft larynx. These lesions are usually associated with severe aspiration.

logic symptoms (Breningstall, 1985; Boyko et al., 1991; Squires et al., 1995). The endocrine symptoms include precocious puberty (common), panhypopituitarism or growth hormone deficiency (less common). Isolated thyroid hormone deficiency has not been associated with hypothalamic hamartoma. The neurologic complications of isolated hypothalamic hamartomas are generally severe and intractable when they do occur. The most common symptom complex is intractable mixed seizure disorder with mid-childhood intellectual decline associated with severe behavioral disorder. Syndromic hypothalamic hamartomas have been reported with a number of disorders other than PHS. They include the oral-facial-digital syndrome (Fujiwara et al., 1999) and the Bardet-Biedl syndrome (Diaz et al., 1991) as well as a number of multiple malformation syndromes that are not classified (Muenke et al., 1991). It is critical to note that the neuroendocrine complications of syndromic hypothalamic hamartomas appear to be distinct from the isolated lesions. Mental retardation and seizures are rare in PHS and, when they do occur, are generally mild. Most patients with PHS do not have endocrine complications, but the few who do are generally abnormal in only one axis (precocious puberty or growth hormone most commonly). Hypothalamic hamartomas can be reliably imaged only using magnetic resonance (Boyko et al., 1991; Biesecker et al., 1996) (Fig. 20–3*C*). They can be subtle and are easily missed if the radiologist is not specifically requested to look for them. Others are startlingly large (>4 cm) but often asymptomatic. Prior publications claim that the hamartomas are isointense to gray matter on all pulse sequences. However, the advent of the FLuid L Attenuated Inversion Recovery (FLAIR) techniques has rendered this criterion obsolete. A number of hypothalamic hamartomas show elevated signal intensity on FLAIR compared to surrounding gray matter. This should not be misinterpreted as a sign of a malignancy. Hypothalamic hamartomas do not enhance with gadolinium contrast agents.

The airway anomalies of PHS are also interesting and relatively specific. The most common manifestation is a bifid epiglottis (Fig. 20–5*A*) (Ondrey et al., 2000). This malformation is nearly always asymptomatic.‖ It is known to occur only in a few other disorders, including Bardet-Biedl syndrome (one case) and oral-facial-digital syndrome (one case) (Matheny et al., 2000). Thus, bifid epiglottis is a highly specific diagnostic sign for PHS. The epiglottis is easy to visualize with a small-caliber, flexible endoscope via the nasal passages. The laryngeal mirror is also effective but cannot be used for photographic documentation. A more severe airway malformation is the laryngeal cleft. These lesions (Fig. 20–5*B*) vary significantly in length but share the attribute of causing intractable aspiration. As mentioned above, it is believed that these lesions contribute to the early demise of the children who are so affected. It has been reported that a number of patients with PHS have atypical lobation of the lungs. This is not known to cause symptoms but may be a useful diagnostic sign. No systematic survey of PHS patients has been done to document the frequency of this manifestation.

The limb anomalies of PHS are also unusual but not as specific as the airway and CNS manifestations mentioned above. The classic manifestation is central polydactyly (also known as *insertional polydactyly* or *mesoaxial polydactyly*). This term intends to describe a limb where there are six well-formed digits with a single normal thumb or great toe, associated with a forked or bifid metacarpal or metatarsal (Fig. 20–4). The designations all presume that the primary defect is a partial duplication of the third or fourth ray; however, this should be treated with some skepticism. There are no data to show that the alternative explanation is not valid: that there is a postaxial duplication with a separate well-formed sixth metacarpal or metatarsal and an abnormal fusion of the proximal third and fourth metacarpal or metatarsal. In spite of this mechanistic conundrum, the so-called central polydactyly is also a rare anomaly, reported in only a few syndromes: PHS, McKusick-Kaufman syndrome (see Chapter 105), Holt-

‖Case reports in the ENT literature would suggest otherwise but suffer from severe ascertainment bias. The only patients who were examined were those who complained of symptoms.

Oram syndrome (see Chapter 69), and oral-facial-digital syndrome type 6 (Winter et al., 1993).

On the basis of these relatively specific malformations, it would appear that PHS is straightforward to diagnose, which is generally true. Simple clinical diagnostic criteria have been published (Biesecker et al., 1996), which take into account the hypothalamic hamartoma and central polydactyly in probands with more relaxed criteria for the relatives of a diagnosed probands. Caution must be exercised when diagnosing patients of west central African descent as postaxial polydactyly is quite common in this group and may lead to false-positive diagnoses.

Although it is straightforward to diagnose PHS, there are a number of challenges that can arise. Like GCPS, the mild end of the spectrum is not defined. A number of cases are known where there are multiple family members with central and postaxial polydactyly with bifid epiglottis but no hypothalamic hamartomas. It is not clear whether this represents a mild form of PHS or a distinct disorder. A further pitfall is that hypothalamic hamartomas and bifid epiglottis, although highly specific, can be very subtle and are often missed. Small hypothalamic hamartomas can be difficult to diagnose on magetic resonance imaging (MRI), and if a patient does not have endocrine or neurologic symptoms, an MRI would probably not be ordered at all. Similarly, since bifid epiglottis is nearly always asymptomatic, it is commonly undiagnosed. This is true even among patients who have undergone placement of an endotracheal tube for anesthetic to repair the polydactyly. Nearly all of our patients with bifid epiglottis had previously undergone endotracheal anesthesia, and none was known to have a bifid epiglottis. Therefore, patients who present with apparently nonsyndromic polydactyly should be evaluated carefully by a clinician familiar with these pitfalls. In addition, patients in the medical literature who are said to have nonsyndromic polydactyly but have not undergone detailed studies to exclude these subtle malformations should be viewed with skepticism. Following the discussion of the molecular data, a model will be presented that takes these factors into account.

IDENTIFICATION OF GENE AND MUTATIONAL SPECTRUM

The original molecular studies on GCPS were performed in the laboratory of Prof. Karl-Heinz Grzeschik in Marburg, Germany. It had been observed by others that there were a number of GCPS patients who had translocations or visible deletions of chromosome 7p13-15 (Drabkin et al., 1989; Wagner et al., 1990). Some of these translocations were associated with familial segregation of GCPS, and it was hypothesized that the gene for GCPS lies in this region of the genome. Three of the translocations were shown to interrupt the *GLI3* gene (Vortkamp et al., 1991), a zinc finger transcription factor gene that had been previously cloned by the Vogelstein group (Ruppert et al., 1990). The *GLI3* gene is a member of the *GLI* gene family, which is in turn a member of the C2H2 family of transcription factors. The prototype is the *krüppel* gene of *Drosophila* (Kinzler et al., 1988; Ruppert et al., 1988). Surprisingly little was accomplished in advancing the understanding of either *GLI3* or GCPS in the intervening 6 years, until the discovery that another pleiotropic developmental anomaly syndrome, PHS, was shown to be allelic to GCPS.

The determination that PHS was allelic to GCPS was based on a positional cloning strategy using a handful of families with mild PHS (Kang et al., 1997a). The candidate region was small and included only two known genes, INHBA (inhibin β-A) and *GLI3*. After excluding INHBA as a candidate, the genomic structure of *GLI3* was determined (Kang et al., 1997c), and sequencing revealed frameshift mutations in the gene in two smaller families (Kang et al., 1997b).

Although there are still only a few published mutations in patients with PHS, we have found a number of additional mutations, all of which are 3′ to the zinc finger–encoding domain. The obvious question posed by this discovery was how mutations in a single transcription factor could be responsible for two distinct disorders. Table 20–1 shows that the mutational spectrum for these two phenotypes is not the same. On the basis of the discussion in the phenotype section above, GCPS and preaxial polydactyly (PPD) are grouped together. Similarly, PHS and postaxial polydactyly type A (PAPA) are grouped together. The former grouping shows a broad range of mutations of all classes and is most simply explained by haploinsufficiency. For the PHS/PAPA phenotype, all known mutations correspond to a single type, frameshift or nonsense mutations in the gene 3′ to the zinc finger–encoding domain (Biesecker, 2001). These data figure prominently in developing a model of GLI3 posttranslational regulation, as discussed below under Developmental Pathogenesis (Biesecker, 1997).

COUNSELING AND TREATMENT

Recurrence Risk Estimation and Counseling

The counseling issues for GCPS, PHS, PPD, and PAPA are similar to many other conditions that manifest developmental anomalies inherited in an autosomal dominant pattern. The families can be divided into two groups for consideration of recurrence risk estimation and counseling. The first group includes those with one of these phenotypes inherited in an autosomal dominant pattern with multiple affected family members, and the second includes families with a single sporadic case. The larger families can be given a fairly precise estimate of the likely severity for future offspring that encompasses the range apparent in the affected members of the family, with a small probability that any future child would exceed this range (either more mild or severe). This is based on the clinical observation that the severity of familial PHS and GCPS varies less within family members than it does among different families. Thus, affected members of a large family with variable polydactyly (central and postaxial), asymptomatic hypothalamic hamartomas, and bifid epiglottis have a 50% risk with each pregnancy of having a similarly affected child and a small chance of having a child affected with severe PHS (panhypopituitarism, gelastic seizures, mental retardation, laryngeal clefts, etc.) and a similarly small chance of having an affected child with postaxial polydactyly type B without hypothalamic hamartoma or bifid epiglottis. There are no known cases of nonpenetrance among families with autosomal dominant PHS or GCPS when they are carefully and fully examined with the appropriate modalities (see Note Added in Proof).

Families who have a child affected with a sporadic case of PHS or GCPS pose a different challenge. As is generally true for dominant inheritance, the phenotype of sporadic cases shows a wider range of severity than that seen in familial cases, with a skew toward the severe end of the spectrum. There is no doubt that severe cases of both PHS and GCPS exist and that these patients have reduced reproductive fitness. There are no known cases of gonadal or germinal mosaicism for either GCPS or PHS; however, there is no reason to assume that this cannot occur. It must be considered as a possibility that a family could harbor mosaicism in one parent with a substantial recurrence risk. In addition, there is no reason to assume that a sporadic proband may be mosaic and, thus, more mildly affected than would be expected were the same mutation present in a nonmosaic form. The latter probands may have a risk of having affected children who are more severely affected than the proband.

Further muddying the water is a case report of a family who have two affected children with an apparent phenocopy of PHS (Ng et al.,

Table 20–1. Human and *Drosophila* GLI3 Mutations

Translocation	Deletion	Missense	Splicing	5′ Frameshift/Nonsense	3′ Frameshift Nonsense	
GCPS/PPD	3	16	4	5	8	6
PHS/PAPA	0	0	0	0	0	3*

*In addition, the author has identified 16 more 3′ frameshift mutations but no mutations of any other type in patients with PHS (Biesecker, unpublished data). GCPS, Greig cephalopolysyndactyly syndrome; PHS, Pallister-Hall syndrome; PPD, preaxial polydactyly; PAPA, postaxial polydactyly type A.

2002). Both parents are completely normal and the manifestations in the children are unusual and severe. The children have insertional polydactyly, hypothalamic hamartomas, and bifid epiglottis with additional atypical features such as severe brachydactyly, intractable complex seizures, progressively deteriorating mental retardation, and a severe behavior disorder. Mutations in *GLI3* have been excluded in this family, suggesting locus heterogeneity in addition to the phenotypic discrepancy with typical PHS. These children were originally diagnosed with PHS, though we argue that they have a genetically and phenotypically distinct disorder. Nevertheless, this case serves as a warning that patients with apparently sporadic PHS must be carefully evaluated and that the small risk of this phenocopy must be included in discussions of natural history and recurrence risk.

Based on these considerations, further development of molecular testing is a priority for these disorders. The ability to determine a molecular lesion in sporadic cases would allow exclusion of the phenocopy and provide reassurance to families. It does not appear that molecular testing for the large autosomal dominant families has much to offer as the mild nature of the phenotype argues against termination as a relevant option. For sporadic cases of PHS and GCPS, molecular testing may be extremely useful to confirm the diagnosis in the newborn period. Such testing can be helpful in GCPS to predict the phenotype, but there is no correlation of mutations and severity of phenotype in PHS. The GCPS correlation is based on the observation that the majority of patients with severe GCPS (mental retardation or learning disabilities and/or seizures) have large deletions that extend well beyond *GLI3* on 7p13 (Johnston et al., in press). These patients can be considered to have a GCPS contiguous gene syndrome, and it is presumed that it is the loss of flanking genes on 7p13 that causes the additional symptomatology. Finally, there is the issue of ACLS described above. Although ACLS appears to be very rare, it should be expected that some children who appear to have severe GCPS actually have autosomal recessive ACLS. As of this writing, there are no identified genes (or any linkage data) or clinical findings to allow ACLS to be distinguished from severe GCPS (Brueton et al., 1992). Again, *GLI3* testing may be the most productive avenue in these cases as a *GLI3* deletion would exclude ACLS.

One key counseling issue is to comprehensively and accurately convey to the family the range of severity (which may be quite different from their prior experience). In most families, this leads to a great deal of consternation and ambiguity as there is often a small probability of having a child with a severe, debilitating condition with mental retardation and/or seizures, a relatively larger probability of having a child with major but correctable malformations (most often polydactyly) without significant neurocognitive sequelae, and a small chance of having a child with trivial manifestations of postaxial polydactyly with no other clinically relevant manifestations. These situations are extremely challenging as the enormous range of severity and the inability to precisely predict the phenotype give little indication to the family as to the proper course of action. Many families and practitioners are exposed to a significantly biased range of severity of these conditions in the medical literature. While we have the advantage in the research setting of seeing large and mildly affected families with excellent outcome, many published cases are severe and lead to bias.

Treatment

PHS

The birth of a child with sporadic PHS can be a medical emergency. As mentioned above, some cases of PHS are severe and can be associated with neonatal death. Although the data are not clear, it appears that early mortality in PHS is primarily attributable to adrenal insufficiency secondary to panhypopituitarism and severe airway malformations. Urgent evaluations and treatment may avert death in such cases. Immediate securing of the airway should be the first priority. Initial examination with a laryngoscope may be all that is necessary if the epiglottis and upper laryngeal structures are visualized and appear normal. Intubation of a child with laryngeal clefts can be difficult and may need to be done with endoscopic guidance. As noted above, bifid epiglottis is usually asymptomatic and should not be treated unless there is additional evidence of airway compromise. Once the airway is secured, panhypopituitarism and its most important immediate consequence, adrenal insufficiency, should be excluded or treated if present. The existence of hypoglycemia, hyponatremia, and hyperkalemia can complicate the treatment of other manifestations and alone can lead to early death. Other medical emergencies include imperforate anus and subsequent bowel obstruction.

After the neonatal period, there are a number of other issues that may need to addressed. Hypothalamic hamartomas should not be removed surgically, ablated by radiation, or biopsied unless there is functional evidence that they are behaving in an atypical manner. The hamartoma is associated with two childhood complications (although they occur in a minority of patients): seizures and other endocrine manifestations. A minority of patients with PHS develop seizures, which are classically gelastic. These are partial complex seizures that manifest as laughing without loss of consciousness or major postictal symptoms. They can be subtle, and there is typically a long delay from onset to diagnosis. Other seizures can occur in patients with PHS as well. Referral and evaluation by a pediatric neurologist familiar with these unusual seizures is indicated. Treatment with commonly prescribed anticonvulsants is often effective (valproic acid, neurontin). Other endocrine axes (in addition to cortisol, addressed above) should be evaluated at appropriate times. Thyroid deficiency should be excluded by specific testing (thyroxine, triiodothyronine, thyroid-stimulating hormone) in addition to the routine newborn screen. Growth hormone (GH) axis function can be screened for by testing the level of IGF-I at an appropriate age. Patients with PHS who are GH-deficient typically respond very well to exogenous GH. The children should also be monitored for precocious puberty by regular examination. Treatment with gonadotropin-releasing hormone antagonists is highly effective when precocious puberty occurs.

Other malformations that need to be addressed in childhood are the limb anomalies present in nearly all PHS patients. Surgical removal of postaxial polydactyly is typically straightforward and can be performed in a nonemergent manner. Central polydactyly can be more complex and should be evaluated by a hand surgeon who has experience with complex hand malformations. The geometry of the hand is usually abnormal, with splaying of the digits attached to the fused metacarpal, making surgery more challenging if function is to be preserved. Correction of polydactyly of the feet may be considered elective in some cases. A postaxial digit may not need to be removed if it is well formed, is aligned with the fifth toe, and does not make the foot especially wide. The public rarely notices feet with such extra toes. However, deviated digits, feet that are too wide to fit extra wide shoes, and other problems may necessitate removal.

GCPS

There are fewer medical treatment issues with GCPS than with PHS. Correction of polydactyly is generally mandatory when it is preaxial as these digits commonly interfere significantly with function (hands) or are incompatible with shoe fit (feet). The hypertelorism of GCPS is rarely severe, and I am unaware of any patients having undergone craniofacial surgery for this indication. Early reports suggested that GCPS was associated with craniosynostosis, but this appears to be either a rare manifestation or a spurious association. Patients with GCPS-contiguous gene syndrome (CGS) have an elevated incidence of mental retardation, speech delay, and probably an elevated incidence of generalized seizures. Patients with GCPS-CGS should be monitored closely during development to detect delays and seizures early in order to institute supportive services and anticonvulsants.

MUTATIONS IN PARALOGOUS GENES

No germline mutations have been identified in either *GLI1* or *GLI2* in humans. This may not be surprising in the case of *GLI1* given that the knockout mice have no discernable phenotype. For *GLI2*, the similarity of the *Gli2* knockout mice and the *Gli3^{XtJ}* mutant suggests that patients with phenotypes similar to PHS, GCPS, or other forms of syndromic or isolated polydactyly may harbor mutations in this gene. The gene is an excellent candidate to study in patients with these disorders who are found to have normal *GLI3* alleles. Somatic alterations in *GLI1* are important in basal cell carcinomas. *GLI1* was originally identified as a candidate oncogene in medulloblastoma as it was amplified in many of these tumors. However, subsequent work showed that this tumor is associated with amplification of MDM2 and or CDK4, genes that lie just telomeric of GLI1 (Elkahloun et al., 1996; Myklebost, 1998).

DEVELOPMENTAL PATHOGENESIS

At the same time that the *GLI3* mutations associated with PHS were discovered, the Kornberg laboratory had made significant progress in the understanding of the ci gene (Aza-Blanc and Kornberg, 1999; Aza-Blanc et al., 1997). This elegant work demonstrated that the ci transcription factor was regulated by an unusual post-translational regulatory process. The ci protein was found to be primarily located in the cytoplasm and subsequently shown to be part of a multiprotein complex, including the proteins fused, costal, suppressor of fused, and protein kinase A. When the cell was exposed to hedgehog ligand, ci was freed from the complex and translocated to the nucleus, where it activated downstream genes, including *decapentaplegic, patched,* and *gooseberry.* Under another stimulus in the absence of hedgehog, the ci protein product was cleaved into a truncated form at a point just after the zinc finger domain and translocated to the nucleus, where it repressed downstream genes. These results showed that ci was bifunctional and that turning off genes was as important in *Drosophila* development as turning them on.

Taking these results in *Drosophila* and overlaying them on the results in the human mutations (Table 20–1) resulted in our model of GLI3 pathogenesis. This model is based on a series of clinical and molecular insights. First, careful review of the clinical data showed that there were two nonoverlapping and broad spectra; GCPS and PHS. As described above, the GCPS spectrum ranges at the mild end from isolated preaxial or crossed polydactyly through typical GCPS and on to severe GCPS with contiguous gene deletion. The PHS spectrum ranges from nonsyndromic postaxial polydactyly through mild familial PHS and finally to severe PHS, which is most often sporadic. There are two key insights here: both spectra are broad but do not overlap in any significant way; furthermore, there are no known patients who have manifestations that include both PHS- and GCPS-specific malformations. There is no linear model of mutations that we can devise that is consistent with these data. Instead, the model proposes that GLI3 has two distinct functional modes and that differential perturbation of these modes of function can generate distinct phenotypic spectra. We hypothesized that GLI3, like ci, was bifunctional and subject to posttranslational processing and that the two classes of mutations perturbed the balance of activator and repressor forms in distinct ways. Mutations of *GLI3* that truncate the protein and generate a stable protein are predicted to generate a constitutive repressor allele that does not respond to sonic hedgehog (SHH) signaling. In these patients, the ability of the SHH signaling pathway to modulate signaling via GLI3 is limited but in an asymmetric manner. Since one allele always, and only, generates the repressor form, activation is effectively limited and cannot attain its maximal level. However, repression can be fully engaged by generation of a repressor form of the normal allele. This is clearly distinct from the functional consequences of *GLI3* haploinsufficiency. With haploinsufficiency, by definition, the mutant allele is a null. However, the normal protein product of the normal allele can be converted to an activator or repressor to an equal degree, although the amplitude of the activator and the repressor signal is reduced by half (Fig. 20–6).

This model has support from several sets of experiments, although significant issues remain to be addressed. GLI3 is sequestered in the cytoplasm and processed into an 83 kDa repressor form (Liu et al., 1998; Wang et al., 2000). Transfected GLI3 that mimics the processed from of ci protein clearly represses *PTCH1* transcription (Shin et al., 1999). Transfected GLI3 also modestly activates *PTCH1*. Overall, however, the evidence for the activator function of GLI3 is weak and complicated by the fact that it may be tissue-specific (Ruiz i Altaba, 1997). In addition, no direct evidence exists that endogenous full-

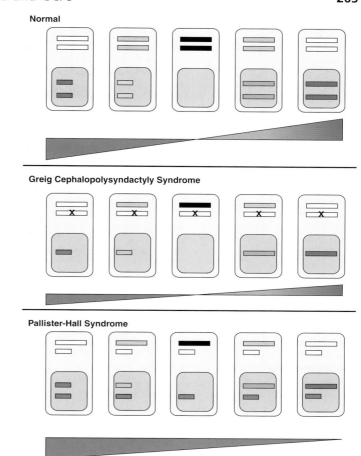

Figure 20–6. Schematic figure of the pathogenic model for GLI3 and Sonic hedgehog (SHH) function and the two phenotypes, Greig cephalopolysyndactyly syndrome (GCPS) and Pallister-Hall syndrome (PHS). The model shows, in a normal cell, two long bars in the cytoplasm that represent GLI3 protein. SHH causes translocation to the nucleus of full-length GLI3, whereas in the absence of SHH, GLI3 is proteolytically processed into an 83 kDa repressor form. The presence of one or two GLI3 proteins in the nucleus is intended to symbolize a hypothesized dosage control of the GLI3 products by the SHH pathway. In the GCPS row, the gradient of GLI3 function is preserved in that SHH still controls the remaining allele, although the mutant null allele cannot contribute to GLI3 function, reducing the amplitude of the gradient. In contrast, PHS is hypothesized to be caused by a shift in the neutral set point of the system because the truncated dominant allele is independent of SHH signaling.

length GLI3 is translocated to the nucleus. Nevertheless, this model remains attractive for several reasons. First, the evolutionary retention of the clearly demonstrated attributes of cytoplasmic sequestration and proteolytic processing would seem peculiar if the other attributes of ci biology were discarded. Second, in spite of opinions to the contrary, the mutational spectra of GCPS and PHS are markedly distinct and correlate extremely well. It has been suggested that there is no genotype–phenotype correlation of PHS and GCPS primarily on the basis of the existence of 3' truncation mutations in both disorders. However, this view ignores the important effect of mRNA processing by the nonsense-mediated mRNA degradation (NMD) machinery. Although much remains to be learned about this system in mammals, what is clear is that mRNAs with premature termination codons (PTCs) are sometimes subjected to degradation. Importantly, not all such PTCs are subjected to this effect and can persist in the cell, generating truncated proteins. Some of these proteins are themselves unstable and can be detected and degraded by the chaperonin/ubiquitination system (see Chapter 80). Again, some of these proteins escape degradation and generate abnormal cellular responses, often via a dominant-negative effect. Taking this into account, it is straightforward to generate a model whereby there are a large variety of mutations in GLI3, most of which generate a completely nonfunctional protein (translocations, deletions, missense mutations, and 5′ PTCs). A small portion of *GLI3* mutations will be 3′ PTCs, and some portion of these will be subjected to NMD or ubiquitin-mediated degradation. These mutations also lead to functional haploinsufficiency and a GCPS phenotype. However, a portion may escape NMD and generate a constitutive repressor. Patients with these mutations would be expected to have PHS. This model takes into account a number of recent observations and is unproven. However, the field of molecular biology is now beyond our previous happily naive state, where we simply assumed that every genomic alteration that *predicts* an altered protein is always associated with the *effect* of such an altered protein *in vivo*. A more sophisticated view of cellular biology is required to take into account our current knowledge of protein processing, mRNA dynamics, and other critical cellular mechanisms of developmental regulation. There is much yet to be learned, which is as true today as when it was recognized originally by Johnson (1967): "Few syndromes known to developmental genetics provide such a range of abnormalities as does extra-toes."

NOTE ADDED IN PROOF

Recently it has been shown that the two affected siblings in this family have the same heterozygous mutation in *GLI3* that occurred on the same parental chromosome, strongly supporting the existence of parental mosaicism (Ng et al., in press). These data supercede the conclusions about phenocapils in the text of this article.

REFERENCES

Aza-Blanc P, Kornberg T (1999). Ci: a complex transducer of the Hedgehog signal. *Trends Genet* 15: 458–462.

Aza-Blanc P, Ramírez-Weber F-A, Laget M-P, Schwartz C, Kornberg TB (1997). Proteolysis that is inhibited by hedgehog targets Cubitus interruptus protein to the nucleus and converts it to a repressor. *Cell* 89: 1043–1053.

Biesecker LG (1997). Strike three for *GLI3*. *Nat Genet* 17: 259–260.

Biesecker LG (2001). Genotype–phenotype correlation in GLI3 disorders. *Eur J Hum Genet* 9(Suppl 1):76.

Biesecker LG, Graham JM Jr (1996). Syndrome of the month: Pallister-Hall syndrome. *J Med Genet* 33: 585–589.

Biesecker LG, Abbott M, Allen J, Clericuzio C, Feuillan P, Graham JM, Jr, Hall J, Kang S, Haskins Olney A, Lefton D, et al. (1996). Report from the workshop on Pallister-Hall syndrome and related disorders. *Am J Med Genet* 65: 76–81.

Bonnemann CG, Lee MM, Krishnamoorthy KS (1995). Pallister-Hall syndrome: further delineation of mild phenotype. *Pediatr Neurol* 11: 146.

Boyko OB, Curnes JT, Oakes WJ, Burger PC (1991). Hamartomas of the tuber cinereum: CT, MR, and pathologic findings. *Am J Neuroradiol* 12: 309–314.

Breningstall GN (1985). Gelastic seizures, precocious puberty, and hypothalamic hamartoma. *Neurology* 35: 1180–1183.

Brueton LA, Chotai KA, van Herwerden L, Schinzel A, Winter RM (1992). The acrocallosal syndrome and Greig syndrome are not allelic disorders. *J Med Genet* 29: 635–637.

Diaz L, Grech K, Prados M (1991). Hypothalamic hamartoma associated with Laurence-Moon-Biedl syndrome. Case report and review of the literature. *Pediatr Neurosurg* 17: 30–33.

Drabkin H, Sage M, Helms C, Green P, Gemmill R, Smith D, Erickson P, Hart I, Ferguson-Smith A, Ruddle F, et al. (1989). Regional and physical mapping studies characterizing the Greig polysyndactyly 3;7 chromosome translocation, t(3;7)(p21.1;p13). *Genomics* 4: 518–529.

Elkahloun A, Bittner M, Hoskins K, Gemmill R, Meltzer P (1996). Molecular cytogenetic characterization and physical mapping of 12q13-15 amplification in human cancers. *Genes Chromosomes Cancer* 17: 205–214.

Fujiwara I, Kondo Y, Iinuma K (1999). Oral-facial-digital syndrome with hypothalamic hamartoma, postaxial ray hypoplasia of the limbs and vaginocystic communication: a new variant? *Am J Med Genet* 83: 77–81.

Gorlin RJ, Cohen MM Jr, Levin LS (1990). Greig cephalopolysyndactyly syndrome: In: *Syndromes of the Head and Neck*. Oxford University Press, New York, pp. 799–800.

Greig DM (1926). Oxycephaly. *Edinb Med J* 33: 189–218.

Hall JG, Pallister SK, Clarren SK, Beckwith JB, Wigglesworth FW, Fraser FC, Benke PJ, Reed SD (1980). Congenital hypothalamic hamartoblastoma, hypopituitarism, imperforate anus, and postaxial polydactyly—a new syndrome? Part I: Clinical, causal, and pathogenetic considerations. *Am J Med Genet* 7: 47–74.

Haskins-Olney A, Plaza S, McComb R (1997). Autosomal dominant Pallister-Hall syndrome in three generations with variable expressivity. Proc Greenwood Genet Cent 16: 126–127.

Hui C-C, Slusarski D, Platt KA, Holmgren R, Joyner A (1994). Expression of three mouse homologs of the *Drosophila* segment polarity gene cubitus interruptus, GLI, GLI-2, and GLI-3, in ectoderm- and mesoderm-derived tissue suggest multiple roles during postimplantation development. *Dev Biol* 162: 402–413.

Johnson DR (1967). Extra-toes: a new mutant gene causing multiple abnormalities in the mouse. *J Embryol Exp Morphol* 17: 543–581.

Johnson DR (1969). Brachyphalangy, an allele of extra-toes in the mouse. *Genet Res* 13: 275–280.

Johnston JJ, Olivos-Glander I, Turner J, Aleck K, Bird LM, Mehta L, Schimke RN, Heilstadt H, Spence JE, Blancato J, Biesecker LG. Clinical and molecular delineation of the Grieg cephalopolysyndactyly contiguous gene deletion syndrome and its distinction from acrocallosal syndrome, *Am J Med Genet* (in press).

Kang S, Allen J, Graham JM Jr, Grebe T, Clericuzio C, Patronas N, Ondrey F, Green E, Schäffer A, Abbott M, et al. (1997a). Linkage mapping and phenotypic analysis of autosomal dominant Pallister-Hall syndrome. *J Med Genet* 34: 441–446.

Kang S, Graham JM Jr, Olney AH, Biesecker LG (1997b). *GLI3* frameshift mutations cause autosomal dominant Pallister-Hall syndrome. *Nat Genet* 15: 266–268.

Kang S, Rosenberg M, Ko VD, Biesecker LG (1997c). Gene structure and allelic expression assay of the human *GLI3* gene. *Hum Genet* 101: 154–157.

Kinzler KW, Ruppert JM, Bigner SH, Vogelstein B (1988). The *GLI* gene is a member of the Kruppel family of zinc finger proteins. *Nature* 332: 371–374.

Lee J, Platt KA, Censullo P, Ruiz i Altaba A (1997). Gli1 is a target of Sonic hedgehog that induces ventral neural tube development. *Development* 124: 2537–2552.

Liu F, Massagué J, Ruiz i Altaba A (1998). Carboxy-terminally truncated Gli3 proteins associate with Smads. *Nat Genet* 20: 325–326.

Matheny M, Hall B, Manaligod JM (2000). Otolaryngologic aspects of oral-facial-digital syndrome. *Int J Pediatr Otorhinolaryngol* 53: 39–44.

Matsumoto N, Fujimoto M, Kato N, Niikawa N (1996). Assignment of the human *Gli2* gene to 2q14 by fluorescence in situ hybridization. *Genomics* 36: 220–221.

Maynard T, Jain M, Balmer C, LaMantia A (2002). High-resolution mapping of the Gli3 mutation Extra-toesJ reveals a 51.5 kb deletion. *Mamm Genome* 13: 58–61.

Mo R, Freer AM, Zinyk DL, Crackower MA, Michaud J, Heng HH, Chik KW, Shi XM, Tsui LC, Cheng SH, et al. (1997). Specific and redundant functions of *Gli2* and *Gli3* zinc finger genes in skeletal patterning and development. *Development* 124: 113–123.

Muenke M, Ruchelli ED, Rorke LB, McDonald-McGinn DM, Orlow MK, Isaacs A, Craparo FJ, Dunn LK, Zackai EH (1991). On lumping and splitting: a fetus with clinical findings of the oral-facial-digital syndrome type VI, the hydrolethalus syndrome, and the Pallister-Hall syndrome. *Am J Med Genet* 41: 548–556.

Myklebost O (1998). *GLI* gene and rhabdomyosarcoma. *Nat Med* 4: 869.

Ng D, Turner JT, Biesecker LG (2003). Genetic heterogeneity of Pallister-Hall syndrome. *Am J Med Genet* (in press).

Ondrey F, Griffith A, Van Waes C, Rudy S, Peters K, McCullagh L, Biesecker LG (2000). Asymptomatic laryngeal malformations are common in patients with Pallister-Hall syndrome. *Am J Med Genet* 94: 64–67.

Penman Splitt M, Wright C, Perry R, Burn J (1994). Autosomal dominant transmission of the Pallister-Hall syndrome. *Clin Dysmorphol* 3: 301–308.

Pohl TP, Mattei M-G, Rüther U (1990). Evidence for allelism of the recessive insertional mutation *add* and the dominant mouse mutation *extra toes (Xt)*. *Development* 110: 1153–1157.

Reifenberger G, Ichimura K, Reifenberger J, Elkahloun AG, Meltzer PS, Collins VP (1996). Refined mapping of 12q13-q15 amplicons in human malignant gliomas suggests CDK4/SAS and MDM2 as independent amplification targets. *Cancer Res* 56: 5141–5145.

Ruiz i Altaba A (1997). Catching a Gli-mpse of Hedgehog. *Cell* 90: 193–197.

Ruppert JM, Kinzler KW, Wong AJ, Bigner SH, Kao F-T, Law ML, Seuanez HN, O'Brien SJ, Vogelstein B (1988). The *GLI*-Kruppel family of human genes. *Mol Cell Biol* 8: 3104–3113.

Ruppert JM, Vogelstein B, Arheden K, Kinzler KW (1990). *GLI3* encodes a 190-kilodalton protein with multiple regions of GLI similarity. *Mol Cell Biol* 10: 5408–5415.

Sama A, Mason JD, Gibbin KP, Young ID, Hewitt M (1994). Familial Pallister-Hall syndrome. *J Med Genet* 31: 740.

Schimmang T, Oda SI, Rüther U (1994). The mouse mutant polydactyly Nagoya (Pdn) defines a novel allele of the zinc finger gene *Gli3*. *Mamm Genome* 5: 384–386.

Schinzel A (1982). Four patients including two sisters with the acrocallosal syndrome (agenesis of the corpus callosum in combination with preaxial hexadactyly). *Hum Genet* 62: 382.

Schinzel A, Kaufmann U (1986). The acrocallosal syndrome in sisters. *Clin Genet* 30: 399–405.

Shin S, Kogerman P, Lindström E, Toftgård R, Biesecker L (1999). *GLI3* mutations in human disorders mimic *Drosophila* Cubitus interruptus protein functions and localization. *Proc Natl Acad Sci USA* 96: 2880–2884.

Sills IN, Rapaport R, Robinson P, Lieber C, Shih LY, Horlick MNB, Schwartz M, Desposito F (1993). Familial Pallister-Hall syndrome: case report and hormonal evaluation. *Am J Med Genet* 47: 321–325.

Squires LA, Constantini S, Miller DC, Wisoff JH (1995). Hypothalamic hamartoma and the Pallister-Hall syndrome. *Pediatr Neurosurg* 22: 303–308.

Topf KF, Kletter GB, Kelch RP, Brunberg JA, Biesecker LG (1993). Autosomal dominant transmission of the Pallister-Hall syndrome. *J Pediatr* 123: 943–946.

Vortkamp A, Gessler M, Grzeschik K-H (1991). *GLI3* zinc finger gene interrupted by translocations in Greig syndrome families. *Nature* 352: 539–540.

Wagner K, Kroisel PM, Rosenkranz W (1990). Molecular and cytogenetic analysis in two patients with microdeletions of 7p and Greig syndrome: hemizygosity for PGAM2 and TCRG genes. *Genomics* 8: 487–491.

Wang B, Fallon J, Beachy P (2000). Hedgehog-regulated processing of Gli3 produces an anterior/poterior repressor gradient in the developing vertebrate limb. *Cell* 100: 423–434.

Wang XQ, Rothnagel JA (2001). Post-transcriptional regulation of the gli1 oncogene by the expression of alternative 5′ untranslated regions. *J Biol Chem* 276: 1311–1316.

Winter RM, Schroer RJ, Meyer LC (1993). Hands and feet. In: *Human Malformations and Related Anomalies*, Volume 2. Stevenson RE, Hall JG, Goodman RM (eds.) Oxford University Press, New York, pp. 805–843.

21 | *SALL1* and the Townes-Brocks Syndrome

JÜRGEN KOHLHASE AND WOLFGANG ENGEL

Townes-Brocks syndrome (TBS, OMIM 107480) is a rare autosomal dominantly inherited malformation syndrome characterized by anal, renal, limb, and ear anomalies. It results from mutations in *SALL1*, a human gene related to the developmental regulator *sal* of *Drosophila melanogaster*. Studies of its chick homologue *Csal1* suggest regulation of *Sall1* expression by the Sonic hedgehog (Shh), Wnt3A/7A, and fibroblast growth factor 4 (FGF4)/8 signaling pathways. The *SALL1* gene product is a zinc finger protein thought to act as a transcription factor. It contains four highly conserved C2H2 double zinc finger domains, which are evenly distributed. A single C2H2 motif is attached to the second domain, and at the amino terminus SALL1 contains a C2HC motif. The protein is exclusively found in the nucleus and localizes to pericentromeric heterochromatin, acting as a transcriptional repressor. Of the 29 known *SALL1* mutations, 28 are located in exon 2, 5′ of the third double zinc finger–encoding region. These are nonsense mutations, one of which causes TBS in nearly half of the sporadic cases; short insertions; short deletions; as well as one gross intraexonic deletion. One mutation within intron 2 creates an aberrant splice site. All mutations lead to preterminal stop codons and are thought to cause the phenotype via haploinsufficiency. However, *Sall1* knockout mice do not show the TBS phenotype, though homozygotes die from kidney malformations commonly seen in TBS.

ROLE OF LOCUS/PATHWAY

SALL1 is the only gene currently known to be mutated in patients with TBS, and mutations of *SALL1* have been found in 64.3%–83.3% of patients with "classical" TBS (Kohlhase et al., 1999c; Marlin et al., 1999). *SALL1* is one of four human genes related to *spalt* (*sal*) of *D. melanogaster* (Kohlhase et al., 1996; Kohlhase et al., 1999a,b; Al-Baradie et al., 2002; Kohlhase et al., 2002). The first indication that *sal* or *sal*-like genes are targets of *hedgehog* signaling came from the observation that in the *Drosophila* wing *sal* is activated in response to *hedgehog* signaling mediated by the transforming growth factor-β (TGF-β)-like protein DPP (de Celis et al., 1996; Lecuit et al., 1996; Nellen et al., 1996; Sturtevant et al., 1997). Köster et al. (1997) showed that in medaka *sal* expression is confined to *hedgehog* signaling centers. Furthermore, *sal* expression domains adjacent to *shh* expression domains are expanded by ectopic SHH, whereas suppression of *shh* expression by overexpression of protein kinase A results in suppression of *sal* expression. While it is not clear whether medaka *sal* is the orthologue of human *SALL1* or *SALL3*, it has been demonstrated that expression of the chick homologue of *SALL1* (*Csal1*) in the limb is activated by ectopic SHH. However, this activation requires signals from the apical ectodermal ridge and involves FGF4/8 as well as Wnt3a and Wnt7a (Farrell and Munsterberg, 2000), showing that *Csal1* expression is under the control of at least three different pathways.

CLINICAL DESCRIPTION

TBS was first described in 1972 as an association of imperforate anus, triphalangeal and supernumerary thumbs, malformed ears, and sensorineural hearing loss, inherited in an autosomal dominant fashion (Townes and Brocks, 1972). Following the first description, several additional families as well as isolated cases have been reported (Reid and Turner, 1976; Kurnit et al., 1978; Walpole and Hockey, 1982; Monteiro de Pina-Neto, 1984; Hersh et al., 1986; Barakat et al., 1988;

de Vries-van der Weerd et al., 1988; Ferraz et al., 1989; König et al., 1990; O'Callaghan and Young, 1990; Cameron et al., 1991; Kotzot et al., 1992; Rossmiller and Pasic, 1994; Parent et al., 1995; Arroyo Carrera et al., 1996; Ishikiriyama et al., 1996; Newman et al., 1997; Wischermann and Holschneider, 1997; Marlin et al., 1998; Doray et al., 1999). The minimal frequency of TBS has been estimated as 1 case per 250,000 liveborns (Martinez-Frias et al., 1999).

The clinical presentation of TBS is highly variable within and between affected families (Powell and Michaelis, 1999). Characteristic features are anorectal abnormalities (imperforate anus, anal stenosis), abnormalities of the hands (preaxial polydactyly [Fig. 21–1], triphalangeal thumbs, rarely hypoplastic thumbs), abnormalities of the feet (syndactyly III/IV, short third toe/metatarsal, overlapping toes [second and fourth overlapping third], pes planus, fused metatarsals), deformities of the outer ear ("lop ears" [Fig. 21–2], microtia, preauricular tags, and hearing loss, which can be sensorineural, conductive, or mixed (Rossmiller and Pasic, 1994). Renal malformations (unilateral or bilateral dysplastic or hypoplastic kidneys, renal agenesis, multicystic kidneys) have also been reported in several cases (Kurnit et al., 1978; Aylsworth, 1985; Barakat et al., 1988; de Vries-van der Weerd et al., 1988; O'Callaghan and Young, 1990; Cameron et al., 1991; Ilyina and Laziuk, 1992) and can lead to renal failure (Rossmiller and Pasic, 1994; Newman et al., 1997). Other genitourinary malformations include dystopic kidneys, hypospadias, posterior urethral valves, vesicoureteral reflux, and meatal stenosis (Kurnit et al., 1978; Hersh et al., 1986; Friedman et al., 1987; de Vries-van der Weerd et al., 1988; Ilyina and Laziuk, 1992; Gabrielli et al., 1993; Lenz, 1993; Rossmiller and Pasic, 1994). Cardiac malformations ranging from mild (persistent ductus arteriosus, atrial septal defect, ventricular septal defect) to severe (tetralogy of Fallot, truncus arteriosus communis, pulmonary valve atresia) are less often reported but clearly part of the TBS phenotypic spectrum, having been observed in several affected members of a TBS family (Surka et al., 2001). Mental retardation is also a less frequent feature (Cameron et al., 1991; Ishikiriyama et al., 1996; Kohlhase et al., 1999c). Reported IQs of TBS patients with mental retardation range from 47 to 60 (Cameron et al., 1991). Other observations suggest, however, that the incidence of mental retardation might be higher, as reflected in the literature because proper IQ testing is not regularly performed in TBS patients (Kohlhase, unpublished data). It is currently not known if the mental retardation is caused by structural brain defects, as might be speculated from the fact that *SALL1* and its murine homologue, *Sall1*, are expressed in distinct areas of the brain during embryonic development (Kohlhase et al., 1996; Buck et al., 2001) (Fig. 21–3).

The eyes can also be affected in TBS patients. Bilateral colobomata of the iris have been reported in a large TBS family (Rossmiller and Pasic, 1994). Two monozygous twins with TBS showed congenital bilateral cataracts (Kohlhase, unpublished data). Another TBS patient suffered from sudden loss of visual acuity due to optic neuropathy (Blanck et al., 2000). While it has been speculated that eye involvement in TBS could be coincidental (Powell and Michaelis, 1999), the expression of mouse *Sall1* in the developing eye (Buck et al., 2001) suggests that *SALL1* mutations could well affect eye development in humans.

In addition, in some families, affected subjects show features typical for both TBS and Goldenhar's syndrome/oculo-auriculovertebral spectrum (Moeschler and Clarren, 1982; Gabrielli et al., 1993; John-

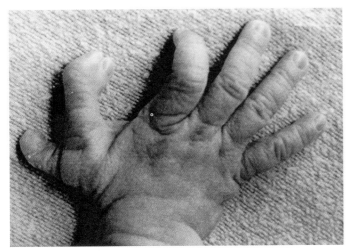

Figure 21–1. Preaxial polydactyly and bifid distal phalanx of thumb with ulnar deviation in a patient with Townes-Brocks syndrome. (From Powell and Michaelis, *J Med Genet* 1999;36:89–93. With kind permission from the BMJ Publishing Group.)

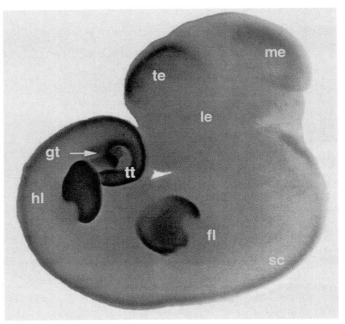

Figure 21–3. Whole-mount in situ hybridization of *Sall1* in a mouse embryo of 11.5 days postconception. In the limbs, a central and a peripheral domain show *Sall1* expression. Note further expression in the genital tubercle (gt), the spinal cord (sc), and the telencephalon (te). fl, forelimb; hl, hindlimb; me, mesencephalon; le, lens endothelium; tt, tail tip. Expression in the olfactory bulbs is not visible in this view.

son et al., 1996). Penetrance seems to be complete in TBS since no unaffected obligate mutation carrier has been reported (Powell and Michaelis, 1999; Kohlhase, unpublished data).

MOLECULAR GENETICS OF THE LOCUS

The first indication of the gene locus mutated in TBS came from cytogenetic findings. The observation of a pericentric inversion, inv(16)(p11.2q12.1) (Friedman et al., 1987), in both an affected father and his affected daughter and the detection of a reciprocal translocation, 46,XX,t(5;16)(p15.3; q12.1), in a girl with TBS suggested that the genetic locus mutated in TBS is at 16q12.1 (Serville et al., 1993). Although several large families were reported following the initial description of the syndrome (Reid and Turner, 1976; Kurnit et al., 1978; O'Callaghan and Young, 1990), no linkage analysis has confirmed the suspected locus or indicated a second gene mutated in TBS patients.

When *SALL1* was mapped to 16q12.1 by fluorescence in situ hybridization (Kohlhase et al., 1996), it became a candidate gene for TBS due to not only its chromosomal position but also its structural relationship to the essential developmental regulator gene *spalt* (*sal*) of *D. melanogaster* (Kühnlein et al., 1994). In *Drosophila*, SAL is required for specification of posterior head and anterior tail segment identity (Jürgens, 1988) as well as for larval tracheal system (Kühnlein and Schuh, 1996) and adult wing (Sturtevant et al., 1997) development.

Prior to the cloning of *SALL1*, *sal*-related genes had been isolated from mouse (*Msal*, now *Sall3* [Ott et al., 1996]) and *Xenopus laevis* (*Xsal-1* [Hollemann et al., 1996]). Both genes are expressed in the developing limbs, heart, kidney, inner ear, and CNS, i.e., in tissues/

organs affected in TBS. The observation that, like *sal* in *Drosophila* (de Celis et al., 1996; Lecuit et al., 1996; Nellen et al., 1996), the *sal* gene in the fish medaka is also activated in response to *Sonic hedgehog* suggested not only that the SAL-like protein structure was conserved in evolution but in addition that SAL-like proteins in vertebrates might likewise act as essential developmental regulators (Köster et al., 1997).

SALL1 is very similar to both *Msal* and *Xsal-1*, and its similar expression in adult tissues (Kohlhase et al., 1996) suggested that it would also be similarly expressed during development. Therefore, *SALL1* was chosen as a TBS candidate gene based on its chromosomal position and the assumption that it functions as a developmental regulator based on information available from other genes of the same family.

SALL1 consists of three coding exons (Kohlhase et al., 1996, 1999c). The first exon carries the most likely initiator methionine and comprises 76 bp of the coding sequence, followed by an intron of about 9 kb. Exon 2 has a length of 3458 bp and is separated from exon 3 by an intron of 1139 bp. Exon 3 contains a 438 bp coding sequence and at least 696 bp of 3′-untranslated region (GenBank accession NM_002968, Y18264, Y18265, X98833).

The open reading frame encodes a protein of 1324 amino acids with four characteristically arranged SAL-like C2H2 double zinc finger domains thought to carry DNA-binding properties (Fig. 21–4). A single zinc finger is attached to the second double zinc finger domain (Kohlhase et al., 1996). The putative protein also contains an additional C2HC zinc finger close to the N terminus, which is present in all known vertebrate SAL-like proteins (Hollemann et al., 1996; Kohlhase et al., 1996; Ott et al., 1996; Köster et al., 1997).

Based on these features, it was assumed that SALL1 acts as a DNA-binding transcription factor, which regulates the expression of specific target genes via binding to specific target sequences within their promoters and interacting with the basal transcription machinery to activate or repress target gene expression. To test if SALL1 is indeed localized in the nucleus as expected for a transcription factor, expression of a GFP-SALL1 fusion protein was examined in NIH3T3 cells. Interestingly, SALL1 was localized in the nucleus in a peculiar pattern but not homogeneously as presumed. The fusion protein was located at pericentromeric heterochromatin (Fig. 21–5) and colocalized in part with the heterochromatin-binding protein M31 (Netzer et al., 2001).

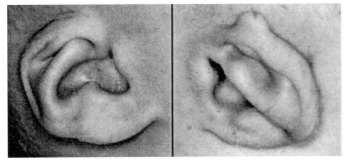

Figure 21–2. Dysplastic ears with overfolded superior helices in a patient with Townes-Brocks syndrome. (Modified from Kohlhase et al., *Nat Genet* 1998;18:81–83. With kind permission from the *Nature* publishing group.)

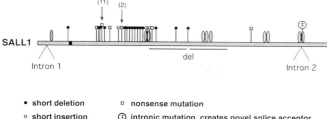

Figure 21–4. Schematic representation of the SALL1 protein (1324 amino acids) and localization of the mutations identified to date. Zinc fingers are indicated as oval symbols. *SALL1* encodes four C2H2 double zinc finger domains distributed over the protein. A single C2H2 domain is attached to the second double zinc finger. At the amino terminus, a single C2HC domain is found. Horizontal bar with *del* shows the position of the combined 1150 bp deletion within exon 2. (*11*) indicates that the 826C>T mutation has been found in 11 unrelated patients. At position 1115, two different nonsense mutations have been detected (*2*). All other mutations have been found only once. Positions of the introns are indicated. (Modified from Kohlhase, *Hum Mutat* 2000;16:460–466. With kind permission from Wiley-Liss, Inc., a subsidiary of John Wiley & Sons, Inc.)

Furthermore, SALL1 was shown to act as a repressor of transcription, raising the question of whether SALL1, like *Ikaros*, a zinc finger transcription factor required for the development of B and T lymphocytes, could exert its repressive function by recruiting its target genes into heterochromatic regions (Brown et al., 1997). More recent studies of *Ikaros* (Sabbattini et al., 2001), however, suggested that the translocation of transcriptionally inactive genes to heterochromatic regions does not result in increased methylation and reduced accessibility of the target genes to nucleases, meaning that the target genes are not heterochromatinized. It is not clear, however, if transcriptionally inactive target genes of SALL1 are indeed likewise translocated into heterochromatic regions.

GENE EXPRESSION

Northern blot analysis showed *SALL1* transcripts in adult placenta, liver, brain, and kidney tissue in increasing amounts (Kohlhase et al., 1996); and by in situ hybridization, transcripts were detected in

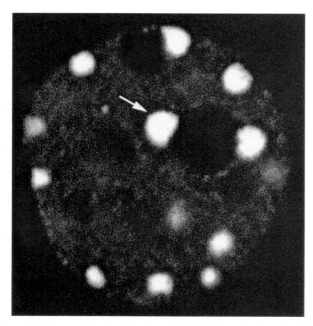

Figure 21–5. Intracellular localization of the SALL1 protein (arrow). (Modified from Netzer et al., *Hum Mol Genet* 2001;10:3017–3024.)

neuronal cells of the developing thalamus (22 weeks). Expression analysis of *SALL1* by reverse-transcription PCR has revealed the presence of *SALL1* transcripts in fetal brain (16–32 weeks), fetal heart (20–25 weeks), fetal kidney, and fetal thymus (both 16–32 weeks), with expression being strongest in fetal kidney (Ma et al., 2001). In fetal kidney of 12 weeks, antibody staining showed SALL1 protein expression in ureteric buds and immature tubules located in the nephrogenic zone near the edge of the developing kidney. Uninduced mesenchyme and glomeruli did not show expression. In 12-week fetal testis, SALL1 protein was detected in Leydig cell precursors; and in 14-week fetal ovaries, it was also expressed, the staining being stronger in the oocytes than in the surrounding follicular and granulosa cells (Ma et al., 2001). In the adult kidney, SALL1 protein is expressed in the cortical tubules around the glomeruli but not in the glomeruli. In adult testis, SALL1 is expressed in Leydig cells, spermatogonia, and Sertoli cells, whereas in the ovary it is found in granulosa cells. In Wilms' tumor, SALL1 expression was detected in condensed blastema and epithelial tubules (Ma et al., 2001).

The orthologous mouse gene *Sall1* is expressed in the neural ectoderm of the prospective head region at day 7.5 postcoitum (pc). *Sall1* expression extends to the neural groove, branchial arches, and the trunk region at day 8.5 pc. At day 9.5 pc, expression is seen at the midbrain–hindbrain boundary, the anterior region of the midbrain, the neural tube, the posterior trunk region, and the mesonephros. At day 10.5 pc, *Sall1* signals are detected in the forelimbs and hindlimbs, the telencephalon, a distinct region of the nasal process, and the lens vesicle (Fig. 21–3). Embryos at 11.5 days show prominent expression in the genital tubercle, the telencephalon, and the olfactory bulbs. At day 12.5 pc, *Sall1* transcripts are observed in cells of the ependymal and mantle layer of the spinal cord; in cells surrounding the lateral, third, and fourth ventricles in the brain; in the epithelium and mesenchyme of the genital tubercle; as well as in the mesenchyme surrounding the branching area of the trachea and esophagus. At this stage, the metanephros shows *Sall1* expression in the cortical region and in mesenchyme cells of the medullar region (Buck et al., 2001).

MUTATIONS

Nineteen different *SALL1* mutations (Marlin et al., 1998; Kohlhase et al., 1998, 1999c; Blanck et al., 2000; Salerno et al., 2000; Surka et al., 2001) have been reported in patients with TBS (Table 21–1). Seven not yet reported mutations have meanwhile been found in TBS patients (Table 21–1) (Kohlhase, unpublished results). One additional mutation was seen in a family whose affected members did not suffer from TBS but showed a branchio-oto-renal (BOR) syndrome-like phenotype (Engels et al., 2000), and the finding of yet another *SALL1* mutation (967C>T) in a family with a similar phenotype confirmed this (Kohlhase, in preparation). An additional mutation was found in a girl who showed features overlapping with TBS and Goldenhar's syndrome (Kohlhase et al., 1999c), adding up to a total of 29 *SALL1* mutations (Table 21–1).

Seven of these are nonsense mutations and occur at six different positions: nucleotides 778, 826, 967, 1115, 1509, and 2779. Interestingly, the 826C>T mutation was found in three unrelated sporadic patients by Marlin et al. (1999), in 7 unrelated sporadic patients by our group (Kohlhase et al., 1999; four unpublished cases), and in one sporadic patient by Keegan et al. (2001). Therefore, this mutation (found in 11 of 39 mutation-positive families) is by far the most common in *SALL1,* and the position represents a true hot spot (Marlin et al., 1999; Keegan et al., 2001). Among sporadic mutation-positive TBS patients (23 cases), this mutation accounts for 47.8% of cases, being detected in 11 patients.

The vast majority of *SALL1* mutations (21) are frameshift mutations, i.e., 16 small deletions of <100 bp, one bigger deletion (1150 bp) within exon 2, and four short insertions (Table 21–1). Initial findings suggested that all point mutations cluster 5′ of the region encoding the first double zinc finger (i.e., nucleotides 1351–1497) (Kohlhase et al., 1999c). However, four point mutations were detected between the coding regions for double zinc fingers 1 and 2 (i.e., nucleotides 2122–2268), and one deletion was found which removes the

Table 21–1. *SALL1* Mutations

Base Change	Amino Acid Change	Position	Phenotype*	Reference
419delC	Frameshift	Exon 2	TBS	Kohlhase et al., 1999c
778C>T	Q260X	Exon 2	TBS	Kohlhase, unpublished data
792-793del2	Frameshift	Exon 2	TBS	Surka et al., 2001
817delG	Frameshift	Exon 2	TBS	Salerno et al., 2000
826C>T	R276X	Exon 2	TBS	Kohlhase, unpublished data; Keegan et al., 2001; Marlin et al., 1999; Kohlhase et al., 1999c
840delC	Frameshift	Exon 2	TBS	Blanck et al., 2000
967C>T	Q323X	Exon 2	BOR-like	Kohlhase, unpublished data
1060-1061insA	Frameshift	Exon 2	TBS	Kohlhase, unpublished data
1115C>A	S372X	Exon 2	TBS	Kohlhase et al., 1999c
1115C>G	S372X	Exon 2	TBS	Kohlhase et al., 1998
1146delT	Frameshift	Exon 2	TBS	Kohlhase et al., 1999c
1200-1206del7	Frameshift	Exon 2	TBS	Kohlhase et al., 1999c
1255delT	Frameshift	Exon 2	TBS	Kohlhase, unpublished data
1262delC	Frameshift	Exon 2	TBS	Kohlhase, unpublished data
1268delC	Frameshift	Exon 2	TBS	Kohlhase et al., 1998
1277-1278delGA	Frameshift	Exon 2	TBS/Goldenhar	Kohlhase et al., 1999c
1291-1300del10	Frameshift	Exon 2	TBS	Kohlhase et al., 1999c
1347-1348delCA	Frameshift	Exon 2	TBS	Marlin et al., 1999
1403-1404insG	Frameshift	Exon 2	TBS	Kohlhase, unpublished data
1411-1412insA	Frameshift	Exon 2	TBS	Marlin et al., 1999
1479-1480insAG	Frameshift	Exon 2	TBS	Marlin et al., 1999
1509C>A	Y503X	Exon 2	TBS	Blanck et al., 2000
1565delC	Frameshift	Exon 2	TBS	Marlin et al., 1999
1819delG	Frameshift	Exon 2	BOR-like	Engels et al., 2000
1966-2005del10	Frameshift	Exon 2	TBS	Marlin et al., 1999
1487del562				
2065del588	Frameshift	Exon 2	TBS	Marlin et al., 1999
2779C>T	Q927X	Exon 2	TBS	Kohlhase, unpublished data
IVS2-19T>A	Aberrant splicing, frameshift	Intron 2	TBS	Blanck et al., 2000

*TBS, Townes-Brocks syndrome; BOR, branchio-oto-renal (syndrome).
Source: Modified from Kohlhase, *Hum Mutat* 2000;16:460-466. With kind permission from Wiley-Liss, Inc., a subsidiary of John Wiley & Sons, Inc.

coding sequence for the first double zinc finger motif partly and for the second completely (Marlin et al., 1999). One nonsense mutation was recently found (2779C>T; Kohlhase, in preparation), which creates a preterminal stop codon 5' to the region encoding the third double zinc finger motif. Another point mutation was detected within intron 2, creating an aberrant splice acceptor site (Blanck et al., 2000).

While *SALL1* mutations resulting in TBS seem to occur all over the gene, most (22/29) *SALL1* mutations are found 5' to or within the region encoding the first double zinc finger, suggesting that this region is especially prone to mutations. The positions of the mutations with respect to the SALL1 protein are shown in Figure 21–4.

The detection rate of *SALL1* mutations in TBS patients varies between the two groups who have reported larger studies (Kohlhase et al., 1999c; Marlin et al., 1999). When typical malformations of the hands, ears, and anus ("classical" TBS) were present, mutations were detected in 64.3% (9 of 14) by Kohlhase et al. (1999) versus 83.3% (10 of 12) of unrelated patients by Marlin et al. (1999). Up to now, *SALL1* mutations have been described in three additional families who did not show the classical picture of TBS or showed no TBS at all (Kohlhase et al., 1999c; Engels et al., 2000). This illustrates that the detection rate is strongly influenced by the diagnostic criteria for TBS and by the fact that TBS overlaps with several dysmorphic conditions, like such as the pattern of vertebral, anal, cardiac, tracheal, esophageal, renal, and limb anomalies (VACTERL), Goldenhar syndrome, oculo-auriculo-vertebral spectrum, and BOR syndrome (Powell and Michaelis, 1999).

Large deletions involving more than one exon or the whole *SALL1* gene have not been detected so far in patients without visible cytogenetic abnormalities. Fluorescence in situ hybridization using an approximately 80 kb PI artificial chromosome (PAC) probe containing the *SALL1* gene has not revealed any deletion (Kohlhase et al., unpublished results). However, heterozygous polymorphisms detected by direct sequencing indicate that by far most patients who do not carry a *SALL1* mutation within the coding region seem to carry no gross *SALL1* deletion (Kohlhase et al., unpublished results).

The failure to detect a *SALL1* mutation in a substantial proportion of patients with a classical TBS phenotype might also suggest locus heterogeneity for TBS. However, there is still no evidence from linkage studies or chromosomal analyses to suggest another gene being mutated in TBS patients without detectable *SALL1* mutation.

No missense mutations in *SALL1* have been reported to date. This might be explained by the fact that point mutations, except for the one true hot spot position at nucleotide 826, occur more rarely than short deletions. Furthermore, based on the current knowledge of *SALL1*, only missense mutations resulting in haploinsufficiency would be expected to cause TBS. Therefore, missense mutations in TBS might only be expected at positions which are essential for SALL1 function. The only amino acids the replacement of which is obviously expected to be deleterious are located within the zinc finger domains. As shown for the transcription factor *Krüppel* in *D. melanogaster*, replacement of an essential cysteine residue within the second of five tandemly arranged zinc finger motifs leads to a functional null allele (Redemann et al., 1988). It might therefore be that similar missense mutations of *SALL1* will be detected with the number of analyzed patients increasing.

However, the question remains of whether missense mutations within other parts of *SALL1* would result in a phenotype different from TBS. While it seems virtually impossible to predict what phenotype might be caused by a missense mutation at any given position within the gene, the identification of two clearly different phenotypes resulting from *SALL1* mutations suggests that other syndromes, possibly sharing some anomalies with TBS, might also be associated with the *SALL1* locus. An example of such a wide phenotypic spectrum is given by the gene *GLI3* (see Chapter 20). While there is controversy as to why certain *GLI3* mutations lead to certain phenotypes (Kalff-Suske et al., 1999; Radhakrishna et al., 1999), it will be interesting to see if *SALL1* mutations might cause a similar range of phenotypes.

POLYMORPHISMS

Twenty-seven polymorphisms have been identified in patients and unaffected parents screened for *SALL1* mutations (Table 21–2). While no clear estimate has been given of the occurrence rates of these sequence variations in normal populations, the most common (Kohlhase,

Table 21–2. *SALL1* Polymorphisms

Base Change	Amino Acid Change	Position	Reference
IVS1+36-37delAC	—	Intron 1	Blanck et al., 2000
IVS1+68T>A	—	Intron 1	Kohlhase, 2000
IVS1+69C>A	—	Intron 1	Kohlhase, 2000
IVS1+118C>G	—	Intron 1	Blanck et al., 2000
IVS1+119G>A	—	Intron 1	Blanck et al., 2000
348C>T	H116H	Exon 2	Kohlhase, 2000
447-448insAGCAGC	SS149-150ins	Exon 2	Kohlhase, 2000
447-448insAGC	S149-150ins	Exon 2	Kohlhase et al., 1999c
448-450delAGC	S150del	Exon 2	Kohlhase et al., 1999c
475A>G	S159G	Exon 2	Kohlhase et al., 1999c
490-492delAGC	S164del	Exon 2	Marlin et al., 1999
1155T>C	S385S	Exon 2	Kohlhase, 2000
1335A>G	A445A	Exon 2	Kohlhase, 2000
2178G>A	R726R	Exon 2	Marlin et al., 1999
2511C>A	I837I	Exon 2	Kohlhase, 2000
2544A>G	Q848Q	Exon 2	Kohlhase, 2000
2574T>C	L858L	Exon 2	Marlin et al., 1999
3456C>T	H1152H	Exon 2	Blanck et al., 2000
IVS2+40C>G	—	Intron 2	Kohlhase, unpublished data
IVS2+274G>C	—	Intron 2	Kohlhase, unpublished data
IVS2+431C>T	—	Intron 2	Kohlhase, unpublished data
IVS2-310C>T	—	Intron 2	Kohlhase, unpublished data
IVS2-207A>G	—	Intron 2	Kohlhase, unpublished data
IVS2-31-32delCT	—	Intron 2	Blanck et al., 2000
3794G>A	G1265E	Exon 3	Marlin et al., 1999
3872A>G	N1291S	Exon 3	Blanck et al., 2000
3915C>T	N1305N	Exon 3	Blanck et al., 2000

Source: Modified from Kohlhase, *Hum Mutat* 2000;16:460-466. With kind permission from Wiley-Liss, Inc., a subsidiary of John Wiley & Sons, Inc.

2000) seem to be variations within the serine/glycine repeat amino-terminal to the first double zinc finger (S149del, S159G, S149-150ins, SS149-150ins) and the two noncoding nucleotide changes, 2574T>C and 3456C>T (all exon 2, see Table 21–2 for further references). While the serine/glycine repeat in most cases consists of 10 serine residues (encoded by an [AGC]10 repeat) followed by 4 glycines (encoded by a [GGC]4 repeat), alleles with 12 serines/4 glycines, 11 serines/4 glycines, 10 serines/5 glycines, 9 serines/5 glycines, and 9 serines/4 glycines have been found in both affected and unaffected people. The serine/glycine repeat is followed again by three serines, one of which has also been deleted without phenotypic consequences (S164del) (Marlin et al., 1999). Other silent changes of the SALL1 amino acid sequences (G1265E, N1291S) have been found in exon 3 but only rarely (Kohlhase et al., 1999c; Marlin et al., 1999).

GENOTYPE–PHENOTYPE CORRELATION

The significant intra- and interfamilial variability in the clinical presentation of patients with TBS has been noted in many reports. Mutation analysis of *SALL1* in TBS patients has so far failed to demonstrate a clear genotype–phenotype correlation. There is no obvious correlation between the clinical presentation and the nature or location of specific point mutations, with the exception of the mutation 1277-1278del causing a phenotype overlapping with Goldenhar's syndrome or 967C>T and 1819delG resulting in a phenotype different from TBS but overlapping with BOR syndrome. Since each of these mutations was found in only one family, it remains unclear whether the different phenotypes are truly caused by different effects of the mutation or more likely due to epigenetic influences.

Mutation analysis of *SALL1* has confirmed that penetrance is complete in TBS. However, there is a significant proportion of germline mosaicism. Our studies have so far revealed two of 39 mutation-positive families in which the unaffected mother either carried the mutation in a detectable mosaic state (Kohlhase et al., 1999c) or gave birth to two affected children while the mutation could not be detected in her DNA from peripheral lymphocytes (Blanck et al., 2000). In the latter, it could be shown that the mutation of both children was inherited from the mother (Kohlhase et al., unpublished results). In another family, the father of an affected child had the second and fourth toes overriding the third. In this man, the mutation causing TBS in his child was found only in mucosa cells but not in lymphocytes (Devriendt et al., 2002).

ESTABLISHING THE DIAGNOSIS

TBS is first diagnosed clinically by the presence of typical malformations (major features) of the hands, ears, and anus. In the presence of only two typical malformations in an affected person, the diagnosis is less secure but becomes substantiated if (*1*) there are typical minor malformations/features (i.e., renal malformations/dysfunction, hearing loss, cardiac defects), (*2*) there are no atypical features (i.e., esophageal atresia or vertebral defects), (*3*) there is more than one affected person in the family (in agreement with autosomal dominant inheritance), and (*4*) the other affected family members show major malformations missing in the index patient. The clinical diagnosis is confirmed by detection of a *SALL1* mutation. Failure to detect a *SALL1* mutation does not, however, exclude the diagnosis. Mutation analysis is currently done by genomic PCR and direct sequencing of PCR products with internal primers.

If the causative mutation is unknown, the diagnosis can be determined prenatally only by high-resolution ultrasound between the 18th and 22nd gestational weeks. Still, this represents a difficult task. The major signs to look for are skeletal malformations, i.e., of the thumbs (triphalangeal thumbs, preaxial polydactyly) or feet. Anal malformations might be assumed by the presence of dilated bowels. Renal malformations are easier to detect, and a severe renal dysfunction will result in an oligohydramnion.

Successful prenatal diagnosis has been obtained in three different families by amplification of *SALL1* from amniotic cell and chorionic villi DNA, respectively, and exclusion/confirmation of mutations 826C>T and 778C>T, respectively (Kohlhase, unpublished results). One prenatal diagnosis has been obtained by amplification of *SALL1* from amniotic cell DNA, and the mutation 826C>T could be excluded (Kohlhase, unpublished results).

MUTATIONS IN ORTHOLOGOUS GENES

Nishinakamura et al. (2001) created a knockout mouse for *Sall1*, the orthologous mouse gene. For this purpose, they replaced exons 2 and 3 by either a neomycin-resistance gene alone or a lacZ–neomycin fusion gene. After homologous recombination, the embryonic stem cells were transferred into C57BL/6N blastocysts. Both *Sall1*-del and *Sall1*-lacZ heterozygous mice showed no detectable phenotype. However, many *Sall1*-lacZ heterozygotes died, presumably from lacZ toxicity. Homozygotes for both *Sall1*-del and *Sall1*-lacZ alleles showed identical phenotypes. All died in the perinatal period and showed severe agenesis or dysgenesis of the kidneys. Remnant kidneys showed a disorganized cortical structure, shrunken glomeruli, necrotic proximal tubules, and multiple cysts. The findings were interpreted to be the result of incomplete outgrowth of the ureteric bud, failure of tubule formation in the mesenchyme, and apoptosis of the mesenchyme (Nishinakamura et al., 2001). It was assumed that the absence of an inductive signal from the ureter primarily caused the phenotype since *Sall1*-deficient mesenchyme was competent for epithelial differentiation.

Apart from this phenotype, neither limb deformities, anorectal anomalies, nor ear anomalies were seen in the mutant mice. Development of other organs, including brain, adrenal glands, bladder, testis, and ovary, was normal. Only the olfactory bulbs showed a slightly disorganized layer structure.

DEVELOPMENTAL PATHOGENESIS

By far, most of the *SALL1* mutations detected in TBS patients to date result in premature stop codons (Table 21–1). Since transcripts carrying a premature stop codon are mostly rapidly degraded, these mutations are likely to cause TBS via SALL1 haploinsufficiency (Culbertson, 1999; Hentze and Kulozik, 1999). This interpretation is supported by the observation that TBS can also result from chromosomal translocations or pericentric inversions. While the breakpoints of the pericentric inversion reported from one family with TBS have not been clarified, the translocation t(5;16)(p15.3;q12.1) in one TBS patient has been shown to result in a breakpoint at least 180 kb downstream of *SALL1*, suggesting a position effect to cause TBS in this patient (Marlin et al., 1999). Another indication for SALL1 haploinsufficiency as the cause for TBS comes from the observation that a fetus with a deletion, del(16)(q11.2;q21), showed malformations overlapping with the TBS phenotype (Knoblauch et al., 2000).

However, the result of two *SALL1* mutations is not easily explained. The mutation IVS2-19T>A results in a stable transcript, which encodes all double zinc finger domains except for the most carboxy-terminal one (Blanck et al., 2000). Further studies will show if this is sufficient to cause loss of *SALL1* gene function.

The mutation 1819delG results in a frameshift and a premature stop codon (Engels et al., 2000). However, the phenotype is overlapping with but different from TBS, suggesting that this mutation has an effect which is different from other short deletions occurring in the same region of the gene (Marlin et al., 1999). A dominant-negative effect for this mutation becomes less likely with the finding of the mutation 967C>T (Kohlhase, in preparation) in a family with a similar phenotype. This mutation is positioned within the hot spot region for TBS mutations, and the diverging phenotype in the family might be explained as a result of different genetic backgrounds, i.e., different states of activity of possible modifier genes.

With SALL1 haploinsufficiency being the most likely explanation as to how SALL1 mutations cause TBS, it was assumed that a knockout for *Sall1*, the murine orthologue (Buck et al., 2000), would create a mouse model for TBS. However, mice heterozygous for a *Sall1* null mutation showed no phenotype at all, whereas homozygous mutant mice showed only severe kidney malformations (Nishinakamura et al., 2001) but not a TBS-like phenotype (see above). It was hypothesized that the relative importance of *SALL1/Sall1* over *SALL2/Sall2* and *SALL3/Sall3* might be higher in humans than in mice, suggesting that these genes might compensate for each other. It remains to be shown by double knock-outs or knock-in mice for these genes if there is indeed any compensation. Also, transgenic mice expressing a truncated *Sall1* gene would be important to test for a dominant-negative effect of *Sall1* mutations, which, however, seems unlikely with respect to the chromosomal aberrations causing TBS (see above).

The pathogenesis of TBS caused by *SALL1* mutations is therefore still unclear. *Sall1* knockout mice might only serve as a model to explain the kidney malformations in TBS patients. The full spectrum of *SALL1* mutations in patients with TBS and overlapping phenotypes is still being delineated. It will be interesting to see if missense mutations at different positions of *SALL1* might also cause TBS or other phenotypes. The identification of such mutations might also help to identify essential functional domains of the SALL1 protein other than the zinc fingers. The identification of SALL1 regulators, interaction partners, and downstream targets and their analysis in patients with identical SALL1 mutations but different phenotypes might help to explain the clinical variability.

REFERENCES

Al-Baradie R, Yamada K, St Hilaire C, Chan WM, Andrews C, McIntosh N, Nakano M, Martonyi EJ, Raymond WR, Okumura S, et al. (2002). Duane Radial Ray Syndrome (Okihiro syndrome) maps to 20q13 and results from mutations in *SALL4*, a new member of the SAL family. *Am J Hum Genet* 71: 1195–1199.

Arroyo Carrera I, Lopez Cuesta MJ, Garcia Garcia MJ, Lozano Rodriguez JA, Carretero Diaz V (1996). The Townes-Brocks syndrome [in Spanish]. *An Esp Pediatr* 44: 364–366.

Aylsworth A (1985). The Townes-Brocks syndrome: a member of the anus-hand-ear family syndromes. *Am J Hum Genet* 37(Suppl): A43.

Barakat A, Butler M, Salter J, Fogo A (1988). Townes-Brocks syndrome: report of three additional patients with previously undescribed renal and cardiac abnormalities. *Dysmorphol Clin Genet* 2: 104–108.

Blanck C, Kohlhase J, Engels S, Burfeind P, Engel W, Bottani A, Patel MS, Kroes HY, Cobben JM (2000). Three novel SALL1 mutations extend the mutational spectrum in Townes-Brocks syndrome. *J Med Genet* 37: 303–307.

Brown K, Guest S, Smale S, Hahm K, Merkenschlager M, Fisher A (1997). Association of transcriptionally silent genes with *Ikaros* complexes at centromeric heterochromatin. *Cell* 91: 845–854.

Buck A, Archangelo L, Dixkens C, Kohlhase J (2000). Molecular cloning, chromosomal localization, and expression of the murine SALL1 ortholog Sall1. *Cytogenet Cell Genet* 89: 150–153.

Buck A, Kispert A, Kohlhase J (2001). Embryonic expression of the murine homologue of *SALL1*, the gene mutated in Townes-Brocks syndrome. *Mech Dev* 104: 143–146.

Cameron TH, Lachiewicz AM, Aylsworth AS (1991). Townes-Brocks syndrome in two mentally retarded youngsters. *Am J Med Genet* 41: 1–4.

Culbertson MR (1999). RNA surveillance. Unforeseen consequences for gene expression, inherited genetic disorders and cancer. *Trends Genet* 15: 74–80.

de Celis J, Barrio R, Kafatos F (1996). A gene complex acting downstream of *dpp* in *Drosophila* wing morphogenesis. *Nature* 381: 421–424.

Devriendt K, Fryns JP, Lemmens F, Kohlhase J, Liebers M (2002). Somatic mosaicism and variable expression of Townes-Brocks syndrome. *Am J Med Genet* 111: 230–231.

de Vries-van der Weerd M-A, Willems P, Mandema H, ten Kate L (1988). A new family with the Townes-Brocks syndrome. *Clin Genet* 34: 195–200.

Doray B, Langer B, Stoll C (1999). Two cases of Townes-Brocks syndrome. *Genet Couns* 10: 359–367.

Engels S, Kohlhase J, McGaughran J (2000). A SALL1 mutation causes a branchio-oto-renal syndrome-like phenotype. *J Med Genet* 37: 458–460.

Farrell ER, Munsterberg AE (2000). csal1 is controlled by a combination of FGF and Wnt signals in developing limb buds. *Dev Biol* 225: 447–458.

Ferraz FG, Nunes L, Ferraz ME, Sousa JP, Santos M, Carvalho C, Maroteaux P (1989). Townes-Brocks syndrome. Report of a case and review of the literature. *Ann Génét* 32: 120–123.

Friedman P, Rao K, Aylsworth A (1987). Six patients with the Townes-Brocks syndrome including five familial cases with a pericentric inversion of chromosome 16. *Am J Hum Genet* 41(Suppl): A60.

Gabrielli O, Bonifazi V, Offidani AM, Cellini A, Coppa GV, Giorgi PL (1993). Description of a patient with difficult nosological classification: Goldenhar syndrome or Townes-Brocks syndrome. *Minerva Pediatr* 45: 459–462.

Hentze MW, Kulozik AE (1999). A perfect message: RNA surveillance and nonsense-mediated decay. *Cell* 96: 307–310.

Hersh J, Jaworski M, Solinger R, Weisskopf B, Donat J (1986). Townes syndrome. A distinct multiple malformation syndrome resembling VACTERL association. *Clin Pediatr (Phila)* 25: 100–102.

Hollemann T, Schuh R, Pieler T, Stick R (1996). *Xenopus Xsal-1*, a vertebrate homolog of the region specific homeotic gene *spalt* of *Drosophila*. *Mech Dev* 55: 19–32.

Ilyina EG, Laziuk GI (1992). Clinical and genetic analysis of the Townes-Brocks syndrome [in Russian]. *Tsitol Genet* 26: 32–35.

Ishikiriyama S, Kudoh F, Shimojo N, Iwai J, Inoue T (1996). Townes-Brocks syndrome associated with mental retardation. *Am J Med Genet* 61: 191–192.

Johnson JP, Poskanzer LS, Sherman S (1996). Three-generation family with resemblance to Townes-Brocks syndrome and Goldenhar/oculoauriculovertebral spectrum. *Am J Med Genet* 61: 134–139.

Jürgens G (1988). Head and tail development of the *Drosophila* embryo involves *spalt*, a novel homeotic gene. *EMBO J* 7: 189–196.

Kalff-Suske M, Wild A, Topp J, Wessling M, Jacobsen EM, Bornholdt D, Engel H, Heuer H, Aalfs CM, Ausems MG, et al. (1999). Point mutations throughout the GLI3 gene cause Greig cephalopolysyndactyly syndrome. *Hum Mol Genet* 8: 1769–1777.

Keegan CE, Mulliken JB, Wu BL, Korf BR (2001). Townes-Brocks syndrome versus expanded spectrum hemifacial microsomia: review of eight patients and further evidence of a "hot spot" for mutation in the *SALL1* gene. *Genet Med* 3: 310–313.

Knoblauch H, Thiel G, Tinschert S, Körner H, Tennstedt C, Chaoui R, Kohlhase J, Dixkens C, Blanck C (2000). Clinical and molecular cytogenetic studies of a large de novo interstitial deletion 16q11.2-16q21 including the putative transcription factor gene SALL1. *J Med Genet* 37: 389–392.

Kohlhase J (2000). *SALL1* mutations in Townes-Brocks syndrome and related disorders. *Hum Mutat* 16: 460–466.

Kohlhase J, Schuh R, Dowe G, Kühnlein R P, Jäckle H, Schroeder B, Schulz-Schaeffer W, Kretzschmar HA, Köhler A, Müller U, et al. (1996). Isolation, characterization, and organ-specific expression of two novel human zinc finger genes related to the *Drosophila* gene *spalt*. *Genomics* 38: 291–298.

Kohlhase J, Wischermann A, Reichenbach H, Froster U, Engel W (1998). Mutations in the *SALL1* putative transcription factor gene cause Townes-Brocks syndrome. *Nat Genet* 18: 81–83.

Kohlhase J, Hausmann S, Stojmenovic G, Dixkens C, Bink K, Schulz-Schaeffer W, Altmann M, Engel W (1999a). *SALL3*, a new member of the human *spalt*-like gene family, maps to 18q23. *Genomics* 62: 216–222.

Kohlhase J, Köhler A, Jäckle H, Engel W, Stick R (1999b). Molecular cloning of a SALL1-related pseudogene and mapping to chromosome Xp11.2. *Cytogenet Cell Genet* 84: 31–34.

Kohlhase J, Taschner P, Burfeind P, Pasche B, Newman B, Blanck C, Breuning M, ten Kate L, Maaswinkel-Mooy P, Mitulla B, et al. (1999c). Molecular analysis of *SALL1* mutations in Townes-Brocks syndrome. *Am J Hum Genet* 64: 435–445.

Kohlhase J, Heinrich M, Schubert L, Liebers M, Kispert A, Laccone F, Turnpenny P, Winter RM, Reardon W (2002). Okihiro syndrome is caused by SALL4 mutations. *Hum Mol Genet* 11: 2979–2987.

König R, Schick U, Fuchs S (1990). Townes-Brocks syndrome. *Eur J Pediatr* 150: 100–103.

Köster R, Stick R, Loosli F, Wittbrodt J (1997). Medaka *spalt* acts as a target gene of *hedgehog* signaling. *Development* 124: 3147–3156.

Kotzot D, Lorenz P, Bieber A, Grobe H (1992). Townes-Brocks-Syndrom. *Monatsschr Kinderheilkd* 140: 343–345.

Kühnlein RP, Schuh R (1996). Dual function of the region specific homeotic gene *spalt* during *Drosophila* tracheal system development. *Development* 122: 2215–2223.

Kühnlein RP, Frommer G, Friedrich M, Gonzalez-Gaitan M, Weber A, Wagner-Bernholz JF, Gehring W, Jäckle H, Schuh R (1994). *spalt* encodes an evolutionary conserved zinc finger protein of novel structure which provides homeotic gene function in the head and tail region of the *Drosophila* embryo. *EMBO J* 13: 168–179.

Kurnit DM, Steele MW, Pinsky L, Dibbins A (1978). Autosomal-dominant transmission of a syndrome of anal, ear, renal, and radial congenital malformations. *J Pediatr* 93: 270–273.

Lecuit T, Brook WJ, Ng M, Calleja M, Sun H, Cohen SM (1996). Two distinct mechanisms for long-range patterning by *Decapentaplegic* in the *Drosophila* wing. *Nature* 381: 387–393.

Lenz W (1993). Comments on contribution by D. Kotzot et al. Townes-Brocks syndrome. *Monatsschr Kinderheilkd* 141: 791–792.

Ma Y, Singer DB, Gozman A, Ford D, Chai L, Steinhoff MM, Hansen K, Maizel AL (2001). Hsal 1 is related to kidney and gonad development and is expressed in Wilms tumor. *Pediatr Nephrol* 16: 701–719.

Marlin S, Toublanc JE, Petit C (1998). Two cases of Townes-Brocks syndrome with previously undescribed anomalies. *Clin Dysmorphol* 7: 295–298.

Marlin S, Blanchard S, Slim R, Lacombe D, Denoyelle F, Alessandri J-L, Calzolari E, Drouin-Garraud V, Ferraz FG, Fourmaintraux A, et al. (1999). Townes-Brocks syndrome: detection of a *SALL1* mutation hotspot and evidence for a position effect in one patient. *Hum Mutat* 14: 377–386.

Martinez-Frias ML, Bermejo Sanchez E, Arroyo Carrera I, Perez Fernandez JL, Pardo Romero M, Buron Martinez E, Hernandez Ramon F (1999). The Townes-Brocks syndrome in Spain: the epidemiological aspects in a consecutive series of cases [in Spanish]. *An Esp Pediatr* 50: 57–60.

Moeschler J, Clarren SK (1982). Familial occurrence of hemifacial microsomia with radial limb defects. *Am J Med Genet* 12: 371–375.

Monteiro de Pina-Neto J (1984). Phenotypic variability in Townes-Brocks syndrome. *Am J Med Genet* 18: 147–152.

Nellen D, Burke R, Struhl G, Basler K (1996). Direct and long-range action of a DPP morphogen gradient. *Cell* 85: 357–368.

Netzer C, Rieger L, Brero A, Zhang C-D, Hinzke M, Kohlhase J, Bohlander S K (2001). *SALL1*, the gene mutated in Townes-Brocks syndrome, encodes a transcriptional repressor which interacts with TRF1/PIN2 and localizes to pericentromeric heterochromatin. *Hum Mol Genet* 10: 3017–3024.

Newman WG, Brunet MD, Donnai D (1997). Townes-Brocks syndrome presenting as end stage renal failure. *Clin Dysmorphol* 6: 57–60.

Nishinakamura R, Matsumoto Y, Nakao K, Nakamura K, Sato A, Copeland N, Gilbert D, Jenkins N, Scully S, Lacey D, et al. (2001). Murine homolog of *SALL1* is essential for ureteric bud invasion in kidney development. *Development* 128: 3105–3115.

O'Callaghan M, Young ID (1990). The Townes-Brocks syndrome. *J Med Genet* 27: 457–461.

Ott T, Kaestner KH, Monaghan AP, Schütz G (1996). The mouse homolog of the region specific homeotic gene *spalt* of *Drosophila* is expressed in the developing nervous system and in mesoderm-derived structures. *Mech Dev* 56: 117–128.

Parent P, Bensaid M, Le Guern H, Colin A, Broussine L, Chabarot A, Cozic A, Jehannin B, de Parscau L (1995). Heterogeneity clinical de syndrome de Townes-Brocks. *Arch Pediatr* 2: 551–554.

Powell CM, Michaelis RC (1999). Townes-Brocks syndrome. *J Med Genet* 36: 89–93.

Radhakrishna U, Bornholdt D, Scott HS, Patel UC, Rossier C, Engel H, Bottani A, Chandal D, Blouin JL, Solanki JY, et al. (1999). The phenotypic spectrum of GLI3 morphopathies includes autosomal dominant preaxial polydactyly type-IV and postaxial polydactyly type-A/B; no phenotype prediction from the position of GLI3 mutations. *Am J Hum Genet* 65: 645–655.

Redemann N, Gaul U, Jäckle H (1988). Disruption of a putative Cys-zinc interaction eliminates the biological activity of the *Krüppel* finger protein. *Nature* 332: 90–92.

Reid IS, Turner G (1976). Familial anal abnormality. *J Pediatr* 88: 992–994.

Rossmiller DR, Pasic TR (1994). Hearing loss in Townes-Brocks syndrome. *Otolaryngol Head Neck Surg* 111: 175–180.

Sabbattini P, Lundgren M, Georgiou A, Chow C, Warnes G, Dillon N (2001). Binding of Ikaros to the lambda5 promoter silences transcription through a mechanism that does not require heterochromatin formation. *EMBO J* 20: 2812–2822.

Salerno A, Kohlhase J, Kaplan BS (2000). Townes-Brocks syndrome and renal dysplasia: a novel mutation in the *SALL1* gene. *Ped Nephrol* 14: 25–28.

Serville F, Lacombe D, Saura R, Billeaud C, Sergent MP (1993). Townes-Brocks syndrome in an infant with translocation t(5;16). *Genet Couns* 4: 109–112.

Sturtevant MA, Biehs B, Marin E, Bier E (1997). The *spalt* gene links the A/P compartment boundary to a linear adult structure in the *Drosophila* wing. *Development* 124: 21–32.

Surka WS, Kohlhase J, Neunert CE, Schneider DS, Proud VK (2001). Unique family with Townes-Brocks syndrome, SALL1 mutation, and cardiac defects. *Am J Med Genet* 102: 250–257.

Townes PL, Brocks ER (1972). Hereditary syndrome of imperforate anus with hand, foot and ear anomalies. *J Pediatr* 8: 321–326.

Walpole IR, Hockey A (1982). Syndrome of imperforate anus, abnormalities of hands and feet, satyr ears, and sensorineural deafness. *J Pediatr* 100: 250–252.

Wischermann A, Holschneider AM (1997). Townes-Brocks-Syndrom. *Monatsschr Kinderheilkd* 145: 382–386.

Part B.
The Wnt (Wingless-Type) Signaling Pathway

22 | Wnt Signaling Pathways

LAIRD C. SHELDAHL AND RANDALL T. MOON

Wingless (Wnt) is a large family of secreted signaling molecules known to play important roles in developmental processes such as cell fate specification, cell migration, and cell proliferation. Misregulation of Wnts can cause a range of developmental defects and is implicated in the genesis of several human cancers. Wnt was initially discovered as a protooncogene, into which the mouse mammary tumor virus integrates and causes mammary tumor formation (Nusse, 1991). The *Drosophila* Wnt-1 ortholog *wingless* (*wg*) had already been discovered; its mutations result in severe patterning defects and embryonic lethality (Nusslein-Volhard and Wieschaus, 1980). There are 18 Wnts in mouse. A current list of known *Wnt* genes along with sequence alignments can be found at the Wnt homepage (http://www.stanford.edu/~rnusse/wntwindow.html).

Wnts are expressed at many stages in development, often overlapping spatially and temporally with other Wnts (reviewed in Miller et al., 1999a). As summarized briefly below, Wnt proteins control development in organisms ranging from nematode worms to humans (Cadigan and Nusse, 1997). Before the name *Wnt* had been coined, mutations in the *Drosophila* ortholog *wg* had been shown to cause embryonic lethality and disruption of proper denticle band patterning. Later, studies in *Xenopus* revealed that ventral overexpression of Wnt-1 led to duplication of the embryonic axis by turning on dorsal-specific genes within ventral regions of the embryo (Sokol et al., 1991).

Wnts play a similar role in the chick organizer (Yamaguchi, 2001), as well as in patterning the limb buds (Tickle, 1995). In the nematode *Caenorhabditis elegans*, the Wnt family member Mom-2 polarizes the embryo at the four-cell stage (Thorpe et al., 1997). Secreted from the P2 cell, the daughter cells of the EMS cell that receives a high Wnt signal will become the E cell while the other cell, receiving a low Wnt signal, forms the MS cell. Loss of Wnt function in vertebrates produces a wide range of developmental defects. The first Wnt knockout mouse, deficient for Wnt-1, had specific midbrain developmental defects (McMahon and Bradley, 1990), while Wnt-3A-deficient mice lack caudal somites and tail bud and have defective notochords (Takada et al., 1994). Wnt-5A-deficient mice have severe defects in the extension of the anterior–posterior axis (Yamaguchi et al., 1999). A complete list of Wnt knockouts can be found at the Wnt homepage.

OVERVIEW OF THE WNT PATHWAYS

Recently, it has become clear that Wnts are capable of activating one of several pathways, yet for many years there was only "the Wnt signaling pathway." The most significant event of this pathway may be the observed increase in β-catenin protein levels; thus the pathway has been called "the Wnt/β-catenin pathway" (Miller et al., 1999a) (Fig. 22–1). In this pathway, Wnt proteins bind to Frizzled (Fz) cell

Figure 22–1. Overview of the Wnt/β-catenin and Wnt/Ca^{2+} pathways. GSK-3, glycogen synthase kinase -3; TCF, T-cell factor; PKC, protein kinase C; PLC, phospholipase C; CamK II, calcium/calmodulin-dependent protein kinase II; PP2A, protein phosphatase 2A; APC, adenomatous polyposis coli; Dsh, Dishevelled; GBP, GSK-3-binding protein; CK, casein kinase; NLK, NEMO-like kinase.

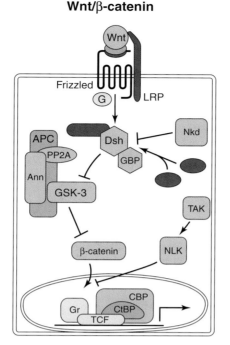

Wnt/β-catenin

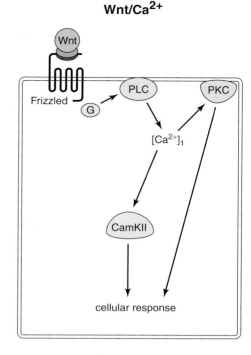

Wnt/Ca^{2+}

surface receptors and activate the cytoplasmic protein Dishevelled (Dsh). Activated Dsh subsequently prevents a group of proteins, known as the destruction complex, from targeting β-catenin for proteosomal degradation. This, in turn, elevates levels of β-catenin, which enters the nucleus and binds members of the lymphoid enhancer factor/T-cell factor (Lef/Tcf) family of transcription factors to activate expression of a variety of genes. In the absence of a Wnt signal, β-catenin is associated with the destruction complex, which includes Axin, adenomatous polyposis coli (APC), and glycogen synthase kinase 3β (GSK3β). Axin and APC form a scaffold, allowing GSK3β to phosphorylate β-catenin, Axin, and APC. Phosphorylation of β-catenin by GSK3β targets β-catenin for ubiquitination and subsequent breakdown by the ubiquitin-proteosome pathway. In the absence of β-catenin, Tcf transcription factors bind DNA and associate with transcriptional corepressors. Thus, Wnts modulate transcription by both relieving repression and activating transcription, in a manner described in greater detail in subsequent sections.

There are an increasing number of examples of Wnts functioning independently of β-catenin. Overexpression of some Wnts and Frizzleds has no effect on β-catenin levels and β-catenin target genes but, instead, elicits intracellular Ca^{2+} flux and activates the Ca^{2+}-responsive enzymes protein kinase C (PKC) and calcium/calmodulin-dependent protein kinase II (CamKII) (reviewed in Kuhl et al., 2000a,b) (Fig. 22–1). This has been called "the Wnt/Ca^{2+} pathway," which can be antagonistic to the Wnt/β-catenin pathway (Kuhl et al., 2001). Whether these are indeed separate signaling pathways or represent two independent arms downstream of the same receptors and ligands is still unclear. Currently, the only example of regulation of cell fate associated with activation of the Wnt/Ca^{2+} pathway is in specification of ventral fate in *Xenopus* embryos (Kuhl et al., 2000a,b), but there are an increasing number of β-catenin-independent Wnt phenotypes whose molecular basis has yet to be determined. Interestingly, this pathway may be involved in regulating cell behavior during gastrulation movements in *Xenopus* development (Torres et al., 1996; Winklbauer et al., 2001).

The Wnt/β-catenin signaling components Dsh and Fz are also required in the planar cell polarity (PCP) pathway, which, among other things, is responsible for the proper alignment of hairs on the *Drosophila* wing (reviewed in Shulman et al., 1998). In vertebrates, there is increasing evidence that homologs of this *Drosophila* pathway exist (reviewed in Sokol, 2000) and, like the Wnt/Ca^{2+} pathway, function in regulating gastrulation movements (Park and Moon, 2002). Moreover, one vertebrate ortholog of the PCP protein Strabismus antagonizes Wnt/β-catenin signaling similar to the Wnt/Ca^{2+} pathway (Park and Moon, 2002). While this is suggestive of a relationship between the PCP and Wnt/Ca^{2+} pathways, these data also point to the need for further study.

THE *WNT* GENE FAMILY

The *Wnt* gene family is defined by sequence homology to *wnt-1* (Nusse and Varmus, 1982) and *wg* (Nusslein-Volhard and Wieschaus, 1980; Rijsewijk et al., 1987). All Wnts contain a conserved pattern of 23 or 24 cysteine residues and are glycosylated prior to secretion. Wnts have been observed to associate with cell surfaces and the extracellular matrix (Papkoff and Schryver, 1990). Glycosaminoglycans found in the extracellular matrix have been shown to act as Wnt cofactors (reviewed in Wells, 2001). Wnts are regarded as somewhat sticky signaling molecules, not as freely diffusible as some other growth factors (Burrus, 1994). Wnts have been shown, though, to act as long-range morphogens (Zecca et al., 1996) as well as signaling to short-range targets, such as neighboring cells in *Drosophila* cuticles (Bejsovec and Martinez Arias, 1991). The *Porcupine* gene is involved in the secretion of Wnts (van den Heuvel et al., 1993; Kadowaki et al., 1996) and may play a role in lipid modification of Wnts (Hofmann, 2000).

There are 18 known mouse *Wnt* genes and seven known in *Drosophila*. These numbers include highly similar A–B pairs within vertebrates. Adding yet another layer of complexity, the zebrafish *Wnt-8* gene encodes two Wnt-8 proteins, expressed in nonidentical patterns (Lekven et al., 2001).

WNT RECEPTORS

The identity of the Wnt receptor remained a mystery for years after many Wnts and Wnt signaling components had been identified. We now know the Frizzled family of seven-transmembrane receptors bind Wnts with high affinity to transduce Wnt signals (Bhanot et al., 1996; Yang-Snyder et al., 1996). This is a large family of proteins, each containing an amino-terminal cysteine-rich domain (Wang et al., 1996).

The intracellular loops of the Fz family of proteins vary significantly in length and lack key domains found in rhodopsin and most other serpentine receptors known to couple to G proteins (Barnes et al., 1998). G proteins are required for Wnt/Ca^{2+} signals (Kuhl et al., 2000b) and Wnt/β-catenin signals (Liu et al., 2001b), but their exact roles in either pathway are currently unclear. A key intracellular domain, located just after the seventh transmembrane domain (Lys-Thr-X-X-X-Trp), is required for activation of the Wnt/β-catenin pathway (Umbhauer et al., 2000). A preliminary sorting of Frizzleds into two groups preferentially coupling to either the Wnt/β-catenin or Wnt/Ca^{2+} pathway has been done (Kuhl et al., 2000b). The caveat on this list is that it is based on basal signaling, without ligands, and in one assay system. One exception so far is *Xenopus* Frizzled 7 (XFz7), which can distinguish between different Wnt ligands to signal via multiple pathways. XFz7 may activate the Wnt/β-catenin pathway in response to Wnt-8B, the PCP pathway in response to Wnt-11, and the Wnt/Ca^{2+} pathway (if it is distinct from the PCP pathway) in response to an unidentified ligand. This suggests that the activation of distinct pathways depends on the specific Wnt/Fz combination (Winklbauer et al., 2001).

Many other transmembrane and extracellular molecules play roles in the reception of Wnt signals. Glypicans are thought to play an important role in presenting Wnts to cell surface receptors as heparin-sulfate mutations impair Wnt signaling (Lin and Perrimon, 2000) and sulfated glycosaminoglycans are required for Wnt/β-catenin signaling in *Drosophila* (Reichsman et al., 1996) and *Xenopus* (Itoh and Sokol, 1994). The glypican Dally has been postulated to act as a coreceptor along with Fz (Lin and Perrimon, 2000; Tsuda et al., 1999). Another coreceptor, the low-density lipoprotein (LDL) receptor–related protein 6 (LRP6) has been identified (Pinson et al., 2000; Tamai et al., 2000; Wehrli et al., 2000) and shown to play a key role in the reception of Wnt signals as well as inhibition of Wnt signals by the secreted molecule Dickkopf (Mao et al., 2001a). In *Drosophila*, loss of the LRP6 homolog *arrow* phenocopies loss of *wg*, indicating that *arrow* is necessary for proper *wg* signaling (Wehrli et al., 2000). Furthermore, overproduction of *wg* is incapable of overcoming loss of *arrow* function (Tamai et al., 2000) but capable of rescuing loss of *dally* (Binari et al., 1997), suggesting that *arrow* is absolutely required for *wg* signaling, whereas proteoglycans facilitate *wg* signaling. While LRP5 and -6 are divergent from other LDL-related protein receptors, other LDL receptor–related proteins endocytose ligand-bound receptors, which suggests that LRP5 and -6 may do more than simply help Wnts bind Frizzleds (Bejsovec, 2000). While not linked to *arrow*, a Wnt link has been observed: Wg protein disappears from alternating stripes in *Drosophila* embryos as it is endocytosed and degraded in lysosomes (Scott, 2001). Lastly, Frizzleds may bind other Frizzleds in order to function properly (Dann et al., 2001).

The function of Wnt signals depends not only on which Wnt a cell is exposed to but also on the receptors and co-receptors present on that cell. In some cases, a tissue is exposed to several Wnt proteins and each Wnt produces a distinct effect. For instance, Wnt-7A regulates dorsal/ventral patterning in the chick limb independent of β-catenin and Lef1, while Wnt-3A functions in the same tissue to affect expression of apical ectodermal ridge-specific genes via β-catenin and Lef1 (Kengaku et al., 1998). Similarly, overexpression of Wnt-5A in *Xenopus* does not lead to stabilization of β-catenin and duplication of the embryonic axis (Torres et al., 1996) and, instead, elicits calcium flux (Slusarski et al., 1997b). However, when coexpressed with human Frizzled 5, a Wnt/β-catenin phenotype is observed as two-headed tadpoles are produced (He et al., 1997). Wnt-5A can also mediate axis duplication when LRP5 is expressed in neighboring cells (Bejsovec, 2000). The latter two experiments suggest that the phenotype produced by a Wnt depends on the particular receptors and coreceptors present.

FRIZZLED INTERACTING PROTEINS

Overexpression of some Frizzled proteins is capable of relocalizing Dsh to the plasma membrane (Yang-Snyder et al., 1996), yet no direct interaction between Fz and Dsh has been shown. Recently, however, two Frizzled-interacting proteins have been identified. Kermit is a cytoplasmic protein with a central PDZ domain that relocalizes to the plasma membrane with overexpression of XFz3 (Tan et al., 2001). While Kermit is required for Xfz3 function in neural crest specification, it has no clear developmental effects prior to gastrulation, which suggests that it is not required for Wnt/β-catenin signaling (Tan et al., 2001). A second Fz-interacting protein has been identified: Golgi-associated PDZ and coiled coil motif containing protein (GOPC), which may be involved in the vesicular transport of Frizzled from the Golgi apparatus to the plasma membrane (Yao et al., 2001).

SECRETED WNT INHIBITORS

There are several families of proteins that interfere with Wnt signaling before or at the stage of Wnts binding to cell surface receptors. These families include the secreted Frizzled-related protein family (FrzB or sFRP for short) (reviewed in Moon et al., 1997), Wnt-inhibitory factor-1 (WIF1) (Hsieh et al., 1999), Cerberus (Bouwmeester et al., 1996; Piccolo et al., 1999), and Dickkopf (Dkk) (Glinka et al., 1998; Fedi et al., 1999). To repress Wnt signaling, Dkk requires LRP5. Perhaps by binding to a part of a Wnt receptor complex, Dkk sterically hinders the binding of Wnts to the Fz/LRP complex (Mao et al., 2001a). FrzB, Wif1, and Cerberus directly bind Wnt proteins, preventing their interaction with Frizzleds. FrzBs look like secreted ligand-binding domains of Frizzleds (Rattner et al., 1997). FrzB, furthermore, can also interact with Frizzleds, suggesting that they may inhibit Wnt signaling by the formation of non-functional Fz/FrzB complexes (Bafico et al., 1999). FrzBs do not bind all Wnt proteins with equal affinity but display specificity in blocking some Wnts but not others (reviewed in Yamaguchi, 2001). Cerberus not only inhibits Wnt signals but is an antagonist of Nodal and bone morphogenetic proteins as well (Piccolo et al., 1999).

THE MULTIFUNCTIONAL PROTEIN DISHEVELLED

To date, no direct interaction between Fz and the next downstream signaling component, Dishevelled, has been described. Furthermore, the exact molecular changes in Dsh that occur upon its activation by Wnt signaling are unclear. Nevertheless, much is known about this unique, if enigmatic, protein. Dsh is a modular protein that contains three identified domains: PDZ, DIX, and DEP. The PDZ domain of Dsh, unlike PDZ domains in many other proteins, does not bind S/TXV motifs (an S/TXV motif is found in the C-terminal region of Fz proteins but is not required for β-catenin signaling [Lee et al., 1999]). Dishevelled's PDZ domain is required for binding to GSK3-binding protein (GBP) (Yost et al., 1998; Li et al., 1999) as well as casein kinase 2 (CK2) (Willert et al., 1997). Deletion of the PDZ domain yields a dominant-negative form that blocks Wnt/β-catenin signaling. The DIX domain (found in **Di**shevelled and **Ax**in [Cadigan and Nusse, 1997]) is required for Dsh dimerization (Rothbacher et al., 2000) and binding to Axin (Smalley et al., 1999). Deletion of this domain abrogates Dsh's functionality in the Wnt/β-catenin pathway yet retains functionality in the PCP pathway. The DEP domain (found in **D**sh, **e**gl-10, and **P**leckstrin) is required for translocation of Dsh to the plasma membrane in response to Fz expression (Axelrod et al., 1998). This event is separable from Wnt/β-catenin function as DEP domain deletion mutants still rescue Wnt/β-catenin signaling, despite being unable to translocate to the plasma membrane (Yanagawa et al., 1995; Boutros et al., 1998).

There are three different Dishevelled proteins in mouse (Dvl1–3) (Lee et al., 1999) but only one in *Xenopus* (Sokol et al., 1995). It is unclear whether different Dsh proteins mediate different known effects of Dsh. A Dvl1$^{-/-}$ mouse has no developmental phenotypes; however, these mice exhibit reduced social interactions and slowed sensorimotor gating similar to mouse models of schizophrenia and Tourette's syndrome (Lijam et al., 1997).

Dsh interacts directly with the destruction complex, binding to Axin, which leads to a decrease in GSK3β-mediated phosphorylation of β-catenin (Kishida et al., 1999; Li et al., 1999a). Dsh recruits GBP (FRAT1 in mammals) to the destruction complex in response to Wnt signaling (Li et al., 1999), and GBP is required for the decrease in phosphorylation of β-catenin in response to Wnt signaling (Yost et al., 1998).

Mouse Dishevelled (Dvl) is phosphorylated in response to signaling by Wg, Wnt-3a, and Fz (Lee et al., 1999). Furthermore, Dsh levels are both enriched and phosphorylated on the prospective dorsal side of 16-128 cell *Xenopus* embryos, the site where β-catenin is known to accumulate and where Dsh would presumably be active if involved in axis specification (Miller et al., 1999b; Rothbacher et al., 2000). Whether this phosphorylation represents the molecular mechanism by which Wnt signaling activates Dsh is unclear. However, deletion analysis suggests that the Dsh domains involved in Wg-induced phosphorylation are distinct from those required for Wnt/β-catenin signaling (Axelrod et al., 1998; Rothbacher et al., 2000). Furthermore, Dsh is phosphorylated by Wnt-11 and Wnt-5A during gastrulation, and this phosphorylation is not concomitant with an increase in β-catenin levels (Tada and Smith, 2000). It is not known whether the sites of Dsh phosphorylation in response to Wnt-5A are the same or different from the sites phosphorylated in response to Wg; but because Wnt-5A can block Wnt/β-catenin signaling (Torres et al., 1996; Kuhl et al., 2001), this suggests that there are multiple phosphorylation sites on Dsh that have distinct roles in regulating Dsh activity.

The protein kinase CK1 phosphorylates Dsh and associates with Axin and the GBP/GSK3β complex (Lee et al., 2001). The protein kinase CK2 (unrelated to CK1) likewise phosphorylates Dsh in vivo (Willert et al., 1997), and PKC phosphorylates Dsh in vitro (Kuhl et al., 2001). The kinase Par-1 also phosphorylates Dishevelled, leading to an increase in Wnt/β-catenin signaling but inhibiting Dsh-mediated activation of Jun N-terminal kinase (JNK) (Sun et al., 2001). Dsh binds protein phosphatase 2C (PP2C), which is capable of dephosphorylating Axin and activating Wnt/β-catenin signaling (Strovel et al., 2000).

Naked Cuticle (Nkd), a newly described Dsh-interacting protein, plays opposing roles in the Wnt/β-catenin pathway and the PCP pathway (reviewed in McEwen and Peifer, 2001). Injection of Nkd disrupts formation of the primary axis and blocks the ability of Wnt-8 to induce a secondary axis in *Xenopus* (Rousset et al., 2001). Blockade of the Wnt/β-catenin pathway occurs upstream of GSK3β (Wharton et al., 2001) and requires and an intact calcium-binding EF hand motif (Yan et al., 2001). Further studies of the Wnt/Ca^{2+} and PCP pathway will need to be undertaken to clarify the relationship between activation of Ca^{2+} and activation of the PCP pathway downstream of Frizzleds.

THE DESTRUCTION COMPLEX OF THE WNT/β-CATENIN PATHWAY

In the absence of a Wnt signal, the destruction complex targets β-catenin for degradation by the ubiquitin-proteosome pathway. Axin and APC are large proteins which act as scaffolds, binding GSK3β and β-catenin. When both are bound to Axin, GSK3β phosphorylates β-catenin on several sites (Yost et al., 1996), targeting β-catenin for ubiquitination and proteosomal degradation (Aberle et al., 1997).

Axin (Zeng et al., 1997) is a negative regulator of β-catenin, serving as a bridge between GSK3β and β-catenin. Axin mutations (in Fused mice) are embryonic lethal and often lead to duplicated embryonic axes (Zeng et al., 1997). Axin contains an N-terminal RGS (regulator of G-protein signaling) domain, which, aptly enough, is found in G-protein signal-regulatory proteins. No evidence exists for Axin interacting with G proteins, but the RGS domain is required for binding to APC (Behrens et al., 1998; Hart et al., 1998; Kishida et al., 1998; Nakamura et al., 1998), the deletion of which leads to a dominant-negative form (Zeng et al., 1997). The central region of Axin binds β-catenin and GSK3β (on distinct sites) (Behrens et al., 1998; Hart et al., 1998; Ikeda et al., 1998; Itoh et al., 1998). At the C terminus, Axin contains a DIX domain, which binds Dsh (Kishida et al., 1999b; Li et al., 1999; Smalley et al., 1999). Dephosphorylation of Axin by PP2A leads to increased β-catenin stability (Willert et al., 1999), while phosphorylation by GSK3β increases the stability of Axin within cells (Yamamoto et al., 1999). Furthermore, phosphorylated Axin binds β-catenin with higher affinity (Willert et al., 1999).

APC was originally identified as a tumor suppressor, and mutations in it are found in the majority of colon cancers (reviewed in Polakis, 1997). These mutations lead to stabilization of β-catenin. APC binds Axin, GSK3β, and β-catenin. APC itself is a target for phosphoryla-

tion by GSK3β, which leads to an increase in affinity for β-catenin (Rubinfeld et al., 1996). Phosphorylation of APC by CK1ϵ also increases its affinity for β-catenin (Rubinfeld et al., 2001). Dephosphorylation by PP2A also increases β-catenin stability (Seeling et al., 1999). While APC is thought of as a negative regulator of Wnt signaling, not all data have consistently suggested this. For instance, overexpression of APC in *Xenopus* activates Wnt signaling and is capable of inducing a second notochord on the ventral side of embryos (Vleminckx et al., 1997). These data, and similar data in *C. elegans* (Rocheleau et al., 1997), have been reconciled with the idea that overexpressed APC may sequester key negative regulatory components without binding β-catenin, thereby leading to stabilization of β-catenin and activation of the Wnt/β-catenin pathway (Miller et al., 1999a). APC resides in the nucleus (Neufeld et al., 2000), at plasma membrane sites involved in cell migration (Nathke, 1999), and in the cytoplasm. Nuclear export of APC can lead to decreases in nuclear β-catenin (Neufeld et al., 2000), although not directly due to APC binding and shuttling β-catenin from the nucleus (Wiechens and Fagotto, 2001).

GSK3β is the central negative regulator of β-catenin stability. Mutations in the *Drosophila* GSK3β ortholog *zeste white-3* (*zw3*) result in accumulation of Armadillo (the β-catenin ortholog) and mimic phenotypes of constitutive Wg signaling (Siegfried et al., 1992; Peifer et al., 1993). Similarly, expression of a dominant-interfering mutant of GSK3β in *Xenopus* leads to stabilization and nuclear accumulation of β-catenin (Yost et al., 1996; Larabell et al., 1997). The potent GSK3β inhibitor lithium has been used to pharmacologically activate Wnt signaling (Hedgepeth et al., 1997). Inhibition of GSK3β by insulin, however, does not affect β-catenin stability (reviewed in Frame and Cohen, 2001), which illustrates that even though the Wnt/β-catenin pathway shares components with other signaling pathways, distinct regulatory mechanisms keep these pathways separate.

GSK3β can phosphorylate several highly conserved serine and threonine residues in β-catenin in vitro (Yost et al., 1996). Mutation of these sites leads to stabilized, constitutively active forms of β-catenin found in a variety of human cancers (reviewed in Polakis, 2001). Phosphorylated β-catenin is a target for B-TrCP/Slimb, a component of the stem cell factor (SCF) ubiquitin ligase complex (Kitagawa et al., 1999; Liu et al., 1999; Winston et al., 1999). Phospho-β-catenin interacts with the SCF ubiquitin ligase complex and becomes ubiquitinated (Kitagawa et al., 1999), which then targets β-catenin for degradation by the 26S proteosome (Orford et al., 1997).

INHIBITION OF THE DESTRUCTION COMPLEX

The mechanism by which Dsh and GBP (and its mammalian homolog FRAT1) reduce GSK-mediated phosphorylation of β-catenin is currently an area of eager study, with two primary hypotheses: via direct down-regulation of GSK3β kinase activity or via alteration of the composition/conformation of the destruction complex. In support of the first hypothesis, treatment of mammalian cells with Wg-conditioned media leads to a twofold reduction in GSK3β activity in a PKC-dependent manner (Cook et al., 1996), and similar results have been seen in *Drosophila* clone8 cells (Ruel et al., 1999). Furthermore, overexpression of Wnt-8 in *Xenopus* leads to a decrease in GSK3β activity that coimmunoprecipitates with Axin (Itoh et al., 1998).

The second model of β-catenin regulation suggests that association of GBP with the destruction complex sterically hinders GSK3β from phosphorylating β-catenin (Fig. 22–2). GBP is recruited to the destruction complex in response to Wnt signaling, binding to the PDZ domain of Dishevelled (Salic et al., 2000). A peptide from GBP was shown to prevent GSK3β–Axin interactions and GSK3β-mediated phosphorylation of Axin and β-catenin (Yost et al., 1998). Furthermore, GBP decreases phosphorylation of β-catenin by GSK3β but does not affect the phosphorylation of a GSK3β-peptide substrate, suggesting that GBP prevents β-catenin from properly associating with the destruction complex, while the much smaller peptide substrate is able to enter and associate with GSK3β (Farr et al., 2000). Reduction of GSK3β activity within the destruction complex may also reduce the amount of β-catenin associated with the destruction complex. Stimulation of C57mg cells with Wnt-3A leads to a reduction in Axin

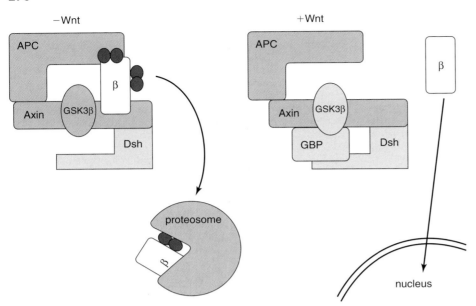

Figure 22–2. The Wnt/β-catenin pathway destruction complex. GSK3β, glycogen synthase kinase 3β; APC, adenomatous polyposis coli; Dsh, Dishevelled; GBP, GSK3-binding protein.

phosphorylation and subsequent decrease in affinity for β-catenin (Willert et al., 1999). However, others have found no changes in Axin's affinity for β-catenin (Salic et al., 2000). Wnt-1 has also been shown to disrupt a quaternary complex composed of Axin, Dvl, APC, and GSK3β (Li et al., 1999). Whether Dishevelled is associated with the active destruction complex and recruits GBP in response to Wnt signals (Li et al., 1999) or whether Dsh associates with the destruction complex in response to Wnt signals and brings GBP along (Salic et al., 2000) is still unclear.

Other Wnt-responsive changes have been observed in destruction-complex proteins. Axin translocates to the plasma membrane and interacts with LRP5 in response to Wnt signaling and is then targeted for degradation (Mao et al., 2001b). Whether Axin translocation and degradation lead to increased β-catenin stability is still unclear.

β-CATENIN AND THE LEF AND TCF TRANSCRIPTION FACTORS

β-Catenin functions both in the transduction of Wnt signals as well as in cell–cell adhesion. When discussing the regulation of β-catenin stability by Wnts, references to "cytoplasmic pools" of β-catenin are made to distinguish free β-catenin and β-catenin bound to the destruction complex from cadherin-bound β-catenin at the plasma membrane. While the cadherin-bound pool of β-catenin has complicated some experimental procedures (Fagotto et al., 1996; Miller and Moon, 1997), there is little evidence of its participation in Wnt signaling. In the presence of Wnt signals, β-catenin is stabilized and accumulates in the cytoplasm and nucleus (reviewed in Sharpe et al., 2001). Nuclear import of β-catenin is independent of importins but dependent on β-catenin's armadillo repeats (reviewed in Akiyama, 2000).

Upon entering the nucleus, β-catenin binds members of the Lef/Tcf family of transcription factors (Cavallo et al., 1997) (Fig. 22–3). There are four mammalian members of the Lef/Tcf family of transcription factors: Lef1, Tcf1, Tcf3, and Tcf4. These are DNA-binding proteins that, through their interaction with other proteins, bend DNA and stimulate transcription (reviewed in Sharpe et al., 2001). Activation of transcription requires transactivation domains in β-catenin for recruitment of other transcriptional cofactors, such as cAMP response element binding protein (CBP) (Takemaru and Moon, 2000) and RNA polymerase. CBP not only plays a role in the activation of Wnt/β-catenin target genes but is also required for repression of Wnt/β-catenin target genes in *Drosophila* and capable of acetylating dTcf and reducing dTcf's affinity for the *Drosophila* β-catenin ortholog Armadillo

(reviewed in Nusse, 1999). While activation of transcription by Tcfs requires the binding of β-catenin to recruit transcriptional activators, Lef1 can activate transcription in certain contexts in the absence of β-catenin (Hsu et al., 1998).

Functional redundancy between Lef/Tcf homologs has been suggested. $Tcf1^{-/-}$, $Tcf4^{-/-}$, and $Lef1^{-/-}$ mice do not show phenotypes that resemble known Wnt functions, whereas double-mutant $Lef1^{-/-}Tcf1^{-/-}$ mice display a phenotype very similar to that of $Wnt-3A^{-/-}$ mice (reviewed in Akiyama, 2000). However, Lef and Tcfs display differences in their ability to act as repressors of Wnt/β-catenin target genes in the absence of Wnt signals (Roose et al., 1998; Brannon et al., 1999), suggesting that functional redundancy is not a steadfast rule.

Lef/Tcf family members bind DNA at conserved regions in the promoters of Wnt-responsive gene promoters, called "Lef-binding sites." One common tool for examination of Wnt signaling is TOPFLASH, or the Tcf-optimal promoter (Korinek et al., 1997). This reporter utilizes the luciferase gene under the control of multiple Lef-binding sites and a basal c-Fos promoter.

In the absence of β-catenin, Lef/Tcf family members bind DNA via their single DNA-binding high-mobility group (HMG) domain and recruit transcriptional corepressors such as Groucho and C-terminal binding protein (CtBP) (Cavallo et al., 1998; Roose et al., 1998; Brannon et al., 1999) (Fig. 22–3). Groucho belongs to a large family of transcriptional corepressors which often convert transcriptional activators to repressors (reviewed in Chen and Courey, 2000). While the mechanism by which Groucho represses transcription is not fully understood, it may involve recruitment of histone deacetylases (Chen and Courey, 2000). Lef1 also associates with the histone deacetylase HDAC1 to repress transcription (Billin et al., 2000).

Wnt/β-catenin signaling can further be regulated by phosphorylation of Lef/Tcf by NEMO-like kinase (NLK, a mitogen-activated protein kinase–related kinase) (Ishitani et al., 1999; Rocheleau et al., 1999). Phosphorylation of Tcf by NLK reduces the ability of Tcf/β-catenin to bind DNA (Ishitani et al., 1999; Meneghini et al., 1999) (Fig. 22–3). In vertebrates, this would reduce the ability of Wnts to activate gene transcription, whereas in *C. elegans*, phosphorylation of Pop1 (Tcf3) by Mom4 (Tak1, the homologue of NLK) interferes with the ability of Pop1 to repress transcription (Shin et al., 1999; Behrens, 2000). Thus, TAK/NLK function in conjunction with Wnt/β-catenin signals to regulate the transcription of genes. Extracellular signals that lead to activation of TAK/NLK have yet to be identified.

Nuclear β-catenin can also be regulated by other HMG-box proteins, such as Xsox17, which directly binds β-catenin and represses

Figure 22–3. Wnt/β-catenin signals in the nucleus. HDAC, histone deacetylase; TCF, T-cell factor; NLK, NEMO-like kinase.

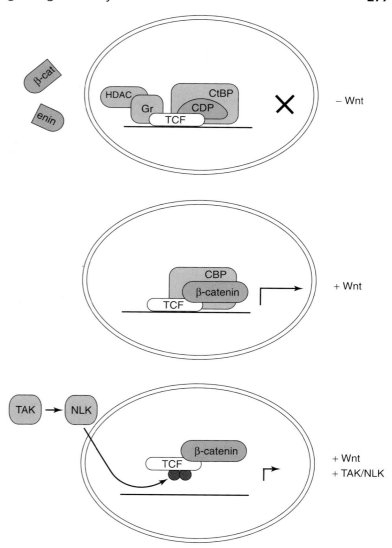

transcription of genes activated by β-catenin, while activating the transcription of other genes (Zorn et al., 1999). Another HMG-box repressor is HBP1, capable of repressing transcription of Wnt/β-catenin target genes (Sampson et al., 2001).

WNT/β-CATENIN TARGET GENES

Among the best-studied target genes of the β-catenin/Tcf/Lef complex are *Xenopus siamois* and *twin*, both required for activation of the Spemann organizer and subsequent development of the embryonic axes (Brannon et al., 1997; Laurent et al., 1997). Other Wnt-responsive genes include developmental regulatory genes such as *Xenopus nodal related-3*; *engrailed* and *ubx* in *Drosophila*; *nacre* in zebrafish; regulators of cell growth and proliferation *c-myc*, *cyclin D1*, and *c-jun*; the cell–cell communication regulator *connexin 43*; and the metalloprotease *matrilysin* (reviewed in Akiyama, 2000). A more complete list can be found at the Wnt homepage.

REGULATION OF β-CATENIN BY WNT-INDEPENDENT MECHANISMS

β-Catenin levels can be regulated by several other signaling pathways. Expression of integrin-linked kinase (ILK) leads to stabilization and nuclear accumulation of β-catenin (Novak et al., 1998), possibly via downregulation of GSK3β activity (Delcommenne et al., 1998).

Degradation of E-cadherins in response to insulin-like growth factor signaling has likewise been shown to increase nuclear β-catenin levels and transcription of Tcf target genes (Morali et al., 2001). Presenilins also affect β-catenin stability as mutations in presenilins associated with rapid-onset Alzheimer's disease decrease the stability of β-catenin in neurons (Zhang et al., 1998). p53 affects β-catenin stability independently of GSK3β and β-transducin repeat containing protein (β-TrCP), via activation of Siah-1, a mediator of cell-cycle arrest, tumor suppression, and apoptosis (Liu et al., 2001a). This process is activated by genotoxic injury, involves APC as well as the F-box protein Ebi, and represents a second mechanism by which β-catenin may be degraded (Matsuzawa and Reed, 2001; Polakis, 2001).

Insulin signaling, while capable of decreasing GSK3β activity, does not alter β-catenin levels or affect transcription of Wnt/β-catenin target genes (reviewed in Weston and Davis, 2001). The insulin-signaling pathway protein Akt, however, has recently been shown to affect the Wnt signaling pathway. Expression of Wnt or Dishevelled increases Akt activity, and activated Akt binds Axin/GSK3β complexes and increases free β-catenin levels (Fukumoto et al., 2001). However, as a constitutively active Akt has no effects on Lef-mediated transcription (Li et al., 1999), it seems unlikely that Akt plays a key role in inhibiting a β-catenin signal. Nevertheless, this once again underlines how a protein's context can determine its function and regulation when shared by multiple signaling pathways.

AXIS FORMATION: AN EXAMPLE OF A ROLE FOR THE WNT/β-CATENIN PATHWAY IN DEVELOPMENT

Wnts play a wide number of roles during development, one example being vertebrate axis specification (reviewed in Moon and Kimelman, 1998). The Wnt/β-catenin signaling pathway has the capability of duplicating the embryonic axis, yet activation of this pathway by Wnts may not be required for specification of the endogenous embryonic axis. Dominant-negative forms of Wnt, capable of blocking secondary axis formation, have no ability to block formation of the endogenous axes (Hoppler et al., 1996). Dominant-negative Frizzleds, as well as wild-type FrzBs, likewise fail to block the endogenous axis in *Xenopus* (reviewed in Sokol, 1999), while in zebrafish, a dominant-negative Fz disrupts the endogenous axis (Nasevicius et al., 1998). Inhibition of posterior Wnt signals by anteriorly localized Wnt antagonists, however, is critical for proper axis formation in chick (reviewed in Yamaguchi, 2001). Thus, while Wnts and Frizzleds capable of activating the Wnt/β-catenin pathway are present in eggs, loss-of-function data are mixed in terms of establishing whether they are required for axis formation.

Dishevelled is a good candidate for participating in axis specification. Levels of Dsh are enriched dorsally at the one-cell stage following cortical rotation and transport along microtubules in *Xenopus* (Miller et al., 1999b). Inhibition of microtubule function blocks not only this enrichment but axis specification as well (Miller et al., 1999b). Furthermore, Dsh is phosphorylated at the right time and place to be involved in axis specification (Rothbacher et al., 2000). A dominant-negative form of Dsh, however, is incapable of inhibiting formation of the endogenous body axis in *Xenopus* (Sokol, 1996), though antisense GBP does inhibit specification of the dorsal/ventral axis (Yost et al., 1998). It is important to note that dominant-negative approaches often fail to abolish interactions of endogenous proteins (Rothbacher et al., 2000), which leaves open the notion that Wnts and/or Dsh function at times in development before these treatments are executed.

While there is only circumstantial evidence for Wnt, Fz, and Dsh function in axis formation, experiments designed to interfere with components downstream of Dsh have shown direct requirements for Wnt signaling components in axis specification. Depletion of maternal β-catenin in *Xenopus* oocytes prevents induction of the primary axis (Heasman et al., 1994, 2000). β-Catenin accumulation, furthermore, has been visualized at the right place and time to be involved in primary axis specification (Larabell et al., 1997). While the latter is consistent with the presence of a Wnt signal, in this same region of the embryo, levels of GSK3β have been reported to be low (Dominguez and Green, 2000). This would account for the localized accumulation of β-catenin, but decreases in GSK3β levels have not been reported in response to Wnt signals. Instead, overexpression of GBP leads to a decrease in levels of GSK3β in a manner dependent on cortical rotation; thus, GBP is a good candidate for an endogenous dorsal determinant.

Overexpression of GSK3β can inhibit accumulation of endogenous β-catenin (Larabell et al., 1997) and formation of the primary axis (Dominguez et al., 1995; He et al., 1995). A dominant-negative Tcf3 likewise represses the endogenous axis (Molenaar et al., 1996), as does a dominant-negative form of a Wnt/β-catenin target gene, *siamois* (Kessler, 1997). Ultimately. the effects of Wnt/β-catenin signaling on axis formation are to induce expression of the regulatory genes *siamois* and *twin*, which in turn promote formation of the Spemann organizer (reviewed in Moon and Kimelman, 1998).

THE WNT/Ca²⁺ PATHWAY

Recently, a second, possibly distinct pathway activated by Wnt and Fz signaling has been identified, the Wnt/Ca²⁺ pathway (reviewed in Kuhl et al., 2000b). Specificity between activation of the Wnt/Ca²⁺ pathway versus the Wnt/β-catenin pathway may be determined by Fz. For instance, Rat Frizzled 1 (Rfz1), but not Rfz2, is capable of activating β-catenin target genes (Yang-Snyder et al., 1996), whereas Rfz2, but not Rfz1, elicits Ca²⁺ flux in zebrafish (Slusarski et al., 1997a) and activates Ca²⁺-the responsive kinases PKC (Sheldahl et

al., 1999) and CamKII (Kuhl et al., 2000b). Activation of the Wnt/Ca²⁺ pathway is sensitive to agents that inhibit G-protein signaling via the $G\alpha_{i/o}$ class of G proteins, although it remains unclear whether G proteins play a direct or indirect role in Wnt/Ca²⁺ signaling.

For many years, the Wnt/Ca²⁺ pathway was referred to as "the Wnt-5A pathway." Wnt-5A along with several other Wnts have very different effects from Wnt-1 and Wg in tissue culture and *Xenopus* experiments. While Wnt-1 and Wg are capable of transforming C57mg mouse mammary cells, Wnt-5A is not (Wong et al., 1994). Antisense Wnt-5a constructs, however, produce morphological changes similar to those in Wnt-1-treated cells, which suggests that the inability of Wnt-5A to transform these cells does not result from a lack of proper receptors but that Wnt-5A plays an active role in inhibiting Wnt/β-catenin signaling (Olson and Gibo, 1998). Similarly, in *Xenopus*, Wnt-1 is capable of duplicating the embryonic axis, while Wnt-5A is not (Torres et al., 1996). Wnt-5a does decrease cell adhesion and is capable of blocking Wnt-8-mediated axis duplication (Torres et al., 1996), further suggesting an antagonistic relationship between the Wnt/Ca²⁺ and Wnt/β-catenin pathways. Wnt-5A is capable of activating the Wnt/β-catenin pathway, however, when coexpressed with human Frizzled 5 (He et al., 1997) or adjacent to cells expressing LRP6 (Bejsovec, 2000), which suggests that specificity between Wnt pathways does not lie solely within the Wnt ligand, and argues against the continued use of the phrase "Wnt-5A pathway."

PKC has been implicated in the Wnt/β-catenin signaling pathway as well. PKC can bind to PDZ domains similar to that in Dsh, and GSK3β is a target for PKC (Saito et al., 1994). Moreover, it has been postulated that Dsh may recruit PKC to the destruction complex to inhibit GSK3β activity (Smalley et al., 1999). PKC activity is required for the transmission of Wg signals to GSK3β (Cook et al., 1996), for the ability of APC to down-regulate β-catenin (Easwaran et al., 1999), and for Dsh to regulate amyloid precursor protein processing (Mudher et al., 2001). Inhibition of PKC activity also abolishes the effects of Wnt-5A and Wnt-7A on rat chondrogenic cell cultures (Bergwitz et al., 2001). These experiments rely upon pharmacological blockade of kinase activity and, thus, may represent changes in the resting state of the cells in question rather than changes in signal transduction. Consistent with this hypothesis, elevation of PKC activity has not been observed upon activation of the Wnt/β-catenin pathway by Wnts and Frizzleds (Sheldahl et al., 1999; Winklbauer et al., 2001). Lastly, Wnt-5A expression affects the transcription of interleukins in rheumatoid arthritic tissues, but whether this involves the Wnt/Ca²⁺ pathway is unclear (Sen et al., 2000).

It is possible that a function of the Wnt/Ca²⁺ pathway is to inhibit the Wnt/β-catenin pathway in vivo, but further study is required. Nevertheless, it is interesting to note that lithium's teratogenic effects involve not only blockade of GSK3β activity and thus activation of the Wnt/β-catenin pathway, but also blockade of the phospholipid signaling required for the generation of Ca²⁺ fluxes. Blockade of the phosphoinositol cycle without blocking GSK3β activity can be achieved, and indeed ventral injection of antibodies to *Xenopus* inositol 1,4,5-trisphosphate receptors induces a secondary axis similar to Li²⁺ treatment (Kume et al., 1997). Furthermore, axis duplication by Li²⁺ can be rescued by treatment with phorbol esters or the phosphatidylinositol cycle intermediate *myo*-inositol (Busa and Gimlich, 1989). This suggests that activation of the Wnt/Ca²⁺ pathway may play an important role in inhibiting the Wnt/β-catenin pathway on the ventral side of the embryo. Concurrent with this idea, expression of the extracellular domain of Fz8 (ECD8) on the ventral side of the embryo leads to secondary axis formation, suggesting that a Wnt (or Wnts) plays an active role on the ventral side of the embryo to suppress dorsal fates (Itoh and Sokol, 1999).

β-CATENIN-INDEPENDENT ROLES OF WNT SIGNALING

In the developing chick limb bud, expression of Wnt-3A activates the Wnt/β-catenin pathway to affect cell differentiation, while Wnt-7A affects the dorsal/ventral polarity of the limb independently of Lef1 (Kengaku et al., 1998). Later in development, Wnt-5A delays maturation of chondrocytes in the appendicular skeleton, while Wnt-4 and a stabilized form of β-catenin accelerate maturation (Hartmann and Tabin, 2000). It remains to be seen whether Wnt-7A or Wnt-5A activates the Wnt/Ca^{2+} pathway to elicit these effects. Experiments in zebrafish and *Xenopus*, however, suggest that some Wnts and Fz may exert their effects via Dsh to control gastrulation. Screens for target genes of a known regulator of gastrulation in *Xenopus*, *brachyury*, revealed that Wnt-11 is required for proper convergent extension movements and gastrulation (Tada and Smith, 2000). Furthermore, blockade of Wnt-11 function by a dominant-negative Wnt is rescued by Dsh. A Dsh deletion construct that does not activate the Wnt/β-catenin pathway (DshΔDIX) likewise rescues the effects of dominant-negative Wnt-11 (Tada and Smith, 2000). The Wnt-11 ortholog in zebrafish, Silberblick, is also necessary for proper convergent extension movements during gastrulation and acts via Dsh but not the Wnt/β-catenin pathway (Heisenberg et al., 2000). Similarly, XFz7 interacts with Wnt-11 to affect convergent extension via a pathway involving Dsh but not β-catenin (Djiane et al., 2000). XFz7 has been shown to activate PKC and CamKII (Kuhl et al., 2000a) as well as the Wnt/β-catenin pathway (Medina and Steinbeisser, 2000) and perhaps the PCP pathway, depending on which Wnt ligand is present (Winklbauer et al., 2001). It is interesting to note that the PCP pathway in *Drosophila* still has no known ligand, Wnt or otherwise (Rulifson et al., 2000).

CONCLUSIONS

The Wnt/β-catenin pathway is quite remarkable in that many of its signaling components are shared by other signaling pathways. Regulating the molecular makeup of a destruction complex is indeed very different from "ordinary" kinase cascades. A little over a decade of research has produced some very detailed understanding of how Wnt proteins signal to cells, yet many gaps remain. How do structurally related Frizzled orthologs "select" activation of the Wnt/β-catenin pathway versus the antagonistic Wnt/Ca^{2+} pathway? What role do G proteins play in Wnt signaling pathways? Do they signal from Frizzleds to Dishevelled? How exactly is the destruction complex regulated? What cellular processes are regulated by the Wnt/Ca^{2+} pathway? Is the PCP pathway a Wnt pathway as well? Wnt signaling is studied in a wide number of experimental systems by an increasing number of researchers; thus, answers to these and other questions should be close at hand.

REFERENCES

Aberle H, Bauer A, Stappert J, Kispert A, Kemler R (1997). Beta-catenin is a target for the ubiquitin-proteasome pathway. *EMBO J* 16(13): 3797–3804.

Akiyama T (2000). Wnt/beta-catenin signaling. *Cytokine Growth Factor Rev* 11(4): 273–282.

Axelrod JD, Miller JR, Shulman JM, Moon RT, Perrimon N (1998). Differential recruitment of Dishevelled provides signaling specificity in the planar cell polarity and Wingless signaling pathways. *Genes Dev* 12(16): 2610–2622.

Bafico A, Gazit A, Pramila T, Finch PW, Yaniv A, Aaronson SA (1999). Interaction of frizzled related protein (FRP) with Wnt ligands and the Frizzled receptor suggests alternative mechanisms for FRP inhibition of Wnt signaling. *J Biol Chem* 274(23): 16180–16187.

Barnes MR, Duckworth DM, Beeley LJ (1998). Frizzled proteins constitute a novel family of G protein–coupled receptors, most closely related to the *secretin* family. *Trends Pharmacol Sci* 19(10): 399–400.

Behrens J (2000). Cross-regulation of the Wnt signalling pathway: a role of MAP kinases. *J Cell Biol* 113 (Pt 6): 911–919.

Behrens J, Jerchow BA, Wurtele M, Grimm J, Asbrand C, Wirtz R, Kuhl M, Wedlich D, Birchmeier W (1998). Functional interaction of an *axin* homolog, *conductin*, with Beta-catenin, APC, and GSK3beta. *Science* 280(5363): 596–599.

Bejsovec A (2000). Wnt signaling: an embarrassment of receptors. *Curr Biol* 10(24): R919–R922.

Bejsovec A, Martinez Arias A (1991). Roles of *wingless* in patterning the larval epidermis of *Drosophila*. *Development* 113(2): 471–485.

Bergwitz C, Wendlandt T, Kispert A, Brabant G (2001). Wnts differentially regulate colony growth and differentiation of chondrogenic rat calvaria cells. *Biochim Biophys Acta* 1538(2–3): 129–140.

Bhanot P, Brink M, Samos CH, Hsieh JC, Wang Y, Macke JP, Andrew D, Nathans J, Nusse R (1996). A new member of the *frizzled* family from *Drosophila* functions as a Wingless receptor. *Nature* 382(6588): 225–230.

Billin AN, Thirlwell H, Ayer DE (2000). Beta-catenin–histone deacetylase interactions regulate the transition of LEF1 from a transcriptional repressor to an activator. *Mol Cell Biol* 20(18): 6882–6890.

Binari RC, Staveley BE, Johnson WA, Godavarti R, Sasisekharan R, Manoukian AS (1997). Genetic evidence that heparin-like glycosaminoglycans are involved in *wingless* signaling. *Development* 124(13): 2623–2632.

Boutros M, Paricio N, Strutt DI, Mlodzik M (1998). Dishevelled activates JNK and dis-

criminates between JNK pathways in planar polarity and Wingless signaling. *Cell* 94(1): 109–118.

Bouwmeester T, Kim S, Sasai Y, Lu B, De Robertis EM (1996). Cerberus is a head-inducing secreted factor expressed in the anterior endoderm of Spemann's organizer. *Nature* 382(6592): 595–601.

Brannon M, Gomperts M, Sumoy L, Moon RT, Kimelman D (1997). A Beta-catenin/XTcf-3 complex binds to the *siamois* promoter to regulate dorsal axis specification in *Xenopus*. *Genes Dev* 11(18): 2359–2370.

Brannon M, Brown JD, Bates R, Kimelman D, Moon RT (1999). XCtBP is a XTcf-3 co-repressor with roles throughout *Xenopus* development. *Development* 126(14): 3159–3170.

Burrus LW (1994). Wnt-1 as a short-range signaling molecule. *Bioessays* 16(3): 155–157.

Busa WB, Gimlich RL (1989). Lithium-induced teratogenesis in frog embryos prevented by a polyphosphoinositide cycle intermediate or a diacylglycerol analog. *Dev Biol* 132(2): 315–324.

Cadigan KM, Nusse R (1997). Wnt signaling: a common theme in animal development. *Genes Dev* 11(24): 3286–3305.

Cavallo R, Rubenstein D, Peifer M (1997). Armadillo and dTCF: a marriage made in the nucleus. *Curr Opin Genet Dev* 7(4): 459–466.

Cavallo RA, Cox RT, Moline MM, Roose J, Polevoy GA, Clevers H, Peifer M, Bejsovec A (1998). *Drosophila* Tcf and Groucho interact to repress Wingless signalling activity. *Nature* 395(6702): 604–608.

Chen G, Courey AJ (2000). Groucho/TLE family proteins and transcriptional repression. *Gene* 249(1–2): 1–16.

Cook D, Fry MJ, Hughes K, Sumathipala R, Woodgett JR, Dale TC (1996). Wingless inactivates glycogen synthase kinase-3 via an intracellular signalling pathway which involves a protein kinase C. *EMBO J* 15(17): 4526–4536.

Dann CE, Hsieh JC, Rattner A, Sharma D, Nathans J, Leahy DJ (2001). Insights into Wnt binding and signalling from the structures of two Frizzled cysteine-rich domains. *Nature* 412(6842): 86–90.

Delcommenne M, Tan C, Gray V, Rue L, Woodgett J, Dedhar S (1998). Phosphoinositide-3-OH kinase-dependent regulation of glycogen synthase kinase 3 and protein kinase B/AKT by the integrin-linked kinase. *Proc Natl Acad Sci USA* 95(19): 11211–11216.

Djiane A, Riou J, Umbhauer M, Boucaut J, Shi D (2000). Role of *frizzled 7* in the regulation of convergent extension movements during gastrulation in *Xenopus* laevis. *Development* 127(14): 3091–3100.

Dominguez I, Green JB (2000). Dorsal downregulation of GSK3beta by a non-Wnt-like mechanism is an early molecular consequence of cortical rotation in early *Xenopus* embryos. *Development* 127(4): 861–868.

Dominguez I, Itoh K, Sokol SY (1995). Role of glycogen synthase kinase 3 beta as a negative regulator of dorsoventral axis formation in *Xenopus* embryos. *Proc Natl Acad Sci USA* 92(18): 8498–8502.

Easwaran V, Song V, Polakis P, Byers S (1999). The ubiquitin-proteasome pathway and serine kinase activity modulate adenomatous polyposis coli protein–mediated regulation of Beta-catenin–lymphocyte enhancer-binding factor signaling. *J Biol Chem* 274(23): 16641–16645.

Fagotto F, Funayama N, Gluck U, Gumbiner BM (1996). Binding to cadherins antagonizes the signaling activity of beta-catenin during axis formation in *Xenopus*. *J Cell Biol* 132(6): 1105–1114.

Farr GH 3rd, Ferkey DM, Yost C, Pierce SB, Weaver C, Kimelman D (2000). Interaction among GSK-3, GBP, axin, and APC in *Xenopus* axis specification. *J Cell Biol* 148(4): 691–702.

Fedi P, Bafico A, Nieto Soria A, Burgess WH, Miki T, Bottaro DP, Kraus MH, Aaronson SA (1999). Isolation and biochemical characterization of the human Dkk-1 homologue, a novel inhibitor of mammalian Wnt signaling. *J Biol Chem* 274(27): 19465–19472.

Frame S, Cohen P (2001). GSK3 takes centre stage more than 20 years after its discovery. *Biochem J* 359(Pt 1): 1–16.

Fukumoto S, Hsieh CM, Maemura K, Layne MD, Yet SF, Lee KH, Matsui T, Rosenzweig A, Taylor WG, Rubin JS, Perrella MA, Lee ME (2001). Akt participation in the Wnt signaling pathway through Dishevelled. *J Biol Chem* 276(20): 17479–17483.

Glinka A, Wu W, Delius H, Monaghan AP, Blumenstock C, Niehrs C (1998). Dickkopf-1 is a member of a new family of secreted proteins and functions in head induction. *Nature* 391(6665): 357–362.

Hart MJ, de los Santos R, Albert IN, Rubinfeld B, Polakis P (1998). Downregulation of Beta-catenin by human Axin and its association with the APC tumor suppressor, Beta-catenin and GSK3 beta. *Curr Biol* 8(10): 573–581.

Hartmann C, Tabin CJ (2000). Dual roles of Wnt signaling during chondrogenesis in the chicken limb. *Development* 127(14): 3141–3159.

He X, Saint-Jeannet JP, Woodgett JR, Varmus HE, Dawid IB (1995). Glycogen synthase kinase-3 and dorsoventral patterning in *Xenopus*. *Nature* 374(6523): 617–622.

He X, Saint-Jeannet JP, Wang Y, Nathans J, Dawid I, Varmus H (1997). A member of the Frizzled protein family mediating axis induction by Wnt-5A. *Science* 275(5306): 1652–1654.

Heasman J, Crawford A, Goldstone K, Garner-Hamrick P, Gumbiner B, McCrea P, Kintner C, Noro CY, Wylie C (1994). Overexpression of cadherins and underexpression of Beta-catenin inhibit dorsal mesoderm induction in early *Xenopus* embryos. *Cell* 79(5): 791–803.

Heasman J, Kofron M, Wylie C (2000). Beta-catenin signaling activity dissected in the early *Xenopus* embryo: a novel antisense approach. *Dev Biol* 222(1): 124–134.

Hedgepeth CM, Conrad LJ, Zhang J, Huang HC, Lee VM, Klein PS (1997). Activation of the Wnt signaling pathway: a molecular mechanism for lithium action. *Dev Biol* 185(1): 82–91.

Heisenberg CP, Tada M, Rauch GJ, Saude L, Concha ML, Geisler R, Stemple DL, Smith JC, Wilson SW (2000). Silberblick/Wnt11 mediates convergent extension movements during zebrafish gastrulation. *Nature* 405(6782): 76–81.

Hofmann K (2000). A superfamily of membrane-bound *O*-acyltransferases with implications for Wnt signaling. *Trends Biochem Sci* 25(3): 111–112.

Hoppler S, Brown JD, Moon RT (1996). Expression of a dominant-negative Wnt blocks induction of MyoD in *Xenopus* embryos. *Genes Dev* 10(21): 2805–2817.

Hsieh JC, Kodjabachian L, Rebbert ML, Rattner A, Smallwood PM, Samos CH, Nusse

R, Dawid IB, Nathans J (1999). A new secreted protein that binds to Wnt proteins and inhibits their activities. *Nature* 398(6726): 431–436.

Hsu SC, Galceran J, Grosschedl R (1998). Modulation of transcriptional regulation by LEF-1 in response to Wnt-1 signaling and association with Beta-catenin. *Mol Cell Biol* 18(8): 4807–4818.

Ikeda S, Kishida S, Yamamoto H, Murai H, Koyama S, Kikuchi A (1998). Axin, a negative regulator of the Wnt signaling pathway, forms a complex with GSK-3beta and beta-catenin and promotes GSK-3beta-dependent phosphorylation of beta-catenin. *EMBO J* 17(5): 1371–1384.

Ishitani T, Ninomiya-Tsuji J, Nagai S, Nishita M, Meneghini M, Barker N, Waterman M, Bowerman B, Clevers H, Shibuya H, et al. (1999). The TAK1-NLK-MAPK-related pathway antagonizes signalling between Beta-catenin and transcription factor TCF. *Nature* 399(6738): 798–802.

Itoh K, Sokol SY (1994). Heparan sulfate proteoglycans are required for mesoderm formation in *Xenopus* embryos. *Development* 120(9): 2703–2711.

Itoh K, Sokol SY (1999). Axis determination by inhibition of Wnt signaling in *Xenopus*. *Genes Dev* 13(17): 2328–2336.

Itoh K, Krupnik VE, Sokol SY (1998). Axis determination in *Xenopus* involves biochemical interactions of axin, glycogen synthase kinase 3 and Beta-catenin. *Curr Biol* 8(10): 591–594.

Kadowaki T, Wilder E, Klingensmith J, Zachary K, Perrimon N (1996). The segment polarity gene *porcupine* encodes a putative multitransmembrane protein involved in Wingless processing. *Genes Dev* 10(24): 3116–3128.

Kengaku M, Capdevila J, Rodriguez-Esteban C, De La Pena J, Johnson RL, Belmonte JC, Tabin CJ (1998). Distinct WNT pathways regulating AER formation and dorsoventral polarity in the chick limb bud. *Science* 280(5367): 1274–1277.

Kessler DS (1997). Siamois is required for formation of Spemann's organizer. *Proc Natl Acad Sci USA* 94(24): 13017–13022.

Kishida M, Koyama S, Kishida S, Matsubara K, Nakashima S, Higano K, Takada R, Takada S, Kikuchi A (1999a). Axin prevents Wnt-3a-induced accumulation of Beta-catenin. *Oncogene* 18(4): 979–985.

Kishida S, Yamamoto H, Hino S, Ikeda S, Kishida M, Kikuchi A (1999b). DIX domains of Dvl and Axin are necessary for protein interactions and their ability to regulate Beta-catenin stability. *Mol Cell Biol* 19(6): 4414–4422.

Kishida S, Yamamoto H, Ikeda S, Kishida M, Sakamoto I, Koyama S, Kikuchi A (1998). Axin, a negative regulator of the wnt signaling pathway, directly interacts with adenomatous polyposis coli and regulates the stabilization of Beta-catenin. *J Biol Chem* 273(18): 10823–10826.

Kitagawa M, Hatakeyama S, Shirane M, Matsumoto M, Ishida N, Hattori K, Nakamichi I, Kikuchi A, Nakayama K (1999). An F-box protein, FWD1, mediates ubiquitin-dependent proteolysis of Beta-catenin. *EMBO J* 18(9): 2401–2410.

Korinek V, Barker N, Morin PJ, van Wichen D, de Weger R, Kinzler KW, Vogelstein B, Clevers H (1997). Constitutive transcriptional activation by a Beta-catenin–Tcf complex in $APC^{-/-}$ colon carcinoma. *Science* 275(5307): 1784–1787.

Kuhl M, Sheldahl LC, Malbon CC, Moon RT (2000a). Ca^{2+}/calmodulin-dependent protein kinase II is stimulated by Wnt and Frizzled homologs and promotes ventral cell fates in *Xenopus*. *J Biol Chem* 275(17): 12701–12711.

Kuhl M, Sheldahl LC, Park M, Miller JR, Moon RT (2000b). The Wnt/Ca^{2+} pathway: a new vertebrate Wnt signaling pathway takes shape. *Trends Genet* 16(7): 279–283.

Kuhl M, Geis K, Sheldahl LC, Pukrop T, Moon RT, Wedlich D (2001). Antagonistic regulation of convergent extension movements in *Xenopus* by Wnt/beta-catenin and Wnt/Ca^{2+} signaling. *Mech Dev* 106(1–2): 61–76.

Kume S, Muto A, Inoue T, Suga K, Okano H, Mikoshiba K (1997). Role of inositol 1,4,5-trisphosphate receptor in ventral signaling in *Xenopus* embryos. *Science* 278(5345): 1940–1943.

Larabell CA, Torres M, Rowning BA, Yost C, Miller JR, Wu M, Kimelman D, Moon RT (1997). Establishment of the dorso-ventral axis in *Xenopus* embryos is presaged by early asymmetries in Beta-catenin that are modulated by the Wnt signaling pathway. *J Cell Biol* 136(5): 1123–1136.

Laurent MN, Blitz IL, Hashimoto C, Rothbacher U, Cho KW (1997). The *Xenopus* homeobox gene *twin* mediates Wnt induction of goosecoid in establishment of Spemann's organizer. *Development* 124(23): 4905–4916.

Lee E, Salic A, Kirschner MW (2001). Physiological regulation of Beta-catenin stability by Tcf3 and CK1ϵ. *J Cell Biol* 154(5): 983–994.

Lee JS, Ishimoto A, Yanagawa S (1999). Characterization of mouse *dishevelled* (Dvl) proteins in Wnt/Wingless signaling pathway. *J Biol Chem* 274(30): 21464–21470.

Lekven AC, Thorpe CJ, Waxman JS, Moon RT (2001). Zebrafish *wnt8* encodes two Wnt-8 proteins on a bicistronic transcript and is required for mesoderm and neuectoderm patterning. *Dev Cell* 1: 103–114.

Li L, Yuan H, Weaver CD, Mao J, Farr GH 3rd, Sussman DJ, Jonkers J, Kimelman D, Wu D (1999). Axin and Frat1 interact with Dvl and GSK, bridging Dvl to GSK in Wnt-mediated regulation of LEF-1. *EMBO J* 18(15): 4233–4240.

Lijam N, Paylor R, McDonald MP, Crawley JN, Deng CX, Herrup K, Stevens KE, Maccaferri G, McBain CJ, Sussman DJ, et al. (1997). Social interaction and sensorimotor gating abnormalities in mice lacking Dvl1. *Cell* 90(5): 895–905.

Lin X, Perrimon N (1999). Dally cooperates with *Drosophila* Frizzled 2 to transduce Wingless signalling. *Nature* 400(6741): 281–284.

Lin X, Perrimon N (2000). Role of heparan sulfate proteoglycans in cell–cell signaling in Drosophila. *Matrix Biol* 19(4): 303–307.

Liu C, Kato Y, Zhang Z, Do VM, Yankner BA, He X (1999). Beta-Trcp couples beta-catenin phosphorylation-degradation and regulates *Xenopus* axis formation. *Proc Natl Acad Sci USA* 96(11): 6273–6278.

Liu J, Stevens J, Rote CA, Yost HJ, Hu Y, Neufeld KL, White RL, Matsunami N (2001a). Siah-1 mediates a novel Beta-catenin degradation pathway linking p53 to the adenomatous polyposis coli protein. *Mol Cell* 7(5): 927–936.

Liu T, DeCostanzo AJ, Liu X, Wang H, Hallagan S, Moon RT, Malbon CC (2001b). G protein signaling from activated rat Frizzled-1 to the Beta-catenin-Lef-Tcf pathway. *Science* 292(5522): 1718–1722.

Mao B, Wu W, Li Y, Hoppe D, Stannek P, Glinka A, Niehrs C (2001a). LDL-receptor-related protein 6 is a receptor for Dickkopf proteins. *Nature* 411(6835): 321–325.

Mao J, Wang J, Liu B, Pan W, Farr GH 3rd, Flynn C, Yuan H, Takada S, Kimelman D, Li L, et al. (2001b). Low-density lipoprotein receptor–related protein-5 binds to Axin and regulates the canonical Wnt signaling pathway. *Mol Cells* 7(4): 801–809.

Matsuzawa SI, Reed JC (2001). Siah-1, SIP, and Ebi collaborate in a novel pathway for beta-catenin degradation linked to p53 responses. *Mol Cells* 7(5): 915–926.

McEwen DG, Peifer M (2001). Wnt signaling: the naked truth? *Curr Biol* 11(13): R524–R526.

McMahon AP, Bradley A (1990). The *Wnt-1* (*int-1*) proto-oncogene is required for development of a large region of the mouse brain. *Cell* 62(6): 1073–1085.

Medina A, Steinbeisser H (2000). Interaction of Frizzled 7 and Dishevelled in *Xenopus*. *Dev Dyn* 218(4): 671–680.

Meneghini MD, Ishitani T, Carter JC, Hisamoto N, Ninomiya-Tsuji J, Thorpe CJ, Hamill DR, Matsumoto K, Bowerman B (1999). MAP kinase and Wnt pathways converge to downregulate an HMG-domain repressor in *Caenorhabditis elegans*. *Nature* 399(6738): 793–797.

Miller JR, Moon RT (1997). Analysis of the signaling activities of localization mutants of Beta-catenin during axis specification in *Xenopus*. *J Cell Biol* 139(1): 229–243.

Miller JR, Hocking AM, Brown JD, Moon RT (1999a). Mechanism and function of signal transduction by the Wnt/Beta-catenin and Wnt/Ca^{2+} pathways. *Oncogene* 18(55): 7860–7872.

Miller JR, Rowning BA, Larabell CA, Yang-Snyder JA, Bates RL and Moon RT (1999b). Establishment of the dorsal–ventral axis in *Xenopus* embryos coincides with the dorsal enrichment of Dishevelled that is dependent on cortical rotation. *J Cell Biol* 146(2): 427–437.

Molenaar M, van de Wetering M, Oosterwegel M, Peterson-Maduro J, Godsave S, Korinek V, Roose J, Destree O, Clevers H (1996). XTcf-3 transcription factor mediates Beta-catenin-induced axis formation in *Xenopus* embryos. *Cell* 86(3): 391–399.

Moon RT, Kimelman D (1998). From cortical rotation to organizer gene expression: toward a molecular explanation of axis specification in *Xenopus*. *Bioessays* 20(7): 536–545.

Moon RT, Brown JD, Yang-Snyder JA, Miller JR (1997). Structurally related receptors and antagonists compete for secreted Wnt ligands. *Cell* 88(6): 725–728.

Morali OG, Delmas V, Moore R, Jeanney C, Thiery JP, Larue L (2001). IGF-II induces rapid Beta-catenin relocation to the nucleus during epithelium to mesenchyme transition. *Oncogene* 20(36): 4942–4950.

Mudher A, Chapman S, Richardson J, Asuni A, Gibb G, Pollard C, Killick R, Iqbal T, Raymond L, Varndell I, et al. (2001). Dishevelled regulates the metabolism of amyloid precursor protein via protein kinase C/mitogen-activated protein kinase and c-Jun terminal kinase. *J Neurosci* 21(14): 4987–4995.

Nakamura T, Hamada F, Ishidate T, Anai K, Kawahara K, Toyoshima K, Akiyama T (1998). Axin, an inhibitor of the Wnt signalling pathway, interacts with beta-catenin, GSK-3beta and APC and reduces the Beta-catenin level. *Genes Cells* 3(6): 395–403.

Nasevicius A, Hyatt T, Kim H, Guttman J, Walsh E, Sumanas S, Wang Y, Ekker SC (1998). Evidence for a Frizzled-mediated Wnt pathway required for zebrafish dorsal mesoderm formation. *Development* 125(21): 4283–4292.

Nathke IS (1999). The adenomatous polyposis coli protein. *Mol Pathol* 52(4): 169–173.

Neufeld KL, Zhang F, Cullen BR, White RL (2000). APC-mediated downregulation of Beta-catenin activity involves nuclear sequestration and nuclear export. *EMBO Rep* 1(6): 519–523.

Novak A, Hsu SC, Leung-Hagesteijn C, Radeva G, Papkoff J, Montesano R, Roskelley C, Grosschedl R, Dedhar S (1998). Cell adhesion and the integrin-linked kinase regulate the LEF-1 and Beta-catenin signaling pathways. *Proc Natl Acad Sci USA* 95(8): 4374–4379.

Nusse R (1991). Insertional mutagenesis in mouse mammary tumorigenesis. *Curr Top Microbiol Immunol* 171: 43–65.

Nusse R (1999). WNT targets. Repression and activation. *Trends Genet* 15(1): 1–3.

Nusse R, Varmus HE (1982). Many tumors induced by the mouse mammary tumor virus contain a provirus integrated in the same region of the host genome. *Cell* 31(1): 99–109.

Nusslein-Volhard C, Wieschaus E (1980). Mutations affecting segment number and polarity in *Drosophila*. *Nature* 287(5785): 795–801.

Olson DJ, Gibo DM (1998). Antisense Wnt-5a mimics Wnt-1-mediated C57MG mammary epithelial cell transformation. *Exp Cell Res* 241(1): 134–141.

Orford K, Crockett C, Jensen JP, Weissman AM, Byers SW (1997). Serine phosphorylation-regulated ubiquitination and degradation of Beta-catenin. *J Biol Chem* 272(40): 24735–24738.

Papkoff J, Schryver B (1990). Secreted Int-1 protein is associated with the cell surface. *Mol Cell Biol* 10(6): 2723–2730.

Park M, Moon RT (2002). The planar cell polarity gene *strabismus* encodes a Dishevelled-associated protein that regulates cell behavior and cell fate in vertebrate embryos. *Nat Cell Biol* 4(1):20–25.

Peifer M, Orsulic S, Pai LM, Loureiro J (1993). A model system for cell adhesion and signal transduction in *Drosophila*. *Dev Suppl* 163–176.

Piccolo S, Agius E, Leyns L, Bhattacharyya S, Grunz H, Bouwmeester T, De Robertis EM (1999). The head inducer Cerberus is a multifunctional antagonist of Nodal, BMP and Wnt signals. *Nature* 397(6721): 707–710.

Pinson KI, Brennan J, Monkley S, Avery BJ, Skarnes WC (2000). An LDL-receptor-related protein mediates Wnt signalling in mice. *Nature* 407(6803): 535–538.

Polakis P (1997). The adenomatous polyposis coli (APC) tumor suppressor. *Biochim Biophys Acta* 1332(3): F127–F147.

Polakis P (2001). More than one way to skin a catenin. *Cell* 105(5): 563–566.

Rattner A, Hsieh JC, Smallwood PM, Gilbert DJ, Copeland NG, Jenkins NA, Nathans J (1997). A family of secreted proteins contains homology to the cysteine-rich ligand-binding domain of *frizzled* receptors. *Proc Natl Acad Sci USA* 94(7): 2859–2863.

Reichsman F, Smith L, Cumberledge S (1996). Glycosaminoglycans can modulate extracellular localization of the Wingless protein and promote signal transduction. *J Cell Biol* 135(3): 819–827.

Rijsewijk F, Schuermann M, Wagenaar E, Parren P, Weigel D, Nusse R (1987). The

Drosophila homolog of the mouse mammary oncogene *int-1* is identical to the segment polarity gene *wingless*. *Cell* 50(4): 649–657.
Rocheleau CE, Downs WD, Lin R, Wittmann C, Bei Y, Cha YH, Ali M, Priess JR, Mello CC (1997). Wnt signaling and an APC-related gene specify endoderm in early *C. elegans* embryos. *Cell* 90(4): 707–716.
Rocheleau CE, Yasuda J, Shin TH, Lin R, Sawa H, Okano H, Priess JR, Davis RJ, Mello CC (1999). WRM-1 activates the LIT-1 protein kinase to transduce anterior/posterior polarity signals in *C. elegans*. *Cell* 97(6): 717–726.
Roose J, Molenaar M, Peterson J, Hurenkamp J, Brantjes H, Moerer P, van de Wetering M, Destree O, Clevers H (1998). The *Xenopus* Wnt effector XTcf-3 interacts with Groucho-related transcriptional repressors. *Nature* 395(6702): 608–612.
Rothbacher U, Laurent MN, Deardorff MA, Klein PS, Cho KW, Fraser SE (2000). Dishevelled phosphorylation, subcellular localization and multimerization regulate its role in early embryogenesis. *EMBO J* 19(5): 1010–1022.
Rousset R, Mack JA, Wharton KA Jr, Axelrod JD, Cadigan KM, Fish MP, Nusse R, Scott MP (2001). Naked cuticle targets dishevelled to antagonize Wnt signal transduction. *Genes Dev* 15(6): 658–671.
Rubinfeld B, Albert I, Porfiri E, Fiol C, Munemitsu S, Polakis P (1996). Binding of GSK3beta to the APC–beta-catenin complex and regulation of complex assembly. *Science* 272(5264): 1023–1026.
Rubinfeld B, Tice DA, Polakis P (2001). Axin dependent phosphorylation of the adenomatous polyposis coli protein mediated by casein kinase 1 epsilon. *J Biol Chem* 3: 3.
Ruel L, Stambolic V, Ali A, Manoukian AS, Woodgett JR (1999). Regulation of the protein kinase activity of Shaggy(Zeste-white3) by components of the Wingless pathway in *Drosophila* cells and embryos. *J Biol Chem* 274(31): 21790–21796.
Rulifson EJ, Wu CH, Nusse R (2000). Pathway specificity by the bifunctional receptor Frizzled is determined by affinity for Wingless. *Mol Cell* 6(1): 117–126.
Saito Y, Vandenheede JR, Cohen P (1994). The mechanism by which epidermal growth factor inhibits glycogen synthase kinase 3 in A431 cells. *Biochem J* 303(Pt 1): 27–31.
Salic A, Lee E, Mayer L, Kirschner MW (2000). Control of beta-catenin stability: reconstitution of the cytoplasmic steps of the wnt pathway in *Xenopus* egg extracts. *Mol Cells* 5(3): 523–532.
Sampson EM, Haque ZK, Ku MC, Tevosian SG, Albanese C, Pestell RG, Paulson KE, Yee AS (2001). Negative regulation of the Wnt–Beta-catenin pathway by the transcriptional repressor HBP1. *EMBO J* 20(16): 4500–4511.
Scott M (2001). Signalling and endocytosis: Wnt breaks down on back roads. *Nat Cell Biol* 3(8): E185–E186.
Seeling JM, Miller JR, Gil R, Moon RT, White R, Virshup DM (1999). Regulation of Beta-catenin signaling by the B56 subunit of protein phosphatase 2A. *Science* 283(5410): 2089–2091.
Sen M, Lauterbach K, El-Gabalawy H, Firestein GS, Corr M, Carson DA (2000). Expression and function of *wingless* and *frizzled* homologs in rheumatoid arthritis. *Proc Natl Acad Sci USA* 97(6): 2791–2796.
Sharpe C, Lawrence N, Martinez Arias A (2001). Wnt signalling: a theme with nuclear variations. *Bioessays* 23(4): 311–318.
Sheldahl LC, Park M, Malbon CC, Moon RT (1999). Protein kinase C is differentially stimulated by Wnt and Frizzled homologs in a G-protein-dependent manner. *Curr Biol* 9(13): 695–698.
Shin TH, Yasuda J, Rocheleau CE, Lin R, Soto M, Bei Y, Davis RJ, Mello CC (1999). MOM-4, a MAP kinase kinase kinase-related protein, activates WRM-1/LIT-1 kinase to transduce anterior/posterior polarity signals in *C. elegans*. *Mol Cells* 4(2): 275–280.
Shulman JM, Perrimon N, Axelrod JD (1998). Frizzled signaling and the developmental control of cell polarity. *Trends Genet* 14(11): 452–458.
Siegfried E, Chou TB, Perrimon N (1992). Wingless signaling acts through Zeste-white 3, the *Drosophila* homolog of glycogen synthase kinase-3, to regulate engrailed and establish cell fate. *Cell* 71(7): 1167–1179.
Slusarski DC, Corces VG, Moon RT (1997a). Interaction of Wnt and a Frizzled homologue triggers G-protein-linked phosphatidylinositol signalling. *Nature* 390(6658): 410–413.
Slusarski DC, Yang-Snyder J, Busa WB, Moon RT (1997b). Modulation of embryonic intracellular Ca^{2+} signaling by Wnt-5A. *Dev Biol* 182(1): 114–120.
Smalley MJ, Sara E, Paterson H, Naylor S, Cook D, Jayatilake H, Fryer LG, Hutchinson L, Fry MJ, Dale TC (1999). Interaction of Axin and Dvl-2 proteins regulates Dvl-2-stimulated TCF-dependent transcription. *EMBO J* 18(10): 2823–2835.
Sokol SY (1996). Analysis of Dishevelled signalling pathways during *Xenopus* development. *Curr Biol* 6(11): 1456–1467.
Sokol SY (1999). Wnt signaling and dorso-ventral axis specification in vertebrates. *Curr Opin Genet Dev* 9(4): 405–410.
Sokol S (2000). A role for Wnts in morphogenesis and tissue polarity. *Nat Cell Biol* 2(7): E124–E125.
Sokol S, Christian JL, Moon RT, Melton DA (1991). Injected Wnt RNA induces a complete body axis in *Xenopus* embryos. *Cell* 67(4): 741–752.
Sokol SY, Klingensmith J, Perrimon N, Itoh K (1995). Dorsalizing and neuralizing properties of Xdsh, a maternally expressed *Xenopus* homolog of *dishevelled*. *Development* 121(6): 1637–1647.
Strovel ET, Wu D, Sussman DJ (2000). Protein phosphatase 2Calpha dephosphorylates Axin and activates LEF-1-dependent transcription. *J Biol Chem* 275(4): 2399–2403.
Sun TQ, Lu B, Feng JJ, Reinhard C, Jan YN, Fantl WJ, Williams LT (2001). PAR-1 is a Dishevelled-associated kinase and a positive regulator of Wnt signalling. *Nat Cell Biol* 3(7): 628–636.
Tada M, Smith JC (2000). Xwnt11 is a target of *Xenopus Brachyury*: regulation of gastrulation movements via Dishevelled, but not through the canonical Wnt pathway. *Development* 127(10): 2227–2238.
Takada S, Stark KL, Shea MJ, Vassileva G, McMahon JA, McMahon AP (1994). Wnt-3a regulates somite and tailbud formation in the mouse embryo. *Genes Dev* 8(2): 174–189.
Takemaru KI, Moon RT (2000). The transcriptional coactivator CBP interacts with Beta-catenin to activate gene expression. *J Cell Biol* 149(2): 249–254.
Tamai K, Semenov M, Kato Y, Spokony R, Liu C, Katsuyama Y, Hess F, Saint-Jeannet JP, He X (2000). LDL-receptor-related proteins in Wnt signal transduction. *Nature* 407(6803): 530–535.
Tan C, Deardorff MA, Saint-Jeannet JP, Yang J, Arzoumanian A and Klein PS (2001). Kermit, a Frizzled interacting protein, regulates Frizzled 3 signaling in neural crest development. *Development* 128(19): 3665–3674.
Thorpe CJ, Schlesinger A, Carter JC, Bowerman B (1997). Wnt signaling polarizes an early *C. elegans* blastomere to distinguish endoderm from mesoderm. *Cell* 90(4): 695–705.
Tickle C (1995). Vertebrate limb development. *Curr Opin Genet Dev* 5(4): 478–484.
Torres MA, Yang-Snyder JA, Purcell SM, DeMarais AA, McGrew LL, Moon RT (1996). Activities of the Wnt-1 class of secreted signaling factors are antagonized by the Wnt-5A class and by a dominant negative cadherin in early *Xenopus* development. *J Cell Biol* 133(5): 1123–1137.
Tsuda M, Kamimura K, Nakato H, Archer M, Staatz W, Fox B, Humphrey M, Olson S, Futch T, Kaluza V, et al. (1999). The cell-surface proteoglycan Dally regulates Wingless signalling in *Drosophila*. *Nature* 400(6741): 276–280.
Umbhauer M, Djiane A, Goisset C, Penzo-Mendez A, Riou JF, Boucaut JC, Shi DL (2000). The C-terminal cytoplasmic Lys-thr-X-X-X-Trp motif in frizzled receptors mediates Wnt/Beta-catenin signalling. *EMBO J* 19(18): 4944–4954.
van den Heuvel M, Harryman-Samos C, Klingensmith J, Perrimon N, Nusse R (1993). Mutations in the segment polarity genes *wingless* and *porcupine* impair secretion of the *wingless* protein. *EMBO J* 12(13): 5293–5302.
Vleminckx K, Wong E, Guger K, Rubinfeld B, Polakis P, Gumbiner BM (1997). Adenomatous polyposis coli tumor suppressor protein has signaling activity in *Xenopus laevis* embryos resulting in the induction of an ectopic dorsoanterior axis. *J Cell Biol* 136(2): 411–420.
Wang Y, Macke JP, Abella BS, Andreasson K, Worley P, Gilbert DJ, Copeland NG, Jenkins NA, Nathans J (1996). A large family of putative transmembrane receptors homologous to the product of the *Drosophila* tissue polarity gene *frizzled*. *J Biol Chem* 271(8): 4468–4476.
Wehrli M, Dougan ST, Caldwell K, O'Keefe L, Schwartz S, Vaizel-Ohayon D, Schejter E, Tomlinson A, DiNardo S (2000). *arrow* encodes an LDL-receptor-related protein essential for Wingless signalling. *Nature* 407(6803): 527–530.
Wells WA (2001). Squeezing in with sugar. *J Cell Biol* 154(5): 905.
Weston CR, Davis RJ (2001). Signal transduction: signaling specificity—a complex affair. *Science* 292(5526): 2439–2440.
Wharton KA Jr, Zimmermann G, Rousset R, Scott MP (2001). Vertebrate proteins related to *Drosophila* Naked Cuticle bind Dishevelled and antagonize Wnt signaling. *Dev Biol* 234(1): 93–106.
Wiechens N, Fagotto F (2001). CRM1- and Ran-independent nuclear export of Beta-catenin. *Curr Biol* 11(1): 18–27.
Willert K, Brink M, Wodarz A, Varmus H, Nusse R (1997). Casein kinase 2 associates with and phosphorylates Dishevelled. *EMBO J* 16(11): 3089–3096.
Willert K, Shibamoto S, Nusse R (1999). Wnt-induced dephosphorylation of Axin releases Beta-catenin from the Axin complex. *Genes Dev* 13(14): 1768–1773.
Winklbauer R, Medina A, Swain RK, Steinbeisser H (2001). Frizzled-7 signalling controls tissue separation during *Xenopus* gastrulation. *Nature* 413(6858): 856–860.
Winston JT, Strack P, Beer-Romero P, Chu CY, Elledge SJ, Harper JW (1999). The SCF-beta-TRCP-ubiquitin ligase complex associates specifically with phosphorylated destruction motifs in IkappaBalpha and beta-catenin and stimulates IkappaBalpha ubiquitination in vitro. *Genes Dev* 13(3): 270–283.
Wong GT, Gavin BJ, McMahon AP (1994). Differential transformation of mammary epithelial cells by Wnt genes. *Mol Cell Biol* 14(9): 6278–6286.
Yamaguchi TP (2001). Heads or tails: Wnts and anterior–posterior patterning. *Curr Biol* 11(17): R713–R724.
Yamaguchi TP, Bradley A, McMahon AP, Jones S (1999). A Wnt5a pathway underlies outgrowth of multiple structures in the vertebrate embryo. *Development* 126(6): 1211–1223.
Yamamoto H, Kishida S, Kishida M, Ikeda S, Takada S, Kikuchi A (1999). Phosphorylation of Axin, a Wnt signal negative regulator, by glycogen synthase kinase-3beta regulates its stability. *J Biol Chem* 274(16): 10681–10684.
Yan D, Wallingford JB, Sun TQ, Nelson AM, Sakanaka C, Reinhard C, Harland RM, Fantl WJ, Williams LT (2001). Cell autonomous regulation of multiple Dishevelled-dependent pathways by mammalian Nkd. *Proc Natl Acad Sci USA* 98(7): 3802–3807.
Yanagawa S, van Leeuwen F, Wodarz A, Klingensmith J, Nusse R (1995). The Dishevelled protein is modified by Wingless signaling in *Drosophila*. *Genes Dev* 9(9): 1087–1097.
Yang-Snyder J, Miller JR, Brown JD, Lai CJ, Moon RT (1996). A *frizzled* homolog functions in a vertebrate Wnt signaling pathway. *Curr Biol* 6(10): 1302–1306.
Yao R, Maeda T, Takada S, Noda T (2001). Identification of a PDZ domain containing Golgi protein, GOPC, as an interaction partner of *frizzled*. *Biochem Biophys Res Commun* 286(4): 771–778.
Yost C, Torres M, Miller JR, Huang E, Kimelman D, Moon RT (1996). The axis-inducing activity, stability, and subcellular distribution of Beta-catenin is regulated in *Xenopus* embryos by glycogen synthase kinase 3. *Genes Dev* 10(12): 1443–1454.
Yost C, Farr GH 3rd, Pierce SB, Ferkey DM, Chen MM, Kimelman D (1998). GBP, an inhibitor of GSK-3, is implicated in Xenopus development and oncogenesis. *Cell* 93(6): 1031–1041.
Zecca M, Basler K, Struhl G (1996). Direct and long-range action of a Wingless morphogen gradient. *Cell* 87(5): 833–844.
Zeng L, Fagotto F, Zhang T, Hsu W, Vasicek TJ, Perry WL, 3rd, Lee JJ, Tilghman SM, Gumbiner BM, Costantini F (1997). The mouse Fused locus encodes Axin, an inhibitor of the Wnt signaling pathway that regulates embryonic axis formation. *Cell* 90(1): 181–192.
Zhang Z, Hartmann H, Do VM, Abramowski D, Sturchler-Pierrat C, Staufenbiel M, Sommer B, van de Wetering M, Clevers H, Saftig P, et al. (1998). Destabilization of Beta-catenin by mutations in presenilin-1 potentiates neuronal apoptosis. *Nature* 395(6703): 698–702.
Zorn AM, Barish GD, Williams BO, Lavender P, Klymkowsky MW, Varmus HE (1999). Regulation of Wnt signaling by Sox proteins: XSox17 alpha/beta and XSox3 physically interact with Beta-catenin. *Mol Cells* 4(4): 487–498.

23 | *WISP3* and Progressive Pseudorheumatoid Dysplasia

WAFAA SUWAIRI AND MATTHEW L. WARMAN

Mutation in *WISP3*, a member of the CCN (CTGF, CEF10/Cyr61, Nov, and, now, WISP1, WISP2, and WISP3) family of secreted growth regulators, causes the autosomal recessive disorder progressive pseudorheumatoid dysplasia (PPD) (Hurvitz et al., 1999). Of the six members of the CCN gene family, only *WISP3* has been associated with a human mendelian disease phenotype. The precise developmental pathway by which *WISP3* causes disease is unknown. Targeted disruptions of *Wisp3*, *Ctgf*, and *Cyr61* in mice suggest that one role for CCN family members is in the regulation of angiogenesis.

THE *WISP3* LOCUS

The CCN gene family encodes cysteine-rich secreted proteins with putative roles in cell/tissue growth and differentiation (Brigstock, 1999; Perbal, 2001). These proteins may be secreted, matrix bound, or membrane bound (Yang and Lau, 1991; Brigstock et al., 1997; Desnoyers et al., 2001). CCN family members are characterized by their conserved modular architecture consisting of domains with similarity to insulin-like growth factor (IGF)-binding proteins, von Willebrand type C repeats, thrombospondin type 1 repeats, and cysteine knots (Bork, 1993) (Figure 23–1). Despite their highly conserved modular organization, individual CCN family members appear to have distinctive patterns of expression and biologic properties.

Cef10/Cyr61 and CTGF, the first members of the CCN family, are proteins that were first described in 1989 and 1991, respectively (Simmons et al., 1989; O'Brien et al., 1990; Bradham et al., 1991). *WISP3* was identified in 1998 through in silico analysis as a paralog of the gene *WISP1* (Pennica et al., 1998). *WISP1* had been isolated by a PCR-based subtraction hybridization strategy as a transcript induced by Wnt-1 (see Chapter 22) stimulation of a mouse mammary epithelial cell line.

CLINICAL DESCRIPTION

Spondyloepiphyseal dysplasia (SED) represents a heterogeneous group of skeletal disorders that are characterized by varying degrees of platyspondyly and abnormal shape and structure of the epiphyses. PPD (OMIM 208230), also referred to as *spondyloepiphyseal dysplasia tarda with progressive arthropathy* and *progressive pseudorheumatoid arthritis of childhood*, is one of the autosomal recessive subtypes of SED (Wynne-Davies et al., 1982; Spranger et al., 1983; el-Shanti et al., 1997).

Patients affected with PPD appear normal at birth and during early infancy. Their onset of symptoms occurs between 2 and 11 years, with most patients presenting before the age of 8 years. The most common presenting complaint is an altered gait. Other presenting complaints include bowing of the legs, muscle weakness, and symmetric swelling of the proximal interphalangeal joints (Figure 23–2). Because of stiff and "swollen" joints, PPD can resemble juvenile rheumatoid arthritis (JRA), which is often the initial diagnosis. However, unlike patients with JRA, patients with PPD show no signs of joint inflammation (i.e., fluid, redness, or warmth). Furthermore, the normal sedimentation rate, negative rheumatoid factor and antinuclear antibodies, and histologically normal appearing synovium are inconsistent with JRA. The diagnosis of PPD is typically made based on radiographic findings that include osseous distention of the ends of the phalanges (Figure 23–3) and platyspondyly.

Clinically and radiologically, patients experience articular cartilage loss and destructive bone changes as they age. The progressive nature of this disease frequently necessitates joint replacement surgery by the second and third decades of life. Pathologic material obtained at the time of joint replacement surgery has changes consistent with common end-stage osteoarthritis (even though these individuals are in their teenage years) (Figure 23–4). Articular cartilage specimens have not been available from patients who are not as advanced in their disease process. However, MRI of affected joints does not reveal significant abnormality of the articular cartilage (Figure 23–5). Consequently, the precise pathogenic mechanism that predisposes articular cartilage to fail in affected individuals is not known.

Extraskeletal manifestations have not been reported in this disorder. Patients have a normal facial appearance and normal intelligence. The disease is autosomal recessive, as there does not appear to be an increased incidence of osteoarthritis among obligate carriers (e.g., parents of affected individuals).

MOLECULAR GENETICS

A single, large, inbred kindred that was segregating PPD was used to assign the disease locus to human chromosome 6q (el-Shanti et al., 1997, 1998). Fine mapping using additional families narrowed the interval (Fischer et al., 1998), leading *WISP3* to be tested as a positional candidate (Hurvitz et al., 1999). Putative loss-of-function mutations in WISP3 have been identified in many patients (Hurvitz et al., 1999; unpublished observations). *WISP3* mutations have been detected only in patients with the typical features of PPD. Mutant alleles include deletions, frameshifts, nonsense, and missense mutations. To date, all identified missense mutations destroy or create cysteine residues and are likely to cause their effect by disrupting normal protein folding; however, this hypothesis has not been formally tested. Mutations in WISP3 have not been detected in every patient with typical disease, but locus homogeneity is suspected because several patients from consanguineous unions with undetectable mutations still appear to be linked to the disease locus on human chromosome 6q. No patient with an atypical form of PPD (e.g., those with

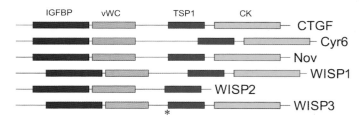

Figure 23–1. The modular architecture of the CCN protein family. Commonly used family member names are at the right, although members may go by other names based on the species and means by which they were identified. Protein sizes vary among family members, ranging from 250 amino acid residues for WISP2 to 381 residues for Cyr61. Motifs common to all family members are the signal peptide and three domains with homology to the insulin-like growth factor–binding proteins (IGFBP), von Willebrand type C (vWC), and thrombospondin 1 (TSP1). All family members, with the exception of WISP2, also have a cystine-knot-like domain (CK) near the carboxyl terminus. Smaller protein fragments have been recovered for several family members, suggesting that protein cleavage will have physiologic relevance.

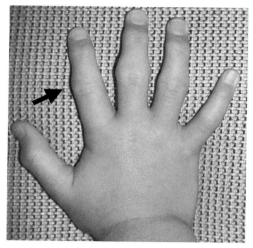

Figure 23–2. Photograph of the right hand of an 8-year-old boy with progressive pseudorheumatoid dysplasia, showing enlargement of the proximal interphalangeal joints (*arrow*). The distal interphalangeal joints are also enlarged.

different clinical or radiologic appearance or those thought to be dominantly inherited) has had a detectable *WISP3* mutation.

ESTABLISHING THE DIAGNOSIS

The diagnosis of PPD is based on clinical and radiographic findings. Molecular genetic identification of *WISP3* mutation has been performed on a research basis and is being transitioned for clinical use. Because clear disease-causing mutations have not been detected in all patients with typical clinical and radiographic features of PPD, failure to find a mutation cannot preclude the diagnosis. Because the signs and symptoms of PPD are not present at birth or during early infancy, prenatal diagnosis by ultrasonography or radiography is not possible. Rather, prenatal diagnosis requires DNA-based mutation detection.

MANAGEMENT

There are no specific management recommendations for patients with PPD. The disease course is that of progressive, painful joint degeneration with no demonstrable prevention, improvement, or slowing of

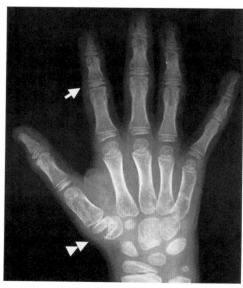

Figure 23–3. Radiograph of the right hand of the child in Figure 23–2, obtained at age 6 years. Shown is widening the distal ends of the proximal phalanges (*arrow*) and advanced bone age, as suggested by the pattern of carpal bone ossification (*double arrowhead*).

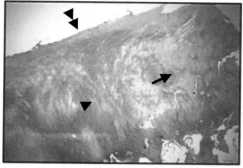

Figure 23–4. Hematoxylin and eosin–stained section (original magnification, ×40) of articular cartilage recovered from the femoral head of an 18-year-old man with progressive pseudorheumatoid dysplasia. The cartilage was obtained at the time of this individual's total hip joint replacement surgery. Shown are fibrillation of the cartilage surface (*double arrowhead*), the abnormal clustering of chondrocytes (*arrow*), and the atypical fibrillar appearance of the cartilage (*arrowhead*). Each of these features is seen in common end-stage osteoarthritis.

disease progression using anti-inflammatory drugs. Reduced mobility of multiple joints and chronic joint pain have been improved with joint replacement surgery. It has not been determined whether restricting physical activities that can be damaging to joints will delay the progression of disease in newly diagnosed patients.

MUTATIONS IN ORTHOLOGOUS AND PARALAGOUS GENES

Wisp3 has been disrupted by homologous recombination in mice (unpublished observations). Surprisingly, targeted disruption of *Wisp3* in the mouse does not recapitulate the human disease. Knockout mice are viable, and fertile, and they do not develop subjective or objective findings of joint disease. Knockout mutations have been created in two other members of the CCN family. Targeted disruption of *Cyr61* causes embryonic lethality due to failed placental implantation in most affected embryos or due to large vessel rupture in embryos that do appear to successfully implant (Mo et al., 2002). Targeted disruption of *Ctgf* causes a neonatal lethal skeletal dysplasia, with histologic findings suggesting defective vascular invasion of calcified cartilage within developing long bones (Ivkovic et al., 2003). Consequently, the site-specific regulation of vascular formation/invasion appears to be one of the functions of CCN family members.

DEVELOPMENTAL PATHOGENESIS

Studies in humans indicate that WISP3 is essential to the maintenance of articular cartilage because genetic deficiency of this protein causes PPD. However, the precise mechanism by which *WISP3* affects car-

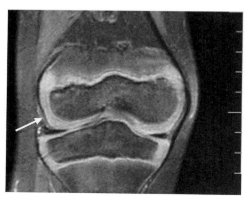

Figure 23–5. MRI, coronal section, of the right knee of the child in Figure 23–2 obtained at age 8 years. The bright-appearing layers of articular cartilage covering the femoral condyles (*arrow*) and tibial plateau appear normal. The growth plate cartilage also appears normal.

tilage homeostasis is unknown. Pathologic material obtained at the time of joint arthroplasty from patients with PPD resembles that from older patients with common, idiopathic, end-stage osteoarthritis. Targeted disruption of the gene in mice has not resulted in joint pathology under normal laboratory mouse living conditions; whether a phenotype can be provoked in laboratory mice has not yet been determined. Therefore, the potential role or roles of WISP3 in human joint development and homeostasis can only be inferred from clinical findings in patients with PPD or extrapolated from biologic studies of other CCN family members.

Several reports have suggested that CCN proteins have roles during skeletal development. The CCN family members Ctgf, Nov, Cyr61, and Wisp2 are expressed in developing skeletal elements (Wong et al., 1997; Kumar et al., 1999; Nakanishi et al., 2000; Nishida et al., 2000; Perbal, 2001). Complicating the study of WISP3 is that it has not been detected in any skeletally derived tissues or cell lines by Northern or Western blot analysis or by in situ hybridization. Expression in a human mammary epithelial cell line has been reported (van Golen et al., 1999; Kleer et al., 2002), and loss of expression has been found in inflammatory breast cancer tumors (van Golen et al., 1999). However, most laboratories that study WISP3 have detected its expression only by RT-PCR and in only a few cell types.

The observation that targeted disruption of the CCN family members *Cyr61* and *Ctgf* causes site-specific abnormalities in vasculogenesis may be relevant to understanding the developmental role of WISP3. Radiographically, patients with PPD have more mature-appearing secondary centers of ossification than do age- and gender-matched control subjects. Although advanced bone age may be a secondary consequence of joint pathology, one may speculate that disrupted timing/progression of secondary center of ossification formation/maturation is the primary underlying cause of joint disease in PPD. In articulating joints, cartilage attaches to the subchondral bone that forms at sites of secondary centers of ossification. Because vascular invasion precedes the formation of secondary centers of ossification, a role of WISP3 may be to regulate the maturation of secondary centers, thereby affecting the long-term stabilization of overlying articular cartilage to underlying subchondral bone.

Several in vitro studies suggest that WISP3 may also be involved in the regulation of tumor growth. Quantitative RT-PCR studies found increased expression of WISP3 in 12 of 19 colon adenocarcinomas compared with normal mucosa (Pennica et al., 1998). WISP3 expression was found by differential display to be lost in inflammatory breast cancer (van Golen et al., 1999). Stable transfection of a WISP3 expression vector into the SUM149 inflammatory breast cancer tumor cell line caused the cells to become less proliferative, invasive, and proangiogenic compared with the untransfected cell line and empty vector transfected cell line (Kleer et al., 2002). Somatic WISP3 frameshift mutations have been found within a significant proportion of mismatch repair defective colon neoplasias (Thorstensen et al., 2003). The frameshift occurs at a polyA(9) tract within the human WISP3 coding sequence, which would be predicted to truncate the protein at the beginning of the TSP1 domain (see asterisk below the WISP3 schematic in Fig. 23-1). The rate of mutation at this locus is higher than at polyA(9) sites within "neutral" locations (introns), suggesting that WISP3 mutation may contribute to the multistep process of colon neoplasia.

The primary, noncompensated role (at least in humans) of WISP3 during development occurs postnatally and involves the formation and/or homeostasis of articular cartilage surfaces. Delineating the precise role of WISP3 in this process and its potential roles in the regulation of tumor growth requires further study.

REFERENCES

Bork P (1993). The modular architecture of a new family of growth regulators related to connective tissue growth factor. *FEBS Lett* 327: 125–130.

Bradham DM, Igarashi A, Potter RL, Grotendorst GR (1991). Connective tissue growth factor: a cysteine-rich mitogen secreted by human vascular endothelial cells is related to the SRC-induced immediate early gene product CEF-10. *J Cell Biol* 114: 1285–1294.

Brigstock DR (1999). The connective tissue growth factor/cysteine-rich 61/nephroblastoma overexpressed (CCN) family. *Endocr Rev* 20: 189–206.

Brigstock DR, Steffen CL, Kim GY, Vegunta RK, Diehl JR, Harding PA (1997). Purification and characterization of novel heparin-binding growth factors in uterine secretory fluids. Identification as heparin-regulated Mr 10,000 forms of connective tissue growth factor. *J Biol Chem* 272: 20275–20282.

Desnoyers L, Arnott D, Pennica D (2001). WISP-1 binds to decorin and biglycan. *J Biol Chem* 276: 47599–47607.

el-Shanti H, Murray JC, Semina EV, Beutow KH, Scherpbier T, al-Alami J (1998). Assignment of gene responsible for progressive pseudorheumatoid dysplasia to chromosome 6 and examination of COL10A1 as candidate gene. *Eur J Hum Genet* 6: 251–256.

el-Shanti HE, Omari HZ, Qubain HI (1997). Progressive pseudorheumatoid dysplasia: report of a family and review. *J Med Genet* 34: 559–563.

Fischer J, Urtizberea JA, Pavek S, Vandiedonck C, Bruls T, Saker S, Alkatip Y, Prud'homme JF, Weissenbach J (1998). Genetic linkage of progressive pseudorheumatoid dysplasia to a 3-cM interval of chromosome 6q22. *Hum Genet* 103: 60–64.

Hurvitz JR, Suwairi WM, Van Hul W, El-Shanti H, Superti-Furga A, Roudier J, Holderbaum D, Pauli RM, Herd JK, Van Hul EV, et al. (1999). Mutations in the CCN gene family member WISP3 cause progressive pseudorheumatoid dysplasia. *Nat Genet* 23: 94–98.

Ivkovic S, Yoon BS, Popoff SN, Safadi FF, Libuda DE, Stephenson RC, Daluiski A, Lyons KM (2003). Connective tissue growth factor coordinates chondrogenesis and angiogenesis during growth and development. *Development* 130: 2779–2791.

Kleer CG, Zhang Y, Pan Q, van Golen KL, Wu ZF, Livant D, Merajver SD (2002). WISP3 is a novel tumor suppressor gene of inflammatory breast cancer. *Oncogene* 21: 3172–3180.

Kumar S, Hand AT, Connor JR, Dodds RA, Ryan PJ, Trill JJ, Fisher SM, Nuttall ME, Lipshutz DB, Zou C, et al. (1999). Identification and cloning of a connective tissue growth factor-like cDNA from human osteoblasts encoding a novel regulator of osteoblast functions. *J Biol Chem* 274: 17123–17131.

Mo FE, Muntean AG, Chen CC, Stolz DB, Watkins SC, Lau LF (2002). CYR61 (CCN1) is essential for placental development and vascular integrity. *Mol Cell Biol* 22: 8709–8720.

Nakanishi T, Nishida T, Shimo T, Kobayashi K, Kubo T, Tamatani T, Tezuka K, Takigawa M (2000). Effects of CTGF/Hcs24, a product of a hypertrophic chondrocyte-specific gene, on the proliferation and differentiation of chondrocytes in culture. *Endocrinology* 141: 264–273.

Nishida T, Nakanishi T, Asano M, Shimo T, Takigawa M (2000). Effects of CTGF/Hcs24, a hypertrophic chondrocyte-specific gene product, on the proliferation and differentiation of osteoblastic cells in vitro. *J Cell Physiol* 184: 197–206.

O'Brien TP, Yang GP, Sanders L, Lau LF (1990). Expression of cyr61, a growth factor-inducible immediate-early gene. *Mol Cell Biol* 10: 3569–3577.

Pennica D, Swanson TA, Welsh JW, Roy MA, Lawrence DA, Lee J, Brush J, Taneyhill LA, Deuel B, Lew M, et al. (1998). WISP genes are members of the connective tissue growth factor family that are up-regulated in wnt-1-transformed cells and aberrantly expressed in human colon tumors. *Proc Natl Acad Sci USA* 95: 14717–14722.

Perbal B (2001). NOV (nephroblastoma overexpressed) and the CCN family of genes: structural and functional issues. *Mol Pathol* 54: 57–79.

Simmons DL, Levy DB, Yannoni Y, Erikson RL (1989). Identification of a phorbol ester-repressible v-src-inducible gene. *Proc Natl Acad Sci USA* 86: 1178–1182.

Spranger J, Albert C, Schilling F, Bartsocas C, Stoss H (1983). Progressive pseudorheumatoid arthritis of childhood (PPAC). A hereditary disorder simulating rheumatoid arthritis. *Eur J Pediatr* 140: 34–40.

Thorstensen L, Holm R, Lothe RA, Trope C, Carvalho B, Sobrinho-Simoes M, Seruca R (2003). WNT-inducible signaling pathway protein 3, WISP-3, is mutated in microsatellite unstable gastrointestinal carcinomas but not in endometrial carcinomas. *Gastroenterology* 124: 270–271.

van Golen KL, Davies S, Wu ZF, Wang Y, Bucana CD, Root H, Chandrasekharappa S, Strawderman M, Ethier SP, Merajver SD (1999). A novel putative low-affinity insulin-like growth factor-binding protein, LIBC (lost in inflammatory breast cancer), and RhoC GTPase correlate with the inflammatory breast cancer phenotype. *Clin Cancer Res* 5: 2511–2519.

Wong M, Kireeva ML, Kolesnikova TV, Lau LF (1997). Cyr61, product of a growth factor-inducible immediate-early gene, regulates chondrogenesis in mouse limb bud mesenchymal cells. *Dev Biol* 192: 492–508.

Wynne-Davies R, Hall C, Ansell BM (1982). Spondylo-epiphysial dysplasia tarda with progressive arthropathy. A "new" disorder of autosomal recessive inheritance. *J Bone Joint Surg Br* 64: 442–445.

Yang GP, Lau LF (1991). Cyr61, product of a growth factor-inducible immediate early gene, is associated with the extracellular matrix and the cell surface. *Cell Growth Differ* 2: 351–357.

Part C.
The Transforming Growth Factor β (TGF-β) Signaling Pathway

24 | An Introduction to TGF-β-Related Signaling

ANNA PETRYK AND MICHAEL B. O'CONNOR

Members of the transforming growth factor-beta (TGF-β) super-family of secreted polypeptides play diverse roles in regulating numerous biological processes in a wide variety of organisms. These factors have been implicated in mediating embryonic development, cell proliferation and differentiation, apoptosis, organogenesis, and wound healing; and when misregulated, they can contribute to carcinogenesis. Phylogenetic considerations suggest that this family is one of the oldest signaling pathways, having arisen before the divergence of a common ancestor of arthropods and vertebrates about 1.3 billion years ago (Newfeld et al., 1999). In this chapter, we will provide an overview of the signal-transduction pathway utilized by these factors and the mechanisms by which the activities of these pathways are regulated. Much of our understanding of the biology of these factors derives from a multidisciplinary experimental approach using biochemical, genetic, and embryological methods as well as numerous model systems such as *Drosophila, Caenorhabditis elegans, Xenopus,* zebrafish, and mice. We will give only selected examples here, and the reader is encouraged to examine other reviews (Massagué, 1998; Masasagué and Chen, 2000) for supplementary information on specific aspects of the biology of these factors. In addition, other chapters in this volume will focus on various human pathologies and developmental disorders that have been linked to defects in different components of this pathway (see Chapters 25–29).

As we currently understand it, the basic signaling mechanism of these factors is rather simple (Fig. 24–1, Table 24–1). Ligands of this family bind to a set of distinct serine/threonine kinase transmembrane proteins known as type I and type II receptors. The type II receptor possesses a constitutively active kinase that phosphorylates the type I receptor within a conserved glycine/serine-rich sequence called the *GS domain*. This phosphorylation event activates the type I receptor through a presumed conformational change, allowing it to recognize its major substrates. These substrates are transcription factors of the Smad family, which, after phosphorylation by type I receptors, move to the nucleus, where they regulate transcription of downstream target genes. Since in most organisms there is a more limited number of receptors and Smad proteins than there are ligands, complex regulatory mechanisms appear to have evolved that endow these factors with the ability to orchestrate a wide variety of biological processes with exquisite specificity. The organization of this chapter follows the fate of a signal beginning with ligand secretion and ending with propagation of the signal to downstream targets in the nucleus. Potential points of regulation within the pathway that have been identified or are likely points of control will be highlighted in the different sections.

LIGANDS

All TGF-β-type ligands are dimeric peptides of approximately 100 amino acids, which are derived by proteolytic processing within the C-terminal portion of a proprotein. The proteases that cleave these

285

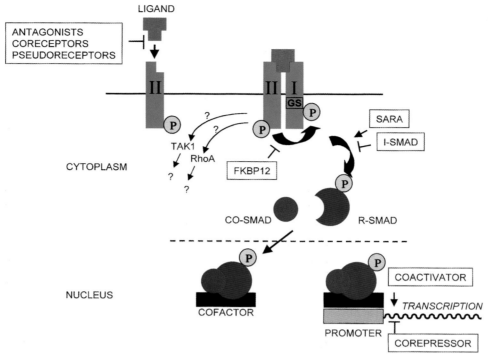

Figure 24–1. Ligands of the TGF-β superfamily signal through two distinct classes of transmembrane serine-threonine kinases, known as types I and II receptors. The accessibility of ligands to receptors is regulated by ligand antagonists, coreceptors, and pseudoreceptors. Ligand binding induces a heteromeric complex in which the constitutively active type II kinase phosphorylates the type I receptor within a conserved glycine/serine-rich sequence, the GS domain. This phosphorylation event activates the type I kinase domain so that it can bind and phosphorylate appropriate receptor-regulated Smads (R-Smad). Once phosphorylated, the R-Smads complex with a common non-phosphorylated Samd (Smad4), translocate to the nucleus, and regulate transcription of downstream target genes. Recruitment of some Smads to type I receptors is facilitated by Smad anchor for receptor activation (SARA). Nonspecific activation of type II receptors is prevented by binding of FKBP12 to the GS domain in the basal state. Once in the nucleus, Smads associate with DNA-binding cofactors, which confer specificity on the interaction of Smads with DNA elements. Binding of the Smad/cofactor complex to the promoter recruits coactivators or corepressors that regulate transcription. TGF-β receptors can also signal via other pathways, e.g., through activation of MAPK kinase kinase (Tak1) or RhoA, which do not involve Smad phosphorylation.

proproteins to liberate the mature ligands are members of the furin family of growth factor convertases. In some cases, activation of the growth factors is limited at this step (Constam and Robertson, 1999). The ligand domain itself is rich in cysteine residues, which exhibit a conserved spacing pattern. Intramolecular disulfide bridges formed by several of these cysteines give rise to a distinct three-dimensional structure, termed the *cysteine knot* (Sun and Davies, 1995), a characteristic feature shared by all ligands of this superfamily. An intermolecular disulfide bridge helps to stabilize the dimer structure for most ligands, and in some cases, heterodimers between two different family members can also form, which can have very different biological activities from either homodimer.

Sequence alignments between, and signaling assays with, different family members have allowed two major subgroups within the TGF-β superfamily to be identified (Newfeld et al., 1999). These are the bone morphogenetic proteins (BMPs) and the TGF-β/activin group. Within these subfamilies, other groupings have been assigned, including the growth and differentiation factors (GDFs) and the nodal family. In addition, there are several outlying factors that include mullerian inhibiting substance (MIS) and a very distant member, glia-derived neurotropic growth factor (GDNF) (see Chapters 35 and 44). However, even though GDNF shares the characteristic cysteine spacing pattern of other TGF-β family members, its signal is propagated via a tyrosine kinase receptor rather than the serine/threonine kinase receptor family utilized by all other TGF-β types (Durbec et al., 1996). Therefore, its inclusion as a member of the TGF-β family is equivocal at this time.

The founding member of the TGF-β superfamily was TGF-β1, a factor originally identified as an activity produced by retrovirally

Table 24–1. Basic TGF-β Family Signaling Mechanisms

Ligand	Type I Receptor	Type II Receptor	Smad	Cofactor
Vertebrates				
TGF-β	TβR-I (ALK5)	TβR-II	Smad2	AP-1, TFE3
Activin	ActR-I (ALK4)	ActR-II	Smad3	FAST, OAZ
		ActR-IIB		Mixer and Milk
BMP	BMPR-IA (ALK3)	BMPR-II	Smad1	Hoxc-8, Hoxa-9
	BMPR-IB (ALK6)	ActR-II	Smad5	PEBP2/CBF
	ActR-I (ALK4)	ActR-IIB	Smad8	SIP1
Drosophila melanogaster				
Activin	babo	Punt	dSmad2	
Dpp	Tkv		Mad	
Scw, Gbb	Sax			

TGF, transforming growth factor; BMP, bone morphogenetic protein; AP-1, activator protein 1; PEBP2/CBF, polyomavirus enhancer binding protein 2/core binding factor; Olf-1/EBF, olfactory neuronal transcription factor; SIP1, Smad-interacting protein 1; OAZ, OIF-1/EBF-associated zinc finger; FAST, Forkhead activin signal transducer.

transformed cells that simulated growth of rat fibroblasts (Roberts et al., 1981). Since that time, it has become clear that the response of cells to these factors in terms of growth stimulation, inhibition, or differentiation is dependent on the cellular context; therefore, the family name is a bit of a misnomer. At present, the TGF-β subgroup has been described only in vertebrates and consists of three members in mammals (TGF-β1–3). These factors are about 65%–70% identical to one another but show different activities and distinct patterns of expression in embryonic and adult tissues, where they play diverse roles in vertebrate embryonic development and human disease. For example, mice deficient in TGF-β2 have multiple developmental abnormalities, including cardiac, lung, craniofacial, limb, and spinal column defects (Sanford et al., 1997). TGF-β2 has been implicated in the pathogenesis of cleft palate in humans (Lidral et al., 1998). TGF-βs also have a role in cancer (primarily functioning as tumor suppressors), angiogenesis, immune function, and tissue repair (Blobe et al., 2000).

BMPs were first described by Urist (1965) as potent inducers of endochondral bone formation after implantation at ectopic sites in rats. Since then, more than 20 members of the BMP/GDF family have been identified in both vertebrate and invertebrate species and shown to have diverse roles in embryonic development from tissue specification in early embryos to organogenesis and skeletal patterning (Hogan, 1996; Chang et al., 2001a). Mutations of BMPs frequently have profound effects on the developing embryo. For example, a mutation in BMP2 is embryonic-lethal and produces defects in amnion/chorion and cardiac development in mice (Zhang and Bradley, 1996). BMP4 deficiency leads to early embryonic death and failure to form mesoderm (Winnier et al., 1995). BMP4 heterozygous null mice exhibit defects in limb formation (Dunn et al., 1997). Doubly heterozygous BMP4 and BMP7 mice have multiple skeletal abnormalities, particularly in the rib cage and the distal part of the limbs (Katagiri et al., 1998).

During early *Xenopus* embryogenesis, BMPs affect axial patterning, promote formation of ventral mesoderm, and antagonize the formation of dorsal tissues such as the nervous system (De Robertis et al., 2000). Members of the nodal family of BMPs form part of a hierarchical network of TGF-β-type factors that regulate left/right asymmetry of internal organ anatomy and physiology (Whitman and Mercola, 2001).

BMPs are also found in invertebrates. In *Drosophila*, the Decapentaplegic (Dpp) product shows 75% amino acid identity within the ligand domain to BMPs 2 and 4. In addition to this sequence conservation, Dpp and BMP2/4 are functionally conserved. Thus, Dpp can produce ectopic bones when implanted into rats, while BMP4 can rescue dpp mutants when expressed in *Drosophila* (Padgett et al., 1994). Two other BMP-type ligands, Screw (Scw) and Glass bottom boat (Gbb, also known as 60A), are also found in *Drosophila*; and these are most closely related to vertebrate the BMP5, -6, and -7 subgroup (Arora et al., 1994; Khalsa et al., 1998). Dpp controls many aspects of *Drosophila* development, including early dorsal/ventral axis specification, gut and tracheal morphogenesis, and appendage growth and patterning (Raftery and Sutherland, 1999). In most processes examined so far, the ligands Scw and Gbb appear to play auxiliary roles as factors that enhance the primary Dpp signal (Haerry et al., 1998; Nguyen et al., 1998; Neul and Ferguson, 1998). This may come about, in part, by heterodimerization among the different BMP ligands. In vertebrates, for example, BMP2 and -7 heterodimers are much more active in a bone-induction assay than either homodimer (Israel et al., 1996). How frequent heterodimerization occurs within a subfamily is not clear nor is it clear, how often heterodimerization might occur between family members. One recent report suggests that BMPs can heterodimerize with Nodal to attenuate the ability of Nodal to propagate a signal (Yeo and Whitman, 2001).

In *C. elegans*, unc-129 encodes a highly divergent BMP family member that appears to provide a guidance cue for pathfinding of certain ventral nerve cord motor neurons (Colavita et al., 1998).

GDFs are closely related to BMPs and may play somewhat overlapping roles during development. GDF5 is expressed at the sites of joint formation, and mutations in the *Gdf5* gene result in brachypodism in mice (Storm et al., 1994). A mutation in its human homo-

logue, *cartilage-derived morphogenetic protein-1* (*CDMP-1*), causes chondrodysplasia Grebe type, characterized by severe limb shortening (Thomas et al., 1997; see Chapter 27).

Nodals play important roles during early embryogenesis in vertebrates, particularly in mesoderm formation and the establishment of left/right asymmetry (Whitman, 2001). They have also been implicated in the formation of the endoderm, the ventral midline of the neural tube, and anterior/posterior patterning (Schier and Shen, 2000) in mice.

Activins/inhibins were first identified for their roles in regulating the production of follicle-stimulating hormone (FSH) from pituitary cells (Ling et al., 1986). Activins are homo- and heterodimers composed of two β chains, βA and βB, while inhibins are heterodimers of either a βA or βB chain with an α chain. Activins and inhibins have opposing biological activities: activin stimulates FSH production, while inhibin antagonizes its production. Activins and inhibins regulate the pituitary/gonadal axis through endocrine, paracrine, and autocrine mechanisms (Matzuk et al., 1996; Ethier and Findlay, 2001). Inhibin is also implicated in the development of gonadal tumors (Matzuk et al., 1992). At least two other activin-like factors have been identified, but their biological roles are not well studied (Lau et al., 2000).

MIS is responsible for the initiation of regression of the mullerian ducts in utero in males through the induction of apoptosis and epithelial–mesenchymal transformation (Allard et al., 2000; see also Chapter 44). The mullerian ducts give rise to the oviducts, uterus, and the upper portion of the vagina in females; therefore, their regression is crucial for male sexual differentiation. Mutations in MIS lead to persistence of the mullerian duct derivatives (Belville et al., 1999). MIS also plays a role in adult germ cell maturation and gonadal function (Ingraham et al., 2000).

One unusual subclass of related ligands is the antivins and leftys. The first member of this class, lefty1, was identified as a novel TGF-β expressed on the left side of gastrulating mouse embryos (Meno et al., 1996). Antivin was identified in zebrafish as a factor that antagonizes activins and nodals for induction of mesendodermal derivatives (Thisse and Thisse, 1999). What sets this subfamily of ligands apart is their lack of the large α-helix segment involved in ligand dimerization and an absence of the cysteine residue required for covalent stabilization of homo- and heterodimers. At present, it is not clear how these molecules antagonize the activity of activins and nodals. One model envisions that they may titrate either a signaling receptor or a coreceptor into an inactive complex. However, there is also recent evidence suggesting that lefty activates a mitogen-activated protein kinase (MAPK) cascade and, therefore, that antagonism of activin/nodal signaling might take place at some downstream level (Ulloa et al., 2001).

Ligand Antagonists: Regulation of Ligand Availability

One emerging theme concerning the biology of these factors is that their activities are often regulated very early within the signal-transduction cascade at the level of ligand accessibility to the receptor (Fig. 24–2). This first became clear during study of the prototypical family member TGF-β1. After cleavage of the proprotein within the Golgi apparatus, TGF-β1 is secreted into the extracellular matrix as an inactive protein, bound noncovalently to the N-terminal propeptide known as latency-associated protein (LAP) (Fig. 24–2A). Frequently, the TFG-β prosegment is also covalently attached through disulfide bonds to one of four fibrillin-like latent TGF-β binding protein (LTBPs) (Oklu and Hesketh, 2000). LTBP-3 knockout mice have bone abnormalities similar to those generated by impairing TGF-β itself, suggesting that these cofactors play significant in vivo roles in regulating TGF-β activity (Dabovic et al., 2002). The present view is that the LTBPs play at least two important roles in modulating TGF-β activity: (*1*) they facilitate folding and secretion (Miyazono et al., 1991) of the latent complex from the source cells and (*2*) they appear to facilitate activation of the latent complex (Gualandris et al., 2000), perhaps by targeting it to appropriate regions within the extracellular matrix. Several different mechanisms have been proposed for activation

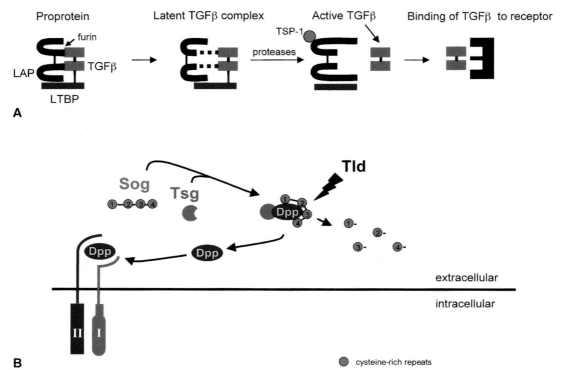

Figure 24–2. (*A*) TGF-β is synthesized as a proprotein. After cleavage of the proprotein within the Golgi apparatus, TGF-β is secreted into the extracellular matrix as an inactive protein, bound noncovalently to the N-terminal propeptide known as the latency-associated protein (LAP), and covalently bound to latent TGF-β-binding protein (LTBPs). Active TGF-β is released from the latent TGF-β complex when LAP associates with thrombospondin-1 (TSP-1), which induces a conformational change, or is processed by proteases. (*B*) Twisted gastrulation (Tsg) and Sog/Chordin form tripartite complexes with Decapentaplegic/bone morphogenetic proteins (Dpp/BMPs) and synergistically inhibit the action of Dpp/BMPs by preventing their binding to receptor. Dpp/BMPs are released from the complex by the action of Tolloid (Tld). Other ligand inhibitors include follistatin, Noggin, and Dan family members.

of the latent TGF-β complex, including processing of LAP by the plasminogen activation complex (Rifkin et al., 1997). However, induction of a conformational change within LAP by association with thrombospondin-1 (TSP-1) may be the primary in vivo mechanism of activation since TSP-1 knockout mice display many phenotypes in common with TGF-β1 knockout mice (Crawford et al., 1998). How common this mechanism of ligand regulation might be among the various subfamilies is not clear. At least one BMP-type factor, myostatin, has been shown to form a latent complex with its N-terminal proprotein (Lee and McPherron, 2001), but how many others do and whether they form bonds to LTBP-type proteins remain to be determined.

Association of ligand with a LAP and LTBP protein is not the only way that ligand–receptor interactions are controlled. A large number of secreted antagonists that have differential affinities toward particular TGF-β family members have also been described. These molecules tend to have cysteine-rich domains that share weak similarity to extracellular matrix molecules. One of the first to be described was follistatin. It functions as an antagonist of activin and causes decreases in FSH secretion by the pituitary gland, whereas activin stimulates FSH secretion (Knight and Glister, 2001). Follistatin binds activin directly and prevents its interactions with cell surface receptors (de Winter et al., 1996). Follistatin can also bind BMPs (Iemura et al., 1998).

Within the BMP family, several additional types of inhibitor have been identified (Fig. 24–2B). These include Chordin (*Drosophila* Sog), twisted gastrulation (Tsg), and differential screening-selected gene aberrative in neuroblastoma (DAN) family members such as cerberus and gremlin. During the development of an organism from an egg to an embryo, embryonic cells, which are initially indistinguishable from each other, organize into recognizable patterns along three axes, anterior/posterior, dorsal/ventral, and left/right. Such cell commitment is controlled, in part, by gradients of secreted TGF-β-type factors. Since the response of cells to these gradients is concentration-dependent, they are often referred to as *morphogens* and the source tissue is given the term *organizer* (Joubin and Stern, 2001). The Spe-

mann organizer, a region of tissue that forms near the blastopore lip, is a classic example in *Xenopus* (DeRobertis et al., 2000), while Hensen's node appears to play an equivalent function in mice.

It is now known that the organizer secretes many different types of antagonist molecules and, in so doing, helps to establish gradients of morphogens. The morphogens then provide spatial cues for further patterning of the developing embryo. One of the best studied examples of morphogen regulation by secreted antagonists is the interplay of BMP/Dpp with the inhibitors Chordin (Sog in flies) and Twisted gastrulation (Tsg). These two factors act synergistically to block BMP/Dpp signaling in frogs, zebrafish, and flies, although the complexity of the interactions is still not entirely understood in vertebrates (Oelgeschläger et al., 2000; C. Chang et al., 2001b; Ross et al., 2001; Scott et al., 2001). In flies, the model that has been proposed suggests that a peak concentration of Dpp needs to be maintained in the dorsal region for the dorsal structures to develop properly. The Dpp peak is achieved through the action of a tripartite complex between Dpp, Sog, and Tsg. Since Sog is secreted from ventral lateral cells and Dpp and Tsg from dorsal cells, the idea is that Sog diffusion toward the dorsal side drives the patterning process. When Sog encounters Dpp and Tsg in dorsal lateral domains, it forms a tripartite complex that prevents the binding of Dpp to its receptor at sites in the dorsal lateral region. By blocking receptor binding, this complex facilitates diffusion of Dpp toward the dorsal side (Ross et al., 2001). Once the concentration of Dpp/Sog/Tsg is enhanced in the dorsalmost cells, Dpp is released from the complex by the action of Tolloid (Marqués et al., 1997), a zinc metalloprotease which cleaves Sog. Sog fragments also appear to have biological activity (Yu et al., 2000). Tolloid (Tld) has several vertebrate homologues, including BMP1, Xolloid, and Tld (Piccollo et al., 1997). A similar mechanism appears to control zebrafish and *Xenopus* dorsal/ventral axis specification, although in these organisms the dorsal/ventral axis is inverted relative to *Drosophila* (DeRobertis and Sasai, 1996). As can be appreciated by this example, morphogen gradients are dependent not only on the binding of the ligand by the antagonists but also on their concentration, site of synthesis, direction, and rates of diffusion.

The role of Chordin and Tsg in mice and humans is currently less well characterized. In mice, Chordin together with another BMP antagonist, Noggin, appear to regulate formation of the forebrain since mice deficient for both proteins display severe defects in forebrain development, resulting in holoprosencephaly (Bachiller et al., 2000).

Noggin, like Chordin, is expressed in the Spemann organizer in amphibian embryos, where it promotes the formation of neural tissue and dorsalization of ventral mesoderm (Piccolo et al., 1996). In mice, noggin is important for skeletal development (Brunet et al., 1998). Mice deficient in noggin have defects within the axial skeleton and fail to form joints properly. Mutations in *NOG* in humans result in proximal symphalangism and multiple synostoses syndrome (Gong et al., 1999; see Chapter 25).

The DAN family of secreted antagonists includes mammalian Dan, Cer1 (cerberus-related), PRDC (protein related to DAN and cerberus), Drm (homologous to *Xenopus* gremlin), Dte (dante), chick Caronte, and *C. elegans* CeCan1 (Pearce et al., 1999; Yokouchi et al., 1999). An additional member of the DAN family, sclerosteosis (SOST), has recently been identified in a search for mutations that result in an autosomal recessive bone dysplasia sclerosteosis (Brunkow et al., 2001). Dan proteins share a cysteine-rich region, which is similar to the cysteine knot of TGF-β.

Cerberus is a potent inducer of ectopic head formation in *Xenopus* embryos (Bouwmeester et al., 1996). It antagonizes not only BMP activity but also Nodal and Wnt signals (Piccolo et al., 1999). In mice, however, it is not essential for head formation (Shawlot et al., 2000).

Both Dan and Drm inhibit cell growth and have tumor-suppressive activity (Ozaki et al., 1995; Topol et al., 2000). Chick Caronte is involved in left/right axis formation by antagonizing BMP signals and inducing the asymmetric expression of Lefty (Yokouchi et al., 1999). In mice, Dante and Nodal are expressed asymmetrically in the node, with Dante predominating on the right and Nodal on the left (Pearce et al., 1999).

RECEPTORS

The TGF-β superfamily of ligands signals through transmembrane type I and type II receptors. Both types of receptor have a cysteine-rich extracellular domain, a hydrophobic transmembrane region, and a cytoplasmic domain with serine/threonine kinase activity. A distinctive feature of type I receptors is the presence of a GS domain just distal to the transmembrane segment, which becomes phosphorylated by the activated type II receptors upon ligand binding (Wrana et al., 1994). Activated type I receptors interact with Smads through the L45 loop of the kinase domain, a region that determines the specificity of the interaction (Feng and Derynck, 1997).

Activation of type I receptors may involve more than simple phosphorylation within the GS box. TGF-β receptors undergo internalization through association with the clathrin adaptor protein AP2, and blocking receptor complex internalization appears to inhibit phosphorylation (Garamszegi et al., 2001). These data suggest that either the microenvironment of the early endosome or some other component within the endosome may be required for type I receptor activation in addition to the type II component.

In vertebrates, type II receptors for four major TGF-β subfamilies include TGF-β type II receptor (TβR-II) for TGF-β, BMP type II receptor (BMPR-II) for BMPs, activin type II and type IIB (ActR-II and ActR-IIB) receptors for activin as well as BMPs, and the anti-mullerian hormone (AMH) type II receptor (AMHR-II) for MIS (Mathews and Vale, 1991; Lin et al., 1992; Mathews et al., 1992; di Clemente et al., 1994; Chang et al., 1997) (Table 24–1). Mutations in the human BMPR-II lead to both sporadic as well as familial cases of primary pulmonary hypertension (Lane et al., 2000; Deng et al., 2000)

Type I receptors, also known as activin receptor-like kinases (ALK), include TβR-I (ALK-5), BMPR-IA (ALK-3), BMPR-IB (ALK-6), ActR-I (ALK-4), as well as Alk-1 and -7 (Yamashita et al., 1994; Koenig et al., 1994; Attisano et al., 1996; Ryden et al., 1996). ActR-I can bind both activin and BMPs (Liu et al., 1995), while Alk-1 binds TGF-β1 but sends a BMP-type signal (see below).

In *Drosophila*, the BMPs, including Dpp, Scw, and Gbb, bind to the type II receptor Punt (Letsou et al., 1995), which activates type I receptors Thick veins (Tkv) and Saxophone (Sax) (Brummel et al., 1994; Neul and Ferguson, 1998; Haerry et al., 1998) and signal through Mad. The type I receptor for the Activin pathway is *baboon* (*babo*) (Brummel et al., 1999), which signals through dSmad2 rather than Mad.

In *C. elegans*, only two type I receptors (Daf-1 and Sma-6) and one type II receptor (Daf-4) appear to mediate signaling by four ligands (Patterson and Padgett, 2000). This organism also appears to have evolved a novel mechanism for signaling at certain developmental stages since in some cases daf-1 can signal in the absence of a functional type II receptor (Gunther et al., 2000).

In the absence of ligand, type I and type II receptors exist in the form of homodimers. The binding of TGF-β to type II receptor induces the formation of a heterotetrameric receptor complex with type I receptor (Yamashita et al., 1994). BMP receptors show more variable oligomerization patterns in the basal state manifested by the formation of both homodimers (e.g., BMPR-IA/BMPR-IA or BMPR-II/BMPR-II) and heterodimers (e.g., BMPR-II/BMPR-IA) (Gilboa et al., 2000).

Coreceptors

Betaglycan and endoglin are cell surface molecules (also known as type III receptors) that bind TGF-βs but do not have signaling capability. Betaglycan is a membrane-bound proteoglycan with a short intracellular tail, while endoglin, although it shares some sequence similarity to betaglycan within the core protein, does not contain additional sites for heparan or chondroitin sulfate sugar chains. These two proteins are thought to primarily regulate the accessibility of TGF-βs to type II receptors and can be either antagonistic or agonistic (Letamendia et al., 1998). For example, TGF-β2 has poor affinity for type I and type II receptors. However, the presence of betaglycan on the cell surface facilitates binding of TGF-β2 to the signaling receptors and improves the responsiveness of cells to this factor (Lopez-Casillas et al., 1993). Betaglycan can also be shed from the cell surface, and in this case it appears to antagonize TGF-β signaling (Lopez-Casillas et al., 1994), perhaps by allowing diffusion of the ligand away from the cell surface. In *Drosophila*, the glypican related proteoglycan Dally may serve a similar coreceptor role in mediating some aspects of Dpp signaling (Jackson et al., 1997).

Betaglycan has also been implicated in mediating inhibin signaling. As outlined above, activins are composed of homo- or heterodimers of βA or βB subunits, while inhibins are heterodimers of a β chain with an α subunit. Inhibins can bind to the activin type II receptor through their β subunit but fail to recruit a type I receptor (Xu et al., 1995). This could potentially explain the antagonistic effects of inhibins on the endocrine system if they simply compete with activins for binding to the type II receptor. However, the affinity of the inhibin heterodimer for the type II receptor is much lower than that of activin. This means that inhibins need to be present in large excess at target tissues for this mechanism to be effective, a scenario at odds with many experimental observations. One possible solution to this dilemma is the finding that betaglycan binds inhibin with high affinity and can enhance the binding of inhibin to the type II receptor (Lewis et al., 2000). The complex formed does not dissociate readily, and activin does not compete for it. This finding potentially explains how inhibins block activin signaling. Whether inhibins also have an independent receptor that activates an intracellular signal-transduction cascade remains to be determined.

Endoglin is highly expressed in endothelial cells, and its elimination in humans results in hereditary hemorrhagic telangiectasia (McAllister et al., 1994; see Chapter 28), characterized by bleeding from dilated blood vessels within the skin and mucous membranes. This phenotype is also seen in patients with mutations in Alk-1, which, until recently, was considered an orphan type I receptor. It has now been shown that Alk-1 can bind and mediate TGF-β1 signaling in endothelial cells, whereas previously Alk-5 was thought to be the primary type I receptor for TGF-β-type ligands (Oh et al., 2000). Expression of endoglin on endotheial cells may therefore help direct

TGF-β1 signaling through Alk-1 instead of Alk-5. Interestingly, Alk-1 does not signal through Smads 2 and 3, as does Alk-5, but rather through Smads 1 and 5, which previously have been implicated only in BMP signaling (see below).

A final example of coreceptor requirement for signal transduction is illustrated by the nodal-type ligands. These molecules bind and signal through ActR-IIB and Alk-4 but require epidermal growth factor (EGF)/TGF-α-like transmembrane proteins of the Cripto/One-eyed pinhead family for effective binding and signaling (Yeo and Whitman, 2001).

Negative Regulators at the Receptor Level

BAMBI is a transmembrane protein which functions as a pseudoreceptor for BMP, activin, and TGF-β (Onichtchouk et al., 1999). It is structurally similar to type I receptors except for the absence of a kinase domain within its intracellular portion. By forming heterodimeric complexes with type I receptors, BAMBI inhibits signaling by TGF-β ligands.

FKBP12 is a cytosolic protein which binds to the GS domain of TGF-β type I receptor, blocking its phosphorylation (Chen et al., 1997a). The fact that FKBP12 binds to TGF-βR-I in the basal state and that this interaction is abolished by ligand binding to TβR-II suggest that FKBP12 may play a protective role, preventing nonspecific activation of the TGF-β pathway. However, its role in vivo is not entirely understood since FKBP12-deficient mice have apparently normal TGF-β signaling (Shou et al., 1998).

Finally, downregulation of TGF-β receptors is induced by Smad7 (see below), which recruits Smad ubiquitination regulatory factor 1 (Smurf1), an E3 ubiquitin ligase, to the receptor complex (Ebisawa et al., 2001), marking it for degradation by the proteosome. In Drosophila, the absence of a Smurf1 homologue leads to a prolonged Dpp signal in the early embryo (Podos et al., 2001). As a result, some cells are not specified correctly during early developmental stages, ultimately leading to defects in gut development at later stages of embryogenesis. Several additional receptor binding proteins, such as TGF-β receptor-interacting protein 1 (TRIP-1) (Chen et al., 1995), serine-threonine kinase receptor-associated protein (STRAP) (Datta et al., 1998), TBR-I-associated protein-1 (TRAP-1) (Charng et al., 1998), and protein phosphatase 2A, have been identified by yeast two-hybrid screens; but little is presently known about the functional significance of these interactions.

SMAD PROTEINS

Cloning of the Drosophila gene mothers against dpp (Mad) was the first step in identifying substrates for TGF-β receptors (Raftery et al., 1995; Sekelsky et al., 1995). Mutations in the Drosophila Mad gene as well as mutations in the small (sma) genes of C. elegans (Savage et al., 1996) produced phenotypes similar to that produced by mutations in TGF-β ligands and receptors, suggesting that these proteins were somehow involved in mediating TGF-β signal transduction in these organisms. Soon, homologues were also identified in vertebrates, and the unified descriptive term Smad was introduced (Derynck et al., 1996).

The Smad proteins contain highly conserved amino- and carboxy-terminal domains (MH1 and MH2, respectively) separated by a linker (Shi et al., 1997, 1998). The MH1 domain has a DNA-binding motif, whereas the MH2 domain interacts with receptors and other proteins/transcription factors and mediates many of the biological effects of Smad proteins. There are three subclasses of Smads: receptor-regulated Smads (R-Smads), common Smads (Co-Smads), and inhibitory Smads (I-Smads) (Itoh et al., 2001). The R-Smads, which are direct substrates of the type I receptor kinase, are phosphorylated on serine residues within a carboxy-terminal SSXS motif (Kretzschmar et al., 1997).

Activation of various R-Smads is ligand-specific. Type I receptors for BMP and GDF interact with Smad1, Smad5, and Smad8 (Hoodless et al., 1996), whereas type I receptors for TGF-β and activin phosphorylate Smad2 and Smad3 (Macias-Silva et al., 1996; Liu et al., 1997b; Brummel et al., 1999). Recruitment of Smad2 to the activin

and TGF-β receptors is facilitated by SARA (Smad anchor for receptor activation), a protein that contains an FYVE domain and binds to both R-Smads and type I and type II receptors (Tsukazaki et al., 1998). Whether additional FYVE-type proteins help recruit the BMP-specific Smads to their respective type I receptors is not clear.

Following phosphorylation, R-Smads associate with Co-Smads, which are Smad4/DPC4 in vertebrates (Lagna et al., 1996; Zhang et al., 1997) and Medea in Drosophila (Hudson et al., 1998; Wisotzkey et al., 1998). The R-Smad/Co-Smad complex then translocates to the nucleus, where it modulates transcription (Liu et al., 1997a). The Co-Smads are not phosphorylated but rely on association with their partner R-Smad for translocation from the cytoplasm to the nucleus. Mutations in Smad4/DPC4 provided one of the first definite links of aberrations in this signaling pathway as causative for certain human cancers (Eppert et al., 1996).

I-Smads (Smad6 and Smad7) antagonize the activity of TGF-β superfamily proteins (Imamura et al., 1997; Nakao et al., 1997; Hayashi et al., 1997). In Drosophila, an inhibitory Smad, Daughters against Dpp (Dad), inhibits Mad signaling (Tsuneizumi et al., 1997). Both Smad6 and Smad7 bind to type I receptors of BMP and TGF-β but do not contain the SSXS phosphorylation sequence within the MH2 domain. As a result, they cannot be phosphorylated and released by the type I receptor, thereby interfering with phosphorylation of R-Smads. Smad6 also inhibits BMP signaling in a non-receptor-dependent way, by either competing with Smad4 for binding to receptor-activated Smad1 (Hata et al., 1998) or acting as a transcriptional corepressor (see DNA-Binding Cofactors). Consistent with a potential negative role for Smad6 in modulating BMP signaling, mice deficient for Smad6 exhibit ossification of the aorta, suggestive of excess BMP signaling (Galvin et al., 2000). While Smad6 can inhibit BMP signaling, its own activity is also inhibited by BMP receptor activation in a reciprocal fashion. The mediator of BMP-induced Smad6 inhibition is a cytoplasmic protein, associated molecule with the SH3 domain of STAM (AMSH), which binds directly to Smad6 (Itoh et al., 2001).

Negative Regulators of Smads

A number of regulatory mechanisms that attenuate TGF-β signaling by interference with nuclear accumulation of Smads have been identified. For example, phosphorylation of R-Smads within the spacer region between the MH1 and MH2 domains by Ras-activated Erk MAPKs causes cytoplasmic retention of R-Smads and, therefore, reduced availability of Smads for TGF-β signaling (Kretzschmar et al., 1999).

Another method of negative regulation is ubiquitination of R-Smads through association with the Smurf proteins. As described above for receptor turnover, ubiquitination of R-Smads can lead to degradation by the proteosome (Zhu et al., 1999; Lo and Massague, 1999).

Transcriptional Regulation of Downstream Genes

Since the binding of the MH1 domain to DNA is non-selective and of low affinity, Smads, upon entry into the nucleus, associate with DNA-binding cofactors that confer specificity on the interaction of Smads with DNA elements. Binding of the Smad/cofactor complex to the promoter recruits coactivators or corepressors that regulate transcription (Massagué and Wotton, 2000). In Drosophila, Mad may also bind directly to an enhancer within the vestigial wing-patterning gene and activate its transcription (Kim et al., 1997).

DNA-Binding Cofactors

The first Smad cofactor identified was the Forkhead activin signal transducer (FAST1), from Xenopus (Chen et al., 1996). This factor is a member of the winged helix family of DNA-binding proteins and was discovered in a search for transcription factors that bind to the Mix.2 activin responsive element (ARE). Mix.2 is an early response gene specific to the activin (nodal) pathway. After receptor activation and phosphorylation of Smad2, Smad2 activates Mix.2 transcription by forming a complex with FAST1 and Smad4 on the ARE (Chen et al., 1997b). Specific residues in both Fast1 and the MH2 domain of Smads 2 and 3 are required for complex formation. A murine homologue, FAST2, also forms a complex with Smad2 to induce the mouse *goosecoid* (*gsc*) promoter (Labbe et al., 1998). Smad3 competes with Smad2 for the binding site on Smad4 and thereby inhibits *gsc* transcription. In *Xenopus*, the homeodomain proteins Mixer and Milk can also recruit Smad2/4 complexes to specific promoters via interactions through a protein motif similar to the Smad binding domain of FAST1 (Germain et al., 2000).

In the TGF-β pathway, the plasminogen activator inhibitor-1 gene (*PAI-1*) requires the activity of transcription factors AP1 (c-Jun and c-Fos) and transcription factor E3 (TFE3). These factors cooperate with Smad3 and Smad4 to activate PAI-1 (Zhang et al., 1998; Hua et al., 1998; Wong et al., 1999). Additional activin and TGF-β responses in other tissues and at other times in development do not seem to involve any of these identified cofactors, suggesting that additional Smad-interacting proteins specific for these pathways remain to be discovered.

For the BMP pathway, several interacting DNA-binding cofactors have also been discovered. In *Xenopus*, the zinc finger transcription factor olfactory neuronal transcription factor 1/early B-cell factor (Olf-1/EBF) associated zinc finger (OAZ) forms complexes with Smad1 and Smad4 to regulate transcription of the BMP2-responsive gene *Xvent-2* (Hata et al., 2000), a transcription factor that controls mesoderm ventralization and suppresses neuralization. In mice, Hoxc-8 and Hoxa-9 bind to the osteopontin (OPN) promoter and repress its transcription. Smad proteins regulate the binding of Hox proteins to the OPN promoter at various levels. Smad6 interacts with Hoxc-8 and Hoxa-9 as a transcriptional corepressor (Bai et al., 2000). Smad1, however, displaces Hoxc-8 from its DNA-binding site, upregulating *OPN* gene expression (Shi et al., 1999). To counteract this effect, Smad6 forms a complex with Hoxc-8, which prevents the interaction between Smad1 and Hoxc-8. Smad3 binds directly to the OPN promoter, activating transcription of the gene, whereas Smad4 acts indirectly through displacement of Hoxa-9 from the DNA (Shi et al., 2001).

Smad-interacting protein 1 (SIP1) is a zinc finger protein which, in *Xenopus*, binds to the promoter of a target gene, *Brachyury*, acting as a transcriptional repressor (Verschueren et al., 1999). SIP1 binds directly to the MH2 domain of R-Smads and recruits them to the DNA. Mutations in human SIP1 result in Hirschsprung's disease (Wakamatsu et al., 2001). Other nuclear factors, such as the polyomavirus enhancer binding protein 2/core binding factor (PEBP2/CBF), bind to R-Smads and activate the Ig Cα promoter (Hanai et al., 1999). The α subunits of PEBP2/CBF contain a Runt domain and, hence, have been renamed the Runt-related transcription factors (Runx), which are essential for hematopoiesis and osteogenesis (Tsui and Noda, 2000). Runt-related gene 2 (*Runx2*) interacts with Smad1, and mutations in the human gene result in cleidocranial dysplasia (Zhang et al., 2000; see Chapter 29). A final Smad-interacting protein is Tob, an antiproliferation factor. In cell culture, Tob associates with BMP Smads and can block transcriptional activation of BMP-responsive promoters (Yoshida et al., 2000). It must be borne in mind, however, that even though these factors can bind to the BMP Smads, in most cases, the physiological significance of these interactions for BMP signaling in vivo during development has not been definitively demonstrated. In contrast, in *Drosophila*, the zinc finger factor Schnurri binds to Mad and appears to displace a negative regulator, Brinker, from various BMP-responsive genes, demonstrating a direct role for this factor in mediating BMP signals in vivo (Marty et al., 2000).

Coactivators

Although both R-Smads and Co-Smads can activate transcription primarily through sequences in their MH2 domains, this activity results, at least in part, from the ability of the MH2 domain to recruit the general transcriptional coactivators p300 and cAMP response element binding protein (CBP). The CBP/p300 proteins activate transcription by either recruiting other transcription factors or by exposing specific promoters via production of chromatin structure alterations through their histone acetylase activity (Janknecht et al., 1998; Pouponnot et al., 1998). One transcription factor that binds to CBP/p300 is melanocyte-specific gene 1 (MSG1) (Yahata et al., 2000). MSG1 is a nuclear protein that induces transcription but does not bind directly to

DNA. Its C-terminal domain binds to CBP/p300, thereby enhancing CBP/p300-mediated transcription. In addition, its N-terminal domain interacts with Smad proteins and further promotes the Smad–CBP/p300 interactions. In some cells, the interaction between CBP and Smad proteins can be inhibited by E1A protein (Topper et al., 1998) or Smad nuclear interacting protein 1 (SNIP1) (Kim et al., 2000).

Corepressors

Corepressors, including TGF-interacting factor (TGIF), c-Ski, and SnoN, interact with the MH2 domain of Smad2 and Smad3 in the TGF-β/activin pathway, whereas Hox proteins interact with both TGF-β and BMP signaling pathways.

TGIF is a DNA-binding homeodomain protein with two identifiable repression domains. One of the domains interacts with histone deacetylases (HDACs) (Wotton et al., 1999a,b). Deacetylation of histones by HDACs leads to chromatin condensation and decreased accessibility of transcriptional activators to their targets. Thus, the interaction of TGIF with HDACs accounts, at least in part, for the activity of TGIF as a transcriptional repressor. In humans, TGIF maps to 18p11.3, which is a minimal critical region for holoprosencephaly and appears to account for some cases of this abnormality (Gripp et al., 2000).

The nuclear oncoprotein Ski and a Ski-related protein, Sno, associate with Smads 2 and 3 in the basal state and repress transcription by recruiting transcriptional corepressors N-CoR and HDACs (Akiyoshi et al., 1999; Luo et al., 1999). While transcriptional repression by TGIF is induced by TGF-β, Ski/Sno proteins undergo degradation upon activation of TGF-β signaling, perhaps setting a threshold for the transcriptional response (Sun et al., 1999).

NON-SMAD SIGNALING PATHWAYS

A number of reports have suggested that TGF-β receptors can, in certain cellular contexts, signal via other pathways that may not involve Smad phosphorylation. The first of these to be reported was the activation of MAPK kinase kinase, known as Tak1, by both TGF-β and BMP ligands (Yamaguchi et al., 1995). Under normal conditions, activation of Tak1 in *Xenopus* leads to apoptosis; but if the apoptotic response is blocked by p35, then activated Tak1 can ventralize embryos, mimicking BMP signaling (Shibuya et al., 1998). In addition, kinase-deficient forms of TAK1 can partially block ectopic BMP signals. A potential direct link of Tak1 to BMP receptors has been uncovered through the two proteins Tak binding protein (Tab) and inhibitor of apoptosis (IAP) (Shibuya et al., 1998; Yamaguchi et al., 1999). Tab binds directly to TAK1 and is involved in activation, while IAP binds to BMP receptors and TAB. The primary function of this pathway might be to mediate the apoptotic response that BMP signals can generate in some tissues, such as the interdigit zone during appendage development or the death of inner mass cells during embryo cavitation. TGF-β signals have also been implicated in activating RhoA, phosphatidylinositol 3-kinase, and Jun kinase (Engel et al. 1999; Bakin et al. 2000; Bhowmick et al. 2001), although how and if activation of these pathways is directly coupled mechanistically to TGF-β receptor activation is unclear.

INTERACTION WITH OTHER PATHWAYS

Wingless (Wnt) Signaling Pathway

Activation of Wnt signaling results in accumulation of β-catenin, its nuclear translocation, binding to the transcription factors lymphoid enhancer binding factor/T-cell factor (LEF/TCF), and activation of target genes, e.g., *Xwnt* (Letamendia et al., 2001). However, TGF-β signaling may also activate *Xwnt* either synergistically with Wnt or even independently of Wnt. Either effect requires the binding of Smad3 and Smad4 to Smad binding elements (SBE) adjacent to LEF1/TCF binding sites (Labbe et al., 2000). The main mechanism that accounts for the synergism is a physical interaction between Smad proteins and LEF1/TCF. Smad4 may also be involved in Wnt signaling independently of TGF-β through the interaction with LEF1/TCF and β-catenin (Nishita et al., 2000).

MAPK Pathway

As mentioned earlier, Ras-activated Erk MAPKs limit the availability of Smad1 for BMP signaling through phosphorylation and cytoplasmic retention of Smad1 (Kretzschmar et al., 1999). At the same time, activation of the MAPK pathway by EGF and hepatocyte growth factor enhances phosphorylation of Smad2, having a positive effect on TGF-β signaling (de Caestecker et al., 1998).

Activin activates not only the Smad pathway but also p38 kinase, which results in phosphorylation of activating transcription factor 2 (ATF2) (Cocolakis et al., 2001).

The interaction between TGF-β and the MAPK pathway also occurs at the level of the TGF-β receptor (Blanchette et al., 2001). Binding of TGF-β1 to its receptor recruits not only Smads but also the p42/p44 MAPK pathway, which enhances nuclear translocation of Smad2 and transactivation of furin. Furin is a proprotein convertase, which cleaves latent precursor molecules such as TGF-βs into biologically active proteins. Therefore, activation of furin by TGF-β1 provides the means for autoregulation of TGF-β1 activity.

Vitamin D Signaling Pathway

Regulation of vitamin D receptor (VDR) activity by TGF-β is mediated through Smad proteins (Yanagi et al., 1999; Yanagisawa et al., 1999). Smad3 enhances transactivation of VDR, while Smad7 prevents the formation of Smad3/VDR complexes.

Cytokine Receptor Pathway

IFN-γ signals through JAK tyrosine kinase receptors, which activate the transcription factor STAT1 (Ulloa et al., 1999). Activation of the IFN-γ pathway inhibits TGF-β signaling through STAT-mediated induction of inhibitory Smad7. BMP and cytokine receptor pathways can also act synergistically to promote differentiation of fetal neural progenitors into astrocytes (Nakashima et al., 1999). In this case, the interaction between STATs and Smads is facilitated by coactivator p300, which binds to both proteins.

In summary, regulation of the TGF-β signaling pathway is remarkably complex and occurs at multiple levels within the signaling cascade. Since this pathway is highly evolutionarily conserved, study of its regulation in various model systems provides important insights into its potential regulation in humans. Throughout this chapter, we have provided numerous examples of diseases resulting from misregulation, although given the complexity that has been unveiled through the study of model organisms, it is likely that many additional pathogenic and congenital conditions will be linked to aberrations in this pathway in the future.

REFERENCES

Akiyoshi S, Inoue H, Hanai J, Kusanagi K, Nemoto N, Miyazono K, Kawabata M (1999). c-Ski acts as a transcriptional co-repressor in transforming growth factor-beta signaling through interaction with smads. J Biol Chem 274: 35269–35277.

Allard S, Adin P, Gouedard L, di Clemente N, Josso N, Orgebin-Crist MC, Picard JY, Xavier F (2000). Molecular mechanisms of hormone-mediated mullerian duct regression: involvement of beta-catenin. Development 127: 3349–3360.

Arora K, Levine M, O'Connor M (1994). The screw gene encodes a ubiquitously expressed member of the TGF-β family required for specification of dorsal cell fates in the Drosophila embryo. Genes Dev 8: 2588–2601.

Attisano L, Wrana JL, Montalvo E, Massague J (1996). Activation of signalling by the activin receptor complex. Mol Cell Biol 16: 1066–1073.

Bachiller D, Klingensmith J, Kemp C, Belo JA, Anderson RM, May SR, McMahon JA, McMahon AP, Harland RM, Rossant J, et al. (2000). The organizer factors Chordin and Noggin are required for mouse forebrain development. Nature 403: 658–661.

Bai S, Shi X, Yang X, Cao X (2000). Smad6 as a transcriptional corepressor. J Biol Chem 275: 8267–8270.

Bakin AV, Tomlinson AK, Bhowmick NA, Moses HL, Arteaga CL (2000). Phosphatidylinositol 3-kinase function is required for transforming growth factor beta–mediated epithelial to mesenchymal transition and cell migration. J Biol Chem 275: 36803–36810.

Belville C, Josso N, Picard JY (1999). Persistence of mullerian derivatives in males. Am J Med Genet 89: 218–223.

Bhowmick NA, Ghiassi M, Bakin A, Aakre M, Lundquist CA, Engel ME, Arteaga CL, Moses HL (2001). Transforming growth factor-beta1 mediates epithelial to mesenchymal transdifferentiation through a RhoA-dependent mechanism. Mol Biol Cell 12: 27–36.

Blanchette F, Rivard N, Rudd P, Grondin F, Attisano L, Dubois CM (2001). Cross-talk between the p42/p44 MAP kinase and Smad pathways in transforming growth factor β1-induced furin gene transactivation. J Biol Chem 276: 33986–33994.

Blobe GC, Schiemann WP, Lodish HF (2000). Role of transforming growth factor beta in human disease. N Engl J Med 342: 1350–1358.

Bouwmeester T, Kim S, Sasai Y, Lu B, De Robertis EM (1996). Cerberus is a head-inducing secreted factor expressed in the anterior endoderm of Spemann's organizer. Nature 382: 595–601.

Brummel T, Abdollah S, Haerry TE, Shimell MJ, Merriam J, Raftery L, Wrana JL, O'Connor MB (1999). The Drosophila activin receptor baboon signals through dSmad2 and controls cell proliferation but not patterning during larval development. Genes Dev 13: 98–111.

Brummel TJ, Twombly V, Marqués G, Wrana JL, Newfeld SJ, Attisano L, Massague J, O'Connor MB, Gelbart WM (1994). Characterization and relationship of Dpp receptors encoded by the saxophone and thick veins genes in Drosophila. Cell 78: 251–261.

Brunet LJ, McMahon JA, McMahon AP, Harland RM (1998). Noggin, cartilage morphogenesis, and joint formation in the mammalian skeleton. Science 280: 1455–1457.

Brunkow ME, Gardner JC, Van Ness J, Paeper BW, Kovacevich BR, Proll S, Skonier JE, Zhao L, Sabo PJ, Fu Y, et al. (2001). Bone dysplasia sclerosteosis results from loss of the SOST gene product, a novel cystine knot-containing protein. Am J Hum Genet 68: 577–589.

Chang C, Wilson PA, Mathews LS, Hemmati-Brivanlou A (1997). A Xenopus type I activin receptor mediates mesodermal but not neural specification during embryogenesis. Development 124: 827–837.

Chang H, Lau AL, Matzuk MM (2001a). Studying TGF-beta superfamily signaling by knockouts and knockins. Mol Cell Endocrinol 180: 39–46.

Chang C, Holtzman DA, Chau S, Chickering T, Woolf EA, Holmgren LM, Bodorova J, Gearing DP, Holmes WE, Brivanlou AH (2001b). Twisted gastrulation can function as a BMP antagonist. Nature 410: 483–487.

Charng MJ, Zhang D, Kinnunen P, Schneider MD (1998). A novel protein distinguishes between quiescent and activated forms of the type I transforming growth factor beta receptor. J Biol Chem 273: 9365–9368.

Chen RH, Miettinen PJ, Maruoka EM, Choy L, Derynck R (1995). A WD-domain protein that is associated with and phosphorylated by the type II TGF-beta receptor. Nature 377: 548–552.

Chen X, Rubock MJ, Whitman M (1996). A transcriptional partner for MAD proteins in TGF-beta signalling. Nature 383: 691–696.

Chen YG, Liu F, Massague J (1997a). Mechanism of TGFbeta receptor inhibition by FKBP12. EMBO J 16: 3866–3876.

Chen X, Weisberg E, Fridmacher V, Watanabe M, Naco G, Whitman M (1997b). Smad4 and FAST-1 in the assembly of activin-responsive factor. Nature 389: 85–89.

Cocolakis E, Lemay S, Ali S, Lebrun JJ (2001). The p38 MAPK pathway is required for cell growth inhibition of human breast cancer cells in response to activin. J Biol Chem 276: 18430–18436.

Colavita A, Krishna S, Zheng H, Padgett RW, Culotti JG (1998). Pioneer axon guidance by UNC-129, a C. elegans TGF-beta. Science 281: 706–709.

Constam DB, Robertson EJ (1999). Regulation of bone morphogenetic protein activity by pro domains and proprotein convertases. J Cell Biol 144: 139–149.

Crawford SE, Stellmach V, Murphy-Ullrich JE, Ribeiro SM, Lawler J, Hynes RO, Boivin GP, Bouck N (1998). Thrombospondin-1 is a major activator of TGF-beta1 in vivo. Cell 93: 1159–1170.

Dabovic B, Chen Y, Colarossi C, Obata H, Zambuto L, Perle MA, Rifkin DB (2002). Bone abnormalities in latent TGFβ binding protein (Ltbp)-3-null mice indicate a role for Ltbp-3 in modulating TGFβ bioavailability. J Cell Biol 156: 227–232.

Datta PK, Chytil A, Gorska AE, Moses HL (1998). Identification of STRAP, a novel WD domain protein in transforming growth factor-beta signaling. J Biol Chem 273: 34671–34674.

de Caestecker MP, Parks WT, Frank CJ, Castagnino P, Bottaro DP, Roberts AB, Lechleider RJ (1998). Smad2 transduces common signals from receptor serine-threonine and tyrosine kinases. Genes Dev 12: 1587–1592.

Deng Z, Morse JH, Slager SL, Cuervo N, Moore KJ, Venetos G, Kalachikov S, Cayanis E, Fischer SG, Barst RJ, et al. (2000). Familial primary pulmonary hypertension (gene PPH1) is caused by mutations in the bone morphogenetic protein receptor-II gene. Am J Hum Genet 67: 737–744.

De Robertis EM, Sasai Y (1996). A common plan for dorsoventral patterning in bilateria. Nature 380: 37–40.

De Robertis EM, Larrain J, Oelgeschlager M, Wessely O (2000). The establishment of Spemann's organizer and patterning of the vertebrate embryo. Nat Rev Genet 1: 171–181.

Derynck R, Gelbart WM, Harland RM, Heldin CH, Kern SE, Massague J, Melton DA, Mlodzik M, Padgett RW, Roberts AB, et al. (1996). Nomenclature: vertebrate mediators of TGFbeta family. Cell 87: 173.

de Winter JP, ten Dijke P, de Vries CJ, van Achterberg TA, Sugino H, de Waele P, Huylebroeck D, Verschueren K, van den Eijnden-van Raaij AJ (1996). Follistatins neutralize activin bioactivity by inhibition of activin binding to its type II receptors. Mol Cell Endocrinol 116: 105–114.

di Clemente N, Wilson C, Faure E, Boussin L, Carmillo P, Tizard R, Picard JY, Vigier B, Josso N, Cate R (1994). Cloning, expression, and alternative splicing of the receptor for anti-mullerian hormone. Mol Endocrinol 8: 1006–1020.

Dunn NR, Winnier GE, Hargett LK, Schrick JJ, Fogo AB, Hogan BLM (1997). Haploinsufficient phenotypes in Bmp4 heterozygous null mice and modification by mutations in Gli3 and Alx4. Dev Biol 188: 235–247.

Durbec P, Marcos-Gutierrez CV, Kilkenny C, Grigoriou M, Wartiowaara K, Suvanto P, Smith D, Ponder B, Costantini F, Saarma M, et al. (1996). GDNF signalling through the Ret receptor tyrosine kinase. Nature 81: 789–793.

Ebisawa T, Fukuchi M, Murakami G, Chiba T, Tanaka K, Imamura T, Miyazono K (2001). Smurf1 interacts with transforming growth factor-beta type I receptor through Smad7 and induces receptor degradation. J Biol Chem 276: 12477–12480.

Engel ME, McDonnell MA, Law BK, Moses HL (1999). Interdependent SMAD and JNK signaling in transforming growth factor-beta–mediated transcription. J Biol Chem 274: 37413–37420.

Eppert K, Scherer SW, Ozcelik H, Pirone R, Hoodless P, Kim H, Tsui LC, Bapat B, Gallinger S, Andrulis IL, et al. (1996). MADR2 maps to 18q21 and encodes a TGFbeta-regulated MAD-related protein that is functionally mutated in colorectal carcinoma. *Cell* 86: 543–552.

Ethier JF, Findlay JK (2001). Roles of activin and its signal transduction mechanisms in reproductive tissues. *Reproduction* 121: 667–675.

Feng XH, Derynck R (1997). A kinase subdomain of transforming growth factor-beta (TGF-beta) type I receptor determines the TGF-beta intracellular signaling specificity. *EMBO J* 16: 3912–3923.

Galvin KM, Donovan MJ, Lynch CA, Meyer RI, Paul RJ, Lorenz JN, Fairchild-Huntress V, Dixon KL, Dunmore JH, Gimbrone MA Jr, et al. (2000). A role for smad6 in development and homeostasis of the cardiovascular system. *Nat Genet* 24: 171–174.

Garamszegi N, Dore JJ Jr, Penheiter SG, Edens M, Yao D, Leof EB (2001). Transforming growth factor beta receptor signaling and endocytosis are linked through a COOH terminal activation motif in the type I receptor. *Mol Biol Cell* 12: 2881–2893.

Germain S, Howell M, Esslemont GM, Hill CS (2000). Homeodomain and winged-helix transcription factors recruit activated Smads to distinct promoter elements via a common Smad interaction. *Genes Dev* 14: 435–451.

Gilboa L, Nohe A, Geissendorfer T, Sebald W, Henis YI, Knaus P (2000). Bone morphogenetic protein receptor complexes on the surface of live cells: a new oligomerization mode for serine/threonine kinase receptors. *Mol Biol Cell* 11: 1023–1035.

Gong Y, Krakow D, Marcelino J, Wilkin D, Chitayat D, Babul-Hirji R, Hudgins L, Cremers CW, Cremers FP, Brunner HG, et al. (1999). Heterozygous mutations in the gene encoding noggin affect human joint morphogenesis. *Nat Genet* 21: 302–304.

Gripp KW, Wotton D, Edwards MC, Roessler E, Ades L, Meinecke P, Richieri-Costa A, Zackai EH, Massague J, Muenke M, et al. (2000). Mutations in TGIF cause holoprosencephaly and link NODAL signalling to human neural axis determination. *Nat Genet* 25: 205–208.

Gualandris A, Annes JP, Arese M, Noguera I, Jurukovski V, Rifkin DB (2000). The latent transforming growth factor-beta-binding protein-1 promotes in vitro differentiation of embryonic stem cells into endothelium. *Mol Biol Cell* 11: 4295–4308.

Gunther CV, Georgi LL, Riddle DL (2000). A *Caenorhabditis elegans* type I TGF beta receptor can function in the absence of type II kinase to promote larval development. *Development* 127: 3337–3347.

Haerry TE, Khalsa O, O'Connor MB, Wharton KA (1998). Synergistic signaling by two BMP ligands through the SAX and TKV receptors controls wing growth and patterning in *Drosophila*. *Development* 125: 3977–3987.

Hanai J, Chen LF, Kanno T, Ohtani-Fujita N, Kim WY, Guo WH, Imamura T, Ishidou Y, Fukuchi M, Shi MJ, et al. (1999). Interaction and functional cooperation of PEBP2/CBF with Smads. Synergistic induction of the immunoglobulin germline Calpha promoter. *J Biol Chem* 274: 31577–31582.

Hata A, Lagna G, Massague J, Hemmati-Brivanlou A (1998). Smad6 inhibits BMP/Smad1 signaling by specifically competing with the Smad4 tumor suppressor. *Genes Dev* 12: 186–197.

Hata A, Seoane J, Lagna G, Montalvo E, Hemmati-Brivanlou A, Massague J (2000). OAZ uses distinct DNA- and protein-binding zinc fingers in separate BMP-Smad and Olf signaling pathways. *Cell* 100: 229–240.

Hayashi H, Abdollah S, Qiu Y, Cai J, Xu YY, Grinnell BW, Richardson MA, Topper JN, Gimbrone MA Jr, Wrana JL, et al. (1997). The MAD-related protein Smad7 associates with the TGFbeta receptor and functions as an antagonist of TGFbeta signaling. *Cell* 89: 1165–1173.

Hogan BLM (1996). Bone morphogenetic proteins: multifunctional regulators of vertebrate development. *Genes Dev* 10: 1580–1594.

Hoodless PA, Haerry T, Abdollah S, Stapleton M, O'Connor MB, Attisano L, Wrana JL (1996). MADR1, a MAD-related protein that functions in BMP2 signaling pathways. *Cell* 85: 489–500.

Hua X, Liu X, Ansari DO, Lodish HF (1998). Synergistic cooperation of TFE3 and smad proteins in TGF-beta-induced transcription of the plasminogen activator inhibitor-1 gene. *Genes Dev* 12: 3084–3095.

Hudson JB, Podos SD, Keith K, Simpson SL, Ferguson EL (1998). The *Drosophila Medea* gene is required downstream of dpp and encodes a functional homolog of human Smad4. *Development* 125: 1407–1420.

Iemura S, Yamamoto TS, Takagi C, Uchiyama H, Natsume T, Shimasaki S, Sugino H, Ueno N (1998). Direct binding of follistatin to a complex of bone-morphogenetic protein and its receptor inhibits ventral and epidermal cell fates in early *Xenopus* embryo. *Proc Natl Acad Sci USA* 95: 9337–9342.

Imamura T, Takase M, Nishihara A, Oeda E, Hanai J, Kawabata M, Miyazono K (1997). Smad6 inhibits signalling by the TGF-beta superfamily. *Nature* 389: 622–626.

Ingraham HA, Hirokawa Y, Roberts LM, Mellon SH, McGee E, Nachtigal MW, Visser JA (2000). Autocrine and paracrine mullerian inhibiting substance hormone signaling in reproduction. *Recent Prog Horm Res* 55: 53–67.

Israel DI, Nove J, Kerns KM, Kaufman RJ, Rosen V, Cox KA, Wozney JM (1996). Heterodimeric bone morphogenetic proteins show enhanced activity in vitro and in vivo. *Growth Factors* 13: 291–300.

Itoh F, Asao H, Sugamura K, Heldin CH, ten Dijke P, Itoh S (2001). Promoting bone morphogenetic protein signaling through negative regulation of inhibitory Smads. *EMBO J* 20: 4132–4142.

Itoh S, Itoh F, Goumans MJ, Ten Dijke P (2000). Signaling of transforming growth factor-beta family members through Smad proteins. *Eur J Biochem* 267: 6954–6967.

Jackson SM, Nakato H, Sugiura M, Jannuzi A, Oakes R, Kaluza V, Golden C, Selleck SB (1997). Dally, a *Drosophila* glypican, controls cellular responses to the TGF-beta-related morphogen, Dpp. *Development* 124: 4113–4120.

Janknecht R, Wells NJ, Hunter T (1998). TGF-beta-stimulated cooperation of smad proteins with the coactivators CBP/p300. *Genes Dev* 12: 2114–2119.

Joubin K, Stern CD (2001). Formation and maintenance of the organizer among the vertebrates. *Int J Dev Biol* 45: 165–175.

Katagiri T, Boorla S, Frendo J-L, Hogan BLM, Karsenty G (1998). Skeletal abnormalities in doubly heterozygous Bmp4 and Bmp7 mice. *Dev Genet* 22: 340–348.

Khalsa O, Yoon JW, Torres-Schumann S, Wharton KA (1998). TGF-beta/BMP superfamily members, Gbb-60A and Dpp, cooperate to provide pattern information and establish cell identity in the *Drosophila* wing. *Development* 125: 2723–2734.

Kim J, Johnson K, Chen HJ, Carroll S, Laughon A (1997). *Drosophila* Mad binds to DNA and directly mediates activation of vestigial by Decapentaplegic. *Nature* 388: 304–308.

Kim RH, Wang D, Tsang M, Martin J, Huff C, de Caestecker MP, Parks WT, Meng X, Lechleider RJ, Wang T, et al. (2000). A novel smad nuclear interacting protein, SNIP1, suppresses p300-dependent TGF-beta signal transduction. *Genes Dev* 14: 1605–1616.

Knight PG, Glister C (2001). Potential local regulatory functions of inhibins, activins and follistatin in the ovary. *Reproduction* 121: 503–512.

Koenig BB, Cook JS, Wolsing DH, Ting J, Tiesman JP, Correa PE, Olson CA, Pecquet AL, Ventura F, Grant RA (1994). Characterization and cloning of a receptor for BMP-2 and BMP-4 from NIH 3T3 cells. *Mol Cell Biol* 14: 5961–5974.

Kretzschmar M, Liu F. Hata A, Doody J, Massague J (1997). The TGF-beta family mediator Smad1 is phosphorylated directly and activated functionally by the BMP receptor kinase. *Genes Dev* 11: 984–995.

Kretzschmar M, Doody J, Timokhina I, Massague J (1999). A mechanism of repression of TGFbeta/Smad signaling by oncogenic Ras. *Genes Dev* 13: 804–816.

Labbe E, Silvestri C, Hoodless PA, Wrana JL, Attisano L (1998). Smad2 and Smad3 positively and negatively regulate TGF beta-dependent transcription through the forkhead DNA-binding protein FAST2. *Mol Cells* 2: 109–120.

Labbe E, Letamendia A, Attisano L (2000). Association of Smads with lymphoid enhancer binding factor 1/T cell-specific factor mediates cooperative signaling by the transforming growth factor-beta and wnt pathways. *Proc Natl Acad Sci USA* 97: 8358–8363.

Lagna G, Hata A, Hemmati-Brivanlou A, Massague J (1996). Partnership between DPC4 and SMAD proteins in TGF-beta signalling pathways. *Nature* 383: 832–836.

Lane KB, Machado RD, Pauciulo MW, Thomson JR, Phillips JA 3rd, Loyd JE, Nichols WC, Trembath RC (2000). Heterozygous germline mutations in BMPR2, encoding a TGF-beta receptor, cause familial primary pulmonary hypertension. The International PPH Consortium. *Nat Genet* 26: 81–84.

Lau AL, Kumar TR, Nishimori K, Bonadio J, Matzuk MM (2000). *Activin betaC* and *betaE* genes are not essential for mouse liver growth, differentiation, and regeneration. *Mol Cell Biol* 20: 6127–6137.

Lee SJ, McPherron AC (2001). Regulation of myostatin activity and muscle growth. *Proc Natl Acad Sci USA* 98: 9306–9311.

Letamendia A, Labbe E, Attisano L (2001). Transcriptional regulation by Smads: crosstalk between the TGF-beta and Wnt pathways. *J Bone Joint Surg Am* 83(Suppl 1, Pt 1): S31–S39.

Letsou A, Arora K, Wrana JL, Simin K, Twombly V, Jamal J, Staehling-Hampton K, Hoffmann FM, Gelbart WM, Massague J (1995). *Drosophila* Dpp signaling is mediated by the *punt* gene product: a dual ligand-binding type II receptor of the TGF beta receptor family. *Cell* 80: 899–908.

Lewis KA, Gray PC, Blount AL, MacConell LA, Wiater E, Bilezikjian LM, Vale W (2000). Betaglycan binds inhibin and can mediate functional antagonism of activin signalling. *Nature* 404: 411–414.

Lidral AC, Romitti PA, Basart AM, Doetschman T, Leysens NJ, Daack-Hirsch S, Semina EV, Johnson LR, Machida J, Burds A, et al. (1998). Association of MSX1 and TGFB3 with nonsyndromic clefting in humans. *Am J Hum Genet* 63: 557–568.

Lin HY, Wang XF, Ng-Eaton E, Weinberg RA, Lodish HF (1992). Expression cloning of the TGF-beta type II receptor, a functional transmembrane serine/threonine kinase. *Cell* 68: 775–785.

Ling N, Ying SY, Ueno N, Shimasaki S, Esch F, Hotta M, Guillemin R (1986). Pituitary FSH is released by a heterodimer of the beta-subunits from the two forms of inhibin. *Nature* 321: 779–782.

Liu F, Ventura F, Doody J, Massague J (1995). Human type II receptor for bone morphogenic proteins (BMPs): extension of the two-kinase receptor model to the BMPs. *Mol Cell Biol* 15: 3479–3486.

Liu F, Pouponnot C, Massague J (1997a). Dual role of the Smad4/DPC4 tumor suppressor in TGFbeta-inducible transcriptional complexes. *Genes Dev* 11: 3157–3167.

Liu X, Sun Y, Constantinescu SN, Karam E, Weinberg RA, Lodish HF (1997b). Transforming growth factor beta–induced phosphorylation of Smad3 is required for growth inhibition and transcriptional induction in epithelial cells. *Proc Natl Acad Sci USA* 94: 10669–10674.

Lo RS, Massague J (1999). Ubiquitin-dependent degradation of TGF-beta-activated Smad2. *Nat Cell Biol* 1: 472–478.

Lopez-Casillas F, Wrana JL, Massague J (1993). Betaglycan presents ligand to the TGF beta signaling receptor. *Cell* 73: 1435–1444.

Lopez-Casillas F, Payne HM, Andres JL, Massague J. (1994). Betaglycan can act as a dual modulator of TGF-beta access to signaling receptors: mapping of ligand binding and GAG attachment *J Cell Biol* 124: 557–568.

Luo K, Stroschein SL, Wang W, Chen D, Martens E, Zhou S, Zhou Q (1999). The Ski oncoprotein interacts with the Smad proteins to repress TGFbeta signaling. *Genes Dev* 13: 2196–2206.

Macias-Silva M, Abdollah S, Hoodless PA, Pirone R, Attisano L, Wrana JL (1996). MADR2 is a substrate of the TGFbeta receptor and its phosphorylation is required for nuclear accumulation and signaling. *Cell* 87: 1215–1224.

Marqués G, Musacchio M, Shimell MJ, Wünnenberg-Stapleton K, Cho KWY, O'Connor MB (1997). Production of a Dpp activity gradient in the early *Drosophila* embryo through the opposing actions of the Sog and Tld proteins. *Cell* 91: 463–473.

Marty T, Muller B, Basler K, Affolter M (2000). Schnurri mediates Dpp-dependent repression of brinker transcription. *Nat Cell Biol* 2: 745–749.

Massagué J (1998). TGF-β signal transduction. *Annu Rev Biochem* 67: 753–791.

Massagué J, Chen, Y-G (2000). Controlling TGF-β signaling. *Genes Dev* 14: 627–644.

Massagué J, Wotton D (2000). Transcription control by the TGf-β/Smad signaling system. *EMBO J* 19: 1745–1754.

Mathews LS, Vale WW (1991). Expression cloning of an activin receptor, a predicted transmembrane serine kinase. *Cell* 65: 973–982.

Mathews LS, Vale WW, Kintner CR (1992). Cloning of a second type of activin receptor and functional characterization in *Xenopus* embryos. *Science* 255: 1702–1705.

Matzuk MM, Finegold MJ, Su JG, Hsueh AJ, Bradley A (1992). *Alpha-inhibin* is a tumour-suppressor gene with gonadal specificity in mice. *Nature* 360: 313–319.
Matzuk MM, Kumar TR, Shou W, Coerver KA, Lau A, Behringer RR, Finegold MJ (1996). Transgenic models to study the roles of inhibins and activins in reproduction, oncogenesis, and development. *Recent Prog Horm Res* 51: 123–154.
McAllister KA, Grogg KM, Johnson DW, Gallione CJ, Baldwin MA, Jackson CE, Helmbold EA, Markel DS, McKinnon WC, Murrell J (1994). Endoglin, a TGF-beta binding protein of endothelial cells, is the gene for hereditary haemorrhagic telangiectasia type 1. *Nat Genet* 8: 345–351.
Meno C, Saijoh Y, Fujii H, Ikeda M, Yokoyama T, Yokoyama M, Toyoda Y, Hamada H (1996). Left–right asymmetric expression of the TGF beta-family member lefty in mouse. *Nature* 381: 151–155.
Miyazono K, Olofsson A, Colosetti P, Heldin CH (1991). A role of the latent TGF-beta 1-binding protein in the assembly and secretion of TGF-beta 1. *EMBO J* 10: 1091–1101.
Nakao A, Afrakhte M, Moren A, Nakayama T, Christian JL, Heuchel R, Itoh S, Kawabata M, Heldin NE, Heldin CH, et al. (1997). Identification of Smad7, a TGFbeta-inducible antagonist of TGF-beta signalling. *Nature* 389: 631–635.
Nakashima K, Yanagisawa M, Arakawa H, Kimura N, Hisatsune T, Kawabata M, Miyazono K, Taga T (1999). Synergistic signaling in fetal brain by STAT3-Smad1 complex bridged by p300. *Science* 284: 479–482.
Neul JL, Ferguson EL (1998). Spatially restricted activation of the SAX receptor by SCW modulates DPP/TKV signaling in *Drosophila* dorsal–ventral patterning. *Cell* 95: 483–494.
Newfeld SJ, Wisotzkey RG, Kumar S (1999). Molecular evolution of a developmental pathway: phylogenetic analyses of TGF-β family ligands, receptors and Smad signal transducers. *Genetics* 152: 783–795.
Nguyen M, Park S, Marques G, Arora K (1998). Interpretation of a BMP activity gradient in *Drosophila* embryos depends on synergistic signaling by two type I receptors, SAX and TKV. *Cell* 95: 495–506.
Nishita M, Hashimoto MK, Ogata S, Laurent MN, Ueno N, Shibuya H, Cho KW (2000). Interaction between Wnt and TGF-beta signalling pathways during formation of Spemann's organizer. *Nature* 403: 781–785.
Oelgeschläger M, Larrain J, Geissert D, De Robertis EM (2000). The evolutionarily conserved BMP-binding protein Twisted gastrulation promotes BMP signalling. *Nature* 405: 757–763.
Oh SP, Seki T, Goss KA, Imamura T, Yi Y, Donahoe PK, Li L, Miyazono K, ten Dijke P, Kim S, et al. (2000). Activin receptor-like kinase 1 modulates transforming growth factor-beta 1 signaling in the regulation of angiogenesis. *Proc Natl Acad Sci USA* 97: 2626–2631.
Oklu R, Hesketh R (2000). The latent transforming growth factor beta binding protein (LTBP) family. *Biochem J* 352: 601–610.
Onichtchouk D, Chen YG, Dosch R, Gawantka V, Delius H, Massague J, Niehrs C (1999). Silencing of TGF-beta signalling by the pseudoreceptor BAMBI. *Nature* 401: 480–485.
Ozaki T, Nakamura Y, Enomoto H, Hirose M, Sakiyama S (1995). Overexpression of *DAN* gene product in normal rat fibroblasts causes a retardation of the entry into the S phase. *Cancer Res* 55: 895–900.
Padgett RW, Wozney JM, Gelbart WM (1994). Human BMP sequences can confer normal dorsal–ventral patterning in the *Drosophila* embryo. *Proc Natl Acad Sci USA* 90: 2905–2906.
Patterson GI, Padgett RW (2000). TGF beta–related pathways. Roles in *Caenorhabditis elegans* development. *Trends Genet* 16: 27–33.
Pearce JJ, Penny G, Rossant J (1999). A mouse *cerberus/DAN-related*•gene family. *Dev Biol* 209: 98–110.
Piccolo S, Sasai Y, Lu B, De Robertis EM (1996). Dorsoventral patterning in *Xenopus*: inhibition of ventral signals by direct binding of chordin to BMP-4. *Cell* 86: 589–598.
Piccolo S, Agius E, Lu B, Goodman S, Dale L, De Robertis EM (1997). Cleavage of Chordin by Xolloid metalloprotease suggests a role for proteolytic processing in the regulation of Spemann organizer activity. *Cell* 91: 407–416.
Piccolo S, Agius E, Leyns L, Bhattacharyya S, Grunz H, Bouwmeester T, De Robertis EM (1999). The head inducer Cerberus is a multifunctional antagonist of Nodal, BMP and Wnt signals. *Nature* 397: 707–710.
Podos SD, Hanson KK, Wang YC, Ferguson EL (2001). The DSmurf ubiquitin-protein ligase restricts BMP signaling spatially and temporally during *Drosophila*. *Dev Cell* 1: 567–578.
Pouponnot C, Jayaraman L, Massague J (1998). Physical and functional interaction of SMADs and p300/CBP. *J Biol Chem* 273: 22865–22868.
Raftery LA, Sutherland DJ (1999). TGF-β family signal transduction in *Drosophila* development: from Mad to Smads. *Dev Biol* 210: 251–268.
Raftery LA, Twombly V, Wharton K, Gelbart WM (1995). Genetic screens to identify elements of the decapentaplegic signaling pathway in *Drosophila*. *Genetics* 139: 241–254.
Rifkin DB, Gleizes PE, Harpel J, Nunes I, Munger J, Mazzieri R, Noguera I (1997). Plasminogen/plasminogen activator and growth factor activation. *Ciba Found Symp* 212: 105–115.
Roberts AB, Anzano MA, Lamb LC, Smith JM, Sporn MB (1981). New class of transforming growth factors potentiated by epidermal growth factor: isolation from non-neoplastic tissues. *Proc Natl Acad Sci USA* 78: 5339–5343.
Ross JJ, Shimmi O, Vilmos P, Petryk A, Kim H, Gaudenz K, Hermanson S, Ekker SC, O'Connor MB, Marsh JL (2001). Twisted gastrulation is a conserved extracellular BMP antagonist. *Nature* 410: 479–483.
Ryden M, Imamura T, Jornvall H, Belluardo N, Neveu I, Trupp M, Okadome T, ten Dijke P, Ibanez CF (1996). A novel type I receptor serine-threonine kinase predominantly expressed in the adult central nervous system. *J Biol Chem* 271: 30603–30609.
Sanford LP, Ormsby I, Gittenberger-de Groot AC, Sariola H, Friedman R, Boivin GP, Cardell EL, Doetschman T (1997). TGFbeta2 knockout mice have multiple developmental defects that are non-overlapping with other TGFbeta knockout phenotypes. *Development* 124: 2659–2670.
Savage C, Das P, Finelli AL, Townsend SR, Sun CY, Baird SE, Padgett RW (1996). *Caenorhabditis elegans* genes sma-2, sma-3, and sma-4 define a conserved family of transforming growth factor beta pathway components. *Proc Natl Acad Sci USA* 93: 790–794.
Schier AF, Shen MM (2000). Nodal signalling in vertebrate development. *Nature* 403: 385–389.
Scott IC, Blitz IL, Pappano WN, Maas SA, Cho KWY, Greenspan DS (2001). Homologues of Twisted gastrulation are extracellular cofactors in antagonism of BMP signalling. *Nature* 410: 475–478.
Sekelsky JJ, Newfeld SJ, Raftery LA, Chartoff EH, Gelbart WM (1995). Genetic characterization and cloning of *mothers against dpp*, a gene required for decapentaplegic function in *Drosophila* melanogaster. *Genetics* 139: 1347–1358.
Shawlot W, Min Deng J, Wakamiya M, Behringer RR (2000). The *cerberus-related* gene, *Cerr1*, is not essential for mouse head formation. *Genesis* 26: 253–258.
Shi X, Yang X, Chen D, Chang Z, Cao X (1999). Smad1 interacts with homeobox DNA-binding proteins in bone morphogenetic protein signaling. *J Biol Chem* 274: 13711–13717.
Shi X, Bai S, Li L, Cao X (2001). Hoxa-9 represses transforming growth factor-beta-induced osteopontin gene transcription. *J Biol Chem* 276: 850–855.
Shi Y, Hata A, Lo RS, Massague J, Pavletich NP (1997). A structural basis for mutational inactivation of the tumour suppressor Smad4. *Nature* 388: 87–93.
Shi Y, Wang YF, Jayaraman L, Yang H, Massague J, Pavletich NP (1998). Crystal structure of a Smad MH1 domain bound to DNA: insights on DNA binding in TGF-beta signaling. *Cell* 94: 585–594.
Shibuya H, Iwata H, Masuyama N, Gotoh Y, Yamaguchi K, Irie K, Matsumoto K, Nishida E, Ueno N (1998). Role of TAK1 and TAB1 in BMP signaling in early *Xenopus* development. *EMBO J* 17: 1019–1028.
Shou W, Aghdasi B, Armstrong DL, Guo Q, Bao S, Charng MJ, Mathews LM, Schneider MD, Hamilton SL, Matzuk MM (1998). Cardiac defects and altered ryanodine receptor function in mice lacking FKBP12. *Nature* 391: 489–492.
Storm EE, Huynh TV, Copeland NG, Jenkins NA, Kingsley DM, Lee S-J (1994). Limb alterations in brachypodism mice due to mutations in a new member of the TGFβ-superfamily. *Nature* 368: 639–643.
Sun PD, Davies DR (1995). The cystine-knot growth-factor superfamily. *Annu Rev Biophys Biomol Struct* 24: 269–291.
Sun Y, Liu X, Ng-Eaton E, Lodish HF, Weinberg RA (1999). SnoN and Ski protooncoproteins are rapidly degraded in response to transforming growth factor beta signaling. *Proc Natl Acad Sci* USA 96: 12442–12447.
Thisse C, Thisse B (1999). Antivin, a novel and divergent member of the TGFbeta superfamily, negatively regulates mesoderm induction. *Development* 126: 229–240.
Thomas JT, Kilpatrick MW, Lin K, Erlacher L, Lembessis P, Costa T, Tsipouras P, Luyten FP (1997). Disruption of human limb morphogenesis by a dominant negative mutation in the CDMP1. *Nat Genet* 17: 58–64.
Topol LZ, Modi WS, Koochekpour S, Blair DG (2000). *DRM/GREMLIN* (*CKTSF1B1*) maps to human chromosome 15 and is highly expressed in adult and fetal brain. *Cytogenet Cell Genet* 89: 79–84.
Topper JN, DiChiara MR, Brown JD, Williams AJ, Falb D, Collins T, Gimbrone MA Jr (1998). CREB binding protein is a required coactivator for Smad-dependent, transforming growth factor beta transcriptional responses in endothelial cells. *Proc Natl Acad Sci USA* 95: 9506–9511.
Tsui K, Noda M (2000). Identification and expression of mouse *Runx1/Pebp2alphaB/Cbfa2/AML1* gene. *Biochem Biophys Res Commun* 274: 171–176.
Tsukazaki T, Chiang TA, Davison AF, Attisano L, Wrana JL (1998). SARA, a FYVE domain protein that recruits Smad2 to the TGFbeta receptor. *Cell* 95: 779–791.
Tsuneizumi K, Nakayama T, Kamoshida Y, Kornberg TB, Christian JL, Tabata T (1997). Daughters against dpp modulates dpp organizing activity in *Drosophila* wing development. *Nature* 389: 627–631.
Ulloa L, Doody J, Massague J (1999). Inhibition of transforming growth factor-beta/SMAD signalling by the interferon-gamma/STAT pathway. *Nature* 397: 710–713.
Ulloa L, Creemers JW, Roy S, Liu S, Mason J, Tabibzadeh S (2001). Lefty proteins exhibit unique processing and activate the MAPK pathway. *J Biol Chem* 276: 21387–21396.
Urist MR (1965). Bone formation by autoinduction. *Science* 150: 893–899.
Verschueren K, Remacle JE, Collart C, Kraft H, Baker BS, Tylzanowski P, Nelles L, Wuytens G, Su MT, Bodmer R, et al. (1999). SIP1, a novel zin finger/homeodomain repressor, interacts with Smad proteins and binds to 5′-CACCT sequences in candidate target genes. *J Biol Chem* 274: 20489–20498.
Wakamatsu N, Yamada Y, Yamada K, Ono T, Nomura N, Taniguchi H, Kitoh H, Mutoh N, Yamanaka T, Mushiake K, et al. (2001). Mutations in SIP1, encoding Smad interacting protein-1, cause a form of Hirschsprung disease. *Nat Genet* 27: 369–370.
Whitman M (2001). Nodal signaling in early vertebrate embryos: themes and variations. *Dev Cell* 1: 605–617.
Whitman M, Mercola M (2001). TGF-β superfamily signaling and left–right asymmetry. *Sci STKE* Jan 9(64): RE1.
Winnier G, Blessing M, Labosky PA, Hogan BL (1995). Bone morphogenetic protein-4 is required for mesoderm formation and patterning in the mouse. *Genes Dev* 9: 2105–2116.
Wisotzkey RG, Mehra A, Sutherland DJ, Dobens LL, Liu X, Dohrmann C, Attisano L, Raftery LA (1998). Medea is a *Drosophila* Smad4 homolog that is differentially required to potentiate DPP responses. *Development* 125: 1433–1445.
Wong C, Rougier-Chapman EM, Frederick JP, Datto MB, Liberati NT, Li JM, Wang XF (1999). Smad3-Smad4 and AP-1 complexes synergize in transcriptional activation of the c-Jun promoter by transforming growth factor beta. *Mol Cell Biol* 19: 1821–1830.
Wotton D, Lo RS, Lee S, Massague J (1999a). A Smad transcriptional corepressor. *Cell* 97: 29–39.
Wotton D, Lo RS, Swaby LA, Massague J (1999b). Multiple modes of repression by the Smad transcriptional corepressor TGIF. *J Biol Chem* 274: 37105–37110.
Wrana JL, Attisano L, Wieser R, Ventura F, Massague J (1994). Mechanism of activation of the TGF-beta receptor. *Nature* 370: 341–347.

Xu J, McKeehan K, Matsuzaki K, McKeehan WL (1995). Inhibin antagonizes inhibition of liver cell growth by activin by a dominant-negative mechanism. *J Biol Chem* 270: 6308–6313.

Yahata T, de Caestecker MP, Lechleider RJ, Andriole S, Roberts AB, Isselbacher KJ, Shioda T (2000). The MSG1 non-DNA-binding transactivator binds to the p300/CBP coactivators, enhancing their functional link to the Smad transcription factors. *J Biol Chem* 275: 8825–8834.

Yamaguchi K, Shirakabe K, Shibuya H, Irie K, Oishi I, Ueno N, Taniguchi T, Nishida E, Matsumoto K (1995). Identification of a member of the MAPKKK family as a potential mediator of TGF-beta signal transduction. *Science* 270: 2008–2011.

Yamaguchi K, Nagai S, Ninomiya-Tsuji J, Nishita M, Tamai K, Irie K, Ueno N, Nishida E, Shibuya H, Matsumoto K (1999). XIAP, a cellular member of the inhibitor of apoptosis protein family, links the receptors to TAB1-TAK1 in the BMP signaling pathway. *EMBO J* 18: 179–187.

Yamashita H, ten Dijke P, Franzen P, Miyazono K, Heldin CH (1994). Formation of hetero-oligomeric complexes of type I and type II receptors for transforming growth factor-beta. *J Biol Chem* 269: 20172–20178.

Yanagi Y, Suzawa M, Kawabata M, Miyazono K, Yanagisawa J, Kato S (1999). Positive and negative modulation of vitamin D receptor function by transforming growth factor-beta signaling through smad proteins. *J Biol Chem* 274: 12971–12974.

Yanagisawa J, Yanagi Y, Masuhiro Y, Suzawa M, Watanabe M, Kashiwagi K, Toriyabe T, Kawabata M, Miyazono K, Kato S (1999). Convergence of transforming growth factor-beta and vitamin D signaling pathways on SMAD transcriptional coactivators. *Science* 283: 1317–1321.

Yeo C, Whitman M (2001). Nodal signals to Smads through Cripto-dependent and Cripto-independent mechanisms. *Mol Cells* 7: 949–957.

Yokouchi Y, Vogan KJ, Pearse RV 2nd, Tabin CJ (1999). Antagonistic signaling by *Caronte*, a novel *cerberus-related* gene, establishes left–right asymmetric gene expression. *Cell* 98: 573–583.

Yoshida Y, Tanaka S, Umemori H, Minowa O, Usui M, Ikematsu N, Hosoda E, Imamura T, Kuno J, Yamashita T, et al. (2000). Negative regulation of BMP/Smad signaling by Tob in osteoblasts. *Cell* 103: 1085–1097.

Yu K, Srinivasan S, Shimmi O, Biehs B, Rashka KE, Kimelman D, O'Connor MB, Bier E (2000). Processing of the *Drosophila* Sog protein creates a novel BMP inhibitory activity. *Development* 127: 2143–2154.

Zhang H, Bradley A (1996). Mice deficient for BMP2 are nonviable and have defects in amnion/chorion and cardiac development. *Development* 122: 2977–2986.

Zhang Y, Musci T, Derynck R (1997). The tumor suppressor Smad4/DPC 4 as a central mediator of Smad function. *Curr Biol* 7: 270–276.

Zhang Y, Feng XH, Derynck R (1998). Smad3 and Smad4 cooperate with c-Jun/c-Fos to mediate TGF-beta-induced transcription. *Nature* 394: 909–913.

Zhang YW, Yasui N, Ito K, Huang G, Fujii M, Hanai J, Nogami H, Ochi T, Miyazono K, Ito Y (2000). A RUNX2/PEBP2alphaA/CBFA1 mutation displaying impaired transactivation and Smad interaction in cleidocranial dysplasia. *Proc Natl Acad Sci USA* 97: 10549–10554.

Zhu H, Kavsak P, Abdollah S, Wrana JL, Thomsen GH (1999). A SMAD ubiquitin ligase targets the BMP pathway and affects embryonic pattern formation. *Nature* 400: 687–693.

25 | *NOG* and Proximal Symphalangisms, Multiple Synostosis Syndrome, Tarsal-Carpal Coalition, and Isolated Stapes Ankylosis

MATTHEW L. WARMAN

Noggin was the first demonstrated antagonist of bone morphogenetic protein (BMP) signaling. A widely expressed, secreted, interchain, disulfide-linked dimer, Noggin binds to several transforming growth factor-β (TGFβ) superfamily members and inhibits their ability to signal through cognate cell surface receptors. Because Noggin is capable of binding to and inhibiting a repertoire of signaling molecules, it has been extensively used in vitro and in model organisms to dissect the diverse roles of the TGFβ superfamily during development. The role of Noggin during development has been evaluated by creating knockout mice and by identifying disease-causing mutations in humans. Mice completely lacking Noggin die at birth with multiple malformations affecting the neural tube, sclerotome, myotome, axial skeleton, and appendicular skeleton. No human phenotype associated with homozygous loss-of-function mutations in *NOG* has been reported. However, four dominantly inherited human syndromes with overlapping phenotypes have been linked to the *NOGGIN* locus on human chromosome 17 and have had heterozygous *NOG* mutations identified. These syndromes are proximal symphalangism (SYM1; OMIM 185800), multiple synostosis syndrome (SYNS1; OMIM 186500), tarsal-carpal coalition (TCC; OMIM 186570), and isolated stapes ankylosis (OMIM 184460). Both *cis*- and *trans*-acting modifier loci have been postulated to account for the different human disease phenotypes that result from heterozygous *NOG* mutations.

THE *NOGGIN* LOCUS

Noggin was initially identified in *Xenopus laevis*, on the ability of its cDNA to rescue normal dorsal development in ventralized embryos (Smith and Harland, 1992). Subsequent studies indicated that Noggin's dorsalizing effect in *X. laevis* was due to its ability to bind and inhibit BMP4 (Zimmerman et al., 1996). Exogenous Noggin could also inhibit DPP signaling in *Drosophila* (Holley et al., 1996). Single Noggin loci have been identified in mice and humans. Three Noggin loci have been identified in zebrafish. The human *NOGGIN* locus maps to chromosome 17q22 and has its entire open reading frame contained within a single exon (Valenzuela et al., 1995; Gong et al., 1999). The noncoding domains that regulate the temporal and spatial expression of Noggin during development have not been described. Human Noggin is a 232-amino-acid residue polypeptide that undergoes *N*-linked glycosylation, contains a cystine-knot motif, and is secreted as an interchain, disulfide-bonded homodimer (Smith et al., 1993; Marcelino et al., 2001; Groppe et al., 2002).

CLINICAL DESCRIPTION

Synostosis syndromes represent a heterogeneous group of skeletal disorders that are characterized based on their patterns of axial and appendicular joint fusion. Proximal SYM1 is an autosomal dominant skeletal disorder in which the most common finding is bony fusion affecting the proximal interphalangeal joint of the fifth digit (Figure 25–1). A large family study of proximal SYM1, in which a *Nog* mutation was subsequently identified, indicated that the phenotype is highly penetrant (Strasburger et al., 1965). The second most common feature in individuals with SYM1 appears to be talonavicular fusion in the foot. Bony fusions involving other carpal and tarsal bones are also common, as is brachydactyly. In addition to the appendicular involvement, a significant proportion of affected family members are deaf due to fusion between the stapes and the petrous part of the tem-

poral bone. Consequently, the name proximal symphalangism syndrome does not fully reflect the diverse extent of skeletal involvement that is present among affected individuals.

SYNS1 has been considered a clinically distinct entity from SYM1, even though the two disorders are dominantly inherited and have significant clinical overlap (Krakow et al., 1998). Common to both syndromes is the pattern of interphalangeal joint fusion, the presence of tarsal and carpal bone coalition, and hearing loss associated with ankylosis of the stapes to the petrous bone. SYNS1 differs from SYM1 with respect to the severity of brachydactyly and bony fusions affecting the axial and proximal appendicular skeleton (elbows and hips). Furthermore, individuals with SYNS1 have been described as having mild facial dysmorphism (cylindrical appearing nose). Despite these differences, allelism between SYM1 and SYNS1 was hypothesized, supported by linkage, and confirmed by detecting *NOG* mutations (Krakow et al., 1998; Gong et al., 1999).

Three families have been described in which proximal symphalangism, tarsal coalition, and carpal coalition are inherited as an autosomal dominant trait (TCC). Similar to SYM1, proximal symphalangism and disabling ankle and foot problems are the most common findings in these families. However, TCC appeared clinically distinct from SYM1 and SYNS1 in that none of the 21 affected individuals among the three families has symptoms or signs of stapes ankylosis (Dixon et al., 2001). In one family, linkage analysis mapped TCC to an interval on chromosome 17q that overlapped the SYM1 and SYNS1 candidate regions, and heterozygous *NOG* mutations were subsequently identified in each of the three families (Dixon et al., 2001).

Three families have also been described in which stapes ankylosis, broad thumbs, broad toes, and hyperopia, with and without other minor anomalies ("cylindrical" nose, cervical fusion, cutaneous syndactyly), are inherited as an autosomal dominant trait (OMIM 184460). Although the stapes ankylosis and facial features were similar to that described in SYM1 or SYNS1, this disorder was considered distinct because only 1 of 15 affected individuals had signs of proximal symphalangism (Brown et al., 2002). Furthermore, hyperopia and broad thumbs and toes had not been noted in families segregating SYM1 or SYNS1. In two of the families, *NOG* was evaluated and disease-causing mutations were identified (Brown et al., 2002).

MOLECULAR GENETICS

A single extended kindred, initially described by Dr. Harvey Cushing during his tenure at the Johns Hopkins Hospital, was used map the SYM1 locus to human chromosome 17q (Polymeropoulos et al., 1995). Based on phenotypic overlap with SYM1, linkage to chromosome 17q was tested and confirmed in a single family with SYNS1 (Krakow et al., 1998). The co-localization of human *NOG* to the SYM1 and SYNS1 candidate intervals and the observation that *Nog* knockout mice had multiple joint fusions (Brunet et al., 1998) led to the sequencing of human *NOG* in patients/families with SYM1 and SYNS1. Among the first seven unrelated patients sequenced, all were found to have unique heterozygous *NOG* missense mutations (Gong et al., 1999). Included among these first seven mutations were individuals from the families that were used to initially map SYM1 and SYNS1. Three additional SYM1 and SYNS1 mutations have been published, including nonsense and frameshift mutations (Takahashi et al., 2001; Mangino et al., 2002). *NOG* coding sequence mutations have not been

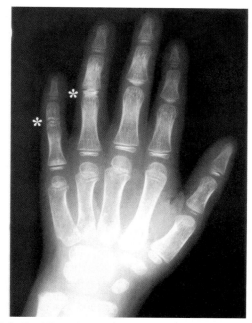

Figure 25–1. Hand X-ray from a child with SYM1. Asterisks indicate abnormally formed proximal interphalangeal joints affecting digits 4 and 5.

detected in all patients referred with a clinical diagnosis of SYM1 and SYNS1 (author's unpublished observations). Whether this reflects misdiagnosis, locus heterogeneity, or *NOG* mutations that are undetectable using current screening strategies is unknown. *NOG* has typically been screened for mutations by PCR amplifying its 696-bp open reading frame and directly sequencing the resulting amplimers. This approach will miss disease-causing mutations that result from microdeletions that involve the *NOG* locus or mutations that affect the noncoding regulatory regions of the gene. The former possibility must be seriously considered because patients with multiple malformations, including symphalangism, and microscopic deletions involving human chromosome 17q22 have been described (Park et al., 1992; Dallapiccola et al., 1993; Khalifa et al., 1993). Also, a second multiple synostosis locus (*SYNS2*) on human chromosome 20, with a putative disease-causing missense mutation in *GDF5*, has been reported in a single large kindred (Akarsu et al., 1999). TCC was also mapped in a single family to an interval that contained the *NOG* locus, and *NOG* mutations were identified in three families with TCC (Dixon et al., 2001). Interestingly, two of the mutations have been previously reported in patients clinically diagnosed as having SYM1, suggesting that *cis-* and *trans-*acting factors likely modify the effects of *NOG* mutations. Because of clinical overlap with SYM1 and SYNS1, *NOG* was also tested as a candidate gene in two families with autosomal dominant stapes ankylosis, broad thumbs, broad toes, and hyperopia syndrome. A nonsense mutation was detected in one family and a frameshift was detected in the other (Brown et al., 2002). The existence of modifier loci was postulated to account for the variable phenotypes that appear to result from similar types of mutations within the *NOG* locus.

ESTABLISHING THE DIAGNOSIS

Surprisingly, among the four disorders that have been associated with *NOG* mutations, there is no single common feature. Therefore, no single clinical symptom or sign can include or preclude *NOG* as the potential disease-causing locus. *NOGGIN* should be considered a strong candidate for causing phenotypes that have proximal symphalangism, tarsal coalition, carpal coalition, or stapes ankylosis as a component feature. Other features, such as cylindrical nose, brachydactyly, short or broad thumbs, and hyperopia, have also been observed in families segregating *NOG* mutations. However, it is not presently known whether any of these features in isolation are likely to be caused by a *NOG* variant. A combination of clinical examination, radiographic study, and formal hearing evaluation will be helpful in diagnosing the aforementioned disorders.

NOG mutation detection is available on a research basis and is being transitioned to clinical testing in several laboratories. Since the most used *NOG* mutation screening methods will miss some disease-causing mutations (see previous section), failure to identify a *NOG* coding sequence mutations does not exclude the locus as being disease causing. Signs and symptoms resulting from *NOG* mutation need not be present at birth or during early infancy. Therefore, prenatal diagnosis by ultrasonography or radiography will not be reliable.

MANAGEMENT

Hearing loss in patients with *NOG* mutations is generally surgically correctable. Orthopedic intervention may be helpful in lessening the morbidity associated with ankle and foot involvement. Decreased life expectancy or poor quality of life was not observed in the one extensively characterized family that is segregating SYM1. Quality and quantity of life are also unlikely to be significantly impacted by the other disorders with heterozygous *NOG* mutations; however, studies have not specifically commented on this aspect of the disease.

MUTATIONS IN ORTHOLOGOUS AND PARALAGOUS GENES

Noggin is a potent inhibitor of BMP signaling; therefore, it has been extensively used in vitro and in model organism studies to explore the consequences of altered BMP signaling on cellular and developmental processes. In model organisms, the consequence of *Nog* mutation has been studied only in mice. Targeted deletion of murine *Nog* caused no obvious phenotype in heterozygous knockout mice but caused an embryonic lethal phenotype in homozygous knockout mice (McMahon et al., 1998). Three studies describe different features in the *Nog* knockout mice. The axial skeleton was noted to have normal-appearing cervical vertebrae, fused thoracic vertebrae with missing neural arches, and absent lumbar vertebrae (Brunet et al., 1998). In the appendicular skeleton, the sizes of the skeletal elements were increased, and there was a generalized failure in the formation of diarthrodal joints (Brunet et al., 1998). Abnormal joint formation is the principal feature associated with heterozygous *NOG* mutations in humans (Gong et al. 1999). Contrary to what might have been predicted based on the original identification of Noggin as a neural inducer in *X. laevis*, normal neural induction occurs in *Nog* null mice (McMahon et al., 1998). However, the patterning of the neural tube and somites is abnormal in *Nog* null embryos. The neural tube fails to close in all embryos, although its extent is modified by genetic background (e.g., C57BL/6J versus 129/Sv strains) (McMahon et al., 1998). Also severely impaired are the patterning and growth of the ventral neural tube and induction of sclerotome and myotome growth (McMahon et al., 1998). A third aspect of Noggin function that has been examined in the *Nog* null mice is the guidance of axons (Dionne et al., 2002). Abnormal branching of cranial nerve VII in the jaw and of motor neurons in the distal forelimb occurs in knockout mice (Dionne et al., 2002). In addition, axons from dorsal root ganglia (DRG) entering the spinal cord are patterned incorrectly in *Nog* null mice (Dionne et al., 2002).

DEVELOPMENTAL PATHOGENESIS

Noggin was initially identified in an expression screen using *X. laevis* embryos that had been ventralized with ultraviolet radiation to identify neural inducers that could mimic the role of the Spemann organizer (Smith and Harland, 1992; Smith et al., 1993). Noggin has this effect in *X. laevis* because of its ability to bind and inhibit BMP4 signaling (Zimmerman et al., 1996). As such, Noggin was the first discovered direct BMP antagonist. Subsequent studies indicate that Noggin is able to bind multiple members of the BMP and GDF subfamilies of the TGFβ superfamily of secreted growth regulators. Noggin has been shown to bind with high affinity to BMP2 and BMP4 and with lower affinity to BMP7 (Zimmerman et al., 1996). The crystal structure of the NOGGIN–BMP7 binding complex has been determined (Groppe et al., 2002). Noggin has a cysteine-knot motif similar to that found in TGFβ superfamily members; it exists in dimeric form and on binding to BMP7, induces a conformational change in BMP7 that blocks the binding sites of BMP for its cognate type I and II cell surface receptors (Groppe et al., 2002). Consequently, Noggin interferes with BMP signaling by blocking the ability of the signaling molecules to bind to their cognate receptors. There is no evidence that Noggin has roles other than as a signaling antagonist.

Through its role as an antagonist, Noggin participates in a wide variety of developmental processes. This is exemplified by studies in mice and humans with *NOG* mutations and by studies in other model organisms in which Noggin has been used as a tool to interfere with BMP signaling. Overexpression of Noggin disrupts limb growth (Capdevila and Johnson, 1998; Pizette and Niswander, 1999, 2000) and feather formation in chickens (Yu et al., 2002) and limb, hair follicle, and cranial suture formation in mice (Kulessa et al., 2000; Warren et al., 2003). Exposure to exogenously applied Noggin affects the formation of limb (Groppe et al., 2002) and facial structures in chickens (Lee et al., 2001). More than 100 articles have been published that report diverse cellular and developmental responses to exogenous Noggin. However, it is unknown which of these effects reflect Noggin's endogenous developmental role or the ability of exogenously expressed, or applied, Noggin to substitute for other naturally occurring BMP signaling antagonists. Although not closely related to Noggin, at least seven other cystine-knot–containing BMP antagonists have been identified, including chordin, follistatin, DAN, Cerberus, Gremlin, Dante, and Sclerostin (Balemans and Van Hul, 2002). Several appear to be able to compensate for the absence of another in the context of specific developmental pathways. For example, in mice the BMP antagonists Chordin and Noggin appear to compensate for each other's absence during early dorsal patterning, because early patterning problems occur only in mice who lack both proteins (Bachiller et al., 2000).

Because exogenously applied, or expressed, Noggin is capable of interfering with BMP signaling that might ordinarily be modulated by other BMP antagonists, the most direct insights into the spatial and temporal roles of Noggin during development are derived from knockout mice. Within the developing neural tube, Noggin is essential for facilitating the continued growth of ventral structures, because increased apoptosis within this region occurs in its absence (McMahon et al., 1998). Within somites, Noggin-mediated inhibition of BMP signaling is required to enable Sonic Hedgehog (SHH) to induce differentiation of sclerotomal and myotomal elements (McMahon et al., 1998). Within the spinal cord, Noggin helps direct ingrowth of dorsal root ganglia axons (Dionne et al., 2002). When DRG explants from wild-type mice are co-cultured with spinal cord explants from knockouts, the DRG axonal ingrowth is abnormal; however, when the converse experiment is performed (DRG explants from knockouts and spinal cord explants from wild-type), the DRG axonal growth appears normal (Dionne et al., 2002). These experiments suggest Noggin acts within the spinal cord to set up morphogenic gradients that direct axonal growth. It is not yet known how Noggin helps to establish this morphogenic gradient. Finally, Noggin has multiple roles during the morphogenesis of appendicular skeletal elements. Multiple BMPs are expressed during the condensation and differentiation of mesenchyme into the chondrocytic anlage of a skeletal element. Noggin expression regulates this BMP-mediated process, because skeletal elements in knockout mice are enlarged at the expense of neighboring nonskeletal structures (Brunet et al., 1998).

As noted in both the knockout mice and in humans with heterozygous *NOG* mutations, Noggin is also important during the formation of diarthrodal joints. Noggin-mediated inhibition of BMP signaling is needed to make cells receptive to other signaling proteins during somite differentiation (McMahon et al., 1998); similar requirements for noggin-mediated BMP inhibition occur during joint morphogenesis. In *Nog* knockout mice, the chondrocytic cells residing at "joint-forming" regions of skeletal anlage fail to express markers associated with early joint patterning such as GDF5 (Brunet et al., 1998). This suggests that Noggin-mediated inhibition of BMP signaling is specifically required at sites of future joints to enable those cells to further differentiate. Interestingly, Noggin seems not to affect the expression of global patterning genes, such as members of the *Hox* complex, or of other genes that are associated with maturation of developing skele-

tal elements, such as *Indian Hedgehog* and *Parathyroid Hormone Related Peptide* (Brunet et al., 1998). However, the expression of other identified upstream signaling factors that can specify sites of joint formation (e.g., Wnt 14) has not yet been evaluated in the *Nog* knockout mice.

The principal role of Noggin during morphogenesis is to inhibit BMP signaling and thereby create a local milieu that enables cells to respond to other signaling molecules. The precision by which Noggin is able to modulate complex developmental processes may be established through several means. First, Noggin has different affinities for members of the BMP/GDF families (Zimmerman et al., 1996). Second, Noggin may bind BMP molecules intracellularly, before their secretion (Marcelino et al., 2001). This can serve to rapidly down-regulate BMP signaling by specific cells or to facilitate the formation of long-range BMP signaling gradients. Third, Noggin can bind sulfated proteoglycans at the cell surface, thereby permitting cells to trap Noggin locally and inhibit BMP signaling in a cell autonomous manner (Paine-Saunders et al., 2002). Fourth, BMP signaling can induce Noggin expression by cells as a means of feedback regulating this activity (Sela-Donenfeld and Kalcheim, 2002).

In humans, the developmental pathway affected in most individuals with heterozygous *NOG* mutations is the formation of appendicular joints. Among single families segregating *NOG* mutations, there are examples of individuals who are nonpenetrant for specific joint malformations (Strasburger et al., 1965). Whether this incomplete penetrance and other examples within families of variable expression result from the effect of modifier loci or random chance is not known. Support for the existence of modifier loci derives from the observation in knockout mice that the penetrance of open cranial neural tube is background dependent (McMahon et al., 1998). Less easy to explain in humans is how identical mutations in different families cause different phenotypes that appear to "breed true," such as heterozygous missense mutations that cause both SYM1 and TCC (Dixon et al., 2001) and nonsense and frameshift mutations that cause SYM1, SYNS1, and autosomal dominant stapes ankylosis (Takahashi et al., 2001; Brown et al., 2002; Mangino et al., 2002). It is possible that families with identical mutations on divergent genetic backgrounds have different polymorphic *cis*-acting elements in their wild-type *NOG* allele or different *trans*-acting elements elsewhere in their genome. Alternatively, families who cluster a specific phenotypic trait could represent a subset of all affected families in which this otherwise randomly distributed (stochastically determined) trait is by chance atypically distributed.

REFERENCES

Akarsu AN, Rezaie T, Demirtas M, Farhud DD, Sarfarazi M (1999). Multiple synostosis type 2 (SYNS2) maps to 20q11.2 and caused by a missense mutation in the growth/differentiation factor 5 (GDF5). *Am J Hum Genet* 65 supplement: A281.

Bachiller D, Klingensmith J, Kemp C, Belo JA, Anderson RM, May SR, McMahon JA, McMahon AP, Harland RM, Rossant J, et al. (2000). The organizer factors Chordin and Noggin are required for mouse forebrain development. *Nature* 403: 658–661.

Balemans W, Van Hul W (2002). Extracellular regulation of BMP signaling in vertebrates: a cocktail of modulators. *Dev Biol* 250: 231–250.

Brown DJ, Kim TB, Petty EM, Downs CA, Martin DM, Strouse PJ, Moroi SE, Milunsky JM, Lesperance MM (2002). Autosomal dominant stapes ankylosis with broad thumbs and toes, hyperopia, and skeletal anomalies is caused by heterozygous nonsense and frameshift mutations in *NOG*, the gene encoding noggin. *Am J Hum Genet* 71: 618–624.

Brunet LJ, McMahon JA, McMahon AP, Harland RM (1998). Noggin, cartilage morphogenesis, and joint formation in the mammalian skeleton. *Science* 280: 1455–1457.

Capdevila J, Johnson RL (1998). Endogenous and ectopic expression of noggin suggests a conserved mechanism for regulation of BMP function during limb and somite patterning. *Dev Biol* 197: 205–217.

Dallapiccola B, Mingarelli R, Digilio C, Obregon MG, Giannotti A (1993). Interstitial deletion del(17) (q21.3q23 or 24.2) syndrome. *Clin Genet* 43: 54–55.

Dionne MS, Brunet LJ, Eimon PM, Harland RM (2002). Noggin is required for correct guidance of dorsal root ganglion axons. *Dev Biol* 251: 283–293.

Dixon ME, Armstrong P, Stevens DB, Bamshad M (2001). Identical mutations in *NOG* can cause either tarsal/carpal coalition syndrome or proximal symphalangism. *Genet Med* 3: 349–353.

Gazzerro E, Gangji V, Canalis E (1998). Bone morphogenetic proteins induce the expression of noggin, which limits their activity in cultured rat osteoblasts. *J Clin Invest* 102: 2106–2114.

Gong Y, Krakow D, Marcelino J, Wilkin D, Chitayat D, Babul-Hirji R, Hudgins L, Cremers CW, Cremers FP, Brunner HG, et al. (1999). Heterozygous mutations in the gene encoding noggin affect human joint morphogenesis. *Nat Genet* 21: 302–304.

Groppe J, Greenwald J, Wiater E, Rodriguez-Leon J, Economides AN, Kwiatkowski W, Affolter M, Vale WW, Belmont JC, Choe S (2002). Structural basis of BMP signalling inhibition by the cystine knot protein Noggin. *Nature* 420: 636–642.

Holley SA, Neul JL, Attisano L, Wrana JL, Sasai Y, O'Connor MB, De Robertis EM, Ferguson EL (1996). The Xenopus dorsalizing factor noggin ventralizes Drosophila embryos by preventing DPP from activating its receptor. *Cell* 86: 607–617.

Khalifa MM, MacLeod PM, Duncan AM (1993). Additional case of de novo interstitial deletion del(17)(q21.3q23) and expansion of the phenotype. *Clin Genet* 44: 258–261.

Krakow D, Reinker K, Powell B, Cantor R, Priore MA, Garber A, Lachman RS, Rimoin DL, Cohn DH (1998). Localization of a multiple synostoses-syndrome disease gene to chromosome 17q21-22. *Am J Hum Genet* 63: 120–124.

Kulessa H, Turk G, Hogan BL (2000). Inhibition of Bmp signaling affects growth and differentiation in the anagen hair follicle. *EMBO J* 19: 6664–6674.

Lee SH, Fu KK, Hui JN, Richman JM (2001). Noggin and retinoic acid transform the identity of avian facial prominences. *Nature* 414: 909–912.

Mangino M, Flex E, Digilio MC, Giannotti A, Dallapiccola B (2002). Identification of a novel *NOG* gene mutation (P35S) in an Italian family with symphalangism. *Hum Mutat* 19: 308.

Marcelino J, Sciortino CM, Romero MF, Ulatowski LM, Ballock RT, Economides AN, Eimon PM, Harland RM, Warman ML (2001). Human disease-causing *NOG* missense mutations: effects on noggin secretion, dimer formation, and bone morphogenetic protein binding. *Proc Natl Acad Sci USA* 98: 11353–11358.

McMahon JA, Takada S, Zimmerman LB, Fan CM, Harland RM, McMahon AP (1998). Noggin-mediated antagonism of BMP signaling is required for growth and patterning of the neural tube and somite. *Genes Dev* 12: 1438–1452.

Paine-Saunders S, Viviano BL, Economides AN, Saunders S (2002). Heparan sulfate proteoglycans retain Noggin at the cell surface: a potential mechanism for shaping bone morphogenetic protein gradients. *J Biol Chem* 277: 2089–2096.

Park JP, Moeschler JB, Berg SZ, Bauer RM, Wurster-Hill DH (1992). A unique de novo interstitial deletion del(17)(q21.3q23) in a phenotypically abnormal infant. *Clin Genet* 41: 54–56.

Pizette S, Niswander L (1999). BMPs negatively regulate structure and function of the limb apical ectodermal ridge. *Development* 126: 883–894.

Pizette S, Niswander L (2000). BMPs are required at two steps of limb chondrogenesis: formation of prechondrogenic condensations and their differentiation into chondrocytes. *Dev Biol* 219: 237–249.

Polymeropoulos MH, Poush J, Rubenstein JR, Francomano CA (1995). Localization of the gene (SYM1) for proximal symphalangism to human chromosome 17q21-q22. *Genomics* 27: 225–229.

Sela-Donenfeld D, Kalcheim C (2002). Localized BMP4-noggin interactions generate the dynamic patterning of noggin expression in somites. *Dev Biol* 246: 311–328.

Smith WC, Harland RM (1992). Expression cloning of noggin, a new dorsalizing factor localized to the Spemann organizer in Xenopus embryos. *Cell* 70: 829–840.

Smith WC, Knecht AK, Wu M, Harland RM (1993). Secreted noggin protein mimics the Spemann organizer in dorsalizing Xenopus mesoderm. *Nature* 361: 547–549.

Strasburger AK, Hawkins MR, Eldridge R, Hargrave RL, McKusick VA (1965). Symphalangism: genetic and clinical aspects. *Bull Johns Hopkins Hosp* 117: 108–127.

Takahashi T, Takahashi I, Komatsu M, Sawaishi Y, Higashi K, Nishimura G, Saito H, Takada G (2001). Mutations of the *NOG* gene in individuals with proximal symphalangism and multiple synostosis syndrome. *Clin Genet* 60: 447–451.

Valenzuela DM, Economides AN, Rojas E, Lamb TM, Nunez L, Jones P, Lp NY, Espinosa R 3rd, Brannan CI, Gilbert DJ, et al. (1995). Identification of mammalian noggin and its expression in the adult nervous system. *J Neurosci* 15: 6077–6084.

Warren SM, Brunet LJ, Harland RM, Economides AN, Longaker MT (2003). The BMP antagonist noggin regulates cranial suture fusion. *Nature* 422: 625–629.

Yu M, Wu P, Widelitz RB, Chuong CM (2002). The morphogenesis of feathers. *Nature* 420: 308–312.

Zimmerman LB, De Jesus-Escobar JM, Harland RM (1996). The Spemann organizer signal noggin binds and inactivates bone morphogenetic protein 4. *Cell* 86: 599–606.

26 | *ZIC3, CFC1, ACVR2B,* and *EBAF* and the Visceral Heterotaxies

STEPHANIE M. WARE AND JOHN W. BELMONT

*H*eterotaxy is a clinical phenotype resulting from a failure to correctly establish left/right (LR) patterning during embryogenesis. Multiple congenital anomalies may result from discordant positioning of normally asymmetrical internal organs and vasculature. Midline defects and anomalies of paired organs can occur, presumably due to a failure to correctly segregate left and right. Mutations in three genes that function in the transforming growth factor-β (TGF-β) signaling pathway, Activin receptor type IIB (*ACVR2B*), the epidermal growth factor-cripto/FRL1(one-eyed pinhead)/cryptii (*EGF-CFC*) family member *CRYPTIC*, and *LEFTYA*, have been found in a small number of patients with heterotaxy. Mutations in the zinc finger transcription factor ZIC3 have been described in four X-linked familial cases and one sporadic case of heterotaxy, as well as in one case of isolated congenital heart disease. The degree to which genes involved in LR patterning may contribute to isolated congenital anomalies as opposed to classic heterotaxy is not currently known, and the incidence of these genetic defects may be underappreciated. A molecular understanding of the important events in the generation of LR patterning, including TGF-β signaling in the node and left lateral plate mesoderm of the gastrulation-stage embryo, is emerging. Studies in mouse, chick, *Xenopus*, and zebrafish are contributing to the delineation of the developmental pathogenesis of these disorders as well as identifying candidate genes for further investigation.

DISORDERS OF LATERALITY

A great deal of progress has been made toward understanding the molecular basis of LR patterning in the past 5 years, with critical contributions emerging from the description of TGF-β signaling in early embryogenesis. Despite a growing appreciation of the early events in LR patterning, much remains to be resolved. In addition, later embryonic events related to the mechanism by which aberrant signaling in early embryogenesis translates into abnormal organogenesis and the development of a wide spectrum of congenital anomalies remain poorly understood.

The term *heterotaxy*, from the Greek for "other arrangement," implies abnormal LR embryonic patterning, rather than a specific final outcome, and refers to an unusual spatial arrangement of thoracic and/or abdominal organs in relationship to each other. The normal LR anatomical arrangement, judged relative to the visceroatrial position, is called *situs solitus*. Complete reversal of asymmetrical structures in the thorax and abdomen is called *situs inversus* and occurs in approximately 1 in 8000–25,000 individuals. If right and left patterns of ordinarily asymmetrical structures are discordant, the resulting disorder is called *situs ambiguus*. A number of names have been used to describe this condition, including isomerism sequence, asplenia syndrome, Ivemark's syndrome, polysplenia syndrome, situs ambiguus, heterotaxia, partial situs inversus, and laterality sequence. A simplistic approach is to describe any arrangement of body symmetry that deviates from normal as heterotaxy, including both situs ambiguus and situs inversus. When referring to specific organs, it is generally more useful to describe the specific anatomy with reference to whether the organ is lateralized, either to the appropriate or opposite side, or is abnormally symmetrical (a loss of lateralization).

Clinically, heterotaxy syndromes are characterized by a wide variety of congenital anomalies of both midline structures as well as lateralized internal organs. Incomplete or failed LR patterning may lead to anatomical discordances (e.g., transposition of the great arteries), loss of structures (e.g., asplenia), or duplication (e.g., right atrial isomerism in which left atrial development is concomitantly lost). An understanding of the spectrum of heterotaxic phenotypes is aided by an appreciation of the embryology of the individual organ systems involved.

All unpaired organs of the chest and abdomen begin development in the midline and subsequently lateralize. The earliest organ asymmetry is detected in the heart tube which undergoes rightward looping on embryonic day 23 (six- to eight-somite stage). Prior to the six-somite stage, the heart is an overtly symmetrical linear tube. The first sign of asymmetry in the developing heart tube is a slight swelling on the left side and a deepening of the left lateral furrow (Biben and Harvey, 1997; Harvey and Rosenthal, 1999; Manner, 2000). Subsequently, the atrioventricular (AV) junction is displaced to the left and the primitive ventricle rotates counterclockwise. The conotruncal portion of the heart tube, consisting of the future right ventricle (bulbus cordis) and outflow tract (truncus arteriosus), initially located on the right side of the pericardial cavity, moves to a more medial position.

The vasculature also exhibits LR asymmetry, but the mechanism by which it is generated differs. Most of the lateralized arteries and veins initially develop as paired vessels with subsequent regression of the mirror-image vessel. Examples include the superior and inferior vena cava as well as the umbilical and vitelline veins.

In the abdomen, LR asymmetry begins and ends later than in the chest. The stomach emerges as a fusiform dilatation caudally from the esophagus, attached to dorsal and ventral mesenteries. Differential growth creates greater (dorsal) and lesser (ventral) curvatures.

The primitive gut tube begins as a symmetrical midline structure formed by folding of the splanchnopleure endoderm and splanchnic mesoderm. The foregut, midgut, and hindgut structures correspond embryologically and physiologically to the arterial distributions of the celiac, superior mesenteric, and inferior mesenteric arteries, respectively. The position of the gut with respect to the superior mesenteric artery is, therefore, indicative of its LR position. The intestine undergoes physiological herniation due to rapid growth of the primitive intestinal loops by embryonic day 36. A 270-degree counterclockwise rotation of the primitive intestinal loop around the superior mesenteric artery occurs over the next month. This rotation causes the small intestine to pass posterior to the superior mesenteric artery. In the process of fixation, the small intestine becomes attached to the posterior abdominal wall by mesentery (from the ligament of Treitz to the ileocecal area).

The liver, gallbladder, and spleen are positioned during the period of physiological gut herniation and gut rotation. The liver is induced from an endodermal thickening of the foregut/midgut at 3 weeks' gestation. It is an asymmetrical but bilateral organ. The developmental processes that regulate the formation of the bile ducts are not clear, and anatomical variations are common. Two diverticula, hepatic and cystic, arise together from the embryonic gut. The intrahepatic bile ducts and the left and right bile ducts arise from the hepatic diverticula. The gallbladder arises from a localized dilatation of the cystic diverticula. The spleen was previously believed to be the only unpaired internal organ to initiate development asymmetrically, but recent data suggest that it develops from paired primordia with regression of the right side (Patterson et al., 2000).

CLINICAL AND ANATOMICAL PATHOLOGY

Although situs ambiguus can have a wide variety of presentations involving a number of different organ systems, historically there have been two broad clinical categories (Table 26–1). The asplenia type represents a predominant bilateral right-sidedness (right isomerism), whereas the polysplenia type represents a predominant bilateral left-sidedness (left isomerism). Although treated separately historically, asplenia and polysplenia are now believed to arise from a common set of morphogenetic errors (Phoon and Neill, 1994; Ruscazio et al., 1998; Ticho et al., 2000). As the underlying molecular defects are elucidated in patients with heterotaxy, it will be important to carefully document the phenotype of affected individuals. It remains to be determined whether specific mutations correlate with the asplenia versus polysplenia phenotype (see below), and controversy exists regarding the clinical utility of these categories (Uemura et al., 1995). In general, organ malformations in patients with heterotaxy appear to arise independently of each other. Overall, the heart defects seen in patients with asplenia or right-sided spleen tend to be more severe and complex than those seen with polysplenia (Peoples et al., 1983; Van Praagh et al., 1990, 1997; Phoon and Neill, 1994; Uemura et al., 1995; Ticho et al., 2000; Aylsworth, 2001).

Table 26–1. Characteristics of Asplenia and Polysplenia

Characteristics	Polysplenia	Asplenia
Sex distribution	Equal	Males
Heart defects	60–90	>97
Heart anatomy		
AV valves		
Common	66	92
Separate	22	6
Solitary	12	2
AV connections		
Biventricular	74	46
Univentricular	26	54
Ventricular morphology		
Single/dominant LV	30	6–14
Single/dominant RV	20	7–10
Indeterminate	4	5–26
Ventriculoarterial connections		
Discordant	2–16	2–62
DORV	15–43	13–43
Common arterial trunk	0	0–10
Concordant	45–69	45
Pulmonary venous return	Partial APVR	TAPVR
All to one atrium	40–48	36–40
Bilateral	39–60	0–60
Extracardiac connection	0–13	42–64
LVOTO (all types)	3–28	Rare
PS/PA	7–34	36–48
Vasculature		
Bilateral SVC	47–62	46–71
Interrupted IVC	0–3	65–80
Bronchi	Hyparterial	Eparterial
Spleen	Multiple	Absent
Gallbladder	Extrahepatic biliary atresia	Normal
Intestine	Malrotation	Malrotation
Other		Microgastria, right-sided stomach Tracheoesophageal fistula Imperforate anus

All numbers represent percentages. APVR, anomalous pulmonary venous return; AV, atrioventricular; DORV, double outlet right ventricle; IVC, inferior vena cava; LV, left ventricle; LVOTO, LV outflow tract obstruction; PA, pulmonic atresia; PS, pulmonic stenosis; RV, right ventricle; SVC, superior vena cava; TAPVR, total anomalous pulmonary venous return.

Sources: Summarized from Peoples et al., 1983; Phoon and Neill, 1994; Uemura et al., 1995; Van Praagh et al., 1990.

Spectrum of Congenital Heart Disease in Patients with Heterotaxy

The heart is the first organ to demonstrate clear differences along the LR axis of the developing embryo. It is not surprising then that disturbances in LR patterning very often adversely affect heart development. Heart defects in heterotaxy represent some of the most complicated types of congenital heart disease (CHD). Included in the list of CHD are malposition and transposition of the great arteries (TGA), atrial septal defects, ventricular septal defects, bilateral superior vena cava, partial anomalous pulmonary venous return, intrahepatic interruption of the inferior vena cava with connection to the azygous or hemiazygous vein, double outlet right ventricle, common atrium, AV canal defects, pulmonary atresia and stenosis, single ventricle, and left ventricular outflow tract obstruction (Table 26–1).

The development of laterality in the heart can be thought of in distinct segments: atrial, ventricular, and outflow tract (future aorta and pulmonary artery). Each of these segments must independently develop LR anatomy and correctly orient with relation to the other regions. Of these segments, only the atria are truly lateralized. Their sidedness can be identified by the different morphology of the right and left appendages. Two autopsy series, consisting of 291 and 1842 congenitally malformed hearts, showed atrial isomerism (in which the left or right asymmetrical structure is duplicated with loss of the alternate) to be relatively common, occurring in 5.2% and 3.1% of cases, repectively (Hegerty et al., 1985; Sharma et al., 1988). In contrast, the ventricles have identifiable right and left chambers, determined primarily by the degree of trabeculation, but isomerism is exceedingly rare. Importantly, the position of the heart within the thorax and the orientation of the apex do not predict the atrial or ventricular arrangement (Brown and Anderson, 1999).

Some of the defects seen in heterotaxy are readily interpreted as arising from abnormal LR specification, such as L-loop with dextrocardia, in which a mirror-image heart resides in the right thoracic compartment but is otherwise completely normal. Other heart defects, like dextro-TGA (d-TGA) may be due to abnormal positioning of the ventricles with respect to the common outflow tract. Alternatively, corrected, or levo-, TGA (l-TGA) may result from a discordant ventricular relationship to the left atrium and aorta, resulting in the anatomical right ventricle pumping the systemic circulation (*ventricular inversion*). Associated cardiac defects, like partial anomalous pulmonary venous return (PAPVR), are presumably secondary, but this is not certain. Congenital heart defects are a major cause of morbidity and mortality in patients with heterotaxy.

Pulmonary Isomerism

Pulmonary manifestations of laterality disorders primarily involve isomerism. Bilateral right isomerism results in a trilobed anatomy bilaterally with bilateral eparterial bronchi. In left isomerism, both lungs have the lobar and hilar anatomy characteristic of a normal left lung. Patients with lung isomerism generally have no pulmonary complications. Patients with primary ciliary disorders have impaired mucociliary clearance and related complications which are covered in Chapter 94. There are case reports of complications from vascular rings in individuals with situs ambiguus (Feingold et al., 2001).

Defects of the Abdominal Viscera: Right-Sided Stomach, Midline Liver, Biliary Atresia, Annular Pancreas, and Intestinal Malrotation

Although some controversy exists about the mechanisms underlying positioning of the stomach, most evidence suggests that "rotation" around its longitudinal axis is primarily extrinsic (Nebot-Cegarra et al., 1999). Displacement of the stomach to the right is seen in heterotaxy and presumably occurs exclusively in the context of abnormal outgrowth of the liver primordium and positional alteration of the dorsal and ventral mesenteries. The stomach may be small in addition to its malposition (Kroes and Festen, 1998).

The liver may reside in the midline or may be reversed in its left and right lobes. Anatomical distinction is made based on the position of the falciform ligament, which separates the right and left lobes. A midline liver suggests that the normal asymmetrical growth induction on the right is disturbed. It is seen not uncommonly in heterotaxy and has little clinical significance. In some cases, a midline liver may be associated with extrahepatic biliary atresia, and the mechanism(s) by which this occurs is unclear (Deveci and Deveci, 2000). It is interesting that the *inv/inv* mouse model, in which situs inversus is the most common finding, consistently exhibits biliary atresia (Mazziotti et al., 1999), but whether this reflects a disturbance in LR patterning or an intrinsic defect in bile duct differentiation is unknown.

The pancreas arises from dorsal (future anterior head, body, and tail) and ventral (future posterior head and uncinate process) primordia. The dorsal pancreas emerges directly from the foregut, but the ventral pancreas appears as an evagination from the bile duct at the biliary duodenal angle. Annular pancreas is an abnormality in which the organ encircles the middle part of the duodenum, leading to constriction and obstruction. The origin of annular pancreas is unknown, but it presumably occurs because of malpositioned duodenum in relation to the ventral and dorsal pancreatic primordia.

Abnormal rotation of the intestinal loop can result in obstruction or *volvulus* (vascular obstruction). In some cases, the primitive intestinal loop undergoes initial rotation but fails to rotate the complete 270 degrees (Ditchfield and Hutson, 1998). In these individuals, as the intestine returns to the abdominal cavity, the later returning loops are positioned more and more to the right due to the lack of rotation. As a result, the colon is located on the left side of the abdomen and the small intestinal loops on the right. In other cases, there is reversed rotation of the intestinal loop (O'Connell and Lynch, 1990). As a result, the transverse colon passes behind the duodenum and behind the superior mesenteric artery.

Midline Malformations

Midline malformations occur in conjunction with heterotaxy, indicating a critical role for the midline in maintaining LR asymmetry dur-

ing embryogenesis (see Developmental Pathogenesis below). CNS abnormalities, axial skeletal defects, anal atresia or stenosis reflecting hindgut deficiency, and urinary tract anomalies have been observed. These anomalies occur equally in asplenia and polyspenia phenotypes (Ticho et al., 2000). In 160 autopsy cases of patients with heterotaxy, midline defects were found in 38% (60/160). In heterotaxy patients with midline defects, genitourinary and musculoskeletal defects were the most common, being found in 26% and 24% of patients, respectively (Ticho et al., 2000). Sacral dysplasia and anorectal anomalies are commonly seen in X-linked pedigrees and have been reported in patients with mutations in *ZIC3*. In pedigrees in which a *ZIC3* mutation was identified, both carrier females as well as affected males were noted to have anal anomalies (Casey et al., 1993; Gebbia et al., 1997).

Nonrandom Associations and Clinical Syndromes with Heterotaxy

Situs ambiguus and situs inversus are nonrandomly associated with a variety of other congenital anomalies and with several discrete clinical syndromes (see Table 26–2). The presence of heterotaxy or related birth defects in a child with a more complex set of defects should raise the diagnostic consideration of one of these disorders. There are no obvious connections between the individual heterotaxy-associated syndromes except that the anatomical defects themselves suggest early disturbances in mesoderm growth, patterning, or allocation. It is also clear that pleiotropic effects are operative in that there is evidence for early embryonic abnormalities but later anomalies in specific tissue growth. Examples of the latter include Ellis-van Creveld syndrome and thiamine-responsive megaloblastic anemia (Donlan et al., 1969; Viana and Carvalho, 1978). In several of the disorders, the associated laterality defects may occur in only a small subset of affected patients, e.g., Goldenhar (Kumar et al., 1993) or Marden-Walker (Temtamy et al., 1975) syndrome. Several potential syndromes are of interest but either have not been observed in more than one family or population or have been observed so rarely that

Table 26–2. Malformations and Syndromes Associated with Heterotaxy and Dextrocardia

OMIM	Syndrome	Abnormality and Reference
—	Aglossia-situs inversus	Situs inversus totalis (Dunham and Austin, 1990; Amor and Craig, 2001)
*202650	Agnathia-holoprosencephaly	Dextrocardia (Ozden et al., 2000; Amor and Craig, 2001)
—	Astley-Kendall (short-limbed dwarfism with extensive stippling)	Dextrocardia (Elcioglu and Hall, 1998)
221950	Aughton (dextrocardia with unusual facies and microphthalmia)	Dextrocardia (Aughton, 1990; Nachlieli and Gershoni-Baruch, 1992)
—	Bonnemann-Meinecke	Dextrocardia (Bonnemann and Meinecke, 1996)
*211890	Cumming (campomelia, lymphocele, polycystic kidneys, polysplenia)	Dextrocardia (Cumming et al., 1986; Ming et al., 1997)
106400	Diffuse idiopathic skeletal hyperostosis	Situs inversus (Carile et al., 1989)
223340	DK-phocomelia	Accessory spleen, abnormal lobation of lungs (Bird et al., 1994)
#225500	Ellis-van Creveld	Dextrocardia (Donlan et al., 1969; Digilio et al., 1999)
*263210	Gillessen-Kaesbach	Dextrocardia (Gillessen-Kaesbach et al., 1993)
*164210	Goldenhar (oculoauriculovertebral dysplasia)	Situs inversus, d-TGA, bilateral SVC (Kumar et al., 1993; Lin et al., 1998)
*243800	Johanson-Blizzard	Dextrocardia, d-TGA (Vanlieferinghen et al., 2001)
*601612	Lung agenesis	Dextrocardia (Fokstuen and Schinzel, 2000)
*248700	Marden-Walker	Dextrocardia (Temtamy et al., 1975)
—	Maternal diabetes	d-TGA, heterotaxia (Morishima et al., 1996; Slavotinek et al., 1996; Lin et al., 2000; Martinez-Frias, 2001)
*157900	Mobius	Dextrocardia (Caravella and Rogers, 1978; Bosch-Banyeras et al., 1984)
—	Mubashir (faciocerebroskeletocardiac)	Situs inversus (Mubashir et al., 1999)
*256540	Galactosialidosis	Dextrocardia (Say et al., 1992)
202660	PAGOD (pulmonary hypoplasia, hypoplasia of the pulmonary artery, agonadism, omphalocele/diaphragmatic defect, and dextrocardia)	Dextrocardia (Kennerknecht et al., 1993; Macayran et al., 2002)
—	Peters' anomaly-CHD	Dextrocardia (Kresca and Goldberg, 1978)
173800	Poland	Dextrocardia (Fraser et al., 1997)
#263200	Renal-hepatic-pancreatic dysplasia	d-TGA, situs ambiguous (Lurie et al., 1991)
#249270	Rogers (thiamine-responsive megaloblastic anemia)	Situs inversus totalis (Viana and Carvalho, 1978)
263510	Short-rib polydactyly type III (Verma-Naumoff)	Dextrocardia (Chen et al., 2002)
185120	Stratton-Parker (growth hormone deficiency, wormian bones, brachycamptodactyly)	Dextrocardia (Stratton and Parker, 1989)
*275210	Tight skin contracture	Dextrocardia (Smitt et al., 1998)

d-TGA, dextrotransposition of the great arteries; SVC, superior vena cava; CHD, congenital heart disease.
*Mode of inheritance proven, gene locus determined.
No symbol, mode of inheritance nuclear.
#Non-locus entry, usually a phenotype.

the proper nosology is uncertain (Bonnemann and Meinecke, 1996; El-cioglu and Hall, 1998; Mubashir et al., 1999).

Situs ambiguus has been described in association with renal-hepatic-pancreatic dysplasia (RHPD) and situs inversus with renal and pancreatic dysplasia (Balci et al., 2000; Aylsworth, 2001). In addition, both situs ambiguus and situs inversus are seen in a proportion of patients with agnathia-holoprosencephaly and the less severe micrognathia/microglossia spectrum of malformations (Pauli et al., 1981; Leech et al., 1988; Hersh et al., 1989; Robinson and Lenke, 1989; Meinecke et al., 1990; Persutte et al., 1990; Stoler and Holmes, 1992; Bonnemann and Meinecke, 1996; Chabrolle et al., 1998; Ozden et al., 2000, 2002; Amor and Craig, 2001; Aylsworth, 2001). The relation of these disorders to one another is not clear, and it remains to be determined if they result from variable expression and allelic heterogeneity at a single locus. A number of case reports detail the association of situs inversus and hyperostosis (Bahrt et al., 1983; Mituszova and Molnar, 1984; Rucco and Zucchi, 1985; Ciocci, 1987; Carile et al., 1989).

There is also a mechanistically informative association of heterotaxy with conjoined twinning. Right-sided conjoined twins may have left or right isomerisms and discordant inversions. The left twin may also have defects of situs. This phenomenon is not observed in craniopagus twins; i.e., defects of situs are probably caused by interactions between the signals emanating from the primitive streak/node or lateral plate mesoderm (Layton, 1989; Lander et al., 1998; Izpisua Belmonte, 1999).

GENETICS AND INHERITANCE OF HETEROTAXY

Epidemiology

Situs inversus occurs in approximately 1 in 8000–25,000 individuals, with ethnic differences and a paternal age effect previously noted (Lian et al., 1986; Correa-Villasenor et al., 1991; Phoon and Neill, 1994). It is much harder to estimate the birth incidence and prevalence of LR patterning defects because of the mechanistic ambiguity of some common birth defects. Congenital heart defects occur in about 5 to 7/1000 live births. Heterotaxy, including l-TGA or ventricular inversion, accounts for about 3% of congenital heart defects (Lin et al., 2000; Loffredo, 2000). However, d-TGA and related malpositioning of the great arteries accounts for 9%–10% of heart defects. It is not yet clear whether the majority of TGA results from early patterning defects or disturbances in the septation of the common outflow tract. Intestinal malrotation, nonrotation, and reverse rotation are also very common birth defects (Rescorla et al., 1990). What percentage of malrotation, in the absence of other clear signs of heterotaxy, might be due to early embryonic axis disturbances versus later abnormalities in intestinal growth is an interesting question for future investigation. The true incidence of birth defects related to anomalies of the embryonic axes may be much higher than currently appreciated.

Inheritance

Familial clustering of situs inversus and situs ambiguus has been reported. The occurrence in siblings of unaffected parents and accompanying consanguinity has been interpreted as evidence for autosomal recessive inheritance (Hurwitz & Caskey, 1982; Cesko et al., 1997, 2001; Kosaki and Casey, 1998). Other pedigrees have been more suggestive of autosomal dominant inheritance with incomplete penetrance (Alonso et al., 1995; Casey et al., 1996). The occurrence of families with X-linked inheritance has been demonstrated by linkage analysis (HTX1, Xq26.2, OMIM 306955) and confirmed by mutant gene identification (ZIC3) (Casey et al., 1993; Gebbia et al., 1997). Most cases of heterotaxy are sporadic, and it has been assumed that mendelian inheritance represented the rare exception. However, approximately 10% of infants with heterotaxy have a family history of a close relative with congenital heart defects (Belmont JW, unpublished data). Some of these might not have been interpreted as LR patterning defects (e.g., hypoplastic left ventricle) outside the context of the index case. Familial clustering of d-TGA has also recently been reassessed, again pointing to the higher than expected occurrence of significant

congenital heart defects in relatives, although not always TGA (Digilio et al., 2001). Assessment of the familiality of LR defects is, therefore, complicated by lack of critical population-based data collection for family history, incomplete penetrance in families with apparent mendelian inheritance, and ambiguity as to the origin of atypical birth defects in close relatives. One may add to the observation of familial clustering some or all of the following factors: occurrence of heterotaxy defects within more complex multisystem syndromes or chromosomal disorders, unknown environmental liability factors, locus heterogeneity, allelic heterogeneity, sex differences, phenocopies, incomplete ascertainment due to fetal loss, and reduced family size due to burden of disease. Taken together, these are all typical of "complex traits." Although very challenging to investigate, there are several approaches, particularly those informed by animal models, that should clarify the inheritance patterns and the genetic causation of LR defects in the future.

Known Heterotaxy Disease Loci

Genes contributing to heterotaxy have been identified in a small but growing subset of sporadic and familial cases. Positional cloning has been utilized to identify the genetic cause of LR axis defects in one sporadic and four familial cases of LR axis malformation. In these cases, intragenic mutations in ZIC3, an X-linked zinc finger transcription factor, were found. ZIC3, which had not previously been implicated in vertebrate LR axis development, was the first gene to be unequivocally associated with human situs abnormalities (Gebbia et al., 1997). In these studies, most males with a ZIC3 mutation were situs ambiguus. The affected males had complex congenital heart defects, including dextrocardia, TGA, pulmonic atresia or stenosis, double outlet right ventricle (DORV), and common AV canal and right aortic arch. Both polysplenia and asplenia were seen. In one family, three of seven carrier females were situs inversus. However, in one unique family, the affected males had d-TGA and various midline defects without other signs of laterality defects. In addition, a maternal uncle bearing the associated ZIC3 mutation was phenotypically normal, thus demonstrating incomplete penetrance for this unique allele (Megarbane et al., 2000).

To date, rare mutations in ZIC3, ACVR2B, LEFTYA, and CRYPTIC have been found in humans with laterality defects; but together these account for fewer than 10% of patients with heterotaxy. Two unrelated patients with LEFTYA mutations were quite similar in their cardiac anatomy: d-looping of the ventricles with normally related great arteries, hypoplastic left ventricle, and complete AV canal defect with a common AV valve. Both had persistence of a left-sided superior vena cava, an unusual anatomical variant. Each had left pulmonary isomerism (Kosaki et al., 1999a). In contrast, patients with ACVR2B mutations had either ventricular inversion or d-TGA, left atrial isomerism, absence of the right superior vena cava, but normal pulmonary venous return. Visceral anomalies included asplenia or polysplenia and midline liver (Kosaki et al., 1999b). Mutations in CRYPTIC were associated with a mixed set of defects. Four patients were found to have heterozygous mutations. The mutations were associated with dextrocardia, TGA, and left atrial isomerism. Noncardiac anomalies included both left and right pulmonary isomerism, right-sided stomach, intestinal malrotation, and either asplenia or polysplenia (Bamford et al., 2000).

As noted below, CRYPTIC and ACVR2B are thought to play necessary roles in NODAL signaling, so one might assume that evidence of L-patterning failure would predominate, i.e. right pulmonary isomerism, asplenia, etc. The more complex picture present in this small number of patients strongly suggests that either earlier NODAL functions are disturbed or that alternative functions of CRYPTIC and ACVR2B are important in the phenotype. CRYPTIC mutations have also recently been detected in 2 of 86 patients with d-TGA or DORV but without other features of heterotaxy (Goldmuntz et al., 2002). This result is supportive of the supposition that patients with isolated forms of the characteristic heterotaxy heart defects or visceral abnormalities have causative mutations in LR patterning genes. More extensive surveys of LR patterning gene mutations in sporadic heterotaxy cases are in preparation, and the data should be available in the next several years.

DIAGNOSIS AND PROGNOSIS

Situs inversus may be asymptomatic and escape notice despite routine physical exam. Heterotaxy-type birth defects, however, most often present in the immediate newborn period because of cardiorespiratory distress or feeding difficulty. Physical examination may reveal dyspnea, cyanosis, and/or cardiac murmur because of CHD. Abnormal position of the point of maximum impact (PMI) and right-sided heart sounds may be present but can be difficult to appreciate. Abnormal oxygen saturation despite maximal inspired oxygen supplementation would strongly suggest malposition of the great arteries. If there is no accompanying ventricular or atrial septal defect, closure of the ductus arteriosus causes rapid deterioration. Chest radiograph may show a normal to minimally enlarged cardiac silhouette with displacement to the middle or right. The classic "egg on a string" appearance of isolated d-TGA may be created by a narrow superior mediastinum (because of the anterior/posterior relationship of the aorta and the main pulmonary artery). The diagnosis of d-TGA is made by echocardiography. An anterior aorta arising from the right ventricle along with a posteriorly positioned pulmonary artery arising from the left ventricle confirm the diagnosis. Because l-TGA or ventricular inversion is most often accompanied by other complex defects, these children most often also present with cardiorespiratory failure.

Intestinal obstruction secondary to malrotation or annular pancreas presents with poor feeding, abdominal distension, and bloody diarrhea. Volvulus may lead rapidly to bowel necrosis and then to sepsis and hypotension. Plain films of the abdomen may show a "double bubble" sign, i.e., distended stomach, little intraluminal gas in the affected segment, and then distended loops of small intestine distal to the obstruction (Long et al., 1996). Upper gastrointestinal series is expected to show abnormal position of the proximal jejunum with possible restriction to the right side. Volvulus is a more severe complication and may show a dilated duodenum terminating in a sharp beak-like or "corkscrew" shape.

The prognosis for patients with heterotaxy varies considerably depending on the specific constellation of congenital anomalies. For many patients, the type of congenital heart defect is the major determinant of long-term prognosis. There is some evidence that children with heterotaxy have increased cardiac-related morbidity and mortality compared to children with isolated heart defects of the same type. Evaluation of patients after bi-directional Glenn anastomosis showed a fourfold increased risk of mortality in patients with heterotaxy (Alejos et al., 1995). A 28-year Toronto study of patients with left atrial isomerism (Gilljam et al., 2000) and a 26-year study of patients with right atrial isomerism (Hashmi et al., 1998) indicated 5-year survival rates of 61% and 35%, respectively. The poor overall outcome prompted Gilljam et al. (2000) to suggest cardiac transplant as an alternative in select cases. At least one recent report suggests that cardiac transplant may offer improved outcome over standard surgical management for some high-risk heterotaxy patients (Larsen et al., 2002).

MANAGEMENT

Medical Management

Medical management in patients with heterotaxy is individualized and based on the underlying congenital malformations. The diagnostic evaluation of a patient with heterotaxy should include a number of imaging studies to document the anatomy. Echocardiogram and/or cardiac magnetic resonance imaging, abdominal and renal ultrasound, as well as vertebral X-rays to evaluate vertebral and rib anomalies should be performed. Consideration should be given to a barium swallow study to exclude malrotation as well as imaging of the CNS. The spleen can be evaluated by ultrasound and spleen function by a peripheral blood smear to document the presence or absence of Howell-Jolly bodies. A spleen scan can also be performed to evaluate spleen function. Current American Heart Association guidelines recommend antibiotic prophylaxis and pneumococcal vaccine for functional asplenia.

Surgical Management

Stabilization of typical d-TGA infants requires that adequate mixing of oxygenated blood for delivery to the systemic circulation be preserved or established. Some patients have either large ventral or atrial septal defects, so only supportive measures are required. A prostaglandin infusion may be needed to maintain patency of the ductus arteriosus. Balloon atrial septostomy via cardiac catheterization can be used to create an atrial septal defect, allowing some mixing of oxygenated blood for the systemic circulation. The Mustard or Senning procedure was considered standard of care until the more difficult arterial switch procedure was introduced (Van Praagh and Jung, 1991). These procedures use an intraatrial baffle to direct deoxygenated blood to the mitral valve and left ventricle, where it can be pumped into the pulmonary artery and lungs. Oxygenated blood from the lungs returns via the pulmonary veins to flow across the baffle to the tricuspid valve and right ventricle and, thus, into the aorta. However, these procedures led to late right ventricular failure due to the difference in right and left myocardial capability to serve the workload of the systemic circulation. In the arterial switch operation, the surgeon transects the aorta and main pulmonary artery, moves the main pulmonary artery anterior, moves the aorta posterior, and then moves the coronary arteries from anterior to posterior. The latter step requires great skill to avoid vessel damage and obstruction. Valvar pulmonary stenosis precludes the use of an arterial switch procedure, and then palliative procedures, such as the Rastelli repair, are employed (Kreutzer et al., 2000).

Volvulus requires detorsion and resection of obviously necrotic areas. Correction of malrotation is called *Ladd's procedure* and involves resection of the attachments of the colon to the abdominal wall (Ladd's bands). The mesentery of the midgut is divided, giving a broader base of attachment and thus making torsion unlikely. An appendectomy is performed on all patients because malposition of the appendix may make later diagnosis of appendicitis difficult. Recent literature suggests the use of less invasive laparoscopic adaptations of this procedure (Bass et al., 1998).

Counseling

Elicitation of a three-generation pedigree is the first requisite in counseling. A history of affected maternal uncles, for example, would strongly suggest X-linked inheritance and the potential diagnosis of HTX1 (ZIC3). Further counseling would then be greatly aided by direct mutation analysis of *ZIC3*, which is now clinically available (B. Casey, Children's and Women's Health Centre of British Columbia, Molecular Diagnostic Laboratory). Examples of both affected females, nonpenetrance in males, and very low sample size, however, make specific counseling more difficult. Bayesian methods that take into account information from the pedigree and mutation testing are preferred but are beyond the scope of this short chapter. In all pedigrees with "dominant" inheritance, there is evidence for variability in severity of the defects (expression) and lack of defects in obligate carriers (nonpenetrance). While the risk of transmission of the mutant allele is 50%, the risk of defects in practice appears to be substantially less. Variable expression and nonpenetrance may be influenced by background genes, specific modifier genes, sex, unknown environmental variables, and stochastic factors.

There have been many methodological limitations in previous studies of sibling recurrence risk for sporadic LR patterning defects. The most serious limitations include suitability of case definition, ascertainment bias, low response rates, and inadequate sample size. Taking into consideration all of these weaknesses, the observed recurrence risk ranges from 2.0% to 4.75% (Boughman et al., 1987; Maestri et al., 1988; Nora and Nora, 1988a,b; Weigel et al., 1989; Pradat, 1994). There are no available estimates of confidence intervals. Standard recurrence risk counseling for sporadic heterotaxy then is about 3%. Offspring recurrence data are even more limited, and no studies have examined heterotaxy defects per se (Rose et al., 1985). Taking into account all congenital heart defects, there is evidence that offspring recurrence risks are somewhat higher than would be expected from a pure multifactorial model (Rose et al., 1985; Nora and Nora, 1987; Whittemore, 1988; Digilio et al., 2001). There is also a consistently higher risk of offspring recurrence in affected mothers. A serious limitation of all of these studies is the inability to distinguish pedigrees in which there is evidence for segregation of a major gene (i.e., mendelian inheritance) from the more common sporadic cases. A significant component of the sibling and offspring recurrences may have originated from HTX1 or dominant families, and the risks to other families may be more modest.

DEVELOPMENTAL PATHOGENESIS

Heterotaxy, both situs ambiguus and situs inversus, results from abnormalities in the generation of the LR axis. Of the three body axes, anterior/posterior (AP), dorsal/ventral (DV) and LR, the LR axis is determined last. This patterning occurs in the embryo during gastrulation and is the result of several sequential developmental events (see Chapter 5 for extensive discussion). Initially, the left and right sides must be specified and oriented in relation to the AP and DV axes. Next, symmetry must be broken. This stage is recognized in animal models by asymmetrical gene expression. Subsequently, this signal must be propagated and transmitted. Pathways of asymmetrical gene expression have been elucidated in a variety of model organisms that result in a cascade of lateralized signaling which specifies morphological asymmetry. This asymmetrical gene expression occurs well before the first morphological sign of LR asymmetry, the rightward looping of the embryonic heart tube. Finally, the asymmetrical signal and positional information must be conferred upon individual organs to regulate asymmetrical and lateralized organogenesis. Conceptually, a breakdown in any of these steps will result in failure to correctly establish the LR axis and ultimately in a spectrum of abnormal morphogenesis varying in severity depending on the specific stage at which the defect occurs. Currently, the majority of insight into these pathways comes from various animal models, with the pathways of asymmetrical gene expression being the best characterized. Less is currently known about early and late events, i.e., the events contributing to the early assignment of the LR axis and the late events translating positional information to developing organs.

Throughout the development of LR asymmetry, at least three regions of the embryo play a key role. First, the node (Hensen's node [chick], Spemann's organizer [*Xenopus*], embryonic shield [zebrafish]) is a key structure involved in the early breaking of symmetry. Second, the embryonic midline, including the notochord and prospective floor plate of the ventral neural tube, plays a critical role in maintaining asymmetry. Third, the lateral plate mesoderm (LPM) is critical for asymmetrical gene expression and propagation of lateralized signaling (Fig. 26–1). Within each of these structures, specific signaling pathways generate and/or maintain LR asymmetry.

Here, we will give an overview of the current understanding of the generation of LR asymmetry with an emphasis on general pathways and relevance to human disease. Excellent reviews summarize more completely the divergent mechanisms of LR asymmetry in various model organisms (Mercola, 1999; Burdine and Schier, 2000; Mercola and Levin, 2001; Hamada et al., 2002).

Establishment of LR Asymmetry

How and where the early bilateral symmetry of the embryo is first broken leading to lateralized signaling and, ultimately, morphological asymmetry is not known. There is evidence that gap junctional communication plays a role in both chick and *Xenopus* prior to asymmetrical gene expression at the node (Levin and Mercola, 1998, 1999). In addition, the requirement has been recently demonstrated for differential ion flux created by H^+/K^+-ATPase activity during the first two cell divisions in *Xenopus* as well as in primitive streak-stage chick embryos in order to generate correct LR asymmetry (Levin et al., 2002). In mouse, targeted deletion of the calcium release channel polycystin-2, which is mutated in autosomal dominant polycystic kidney disease, results in LR patterning abnormalities, including right pulmonary isomerism (Pennekamp et al., 2002).

In the mouse, the node is the site of the earliest known molecular asymmetries and is essential for the development of LR asymmetry. Node cells have specialized monocilia that can generate a leftward flow of extraembryonic fluid via vortical ciliary motion (Sulik et al., 1994; Bellomo et al., 1996; Nonaka et al., 1998; Okada et al., 1999). A "nodal flow" hypothesis, in which the cilia at the node are responsible for initiating LR asymmetry by concentrating secreted factor(s) to the left, has been proposed. Recent data provide direct evidence for this model. In addition, node monocilia as well as LR dynein (LRD), a protein required for beating cilia, are conserved in mouse, chick, *Xenopus*, and zebrafish (Essner et al., 2002; Nonaka et al., 2002). This suggests the possibility of a shared mechanism of establishing asymmetry. However, it remains to be determined whether ciliary movement of particles is responsible for the initial symmetry breaking in all or any organisms. There are a number of observations, in addition to those mentioned previously, which suggest that divergent mechanisms for the initial establishment of LR asymmetry may exist, including the fact that the mechanics and timing of gastrulation differ by model organism, the timing of asymmetrical gene expression differs by model organism, and asymmetrical gene expression is not conserved. Further studies will be required to resolve the shared and unique molecular mechanisms underlying symmetry breaking in different model organisms.

Recent mouse gene-targeting experiments resulting in absent (kinesin *Kif3A/Kif3B, Tg737*/polaris, and winged helix factor *hepatocyte nuclear factor/forkhead homologue 4*) or immotile (*lrd*, the mutated gene in *iv* mice) nodal cilia result in mice with a randomized LR axis and further support the importance of node monocilia (Chen et al., 1998; Nonaka et al., 1998; Marszalek et al., 1999; Supp et al., 1999; Takeda et al., 1999; Murcia et al., 2000). Furthermore, disruption of the lateralized signaling cascade (see below) is noted in these mice, again suggesting that ciliary function is critical for the generation of LR asymmetry.

Study of the steps required for LR axis specification has been complicated by the fact that numerous genes which display asymmetrical expression in the chick are expressed symmetrically in the mouse and have an unclear role in LR patterning. In 1995, four genes, *Sonic hedgehog (Shh), nodal, HNF3β,* and *activin receptor IIA (ActRIIA)*, were identified as being expressed asymmetrically in the chick embryo (Levin et al., 1995). Only one of these, *nodal*, is expressed asymmetrically in mouse. The functional significance of this is unclear. In chick, expression of *ActRIIA* on the right of the embryo is the earliest known asymmetry. Other signaling centers, such as the LR coordinator, may play roles in vertebrates such as *Xenopus* (Hyatt and Yost, 1998).

Table 26–3 summarizes the animal models showing abnormalities in genes expressed within or near the node. In humans, the only known

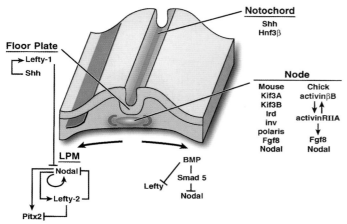

Figure 26–1. Overview of genetic pathways for left/right (LR) development. A schematic of a neural fold-stage embryo is shown. Embryonic ectoderm, node and notochord, and left lateral plate mesoderm (LPM) and perinodal endoderm are shown. Early asymmetric gene expression occurs around the node, differs in mouse and chick, and results in left-sided expression of *nodal.* Nodal monocilia are responsible for a leftward flow of morphogens. Expression of *lefty-1* in the midline provides a molecular barrier to maintain asymmetric left-sided morphogen expression. *Nodal* expression in the left LPM is limited by *lefty-2* and *lefty-1.* In chick, *caronte* transfers LR asymmetric information to repress bone morphogenetic protein (*BMP*)–mediated inhibition on the left and suppresses bone morphogenetic protein (*BMP*)–mediated inhibition on the left. The *nodal* signal on the left generates situs-specific morphogenesis via the transcription factor *pitx2.*

Table 26–3. Mutations in Model Organisms Affecting Left/Right and/or Axial Patterning

Gene	Role	Model	Phenotype	Reference
Node				
Kif3A	Kinesin superfamily	M	No nodal cilia, situs inversus or delayed looping, axial defects	Marszalek et al., 1999; Takeda et al., 1999
Kif3B	Kinesin superfamily	M	Defects similar to *Kif3A*, bilateral *pitx2*	Nonaka et al., 1998
T-brachyury	Transcription factor	M	Node, notochord defects; abn heart looping; nodal absent	King et al., 1998
iv/lrd	Axonemal dynein	M	Situs inversus/ambiguus/solitus; abn lefty, nodal; immotile cilia	Supp et al., 1997, 1999
Polaris/Tg737	Allelic to *orpk* insertional mutant	M	Mid-gestation arrest, NTD, pericardial enlargement, randomized looping, loss of node monocilia	Murcia et al., 2000
fgf8 −/neo	FGF signaling family	M	Situs inversus/no looping/R pulm isomerism, hypomorphic with variable phenotype	Meyers and Martin, 1999
HNF3β	Transcription factor	M	Lack of node and notochord, failure of turning and heart loopings	Ang and Rossant, 1994; Weinstein et al., 1994
inversin	Ankyrin repeat	M	90% situs inversus, 10% situs ambiguus, abn nodal flow	Yokoyama et al., 1993; Mochizuki et al., 1998; Morgan et al., 1998; Okada et al., 1999
Hfh-4/fkh	Transcription factor	M	Absence of cilia, lack of lrd; situs ambiguus	Chen et al., 1998
Gdf-1	TGF-β signaling	M	R pulm isomerism, heart defects	Rankin et al., 2000
Smoothened, Shh/Ihh	Hedgehog signaling	M	Failure to establish asymmetry; cyclopia; failure to turn; hedgehog signaling in node required for *Gdf-1*	Zhang et al., 2001
Midline				
HNF3β/nodal	Transcription factor/TGF-β	M	Situs ambiguus in compound heterozygotes, nodal bilateral	Collignon et al. 1996
Lefty-1	TGF-β signaling	M	Situs ambiguus; L pulm isomerism; bilateral *nodal, lefty2, pitx2*	Meno et al. 1998
SIL	Early response gene	M	Axial defects, randomized looping	Izraeli et al. 1999
Shh	Hedgehog signaling	M,C	L pulm isomerism; leftward heart, notochord degeneration, cyclopia; heterotaxia with misexpression in chick	Chiang et al. 1996; Levin et al. 1997; Izraeli et al. 1999; Meyers and Martin, 1999; Tsukui et al. 1999
No turning	Unknown	M	Notochord degeneration, caudal truncation, NTD, situs ambiguus	Melloy et al. 1998
Floating head	Transcription factor	Z	Absent notochord, randomized heart and gut looping	Halpern et al. 1995; Talbot et al. 1995; Danos and Yost, 1996
Pdi-p5	Protein disulfide isomerase	Z	Brain, heart, liver, pancreatic defects; bilat *lefty-1, lefty-2*	Hoshijima et al. 2002
Nodal Signaling Pathway				
Nodal −flloxed	TGF-β signaling	M	Hypomorphic nodal; phenotypic variability, least severe with situs ambiguus/TGA	Lowe et al. 2001
Cryptic/oep	EGF-CFC	M,Z	R pulm isomerism; asplenia: absent *nodal, lefty-2, pitx2*	Gaio et al. 1999; Yan et al. 1999
Lefty-2	TGF-β signaling	M	L isomerism, increased nodal diffusion	Meno et al. 1999, 2001

Gene	Function	Species	Phenotype	References
FoxH1(Fast)	TGF-β signaling	M	Lack of definitive node and derivatives, similar to HNF3β	Hoodless et al., 2001; Yamamoto et al., 2001
ActRIIB	TGF-β signaling	M	Situs ambiguus, R pulm isomerism, homeotic transformations of vertebral column	Oh and Li, 1997
Smad5	TGF-β signaling	M	Lethal by e11.5; loss of lefty-1, bilateral nodal, pitx2; heart looping defects; R pulm isomerism	Chang et al., 2000
Pitx2	Transcription factor	M,C,X	R pulm isomerism; situs inversus with misexpression in C, X	Gage et al., 1999; Kitamura et al., 1999; Lin et al., 1999; Liu et al., 2001
Smad2/nodal	TGF-β signaling	M	Abn gastrulation, holoprosenchephaly, R pulm isomerism; TGA	Nomura and Li, 1998
Cyclops(nodal)	TGF-β signaling	Z	Cyclopia, absent floor plate, randomized heart and gut looping	Hatta et al., 1991; Sampath et al., 1997; Schilling et al., 1999
caronte	TGF-β signaling	C	Randomized heart situs; misexpression induces ectopic lefty in R midline	Rodriguez Esteban et al., 1999; Yokouchi et al., 1999
BMP4	TGF-β signaling	M,C,X,Z	Early embryonic-lethal in mouse, situs ambiguus with overexpression, required for heart looping in Z	Winnier et al., 1995; Chen et al., 1997; Levin et al., 1997; Breckenridge et al., 2001
Derriere	TGF-β signaling	X	R ectopic expression gives situs inversus, dominant-negative situs ambiguus	Hanafusa et al., 2000
Other				
Mgat-1	GlcNAc transferase	M	Situs ambiguus with lethality e10.5	Metzler et al., 1994
Furin	Serine protease	M	Failure to turn; failure of heart looping; L pulm isomerism; cyclopia, craniofacial malformation	Constam and Robertson, 2000a,b
N-cadherin	Adhesion	C	Randomized heart looping; altered Snail, pitx2 expression	Garcia-Castro et al., 2000
Rotatin	Unknown	M	Randomized heart looping, delayed NT closure, failed axial rotation	Faisst et al., 2002
Claudin	Tight junction protein	X	Visceral situs randomization with overexpression	Brizuela et al., 2001
Fused toes/Fatso	Unknown	M	Random LR, craniofacial abnormality, thymic hyperplasia, partial syndactyly	Heymer et al., 1997; Peters et al., 1999
Zic3	Transcription factor	M,X	Gastrulation defects; vertebral defects; NTD, R/L pulm isomerism and inversion; randomized looping	Kitaguchi et al., 2000, 2002; Purandare et al., 2002
Bent tail	Microdeletion	M	Microdeletion encompasses Zic3 locus, LR patterning defects, omphalocele, orofacial clefting	Carrel et al., 2000; Klootwijk et al., 2000

Not all left/right (LR) defects or asymmetrically expressed genes are included in this table; several genes function in two or more categories; abn, abnormal; C, chick; e, embryonic day; L pulm, left pulmonary; M, mouse; NTD, neural tube defect; *oep*, one-eyed pinhead; *orpk*, Oak Ridge polycystic kidney; R pulm, right pulmonary; TGA, transposition of the grat arteries; X, *Xenopus*; Z, zebrafish.

defects associated with the specification stage of the LR axis are those associated with primary ciliary dysfunction (see Chapter 94). *Zic3* mutation carriers should be included in the molecular differential for patients with situs inversus (Gebbia et al., 1997). The *Zic3* mouse model corroborates a role for *Zic3* in axis specification (Purandare et al., 2002).

Propagation of Asymmetrical Gene Expression: Role of the Midline and LPM

Nodal is a critical member of the TGF-β family that initiates asymmetrical signaling from the node (Brennan et al., 2002). In the mouse and chick, *nodal* is initially expressed symmetrically in the perinodal region (Fig. 26–1). Subsequently, presumably as a result of the action of node monocilia, nodal expression becomes lateralized to the left side of the node between the two- to three-somite stage. This asymmetrical nodal expression at the node is followed by asymmetrical expression in the left LPM. *Nodal* signals appear to be determinants for left-sidedness in all vertebrates, and aberrant *nodal* expression, either at the node or in the LPM, will result in situs abnormalities (Collignon et al., 1996; Lowe et al., 1996; Meno et al., 1996; Sampath et al., 1997) (Table 26–3).

Thus far, signaling in the LPM appears to be the most highly conserved step of LR axis formation. Several genes in the LR pathway are expressed primarily in the LPM during gastrulation and are evolutionarily conserved among vertebrates, including *nodal* and *lefty-2*, members of the TGF-β family, and *pitx2*, a homeobox transcription factor. In addition, *lefty-1*, another TGF-β family member, is expressed primarily in the left prospective floor plate in mouse and chick (Fig. 26–1) (Meno et al., 1996).

The pathways required for the propagation of *nodal* signaling in the left LPM are beginning to be elucidated. In the presence of an EGF-CFC (*cryptic, one-eyed pinhead, cripto*) protein cofactor, *nodal* signals via Alk4 and Alk7 type I receptors and ActRIIA and ActRIIB type II receptors to activate Smad2 (and presumably Smad3), Smad4, and FAST (FoxHI) transcription factors (Fig. 26–2; also see Chapter 24) (reviewed in Schier and Shen, 2000; Schier and Talbot, 2001; Whitman, 2001). Cripto interaction with Alk4 is required for nodal binding to the Alk4/ActRIIB receptor complex and for activation of Smad2. Furthermore, heterodimers between nodal and bone morphogenetic proteins (BMPs) can inhibit BMP signaling, thus providing an additional mechanism for the generation of differential gene expression (Yeo and Whitman, 2001). In mouse, the potential targets of nodal signaling via FAST/FoxHI include *nodal, lefty-2, goosecoid, HNF3β* (*Foxa2*), and *pitx2*. Targeted deletion of *FAST/FoxH1* in the mouse causes a range of defects, consistent with the the broad role of *nodal* during development of the AP axis, the node, and LR asymmetry (Hoodless et al., 2001; Yamamoto et al., 2001).

Asymmetrical *nodal* signaling activates *Pitx2* transcription via the Smad–Fast pathway. In addition, *nodal* positively regulates its own tran-

scription as well as that of *lefty-2*. Both *lefty-1* and *lefty-2* inhibit *nodal* signaling, most likely by blocking nodal receptors, thereby serving to delimit the boundaries of "leftness" (Meno et al., 1996, 1998, 1999; Cheng et al., 2000). The limitation of both the range and duration of *nodal* expression appears to be critical to the establishment of correct LR asymmetry (Meno et al., 2001). In this cascade, *Pitx2* appears to be the most downstream gene and is expressed asymmetrically in the LPM as well as in developing organs, including the heart and visceral progenitors. The pathway including *nodal, lefty,* and *Pitx2* has been demonstrated in all four model organisms; and signal transduction via Smad and FAST has been demonstrated in mouse and *Xenopus*.

Failure to maintain asymmetrical expression of the *nodal, lefty,* and *pitx2* genes results in situs ambiguus. For example, in the mouse *iv* mutation, the genes are expressed randomly on the right, on the left, bilaterally, or not at all. Correspondingly, the mice show situs inversus, situs solitus, and situs ambiguus. In the *inv* mouse, in which situs inversus is seen, the *nodal* pathway genes are expressed on the right. Studies in mouse null mutants or hypomorphs indicate that absent expression of *nodal, lefty-2,* and *Pitx2* results in a "right-sided" phenotype, with right pulmonary isomerism, cardiac looping defects, and asplenia, whereas bilateral expression of the genes *lefty-1* and *Shh* results in a "left-sided" phenotype (Collignon et al., 1996; Lowe et al., 1996; Meno, 1996, 1998, 1999; Sampath et al., 1997; Meyers and Martin, 1999; Tsukui et al., 1999; Saijoh et al., 2000).

An understanding of the signaling pathways in the left LPM provides insight into the pathogenesis of the mutations described in human heterotaxy patients. In mice, null mutations in *ActRIIB* and *CRYPTIC/EFG-CFC* result in a failure of *nodal* signaling and, predictably, right isomerism (failure to establish leftness) (Table 26–3). Null mutations in *lefty-1* result in failure to restrict *nodal* to the left and, therefore, in left isomerism. However, the phenotypes found in patients with *EFG-CFC* and *ACVR2B* mutations, in which examples of both right isomerism and left isomerism are seen, are not so straighforward. There are a number of possible explanations for the discrepancies between mouse and human, including differences resulting from haploinsufficiency (human) vs. null (mouse) mutations, alternative functions of *CRYPTIC* and *ACVR2B,* a requirement for earlier *NODAL* functions, and differential effect of modifier genes. Closer analysis of the molecular phenotype of the model organisms shows that in both mouse and chick loss of *cryptic* results in loss of *lefty-1* expression, in addition to its other effects (Gaio et al., 1999; Yan et al., 1999; Schlange et al., 2001). This result would predict the development of left isomerism and provides a potential explanation for the variable LR phenotypes in patients. These results highlight the complexity of the signaling pathways and regulatory interactions involved in LR patterning. Further complexity arises from developmental stage-specific and threshold-specific differential responses. Because of the small number of patients identified, it is not yet possible to determine whether specific genotypes will be predictive of a given laterality spectrum.

Just as *nodal* signaling must be maintained and propagated on the left of the embryo, so must it be repressed on the right side. Recent evidence suggests that BMP signaling on the right side plays a role. In chick, suppression of BMP signaling on the left is required for nodal expression and BMP expression on the right inhibits nodal signaling. In mice lacking *Smad5,* a mediator of BMP signaling, *nodal* is expressed bilaterally (Chang et al., 2000). The zinc finger transcription factor *Snail* is another candidate for mediating right-sided gene expression. It is expressed asymmetrically on the right in chick and, to a lesser degree, in mouse. Its transcription is repressed by nodal signaling (Isaac et al., 1997; Patel et al., 1999; Nieto, 2002). Further delineation of its role in mediating right-sided gene expression will require identification of its downstream targets. *Dante,* a member of the mouse *Cerberus/Dan-related* gene family, is expressed on the right side of the node; but the significance of this asymmetrical expression is not yet known (Pearce et al., 1999).

Midline

The notochord and the prospective floor plate of the neural tube have also been implicated as playing a role in LR axis specification. As cells of the epiblast delaminate and invaginate during gastrulation, the

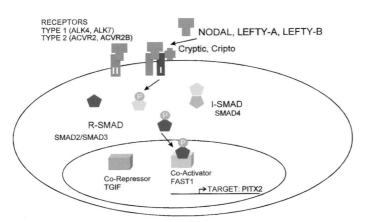

Figure 26–2. *Nodal* signal-transduction pathway follows the basic pattern of all TGF-β signaling (see Chapter 24). The known pathway-specific components are shown. The molecules highlighted in yellow are those in which human mutations have been demonstrated. However, patients with mutations in *TGIF* and *PITX2* do not exhibit obvious defects in left/right patterning.

mesodermal layer is established. Cells that migrate through the node during gastrulation establish the midline of the embryo, including the notochord. Inductive interactions subsequently occur between the notochord and ventral neural tube. Models that produce disruption of axial patterning of the mesoderm, either surgically or genetically, result in a concomitant disruption of LR axis formation, indicating that the midline plays a key role in separating the left from the right (Table 26–3). In addition, experiments in various model organisms suggest that key processes occur coincidentally with mesoderm induction and specification that are responsible for both the correct alignment of the midline axis as well as the assignment of left and right in relation to it.

As mentioned above, *lefty-1* expression in the mouse embryonic midline plays a critical role in generating LR asymmetry by restricting nodal expression. To date, there are no mouse mutants with midline defects that retain normal *lefty-1* expression in the prospective floor plate. The lefty proteins are divergent TGF-β family ligands. Humans and mice have two lefty genes each (*LEFTYA* and *LEFTYB* in humans, *lefty-1* and *lefty-2* in mice). *Xenopus* has a single lefty gene (*antivin*) (Kosaki et al., 1999a; Cheng et al., 2000). *Lefty* expression in the notochord and/or floor plate is conserved among vertebrates. In mouse and chick, *lefty-1* expression is induced by *sonic hedgehog.* In addition to a molecular barrier, the ventral side of the notochord contains monociliated cells that could theoretically contribute to a structural barrier function. It is not completely clear how the midline barrier functions and what additional genes play a role in its structural and molecular maintenance. Defects in the midline barrier and/or structural defects in the midline provide a potential explanation for the frequency of midline anomalies seen in human heterotaxy patients. In support of this, many midline defects, including CNS anomalies and vertebral anomalies, have been seen in animal models with LR patterning defects affecting this stage of LR axis patterning (Table 26–3).

Other Important Mediators of LR Asymmetry

In addition to the TGF-β family, there are a number of other important mediators of laterality. In general, the function of these genes is less well conserved between organisms. Genes belonging to families such as *Wnt,* fibroblast growth factor (*Fgf*), and *sonic hedgehog* (*Shh*) play roles not only in DV and AP patterning but also in the generation of LR asymmetry (see Chapters 16, 22, and 32). In chick, *Shh* is expressed asymmetrically and is a key signaling intermediate acting upstream of *nodal* and *lefty-1. Shh* induces *caronte,* a *Bmp2* and *Bmp4* antagonist, that allows activation of *nodal* and *lefty-1* both at the node and in the left LPM by relieving BMP-mediated repression (Burdine and Schier, 2000; Mercola and Levin, 2001). In both chick and mouse, *Shh* is able to induce *lefty-1* in the midline (see Fig. 26–1). In mouse, *Shh* is symmetrically expressed and has been proposed as a right determinant that functions to repress left-sided determinants on the right. Consistent with this, *Shh*[−/−] mice show bilateral *Pitx2* expression and no *lefty-1* expression. In addition, *Shh*[−/−] mice show axial patterning defects, consistent with a midline role via *lefty-1* (Chiang et al., 1996; Izraeli et al., 1999, 2001; Meyers and Martin, 1999; Tsukui et al., 1999).

In the mouse, *fgf8* is important for left-sidedness, acting upstream of nodal in the node. In chick, however, *fgf8* is expressed on the right side of the node and acts to suppress *caronte,* thereby allowing *BMP*-mediated repression of nodal signaling (Boettger et al., 1999; Meyers and Martin, 1999; Monsoro-Burq & Le Douarin, 2001).

Zic3 has been studied in both mouse and *Xenopus.* In mouse, it is dispensable for the initiation of *nodal* expression at the node but is required for the maintenance of *nodal* expression (Purandare et al., 2002). The wide phenotypic variability in mice as well as the finding of right isomerism, left isomerism, and situs inversus in both the mouse model and human patients with *Zic3* mutations suggests that *Zic3* acts at multiple stages within the LR asymmetry pathway (Gebbia et al., 1997; Purandare et al., 2002). In *Xenopus,* studies have suggested that *Zic3* acts upstream of *nodal* in the signaling cascade of LR asymmetry, and it has been suggested that *Zic3* may play a role in the specification of cells as either mesoderm or neuroectoderm. Overexpression of *Zic3* induces proneural genes as well as neural crest markers (Nakata et al., 1997; Kitaguchi et al., 2000; Koyabu et al., 2001). *Zic3*

can physically and functionally interact with members of the *Gli* superfamily, and the *Zic* gene family has been proposed to interact with genes important for patterning, including (*Shh*) (via Gli-dependent signaling) (Koyabu et al., 2001; Mizugishi et al., 2001) and *Fgf8.* However, there has been no definitive demonstration of these regulatory interactions in vivo.

Asymmetrical Organ Morphogenesis

The lateralized signaling that occurs in the left LPM must be translated to the individual internal organs. Very little is known about how these processes are coordinated. *Pitx2,* the most downstream component of the signaling pathway, is expressed in the left LPM in mouse, chick, *Xenopus,* and zebrafish and is the transcriptional target of *nodal* signaling. During organogenesis, *Pitx2* expression remains asymmetrical in the developing heart and gut (Logan et al., 1998; Piedra et al., 1998; Campione et al., 1999, 2001). There are three isoforms of pitx2 in the mouse (pitx2a, pitx2b, and pitx2c). Mouse embryos lacking *pitx2* exhibit right pulmonary isomerism and complex heart defects. In addition, the embryos fail to undergo proper embryonic turning (Gage et al., 1999; Kitamura et al., 1999; Lin et al., 1999; Lu et al., 1999). Targeting of the pitx2c isoform indicates that the dosage of pitx2c is critical for proper cardiac morphogenesis and that the atrial, ventricular, and outflow tract segments have a differential requirement for pitx2c, as does the developing lung (Liu et al., 2001).

The mechanisms by which *pitx2* mediates asymmetrical organogenesis are largely unknown. *Nodal* is a target of *pitx2* and regulates its own expression. In addition, procollagen lysyl hydroxylase (PLOD)-1, mutated in Ehlers-Danlos type 6, kyphoscoliosis type, and PLOD-2 are potential targets but unlikely candidates for LR patterning defects. It is also interesting to note that haploinsufficiency of *pitx2* is found in Rieger's syndrome, a genetically and phenotypically heterogeneous disorder characterized by anterior eye chamber abnormalities, hypodontia, and umbilical hernia. Heart defects can be seen in Rieger's syndrome, but heterotaxy is not characteristic.

Recent experiments have indicated a role for *BMP4* in mediating asymmetrical organogenesis in the heart. The function of *BMP4* is not yet clear and appears to differ by model organism. In both *Xenopus* and zebrafish, *BMP4* is expressed in the left linear heart and required for looping morphogenesis. Alterations in *BMP4* expression result in randomization or failure of looping (Chen et al., 1997; Branford et al., 2000; Breckenridge et al., 2001). Furthermore, in zebrafish, LR patterning of the heart is affected but the visceral organs are not (Schilling et al., 1999). This finding provides some insight into the discordant organ arrangements found in heterotaxy and suggests that each organ interprets signal independently. One would predict that additional signaling molecules will be identified which influence the LR patterning of individual organs and will result in further identification of differing thresholds of responsiveness, both within and between organs, during critical developmental windows. In chick, *BMP4* is critical for the maintenance of *Shh* asymmetry within the node. *BMP4* regulates expression of both *Fgf8* and *Shh* and, thus, is a critical coordinator of LR patterning (Monsoro-Burq and Le Douarin, 2000, 2001). Its role in asymmetrical organogenesis, however, is less clear. The role of *BMP4* in mouse LR asymmetry is also unclear due to early embryonic lethality in homozygotes (Winnier et al., 1995). Recent mouse models which circumvent the early lethality seen in *BMP4* knockout mice should facilitate further investigation of this gene's function (Fujiwara et al., 2002; Piedra and Ros, 2002). Further work will be required to better understand the molecular mechanisms by which aberrant early LR signals are translated into abnormal organogenesis. Investigations in this area show significant potential for further contributions to a molecular and mechanistic understanding of the development of heterotaxy.

One of the challenges for future studies of LR axis patterning will be to further delineate the shared and divergent mechanisms utilized by the various model organisms to achieve LR specification. In addition, investigation of the mechanisms underlying differential utilization and regulation of shared DV, AP, and LR signaling pathways will provide further insight into both the development of body pattern as well as the heterotaxy spectrum.

REFERENCES

Alejos JC, Williams RG, Jarmakani JM, Galindo AJ, Isabel-Jones JB, Drinkwater D, Laks H, Kaplan S (1995). Factors influencing survival in patients undergoing the bidirectional Glenn anastomosis. *Am J Cardiol* 75: 1048–1050.

Alonso S, Pierpont ME, Radtke W, Martinez J, Chen SC, Grant JW, Dahnert I, Taviaux S, Romey MC, Demaille J, et al. (1995). Heterotaxia syndrome and autosomal dominant inheritance. *Am J Med Genet* 56: 12–15.

Amor DJ, Craig JE (2001). Situs inversus totalis and congenital hypoglossia. *Clin Dysmorphol* 10: 47–50.

Ang SL, Rossant J (1994). *HNF-3 beta* is essential for node and notochord formation in mouse development. *Cell* 78: 561–574.

Aughton DJ (1990). Clinical anophthalmia, dextrocardia, and skeletal anomalies in an infant born to consanguineous parents. *Am J Med Genet* 37: 178–181.

Aylsworth AS (2001). Clinical aspects of defects in the determination of laterality. *Am J Med Genet* 101: 345–355.

Bahrt KM, Nashel DJ, Haber G (1983). Diffuse idiopathic skeletal hyperostosis in a patient with situs inversus. *Arthritis Rheum* 26: 811–812.

Balci S, Bostanoglu S, Altinok G, Ozaltin F (2000). New syndrome? Three sibs diagnosed prenatally with situs inversus totalis, renal and pancreatic dysplasia, and cysts. *Am J Med Genet* 90: 185–187.

Bamford RN, Roessler E, Burdine RD, Saplakoglu U, dela Cruz J, Splitt M, Goodship JA, Towbin J, Bowers P, Ferrero GB, et al. (2000). Loss-of-function mutations in the EGF-CFC gene *CFC1* are associated with human left–right laterality defects. *Nat Genet* 26: 365–369.

Bass KD, Rothenberg SS, Chang JH (1998). Laparoscopic Ladd's procedure in infants with malrotation. *J Pediatr Surg* 33: 279–281.

Bellomo D, Lander A, Harragan I, Brown NA (1996). Cell proliferation in mammalian gastrulation: the ventral node and notochord are relatively quiescent. *Dev Dyn* 205: 471–485.

Biben C, Harvey RP (1997). Homeodomain factor Nkx2-5 controls left/right asymmetric expression of bHLH gene *eHand* during murine heart development. *Genes Dev* 11: 1357–1369.

Bird LM, Newbury RO, Ruiz-Velasco R, Jones MC (1994). Recurrence of diaphragmatic agenesis associated with multiple midline defects: evidence for an autosomal gene regulating the midline. *Am J Med Genet* 53: 33–38.

Boettger T, Wittler L, Kessel M (1999). FGF8 functions in the specification of the right body side of the chick. *Curr Biol* 9: 277–280.

Bonnemann CG, Meinecke P (1996). Bilateral porencephaly, cerebellar hypoplasia, and internal malformations: two siblings representing a probably new autosomal recessive entity. *Am J Med Genet* 63: 428–433.

Bosch-Banyeras JM, Zuasnabar A, Puig A, Catala M, Cuatrecasas JM (1984). Poland-Mobius syndrome associated with dextrocardia. *J Med Genet* 21: 70–71.

Boughman JA, Berg KA, Astemborski JA, Clark EB, McCarter RJ, Rubin JD, Ferencz C (1987). Familial risks of congenital heart defect assessed in a population-based epidemiologic study. *Am J Med Genet* 26: 839–849.

Branford WW, Essner JJ, Yost HJ (2000). Regulation of gut and heart left–right asymmetry by context-dependent interactions between *Xenopus* lefty and BMP4 signaling. *Dev Biol* 223: 291–306.

Breckenridge RA, Mohun TJ, Amaya E (2001). A role for BMP signalling in heart looping morphogenesis in *Xenopus*. *Dev Biol* 232: 191–203.

Brennan J, Norris DP, Robertson EJ (2002). Nodal activity in the node governs left–right asymmetry. *Genes Dev* 16: 2339–2344.

Brizuela BJ, Wessely O, De Robertis EM (2001). Overexpression of the *Xenopus* tight-junction protein claudin causes randomization of the left–right body axis. *Dev Biol* 230: 217–229.

Brown NA, Anderson RH (1999). Symmetry and laterality in the human heart: developmental implications. In: *Heart Development*. Harvey RP, Rosenthal N (eds.) Academic Press, San Diego, pp. 447–461.

Burdine RD, Schier AF (2000). Conserved and divergent mechanisms in left–right axis formation. *Genes Dev* 14: 763–776.

Campione M, Steinbeisser H, Schweickert A, Deissler K, van Bebber F, Lowe LA, Nowotschin S, Viebahn C, Haffter P, Kuehn MR, et al. (1999). The homeobox gene Pitx2: mediator of asymmetric left–right signaling in vertebrate heart and gut looping. *Development* 126: 1225–1234.

Campione M, Acardo JM, Piedra E, Christoffels VM, Schweickert A, Blum M, Franco D, Moorman AF (2001). Pitx2 expression defines a left cardiac lineage of cells: evidence for atrial and ventricular molecular isomerism in the *iv/iv* mice. *Dev Biol* 231: 252–264.

Caravella L, Rogers GL (1978). Dextrocardia and ventricular septal defect in the Mobius syndrome. *Ann Ophthalmol* 10: 572–575.

Carile L, Verdone F, Aiello A, Buongusto G (1989). Diffuse idiopathic skeletal hyperostosis and situs viscerum inversus. *J Rheumatol* 16: 1120–1122.

Carrel T, Purandare SM, Harrison W, Elder F, Fox T, Casey B, Herman GE (2000). The X-linked mouse mutation Bent tail is associated with a deletion of the *Zic3* locus. *Hum Mol Genet* 9: 1937–1942.

Casey B, Devoto M, Jones K, Ballabio A (1993). Mapping a gene for familial situs abnormalities to human chromosome Xq24-q27.1. *Nat Genet* 5: 403–407.

Casey B, Cuneo B, Vitali C, van Hecke H, Barrish J, Hicks J, Ballabio A, Hoo J (1996). Autosomal dominant transmission of familial laterality defects. *Am J Med Genet* 61: 325–328.

Cesko I, Hajdu J, Toth T, Marton T, Papp C, Papp Z (1997). Ivemark syndrome with asplenia in siblings. *J Pediatr* 130: 822–824.

Cesko I, Hajdu J, Marton T, Tarnai L, Papp Z (2001). Polysplenia and situs inversus in siblings. Case reports. *Fetal Diagn Ther* 16: 1–3.

Chabrolle JP, Labenne M, Cailliez D, Poinsot J, Bruel H, Vercoustre L (1998). Hypoglossia, situs inversus and absence of the pituitary in a neonate: teratogenic effect of maternal hyperthermia? [in French]. *Arch Pediatr* 5: 163–166.

Chang H, Zwijsen A, Vogel H, Huylebroeck D, Matzuk MM (2000). *Smad5* is essential for left–right asymmetry in mice. *Dev Biol* 219: 71–78.

Chen CP, Chang TY, Tzen CY, Lin CJ, Wang W (2002). Sonographic detection of situs inversus, ventricular septal defect, and short-rib polydactyly syndrome type III (Verma-Naumoff) in a second-trimester fetus not known to be at risk. *Ultrasound Obstet Gynecol* 19: 629–631.

Chen J, Knowles H, Hebert J, Hackett B (1998). Mutation of the mouse hepatocyte nuclear factor/forkhead homologue 4 gene results in an absence of cilia and random left–right asymmetry. *J Clin Invest* 102: 1077–1082.

Chen JN, van Eeden FJ, Warren KS, Chin A, Nusslein-Volhard C, Haffter P, Fishman MC (1997). Left–right pattern of cardiac BMP4 may drive asymmetry of the heart in zebrafish. *Development* 124: 4373–4382.

Cheng AM, Thisse B, Thisse C, Wright CV (2000). The lefty-related factor Xatv acts as a feedback inhibitor of nodal signaling in mesoderm induction and L-R axis development in *Xenopus*. *Development* 127: 1049–1061.

Chiang C, Litingtung Y, Lee E, Young K, Corden J, Westphal H, Beachy P (1996). Cyclopia and defective axial patterning in mice lacking *Sonic hedgehog* gene function. *Nature* 383: 407–413.

Ciocci A (1987). Diffuse idiopathic skeletal hyperostosis (DISH) and situs viscerum inversus. Report of a single case. *Clin Exp Rheumatol* 5: 159–160.

Collignon J, Varlet I, Robertson EJ (1996). Relationship between asymmetric nodal expression and the direction of embryonic turning. *Nature* 381: 155–158.

Constam DB, Robertson EJ (2000a). SPC4/PACE4 regulates a TGFbeta signaling network during axis formation. *Genes Dev* 14: 1146–1155.

Constam DB, Robertson EJ (2000b). Tissue-specific requirements for the proprotein convertase furin/SPC1 during embryonic turning and heart looping. *Development* 127: 245–254.

Correa-Villasenor A, McCarter R, Downing J, Ferencz C (1991). White–black differences in cardiovascular malformations in infancy and socioeconomic factors. The Baltimore–Washington Infant Study Group. *Am J Epidemiol* 134: 393–402.

Cumming WA, Ohlsson A, Ali A (1986). Campomelia, cervical lymphocele, polycystic dysplasia, short gut, polysplenia. *Am J Med Genet* 25: 783–790.

Danos MC, Yost HJ (1996). Role of notochord in specification of cardiac left–right orientation in zebrafish and Xenopus. *Dev Biol* 177: 96–103.

Deveci MS, Deveci G (2000). Biliary atresia splenic malformation syndrome—is it a result of embryonically midline rotational defects? A case report. *J Pediatr Surg* 35: 1377–1380.

Digilio MC, Marino B, Ammirati A, Borzaga U, Giannotti A, Dallapiccola B (1999). Cardiac malformations in patients with oral-facial-skeletal syndromes: clinical similarities with heterotaxia. *Am J Med Genet* 84: 350–356.

Digilio MC, Casey B, Toscano A, Calabro R, Pacileo G, Marasini M, Banaudi E, Giannotti A, Dallapiccola B, Marino B (2001). Complete transposition of the great arteries: patterns of congenital heart disease in familial precurrence. *Circulation* 104: 2809–2814.

Ditchfield MR, Hutson JM (1998). Intestinal rotational abnormalities in polysplenia and asplenia syndromes. *Pediatr Radiol* 28: 303–306.

Donlan MA, Murphy JJ, Brakel CA (1969). Ellis-van Creveld syndrome associated with complete situs inversus. *Clin Pediatr (Phila)* 8: 366–368.

Dunham ME, Austin TL (1990). Congenital aglossia and situs inversus. *Int J Pediatr Otorhinolaryngol* 19: 163–168.

Elcioglu N, Hall CM (1998). A lethal skeletal dysplasia with features of chondrodysplasia punctata and osteogenesis imperfecta: an example of Astley-Kendall dysplasia. Further delineation of a rare genetic disorder. *J Med Genet* 35: 505–507.

Essner JJ, Vogan KJ, Wagner MK, Tabin CJ, Yost HJ, Brueckner M (2002). Conserved function for embryonic nodal cilia. *Nature* 418: 37–38.

Faisst AM, Alvarez-Bolado G, Treichel D, Gruss P (2002). *Rotatin* is a novel gene required for axial rotation and left–right specification in mouse embryos. *Mech Dev* 113: 15–28.

Feingold B, O'Sullivan B, del Nido P, Pollack P (2001). Situs inversus totalis and corrected transposition of the great arteries [I,D,D] in association with a previously unreported vascular ring. *Pediatr Cardiol* 22: 338–342.

Fokstuen S, Schinzel A (2000). Unilateral lobar pulmonary agenesis in sibs. *J Med Genet* 37: 557–559.

Fraser FC, Teebi AS, Walsh S, Pinsky L (1997). Poland sequence with dextrocardia: which comes first? *Am J Med Genet* 73: 194–196.

Fujiwara T, Dehart DB, Sulik KK, Hogan BL (2002). Distinct requirements for extra-embryonic and embryonic bone morphogenetic protein 4 in the formation of the node and primitive streak and coordination of left–right asymmetry in the mouse. *Development* 129: 4685–4696.

Gage PJ, Suh H, Camper SA (1999). Dosage requirement of Pitx2 for development of multiple organs. *Development* 126: 4643–4651.

Gaio U, Schweickert A, Fischer A, Garratt AN, Muller T, Ozcelik C, Lankes W, Strehle M, Britsch S, Blum M, et al. (1999). A role of the *cryptic* gene in the correct establishment of the left–right axis. *Curr Biol* 9: 1339–1342.

Garcia-Castro MI, Vielmetter E, Bronner-Fraser M (2000). N-Cadherin, a cell adhesion molecule involved in establishment of embryonic left–right asymmetry. *Science* 288: 1047–1051.

Gebbia M, Ferrero GB, Pilia G, Bassi MT, Aylsworth AS, Penman-Splitt M, Bird LM, Bamford JS, Burn J, Schlessinger D, et al. (1997). X-linked situs abnormalities result from mutations in *ZIC3*. *Nat Genet* 17: 305–308.

Gillessen-Kaesbach G, Meinecke P, Garrett C, Padberg BC, Rehder H, Passarge E (1993). New autosomal recessive lethal disorder with polycystic kidneys type Potter I, characteristic face, microcephaly, brachymelia, and congenital heart defects. *Am J Med Genet* 45: 511–518.

Gilljam T, McCrindle BW, Smallhorn JF, Williams WG, Freedom RM (2000). Outcomes of left atrial isomerism over a 28-year period at a single institution. *J Am Coll Cardiol* 36: 908–916.

Goldmuntz E, Bamford R, Karkera JD, dela Cruz J, Roessler E, Muenke M (2002). *CFC1* mutations in patients with transposition of the great arteries and double-outlet right ventricle. *Am J Hum Genet* 70: 776–780.

Halpern ME, Thisse C, Ho RK, Thisse B, Riggleman B, Trevarrow B, Weinberg ES, Postlethwait JH, Kimmel CB (1995). Cell-autonomous shift from axial to paraxial mesodermal development in zebrafish floating head mutants. *Development* 121: 4257–4264.

Hamada H, Meno C, Watanabe D, Saijoh Y (2002). Establishment of vertebrate left–right asymmetry. *Nat Rev Genet* 3: 103–113.

Hanafusa H, Masuyama N, Kusakabe M, Shibuya H, Nishida E (2000). The TGF-beta family member derriere is involved in regulation of the establishment of left–right asymmetry. *EMBO Rep* 1: 32–39.

Harvey RP, Rosenthal N (1999). *Heart Development*. Academic Press, San Diego, 530 pp.

Hashmi A, Abu-Sulaiman R, McCrindle BW, Smallhorn JF, Williams WG, Freedom RM (1998). Management and outcomes of right atrial isomerism: a 26-year experience. *J Am Coll Cardiol* 31: 1120–1126.

Hatta K, Kimmel C, Ho R, Walker C (1991). The cyclops mutation blocks specification of the floor plate of the zebrafish central nervous system. *Nature* 350: 339–341.

Hegerty AS, Anderson RH, Ho SY (1985). Congenital heart malformations in the first year of life—a necropsy study. *Br Heart J* 54: 583–592.

Hersh JH, McChane RH, Rosenberg EM, Powers WH Jr, Corrigan C, Pancratz L (1989). Otocephaly–midline malformation association. *Am J Med Genet* 34: 246–249.

Heymer J, Kuehn M, Ruther U (1997). The expression pattern of *nodal* and *lefty* in the mouse mutant Ft suggests a function in the establishment of handedness. *Mech Dev* 66: 5–11.

Hoodless PA, Pye M, Chazaud C, Labbe E, Attisano L, Rossant J, Wrana JL (2001). FoxH1 (Fast) functions to specify the anterior primitive streak in the mouse. *Genes Dev* 15: 1257–1271.

Hoshijima K, Metherall JE, Grunwald DJ (2002). A protein disulfide isomerase expressed in the embryonic midline is required for left/right asymmetries. *Genes Dev* 16: 2518–2529.

Hurwitz RC, Caskey CT (1982). Ivemark syndrome in siblings. *Clin Genet* 22: 7–11.

Hyatt B, Yost HJ (1998). The left–right coordinator: the role of Vg1 in organizing left–right axis formation. *Cell* 93: 37–48.

Isaac A, Sargent MG, Cooke J (1997). Control of vertebrate left–right asymmetry by a *snail*-related zinc finger gene. *Science* 275: 1301–1304.

Izpisua Belmonte JC (1999). How the body tells left from right. *Sci Am* 280: 46–51.

Izraeli S, Lowe LA, Bertness VL, Good DJ, Dorward DW, Kirsch IR, Kuehn MR (1999). The *SIL* gene is required for mouse embryonic axial development and left–right specification. *Nature* 399: 691–694.

Izraeli S, Lowe LA, Bertness VL, Campaner S, Hahn H, Kirsch IR, Kuehn MR (2001). Genetic evidence that *Sil* is required for the Sonic Hedgehog response pathway. *Genesis* 31: 72–77.

Kennerknecht I, Sorgo W, Oberhoffer R, Teller WM, Mattfeldt T, Negri G, Vogel W (1993). Familial occurrence of agonadism and multiple internal malformations in phenotypically normal girls with 46,XY and 46,XX karyotypes, respectively: a new autosomal recessive syndrome. *Am J Med Genet* 47: 1166–1170.

King T, Beddington RS, Brown NA (1998). The role of the *brachyury* gene in heart development and left–right specification in the mouse. *Mech Dev* 79: 29–37.

Kitaguchi T, Nagai T, Nakata K, Aruga J, Mikoshiba K (2000). *Zic3* is involved in the left–right specification of the *Xenopus* embryo. *Development* 127: 4787–4795.

Kitaguchi T, Mizugishi K, Hatayama M, Aruga J, Mikoshiba K (2002). *Xenopus Brachyury* regulates mesodermal expression of *Zic3*, a gene controlling left–right asymmetry. *Dev Growth Differ* 44: 55–61.

Kitamura K, Miura H, Miyagawa-Tomita S, Yanazawa M, Katoh-Fukui Y, Suzuki R, Ohuchi H, Suehiro A, Motegi Y, Nakahara Y, et al. (1999). Mouse Pitx2 deficiency leads to anomalies of the ventral body wall, heart, extra- and periocular mesoderm and right pulmonary isomerism. *Development* 126: 5749–5758.

Klootwijk R, Franke B, van der Zee CE, de Boer RT, Wilms W, Hol FA, Mariman EC (2000). A deletion encompassing *Zic3* in bent tail, a mouse model for X-linked neural tube defects. *Hum Mol Genet* 9: 1615–1622.

Kosaki K, Casey B (1998). Genetics of human left–right axis malformations. *Semin Cell Dev Biol* 9: 89–99.

Kosaki K, Bassi MT, Kosaki R, Lewin M, Belmont J, Schauer G, Casey B (1999a). Characterization and mutation analysis of human *LEFTY A* and *LEFTY B*, homologues of murine genes implicated in left–right axis development. *Am J Hum Genet* 64: 712–721.

Kosaki R, Gebbia M, Kosaki K, Lewin M, Bowers P, Towbin JA, Casey B (1999b). Left–right axis malformations associated with mutations in *ACVR2B*, the gene for human activin receptor type IIB. *Am J Med Genet* 82: 70–76.

Koyabu Y, Nakata K, Mizugishi K, Aruga J, Mikoshiba K (2001). Physical and functional interactions between Zic and Gli proteins. *J Biol Chem* 276: 6889–6892.

Kresca LJ, Goldberg MF (1978). Peters' anomaly: dominant inheritance in one pedigree and dextrocardia in another. *J Pediatr Ophthalmol Strabismus* 15: 141–146.

Kreutzer C, De Vive J, Oppido G, Kreutzer J, Gauvreau K, Freed M, Mayer JE Jr, Jonas R, del Nido PJ (2000). Twenty-five-year experience with rastelli repair for transposition of the great arteries. *J Thorac Cardiovasc Surg* 120: 211–223.

Kroes EJ, Festen C (1998). Congenital microgastria: a case report and review of literature. *Pediatr Surg Int* 13: 416–418.

Kumar A, Friedman JM, Taylor GP, Patterson MW (1993). Pattern of cardiac malformation in oculoauriculovertebral spectrum. *Am J Med Genet* 46: 423–426.

Lander A, King T, Brown NA (1998). Left–right development: mammalian phenotypes and conceptual models. *Semin Cell Dev Biol* 9: 35–41.

Larsen R, Eguchi J, Mulla N, Johnston J, Fitts J, Kuhn M, Razzouk A, Chinnock R, Bailey L (2002). Usefulness of cardiac transplantation in children with visceral heterotaxy (asplenic and polysplenic syndromes and single right-sided spleen with levocardia) and comparison of results with cardiac transplantation in children with dilated cardiomyopathy. *Am J Cardiol* 89: 1275–1279.

Layton WM (1989). Situs inversus in conjoined twins. *Am J Med Genet* 34: 297.

Leech RW, Bowlby LS, Brumback RA, Schaefer GB Jr (1988). Agnathia, holoprosencephaly, and situs inversus: report of a case. *Am J Med Genet* 29: 483–490.

Levin M, Mercola M (1998). Gap junctions are involved in the early generation of left–right asymmetry. *Dev Biol* 202: 90–105.

Levin M, Mercola M (1999). Gap junction–mediated transfer of left–right patterning signals in the early chick blastoderm is upstream of Shh asymmetry in the node. *Development* 126: 4703–4714.

Levin M, Johnson RL, Stern CD, Kuehn M, Tabin C (1995). A molecular pathway determining left–right asymmetry in chick embryogenesis. *Cell* 82: 803–814.

Levin M, Pagan S, Roberts DJ, Cooke J, Kuehn MR, Tabin CJ (1997). Left/right patterning signals and the independent regulation of different aspects of situs in the chick embryo. *Dev Biol* 189: 57–67.

Levin M, Thorlin T, Robinson KR, Nogi T, Mercola M (2002). Asymmetries in H^+/K^+-ATPase and cell membrane potentials comprise a very early step in left–right patterning. *Cell* 111: 77–89.

Lian ZH, Zack MM, Erickson JD (1986). Paternal age and the occurrence of birth defects. *Am J Hum Genet* 39: 648–660.

Lin AE, Ticho BS, Houde K, Westgate MN, Holmes LB (2000). Heterotaxy: associated conditions and hospital-based prevalence in newborns. *Genet Med* 2: 157–172.

Lin CR, Kioussi C, O'Connell S, Briata P, Szeto D, Liu F, Izpisua-Belmonte JC, Rosenfeld MG (1999). Pitx2 regulates lung asymmetry, cardiac positioning and pituitary and tooth morphogenesis. *Nature* 401: 279–282.

Lin HJ, Owens TR, Sinow RM, Fu PC Jr, DeVito A, Beall MH, Lachman RS (1998). Anomalous inferior and superior venae cavae with oculoauriculovertebral defect: review of Goldenhar complex and malformations of left–right asymmetry. *Am J Med Genet* 75: 88–94.

Liu C, Liu W, Lu MF, Brown NA, Martin JF (2001). Regulation of left–right asymmetry by thresholds of Pitx2c activity. *Development* 128: 2039–2048.

Loffredo CA (2000). Epidemiology of cardiovascular malformations: prevalence and risk factors. *Am J Med Genet* 97: 319–325.

Logan M, Pagan-Westphal SM, Smith DM, Paganessi L, Tabin CJ (1998). The transcription factor Pitx2 mediates situs-specific morphogenesis in response to left–right asymmetric signals. *Cell* 94: 307–317.

Long FR, Kramer SS, Markowitz RI, Taylor GE (1996). Radiographic patterns of intestinal malrotation in children. *Radiographics* 16: 547–560.

Lowe LA, Supp DM, Sampath K, Yokoyama T, Wright CV, Potter SS, Overbeek P, Kuehn M (1996). Conserved left–right asymmetry of *nodal* expression and alterations in murine situs inversus. *Nature* 381: 158–161.

Lowe LA, Yamada S, Kuehn MR (2001). Genetic dissection of *nodal* function in patterning the mouse embryo. *Development* 128: 1831–1843.

Lu MF, Pressman C, Dyer R, Johnson RL, Martin JF (1999). Function of Rieger syndrome gene in left–right asymmetry and craniofacial development. *Nature* 401: 276–278.

Lurie IW, Kirillova IA, Novikova IV, Burakovski IV (1991). Renal-hepatic-pancreatic dysplasia and its variants. *Genet Couns* 2: 17–20.

Macayran JF, Doroshow RW, Phillips J, Sinow RM, Furst BA, Smith LM, Lin HJ (2002). PAGOD syndrome: eighth case and comparison to animal models of congenital vitamin A deficiency. *Am J Med Genet* 108: 229–234.

Maestri NE, Beaty TH, Liang KY, Boughman JA, Ferencz C (1988). Assessing familial aggregation of congenital cardiovascular malformations in case-control studies. *Genet Epidemiol* 5: 343–354.

Manner J (2000). Cardiac looping in the chick embryo: a morphological review with special reference to terminological and biomechanical aspects of the looping process. *Anat Rec* 259: 248–262.

Marszalek JR, Ruiz-Lozano P, Roberts E, Chien KR, Goldstein LS (1999). Situs inversus and embryonic ciliary morphogenesis defects in mouse mutants lacking the KIF3A subunit of kinesin-II. *Proc Natl Acad Sci USA* 96: 5043–5048.

Martinez-Frias ML (2001). Heterotaxia as an outcome of maternal diabetes: an epidemiological study. *Am J Med Genet* 99: 142–146.

Mazziotti MV, Willis LK, Heuckeroth RO, LaRegina MC, Swanson PE, Overbeek PA, Perlmutter DH (1999). Anomalous development of the hepatobiliary system in the Inv mouse. *Hepatology* 30: 372–378.

Megarbane A, Salem N, Stephan E, Ashoush R, Lenoir D, Delague V, Kassab R, Loiselet J, Bouvagnet P (2000). X-linked transposition of the great arteries and incomplete penetrance among males with a nonsense mutation in *ZIC3*. *Eur J Hum Genet* 8: 704–708.

Meinecke P, Padberg B, Laas R (1990). Agnathia, holoprosencephaly, and situs inversus: a third report. *Am J Med Genet* 37: 286–287.

Melloy P, Ewart J, Cohen M, Desmond M, Kuehn M, Lo C (1998). *No turning*, a mouse mutation causing left-right and axial patterning defects. *Dev Biol* 193: 77–89.

Meno C, Saijoh Y, Fujii H, Ikeda M, Yodoyama T, Yokoyama M, Toyoda Y, Hamada H (1996). Left–right asymmetric expression of the TGFβ family member lefty in mouse embryos. *Nature* 381: 151–155.

Meno C, Shimono A, Saijoh Y, Yashiro K, Mochida K, Ohishi S, Noji S, Kondoh H, Hamada H (1998). lefty-1 is required for left–right determination as a regulator of lefty-2 and nodal. *Cell* 94: 287–297.

Meno C, Gritsman K, Ohishi S, Ohfuji Y, Heckscher E, Mochida K, Shimono A, Kondoh H, Talbot WS, Robertson EJ, et al. (1999). Mouse Lefty2 and zebrafish antivin are feedback inhibitors of nodal signaling during vertebrate gastrulation. *Mol Cells* 4: 287–298.

Meno C, Takeuchi J, Sakuma R, Koshiba-Takeuchi K, Ohishi S, Saijoh Y, Miyazaki J, ten Dijke P, Ogura T, Hamada H (2001). Diffusion of nodal signaling activity in the absence of the feedback inhibitor Lefty2. *Dev Cell* 1: 127–138.

Mercola M (1999). Embryological basis for cardiac left–right asymmetry. *Semin Cell Dev Biol* 10: 109–116.

Mercola M, Levin M (2001). Left–right asymmetry determination in vertebrates. *Annu Rev Cell Dev Biol* 17: 779–805.

Metzler M, Gertz A, Sarkar M, Schachter H, Schrader J, Marth J (1994). Complex asparagine-linked oligosaccharides are required for morphogenic events during post-implantation development. *EMBO J* 13: 2056–2065.

Meyers EN, Martin GR (1999). Differences in left-right axis pathways in mouse and chick: functions of *FGF8* and *SHH*. *Science* 285: 403–406.

Ming JE, McDonald-McGinn DM, Markowitz RI, Ruchelli E, Zackai EH (1997). Heterotaxia in a fetus with campomelia, cervical lymphocele, polysplenia, and multicystic dysplastic kidneys: expanding the phenotype of Cumming syndrome. *Am J Med Genet* 73: 419–424.

Mituszova M, Molnar E (1984). Another report of diffuse idiopathic skeletal hyperostosis. *Arthritis Rheum* 27: 1074.

Mizugishi K, Aruga J, Nakata K, Mikoshiba K (2001). Molecular properties of Zic proteins as transcriptional regulators and their relationship to GLI proteins. *J Biol Chem* 276: 2180–2188.

Mochizuki T, Saijoh Y, Tsuchiya K, Shirayoshi Y, Takai S, Taya C, Yonekawa H, Yamada K, Nihei H, Nakatsuji N, et al. (1998). Cloning of *inv*, a gene that controls left/right asymmetry and kidney development. *Nature* 395: 177–181.

Monsoro-Burq A, Le Douarin N (2000). Left–right asymmetry in BMP4 signalling pathway during chick gastrulation. *Mech Dev* 97: 105–108.

Monsoro-Burq A, Le Douarin NM (2001). BMP4 plays a key role in left–right patterning in chick embryos by maintaining Sonic Hedgehog asymmetry. *Mol Cell* 7: 789–799.

Morgan D, Turnpenny L, Goodship J, Dai W, Majumder K, Matthews L, Gardner A, Schuster G, Vien L, Harrison W, et al. (1998). *Inversin*, a novel gene in the vertebrate left–right axis pathway, is partially deleted in the *inv* mouse. *Nat Genet* 20: 149–156.

Morishima M, Yasui H, Ando M, Nakazawa M, Takao A (1996). Influence of genetic and maternal diabetes in the pathogenesis of visceroatrial heterotaxy in mice. *Teratology* 54: 183–190.

Mubashir MA, Sabry MA, Farah S, Haseeb N, Quasrawi B, al-Busairi W, al-Dabbous R, al-Awadi SA, Farag TI (1999). New syndromic entity of situs inversus totalis. *Clin Dysmorphol* 8: 23–27.

Murcia NS, Richards WG, Yoder BK, Mucenski ML, Dunlap JR, Woychik RP (2000). The Oak Ridge polycystic kidney (*orpk*) disease gene is required for left–right axis determination. *Development* 127: 2347–2355.

Nachlieli T, Gershoni-Baruch R (1992). Dextrocardia, microphthalmia, cleft palate, choreoathetosis, and mental retardation in an infant born to consanguineous parents. *Am J Med Genet* 42: 458–460.

Nakata K, Nagai T, Aruga J, Mikoshiba K (1997). *Xenopus Zic3*, a primary regulator both in neural and neural crest development. *Proc Natl Acad Sci USA* 94: 11980–11985.

Nebot-Cegarra J, Maraculla-Sanz E, Reina-De La Torre F (1999). Factors involved in the "rotation" of the human embryonic stomach around its longitudinal axis: computer-assisted morphometric analysis. *J Anat* 194(Pt 1): 61–69.

Nieto MA (2002). The snail superfamily of zinc-finger transcription factors. *Nat Rev Mol Cell Biol* 3: 155–166.

Nomura M, Li E (1998). Smad2 role in mesoderm formation, left–right patterning and craniofacial development. *Nature* 393: 786–790.

Nonaka S, Tanaka Y, Okada Y, Takeda S, Harada A, Kanai Y, Kido M, Hirokawa N (1998). Randomization of left–right asymmetry due to loss of nodal cilia generating leftward flow of extraembryonic fluid in mice lacking KIF3B motor protein. *Cell* 95: 829–837.

Nonaka S, Shiratori H, Saijoh Y, Hamada H (2002). Determination of left–right patterning of the mouse embryo by artificial nodal flow. *Nature* 418: 96–99.

Nora JJ, Nora AH (1987). Maternal transmission of congenital heart diseases: new recurrence risk figures and the questions of cytoplasmic inheritance and vulnerability to teratogens. *Am J Cardiol* 59: 459–463.

Nora JJ, Nora AH (1988a). Familial risk of congenital heart defect. *Am J Med Genet* 29: 231–233.

Nora JJ, Nora AH (1988b). Update on counseling the family with a first-degree relative with a congenital heart defect. *Am J Med Genet* 29: 137–142.

O'Connell PR, Lynch G (1990). Reversed intestinal rotation associated with anomalous mesenteric venous drainage. Report of a case. *Dis Colon Rectum* 33: 883–885.

Oh S, Li E (1997). The signaling pathway mediated by the type IIB activin receptor controls axial patterning and lateral asymmetry in the mouse. *Genes Dev* 11: 1812–1826.

Okada Y, Nonaka S, Tanaka Y, Saijoh Y, Hamada H, Hirokawa N (1999). Abnormal nodal flow precedes situs inversus in iv and inv mice. *Mol Cells* 4: 459–468.

Ozden S, Ficicioglu C, Kara M, Oral O, Bilgic R (2000). Agnathia-holoprosencephaly-situs inversus. *Am J Med Genet* 91: 235–236.

Ozden S, Bilgic R, Delikara N, Basaran T (2002). The sixth clinical report of a rare association: agnathia-holoprosencephaly-situs inversus. *Prenat Diagn* 22: 840–842.

Patel K, Isaac A, Cooke J (1999). Nodal signalling and the roles of the transcription factors SnR and Pitx2 in vertebrate left–right asymmetry. *Curr Biol* 9: 609–612.

Patterson KD, Drysdale TA, Krieg PA (2000). Embryonic origins of spleen asymmetry. *Development* 127: 167–175.

Pauli RM, Graham JM Jr, Barr M Jr (1981). Agnathia, situs inversus, and associated malformations. *Teratology* 23: 85–93.

Pearce JJ, Penny G, Rossant J (1999). A mouse cerberus/Dan-related gene family. *Dev Biol* 209: 98–110.

Pennekamp P, Karcher C, Fischer A, Schweickert A, Skryabin B, Horst J, Blum M, Dworniczak B (2002). The ion channel polycystin-2 is required for left–right axis determination in mice. *Curr Biol* 12: 938–943.

Peoples WM, Moller JH, Edwards JE (1983). Polysplenia: a review of 146 cases. *Pediatr Cardiol* 4: 129–137.

Persutte WH, Yeasting RA, Kurczynski TW, Lenke RR, Robinson H (1990). Agnathia malformation complex associated with a cystic distention of the oral cavity and hydranencepahly. *J Craniofac Genet Dev Biol* 10: 391–397.

Peters T, Ausmeier K, Ruther U (1999). Cloning of Fatso (*Fto*), a novel gene deleted by the Fused toes (*Ft*) mouse mutation. *Mamm Genome* 10: 983–986.

Phoon CK, Neill CA (1994). Asplenia syndrome: insight into embryology through an analysis of cardiac and extracardiac anomalies. *Am J Cardiol* 73: 581–587.

Piedra ME, Ros MA (2002). BMP signaling positively regulates Nodal expression during left right specification in the chick embryo. *Development* 129: 3431–3440.

Piedra ME, Icardo JM, Albajar M, Rodriguez-Rey JC, Ros MA (1998). Pitx2 participates in the late phase of the pathway controlling left-right asymmetry. *Cell* 94: 319–324.

Pradat P (1994). Recurrence risk for major congenital heart defects in Sweden: a registry study. *Genet Epidemiol* 11: 131–140.

Purandare SM, Ware SM, Kwan KM, Gebbia M, Bassi MT, Deng JM, Vogel H, Behringer RR, Belmont JW, Casey B (2002). A complex syndrome of left–right axis, central nervous system and axial skeleton defects in *Zic3* mutant mice. *Development* 129: 2293–2302.

Rankin CT, Bunton T, Lawler AM, Lee SJ (2000). Regulation of left–right patterning in mice by growth/differentiation factor-1. *Nat Genet* 24: 262–265.

Rescorla FJ, Shedd FJ, Grosfeld JL, Vane DW, West KW (1990). Anomalies of intestinal rotation in childhood: analysis of 447 cases. *Surgery* 108: 710–716.

Robinson HB Jr, Lenke R (1989). Agnathia, holoprosencephaly, and situs inversus. *Am J Med Genet* 34: 266–267.

Rodriguez Esteban C, Capdevila J, Economides AN, Pascual J, Ortiz A, Izpisua Belmonte JC (1999). The novel Cer-like protein Caronte mediates the establishment of embryonic left–right asymmetry. *Nature* 401: 243–251.

Rose V, Gold RJ, Lindsay G, Allen M (1985). A possible increase in the incidence of congenital heart defects among the offspring of affected parents. *J Am Coll Cardiol* 6: 376–382.

Rucco V, Zucchi A (1985). Ankylosing vertebral hyperostosis and dextrocardia. Apropos of a case [in French]. *Rev Rhum Mal Osteoartic* 52: 649.

Ruscazio M, Van Praagh S, Marrass AR, Catani G, Iliceto S, Van Praagh R (1998). Interrupted inferior vena cava in asplenia syndrome and a review of the hereditary patterns of visceral situs abnormalities. *Am J Cardiol* 81: 111–116.

Saijoh Y, Adachi H, Sakuma R, Yeo CY, Yashiro K, Watanabe M, Hashiguchi H, Mochida K, Ohishi S, Kawabata M, et al. (2000). Left–right asymmetric expression of lefty2 and nodal is induced by a signaling pathway that includes the transcription factor FAST2. *Mol Cells* 5: 35–47.

Sampath K, Cheng AMS, Frisch A, Wright CV (1997). Functional differences among *Xenopus nodal-related* genes in left–right axis determination. *Development* 124: 3293–3302.

Say B, Hommes FA, Malik SA, Carpenter NJ (1992). An infant with multiple congenital abnormalities and biochemical findings suggesting a variant of galactosialidosis. *J Med Genet* 29: 423–424.

Schier AF, Shen MM (2000). Nodal signalling in vertebrate development. *Nature* 403: 385–389.

Schier AF, Talbot WS (2001). Nodal signaling and the zebrafish organizer. *Int J Dev Biol* 45: 289–297.

Schilling TF, Concordet JP, Ingham PW (1999). Regulation of left–right asymmetries in the zebrafish by Shh and BMP4. *Dev Biol* 210: 277–287.

Schlange T, Schnipkoweit I, Andree B, Ebert A, Zile MH, Arnold HH, Brand T (2001). Chick CFC controls Lefty1 expression in the embryonic midline and nodal expression in the lateral plate. *Dev Biol* 234: 376–389.

Sharma S, Devine W, Anderson RH, Zuberbuhler JR (1988). The determination of atrial arrangement by examination of appendage morphology in 1842 heart specimens. *Br Heart J* 60: 227–231.

Slavotinek A, Hellen E, Gould S, Coghill SB, Huson SM, Hurst JA (1996). Three infants of diabetic mothers with malformations of left–right asymmetry—further evidence for the aetiological role of diabetes in this malformation spectrum. *Clin Dysmorphol* 5: 241–247.

Smitt JH, van Asperen CJ, Niessen CM, Beemer FA, van Essen AJ, Hulsmans RF, Oranje AP, Steijlen PM, Wesby-van Swaay E, Tamminga P, et al. (1998). Restrictive dermopathy. Report of 12 cases. Dutch Task Force on Genodermatology. *Arch Dermatol* 134: 577–579.

Stoler JM, Holmes LB (1992). A case of agnathia, situs inversus, and a normal central nervous system. *Teratology* 46: 213–216.

Stratton RF, Parker MW (1989). Growth hormone deficiency, wormian bones, dextrocardia, brachycamptodactyly, and other midline defects. *Am J Med Genet* 32: 169–173.

Sulik K, Dehart DB, Iangaki T, Carson JL, Vrablic T, Gesteland K, Schoenwolf GC (1994). Morphogenesis of the murine node and notochordal plate. *Dev Dyn* 201: 260–278.

Supp DM, Witte DP, Potter SS, Brueckner M (1997). Mutation of an axonemal dynein affects left–right asymmetry in inversus viscerum mice. *Nature* 389: 963–966.

Supp DM, Brueckner M, Kuehn MR, Witte DP, Lowe LA, McGrath J, Corrales J, Potter SS (1999). Targeted deletion of the ATP binding domain of *left–right dynein* confirms its role in specifying development of left–right asymmetries. *Development* 126: 5495–5504.

Takeda S, Yonekawa Y, Tanaka Y, Okada Y, Nonaka S, Hirokawa N (1999). Left–right asymmetry and kinesin superfamily protein KIF3A: new insights in determination of laterality and mesoderm induction by $kif3A^{-/-}$ mice analysis. *J Cell Biol* 145: 825–836.

Talbot WS, Trevarrow B, Halpern ME, Melby AE, Farr G, Postlethwait JH, Jowett T, Kimmel CB, Kimelman D (1995). A homeobox gene essential for zebrafish notochord development. *Nature* 378: 150–157.

Temtamy SA, Shoukry AS, Raafat M, Mihareb S (1975). Probable Marden-Walker syndrome: evidence for autosomal recessive inheritance. *Birth Defects Orig Artic Ser* 11: 104–108.

Ticho BS, Goldstein AM, Van Praagh R (2000). Extracardiac anomalies in the heterotaxy syndromes with focus on anomalies of midline-associated structures. *Am J Cardiol* 85: 729–734.

Tsukui T, Capdevila J, Tamura K, Ruiz-Lozano P, Rodriguez-Esteban C, Yonei-Tamura S, Magallon J, Chandraratna RA, Chien K, Blumberg B, et al. (1999). Multiple left–right asymmetry defects in $Shh^{-/-}$ mutant mice unveil a convergence of the shh and retinoic acid pathways in the control of Lefty-1. *Proc Natl Acad Sci USA* 96: 11376–11381.

Uemura H, Ho SY, Devine WA, Anderson RH (1995). Analysis of visceral heterotaxy according to splenic status, appendage morphology, or both. *Am J Cardiol* 76: 846–849.

Vanlieferinghen PH, Borderon C, Francannet CH, Gembara P, Dechelotte P (2001). Johanson-Blizzard syndrome. A new case with autopsy findings. *Genet Couns* 12: 245–250.

Van Praagh R, Jung WK (1991). The arterial switch operation in transposition of the great arteries: anatomic indications and contraindications. *Thorac Cardiovasc Surg* 39(Suppl 2): 138–150.

Van Praagh S, Kreutzer J, Alday L, Van Praagh R (1990). Systemic and pulmonary venous connections in visceral heterotaxy, with emphasis on the diagnosis of the atria situs: a study of 109 postmortem cases. In: *Developmental Cardiology, Morphogenesis and Function.* Clark E, Takao A (eds.) Futura, Mt. Kisco, NY, pp. 671–721.

Van Praagh S, Geva T, Friedberg DZ, Oechler H, Colli A, Frigiola A, Van Praagh R (1997). Aortic outflow obstruction in visceral heterotaxy: a study based on twenty postmortem cases. *Am Heart J* 133: 558–569.

Viana MB, Carvalho RI (1978). Thiamine-responsive megaloblastic anemia, sensorineural deafness, and diabetes mellitus: a new syndrome? *J Pediatr* 93: 235–238.

Weigel TJ, Driscoll DJ, Michels VV (1989). Occurrence of congenital heart defects in siblings of patients with univentricular heart and tricuspid atresia. *Am J Cardiol* 64: 768–771.

Weinstein DC, Ruiz i Altaba A, Chen WS, Hoodless P, Prezioso VR, Jessell TM, Darnell JE Jr (1994). The winged-helix transcription factor HNF-3 beta is required for notochord development in the mouse embryo. *Cell* 78: 575–588.

Whitman M (2001). Nodal signaling in early vertebrate embryos: themes and variations. *Dev Cell* 1: 605–617.

Whittemore R (1988). Maternal transmission of congenital heart disease. *Am J Cardiol* 61: 499–500.

Winnier G, Blessing M, Labosky P, Hogan BL (1995). Bone morphogenetic protein-4 is required for mesoderm formation and patterning in the mouse. *Genes Dev* 9: 2105–2116.

Yamamoto M, Meno C, Sakai Y, Shiratori H, Mochida K, Ikawa Y, Saijoh Y, Hamada H (2001). The transcription factor FoxH1 (FAST) mediates Nodal signaling during anterior–posterior patterning and node formation in the mouse. *Genes Dev* 15: 1242–1256.

Yan YT, Gritsman K, Ding J, Burdine RD, Corrales JD, Price SM, Talbot WS, Schier AF, Shen MM (1999). Conserved requirement for *EGF-CFC* genes in vertebrate left–right axis formation. *Genes Dev* 13: 2527–2537.

Yeo C, Whitman M (2001). Nodal signals to Smads through Cripto-dependent and Cripto-independent mechanisms. *Mol Cell* 7: 949–957.

Yokouchi Y, Vogan KJ, Pearse RV 2nd, Tabin CJ (1999). Antagonistic signaling by *Caronte,* a novel *Cerberus*-related gene, establishes left–right asymmetric gene expression. *Cell* 98: 573–583.

Yokoyama T, Copeland N, Jenkins N, Montgomery C, Elder F, Overbeek P (1993). Reversal of left–right asymmetry: a situs inversus mutation. *Science* 260: 679–682.

Zhang XM, Ramalho-Santos M, McMahon AP (2001). *Smoothened* mutants reveal redundant roles for Shh and Ihh signaling including regulation of L/R symmetry by the mouse node. *Cell* 106: 781–792.

27 | *CDMP1* and Chondrodysplasia (Grebe, Hunter-Thompson, and Du Pan Types) and Brachydactyly, Type C

MICHAEL W. KILPATRICK AND PETROS TSIPOURAS

The human osteochondrodysplasias comprise a large and heterogeneous group of inherited disorders affecting skeletal morphogenesis. Grebe type chondrodysplasia (OMIM 200700) is characterized by a normal axial skeleton and severely shortened and deformed extremities exhibiting a proximodistal gradient of severity. This condition is classified as a form of acromesomelic dysplasia. Two other phenotypically similar conditions are the Hunter-Thompson (OMIM 201250) and Du Pan (OMIM 228900) types of chondrodysplasia. Brachydactyly type C (OMIM 113100) is characterized primarily by shortening and hypersegmentation of phalangeal and metacarpal bones and occasionally polydactyly and other skeletal abnormalities. In contrast to the autosomal-recessive Grebe, Hunter-Thompson, and Du Pan types of chondrodysplasia, brachydactyly type C is inherited in an autosomal-dominant manner. These conditions are caused by mutations in the gene encoding cartilage-derived morphogenetic protein-1 (*CDMP1*) (OMIM 601146), and they together comprise the spectrum of *CDMP1* morphopathies. *CDMP1* encodes a signaling molecule, which is a member of the transforming growth factor-β (TGF-β) superfamily.

CDMP1

The TGF-β superfamily comprises a large group of functionally diverse secreted signaling molecules that regulate an array of cellular processes, including cell proliferation, lineage determination, differentiation, motility, adhesion, and death (Massague, 1998; Massague and Chen, 2000). They elicit their response through binding to specific transmembrane serine/threonine kinase receptors and activating Smad transcription factors (Massague et al., 1994; Massague and Wotton, 2000).

CDMP1 and its mouse homologue growth and differentiation factor-5 (Gdf5) were discovered independently in screening for bone morphogenetic proteins (BMPs) (Chang et al., 1994; Storm et al., 1994). CDMP1/Gdf5 is closely related to the BMPs (Kingsley, 1994; Hogan, 1996) and is expressed predominantly in the cartilaginous cores of the developing long bones and the more distal elements of the extremities that develop from the limb bud. It is also expressed at the position of future joint spaces, suggesting a role in the restriction of joint formation to the appropriate location (Chang et al., 1994; Storm et al., 1994; Storm and Kingsley, 1996). CDMP1 is one of several molecules identified as regulators of limb skeletogenesis and appendicular bone development.

The *CDMP1* gene comprises two exons that encode a 56 kDa precursor polypeptide. Exon 1 contains the 5′-untranslated region (UTR) and 681 bases of coding sequence, and exon 2 contains the remaining 873 bases of coding sequence, including the sequence encoding the 14 kDa active domain of the protein and 557 bases of the 3′-UTR (Fig. 27–1) (Thomas et al., 1996). The CDMP1 precursor polypeptide dimerizes through formation of a single inter-chain disulfide bond between one of seven highly conserved cysteine residues. The dimerized precursor undergoes proteolysis at an R-X-X-R cleavage site to produce the biologically active mature protein that is secreted from the cell (Luyten, 1997). Mapping analysis demonstrated that the *CDMP1* gene was located on 20q11.2 (Lin et al., 1996). The *Gdf5* gene has been localized in a syntenic region of mouse chromosome 2 (Storm et al., 1994; Chang et al., 1994).

CLINICAL PHENOTYPES

What is presently recognized as a phenotypic continuum of *CDMP1*-associated morphopathies comprises three chondrodysplasias, Grebe type, Hunter-Thompson type, and Du Pan type, characterized by short stature, acromesomelic pattern of shortening, and bone aplasias/hypoplasias. The most severe phenotypic manifestations are observed in the Grebe type. Affected individuals with any of the three chondrodysplasias are homozygotes or compound heterozygotes for mutations in the *CDMP1* gene. However, obligate carriers of Grebe type chondrodysplasia express a phenotype including brachydactyly. It is therefore not surprising that *CDMP1* gene mutations have been identified in brachydactyly type C, a condition inherited as an autosomal-dominant trait. The aforementioned phenotypes have been reported in several populations (Bell, 1951; Scott, 1969; Garcia-Castro and Perez-Comas, 1975; Meera Khan and Khan, 1982; Kumar et al., 1984; Feng et al., 1985; Teebi et al., 1986; Curtis, 1986; Romeo et al., 1997).

Grebe Type

Following the initial description by Grebe (1952), Quelce-Salgado (1964) reported several cases originating in a geographically remote area in Bahia state, Brazil. This population was revisited and phenotypically delineated by Costa et al. (1998). Affected homozygotes present with short stature, average adult height 100 cm, bone aplasias and hypoplasias, polydactyly, and lack of joint formation (Fig. 27–2). The extremities are shortened and malformed, displaying a proximodistal gradient of severity in contrast to normal craniofacies and axial skeleton. There is striking shortness of the forearms and shanks. Fingers and toes are replaced by knob-like appendages. Postaxial polydactyly is a consistent finding. Imaging studies have revealed malformation or absence of several joints in the carpus, tarsus, hand, and foot (Fig. 27–2). Radiologically, the humeri and femora are relatively normal, the radii/ulnae and tibiae/fibulae are shortened and hypoplastic, and several bones in the carpal/tarsal rows and metacarpals/metatarsals are absent or fused. The proximal and middle phalanges of the fingers and toes are invariably missing, while the distal phalanges are present (Fig. 27–2). Costa et al., (1998) phenotypically studied several heterozygotes and found a skeletal phenotype whose manifestations included polydactyly, brachydactyly, hallux valgus, metatarsus adductus, and delayed appearance of ossification centers.

Hunter-Thompson Type

The acromesomelic pattern of severity is also observed in the Hunter-Thompson type chondrodysplasia; however, the overall phenotype is less pronounced than in the Grebe type (Hunter and Thompson, 1976). Langer et al., (1989) first drew attention to the phenotypic similarity between the Grebe and Hunter-Thompson types of chondrodysplasia. Affected individuals are short-statured, and adult height is approximately 120 cm. Unlike what is observed in the Grebe type, the anatomical structures of the distal extremities are better delineated (Table 27–1). The forearms and shanks are shortened, and the fingers and toes are brachydactylous. Joint dislocations are common. As in Grebe type chondrodysplasia, the craniofacies and trunk are normal. Radiologically, the bones of the middle and distal segments of the extremities are hypoplastic. Fusion and/or segmentation defects have been observed in the carpal/tarsal, metacarpal/metatarsal, and phalangeal bones. Heterozygotes do not express a phenotype.

Figure 27–1. Schematic diagram of *CDMP-1/Gdf5*. The genomic structure is shown on top, with the cDNA shown underneath. The regions encoding the signal peptide (S), propeptide (P), and active domain (gray rectangle) are designated. The positions of the seven cysteine residues (C) conserved among transforming growth factor-β superfamily members, which are required for dimerization and correct folding of the molecule, are shown in the active domain. The mutations responsible for Hunter-Thompson (HT), Grebe type and Du Pan type chondrodysplasia, and brachydactyly type C (BTC) are shown, along with the lesions identified in the three independent *bp* mutant strains (*bp*, *bp^J*, and *bp^{3j}*). The mutation identified in a kindred with a Grebe-like phenotype is indicated by an asterisk. Nucleotide numbers are normalized to the *CDMP-1* sequence.

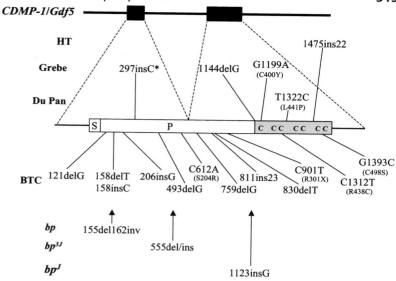

Du Pan Type

Du Pan type chondrodysplasia was originally described by Du Pan in 1924. It is characterized by short stature, brachydactyly, and fibular hypoplasia. Further delineation of the phenotype was offered by Ahmad et al., (1990) based on a large Pakistani kindred. The condition is inherited as an autosomal-recessive trait, and heterozygotes do not appear to express any phenotypic manifestations. A comparison of the Grebe, Hunter-Thompson, and Du Pan phenotypes is provided in Table 27–1.

Brachydactyly Type C

Shortness of fingers is the cardinal manifestation of brachydactyly type C; however, polydactyly, Madelung deformity, talipes, shortness of toes, hip dysplasia, and short stature have been described as occasional findings. Following the original description by Bell (1951), several reports delineated the condition (Haws, 1963). Shortness of the middle phalanx of the second, third, and fifth fingers and of the first metacarpal is invariably present along with hypersegmentation and/or fusion of phalanges (Fig. 27–3).

MOLECULAR GENETICS

Individuals with Hunter-Thompson type acromesomelic dysplasia harbor a frameshift mutation resulting from a 22 bp insertion at nucleotide 1448 of the *CDMP1* gene (Thomas et al., 1996). The insertion is a tandem duplication of nucleotides 1453–1474 in the mature region of the *CDMP1* molecule, predicting an altered reading frame of 43 amino acids ending in a premature stop codon (Fig. 27–1).

Thomas et al., (1997) identified a common haplotype in 13 of 14 chromosomes from affected individuals of the family segregating Grebe-type chondrodysplasia originally described by Quelce-Salgado (1964). Additionally, all obligate carriers analyzed possessed a single copy of the common haplotype. Sequence analysis of the *CDMP1* coding sequence in genomic DNA from affected individuals homozygous for this haplotype identified a G-to-A transition, predicting a tyrosine-for-cysteine substitution at amino acid 400 in the active domain of *CDMP1* (Fig. 27–1) (Thomas et al., 1997). The affected individual with only a single copy of this haplotype was a compound heterozygote, possessing a single copy of the G1199A mutation and a second allele with a deletion of a guanine nucleotide at position 1144. The del1144G mutation predicts a frameshift and premature stop codon 70 amino acids downstream (Fig. 27–1). This individual was phenotypically identical to homozygotes for the G1199A mutation. The *CDMP1* gene was analyzed in three additional unrelated families from Brazil. All affected individuals were homozygous for the G1199A mutation (Thomas et al., 1997).

A kindred with a Grebe-like phenotype segregated a frameshift mutation in the *CDMP1* gene (Faiyaz-Ul-Haque et al., 2002a). Affected individuals carried two copies of a single nucleotide insertion of a C at residue 297 in the coding region of the *CDMP1* gene. This produces a frameshift in codon 99 that is predicted to result in premature termination of the polypeptide six amino acids downstream (Fig. 27–1).

Brachydactyly type C follows an autosomal-dominant pattern of inheritance, with marked variability in expression. Brachydactyly type C was mapped to 20q11.2 by genetic linkage analysis (Polinkovsky et al., 1997). Sequence analysis of the *CDMP1* gene in this family identified a heterozygous nonsense mutation: a C-to-T transition at position 901 of the coding sequence predicting the conversion of the arginine at position 301 to a stop codon (Fig. 27–1) (Polinkovsky et al., 1997). Subsequent analyses of individuals with brachydactyly type C have demonstrated locus homogeneity and identified *CDMP1* mutations in all affected individuals (Polinkovsky et al., 1997; Galjaard et al., 2001; Everman et al., 2002). A variety of heterozygous *CDMP1* mutations have been described, including frameshift and nonsense mutations in the *CDMP1* prodomain and missense mutations in the active domain (Fig. 27–1).

Similarities of the phenotype observed in Du Pan syndrome to that of the Hunter-Thompson and Grebe types of acromesomelic chondrodysplasia prompted Faiyaz-Ul-Haque et al. (2002b) to examine genomic DNA from a Pakistani family with Du Pan syndrome for mutations in the *CDMP1* gene. Homozygosity for a missense mutation, T-to-C at nucleotide 1322 of the coding sequence predicting a L441P substitution in the active domain, was identified (Fig. 27–1).

ANIMAL MODELS

The autosomal-recessive mouse *brachypodism (bp)* mutation was first reported by Landauer in 1952 and resembles the human Hunter-Thompson phenotype. The mutation affects exclusively the appendicular skeleton, with abnormalities that include a decrease in the length of the long bones of the limbs, abnormal joint development in the limb and sternum, and a reduction in the number of bones in digits 2–5 (Fig. 27–4) (Grüneberg and Lee, 1973; Storm and Kingsley, 1996).

Three distinct mutations in the *Gdf5* gene were identified in three independent *bp* mutant strains. All three mutant alleles, *bp*, *bp^J*, and *bp^{3j}*, contained frameshifts in the *Gdf5* coding sequence (Storm et al., 1994) (Fig. 27–1). In *bp* mice, bases 155–161 of the normal *Gdf5* sequence are deleted and this deletion is accompanied by an inversion of bases 162–174. This causes a frameshift that results in creation of a premature stop codon 62 amino acids downstream. In *bp^J* mice, insertion of a G at position 1123 causes a frameshift that predicts a premature stop codon 41 amino acids downstream. In *bp^{3j}* mice, a deletion/insertion at position 555 causes a frameshift that results in a premature termination immediately 3′ to the insertion. All three frameshift mutations occur prior to the mature signaling portion of

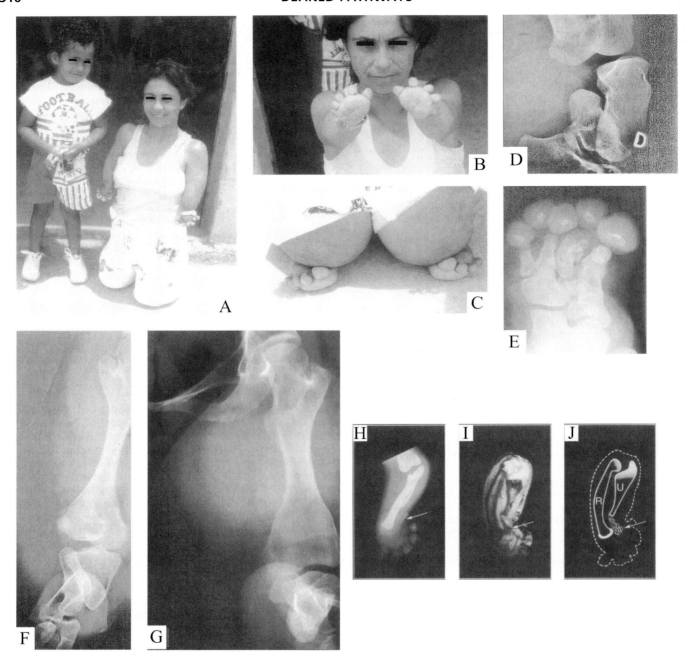

Figure 27–2. Clinical and radiographic features of Grebe type chondrodysplasia. *A*: Affected woman with her unaffected 4-year-old son. Close-up of the palms of the hands (*B*) and feet (*C*). Note markedly short limbs, knob-like fingers and toes, polydactyly, and oligodactyly of the right foot due to autoamputation. *D–G*: Radiographs of the lower limbs of affected adults. *D*: Short metatarsals ectopically located and fused; absent proximal and middle phalanges. *E*: Abnormally shaped and misplaced tarsal bones. *F, G*: Short femoral neck and diaphysis. Short and triangularly shaped tibia, short fibula. *H–J*: Radiograph (*H*), magnetic resonance (MR) scan (*I*), and schematic representation (*J*) of the right arm and hand of a 10-year-old male. *H, I*: Hypoplastic and angulated radius. *I, J*: The ulnar diaphysis terminates abruptly, and its distal segment is composed of fibrous tissue, as indicated by arrow. *I*: MR scan shows cartilage in the articular surfaces of the elbow but not between the remaining skeletal structures. (Modified from Costa et al., 1998.)

Gdf5 and are therefore expected to represent functional null mutations (Fig. 27–1).

PATHOGENIC MECHANISMS

The recessive mouse *bp* phenotype is caused by null mutations in the *Gdf5* gene. Studies of digit development in *bp* mice suggest that mutations leading to lack of functional *Gdf5* disrupt the initial cleavage of digital rays into separate elements (Milaire, 1965; Grüneberg and Lee, 1973). The early limb bud in *bp* mice is normal in size and shape, and the initial digital ray condensations are as long as in wild type, although somewhat thinner. Major differences in development are first observed between embryonic days 12.5 and 14.5, when the digital ray is beginning to segment. In *bp* mice, the central part of the digital ray fails to develop an interzone and there is a subsequent failure to separate the proximal and medial phalanges, thus producing a single combined element (Grüneberg and Lee, 1973). This early segmentation defect is observed at a site where *Gdf5* is highly expressed, strongly suggesting that the *Gdf5* gene product plays a direct role in this segmentation process. It has been speculated (Hinchliffe and Johnson, 1980) that mutations at the *bp* locus cause a disruption in the usual pattern that determines where joints are to occur in the limb. This is strongly supported by the striking expression pattern of the *Gdf5* gene (Storm and Kingsley, 1996). Investigation of the response of developing mouse and chick limbs to the effect of exogenous Gdf5 protein confirmed the multiple functions of *Gdf5* in skeletogenesis, including

Table 27–1. Phenotypic Comparison of the Grebe, Hunter-Thompson, and Du Pan Types of Acromesomelic Chondrodysplasia

	Grebe Type	Hunter-Thompson Type	Du Pan Type
Upper limb			
Proximal and middle segments	Short and bowed middle segment Short and bowed radius Shorter ulna than radius Radio-ulnar dislocation Limited elbow movement	Shorter middle than proximal segment Short and mildly bowed radius Slightly shorter ulna than radius Radio-ulnar dislocation	Normal middle segment Normal length of radius and ulna Almost normal radio-ulnar joint
Distal segment	Severe shortness of hand Knob-like fingers/single phalangeal bone (distal) Fusion of carpal bones Short abnormal metacarpal Occasional polydactyly	Less severe shortness of hands Abnormal carpal bones Metacarpals short and cuboidal Proximal and middle phalanges short Relatively normal distally	Mild shortness of hand Mis-aligned carpal bones Relatively short metacarpals with normal length Second metacarpal Hypoplastic phalanges All phalangeal bones present
Lower limb			
Proximal and middle segments	Short proximal segment Severe shortness of middle segment Limited knee movement Short deformed tibiae/fibulae Absent or hypoplastic patellae	Short proximal segment, shorter middle segment Dislocated ankle Shortened tibia, very short fibula	Short proximal segment Relatively normal middle segment with complete absence of fibulae Posterior dislocation of femur and tibia Displaced patella Deformed ankle joints
Distal segment	Small feet with short toes Limited movement of ankle Deformed tarsal bones Fused metatarsals Absent proximal and middle phalanges	Very short, everted foot Globular third, forth and fifth toes	Tarsal bones present but deformed Short and mis-aligned metatarsals Short, knob-like toes with some missing Hypoplastic nails
Heterozygous phenotype	Brachydactyly Polydactyly Malpositioning of the digits	None detected	None detected

Source: Faiyaz-Ul-Haque et al. (2002b).

its role in joint development (Storm and Kingsley, 1999). Interestingly, although *Gdf5* is expressed in nearly all synovial joints of the limb, only a subset of the joints is disrupted by *bp* null mutations. Thus, it is possible that other members of the BMP family may provide partially overlapping functions that compensate for loss of *Gdf5* at some locations. In this regard, the mature signaling region of the Gdf5 protein shares 80%–90% amino acid sequence identity with gdf6 and gdf7 and approximately 50%–60% identity with BMPs 2, 4, 5, 6, 7, and 8 (Storm et al., 1994). The *Gdf6* and *Gdf7* genes are also expressed in and around developing joints (Hattersley et al., 1995; Wolfman et al., 1995) and are the most obvious candidates for overlapping functions.

The *CDMP1* mutation responsible for Hunter-Thompson type chondrodysplasia is, in all probability, a null mutation that leads to the production of no active CDMP1 protein (Thomas et al., 1996).

Comparison of the Hunter-Thompson and Grebe types, along with the mild phenotype observed in Grebe heterozygotes, suggests that the C400Y substitution produces a dominant-negative effect. The C400Y mutation substitutes a tyrosine for the first of seven highly conserved cysteine residues in the active domain of the protein affecting processing and secretion (Thomas et al., 1997). Immunoprecipitation experiments demonstrated that both mutant C400Y and wild-type *CDMP1* protein can form heterodimers with other BMP family members and can inhibit their secretion. Thus, the dominant-negative effect of the C400Y mutation may occur through the formation of nonfunctional bmp/C400Y CDMP1 heterodimers. The potency of the C400Y mutation in disrupting the function of related BMP family members was demonstrated by the individual who was a compound heterozygote for the C400Y mutation and a null *CDMP1* allele (Thomas et al., 1997). The phenotype in this individual is indistinguishable from that ob-

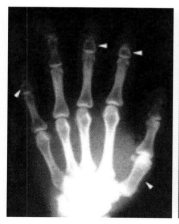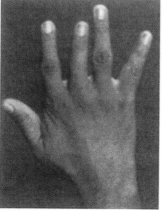

Figure 27–3. Radiographic and clinical features of brachydactyly type C (BTC). *Left*: Radiograph of the left hand of individual with BTC, with arrows indicating disproportionate shortening of the first metacarpal bone and the second, third, and fifth middle phalangeal bones. *Right*: Right hand of an individual with BTC, with disproportionate shortening of the second and third fingers. (Modified from Warman, 2000, and Everman et al., 2002).

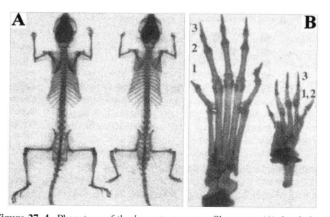

Figure 27–4. Phenotype of the *bp* mutant mouse. Shown are (*A*) the skeleton and (*B*) the right hind feet of a *bp^j* homozygote (*right*) alongside an age-matched wild-type animal (*left*). The long bones are reduced and the fibula shortened proximally (*A*). The number of phalanges is reduced and the tarsals shortened and irregular in shape (*B*). The phalanges are numbered for comparison. (Modified from Storm et al., 1994.)

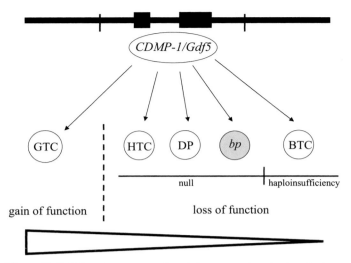

Figure 27–5. Schematic representation of the proposed mechanism for loss-of-function or gain-of-function *CDMP1/Gdf5* mutations. Human and mouse mutations are depicted as white and gray circles, respectively. GTC, HTC, DP, *bp*, and BTC refer to Grebe type, Hunter-Thompson, and Du Pan type chondrodysplasias; brachypodism; and brachydactyly type C, respectively. The gradient of phenotypic severity is represented by the arrow underneath.

served in homozygotes for the C400Y mutation. The C400Y *CDMP1* mutation and its proposed mechanism of action provided the first human genetic indication that composite expression patterns of different BMPs dictate limb and digit morphogenesis.

Brachydactyly type C is caused by a diverse group of heterozygous *CDMP1* mutations, which are predicted to result in either a truncated protein, a protein whose mature domain cannot be efficiently cleaved by endogenous endopeptidases, or a protein that contains an abnormal disulfide-bonded mature domain (Fig. 27–1) (Everman et al., 2002). Each of these situations is likely to result in a nonfunctional protein, supporting the hypothesis that haploinsufficiency of *CDMP1* is the underlying mechanism of brachydactyly type C (Warman 2000; Everman et al., 2002). Observation of families with nonpenetrant carriers of brachydactyly type C mutations has led to the suggestion that brachydactyly type C–causing mutations reduce CDMP1 protein levels just below the biological threshold required for normal digit development and that modifier loci, environmental influences, and/or stochastic events that contribute to the variable expression in brachydactyly type C may also contribute to its nonpenetrance (Everman et al., 2002).

In summary, abnormal phenotypes have been associated with presumable loss-of-function, gain-of-function, and haploinsufficiency mutations of the *CDMP1/Gdf5* locus in human and mouse (Fig. 27–5). *In vitro* studies offer a paradigm of the operative model during development; however, additional factors might be involved. There is functional overlap between the various CDMPs and the larger family of BMPs, which is not sufficient to ablate the effects of particular mutations. Gain-of-function mutations result in the most severe phenotype (Grebe type chondrodysplasia). At the opposite end of the phenotypic spectrum, haploinsufficiency results in brachydactyly type C. Detailed comparison of the various phenotypic entities cannot shed further light on the pathogenic mechanisms. These might be further elucidated by the study of transgenic animal models.

REFERENCES

Ahmad M, Abbas H, Wahab A, Haque S (1990). Fibular hypoplasia and complex brachydactyly (Du Pan syndrome) in an inbred Pakistani kindred. *Am J Med Genet* 36: 292–296.
Bell J (1951). On brachydactyly and symphalangism. In: *The Treasury of Human Inheritance*, Volume 5. Penrose LS (ed.) Cambridge University Press, London, pp. 1–31.
Chang SC, Hoang B, Thomas JT, Vukicevic S, Luyten FP, Ryba NJ, Kozak CA, Reddi AH, Moos M Jr (1994). Cartilage-derived morphogenetic proteins. New members of the transforming growth factor-beta superfamily predominantly expressed in long bones during human embryonic development. *J Biol Chem* 269: 28227–28234.
Costa T, Ramsby G, Cassia F, Peters K-R, Soares J, Correa J, Quelce-Salgado A, Tsipouras P (1998). Grebe syndrome: clinical and radiographic findings in affected individuals and heterozygous carriers. *Am J Med Genet* 75: 523–529.
Curtis D (1986). Heterozygote expression in Grebe chondrodysplasia. *Clin Genet* 29: 455–456.

Du Pan CM (1924). Absence congenitale du perone sans deformation du tibia: curieuses deformations congenitales des mains. *Rev Orthop* 11: 227–234.
Everman DB, Bartels CF, Yang Y, Yanamandra N, Goodman FR, Mendoza-Londono JR, Savarirayan R, White SM, Graham JM Jr, Gale RP, et al. (2002). The mutational spectrum of brachydactyly type C. *Am J Med Genet* 112: 291–296.
Faiyaz-Ul-Haque M, Ahmad W, Wahab A, Haque S, Azim AC, Zaidi SHE, Teebi AS, Ahmad M, Cohn DH, Siddique T, et al. (2002a). A frameshift mutation in the cartilage derived morphogenetic protein 1 (*CDMP1*) gene and severe acromesomelic chondrodysplasia resembling Grebe type chondrodysplasia. *Am J Med Genet* 111: 31–37.
Faiyaz-Ul-Haque M, Ahmad W, Zaidi SHE, Haque S, Teebi AS, Ahmad M, Cohn DH, Tsui LC (2002b). Mutation in the cartilage-derived morphogenetic protein-1 (*CDMP1*) gene in a kindred affected with fibular hypoplasia and complex brachydactyly (DuPan syndrome). *Clin Genet* 61: 454–458.
Feng B, Chen RB, Luo JG, Chen RG, Zheng YM (1985). A kindred of Miao nationality affected with Grebe-Quelce-Salgado achondrogenesis. *Acta Genet Sinica* 12: 378–386.
Galjaard RJH, van der Ham LI, Posch NAS, Dijkstra PF, Oostra BA, Hovius SER, Timmenga EJF, Sonneveld GJ, Hoogeboom AJM, Heutink P (2001). Differences in complexity of isolated brachydactyly type C cannot be attributed to locus heterogeneity alone. *Am J Med Genet* 98: 256–262.
Garcia-Castro JM, Perez-Comas A (1975). Nonlethal achondrogenesis (Grebe-Quelce-Salgado type) in two Puerto Rico sibships. *J Pediat* 87: 948–952.
Grebe H (1952). Die Achondrogenesis: ein einfach rezessives Erbmerkmal. *Folia Hered Pathol* 2: 23–28.
Grüneberg H, Lee AJ (1973). The anatomy and development of brachypodism in the mouse. *J Embryol Exp Morphol* 30: 119–141.
Hattersley G, Hewick R, Rosen V (1995). In situ localization and in vitro activity of BMP-13. *J Bone Min Res* 10: S163.
Haws DV (1963). Inherited brachydactyly and hypoplasia of the bones of the extremities. *Ann Hum Genet* 26: 201–212.
Hinchliffe JR, Johnson DR (1980). *The Development of the Vertebrate Limb*. Clarendon Press, Oxford, 1980.
Hogan BLM (1996). Bone morphogenetic proteins: multifunctional regulators of vertebrate development. *Genes Dev* 10: 1580–1594.
Hunter AGW, Thompson MW (1976). Acromesomelic dwarfism: description of a patient and comparison with previously reported cases. *Hum Genet* 34: 107–113.
Kingsley DM (1994). What do BMPs do in mammals? Clues from the mouse short-ear mutation. *Trends Genet* 10: 16–21.
Kumar D, Curtis D, Blank CE (1984). Grebe chondrodysplasia and brachydactyly in a family. *Clin Genet* 25: 68–72.
Landauer W (1952). Brachypodism, a recessive mutation of house mice. *J Hered* 43: 293–298.
Langer LO, Cervenka J, Camargo M (1989). A severe autosomal recessive acromesomelic dysplasia, the Hunter-Thompson type, and comparison with the Grebe type. *Hum Genet* 81: 323–328.
Lin K, Thomas JT, McBride OW, Luyten FP (1996). Assignment of a new TGF-beta superfamily member, human cartilage-derived morphogenetic protein-1, to chromosome 20q11.2. *Genomics* 34: 150–151.
Luyten FP (1997). Cartilage-derived morphogenetic protein-1. *Int J Cell Biol* 29: 1241–1244.
Massague J (1998). TGFβ signal transduction. *Annu Rev Biochem* 67: 753–791.
Massague J, Chen YG (2000). Controlling TGF-beta signaling. *Genes Dev* 15: 627–644.
Massague J, Wotton D (2000). Transcriptional control by the TGF-beta/Smad signaling system. *EMBO J* 19: 1745–1754.
Massague J, Attisano L, Wrana JL (1994). The TGF-β family and its composite receptors. *Trends Genet* 18: 172–178.
Meera Khan P, Khan A (1982). Grebe chondrodysplasia in three generations of an Andhra family in India. *Prog Clin Biol Res* 104: 69–80.
Milaire J (1965). Étude morphogénétique de trois malformations congénitales de l'autopode chez la souris (syndactylisme–brachypodisme–Hémimélie dominante) par des méthodes cytochimiques. *Acad R Belg Classe Sci Mem* 16: 1–120.
Polinkovsky A, Robin NH, Thomas JT, Irons M, Lynn A, Goodman FR, Reardon W, Kant SG, Brunner HG, van der Burgt I, et al. (1997). Mutations in CDMP1 cause autosomal dominant brachydactyly type C. *Nat Genet* 17: 18–19.
Quelce-Salgado A (1968). A rare genetic syndrome. *Lancet* I: 1430.
Romeo G, Zonana J, Lachman RS, Opitz JM, Scott CI Jr, Spranger JW, Rimoin DL (1977). Grebe chondrodysplasia and similar forms of severe short-limbed dwarfism. *Birth Defects* XIII(3C): 109–115.
Scott CI Jr (1969). Discussion. The clinical delineation of birth defects. IV. Skeletal dysplasias. *Birth Defects* 4: 14–16.
Storm EE, Kingsley DM (1996). Joint patterning defects caused by single and double mutations in members of the bone morphogenetic protein (BMP) family. *Development* 122: 3969–3979.
Storm EE, Kingsley DM (1999). GDF5 coordinates bone and joint formation during digit development. *Dev Biol* 209: 11–27.
Storm EE, Huynh TV, Copeland NG, Jenkins NA, Kingsley DM, Lee SJ (1994). Limb alterations in brachypodism mice due to mutations in a new member of the TGF-beta superfamily. *Nature* 368: 639–643.
Teebi AS, Al-Awadi SA, Opitz JM, Spranger J (1986). Severe short-limb dwarfism resembling Grebe chondrodysplasia. *Hum Genet* 74: 386–390.
Thomas JT, Lin K, Nandekar M, Camargo M, Cervenka J, Luyten FP (1996). A human chondrodysplasia due to a mutation in a TGF-beta superfamily member. *Nat Genet* 12: 315–317.
Thomas JT, Kilpatrick MW, Lin K, Erlacher L, Lembessis P, Costa T, Tsipouras P, Luyten FP (1997). Disruption of human limb morphogenesis by a dominant negative mutation in CDMP1. *Nat Genet* 58–64.
Warman ML (2000). Human genetic insights into skeletal development, growth and homeostasis. *Clin Orthop* 1: S40–S54.
Wolfman NM, Celeste AJ, Cox K, Hattersley G, Nelson R, Yamaji N, DiBlasio-Smith E, Nova J, Song JJ, Wozney JM, et al. (1995). Preliminary characterization of the biological activities of rhBMP-12. *J Bone Miner Res* 10: S148.

28 | *ENG* and *ALK1* and Hereditary Hemorrhagic Telangiectasia (Osler-Weber-Rendu Syndrome) and Vascular Morphogenesis

DOUGLAS A. MARCHUK AND JONATHAN N. BERG

Although first described 100 years ago, until recently little was known about the molecular basis of hereditary hemorrhagic telangiectasia (HHT). Thus far, two genes have been identified that, when mutated, give rise to this disorder. *Endoglin* maps to chromosome 9q33-q34 and is mutated in type 1 HHT. HHT1 families show a higher incidence of pulmonary involvement than families with other types of HHT. A second gene for HHT maps to chromosome 12q13, and this locus has been termed type 2 HHT. The *ALK1* gene, encoding activin receptor-like kinase 1, is mutated in HHT2. These families exhibit a lower incidence of pulmonary involvement and later onset of symptoms. There is suggestive evidence for a third gene with, thus far, two families that appear to exclude linkage to *endoglin* and *ALK1*.

Mutations in both the *endoglin* and *ALK1* genes are for the most part family-specific. Numerous mutations have been described in both genes that would potentially abrogate function and, in many cases, result in no protein product at all. DNA sequence analysis of individual coding exons for diagnosis is possible but labor-intensive. A diagnostic test for newborns measuring endoglin levels in umbilical vein endothelial cells, and monocytes in children or adults, may hold promise for HHT1.

Endoglin and ALK1 are endothelially expressed binding proteins of the family of transforming growth factor-β (TGF-β) ligands. It is likely that HHT pathology is caused by a defective response of endothelial cells to TGF-β due to mutations in either protein. Endoglin is an accessory protein that can negatively regulate TGF-β signaling. ALK1 is a true receptor with a TGF-β signaling function. Thus, ALK1 and endoglin may interact at the endothelial cell surface in a common signal-transduction pathway involving TGF-β. Recent evidence suggests that the genes for HHT are involved in the angiogenic switch of capillary morphogenesis. Genes regulated by ALK1 signaling appear to promote the activation phase, characterized by endothelial cell proliferation, invasion, and migration. Genes regulated by the ubiquitously expressed TGF-β receptor type I (TβRI) appear to promote the resolution phase, characterized by vessel maturation. Endoglin also has a negative modulatory role, at least for TβRI.

The vascular lesions in HHT are localized to discrete regions within the affected tissue, with no evidence of abnormal vascular structure or pathology outside the lesions themselves. This suggests that some genetic, physiologic, or mechanical event initiates the formation of each vascular lesion. The pathobiology of the disease may be related to remodeling of the vascular endothelium following an unknown initiating event. TGF-β mediates vascular remodeling through effects on extracellular matrix production by endothelial cells, stromal interstitial cells, smooth muscle cells, and pericytes. Perturbations in the TGF-β signaling pathway in HHT may lead to altered repair of vascular endothelium and remodeling of the vascular tissue via changes in expression profiles of extracellular matrix proteins.

ROLE OF SPECIFIC LOCI

TGF-β Signaling

Endoglin and ALK1 are receptors for members of the TGF-β superfamily of ligands. TGF-β is the prototypical member of this family of ligands, which includes activins, bone morphogenetic proteins (BMPs), and mullerian inhibitory substance. These cytokines regulate many aspects of cellular function, such as proliferation, differentiation, adhesion, migration, and extracellular matrix formation (Sporn and Roberts, 1992; Kingsley, 1994; Massague, 1998). TGF-β has three distinct isoforms: β1, β2, and β3.

Signaling through TGF-β occurs via different ligand-induced heteromeric receptor complexes consisting of type I and type II transmembrane serine/threonine kinase receptors. Models for TGF-β and activin signaling have been proposed by several authors (reviewed in Wrana et al., 1994; Massague, 1998; Piek et al., 1999). TGF-β or activin initially binds the constitutively phosphorylated type II receptor, thereby recruiting the type I receptor into the ligand/type II receptor complex. The type I receptor is subsequently phosphorylated by the type II receptor on serine and threonine residues in its cytoplasmic juxtamembrane glycine/serine-rich (GS) domain (Wieser et al., 1995). The type I receptor then phosphorylates downstream signaling mediators such as members of the recently identified Smad family, which translocate to the nucleus to effect changes in gene expression (reviewed in Heldin et al., 1997; Attisano and Wrana, 1998; Kretzschmar and Massague, 1998).

Smads 6 and 7, which were first identified in endothelial cells in response to fluid laminar shear stress (Topper et al., 1997), are now known to be anti-Smads. These Smads can act as negative regulators of signaling by stable interactions with TβRI, preventing association with the other Smads (Hayashi et al., 1997; Nakao et al., 1997a). Whether these endothelial Smads have any role in the pathophysiology of HHT remains to be elucidated.

Function of Endoglin

Endoglin, also called CD105, was initially identified as a surface antigen of acute lymphoblastic leukemia cells (Quackenbush and Letarte, 1985; Haruta and Seon, 1986). It was later determined that this antigen is primarily expressed on the cell membrane of endothelial cells from all blood vessels, including capillaries, arterioles, small arteries, venules, and high endothelial venules, and in umbilical cord veins (Gougos and Letarte, 1988). Additional cell types that express endoglin include syncytiotrophoblasts, stromal cells, smooth muscle cells, activated monocytes/macrophages, and a subpopulation of bone marrow cells (Haruta and Seon, 1986; Buhring et al., 1991; Gougos et al., 1992; Lastres et al., 1992; St-Jacques et al., 1994; Rokhlin et al., 1995; Robledo et al., 1996; H. Zhang et al., 1996; Caniggia et al., 1997; Adam et al., 1998).

Endoglin is a homodimeric integral membrane protein (Gougos and Letarte, 1990). The 90 kDa endoglin protein contains 658 amino acids comprising a single transmembrane domain, a short 47 aa cytoplasmic domain, and a 586 aa extracellular domain including the signal peptide. The extracellular domain contains 16 cysteine residues that are involved in both inter- and intramolecular disulfide bridges. Cysteine residues between residues 330 and 412 are involved in disulfide bond-aided endoglin dimerization (Raab et al., 1999; Lux et al., 2000). There are at least four confirmed *N*-linked glycosylation sites (aa 58–60, aa 121–123, aa 134–136, aa 307–309) (Lo et al., 1998) and one or more *O*-linked glycosylation sites (Gougos and Letarte, 1990). Mutation analyses of the *N*-linked glycosylation sites demonstrate that glycosylation is not a major factor in endoglin protein trafficking. One function of *N*-linked glycosylation of endoglin might be to stabilize the secondary and/or tertiary structure of the protein during the folding and trafficking process.

The endoglin protein is encoded by a gene comprising 15 exons (Shovlin et al., 1997; Gallione et al., 1998). In addition to the originally identified endoglin cDNA, a splice variant was detected called S-endoglin (for short endoglin), coding for an 85 kDa protein (Bellon et al., 1993). The extracellular and transmembrane domains of S-endoglin and the longer endoglin version (L-endoglin) are identical, while alternative splicing creates a novel 14 aa residue cytoplasmic domain for S-endoglin. These two isoforms are coexpressed in different cell types, although the majority of the transcripts correspond to L-endoglin. Although the physiologic distinctions between L- and S-endoglin are not completely known, in at least two assays of signaling, they differ in their response to ligand (Lastres et al., 1996).

Endoglin is classified as a TGF-β type III receptor based on its sequence homology to the proteoglycan betaglycan (Lopez-Casillas et al., 1991; Wang et al., 1991; Moren et al., 1992). Both are transmembrane receptor proteins with short cytoplasmic domains and no known active signaling function. Their transmembrane and cytoplasmic domains are 74% identical at the amino acid level (Wang et al., 1991). Betaglycan is expressed on many different cell types, including mesenchymal cells, epithelial cells, and neuronal cells (Wang et al., 1991). Betaglycan binds all three TGF-β isoforms and presents the ligands to the signaling receptors TβRII and TβRI, increasing the signaling activity of the type I receptor (Lopez-Casillas et al., 1993). Because of its sequence homology to betaglycan, a similar function was originally proposed for endoglin.

Endoglin is the most abundant TGF-β binding protein on endothelial cells (Cheifetz et al., 1992) and binds the β1 and β3 isoforms but not β2. Only 1% of the total endoglin molecules on the endothelial cell surface bind to TGF-β (Cheifetz et al., 1992). Despite its sequence similarities with betaglycan, endoglin appears to be an inhibitor of TGF-β signaling. In stable endoglin-transfected L6 cells, endoglin blocks both the TGF-β1-induced activation of a plasminogen activator inhibitor-1 (PAI-1) promoter reporter construct and the cell proliferation inhibitory effect of TGF-β1 (Letamendia et al., 1998). Furthermore, when overexpressed in the monocyte cell line U937, endoglin inhibits the TGF-β1-induced expression of fibronectin as well as the TGF-β1-induced downregulation of c-myc expression (Lastres et al., 1996).

Although endoglin exists primarily as a homodimer on the cell surface, it can also be found in a heteromeric complex with TβRI, TβRII, and ALK1 (Lastres et al., 1996; H. Zhang et al., 1996a; Lux et al., 1999; Pece-Barbara et al., 1999). When coexpressed with ActRII and ActRIIB, endoglin can also be an activin and BMP7 receptor, respectively (Pece-Barbara et al., 1999).

Endoglin is constitutively phosphorylated on its serine residues, and incubation with the protein kinase C inhibitor H-7 prevents endoglin phosphorylation (Lastres et al., 1994). After TGF-β1 treatment, endoglin becomes rapidly dephosphorylated. The regulatory role of these changes, if any, is unknown. The endoglin amino acid sequence also contains an RGD tripeptide (Gougos and Letarte, 1990), a key recognition motif found on extracellular matrix proteins such as fibronectin, von Willebrand's factor, fibrinogen, type I collagen, and vitronectin. This tripeptide is recognized by integrins (Ruoslahti and Pierschbacher, 1987; Hynes, 1987), which are important factors in cell–cell adhesion. The RGD sequence of endoglin may be involved in monocyte adhesion to endothelial cells (Gougos et al., 1992). Endoglin overexpression also inhibits the migratory capacity of NCTC929 fibroblasts. This may be a consequence of reduced PAI-1 and fibronectin production, impairing cell motility. Alternatively, high levels of endoglin might favor cell–cell interactions rather than migration (Guerrero-Esteo et al., 1999).

Several reports suggest that endoglin plays a key role in tumor-related angiogenesis. Elevated expression of endoglin correlates with proliferation of tumor endothelial cells (Miller et al., 1999), and higher levels of endoglin correlate with poor prognosis in breast carcinoma (Kumar et al., 1999). In vitro as well as in vivo studies demonstrate that anti-endoglin antibodies inhibit endothelial cell growth (Maier et al., 1997; Matsuno et al., 1999). In a therapeutic study, SCID mice were inoculated subcutaneously with MCF-7 human breast cancer cells and left untreated until palpable tumors of 4–6 mm in diameter appeared (Matsuno et al., 1999). These mice were then treated three times with two different conjugated monoclonal antiendoglin antibodies. Long-lasting, complete tumor regression (for at least 100 days) without further therapy was induced in the majority of tumor-bearing mice.

In view of the potential therapeutic applications of modulating endoglin gene expression for both HHT and possibly cancer, it is important to understand its tissue-specific expression. Two reports investigated the endoglin promoter structure (Rius et al., 1998; Graulich et al., 1999). There are several major and minor initiation transcription sites located approximately 350–420 nucleotides upstream of the ATG start codon. In the immediate upstream region of these initiation sites, no consensus TATA or CAAT boxes were found. The 5'-flanking region of endoglin contains several putative regulatory elements also present in other endothelium-specific genes, such as those for vWF, P-selectin, E-selectin, vascular cell adhesion molecule-1 (VCAM-1), platelet/endothelial cell adhesion molecule (PECAM), very late activation protein 4 receptor, alpha-4 subunit (VLA-4), and endothelin-1 (Pugh and Tjian, 1990; Williams and Tjian, 1991; Baeuerle and Henkel, 1994; Bassuk and Leiden, 1997; Orkin and Zon, 1997). These consensus elements include activator protein-2 (AP-2) sites, motifs of the ets family of transcription factors, one GATA site, two nuclear factor κB (NFκB) sites, five SP1 sites, and several TGF-β response elements including two putative SMAD sites. Various steroid-responsive elements have also been identified, and a Myc/Max site and several AP-1 and activating transcription factor/cAMP response element binding protein (ATF/CREB) sites are located further upstream (Graulich et al., 1999).

Reporter constructs using the endoglin promoter have been tested in several cell types. These constructs display endothelium-specific activity with no or only basal expression in porcine and human keratinocytes, the human hepatoma cell line HepG2, the human erythroleukemia cell line K562, mouse NIH3T3 fibroblasts, and the human cervical carcinoma cell line HeLa. The endoglin promoter is induced in the presence of TGF-β1, as suggested by the presence of the different TGF-β response elements. In monocytes, endoglin expression can be induced by either TGF-β1 or the phorbol ester phorbol myristate acetate (PMA). In light of the putative SMAD binding sites, it is interesting to note that SMAD3-mediated transcription can be induced by PMA. PMA addition to hematopoietic cells was found to activate a GAL4/SMAD-dependent promoter and a TGF-β-responsive promoter (Biggs and Kraft, 1999).

Endoglin expression is also upregulated by estradiol (Rius et al., 1998). This is intriguing in light of the therapeutic use of estrogens to control epistaxis and gastrointestinal bleeding in HHT patients. Estrogens are thought to control hemorrhage by inducing metaplasia of normal nasal mucosa to thick layers of keratinizing squamous epithelium (Harrison, 1964). This presumably covers the telangiectases and protects them against local trauma. Estrogens may also modulate the expression levels of coagulation factors (Geland, 1983). However, direct modulation of endoglin levels by estrogen may play a role in its efficacy at controlling bleeding in HHT patients.

Function of ALK1

ALK1 is a type I cell-surface receptor of the TGF-β superfamily of ligands. The protein is expressed primarily on endothelial cells and in highly vascularized tissues (Attisano et al., 1993). The ALK1 gene contains 10 exons, nine of which encode the protein sequence (Berg et al., 1997). ALK1 (also called TSR1, -R3) was cloned independently by three different groups (Attisano et al., 1993; ten Dijke et al., 1993; He et al., 1993). ALK1 has a molecular weight of approximately 60–70 kDa depending on its glycosylation status. Initial analyses of the newly described ALK1 receptor did not yield clear information about the corresponding ligand, the type II receptor, or the function of ALK1 in the cell. In coexpression studies in COS cells, ALK1 is able to bind TGF-β1 or Activin when coexpressed with TβRII and ActRII, respectively. However, neither of these complexes elicits a signal, as determined by a number of outcomes, including proliferation response, alteration in fibronectin expression, or ability to activate a PAI-1 promoter-based reporter gene in the mink lung cell line Mv1Lu. Nonetheless, these observations could not exclude TGF-β and activin as ALK1 ligands because ALK1 signaling initiated by these cytokines might activate other cellular responses. Using a chimeric ALK1 receptor comprising the extracellular ligand-binding domain of ALK1 fused to the intracellular signaling domain of TβRI, ALK1 was shown to be a receptor for TGF-β1 and -β3 ligands but not -β2 (Lux et al., 1999). This ligand specificity parallels that of endoglin (Cheifetz et al., 1992). This chimeric receptor can also signal through a third, yet unidentified ligand, present in human serum, which was shown not to be Activin A, BMP2, BMP7, or Inhibin (Lux et al., 1999). Signaling assays with coexpressed receptor pairs (Lux et al., 1999) and cross-linking studies (Oh et al., 2000) show that the corresponding type II receptor for ALK1 for TGF-β signaling is TβRII, while for signal induction by the unidentified ligand ALK1 probably complexes with ActRII or ActRIIB. ALK1 appears to have a lower affinity to the TGF-βs than TβRI (ALK-5), as suggested by the lower signaling activity of ALK1 compared to TβRI (ten Dijke et al., 1993; Lux et al., 1999). ALK1 signaling can inhibit the TGF-β1-induced activation of the PAI-1 promoter reporter construct (Lux et al., 1999).

These data suggest that one ALK1 function is to inhibit TGF-β1-induced cellular responses in endothelial cells. With few exceptions, endothelial cell turnover in a healthy adult organism is very low. Maintenance of the quiescent state is regulated by endogenous negative regulators. During angiogenesis, the balance between negative and positive regulators is shifted toward the positive regulators. TGF-β1 can be either a negative or a positive regulator, and this biphasic effect on angiogenesis is dependent on TGF-β1 concentration. Therefore, the endothelial response to TGF-β1 may also be concentration-dependent. This biphasic effect may be established by the use of two different receptors, such as TβRI and ALK1, which may have different affinities for TGF-β1.

TGF-β and activin signaling are usually mediated by Smad2 and Smad3 (Eppert et al., 1996; Macias-Silva et al., 1996; Y. Zhang et al., 1996; Nakao et al., 1997b,c). Smad1 and Smad5 were thought to be primarily BMP signal mediators. However, these two Smads may also be involved in TGF-β1 and TGF-β3 signaling (Liu et al., 1998; Yue et al., 1999). Murine Smad5 becomes phosphorylated after TGF-β1 induction, and overexpression of murine Smad5 in L6 cells results in growth arrest (Yingling et al., 1996). This is a typical effect of TGF-β on these cells. Smad5 is also involved in the signaling pathway by which TGF-β inhibits primitive human hematopoietic progenitor cell proliferation, and Smad5 antisense oligonucleotides can interrupt this signal (Bruno et al., 1998). Although ALK1 is a TGF-β receptor, the ALK1 downstream targets are Smad1 and Smad5. A constitutively active ALK1 receptor phosphorylates Smad1 (Macias-Silva et al., 1998; Chen and Massague, 1999). Furthermore, TGF-β1 is able to induce Smad1 and Smad5 phosphorylation via ALK1 (ten Dijke et al., 1993; also reported as unpublished data in Macias-Silva et al., 1998; Piek et al., 1999; Chen and Massague, 1999). Studies in breast cancer cells demonstrated that TGF-β3 responses are mediated by Smad1 (Liu et al., 1998). It is possible that some of the reported Smad1 and Smad5 effects are induced by TGF-β1 via ALK1 signaling, rather than TβRI. Therefore, it is important to further elucidate the role of Smad1 and Smad5 in the ALK1 signaling pathway.

CLINICAL DESCRIPTION

Historical Perspective

HHT is an autosomal dominant disease characterized by recurrent epistaxis, mucocutaneous telangiectasis, and arteriovenous malformations, particularly of the pulmonary and cerebral circulation. The original name of the disorder, Osler-Rendu-Weber syndrome, originates from three physicians who wrote early descriptions of the disease. A paper by Rendu (1896) entitled "Epistaxis répétées chez un sujet porteur de petits angiomes cutanes et muqueux" ("Recurring nosebleeds in a patient with small cutaneous angiomas of the skin and mucous membranes") remains one of the best descriptions of the disease. Rendu described a 52-year-old man admitted with a prolonged nosebleed. He had a history of epistaxis occurring several times a day, which started at the age of 12 and became much more frequent after the age of 35. He described facial lesions:

Il existe sur la peau du nez, des joues, de la levre superieure et du menton de petites taches pourprees . . . les plus grosses atteignant les dimensions d'une lentille, et qui sont de veritables angiome cutanes, produit par une dilatation des vaisseaux superficiels de la peau.

On the skin of the nose, cheeks, upper lip and chin, there are small purple marks . . . the largest approach the size of a lentil, and these are true cutaneous angiomas produced by a dilatation of the superficial vessels of the skin (Rendu, 1896).

Earlier descriptions of the syndrome exist, and these include one by H.G. Sutton in the *Medical Mirror* in 1864 and a discussion of the association between hemoptysis and epistaxis by C. Rattray in a dissertation presented to the Royal Medical Society in Edinburgh in 1800. The more descriptive name *hereditary hemorrhagic telangiectasia* originated in a comprehensive discussion of the disorder written by Hanes in 1909, while a resident at Johns Hopkins Hospital.

Prevalence of HHT

Two studies have attempted to estimate the incidence of HHT based on epidemiologic recruitment of cases. A study of the French population (Bideau et al., 1980, 1992) estimated an overall prevalence of 1 in 8345 people. However, several areas had a much higher local prevalence, such as the Jura region (1 in 5062) and Deux-Sevres (1 in 4287). The minimum point prevalence in the north of England was estimated at 1 in 39,216 based on questionnaires sent to general practitioners; ear, nose, and throat surgeons; and hematologists, revealing a minimum reported incidence of 79 cases in a population of 3.1 million (Porteous et al., 1992). A further study in Vermont based on known cases of HHT estimated the minimum prevalence at approximately 1 in 16,500 (Guttmacher et al., 1994). This wide variation in estimates of prevalence is likely to be due in part to underdiagnosis, with many cases in the population unidentified, and in part to a high incidence in some isolated populations.

CLINICAL FEATURES

Mucocutaneous Telangiectases

The classical mucocutaneous lesions, as described by Rendu in 1896, are small, purple marks of variable size with a characteristic distribution. These blanche on pressure and refill immediately. Classical lesions are shown in Figure 28–1. As described by several authors (Osler, 1901; Bird et al., 1957), the telangiectases can become raised and nodular, usually in later life. Spider angiomas have been reported (Bird et al., 1957) but are not as characteristic.

A study in the French population found telangiectases in 74% of 240 patients on careful examination (Plauchu et al., 1989). About half of all patients who could remember the time of onset of lesions reported first appearance before the age of 30. They reported the most common site of telangiectases as the face (63% of patients) followed by the mouth (48%) and hands (37%). Lesions on the trunk, arms, and lower limbs were much less common (fewer than 10% of patients), with many fewer lesions at these sites. For patients with oral involvement, the lower lip and tongue were most frequently involved. The palate was involved in 13% of patients, as were the ears. The floor of the mouth, conjunctiva, eyelids, and gums were involved in 5% or fewer of patients.

In a British study (Porteous et al., 1992), the sites most frequently affected with telangiectases were the palm and nailbed (71% of all patients), lips and tongue (66%), and the face (20%).

Epistaxis

Epistaxis is usually the first symptom of HHT to occur, although the frequency and severity are very variable. Some people are only ever mildly affected, whereas in others epistaxis can be prolonged and at times life-threatening. Plauchu et al. (1989) found more than half of patients had epistaxis before the age of 20, with 90% complaining of the symptom by age 45. Of those between the ages of 45 and 60, 70% had heavy episodes lasting more than 10 minutes. Porteous et al.

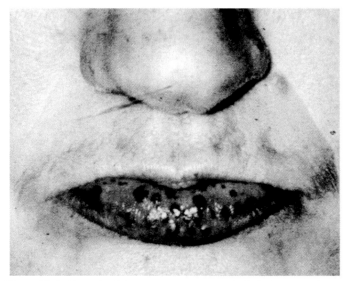

Figure 28–1. Example of the mucocutaneous vascular lesions commonly observed in hereditary hemorrhagic telangiectasia. Multiple telangiectasias are evident on the lower lip.

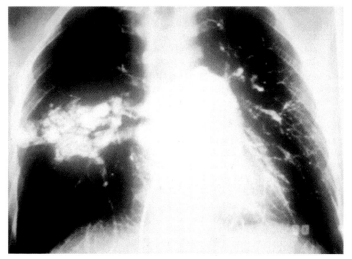

Figure 28–2. Pulmonary angiograph showing a large pulmonary arteriovenous malformation in the right mid-zone with smaller lesions around the left hilum. Over 50% of the cardiac output was passing through the lesions, leading to cyanosis, finger-clubbing, and severely restricted exercise tolerance.

(1992) reported that 16 of 40 patients over the age of 50 said the epistaxis had stayed the same, 16 said it had deteriorated, and 8 said it had improved. In a study of patients screened for pulmonary arteriovenous malformations (Assar et al., 1991), an increase in the frequency of epistaxis with age was seen, from an average of 8 per month under age 20 to 22 per month over age 40.

Gastrointestinal Hemorrhage

Gastrointestinal hemorrhage has been less commonly encountered in population-based studies and usually starts in later life. In the French study (Plauchu et al., 1989), 16% of patients were affected but half were over age 58; only 1.5% of those under the age of 30 had gastrointestinal hemorrhage. Porteous et al. (1992) reported 16 patients out of 56 suffering this complication, mainly from the upper gastrointestinal tract. A Danish study (Vase and Grove, 1986) found gastro-intestinal hemorrhage in 35 of 139 patients, only two of whom were under age 40. Median age at onset was 55 compared to a median age of 11 for the onset of epistaxis. These patients had predominantly gastric and duodenal telangiectases, although five also had colonic telangiectases.

Hepatic Complications

The incidence of symptomatic hepatic lesions is low. In a French cohort (Plauchu et al., 1989), 8% of patients exhibited hepatomegaly, jaundice, cirrhosis or a hepatic murmur. Onset of symptoms was usually in later life. Several families have been reported with a much higher incidence of hepatic involvement than expected. A family with a father, three daughters, and a grandson with symptomatic liver lesions and other classical features of HHT has been reported (Martini, 1978). His review of all autopsy evidence to date suggested that fibrovascular lesions were a common finding in HHT, with evidence of cirrhosis in some patients. Angiographic findings in those with symptomatic hepatic lesions usually show diffuse small arteriovenous communications.

Pulmonary Complications

Pulmonary arteriovenous malformations (PAVMs) are one of the most characteristic lesions of HHT. They vary in size from insignificantly small to very large and may be single or very numerous. An angiogram showing a PAVM is given in Figure 28–2. Complications of PAVMs can arise as a result of a large pulmonary shunt. This manifests as cyanosis and hypoxia with finger clubbing and exercise limitation. More commonly, PAVMs are asymptomatic until they present with hemoptysis, stroke, or cerebral abscess. Hemoptysis or hemothorax

has been reported as a complication in 11 of 143 patients with PAVMs and HHT (Ference et al., 1994). Bleeding in some of these cases may have come from endobronchial telangiectases (Wirth et al., 1996). In an unpublished study (L. Charnas personal communication), 102 patients referred for embolization of PAVMs were screened by computed tomography (CT) or magnetic resonance imaging (MRI). Nine patients had clinically silent infarctions, 13 had subtle focal neurologic findings, and 21 had a history of stroke confirmed on scanning. PAVMs may therefore have been causative of cerebral infarcts in up to 43 of 102 patients. In 11 patients, the stroke predated the diagnosis of PAVM. Cerebral abscesses had affected nine of this patient series.

Presence of a PAVM also confers a higher risk of complication in pregnancy, although it is difficult to accurately quantify this. Worsening of the pulmonary shunt is well documented and improves to some extent after delivery (Swinburne et al., 1986). There is also a high incidence of stroke and pulmonary hemorrhage documented in women who become pregnant who are known to have a preexisting PAVM. A series of 161 pregnancies in 47 women with HHT (Shovlin et al., 1995) showed worsening shunt in six patients, stroke in three, and fatal pulmonary hemorrhage in two. In all but one case, complications occurred in the 12 mothers with known PAVMs, suggesting a much lower risk in mothers who have screened negative for a PAVM.

Different reports give varied estimates of the incidence of PAVMs. Plauchu et al. (1989) estimated that 4.6% of their population had PAVMs. In the north of England (Porteous et al., 1992), PAVMs were reported in 13 of 56 individuals. A Danish study (Vase et al., 1985), found that 16 of 95 patients had PAVMs on screening by chest X-ray. In a study of patients and their first degree relatives in Holland (Haitjema et al., 1995a,b), PAVMs were seen in 12 of 36 patients. Some early case reports found no PAVMs in families (Bird et al., 1957; Hodgson et al., 1959), whereas a high incidence has been seen in other families (Hodgson et al., 1959; Shovlin et al., 1994).

CNS Complications

Some complications affecting the CNS, such as embolic stroke and cerebral abscess, result directly from loss of the pulmonary filtering capability caused by a PAVM. Cerebral arteriovenous malformations (CAVMs) were found in 4 or 36 Dutch patients on CT scanning (Haitjema et al., 1995b). Most lesions are asymptomatic, but complications of epilepsy or hemorrhage can develop without warning. Reports of CAVMs often show clustering within a family (King et al., 1977; Lesser et al., 1986; Kikuchi et al., 1994). This may be due to genetic background or specific gene mutations predisposing to such lesions. Treatment of asymptomatic CAVMs is controversial, and whether or not to operate on a lesion depends on its size, position, and estimated likelihood of bleeding.

Migraine occurs more commonly in HHT (Steele et al., 1993). The reason for this is unknown; possibly, small asymptomatic cerebral arteriovenous malformations cause migrainous symptoms, or loss of pulmonary filtering capacity allows vascular mediators to circulate in abnormal concentrations to the cerebral circulation, producing migrainous symptoms.

To date, the only assessment of HHT penetrance is based on clinical criteria and incidence in unaffected obligate carriers of the disease. Three asymptomatic obligate carriers were seen in the French series of 103 patients (Plauchu et al., 1989). When looking at penetrance in relation to age in this cohort, it was estimated to be 75% by age 25 and 90% by age 45. In the British series (Porteous et al., 1992), 83% were symptomatic by age 26 and all by age 40.

Pathologic Findings in HHT

Three studies have looked at the microscopic structure of skin lesions. The most recent and systematic study (Braverman et al., 1990) was performed by microscopy of a series of skin lesion biopsies. This has built up a picture of lesion development over time. Very early lesions showed dilatation of the postcapillary venule with preservation of the capillary bed. As the lesions increased in size, the capillary segments disappeared, leaving a direct arteriovenous connection, which enlarged under pressure. The lesions were associated with a perivascular cell infiltrate, which consisted of a mixture of lymphocytes and monocytic cells (Fig. 28–3).

Electron microscopy on a number of mucosal and cutaneous telangiectases showed that the lesions were dilated small venules with a thin endothelial cell wall (Hashimoto and Pritzker, 1972). There was some evidence of weakness of junctions between endothelial cells. Often, dilatation resulted in cavernous spaces filled with fibrin and erythrocytes. The abnormal regions were not in association with smooth muscle cells or fibroblasts.

A further study (Menefee et al., 1975) confirmed the presence of dilated post-capillary venules but noted that the basal lamina was often duplicated and thickened. This suggested that there was considerable endothelial cell death and regeneration. This might also be due to abnormal turnover of old basal membrane. Evidence of extravasation of blood was seen, including erythrocytes and deposition of fibrin, which could form the basis for new capillary sprouts, although no such sprouts were noted.

The triggering factor that initiates formation of a telangiectasis is unknown, and the reasons that only specific areas of skin and mucous membranes are affected are also unclear. It has been suggested that thermal insult, ultraviolet light, or a second genetic mutation may initiate lesion formation.

MOLECULAR GENETICS

Endoglin, the HHT1 Gene

In the absence of clear candidate genes for HHT, a positional cloning approach was used to identify the molecular defect. Genetic linkage for some families was established to markers on 9q33-q34 (McDonald et al., 1994; Shovlin et al., 1994). The identification of key obligate recombinants in affected individuals from families linked to this region allowed refinement of the HHT1 locus. The most likely position of the HHT1 gene was defined within a 2–3 cM interval between D9S60 and D9S61 (Shovlin et al., 1994; Heutink et al., 1994; McAllister et al., 1994a). *Endoglin* was considered a strong candidate gene based on its location on human chromosome 9q34 (Fernandez-Ruiz et al., 1993), its precise position in the syntenic region of the mouse genome (Pilz et al., 1995), and its biologic properties as a TGF-β binding protein expressed predominantly in endothelial cells. Mutations in *endoglin* were subsequently identified in HHT1 kindreds (McAllister et al., 1994a). More recent physical mapping shows that the *endoglin* gene maps between genetic markers D9S60 and D9S61, near D9S315 and D9S112. These latter markers are useful to establish or exclude linkage to this locus in new HHT families.

ALK1, the HHT2 Gene

Locus heterogeneity for HHT was indicated by families which excluded linkage to chromosome 9q3 (Shovlin et al., 1994; Heutink, et al., 1994; McAllister et al., 1994b). A second HHT locus (HHT2) was subsequently identified in the pericentromeric region of chromosome 12 (Vincent et al., 1995; Johnson et al., 1996). Based on haplotype analysis and crossovers in these 12q-linked families, a 1 cM candidate interval was established between D12S347 and D12S368. These markers are useful to establish or exclude linkage to this locus in new HHT families. A potential candidate gene, *ALK1*, was shown to map within this interval. ALK1 is a type I cell-surface receptor for the TGF-β superfamily of ligands. The protein is expressed primarily on endothelial cells and in highly vascularized tissues (Attisano et al., 1993; ten Dijke et al., 1993). Mutations were identified within this gene in HHT2 families (Johnson et al., 1996; Berg et al., 1997). Recently, mutations in *ALK1* were also identified in families with vascular dilatation characteristic of HHT and occlusion of small pulmonary arteries typical of primary pulmonary hypertension (Trembath et al., 2001). Thus, pulmonary hypertension in association with HHT can be caused by mutations in *ALK1*.

Evidence for Further HHT Loci

Two reports have suggested the existence of a third locus for HHT. Wallace and Shovlin (2000) reported convincing exclusion of both

Figure 28–3. Development of cutaneous vascular malformations (telangiectasia) in hereditary hemorrhagic telangiectasia. *Left*: In normal skin, arterioles (A) in the papillary dermis connect to venules (V) through multiple capillaries (C). A normal postcapillary venule (shown in cross section in the inset) consists of the lumen (L), a single layer of endothelial cells (blue), and two to three layers of pericytes. *Center*: In the early stage of telangiectasia development, a single venule becomes dilated but is still connected to an arteriole through one or more capillaries. A perivascular lymphocytic infiltrate is present. *Right*: In fully developed telangiectasias, the venule and its branches become markedly dilated, elongated, and convoluted throughout the dermis. The connecting arterioles also become dilated, and these communicate directly with the venules without an intervening capillary bed. The perivascular infiltrate is still present. The dilated descending venule is markedly thickened with as many as 11 layers of smooth muscle cells. (Adapted from Braverman et al., 1990.)

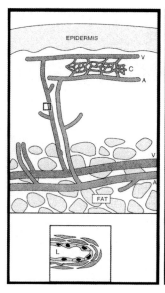
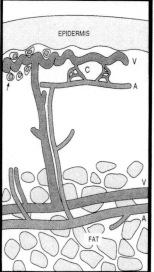
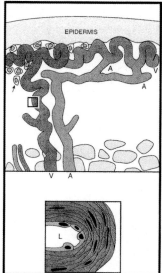

HHT1 and HHT2 loci in a large family with a high incidence of PAVMs. Piantanida et al. (1996) reported a large family with a high incidence of hepatic involvement, for which the two known loci had also been excluded. To date, however, no evidence of linkage to a third locus has been published and no other gene identified.

Genotype–Phenotype Correlation

Few clinical studies have examined the phenotypic differences between patients with HHT1 (*endoglin* mutations) and those with HHT2 (*ALK1* mutations). No study has examined the differences in the pathology of lesions between these two groups.

Incidence of PAVMs

An initial subjective observation was made that the families linked to *endoglin* on 9q34 seemed to have a much higher incidence of PAVMs than families for whom this locus was excluded (Porteous et al., 1994; McAllister et al., 1994b). Further analysis confirmed that this difference was genuine (Berg et al., 1996). This study showed that for patients in whom HHT can be attributed to *endoglin* mutation, there is an incidence of PAVMs of approximately 30% but that the incidence of PAVMs was <5% in patients for whom the *endoglin* locus had been excluded.

More recent studies of families with known *ALK1* mutations have shown PAVMs in some affected individuals. In one large family, the incidence was at a lower rate (around 6%) than for patients with *endoglin* mutations (McDonald et al., 2000); in another family, HHT was caused by a specific missense mutation in *ALK1* (Kjeldsen et al., 2000).

It is now accepted that, on the whole, patients with HHT2 have a lower incidence of PAVMs than patients with HHT1. The reason why occasional HHT2 families show a high incidence of PAVMs is not understood but may be related to a locus-specific effect or other as yet unidentified modifier loci.

Difference in Severity of Disease

Only one unpublished study (Berg et al., unpublished data) has looked at age at onset and presence or absence of other clinical features for patients with known *endoglin* or *ALK1* mutations. This study, based on a questionnaire survey of patients with known mutations, has shown significantly younger onset of epistaxis ($P < 0.01$) and earlier appearance of telangiectases ($P < 0.001$) in patients with HHT1 compared to those with HHT2.

Endoglin MUTATIONS IN HHT1

Over 50 distinct mutations have been identified in the *endoglin* gene in HHT families. In all but a few cases, these mutations appear to be family-specific. These include missense mutations, nonsense mutations, larger genomic deletions, splice site changes, and small nucleotide insertions and deletions leading to frameshifts and premature stop codons. Nonsense mutations and frameshift mutations have been identified in exons 3–12, which, if translated, would produce severely truncated proteins. Expression data from a number of frameshift and nonsense mutations show that many of these create unstable messages (Pece et al., 1997; Gallione et al., 1998); therefore, little to no mutant proteins would be produced. Thus, these mutations are assumed to create null alleles. The identical missense mutation within the start codon of the *endoglin* gene has been identified in two unrelated families (Gallione et al., 1998). This mutation appears to be a null allele that eliminates the translation of the endoglin protein, similar to start codon mutations in other genetic disorders (John et al., 1992; Sligh et al., 1992; Conley et al., 1994; Lastres et al., 1996). Large and small deletions of the coding region have also been described (Shovlin et al., 1997), some of which are not transcribed. These are also clear examples of null alleles.

As in many genetic disorders, the missense mutations in *endoglin* can be instructive for understanding endoglin structure and function (Gallione et al., 1998). Two missense mutations in *endoglin* are within or adjacent to Cys[53], suggesting that this is a critical residue involved in intra- or intermolecular disulfide bridging. In another HHT family,

a conserved tryptophan at codon 149 is mutated to a cysteine. It may be significant that this mutation creates, rather than destroys, a cysteine as this substitution might cause aberrant disulfide linkages. In another family, a Leu-to-Pro substitution disrupts a predicted α helix in the extracellular domain. These missense mutations suggest that in these cases the mutant *endoglin* is misfolded and thus potentially nonfunctional. Expression studies show that this is the case (Pece-Barbara et al., 1999; Lux et al., 2000). In general, these missense mutations show no cell-surface expression. Thus, each of the *endoglin* mutations would be predicted to lead to reduced levels of functional *endoglin* at the endothelial cell surface.

ALK1 MUTATIONS IN HHT2

Over 20 mutations have been identified in the *ALK1* gene in different HHT families, indicating that, like *endoglin* mutations, *ALK1* mutations are for the most part family-specific. Mutations are found throughout the gene and fall into classes of nonsense, frameshift, and missense mutations. The nonsense and frameshift mutations are found in the extracellular domain as well as in the kinase domain. If translated, these would create truncated proteins. The strongest candidate for a null allele in the *ALK1* gene is a 1 bp insertion mutation in exon 3 (140insG) (Klaus et al., 1998). This theoretical polypeptide would lack a large portion of the extracellular domain, the entire transmembrane and GS domains, and the entire serine-threonine kinase domain. RNA expression data for some of the *ALK1* nonsense and frameshift mutations show that little or no message can be detected from the mutant allele (Berg et al., 1997). Five distinct missense mutations have been identified within the kinase domain of *ALK1*. These appear at residues that are conserved in the *ALK* gene family and more generally in most serine-threonine kinase receptors. These data suggest that these mutations reduce or abrogate *ALK1* signaling, although this has not formally been tested in a signaling assay. Five distinct missense mutations have also been identified in the extracellular domain of *ALK1*. Intriguingly, all are within or near conserved cysteine residues in the extracellular domain, suggesting that amino acid substitutions at or near these residues might interfere with critical intra- or intermolecular disulfide bridges. Three of the missense mutations in the extracellular domain were tested in a signaling assay using a chimeric *ALK1* receptor, and these mutations abrogated signaling (Lux et al., 1999). These data, in combination with the sum of the mutation data, suggest that most mutations create null alleles, leading to reduced signaling through the *ALK1* receptor.

ESTABLISHING THE DIAGNOSIS

Clinical diagnosis has always been based on combinations of the presence of affected first-degree relatives, frequent epistaxis, presence of a PAVM, and classical telangiectases. Recently, the Medical Advisory Board of the HHT Foundation International recommended the following consensus clinical diagnostic criteria (Shovlin et al., 2000), diagnosis requiring three of the following four criteria: presence of epistaxes, telangiectasia, visceral lesions, and an appropriate family history. The presence of two of these should be considered as a possible or suspect status. However, given the frequency of nosebleeds in the general population, Shovlin et al. (1994) recommended that frequent epistaxis with an affected relative should not be sufficient for a diagnosis in a research setting. In a clinical setting, it may be appropriate to have a higher index of suspicion.

Screening of patients with HHT for asymptomatic PAVMs is advocated by most authors. However, not all authors agree on the best method of screening. Chest X-ray and pulse oximetry, measuring the saturation drop between supine and erect positioning, has been advocated as a simple test (Hughes, 1994) but never truly validated (Kjeldsen et al., 1996). The use of lung perfusion scan, when a right-to-left shunt would lead to increased deposition of radiolabeled macroaggregates in the kidneys, may prove to be a more useful test (White, 1992). Measurement of arterial oxygen saturation and right-to-left shunt have been shown to be both sensitive and specific as screening tests (Haitjema et al., 1995a). Contrast echocardiography has been advocated as a sensitive screening test, although it remains to be fully assessed in this role (Kjeldsen et al., 1996). Helical CT scanning is expensive but allows demonstration of the architecture of complex lesions. Angiography remains the gold standard for investigation of suspected lesions (Hughes, 1994; Wirth and White, 1996).

PROSPECTS FOR A MOLECULAR DIAGNOSTIC TEST FOR HHT

Since the genomic structures for the *endoglin* and *ALK1* genes are known (McAllister et al., 1994a; Shovlin et al., 1997; Berg et al., 1997), amplification of individual exons and DNA sequence analysis could be performed as a diagnostic test for HHT. The family-specific nature of mutations suggests that this would be labor-intensive. In addition, the possibility of large deletions would need to be investigated thoroughly before any negative result could be confirmed in new families (Shovlin et al., 1997).

Measurement of endoglin expression from appropriate tissues has been exploited for diagnostic assays for HHT1. Protein expression assays have been performed on human umbilical vein endothelial cells isolated from newborns of affected mothers (Eiken et al., 1992; Cymerman et al., 2000). This tissue is one of the few available from living patients that expresses high levels of endoglin protein. Using a monoclonal antibody to the endoglin protein, these studies revealed reduced endoglin protein levels in mutation carriers. This human umbilical vein endothelial cell endoglin protein expression assay has been suggested as a simple screening test for newborns in HHT kindreds (Cymerman et al., 2000). Macrophages, or activated monocytes, express endoglin on the cell surface, albeit at levels greatly reduced from those of endothelial cells. Nonetheless, peripheral blood can be obtained from children or adults; and after activation of the monocytes by adherence to a plastic culture dish for approximately 24 hours, these can be assayed for endoglin protein levels. This offers the possibility of diagnosis for individuals in HHT kindreds other than newborns. When these cells are isolated from known HHT1 patients, endoglin levels are approximately 50% of normal values (Eiken et al., 1992; Pece et al., 1997). Thus, a protein assay for HHT1 screening might also be possible for children and adults. However, endoglin levels on activated monocytes can vary widely as these are modulated by hormones and other factors. This may limit the use of the monocyte endoglin assay as a diagnostic tool.

MANAGEMENT

Management of HHT is related to the organ systems affected in the individual patient and the extent of symptoms. Embolization of PAVMs is advocated for all lesions, with feeding vessels greater than 3 mm (White, 1992; White et al., 1996). Rare complications of treatment include localized pleurisy, arrhythmia, and rarely paradoxical embolism of occluding device (Haitjema et al., 1995b, 1996; White, et al., 1996). Early recurrence of an AVM can be due to failure to occlude all feeding vessels; late recurrence can occur following recanalization of a lesion (White et al., 1996). Small, previously unidentified PAVMs may also increase in size and become significant during follow-up. Not all lesions are amenable to embolization; some are still too large for embolization and can be safely removed surgically. Treatment of patients with multiple small PAVMs remains difficult (Wirth and White, 1996). Diffuse, small hepatic arteriovenous malformations often preclude treatment by transcutaneous embolization. Occasionally, liver transplant has proved the only available treatment (Bauer et al., 1995).

Various treatments for gastrointestinal hemorrhage are available. Laser treatment can be effective if lesions are few in number (Bown et al., 1985), but the long-term results may be less promising (Naveau et al., 1990). Desmopressin has been used with success to control acute bleeds refractory to normal management (Quitt et al., 1990). Successful treatment of those with severe hemorrhage using estrogens is now established (Van Cutsem et al., 1988, 1990; Van Cutsem and Piessevaux, 1996).

ANIMAL MODELS OF HHT

Studies on TGF-β1 and TβRII knockout mice demonstrate the importance of TGF-β signaling for vascular development. Targeted disruption of the TGF-β ligand results in defects of yolk sac vasculature, specifically disruption of cellular adhesion between the two endothelial layers of the yolk sac. Leakage of blood cells into the yolk sac is reminiscent of the HHT hemorrhage defect. This defect occurs in only 50% of the offspring due to strain differences that affect the stage of development where lethality occurs, indicating that the phenotype of TGF-β1 null mice is dependent on modification by other genes (Bonyadi et al., 1997). TβRII is also critical for angiogenesis in the yolk sac but not in primary vasculogenesis (Dickson et al., 1995; Oshima et al., 1996). TβRII overexpression as well as TβRII inhibition lead to phenotypes similar to those in TβRII and TGF-β1 knockout mice (Goumans et al., 1999). These data suggest that TGF-β1 is necessary for the organization and maintenance of the vascular network. Furthermore, TGF-β1 is responsible for the deposition of fibronectin in the extracellular matrix, to guarantee yolk sac integrity. Thus, TGF-β1 signaling must be optimal and exactly balanced for normal yolk sac development. How this is achieved, either through different TGF-β receptors such as TβRI and ALK1 or by specific Smad signaling pathways, is yet unknown. The early-death phenotype due to defects in yolk sac vascularization may mask later effects on vasculogenesis in the embryo proper. Thus, these mouse models, while providing some clues as to the role of TGF-β signaling in angiogenesis, do not explain the nature of the defect seen in HHT.

The roles of the *endoglin* and *ALK1* genes in vascular development have also been probed by their disruption in the mouse. For both genes, homozygous knockout mice exhibit embryonic lethality due to arrested endothelial remodeling. Three different groups have disrupted the *endoglin* gene (Li et al., 1999; Bourdeau et al., 1999; Arthur et al., 2000). The primary defect is maturation arrest of the primitive vascular plexus of the yolk sac into defined vessels, leading to channel dilatation and rupture. Embryos show distended blood yolk sac vessels by embryonic day (e) 9.5, a lack of vascular organization by e10.5, and embryos resorption by e11.5. Smooth muscle cell differentiation and recruitment to the vessels are also defective. Various heart defects have been reported, including abnormal cardiac looping and enlarged cardiac ventricles and pericardical sac. Heart valve formation is also disrupted, with reduction in the size of the atrioventricular endocardial cushions and disorganization of the endothelial surface of the cushions. Thus, *endoglin* plays a crucial role in heart development.

ALK1 homozygous null embryos also exhibit embryonic lethality due to defects in vascular development. By e9.5 they show absence of mature blood vessels in the yolk sac, and the embryos are resorbed by e10.5. Histologic analysis of the mutant embryos shows excessive fusion of capillary plexus into cavernous vessels. Hyperdilatation of large vessels and deficient differentiation and recruitment of smooth muscle cells are also evident. The endocardium and myocardium are also immature, suggesting a role for *ALK1* in heart development. Transcript levels of tissue-type plasminogen activator, urokinase-type plasminogen activator, and PAI-1 are elevated in the embryos, in keeping with a role of the plasminogen–plasmin system in the proteolysis of perivascular matrix during angiogenesis (Saksela and Rifkin, 1988; Carmeliet et al., 1994).

Preliminary analyses of heterozygotes for both *ALK1* and *endoglin* knockout mice, the proper genetic model for the HHT phenotype, suggest that a phenotype will be less obvious and may be strain-specific. A subtle phenotype of vessel dilatation under the abdominal skin was noted in a few mice in one study of *endoglin* heterozygotes (Arthur et al., 2000). In another study, a phenotype of epistaxis, cutaneous telangiectases, and disease sequelae including stroke and congestive heart failure was observed for *endoglin* heterozygotes when crossed into the inbred mouse strain background 129/Ola (Bourdeau, et al., 1999, 2001). *ALK1* heterozyotes also exhibit vascular lesions in a mixed genetic background (Srinivasan and Marchuk, unpublished observations). As previously described, strain-specific phenotypes are also seen with TGF-β1-deficient mice (Bonyadi et al., 1997). The existence of genetic modifiers of the mouse phenotypes is consistent with the phenotypic data in human HHT kindreds, where the phenotype can vary widely even in the same family, suggesting that other genetic and environmental factors modify the phenotype. The identification of modifier genes in the mouse should eventually lead to examination of their human homologues in HHT kindreds.

DEVELOPMENTAL PATHOGENESIS OF HHT

Physiologic Effects of TGF-β on Vascular Morphogenesis

TGF-β inhibits the division and migration of endothelial cells (Sato and Rifkin, 1989). TGF-β-induced suppression of endothelial growth is important in branching morphogenesis of capillaries (Roberts, 1998). This growth-inhibitory effect may also be important in the remodeling seen in vascular lesion formation in HHT. TGF-β also induces changes in gene expression of a number of extracellular matrix proteins. Genes that are upregulated (in mesechymal cells) by TGF-β include fibronectin, a number of collagen types, biglycan, and decorin. Other known genes that are upregulated in response to TGF-β include inhibitors of metalloproteinases such as PAI-1 and tissue inhibitor of metalloproteinase-1. TGF-β1 is upregulated in repair of injury, in response to stress, and during virus-induced pathogenesis; any of these might be a trigger for lesion formation. TGF-β1 also upregulates the synthesis and secretion of endothelin by vascular endothelial cells cultured in vitro (Kurihara et al., 1989). Endothelin-1 is a potent vasoconstrictor implicated in the pathogenesis of hypertension and vascular remodeling, but its role in HHT has not been addressed.

Genes that are downregulated in response to TGF-β include plasminogen activator, collagenase, elastase, stromelysin, and c-myc. It is intriguing that HHT-associated lesions show increased plaminogen activator levels, as measured by a histochemical fibrin slide assay (Kwaan and Silverman, 1973). The fibrinolysis inhibitor aminocaproic acid has therefore been used with limited success to control hemorrhage in HHT. As it appears that ALK1 and endoglin inhibit TGF-β signaling, an endoglin or ALK1 mutation would be expected to lead to increased levels of plasminogen activator, especially at the site of a vascular lesion. This is supported by the mouse knockout of ALK1, where mutant embryos show increased levels of plasminogen activator (Oh et al., 2000).

The only analysis of extracellular matrix gene expression patterns in HHT was a comparative study of fibroblasts from HHT and ataxia-telangiectasia patients (Becker and Tabor, 1989). Although HHT fibroblasts showed a high level of fibronectin and increased levels of integrin and β-actin mRNA expression, it is not clear whether fibroblasts would show the same effects as endothelial cells. Nonetheless, increased levels of fibronectin would be expected in HHT patient tissue if endoglin and ALK1 play negative roles in TGF-β signaling.

The combined biochemical data suggest that ALK1 and endoglin play crucial roles in regulating capillary morphogenesis. Endothelial cells can exist in either an activation phase or a resolution phase during angiogenesis (Fig. 28–4). The activation phase is characterized by endothelial cell invasion, migration into the extracellular space, subsequent proliferation, and capillary tube formation. Proteolytic degradation of the basement membrane is required to initiate this process. The resolution phase is characterized by cessation of migration and proliferation and reestablishment of the basement membrane. Analysis of the TGF-β response of endothelial cells with ALK1 or ALK-5 removed by antisense RNA suggests that the two receptors are involved in the balance between the activation and resolution phases of angiogenesis (Goumans et al., 2002). Infection of endothelial cells with constitutively active ALK1 leads to increased cell migration and proliferation. In contrast, constitutively active ALK-5 leads to decreased cell migration and proliferation. In addition, activated ALK-5 induces PAI-1, suggesting a role in vessel maturation. The combined biochemical and mouse knockout data suggest a model for the roles of endoglin and ALK1 in angiogenesis and in the pathogenesis of HHT (Fig. 28–5). The vascular abnormalities in the ALK1 null mice

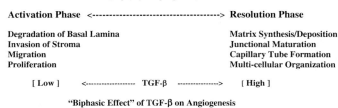

Figure 28–4. The angiogenic switch, capillary morphogenesis, and TGF-β. Endothelial cells go through two distinct phases during capillary morphogenesis, as described in the text. TGF-β may play a critical role in this angiogenic switch as in vitro data suggest that low concentrations of ligand favor events associated with the activation phase, whereas high concentrations favor events associated with the resolution phase.

may result from inappropriate persistence of the resolution phase of angiogenesis. Thus, ALK1 may regulate the transition of endothelial cells from the activation to the resolution phase of angiogenesis. The biphasic effect of TGF-β on endothelial cells may also be part of this transition (Pepper et al., 1996). Low concentration of TGF-β may favor binding to the higher-affinity TβRI receptor, which may modulate genes involved in the resolution phase of angiogenesis. Higher concentrations of the TGF-β ligand may be required for binding to the lower-affinity ALK1 receptor, which inhibits the TβRI pathway and, thus, may shift the gene expression profile to favor the activation phase of angiogenesis.

Mutations in the ALK1 gene would reduce signaling through this receptor, thus favoring signaling through TβRI and the resolution phase of angiogenesis. Mutations in endoglin would have a similar effect, removing the negative modulation of TGF-β through TβRI, thereby shifting the balance of signal to favor the activation phase. This model assumes that endoglin enhances (or at least does not inhibit) ALK1 receptor–mediated signaling.

Another possibility is that altered TGF-β signaling may not be the underlying cause of HHT. Since ALK1 can signal through a yet unidentified ligand and endoglin might modulate this signal, these data suggest that a different ligand could be involved. One scenario is that the TGF-β signaling pathway competes with an alternative pathway for a common downstream effector. In this way, signaling through ALK1 may inhibit TGF-β signaling. It has been demonstrated that high levels of BMP signaling titrate Smad4 and compete with activin signaling (Candia et al., 1997). A similar competition for ALK1 and endoglin may occur by the TGF-β ligand and another ligand.

Vascular Lesion Development in HHT

Although the mechanisms by which mutations affect endoglin and ALK1 function are being elucidated, the factor(s) responsible for vascular lesion formation remains unknown. A reduction to 50% of functional endoglin or ALK1 levels is compatible with development of a normal vascular system in utero since there is no evidence of increased miscarriage in HHT families (W. McKinnon and A. Guttmacher, personal communication). However, mutation carriers are at nearly 100% risk of developing the vascular lesions observed in HHT. Significantly, one of the most crucial aspects of lesion development, that is, whether the lesions are congenital or not, has yet to be determined. Although the cutaneous lesions suggest the contrary, it is possible that the lesions may be congenital and microscopic in size at birth and increase in size with time. Whether an increase in size or de novo development, it appears from studies of PAVMs that a number of factors can influence the growth and/or development of vascular lesions.

Hormonal influences are one possible factor in HHT pathogenesis. Women with HHT exhibit increased epistaxis when circulating levels of endogenous estrogen are low, such as during menopause, after ovariectomy, and at the end of menstruation (Koch et al., 1952). Estrogen–progesterone therapy reduces gastrointestinal hemorrhage and epistaxis, although these observations may relate more to hemorrhage than actual lesion development. Females are also at risk for developing PAVMs during pregnancy, which suggests a more direct hor-

Figure 28–5. Model for the role of ALK1 and endoglin (ENG) in the angiogenic switch observed during capillary morphogenesis. TGF-*β* can signal via two distinct receptor-mediated pathways in endothelial cells. T*β*RI is a ubiquitously expressed type I receptor, which in concert with ligand binding to T*β*RII (type II receptor), activates a pathway that includes Smad2/3 and Smad4 complexes. This pathway leads to transcriptional activation of genes involved in the activation phase of angiogenesis. ALK1 is an endothelium-specific type I receptor for TGF-*β*, which, in concert with ligand binding to T*β*RII (type II receptor), signals through a pathway that includes Smad1/5 and Smad4. This pathway leads to transcriptional activation of genes involved in the resolution phase of angiogenesis. Endoglin is a negative modulator of TGF-*β* signaling through T*β*RI, though its role in signaling via the ALK1 receptor is less clear. Modulation of TGF-*β* concentrations in the surrounding tissue would favor signaling through one or the other receptor, thus promoting the activation or resolution phase.

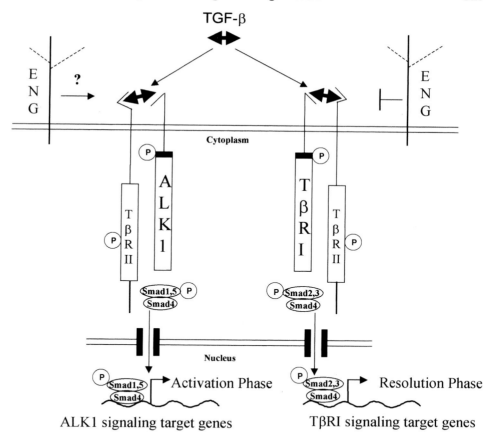

monal influence on lesion development. Hemodynamic influences are also likely to play a role in the pathogenesis of HHT. Pregnancy induces profound changes in hemodynamic flow, and these might relate to the development or exacerbation of PAVMs, especially during the third trimester.

Endothelial damage has been postulated as a trigger for lesion formation. Menefee and colleagues (1975) carried out an electron microscopic study of vascular lesions in HHT before and after therapy with synthetic estrogen–progesterone. Prior to treatment, the authors noted a defect in the junctions of the endothelial cells, as did Hashimoto and Pritzker (1972) but not Jahnke (1970). In addition, they found evidence for extravasation of blood in the form of erythrocytes and thrombi in the connective tissue near the vascular lesion. Since fibrin can be a matrix for endothelial budding, they proposed that repeated episodes of the sequence, endothelial break–blood leakage–fibrin framework–new endothelial outgrowth from an affected vessel, might explain the development of new vascular lesions with increasing age. They identified what appeared to be degenerating or damaged endothelial cells in the vascular lesions. These sites of degeneration were proposed to result in gaps in the lesion, where extravasation would commence. Reduced levels of surface endoglin or ALK1 protein might interfere with normal repair of the vessel wall, resulting in a cascade of effects that ultimately change the vascular architecture. Interestingly, after treatment with norethynodrel and mestranol, vascular integrity appeared to be restored without residual endothelial gaps or degenerative changes (Menefee et al., 1975). The mechanism whereby estrogenic hormones might influence endothelial integrity is unclear. However, it may be that upregulation of endoglin plays some role in this process (Rius et al., 1998).

Another possible trigger for lesion development might be changes in hemodynamics due to obstruction of venules. This is similar to what has been proposed for vascular ectasias of the colon. Vascular ectasias of the colon are a cause of lower intestinal hemorrhage in the elderly. One theory, based on a study of cleared and injected tissues from colon specimens, suggests a model where ectasias are formed by chronic in-

termittent low-grade obstruction of submucosal veins (Boley et al., 1977). The authors proposed that the initial effects of this obstruction were dilatation and tortuosity of submucosal veins extending to venules, capillaries, and arteries of the vascular unit. The eventual loss of competence of the precapillary sphincters can result in an arteriovenous shunt. Prolonged increased flow through this shunt can lead to alterations in the arteries supplying the shunt and the veins draining it. If a similar course of events is involved in arteriovenous malformation development in HHT, it may be that the initial event is chronic low-grade obstruction of the veins or venules.

Another model for lesion formation involves complete loss of endoglin or ALK1 due to somatic mutation of the normal endoglin or ALK1 allele in an endothelial cell. This two-hit hypothesis is similar to a Knudson tumor-suppressor model but with some distinct differences. Since TGF-*β* signaling in endothelial cells modulates vascular remodeling by inducing changes in the extracellular matrix (Madri et al., 1989; Merwin et al., 1990), complete loss of signaling may induce remodeling of the capillary bed to form larger vessels, rather than directly affecting the rate of endothelial cell proliferation. Additional changes in the vascular architecture, such as arterialization of the venous side of the lesion, may occur as a secondary response to the hemodynamic changes due to direct shunting of arterial blood into the venous return (Braverman et al., 1990). Therefore, the resulting lesion would not be clonal expansion of the cell harboring the original somatic mutation; thus, loss of heterozygosity or lack of endoglin (or ALK1) protein might not be evident. Neither loss of heterozygosity nor absence of endoglin immunostaining has been observed in a small number of HHT1-associated PAVMs (Stenzel and Marchuk, unpublished observations).

CONCLUSION

HHT is an autosomal dominant syndrome characterized by multisystem vascular dysplasia. Apart from its importance as a disease of considerable morbidity, the microanatomy of the associated vascular lesions suggested that study of the syndrome would yield important information about vascular morphogenesis. Research conducted over the past decade has borne this out. The explosion of information concerning HHT began with the identification of the two genes mutated in what is now known as type I and type II HHT. Mutations identified in the *endoglin* and *ALK1* genes demonstrated that the underlying pathogenesis of HHT involves perturbation of TGF-β signaling in vascular endothelial cells. Biochemical analyses combined with mouse models of the disease suggest that the two genes are crucial members of the angiogenic switch, regulating the shift from the activation phase to the resolution phase of blood vessel formation. Continued research on these proteins and their role in angiogenesis should shed light on the complex process of angiogenesis. It is likewise hoped that continued research will suggest novel approaches to therapy for this intriguing genetic disorder.

REFERENCES

Adam PJ, Clesham GJ, Weissberg PL (1998). Expression of endoglin mRNA and protein in human vascular smooth muscle cells. *Biochem Biophys Res Commun* 247: 33–37.

Arthur HM, Ure J, Smith AJ, Renforth G, Wilson DI, Torsney E, Charlton R, Parums DV, Jowett T, Marchuk DA, et al. (2000). Endoglin, an ancillary TGFbeta receptor, is required for extraembryonic angiogenesis and plays a key role in heart development. *Dev Biol* 217: 42–53.

Assar OS, Friedman CM, White RI Jr (1991). The natural history of epistaxis in hereditary hemorrhagic telangiectasia. *Laryngoscope* 101: 977–980.

Attisano L, Wrana JL (1998). Mads and Smads in TGF beta signalling. *Curr Opin Cell Biol* 10: 188–194.

Attisano L, Carcamo J, Ventura F, Weis FM, Massague J, Wrana JL (1993). Identification of human activin and TGF beta type I receptors that form heteromeric kinase complexes with type II receptors. *Cell* 75: 671–680.

Baeuerle PA, Henkel T (1994). Function and activation of NF-kappa B in the immune system. *Annu Rev Immunol* 12: 141–179.

Bassuk AG, Leiden JM (1997). The role of Ets transcription factors in the development and function of the mammalian immune system. *Adv Immunol* 64: 65–104.

Bauer T, Britton P, Lomas D, Wight DG, Friend PJ, Alexander GJ (1995). Liver transplantation for hepatic arteriovenous malformation in hereditary haemorrhagic telangiectasia. *J Hepatol* 22: 586–590.

Becker Y, Tabor E (1989). Skin fibroblasts from patients with the genetic disorder hereditary hemorrhagic telangiectasia share features with ataxia-telangiectasia fibroblasts in their response to the radiomimetic drug neocarzinostatin. *Isr J Med Sci* 25: 81–86.

Bellon T, Corbi A, Lastres P, Cales C, Cebrian M, Vera S, Cheifetz S, Massague J, Letarte M, Bernabeu C (1993). Identification and expression of two forms of the human transforming growth factor-beta-binding protein endoglin with distinct cytoplasmic regions. *Eur J Immunol* 23: 2340–2345.

Berg JN, Guttmacher AE, Marchuk DA, Porteous ME (1996). Clinical heterogeneity in hereditary haemorrhagic telangiectasia: are pulmonary arteriovenous malformations more common in families linked to endoglin? *J Med Genet* 33: 256–257.

Berg JN, Gallione CJ, Stenzel TT, Johnson DW, Allen WP, Schwartz CE, Jackson CE, Porteous ME, Marchuk DA (1997). The activin receptor-like kinase 1 gene: genomic structure and mutations in hereditary hemorrhagic telangiectasia type 2. *Am J Hum Genet* 61: 60–67.

Bideau A, Plauchu H, Jacquard A, Robert JM, Desjardins B (1980). Genetic aspects of Rendu-Osler disease in Haut-Jura: convergence of methodological approaches of historic demography and medical genetics [in French]. *J Genet Hum* 28: 127–147.

Bideau A, Brunet G, Heyer E, Plauchu H, Robert JM (1992). An abnormal concentration of cases of Rendu-Osler disease in the Valserine Valley of the French Jura: a genealogical and demographic study. *Ann Hum Biol* 19: 233–247.

Biggs JR, Kraft AS (1999). The role of the Smad3 protein in phorbol ester–induced promoter expression. *J Biol Chem* 274: 36987–36994.

Bird RM, Hammarsten JF, Marshall R, Robinson RR (1957). A family reunion. A study of hereditary hemorrhagic telangiectasia. *N Engl J Med* 257: 105–109.

Boley SJ, Sammartano R, Adams A, DiBiase A, Kleinhaus S, Sprayregen S (1977). On the nature and etiology of vascular ectasias of the colon. Degenerative lesions of aging. *Gastroenterology* 72: 650–660.

Bonyadi M, Rusholme SA, Cousins FM, Su HC, Biron CA, Farrall M, Akhurst RJ (1997). Mapping of a major genetic modifier of embryonic lethality in TGF beta 1 knockout mice. *Nat Genet* 15: 207–211.

Bourdeau A, Dumont DJ, Letarte M (1999). A murine model of hereditary hemorrhagic telangiectasia. *J Clin Invest* 104: 1343–1351.

Bourdeau A, Faughnan ME, McDonald ML, Paterson AD, Wanless IR, Letarte M (2001). Potential role of modifier genes influencing transforming growth factor-beta1 levels in the development of vascular defects in endoglin heterozygous mice with hereditary hemorrhagic telangiectasia. *Am J Pathol* 158: 2011–2020.

Bown SG, Swain CP, Storey DW, Collins C, Matthewson K, Salmon PR, Clark CG (1985). Endoscopic laser treatment of vascular anomalies of the upper gastrointestinal tract. *Gut* 26: 1338–1348.

Braverman IM, Keh A, Jacobson BS (1990). Ultrastructure and three-dimensional organization of the telangiectases of hereditary hemorrhagic telangiectasia. *J Invest Dermatol* 95: 422–427.

Bruno E, Horrigan SK, Van Den Berg D, Rozler E, Fitting PR, Moss ST, Westbrook C, Hoffman R (1998). The *Smad5* gene is involved in the intracellular signaling pathways that mediate the inhibitory effects of transforming growth factor-beta on human hematopoiesis. *Blood* 91: 1917–1923.

Buhring HJ, Muller CA, Letarte M, Gougos A, Saalmuller A, van Agthoven AJ, Busch FW (1991). Endoglin is expressed on a subpopulation of immature erythroid cells of normal human bone marrow. *Leukemia* 5: 841–847.

Candia AF, Watabe T, Hawley SH, Onichtchouk D, Zhang Y, Derynck R, Niehrs C, Cho KW (1997). Cellular interpretation of multiple TGF-beta signals: intracellular antagonism between activin/BVg1 and BMP-2/4 signaling mediated by Smads. *Development* 124: 4467–4480.

Caniggia I, Taylor CV, Ritchie JW, Lye SJ, Letarte M (1997). Endoglin regulates trophoblast differentiation along the invasive pathway in human placental villous explants. *Endocrinology* 138: 4977–4988.

Carmeliet P, Schoonjans L, Kieckens L, Ream B, Degen J, Bronson R, De Vos R, van den Oord JJ, Collen D, Mulligan RC (1994). Physiological consequences of loss of plasminogen activator gene function in mice. *Nature* 368: 419–424.

Cheifetz S, Bellon T, Cales C, Vera S, Bernabeu C, Massague J, Letarte M (1992). Endoglin is a component of the transforming growth factor-beta receptor system in human endothelial cells. *J Biol Chem* 267: 19027–19030.

Chen YG, Massague J (1999). Smad1 recognition and activation by the ALK1 group of transforming growth factor-beta family receptors. *J Biol Chem* 274: 3672–3677.

Conley ME, Fitch-Hilgenberg ME, Cleveland JL, Parolini O, Rohrer J (1994). Screening of genomic DNA to identify mutations in the gene for Bruton's tyrosine kinase. *Hum Mol Genet* 3: 1751–1756.

Cymerman U, Vera S, Pece-Barbara N, Bourdeau A, White RI Jr, Dunn J, Letarte M (2000). Identification of hereditary hemorrhagic telangiectasia type 1 in newborns by protein expression and mutation analysis of endoglin. *Pediatr Res* 47: 24–35.

Dickson MC, Martin JS, Cousins FM, Kulkarni AB, Karlsson S, Akhurst RJ (1995). Defective haematopoiesis and vasculogenesis in transforming growth factor-beta 1 knock out mice. *Development* 121: 1845–1854.

Eiken HG, Knappskog PM, Apold J, Skjelkvale L, Boman H (1992). A de novo phenylketonuria mutation: ATG (Met) to ATA (Ile) in the start codon of the phenylalanine hydroxylase gene. *Hum Mutat* 1: 388–391.

Eppert K, Scherer SW, Ozcelik H, Pirone R, Hoodless P, Kim H, Tsui LC, Bapat B, Gallinger S, Andrulis IL, et al. (1996). MADR2 maps to 18q21 and encodes a TGFbeta-regulated MAD-related protein that is functionally mutated in colorectal carcinoma. *Cell* 86: 543–552.

Ference BA, Shannon TM, White RI Jr, Zawin M, Burdge CM (1994). Life-threatening pulmonary hemorrhage with pulmonary arteriovenous malformations and hereditary hemorrhagic telangiectasia. *Chest* 106: 1387–1390.

Fernandez-Ruiz E, St-Jacques S, Bellon T, Letarte M, Bernabeu C (1993). Assignment of the human endoglin gene (*END*) to 9q34 → qter. *Cytogenet Cell Genet* 64: 204–207.

Gallione CJ, Klaus DJ, Yeh EY, Stenzel TT, Xue Y, Anthony KB, McAllister KA, Baldwin MA, Berg JN, Lux A, et al. (1998). Mutation and expression analysis of the endoglin gene in hereditary hemorrhagic telangiectasia reveals null alleles. *Hum Mutat* 11: 286–294.

Geland J (1983). Exploiting sex for therapeutic purposes. *N Engl J Med* 308: 1417–1419.

Gougos A, Letarte M (1988). Identification of a human endothelial cell antigen with monoclonal antibody 44G4 produced against a pre-B leukemic cell line. *J Immunol* 141: 1925–1933.

Gougos A, Letarte M (1990). Primary structure of endoglin, an RGD-containing glycoprotein of human endothelial cells. *J Biol Chem* 265: 8361–8364.

Gougos A, St Jacques S, Greaves A, O'Connell PJ, d'Apice AJ, Buhring HJ, Bernabeu C, van Mourik JA, Letarte M (1992). Identification of distinct epitopes of endoglin, an RGD-containing glycoprotein of endothelial cells, leukemic cells, and syncytiotrophoblasts. *Int Immunol* 4: 83–92.

Goumans MJ, Zwijsen A, van Rooijen MA, Huylebroeck D, Roelen BA, Mummery CL (1999). Transforming growth factor-beta signalling in extraembryonic mesoderm is required for yolk sac vasculogenesis in mice. *Development* 126: 3473–3483.

Goumans MJ, Valdimarsdottir G, Itoh S, Rosendahl A, Sideras P, ten Dijke P (2002). Balancing the activation state of the endothelium via two distinct TGF-beta type I receptors. *EMBO J* 21: 1743–1753.

Graulich W, Nettelbeck DM, Fischer D, Kissel T, Muller R (1999). Cell type specificity of the human endoglin promoter. *Gene* 227: 55–62.

Guerrero-Esteo M, Lastres P, Letamendia A, Perez-Alvarez MJ, Langa C, Lopez LA, Fabra A, Garcia-Pardo A, Vera S, Letarte M, et al. (1999). Endoglin overexpression modulates cellular morphology, migration, and adhesion of mouse fibroblasts. *Eur J Cell Biol* 78: 614–623.

Guttmacher AE, McKinnon WC, Upton MD (1994). Hereditary hemorrhagic telangiectasia: a disorder in search of the genetics community. *Am J Med Genet* 52: 252–253.

Haitjema T, Disch F, Overtoom TT, Westermann CJ, Lammers JW (1995a). Screening family members of patients with hereditary hemorrhagic telangiectasia. *Am J Med* 99: 519–524.

Haitjema TJ, Overtoom TT, Westermann CJ, Lammers JW (1995b). Embolisation of pulmonary arteriovenous malformations: results and follow up in 32 patients. *Thorax* 50: 719–723.

Haitjema T, ten Berg JM, Overtoom TT, Ernst JM, Westermann CJ (1996). Unusual complications after embolization of a pulmonary arteriovenous malformation. *Chest* 109: 1401–1404.

Harrison DFN (1964). Familial haemorrhagic telangiectases: 20 cases treated with systemic oestrogen. *Q J Med* 33: 25–38.

Haruta Y, Seon BK (1986). Distinct human leukemia-associated cell surface glycoprotein GP160 defined by monoclonal antibody SN6. *Proc Natl Acad Sci USA* 83: 7898–7902.

Hashimoto K, Pritzker MS (1972). Hereditary hemorrhagic telangiectasia. An electron microscopic study. *Oral Surg Oral Med Oral Pathol* 34: 751–768.

Hayashi H, Abdollah S, Qiu Y, Cai J, Xu YY, Grinnell BW, Richardson MA, Topper JN, Gimbrone MA Jr, Wrana JL, et al. (1997). The MAD-related protein Smad7 associates with the TGFbeta receptor and functions as an antagonist of TGFbeta signaling. *Cell* 89: 1165–1173.

He WW, Gustafson ML, Hirobe S, Donahoe PK (1993). Developmental expression of four novel serine/threonine kinase receptors homologous to the activin/transforming growth factor-beta type II receptor family. *Dev Dyn* 196: 133–142.

Heldin CH, Miyazono K, ten Dijke P (1997). TGF-beta signalling from cell membrane to nucleus through SMAD proteins. *Nature* 390: 465–471.

Heutink P, Haitjema T, Breedveld GJ, Janssen B, Sandkuijl LA, Bontekoe CJ, Westerman CJ, Oostra BA (1994). Linkage of hereditary haemorrhagic telangiectasia to chromosome 9q34 and evidence for locus heterogeneity. *J Med Genet* 31: 933–936.

Hodgson CHBH, Good CA, Clagett OT (1959). Hereditary haemorrhagic telangiectasia and pulmonary arteriovenous fistula. *N Engl J Med* 261: 625–635.

Hughes JM (1994). Intrapulmonary shunts: coils to transplantation. *J R Coll Physicians Lond* 28: 247–253.

Hynes RO (1987). Integrins: a family of cell surface receptors. *Cell* 48: 549–554.

Jahnke V (1970). Ultrastructure of hereditary telangiectasia. *Arch Otolaryngol* 91: 262–265.

John SW, Scriver CR, Laframboise R, Rozen R (1992). In vitro and in vivo correlations for I65T and M1V mutations at the phenylalanine hydroxylase locus. *Hum Mutat* 1: 147–153.

Johnson DW, Berg JN, Baldwin MA, Gallione CJ, Marondel I, Yoon SJ, Stenzel TT, Speer M, Pericak-Vance MA, Diamond A, et al. (1996). Mutations in the activin receptor-like kinase 1 gene in hereditary haemorrhagic telangiectasia type 2. *Nat Genet* 13: 189–195.

Kikuchi K, Kowada M, Sasajima H (1994). Vascular malformations of the brain in hereditary hemorrhagic telangiectasia (Rendu-Osler-Weber disease). *Surg Neurol* 41: 374–380.

King CR, Lovrien EW, Reiss J (1977). Central nervous system arteriovenous malformations in multiple generations of a family with hereditary hemorrhagic telangiectasia. *Clin Genet* 12: 372–381.

Kingsley DM (1994). The TGF-beta superfamily: new members, new receptors, and new genetic tests of function in different organisms. *Genes Dev* 8: 133–146.

Kjeldsen AD, Vase P, Oxhoj H (1996). Hereditary hemorrhagic telangiectasia. *N Engl J Med* 334: 331–332.

Kjeldsen AD, Oxhoj H, Andersen PE, Green A, Vase P (2000). Prevalence of pulmonary arteriovenous malformations (PAVMs) and occurrence of neurological symptoms in patients with hereditary haemorrhagic telangiectasia (HHT). *J Intern Med* 248: 255–262.

Klaus DJ, Gallione CJ, Anthony K, Yeh EY, Yu J, Lux A, Johnson DW, Marchuk DA (1998). Novel missense and frameshift mutations in the activin receptor-like kinase-1 in HHT. Hum Mutat Online Mutations in Brief #164 Brief #164. http://interscience.wiley.com/jpages/1059-7794/html/mutation/Klautext.htm

Koch H, Escher G, Lewis J (1952). Hormonal management of hereditary haemorrhagic telangiectasis. *JAMA* 149: 1376–1380.

Kretzschmar M, Massague J (1998). SMADs: mediators and regulators of TGF-beta signaling. *Curr Opin Genet Dev* 8: 103–111.

Kumar S, Ghellal A, Li C, Byrne G, Haboubi N, Wang JM, Bundred N (1999). Breast carcinoma: vascular density determined using CD105 antibody correlates with tumor prognosis. *Cancer Res* 59: 856–861.

Kurihara H, Yoshizumi M, Sugiyama T, Takaku F, Yanagisawa M, Masaki T, Hamaoki M, Kato H, Yazaki Y (1989). Transforming growth factor-beta stimulates the expression of endothelin mRNA by vascular endothelial cells. *Biochem Biophys Res Commun* 159: 1435–1440.

Kwaan HC, Silverman S (1973). Fibrinolytic activity in lesions of hereditary hemorrhagic telangiectasia. *Arch Dermatol* 107: 571–573.

Lastres P, Bellon T, Cabanas C, Sanchez-Madrid F, Acevedo A, Gougos A, Letarte M, Bernabeu C (1992). Regulated expression on human macrophages of endoglin, an Arg-Gly-Asp-containing surface antigen. *Eur J Immunol* 22: 393–397.

Lastres P, Martin-Perez J, Langa C, Bernabeu C (1994). Phosphorylation of the human-transforming-growth-factor-beta-binding protein endoglin. *Biochem J* 301: 765–768.

Lastres P, Letamendia A, Zhang H, Rius C, Almendro N, Raab U, Lopez LA, Langa C, Fabra A, Letarte M, et al. (1996). Endoglin modulates cellular responses to TGF-beta 1. *J Cell Biol* 133: 1109–1121.

Lesser BA, Wendt D, Miks VM, Norum RA (1986). Identical twins with hereditary hemorrhagic telangiectasia concordant for cerebrovascular arteriovenous malformations. *Am J Med* 81: 931–934.

Letamendia A, Lastres P, Botella LM, Raab U, Langa C, Velasco B, Attisano L, Bernabeu C (1998). Role of endoglin in cellular responses to transforming growth factor-beta. A comparative study with betaglycan. *J Biol Chem* 273: 33011–33019.

Li DY, Sorensen LK, Brooke BS, Urness LD, Davis EC, Taylor DG, Boak BB, Wendel DP (1999). Defective angiogenesis in mice lacking endoglin. *Science* 284: 1534–1537.

Liu X, Yue J, Frey RS, Zhu Q, Mulder KM (1998). Transforming growth factor beta signaling through Smad1 in human breast cancer cells. *Cancer Res* 58: 4752–4757.

Lo RS, Chen YG, Shi Y, Pavletich NP, Massague J (1998). The L3 loop: a structural motif determining specific interactions between SMAD proteins and TGF-beta receptors. *EMBO J* 17: 996–1005.

Lopez-Casillas F, Cheifetz S, Doody J, Andres JL, Lane WS, Massague J (1991). Structure and expression of the membrane proteoglycan betaglycan, a component of the TGF-beta receptor system. *Cell* 67: 785–795.

Lopez-Casillas F, Wrana JL, Massague J (1993). Betaglycan presents ligand to the TGF beta signaling receptor. *Cell* 73: 1435–1444.

Lux A, Attisano L, Marchuk DA (1999). Assignment of transforming growth factor beta1 and beta3 and a third new ligand to the type I receptor ALK1. *J Biol Chem* 274: 9984–9992.

Lux A, Gallione CJ, Marchuk DA (2000). Expression analysis of endoglin missense and truncation mutations: insights into protein structure and disease mechanisms. *Hum Mol Genet* 9: 745–755.

Macias-Silva M, Abdollah S, Hoodless PA, Pirone R, Attisano L, Wrana JL (1996). MADR2 is a substrate of the TGFbeta receptor and its phosphorylation is required for nuclear accumulation and signaling. *Cell* 87: 1215–1224.

Macias-Silva M, Hoodless PA, Tang SJ, Buchwald M, Wrana JL (1998). Specific activation of Smad1 signaling pathways by the BMP7 type I receptor, ALK2. *J Biol Chem* 273: 25628–25636.

Madri JA, Reidy MA, Kocher O, Bell L (1989). Endothelial cell behavior after denudation injury is modulated by transforming growth factor-beta1 and fibronectin. *Lab Invest* 60: 755–765.

Maier JA, Delia D, Thorpe PE, Gasparini G (1997). In vitro inhibition of endothelial cell growth by the antiangiogenic drug AGM-1470 (TNP-470) and the anti-endoglin antibody TEC-11. *Anticancer Drugs* 8: 238–244.

Martini GA (1978). The liver in hereditary haemorrhagic teleangiectasia: an inborn error of vascular structure with multiple manifestations: a reappraisal. *Gut* 19: 531–537.

Massague J (1998). TGF-beta signal transduction. *Annu Rev Biochem* 67: 753–791.

Matsuno F, Haruta Y, Kondo M, Tsai H, Barcos M, Seon BK (1999). Induction of lasting complete regression of preformed distinct solid tumors by targeting the tumor vasculature using two new anti-endoglin monoclonal antibodies. *Clin Cancer Res* 5: 371–382.

McAllister KA, Grogg KM, Johnson DW, Gallione CJ, Baldwin MA, Jackson CE, Helmbold EA, Markel DS, McKinnon WC, Murrell J, et al. (1994a). Endoglin, a TGF-beta binding protein of endothelial cells, is the gene for hereditary haemorrhagic telangiectasia type 1. *Nat Genet* 8: 345–351.

McAllister KA, Lennon F, Bowles-Biesecker B, McKinnon WC, Helmbold EA, Markel DS, Jackson CE, Guttmacher AE, Pericak-Vance MA, Marchuk DA (1994b). Genetic heterogeneity in hereditary haemorrhagic telangiectasia: possible correlation with clinical phenotype. *J Med Genet* 31: 927–932.

McDonald JE, Miller FJ, Hallam SE, Nelson L, Marchuk DA, Ward KJ (2000). Clinical manifestations in a large hereditary hemorrhagic telangiectasia (HHT) type 2 kindred. *Am J Med Genet* 93: 320–327.

McDonald MT, Papenberg KA, Ghosh S, Glatfelter AA, Biesecker BB, Helmbold EA, Markel DS, Zolotor A, McKinnon WC, Vanderstoep JL, et al. (1994). A disease locus for hereditary haemorrhagic telangiectasia maps to chromosome 9q33-34. *Nat Genet* 6: 197–204.

Menefee MG, Flessa HC, Glueck HI, Hogg SP (1975). Hereditary hemorrhagic telangiectasia (Osler-Weber-Rendu disease). An electron microscopic study of the vascular lesions before and after therapy with hormones. *Arch Otolaryngol* 101: 246–251.

Merwin JR, Anderson JM, Kocher O, Van Itallie CM, Madri JA (1990). Transforming growth factor beta 1 modulates extracellular matrix organization and cell–cell junctional complex formation during in vitro angiogenesis. *J Cell Physiol* 142: 117–128.

Miller DW, Graulich W, Karges B, Stahl S, Ernst M, Ramaswamy A, Sedlacek HH, Muller R, Adamkiewicz J (1999). Elevated expression of endoglin, a component of the TGF-beta-receptor complex, correlates with proliferation of tumor endothelial cells. *Int J Cancer* 81: 568–572.

Moren A, Ichijo H, Miyazono K (1992). Molecular cloning and characterization of the human and porcine transforming growth factor-beta type III receptors. *Biochem Biophys Res Commun* 189: 356–362.

Nakao A, Afrakhte M, Moren A, Nakayama T, Christian JL, Heuchel R, Itoh S, Kawabata M, Heldin NE, Heldin CH, et al. (1997a). Identification of Smad7, a TGFbeta-inducible antagonist of TGF-beta signalling. *Nature* 389: 631–635.

Nakao A, Imamura T, Souchelnytskyi S, Kawabata M, Ishisaki A, Oeda E, Tamaki K, Hanai J, Heldin CH, Miyazono K, et al. (1997b). TGF-beta receptor-mediated signalling through Smad2, Smad3 and Smad4. *EMBO J* 16: 5353–5362.

Nakao A, Roijer E, Imamura T, Souchelnytskyi S, Stenman G, Heldin CH, ten Dijke P (1997c). Identification of Smad2, a human Mad-related protein in the transforming growth factor beta signaling pathway. *J Biol Chem* 272: 2896–2900.

Naveau S, Aubert A, Poynard T, Chaput JC (1990). Long-term results of treatment of vascular malformations of the gastrointestinal tract by neodymium YAG laser photocoagulation. *Dig Dis Sci* 35: 821–826.

Oh SP, Seki T, Goss KA, Imamura T, Yi Y, Donahoe PK, Li L, Miyazono K, ten Dijke P, Kim S, et al. (2000). Activin receptor-like kinase 1 modulates transforming growth factor-beta 1 signaling in the regulation of angiogenesis. *Proc Natl Acad Sci USA* 97: 2626–2631.

Orkin SH, Zon LI (1997). Genetics of erythropoiesis: induced mutations in mice and zebrafish. *Annu Rev Genet* 31: 33–60.

Oshima M, Oshima H, Taketo MM (1996). TGF-beta receptor type II deficiency results in defects of yolk sac hematopoiesis and vasculogenesis. *Dev Biol* 179: 297–302.

Osler W (1901). On a family form of recurring epistaxis, associated with multiple telangiectases of the skin and mucous membranes. *Bull Johns Hopkins Hosp* 12: 333–337.

Pece N, Vera S, Cymerman U, White RI Jr, Wrana JL, Letarte M (1997). Mutant endoglin in hereditary hemorrhagic telangiectasia type 1 is transiently expressed intracellularly and is not a dominant negative. *J Clin Invest* 100: 2568–2579.

Pece-Barbara N, Cymerman U, Vera S, Marchuk DA, Letarte M (1999). Expression analysis of four endoglin missense mutations suggests that haploinsufficiency is the predominant mechanism for hereditary hemorrhagic telangiectasia type 1. *Hum Mol Genet* 8: 2171–2181.

Pepper MS, Montesano R, Mandriota SJ, Orci L, Vassalli JD (1996). Angiogenesis: a paradigm for balanced extracellular proteolysis during cell migration and morphogenesis. *Enzyme Protein* 49: 138–162.

Piantanida M, Buscarini E, Dellavecchia C, Minelli A, Rossi A, Buscarini L, Danesino C (1996). Hereditary haemorrhagic telangiectasia with extensive liver involvement is not caused by either HHT1 or HHT2. *J Med Genet* 33: 441–443.

Piek E, Westermark U, Kastemar M, Heldin CH, van Zoelen EJ, Nister M, Ten Dijke P (1999). Expression of transforming-growth-factor (TGF)-beta receptors and Smad proteins in glioblastoma cell lines with distinct responses to TGF-beta1. *Int J Cancer* 80: 756–763.

Pilz A, Woodward K, Povey S, Abbott C (1995). Comparative mapping of 50 human chromosome 9 loci in the laboratory mouse. *Genomics* 25: 139–149.

Plauchu H, de Chadarevian JP, Bideau A, Robert JM (1989). Age-related clinical profile of hereditary hemorrhagic telangiectasia in an epidemiologically recruited population. *Am J Med Genet* 32: 291–297.

Porteous ME, Burn J, Proctor SJ (1992). Hereditary haemorrhagic telangiectasia: a clinical analysis. *J Med Genet* 29: 527–530.

Porteous ME, Curtis A, Williams O, Marchuk D, Bhattacharya SS, Burn J (1994). Genetic heterogeneity in hereditary haemorrhagic telangiectasia. *J Med Genet* 31: 925–926.

Pugh BF, Tjian R (1990). Mechanism of transcriptional activation by Sp1: evidence for coactivators. *Cell* 61: 1187–1197.

Quackenbush EJ, Letarte M (1985). Identification of several cell surface proteins of non-T, non-B acute lymphoblastic leukemia by using monoclonal antibodies. *J Immunol* 134: 1276–1285.

Quitt M, Froom P, Veisler A, Falber V, Sova J, Aghai E (1990). The effect of desmopressin on massive gastrointestinal bleeding in hereditary telangiectasia unresponsive to treatment with cryoprecipitate. *Arch Intern Med* 150: 1744–1746.

Raab U, Velasco B, Lastres P, Letamendia A, Cales C, Langa C, Tapia E, Lopez-Bote JP, Paez E, Bernabeu C (1999). Expression of normal and truncated forms of human endoglin. *Biochem J* 339: 579–588.

Rendu HJ (1896). Epistaxis répétées chez un sujet porteur de petits angiomes cutanés et muqueux. *Gaz des Hôpitaux* 1896: 1322–1323.

Rius C, Smith JD, Almendro N, Langa C, Botella LM, Marchuk DA, Vary CPH, Bernabeu C (1998). Cloning of the promoter region of human endoglin, the target gene for hereditary hemorrhagic telangiectasia type 1. *Blood* 92: 4677–4690.

Roberts AB (1998). Molecular and cell biology of TGF-beta. *Miner Electrolyte Metab* 24: 111–119.

Robledo MM, Hidalgo A, Lastres P, Arroyo AG, Bernabeu C, Sanchez-Madrid F, Teixido J (1996). Characterization of TGF-beta 1-binding proteins in human bone marrow stromal cells. *Br J Haematol* 93: 507–514.

Rokhlin OW, Cohen MB, Kubagawa H, Letarte M, Cooper MD (1995). Differential expression of endoglin on fetal and adult hematopoietic cells in human bone marrow. *J Immunol* 154: 4456–4465.

Ruoslahti E, Pierschbacher MD (1987). New perspectives in cell adhesion: RGD and integrins. *Science* 238: 491–497.

Saksela O, Rifkin DB (1988). Cell-associated plasminogen activation: regulation and physiological functions. *Annu Rev Cell Biol* 4: 93–126.

Sato Y, Rifkin DB (1989). Inhibition of endothelial cell movement by pericytes and smooth muscle cells: activation of a latent transforming growth factor-beta 1-like molecule by plasmin during co-culture. *J Cell Biol* 109: 309–315.

Shovlin CL, Hughes JM, Tuddenham EG, Temperley I, Perembelon YF, Scott J, Seidman CE, Seidman JG (1994). A gene for hereditary haemorrhagic telangiectasia maps to chromosome 9q3. *Nat Genet* 6: 205–209.

Shovlin CL, Winstock AR, Peters AM, Jackson JE, Hughes JM (1995). Medical complications of pregnancy in hereditary haemorrhagic telangiectasia. *QJM* 88: 879–887.

Shovlin CL, Hughes JM, Scott J, Seidman CE, Seidman JG (1997). Characterization of endoglin and identification of novel mutations in hereditary hemorrhagic telangiectasia. *Am J Hum Genet* 61: 68–79.

Shovlin CL, Guttmacher AE, Buscarini E, Faughnan ME, Hyland RH, Westermann CJ, Kjeldsen AD, Plauchu H (2000). Diagnostic criteria for hereditary hemorrhagic telangiectasia (Rendu-Osler-Weber syndrome). *Am J Med Genet* 91: 66–67.

Sligh JE Jr, Hurwitz MY, Zhu CM, Anderson DC, Beaudet AL (1992). An initiation codon mutation in CD18 in association with the moderate phenotype of leukocyte adhesion deficiency. *J Biol Chem* 267: 714–718.

Sporn MB, Roberts AB (1992). Autocrine secretion—10 years later. *Ann Intern Med* 117: 408–414.

Steele JG, Nath PU, Burn J, Porteous ME (1993). An association between migrainous aura and hereditary haemorrhagic telangiectasia. *Headache* 33: 145–148.

St-Jacques S, Cymerman U, Pece N, Letarte M (1994). Molecular characterization and in situ localization of murine endoglin reveal that it is a transforming growth factor-beta binding protein of endothelial and stromal cells. *Endocrinology* 134: 2645–2657.

Swinburne AJ, Fedullo AJ, Gangemi R, Mijangos JA (1986). Hereditary telangiectasia and multiple pulmonary arteriovenous fistulas. Clinical deterioration during pregnancy. *Chest* 89: 459–460.

ten Dijke P, Ichijo H, Franzen P, Schulz P, Saras J, Toyoshima H, Heldin CH, Miyazono K (1993). Activin receptor-like kinases: a novel subclass of cell-surface receptors with predicted serine/threonine kinase activity. *Oncogene* 8: 2879–2887.

Topper JN, Cai J, Qiu Y, Anderson KR, Xu YY, Deeds JD, Feeley R, Gimeno CJ, Woolf EA, Tayber O, et al. (1997). Vascular MADs: two novel MAD-related genes selectively inducible by flow in human vascular endothelium. *Proc Natl Acad Sci USA* 94: 9314–9319.

Trembath RC, Thomson JR, Machado RD, Morgan NV, Atkinson C, Winship I, Simonneau G, Galie N, Loyd JE, Humbert M, et al. (2001). Clinical and molecular genetic features of pulmonary hypertension in patients with hereditary hemorrhagic telangiectasia. *N Engl J Med* 345: 325–334.

Van Cutsem E, Piessevaux H (1996). Pharmacologic therapy of arteriovenous malformations. *Gastrointest Endosc Clin N Am* 6: 819–832.

Van Cutsem E, Rutgeerts P, Geboes K, Van Gompel F, Vantrappen G (1988). Estrogen-progesterone treatment of Osler-Weber-Rendu disease. *J Clin Gastroenterol* 10: 676–679.

van Cutsem E, Rutgeerts P, Vantrappen G (1990). Treatment of bleeding gastrointestinal vascular malformations with oestrogen-progesterone. *Lancet* 335: 953–955.

Vase P, Grove O (1986). Gastrointestinal lesions in hereditary hemorrhagic telangiectasia. *Gastroenterology* 91: 1079–1083.

Vase P, Holm M, Arendrup H (1985). Pulmonary arteriovenous fistulas in hereditary hemorrhagic telangiectasia. *Acta Med Scand* 218: 105–109.

Vincent P, Plauchu H, Hazan J, Faure S, Weissenbach J, Godet J (1995). A third locus for hereditary haemorrhagic telangiectasia maps to chromosome 12q [erratum appears in *Hum Mol Genet* 1995;4(7):1243]. *Hum Mol Genet* 4: 945–949.

Wallace GM, Shovlin CL (2000). A hereditary haemorrhagic telangiectasia family with pulmonary involvement is unlinked to the known HHT genes, endoglin and ALK1. *Thorax* 55: 685–690.

Wang XF, Lin HY, Ng-Eaton E, Downward J, Lodish HF, Weinberg RA (1991). Expression cloning and characterization of the TGF-beta type III receptor. *Cell* 67: 797–805.

White RI Jr (1992). Pulmonary arteriovenous malformations: how do we diagnose them and why is it important to do so? *Radiology* 182: 633–635.

White RI Jr, Pollak JS, Wirth JA (1996). Pulmonary arteriovenous malformations: diagnosis and transcatheter embolotherapy. *J Vasc Interv Radiol* 7: 787–804.

Wieser R, Wrana JL, Massague J (1995). GS domain mutations that constitutively activate T beta R-I, the downstream signaling component in the TGF-beta receptor complex. *EMBO J* 14: 2199–2208.

Williams T, Tjian R (1991). Analysis of the DNA-binding and activation properties of the human transcription factor AP-2. *Genes Dev* 5: 670–682.

Wirth JA, Pollak JS, White RI Jr (1996). Pulmonary arteriovenous malformations. In: *Current Pulmonology and Critical Care Medicine, vol. 17.* George RB, Campbell GD, Jenkinson SG, Matthay RA (eds). Mosby, St. Louis, pp. 261–297.

Wrana JL, Attisano L, Wieser R, Ventura F, Massague J (1994). Mechanism of activation of the TGF-beta receptor. *Nature* 370: 341–347.

Yingling JM, Das P, Savage C, Zhang M, Padgett RW, Wang XF (1996). Mammalian dwarfins are phosphorylated in response to transforming growth factor beta and are implicated in control of cell growth. *Proc Natl Acad Sci USA* 93: 8940–8944.

Yue J, Frey RS, Mulder KM (1999). Cross-talk between the Smad1 and Ras/MEK signaling pathways for TGFbeta. *Oncogene* 18: 2033–2037.

Zhang H, Shaw AR, Mak A, Letarte M (1996). Endoglin is a component of the transforming growth factor (TGF)-beta receptor complex of human pre-B leukemic cells. *J Immunol* 156: 564–573.

Zhang Y, Feng X, We R, Derynck R (1996). Receptor-associated Mad homologues synergize as effectors of the TGF-beta response. *Nature* 383: 168–172.

29 | *RUNX2* and Cleidocranial Dysplasia

BRENDAN LEE AND GUANG ZHOU

RUNX2 is a RUNT-domain transcription factor that is required for osteoblast cell fate commitment and chondrocyte maturation. Hence, it serves as a central regulator of intramembranous and endochondral ossification during embryonic skeletogenesis and during the postnatal period. *Runx2* directs the expression of multiple genes, including matrix components of bone and hypertrophic cartilage, and regulates the transition of hypertrophic chondrocyte to primary spongiosa. It acts in a context-dependent fashion that is specified by both upstream transcriptional regulators of *Runx2* expression and direct protein–protein interactions that regulate *Runx2* transactivation of target genes. Haploinsufficiency of *RUNX2* in humans causes a dominantly inherited skeletal dysplasia, cleidocranial dysplasia (CCD). CCD is characterized by delayed intramembranous ossification and defective chondrocyte maturation in some (but not all) bones. The clinical spectrum includes classic CCD, which is characterized by the triad of delayed closure of the fontanel, hypoplastic clavicles, and dental anomalies. However, genotype–phenotype studies show that *RUNX2* mutations can also be associated with mild CCD that is predominated by dental features, as well as with severe CCD that is complicated by significant osteoporosis. The clinical diagnosis can usually be confirmed by finding pathognomonic features on radiographic studies. Management is conservative for the skeletal complications. In contrast, the significant morbidity associated with dental anomalies dictates an aggressive multidisciplinary approach. Both in vitro cell studies and mouse models have identified regulators of RUNX2 function, while the description of CCD-related conditions raise interesting questions about their potential relation to components of the RUNX2 transcriptional network.

HISTORY OF RUNX2 AND ROLE IN DIFFERENTIATION

RUNX2 is one of three mammalian orthologs (*RUNX1, RUNX2, RUNX3*) of the *Drosophila Runt* gene (Wheeler et al., 2000; Karsenty, 2001) that have in common a highly conserved 128 amino acid RUNT domain which uniquely mediates DNA binding and protein–protein interactions. *Drosophila* Runt is a transcription factor that specifies cell fate and pattern formation in multiple developmental programs, including sexual differentiation, segmentation, and neurogenesis (Canon and Banerjee, 2000). In the early 1990s, interest in the vertebrate ortholog RUNT protein first described, RUNX1 (also called AML1 and CBFA2), peaked with its implication in the fusion gene product AML1/ETO generated by translocation of chromosomes 8 to 21 that occur in acute myelogenous leukemia (AML) (Erickson et al., 1992). From studies in *Drosophila*, it was well known that Runt functioned in a context-dependent manner, interacting with multiple proteins such as *Drosophila* Brother and Big brother or its vertebrate ortholog core-binding factor β (CBFβ) (Adya et al., 2000). The importance of this interaction in vivo was underscored by the description of another fusion gene product, CBFβ, with the myosin heavy chain (MYH) that was generated by chromosome 16 inversions in cases of AML (Claxton et al. 1994). In fact, loss of function of Runx1 and Cbfβ in mice produces similar phenotypes, and both phenotypes exhibit embryonic lethality by E11.5–12.5 due to loss of definitive hematopoiesis (Castilla et al., 1996; Okuda et al., 1996; Sasaki et al., 1996; Wang et al., 1996a). Human and mouse studies thus demonstrate that these two interacting proteins (RUNX1 and CBFβ) are required for differentiation of hematopoietic cells. Very recently, the *RUNX3* gene has been implicated in diverse processes such as neurogenesis and gastric epithelial proliferation (Levanon et al., 2002; Li et al., 2002).

By the mid-1990s, another vertebrate RUNT domain protein, RUNX2 (also called AML3, PEBP2αA, OSF2, and CBFA1), became the focus of studies unrelated to hematopoiesis. A series of converging studies pointed to the critical function of RUNX2 during skeletal morphogenesis and, especially, osteoblast differentiation (Karsenty et al., 1999). During mouse embryogenesis *Runx2* was noted to be expressed in mesenchymal condensates which are the precursors to chondroprogenitor and osteoprogenitor cells (Ducy et al., 1997). Moreover, RUNX2 was identified as a unique transcription factor that bound to *cis* elements in the promoter of osteoblastic genes such as *osteocalcin, BSP, Col1a1,* and *osteopontin*. Both mouse genetics and tissue culture studies demonstrate that RUNX2 directly upregulates these genes during osteoblast differentiation. Its requirement during skeletogenesis was further proven with the generation of the *Runx2* null mouse model (Komori et al., 1997; Otto et al., 1997). *Runx2* null mice exhibit neonatal lethality due to absence of bone. They have a skeletal anlage made of only cartilage.

The vertebrate skeleton arises from mesenchymal condensations of cells that differentiate into either osteoblasts or chondrocytes (Ducy and Karsenty, 1998). Direct differentiation into osteoblasts occurs with intramembranous ossification that involves primarily the neurocranium—the parietal, occipital, frontal, and temporal bones of the skull. These bones are completely missing in the *Runx2* null mice, thus demonstrating an absolute requirement for RUNX2 in this process. During endochondral ossification of the chondrocranium—base of the skull—and of the axial (vertebral) and appendicular (limbs) skeleton, mesenchymal condensates differentiate into proliferating chondrocytes. These chondrocytes terminally differentiate into hypertrophic chondrocytes which undergo apoptosis. Finally, they are replaced by bony spongiosa at primary and secondary centers of ossification.

The *Runx2* null mice fail to undergo ossification and associated mineralization. Histochemical analysis showed absence of osteoblasts (Hoshi et al., 1999). Together these studies show that RUNX2 is absolutely required for osteoblast cell fate commitment. Further analyses (see below) demonstrate that the *Runx2* null mice also have defects in chondrocyte maturation, suggesting an additional role for RUNX2 in the transition from hypertrophic chondrocyte to primary spongiosa of the bone (Kim et al., 1999; Enomoto et al., 2000; Leboy et al., 2001; Takeda et al., 2001; Ueta et al., 2001). Still not completely clear however, is the effect of RUNX2 on osteoclastogenesis (Thirunavukkarasu et al., 2001). In vitro studies and mouse studies suggest a defect in osteoclastogenesis, though whether this is a cell-autonomous effect in osteoclasts or a non-cell-autonomous effect via alteration of the secreted signals from osteoblasts is not yet clear (O'Brien et al., 2002).

Significant structure–function studies have been performed on RUNX2 (Fig. 29–1). This protein has in common with the other vertebrate RUNT proteins the conserved RUNT domain, as well as a carboxy-terminal proline/serine/threonine-rich (PST) domain (Geoffroy et al., 1998; Thirunavukkarasu et al., 1998; Xiao et al., 1998). However, the presence of a unique stretch of glutamines (Q) followed by alanines (A) constitutes a Q/A domain at its amino terminus, but this domain is not found in either RUNX1 or RUNX3. There are 23 consecutive glutamines and 17 consecutive alanines in RUNX2.

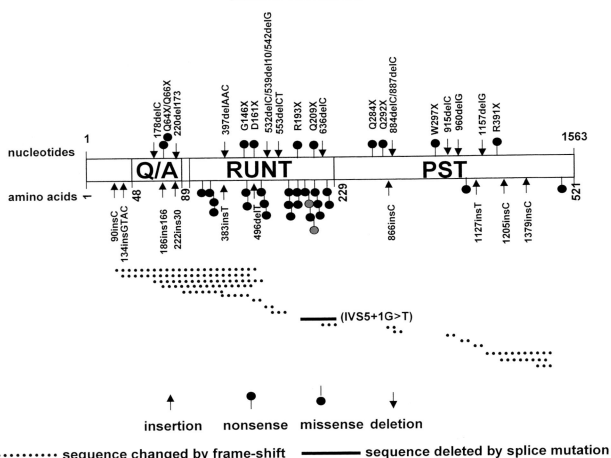

Figure 29–1. Schematic of RUNX2 domains. Q/A domain, 23 consecutive glutamines followed by 17 consecutive alanine residues (in humans); RUNT, Runt DNA binding and protein interaction domain; PST, proline/serine/threo-nine-rich transactivation and protein interaction domain. Nucelotide and amino acid positions are shown above and below, respectively. Positions and type of mutations reported in cleidocranial dysplasia (CCD) are also shown.

Finally, there is a unique valine/tryptophan/arginine/proline/tyrosine (VWRPY) pentanucleotide motif in the carboxy terminus of the PST domain that has been implicated in the interaction with the Groucho family of transcriptional repressors (Aronson et al., 1997; Levanon et al., 1998; Thirunavukkarasu et al., 1998). In fact, multiple proteins have been reported to interact with RUNX2 (Table 29–1). The in vivo relevance of many such interactions remains to be elucidated in most cases.

One of the best-studied interactors of the RUNT domain is CBFβ (Ogawa et al., 1993; Fujioka et al., 1996). Primarily studied with re-spect to RUNX1 and CBFβ, the interaction domains have been well documented by X-ray crystallographic studies (Warren et al., 2000; Tahirov et al., 2001). However, because of the early embryonic lethal-ity (prior to skeletogenesis) of the *Cbfβ* mouse null mutants, until re-cently it has been unclear whether this interaction is important for RUNX2 (Castilla et al., 1996; Wang et al., 1996b). The mutation data in humans support such an interaction (see later in this chapter) (Zhou et al., 1999). Data from in vitro transfection studies and from human mutation analyses suggest that the Q/A domain contributes to the trans-

Table 29–1. Proteins That Interact with RUNX2

RUNX2 interactor	Target*	Reference
Androgen receptor	SLP	Ning and Robins, 1999
AP1(c-Fos/c-Jun)	MMP13	D'Alonzo et al., 2002
Cbfβ	ALP, COL1A1, BGLAP, OPN	Ogawa et al., 1993; Harada et al., 1999
C/EBP	BGLAP	Gutierrez et al., 2002
ERK	RUNX2	Wang et al., 2002; Ziros et al., 2002
ETS1	OPN	Sato et al., 1998
TLE2/Groucho	BGLAP	Thirunavukkarasu et al., 1998
HES-1	BGLAP	McLarren et al., 2000
Glucocorticoid receptor	SLP	Ning and Robins, 1999
MAPK	BGLAP	Xiao et al., 2000
Msx2	BGLAP	Shirakabe et al., 2001
MOZ/MOZF	BGLAP	Pelletier et al., 2002
PKA	MMP13	Selvamurugan et al., 2000
Retinoblastoma protein (RB)	BGLAP	Thomas et al., 2001
Smad3	BGLAP	Alliston et al., 2001
Smad5	ALP	Lee et al., 2000
YAP	N/A	Yagi et al., 1999

*SLP, sex-limited protein; MMP13, collagenase 3; ALP, alkaline phosphatase; Colla1, type I collagen; BGLAP, osteocalcin; OPN, os-teopontin; RUNX2, Runt-related transcription factor 2; N/A, not determined.

activation by RUNX2, but other functions have not yet been identified (Mundlos et al., 1997; Thirunavukkarasu et al., 1998). Clearly, the context-dependent activity of RUNX2 during osteoblast differentiation and during chondrogenesis is a function of specific interactions with coactivators and repressors.

At present, *RUNX2* regulation by upstream and downstream factors is less defined. A novel zinc finger–containing transcription factor Osterix (*Osx*) was found to be expressed specifically in osteoblast progenitors, and its absence resulted in a phenotype similar to *Runx2* deficiency (Nakashima et al., 2002). The fact that *Osx* is not expressed in *Runx2*-null mice while *Runx2* is expressed in *Osx*-null mice strongly suggests that *Osx* is an essential downstream effector of *Runx2*. Several homeobox-containing proteins have also been identified as possible regulators of *Runx2* expression in different skeletal elements by mouse genetic studies. *Hoxa2*-deficient mice exhibited ectopic bone formation associated with ectopic *Runx2* expression in the second branchial arch (Kanzler et al., 1998). In contrast, down-regulation of *Runx2* in both *Msx2*- and *Bapx1*-deficient mice was observed with delayed osteoblast differentiation (Tribioli and Lufkin, 1999; Akazawa et al., 2000). Interestingly, while the defect in *Bapx1*-deficient mice is localized to the axial skeleton, the skeletal abnormality in *Msx2*-deficient mice is observed in the skull and long bones (Satokata et al. 2000). Cell studies have supported a direct regulation of *Runx2* by both *Msx2* and *Dlx5* (Shirakabe et al., 2001). Secreted factors or their receptors have also been shown to regulate *Runx2* expression. *Indian hedgehog (Ihh)*–deficient mice lacked differentiated osteoblasts in long bones with absence of *Runx2* expression (St-Jacques et al., 1999). In a mouse FGF receptor 1 (FGFR1) model for Pfeiffer syndrome, accelerated osteoblast differentiation was observed in the sutures of the mutant mice with increased *Runx2* expression (Zhou et al., 2000). Cell culture studies suggest that RUNX2 is phosphorylated by MAP kinase (MAPK) which integrates bone morphogenetic proteins (BMP) and integrin-matrix signals from the extracellular matrix (Xiao et al., 2002). Furthermore, parathyroid hormone (PTH) has been shown to directly regulate osteoblast proliferation in part by acting on RUNX2 via protein kinase C (PKC) (Swarthout et al., 2002). Posttranslational regulation of RUNX2 also occurs in ubiquitin-mediated degradation (Tintut et al., 1999).

The *RUNX2* gene maps to human chromosome 6p12–21 (Lee et al., 1997; Mundlos et al., 1997). It is encoded by 9 exons. The major RUNX2 protein expressed by osteoblasts is 521 amino acids long, with the initiation codon at the first in-frame methionine present in the second exon (Geoffroy et al., 1998; Xiao et al., 1998). The entire gene spans more than 200 kb (Otto et al., 2002). During mouse embryogenesis, *Runx2* expression is detected at 9.5 days postcoitum (dpc) only in the notochord, and at 10.5 dpc in condensing mesenchymal cells such as the primordia of the shoulder bone (Ducy, 2000). At 12.5 dpc, *Runx2* is strongly expressed in every forming skeletal condensation, including ribs, vertebral bodies, and developing bones of limbs and pelvic girdles, as well as in jaws and skull (Ducy et al., 1997). By 14.5 dpc, it begins to be restricted to areas of the perichondrium during endochondral ossification and is strongly expressed in osteoblasts and somewhat less so in hypertrophic chondrocytes (Ducy et al., 1997; Takeda et al., 2001). This expression pattern correlates with its function during osteogenesis and chondrocyte maturation. The specific *cis* regulatory elements that define *RUNX2* expression are still poorly defined, although transgenic mouse and tissue culture studies suggest that autoactivation contributes to *Runx2* expression (Ducy et al., 1999; Drissi et al., 2000; Xiao et al., 2001).

CLINICAL FEATURES AND NATURAL HISTORY OF CLEIDOCRANIAL DYSPLASIA

Three converging lines of research highlighted the importance of RUNX2 in skeletogenesis in the mid-1990s. The first described its ability to direct the expression of osteoblast-specific genes (Ducy et al., 1997). The second reported the consequences of its loss of function in mouse (Komori et al., 1997; Otto et al., 1997). The third was the discovery of *RUNX2* mutations in the human skeletal dysplasia cleidocranial dysplasia (CCD) (Lee et al., 1997; Mundlos et al., 1997).

CCD is characterized by pathognomonic features, including delayed ossification of the fontanel, hypoplastic or aplastic clavicles, and dental anomalies. Although the original description is often credited to French neurologists in 1896 (Marie and Sainton, 1898), historians have hypothesized that the original description of CCD may date back to the writings of Homer in the *Illiad* and the *Odyssey* (Altschuler 2001). Multiple reports have added significantly to the clinical and radiographic delineation of the syndrome (Jarvis and Keats 1974; Chitayat et al., 1992; Jones, 1997). Recently, a retrospective natural history study elucidated additional features in this condition that primarily affects the skeletal system (Cooper et al., 2001).

The further delineation of the syndrome has made it clear that CCD is a generalized dysplasia and not a dysostosis that affects specific skeletal elements. While the most affected bones involve elements that ossify by intramembranous ossification, skeletal elements such as the phalanges that ossify by endochondral ossification are also affected. In fact, short stature and brachydactyly are significant components of this syndrome. In the natural history study by Cooper et al., the mean adult male and female heights were 165 ± 8 cm and 156 ± 10 cm, respectively. The significant effect on clavicular development supports the presence of a generalized dysplasia since it is among the first bones to ossify and does so via both intramembranous ossification and (secondarily) endochondral ossification during the embryonic period (Gardner, 1968; Hall, 2001). The prevalence of CCD is unclear, but estimates of 1 in 1 million have been made, though this is likely an underestimate. There is no sex or ethnic predilection, and the new mutation rate varies among different studies from 16% to 40% (Siggers, 1975). The condition is dominantly inherited and exhibits high penetrance with variable expressivity.

CCD patients are often diagnosed by finding wide open sutures and fontanels, along with hypoplastic clavicles that enable the patient to appose their shoulders. However, because there is little initial morbidity associated with these symptoms, patients may escape diagnosis until they are seen for dental complications by pediatric dentists. Patients have delayed loss of primary dentition, delayed eruption of permanent dentition, dentigerous cysts, and supernumerary teeth (Becker et al., 1997a, 1997b). In additional, they may have malocclusion. The dental findings are part of a constellation of craniofacial features that also include brachycephaly, frontal bossing with relative macrocephaly, depressed nasal ridge, underdevelopment of the zygomatic and lacrimal bones, and relative prognathism (Jensen and Kreiborg, 1993a, 1993b, 1995; Kreiborg et al., 1999). There is delayed closure of the fontanel and of sutures, and the open fontanel may persist even until adulthood (Cooper et al., 2001). The clavicles may be hypoplastic or aplastic, and in experienced centers, prenatal ultrasonographic diagnosis based on this may be performed as early as 15 weeks (Hamner et al., 1994; Hassan et al., 1997; Stewart et al., 2000). Additional skeletal features that may develop throughout life include genu valgum, pes planus, and scoliosis (Cooper et al., 2001). While patients in general do not have an increased risk of fractures or decreased bone mineral density, a subset of patients has been described to have recurrent fractures and osteopenia (see Table 29–2) (Quack et al., 1999; Bergwitz et al., 2001; Cooper et al., 2001; Otto et al., 2002). Patients have an increased incidence of upper respiratory complications such as loud breathing, chronic congestion, and snoring. Associated with this are increased incidences of hearing loss and childhood otitis. While patients with CCD may have an increased incidence of learning disabilities, there was no significant difference regarding ultimate level of education attained when compared to their sibs. Finally, the incidence of primary caesarian section is significantly higher in women with CCD, and this may be due in part to cephalopelvic disproportion (Cooper et al., 2001).

The radiographic features of CCD reflect the presence of a generalized dysplasia that affects bone and cartilage (Fig. 29–2) (Taybi and Lachman, 1996). Delayed or absent ossification reflects the former, and shortened long bones reflect the latter. Alterations of the axial skeleton can be found in the skull, the vertebrae, the pelvis, and the clavicles. The appendicular skeleton is affected primarily with alterations, especially of acromelic elements. Patients have a brachecephalic skull with frontal bossing, wide sutures, wormian bones, and

Table 29–2. *RUNX2* Mutations in Cleidocranial Dysplasia (CCD)

Location	Mutation*	Type†	Comment	Reference‡
N terminus	90insC (stop in runt)	F	Mild CCD	Zhou
	134insGTAC (stop in runt)	F		Otto
Q/A domain	178delC (stop in runt)	F		Otto
	186ins16 (stop in runt)	F		Mundlos
	Q64X	N		Otto
	Q66X	N		Otto
	220del173 (stop in runt)	F		Zhou
	222ins30	I	In-frame duplication of 10 alanines, which abolishes transactivation	Mundlos
Runt domain	L113R	M		Quack
	S118R	M		Quack
	F121C	M	Mild CCD, but classic CCD when found as compound heterozygote with G511S	Quack
	C123R	M		Quack
	383insT (stop in runt)	F		Yokozeki
	397delAAC	D	Abolished DNA binding	Zhou
	IVS3+1G>C	S		Otto
	G146X	N		Zhou
	R148G	M	One family member with classic CCD; one with dental anomalies only	Golan
	V156G	M		Otto
	D161X	N		Quack
	495delT (stop in runt)	F		Otto
	R169P	M		Otto
	R169Q	M		Zhou
	M175R	M	Abolishes DNA binding and transactivation	Lee
	532delC	F		Zhang
	539del10	F		Mundlos
	542delG (stop in runt)	F	CCD plus fractures	McBride
	553delCT (stop in runt)	F		Zhou
	R190P	M		McBride
	R190Q	M	Abolishes DNA binding	Zhou
	R190W	M	CCD plus osteoporosis	Giannoti; Bergwitz; Otto
	S191N	M	Abolishes DNA binding and transactivation	Lee
	R193L	M		McBride
	R193X	N		Zhang; Quack; Otto
	F197S	M		Zhang
	L199F	M	Abolishes DNA binding and transactivation	Zhou
	T200A	M	Father with dental anomalies and two children with classic CCD; no effect on DNA binding and transactication; partially decreases potential Cbfβ interaction	Zhou
	I201K	M		Otto
	T205R	M		Quack
	Q209R	M		Zhou
	Q209H	M		McBride
	Q209X	N	CCD and cleft lip	Yamachika
	636delC (stop in runt)	F		Zhou
	R225Q	M	Abolishes DNA binding	Zhou; Quack; Otto
	R225W	M	Interferes with nuclear accumulation	Quack; Sakai; Otto
	IVS5+1 G>T in-frame exon skipping	S	In-frame deletion of last 35 amino acids of RUNT domain	Zhou; Zhang
	IVS5+2T>C	S		Otto
	IVS5+4delAAGT	S		Otto
PST domain	821delC (stop in PST)	F	CCD plus osteoporosis	Bergwitz
	824delG (stop in PST)	F		Quack
	Q280X	N		Otto
	Q284X	N		McBride
	Q292X	N		McBride
	866insC (stop in PST)	F		McBride
	884delC (stop in PST)	F		Zhou
	887delC (stop in PST)	F		Quack
	W297X	N		Mundlos
	915delC (stop in PST)	M		Quack
	960delG (stop in PST)	F		McBride
	A362V	M		Otto
	1127insT (stop in PST)	F		Quack
	1157delG (stop in PST)	F		Quack
	R391X	N	Classic CCD plus brachydactyly (Tsai); abolishes SMAD interaction; residual transactivation potential	Zhou; Zhang; Tsai
	1205insC (stop in PST)	F	Severe CCD with fractures	Quack
	1379insC (stop in PST)	F	Mild CCD	Quack
	G511S	M	No phenotype alone (may be neutral polymorphism)	Quack

*Mutation numbering begins with the ATG codon in exon 2 as number 1, which corresponds to the major osteoblast-specific RUNX2 protein product starting with MASNSL (Lee et al., 1997).

†Mutations are grouped according to RUNX2 functional domains with mutation types as listed: F, frameshift; M, missense; N, nonsense; D, deletion; I, insertion; S, splicing.

‡First author only listed: Lee et al., 1997; Mundlos et al., 1997; Zhou et al., 1999; Quack et al., 1999; Giannotti et al., 2000; Golan et al., 2000; Tsai et al., 2000; Yokozeki et al., 2000; Zhang et al., 2000b; Bergwitz et al., 2001; Yamachika et al., 2001; Otto et al., 2002; Sakai et al., 2002; McBride et al., 2002.

Figure 29–2. Radiographic findings in cleidocranial dysplasia (CCD). (*A*) Lateral skull series of a 5-month-old female, (*left*), a 13-year-old female (middle), and a 41-year-old male (right), each with CCD. Note open fontanel, wormian bones, supernumerary dentition, midfacial hypoplasia, and prognathism. (*B*) Chest series of the same CCD patients. Note hypoplastic clavicles and downsloping ribs. (*C*) Hand series of a 5-month-old female (left), an 11-year-old female (middle), and a 41-year-old male, each with CCD. Note especially the coned epiphyses in the 11-year-old.

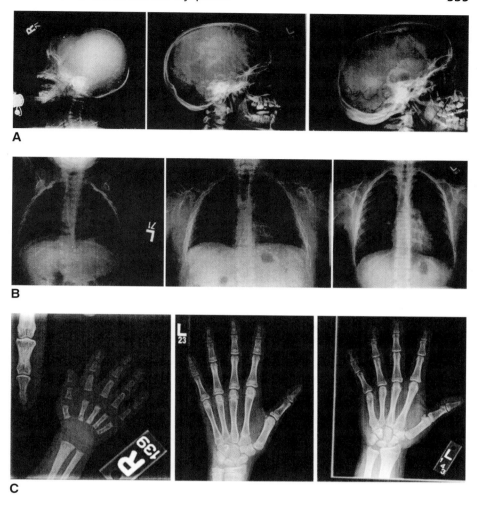

widely open and persistent anterior fontanel. There is midface hypoplasia and prognathism. Delayed ossification of the hyoid is often seen. Vertebral findings include posterior wedging, scoliosis, and spondylolysis. There is often hypoplasia or total aplasia of the clavicles with small scapulae. Finally, there may be absent or delayed ossification of the symphysis pubis and hypoplastic iliac wings. Distal findings include short phalanges, pseudoepiphyses of the metacarpals, and pseudoepiphyses of the phalanges. Both coxa vara and valga may be found and reflect undermodeling of long bones. Characteristic dental findings contribute to the morbidity of this condition. Patients often exhibit supernumerary dentition on radiographic studies (McNamara et al., 1999).

MOLECULAR GENETICS OF *RUNX2* MUTATIONS IN CCD

Over 60 different *RUNX2* mutations have been described in CCD patients from all ethnic backgrounds (Fig. 29–1, Table 29–2) (McBride et al., 2002; Otto et al., 2002). Deletions of the gene, as well as all types of subtle mutations, have been described. While some mutations have been recurrent and the majority of them are missense and cluster in the RUNT domain, no single mutation represents a significant proportion of total mutations. The majority of mutations produce haploinsufficiency of RUNX2 (Lee et al., 1997; Mundlos et al., 1997). This may be due to premature termination of the protein or abolition of its DNA binding (Zhou et al., 1999).

Extensive functional studies have been performed on mutations in the RUNT domain, and almost all exhibit disrupted DNA binding in electrophoretic mobility shift assays (EMSA) using the RUNX2 binding site–containing OSE2 enhancer element from the osteocalcin pro-

moter as a probe (Lee et al., 1997). Similarly, mutant RUNX2 proteins do not transactivate a reporter construct containing the OSE2 element in co-transfection studies (Zhou et al., 1999). The best genetic proof of haploinsufficiency as the predominant mechanism in the pathogenesis of CCD is the description of patients with complete deletion of *RUNX2* (Mundlos et al., 1995). However, some genotype–phenotype correlations do exist. For example, a unique mutation in the RUNT domain, T200A, has been described in a family with mild CCD and individuals who have primarily isolated dental anomalies (Zhou et al., 1999). Interestingly, this mutation does not affect its DNA binding or transactivation in vitro. Instead, it is the one of the few mutations described to date which map to an amino acid stretch that is reported to be critical for RUNT domain–CBFβ interaction. Mutation of this residue in a RUNT peptide partially impairs its interaction with CBFβ in vitro (Tahirov et al., 2001). These data suggest that the CCD-like phenotype may be generated by disruption of RUNT interaction with CBFβ, and, by extension, CBFβ–RUNX2 interaction may be important in vivo for skeletogenesis. Recent studies of a hypomorphic mutation of murine *Cbfβ* (which has sufficient activity to support embryonic hematopoiesis and late embryonic survival) appears to support the requirement of Cbfβ for skeletogenesis (Paul Liu, NIH, personal communication).

In contrast to the mild phenotype associated with the T200A mutation, severe CCD associated with significant osteopenia and recurrent fractures has also been described (see Table 29–2) (Quack et al., 1999; Bergwitz et al., 2001). These cases may be associated with late-truncating mutations in the PST domain. Mutations in the last exon may escape nonsense mediated decay, and truncated proteins may be generated that may have either dominant-negative or gain-of-function effects. For example, overexpression of the Runt domain alone acts in a dominant negative fashion in transgenic mice that exhibit transient osteopenia. One late-truncation mutation in RUNX2 has been shown to be unable to interact with SMAD proteins and to exhibit decreased transactivation in vitro (Zhang et al., 2000a; Ito and Zhang 2001). Mutations of the Q/A domain have also been associated with CCD. While contraction of the 17 consecutive alanines stretch to 11 alanines is a neutral polymorphic variant in the population, expansion or duplication of this stretch causes a loss of transactivation and CCD—hence, the assignment of a transactivation function to this domain (Mundlos et al., 1997; Thirunavukkarasu et al., 1998). Interestingly, the length of 23 consecutive polyglutamines is not polymorphic, and no expansion or missense mutations have yet been associated with this region. The lack of polymorphic expansion is likely due to interruption of the pure CAG repeat with CAA codons. However, the effects of potential expansions are still unknown.

ESTABLISHING THE DIAGNOSIS

CCD is a clinical diagnosis that is often considered in the neonatal and infant period when large fontanel and widely separated sutures are noted. A subsequent chest radiograph will show hypoplastic clavicles (Fig. 29–2). Other suggestive radiographic signs include underossification of the pubic symphysis and hyoid bones. Brachydactyly may not be evident in the neonatal period. Classic CCD in the older child and adolescent is more straightforward to diagnosis because of prominent dental symptoms, including delayed loss of primary dentition and delayed eruption of permanent and supernumerary teeth, in addition to short stature. Classically, children will also be able to appose their shoulders. While learning disability may be found, children are usually of normal intelligence. In general, any time either hypoplastic clavicles or a large open fontanel (or both) are found, CCD should be considered. Common causes of large fontanel such as hypothyroidism should be ruled out. A complete radiographic survey of the skeleton, including hands and feet, should be performed. Chromosome analysis may be indicated especially if there is associated developmental delay. A rare CCD-like phenotype has been reported; it is associated with duplication and translocation of chromosome 8q22 (Brueton et al., 1992).

Whenever CCD is considered, careful examination of the parents should be performed. Because of significant variable expressivity, features in affected parents may be subtle. The dental findings exhibit the highest penetrance, and clinical history of delayed eruption or loss of dentition should be ascertained; if the results are in doubt, radiographic studies should be performed. If no history or clinical signs of CCD are found in the family, then the proband is likely the result of a de novo dominant mutation.

While the possibility of germline mosaicism has been reported in CCD, this has not been proven on a molecular level (Zackai et al., 1997). The incidence of germline mosaicism in CCD is likely low (<1%). In at-risk pregnancies, prenatal ultrasonographic diagnoses can be attempted in experienced centers by 15 weeks (Hamner et al., 1994; Hassan et al., 1997). Molecular analysis is available on a research basis by direct sequencing of PCR-amplified exons. This approach has a yield of between 50% and 70% (Quack et al., 1999; Zhou et al., 1999). Because relatively few exons are spread over a large genomic region, Southern analyses with cDNA probes may also fail to detect large deletions. Because of the restricted expression to skeletal tissues, RT-PCR sequence analysis is generally not feasible. Prenatal DNA diagnosis can be attempted if the mutation in the proband is found by analysis of genomic DNA.

Several rarer conditions should be considered in the differential diagnosis for CCD. CCD has been reported to occur in conjunction with parietal foramina (PFM) (Golabi et al., 1984). The status of RUNX2 in these patients is unknown, but the association of CCD and parietal foramina is intriguing. Isolated PFM has been associated with loss of function of either of two transcription factors, ALX4 and MSX2 (Wilkie et al., 2000; Wu et al., 2000; Wuyts et al., 2000; Mavrogiannis et al., 2001). Moreover, MSX2 has been shown in tissue culture studies to interact with RUNX2 and to repress is its activity (Shirakabe et al., 2001). These data raise the question of whether a dysregulation of

RUNX2 and MSX2 interaction contributes to PFM/CCD. Other conditions in the differential diagnosis include more severe Crane-Heise syndrome, which is also associated with mineralization defects of the axial skeleton (Crane and Heise, 1981). Similarly, Yunis-Varon syndrome is associated with distal limb defects (absent thumbs and aphalangia) in addition to the features of CCD (Yunis and Varon, 1980). There is also significant undermineralization of the skeleton in this condition. Mandibuloacral dysplasia is associated with clavicular hypoplasia, wide sutures, and skin abnormalities (Young et al., 1971; Zina et al., 1981). Perhaps the greatest clinical overlap is with pycnodystostosis with similar fontanel, clavicular, and dental findings (Soliman et al., 2001). However, CCD and pycnodystostosis can be easily distinguished by radiographic studies which will show osteosclerosis in the latter.

MANAGEMENT, TREATMENT, AND COUNSELING

Patients with CCD should receive regular hearing evaluations and routine orthopedic follow-up for the skeletal complications, though a conservative management approach is indicated (Richie and Johnston, 1989; Cooper et al., 2001; Dhooge et al., 2001). This is in contrast to the dental complications that require more aggressive intervention. Ultimately, primary dentition should be removed and permanent dentition exposed. Since multiple dental surgeries are usually required, it is critical to have a team of pediatric dentists and oral surgeons experienced in management of craniofacial disorders (Becker et al., 1997a, 1997b). The overall aim is to achieve functioning occlusion by late adolescence. Because of delayed craniofacial development and midfacial hypoplasia, symptoms of upper airway obstruction and sleep apnea should prompt an evaluation that includes a formal sleep study (Cooper et al., 2001). Symptoms of upper airway obstruction, as well as a history of persistent sinusitis or otitis, may indicate the need for surgical intervention that ranges from adenoidectomy to craniofacial reconstruction in severe cases where medical therapy has failed. Children should be evaluated for signs of submucous cleft palate, and women with the disease should be aware of their increased risk for cesarean section (Cooper et al., 2001). Recurrence risk counseling should be for a dominantly transmitted condition with high penetrance, variable expressivity, and low empirical incidence for germline mosaicism.

MOUSE MODELS OF *Runx2* FUNCTION

Several mouse models regarding *Runx2* function have already been generated. The first described model for loss of *Runx2* function in mouse is the *Ccd* mouse (Sillence et al., 1987). This semidominant mouse mutant carries a microdeletion involving the *Runx2* locus and has many of the features of CCD. A specific *Runx2* null mouse mutation was generated by homologous recombination by two groups, and it confirmed the CCD phenotype in heterozygous mice (Komori et al., 1997; Otto et al., 1997); these mice had delayed ossification of the fontanel and hypoplastic clavicles (Huang et al., 1997). Later studies correlated the long bone dysplasia in patients with the finding of defects of chondrocyte maturation, especially in null mice (Zheng et. al., unpublished manuscript; Stricker et al., 2002). Dramatically, *Runx2* null mice have only a cartilage anlage of the skeleton, and there are no osteoblasts or mineralization. The critical balance between bone formation and resorption is perturbed during the transition from chondrogenesis to osteoblastogenesis in *Runx2* null mice. The process of vascular invasion, osteoclast formation, and periosteal bone formation is also perturbed (Inada et al., 1999; Jimenez et al., 1999, 2001; Kim et al., 1999; Zelzer et al., 2001).

The requirement for Runx2 during chondrogenesis is underscored by additional transgenic mice which show that constitutive expression of Runx2 in nonhypertrophic chondrocytes using a type II collagen promoter can induce chondrocyte hypertrophy and partially rescue the chondrocyte maturation and vascular invasion defects in *Runx2* null mice (Takeda et al., 2001; Ueta et al., 2001). A *Runx2* mutant mouse model similar to a nonsense mutation R391X in CCD has also been generated. Interestingly, mice heterozygous for the deletion do not de-

Figure 29–3. Regulation of RUNX2 during skeletogenesis. Upstream regulators of RUNX2 expression is shown. Direct regulator of RUNX2 protein and its transactivation targets are shown. Negative vs. positive effects are shown above and below, respectively.

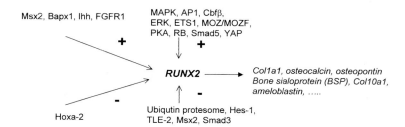

velop clavicles, while homozygotes do not form bone due to maturational arrest of osteoblasts (Choi et al., 2001). Thus the carboxy-terminal portion of Runx2 is essential for osteoblast differentiation during embryonic development, perhaps by directing intranuclear targeting. Transgenic mice models have also demonstrated that *Runx2* is also required for bone formation beyond embryonic development. When an osteocalcin promoter was used to force expression of a dominant-negative form of *Runx2* in fully differentiated osteoblasts postnatally, transient osteopenia resulted, due to the altered function of osteoblasts and autoregulation of the *Runx2* promoter (Ducy et al., 1999; Drissi et al., 2000). Interestingly, overexpression of wild-type Runx2 in differentiating osteoblasts using a type I collagen promoter *Col1a1* caused osteopenia and recurrent fractures in transgenic mice (Liu et al., 2001). The effect is due in part to maturational arrest of osteoblast differentiation. These data point to the pleiotropic effect of *Runx2* during endochondral and intramembranous ossification, which is context dependent and specified by a fine balance between the levels of Runx2 expression and interaction with coactivators and repressors.

PATHOGENESIS OF CCD AND IMPORTANT QUESTIONS

The clinical and radiographic delineation of CCD clearly reveals the consequences of disturbed endochondral and intramembranous ossification. The epiphyseal findings (often in the hands) and the short stature underscore the former, while the delayed ossification of the clavicle and skull bones reflect the latter. The delayed ossification reflects the requirement for *Runx2* for osteoblast cell fate commitment. It is required for differentiation of the mesenchymal cell into the osteoblast lineage. A host of genes found in osteoblasts—including osteocalcin, type I collagen, alkaline phosphatase, and osteopontin—contribute to the transcriptional network specified by *Runx2* in osteoblast differentiation and maintenance (Fig. 29–3). Interaction with multiple proteins in the transcriptional apparatus contributes to the full differentiation and maintenance of this cell type and indirectly to the balance of bone formation with resorption (Fig. 29–3).

Mouse studies show a requirement for Runx2 during chondrocyte maturation at least in some skeletal elements. This has been borne out by the histological study of one fetal case of CCD in which the growth plate demonstrates a shortened zone of hypertrophy with a qualitative decrease of type X collagen (Zheng et al., unpublished manuscript). The defect in endochondral ossification reflects the importance of *Runx2* for induction of chondrocyte hypertrophy and the subsequent transition to primary spongiosa. Some important genes within this transcriptional network include VEGF, MMP13/collagenase 3, and type X collagen (Zheng et al., unpublished manuscript). The fact that not all bones in CCD patients or in the *Runx2* null mice are affected suggests that Runx2 is required but not sufficient for chondrocyte maturation. Other transcription factors that may specify this process remain to be elucidated.

The dental phenotype in CCD points to an alternative function for Runx2 during development. It is up-regulated in ectodermally derived ameloblasts and down-regulated in fully differentiated odontoblasts. It is expressed in dental mesenchyme, stimulates epithelial morphogenesis, and contributes to the transactivation of tooth-specific genes

such as ameloblastin (Bronckers et al., 2001; Dhamija and Krebsbach, 2001). However, studying the human phenotype using the mouse model has been more difficult since mice do not have the equivalent of deciduous and permanent dentition. Its expression pattern suggests that Runx2 may regulate epithelial mesenchymal interactions during dentinogenesis (D'Souza et al., 1999).

The study of CCD and CCD-related phenotypes has generated new questions that are important for understanding skeletogenesis, the pathogenesis of this and other skeletal dysplasias, and the relevance of these genetic determinants in more common diseases such as osteoporosis. CCD-related conditions raise the possibility that they may be caused by either gain of function or dominant-negative mutations in *RUNX2* and by mutations in genes that regulate RUNX2 action such as *CBFβ*. Alternatively, they may be due to mutations in target genes of *RUNX2* transcriptional regulation. Additional loci for CCD-like conditions is suggested by the finding of patients with chromosomal alterations involving 8q22 (Brueton et al., 1992). The fact that no linkage studies have identified locus heterogeneity in families with classic CCD suggests that the CCD-like condition associated with 8q22 may be due to a gain-of-function-type mutation, as opposed to a simple loss of function. Given that haploinsufficiency produces CCD—while mild mutations that do not affect binding or transactivation can cause mild CCD and a primary dental phenotype—begs the question of whether isolated supernumerary teeth, delayed eruption, or loss of dentition might be associated with hypomorphic *RUNX2* alleles. In contrast, clinical studies show that subsets of CCD patients have osteopenia and mice overexpressing wild-type Runx2 have osteopenia (Cooper et al., 2001; Liu et al., 2001). These data raise the hypothesis that extreme imbalance of *RUNX2* activity either by a dominant-negative mutation or gain-of-function mutation may produce an osteopenic phenotype. Since it is clear that genes such as type I collagen are targets of *Runx2*, it must be determined whether subtle alterations in *Runx2* expression caused by SNP variants in its promoter will be important genetic determinants for postmenopausal osteoporosis, much like the effects of the SpI polymorphism of the type I collagen gene (Ralston, 2002). By studying rare genetic diseases such as CCD, we may gain knowledge about the structure–function correlation of the mutant gene, as well as the components of the genetic pathway in which it acts.

ACKNOWLEDGMENTS

The authors thank O. Hernandez for administrative assistance and S. Carter, R.N., for clinical assistance. Portions of this work were supported by the National Institutes of Health, the March of Dimes, and the Arthritis Foundation.

REFERENCES

Adya N, Castilla LH, Liu PP (2000). Function of CBFβ/Bro proteins. *Semin Cell Dev Biol* 11: 361–368.
Akazawa H, Komuro I, Sugitani Y, Yazaki Y, Nagai R, Noda T (2000). Targeted disruption of the homeobox transcription factor Bapx1 results in lethal skeletal dysplasia with asplenia and gastroduodenal malformation. *Genes Cells* 5: 499–513.
Alliston T, Choy L, Ducy P, Karsenty G, Derynck R (2001). TGF-β-induced repression of CBFA1 by Smad3 decreases cbfa1 and osteocalcin expression and inhibits osteoblast differentiation. *EMBO J* 20: 2254–2272.
Altschuler EL (2001). Cleidocranial dysostosis and the unity of the Homeric epics: an essay. *Clin Orthop* Feb. (383): 286–289.
Aronson BD, Fisher AL, Blechman K, Caudy M, Gergen JP (1997). Groucho-dependent and -independent repression activities of runt domain proteins. *Mol Cell Biol* 17: 5581–5587.

Becker A, Lustmann J, Shteyer A (1997a). Cleidocranial dysplasia: 1. General principles of the orthodontic and surgical treatment modality. *Am J Orthod Dentofacial Orthop* 111: 28–33.
Becker A, Shteyer A, Bimstein E, Lustmann J (1997b). Cleidocranial dysplasia: 2. Treatment protocol for the orthodontic and surgical modality. *Am J Orthod Dentofacial Orthop* 111: 173–183.
Bergwitz C, Prochnau A, Mayr B, Kramer FJ, Rittierodt M, Berten HL, Hausamen JE, Brabant G (2001). Identification of novel *CBFA1/RUNX2* mutations causing cleidocranial dysplasia. *J Inherit Metab Dis* 24: 648–656.
Bronckers AL, Engelse MA, Cavender A, Gaikwad J, D'Souza RN (2001). Cell-specific patterns of Cbfa1 mRNA and protein expression in postnatal murine dental tissues. *Mech Dev* 101: 255–258.
Brueton LA, Reeve A, Ellis R, Husband P, Thompson EM, Kingston HM (1992). Apparent cleidocranial dysplasia associated with abnormalities of 8q22 in three individuals. *Am J Med Genet* 43: 612–618.
Canon J, Banerjee U (2000). Runt and Lozenge function in *Drosophila* development. *Semin Cell Dev Biol* 11: 327–336.
Castilla LH, Wijmenga C, Wang Q, Stacy T, Speck NA, Eckhaus M, Marin-Padilla M, Collins FS, Wynshaw-Boris A, Liu PP (1996). Failure of embryonic hematopoiesis and lethal hemorrhages in mouse embryos heterozygous for a knocked-in leukemia gene *CBFB-MYH11*. *Cell* 87: 687–696.
Chitayat D, Hodgkinson KA, Azouz EM (1992). Intrafamilial variability in cleidocranial dysplasia: a three generation family. *Am J Med Genet* 42: 298–303.
Choi JY, Pratap J, Javed A, Zaidi SK, Xing L, Balint E, Dalamangas S, Boyce B, van Wijnen AJ, Lian JB, et al. (2001). Subnuclear targeting of Runx/Cbfa/AML factors is essential for tissue-specific differentiation during embryonic development. *Proc Natl Acad Sci USA* 98: 8650–8655.
Claxton DF, Liu P, Hsu HB, Marlton P, Hester J, Collins F, Deisseroth AB, Rowley JD, Siciliano MJ (1994). Detection of fusion transcripts generated by the inversion 16 chromosome in acute myelogenous leukemia. *Blood* 83: 1750–1756.
Cooper SC, Flaitz CM, Johnston DA, Lee B, Hecht JT (2001). A natural history of cleidocranial dysplasia. *Am J Med Genet* 104: 1–6.
Crane JP, Heise RL (1981). New syndrome in three affected siblings. *Pediatrics* 68: 235–237.
D'Alonzo RC, Selvamurugan N, Karsenty G, Partridge NC (2002). Physical interaction of the activator protein-1 factors c-Fos and c-Jun with Cbfa1 for collagenase-3 promoter activation. *J Biol Chem* 277: 816–822.
Dhamija S, Krebsbach PH (2001). Role of Cbfa1 in ameloblastin gene transcription. *J Biol Chem* 276: 35159–35164.
Dhooge I, Lantsoght B, Lemmerling M, Vanzieleghem B, Mortier G (2001). Hearing loss as a presenting symptom of cleidocranial dysplasia. *Otol Neurotol* 22: 855–857.
Drissi H, Luc Q, Shakoori R, Chuva De Sousa Lopes S, Choi JY, Terry A, Hu M, Jones S, Neil JC, Lian JB, et al (2000). Transcriptional autoregulation of the bone related *CBFA1/RUNX2* gene. *J Cell Physiol* 184: 341–350.
D'Souza RN, Berg T, Gaikwad J, Cavender A, Owen M, Karsenty G, Thesleff I (1999). Cbfa1 is required for epithelial–mesenchymal interactions regulating tooth development in mice. *Development* 126: 2911–2920.
Ducy P (2000). Cbfa1: a molecular switch in osteoblast biology. *Dev Dyn* 219: 461–471.
Ducy P, Karsenty G (1998). Genetic control of cell differentiation in the skeleton. *Curr Opin Cell Biol* 10: 614–619.
Ducy P, Zhang R, Geoffroy V, Ridall AL, Karsenty G (1997). Osf2/Cbfa1: a transcriptional activator of osteoblast differentiation. *Cell* 89: 747–754.
Ducy P, Starbuck M, Priemel M, Shen J, Pinero G, Geoffroy V, Amling M, Karsenty G (1999). A Cbfa1-dependent genetic pathway controls bone formation beyond embryonic development. *Genes Dev* 13: 1025–1036.
Enomoto H, Enomoto-Iwamoto M, Iwamoto M, Nomura S, Himeno M, Kitamura Y, Kishimoto T, Komora T (2000). Cbfa1 is a positive regulatory factor in chondrocyte maturation. *J Biol Chem* 275: 8695–8702.
Erickson P, Gao J, Chang KS, Look T, Whisenant E, Raimondi S, Lasher R, Trujillo J, Rowley J, Drabkin H (1992). Identification of breakpoints in t (8;21) acute myelogenous leukemia and isolation of a fusion transcript, AML1/ETO, with similarity to *Drosophila* segmentation gene, runt. *Blood* 80: 1825–1831.
Fujioka M, Yusibova GL, Sackerson CM, Tillib S, Mazo A, Satake M, Goto T (1996). Runt domain partner proteins enhance DNA binding and transcriptional repression in cultured *Drosophila* cells. *Genes Cells* 1: 741–754.
Gardner E (1968). The embryology of the clavicle. *Clin Orthop* 58: 9–16.
Geoffroy V, Corral DA, Zhou L, Lee B, Karsenty G (1998). Genomic organization, expression of the human *CBFA1* gene, and evidence for an alternative splicing event affecting protein function. *Mamm Genome* 9: 54–57.
Giannotti A, Tessa A, Patrono C, Florio LD, Velardo M, Dionisi-Vici C, Bertini E, Santorelli FM (2000). A novel *CBFA1* mutation (R190W) in an Italian family with cleidocranial dysplasia. *Hum Mutat* 16: 277.
Golabi M, Carey J, Hall BD (1984). Parietal foramina clavicular hypoplasia: an autosomal dominant syndrome. *Am J Dis Child* 138: 596–599.
Golan I, Preising M, Wagener H, Baumert U, Niederdellmann H, Lorenz B, Mussig D (2000). A novel missense mutation of the CBFA1 gene in a family with cleidocranial dysplasia (CCD) and variable expressivity. *J Craniofac Genet Dev Biol* 20: 113–120.
Gutierrez S, Javed A, Tennant DK, van Rees M, Montecino M, Stein GS, Stein JL, et al. (2002). CCAAT/enhancer-binding proteins (C/EBP) β and δ activate osteocalcin gene transcription and synergize with Runx2 at the C/EBP element to regulate bone-specific expression. *J Biol Chem* 277: 1316–1323.
Hall BK (2001). Development of the clavicles in birds and mammals. *J Exp Zool* 289: 153–161.
Hamner LH 3rd, Fabbri EL, Browne PC (1994). Prenatal diagnosis of cleidocranial dysostosis. *Obstet Gynecol* 83: 856–857.
Harada H, Tagashira S, Fujiwara M, Ogawa S, Katsumata T, Yamaguchi A, Komori T, Nakatsuka M (1999). Cbfa1 isoforms exert functional differences in osteoblast differentiation. *J Biol Chem* 274: 6972–6978.
Hassan J, Sepulveda W, Teixeira J, Garrett C, Fisk NM (1997). Prenatal sonographic diagnosis of cleidocranial dysostosis. *Prenat Diagn* 17: 770–772.
Hoshi K, Komori T, Ozawa H (1999). Morphological characterization of skeletal cells in Cbfa1-deficient mice. *Bone* 25: 639–651.
Huang LF, Fukai N, Selby PB, Olsen BR, Mundlos S (1997). Mouse clavicular development: analysis of wild-type and cleidocranial dysplasia mutant mice. *Dev Dyn* 210: 33–40.
Inada M, Yasui T, Nomura S, Miyake S, Deguchi K, Himeno M, Sato M, Yamagiwa H, Kimura T, Yasui N, et al. (1999). Maturational disturbance of chondrocytes in Cbfa1-deficient mice. *Dev Dyn* 214: 279–290.
Ito Y, Zhang YW (2001). A RUNX2/PEBP2αA/CBFA1 mutation in cleidocranial dysplasia revealing the link between the gene and Smad. *J Bone Miner Metab* 19: 188–194.
Jarvis JL, Keats TE (1974). Cleidocranial dysostosis: a review of 40 new cases. *Am J Roentgenol Radium Ther Nucl Med* 121: 5–16.
Jensen BL, Kreiborg S (1993a). Craniofacial abnormalities in 52 school-age and adult patients with cleidocranial dysplasia. *J Craniofac Genet Dev Biol* 13: 98–108.
Jensen BL, Kreiborg S (1993b). Development of the skull in infants with cleidocranial dysplasia. *J Craniofac Genet Dev Biol* 13: 89–97.
Jensen BL, Kreiborg S (1995). Craniofacial growth in cleidocranial dysplasia—a roentgencephalometric study. *J Craniofac Genet Dev Biol* 15: 35–43.
Jimenez MJ, Balbin M, Lopez JM, Alvarez J, Komori T, Lopez-Otin C (1999). Collagenase 3 is a target of Cbfa1, a transcription factor of the runt gene family involved in bone formation. *Mol Cell Biol* 19: 4431–4442.
Jimenez MJ, Balbin M, Alvarez J, Komori T, Bianco P, Holmbeck K, Birkedal-Hansen H, Lopez JM, Lopez-Otin C (2001). A regulatory cascade involving retinoic acid, Cbfa1, and matrix metalloproteinases is coupled to the development of a process of perichondrial invasion and osteogenic differentiation during bone formation. *J Cell Biol* 155: 1333–1344.
Jones KL (1997). *Smith's Recognizable Patterns of Human Malformation.* W. B. Saunders, Philadelphia, pp. 408–409.
Kanzler B, Kuschert SJ, Liu YH, Mallo M (1998). Hoxa-2 restricts the chondrogenic domain and inhibits bone formation during development of the branchial area. *Development* 125: 2587–2597.
Karsenty G (2001). Minireview: transcriptional control of osteoblast differentiation. *Endocrinology* 142: 2731–2733.
Karsenty G, Ducy P, Starbuck M, Priemel M, Shen J, Geoffroy V, Amling M (1999). Cbfa1 as a regulator of osteoblast differentiation and function. *Bone* 25: 107–108.
Kim IS, Otto F, Zabel B, Mundlos S (1999). Regulation of chondrocyte differentiation by Cbfa1. *Mech Dev* 80: 159–170.
Komori T, Yagi H, Nomura S, Yamaguchi A, Sasaki K, Deguchi K, Shimizu Y, Bronson RT, Gao YH, Inada M, et al. (1997). Targeted disruption of Cbfa1 results in a complete lack of bone formation owing to maturational arrest of osteoblasts. *Cell* 89: 755–764.
Kreiborg S, Jensen BL, Larsen P, Schleidt DT, Darvann T (1999). Anomalies of craniofacial skeleton and teeth in cleidocranial dysplasia. *J Craniofac Genet Dev Biol* 19: 75–79.
Leboy P, Grasso-Knight G, D'Angelo M, Volk SW, Lian JV, Drissi H, Stein GS, Adams SL (2001). Smad-Runx interactions during chondrocyte maturation. *J Bone Joint Surg Am* 83A: S15–S22.
Lee B, Thirunavukkarasu K, Zhou L, Pastore L, Baldini A, Hecht J, Geoffroy V, Ducy P, Karsenty G (1997). Missense mutations abolishing DNA binding of the osteoblast-specific transcription factor Osf2/Cbfa1 in cleidocranial dysplasia. *Nat Genet* 16: 307–310.
Lee KS, Kim HJ, Li QL, Chi XZ, Ueta C, Komori T, Wozney JM, Kim EG, Choi JY, Ryoo HM, Bae SC (2000). Runx2 is a common target of transforming growth factor β1 and bone morphogenetic protein 2, and cooperation between Runx2 and Smad5 induces osteoblast-specific gene expression in the pluripotent mesenchymal precursor cell line C2C12. *Mol Cell Biol* 20: 8783–8792.
Levanon D, Goldstein RE, Bernstein Y, Tang H, Goldenberg D, Stifani S, Paroush Z, Groner Y (1998). Transcriptional repression by AML1 and LEF-1 is mediated by the TLE/Groucho corepressors. *Proc Natl Acad Sci USA* 95: 11590–11595.
Levanon D, Bettoun D, Harris-Cerruti C, Woolf E, Negreanu V, Eilam R, Bernstein Y, Goldenberg D, Xiao C, Flieganf M, et al (2002). The Runx3 transcription factor regulates development and survival of TrkC dorsal root ganglia neurons. *EMBO J* 21: 3454–3463.
Li QL, Ito K, Sakakura C, Fukamachi H, Inoue K, Chi XZ, Lee KY, Nomura S, Lee CW, Han SB, et al. (2002). Causal relationship between the loss of RUNX3 expression and gastric cancer. *Cell* 109: 113–124.
Liu W, Toyosawa S, Furuichi T, Kanatani N, Yoshida C, Liu Y, Himeno M, Narai S, Yamaguchi A, Komori T (2001). Overexpression of Cbfa1 in osteoblasts inhibits osteoblast maturation and causes osteopenia with multiple fractures. *J Cell Biol* 155: 157–166.
Marie P, Sainton P (1898). Sur la dysostose cleido-cranienne herediataire. *Rev Neurol* 6: 835.
Mavrogiannis LA, Antonopoulou I, Baxova A, Kutilek S, Kim CA, Sugayama SM, Salamanca A, et al. (2001). Haploinsufficiency of the human homeobox gene *ALX4* causes skull ossification defects. *Nat Genet* 27: 17–18.
McBride K, Napierala D, Chen Y, Zheng Q, Zhou G, Lee B (2002). *RUNX2/CBFA1* mutations in cleidocranial dysplasia: phenotypic and structure/function correlations. In *The Growth Plate*, eds. Shapiro IM, Boyan B, Anderson HC (Amsterdam, IOS Press), pp. 213–222.
McLarren KW, Lo R, Grbavec D, Thirunavukkarasu K, Karsenty G, Stifani S (2000). The mammalian basic helix loop helix protein HES-1 binds to and modulates the transactivating function of the runt-related factor Cbfa1. *J Biol Chem* 275: 530–538.
McNamara CM, O'Riordan BC, Blake M, Sandy JR (1999). Cleidocranial dysplasia: radiological appearances on dental panoramic radiography. *Dentomaxillofac Radiol* 28: 89–97.
Mundlos S, Mulliken JB, Abramson DL, Warman ML, Knoll JH, Olsen BR (1995). Genetic mapping of cleidocranial dysplasia and evidence of a microdeletion in one family. *Hum Mol Genet* 4: 71–75.
Mundlos S, Otto F, Mundlos C, Mulliken JB, Aylsworth AS, Albright S, Lindhout D,

Cole WG, Henn W, Knoll JH, et al (1997). Mutations involving the transcription factor CBFA1 cause cleidocranial dysplasia. *Cell* 89: 773–779.

Nakashima K, Zhou X, Kunkel G, Zhang Z, Deng JM, Behringer RR, de Crombrugghe B (2002). The novel zinc finger–containing transcription factor osterix is required for osteoblast differentiation and bone formation. *Cell* 108: 17–29.

Ning YM, Robins DM (1999). AML3/CBFα1 is required for androgen-specific activation of the enhancer of the mouse *sex-limited protein* (*Slp*) gene. *J Biol Chem* 274: 30624–30630.

O'Brien CA, Kern B, Gubrij I, Karsenty G, Manolagas SC (2002). Cbfa1 does not regulate RANKL gene activity in stromal/osteoblastic cells. *Bone* 30: 453–462.

Ogawa E, Inuzuka M, Maruyama M, Satake M, Naito-Fujimoto M, Ito Y, Shigesada K (1993). Molecular cloning and characterization of PEBP2 β, the heterodimeric partner of a novel *Drosophila* runt-related DNA binding protein PEBP2 α. *Virology* 194: 314–331.

Okuda T, van Deursen J, Hiebert SW, Grosveld G, Downing JR (1996). AML1, the target of multiple chromosomal translocations in human leukemia, is esential for normal fetal liver hematopoiesis. *Cell* 84: 321–330.

Otto F, Thornell AP, Crompton T, Denzel A, Gilmour KC, Rosewell IR, Stamp GWH, Beddington RS, Mundlos S, Olsen BP, et al. (1997). *Cbfa1*, a candidate gene for cleidocranial dysplasia syndrome, is essential for osteoblast differentiation and bone development. *Cell* 89: 765–771.

Otto F, Kanegane H, Mundlos S (2002). Mutations in the *RUNX2* gene in patients with cleidocranial dysplasia. *Hum Mutat* 19: 209–216.

Pelletier N, Champagne N, Stifani S, Yang XJ (2002). MOZ and MORF histone acetyltransferases interact with the Runt-domain transcription factor Runx2. *Oncogene* 21: 2729–2740.

Quack I, Vonderstrass B, Stock M, Aylsworth AS, Becker A, Brueton L, Lee PJ, Majeswki F, Mulliken JE, Suri M, et al. (1999). Mutation analysis of core binding factor A1 in patients with cleidocranial dysplasia. *Am J Hum Genet* 65: 1268–1278.

Ralston SH (2002). Genetic control of susceptibility to osteoporosis. *J Clin Endocrinol Metab* 87: 2460–2466.

Richie MF, Johnston CE (1989). Management of developmental coxa vara in cleidocranial dysostosis. Orthopedics 12: 1001–1004.

Sakai N, Hasegawa H, Yamazaki Y, Ui K, Tokunaga K, Hirose R, Uchinuma E, Susami T, Takato T (2002). A case of a Japanese patient with cleidocranial dysplasia possessing a mutation of *CBFA1* gene. *J Craniofac Surg* 13: 31–34.

Sasaki K, Yagi H, Bronson RT, Tominaga K, Matsunashi T, Deguchi K, Tani Y, Kishimoto T, Komori T (1996). Absence of fetal liver hematopoiesis in mice deficient in transcriptional coactivator core binding factor β. *Proc Natl Acad Sci USA* 93: 12359–12363.

Sato M, Morii E, Komori T, Kawahata H, Sugimoto M, Terai K, Shimizu H, Yasui T, Ogihara H, Yasui N, et al. (1998). Transcriptional regulation of *osteopontin* gene in vivo by PEBP2αA/CBFA1 and ETS1 in the skeletal tissues. *Oncogene* 17: 1517–1525.

Satokata I, Ma L, Ohshima H, Bei M, Woo I, Nishizawa K, Maeda T, Takano Y, Uchiyama M, Heaney S, et al. (2000). Msx2 deficiency in mice causes pleiotropic defects in bone growth and ectodermal organ formation. *Nat Genet* 24: 391–395.

Selvamurugan N, Pulumati MR, Tyson DR, Partridge NC (2000). Parathyroid hormone regulation of the rat collagenase-3 promoter by protein kinase A-dependent transactivation of core binding factor α1. *J Biol Chem* 275: 5037–5042.

Shirakabe K, Terasawa K, Miyama K, Shibuya H, Nishida E (2001). Regulation of the activity of the transcription factor Runx2 by two homeobox proteins, Msx2 and Dlx5. *Genes Cells* 6: 851–856.

Siggers DC (1975). Cleidocranial dysostosis. *Dev Med Child Neurol* 17: 522–524.

Sillence DO, Ritchie HE, Selby PB (1987). Animal model: skeletal anomalies in mice with cleidocranial dysplasia. *Am J Med Genet* 27: 75–85.

Soliman AT, Ramadan MA, Sherif A, Aziz Bedair ES, Rizk MM (2001). Pycnodysostosis: clinical, radiologic, and endocrine evaluation and linear growth after growth hormone therapy. *Metabolism* 50: 905–911.

Stewart PA, Wallerstein R, Moran E, Lee MJ (2000). Early prenatal ultrasound diagnosis of cleidocranial dysplasia. *Ultrasound Obstet Gynecol* 15: 154–156.

St-Jacques B, Hammerschmidt M, McMahon AP (1999). Indian hedgehog signaling regulates proliferation and differentiation of chondrocytes and is essential for bone formation. *Genes Dev* 13: 2072–2086.

Stricker S, Fundele R, Vortkamp A, Mundlos S (2002). Role of *runx* genes in chondrocyte differentiation. *Dev Biol* 245: 95–108.

Swarthout JT, D'Alonzo RC, Selvamurugan N, Partridge NC (2002). Parathyroid hormone-dependent signaling pathways regulating genes in bone cells. *Gene* 282: 1–17.

Tahirov TH, Inoue-Bungo T, Morii H, Fujikawa A, Sasaki M, Kimura K, Shiina M, Sato K, Kumasaka T, Yamamoto M, et al. (2001). Structural analyses of DNA recognition by the AML1/Runx-1 Runt domain and its allosteric control by CBFβ. *Cell* 104: 755–767.

Takeda S, Bonnamy JP, Owen MJ, Ducy P, Karsenty G (2001). Continuous expression of Cbfa1 in nonhypertrophic chondrocytes uncovers its ability to induce hypertrophic chondrocyte differentiation and partially rescues Cbfa1-deficient mice. *Genes Dev* 15: 467–481.

Taybi H, Lachman RS (1996). *Radiology of Syndromes, Metabolic Disorders, and Skeletal Dysplasias.* Mosby-Year Book, St. Louis, pp. 788–790.

Thirunavukkarasu K, Mahajan M, McLarren KW, Stifani S, Karsenty G (1998). Two domains unique to osteoblast-specific transcription factor Osf2/Cbfa1 contribute to its transactivation function and its inability to heterodimerize with Cbfβ. *Mol Cell Biol* 18: 4197–4208.

Thirunavukkarasu K, Miles RR, Halladay DL, Yang X, Galvin RJ, Chandrasekhar S, Martin TJ, Onvia JE (2001). Stimulation of osteoprotegerin (OPG) gene expression by transforming growth factor-β (TGF-β): mapping of the OPG promoter region that mediates TGF-β effects. *J Biol Chem* 276: 36241–36250.

Thomas DM, Carty SA, Piscopo DM, Lee JS, Wang WF, Forrester WC, Hinds PW (2001). The retinoblastoma protein acts as a transcriptional coactivator required for osteogenic differentiation. *Mol Cell* 8: 303–316.

Tintut Y, Parhami F, Le V, Karsenty G, Demer LL (1999). Inhibition of osteoblast-specific transcription factor Cbfa1 by the cAMP pathway in osteoblastic cells: ubiquitin/proteasome-dependent regulation. *J Biol Chem* 274: 28875–28879.

Tribioli C, Lufkin T (1999). The murine Bapx1 homeobox gene plays a critical role in embryonic development of the axial skeleton and spleen. *Development* 126: 5699–5711.

Tsai FJ, Wu JY, Lin WD, Tsai CH (2000). A stop codon mutation in the *CBFA 1* gene causes cleidocranial dysplasia. *Acta Paediatr* 89: 1262–1265.

Ueta C, Iwamoto M, Kanatani N, Yoshida C, Liu Y, Enomoto-Iwamoto M, Ohmori T, Enomoto H, Nakata K, Takeda K, et al. (2001). Skeletal malformations caused by overexpression of Cbfa1 or its dominant negative form in chondrocytes. *J Cell Biol* 153: 87–100.

Wang FS, Wang CJ, Sheen-Chen SM, Kuo YR, Chen RF, Yang KD (2002). Superoxide mediates shock wave induction of ERK-dependent osteogenic transcription factor (CBFA1) and mesenchymal cell differentiation toward osteoprogenitors. *J Biol Chem* 277: 10931–10937.

Wang Q, Stacy T, Binder M, Marin-Padilla M, Sharpe AH, Speck NA (1996a). Disruption of the *Cbfa2* gene causes necrosis and hemorrhaging in the central nervous system and blocks definitive hematopoiesis. *Proc Natl Acad Sci USA* 93: 3444–3449.

Wang Q, Stacy T, Miller JD, Lewis AF, Gu TL, Huang X, Bushweller JH, Bories JC, Alt FW, Ryan G, et al. (1996b). The CBFβ subunit is essential for CBFα2 (AML1) function in vivo. *Cell* 87: 697–708.

Warren AJ, Bravo J, Williams RL, Rabbitts TH (2000). Structural basis for the heterodimeric interaction between the acute leukaemia-associated transcription factors AML1 and CBFβ. *EMBO J* 19: 3004–3015.

Wheeler JC, Shigesada K, Gergen JP, Ito Y (2000). Mechanisms of transcriptional regulation by Runt domain proteins. *Semin Cell Dev Biol* 11: 369–375.

Wilkie AO, Tang Z, Elanko N, Walsh S, Twigg SR, Hurst JA, Wall SA, Chrzanowska KH, Maxron RE Jr. (2000). Functional haploinsufficiency of the human homeobox gene *MSX2* causes defects in skull ossification. *Nat Genet* 24: 387–390.

Wu YQ, Badano JL, McCaskill C, Vogel H, Potocki L, Shaffer LG (2000). Haploinsufficiency of *ALX4* as a potential cause of parietal foramina in the 11p11.2 contiguous gene-deletion syndrome. *Am J Hum Genet* 67: 1327–1332.

Wuyts W, Reardon W, Preis S, Homfray T, Rasore-Quartino A, Christians H, Willems PJ, Van Hul W (2000). Identification of mutations in the *MSX2* homeobox gene in families affected with foramina parietalia permagna. *Hum Mol Genet* 9: 1251–1255.

Xiao G, Jiang D, Thomas P, Benson MD, Guan K, Karsenty G, Franceschi RT (2000). MAPK pathways activate and phosphorylate the osteoblast-specific transcription factor, Cbfa1. *J Biol Chem* 275: 4453–4459.

Xiao G, Gopalakrishnan R, Jiang D, Reith E, Benson MD, Franceschi RT (2002). Bone morphogenetic proteins, extracellular matrix, and mitogen-activated protein kinase signaling pathways are required for osteoblast-specific gene expression and differentiation in MC3T3-E1 cells. *J Bone Miner Res* 17: 101–110.

Xiao ZS, Thomas R, Hinson TK, Quarles LD (1998). Genomic structure and isoform expression of the mouse, rat and human Cbfa1/Osf2 transcription factor. *Gene* 214: 187–197.

Xiao ZS, Liu SG, Hinson TK, Quarles LD (2001). Characterization of the upstream mouse *Cbfa1/Runx2* promoter. *J Cell Biochem* 82: 647–659.

Yagi R, Chen LF, Shigesada K, Murakami Y, Ito Y (1999). A WW domain-containing yes-associated protein (YAP) is a novel transcriptional co-activator. *EMBO J* 18: 2551–2562.

Yamachika E, Tsujigiwa H, Ishiwari Y, Mizukawa N, Nagai N, Sugahara T (2001). Identification of a stop codon mutation in the *CBFA1* runt domain from a patient with cleidocranial dysplasia and cleft lip. *J Oral Pathol Med* 30: 381–383.

Yokozeki M, Ohyama K, Tsuji M, Goseki-Sone M, Oida S, Orimo H, Moriyama K, Kuroda T (2000). A case of Japanese cleidocranial dysplasia with a *CBFA1* frameshift mutation. *J Craniofac Genet Dev Biol* 20: 121–126.

Young LW, Radebaugh JF, Rubin P, Sensenbrenner JA, Fiorelli G, McKusick VA (1971). New syndrome manifested by mandibular hypoplasia, acroosteolysis, stiff joints and cutaneous atrophy (mandibuloacral dysplasia) in two unrelated boys. *Birth Defects Orig Artic Ser* 7: 291–297.

Yunis E, Varon H (1980). Cleidocranial dysostosis, severe micrognathism, bilateral absence of thumbs and first metatarsal bone, and distal aphalangia: a new genetic syndrome. *Am J Dis Child* 134: 649–653.

Zackai EH, Robin NH, McDonaldmcginn DM (1997). Sibs with cleidocranial dysplasia born to normal parents: germ line mosaicism. *Am J Med Genet* 69: 348–351.

Zelzer E, Glotzer DJ, Hartmann C, Thomas D, Fukai N, Soker S, Olsen BR (2001). Tissue specific regulation of VEGF expression during bone development requires Cbfa1/Runx2. *Mech Dev* 106: 97–106.

Zhang YW, Yasui N, Ito K, Huang G, Fujii M, Hanai J, Nogami H, Ochi T, Miyazono K, Ito Y (2000a). A *RUNX2/PEBP2αA/CBFA1* mutation displaying impaired transactivation and Smad interaction in cleidocranial dysplasia. *Proc Natl Acad Sci USA* 97: 10549–10554.

Zhang YW, Yasui N, Kakazu N, Abe T, Takada K, Imai S, Sato M, Nomura S, Ochi T, Okuzumi S, et al. (2000b). PEBP2αA/CBFA1 mutations in Japanese cleidocranial dysplasia patients. *Gene* 244: 21–28.

Zheng Q, Zhou G, Chen Y, Morello R, Krakow D, Wilcox W, Lee B (2003). Type X collagen gene regulation by *Runx2* contributes to its hypertrophic chondrocyte-specific expression in vivo. (Unpublished manuscript).

Zhou G, Chen Y, Zhou L, Thirunavukkarasu K, Hecht J, Chitayat D, Gelb BD, Pirinen S, Berry SA, Greenberg CR, et al. (1999). *CBFA1* mutation analysis and functional correlation with phenotypic variability in cleidocranial dysplasia. *Hum Mol Genet* 8: 2311–2316.

Zhou YX, Xu X, Chen L, Li C, Brodie SG, Deng CX (2000). A Pro250Arg substitution in mouse Fgfr1 causes increased expression of Cbfa1 and premature fusion of calvarial sutures. *Hum Mol Genet* 9: 2001–2008.

Zina AM, Cravario A, Bundino S (1981). Familial mandibuloacral dysplasia. *Br J Dermatol* 105: 719–723.

Ziros PG, Gil AP, Georgakopoulos T, Habeos I, Kletsas D, Basdra EK, Papavassiliou AG (2002). The bone-specific transcriptional regulator Cbfa1 is a target of mechanical signals in osteoblastic cells. *J Biol Chem* 277: 23934–23941.

Part D.
The Tumor Necrosis Factor Signaling Pathway

30 | Signaling by TNF and Related Ligands

PASCAL SCHNEIDER

Family members of the tumor necrosis family receptors (TNFR) engage two main signaling pathways: activation of kinases and transcription factors on the one hand, and caspase activation and cell death on the other hand. Although each of these pathways uses distinct mechanisms of action and unrelated executers, they are highly cross-regulated. In this chapter, the structure and function of ligands and receptors of the TNF and TNFR families are discussed; then the cell death, MAPK, and NF-κB signaling pathways are described. Emphasis is placed on the description of the primary (Figs. 30–1 and 30–3) and ternary structure (Fig. 30–2) of many proteins involved in these pathways. Their site of action and their interaction partners (Fig. 30–4), as well as their function in vivo (Table 30–1) are also stressed. The following reviews are of particular interest regarding different aspects of this chapter: TNFR family (Locksley et al., 2001; Bodmer et al., 2002), TNF signaling (Baud and Karin, 2001), NF-κB activation (Karin and Ben-Neriah, 2000), and MAPK pathways (Widmann et al., 1999).

BIOLOGY OF TNF AND TNF RECEPTOR FAMILY MEMBERS

In the human, 29 receptors and 18 ligands have been described in the TNF and TNFR families (Fig. 30–1), and the function of most of them has been explored in gene deletion experiments (Table 30–1; please note that knockouts referenced in this table are not further referenced

in the text). Table 30–2 is a compilation of the usual synonyms for molecules cited in this chapter.

The FasL–Fas pair is an efficient trigger of the apoptotic cell death machinery. Inactivation of either FasL or Fas is a major genetic cause of autoimmune lymphoproliferative syndrome (ALPS) in humans and causes lymphoproliferation and autoimmunity in mice with a susceptible genetic background (Fisher et al., 1995; Rieux-Laucat et al., 1999). TRAIL engages a complex array of receptors, two of them being potent death inducers that appear to be especially active in transformed cells (Griffith and Lynch, 1998). Inhibition of endogenous TRAIL with neutralizing antibodies favors lung metastasis of various tumor cells in an experimental model (Takeda et al., 2001). Tumor surveillance may be the prime role of TRAIL, as $Trail^{-/-}$ mice have been reported to be largely normal.

Knockouts of TRAMP and DR6, two orphan receptors that potently induce cell death in transfected cells, display rather mild phenotypes that affect T-cell negative selection and Th2 T-cell responses, respectively. TL1A, the ligand of TRAMP, stimulates IL-2 responsiveness and allogeneic responses of activated T cells (Migone et al., 2002). DCR3 is a soluble decoy receptor for TL1A, and possibly FasL, and may therefore regulate signaling through certain death receptors. NGFR, the only receptor with demonstrated involvement in neuronal cell death, also negatively regulates hair follicle development. NGFR is unique in the TNFR family in that it interacts, albeit with low affinity, with ligands of the

Figure 30–1. The TNF and TNFR family of ligands and receptors. Ligands are shown in the upper part of the figure, with the TNF homology domain (THD) in green. Receptors are drawn in the lower part of the figure. The modular organization of the extracellular domain is represented with a code, as described in the insert. Intracellular motifs are also represented, including death domain and the consensus TRAF-binding sites, P/S/A/T-x-Q/E-E and P-x-Q-x-T/S. For receptors characterized in several species, only the conserved sites are shown. A checkmark identifies TRAF-binding sites for which there is biochemical evidence. Intracellular interacting proteins are listed below the receptors, with numerals referring to TRAF molecules. The official TNF and TNFR superfamily numbers are indicated, when available. Proteins are drawn to scale, with the exception of the THD, which should appear two times larger.

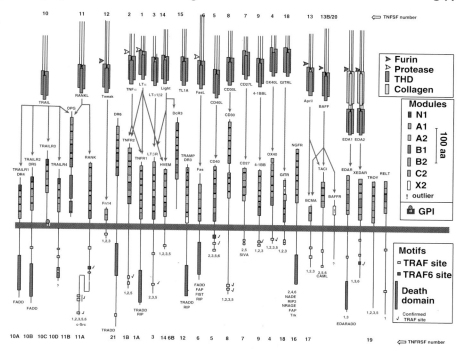

neurotrophin family—such as nerve growth factor (NGF), brain-derived neurotrophic factor (BDNF), and other neurotrophins (NTs)—which are structurally unrelated to TNF. In addition to NGFR, neurotrophins engage with high affinity a family of Trk receptor tyrosine kinases (Yano and Chao, 2000). NGFR physically interacts with Trks and fails to induce cell death in cells that coexpress these receptors.

TNFR1, TNFR2, and their ligands are intimately implicated in the inflammatory response. In humans, TNF receptor–associated periodic fever syndrome (TRAPS) is associated with mutations of TNFR1 that prevent the down-regulation of the inflammatory response, possibly by interfering with its shedding from the cell surface after TNF engagement (McDermott et al., 1999; Galon et al., 2000). TNF deregulation contributes to autoimmune manifestations such as rheumatoid arthritis and Crohn's disease, and its inhibition is of great therapeutic benefit for these conditions (Feldmann, 2001). Under physiological conditions, TNF is necessary for proper development of follicular dendritic cells and germinal centers, and therefore it impinges on humoral immune responses. TNFR1 is a potent inducer of cell death, but this property is generally obliterated by its concomitant ability to induce strong anti-apoptotic responses. As TNF is transiently but highly expressed in fetal liver, disruption of the anti-apoptotic NF-κB pathway uncovers the pro-apoptotic activity of TNFR1, leading to liver injury and embryonic cell death. This phenotype is largely rescued by concomitant deletion of TNFR1.

RANK and LTβR are two receptors that are crucially involved in secondary lymphoid organ formation (Fu and Chaplin, 1999; Kim et al., 2000). RANK is necessary for the emergence of CD3$^-$ CD4$^+$ cells from hematopoietic precursors. During embryogenesis, these cells are attracted by chemokines to the location of the future lymph node. At this site, CD3$^-$ CD4$^+$ cells engage LTβR expressed on stromal cells, which respond by producing B lymphocyte chemoattractant (BLC) and other chemokines. B cells are recruited to the rudimentary lymph node and can substitute for CD3$^-$ CD4$^+$ cells in providing LTβR signal to stromal cells. Follicular dendritic cells and T cells are recruited at a subsequent stage. LTβR, but not RANK, is also required for the formation of Peyer's patches. In addition to its role in lymph node formation, RANK is absolutely required for osteoclastogenesis, and its absence leads to increased mineral bone formation (osteopetrosis). In familial expansile osteolysis, duplication of a short hydrophobic segment converts the signal peptide of RANK into a membrane anchor. The modified receptor apparently gains constitutive activity, thus leading to local increase in bone remodeling. This results in the formation of bone with poor mechanical

properties (Hughes et al., 2000). The osteoclastogenic activity of RANKL is modulated by a soluble receptor, OPG, which acts as a physiologic inhibitor (Simonet et al., 1997). RANK is also implicated in the development of the mammary gland (Fata et al., 2000). RANKL is expressed by osteoblasts in response to various bone resorption signals, and also by activated T lymphocytes at an inflammatory site. TNF produced at an inflammatory site has a potent, TNFR1-mediated co-stimulatory effect on osteoclast formation (Lam et al., 2000; Zhang et al., 2001). In rheumatoid arthritis, the chronic conjugate action of TNF and RANKL on osteoclast activation is believed to be the main cause of cartilage and bone erosion (Kong et al., 1999a).

CD40L and BAFF both have a strong influence on B-cell biology. CD40L is essential for dendritic cell and B-cell activation by T helper cells and is further required for B-cell proliferation, antibody production, and isotype switch in T-dependent humoral responses. Genetic inactivation of CD40L has been identified in a range of patients with X-linked immunodeficiency and hyper-IgM syndrome (Grewal and Flavell, 1998). BAFF acting through BAFFR provides survival signals and allows B-cell maturation in the periphery. A second BAFF receptor, TACI, is required for efficient T-independent humoral responses. Interestingly, TACI also binds to APRIL, a ligand that has been implicated in tumor cell growth. However, APRIL's effect on tumor cell growth is probably mediated by another, unidentified, APRIL receptor (Rennert et al., 2000).

In the immune system, a distinct set of receptors is important for T-cell function. CD27 activates effector T cells and promotes formation of memory T cells. 4-1BB is a co-stimulator of the cytotoxic T-cell response, and OX40 induces the anti-apoptotic pathways that are required for long-term T-cell survival after priming by dendritic cells. In contrast, CD30 negatively regulates the proliferation of activated T cells to prevent the emergence of autoreactive cells. In particular, CD30 activation leads to the down-regulation of three toxic proteins used by effector T cells—namely, granzyme B, perforin, and FasL (Muta et al., 2000). Little is known about GITR and RELT, but these receptors are likely to function in lymphoid cells. There are several ligands of the TNF family that do not seem to play a role in the immune system. TWEAK has been implicated in triggering vascularization (Lynch et al., 1999; Wiley et al., 2001). EDA and EDAR are crucially involved in the formation of epidermal appendages such as hair, teeth, and eccrine sweat glands (see Chapter 31). Although the function of XEDAR and of the orphan receptor TROY awaits discovery, their expression pattern re-

Table 30–1. Major Features of Knockout and of Some Other Mice in Relation to the Tumor Necrosis Factor Receptor (TNFR) Family and Signaling Pathways

Protein	Type	Viability	Phenotype	References
TRAIL	−/−	Viable	No abnormal phenotype	Sedger et al., 2000
RANKL	−/−	Viable	Osteopetrosis; no osteoclast formation; alymphoplasia; mammary gland defects	Kong et al., 1999; Fata et al., 2000
RANK	−/−	Viable	Osteopetrosis; no osteoclast formation; alymphoplasia; mammary gland defects	Dougall et al., 1999; Fata et al., 2000
OPG	−/−	Viable	Severe osteoporosis; vascular calcification	Bucay et al., 1998
TRAMP	−/−	Viable	Mild impairment of thymocyte negative selection	Wang et al., 2001b
DR6	−/−	Viable	Attenuation of JNK-mediated TH-2 responses	Zhao et al., 2001
TNF	−/−	Viable	Lack of FDCs; impaired germinal center formation and humoral responses	Pasparakis et al., 1996
TNFR1	−/−	Viable	Resistant to septic shock (LPS); susceptible to infections; altered FDC and B-cell architecture	Pfeffer et al., 1993; Rothe et al., 1993; Pasparakis et al., 1997
TNFR2	−/−	Viable	Resistant to subcutaneous necrotic effect of TNF; increased resistance to TNF-induced death	Erickson et al., 1994
LTα	−/−	Viable	Alymphoplasia; disrupted splenic architecture	De Togni et al., 1994; Banks et al., 1995
RANKL Tg × LTα	Tg in −/−	Viable	No rescue of lymph node formation	Kim et al., 2000
LTβ	−/−	Viable	Alymphoplasia; disrupted splenic architecture	Alimzhanov et al., 1997; Koni et al., 1997
LTβR	−/−	Viable	Alymphoplasia; disrupted splenic architecture (no marginal zone, no FDC, no T-B segregation)	Futterer et al., 1998
FasL	Def*	Viable	*gld* mice; generalized lymphoproliferation	Takahashi et al., 1994
Fas	Def*	Viable	*lpr* mice; lymphoproliferation; resistance to α-Fas-mediated apoptosis	Watanabe-Fukunaga et al., 1992
Fas	−/−	Viable	Hyperplasia in peripheral lymphoid organs and liver	Adachi et al., 1995
CD40L	−/−	Viable	Impaired T-dependent responses	Renshaw et al., 1994; Xu et al., 1994
CD40	−/−	Viable	Impaired T-dependent responses; no isotype switch in T-dependent responses	Kawabe et al., 1994
CD30	−/−	Viable	Impaired negative selection of T cells; unlimited proliferation of autoreactive T cells	Amakawa et al., 1996; Kurts et al., 1999
CD27L	Tg in B cells	Viable	Increased number of effector T cells and IFNγ production, leading to decreased B-cell number	Arens et al., 2001
CD27	−/−	Viable	Impaired CD4 and CD8 T-cell responses; impaired T-cell memory	Hendriks et al., 2000
4-1BBL	−/−	Viable	Impaired cytotoxic T-cell responses	DeBenedette et al., 1999
OX40L	−/−	Viable	Impaired T-cell priming by dendritic cells	Chen et al., 1999; Murata et al., 2000
OX40	−/−	Viable	Failure of activated T cells to up-regulate Bcl-2 and Bcl-X_L, leading to early death	Rogers et al., 2001
NGFR	−/−	Viable	Defect in sensory neurons; excess survival of TrkA-negative neurons; enhanced hair follicle development	Lee, 1992; Van der Zee, 1996; Botchkareva et al., 1999
BAFF	−/−	Viable	Impaired peripheral B-cell maturation at transitional type-2 stage	Gross et al., 2001; Schiemann et al., 2001
BCMA	−/−	Viable	No detectable lymphocyte dysfunction	Schiemann et al., 2001; Xu and Lam, 2001
TACI	−/−	Viable	B-cell accumulation; impaired T-independent responses	von Bulow et al., 2001; Yan et al., 2001
BAFFR	Def	Viable	A/WySnJ mice; impaired peripheral B-cell maturation at transitional type-2 stage	Thompson et al., 2001; Yan et al., 2001
EDA	Def	Viable	*Tabby* mice; hypoplastic hair, teeth, eccrine sweat glands	Ferguson, 1997; Srivastava, 1997
EDAR	Def	Viable	*Downless* mice; hypoplastic hair, teeth, eccrine sweat glands	Headon and Overbeek, 1999
TRAF-1	−/−	Viable	Enhanced TNFR2 signaling; resistant to subcutaneous necrotic effect of TNF	Tsitsikov et al., 2001
TRAF-2	−/−	Die d 10–14	Runted; no JNK activation by TNF; TNF hypersensitivity; fewer pre-B cells	Lee et al., 1997; Yeh et al., 1997
TRAF-2 × TNFR1	−/−	Viable	No NF-κB activation by TNF	Nguyen et al., 1999
TRAF-3	−/−	Die d 10	White blood cell hypoplasia; in RC, impaired T-cell and TD responses; normal CD40 responses of B cells	Xu et al., 1996
TRAF-4	−/−	Viable	Constricted upper trachea	Shiels et al., 2000
TRAF-5	−/−	Viable	Impaired CD40 and CD27 lymphocyte activation	Nakano et al., 1999
TRAF-2 × TRAF-5	D−/−	Die 2–3w	Runted; impaired JNK and NF-κB activation in response to TNF	Tada et al., 2001
TRAF-6	−/−	Die d 19	Runted; osteopetrosis; impaired LPS, IL-1, and CD40 signaling; alymphoplasia	Lomaga et al., 1999; Naito et al., 1999
RIP	−/−	Die 1–3 d	Apoptosis in lymphoid and adipose tissue; TNF hypersensitivity; impaired TNF-induced NF-κB	Kelliher et al., 1998
EDARADD	Def	Viable	Crinkled mice; hypoplastic hair, teeth, eccrine sweat glands	Headon et al., 2001
FADD	−/−	Die E10	Heart defect; in radiation chimera, impaired activation-induced T-cell proliferation	Zhang et al., 1998
FLIP	−/−	Die E10	Heart defect; hypersensitivity to death ligands	Yeh et al., 2000
Caspase-8	−/−	Die E10	Heart defect; impaired apoptosis via death receptors	Varfolomeev et al., 1998
Caspase-10	Def	Viable	Autoimmune lymphoproliferative syndrome in humans (no Caspase-10 in mouse)	Wang et al., 1999
PEA-15	−/−	Viable	Hypersensitivity of actinomycin D-treated astrocytes to TNF	Kitsberg et al., 1999
Caspase-1	−/−	Viable	Resistance to LPS; defective IL-1 processing	Kuida et al., 1995
Caspase-2	−/−	Viable	Excess germ cells; impaired granzyme B / perforin-mediated cell death	Bergeron et al., 1998
Caspase-3	−/−	Die 1–3 w	Brain hyperplasia; normal sensitivity of thymocytes to various death stimuli	Kuida et al., 1996

(Continued)

Table 30–1. *Continued*

Protein	Type	Viability	Phenotype	References
Caspase-9	−/−	Perinatal death	Brain hyperplasia; no cytochrome c-dependent activation of caspase-3	Kuida et al., 1998
Caspase-11	−/−	Viable	Resistant to LPS; impaired caspase-1 activation	Wang et al., 1998
Apaf-1	−/−	Die E16; 5% are	Brain hyperplasia; impaired caspase-3 and -9 activation; normal Fas-induced death in activated T cells; defective spermatogenesis viable	Cecconi et al., 1998; Yoshida et al., 1998; Honarpour et al., 2000
Cyto c	−/−	Die E9	Resistance of embryonic cells to serum withdrawal and UV; TNF hypersensitivity	Li et al., 2000
RAIDD	500 kb del	Viable	High growth (30–50%); other genes may be affected	Horvat and Medrano, 1998
IKKα	−/−	Die d 1	Thick epidermis, abnormal skeleton; no defect in IκB degradation; in radiation chimera, no PP or impaired LTβR signaling	Hu et al., 1999; Li et al., 1999
IKKαKD	Ki in −/−	Viable	Alymphoplasia; impaired B-cell maturation; impaired NF-κB2 processing	Senftleben et al., 2001
IKKβ	−/−	Die E14	Liver apoptosis; TNF hypersensitivity and defective NF-κB activation by IL-1 or TNF	Li et al., 1999; Tanaka et al., 1999
NEMO	−/−	Die E13 +/− females viable	Liver apoptosis; TNF hypersensitivity and defective NF-κB activation by IL-1 or TNF; +/− females have incontinentia pigmenti	Makris et al., 2000; Rudolph et al., 2000; Schmidt-Supprian et al., 2000
c-Rel	−/−	Viable	Impaired humoral responses, CD3/CD28 T cell pathway, and macrophage function	Kontgen et al., 1995; Gerondakis et al., 1996; Grigoriadis et al., 1996
RelA	−/−	Die E15	Liver hypersensitivity to TNF; defect in inducible but not constitutive NF-κB activity	Beg et al., 1995; Beg and Baltimore, 1996
RelA × TNFR1	D−/−	Viable	Highly susceptible to infections; defective neutrophil recruitment to lungs	Alcamo et al., 2001
c-REl × RelA	D−/−	Die E13	Liver apoptosis; in radiation chimera + bone marrow, impaired T-cell and peripheral B-cell maturation; partly rescued by Bcl2 in B cells	Grossmann et al., 2000
RelB	−/−	Viable	Impaired APC function; lack of thymic medullary epithelial cells	Burkly et al., 1995
NF-κB1	−/−	Viable	B-cell defect (proliferation but no Ig production in response to CD40L; no switch to IgG3 and IgE); increased B-cell death in G0	Sha et al., 1995; Snapper et al., 1996; Grumont et al., 1998
NF-κB2	−/−	Viable	Decreased B cells, altered B-cell architecture, T-dependent and T-independent responses; impaired germinal centers, but Ig switch occurs	Caamano et al., 1998; Franzoso et al., 1998
RelA × NF-κB1	D−/−	Die E13	Liver apoptosis; in radiation chimera + bone marrow, impaired peripheral B-cell maturation	Horwitz et al., 1997
NF-κB1 × NF-κB2	D−/−	Viable	Osteopetrosis (not seen in single −/−); no mature osteoclasts and B cells; impaired macrophage function, spleen, and thymus architecture	Franzoso et al., 1997b
Bcl-3	−/−	Viable	Impaired TH1 and T-dependent responses, secondary lymphoid organ architecture, and germinal center formation; decreased B-cell number	Franzoso et al., 1997
IκBα	−/−	Die d 8	Runted; skin defects; granulopoiesis; constitutive NF-κB in hemopoietic cells but not fibroblasts; lack of NF-κB repression postinduction in fibroblasts	Beg et al., 1995; Klement et al., 1996
IκBα × NF-κB1	D−/−	Die 2–4 w	Significant rescue of IκBα−/− phenotype	Beg et al., 1995
IκBβ	Ki in IκBα−/−	Viable	Total rescue of IκBα−/− phenotype	Cheng et al., 1998
MEKK1	−/−	Viable	Defective eyelid closure due to impaired epithelial cell migration; impaired JNK activation in response to TNF, IL-1, dsRNA, and LPS in embryonic stem cells, but not macrophages or fibroblasts; NF-κB unaffected	Yujiri et al., 1998, 2000; Xia et al., 2000
MEKK3	−/−	Die E11	In embryonic fibroblasts, defective NF-κB signal downstream of RIP and TRAF2	Yang et al., 2001
NIK	Def	Viable	*Aly* mice; alymphoplasia; impaired T-dependent humoral responses; B-lymphocytopenia, altered splenic, and thymic architecture	Shinkura et al., 1999
NIK	−/−	Viable	Alymphoplasia; disrupted NF-κB signal; impaired transcriptional activity of NF-κB in LTβR (but not TNF) signaling	Yin et al., 2001
TBK	−/−	Die	Liver degeneration; normal lymphocytes; impaired NF-κB-dependent transcription in response to TNF and IL-1	Bonnard et al., 2000
PKCζ	−/−	Viable	Altered splenic FDC and B-cell architecture (similar to TNFR1−/−); impaired TNF and α-LTβR NF-κB activation in lung but not in liver	Leitges et al., 2001
GSK3-β	−/−	Die mid gestation	Liver hypersensitivity to TNF; rescued by anti-TNF; transactivation of NF-κB is defective	Hoeflich et al., 2000
A20	−/−	Viable	Inflammation, cachexia; hypersensitivity to TNF and LPS; failure to terminate NF-κB-mediated responses	Lee et al., 2000
Akt1	−/−	Viable	Smaller size; increased thymic apoptosis; embryonic fibroblasts are more sensitive to TNF and anti-Fas-mediated apoptosis	Chen et al., 2001

(Continued)

Table 30–1. Major Features of Knockout and of Some Other Mice in Relation to the Tumor Necrosis Factor Receptor (TNFR) Family and Signaling Pathways (*Continued*)

Protein	Type	Viability	Phenotype	References
MKK4	−/−	Die E13	Abnormal liver development, impaired JNK activation in response to TNF or IL-1; in radiation chimera, frequent B- and T-cell expansions	Nishina et al., 1997; Ganiatsas et al., 1998; Swat et al., 1998
JNK1	−/−	Viable	T-cell hyperproliferation; decreased AICD	Dong et al., 1998
JNK2	−/−	Viable	Impaired CD3-mediated death of thymocytes; normal anti-Fas death and AICD; impaired T-cell activation	Sabapathy et al., 1999
JNK3	−/−	Viable	Hippocampal neurons resistant to glutamate receptor agonist–induced apoptosis	Yang et al., 1997
JNK1 × JNK2	D$^{-/-}$	Die E11	Reduced apoptosis in hindbrain; excess apoptosis and caspase activation in forebrain	Kuan et al., 1999
JNK1 × JNK3	D$^{-/-}$	Viable	†	Kuan et al., 1999
JNK2 × JNK3	D$^{-/-}$	Viable	†	Kuan et al., 1999
c-Jun	−/−	Die E13	Hepatogenesis defect	Hilberg et al., 1993; Eferl et al., 1999
c-Fos	−/−	Die in weeks	Growth retardation, osteopetrosis, impaired tooth eruption	Wang et al., 1992
JIP	−/−	Die early	Embryonic death prior to blastocyst implantation, probably due to accelerated cell death during the first cell cycles	Thompson et al., 2001b
SHP2	−/−Δ46-110	Die E10	Impaired NF-κB but normal MAPK activation (JNK, ERK, p38) in response to TNF and IL-1 in embryonic fibroblasts	Saxton et al., 1997; You et al., 2001
c-Src	−/−	Die in weeks	Osteopetrosis, no tooth eruption (up to 6-month survival if mice are on a liquid diet); osteoclastogenesis occurs, but osteoclast function is impaired	Soriano et al., 1991; Amling et al., 2000
c-Src	Tg in −/−	Viable	Tg expression of wt c-Src in osteoclasts rescues c-Src$^{-/-}$ phenotype; partial rescue with kinase-dead c-Src	Schwartzberg et al., 1997
XIAP	−/−	Viable	No detectable defect; increased c-IAP1 and 2 expression	Harlin et al., 2001
Bcl-2	−/−	Viable	Growth retardation; lymphoid cell and melanocyte apoptosis, polycystic kidney; impaired life span of immature but not activated T and B cells (IL4 + CD40L rescue B cells)	Veis et al., 1993; Nakayama et al., 1995
Bcl-2 × Bax	D$^{-/-}$	Viable	Rescue of Bcl-2$^{-/-}$ lymphocyte deficit	Knudson and Korsmeyer, 1997
Bcl-X	−/−	Die E13	Neuronal and hematopoietic cell apoptosis; in radiation chimera, impaired T and B maturation; impaired life span of immature but not mature lymphocytes	Motoyama et al., 1995
Bcl-X × Bax	D$^{-/-}$	Die before birth	Partial rescue of Bax$^{-/-}$ neuronal cell death	Shindler et al., 1997
Bcl-X × caspase-9	D$^{-/-}$	Die before birth	Brain hyperplasia (Casp-9$^{-/-}$ dominant over Bax$^{-/-}$ phenotype)	Zaidi et al., 2001
Bax	−/−	Viable	Thymocyte and B-cell hyperplasia; deficient spermatogenesis; accelerated tumor growth with decreased p53-dependent apoptosis	Knudson et al., 1995; Yin et al., 1997
Bak	−/−	Viable	No gross defect; Bak$^{-/-}$ cells are resistant to granzyme B-mediated death	Lindsten et al., 2000; Wang et al., 2001
Bax × Bak	D$^{-/-}$	Perinatal death, 10% survive	In surviving adults, neuron and lymphocyte hyperplasia; imperforate vaginal canal, remnant interdigital webs; resistance to tBid-mediated apoptosis	Lindsten et al., 2000; Wei et al., 2001
Mcl-1	−/−	Die E4	Trophectoderm defect, no implant in uterus	Rinkenberger et al., 2000
Bcl-w	−/−	Viable	Male sterility; reduced germ and Sertoli cells in testis	Print et al., 1998
Bid	−/−	Viable	Resistant to anti-Fas-induced liver apoptosis; impaired Fas and TNF-mediated apoptosis	Yin et al., 1999
Bim	−/−	Viable	B and other cells hyperplasia; hyperglobulinemia; cells resistant to cytokine deprivation–induced apoptosis	Bouillet et al., 1999
Bim × Bcl-2	D$^{-/-}$	Viable	Rescue of Bcl-2$^{-/-}$ phenotype	Bouillet et al., 2001
DAXX	−/−	Die E10	Increased spontaneous apoptosis	Michaelson et al., 1999
AIF	−/−	Die early	Resistance to growth factor withdrawal; defective cell death in embryoid bodies	Joza et al., 2001
Acid sphingo-myelinase	−/−	Viable	Niemann-Pick disease; resistance to radiation-induced apoptosis, suppression of oocyte apoptosis; TNF-induced NF-κB unaffected	Otterbach and Stoffel, 1995; Santana et al., 1996; Zumbansen and Stoffel, 1997; Morita et al., 2000

*Def, deficient (natural mutants in which function of protein is impaired).
†Blank entries denote that phenotype has not been fully analyzed.

sembles that of EDAR, predicting a function in the epidermis (Kojima et al., 2000; Yan et al., 2000).

STRUCTURAL FEATURES AND PROCESSING OF TNF FAMILY LIGANDS

Ligands of the TNF family are type II transmembrane proteins (extracellular COOH terminus) characterized by a C-terminal domain that is coined THD (TNF homology domain) (Fig. 30–2A). Crystallographic studies show that the THDs of TNF (Eck and Sprang, 1989), LTα (Eck et al., 1992), CD40L (Karpusas et al., 1995), TRAIL (Hymowitz et al., 2000), RANKL (Ito et al., 2002; Lam et al., 2001), and BAFF (Karpusas et al., 2002) have a homotrimeric structure which, in the case of TRAIL, is stabilized by a structural zinc atom. The heterotrimeric LTα1β2 ligand is a notable exception to the homotrimer rule. In most ligands, the C-terminal THD domain is linked to the transmembrane region by a stalk of variable length, which is frequently the target of proteolytic cleavage in ligands that are entirely or partially released in a soluble form. Prote-

Table 30–2. Usual Synonyms for TNF and TNFR Family Proteins and for Intracellular Signaling Molecules

TNF AND TNFR FAMILIES	INTRACELLULAR SIGNALING MOLECULES
4-1BB/CD137	ABIN1/NAF1
APRIL/TRDL1	Akt/PKB
BAFF/BLyS/THANK/TALL-1/zTNF4	ASK1/MAP3K5
CD27L/CD70	Bim/Bod
CD40L/gp39/CD145	Caspase-8/FLICE
DcR3/TR6	c-IAP1/HIAP-2/MIHB
Fas/Apo-1/CD95	c-IAP2/HIAP-1/MIHC
FasL/CD95L	Diablo/Smac
GITR/AITR	EDARADD/Crinkled
GITRL/AITRL/TL6	ERK1/MAPK3
HVEM/ATAR/TR2	ERK2/MAPK1
LIGHT/HVEML	FADD/MORT1
LTα/TNFβ	FLIP/Casper/
LTβR/CD18	I-FLICE/FLAME/CASH/CLARP
NGFR/p75NTR	GCK/MAP4K2
OPG/OCIF	GCKR/MAP4K5
OX40/CD134	HIPK3/FIST3
OX40L/gp34	IKKα/IKK1
RANK/ODFR	IKKβ/IKK2
RANKL/TRANCE/ODF/OPGL	IKKε/IKKi
TNF/TNFα	IκBα/MAD3
TNFR1/p55/CD120a	JNK1/MAPK8
TNFR2/p75/CD120b	JNK2/MAPK9
TRAIL/Apo2L	JNK3/MAPK10
TRAILR1/DR4/Apo-2	MEK1/MAP2K1
TRAILR2/DR5/Killer	MEK2/MAP2K2
TRAILR3/DcR1/TRID	MEKK1/MAP3K1
TRAILR4/DcR2/TRUNDD	MEKK3/MAP3K3
TRAMP/DR3/Wsl/Apo-3	MKK3/MAP2K3
TROY/TAJ	MKK4/MAP2K4/SEK1/JNKK1
VEGI/TL1	MKK4/MAP2K4/SEK1/JNKK1
	MKK5/MAP2K5
	MKK6/MAP2K6
	MKK7/MAP2K7/JNKK2
	NEMO/IKKγ
	NF-kB1/p105 (p50)
	NF-kB2/p100 (p52)
	Omi/HtrA2
	P38/SAPK/MAPK14
	P60/p62/Zip/Osi
	RAIDD/CRADD
	RelA/p65
	RIP2/CARDIAK/RICK
	SHP1/PTP1C
	SHP2/PTP2C
	TAK1/MAP3K7
	TANK/I-TRAF
	TBK/T2K/NAK
	XIAP/MIAP3/MIHA

olytic cleavage is mediated either by metalloproteases—TNF (Black et al., 1997), RANKL (Schlondorff et al., 2001), and FasL (Tanaka et al., 1998)—or by members of the furin pro-protein convertase family of serine proteases: EDA (Chen et al., 2001b), BAFF (Schneider et al., 1999), APRIL (Lopez-Fraga et al., 2001), and TWEAK. The biological activity of ligands is affected by solubilization, but in very different ways. EDA and its receptor EDAR are expressed at distinct sites, and it is therefore not surprising that proteolytic processing of EDA is required for its biological activity (Headon and Overbeek, 1999). Consequently, both mutations that affect the furin cleavage site of EDA and mutations that delete its entire extracellular domain lead to indistinguishable phenotypes in human patients (Monreal et al., 1998). In contrast, processing of FasL to its soluble form decreases its pro-apoptotic activity, indicating that apoptosis is mediated by membrane-bound FasL (Schneider et al., 1998; Tanaka et al., 1998). Similarly, the biological activity of CD40L is associated with its membrane-bound form, which can be mimicked by aggregation of several soluble trimers. In the case of TNF, the soluble form acts systemically on TNFR1, but membrane-bound TNF is the prime activating ligand of TNFR2 (Grell et al., 1995).

STRUCTURAL FEATURES OF THE TNF RECEPTOR FAMILY

The signature of the TNFR family resides in the cysteine-rich extracellular moiety, and the molecular architecture of this domain has been reviewed recently (Naismith and Sprang, 1998; Bodmer et al., 2002). The intracellular signaling domains of TNFR family members are much more heterogenous, reflecting their ability to engage different signaling pathways (Fig. 30–1). Members of the TNF receptor family are generally type I transmembrane proteins, which contain a signal peptide and therefore exhibit their mature N terminus outside the cell. They are more rarely secreted proteins (DcR3, OPG) or type III transmembrane proteins (XEDAR, BAFFR, BCMA, and TACI, which are devoid of signal peptide and have their N terminus outside the cell). Soluble or signaling-incompetent receptors can also be generated by alternative splicing that removes the transmembrane domain or part of the intracellular domain (Cascino et al., 1995; Jenkins et al., 2000).

TNFRs, Extracellular Moiety

TNF receptors are characterized by the presence of two to eight elementary structural modules, each of which is stabilized by one or two disulfide bridges. The successive arrangement of modules confers receptors with their elongated shape, and the disulfide bridges are arranged like steps of a slightly twisted ladder (Fig. 30–2B). Although the modules are necessary and sufficient for ligand recognition and binding, structural examination of two ligand–receptor complexes reveals that only three out of five (TRAILR2) or eight (TNFR1) modules are directly involved in ligand binding (Fig. 30–2A). According to crystallographic studies, the receptor–ligand complex exists in a 3–3 stoichiometry, with each of the three monomeric receptors binding the interface formed by two ligand subunits of the trimeric ligand (Fig. 30–2A). However, there is some genetic evidence that receptors may not always be monomeric. The soluble, N-terminal portion of Fas appears to act as a dominant negative inhibitor of Fas signaling in a patient with ALPS, although this truncated form of Fas cannot bind to FasL. These data inspired a model in which the N-terminal domain of Fas (called PLAD, for pre-ligand association domain) mediates self-association of Fas to generate a signaling-competent receptor (Chan et al., 2000; Siegel et al., 2000). Ligand-independent association of TNFR1 is also suggested by the fact that TNFR1 can crystallize as head-to-tail or head-to-head dimers (Rodseth et al., 1994). In the head-to-head dimer, the ligand-binding site remains accessible. This may provide a structural hint of how PLAD-mediated receptor association occurs.

TNFRs, Intracellular Moiety

The death domain is an intracellular structure of about 80 amino acids found in eight TNF receptor family members. Death domains typically mediate homotypic interactions with other death domain–containing proteins (FADD, TRADD, RIP, EDARADD) (Fig. 30–2C). Despite their exclusive name, death domains not only signal cell death but also can activate NF-κB and MAPK, depending on the receptor. The majority of TNFRs also interact directly with the TRAF family of proteins, via short linear motifs of up to 18 amino acids (Fig. 30–2A). The identification of TRAF2- and TRAF3-binding sites in several receptors yielded the following consensus sequences: P/S/A/T-x-Q/E-E and P-x-Q-x-T/S, but the actual binding site extends beyond these motifs. The occurrence of these consensus sequences is indicated in Figure 30–1, but others may exist. Although TRAF2 and TRAF3 recognize identical consensus sequences, they bind overlapping but distinct sequences of CD40 (Ni et al., 2000). TRAF6 binds distinct sites that have been identified in CD40, RANK and XEDAR, yielding no clear consensus sequence (P-x-E) (Darnay et al., 1999; Yan et al., 2000). A 3 amino acid sequence at the extreme C terminus of Fas, NGFR, and possibly TRAILR4 corresponds to the specificity (S/T-x-V/L/I) of the third PDZ domain of FAP-1, a protein tyrosine phosphatase that appears to negatively regulate the apoptotic function of Fas (Fig. 30–2C). A potential substrate of FAP-1 is the Tyr42 of IκBα, but the significance of these interactions remains to be demonstrated (Yanagisawa et al., 1997; Nakai et al., 2000).

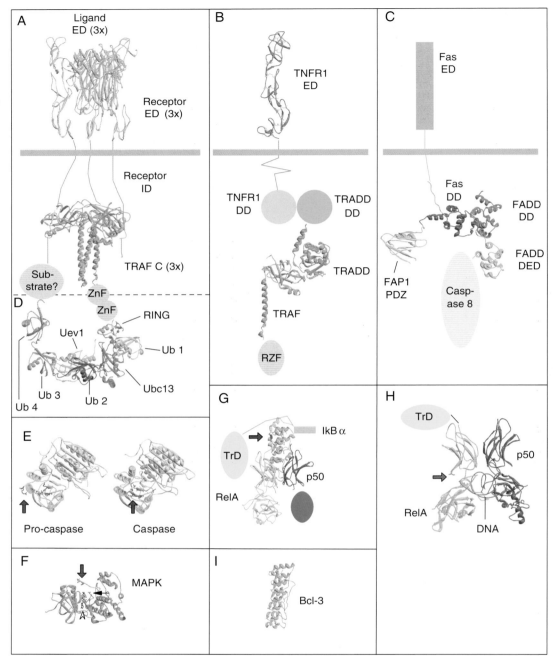

Figure 30–2. Structural features of proteins relevant to TNFR signaling. The structure of various proteins (or protein domains) relevant to TNFR signaling is depicted. Domains for which no structural data are available are schematized. (*A*) Receptor-ligand complex (TNFR1 and LTα) and TRAF-2 bound to CD40 peptides (pdb ID 1TNR and 1CZZ). (*B*) TNFR1, TRADD, and TRAF2 (pdb ID 1EXT and 1F3V). (*C*) Fas, FADD, and PDZ domain of FAP1 (pdb ID 1FAD, 1DDF, 1A1W, and 2PDZ). The death domains of Fas and FADD were positioned using 3YGS (CARD–CARD) as a template. As the structure of the PDZ domain of FAP1 has not been determined, the PDZ domain of syntrophin is shown instead. Different PDZ domains have virtually superimposable structures. The PDZ domain of syntrophin is complexed to a peptide whose C-terminal LSV sequence is identical to that of Fas. The DD and DED of FADD originate from two separate structures). (*D*) Model of the RING domain of TRAF6 complexed to Ubc13 and Uev1, with a nascent chain of K63-linked polyubiquitin. The interaction between the RING domain of TRAF6 and the ubiquitin-conjugating enzyme Ubc13 was modeled on the structure of c-Cbl complexed to UbcH7 (pdb ID 1FBV). The Ubc13–Uev1 interaction was inferred from the structure of Ubc13 complexed to the Uev1 homolog Mms2 (pdb ID 1J7D). Ubiquitins (pdb ID 1AAR) were positioned on the Ubc13–Uev1 complex according to a published model (Chan and Hill, 2001). (*E*) Structure of procaspase-7 and of active caspase-7 (pdb ID 1K88 and 1K86). Arg_{233}, which is part of the S1 specificity pocket that accommodates the P1 Asp residue of the substrate, is shown with an arrow. This residue undergoes a dramatic repositioning in the active caspase. (*F*) Structure of the MAPK JNK3 complexed to an ATP analogue (arrowhead) (Pdb ID 1JNK). The thick arrow points to the phosphorylation targets Tyr and Thr in the activation loop. The thin arrow indicates the active site Asp which is shown in red. (*G*) NF-κB complexed to its inhibitor IκBα (pdb ID 1NFI). The arrow points to the nuclear localization signal. TrD, transactivation domain of RelA. The N-terminal regulatory region of IκBα is shown as a pink box. (*H*) NF-κB complexed to DNA (pdb ID 1VKX). The arrow points to Ser_{276}, whose phosphorylation favors interaction with the transcriptional coactivators CBP and p300. (*I*) Structure of Bcl-3, an NF-κB-binding protein with transactivating activity (pdb ID 1K1A).

The protein tyrosine phosphatases SHP-1 and SHP-2 have recently been reported to bind to a phosphotyrosine site (Y-x-x-L) conserved in all death receptors (Daigle et al., 2002). While this "conserved" sequence is located on helix 4 of the death domain in most receptors and is predicted to be exposed to the surface, it is found on helix 5 in Fas, where the Tyr residue is deeply buried, most probably precluding phosphorylation (Huang et al., 1996). Several other proteins interact with TNFRs, but the significance of these interactions is currently unclear. CD27 binds SIVA, a death-promoting protein with a unique C-terminal motif of 12 cysteines, also found in a SIVA-like protein (Prasad et al., 1997). NADE and NRAGE interact with the death domain of NGFR to mediate proapoptotic functions, but NRAGE only does so if NGFR is not physically associated to TrkA (Mukai et al., 2000; Salehi et al., 2000). Curiously, the CARD-containing kinase RIP2 interacts with the DD of NGFR and can reconstitute NGF-dependent NF-κB activation in RIP2-deficient Schwann's cells, despite the fact that DD usually do not interact with CARD domains (Khursigara et al., 2001).

CELL DEATH PATHWAYS

Caspases are Asp-specific cysteine proteases that function in two main pathways: inflammation (caspase-1, 4, 5, and 11) and apoptosis (caspase-2, 3, 6, 7, 8, 9, and 10), the latter being relevant to TNFR signaling (Nicholson, 1999). Further distinction is made between effector caspases that are devoid of large prodomains, and which cannot undergo auto-catalytic activation, and apical caspases. The latter can be aggregated and auto-activated by their N-terminal prodomain, which contains either death effector (DED) or caspase recruitment (CARD) domains (Fig. 30–3). The active site of procaspases is folded in an inactive conformation but rearranges into a (much more) active form upon proteolytic cleavage between the p20 and p10 caspase subunits (Fig. 30–2) (Chai et al., 2001). Procaspase-8 and procaspase-10 are recruited to the death domains of Fas, TRAILR1, and TRAILR2 through a single intermediate adapter protein, FADD (Fig. 30–2C) Kischkel et al., 2001; Walczak and Sprick, 2001). Genetic evidence demonstrates that FADD and caspase-8 also mediate caspase-dependent cell death induced by TNFR1 (Zhang et al., 1998), although the biochemical connection between FADD and TNFR1 is not fully understood. TNFR1 interacts with TRADD (Fig. 30–2B), TRADD with FADD, and FADD with Caspase 8 and 10. However, unlike TRADD, endogenous FADD is not found associated with the signaling complex of TNFR1, suggesting that a secondary apoptotic complex may form (Kischkel et al., 2000). This hypothesis is consistent with the slower kinetics of caspase activation by TNFR1, compared with its activation of NF-κB or caspase activation by Fas.

Caspase-8 activation is potently inhibited by FLIP, a caspase-8-related but catalytically inactive protein that interacts with both FADD and caspase-8. Although FLIP is expressed at lower levels than is caspase-8, it is preferentially co-recruited to the receptor upon activation (Irmler et al., 1997; Thome and Tschopp, 2001). Thus, the ratio between the amount of death receptors engaged by the ligand on one hand and of FLIP on the other hand determines the outcome of caspase-8 activation (Kataoka et al., 2002). FLIP not only prevents caspase-8 activation but also triggers NF-κB and MAPK signaling. Because of these properties, FLIP can potentially divert a death signal into either a survival or a differentiation signal, or both (Kataoka et al., 2000). The idea that a complex containing FADD, caspase-8, and FLIP may lead to proliferation instead of cell death is consistent with the phenotypes of $FADD^{-/-}$, $caspase-8^{-/-}$, and $FLIP^{-/-}$ mice, all of which die from developmental heart defects. It also helps explain the phenotype of $FADD^{-/-}$ T cells, which display impaired proliferation.

In some cells activated caspase-8 can directly process and activate effector caspases, but in other cells insufficient amounts of caspase-8 are generated. In the latter case, an amplification loop involving the mitochondrial pro-apoptotic pathway is required (Fig. 30–4). The amplification loop probably helps to overcome the action that endogenous inhibitors of apoptosis (IAPs) exert on effector caspases. In addition, a proportion of active caspase-8 appears to be sequestered on the outer mitochondrial membrane in a way that prevents access to the substrate, possibly through interactions with the protein BAR (Stegh et al., 2001).

Bax and Bak are two potent activators of the mitochondrial apoptotic pathway. They are kept in check by anti-apoptotic members of the Bcl-2 family (Bcl-2, Bclw, BclX$_L$), which are themselves negatively regulated by BH3-only proteins such as Bid and Bim. Caspase-8 processes Bid to a truncated, pro-apoptotic form that can be myristoylated on the newly generated N terminus, perhaps contributing to its relocalization to the mitochondria (Zha et al., 2000). Interestingly, Bid is also the prime target of the serine protease granzyme B that is produced by cytotoxic T cells (Wang et al., 2001). Anti-Fas antibody-induced fulminant liver apoptosis is greatly diminished in $Bid^{-/-}$ mice, supporting the involvement of the amplification loop in mediating the Fas death signal in hepatocytes (Yin et al., 1999). The amplification loop is also required for TRAIL-mediated cell death, at least in certain cell types (Deng et al., 2002). Interestingly, phosphorylated Bid is a poor caspase-8 substrate, implicating kinases in the control of death receptor–mediated cell death (Desagher et al., 2001). Bid phosphorylation may occur in response to specific growth factors, which also up-regulate anti-apoptotic Bcl-2 family members (Kosai et al., 1998).

Truncated Bid leads to the inactivation of Bcl-2 family members, to the activation of Bax and Bak (Wei et al., 2001), and to the subsequent release of several periplasmic mitochondrial proteins into the cytoplasm, among which are cytochrome c, Diablo, Omi/HtrA2 (Verhagen et al., 2002), and AIF. Cytochrome c serves as a ligand that activates procaspase-9 in an Apaf-1-dependent manner, amplifying the action of apical caspases on effector caspases. Diablo and Omi compete for the binding of caspases to IAPs, liberating active caspase-3, 7, and 9 from their inhibitor. Interestingly, Omi has a serine protease domain whose activity is required to induce atypical, caspase-independent cell death (Suzuki et al., 2001). AIF induces a poorly characterized, caspase-independent death pathway, but genetic evidence indicates its relevant role, at least in early embryonic development. The importance of cytochrome c, Apaf-1, caspase-9, and caspase-3 in neuronal cell death is obvious from knockout mice studies, but their function appears to be redundant in most other cell types, as witnessed by the fairly normal phenotype of the few $Apaf-1^{-/-}$ that escape embryonic death (Honarpour et al., 2000).

In this respect, it is worth mentioning that work performed in C. elegans predicts the existence of a mammalian homolog of CED4 (mCDE4), distinct from Apaf-1, that would directly connect Bcl-2 family members to caspase activation in a cytochrome c–independent manner. In addition, caspase-independent pathways are likely to provide an important contribution to cell death. For example, Fas can engage a caspase-independent cell death pathway that relies on FADD and RIP. This latter pathway, however, seems to be restricted to T cells (Holler et al., 2000). Fas-induced apoptosis may require formation of macroscopic signaling structures that are characterized by modifications of Fas and capping (Algeciras-Schimnich et al., 2002). Ceramide generation may be required for this process, as this does not happen in acid sphingomyelinase–deficient cells (Cremesti et al., 2001). Other modifications—for example, with the ubiquitin homolog SUMO—are likely to be linked to death receptor signaling, but the molecular mechanism by which this may happen remains unclear. Fas also interacts with FAF1, another protein that is potentially involved in the regulation of ubiquitination (Ryu et al., 1999; Buchberger et al., 2001).

TRAF PROTEINS: ESSENTIAL COMPONENTS OF NONAPOPTOTIC SIGNALING BY TNFRs

The TRAF family of proteins plays a central role in the activation of MAPK pathways and NF-κB and AP-1 transcription factors in response to activation of TNFR, IL-1R, and Toll-R families (Inoue et al., 2000). The six mammalian TRAFs have a common structural organization with an N-terminal ring domain (containing two zinc atoms), two or three TRAF-type zinc fingers (each containing two zinc atoms), a coiled-coil region, and a C-terminal globular TRAF-C domain. TRAF-1 is a notable exception in that it contains neither a ring domain nor TRAF-type zinc fingers. Although zinc fingers are fre-

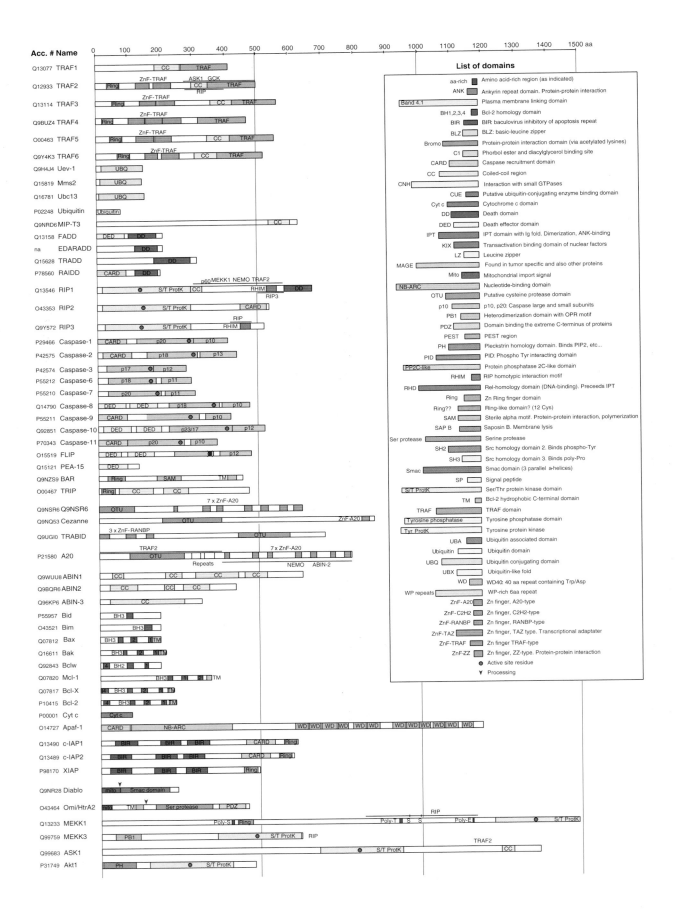

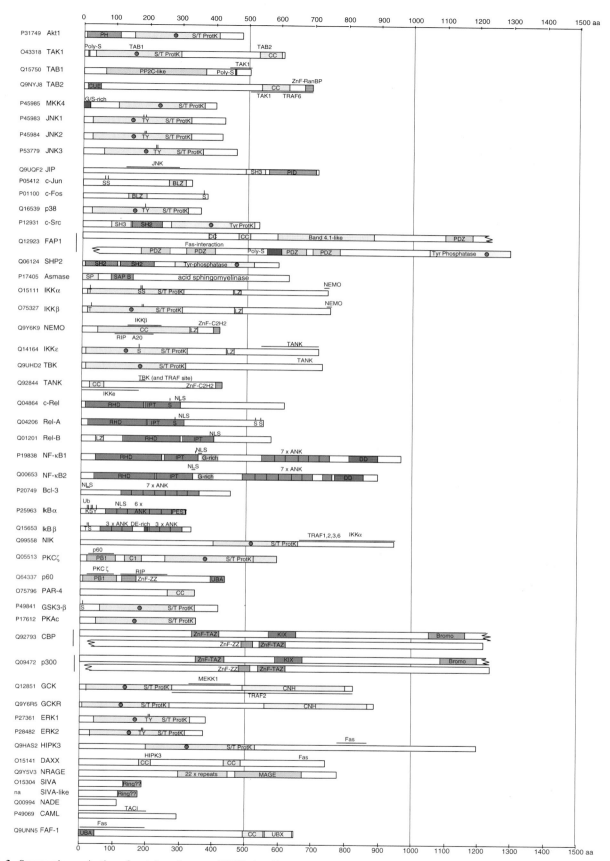

Figure 30–3. Structural organization of proteins relevant to TNFR signaling. This figure shows selected structural features of proteins that are involved in TNFR signaling or that are mentioned in the text. The proteins are drawn to scale, and protein accession numbers identify their sequences. In some instances, phosphorylation sites or interaction regions with defined partners are indicated, in a nonexhaustive fashion. A brief description of the different domains and of their function is given in the insert. Domains were drawn according to SMART, Swiss-Prot entries, and other sources.

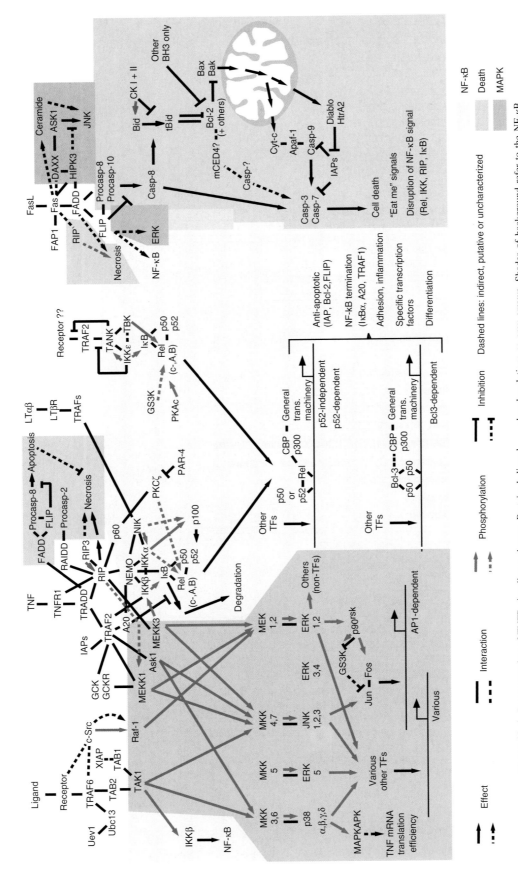

Figure 30–4. Representation of TNFR signaling pathways. Proteins believed to be involved in the signaling pathways of various TNFR are shown in this scheme. Reported protein–protein interactions are shown as black lines and phosphorylations as grey arrows. Shades of background refer to the NF-κB (pale), death (medium) and MAPK (dark) activation pathways. CKI + II: casein kinase I + II.

quently involved in the interaction of proteins with nucleic acids, this appears not to be the case for most, if not all, of the many zinc finger–containing proteins involved in TNFR signaling (Fig. 30–3). In this case, zinc fingers usually mediate protein–protein interactions. Zinc fingers that contain several zinc atoms can organize into compact, knotlike structures, such as that of the transcriptional adapter zinc (TAZ) finger domain in the transcriptional activator CBP. Interestingly, the TAZ-type zinc finger is one of the closest homologs of the TRAF-type zinc fingers, but no structural data are available (Laity et al., 2001). TRAFs form homo- and heterotrimeric structures via their coiled-coil and TRAF-C regions (Fig. 30–2A) and can be recruited to TNFRs, either directly or indirectly. A cleft in the TRAF-C domain accommodates linear TRAF-binding sequences of receptors such as TNFR2, CD40, CD30, OX40, 4-1BB, CD27, LTβR, RANK, XEDAR, and TROY (Ni et al., 2000; Ye and Wu, 2000). The affinity of this interaction is low, and recruitment of TRAFs to the receptors requires an avidity effect that is provided by ligand-induced oligomerization of receptors (Ye and Wu, 2000). TRAF2 is recruited to TNFR1 via the adapter molecule TRADD, the N-terminal domain of which makes extensive contacts with the TRAF-C domain of TRAF2 (Park et al., 2000) (Fig. 30–2B). In EDAR signaling, TRAFs are recruited by the adapter molecule EDARADD, which itself contains a linear TRAF-binding segment (Headon et al., 2001).

TRAF2 and TRAF5 are closely related and have partially redundant and overlapping functions. Together with TRAF6, they are implicated in the activation of NF-κB through IκB kinase (IKK) and of AP-1 through Jun kinases (JNKs) and extracellular regulated kinases (ERKs) (Fig. 30–4). Neither TRAF3 nor TRAF4 seems to readily activate these pathways (Arch et al., 1998). TRAF4 appears to play no or only a minor role in TNFR family signaling, whereas TRAF3 has been implicated in mediating cell death components of LTβR signaling (Force et al., 2000) but is apparently dispensable for signaling through CD40. The phenotype of TRAF3-deficient mice points to vital functions of TRAF3, but it is unclear how these are mediated. Interestingly, TRAF3 can be sequestered to microtubules by the protein MIP-T3 and then can be released upon CD40 engagement (Ling and Goeddel, 2000). Finally, TRAF1 is an NF-κB-inducible gene, which participates in the shutdown of NF-κB responses, possibly by "poisoning" signaling of other TRAFs by heteromer formation. TRIP, a direct TRAF interactor that inhibits the function of TRAF2, may have a similar mode of action (Lee and Choi, 1997).

Other TRAF interaction partners are discussed in the following sections.

RIP KINASES

The kinase RIP1, which is linked to TNFR1 either directly through DD–DD interactions or through the death domain (DD) of TRADD, is an essential component of the TNFR1-mediated NF-κB signaling pathway. RIP1 has several interaction partners and appears to function as a scaffolding protein rather than as a kinase in the NF-κB pathway, for which its kinase activity is dispensable. It is not uncommon that kinases fulfill functions independent of their kinase activity, as exemplified by the role of c-Src in osteoclast activation (Schwartzberg et al., 1997), IKKα in skin differentiation (Hu et al., 2001), or GCK in MEKK1 activation (Chadee et al., 2002). Kinase domains related to that of RIP are found in the proteins coined RIP2 (which contains a CARD domain) and RIP3 (which contains neither DD nor CARD). RIP3 and RIP associate through a short homotypic domain, and the phosphorylation of RIP by RIP3 decreases RIP's ability to signal NF-κB (Sun et al., 2002). RIP appears to be connected to caspase-2 by the adapter protein RAIDD, but the relevance of this interaction has not been clarified, even though caspase-2 and RAIDD-deficient mice are available.

MAP KINASE ACTIVATION PATHWAYS

The backbone of a typical MAPK activation pathway comprises three kinases: the MAP kinase itself (MAPK); an upstream MAPK kinase (MKK), which is physically associated to a given MAPK and highly specific for its cognate substrate; and an apical MKK kinase (MAP3K),

which may activate different MKKs (Widmann et al., 1999). There are five groups of MAPK. At least three are common targets of TNFR signaling—namely, the p38 MAPKs, the JNKs, and the ERK1/2 group. MAPKs typically induce proliferation, differentiation, adaptation to environmental stress, and apoptotic responses. In general, the protein kinases are activated by phosphorylation of an activation loop that covers the active site (Fig. 30–2F). This loop is displaced upon phosphorylation with concomitant repositioning of the active site in its active conformation. The activation loops of MAPKs are phosphorylated on Tyr and Thr residues by dual-specificity kinases (the MKKs) that require additional structural recognition elements in their substrates, and which are therefore highly specific. The activation loops of MKKs are phosphorylated on Ser/Thr residues by the less-specific MAP3Ks. Activation loops of inhibitor of NF-κB kinases (IKKs) resemble that of the MKKs and are also targets of MAP3Ks. The identification of physiologic activators of IKKs and MKKs is a delicate task, because overexpression of a MAP3K often leads to the activation of these pathways, even if they are not relevant to the function of the endogenous MAP3K. Channeling MAP3K activity into a specific MAPK pathway is performed by scaffolding proteins that assemble a MAPK, a MKK, and a MAP3K into a single complex (for example the scaffolding protein JIP interacts with JNK, MKK7, and the MAP3K MLK) (Thompson et al., 2001b).

Several MAP3Ks are involved in TNF signaling pathways. TRAF2 interacts with both the MAP3K MEKK1 and the germinal center kinase (GCK), an activator of MEKK1 (Yuasa et al., 1998). MEKK1 activation occurs by oligomerization and autophosphorylation, a process that requires oligomerization of TRAF2 (the RING domain is essential) and GCK (the kinase activity is not required) in reconstituted systems (Baud et al., 1999; Chadee et al., 2002). GCK-related kinase (GCKR) seems to play a role similar to GCK in this respect (Shi and Kehrl, 1997). In addition, RIP participates in MEKK1 activation through phosphorylation of two Ser residues outside of the kinase domain, as deduced from a study using RIP-deficient Jurkat T cells (Kim et al., 2001). TRAF-2 also interacts with the C terminus of the MAP3K Ask1 and mediates its activation in a RING domain–dependent manner (Nishitoh et al., 1998). These data are consistent with the abrogation of TNF-induced JNK responses in $TRAF2^{-/-}$ cells, and, taking into account that Ask1 or additional MAP3K contribute to JNK activation, they also fit with the partial and cell type dependent JNK defect in $MEKK1^{-/-}$ cells (Xia et al., 2000). The MAP3K MEKK3 interacts with RIP and mediates NF-κB signals through phosphorylation of IKK, in agreement with the observation that $MEKK3^{-/-}$ fibroblasts fail to activate NF-κB in response to TNF (Yang et al., 2001). Thus, MEKK3 might be one of the relevant physiological IKK activators that mediate the previously recognized essential function of RIP in NF-κB signaling (Kelliher et al., 1998).

Different TRAF molecules can engage different MAP3Ks. Thus, TRAF6 recruits and activates the MAP3K TAK1 through interaction with TAB2 (Takaesu et al., 2000). Although TAK1 requires the activator TAB1, whose C-terminal α helix is believed to displace an intrinsic inhibitory helix in the active site of TAK1 (Ono et al., 2001), its activation by TRAF6 also depends on K63-linked polyubiquitin, which is functionally very different from the classical K48-linked polyubiquitin that targets proteins to degradation. TRAF6 and its RING domain function as an E3 ligase in this reaction, which utilizes the E2 enzyme Ubc13 in complex with the ubiquitin-E2 variant Uev1 (Fig. 30–2D) (Wang et al., 2001). Although the target of K63-polyubiquitination is currently unknown, it is required for TAK1 activation, which, in turn, activates JNK and p38 pathways, as well as NF-κB activation through IKK phosphorylation (Wang et al., 2001).

Ubiquitin is first activated by a unique ubiquitin-activating enzyme (E1) and transferred to several ubiquitin-conjugating enzymes (E2s) harboring distinct functions. In turn, a particular E2 interacts with several ubiquitin-protein ligases (E3s) via the HECT or RING domain of the E3 protein. In addition to the E2-recruiting RING domain, E3 proteins provide specificity for the substrate by recognizing ubiquitination signals on the target protein. E3 can be either a single polypeptide or a protein complex in which the RING and the substrate recognition units are part of different proteins (Pickart, 2001). Although it has not yet been demonstrated, it appears likely that TRAF6 will mediate K63 polyubiquitination functions in CD40 and RANK signaling. Indeed, osteoclast formation from precursor cells lacking the RING of TRAF6 is impaired, although this TRAF6 mutant can signal NF-κB and, to a lesser extent, MAPK activation in TRAF6-deficient fibroblasts (Kobayashi et al., 2001). This also demonstrates that, in addition to the RING domain–dependent MAP3K TAK1, TRAF6 can signal NF-κB through other RING domain–independent MAP3K (Kobayashi et al., 2001). PP2Cb, a protein phosphatase, inactivates TAK1 by dephosphorylation. Interestingly, the protein phosphatase domain of TAB1 does not appear to be involved in this process (Hanada et al., 2001).

It will be of interest to determine whether the RING domain–containing TRAF2, 3, and 5 can also function as E3 enzymes. However, the RING domains of the different TRAFs are not equivalent, and exchanging the RING domain of TRAF2 for that of TRAF3 abolishes its ability to activate NF-κB (Takeuchi et al., 1996). In the context of ubiquitination, it is noteworthy that RIP interacts with p60, a protein that contains an UBA domain which has been shown to interact noncovalently with ubiquitin. p60 interacts with PKCζ (and other atypical PKCs) via homotypic interactions involving PB1 domains, and knockouts of *PKCζ* have defective NF-κB signaling in response to TNF and LTβR stimulation in tissues that normally express PKCζ. This defect leads to a phenotype similar to that observed in *TNFR1*$^{-/-}$ mice (Leitges et al., 2001). These results predict that Par-4, a natural inhibitor of PKCζ, should increase cellular sensitivity to TNF-induced apoptosis, which is indeed the case (Diaz-Meco et al., 1999).

In addition to mediating apoptotic responses, Fas also induces JNK activation by one or more of several proposed pathways:

1. Ceramide generation—but this hypothesis has been challenged (Verheij et al., 1996; Watts et al., 1997)
2. Caspase-dependent activation of MEKK1 by cleavage at Asp68 (Deak et al., 1998)
3. DAXX-dependent Ask1 activation (Yang et al., 1997b; Chang et al., 1998)

However, genetic evidence points to a prosurvival rather than a proapoptotic role for DAXX (Michaelson et al., 1999), and JNK induction by FasL apparently occurs independently of DAXX (Villunger et al., 2000). Whatever the mechanism of JNK activation by Fas, it is negatively regulated by the Fas- (and DAXX)-interacting kinase HIPK3 (Rochat-Steiner et al., 2000). *JNK1*$^{-/-}$ mice show T-cell hyperproliferation and decreased activation-induced cell death (AICD) (Dong et al., 1998). As AICD requires Fas and FasL, the phenotype is consistent with the effect of JNK being to induce FasL as one of its downstream target genes (Morishima et al., 2001). JNK1, 2, and 3 have partially overlapping functions. Double knockout of JNK1 and JNK2, but not of individual JNK or any other combination of two JNKs, is lethal and displays apoptosis deregulation in the brain.

Genetic analyses suggest important links between RANK, TRAF6, NF-κB1/2, the kinase c-Src, and the transcription factor Fos. Mice deficient in any of these proteins develop severe osteopetrosis (see Table 30–1), which has at least two different causes. Osteoclasts develop but fail to resorb bone in c-Src- and Fos-deficient mice, whereas they fail to form in RANK, NF-κB1/2, and TRAF6 knockouts. Interestingly, *TRAF6*$^{-/-}$ osteoclast precursors reconstituted with full-length TRAF6 give rise to functional osteoclasts, but this rescue is only partial with a TRAF6 mutant lacking the RING domain (Kobayashi et al., 2001). In the latter case, osteoclasts are formed but not activated, similar to the situation in *c-Src* and *Fos*$^{-/-}$. Thus, TRAF6 and RANK are likely to activate a kinase-independent function of c-Src that, in turn, is important for Fos activation, possibly through the MAP3K Raf-1, the ERK pathway and its downstream target p90rsk that phosphorylates Fos and GSK3-β (Fig. 30–4). Fos is activated by phosphorylation, whereas GSK3-β is inhibited and therefore releases its inhibitory action on Jun. Thus, the ERK1/2 pathway allows activation of Jun and Fos, two important subunits of the transcription factor AP-1 (Fig. 3–2J).

ACTIVATION OF NF-κB

There is a striking overlap between tissues that express members of the TNF family and tissues with active NF-κB-driven transcription (Carlsen et al., 2002). In addition, genetic impairment of NF-κB re-

produces, at least partially, the phenotype generated by the deficit of many TNFRs, including EDAR, LTβR, TNFR1, RANK, and CD40 (Schmidt-Ullrich et al., 2001) (Table 30–1). NF-κB is kept inactive in the cytoplasm through association with an inhibitor, IκB, of which there are several species with different tissue distributions. The different IκBs fullfill the same function and are interchangeable (Cheng et al., 1998). IκBs are inactivated through sequential events of phosphorylation, K48-polyubiquitination, and proteasomal degradation, thus, allowing the release of translocation- and DNA binding-competent NF-κB.

IκB is phosphorylated by the IκB kinase (IKK) complex, which contains two kinases, IKKα and IKKβ, and a third essential but non-kinase protein called NEMO. IKKβ is the physiologic kinase of IκB, whereas the kinase activity of IKKα acts at the level of regulation and activation of the NF-κB transcription factor itself. IKKα also plays important, kinase-independent functions in skin development. Finally, NEMO is essential for the function of the IKK complex, and genetic deficiencies of this X-linked gene cause incontinentia pigmenti in heterozygote females and are generally lethal in males (Smahi et al., 2000). However, a non-lethal, combined phenotype of ectodermal dysplasia and immunodeficiency is observed in males with apparently "milder" mutations of NEMO, thus pointing to the essential role of NF-κB downstream of several TNFRs such as EDAR and CD40 (Zonana et al., 2000; Jain et al., 2001). Recruitment of the IKK complex to activated TNFR1 depends on the presence of oligomerized TRAF2 which harbors an intact RING domain. The complex may be stabilized by RIP–NEMO interactions, although this does not seem to be essential. One of the crucial functions of NEMO is to recruit and position IκB, the substrate of IKKβ (Yamamoto et al., 2001).

There is a striking homology between components of the IKK complex on the one hand and IKKε, TBK, and TANK on the other hand (Fig. 30–3), both at the level of structural organization and mode of interaction and at the level of functional implication in NF-κB activation. IKKε is part of an inducible IκB kinase complex that can phosphorylate IκBα on both critical Ser residues (Peters et al., 2000). TANK has a consensus TRAF-binding sequence and competes with receptors for TRAF binding, but signals that trigger TANK aggregation are not known. Although the biochemical implication of the putative IKKε–TBK–TANK complex in TNFR signaling is unclear, its functional significance is highlighted by the phenotype of *TBK*$^{-/-}$ mice that die from excess liver apoptosis during embryogenesis, just as *IKKβ* and *RelA* knockouts do.

The IKK-mediated degradation of IκB is insufficient to promote efficient transcription of NF-κB-dependent genes. Indeed, NF-κB requires further modifications to recruit transcriptionnal coactivators such as CBP and p300, which connect NF-κB and other transcription factors to the general transcription machinery (Zhong et al., 1998) (Fig. 30–4). NF-κB activating events include either phosphorylation at different sites or recruitment of Bcl-3, a protein structurally related to the inhibitor IκB, but with transactivating activity (Michel et al., 2001) (Fig. 30–2I). Kinases with direct or indirect involvement in positive regulation of NF-κB include PKAc, GSK3-β, PKCζ, TBK, and IKKα, whose relevance has been supported in knockout animals (with the exception of PKAc). The transcription factor NF-κB is a heterodimer consisting of one Rel and one NF-κB protein, both of which contain a DNA-binding Rel homology domain and a dimerization domain (Fig. 30–2H). The three Rel proteins (c-Rel, RelA, and RelB) also contain a C-terminal transactivation domain. There are two NF-κB proteins, NF-κB1 and NF-κB2, with molecular masses of 105 and 100 kDa, respectively. After processing, their N-terminal portions give rise to the p50 and p52 subunits of NF-κB that lack a transactivation domain. Both p50 and p52 can also form homodimers that are believed to act as transcription inhibitors, unless they are complexed with Bcl-3. Transcriptional activity of a given NF-κB-dependent gene is regulated with very different stringencies by the composition of NF-κB itself, but also by the action of distinct transcription factors at their respective sites. For example, generation of sterile germline transcripts of the IgE heavy chain, a prerequisite for isotype switch to this isotype, depends on the conjugated action of CD40L (inducing NF-κB) and of IL-4 (inducing STAT6) (Messner et al., 1997).

The kinase NIK is an essential mediator of LTβR, but not TNFR1 signals, and also plays a role in peripheral B-cell maturation (Matsushima et al., 2001). Natural or targeted disruption of NIK abrogates LTβR-mediated NF-κB signals and results in alymphoplasia and B-cell lymphocytopenia. These phenotypes are also observed in mice that express a kinase dead version of IKKα, suggesting that activation of IKKα might be the prime target of NIK, and this is consistant with the reported interaction of NIK with phosphorylated IKKα (Luftig et al., 2001). Interestingly, IKKα is required for the processing of NF-κB2 to its p52 subunit in B cells, and therefore it controls the expression of p52-dependent genes (Senftleben et al., 2001). As B cells do not express LTβR, it is likely that NIK and IKKα might be under the control of BAFFR in these cells.

TERMINATION OF NF-κB SIGNALS

NF-κB controls expression of many genes involved in cellular activation—cell type–specific differentiation and inflammatory and anti-apoptotic responses—but also in the termination of the NF-κB signal. Induction of IκBα, TRAF1, and A20 serves the latter function. In particular, A20 interacts with TRAF2 and NEMO in the TNFR1 signaling complex to prevent IκB degradation, although the biochemical basis for this inhibition is not clear (Zhang et al., 2000). A20 binds several other partners with coiled-coil domain called ABIN. ABINs also interact with TRAFs and are believed to stimulate the inhibitory activity of A20 and possibly other A20-related molecules such as Cezanne, TRABID, and Q9NSR6 (Heyninck et al., 1999; Evans et al., 2001).

Another mechanism that regulates termination of the NF-κB response seems to involve proteasome-dependent degradation of TRAF2 (and TRAF3) and is inferred from the comparison of signaling ability of CD40 and LMP1. The Epstein-Barr virus protein LMP-1 is a membrane protein with six transmembrane domains and a C-terminal signaling portion. Although LMP-1 is structurally unrelated to the TNFR family, it is able to mimic most of the CD40 signaling events, including NF-κB activation. In this case, however, the NF-κB is not down-regulated, suggesting that CD40 (and CD30 and TNFR2) not only signals via TRAFs (like LMP-1 does) but also is able to induce termination of the response, possibly by initiating pathways that lead to ubiquitination and degradation of the TRAFs (Brown et al., 2001).

CROSS-TALK BETWEEN NF-κB AND CELL DEATH PATHWAYS

Proliferation and differentiation signals transmitted by TNFRs also negatively regulate cell death by up-regulating anti-apoptotic proteins such as FLIP, IAPs, and anti-apoptotic Bcl-2 family members, or by rendering the caspase substrate resistant to cleavage (Desagher et al., 2001; Micheau et al., 2001). Not surprisingly, activation of death programs leads to the shutdown of the NF-κB and other prosurvival pathways, most often by caspase-dependant cleavage of key regulators into inactive or dominant-negative molecules. Thus, proteolytic processing of RIP (Martinon et al., 2000), IKKβ (Tang et al., 2001), and IκBα (Levkau et al., 1999) all impair NF-κB signaling and promote cell death. In the case of IκBα, removal of a short N-terminal fragment containing the Lys residues that are targets of ubiquitination precludes IκBα degradation and NF-κB activation (Levkau et al., 1999). Caspases also cleave and inactivate the kinase Akt (Rokudai et al., 2000), which is an important mediator of anti-apoptotic signals downstream of growth factor receptors, and this is consistent with the observation that Akt$^{-/-}$ fibroblasts display higher susceptibility to TNF and FasL-induced cell death.

CONCLUDING REMARKS

Our understanding of the function of TNF and TNFR family members and of their mode of signaling has progressed considerably over the past 10 years. Many different investigation techniques have proved very useful and complementary in characterizing structural, mechanistic, and physiological aspects of TNF signaling. However, many potentially important issues remain to be explored in greater detail. These include the function of intracellular receptor pools, the identification of silencers, the role of ubiquitin and ubiquitin-like molecules, the extent of cross-talk between different receptors, the importance of lipid rafts in TNF signaling, and the characterization of the large signaling complexes induced by capping. Moreover, more work is required to investigate the physiological relevance of many protein–protein interactions that have been or will be detected in yeast two-hybrid or overexpression experiments.

Ligands and receptors of the TNF family are intimately involved in the biology of peripheral leucocytes and therefore have major effects on both the physiologic and the pathologic immune responses. A subset of TNF receptors controls developmental aspects within or outside of the immune system. The basic features of TNF receptor activation by TNF ligands are remarkably conserved. Despite this apparent homogeneity, TNF receptors can signal activation of cell death pathways or activation of survival and differentiation programs. These opposite outcomes appear to be carefully cross-regulated.

ACKNOWLEDGMENTS

I thank Jurg Tschopp, Fabio Martinon, Kim Burns, and Olivier Gaide for support and for their careful reading of the manuscript. I am grateful to Naohiro Inohara for the creation and maintenance of a most useful site on apoptosis regulators (http://www.personal.umich.edu/~ino/List/AList.html). This work was supported by grants from the Swiss National Foundation for Scientific Research.

REFERENCES

Adachi M, Suematsu S, Kondo T, Ogasawara J, Tanaka T, Yoshida N, Nagata S (1995). Targeted mutation in the *Fas* gene causes hyperplasia in peripheral lymphoid organs and liver. *Nat Genet* 11: 294–300.

Alcamo E, Mizgerd JP, Horwitz BH, Bronson R, Beg AA, Scott M, Doerschuk CM, Hynes RO, Baltimore D (2001). Targeted mutation of TNF receptor I rescues the RelA-deficient mouse and reveals a critical role for NF-κB in leukocyte recruitment. *J Immunol* 167: 1592–1600.

Algeciras-Schimnich A, Shen L, Barnhart BC, Murmann AE, Burkhardt JK, Peter ME (2002). Molecular ordering of the initial signaling events of CD95. *Mol Cell Biol* 22: 207–220.

Alimzhanov MB, Kuprash DV, Kosco-Vilbois MH, Luz A, Turetskaya RL, Tarakhovsky A, Rajewsky K, Nedospasov SA, Pfeffer K (1997). Abnormal development of secondary lymphoid tissues in lymphotoxin β-deficient mice. *Proc Natl Acad Sci USA* 94: 9302–9307.

Amakawa R, Hakem A, Kundig TM, Matsuyama T, Simard JJ, Timms E, Wakeham A, Mittruecker HW, Griesser H, Takimoto H, et al. (1996). Impaired negative selection of T cells in Hodgkin's disease antigen CD30-deficient mice. *Cell* 84: 551–562.

Amling M, Neff L, Pfiemel M, Schilling AF, Rueger JM, Baron R (2000). Progressive increase in bone mass and development of odontomas in aging osteopetrotic c-src-deficient mice. *Bone* 27: 603–610.

Arch RH, Gedrich RW, Thompson CB (1998). Tumor necrosis factor receptor-associated factors (TRAFs): a family of adapter proteins that regulates life and death. *Genes Dev* 12: 2821–2830.

Arens R, Tesselaar K, Baars PA, van Schijndel GM, Hendriks J, Pals ST, Krimpenfort P, Borst J, van Oers MH, van Lier RA (2001). Constitutive CD27/CD70 interaction induces expansion of effector-type T cells and results in IFNγ-mediated B cell depletion. *Immunity* 15: 801–812.

Banks RE, Rouse BT, Kerley MK, Blair PJ, Godfrey VL, Kulin NA, Bouley DM, Thomas J, Kanangat S, Mucenski ML (1995). Lymphotoxin-α-deficient mice: effects on secondary lymphoid organ development and humoral immune responsiveness. *J Immunol* 155: 1685–1693.

Baud V, Karin M (2001). Signal transduction by tumor necrosis factor and its relatives. *Trends Cell Biol* 11: 372–377.

Baud V, Liu ZG, Bennett B, Suzuki N, Xia Y, Karin M (1999). Signaling by proinflammatory cytokines: oligomerization of TRAF2 and TRAF6 is sufficient for JNK and IKK activation and target gene induction via an amino-terminal effector domain. *Genes Dev* 13: 1297–1308.

Beg AA, Baltimore D (1996). An essential role for NK-κB in preventing TNF-α-induced cell death. *Science* 274: 782–784.

Beg AA, Sha WC, Bronson RT, Baltimore D (1995a). Constitutive NF-κB activation, enhanced granulopoiesis, and neonatal lethality in IκB α-deficient mice. *Genes Dev* 9: 2736–2746.

Beg AA, Sha WC, Bronson RT, Ghosh S, Baltimore D (1995b). Embryonic lethality and liver degeneration in mice lacking the RelA component of NF-κB. *Nature* 376: 167–170.

Bergeron L, Perez GI, Macdonald G, Shi L, Sun Y, Jurisicova A, Varmuza S, Latham KE, Flaws JA, Salter JC, et al. (1998). Defects in regulation of apoptosis in caspase-2-deficient mice. *Genes Dev* 12: 1304–1314.

Black RA, Rauch CT, Kozlosky CJ, Peschon JJ, Slack JL, Wolfson MF, Castner BJ, Stocking KL, Reddy P, Srinivasan S, et al. (1997). A metalloproteinase disintegrin that release tumour-necrosis factor-α from cells. *Nature* 385: 729–733.

Bodmer JL, Schneider P, Tschopp J (2002). The molecular architecture of the TNF superfamily. *Trends Biochem Sci* 27: 19–26.

Bonnard M, Mirtsos C, Suzuki S, Graham K, Huang J, Ng M, Itie A, Wakeham A, Shahin-

ian A, Henzel WJ, et al. (2000). Deficiency of T2K leads to apoptotic liver degeneration and impaired NF-κB-dependent gene transcription. *EMBO J* 19: 4976–4985.
Botchkareva NV, Botchkarev VA, Chen LH, Lindner G, Paus R (1999). A role for p75 neurotrophin receptor in the control of hair follicle morphogenesis. *Dev Biol* 216: 135–153.
Bouillet P, Metcalf D, Huang DC, Tarlinton DM, Kay TW, Kontgen F, Adams JM, Strasser A (1999). Proapoptotic Bcl-2 relative Bim required for certain apoptotic responses, leukocyte homeostasis, and to preclude autoimmunity. *Science* 286: 1735–1738.
Bouillet P, Cory S, Zhang LC, Strasser A, Adams JM (2001). Degenerative disorders caused by Bcl-2 deficiency prevented by loss of its BH3-only antagonist Bim. *Dev Cell* 1: 645–653.
Brown KD, Hostager BS, Bishop GA (2001). Differential signaling and tumor necrosis factor receptor-associated factor (TRAF) degradation mediated by CD40 and the Epstein-Barr virus oncoprotein latent membrane protein 1 (LMP1). *J Exp Med* 193: 943–954.
Bucay N, Sarosi I, Dunstan CR, Morony S, Tarpley J, Capparelli C, Scully S, Tan HL, Xu W, Lacey DL, et al. (1998). Osteoprotegerin-deficient mice develop early onset osteoporosis and arterial calcification. *Genes Dev* 12: 1260–1268.
Buchberger A, Howard MJ, Proctor M, Bycroft M (2001). The UBX domain: a widespread ubiquitin-like module. *J Mol Biol* 307: 17–24.
Burkly L, Hession C, Ogata L, Reilly C, Marconi LA, Olson D, Tizard R, Cate R, Lo D (1995). Expression of relB is required for the development of thymic medulla and dendritic cells. *Nature* 373: 531–536.
Caamano JH, Rizzo CA, Durham SK, Barton DS, Raventos-Suarez C, Snapper CM, Bravo R (1998). Nuclear factor (NF)-κ B2 (p100/p52) is required for normal splenic microarchitecture and B cell–mediated immune responses. *J Exp Med* 187: 185–196.
Carlsen H, Moskaug JO, Fromm SH, Blomhoff R (2002). In vivo imaging of NF-κB activity. *J Immunol* 168: 1441–1446.
Cascino I, Fiucci G, Papoff G, Ruberti G (1995). Three functional soluble forms of the human apoptosis-inducing Fas molecule are produced by alternative splicing. *J Immunol* 154: 2706–2713.
Cecconi F, Alvarez-Bolado G, Meyer BI, Roth KA, Gruss P (1998). Apaf1 (CED-4 homolog) regulates programmed cell death in mammalian development. *Cell* 94: 727–737.
Chadee DN, Yuasa T, Kyriakis JM (2002). Direct activation of mitogen-activated protein kinase kinase kinase MEKK1 by the Ste20p homologue GCK and the adapter protein TRAF2. *Mol Cell Biol* 22: 737–749.
Chai J, Wu Q, Shiozaki E, Srinivasula SM, Alnemri ES, Shi Y (2001). Crystal structure of a procaspase-7 zymogen: mechanisms of activation and substrate binding. *Cell* 107: 399–407.
Chan FK, Chun HJ, Zheng L, Siegel RM, Bui KL, Lenardo MJ (2000). A domain in TNF receptors that mediates ligand-independent receptor assembly and signaling. *Science* 288: 2351–2354.
Chan NL, Hill CP (2001). Defining polyubiquitin chain topology. *Nat Struct Biol* 8: 650–652.
Chang HY, Nishitoh H, Yang X, Ichijo H, Baltimore D (1998). Activation of apoptosis signal-regulating kinase 1 (ASK1) by the adapter protein Daxx. *Science* 281: 1860–1863.
Chen AI, McAdam AJ, Buhlmann JE, Scott S, Lupher ML Jr, Greenfield EA, Baum PR, Fanslow WC, Calderhead DM, Freeman GJ, Sharpe AH (1999). Ox40-ligand has a critical costimulatory role in dendritic cell : T cell interactions. *Immunity* 11: 689–698.
Chen WS, Xu PZ, Gottlob K, Chen ML, Sokol K, Shiyanova T, Roninson I, Weng W, Suzuki R, Tobe K, et al. (2001a). Growth retardation and increased apoptosis in mice with homozygous disruption of the *Akt1* gene. *Genes Dev* 15: 2203–2208.
Chen Y, Molloy SS, Thomas L, Gambee J, Bachinger HP, Ferguson B, Zonana J, Thomas G, Morris NP (2001b). Mutations within a furin consensus sequence block proteolytic release of ectodysplasin-A and cause X-linked hypohidrotic ectodermal dysplasia. *Proc Natl Acad Sci USA* 98: 7218–7223.
Cheng JD, Ryseck RP, Attar RM, Dambach D, Bravo R (1998). Functional redundancy of the nuclear factor κB inhibitors IκBα and IκBβ. *J Exp Med* 188: 1055–1062.
Cremesti A, Paris F, Grassme H, Holler N, Tschopp J, Fuks Z, Gulbins E, Kolesnick R (2001). Ceramide enables fas to cap and kill. *J Biol Chem* 276: 23954–23961.
Daigle I, Yousefi S, Colonna M, Green DR, Simon HU (2002). Death receptors bind SHP-1 and block cytokine-induced anti-apoptotic signaling in neutrophils. *Nat Med* 8: 61–67.
Darnay BG, Ni J, Moore PA, Aggarwal BB (1999). Activation of NF-κB by RANK requires tumor necrosis factor receptor-associated factor (TRAF) 6 and NF-κB-inducing kinase: identification of a novel TRAF6 interaction motif. *J Biol Chem* 274: 7724–7731.
Deak JC, Cross JV, Lewis M, Qian Y, Parrott LA, Distelhorst CW, Templeton DJ (1998). Fas-induced proteolytic activation and intracellular redistribution of the stress-signaling kinase MEKK1. *Proc Natl Acad Sci USA* 95: 5595–5600.
DeBenedette MA, Wen T, Bachmann MF, Ohashi PS, Barber BH, Stocking KL, Peschon JJ, Watts TH (1999). Analysis of 4-1BB ligand (4-1BBL)-deficient mice and of mice lacking both 4-1BBL and CD28 reveals a role for 4-1BBL in skin allograft rejection and in the cytotoxic T cell response to influenza virus. *J Immunol* 163: 4833–4841.
Deng Y, Lin Y, Wu X (2002). TRAIL-induced apoptosis requires Bax-dependent mitochondrial release of Smac/DIABLO. *Genes Dev* 16: 33–45.
Desagher S, Osen-Sand A, Montessuit S, Magnenat E, Vilbois F, Hochmann A, Journot L, Antonsson B, Martinou JC (2001). Phosphorylation of bid by casein kinases I and II regulates its cleavage by caspase 8. *Mol Cell* 8: 601–611.
De Togni P, Goellner J, Ruddle NH, Streeter PR, Fick A, Mariathasan S, Smith SC, Carlson R, Shornick LP, Strauss-Schoenberger J, et al. (1994). Abnormal development of peripheral lymphoid organs in mice deficient in lymphotoxin. *Science* 264: 703–707.
Diaz-Meco MT, Lallena MJ, Monjas A, Frutos S, Moscat J (1999). Inactivation of the inhibitory κB protein kinase/nuclear factor κB pathway by Par-4 expression potentiates tumor necrosis factor α-induced apoptosis. *J Biol Chem* 274: 19606–19612.
Doffinger R, Smahi A, Bessia C, Geissmann F, Feinberg J, Durandy A, Bodemer C, Kenwrick S, Dupuis-Girod S, Blanche S, et al. (2001). X-linked anhidrotic ectodermal dysplasia with immunodeficiency is caused by impaired NF-κB signaling. *Nat Genet* 27: 277–285.
Dong C, Yang DD, Wysk M, Whitmarsh AJ, Davis RJ, Flavell RA (1998). Defective T cell differentiation in the absence of Jnk1. *Science* 282: 2092–2095.
Dougall WC, Glauccum M, Charrier K, Rohrbach K, Brasel K, De Smedt T, Daro E, Smith J, Tometsko ME, Maliszewski CR, et al. (1999). RANK is essential for osteoclast and lymph node development. *Genes Dev* 13: 2412–2424.
Eck MJ, Sprang SR (1989). The structure of tumor necrosis factor-α at 2.6 Å resolution: implications for receptor binding. *J Biol Chem* 264: 17595–17605.
Eck MJ, Ultsch M, Rinderknecht E, de Vos AM, Sprang SR (1992). The structure of human lymphotoxin (tumor necrosis factor-β) at 1.9-A resolution. *J Biol Chem* 267: 2119–2122.
Eferl R, Sibilia M, Hilberg F, Fuchsbichler A, Kufferath I, Guertl B, Zenz R, Wagner EF, Zatloukal K (1999). Function of c-Jun in liver and heart development. *J Cell Biol* 145: 1049–1061.
Erickson SL, de Sauvage FJ, Kikly K, Carver-Moore K, Pitts-Meek S, Gillett N, Sheehan KC, Schreiber RD, Goeddel DV, Moore MW (1994). Decreased sensitivity to tumour-necrosis factor but normal T-cell development in TNF receptor-2-deficient mice. *Nature* 372: 560–563.
Evans PC, Taylor ER, Coadwell J, Heyninck K, Beyaert R, Kilshaw PJ (2001). Isolation and characterization of two novel A20-like proteins. *Biochem J* 357: 617–623.
Fata JE, Kong YY, Li J, Sasaki T, Irie-Sasaki J, Moorehead RA, Elliott R, Scully S, Voura EB, Lacey DL, et al. (2000). The osteoclast differentiation factor osteoprotegerin-ligand is essential for mammary gland development. *Cell* 103: 41–50.
Feldmann M (2001). Pathogenesis of arthritis: recent research progress. *Nat Immunol* 2: 771–773.
Ferguson BM, Brockdorff N, Formstone E, Ngyuen T, Kronmiller JE, Zonana J (1997). Cloning of Tabby, the murine homolog of the human EDA gene: evidence for a membrane-associated protein with a short collagenous domain. *Hum Mol Genet* 6: 1589–1594.
Fisher GH, Rosenberg FJ, Straus SE, Dale JK, Middleton LA, Lin AY, Strober W, Lenardo MJ, Puck JM (1995). Dominant interfering *Fas* gene mutations impair apoptosis in a human autoimmune lymphoproliferative syndrome. *Cell* 81: 935–946.
Force WR, Glass AA, Benedict CA, Cheung TC, Lama J, Ware CF (2000). Discrete signaling regions in the lymphotoxin-β receptor for tumor necrosis factor receptor-associated factor binding, subcellular localization, and activation of cell death and NF-κB pathways. *J Biol Chem* 275: 11121–11129.
Franzoso G, Carlson L, Scharton-Kersten T, Shores EW, Epstein S, Grinberg A, Tran T, Shacter E, Leonardi A, Anver M, et al. (1997a). Critical roles for the Bcl-3 oncoprotein in T cell–mediated immunity, splenic microarchitecture, and germinal center reactions. *Immunity* 6: 479–490.
Franzoso G, Carlson L, Xing L, Poljak L, Shores EW, Brown KD, Leonardi A, Tran T, Boyce BF, Siebenlist U (1997b). Requirement for NF-κB in osteoclast and B-cell development. *Genes Dev* 11: 3482–3496.
Franzoso G, Carlson L, Poljak L, Shores EW, Epstein S, Leoanrdi A, Grinberg A, Tran T, Scharton-Kersten T, Anver M, et al. (1998). Mice deficient in nuclear factor (NF)-κB/p52 present with defects in humoral responses, germinal center reactions, and splenic microarchitecture. *J Exp Med* 187: 147–159.
Fu YX, Chaplin DD (1999). Development and maturation of secondary lymphoid tissues. *Annu Rev Immunol* 17: 399–433.
Futterer A, Mink K, Luz A, Kosco-Vilbois MH, Pfeffer K (1998). The lymphotoxin β receptor controls organogenesis and affinity maturation in peripheral lymphoid tissues. *Immunity* 9: 59–70.
Galon J, Aksentijevich I, McDermott MF, O'Shea JJ, Kastner DL (2000). TNFRSF1A mutations and autoinflammatory syndromes. *Curr Opin Immunol* 12: 479–486.
Ganiatsas S, Kwee L, Fujiwara Y, Perkins A, Ikeda T, Labow MA, Zon LI (1998). SEK1 deficiency reveals mitogen-activated protein kinase cascade crossregulation and leads to abnormal hepatogenesis. *Proc Natl Acad Sci USA* 95: 6881–6886.
Gerondakis S, Strasser A, Metcalf D, Grigoriadis G, Scheerlinck JY, Grumont RJ (1996). Rel-deficient T cells exhibit defects in production of interleukin 3 and granulocyte-macrophage colony-stimulating factor. *Proc Natl Acad Sci USA* 93: 3405–3409.
Grell M, Douni E, Wajant H, Lohden M, Clauss M, Maxeiner B, Georgooulos S, Lesslauer W, Kollias G, Pfizenmaier K, et al. (1995). The transmembrane form of tumor necrosis factor is the prime activating ligand of the 80 kDa tumor necrosis factor receptor. *Cell* 83: 793–802.
Grewal IS, Flavell RA (1998). CD40 and CD154 in cell-mediated immunity. *Annu Rev Immunol* 16: 111–135.
Griffith TS, Lynch DH (1998). TRAIL: a molecule with multiple receptors and control mechanisms. *Curr Opin Immunol* 10: 559–563.
Grigoriadis G, Zhan Y, Grumont RJ, Metcalf D, Handman E, Cheers C, Gerondakis S (1996). The Rel subunit of NA-κB-like transcription factors is a positive and negative regulator of macrophage gene expression: distinct roles for Rel in different macrophage populations. *EMBO J* 15: 7099–7107.
Gross JA, Dillon SR, Mudri S, Johnston J, Littau A, Roque R, Rixon M,Schou O, Foley KP, Haugen H, et al. (2001). TACI-Ig neutralizes molecules critical for B cell development and autoimmune disease: impaired B cell maturation in mice lacking BLyS. *Immunity* 15: 289–302.
Grossman M,O'Reilly LA, Gugasyan R, Strasser A, Adams JM, Gerondakis S (2000). The anti-apoptotic activities of Rel and RelA required during B-cell maturation involve the regulation of Bcl-2 expression. *EMBO J* 19: 6351–6360.
Grumont RJ, Rourke IJ, O'Reilly LA, Strasser A, Miyake K, Sha W, Gerondakis S (1998). B lymphocytes differentially use the Rel and nuclear factor κB1 (NF-κB1) transcription factors to regulate cell cycle progression and apoptosis in quiescent and mitogen-activated cells. *J Exp Med* 187: 663–674.
Hanada M, Ninomiya-Tsuji J, Komaki K, Ohnishi M, Katsura K, Kanamaru R, Matsumoto K, Tamura S (2001). Regulation of the TAK1 signaling pathway by protein phosphatase 2C. *J Biol Chem* 276: 5753–5759.
Harlin H, Reffey SB, Duckett CS, Lindsten T, Thompson CB (2001). Characterization of XIAP-deficient mice. *Mol Cell Biol* 21: 3604–3608.
Haswell LE, Glennie MJ, Al-Shamkhani A (2001). Analysis of the oligomeric requirement for signaling by CD40 using soluble multimeric forms of its ligand, CD154. *Eur J Immunol* 31: 3094–3100.

Headon DJ, Overbeek PA (1999). Involvement of a novel Tnf receptor homologue in hair follicle induction. *Nat Genet* 22: 370–374.
Headon DJ, Emmal SA, Ferguson BM, Tucker AS, Justice MJ, Sharpe PT, Zonana J, Overbeek PA (2001). Gene defect in ectodermal dysplasia implicates a death domain adapter in development. *Nature* 414: 913–916.
Hendriks J, Gravestein LA, Tesselaar K, van Lier RA, Schumacher TN, Borst J (2000). CD27 is required for generation and long-term maintenance of T cell immunity. *Nat Immunol* 1: 433–440.
Heyninck K, De Valck D, Vanden Berghe W, Van Criekinge W, Contreras R, Fiers W, Haegeman G, Beyaert R (1999). The zinc finger protein A20 inhibits TNF-induced NF-κB-dependent gene expression by interfering with an RIP- or TRAF2-mediated transactivation signal and directly binds to a novel NF-κB-inhibiting protein ABIN. *J Cell Biol* 145: 1471–1482.
Hilberg F, Aguzzi A, Howells N, Wagner EF (1993). c-jun is essential for normal mouse development and hepatogenesis. *Nature* 365: 179–181.
Hoeflich KP, Luo J, Rubie EA, Tsao MS, Jin O, Woodgett JR (2000). Requirement for glycogen synthase kinase-3β in cell survival and NF-κB activation. *Nature* 406: 86–90.
Holler N, Zaru R, Micheau O, Thome M, Attinger A, Valitutti S, Bodmer JL, Schneider P, Seed B, Tschopp J (2000). Fas triggers an alternative, caspase-8-independent cell death pathway using the kinase RIP as effector molecule. *Nat Immunol* 1: 489–495.
Honarpour N, Du C, Richardson JA, Hammer RE, Wang X, Herz J (2000). Adult Apaf-1-deficient mice exhibit male infertility. *Dev Biol* 218: 248–258.
Horvat S, Medrano JF (1998). A 500-kb YAC and BAC contig encompassing the high-growth deletion in mouse chromosome 10 and identification of the murine Raidd/Cradd gene in the candidate region. *Genomics* 54: 159–164.
Horwitz BH, Scott ML, Cherry SR, Bronson RT, Baltimore D (1997). Failure of lymphopoiesis after adoptive transfer of NF-κB-deficient fetal liver cells. *Immunity* 6: 765–772.
Hu Y, Baud V, Delhase M, Zhang P, Deerinck T, Ellisman M, Johnson R, Karin M (1999). Abnormal morphogenesis but intact IKK activation in mice lacking the IKKα subunit of IκB kinase. *Science* 284: 316–320.
Hu Y, Baud V, Oga T, Kim KI, Yoshida K, Karin M (2001). IKKα controls formation of the epidermis independently of NF-κB. *Nature* 410: 710–714.
Huang B, Eberstadt M, Olejniczak ET, Meadows RP, Fesik SW (1996). NMR structure and mutagenesis of the Fas (APO-1/CD95) death domain. *Nature* 384: 638–641.
Hughes AE, Ralston SH, Marken J, Bell C, MacPherson H, Wallace RG, van Hul W, Whyte MP, Nakatsuka K, Hovy L, Anderson DM (2000). Mutations in TNFRSF11A, affecting the signal peptide of RANK, cause familial expansile osteolysis. *Nat Genet* 24: 45–48.
Hymowitz SG, O'Connell MP, Ultsch MH, Hurst A, Totpal K, Ashkenazi A, de Vos AM, Kelley RF (2000). A unique zinc-binding site revealed by a high-resolution X-ray structure of homotrimeric Apo2L/TRAIL. *Biochemistry* 39: 633–640.
Inoue J, Ishida T, Tsukamoto N, Kobayashi N, Naito A, Azuma S, Yamamoto T (2000). Tumor necrosis factor receptor-associated factor (TRAF) family: adapter proteins that mediate cytokine signaling. *Exp Cell Res* 254: 14–24.
Irmler M, Thome M, Hahne M, Schneider P, Hofmann K, Steiner V, Bodmer JL, Schroter M, Burns K, Mattmann C, et al. (1997). Inhibition of death receptor signals by cellular FLIP. *Nature* 388: 190–195.
Ito S, Wakabayashi K, Ubukata O, Hayashi S, Okada F, Hata T (2002). Crystal structure of the extracellular domain of mouse RANK ligand at 2.2 Å resolution. *J Biol Chem* 277: 6631–6636.
Jain A, Ma CA, Liu S, Brown M, Cohen J, Strober W (2001). Specific missense mutations in NEMO result in hyper-IgM syndrome with hypohydrotic ectodermal dysplasia. *Nat Immunol* 2: 223–228.
Jenkins M, Keir M, McCune JM (2000). A membrane-bound Fas decoy receptor expressed by human thymocytes. *J Biol Chem* 275: 7988–7993.
Joza N, Susin SA, Daugas E, Stanford WL, Cho SK, Li CY, Sasaki T, Elia AJ, Cheng HY, Ravagnan L, et al. (2001). Essential role of the mitochondrial apoptosis-inducing factor in programmed cell death. *Nature* 410: 549–554.
Karin M, Ben-Neriah Y (2000). Phosphorylation meets ubiquitination: the control of NF-κB activity. *Annu Rev Immunol* 18: 621–663.
Karpusas M, Hsu YM, Wang JH, Thompson J, Lederman S, Chess L, Thomas D (1995). 2 A crystal structure of an extracellular fragment of human CD40 ligand. *Structure* 3: 1426.
Karpusas M, Cachero TG, Qian F, Boriack-Sjodin A, Mullen C, Strauch K, Hsu YM, Kalled SL (2002). Crystal structure of extracellular human BAFF, a TNF family member that simulates B lymphocytes. *J Mol Biol* 315: 1145–1154.
Kataoka T, Budd RC, Holler N, Thome M, Martinon F, Irmler M, Burns K, Hahne M, Kennedy N, Kovacsovics M, Tschopp J (2000). The caspase-8 inhibitor FLIP promotes activation of NF-κB and Erk signaling pathways. *Curr Biol* 10: 640–648.
Kataoka T, Ito M, Budd RC, Tschopp J, Nagai K (2002). Expression level of c-FLIP versus Fas determines susceptibility to FasL-induced cell death in murine thymoma EL-4 cells. *Exp Cell Res* 273: 256–264.
Kawabe T, Naka T, Yoshida K, Tanaka T, Fujiwara H, Suematsu S, Yoshida N, Kishimoto T, Kikutani H (1994). The immune responses in CD40-deficient mice: impaired immunoglobulin class switching and germinal center formation. *Immunity* 1: 167–178.
Kelliher MA, Grimm S, Ishida Y, Kuo F, Stanger BZ, Leder P (1998). The death domain kinase RIP mediates the TNF-induced NF-κB signal. *Immunity* 8: 297–303.
Khursigara G, Bertin J, Yano H, Moffett H, DiStefano PS, Chao MV (2001). A prosurvival function for the p75 receptor death domain mediated via the caspase recruitment domain receptor-interacting protein 2. *J Neurosci* 21: 5854–5863.
Kim D, Mebius RE, MacMicking JD, Jung S, Cupedo T, Castellanos Y, Rho J, Wong BR, Josien R, Kim N, et al. (2000). Regulation of peripheral lymph node genesis by the tumor necrosis factor family member TRANCE. *J Exp Med* 192: 1467–1478.
Kim JW, Joe CO, Choi EJ (2001). Role of receptor-interacting protein in tumor necrosis factor-α-dependent MEKK1 activation. *J Biol Chem* 276: 27064–27070.
Kischkel FC, Lawrence DA, Chuntharapai A, Schow P, Kim KJ, Ashkenazi A (2000). Apo2L/TRAIL-dependent recruitment of endogenous FADD and caspase-8 to death receptors 4 and 5. *Immunity* 12: 611–620.
Kischkel FC, Lawrence DA, Tinel A, LeBlanc H, Virmani A, Schow P, Gazdar A, Blenis J, Arnott D, Ashkenazi A (2001). Death receptor recruitment of endogenous caspase-10 and apoptosis initiation in the absence of caspase-8. *J Biol Chem* 276: 46639–46646.
Kitsberg D, Formstecher E, Fauquet M, Kubes M, Cordier J, Canton B, Pan G, Rolli M, Glowinski J, Chneiweiss H (1999). Knock-out of the natural death effector domain protein PEA-15 demonstrates that its expression protects astrocytes from TNFα-induced apoptosis. *J Neurosci* 19: 8244–8251.
Klement JF, Rice NR, Car BD, Abbondanzo SJ, Powers GD, Bhatt PH, Chen CH, Rosen CA, Stewart CL (1996). IκBα deficiency results in a sustained NF-κB response and severe widespread dermatitis in mice. *Mol Cell Biol* 16: 2341–2349.
Knudson CM, Korsmeyer SJ (1997). Bcl-2 and Bax function independently to regulate cell death. *Nat Genet* 16: 358–363.
Knudson CM, Tung KS, Tourtellotte WG, Brown GA, Korsmeyer SJ (1995). Bax-deficient mice with lymphoid hyperplasia and male germ cell death. *Science* 270: 96–99.
Kobayashi N, Kadono Y, Naito A, Matsumoto K, Yamamoto T, Tanaka S, Inoue J (2001). Segregation of TRAF6-mediated signaling pathways clarifies its role in osteoclastogenesis. *EMBO J* 20: 1271–1280.
Kojima T, Morikawa Y, Copeland NG, Gilbert DJ, Jenkins NA, Senba E, Kitamura T (2000). TROY, a newly identified member of the tumor necrosis factor receptor superfamily, exhibits a homology with Edar and is expressed in embryonic skin and hair follicles. *J Biol Chem* 275: 20742–20747.
Kong YY, Feige U, Sarosi I, Bolon B, Tafuri A, Morony S, Capparelli C, Li J, Elliott R, McCabe S, et al. (1999a). Activated T cells regulate bone loss and joint destruction in adjuvant arthritis through osteoprotegerin ligand. *Nature* 402: 304–309.
Kong YY, Yoshida H, Sarosi I, Tan HL, Timms E, Capparelli C, Morony S, Oliveira-dos-Santos AJ, Van G, Itie A, Khoo W, et al. (1999b). OPGL is a key regulator of osteoclastogenesis, lymphocyte development and lymph-node organogenesis. *Nature* 397: 315–323.
Koni PA, Sacca R, Lawton P, Browning JL, Ruddle NH, Flavell RA (1997). Distinct roles in lymphoid organogenesis for lymphotoxins α and β revealed in lymphotoxin β-deficient mice. *Immunity* 6: 491–500.
Kontgen F, Grumont RJ, Strasser A, Metcalf D, Li R, Tarlinton D, Gerondakis S (1995). Mice lacking the c-rel proto-oncogene exhibit defects in lymphocyte proliferation, humoral immunity, and interleukin-2 expression. *Genes Dev* 9: 1965–1977.
Kosai K, Matsumoto K, Nagata S, Tsujimoto Y, Nakamura T (1998). Abrogation of Fas-induced fulminant hepatic failure in mice by hepatocyte growth factor. *Biochem Biophys Res Commun* 244: 683–690.
Kuan CY, Yang DD, Samanta Roy DR, Davis RJ, Rakic P, Flavell RA (1999). The Jnk1 and Jnk2 protein kinases are required for regional specific apoptosis during early brain development. *Neuron* 22: 667–676.
Kuida K, Lippke JA, Ku G, Harding MW, Livingston DJ, Su MS, Flavell RA (1995). Altered cytokine export and apoptosis in mice deficient in interleukin-1 β-converting enzyme. *Science* 267: 2000–2003.
Kuida K, Zheng TS, Na S, Kuan C, Yang D, Karasuyama H, Rakic P, Flavell RA (1996). Decreased apoptosis in the brain and premature lethality in CPP32-deficient mice. *Nature* 384: 368–372.
Kuida K, Haydar TF, Kuan CY, Gu Y, Tana C, Karasuyama H, Su MS, Rakic P, Flavell RA (1998). Reduced apoptosis and cytochrome c–mediated caspase activation in mice lacking caspase 9. *Cell* 94: 325–337.
Kurts C, Carbone FR, Krummel MF, Koch KM, Miller JF. Heath WR (1999). Signalling through CD30 protects against autoimmune diabetes mediated by CD8 T cells. *Nature* 398: 341–344.
Laity JH, Lee BM, Wright PE (2001). Zinc finger proteins: new insights into structural and functional diversity. *Curr Opin Struct Biol* 11: 39–46.
Lam J, Takeshita S, Barker JE, Kanagawa O, Ross FP, Teitelbaum SL (2000). TNF-α induces osteoclastogenesis by direct stimulation of macrophages exposed to permissive levels of RANK ligand. *J Clin Invest* 106: 1481–1488.
Lam J, Nelson CA, Ross FP, Teitelbaum SL, Fremont DH (2001). Crystal structure of the TRANCE/RANKL cytokine reveals determinants of receptor-ligand specificity. *J Clin Invest* 108: 971–979.
Lee EG, Boone DL, Chai S, Libby SL, Chien M, Lodolce JP, Ma A (2000). Failure to regulate TNF-induced NF-κB and cell death responses in A20-deficient mice. *Science* 289: 2350–2354.
Lee KF, Li E, Huber LJ, Landis SC, Sharpe AH, Chao MV, Jaenisch R (1992). Targeted mutation of the gene encoding the low affinity NGF receptor p75 leads to deficits in the peripheral sensory nervous system. *Cell* 69: 737–749.
Lee SY, Choi Y (1997). TRAF-interacting protein (TRIP): a novel component of the tumor necrosis factor receptor (TNFR)- and CD30-TRAF signaling complexes that inhibits TRAF2-mediated NF-κB activation. *J Exp Med* 185: 1275–1285.
Lee SY, Reichlin A, Santana A, Sokol KA, Nussenzweig MC, Choi Y (1997). TRAF2 is essential for JNK but not NF-κB activation and regulates lymphocyte proliferation and survival. *Immunity* 7: 703–713.
Leitges M, Sanz L, Martin P, Duran A, Braun U, Garcia JF, Camacho F, Diaz-Meco MT, Rennert PD, Moscat J (2001). Targeted disruption of the *ζPKC* gene results in the impairment of the NF-κB pathway. *Mol Cell* 8: 771–780.
Levkau B, Scatena M, Giachelli CM, Ross R, Raines EW (1999). Apoptosis overrides survival signals through a caspase-mediated dominant-negative NF-κB loop. *Nat Cell Biol* 1: 227–233.
Li K, Li Y, Shelton JM, Richardson JA, Spencer E, Chen ZJ, Wang X, Williams RS (2000). Cytochrome c deficiency causes embryonic lethality and attenuates stress-induced apoptosis. *Cell* 101: 389–399.
Li Q, Lu Q, Hwang JY, Buscher D, Lee KF, Izpisua-Belmonte JC, Verma IM (1999a). IKK1-deficient mice exhibit abnormal development of skin and skeleton. *Genes Dev* 13: 1322–1328.
Li ZW, Chu W, Hu Y, Delhase M, Deerinck T, Ellisman M, Johnson R, Karin M (1999b).

The IKKβ subunit of IκB kinase (IKK) is essential for nuclear factor κB activation and prevention of apoptosis. *J Exp Med* 189: 1839–1845.

Lindsten T, Ross AJ, King A, Zong WX, Rathmell JC, Shiels HA, Ulrich E, Waymire KG, Mahar P, Frauwirth K, et al. (2000). The combined functions of proapoptotic Bcl-2 family members bak and bax are essential for normal development of multiple tissues. *Mol Cell* 6: 1389–1399.

Ling L, Goeddel DV (2000). MIP-T3, a novel protein linking tumor necrosis factor receptor-associated factor 3 to the microtubule network. *J Biol Chem* 275: 23852–23860.

Liou ML, Liou HC (1999). The ubiquitin-homology protein, DAP-1, associates with tumor necrosis factor receptor (p60) death domain and induces apoptosis. *J Biol Chem* 274: 10145–10153.

Locksley RM, Killeen N, Lenardo MJ (2001). The TNF and TNF receptor superfamilies: integrating mammalian biology. *Cell* 104: 487–501.

Lomaga MA, Yeh WC, Sarosi I, Duncan GS, Furlonger C, Ho A, Morony S, Capparelli C, Van G, Kaufman S, et al. (1999). TRAF6 deficiency results in osteopetrosis and defective interleukin-1, CD40, and LPS signaling. *Genes Dev* 13: 1015–1024.

Lopez-Fraga M, Fernandez R, Albar JP, Hahne M (2001). Biologically active APRIL is secreted following intracellular processing in the Golgi apparatus by furin convertase. *EMBO Rep* 2: 945–951.

Luftig MA, Cahir-McFarland E, Mosialos G, Kieff E (2001). Effects of the NIK *aly* mutation on NF-κB activation by the Epstein-Barr virus latent infection membrane protein, lymphotoxin β receptor, and CD40. *J Biol Chem* 276: 14602–14606.

Lynch CN, Wang YC, Lund JK, Chen YW, Leal JA, Wiley SR (1999). TWEAK induces angiogenesis and proliferation of endothelial cells. *J Biol Chem* 274: 8455–8459.

Makris C, Godfrey VL, Krahn-Senftleben G, Takahashi T, Roberts JL, Schwartz T, Feng L, Johnson RS, Karin M (2000). Female mice heterozygous for IKK γ/NEMO deficiencies develop a dermatopathy similar to the human X-linked disorder incontinentia pigmenti. *Mol Cell* 5: 969–979.

Martinon F, Holler N, Richard C, Tschopp J (2000). Activation of a pro-apoptotic amplification loop through inhibition of NF-κB-dependent survival signals by caspase-mediated inactivation of RIP. *FEBS Lett* 468: 134–136.

Matsushima A, Kaisho T, Rennert PD, Nakano H, Kurosawa K, Uchida D, Takeda K, Akira S, Matsumoto M (2001). Essential role of nuclear factor (NF)-κB-inducing kinase and inhibitor of κB (IκB) kinase α in NF-κB activation through lymphotoxin β receptor, but not through tumor necrosis factor receptor I. *J Exp Med* 193: 631–636.

McDermott MF, Aksentijevich I, Galon J, McDermott EM, Ogunkolade BW, Centola M, Mansfield E, Gadina M, Karenko L, Pettersson T, et al. (1999). Germline mutations in the extracellular domains of the 55 kDa TNF receptor, TNFR1, define a family of dominantly inherited autoinflammatory syndromes. *Cell* 97: 133–144.

Messner B, Stutz AM, Albrecht B, Peiritsch S, Woisetschlager M (1997). Cooperation of binding sites for STAT6 and NFκB/rel in the IL-4-induced up-regulation of the human IgE germline promoter. *J Immunol* 159: 3330–3337.

Michaelson JS, Bader D, Kuo F, Kozak C, Leder P (1999). Loss of Daxx, a promiscuously interacting protein, results in extensive apoptosis in early mouse development. *Genes Dev* 13: 1918–1923.

Micheau O, Lens S, Gaide O, Alevizopoulos K, Tschopp J (2001). NF-κB signals induce the expression of c-FLIP. *Mol Cell Biol* 21: 5299–5305.

Michel F, Soler-Lopez M, Petosa C, Cramer P, Siebenlist U, Muller CW (2001). Crystal structure of the ankyrin repeat domain of Bcl-3: a unique member of the IκB protein family. *EMBO J* 20: 6180–6190.

Migone TS, Zhang J, Luo X, Zhuang L, Chen C, Hu B, Hong JS, Perry JW, Chen SF, Zhou JX, et al. (2002). TL1A is a TNF-like ligand for DR3 and TR6/DcR3 and functions as a T cell costimulator. *Immunity* 16: 479–492.

Monreal AW, Zonana J, Ferguson B (1998). Identification of a new splice form of the EDA1 gene permits detection of nearly all X-linked hypohidrotic ectodermal dysplasia mutations. *Am J Hum Genet* 63: 380–389.

Morishima Y, Gotoh Y, Zieg J, Barrett T, Takano H, Flavell R, Davis RJ, Shirasaki Y, Greenberg ME (2001). β-amyloid induces neuronal apoptosis via a mechanism that involves the c-Jun N-terminal kinase pathway and the induction of Fas ligand. *J Neurosci* 21: 7551–7560.

Morita Y, Perez GI, Paris F, Miranda SR, Ehleiter D, Haimovitz-Friedman A, Fuks Z, Xie Z, Reed JC, Schuchman EH, et al. (2000). Oocyte apoptosis is suppressed by disruption of the acid sphingomyelinase gene or by sphingosine-1-phosphate therapy. *Nat Med* 6: 1109–1114.

Motoyama N, Wang F, Roth KA, Sawa H, Nakayama K, Negishi I, Senju S, Zhang Q, Fujii S, et al. (1995). Massive cell death of immature hematopoietic cells and neurons in Bcl-x-deficient mice. *Science* 267: 1506–1510.

Mukai J, Hachiya T, Shoji-Hoshino S, Kimura MT, Nadano D, Suvanto P, Hanaoka T, Li Y, Irie S, Greene LA, Sato TA (2000). NADE, a p75NTR-associated cell death executor, is involved in signal transduction mediated by the common neurotrophin receptor p75NTR. *J Biol Chem* 275: 17566–17570.

Murata K, Ishii N, Takano H, Miura S, Ndhlovu LC, Nose M, Noda T, Sugamura K (2000). Impairment of antigen-presenting cell function in mice lacking expression of OX40 ligand. *J Exp Med* 191: 365–374.

Muta H, Boise LH, Fang L, Podack ER (2000). CD30 signals integrate expression of cytotoxic effector molecules, lymphocyte trafficking signals, and signals for proliferation and apoptosis. *J Immunol* 165: 5105–5111.

Naismith JH, Sprang SR (1998). Modularity in the TNF-receptor family. *Trends Biochem Sci* 23: 74–79.

Naito A, Azuma S, Tanaka S, Miyazaki T, Takaki S, Takatsu K, Nakao K, Nakamura K, Katsuki M, Yamamoto T, Inoue J (1999). Severe osteopetrosis, defective interleukin-1 signalling and lymph node organogenesis in TRAF6-deficient mice. *Genes Cells* 4: 353–362.

Nakai Y, Irie S, Sato TA (2000). Identification of IκBα as a substrate of FAP-1. *Eur J Biochem* 267: 7170–7175.

Nakano H, Sakon S, Koseki H, Takemori T, Tada K, Matsumoto M, Munechika E, Sakai T, Shirasawa T, Akiba H, et al. (1999). Targeted disruption of *Traf5* gene causes defects in CD40- and CD27-mediated lymphocyte activation. *Proc Natl Acad Sci USA* 96: 9803–9808.

Nakayama K, Dustin LB, Loh DY (1995). T–B cell interaction inhibits spontaneous apoptosis of mature lymphocytes in Bcl-2-deficient mice. *J Exp Med* 182: 1101–1109.

Nguyen LT, Duncan GS, Mirtsos C, Ng M, Speiser DE, Shahinian A, Marino MW, Mak TW, Ohashi PS, Yeh WC (1999). TRAF2 deficiency results in hyperactivity of certain TNFR1 signals and impairment of CD40-mediated responses. *Immunity* 11: 379–389.

Ni CZ, Welsh K, Leo E, Chiou CK, Wu H, Reed JC, Ely KR (2000). Molecular basis for CD40 signaling mediated by TRAF3. *Proc Natl Acad Sci USA* 97: 10395–10399.

Nicholson DW (1999). Caspase structure, proteolytic substrates, and function during apoptotic cell death. *Cell Death Differ* 6: 1028–1042.

Nishina H, Fischer KD, Radvanyi L, Shahinian A, Hakem R, Rubie EA, Bernstein A, Mak TW, Woodgett JR, Penninger JM (1997). Stress-signaling kinase Sek1 protects thymocytes from apoptosis mediated by CD95 and CD3. *Nature* 385: 350–353.

Nishitoh H, Saitoh M, Mochida Y, Takeda K, Nakano H, Rothe M, Miyazono K, Ichijo H (1998). ASK1 is essential for JNK/SAPK activation by TRAF2. *Mol Cell* 2: 389–395.

Okura T, Gong L, Kamitani T, Wada T, Okura I, Wei CF, Chang HM, Yeh ET (1996). Protection against Fas/APO-1- and tumor necrosis factor–mediated cell death by a novel protein, sentrin. *J Immunol* 157: 4277–4281.

Ono K, Ohtomo T, Sato S, Sugamata Y, Suzuki M, Hisamoto N, Ninomiya-Tsuji J, Tsuchiya M, Matsumoto K (2001). An evolutionarily conserved motif in the TAB1 C-terminal region is necessary for interaction with and activation of TAK1 MAPKKK. *J Biol Chem* 276: 24396–24400.

Otterbach B, Stoffel W (1995). Acid sphingomyelinase-deficient mice mimic the neurovisceral form of human lysosomal storage disease (Niemann-Pick disease). *Cell* 81: 1053–1061.

Park YC, Ye H, Hsia C, Segal D, Rich RL, Liou HC, Myszka DG, Wu H (2000). A novel mechanism of TRAF signaling revealed by structural and functional analyses of the TRADD–TRAF2 interaction. *Cell* 101: 777–787.

Pasparakis M, Alexopoulou L, Episkopou V, Kollias G (1996). Immune and inflammatory responses in TNF α-deficient mice: a critical requirement for TNF α in the formation of primary B cell follicles, follicular dendritic cell networks and germinal centers, and in the maturation of the humoral immune response. *J Exp Med* 184: 1397–1411.

Pasparakis M, Alexopoulou L, Grell M, Pfizenmaier K, Bluethmann H, Kollias G (1997). Peyer's patch organogenesis is intact yet formation of B lymphocyte follicles is defective in peripheral lymphoid organs of mice deficient for tumor necrosis factor and its 55-kDa receptor. *Proc Natl Acad Sci USA* 94: 6319–6323.

Peters RT, Liao SM, Maniatis T (2000). IKKϵ is part of a novel PMA-inducible IκB kinase complex. *Mol Cell* 5: 513–522.

Pfeffer K, Matsuyama T, Kundig TM, Wakeham A, Kishihara K, Shahinian A, Wiegmann K, Ohashi PS, Kronke M, Mak TW (1993). Mice deficient for the 55 kd tumor necrosis factor receptor are resistant to endotoxic shock, yet succumb to *L. monocytogenes* infection. *Cell* 73: 457–467.

Pickart CM (2001). Mechanisms underlying ubiquitination. *Annu Rev Biochem* 70: 503–533.

Prasad KV, Ao Z, Yoon Y, Wu MX, Rizk M, Jacquot S, Schlossman SF (1997). CD27, a member of the tumor necrosis factor receptor family, induces apoptosis and binds to Siva, a proapoptotic protein. *Proc Natl Acad Sci USA* 94: 6346–6351.

Print CG, Loveland KL, Gibson L, Meehan T, Stylianou A, Wreford N, de Kretser D, Metcalf D, Kontgen F, Adams JM, Cory S (1998). Apoptosis regulator bcl-w is essential for spermatogenesis but appears otherwise redundant. *Proc Natl Acad Sci USA* 95: 12424–12431.

Rennert P, Schneider P, Cachero TG, Thompson J, Trabach L, Hertig S, Holler N, Qian F, Mullen C, Strauch K, et al. (2000). A soluble form of B cell maturation antigen, a receptor for the tumor necrosis factor family member APRIL, inhibits tumor cell growth. *J Exp Med* 192: 1677–1684.

Renshaw BR, Fanslow WC 3rd, Armitage RJ, Campbell KA, Liggitt D, Wright B, Davison BL, Maliszewski CR (1994). Humoral immune responses in CD40 ligand-deficient mice. *J Exp Med* 180: 1889–1900.

Rieux-Laucat F, Blachere S, Danielan S, De Villartay JP, Oleastro M, Solary E, Bader-Meunier B, Arkwright P, Pondare C, Bernaudin F, et al. (1999). Lymphoproliferative syndrome with autoimmunity: a possible genetic basis for dominant expression of the clinical manifestations. *Blood* 94: 2575–2582.

Rinkenberger JL, Horning S, Klocke B, Roth K, Korsmeyer SJ (2000). Mcl-1 deriency results in peri-implantation embryonic lethality. *Genes Dev* 14: 23–27.

Rochat-Steiner V, Becker K, Micheau O, Schneider P, Burns K, Tschopp J (2000). FIST/HIPK3: a Fas/FADD-interacting serine/threonine kinase that induces FADD phosphorylation and inhibits fas-mediated Jun NH(2)-terminal kinase activation. *J Exp Med* 192: 1165–1174.

Rodseth LE, Brandhuber B, Devine TQ, Eck MJ, Hale K, Naismith JH, Sprang SR (1994). Two crystal forms of the extracellular domain of type I tumor necrosis factor receptor. *J Mol Biol* 239: 332–335.

Rogers PR, Song J, Gramaglia I, Killeen N, Croft M (2001). OX40 promotes Bcl-xL and Bcl-2 expression and is essential for long-term survival of CD4 T cells. *Immunity* 15: 445–455.

Rokudai S, Fujita N, Hashimoto Y, Tsuruo T (2000). Cleavage and inactivation of antiapoptotic Akt/PKB by caspases during apoptosis. *J Cell Physiol* 182: 290–296.

Rothe J, Lesslauer W, Lotscher H, Lang Y, Koebel P, Kontgen F, Althage A, Zinkernagel R, Steinmetz M, Bluethmann H (1993). Mice lacking the tumour necrosis factor receptor 1 are resistant to TNF-mediated toxicity but highly susceptible to infection by *Listeria monocytogenes*. *Nature* 364: 798–802.

Rudolph D, Yeh WC, Wakeham A, Rudolph B, Nallainathan D, Potter J, Elia AJ, Mak TW (2000). Severe liver degeneration and lack of NF-κB activation in NEMO/IKKγ-deficient mice. *Genes Dev* 14: 854–862.

Ryu SW, Chae SK, Lee KJ, Kim E (1999). Identification and characterization of human Fas associated factor 1, hFAF1. *Biochem Biophys Res Commun* 262: 388–394.

Sabapathy K, Hu Y, Kallunki T, Schreiber M, David JP, Jochum W, Wagner EF, Karin M (1999). JNK2 is required for efficient T-cell activation and apoptosis but not for normal lymphocyte development. *Curr Biol* 9: 116–125.

Salehi AH, Roux PP, Kubu CJ, Zeindler C, Bhakar A, Tannis LL, Verdi JM, Barker PA (2000). NRAGE, a novel MAGE protein, interacts with the p75 neurotrophin receptor and facilitates nerve growth factor–dependent apoptosis. *Neuron* 27: 279–288.

Santana P, Pena LA, Haimovitz-Friedman A, Martin S, Green D, McLoughlin M, Cordon-Cardo C, Schuchman EH, Fuks Z, Kolesnick R (1996). Acid sphingomyelinase-deficient human lymphoblasts and mice are defective in radiation-induced apoptosis. *Cell* 86: 189–199.

Saxton TM, Henkemeyer M, Gasca S, Shen R, Rossi DJ, Shalaby F, Feng GS, Pawson T (1997). Abnormal mesoderm patterning in mouse embryos mutant for the SH2 tyrosine phosphatase Shp-2. *EMBO J* 16: 2352–2364.

Schiemann B, Gommerman JL, Vora K, Cachero TG, Shulga-Morskaya S, Dobles M, Frew E, Scott ML (2001). An essential role for BAFF in the normal development of B cells through a BCMA-independent pathway. *Science* 293: 2111–2114.

Schlondorff J, Lum L, Blobel CP (2001). Biochemical and pharmacological criteria define two shedding activities for TRANCE/OPGL that are distinct from the tumor necrosis factor α convertase. *J Biol Chem* 276: 14665–14674.

Schmidt-Supprian M, Bloch W, Courtois G, Addicks K, Israel A, Rajewsky K, Pasparakis M (2000). NEMO/IKK γ-deficient mice model incontinentia pigmenti. *Mol Cell* 5: 981–992.

Schmidt-Ullrich R, Aebischer T, Hulsken J, Birchmeier W, Klemm U, Scheidereit C (2001). Requirement of NF-κB/Rel for the development of hair follicles and other epidermal appendices. *Development* 128: 3843–3853.

Schneider P, Holler N, Bodmer JL, Hahne M, Frei K, Fontana A, Tschopp J (1998). Conversion of membrane-bound Fas (CD95) ligand to its soluble form is associated with downregulation of its proapoptotic activity and loss of liver toxicity. *J Exp Med* 187: 1205–1213.

Schneider P, MacKay F, Steiner V, Hofmann K, Bodmer JL, Holler N, Ambrose C, Lawton P, Bixler S, Acha-Orbea H, et al. (1999). BAFF, a novel ligand of the tumor necrosis factor family, stimulates B cell growth. *J Exp Med* 189: 1747–1756.

Schwartzberg PL, Xing L, Hoffmann O, Lowell CA, Garrett L, Boyce BF, Varmus HE (1997). Rescue of osteoclast function by transgenic expression of kinase-deficient Src in *src*$^{-/-}$ mutant mice. *Genes Dev* 11: 2835–2844.

Sedger L, Glaccum M, Dougall WC, Schuh J, Gliniak B, Peschon JJ (2000). Characterization of mice with targeted disruption of *TRAIL/Apo2L* gene. *Scand J Immunol* 51: 92.

Senftleben U, Cao Y, Xiao G, Greten FR, Krahn G, Bonizzi G, Chen Y, Hu Y, Fong A, Sun SC, Karin M (2001). Activation by IKKα of a second, evolutionary conserved, NF-κ B signaling pathway. *Science* 293: 1495–1499.

Sha WC, Liou HC, Tuomanen EI, Baltimore D (1995). Targeted disruption of the p50 subunit of NF-κB leads to multifocal defects in immune responses. *Cell* 80: 321–330.

Shi CS, Kehrl JH (1997). Activation of stress-activated protein kinase/c-Jun N-terminal kinase, but not NF-κB, by the tumor necrosis factor (TNF) receptor 1 through a TNF receptor-associated factor 2- and germinal center kinase related-dependent pathway. *J Biol Chem* 272: 32102–32107.

Shiels H, Li X, Schumacker PT, Maltepe E, Padrid PA, Sperling A, Thompson CB, Lindsten T (2000). TRAF4 deficienty leads to tracheal malformation with resulting alterations in air flow to the lungs. *Am J Pathol* 157: 679–688.

Shindler KS, Latham CB, Roth KA (1997). Bax deficiency prevents the increased cell death of immature neurons in bcl-x-deficient mice. *J Neurosci* 17: 3112–3119.

Shinkura R, Kitada K, Matsuda F, Tashiro K, Ikuta K, Suzuki M, Kogishi K, Serikawa T, Honjo T (1999). Alymphoplasia is caused by a point mutation in the mouse gene encoding Nf-κ b-inducing kinase. *Nat Genet* 22: 74–77.

Siegel RM, Frederiksen JK, Zacharias DA, Chan FK, Johnson M, Lynch D, Tsien RY, Lenardo MJ (2000). Fas preassociation required for apoptosis signaling and dominant inhibition by pathogenic mutations. *Science* 288: 2354–2357.

Simonet WS, Lacey DL, Dunstan CR, Kelley M, Chang MS, Luthy R, Nguyen HQ, Wooden S, Bennett L, Boone T, et al. (1997). Osteoprotegerin: a novel secreted protein involved in the regulation of bone density. *Cell* 89: 309–319.

Smahi A, Courtois G, Vabres P, Yamaoka S, Heuertz S, Munnich A, Israel A, Heiss NS, Klauck SM, Kioschis P, et al. (2000). Genomic rearrangement in NEMO impairs NF-κB activation and is a cause of incontinentia pigmenti. *Nature* 405: 466–472.

Snapper CM, Zelazowski P, Rosas FR, Kehry MR, Tian M, Baltimore D, Sha WC (1996). B cells from p50/NF-κB knockout mice have selective defects in proliferation, differentiation, germ-line CH transcription, and Ig class switching. *J Immunol* 156: 183–191.

Soriano P, Montgomery C, Geske R, Bradley A (1991). Targeted disruption of the c-src proto-oncogene leads to osteopetrosis in mice. *Cell* 64: 693–702.

Srivastava AK, Pispa J, Hartung AJ, Du Y, Ezer S, Jenks T, Shimada T, Pekkanen M, Mikkola ML, Ko MS, et al. (1997). The Tabby phenotype is caused by mutation in a mouse homologue of the EDA gene that reveals novel mouse and human exons and encodes a protein (ectodysplasin-A) with collagenous domains. *Proc Natl Acad Sci USA* 94: 13069–13074.

Stegh AH, Barnhart BC, Volkland J, Algeciras-Schimnich A, Ke N, Reed JC, Peter ME (2001). Inactivation of caspase-8 on mitochondria of Bcl-xL-expressing MCF7-Fas cells: role for the bifunctional apoptosis regulator protein. *J Biol Chem* 277: 4351–4360.

Sun X, Yin J, Starovasnik MA, Fairbrother WJ, Dixit VM (2002). Identification of a novel homotypic interaction motif required for the phosphorylation of receptor interacting protein (RIP) by RIP3. *J Biol Chem* 277: 9505–9511.

Suzuki Y, Imai Y, Nakayama H, Takahashi K, Takio K, Takahashi R (2001). A serine protease, HtrA2, is released from the mitochondria and interacts with XIAP, inducing cell death. *Mol Cell* 8: 613–621.

Swat W, Fujikawa K, Ganiatsas S, Yang D, Xavier RJ, Harris NL, Davidson L, Ferrini R, Davis RJ, Labow MA, et al. (1998). SEK1/MKK4 is required for maintenance of a normal peripheral lymphoid comaprtment but not for lymphocyte development. *Immunity* 8: 625–634.

Tada K, Okazaki T, Sakon S, Kobarai T, Kurosawa K, Yamaoka S, Hashimoto H, Mak TW, Yagita H, Okumura K, et al. (2001). Critical roles of TRAF2 and TRAF5 in tumor necrosis factor–induced NF-κB activation and protection from cell death. *J Biol Chem* 276: 36530–36534.

Takaesu G, Kishida S, Hiyama A, Yamaguchi K, Shibuya H, Irie K, Ninomiya-Tsuji J, Matsumoto K (2000). TAB2, a novel adaptor protein, mediates activation of TAK1 MAPKKK by linking TAK1 to TRAF6 in the IL-1 signal transduction pathway. *Mol Cell* 5: 649–658.

Takahashi T, Tanaka M, Brannan CI, Jenkins NA, Copeland NG, Suda T, Nagata S (1994). Generalized lymphoproliferative disease in mice, caused by a point mutation in the Fas ligand. *Cell* 76: 969–976.

Takeda K, Hayakawa Y, Smyth MJ, Kayagaki N, Yamaguchi N, Kakuta S, Iwakura Y, Yagita H, Okumura K (2001). Involvement of tumor necrosis factor–related apoptosis-inducing ligand in surveillance of tumor metastasis by liver natural killer cells. *Nat Med* 7: 94–100.

Takeuchi M, Rothe M, Goeddel DV (1996). Anatomy of TRAF2: distinct domains for NF-κB activation and association with TNF signaling proteins. *J Biol Chem* 271: 19935–19942.

Tanaka M, Itai T, Adachi M, Nagata S (1998). Downregulation of Fas ligand by shedding. *Nat Med* 4: 31–36.

Tanaka M, Fuentes ME, Yamaguchi K, Durnin MH, Dalrymple SA, Hardy KL, Goeddel DV (1999). Embryonic lethality, liver degeneration, and impaired NF-κ B activation in IKK-β-deficient mice. *Immunity* 10: 421–429.

Tang G, Yang J, Minemoto Y, Lin A (2001). Blocking caspase-3-mediated proteolysis of IKKβ suppresses TNF-α-induced apoptosis. *Mol Cell* 8: 1005–1016.

Thome M, Tschopp J (2001). Regulation of lymphocyte proliferation and death by FLIP. *Nature Reviews Immunol* 1: 50–58.

Thompson JS, Bixler SA, Qian F, Vora K, Scott ML, Cachero TG, Hession C, Schneider P, Sizing ID, Mullen C, et al. (2001a). BAFF-R, a newly identified TNF receptor that specifically interacts with BAFF. *Science* 293: 2108–2111.

Thompson NA, Haefliger JA, Senn A, Tawadros T, Magara F, Ledermann B, Nicod P, Waeber G (2001b). Islet-brain1/JNK-interacting protein-1 is required for early embryogenesis in mice. *J Biol Chem* 276: 27745–27748.

Tsitsikov EN, Laouini D, Dunn IF, Sannikova TY, Davidson L, Alt FW, Geha RS (2001). TRAF1 is a negative regulator of TNF signaling: enhance TNF signaling in TRAF1-deficient mice. *Immunity* 15: 647–657.

Van der Zee CE, Ross Gm, Riopelle RJ, Hagg T (1996). Survival of cholinergikc forebrain neurons in developing p75NGFR-deficient mice. *Science* 274: 1729–1732.

Van Huffel S, Delaei F, Heyninck K, De Valck D, Beyaert R (2001). Identification of a novel A20-binding inhibitor of nuclear factor-κ B activation termed ABIN-2. *J Biol Chem* 276: 30216–30223.

Varfolomeev EE, Schuchmann M, Luria V, Chiannilkulchai N, Beckmann JS, Mett IL, Rebrokov D, Brodianski VM, Kemper OC, Kollet O, et al. (1998). Targeted disruption of the mouse Caspase 8 gene ablates cell death induction by the TNF receptors, Fas/Apo1, and DR3 and is lethal prenatally. *Immunity* 9: 267–276.

Veis DJ, Sorenson CM, Shutter JR, Korsmeyer SJ (1993). Bcl-2-deficient mice demonstrate fulminant lymphoid apoptosis, polycystic kidneys, and hypopigmented hair. *Cell* 75: 229–240.

Verhagen AM, Silke J, Ekert PG, Pakusch M, Kaufmann H, Connolly LM, Day CL, Tikoo A, Burke R, Wrobel C, et al. (2002). HtrA2 promotes cell death through its serine protease activity and its ability to antagonize inhibitor of apoptosis proteins. *J Biol Chem* 277: 445–454.

Verheij M, Bose R, Lin XH, Yao B, Jarvis WD, Grant S, Birrer MJ, Szabo E, Zon LI, Kyriakis JM, et al. (1996). Requirement for ceramide-initiated SAPK/JNK signalling in stress-induced apoptosis. *Nature* 380: 75–79.

Villunger A, Huang DC, Holler N, Tschopp J, Strasser A (2000). Fas ligand–induced c-Jun kinase activation in lymphoid cells requires extensive receptor aggregation but is independent of DAXX, and Fas-mediated cell death and does not involve DAXX, RIP, or RAIDD. *J Immunol* 165: 1337–1343.

von Bulow GU, van Deursen JM, Bram RJ (2001). Regulation of the T-independent humoral response by TACI. *Immunity* 14: 573–582.

Walczak H, Sprick MR (2001). Biochemistry and function of the DISC. *Trends Biochem Sci* 26: 452–453.

Wang C, Deng L, Hong M, Akkaraju GR, Inoue J, Chen ZJ (2001). TAK1 is a ubiquitin-dependent kinase of MKK and IKK. *Nature* 412: 346–351.

Wang EC, Thern A, Denzel A, Kitson J, Farrow SN, Owen MJ (2001b). DR3 regulates negative selection during thymnocyte development. *Mol Cell Biol* 21: 3451–3461.

Wang GQ, Wieckowski E, Goldstein LA, Gastman BR, Rabinovitz A, Gambotto A, Li S, Fang B, Yin XM, Rabinowich H (2001c). Resistance to granzyme B-mediated cytochrome c release in Bak-deficient cells. *J Exp Med* 194: 1325–1337.

Wang J, Zheng L, Lobito A, Chan FK, Dale J, Sneller M, Yao X, Puck JM, Straus SE, Lenardo MJ (1999). Inherited human Caspase 10 mutations underlie defective lymphocyte and dendritic cell apoptosis in autoimmune lymphoproliferative syndrome type II. *Cell* 98: 47–58.

Wang S, Miura M, Jung YK, Zhu H, Li E, Yuan J (1998). Murine caspase-11, an ICE-interacting protease, is essential for the activation of ICE. *Cell* 92: 501–509.

Wang ZQ, Ovitt C, Grigoriadis AE, Mohle-Steinlein U, Ruther U, Wagner EF (1992). Bone and haematopoietic defects in mice lacking c-fos. *Nature* 360: 741–745.

Watanabe-Fukunaga R, Brannan CI, Copeland NG, Jenkins NA, Nagata S (1992). Lymphoproliferation disorder in mice explained by defects in Fas antigen that mediates apoptosis. *Nature* 356: 314–317.

Watts JD, Gu M, Polverino AJ, Patterson SD, Aebersold R (1997). Fas-induced apoptosis of T cells occurs independently of ceramide generation. *Proc Natl Acad Sci USA* 94: 7292–7296.

Wei MC, Zong WX, Cheng EH, Lindsten T, Panoutsakopoulou V, Ross AJ, Roth KA, MacGregor GR, Thompson CB, Korsmeyer SJ (2001). Proapoptotic BAX and BAK: a requisite gateway to mitochondrial dysfunction and death. *Science* 292: 727–730.

Widmann C, Gibson S, Jarpe MB, Johnson GL (1999). Mitogen-activated protein kinase: conservation of a three-kinase module from yeast to human. *Physiol Rev* 79: 143–180.

Wiley SR, Cassiano L, Lofton T, Davis-Smith T, Winkles JA, Lindner V, Liu H, Daniel TO, Smith CA, Fanslow WC (2001). A novel TNF receptor family member binds TWEAK and is implicated in angiogenesis. *Immunity* 15: 837–846.

Xia Y, Makris C, Su B, Li E, Yang J, Nemerow GR, Karin M (2000). MEK kinase 1 is critically required for c-Jun N-terminal kinase activation by proinflammatory stimuli and growth factor–induced cell migration. *Proc Natl Acad Sci USA* 97: 5243–5248.

Xu J, Foy TM, Laman JD, Elliott EA, Dunn JJ, Waldschmidt TJ, Elsemore J, Noelle RJ, Flavell RA (1994). Mice deficient for the CD40 ligand. *Immunity* 1: 423–431.

Xu S, Lam KP (2001). B-cell maturation protein, which binds the tumor necrosis factor family members BAFF and APRIL, is dispensable for humoral immune responses. *Mol Cell Biol* 21: 4067–4074.

Xu Y, Cheng G, Baltimore D (1996). Targeted disruption of TRAF3 leads to postnatal lethality and defective T-dependent immune responses. *Immunity* 5: 407–415.

Yamamoto Y, Kim DW, Kwak YT, Prajapati S, Verma U, Gaynor RB (2001). IKKγ/NEMO facilitates the recruitment of the Iκ proteins into the IκB kinase complex. *J Biol Chem* 276: 36327–36336.

Yan M, Wang LC, Hymowitz SG, Schilbach S, Lee J, Goddard A, de Vos AM, Gao WQ, Dixit VM (2000). Two-amino acid molecular switch in an epithelial morphogen that regulates binding to two distinct receptors. *Science* 290: 523–527.

Yan M, Brady JR, Chan B, Lee WP, Hsu B, Harless S, Cancro M, Grewal IS, Dixit VM (2001a). Identification of a novel receptor for B lymphocyte stimulator that is mutated in a mouse strain with severe B cell deficiency. *Curr Biol* 11: 1547–1552.

Yan M, Wang H, Chan B, Roose-Girma M, Erickson S, Baker T, Tumas D, Grewal IS, Dixit VM (2001b). Activation and accumulation of B cells in TACI-deficient mice. *Nat Immunol* 2: 638–643.

Yanagisawa J, Takahashi M, Kanki H, Yano-Yanagisawa H, Tazunoki T, Sawa E, Nishitoba T, Kamishohara M, Kobayashi E, Kataoka S, Sato T (1997). The molecular interaction of Fas and FAP-1: a tripeptide blocker of human Fas interaction with FAP-1 promotes Fas-induced apoptosis. *J Biol Chem* 272: 8539–8545.

Yang DD, Kuan CY, Whitmarsh AJ, Rincon M, Zheng TS, Davis RJ, Takic P, Flavell RA (1997a). Absence of excitotoxicity-induced apoptosis in the hippocampus of mice lacking the *Jnk3* gene. *Nature* 389: 865–870.

Yang J, Lin Y, Guo Z, Cheng J, Huang J, Deng L, Liao W, Chen Z, Liu Z, Su B (2001). The essential role of MEKK3 in TNF-induced NF-κB activation. *Nat Immunol* 2: 620–624.

Yang X, Khosravi-Far R, Chang HY, Baltimore D (1997b). Daxx, a novel Fas-binding protein that activates JNK and apoptosis. *Cell* 89: 1067–1076.

Yano H, Chao MV (2000). Neurotrophin receptor structure and interactions. *Pharm Acta Helv* 74: 253–260.

Ye H, Wu H (2000). Thermodynamic characterization of the interaction between TRAF2 and tumor necrosis factor receptor peptides by isothermal titration calorimetry. *Proc Natl Acad Sci USA* 97: 8961–8966.

Yeh WC, Shahinian A, Speiser D, Kraunus J, Billia F, Wakeham A, de la Pompa JL, Ferrick D, Hum B, Iscove N, et al. (1997). Early lethality, functional NF-κB activation, and increased sensitivity to TNF-induced cell death in TRAF2-deficient mice. *Immunity* 7: 715–725.

Yeh WC, Itie A, Elia AJ, Ng M, Shu HB, Wakeham A, Mirtsos C, Suzuki N, Bonnard M, Goeddel DV, Mak TW (2000). Requirement for Casper (c-FLIP) in regulation of death receptor–induced apoptosis and embryonic development. *Immunity* 12: 633–642.

Yin C, Knudson CM, Korsmeyer SJ, Van Dyke T (1997). Bax suppresses tumorigenesis and stimulates apoptosis in vivo. *Nature* 385: 637–640.

Yin L, Wu L, Wesche H, Arthur CD, White JM, Goeddel DV, Schreiber RD (2001). De-fective lymphotoxin-β receptor-induced NF-κB transcriptional activity in NIK-deficient mice. *Science* 291: 2162–2615.

Yin XM, Wang K, Gross A, Zhao Y, Zinkel S, Klocke B, Roth KA, Korsmeyer SJ (1999). Bid-deficient mice are resistant to Fas-induced hepatocellular apoptosis. *Nature* 400: 886–891.

Yoshida H, Kong YY, Yoshida R, Elia AJ, Hakem A, Hakem R, Penninger JM, Mak TW (1998). Apaf1 is required for mitochondrial pathways of apoptosis and brain development. *Cell* 94: 739–750.

You M, Flick LM, Yu D, Feng GS (2001). Modulation of the nuclear factor κ B pathway by Shp-2 tyrosine phosphatase in mediating the induction of interleukin (IL)-6 by IL-1 or tumor necrosis factor. *J Exp Med* 193: 101–110.

Yuasa T, Ohno S, Kehrl JH, Kyriakis JM (1998). Tumor necrosis factor signaling to stress-activated protein kinase (SAPK)/Jun NH2-terminal kinase (JNK) and p38: germinal center kinase couples TRAF2 to mitogen-activated protein kinase/ERK kinase kinase 1 and SAPK while receptor interacting protein associates with a mitogen-activated protein kinase kinase kinase upstream of MKK6 and p38. *J Biol Chem* 273: 22681–22692.

Yujiri T, Sather S, Fanger GR, Johnson GL (1998). Role of MEKK1 in cell survival and activation of JNK and ERK pathways defined by targeted gene disruption. *Science* 282: 1911–1914.

Yujiri T, Ware M, Widmann C, Over R, Russell D, Chan E, Zaitsu Y, Clarke P, Tyler K, Oka Y, et al. (2000). MEK kinase 1 gene disruption alters cell migration and c-Jun NH2-terminal kinase regulation but does not cause a measurable defect in NF-κB activation. *Proc Natl Acad Sci USA* 97: 7272–7277.

Zaidi AU, D'Sa-Eipper C, Brenner J, Kuida K, Zheng TS, Flavell RA, Rakic P, Roth KA (2001). Bcl-X(L)-caspase-9 interactions in the developing nervous system: evidence for multiple death pathways. *J Neurosci* 21: 169–175.

Zha J, Weiler S, Oh KJ, Wei MC, Korsmeyer SJ (2000). Posttranslational N-myristoylation of BID as a molecular switch for targeting mitochondria and apoptosis. *Science* 290: 1761–1765.

Zhang J, Cado D, Chen A, Kabra NH, Winoto A (1998). Fas-mediated apoptosis and activation-induced T-cell proliferation are defective in mice lacking FADD/Mort1. *Nature* 392: 296–300.

Zhang SQ, Kovalenko A, Cantarella G, Wallach D (2000). Recruitment of the IKK signalosome to the p55 TNF receptor: RIP and A20 bind to NEMO (IKKγ) upon receptor stimulation. *Immunity* 12: 301–311.

Zhang YH, Heulsmann A, Tondravi MM, Mukherjee A, Abu-Amer Y (2001). Tumor necrosis factor-α (TNF) stimulates RANKL-induced osteoclastogenesis via coupling of TNF type 1 receptor and RANK signaling pathways. *J Biol Chem* 276: 563–568.

Zhao H, Yan M, Wang H, Erickson S, Grewal IS, Dixit VM (2001). Impaired c-Jun amino terminal kinase activity and T cell differentiation in death receptor 6-deficient mice. *J Exp Med* 194: 1441–1448.

Zhong H, Voll RE, Ghosh S (1998). Phosphorylation of NF-κ B p65 by PKA stimulates transcriptional activity by promoting a novel bivalent interaction with the coactivator CBP/p300. *Mol Cell* 1: 661–671.

Zonana J, Elder ME, Schneider LC, Orlow SJ, Moss C, Golabi M, Shapira SK, Farndon PA, Wara DW, Emmal SA, Ferguson BM (2000). A novel X-linked disorder of immune deficiency and hypohidrotic ectodermal dysplasia is allelic to incontinentia pigmenti and due to mutations in IKK-γ (NEMO). *Am J Hum Genet* 67: 1555–1562.

Zumbansen M, Stoffel W (1997). Tumor necrosis factor α activates NF-κB in acid sphingomyelinase-deficient mouse embryonic fibroblasts. *J Biol Chem* 272: 10904–10909.

31 | ED1, EDAR, and EDARADD and the Hypohidrotic Ectodermal Dysplasias and the Ectodysplasin Signaling Pathway

JONATHAN ZONANA

The ectodermal dysplasia syndromes are a group of heterogeneous inherited disorders that display different combinations of congenital defects of the hair, teeth, nails, and sweat glands (Pinheiro and Freire-Maia, 1994). These structures are all appendages derived from oral and epidermal ectoderm and are formed during development by reciprocal molecular interactions between the epithelium and the mesenchyme (see Chapter 15) (Tucker and Sharpe, 1999; Thesleff, 2000; Fuchs et al., 2001). The pathology seen in these conditions ranges from aplasia or hypoplasia to dysplasia of the affected structures. The defects are secondary to the abnormal induction, proliferation, or differentiation of the epidermal appendages during morphogenesis. The hypohidrotic, or anhidrotic, ectodermal dysplasias (HED or EDA), are a subgroup of the ectodermal dysplasias that have in common significant abnormalities of the eccrine sweat glands, resulting in diminished or lack of sweating (hypohidrosis or anhidrosis) and abnormalities of teeth and hair (Table 31–1). Positional cloning studies in both humans and mice have revealed that the genetic loci responsible for these disorders form a previously unknown developmental pathway. The protein products of each of these loci are expressed in the epithelial cells of developing teeth, hair follicles, and eccrine sweat glands during embryonic development, and loss of their function results in abnormal morphogenesis.

This new developmental pathway, named the ectodysplasin (Eda) pathway, consists of a ligand and a receptor belonging to the tumor necrosis factor–like (TNF) superfamily and their associated intracellular proteins (Kere et al., 1996; Monreal et al., 1998, 1999; Headon et al., 2001). The receptor complex transduces a signal to the nucleus by means of a transcription factor NF-κB, which ultimately leads to the appropriate cellular response (Schmidt-Ullrich et al., 2001). The ectodysplasin pathway shares several downstream elements (NF-κB, IKK complex) with other TNF signal-transduction pathways (Israel, 2000). Mutations at three separate loci within the ectodysplasin pathway are responsible for clinically indistinguishable forms of hypohidrotic ectodermal dysplasia.

CLINICAL DISORDERS

X-linked Hypohidrotic Ectodermal Dysplasia

X-linked recessive hypohidrotic ectodermal dysplasia (XLHED) is the most common form of ectodermal dysplasia (Fig. 31–1). Significant intra- and interfamilial variability exist in the degree of hypohidrosis and hypodontia seen in affected individuals, but the nails of affected individuals are normal (Clarke et al., 1987). Affected males are usually missing a majority of their primary and secondary dentition (Nakata et al., 1980; Crawford et al., 1991). If present, the maxillary central incisors and canines may be conical in shape. Hypotrichosis occurs, with a diminished amount of frequently lightly pigmented scalp hair in childhood, which is lost prematurely, thus resulting in early balding. Body hair and eyebrows are sparse, but facial and pubic hair are normal. The skin is generally thin, with susceptibility to eczema and with periorbital wrinkling and hyperpigmentation. Involvement of the nasal and respiratory mucosa lead to problems of atrophic rhinitis with ozena, as well as to frequent respiratory infections. There may be an increased incidence of gastroesophageal reflux and feeding problems during infancy. Craniofacial features frequently include a depressed nasal bridge and everted lips.

Heterozygous female carriers have variable degrees of clinical involvement. Findings range from no manifestations to clinically significant hypodontia, hypotrichosis, and unilateral or bilateral hypoplasia of the breasts (Pinheiro et al., 1981; Clarke and Burn, 1991). The majority of carrier females, even those with significant hypodontia, are not identified until a fully affected male is born into the family. The wide clinical variability seen in carrier females is due to the process of X inactivation (lyonization), which limits carrier detection based on physical examination. Thus, female carriers of XLHED are mosaics of functionally normal and abnormal cells, and their clinical findings depend on the percentage of abnormal progenitor cells that give rise to their hair, teeth, and sweat glands.

Autosomal Recessive Hypohidrotic Ectodermal Dysplasia

The existence of an autosomal recessive form of HED—ARHED—was suspected for a number of years by several investigators (Gorlin et al., 1970). This hypothesis was supported by linkage analysis (Munoz et al., 1997) and ultimately confirmed by the isolation of genes from two separate autosomal loci (Headon and Overbeek, 1999; Monreal et al., 1999; Headon et al., 2001). The clinical phenotype of patients with the autosomal recessive form of HED is indistinguishable from the signs and symptoms in males with the X-linked recessive form. The major clinical distinction between the autosomal and X-linked recessive forms is the occurrence of complete manifestations in affected females: affected females with ARHED are usually more severely affected than the majority of carrier females with the X-linked form, although rare carriers of the X-linked form may have marked manifestations. Heterozygote parents and siblings of ARHED probands have no ectodermal defects. ARHED is far less common than XLHED, but its true incidence awaits molecular analysis of a larger group of patients. Consanguinity has been noted in multiple families with ARHED.

Autosomal Dominant Hypohidrotic Ectodermal Dysplasia

Few families with autosomal dominant form of hypohidrotic ectodermal dysplasia (ADHED) have been published (Jorgenson et al., 1987; Aswegan et al., 1997). The phenotype as described in one large family with four affected generations showed intrafamilial variability, but nearly all individuals had fine, slow-growing scalp and body hair with sparse eyebrows (Jorgenson et al., 1987; Aswegan et al., 1997). All affected individuals were missing some of their primary or secondary dentition, with nearly all of them missing their four lower permanent incisors. The maxillary primary incisors were frequently conical. Almost all had reduced sweating, and many had clinical heat intolerance. The nails were usually normal.

MOLECULAR GENETICS

ED1

ED1 maps to Xq12–q13.1 and contains nine exons, which are alternatively spliced (Bayes et al., 1998; Monreal et al., 1998). Although multiple splice forms have been detected, only two forms have been shown to have biological activity in vitro (Yan et al., 2000). *ED1* codes for ectodysplasin (EDA), a member of the TNF ligand family. The

Table 31–1. The Hypohidrotic Ectodermal Dysplasias (HED)

OMIM Number	Clinical Disorder	Gene	Chromosome Location	Protein	Function
305100	X linked HED (XLHED)	*ED1*	Xq12–q13.1	Ectodysplasin (EDA)	Ligand
224900	Autosomal recessive HED (ARHED)	*EDAR*	2q11–q13	Ectodysplasin receptor (EDAR)	Receptor for EDA ligand
224900	Autosomal recessive HED (ARHED)	*EDARADD*	1q42.2–q43	Ectodysplasin receptor–associated death domain (EDARADD)	Adapter protein; binds to the cytoplasmic domain of receptor
129490	Autosomal dominant HED (ED3; ADHED)	*EDAR*	2q11–q13	Ectodysplasin receptor (EDAR)	Receptor for EDA ligand
300291	HED with immune deficiency (HED-ID)	*NEMO (IKK-γ)*	Xq28	NEMO	Regulator of NFκB signaling

originally isolated splice form (EDA-O) contains only exons 1 and 2, and its biological significance, if any, remains unclear. Subsequently, additional splice forms were identified. Both EDA-A1 and A2 contain eight exons, each lacking exon 2, and code for proteins of 391 and 389 amino acids, respectively (Yan et al., 2000). The two isoforms differ by the use of an alternate donor splice site within IVS8. Exon 8 of EDA-A1 contains six more nucleotides than exon 8 of EDA-A2 and codes for two amino acids (Val307 and Glu308). Molecular modeling of these two amino acids places them at the surface of the ligand's binding domain, with the alternate splice forms conferring receptor specificity (Yan et al., 2000).

Ectodysplasin, the product of the *ED1* locus, is expressed by epithelial cells of the developing tooth, hair follicle, and eccrine sweat gland (Montonen et al. 1998). EDA-A1 binds exclusively to the EDA-A1 receptor (EDAR), and is essential for normal morphogenesis of ectodermal appendages (Kumar et al., 2001; Schneider et al., 2001; Srivastava et al., 2001). EDA-A2 binds solely to a distinct receptor, the EDA-A2 receptor (XEDAR), which maps to the X chromosome. Mutations in *XEDAR* have not been identified or associated with human disorders. Both EDA isoforms are type II transmembrane proteins that contain a short intracellular domain, a single transmembrane domain, and an extracellular domain which is cleaved by a protease, most likely furin (Bayes et al., 1998; Monreal et al., 1998; Ezer et al., 1999; Mikkola et al., 1999; Chen et al., 2001b; Elomaa et al., 2001; Laurikkala et al., 2001; Schneider et al., 2001). Epithelial cells can secrete the extracellular portion of the ligand and thus function in either a paracrine or a juxtacrine manner. In situ hybridization data in the developing murine tooth indicate that the secreted ligand must be transported to interact with its receptor. The processed ligand contains a collagen-like repeat (GlyXY)$_{19}$ with a single interruption, as well as a C-terminal domain with TNF family homology. This domain is re-

sponsible for binding to the extracellular domain of the receptors. The TNF superfamily ligands form homotrimers and bind to a trimerized receptor molecule at each monomer–monomer interface (Baud and Karin, 2001; Locksley et al., 2001).

Several groups, surveying over 100 patients with presumed XLHED, have identified numerous mutations in *ED1* (Paakkonen et al., 2001; Schneider et al., 2001; Vincent et al., 2001). Mutation detection rates varied from 95% to 63%, due to detection methods utilized and patient selection. As expected, direct sequencing had the highest yield of mutations and single-stranded conformational polymorphism (SSCP) analysis had the lowest. In addition, mutation detection rates were higher in typically affected male patients and in families with more than one affected generation. This reflects the increased like-lihood of autosomal forms of the disorder in families with severely affected females, and those with sporadic cases or a single affected sibship.

All types of mutations have been noted at the *ED1* locus. Large genomic rearrangements with deletion of single exons or of the entire gene occur but are uncommon. Mutations within the small intracellular cytoplasmic domain usually result in premature truncation of the protein due to either nonsense mutations or in small insertions or deletions, resulting in frameshifts. Missense mutations occur either within the transmembrane domain or in the residues proximate to it, changing polarity and likely affecting insertion of the protein into the membrane. The largest cluster of mutations identified in *ED1* occur within exon 3 in the codons for the protease cleavage site within the extracellular domain (Arg156-Asn-Lys-Arg159) (Chen et al., 2001b). These missense mutations replace the basic amino acids arginine and lysine within the cleavage site for the proprotein convertase furin. Missense mutations within this domain are recurrent and represent 20% to 30% of the changes detected in individuals with XLHED (Schneider et al., 2001; Vincent et al., 2001). The frequent mutations at Arg156 and Arg159 are due to C-to-T transitions at CpG dinucleotides, and they are independent events rather than ancestral mutations. In vitro studies confirm that the ectodysplasin-A protein is cleaved between residues 159 and 160 and that the common mutations within exon 3 prevent normal processing (Chen et al., 2001b; Schneider et al., 2001). Another recurrent missense mutation, R153C, leads to the formation of an interchain disulfide bridge that likely interferes with normal processing.

Another cluster of recurrent mutations is found within exon 5 and involves the GlyXY$_{19}$ collagen domain. These mutations consist of in-frame deletions of two to four GlyXY repeats and may affect trimerization of the ligand, multimerization of the trimerized ligands, or some yet to be defined interaction between the EDA collagen domain and other extracellular matrix proteins (Bayes et al., 1998; Schneider et al., 2001). Similar to other collagen-like molecules, missense mutations that affect glycine or proline residues are seen within the GlyXY domain and likely disrupt triple helix formation.

Missense mutations also occur within the TNF homology domain of the EDA-A extracellular domain. The mutations affect residues within the conserved β-sheet structures or less conserved loops, as defined by a homology comparison of the EDA-A ligand and its closest relatives within the TNF ligand superfamily BAFF, April, and Tweak (Bodmer et al., 2002). A number of these mutations have been shown in vitro to impair proper folding or secretion, or binding to the EDA and XEDAR receptors (Schneider et al., 2001).

Finally, a number of splice site mutations have been identified. One

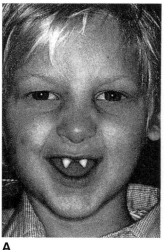 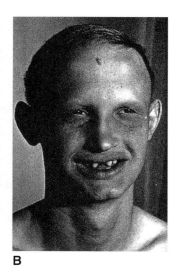

A **B**

Figure 31–1. Child (A) and adult (B) with hypohidrotic ectodermal dysplasia. Note missing and dysplastic teeth, periorbital darkening and wrinkling, as well as light-colored and sparse scalp hair. (From Figure 3.78, page 254, *Genetic Skin Disorders*, Virginia Sybert, Oxford University Press.)

that is particularly instructive affects IVS8, the intron splice donor site that is utilized for the EDA-A1 isoform, but not for EDA-A2 (Schneider et al., 2001). This mutation eliminates the EDA-A1, but not the EDA-A2, splice variant and provides evidence that EDA-A1 is the critical splice form needed for normal morphogenesis. This conclusion has been confirmed by the transgenic rescue of the *Tabby* mouse, a spontaneous mouse mutant that lacks EDA function, with a cDNA for the EDA-A1 isoform alone (Srivastava et al., 2001).

All of the known mutant forms of the EDA protein result in loss of function in vivo. No genotype–phenotype correlation exists for the mutations that affect the EDA-A1 splice form. It is possible that mutations that affect only the EDA-A2 splice form or its receptor XEDAR will have a phenotype distinct from that seen in the hypohidrotic ectodermal dysplasias.

EDAR

EDAR (ectodysplasin 1, anhidrotic receptor [ectodysplasin A-1 receptor]) is a new member of the TNF receptor superfamily and is a type I transmembrane protein with a single transmembrane domain (Headon and Overbeek, 1999; Monreal et al., 1999). The gene consists of 12 exons and codes for a 488 amino acid protein. The extracellular domain contains cysteine-rich repeats, which are characteristic of other members of the TNFR superfamily and are involved in ligand binding. The extracellular domain of EDAR exclusively binds the ectodysplasin A-1 form of the EDA ligand (Yan et al., 2000). Upon ligand binding, the receptor is believed to trimerize and a signal is transduced (Locksley et al., 2001). An intracellular death domain (Weber and Vincenz, 2001) within the cytoplasmic portion of the receptor serves as a platform for the transduction of signals to downstream molecules.

Missense mutations within different domains of the receptor can result in different patterns of inheritance for the disorder. Two missense mutations within the extracellular ligand-binding domain (C87R and R89H) cause autosomal recessive hypohidrotic ectodermal dysplasia (Monreal et al., 1999). The mutations abolished or severely diminished EDAR in vitro binding to EDA-A1 (Schneider et al., 2001). In addition, the EDAR C87R protein construct was poorly recovered when it was expressed in cell culture, suggesting a defect in protein folding or solubility. A third family with ARHED resulted from compound heterozygosity for a deletion of exon 4 and a missense mutation (Arg89His) within the extracellular domain, and a fourth family was homozygous for an acceptor splice site mutation within IVS2. Thus, all of the recessive mutations result in loss of function.

Heterozygous mutations within exon 12 of the intracellular domain may result in autosomal dominant hypohidrotic ectodermal dysplasia (ADHED) (Monreal et al., 1999). Exon 12 codes for the most carboxy-terminal portion of the EDAR receptor protein and contains the death domain that is critical for signal transduction. Two unrelated families had a common nonsense mutation (Arg358Ter), which is predicted to truncate the cytoplasmic portion of the protein and eliminate the death domain. This is identical to the effect of the dominant mutation involving the *Edar* gene (*Dl^slk*) seen in the mouse, which also results in a truncated protein prior to the death domain. The loss of the death domain results in a dominant-negative effect on function, presumably due to interference with homotrimerization of the receptor or proper interaction of the death domains with their cytoplasmic adapter proteins. Similar dominant-negative mutations have been described in other members of the TNFR family, as in mutations of the Fas antigen in the autoimmune lymphoproliferative syndrome (Mullauer et al., 2001). An additional mutation in a third family involves a nonconserved missense mutation (Arg420Gln) within the death domain. All of the mutations involving the death domain have been shown in vitro to drastically reduce NF-κB signaling (Kumar et al., 2001). Dominantly inherited mutations may have a less severe phenotype than complete loss of function seen in the X-linked or autosomal recessive forms. However, an inadequate number of families have been analyzed to form any firm conclusion about this.

EDARADD

The EDAR-associated death domain (EDARADD) protein (ectodysplasin 1, anhidrotic receptor–associated death domain) maps to chromosome 1q42.2–q43, a region syntenic with mouse chromosome 13 where one of the murine autosomal HED loci (*crinkled*) had been located. The protein is encoded by six exons and consists of 205 amino acids (Headon et al., 2001). It contains a carboxy-terminal death domain, which interacts with the intracellular death domain of the EDA receptor (EDAR). In addition, the amino terminal end contains the sequence Pro-Ile-Gln-Asp-Thr, which corresponds to a Traf interaction motif. This domain interacts in vitro with Traf1, 2, and 3, but deletion of the domain does not abolish NF-κB signaling. EDARADD is a cytoplasmic adapter protein that links the ectodysplasin receptor with downstream signaling proteins such as NF-κB (Courtois et al., 2001).

A single consanguineous family with ARHED (Muñoz et al., 1997), has been found to have a mutation in EDARADD (424G>A) (Headon et al., 2001). The phenotype seen with this recessive loss of function mutation is identical to that seen with loss of function of either the ligand or the receptor. The mutation produces a nonconservative change, substituting a lysine for a glutamic acid (E142K) within the death domain. This residue is conserved in both mouse and humans, and in vitro testing shows that the mutation greatly reduced the binding of EDARADD to EDAR.

ESTABLISHING THE DIAGNOSIS

The initial step in establishing the diagnosis of hypohidrotic ectodermal dysplasia is by careful clinical examination of all affected and at-risk individuals in the family. There is a considerable degree of inter- and intrafamilial variability in families with XLHED. The number and shape of the primary and secondary dentition should be noted, and dental records should be consulted as necessary. Affected males with XLHED are missing most of their dentition, with a mean of four primary or secondary teeth (Crawford et al., 1991; Guckes et al., 1998). Examination and classification of carrier females of XLHED is problematic. Although about 75% of carrier females will be missing one or more teeth (excluding the third molars), there is overlap with the dentition of the general population (Pinheiro et al., 1981). Knowledge of the prevalence and distribution of absent teeth in the general population is essential. Absence of the third molars cannot be counted since they are absent in 20% of the population. Although the upper lateral incisors are frequently absent in carriers, incisor-premolar hypodontia (IPH) occurs in 8% to 10% of the population. IPH may be inherited as an autosomal dominant or recessive nonsyndromic disorder (Arte et al., 2001; Pirinen et al., 2001).

Hypoplasia of the mammary glands is seen in females affected with HED, and possible carriers should be questioned about breast asymmetry or difficulties with lactation (Burck and Held, 1981; Taylor and Clugston, 1999). Due to lyonization in X-linked disorders, one cannot rule out a woman being a carrier based on a normal physical exam. Fully manifesting females can rarely be seen in X-linked recessive disorders due to extreme skewing of the otherwise usually random X inactivation pattern (Puck and Willard, 1998). Identification of the carrier status of at-risk females with XLHED is possible by physical examination, when the findings are unambiguously abnormal. Heterozygous carriers of ARHED do not have clinical manifestations.

Close examination of the nails and hair should be performed, and females should be examined for patches of alopecia, indicating possible mosaicism and X-linked inheritance. There is no simple way to examine individuals for the number or distribution of sweat pores (Berg et al., 1990). Several methods have been utilized, including starch-iodine application and thermal imaging, to detect a mosaic pattern of sweating in potential female carriers, but their clinical utility is quite limited. Skin biopsy to quantitate the number of sweat glands is unnecessary and may be misleading because of the irregularity of sweat gland distribution and the difficulty of identifying them even in skin biopsies from normal controls. A history of hypohidrosis may also be difficult to judge due to the normal variation of heat tolerance among the general population. Documentation of clinical episodes of hyperthermia is extremely helpful in the young child.

Once it has been established that an individual has a combination of hypotrichosis, hypohidrosis, and hypodontia, the disease likely falls within one of the hypohidrotic ectodermal dysplasias. Presence of additional congenital malformations that do not involve the ectodermal appendages, such as cleft palate, should make one consider other ectodermal dysplasias, including the Rapp-Hodgkin and the EEC syndromes (Rapp and Hodgkin, 1968; Celli et al., 1999).

Attention should be paid to any history of significant recurrent infections, since males may be affected with the related disorder of hypohidrotic ectodermal dysplasia with immunodeficiency (HED-ID)—also known as anhidrotic ectodermal dysplasia with immune deficiency (EDA-ID) or X-linked hyper-IGM immunodeficiency with hypohidrotic ectodermal dysplasia (XHM-ED) (Zonana et al., 2000; Aradhya et al., 2001a; Doffinger et al., 2001; Jain et al., 2001). These syndromes are allelic disorders and are due to mutations within NEMO (IKK-γ), a signaling molecule downstream of the ectodysplasin pathway that regulates NF-κB signaling (see Chapter 30). HED-ID is an X-linked disorder, and the abnormalities of hair, teeth, and eccrine sweat glands of affected males can be identical to those in individuals with XLHED, ARHED, or ADHED. The NEMO mutations in HED-ID retain some residual protein function since complete loss of function of NEMO causes prenatal lethality in affected males and causes the allelic disorder incontinentia pigmenti in females (Smahi et al., 2000; Aradhya et al., 2001b).

Since clinical manifestations are indistinguishable in fully affected individuals with XLHED, ARHED, and ADHED, one seeks help from the pedigree to establish a possible mode of inheritance. The presence of a severely affected female or consanguinity increases the likelihood of the autosomal recessive form. However, X-autosome translocations may also result in a fully affected female. In balanced X-autosome translocation carriers, the normal X chromosome is preferentially inactivated, and—if the female has signs of an X-linked condition—the assumption is that the break in the translocated X chromosome has disrupted the gene, leaving the female with no functional copy. Multiple affected females with X-autosome balanced translocations have been identified, all with breakpoints in the Xq12–q13.1 region, which disrupts the *ED1* gene (Zonana et al., 1988; Turleau et al., 1989; Limon et al., 1991; Plougastel et al., 1992; Kere et al., 1993; Thomas et al., 1993). Therefore, fully affected females should be karyotyped unless the pedigree reveals a clear mode of inheritance. Sporadic cases of HED present the greatest diagnostic difficulty. Although XLHED is the most likely diagnosis when there is an isolated affected male because of its higher frequency, a small number of these individuals will have an autosomal form of the disorder.

Molecular Testing

Molecular testing can help in diagnosing the type of HED disorders an individual is affected with, and whether females are carriers of XLHED. Sporadic females with isolated hypodontia may be carriers of XLHED, and molecular analysis of ED1 may be helpful. Since XLHED is the most common of the disorders, *ED1* should be analyzed first, unless there are indications from the pedigree of autosomal inheritance. Clinical molecular testing is available for *ED1*, and sequencing of the complete gene should detect greater than 90% of mutations in families with clear X-linked inheritance (Monreal et al., 1998). Screening by other mutation detection methods, such as SSCP, is less sensitive. Exons 3, 5, and 9 (which contain recurrent mutations) should be screened first, followed by the other exons (Monreal et al., 1998; Paakkonen et al., 2001; Schneider et al., 2001; Vincent et al., 2001). Linkage analysis can also be applied to XLHED by utilizing flanking microsatellite markers (Zonana et al., 1992). Clinical testing for *EDAR* mutations is available for cases of possible ARHED or ADHED. Exon 12 should be screened first in families with possible dominant inheritance. Clinical testing is not currently available for EDARADD because of the rarity of the disorder. As with most clinical molecular testing, inability to find a mutation in a family reduces the probability that the family has a specific form of HED, but does not eliminate it. Mutations within intronic regions or promoters may affect gene expression, and their detection would require RNA analysis.

Prenatal Diagnosis

Female carriers of XLHED have undergone prenatal diagnosis, while others have opted for testing of their newborn males for the purpose of early identification and management of the disorder. The earliest attempts at prenatal diagnosis of an affected male fetus were done by fetoscopy with the histologic analysis of multiple fetal skin biopsies (Anton-Lamprecht et al., 1982; Blanchet-Bardon and Nazzaro, 1987). However, this diagnostic technique had limitations due to its timing, availability, and the risk of the procedure to the pregnancy. The test could not be performed until well into the second trimester at 20 weeks gestation, since neither eccrine sweat glands nor hair follicles can be readily observed before that time. Prenatal diagnosis of XLHED is now possible by linkage analysis in informative families (Zonana et al., 1990), and direct DNA-based diagnostic testing of potentially affected males can be done if the mutation in the family is known. Although molecular diagnosis of carrier females is possible, the degree of clinical involvement, if any, is impossible to predict. Thus, the only useful information would be the determination of carrier status. Testing and counseling of at-risk females who are minors, including the fetus, are best deferred until reproductive age (American Society of Human Genetics Board of Directors and American College of Medical Genetics Board of Directors, 1995). Prenatal diagnosis of ADHED or ARHED is possible by molecular analysis of *EDAR* if the mutation is known.

MANAGEMENT AND COUNSELING

Undiagnosed, hypohidrotic ectodermal dysplasia can cause significant morbidity and mortality during early childhood. When it is promptly recognized and management is initiated, HED is compatible with a normal life span, lifestyle, and intelligence. The National Foundation for Ectodermal Dysplasias (NFED), a lay family support group, has produced extensive educational materials on the management of all aspects of these disorders for patients, their families, and physicians (see http://www.nfed.com).

Early identification of the disorder is of importance in ensuring that the appropriate environmental and medical measures are taken to avoid uncontrolled hyperthermia due to the lack of sweating. Mortality has been reported to be as high as 20% during infancy, presumably due to unrecognized episodes of hyperthermia (Clarke et al., 1987). Some unexplained "sudden infant deaths" in these families are likely due to undiagnosed episodes of hyperthermia. Since teeth, hair, and sweating are usually absent or scant in normal newborns, signs and symptoms of HED are usually inapparent in affected neonates, except for extensive peeling of the skin in some infants (Executive and Scientific Advisory Boards, 1989). Thus early diagnosis and treatment of the disorder is difficult, especially for sporadic cases. Affected individuals, chiefly males with XLHED, are commonly identified during infancy or early childhood because of their recurrent unexplained fevers or by absent or delayed eruption of their primary dentition.

Heat intolerance persists into later childhood and adulthood but, can be managed by environmental interventions. Fevers and hot environments should be controlled with the appropriate antipyretics or by environmental cooling measures, including air conditioning. Dry skin and eczema, frequently seen in affected individuals, should be appropriately treated. Problems of the nasal mucosa result in crusting and ozena that can be treated with the application of appropriate nasal solutions. Early and extensive dental treatment is needed throughout childhood, due to the absence of the majority of the deciduous and permanent dentition. Treatment of hypodontia should begin early in life with dentures as early as 3 years of age. Dental implants are a treatment option in older individuals (Guckes et al., 1998; Kearns et al., 1999).

A medical genetics evaluation for families with hypohidrotic ectodermal dysplasia is beneficial in establishing a specific diagnosis, ascertaining mode of inheritance, and defining recurrence risks. The presence of nonallelic genetic heterogeneity complicates counseling. In families with XLHED, affected individuals may have a prior family history of the disorder, but in many cases there is only a single affected individual. In both instances, the disorder is the result of mutations within *ED1*, but in the latter situation, a recent mutation may have occurred during oogenesis in the mother or maternal grandmother, or during spermatogenesis in the maternal grandfather (Zonana et al., 1993, 1994). Molecular testing of the affected proband, with subsequent testing of the mother if a mutation is detected, can help clarify the mother's carrier status. XLHED carriers have a 25% risk of having an affected son and a 25% risk of having a carrier daughter with each pregnancy. Affected males cannot pass the trait on to their sons, but all of their daughters are obligate carriers. The risk of having an affected male in the offspring of aunts, sisters, and daughters of an affected individual will be negligible if the condition is inherited as an autosomal recessive trait, but the risk may be as high as 25% if the trait is X linked. When no additional clues are present—such as the presence of a severely affected female or consanguinity indicating likelihood of autosomal recessive inheritance—molecular testing of ED1 and EDAR may help determine the mode of inheritance, if a clear pathogenic mutation is found.

MUTATIONS IN ORTHOLOGOUS GENES

The teeth, hair, and eccrine sweat glands are all mammalian epidermal appendages that develop by reciprocal interaction of the epithelium and mesenchyme. Analysis of the orthologous genes in the mouse played a key role in the delineation of the human ectodysplasin pathway. Mutant mice with congenital malformations of the teeth, hair, and eccrine sweat glands had been characterized and the traits mapped to three separate loci (*Ta, cr, dl*) (Sundberg, 1994). Similar to the human disorders, the affected mice from all three mutant loci were phenotypically indistinguishable from one another. Affected structures were analogous to those in humans with HED (Blecher, 1986). Affected mice have focal alopecia behind the ears and on the tail, along with an abnormal coat texture due to the absence of two of the four types of pelage hairs, the guard, and zigzag hairs. Tooth abnormalities include absent or small incisors and molars, with a lesser number of cusps. Eccrine sweat glands are present only on the footpads of mice, and they are absent or reduced in the mutant lines.

The genes from each of the murine disorders have been cloned, and they correspond to the known loci in the human ectodsyplasin pathway *Ta/Eda* (Ferguson et al., 1997; Srivastava et al., 1997), *dl/Edar* (Headon and Overbeek, 1999), and *cr/Edaradd* (Headon et al., 2001). The murine proteins have a very high degree of amino acid sequence conservation when compared to their human orthologs. The amino acid identity is 94% for ED1/Eda, 91% for EDAR/Edar, and 80% for EDARADD/Edaradd. The identity of the residues approaches 100% within the known critical functional domains.

The scales of fish and the feathers of birds are additional examples of epidermal appendages in vertebrates (Chuong et al., 2001; Sharpe, 2001). Although fish scales and mammalian hair have somewhat analogous functions, they have dissimilar biochemical compositions and structural forms. The ectodysplasin pathway appears to have a similar role in the developing integument of both mammals and fish during the initiation and patterning of epidermal appendage formation (Kondo et al., 2001). This evolutionary conservation is similar to the developmental role of Pax6 during eye development in *Drosophila* and mammals, even though the structures themselves are dissimilar (Quiring et al., 1994).

ED1

The *Tabby* and human *ED1* loci mapped to regions of known synteny on the X chromosomes of each species. Although *ED1* was identified by positional cloning in the human (Kere et al., 1996), the initial splice form identified (Eda-O) was incomplete and missed most of the extracellular domain, including the TNF-binding domain. Only by the isolation of the murine ortholog were the larger biologically active isoforms (EDA-A1 and A2) identified (Ferguson et al., 1997; Srivastava et al., 1997). The Eda-O splice form has not been detected in the mouse. The disorder of hypohidrotic ectodermal dysplasia has been observed in dogs and cows, where it is also inherited as an X-linked recessive trait (Casal et al., 1997; Drogemuller et al., 2001). The bovine *ED1* gene is highly conserved in comparison to that in the human and mouse sequence, and affected cattle have a deletion of exon 3 (Drogemuller et al., 2001). The genome sequence database for the pufferfish *Fugu rubripes* (http://fugu.hgmp.mrc.ac.uk/PFW/) argues for the conservation of the ectodysplasin gene among other nonmammalian vertebrates.

EDAR

An autosomal locus in the mouse (*downless*), with an HED phenotype, was positionally cloned and found to code for the ectodysplasin receptor (EDAR) (Headon et al., 2001). Abnormal alleles in the mouse can produce both autosomal recessive and dominant HED. This is analogous to mutations in human *EDAR*. The mutation of the dominant allele of the *downless sleek* mouse (*Dl^{slk}*) truncates the intracellular domain of the receptor prior to the death domain. This is a dominant-negative mechanism analogous to the mutations detected in human ADHED.

Of evolutionary interest, a spontaneous mutant, reduced scale-3 (*rs3*) in the teleost fish medaka (*Oryzias latipes*), lacks scales. This recessive trait was mapped to a linkage group syntenic to human chromosome 2, and investigators were able to clone an ortholog with 56% amino acid identity to human *EDAR* (Kondo et al., 2001). The mutant allele had a transposon insertion within intron 1 and led to abnormal splicing and lack of *EDAR* production. *EDAR* was expressed in wild-type fish during early stages of scale development. The embryonic pattern of *EDAR* expression in the epithelium during scale placode development shows a pattern identical to that seen in the mouse epithelium during hair follicle formation. An *EDAR* ortholog is also predicted in the pufferfish *Fugu rubripes*.

EDARADD

The murine mutant *crinkled* is the ortholog of the gene coding for the human ectodysplasin receptor–associated death domain protein. Its positional cloning led to identification of the human gene. The only known mutant allele in the mouse was detected in the progeny of a male mouse that had been treated with nitrogen mustard. The murine locus is on chromosome 13, and the *cr* mutation is caused by a complete genomic deletion of the *Edaradd* gene (Headon et al., 2001).

DEVELOPMENTAL PATHOGENESIS

The teeth, hair, and eccrine sweat glands are all mammalian epidermal appendages that initially develop by reciprocal interaction of the epithelium and mesenchyme. All of the appendages go through similar sequential stages of induction, morphogenesis, and differentiation (Chuong and Noveen, 1999; Chuong et al., 2001). Some appendages, such as mammalian hair, have continued cycles of cell death and regeneration throughout adult life, and thus they maintain a stem cell population (Fuchs et al., 2001). The proteins of the ectodysplasin pathway continue to be expressed in the mature hair follicle, and pathway defects may be responsible for the premature balding seen in HED. The proteins EDA, EDAR, and EDARADD are all expressed in epithelial but not mesenchymal cells of the developing hair follicle and tooth. EDAR and EDARADD are coexpressed in the same subset of epithelial cells (Headon et al., 2001), while EDA is expressed in the alternate cells, thus creating a reciprocal pattern of epithelial cell expression (Tucker et al., 2000; Laurikkala et al., 2001). This would indicate that the mode of action of the ligand is not autocrine in nature but is likely juxtacrine or paracrine. The processed and secreted form of the ligand is essential for normal morphogenesis (Chen et al., 2001b).

At what stage of appendage development are the defects seen in HED most likely to occur? Defects in the appendages are variable both in any one individual and between individuals. The defects range from complete absence of a structure—indicating a likely defect in the early stages of epithelial or mesenchymal induction—to hypoplasia or dysplasia, as in a conical tooth. These latter defects are more likely to be due to a defect in cellular proliferation or differentiation. It is still unknown whether the pathogenesis of the defects in teeth, hair follicle and eccrine sweat glands are identical. Data from the mouse suggest that defects in the ectodysplasin pathway may affect hair follicle and teeth at different developmental stages. Tooth morphogenesis in the mouse is initiated by signals from the early oral epithelium (E9–11) to the underlying mesenchyme. Stages include thickening of the oral epithelium progressing to the bud, cap, and bell stages (Thesleff, 2000). The enamel knot, an epithelial signaling center that expresses at least 10 signaling molecules, first appears at the tip of the tooth bud and is fully developed by the cap stage. The enamel knot subsequently disappears by apoptosis.

Ed1 transcripts are observed at E10 in the simple epithelium that covers the mandibular arch before tooth bud formation (Tucker et al., 2000; Laurikkala et al., 2001). Eda expression is intense in the basal cells of the tooth bud except in the area of the developing enamel knot. At the cap stage E14, Eda expression is intense in the outer enamel epithelium and persists into the bell stage and postnatally. Edar expression is absent until the initiation of tooth development at E11 in the budding epithelial cells, and its expression is then restricted to the enamel knot throughout the cap stage (E14). The enamel knot is either hypoplastic or abnormally spread out (or both) in the developing teeth of *Tabby* and *downless* mice. However, expression of all of the usual signaling molecules by the hypoplastic enamel knot is normal (Tucker and Sharpe, 1999). The EDA pathway is not visibly involved in the early induction of tooth development during murine tooth development, but likely it is needed for the proliferation and survival of the cells of the enamel knot. The in vitro administration of various signaling molecules in tooth explant cultures suggests that expression of Wnt6 in epithelial cells may up-regulate Eda expression and that mesenchymal expression of activinβA may up-regulate Edar expression in adjoining epithelial cells (Laurikkala et al., 2001).

Human hair follicles begin to form at 80 days estimated gestational age (EGA), and proliferation and differentiation continues during the second trimester (Holbrook, 1988; Holbrook and Minami, 1991). Eccrine sweat gland anlagen appear on the volar surfaces of the body at 3 to 4 months EGA and elsewhere during the fifth month of gestation. Minimal data exist as to the expression patterns of EDA during human embryonic and fetal development. EDA expression was detected in a study of human fetal tissues in the epidermis at 8 weeks EGA and at 18 weeks EGA in hair follicles (Montonen et al., 1998). EDA expression was not limited to the skin and its appendages but was also seen in osteoblasts, thymus, and neuroectoderm, even though these cells and organs are not obviously affected in these disorders. Ectodysplasin is expressed postnatally in the epidermis, in the eccrine sweat glands, and in the epithelial cells of the matrix and outer root sheath of hair follicles. No signal is present in the dermis or in the dermal papilla of the hair follicle (Kere et al., 1996). The role of the ectodysplasin pathway in hair follicle development is well described in the mouse. EDAR expression is uniformly present in the basal cells of the epidermis before follicle initiation (E13) (Headon and Overbeek, 1999). Expression is then up-regulated at the sites in the epidermis where hair follicles will form, prior to the morphological appearance of the placodes (E15). It is simultaneously down-regulated in the epithelial cells that surround the sites of future hair follicles. Thus, *EDAR* signaling is required at the very earliest stages of hair follicle induction, and lateral inhibition of its expression may have a role in hair follicle patterning. Unlike the focal pattern of expression of EDAR at the sites of future hair placode formation, Eda is initially expressed at low levels in fetal epidermis but is then down-regulated in the developing cells of the hair follicle placode (Montonen et al., 1998).

During hair follicle development, Sonic hedgehog (Shh) is normally expressed at E15 in epidermal cells, and bone morphogenic protein 4 (Bmp4) is expressed in the preplacode clusters of mesenchymal cells. In *downless* mice that lack EDAR function, neither *Shh* nor *Bmp4* expression is detected at E15 (Headon and Overbeek, 1999). Shh is a key signaling molecule in hair follicle formation, and the data suggest that its expression is downstream of the EDA signaling pathway. β-Catenin expression has also been shown to be essential for hair placode development, but mutants with loss of β-catenin function express normal levels of *EDAR*. Therefore, β-catenin is genetically downstream of *EDA/EDAR* and has been shown to be upstream of *bmp* and *shh* during follicle placode formation (Huelsken et al., 2001). β-Catenin function is also essential for the differentiation of stem cells into follicular keratinocytes in the postnatal hair follicle cycle. How this relates to a possible role of the EDA pathway in the postnatal hair cycle is undetermined.

Stimulation of the ectodysplasin pathway in vitro by ligand binding to its receptor results in activation of NF-κB (Yan et al., 2000;

Kumar et al., 2001). The NF-κB/Rel family is a group of transcriptional activators, employed by multiple signaling pathways, to induce the expression of a large number of genes that are involved in cell survival, proliferation, and host defense. The activators of NF-κB, as well as the genes induced by it, are specific to tissue and context. NF-κB is composed of hetero- and homodimers of a group of related proteins (p50, p65, p52, Rel, and RelB) that are sequestered by the cytoplasmic IκB proteins (Chen et al., 2001a). Upon activation of the EDA pathway, NF-κB is translocated from the cytoplasm to the nucleus by the phosphorylation and subsequent degradation of the IκB proteins by the IKK complex (Israel, 2000). IKKγ (NEMO), part of the IKK complex, is mutated in HED-ID, and the complex is utilized for signaling by other pathways, including CD40 and RANK. Defective signaling of these latter pathways is likely responsible for the immunodeficiency and occasional osteopetrosis seen in HED-ID (Zonana et al., 2000; Doffinger et al., 2001; Jain et al., 2001).

NF-κB translocation to the nucleus can be blocked in vivo by the expression of a superrepressor of NF-κB activation, a mutant form of IκB that cannot be phosphorylated. When the superrepressor was inserted transgenically in mice, it produced defects of the ectodermal appendages identical to those seen in *Eda (Tabby)* and *Edar (downless)* mutant mice (Schmidt-Ullrich et al., 2001). Although inhibition of NF-κB function appeared to increase cellular apoptosis in the developing hair follicle, increased apoptosis has not been observed in the developing hair follicles or teeth of mutant *Eda* or *Edar* mice.

None of the downstream genes stimulated by the EDA pathway are currently known, and their discovery awaits expression analyses in wild-type and mutant tissues and cells. The EDA pathway may well utilize additional signaling pathways such as the c-Jun pathway, although the data for c-Jun involvement are unclear. The disruption of the NF-κB pathway alone appears sufficient to cause all of the structural defects seen with loss of EDA ligand or receptor function. The anomalies seen in HED are due to functional defects at various stages of development, including problems of induction of the hair follicle, or of proliferation and cell survival, as seen during tooth development in the enamel knot.

REFERENCES

American Society of Human Genetics Board of Directors and American College of Medical Genetics Board of Directors (1995). Points to consider: ethical, legal, and psychosocial implications of genetic testing in children and adolescents. *Am J Hum Genet* 57: 1233–1241.

Anton-Lamprecht I, Arnold M, Rauskolb R, Schinzel A, Schmid W, Schnyder U (1982). Prenatal diagnosis of anhidrotic ectodemal dysplasia. *Hum Genet* 62: 180.

Aradhya S, Courtois G, Rajkovic A, Lewis R, Levy M, Israel A, Nelson D (2001a). Atypical forms of incontinentia pigmenti in male individuals result from mutations of a cytosine tract in exon 10 of NEMO (IKK-γ). *Am J Hum Genet* 68: 765–771.

Aradhya S, Woffendin H, Jakins T, Bardaro B, Esposito T, Smahi A, Shaw C, Levy M, Munnich A, D'Urso M, et al. (2001b). A recurrent deletion in the ubiquitously expressed *NEMO* (IKK-γ) gene accounts for the vast majority of incontinentia pigmenti mutations. *Hum Mol Genet* 10: 2171–2179.

Arte S, Nieminen P, Apajalahti S, Haavikko K, Thesleff I, Pirinen S (2001). Characteristics of incisor-premolar hypodontia in families. *J Dent Res* 80: 1445–1450.

Aswegan AL, Josephson KD, Mowbray R, Pauli RM, Spritz RA, Williams MS (1997). Autosomal dominant hypohidrotic ectodermal dysplasia in a large family. *Am J Med Genet* 72: 462–467.

Baud V, Karin M (2001). Signal transduction by tumor necrosis factor and its relatives. *Trends Cell Biol* 11: 372–377.

Bayes M, Hartung AJ, Ezer S, Pispa J, Thesleff I, Srivastava AK, Kere J (1998). The anhidrotic ectodermal dysplasia gene (*EDA*) undergoes alternative splicing and encodes ectodysplasin-A with deletion mutations in collagenous repeats. *Hum Mol Genet* 7: 1661–1669.

Berg D, Weingold DH, Abson KG, Olsen EA (1990). Sweating in ectodermal dysplasia syndromes: a review. *Arch Dermatol* 126: 1075–1079.

Blanchet-Bardon C, Nazzaro V (1987). Use of morphological markers in carriers as an aid in genetic counseling and prenatal diagnosis. *Curr Probl Dermatol* 16: 109–119.

Blecher SR (1986). Anhidrosis and absence of sweat glands in mice hemizygous for the Tabby gene: supportive evidence for the hypothesis of homology between *Tabby* and human anhidrotic (hypohidrotic) ectodermal dysplasia (Christ-Siemens-Touraine syndrome). *J Invest Dermatol* 87: 720–722.

Bodmer JL, Schneider P, Tschopp J (2002). The molecular architecture of the TNF superfamily. *Trends Biochem Sci* 27: 19–26.

Burck U, Held KR (1981). Athelia in a female infant heterozygous for anhidrotic ectodermal dysplasia. *Clin Genet* 19: 117–121.

Casal ML, Jezyk PF, Greek JM, Goldschmidt MH, Patterson DF (1997). X-linked ectodermal dysplasia in the dog. *J Hered* 88: 513–517.

Celli J, Duijf P, Hamel BC, Bamshad M, Kramer B, Smits AP, Newbury-Ecob R, Hennekam RC, Van Buggenhout G, van Haeringen A, et al. (1999). Heterozygous germline mutations in the p53 homolog *p63* are the cause of EEC syndrome. *Cell* 99: 143–153.

Chen F, Castranova V, Shi X (2001a). New insights into the role of nuclear factor-κB in cell growth regulation. *Am J Pathol* 159: 387–397.

Chen Y, Molloy SS, Thomas L, Gambee J, Bachinger HP, Ferguson B, Zonana J, Thomas G, Morris NP (2001b). Mutations within a furin consensus sequence block proteolytic release of ectodysplasin-A and cause X-linked hypohidrotic ectodermal dysplasia. *Proc Natl Acad Sci USA* 98: 7218–7223.

Chuong CM, Noveen A (1999). Phenotypic determination of epithelial appendages: genes, developmental pathways, and evolution. *J Investig Dermatol Symp Proc* 4: 307–311.

Chuong CM, Hou I, Chen PI, Wu P, Patel N, Chen Y (2001). Dinosaur's feather and chicken's tooth? Tissue engineering of the integument. *Eur J Dermatol* 11: 286–292.

Clarke A, Burn J (1991). Sweat testing to identify female carriers of X linked hypohidrotic ectodermal dysplasia. *J Med Genet* 28: 330–333.

Clarke A, Phillips DJ, Brown R, Harper PS (1987). Clinical aspects of X-linked hypohidrotic ectodermal dysplasia. *Arch Dis Child* 62: 989–996.

Courtois G, Smahi A, Israel A (2001). NEMO/IKK γ: linking NF-κB to human disease. *Trends Mol Med* 7: 427–430.

Crawford PJM, Aldred MJ, Clarke A (1991). Clinical and radiographic dental findings in X linked hypohidrotic ectodermal dysplasia. *J Med Genet* 28: 181–185.

Doffinger R, Smahi A, Bessia C, Geissmann F, Feinberg J, Durandy A, Bodemer C, Kenwrick S, Dupuis-Girod S, Blanche S, et al. (2001). X-linked anhidrotic ectodermal dysplasia with immunodeficiency is caused by impaired NF-κB signaling. *Nat Genet* 27: 277–285.

Drogemuller C, Distl O, Leeb T (2001). Partial deletion of the bovine *ED1* gene causes anhidrotic ectodermal dysplasia in cattle. *Genome Res* 11: 1699–1705.

Elomaa O, Pulkkinen K, Hannelius U, Mikkola M, Saarialho-Kere U, Kere J (2001). Ectodysplasin is released by proteolytic shedding and binds to the EDAR protein. *Hum Mol Genet* 10: 953–962.

Executive and Scientific Advisory Boards of the National Foundation for Ectodermal Dysplasias (1989). Scaling skin in the neonate: a clue to the early diagnosis of X-linked hypohidrotic ectodermal dysplasia (Christ-Siemens-Touraine syndrome). *J Pediatr* 114: 600–602.

Ezer S, Bayes M, Elomaa O, Schlessinger D, Kere J (1999). Ectodysplasin is a collagenous trimeric type II membrane protein with a tumor necrosis factor–like domain and co-localizes with cytoskeletal structures at lateral and apical surfaces of cells. *Hum Mol Genet* 8: 2079–2086.

Ferguson BM, Brockdorff N, Formstone E, Ngyuen T, Kronmiller JE, Zonana J (1997). Cloning of *Tabby*, the murine homolog of the human *EDA* gene: evidence for a membrane-associated protein with a short collagenous domain. *Hum Mol Genet* 6: 1589–1594.

Fuchs E, Merrill BJ, Jamora C, DasGupta R (2001). At the roots of a never-ending cycle. *Dev Cell* 1: 13–25.

Gorlin RJ, Old T, Anderson VE (1970). Hypohidrotic ectodermal dysplasia in females: a critical analysis and argument for genetic heterogeneity. *Z Kinderheilkd* 108: 1–11.

Guckes AD, Roberts MW, McCarthy GR (1998). Pattern of permanent teeth present in individuals with ectodermal dysplasia and severe hypodontia suggests treatment with dental implants. *Pediatr Dent* 20: 278–280.

Headon DJ, Overbeek PA (1999). Involvement of a novel Tnf receptor homologue in hair follicle induction. *Nat Genet* 22: 370–374.

Headon DJ, Emmal SA, Ferguson BM, Tucker AS, Justice MJ, Sharpe PT, Zonana J, Overbeek PA (2001). Gene defect in ectodermal dysplasia implicates a death domain adapter in development. *Nature* 414: 913–916.

Holbrook KA (1988). Structural abnormalities of the epidermally derived appendages in skin from patients with ectodermal dysplasia: insight into developmental errors. *Birth Defects* 24: 15–44.

Holbrook KA, Minami SI (1991). Hair follicle embryogenesis in the human: characterization of events in vivo and in vitro. *Ann NY Acad Sci* 642: 167–196.

Huelsken J, Vogel R, Erdmann B, Cotsarelis G, Birchmeier W (2001). β-Catenin controls hair follicle morphogenesis and stem cell differentiation in the skin. *Cell* 105: 533–545.

Israel A (2000). The IKK complex: an integrator of all signals that activate NF-κB? *Trends Cell Biol* 10: 129–133.

Jain A, Ma CA, Liu S, Brown M, Cohen J, Strober W (2001). Specific missense mutations in *NEMO* result in hyper-IgM syndrome with hypohydrotic ectodermal dysplasia. *Nat Immunol* 2: 223–228.

Jorgenson RJ, Dowben JS, Dowben SL (1987). Autosomal dominant ectodermal dysplasia. *J Craniofac Genet Dev Biol* 7: 403–412.

Kearns G, Sharma A, Perrott D, Schmidt B, Kaban L, Vargervik K (1999). Placement of endosseous implants in children and adolescents with hereditary ectodermal dysplasia. *Oral Surg Oral Med Oral Pathol Oral Radiol Endod* 88: 5–10.

Kere J, Grzeschik KH, Limon J, Gremaud M, Schlessinger D, de la Chapelle A (1993). Anhidrotic ectodermal dysplasia gene region cloned in yeast artificial chromosomes. *Genomics* 16: 305–310.

Kere J, Srivastava AK, Montonen O, Zonana J, Thomas N, Ferguson B, Munoz F, Morgan D, Clarke A, Baybayan P, et al. (1996). X-linked anhidrotic (hypohidrotic) ectodermal dysplasia is caused by mutation in a novel transmembrane protein. *Nat Genet* 13: 409–416.

Kondo S, Kuwahara Y, Kondo M, Naruse K, Mitani H, Wakamatsu Y, Ozato K, Asakawa S, Shimizu N, Shima A (2001). The medaka *rs-3* locus required for scale development encodes ectodysplasin-A receptor. *Curr Biol* 11: 1202–1206.

Kumar A, Eby MT, Sinha S, Jasmin A, Chaudhary PM (2001). The ectodermal dysplasia receptor activates the nuclear factor-κB, JNK, and cell death pathways and binds to ectodysplasin A. *J Biol Chem* 276: 2668–2677.

Laurikkala J, Mikkola M, Mustonen T, Aberg T, Koppinen P, Pispa J, Nieminen P, Galceran J, Grosschedl R, Thesleff I (2001). TNF signaling via the ligand–receptor pair ectodysplasin and edar controls the function of epithelial signaling centers and is regulated by Wnt and activin during tooth organogenesis. *Dev Biol* 229: 443–455.

Limon J, Filipiuk J, Nedoszytko B, Mrozek K, Castren M, Larramendy M, Roszkiewicz J (1991). X-linked anhidrotic ectodermal dysplasia and de novo t(X;1) in a female. *Hum Genet* 87: 338–340.

Locksley RM, Killeen N, Lenardo MJ (2001). The TNF and TNF receptor superfamilies: integrating mammalian biology. *Cell* 104: 487–501.

Mikkola ML, Pispa J, Pekkanen M, Paulin L, Nieminen P, Kere J, Thesleff I (1999). Ectodysplasin, a protein required for epithelial morphogenesis, is a novel TNF homologue and promotes cell-matrix adhesion. *Mech Dev* 88: 133–146.

Monreal AW, Zonana J, Ferguson B (1998). Identification of a new splice form of the *EDA1* gene permits detection of nearly all X-linked hypohidrotic ectodermal dysplasia mutations. *Am J Hum Genet* 63: 380–389. [published erratum appears in *Am J Hum Genet* 1998 63(4):1253–1255].

Monreal AW, Ferguson BM, Headon DJ, Street SL, Overbeek PA, Zonana J (1999). Mutations in the human homologue of mouse *dl* cause autosomal recessive and dominant hypohidrotic ectodermal dysplasia. *Nat Genet* 22: 366–369.

Montonen O, Ezer S, Saarialho-Kere UK, Herva R, Karjalainen-Lindsberg ML, Kaitila I, Schlessinger D, Srivastava SK, Thesleff I, Kere J (1998). The gene defective in anhidrotic ectodermal dysplasia is expressed in the developing epithelium, neuroectoderm, thymus, and bone. *J Histochem Cytochem* 46: 281–289.

Mullauer L, Gruber P, Sebinger D, Buch J, Wohlfart S, Chott A (2001). Mutations in apoptosis genes: a pathogenetic factor for human disease. *Mutat Res* 488: 211–231.

Muñoz F, Lestringant G, Sybert V, Frydman M, Alswaini A, Frossard PM, Jorgenson R, Zonana J (1997). Definitive evidence for an autosomal recessive form of hypohidrotic ectodermal dysplasia clinically indistinguishable from the more common X-linked disorder. *Am J Hum Genet* 61: 94–100.

Nakata M, Koshiba H, Eto K, Nance WE (1980). A genetic study of anodontia in X-linked hypohidrotic ectodermal dysplasia. *Am J Hum Genet* 32: 908–919.

Paakkonen K, Cambiaghi S, Novelli G, Ouzts LV, Penttinen M, Kere J, Srivastava AK (2001). The mutation spectrum of the *EDA* gene in X-linked anhidrotic ectodermal dysplasia. *Hum Mutat* 17: 349.

Pinheiro M, Freire-Maia N (1994). Ectodermal dysplasias: a clinical classification and a causal review. *Am J Med Genet* 53: 153–162.

Pinheiro M, Ideriha M, Chautard-Freire-Maia E, Freire-Maia N, Primo-Parmo S (1981). Christ-Siemens-Touraine syndrome: investigations on two large Brazilian kindreds with a new estimate of the manifestation rate among carriers. *Hum Genet* 57: 428–431.

Pirinen S, Kentala A, Nieminen P, Varilo T, Thesleff I, Arte S (2001). Recessively inherited lower incisor hypodontia. *J Med Genet* 38: 551–556.

Plougastel B, Couillin P, Blanquet V, Le Guern E, Bakker E, Turleau C, De Grouchy J, Creau-Goldberg N (1992). Mapping around the Xq13.1 breakpoints of two X/A translocations in hypohidrotic ectodermal dysplasia (EDA) female patients. *Genomics* 14: 523–525.

Puck JM, Willard HF (1998). X inactivation in females with X-linked disease. *N Engl J Med* 338: 325–328.

Quiring R, Walldorf U, Kloter U, Gehring WJ (1994). Homology of the eyeless gene of *Drosophila* to the *Small eye* gene in mice and *Aniridia* in humans. *Science* 265: 785–789.

Rapp RS, Hodgkin WE (1968). Anhidrotic ectodermal dysplasia: autosomal dominant inheritance with palate and lip anomalies. *J Med Genet* 5: 269–272.

Schmidt-Ullrich R, Aebischer T, Hulsken J, Birchmeier W, Klemm U, Scheidereit C (2001). Requirement of NF-κB/Rel for the development of hair follicles and other epidermal appendices. *Development* 128: 3843–3853.

Schneider P, Street SL, Gaide O, Hertig S, Tardivel A, Tschopp J, Runkel L, Alevizopoulos K, Ferguson BM, Zonana J (2001). Mutations leading to X-linked hypohidrotic ectodermal dysplasia affect three major functional domains in the TNF family member EDA. *J Biol Chem* 14: 14.

Sharpe PT (2001). Fish scale development: hair today, teeth and scales yesterday? *Curr Biol* 11: R751–752.

Smahi A, Courtois G, Vabres P, Yamaoka S, Heuertz S, Munnich A, Israel A, Heiss NS, Klauck SM, Kioschis P, et al. (2000). Genomic rearrangement in *NEMO* impairs NF-κB activation and is a cause of incontinentia pigmenti. *Nature* 405: 466–472.

Srivastava AK, Pispa J, Hartung AJ, Du Y, Ezer S, Jenks T, Shimada T, Pekkanen M, Mikkola ML, Ko MS, et al. (1997). The Tabby phenotype is caused by mutation in a mouse homologue of the *EDA* gene that reveals novel mouse and human exons and encodes a protein (ectodysplasin-A) with collagenous domains. *Proc Natl Acad Sci USA* 94: 13069–13074.

Srivastava AK, Durmowicz MC, Hartung AJ, Hudson J, Ouzts LV, Donovan DM, Cui CY, Schlessinger D (2001). Ectodysplasin-A1 is sufficient to rescue both hair growth and sweat glands in *Tabby* mice. *Hum Mol Genet* 10: 2973–2981.

Sundberg JP (1994). Handbook of mouse mutations with skin and hair abnormalities. Animal models and biomedical tools. In *Dermatology: Clinical and Basic Science*. Maibach HI (ed.) CRC Press, Boca Raton, pp. 221–230, 241–246, 455–462.

Taylor CD, Clugston PA (1999). Breast reconstruction in ectodermal dysplasia. *Ann Plast Surg* 43: 36–41.

Thesleff I (2000). Genetic basis of tooth development and dental defects. *Acta Odontol Scand* 58: 191–194.

Thomas NST, Chelly J, Zonana J, Davies KJP, Morgan S, Gault J, Rack KA, Buckle VJ, Brockdorff N, Clarke A, Monaco A (1993). Characterisation of molecular DNA rearrangements within the Xq12–q13.1 region, in three patients with X-linked hypohidrotic ectodermal dysplasia (EDA). *Hum Mol Genet* 2: 1679–1685.

Tucker AS, Sharpe PT (1999). Molecular genetics of tooth morphogenesis and patterning: the right shape in the right place. *J Dent Res* 78: 826–834.

Tucker AS, Headon DJ, Schneider P, Ferguson BM, Overbeek P, Tschopp J, Sharpe PT (2000). Edar/Eda interactions regulate enamel knot formation in tooth morphogenesis. *Development* 127: 4691–4700.

Turleau C, Niaudet P, Cabanis MO, Plessis G, Cau D, de Grouchy J (1989). X-linked hypohidrotic ectodermal dysplasia and t(X;12) in a female. *Clin Genet* 35: 462–466.

Vincent MC, Biancalana V, Ginisty D, Mandel JL, Calvas P (2001). Mutational spectrum of the *ED1* gene in X-linked hypohidrotic ectodermal dysplasia. *Eur J Hum Genet* 9: 355–363.

Weber CH, Vincenz C (2001). The death domain superfamily: a tale of two interfaces? *Trends Biochem Sci* 26: 475–481.

Yan M, Wang LC, Hymowitz SG, Schilbach S, Lee J, Goddard A, de Vos AM, Gao WQ, Dixit VM (2000). Two-amino acid molecular switch in an epithelial morphogen that regulates binding to two distinct receptors. *Science* 290: 523–527.

Zonana J, Roberts SH, Thomas NS, Harper PS (1988). Recognition and reanalysis of a cell line from a manifesting female with X linked hypohidrotic ectodermal dysplasia and an X; autosome balanced translocation. *J Med Genet* 25: 383–386.

Zonana J, Schinzel A, Upadhyaya M, Thomas NS, Anton-Lamprecht I, Harper PS (1990). Prenatal diagnosis of X-linked hypohidrotic ectodermal dysplasia by linkage analysis. *Am J Med Genet* 35: 132–135.

Zonana J, Jones M, Browne D, Litt M, Kramer P, Becker HW, Brockdorff N, Rastan S, Davies KP, Clarke A, et al. (1992). High-resolution mapping of the X-linked hypohidrotic ectodermal dysplasia (*EDA*) locus. *Am J Hum Genet* 51: 1036–1046.

Zonana J, Jones M, Clarke A, Gault J, Muller B, Thomas NS (1994). Detection of de novo mutations and analysis of their origin in families with X linked hypohidrotic ectodermal dysplasia. *J Med Genet* 31: 287–292.

Zonana J, Elder ME, Schneider LC, Orlow SJ, Moss C, Golabi M, Shapira SK, Farndon PA, Wara DW, Emmal SA, Ferguson BM (2000). A novel X-linked disorder of immune deficiency and hypohidrotic ectodermal dysplasia is allelic to incontinentia pigmenti and due to mutations in IKK-γ (NEMO). *Am J Hum Genet* 67: 1555–1562.

Part E.
The Fibroblast Growth Factor Signaling Pathway

32 | Molecular and Cellular Biology of FGF Signaling

DAVID GIVOL, VERARAGAVAN P. ESWARAKUMAR, AND PETER LONAI

COMPONENTS OF THE FGF SYSTEM

The FGF Ligands

To date, 23 mammalian fibroblast growth factors (FGFs) are known. The first was discovered in the 1970s as a mitogen that can stimulate the growth of fibroblasts (Gospodarowicz, 1974). The FGFs range in size between 17 and 34 kDa in vertebrates, and they share a conserved core region of 120 amino acids that show 40% to 60% identity. Their most important common property is the binding of heparan sulfate proteoglycan (HSPG) and high affinity for the glycosaminoglycan heparin (Burgess and Maciag, 1989). This property served as the basis for methods to purify the various FGFs, and, as will be shown later, the binding of heparan sulfate is required for signaling by FGF (for a recent review, see Ornitz and Itoh, 2001). FGFs are present also in invertebrates. *Drosophila* has only one FGF (*branchless*), and *C. elegans* has two FGFs (*egl*-17 and *let*-756), suggesting extensive gene duplication during vertebrate development (Coulier et al., 1997).

The multiplicity of functions of FGFs is reflected in their tissue localization and temporal expression. Some of these proteins are expressed only during embryonal development (FGF3, 4, 8, 15, 17, and 19), whereas others (FGF1, 2, 5–7, 9–14, 16, 18, 20–23) are expressed in embryonic and adult tissues. All FGFs are found in the extracellular matrix (ECM); FGF3–8, 10, 15, 17–19, and 21–23 have signal peptides and are secreted proteins. Although they have no definable signal peptides, FGF9, 16, and 20 are still secreted, whereas FGF1 and 2, which are found bound to the ECM, seem to be released either by damaged cells or by an exocytic mechanism (Mignatti et al., 1992). FGF1 is also known as acidic FGF (aFGF) and FGF2 as basic FGF (bFGF), and they were used in most studies as the prototype of FGF. FGF1 is a universal ligand, which binds to all FGF receptors (FGFR).

The expression pattern of FGFs indicates their importance in early embryonal development and in organogenesis—in particular, in limb, lung, bone, and brain development. In some organs (e.g., limb) it was shown that FGFs signal across epithelial–mesenchymal boundaries in a vectorial way, and different FGFs (e.g., FGF8 and 10) form a reciprocal loop in organizing the limb development. This requires delicate control of the specificity and affinity between different FGFs and their receptors.

The diversity of FGF functions has also been probed by gene targeting and spontaneous mutations. Gene disruption (knockout) has been performed with 15 FGF genes. Knockouts of six FGFs were lethal (FGF4, 8–10, 15, and 18), whereas various defects were found in the viable mutants. In mouse the angora (hair growth) mutation is allelic to FGF5, and in humans the mutation of FGF23 caused hypophosphatemic rickets (ADHR), which is characterized by short stature, bone pain, deformation of lower extremities, and dental abscesses.

FGF Structure and Heparin Binding

The structure of several FGFs (FGF1, FGF2, FGF4, and FGF9) was determined by X-ray crystallography, some in complexes with sulfated oligosaccharides (for review, see Faham et al., 1998). This helped identify the heparan sulfate (HS–binding residues in FGF (Fig. 32–1). The structure of FGF contains four-stranded β sheets arranged in a triangular array to form a β trefoil structure, which consists of three copies of a basic four-stranded antiparallel β sheet (Zhu et al., 1991; Faham et al., 1998). Several basic amino acids in the loop between β strands 10 and 11 (Arg120, Lys125, Gln134, Lys135) and the loop between strands 1 and 2 (Lys26 and Asn27), form the heparan-binding site in FGF2 (Faham et al., 1998; Plotnikov et al., 1999). Crystal structure of FGF and HS show dimers of FGFs in *trans* orientation that are stabilized by the sulfated octosaccharide chain (DiGabriele et al., 1998). It should be noted, however, that this orientation is not reflected in FGF dimers in the ternary complex formed between the FGF receptor, FGF, and HS (Schlessinger et al., 2000). Rather, the HS forms a bridge between FGF and FGFR. It appears that FGF interacts with two types of receptors on the cell surface. One is the low-affinity receptor HSPG ($\sim 10^{-9}$ Kd), and the second group contains the high-affinity membrane-bound FGF receptors ($\sim 10^{-11}$ K_d). The interaction between FGFs and the two classes of receptors in relation to signaling into the cell was a puzzle for many years and the subject of many investigations (Ornitz, 2000). This puzzle was solved to a large extent by a recent crystallization and structure determination of the FGF : HS : FGFR complex.

Heparin has long been recognized as necessary for efficient signal transduction by FGFs in cells (Klagsbrun, 1990). Cells deficient in HSPG will respond to FGF only after the addition of heparin (Rapraeger et al., 1991; Yayon et al., 1991). Heparan sulfates are long polymers of repeating disaccharides consisting of L-iduronic acid (IdoA) (or D-glucuronic acid) and D-glucosamine (GlcN) joined by α 1–4 linkages, which are covalently linked to a core protein and located in the extracellular matrix. The disaccharide subunit can undergo sulfation at three positions—one at the 2-O of IdoA, and two at the O-6 and 2-NH2 of GlcN (Fig. 32–2). These sulfate groups are essential for the binding to the positive amino acids in FGFs, as well as in FGFRs, and are required for binding and signaling in cells. Heparin

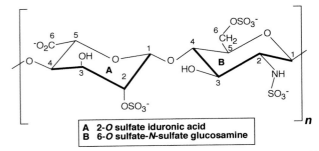

Figure 32–2. Structure of the repeating disaccharide unit of heparan sulfate with O- and N-sulfate groups.

is a type of heparan sulfate made by mast cells that has the highest amount of iduronic acid and N- and O-sulfate residues. Quantitative variations in the extent of sulfation influence the affinity of HS to FGF. The binding specificity of HSPG by different FGFs may play an important role in signaling by FGF since large tissue variation in the extent of O-sulfation was found. It is suggested that some of the activity of FGFs depends on the local concentration of HS and its extent of sulfation.

FGF Receptors: Isoforms and Alternative Splicing Variants

Despite the importance of HSPG and HS in regulating FGF signaling, the high-affinity receptors for FGF, which signal into the cell, are membrane-bound receptor tyrosine kinases (RTKs). Four FGF receptors (FGFR 1–4) have been cloned and characterized in terms of their binding affinity and specificity to FGFs. Initially, partial cDNA clones of FGFR were isolated in 1988 by cross-hybridization with the oncogenes *fms* (denoted *flg*) (Ruta et al., 1988) and by expression as tyrosine kinase in bacteria (denoted *bek*) (Kornbluth et al., 1988). A full-length cDNA identified as FGFR was published in 1989 (Lee et al., 1989). By 1991, four distinct FGFRs had been identified in mouse, humans, and chicken (for reviews, see Givol and Yayon, 1992; Jaye et al., 1992).

FGF receptors are membrane-bound and belong to the large family of receptor tyrosine kinases (Hunter, 2000). They contain an extracellular ligand-binding portion consisting of three immunoglobulin (Ig)-like domains (DI, DII, and DIII), a single transmembrane region of ~22 amino acids, and a cytoplasmic split kinase domain. FGFR also contains an acidic domain—a stretch of 7 to 8 acidic residues between DI and DII (Fig. 32–3). The transcript of FGFRs results in the expression of many variants due to various alternative splicing events, which determine the number of Ig-like domains (three or two domains), the formation of soluble secreted forms of the extracellular portion, and, most significantly, alternative splicing at DIII that may change the ligand-binding properties of the receptor (Givol and Yayon, 1992). The ligand binding by FGFR with only two Ig domains (DII and DIII) is similar to that of the intact receptor with three Ig domains, (DI–DIII), suggesting that DI may not be involved in binding of FGF. Both DII and DIII are encoded by two exons. DII is encoded by exons 5 and 6. In DIII, exon 7 encodes the N-terminal half (denoted IIIa), and two alternative exons, exon 8 and 9, encode the C-terminal half of DIII (denoted IIIb and IIIc, respectively) (Johnson et al., 1991). Since DIII contributes significantly to the binding specificity, two alternative FGFRs are formed by this alternative splicing, denoted the IIIb and the IIIc forms (Fig. 32–3).

The critical role of the second half of DIII in determining the FGFR specificity was best exemplified with FGFR2. FGFR2IIIc binds FGF1 and 2, but not FGF7 (KGF), whereas FGFR2IIIb binds FGF1 and FGF7, but not FGF2, and is therefore denoted as KGFR (Miki et al., 1992; Yayon et al., 1992). Recent structure determination provides a molecular basis for this specificity. This alternative usage of either IIIb or IIIc is shared by FGFR1–3, but not by FGFR4. Thus, the number of FGFRs may be increased to seven, since three of the genes may each be translated into two distinct receptors as far as ligand speci-

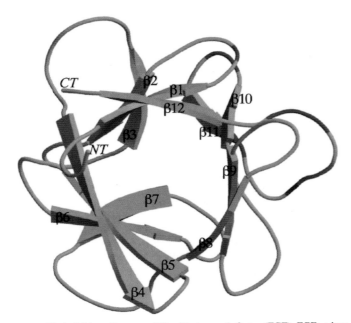

Figure 32–1. Ribbon diagram of fibroblast growth factor (FGF). FGFs adopt a β-trefoil fold, which consists of three bundles of four antiparallel β-sheets. The view is chosen to best illustrate the internal symmetry of the β-trefoil fold. NT and CT denote amino and carboxy termini, respectively. The location of residues that interact with heparan sulfate are indicated in blue. (Image provided by Dr. M. Mohammadi.)

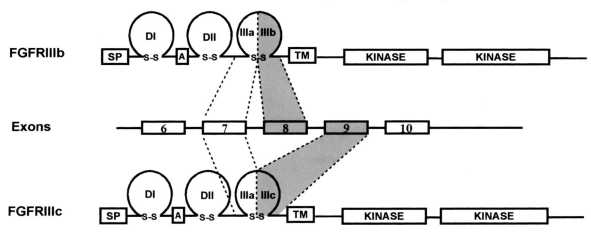

Figure 32–3. The two forms of fibroblast growth factor receptor (FGFR) produced by alternative splicing of exons 8 and 9. The structure of FGFR shows the three disulfide-linked Ig domains (DI–III), the acidic box (A), the transmembrane domain (TM), and the intracellular bipartite kinase domain. Part of the FGFR gene containing exons 6–10 is shown. Note that due to alternative splicing the C-terminal half of domain III is encoded by exon 8 in FGFRIIIb and by exon 9 in FGFRIIIc. The N-terminal half (IIIa) is encoded by exon 7 in both.

ficity is concerned. An important cellular aspect of this alternative splicing event was established when it was found that the expression of the IIIb and IIIc forms is cell-type specific and mutually exclusive (Orr-Urteger et al., 1993). For example, in the case of FGFR2, epithelial cell lineage expresses KGFR (FGFR2IIIb), and mesenchymal cell lineage expresses FGFR2IIIc. This holds true also for the other FGFRs (Avivi et al., 1993) and generates a mechanism for the formation of specific ligand–receptor pairs across epithelial–mesenchymal layers at critical stages of organogenesis.

What may happen if this mechanism goes wrong? Recent studies show that a switch from expression of IIIb to IIIc is associated with the transition from nonmalignant prostate tumor epithelial cells to a malignant tumor (Jones et al., 2001), and aberrant FGFR3 splicing was reported in colon cancer (Jang et al., 2000). This switch in FGFR forms may create an autocrine loop, whereby the growth factor and the receptor are produced in the same cell, and provides growth advantage to the cancer cell. Table 32–1 illustrates some aspects of the FGFRs ligand specificity as analyzed for 14 FGFs. The specificity was analyzed by the relative mitogenic activity on Baf3 cells in the presence of equal amounts of heparin and illustrates the distinction in signaling between the IIIb and IIIc forms of FGFR1–3 (Ornitz et al., 1996).

Structural Basis for Dimerization and Activation of FGFR

RTKs play important roles in the control of a variety of developmental and cellular processes, including cell proliferation, motility, and differentiation (Hunter, 2000). A key and universal event in cell signaling by RTK is ligand-induced dimerization, which activates the kinase domain and leads to auto-transphosphorylation of tyrosine residues on the intracellular portion of the receptor (Lemmon and Schlessinger, 1994). In some RTKs the dimerization step takes place due to dimeric ligand (e.g., platelet-derived growth factor [PDGF], vascular endothelial growth factor [VEGF]), or the receptor itself may be a covalent dimer (e.g., insulin receptor). However, both FGF and its receptor are monomeric, and, although FGF binds to FGFR, receptor dimerization takes place only after the addition of heparin (Spivak-Kroizman et al., 1994). Recent crystallographic analysis of the extracellular domain (only DI and DII domains) of FGFR1 or FGFR2 with FGF and sulfated oligosaccharide produced a model that explains the dimerization of FGFRs (Plotnikov et al., 1999; Schlessinger et al., 2000; Stauber et al., 2000). It appears that heparin binding is not limited to FGFs; rather, the FGFR also binds heparin to a lysine-rich sequence in DII that has been implicated as a heparin-binding site (Kan et al., 1993) and is denoted the "canyon" (Plotnikov et al., 1999).

The crystal structure of the dimer of FGFR1 and FGF2 (Fig. 32–4) showed the following features: the dimeric complex contains two FGFRs and two FGFs (1:1 ratio) and is stabilized mainly by interdomain interactions of DII from the two FGFRs. The two FGF monomers do not interact with each other, but each FGF interacts with residues from both DII and DIII of one receptor, as was shown previously by studies with chimeric receptors (Zimmer et al., 1993). In addition, each FGF shows secondary interactions with DII of the other receptor. Thus, FGF displays some bivalency, although this secondary interaction is not strong enough to form a stable dimer. Several residues from the linker between DII and DIII strongly participate in FGF binding.

Table 32–1. Relative Mitogenic Activity of Fibroblast Growth Factors (FGFs) in Baf3 Cells Expressing Various FGFRs

	FGFR1IIIb	FGFR2IIIb	FGFR3IIIb	FGFR1IIIc	FGFR2IIIc	FGFR3IIIc	FGFR4
FGF1	100	100	100	100	100	100	100
FGF2	60	—	—	100	65	107	110
FGF3	35	45	—	—	—	—	—
FGF4	15	15	—	100	100	70	110
FGF5	—	—	—	60	25	12	—
FGF6	—	—	—	55	60	—	80
FGF7	—	80	—	—	—	—	—
FGF8	—	—	—	—	20	40	75
FGF9	—	—	40	20	90	95	75
FGF10	—	100	—	—	—	—	—
FGF16	—	—	—	—	—	—	70
FGF17	—	—	—	—	54	90	95
FGF18	—	—	—	25	100	100	80
FGF19	—	—	—	—	—	—	90

Source: Adapted from Ornitz et al., 1996, and Xu et al., 2000.
Assay was by [³H]thymidine incorporation in the presence of 2 μg/ml heparin. Values were rounded up and represent the percentage of incorporation relative to FGF1. Values below 10% were not included. FGF7 and 10 are considered to be mesenchymally expressed, and FGF 2, 4, 6, 8, 9, and 17 are considered to be expressed in epithelia.

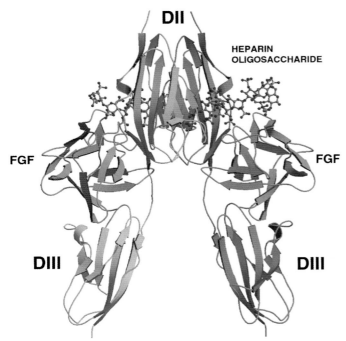

Figure 32–4. Ribbon diagram of the dimeric FGF : FGFR : heparin complex. Both FGFs are colored brown, and FGFR protomers are colored green and blue. The dimer is stabilized by interactions of FGF, FGFR, and heparin from each ternary complex with FGFR in the other ternary complex. The heparin oligosaccharides are rendered in ball and stick. Oxygen and nitrogen are red and blue, respectively, and sulfur is yellow. See text for more details. (Image provided by Dr. M. Mohammadi.)

In the ternary complex of FGF : HS : FGFR, on the surface of DII, in the region called canyon, lysines 160, 163, 172, 175, and 177 make hydrogen bonds with the sulfate groups of HS. The sulfated oligosaccharide binds to the heparin-binding site in DII of the receptor and to the two FGFs and acts like a "seat belt" in holding together the DII domains and the two FGFs (Fig. 32–4). The FGF interacts with HS through Asn27, Arg120, Lys125, Lys129, Gln134, and Lys135. In fact, two decasaccharides were found in the complex along the canyon, making a complex of FGF : FGFR : HS with a 2:2:2 ratio for the components (Schlessinger et al., 2000).

This structure may explain a large body of evidence on the involvement of both FGF and heparin in signaling through FGFR. Thus, heparin is bridging FGF and FGFR rather than the two FGFs, and the stable signaling complex contains two FGFs, two FGFRs, and two HSs in a ternary complex. Heparin increases the affinity of FGF to FGFR by stabilizing the complex. The comparison of the three structures of FGF1 : FGFR1, FGF2 : FGFR1, and FGF2 : FGFR2 also allows us to explain some of the specificity of FGFs to their receptors. For example, FGF1, which is the nondiscriminatory ligand, binds to all FGFRs. In contrast, FGF2 and FGF4 show more specific binding, and this is due to additional interactions between DIII of FGFR and the N-terminal portion of these FGFs. Furthermore, the region in DIII, which interacts with these FGFs, is subject to alternative splicing. Consequently, FGF2, but not FGF1, discriminates between the IIIc and IIIb variants.

The crystal structures also may point to the importance of the sulfated positions on HS (Fig. 32–2), which are involved in binding and indicate the possibility of novel sulfated molecules as inhibitors for FGF signaling. This understanding of the role of HS in the signaling complex opens the way to analyze differential binding and regulation of FGFR signaling by HS. HS oligosaccharides of defined size and sulfation were found to modulate the specificity of ligand–receptor interaction in FGFR signaling. Such an assay using Baf3 cells expressing FGFR1–3 shows dramatic differences in the proliferation response using FGF and 25 different heparin-derived oligosaccharides. Some of the oligosaccharides were more potent than heparin for FGFR2, and

some were even inhibitory (Guimond and Turnbull, 1999). Selectively desulfated heparin at the 6-O position inhibits FGF2-induced mitogenic and angiogenic response (Lundin et al., 2000). It is possible that in the future such saccharides or other small molecules with defined sulfation sites will be utilized as modulators of FGFR signaling (Gallagher, 2001). Furthermore, changes in the extra cellular matrix during development may influence signaling by FGF.

SIGNALING PATHWAYS

Tyrosine Phosphorylation and Signaling Proteins

Ligand binding (FGF and HS) to the extracellular portion of FGFR leads to dimerization and stimulation of auto-transphosphorylation by activating the kinase domain. The phosphotyrosines (pTyr) generated by the autophosphorylation are located in the cytoplasmic domain and become docking sites for a variety of signaling proteins (for reviews, see Klint and Claesson-Welsh, 1999; Schlessinger, 2000). The signaling proteins are structurally modular, and one of their modules (either the SH2 or the PTB domain) binds to pTyr. The specificity of this binding is determined by the amino acids adjacent to the pTyr on the N-terminal side (PTB domain) or on the C-terminal side (SH2 domain) of the pTyr. Other modules in these signaling molecules may bind to a proline-rich sequence motif like ProXXPro (SH3 domain) or ProXProX (WW domain). Other modules (PH domain) bind to different phosphoinositides—some of which are products of PI-3 kinase—and are targeted to membranes and a module containing the PDZ domain binds to hydrophobic amino acids at the C terminus of proteins. These modules or domains transmit the signal by forming a bridge between the pTyr on the receptors and other cellular targets. In addition to these binding modules, most signaling molecules contain enzymatic activity such as phosphorylation, dephosphorylation, phospholipase C, or RasGAP activity, which is being used to modify downstream cellular targets. Some pTyr-binding proteins contain only SH2 and SH3 domains (e.g., Grb2, Nck, Crk, Shc) and serve as adaptors that link the receptor pTyr to other proteins in the signaling cascade.

Another mode of signaling is by an alternative indirect mechanism that recruits signaling molecules to pTyr, which are not located on the RTK itself but on another non-receptor protein (docking protein) which is anchored to the membrane and is phosphorylated by the FGFR. The multiple pTyr generated are docking sites for SH2 domains. The main docking protein for FGFR is FRS2 (also denoted SNT), a 90 kDa molecule which is a substrate for FGFR that phosphorylates several tyrosines on FRS2. This generates four binding sites for Grb2 and two sites for Shp2 (pTyrphosphatase). The FRS2 lacks SH2 domain but is bound to FGFR through a PTB domain and can be directly phosphorylated as a substrate of FGFR kinase. It appears that most of the signaling molecules recruited by FGF stimulation are doing so through FRS2 and not FGFR itself. Targeted disruption of FRS2 resulted in impairment of FGF signaling and in embryonal lethality (Hadari et al., 2001).

Phosphorylated Tyrosines on FGFR

The cytoplasmic portion of FGFR1 contains eight tyrosines, which are potential phosphorylation sites, and five of them are conserved in all receptors, as shown in Table 32–2 (for review, see Klint and Claesson-Welsh, 1999). The main function of each Tyr after phosphorylation was studied in FGFR1 and FGFR3. Tyr776, although conserved in FGFR1–4, is not phosphorylated. The two residues Tyr653

Table 32–2. Conserved Tyrosine Residues in the Cytoplasmic Domain of FGFRs

FGFR1	FGFR2	FGFR3	FGFR4
Tyr463	Tyr466		
Tyr583/585	Tyr586/588	Tyr577	
Tyr653/654	Tyr656/657	Tyr647/648	Tyr642/643
Tyr730	Tyr733	Tyr724	Tyr719
Tyr766	Tyr769	Tyr760	Tyr754
Tyr776	Tyr779	Tyr770	Tyr764

and Tyr654 are part of the activation loop controlling the kinase active site, and they are also conserved in all FGFRs (see Table 32–2). Mutation of these tyrosines to phenylalanine abolishes the kinase activity of FGFR1 (Mohammadi et al., 1996). When phosphorylated, Tyr766 creates the binding site for PLCγ in FGFR1 (Mohammadi et al., 1991) and FGFR3 (Hart et al., 2001). The pTyr724 is the binding site for PI-3K, as well as for STAT1 and 3 and Shp2, at least in FGFR3 (Hart et al., 2001). Figure 32–5 shows the position and presumed functions of pTyr in the cytoplasmic domain, as analyzed in FGFR3. The requirement of tyrosine phosphorylation for signaling in FGFR3 was studied by introducing a mutation (Lys650Glu) that makes the kinase constitutively active. This was followed by mutation of all tyrosines to phenylalanine, which resulted in complete inactivation of the cellular functions of the receptor. Adding back of the original tyrosines one at a time by Phe to Tyr back-mutation showed that Tyr724 (homolog of Tyr 730 in FGFR1) can restore all the cellular functions tested, such as PI-3K activation, STAT and MAPK phosphorylation and cell transformation (Hart et al., 2001). The list of homologous tyrosines in FGFR1–4, as shown in Table 32–2 allows the comparison of various FGFRs with Figure 32–5, which describes the tyrosines of FGFR3.

Signaling Pathways Activated by the Signaling Molecules

The intracellular signaling downstream from the FGFR may split into several pathways (for reviews, see Klint and Claesson-Welsh, 1999; Schlessinger, 2000). The most common one is the stimulation of Ras by activating the GTP for GDP exchange. In this process Grb2 binds to pTyr through its SH2 and to Sos through its SH3, thus recruiting Sos to the membrane where it can stimulate Ras by catalyzing the exchange of GDP for GTP. The activated Ras now interacts with Raf (a serine kinase), and Raf stimulates MAP kinase kinase (MAPKK) by phosphorylating a key Ser residue. MAPKK phosphorylates and activates MAPK (ERK), and MAPK crosses the nuclear membrane into the nucleus, where it phosphorylates and activates various transcription factors which then activate genes responding to FGF. This signaling cascade is highly conserved throughout evolution and has an important role in the control of cell differentiation and proliferation.

Another intracellular signaling pathway is the activation through the STAT pathway. STAT (signal transduction and activation of transcription) binds to pTyr through its SH2 domain, and this is followed by the formation of dimeric STAT, which is translocated directly into the nucleus and binds to the target DNA sequence to activate target genes as a transcription factor (Darnell, 1997).

Additional intracellular signaling is through the phosphoinositol pathway, which generates second messengers. The SH2 domain of pLCγ binds to pTyr on the receptor. The activated pLCγ hydrolyzes phosphatidylinositol-(4,5)-diphosphate into diacylglycerol and inositol diphosphate. Diacylglycerol activates the family of protein kinase C, which regulates gene activity. The inositol-(4,5)-diphosphate stimulates the release of Ca^{2+} which binds calmodulin and activates calmodulin-dependent kinases. The PI-3 kinase (PI-3K) is also activated by FGFR, when the PI-3K binds to pTyr through the SH2 domain of its p85 subunit. The activated PI-3K phosphorylates phosphatidylinositol phosphate to the triphosphate form, which serves as a second messenger to recruit signaling molecules to the membrane. For example, PI-3K-activated PKB (Akt) phosphorylates BAD, an anti-apoptotic protein, or Fork Head (FKH), which down-regulates the TNF pathway and thus increases cell survival.

Cell Signaling Depends on Cell Context

The complexity of signaling pathways due to recruitment of multiple proteins within a short time after FGF stimulation raises the question of the specificity of the signal. Why does stimulation of FGFR in fibroblasts result in proliferation, whereas in chondrocytes the outcome is growth inhibition, and in early development FGFR1 controls yet another function like cell migration?

This paradox was reconciled by demonstrating that FGFR3 signaling can operate at least along two different pathways. One, the Ras-MAPK pathway, leads to cell proliferation, whereas the other pathway, operating through STAT1, induces cell cycle inhibitors. The chosen pathway depends on the cellular context. Recent experiments comparing the effect of FGF on a rat chondrosarcoma cell line (RCS) that expresses FGFR3 versus its effect on NIH3T3 fibroblasts shed more light on the utilization of these two signaling pathways by FGFR3 (Sahni et al., 1999). Surprisingly, FGF1 treatment of RCS cells resulted in marked inhibition of cell proliferation and DNA synthesis, whereas FGF1 had a proliferative effect on NIH3T3 cells. In addition, FGF1 treatment of RCS cells significantly increased the phosphorylation of STAT1 and its translocation to the nucleus. Similar results were reported previously using the TDII mutant (Lys650Glu) of FGFR3 expressed in 293 cells (Su et al., 1997).

STAT1 is known to be activated in the interferon-induced pathway by tyrosine phosphorylation and nulcear translocation where it functions as a transcription factor (Darnell, 1997). One of the targets for STAT1 activation is p21[waf1] (Chin et al., 1996), a general inhibitor of cyclin-dependent kinases, which is also a major mediator of p53-induced growth arrest. Comparison of RCS cells with transfected NIH3T3 cells expressing either wild-type FGFR3 or the activated mutant receptor present in achondroplasia (FGFR3[ach]) demonstrated different routes of FGFR3 activation in the two cellular contexts. The activation of FGFR3 in RCS cells increased STAT1 phosphorylation and p21[waf1] expression, whereas such effects were not observed in NIH3T3 cells expressing either FGFR3 or FGFR3[ach]. Thus the growth inhibitory effect of FGFR3 is specific to the cell type and utilizes a signaling pathway in chondrocytes that is different from the one in fibroblasts.

These results were confirmed in experiments with cells derived from STAT1[−/−] mice (Sahni et al., 1999). FGF treatment of primary chondrocytes from STAT1[−/−] mice did not inhibit DNA synthesis or cell

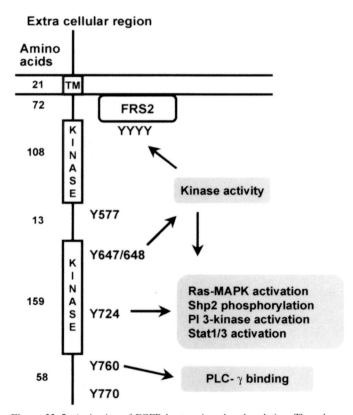

Figure 32–5. Activation of FGFR by tyrosine phosphorylation. The scheme shows the position of major tyrosines that are phosphorylated in the kinase domain of FGFR3 and the signaling molecules that bind to them (Hart et al., 2001). Homologous tyrosines are phosphorylated in other FGFRs (see Table 32–2 for comparison of conservative tyrosines). Also shown is the membrane-bound FRS2, which is phosphorylated by FGFR and serves as a platform to recruit signaling molecules in response to FGF stimulation (see text for explanation).

proliferation. Similar results were observed when metatarsal bone culture was used. Treatment of wild-type metatarsal bones with FGF1 led to inhibition of chondrocyte growth, whereas in metatarsals from STAT1-deficient mice, no inhibition of chondrocyte proliferation was observed. These experiments indicate that the inhibitory effect of FGFR3 in chondrocytes depends on activation of the STAT1 pathway. The different signaling pathways chosen by FGF/FGFR are important to understanding the effect of FGFR mutation. It appears that FGFRs contain many germline mutations, which affect mainly skeletal development.

FGFR MUTATIONS

Functional Classification of Mutations

The first germline mutation in the FGFR was identified in 1994 as a point mutation (G to A) resulting in a Gly to Arg replacement in codon 380, located in the transmembrane region of FGFR3. This mutation is responsible for over 97% of achondroplasia, the common form of dwarfism (Rousseau et al., 1994; Shiang et al., 1994). This was followed by a rapid discovery of many more mutations in FGFR2 and FGFR3 and one mutation in FGFR1, and today close to 100 mutations are known, most of them are associated with bone formation.

Almost all the mutations in FGFR2 are located in DIII or in the linker between DII and DIII, whereas FGFR3 also contains mutations in the transmembrane and cytoplasmic domains (for review, see Naski and Ornitz, 1998; Kannan and Givol, 2000). All the mutations in the coding regions are missense mutations and exhibit a dominant phenotype, suggesting gain of function. These mutations can be divided into four groups. The first group consists of mutations that alter the number of cysteine residues within the extracellular domain into an uneven number. This prevents the formation of intrachain disulfide bonds within the Ig-like domains (Fig. 32–3) and may facilitate interchain disulfide bond formation, thus resulting in ligand-independent dimerization and signaling. For example, in ~40% of the Pfeiffer's syndrome cases, Cys342 is changed into one of six possible amino acids (Ser, Arg, Gly, Trp, Phe, and Tyr). Most of these substitutions were observed in patients with craniosynostosis. Hence, the phenotype is very likely independent of the new amino acid but may result from the loss of the cysteine residue. In addition, many of the observed mutations in DIII of FGFR2 introduce an additional cysteine residue, also leading to the possibility of interchain disulfide bond formation (Wilkie, 1997; Cornejo-Roldan et al., 1999). These examples classify the phenotypes resulting from these FGFR mutations as a "receptor dimerization syndrome," a signaling terminology for human disease. Other mutations that do not directly involve a Cys residue may also result in a similar effect. For example, Tyr340His or Thr341Pro, both of which are adjacent to Cys342, may also interfere with the formation of an intrachain disulfide bond in DIII and allow the formation of interchain disulfide bond.

The next class of mutations includes those that increase the affinity of the receptor to FGF ligands and appear in homologous position in all three FGFRs (Bellus et al., 1996). Examples are Pro252Arg in FGFR1, Pro253Arg in FGFR2, and Pro250Arg in FGFR3. This proline may be considered as part of the DII-DIII linker, and it is located in a highly conserved stretch of 16 amino acids that are identical in FGFR1–3. This proline is also a contact residue in the FGF–FGFR complex (Plotnikov et al., 1999). The resulting phenotype is different for each mutation, resulting in Pfeiffer's syndrome with Pro252Arg in FGFR1, Apert's syndrome with Pro253Arg in FGFR2, and Muenke's syndrome or craniosynostosis with Pro250Arg in FGFR3 (Bellus et al., 1996). This suggests that the phenotype of the mutation depends on the time and tissue expression of the particular FGFR mutated. Other mutations that appear in both FGFR2 and 3 with different phenotypes include Ser372Cys, Tyr375Cys, and Gly384Arg (Passos-Bueno et al., 1999).

The third group of mutations is more diverse and includes nucleotide changes in the intron, mainly at the splice acceptor site of exon 9 (Cornejo-Roldan et al., 1999). In addition, this group includes mutations that contain a small deletion or insertion in DIII (Wilkie, 1997)

and a mutation in FGFR3, which cancels the termination codon (X807) and leads to extension of the receptor by 141 amino acids (Rousseau et al., 1995).

Unlike FGFR1-2, the mutations in FGFR3 are not confined only to the ectodomain. The most common mutation in FGFR3 is Gly380Arg in the transmembrane domain (Passos-Bueno et al., 1999). A mouse model generated by gene targeting of this mutation into FGFR3 produced achondroplastic mouse and provided direct evidence that the Gly380Arg mutation is the cause of achondroplasia (Wang et al., 1999). This mutation introduces a charged amino acid into the hydrophobic transmembrane domain and is in a homologous position to that of the Val664Glu mutation in *Neu* (*HER2*), which activates the Neu kinase and converts HER2 into an oncogene (Bargmann et al., 1986). Studies from the Neu oncogene indicated that the Val664Glu mutation induces ligand-independent receptor dimerization and suggested that achondroplastic FGFR3 may also exhibit some receptor dimerization (Webster and Donoghue, 1996). The Gly380Arg mutation is dominant and causes achondroplasia in the heterozygous state.

The fourth type of mutation is the Lys650Glu mutation in the cytoplasmic portion of the receptor that leads to strong constitutive ligand-independent activity, without dimerization. Lys650Met (Tavormina et al., 1999) shows the strongest constitutive activation out of the known mutants of FGFR3, thus demonstrating that the replacing amino acid determines the extent of receptor activation.

Correlation between Mutation, Receptor Activation, and Disease Severity

The kinase activity of RTK is regulated by ligand binding that leads to receptor dimerization (Lemmon and Schlessinger, 1994). The discovery of mutation Gly380Arg in FGFR3 in achondroplasia prompted experiments to understand the relationship between this or other mutations and the kinase activity of FGFR. To this end, many chimeric receptor constructs were tested for kinase and transforming activity. Some experiments utilized FGFR3 (Li et al., 1997), but others used a chimera that contains the stronger kinase domain from FGFR1 (Naski et al., 1996) or from Neu (Galvin et al., 1996) fused to the transmembrane and ectodomain from the mutant FGFR3. The results showed that the Gly380Arg mutation activated the receptor kinase activity (by 18%) in a ligand-independent manner. Furthermore, other charged residues at position 380 (e.g., Glu and Asp) also activated the receptor (Webster and Donoghue, 1997). The mutant chimera also stimulated cell proliferation and transformed NIH3T3 cells in a manner similar to the *Neu* oncogene. Thus, the transmembrane region can regulate the kinase activity of FGFR3, similar to the analogous mutation Val664Glu in Neu where the activation was due to stabilization of dimer formation (Weiner et al., 1989).

The Arg248Cys mutation activates FGFR3 in a ligand-independent manner, as shown by receptor self-phosphorylation and increased cell proliferation (Galvin et al., 1996). It was also demonstrated that the mutant receptor forms a disulfide-linked homodimer, which results in ligand-independent activation. This stronger receptor activation leads to the more severe phenotype of TDI. Mutations that do not involve a cysteine residue may operate through changes in ligand binding. For example, Pro253Arg and Ser252Trp, respectively, cause a 2- and 6-fold increased affinity of FGFR2 to FGF2 by decreasing the dissociation constant (Anderson et al., 1998). Pro253 is a contact residue in the FGF–FGFR complex (Plotnikov et al., 1999). Both mutations cause Apert syndrome and provide another mechanism for FGFR activation, allowing the receptor to bind FGF at lower concentration. Indeed, the recent crystal structure of these FGFR2 mutants with FGF2 indicates that the Pro253Arg mutation will enable FGFR2 to bind indiscriminately any FGF, while both the Ser252Trp and Pro253Arg mutations will increase the interactions and contacts between FGF2 and FGFR2, which then enhance ligand affinity (Ibrahimi et al., 2001). We reached the stage of disease diagnosis by molecular contacts in crystal structure.

Another type of mutation in FGFR3 is the Lys650Glu mutation in the kinase-activating loop (Tavormina et al., 1995). This activating loop is a conserved sequence in tyrosine kinases, which inhibits the kinase activity of the receptor, and this auto inhibition is relieved upon phosphorylation of Tyr647 and Tyr648 due to the ligand-induced dimerization (Mohammadi et al., 1996). The Lys650Glu mutation removes the constraints conferred on the active site by this activating loop and activates the kinase about 100-fold, compared to the wild-type receptor, and this is about 20-fold more than activation by the Gly380Arg mutation (Webster et al., 1996). The Lys650Glu mutant results in a ligand-independent kinase activity that is almost one-half that of the maximal ligand-induced kinase activity and does not require dimerization. The phenotype of this mutation, thanatophoric dysplasia II (TDII), is much more severe than that of achondroplasia and results in death soon after birth. The Lys650Met mutation exhibits 3-fold higher kinase activity than does Lys650Glu and results in a different syndrome—TDI, or SADDAN (Tavormina et al., 1999). This is an example of how different amino acids at the same position can determine the degree of activation and the severity of the disease. The degree of kinase activity by some of the mutations can be graded as follows: ligand-induced kinase = Arg248Cys = Lys650Met > Lys650Glu > Gly380Arg.

The examples discussed above demonstrate three mechanisms for activation of FGFRs by mutations: (*1*) dimerization by unpaired cysteines, leading to constitutive receptor activation, (*2*) increased receptor signaling due to increased affinity for the ligand, and (*3*) activation by removal of inhibition by the activating loop in the kinase domain. The constitutive kinase activity of the mutant receptors ranges from only several percentage of full activation to close to 100% of ligand-induced activity. The disease phenotype correlates with the timing and tissue localization of the ligand-independent kinase activity, and the severity of the disease is proportional to the degree of kinase activation.

FUNCTIONS ASSOCIATED WITH THE FGF SYSTEM

Localization and Genetic Analysis

The present interest in the developmental role of the FGF system arose during the late 1980s with the discovery that FGF1 and 2 and their receptors contribute to mesoderm induction during amphibian gastrulation (Smith, 1989; Amaya et al., 1991). Two additional findings enhanced this interest. An integration site of the mouse mammary tumor virus was found to localize with a gene for FGF4 (Dickson et al., 1989), suggesting the possible involvement of this gene family with cancer. In addition, the angiogenic effects of FGFs were demonstrated (Flamme and Risau, 1992). Thus, already the early research mapped out a broad field for the activity of these growth factors and receptors. The last 15 years have seen great progress in all branches of this field.

The list of FGFs, defined by functional homology, reaches 23, and the four FGFRs with their mutually exclusive splice variants constitute seven receptors with individual expression patterns and binding specificity. FGFs are expressed during most stages of development and organogenesis. FGF4 is already transcribed in the internal cell mass (ICM) of the blastocyst, from which all the embryonic cell lineages develop, and it also has roles during gastrulation (Niswander and Martin, 1992). Other isotypes are active only from mid-gestation onward and are restricted to a few cell lineages and organs, such as FGF6 to myogenesis (deLapeyriere et al., 1993) or FGF17 to the brain, developing skeleton, and arteries (Xu et al., 1999a, 2000).

The expression pattern of most FGFRs covers a broad temporal-spatial scale. FGFR2IIIc, for example, is already expressed both in the unfertilized egg (Haffner-Krausz et al., 1999) and during late osteogenesis (Orr-Urtreger et al., 1993; Lonai, 1996). There is evidence that FGFR2 is expressed by the nascent trophectoderm of compacted morulae (Haffner-Krausz et al., 1999), and most FGFRs are transcribed by the pre-gastrulation egg cylinder stage (Rappolee et al., 1998; Chen et al., 2000). Reviewing the detailed expression pattern of FGF and FGFR is beyond the scope of this chapter, and a number of contemporary reviews are available. The multiplicity and function of FGFs was reviewed recently (Ornitz and Itoh, 2001), while the structure and function of FGFRs were summarized in somewhat earlier reviews (Givol and Yayon, 1992; Jaye et al., 1992; Johnson and Williams, 1993; Kannan and Givol, 2000). Specific reviews describe the role of FGFs in limb development (Martin, 1998; Xu et al., 1999c), osteogenesis (Naski and Ornitz, 1998), odontogenesis (Thesleff and Sharpe, 1997), brain development (Crossley et al., 1996; Lee et al., 1997), angiogenesis (Risau and Flamme, 1995), and wound healing (Werner, 1998). Good summaries of this material are now available online at various URLs, including http://www.informatics.jax.org/searches/expression_form.shtml and http://genex.hgu.mrc.ac.uk/.

Most information regarding the function of the FGF system comes from studying specific developmental mechanisms and gene targeting. Gene targeting is the most powerful technique for the characterization of mammalian gene function, and the bulk of present knowledge comes from targeted loss-of-function mutations. They provide the basis for a close to comprehensive analysis when the targeted mutation is viable, such as the mutations of FGF3, 5, 7, and 17 (Table 32–3) or of FGFR2c and FGFR3 and 4 (Table 32–4). In contrast, embryonic lethal mutations may preclude the analysis of the gene's function beyond a certain stage of embryogenesis. FGF8 may serve as an example. Targeted disruption of this gene leads to lethality during gastrulation (Sun et al., 1999). This phenotype hides the role of FGF8 in limb development, which has been clarified with promoters specific for the apical ectodermal ridge (AER) of the limb bud, where FGF8 is synthesized. The AER and its FGFs are responsible for proximal–distal limb outgrowth. The role of FGF8 in limb development has been demonstrated by conditional gene targeting, using the Cre-loxP and flp systems (Lewandoski et al., 2000; Moon and Capecchi, 2000).

Early embryonic lethality, among other reasons, may be due to placentation defects, which can be corrected by aggregating homozygous

Table 32–3. Targeted Mutagenesis of Fibroblast Growth Factor (FGF) Isotypes

Gene	Mutation	Survival*	Phenotype	Reference
FGF1	Recessive/null	Viable	No obvious defect	Miller et al., 2000
FGF2	Recessive/null	Viable	Neuronal, skeletal, mild cardiovascular, skin wound healing and thrombocytosis	Dono et al., 1998
FGF3	Recessive/null	Viable	Inner ear, tail outgrowth	Mansour et al., 1993
FGF4	Recessive/null	Lethal, E5.5	Inner cell mass (ICM) proliferation	Feldman et al., 1995
FGF5	Recessive/null	Viable	Long hair, mouse *Angora* mutation	Hebert et al., 1994
FGF6	Recessive/null	Viable	Muscle regeneration	Floss et al., 1997
FGF7	Recessive/null	Viable	Hair follicle and kidney defect	Guo et al., 1996
FGF8	Recessive/null	Lethal, E8.5	Gastrulation, cardiac, craniofacial, forebrain, midbrain, and cerebellar development	Meyers et al., 1998
FGF9	Recessive/null	Lethal, P0	Lung mesenchyme, XY sex reversal	Colvin et al., 2001
FGF10	Recessive/null	Lethal, P0	Absence of limbs, lungs, thyroid, pituitary, salivary glands; defects in teeth, kidneys, hair follicles, and digestive organs	Min et al., 1998 Sekine et al., 1999
FGF14	Recessive/null	Viable	Neurological phenotype	Wang et al., 2000
FGF17	Recessive/null	Viable	Midline cerebellar development	Xu et al., 2000
FGF18	Recessive/null	Lethal P1	Chondrogenesis and osteogenesis FGFR3-like	Liu et al., 2002

E, embryonic day; P, postnatal day.

Table 32–4. Targeted Mutagenesis of Fibroblast Growth Factor Receptor (FGFR) Isotypes: Loss of Function

Gene	Mutation	Survival*	Phenotype	Reference
FGFR1	Recessive/null	Lethal, E9.5–E12.5	Defective cell migration through primitive streak; posterior axis defect	Yamaguchi et al., 1994 Deng et al., 1994
FGFR1α	Recessive/null	Lethal, E9.5–E12.5	Distal truncation of limbs; posterior embryonic defect	Xu et al., 1999b
FGFR1-IIIb	Recessive/null	Viable	No obvious phenotype	Partanen et al., 1998
FGFR1-IIIc	Recessive/null	Lethal, E9.5	Defective cell migration through primitive streak; posterior axis defect	Partanen et al., 1998
FGFR2	Recessive/null	Lethal, E10.5	Defect in placenta and limb bud formation; absence of lungs	Xu et al., 1998 Arman et al., 1999
FGFR2	Inhibitory/recessive	Lethal E4.5	Trophoblast defect at implantation; inhibits additional FGFR	Arman et al., 1998
FGFR2-IIIb	Recessive/null	Lethal, P0	Agenesis of lungs, anterior pituitary, thyroid, teeth, and limbs; dysgenesis of kidneys, salivary glands, adrenal glands, thymus, pancreas, skin, otic vesicles, glandular stomach, and hair follicle	De Moerlooze et al., 2000 Revest et al., 2001
FGFR2-IIIc	Recessive/null	Viable	Craniosynostosis of skull base (chondrocranium); dwarf	Eswarakumar et al., 2002
FGFR3	Recessive/null	Viable	Bone over growth; inner ear defect	Colvin et al., 1996 Deng et al., 1996
FGFR4	Recessive/null	Viable	No obvious phenotype; growth retardation and lung defects in double mutant with FGFR3	Weinstein et al., 1998a

*E, embryonic day; P, postnatal day.

mutant embryonic stem (ES) cells with tetraploid wild-type embryos. This method was used to reveal the full effect of an FGFR2 mutation on limb development and branching morphogenesis (Arman et al., 1999). Closely related members of gene families may replace the function of a single mutated isotype. This maybe the situation in pre-gastrulation embryogenesis, which is not affected by null mutations of FGFR1 (Deng et al., 1994; Yamaguchi et al., 1994), FGFR2 (Xu et al., 1998), FGFR3 (Colvin et al., 1996; Deng et al., 1996), or FGFR4 (Weinstein et al., 1998b). However, all four FGFRs are expressed in the preimplantation, early postimplantation mouse embryo or embryoid body (Chen et al., 2000). In contrast, dominant negative FGFR4 (Chai et al., 1998) and inhibitory mutations of FGFR2 (Arman et al., 1998), which presumably affect multiple receptor isotypes, are lethal in the blastocyst stage or shortly after implantation. Redundancy has also been observed. In the targeted mutagenesis of FGFR4, no phenotype was observed, because other FGFR isotypes may rescue the function of the disrupted one. Double mutants of FGFR4 and FGFR3, however, revealed lung alveogenesis defects (Weinstein et al., 1998a). The results of gene targeting of mouse FGFs is given in Table 32–3, and the results of gene targeting of FGFRs are summarized in Table 32–4.

Recent research in the field of FGF receptors was influenced by their human gain-of-function mutation. Besides their clinical importance, the analysis of these mutations revealed important molecular aspects of bone development. FGFR3 was shown to be involved in achondroplasia (Rousseau et al., 1994), whereas FGFR2 and to a smaller extent FGFR1 are involved in craniosynostosis (Muenke and Schell, 1995; Wilkie, 1997; Hehr and Muenke, 1999). Most of these congenital anomalies are due to the stabilization of receptor dimers, which leads to ligand-independent stimulation or increased affinity and broadening specificity of the FGFR.

Experimental mouse models of achondroplasia (Chen et al., 1999; Wang et al., 1999), Pfeiffer-type craniosynostosis (Zhou et al., 2000), and thanatophoric dysplasia (Li et al., 1999) were produced by a "knockin" methodology that generates single-point mutations (Table 32–5). These animal models may become useful for screening potential drugs that inhibit receptor tyrosine kinase activity, and they may also help clarify the role of FGF signaling in bone development. The mutant mice provide the opportunity for testing the findings from cellular work on the mechanism of FGFR3 function.

Analysis by in situ hybridization and immunohistochemistry shows that both STAT1 and STAT5 are overexpressed in the chondrocytes and are translocated to the nucleus. Although p21[waf1] is only slightly increased, other cell cycle inhibitors (p16, p18, and p19) are overexpressed in the mutant growth plate and may be the mediators of FGFR3 activity in chondrocytes (Li et al., 1999). Another pathway has been indicated through inhibition of Indian hedgehog (Ihh) signaling and BMP4 (bone morphogenic protein 4) expression in chondrocytes by mutant FGFR3, suggesting that FGFR3 can coordinate skeletal growth by controlling the growth of both bone and cartilage (Naski et al., 1998). Interestingly, the loss-of-function mutation of FGFR3 (Table 32–4) causes long bone overgrowth and down-regulation of the molecules that mediate chondrogenesis (Colvin et al., 1996; Deng et al., 1996); thus, FGFR3 seems to be a negative regulator of bone growth, which functions by inhibiting chondrocyte proliferation and enhancing their differentiation and finally their takeover by osteoblasts and mineralization.

Recent genetic analysis of the IIIc splice variant of FGFR2 sheds additional light on the mechanism of osteogenesis. A point mutation in exon 9—the specific exon of FGFR2IIIc—caused translational stop codons. This recessive viable mutation displayed shortening of the endochondral skull base and reduced mineralization of both the skull base and the skull vault, as well as the axial and appendicular skeleton, with a decrease in the transcription of Ssp1 (osteopontin) and Cbfa1/Runx2 expressed by the osteocyte lineage. Somewhat less reduction in the transcription of the chondrocyte-specific PTHrP and Shh was also observed (Eswarakumar et al., 2002). It appears, therefore, that the function of FGFR2IIIc is formally opposite to that of FGFR3, inasmuch as it is a positive regulator of osteogenesis mainly by its positive control on the osteocyte lineage. A recent report on the role of FGF18 (Liu et al., 2002) suggests that it may be the ligand of FGFR2IIIc, at least in part of its osteogenic roles. It follows that the FGF system forms an interaction loop between FGFR3 and FGFR2IIIc, where the former controls bone elongation and growth by supporting chondrocyte differentiation, and the latter enhances the activity of the osteocyte lineage, thus promoting ossification and finally mineralization.

Comprehensive functional analysis of a gene family by gene targeting is still a daunting task. Conditional activation of targeted mutations by site-specific recombinases, such as Cre and flp, can activate a mutation at a chosen site. Such mutations can clarify specific gene activity, especially in cases when early lethality covers later activities of a target gene. Conditional gene targeting, however, requires appropriate

Table 32–5. Targeted Mutagenesis of Fibroblast Growth Factor Receptors (FGFRs): Gain of Function and Animal Models

Gene	Mutation	Survival	Phenotype	Reference
FGFR1	Pro250Arg dominant/heterozygote	Viable	Pfeiffer syndrome	Zhou et al., 2000
FGFR3	Gly374Arg dominant/heterozygote	Viable	Achondroplasia, fertility defects	Wang et al., 1999
FGFR3	Gly369Cys dominant/heterozygote	Viable	Achondroplasia	Chen et al., 1999
FGFR3	Lys644Glu dominant/homozygote	Viable	Thanatophoric dysplasia II (TDII)	Iwata et al., 2000
FGFR3	Lys644Met dominant/heterozygote	Viable	SADDAN (TDI)	Iwata et al., 2001

spatially restricted promoters, which are not always available. Double mutant crosses that can also clarify redundancy are rather time-consuming. Thus, a comprehensive analysis of the FGF system is not yet available. Progress of the genome projects requires more and faster assays of gene function. This led to an upswing of large mutant screens (Hrabé de Angelis et al., 2000). Newer and faster methods of targeted mutagenesis, such as creating mouse strains with megabase size functionally haploid chromosome stretches (Mills and Bradley, 2001) are also emerging. These new large-scale techniques will speed up the detailed understanding of the FGF, FGFR, and other gene families. The presently available information, however, already points to a number of common characteristics of the FGF system. Here we will discuss the feature of coordinated localization and ligand-binding specificity of FGFs and FGFR splicing alternatives and will analyze the relationship between the FGF system and the extracel-lular matrix, the basement membrane, and epithelial mesenchymal interactions.

Coordinated Control of Localization and Binding Specificity

Three of the four receptors—FGFR1, 2, and 3—have splicing alternatives, based on mutually exclusive usage of the exons that encode the C-terminal half of the third Ig-like loop of the extracellular domain (Fig. 32–3). These changes confer unique binding specificity to the transcriptional alternatives, as was first demonstrated for FGFR2, where it was found that the IIIb alternative of FGFR2 binds keratinocyte growth factor (KGF) (i.e., it is the KGF receptor [KGFR]) whereas the IIIc alternative does not bind KGF but does bind FGFR2 (Miki et al., 1992; Yayon et al., 1992). Studying the localized expression of FGFR2 alternatives revealed that FGFR2IIIb is expressed not only in keratinocytes of the skin and surface ectoderm (Aaronson et al., 1991) but also in internal epithelia, such as the gut and blood vessels. Its IIIc alternative, in contrast, was found in mesenchymes, in the paraxial and lateral mesoderm, and in developing bones and muscle. The detailed expression pattern of FGFR1 and FGFR3 is less well known; nevertheless, it seems to be a general rule that IIIb-type alternatives are expressed in epithelia, whereas IIIc-type alternatives are found in the mesenchyme (Orr-Urtreger et al., 1993). The unique expression pattern of IIIb and IIIc alternatives of FGFR1, 2, and 3 was confirmed in tooth (Kettunen et al., 1998) and calvarial bone and suture development (Rice et al., 2000). Although gene targeting of FGFR1IIIb and FGFR1IIIc suggested that most of the activity of FGFR1 is associated with the IIIc alternative (Rossant et al., 1997), recent results suggest that FGFR1IIIb may also have specific roles. FGFR1IIIb cloned from a murine skin wound cDNA library is expressed in sebaceous glands of the skin and in neurons of the hippocampus and cerebellum, and, like other IIIb-type FGF receptors, it interacts with FGF10 in the mesenchyme (Beer et al., 2000).

The IIIb and IIIc alternatives of FGFR1, FGFR2, and FGFR3 transfected to Baf3 cells show differential binding specificity to mesenchymal and epithelial FGFs (Ornitz et al., 1996; see Table 32–1), as was suggested for the splicing alternatives of FGFR2 on the basis of their expression patterns (Orr-Urtreger et al., 1993). Taken together, mesenchymal FGF isotypes are recognized by epithelial IIIb-type receptors, while epithelial FGF isotypes activate mesenchymal IIIc-type FGF receptors. This coordinated regulation appears to be eminently suitable to mediate cross-talk between adjacent cell sheets, such as the epithelia and the mesenchymes. It appears that this complex mechanism relies largely on the cellular environment. Alternative exon usage depends on the availability of the specific splicing factors in the relevant cell (Del Gatto et al., 1997; Carstens et al., 1998). It follows that localized expression of an FGFR variant depends on internal processes of the cell expressing it, and expression may be subject to changes induced by normal or malignant differentiation. With the progress of the genome projects, it is becoming clear that alternative splicing and mutually exclusive exon usage is shared by multiple mammalian gene families.

Evolution of coordinated regulation of cell-specific splicing and the selective localization of their ligands had to develop through complex steps during evolution (Coulier et al., 1997). It is noteworthy that in *Drosophila*, breathless, the FGFR of the fly, is expressed in the ep-

ithelium of the tracheal primordium, and its ligand branchless is found in its mesenchymal environment (Klambt et al., 1992; Sutherland et al., 1996). It follows that the coordinated regulation of FGF and FGFR is conserved during evolution. Since the organs of most higher animals and humans are built on adjacent epithelia and mesenchymes (or on other consecutive cell sheets), this paradigm should be important for a better understanding of morphogenesis and organogenesis.

Coordinated spatial regulation of the FGF–FGFR interaction has been demonstrated in a number of developmental mechanisms. The prime example is vertebrate limb development (for reviews, see Martin, 1998; Xu et al., 1999c). Limb outgrowth is mediated by the apical ectodermal ridge (AER), a multilayered epithelial organ on the edge of the developing limb bud. After being removed, the function of the AER can be replaced by externally added FGF (Niswander et al., 1993). This important finding is supported by the direct effect of FGFs on limb outgrowth. Overexpressing FGFs by implanting FGF-Sepharose beads in chick—or, to a lesser extent, in transgenic mouse embryos—results in de novo limb outgrowth (Cohn et al., 1995; Abud et al., 1996). Later genetic studies indicate that the major epithelial mediator of limb outgrowth is FGF8 (Lewandoski et al., 2000; Moon and Capecchi, 2000), which is expressed in the AER-forming epithelium and in mature AER (Heikinheimo et al., 1994).

The epithelial FGFR2IIIb receptor is also expressed in the AER (Orr-Urtreger et al., 1991, 1993). Targeted mutagenesis of FGFR2 (Xu et al., 1998; Arman et al., 1999), or specifically that of its IIIb form (De Moerlooze et al., 2000; Revest et al., 2001), abrogates limb outgrowth and branching morphogenesis of many organs. The epithelial FGFR2IIIb splice variant has affinity for FGF7 and FGF10 in the mesenchyme. Indeed, FGF10 is required for limb outgrowth, and its loss-of-function phenotype is similar to that of FGFR2IIIb (Min et al., 1998; Sekine et al., 1999). Thus as it has been suggested (Ohuchi et al., 1997; Xu et al., 1998), FGFR2 in the AER forms an interaction loop with FGF10 in the mesenchyme (Fig. 32–6).

The FGFR2IIIb–FGF10 interaction does not indicate which receptor may mediate the epithelial FGF8 signal that is essential for limb development (Fig. 32–5). FGR2IIIc is expressed in the limb bud mesenchyme (Orr-Urtreger et al., 1993), but as a recent gene-targeting experiment shows, this receptor is involved in osteogenesis and has only secondary and general effects on the limb skeleton (Eswarakumar et al., 2002). Loss of FGFR1 results in lethality during late gastrulation and early organogenesis (Deng et al., 1994; Yamaguchi et al., 1994), but a chimera experiment revealed that it affects limb development (Deng et al., 1996) and that a hypomorph mutation of FGFR1IIIc creates overt limb defects (Rossant et al., 1997; Partanen et al., 1998). It is therefore likely that the mesenchymal receptor for AER-derived FGFs may be FGFR1IIIc (Fig. 32–6).

The FGF system's involvement in limb development reflects the role of its coordinated regulation of localization and binding specificity in epithelial mesenchymal interaction. FGF signaling is one of the earliest inducers of limb development, and up to recently there was little indication of what induces FGF signaling in the limb fields. A recent study suggests that FGF8 in the chick embryo is activated by Wnt-3a, whereas FGF10 in the forelimb is activated by Wnt-2b and in the hind limb by Wnt-8c (Kawakami et al., 2001; reviewed by Tickle and Munsterberg, 2001).

Limb development is not the only example of coordinate regulation of localization and binding specificity. In the blastocyst, FGF4 is expressed in the inner cell mass, which gives rise to the embryo (Niswander and Martin, 1992), and its disruption causes early lethality (Feldman et al., 1995). FGFR2, in contrast, is restricted to the trophectoderm from which the extraembryonic membranes develop (Haffner-Krausz et al., 1999). Transgenic embryos expressing dominant-negative FGFR4 cDNA die as blastocysts. The present data suggest that multiple FGFRs are active in the early embryo (Chai et al., 1998), and it is not exactly clear which splice alternatives interact with FGF4. Additional examples for interactions between cell layers include FGF–FGFR signaling in odontogenesis (Harada et al., 1999) and liver development (Jung et al., 1999).

It is of clinical interest that ectopic expression of FGFR alternatives, or broadening of their binding specificity, facilitates recep-

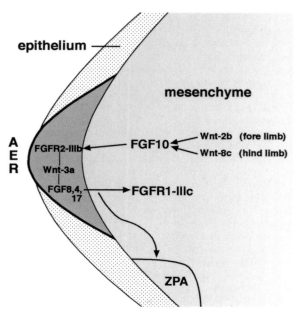

Figure 32–6. FGF–FGFR interactions in the developing vertebrate limb. Cross-section along the dorsal–ventral axis of the early limb bud. Limb outgrowth is a result of epithelial–mesenchymal interactions. Proximal-distal limb outgrowth is regulated by the apical ectodermal ridge (AER), a specialized epithelium at the dorsal–ventral interface of the paddle-shaped early limb bud. Anterior–posterior (thumb to little finger) specification is dictated from an area in the distal mesenchyme, the zone of polarizing activity (ZPA). The AER interacts with the ZPA and with an area in the mesenchyme, the progress zone, immediately beneath the AER. The function of the surgically removed AER can be replaced by FGF, and the AER indeed produces FGF8 and other FGF isotypes. FGFR2IIIb is expressed in the AER, whereas FGF10 (its ligand) in the limb mesenchyme. Targeted disruption of FGFR2IIIb and FGF10 result in similar phenotypes of complete absence of limbs (tetraamelia) and branching lung morphogenesis. FGFR1IIIc is required for the progress zone mesenchyme. Thus FGFR2IIIb with FGF10 and FGFR1IIIc with FGF8 and FGF4 describe an epithelial mesenchymal interaction loop. The figure also shows that FGF10 (in the chick embryo) is activated by the signaling molecules Wnt-2b or Wnt-8c, whereas FGF8 in the AER is probably activated by Wnt-3a.

tor–ligand interaction in the same cell layer. This interference with the coordinate regulation of receptor alternatives and their ligands may lead to pathological results. Apert's syndrome is the most severe form of craniosynostosis (premature fusion of cranial sutures), with excessive fusion of fingers and toes, brain malformations, and mental retardation. Two mutations cause this phenotype: Ser252Trp and Pro253Arg in the linker between DII and DIII. They are associated with increased ligand affinity or change of specificity (Anderson et al., 1998; Yu et al., 2000; Ibrahimi et al., 2001), and the mesenchymal tissues of these patients express mutant FGFR2IIIc that can be activated by mesenchymally expressed ligands (FGF7 and 10). Similarly, the mutant FGFR2IIIb expressed in epithelium can be abnormally activated by epithelial ligands (FGF2, 6, and 9). The other, much rarer, cases of Apert's syndrome contain Alu insertions upstream or within exon 9 which encodes the FGFR2IIIc alternative. Here (Oldridge et al., 1999), as well as in a new mouse model where exon 9 was deleted, the result is expression of the IIIb form in tissues where the IIIc is normally expressed (Hajihosseini et al., 2001). This mesenchymal expression of FGFR2IIIb results in defects like Apert's syndrome. Both types of mutation are associated with abnormal mesenchymal differentiation, including bone and parenchymal tissue defects.

Considering the multiplicity of physiological processes that are controlled by the FGF system, these types of splicing defect may be involved in additional, hitherto unrecognized pathologies. Abnormal splicing has been observed in hormone-resistant prostate cancer cell lines (Yan, 1993; Carstens et al., 1998), and a subgroup of prostate cancer patients was characterized by abnormal splicing of FGFR2

(Kwabi-Addo et al., 2001). We assume that additional pathologies will be found to be associated with the disturbed localization and binding specificity of FGFR variants. Common to these mutations is that either the mutant receptor becomes expressed in an ectopic cell layer or its binding specificity is altered. Both changes break the coordinated control of FGFR localization and binding specificity, as much as mesenchymal receptors now also bind mesenchymal ligands and normally epithelial receptors also bind epithelial ligands. This change disrupts the epithelial mesenchymal interactions that are required for the normal control of cell differentiation and organogenesis and may have serious pathological consequences.

Interactions of FGFs and FGFRs with the Extracellular Matrix

The present view of FGF signaling suggests that heparan sulfates of the extracellular matrix not only bind and accumulate FGF but also contribute to receptor dimerization (Spivak-Kroizman et al., 1994) and are essential components of the signaling complex (Plotnikov et al., 1999). Some HSPGs associate with the cell surface, such as syndecans and glypicans, which are integral membrane proteins, whereas perlecan and agrin bind to laminin and collagen IV isotypes, the network-forming proteins of the basement membrane (Timpl and Brown, 1996; Perrimon and Bernfield, 2000). Introduction of various sugar moieties into heparan sulfates can create a very high degree of structural variability (Turnbull et al., 2001). There is evidence to suggest that the structure of heparan sulfates contributes to the specificity of FGF signaling. The binding of FGF2 in situ to its receptors may be modified by locally available HSPGs (Chang et al., 2000). Heparan sulfate biosynthesis is template independent, and the same protein core could carry diverse heparan sulfates; thus, one can foresee that these sulfates may introduce a degree of local variation to the specificity of FGF signaling and modify cell differentiation and development to a yet-unknown extent.

Recent genetic analysis of the complex synthesis of HSPG saccharides provided new insights. Mutations in enzymes of heparan sulfate biosynthesis and in the core proteins of HSPG are connected to developmental defects (for review, see Perrimon and Bernfield, 2000). The phenotypes of *sugarless* and *sulfateless,* mutations of *Drosophila* genes that encode enzymes of heparan sulfate biosynthesis, are similar to mutations of the *Drosophila* FGFR *breathless.* Moreover, overexpression of *Drosophila* FGFR could partially rescue the *sugarless* and *sulfateless* phenotype (Lin et al., 1999), suggesting that HSPG biosynthesis and FGFRs are functionally connected.

Besides intimate involvement of FGF signaling with heparan sulfates, it was recently acknowledged that other polypeptide growth factors also display affinity to heparin and the extracellular matrix. To this group belong heparin-binding EGF and members of the important *hedgehog* and wnt families of signaling factors (for reviews, see Perrimon and Bernfield, 2000; Selleck, 2000; see Chapters 16 and 22). The emerging paradigm suggests that the extracellular matrix through its HSPGs is a central mediator of differentiation and developmental signaling. Thus cell to cell interactions take place through the extracellular matrix as its intermediary, which sorts and presents growth factors, but participates, as in the case of the FGF system, in the receptor–ligand interactions as well. Cell surface HSPGs contribute to cell to cell signaling, whereas the basement membrane, a mat-like modification of the extracellular matrix that separates cell layers, mediates interactions between cell sheets, such as epithelia and mesenchymes. The laminin and collagen IV isotypes of the basement membrane are required for epithelial morphogenesis in various organs (for review, see Ekblom et al., 1998).

Connection between FGF signaling and basement membrane formation was demonstrated by experiments with ES cell–derived embryoid bodies that expressed truncated FGFR2 cDNA. This dominant-negative mutation, which may abrogate the function of most FGFR isotypes, failed to differentiate into the two epithelial layers of the embryoid body and did not form basement membrane. The mutation was characterized by abrogation of PI3K signaling via the inhibition of Akt/PKB phosphorylation (Chen et al., 2000). Embryoid bodies with defective FGF signaling failed to express laminin and collagen IV isotypes, but this loss-of-function phenotype could be partially restored by externally added purified laminin-1, suggesting a role for FGF signaling in laminin and collagen biosynthesis and basement membrane assembly (Li et al., 2001a). This suggestion was validated by showing that constitutively active Akt/PKB activates laminin and collagen IV transcription, whereas dominant-negative Akt/PKB inhibits it (Li et al. 2001b). It follows that FGF signaling may directly affect basement membrane assembly through activating the PI3K-Akt/PKB pathway.

Laminin isotypes bind proteoglycans and other basement membrane proteins, as they are at the core of basement membrane self assembly (Cheng et al., 1997). Basement membrane assembly activated by FGF signaling may be a powerful amplifier of HSPG-associated signaling. Basement membranes are at the interface of cell sheets, and, as such, they are eminent candidates to convey epithelial mesenchymal interactions. Therefore, the two functional characteristics of the FGF system discussed here—coordinated localization and binding specificity of FGFs and FGFRs—as well as regulation of basement membrane assembly, can explain important aspects of developmental and physiological signaling.

A somewhat similar functional connection was found between FGF signaling and cell to cell or cell to matrix adhesion. FGFR1 and Shp2 and associated phosphatase are expressed in the progress zone mesenchyme of the developing limb bud, and their loss-of-function mutations lead to cell shape changes and changes in cell to cell adhesion (Saxton et al., 2000). In the early embryo, FGFR1 is required for migration of the presumptive mesoderm across the primitive streak. Ciruna and Rossant (2001) have shown that FGFR1 orchestrates this epithelium to mesenchyme transition through the control of Snail and E-cadherin, which also involves the β-catenin control of the wnt–cadherin interaction.

As described in this chapter, recent molecular analysis delineates the requirement for an FGF–FGFR–heparin sulfate complex for receptor activation; the role of heparin sulfates in embryonic development; and the relationship between cell adhesion, the extracellular matrix, and FGF signaling. It is likely that this type of research presents an opening toward a common mechanism for the role of the FGF system in development and differentiation.

ACKNOWLEDGMENTS

We thank J. Krishnamurthy for his help in preparation and editing of this manuscript. We are indebted to Dr. Moosa Mohammadi for the production of the ribbon models of FGF and the complex FGF : FGFR : Heparin.

REFERENCES

Aaronson SA, Bottaro DP, Miki T, Ron D, Finch PW, Fleming TP, Ahn J, Taylor WG, Rubin JS (1991). Keratinocyte growth factor: a fibroblast growth factor family member with unusual target cell specificity. *Ann NY Acad Sci* 638: 62–77.

Abud H, Skinner JA, McDonald FJ, Bedford MT, Lonai P, Heath JK (1996). Ectopic expression of FGF-4 in chimeric mouse embryos induces the expression of early markers of limb development in the lateral ridge. *Dev Genet* 181: 51–65.

Amaya E, Musci TJ, Kirschner MW (1991). Expression of a dominant negative mutant of the FGF receptor disrupts mesoderm formation in *Xenopus* embryos. *Cell* 66: 257–270.

Anderson J, Burns HD, Enriquez-Harris P, Wilkie AOM, Heath JK (1998). Apert syndrome mutations in fibroblast growth factor receptor 2 exhibit increased affinity for FGF ligand. *Hum Mol Genet* 7: 1475–1483.

Arman E, Haffner-Krausz R, Chen Y, Heath JK, Lonai P (1998). Targeted disruption of FGFR2 suggests a role for FGF signaling in pre-gastrulation mammalian development. *Proc Natl Acad Sci USA* 95: 5082–5087.

Arman E, Haffner-Krausz R, Gorivodsky M, Lonai P (1999). FGFR2 is required for limb outgrowth and lung branching morphogenesis. *Proc Natl Acad Sci USA* 96: 11895–11899.

Avivi A, Yayon A, Givol D (1993). A novel form of FGF receptor-3 using an alternative exon in the immunoglobulin domain III. *FEBS Lett* 330: 249–252.

Bargmann CI, Hung MC, Weinberg RA (1986). Multiple independent activations of the neu oncogene by a point mutation altering the transmembrane domain of p185. *Cell* 45: 649–657.

Beer HD, Vindevoghel L, Gait MJ, Revest JM, Duan DR, Mason I, Dickson C, Werner S (2000). Fibroblast growth factor (FGF) receptor 1-IIIb is a naturally occurring functional receptor for FGFs that is preferentially expressed in the skin and the brain. *J Biol Chem* 275: 16091–16097.

Bellus GA, Gaudenz K, Zackai EH, Clarke LA, Szabo J, Francomano CA, Muenke M (1996). Identical mutations in three different fibroblast growth factor receptor genes in autosomal dominant craniosynostosis syndromes. *Nat Genet* 14: 174–176.

Burgess WH, Maciag T (1989). The heparin binding (fibroblast) growth factor family of proteins. *Annu Rev Biochem* 58: 575–606.

Carstens RP, McKeehan WL, Garcia-Blanco MA (1998). An intronic sequence element mediates both activation and repression of rat fibroblast growth factor receptor 2 pre-mRNA splicing. *Mol Cell Biol* 18: 2205–2217.

Chai N, Patel Y, Jacobson K, McMahon J, McMahon A, Rappolee DA (1998). FGF is an essential regulator of the fifth cell division in preimplantation mouse embryos. *Dev Biol* 198: 105–115.

Chang Z, Meyer K, Rapraeger AC, Friedl A (2000). Differential ability of heparan sulfate proteoglycans to assemble the fibroblast growth factor receptor complex in situ. *FASEB J* 14: 137–144.

Chen L, Adar R, Yang X, Monsonego EO, Li C, Hauschka PV, Yayon A, Deng CX (1999). Gly369Cys mutation in mouse FGFR3 causes achondroplasia by affecting both chondrogenesis and osteogenesis. *J Clin Invest* 104: 1517–1525.

Chen Y, Li X, Eswarakumar VP, Seger R, Lonai P (2000). Fibroblast growth factor (FGF) signaling through PI 3-kinase and Akt/PKB is required for embryoid body differentiation. *Oncogene* 19: 3750–3756.

Cheng YS, Champliaud MF, Burgeson RE, Marinkovich MP, Yurchenco PD (1997). Self-assembly of laminin isoforms. *J Biol Chem* 272: 31525–31532.

Chin YE, Kitagawa M, Su WC, You ZH, Iwamoto Y, Fu XY (1996). Cell growth arrest and induction of cyclin-dependent kinase inhibitor p21$^{WAF1/Cip1}$ mediated by STAT1. *Science* 272: 719–722.

Ciruna B, Rossant J (2001). FGF signaling regulates mesoderm cell fate specification and morphogenetic movement at the primitive streak. *Dev Cell* 1: 37–49.

Cohn MJ, Izpisua-Belmonte JC, Abud H, Heath JK, Tickle C (1995). Fibroblast growth factors induce additional limb development from the flank of chick embryos. *Cell* 80: 739–746.

Colvin JS, Bohne BA, Harding GW, McEwen DG, Ornitz DM (1996). Skeletal overgrowth and deafness in mice lacking fibroblast growth factor receptor 3. *Nat Genet* 12: 390–397.

Colvin JS, White AC, Pratt SJ, Ornitz DM (2001). Lung hypoplasia and neonatal death in FGF9-null mice identify this gene as an essential regulator of lung mesenchyme. *Development* 128: 2095–2106.

Cornejo-Roldan LR, Roessler E, Muenke M (1999). Analysis of the mutational spectrum of the *FGFR2* gene in Pfeiffer syndrome. *Hum Genet* 104: 425–431.

Coulier F, Pontarotti P, Roubin R, Hartung H, Goldfarb M, Birnbaum D (1997). Of worms and men: an evolutionary perspective on the fibroblast growth factor (FGF) and FGF families. *J Mol Evol* 44: 43–56.

Crossley PH, Martinez S, Martin GR (1996). Midbrain development induced by FGF8 in the chick embryo. *Nature* 380: 66–68.

Darnell JE Jr (1997). STATs and gene regulation. *Science* 277: 1630–1635.

Del Gatto F, Plet A, Gesnel MC, Fort C, Breathnach R (1997). Multiple interdependent sequence elements control splicing of a fibroblast growth factor receptor 2 alternative exon. *Mol Cell Biol* 17: 5106–5116.

deLapeyriere O, Ollendorff V, Planche J, Ott MO, Pizette S, Coulier F, Birnbaum D (1993). Expression of the *FGF6* gene is restricted to developing skeletal muscle in the mouse embryo. *Development* 118: 601–611.

De Moerlooze L, Spencer-Dene B, Revest J, Hajihosseini M, Rosewell I, Dickson C (2000). An important role for the IIIb isoform of fibroblast growth factor receptor 2 (FGFR2) in mesenchymal-epithelial signalling during mouse organogenesis. *Development* 127: 483–492.

Deng C, Wynshaw-Boris A, Zhou F, Kuo A, Leder P (1996). Fibroblast growth factor receptor-3 is a negative regulator of bone growth. *Cell* 84: 911–921.

Deng CX, Wynshaw-Boris A, Shen MM, Daugherty C, Ornitz DM, Leder P (1994). Murine FGFR-1 is required for early postimplantation growth and axial organization. *Genes Dev* 8: 3045–3057.

Dickson C, Deed R, Dixon M, Peters G (1989). The structure and function of the int-2 oncogene. *Prog Growth Factor Res* 1: 123–132.

DiGabriele AD, Lax I, Chen DI, Svahn CM, Jaye M, Schlessinger J, Hendrickson WA (1998). Structure of a heparin-linked biologically active dimer of fibroblast growth factor. *Nature* 393: 812–817.

Dono R, Texido G, Dussel R, Ehmke H, Zeller R (1998). Impaired cerebral cortex development and blood pressure regulation in FGF-2-deficient mice. *EMBO J* 17: 4213–4225.

Ekblom M, Falk M, Salmivirta K, Durbeej M, Ekblom P (1998). Laminin isoforms and epithelial development. *Ann NY Acad Sci* 857: 194–211.

Eswarakumar VP, Monsonego-Ornan E, Pines M, Antonopoulou I, Morriss-Kay GM, Lonai P (2002). The IIIc alternative of Fgfr2 is a positive regulator of bone formation *Development* 129: 3783–3793.

Faham S, Linhardt RJ, Rees DC (1998). Diversity does make a difference: fibroblast growth factor–heparin interactions. *Curr Opin Struct Biol* 8: 578–586.

Feldman B, Poueymirou W, Papaioannou VE, DeChiara TM, Goldfarb M (1995). Requirement of FGF4 for postimplantation mouse development. *Science* 267: 246–249.

Flamme I, Risau W (1992). Induction of vasculogenesis and hematopiesis in vitro. *Development* 116: 435–439.

Floss T, Arnold HH, Braun T (1997). A role for FGF-6 in skeletal muscle regeneration. *Genes Dev* 11: 2040–2051.

Gallagher JT (2001). Heparan sulfate: growth control with a restricted sequence menu. *J Clin Invest* 108: 357–361.

Galvin BD, Hart KC, Meyer AN, Webster MK, Donoghue DJ (1996). Constitutive receptor activation by Crouzon syndrome mutations in fibroblast growth factor receptor FGFR2 and FGFR2/Neu chimeras. *Proc Natl Acad Sci USA* 93: 7894–7899.

Givol D, Yayon A (1992). Complexity of FGF receptors: genetic basis for structural diversity and functional specificity. *FASEB J* 6: 3362–3369.

Gospodarowicz D (1974). Localisation of a fibroblast growth factor and its effect alone and with hydrocortisone on 3T3 cell growth. *Nature* 249: 123–127.

Guimond SE, Turnbull JE (1999). Fibroblast growth factor receptor signalling is dictated by specific heparan sulphate saccharides. *Curr Biol* 9: 1343–1346.

Guo L, Degenstein L, Fuchs E (1996). Keratinocyte growth factor is required for hair development but not for wound healing. *Genes Dev* 10: 165–175.

Hadari YR, Gotoh N, Kouhara I, Lax I, Schlessinger J (2001). Critical role for the docking-protein FRS2 alpha in FGF receptor-mediated signal transduction pathways. *Proc Natl Acad Sci USA* 98: 8578–8583.

Haffner-Krausz R, Gorivodsky M, Chen Y, Lonai P (1999). Expression of FGFR2 during oogenesis, preimplantation and early postimplantation embryogenesis. *Mech Dev* 85: 167–172.

Hajihosseini MK, Wilson S, De Moerlooze L, Dickson C (2001). A splicing switch and gain-of-function mutation in FGFR2-IIIc hemizygotes causes Apert/Pfeiffer-syndrome-like phenotypes. *Proc Natl Acad Sci USA* 98: 3855–3860.

Harada H, Kettunen P, Jung HS, Mustonen T, Wang YA, Thesleff I (1999). Localization of putative stem cells in dental epithelium and their association with Notch and FGF signaling. *J Cell Biol* 147: 105–120.

Hart KC, Robertson SC, Donoghue DJ (2001). Identification of tyrosine residues in constitutively activated fibroblast growth factor receptor 3 involved in mitogenesis, Stat activation, and phosphatidylinositol 3-kinase activation. *Mol Biol Cell* 12: 931–942.

Hebert JM, Rosenquist T, Gotz J, Martin GM (1994). FGF5 as a regulator of the hair growth cycle: evidence from targeted and spontaneous mutations. *Cell* 78: 1017–1025.

Hehr U, Muenke M (1999). Craniosynostosis syndromes: from genes to premature fusion of skull bones. *Mol Genet Metab* 68: 139–151.

Heikinheimo M, Lawshe A, Shackleford GM, Wilson DB, MacArthur CA (1994). FGF-8 expression in the post-gastrulation mouse suggests roles in the development of the face, limbs and central nervous system. *Mech Dev* 48: 129–138.

Hrabé de Angelis MH, Flaswinkel H, Fuchs H, Rathkolb B, Soewarto D, et al. (2000). Genome-wide, large-scale production of mutant mice by ENU mutagenesis. *Nat Genet* 25: 444–447.

Hunter T (2000). Signaling-2000 and beyond. *Cell* 100: 113–127.

Ibrahimi OA, Eliseenkova AV, Plotnikov AN, Yu K, Ornitz DM, Mohammadi M (2001). Structural basis for fibroblast growth factor receptor 2 activation in Apert syndrome. *Proc Natl Acad Sci USA* 98: 7182–7187.

Iwata T, Chen L, Li C, Ovchinnikov DA, Behringer RR, Francomano CA, Deng CX (2000). A neonatal lethal mutation in FGFR3 uncouples proliferation and differentiation of growth plate chondrocytes in embryos. *Hum Mol Genet* 9: 1603–1613.

Iwata T, Li CL, Deng CX, Francomano CA (2001). Highly activated Fgfr3 with the K644M mutation causes prolonged survival in severe dwarf mice. *Hum Mol Genet* 10: 1255–1264.

Jang JH, Shin KH, Park YJ, Lee RJ, McKeehan WL, Park JG (2000). Novel transcripts of fibroblast growth factor receptor 3 reveal aberrant splicing and activation of cryptic splice sequences in colorectal cancer. *Cancer Res* 60: 4049–4052.

Jaye M, Schlessinger J, Dionne CA (1992). Fibroblast growth factor receptor tyrosine kinases: molecular analysis and signal transduction. *Biochim Biophys Acta* 1135: 185–199.

Johnson DE, Williams LT (1993). Structural and functional diversity in the FGF receptor multigene family. *Adv Cancer Res* 60: 1–41.

Johnson DE, Lu J, Chen H, Werner S, Williams LT (1991). The human fibroblast growth factor receptor genes: a common structural arrangement underlies the mechanisms for generating receptor forms that differ in their third immunoglobulin domain. *Mol Cell Biol* 11: 4627–4634.

Jones RB, Wang F, Luo Y, Yu C, Jin C, Suzuki T, Kan M, McKeehan WL (2001). The nonsense-mediated decay pathway and mutually exclusive expression of alternatively spliced FGFR2IIIB and -IIIc mRNAs. *J Biol Chem* 276: 4158–4167.

Jung J, Zheng M, Goldfarb M, Zaret KS (1999). Initiation of mammalian liver development from endoderm by fibroblast growth factors. *Science* 284: 1998–2003.

Kan M, Wang F, Xu J, Crabb JW, Hou J, McKeehan WL (1993). An essential heparin binding domain in the fibroblast growth factor receptor kinase. *Science* 259: 1918–1921.

Kannan K, Givol D (2000). FGF receptor mutations: dimerization syndromes, cell growth suppression, and animal models. *IUBMB Life* 49: 197–205.

Kawakami Y, Capdevila J, Buscher D, Itoh T, Rodriguez Esteban C, Izpisua Belmonte JC (2001). WNT signals control FGF-dependent limb initiation and AER induction in the chick embryo. *Cell* 104: 891–900.

Kettunen P, Karavanova I, Thesleff I (1998). Responsiveness of developing dental tissues to fibroblast growth factors: expression of splicing alternatives of FGFR1, -2, -3, and of FGFR4; and stimulation of cell proliferation by FGF-2, -4, -8, and -9. *Dev Genet* 22: 374–385.

Klagsburn M (1990). The affinity of fibroblast growth factors for heparin; FGF–heparan sulfate interactions in cells and extracellular matrix. *Curr Biol* 2: 857–863.

Klambt C, Glazer L, Shilo B-Z (1992). *breathless*, a *Drosophila* FGF receptor homolog, is essential for migration of tracheal and specific midline glial cells. *Genes Dev* 6: 1668–1678.

Klint P, Claesson-Welsh L (1999). Signal transduction by fibroblast growth factor receptors. *Front Biosci* 4: D165.

Kornbluth S, Paulson KE, Hanafusa H (1988). Novel tyrosine kinase identified by phosphotyrosine antibody screening of cDNA libraries. *Mol Cell Biol* 8: 5541–5544.

Kwabi-Addo B, Ropiquet F, Giri D, Ittmann M (2001). Alternative splicing of fibroblast growth factor receptors in human prostate cancer. *Prostate* 46: 163–172.

Lee PL, Johnson DE, Cousens LS, Fried VA, Williams LT (1989). Purification and cDNA cloning of a receptor for basic fibroblast growth factor. *Science* 245: 57–60.

Lee SMK, Danielian PS, Fritzsch B, McMahon AP (1997). Evidence that FGF8 signaling from the midbrain–hindbrain junction regulates growth and polarity in the developing brain. *Development* 124: 959–969.

Lemmon MA, Schlessinger J (1994). Regulation of signal transduction and signal diversity by receptor oligomerization. *Trends Biochem Sci* 19: 459–463.

Lewandoski M, Sun X, Martin GR (2000). FGF8 signalling from the AER is essential for normal limb development. *Nat Genet* 26: 460–463.

Li C, Chen L, Iwata T, Kitagawa M, Fu XY, Deng CX (1999). A Lys644Glu substitution in fibroblast growth factor receptor 3 (FGFR3) causes dwarfism in mice by activation of STATs and ink4 cell cycle inhibitors. *Hum Mol Genet* 8: 35–44.

Li X, Chen Y, Scheele S, Arman E, Haffner-Krausz R, Ekblom P, Lonai P (2001a). FGF signaling and basement membrane assembly are connected during epithelial morphogenesis of the embryoid body. *J Cell Biol* 153: 811–822.

Li X, Talts U, Talts JF, Arman E, Ekblom P, Lonai P (2001b). Akt/PKB regulates laminin and collagen IV isotypes of the basement membrane. *Proc Natl Acad Sci USA* 98: 14416–14421.

Li Y, Mangasarian K, Mansukhani A, Basilico C (1997). Activation of FGF receptors by mutations in the transmembrane domain. *Oncogene* 14: 1397–1406.

Lin X, Buff EM, Perrimon N, Michelson AM (1999). Heparan sulfate proteoglycans are essential for FGF receptor signaling during *Drosophila* embryonic development. *Development* 126: 3715–3723.

Liu Z, Xu J, Colvin JS, Ornitz DM (2002). Coordination of chondrogenesis and osteogenesis by fibroblast growth factor 18. *Genes Dev* 16: 859–869.

Lonai P (1996). Functional analysis of the FGF system. In *Mammalian Development*. Lonai P (ed.) Harwood Academic Publishers, Amsterdam, pp. 217–231.

Lundin L, Larsson H, Kreuger J, Kanda S, Lindahl U, Salmivirta M, Claesson-Welsh L (2000). Selectively desulfated heparin inhibits fibroblast growth factor–induced mitogenicity and angiogenesis. *J Biol Chem* 275: 24653–24660.

Mansour SL, Goddard JM, Capecchi MR (1993). Mice homozygous for a targeted disruption of the proto-oncogene int-2 have developmental defects in the tail and inner ear. *Development* 117: 13–28.

Martin GR (1998). The roles of FGFs in the early development of vertebrate limbs. *Genes Dev* 12: 1571–1586.

Meyers EN, Lewandoski M, Martin GR (1998). An FGF8 mutant allelic series generated by Cre- and Flp-mediated recombination. *Nat Genet* 18: 136–141.

Mignatti P, Morimoto T, Rifkin DB (1992). Basic fibroblast growth factor, a protein devoid of secretory signal sequence, is released by cells via a pathway independent of the endoplasmic reticulum–Golgi complex. *J Cell Physiol* 151: 81–93.

Miki T, Bottaro DP, Fleming TP, Smith CL, Burgess WH, Chan AM, Aaronson SA (1992). Determination of ligand-binding specificity by alternative splicing: two distinct growth factor receptors encoded by a single gene. *Proc Natl Acad Sci USA* 89: 246–250.

Miller DL, Ortega S, Bashayan O, Basch R, Basilico C (2000). Compensation by fibroblast growth factor 1 (FGF1) does not account for the mild phenotypic defects observed in FGF2 null mice. *Mol Cell Biol* 20: 2260–2268.

Mills AA, Bradley A (2001). From mouse to man: generating megabase chromosome rearrangements. *Trends Genet* 17: 331–339.

Min H, Danilenko DM, Scully SA, Bolon B, Ring BD, Tarpley JE, DeRose M, Simonet WS (1998). FGF-10 is required for both limb and lung development and exhibits striking functional similarity to *Drosophila branchless*. *Genes Dev* 12: 3156–3161.

Mohammadi M, Honegger AM, Rotin D, Fischer R, Bellot F, Li W, Dionne CA, Jaye M, Rubinstein M, Schlessinger J (1991). A tyrosine-phosphorylated carboxy-terminal peptide of the fibroblast growth factor receptor (Flg) is a binding site for the SH2 domain of phospholipase C-γ 1. *Mol Cell Biol* 11: 5068–5078.

Mohammadi M, Schlessinger J, Hubbard SR (1996). Structure of the FGF receptor tyrosine kinase domain reveals a novel autoinhibitory mechanism for receptor tyrosine kinases. *Cell* 86: 577–587.

Moon AM, Capecchi MR (2000). Fgf8 is required for outgrowth and patterning of the limbs. *Nat Genet* 4: 455–459.

Muenke M, Schell U (1995). Fibroblast-growth-factor receptor mutations in human skeletal disorders. *Trends Genet* 11: 308–313.

Naski MC, Ornitz DM (1998). FGF signaling in skeletal development. *Front Biosci* 3: d781–794.

Naski MC, Wang Q, Xu J, Ornitz DM (1996). Graded activation of fibroblast growth factor receptor 3 by mutations causing achondroplasia and thanatophoric dysplasia. *Nat Genet* 13: 233–237.

Naski MC, Colvin JS, Coffin JD, Ornitz DM (1998). Repression of hedgehog signaling and BMP4 expression in growth plate cartilage by fibroblast growth factor receptor 3. *Development* 125: 4977–4988.

Niswander L, Martin GR (1992). FGF-4 expression during gastrulation, myogenesis, limb and tooth development in the mouse. *Development* 114: 755–768.

Niswander L, Tickle C, Vogel A, Booth I, Martin GR (1993). FGF-4 replaces the apical ectodermal ridge and directs outgrowth and patterning of the limb. *Cell* 75: 579–587.

Ohuchi H, Nakagawa T, Yamamoto A, Araga A, Ohata T, Ishimaru Y, Yoshioka H, Kuwana T, Nohno T, Yamasaki M, et al. (1997). The mesenchymal factor, FGF10, initiates and maintains the outgrowth of the chick limb bud through interaction with FGF8, an apical ectodermal factor. *Development* 124: 2235–2244.

Oldridge M, Zackai EH, McDonald-McGinn DM, Iseki S, Morriss-Kay GM, Twigg SR, Johnson D, Wall SA, Jiang W, Theda C, et al. (1999). De novo alu-element insertions in FGFR2 identify a distinct pathological basis for Apert syndrome. *Am J Hum Genet* 64: 446–461.

Ornitz DM (2000). FGFs, heparan sulfate and FGFRs: complex interactions essential for development. *Bioessays* 22: 108.

Ornitz DM, Itoh N (2001). Fibroblast growth factors. *Genome Biol* 2: REVIEWS3005.

Ornitz DM, Xu J, Colvin JS, McEwen DG, McArthur CA, Coulier F, Gao G, Goldfarb M (1996). Receptor specificity of the fibroblast growth factor family. *J Biol Chem* 271: 15292–15297.

Orr-Urtreger A, Givol D, Yayon A, Yarden Y, Lonai P (1991). Developmental expression of two murine fibroblast growth factor receptors, flg and bek. *Development* 113: 1419–1434.

Orr-Urtreger A, Bedford MT, Burakova T, Arman E, Zimmer Y, Yayon A, Givol D, Lonai P (1993). Developmental localization of the splicing alternatives of fibroblast growth factor receptor-2 (FGFR2). *Dev Biol* 158: 475–486.

Partanen J, Schwartz L, Rossant J (1998). Opposite phenotypes of hypomorphic and Y766 phosphorylation site mutations reveal a function for FGFR1 in anteroposterior patterning of mouse embryos. *Genes Dev* 12: 2332–2344.

Passos-Bueno MR, Wilcox WR, Jabs EW, Sertie AL, Alonso LG, Kitoh H (1999). Clinical spectrum of fibroblast growth factor receptor mutations. *Hum Mutat* 14: 115–125.

Perrimon N, Bernfield M (2000). Specificities of heparan sulfate proteoglycans in developmental processes. *Nature* 404: 725–728.

Plotnikov AN, Schlessinger J, Hubbard SR, Mohammadi M (1999). Structural basis for FGF receptor dimerization and activation. *Cell* 98: 641–650.

Rappolee DA, Patel Y, Jacobson K (1998). Expression of fibroblast growth factor receptors in peri-implantation mouse embryos. *Mol Reprod Dev* 51: 254–264.

Rapraeger AC, Krufka A, Olwin BB (1991). Requirement of heparan sulfate for bFGF-mediated fibroblast growth and myoblast differentiation. *Science* 252: 1705–1708.

Revest JM, Spencer-Dene B, Kerr K, De Moerlooze L, Rosewell I, Dickson C (2001). Fibroblast growth factor receptor 2-IIIb acts upstream of Shh and FGF4 and is required for limb bud maintenance but not for the induction of FGF8, FGF10, Msx1, or Bmp4. *Dev Biol* 231: 47–62.

Rice DP, Aberg T, Chan Y, Tang Z, Kettunen PJ, Pakarinen L, Maxson RE, Thesleff I (2000). Integration of FGF and TWIST in calvarial bone and suture development. *Development* 127: 1845–1855.

Risau W, Flamme I (1995). Vasculogenesis. *Annu Rev Cell Dev Biol* 11: 73–91.

Rossant J, Ciruna B, Partanen J (1997). FGF signaling in mouse gastrulation and antero-posterior patterning. *Cold Spring Harb Symp Quant Biol* 62: 127–133.

Rousseau F, Bonaventure J, Legeai-Mallet L, Pelet A, Rozet JM, Maroteaux P, Le Merrer M, Munnich A (1994). Mutations in the gene encoding fibroblast growth factor receptor 3 in achondroplasia. *Nature* 371: 252–254.

Rousseau F, Saugier P, Le Merrer M, Munnich A, Delezoide AL, Maroteaux P, Bonaventure J, Narcy F, Sanak M (1995). Stop codon FGFR3 mutations in thanatophoric dwarfism type I. *Nat Genet* 10: 11–12.

Ruta M, Howk R, Ricca G, Drohan W, Labelshansky M, Laureys G, Barton E, Francke U, Schlessinger J, Givol D (1988). A novel protein–tyrosine kinase gene whose expression is modulated during embryonic development. *Oncogene* 3: 9–15.

Sahni M, Ambrosetti DC, Mansukhani A, Gertner R, Levy D, Basilico C (1999). FGF signaling inhibits chondrocyte proliferation and regulates bone development through the STAT-1 pathway. *Genes Dev* 13: 1361–1366.

Saxton TM, Ciruna BG, Holmyard D, Kulkarni S, Harpal K, Rossant J, Pawson T (2000). The SH2 tyrosine phosphatase shp2 is required for mammalian limb development. *Nat Genet* 4: 420–423.

Schlessinger J (2000). Cell signaling by receptor tyrosine kinases. *Cell* 103: 211–225.

Schlessinger J, Plotnikov AN, Ibrahimi OA, Eliseenkova AV, Yeh BK, Yayon A, Linhardt RJ, Mohammadi M (2000). Crystal structure of a ternary FGF-FGFR-heparin complex reveals a dual role for heparin in FGFR binding and dimerization. *Mol Cell* 6: 743–750.

Sekine T, Ohuchi H, Fujiwara M, Yamasaki M, Yoshizawa T, Sato T, Yagishita N, Matsui D, Koga Y, Itoh N, Kato S (1999). FGF10 is essential for limb and lung formation. *Nat Genet* 21: 138–141.

Selleck SB (2000). Proteoglycans and pattern formation: sugar biochemistry meets developmental genetics. *Trends Genet* 16: 206–212.

Shiang R, Thompson LM, Zhu YZ, Church DM, Fielder TJ, Bocian M, Winokur ST, Wasmuth JJ (1994). Mutations in the transmembrane domain of FGFR3 cause the most common genetic form of dwarfism, achondroplasia. *Cell* 787: 335–342.

Smith JC (1989). Mesoderm induction and mesoderm-inducing factors in early amphibian development. *Development* 105: 665–677.

Spivak-Kroizman T, Lemmon MA, Dikic I, Ladbury JE, Pinchasi J, Huang J, Jaye M, Crumley G, Schlessinger J, Lax I (1994). Heparin induced oligomerization of FGF molecules is responsible for FGF receptor dimerization, activation and cell proliferation. *Cell* 79: 1015–1024.

Stauber DJ, DiGabriele AD, Hendrickson WA (2000). Structural interactions of fibroblast growth factor and its ligands. *Proc Natl Acad Sci* 97: 49–54.

Su WC, Kitagawa M, Xue N, Xie B, Garofalo S, Cho J, Deng C, Horton WA, Fu XY (1997). Activation of Stat1 by mutant fibroblast growth factor receptor in thanatophoric dysplasia type II dwarfism. *Nature* 386: 288–292.

Sun X, Meyers EN, Lewandoski M, Martin GR (1999). Targeted disruption of FGF8 causes failure of cell migration in the gastrulating mouse embryo. *Genes Dev* 13: 1834–1846.

Sutherland D, Samakovlis C, Krasnow M (1996). *branchless* encodes a *Drosophila* FGF homolog that controls tracheal cell migration and the pattern of branching. *Cell* 87: 1091–1101.

Tavormina PL, Shiang R, Thompson LM, Zhu YZ, Wilkin DJ, Lachman RS, Wilcox WR, Rimoin DL, Cohn DH, Wasmuth JJ (1995). Thanatophoric dysplasia (types I and II) caused by direct mutations in fibroblast growth factor receptor 3. *Nat Genet* 9: 321–328.

Tavormina PL, Bellus GA, Webster MK, Bamshad MJ, Fraley AE, McIntosh I, Szabo J, Jiang W, Jabs EW, Wilcox WR, et al. (1999). A novel skeletal dysplasia with developmental delay and acanthosis nigricans is caused by a Lys-650-Met mutation in fibroblast growth factor receptor 3 gene. *Am J Hum Genet* 64: 722–731.

Thesleff I, Sharpe P (1997). Signalling networks regulating dental development. *Mech Dev* 67: 111–123.

Tickle C, Munsterberg A (2001). Vertebrate limb development: the early stages in chick and mouse. *Curr Opin Genet Dev* 11: 476–481.

Timpl R, Brown JC (1996). Supramolecular assembly of basement membranes. *BioEssays* 18: 123–132.

Turnbull J, Powell A, Guimond S (2001). Heparan sulfate: decoding a dynamic multifunctional cell regulator. *Trends Cell Biol* 11: 75–82.

Wang Q, McEwen DG, Ornitz DM (2000). Subcellular and developmental expression of alternatively spliced forms of fibroblast growth factor 14. *Mech Dev* 90: 283–287.

Wang Y, Spatz ML, Kannan K, Hayk H, Avivi A, Gorivodsky M, Pines M, Yayon A, Lonai P, Givol D (1999). A mouse model for achondroplasia produced by targeting fibroblast growth factor receptor 3. *Proc Natl Acad Sci USA* 96: 4455–4460.

Webster MK, Donoghue DJ (1996). Constitutive activation of fibroblast growth factor receptor 3 by the transmembrane domain point mutation found in achondroplasia. *EMBO J* 15: 520.

Webster MK, Donoghue DJ (1997). FGFR activation in skeletal disorders: too much of a good thing. *Trends Genet* 13: 178–182.

Webster MK, D'Avis PY, Robertson SC, Donoghue DJ (1996). Profound ligand-independent kinase activation of fibroblast growth factor receptor 3 by the activation loop mutation responsible for a lethal skeletal dysplasia, thanatophoric dysplasia type II. *Mol Cell Biol* 16: 4081–4087.

Weiner DB, Liu J, Cohen JA, Williams WV, Greene MI (1989). A point mutation in the neu oncogene mimics ligand induction of receptor aggregation. *Nature* 339: 230–231.

Weinstein M, Xu X, Ohyama K, Deng C-X (1998a). FGFR3 and FGFR4 function cooperatively to direct alveogenesis in the murine lung. *Development* 125: 3615–3623.

Weinstein M, Yang X, Li C, Xu X, Gotay J, Deng C-X (1998b). Failure of egg cylinder elongation and mesoderm induction in mouse embryos lacking the tumor suppressor smad2. *Proc Natl Acad Sci USA* 95: 9378–9383.

Werner S (1998). Keratinocyte growth factor: a unique player in epithelial repair processes. *Cytokine Growth Factor Rev* 9: 153–165.

Wilkie AO (1997). Craniosynostosis: genes and mechanisms. *Hum Mol Gen* 6: 1647–1656.

Xu X, Weinstein M, Li C, Naski M, Cohen RI, Ornitz DM, Leder P, Deng C (1998). Fibroblast growth factor receptor 2 (FGFR2)-mediated reciprocal regulation loop between FGF8 and FGF10 is essential for limb induction. *Development* 125: 753–765.

Xu J, Lawshe A, MacArthur CA, Ornitz DM (1999a). Genomic structure, mapping, activity and expression of fibroblast growth factor 17. *Mech Dev* 83: 165–178.

Xu X, Li C, Takahashi K, Slavkin HC, Shum L, Deng CX (1999b). Murine fibroblast growth factor 1α isoforms mediate node regression and are essential for posterior mesoderm development. *Dev Biol* 208: 293–306.

Xu X, Weinstein M, Li C, Deng C (1999c). Fibroblast growth factor receptors (FGFRs) and their roles in limb development. *Cell Tissue Res* 296: 33–43.

Xu J, Liu Z, Ornitz DM (2000). Temporal and spatial gradients of FGF8 and FGF17 regulate proliferation and differentiation of midline cerebellar structures. *Development* 127: 1833–1843.

Yamaguchi TP, Harpal K, Henkemeyer M, Rossant J (1994). FGR-1 is required for embryonic growth and mesodermal patterning during mouse gastrulation. *Genes Dev* 8: 3032–3044.

Yan G, Fukabori Y, McBride G, Nikolaropolous S, McKeehan WL (1993). Exon switching and activation of stromal and embryonic fibroblast growth factor (FGF)-FGF receptor genes in prostate epithelial cells accompany stromal independence and malignancy. *Mol Cell Biol* 13: 4513–4522.

Yayon A, Klagsburn M, Esko JD, Ledeer P, Ornitz DM (1991). Cell surface, heparin-like molecules are required for binding of basic fibroblast growth factor to its high affinity receptor. *Cell* 64: 841–848.

Yayon A, Zimmer Y, Hong SG, Avivi A, Yarden Y, Givol D (1992). A confined variable region confers ligand specificity to fibroblast growth factor receptor. *EMBO J* 11: 1885–1890.

Yu K, Herr AB, Waksman G, Ornitz DM (2000). Loss of fibroblast growth factor receptor 2 ligand-binding specificity in Apert syndrome. *Proc Natl Acad Sci USA* 97: 14536–14541.

Zhou YX, Xu X, Chen L, Li C, Brodie SG, Deng CX (2000). A Pro250Arg substitution in mouse Fgfr1 causes increased expression of Cbfa1 and premature fusion of calvarial sutures. *Hum Mol Genet* 9: 2001–2008.

Zhu X, Komiya H, Chirino A, Faham S, Fox GM, Arakawa T, Hsu BT, Rees DC (1991). Three-dimensional structures of acidic and basic fibroblast growth factors. *Science* 251: 90–93.

Zimmer Y, Givol D, Yayon A (1993). Multiple structural elements determine ligand binding of fibroblast growth factors. *J Biol Chem* 268: 7899–7903.

33 | FGFs/FGFRs and Associated Disorders

M. MICHAEL COHEN, JR.

Topics covered in this chapter are organized under the following headings: fibroblast growth factor/fibroblast growth factor receptor (FGF/FGFR) biology; FGFRs; relationship between Fgfr3 and Twist; other FGFRs of uncertain physiological roles; FGFs; intracellular FGFs and FGFRs; cell adhesion molecule (CAM) homology domain (CHD); heparan sulfate proteoglycans (HSPGs); intracellular signaling; clinical phenotypes; FGFR mutations of short-limb skeletal dysplasias and craniosynostosis syndromes; FGF/FGFR alterations in neoplasia; misguided interpretations; prenatal diagnosis and genetic counseling; management; and mechanisms.

Some major short-limb skeletal dysplasias and some craniosynostosis syndromes are caused by mutations in fibroblast growth factor receptors (Cohen, 1997b) (Table 33–1). In a disorder such as thanatophoric dysplasia, however, both short limbs and craniosynostosis occur.

FGF/FGFR BIOLOGY

FGFRs are a subset of receptor tyrosine kinases, each composed of an extracellular ligand-binding domain, a single-pass transmembrane domain, and a split intracellular kinase domain. Activation takes place when a trimolecular complex—FGF/FGFR/HSPG—results in receptor dimerization, autophosphorylation, and downstream signaling (Givol and Yayon, 1992; Johnson and Williams, 1993; Mason, 1994a; Spivak-Kroizman et al., 1994). There are four known FGFRs (Ullrich and Schlessinger, 1990; Jaye et al., 1992; Kostrzewa and Müller, 1998; Miki et al., 1992; Johnson and Williams, 1993) (Table 33–2). Twenty-two human FGFs are known at this writing (Smallwood et al., 1996; Coulier et al., 1997; Martin, 1998; Ornitz and Itoh, 2001) (Table 33–3).

The biology of FGFs and FGFRs is complex because of different receptors with alternative splicing, multiple ligands (some having different isoforms), and different HSPGs. During embryogenesis and subsequent development, their expressions occur differentially in terms of location, timing, and kinetic factors. Several other considerations complicate FGF and FGFR biology even further: (*a*) fifth and sixth FGFRs of uncertain physiological roles (see Table 33–2); (*b*) FGFR cell adhesion molecule homology domain; and (*c*) several different gain-of-function mechanisms for FGFR mutations (Burrus et al., 1992; Givol and Yayon, 1992; Johnson and Williams, 1993; Mason, 1994a, 1994b; Galvin et al., 1996; Green et al., 1996; Neilson and Friesel, 1996; Webster and Donoghue, 1997; Anderson et al., 1998; Robertson et al., 1998; Oldridge et al., 1999; Wiedemann and Trueb, 2000; Yu et al., 2000; Wilkie et al., 2002).

FIBROBLAST GROWTH FACTOR RECEPTORS

Four high-affinity FGFRs have been identified that encode transmembrane tyrosine kinases (Table 33–2). The primary structure of FGFRs consists of a signal peptide; three immunoglobulin-like loops (IgI, IgII, and IgIII); an acidic amino acid domain (acid box) located between IgI and IgII; a cell adhesion molecule (CAM) homology domain (CHD) also located between IgI and IgII; a single-pass transmembrane domain; a split kinase domain with a unique 14 amino acid insert; and a carboxy-terminal tail (Fig. 33–1). Each loop has a disulfide bond. The degree to which the four FGFRs are similar is shown as the "average amino acid percentage identity" in Figure 33–1. The intracellular kinase domains are the most highly conserved. In the ex-

tracellular domain, IgIII is the most highly conserved of the three loops (Givol and Yayon, 1992; Johnson and Williams, 1993).

The double loop on the second half of IgIII (Fig. 33–2) indicates that all FGFRs except FGFR4 have alternatively spliced forms in this region. Spliced form IIIc is the most abundant and is expressed primarily in mesenchymal tissues (Fig. 33–2). Spliced form IIIb is less abundant and is expressed primarily in epithelial tissues (Ornitz et al., 1996; Ornitz and Itoh, 2001). IIIa refers to the first half of the IgIII loop, and it is always present. Thus, there are two possible forms—IIIa/IIIc or IIIa/IIIb—except in FGFR4, which has only the IIIa/IIIc form.

There are other types of alternatively spliced forms (Fig. 33–3). For example, IgI can be skipped in the FGFRs, resulting in a short receptor form with only two Ig loops (IgII and IgIII). Receptors lacking IgI do not have altered ligand-binding specificities (Johnson and Williams, 1993). Thus, intracellular signaling can take place with the short form. There is a IIIa form of FGFR1 (neither IIIc nor IIIb is present) that terminates within IgIII, resulting in a secreted form (Givol and Yayon, 1992; Johnson and Williams, 1993). There are many other splice variants. Xu et al. (1992) estimated 96 possible variants that may occur among the four genes that code for the FGFRs. Twig et al. (1998) identified a highly conserved divergent 5′ splice site in FGFR1, FGFR2, and FGFR3. Alternative splicing of a hexanucleotide sequence encodes ValThr at the end of exon 11. ValThr+/ValThr− splicing may play a significant role in controling FGFR signaling through the MAP kinase pathway.

RELATIONSHIP BETWEEN Fgfr3 AND Twist

Bone formation at the osteogenic fronts of the presumptive cranial sutures involves at least two distinct steps: (*1*) proliferation of pre-osteoblasts followed by cell cycle arrest and (*2*) differentiation of osteoblasts proper (Fig. 33–4). p21, which arrests the cell cycle of osteoblastic precursors, and *Fgfr3*, which generates signals resulting in osteoblastic differentiation, are controlled by the same transcription factor, E2A, which is a basic helix–loop–helix (bHLH) gene that encodes two alternatively spliced products, E12 and E47, which differ in their bHLH domains and DNA-binding properties. E2A and co-activator CBP can be blocked by bHLH Twist and by the dominant-negative HLH proteins Id1 and Id2. Twist and Fgfr3 expression are mutually exclusive: Twist is expressed in pre-osteoblasts, and Fgfr3 leads to osteoblastic differentiation. Although wild-type Twist inhibits p21, *Twist* mutations, which show haploinsufficiency, fail to inhibit p21; cell cycle arrest is followed by early differentiation of the sutural osteogenic fronts. Thus, there is a link between Twist and Fgfr3 pathways. Dysfunction of Twist and overactivation of Fgfr3 signaling result in craniosynostosis because of acceleration in bone differentiation (Funato et al., 2001).

OTHER FGFRs OF UNCERTAIN PHYSIOLOGICAL ROLES

A fifth receptor, cysteine-rich FGF (CFR), is highly conserved among vertebrates. The extracellular domain is composed of 16 cysteine-rich repeat units. The intracellular domain is extremely short, containing only 13 amino acids. Receptor binding occurs with FGF1, FGF2, and FGF4. Since the cytoplasmic domain is short, a role in signal transduction is unlikely. Although the function of cysteine-rich FGFR is

Table 33–1. Genes Bearing Known Mutations on Fibroblast Growth Factor Receptors (FGFRs)

FGFRs	Disorders	Craniosynostosis	Short-Limb Skeletal Dysplasia
FGFR1	Pfeiffer syndrome	+	
FGFR2	Apert syndrome	+	(+)*
	Pfeiffer syndrome	+	
	Crouzon syndrome	+	
	Jackson-Weiss syndrome	+	
	Beare-Stevenson cutis gyrata syndrome	+	
	Nonclassifiable craniosynostosis	+	
FGFR3	Achondroplasia		+
	Hypochondroplasia†		+
	Thanatophoric dysplasia, type 1	+	+
	Thanatophoric dysplasia, type 2	+	+
	SADDAN		+
	Crouzonodermoskeletal syndrome	+	
	Muenke syndrome	+	

Source: From Cohen (2000a).

Some craniosynostosis syndromes are caused by mutations in other genes. *TWIST* mutations cause Saethre-Chotzen syndrome. One *MSX2* mutation causes Boston-type craniosynostosis.

*Although not a short-limb skeletal dysplasia, the limbs are shorter than normal; mild rhizomelia is evident by measurement of the femora and humeri.

†Only one patient with hypochondroplasia has been reported with craniosynostosis.

unknown, it may have more than one function. Cellular uptake of FGF is one possibility. The receptor is primarily located in the Golgi apparatus, so it may regulate the secretion of FGF3 (Burrus et al., 1992; Zhou et al., 1997; Köhl et al., 2000).

A sixth receptor, FGFR-like 1 (FGFRL1), has a large extracellular domain with three immunoglobulin-like loops, a transmembrane domain, and a short intracellular domain of about 100 amino acids. A role in intracellular signaling is unlikely. FGFRL1 maps to 4p16 in close proximity to FGFR3. The transcript is preferentially expressed in cartilage. Although its function is unknown, dimerization with a true FGFR could inhibit signaling by blocking transphosphorylation (Wiedemann and Trueb, 2000).

FIBROBLAST GROWTH FACTORS

At this writing, FGFs are a family of 22 human structurally related polypeptide mitogens (Table 33–3) and others can be anticipated in the future. FGFs encode proteins with a molecular weight of 17 to 34 kDa. They have a 13% to 71% amino acid identity and share an internal core region of 28 highly conserved and 6 identical amino acids (Ornitz and Itoh, 2001).

Although initially shown to be mitogenic for cells of mesodermal origin, FGFs were later shown to be mitogenic for cells of ectodermal, neuroectodermal, and endodermal derivations. FGFs are involved in developmental induction and differentiation, cell growth and migration, bone growth and development, neuronal differentiation, angiogenesis, wound healing, and tumorigenesis (Givol and Yayon, 1992; Johnson and Williams, 1993; Mason, 1994a; Burke et al., 1998). Chromosome locations are known for all 22 FGFs except *FGF16* (Table 33–3). Human *FGF19* may be the ortholog of mouse *Fgf15*. Some FGFs are expressed during embryonic development, and some are expressed in both embryonic and adult tissues (Table 33–3). *FGF1* and *FGF2* are the most

abundant of the FGFs. A subset of the FGF family, expressed in adult tissues, is important for neuronal signal transduction in the central and peripheral nervous systems (Ornitz and Itoh, 2001).

For FGFR2, ligand-binding properties are very specific: FGF7 and FGF10 for the IgIIIb isoform are expressed in epithelial tissues, and FGF2, FGF4, FGF6, FGF8, and FGF9 for the IgIIIc isoform are expressed in mesenchymal tissues.[a]

INTRACELLULAR FGFs AND FGFRs

FGFs or FGFRs, or both, can be internalized in the intracellular compartments, including the nucleus. Among FGFs are FGF1, FGF2, higher molecular weight FGF2 and FGF3, and also FGF11, FGF12, FGF13, and FGF14 (Goldfarb, 2001). It has been suggested that

[a]IgIIIb and IgIIIc isoforms are also found with FGFR1 and FGFR3. FGFR4 has only the IgIIIc isoform.

Table 33–2. FGFR Genes and Their Chromosomal Locations

Genes	Chromosome Locations
High-affinity FGFRs	
FGFR1	8p12
FGFR2	10q22.3–q26
FGFR3	4p16.3
FGFR4	5q33–qter
FGFRs of uncertain physiological roles*	
CFR†	16q22–q23
FGFRL1‡	4p16

*Short cytoplasmic domains; intracellular signaling roles unlikely. See section titled "Two Other FGFRs of Uncertain Physiological Roles."

†Cysteine-rich FGF receptor.

‡FGFR-like 1.

Table 33–3. *FGF* Genes: Chromosomal Locations and Expressions

FGF Genes	Chromosomal Locations	Embryonic Expression	Embryonic and Adult Expression
FGF1	5q31		+
FGF2	4q26–q27		+
FGF3	11q13	+	
FGF4	11q13.3	+	
FGF5	4q21		+
FGF6	12p13		+
FGF7	15q15–q21.1		+
FGF8	10q24	+	
FGF9	13q11–q12		+
FGF10	5p12–p13		+
FGF11	17p13.1		+
FGF12	3q28		+
FGF13	Xq26		+
FGF14	13q34		+
*Fgf15**		+	
FGF16	?†		+
FGF17	8p21	+	
FGF18	5q34		+
*FGF19**	11q13.1	+	
FGF20	8p21.3–p22		+
FGF21	19q13.1–qter		+
FGF22	19p13.3		+
FGF23	12p13.3		+

Source: Data from GenBank, HUGO, Cytokine Family cDNA Database, LocusLink, and Yamashita et al. (2000).

*Human *FGF19* may be the ortholog of mouse *Fgf15*.

†In humans, chromosomal locations have been identified in 22 *FGF* genes. Only the chromosomal location of *FGF16* is unknown to date.

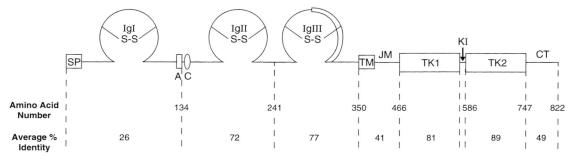

Figure 33–1. Basic structure of fibroblast growth factor receptors (FGFRs). SP, signal peptide. Three immunoglobulin-like loops (IgI, IgII, IgIII). Note double loop on second half of IgIII, which has alternatively spliced forms, except on FGFR4. Each immunoglobulin-like loop has a disulfide bond, S–S. A, acid box; C, CAM (cell adhesion molecule) homology domain; TM, transmembrane domain; JM, juxtamembrane region. Split kinase domain (TK1, TK2) with kinase insert (KI) between them. CT, COOH tail. Note amino acid numbers. Also note average percent amino acid identity of all four FGFRs. The intracellular kinase domain is the most highly conserved. In the extracellular domain, IgIII is the most highly conserved of the three loops. (From Cohen, 2000a.)

FGFRs deliver FGFs to the intracellular compartments where they can interact with other targets to trigger biological responses (Wiedlocha et al., 1994, 1996). It has also been suggested that FGFRs translocate to the nucleus to promote FGF-mediated biological responses (Peng et al., 2001; Reilly and Mahler, 2001).

CELL ADHESION MOLECULE HOMOLOGY DOMAIN

Neural cell adhesion molecules (CAMs) are widely expressed and may act as putative ligands for FGFRs and result in FGFR activation and signaling (Mason, 1994b; Green et al., 1996). CAMs, occurring on the cell surface of neurons, guide growing axons to their target cells by acting as a kind of "railway switching system." A CAM homology domain (CHD), a linear stretch of 20 amino acids containing the same sequences found in three CAMs (L1, N-CAM, and N-Cadherin), is found between IgI and IgII in FGFR1, FGFR2, and FGFR3 (Williams et al., 1994) (Fig. 33–5).

CAM–FGFR interaction might be direct or indirect and might occur in *cis* or *trans*. A possible model for direct CAM–FGFR interaction has been proposed, based on the common motifs in CAMs and in the CHD of FGFRs. Homophilic binding between the CAMs might result in a clustering of CAMs together with a co-clustering of FGFRs with CAM–FGFR interaction being in *cis* (Doherty et al., 1995; Green et al., 1996).

HEPARAN SULFATE PROTEOGLYCANS

All members of the FGF family (Table 33–3) are known to bind to the glycosaminoglycan heparan sulfate (HS). Heparan sulfate proteoglycans (HSPGs) are located on the cell surface and in the extracellular matrix (Givol and Yayon, 1992). Cell surface HSPGs include the glypican and syndecan families. Perlecan is a secreted HSPG that is abundant in the basement membranes. All three have been implicated in FGF signaling and, although this seems somewhat contradictory, they may be explained by cell source and context, which might be more important determinants of HS chain structures and function than the identity of the core protein (Chang et al., 2000).

FGFs bind to HSPGs with lower affinity than they do to FGFRs (Mason, 1994a). The trimolecular complex between FGF, HSPG, and FGFR results in receptor activation. The affinity of FGFs for HSPGs may limit diffusion of growth factors. Thus, FGFs may produce their effects close to their site of production, making spatial and temporal patterns of the FGF/FGFR/HSPG complex an important biological regulatory mechanism (Naski and Ornitz, 1998).

In many studies, HS is used instead of HSPG. HS is more extensively sulfated and is produced by a few specialized cells in vivo, such as mast cells. In contrast, HSPG is less extensively sulfated but more abundant in vivo. Based on different HS-binding requirements of FGFs and FGFRs, HS can be either stimulators or inhibitors of FGF signaling (Chang et al., 2000).

INTRACELLULAR SIGNALING

Significant FGF ligand binding and subsequent conformational changes of the FGFR extracellular domain result in dimerization, autophosphorylation—specifically generating phosphotyrosine (pTyr)—and the initiation of downstream signaling. Several conserved protein molecules regulate signal transduction by mediating protein–protein interactions. The Src homology (SH) domains explicitly recognize pTyr, which acts as an all-or-nothing switch for SH binding. Residues C-terminal to pTyr determine which SH domains, and therefore which SH proteins, are bound (Ullrich and Schlessinger, 1990; Pawson and Gish, 1992; Mason, 1994a; Pawson, 1995). FGFR intracellular signaling pathways are shown in Figure 33–6.

Mitogen-Activating Protein (MAP) Kinase Pathway

The MAP kinase pathway, shown on the right side of Figure 33–6, plays a major role in cell differentiation and proliferation. FRS2 is a lipid-anchored docking protein that targets signaling molecules to the plasma membrane. GRB2 is an adaptor protein that couples the activated receptor to other signaling molecules but has no intrinsic signaling properties of its own. Its SH2 domain binds to a phosphotyrosine residue on the activated FGFR receptor. Its SH3 domain binds to Sos, a guanine nucleotide exchange factor, which thereby becomes lo-

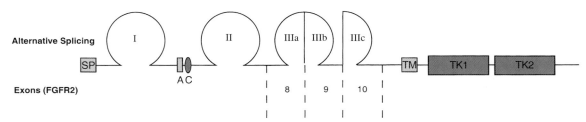

Figure 33–2. Diagram of a fibroblast growth factor receptor, specifically FGFR2, illustrating alternative splicing of the second half of IgIII. The NH₂-terminal half of IgIII is encoded by one exon (IIIa or 8), and is thus constant. The COOH terminal half of IgIII may be alternatively coded by either of two exons: IIIb (or 9) and IIIc (or 10). SP, signal peptide; A, acid box; C, CAM homology domain. Ig loops I, II, and III. Constant half of IgIII (IIIa). Alternative half of IgIII (IIIb or IIIc). TM, transmembrane domain. TK1 and TK2, split kinase domain. (From Cohen, 2000a.)

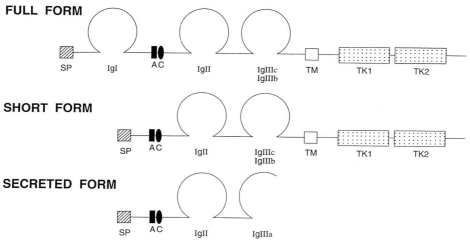

FULL FORM

SP IgI AC IgII IgIIIc IgIIIb TM TK1 TK2

SHORT FORM

SP AC IgII IgIIIc IgIIIb TM TK1 TK2

SECRETED FORM

SP AC IgII IgIIIa

Figure 33–3. Full, short, and secreted forms of FGFRs. IgI is missing from the short form. The secreted form is not membrane bound. FGFR1 and FGFR2 can both have full and short forms. FGFR1 can have a secreted form. SP, Signal peptide; A, acid box; C, CAM homology domain. Immunoglobulin-like loops IgI, IgII, and IgIII. Alternatively spliced second half of IgIII, IgIIIc and IgIIIb. Secreted form has NH_2 terminal half of IgIII, IgIIIa. TM, transmembrane domain; TK1 and TK2, split kinase domains. (From Cohen, 2000a.)

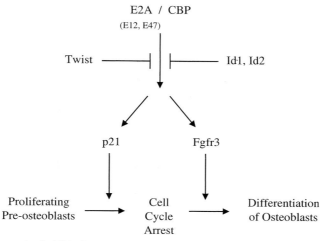

E2A / CBP
(E12, E47)

Twist ———⊣   ⊢——— Id1, Id2

p21   Fgfr3

Proliferating
Pre-osteoblasts → Cell Cycle Arrest → Differentiation of Osteoblasts

Figure 33–4. Regulation of p21 and Fgfr3 expression by E2A, CBP, Twist, Id1, and Id2. Dysfunction of Twist and overactivation of Fgfr3 signaling result in craniosynostosis because of acceleration in bone differentiation. Thus, there is a link between the Twist and Fgfr3 pathways. (Modified from Funato et al. 2001.)

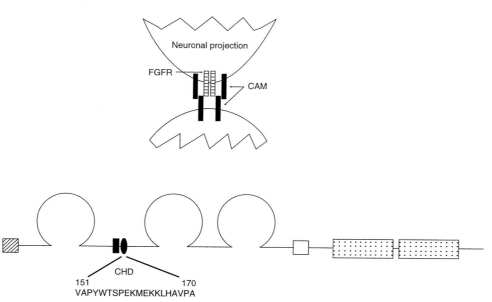

Neuronal projection

FGFR   CAM

CHD

151   170
VAPYWTSPEKMEKKLHAVPA

Figure 33–5. *Top*: Neuronal projection moving toward functional contact with target cell. Movement guided by cell adhesion molecules (CAM) on neuronal projection (black) and on target cell (black). Fibroblast growth factor receptor (FGFR) is membrane bound to neuronal projection (striped). *Bottom*: FGFR showing CAM homology domain (CHD) with linear stretch (151–170) of 20 amino acids (black oval). Hatched box is the signal peptide; black oblong is the acid box; open box is the transmembrane domain. Dotted oblongs are the split kinase domain. (From Cohen, 2000a.)

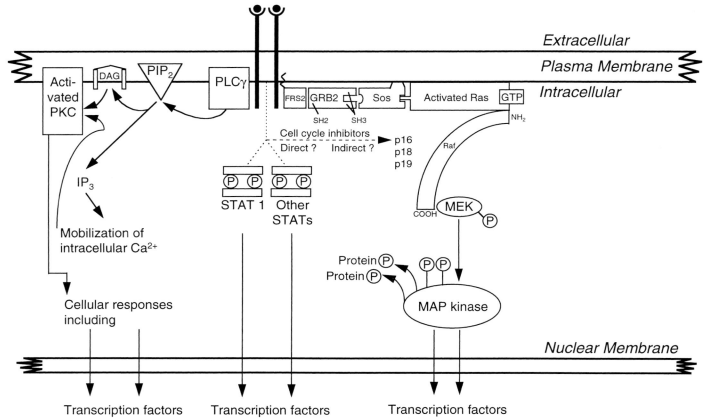

Figure 33–6. FGFR intracellular signaling. Bold black lines with cups represent FGFRs. Solid black circles in cups represent FGF ligands. *Right side*, MAP kinase pathway; *left side*, PKC pathway; center, STAT activation. (From Cohen, 2000a.) See text for details.

calized to the plasma membrane. Sos then binds to Ras/GDP, leading to the release of GDP and becoming activated by GTP, which results in the tethering of Ras to the plasma membrane. Raf, a serine/threonine kinase, is bound by its N-terminal domain to Ras. The C-terminal end of Raf, in turn, binds to and phosphorylates MEK, a protein kinase that phosphorylates tyrosine and serine residues. MEK then phosphorylates and activates MAP kinase, which has serine and threonine residues. Finally, MAP kinase itself phosphorylates many different proteins, including intranuclear transcription factors, thereby modulating their activity (Marshall, 1995; Park et al., 1995a; Kouhara et al., 1997).

Protein Kinase C (PKC) Pathway

The PKC (protein kinase C) pathway is shown on the left side of Figure 33–6. PKC is the collective term for a family of protein kinases that are soluble and cytosolic when inactive. PKC, bound to the plasma membrane when activated, produces varied responses in different cells, indicating a key role for many aspects of cellular growth and metabolism. PKC can also phosphorylate various transcription factors that, depending on cell type, induce or repress synthesis of certain mRNAs.

After being activated by pTyr, phospholipase Cγ (PLCγ) cleaves membrane component phosphatidylinositol bisphosphate (PIP2). This generates two potent intracellular messengers: diacylglycerol (DAG) and inositol trisphosphate (IP3). The latter triggers the release of sequestered calcium ions (Ca^{2+}) that, together with DAG, activate PKC (Nishizuka, 1995).

Signal Transducers and Activators of Transcription (STATs)

STATs (signal transducers and activators of transcription) are a family of latent cytoplasmic transcription factors. STAT activation is shown in the center of Figure 33–6. Seven STATs have been identified at this writing. Ligand-activated receptors with kinase activity cat-

alyze phosphorylation at the single tyrosine site of any STAT, which then dimerizes with a partner molecule by reciprocal SH2 phosphotyrosine interaction. Following activation, STAT homodimers translocate to the nucleus. STATs are known to have various biological functions (Darnell, 1997), including the regulation of apoptosis (Schindler, 1998). FGFR3 mutations for types 1 and 2 thanatophoric dysplasia (*vide infra*) have been shown to involve activation of STAT1 and, by extension, STAT5a and STAT5b (Su et al., 1997; Legeai-Mallet et al., 1998; Li et al., 1999).

CLINICAL PHENOTYPES

Clinical phenotypes of various craniosynostosis syndromes and short-limb skeletal dysplasias are summarized in Table 33–4. Some of these are illustrated: Apert syndrome (Figs. 33–7 to 33–9), Crouzon syndrome (Fig. 33–10), Pfeiffer syndrome (Figs. 33–11 to 33–13), achondroplasia (Fig. 33–14), hypochondroplasia (Fig. 33–15), type 1 thanatophoric dysplasia (Figs. 33–16 and 33–17), and type 2 thanatophoric dysplasia (Figs. 33–18 and 33–19).

FGF/FGFR MUTATIONS

FGFR mutations in various craniosynostosis syndromes and short-limb skeletal dysplasias are summarized in Table 33–4 and illustrated in Figure 33–20. Most mutations for major craniosynostosis syndromes are found on *FGFR2*, but only one is located on *FGFR1*. Craniosynostosis syndromes with mutations on *FGFR2* can have overlapping phenotypes (Wilkie et al., 2002). Mutations for short-limb skeletal dysplasias such as achondroplasia, hypochondroplasia, and SADDAN are located on *FGFR3*, but craniosynostosis is not a feature; thanatophoric dysplasia, however, is associated with craniosynostosis. Muenke syndrome is also associated with craniosynostosis, but short limbs are not part of the phenotype. At this writing,

Table 33–4. FGFR/FGF Mutations[a]

Syndrome	Phenotype	Chromosome Localization	Gene	Exon/Domain[b]	Nucleotide Change[c]	Amino Acid Substitution
Apert syndrome	Craniosynostosis, symmetric syndactyly of hands and feet, other anomalies	10q25.3–q26	*FGFR2*	8/Linker:IgII-IgIII	755C → G	Ser252Trp
					758C → G	Pro253Arg
					755_756CG → TT	Ser252Phe[d]
				Intron 9	940-2A → G[d]	Splicing
					940-3_ -4ins*Alu*[d]	(Acceptor)
				10/IgIIIc	1041_1042ins*Alu*[d]	
Crouzon syndrome	Craniosynostosis, midface deficiency, ocular proptosis	10q25.3–q26	*FGFR2*	3/IgI	314A → G	Tyr105Cys[d]
				8/Linker:IgII-IgIII	755C → T	Ser252Leu[d]
					760C → T	His254Tyr
					788C → T	Pro263Leu
					799T → C	Ser267Pro[e]
				8/IgIIIa	803insTGG	Thr268ThrGly[d]
					826T → G	Phe276Val[e]
					833G → T	Cys278Phe[e]
					833G → A	Cys278Tyr
					842A → G	Tyr281Cys
					858_866delCCACATCCA	His287_Glndel[d]
					863T → C	Ile288Ser
					866A → C	Gln289Pro
					868T → G	Trp290Gly
					868T → C	Trp290Arg
					874A → G	Lys292Glu
					902A → G	Tyr301Cys
				10/IgIIIc	983A → G	Tyr328Cys
					992A → T	Asp331Ile
					1009G → C	Ala337Pro
					1011_1012insGACGCT	AspAla377_378ins[d]
					1012G → C	Gly338Arg
					1013G → A	Gly338Glu
					1018T → C	Tyr340His
					1024T → A	Cys342Ser[e]
					1024T → C	Cys342Arg[e]
					1025G → A	Cys342Tyr[e]
					1025G → C	Cys342Ser[e]
					1025G → C	Cys342Phe
					1026C → G	Cys342Trp
					1031C → G	Ala344Gly[f]
					1032G → A	Ala344Ala[g]
					1040C → G	Ser347Cys
					1061C → G	Ser354Cys
					1061C → A[h]	Ser354Tyr
					1061C → T	Ser354Phe
					1066-1074delTGGTTGACA	Trp356_Thr358del[d]
				14/TK1	1645A → C	Asn549His
				17/TK2	2032A → G	Arg678Gly
Pfeiffer syndrome	Craniosynostosis, broad thumbs, broad great toes, other anomalies	8p11.2–p12	*FGFR1*	7/Linker:IgII-IgIII	755C → G	Pro252Arg
		10q25.3-q26	*FGFR2*	5/IgII	514_515GC → TT	Ala172Phe[d]
				8/Linker:IgII-IgIII	755C → G	Ser252Trp[d]
				8/IgIIIa	755_757CGC → TCT	Ser252Phe/Pro253Ser[d]
					799T → C	Ser267Pro[e]
					826T → G	Phe276Val[e]
					833G → T	Cys278Phe[e]
					864_881del	Ile288Met; Gln289_Val294del[d]
					870G → T	Trp290Cys
					870G → C	Trp290Cys
				Intron 9	940-3T → G	Splicing
					940-2A → G	(Acceptor)
					940-2A → T	
					940-1G → C	
					940-1G → A	
					c.940-3_946del10insACC	
					940G → T	Ala314Ser
				10/IgIIIc	966A → C	Asp321Ala
					1019A → G	Tyr340Cys
					1021A → C	Thr341Pro
					1024T → C	Cys342Arg[e]
					1024T → G	Cys342Gly
					1024T → A	Cys342Ser[e]

(Continued)

Table 33–4. FGFR/FGF Mutations[a] (*Continued*)

Syndrome	Phenotype	Chromosome Localization	Gene	Exon/Domain[b]	Nucleotide Change[c]	Amino Acid Substitution
					1025G → A	Cys342Tyr[e]
					1025G → C	Cys342Ser[e]
					1025_1026GC → CT	Cys342Ser
					1026C → G	Cys342Trp
					1030G → C	Ala344Pro
					1052C → G	Ser351Cys
					1075G → T	Val359Phe
					1084_1085ins TCAACA	Gly345_Pro361del[d,i]
					1084+1G → T	Splicing
					1084+3A → G	(Donor)
				11/IgIII-TM	1124A → G	Tyr375Cys[j]
				15/TK1	1694A → G	Glu565Gly
				16/TK2	1922A → G	Lys641Arg
				17/TK2	1988G → A	Gly663Glu
Syndactyly	Apert-like hands and feet without cranio-synostosis; normal craniofacial appearance except for broad forehead		FGFR2	8/IIIa:10/IIIc	Two heterozygous mutations[d]	
					755C → T	Ser252Lys
					943G → T	Ala315Ser
Jackson-Weiss syndrome	Tarsal/metatarsal coalitions and, variably, craniosynostosis and broad great toes	10q25.3–q26	FGFR2	10/IgIIIc	1031C → G	Ala344Gly[f]
Beare-Stevenson cutis gyrata syndrome	Cloverleaf or Crouzonoid skull, cutis gyrata, furrowed palms and soles, cutaneous/mucosal tags, prominent umbilical stump	10q25.3–q26	FGFR2	11/IgIII-TM	1115C → G	Ser372Cys
					1124A → G	Tyr375Cys[j]
		4p16	FGFR3	7:Linker:IgII-IgIII	749C → G	Pro250Arg[k]
Nonclassifiable disorders with craniosynostosis	Variable phenotypes	10q25.3-q26	FGFR2	8/IgIIIa	804_809delGTGGTC	Val269_Val270del[d]
					870G → T	Trp290Cys
				10/IgIIIc	943G → T	Ala315Ser
					1113G → A	Gly338Glu
					1032G → A	Ala344Ala[g]
				11/TM	1150G → A	Gly384Arg
				16/TK2	1977G → T	Lys659Asn
Muenke syndrome	Unilateral or bilateral coronal synostosis, radiographic thimble-like middle phalanges (hands), other anomalies	4p16	FGFR3	7/Linker:IgII-IgIII	749C → G	Pro250Arg
Crouzonodermo-skeletal syndrome	Craniofacial dysostosis, acanthosis nigricans, cementomas, vertebral alterations	4p16	FGFR3	10/TM	1172C → A	Ala391Glu
Achondroplasia	Rhizomelic shortening of limbs, trident hands, midface deficiency	4p16	FGFR3	10/TM	1037G → A	Gly346Glu
					1125G → T	Gly375Cys
					1138G → C	Gly380Arg
					1138G → A	Gly380Arg
					742C → T	Arg248Cys[l]
					1620C → G	Asn540Lys[l]
Hypochondroplasia	Short limbs albeit longer than in achondroplasia, large head circumference	4p16	FGFR3	9/IgIII-TM	983A → T	Asn328Ile
				13/TK1	1612A → G	Ile538Val
					1619A → C	Asn540Thr
					1619A → G	Asn540Ser
					1620C → A	Asn540Lys[m]
					1620C → G	Asn540Lys
				15/TK2	1948A → C	Lys650Gln
					1950A → T	Lys650Asn
					1950G → C	Lys650Asn
Thanatophoric dysplasia		4p16	FGFR3			
	Type I (curved humeri and femora; may have cloverleaf skull)			7/Linker:IgII-IgIII	742C → T	Arg248Cys
					746C → G	Ser249Cys
				10/IgIII-TM	1108G → T	Gly370Cys
					1111A → T	Ser371Cys
					1118A → G	Tyr373Cys
				15/TK2	1949A → T	Lys650Met[n]
				19/C-tail	2458T → G	Stop807Gly
					2458T → A	Stop807Arg
					2460A → T	Stop807Cys
	Type II (straight humeri and femora; cloverleaf skull more commonly found)			15/TK2	1948A → G	Lys650Glu

(*Continued*)

Table 33–4. *Continued*

Syndrome	Phenotype	Chromosome Localization	Gene	Exon/Domain[b]	Nucleotide Change[c]	Amino Acid Substitution
SADDAN	Short-limb skeletal dysplasia, developmental delay, acanthosis nigricans	4p16	*FGFR3*	15/TK2	1949A → T	Lys650Met[n]
Autosomal dominant cerebellar ataxia	Early-onset tremor, dyskinesia, slowly progressive cerebellar ataxia	13q34		4/-	434T → C	Phe145Ser
Autosomal dominant hypophosphatemic rickets	Low serum phosphorus, rickets, osteomalacia, lower limb anomalies, short stature, bone pain, dental abscesses	12p13.3	*FGF23*	1/-	527G → A 535C → T 536G → A	Arg176Gln Arg179Trp Arg179Gln

[a]This table is updated from Cohen (2000a). In constructing the table, I have relied on the work of many authors who are cited in the text.

[b]IgI, IgII, IgIII = immunoglobulin-like loops. Linker:IgII-IgIII = linker region between IgII and IgIII. IgIIIa = first half of IgIII. IgIIIc = alternatively spliced second half of IgIII (most common form and transcripts highly expressed in mesenchyme). TM = transmembrane domain. TK1 = first kinase domain. C-tail = carboxy-terminal tail. FGFR2 exon numbers are based on Ingersoll et al. (2002) and supersede the exon numbers of Givol and Yayon (1992).

[c]Numbering of nucleotides is based on the recommendations of Antonarakis and the Nomenclature Working Group Publication (1998). To convert nucleotide numbers based on FGFR2 cDNA sequence reported by Dionne et al. (1990), subtract 179. To convert the original numbers based on the sequence reported by Houssaint et al. (1990), subtract 12. Nomenclature for the description of human sequence variations is based on the recommendations of den Dunnen and Antonarakis (2001).

[d]"Rare" mutation (Meyers et al., 1995; Oldridge et al., 1995, 1997, 1999; Pulleyn et al., 1996; Passos-Bueno et al., 1997, 1998b; Kan et al., 2002; Teebi et al., 2002; Wilkie et al., 2002).

[e]Mutations reported in both Crouzon syndrome and Pfeiffer syndrome (see Cohen, 2000a).

[f]Mutation reported in both Jackson-Weiss syndrome and Crouzon syndrome (Jabs et al., 1994; Gorry et al., 1995). Ala344Gly reported for Jackson-Weiss syndrome (Jabs et al., 1994) has been misprinted as Arg344Gly and as Ala342Gly (Jabs, 1995). The first of these misprints also appears in Mulvihill (1995).

[g]Ala344Ala obviously does not involve an amino acid change, but the G → A transition creates a donor splice site, causing a 17 amino acid deletion (Li et al., 1995).

[h]1061C → A is misprinted as 1061T → A in Kress et al. (2000).

[i]Insertion activates cryptic donor splice site (Meyers et al., 1996).

[j]Mutation for several cases of Beare-Stevenson cutis gyrata syndrome. One case of severe Pfeiffer syndrome with this mutation has been recorded, but cutis gyrata and acanthosis nigricans were not features (Kan et al., 2002).

[k]Mutation very atypical for Beare-Stevenson cutis gyrata syndrome (Roscioli et al., 2001). This mutation is associated with Muenke syndrome (Muenke et al., 1997).

[l]Patients with classic achondroplasia but with mutations for thanatophoric dysplasia, type 1 (Arg248Cys), and hypochondroplasia (Arg540Lys) (Camera et al., 2001). This is a rare occurrence.

[m]Only one patient with hypochondroplasia has been reported with craniosynostosis (Angle et al., 1998), but cloverleaf skull, also reported by these authors, is not present.

[n]Rare mutation for thanatophoric dysplasia, type 1 (Kitoh et al., 1998). Mutation is usually for SADDAN (Bellus et al., 1999; Tavormina et al., 1999).

no mutations are known on *FGFR4*. Gaudenz et al. (1998) analyzed patients with craniosynostosis for the possibility of a Pro246Arg mutation in the linker region between IgII and IgIII on *FGFR4* with negative results.

Mutations identified on *FGFR2* and *FGFR3* may be located extracellularly or intracellularly. Almost all nucleotide changes are of the missense or splice-site types. Occasionally, small in-frame insertions and deletions are reported (Table 33–4). *FGFR* mutations involve gain of function, in contrast to *TWIST* mutations for Saethre-Chotzen syndrome, which involve haploinsufficiency (Cohen, 2000a).

All human mutations on FGFRs known to date allow early human development to proceed normally but interfere with later development, particularly bone. When mesenchyme is converted to bone, the molecular cross-talk is highly complex and only partially understood. Much work remains to be done in unraveling the pathogenesis of these phenotypes (Cohen, 2000a).

Apert Syndrome

Wilkie et al. (1995a) discovered two mutations in the linker region between IgII and IgIII on FGFR2: 755C → G, resulting in Ser252Trp, and 758C → G, resulting in Pro253Arg (Table 33–4). Confirmation of the two major mutations for Apert syndrome has come from other sources (Park et al., 1995c; Passos-Bueno et al., 1998a; Tsai et al.,

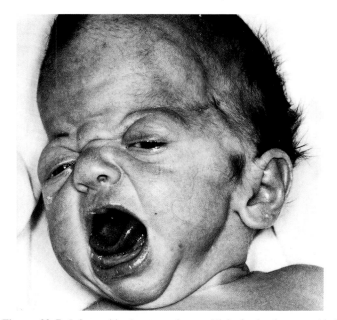

Figure 33–7. Infant with Apert syndrome. High forehead, supraorbital grooves, and ocular proptosis. (From Cohen and Kreiborg, 1993.)

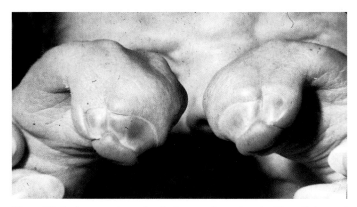

Figure 33–8. Apert syndrome hands. Symmetric syndactyly. (From Cohen and Kreiborg, 1993.)

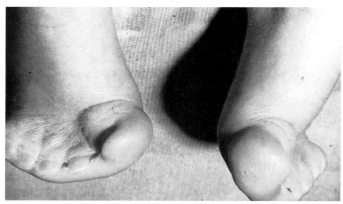

Figure 33–9. Apert syndrome feet. Symmetric syndactyly. (From Cohen and Kreiborg 1993.)

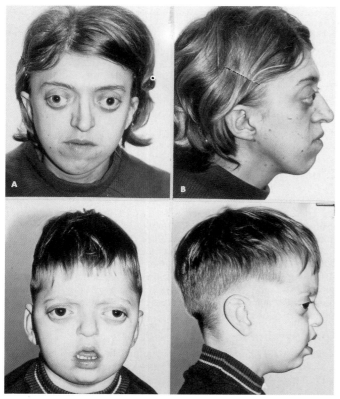

Figure 33–10. Crouzon syndrome in a mother and her son. (A–D) brachycephaly, ocular proptosis, and maxillary hypoplasia. (From Cohen, 1975.)

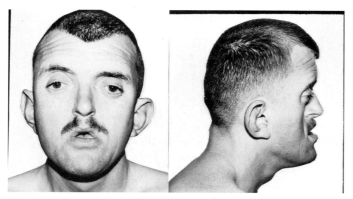

Figure 33–11. Pfeiffer syndrome. Turribrachycephaly, ocular proptosis, downslanting palpebral fissures, and midface deficiency. (From Cohen, 1975.)

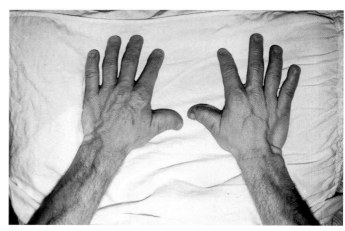

Figure 33–12. Pfeiffer syndrome. Brachydactyly and broad thumbs that deviate radially. (From Cohen, 1975.)

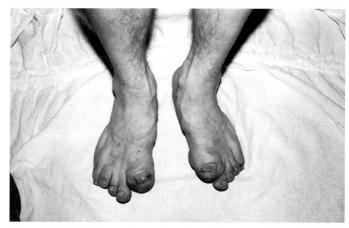

Figure 33–13. Pfeiffer syndrome. Short, broad, deviated halluces and soft tissue syndactyly between left second and third toes and between right second, third, and fourth toes. (From Cohen, 1975.)

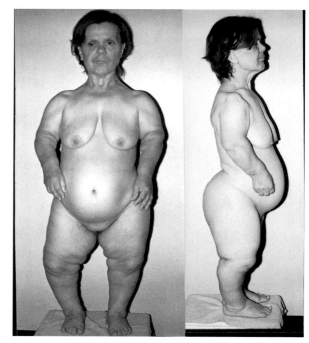

Figure 33–14. Achondroplasia. Rhizomelic shortening of limbs, lumbar lordosis, and protuberant addomen. (From Cohen, 1997d.)

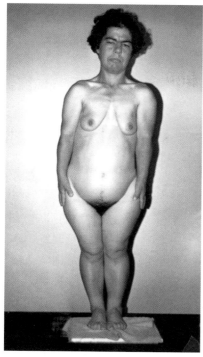

Figure 33–15. Hypochondroplasia. Short limbs, albeit longer than in achondroplasia. (From Cohen, 1997d.)

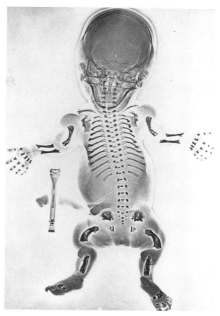

Figure 33–17. Xeroradiograph of type 1 thanatophoric dysplasia. Abnormal skull, hypoplastic vertebrae, abnormally shaped clavicles, bell-shaped rib cage, short bowed humeri and femora, and thin fibulae and tibiae. (From Elejalde and de Elejalde, 1985.)

1998; Lajeunie et al., 1999a). Origin of new mutations is exclusively of paternal origin (Moloney et al., 1996).

On occasion, other types of mutations have been recorded (Passos-Bueno et al., 1997; Oldridge et al., 1997, 1999; Lajeunie et al., 1999a). Oldridge et al. (1997) and Lajeunie et al. (1999a) found a 755_756CG → TT nucleotide change, resulting in Ser252Phe; its rarity is based on the requirement of two nucleotide substitutions (Table 33–4). Passos-Bueno et al. (1997) observed an acceptor splice site mutation (940-2A → G) in an Apert syndrome patient; the mutation is usually associated with Pfeiffer syndrome. Oldridge et al. (1999) reported two *Alu* insertions that arose in the paternal germline (Table 33–4). By analyzing FGFR2 expression in keratinocyte and fibroblast cell lines from an Apert *Alu* patient, Oldridge et al. (1999) observed ectopic expression of the alternative spliceform, IgIIIb (exon 9), suggesting that signaling through IgIIIb causes the syndactyly of Apert syndrome.

The frequency extimates of various mutations in Apert syndrome ($n = 289$) are as follows: Ser252Trp (66%), Pro253Arg (32.2%), and rare mutations (1.8%)† (Wilkie and Wall, 1996; Oldridge et al., 1997, 1999; Passos-Bueno et al., 1998a).

Genotype–phenotype correlations have been reported by Slaney et al. (1996). Ser252Trp is more frequently associated with cleft palate, and Pro253Arg is more frequently found with severe syndactyly. Confirmatory studies were provided by Lajeunie et al. (1999a) and von Gernet et al. (2000).

†1.8% is probably an overestimate due to reporting bias.

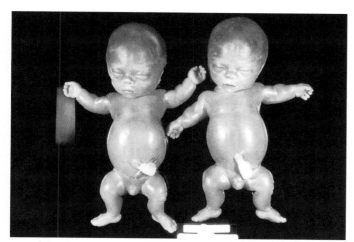

Figure 33–16. Identical twins with type 1 thanatophoric dysplasia. Disproportionately large heads, bell-shaped chests, and micromelia. (From Cohen, 2000b.)

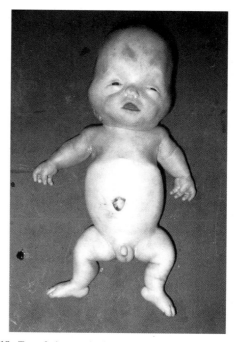

Figure 33–18. Type 2 thanatophoric dysplasia. Cloverleaf skull, bell-shaped chest, and micromelia. (From Cohen, 2000b.)

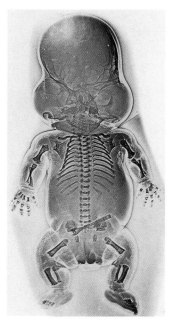

Figure 33–19. Xeroradiograph of type 2 thanatophoric dysplasia. Cloverleaf skull, short ribs, hypoplastic vertebrae, small pelvic bones, and short limbs with straight long bones. (From Elejalde and de Elejalde, 1985.)

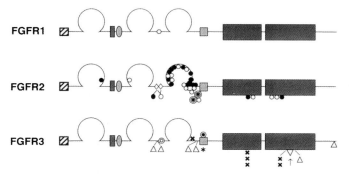

◇ Apert syndrome
○ Pfeiffer syndrome
● Crouzon syndrome
□ Jackson-Weiss syndrome
◉ Beare-Stevenson cutis gyrata syndrome

△ Thanatophoric dysplasia, Type I
▽ Thanatophoric dysplasia, Type II
↑ SADDAN
✱ Achondroplasia
✖ Hypochondroplasia
◎ Crouzonodermoskeletal syndrome
◉ Muenke syndrome

Figure 33–20. Most mutations for major craniosynostosis syndromes are on FGFR2 with only one known mutation on FGFR1. Mutations for major short-limb skeletal dysplasias are on *FGFR3*. Fibroblast growth factor receptors 1, 2, 3. Hatched square is the signal peptide; solid oblong is the acid box; solid oval is the CAM homology domain; solid square is the transmembrane domain; long oblongs are kinase domains 1 and 2. Three loops from left to right are immunoglobulin-like domains (IgI, IgII, IgIII). IIIc is an alternatively spliced form of the second half of IgIII. Because the three receptor diagrams are small and the mutation symbols are large, specific locations of the mutations are only approximate. For clarity, only a few of the many mutations for Crouzon syndrome and Pfeiffer syndrome are shown on FGFR2. (From Cohen, 2000a.) See Table 33–4.

Munro and Wilkie (1998) reported a 14-year-old normal boy who had unremarkable acne vulgaris, but severe acne with comedones was found extending down his left arm. DNA extracted from this severe lesion was shown to have a somatic mutation on *FGFR2*, Ser252Trp, the same mutation that causes Apert syndrome when present in the germline.

Pfeiffer Syndrome

Mutations causing Pfeiffer syndrome are found on FGFR1 (only one mutation) and FGFR2 (many mutations) (Muenke et al., 1994; La-jeunie et al., 1995; Rutland et al., 1995; Schell et al., 1995; Tartaglia et al., 1997; Gripp et al., 1998b; Schaefer et al., 1998; Cornejo-Roldan et al., 1999; Oldridge et al., 1999; Kress et al., 2000; Kan et al., 2002; Teebi et al., 2002; Wilkie, 2002). The one *FGFR1* mutation is in the linker region between IgII and IgIII:755C → G, resulting in Pro252Arg. Most *FGFR2* mutations cluster on IgIII (exons 8 and 10), but others have been found, including one on IgII, one near the transmembrane domain, and several in the split tyrosine kinase domain (Table 33–4, Fig. 33–20).

New mutations are exclusively of paternal origin (Glaser et al., 2000). Over 30 different mutations have been reported at this writing (Table 33–4). To date, about half a dozen of these mutations have also been found with Crouzon syndrome, and one 18 bp deletion overlaps with a 9 bp deletion noted with Crouzon syndrome (Oldridge et al., 1995) (Table 33–4). For about 45% of patients with Pfeiffer syndrome, no mutation has been identified (*n* = 78). Among 40 patients with mutations, 42.5% involve Cys278 and particularly Cys342. Splice site mutations account for perhaps 10% of mutations (Cornejo-Roldan et al., 1999).

A mutation with a severe Pfeiffer phenotype is 1052C → G, resulting in Ser351Cys (Gripp et al., 1998b).‡ Another mutation with severe Pfeiffer syndrome is 870G → T, resulting in Trp290Cys (Schaefer et al., 1998).§ Still another severe Pfeiffer phenotype was

‡More than a dozen instances of Ser351Cys are known (M. Muenke, personal communication, 1999). Although the phenotype is always severe, not all patients have either broad thumbs or broad great toes. Therefore, by clinical definition, some patients have Pfeiffer syndrome and others do not.
§A severe nonclassifiable craniosynostosis syndrome with the same mutation was reported by Shotelersuk et al. (2002) and commented on by Cohen (2002b). See section titled "Nonclassifiable FGFR2 Disorders with Craniosynostosis."

found with an 1124A → G nucleotide change, resulting in Tyr375Cys (Kan et al., 2002); this mutation is associated with several cases of Beare-Stevenson cutis gyrata syndrome (*vide infra*). Cutis gyrata and acanthosis nigricans, features of Beare-Stevenson syndrome, however, were not associated with the severe case of Pfeiffer reported by Kan et al. (2002). The 940-2A → G substitution of the 3′ splice site up-stream of exon 9 is associated with a relatively severe phenotype, particularly with respect to the hands and feet (Oldridge et al., 1999). Passos-Bueno et al. (1997) reported a Pfeiffer splice site mutation with an Apert-like phenotype. The same group also observed a Pfeiffer-like phenotype with a nucleotide change of 755C → G, resulting in Ser252Trp (Passos-Bueno et al., 1998b), the most common mutation for Apert syndrome. Ser252Phe/Pro253Ser, resulting in Pfeiffer syndrome, is extremely rare because it requires three nucleotide substitutions (755_757CGC → TCT) (Oldridge et al., 1997). One unusual Pfeiffer mutation is an insertion (1084_1085insTCAACA) that activates a cryptic donor splice site (Gly345_Pro361del) (Meyers et al., 1996).

Rutland et al. (1995), Schell et al. (1995), and Robin et al. (1998a) suggested that clinical differences might exist between the mutation on *FGFR1* and those on *FGFR2*. Roscioli et al. (2000) reviewed the clinical findings associated with the *FGFR1* mutation. Severe craniosynostosis and midface hypoplasia, more pronounced ocular prop-tosis, and perhaps broader thumbs are more likely to be associated with mutations on *FGFR2* than with the single mutation on *FGFR1*, although there is some overlap (Rutland et al., 1995; Schell et al., 1995). Abnormalities of the hands and feet tend to be more severe in cases with splice site mutations. A severe limb phenotype with very broad thumbs and great toes, together with cutaneous syndactyly of digits 2 to 5, has been found with an IgII mutation, Ala172Phe. Mutations in the split tyrosine kinase domain tend to exhibit mild broadening of the thumbs and great toes (Kan et al., 2002; Wilkie et al., 2002).

Crouzon Syndrome

New mutations are of paternal origin (Glaser et al., 2000). At this writing, more than 30 mutations for Crouzon syndrome are known (Table

33–4). Most are located on IgIII of FGFR2 (exons 8 and 10). To date, about half a dozen mutations are identical to those that cause Pfeiffer syndrome and one 9 bp deletion overlaps with an 18 bp deletion in Pfeiffer syndrome (Reardon et al., 1994; Oldridge et al., 1995; Meyers et al., 1996; Cohen, 1997a, 1997b, 1997c; Kress et al., 2000, Chun et al., 2002). One common Crouzon mutation, 1032G → A, does not result in an amino acid substitution (Ala344Ala), but it does produce a cryptic donor splice site, causing a deletion of 17 amino acids and shortening the distance from the disulfide bond of IgIIIc to the transmembrane domain (Li et al., 1995). Other mutations have been reported. Two rare Crouzon mutations are found, respectively, on IgI, 314A → G, resulting in Tyr105Cys (Pulleyn et al., 1996; Kan et al., 2002), and in the linker region between IgII and IgIII (755C → T, resulting in Ser252Leu) (Oldridge et al., 1997). In the latter mutation, the Crouzon phenotype was very mild. Other family relatives with this mutation were normal (Oldridge et al., 1997). Kan et al. (2002) reported mutations in the split tyrosine kinase domain. One mutation was found in the first kinase domain: 1645A → C, resulting in Asn549His, which occurs at the equivalent residue to the FGFR3 540 residue, a mutational hotspot for hypochondroplasia (Table 33–4, Fig. 33–20). Another mutation was found in the second kinase domain, 2032A → G, resulting in Arg678Gly.

Jackson-Weiss Syndrome

Jabs et al. (1994) reported an *FGFR2* mutation in the Jackson-Weiss family: 1031C → G, resulting in Ala344Gly (Table 33–4). This has been misprinted as Arg344Gly (Jabs, 1995) and also as Ala342Gly (Mulvihill, 1995). The Jackson-Weiss syndrome mutation has also been found in a family with Crouzon syndrome (Gorry et al., 1995). A family reported as having "Jackson-Weiss syndrome" (Adès et al., 1994) and also called "Adelaide type craniosynostosis" (Hollway et al., 1995) is known to have Muenke syndrome (FGFR3 Pro250Arg) (Muenke et al., 1997). Cohen (2001) compared the original Jackson-Weiss family with other reported cases harboring *FGFR2* mutations said to be associated with a Jackson-Weiss phenotype. He found other phenotypes with identical mutations, particularly Crouzon and Pfeiffer syndromes. Thus, the term "Jackson-Weiss syndrome" at this writing is best applied to the original Jackson-Weiss family (Jackson et al., 1976; Heike et al., 2001).

Beare-Stevenson Cutis Gyrata Syndrome

Przylepa et al. (1996) and Krepelová et al. (1998) reported mutations for Beare-Stevenson cutis gyrata syndrome on FGFR2: 1124A → G, resulting in Tyr375Cys near the transmembrane domain, and 1115C → G, resulting in Ser372Cys in the carboxy-terminal end of the linker region between IgIII and the transmembrane domain (Table 33–4). Most cases of the syndrome are associated with Tyr375Cys. *FGFR3* Pro250Arg has been associated with Beare-Stevenson-like anomalies in a single case (Roscioli et al., 2001) (*vide infra*).

Nonclassifiable FGFR2 Disorders with Craniosynostosis

Steinberger et al. (1996), Pulleyn et al. (1996), Johnson et al. (2000), Kan et al. (2002), and Shotelersuk et al. (2002) reported some *FGFR2* mutations with craniosynostosis that were not classifiable into clinically known syndrome categories (Table 33–4).

The common Crouzon mutation 1032G → A does not result in an amino acid substitution (Ala344Ala) but produces a cryptic donor splice site that causes a 17 amino acid deletion. In the family reported by Steinberger et al. (1996), however, a variable phenotype was observed through three generations that could not be classified as any of the syndromes known to be associated with *FGFR2* mutations. Kan et al. (2002) reported four of eight cases with vertical transmission of Ala344Ala; in two of the four families, the phenotype was unclassifiable.

Pulleyn et al. (1996) reported five patients. Two had the same mutation: Gly338Glu (their cases 1 and 2). One of these (their case 1) is found in Table 33–4. In my view, their case 2 is an example of Crouzon syndrome. Midface deficiency and ocular proptosis are present, but craniosynostosis is absent. However, other such cases have been reported. Shiller (1959) described a family in which the proband had

cloverleaf skull; some of the other affected members of the family had classic Crouzon syndrome with craniosynostosis; still others had ocular proptosis and midface deficiency without synostosis. Park et al. (1995b) noted a mother and son associated with Trp290Gly; neither had craniosynostosis per se.

In my view, case 3 of Pulleyn et al. (1996) is also an example of Crouzon syndrome with scaphocephaly. Their patient had an unusual mutation on IgI (Tyr105Cys). In Crouzon syndrome, head shape depends on the order and rate of progression of sutural synostosis. Brachycephaly is most commonly observed, but scaphocephaly, trigonocephaly, and cloverleaf skull may also be found in some instances. S. Kreiborg and I (unpublished) have two Crouzon families with scaphocephaly.

Pulleyn et al. (1996) also reported a patient with cloverleaf skull and fixed elbow joints. However, I regard this as a defined syndrome with a severe phenotype (Cohen and MacLean, 2000).

Johnson et al. (2000) and Kan et al. (2002) reported an unclassifiable case: 943G → T, resulting in Ala315Ser (exon 10). Kan et al. (2002) found another unclassifiable case: 1977G → T, resulting in Lys659Asn (exon 16), a mutation that occurs at an equivalent residue to the FGFR3 650 residue for mutations in thanatophoric dysplasia, types 2 and SADDAN.

Shotelersuk et al. (2000) observed a unique unclassifiable patient with an 870G → T change, resulting in Trp290Cys.‖

Paznekas et al. (1998) reported a study of *TWIST* mutations for Saethre-Chotzen syndrome. They included one patient (their Fig. 1F) with an *FGFR2* mutation who lacks many features of Saethre-Chotzen syndrome. I think their patient has an unclassifiable type of craniosynostosis.

Muenke Syndrome

Muenke et al. (1997) reported 61 cases of *FGFR3* Pro250Arg (Table 33–4). Autosomal dominant inheritance was observed in 12 of the families. Expressivity is extremely variable. Golla et al. (1996) described a patient with cloverleaf skull; another affected member of the family had unilateral coronal synostosis with marked facial asymmetry. Muenke et al. (1997) described two sibs with bilateral coronal synostosis; the affected father had macrocephaly only. Roscioli et al. (2001) reported a patient with Beare-Stevenson-like anomalies.

Gripp et al. (1998a) found four mutations among 37 sporadic cases of unicoronal synostosis (11%). It is particularly noteworthy that three fathers of unicoronal probands tested positive for the mutation themselves. None of the three fathers had craniosynostosis and had never come to medical attention previously. They were unaware of their 50% risk of passing the mutation on to their other children. Nonpenetrance was also found by Robin et al. (1998b). It must be emphasized that the 50% recurrence risk is for the mutation per se, not for the phenotype. The prevalence of the abnormal phenotype in mutation carriers is unknown at present. It is possible that Muenke syndrome may account for a significant proportion of familial instances of coronal synostosis. For example, in a study of 26 patients with apparently nonsyndromic coronal synostosis, Moloney et al. (1997) found 8 patients (31%) with the *FGFR3* Pro250Arg mutation.

Muenke et al. (1997) found a C → G transversion at position 749, resulting in Pro250Arg (Bellus et al., 1996; Muenke et al., 1997; Reardon et al., 1997). Moloney et al. (1997) estimated that this transversion rate is the highest currently known in the human genome. The only ones showing somewhat comparable frequencies are 1138G → A on FGFR3, resulting in achondroplasia, and 755C → G on FGFR2, resulting in Apert syndrome.

Borderline intelligence was found in about 30% of patients (Muenke et al., 1997), and either developmental delay or mental deficiency was noted in a minority of cases (Muenke et al., 1997; Reardon et al., 1997). Lajeunie et al. (1999b) demonstrated variation in expression by gender, and Muenke et al. (1997) found an increased frequency of sensorineural hearing loss.

‖Craniosynostosis, hydrocephalus, mental deficiency, non-Pfeiffer-like broad thumbs and great toes, severe multiple bony abnormalities of the limbs and spine, and acanthosis nigricans (see Cohen, 2002b).

Crouzonodermoskeletal Syndrome

To call this disorder "Crouzon syndrome with acanthosis nigricans" shows that we are prisoners of our own conventional terminology. In addition to acanthosis nigricans, cementomas of the jaws and alterations of the vertebral column have been found in a number of patients, both reported and unreported. At this writing, the frequency with which they occur in this syndrome is unknown because clinical manifestations have not been evident. Certainly, when a diagnosis of Crouzonoid phenotype and acanthosis nigricans is made, radiographic study should be instituted. It seems clear that this condition is completely separate from Crouzon syndrome. It is caused by a *highly specific* mutation that is 11 amino acids away from the common mutation for achondroplasia. An *FGFR3* transmembrane mutation, 1172C → A, resulting in Ala391Glu, has been recorded (Meyers et al., 1995; Wilkes et al., 1996; Schweitzer et al., 2001) (Table 33–4). A specific mutation with a specific phenotype requires a specific name. Elsewhere (Cohen, 1999), I have proposed the name "Crouzonodermoskeletal syndrome." The term includes the Crouzonoid phenotype (*Crouzono*) acanthosis nigricans (*dermo*), and jaw cementomas and vertebral alterations (*skeletal*).

Achondroplasia

More than 80% of achondroplasia cases are sporadic; increased paternal age has been demonstrated, and mutations are exclusively of paternal origin (Wilkin et al., 1998). The most common *FGFR3* mutation is 1138G → A, resulting in Gly380Arg. Another nucleotide change, 1138G → C, also results in the same amino acid substitution. Other rare mutations have been recorded: 1125G → T, resulting in Gly375Cys, and 1037G → A, resulting in Gly346Glu (Shiang et al., 1994; Bellus et al., 1995a; Prinos et al., 1995; Superti-Furga et al., 1995; Bonaventure et al., 1996; Cohen, 1997b, 1998; Szabo et al., 1997; Muenke et al., 1998). Camera et al. (2001) reported two patients with classic achondroplasia but with mutations for thanatophoric dysplasia, type 1 (742C → T, resulting in Arg248Cys), and hypochondroplasia (1620C → G, resulting in Asn540Lys) (Table 33–4).

Hypochondroplasia

Hypochondroplasia is a common skeletal dysplasia with radiographic features similar to those found in achondroplasia, although milder in degree. Short stature is not usually recognized until about 22 months of age. Diagnosis is not commonly made in the newborn period, although macrocephaly is a common feature at birth; the face is normal.

Mutations have been reported in exon 9 and in the split tyrosine kinase domain (exon 13 and exon 15) (Table 33–4). Two recurrent mutations in exon 13, 1620C → A and 1620C → G, result in Asn540Lys and account for about 50% to 70% of all cases of hypochondroplasia (Bellus et al., 1995b, 1996, 2000; Prinster et al., 1998; Ramaswami et al., 1998; Grigelioniene et al., 2000). A Crouzon syndrome mutation in the first kinase domain occurs at the equivalent residue on *FGFR2* (Kan et al., 2002) (*vide supra*).

Genetic heterogeneity has been found in some families by excluding linkage to 4p16.3 (Stoilov et al., 1995; Rousseau et al., 1996a; Grigelioniene et al., 1998). Other mutations have been found in isolated families, including Ile538Val (Grigelioniene et al., 1998), Asn540Thr (Deutz-Terlouw et al., 1998), Asn328Ile (Winterpacht et al., 2000), and Asn540Ser (Mortier et al., 2000) (Table 33–4, Fig. 33–20).

Mutations in the second kinase domain include 1948A → C, resulting in Lys650Gln, and both 1950G → T and 1950G → C, resulting in Lys650Asn (Bellus et al., 2000) (Table 33–4, Fig. 33–20). The Lys650Asn/Gln mutations have a milder phenotype than patients with the common Asn540Lys mutation. The 650 amino acid residue is the same one affected in thanatophoric dysplasia, type 2, in SADDAN, and rarely in thanatophoric dysplasia, type 1 (*vide infra*).

Thanatophoric Dysplasia

In thanatophoric dysplasia, type 2, a single mutation in the second kinase domain of *FGFR3*, 1948A → G, resulting in Lys650Glu, accounts for all cases to date. Type 1 has been associated with several different *FGFR3* mutations, both extracellular and intracellular. The most common of these is found in the linker region between IgII and IgIII: 742C → T, resulting in Arg248Cys. The second most common mutation is

1118A → G, resulting in Tyr373Cys. Intracellular stop codon mutations at amino acid residue 807 result in a receptor elongated by 141 amino acids, producing a hydrophobic domain near the carboxy terminus (Rousseau et al., 1995, 1996b; Tavormina et al., 1995a, 1995b; Cohen, 1997b, 1998; Wilcox et al., 1998) (Table 33–4, Fig. 33–20). Of all the mutations in thanatophoric dysplasia, the most frequent substitutions are transitions, accounting for 85% of all cases (Wilcox et al., 1998). Rarely, type 1 been reported with the same mutation that results in SADDAN: 1949A → T, resulting in Lys650Met (Kitoh et al., 1998) (*vide infra*).

Brodie et al. (1999) reported 17 cases of platyspondylic lethal skeletal dysplasia of the San Diego type with *FGFR3* mutations identical to those found in type 1 thanatophoric dysplasia. Large inclusion bodies were observed in the rough endoplasmic reticulum. In contrast, large inclusion bodies were rare in type 1, and small-to-medium inclusions were observed in only 32% of type 1 cases.

Brodie et al. (1999) suggested that the radiographic appearance of the San Diego type may evolve into type 1 thanatophoric dysplasia at a later gestational age. The presence of inclusion bodies may explain the radiographic differences and decreased severity of the morphologic changes in the San Diego type because less mutant FGFR3 may reach the cell surface and participate in signaling.

In type 1 cases, only 27.6% have craniosynostosis ($n = 58$), involving particularly Arg248Cys and Tyr373Cys, occurring more frequently with the latter mutation (Wilcox et al., 1998) (Table 33–4). Cloverleaf skull of mild degree accounts for 3.4% of these cases. In contrast, type 2 cases are associated with craniosynostosis in 93% ($n = 15$), all involving Lys650Glu (Tavormina et al., 1995b). Cloverleaf skull of severe degree accounts for 53% of these cases.

SADDAN

Tavormina et al. (1999) and Bellus et al. (1999) described what they called SADDAN, standing for *severe achondroplasia, developmental delay*, and *acanthosis nigricans*. The severity of the phenotype can perhaps be thought of as less than that of thanatophoric dysplasia but greater than that of achondroplasia. The term SADDAN will become established because the precedent has been set. However, I am concerned that the term "severe achondroplasia" may be misleading to the uninitiated because they might gain the impression that the disorder is really achondroplasia but of more severe degree than usual.

The mutation involves the same FGFR3 amino acid residue (650) affected in thanatophoric dysplasia, type 2, but instead of the usual thanatophoric dysplasia, type 2 mutation (Lys650Glu), the mutation substitutes a methionine (Lys650Met). The nucleotide change (1949A → T) is adjacent to the one for thanatophoric dysplasia, type 2 (1948A → G) (Table 33–4).

Autosomal Dominant Cerebellar Ataxia

Hereditary spinocerebellar ataxias are clinically and genetically heterogenous. More than 14 different genetic loci have been identified. An autosomal dominant type is characterized by early-onset tremor, dyskinesia, and slowly progressive cerebellar ataxia. A mutation in FGF14, which maps to 13q34, has been identified: 434T→C, resulting in Phe145Ser (van Swieten et al., 2003).

Autosomal Dominant Hypophosphatemic Rickets

FGF23 missense mutations were identified in autosomal dominant hypophosphatemic rickets (ADHR Consortium, 2000) (Table 33–4); they involved Arg176 and Arg179 in exon 1. Shimada et al. (2001) cloned and characterized *FGF23* as a cause of tumor-induced osteomalacia. Renal wasting results in hypophosphatemia in tumor-induced osteomalacia; removal of the tumor normalizes phosphate metabolism (Strewler, 2001; White et al., 2001). Overproduction of FGF23 causes tumor-induced osteomalacia, whereas *FGF23* mutations result in autosomal dominant hypophosphatemic rickets, possibly by preventing proteolytic cleavage, which enhances the biologic activity of FGF23 (Shimada et al., 2001; Carpenter, 2003; Jonsson et al., 2003).

FGF/FGFR ALTERATIONS IN NEOPLASIA

FGF/FGFR alterations in neoplasm have been discussed by Cohen (2003). Some FGFs were initially isolated as oncogenes—for exam-

Table 33–5. 8p11 Myeloproliferative Syndrome

Proteins (Alternative Terms)	Meaning of Acronyms	Protein Motifs	Chromosome Localization	Translocations Involving FGFR1	FGFR1/Protein Fusions
ZNF198 (RAMP) (FIM)	Zinc finger 198 (*Rearranged in an atypical myeloproliferative disorder*) (*Fused in myeloproliferative disorder*)	Four atypical zinc fingers (Cys-X$_2$-Cys-X$_{19-20}$-Cys-X$_3$-Cys)	13q12	t(8;13)(p11;q12)	FGFR1 (exon 9); ZNF198 (exon 17)
CEP110	*Centromere protein 110*	Four consensus leucine zippers [L-X(6)-L-X(6)-L]	9q33	t(8;9)(p11;q33)	FGFR1 (exon 9); CEP110 (exon 15)
FOP	*FGFR1 oncogene protein*	Two regions of leucine-rich repeats	6q27	t(6;8)(q27;p11)	FGFR1 (exon 9); FOP (exon 5 or exon 9)

Source: Data from Popovici et al. (1998, 1999), Smedley et al. (1998), Xiao et al. (1998), Kulkarni et al. (1999), Ollendorff et al. (1999), Guasch et al. (2000), Sohal et al. (2001).

ple, FGF3 (Dickson et al., 1991), FGF4 (Yoshida et al., 1991), FGF5 (Goldfarb et al., 1991), and FGF6 (Coulier et al. (1991). FGF7 was isolated from mouse mammary carcinoma cells as an androgen-induced growth factor (Tanaka et al., 1992), and FGF9 was isolated from human glioma cells as a glia-activating factor (Miyamoto et al., 1993).

FGFR1 is involved in the 8p11 myeloproliferative syndrome characterized by chronic myeloid hyperplasia, eosinophilia, T- or B-cell lymphoblastic lymphoma, and acute myelogenous leukemia. The syndrome is associated with at least three different genes that are fused to *FGFR1: ZNF198, CEP110*, and *FOP* (Popovici et al., 1998; Smedley et al., 1998; Xiao et al., 1998; Kulkarni et al., 1999; Ollendorf et al., 1999; Popovici et al., 1999; Guasch et al., 2000; Sohal et al., 2001). The genes, the meaning of their acronyms, their chromosome localizations, their protein motifs, types of translocations, and exons involved in the fusions are summarized in Table 33–5.

FGFR3 mutations—the same ones that cause thanatophoric dysplasia—have been identified in 40% to 50% of all bladder cancers (Cappellen et al., 1999; Sibley et al., 2001; van Rhijn et al., 2001). Cancer recurrence rates have been shown to be dramatically lower for tumors with mutant *FGFR3* genes, suggesting that the frequency of cystoscopic monitoring may be reduced in patients with *FGFR3*-positive tumors (Kimura et al., 2001; van Rhijn et al., 2001). *FGFR3* mutations in cervical cancers are found with low frequency (Capellen et al., 1999; Wu et al., 2000; Sibley et al., 2001). Aberrant splicing and activation of cryptic splice sequences in FGFR3 have been identified in colorectal cancer (Jang et al., 2000, 2001). In multiple myeloma, a frequent translocation, t(4;14)(p16.3;q32.3), is associated with activating *FGFR3* mutations for thanatophoric dysplasia, type 2, and SADDAN (Chesi et al., 1997). Gastric cancer has been reported with *FGFR2* mutations for Crouzon and Pfeiffer syndromes (Jang et al., 2001). Other FGF/FGFR alterations in neoplasia have also been reported (Kobrin et al., 1993; Yamaguchi et al., 1994; Maerz et al., 1998; Jang et al., 2001; Kwabi-Addo et al., 2001; Shah et al., 2002) (Table 33–6).

MISGUIDED INTERPRETATIONS

Antley-Bixler syndrome is characterized by craniosynostosis, dysplastic ears, arachnodactyly, radiohumeral synostosis, femoral bowing, and joint contractures. Cardiovascular and urogenital anomalies have occurred in some patients. It should be noted, however, that *most reported genital anomalies in Antley-Bixler syndrome do not include ambiguous genitalia* despite assertions to the contrary (Kelley et al., 2002). The syndrome has been observed in sibs four times, and consanguinity has been noted in a number of instances (see Cohen, 2000c). Thus, autosomal recessive inheritance is supported. Although genetic heterogeneity is common in many disorders, there is no convincing evidence *to date* to suggest genetic heterogeneity in Antley-Bixler syndrome.

Several articles have claimed that Antley-Bixler syndrome is caused by mutations in *FGFR2* (e.g., Chun et al., 1998; Okajima et al., 1999; Reardon et al., 2000; Tsai et al., 2001; Kelley et al., 2002) by defining the combination of craniosynostosis and elbow ankylosis as the cardinal features of the syndrome. However, elbow ankylosis is nonspecific in craniosynostosis syndromes and can be found in a number of them besides Antley-Bixler syndrome including Pfeiffer syndrome,

Apert syndrome, Ives-Houston syndrome, Berant syndrome, and cloverleaf skull (Cohen and MacLean, 2000). Gripp et al. (1999) showed that the overall pattern of anomalies exhibited by the patient of Chun et al. (1998) was at variance with Antley-Bixler syndrome. Other presumed cases represent Pfeiffer syndrome or cloverleaf skull with elbow ankylosis. The statement that "there is evidence for at least four different causes of the Antley-Bixler phenotype" (Kelley et al., 2002) is unwarranted. No patient with an *FGFR2* mutation reported to date has Antley-Bixler syndrome. That Antley-Bixler syndrome can be caused by the teratogen fluconazole (Kelley et al., 2002) is in conflict with the report of Aleck and Bartley (1997): they noted that although fluconazole embryopathy has some features in common with Antley-Bixler syndrome, *the conditions are clinically distinguishable.*

At least at the present time, no classical patients with Antley-Bixler syndrome have been shown to harbor an FGFR2 mutation. To say and to repeat that Antley-Bixler syndrome can also be caused by FGFR2 mutations does not make it so. Unfortunately, many reviews of FGFRs perpetuate the Antley-Bixler/*FGFR2* inaccuracy. The use of the term "Antley-Bixler-*like* syndrome" is not helpful either and leads to confusion.

Tsukuno et al. (1999) reported two Pfeiffer syndrome patients with an *FGFR2* acceptor splice site mutation, 940-2A → G, which they interpreted as resulting in haploinsufficiency. Such an interpretation goes against the well-established gain of function known to characterize *FGFR* mutations (Johnson and Wilkie, 2000).

PRENATAL DIAGNOSIS AND GENETIC COUNSELING

All *FGFR* mutations for craniosynostosis syndromes and short-limb skeletal dysplasias are autosomal dominant, and if one parent is affected, genetic counseling is straightforward and prenatal molecular diagnosis is possible by CVS or amniocentesis (Cohen and MacLean, 2000). Instances in which one parent has achondroplasia and the other hypochondroplasia have been reported (Chitayat et al., 1999; Huggins et al., 1999a, 1999b). Pregnancy following preimplantation genetic diagnosis for Crouzon syndrome has been described (Abou-Sleiman et al., 2002).

Prenatal molecular diagnosis in sporadic cases is more problematic. Often ultrasonograms are carried out for other reasons and diagnosis is made coincidently and too late to offer the option of pregnancy termination. In achondroplasia, short limbs may be evident on ultrasound. Macrocephaly and/or mild shortening of the limbs interpreted by ultrasonography may suggest the possibility of hypochondroplasia. Clinical diagnosis of hypochondroplasia during early infancy is usually difficult and is often made at a later time. The limited number of mutations for achondroplasia and Apert syndrome facilitate molecular confirmation, whereas Crouzon syndrome and Pfeiffer syndrome each have more than 30 known mutations (Cohen and MacLean, 2000).

For molecularly diagnosed conditions that sometimes appear to be sporadic, such as *FGFR3* Pro250Arg, a parent may harbor the mutation and yet be clinically silent. Thus, once the mutation has been identified, parental studies are essential for recurrence risk counseling (Zackai et al., 2000).

All cases of thanatophoric dysplasia essentially occur sporadically. The recurrence risk is extremely low, with rare exceptions explain-

Table 33–6. Other FGF/FGFR Alterations in Neoplasia

Tumors	Findings	Comments	References
Bladder cancer	Frequent *FGFR3* activating mutations 742C → T, resulting in Arg248Cys 746C → G, resulting in Ser249Cys 1114G → T, resulting in Gly372Cys 1954A → G, resulting in Lys652Glu	First three mutations are the same as those for thanatophoric dysplasia, type 1. The fourth mutation is the same as that for thanatophoric dysplasia, type 2. The amino acid markers are increased by 2 because the IIIb isoform contains 2 more amino acids than IIIc. Dramatically lower recurrence rates are found for tumors with mutant *FGFR3* genes	Cappellen et al., 1999; Kimura et al., 2001; Sibley et al., 2001; van Rhijn et al., 2001
Cervical cancer	Low frequency of an *FGFR3* activating mutation 746C → G, resulting in Ser249Cys	Mutation is the same as that for thanatophoric dysplasia, type 1	Cappellen et al., 1999; Wu et al., 2000; Sibley et al., 2001
Colorectal cancer	*FGFR3* novel mutations 849delC, resulting in His284fs292X 964G → A, resulting in Glu322Lys FGFR3 frequently inactivated by aberrant splicing and activation of cryptic splice donor sites within exon 7		Jang et al., 2000, 2001
Multiple myeloma	Frequent translocation t(4;14)(p16.3;q32.3) associated with activating mutations in *FGFR3* 1948A → G, resulting in Lys650Glu 1949A → T, resulting in Lys650Met	The former mutation is the same as that for thanatophoric dysplasia, type 2; the latter is the same as that for SADDAN	Chesi et al., 1997
Gastric cancer	*FGFR2* mutations 799T → C, resulting in Ser267Pro 940-2A → G	First mutation same as one causing Crouzon syndrome and Pfeiffer syndrome as well. Second mutation is splice type, causing Pfeiffer syndrome	Jang et al., 2001
Prostate cancer	FGFR1 not expressed in normal prostate epithelial cells but is expressed in the IIIc form in 20% of prostate cancers. FGFR2 expressed in IIIb form in normal prostate epithelial cells and is expressed as the IIIb form predominantly or exclusively in prostatic cancer but in a subset, the IIIc form is increased	FGFR3 in the IIIb form in normal epithelial cells and in prostatic cancer are similarly expressed	Kwabi-Addo et al., 2001
Astrocytoma	FGFR2 is abundant in normal white matter and in low-grade astrocytomas, but is not found in highly malignant astrocytomas. Conversely, FGFR1, barely detectable in normal white matter, is elevated in highly malignant astrocytomas		Yamaguchi et al., 1994
Pancreatic adenocarcinoma	FGF1, FGF2, and FGFR1 are often overexpressed in tumor. When FGF2 is present and FGF1 is absent, postoperative patient survival is shorter. Overexpressed FGFR4 is mediated by an intronic enhancer activated by HNF1α	FGFR1 is normally expressed in acinar cells but not in ductal cells. Tumors overexpress FGFR1 and yet are of ductal origin	Kobrin et al., 1993; Shah et al., 2002
Male germ cell tumors, subset	Increased FGF4 expression, particularly in embryonal carcinomas		Maerz et al., 1998

able as examples of gonadal mosaicism. It has been estimated that among women receiving prenatal care, about 80% to 90% of various lethal skeletal dysplasias can be detected in utero. However, accurate antenatal diagnosis per se rather than simply nonspecific identification has only been made approximately 48% of the time. Pregnancies have been terminated with an average detection of about 21 weeks. When fetal ultrasonic identification of a nonspecific lethal skeletal dysplasia leads to pregnancy termination, clinical examination, radiographs, and autopsy are mandatory for making a specific diagnosis. For thanatophoric dysplasia per se, if specific prenatal detection with molecular confirmation is not possible, molecular diagnosis should be made following termination or following birth (Cohen and MacLean, 2000).

MANAGEMENT

Management issues in FGFR short-limb skeletal dysplasias and in craniosynostosis syndromes are complex, and treatments are individualized. These issues have been discussed in detail elsewhere (Cohen and MacLean, 2000; Pauli, 2001). Only the essentials can be outlined here.

The management of achondroplasia, the most common short-limb skeletal dysplasia, is summarized in Table 33–7. Although thanatophoric dysplasia is lethal, modern neonatal care, long-term medical care, and chronic ventilator dependence have made long-term survival possible in a few cases. The justification of respiratory care in such cases has been debated.

For craniosynostosis syndromes, evaluation and various surgical procedures require proper timing and coordination. Management is outlined in Table 33–8.

ORTHOLOGOUS GENES AND ANIMAL MODELS

For a discussion of orthologous genes, animal models, specific tissue expression of various transcripts, and tertiary structure, see Chapter 32.

MECHANISMS

Gain-of-function mechanisms for FGFR mutations include (*a*) ligand independent dimerization, (*b*) enhanced ligand-binding affinity, (*c*) loss of ligand-binding specificity, (*d*) ectopic spliceform expression, (*e*) chimeric FGFR proteins resulting from translocation, and (*f*) loss of dimerization dependence. A model for the effect of point mutations on FGFR function (Webster and Donoghue, 1997) is shown in Figure 33–21.

FGFR mutations may create or destroy cysteine residues, leaving an unpaired cysteine that can produce intermolecular disulfide bonding and constitutive receptor activation (Neilson and Friesel, 1996).

Table 33–7. Management of Achondroplasia

Adaptive modifications
  E.g., appropriately placed stepstools, modifications for toileting, automobile foot extensions
Short stature (no effective treatment)
  Growth hormone therapy, osteodistraction/leg lengthening, C-type natriuretic peptide (experimental FGFR3^{ACH} mouse model only; 75% rescue of bone length)
Symptomatic hydrocephalus (not compensatory hydrocephalus [benign ventriculomegaly] which is common)
  Ventriculoperitoneal shunting
Small foramen magnum with significant neurological findings (persistent hypotonia, increased reflexes or clonus in the legs)
  Suboccipital and cervical decompressive surgery
Severe and/or progressive spinal stenosis
  Surgical intervention
Obstructive sleep apnea (snoring is virtually a uniform feature; 60% history suggestive of airway obstruction with 38% clinically confirmed cases)
  Graded series of options (T & A, weight loss, CPAP, BiPAP, modified uvulopharyngopalatoplasty, tracheostomy)
Obesity (common)
  Nutritional counseling
Varus deformity (common)
  Appropriate management
Thoracolumbar abnormalities (significant ones)
  Bracing, surgical intervention

Source: Data from Pauli (2001). See also Weber et al. (1996), Yasoda et al. (1998, 2002), and Cohen (2002a).

Table 33–8. Management of Craniosynostosis Syndromes

EVALUATION

CNS
  MRI to define possible CNS abnormalities in Apert, Pfeiffer, and Crouzon syndromes
  DQ/IQ at appropriate times
Skull
  Radiographs, CTs, and three-dimensional CTs to define which sutures are involved
Airway
  Assessment for upper and lower respiratory compromise; in Apert, Pfeiffer, and Crouzon syndromes, lower respiratory compromise is rarely due to solid cartilaginous trachea
Cardiovascular and genitourinary system
  Apert syndrome (cardiovascular anomalies,10%; genitourinary anomalies, 10%)
Eyes
  Assessment for degree of ocular proptosis in Apert, Pfeiffer, and Crouzon syndromes
Hearing
  Possible ossicular ankylosis in Apert syndrome; also hearing impairment secondary to cleft or high-arched palate
Hands and feet
  Radiographic assessment of hands and feet in Apert syndrome; hands in Pfeiffer syndrome
Vertebrae
  Radiographic assessment for fusions in Apert, Pfeiffer, and Crouzon syndromes

SURGERY

Skull
  Early frontal bone advancement in Apert, Pfeiffer, and Crouzon syndromes
  Relief of fused sutures
Face
  Le Fort III surgical advancement for Apert, Pfeiffer, and Crouzon syndromes
  Surgical and orthodontic treatment for jaws and teeth
Hands
  Surgical separation of digits in Apert syndrome, but feet treated only symptomatically
  Soft tissue syndactyly in some cases of Pfeiffer syndrome may need attention
Management
  Various other problems based on evaluation

Source: Adapted from Cohen and MacLean (2000).

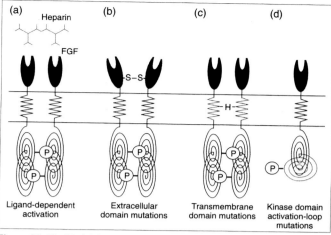

Figure 33–21. Model for the effect of point mutations on FGFR function. (*a*) Normal ligand-dependent activation leads to regulated signals for proliferation and differentiation of bones. (*b*) Certain extracellular domain mutations activate the receptors through the formation of aberrant disulfide bonds (indicated by S–S) leading to ligand-independent dimerization. (*c*) Transmembrane domain mutations result in hydrogen (H)-bonded FGFR dimers. (*d*) Mutations in the activation loop of the kinase domain result in conformational changes that activate receptor tyrosine kinase activity. (From Webster and Donoghue, 1997.)

In FGFR2, the disulfide bond of IgIII is formed by Cys278 and Cys342, both of which are involved in many Crouzon and Pfeiffer syndrome mutations; Cys342 is involved more commonly of the two. Many mutations to cysteine occur with Crouzon and Pfeiffer syndromes, thanatophoric dysplasia, type 1, and Beare-Stevenson cutis gyrata syndrome (Table 33–9). Some noncysteine mutations, particu-

Table 33–9. Mutations Involving Cysteine

Crouzon syndrome (FGFR2)
  Tyr105Cys (IgI)
  Cys278Phe (IgIIIa)
  Tyr281Cys (IgIIIc)
  Tyr301Cys (IgIIIa)
  Tyr328Cys (IgIIIc)
  Cys342Ser (IgIIIc)1024T → A
  Cys342Ser (IgIIIc)1025G → C
  Cys342Arg (IgIIIc)
  Cys342Tyr (IgIIIc)
  Cys342Phe (IgIIIc)
  Cys342Trp (IgIIIc)
  Ser347Cys (IgIIIc)
  Ser354Cys (IgIIIc)
Pfeiffer syndrome (FGFR2)
  Cys278Phe (IgIIIa)
  Trp290Cys (IgIIIa) 870G → T
  Trp290Cys (IgIIIa) 870G → C
  Tyr340Cys (IgIIIc)
  Cys342Arg (IgIIIc)
  Cys342Gly (IgIIIc)
  Cys342Tyr (IgIIIc)
  Cys342Ser (IgIIIc)1024T → A
  Cys342Ser (IgIIIc)1025G → C
  Cys342Ser (IgIIIc)1025_1026GC → CT
  Cys342Trp (IgIIIc)
  Ser351Cys (IgIIIc)
Beare-Stevenson cutis gyrata syndrome (FGFR2)
  Ser372Cys (IgIIIc-TM)
  Tyr375Cys (IgIIIc-TM)
Thanatophoric dysplasia, type 1 (FGFR3)
  Arg248Cys (Linker:IgII-IgIIIa)
  Ser249Cys (Linker:IgII-IgIIIa)
  Gly370Cys (IgIIIc-TM)
  Ser371Cys (IgIIIc-TM)
  Tyr373Cys (IgIIIc-TM)
  Stop807Cys (C-tail)

Source: From Cohen (2000a).

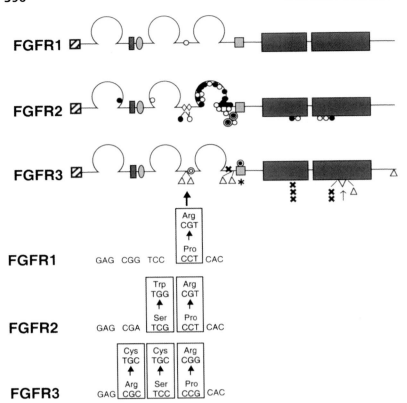

Figure 33–22. Mutations in the linker region between IgII and IgIII on *FGFR1*, *FGFR2*, and *FGFR3*. Mutations for Apert syndrome on *FGFR2* (Ser252Trp and Pro253Arg) have been shown to have enhanced ligand-binding affinity. It is probable that the mutations for Pfeiffer syndrome on *FGFR1* (Pro252Arg) and for Muenke syndrome on *FGFR3* (Pro250Arg) also have enhanced ligand-binding affinity. *FGFR3* mutations to cysteine for thanatophoric dysplasia, type 1 (Arg248Cys and Ser249Cys) have ligand-independent activation. (From Cohen, 2000a.)

larly those near cysteine residues that stabilize the IgIII loop structure, can disrupt intramolecular disulfide bonds, resulting in intermolecular disulfide bonding and ligand-independent activation (Robertson et al., 1998).

Naski et al. (1996) showed that the *FGFR3* transmembrane mutation for achondroplasia, Gly380Arg, was weakly activating compared to the Arg248Cys mutation for thanatophoric dysplasia, type 1, which was strongly activating. The former mutation may result from hydrogen-bonded FGFR dimers (Webster and Donoghue, 1996) while the latter is based on intermolecular disulfide-bonded dimers (Fig. 33–21). The Lys650Glu mutation for thanatophoric dysplasia, type 2 is strongly activating, but less so than the Arg248Cys mutation for type 1. Bellus et al. (2000) showed that the Lys650Asn/Gln and Lys650Thr mutations for hypochondroplasia had *FGFR3* tyrosine kinase activation approximately 3- to 5-five fold greater than the wild type, the Lys650Gln mutation for thanatophoric dysplasia, type 2 being about 10-fold greater, and the Lys650Met mutation for SADDAN being about 18-fold greater. The Lys650 residue, located within the activation loop of the *FGFR3* tyrosine kinase domain (Mohammadi et al., 1996), plays an important role in stabilizing the loop in an inactive conformation (Webster et al., 1996). Activating mutations of this residue may pre-

clude the need for receptor dimerization (Webster and Donoghue, 1997) (Fig. 33–21).

The linker region between IgII and IgIII has mutations on *FGFR1* (Pfeiffer syndrome), *FGFR2* (Apert syndrome), and *FGFR3* (Muenke syndrome) (Fig. 33–22). Apert mutations are ligand dependent, unlike mutations in Crouzon syndrome (Table 33–10). Anderson et al. (1998) studied the ectodomain of *FGFR2* Apert mutations (Ser252Trp and Pro253Arg) in solution. Using FGF2 as a ligand, *FGFR2* Apert mutations were compared to the *FGFR2* wild type. Apert mutations showed a selective decrease in the kinetics of ligand dissociation. The rate of dissociation was slower for Ser252Trp than for Pro253Arg. Thus, enhanced FGFR2 occupancy occurs at low concentrations of FGF2 (Anderson et al., 1998).

The evidence for gain of function based on accentuated ligand binding is most compelling for Apert syndrome and appears to be related to the bulky amino acid substitutions (Ser252Trp, Pro253Arg) that alter the relative orientation of IgII and IgIII (Anderson et al., 1998; Wilkie et al., 1995b). It is probable that linker mutations on *FGFR1* (Pfeiffer syndrome) and *FGFR3* (Muenke syndrome) behave similarly. Neilsen and Friesel (1996) demonstrated constitutive activation by analyzing FGFR1 and FGFR2 mutant receptor proteins expressed in

Table 33–10. Differences in FGFR2 Molecular Biology in Apert and Crouzon Syndromes

	Apert Syndrome	Crouzon Syndrome
Physical clustering of mutations	Two specific mutations in adjacent amino acids in linker region between IgII and IgIII	More than 30 widely dispersed mutations on IgIII and a few elsewhere
Types of mutations	Bulky amino acid substitutions (Ser252Trp, Pro253Arg)	Frequently involve cysteine residues
Consequences of mutations	Gain-of-function mechanism with specific on effects skeletogenesis	Gain-of-function mechanism with specific effects on skeletogenesis
Mechanisms	Enhanced ligand-binding affinity, loss of ligand-binding specificity, ectopic splice-form expression*	Ligand-independent receptor activation
Phenotypic/molecular correlations	Yes	No

*Apert limb abnormalities can be caused by either having an abnormal receptor in its normal place or a normal receptor in the wrong place.
Source: Modified from Cohen (2000a).

Xenopus oocytes. All but one—a mutant that was equivalent to the *FGFR1* linker mutation for Pfeiffer syndrome (Pro252Arg)—showed increased tyrosine kinase activity. This is indirect evidence for ligand dependence for the linker mutation on FGFR1 for Pfeiffer syndrome. At this writing, no evidence, either direct or indirect, is available for the FGFR3 Pro250Arg linker mutation for Muenke syndrome. Two of the type I thanatophoric dysplasia mutations are also in the linker region of FGFR3 (Fig. 33–22). However, they are mutations to cysteine (Arg248Cys and Ser249Cys) and therefore result in ligand-independent activation.

Oldridge et al. (1999) studied *Alu* insertions in two Apert syndrome patients who lacked the canonical missense mutations (Ser252Trp and Pro253Arg) and showed that the limb abnormalities in the syndrome are caused by aberrant FGFR2 IgIIIa/b signaling. They also studied splice site mutations (940-2A → G and 940-2A → T) in two Pfeiffer syndrome patients with relatively severe limb defects: radial deviation of the thumbs, varus deviation of the halluces, marked broadening of all four first digits, and some degree of soft tissue syndactyly. The level of ectopic IgI-IIb expression was found to be highest in an Apert syndrome patient with an *Alu* insertion, intermediate in a Pfeiffer syndrome patient with 940-2A → G, and lowest in a Pfeiffer syndrome patient with 940-2A → T.

Yu et al. (2000) showed that the *FGFR2* Apert mutation Ser252Trp broke the cardinal rule governing ligand specificity: the IgIIIc isoform allowed activation by FGF7 and FGF10, and the IgIIIb isoform allowed activation by FGF2, FGF6, and FGF9, permitting autocrine signaling in tissues that express these ligands. Although ligand specificity is lost, ligand dependence for receptor activation is retained. Apert limb abnormalities can be caused by either having an abnormal receptor in its normal place or a normal receptor in the wrong place (Oldridge et al., 1999; Yu and Ornitz, 2001; Wilkie et al., 2002).

Based on the crystal structure of the mutant proteins, Ibrahami et al. (2001) showed additional interactions between FGFR2 and FGF2 that increased FGFR2/FGF2 affinity. They proposed that Pro253Arg increased the affinity for a limited subset of FGFs. A radically different model was proposed by Pellegrini et al. (2000). Based on the crystal structure of FGFR2 and, instead, FGF1, they suggested that *cis/trans* isomerization at the Pro253 residue might explain the differences in FGFR2 activation.

ACKNOWLEDGMENTS

I am grateful to Andrew O. M. Wilkie (Weatherall Institute of Molecular Medicine, Oxford) for helpful discussion. I also wish to acknowledge the administrative skill of Ruth E. MacLean (Dalhousie University, Halifax) without whose expertise this chapter would not have been possible.

REFERENCES

Abou-Sleiman PM, Apessos A, Harper JC, Serhal P, Delhanty JD (2002). Pregnancy following preimplementation genetic diagnosis for Crouzon syndrome. *Hum Mol Reprod* 8: 304–309.

Adès LC, Mulley JC, Senga IP, Morris LL, David DJ, Haan EA (1994). Jackson-Weiss syndrome: clinical and radiological findings in a large kindred and exclusion of the gene from 7p21 and 5qter. *Am J Med Genet* 51: 121–130.

ADHR Consortium (2000). Autosomal dominant hypophosphataemic rickets is associated with mutations in *FGF23*. *Nat Genet* 26: 345–348.

Aleck KA, Bartley DL (1997). Multiple malformation syndrome following fluconazole use in pregnancy: report of an additional patient. *Am J Med Genet* 72: 253–256.

Anderson J, Burns HD, Enriquez-Harris P, Wilkie AOM, Heath JK (1998). Apert syndrome mutations in fibroblast growth factor receptor 2 exhibit increased affinity for FGF ligand. *Hum Mol Genet* 7: 1475–1483.

Angle B, Herch JM, Christensen KM (1998). Molecularly proven hypochondroplasia with cloverleaf skull deformity: a novel association. *Clin Genet* 54: 417–420.

Antonarakis SE and the Nomenclature Working Group (1998). Recommendations for a nomenclature system for human gene mutations. *Hum Mutat* 11: 1–3.

Bellus GA, Hefferon TW, Ortiz DE, Luna RI, Hecht JT, Horton WA, Machado M, Kaitila I, McIntosh I, Francomano CA (1995a). Achondroplasia is defined by recurrent G380R mutations of FGFR3. *Am J Hum Genet* 56: 368.

Bellus GA, McIntosh I, Smith EA, Aylsworth AS, Kaitila I, Horton WA, Greenaw GA, Hecht JT, Francomano CA (1995b). A recurrent mutation in the tyrosine kinase domain of fibroblast growth factor receptor 3 causes hypochondroplasia. *Nat Genet* 10: 357–359.

Bellus GA, Gaudenz K, Zackai EH, Clarke LA, Szabo J, Francomano CA, Muenke M (1996). Identical mutations in three different fibroblast growth factor receptor genes in autosomal dominant craniosynostosis syndromes. *Nat Genet* 14: 174–176.

Bellus GA, Bamshed MJ, Przylepa KA, Dorst J, Lee RR, Hurko O, Jabs EW, Curry CJR, Wilcox WR, Lachman RS, et al. (1999). Severe achondroplasia with developmental delay and acanthosis nigricans (SADDAN): phenotypic analysis of a new skeletal dysplasia caused by a Lys650Met mutation in fibroblast growth factor receptor 3. *Am J Med Genet* 85: 53–65.

Bellus GA, Spector EB, Speiser PW, Weaver CA, Garber AT, Bryke CR, Israel J, Rosengren SS, Webster MK, Donoghue DJ, Francomano CA (2000). Distinct missense mutations of the FGFR3 Lys650 codon modulate receptor kinase activation and the severity of the skeletal dysplasia phenotype. *Am J Hum Genet* 67: 1411–1421.

Bonaventure J, Rousseau F, Legeai-Mallet L, Le Merrer M, Munnich A, Maroteaux P (1996). Common mutations in the fibroblast growth factor receptor 3 (*FGFR3*) gene account for achondroplasia, hypochondroplasia and thanatophoric dwarfism. *Am J Med Genet* 63: 148–154.

Brodie SG, Kitoh H, Lachman RS, Nolasco LM, Mekikian PB, Wilcox WR (1999). Platyspondylic lethal skeletal dysplasia, San Diego type, is caused by FGFR3 mutations. *Am J Med Genet* 84: 476–480.

Burke D, Wilkes D, Blundell TL, Malcolm S (1998). Fibroblast growth factor receptors: lessons from the genes. *Trends Biochem* 23: 59–62.

Burrus LW, Zuber ME, Lueddecke BA, Olwin BB (1992). Identification of a cysteine-rich receptor for fibroblast growth factors. *Mol Cell Biol* 12: 5600–5609.

Camera G, Baldi M, Strisciuglio G, Concolino D, Mastroiacovo P, Baffico M (2001). Occurrence of thanatophoric dysplasia type I (R248C) and hypochondroplasia (N540K) mutations in two patients with achondroplasia phenotype. *Am J Med Genet* 104: 277–281.

Cappellen D, De Oliveira C, Ricol D, de Medina S, Bourdin J, Sastre-Garau X, Chopin D, Thiery JP, Radvanyi F (1999). Frequent activating mutations of FGFR3 in human bladder and cervix carcinomas. *Nat Genet* 23: 18–20.

Carpenter TO (2003). Oncogenic osteomalacia—a complex dance of factors. *N Engl J Med* 348: 1705–1708.

Chang Z, Meyer K, Rapraeger AC, Friedl A (2000). Differential ability of heparan sulfate proteoglycans to assemble the fibroblast growth factor receptor complex in situ. *FASEB J* 14: 137–144.

Chesi M, Nardini E, Brents LA, Schrock E, Ried T, Kuehl WM, Bergsagel PL (1997). Frequent translocation t(4;14)(p16.3;q32.3) in multiple myeloma is associated with increased expression and activating mutations of fibroblast growth factor receptor 3. *Nat Genet* 16: 260–264.

Chitayat D, Fernandez B, Gardner A, Moore L, Glance P, Dunn M, Chun K, Sgro M, Ray P, Allingham-Hawkins D (1999). Compound heterozygosity for the achondroplasia-hypochondroplasia FGFR3 mutations: prenatal diagnosis and postnatal outcome. *Am J Med Genet* 84: 401–405.

Chun K, Siegel-Bartelt J, Chitayat D, Phillips J, Ray PN (1998). FGFR2 mutation associated with clinical manifestations consistent with Antley-Bixler syndrome. *Am J Med Genet* 77: 219–224.

Chun K, Steele L, Ray PN (2003). Graduated strategy for the molecular diagnosis of craniosynostosis syndromes. *Am J Med Genet*, in press.

Cohen MM Jr (1975). An etiologic and nosologic overview of craniosynostosis syndromes. *Birth Defects* 11(2): 137–189.

Cohen MM Jr (1997a). Molecular biology of craniosynostosis with special emphasis on fibroblast growth factor receptors. In *Studies in Stomatology and Craniofacial Biology*. Cohen MM Jr, Baum BJ, (eds.) IOS Press, Amsterdam, pp. 307–329.

Cohen MM Jr (1997b). Short limb skeletal dysplasias and craniosynostoses: what do they have in common? *Pediatr Radiol* 27: 442–446.

Cohen MM Jr (1997c). Transforming growth factor βs and fibroblast growth factors and their receptors: role in sutural biology and craniosynostosis. *J Bone Min Res* 12: 322–331.

Cohen MM Jr (1997d). *The Child with Multiple Birth Defects, 2nd Edition*. Oxford University Press, New York.

Cohen MM Jr (1998). Achondroplasia, hypochondroplasia, and thanatophoric dysplasia: clinically related skeletal dysplasias that are also related at the molecular level. *Int J Oral Maxfac Surg* 27: 451–455.

Cohen MM Jr (1999). Let's call it "Crouzonodermoskeletal syndrome" so we won't be prisoners of our own conventional terminology. *Am J Med Genet* 84: 74.

Cohen MM Jr (2000a). Fibroblast growth factor receptor mutations. In: *Craniosynostosis: Diagnosis, Evaluation, and Management, 2nd Edition*. Cohen MM Jr., MacLean RE (eds.) Oxford University Press, New York, pp. 77–94.

Cohen MM Jr (2000b). Thanatophoric dysplasia. In: *Craniosynostosis: Diagnosis, Evaluation, and Management, 2nd Edition*. Cohen MM Jr, MacLean RE (eds.) Oxford University Press, New York, pp. 366–373.

Cohen MM Jr (2000c). Other syndromes with craniosynostosis. In: *Craniosynostosis: Diagnosis, Evaluation, and Management, 2nd Edition*. Cohen MM Jr, MacLean RE (eds.) Oxford University Press, New York, pp. 385–440.

Cohen MM Jr (2001). Jackson-Weiss syndrome. *Am J Med Genet* 100: 325–329.

Cohen MM Jr (2002a). Bone morphogenetic proteins with some comments on fibrodysplasia ossificans progressiva and *NOGGIN*. *Am J Med Genet* 109: 87–92.

Cohen MM Jr (2002b). Unclassifiable craniosynostosis phenotypes, FGFR2 Trp290 mutations, acanthosis nigricans, and unpaired cysteine mutations. *Am J Med Genet* 113: 1–3.

Cohen MM Jr (2003). Neoplasms associated with alterations in fibroblast growth factor receptors. *Am J Med Genet* 119A: 97–100.

Cohen MM Jr, Kreiborg S (1993). An updated pediatric perspective on the Apert syndrome. *Am J Dis Child* 147: 989–993.

Cohen MM Jr, MacLean RE (2000). *Craniosynostosis: Diagnosis, Evaluation, and Management, 2nd Edition*. Oxford University Press, New York.

Cornejo-Roldan LR, Roessler E, Muenke M (1999). Analysis of the mutational spectrum of the *FGFR2* gene in Pfeiffer syndrome. *Hum Genet* 104: 425–431.

Coulier F, Ollendorff V, Marics I, Rosnet O, Batoz M, Planche J, Marchetto S, Pebusque M-J, DeLapeyriere O, Birnbaum D (1991). The *FGF6* gene within the *FGF* multigene family. *Ann NY Acad Sci* 638: 53–61.

Coulier F, Pontarotti P, Roubin R, Hartung H, Goldfarb M, Birnbaum D (1997). Of worms and men: an evolutionary perspective on the fibroblast growth factor (FGF) and FGF receptor families. *J Mol Evol* 44: 43–56.

Cytokine Family cDNA Database. Available at http: //ctokine.medic.kumamoyo-u.ac.jp/ CFC/FGF/FGF.html

Darnell JE Jr (1997). STATs and gene regulation. *Science* 277: 1630–1635.

den Dunnen JT, Antonarakis E (2001). Nomenclature for the description of human sequence variations. *Hum Genet* 109: 121–124.

Deutz-Terlouw PP, Losekoot M, Aalfs CM, Hennekam RC, Bakker E (1998). Asn540Thr substitution in the fibroblast growth factor receptor 3 tyrosine kinase domain causing hypochondroplasia. *Hum Mutat Suppl* 1: S62–S65.

Dickson C, Fuller-Pace F, Kiefer P, Acland P, MacAllan D, Peters G (1991). Expression, processing, and properties of *int-2*. *Ann NY Acad Sci* 638: 18–26.

Dionne CA, Crumley G, Bellot F, Kaplow JM, Searfoss G, Ruta M, Burgess WH, Jaye M, Schlessinger J (1990). Cloning and expression of two distinct high-affinity receptors cross-reacting with acidic and basic fibroblast growth factors. *EMBO J* 9: 2685–2692.

Doherty P, Williams EJ, Walsh FS (1995). A soluble chimeric form of the L1 glycoprotein stimulates neurite outgrowth. *Neuron* 14: 1–20.

Elejalde BR, de Elejalde MM (1985). Thanatophoric dysplasia: fetal manifestations and prenatal diagnosis. *Am J Med Genet* 22: 669–683.

Funato N, Ohtani K, Ohyama K, Kuroda T, Nakamura M (2001). Common regulation of growth arrest and differentiation of osteoblasts by helix–loop–helix factors. *Mol Cell Biol* 21: 7416–7428.

Galvin BD, Hart KC, Meyer AN, Webster MK, Donoghue DJ (1996). Constitutive receptor activation by Crouzon syndrome mutations in fibroblast growth factor receptor (FGFR)2 and FGFR2/Neu chimeras. *Proc Natl Acad Sci USA* 93: 7894–7899.

Gaudenz K, Roessler E, Vainikka S, Alitalo K, Muenke M (1998). Analysis of patients with craniosynostosis syndromes for a Pro246Arg mutation in FGFR4. *Mol Genet Metabol* 64: 76–79.

GenBank. Available at http: //www.ncbi.nkm.nih.gov/Genbank/index.html

Givol D, Yayon A (1992). Complexity of FGF receptors: genetic basis for structural diversity and functional specificity. *FASEB J* 6: 3362–3369.

Glaser RL, Jiang W, Boyadjiev SA, Tran AK, Zachary AA, Johnson D, Walsh S, Oldridge M, Wall SA, Wilkie AOM, Jabs EW (2000). Paternal origin of FGFR2 mutations in sporadic cases of Crouzon and Pfeiffer syndromes. *Am J Hum Genet* 66: 768–777.

Goldfarb M (2001). Signaling by fibroblast growth factors: the inside story. Available at http://www.stke.org/ogi/content/full/OC_sigtrans;2001

Goldfarb M, Bates B, Drucker B, Hardin J, Haub O (1991). Expression and possible functions of the FGF-5 gene. *Ann NY Acad Sci* 638: 38–52.

Golla A, Lichtner P, von Gernet S, Winterpacht A, Fairley J, Murken J, Schuffenhauer S (1996). Phenotypic expression of the fibroblast growth factor receptor 3 (FGFR3) mutation P250R in a large craniosynostosis family. *J Med Genet* 34: 683–684.

Gorry MC, Preston RA, White GJ, Zhang Y, Singhal VK, Losken HW, Parker MG, Nwokoro NA, Post JC, Ehrlich GD (1995). Crouzon syndrome: mutations in two spliceoforms of FGFR2 and a common point mutation shared with Jackson-Weiss syndrome. *Hum Mol Genet* 4: 1387–1390.

Green PJ, Walsh FS, Doherty P (1996). Promiscuity of fibroblast growth factor receptors. *Bioessays* 18: 639–646.

Grigelioniene G, Hagenas L, Eklof O, Neumeyer L, Haereid PE, Anvret M (1998). A novel missense mutation Ile538Val in the fibroblast growth factor receptor 3 in hypochondroplasia. *Hum Mutat* 11: 333.

Grigelioniene G, Eklof O, Aurencikas E, Ollars B, Hertel NT, Dumanski JP, Hagenas L (2000). The Asn540Lys mutation in FGR3 and phenotype in hypochondroplasia. *Acta Paediatr* 89: 1072–1076.

Gripp KW, McDonald-McGinn DM, Gaudenz K, Whitaker LA, Bartlett SP, Glat PM, Cassileth LB, Mayro R, Zackai EH, Muenke M (1998a). Identification of the first genetic cause for isolated unilateral coronal synostosis: a unique mutation in the fibroblast growth factor receptor 3 (FGFR3). *J Pediatr* 132: 714–716.

Gripp KW, Stolle CA, McDonald-McGinn DM, Markowitz RI, Bartlett SP, Whitaker LA, Katowitz JA, Muenke M, Zackai EH (1998b). Phenotype of the fibroblast growth factor receptor 2 Ser351Cys mutation: Pfeiffer syndrome type III. *Am J Med Genet* 78: 356–360.

Gripp KW, Zackai EH, Cohen MM Jr (1999). Not Antley-Bixler syndrome. *Am J Med Genet* 83: 65–66.

Guasch G, Mack GJ, Popovici C, Dastugue N, Birnbaum D, Rattner JB, Pebusque MJ (2000). FGFR1 is fused to the centrosome-associated protein CEP110 in the 8p12 stem cell myeloproliferative disorder with t(8;9)(p12;q33). *Blood* 95: 1788–1796.

Heike C, Seto M, Hing A, Paladin A, Cunningham M (2001). A century of Jackson-Weiss syndrome: further delineation of clinical and radiographic findings in "lost" descendants of the original JWS kindred. *Am J Med Genet* 100: 315–324.

Hollway GE, Phillips HA, Adès LC, Haan EA, Mulley JC (1995). Localization of craniosynostosis Adelaide type to 4p16. *Hum Molec Genet* 4: 681–683.

Houssaint E, Blanquet PR, Champion-Arnaud P, Gesnel MC, Torriglia A, Courtois Y, Breathnach R (1990). Related fibroblast growth factor receptor genes exist in the human genome. *Proc Natl Acad Sci* 87: 8180–8184.

Huggins MJ, Mernagh JR, Steele L, Smith JR, Nowaczyk MJM (1999a): Brief clinical report: prenatal sonographic diagnosis of hypochondroplasia in a high-risk fetus. *Am J Med Genet* 87: 226–229.

Huggins MJ, Smith JR, Chun K, Ray PN, Shah JK, Whelan DT (1999b). Achondroplasia–hypochondroplasia complex in a newborn infant. *Am J Med Genet* 84: 396–400.

HUGO Gene Nomenclature Database. Available at http://www.gene.ucl.ac.uk/nomenclature/

Ibrahimi OA, Eliseenkova AV, Plotnikov AN, Ornitz DM, Mohammadi M (2001). Structural basis for fibroblast growth factor receptor 2 activation in Apert syndrome. *Proc Natl Acad Sci USA* 98: 7182–7187.

Jabs EW (1995). Jackson-Weiss and Crouzon syndromes are allelic with mutations in fibroblast growth factor receptor 2. *Nat Genet* 9: 451.

Jabs EW, Li X, Scott AF, Meyers G, Chen W, Eccles M, Mao J, Carnas LR, Jackson CE, Jaye M (1994). Jackson-Weiss and Crouzon syndromes are allelic with mutations in fibroblast growth factor receptor 2. *Nat Genet* 8: 275–279.

Jackson CE, Weiss L, Reynolds WA, Forman TF, Peterson JA (1976). Craniosynostosis, midface hypoplasia, and foot abnormalities: an autosomal dominant phenotype in a large Amish kindred. *J Pediatr* 88: 963–968.

Jang J-H, Shin K-H, Park Y-J, Lee RJ, McKeehan WL, Park J-G (2000). Novel transcripts of *fibroblast growth factor receptor 3* reveal aberrant splicing and activation of cryptic splice sequences in colorectal cancer. *Cancer Res* 60: 4049–4052.

Jang J-H, Shin K-H, Park J-G (2001). Mutations in *fibroblast growth factor receptor 2* and *fibroblast growth factor receptor 3* genes associated with human gastric and colorectal cancers. *Cancer Res* 61: 3541–3543.

Jaye M, Schlessinger J, Dionne CA (1992). Fibroblast growth factor receptor tyrosine kinases: molecular analysis and signal transduction. *Biochim Biophys Acta* 1135: 185–199.

Johnson D, Wilkie AOM (2000). Pfeiffer syndrome is *not* caused by haploinsufficient mutations of *FGFR2*. *J Craniofac Genet Dev Biol* 20: 109–111.

Johnson D, Wall SA, Mann S, Wilkie AOM (2000). A novel mutation, Ala315Ser, in FGFR2: gene–environment interaction leading to craniosynostosis. *Eur J Hum Genet* 8: 571–577.

Johnson DE, Williams LT (1993). Structural and functional diversity in the FGF receptor multigene family. *Adv Cancer Res* 60: 1–41.

Jonsson KB, Zahradnik R, Larsson T, White KE, Sugimoto T, Imanishi Y, Yamamoto T, Hampson G, Koshiyama H, Ljuggren O, Oba K, Yang IM, Miyauchi A, Econs MJ, Lavigne J, Jüppner H (2003). Fibroblast growth factor 23 in oncogenic osteomalacia and X-linked hypophosphatemia. *N Engl J Med* 348: 1656–1661.

Kan S-h, Elanko N, Johnson D, Cornejo-Roldan L, Cook J, Reich EW, Tomkins S, Verloes A, Twigg SRF, Rannan-Eliya S, et al. (2002). Genomic screening of fibroblast growth factor receptor 2 reveals a wide spectrum of mutations in patients with syndromic craniosynostosis. *Am J Hum Genet* 70: 472–486.

Kelley RI, Kratz LE, Glaser RL, Netzloff ML, Wolf LM, Jabs EW (2002). Abnormal sterol metabolism in a patient with Antley-Bixler syndrome and ambiguous genitalia. *Am J Med Genet* 110: 95–102.

Kimura T, Suzuki H, Ohashi T, Asano K, Kiyota H, Eto Y (2001). The incidence of thanatophoric dysplasia mutations in *FGFR3* gene is higher in low-grade or superficial bladder carcinomas. *Cancer* 92: 2555–2561.

Kitoh H, Brodie SG, Kupke KG, Lachman RS, Wilcox WR (1998). Lys650Met substitution in the tyrosine kinase domain of the fibroblast growth factor receptor gene causes thantophoric dysplasia type 1. *Hum Mutat* 12: 362–363.

Kobrin MS, Yamanaka Y, Friess H, Lopez ME, Korc M (1993). Aberrant expression of type I fibroblast growth factor receptor in human pancreatic adenocarcinomas. *Cancer Res* 53: 4741–4744.

Köhl R, Antoine M, Olwin BB, Dickson C, Kiefer P (2000). Cysteine-rich fibroblast growth factor receptor alters secretion and intracellular routing of fibroblast growth factor 3. *J Biol Chem* 275: 15741–15748.

Kostrzewa M, Müller U (1998). Genomic structure and complete sequence of the human FGFR4 gene. *Mamm Genome* 9: 131–135.

Kouhara H, Hadari YR, Spivak-Kroizman T, Schilling J, Bar-Sagi D, Lax I, Schlessinger J (1997), A lipid-anchored Grb2-binding protein that links FGF-receptor activation to the Ras/MAPK signaling pathway. *Cell* 89: 693–702.

Krepelová A, Baxová A, Calda P, Plavka R, Kapras J (1998). FGFR2 gene mutation (Tyr375Cys) in a new case of Beare-Stevenson syndrome. *Am J Med Genet* 76: 362–364.

Kress W, Collmann H, Büsse M, Halliger-Keller B, Mueller CR (2000). Clustering of FGFR2 gene mutations in patients with Pfeiffer and Crouzon syndromes (FGFR2-associated craniosynostoses). *Cytogenet Cell Genet* 91: 134–137.

Kulkarni S, Reiter A, Smedley D, Goldman JM, Cross NC (1999). The genomic structure of ZNF198 and location of breakpoints in the t(8;13) myeloproliferative syndrome. *Genomics* 51: 118–121

Kwabi-Addo B, Ropiquet F, Giri D, Ittmann M (2001). Alternative splicing of fibroblast growth factor receptors in human prostate cancer. *Prostate* 46: 163–172.

Lajeunie E, Wei Ma H, Bonaventure J, Munnich A, Le Merrer M, Renier D (1995). *FGFR2* mutations in Pfeiffer syndrome. *Nat Genet* 9: 108.

Lajeunie E, Cameron R, El Ghouzzi V, de Parseval N, Journeau P, Gonzales M, Delezoide A-L, Bonaventure J, Le Merrer M, Renier D (1999a). Clinical variability in patients with Apert's syndrome. *J Neurosurg* 90: 443–447.

Lajeunie E, El Ghouzzi V, Le Merrer M, Munnich A, Bonaventure J, Renier D (1999b). Sex related expressivity of the phenotype in coronal craniosynostosis caused by the recurrent P250R *FGFR3* mutation. *J Med Genet* 36: 9–13.

Li C, Chen L, Iwata T, Kitagawa M, Fu X-Y, Deng C-X (1999). A Lys644Glu substitution in fibroblast growth factor receptor 3 (FGFR3) causes dwarfism in mice by activation of STATs and ink4 cell cycle inhibitors. *Hum Mol Genet* 8: 35–44.

Li X, Park W-J, Pyeritz RE, Jabs EW (1995). Effect on splicing of a silent FGFR2 mutation in Crouzon syndrome. *Nat Genet* 9: 232–233.

LocusLink. Available at http://ncbi.nlm.nih.gov/LocusLink/

Maerz WJ, Baselga J, Reuter VE, Mellado B, Myers ML, Bosl GJ, Spinella MJ, Dmitrovsky E (1998). FGF4 dissociates anti-tumorigenic from differentiation signals of retinoic acid in human embryonal carcinomas. *Oncogene* 17: 761–767.

Marshall CJ (1995). Specificity of receptor tyrosine kinase signaling: transient versus sustained extracellular signal-regulated kinase activation. *Cell* 80: 179–185.

Martin GR (1998). The roles of FGFs in the early development of vertebrate limbs. *Genes Dev* 12: 1571–1586.

Mason I (1994a). The ins and outs of fibroblast growth factors. *Cell* 78: 547–552.

Mason I (1994b). Do adhesion molecules signal via FGF receptors? *Curr Biol* 4: 1158–1161.

Meyers GA, Orlow SJ, Munro IR, Przylepa KA, Jabs EW (1995). Fibroblast growth factor receptor 3 (FGFR3) transmembrane mutation in Crouzon syndrome with acanthosis nigricans. *Nat Genet* 11: 462–464.

Meyers GA, Day D, Goldberg R, Daentl DL, Przylepa KA, Abrams LJ, Graham JM Jr, Feingold M, Moeschler JB, Rawnsley E, et al. (1996). FGFR2 exon IIIa and IIIc mutations in Crouzon, Jackson-Weiss, and Pfeiffer syndromes: evidence for missense changes, insertions, and a deletion due to alternative RNA splicing. *Am J Hum Genet* 58: 491–498.

Miki T, Bottaro DP, Fleming TP, Smith CL, Burgess WH, Chan AM-L, Aaronson SA (1992). Determination of ligand-binding specificity by alternative splicing: two distinct growth factor receptors encoded by a single gene. *Biochem* 89: 246–250.

Miyamoto M, Naruo K-I, Seko C, Matsumoto S, Kondo T, Kurokawa T (1993). Molecular cloning of a novel cytokine cDNA encoding the ninth member of the fibroblast growth factor family, which has a unique secretion property. *Mol Cell Biol* 13: 4251–4259.

Mohammadi M, Schlessinger J, Hubbard SR (1996). Structure of the FGF receptor tyrosine kinase domain reveals a novel autoinhibitory mechanism. *Cell* 86: 577–587.

Moloney DM, Slaney SF, Oldridge M, Wall SA, Sahlin P, Stenman G, Wilkie AOM (1996). Exclusive paternal origin of new mutations in Apert syndrome. *Nat Genet* 13: 48–53.

Moloney DM, Wall SA, Ashworth GJ, Oldridge M, Francomano CA, Muenke M, Wilkie AOM (1997). Prevalence of Pro250Arg mutation of fibroblast growth factor receptor 3 in coronal craniosynostosis. *Lancet* 349: 1059–1062.

Mortier G, Nuytinck L, Craen M, Renard J-P, Leroy JG, De Paepe A (2000). Clinical and radiographic features of a family with hypochondroplasia owing to a novel Asn540Ser mutation in the fibroblast growth factor receptor 3 gene. *J Med Genet* 37: 220–224.

Muenke M, Schell T, Hehr A, Robin NH, Losken HW, Schinzel A, Pulleyn LJ, Rutland P, Reardon W, Malcolm S, Winter RM (1994). A common mutation in the fibroblast growth factor receptor 1 gene in Pfeiffer syndrome. *Nat Genet* 8: 269–273.

Muenke M, Gripp KW, McDonald-McGinn DM, Gaudenz K, Whitaker LA, Bartlett SP, Markowitz RI, Robin NH, Nwokoro N, Mulvihill JJ, et al. (1997). A unique point mutation in the fibroblast growth factor receptor 3 (*FGFR3*) gene defines a new craniosynostosis syndrome. *Am J Hum Genet* 60: 555–564.

Muenke M, Francomano CA, Cohen MM Jr, Jabs EW (1998). Fibroblast growth factor receptor-related skeletal disorders. In: *Principles of Molecular Medicine*. Jameson JL (ed.) Humana Press, Totowa, N.J., pp. 1029–1038.

Mulvihill JJ (1995). Craniofacial syndromes: no such thing as a single gene disease. *Nat Genet* 9: 101–103.

Munro CS, Wilkie AOM (1998). Epidermal mosaicism producing localised acne: somatic mutation in FGFR2. *Lancet* 352: 704–705.

Naski MC, Ornitz DM (1998). FGF signaling in skeletal development. *Front Biosci* 3: 781–794.

Naski MC, Wang Q, Xu J, Ornitz DM (1996). Graded activation of fibroblast growth factor receptor 3 by mutations causing achondroplasia and thanatophoric dysplasia. *Nat Genet* 13: 233–237.

Neilson KM, Friesel RE (1996). Ligand-independent activation of fibroblast growth factor receptors by point mutations in the extracellular, transmembrane, and kinase domains. *J Biol Chem* 271: 25049–25057.

Nishizuka Y (1995). Protein kinase C and lipid signaling for sustained cellular responses. *FASEB J* 9: 484–492.

Okajima K, Robinson LK, Hart MA, Abuelo DN, Cowan LS, Hasega T, Maumenee IH, Jabs EW (1999). Ocular anterior chamber dysgenesis in craniosynostosis syndromes with a fibroblast growth factor receptor 2 mutation. *Am J Med Genet* 85: 160–170.

Oldridge M, Wilkie AOM, Slaney SF, Poole MD, Pulleyn LJ, Rutland P, Hockley AD, Wake MJC, Goldin JH, Winter RM, et al. (1995). Mutations in the third immunoglobulin domain of the fibroblast growth factor receptor-2 gene in Crouzon syndrome. *Hum Mol Genet* 4: 1077–1082.

Oldridge M, Lunt PW, Zackai EH, McDonald-McGinn DM, Muenke M, Moloney DM, Twigg SRF, Heath JK, Howard TD, Hoganson G, et al. (1997). Genotype–phenotype correlations for nucleotide substitutions in the IgII-IgIII linker of FGFR2. *Hum Mol Genet* 6: 137–143.

Oldridge M, Zackai EH, McDonald-McGinn DM, Iseki S, Morriss-Kay GM, Twigg SRF, Johnson D, Wall SA, Jiang W, Theda C, et al. (1999). *De novo Alu* element insertions in *FGFR2* identify a distinct pathological basis for Apert syndrome. *Am J Hum Genet* 64: 446–461.

Ollendorff V, Guasch G, Isnardon D, Galindo R, Birnbaum D, Pebusque MJ (1999). Characterization of FIM-FGFR1, the fusion product of the myeloproliferative disorder-associated t(8;13) translocation. *J Biol Chem* 274: 26922–26930.

Ornitz DM, Itoh N (2001). Protein family review: fibroblast growth factors. *Genome Biol* 2: 3005.1–3005.12.

Ornitz DM, Xu J, Colvin JS, McEwen DG, MacArthur CA, Coulier F, Gao G, Goldfarb M (1996). Receptor specificity of the fibroblast growth factor family. *J Biol Chem* 271: 15292–15297.

Park W-J, Bellus GA, Jabs EW (1995a). Mutations in fibroblast growth factor receptors: phenotypic consequences during eukaryotic development. *Am J Hum Genet* 57: 748–754.

Park W-J, Meyers GA, Li X, Theda C, Day D, Orlow SJ, Jones MC, Jabs EW (1995b). Novel FGFR2 mutations in Crouzon and Jackson-Weiss syndromes show allelic heterogeneity and phenotypic variability. *Hum Mol Genet* 4: 1229–1233.

Park W-J, Theda C, Maestri NE, Meyers GA, Fryburg JS, Dufresne C, Cohen MM Jr, Jabs EW (1995c). Analysis of phenotypic features and *FGFR2* mutations in Apert syndrome. *Am J Hum Genet* 57: 321–328.

Passos-Bueno MR, Sertié AL, Zatz M, Richieri-Costa A (1997). Pfeiffer mutation in an Apert patient: how wide is the spectrum of variability due to mutations in the FGFR2 gene? *Am J Med Genet* 71: 243–245.

Passos-Bueno MR, Sertié AL, Richieri-Costa A, Alonso LG, Zatz M, Alonso N, Brunoni D, Ribeiro SFM (1998a). Description of a new mutation and characterization of *FGFR1*, *FGFR2*, and *FGFR3* mutations among Brazilian patients with syndromic craniosynostoses. *Am J Med Genet* 78: 237–241.

Passos-Bueno MR, Richieri-Costa A, Sertié AL, Kneppers A (1998b). Presence of the Apert canonical S252W FGFR2 mutation in a patient without severe syndactyly. *J Med Genet* 35: 677–679.

Pauli RM (2001). Achondroplasia. In: *Management of Genetic Syndromes*. Cassidy SB, Allanson JE (eds.) Wiley, New York, pp. 9–32.

Pawson T (1995). Protein modules and signalling networks. *Nature* 373: 573–580.

Pawson T, Gish GD (1992). SH2 and SH3 domains: from structure to function. *Cell* 71: 359–362.

Paznekas WA, Cunningham ML, Howard TD, Korf BR, Lipson MH, Grix AW, Feingold M, Goldberg R, Borochowitz Z, Aleck K, et al. (1998). Genetic heterogeneity of Saethre-Chotzen syndrome, due to *TWIST* and *FGFR* mutations. *Am J Hum Genet* 62: 1370–1380.

Pellegrini L, Burke DF, von Delft F, Mulloy B, Blundell TL (2000). Crystal structure of fibroblast growth factor receptor ectodomain bound to ligand and heparin. *Nature* 407: 1029–1034.

Peng H, Moffett J, Myers J, Fang X, Stachowiak EK, Maher P, Kratz E, Hines J, Fluharty SJ, Mizukoshi E, et al. (2001). Novel nuclear signaling pathway mediates activation of fibroblast growth factor-2 gene by type 1 and type 2 angiotensin II receptors. *Mol Biol Cell* 12: 449–462.

Popovici C, Adelaide J, Ollendorff V, Chaffanet M, Guasch G, Jacrot M, Leroux D (1998). Fibroblast growth factor receptor 1 is fused to FIM in stem-cell myeloproliferative disorder with t(8;13). *Proc Natl Acad Sci USA* 95: 5712–5717.

Popovici C, Zhang B, Gregoire MJ, Jonveaux P, Lafage-Pochitaloff M, Birnbaum D, Pebusque MJ (1999). The t(6;8)(q27;p11) translocation in a stem cell myeloproliferative disorder fuses a novel gene, FOP, to fibroblast growth factor receptor 1. *Blood* 93: 1381–1389.

Prinos P, Kilpatrick MW, Tsipouras P (1995). A novel G346E *FGFR3* mutation in achondroplasia. *Pediatr Res* 37: pt.2: 151 A.

Prinster C, Carrera P, Delmaschio M, Weber G, Maghnie M, Vigone MC, Mora S, Tonini G, Rigon F, Beluffi G, et al. (1998). Comparison of clinical-radiological and molecular findings in hypochondroplasia. *Am J Med Genet* 75: 109–112.

Przylepa KA, Paznekas W, Zhang M, Golabi M, Bias W, Bamshad MJ, Carey JC, Hall BD, Stevenson R, Orlow SJ, et al. (1996). Fibroblast growth factor receptor 2 mutations in Beare-Stevenson cutis gyrata syndrome. *Nat Genet* 13: 492–494.

Pulleyn LJ, Reardon W, Wilkes D, Rutland P, Jones BM, Hayward R, Hall CM, Brueton L, Chun N, Lammer E, et al. (1996). Spectrum of craniosynostosis phenotypes associated with novel mutations at the fibroblast growth factor receptor 2 locus. *Eur J Hum Genet* 4: 283–291.

Ramaswami U, Rumsby G, Hindmarsh PC, Brook CG (1998). Genotype and phenotype in hypochondroplasia. *J Pediatr* 133: 99–102.

Reardon W, Winter RM, Rutland P, Pulleyn LJ, Jones BM, Malcolm S (1994). Mutations in the fibroblast growth factor receptor 2 gene cause Crouzon syndrome. *Nat Genet* 8: 98–103.

Reardon W, Wilkes D, Rutland P, Pulleyn LJ, Malcolm S, Dean JCS, Evans RD, Jones BM, Hayward R, Hall CM, et al. (1997). Craniosynostosis associated with *FGFR3* Pro250Arg mutation results in a range of clinical presentations including unisutural sporadic craniosynostosis. *J Med Genet* 34: 632–636.

Reardon W, Smith A, Honour JW, Hindmarsh P, Das D, Rumsby G, Nelson I, Malcolm S, Adès L, Sillence D, et al. (2000). Evidence for digenic inheritance in some cases of Antley-Bixler syndrome? *J Med Genet* 37: 26–32.

Reilly JF, Maher PA. (2001). Importin beta-mediated nuclear import of fibroblast growth factor receptor: role in cell proliferation. *J Cell Biol* 152: 1307–1312.

Robertson SC, Meyer AN, Hart KC, Galvin BD, Webster MK, Donoghue DJ (1998). Activating mutations in the extracellular domain of the fibroblast growth factor receptor 2 function by disruption of the disulfide bond in the third immunoglobulin-like domain. *Proc Natl Acad Sci USA* 95: 4567–4572.

Robin NH, Scott JA, Arnold JE, Goldstein JA, Shilling BB, Marion RW, Cohen MM Jr (1998a). Favorable prognosis for children with Pfeiffer syndrome types 2 and 3: implications for classification. *Am J Med Genet* 75: 240–244.

Robin NH, Scott JA, Cohen AR, Goldstein JA (1998b). Nonpenetrance in FGFR3-associated coronal synostosis syndrome. *Am J Med Genet* 80: 296–297.

Roscioli T, Flanagan S, Kumar P, Masel J, Gattas M, Hyland VJ, Glass IA (2000). Clinical findings in a patient with *FGFR1* P252R mutation and comparison with the literature. *Am J Med Genet* 93: 22–28.

Roscioli T, Flanagan S, Mortimore RJ, Kumar P, Weedon D, Masel J, Lewandowski R, Hyland V, Glass IA (2001). Premature calvarial synostosis and epidermal hyperplasia (Beare-Stevenson syndrome-like anomalies) resulting from a P250R missense mutation in the gene encoding fibroblast growth factor receptor 3. *Am J Med Genet* 101: 187–194.

Rousseau F, Saugier P, Le Merrer M, Munnich A, Delezoide A-L, Maroteaux P, Bonaventure J, Narcy F, Sanak M (1995). Stop codon FGFR3 mutations in thanatophoric dwarfism type 1. *Nat Genet* 10: 11–12.

Rousseau F, Bonaventure J, Legeai-Mallet L, Schmidt H, Weissenbach J, Maroteaux P, Munnich A, Le Merrer F (1996a). Clinical and genetic heterogeneity of hypochondroplasia. *J Med Genet* 33: 749–752.

Rousseau F, El Ghouzzi V, Delezoide AL, Legeai-Mallet L, Le Merrer M, Munnich A, Bonaventure J (1996b). Missense FGFR3 mutations create cysteine residues in thanatophoric dwarfism type I (TD1). *Hum Mol Genet* 5: 509–512.

Rutland P, Pulleyn LJ, Reardon W, Baraitser M, Hayward R, Jones B, Malcolm S, Winter RM, Oldridge M, Slaney SF, et al. (1995). Identical mutations in the *FGFR2* gene cause both Pfeiffer and Crouzon syndrome phenotypes. *Nat Genet* 9: 173–176.

Schaefer F, Anderson C, Can B, Say B (1998). Novel mutation in the *FGFR2* gene at the same codon as the Crouzon syndrome mutations in a severe Pfeiffer syndrome type 2 case. *Am J Med Genet* 75: 252–255.

Schell U, Hehr A, Feldman GJ, Robin NH, Zackai EH, de Die-Smulders C, Viskochil DH, Stewart JM, Wolff G, Ohashi H, et al. (1995). Mutations in FGFR1 and FGFR2 cause familial and sporadic Pfeiffer syndrome. *Hum Mol Genet* 4: 323–328.

Schweitzer DN, Graham JM Jr, Lachman RS, Jabs EW, Okajima K, Przylepa KA, Shanske A, Chen K, Neidich JA, Wilcox WR (2001). Subtle radiographic findings of achondroplasia in patients with Crouzon syndrome with acanthosis nigricans due to an Ala391Glu substitution in FGFR3. *Am J Med Genet* 98: 75–91.

Shah RNH, Ibbitt JC, Alitalo K, Hurst HC (2002). FGFR4 overexpression in pancreatic cancer is mediated by an intronic enhancer activated by HNF1α. *Oncogene* 21: 8251–8261.

Shiang R, Thompson LM, Zhu Y-Z, Church DM, Fielder TJ, Bocian M, Winokur ST, Wasmuth JJ (1994). Mutations in the transmembrane domain of FGFR3 cause the most common genetic form of dwarfism, achondroplasia. *Cell* 78: 335–342.

Shiller JG (1959). Craniofacial dysostosis of Crouzon: a case report and pedigree with emphasis on heredity. *Pediatrics* 23: 107–112.

Shimada T, Mizutani S, Muto T, Yoneya T, Hino R, Takeda S, Takeuchi Y, Fujita T, Fukumoto S, Yamashita T (2001). Cloning and characterization of FGF23 as a causative factor of tumor-induced osteomalacia. *Proc Natl Acad Sci USA* 98: 6500–6505.

Shotelersuk V, Ittiwut C, Srivuthana S, Mahatumarat C, Lerdlum S, Wacharasindhu S (2002). Distinct craniofacial-skeletal-dermatological dysplasia in a patient with W290C mutation in *FGFR2*. *Am J Med Genet* 113: 4–8.

Sibley K, Stern P, Knowles MA (2001). Frequency of fibroblast growth factor receptor 3 mutations in sporadic tumours. *Oncogene* 20: 4416–4418.

Slaney SF, Oldridge M, Hurst JA, Morriss-Kay GM, Hall CM, Poole MD, Wilkie AOM (1996). Differential effects of *FGFR2* mutations on syndactyly and cleft palate in Apert syndrome. *Am J Hum Genet* 58: 923–932.

Smallwood PM, Muñoz-Sanjuan I, Tong P, Macke JP, Hendry SHC, Gilbert DJ, Copeland NG, Jenkins NA, Nathans J (1996). Fibroblast growth factor (FGF) homologous factors: new members of the FGF family implicated in nervous system development. *Proc Natl Acad Sci USA* 93: 9850–9857.

Smedley D, Hamoudi R, Clark J, Warren W, Abdul-Rauf M, Somers G, Venter D (1998). The t(8;13)(p11;q11–12) rearrangement associated with an atypical myeloproliferative disorder fuses the fibroblast growth factor receptor 1 gene to a novel gene RAMP. *Hum Mol Genet* 74: 637–642.

Sohal J, Chase A, Mould S, Corcoran M, Oscier D, Iqbal S, Parker S (2001). Identification of four new translocations involving *FGFR1* in myeloid disorders. *Genes Chromosomes Cancer* 32: 155–163.

Spivak-Kroizman, Lemmon MA, Dikic I, Ladbury JE, Pinchasi D, Huang J, Jaye M (1994). Heparin-induced oligomerization of FGF molecule is responsible for FGF receptor dimerization activation and cell proliferation. *Cell* 79: 1015–1024.

Steinberger D, Reinhartz T, Unsöld R, Müller U (1996). FGFR2 mutation in clinically nonclassifiable autosomal dominant craniosynostosis with pronounced phenotypic variation. *Am J Med Genet* 66: 81–86.

Stoilov I, Kilpatrick MW, Tsipouras P, Costa T (1995). Possible genetic heterogeneity in hypochondroplasia. *J Med Genet* 32: 492–493.

Strewler GJ (2001). FGF23, hypophosphatemia, and rickets: has phosphorylation been found? *Proc Natl Acad Sci USA* 98: 5945–5946.

Superti-Furga A, Eich G, Bucher HU, Wisser J, Giedion A, Gitzelmann R, Steinmann B (1995). A glycine 375-to-cysteine substitution in the transmembrane domain of the fibroblast growth factor receptor-3 in a newborn with achondroplasia. *Eur J Pediatr* 154:215.

Szabo JK, Wilkin DJ, Cameron R, Henderson S, Bellus G, Kaitila I, Loughlin J, Munnich A, Sykes B, Bonaventure J, Francomano CA. (1997). The achondroplasia mutation occurs exclusively on the paternally derived fibroblast growth factor receptor 3 (*FGFR3*) allele. *Am J Hum Genet* 60 (Suppl): Abstract No. 2040.

Tanaka A, Miyamoto K, Minamino N, Takeda M, Sato B, Matsuo H, Matsumoto K (1992). Cloning and characterization of an androgen-induced growth factor essential for the androgen-dependent growth of mouse mammary carcinoma cells. *Proc Natl Acad Sci USA* 89: 8928–8932.

Tartaglia M, Valeri S, Velardi F, Di Rocco C, Battaglia PA (1997). Trp290Cys mutation in exon IIIa of the fibroblast growth factor receptor 2 (*FGFR2*) gene is associated with Pfeiffer syndrome. *Hum Genet* 99: 602–606.

Tavormina PL, Rimoin DL, Cohn DH, Zhu Y-Z, Shiang R, Wasmuth JJ (1995a). Another mutation that results in the substitution of an unpaired cysteine residue in the extracellular domain of FGFR3 in thanatophoric dysplasia type I. *Hum Mol Genet* 4: 2175–2177.

Tavormina PL, Shiang R, Thompson LM, Zhu Y-Z, Wilkin DJ, Lachman RS, Wilcox WR, Rimoin DL, Cohn DH, Wasmuth JJ (1995b). Thanatophoric dysplasia (types I and II) caused by distinct mutations in fibroblast growth factor receptor 3. *Nat Genet* 9: 321–328.

Tavormina PL, Bellus GA, Webster MK, Bamshad MJ, Fraley AE, McIntosh I, Szabo J, Jiang W, Jabs EW, Wilcox WR, et al. (1999). A novel skeletal dysplasia with developmental delay and acanthosis nigricans is caused by a Lys650Met mutation in the fibroblast growth factor receptor 3 gene. *Am J Hum Genet* 64: 722–731.

Teebi AS, Kennedy S, Chun K, Ray PN (2002). Severe and mild phenotypes in Pfeiffer syndrome with splice acceptor mutations in exon IIIc of *FGFR2*. *Am J Med Genet* 107: 43–47.

Tsai F-J, Hwu W-L, Lin S-P, Chang J-G, Wang T-R, Tsai C-H (1998). Mutation in brief: two common mutations 934C to G and 937C to G of *fibroblast growth factor receptor 2 (FGFR2)* gene in Chinese patients with Apert syndrome. *Hum Mutat Suppl* 1: S18–S19.

Tsai F-J, Wu J-Y, Yang C-F, Tsai C-H (2001). Further evidence that fibroblast growth factor receptor 2 mutations cause Antley-Bixler syndrome. *Acta Paediatr* 90: 595–597.

Tsukuno M, Suzuki H, Eto T (1999). Pfeiffer syndrome caused by haploinsufficient mutation of *FGFR2*. *J Craniofac Genet Dev Biol* 19: 183–188.

Twigg SRF, Burns HD, Oldridge M, Heath JK, Wilkie AOM (1998). Conserved use of a non-canonical 5′ splice site (*IGA*) in alternative splicing by fibroblast growth factor-receptors 1, 2 and 3. *Hum Mol Genet* 7: 685–691.

Ullrich A, Schlessinger J (1990). Signal transduction by receptors with tyrosine kinase activity. *Cell* 61: 203–212.

van Rhijn BW, Lurkin I, Radvanyi F, Kirkels WJ, van der Kwast TH, Zwarthoff EC (2001). The fibroblast growth factor receptor 3 (*FGFR3*) mutation is a strong indicator of superficial bladder cancer with low recurrence rate. *Cancer Res* 61: 1265–1268.

van Swieten JC, Brusse E, de Graaf BM, Krieger E, van de Graaf R, de Koning I, Maat-Kievit A, Leegwater P, Dooijes D, Oostra BA, Heutink P (2003). A mutation in the fibroblast growth factor 14 gene is associated with autosomal dominant cerebellar ataxia. *Am J Hum Genet* 72: 191–199.

von Gernet S, Golla A, Ehrenfels Y, Schuffenhauer S, Fairley JD (2000). Genotype–phenotype analysis in Apert syndrome suggests opposite effects of the two recurrent mutations on syndactyly and outcome of craniofacial surgery. *Clin Genet* 57: 137–139.

Weber G, Prinster C, Meneghel M, Russo F, Mora S, Puzzovio M, Del Maschio M, Chiumello G (1996). Human growth hormone treatment in prepubertal children with achondroplasia. *Am J Med Genet* 61: 396–400.

Webster MK, Donoghue DJ (1996). Constitutive activation of fibroblast growth factor receptor 3 by the transmembrane domain point mutation found in achondroplasia. *EMBO J* 15: 520–527.

Webster MK, Donoghue DJ (1997). FGFR activation in skeletal disorders: too much of a good thing. *Trends Genet* 13: 178–182.

Webster MK, d'Avis PY, Robertson SC, Donoghue DJ (1996). Profound ligand-independent kinase activation of fibroblast growth factor receptor 3 by the activation loop mutation responsible for a lethal skeletal dysplasia, thanatophoric dysplasia type II. *Mol Cell Biol* 16: 4081–4087.

White KE, Jonsson KB, Carn G, Hampson G, Spector TD, Mannstadt M, Lorenz-Depiereux B, Miyauchi A, Yang IM, Ljunggren O, et al. (2001). The autosomal dominant hypophosphatemic rickets (ADHR) gene is a secreted polypeptide overexpressed by tumors that cause phosphate wasting. *J Clin Endocr Metab* 86: 497–500.

Wiedemann M, Trueb B (2000). Characterization of a novel protein (FGFRL1) from human cartilage related to FGF receptors. *Genomics* 69: 275–279.

Wiedlocha A, Falnes PO, Madshus IH, Sandvig, K, Olsnes S (1994). Dual mode of signal transduction by externally added acidic fibroblast growth factor. *Cell* 76: 1039–1051.

Wiedlocha A, Falnes PO, Rapak A, Muñoz R, Klingenberg O, Olsnes S (1996). Stimulation of proliferation of a human osteosarcoma cell line by exogenous acidic fibroblast growth factor requires both activation of receptor tyrosine kinase and growth factor internalization. *Mol Biol Cell* 12: 449–462.

Wilcox WR, Tavormina PL, Krakow D, Kitoh H, Lachman RS, Wasmuth JJ, Thompson LM, Rimoin DL (1998). Molecular, radiologic, and histopathologic correlations in thanatophoric dysplasia. *Am J Med Genet* 78: 274–281.

Wilkes D, Rutland P, Pulleyn LJ, Reardon W, Moss C, Ellis JP, Winter RM, Malcolm S (1996). A recurrent mutation, ala391glu, in the transmembrane region of FGFR3 causes Crouzon syndrome and acanthosis nigricans. *J Med Genet* 33: 744–748.

Wilkie AOM, Slaney SF, Oldridge M, Poole MD, Ashworth GJ, Hockley AD, Hayward RD, David DJ, Pulleyn LJ, Rutland P, et al. (1995a). Apert syndrome results from localized mutations of *FGFR2* and is allelic with Crouzon syndrome. *Nat Genet* 9: 165–172.

Wilkie AOM, Morriss-Kay GM, Jones EY, Heath JK (1995b). Functions of fibroblast growth factors and their receptors. *Curr Biol* 5: 500–507.

Wilkie AOM, Wall SA (1996). Craniosynostosis: novel insights into pathogenesis and treatment. *Curr Opin Neurol* 9: 146–152.

Wilkie AOM, Patey SJ, Kan S-h, van den Ouweland AMW, Hamel BCJ (2002). FGFs, their receptors, and human limb malformations: clinical and molecular correlations. *Am J Med Genet* 112: 266–278.

Wilkie AOM (2002). Abnormal spliceform expression associated with splice acceptor mutations in exon IIIc of FGFR2. *Am J Med Genet* 111: 105.

Wilkin DJ, Szabo JK, Cameron R, Henderson S, Bellus GA, Mack ML, Kaitila I, Loughlin J, Munnich A, Sykes B, et al. (1998). Mutations in fibroblast growth-factor receptor 3 in sporadic cases of achondroplasia occur exclusively on the paternally derived chromosome. *Am J Hum Genet* 63: 711–716.

Williams EJ, Furness J, Walsh FS, Doherty P (1994). Activation of the FGF receptor underlies neurite outgrowth stimulated by L1, N-CAM, and N-Cadherin. *Neuron* 13: 583–594.

Winterpacht A, Hilbert K, Stelzer C, Schweikardt T, Decker H, Spranger J, Zabel B (2000). A novel mutation in *FGFR-3* disrupts a putative *N*-glycosylation site and results in hypochondroplasia. *Physiol Genomics* 2: 9–12.

Wu B, Connolly D, Ngelangel C, Bosch FX, Muñoz N, Cho KR (2000). Somatic mutations of fibroblast growth factor receptor 3 (FGFR3) are uncommon in carcinomas of the uterine cervix. *Oncogene* 19: 5543–5546.

Xiao S, Nalabolu SR, Aster JC, Ma J, Abruzzo L, Jaffe ES, Stone R, Weissman SM, Hudson TJ, Fletcher JA (1998). *FGFR1* is fused with a novel zinc-finger gene, *ZNF198*, in the t(8;13) leukaemia/lymphoma syndrome. *Nat Genet* 18: 84–87.

Xu J, Nakahara M, Crabb JW, Shi E, Matuo Y, Fraser M, Kan M, Hou J, McKeehan WL (1992). Expression and immunochemical analysis of rat and human fibroblast growth factor receptor (flg) isoforms. *J Biol Chem* 267: 17792–17803.

Yamaguchi F, Saya H, Bruner JM, Morrison RS (1994). Differential expression of two fibroblast growth factor–receptor genes is associated with malignant progression in human astrocytomas. *Proc Natl Acad Sci USA* 91: 484–488.

Yamashita T, Yoshioka M, Itoh N (2000). Identification of a novel fibroblast growth factor, FGF-23, preferentially expressed in the ventrolateral thalamic nucleus of the brain. *Biochem Biophys Res Commun* 277: 494–498.

Yasoda A, Ogawa Y, Suda M, Tamura N, Mori K, Sakuma Y, Chusho H, Shiota K, Tanaka K, Nakao K (1998). Natriuretic peptide regulation of endochondral ossification. *J Biol Chem* 273: 11695–11700.

Yasoda A, Komatsu Y, Chusho H, Miyazawa T, Miura M, Ozasa A, Kurihara T, Rogi T, Tanaka S, Suda M, et al. (2002). Targeted overexpression of C-type natriuretic peptide in chondrocytes corrects the dwarfism in achondroplasia, caused by the constitutive active mutation of FGF receptor 3. *Nat Med* (in press).

Yoshida T, Sakamoto H, Miyagawa K, Sugimura T, Terada M (1991). Characterization of the *hst-1* gene and its product. *Ann NY Acad Sci* 638: 27–37.

Yu K, Ornitz DM. (2001). Uncoupling fibroblast growth factor receptor 2 ligand binding specificity leads to Apert syndrome-like phenotypes. *Proc Natl Acad Sci USA* 98: 3641–3643.

Yu K, Herr AB, Waksman G, Ornitz DM (2000). Loss of fibroblast growth factor receptor 2 ligand-binding specificity in Apert syndrome. *Proc Natl Acad Sci USA* 97: 14536–14541.

Zackai EH, Gripp KW, Stolle CA (2000). Craniosynostosis: molecular testing—a necessity for counseling. *Am J Med Genet* 92: 157.

Zhou Z, Zuber ME, Burrus LW, Olwin BB (1997). Identification and characterization of a fibroblast growth factor (FGF) binding domain in the cysteine-rich FGF receptor. *J Biol Chem* 372: 5167–5174.

34 | *TWIST* and the Saethre-Chotzen Syndrome

ETHYLIN WANG JABS

Saethre-Chotzen syndrome (OMIM 101400) is dominantly inherited with high penetrance and variable expressivity. The incidence is approximately 1/25,000 to 1/65,000. The most frequently observed features are craniosynostosis (primarily of the coronal sutures resulting in brachycephaly), low frontal hairline, facial asymmetry, ptosis of the eyelids, prominent helical crus, syndactyly, and broad great toe. This craniosynostosis syndrome is caused by mutations in the basic helix-loop-helix (bHLH) transcription factor TWIST (OMIM 601622). At least 73 different mutations, including missense, nonsense, small insertions, deletions leading to frameshifts, and duplications, have been identified in patients. These mutations lead to loss of the ability of the HLH domain to dimerize or of the basic region to bind to its target(s). Haploinsufficiency of *TWIST* due to chromosomal rearrangements or deletions involving the 7p21-22 region is found in Saethre-Chotzen patients who also have mental retardation. Twist heterozygous null mice with craniofacial and limb abnormalities that resemble Saethre-Chotzen syndrome further support loss of function as the mechanism by which mutant TWIST yields the Saethre-Chotzen phenotype. Previously, patients with Saethre-Chotzen-like features and duplication of the great toe or radial ray hypoplasia were clinically diagnosed as having separate entities, Robinow-Sorauf or Baller-Gerold syndrome, respectively. These patients also have TWIST mutations and are now thought to represent variability in the expression of Saethre-Chotzen syndrome. TWIST normally has an inhibitory role in osteoblast and myocyte differentiation, and craniosynostosis in Saethre-Chotzen is secondary to increased cell proliferation and maturation. Modifiers of TWIST mutations include components of developmental pathways especially those involved in osteoblast differentiation, and are likely to include the fibroblast growth factor receptors (FGFRs) and the homoeobox domain–containing transcription factor MSX2.

LOCUS AND DEVELOPMENTAL PATHWAY

The human *TWIST* gene codes for a transcription factor belonging to the bHLH family of proteins, the prototypes being E12 and E47 (Murre et al., 1989; Jan and Jan, 1993). The gene maps to chromosome 7p21 and produces a transcript with a single coding region in the first exon and a nontranslated second exon (Howard et al., 1997; Wang et al., 1997). The TWIST protein contains 202 amino acids with a molecular weight of 20.96 kDa. The protein has a basic DNA-binding region, followed by a region of dimerization composed of two amphipathic α helices separated by an intervening loop domain (Fig. 34–1). The HLH region is necessary and sufficient for protein dimerization, and dimerization is needed prior to DNA binding. The basic amino acid–rich region is required for DNA binding. Several in vitro and in vivo studies have shown that the basic region of homo- or heterodimers of twist binds preferentially to E-box sequences 5′CATATG3′ (Castanon et al., 2001).

The amino acid residues of the bHLH region have at least 68% identity, and the loop region alone is 100% identical among *Drosophila*, *Xenopus*, mouse, and human. Nuclear localization sequences are located within the HLH region and at other positions. The twist-specific WR motif, ERLSYAFSVWRMEG, located 20–55 amino acids beyond the second helix, is also highly conserved among vertebrates (Spring et al., 2000). In *Drosophila*, the N-terminal region interacts directly with the basal transcriptional machinery and other transcriptional regulators such as dorsal, a member of the rel family of transcription factors (Shirokawa and Courey, 1997; Pham et al., 1999). These two proteins work synergistically to regulate downstream targets such as snail, a zinc-finger protein that is crucial for gastrulation and maintenance of twist expression. Direct binding of mouse Twist between amino acids 30 and 60 (equivalent to human amino acids 30 and 63) occurs at two independent domains of the histone acetyltransferases P300 and p300/CBP-associated factor, whose epigenetic effect can alter transcriptional activity (Hamamori et al., 1999). The C-terminal domain of mouse Twist is necessary for repression of Mef2 myogenic activity in cell culture (Spicer et al., 1996).

The mouse and human *TWIST* genes have 71% nucleotide sequence identity in the promoter region from the cap site to approximately 300 bp upstream. When the putative human promoter sequence upstream of the transcription-initiation site (up to −824) is screened for DNA consensus sequence motifs, binding sites for many transcription factors are found. Of interest are potential binding sites for nuclear factor κB (NF-κB) (GGGRHTYYHC at position −89 to −99) and engrailed (HCWATHAAA at position −112 to −104). These sites are 100% conserved in the corresponding region of the mouse *Twist* gene. Other consensus sequences, such as those that bind AP-2, Sp1, RB, and ATF cAMP response element–binding protein (CREB), are present in the 5′ regulatory region of the human *TWIST* gene. Thus, twist uses several mechanisms to implement its function. Twist N terminus, C terminus, and other regions interacting with other proteins and the HLH region allows for different homodimer and heterodimer combinations that can alter binding activity, target preference site, and biologic activities.

Human *TWIST* is expressed as a 1.6 kb mRNA in placenta, which is largely fetal in origin and mostly derived from mesoderm (Wang et al., 1997). It is also expressed in fetal lung-derived fibroblasts, peritoneal mesothelial cells, and endometrial fibroblasts (the latter represent mesodermal cells derived from young adults). It is less expressed in adult heart, skeletal muscle, kidney, pancreas, and fibroblasts. Expression has not been observed in brain, fetal astrocytes, retinal pigmented epithelial, mammary epithelial cells that are ectodermal in origin, and lung or liver, which are primarily derived from the endoderm. It is also not expressed in T lymphocytes, whose primary cells are derived from mesodermal tissue. These results indicate that in human fetuses and adults *TWIST* is expressed preferentially in mesodermally derived tissues but only in a subset of mesodermal tissues, as has been documented in *Xenopus* (Hopwood et al., 1989) and mouse (Fuchtbauer, 1995; Stoetzl et al., 1995).

Several proteins have been proposed to interact with and be targets of TWIST. Members of the bHLH family of proteins are potential TWIST dimerization partners, such as E proteins, MYOD (muscle developmental protein), MYC (growth and regulation), DERMO1 (osteoblast development), and ID (general inhibitor of HLH proteins because it lacks a basic region). The basic domain of the myogenic factor MyoD is reported to physically interact with the basic domain of mouse Twist (Hamamori et al., 1997). The association between these basic regions is implicated as one mechanism by which Twist can regulate myogenesis in vertebrates.

Msh2 and *DFR1* have been suggested as targets because mesodermal expression of these genes is disrupted in *twist* mutant embryos of *Drosophila* (Bodmer et al., 1990; Shishido et al., 1993). The presence

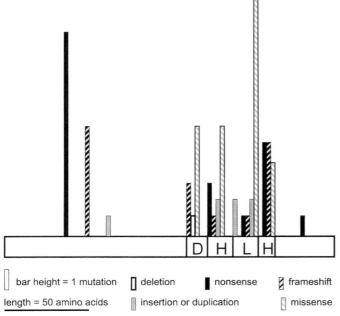

Figure 34–1. Diagram of TWIST mutations found in Saethre-Chotzen syndrome. The total number of different intragenic mutations in each domain (5′ DNA binding; D, DNA binding; H, helix 1; L, loop; H, helix 2; 3′ helix-loop-helix) is represented by the bar height.

of binding sites of Msx and HLH proteins at the rat *Osteocalcin* promoter suggests potential interactions (Heinrichs et al., 1993; Tamura and Noda, 1994). *Cbfa1*/Runx2 transcription factor also binds to the *Osteocalcin* promoter, encodes an osteoblast-specific transcription factor, and regulates osteoblastic differentiation (Ducy and Karsenty, 1995). Human homologues of these four genes are also implicated in a common signaling pathway(s) for calvarial development. Loss-of-function mutations of *TWIST* and gain-of-function mutations of *FGFR1*, *FGFR2*, *FGFR3*, and *MSX2*, a homeobox domain–containing transcription factor, have been described in other craniosynostosis syndromes (see Chapters 33 and 52). Loss of function of CBFA1 has been described in a condition with delayed closure of the sutures, cleidocranial dysostosis (see Chapter 29) (Mundlos et al., 1997). Snail, a member of the snail family of zinc-finger proteins that also includes slug, and twist are thought to be in the same genetic pathway, with

the former downstream of the latter because *snail* transcription is absent in *Drosophila* twist mutants (Simpson, 1983).

CLINICAL FEATURES

Saethre-Chotzen syndrome (acrocephalosyndactyly type III) is one of the more commonly inherited craniosynostosis syndromes in humans (Saethre, 1931; Chotzen, 1932). It is characterized by craniosynostosis, facial dysmorphisms, and hand and foot abnormalities (Fig. 34–2, Table 34–1) (Cohen, 2000; Gorlin et al., 2001). Coronal synostosis resulting in brachycephaly is the most frequent cranial abnormality found in this condition. Surgical intervention to allow brain growth and to prevent neurologic sequelae is required in moderate to severe cases. The most common facial features are asymmetry, hypertelorism, and maxillary hypoplasia. Other features include a high forehead, low frontal hairline, late closing fontanelle, strabismus, ptosis, lacrimal duct stenosis, prominent ear crus, lowest posteriorly rotated small ears, hearing loss, and deviated nasal septum. Oral manifestations include high arch or cleft palate, class III malocclusion, and enamel hypoplasia. The limb anomalies consist of brachydactyly, cutaneous syndactyly (especially of the second and third fingers and toes), hallux valgus, short stature, radioulnar synostosis, and vertebral fusion. Mild to moderate mental retardation has been noted in some cases. The more common craniofacial and limb anomalies in humans are reminiscent of those observed in *Twist* heterozygote knockout mice (Fig. 34–3; see below, Animal Models). The inter- and intrafamilial variability is significant, with some patients having fusion of other sutures or no apparent craniosynostosis but abnormal skull morphology. The degree of syndactyly is variable, or digital abnormalities can be absent. As an example, a patient with Crouzon-like features, craniosynostosis, and no limb involvement had a *TWIST* mutation (Carbonara et al., 1999).

IDENTIFICATION OF GENE AND MUTATIONAL SPECTRUM

Several lines of experimental evidence led to the discovery that *TWIST* is the disease gene for Saethre-Chotzen syndrome. First, craniosynostosis is a feature of the chromosome del7p syndrome and occurred if the deletion involved the distal portion of band 7p21 and included 7p22 (Schomig-Spingler et al., 1986; Cohen and MaClean, 2000). Second, the locus for the Saethre-Chotzen syndrome, which has craniosynostosis as a prominent feature, was also mapped to human chromosome 7p21-p22, using associated chromosome 7p deletions and rearrangements and linkage analysis (Brueton et al., 1992; Reardon et

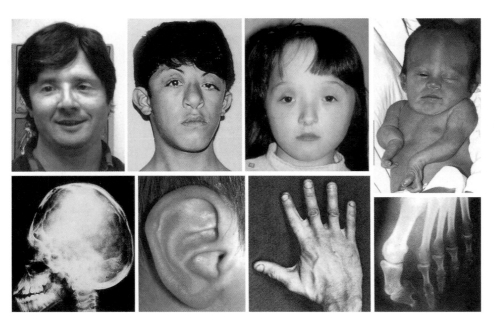

Figure 34–2. Saethre-Chotzen phenotype. Note variability of craniofacial features with brachycephaly, facial asymmetry, midfacial hypoplasia, ptosis, downward slanting palpebral fissures, prominent ear crus, and syndactyly. On the *top far right*, the patient with metopic ridging, overlapping helix, and preaxial reduction of upper limbs was diagnosed with Baller-Gerold syndrome. On the *bottom far right*, X-rays of the duplication of the distal phalanx of the great toe were found in a patient diagnosed with Robinow-Sorauf. The first three individuals on the *top row* from left to right and the patient with the toe duplication had the following TWIST mutations: 356A>C, 384_385insC, 416_417dup21, and 460-461insA, respectively. (Photos were previously published: *top left to right*, Howard et al., 1997 [male]; Paznekas et al., 1998 [adult male and female child]; Cohen, 1975 [infant]; *bottom left to right*, Howard et al., 1997 [skull]; Cohen, 2000 [ear]; Bartsocas et al., 1970 [hand]; Kunz et al., 1999 [foot].)

Legend for Figure 34–1:
bar height = 1 mutation | deletion | nonsense ■ | frameshift ▨
length = 50 amino acids | insertion or duplication ▩ | missense

Table 34–1. Clinical Features in Saethre-Chotzen and Phenotypically Related Syndromes

Characteristics	TWIST Gene* (n = 50)	Deletion (n = 7)	Robinow-Sorauf (n = 8)	Baller-Gerold (n = 5)	FGFR3 P250R (n = 14)
Age (years)	1/12–62	2.5–13	8/12–adult	Birth–adult	1.5–41
Sex ratio (F:M)	22:20	3:0	5:3	2:3	8:6
Abnormal karyotype	0%	100%	0%	0%	0%
Craniosynostosis	70	100	63	40	64
Coronal synostosis	58	71	63	40	64
Lambdoidal synostosis	14	0	13	0	14
Sagittal synostosis	10	0	25	20	7
Metopic synostosis	10	29	13	20	7
Acrobrachycephaly	57	100	50	—	43
Plagiocephaly	29	100	38	—	36
Large fontanelle	31	0	13	20	7
Low frontal hairline	48	71	—	40	14
Facial asymmetry	48	86	13	40	29
Eyebrow irregularity	20	50	—	—	7
Ptosis	64	100	38	0	21
Downslanting eyes	30	71	25	0	36
Epicanthal folds	33	57	—	60	29
Hypertelorism	38	43	—	20	57
Strabismus	26	29	—	20	21
Ear anomalies	34	86	—	40	7
Syndactyly	34	57	63	20	21
Brachydactyly or other upper limb abnormalities	26	71	38 Broad, valgus thumbs	60 Pedunculated thumb, radial hypoplasia	36
Broad great toe or other lower limb abnormalities	54	71	75 Hallux valgus, duplication of distal phalanx	80 Hallux valgus	21
Clinodactyly	36	71	—	20	21
Short stature	17	50	—	—	7
Learning disabilities/ mental retardation	10	71	0	—	7
Hearing loss	10	50	—	—	21
Reference	Paznekas et al., 1998; Johnson et al., 1998; Chun et al., 2002	Johnson et al., 1998; Chun et al., 2002	Kunz et al., 1999; Cai et al., in press	Gripp et al., 1999; Seto et al., 2001	Paznekas et al., 1998; Chun et al., 2002

*Patients with intragenic *TWIST* mutations.

n, number of individuals; there may be more than one affected individual per family. —, not noted in report.

al., 1993; Reid et al., 1993; Lewanda et al., 1994; Rose et al., 1994; Tsuji et al., 1994; Van Herwerden et al., 1994; Wilkie et al., 1995). Third, the mouse *Twist* gene was mapped to chromosome 12 in the region B-C1, which is homologous to human chromosome 7p21-22. Finally, when the phenotype of the *Twist* heterozygous null mouse was noted to be similar to Saethre-Chotzen syndrome and the human *TWIST* gene was mapped to 7p21-p22, *TWIST* became the leading candidate gene for Saethre-Chotzen.

As predicted, *TWIST* was found to contain mutations in Saethre-Chotzen syndrome patients (El Ghouzzi et al., 1997; Howard et al., 1997), and now at least 73 different mutations are known in the first exon and clustered in regions coding for important functional domains (Fig. 34–1, Table 34–2) (Gripp et al., 2000a). Approximately three-fourths of the mutations (77%) occur in the DNA-binding, helix 1, loop, and helix 2 domains. The rest occur 5′ of the DNA-binding and HLH domains, suggesting that this region is also important for protein function. The majority (63%, 46/73) are single base pair substitutions. Twenty-two percent (16/73) are small deletions, and 8% (6/73) are small insertions. Two mutations are a combination of a deletion and insertion or a deletion and a nucleotide change. Ten percent (7/73) are duplications, and almost all are 21 bp duplications thought to result from unequal crossover due to the presence of flanking 6 bp repeat sequences occurring at 21 bp intervals. The 416_417dup21 at the junction of the helix 1 and loop domains is the most frequent recurrent mutation, reported in at least seven unrelated families. The most likely effect of such a large insertion is disruption of the tertiary structure of the HLH critical for dimerization. The missense mutations occurring in the helix and loop domains are also likely to affect dimerization. Single mutations 5′ of the HLH region may weaken or destroy

DNA binding. No splice site, intronic mutations, or changes within the untranslated second exon have been reported.

Sixteen large deletions involving *TWIST* and 9 chromosome rearrangements with 5 cases occurring 3′ of the *STOP* codon of *TWIST* have been identified in patients with Saethre-Chotzen-like features. Eight cases have documented translocations involving another chromosome. A comprehensive survey using sequencing of the *TWIST* gene, chromosome analysis, fluorescent *in situ* hybridization, and Southern blot analysis detected approximately 80% of gene mutations, 37% of which were large deletions (Table 34–3) (Johnson et al., 1998). Definitive phenotype–genotype correlations have not been found, with the exception of Saethre-Chotzen syndrome patients who have a similar but more complex phenotype and mild to moderate mental retardation. This subgroup of patients usually has large deletions encompassing the *TWIST* gene and several megabases of flanking sequence (Table 34–3). Haploinsufficiency of the intergenic region or gene(s) around *TWIST* may contribute to developmental delay. It has been suggested that *TWIST* mutations may be specific to Saethre-Chotzen syndrome because no *TWIST* mutations have been detected in more than 50 cases of isolated coronal synostosis (El Ghouzzi et al., 1999; Boyd et al., 2002).

Two syndromes previously described to be distinct acrocephaly-syndactyly entities, Robinow-Sorauf syndrome (OMIM 180750) and Baller-Gerold syndrome (OMIM 218600) have mutations in *TWIST* (Fig. 34–2, Table 34–1). The former condition was previously distinguished on the basis of having bifid halluces, and the latter condition has hypoplastic or aplastic thumb and radii. Based on molecular evidence, it has been proposed that these conditions represent the variability of abnormal limb manifestations in families with *TWIST* mutations (Zackai et al., 1998).

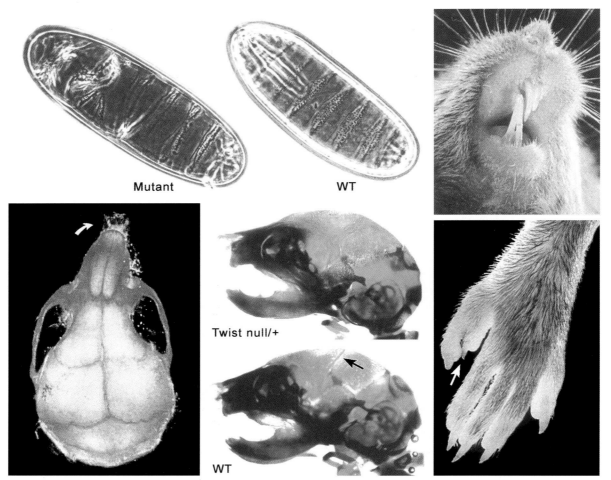

Figure 34–3. *Drosophila* null and mouse heterozygote null mutant phenotypes. *Top left* and *middle* panels show 24-hour-old mutant *Drosophila* embryo with the head end twisted in the egg case and the gastrulating wild-type embryo. Other panels show the mutant mouse with twisted skull and duplicated great toe. Dark arrow pointing to the open coronal suture of the wild-type mouse is compared to the synostosed suture in the mutant mouse of middle panels. (Photos previously published: *top left to right*, Simpson, 1983 [left and middle]; Bourgeois et al., 1998; *bottom left to right*, Bourgeois et al., 1998; El Ghouzzi et al., 1997.)

Table 34–2. Mutations in the *TWIST* Gene

Nucleotide Change[†,‖]	Amino Acid Change[‡,§,‖]	Functional Domain	Number of Cases*	Reference
7C>T	Q3X	5′ DNA binding	2	Elanko et al., 2001, and Cai et al., submitted
82C>T	Q28X	5′ DNA binding	1	Dollfus et al., 2002
106G>T	G36X	5′ DNA binding	1	Elanko et al., 2001
127_137del11	R43fsX233	5′ DNA binding	1	Boeck et al., 2001
128_138del11	R44fsX233	5′ DNA binding	1	Cai et al., submitted
181G>T	G61X	5′ DNA binding	1	Rose et al., 1997
193G>T	E65X	5′ DNA binding	3	Rose et al., 1997; Kasparcova et al., 1998; El Ghouzzi et al., 1999
211C>T	Q71X	5′ DNA binding	1, R-S	Cai et al., in press
230delA;232T>C	K77fsX124	5′ DNA binding	1	Rose et al., 1997; Johnson et al., 1998
263delG	G88fsX124	5′ DNA binding	1	Gripp et al., 2000a
272_273ins10	S93fsX292	5′ DNA binding	1	Kasparcova et al., 1998
276_277dup21	G92_S93insGAGGGGG	5′ DNA binding	2	Kasparcova et al., 1998, and Cai et al., submitted
283delAinsCG	S95fsX237	5′ DNA binding	1	Elanko et al., 2001
308_309insA	Y103X	5′ DNA binding	1	Howard et al., 1997; Paznekas et al., 1998
309C>A/G	Y103X	5′ DNA binding	8	El Ghouzzi et al., 1997; Paznekas et al., 1998; El Ghouzzi et al., 1999, and Cai et al., submitted
309delC	Y103X	5′ DNA binding	1	Cai et al., submitted
310G>T	E104X	5′ DNA binding	2	Johnson et al., 1998; El Ghouzzi et al., 1999
340A>G	N114D	DNA binding	1	Carbonara et al., 1999
346C>T	R116W	DNA binding	1	Paznekas et al., 1998
348del17	R116fsX231	DNA binding	1	Chun et al., 2002
352C>T	R118C	DNA binding	1	Bonaventure, unpublished
352_354del3	R118del	DNA binding	1	El Ghouzzi et al., 1998

(continued)

Table 34–2. *Continued*

Nucleotide Change[†,‡]	Amino Acid Change[‡,§,‖]	Functional Domain	Number of Cases*	Reference
353G>A	R118H	DNA binding	2	Rose et al., 1997; Muenke and Wilkie, 2001
353_360del8	R118fsX234	DNA binding	1	El Ghouzzi et al., 1999
355delC	Q119fsX124	DNA binding	1	Elanko et al., 2001
356A>C	Q119P	DNA binding	1	Howard et al., 1997
359G>C	R120P	DNA binding	1	Kasparcova et al., 1998
364C>T	Q122X	Helix I	2	Paznekas et al., 1998, and Cai et al., submitted
368C>A	S123X	Helix I	1	El Ghouzzi et al., 1997
368C>G	S123W	Helix I	1	Johnson et al., 1998
376G>T	E126X	Helix I	4	El Ghouzzi et al., 1997, 1999; Rose et al., 1997; Kasparcova et al., 1998
379_381dup	A127_F128insA	Helix I	1	Elanko et al., 2001
384_385insC	A129fsX237	Helix I	1	Paznekas et al., 1998
385G>C	A129P	Helix I	1	Bonaventure, unpublished
392T>C	L131P	Helix I	1	El Ghouzzi et al., 1997
395G>C	R132P	Helix I	1	Paznekas et al., 1998
402C>G	I134M	Helix I	1	Rose et al., 1997
405_406dup21	I135_P136ins AALRKII	Helix I	2	Howard et al., 1997; Lee et al., 2002
407C>T	P136L	Helix I	2	Johnson et al., 1998; Kasparcova et al., 1998
415C>T	P139S	Loop	1	Paznekas et al., 1998
416C>A	P139H	Loop	1	Elanko et al., 2001
416C>T	P139L	Loop	1	Chun et al., 2002
416_417dup21	P139_S140ins KIIPTLP	Loop	7	El Ghouzzi et al., 1997; Howard et al., 1997; Johnson et al., 1998; Paznekas et al., 1998; Elanko et al., 2001, and Cai et al., submitted
417_418dup21	P139_S140ins KIIPTLP	Loop	2	El Ghouzzi et al., 1997; Rose et al., 1997
418_419dup21	S140X	Loop	1	Rose et al., 1997
420_421dup21	S140_D141insIIPTLPS	Loop	2	Rose et al., 1997, and Cai et al., submitted
421G>T	D141Y	Loop	2	Johnson et al., 1998; Paznekas et al., 1998
422A>G	D141G	Loop	1	Rose et al., 1997
423_424ins25	D141_K142insDHPHAALGfsX297	Loop	1	El Ghouzzi et al., 1999
430A>C	S144R	Loop	2	El Ghouzzi et al., 1999
433A>G	K145E	Loop	1	El Ghouzzi et al., 1999
433_455del23	K145fsX229	Loop	1	Howard et al., 1997
435G>C	K145N	Loop	1	Rose et al., 1997
442A>G	T148A	Loop	1	Kasparcova et al., 1998
443C>A	T148N	Loop	1	Ray et al., 1997; Chun et al., 2002
445C>T	L149F	Loop	2	Paznekas et al., 1998, and Cai et al., submitted
454G>C	A152P	Loop	1	Elanko et al., 2001
455C>T	A152V	Loop	1	Paznekas et al., 1998
460A>G	R154G	Helix 2	1	Rose et al., 1997
460_461insA	R154fsX237	Helix 2	1, R-S	Kunz et al., 1999
464_469del5	Y155X	Helix 2	1	El Ghouzzi et al., 1999
465C>A	Y155X	Helix 2	1	Elanko et al., 2001
466A>G	I156V	Helix 2	1, B-G	Seto et al., 2001
472T>C	F158L	Helix 2	1	Elanko et al., 2001
475C>T	L159F	Helix 2	1	El Ghouzzi et al., 1999
480C>G	Y160X	Helix 2	1	Kasparcova et al., 1998
481C>T	Q161X	Helix 2	2	El Ghouzzi et al., 1999
481delC	Q161fsX230	Helix 2	1	Elanko et al., 2001
482_488del7	Q161fsX228	Helix 2	1	Cai et al., submitted
485_488del4	V162fsX229	Helix 2	1	Elanko et al., 2001
487delC	L163fsX230	Helix 2	1	El Ghouzzi et al., 1999
490C>T	Q164X	Helix 2	1	Gripp et al., 2000b
541G>T	E181X	3' Helix 2	1, B-G	Gripp et al., 1999

*R-S/B-G, Case has diagnosis of Robinow-Sorauf or Baller-Gerold syndrome.
†Genomic sequence based on GenBank numbers U80998 and NT_007819.
‡Protein sequence derived from GenBank number 1769550.
§Amino acid number 1 is the initiator methionine.
‖Mutation nomenclature based on Den Dunnen and Antonarakis (2000).

In addition to mutations in *TWIST*, there are several cases with the FGFR3 Pro250Arg mutation and features that resemble Saethre-Chotzen syndrome (Table 34–1). These patients provide clinical evidence that Saethre-Chotzen syndrome is genetically heterogeneous and that these two disease genes are components of a common developmental pathway (Bellus et al., 1996; Golla et al., 1997; Muenke et al., 1997; Paznekas et al., 1998; El Ghouzzi et al., 1999; Chun et al., 2002). No mutations have been found in candidate genes implicated as potential components of the same developmental pathway, including *SNAIL, SLUG,* and *DERMO1* (Paznekas et al., 1998; Boyd et al., 2002; Wang et al., 2002).

COUNSELING AND TREATMENT

Clinical diagnosis for Saethre-Chotzen syndrome can be challenging, even though this condition has high penetrance, because the variability is extreme. Patients are brought to medical attention as early as the newborn period on account of the abnormal shape of the skull and limb abnormalities. Other individuals are unaware that they have the condition until they have a child who is severely affected. Dysmorphologic, radiologic, ophthalmologic, and neurologic evaluations are usually performed; and three-dimensional computed tomographic scan is the standard for diagnosis of craniosynostosis. Diagnostic confir-

Table 34–3. Chromosomal Mutations in Saethre-Chotzen-like Patients

Features	Karyotype	Microdeletion	Reference
Saethre-Chotzen	Normal	Deletion of *TWIST* gene 5.5 kb–7.8 Mb	Cai et al., submitted
Saethre-Chotzen, developmental delay	Normal	Deletion of *TWIST* gene with insGT 2.924 kb	Johnson et al., 1998
Saethre-Chotzen, developmental delay	Normal	Deletion of *TWIST* gene 3.5–5.6 Mb	Johnson et al., 1998
Saethre-Chotzen, developmental delay	Normal	Deletion of *TWIST* gene 5.5–10.16 Mb	Johnson et al., 1998
Saethre-Chotzen, developmental delay	Normal	Deletion of *TWIST* gene > 7.7 kb	Gripp et al., 2001
Saethre-Chotzen, developmental delay	Normal	Deletion of *TWIST* gene > 45 kb	Gripp et al., 2001
Saethre-Chotzen, developmental delay	Normal	Deletion of *TWIST* gene > 45 kb	Gripp et al., 2001
Saethre-Chotzen, developmental delay	Normal	Deletion of *TWIST* gene > 7.7 kb	Gripp et al., 2001
Saethre-Chotzen, developmental delay	Normal	Deletion of *TWIST* gene 797 bp 510 kb	Cai et al., submitted
Saethre-Chotzen, developmental delay	Normal	Deletion of *TWIST* gene > 600 kb	Cai et al., submitted
Saethre-Chotzen	t(6;7)(q16.2;p15.3)	518 bp deletion 5 kb 3′ of *TWIST* gene	Tsuji et al., 1994, 1995 Krebs et al., 1997
Saethre-Chotzen	inv(7)(p21.3q34)	Inversion breakpoint in 10 kb region 260 kb 3′ of *TWIST* gene	Cai et al., submitted
Saethre-Chotzen	t(7;10)(p21.2;q21.2)	Translocation breakpoint in 1.1 Mb region, 70–250 kb 3′ of *TWIST* gene	Reardon et al., 1993; Rose et al., 1997
Saethre-Chotzen	t(2;7)(q21.1;p21.2)	Translocation breakpoint in 1.1 Mb region, 70–250 kb 3′ of *TWIST* gene	Wilkie et al., 1995; Rose et al., 1997
Saethre-Chotzen, developmental delay	t(7;18)(p21.2;q23)	Translocation breakpoint in 1.1 Mb region, 70–250 kb 3′ of *TWIST* gene	Wilkie et al., 1995; Rose et al., 1997
Saethre-Chotzen, growth hormone deficiency	t(5;7)(p15.3;p21.2)	Translocation breakpoint in Mb region	Wilkie et al., 1995; Rose et al., 1997
Saethre-Chotzen-like, epigastric and umbilical hernias, developmental delay	t(7;8)(p21;q13)	Deletion of *TWIST* gene > 11.56 Mb	Johnson et al., 1998
Saethre-Chotzen, developmental delay	del(7)(p15.1p21.3)	Deletion of *TWIST* gene 510 kb–16 Mb	Cai et al., submitted
Saethre-Chotzen, skeletal abnormalities, developmental delay	del(7)(p15.3p21.3)	Deletion of *TWIST* gene > 45 kb	Chun et al., 2002
Saethre-Chotzen, blepharophimosis, VSD, anal malposition/stenosis, developmental delay	del(7)(p15.3p21.3)	Deletion of *TWIST* gene > 45 kb	Chun et al., 2002
Saethre-Chotzen, VSD, ASD, cryptorchidism	der(1)t(1;2;7;18)(q31.1;q24.3;p21.1;p11.3), der(2)t(1;2;7;18), der(7)t(1;2;7;18)t(7;18)(q21.2;q21.31), der(18)t(1;2;7;18)t(7;18)	Translocation breakpoint < 45 kb region	Gripp et al., 2001
Saethre-Chotzen, coarctation of the aorta, developmental delay	t(2;7)(p23;p22)	Translocation breakpoint >260 kb 3′ to *TWIST* gene	Reid et al., 1993; Lewanda et al., 1994, and Cai et al., submitted
Craniosynostosis, metopic synostosis, facial and hand dysmorphisms, developmental delay	del(7)(p15.3p21.3)	Deletion of *TWIST* gene 797 bp–14.4 Mb	Cai et al., submitted
Coronal synsostosis; cutis aplasia; facial, hand, and foot anomalies; constriction band of left arm; developmental delay	Normal	Deletion of *TWIST* gene 600 kb–8.7 Mb	Cai et al., submitted

VSD, ventricular septal defect; ASD, atrial septal defect.

mation of Saethre-Chotzen syndrome is possible by identifying a *TWIST* mutation including large deletions of the chromosome 7p2 region. If patients with Saethre-Chotzen syndrome-like features are *TWIST*-negative, they should be tested for the FGFR3 Pro[250]Arg mutation. Prenatal molecular diagnosis is possible if the mutation is known for an affected parent. Affected individuals are counseled that they have a 50% risk of passing on the mutation to their offspring, but the degree of phenotypic severity may not breed true.

Treatment requires a multidisciplinary team approach tailored to the specific craniofacial, ocular, audiologic, dental, and skeletal malformations present. Surgical release of the synostosed sutures is needed for moderate to severe cases, to allow continued brain growth and development and to prevent neurologic sequelae. When craniofacial surgery is required, a series of procedures may be necessary, with the first occurring usually before 6 months of age. Surgical procedures for limb abnormalities may be needed to improve function. Monitoring of intellectual development is needed should an affected individual need special educational assistance.

ANIMAL MODELS

The *twist* gene was first identified in a *Drosophila* homozygous null mutant with a lethal phenotype (Simpson, 1983; Thisse et al., 1988). Gastrulation was disrupted, with failure of the ventral furrow and the mesoderm layer to develop. The anterior end of the embryo was "twisted" in the egg, from which the name of the mutated gene was derived (Fig. 34–3). In mouse, *Twist* is also expressed during mesodermal development of the embryonic head and limbs (Fuchtbauer, 1995; Stoetzel et al., 1995). *Twist* expression first occurs along a dorsoventral gradient until the headfold stage, and then it is observed along the rostrocaudal axis as development proceeds in the mesoderm and in neural crest cell derivatives. At day 7 postcoitum, *Twist* is present in the mesoderm outside the primitive streak, and later it is found in the somites, head mesenchyme, first aortic arches, second through fourth branchial arches, limb buds, and the mesenchyme beneath the epidermis. At day 8 postcoitum, *Twist* is primarily expressed in the undifferentiated cells and may inhibit muscle and cartilage differentiation. During organogenesis, *Twist* is expressed within areas of mesenchymal–epithelial interaction. *Twist* transcripts have been detected in osteoblastic cells from newborn mouse calvaria (Murray et al., 1992).

Mouse homozygous knockouts for *Twist* die at embryonic day 11.5 and exhibit a failure of neural tube closure specifically in the cranial region (Chen and Behringer, 1995). As predicted by expression studies, these mutants also have defects in head mesenchyme, branchial arches, somites, and limb buds. Disorganization of surrounding mesenchymal cells in the cranial region compromise the integrity of the blood vessels, leading to improper blood circulation, a probable cause of embryonic death. No apical ectodermal ridge is found in the mutant buds, thus affecting limb bud outgrowth.

Mice heterozygous for *Twist* null mutations display skull defects of coronal synostosis and poorly developed squamosal bones (derivatives from the first branchial arch) as well as overdeveloped interparietal bones and duplication of hind leg digits involving a metatarus and one to three phalanges (Fig. 34–3) (El Ghouzzi et al., 1997; Bourgeois et al., 1998; Carver et al., 2002). In addition, other malformations are observed, such as defects of middle ear formation and xiphoid process. The expressivity of the mouse mutant heterozygous phenotype varies depending on the genetic background. The mouse phenotype is consistent with the human Saethre-Chotzen syndrome phenotype of "overossification" leading to craniosynostosis, premature fusion of skull bones, and broad or duplicated digits (Fig. 34–2). The clinical features of facial asymmetry and ptosis observed in humans could be due to vascular, muscular, or neural involvement.

DEVELOPMENTAL PATHOGENESIS

The prominent feature of craniosynostosis in Saethre-Chotzen syndrome suggests that the *TWIST* gene plays a crucial role in cranial osteogenesis. Calvarial bone formation occurs by membranous ossification, characterized by direct formation of bone matrix synthesized by osteoblasts. Sutures present at the junction of ossification plaques are composed of two adjacent membranous bony fronts formed by osteoblasts arising from the differentiation of preosteoblasts originating from mesenchymal cells (Opperman et al., 2000). During membranous ossification, *TWIST* is expressed early during osteoblast differentiation, suggesting that it is involved in osteoblast maturation (Alborzi et al., 1996).

The gene deletions and nonsense mutations in humans and the similarity of the human disease and knockout mouse phenotypes point to haploinsufficiency as the major etiologic mechanism of the disease. Loss of TWIST protein function is induced by loss of the ability to dimerize due to mutations in the HLH region, loss of the ability of a dimerized complex to bind DNA due to mutations of the DNA-binding region, protein degradation, or subcellular mislocalization (El Ghouzzi et al., 2000, 2001). Deletions 3' of the gene suggest that there are important regulatory factors in this region, and translocations involving other chromosomes may exert a positional effect. However,

a dominant-negative effect may be the mechanism for some mutations because it has been shown that *Caenorhabditis elegans* twist mutant protein (E29K) can bind to target promoters as a dimer then block transcription (Corsi et al., 2002). Conversely, duplication of chromosome 7p21 in humans has been associated with an unusually large, late closing fontanelle in several patients; and in one case, three copies of the *TWIST* gene were present, suggesting that TWIST lies in a dosage-sensitive pathway controlling the differentiation of sutural mesenchymal cells into definitive osteoblasts (Caiulo et al., 1989; Lurie et al., 1995; Cai et al., 1999; Megarbane et al., 2001; Stankiewicz et al., 2001).

It is thought that TWIST has an inhibitory effect on tissue differentiation, namely osteogenesis and myogenesis, based on the observation that markers for these tissue precursors and TWIST have mutually exclusive patterns of expression (Sandell et al., 1991; Hebrok et al., 1994). In the case of myogenesis, TWIST acts as a negative regulator of transcription. The inhibitory action of TWIST may be mediated in part by the maintenance of condensed chromatin through inhibition of histone acetylation as TWIST binds to histone acetyltransferase domains (Hamamori et al., 1999). Consistent with this hypothesis, Twist haploinsufficiency in Saethre-Chotzen syndrome with the Y103X mutation results in increased growth, type I collagen expression, and osteogenic capability of human calvarial osteoblasts (Yousfi et al., 2001), indicating that cell overproliferation and abnormal maturation of osteoblasts result in coronal synostosis (Jabs, 2001). Twist haploinsufficiency in Saethre-Chotzen syndrome with the Y103X, Q109X, or R118C mutation promotes apoptosis in human calvarial osteoblasts through a tumor necrosis factor-α–caspase-2–caspase-8–caspases3, 6, and 7 cascade (Yousfi et al., 2002). Also consistent with these data is the "massive wave" of apoptosis seen in Twist null mice during development. These observations demonstrate the complex balancing act Twist plays as it is involved in cell proliferation, maturation, and antiapoptosis in human calvarial osteoblasts.

With the identification of other genes expressed in the calvarial sutures and limbs, information is emerging regarding the epistatic interaction of these various genes and whether their products act either upstream or downstream from one another in the molecular pathway(s) of calvarial and limb development. DERMO1 and ID1, along with TWIST, are expressed in osteoblasts and are negative regulators of osteoblast differentiation (Murray et al., 1992; Tamura and Noda, 1999; Lee et al., 2000). With loss of function of TWIST in Saethre-Chotzen patients, there would be loss of its inhibitory effect on its downstream targets such as FGFRs and CBFA1/RUNX2.

One would hypothesize that in humans FGFRs lie downstream of TWIST in the same developmental pathway of skull and limb development because of overlapping clinical phenotypes of the conditions caused by mutations in these two gene families. Further evidence from developmental biology supports the premise. In *Drosophila*, *twist* regulates the expression of *DFR1*, an FGFR homologue. The *Drosophila* TWIST protein is required for proper formation of mesodermal tissues, and expression patterns of twist and *Dfr1* are similar in the wing and leg disc. In *Drosophila* embryos, *DFR1* expression was not detected in twist mutants (Shishido et al., 1993). In turn, *DFR1*-negative embryos showed the same phenotype as *twist*-negative mutants. Similarly, during *Xenopus* development, *twist* is detected initially at the early gastrula stage, specifically in mesoderm (Hopwood et al., 1989). A *Xenopus* dominant-negative FGFR mutant causes specific defects in gastrulation and posterior/lateral mesoderm formation (Amaya et al., 1991). In still another organism, *C. elegans*, a *twist* homologue, designated *hlh-8*, has been identified (Harfe et al., 1998). Early hlh-8 promoter activity requires the homeobox protein MAB-5, and hlh-8 apparently acts as a transcriptional activator and *in vivo* can activate the promoter of a FGFR homologue, *egl-15*.

Most relevant and analogous to the human situation of loss of function in TWIST and gain of function in FGFRs leading to craniosynostosis is evidence derived from mouse. Unlike the situation in *Drosophila* and *C. elegans*, where loss of function of the twist homologue leads to loss of the fgfr homologue DFR1 or the twist homologue activates the fgfr homologue egl-15, respectively, in mouse

Twist expression precedes that of *Fgfr* genes during the initiation of coronal suture development and *Twist* heterozygous knockouts develop ectopic expression of *Fgfr2* at the suture (Rice et al., 2000). Thus, Twist loss of function leads to gain of function of Fgfr2 in mouse, and mouse Twist normally represses Fgfr activity in osteoblast as well as in muscle differentiation.

Our laboratory found that another craniosynostosis condition, craniosynostosis, Boston type (OMIM 123101), has a mutation in a homeobox gene, *MSX2*, which is expressed in the neural crest–derived mesenchyme of the first through fourth branchial arches and in developing calvarial sutures, teeth, and limb buds. A missense mutation in the homeodomain, Pro148His, was found in a large family with variable phenotypic features, ranging from cloverleaf skull deformity to mild frontal orbital recession (Jabs et al., 1993). This mutation exerts its effect by a gain-of-function mechanism because there is increased binding affinity of mutant Msx2 to a target (Semenza et al., 1995; Ma et al., 1996), and overexpression of Msx2 in a transgenic mouse leads to premature closure of clavarial sutures (Liu et al., 1995). It is likely that this homeodomain protein is a component of the same developmental pathway(s) as TWIST and FGFR. MSX2 in humans could perform a function similar to the homeobox-containing protein MAB-5 in *C. elegans* and function as an upstream activator of TWIST or, perhaps, as a downstream nuclear transcription factor activated by the FGFR signaling pathway involving ras/raf signal transduction.

Elucidation of other components in this pathway will assist in the identification of additional candidate genes for craniosynostosis and modifying genes that will define at the molecular level descriptive terms such as *degree of penetrance* and *variability in phenotype*. Delineation of the precise modulation of gene and protein expression secondary to interactions among the components of the pathway(s) will determine the molecular basis for the phenotypic differences among individual Saethre-Chotzen syndrome patients. Transcription profiling of *twist* loss of function in *Drosophila* embryos implicating hundreds of genes, many with vertebrate homologues, sets the stage for the future comprehensive view of the developmental pathway(s) involving twist (Furlong et al., 2001).

ACKNOWLEDGMENTS

Supported by National Institutes of Health grant P60 DE13078.

REFERENCES

Alborzi A, Mac K, Glackin CA, Murray SS, Zernik JH (1996). Endochondral and intramembranous fetal bone development: osteoblastic cell proliferation, and expression of alkaline phosphatase, m-twist, and histone H4. *J Craniofac Genet Dev Biol* 16: 94–106.

Amaya E, Musci TJ, Kirschner MW (1991). Expression of a dominant negative mutant of the FGF receptor disrupts mesoderm formation in *Xenopus* embryos. *Cell* 66(2):257–270.

Bartsocas CS, Weber AL, Crawford JD (1970). Acrocephalosyndactyly type III: Chotzen's syndrome. *J Pediatr* 77(2): 267–272.

Bellus GA, Gaudenz K, Zackai EH, Clarke LA, Szabo J, Francomano CA, Muenke M (1996). Identical mutations in three different fibroblast growth factor receptor genes in autosomal dominant craniosynostosis syndromes. *Nat Genet* 14: 174–176.

Bodmer R, Jan LY, Jan YN (1990). A new homeobox-containing gene, *msh-2*, is transiently expressed early during mesoderm formation of *Drosophila*. *Development* 110(3): 661–669.

Boeck A, Kosan C, Ciznar P, Kunz J (2001). Saethre-Chotzen syndrome and hyper IgE syndrome in a patient with a novel 11 bp deletion of the *TWIST* gene. *Am J Med Genet* 104: 53–56.

Bourgeois P, Bolcato-Bellemin AL, Danse JM, Bloch-Zupan A, Yoshiba K, Stoetzel C, Perrin-Schmitt F (1998). The variable expressivity and incomplete penetrance of the twist-null heterozygous mouse phenotype resemble those of human Saethre-Chotzen syndrome. *Hum Mol Genet* 7(6): 945–957.

Boyd SAB, Zhang G, Ingersoll R, Isaac N, Kasch L, Hur D, Jabs EW, Beaty T, Scott AF (2002). Analysis of candidate genes for non-syndromic craniosynostosis. *Am J Hum Genet* 71(4): A1795.

Brueton LA, Van Herwerden L, Chotai KA, Winter RM (1992). The mapping of a gene for craniosynostosis: evidence for linkage of the Saethre-Chotzen syndrome to distal chromosome 7p. *J Med Genet* 29(10): 681–685.

Cai T, Ping Y, Tagle DA, Xia JH (1999). Duplication of 7p21.2->pter due to maternal 7p;21q translocation: implication for critical segment assignment in the 7p duplication syndrome. *Am J Med Genet* 86: 305–311.

Cai J, Shoo BA, Sorauf T, Jabs EW (in press). A novel mutation in the *TWIST* gene, implicated in Saethre-Chotzen syndrome, is found in the original case of "Robinow-Sorauf syndrome". *Clin Genet*.

Cai J, Goodman BK, Patel AS, Mulliken J, Van Maldergem L, Hoganson GE, Paznekas WA, Ben-Neriah Z, Sheffer R, Cunningham ML, Daentl DL, Jabs EW (submitted). Increased risk for developmental delay in Saethre-Chotzen syndrome is associated with *TWIST* deletions: an improved strategy for *TWIST* mutation screening.

Caiulo A, Bardoni B, Camerino G, Guioli S, Minelli A, Piantanida M, Crosato F, Dalla Fior T, Maraschio P (1989). Cytogenetic and molecular analysis of an unbalanced translocation (X;7)(q28;p15) in a dysmorphic girl. *Hum Genet* 84: 51–54.

Carbonara C, Snaiz L, Genitori L, Peretta P, Mussa F, Nurisso C, Restagno G, Belli S, Ferrero GB (1999). A novel N114D TWIST mutation in a Crouzon-like patient. *Am J Hum Genet* 65(Suppl): A144.

Carver EA, Oram KF, Gridley T (2002). Craniosynostosis in *Twist* heterozygous mice: a model for Saethre-Chotzen syndrome. *Anat Rec* 268(2): 90–92.

Castanon I, Von Stetina S, Kass J, Baylies MK (2001). Dimerization partners determine the activity of the Twist bHLH protein during *Drosophila* mesoderm development. *Development* 128: 3145–3159.

Chen ZF, Behringer RR (1995). Twist is required in head mesenchyme for cranial neural tube morphogenesis. *Genes Dev* 9(6): 686–699.

Chotzen F (1932). Eine eigenartige familiare entwicklungsstorung (akrocephalosyndaktylie, dysostosis craniofacialis und hypertelorismus). *Monatschr Kinderheilkd* 55: 97–122.

Chun K, Teebi AS, Jung JH, Kennedy S, Laframboise R, Meschino WS, Nakabayashi K, Scherer SW, Ray PN, Teshima I (2002). Genetic analysis of patients with the Saethre-Chotzen phenotype. *Am J Med Genet* 110: 136–143.

Cohen MM Jr (1975). An etiologic and nosologic overview of craniosynostosis syndromes. *Birth Defects* 11(2): 137–189.

Cohen MM Jr. (2000). Saethre-Chotzen syndrome. In: Cohen MM Jr, MaClean RE (eds). *Craniosynostosis: Diagnosis, Evaluation, and Management, 2nd Edition.* Oxford University Press, Oxford, pp. 374–376.

Corsi AK, Brodigan TM, Jorgensen EM, Krause M (2002). Characterization of a dominant negative *C. elegans* Twist mutant protein with implications for human Saethre-Chotzen syndrome. *Development* 129: 2761–2772.

Den Dunnen JT, Antonarakis SE (2000). Mutation nomenclature extensions and suggestions to describe complex mutations: a discussion. *Hum Mutat* 15: 7–12.

Dollfus H, Kumaramanickavel G, Biswas P, Stoetzel C, Quillet R, Denton M, Maw M, Perrin-Schmitt F (2001). Identification of a new *TWIST* mutation (7p21) with variable eyelid manifestations supports locus homogeneity of BPES at 3q22. *Am J Med Genet* 38: 470–472.

Ducy P, Karsenty G (1995). Two distinct osteoblast-specific *cis*-acting elements control expression of a mouse osteocalcin gene. *Mol Cell Biol* 15: 1858–1869.

Elanko N, Sibbring JS, Metcalfe KA, Clayton-Smith J, Donnai D, Temple IK, Wall SA, Wilkie AOM (2001). A survey of *TWIST* for mutations in craniosynostosis reveals a variable length polyglycine tract in asymptomatic individuals. *Hum Mutat* 18: 535–541.

El Ghouzzi V, Le Merrer M, Perrin-Schmitt F, Lajeunie E, Benit P, Renier D, Bourgeois P, Bolcato-Bellemin AL, Munnich A, Bonaventure J (1997). Mutations of the *TWIST* gene in the Saethre-Chotzen syndrome. *Nat Genet* 15(1): 42–46.

El Ghouzzi V, Lajeunie M, Le Merrer M, Cormier R, Renier D, Munnich A, Bonaventure J (1998). TWIST mutations disrupting the b-HLH domain are specific to Saethre-Chotzen syndrome. *Am J Hum Genet* Suppl. 61: A332.

El Ghouzzi V, Lajeunie E, Le Merrer M, Cormier-Daire V, Renier D, Munnich A, Bonaventure J (1999). Mutations within or upstream of the basic helix-loop-helix domain of the *TWIST* gene are specific to Saethre-Chotzen syndrome. *Eur J Hum Genet* 7(1): 27–33.

El Ghouzzi V, Legeai-Mallet L, Aresta S, Benoist C, Munnich A, de Gunzburg J, Bonaventure J (2000). Saethre-Chotzen mutations cause TWIST protein degradation or impaired nuclear location. *Hum Mol Genet* 9: 813–819.

El Ghouzzi V, Legeai-Mallet L, Benoist-Lasselin C, Lajeunie E, Renier D, Munnich A, Bonaventure J (2001). Mutations in the basic domain and the loop-helix II junction of TWIST abolish DNA binding in Saethre-Chotzen syndrome. *FEBS Lett* 492: 112–118.

Fuchtbauer EM (1995). Expression of M-twist during postimplantation development of the mouse. *Dev Dyn* 204(3): 316–322.

Furlong EEM, Andersen EC, Null B, White KP, Scott MP (2001). Patterns of gene expression during *Drosophila* mesoderm development. *Science* 293: 1629–1633.

Golla A, Lichtner P, von Gernet S, Winterpacht A, Fairley J, Murken J, Schuffenhauer S (1997). Phenotypic expression of the fibroblast growth factor receptor 3 (FGFR3) mutation P250R in a large craniosynostosis family. *J Med Genet* 34: 683–684.

Gorlin RJ, Cohen MM Jr, Hennekam RCM (2001). Saethre-Chotzen. In: *Syndromes of the Head and Neck, 4th edition.* Oxford University Press, Oxford, pp. 664–665.

Gripp KW, Stolle CA, Celle L, McDonald-McGinn DM, Whitaker LA, Zackai EH (1999). *TWIST* gene mutation in a patient with radial aplasia and craniosynostosis: further evidence for heterogeneity of Baller-Gerold syndrome. *Am J Med Genet* 82(2): 170–176.

Gripp KW, Zackai EH, Stolle CA (2000a). Mutations in the human *TWIST* gene. *Hum Mutat* 15: 150–155.

Gripp KW, Zackai EH, Stolle CA (2000b). Erratum. Mutations in the human *TWIST* gene. *Hum Mutat* 15: 479.

Gripp KW, Kasparcova V, McDonald-McGinn DM, Bhatt S, Bartlett SP, Storm AL, Drumheller TC, Emanuel BS, Zackai EH, Stolle CA (2001). A diagnostic approach to identifying submicroscopic 7p21 deletions in Saethre-Chotzen syndrome: fluorescence in situ hybridization and dosage-sensitive Southern blot analysis. *Genet Med* 3: 102–108.

Hamamori Y, Wu HY, Sartorelli V, Kedes L (1997). The basic domain of myogenic basic helix-loop-helix (bHLH) proteins is the novel target for direct inhibition by another bHLH protein, Twist. *Mol Cell Biol* 17(11): 6563–6573.

Hamamori Y, Sartorelli V, Ogryzko V, Puri PL, Wu HY, Wang JYJ, Nakatani Y, Kedes L (1999). Regulation of histone acetyltransferases p300 and PCAF by the bHLH protein Twist and adenoviral oncoprotein E1A. *Cell* 96: 405–413.

Harfe BD, Vaz Gomes A, Kenyon C, Liu J, Krause M, Fire A (1998). Analysis of a *Caenorhabditis elegans* Twist homolog identifies conserved and divergent aspects of mesodermal patterning. *Genes Dev* 12(16): 2623–2635.

Hebrok M, Wertz K, Fuchtbauer EM (1994). M-twist is an inhibitor of muscle differentiation. *Dev Biol* 165: 537–544.

Heinrichs AA, Banerjee C, Bortell R, Owen TA, Stein JL, Stein GS, Lian JB (1993). Identification and characterization of two proximal elements in the rat osteocalcin gene promoter that may confer species-specific regulation. *J Cell Biochem* 53(3): 240–250.

Hopwood ND, Pluck A, Gurdon JB (1989). A *Xenopus* mRNA related to *Drosophila* twist is expressed in response to induction in the mesoderm and the neural crest. *Cell* 59(5): 893–903.

Howard TD, Paznekas WA, Green ED, Chiang LC, Ma N, Ortiz de Luna RI, Garcia Delgado C, Gonzalez-Ramos M, Kline AD, Jabs EW (1997). Mutations in TWIST, a basic helix-loop-helix transcription factor, in Saethre-Chotzen syndrome. *Nat Genet* 15(1): 36–41.

Jabs EW (2001). A Twist in the fate of human osteoblasts identifies signaling molecules involved in skull development. *J Clin Invest* 107: 1075–1077.

Jabs EW, Muller U, Li X, Ma L, Luo W, Haworth IS, Klisak I, Sparkes R, Warman ML, Mulliken JB, et al. (1993). A mutation in the homeodomain of the human *MSX2* gene in a family affected with autosomal dominant craniosynostosis. *Cell* 75(3): 443–450.

Jan YN, Jan LY (1993). HLH proteins, fly neurogenesis, and vertebrate myogenesis. *Cell* 75(5): 827–830.

Johnson D, Horsley SW, Moloney DM, Oldridge M, Twigg SR, Walsh S, Barrow M, Njolstad PR, Kunz J, Ashworth GJ, et al. (1998). A comprehensive screen for *TWIST* mutations in patients with craniosynostosis identifies a new microdeletion syndrome of chromosome band 7p21.1. *Am J Hum Genet* 63(5): 1282–1293.

Kasparcova V, Stolle CA, Gripp KW, Celle L, McDonald-McGinn D, Bartlett S, Whitaker L, Zackai EH (1998). Molecular analysis of patients with Saethre-Chotzen syndrome; novel mutations and polymorphisms in the *TWIST* gene. *Am J Hum Genet Suppl* 63(4): A367.

Krebs I, Weis I, Hudler M, Rommens JM, Roth H, Scherer SW, Tsui LC, Fuchtbauer EM, Grzeschik KH, Tsuji K, et al. (1997). Translocation breakpoint maps 5 kb 3′ from *TWIST* in a patient affected with Saethre-Chotzen syndrome. *Hum Mol Genet* 6(7): 1079–1086.

Kunz J, Hundler M, Fritz B, Gillessen-Kaesbach G, Passarge E (1999). Identification of a frameshift mutation in the gene *TWIST* in a family affected with Robinow-Sorauf syndrome. *J Med Genet* 36(8): 650–652.

Lee MS, Lowe G, Flanagan S, Kuchler K, Glackin CA (2000). Human Dermo-1 has attributes similar to twist in early bone development. *Bone* 27(5): 591–602.

Lee S, Seto M, Sie K, Cunningham M (2002). A child with Saethre-Chotzen syndrome, sensorineural hearing loss, and a *TWIST* mutation. *Cleft Palate Craniofac J* 39(1): 110–114.

Lewanda AF, Green ED, Weissenbach J, Jerald H, Taylor E, Summar ML, Phillips JA III, Cohen M, Feingold M, Mouradian W, et al. (1994). Evidence that the Saethre-Chotzen syndrome locus lies between D7S664 and D7S507, by genetic analysis and detection of a microdeletion in a patient. *Am J Hum Genet* 55(6): 1195–1201.

Liu YH, Kundu R, Wu L, Luo W, Ignelzi MA Jr, Snead ML, Maxson RE Jr (1995). Premature suture closure and ectopic cranial bone in mice expressing *Msx2* transgenes in the developing skull. *Proc Natl Acad Sci USA* 92(13): 6137–6141.

Lurie IW, Schwartz MF, Schwartz S, Cohen MM (1995). Trisomy 7p resulting from isochromosome formation and whole-arm translocation. *Am J Med Genet* 55: 62–66.

Ma L, Golden S, Wu L, Maxson R (1996). The molecular basis of Boston-type craniosynostosis: the Pro148His mutation in the N-terminal arm of the MSX2 homeodomain stabilizes DNA binding without altering nucleotide sequence preferences. *Hum Mol Genet* 5(12): 1915–1920.

Megarbane A, Le Lorc'H M, Elghezal H, Joly G, Gosset P, Souraty N, Samaras L, Prieur M, Vekemans M, Turleau C, et al. (2001). Pure partial 7p trisomy including the *TWIST, HOXA,* and *GLI3* genes. *J Med Genet* 38: 178–182.

Muenke M, Wilkie AOM (2001). Craniosynostosis syndromes in: Scrivner CR, Beudet AL, Sly WS, Valle D (eds) *The Metabolic and Molecular Bases of Inherited Disease, 8th Edition.* McGraw-Hill, New York, pp. 6128–6139.

Muenke M, Gripp KW, McDonald-McGinn DM, Gaudenz K, Whitaker LA, Bartlett SP, Markowitz RI, Robin NH, Nwokoro N, Mulvihill JJ, et al. (1997). A unique point mutation in the fibroblast growth factor receptor 3 gene (*FGFR3*) defines a new craniosynostosis syndrome. *Am J Hum Genet* 60: 555–564.

Mundlos S, Otto F, Mundlos C, Mulliken JB, Aylsworth AS, Albright S, Lindhout D, Cole WG, Henn W, Knoll JH, Owen MJ, Mertelsmann R, Zabel BU, Olsen BR (1997). Mutations involving the transcription factor CBFA1 cause cleidocranial dysplasia. *Cell* 89: 773–779.

Murray SS, Glackin CA, Winters KA, Gazit D, Kahn AJ, Murray EJ (1992). Expression of helix-loop-helix regulatory genes during differentiation of mouse osteoblastic cells. *J Bone Miner Res* 7(10): 1131–1138.

Murre C, McCaw PS, Baltimore D (1989). A new DNA binding and dimerization motif in immunoglobulin enhancer binding, daughterless, MyoD, and myc proteins. *Cell* 56: 777–783.

Opperman L, Adab K, Gakunga P (2000). Transforming growth factor-β2 and TGF-β3 regulate fetal rat cranial suture morhpogenesis by regulating rates of cell proliferation and apoptosis. *Dev Dyn* 219: 237–247.

Paznekas WA, Cunningham ML, Howard TD, Korf BR, Lipson MH, Grix AW, Feingold M, Goldberg R, Borochowitz Z, Aleck K, et al. (1998). Genetic heterogeneity of Saethre-Chotzen syndrome, due to TWIST and FGFR mutations. *Am J Hum Genet* 62(6): 1370–1380.

Pham AD, Muller S, Sauer F (1999). Mesoderm-determining transcription in *Drosophila* is alleviated by mutations in *TAF(II)60* and *TAF(II)110. Mech Dev* 84: 3–16.

Ray PN, Siegel-Bartelt J, Chun K (1997). A unique mutation in *TWIST* causes Saethre-Chotzen syndrome. *Am J Hum Genet Suppl* 61: A344.

Reardon W, McManus SP, Summers D, Winter RM (1993). Cytogenetic evidence that the Saethre-Chotzen gene maps to 7p21.2. *Am J Med Genet* 47(5): 633–636.

Reid CS, McMorrow LE, McDonald-McGinn DM, Grace KJ, Ramos FJ, Zackai EH, Co-

hen MM Jr, Jabs EW (1993). Saethre-Chotzen syndrome with familial translocation at chromosome 7p22. *Am J Med Genet* 47(5): 637–639.

Rice DP, Aberg T, Chan Y, Tang Z, Kettunen PJ, Pakarinen L, Maxson RE, Thesleff L (2000). Integration of FGF and TWIST in calvarial bone and suture development. *Development* 127(9): 1845–1855.

Rose CS, King AA, Summers D, Palmer R, Yang S, Wilkie AO, Reardon W, Malcolm S, Winter RM (1994). Localization of the genetic locus for Saethre-Chotzen syndrome to a 6 cM region of chromosome 7 using four cases with apparently balanced translocations at 7p21.2. *Hum Mol Genet* 3(8): 1405–1408.

Rose CSP, Patel P, Reardon W, Malcolm S, Winter RM (1997). The *TWIST* gene, although not disrupted in Saethre-Chotzen patients with apparently balanced translocations of 7p21, is mutated in familial and sporadic cases. *Hum Mol Genet* 6(8): 1369–1373.

Saethre H (1931). Ein eitrag zum turmschadelproblem (pathogeneses, erbuchkeit und symptomologie). *Dtsch Z Nervenheikd* 117: 533–555.

Sandell LJ, Morris N, Robbins JR, Goldring MB (1991). Alternatively spliced type II procollagen mRNAs define distinct populations of cells during vertebral development: differential expression of the amino-propeptide. *J Cell Biol* 114: 1307–1319.

Schomig-Spingler M, Schmid M, Brosi W, Grimm T (1986). Chromosome 7 short arm deletion, 7p21-pter. *Hum Genet* 74(3): 323–325.

Semenza GL, Wang GL, Kundu R (1995). DNA binding and transcriptional properties of wild-type and mutant forms of the homeodomain protein Msx2. *Biochem Biophys Res Commun* 209(1): 257–262.

Seto ML, Lee SJ, Sze RW, Cunningham ML (2001). Another TWIST on Baller-Gerold syndrome. *Am J Med Genet* 104: 323–330.

Shirokawa JM, Courey AJ (1997). A direct contact between the dorsal rel homology domain and Twist may mediate transcriptional synergy. *Mol Cell Biol* 17(6): 3345–3355.

Shishido E, Higashijima S, Emori Y, Saigo K (1993). Two FGF-receptor homologues of *Drosophila:* one is expressed in mesodermal primordium in early embryos. *Development* 117(2): 751–761.

Simpson P (1983). Maternal–zygotic gene interactions during formation of the dorsoventral pattern in *Drosophila* embryos. *Genetics* 105: 615–632.

Spicer DB, Rhee J, Cheung WL, Lassar AB (1996). Inhibition of myogenic bHLH and MEF2 transcription factors by the bHLH protein Twist. *Science* 272: 1476–1480.

Spring J, Yanze N, Middel AM, Stierwald M, Groger H, Schmid V (2000). The mesoderm specification factor twist in the life cycle of jellyfish. *Dev Biol* 228: 363–375.

Stankiewicz P, Thiele H, Baldermann C, Kruger A, Giannakudis I, Dorr S, Werner N, Kunz J, Rappold GA, Hansmann I (2001). Phenotypic findings due to trisomy 7p15.3-pter including the *TWIST* locus. *Am J Med Genet* 103: 56–62.

Stoetzel C, Weber B, Bourgeois P, Bolcato-Bellemin AL, Perrin-Schmitt F (1995). Dorsoventral and rostro-caudal sequential expression of M-twist in the postimplantation murine embryo. *Mech Dev* 51(2–3): 251–263.

Tamura M, Noda M (1994). Identification of a DNA sequence involved in osteoblast-specific gene expression via interaction with helix-loop-helix (HLH)-type transcription factors. *J Cell Biol* 126(3): 773–782.

Tamura M, Noda M (1999). Identification of DERMO-1 as a member of helix-loop-helix type transcription factors expressed in osteoblastic cells. *J Cell Biochem* 72(2): 167–176.

Thisse B, Stoetzel C, Gorostiza-Thisse C, Perrin-Schmitt F (1988). Sequence of the *twist* gene and nuclear localization of its protein in endomesodermal cells of early *Drosophila* embryos. *EMBO J* 7: 2175–2183.

Tsuji K, Narahara K, Kikkawa K, Murakami M, Yokoyama Y, Ninomiya S, Seino Y (1994). Craniosynostosis and hemizygosity for D7S135 caused by a de novo and apparently balanced t(6;7) translocation. *Am J Med Genet* 49(1): 98–102.

Tsuji K, Narahara K, Yokoyama Y, Grzeschik KH, Kunz J (1995). The breakpoint on 7p in a patient with t(6;7) and craniosynostosis is spanned by a YAC clone containing the *D7S503* locus. *Hum Genet* 95: 303–307.

Van Herwerden L, Rose CS, Reardon W, Brueton LA, Weissenbach J, Malcolm S, Winter RM (1994). Evidence for locus heterogeneity in acrocephalosyndactyly: a refined localization for the Saethre-Chotzen syndrome locus on distal chromosome 7p and exclusion of Jackson-Weiss syndrome from craniosynostosis loci on 7p and 5q. *Am J Hum Genet* 54(4): 669–674.

Wang SM, Coljee VW, Pignolo RJ, Rotenberg MO, Cristofalo VJ, Sierra F (1997). Cloning of the human *TWIST* gene: its expression is retained in adult mesodermally-derived tissues. *Gene* 187(1): 83–92.

Wang YL, Paznekas WA, Kotch LE, Jabs EW (2002). Basic helix-loop-helix transcription factors Twist and Dermo1 during palatal, tooth, and calvarial development. *Am J Hum Genet* 71(4): A846.

Wilkie AO, Yang SP, Summers D, Poole MD, Reardon W, Winter RM (1995). Saethre-Chotzen syndrome associated with balanced translocations involving 7p21: three further families. *J Med Genet* 32(3): 174–180.

Yousfi M, Lasmoles F, Lomri A, Delannoy P, Marie PJ (2001). Increased bone formation and decreased osteocalcin expression induced by reduced Twist dosage in the Saethre-Chotzen syndrome. *J Clin Invest* 107: 1153–1161.

Yousfi M, Lasmoles F, El Ghouzzi V, Marie PJ (2002). Twist haploinsufficiency in Saethre-Chotzen syndrome induces calvarial osteoblast apoptosis due to increased TNFα expression and caspase-2 activation. *Hum Mol Genet* 11(4): 359–369.

Zackai EH, Gripp KW, McDonald-McGinn DM, Celle L, Whitaker R L, Bartlett S, Stolle CA (1998). The likely demise of the Robinow-Sorauf (MIM180750) and Baller-Gerold (MIM 218600) syndromes: *TWIST* mutations identified. *Am J Hum Genet Suppl.* 63:A18.

Part F.
The Glial Cell–Derived Neurotrophic Factor Signaling Pathway

35 | Signaling Pathways of Glial Cell–Derived Neurotrophic Factor

LOUIS F. REICHARDT

Glial cell–derived neurotrophic factor (GDNF), a distant relative of transforming growth factor-β (TGFβ), was purified as a factor that promotes the survival and differentiation of embryonic mesencephalic dopaminergic neurons (Lin et al., 1993). A closely related protein, neurturin, was purified as a factor that promotes the survival of sympathetic neurons (Kotzbauer et al., 1996). Subsequently, two additional members of the GDNF family of ligands—artemin and persephin—were identified in EST databases (Baloh et al., 1998; Milbrandt et al., 1998; Masure et al., 1999). Each of these proteins has been shown to function as a survival and differentiation factor for subpopulations of cultured neurons (reviewed in Airaksinen et al., 1999; Baloh et al., 2000a; Bennett, 2001; Butte, 2001; Manie et al., 2001; Takahashi, 2001).

The search for GDNF receptors was initially frustrating and led to the characterization of a glycosylphosphatidylinositol (GPI)-anchored binding protein now named GFRα1 that seemed unlikely to function as a single subunit receptor for this neurotrophic factor (Treanor et al., 1996). But when mice lacking GDNF were examined (Moore et al., 1996; Pichel et al., 1996), they proved to have an almost identical phenotype to mice that lacked the orphan receptor tyrosine kinase c-ret (Schuchardt et al., 1994). In each instance, severe deficits were seen in development of the metanephric kidney and the enteric nervous system, suggesting that they act through the same signaling pathway. Indeed, it was rapidly demonstrated that GFRα1 is the major ligand-binding subunit in a signaling complex that includes c-ret (e.g. Durbec et al., 1996a; Jing et al., 1996). More recent work has demonstrated the existence of four members of the GFRα family (GFRα1–4) that, after ligand engagement, activate the c-ret tyrosine kinase (Airaksinen et al., 1999; Klein et al., 1997; Enokido et al., 1998; Lindahl et al., 2001) with GDNF, neurturin, artemin, and persephin functioning as reasonably specific ligands for GFRα1, GFRα2, GFRα3, and GFRα4, respectively. In prior work, inactivating mutations of c-ret had been shown to be responsible for many cases of Hirschsprung disease, which is caused by a failure of enteric neuron precursors to populate normally the intestine (Edery et al., 1994). In addition, mutations or gene fusions that activate the tyrosine kinase activity of c-ret had been shown to be oncogenic, resulting in multiple endocrine neoplasia and medullary thyroid carcinoma (Goodfellow, 1994). Consequently, the signaling pathways activated by GDNF have been of keen interest to both developmental biologists and oncologists.

LIGAND–RECEPTOR INTERACTIONS

The members of the GDNF family are secreted disulfide-bonded homodimers that are distant relatives of TGFβ (Lin et al., 1993; Kotzbauer et al., 1996; Baloh et al., 1998; Milbrandt et al., 1998; Masure et al., 1999; Rosenblad et al., 2000). The three-dimensional structure of GDNF has been determined at high resolution (Eigenbrot and Gerber, 1997). This structural information has made it possible to identify the surface residues in GDNF that are responsible for mediating interactions with GFRα1. The structural information has guided experiments in which domains are swapped between GDNF family members. Individual amino acids within domains involved in receptor interactions have been mutated to confirm their functions (Baloh et al., 2000b; Eketjall et al., 1999).

The GFRα family (GFRα1–4) consists of four glycosylphosphatidylinositol (GPI)-anchored membrane proteins that bind preferentially to GDNF, neurturin, artemin, and persephin, respectively (Airaksinen et al., 1999; Scott and Ibanez, 2001). Although each member of this family has a single preferred ligand, several have been shown to bind to additional members of the GFRα family with lower affinity. While association of a GFRα receptor with c-ret is promoted by ligand engagement (Treanor et al., 1996), in the absence of ligand some of the GFRα receptors also interact with c-ret with lower affinities (Sanicola et al., 1997; Eketjall et al., 1999). Association between a GFRα subunit and c-ret has been shown to broaden the ligand-binding ability of the complex (Sanicola et al., 1997). For example, some mutants of GDNF are defective in binding to GFRα1 and are able to bind and activate signaling in cells that express both GFRα1 and c-ret (Eketjall et al., 1999).

When first isolated, clones of GFRα1 were shown to encode a 461 amino acid long protein that includes a cleavable signal sequence. The presence of a C-terminal hydrophobic sequence without any C-terminal hydrophilic region, preceded by a group of three small amino acids, defined a cleavage and recognition site for possible addition of a glycosylphosphatidylinositol (GPI)-linked membrane anchor (Jing et al., 1996; Treanor et al., 1996). GFRα1 was shown to be associated with the membrane from which it was released by phosphatidylinositol-specific phospholipase C. The presence of GFRα1 was essential for autophosphorylation of c-ret by GDNF. Interestingly, both soluble and membrane-attached GFRα1 were effective in mediating GDNF-promoted c-ret autophosphorylation, suggesting that GFRα receptors can act in *trans*. Each of the other members of the GFRα family has subsequently been shown to have similar properties (Buj-Bello et al., 1997; Thompson et al., 1998). In addition, transcription of the mouse GFRα4 gene generates interesting developmentally regulated and tissue-specific splice variants, several of which are predicted to result in expression of secreted soluble proteins and one of which is predicted to generate a *trans*-membrane isoform (Lindahl et al., 2000). Splice variants predicted to result in expression of both GPI-attached and secreted receptors have also been reported in rat and human tissues (Masure et al., 2000; Lindahl et al., 2001). The functional importance of these variants has not yet been investigated.

In initial characterizations, the extracellular domains of GFRα subunits were observed to be cysteine-rich. In subsequent analyses, three domains in the extracellular portions of the GFRα receptors have been defined (Lindahl et al., 2000; Scott and Ibanez, 2001). The central domain, which is the most conserved, has been shown to determine ligand-binding specificity for GDNF and for neurturin. Because there are different crucial ligand-binding determinants for these two trophic factors, it was possible to construct a GFRα1–GFRα2 chimeric receptor that binds both ligands with similar efficiency (Scott and Ibanez, 2001). Although GFRα1–3 in mammals and GFRα1–4 in chick share these three domains, the mouse, rat, and human GFRα4 receptors lack the most N-terminal cysteine-rich domain (Lindahl et al., 2000, 2001; Masure et al., 2000; Zhou et al., 2001). None of the splice variants of GFRα4 alter the central domain.

RET was originally identified as an oncogene activated by fusion of a tyrosine kinase domain to other proteins (Takahashi et al., 1985). When first sequenced, the protooncogene c-ret appeared to be a receptor tyrosine kinase that contained a cleavable signal sequence, an approximately 600 amino acid extracellular domain, a transmembrane domain, and a cytoplasmic domain with a tyrosine kinase plus several tyrosines that could potentially serve after phosphorylation as recruitment sites for signaling proteins (Takahashi et al., 1988, 1989) (Fig. 35–1). C-ret was unusual because it lacked the immunoglobu-

lin, leucine-rich repeats and the fibronectin-type III repeats that are present in the extracellular domains of other members of the receptor tyrosine kinase family (Schneider, 1992; Iwamoto et al., 1993). In addition, differential splicing 3' of exon 19 generates short (9 a.a.), medium (43 a.a.), and long (51 a.a.) isoforms of the cytoplasmic domain, all of which contain a functional tyrosine kinase but differ in their docking sequences for adapter proteins (Tahira et al., 1990; Lorenzo et al., 1995, 1997). Of these, only the short and long isoforms are expressed at significant levels in vivo.

Initial analyses indicated that the approximately 600 amino acid long extracellular domain lacked homology to known proteins. Subsequent analysis, though, indicated the presence of conserved repeats homologous in position and sequence to the Ca^{2+}-binding domains of cadherins (Schneider, 1992; Hill et al., 2001). Recent molecular modeling of the extracellular domain of c-ret has confirmed the presence of four cadherin-like domains, followed by a cysteine-rich, membrane-proximal domain that is similar to the membrane-proximal domain of the cadherin-related protein flamingo (Anders et al., 2001). Similar to cadherins, c-ret binds Ca^{2+}, and the presence of Ca^{2+} is essential for crosslinking of ^{125}I-GDNF to c-ret, but not to GFRα1, on cells that express both receptor subunits (Anders et al., 2001). This suggested that Ca^{2+} stabilizes the structure of the c-ret extracellular domain. The presence of Ca^{2+} is also essential for surface expression of c-ret, suggesting that Ca^{2+} is essential for stabilization of c-ret inside the endoplasmic reticulum (van Weering et al., 1998). Since GFRα and GDNF homologs have not been identified in the *Drosophila* genome, c-ret may have evolved from a cell adhesion molecule.

Although GDNF family ligands provide the most direct pathway for activation through GFRα subunits of c-ret, an alternative pathway has recently been described in neurons that coexpress trkA, a receptor tyrosine kinase that is activated by nerve growth factor (NGF) (Tsui-Pierchala et al., 2002). Mature sympathetic neurons have lost their dependence on NGF for survival, but they continue to require it for process outgrowth and differentiation. NGF-mediated activation of TrkA results in delayed phosphorylation of c-ret in mature sympathetic neurons both in vitro and in vivo (Tsui-Pierchala et al., 2002). Only the long isoform Ret51, not the short isoform Ret9, is phosphorylated in response to NGF. Optimal responses to NGF in vitro by these neurons depends on c-ret, but not on the GFRα subunit function. Thus, in some neurons NGF transactivates the long isoform of c-ret, which, in turn, facilitates the normal maturation of these cells. The mechanism by which this occurs is not known, but the slow kinetics of c-ret phosphorylation suggest that trkA does not directly phosphorylate c-ret.

SIGNALING ACTIVATED BY C-RET

Because of its important roles in normal development and in oncogenesis, signaling pathways regulated by c-ret and oncogenic ret variants have been intensely studied and are frequently reviewed (van Weering and Bos, 1998; Mason, 2000; Saarma, 2000; Manie et al., 2001; Takahashi, 2001). Ligand engagement of a GFRα receptor in cells that also express c-ret results in dimerization and activation of the c-ret tyrosine kinase activity. Immediate substrates of this kinase include six tyrosines in the c-ret cytoplasmic domain (Liu et al., 1996) (Fig. 35–1). Of these, four tyrosines (Y-905, Y-1015, Y-1062, Y-1096) have been shown to provide docking sites for cytoplasmic signaling proteins (Hayashi et al., 2000; Coulpier et al., 2002). Phosphorylated Y905 has been shown to provide a docking site for Grb7 and Grb10 (Pandey et al., 1995, 1996). It is not certain what roles the Grb7/10/14 family of adaptor proteins play in c-ret-mediated signaling, but these proteins have been shown to regulate cell migration and survival (Han et al., 2001). Recent work, for example, indicates that Grb10 functions as a coactivator of Akt (Jahn et al., 2002). Y-1096 is present in the long, but not in the short or middle, isoforms of c-ret and has been shown to provide a docking site for the adaptor Grb2 (Liu et al., 1996). Recruitment of Grb2 provides a potential mechanism for activation of the PI3 kinase–Akt and Ras–Map kinase pathways.

Phosphorylated Y-1015 mediates docking of PLCγ1, which is activated by phosphorylation and then acts to hydrolyze phosphatidy-

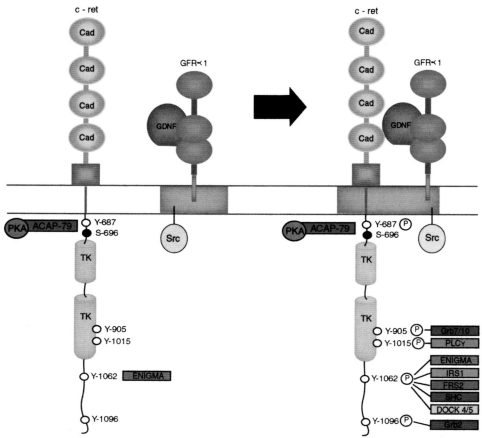

Figure 35–1. Interactions of GDNF with GFRα1 and c-ret. Depicted on the left is GDNF binding to GFRα1 that is preferentially localized in cholesterol and sphingolipid-rich lipid rafts. GDNF binding to GFRα1 results in activation of src-family tyrosine kinases that are also present in lipid rafts. Downstream signaling events (not shown) include activation of MAP kinase, CREB, and phospholipase-C. Shown also in the left panel is c-ret attached to two proteins—ACAP and ENIGMA—that associate with this receptor irrespective of its activation state. ACAP provides a docking site for protein kinase A that has been shown to phosphorylate S-696, thereby regulating signaling through Y-687. Depicted on the right is the recruitment by the GDNF–GFRα1 complex of c-ret to the lipid raft. Recruitment of c-ret results in activation of its tyrosine kinase and phosphorylation of several tyrosines in its cytoplasmic domain. Phosphorylation of Y-905 results in recruitment of two adapters Grb7 and Grb10 that activate poorly characterized downstream signaling pathways. Phosphorylation of Y-1015 permits recruitment and activation of phospholipase-Cγ1. Activation of PLC results in increased cytoplasmic Ca²⁺ and activation of Ca²⁺- and diacylglycerol-regulated protein kinases. Phosphorylation of Y-1062 results in recruitment of several different adaptors, including IRS1, FRS2, Shc, Dok4, and Dok5. These adaptors have been shown to activate several intracellular signaling pathways, including cascades controlled by Ras, Erk-1/2, Erk-5, PI3 kinase, and rac (see text for details). Phosphorylation of Y-1096 permits recruitment of Grb2 and results in activation of ras through SOS. Localization of c-ret in lipid rafts has been shown to promote the recruitment of FRS2. Localization of c-ret to rafts is essential for normal activation of several of the signaling pathways summarized above and described in more detail in the text.

linositides to generate inositol *tris*-phosphate and diacylglycerol. Inositol *tris*-phosphate induces release of Ca^{2+} stores, increasing levels of cytoplasmic Ca^{2+}. This results in activation of the various enzymes that are regulated by cytoplasmic Ca^{2+}, including Ca^{2+}-calmodulin-regulated protein kinases and phosphatases and Ca^{2+}-regulated isoforms of protein kinase C. Formation of diacylglycerol (DAG) stimulates the activities of DAG-regulated isoforms of protein kinase C. One of these DAG-regulated isoforms, PKCδ, is required for activation of the mitogen activated protein kinase (ERK) cascade and ERK-dependent differentiation in many neuronal cells (Corbit et al., 1999, 2000). It appears to act between Raf and MEK in the ERK signaling cascade. Activation of PLCγ1 through Y-1015 is essential to observe the full oncogenic and proliferative activities of ret (Borrello et al., 1996).

By far the most important mediator of signaling by c-ret appears to be Y-1062 (Fig. 35–1). Interestingly, while Y-1062 is present in the long, medium, and short isoforms of c-ret, splicing introduces different sequences immediately 3′ of the codon for Y-1062, so the amino acid sequence immediately C-terminal of Y-1062 differs between the RET 9, RET 43, and RET 51 isoforms, thus providing the potential for differential recognition of signaling proteins at this site (Tahira et al., 1990; Myers et al., 1995; Lorenzo et al., 1997). The presence of Y-1062 is required for the oncogenic and proliferative activities of c-ret isoforms (Melillo et al., 2001b). The signaling pathways activated by phosphorylation of this site are extensive and include the Ras, PI3 kinase, Jun kinase, p38MAP kinase, Erk-1/2 and Erk-5 kinases, and Rac (Hayashi et al., 2001; Fukuda et al., 2002). Depending on cell type, phosphorylation of this site promotes cell survival, proliferation, differentiation, motility, or oncogenesis. When phosphorylated, this site has been shown to recruit several different adaptor proteins, including IRS1, FRS2, Shc, Dok4 and Dok5 (Arighi et al., 1997; Hayashi et al., 2000; Grimm et al., 2001; Melillo et al., 2001a, 2001b). Shc recruitment provides pathways through Grb2 and the Ras exchange factor SOS (son of sevenless) for activation of Ras. Activation of Ras by SOS has many downstream consequences, including stimulation of PI3 kinase, activation of the c-raf/ERK pathway, and stimulation of the p38MAP kinase pathway (Xing et al., 1998).

Alternatively, Shc recruitment of Grb2 has also been shown to promote association of the adapter Gab1, which, in turn, binds and facilitates activation through phosphorylation of PI3 kinase and the downstream signaling pathways. Recruited IRS1 has been shown to associate directly with, thereby facilitating, activation of PI3 kinase

(Melillo et al., 2001a). FRS2 recruitment and phosphorylation provides multiple docking sites for the Grb2–SOS complex, thereby promoting activation of RAS, the ERKs, and PI3 kinase (Melillo et al., 2001b). FRS2 also provides a site for recruitment of Crk that, in turn, recruits the exchange factor C3G, thereby activating the small G protein Rap1 (York et al., 2000). This provides a mechanism for activation of B-raf and the ERKs that does not depend on Ras. Because Rap1 is localized to endosomes, efficient activation of this pathway appears to require endocytosis of ligand–receptor complexes (York et al., 2000; Howe et al., 2001). In PC-12 cells, FRS2-mediated signaling has been shown to be essential for the prolonged activation of the ERK cascade that is required to promote differentiation of these cells (Grewal et al., 1999; York et al., 2000). FRS2 also provides a docking site for the tyrosine phosphatase Shp2 (Hadari et al., 1998). Shp2 has been shown to enhance activation of the Ras-Raf-MEK-ERK pathway by a mechanism that is not clear. Gab1 also has been shown to nucleate formation of a complex that includes Shp2 (Shi et al., 2000).

P62^{dok} is an adaptor protein that has been shown to associate with several receptor tyrosine kinases. P62^{dok} also associates with RasGAP and has been shown to inhibit ERK kinase activation. There are at least five dok homologs that associate with c-ret in a two-hybrid assay (Grimm et al., 2001). Two of these, dok4 and dok5, are novel. Association of these adaptors with c-ret depends on phosphorylation of Y-1062. In contrast to p62^{dok}, these two adaptors do not interact with RasGAP, and overexpression enhances rather than inhibits ERK activation. Ligand engagement of c-ret in PC-12 cells results in neurite outgrowth that requires Y-1062. Fusion of sequences from either dok4 or dok5, but not dok2, to a mutated c-ret lacking Y-1062 also permits GDNF-dependent neurite outgrowth by PC-12 cells (Grimm et al., 2001). The same fusions also are able to mediate GDNF-dependent survival of these cells in a serum-free medium. Thus these two adaptors are likely to be important in mediating neuronal responses to GDNF and its family members.

The differentiation-promoting responses observed in PC-12 cells and neurons differ fundamentally from the proliferative responses observed in other cells. Clearly, responses to c-ret activation are cell-type specific, depending on the repertoires of the intracellular signaling proteins that are present in different cell types. Responses of different cell types to neurotrophins also depend on cell type, with some cells showing proliferative and others differentiative responses (Huang and Reichardt, 2001). Among other targets of probable importance for promoting differentiation, activation of c-ret has been shown to up-regulate the cyclin-dependent kinase inhibitor p27^{kip1} (Baldassarre et al., 2002).

In addition to classical adaptors, the Y-1062 site is also essential for recruiting a PDZ protein named ENIGMA (Durick et al., 1996, 1998). ENIGMA is an interesting protein that consists of an N-terminal PDZ domain plus three Lim domains, one of which associates specifically with c-ret in an interaction that depends on Y-1062. This interaction does not depend on phosphorylation of this tyrosine, however. While the function of ENIGMA in c-ret signaling is uncertain, it is essential for the mitogenic activity of a cAMP-dependent kinase RIα–c-ret fusion protein named Ret/Ptc2 that causes papillary thyroid carcinoma (Durick et al., 1998). ENIGMA is believed to promote mitogenesis and oncogenesis by localizing Ret/Ptc2 to the membrane through its PDZ domain. Since Y-1062 is essential for recruitment of adaptors, such as Shc, that are essential for the mitogenic and oncogenic activities of Ret/Ptc2, dimerization is essential not only to activate the tyrosine kinase activity but also to permit simultaneous localization of Ret/Ptc2 to the membrane through ENIGMA and recruitment of these adaptors. Because Y-1062 recruits so many different adaptors, which, in turn, nucleate formation of different signaling complexes that affect cell function, it will be a major challenge for future scientists to understand the factors that bias c-ret-mediated signaling responses into specific pathways, such as proliferation versus differentiation.

The protein kinase A–anchoring protein ACAP-79 also associated with c-ret in a ligand-independent manner (Fukuda et al., 2002). ACAP-79 provides a high-affinity docking site for the type II regulatory subunit of cAMP-dependent protein kinase. In response to cAMP, S-696 in the cytoplasmic domain of c-ret is phosphorylated, and phosphorylation at this site promotes a guanine nucleotide exchange factor activity for Rac-1 and promotes lamellipodia formation in the presence of GDNF. Mutation of S-696 or Y-1062 decreases Rac-1 guanine nucleotide exchange factor activity, but mutation of Y-687 rescues the phenotype of the S-696 mutation. These data suggest that guanine nucleotide exchange factor activity is promoted by signals depend on phosphorylation of Y-1062, but is inhibited by a signal that emanates from phosphorylated Y-687. cAMP-dependent phosphorylation of S-696 prevents signaling from phosphorylated Y-687. These data illuminate a novel mechanism through which cAMP regulates a tyrosine kinase–mediated signaling pathway.

SIGNALING THROUGH GFRα SUBUNITS

GFRα subunits function in large part as binding partners for GDNF family ligands. Initially, GFRα subunits were believed to only function as binding subunits of the c-ret receptor complex. However, recent work has demonstrated that these subunits have broader and more direct roles in mediating signaling by GDNF (Saarma, 2001). Among other functions, the presence of a GFRα subunit appears to inhibit basal activation of the c-ret kinase in the absence of physiological ligands (Trupp et al., 1998). Since inhibition has only been observed in COS cells in which c-ret was overexpressed alone or in combination with a GFRα subunit, the physiological significance of this observation is uncertain.

Similar to other GPI-anchored membrane proteins, GFRα subunits are preferentially localized to cholesterol and sphingolipid-rich lipid rafts (Poteryaev et al., 1999; Trupp et al., 1999), where src-family kinases are also concentrated (Lee et al., 2001). GDNF application to cells expressing GFRα1, but not c-ret, has been shown to activate src kinase (Trupp et al., 1999). In turn, GFRα1-mediated src kinase promotes phosphorylation of MAP kinase, CREB, and phospholipase-Cγ1 (Trupp et al., 1998; Poteryaev et al., 1999). Activation of the pathways through GFRα1 alone is much less prolonged than activation through c-ret (Trupp et al., 1998), but since many cells express GFRα subunits that do not coexpress c-ret, this signaling pathway probably has physiological consequences. A recent report suggests that ligand engagement of GFRα2 does not activate the signaling pathways that are activated by ligand engagement of GFRα1 in the absence of c-ret (Pezeshki et al., 2001), so it is not certain that c-ret-independent signaling is promoted by all four of the GFRα subunits.

One of the most important functions of ligand-bound GFRα subunits now appears to be recruitment of c-ret to lipid rafts, where it acquires new signaling properties. Disruption of the specialized lipid raft domains by cholesterol depletion has been shown to severely attenuate c-ret-dependent GDNF signaling (Tansey et al., 2000). GDNF binding to the GFRα1 subunit results in relocalization of c-ret from the bulk membrane to the detergent-resistant lipid raft domain (Tansey et al., 2000). In this specialized domain, c-ret interacts with signaling proteins that it does not associate with outside of the rafts. For example, c-ret outside of rafts is found in association with Shc, but not FRS2, while the c-ret in rafts is preferentially associated with FRS2, but not Shc (Paratcha et al., 2001). In addition, raft-associated c-ret interacts with and activates c-src, but not other src-related tyrosine kinases. Despite the theoretical existence of other pathways to PI3 kinase through Y-1062, c-src is essential in neurons for activation of the PI3 kinase–Akt pathway and GDNF-dependent survival and neurite outgrowth (Tansey et al., 2000; Encinas et al., 2001). Intriguingly, both soluble and membrane-tethered GFRα subunits are able to recruit c-ret to lipid rafts and potentiate downstream signaling by GDNF (Paratcha et al., 2001). The mechanism by which ligand-bound GFRα in *trans* recruits c-ret to rafts is not certain, but it must differ from the mechanism through which ligand-bound, membrane-tethered GFRα subunits recruit c-ret in *cis*, because *trans* recruitment requires an active c-ret kinase, while *cis*-recruitment does not. Since GFRα subunits have been shown to be released from cells that do not express c-ret (Trupp et al., 1997; Yu et al., 1998; Worley et al., 2000; Paratcha et al., 2001), the ability of a ligand-bound GFRα subunit to promote activation and localization of c-ret to lipid rafts is very likely to be biologically important.

FUNCTIONS OF GDNF FAMILY-MEDIATED SIGNALING PATHWAYS

GDNF is strongly expressed in the developing gut (Moore et al., 1996). In GDNF, GFRα1, and c-ret mutants, enteric neurons fail to populate the intestine, and only a few of these neurons are present in the stomach and esophagus (Schuchardt et al., 1994; Durbec et al., 1996b; Moore et al., 1996; Pichel et al., 1996; Sanchez et al., 1996; Cacalano et al., 1998; Enomoto et al., 1998). The phenotypes of these mice are similar to, but more severe than, those of humans with Hirschsprung disease in which deficits in enteric neuron populations in the lower intestine result in intestinal obstruction (Edery et al., 1997; Gabriel et al., 2002). Indeed, Hirschsprung disease is often associated with heterozygous mutations that result in deficits in signaling through c-ret or components of the c-ret signaling pathway (Edery et al., 1994; Romeo et al., 1994; Amiel et al., 1996; Attie et al., 1996; Kusafuka and Puri, 1998; Parisi and Kapur, 2000; Gabriel et al., 2002). Mice heterozygous for GDNF have been shown to have frequent obstructions of the lower intestine that result in very high levels of postnatal lethality (Shen et al., 2002), and some humans with Hirschsprung disease also have mutations in GDNF (Eketjall and Ibanez, 2002).

The GDNF to c-ret signaling pathway appears to act at many steps in differentiation of the enteric nervous system (Gershon, 1998; Pachnis et al., 1998). A pool of neural crest cells from the hindbrain gives rise to most of the enteric nervous system. In the absence of GDNF signaling, there are deficits in the initial appearance of these cells in the gut anlage, reflecting defects in migration, as well as increases in apoptosis of this pool (Durbec et al., 1996b; Taraviras et al., 1999). In culture and in intestinal explants, GDNF and neurturin have been shown to promote survival, proliferation, and differentiation of enteric neuron precursors (Hearn et al., 1998; Heuckeroth et al., 1998; Taraviras et al., 1999). Localized extrinsic sources of GDNF also attract these cells in what is most likely a chemotropic response (Young et al., 2001). Activation of the PI3 kinase/Akt pathway has been shown to be essential for the proliferative response of quail enteric precursors (Focke et al., 2001). In transplantation experiments it has been possible to show that c-ret-expressing neural precursors can invade the gut and populate it efficiently from a c-ret mutant embryo, demonstrating that the GDNF to c-ret pathway is required in the neural crest–derived progenitor cells and not in the nonneural cells of the developing gut (Natarajan et al., 1999). Intriguingly, with development, enteric precursors shift from a proliferative to a trophic and differentiative response to GDNF (Worley et al., 2000). At later stages of development, c-ret expression is restricted to a population of enteric precursors that is committed to differentiate into neurons (Lo and Anderson, 1995).

Interestingly, the short and long isoforms of c-ret differ in their abilities to support development of the enteric nervous system (de Graaff et al., 2001). By targeted exon deletion, mice have been generated that only express the short or long isoform. Animals that express RET51, but not RET9, lack enteric neurons in the colon, while animals that only express RET9 appear completely normal. During development, enteric neural precursors expressing only RET51 never populate the distal gut. This is not simply because they migrate more slowly than normal precursors. The same deficit is observed in organ cultures of the embryonic gut in which the overall growth and elongation of the gut is quite limited. Consequently, the observations suggest that there are differences in the signaling required to permit invasion of the proximal and distal segments of the gut.

Absence of signaling by GDNF family members also results in deficits in additional neuronal populations, including sensory, motor, and autonomic populations (Moore et al., 1996; Sanchez et al., 1996; Heuckeroth et al., 1999; Nishino et al., 1999; Rossi et al., 1999, 2000; Enomoto et al., 2000, 2001; Laurikainen et al., 2000; Hashino et al., 2001). Analyses of targeted mutants have demonstrated survival requirements for c-ret, two of the GDNF family members, and three of

the GFRα subunits. GDNF family members can be transported retrogradely from targets (Leitner et al., 1999) and can function as target-derived trophic factors, similar to nerve growth factor (Oppenheim et al., 1995; Hashino et al., 2001).

In addition, c-ret signaling has been shown to be required for migration of neural precursors of sympathetic neurons (Enomoto et al., 2001). As a result, the superior cervical ganglion is misplaced in both the GFRα3 and c-ret mutants (Nishino et al., 1999; Enomoto et al., 2001). Deficits in neuronal number and delays in neuronal differentiation are seen throughout the sympathetic chain in the c-ret mutant (Enomoto et al., 2001). In addition, sympathetic axons are misrouted, almost certainly because the axons fail to respond to artemin. Artemin is expressed in the vasculature that provides an initial guidance cue for these axons and has been shown to be chemotropic for these axons in vitro. In both wild-type and mutant embryos, almost all cell death in sympathetic ganglia occurs after down-regulation of c-ret expression. In the mutant, there is a similar elevation in cell death in both c-ret-expressing and non-expressing neurons. As a result, the elevated cell death observed in the mutant has been attributed to failure of neurons to contact sources of other trophic factors. It does not appear to be caused by direct dependence on artemin or other members of the GDNF family.

Both GDNF and neurturin are required for normal development of several parasympathetic ganglia, with GDNF required early and neurturin later in development (Enomoto et al., 2000; Rossi et al., 2000; Hashino et al., 2001). The sequential requirement for GDNF and neurturin correlates with changes in their expression in target tissues and with changes in expression of the GFRα1 and GFRα2 receptors in the neurons that innervate these tissues (Rossi et al., 2000; Hashino et al., 2001).

In addition to these striking effects on development of sympathetic and parasympathetic neurons, GDNF mutants have been shown to have deficits in both neural crest–derived and placode-derived sensory ganglia (Moore et al., 1996; Sanchez et al., 1996). It is not certain whether these deficits reflect a requirement for trophic factor support by either neural precursors or mature neurons, or both.

GDNF also regulates the survival of motor and autonomic neurons in the spinal cord. In the GDNF mutant, deficits were seen in some, but not all, cranial motor nuclei and in motor neurons in the spinal cord (Moore et al., 1996). Because there are distinct profiles of GFRα subunit expression in various motor neuron populations, it has seemed attractive to imagine that different muscles express different GDNF family members that provide trophic support for specific populations of motor neurons (Mikaels et al., 2000). Absence of GDNF or GFRα1 has been shown to result in selective loss of defined subpopulations of motor neurons that express GFRα1 and c-ret (Garces et al., 2000; Oppenheim et al., 2000). Interestingly, no deficits were observed in GFRα2 mutants (Garces et al., 2000). In zebrafish, GFRα1 is expressed in a specific primary motor neuron, CaP, while GDNF is expressed specifically in the muscle that it innervates (Shepherd et al., 2001). Ectopic expression of GDNF results in perturbations in growth by the CaP axon. Depletion of GDNF with morpholino antisense oligos did not, though, result in death or abnormal axon growth by the CaP neuron. GDNF also has been shown to prevent the death of preganglionic neurons in the intermediolateral column of the spinal cord after the removal of their target, the adrenal gland (Schober et al., 1999). Since GDNF is expressed in adrenal chromaffin cells, it is almost certainly functioning as a target-derived trophic factor.

GDNF-dependent survival of chick motor neurons depends on signaling through the PI3 kinase–Akt pathway, similar to survival of other neurons promoted by neurotrophins, such as nerve growth factor (NGF) or brain derived growth factor (BDNF) (Soler et al., 1999; Huang and Reichardt, 2001). There are differences in the essential survival pathways activated by GDNF and neurotrophins, however. In contrast to BDNF, GDNF has been shown to elevate levels of X-linked inhibitor of apoptosis (XIAP) and neuronal inhibitor of apoptosis (NAIP) proteins in motor neurons after sciatic nerve axotomy (Perrelet et al., 2002). Inhibition of NAIP or XIAP activity prevents GDNF-, but not BDNF-mediated neuroprotective effects.

The GDNF family of ligands has numerous additional effects that are of functional importance in the mature nervous system. They have been shown to protect neuronal subpopulations from excitotoxicity (Pérez-Navarro et al., 1999; Bonde et al., 2000; Gratacos et al., 2001; Marco et al., 2002). As described, they are also neuroprotective after axotomy (Perrelet et al., 2002). In cell culture they have been shown to promote synapse formation (Wang et al., 2002). In vivo, overexpression of GDNF in muscle increases the number of fibers innervated by single motor neurons and promotes constant remodeling of neuromuscular junctions (Keller-Peck et al., 2001).

Similar to neurotrophins, GDNF and its relatives have been shown to regulate expression of a variety of ion channels and receptors (Bradbury et al., 1998; Fjell et al., 1999; Brene et al., 2000; Cummins et al., 2000; Boettger et al., 2002). In some instances, GDNF appears to regulate the same channels as neurotrophins, but there are also numerous examples of differential regulation. Of potential clinical importance, GDNF has been shown to be analgesic in a model of neuropathic pain and is believed to act by regulating expression of Na^+ channels in nociceptive sensory neurons (Boucher et al., 2000). In addition to chronic effects, which are mediated largely through gene expression, GDNF has been shown to acutely regulate the activity of channels in subpopulations of neurons. For example, GDNF has been shown to potentiate the excitability of cultured midbrain dopaminergic neurons through reversible inhibition of transient A-type K^+ channels (Yang et al., 2001). GDNF activates the MAP kinase cascade in these neurons, and MAP kinase has been shown to directly phosphorylate these channels. Inhibition of the MAP kinase cascade prevents the effect of GDNF, so it is likely that phosphorylation by MAP kinase directly regulates the activity of these channels. Similar to BDNF, GDNF has been shown to enhance Ca^{2+} entry and potentiate release of acetylcholine in *Xenopus* spinal cord–skeletal muscle co-cultures (Wang et al., 2001). Long-term exposure to GDNF increases expression of a Ca^{2+}-binding protein, frequenin. Interestingly, inhibition of frequenin expression with anti-sense oligos or of its function with a specific antibody prevents the effects of GDNF on Ca^{2+} entry. Overexpression of frequenin results in a similar phenotype to that observed following GDNF application, and the response to each occludes the response to the other. Both GDNF and frequenin have been shown to increase the opening probability of N-type, but not L-type, Ca^{2+} channels. Thus GDNF acts through frequenin to regulate Ca^{2+} channel function by a mechanism that is not yet understood.

Signaling mediated by GDNF family members also is important for development outside of the nervous system. In particular, GDNF signaling through GFRα1 and c-ret is essential for normal development of the metanephric kidney where GDNF is expressed at high levels in the metanephric mesenchyme while GFRα1 and c-ret are expressed in the ureteric bud (Pachnis et al., 1993; Hellmich et al., 1996; Kreidberg, 1996; Moore et al., 1996). In the absence of any of these three proteins, the ureteric bud fails to invade and branch within the metanephric mesenchyme, so mature kidneys are absent from the vast majority of animals (Schuchardt et al., 1994, 1996; Moore et al., 1996; Pichel et al., 1996; Sanchez et al., 1996; Cacalano et al., 1998; Enomoto et al., 1998; Tomac et al., 2000). Even mice with only one copy of the GDNF gene have frequent unilateral kidney agenesis, and the average size of their kidneys is reduced by 25% with fewer nephrons and a reduced ureteric duct volume (Moore et al., 1996; Cullen-McEwen et al., 2001).

Intriguingly, despite the similarities in inductive interactions in formation of the pro, meso, and metanephric kidneys, in mice GDNF/GFRα1/c-ret signaling is essential only for development of the metanephros. Consistent with this, no deficit in pronephric kidney development is observed following GDNF depletion in zebrafish using anti-sense morpholino-oligonucleotides (Shepherd et al., 2001). In contrast, GDNF signaling through GFRα1 has been shown to be essential for normal migration of pronephric duct cell precursors in axolotl (Drawbridge et al., 2000). The observations in axolotl suggest that GDNF may contribute to pronephric development in other species, but that other factors may compensate when it is absent or present at abnormally low concentrations.

In rodents, GDNF signaling appears to regulate initial formation of the ureteric bud because application of GDNF is capable of inducing

bud formation from other regions of the wolffian duct (Sainio et al., 1997). GDNF signaling through GFRα1 and c-ret, however, is important throughout kidney development, not just during initial invasion of the ureteric bud. In organ culture, interference with GDNF signaling inhibits branching of the ureteric bud, while application of exogenous GDNF strongly promotes ureteric bud growth and branching (Vega et al., 1996; Pepicelli et al., 1997; Ehrenfels et al., 1999). Interestingly, the short and long isoforms of c-ret also differ in their abilities to support kidney development (de Graaff et al., 2001). In the presence of only RET51 the ureteric bud initiates invasion of the metanephric mesenchyme, but later steps in kidney development do not occur normally. In contrast, expression of RET9 alone supports all steps in kidney development. In the c-ret mutant background, forced expression of ligand-dependent or constitutively active RET9, but not RET51, rescues kidney development. Thus there must be differences in the essential c-ret-mediated signaling pathways at various stages of kidney development.

GDNF acts in part by stimulating and directing cell motility. GDNF has been shown to be chemotactic, attracting ureteric buds to localized sources of GDNF (Sainio et al., 1997). GDNF also stimulates the motility of kidney-derived epithelial cells (Tang et al., 1998). Some groups have observed that GDNF increases cell proliferation in the tips of the branches of the ureteric bud (Pepicelli et al., 1997). Activation of the PI3 kinase pathway is required for the responses of both kidney-derived epithelial cells and ureteric buds to GDNF (Tang et al., 2002).

Many of the growth factors and transcription factors that regulate kidney development act, at least partly, through regulation of GDNF or c-ret expression. Once the primary ureteric bud invades the metanephric mesenchyme, expression of c-ret is focused in the tips of the branches of the ureteric bud, while GDNF expression is induced in the mesenchyme surrounding these tips. Ectopic expression of c-ret throughout the ureteric bud–derived epithelia, for example, alters the normal pattern of kidney morphogenesis, possibly because inappropriately localized c-ret competes with bud-tip-localized c-ret for GDNF (Srinivas et al., 1999). Expression of GDNF or c-ret (or both) is strongly reduced in several mutants that prevent normal kidney development, such as Emx2 (Miyamoto et al., 1997), Eya1 (Xu et al., 1999), Pax2 (Brophy et al., 2001), double mutants of Hoxa11 and Hoxd11 (Patterson et al., 2001), and a double mutant of two retinoic acid receptors Rara and Rarb2 (Batourina et al., 2001). In the latter instance, c-ret expression in the ureteric bud has been shown to depend indirectly on vitamin A–mediated signaling through receptors localized in the metanephric stromal cells (Lelievre-Pegorier et al., 1998; Moreau et al., 1998; Mendelsohn et al., 1999; Batourina et al., 2001). Forced Hoxb7 promoter-driven expression of c-ret in the kidney anlage rescues kidney development in the absence of normal vitaminA–mediated signaling. Therefore, the reduction in c-ret expression clearly explains the deficits observed in vitamin A–deficient animals and in animals that lack the two retinoic acid receptors. In contrast, the domain of expression of GDNF in the intermediate mesenchyme is expanded anteriorly in double Foxc1 and Foxc2 mutants, resulting in frequent presence of duplex kidneys and double ureters (Kume et al., 2000). Expression of several genes believed to be important in kidney development, including *Wnt11*, *Wnt4*, and *Ld* (limb deformity), are down-regulated when GDNF to c-ret signaling in the kidney is inhibited through use of a Ret–Ig fusion protein (Pepicelli et al., 1997; Ehrenfels et al., 1999). By combined use of expression analysis and genetics, signaling pathways upstream and downstream of GDNF signaling are gradually being assembled.

Signaling mediated by GDNF family members is also essential for normal differentiation of other tissues. For example, GDNF and its receptors are expressed in the anlage of teeth, and GDNF has recently been shown to be essential for their normal development (de Vicente et al., 2002). In its absence, ameloblasts and odontoblasts fail to develop fully, resulting in an absence of the enamel matrix and predentin layers. Expression of GDNF, neurturin, and their receptors in skin changes in correlation with different phases of hair follicle growth and regression (Botchkareva et al., 2000). Hair follicle regression is delayed by exogenous GDNF or neurturin and is accelerated in

GFRα1$^{+/-}$ and GFRα2$^{-/-}$ mice (Botchkareva et al., 2000), indicating that these factors control the phase shift from growth to regression. As a final example of special interest, GDNF is expressed in Sertoli cells in the testes, where it is induced by follicle-stimulating hormone (Meng et al., 2000; Tadokoro et al., 2002). GDNF promotes proliferation of undifferentiated spermatogonia and decreases their sensitivity to differentiation signals. As a result, the testes of mice with one copy of a GDNF null allele are depleted in stem cell reserves, while the testes of males in which GDNF is overexpressed accumulate undifferentiated spermatogonia (Meng et al., 2000). In older mice, this results in development of malignant tumors expressing germ cell markers (Meng et al., 2001).

GDNF SIGNALING PATHWAYS AND HUMAN DISEASE

The human genetics of the GDNF signaling pathway has provided interesting insights of general interest into the anatomy of receptor tyrosine kinase signaling. This has been possible because abnormalities in this signaling pathway are associated with Hirschsprung disease, which is caused by deficiencies in signaling through this pathway, and several forms of cancer, which are associated with excessive activation of this pathway (reviewed in Hansford and Mulligan, 2000; Jhiang, 2000; Manie et al., 2001; Takahashi, 2001; Gabriel et al., 2002; McCabe, 2002; Passarge, 2002; see Chapter 36). Hirschsprung disease is a human disorder caused by failure of enteric neurons to populate the caudal intestine. Long-segment and short-segment Hirschsprung disease are distinguished by the length of intestine not populated by enteric neurons (Gabriel et al., 2002). Four classes of mutations in c-ret have been identified that are associated with Hirschsprung disease. Each reduces or compromises signaling through this receptor tyrosine kinase. One class of mutations alters important amino acid residues in the extracellular domain of c-ret that reduce c-ret maturation and transport to the surface membrane (Iwashita et al., 1996; Ito et al., 1997; Takahashi et al., 1999; Manie et al., 2001). Molecular modeling of the cadherin domains indicates that each of the amino acids mutated in this class of Hirschsprung disease is important for stabilizing the structure of a domain, so these mutations almost certainly reduce maturation and surface expression through effects on protein folding (Anders et al., 2001). Thus there is comparatively little c-ret available to be activated by GDNF family members.

Not surprisingly, the severity of Hirschsprung disease correlates inversely with the amount of mutant ret transport to the surface with the transport of mutants resulting in long-segment disease being more severely impaired than the transport of mutants giving rise to short-segment disease (Iwashita et al., 1996). A second class of mutants is located in the kinase domain of c-ret; they reduce or abolish c-ret's tyrosine kinase activity (reviewed in Takahashi, 2001). These mutations occur in conserved amino acids shared with other tyrosine kinases. Finally, two classes of mutations affect signal transduction initiated by c-ret. Several have been shown to inhibit the activation of PLCγ1. Others affect amino acid residues close to the crucial Y-1062 site and have been shown to inhibit Shc, FRS2, and IRS1 binding to this site and to impair activation of the PI3 kinase–Akt and Ras–Erk pathways (Geneste et al., 1999; Ishiguro et al., 1999; Melillo et al., 2001a, 2001b). It seems likely that they also affect binding by some of the other adaptor proteins known to recognize this site, such as Dok4 and Dok5. Thus, analysis of a genetically inherited human disease has resulted in dissection of the essential domains of a receptor tyrosine kinase.

Finally, recent work indicates that overexpression of c-ret induces apoptosis in some cells, which is suppressed by the presence of GDNF (Bordeaux et al., 2000). Overexpression of several of the mutants associated with Hirschsprung disease also promotes apoptosis, but the apoptosis induced by these mutants cannot be suppressed by GDNF. C-ret-promoted apoptosis appears to involve cleavage of the cytoplasmic domain by a caspase-dependent mechanism. The molecular details of this signaling pathway are not yet understood.

Mutations in other components of the GDNF signaling pathway may also contribute to appearance of a Hirschsprung disease phenotype (Gabriel et al., 2002). Several mutations in GDNF and neur-turin have been identified in patients with Hirschsprung disease, and some of the GDNF mutants have been shown to result in expression of a GDNF with reduced binding affinity for GFRα1 (Doray et al., 1998; Eketjall and Ibanez, 2002). While none of these alone seems likely to cause Hirschsprung disease, they may contribute to pathogenesis in collaboration with other genetic alterations. It seems possible that contributions to the Hirschsprung disease phenotype could also be made by alleles of genes encoding proteins in the c-ret signaling pathway.

Ret was first identified as an oncogene present in a human lymphoma that was the product of recombination between two unlinked DNA segments, generating a fusion protein including a tyrosine kinase (Takahashi et al., 1985; Takahashi and Cooper, 1987). Since this initial discovery, mutations or fusions of c-ret have been associated with several different types of cancer, including papillary thyroid carcinomas (PTC), multiple endocrine neoplasia type 2 (MEN2), pheochromocytoma, and parathyroid hyperplasia (Jhiang, 2000). Analysis of oncogenic forms of c-ret has identified several classes of mechanisms that render the activity of its tyrosine kinase partially or completely independent of the ligand. In the first, the cytoplasmic domain of c-ret is fused to the product of another gene, resulting in formation of a constitutively dimerized fusion protein (Takahashi et al., 1985). Eight different genes have been identified that are rearranged to form fusions with ret in PTCs (Jhiang, 2000). Approximately 5% to 30% of spontaneous papillary thyroid carcinomas are associated with gene fusions of this type. As discussed previously, proliferative and oncogenic responses by one of these fusion proteins have been shown to depend on interaction of the soluble fusion protein with the LIM and PDZ-domain-containing protein ENIGMA that relocalizes ret from the cytoplasm to the membrane (Durick et al., 1996, 1998). It seems likely that other fusion proteins of this type also require ENIGMA to promote oncogenesis efficiently.

A second type of mutation generates an unpaired cysteine in the extracellular domain of c-ret that results in the constitutive dimerization and activation of membrane-associated ret (Santoro et al., 1995). These are dominant oncogenic mutations that result in MEN2 class A disease. In at least some cases, full activation of the mutant receptor requires the presence of a GDNF ligand, indicating that dimerization alone does not create an optimal conformation for activation of the ret tyrosine kinase activity (Mograbi et al., 2001).

In the third class of mutation, an alteration in the c-ret kinase domain (M918T) increases the basal kinase activity of c-ret and alters its substrate preferences without promoting constitutive dimerization and results in MEN2 class B disease (Santoro et al., 1995; Liu et al., 1996). Ret (M918T) can be further activated by GDNF family ligands, so the pattern of expression of these ligands may contribute to the neoplastic phenotype. Not unexpectedly, many of the tyrosines phosphorylated in c-ret in response to GDNF application are also phosphorylated in these oncogenic ret proteins, including notably Y-1062 (Liu et al., 1996). Phosphorylation of Y-1096 is not observed in the MEN2B mutant (M918T), but there is increased phosphorylation of Y-1062, and a new phosphorylation site is created (Liu et al., 1996; Salvatore et al., 2001). Thus, differences in tyrosine kinase activity and substrate specificity are both thought to contribute to differences in the cancers that are associated with different ret mutations. Many studies have shown that adapters such as Shc, Grb2, FRS2, IRS1, and PLCγ1 are recruited by oncogenic mutants of Ret protein, thereby activating the Ras-Map kinase, PI3 kinase–Akt, PLC, and other signaling pathways within affected cells (Hansford and Mulligan, 2000; Jhiang, 2000; Takahashi, 2001).

CONCLUSION

GDNF and its relatives have proven to have unusually interesting signaling pathways that are important in normal development of the nervous system and other organs. Because of its involvement in both development and oncogenesis, studies have provided a model of how human genetics can contribute to an understanding of receptor function, cell biology, and disease. Characterization of mouse mutants lacking these proteins or their receptors have illuminated the diversity of mechanisms through which trophic factors regulate cell behavior and development, both inside and outside of the nervous system. These proteins have also been shown to regulate the electrical properties of neurons through control of transmitter receptors and ion channels. Because they protect neurons against a variety of toxic insults, they are strong candidates to be developed as therapeutic agents to treat Parkinson's and other diseases. Uncontrolled activity of the common receptor c-ret contributes to development of several different cancers. The signaling cascades characterized as part of the effort to understand the oncogenic activity of ret have proven to be of general interest and, in the future, may provide targets for therapeutic treatments of many cancers in addition to those involving c-ret and the GDNF signaling pathway.

ACKNOWLEDGMENTS

I wish to thank Drs. Ursula Funfschilling, Beatriz Rico, and Sam Pleasure for critical review of the manuscript. I also thank Ms. Sonia Brown for design of Figure 35–1. Work in my laboratory has been supported by grants from the National Institutes of Health and Howard Hughes Medical Institute. I am an investigator in the Howard Hughes Medical Institute.

REFERENCES

Airaksinen MS, Titievsky A, Saarma M (1999). GDNF family neurotrophic factor signaling: four masters, one servant? *Mol Cell Neurosci* 13: 313–325.

Amiel J, Attie T, Jan D, Pelet A, Edery P, Bidaud C, Lacombe D, Tam P, Simeoni J, Flori E, et al. (1996). Heterozygous endothelin receptor B (EDNRB) mutations in isolated Hirschsprung disease. *Hum Mol Genet* 5: 355–357.

Anders J, Kjar S, Ibanez CF (2001). Molecular modeling of the extracellular domain of the RET receptor tyrosine kinase reveals multiple cadherin-like domains and a calcium-binding site. *J Biol Chem* 276: 35808–35817.

Arighi E, Alberti L, Torriti F, Ghizzoni S, Rizzetti MG, Pelicci G, Pasini B, Bongarzone I, Piutti C, Pierotti MA, Borrello MG (1997). Identification of Shc docking site on Ret tyrosine kinase. *Oncogene* 14: 773–782.

Attie T, Amiel J, Jan D, Edery P, Pelet A, Salomon R, Munnich A, Lyonnet S, Nihoul-Fekete C (1996). [Genetics of Hirschsprung disease]. *Ann Chir* 50: 538–541.

Baldassarre G, Bruni P, Boccia A, Salvatore G, Melillo RM, Motti ML, Napolitano M, Belletti B, Fusco A, Santoro M, Viglietto G (2002). Glial cell line-derived neurotrophic factor induces proliferative inhibition of NT2/D1 cells through RET-mediated up-regulation of the cyclin-dependent kinase inhibitor p27(kip1). *Oncogene* 21: 1739–1749.

Baloh RH, Tansey MG, Lampe PA, Fahrner TJ, Enomoto H, Simburger KS, Leitner ML, Araki T, Johnson EM Jr, Milbrandt J (1998). Artemin, a novel member of the GDNF ligand family, supports peripheral and central neurons and signals through the GFRα3-RET receptor complex. *Neuron* 21: 1291–1302.

Baloh RH, Enomoto H, Johnson EM Jr, Milbrandt J (2000a). The GDNF family ligands and receptors: implications for neural development. *Curr Opin Neurobiol* 10: 103–110.

Baloh RH, Tansey MG, Johnson EM Jr, Milbrandt J (2000b). Functional mapping of receptor specificity domains of glial cell line-derived neurotrophic factor (GDNF) family ligands and production of GFRα1 RET-specific agonists. *J Biol Chem* 275: 3412–3420.

Batourina E, Gim S, Bello N, Shy M, Clagett-Dame M, Srinivas S, Costantini F, Mendelsohn C (2001). Vitamin A controls epithelial/mesenchymal interactions through Ret expression. *Nat Genet* 27: 74–78.

Bennett DL (2001). Neurotrophic factors: important regulators of nociceptive function. *Neuroscientist* 7: 13–17.

Boettger MK, Till S, Chen MX, Anand U, Otto WR, Plumpton C, Trezise DJ, Tate SN, Bountra C, Coward K, et al. (2002). Calcium-activated potassium channel SK1- and IK1-like immunoreactivity in injured human sensory neurones and its regulation by neurotrophic factors. *Brain* 125: 252–263.

Bonde C, Kristensen BW, Blaabjerg M, Johansen TE, Zimmer J, Meyer M (2000). GDNF and neublastin protect against NMDA-induced excitotoxicity in hippocampal slice cultures. *Neuroreport* 11: 4069–4073.

Bordeaux MC, Forcet C, Granger L, Corset V, Bidaud C, Billaud M, Bredesen DE, Edery P, Mehlen P (2000). The RET proto-oncogene induces apoptosis: a novel mechanism for Hirschsprung disease. *EMBO J* 19: 4056–4063.

Borrello MG, Alberti L, Arighi E, Bongarzone I, Battistini C, Bardelli A, Pasini B, Piutti C, Rizzetti MG, Mondellini P, et al. (1996). The full oncogenic activity of Ret/ptc2 depends on tyrosine 539, a docking site for phospholipase Cγ. *Mol Cell Biol* 16: 2151–2163.

Botchkareva NV, Botchkarev VA, Welker P, Airaksinen M, Roth W, Suvanto P, Muller-Rover S, Hadshiew IM, Peters C, Paus R (2000). New roles for glial cell line-derived neurotrophic factor and neurturin: involvement in hair cycle control. *Am J Pathol* 156: 1041–1053.

Boucher TJ, Okuse K, Bennett DL, Munson JB, Wood JN, McMahon SB (2000). Potent analgesic effects of GDNF in neuropathic pain states. *Science* 290: 124–127.

Bradbury EJ, Burnstock G, McMahon SB (1998). The expression of P2X3 purinoceptors in sensory neurons: effects of axotomy and glial-derived neurotrophic factor. *Mol Cell Neurosci* 12: 256–268.

Brene S, Messer C, Okado H, Hartley M, Heinemann SF, Nestler EJ (2000). Regulation of GluR2 promoter activity by neurotrophic factors via a neuron-restrictive silencer element. *Eur J Neurosci* 12: 1525–1533.

Brophy PD, Ostrom L, Lang KM, Dressler GR (2001). Regulation of ureteric bud outgrowth by Pax2-dependent activation of the glial derived neurotrophic factor gene. *Development* 128: 4747–4756.

Buj-Bello A, Adu J, Pinon LG, Horton A, Thompson J, Rosenthal A, Chinchetru M, Buch-

man VL, Davies AM (1997). Neurturin responsiveness requires a GPI-linked receptor and the Ret receptor tyrosine kinase. *Nature* 387: 721–724.

Butte MJ (2001). Neurotrophic factor structures reveal clues to evolution, binding, specificity, and receptor activation. *Cell Mol Life Sci* 58: 1003–1013.

Cacalano G, Fariñas I, Wang LC, Hagler K, Forgie A, Moore M, Armanini M, Phillips H, Ryan AM, Reichardt LF, et al. (1998). GFRα1 is an essential receptor component for GDNF in the developing nervous system and kidney. *Neuron* 21: 53–62.

Corbit KC, Foster DA, Rosner MR (1999). Protein kinase Cδ mediates neurogenic but not mitogenic activation of mitogen-activated protein kinase in neuronal cells. *Mol Cell Biol* 19: 4209–4218.

Corbit KC, Soh JW, Yoshida K, Eves EM, Weinstein IB, Rosner MR (2000). Different protein kinase C isoforms determine growth factor specificity in neuronal cells. *Mol Cell Biol* 20: 5392–5403.

Coulpier M, Anders J, Ibanez CF (2002). Coordinated activation of autophosphorylation sites in the RET receptor tyrosine kinase: importance of tyrosine 1062 for GDNF mediated neuronal differentiation and survival. *J Biol Chem* 277: 1991–1999.

Cullen-McEwen LA, Drago J, Bertram JF (2001). Nephron endowment in glial cell line-derived neurotrophic factor (GDNF) heterozygous mice. *Kidney Int* 60: 31–36.

Cummins TR, Black JA, Dib-Hajj SD, Waxman SG (2000). Glial-derived neurotrophic factor upregulates expression of functional SNS and NaN sodium channels and their currents in axotomized dorsal root ganglion neurons. *J Neurosci* 20: 8754–8761.

de Graaff E, Srinivas S, Kilkenny C, D'Agati V, Mankoo BS, Costantini F, Pachnis V (2001). Differential activities of the RET tyrosine kinase receptor isoforms during mammalian embryogenesis. *Genes Dev* 15: 2433–2444.

de Vicente JC, Cabo R, Ciriaco E, Laura R, Naves FJ, Silos-Santiago I, Vega JA (2002). Impaired dental cytodifferentiation in glial cell-line derived growth factor (GDNF) deficient mice. *Ann Anat* 184: 85–92.

Doray B, Salomon R, Amiel J, Pelet A, Touraine R, Billaud M, Attie T, Bachy B, Munnich A, Lyonnet S (1998). Mutation of the RET ligand, neurturin, supports multigenic inheritance in Hirschsprung disease. *Hum Mol Genet* 7: 1449–1452.

Drawbridge J, Meighan CM, Mitchell EA (2000). GDNF and GFRα-1 are components of the axolotl pronephric duct guidance system. *Dev Biol* 228: 116–124.

Durbec P, Marcos-Gutierrez CV, Kilkenny C, Grigoriou M, Wartiowaara K, Suvanto P, Smith D, Ponder B, Costantini F, Saarma M, et al. (1996a). GDNF signalling through the Ret receptor tyrosine kinase. *Nature* 381: 789–793.

Durbec PL, Larsson-Blomberg LB, Schuchardt A, Costantini F, Pachnis V (1996b). Common origin and developmental dependence on c-ret of subsets of enteric and sympathetic neuroblasts. *Development* 122: 349–358.

Durick K, Wu RY, Gill GN, Taylor SS (1996). Mitogenic signaling by Ret/ptc2 requires association with enigma via a LIM domain. *J Biol Chem* 271: 12691–12694.

Durick K, Gill GN, Taylor SS (1998). Shc and Enigma are both required for mitogenic signaling by Ret/ptc2. *Mol Cell Biol* 18: 2298–2308.

Edery P, Lyonnet S, Mulligan LM, Pelet A, Dow E, Abel L, Holder S, Nihoul-Fekete C, Ponder BA, Munnich A (1994). Mutations of the RET proto-oncogene in Hirschsprung disease. *Nature* 367: 378–380.

Edery P, Eng C, Munnich A, Lyonnet S (1997). RET in human development and oncogenesis. *Bioessays* 19: 389–395.

Ehrenfels CW, Carmillo PJ, Orozco O, Cate RL, Sanicola M (1999). Perturbation of RET signaling in the embryonic kidney. *Dev Genet* 24: 263–272.

Eigenbrot C, Gerber N (1997). X-ray structure of glial cell–derived neurotrophic factor at 1.9 A resolution and implications for receptor binding. *Nat Struct Biol* 4: 435–438.

Eketjall S, Ibanez CF (2002). Functional characterization of mutations in the GDNF gene of patients with Hirschsprung disease. *Hum Mol Genet* 11: 325–329.

Eketjall S, Fainzilber M, Murray-Rust J, Ibanez CF (1999). Distinct structural elements in GDNF mediate binding to GFRα1 and activation of the GFRα1-c-Ret receptor complex. *EMBO J* 18: 5901–5910.

Encinas M, Tansey MG, Tsui-Pierchala BA, Comella JX, Milbrandt J, Johnson EM Jr. (2001). c-Src is required for glial cell–derived neurotrophic factor (GDNF) family ligand-mediated neuronal survival via a phosphatidylinositol-3 kinase (PI3K)-dependent pathway. *J Neurosci* 21: 1464–1472.

Enokido Y, de Sauvage F, Hongo JA, Ninkina N, Rosenthal A, Buchman VL, Davies A. M (1998). GFR α-4 and the tyrosine kinase Ret form a functional receptor complex for persephin. *Curr Biol* 8: 1019–1022.

Enomoto H, Araki T, Jackman A, Heuckeroth RO, Snider WD, Johnson EM Jr., Milbrandt J (1998). GFR α1-deficient mice have deficits in the enteric nervous system and kidneys. *Neuron* 21: 317–324.

Enomoto H, Heuckeroth RO, Golden JP, Johnson EM, Milbrandt J (2000). Development of cranial parasympathetic ganglia requires sequential actions of GDNF and neurturin. *Development* 127: 4877–4889.

Enomoto H, Crawford PA, Gorodinsky A, Heuckeroth RO, Johnson EM Jr., Milbrandt J (2001). RET signaling is essential for migration, axonal growth and axon guidance of developing sympathetic neurons. *Development* 128: 3963–3974.

Fjell J, Cummins TR, Dib-Hajj SD, Fried K, Black JA, Waxman SG (1999). Differential role of GDNF and NGF in the maintenance of two TTX-resistant sodium channels in adult DRG neurons. *Brain Res Mol Brain Res* 67: 267–282.

Focke PJ, Schiltz CA, Jones SE, Watters JJ, Epstein ML (2001). Enteric neuroblasts require the phosphatidylinositol 3-kinase pathway for GDNF-stimulated proliferation. *J Neurobiol* 47: 306–317.

Fukuda T, Kiuchi K, Takahashi M (2002). Novel mechanism of regulation of Rac activity and lamellipodia formation by RET tyrosine kinase. *J Biol Chem* 277: 19114–19121.

Gabriel SB, Salomon R, Pelet A, Angrist M, Amiel J, Fornage M, Attie-Bitach T, Olson JM, Hofstra R, Buys C, et al. (2002). Segregation at three loci explains familial and population risk in Hirschsprung disease. *Nat Genet* 31: 89–93.

Garces A, Haase G, Airaksinen MS, Livet J, Filippi P, deLapeyriere O (2000). GFRα 1 is required for development of distinct subpopulations of motoneuron. *J Neurosci* 20: 4992–5000.

Geneste O, Bidaud C, De Vita G, Hofstra RM, Tartare-Deckert S, Buys CH, Lenoir GM,

Santoro M, Billaud M (1999). Two distinct mutations of the RET receptor causing Hirschsprung disease impair the binding of signalling effectors to a multifunctional docking site. *Hum Mol Genet* 8: 1989–1999.

Gershon MD (1998). Genes, lineages, and tissue interactions in the development of the enteric nervous system. *Am J Physiol* 275: G869–873.

Goodfellow PJ (1994). Inherited cancers associated with the RET proto-oncogene. *Curr Opin Genet Dev* 4: 446–452.

Gratacos E, Perez-Navarro E, Tolosa E, Arenas E, Alberch J (2001). Neuroprotection of striatal neurons against kainate excitotoxicity by neurotrophins and GDNF family members. *J Neurochem* 78: 1287–1296.

Grewal SS, York RD, Stork PJ (1999). Extracellular-signal-regulated kinase signalling in neurons. *Curr Opin Neurobiol* 9: 544–553.

Grimm J, Sachs M, Britsch S, Di Cesare S, Schwarz-Romond T, Alitalo K, Birchmeier W (2001). Novel $p62^{dok}$ family members, dok4 and dok5, are substrates of the c-Ret receptor tyrosine kinase and mediate neuronal differentiation. *J Cell Biol* 154: 345–354.

Hadari YR, Kouhara H, Lax I, Schlessinger J (1998). Binding of Shp2 tyrosine phosphatase to FRS2 is essential for fibroblast growth factor–induced PC12 cell differentiation. *Mol Cell Biol* 18: 3966–3973.

Han DC, Shen TL, Guan JL (2001). The Grb7 family proteins: structure, interactions with other signaling molecules and potential cellular functions. *Oncogene* 20: 6315–6321.

Hansford JR, Mulligan LM (2000). Multiple endocrine neoplasia type 2 and RET: from neoplasia to neurogenesis. *J Med Genet* 37: 817–827.

Hashino E, Shero M, Junghans D, Rohrer H, Milbrandt J, Johnson EM Jr. (2001). GDNF and neurturin are target-derived factors essential for cranial parasympathetic neuron development. *Development* 128: 3773–3782.

Hayashi H, Ichihara M, Iwashita T, Murakami H, Shimono Y, Kawai K, Kurokawa K, Murakumo Y, Imai T, Funahashi H, et al. (2000). Characterization of intracellular signals via tyrosine 1062 in RET activated by glial cell line-derived neurotrophic factor. *Oncogene* 19: 4469–4475.

Hayashi Y, Iwashita T, Murakamai H, Kato Y, Kawai K, Kurokawa K, Tohnai I, Ueda M, Takahashi M (2001). Activation of BMK1 via tyrosine 1062 in RET by GDNF and MEN2A mutation. *Biochem Biophys Res Commun* 281: 682–689.

Hearn CJ, Murphy M, Newgreen D (1998). GDNF and ET-3 differentially modulate the numbers of avian enteric neural crest cells and enteric neurons in vitro. *Dev Biol* 197: 93–105.

Hellmich HL, Kos L, Cho ES, Mahon KA, Zimmer A (1996). Embryonic expression of glial cell-line derived neurotrophic factor (GDNF) suggests multiple developmental roles in neural differentiation and epithelial–mesenchymal interactions. *Mech Dev* 54: 95–105.

Heuckeroth RO, Lampe PA, Johnson EM, Milbrandt J (1998). Neurturin and GDNF promote proliferation and survival of enteric neuron and glial progenitors in vitro. *Dev Biol* 200: 116–129.

Heuckeroth RO, Enomoto H, Grider JR, Golden JP, Hanke JA, Jackman A, Molliver DC, Bardgett ME, Snider WD, Johnson EM Jr, Milbrandt J (1999). Gene targeting reveals a critical role for neurturin in the development and maintenance of enteric, sensory, and parasympathetic neurons. *Neuron* 22: 253–263.

Hill E, Broadbent ID, Chothia C, Pettitt J (2001). Cadherin superfamily proteins in *Caenorhabditis elegans* and *Drosophila melanogaster*. *J Mol Biol* 305: 1011–1024.

Howe CL, Valletta JS, Rusnak AS, Mobley WC (2001). NGF signaling from clathrin-coated vesicles: evidence that signaling endosomes serve as a platform for the Ras-MAPK pathway. *Neuron* 32: 801–814.

Huang EJ, Reichardt LF (2001). Neurotrophins: roles in neuronal development and function. *Annu Rev Neurosci* 24: 677–736.

Ishiguro Y, Iwashita T, Murakami H, Asai N, Iida K, Goto H, Hayakawa T, Takahashi M (1999). The role of amino acids surrounding tyrosine 1062 in ret in specific binding of the shc phosphotyrosine-binding domain. *Endocrinology* 140: 3992–3998.

Ito S, Iwashita T, Asai N, Murakami H, Iwata Y, Sobue G, Takahashi M (1997). Biological properties of Ret with cysteine mutations correlate with multiple endocrine neoplasia type 2A, familial medullary thyroid carcinoma, and Hirschsprung disease phenotype. *Cancer Res* 57: 2870–2872.

Iwamoto T, Taniguchi M, Asai N, Ohkusu K, Nakashima I, Takahashi M (1993). cDNA cloning of mouse ret proto-oncogene and its sequence similarity to the cadherin superfamily. *Oncogene* 8: 1087–1091.

Iwashita T, Murakami H, Asai N, Takahashi M (1996). Mechanism of ret dysfunction by Hirschsprung mutations affecting its extracellular domain. *Hum Mol Genet* 5: 1577–1580.

Jahn T, Seipel P, Urschel S, Peschel C, Duyster J (2002). Role for the adaptor protein Grb10 in the activation of Akt. *Mol Cell Biol* 22: 979–991.

Jhiang SM (2000). The RET proto-oncogene in human cancers. *Oncogene* 19: 5590–5597.

Jing S, Wen D, Yu Y, Holst PL, Luo Y, Fang M, Tamir R, Antonio L, Hu Z, Cupples R, et al. (1996). GDNF-induced activation of the ret protein tyrosine kinase is mediated by GDNFR-α, a novel receptor for GDNF. *Cell* 85: 1113–1124.

Keller-Peck CR, Feng G, Sanes JR, Yan Q, Lichtman JW, Snider WD (2001). Glial cell line–derived neurotrophic factor administration in postnatal life results in motor unit enlargement and continuous synaptic remodeling at the neuromuscular junction. *J Neurosci* 21: 6136–6146.

Klein RD, Sherman D, Ho WH, Stone D, Bennett GL, Moffat B, Vandlen R, Simmons L, Gu Q, Hongo JA, et al. (1997). A GPI-linked protein that interacts with Ret to form a candidate neurturin receptor. *Nature* 387: 717–721.

Kotzbauer PT, Lampe PA, Heuckeroth RO, Golden JP, Creedon DJ, Johnson EM, Jr, Milbrandt J (1996). Neurturin, a relative of glial-cell-line-derived neurotrophic factor. *Nature* 384: 467–470.

Kreidberg JA (1996). Gene targeting in kidney development. *Med Pediatr Oncol* 27: 445–452.

Kume T, Deng K, Hogan BL (2000). Murine forkhead/winged helix genes Foxc1 (Mf1) and Foxc2 (Mfh1) are required for the early organogenesis of the kidney and urinary tract. *Development* 127: 1387–1395.

Kusafuka T, Puri P (1998). Genetic aspects of Hirschsprung disease. *Semin Pediatr Surg* 7: 148–155.

Laurikainen A, Hiltunen JO, Thomas-Crusells J, Vanhatalo S, Arumae U, Airaksinen MS, Klinge E, Saarma M (2000). Neurturin is a neurotrophic factor for penile parasympathetic neurons in adult rat. *J Neurobiol* 43: 198–205.

Lee H, Woodman SE, Engelman JA, Volonte D, Galbiati F, Kaufman HL, Lublin DM, Lisanti MP (2001). Palmitoylation of caveolin-1 at a single site (Cys-156) controls its coupling to the c-Src tyrosine kinase: targeting of dually acylated molecules (GPI-linked, transmembrane, or cytoplasmic) to caveolae effectively uncouples c-Src and caveolin-1 (TYR-14). *J Biol Chem* 276: 35150–35158.

Leitner ML, Molliver DC, Osborne PA, Vejsada R, Golden JP, Lampe PA, Kato AC, Milbrandt J, Johnson EM Jr (1999). Analysis of the retrograde transport of glial cell line–derived neurotrophic factor (GDNF), neurturin, and persephin suggests that in vivo signaling for the GDNF family is GFRα coreceptor-specific. *J Neurosci* 19: 9322–9331.

Lelievre-Pegorier M, Vilar J, Ferrier ML, Moreau E, Freund N, Gilbert T, Merlet-Benichou C (1998). Mild vitamin A deficiency leads to inborn nephron deficit in the rat. *Kidney Int* 54: 1455–1462.

Lin LF, Doherty DH, Lile JD, Bektesh S, Collins F (1993). GDNF: a glial cell line-derived neurotrophic factor for midbrain dopaminergic neurons. *Science* 260: 1130–1132.

Lindahl M, Timmusk T, Rossi J, Saarma M, Airaksinen MS (2000). Expression and alternative splicing of mouse Gfra4 suggest roles in endocrine cell development. *Mol Cell Neurosci* 15: 522–533.

Lindahl M, Poteryaev D, Yu L, Arumae U, Timmusk T, Bongarzone I, Aiello A, Pierotti MA, Airaksinen MS, Saarma M (2001). Human glial cell line–derived neurotrophic factor receptor α 4 is the receptor for persephin and is predominantly expressed in normal and malignant thyroid medullary cells. *J Biol Chem* 276: 9344–9351.

Liu X, Vega QC, Decker RA, Pandey A, Worby CA, Dixon JE (1996). Oncogenic RET receptors display different autophosphorylation sites and substrate binding specificities. *J Biol Chem* 271: 5309–5312.

Lo L, Anderson DJ (1995). Postmigratory neural crest cells expressing c-RET display restricted developmental and proliferative capacities. *Neuron* 15: 527–539.

Lorenzo MJ, Eng C, Mulligan LM, Stonehouse TJ, Healey CS, Ponder BA, Smith DP (1995). Multiple mRNA isoforms of the human RET proto-oncogene generated by alternate splicing. *Oncogene* 10: 1377–1383.

Lorenzo MJ, Gish GD, Houghton C, Stonehouse TJ, Pawson T, Ponder BA, Smith DP (1997). RET alternate splicing influences the interaction of activated RET with the SH2 and PTB domains of Shc, and the SH2 domain of Grb2. *Oncogene* 14: 763–771.

Manie S, Santoro M, Fusco A, Billaud M (2001). The RET receptor: function in development and dysfunction in congenital malformation. *Trends Genet* 17: 580–589.

Marco S, Perez-Navarro E, Tolosa E, Arenas E, Alberch J (2002). Striatopallidal neurons are selectively protected by neurturin in an excitotoxic model of Huntington's disease. *J Neurobiol* 50: 323–332.

Mason I (2000). The RET receptor tyrosine kinase: activation, signalling and significance in neural development and disease. *Pharm Acta Helv* 74: 261–264.

Masure S, Geerts H, Cik M, Hoefnagel E, Van Den Kieboom G, Tuytelaars A, Harris S, Lesage AS, Leysen JE, Van Der Helm L, et al. (1999). Enovin, a member of the glial cell-line-derived neurotrophic factor (GDNF) family with growth promoting activity on neuronal cells: existence and tissue-specific expression of different splice variants. *Eur J Biochem* 266: 892–902.

Masure S, Cik M, Hoefnagel E, Nosrat CA, Van der Linden I, Scott R, Van Gompel P, Lesage AS, Verhasselt P, Ibanez CF, Gordon RD (2000). Mammalian GFRα-4, a divergent member of the GFRα family of coreceptors for glial cell line-derived neurotrophic factor family ligands, is a receptor for the neurotrophic factor persephin. *J Biol Chem* 275: 39427–39434.

McCabe ER (2002). Hirschsprung disease: dissecting complexity in a pathogenetic network. *Lancet* 359: 1169–1170.

Melillo RM, Carlomagno F, De Vita G, Formisano P, Vecchio G, Fusco A, Billaud M, Santoro M (2001a). The insulin receptor substrate (IRS)-1 recruits phosphatidylinositol 3-kinase to Ret: evidence for a competition between Shc and IRS1 for the binding to Ret. *Oncogene* 20: 209–218.

Melillo RM, Santoro M, Ong SH, Billaud M, Fusco A, Hadari YR, Schlessinger J, Lax I (2001b). Docking protein FRS2 links the protein tyrosine kinase RET and its oncogenic forms with the mitogen-activated protein kinase signaling cascade. *Mol Cell Biol* 21: 4177–4187.

Mendelsohn C, Batourina E, Fung S, Gilbert T, Dodd J (1999). Stromal cells mediate retinoid-dependent functions essential for renal development. *Development* 126: 1139–1148.

Meng X, Lindahl M, Hyvonen ME, Parvinen M, de Rooij DG, Hess MW, Raatikainen-Ahokas A, Sainio K, Rauvala H, Lakso M, et al. (2000). Regulation of cell fate decision of undifferentiated spermatogonia by GDNF. *Science* 287: 1489–1493.

Meng X, de Rooij DG, Westerdahl K, Saarma M, Sariola H (2001). Promotion of seminomatous tumors by targeted overexpression of glial cell line-derived neurotrophic factor in mouse testis. *Cancer Res* 61: 3267–3271.

Mikaels A, Livet J, Westphal H, De Lapeyriere O, Ernfors P (2000). A dynamic regulation of GDNF-family receptors correlates with a specific trophic dependency of cranial motor neuron subpopulations during development. *Eur J Neurosci* 12: 446–456.

Milbrandt J, de Sauvage FJ, Fahrner TJ, Baloh RH, Leitner ML, Tansey MG, Lampe PA, Heuckeroth RO, Kotzbauer PT, Simburger KS, et al. (1998). Persephin, a novel neurotrophic factor related to GDNF and neurturin. *Neuron* 20: 245–253.

Miyamoto N, Yoshida M, Kuratani S, Matsuo I, Aizawa S (1997). Defects of urogenital development in mice lacking Emx2. *Development* 124: 1653–1664.

Mograbi B, Bocciardi R, Bourget I, Juhel T, Farahi-Far D, Romeo G, Ceccherini I, Rossi B (2001). The sensitivity of activated Cys Ret mutants to glial cell line–derived neurotrophic factor is mandatory to rescue neuroectodermic cells from apoptosis. *Mol Cell Biol* 21: 6719–6730.

Moore MW, Klein RD, Fariñas I, Sauer H, Armanini M, Phillips H, Reichardt LF, Ryan AM, Carver-Moore K, Rosenthal A (1996). Renal and neuronal abnormalities in mice lacking GDNF. *Nature* 382: 76–79.

Moreau E, Vilar J, Lelievre-Pegorier M, Merlet-Benichou C, Gilbert T (1998). Regulation of c-ret expression by retinoic acid in rat metanephros: implication in nephron mass control. *Am J Physiol* 275: F938–945.

Myers SM, Eng C, Ponder BA, Mulligan LM (1995). Characterization of RET proto-oncogene 3′ splicing variants and polyadenylation sites: a novel C-terminus for RET. *Oncogene* 11: 2039–2045.

Natarajan D, Grigoriou M, Marcos-Gutierrez CV, Atkins C, Pachnis V (1999). Multipotential progenitors of the mammalian enteric nervous system capable of colonising aganglionic bowel in organ culture. *Development* 126: 157–168.

Nishino J, Mochida K, Ohfuji Y, Shimazaki T, Meno C, Ohishi S, Matsuda Y, Fujii H, Saijoh Y, Hamada H (1999). GFR α3, a component of the artemin receptor, is required for migration and survival of the superior cervical ganglion. *Neuron* 23: 725–736.

Oppenheim RW, Houenou LJ, Johnson JE, Lin LF, Li L, Lo AC, Newsome AL, Prevette DM, Wang S (1995). Developing motor neurons rescued from programmed and axotomy-induced cell death by GDNF. *Nature* 373: 344–346.

Oppenheim RW, Houenou LJ, Parsadanian AS, Prevette D, Snider WD, Shen L (2000). Glial cell line–derived neurotrophic factor and developing mammalian motoneurons: regulation of programmed cell death among motoneuron subtypes. *J Neurosci* 20: 5001–5011.

Pachnis V, Mankoo B, Costantini F (1993). Expression of the c-ret proto-oncogene during mouse embryogenesis. *Development* 119: 1005–1017.

Pachnis V, Durbec P, Taraviras S, Grigoriou M, Natarajan D (1998). Role of the RET signal transduction pathway in development of the mammalian enteric nervous system. *Am J Physiol* 275: G183–186.

Pandey A, Duan H, Di Fiore PP, Dixit VM (1995). The Ret receptor protein tyrosine kinase associates with the SH2-containing adapter protein Grb10. *J Biol Chem* 270: 21461–21463.

Pandey A, Liu X, Dixon JE, Di Fiore PP, Dixit VM (1996). Direct association between the Ret receptor tyrosine kinase and the Src homology 2-containing adapter protein Grb7. *J Biol Chem* 271: 10607–10610.

Paratcha G, Ledda F, Baars L, Coulpier M, Besset V, Anders J, Scott R, Ibanez CF (2001). Released GFRα1 potentiates downstream signaling, neuronal survival, and differentiation via a novel mechanism of recruitment of c-Ret to lipid rafts. *Neuron* 29: 171–184.

Parisi MA, Kapur RP (2000). Genetics of Hirschsprung disease. *Curr Opin Pediatr* 12: 610–617.

Passarge E (2002). Dissecting Hirschsprung disease. *Nat Genet* 31: 11–12.

Patterson LT, Pembaur M, Potter SS (2001). Hoxa11 and Hoxd11 regulate branching morphogenesis of the ureteric bud in the developing kidney. *Development* 128: 2153–2161.

Pepicelli CV, Kispert A, Rowitch DH, McMahon AP (1997). GDNF induces branching and increased cell proliferation in the ureter of the mouse. *Dev Biol* 192: 193–198.

Pérez-Navarro E, Arenas E, Marco S, Alberch J (1999). Intrastriatal grafting of a GDNF-producing cell line protects striatonigral neurons from quinolinic acid excitotoxicity in vivo. *Eur J Neurosci* 11: 241–249.

Perrelet D, Ferri A, Liston P, Muzzin P, Korneluk RG, Kato AC (2002). IAPs are essential for GDNF-mediated neuroprotective effects in injured motor neurons in vivo. *Nat Cell Biol* 4: 175–179.

Pezeshki G, Franke B, Engele J (2001). Evidence for a ligand-specific signaling through GFRα-1, but not GFRα-2, in the absence of Ret. *J Neurosci Res* 66: 390–395.

Pichel JG, Shen L, Sheng HZ, Granholm AC, Drago J, Grinberg A, Lee EJ, Huang SP, Saarma M, Hoffer BJ, et al. (1996). Defects in enteric innervation and kidney development in mice lacking GDNF. *Nature* 382: 73–76.

Poteryaev D, Titievsky A, Sun YF, Thomas-Crusells J, Lindahl M, Billaud M, Arumae U, Saarma M (1999). GDNF triggers a novel ret-independent Src kinase family-coupled signaling via a GPI-linked GDNF receptor α1. FEBS Lett 463: 63–66.

Romeo G, Ronchetto P, Luo Y, Barone V, Seri M, Ceccherini I, Pasini B, Bocciardi R, Lerone M, Kaariainen H, et al. (1994). Point mutations affecting the tyrosine kinase domain of the RET proto-oncogene in Hirschsprung disease. *Nature* 367: 377–378.

Rosenblad C, Gronborg M, Hansen C, Blom N, Meyer M, Johansen J, Dago L, Kirik D, Patel UA, Lundberg C, et al. (2000). In vivo protection of nigral dopamine neurons by lentiviral gene transfer of the novel GDNF-family member neublastin/artemin. *Mol Cell Neurosci* 15: 199–214.

Rossi J, Luukko K, Poteryaev D, Laurikainen A, Sun YF, Laakso T, Eerikainen S, Tuominen R, Lakso M, Rauvala H, et al. (1999). Retarded growth and deficits in the enteric and parasympathetic nervous system in mice lacking GFR alpha2, a functional neurturin receptor. *Neuron* 22: 243–252.

Rossi J, Tomac A, Saarma M, Airaksinen MS (2000). Distinct roles for GFRα1 and GFRα2 signalling in different cranial parasympathetic ganglia in vivo. *Eur J Neurosci* 12: 3944–3952.

Saarma M (2000). GDNF: a stranger in the TGF-β superfamily? *Eur J Biochem* 267: 6968–6971.

Saarma M (2001). GDNF recruits the signaling crew into lipid rafts. *Trends Neurosci* 24: 427–429.

Sainio K, Suvanto P, Davies J, Wartiovaara J, Wartiovaara K, Saarma M, Arumae U, Meng X, Lindahl M, Pachnis V, Sariola H (1997). Glial-cell-line-derived neurotrophic factor is required for bud initiation from ureteric epithelium. *Development* 124: 4077–4087.

Salvatore D, Melillo RM, Monaco C, Visconti R, Fenzi G, Vecchio G, Fusco A, Santoro M (2001). Increased in vivo phosphorylation of ret tyrosine 1062 is a potential pathogenetic mechanism of multiple endocrine neoplasia type 2B. *Cancer Res* 61: 1426–1431.

Sanchez MP, Silos-Santiago I, Frisen J, He B, Lira SA, Barbacid M (1996). Renal agenesis and the absence of enteric neurons in mice lacking GDNF. *Nature* 382: 70–73.

Sanicola M, Hession C, Worley D, Carmillo P, Ehrenfels C, Walus L, Robinson S, Jaworski G, Wei H, Tizard R, et al. (1997). Glial cell line–derived neurotrophic factor-dependent RET activation can be mediated by two different cell-surface accessory proteins. *Proc Natl Acad Sci USA* 94: 6238–6243.

Santoro M, Carlomagno F, Romano A, Bottaro DP, Dathan NA, Grieco M, Fusco A, Vecchio G, Matoskova B, Kraus MH, et al. (1995). Activation of RET as a dominant transforming gene by germline mutations of MEN2A and MEN2B. *Science* 267: 381–383.

Schneider R (1992). The human protooncogene ret: a communicative cadherin? *Trends Biochem Sci* 17: 468–469.

Schober A, Hertel R, Arumae U, Farkas L, Jaszai J, Krieglstein K, Saarma M, Unsicker K (1999). Glial cell line–derived neurotrophic factor rescues target-deprived sympathetic spinal cord neurons but requires transforming growth factor-β as cofactor in vivo. *J Neurosci* 19: 2008–2015.

Schuchardt A, D'Agati V, Larsson-Blomberg L, Costantini F, Pachnis V (1994). Defects in the kidney and enteric nervous system of mice lacking the tyrosine kinase receptor Ret. *Nature* 367: 380–383.

Schuchardt A, D'Agati V, Pachnis V, Costantini F (1996). Renal agenesis and hypodysplasia in ret-k-mutant mice result from defects in ureteric bud development. *Development* 122: 1919–1929.

Scott RP, Ibanez CF (2001). Determinants of ligand binding specificity in the glial cell line–derived neurotrophic factor family receptor α S. *J Biol Chem* 276: 1450–1458.

Shen L, Pichel JG, Mayeli T, Sariola H, Lu B, Westphal H (2002). Gdnf haploinsufficiency causes Hirschsprung-like intestinal obstruction and early-onset lethality in mice. *Am J Hum Genet* 70: 435–447.

Shepherd IT, Beattie CE, Raible DW (2001). Functional analysis of zebrafish GDNF. *Dev Biol* 231: 420–435.

Shi ZQ, Yu DH, Park M, Marshall M, Feng GS (2000). Molecular mechanism for the Shp-2 tyrosine phosphatase function in promoting growth factor stimulation of Erk activity. *Mol Cell Biol* 20: 1526–1536.

Soler RM, Dolcet X, Encinas M, Egea J, Bayascas JR, Comella JX (1999). Receptors of the glial cell line–derived neurotrophic factor family of neurotrophic factors signal cell survival through the phosphatidylinositol 3-kinase pathway in spinal cord motoneurons. *J Neurosci* 19: 9160–9169.

Srinivas S, Wu Z, Chen CM, D'Agati V, Costantini F (1999). Dominant effects of RET receptor misexpression and ligand-independent RET signaling on ureteric bud development. *Development* 126: 1375–1386.

Tadokoro Y, Yomogida K, Ohta H, Tohda A, Nishimune Y (2002). Homeostatic regulation of germinal stem cell proliferation by the GDNF/FSH pathway. *Mech Dev* 113: 29–39.

Tahira T, Ishizaka Y, Itoh F, Sugimura T, Nagao M (1990). Characterization of ret proto-oncogene mRNAs encoding two isoforms of the protein product in a human neuroblastoma cell line. *Oncogene* 5: 97–102.

Takahashi M (2001). The GDNF/RET signaling pathway and human diseases. *Cytokine Growth Factor Rev* 12: 361–373.

Takahashi M, Cooper GM (1987). ret transforming gene encodes a fusion protein homologous to tyrosine kinases. *Mol Cell Biol* 7: 1378–1385.

Takahashi M, Ritz J, Cooper GM (1985). Activation of a novel human transforming gene, ret, by DNA rearrangement. *Cell* 42: 581–588.

Takahashi M, Buma Y, Iwamoto T, Inaguma Y, Ikeda H, Hiai H (1988). Cloning and expression of the ret proto-oncogene encoding a tyrosine kinase with two potential transmembrane domains. *Oncogene* 3: 571–578.

Takahashi M, Buma Y, Hiai H (1989). Isolation of ret proto-oncogene cDNA with an amino-terminal signal sequence. *Oncogene* 4: 805–806.

Takahashi M, Iwashita T, Santoro M, Lyonnet S, Lenoir GM, Billaud M (1999). Co-segregation of MEN2 and Hirschsprung disease: the same mutation of RET with both gain and loss-of-function? *Hum Mutat* 13: 331–336.

Tang MJ, Worley D, Sanicola M, Dressler GR (1998). The RET-glial cell-derived neurotrophic factor (GDNF) pathway stimulates migration and chemoattraction of epithelial cells. *J Cell Biol* 142: 1337–1345.

Tang MJ, Cai Y, Tsai SJ, Wang YK, Dressler GR (2002). Ureteric bud outgrowth in response to RET activation is mediated by phosphatidylinositol 3-kinase. *Dev Biol* 243: 128–136.

Tansey MG, Baloh RH, Milbrandt J, Johnson EM Jr. (2000). GFRα-mediated localization of RET to lipid rafts is required for effective downstream signaling, differentiation, and neuronal survival. *Neuron* 25: 611–623.

Taraviras S, Marcos-Gutierrez CV, Durbec P, Jani H, Grigoriou M, Sukumaran M, Wang LC, Hynes M, Raisman G, Pachnis V (1999). Signalling by the RET receptor tyrosine kinase and its role in the development of the mammalian enteric nervous system. *Development* 126: 2785–2797.

Thompson J, Doxakis E, Pinon LG, Strachan P, Buj-Bello A, Wyatt S, Buchman VL, Davies AM (1998). GFRα-4, a new GDNF family receptor. *Mol Cell Neurosci* 11: 117–126.

Tomac AC, Grinberg A, Huang SP, Nosrat C, Wang Y, Borlongan C, Lin SZ, Chiang YH, Olson L, Westphal H, Hoffer BJ (2000). Glial cell line–derived neurotrophic factor receptor α1 availability regulates glial cell line–derived neurotrophic factor signaling: evidence from mice carrying one or two mutated alleles. *Neuroscience* 95: 1011–1023.

Treanor JJ, Goodman L, de Sauvage F, Stone DM, Poulsen KT, Beck CD, Gray C, Armanini MP, Pollock RA, Hefti F, et al. (1996). Characterization of a multicomponent receptor for GDNF. *Nature* 382: 80–83.

Trupp M, Belluardo N, Funakoshi H, Ibanez CF (1997). Complementary and overlapping expression of glial cell line–derived neurotrophic factor (GDNF), c-ret proto-oncogene, and GDNF receptor-α indicates multiple mechanisms of trophic actions in the adult rat CNS. *J Neurosci* 17: 3554–3567.

Trupp M, Raynoschek C, Belluardo N, Ibanez CF (1998). Multiple GPI-anchored receptors control GDNF-dependent and independent activation of the c-Ret receptor tyrosine kinase. *Mol Cell Neurosci* 11: 47–63.

Trupp M, Scott R, Whittemore SR, Ibanez CF (1999). Ret-dependent and -independent mechanisms of glial cell line-derived neurotrophic factor signaling in neuronal cells. *J Biol Chem* 274: 20885–20894.

Tsui-Pierchala BA, Milbrandt J, Johnson EM Jr. (2002). NGF utilizes c-Ret via a novel GFL-independent, inter-RTK signaling mechanism to maintain the trophic status of mature sympathetic neurons. *Neuron* 33: 261–273.

van Weering DH, Bos JL (1998). Signal transduction by the receptor tyrosine kinase Ret. *Recent Results Cancer Res* 154: 271–281.

van Weering DH, Moen TC, Braakman I, Baas PD, Bos JL (1998). Expression of the receptor tyrosine kinase Ret on the plasma membrane is dependent on calcium. *J Biol Chem* 273: 12077–12081.

Vega QC, Worby CA, Lechner MS, Dixon JE, Dressler GR (1996). Glial cell line–derived neurotrophic factor activates the receptor tyrosine kinase RET and promotes kidney morphogenesis. *Proc Natl Acad Sci USA* 93: 10657–10661.

Wang CY, Yang F, He X, Chow A, Du J, Russell JT, Lu B (2001). Ca^{2+} binding protein frequenin mediates GDNF-induced potentiation of Ca^{2+} channels and transmitter release. *Neuron* 32: 99–112.

Wang CY, Yang F, He XP, Je HS, Zhou JZ, Eckermann K, Kawamura D, Feng L, Shen L, Lu B (2002). Regulation of neuromuscular synapse development by glial cell line–derived neurotrophic factor and neurturin. *J Biol Chem* 277: 10614–10625.

Worley DS, Pisano JM, Choi ED, Walus L, Hession CA, Cate RL, Sanicola M, Birren SJ (2000). Developmental regulation of GDNF response and receptor expression in the enteric nervous system. *Development* 127: 4383–4393.

Xing J, Kornhauser JM, Xia Z, Thiele EA, Greenberg ME (1998). Nerve growth factor activates extracellular signal-regulated kinase and p38 mitogen-activated protein kinase pathways to stimulate CREB serine 133 phosphorylation. *Mol Cell Biol* 18: 1946–1955.

Xu PX, Adams J, Peters H, Brown MC, Heaney S, Maas R (1999). Eya1-deficient mice lack ears and kidneys and show abnormal apoptosis of organ primordia. *Nat Genet* 23: 113–117.

Yang F, Feng L, Zheng F, Johnson SW, Du J, Shen L, Wu CP, Lu B (2001). GDNF acutely modulates excitability and A-type K^+ channels in midbrain dopaminergic neurons. *Nat Neurosci* 4: 1071–1078.

York RD, Molliver DC, Grewal SS, Stenberg PE, McCleskey EW, Stork PJ (2000). Role of phosphoinositide 3-kinase and endocytosis in nerve growth factor–induced extracellular signal-regulated kinase activation via Ras and Rap1. *Mol Cell Biol* 20: 8069–8083.

Young HM, Hearn CJ, Farlie PG, Canty AJ, Thomas PQ, Newgreen DF (2001). GDNF is a chemoattractant for enteric neural cells. *Dev Biol* 229: 503–516.

Yu T, Scully S, Yu Y, Fox GM, Jing S, Zhou R (1998). Expression of GDNF family receptor components during development: implications in the mechanisms of interaction. *J Neurosci* 18: 4684–4696.

Zhou B, Bae SK, Malone AC, Levinson BB, Kuo YM, Cilio MR, Bertini E, Hayflick SJ, Gitschier JM (2001). hGFRα-4: a new member of the GDNF receptor family and a candidate for NBIA. *Pediatr Neurol* 25: 156–161.

36 | *RET* and Hirschsprung Disease and Multiple Endocrine Neoplasia Type 2

ANDREW S. MCCALLION AND ARAVINDA CHAKRAVARTI

RET signaling is an integral component of normal embryonic development and neuronal maintenance. Mutations in the *RET* gene play a central role in two common heritable pathologies affecting neural crest–derived tissues: constitutive activating mutations lead to multiple endocrine neoplasia type 2 (MEN2; OMIM 171400 and 162300), a dominantly inherited cancer predisposition, and loss-of-function mutations lead to Hirschsprung disease (HSCR; OMIM 142623), a developmental defect resulting in functional intestinal obstruction in neonates. Genetic analyses of this pathway in human patients and model organisms have resulted in an understanding of the molecular mechanisms that underlie MEN2 and HSCR, and in changes to the clinical care and counseling of patients. In this chapter we review the progress made in elucidating the multiple roles of this pathway in normal human development and inherited disease.

Mutations in or misregulation of several genes with critical roles in mammalian development are now known to be central to the genesis of neoplastic and developmental disease. The protooncogene *RET* (Rearranged during transfection), encoding a receptor tyrosine kinase (RTK) (Takahashi et al., 1985; Takahashi and Cooper, 1987), is primarily expressed (*a*) in neural crest (NC), urogenital precursors, adrenal medulla, and thyroid during embryogenesis and (*b*) in cell populations of the CNS (central nervous system), PNS (peripheral nervous system), and endocrine systems throughout postnatal life. The gene comprises 21 exons encompassing approximately 55 kb of human genomic DNA on chromosome 10q11.1, and generates a transcript that is subject to alternative splicing at the 5′ and 3′ termini, resulting in the expression of multiple isoforms. The largest of these isoforms encodes a 1114-residue protein (RET51) and possesses 51 C-terminal residues. The majority of the 1114 amino acids are shared among all RET isoforms, although they differ in the composition of their most C-terminal residues. The C-termini of RET43 and RET9 comprise 43 and 9 amino acids, respectively (*Lorenzo et al., 1995; *Hansford and Mulligan, 2000). *RET* mRNA species that are subject to 5′ alternative splicing events are predicted to encode transmembrane isoforms with truncated extracellular domains and a variant predicted to be a soluble form of RET (Hansford and Mulligan, 2000). RET spans the cell membrane, transducing signals upon activation by members of the glial cell-line-derived neurotrophic factor (GDNF) family of ligands, which includes: GDNF, artemin (ARTN), neurturin (NRTN), and persephin (PSPN). Ligand binding by RET is mediated by glycosyl phosphoinositol–linked GFRA coreceptors (Airaksinen et al., 1999), resulting in signal transduction through multiple intracellular pathways (see Chapter 35).

THE RET RECEPTOR TYROSINE KINASE

RET was originally identified as a protooncogene in a classic cell transformation study (Takahashi et al., 1985; Takahashi and Cooper, 1987) and subsequently in a proportion of papillary thyroid carcinomas (PTC) (*Bongarzone et al., 1989). The *RET* gene encodes a receptor tyrosine kinase (RTK) that comprises a signal peptide, a cysteine-rich region, a transmembrane region, a conserved intracellular tyrosine kinase (TK) catalytic domain, and an extracellular (cadherin-related) ligand-binding domain (Fig. 36–1). Cadherins are Ca^{2+}-dependent cell-

*All reference citations marked with an asterisk will be found at http://chakravarti.som.jhmi.edu/resume/andy_chap36_ref.htm

adhesion molecules whose adhesive properties are imputed by tandem repeat motifs of approximately 110 amino acids.

The extracellular region is extended and stabilized upon binding Ca^{2+} between these domains; consequently, it is protected from proteolytic degradation. Similarly, the RET extracellular domain comprises four tandemly repeated cadherin-like domains (Anders et al., 2001) known to bind Ca^{2+} ions. RET is also relatively resistant to proteolytic cleavage by trypsin in the presence of Ca^{2+} (*Takahashi et al., 1993); its ligand binding is calcium-dependent (*Nozaki et al., 1998), and reduction in the levels of extracellular calcium interferes with RET folding in the endoplasmic reticulum (*van Weering et al., 1998). These data are consistent with the hypothesis that Ca^{2+} binding in the extracellular domain induces or stabilizes conformational change, which is required for receptor–ligand interaction.

RET is expressed throughout the developing central and peripheral nervous systems (enteric, sensory, and autonomic ganglia) and the excretory system, mediating signals that are proposed to influence cell proliferation, differentiation, migration, and apoptosis. It is activated by members of the glial cell-line-derived neurotrophic factor (GDNF) family, a recently identified family of ligands (Durbec et al., 1996; Trupp et al., 1996) which share a structural configuration comprising three disulfide bridges (the cysteine knot). These transforming growth factor-β (TGF-β)-related proteins include GDNF, neurturin (NRTN), artemin (ARTN), and persephin (PSPN) (*Milbrandt et al., 1998) and play a critical role in neuronal maintenance. GDNF, ARTN, and NRTN are known to support the survival of CNS and PNS neurons in vitro (Henderson et al., 1994; Baloh et al., 1998; *Heuckeroth et al., 1998; *Nishino et al., 1999). PSPN has thus far only been shown to support survival of nigrostriatal and motor neurons (Milbrandt et al., 1998).

Members of the GDNF family are unusual RTK ligands. The activation targets of other TGF-β family members are not receptor tyrosine kinases but, rather, receptor serine/threonine kinases. RET activation by these ligands requires the formation of a receptor complex with a glycosyl phosphatidylinositol (GPI)-linked coreceptor. Termed GDNF family receptors α1–4 (GFRA1–4), these coreceptor proteins mediate RET activation by GDNF, NTRN, ARTN, and PSPN, with varying specificity. Data from multiple in vitro studies clearly demonstrate the potential for promiscuity in these relationships (see Chapter 35 for detail). However, studies utilizing targeted mutations in the mouse indicate that specific combinations of GDNF family ligands (GFL) and accessory proteins are necessary for the correct development and maintenance of populations of central and peripheral neurons; they require tight control of regulation of expression to exert their effect (see "Lessons from Model Organisms" in this chapter.) It is now clear that distinct in vivo roles may exist for specific receptor–ligand complexes.

Signaling Downstream from RET

All receptor tyrosine kinases have a basic topology in common: an extracellular ligand-binding domain, a single transmembrane domain, and a cytoplasmic domain that harbors kinase activity (see Chapter 35). Ligand binding elicits phosphorylation of tyrosine residues within intracellular domains, resulting in receptor dimerization, autophosphorylation, phosphorylation of other intracellular substrates, and the subsequent activation of a variety of signal transduction pathways. RET can signal through a range of pathways, including RAS/ERK (extracellular signal-regulated kinase) (*Besset et al., 2000), p38

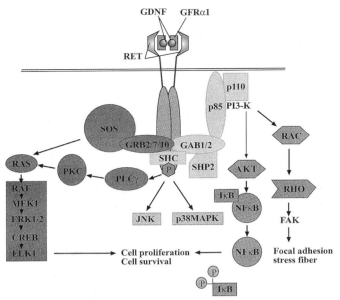

Figure 36–1. Biochemical pathways used by RET signaling. SOS, son of sevenless guanine nucleotide exchange factor; RAS, rat sarcoma virus oncogene homolog; ERK, extracellular signal regulated kinase; PKC, protein kinase C; PLCgamma, phospholipase C gamma; MEK1, MAP kinase kinase; CREB, cAMP response binding protein; ELK1, ETS oncogene family member; JNK, c-Jun N-terminal kinase; p38 MAPK, mitogen activated protein kinase; GAB1/2, GRB2-associated adaptor proteins 1 and 2; SHP2, tyrosine phosphatase SHP2; PI3K, phosphatidylinositol 3-kinase; NFκB, nuclear factor of kappa light polypeptide gene enhancer in B-cells; IκB, inhibitor of kappa light chain in B cells; AKT, v-akt murine thymoma viral oncogene homolog 1; RAC, ras-related C3 botulinum toxin substrate (rho family, small GTP binding protein RAC); RHO, rhodopsin related GTPases; FAK, focal adhesion kinase; GRB10/GRB2, growth factor receptor-bound proteins 10 and 2; SHC, signaling and transforming protein containing Src homology. (Adapted from Takahashi, 2001, with permission of Elsevier Science.)

MAPK (mitogen-activated protein kinase) (*Ohiwa et al., 1997), NF-κB (*Ludwig et al., 2001), PI3K/AKT (phosphatidylinositol 3-kinase) (*Hayashi et al., 2000), and JNK (c-Jun N-terminal kinase) (*Chiariello et al., 1998), thus driving cell proliferation, survival, migration, or differentiation.

Most RET isoforms have 16 tyrosine residues in their intracellular domain, but RET51, the longest isoform, contains an additional two tyrosines within the carboxy-terminal domain. Certain tyrosine residues in particular should be noted: residues Y905, Y1015, and Y1062 are shared by all isoforms. Y905 is the site for RET autophosphorylation within the activation loop, and Y1015 and Y1062 comprise binding sites for the adaptor proteins GRB10 and SHC/SNT(FRS2)/Enigma, respectively (Pandey et al., 1995; Asai et al., 1996; *Ohiwa et al., 1997; van Weering and Bos, 1998). Tyrosine 1096 (RET Y1096), which is present only in the longest RET isoform, represents a binding site for GRB2 (Alberti et al., 1998) (see Chapter 35).

The Role of RET in Human Disease

The relevance of the *RET* gene to clinical pathology was first revealed when mutations were identified in patients with papillary thyroid carcinoma (PTC) and then in MEN2 (Donis-Keller et al., 1993; *Mulligan et al., 1993; Hofstra et al., 1994). Germline *RET* mutations are now known to be responsible for almost all cases of MEN2 (see "Activating RET Mutations in MEN2" in this chapter). Two critical observations—the cooccurrence of HSCR and MEN2 (both of which map to proximal human chromosome 10q) and deletions of this region in some HSCR patients—led to the genetic mapping and identification of *RET* mutations in patients with HSCR (Luo et al., 1993; Edery et al., 1994; Fewtrell et al., 1994; Romeo et al., 1994). This vital receptor tyrosine kinase (RTK) pathway is now the focus of fervent study and has yielded substantial insight into the fields of cancer biology, congenital malformations, and development of the nervous, endocrine, and urogenital sys-

tems. One critical element of these analyses has been the examination of RET expression during development.

RET Expression during Embryogenesis

The temporal and spatial patterns of RET expression in the mouse, rat, chicken, and humans are consistent with proposed roles for this receptor-mediated pathway in kidney organogenesis, and in the development of the CNS and PNS. The temporal and spatial patterns of RET expression during development have been extensively studied in the mouse (Pachnis et al., 1993; *Golden et al., 1998, 1999). Other studies have examined RET expression during embryogenesis in humans, in teleosts, and in *Drosophila melanogaster* (*Sugaya et al., 1994; *Bisgrove et al., 1997; Marcos-Gutierrez et al., 1997; *Attie-Bitach et al., 1998; Hahn and Bishop, 2001). The temporal and spatial distribution of human *RET* mRNA encoding the different RET isoforms has also been reported (*Ivanchuk et al., 1997). RET9 and RET51 mRNA are generated in concert and are generally among the most abundant transcripts in the tissues in which they are expressed. RET9 and RET51 are thus far the only RET isoforms that are known to be expressed in vivo. It remains unclear whether the other putative isoforms are actually expressed.

In the Developing Autonomic Nervous System

The enteric nervous system comprises the ganglia of the Auerbach (myenteric) and Meissner (submucosal) plexuses of the intestinal tract. Enteric neuron precursors are primarily contributed by the vagal NC emigrés, which migrate ventrally through the posterior branchial arches into the foregut mesenchyme (see Chapter 12), although lesser contributions are also made by anterior truncal and sacral NC populations. Strong signal corresponding to RET is present in the mesenchymal cells at the level of the third and fourth branchial arches between 9 and 9.5 days post coitus, along the migratory path of enteric neuron precursors. By 9.5 dpc diffuse signal is detectable between the surface ectoderm and the neural tube (NT), and in the sclerotome at the truncal level indicative of migrating neural crest (NC) forming the dorsal root ganglia (DRG) (Pachnis et al., 1993; *Young et al., 1999). At 10 dpc these RET-positive neural crest emigrés exit from the posterior branchial arch, enter the foregut mesenchyme, and begin to migrate in a cranio–caudal direction. Migration of these neuronal precursors continues, until the entire myenteric plexus is populated at 13.5–14.5 dpc (Pachnis et al., 1993; Young et al., 1999).

This pattern of RET expression is paralleled in human embryogenesis. Human *RET* mRNAs are first detected in the NC-derived precursors of the developing enteric nervous system (ENS) at Carnegie 12 (embryonic days 27–30) (Attie-Bitach et al., 1998). RET expression progresses caudally with a wave front of crest emigrés and is subsequently detected in the midgut and hindgut until Carnegie 16. RET-positive migrating NC, corresponding to sympathetic ganglia anlage in the mouse, begin to coalesce alongside the dorsal aorta at 9.5 dpc (Pachnis et al., 1993). RET expression is detected throughout the establishment of this autonomic component and is maintained after completion of sympathetic gangliogenesis (14.5 dpc), which is consistent with a proposed role for RET in the maintenance of both sympathetic and parasympathetic neuronal populations.

In the Developing Central Nervous System

RET expression is also detected in the developing central nervous system (CNS). Signals corresponding to *Ret* mRNAs are detected along the ventrolateral margins of the spinal cord between 10.5 and 14.5 dpc (Pachnis et al., 1993). *Ret* mRNAs are present in the ventral margins along the entire length of the anterior/posterior axis. Human *RET* mRNA is also present along the anterior/posterior axis of the neural tube between Carnegie stages 13 and 16 (Attie-Bitach et al., 1998). The ventral location of RET-positive cells in the developing spinal cord is consistent with the topographical position of presumptive motor neurons.

In the Developing Excretory System

Vertebrate renal genesis comprises sequential establishment of three organ stages—pronephros, mesonephros, and metanephros (Saxen and Sariola, 1987)—resulting from reciprocal epithelial–mesenchymal inductive interactions (see Chapter 10). RET is expressed in the developing mouse nephric duct between 9 and 10.5 dpc and, subsequently, in the forming ureteric bud upon the invasion of the metanephric mesenchyme (Pachnis et al., 1993). At this point (11.5 dpc) the metanephric kidney develops, as the ureteric bud (caudal nephric duct) branches from the wolffian duct into the metanephric blastema, triggered by inductive signals from blastemal cells. RET expression continues in the nephrogenic zone, and by 13.5 dpc may be detected at the outer margins of the nascent kidney but is absent from more central regions (Pachnis et al., 1993).

Once again this pattern is consistent with the detection of *RET* mRNA in the human mesonephric duct at Carnegie 11 (embryonic days 23–26) (Attie-Bitach et al., 1998). At this stage *RET* transcripts are also present in the mesonephric tubules and the wolffiann duct and, subsequently, in the ureteric bud (Carnegie 16, embryonic days 37–42) (Attie-Bitach et al., 1998).

Between Vertebrate and Invertebrate Species

The *RET* gene and spatial expression patterns of its products appear to be widely conserved among vertebrates and invertebrates. In teleosts, mRNAs corresponding to the zebrafish otholog (*ret1*) are found in the presumptive brain (3-somite stage), the hypothalamus (12- and 18-somite stage), and the primary sensory and motor neurons of the developing nervous system (Bisgrove et al., 1997; Marcos-Gutierrez et al., 1997). A *ret1* transcript is also detected among the NC emigrés. At the 12-somite stage, *ret1*-positive cells are present dorsal to the hindbrain between rhombomeres 3 and 5 (r 3–5), and by the 18- to 24-somite stages these cells are present among discrete subpopulations of PNS cranial ganglia. This is in close correspondence to embryonic studies in mouse and humans (see "RET Expression during Embryogenesis"). The *ret1*-positive cells have also been observed in the gut wall of teleost larvae (3- to 8-day stage). Their localization and punctate patterns mirror the appearance of NC-derived enteric neuroblasts in higher vertebrates (Bisgrove et al., 1997; Marcos-Gutierrez et al., 1997). Consistent with expression analyses in mammalian species, *ret1*-positive cells are also present in the pronephric ducts of 4- to 6-somite stage embryos and are detected along the wolffian duct up to the 18-somite stage until it is down-regulated and restricted to the posterior nephric duct (26-somite stage) (Bisgrove et al., 1997; Marcos-Gutierrez et al., 1997).

Identification of a *RET* ortholog in *Drosophila* further illustrates the extent of conservation of this remarkable protein. Although *Drosophila* lack both a neural crest and an enteric nervous system, *D-ret* mRNA is detected in the forming somatogastric nervous system (Sugaya et al., 1994; Hahn and Bishop, 2001). *D-ret* mRNAs are also present in the forming malpighian tubules of the developing excretory system, in a manner consistent with RET expression in the pronephric and mesonephric ducts of vertebrate species. Thus, most species in which *RET* orthologs have been identified and studied express their corresponding *RET* gene product in tissues and organ systems that are analogous. These data underscore the critical nature of this gene across vertebrate and invertebrate development.

CLINICAL DESCRIPTION OF HIRSCHSPRUNG DISEASE

Hirschsprung disease (HSCR), or aganglionic megacolon, is a congenital malformation characterized by an absence of neural crest–derived enteric neurons along a variable length of the distal large intestine. Patients typically present in the neonatal period with intestinal obstruction and abdominal distension resulting from an inability to propagate peristaltic waves in the distal gut (Table 36–1). In the 1940s, Swenson and Bill (1948) demonstrated that the affected segment was not the proximal dilated segment but, rather, the distal grossly normal intestine. Their work, and other studies, revealed that this peristaltic failure was caused by a regional absence of enteric ganglia from the myenteric (Auerbach) and submucosal (Meissner) plexuses (Swenson and Bill, 1948; Whitehouse and Kernohan, 1948) and was the pathological origin of HSCR. Mortality among affected individuals was nearly 100% until the advent of corrective surgical procedures in which the affected bowel is resected and the integrity of the bowel reestablished by abdomino-anal pull-through (Swenson and Bill, 1948; *Swenson, 1996) (see "HSCR Clinical Presentation and Surgical Intervention" in this chapter). The resulting decrease in the mortality rate revealed the heritability of HSCR in the offspring of affected individuals (Meier-Ruge et al., 1972; Swenson, 1996).

HSCR is the most common form of functional intestinal obstruction in neonates, with an incidence of 1 in 5000 livebirths; it demonstrates complex patterns of inheritance. Although mendelian forms of HSCR have been described, the majority of patients are probably the result of oligogenic inheritance (Chakravarti and Lyonnet, 2000). Mutations in multiple genes encoding members of the receptor tyrosine kinase, the endothelin receptor type B (EDNRB) and the SOX10 transcription factor pathways have been reported in patients with HSCR (Table 36–2). Targeted and spontaneous mutations of these and related genes in mice, embryologic analyses of enteric development, and functional analyses of gene mutations have also illuminated the molecular and pathological processes involved in HSCR. It is now becoming increasingly clear that the *RET* gene may be central to the genesis of most HSCR cases. This hypothesis is supported by several recent studies that affirm the multifactorial nature of the disease, largely in concert with mutations at *RET* (Bolk et al., 2000; Carrasquillo et al., 2002; Gabriel et al., 2002).

Pathological Classification of HSCR

HSCR is generally classified based on the extent of aganglionosis. Although the rectum is always affected, the upper limit of correct innervation is highly variable. Short-segment disease (S-HSCR) comprises the vast majority of HSCR cases (67%–82%) and is defined as aganglionosis extending between the rectum and the upper sigmoid colon (Badner et al., 1990; Chakravarti and Lyonnet, 2000) (Fig. 36–2). Long-segment disease (L-HSCR) is defined as intestinal aganglionosis that involves and extends beyond the splenic flexure (*Weinberg, 1975) (Fig. 36–2). However, pathological examination has resulted in attempts to refine the definition by establishing multiple categories, in-

Table 36–1. Clinical Indicators and Selected Syndromic Features Associated with Hirschsprung Disease

Clinical Indicator	Frequency (%)	Syndromic Association
Age at diagnosis ≤ 1 month	61	
Failure to pass meconium*	60	
Retarded passage of meconium*	40	
Constipation	68	
Abdominal distension	30–90	
Vomiting	37	
Hypopigmentation	N/A	Shah-Waardenburg syndrome (WS4)
Sensorineural deafness	N/A	Shah-Waardenburg syndrome (WS4)
Medullary thyroid carcinoma	N/A	MEN2A, FMTC†
Pigmentary retinopathy	N/A	Bardet-Biedl syndrome
Skeletal dyplasia	N/A	cartilage-hair hypoplasia
Microcephaly/growth retardation	N/A	Smith-Lemli-Opitz syndrome types 1 and 2

*First 48 hours postnatal life.

†MEN2A, multiple endocrine neoplasia type 2A; FMTC, familial medullary thyroid carcinoma.

N/A, not available.

Table 36–2. Human Hirschsprung Disease (HSCR) Genes, Associated Phenotypes, and Penetrance Values

Human Gene	Map Location	No. of Mutations	Phenotype in Mutant Homozygotes	Phenotype in Mutant Heterozygotes	Penetrance %
RET	10q11	89	Unobserved	HSCR	51–72
GDNF	5p13	5	Unobserved	HSCR	N/A
NTN	19p13	1	Unobserved	HSCR	N/A
EDNRB	13q22	15	HSCR*	HSCR	8–85
EDN3	20q13	2	HSCR*	HSCR	N/A
ECE-1	1p36	1	Unobserved	HSCR†	N/A

*Shah-Waardenburg syndrome (WS4/HSCRII).
†Cardiac defects, craniofacial abnormalities, and dysmorphic features.
N/A, not available.

cluding ultra-short (anal aganglionosis), short, colonic (classical), long, and total colonic HSCR (*Neilson and Yazbeck, 1990).

HSCR may occur as an isolated malformation or is found in association with other neurocristopathy syndromes such as Waardenburg's syndrome type 4 (WS4) (reviewed in McCallion and Chakravarti, 2001) or multiple endocrine neoplasia type 2 (MEN2) (see below). Other syndromic associations include Goldberg-Shprintzen syndrome, distal limb abnormalities, Bardet-Biedl syndrome (BBS), Smith-Lemli-Opitz (SLO) syndrome types 1 and 2, and cartilage-hair hypoplasia (reviewed in Chakravarti and Lyonnet, 2000). Some of these associations reflect the common NC ancestry of affected tissues, including the pigmentary, cardiac, and craniofacial abnormalities associated with WS4, BBS, and SLO. In general, however, these associations suggest that at least some of the additional HSCR susceptibility loci comprise genes with pleiotropic effects.

Genetics of HSCR

HSCR is considered to be a sex-modified, multigenic trait. A full review of the classical and molecular genetics of HSCR has recently been published (Chakravarti and Lyonnet, 2000). However, several characteristics are noteworthy. Early genetic studies of HSCR revealed the heritablity of the disorder and emphasized the elevated risk to relatives compared with the general population. This recurrence risk was demonstrated to be dependent on the sex of both the affected individual and the relative (see Chakravarti and Lyonnet, 2000). HSCR exhibits a marked sex bias, which depends on the length of the aganglionic segment and is manifested in the observation that both incidence and penetrance is approximately 2-fold to 4-fold higher in males. It has been noted that both penetrance of known mutations and the compatible models of inheritance vary with the presence or absence of associated syndromic features—a hallmark of complex disorders.

CLINICAL DESCRIPTION OF MEN TYPE 2

Multiple endocrine neoplasia type 2 (MEN2) is an autosomal dominant cancer syndrome characterized by medullary thyroid carcinoma (MTC), accompanied or not by HPT (hyperparathyroidism) and PC (pheochromocytoma) (Schimke et al., 1968). MEN2A and 2B demonstrate similar incidence of MTC (100%) and PC (50%), but MEN2A patients demonstrate HPT with moderate frequency (15%–30%), and MEN2B is characterized by the additional occurrence of developmental abnormalities (Table 36–3) (*Gorlin et al., 1968; Ponder, 1999; *Jhiang, 2000). Patients with familial MTC (FMTC) develop MTC as the sole clinical feature (Table 36–3).

Pathological Classification of MEN2

MTC is the clinical hallmark of MEN2, and its cellular origin is believed to lie in the calcitonin-producing, neuroendocrine, thyroid C-cell population. Approximately 25% of MTC cases are familial and comprise the MEN2 group of cancer syndromes. MEN2 may be subclassified as type 2A (MEN2A), type 2B (MEN2B) or familial medullary thyroid carcinoma (FMTC), depending on which organs are affected (Table 36–3) (Schimke et al., 1968), although MTC is common in all subtypes. MEN2A is characterized by the association of MTC, PC, and HPT (*Schimke, 1984) and accounts for almost 90% of the incidence of MEN2. Approximately 30% of individuals with MEN2 will be asymptomatic for MTC, PC, or HPT by age 70 (*Easton et al., 1989). Thus, the incomplete penetrance of the causative mutations may have implications for our capacity to detect clinical onset and follow-up in the families of affected individuals. FMTC is diagnosed in families, with multiple affected individuals in two or more generations, in which MTC segregates as a sole disease indicator.

Some 5% of all cases of MEN2 present as MEN2B. Although MEN2B and MEN2A share the presentation of MTC in affected individuals, type 2B disease lacks HPT as a clinical feature but often presents additional developmental abnormalities, such as intestinal ganglioneuromatosis; medullated corneal nerves; neuromas of the lips, tongue, and conjunctiva; and *marfanoid habitus* (see Table 36–3 and below) (Gorlin et al., 1968; Schimke et al., 1968).

Genetics of MEN2

Multiple endocrine neoplasia demonstrates an autosomal dominant pattern of inheritance and arises from mutations at the RET locus (Donis-Keller et al., 1993; *Mulligan et al., 1993; Eng et al., 1996). No sex bias or parent of origin effect has been reported in any of the MEN2 syndromes. Incomplete penetrance of PC and HPT is a clinical characteristic of MEN2A.

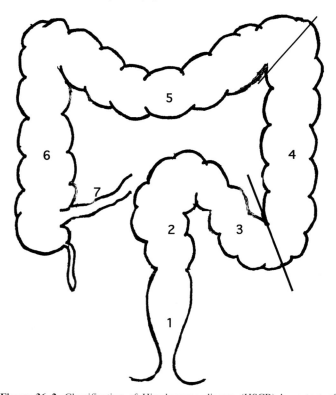

Figure 36–2. Classification of Hirschsprung disease (HSCR) by extent of aganglionosis. 1: ultra-short-segment; 2–3: short-segment HSCR; 4: colonic-segment HSCR; 5–6: long-segment HSCR; 6–7: total colonic. The bars represent points of transition in classification. Involvement of segment 4 may result in classification of HSCR as either S- or L-HSCR dependent on proximity to sigmoid colon or splenic flexure, respectively.

Table 36–3. Diagnostic Indicators (in percent) of MEN2 and HSCR

	MTC	HPT	PC	Aganglionosis	Associated features
MEN2A	100	15–35	40	0	None*
MEN2B	100	0	50	0	Intestinal ganglioneuromatosis, neuroma, *marfanoid habitus*
FMTC	100	0	0	0	Indolent disease progression*
HSCR	0	0	0	100	Megacolon

MTC, medullary thyroid carcinoma; HPT, hyperparathyroidism; PC, pheochromocytoma. MEN2A, 2B, multiple endocrine neoplasia type 2A and type 2B; FMTC, familial MTC; HSCR, Hirschsprung disease.
*Infrequent co-incidence of indicators.

RET MUTATIONS AND GENOTYPE–PHENOTYPE CORRELATION

RET mutations resulting in HSCR and MEN2 may be broadly categorized. HSCR results from mutations that compromise the developmental expression or activity of the RET pathway (Pasini et al., 1995; Iwashita et al., 1996; *Pelet et al., 1998), and this is consistent with a role for RET in the proliferation, differentiation, or survival (or all three) of neuronal precursors. MEN2 is generally considered to result from *RET* mutations that render the pathway constitutively active, and this is consistent with a role in neoplastic transformation (*Rossel et al., 1997). *RET* is also constitutively activated by rearrangement in 5% to 30% of papillary thyroid carcinoma (PTC) (*Jhiang and Mazzaferri, 1994), although presentation of PTC is seldom associated with MEN2.

Although HSCR and MEN2A both result from mutations within the *RET* gene, they are normally observed in isolation and are believed to result from different mutation types and cellular mechanisms. Inactivating mutations are associated with HSCR, whereas MEN2 results from activating mutations, resulting in cellular transformation. Therefore, the identification of *RET* mutations (C618 and C620) in families that segregate both HSCR and MEN2 (FMTC or MEN2A) has resulted in speculation about which mechanisms may be compatible with both disorders (*Mulligan et al., 1994; *Decker et al., 1998). Furthermore, a number of families have now been reported in which HSCR segregates as a sole clinical feature, yet the affected individuals harbor MEN2-causative *RET* mutations (Ito et al., 1997).

Inactivating *RET* Mutations and Hirschsprung Disease

The frequency of detection of *RET* mutations in HSCR patients is variable (10%–50%) among different studies and is highly dependent on family history and the extent of disease in the individual patient (Chakravarti and Lyonnet, 2000). Studies that have selected for individuals with extensive family history of HSCR or sporadic incidence of L-HSCR result in an elevated rate of detection of *RET* mutations (Angrist et al., 1995; Attie et al., 1995; Seri et al., 1997). *RET* mutations are more frequently found in patients with familial (49%) rather than sporadic (35%) disease, and in individuals with L-HSCR (57%) rather than S-HSCR (32%) (Chakravarti and Lyonnet, 2000). At least 89 unique *RET* mutations have been identified among individuals with HSCR; they include nonsense mutations, missense mutations, small insertions, and deletions (Chakravarti and Lyonnet, 2000) (Fig. 36–3). *RET* mutations associated with HSCR occur throughout the entire gene and are in stark contrast with the domain-specific mutations identified with MEN2.

HSCR mutations in the *RET* gene are generally loss-of-function alleles. Affected individuals are heterozygotes for mutations at *RET*, suggesting that HSCR results from haploinsufficiency. The complex

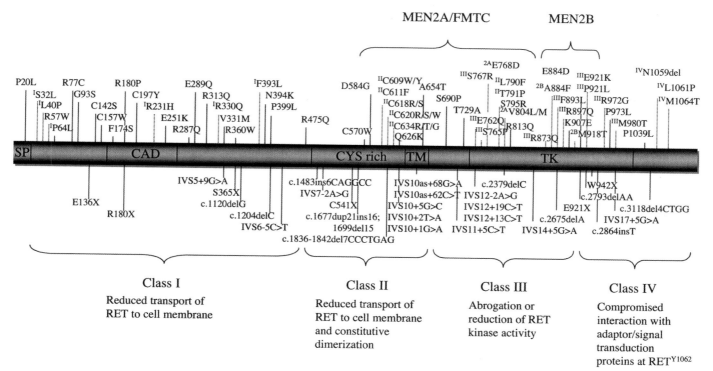

Figure 36–3. Schematic representation of the RET protein and mutations associated with MEN type 2 and HSCR. I, HSCR class I *RET* mutations; II, HSCR class II and FMTC/MEN2A *RET* mutations; 2A, *RET* mutations uniquely associated with MEN2A; III, HSCR class III *RET* mutations; IV, HSCR class IV *RET* mutations; 2B, MEN2B *RET* mutations. All classified mutations are listed above the schematic of the *RET* gene. Mutations lacking superscript symbols correspond to HSCR mutations for which detailed functional information was not available. SP, signal peptide; CAD, cadherin domain; CYS rich, cysteine-rich domain; TM, transmembrane domain; TK, tyrosine kinase domain. (Adapted from Chakravarti and Lyonnet, 2000, and Manié et al., 2001, with permission of McGraw-Hill Companies and Elsevier Science.)

nature of HSCR inheritance and associated phenotypic variation is reflected in the observed relationship between *RET* genotype and phenotype. Coding-sequence mutations (missense and nonsense) are more frequently associated with L-HSCR and are often compatible with mendelian patterns of HSCR inheritance. However, even when *RET* mutations are identified, they display markedly reduced penetrance (50%–70%) and gender bias.

The known RET mutations are postulated to comprise four functional subclasses (Pelet et al., 1998; Iwashita et al., 2001). Class I mutations lie within the extracellular domain and are proposed to interfere with RET maturation and its translocation to the plasma membrane. Class II mutations are shared with MEN2A/FMTC, replacing Cys609, 611, 618, or 620 with another residue (see "*RET* Mutations Common to Both HSCR and MEN2" in this chapter), and are hypothesized to result in constitutive activation of the receptor and reduction in the number of mature receptors at the cell surface (Takahashi et al., 1999). Class III mutations occur in codons of the TK domain, reducing the catalytic activity of the receptor, but only those mutations disrupting residues shared by most TK members completely abolish catalytic activity. Mutations in nonconserved sequence are reported only to diminish activity of the PLCγ-pathway (Iwashita et al., 2001). Class IV mutations are found in the region around RET^{Y1062} and compromise the efficiency with which RET binds to its effector molecules—for example, Shc, IRS1 (insulin receptor substrate-1), and FRS2 (fibro-blast growth factor [FGF] receptor substrate-2) (Geneste et al., 1999; *Melillo et al., 2001a,b) Fig. 36–3 shows all four classes discussed in this paragraph.

The majority of HSCR families demonstrating linkage to the *RET* locus fail to reveal coding-sequence mutations in the gene (Chakravarti and Lyonnet, 2000). These families, in whom segregation of the disease phenotype is compatible with non-mendelian models of inheritance, comprise mostly S-HSCR probands. Several reports have attempted to reduce the complexity of genetic analysis, in these families, by selecting HSCR pedigrees comprising affected individuals who meet more precisely defined phenotype or genotype criteria. Bolk et al. (2000) conducted a genome scan in large multicase families, comprising >3 affected individuals, in multiple generations. This study revealed a new HSCR susceptibility locus on human chromosome 9q31, which segregated with HSCR only in families in which affected individuals did not harbor a coding-sequence mutation in *RET*. In a more recent study, Gabriel et al. (2002) conducted a genome-wide linkage analysis in a collection of multicase S-HSCR families. This approach identified two further HSCR loci (3p21 and 19q12) which, in combination with alleles at *RET*, were sufficient to explain S-HSCR recurrence risk in these families (Gabriel et al., 2002). These data clearly demonstrate that grouping families according to phenotypic classes or mutation type at known susceptibility loci may facilitate genetic dissection HSCR.

Several explanations exist for those HSCR families that do not harbor *RET* coding-sequence mutations. First, *RET* linkage may appear by chance in small families. This is true in at least rare cases but is insufficient to explain the vast majority of families (Bolk et al., 2000). Second, mutations in a closely linked gene may be the genesis of HSCR. However, analysis of human genomic sequence around *RET* (0.5 Mb 5' and 3') have failed to reveal another candidate gene (Carrasquillo et al., 2002). Third, mutations in as-yet-unidentified *RET* regulatory sequences may compromise RET expression. In addition, *RET* may be subject to epigenetic regulation.

The latter two explanations appear the most feasible, both implicating *RET* misregulation in HSCR and consistent with a *RET*-modifying role for additional susceptibility loci in these families. It is noteworthy, therefore, that several studies have now identified a role for *RET* and *EDNRB* in combination, in the causation of HSCR. Auricchio et al. (1999) reported an HSCR patient who was heterozygous for hypomorphic mutations within *RET* and *EDNRB*: each parent was heterozygous for one mutation, yet neither parent was affected. This suggests a direct genetic, if not biochemical, interaction between the pathways.

Moreover, in a series of recent studies conducted in our laboratory, we have demonstrated genetic interaction between *RET* and *EDNRB* (endothelin receptor type B) in HSCR families of a large Mennonite kindred (Carrasquillo et al., 2002; McCallion et al., 2003; Puffenberger et al., 1994). In 1994 we reported a missense (W276C) mutation in *EDNRB* shared among the majority of affected individuals in this population. Our data also revealed non-random segregation of polymorphisms within *RET* with the HSCR phenotype (Puffenberger et al., 1994). We have now demonstrated that HSCR penetrance in this isolate depends on the combined influence of alleles at *RET* and *EDNRB*. Furthermore, we have recapitulated these findings in the mouse (see "Lessons from Model Organisms" in this chapter). These results clearly illustrate how genetic interaction between *RET* and other susceptibility loci comprise a mechanism for HSCR and emphasize the central role played by *RET* in HSCR genesis.

RET mutations in HSCR are generally accepted to reduce the expression or signaling capacity of the receptor. However, it is noteworthy that a small but significant number of families present with cooccurrence of MEN2 and HSCR. Thus, mutations previously defined as RET-activating in neoplastic MEN2 syndromes may also result in HSCR (see "*RET* Mutations Common to Both HSCR and MEN2" in this chapter).

Activating *RET* Mutations in MEN2

Identification of *RET* mutations has provided some insight into the mechanisms of receptor activation that result in MEN2. MEN2 is caused by missense mutations in specific codons, resulting in the elimination of a cysteine or the addition of a tyrosine residue. Mutations in cysteine codons C609, C611, C618, C620 (*RET* exon 10), or C634 (*RET* exon 11) have been identified in 98% of unrelated MEN2A and in 85% of FMTC families (Mulligan and Ponder, 1995) (Fig. 36–3).

C634 is the most frequently mutated codon in MEN2A (C634R, C634T and C634G), accounting for 80% to 90% of patients (Mulligan and Ponder, 1995; Eng et al., 1996). The paired cysteine residues of the RET extracellular domain are believed to mediate the intramolecular binding that is required to determine the tertiary structure of the receptor. Mutation of one of these cysteines results in the generation of an unpaired residue, which subsequently mediates the establishment of an illegitimate disulfide bond with an adjacent RET molecule, receptor dimerization, and constitutive activation of the signaling pathway. This mechanism is also proposed to explain the activating influence of mutations in other cysteine residues. Three novel mutations have also been identified in the region that encodes the TK domain of RET, in patients with FMTC (Bolino et al., 1995; *Eng et al., 1995b; *Boccia et al., 1997). The position of these mutations, within the kinase domain, suggests that they may result in promiscuous use of substrates that are not normally available to RET-mediated signaling or that they disrupt the autoregulation of the kinase domain in a manner that relieves normal autoinhibition mediated by the activation loop. Mutations in these codons account for 10% to 20% of FMTC cases (Hansford and Mulligan, 2000).

The *RET* mutation M918T (exon 16) is responsible for 95% of cases of MEN2B (*Eng et al., 1994; Mulligan and Ponder, 1995) (Fig. 36–3). M918T mutations are believed to disrupt the substrate recognition of the TK catalytic core (*Songyang et al., 1995), resulting in constitutive activation and altered recognition of intracellular substrates such as the non-receptor tyrosine kinase substrates *c-abl* and *c-src* (*Bocciardi et al., 1997; *Murakami et al., 1999), although one may also envisage M918T compromising RET autoregulation by disrupting the autoinhibitory function of the activation loop.

RET Mutations Common to Both HSCR and MEN2

Studies using in vitro biochemical and transfection assays have revealed that cysteine codon mutations in *RET* result in constitutive dimerization and activation of the receptor (Borrello et al., 1995; Santoro et al., 1995). Mutations in codons C609 and C611 are more frequently associated with FMTC than are C634 mutations, which are strongly associated with MEN2A. One suggestion is that C634 mutations have a greater activating influence on the resulting receptor than do mutations in the more 5' coding sequence. Transfection studies and biochemical assays of kinase activity have shown that non-C634 mutations have a weaker transforming influence on receptor activity. Furthermore, mutations at more 5' positions (e.g., C609, C611, C618, and C620) also appear to result in a reduction in the number of functional receptors at the cell surface (*Carlomagno et al., 1997; Ito et al., 1997; Takahashi et al., 1999) (Fig. 36–3). These data influence two unaddressed issues. First, the data are compatible with the hypothesis that MEN2A and FMTC represent the same entity—and that the variation in clinical presentation may be explained by differences in RET signaling and thus the penetrance of mutations. Second, the data are also compatible with a causative role for C618R and C620R mutations in the cooccurrence of HSCR and MEN2A. These mutations may reduce the numbers of mature RET receptors at the cell surface beneath a threshold number required for enteric gangliogenesis during development. However, constitutive activation of these mature receptors may still be sufficient for the genesis of MTC and PC.

HSCR CLINICAL PRESENTATION AND SURGICAL INTERVENTION

The vast majority of HSCR is diagnosed in the neonatal period and in term-born infants of normal birth weight. As many as 61% of affected infants are diagnosed within the first month of life with a range of characteristic symptoms, including failure to pass meconium in the first 48 hours of life (60%), abdominal distension (30%–90%), vomiting (37%) accompanied by bile or blood, and diarrhea (Table 36–1). One important and helpful symptom is the vacuity of the rectal ampulla, along with the associated explosive release of meconium and flatus upon rectal examination. Clinical features pertinent to the post-newborn period include constipation (68%); chronic, albeit variable, abdominal distension; retarded passage of meconium, and vomiting (37%) (Table 36–1). Individuals with a late or adult diagnosis of HSCR often have a history of gastrointestinal dysfunction, motility problems, or failure to thrive. Diagnostic investigation may include abdominal X-ray, barium enema, and anorectal manometry. However, definitive diagnosis requires rectal biopsy and examination of parasympathetic innervation by acetylcholinesterase staining (Meier-Ruge et al., 1972). Aganglionic intestine is characterized by the absence of the normal reticulate pattern of enteric innervation and its replacement by a sparse pattern of hypertrophic neurites that extend through the aganglionic distal gut.

Surgical correction follows a simple principle: by resecting the affected region and placing the normal bowel at the rectum, one may remove the potential for tonic contraction of the affected segment. Corrective procedures, termed ano-rectal pull-through, were developed by Swenson and Soave (Swenson and Bill, 1948; *Swenson, 1967; Soave, 1966). Earlier diagnosis has now ameliorated the prior need for interim colostomy, to allow recovery of the proximal bowel. Although prognosis continues to improve, HSCR remains life-threatening. The mortality associated with corrective surgery has dropped from 19% in the 1960s to 6% in the 1980s and now <1% (Chakravarti and Lyonnet, 2000). The current morbidity and mortality of HSCR results largely from sepsis, enterocolitis, or post-operative perforation but is also subject to complications imputed by associated syndromic features (Moore SW et al., 1996).

Most HSCR patients experience postoperative motility problems throughout life. It is not clear whether RET signaling is required in the gut during postnatal development and adult life, although a clear role exists for the enteric nervous system in regulating intestinal secretions—for example, through the release of VIP (vasoactive intestinal polypeptide) (Le Douarin and Kalcheim, 1999). Furthermore, neurturin is expressed in the gut throughout adult life (Golden et al., 1998), suggesting that RET signaling may play a role in the normal function or maintenance of the ENS. Consequently, surgical resection of the aganglionic segment in HSCR patients may remove the obvious incapacity for normal peristalsis, but compromised RET signaling in the gut may continue to interfere with the normal function of the remaining intestinal tract.

MEN2 CLINICAL PRESENTATION AND SURGICAL INTERVENTION

Almost all individuals with MEN2A present with multifocal MTC, in the second to fourth decade of life (Table 36–3), contrasting with the later onset of sporadic MTC (sixth decade) (Brandi et al., 2001). Clin-

ical presentation may be as a mass in the neck or as metastatic disease. Histological examination is essential to confirm the diagnosis before surgery is performed and is usually conducted by fine-needle biopsy. MTC originates in the parafollicular calcitonin-producing C cells of the thyroid—a population of neuroendocrine amine precursor uptake and decarboxylation (APUD) cells. C-cell hyperplasia (CCH) is generally accepted as the precursor to MTC. Calcitonin is also produced by MTCs and serves as an important tumor marker for MEN2.

The identification of RET as the causative gene in MEN2 allows DNA-based testing in patients and their family members, and this comprises the diagnostic gold standard (See "Surveillance and Counseling in MEN2 and HSCR" in this chapter). Less frequent but associated indicators include HSCR (see "HSCR Clinical Presentation and Surgical Intervention") and cutaneous lichen amyloidosis (brownish plaques in the intrascapular area). The identification of four or more family members with MTC, in the absence of PC, is usually sufficient to diagnose FMTC. Unfortunately, in smaller families (three or fewer affected individuals) it becomes difficult to distinguish between FMTC or MEN2A (before the identification of PC) and coincidental sporadic cases. Thus, RET testing may help resolve the diagnosis in some families.

The elucidation of the genetic causes of MEN2A dramatically improved the capacity to diagnose and manage the disease. Prognosis is generally good with early detection and surgical intervention. Cases in which patients are diagnosed with MTC before it is palpable are rarely complicated by lymph node metastases (*Wells et al., 1994). Surgical intervention in MTC tends to be the preferred treatment for many reasons: radiation and chemotherapy are ineffective, and MTC cells fail to take up radioactive iodine; surgical treatment of primary MTC normally involves total thyroidectomy, parathyroidectomy (*Dralle et al., 1994), and autotransplantation of parathyroid tissue into the muscle of the nondominant forearm of the patient (Olson et al., 1996).

MEN2B is more aggressive and is frequently diagnosed early in life—by facial appearance, ganglioneuromas on the lips, mucosal neuromas, intestinal dysfunction, and ganglioneuromatosis of the gut (Table 36–3). Molecular confirmation of diagnosis relies, preferably, on mutation detection in the RET gene, or by the elevation of pentagastrin-induced calcitonin levels beyond normative baseline levels. Diagnosis of type 2B disease is also facilitated by clinical presentation of *marfanoid habitus*, midface hypergnathism, and hyperflexible joints (Gorlin et al., 1968). Surgical intervention in MEN2B individuals is recommended during infancy because of the aggressive nature and early onset of MTC in these patients (Wells et al., 1994).

Surveillance and Counseling in MEN2 and HSCR

HSCR is a sex-modified multifactorial disorder, and genetic counseling has primarily been limited to assigning an overall risk of 4% to siblings and other first-degree relatives of a proband. In isolated HSCR, more precise estimates of risk may be established, based on the known variation in recurrence risk by sex of proband and consultand, and by extent of aganglionosis (Badner et al., 1990). To date, genetic testing in isolated HSCR has been restricted to research protocols and is currently rarely considered for evaluation of clinical risk. Continued surveillance or biochemical testing may be warranted in HSCR patients who harbor MEN2A mutations to ascertain whether they are predisposed to neuroendocrine tumors (see "RET Mutations Common to Both HSCR and MEN2" in this chapter). Recent studies emphasize the central role of RET in the oligogenic inheritance of HSCR in association with loci at 3p21, 9q31, and 19q12, with estimates of a 4.2-, 5.0-, and 8.3-fold risk increase, respectively. These studies show the potential for more informative molecular testing in familial cases and estimation of the recurrence risk increase to siblings, although the utility of this approach is untested.

Predictive testing for MEN type 2 is made feasible by the high frequency of detectable mutations (95%). Testing may be facilitated by direct DNA sequencing of RET exons 8, 10, 11, and 13–16 (Van Heurn et al., 1996), although other PCR-based mutation detection assays are also frequently used to screen for the presence of sequence variants (*Lips et al., 1994; Neumann et al., 1995). DNA testing should eliminate unnecessary surgical intervention and permit identification, counseling, surveillance, and clinical management of individuals who may otherwise have been missed.

LESSONS FROM MODEL ORGANISMS

The mouse is an experimental genetic system in which mutations can be generated at will and their in vivo effects studied (Table 36–4). The mouse permits analysis of mutations in isolation or in combination, provides access to all tissues, and facilitates correlation with human disease. Targeted mutations generated in genes that encode RET pathway components have been central to the elucidation of their critical roles in development and disease. Null mutations in *Ret* result in intestinal aganglionosis and renal agenesis, whereas transgenic mice that express MEN2A and MEN2B mutated forms of the RET protein present with MTC and renal anomalies. These strains represent many features of the human disease.

The RET-Mediated Pathway and HSCR Models

The majority of neurons and glia of the ENS are contributed by the vagal NC emigrés that migrate ventromedially into the foregut, and then caudally to innervate the entire length of the intestinal tract (see Chapter 12) (Le Douarin and Kalcheim, 1999). Developmental studies in mice deficient in RET or GDNF have demonstrated a role for these proteins in the survival and correct migration of enteric neuroblasts (Schuchardt et al., 1994; Moore MW, et al., 1996; Pichel et al., 1996; Sanchez et al., 1996). The role of RET in neural crest and renal development was clarified by the expression pattern of RET during mouse embryogenesis and the phenotype of *Ret* null mice (Pachnis et al., 1993).

Mice harboring homozygous null mutations in the genes that encode RET, GDNF, and GFRα1 display total enteric aganglionosis and renal agenesis (Schuchardt et al., 1994; Moore MW, et al., 1996; Pichel et al., 1996; Sanchez et al., 1996) (Table 36–5). These mice develop to term and die within the first 24 hours postpartum. In addition, *Ret* null mice exhibit pyloric stenosis, dilated proximal intestine, and an empty bladder. Their inability to propagate peristaltic waves results in the accumulation of milk in the stomach (Schuchardt et al., 1994).

Likewise *Gdnf* and *Gfrα1* null mice demonstrate peristaltic failure, which correlates with the lack of enteric ganglia. Thus the RET-mediated pathway is vital for normal development of the ENS, but notable differences are observed between mice deficient in RET and those deficient in the GDNF ligand family members or their accessory proteins. Intestinal aganglionosis observed in *Ret* null mice extends from the rectum to the stomach (Schuchardt et al., 1994), whereas *Gdnf* null mice lack enteric neurons below the midesophagus (Moore MW, et al., 1996; Pichel et al., 1996; Sanchez et al., 1996) (Table 36–5). $Ret^{-/-}$ mice lack superior cervical ganglia (SCG), which contrasts with observations in $Gdnf^{-/-}$ (35% reduction) and $Gfrα1^{-/-}$ mice in which these ganglia were either normal or only moderately affected (Moore MW, et al., 1996; Pichel et al., 1996; Sanchez et al., 1996; *Cacalano et al., 1998; Enomoto et al., 1998). SCG defects were also identified in mice deficient in GFRA3, although other ganglia appeared normal (Nishino et al., 1999). Also mice deficient in GDNF exhibit significantly more neuronal loss than do *Gfrα1* null mice, which is consistent with the observation in vitro that GDNF can elicit

its signal in the absence of GFRA1. These data suggest that GDNF may also signal through other accessory receptor proteins (e.g. GFRA2), or that further redundancy among the receptors and accessory proteins facilitating signaling through RET may exist.

Mice deficient in NTRN or GFRA2 are viable, but they demonstrate dramatic reduction in the numbers of parasympathetic cholinergic neurons in the intestine and in the lacrimal and submandibular glands (*Heuckeroth et al., 1999; *Rossi et al., 1999) (Table 36–5). This indicates that these structures depend more on RET-mediated signaling than on *Gdnf* effects. The significant overlap in the phenotype of *Nrtn* and *Gfrα1* null mice may indicate their in vivo physiological relationship and confirms the critical role of NRTN in the normal development of cranial parasympathetic neurons. The postnatal development of these mice is also dramatically retarded (Airaksinen et al., 1999; Heuckeroth et al., 1999; Rossi et al., 1999). Null mutations in *Artn*, *Pspn*, and *Gfrα4* have not yet been reported, but it is clear that distinct in vivo roles may exist for specific receptor–ligand complexes.

Mice deficient in either *Ret* or *Gdnf* also demonstrate renal agenesis due to a lack of induction of the ureteric bud. The metanephric kidney develops at E11 when the ureteric bud branches from the wolffian duct into the metanephric blastema, induced by signals from blastemal cells (Saxen and Sariola, 1987). Thus, this pathway plays an important role in the epithelial–mesenchymal interaction of ureteric bud induction in kidney development. A number of these studies (Schuchardt et al., 1994; Moore et al., 1996) have also reported that *Ret* and *Gdnf* heterozygote animals occasionally demonstrate unilateral or bilateral renal agenesis, suggesting that 50% of wild-type RET protein approaches the threshold required for normal renal organogenesis.

HSCR MODELS, DISEASE MECHANISMS, AND CLINICAL RELEVANCE

The regional absence of enteric ganglia observed in the distal gut of HSCR patients and corresponding mouse models is consistent with the cranio–caudal migration of vagal NC–derived enteric neuron precursors. It is clear that failure in the mechanisms of proliferation, migration, survival, homing, or differentiation associated with these NC-derived populations may result in the early cessation or incomplete colonization of the developing gut. Embryonic analyses in the mouse have provided clues concerning the pathological mechanisms induced in these populations, resulting from functional defects of the RET pathway, as seen in *Gdnf* and *Ret* null mice. The foregut (esophagus and stomach wall) of *Gdnf* null homozygotes is colonized by enteric neuroblast precursors at embryonic day 12.5 (12.5 dpc), but in mice examined at birth these neurons are absent (Sanchez et al., 1996). TUNEL analysis of these embryos at 12.5 dpc confirmed the presence of apoptotic nuclei, which is consistent with the original location of the absent precursor.

This cellular loss is paralleled in the development of the SCG, wherein the SCG anlage is formed by 10.5 dpc but absent at 12.5 dpc (Sanchez et al., 1996). The presence of these cell populations in the foregut and SCG anlage suggests that the corresponding NC-derived populations are competent to migrate into these locations and that their identity is consistent with their position, yet their subsequent apoptosis reveals that cell death is aberrantly imposed on a proportion of this

Table 36–4. Mouse Hirschsprung Disease Genes, Associated Phenotypes, and Penetrance Values

Mouse Gene	Mouse Chromosome	Mutation Type*	Enteric Phenotype in Mutant Heterozygotes	Enteric Phenotype in Mutant Homozygotes
Ret	6	KO	None	L-HSCR*†
Gdnf	15	KO	None	L-HSCR*†
Ednrb	14	KO, s^l	None	S-HSCR‡
Ednrb	14	s	None	None
Edn	2	KO	None	S-HSCR‡
Ece1	?	KO	None	S-HSCR‡§

KO, Knockout (targeted mutation). *s*, piebald; s^l, piebald lethal.
*Unilateral renal agenesis/dysgenesis at low frequency.
†Bilateral renal agenesis.
‡Pigmentary abnormalities.
§Cardiac defects, craniofacial abnormalities, dysmorphic features.

Table 36–5. Phenotype Comparison (in percent) of Targeted Mutations in Mouse Genes that Encode RET Receptor Complex Proteins

Cell Population	$Ret^{-/-}$	$Gdnf^{-/-}$	$Gfr\alpha1^{-/-}$	$Gfr\alpha2^{-/-}$	$Gfr\alpha3^{-/-}$	$Ntrn^{-/-}$
CNS neurons						
Dopaminergic	0	0	0			
Spinal lumbar	ND	22–31	24	ND	ND	ND
Noradrenergic	0	0	0			
Sensory ganglia						
Vestibular		0	0			
Petrosal-nodose	ND	40	15	Reduced (NS)	ND	0
L5 dorsal root (DRG)	ND	23	0	Reduced (NQ)	NS	NS
Motor nuclei						
Facial		0	0			
Trigeminal	ND	19	22	Reduced (NQ)	NS	69
Sympathetic neurons						
Superior cervical	100	35	0	0	20–40	0
Parasympathetic neurons						
Enteric neurons	s–r	e–r	s–r	15–45*	NS	15#
Submandibular gland	ND	ND	45	81	NS	ND
Other phenotypes						
Renal agenesis/dysgenesis	Yes	Yes	Yes	NS	NS	NS
Viability	Dead P0	Dead P0	Dead P0	Viable	Viable	Viable

ND, not done; NS, not significant; NQ, not quantified; SI, small intestine; P0, postnatal day zero; s–r, ENS absent from stomach to rectum; e–r, ENS absent from stomach to rectum; *, reduction in numbers of ENS fine fibers of small intestine; #, reduction in numbers of enteric ganglia throughout the intestinal tract.

population. This may result from a loss of proliferative capacity, enforced cessation of migration by the cellular microenvironment, or a simple loss of survival signaling, and it may conceivably result in an inappropriate halt of migration and the subsequent inability of this population to colonize the developing midgut and hindgut.

These studies reveal several features of RET signaling in ENS development. First, RET signaling is critical for normal development of the ENS. Second, the ENS of the mammalian foregut receives a significant contribution from a RET-independent truncal NC population, which is consistent with the observation that this neuronal population is dramatically less affected than the midgut and hindgut of *Ret* null animals. Third, the early stages of RET-positive vagal NC migration also appear to be independent of RET-mediated signaling, thus permitting migration into the foregut mesenchyme and contribution to esophageal innervation. However, RET-mediated signaling is required for subsequent colonization and gangliogenesis in the more distal gut.

Whether this signaling is required for the survival, maintenance, or proliferation of precursor populations—or the migration and differentiation of precursors—is as yet unclear. The ligand-independent apoptosis observed in GDNF-deficient mice requires caspase cleavage of the intracellular portion of RET. Although the mechanism and its relevance to HSCR pathology is still unclear, this observation does require further examination and suggests that RET signaling is required for neuronal maintenance during embryogenesis (*Bordeaux et al., 2000). Finally, labeling of migrating cell populations using lipophillic fluors (e.g., DiI) have confirmed that the enteric and SCG precursor populations originate within the same pool of bipotential progenitor cells (Durbec et al., 1996b).

Human HSCR and Mouse Models

Mouse models, which carry mutations in genes encoding RET pathway components, demonstrate three distinct discrepancies with human disease. First, aganglionosis in mice is restricted to the homozygous null genotypes in *Ret* and *Gdnf*, yet HSCR patients are heterozygotes for mutations within the orthologs. Second, phenotypic penetrance is complete in most mouse models, but human mutations display reduced penetrance. Third, phenotypic expression in mice demonstrates no sex bias, whereas human mutations in the same genes result in a 2-fold higher penetrance in males versus females.

These phenotypic differences between human HSCR and mouse models are not unexpected. First, the mouse mutations are observed in a homogenous genome, whereas the human genome is highly variable: phenotypic expression is, therefore, likely to be sensitive to genetic background. Second, while the mouse mutations are complete nulls, the majority of human mutations are weak hypomorphs. Third, there may be intrinsic differences between mice and humans in enteric development.

Consequently, our studies of HSCR in a Mennonite isolate, in which clinical expression depends on the combined influence of alleles at *RET* and *EDNRB*, prompted us to examine the potential for modification and noncomplementation between these loci in the mouse (see "Genetics of HSCR" in this chapter). Significantly, although $Ret^{-/+}$ (Schuchardt et al., 1994) and $Ednrb^{s/s}$ (s, hypomorphic allele of *Ednrb*) do not, in isolation, result in aganglionosis (Carrasquillo et al., 2002; McCallion et al., 2003) (Table 36–2), $Ret^{-/+}/Ednrb^{s/s}$ mice present with a stark HSCR phenotype (see "Lessons from Models Organisms" in this chapter). These mice are severely affected, present with abdominal distension or distress by weaning (3–4 weeks postpartum) (or both) and acetylcholinesterase staining of the intestinal tracts of $Ret^{-/+}/Ednrb^{s/s}$ mice reveals severe aganglionosis, involving the region between the rectum and the splenic flexure (Carrasquillo et al., 2002; McCallion et al., 2003). The extent of aganglionosis observed represents an intermediate phenotype between *Ret* homozygous null mice (rectum to stomach, inclusive) (Schuchardt et al., 1994) and the naturally occurring deletion piebald lethal $Ednrb^s-1/Ednrb^s-1$ (terminal colon) (Webster, 1974; Hosoda et al., 1994). The extent of a ganglionosis also more faithfully represents the extent and variation in length of aganglionic segment observed in human HSCR patients. Furthermore, penetrance of the phenotype of $Ret^{-/+}/Ednrb^{s/s}$ mice is greater in males than in females. Thus, our data recapitulate the clinical observation in human patients and are consistent with the hypothesis that genetic interaction between mutant alleles of the mouse genes *Ret* and *Ednrb* may be a causative mechanism in HSCR.

RET and EDNRB act through signal transduction pathways which, until recently, had been considered biochemically independent. Receptor tyrosine kinase (RTK) pathways transduce signals from growth factors, regulating proliferation and differentiation. G protein–coupled receptors (GPCR) mediate signals that result in alteration of intracellular Ca^{2+}, cellular contraction or secretion, or the activation of mitogen-activated protein (MAP) kinases. However, RTKs, like EGFR, can be required for GPCR-mediated mitogenic signaling, and RTK phosphorylation occurs only after GPCR activation (van Biesen et al., 1995; *Prenzel et al., 1999). Heterotrimeric G proteins dissociate to yield G_α-GTP and the $G_{\beta\gamma}$ subunits upon GPCR activation, resulting in activation of unknown effectors. These $G_{\beta\gamma}$ subunit–regulated molecules then induce RTK phosphorylation, resulting in Ras activation of the MAP kinase cascade (Luttrell et al., 1999).

These data are consistent with the hypothesis that *EDNRB* modulates *RET* in the genesis of HSCR. Pathways compromised in HSCR are subject to mutation dosage effects, and our data suggest that these two pathways may interact. This may be the first demonstration of interaction between genes encoding two major signaling pathways as a mechanism for a complex human disease. Furthermore, the observed phenotype and sex differences clearly indicate that the variation in

HSCR phenotype expression and sex bias observed in humans can be recapitulated in the mouse.

MEN2 MODELS, DISEASE MECHANISMS, AND CLINICAL RELEVANCE

Several of the activating *RET* mutations observed in patients with MEN type 2 have now been established and studied in transgenic mouse strains (Table 36–6). Transgenes harboring the MEN2A-like *RET* C634R mutation have been established, and their phenotypic effects have been scrutinized (Michiels et al., 1997; *Kawai et al., 2000; *Reynolds et al., 2001). Mice expressing the C634R mutant short isoform of RET (RET9-2A), under the control of the calcitonin gene-related protein/calcitonin (CGRP/CT) promoter, develop bilateral C-cell hyperplasia (CCH) and subsequently multifocal MTC (Michiels et al., 1997). Mice expressing the long form of the same mutant allele (RET51-2A) display MTC, PTC, and defects in thyroid follicular structure (Reynolds et al., 2001). The diffuse CCH observed in juvenile mice of these strains is considered a genuine pre-neoplastic state, and a precursor for the multifocal MTC observed in more mature animals. Multifocal follicular thyroid tumors are the clinical hallmark of hereditary MTC in humans. The tumors observed in these mice displayed strong calcitonin and RET immunoreactivity. Penetrance of these tumors was 93% (42 of 45) in RET9-MEN2A mice and 52% (51 of 78) in RET51-MEN2A mice at 1 year of age. Discrepancies in the penetrance of MTC between these reports must be tempered by the differences in the promoters (rat versus human CGRP/CT) and mouse strains (DBA2 versus CBA/B6/FVB) used (Table 36–6).

The delayed onset of neoplastic disease may indicate that hyperplastic C cells require additional genetic lesions. This hypothesis is consistent with the observed loss of chromosome arms 1p, 3q, and 22q in MTC tumors in human subjects (*Eng et al., 1996b), and additional M918T mutations in 3 of 15 tumors resected from FMTC patients who harbored germline mutations at one of the five critical cysteines in RET. Transgenic mice expressing RET-2A fused to the MMLV^{LTR} exhibit in CCH or MTC in with 100% penetrance and mammary/parotid gland tumors with 50% penetrance (Table 36–6).

Mice harboring a targeted MEN2B mutation (M919T, mouse *Ret*) have also been established, recreating the genetic lesion observed in MEN2B patients in vivo (Smith-Hicks et al., 2000). Ret^{M919T}/Ret^+ mice display CCH (31%, <7 months; 41%, <12 months), and with decreased age of onset, expression is decreased in homozygote mutant mice (Table 36–6). Tyrosine hydroxylase (TH) and Chromogranin A (CGA) positive PC was also detected (100%, 6 months), consistent with the human equivalent. However, unlike human PC, they fail to express the phenylethanolamine-*N*-methyltransferase (PMNT) that is required for epinephrine production from norepinephrine. Absence of intestinal ganglioneuroma and oral neuroma in homozygotes suggested that the alteration of substrate specificity mediated by the Ret^{M919T} mutation may render both partial loss-of-function and gain-of-function effects. Thus one might expect to observe intestinal aganglionosis and renal agenesis in these mice. However, generation of a Ret^{M919T}/Ret^- mouse strain yielded no such observation. Thus, one must deduce that the observed pathological effects in these mice result only from a mutation dosage effect of the gain-of-function allele Ret^{M919T}. Furthermore, as RET gains access to new substrates through the Ret^{M919T} mutation, it must retain access to all normal RET substrates or only lose access to the substrates that are not essential for ENS and renal development.

Mouse models have also been established expressing the M918T mutation under the control of the dopamine β-hydroxylase (DβH) (Gestblom et al., 1999; *Sweetser et al., 1999) and calcitonin (CALC) (*Acton et al., 2000) promoters (Table 36–6). CALC-MEN2B-RET mice present with CCH and MTC (13%). DβH-RET-MEN2B mice exhibit benign neuroglial tumors in their sympathetic nervous systems and adrenal glands, consistent with ganglioneuromas observed in MEN2B patients (Table 36–6). However, no metastatic or malignant neoplasms were ever observed among these mice. Discrepancies between these models and human MEN2B are not altogether surprising and may actually reflect differences in the level and timing of RET-MEN2B expression driven by endogenous versus exogenous promoters, transgene copy number, differences in mouse–human physiology, or the use of the short versus all mutated isoforms of RET. The clinical features of MEN2B also include intestinal mucosal ganglioneuroma along the length of the gastrointestinal tract. Their absence in these mice implies that the human ENS is more sensitive to this pathological outcome than is that of the mouse.

PERSPECTIVES AND CONCLUDING REMARKS

It may be of little surprise that mutations within the same gene can result in such distinct and unrelated phenotypes as MEN2 and HSCR. These differences probably arise from the distinct effects of loss-of-function versus activating mutations, and how different cell types react to increases and decreases in RET protein or signaling. It is more difficult to understand how the same mutation can result in both disorders. *RET* mutations underlying HSCR require germline mutations at additional loci for disease expression, yet MEN2 tumors likely acquire additional somatic mutation in RET over time. Thus, these additional genetic events probably play critical roles in the resulting phenotypes. Furthermore, sensitivity to RET signaling among cell types and developmental stages—along with signal transduction, which uses distinct downstream pathways in each cell type—also contributes to the different outcomes.

Mouse models are critical to the dissection of human disease. Many "models" are able to mirror specific aspects of a particular pathology but are often unable to recapitulate the observed variation in clinical presentation, penetrance, sex bias, and so on. It is clear from the mod-

Table 36–6. Comparison of the Clinical Features of MEN2 Syndromes with the Phenotypes Observed in MEN2 Transgenic Mice

	CCH	MTC	HPT	PC	PTC	NH	IGN	PCA	M/PA	Kidney Defect	Isoforms	Mutation	Promoter
HUMAN PATHOLOGY													
MEN2A	+	+	+	+	+^{rare}							Fig. 36–3	
MEN2B	+	+	-	+	+^{rare}		+					Fig. 36–3	
FMTC	+	+	-							+ (Lore et al., 2001)		Fig. 36–3	
TRANSGENIC MOUSE STRAIN													
RET9-MEN2A	+	+	−	−	−						RET9	C634R	rCGRP/CT
RET51-MEN2A	+	+	−	−	+		+				RET51	C634R	hCGRP/CT
MMLV^{LTR}-MEN2A	+	+	−	−	−	+		+			RET51	C634R	MMLV^{LTR}
$Ret^{M919T/M919T}$	+	−	−	+	−						All	Ret^{M919T}	*Ret*
CALC-MEN2B-*RET*	+	+	−	−	−					Cysts	RET9	M918T	h*CALC-1*
DβH-RET-MEN2B	+	+	−	−	−					Agenesis	RET9	M918T	DβH

CCH, C-cell hyperplasia; MTC, medullary thyroid carcinoma; HPT, hyperparathyroidism; PC, pheochromocytoma; PTC, parathyroid carcinoma; NH, neuroglial hyperplasia; IGN, intestinal ganglioneuroma; PCA, pancreatic cyst-adenocarcinoma; M/PA, mammary/parotid carcinoma. +, present (frequency in text); +^{rare}, present as a rare association. *Promoters:* rCGRP/CT, rat calcitonin gene-related protein/calcitonin promoter; hCGRP/CT, human calcitonin gene-related protein/calcitonin promoter; MMLV^{LTR}, Moloney murine leukemia virus—long terminal repeat; CALC-1, human calcitonin gene promoter; DβH, dopamine β hydroxylase.

els of HSCR that targeted or spontaneous null mutations in a single gene fail, except in gross terms, to recapitulate clinical observations in patients. Perhaps our expectations of mouse models are inappropriate. Generation of a more valid HSCR model has required the combination of multiple alleles of *Ret* and *Ednrb* in the same mouse. Disease modeling in mice may benefit greatly from this paradigm of combining the effects at different loci. Furthermore, one can see how the study of other model organisms, particularly *Drosophila*, has benefited greatly from the availability of allelic series comprising a range of hypomorphs, hypermorphs, and neomorphs. The generation of allelic series including hypomorphic mutations in multiple genes known to be involved in a disease process, may, in general, produce better mouse models of human disease.

ACKNOWLEDGMENTS

We acknowledge the great debt owed, by all investigators in these fields, to the many HSCR and MEN2 families across the world, and to the Chakravarti laboratory members, past and present, whose contributions have made possible many of the studies discussed in this review. We thank Minerva Carrasquillo, Eileen Emisson, Renee Read, and Anirban Maitra for their critical reading of the manuscript, and we are indebted to Ron Conlon for guidance concerning mouse embryology and many helpful discussions on the manuscript.

REFERENCES

Unabridged reference list may be found at http://chakravarti.som.jhmi.edu/resume/andy_chap36_ref.htm

Airaksinen MS, Titievsky A, Saarma M (1999). GDNF family neurotrophic factor signaling: four masters, one servant? *Mol Cell Neurosci* 13: 313–325.

Angrist M, Bolk S, Thiel B, Puffenberger EG, Hofstra RM, Buys CH, Cass DT, Chakravarti A (1995). Mutation analysis of the RET receptor tyrosine kinase in Hirschsprung disease. *Hum Mol Genet* 4: 821–830.

Attie T, Pelet A, Edery P, Eng C, Mulligan LM, Amiel J, Boutrand L, Beldjord C, Nihoul-Fekete C, Munnich A, et al. (1995). Diversity of RET proto-oncogene mutations in familial and sporadic Hirschsprung disease. *Hum Mol Genet* 4: 1381–1386.

Auricchio A, Griseri P, Carpentieri ML, Betsos N, Staiano A, Tozzi A, Priolo M, Thompson H, Bocciardi R, Romeo G, et al. (1999). Double heterozygosity for a RET substitution interfering with splicing and an EDNRB missense mutation in Hirschsprung disease. *Am J Hum Genet* 64: 1216–1221.

Badner JA, Sieber WK, Garver KL, Chakravarti A (1990). A genetic study of Hirschsprung disease. *Am J Hum Genet* 46: 568–580.

Baloh RH, Tansey MG, Lampe PA, Fahrner TJ, Enomoto H, Simburger KS, Leitner ML, Araki T, Johnson EM Jr, Milbrandt J (1998). Artemin, a novel member of the GDNF ligand family, supports peripheral and central neurons and signals through the GFRα3-RET receptor complex. *Neuron* 21: 1291–1302.

Bolino A, Schuffenecker I, Luo Y, Seri M, Silengo M, Tocco T, Chabrier G, Houdent C, Murat A, Schlumberger M, et al. (1995). RET mutations in exons 13 and 14 of FMTC patients. *Oncogene* 10: 2415–2419.

Bolk S, Pelet A, Hofstra RM, Angrist M, Salomon R, Croaker D, Buys CH, Lyonnet S, Chakravarti A (2000). A human model for multigenic inheritance: phenotypic expression in Hirschsprung disease requires both the RET gene and a new 9q31 locus. *Proc Natl Acad Sci USA* 97: 268–273.

Borrello MG, Smith DP, Pasini B, Bongarzone I, Greco A, Lorenzo MJ, Arighi E, Miranda C, Eng C, Alberti L, et al. (1995). RET activation by germline MEN2A and MEN2B mutations. *Oncogene* 11: 2419–2427.

Brandi ML, Gagel RF, Angeli A, Bilezikian JP, Beck-Peccoz P, Bordi C, Conte-Devolx B, Falchetti A, Gheri RG, Libroia A, et al. (2001). Guidelines for diagnosis and therapy of MEN type 1 and type 2. *J Clin Endocrinol Metab* 86: 5658–5671.

Carrasquillo M, McCallion AS, Puffenberger EG, Kashuk CS, Nouri N, Chakravarti A (2002). Genome-wide association study and mouse model identify interaction between RET and EDNRB pathways in Hirschsprung disease. *Nat Genet* 32: 237–244.

Chakravarti A, Lyonnet S (2000). Hirschsprung Disease. In: *The Metabolic and Molecular Bases of Inherited Disease, 8th edition*. Scriver CR, Beaudet AL, Valle D, Sly W (eds.) McGraw-Hill, New York.

Donis-Keller H, Dou S, Chi D, Carlson KM, Toshima K, Lairmore TC, Howe JR, Moley JF, Goodfellow P, Wells SA Jr. (1993). Mutations in the RET proto-oncogene are associated with MEN 2A and FMTC. *Hum Mol Genet* 2: 851–856.

Durbec P, Marcos-Gutierrez CV, Kilkenny C, Grigoriou M, Wartiowaara K, Suvanto P, Smith D, Ponder B, Costantini F, Saarma M, et al. (1996a). GDNF signalling through the Ret receptor tyrosine kinase. *Nature* 381: 789–793.

Edery P, Lyonnet S, Mulligan LM, Pelet A, Dow E, Abel L, Holder S, Nihoul-Fekete C, Ponder BA, Munnich A (1994). Mutations of the RET proto-oncogene in Hirschsprung's disease. *Nature* 367: 378–380.

Eng C, Mulligan LM, Smith DP, Healey CS, Frilling A, Raue F, Neumann HP, Ponder MA, Ponder BA (1995). Low frequency of germline mutations in the RET proto-oncogene in patients with apparently sporadic medullary thyroid carcinoma. *Clin Endocrinol* 43: 123–127.

Eng C, Clayton D, Schuffenecker I, Lenoir G, Cote G, Gagel RF, van Amstel HK, Lips CJ, Nishisho I, Takai SI, et al. (1996). The relationship between specific RET proto-oncogene mutations and disease phenotype in multiple endocrine neoplasia type 2: International RET Mutation Consortium analysis. *JAMA* 276: 1575–1579.

Enomoto H, Araki T, Jackman A, Heuckeroth RO, Snider WD, Johnson EM Jr, Milbrandt

J (1998). GFR α-deficient mice have deficits in the enteric nervous system and kidneys. *Neuron* 21: 317–324.

Fewtrell MS, Tam PK, Thomson AH, Fitchett M, Currie J, Huson SM, Mulligan LM (1994). Hirschsprung's disease associated with a deletion of chromosome 10 (q11.2q21.2): a further link with the neurocristopathies? *J Med Genet* 31: 325–327.

Gabriel SB, Salomon R, Pelet A, Angrist M, Amiel J, Fornage M, Attie-Bitach T, Olson JM, Hofstra R, Buys C, et al. (2002). Segregation at three loci explains familial and population risk in Hirschsprung disease. *Nat Genet* 31: 89–93.

Gestblom C, Sweetser DA, Doggett B, Kapur RP (1999). Sympathoadrenal hyperplasia causes renal malformations in Ret (MEN2B)-transgenic mice. *Am J Pathol* 155: 2167–2179.

Hahn M, Bishop J (2001). Expression pattern of *Drosophila* ret suggests a common ancestral origin between the metamorphosis precursors in insect endoderm and the vertebrate enteric neurons. *Proc Natl Acad Sci USA* 98: 1053–1058.

Henderson CE, Phillips HS, Pollock RA, Davies AM, Lemeulle C, Armanini M, Simmons L, Moffet B, Vandlen RA, Simpson LC, et al. (1994). GDNF: a potent survival factor for motoneurons present in peripheral nerve and muscle. *Science* 266: 1062–1064.

Hofstra RM, Landsvater RM, Ceccherini I, Stulp RP, Stelwagen T, Luo Y, Pasini B, Hoppener JW, van Amstel HK, Romeo G (1994). A mutation in the RET proto-oncogene associated with multiple endocrine neoplasia type 2B and sporadic medullary thyroid carcinoma. *Nature* 367: 375–376.

Hosoda K, Hammer RE, Richardson JA, Baynash AG, Cheung JC, Giaid A, Yanagisawa M (1994). Targeted and natural (piebald-lethal) mutations of endothelin-B receptor gene produce megacolon associated with spotted coat color in mice. *Cell* 79: 1267–1276.

Ito S, Iwashita T, Asai N, Murakami H, Iwata Y, Sobue G, Takahashi M (1997). Biological properties of Ret with cysteine mutations correlate with multiple endocrine neoplasia type 2A, familial medullary thyroid carcinoma, and Hirschsprung's disease phenotype. *Cancer Res* 57: 2870–2872.

Iwashita T, Murakami H, Asai N, Takahashi M (1996). Mechanism of ret dysfunction by Hirschsprung mutations affecting its extracellular domain. *Hum Mol Genet* 5: 1577–1580.

Iwashita T, Kurokawa K, Qiao S, Murakami H, Asai N, Kawai K, Hashimoto M, Watanabe T, Ichihara M, Takahashi M (2001). Functional analysis of RET with Hirschsprung mutations affecting its kinase domain. *Gastroenterology* 121: 24–33.

Le Douarin N, Kalcheim C (1999). *The Neural Crest, 2nd edition*. Cambridge University Press, Cambridge.

Luo Y, Ceccherini I, Pasini B, Matera I, Bicocchi MP, Barone V, Bocciardi R, Kaariainen H, Weber D, Devoto M, et al. (1993). Close linkage with the RET protooncogene and boundaries of deletion mutations in autosomal dominant Hirschsprung disease. *Hum Mol Genet* 2: 1803–1808.

Luttrell LM, Daaka Y, Lefkowitz RJ (1999). Regulation of tyrosine kinase cascades by G-protein-coupled receptors. *Curr Opin Cell Biol* 11: 177–183.

Manié S, Santoro M, Fusco A, Billaud M (2001). The RET receptor: function in development and dysfunction in congenital malformation. *Trends Genet* 17: 580–589.

Marcos-Gutierrez CV, Wilson SW, Holder N, Pachnis V (1997). The zebrafish homologue of the ret receptor and its pattern of expression during embryogenesis. *Oncogene* 14: 879–889.

McCallion AS, Chakravarti A (2001). EDNRB/EDN3 and Hirschsprung disease type II. *Pigment Cell Res* 14: 161–169.

McCallion AS, Stames E, Conlon RA, Chakravarti A (2003). Phenotype variation in two-locus mouse models of Hirschsprung disease: Tissue specific interaction between Ret and *Ednrb*. *Proc Natl Acad Sci USA* 100: 1826–1831.

Meier-Ruge W, Hunziker O, Tobler HJ, Walliser C (1972). The pathophysiology of aganglionosis of the entire colon (Zuelzer-Wilson syndrome): morphometric investigations of the extent of sacral parasympathetic innervation of the circular muscles of the aganglionic colon. *Beitr Pathol* 147: 228–236.

Michiels FM, Chappuis S, Caillou B, Pasini A, Talbot M, Monier R, Lenoir GM, Feunteun J, Billaud M (1997). Development of medullary thyroid carcinoma in transgenic mice expressing the RET protooncogene altered by a multiple endocrine neoplasia type 2A mutation. *Proc Natl Acad Sci USA* 94: 3330–3335.

Moore MW, Klein RD, Farinas I, Sauer H, Armanini M, Phillips H, Reichardt LF, Ryan AM, Carver-Moore K, Rosenthal A (1996). Renal and neuronal abnormalities in mice lacking GDNF. *Nature* 382: 76–79.

Moore SW, Albertyn R, Cywes S (1996). Clinical outcome and long-term quality of life after surgical correction of Hirschsprung's disease. *J Pediatr Surg* 31: 1496–1502.

Mulligan LM, Ponder BA (1995). Genetic basis of endocrine disease: multiple endocrine neoplasia type 2. *J Clin Endocrinol Metab* 80: 1989–1995.

Neumann HP, Eng C, Mulligan LM, Glavac D, Zauner I, Ponder BA, Crossey PA, Maher EU, Brauch H (1995). Consequences of direct genetic testing for germline mutations in the clinical management of families with multiple endocrine neoplasia, type II. *JAMA* 274: 1149–1151.

Olson JA Jr, DeBenedetti MK, Baumann DS, Wells SA Jr (1996). Parathyroid autotransplantation during thyroidectomy. Results of long-term follow-up. *Ann Surg* 223: 472–478; discussion 478–480.

Pachnis V, Mankoo B, Costantini F (1993). Expression of the c-ret proto-oncogene during mouse embryogenesis. *Development* 119: 1005–1017.

Pasini B, Borrello MG, Greco A, Bongarzone I, Luo Y, Mondellini P, Alberti L, Miranda C, Arighi E, Bocciardi R, et al. (1995). Loss of function effect of RET mutations causing Hirschsprung disease. *Nat Genet* 10: 35–40.

Pichel JG, Shen L, Sheng HZ, Granholm AC, Drago J, Grinberg A, Lee EJ, Huang SP, Saarma M, Hoffer BJ, et al. (1996a). Defects in enteric innervation and kidney development in mice lacking GDNF. *Nature* 382: 73–76.

Ponder BA (1999). The phenotypes associated with ret mutations in the multiple endocrine neoplasia type 2 syndrome. *Cancer Res* 59: 1736s–1741s; discussion 1742s.

Puffenberger EG, Kauffman ER, Bolk S, Matise TC, Washington SS, Angrist M, Weissenbach J, Garver KL, Mascari M, Ladda R, et al. (1994). Identity-by-descent and association mapping of a recessive gene for Hirschsprung disease on human chromosome 13q22. *Hum Mol Genet* 3: 1217–1225.

Romeo G, Ronchetto P, Luo Y, Barone V, Seri M, Ceccherini I, Pasini B, Bocciardi R, Lerone M, Kaariainen H, et al. (1994). Point mutations affecting the tyrosine kinase domain of the RET proto-oncogene in Hirschsprung's disease. *Nature* 367: 377–378.

Sanchez MP, Silos-Santiago I, Frisen J, He B, Lira SA, Barbacid M (1996). Renal agenesis and the absence of enteric neurons in mice lacking GDNF. *Nature* 382: 70–73.

Santoro M, Carlomagno F, Romano A, Bottaro DP, Dathan NA, Grieco M, Fusco A, Vecchio G, Matoskova B, Kraus MH, et al. (1995). Activation of RET as a dominant transforming gene by germline mutations of MEN2A and MEN2B. *Science* 267: 381–383.

Saxen L, Sariola H (1987). Early organogenesis of the kidney. *Pediatr Nephrol* 1: 385–392.

Schimke RN, Hartman WH, Prout TW, Rimoin DL (1968). Syndrome of bilateral pheochromocytoma, medullary thyroid carcinoma and multiple neuroma. *N Engl J Med* 279: 1–7.

Schuchardt A, D'Agati V, Larsson-Blomberg L, Costantini F, Pachnis V (1994). Defects in the kidney and enteric nervous system of mice lacking the tyrosine kinase receptor Ret. *Nature* 367: 380–383.

Seri M, Yin L, Barone V, Bolino A, Celli I, Bocciardi R, Pasini B, Ceccherini I, Lerone M, Kristoffersson U, et al. (1997). Frequency of RET mutations in long- and short-segment Hirschsprung disease. *Hum Mutat* 9: 243–249.

Smith-Hicks CL, Sizer KC, Powers JF, Tischler AS, Costantini F (2000). C-cell hyperplasia, pheochromocytoma and sympathoadrenal malformation in a mouse model of multiple endocrine neoplasia type 2B. *EMBO J* 19: 612–622.

Soave F (1966). Hirschsprung's disease: technique and results of Soave's operation. *Br J Surg* 53: 1023–1027.

Swenson O, Bill A (1948). Resection of rectum and rectosigmoid with preservation of sphincter for benign spastic lesions producing megacolon. *Surgery* 24: 212.

Takahashi M (2001). RET-GDNF signaling in human diseases. *Cytokine Growth Factor Rev* 12: 361–373.

Takahashi M, Cooper GM (1987). ret transforming gene encodes a fusion protein homologous to tyrosine kinases. *Mol Cell Biol* 7: 1378–1385.

Takahashi M, Ritz J, Cooper GM (1985). Activation of a novel human transforming gene, ret, by DNA rearrangement. *Cell* 42: 581–588.

Takahashi M, Iwashita T, Santoro M, Lyonnet S, Lenoir GM, Billaud M (1999). Co-segregation of MEN2 and Hirschsprung's disease: the same mutation of RET with both gain and loss-of-function? *Hum Mutat* 13: 331–336.

Trupp M, Arenas E, Fainzilber M, Nilsson AS, Sieber BA, Grigoriou M, Kilkenny C, Salazar-Grueso E, Pachnis V, Arumae U (1996). Functional receptor for GDNF encoded by the c-ret proto-oncogene. *Nature* 381: 785–789.

van Biesen T, Hawes BE, Luttrell DK, Krueger KM, Touhara K, Porfiri E, Sakaue M, Luttrell LM, Lefkowitz RJ (1995). Receptor-tyrosine-kinase- and Gβγ-mediated MAP kinase activation by a common signalling pathway. *Nature* 376: 781–784.

van Heurn LW, Schaap C, Sie G, Haagen AA, Gerver WJ, Freling G, van Amstel HK, Heineman E (1999). Predictive DNA testing for multiple endocrine neoplasia 2: a therapeutic challenge of prophylactic thyroidectomy in very young children. *J Pediatr Surg* 34: 568–571.

Webster W (1974). Aganglionic megacolon in piebald-lethal mice. *Arch Pathol* 97: 111–117.

Whitehouse F, Kernohan J (1948). Myenteric plexuses in congenital megacolon: study of 11 cases. *Arch Intern Med* 82: 75.

Part G.
The Endothelin Signaling Pathway

37 | Introduction to Endothelin-3/Endothelin-B Receptor and *SOX10* Signaling Pathways

CHERYL E. GARIEPY AND MASASHI YANAGISAWA

Hirschsprung disease (congenital absence of the distal enteric nervous system [ENS]) and Waardenburg syndrome (pigment abnormalities and sensorineural deafness) result from abnormal embryonic development of neural crest–derived cells. These developmental abnormalities occur together in humans (Shah-Waardenburg syndrome) and in several species of animals. The Shah-Waardenburg syndrome is caused by mutations in the genes that encode the endothelin-B receptor (*EDNRB*), one of its ligands, endothelin-3 (*EDN3*), and the transcription factor *SOX10* (see Chapter 38). A similar phenotype occurs in animals homozygous for targeted or naturally occurring disruption of *ednrb* and *edn3* or heterozygous for targeted or naturally occurring disruption of *sox10* (Baynash et al., 1994; Hosoda et al., 1994; Herbarth et al., 1998; Southard-Smith et al., 1998; Britsch et al., 2001).

These mutant mice are important tools for studying melanocyte and ENS development. The roles of edn3/ednrb and sox10 signaling in development of pigment cells and the ENS are just beginning to emerge. Despite the similarities of the skin and enteric phenotypes observed in *sox10*, *edn3*, and *ednrb* mutant animals and humans, a clear connection between the two signaling systems has not yet been established.

During development, *ednrb* and *sox10* are expressed by early melanocyte precursors (Gariepy et al., 1998; Herbarth et al., 1998;

Kuhlbrodt et al., 1998; Pusch et al., 1998). An absence of ednrb activation on the neural crest (NC) cell leads to an early reduction in melanoblast number and a failure of migration. It is not yet clear whether this abnormality results from a failure of NC cell proliferation, migration, or differentiation. Several lines of evidence suggest that edn3/ednrb signaling may be required near the time of initiation of melanoblast migration (Opdecamp et al., 1998; Shin et al., 1999). In vitro, edn3/ednrb signaling affects NC cell proliferation early in the melanocyte lineage and differentiation in melanoblasts (Reid et al., 1996; Opdecamp et al., 1998; Dupin et al., 2000). Sox10 appears to be a transcriptional regulator of other early melanoblast markers (Potterf et al., 2000, 2001). Homozygous *sox10* mutant embryos exhibit early, near-complete apoptotic loss of melanoblasts. Heterozygous *sox10* mutant embryos exhibit delayed melanoblast development and sharp apoptotic reductions in early melanoblast numbers (Potterf et al., 2001). Despite this, skin pigmentation may be nearly complete, suggesting that a later population of melanoblasts is less effected by sox10 deficiency.

Ednrb and *sox10* are also expressed in early ENS precursors. In the absence of ednrb activation, ENS precursors in the mouse show abnormalities in gut colonization beginning in the region of the cecum, and several lines of evidence suggest that ednrb activation during intestinal colonization is critical for complete colonization of the distal gut (Coventry et al., 1994; Shin et al., 1999; Woodward et al., 2000; Sidebotham et al., 2002). In vitro evidence indicates that edn3/endrb signaling maintains ENS precursors in an undifferentiated state (Hearn et al., 1998; Wu et al., 1999). ENS precursors in homozygous *sox10* mutant mice undergo apoptosis before they reach the gut. ENS precursors in heterozygous *sox10* mutant mice exhibit early delays in migration and apoptosis, though final gut colonization may be complete, suggesting that haploinsufficiency for *sox10* selectively affects an early subset of ENS precursors (Southard-Smith et al., 1998; Kapur 1999a).

Our understanding of the complex mechanisms by which edn3/endrb and sox10 signaling bring about normal development of the ENS and epidermal melanocytes is only in its infancy. The interaction of these pathways in vivo is not yet defined, modifying genes are just beginning to be described, and downstream mediators of these signaling pathways are largely unknown.

NEURAL CREST ORIGIN OF EPIDERMAL MELANOCYTES AND THE ENS

Melanocytes, enteric neurons, and enteric glia are neural crest (NC)–derived tissues. The NC is a group of cells that detach from the neuroepithelium of the folding neural tube and migrate into the embryo in two, loosely organized streams. One stream spreads dorsally under the ectoderm and gives rise to pigment cells. The other stream spreads ventrally along the sides of the neural tube and gives rise to most of the peripheral nervous system, adrenal chromaffin cells, C cells of the thyroid, skeletal and muscular components of the head and neck, and portions of the cardiac outflow tract (Garcia-Castro and Bronner-Fraser, 1999; Le Dourarin and Kalcheim, 1999) (see Chapter 6).

In the mouse, NC migration begins around embryonic day 8 (E8), and melanoblasts can be detected along the dorsal migration pathway shortly thereafter (Matsui et al., 1990; Keshet et al., 1991; Pavan and Tilghman, 1994). Melanoblasts invade the epidermis at approximately E12 (Yoshida et al., 1996), proliferate extensively, and differentiate into mature melanocytes beginning at E16 (Hirobe, 1984). Although melanocytes are derived from all axial levels of the NC, the majority of them are derived from trunk regions of the embryo (Le Douarin and Dupin, 1993).

The enteric nervous system (ENS) is derived from specific axial levels of the NC. Vagal (somites 1–5), truncal (somites 6–7), and sacral (caudal to somite 28) NC cells colonize the gut. Vagal- and truncal-derived ENS precursors follow a ventral migration pathway, enter the foregut mesenchyme (mouse E9.5), and colonize the developing gut in a rostral-to-caudal progression (Kapur et al., 1991). The entire colonization process, from NC to rectum, takes 5 days in the mouse and more than 6 weeks in humans. Colonization of the hindgut by vagal NC–derived cells is complete around E14 in the mouse (Kapur et al., 1992; Young et al., 1998). Ganglia throughout the length of the gut originate in the vagal NC. The esophagus and proximal stomach are also populated by cells derived from the truncal NC (Durbec et al., 1996). The colonization of the gut by sacral NC–derived cells and the contribution of these cells to the ENS in the mouse are controversial. Recent evidence indicates that sacral NC cells emigrate from the neural plate after E10 and form extraenteric pelvic ganglia. Renal subcapsular hindgut graft experiments suggest that these NC–derived cells are able to colonize the gut (after E14) and contribute to the ENS, even in the absence of vagal NC–derived cells (Kapur, 2000). However, evidence suggests that only a minority of hindgut neurons may be sacral NC–derived, and genetic abnormalities that interfere with complete colonization of the gut by vagal NC–derived cells usually lead to complete aganglionosis of the terminal hindgut.

MOUSE MODELS OF SHAH-WAARDENBURG SYNDROME

Development of melanocytes and the ENS involves common signaling pathways, as evidenced by the frequency of coexpression of congenital abnormalities in pigmentation and enteric ganglia. In humans, areas of deficient skin, hair, or eye pigmentation (Waardenburg syndrome) combined with an absence of the ENS in a variable length of distal gut (Hirschsprung disease) is termed the Shah-Waardenburg syndrome. The Shah-Waardenburg syndrome is caused by mutations in the genes that encode the endothelin-B receptor (*EDNRB*), one of its ligands, endothelin–3 (*EDN3*), and the transcription factor *SOX10* (see Chapter 38). A similar phenotype occurs in animals homozygous for targeted or naturally occurring disruption of *ednrb* and *edn3* or heterozygous for targeted or naturally occurring disruption of *sox10* (see Table 37–1). Naturally occurring mouse mutations of *ednrb* include complete deletion of *ednrb*, *piebald lethal* (s^l), and a mutation leading to a reduced level of normal *ednrb* expression, *piebald* (*s*). *Ednrb*$^{s/s}$ mice have approximately 27% of the wild-type level of ednrb receptors (Hosoda, et al., 1994). The naturally occurring mouse mutation of *edn3*, *lethal spotting* (*ls*), results in a single amino acid substitution in the edn3 propeptide that prevents the proteolytic activation of the peptide. The naturally occurring mouse mutation of *sox10* is *dominant megacolon*, *Dom*. *Sox10*^{Dom} is a single bp insertion that produces a truncated product with an abnormal carboxy terminus (Herbarth et al., 1998; Southard-Smith et al., 1998). The similarity of phenotype between *sox10*$^{Dom/+}$ and *sox10*$^{LacZ/+}$ mice suggests that *sox10*^{Dom} is a null mutation (Britsch et al., 2001).

Mice that lack functional ednrb (*ednrb*$^{s/s}$ and *ednrb*$^{-/-}$) exhibit pigment in <10% of the skin surface. Pigmentation is restricted to small areas along the back, generally in the head and hip regions only. These animals uniformly have distal colonic aganglionosis. Mice that lack functional edn3 (*edn3*$^{ls/ls}$ and *edn3*$^{-/-}$) have large areas of abnormal pigmentation but tend to be more pigmented than *ednrb*-deficient animals; they uniformly exhibit distal colonic aganglionosis. On the most commonly studied genetic background (mixed C57Bl/6J × C3HeB/FeJ), *sox10*$^{Dom/+}$ individuals uniformly show an absence of epidermal melanocytes in the distal extremities and in a spot on the abdomen, as well as distal colonic deficiency in the ENS (Kapur et al., 1996). The expression and penetrance of the *ednrb*$^{s/s}$ and *sox10*$^{Dom/+}$ phenotypes are strongly influenced by other genes (Lane and Liu, 1984; Pavan et al., 1995). The roles of edn3/ednrb and sox10 signaling in the development of pigment cells and the ENS are beginning to be defined, largely through studies that take advantage of mutant mice.

THE ENDOTHELIN SYSTEM

Endothelins are a family of 21-amino acid vasoactive isopeptides: EDN1, EDN2, and EDN3. Each isopeptide contains two intrachain disulfide bonds and is encoded by a separate gene. The three isopeptides vary by not more than six amino acids (Inoue et al., 1989). Each peptide is produced as an inactive preproendothelin that is cleaved by dibasic pair-specific endopeptidases to yield the biologically inactive propeptide (38–41 amino acids), known as "big endothelin." Mature endothelins are produced through the action of phosphoramindon-inhibitable metaloproteases termed "endothelin-converting enzymes" (ECEs). There are two major classes of ECEs—ECE1 and ECE2—that vary in their cellular localization and pH of optimal activity (Xu et al., 1994; Emoto and Yanagisawa 1995).

The two endothelin receptors—EDNRA and EDNRB—are G protein–coupled, heptahelical membrane receptors and encoded by separate genes. EDNRB is nonselective for the three endothelins, whereas EDNRA shows highest affinity to EDN1 (Arai et al., 1990; Sakurai et al., 1990). *EDNRB* is located on human chromosome 13q22, and *EDN3* is located on human chromosome 20q13.2–q13.3.

Targeted disruption of genes in the endothelin system in mice establishes that the physiologically relevant ligand for ednrb in development is edn3. Although ednrb accepts edn1 and edn2 with equally high affinity as edn3, *edn3*$^{-/-}$ mice exhibit a developmental phenotype very similar to *ednrb*$^{-/-}$ mice (Baynash et al., 1994; Hosoda et al., 1994). This finding also demonstrates that endothelins function largely in an autocrine or paracrine manner during development. The milder coat color and enteric phenotype in *edn3*$^{-/-}$ mice compared to *ednrb*$^{-/-}$ mice suggests that edn1 and edn2 may partially compensate for edn3 deficiency. *Ece1*$^{-/-}$ mice exhibit craniofacial and cardiac outflow abnormalities (caused by failure of active edn1 pro-

Table 37–1. Animal Models of Abnormal edn3/ednrb or sox10 Signaling

Gene	Species	Mutation Name or Designation	Autosomal Dominant (D) or Recessive (r)	Mutation	Pigment Phenotype	Enteric Phenotype	Other Phenotypes	References
ednrb	Mouse	Piebald lethal, s^l	r	Gene deletion	<5% pigmented (dorsal head and hips) with black eyes	Absent ENS in distal colon and rectum		Hosoda et al., 1994; Pavan 1994; Silvers, 1979
		Piebald, s	r	Disruption of enhancer element	>80% pigmented; distal extremities and ventral spot not pigmented	None		Pavan and Tilghman, 1994; Silvers, 1979
		Knockout, —	r	Deletion of exon 3	<10% pigmented (see piebald lethal)	See s^l		Hosoda et al., 1994
	Rat	Spotting lethal, sl	r	Deletion of 3' end of first exon	<10% pigmented with black eyes; dorsal head with decreased pigment density	Absent ENS in distal ileum through rectum		Ikadai et al., 1979
	Horse	Overo-lethal-white	r	Dinucleotide substitution	<10% pigmented with blue eyes and clear hooves	Absent ENS from mid-small intestine to rectum	Deafness	McCabe et al., 1990; Metallinos et al., 1998; Santschi et al., 1998; Vonderfecht et al., 1983
	Zebrafish	Rose	r	Several described, including premature stop codons	Disruption of ventral stripes; iridophore defect	None described	Runting observed in some mutants	Parichy et al., 2000
ecel	Mouse	Knockout, —	r	Exon 5' to zinc-binding motif replaced	Absent epidermal melanocytes	Absent ENS in at least distal colon	Embryonic lethal with craniofacial defects and cardiac outflow anomalies	Yanagisawa et al., 1998
edn3	Mouse	Lethal spotting, ls	r	Point missense mutation	20–30% pigmented with black eyes; pigmentation in dorsal head and hip	Absent ENS in distal colon and rectum; ~15% survive into adulthood		Baynash et al., 1994
		Knockout, —	r	Deletion of edn3-encoding portion of exon 2	See ls	See ls		Baynash et al., 1994
sox10	Mouse	Dominant megacolon, Dom	D	Single base insertion giving rise to abnormal product	Ventral white spot with white paws	Heterozygotes: Absent ENS in distal colon and rectum; normal ENS development observed on some genetic backgrounds		Herbarth et al., 1998; Lane and Liu, 1984; Kapur et al., 1996; Southard-Smith et al., 1998
		Knockout, LacZ	D	Replacement of exons 3–5 with LacZ	Ventral white spot with black eyes	Heterozygotes: Distal ENS absent		Britsch et al., 2001

duction), as well as an absence of epidermal melanocytes and distal enteric neurons (Yanagisawa et al., 1998). Therefore, ece1 is the protease responsible for the formation of active edn3 in the developing embryo. *ECE1* is located on human chromosome 1p36.1.

EDNRB/EDN3 SIGNALING DURING DEVELOPMENT

In the developing embryo, *ednrb* is expressed in the neural tube before the initiation of NC migration (Brand et al., 1998; Gariepy et al., 1998; Yanagisawa et al., 1998). *Ednrb* continues to be expressed by early melanoblasts and ENS precursors as they begin to migrate. Data from human embryos indicate that once two topographically distinct subpopulations form, melanocyte precursors stop expressing *EDNRB* (Brand et al., 1998). However, in rats, a distinct population of cells, consistent with the temporal and spacial localization of melanoblasts, express *ednrb* (Gariepy et al., 1998). *Ednrb* is expressed by ENS precursors as they colonize the gut mesenchyme (Brand et al., 1998; Gariepy et al., 1998). *Ednrb* expression is also reported in enteric mesenchymal cells (Wu et al., 1999; Lang et al., 2000). *Edn3* and *ece1* are expressed by the mesenchyme surrounding the neural tube, along the dorsal migration pathway of the melanoblasts and in the developing gut mesoderm (Yanagisawa et al., 1998; Lang et al., 2000). Enteric EDN3 expression is highest in the embryonic cecum (Leibl et al., 1999).

Melanocyte Development

Ednrb^{s1/s} mice (with approximately 12.5% of the wild-type level of *ednrb* expression) are approximately 50% pigmented, while *ednrb^{s/s}* mice (with approximately 25% of the wild-type level of *ednrb* expression) are approximately 80% pigmented (Hosoda et al., 1994). Therefore, it appears that there is an ednrb "dose–response" relationship in melanocyte development and that normal pigmentation on this genetic background requires >25% of the wild-type level of *ednrb* expression.

Expression of the melanoblast-specific marker dopachrome tautomerase, *dct*, is delayed, and the number of cells expressing *dct* is reduced in *ednrb^{s1/s1}* mice at E10.5. *Dct*-expressing cells are also abnormally restricted in location. These findings have led to the suggestion that ednrb is important at or immediately before melanoblast proliferation and migration. However, because *ednrb^{-/-}* mice exhibit some pigmentation, ednrb is apparently not absolutely required for this process (Pavan and Tilghman, 1994; Reid et al., 1996; Opdecamp et al., 1998).

Shin et al (1999) used a tetracycline-inducible system to generate strains of mice in which *ednrb* expression could be limited to specific stages of embryogenesis. They found that normal melanocyte development required *ednrb* expression between E10 and E12.5, corresponding to an initial melanoblast migration stage. These investigators suggest that *ednrb* is required by melanoblasts for the transition from premigratory to migratory cells and/or for the initiation of migration.

In vitro studies using quail cells demonstrate that edn3 markedly increases the proliferation of pluripotent NC cells and stimulates an increase in the number of melanocytes (Lahav et al., 1996; Stone et al., 1997). In primary mouse NC cell cultures, edn3 treatment leads to expansion of the melanocyte progenitor pool, beginning at approximately E10, and differentiation of progenitors into mature melanocytes, beginning at approximately E14 (Reid et al., 1996; Opdecamp et al., 1997, 1998). Yoshida et al. (1996) suggest that edn3 may be required for melanocyte proliferation within the epidermis. Edn3 not only increases the number of postmigratory melanocytes in vitro but also can induce the differentiation of melanocytes and glia from a clonal population of melanocytes (Dupin et al., 2000). Edn3 may play a role in terminal differentiation of melanocytes both pre- and perinatally (Reid et al., 1996; Opdecamp et al., 1998; Sviderskaya et al., 1998).

ENS Development

Distal ENS deficiency occurs only in mice with severe ednrb deficiency. That is, distal intestinal aganglionosis is routinely found in *ednrb^{s1/s1}*, *ednrb^{s1/-}*, or *ednrb^{-/-}* mice but is almost never found in *ednrb^{s1/s}* or *ednrb^{s/s}* mice. This is compatible with the idea that a very low level of ednrb—estimated at 12.5% of wild-type levels in *ednrb^{s1/sl}* mice (Hosoda, et al., 1994)—is sufficient for normal development of the ENS.

Most, if not all, vagal NC cells are transiently catecholaminergic (i.e., express dopamine-β-hydroxylase; DβH) during their colonization of the developing gut mesenchyme. Using a *DβH-lacZ* transgene and β-galactosidase staining to visualize the ENS precursors, abnormalities in ENS colonization of the developing gut are first noted in the cecum of *ednrb^{s1/s1}* mice at E12 (Coventry et al., 1994). Genetic studies allowing for time-controlled expression of *ednrb* in developing mice found that the critical period in ENS development for *ednrb* expression is E10 to E12.5 (Shin et al., 1999). This corresponds to the period when the vagal NC–derived cells colonize the distal ileum through proximal colon. Organ-culture experiments demonstrate failure of colonization by NC cells when mouse embryonic gut explants are treated with an ednrb-selective antagonist during a similar time frame (E11.5–E12.5) (Woodward et al., 2000). Sidebotham and colleagues (2002) isolated E11.5 mouse colons and detected only a very small number of NC-derived cells in the proximal portion, at the leading edge of the ENS precursor colonization front. Using organ culture, they found that this small group of cells was able to populate the entire colon with normal appearing ganglia. However, they observed terminal aganglionosis in colons cultured in the presence of an ednrb-selective antagonist. They conclude that the cells at the leading edge of colonization are NC stem cells and that normal development of these cells depends on edn3/ednrb signaling within the colon, after E11.5. Taken together, these findings suggest that an absence of ednrb signaling as the ENS precursors colonize the pericecal (distal ileum to proximal colon) region leads to ENS deficits in the distal colon. This localization may be modified by the genetic background as rats, horses, and humans with *EDNRB/ednrb* or *EDN3/edn3* mutations exhibit ENS deficits well proximal to the ileocecal junction, indicating that ENS deficits in ednrb deficiency have the potential of being very extensive (see Table 37–1 this chapter and Tables 38–1 and 38–3 of the following chapter).

Studies using tissue-specific expression of *ednrb* or *edn3* via a transgene in rodents demonstrate that activation of ednrb on NC-derived cells allows for apparently normal ENS development. In the ednrb-null (*ednrb^{sl/sl}*) rat, expression of a *DβH-ednrb* transgene results in rats that live and grow well into adulthood with no obvious abnormalities in intestinal function (Gariepy et al., 1998). The *DβH* promoter has also been used to drive *edn3* expression specifically in NC-derived cells in the developing gut of *edn3^{-/-}* mice. Mice expressing *edn3* only under the control of the *DβH* promoter develop a functionally normal ENS and live well into adulthood (Rice et al., 2000). Thus, ectopic expression of the ligand on the receptor-expressing cells is sufficient to allow complete colonization of the gut. The ability of *DβH* transgenes to "rescue" ednrb-null and edn3-null animals from their intestinal abnormality suggests that the critical location for ednrb activation in ENS development is on the NC-derived cell itself, and that ednrb activation on other cell types is not necessary for NC colonization of the developing gut.

DβH promoter–driven expression does not begin until the NC cells have entered the foregut mesenchyme (Kapur et al., 1992), and the *DβH-ednrb* transgene does not alter the coat color phenotype of the *ednrb^{sl/sl}* rat (Gariepy et al., 1998). These findings indicate that the critical period for ednrb activation in gut development is after the separation of the enteric and melanocyte lineages. Coat color in *edn3^{-/-}* mice is partially "rescued" by the *DβH-edn3* transgene. This is likely to be through diffusion of transgene-produced edn3 to melanocyte precursors (Rice et al., 2000).

Kapur and colleagues (1995) reported aggregation chimera studies in ednrb-null (*ednrb^{sl/sl}*) mice. They found that the ENS precursors could successfully colonize the distal hindgut if the majority of cells were wildtype. Conversely, wild-type ENS precursors were unsuccessful in colonizing the distal hindgut if the majority of cells were ednrb-null. The non-cell-autonomous nature of ednrb signaling described in this study suggests that activation of ednrb on the ENS precursor is communicated to neighboring ENS precursors. This communication may be in the form of direct cell–cell contact, secretion of specific signaling molecules, or alterations to the extracellular matrix.

To investigate intracellular signaling events in ENS precursors during gut colonization, the *DβH* promoter was used to direct expression of constitutively active mutant forms of G protein α-subunits (including $G\alpha_i$, $G\alpha_z$, $G\alpha_s$, $G\alpha_q$, $G\alpha_0$, and $G\alpha_{12}$) and two MAP kinase pathway molecules—Δ MEK1 and Raf1-KAAX—in *ednrb*$^{-/-}$ mice (Leevers et al., 1994; Mansour et al., 1994; Dhanasekaran et al., 1995). *Ednrb*$^{-/-}$ mice were rescued from their intestinal phenotype by *DβH*-$G\alpha_z$Q205L and, with decreased frequency, by *Dβ*-$G\alpha_i$Q205L. The other transgenes had no effect on survival of *ednrb*$^{-/-}$ mice. In vitro assays confirm that $G\alpha_z$ can couple to ednrb in transfected cells (M. Yanagisawa, unpublished observation). Interestingly, $G\alpha_z$ is a unique G protein with low intrinsic GTPase activity and a relatively restricted expression pattern in neurons and neuroendocrine cells. These findings suggest that $G\alpha_z$ may mediate the transduction of ednrb activation in ENS precursors during development.

Pax3 is a member of the paired-box-containing family of nuclear transcription factors. Individuals heterozygous for *PAX3* mutations exhibit Waardenburg's syndrome (see Chapter 61). Homozygous loss of function of *pax3* in the mouse is embryonic lethal (Epstein et al., 1991, 1993; Ayme and Philip, 1995) with no NC-cell colonization of the gut distal to the stomach (Lang et al., 2000). *Ednrb* mRNA is absent in the few NC-derived cells that successfully form enteric ganglia in *pax3*-null embryos at E12.5, indicating that *pax3* may regulate *ednrb* expression. Clearly, however, the decrease in *ednrb* expression cannot fully explain the observed defects in *pax3*$^{-/-}$ embryos.

Edn3$^{ls/ls}$ embryonic hindgut shows increased extracellular matrix components, including laminin, compared to wild-type embryonic hindgut (Tennyson et al., 1986, 1990; Gershon and Tennyson, 1991). This alteration is not seen in another mouse model of Hirschsprung's disease (the *ret*$^{-/-}$ mouse, see Chapter 36) but is reported in the aganglionic gut of humans with Hirschsprung's disease (Parikh et al., 1992). Vagal NC cells express LBP-110, a laminin-binding protein (Pomeranz et al., 1991; Howard and Gershon, 1998), and it has been suggested that interaction of the laminin α-chain in the distal hindgut with LBP-110 contributes to the failure of NC cells to colonize the distal gut (Gershon, 1997). In vitro, NC cells expressing LBP-110 show enhanced neural differentiation in response to laminin (Pomeranz et al., 1993; Chalazonitis et al., 1997). Edn3 also affects the maturation and differentiation of mesenchymal cells isolated from the gut at E13, thus promoting the development of smooth muscle and inhibiting the expression of laminin α1 (Wu et al., 1999).

In addition, edn3/ednrb signaling on the NC cell directly affects NC cell differentiation. Activation of ednrb on NC cells isolated from the gut appears to maintain the cells in a proliferation competent and undifferentiated state. Edn3 does not have an effect on cell proliferation. Neural differentiation could promote premature termination of gut colonization by NC cells. Edn3/ednrb signaling may support complete colonization of the developing gut by inhibiting differentiation and thus allowing continued cell proliferation and migration (Hearn et al., 1998; Wu et al., 1999).

THE SOX10 TRANSCRIPTION FACTOR

Members of the sox family of transcription factors are characterized by the presence of a DNA-binding HMG (high mobility group) domain and are involved in a wide range of developmental processes (Bowles et al., 2000). Sox10 contains 466 amino acids with a potent transcription activation domain at its C terminus (Kuhlbrodt et al., 1998). Peirano and Wegner (2000) report that sox10 functions through two different types of DNA response elements—one that binds sox10 monomers, and a second that favors sox10 dimer binding. The interaction between sox10 monomers and DNA is significantly different from that of sox10 dimers with DNA, suggesting that these two different modes of binding are functionally important. *SOX10* is located on human chromosome 22q13.1

Humans heterozygous for mutations of *SOX10* exhibit Shah-Waardenburg syndrome (see Chapter 38). Myelination defects are also noted in some patients heterozygous for *SOX10* mutations (Pingault et al., 1998; Inoue et al., 1999). Mice homozygous for spontaneous (*sox10*^{Dom}) or targeted (*sox10*^{lacz}) mutations in *sox10* display severe deficits in the peripheral nervous system, including enteric ganglia and the sympathetic chain (Lane 1984; Herbarth et al., 1998; Southard-Smith et al., 1998; Kapur 1999b; Britsch et al., 2001). Sensory neurons (but not satellite cells or Schwann cells) develop in dorsal root ganglia in *sox10*$^{Dom/Dom}$ homozygotes. Sensory and motor neurons degenerate in these animals, supporting the notion of a critical role for glia in neuronal survival (Britsch et al., 2001; Lemke, 2001). Mice homozygous for *sox10* mutations die before or shortly after birth. These mice do not demonstrate respiratory effort at birth and do not move or react to tactile simulation (Britsch et al., 2001).

Sox10 in Development

Sox10 is expressed in NC cells as they leave the neural tube, and expression continues during NC cell migration (Herbarth et al., 1998; Kuhlbrodt et al., 1998; Pusch et al., 1998). Expression is maintained in the ENS and melanocyte lineages, but is not maintained in other NC derivatives (Bondurand et al., 1998; Pusch et al., 1998). Sox10 expression becomes restricted to glia in the PNS and gradually decreases in the ENS during embryonic development (Kuhlbrodt et al., 2001). Both neurons and glia of the ENS express *SOX10* in infants (Sham et al., 2001). In *sox10*$^{Dom/Dom}$ mice, *sox10*-expressing NC cells develop along the dorsal portion of the neural tube, but by E10.5 NC cells are greatly reduced and by E11.5 *sox10*-expressing cells are almost all gone, likely due to increased apoptosis (Southard-Smith et al., 1998; Kapur, 1999b).

Melanocyte Development

Evidence suggests that sox10 plays a critical role in initial melanoblast determination. There is no pigmentation or melanoblast marker expression at E11.5 in *sox10*$^{Dom/Dom}$ mice. Potterf et al. (2001) describe an almost complete absence of *dct*-expressing melanoblasts in E10.5 to E13.5 *sox10*$^{Dom/+}$ mice, despite the fact that adult *sox10*$^{Dom/+}$ mice are almost entirely pigmented. The pigmentation in the adult is thought to be due to a late-migrating population of melanoblasts that arise from the small population of *dct*-expressing cells in early *sox10*$^{Dom/+}$ embryos. However, it is also possible that melanoblasts develop later from another population of cells. The normal timing of expression of other markers of melanoblasts suggests that the lack of *dct* expression is not the result of a general developmental delay in melanocyte development. These data suggest that sox10 affects melanoblast development transiently, until approximately E12.5–13.5.

In vitro evidence supports the concept that sox10 is the head of a transcriptional hierarchy with downstream targets that include the early melanoblast markers, *dct* and *mift* (the microophthalmia-associated transcription factor) (Bondurand et al., 2000; Lee et al., 2000; Potterf et al., 2000, 2001; Verastegui et al., 2000). Sox10 is capable of transactivating the *dct* promoter (Potterf et al., 2001). Promoter deletion and mutational analysis demonstrate that sox10 is a strong activator of *MITF* expression through binding to a region that is evolutionarily conserved between mouse and humans (Potterf et al., 2000; Verastegui et al., 2000). Mutation of *sox10* may lead to a dominant negative effect on *mitf* expression (Lee et al., 2000; Potterf et al., 2000).

ENS Development

Sox10$^{Dom/Dom}$ and *sox10*$^{LacZ/LacZ}$ mice have no ENS in any region of the gastrointestinal tract, and their NC cells undergo apoptosis before they reach the gut (Southard-Smith et al., 1998; Kapur, 1999a; Britsch et al., 2001). *Sox10*$^{Dom/+}$ mice exhibit distal intestinal aganglionosis, though the penetrance of the heterozygous phenotype is strongly influenced by genetic background (Kapur et al., 1996).

The mechanism of action of sox10 in ENS development in not yet clear. *Ednrb*-positive migrating NC cells are detected at E10.5 in both *sox10*^{Dom} homozygous and heterozygous embryos. However, these cells are delayed in their migration. By E11.5, *ednrb* expression along the ventral NC migratory pathway is minimal in *sox10*$^{Dom/Dom}$ embryos and dramatically reduced in heterozygous embryos (Southard-Smith et al., 1998; Kapur 1999a). It is unclear whether the reduced *ednrb* expression noted in *sox10*$^{Dom/+}$ embryos results from a direct effect of the transcription factor or an indirect effect on a common subset of ENS precursors. Increased apoptosis of NC cells is noted in homozygous mutant animals (Southard-Smith et al., 1998; Kapur, 1999a). Sox10 is also reported to regulate *ret* expression (Lang et al., 2000). Given the severity of the *sox10^{Dom/Dom}* (and *sox10^{LacZ/LacZ}*) phenotype, Sox10 clearly has additional roles in NC-derived cell development beyond the regulation of *ednrb* and *ret* Expression of *ednrb* in the neural tube is less affected by the *sox10^{Dom}* mutation (Southard-Smith et al., 1998).

The apparent early delay in NC migration in *sox10^{Dom/+}* embryos is in contrast to delayed colonization beginning in the region of the cecum in ednrb- or edn3-deficient embryos (Coventry et al., 1994). Despite the consistent early delay in colonization, depending on the genetic background, not all *sox10^{Dom/+}* pups have ENS defects. This finding is somewhat analogous to that of nearly normal pigmentation in *sox10^{Dom/+}* mice despite severe, early abnormalities in melanoblast development. Normal ENS development in some *sox10^{Dom/+}* mice suggest that deficiency (but not absence) of sox10 signaling affects only early gut NC colonization and may have little effect on a late-migrating group of ENS precursors (Kapur et al., 1996).

Analysis of aggregation *sox10^{+/+}/sox10^{Dom/+}* chimera embryos suggests that sox10 deficiency directly or indirectly affects microenvironmental signals that influence ENS precursors (Kapur et al., 1996). Non-cell autonomous or community effects of sox10 signaling in postmigratory NC-derived cells from the dorsal root ganglia of *sox10^{+/-}* mice are also described in vitro (Paratore et al., 2001). In vivo, Paratore et al. (2002) report that *sox10^{+/-}* mice exhibit a decreased pool of multipotent NC-derived cells due to acquisition of neuronal traits by these cells. They suggest that, as has been hypothesized in *ednrb^{-/-}* mice, premature neuronal differentiation of multipotent enteric NC cells leads to colonization failure in the distal bowel.

CONCLUSIONS

Investigations into the role of edn3/ednrb and sox10 signaling in the developing embryo are just beginning. Several recent studies suggest that edn3/ednrb signaling maintains migrating ENS precursors in an undifferentiated, colonization competent state (Hearn et al., 1998; Wu et al., 1999; Sidebotham et al., 2002). Early failures of melanoblast development occur in ednrb^{sl/sl} mice, but the mechanism remains unclear (Pavan and Tilghman, 1994). Edn3/ednrb signaling has developmental stage–specific effects in the melanocyte lineage (Reid et al., 1996; Opdecamp et al., 1998). Haploinsufficiency for sox10 appears to interfere with the development and survival of an early subset of melanocyte and ENS precursors. Sox10 appears to be an important transcriptional regulator of several other genes known to be developmentally important in the melanocyte and ENS lineages. Evidence suggests that, in vivo, both these signaling pathways function in a non-cell-autonomous fashion (Kapur et al., 1995, 1996).

Mutation in genes involved in edn3/ednrb and sox10 signaling result in some shared cellular defects. Many key questions regarding edn3/ednrb and sox10 signaling in normal development and the pathogenesis of Shah-Waardenburg syndrome remain unanswered. What is the relationship between these two signaling pathways? The in vivo interaction of these signaling systems has not yet been fully explored. What are the genes capable of modifying the pigment and ENS phenotypes of individuals deficient in edn3/ednrb and sox10 signaling? No doubt, mouse mutants will continue to be invaluable in the identification and characterization of these genes. Finally, what intracellular and intercellular signals lay downstream of edn3/ednrb and sox10 signaling? Gene expression analysis aided by DNA chip technology comparing NC-derived cell populations from mutant and wild-type mice will likely yield important clues in the near future (McCallion and Chakravarti, 2001).

REFERENCES

Arai H, Hori S, Aramori I, Ohkubo H, Nakanishi S (1990). Cloning and expression of a cDNA encoding an endothelin receptor. *Nature* 348: 730–732.

Ayme S, Philip N (1995). Possible homozygous Waardenburg syndrome in a fetus with exencephaly. *Am J Med Genet* 59: 263–265.

Baynash AG, Hosoda K, Giaid A, Richardson JA, Emoto N, Hammer RE, Yanagisawa

M (1994). Interaction of endothelin-3 with endothelin-B receptor is essential for development of neural crest-derived melanocytes and enteric neurons: missense mutation of endothelin-3 gene in lethal spotting mice. *Cell* 79: 1277–1285.

Bondurand N, Kobetz A, Pingault V, Lemort N, Encha-Razavi F, Couly G, Goerich DE, Wegner M, Abitbol M, Goossens M (1998). Expression of the SOX10 gene during human development. *FEBS Lett* 432: 168–172.

Bondurand N, Pingault V, Goerich DE, Lemort N, Sock E, Caignec CL, Wegner M, Goossens M (2000). Interaction among SOX10, PAX3 and MITF, three genes altered in Waardenburg syndrome. *Hum Mol Genet* 9: 1907–1917.

Bowles J, Schepers G, Koopman P (2000). Phylogeny of the SOX family of developmental transcription factors based on sequence and structural indicators. *Dev Biol* 227: 239–255.

Brand M, Le Moullec JM, Corvol P, Gasc JM (1998). Ontogeny of endothelins-1 and -3, their receptors, and endothelin converting enzyme-1 in the early human embryo. *J Clin Invest* 101: 549–559.

Britsch S, Goerich DE, Riethmacher D, Peirano RI, Rossner M, Nave KA, Birchmeier C, Wegner M (2001). The transcription factor Sox10 is a key regulator of peripheral glial development. *Genes Dev* 15: 66–78.

Chalazonitis A, Tennyson VM, Kibbey MC, Rothman TP, Gershon MD (1997). The α1 subunit of lamini-1 promotes the development of neurons by interacting with LBP110 expressed by neural crest-derived cells immunoselected from the fetal mouse gut. *J Neurobiol* 33: 118–138.

Coventry S, Yost C, Palmiter RD, Kapur RP (1994). Migration of ganglion cell precursors in the ileoceca of normal and lethal spotted embryos, a murine model for Hirschsprung disease. *Lab Invest* 71: 82–93.

Dhanasekaran N, Heasley LE, Johnson GL (1995). G protein–coupled receptor systems involved in cell growth and oncogenesis. *Endocr Rev* 16: 259–270.

Dupin E, Glavieux C, Vaigot P, Le Douarin NM (2000). Endothelin 3 induces the reversion of melanocytes to glia through a neural crest-derived glial-melanocytic progenitor. *Proc Natl Acad Sci USA* 97: 7882–7887.

Durbec PL, Larsson-Blomber LB, Schuchardt A, Costantini F, Pachnis V (1996). Common origin and developmental dependence on c-ret of subsets of enteric and sympathetic neuroblasts. *Development* 122: 349–358.

Emoto N, Yanagisawa M (1995). Endothelin-converting enzyme-2 is a membrane-bound, phosphoramidon-sensitive metalloprotease with acidic pH optimum. *J Biol Chem* 270: 15262–15268.

Epstein DJ, Vekemans M, Gros P (1991). Splotch (Sp2H), a mutation affecting development of the mouse neural tube, shows a deletion within the paired homeodomain of Pax-3. *Cell* 67: 767–774.

Epstein DJ, Vogan KJ, Trasler DG, Gros P (1993). A mutation within intron 3 of the Pax-3 gene produces aberrantly spliced mRNA transcripts in the splotch (Sp) mouse mutant. *Proc Natl Acad Sci USA* 90: 532–536.

Garcia-Castro M, Bronner-Fraser M (1999). Induction and differentiation of the neural crest. *Curr Opin Cell Biol* 11: 695–698.

Gariepy C, Williams S, Richardson J, Hammer R, Yanagisawa M (1998). Transgenic expression of the endothelin-B receptor prevents congenital intestinal aganglionosis in a rat model of Hirschsprung disease. *J Clin Invest* 102: 1092–1101.

Gershon MD (1997). Genes and lineages in the formation of the enteric nervous system. *Curr Opin Neurobiol* 7: 101–109.

Gershon MD, Tennyson VM (1991). Microenvironmental factors in the normal and abnormal development of the enteric nervous system. *Prog Clin Biol Res* 373: 257–276.

Hearn CJ, Murphy M, Newgreen D (1998). GDNF and ET-3 differentially modulate the numbers of avian enteric neural crest cells and enteric neurons in vitro. *Dev Biol* 197: 93–105.

Herbarth B, Pingault V, Bondurand N, Kuhlbrodt K, Hermans-Borgmeyer I, Puliti A, Lemort N, Goossens M, Wegner M (1998). Mutation of the Sry-related Sox10 gene in Dominant megacolon, a mouse model for human Hirschsprung disease. *Proc Natl Acad Sci USA* 95: 5161–5165.

Hirobe T (1984). Histochemical survey of the distribution of the epidermal melanoblasts and melanocytes in the mouse during fetal and postnatal periods. *Anat Rec* 208: 589–594.

Hosoda K, Hammer RE, Richardson JA, Greenstein Baynash A, Cheung JC, Giaid A, Yanagisawa M (1994). Targeted and natural (piebald-lethal) mutations of endothelin-B receptor gene produce aganglionic megacolon associated with white-spotted coat color in mice. *Cell* 79: 1267–1276.

Howard MJ, Gershon MD (1998). Development of LBP110 expression by neural crest-derived enteric precursors: migration and differentiation potential in ls/ls mutant mice. *J Neurobiol* 35: 341–354.

Ikadai H, Fujita H, Agematsu Y, Imanichi T (1979). Observation of congenital aganglionosis rat (Hirschsprung's disease) and its genetical analysis. (in Japanese). *Cong Anom* 19: 31–36.

Inoue A, Yanagisawa M, Kimura S, Kasuya Y, Miyauchi T, Goto K, Masaki T (1989). The human endothelin family: three structurally and pharmacologically distinct isopeptides predicted by three separate genes. *Proc Natl Acad Sci USA* 86: 2863–2867.

Inoue K, Tanabe Y, Lupski JR (1999). Myelin deficiencies in both the central and the peripheral nervous systems associated with a SOX10 mutation. *Ann Neurol* 46: 313–318.

Kapur RP (1999a). Early death of neural crest cells is responsible for total enteric aganglionosis in Sox10Dom/sox10Dom mouse embryos. *Pediatr Dev Pathol* 2: 559–569.

Kapur RP (1999b). Hirschsprung disease and other enteric dysganglionoses. *Crit Rev Clin Lab Sci* 36: 225–273.

Kapur RP (2000). Colonization of the murine hindgut by sacral crest-derived neural precursors: experimental support for an evolutionarily conserved model. *Dev Biol* 227: 146–155.

Kapur RP, Hoyle GW, Mercer EH, Brinster RL, Palmiter RD (1991). Some neuronal cell populations express human dopamine β-hydroxylase-lacZ transgenes transiently during embryonic development. *Neuron* 7: 717–727.

Kapur RP, Yost C, Palmiter RD (1992). A transgenic model for studying development of the enteric nervous system in normal and aganglionic mice. *Development* 116: 167–175.

Kapur RP, Sweetser DA, Doggett B, Siebert JR, Palmiter RD (1995). Intracellular signals downstream of endothelin receptor-B mediate colonization of the large intestine by enteric neuroblasts. *Development* 121: 3787–3795.

Kapur RP, Livingston R, Doggett B, Sweetser DA, Siebert JR, Palmiter RD (1996). Abnormal microenvironmental signals underlie intestinal aganglionosis in Dominant megacolon mutant mice. *Dev Biol* 174: 360–369.

Keshet E, Lyman SD, Williams DE, Anderson DM, Jenkins NA, Copeland NG, Parada LF (1991). Embryonic RNA expression patterns of the c-kit receptor and its cognate ligand suggest multiple functional roles in mouse development. *EMBO J* 10: 2425–2435.

Kuhlbrodt K, Herbarth B, Sock E, Hermans-Borgmeyer I, Wegner M (1998). Sox10, a novel transcriptional modulator in glial cells. *J Neurosci* 18: 237–250.

Lahav R, Ziller C, Dupin E, Le Douarin NM (1996). Endothelin 3 promotes neural crest cell proliferation and mediates a vast increase in melanocyte number in culture. *Proc Natl Acad Sci USA* 93: 3892–3897.

Lane PW, Liu HM (1984). Association of megacolon with a dominant spotting gene (Dom) in the mouse. *J Hered* 75: 435–439.

Lang D, Chen F, Milewski R, Li J, Lu MM, Epstein JA (2000). Pax3 is required for enteric ganglia formation and functions with Sox10 to modulate expression of c-ret. *J Clin Invest* 106: 963–971.

Le Douarin NM, Dupin E (1993). Cell lineage analysis in neural crest ontogeny. *J Neurobiol* 24: 146–161.

Le Douarin NM, Kalcheim C (1999). *The Neural Crest, 2nd Edition*. Cambridge University Press, Cambridge.

Lee M, Goodall J, Verastegui C, Ballotti R, Goding CR (2000). Direct regulation of the Microphthalmia promoter by Sox10 links Waardenburg-Shah syndrome (WS4)-associated hypopigmentation and deafness to WS2. *J Biol Chem* 275: 37978–37983.

Leevers SJ, Paterson HF, Marshall CJ (1994). Requirement for Ras in Raf activations overcome by targeting Raf to the plasma membrane. *Nature* 369: 411–414.

Leibl MA, Ota T, Woodward MN, Kenny SE, Lloyd DA, Vaillant CR, Egar DH (1999). Expression of endothelin 3 by mesenchymal cells of embryonic mouse caecum. *Gut* 44: 246–252.

Lemke G (2001). Glial control of neuronal development. *Annu Rev Neurosci* 24: 87–105.

Mansour SJ, Matten WT, Hermann AS, Candia JM, Rong S, Fukasawa K, Vande Woude GF, Ahn NG (1994). Transformation of mammalian cells by constitutively active MAP kinase kinase. *Science* 265: 966–970.

Matsui Y, Zsebo KM, Hogan BL (1990). Embryonic expression of a haematopoietic growth factor encoded by the Sl locus and the ligand for c-kit. *Nature* 347: 667–669.

McCabe L, Griffin LD, Kinzer A, Chandler M, Beckwith JB, McCabe ER (1990). Overo lethal white foal syndrome: equine model of aganglionic megacolon (Hirschsprung Disease). *Am J Med Genet* 36: 336–340.

McCallion AS, Chakravarti A (2001). EDNRB/EDN3 and Hirschsprung disease type II. *Pigment Cell Res* 14: 161–169.

Metallinos DL, Bowling AT, Rine J (1998). A missense mutation in the endothelin-b receptor gene is associated with Lethal White Foal Syndrome: an equine version of Hirschsprung disease. *Mamm Genome* 9: 426–431.

Opdecamp K, Nakayama A, Nguyen MT, Hodgkinson CA, Pavan WJ, Arnheiter H (1997). Melanocyte development in vivo and in neural crest cell cultures: crucial dependence on the Mitf basic–helix–loop–helix–zipper transcription factor. *Development* 124: 2377–2386.

Opdecamp K, Kos L, Arnheiter H, Pavan WJ (1998). Endothelin signalling in the development of neural crest-derived melanocytes. *Biochem Cell Biol* 76: 1093–1099.

Paratore C, Goerich DE, Suter U, Wegner M, Sommer L (2001). Survival and glial fate acquisition of neural crest cells are regulated by an interplay between the transcription factor Sox10 and extrinsic combinatorial signaling. *Development* 128: 3949–3961.

Paratore C, Eichenberger C, Suter U, Sommer L (2002). *Sox10* haploinsufficiency affects maintenance of progenitor cells in a mouse model of Hirschsprung disease. *Hum Mol Gene* 11: 3075–3085.

Parichy DM, Mellgren EM, Rawls JF, Lopes SS, Kelsh RN, Johnson SL (2000). Mutational analysis of endothelin receptor b1 (rose) during neural crest and pigment pattern development in the zebrafish *Danio rerio*. *Dev Biol* 227: 294–306.

Parikh DH, Tam PK, Lloyd DA, Van Velzen D, Edgar DH (1992). Quantitative and qualitative analysis of the extracellular matrix protein, laminin, in Hirschsprung's disease. *J Pediatr Surg* 27: 991–995.

Pavan WJ, Tilghman SM (1994). Piebald lethal (sl) acts early to disrupt the development of the neural crest-derived melanocytes. *Proc Natl Acad Sci USA* 91: 7159–7163.

Pavan WJ, Mac S, Cheng M, Tilghman SM (1995). Quantitative trait loci that modify the severity of spotting in piebald mice. *Genome Res* 5: 29–41.

Peirano RI, Wegner M (2000). The glial transcription factor Sox10 binds to DNA both as monomer and dimer with different functional consequences. *Nucleic Acids Res* 28: 3047–3055.

Pingault V, Bondurand N, Kuhlbrodt K, Goerich DE, Prehu MO, Puliti A, Herbarth B, Hermans-Borgmeyer I, Legius E, Matthijs G, et al (1998). SOX10 mutations in patients with Waardenburg-Hirschsprung disease. *Nat Genet* 18: 171–173.

Pomeranz HD, Sherman DL, Smalheiser NR, Tennyson VM, Gershon MD (1991). Expression of a neurally related laminin binding protein by neural crest–derived cells that colonize the gut: relationship to the formation of enteric ganglia. *J Comp Neurol* 13: 625–642.

Pomeranz HD, Rothman TP, Chalazonitis A, Tennyson VM, Gershon MD (1993). Neural crest–derived cells isolated from the guy by immunoselection develop neuronal and glial phenotypes when cultured on laminin. *Dev Biol* 156: 341–361.

Potterf SB, Furumura M, Dunn KJ, Arnheiter H, Pavan WJ (2000). Transcription factor hierarchy in Waardenburg syndrome: regulation of MITF expression by SOX10 and PAX3. *Hum Genet* 107: 1–16.

Potterf SB, Mollaaghaba R, Hou L, Southard-Smith EM, Hornyak TJ, Arnheiter H, Pavan WJ (2001). Analysis of SOX10 function in neural crest–derived melanocyte development: SOX10-dependent transcriptional control of dopachrome tautomerase. *Dev Biol* 237: 245–257.

Pusch C, Hustert E, Pfeifer D, Sudbeck P, Kist R, Roe B, Wang Z, Balling R, Blin N, Scherer G (1998). The SOX10/Sox10 gene from human and mouse: sequence, expression, and transactivation by the encoded HMG domain transcription factor. *Hum Genet* 103: 115–123.

Reid K, Turnley AM, Maxwell GD, Kurihara Y, Kurihara H, Bartlett PF, Murphy M (1996). Multiple roles for endothelin in melanocyte development: regulation of progenitor number and stimulation of differentiation. *Development* 122: 3911–3919.

Rice J, Doggett B, Sweetser DA, Yanagisawa H, Yanagisawa M, Kapur RP (2000). Transgenic rescue of aganglionosis and piebaldism in lethal spotted mice. *Dev Dyn* 217: 120–132.

Sakurai T, Yanagisawa M, Takuwa Y, Miyazaki H, Kimura S, Goto K, Masaki T (1990). Cloning of a cDNA encoding a non-isopeptide-selective subtype of the endothelin receptor. *Nature* 348: 732–735.

Santschi EM, Purdy AK, Valberg SJ, Vrotsos PD, Kaese H, Mickelson JR (1998). Endothelin receptor B polymorphism associated with lethal white foal syndrome in horses. *Mamm Genome* 9: 306–309.

Sham MH, Lui VC, Fu M, Chen B, Tam PK (2001). SOX10 is abnormally expressed in aganglionic bowel of Hirschsprung's disease infants. *Gut* 49: 220–226.

Shin MK, Levorse JM, Ingram RS, Tilghman SM (1999). The temporal requirement for endothelin receptor-B signalling during neural crest development. *Nature* 402: 496–501.

Sidebotham EL, Woodward MN, Kenny SE, Lloyd DA, Vaillant CR, Edgar DH (2002). Localization and endothelin-3 dependence of stem cells for the enteric nervous system in the embryonic colon. *J Pediatr Surg* 37: 145–150.

Southard-Smith EM, Kos L, Pavan WJ (1998). Sox10 mutation disrupts neural crest development in Dom Hirschsprung mouse model. *Nat Genet* 18: 60–64.

Stone JG, Spirling LI, Richardson MK (1997). The neural crest population responding to endothelin-3 in vitro includes multipotent cells. *J Cell Sci* 110: 1673–1682.

Sviderskaya EV, Easty DJ, Bennett DC (1998). Impaired growth and differentiation of diploid but not immortal melanoblasts from endothelin receptor B mutant (piebald) mice. *Dev Dyn* 213: 452–463.

Tennyson VM, Pham TD, Rothman TP, Gershon MD (1986). Abnormalities of smooth muscle, basal laminae, and nerves in the aganglionic segments of the bowel of lethal spotted mutant mice. *Anat Rec* 215: 267–287.

Tennyson VM, Payetter RF, Rothman TP, Gershon MD (1990). Distribution of hyaluronic acid and chondroitin sulfate proteoglycans in the presumptive aganglionic terminal bowel of ls/ls fetal mice: an ultrastructural analysis. *J Comp Neurol* 291: 345–362.

Verastegui C, Bille K, Ortonne JP, Ballotti R (2000). Regulation of the microphthalmia-associated transcription factor gene by the Waardenburg syndrome type 4 gene, SOX10. *J Biol Chem* 275: 30757–30760.

Vonderfecht S, Bowling AT, Cohen M (1983). Congenital intestinal megacolon in white foals. *Vet Pathol* 20: 65–70.

Woodward MN, Kenny SE, Vaillant C, Lloyd DA, Edgar DH (2000). Time-dependent effects of endothelin-3 on enteric nervous system development in an organ culture model of Hirschsprung's disease. *J Pediatr Surg* 35: 25–29.

Wu JJ, Chen JX, Rothman TP, Gershon MD (1999). Inhibition of in vitro enteric neuronal development by endothelin-3: mediation by endothelin B receptors. *Development* 126: 1161–1173.

Xu D, Emoto N, Giaid A, Slaughter C, Kaw S, de Wit D, Yanagisawa M (1994). ECE-1: a membrane-bound metalloprotease that catalyzes the proteolytic activation of big endothelin-1. *Cell* 78: 473–485.

Yanagisawa H, Yanagisawa M, Kapur RP, Richardson JA, Williams SC, Clouthier DE, de Wit D, Emoto N, Hammer RE (1998). Dual genetic pathways of endothelin-mediated intercellular signaling revealed by targeted disruption of endothelin converting enzyme-1 gene. *Development* 125: 825–836.

Yoshida H, Kunisada T, Kusakabe M, Nishikawa S, Nishikawa SI (1996). Distinct stages of melanocyte differentiation revealed by analysis of nonuniform pigmentation patterns. *Development* 122: 1207–1214.

Young HM, Hearn CJ, Ciampoli D, Southwell BR, Brunet JF, Newgreen DF (1998). A single rostrocaudal colonization of the rodent intestine by enteric neuron precursors is revealed by the expression of Phox2b, Ret, and p75 and by explants grown under the kidney capsule or in organ culture. *Dev Biol* 202: 67–84.

38 | *EDNRB, EDN3,* and *SOX10* and the Shah-Waardenburg Syndrome

JOKE B. G. M. VERHEIJ AND ROBERT M. W. HOFSTRA

Shah-Waardenburg syndrome is a rare congenital disorder with variable expression and is characterized by the combination of Hirschsprung disease (HSCR) and features of Waardenburg syndrome (WS): pigmentary abnormalities and sensorineural deafness. The pigmentary abnormalities consist of patchy areas of depigmentation of the skin, depigmentations of hair, and heterochromia or pale blue irides with hypopigmented fundi. Both HSCR and WS are regarded as neurocristopathies caused by an abnormal migration of neural crest cells during embryonic development toward either the enteric nervous system (ENS) or the skin, hair, and stria vascularis of the inner ear (melanocytes) or abnormal differentiation of these neural crest cells.

To date, mutations in three genes have been found in patients with Shah-Waardenburg syndrome: the gene that encodes the endothelin receptor-B gene (*EDNRB*); the gene that encodes one of the ligands of the endothelin receptor, endothelin-3 (*EDN3*); and a gene that encodes a transcription factor, *SOX10*.

Patients homozygous for *EDNRB* or *EDN3* mutations express full-blown features of Shah-Waardenburg syndrome, whereas patients heterozygous for such mutations may have either isolated HSCR or symptoms of Waardenburg syndrome, or both. The clinical phenotype associated with *SOX10* mutations seems to be much more variable, more frequently displaying short-segment HSCR and hypoganglionosis. Moreover, the majority of patients with *SOX10* mutations show neurological disorders with involvement of both central and peripheral nervous systems. Mutations in one of these three genes are not found in all patients with Shah-Waardenburg syndrome, implying further genetic heterogeneity.

In the case of patients homozygous for *EDNRB* or *EDN3* mutations and with absence of features of Shah-Waardenburg syndrome in heterozygous parents and sibs, autosomal recessive inheritance with a recurrence risk for sibs of 25% seems obvious. With *SOX10* mutations, autosomal dominant inheritance can be assumed, implying a recurrence risk of 50% for offspring of patients. Since two cases of mosaicism have been reported, even though the mutation seems to occur de novo in the patient, for sibs a recurrence risk of about 15% to 20% might apply. Prenatal diagnosis by DNA investigation is possible if the mutation (or mutations) is known.

SHAH-WAARDENBURG SYNDROME

Hirschsprung disease (HSCR) is a congenital disorder that is clinically characterized by intestinal obstruction due to the absence of intramural ganglion cells (aganglionosis) along variable lengths of the colon. In around 80% of cases the aganglionosis is restricted to the rectosigmoid (short-segment HSCR). The mode of inheritance of HSCR can be dominant, recessive, or multifactorial with major and minor genes involved. Mutations in several genes—alone or in combination—are associated with HSCR, the major gene being the *RET* protooncogene (see Chapters 39–41 for a comprehensive review).

Waardenburg syndrome (WS) is a rare congenital disorder that is characterized by a combination of pigmentary abnormalities and sensorineural deafness, with highly variable expression and incomplete penetrance. The pigmentary abnormalities consist of patchy areas of depigmentation of the skin; depigmentations of hair, such as a white forelock (either at birth or later) and premature graying; and heterochromia, or pale blue irides with hypopigmented fundi. Deafness can be uni- or bilateral, and severity ranges from mild to profound. Dysmorphic features like dystopia canthorum and synophrys can be

found as well (Waardenburg, 1951). Clinically and genetically, WS is heterogeneous. Up to now, four types of Waardenburg syndrome have been distinguished: WS1 is WS associated with dystopia canthorum (see Chapter 61), WS2 is WS without dystopia (see Chapter 77), WS3 is WS with limb abnormalities (also called Klein-Waardenburg syndrome), and WS4 or Shah-Waardenburg syndrome is WS associated with HSCR (Read and Newton, 1997).

Both HSCR and WS are regarded as neurocristopathies caused by an abnormal migration of neural crest cells toward either the enteric nervous system (ENS) or the skin and hair (melanocytes) or abnormal differentiation of these cells during embryonic development (5th to 12th week of gestation). Deafness is caused by the absence of melanocytes from the stria vascularis of the inner ear.

Mutations in three genes have been found in patients with Shah-Waardenburg syndrome: the gene encoding the endothelin receptor B gene, *EDRNB*; the gene encoding one of the ligands of the endothelin receptor, endothelin-3, *EDN3*; and a gene encoding a transcription factor possibly related to the endothelin pathway, *SOX10* (see Chapter 37 for a review of the pathways of these genes). However, mutations in one of these three genes are not found in all patients with this rare syndrome, suggesting further genetic heterogeneity.

HISTORICAL PERSPECTIVE

Goldberg (1966) reported the first case of WS and HSCR. McKusick (1973) recognized that there might be a connection between these diseases. He hypothesized that, during gestation, a defect in the migration of pigment cells and nerve cells from the neural crest could cause both disorders. Omenn and McKusick (1979) described four more families with the combination of HSCR and WS, strengthening the idea of a specific entity. In these four families, six patients had HSCR; bilateral profound deafness; and pigmentary abnormalities of hair, eyebrows, skin, and irides. Other family members showed one or more signs of WS. In 1981, Shah and colleagues described 12 babies born to five families in India with long-segment HSCR, white forelock, white eyebrows and eyelashes, and isochromia irides (light brown irides with mosaic pattern). Hearing was not tested, because all babies died in the neonatal period. One of these families also had children with features of Waardenburg's syndrome (heterochromia irides and white forelock) without HSCR.

Besides these families, several other cases with the combination of HSCR and WS have been published by authors from a variety of disciplines: ophthalmology, otorhinolaryngology, pediatric surgery, dermatology, and genetics (Branski et al., 1979; Omenn and McKusick, 1979; Fried and Beer, 1980; Goldberg, 1981; Kelley and Zackai, 1981; Shah et al., 1981; Ambani, 1983; Farndon and Bianchi, 1983; Rarey and Davis, 1984; Mallory et al., 1986; Meire et al., 1987; Ariturk et al., 1992; Attie et al., 1995b; Van Camp et al., 1995; Bonnet et al., 1996).

The association of Hirschsprung disease (both short and long segment) with features of Waardenburg syndrome now bears various names: Shah-Waardenburg syndrome, Waardenburg-Hirschsprung syndrome, and type IV Waardenburg syndrome—or WS4 (OMIM #277580). In this chapter we refer to this disease as Shah-Waardenburg syndrome.

Families with similar phenotypes have been reported, but without deafness or depigmentation (Weinberg et al., 1977; Mahakrishnan and Srinivasan, 1980). A consanguineous Mexican family was described in which bicolored irides and HSCR were the sole manifestations in siblings (Liang et al., 1983). Gross and colleagues (1995) described a consanguineous Shah-Waardenburg-like family, with a syndrome they called

ABCD syndrome. This acronym stands for albinism, black lock, cell migration disorder of the neurocytes of the gut (read: HSCR) and deafness.

CLINICAL DESCRIPTION

HSCR, or colonic aganglionosis, is a congenital disorder that is characterized by intestinal obstruction due to an absence of intramural ganglia along variable lengths of the colon. In around 80% of cases of isolated HSCR, the aganglionosis is restricted to the rectosigmoid (short-segment HSCR). In Shah-Waardenburg syndrome, the length of aganglionosis varies, but in contrast with isolated HSCR, most patients with Shah-Waardenburg syndrome have long-segment or even total intestinal aganglionosis. Clinical features of HSCR are due to intestinal obstruction. For a definite diagnosis a suction rectal biopsy or a full-thickness rectal biopsy is needed.

Iris heterochromia may be complete or partial. In complete heterochromia, each iris has a different color. In partial heterochromia, the different colored area of the iris is sharply demarcated from the remainder and can be unilateral or bilateral. If bilateral, this area may be symmetrical or asymmetrical. Hypoplastic blue irides are characterized by a sapphire blue color (Read and Newton, 1997). In Shah-Waardenburg the majority of patients have one of these pigmentary disturbances of the eyes.

Most patients have a distinctive transient white forelock in infancy, usually in the midline, or strands of white hair elsewhere on the head. The affected area may vary in size from a few hairs to most of the scalp hair (Fig. 38–1). Another feature is premature graying of the hair, meaning that there is a predominance of white hairs appearing in the midline before the age of 30 years. Pigmentation defects can also affect the eyebrows and eyelashes. Patches of depigmentation of the skin are congenital and may be found on the face, trunk, or limbs. However, this is not a frequent finding in Shah-Waardenburg syndrome.

Usually, patients with Shah-Waardenburg syndrome have profound bilateral sensorineural hearing loss. However, cases with mild hearing loss have also been described (Branski et al., 1979).

The existence of dystopia canthorum (lateral displacement of the inner eye canthi) distinguishes WS1 from WS2. Patients with Shah-Waardenburg syndrome do not have dystopia canthorum. Some patients have either a broad nasal root or synophrys, or both.

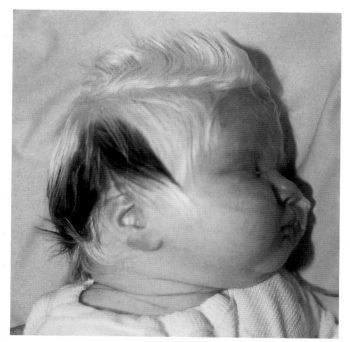

Figure 38–1. Side view of a Turkish girl with Shah-Waardenburg syndrome showing white eyebrows, lashes, and hair, with a black lock at the right temporo-occipital region. (From Gross et al., 1995; Verheij et al., 2002.)

Some patients with Shah-Waardenburg syndrome show additional features, such as rotatory nystagmus, bilateral anomaly of the ureters, and encephalopathy (de Lumley et al., 1980); left pulmonic artery stenosis, ocular ptosis, and unilateral duplication of the renal collecting system (Kaplan and de Chaderevian, 1988); a demyelinating peripheral neuropathy (Jacobs and Wilson, 1992); and cleft lip or palate (Pierpont et al., 1995). These features most likely represent random associations.

However, several patients with Shah-Waardenburg syndrome have neurological symptoms of both central and peripheral nervous systems (mental retardation, hypotonia, ataxia, spasticity, hypotonia, arthrogryposis, alacrima, asialia, and reduced sweating), which may be caused by mutations in *SOX10* (see later in this chapter) (Inoue et al., 1999; Southard-Smith et al., 1999; Touraine et al., 2000; Sham et al., 2001b).

GENETIC ASPECTS OF SHAH-WAARDENBURG SYNDROME

In the first family described with Shah-Waardenburg syndrome (Omenn and McKusick, 1979), patients occurred in three generations, making a dominant mode of inheritance most likely. In contrast to this family, most families described after this suggested an autosomal recessive mode of inheritance, since several families demonstrated parental consanguinity and multiple affected sibs of both sexes (Shah et al., 1981; Farndon and Bianchi, 1983; Attie et al., 1995b). Badner and Chakravarti (1990) discussed a pleiotropic effect of a single dominant gene. This hypothesis proved correct in a large Mennonite family with HSCR and features of WS, where the clinical phenotype appeared gene dosage dependent (see "*EDNRB* Mutations in Shah-Waardenburg Syndrome" in this chapter) (Puffenberger et al., 1994a). All these data support the idea that Shah-Waardenburg syndrome is a genetically heterogeneous condition that displays both recessive and dominant modes of inheritance (with or without reduced penetrance).

GENES INVOLVED

The Endothelin-B Receptor Gene

The finding of the first gene involved in Shah-Waardenburg syndrome followed a classical route. A first clue came from cytogenetic studies. Several patients with HSCR in combination with mental retardation and dysmorphic features proved to have an interstitial deletion of chromosome 13q (Kiss and Osztovics, 1989; Lamont et al., 1989; Bottani et al., 1991). Besides these patients, linkage analysis in a large inbred Mennonite pedigree also pointed at the 13q22 region (Puffenberger et al., 1994b). Moreover, the spontaneous mouse mutant *piebald lethal* with a phenotype of aganglionic megacolon and coat color spotting was mapped to mouse chromosome 14 (Metallinos et al., 1994), a region homologous to human chromosome 13. Hosoda and colleagues (1994) generated a knockout mouse for the endothelin-B receptor (*EDNRB*) gene, which exhibited a phenotype with aganglionic megacolon associated with coat color spotting, identical to the *piebald lethal* mouse. They showed that *EDNRB* was allelic to the *piebald-lethal* locus. These findings indicated an essential role for *EDNRB* in the development of two neural crest–derived cell lineages: the myenteric ganglion neurons and the epidermal melanocytes. Subsequently, the susceptibility locus for HSCR on human chromosome 13q22 was demonstrated to be indeed the *EDNRB* gene, and a missense mutation in exon 4 (W276C) was identified in the previously mentioned large Mennonite kindred with Shah-Waardenburg syndrome (Puffenberger et al., 1994a).

The *EDN3* Gene

The endothelin-B receptor is activated by endothelins, a family of peptides that are 21 amino acids long. Three mammalian endothelins are known: EDN1, EDN2, and EDN3. They are all encoded by a separate gene and are expressed in a variety of vascular and nonvascular tissues (Rubanyi and Polokoff, 1994). Baynash and colleagues (1994) demonstrated that *Edn3*-deficient mice exhibit a phenotype identical to that of *Ednrb* knockout mice—namely, coat color spotting and aganglionic megacolon. By identifying a homozygous *Edn3* missense mutation in the *lethal spotting* mice, they showed that *lethal spotting* is allelic to *Edn3*, suggesting that *EDN3* was a good candidate gene in Shah-Waardenburg syndrome. Indeed, the first reports of homozygous substitution/deletion mutations of the *EDN3* gene in patients with Shah-Waardenburg syndrome appeared 2 years later (Edery et al., 1996; Hofstra et al., 1996).

SOX10

It was the *Dom* mice that provided the clue to the third gene involved in Shah-Waardenburg. Heterozygous *Dom* mice show white spotting and a deficiency of myenteric cells in the colon, with a dominant mode of inheritance. Linkage analysis using inbred *Dom* mice showed that the locus for the phenotype was located on chromosome 15 in a region homologous to the human chromosome region 22q13 (Lane and Liu, 1984; Puliti et al., 1995). Two research groups simultaneously identified the genetic defect in this mouse strain by showing that the phenotype was caused by a mutation of the *Sox10* gene (Herbarth et al., 1998; Southard-Smith et al., 1998). Subsequently, the first heterozygous mutations of *SOX10* in patients with Shah-Waardenburg syndrome were reported (Pingault et al., 1998). Human *SOX10* is a member of the SOX gene family of transcriptional regulators. *SOX10* is selectively expressed in neural crest cells during early stages of development and in glial cells of the peripheral and central nervous system during late development and in the adult (Kuhlbrodt et al., 1998a).

MUTATIONS IN *EDNRB*, *EDN3*, AND *SOX10*

EDNRB Mutations in Shah-Waardenburg Syndrome

As already mentioned, the first human EDNRB mutation was found in the large Mennonite kindred with patients with (a mild variant of) Shah-Waardenburg syndrome in three branches of the kindred. Affected individuals had a homozygous exon 4 mutation (W276C). The phenotype, however, appeared to be not the same for all mutation carriers. Out of 17 homozygotes, 5 showed only nonenteric features of Shah-Waardenburg syndrome, such as bicolored irides, deafness, hypopigmentation, white forelock or premature graying; 3 showed both nonenteric features of Shah-Waardenburg syndrome and HSCR; and 2 had only HSCR (Puffenberger et al., 1994a).

To date, four other patients and families have been described with Shah-Waardenburg syndrome and mutations in the *EDNRB* gene (Attie et al., 1995a; Syrris et al., 1999; Boardman et al., 2001; Verheij et al., 2002) (see Table 38–1). In three of these families patients were homozygous for the mutation found. Heterozygotes did not show any abnormalities related to Shah-Waardenburg syndrome. However, in the fourth family a nonsense mutation of exon 3 of the *EDNRB* gene

(R253X) was detected. All affected individuals in three generations were heterozygous for this mutation and showed a variety of manifestations (one or more of heterochromia, hearing loss, and HSCR). Only one of these patients had HSCR (representing a heterozygous patient with a severe phenotype); none of them showed all three features (Syrris et al., 1999).

EDNRB in Isolated Hirschsprung Disease

Multiple studies have shown that mutations of the *EDNRB* gene also play a role in the development of isolated HSCR. Mutations of *EDNRB* are found in around 3% to 10% of sporadic isolated cases of HSCR (Amiel et al., 1996; Auricchio et al., 1996; Hofstra et al., 1996; Kusafuka et al., 1996, 1997; Inoue et al., 1998; Tanaka et al., 1998; Svensson, et al., 1999a; Sakai et al., 2000). In total, these studies comprise 513 isolated HSCR patients for 24 of whom (almost 5%) truncating mutations were found (see Table 38–2). Besides these, many missense mutations were identified. The pathogenic nature of these missense mutations is less clear. It is important to determine their effects on signal transduction by *EDNRB*. Five of the described missense mutations (A183G, W276C, R319W, M374I, and P383L) were shown to cause a loss of function, confirming their pathogenic nature (Abe et al., 2000).

In the earlier described Mennonite kindred with Shah-Waardenburg syndrome, isolated HSCR also occurs. Both homozygotes and heterozygotes for the missense mutation (W276C) proved to be at risk for developing HSCR, but the penetrance of the homozygotes (74%) was much higher than of heterozygotes (21%), and at least five patients with HSCR did not have this mutation. In the Mennonite kindred, besides linkage to *EDNRB*, significant evidence of non-random transmission of *RET* marker haplotypes in HSCR patients was found (Puffenberger et al., 1994a). Several isolated HSCR patients have been described in which a combination of mutations of two genes was found. Two patients have been reported with coexistence of two functionally significant *EDNRB* and *RET* mutations (one patient with a combination of S305N and I647I, the other 26G → A and IVS10+2T → A; this patient also had Down syndrome)(Auricchio et al., 1999; Sakai et al., 1999). These findings may suggest a direct interaction between these two distinct transmembrane receptors, supporting the assumption of the polygenic nature of HSCR. Svensson and colleagues (1998) described a family with missense mutations in both the *RET* gene (R982C) and the *EDNRB* gene (G57S). In this family, three out of five members had both mutations, but only one boy had isolated HSCR. However, it has been argued that both mutations most likely represent rare polymorphisms (Hofstra et al., 1997).

EDN3 Mutations in Shah-Waardenburg Syndrome and in Isolated HSCR

Mutations in the *EDN3* gene were found in four families with Shah-Waardenburg syndrome (see Table 38–3) (Edery et al., 1996; Hofstra et al., 1996; Bidaud et al., 1997; Pingault et al., 2001). In three fam-

Table 38–1. Clinical Findings in Patients with Shah-Waardenburg Syndrome Caused by Mutations in *EDNRB*

| EDNRB Mutation | Clinical Findings | | Family Description | Reference |
	Homozygous	Heterozygous		
A183G	Iris heterochromia, white forelock, skin pigmentary defects (in one of the sisters), deafness, HSCR	No abnormalities	Two sisters with WS; healthy heterozygous consanguineous parents and brothers	Attie et al., 1995a
R253X	None	Heterochromia and/or deafness and/or long-segment HSCR	Eight affected individuals in three generations; no one with all three features; only one with HSCR	Syrris et al., 1999
G186R	Segmental hypopigmentation face, trunk and upper limb, white scalp hair, total intestinal aganglionosis; hearing not tested	No abnormalities	Patient with Down syndrome, died 3 weeks old; parents and sibs healthy (no DNA available)	Boardman et al., 2001
R201X	Pale blue irides, white eyelashes and brows, white hair with black lock, deafness, total intestinal aganglionosis	No abnormalities	Five sibs (girls and boys) with WS; healthy consanguineous parents and sibs (no DNA available)	Verheij et al., 2002

Table 38–2. Overview of the *EDNRB* Mutation Screening in Patients with Isolated HSCR (numbers)

Reference	Patients Screened	Families	Mutations in Families	Sporadic Patients	Mutations in Sporadic Patients
Amiel et al., 1996	165	80	2	85	5
Auricchio et al., 1996	50		1	50	1
Kusafuka et al., 1997	41		0	41	2
Inoue et al., 1998	37		0	37	1
Tanaka et al., 1998	31		0	31	2
Svensson et al., 1999a	69	7	0	62	3
Sakai et al., 2000	28		0	28	3
Munnes et al., 2000	6	5	0	1	0
Gath et al., 2001	29			29	0
Hofstra (unpublished data)*	86	16	2	70	2
Totals	542	108	5 (4.6%)	434	19 (4.4%)

Only those studies are mentioned that described screening of a number of unselected HSCR patients (unclear mutations/probable polymorphisms excluded).

ilies the patients were homozygous for the mutation. In one of these, the family history suggested that heterozygotes might have hearing loss or depigmentation (Hofstra et al., 1996). In the fourth family patients were heterozygous for a missense mutation. A brother of this mother died shortly after birth from congenital intestinal obstruction (no medical records or DNA available). However, a healthy grandfather, mother, and sib were also heterozygous for this mutation, making it likely that other genes play a role in determining the clinical phenotype (Pingault et al., 2001).

In contrast with mutations of *EDNRB*, *EDN3* mutations are rarely found in isolated HSCR patients. Among 174 patients screened, Bidaud and colleagues (1997) found two missense mutations (A17T and A224T) in two patients with isolated HSCR. In both cases, the mutation was inherited from the asymptomatic mother. A heterozygous frameshift mutation in exon 2 (E90X) was identified in a sporadic patient with short-segment HSCR without any Waardenburg features (Svensson et al., 1999b). Until now, screening has been reported for 290 patients with isolated HSCR. Only three (1%) mutations have been found: two missense mutations and one frameshift mutation (Hofstra et al., 1996; Bidaud et al., 1997; Svensson et al., 1999b). A heterozygous frameshift mutation in exon 4 of *EDN3* was also found in a patient with isolated congenital central hypoventilation syndrome (CCHS). CCHS is associated with HSCR in 16% of patients. Although the mutation seems to result in a functionally inactive protein (E198X), this could not be demonstrated (Bolk et al., 1996). Furthermore, this mutation was also found in patients with isolated HSCR (Bidaud et al., 1997; Svensson et al., 1999b) and in control individuals (Kenny et al., 2000). These considerations make it unlikely that the E198X mutation is a causative one.

ECE-1: An Endothelin-Related Gene

ECE-1 (endothelin-converting enzyme-1) is involved in the proteolytic processing of endothelins 1, 2, and 3, which are encoded by the *EDN1*, *EDN2*, and *EDN3* genes. ECE-1 converts these endothelins to their biologically active peptides, ET1, ET2, and ET3. *Ece1* knockout mice seem to present a combination of features characteristic for the *Edn1* and *Edn3* knockout mice: craniofacial and cardiac defects, in combination with lack of enteric ganglia in the terminal colon. Hofstra and colleagues (Hofstra et al., 1999) scanned the human *ECE-1* gene for mutations in a large number of patients with HSCR, including patients with complete or partial features of Shah-Waardenburg syndrome. A heterozygous missense mutation (R742C) was detected in a patient with HSCR, cardiac defects, craniofacial abnormalities, micropenis, deformities of hands, autonomic dysfunction, and status epilepticus. This mutation was not found in 100 control individuals and 110 HSCR patients (none with the same phenotype). Furthermore, the activity of this mutant *ECE-1* was only 4.7% of that of the wild-type *ECE-1*. It was concluded that this R742C mutation caused or at least contributed to the phenotype of this patient by producing reduced levels of ET1 and ET3.

SOX10 Mutations in Patients with Shah-Waardenburg Syndrome

Pingault and colleagues (1998) reported the screening of *SOX10* in 15 individuals with Shah-Waardenburg syndrome. They found a heterozygous mutation in 4 of them. An in vitro study of these mutations was performed to analyze their effect on *SOX10* function. It was concluded that each of the mutations is likely to lead to functional inactivation of the protein (Kuhlbrodt et al., 1998b). A study by Southard-Smith and colleagues (1999) on 9 patients with HSCR and Waardenburg-associated phenotypes revealed two new nonsense mutations. One of these patients also had neurological abnormalities. Other *SOX10* mutations were also found in patients with WS and neurological involvement of both central and peripheral nervous systems (Inoue et al., 1999; Touraine et al., 2000; Sham et al., 2001b; J. Verheij, unpublished observation) (see Table 38–4). Patients with *SOX10* mutations display less severity in the extent of intestinal agangliono-

Table 38–3. Clinical Findings in Patients with Shah-Waardenburg Syndrome Caused by Mutations in *EDN3*

EDN3 Mutation	Clinical Findings Homozygous	Heterozygous	Family Description	Reference
262GC → T	Pale blue retina, white eyelashes, achromic skin patches, deafness, total colonic aganglionosis	No abnormalities	Unrelated healthy heterozygous parents	Edery et al., 1996
C159F	Brother and sister with hypoplastic blue eyes, pigmentary defects, deafness and total colonic aganglionosis	No abnormalities; family history suggests heterozygous status can give hearing loss or depigmentation	Sister no DNA available; healthy heterozygous parents	Hofstra et al., 1996
E55X	WS (no further description)	No abnormalities	Older brother died with WS, no DNA available; healthy heterozygous consanguineous parents	Bidaud et al., 1997
C169X	None	*Sister*: white forelock, progressive hearing loss, hypopigmentation on hands, long-segment HSCR; *brother*: intestinal obstruction (echo, pregnancy terminated)	Heterozygous mother and sib healthy, brother of mother died of intestinal obstruction (no DNA or medical record)	Pingault et al., 2001

Table 38–4. Clinical Findings in Patients with Shah-Waardenburg Syndrome Caused by Heterozygous Mutations in *SOX10*

| | Clinical Findings | | | |
SOX10 Mutation	Shah-Waardenburg	Neurological Abnormalities	Family Description	Reference
E189X	White hair, blue irides with grey speckles, depigmented skin patches, bilateral deafness, short-segment HSCR	None	De novo mutation	Pingault et al., 1998
Y83X	Fair hair, vivid blue eyes, bilateral deafness, chronic bowel problems	None	De novo mutation	Pingault et al., 1998
482ins6 (GCTCCG)	Deafness, short-segment HSCR	None	Sporadic mutation (no information about parents)	Pingault et al., 1998
1076delGA	Hypopigmentation, deafness, HSCR	None	Mother (no HSCR), son (all three) and daughter (no deafness) with mutation	Pingault et al., 1998
Y207X	Hypopigmentation abdomen and neck, short-segment HSCR		Phenotypically normal parents and sister, de novo mutation	Southard-Smith et al., 1999
Q377X	Brother deafness and long-segment HSCR; sister deafness	Nystagmus plus ataxic cerebral palsy (both sibs)	Sequence analysis of the healthy father shows possible mosaicism	Southard-Smith et al., 1999
1400del12	Iris heterochromia, deafness, long-segment HSCR, dystopia canthorum	Severe leukodystrophy and peripheral neuropathy	De novo mutation; healthy parents and siblings	Inoue et al., 1999
Y313X	Iris heterochromia, deafness, hypomelanotic skin patches, total intestinal aganglionosis	Severe mental retardation, spasticity, nystagmus, myopia, hypogonadism, reduced tear production, growth deficiency	Three sibs (boys) with WS died soon after birth, healthy heterozygous mother, probably somatic mosaicism	Touraine et al., 2000
Y313X	Iris heterochromia, deafness, short-segment HSCR	Mild mental retardation, ataxia, nystagmus, spasticity, seizures, growth retardation, impairment of autonomous system (alacrima, asialia, and reduced sweating)	Healthy parents, mother no carrier, father not available for study	Touraine et al., 2000
S251X	White forelock, deafness, total intestinal aganglionosis	Hypotonia and arthro-gryposis; died soon after birth	De novo mutation	Touraine et al., 2000
168delG	Light brown hair, vivid blue eyes with grey speckles, deafness, short-segment HSCR		De novo mutation	Sham et al., 2001b
X457K	Blue eyes, white forelock, deaf-ness, total colonic aganglionosis	Ptosis right eye, mental and global developmental retardation	De novo mutation	Sham et al., 2001b
S384X	Blue eyes, red hair, deafness, short-segment HSCR	Mild mental retardation, distal arthrogryposis, growth retardation, peripheral neuropathy, delayed myelinization	De novo mutation	Verheij, unpublished observation

sis (more short-segment HSCR and hypoganglionosis). Sham and colleagues (2001b) suggest that mutations in *SOX10* around the HMG domain lead to a milder phenotype (hypoganglionosis, or short-segment HSCR), whereas mutations that affect the C-terminal transactivation domain cause a more severe intestinal aganglionosis phenotype (long-segment HSCR, or total intestinal aganglionosis).

In addition, a *SOX10* missense mutation (S135T) has been reported for a patient with the mild form of Yemenite syndrome (congenital sensorineural hearing loss, nystagmus, hypopigmentation, multiple frecklings, patchy white hair, and dental abnormalities, but no constipation). An in vitro functional study proved that this is a deleterious mutation. However, in another patient with a severe form of Yemenite syndrome, no *SOX10* mutation or deletion could be detected (Bondurand et al., 1999). A single nucleotide deletion (795delG) in *SOX10* has been found in a patient with peripheral neuropathy with hypomyelination, deafness, and chronic intestinal pseudoobstruction (Pingault et al., 2000).

Taken together, *SOX10* mutations are associated with Shah-Waardenburg syndrome. In some cases, the clinical phenotype appears as an incomplete Shah-Waardenburg syndrome with or without neurological features. So far, in 31 unrelated Shah-Waardenburg patients, 12 mutations have been found. The prevalence of *SOX10* mutations

in patients with Shah-Waardenburg syndrome, combined with neurological features, seems high. In 34 unrelated patients with isolated sporadic or familial HSCR, no *SOX10* mutations were found (Pingault et al., 1998).

In summary, mutations in *EDNRB, EDN3,* and *SOX10* are found in a large proportion of patients with Shah-Waardenburg syndrome, but not in all. It is not possible to get a complete picture about the percentage of patients with Shah-Waardenburg syndrome with confirmed mutations in one of these genes. In particular, publications about *EDNRB* and *EDN3* mutations do not report systematic screening of patients. However, we estimate that at least 50% of patients with Shah-Waardenburg syndrome will have one or more mutations in one of these genes.

THERAPY

The treatment of HSCR is resection of the entire aganglionic segment of the colon with anastomosis of the healthy part at the anus. Pigmentary abnormalities of eyes and hair do not need treatment. The patient can use colored lenses or hair dye for cosmetic reasons. Depigmentations of the skin need protection from exposure to ultraviolet light, and avoidance of sunburning is important. Early detection of hearing loss is important, to be followed by appropriate intervention with hearing aids or even by evaluation for a cochlear implant operation if patients are profoundly deaf.

PROGNOSIS

The survival in patients with Shah-Waardenburg syndrome is primarily determined by the severity of HSCR. Mortality for HSCR is under 6%; in particular, however, children with total colonic aganglionosis have a high morbidity. They often need multiple surgical procedures. Moreover, many long-term complications are encountered, such as fecal incontinence and low body weight (Tsuji et al., 1999). Most patients with mutations of the *SOX10* gene show neurological manifestations and mental retardation, varying from mild to severe. However, too few clinical data and insufficient follow-up information are available at present.

GENETIC COUNSELING

Clearly, genetic counseling in families with Shah-Waardenburg syndrome is not straightforward. Clinical investigation of the index patient, parents, and sibs is always necessary. Subsequently, a thorough search for mutations in *EDNRB*, *EDN3*, and *SOX10* (this last gene especially in the presence of neurological features) should be performed. In the case of homozygous mutations of *EDNRB* or *EDN3* and no features of Shah-Waardenburg syndrome in heterozygous parents and sibs, autosomal recessive inheritance with a recurrence risk of 25% seems obvious. In families with *EDN3* or *EDNRB* mutations causing features of Shah-Waardenburg syndrome in heterozygotes in more than one generation, a recurrence risk of 50% for sibs and offspring has to be given, but with a highly variable expression. When a heterozygous mutation is identified in a sporadic patient, a recurrence risk is hard to give, as no hard evidence is present to assume a truly dominant nature of such a mutation. In case of an already described mutation, information available from the literature should be discussed with the parents and patients.

For *SOX10* mutations, autosomal dominant inheritance can be assumed, giving a recurrence risk of 50% for offspring of patients. Although most mutations arise de novo, two cases of somatic mosaicism have been reported (Southard-Smith et al., 1999; Touraine et al., 2000). This means that for sibs, a recurrence risk of about 15% to 20% (2 of 11 families described) might apply, even though in the patient the mutation seems to occur de novo. One should keep in mind that the numbers reported so far are small and therefore inconclusive.

Prenatal diagnosis by DNA investigation is possible if the mutation is known. However, variable expression is described for several mutations in the *SOX10* gene (see Table 38–4), making it difficult for parents to make decisions. Sometimes intestinal obstruction can be identified sonographically but not, in general, in early pregnancy.

ANIMAL MODELS FOR SHAH-WAARDENBURG SYNDROME

The heterogeneous nature of Shah-Waardenburg syndrome is reflected by the number of spontaneous mouse mutants with phenotypes similar to Shah-Waardenburg syndrome—namely, *piebald lethal* (*EDNRB*), *lethal spotting* (*EDN3*) (Lane, 1966), and *dominant megacolon* (*SOX10*) (Lane and Liu, 1984), all mentioned before. Furthermore, the *EDNRB* gene is partially deleted in the autosomal recessive rat mutant *lethal-spotting*, which also has the phenotype of white spotting and congenital aganglionosis (Ceccherini et al., 1995).

Another model resembling Shah-Waardenburg is found in horses and is named lethal white foal syndrome. Horses that were heterozygous for a missense mutation in the first exon of the *EDNRB* gene (I118K) showed white coat spotting patterns. Horses homozygous for this mutation were all white with long-segment aganglionosis (Metallinos et al., 1998; Santschi et al., 1998).

A chicken Sox10 ortholog (cSox10) was cloned to study its role in neural crest cell development (Cheng et al., 2000). Another mouse model for *Sox10* was generated, Sox10[lacZ] mice, demonstrating that haploinsufficiency can explain the phenotype observed in Sox10[Dom] mice (Britsch et al., 2001). The zebrafish colorless mutant phenotype can also be used as a model for Shah-Waardenburg syndrome, showing a combination of defects in both melanocytes and the enteric nervous system (Kelsh and Eisen, 2000).

REFERENCES

Abe Y, Sakurai T, Yamada T, Nakamura T, Yanagisawa M, Goto K (2000). Functional analysis of five endothelin-B receptor mutations found in human hirschsprung disease patients. *Biochem Biophys Res Commun* 275: 524–531.

Ambani LM (1983). Waardenburg and Hirschsprung syndromes. *J Pediatr* 102: 802.

Amiel J, Attie T, Jan D, Pelet A, Edery P, Bidaud C, Lacombe D, Tam P, Simeoni J, Flori E, et al. (1996). Heterozygous endothelin receptor B (EDNRB) mutations in isolated Hirschsprung disease. *Hum Mol Genet* 5: 355–357.

Ariturk E, Tosyali N, Ariturk N (1992). A case of Waardenburg syndrome and aganglionosis. *Turk J Pediatr* 34: 111–114.

Attie T, Till M, Pelet A, Amiel J, Edery P, Boutrand L, Munnich A, Lyonnet S (1995a). Mutation of the endothelin-receptor B gene in Waardenburg-Hirschsprung disease. *Hum Mol Genet* 4: 2407–2409.

Attie T, Till M, Pelet A, Edery P, Bonnet JP, Munnich A, Lyonnet S (1995b). Exclusion of RET and Pax 3 loci in Waardenburg-Hirschsprung disease. *J Med Genet* 32: 312–313.

Auricchio A, Casari G, Staiano A, Ballabio A (1996). Endothelin-B receptor mutations in patients with isolated Hirschsprung disease from a non-inbred population. *Hum Mol Genet* 5: 351–354.

Auricchio A, Griseri P, Carpentieri ML, Betsos N, Staiano A, Tozzi A, Priolo M, Thompson H, Bocciardi R, Romeo G, et al. (1999). Double heterozygosity for a RET substitution interfering with splicing and an EDNRB missense mutation in Hirschsprung disease. *Am J Hum Genet* 64: 1216–1221. (Letter).

Badner JA, Chakravarti A (1990). Waardenburg syndrome and Hirschsprung disease: evidence for pleiotropic effects of a single dominant gene. *Am J Med Genet* 35: 100–104.

Baynash AG, Hosoda K, Giaid A, Richardson JA, Emoto N, Hammer RE, Yanagisawa M (1994). Interaction of endothelin-3 with endothelin-B receptor is essential for development of epidermal melanocytes and enteric neurons. *Cell* 79: 1277–1285.

Bidaud C, Salomon R, Van Camp G, Pelet A, Attie T, Eng C, Bonduelle M, Amiel J, Nihoul-Fekete C, Willems PJ, et al. (1997). Endothelin-3 gene mutations in isolated and syndromic Hirschsprung disease. *Eur J Hum Genet* 5: 247–251.

Boardman JP, Syrris P, Holder SE, Robertson NJ, Carter N, Lakhoo K (2001). A novel mutation in the endothelin B receptor gene in a patient with Shah-Waardenburg syndrome and Down syndrome. *J Med Genet* 38: 646–647.

Bolk S, Angrist M, Xie J, Yanagisawa M, Silvestri JM, Weese-Mayer DE, Chakravarti A (1996). Endothelin-3 frameshift mutation in congenital central hypoventilation syndrome. *Nat Genet* 13: 395–396.

Bondurand N, Kuhlbrodt K, Pingault V, Enderich J, Sajus M, Tommerup N, Warburg M, Hennekam RC, Read AP, Wegner M, Goossens M (1999). A molecular analysis of the yemenite deaf–blind hypopigmentation syndrome: SOX10 dysfunction causes different neurocristopathies. *Hum Mol Genet* 8: 1785–1789.

Bonnet JP, Till M, Edery P, Attie T, Lyonnet S (1996). Waardenburg-Hirschsprung disease in two sisters: a possible clue to the genetics of this association? *Eur J Pediatr Surg* 6: 245–248.

Bottani A, Xie YG, Binkert F, Schinzel A (1991). A case of Hirschsprung disease with a chromosome 13 microdeletion, del(13) (q32.3q33.2): potential mapping of one disease locus. *Hum Genet* 87: 748–750.

Branski D, Dennis NR, Neale JM, Brooks LJ (1979). Hirschsprung's disease and Waardenburg's syndrome. *Pediatrics* 63: 803–805.

Britsch S, Goerich DE, Riethmacher D, Peirano RI, Rossner M, Nave KA, Birchmeier C, Wegner M (2001). The transcription factor Sox10 is a key regulator of peripheral glial development. *Genes Dev* 15: 66–78.

Ceccherini I, Zhang AL, Matera I, Yang G, Devoto M, Romeo G, Cass DT (1995). Interstitial deletion of the endothelin-B receptor gene in the spotting lethal (sl) rat. *Hum Mol Genet* 4: 2089–2096.

Cheng Y, Cheung M, Abu-Elmagd MM, Orme A, Scotting PJ (2000). Chick sox10, a transcription factor expressed in both early neural crest cells and central nervous system. *Brain Res Dev Brain Res* 121: 233–241.

de Lumley WL, Boulesteix J, Rutkowski J, Umdenstock R (1980). Waardenburg syndrome associated with Hirschsprung disease and other abnormalities. *Pediatrics* 65: 368–369.

Edery P, Attie T, Amiel J, Pelet A, Eng C, Hofstra RM, Martelli H, Bidaud C, Munnich A, Lyonnet S (1996). Mutation of the endothelin-3 gene in the Waardenburg-Hirschsprung disease (Shah-Waardenburg syndrome). *Nat Genet* 12: 442–444.

Farndon PA, Bianchi A (1983). Waardenburg's syndrome associated with total aganglionosis. *Arch Dis Child* 58: 932–933.

Fried K, Beer S (1980). Waardenburg's syndrome and Hirschsprung's disease in the same patient. *Clin Genet* 18: 91–92.

Gath R, Goessling A, Keller KM, Koletzko S, Coerdt W, Muntefering H, Wirth S, Hofstra RM, Mulligan L, Eng C, von Deimling A (2001). Analysis of the RET, GDNF, EDN3, and EDNRB genes in patients with intestinal neuronal dysplasia and Hirschsprung disease. *Gut* 48: 671–675.

Goldberg M (1966). Waardenburg's syndrome with fundus and other anomalies. *Arch Ophthalmol* 76: 797–809.

Goldberg M (1981). Piebaldness and Hirschsprung's disease. *Arch Dermatol* 117: 451.

Gross A, Kunze J, Maier RF, Stoltenburg-Didinger G, Grimmer I, Obladen M (1995). Autosomal-recessive neural crest syndrome with albinism, black lock, cell migration disorder of the neurocytes of the gut, and deafness: ABCD syndrome. *Am J Med Genet* 56: 322–326.

Herbarth B, Pingault V, Bondurand N, Kuhlbrodt K, Hermans-Borgmeyer I, Puliti A, Lemort N, Goossens M, Wegner M (1998). Mutation of the Sry-related Sox10 gene in

Dominant megacolon, a mouse model for human Hirschsprung disease. *Proc Natl Acad Sci USA* 95: 5161–5165.

Hofstra RM, Osinga J, Tan-Sindhunata G, Wu Y, Kamsteeg EJ, Stulp RP, Ravenswaaij-Arts C, Majoor-Krakauer D, Angrist M, Chakravarti A, et al. (1996). A homozygous mutation in the endothelin-3 gene associated with a combined Waardenburg type 2 and Hirschsprung phenotype (Shah-Waardenburg syndrome). *Nat Genet* 12: 445–447.

Hofstra RM, Osinga J, Buys CH (1997). Mutations in Hirschsprung disease: when does a mutation contribute to the phenotype? *Eur J Hum Genet* 5: 180–185.

Hofstra RM, Valdenaire O, Arch E, Osinga J, Kroes H, Loffler BM, Hamosh A, Meijers C, Buys CH (1999). A loss-of-function mutation in the endothelin-converting enzyme 1 (ECE-1) associated with Hirschsprung disease, cardiac defects, and autonomic dysfunction. *Am J Hum Genet* 64: 304–308. (Letter).

Hosoda K, Hammer RE, Richardson JA, Baynash AG, Cheung JC, Giaid A, Yanagisawa M (1994). Targeted and natural (piebald-lethal) mutations of endothelin-B receptor gene produce megacolon associated with spotted coat color in mice. *Cell* 79: 1267–1276.

Inoue K, Tanabe Y, Lupski JR (1999). Myelin deficiencies in both the central and the peripheral nervous systems associated with a SOX10 mutation. *Ann Neurol* 46: 313–318.

Inoue M, Hosoda K, Imura K, Kamata S, Fukuzawa M, Nakao K, Okada A (1998). Mutational analysis of the endothelin-B receptor gene in Japanese Hirschsprung's disease. *J Pediatr Surg* 33: 1206–1208.

Jacobs JM, Wilson J (1992). An unusual demyelinating neuropathy in a patient with Waardenburg's syndrome. *Acta Neuropathol (Berl)* 83: 670–674.

Kaplan P, de Chaderevian JP (1988). Piebaldism-Waardenburg syndrome: histopathologic evidence for a neural crest syndrome. *Am J Med Genet* 31: 679–688.

Kelley R, Zackai E (1981). Congenital deafness, Hirschsprung's and Waardenburg syndrome. *Am J Hum Genet* 33: 65A.

Kelsh RN, Eisen JS (2000). The zebrafish colourless gene regulates development of non-ectomesenchymal neural crest derivatives. *Development* 127: 515–525.

Kenny SE, Hofstra RM, Buys CH, Vaillant CR, Lloyd DA, Edgar DH (2000). Reduced endothelin-3 expression in sporadic Hirschsprung disease. *Br J Surg* 87: 580–585.

Kiss P, Osztovics M (1989). Association of 13q deletion and Hirschsprung's disease. *J Med Genet* 26: 793–794.

Kuhlbrodt K, Herbarth B, Sock E, Hermans-Borgmeyer I, Wegner M (1998a). Sox10, a novel transcriptional modulator in glial cells. *J Neurosci* 18: 237–250.

Kuhlbrodt K, Schmidt C, Sock E, Pingault V, Bondurand N, Goossens M, Wegner M (1998b). Functional analysis of Sox10 mutations found in human Waardenburg-Hirschsprung patients. *J Biol Chem* 273: 23033–23038.

Kusafuka T, Wang Y, Puri P (1996). Novel mutations of the endothelin-B receptor gene in isolated patients with Hirschsprung's disease. *Hum Mol Genet* 5: 347–349.

Kusafuka T, Wang Y, Puri P (1997). Mutation analysis of the RET, the endothelin-B receptor, and the endothelin-3 genes in sporadic cases of Hirschsprung's disease. *J Pediatr Surg* 32: 501–504.

Lamont MA, Fitchett M, Dennis NR (1989). Interstitial deletion of distal 13q associated with Hirschsprung's disease. *J Med Genet* 26: 100–104.

Lane PW (1966). Association of megacolon with two recessive spotting genes in the mouse. *J Hered* 57: 29–31.

Lane PW, Liu HM (1984). Association of megacolon with a new dominant spotting gene (Dom) in the mouse. *J Hered* 75: 435–439.

Liang JC, Juarez CP, Goldberg MF (1983). Bilateral bicolored irides with Hirschsprung's disease: a neural crest syndrome. *Arch Ophthalmol* 101: 69–73.

Mahakrishnan A, Srinivasan MS (1980). Piebaldness with Hirschsprung's disease. *Arch Dermatol* 116: 1102.

Mallory SB, Wiener E, Nordlund JJ (1986). Waardenburg's syndrome with Hirschsprung's disease: a neural crest defect. *Pediatr Dermatol* 3: 119–124.

McKusick V (1973). Congenital deafness and Hirschsprung's disease. *N Engl J Med* 288: 691.

Meire F, Standaert L, De Laey JJ, Zeng LH (1987). Waardenburg syndrome, Hirschsprung megacolon, and Marcus Gunn ptosis. *Am J Med Genet* 27: 683–686.

Metallinos DL, Oppenheimer AJ, Rinchik EM, Russell LB, Dietrich W, Tilghman SM (1994). Fine structure mapping and deletion analysis of the murine piebald locus. *Genetics* 136: 217–223.

Metallinos DL, Bowling AT, Rine J (1998). A missense mutation in the endothelin-B receptor gene is associated with Lethal White Foal Syndrome: an equine version of Hirschsprung disease. *Mamm Genome* 9: 426–431.

Munnes M, Fanaei S, Schmitz B, Muiznieks I, Holschneider AM, Doerfler W (2000). Familial form of Hirschsprung disease: nucleotide sequence studies reveal point mutations in the RET proto-oncogene in two of six families but not in other candidate genes. *Am J Med Genet* 94: 19–27.

Omenn GS, McKusick VA (1979). The association of Waardenburg syndrome and Hirschsprung megacolon. *Am J Med Genet* 3: 217–223.

Pierpont JW, St Jacques D, Seaver LH, Erickson RP (1995). A family with unusual Waardenburg syndrome type I (WSI), cleft lip (palate), and Hirschsprung disease is not linked to PAX 3. *Clin Genet* 47: 139–143.

Pingault V, Bondurand N, Kuhlbrodt K, Goerich DE, Prehu MO, Puliti A, Herbarth B, Hermans-Borgmeyer I, Legius E, Matthijs G, et al. (1998). SOX10 mutations in patients with Waardenburg-Hirschsprung disease. *Nat Genet* 18: 171–173.

Pingault V, Guiochon-Mantel A, Bondurand N, Faure C, Lacroix C, Lyonnet S, Goossens M, Landrieu P (2000). Peripheral neuropathy with hypomyelination, chronic intestinal pseudo-obstruction and deafness: a developmental "neural crest syndrome" related to a SOX10 mutation. *Ann Neurol* 48: 671–676.

Pingault V, Bondurand N, Lemort N, Sancandi M, Ceccherini I, Hugot JP, Jouk PS, Goossens M (2001). A heterozygous endothelin 3 mutation in Waardenburg-Hirschsprung disease: is there a dosage effect of EDN3/EDNRB gene mutations on neurocristopathy phenotypes? *J Med Genet* 38: 205–209.

Puffenberger EG, Hosoda K, Washington SS, Nakao K, deWit D, Yanagisawa M, Chakravart A (1994a). A missense mutation of the endothelin-B receptor gene in multigenic Hirschsprung's disease. *Cell* 79: 1257–1266.

Puffenberger EG, Kauffman ER, Bolk S, Matise TC, Washington SS, Angrist M, Weissenbach J, Garver KL, Mascari M, Ladda R (1994b). Identity-by-descent and association mapping of a recessive gene for Hirschsprung disease on human chromosome 13q22. *Hum Mol Genet* 3: 1217–1225.

Puliti A, Prehu MO, Simon-Chazottes D, Ferkdadji L, Peuchmaur M, Goossens M, Guenet JL (1995). A high-resolution genetic map of mouse chromosome 15 encompassing the Dominant megacolon (Dom) locus. *Mamm Genome* 6: 763–768.

Rarey KE, Davis LE (1984). Inner ear anomalies in Waardenburg's syndrome associated with Hirschsprung's disease. *Int J Pediatr Otorhinolaryngol* 8: 181–189.

Read AP, Newton VE (1997). Waardenburg syndrome. *J Med Genet* 34: 656–665.

Rubanyi GM, Polokoff MA (1994). Endothelins: molecular biology, biochemistry, pharmacology, physiology, and pathophysiology. *Pharmacol Rev* 46: 325–415.

Sakai T, Wakizaka A, Nirasawa Y, Ito Y (1999). Point nucleotidic changes in both the RET proto-oncogene and the endothelin-B receptor gene in a Hirschsprung disease patient associated with Down syndrome. *Tohoku J Exp Med* 187: 43–47.

Sakai T, Nirasawa Y, Itoh Y, Wakizaka A (2000). Japanese patients with sporadic Hirschsprung: mutation analysis of the receptor tyrosine kinase proto-oncogene, endothelin-B receptor, endothelin-3, glial cell line-derived neurotrophic factor and neurturin genes: a comparison with similar studies. *Eur J Pediatr* 159: 160–167.

Santschi EM, Purdy AK, Valberg SJ, Vrotsos PD, Kaese H, Mickelson JR (1998). Endothelin receptor B polymorphism associated with lethal white foal syndrome in horses. *Mamm Genome* 9: 306–309.

Shah KN, Dalal SJ, Desai MP, Sheth PN, Joshi NC, Ambani LM (1981). White forelock, pigmentary disorder of irides, and long segment Hirschsprung disease: possible variant of Waardenburg syndrome. *J Pediatr* 99: 432–435.

Sham MH, Lui VC, Fu M, Chen B, Tam PK (2001a). SOX10 is abnormally expressed in aganglionic bowel of Hirschsprung's disease infants. *Gut* 49: 220–226.

Sham MH, Lui V, Chen B, Fu M, Tam P (2001b). Novel mutations of SOX10 suggest a dominant negative role in Shah-Waardenburg syndrome. *J Med Genet* 38: E30.

Southard-Smith EM, Kos L, Pavan WJ (1998). Sox10 mutation disrupts neural crest development in Dom Hirschsprung mouse model. *Nat Genet* 18: 60–64.

Southard-Smith EM, Angrist M, Ellison JS, Agarwala R, Baxevanis AD, Chakravarti A, Pavan WJ (1999). The Sox10(Dom) mouse: modeling the genetic variation of Waardenburg-Shah (WS4) syndrome. *Genome Res* 9: 215–225.

Svensson PJ, Anvret M, Molander ML, Nordenskjold A (1998). Phenotypic variation in a family with mutations in two Hirschsprung-related genes (RET and endothelin receptor B). *Hum Genet* 103: 145–148.

Svensson PJ, Tapper-Persson M, Anvret M, Molander ML, Eng C, Nordenskjold A (1999a). Mutations in the endothelin-receptor B gene in Hirschsprung disease in Sweden. *Clin Genet* 55: 215–217. (Letter).

Svensson PJ, Von Tell D, Molander ML, Anvret M, Nordenskjold A (1999b). A heterozygous frameshift mutation in the endothelin-3 (EDN-3) gene in isolated Hirschsprung's disease. *Pediatr Res* 45: 714–717.

Syrris P, Carter ND, Patton MA (1999). Novel nonsense mutation of the endothelin-B receptor gene in a family with Waardenburg-Hirschsprung disease. *Am J Med Genet* 87: 69–71.

Tanaka H, Moroi K, Iwai J, Takahashi H, Ohnuma N, Hori S, Takimoto M, Nishiyama M, Masaki T, Yanagisawa M, et al. (1998). Novel mutations of the endothelin B receptor gene in patients with Hirschsprung's disease and their characterization. *J Biol Chem* 273: 11378–11383.

Touraine RL, Attie-Bitach T, Manceau E, Korsch E, Sarda P, Pingault V, Encha-Razavi F, Pelet A, Auge J, Nivelon-Chevallier A, et al. (2000). Neurological phenotype in Waardenburg syndrome type 4 correlates with novel SOX10 truncating mutations and expression in developing brain. *Am J Hum Genet* 66: 1496–1503.

Tsuji H, Spitz L, Kiely EM, Drake DP, Pierro A (1999). Management and long-term follow-up of infants with total colonic aganglionosis. *J Pediatr Surg* 34: 158–161.

Van Camp G, Van Thienen MN, Handig I, Van Roy B, Rao VS, Milunsky A, Read AP, Baldwin CT, Farrer LA, Bonduelle M, et al. (1995). Chromosome 13q deletion with Waardenburg syndrome: further evidence for a gene involved in neural crest function on 13q. *J Med Genet* 32: 531–536.

Verheij JBGM, Kunze J, Osinga J, Buys CH, van Essen AJ, Hofstra RMW (2002). ABCD syndrome is caused by a homozygous mutation in the EDNRB gene. *Am J Med Genet* 108: 223–225.

Waardenburg P (1951). A new syndrome combining developmental anomalies of the eyelids, eyebrows and nose root with pigmentary defects of the iris and head hair and with congenital deafness. *Am J Hum Genet* 3: 195–253.

Weinberg AG, Currarino G, Besserman AM (1977). Hirschsprung's disease and congenital deafness. Familial association. *Hum Genet* 38: 157–161.

Part H.
The Notch Signaling Pathway

39 | Introduction to Notch Signaling

ALISON MIYAMOTO AND GERRY WEINMASTER

Notch signal transduction regulates a wide variety of cell types during specification, patterning, and morphogenesis of different tissues and structures throughout the development of both vertebrates and invertebrates (Gridley, 1997; Weinmaster, 1997; Artavanis-Tsakonas et al., 1999). Notch activation involves interactions between a DSL (Delta, Serrate, LAG-2) ligand on a signaling cell and a Notch receptor present on the surface of a responding cell. Genetic studies in *C. elegans* and *Drosophila* indicate that cell fates regulated by Notch signaling require direct cell–cell interactions. However, Notch is unique in that it functions not only as a cell surface receptor for a ligand but also as a signal transducer downstream of ligand binding.

Notch signaling is induced in lateral signaling where initially equivalent cells communicate and take on different developmental fates, as well as in inductive signaling where interactions between nonequivalent cells regulate Notch target gene expression and cellular phenotypes. In many instances Notch-regulated gene expression prevents undifferentiated cells from obtaining a more differentiated state as occurs in neurogenesis, myogenesis, and hematopoiesis, thus suggesting a role for this signaling system in maintaining a pool of immature precursor cells (Gridley, 1997; Weinmaster, 1997; Osborne and Miele, 1999). However, Notch activation can also produce inductive signals to promote the differentiation of certain cell types, including keratinocytes, granulocytes, and glia (Lowell et al., 2000; Schroeder and Just, 2000; Wang and Barres, 2000; Rangarajan et al., 2001). Moreover, Notch signaling in some cells has been reported to cause cell-cycle arrest and to induce apoptosis, while in other cell types Notch signaling protects against apoptosis and is associated with enhanced proliferation (Miele and Osborne, 1999; Osborne and Miele, 1999). Such pleiotropic effects described for Notch signaling likely reflect differences in cell context that serve to modulate ligand-induced Notch signaling. Both the core components and the modulators of the Notch signaling pathway have been identified from a large number of metazoans, and studies using flies, worms, sea urchins, frogs, fish, chickens, rodents, and humans have contributed to the genetic, cellular, and biochemical characterization of this highly conserved, ubiquitous signaling system.

THE NOTCH FAMILY OF RECEPTORS

The prototypic Notch receptor, *Drosophila* Notch (dNotch), is a >300 kDa type 1 transmembrane, cell surface protein (Greenwald, 1994; Weinmaster, 1997) (Fig. 39–1). Structure and function analyses indicate that the extracellular domain functions in ligand binding and repression of the signaling activity intrinsic to the intracellular domain. In fact, expression of constructs that encode only the intracellular domain are constitutively active in the absence of ligand. The Notch-

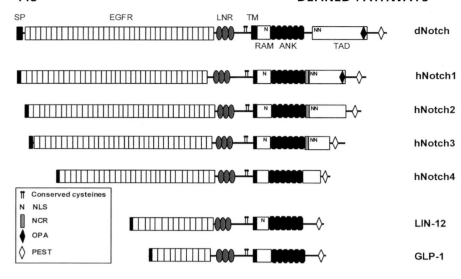

Figure 39–1. The Notch family of receptors. The schematic is based on the following protein sequences from GenBank: *Drosophila* Notch, P07207; human Notch1, P46531; human Notch2, Q04721; human Notch3, Q9UM47; human Notch4, Q99466; *C. elegans* LIN-12, P14585; *C. elegans* GLP-1, P13508. See text for details. Drawing is approximately to scale. SP, signal peptide; EGFR, epidermal growth factor–like repeat; LNR, LIN-12/Notch-related repeat; TM, transmembrane domain; RAM, CSL interaction domain; ANK, ankyrin-like repeats; TAD, transactivation domain; NLS, nuclear localization sequence; NCR, Notch cytokine response domain; OPA, glutamine-rich region; PEST, motif rich in proline, glutamine, serine, and threonine residues that is important in protein turnover.

related *C. elegans* proteins, GLP-1 and LIN-12, exhibit the same overall structure (Fig. 39–1).

Notch-related genes have been identified from a number of metazoans from sea urchin to humans. Four Notch genes have been isolated and studied in mammals (*Notch1*, *Notch2*, *Notch3*, and *Notch4*), and the structures of the proteins encoded by these genes are strikingly similar to dNotch (Greenwald, 1994; Artavanis-Tsakonas et al., 1995; Lardelli et al., 1995; Uyttendaele et al., 1996). A hallmark of the Notch extracellular domain is the presence of multiple, tandemly arrayed epidermal growth factor–like repeats (EGFR). Like dNotch, the Notch1 and Notch2 proteins contain 36 EGFRs, while Notch3 and Notch4 have 34 and 29, respectively. The order of the EGFRs has been conserved among the Notch proteins, suggesting that the spatial arrangement of these repeats is important for function.

Consistent with this idea, mutations in different EGFRs of dNotch produce quite different developmental phenotypes (Hartley et al., 1987; Kelley et al., 1987; Markopoulou and Artavanis-Tsakonas, 1989; Xu et al., 1990). EGFRs are a distinctive motif found in a diverse array of proteins and contain six highly conserved cysteine residues that influence protein structure through disulfide bond formation (Davis, 1990). Although EGFRs 11 and 12 are necessary and sufficient for ligand–receptor interactions, other EGFRs may function in posttranslational modifications to modulate Notch interactions with ligands and/or other extracellular proteins and regulate activation of downstream signaling events. EGFRs can be modified by both *N*- and *O*-linked glycosylation, as well as by hydroxylation, and some bind calcium. Interestingly, mutations in certain Notch3 EGFRs are associated with an inherited vascular dementia, CADASIL (Joutel and Tournier-Lasserve, 1998) discussed in Chapter 40. All CADASIL mutations characterized to date result in either a loss or a gain of a single cysteine residue; however, whether these changes result in gains or losses in Notch3 activity is currently unknown.

As is common with other cell surface receptors, in the absence of ligand the Notch ectodomain prevents receptor activation, and signaling is induced only after ligand binding. The LNR (for LIN-12/Notch-related region) is a cysteine-rich region located immediately downstream of the EGFRs that appears to negatively regulate receptor activation. Deletion of the LNR or missense mutations in this motif in dNotch, LIN-12, and Notch1 produce receptor proteins that are constitutively active in the absence of ligand (Greenwald and Seydoux, 1990; Lieber et al., 1993; Lyman and Young, 1993; Rand et al., 2000). As found for some of the Notch EGFRs, the LNRs bind calcium, which is required for both the stabilization of cell surface Notch and ligand binding. Constitutively active forms of dNotch, LIN-12, and GLP-1 also map to the region between the LNR and the transmembrane (TM) domain (Greenwald and Seydoux, 1990; Lieber et al., 1993; Berry et al., 1997). These mutants foreshadowed the importance of this region, which contains recognition sequences for the

two distinct proteases that are required for ligand-induced activation of the receptors (discussed later in this chapter). In addition, between these proteolytic cleavage sites reside a pair of cysteine residues that have been identified in all Notch-related proteins isolated to date, which when mutated also result in receptor activation. Even though genetic and biochemical studies have proposed roles for these highly conserved cysteines in either receptor oligomerization (Greenwald and Seydoux, 1990) or full-length heterodimeric formation through disulfide bonding (Blaumueller et al., 1997; Pan and Rubin, 1997), their function remains elusive.

The Notch protein is predicted to span the plasma membrane once, and structure and function analyses have identified several regions of the intracellular domain (ICD) that function in downstream signaling events. Juxtaposed to the TM is the so-called RAM domain, which is responsible for strong interactions with the major effector of Notch signaling known as CSL for CBF1 (Honjo, 1996) in mammals, Suppressor of Hairless [Su(H)] in flies and frogs, and LAG-1 in *C. elegans*. In addition to the RAM domain, CSL proteins also interact with the ankyrin (ANK) repeats, of which there are six located immediately next to the RAM domain. The ANK repeats also interact with a number of proteins that function in activation and modulation of Notch signaling, and thus it is not surprising that these repeats have been shown to be both necessary and sufficient for Notch activity.

Flanking the ANK are two nuclear localization signals (NLS). The first is composed of a short stretch of basic amino acids (N), and the second is bipartite with two basic motifs separated by a 10-residue spacer (NN). Both function in targeting the Notch ICD (NICD) to the nucleus. NN is located in a region of high homology that functions in transcriptional activation (TA) through recruitment of a coactivator complex (discussed later in this chapter). In dNotch and Notch1, the TAD contains an OPA sequence that is not retained in the other family members. The C terminus contains a PEST sequence that regulates the intensity and duration of activity in the nucleus through phosphorylation and ubiquitin-targeted NICD proteolysis, as well as binding sites for a number of modulators (described later in this chapter). The number of amino acids between the ANK repeats and the PEST domain is variable among the different Notch proteins, thus accounting for the differently sized cytoplasmic domains. Because different modulators and regulators bind within this region, the sequence differences likely reflect differences in Notch receptor function.

THE DSL FAMILY OF LIGANDS

The DSL ligands that bind and activate the Notch/LIN-12/GLP-1 receptors comprise a family of proteins that are either Delta-like or Serrate-like, based on the structure of the two *Drosophila* ligands, Delta (dDelta) and Serrate (Weinmaster, 1997) (Fig. 39–2). As found with Notch, the DSL ligands are single-pass cell surface proteins that

Figure 39–2. The DSL family of ligands. Structures are based on the following protein sequences from GenBank: *Drosophila* Serrate, P18168; *Drosophila* Delta, P10041; human Jagged1, XP056118; human Jagged2, Q9Y219; human Delta1, O00548; *Xenopus* X-Delta-2, AAB37131; human Delta3, Q9NYJ7; human Delta4, Q9NR61; *C. elegans* LAG-2, P45442; *C. elegans* APX-1, P41990; *C. elegans* ARG-1, T16213. See text for details. The inclusion of ARG-1 is based on sequence homology to other DSL ligands as no studies on ARG-1 have been published to date. The drawing is approximately to scale. SP, signal peptide; NT, N-terminal domain; DSL, Delta/Serrate/LAG-2 domain; EGFR, epidermal growth factor–like repeat; CR, cysteine-rich region; TM, transmembrane domain.

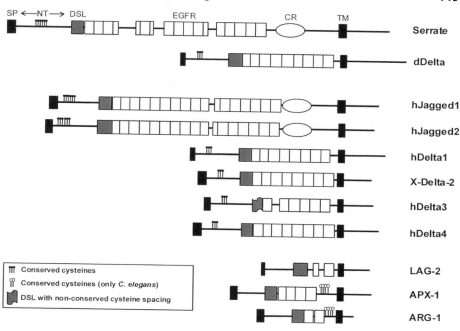

contain multiple EGFRs in their extracellular domains. N-terminal to the EGFRs is the DSL signature motif, which is a degenerate EFGR (Tax et al., 1994). Mutagenesis of LAG-2, APX-1, and Jagged1 have indicated that the DSL domain is important for interactions with the receptor (Fitzgerald and Greenwald, 1995; Henderson et al., 1997; Shimizu et al., 1999). Sequences N-terminal to the DSL domain are also important for interactions with Notch and together with the DSL motif constitute the ligand-binding domain. The N terminus contains a number of cysteine residues conserved between *Drosophila* and vertebrate DSL ligands. The Serrate-like ligands have roughly twice the number of EGFRs as Delta-like proteins and also contain a cysteine-rich region (CR). The EGFRs of Serrate contain inserts that map to the fourth, sixth, and eleventh repeats. The CR region may modulate the binding of ligand to Notch as cell aggregates formed between Delta and Notch-expressing cells are more stable than are aggregates composed of Serrate- and Notch-expressing cells (Rebay et al., 1991).

LAG-2, APX-1, and ARG-1 have been identified as ligands for the LIN-12 and GLP-1 receptors and are Delta-like in that they have a DSL domain followed by a series of EGFRs and lack a CR domain (Fig. 39–2). These ligands have the fewest numbers of EGFRs, and deletion analysis indicates that these repeats are not required for activity. In mammals, three Delta-like genes have been identified: Delta1, 3, and 4. Delta2 has only been identified in *Xenopus*, and four Delta genes have been reported for zebrafish (DeltaA, B, C, and D) of which DeltaD is most similar to Delta1. Delta3 is a highly divergent DSL protein lacking the GW (GWXGXXC) motif within the DSL that is present in all other DSL family members. In addition, in contrast to the tandem array of EGFRs in all Delta-like proteins, Delta3 has an insert following the first EFGR and contains six EGFRs compared to nine in dDelta and eight in the other Delta-like proteins. Mutations in Delta3 are associated with spondylocostal dysostosis and pudgy mice (Kusumi et al., 1998; Bulman et al., 2000), discussed in Chapter 41.

Only two Serrate-like subtypes (Serrate1/Jagged1 and Serrate2/Jagged2) have been isolated from humans, rats, mice, chickens, and frogs. As with Serrate, Jagged1 and Jagged2 are larger than the Delta-like proteins having 16 EGFRs with a single insert in the tenth repeat and a CR region. Binding studies with Jagged1 suggest that the DSL is necessary for Notch binding and that the EGFRs serve to stabilize ligand–receptor interactions (Shimizu et al., 1999). Mutations in Jagged1 are associated with Alagille syndrome (Li et al., 1997), discussed in Chapter 40.

Although the ICD of the ligands are short and do not contain any known motifs, deletion of these sequences in Delta or Serrate produce dominant–negative phenotypes, indicating that these sequences are re-

quired for normal ligand function (Chitnis et al., 1995; Sun and Artavanis-Tsakonas, 1996). Interestingly, deletion of the LAG-2 ICD increases its activity (Henderson et al., 1997). In contrast to the truncated, membrane-bound ligands, secreted extracellular forms of either LAG-2 or APX-1 can activate either LIN-12 or GLP-1; however, another study has found that LAG-2 membrane association is critical for mutant rescue (Fitzgerald and Greenwald, 1995; Henderson et al., 1997).

Consistent with this, soluble forms of dDelta or Serrate expressed in *Drosophila* produce phenotypes that are indicative of a loss in Notch signaling, as found for ICD truncations (Fleming et al., 1997; Hukriede and Fleming, 1997; Hukriede et al., 1997; Sun and Artavanis-Tsakonas, 1997). However, by using a number of different assay systems, various soluble forms of mammalian DSL ligands have been shown to bind Notch, activate signaling, and regulate cellular phenotype (Li et al., 1998; Varnum-Finney et al., 1998; Wang et al., 1998; Sestan et al., 1999; Morrison et al., 2000; Ohishi et al., 2000). Because the antagonistic and agonistic activities described for DSL ligands lack TM and ICD sequences, it would be interesting to know whether soluble DSL ligands normally function in vivo. In this regard, soluble forms of dDelta have been identified from embryos and cultured S2 cells. Furthermore, the ADAM (a disintegrin and metalloproteinase) Kuzbanian has been shown to effect the shedding of a biologically active extracellular domain of dDelta (Qi et al., 1999; Sestan et al., 1999).

The ability of soluble DSL ligands to bind and activate Notch signaling may depend on their oligomerized state (Varnum-Finney et al., 2000; Hicks et al., 2002; Shimizu et al., 2002). When truncated membrane-bound and soluble forms of Delta1 are compared with wild-type (WT) Delta1, the truncated forms are less active (Shimizu et al., 2002). Moreover, the ability of a soluble form of Delta1 to either activate or inhibit Notch signaling depends on the particular multimeric state, thus suggesting that oligomerization of the ligand is involved in receptor activation (Varnum-Finney et al., 2000; Hicks et al., 2002). The mechanism of ligand multimerization within the membrane and the role that the ICD plays in receptor activation are currently unknown. More recently, the ICD of Delta has been shown to be ubiquitinated by Neuralized, which regulates the level of cell surface expression and influences the ability of a cell to send or receive a signal (Kramer, 2001) (discussed later in this chapter).

LIGAND-INDUCED NOTCH SIGNAL TRANSDUCTION

The membrane nature of Notch is consistent with roles in cell fate specification, either as a cell-adhesion molecule or as a receptor for a signaling pathway. To differentiate between these two possibilities,

Struhl and colleagues (1993) engineered soluble forms of LIN-12 and dNotch to encode only the intracellular sequences of these proteins. When these truncated LIN-12 or dNotch proteins were expressed in mutant embryos, both rescued their respective loss-of-function mutant phenotypes, indicating that these truncated forms represent gain-of-function mutant proteins that are constitutively active independent of ligand. These findings support a role for LIN-12/Notch as receptors for a signaling pathway; however, they do not rule out a role for Notch in cell adhesion in other contexts. Importantly, this study was the first to identify a signal for Notch in the nucleus, and studies from other groups find that truncated forms of Notch function as constitutively active proteins and are similarly localized to the nucleus (Fortini et al., 1993; Lieber et al., 1993). Moreover, deletion analyses demonstrate a correlation between the presence of an NLS, a signal for Notch in the nucleus, and functional Notch activity, suggesting that nuclear localization of NICD is an important aspect of Notch signaling (Lieber et al., 1993; Kopan et al., 1994). Together these findings suggest a model for Notch signaling in which Notch functions both at the cell surface and in the nucleus.

Consistent with a role for Notch in the nucleus, the intracellular domains of dNotch, GLP-1, *Xenopus* Notch, and all four mammalian Notch proteins have been shown to physically interact with the CSL DNA-binding proteins (Mumm and Kopan, 2000). In the absence of Notch signaling, CSL proteins function as transcriptional repressors; however, upon activation of Notch signaling, they are converted from repressors into activators of transcription (Hsieh et al., 1996). Moreover, complexes containing NICD and CSL physically associate with DNAs containing CSL-binding sites, and these interactions correlate with transcriptional activation of Notch target genes such as E(spl)/HES (Jarriault et al., 1995)(discussed in detail below).

Even though expression of both membrane-bound and soluble NICD forms result in a signal for Notch in the nucleus, nuclear Notch has not been detected in cells undergoing Notch-mediated cell fate determinations in *Drosophila* or *C. elegans* (Johansen et al., 1989; Kooh et al., 1993). The inability to readily detect a signal for endogenous Notch in the nucleus raised the suspicion that nuclear NICD expression might be an aberrant activity unique to ectopic expression of truncated, mutant forms of Notch. In fact, *TAN-1* and *int-3* are oncogenic versions of the *Notch1* and *Notch4* genes, respectively; both have arisen through gene rearrangements (Gridley, 1997). Curiously, brain sections stained for Notch show a signal in the nucleus of postmitotic neurons, and nuclear Notch is detected in cultured neurons treated with ligand (Sestan et al., 1999; Redmond et al., 2000).

Why Notch is easily detected in nuclei of neurons and not in other cell types is unknown. The difficulty in detecting nuclear Notch produced from endogenous Notch in response to ligand binding may reflect either NICD interactions with other proteins that mask immunodetection or, more likely, regulated turnover of NICD. Alternatively, it has been suggested that the levels of NICD required to activate target genes and effect changes in cellular phenotype are below the level of detection when using conventional cellular imaging techniques (Schroeter et al., 1998). In fact, transfection of Notch DNA in mammalian cells at concentrations that activate gene transcription do not allow direct detection of Notch protein in the nucleus, while a signal for nuclear Notch is detected when higher concentrations of DNA are transfected.

Genetic and biochemical studies using invertebrate and mammalian systems have provided additional support for Notch functioning, both as a ligand-binding receptor and as a direct activator of gene expression (Mumm et al., 2000; Weinmaster, 2000). Of course, this duality of function presents something of a dilemma: subsequent to ligand binding, how does the transmembrane protein Notch get to the nucleus to modify the transcriptional machinery? Does the entire Notch protein enter the nucleus following ligand binding, or is the NICD released from the plasma membrane to allow nuclear translocation as suggested by the dominant–active truncated forms of Notch?

To address these aspects, Gal4VP16 (GV) sequences were inserted into WT dNotch, in either the extracellular or the intracellular domain (Lecourtois and Schweisguth, 1998; Struhl and Adachi, 1998). Expression of these dNotchGV chimeric proteins in Notch mutant em-

bryos rescues the Notch mutant phenotype, indicating that these proteins are functional. However, only chimeric proteins with GV sequences in the cytoplasmic domain of dNotch activate lacZ expression when expressed in embryos carrying a UAS-lacZ transgene. Moreover, lacZ is not activated in dDelta mutant embryos, demonstrating that UAS-lacZ transgene activation requires ligand.

These studies suggest that lacZ expression results from ligand-induced activation of Notch that involves cleavage, release, and translocation of the Notch cytoplasmic domain to the nucleus. Although direct demonstration of ligand-induced proteolysis of Notch was not demonstrated in these studies, biochemical and cellular approaches in mammalian and *Drosophila* tissue culture systems have characterized the proteolytic events that allow Notch to function with CSL to activate transcription of Notch target genes (Mumm et al., 2000; Weinmaster, 2000).

The full complement of factors and precise sequence of events and mechanisms that regulate ligand-dependent proteolysis of Notch remain to be defined. As with other signal transduction schemes, the final pathway is likely to be considerably more complex than current models predict and data support. To date, three proteolytic cleavage sites have been identified in mammalian Notch, designated Site 1 (S1), Site 2 (S2), and Site 3 (S3), and transcriptional studies indicate that proteolysis at all three sites is required for Notch activation of CSL (Fig. 39–3).

CLEAVAGE OF NOTCH AT S1

The primary translational product of the mammalian Notch gene is proteolytically processed in the *trans*-Golgi by a furin-like convertase that cleaves full-length Notch (N^{FL}) at the consensus sequence RXRR ~75 amino acids N-terminal to the TM domain (S1) (Logeat et al., 1998). Cleavage at S1 yields N-terminal 180–200 kDa (N^{EC}) and C-terminal 120 kDa (N^{TM}) fragments that remain associated via divalent cation-dependent, noncovalent interactions and are presented at the cell surface as a heterodimer. The LNR motif upstream of the furin-cleavage site is essential for stable N^{EC}-N^{TM} heterodimeric formation. Deletion of the LNR leads to shedding of N^{EC}, and this mutation results in constitutive signaling activity (Rand et al., 2000).

Interestingly, treatment of Notch1-expressing cells with chelators of divalent cations also results in release of N^{EC} into the culture medium and resultant proteolysis of membrane-bound N^{TM} to generate NICD that transits to the nucleus to activate transcription (Rand et al., 2000). Mutation of the Notch1 furin-recognition sequences or coexpression of a global furin inhibitor prevents the generation of N^{EC} and N^{TM} from N^{FL} and leads to loss in ligand-induced activation of CSL reporters, suggesting that heterodimeric Notch is required for signaling via CSL (Bush et al., 2001).

NICD and Intramembrane Cleavage of Notch

Evidence that Notch is cleaved at the cell surface was first obtained through pulse-chase analysis of a constitutively active, membrane-bound form of Notch1 (ΔEN) lacking extracellular sequences 20 amino acids N-terminal of the TM (Schroeter et al., 1998). A Notch-derived peptide similar in molecular weight to NICD can be detected in ΔEN-expressing cells, and the appearance of this fragment is blocked by both protease inhibitors and drugs that disrupt protein trafficking to the cell surface. This key finding provided the first evidence that Notch could be proteolytically cleaved at the cell surface. Importantly, the appearance of this NICD-like proteolytic fragment correlates with the appearance of Notch in the nucleus and transcriptional activation of CSL.

Sequencing of this NICD-like cleavage fragment identifies a conserved valine residue within the TM domain as a putative cleavage site. In support of this, Notch proteolytic cleavage fragments can be generated in response to the Notch ligand Jagged1, and mutation of the S3 valine prevents the appearance of this cleavage fragment. Further evidence that this valine residue and the S3 cleavage are biologically relevant to Notch function comes from a knockin mouse model where mutation of this valine in both copies of Notch1 phenocopies to a large extent mice deficient in both alleles of WT Notch1 (Huppert et al., 2000).

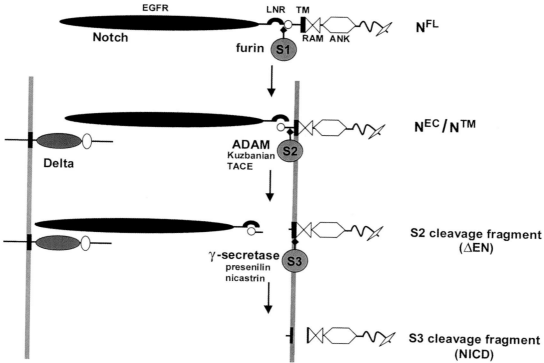

Figure 39–3. Proteolytic cleavage of the Notch receptor. Late in the *trans*-Golgi compartment, Notch is cleaved by a furin-like convertase at a site (S1) C-terminal to the LNR domain to produce a heterodimer (N^EC/N^TM) that is presented on the cell surface. Binding of ligand (in this case, Delta) on a neighboring cell is required before the second cleavage event. Following ligand activation, Notch is cleaved by an ADAM (a disintegrin and metalloprotease) protein, either Kuzbanian in *Drosophila* (Lieber et al., 2002) or TNF-α converting enzyme (TACE) in mammals (Brou et al., 2000; Mumm et al., 2000), at a site 12 amino acids from the transmembrane domain (S2). This cleavage is thought to release N^EC and its associated N^TM stub, although this product has yet to be seen experimentally in response to ligand. The other S2 cleav-age product (structurally similar to ΔE-like Notch constructs) remains associated with the membrane. Cleavage at S2 is currently thought to be the only prerequisite for the third cleavage event to occur. Mediated by γ-secretase (known components of γ-secretase include presenilin 1, presenilin 2, and nicastrin), the third cleavage is at a site internal to the transmembrane domain (S3). The S3 cleavage produces the full intracellular domain of Notch attached to a few amino acids of the transmembrane domain, as well as a small transmembrane stub that has not yet been confirmed experimentally. N^FL, full-length Notch; N^EC/N^TM, noncovalent heterodimer of the Notch extracellular domain with the Notch transmembrane and intracellular domain; ΔEN, deleted extracellular domain Notch; NICD, Notch intracellular domain.

The protease responsible for NICD generation has not been definitively identified; however, a number of findings suggest that presenilins participate in this proteolytic event (Selkoe, 2000; Fortini, 2001). The human presenilin (PS) genes *PS1* and *PS2* were first identified in an inherited, early-onset form of Alzheimer's disease (AD) (Selkoe, 2000). Neurodegeneration characteristic of AD is associated with the accumulation of amyloid peptides (Aβ) produced through aberrant proteolysis of β-amyloid precursor protein (APP). APP is a type 1 transmembrane protein of unknown function that is proteolytically processed by three proteases known as α-, β-, and γ-secretases; however, only the β- and γ-secretases produce neurotoxic Aβ peptides. Mutations in human PS proteins result in aberrant processing of APP within its single TM domain, thereby increasing production of pathogenic Aβ peptides, and loss of either PS1 or PS2 activity in mice impairs intramembrane cleavage of APP.

The findings that PS proteins can be cross-linked to drugs designed to inhibit γ-secretases and that PS proteins share a conserved catalytic center with bacterial-type prepilin peptidases suggests that they function enzymatically as γ-secretases or cofactors of this protease. However, definitive proof that PS proteins function as intramembrane proteases will require demonstration of specific protease activity in vitro, but because γ-secretase activity is associated with a large multiprotein complex dubbed the "secretasome," this may be difficult to achieve.

Homology between PS1 and Sel12, a *C. elegans* protein that facilitates LIN-12 signaling, provided the first connection between PS proteins and Notch/LIN-12 signaling (Levitan and Greenwald, 1995). Corroborating this notion, PS-deficient mutants in *Drosophila* and mice have phenotypes similar to those produced through loss of Notch signaling (Mumm and Kopan, 2000; Selkoe, 2000; Fortini, 2001). Im-portantly, PS activity is required for nuclear access and signaling by both WT Notch and ligand-independent membrane-bound forms of Notch, while the activity of soluble, NICD-like, constitutively active forms of Notch are completely unaffected by losses in PS. Furthermore, NICD is not produced in cells deficient in PS1 and PS2, and the Notch processing defect can be rescued through expression of WT PS1.

The dependence of Notch processing on PS has also been demonstrated through use of γ-secretase inhibitors, as well as a dominant–negative (DN) form of PS1. DN PS1 impairs Notch cleavage without altering cell surface expression of Notch, suggesting that PS1 is not required for Notch stability or targeting to the plasma membrane. Instead, coexpression and cell surface complexes of Notch and PS have been demonstrated in both *Drosophila* and mammalian cells, and this is consistent with the idea that PS is involved in the intramembrane cleavage of Notch that generates NICD. Taken together, these studies support the idea that PS proteins function in the proteolytic processing of Notch and that Notch function is critically dependent on proteolysis and subsequent transport to the nucleus.

Although loss-of-function mutations of presenilin impair both APP and Notch processing, AD-associated mutations of PS1 do not similarly affect cleavage of APP and Notch. Where mutations in PS1 are associated with aberrant cleavage of APP at the γ-secretase site with enhanced production of APP cleavage products, not all AD-associated PS1 mutations are defective in Notch cleavage, and drugs have been developed that prevent γ-secretase cleavage of APP but not Notch (Petit et al., 2001). Whether these differences in APP and Notch processing represent differences in regulation of PS-dependent γ-secretase proteolysis is unclear, but they may allow treatment of AD with drugs that target this protease without compromising Notch function.

As found for PS proteins, genetic and biochemical studies have identified another component of γ-secretase activity that is required for Notch signaling in worms, flies, and mammals (Kopan and Goate, 2002). The gene encoding this protein was first identified through its association with an extended familial AD kindred from the Italian village Nicastro and was thus named Nicastrin. Genetic interactions with Sel12 and the two Notch-related genes, LIN-12 and GLP-1, have identified a related gene from *C. elegans* termed aph-2 (for anterior-pharynx defect), and the *Drosophila* Nicastrin homolog is required for Notch signaling. Nicastrin has been found complexed with PS, Notch, and APP, and roles in γ-secretase cleavage events, as well as protein trafficking, have been suggested for this unique type 1 transmembrane protein.

Intramembrane Cleavage of Notch and Prior Cleavage at S2

Although furin cleavage of full-length Notch1 at S1 does not require ligand, cleavage at the intramembrane S3 site occurs only in response to ligand binding (Mumm and Kopan, 2000). It has also been suggested that cleavage within the membrane can occur only after the majority of the Notch extracellular domain has been removed. Consistent with this idea, a candidate S2 cleavage site in Notch1 maps to a conserved valine that is located 12 amino acids N-terminal to the TM domain, and cleavage at this site is a prerequisite for S3 intramembrane proteolysis.

Purification of the S2 proteolytic activity from cell membranes identifies a protease with characteristics of a metalloprotease known as TACE for its proteolysis of tumor necrosis factor-α (TNF-α). TACE is an ADAM with known "sheddase" activity that functions in the generation (as well as down-regulation) of ligands for receptors through cleavage at the cell surface. Although originally thought to be specific for TNF-α, analyses of mice deficient in TACE activity indicate that a number of different cell surface proteins, including APP, are cleaved by TACE. Mutagenesis of the valine at S2 or treatment with TACE inhibitors leads to decreases in both S2 and S3 cleavage fragments, confirming the identity of the S2 cleavage site and its obligate role in S3 cleavage. Inhibition of S3 cleavage leads to accumulation of the S2 cleavage fragment, and this is consistent with the idea that ligand-induced Notch signaling proceeds via a proteolytic cascade in which cleavage at S3 requires prior cleavage at S2.

In the absence of ligand, the Notch S2 cleavage fragment is not detected, suggesting that this cleavage event is regulated by ligand binding. In contrast, extracellular domain shedding of APP, TNF-α, TGF-α, and ErbB4 induced by TACE can occur in the absence of apparent stimulators. Treatment of cells expressing either APP, TNF-α, TGF-α, or ErbB4 with phorbol esters greatly enhances ectodomain shedding by TACE, but Notch1 is not cleaved by TACE in response to TPA. However, a number of mutations within the LNR and sequences in and around the S1, S2, and S3 cleavage sites in Notch and LIN-12 result in constitutively active proteins (Greenwald and Seydoux, 1990; Weinmaster, 2000). In some cases these mutations promote ectodomain shedding and subsequent intramembrane proteolysis of Notch independent of ligand binding, suggesting that these activating mutations result in changes in protein conformation that are similar to those produced by ligand binding.

Taken together, these observations suggest that ligand binding leads to conformational changes in the Notch ectodomain that function to either unmask the ADAM recognition site or facilitate proteolysis. Although TACE activity normally leads to shedding of cell surface proteins, direct evidence of ligand-induced Notch ectodomain shedding has yet to be reported. One report in *Drosophila* has proposed that internalization of the Notch extracellular domain into the ligand-presenting cell may provide the "force" behind ligand-induced removal of the Notch ectodomain (Parks et al., 2000). Perhaps such ligand-mediated trans-endocytosis precludes detection of the shed Notch ectodomain.

Genetic studies in *Drosophila* and *C. elegans* support a role for additional ADAM family members, Kuzbanian (Kuz, ADAM10) and Sup-17, respectively, in Notch/LIN-12 signaling (Mumm and Kopan, 2000; Weinmaster, 2000). Although transgenic mice deficient in ei-

ther Kuz or Notch1 display similar phenotypes, the exact function of Kuz in Notch signaling remains unclear. Originally proposed as the protease involved in heterodimeric Notch formation, Kuz has more recently been reported to mediate S2 cleavage of dNotch (Blaumueller et al., 1997; Pan and Rubin, 1997; Lieber et al., 2002). Even though TACE can cleave truncated, chimeric Notch proteins in vitro, genetic data supporting a role for TACE in Notch signaling are not as strong as those reported for Kuz. The TACE knockout phenotype is very different from that described for mice deficient in Notch1; however, given the large number of TACE substrates, this is probably not surprising (Swiatek et al., 1994; Conlon et al., 1995; Peschon et al., 1998). That TACE (rather than Kuz) cleaves mammalian Notch at S2 is supported by the observation that Kuz protein does not co-purify with S2 proteolytic activity. Moreover, Notch processing at S2 occurs in cells deficient in Kuz, but not in cells lacking TACE (Brou et al., 2000; Mumm et al., 2000). Since both TACE and Kuz have been reported to cleave APP at the α-secretase site, however, the possibility remains that both of these ADAMs cleave Notch at S2 (Buxbaum et al., 1998).

Although cleavage of Notch at S2 and S3 is thought to occur at the cell surface, definitive data to support this supposition are lacking. Both APP and Notch are found associated with PS at the cell surface; however, PS has been localized to early endosomes, thus suggesting that there are other cellular locations for S3 cleavage (Lah and Levey, 2000). Even if S3 cleavage occurs at the cell surface, it is possible that internalization into endosomes is required to effect release of the S3 cleavage fragment from the membrane, freeing it to translocate to the nucleus.

SIGNALING THROUGH INTRAMEMBRANE PROTEOLYSIS

Notch proteolysis and translocation to the nucleus seems, at first glance, to be a novel signal transduction mechanism. However, a number of recent reports describe similar regulated intramembrane proteolysis (RIP) in species from bacteria to man, which serve to regulate fundamental homeostatic processes such as cellular differentiation, lipid metabolism, and response to unfolded proteins (Brown et al., 2000). In all cases of RIP, membrane proteins are cleaved at multiple sites, with the final cleavage site residing within the membrane-spanning region. Intramembrane cleavage cannot take place until the upstream sequences are removed or shortened to less than 30 residues.

Consistent with these RIP requirements, S3 intramembrane cleavage of both APP and Notch are regulated by PS/γ-secretase that requires prior cleavage by TACE at an S2 site 12 residues upstream of the TM domains. The release of a signaling ICD from Notch is well documented, but it is only recently that the ICD of APP (AICD) has been identified and shown to have transcriptional activity associated with cellular changes (Leissring et al., 2002). A member of the EGF receptor family, ErbB4, has also been reported as an RIP substrate for TACE and PS/γ-secretase, and its ICD likewise shows transcriptional activity (Ni et al., 2001).

CSL-Dependent Signaling

Genetic studies indicate that the CSL genes, *Su(H)* and *lag-1*, are required for normal Notch/LIN-12/GLP-1 function but act downstream of the receptors to positively regulate signaling. Biochemical studies indicate that CSL proteins directly interact with cytoplasmic sequences of Notch and LIN-12/GLP-1. Normally, the CSL proteins function as transcriptional repressors; however, activation of Notch signaling in cells converts these DNA-binding proteins into transcriptional activators (Honjo, 1996). The CSL proteins positively regulate the expression of *Enhancer of split* [*E(spl)*] and the homologous vertebrate genes *ESR1*, *HES-1*, and *HES-5* (Kageyama and Nakanishi, 1997). In fact, induced expression of *E(spl)* and its homologs is a convenient marker to monitor and identify cells that are undergoing Notch signal transduction. Multiple cofactors have been identified for CSL-mediated repression and activation. As sequence-specific DNA-binding proteins, it now appears that CSL proteins serve a "docking" function for multiprotein complexes that function either in transcriptional activation or repression.

CSL transcriptional repression in the absence of activated Notch has been linked to a number of corepressor proteins and their associated histone deacetylases (HDACs) (Fig. 39–4). CSL proteins physically interact with two different corepressor complexes, one containing SMRT (silencing mediator of retinoid and thyroid hormone receptors) and HDAC-1, and the other consisting of corepressors CIR (CBF1-interacting corepressor), SAP30, and HDAC-2. The CSL repression domain is required for these interactions, and SMRT or CIR can compete with NICD for binding to CSL, which results in a suppression of NICD-mediated CSL activation (Kao et al., 1998; Hsieh et al., 1999).

In *Drosophila*, a similar Su(H)/corepressor complex has been found that contains Hairless, a protein previously shown to bind to Su(H), and dCTBP, a known transcriptional corepressor (Morel et al., 2001). CSL proteins can also repress transcription through direct binding to two members of the general transcription machinery—TFIIA and a subunit of TFIID, dTAFII110. CSL binding to either TFIIA or dTAFII110 disrupts the interaction between TFIIA and TFIID that is necessary for transcription from a natural viral promoter (Olave et al., 1998).

Activation of Notch signaling begins the transition of CSL from a repressor to an activator of transcription, and two viruses—Epstein-Barr virus (EBV) and adenovirus—are known to usurp the Notch/CSL pathway to activate transcription of both cellular and viral genes. Studies with these viruses indicate that the EBNA2 protein from EBV and the 13SE1A protein from adenovirus both bind to CSL and activate transcription via a mechanism similar to that described for NICD (Henkel et al., 1994; Ansieau et al., 2001). In fact, studies on EBNA2 were the first to demonstrate that CSL proteins functioned as transcriptional repressors and that through direct interactions with EBNA2 they could be converted into activators of transcription.

Studies on CSL-interacting proteins have further led to the identification of SKIP (Ski-interacting protein) as a mediator of the conversion of CSL from a repressor to an activator. SKIP was identified in a yeast two-hybrid screen for CBF1-interacting proteins and is a member of the CSL/SMRT corepressor complex. SKIP binds to CSL at a site distinct from that for SMRT binding, and SKIP can also bind directly to SMRT. Interestingly, SKIP can also bind to NICD through its ANK repeats, and studies have shown that binding of NICD or SMRT to SKIP is mutually exclusive. This competition between corepressor (SMRT) and activator (NICD) for CSL interaction through SKIP binding (Fig. 39–4), may allow SKIP to act as the "switch" mechanism (Zhou et al., 2000).

NICD/CSL activation complexes also feature other coactivators. Mastermind (mam)—a protein with functional homologs in *Drosophila*, *C. elegans* (LAG-3/sel-8), and vertebrates—interacts with an NICD/CSL complex in a modified two-hybrid assay and can increase NICD-mediated activation of a CSL-reporter construct (Mumm and Kopan, 2000). These findings are consistent with the genetics in *Drosophila* and *C. elegans* that indicate that mam is a positive modulator of Notch signaling. Enhanced CSL activity may be due to the observation that NICD/CSL complexes containing mam are stabilized on DNA relative to complexes lacking mam (Kitagawa et al., 2001). Mam binds to the ANK repeats of Notch and may overlap the binding site for SKIP, as the same two-amino acid mutation in the fourth ANK repeat of Notch1 that abrogates the ability of SKIP to interact with NICD also blocks the interaction of both mouse and *Drosophila* mam with NICD.

No studies have addressed the potential formation of an activation complex including both mam and SKIP, but it is possible to envision that SKIP may have a dual role in recruiting both NICD and mam. NICD also physically interacts with coactivators PCAF, GCN5, and p300/CBP—histone acetyltransferases (HATs) that are associated with transcriptionally active chromatin (Mumm and Kopan, 2000). Consistent with these interactions, HAT inhibitors can block NICD transactivation of a CSL-reporter construct.

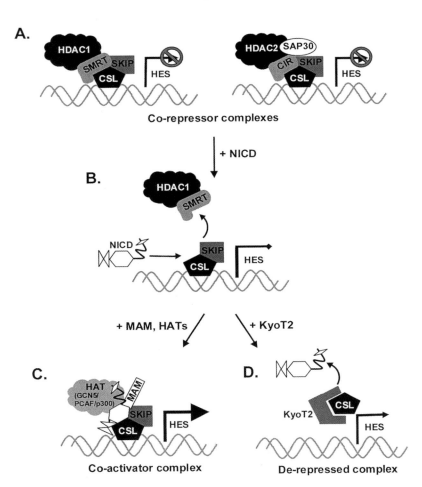

Figure 39–4. CSL proteins mediate corepression and coactivation complexes on DNA. CSL and SKIP proteins are common to both repression and activation complexes. (*A*) In the absence of activated Notch, CSL and SKIP interact with known co-repressor proteins SMRT or CIR and SAP30. These corepressors recruit histone deacetylases (HDAC1 or 2) to the complex, consistent with the correlation between silencing and deacetylated DNA. (*B*) Upon Notch activation, NICD enters the nucleus and displaces the corepressor complex. NICD can physically interact with both CSL and SKIP, in a manner analogous to SMRT, although the Notch ICD and SMRT contain no identifiable sequence similarities. (*C*) Activation complexes also contain the coactivator mastermind (MAM) and histone acetyltransferases (HAT), again consistent with the correlation between acetylated DNA and transcriptional activation. (*D*) Loss of CSL's ability to bind DNA, either through interaction with KyoT2 or mutation of CSL itself, leads to a state of "derepression" where neither activation or repression complexes can be brought to CSL DNA-binding sites. The inability to repress CSL-mediated transcription leads to small increases in transcriptional activation.

Alleviation of CSL-mediated repression can also be "derepressed" in the absence of Notch signaling through removal of CSL from its DNA-binding sites, which leads to a modest transcriptional activation. From a yeast two-hybrid screen, KyoT2, a LIM-only protein, has been isolated that may act in this fashion, as it both blocks DNA binding by CSL in EMSA (electrophoretic mobility shift assay) and competes with activated Notch1 for binding to CSL (Taniguchi et al., 1998).

The three states of transcriptional activity mediated by CSL proteins—repressed, derepressed, and activated—are illustrated by *single-minded* (*sim*) gene expression in *Drosophila* (Morel and Schweisguth, 2000). In the developing *Drosophila* embryo, a single row of cells in the mesoectoderm express the *sim* gene, and this expression can be perturbed by mutation of either *Notch* or *Su(H)*, but the consequences of the mutations are not equivalent. Where *Notch* loss-of-function mutations lead to a severe down-regulation of *sim* expression, an expansion of *sim* expression to two to three cell rows is seen in loss-of-function *Su(H)* mutants. Deletion of Su(H)-binding sites from the *sim* regulatory region also lead to the expansion of sim expression, suggesting that Su(H) is required to limit sim expression. Notch signaling through Su(H) is required to both reverse the repression by Su(H) in the single row of cells and actively drive sim expression. This study highlights an important feature of CSL proteins: that CSL proteins are not "neutral" in the absence of Notch but are actively repressing transcription.

Although a number of Notch target genes have been reported, the best genetically and biochemically characterized direct targets are the *E(spl)/HES/ESR* genes. These genes encode bHLH transcription factors that, in response to Notch signaling, repress both the expression and function of genes that encode activating bHLH transcription factors, such as the *achaete-scute complex (AS-C)* in *Drosophila* and the vertebrate homologs of the *AS-C* genes—*MASH, neuroD, neurogenin,* and *MATH* (Lewis, 1996).

In addition to activating genes involved in neurogenesis, *AS-C* genes also drive *Delta* expression and thus the inhibitory effects of Notch signaling on AS-C proteins produce decreases in ligand expression. Notch signaling can also up-regulate its own expression through CSL activation. Evidence from several organisms supports the idea that Notch/LIN-12/GLP-1 signaling functions in a positive feedback system to regulate receptor expression (Wilkinson et al., 1994; Girard et al., 1996; Heitzler et al., 1996; Berry et al., 1997; Deftos et al., 1998). Feedback loops induced and regulated by Notch signaling are critical to the process of lateral inhibition during neurogenesis, in which a small number of regularly spaced proneural precursors develop within a field of equivalent cells (Greenwald, 1998).

Notch signaling is integral to this process, and it is thought that small differences in ligand and receptor expression among interacting cells are amplified through feedback loops to single out precursors to take on the neural fate. Accordingly, cells that do not receive a Notch inhibitory signal maintain both AS-C expression required for neural determination and high Delta expression. However, high Notch-expressing cells contacted by ligand-signaling cells receive an inhibitory signal that extinguishes AS-C expression, and, as a consequence, they do not become neural and lose Delta expression. Reiteration of the Notch inhibitory signal in a field of progenitors leads to waves of neurogenesis, which ensure the proper spacing, number, and patterning of neurons.

CSL-Independent Signaling

Notch signal transduction is not limited to the "core" CSL-mediated pathway, as studies in vertebrates and invertebrates have observed CSL-independent activities of Notch (Shawber et al., 1996; Wang et al., 1997; Rusconi and Corbin, 1998; Nofziger et al., 1999; Zecchini et al., 1999). Moreover, activation of CSL in the absence of Notch signaling has also been reported (Barolo et al., 2000), indicating that while Notch and CSL often interact they can also function independently of each other. In some cases CSL-independent signaling has been proposed to involve effectors such as ras, JNK, or Deltex.

Ligand-induced Notch signaling, as well as expression of constitutively active forms of Notch1 and Notch2, blocks myogenic differentiation in the absence of CSL activation (Shawber et al., 1996; Nofziger

et al., 1999; Bush et al., 2001). In addition, ligand-independent, activated forms of Notch that lack CSL-interaction domains induce transformation of bone marrow precursors and fibroblasts, thus implicating a novel, CSL-independent Notch signaling pathway in oncogenesis as well (Aster et al., 1997, 2000; Jeffries and Capobianco, 2000). Transcriptional activation of the E2A factor that directs B-cell development is also inhibited by Notch signaling in an apparent CSL-independent manner (Ordentlich et al., 1998). In contrast to CSL-dependent signaling that is induced from a furin-processed heterodimeric Notch, ligand-induced CSL-independent signaling in myoblasts can be triggered from a full-length, furin-resistant, uncleaved Notch receptor (Bush et al., 2001).

Importantly, biochemical studies have documented that a similar uncleaved, full-length Notch protein is endogenously expressed on the surface of a number of different mammalian cell types, and this form appears to be the major species found in *Drosophila* cells. The presence of both furin-processed heterodimeric and unprocessed full-length forms of Notch on the cell surface provides opportunity for DSL ligands, through interaction with two structurally distinct cell surface receptors, to direct separate signaling pathways: one that requires CSL, and one that does not. Although Notch activity in the absence of CSL activation has been reported for a number of different processes, the mechanism of CSL-independent signal transduction is still a mystery.

Modulators of Ligand-Induced Notch Signaling

While gene expression patterns sometimes provide clues as to which ligand–receptor pairs are involved in certain developmental processes, expression studies have indicated that more often than not there is overlapping expression of two or more receptors or ligands within a tissue or cell type, thus underscoring the complexities of ligand-induced Notch signaling. In addition to feedback loops that regulate expression of both the ligand and receptor in interacting cells, the level of ligand-induced Notch signaling ultimately achieved can be regulated by modifiers that serve to control induction, intensity, and duration of signaling.

Consistent with this idea, genetic studies in flies and worms have identified a number of Notch-interacting genes that encode potential modulators of Notch signaling (Panin and Irvine, 1998). Because of the direct and rather simplistic nature of Notch signaling, it seems likely that modifiers provide a means by which this signaling system could mediate a wide variety of cellular responses. In particular, post-translational modifications of Notch, as well as its DSL ligands, have been shown to affect receptor activation, cell surface expression, and protein turnover to modulate ligand-induced downstream signaling events (Fig. 47–5).

POSTTRANSLATIONAL MODIFICATIONS OF NOTCH AND DSL LIGANDS AS REGULATORS OF SIGNALING

Glycosylation

The *Fringe* (*Fng*) gene encodes a modulator of Notch signaling that was first characterized genetically in *Drosophila*, where the ligands Delta and Serrate show overlapping patterns of gene expression and Notch signaling needs to be restricted (Blair, 1997; Irvine, 1999). In these contexts, Fng appears to restrict Notch signaling in a cell-autonomous fashion by inhibiting Serrate- and potentiating Delta-induced activation of Notch. Vertebrates have three *Fringe*-related genes—*Lunatic fringe* (*Lfng*), *Manic fringe* (*Mfng*), and *Radical fringe* (*Rfng*)—which display overlapping patterns of expression with members of the *Notch* and *DSL* gene families, consistent with a conserved function for fringe in modulating Notch signaling (Wu and Rao, 1999). Genetic and biochemical studies indicate that fringe proteins are not absolutely required for Notch signaling and that they function as modulators in some but not all processes mediated by Notch signaling. A potential mechanism by which fringe proteins modulate ligand-induced Notch signaling has only recently become clear.

Two protein motifs provide clues to the biochemical function of fringe (Munro and Freeman, 2000). Fringe proteins contain an N-

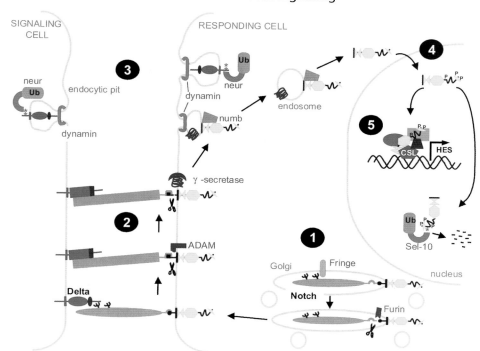

SIGNALING CELL

RESPONDING CELL

Figure 39–5. Modulation of Notch signaling. (*1*) Maturation of the Notch receptor includes posttranslational modifications such as glycosylation by fringe and cleavage by a furin-like convertase that results in the Notch heterodimer found on the cell surface. (*2*) At the cell surface, receptor activation requires binding of ligand, here Delta, from the signaling cell. Binding leads to a conformational change in the receptor (depicted as an oval-to-rectangle transition), which sets up Notch for the ADAM and γ-secretase cleavages. The location of the γ-secretase cleavage is unclear, and shown here are the two possibilities based on the subcellular localization of both presenilins and Notch, either at the cell surface or in early endosomes. (*3*) A number of genetic modifiers of Notch are associated with the endocytic machinery or affect internalization. The E3 ligase neuralized ubiquitinates (**) the Notch ligand Delta, leading to the removal of the ligand from the cell surface. Dynamin, which forms a ring around the neck of endocytic pits and is involved in "pinching off" of endocytic vesicles, is required in both the signaling and responding cell for Notch signaling to occur. When it is ectopically expressed, numb, a negative modulator of Notch signaling, can both bind directly to Notch and block endocytosis. (*4*) The nuclear translocation of Notch may also be regulated by numb, as studies indicate that numb can keep activated forms of Notch out of the nucleus and in the cytosol. Phosphorylation (P) differences of nuclear and cytoplasmic forms of NICD proteins also implicate as yet unknown kinases in the regulation of Notch subcellular localization. (*5*) In the nucleus, NICD interacts with the CSL DNA-binding repressor complex and converts it to a transcriptional activation complex, stimulating expression of downstream target genes such as HES. NICD can also be targeted to ubiquitination machinery by the E3 ligase, Sel10, which leads to NICD degradation.

terminal hydrophobic sequence, and ectopic expression of Fringe in both flies and tissue culture cells results in secretion, suggesting a role for fringe extracellularly. However, secretion of fringe proteins appears to be an artifact of overexpression since replacement of the Fringe hydrophobic sequence with a signal peptide from a known secreted protein results in loss of the fringe effect. Complementing this finding, replacement of the putative signal peptide of Fringe with a Golgi retention signal produces a protein with activity similar to WT Fringe, both in ectopic border formation in the wing and enhanced Delta binding to Notch (Bruckner et al., 2000; Munro and Freeman, 2000).

An important clue to the function of Fringe came from protein sequence analysis that identified a weak homology between Fringe homologs and a family of bacterial glycosyltransferases (Yuan et al., 1997). That Fringe proteins might functionally encode such activity came from the finding that Fringe binds radioactively-labeled UDP, an important property of glycosyltransferases. In addition, a DxD motif is required for catalytic activity, and mutation of the conserved DxD motif in fringe destroyed its ability to modulate ligand-induced Notch signaling (Munro and Freeman, 2000). Additional support for fringe functioning through glycosylation of Notch comes from experiments in mammalian cells where Lfng modulates ligand-induced Notch signaling only when expressed in the Notch-responding cell and not when present in either the extracellular space or the ligand-presenting cell (Hicks et al., 2000). Moreover, immunolocalization studies identify both fly and mammalian fringe exclusively in the Golgi.

These studies support the view that Fringe exerts its biochemical effect on Notch signaling by acting as a gycosyltransferase that modifies Notch proteins as they transit the Golgi apparatus (Blair, 2000).

Consistent with this, work from several groups in both fly and mammalian cells have shown that Notch proteins are modified by both *O*-linked fucose and *O*-linked glucose saccharides. These unusual forms of *O*-linked glycosylation have so far been seen only on EGF-like modules, and biochemical studies indicate that fringe is an *O*-fucose β1,3-*N*-acetylglucosaminyltransferase that extends *O*-fucose moieties on Notch. Consensus sequences for *O*-fucose modification have been identified for serine/threonine residues between the second and third conserved cysteine residues of certain EGFRs (Moloney et al., 2000). Since Fringe extends sites of *O*-fucose modification, *O*-fucosyltransferase-1 (which catalyzes the addition of fucose to Notch) is also required for modulation of ligand-induced Notch signaling by Fringe.

Structural analysis of the *O*-glycans released from Notch identifies di-, tri-, and tetrasaccharides. However, studies with CHO glycosylation mutant cells indicate that β4galactosyltransferase-1 (but not sialyltransferase) is required for fringe to inhibit Jagged1-induced Notch signaling (Chen et al., 2001). These findings indicate that the Galβ4GlcNAcβFuc trisaccharide is the minimum *O*-fucose glycan required for fringe to modulate ligand-induced Notch signaling. In addition, a UDP transporter named "fringe connection" acts genetically upstream of fringe and phenocopies mutants that are defective in Notch-signaling elements (Selva et al., 2001).

Taken together, these studies indicate that fringe is necessary but not sufficient for modification of Notch signaling through glycosylation. Although many Notch EGFRs have potential *O*-linked glycosylation sites, the EGFRs modified by fringe that confer differential ligand activation of Notch are currently unknown. Some of the DSL ligand EGFRs also have consensus sequences for *O*-fucose modification, thus raising the interesting possibility that glycosylation of the ligands may also play a part in modulating Notch signaling in some contexts.

The inhibitory effects of fringe on Serrate-induced Notch signaling were proposed to be through Fringe, preventing Serrate binding to Notch; however, Lfng enhances rather than inhibits binding of Jagged1 to Notch1 in mammalian cells (Hicks et al., 2000). In agreement, Fng does not disrupt Serrate–Notch interactions measured in insect cell aggregations assays and enhances binding of Delta to both mammalian and *Drosophila* cells (Klueg and Muskavitch, 1999; Bruckner et al., 2000).

Since Lfng does not prevent Jagged1 binding to Notch1, what events downstream of ligand binding are affected by Notch glycosylation to inhibit downstream signaling? The constitutive signaling activities of extracellular truncated forms of Notch1 are not altered by Lfng. This finding suggests that the ligand-binding, extracellular domain is required for the fringe effect and that Lfng does not affect downstream signaling events. This places the Fringe effect downstream of ligand binding and upstream of signaling. Together, these findings suggest that Fringe glycosylation affects activation of Notch induced by ligand binding, perhaps through conformational changes in the receptor that either positively or negatively affect extra- and/or intramembrane proteolysis of Notch.

Phosphorylation

Another potential mechanism of Notch regulation is through phosphorylation. Although phosphorylation of the Notch intracellular domain in both *Drosophila* and mammals (Kidd et al., 1998; Foltz and Nye, 2001; Gupta-Rossi et al., 2001; Oberg et al., 2001; Wu et al., 2001) has been reported, the exact sites of phosphorylation and the specific protein kinases involved—as well as the role that phosphorylation plays in ligand-induced Notch signaling—are not well characterized. Phosphorylation of NICD correlates with enhanced binding of the E3 ubiquitin ligase Sel10, suggesting a role for phosphorylation in targeted degradation of NICD. Through these effects, differential phosphorylation of NICD might regulate the intensity or the duration of the Notch signal in the nucleus (discussed below).

Phosphorylation has also been implicated in integrating cellular responses to both Notch signaling and cytokines (Bigas et al., 1998). Signaling from activated forms of Notch1 or Notch2 can prevent myeloid differentiation induced by the cytokine GM-CSF. However, in the case of G-CSF, Notch1 but not Notch2 can prevent promyeloid cells from differentiating in response to this cytokine. These differential responses of Notch1 and Notch2 to G-CSF map to a region downstream of the ANK, designated NCR for Notch Cytokine Response, in which phosphorylation correlates with the ability of Notch2 to block G-CSF-induced differentiation.

When a single serine residue at 2078 is mutated to an alanine, Notch2 can block myeloid differentiation in the presence of G-CSF (Ingles-Esteve et al., 2001). These findings imply that signaling downstream of G-CSF results in Notch2 phosphorylation that prevents Notch2 signaling from blocking differentiation. The NCR also appears to be a major site of phosphorylation in Notch1, suggesting that this region may represent an important phosphoregulatory domain (Foltz and Nye, 2001). However, it is as yet unclear which kinases mediate phosphorylation of Notch1 and Notch2 and how this modification regulates Notch activity.

Ubiquitination

Modification of proteins by ubiquitination is quickly gaining stature as a means of protein regulation, and it is now thought to be as commonplace as phosphorylation (Hicke, 2001). In general, protein ubiquitination is mediated by a complex of at least three enzymes: E1, a ubiquitin-activating enzyme; E2, a ubiquitin-conjugating enzyme; and E3, a ubiquitin ligase that transfers the ubiquitin moiety from E2 to lysine residues on a wide variety of substrates. Ubiquitination is classically associated with targeting modified proteins for proteasome-mediated degradation, but additional roles in endocytosis, cellular trafficking, transcriptional regulation, and even signal transduction have been reported for this ubiquitous protein modification. In addition to glycosylation and phosphorylation, Notch is also modified by ubiquitination by at least two different E3 ligases and is genetically linked to additional E3 ligases, some of which modulate Notch signaling through modifying the DSL ligands.

Neuralized (*neur*) has long been known to genetically interact with Notch signaling elements in *Drosophila*, but its function in modulating ligand-induced signaling was unclear. Although neur contains a RING finger motif, a hallmark of E3 ubiquitin ligases, only recently has neur been shown to function in ubiquitination of proteins. Functional studies in both flies and frogs indicate that Neuralized does not ubiquitinate the Notch receptor, but rather modifies the ligand (Kramer, 2001). The Delta ICD is monoubiquitinated, resulting in internalization and removal of the ligand from the cell surface, and this is consistent with a role for monoubiquitination in endocytosis rather than recognition and degradation by the proteasome as for polyubiquitination.

Although rather paradoxical, low levels of *neur* expression in flies increases Notch signaling, while high levels of neur lead to decreases in signaling. To understand the basis of these findings, it is important to consider that, in addition to activating Notch signaling, DSL ligands can block Notch signaling. Ligands expressed in *cis*, in Notch-responding cells, can block signaling induced by ligands presented in *trans* by neighboring cells (Dorsky et al., 1997; Henrique et al., 1997; Jacobsen et al., 1998). Although the exact basis of the *cis*-dominant negative (DN) effects are unknown, such antagonism by ligand is strictly cell autonomous and likely represents a natural mechanism of Notch modulation. Accordingly, the neur enhancement of ligand-induced Notch signaling is thought to be a consequence of Neur's removing Delta from the cell surface of the Notch-responding cell, thereby alleviating the *cis*-DN effects of ligand on Notch signaling.

However, high levels of Neur overexpression would effectively promote endocytosis of all cell surface Delta, thereby removing all signaling ligand and leading to loss of Notch signaling. The fate of ubiquitinated Delta following endocytosis from the cell surface is less clear, and both lysosomal degradation and rerouting within the cell are possibilities. Nonetheless, through regulating the level of Delta protein at the cell surface, Neur is an effective modulator of Notch signaling. It has also been proposed that neur-regulated ubiquitination/endocytosis of Delta is the driving force behind selection of the ligand-signaling cell during the process of lateral inhibition.

Sel10, like neuralized, modulates Notch signaling through ubiquitination; however, Sel10 contains an F-box that interacts with the ubiquitination complex and seven WD40 repeats that bind phosphorylated target proteins (Gupta-Rossi et al., 2001; Oberg et al., 2001; Wu et al., 2001). First identified in *C. elegans* as a negative modifier of LIN-12 receptor activity, Sel10 physically associates with LIN-12 and mouse Notch4 (Hubbard et al., 1997). Sel10 preferentially interacts with soluble, phosphorylated NICD-like proteins in the nucleus, consistent with where the majority of Sel10 is located. Ubiquitinated-nuclear NICD is not an effective activator of CSL and can be degraded by the proteasome, which together result in losses in Notch signaling. Both proteasome inhibitors and mutations in components of the proteasome lead to enhanced NICD expression and Notch signaling (Schweisguth, 1999). As with other E3 ligases, deletion of the interaction/ligation domain results in loss of ubiquitination, and Sel10 (lacking the F-box) causes an increase in CSL-dependent Notch signaling induced by ligand or constitutively active forms of Notch.

Suppressor of deltex [Su(dx)] represents another class of E3 ligases defined by the presence of a HECT (homologous to the E6-associated protein carboxyl terrminus) ligase domain that is a negative regulator of Notch signaling (Fostier et al., 1998). A mammalian Su(dx)-like protein, called Itch, has been identified from the Itchy mouse that suffers immune defects and constant itching of the skin. Although the exact defect is unknown, Itch has been shown to both bind to ΔEN and to ubiquitinate it (Qiu et al., 2000). Unlike Sel10, where sequences downstream of the ANK are important for NICD ubiquitination, deletion analysis maps the Itch–interaction domain to the N terminus of NICD. Given the negative effects of Su(dx) on Notch signaling in *Drosophila*, it is hypothesized that Itch-mediated ubiquitination of Notch functions to down-regulate signaling, but the exact mechanism and functional relevance of Itch-like ubiquitination to Notch signaling remains to be discovered.

The Deltex gene in *Drosophila* interacts genetically with Notch and other genes in the Notch signaling pathway (Xu and Artavanis-Tsakonas, 1990; Busseau et al., 1994) to positively regulate Notch signaling; however, both positive and negative effects have been reported for its mammalian homologs (Ordentlich et al., 1998; Sestan et al., 1999; Yamamoto et al., 2001). Although Deltex does not activate CSL on its own, it can either enhance or inhibit NICD activation of CSL, depending on the cell type.

Both Deltex and CSL proteins bind within the ANK, and as such the different activities reported for Deltex could be due to competition for Notch binding (Diederich et al., 1994; Matsuno et al., 2002). While contradictory to the role of Deltex as a positive modulator of Notch signaling, it may be that in some contexts Deltex functions as an alternative to CSL proteins as a Notch effector. Conversely, in some circumstances, Deltex may function independently of Notch to produce the same end result. In some cell types Notch signaling increases Deltex expression, suggesting that Deltex functions in a feedback mechanism to regulate the intensity and duration of the Notch signal (Deftos et al., 1998). The findings that Deltex both promotes and inhibits Notch signaling is also in keeping with opposing activities being described for Notch in different cell types.

While the molecular basis of Deltex modulation of Notch signaling is unknown, it is interesting to note that Deltex proteins contain a number of motifs that are found in ubiquitinating proteins such as a RING-H2 finger which is known to interact with the ubiquitinylation complex, and two WWE domains present in HECT and RING domain–containing E3 ligases (Aravind, 2001). In support of Deltex functioning in ubiquitination, deletion of its RING finger produces DN effects as found for other mutated E3 ubiquitin ligases. Furthermore, the E3 ubiquitin ligase Su(dx)/Itch was first identified as an antagonist of Deltex, and the WW motifs in Su(dx)/Itch bind proline-rich regions similar to those present in Deltex. Although direct interactions between Deltex and Su(dx) have not been reported, the positive effects of Deltex on Notch signaling could be through alleviating the negative effects of Su(dx).

The role of ubiquitination modifications and the ever-increasing numbers of E3 ubiqitin ligases are only beginning to be appreciated for the Notch signaling system. It is possible that ubiquitination of Notch by Sel10, Itch, and (potentially) Deltex all lead to different consequences. Further complications arise from the existence of de-ubiuitinating enzymes such as Fat facets in *Drosophila* and the presence of ubiquitin-like proteins that cannot be polymerized like ubiquitin (e.g., SUMO). It is important to note that the majority of evidence for ubiquitination comes from the use of exogenously added, labeled ubiquitin or ubiquitin antibodies that may not distinguish ubiquitin-like proteins from ubiquitin, and as such, it is not yet known what specific endogenous modifications are mediated by E3 ligases.

Modulation of Notch Signaling Through Endocytosis

Although ubiquitination often results in degradation of modified proteins by the proteasome, roles for ubiquitination have been described for multiple steps in the endocytic pathway (Hicke, 2001). The importance of endocytosis in Notch signaling has long been appreciated from the neurogenic phenotype and genetic interactions with Notch demonstrated for *shibire*, the fly homolog of dynamin. Dynamin is a GTPase that localizes to the rim of endocytic pits where it functions in the pinching off of a vesicle from the cell surface; inhibition of dynamin produces defects in endocytosis (Danino and Hinshaw, 2001). Consistent with dynamin's proposed role, ultrastructural studies of *shibire* mutants indicate that coated pits form normally, but the vesicles remain associated with the cell surface.

Interestingly, constitutively active membrane forms of Notch rescue the *shibire* mutant phenotype, indicating that *shibire* is not required for downstream Notch signaling (Struhl and Adachi, 2000). However in the case of ligand-induced activation of Notch, shibire is required in both the ligand-signaling and Notch-receiving cells (Seugnet et al., 1997). The *shibire* requirement in the Notch-responding cell is in keeping with the identification of Delta–Notch complexes in multivesicular bodies in cells that are undergoing cell fate determinations regulated by Notch signaling (Fehon et al., 1991; Klueg and Muskavitch, 1999; Parks et al., 2000).

Moreover, similar ligand–receptor complexes are found in *C. elegans* in cells that specifically express GLP-1 but not LAG-2, suggesting that the ligand is internalized along with the receptor during cell fate determinations mediated by GLP-1 signaling (Fitzgerald and Greenwald, 1995; Henderson et al., 1997). Whether this internalization represents removal of ligand–receptor complexes to allow signaling to continue or is an important aspect of receptor activation and NICD release from the membrane is unknown.

In addition, there is a report of ligand–Notch complexes in the ligand-signaling cell (Parks et al., 2000). Since intramembrane cleavage of Notch requires prior removal of the ectodomain, it has been proposed that trans-endocytosis of the Notch ectodomain into the ligand-presenting cell promotes intramembrane proteolysis and downstream signaling. These findings suggest that in addition to providing ligand for Notch activation, the ligand-signaling cell plays an active role in removal of the repressive Notch ectodomain. Such a role may reflect the requirement for shibire in the ligand-presenting cell. However since *neuralized* regulates the level of cell surface Delta in both ligand and receptor interacting cells, it is difficult in whole animal studies to dissect out how losses in endocytosis lead to losses in ligand-induced Notch signal transduction.

Another modulator of Notch signaling associated with endocytosis is Numb, a determinant of asymmetric division (Guo et al., 1996). Genetic studies indicate that Numb is antagonistic to Notch signaling; however, the molecular basis of this inhibition is unknown. Homologs of *Drosophila Numb* have been isolated from a number of different vertebrates, suggesting a conserved function for Numb proteins in regulating Notch signaling. Numb expression is highly regulated at many levels, including alternative splicing of mRNA, translational repression by the Musashi RNA-binding protein, phosphorylation by Numb-associated kinase, and ubiquitin-mediated degradation by LNX. Loss of any of these regulatory mechanisms leads to increases in Notch activity in genetic assays, which is onsistent with a role for Numb as a negative modulator of Notch signaling.

Numb has been shown to decrease both nuclear translocation of NICD and NICD-mediated transcriptional activation of CSL-based reporter genes (Frise et al., 1996; Sestan et al., 1999). Since Numb is known to interact with a number of different E3 ubiquitin ligases it is possible that Numb may target NICD for degradation through ubiquitination, as described for Sel10. Given the link between ubiquitination and endocytosis, as well as the observation that Numb interacts with both endocytic proteins and Notch (Santolini et al., 2000), it is tempting to speculate that Numb physically links Notch to the endocytic machinery to regulate cellular trafficking of Notch. Perhaps Numb regulates the level of cell surface Notch through stimulating endocytosis of full-length Notch receptors at the cell surface to down-regulate signaling. Alternatively, Numb could prevent the release of NICD from the plasma membrane or its transport to the nucleus, as movement of NICD through the cytoplasm may be a regulated process using endocytic vesicles.

ADDITIONAL REGULATION OF NOTCH SIGNALING

Scabrous (*sca*) is a secreted protein that modulates ligand-induced Notch signaling during border formation in the fly wing (Lee et al., 2000). As found for *Fringe*, *sca* appears to modulate ligand-induced Notch signaling without affecting the levels of the two activating ligands, Delta and Serrate. However unlike *Fringe*, *sca* reduces signaling from both ligands. Although *sca* appears to stablize cell surface expression of Notch (Powell et al., 2001), the mechanism by which *sca* negatively regulates ligand-induced Notch signaling is currently unknown. *Wingless* (*wg*) encodes another secreted protein that both binds to Notch and is antagonistic to Notch signaling (Panin and Irvine, 1998). *Wg* may antagonize Notch signaling by stimulating removal of the Delta-binding site in Notch or through activation of disheveled (dsh) in response to wg signaling (Wesley, 1999). Dsh binds to the Notch cytoplasmic domain, but whether this binding accounts for inhibition in ligand-induced Notch signaling is unclear.

Other genetic modifiers of Notch/LIN-12 have been identified, such as *big brain, pecanex, sanpodo, strawberry notch, Notchless, Nubbin, warthog, sel-1, emb5, abl,* and *dab.* In some cases, direct interactions between these gene products and the receptors have been seen, but their mechanism of action is mostly unknown. Also, signaling from certain growth factor receptors and activation of ras, MAP kinase, and NFκB enhance DSL ligand expression, which could also modulate ligand-induced Notch signaling. Finally, the identification of an internal ribosome entry site within the Notch2 coding sequences offers the intriguing possibility that activated forms of Notch could be produced independent of ligand and proteolytic cleavage to effect downstream signaling (Lauring and Overbaugh, 2000).

SUMMARY

Over the past decade the Notch signaling pathway has established itself as a major signaling system that controls multiple aspects of vertebrate development. Given the large repertoire of cellular processes ascribed to Notch signaling, it is not surprising that mutations in components of this signaling pathway have been linked to inherited human diseases and cancer. The level of uncertainty for how alterations in Notch signaling contribute to human disease underscores the importance of defining the basic mechanisms of Notch signal transduction. Although considerable progress in our understanding of Notch signal transduction and cell types and processes regulated by this signaling system have been made, many of the details remain to be defined. However, it is clear that in addition to regulating cell fate decisions, Notch signaling also influences additional aspects of cellular differentiation, as well as proliferation, morphogenesis, and interactions with other cell types.

It is generally accepted that the DSL ligands activate the Notch receptors, but the specificity and structure of the ligand–receptor interactions at the cell surface (as well as the fate of intracellular ligand–receptor complexes, including their role in Notch signaling) are unknown. Studies with soluble DSL ligands have suggested that the oligomeric state of both the ligand and receptor likely influence downstream signaling; however, the molecular events that regulate ligand–receptor interactions and subsequent proteolysis of Notch to generate a biologically active signal transducer are not fully characterized. Although some of the proteases that effect ligand-induced proteolysis of Notch have been identified, the subcellular locale of proteolysis—as well as the mechanisms regulating release of the cleaved NICD from the membrane and its translocation to the nucleus—has yet to be described.

Even though multiple modulators and feedback loops have been proposed to regulate induction, intensity, and duration of Notch signaling, the molecular details of such controls are lacking. Moreover, a detailed understanding of Notch signal transduction requires identifying downstream effectors, modulators, and targets genes, as well as determining how these genes influence cellular physiology. Finally, the proteins required for the Notch signaling pathway that function independently of the CSL proteins are not well understood. Future studies designed to investigate interactions between the Notch signaling pathway and other signaling pathways that regulate cellular phenotypes are likely to identify additional mechanisms that function to modulate this multipurpose signaling system.

REFERENCES

Ansieau S, Strobl LJ, Leutz A (2001). Activation of the Notch-regulated transcription factor CBF1/RBP-Jκ through the 13SE1A oncoprotein. *Genes Dev* 15: 380–385.

Aravind L (2001). The WWE domain: a common interaction module in protein ubiquitination and ADP ribosylation. *Trends Biochem Sci* 26: 273–275.

Artavanis-Tsakonas S, Matsuno K, Fortini ME (1995). Notch signaling. *Science* 268: 225–232.

Artavanis-Tsakonas S, Rand MD, Lake RJ (1999). Notch signaling: cell fate control and signal integration in development. *Science* 284: 770–776.

Aster JC, Robertson ES, Hasserjian RP, Turner JR, Kieff E, Sklar J (1997). Oncogenic forms of NOTCH1 lacking either the primary binding site for RBP-Jκ or nuclear localization sequences retain the ability to associate with RBP-Jκ and activate transcription. *J Biol Chem* 272: 11336–11343.

Aster JC, Xu L, Karnell FG, Patriub V, Pui JC, Pear WS (2000). Essential roles for ankyrin repeat and transactivation domains in induction of T-cell leukemia by notch1. *Mol Cell Biol* 20: 7505–7515.

Barolo S, Walker RG, Polyanovsky AD, Freschi G, Keil T, Posakony JW (2000). A notch-independent activity of suppressor of hairless is required for normal mechanoreceptor physiology. *Cell* 103: 957–969.

Berry LW, Westlund B, Schedl B (1997). Germ-line tumor formation caused by activation of glp-1, a *Caenorhabditis elegans* member of the Notch family of receptors. *Development* 124: 925–936.

Bigas A, Martin DI, Milner LA (1998). Notch1 and Notch2 inhibit myeloid differentiation in response to different cytokines. *Mol Cell Biol* 18: 2324–2333.

Blair SS (1997). Limb development: marginal fringe benefits. *Curr Biol* 7: R686–690.

Blair SS (2000). Notch signaling: Fringe really is a glycosyltransferase. *Curr Biol* 10: R608–612.

Blaumueller CM, Qi H, Zagouras P, Artavanis-Tsakonas S (1997). Intracellular cleavage of Notch leads to a heterodimeric receptor on the plasma membrane. *Cell* 90: 281–291.

Brou C, Logeat F, Gupta N, Bessia C, LeBail O, Doedens JR, Cumano A, Roux P, Black RA, Israel A (2000). A novel proteolytic cleavage involved in Notch signaling: the role of the disintegrin-metalloprotease TACE. *Mol Cell* 5: 207–216.

Brown MS, Ye J, Rawson RB, Goldstein JL (2000). Regulated intramembrane proteolysis: a control mechanism conserved from bacteria to humans. *Cell* 100: 391–398.

Bruckner K, Perez L, Clausen H, Cohen S (2000). Glycosyltransferase activity of Fringe modulates Notch–Delta interactions. *Nature* 406: 411–415.

Bulman MP, Kusumi K, Frayling TM, McKeown C, Garrett C, Lander ES, Krumlauf R, Hattersley AT, Ellard S, Turnpenny PD (2000). Mutations in the human delta homologue, DLL3, cause axial skeletal defects in spondylocostal dysostosis. *Nat Genet* 24: 438–441.

Bush G, diSibio G, Miyamoto A, Denault JB, Leduc R, Weinmaster G (2001). Ligand-induced signaling in the absence of furin processing of Notch1. *Dev Biol* 229: 494–502.

Busseau I, Diederich RJ, Xu T, Artavanis-Tsakonas S (1994). A member of the Notch group of interacting loci, deltex encodes a cytoplasmic basic protein. *Genetics* 136: 585–596.

Buxbaum JD, Liu KN, Luo Y, Slack JL, Stocking KL, Peschon JJ, Johnson RS, Castner BJ, Cerretti DP, Black RA (1998). Evidence that tumor necrosis factor α converting enzyme is involved in regulated α-secretase cleavage of the Alzheimer amyloid protein precursor. *J Biol Chem* 273: 27765–27767.

Chen J, Moloney DJ, Stanley P (2001). Fringe modulation of Jagged1-induced Notch signaling requires the action of β-4-galactosyltransferase-1. *Proc Natl Acad Sci USA* 98: 13716–13721.

Chitnis A, Henrique D, Lewis J, Ish-Horowicz D, Kintner C (1995). Primary neurogenesis in *Xenopus* embryos regulated by a homologue of the *Drosophila* neurogenic gene Delta. *Nature* 375: 761–766.

Conlon RA, Reaume AG, Rossant J (1995). Notch1 is required for the coordinate segmentation of somites. *Development* 121: 1533–1545.

Danino D, Hinshaw JE (2001). Dynamin family of mechanoenzymes. *Curr Opin Cell Biol* 13: 454–460.

Davis CG (1990). The many faces of epidermal growth factor repeats. *New Biol* 2: 410–419.

Deftos ML, He YW, Ojala EW, Bevan MJ (1998). Correlating notch signaling with thymocyte maturation. *Immunity* 9: 777–786.

Diederich RJ, Matsuno K, Hing H, Artavanis-Tsakonas S (1994). Cytosolic interaction between deltex and Notch ankyrin repeats implicates deltex in the Notch signaling pathway. *Development* 120: 473–481.

Dorsky RI, Chang WS, Rapaport DH, Harris WA (1997). Regulation of neuronal diversity in the *Xenopus* retina by Delta signalling. *Nature* 385: 67–70.

Fehon RG, Johansen K, Rebay I, Artavanis-Tsakonas S (1991). Complex cellular and subcellular regulation of notch expression during embryonic and imaginal development of *Drosophila*: implications for notch function. *J Cell Biol* 113: 657–669.

Fitzgerald K, Greenwald I (1995). Interchangeability of *Caenorhabditis elegans* DSL proteins and intrinsic signalling activity of their extracellular domains in vivo. *Development* 121: 4275–4282.

Fleming RJ, Gu Y, Hukriede NA (1997). Serrate-mediated activation of Notch is specifically blocked by the product of the gene fringe in the dorsal compartment of the *Drosophila* wing imaginal disc. *Development* 124: 2973–2981.

Foltz DR, Nye JS (2001). Hyperphosphorylation and association with RBP of the intracellular domain of Notch1. *Biochem Biophys Res Commun* 286: 484–492.

Fortini ME (2001). Notch and presenilin: a proteolytic mechanism emerges. *Curr Opin Cell Biol* 13: 627–634.

Fortini ME, Rebay I, Caron LA, Artavanis-Tsakonas S (1993). An activated Notch receptor blocks cell-fate commitment in the developing *Drosophila* eye. *Nature* 365: 555–557.

Fostier M, Evans DA, Artavanis-Tsakonas S, Baron M (1998). Genetic characterization of the *Drosophila melanogaster* Suppressor of deltex gene: a regulator of notch signaling. *Genetics* 150: 1477–1485.

Frise E, Knoblich JA, Younger-Shepherd S, Jan LY, Jan YN (1996). The *Drosophila* Numb protein inhibits signaling of the Notch receptor during cell–cell interaction in sensory organ lineage. *Proc Natl Acad Sci USA* 93: 11925–11932.

Girard L, Hanna Z, Beaulieu N, Hoemann CD, Simard C, Kozak CA, Jolicoeur P (1996). Frequent provirus insertional mutagenesis of Notch1 in thymomas of MMTVD/myc transgenic mice suggests a collaboration of c-myc and Notch1 for oncogenesis. *Genes Dev* 10: 1930–1944.

Greenwald I (1994). Structure/function studies of lin-12/Notch proteins. *Curr Opin Genet Dev* 4: 556–562.

Greenwald I (1998). LIN-12/Notch signaling: lessons from worms and flies. *Genes Dev* 12: 1751–1762.

Greenwald I, Seydoux G (1990). Analysis of gain-of-function mutations of the lin-12 gene of *Caenorhabditis elegans*. *Nature* 346: 197–199.

Gridley T (1997). Notch signaling in vertebrate development and disease. *Mol Cell Neurosci* 9: 103–108.

Guo M, Jan LY, Jan YN (1996). Control of daughter cell fates during asymmetric division: interaction of Numb and Notch. *Neuron* 17: 27–41.

Gupta-Rossi N, Le Bail O, Gonen H, Brou C, Logeat F, Six E, Ciechanover A, Israel A (2001). Functional interaction between SEL-10, an F-box protein, and the nuclear form of activated Notch1 receptor. *J Biol Chem* 276: 34371–34378.

Hartley DA, Xu TA, Artavanis-Tsakonas S (1987). The embryonic expression of the Notch locus of *Drosophila melanogaster* and the implications of point mutations in the extracellular EGF-like domain of the predicted protein. *EMBO J* 6: 3407–3417.

Heitzler P, Bourouis M, Ruel L, Carteret C, Simpson P (1996). Genes of the Enhancer of split and achaete–scute complexes are required for a regulatory loop between Notch and Delta during lateral signalling in *Drosophila*. *Development* 122: 161–171.

Henderson ST, Gao D, Christensen S, Kimble J (1997). Functional domains of LAG-2, a putative signaling ligand for LIN-12 and GLP-1 receptors in *Caenorhabditis elegans*. *Mol Biol Cell* 8: 1751–1762.

Henkel T, Ling PD, Hayward SD, Peterson MG (1994). Mediation of Epstein-Barr virus EBNA2 transactivation by recombination signal-binding protein Jκ. *Science* 265: 92–95.

Henrique D, Hirsinger E, Adam J, Le Roux I, Pourquie O, Ish-Horowicz D, Lewis J (1997). Maintenance of neuroepithelial progenitor cells by Delta-Notch signalling in the embryonic chick retina. *Curr Biol* 7: 661–670.

Hicke L (2001). Protein regulation by monoubiquitin. *Nat Rev Mol Cell Biol* 2: 195–201.

Hicks C, Johnston SH, diSibio G, Collazo A, Vogt TF, Weinmaster G (2000). Fringe differentially modulates Jagged1 and Delta1 signalling through Notch1 and Notch2. *Nat Cell Biol* 2: 515–520.

Hicks C, Ladi E, Lindsell C, Hsieh J, Hayward S, Collazo A, Weinmaster G (2002). A secreted Delta1-Fc fusion protein functions both as an activator and inhibitor of Notch1 signaling. *J Neurosci Res* 69: 60–71.

Honjo T (1996). The shortest path from the surface to the nucleus: RBP-JK/Su(H) transcription factor. *Genes Cells* 1: 1–9.

Hsieh JJ, Henkel T, Salmon P, Robey E, Peterson MG, Hayward SD (1996). Truncated mammalian Notch1 activates CBF1/RBPJk-repressed genes by a mechanism resembling that of Epstein-Barr virus EBNA2. *Mol Cell Biol* 16: 952–959.

Hsieh JJ, Zhou S, Chen L, Young DB, Hayward SD (1999). CIR, a corepressor linking the DNA binding factor CBF1 to the histone deacetylase complex. *Proc Natl Acad Sci USA* 96: 23–28.

Hubbard EJ, Wu G, Kitajewski J, Greenwald I (1997). sel-10, a negative regulator of lin-12 activity in *Caenorhabditis elegans*, encodes a member of the CDC4 family of proteins. *Genes Dev* 11: 3182–3193.

Hukriede NA, Fleming RJ (1997). Beaded of Goldschmidt, an antimorphic allele of Serrate, encodes a protein lacking transmembrane and intracellular domains. *Genetics* 145: 359–374.

Hukriede NA, Gu Y, Fleming RJ (1997). A dominant-negative form of Serrate acts as a general antagonist of Notch activation. *Development* 124: 3427–3437.

Huppert SS, Le A, Schroeter EH, Mumm JS, Saxena MT, Milner LA, Kopan R (2000). Embryonic lethality in mice homozygous for a processing-deficient allele of Notch1. *Nature* 405: 966–970.

Ingles-Esteve J, Espinosa L, Milner LA, Caelles C, Bigas A (2001). Phosphorylation of Ser2078 modulates the Notch2 function in 32D cell differentiation. *J Biol Chem* 276: 44873–44880.

Irvine KD (1999). Fringe, Notch, and making developmental boundaries. *Curr Opin Genet Dev* 9: 434–441.

Jacobsen TL, Brennan K, Arias AM, Muskavitch MA (1998). *Cis*-interactions between Delta and Notch modulate neurogenic signalling in *Drosophila*. *Development* 125: 4531–4540.

Jarriault S, Brou C, Logeat F, Schroeter EH, Kopan R, Israel A (1995). Signalling downstream of activated mammalian Notch. *Nature* 377: 355–358.

Jeffries S, Capobianco AJ (2000). Neoplastic transformation by Notch requires nuclear localization. *Mol Cell Biol* 20: 3928–3941.

Johansen KM, Fehon RG, Artavanis-Tsakonas S (1989). The *Notch* gene product is a glycoprotein expressed on the cell surface of both epidermal and neuronal precursor cells during *Drosophila* development. *J Cell Biol* 109: 2427–2440.

Joutel A, Tournier-Lasserve E (1998). Notch signalling pathway and human diseases. *Cell Dev Biol* 9: 619–625.

Kageyama R, Nakanishi S (1997). Helix–loop–helix factors in growth and differentiation of the vertebrate nervous system. *Curr Opin Genet Dev* 7: 659–665.

Kao HY, Ordentlich P, Koyano-Nakagawa N, Tang Z, Downes M, Kintner CR, Evans RM, Kadesch T (1998). A histone deacetylase corepressor complex regulates the Notch signal transduction pathway. *Genes Dev* 12: 2269–2277.

Kelley MR, Kidd S, Deutsch WA, Young MW (1987). Mutations altering the structure of epidermal growth factor-like coding sequences at the *Drosophila* Notch locus. *Cell* 51: 539–548.

Kidd S, Lieber T, Young MW (1998). Ligand-induced cleavage and regulation of nuclear entry of Notch in *Drosophila melanogaster* embryos. *Genes Dev* 12: 3728–3740.

Kitagawa M, Oyama T, Kawashima T, Yedvobnick B, Kumar A, Matsuno K, Harigaya K (2001). A human protein with sequence similarity to *Drosophila* mastermind coordinates the nuclear form of notch and a CSL protein to build a transcriptional activator complex on target promoters. *Mol Cell Biol* 21: 4337–4346.

Klueg KM, Muskavitch MA (1999). Ligand–receptor interactions and *trans*-endocytosis of Delta, Serrate and Notch: members of the Notch signalling pathway in *Drosophila*. *J Cell Sci* 112: 3289–3297.

Kooh PJ, Fehon RG, Muskavitch MA (1993). Implications of dynamic patterns of Delta and Notch expression for cellular interactions during *Drosophila* development. *Development* 117: 493–507.

Kopan R, Goate A (2002). Aph-2/Nicastrin: an essential component of γ-secretase and regulator of Notch signaling and Presenilin localization. *Neuron* 33: 321–324.

Kopan R, Nye JS, Weintraub H (1994). The intracellular domain of mouse Notch: a constitutively activated repressor of myogenesis directed at the basic helix–loop–helix region of MyoD. *Development* 120: 2385–2396.

Kramer H (2001). Neuralized: regulating notch by putting away delta. *Dev Cell* 1: 725–726.

Kusumi K, Sun ES, Kerrebrock AW, Bronson RT, Chi DC, Bulotsky MS, Spencer JB, Birren BW, Frankel WN, Lander ES (1998). The mouse pudgy mutation disrupts Delta homologue Dll3 and initiation of early somite boundaries. *Nat Genet* 19: 274–278.

Lah JJ, Levey AI (2000). Endogenous presenilin-1 targets to endocytic rather than biosynthetic compartments. *Mol Cell Neurosci* 16: 111–126.

Lardelli M, Williams R, Lendahl U (1995). Notch-related genes in animal development. *Int J Dev Biol* 39: 769–780.

Lauring SA, Overbaugh J (2000). Evidence that an IRES within the Notch2 coding region can direct expression of a nuclear form of the protein. *Mol Cell* 6: 939–945.

Lecourtois M, Schweisguth F (1998). Indirect evidence for Delta-dependent intracellular processing of Notch in *Drosophila* embryos. *Curr Biol* 8: 771–774.

Lee EC, Yu SY, Baker NE (2000). The scabrous protein can act as an extracellular antagonist of notch signaling in the *Drosophila* wing. *Curr Biol* 10: 931–934.

Leissring MA, Murphy MP, Mead TR, Akbari Y, Sugarman MC, Jannatipour M, Anliker B, Muller U, Saftig P, De Strooper B, et al. (2002). A physiologic signaling role for the γ-secretase-derived intracellular fragment of APP. *Proc Natl Acad Sci USA* 99: 4697–4702.

Levitan D, Greenwald I (1995). Facilitation of lin-12-mediated signalling by sel-12, a *Caenorhabditis elegans* S182 Alzheimer's disease gene. *Nature* 377: 351–354.

Lewis J (1996). Neurogenic genes and vertebrate neurogenesis. *Curr Opin Neurobiol* 6: 3–10.

Li L, Krantz ID, Deng Y, Genin A, Banta AB, Collins CC, Qi M, Trask BJ, Kuo WL, Cochran J, et al. (1997). Alagille syndrome is caused by mutations in human Jagged1, which encodes a ligand for Notch1. *Nat Genet* 16: 243–251.

Li L, Milner LA, Deng Y, Iwata M, Banta A, Graf L, Marcovina S, Friedman C, Trask BJ, Hood L, Torok-Storb B (1998). The human homolog of rat Jagged1 expressed by marrow stroma inhibits differentiation of 32D cells through interaction with Notch1. *Immunity* 8: 43–55.

Lieber T, Kidd S, Alcamo E, Corbin V, Young MW (1993). Antineurogenic phenotypes induced by truncated Notch proteins indicate a role in signal transduction and may point to a novel function for Notch in nuclei. *Genes Dev* 7: 1949–1965.

Lieber T, Kidd S, Young MW (2002). kuzbanian-mediated cleavage of *Drosophila* Notch. *Genes Dev* 16: 209–221.

Logeat F, Bessia C, Brou C, LeBail O, Jarriault S, Seiday N, Israel A (1998). The Notch1 receptor is cleaved constitutively by a furin-like convertase. *Proc Natl Acad Sci USA* 95: 8108–8112.

Lowell S, Jones P, Le Roux I, Dunne J, Watt FM (2000). Stimulation of human epidermal differentiation by delta-notch signalling at the boundaries of stem-cell clusters. *Curr Biol* 10: 491–500.

Lyman D, Young MW (1993). Further evidence for function of the *Drosophila* Notch protein as a transmembrane receptor. *Proc Natl Acad Sci USA* 90: 10395–10399.

Markopoulou K, Artavanis-Tsakonas S (1989). The expression of the neurogenic locus *NOTCH* during the postembryonic development of *Drosophila melanogaster* and its relationship to mitotic activity. *J Neurogenet* 6: 11–26.

Matsuno K, Ito M, Hori K, Miyashita F, Suzuki S, Kishi N, Artavanis-Tsakonas S, Okano H (2002). Involvement of a proline-rich motif and RING-H2 finger of Deltex in the regulation of Notch signaling. *Development* 129: 1049–1059.

Miele L, Osborne B (1999). Arbiter of differentiation and death: Notch signaling meets apoptosis. *J Cell Physiol* 181: 393–409.

Moloney DJ, Shair LH, Lu FM, Xia J, Locke R, Matta KL, Haltiwanger RS (2000). Mammalian Notch1 is modified with two unusual forms of *O*-linked glycosylation found on epidermal growth factor–like modules. *J Biol Chem* 275: 9604–9611.

Morel V, Schweisguth F (2000). Repression by suppressor of hairless and activation by Notch are required to define a single row of single-minded expressing cells in the *Drosophila* embryo. *Genes Dev* 14: 377–388.

Morel V, Lecourtois M, Massiani O, Maier D, Preiss A, Schweisguth F (2001). Transcriptional repression by suppressor of hairless involves the binding of a hairless-dCtBP complex in *Drosophila*. *Curr Biol* 11: 789–792.

Morrison SJ, Perez SE, Qiao Z, Verdi JM, Hicks C, Weinmaster G, Anderson DJ (2000). Transient Notch activation initiates an irreversible switch from neurogenesis to gliogenesis by neural crest stem cells. *Cell* 101: 499–510.

Mumm, J. S, and Kopan, R (2000). Notch signaling: from the outside in. *Dev Biol* 228: 151–165.

Mumm JS, Schroeter EH, Saxena MT, Griesemer A, Tian X, Pan DJ, Ray WJ, Kopan R (2000). A ligand-induced extracellular cleavage regulates γ-secretase-like proteolytic activation of Notch1. *Mol. Cell* 5: 197–206.

Munro S, Freeman M (2000). The notch signalling regulator fringe acts in the Golgi apparatus and requires the glycosyltransferase signature motif DXD. *Curr Biol* 10: 813–820.

Ni CY, Murphy MP, Golde TE, Carpenter G (2001). γ-Secretase cleavage and nuclear localization of ErbB-4 receptor tyrosine kinase. *Science* 294: 2179–2181.

Nofziger D, Miyamoto A, Lyons KM, Weinmaster G (1999). Notch signaling imposes two distinct blocks in the differentiation of C2C12 myoblasts. *Development* 126: 1689–1702.

Oberg C, Li J, Pauley A, Wolf E, Gurney M, Lendahl U (2001). The Notch intracellular domain is ubiquitinated and negatively regulated by the mammalian Sel-10 homolog. *J Biol Chem* 276: 35847–35853.

Ohishi K, Varnum-Finney B, Flowers D, Anasetti C, Myerson D, Bernstein ID (2000). Monocytes express high amounts of Notch and undergo cytokine specific apoptosis following interaction with the Notch ligand, Delta-1. *Blood* 95: 2847–2854.

Olave I, Reinberg D, Vales LD (1998). The mammalian transcriptional repressor RBP (CBF1) targets TFIID and TFIIA to prevent activated transcription. *Genes Dev* 12: 1621–1637.

Ordentlich P, Lin A, Shen CP, Blaumueller C, Matsuno K, Artavanis-Tsakonas S, Kadesch T (1998). Notch inhibition of E47 supports the existence of a novel signaling pathway. *Mol Cell Biol* 18: 2230–2239.

Osborne B, Miele L (1999). Notch and the immune system. *Immunity* 11: 653–663.

Pan D, Rubin GM (1997). Kuzbanian controls proteolytic processing of Notch and mediates lateral inhibition during *Drosophila* and vertebrate neurogenesis. *Cell* 90: 271–280.

Panin VM, Irvine KD (1998). Modulators of Notch signaling. *Semin Cell Dev Biol* 9: 609–617.

Parks AL, Klueg KM, Stout JR, Muskavitch MA (2000). Ligand endocytosis drives receptor dissociation and activation in the Notch pathway. *Development* 127: 1373–1385.

Peschon JJ, Slack JL, Reddy P, Stocking KL, Sunnarborg SW, Lee DC, Russell WE, Castner BJ, Johnson RS, Fitzner JN, et al. (1998). An essential role for ectodomain shedding in mammalian development. *Science* 282: 1281–1284.

Petit A, Bihel F, Alves da Costa C, Pourquie O, Checler F, Kraus JL (2001). New protease inhibitors prevent γ-secretase-mediated production of Aβ40/42 without affecting Notch cleavage. *Nat Cell Biol* 3: 507–511.

Powell PA, Wesley C, Spencer S, Cagan RL (2001). Scabrous complexes with Notch to mediate boundary formation. *Nature* 409: 626–630.

Qi H, Rand MD, Wu X, Sestan N, Wang W, Rakic P, Xu T, Artavanis-Tsakonas S (1999). Processing of the notch ligand delta by the metalloprotease Kuzbanian. *Science* 283: 91–94.

Qiu L, Joazeiro C, Fang N, Wang HY, Elly C, Altman Y, Fang D, Hunter T, Liu YC (2000). Recognition and ubiquitination of Notch by Itch, a hect-type E3 ubiquitin ligase. *J Biol Chem* 275: 35734–35737.

Rand MD, Grimm LM, Artavanis-Tsakonas S, Patriub V, Blacklow SC, Sklar J, Aster JC (2000). Calcium depletion dissociates and activates heterodimeric notch receptors. *Mol Cell Biol* 20: 1825–1835.

Rangarajan A, Talora C, Okuyama R, Nicolas M, Mammucari C, Oh H, Aster JC, Krishna S, Metzger D, Chambon P, et al. (2001). Notch signaling is a direct determinant of keratinocyte growth arrest and entry into differentiation. *EMBO J* 20: 3427–3436.

Rebay I, Fleming RJ, Fehon RG, Cherbas L, Cherbas P, Artavanis-Tsakonas S (1991). Specific EGF repeats of Notch mediate interactions with Delta and Serrate: implications for Notch as a multifunctional receptor. *Cell* 67: 687–699.

Redmond L, Oh SR, Hicks C, Weinmaster G, Ghosh A (2000). Nuclear Notch1 signaling and the regulation of dendritic development. *Nat Neurosci* 3: 30–40.

Rusconi JC, Corbin V (1998). Evidence for a novel Notch pathway required for muscle precursor selection in *Drosophila*. *Mech Dev* 79: 39–50.

Santolini E, Puri C, Salcini AE, Gagliani MC, Pelicci PG, Tacchetti C, Di Fiore PP (2000). Numb is an endocytic protein. *J Cell Biol* 151: 1345–1352.

Schroeder T, Just U (2000). Notch signalling via RBP-J promotes myeloid differentiation. *EMBO J* 19: 2558–2568.

Schroeter E, Kisslinger J, Kopan R (1998). Notch1 signalling requires ligand-induced proteolytic release of the intracellular domain. *Nature* 393: 382–386.

Schweisguth F (1999). Dominant–negative mutation in the β2 and β6 proteasome subunit genes affect alternative cell fate decisions in the *Drosophila* sense organ lineage. *Proc Natl Acad Sci USA* 96: 11382–11386.

Selkoe DJ (2000). Notch and presenilins in vertebrates and invertebrates: implications for neuronal development and degeneration. *Curr Opin Neurobiol* 10: 50–57.

Selva EM, Hong K, Baeg GH, Beverley SM, Turco SJ, Perrimon N, Hacker U (2001). Dual role of the fringe connection gene in both heparan sulphate and fringe-dependent signalling events. *Nat Cell Biol* 3: 809–815.

Sestan N, Artavanis-Tsakonas S, Rakic P (1999). Contact-dependent inhibition of cortical neurite growth mediated by notch signaling. *Science* 286: 741–746.

Seugnet L, Simpson P, Haenlin M (1997). Requirement for dynamin during Notch signaling in *Drosophila* neurogenesis. *Dev Biol* 192: 585–598.

Shawber C, Nofziger D, Hsieh JJ-D, Lindsell C, Bogler O, Hayward D, Weinmaster G (1996). Notch signaling inhibits muscle cell differentiation through a CBF1-independent pathway. *Development* 122: 3765–3773.

Shimizu K, Chiba S, Kumano K, Hosoya N, Takahashi T, Kanda Y, Hamada Y, Yazaki Y, Hirai H (1999). Mouse Jagged1 physically interacts with Notch2 and other Notch receptors: assessment by quantitative methods. *J Biol Chem* 274: 32961–32969.

Shimizu K, Chiba S, Saito T, Takahashi T, Kumano K, Hamada Y, Hirai H (2002). Integrity of intracellular domain of Notch ligand is indispensable for cleavage required for release of the Notch2 intracellular domain. *EMBO J* 21: 294–302.

Struhl G, Adachi A (1998). Nuclear access and action of notch in vivo. *Cell* 93: 649–660.

Struhl G, Adachi A (2000). Requirements for presenilin-dependent cleavage of notch and other transmembrane proteins. *Mol Cell* 6: 625–636.

Struhl G, Fitzgerald K, Greenwald I (1993). Intrinsic activity of the Lin-12 and Notch intracellular domains in vivo. *Cell* 74: 331–345.

Sun X, Artavanis-Tsakonas S (1996). The intracellular deletions of Delta and Serrate define dominant negative forms of the *Drosophila* Notch ligands. *Development* 122: 2465–2474.

Sun X, Artavanis-Tsakonas S (1997). Secreted forms of DELTA and SERRATE define antagonists of Notch signaling in *Drosophila*. *Development* 124: 3439–3448.

Swiatek PJ, Lindsell CE, del Amo FF, Weinmaster G, Gridley T (1994). Notch1 is essential for postimplantation development in mice. *Genes Dev* 8: 707–719.

Taniguchi Y, Furukawa T, Tun T, Han H, Honjo T (1998). LIM protein KyoT2 negatively regulates transcription by association with the RBP-J DNA-binding protein. *Mol Cell Biol* 18: 644–654.

Tax FE, Yeargers JJ, Thomas JH (1994). Sequence of *C. elegans* lag-2 reveals a cell-signalling domain shared with Delta and Serrate of *Drosophila*. *Nature* 368: 150–154.

Uyttendaele H, Marazzi G, Wu G, Yan Q, Sassoon D, Kitajewski J (1996). Notch4/int-3, a mammary proto-oncogene, is an endothelial cell-specific mammalian Notch gene. *Development* 122: 2251–2259.

Varnum-Finney B, Purton LE, Yu M, Brashem-Stein C, Flowers D, Staats S, Moore KA, Le Roux I, Mann R, Gray G, et al. (1998). The Notch ligand, Jagged-1, influences the development of primitive hematopoietic precursor cells. *Blood* 91: 4084–4091.

Varnum-Finney B, Wu L, Yu M, Brashem-Stein C, Staats S, Flowers D, Griffin JD, Bernstein ID (2000). Immobilization of Notch ligand, Delta-1, is required for induction of notch signaling. *J Cell Sci* 113 Pt 23: 4313–4318.

Wang S, Barres BA (2000). Up a notch: instructing gliogenesis. *Neuron* 27: 197–200.

Wang S, Younger-Shepherd S, Jan LY, Jan YN (1997). Only a subset of the binary cell fate decisions mediated by Numb/Notch signaling in *Drosophila* sensory organ lineage requires Suppressor of Hairless. *Development* 124: 4435–4446.

Wang S, Sdrulla AD, diSibio G, Bush G, Nofziger D, Hicks C, Weinmaster G, Barres B (1998). Notch receptor activation inhibits oligodendrocyte differentiation. *Neuron* 21: 63–75.

Weinmaster G (1997). The ins and outs of notch signaling. *Mol Cell Neurosci* 9: 91–102.

Weinmaster G (2000). Notch signal transduction: a real rip and more. *Curr Opin Genet Dev* 10: 363–369.

Wesley CS (1999). Notch and wingless regulate expression of cuticle patterning genes. *Mol Cell Biol* 19: 5743–5758.

Wilkinson HA, Fitzgerald K, Greenwald I (1994). Reciprocal changes in expression of the receptor lin-12 and its ligand lag-2 prior to commitment in a *C. elegans* cell fate decision. *Cell* 79: 1187–1198.

Wu G, Lyapina S, Das I, Li J, Gurney M, Pauley A, Chui I, Deshaies RJ, Kitajewski J (2001). SEL-10 is an inhibitor of notch signaling that targets notch for ubiquitin-mediated protein degradation. *Mol Cell Biol* 21: 7403–7415.

Wu JY, Rao Y (1999). Fringe: defining borders by regulating the Notch pathway. *Curr Opin Neurobiol* 9: 537–543.

Xu T, Artavanis-Tsakonas S (1990). deltex, a locus interacting with the neurogenic genes, Notch, Delta and mastermind in *Drosophila melanogaster*. *Genetics* 126: 665–677.

Xu T, Rebay I, Fleming RJ, Scottgale TN, Artavanis-Tsakonas S (1990). The Notch locus and the genetic circuitry involved in early *Drosophila* neurogenesis. *Genes Dev* 4: 464–475.

Yamamoto N, Yamamoto S, Inagaki F, Kawaichi M, Fukamizu A, Kishi N, Matsuno K, Nakamura K, Weinmaster G, Okano H, Nakafuku M (2001). Role of Deltex-1 as a transcriptional regulator downstream of the Notch receptor. *J Biol Chem* 276: 45031–45040.

Yuan YP, Schultz J, Mlodzik M, Bork P (1997). Secreted fringe-like signaling molecules may be glycosyltransferases. *Cell* 88: 9–11. (Letter).

Zecchini V, Brennan K, Martinez-Arias A (1999). An activity of Notch regulates JNK signalling and affects dorsal closure in *Drosophila*. *Curr Biol* 9: 460–469.

Zhou S, Fujimuro M, Hsieh JJ, Chen L, Miyamoto A, Weinmaster G, Hayward SD (2000). SKIP, a CBF1-associated protein, interacts with the ankyrin repeat domain of NotchIC To facilitate NotchIC function. *Mol Cell Biol* 20: 2400–2410.

40 | *JAG1* and the Alagille Syndrome

NANCY B. SPINNER AND IAN D. KRANTZ

Alagille syndrome (AGS)—also known as syndromic bile duct paucity or arteriohepatic dysplasia—is a multisystem, autosomal dominant, developmental disorder. This syndrome was first reported by Alagille et al. in 1969 with emphasis on the hepatic manifestations. Focusing more on the cardiac findings, Watson and Miller (1973) described the same entity. In 1975 Alagille and his colleagues formally described the syndrome that carries his name and established specific diagnostic criteria.

AGS is the most common form of familial cholestatic liver disease. In addition to affecting the liver, AGS involves abnormalities of the heart, eye, and skeleton and has a characteristic facial appearance. The kidney and central nervous system are also affected in a smaller percentage of patients (Emerick et al., 1999). The prevalence of AGS has been reported as 1 in 100,000 live births, although this is most likely an underestimate as these patients were ascertained based solely on the finding of neonatal liver disease (Danks et al. 1977).

AGS is characterized by highly variable expressivity (Krantz et al., 1999a,b), and the wide range of phenotypic presentations has been better appreciated since the identification of *Jagged1* (*JAG1*) as the disease-causing gene (Li et al., 1997; Oda et al., 1997). *JAG1* was identified as the AGS disease gene by positional cloning, after a group of AGS patients with deletions of chromosome 20 was found. Mapping of these deletions defined a critical region that contained the putative disease gene, and *JAG1* was localized within this region. Patients without deletions were found to have mutations in *JAG1*. JAG1 is a cell surface protein that functions in the Notch signaling pathway (see Chapter 39). This pathway was first described in *Drosophila melanogaster*, and the name "Notch" derives from the characteristic notched wing found in flies that carry only one functioning copy of the gene.

Currently, *JAG1* mutations can be identified in approximately 70% of patients (Krantz et al., 1998; Crosnier et al., 1999; Spinner et al., 2001). The spectrum of mutations identified, and the presence of total gene deletions in some affected individuals, is consistent with haploinsufficiency for JAG1 being a mechanism for AGS.

CLINICAL FEATURES

With the availability of molecular testing for mutations in *JAG1*, the broad phenotypic variability of AGS is just recently being fully appreciated. Traditionally, the clinical diagnosis of AGS has been based on the criteria established by Alagille et al. (1975, 1987) and includes the histological finding of paucity of the interlobular bile ducts on liver biopsy, in association with a minimum of three of five major clinical features: chronic cholestasis, cardiac disease, skeletal abnormalities, ocular abnormalities, and characteristic facial features. While these characteristic findings used for establishing a clinical diagnosis are seen in the majority of AGS individuals, several other organs and structures have been noted to be involved to a lesser degree—kidney, pancreas, cerebrovascular system, and the extremities. An even wider spectrum of clinical involvement—including intestinal abnormalities, orofacial clefts, hearing loss, and mental retardation—may be seen in those AGS individuals with deletions of chromosome 20p12, encompassing *JAG1* and other genes (Krantz et al., 1997). The incidence of these larger deletions among AGS patients is less than 7% (Desmaze et al., 1992; Krantz et al., 1997).

Familial studies, and more recently molecular testing, have identified individuals with very subtle or isolated findings of the types seen in individuals who meet the full clinical diagnostic criteria of AGS (Krantz et al., 1999b). It is now recognized that the clinical manifestation of AGS can range from subtle, subclinical findings to life-threatening liver or heart disease, or both. This variability has been observed both within and between families.

Hepatic Manifestations

As is true for all of the clinical manifestations of AGS, there is great variability in the degree of hepatic involvement. Most symptomatic patients will present in infancy with mild cholestasis, jaundice (typically a conjugated hyperbilirubinemia), and pruritus that may progress to liver failure accompanied by failure to thrive. However, some mutation carriers may not have any detectable hepatic manifestations (Greenwood et al., 1976; Henrikens et al., 1977; Emerick et al., 1999). This lack of liver abnormalities was demonstrated in two incidences of apparently unaffected living-related transplant donors who were found intraoperatively to be unsuitable due to bile duct paucity (Gurkan et al., 1999). This underscores the importance of a thorough clinical, biochemical, and molecular (if available) examination of an AGS individual's family members as features may be extremely mild.

Jaundice presents as a conjugated hyperbilirubinemia in the neonatal period. Cholestasis is manifested by growth failure, pruritus, and xanthomas (typically forming on extensor surfaces, flexion creases, buttocks, ears, and sites of repetitive friction or trauma) (Fig. 40–1). Laboratory findings most commonly include elevations of serum bile acids, conjugated bilirubin, alkaline phosphatase, cholesterol, and γ-glutamyl transpeptidase (GGT), which indicate a defect in biliary excretion. Less frequently, elevations of serum aminotransferases and triglycerides may be present. Hypercholesterolemia and triglyceridemia may be profound in severe cholestasis.

Liver biopsy classically shows intrahepatic bile duct paucity, although the diagnostic histopathological lesion of intralobular bile duct paucity is progressive and may not be evident in the newborn period. Depending on when a biopsy is performed, there may be a broad range of histologic findings, including portal fibrosis and, rarely, bile duct proliferation (Novotny et al., 1981). Identifying bile duct paucity on biopsy therefore depends on the age of the patient at the time of biopsy, the site the biopsy is taken from, and the expertise of the pathologist. Bile duct paucity is present in from 80% to 100% of liver biopsies from individuals with AGS (Alagille et al., 1987; Deprettere et al., 1987; Hoffenberg et al., 1995; Emerick et al., 1999; Quiros-Tejeira et al., 1999; Crosnier et al., 2000b). Progression to cirrhosis and liver failure occurs in a significant proportion of patients, with 21% to 50% of children with hepatic symptoms in infancy requiring transplantation (Hoffenberg et al., 1995; Emerick et al., 1999).

There is currently no way to predict which patients with neonatal liver disease will progress to end-stage liver disease and require transplantation. Indications for transplantation include synthetic liver dysfunction, intractable portal hypertension, bone fractures, severe pruritus, xanthomata, and growth failure (Piccoli and Spinner, 2001). Results of transplantation have been encouraging, with survival rates ranging from 79% to 100% (Cardona et al., 1995; Hoffenberg et al., 1995; Emerick et al., 1999); but at times transplantation survival is complicated by complex congenital heart disease.

Growth failure has been reported in 50% to 90% of patients (Alagille et al., 1987; Deprettere et al., 1987; Emerick et al., 1999), most likely as a result of malnutrition caused by poor solubilization and

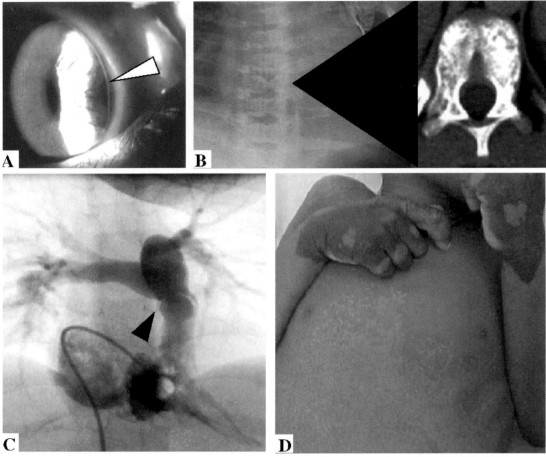

Figure 40–1. Clinical features of Alagille syndrome (AGS). (*A*) Arrowhead indicates posterior embryotoxon (prominent Schwalbe's line). Slit lamp photograph of an anterior segment. (*B*) Arrowhead points to an anterior–posterior radiograph of a thoracic butterfly vertebra, with a magnetic resonance cross-sectional view demonstrating the midline defect in the vertebral body. (*C*) An-giogram, with catheter in right ventricle injecting contrast, demonstrating valvar pulmonic stenosis with diffuse branch pulmonary artery hypoplasia. Note thickened valve leaflets that do not open completely in systole (arrowhead). (*D*) Diffuse xanthomata on the trunk and hands of a young boy with AGS.

absorption of dietary lipids, essential fatty acids, and fat-soluble vitamins.

Cardiac Manifestations

Larger studies have reported congenital heart disease to be present in 81% to 100% of individuals with AGS (Alagille et al., 1987; Deprettere et al., 1987; Emerick et al., 1999). The pulmonary vasculature (pulmonary valve, artery, and arterial branches) is most commonly involved, with peripheral pulmonic stenosis being the most prevalent (Fig. 40–1). Intracardiac lesions are seen in 24% of patients (Emerick et al., 1999). The most frequent complex cardiac malformation seen in these patients is tetralogy of Fallot (TOF) (7%–10%) (Alagille et al., 1987; Deprettere et al., 1987; Emerick et al., 1999). Other cardiac defects seen in association with AGS, listed in order of decreasing frequency, include ventricular septal defects, atrial septal defects, aortic stenosis, and coarctation of the aorta (Silberbach et al., 1994).

While the majority of cardiovascular malformations are hemodynamically insignificant, the more severe malformations have accounted for the majority of early mortality in some series (Deprettere et al., 1987; Emerick et al., 1999). In the series reported by Emerick et al. (1999), the mortality rate was 33% for TOF and 75% for TOF with pulmonary atresia. This is significantly higher than mortality rates for TOF patients who do not have AGS (11% for TOF alone, and 42% for TOF with pulmonary atresia) (Vobecky et al., 1993). This higher rate may be biased due to the cooccurrence of significant hepatic disease in many of the patients reported in these series. It has become clear, from family studies and mutational analysis in individuals with isolated heart defects of the type seen in AGS, that many individuals with *JAG1* mutations

may have isolated congenital heart defects and do not have clinically relevant hepatic involvement (Krantz et al., 1999b).

Interestingly, a large family has been identified in which a mutation in *JAG1* segregates with cardiac disease in the absence of hepatic involvement (discussed later in this chapter) (Eldadah et al., 2001). Mortality and morbidity in individuals with *JAG1* mutations with apparently isolated congenital heart differences has not been formally evaluated and may be better than that noted here. The prevalence of *JAG1* mutations among a large cohort of nonsyndromic TOF patients has been reported as 4% (Smith et al., 1998). The contribution of this gene to other isolated cardiac defects (of the types seen in AGS), such as pulmonic and peripheral pulmonic stenosis, has not been fully evaluated at this time.

Ophthalmologic Manifestations

Larger studies have reported the prevalence of ophthalmologic findings in patients with AGS to be 56% to 88%. The majority of these involve defects of the anterior chamber (posterior embryotoxon, Axenfeld's anomaly, Rieger's anomaly), and retinal pigmentary changes (Alagille et al., 1987; Deprettere et al., 1987; Puklin et al., 1981; Emerick et al., 1999; Hingorani et al., 1999). Posterior embryotoxon (a prominent centrally positioned Schwalbe's ring) (Fig. 40–1), best visualized by slit-lamp examination, has been reported in 56% to 95% of AGS probands (Alagille et al., 1987; Deprettere et al., 1987; Hoffenberg et al., 1995; Emerick et al., 1999). This finding is generally not of clinical significance to the patients, although it is important diagnostically. Posterior embryotoxon occurs in the general population with a frequency of 8% to 15% (Waring et al., 1975), which may result in diagnostic dilemmas in otherwise unaffected family members of AGS probands. Posterior embryotoxon has also been reported in 69% of patients with the velocardiofacial DiGeorge's syndrome (McDonald-McGinn et al., 1999).

In one series, ocular ultrasound examination was performed on 20 children with AGS, and optic disc drusen was seen in 90%, suggesting that ocular ultrasound might aid in clinical diagnosis (Nischal et al., 1997). A spectrum of retinal pigmentary changes has been reported in AGS patients. Although initially assumed to be due to dietary deficiency, these changes are also present in patients with normal serum levels of vitamin A and E (Alagille et al., 1987; Deprettere et al., 1987). In the majority of patients, visual prognosis is good, although mild decreases in acuity have been reported. Other ocular findings have been reported less frequently, including microcornea, keratoconus, congenital macular dystrophy, exotropia, ectopic pupil, band keratopathy, cataracts, strabismus, iris hypoplasia, choroidal folds, and anomalous optic discs (Puklin et al., 1981; Romanchuk et al., 1981; Johnson, 1990; Brodsky and Cunniff, 1993; Wells et al., 1993; Hingorani et al., 1999).

Skeletal Manifestations

Butterfly vertebrae, which result from clefting abnormalities of the vertebral body (Fig. 40–1B, photo B), are the most common skeletal abnormality reported in AGS. Butterfly vertebrae are usually asymptomatic radiologic findings. The frequency of butterfly vertebrae ranges from 22% to 87% in reported cases of AGS (Rosenfield et al., 1980; Alagille et al., 1987; Deprettere et al., 1987; Emerick et al., 1999), while the incidence in the general population is unknown but presumed to be very rare. Other reported skeletal anomalies include narrowing of interpeduncular spaces in the lumbar spine (50%), pointed anterior process of C1, spina bifida occulta, fusion of adjacent vertebrae, hemivertebrae, bony connections between ribs, and short fingers (Watson and Miller, 1973; Rosenfield et al., 1980; Alagille et al., 1987; Deprettere et al., 1987).

Individuals with AGS may also have decreased bone density (osteopenia) and be more prone to fractures and rickets. Contributory factors include severe chronic malnutrition, vitamin D and K deficiency (secondary to fat malabsorption), chronic hepatic and renal disease, magnesium deficiency, and pancreatic insufficiency (Heubi et al., 1997; Piccoli and Spinner, 2001).

Facial Features

The constellation of facial features seen in AGS patients include a prominent forehead, deep-set eyes with moderate hypertelorism, pointed chin, and saddle or straight nose with a bulbous tip. The combination of these features gives the face a triangular appearance (Fig. 40–2). The facies are dynamic and evolve with age, with some of the features being obscured in the newborn period secondary to subcutaneous facial adipose tissue. The features are most characteristic in the toddler to preadolescent period, but begin to change around adolescence to a very typical, but perhaps less recognized, appearance in adulthood (Fig. 40–2) (Kamath et al., 2002a). The chin in the adult becomes prognathic, with less prominence to the forehead, almost inverting the emphasis of the features seen in childhood.

It has been suggested that there is interobserver variability in identification of these features and that they are not specific to AGS syndrome but, rather, are possibly due to cholestasis ("cholestasis facies") (Sokol et al., 1983). A study of the ability of dysmorphologists to differentiate the facies of individuals with AGS from other forms of congenital cholestasis indicates that the facial features in AGS are readily distinguishable from those of other forms of cholestasis (Kamath et al., 2002a).

Minor Features

Renal

Renal anomalies, although clinically diverse, have been reported in 23% to 74% of AGS patients and as such should be considered a major clinical manifestation of AGS. Reported renal abnormalities have included solitary kidney, ectopic kidney, bifid pelvis and duplicated ureters, small kidneys, and unilateral and bilateral multicystic and dysplastic kidneys. Additionally, renal tubular acidosis in infancy, neonatal renal insufficiency, fatal juvenile nephronophthisis, "lipidosis" of the glomeruli, tubulointerstitial nephropathy, and adult-onset renal insufficiency and failure have all been reported (Watson and Miller 1973; LaBrecque et al., 1982; Hyams et al., 1983; Alagille et al., 1987; Habib et al., 1987; Russo et al., 1987; Tolia et al., 1987; Martin et al., 1996; Schonck et al., 1998; Emerick et al., 1999).

Renal vascular disease (arterial stenosis), which may result in systemic hypertension, has also been reported (Berard et al., 1998; Quiros-Tejeira et al., 1999). Other vascular abnormalities that have been reported in AGS are discussed below.

Vascular

Intracranial bleeding is becoming increasingly recognized as a significant cause of morbidity and mortality in AGS, with occurrences as high as 15% (Hoffenberg et al., 1995; Emerick et al., 1999). Fatality rates were between 30% and 50% for these events. Bleeds have been reported to be epidural, subdural, subarachnoid, and intraparenchymal. The majority are spontaneous and not associated with a clear predisposing event, although some have been temporally related to minor head trauma or coagulopathy.

Additional reports have noted the association of various vascular malformations with AGS, including renovascular anomalies (Berard et al., 1998), middle aortic syndrome (Shefler et al., 1997), and "moyamoya syndrome" (Rachmel et al., 1989; Woolfenden et al., 1999). This may indicate that there is an underlying "vasculopathy" present in some individuals with *JAG1* mutations that may be the cause of the intracranial hemorrhages.

Mutations in a gene coding for another member of the Notch signaling pathway, the Notch 3 receptor, result in CADASIL (cerebral autosomal-dominant arteriopathy with subcortical infarcts and leukoencephalopathy) syndrome. CADASIL is an autosomal dominant, adult-onset disorder characterized by strokes and dementia that result from an angiopathy involving primarily the small cerebral arteries (Joutel et al., 1996). Furthermore, the Jagged1 knockout mouse is lethal in the early embryonic period secondary to vascular anomalies of the developing yolk sac (Xue et al., 1999). These findings in association with the increasing number of reports of vascular abnormalities in AGS may indicate that disruptions of the Notch signaling pathway may interfere with either vasculogenesis or the maintenance of vascular integrity, or both.

Cognitive Functioning

In the earlier reports of this syndrome, Alagille et al. (1975) noted significant mental retardation (IQ 60 to 80) in 9 of 30 patients studied. A recent study (Emerick et al., 1999) demonstrated mild delays in gross motor skills in 16% and mild mental retardation in only 2%. This decreased incidence of developmental and cognitive involvement in the later studies is most likely secondary to earlier disease recognition and more aggressive medical, surgical, and nutritional management and intervention.

Other Findings

Other consistently reported findings in AGS have included the following: delayed puberty and high-pitched voice (Alagille et al., 1987), hearing loss (LaBrecque et al., 1982; Hingorani et al., 1999), pancreatic insufficiency (Chong et al., 1989; Emerick et al., 1999), supernumerary digital "flexion" creases (Kamath et al., 2002b), and craniosynostosis (Kamath et al., 2002c). Several other findings have been reported, including tracheal and bronchial stenosis, jejunal and ileal atresia and stenosis, malrotation, microcolon, otitis media, chronic sinusitis, macrocephaly, hypothyroidism, and insulin-dependant diabetes (Piccoli and Spinner, 2001). Many of these manifestations have been reported in individuals with AGS who have a deletion of chromosome 20p12 that encompasses the *JAG1* gene and other genes in the region. In any child with an expanded AGS phenotype, one should always consider the possibility of a 20p12 deletion as the underlying cause, and this should be investigated before mutational analysis of the *JAG1* gene is undertaken.

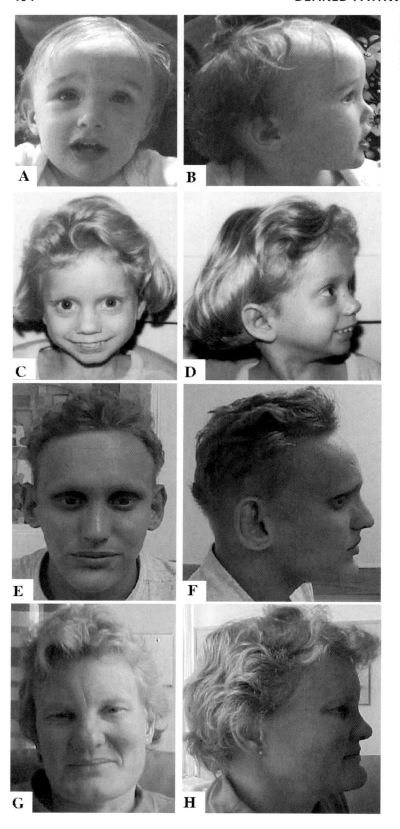

Figure 40–2. Evolution of the facial features in AGS. Note prominent forehead and pointed chin in the younger children: (*A, B*) 3-month-old female and (*C, D*) 7-year-old female. There is a transition to a larger prognathic chin in the adults: (*E, F*) 22-year-old male and (*G, H*) 42-year-old female.

OUTCOMES

The outcome and prognosis for an individual with AGS is highly variable and is directly related to the severity of the liver or cardiac involvement. Mortality is estimated at 15% to 20% and is equally attributable to both of these organs. Complex congenital heart disease is responsible for most of the neonatal deaths, while liver failure accounts for most of the later morbidity and mortality. Intracranial hemorrhage is becoming an increasingly recognized cause of morbidity and mortality in this syndrome.

Although several studies have looked at the long-term survival of individuals with AGS, the numbers are complicated by the clinical variability among the various study populations and the percentage that have undergone liver transplantation. At a mean of 4.4 years post-transplant, Tzakis et al. (1993) found that 13 of 23 patients (57%) were alive with normal liver function. Increased mortality was noted in patients with more severe cardiac disease or those who had a previous Kasai procedure. A study by Hoffenberg et al. (1995) followed 26 patients and demonstrated a predicted long-term survival rate of 50% without transplantation and 87% with transplantation. In this study, three children died at 3, 6, and 24 months of age—one from a complex congenital heart defect, and two from intracranial hemorrhages. Eight of the study subjects underwent liver transplantation, and all were still alive at a median of 5.4 years posttransplantation. A study by Quiros-Tejeira et al. (1999) demonstrated a 72% survival rate among a cohort of 43 AGS patients (47% of which had received a liver transplant) at a mean follow-up of 8.9 years. Emerick et al. (1999) estimated the 20-year survival rate to be 75% overall (60% in the transplanted patients and 80% in the nontransplanted patients) for a cohort of 92 AGS patients, in which 21% had a liver transplant. In this study, 15 of the 92 patients died: 4 deaths were from hepatic causes (3 posttransplant) (age 3.3–11.5 years); 2 from nontraumatic head bleeds (1 posttransplant) (age 2 and 6 years); 2 from traumatic head bleeds (ages 1 and 2.5 years); 3 from multisystem/cardiac failure (age 1.2–2 years); 1 from squamous cell carcinoma at 30 years; 1 from infection at 10.1 years; 1 from pneumonia at 1.5 years; and 1 of unknown cause at 1.7 years.

TREATMENT

The management of individuals with AGS varies, depending on the severity of their clinical manifestations. Other than surgical and medical care for congenital heart defects, gastroenterologists will be the most helpful in supervising ongoing care and management.

As a result of the intrahepatic cholestasis, there may be significant jaundice, fat malabsorption, and pruritus. The majority of symptomatic patients will present in infancy and may improve with time, or they may progressively worsen with the development of cirrhosis and hepatic failure requiring liver transplantation. Fat malabsorption can result in caloric deprivation and fat-soluble vitamin deficiencies. The cholestasis and related elevation in serum bile acid concentrations result in severe pruritus in many affected children and adults. The pruritus seen in AGS is among the worst of any form of chronic liver disease. It is rarely present before 3–5 months of age but is seen in nearly all children with AGS by 3 years of age, even in those who are anicteric (Collins et al., 1981; Alagille et al., 1987; Deprettere et al., 1987; Piccoli and Witzleben, 2000). Pharmacologic and dietary treatment modalities are summarized in Table 40–1.

Liver transplantation is indicated in those patients with synthetic liver dysfunction, intractable portal hypertension, bone fractures, severe pruritus, xanthomata, and growth failure (Piccoli and Spinner, 2001). Transplantation becomes necessary in 21% to 50% of patients with hepatic

manifestations in infancy (Hoffenberg et al., 1995; Emerick et al., 1999) with posttransplant survival ranging from 79% to 100% (Cardona et al., 1995; Hoffenberg et al., 1995; Emerick et al., 1999). These results indicate that individuals with AGS are good candidates for transplantation, although morbidity and mortality posttransplant are influenced by the degree of cardiopulmonary involvement.

GENETICS

The familial nature of AGS was recognized from the first descriptions of the disorder. Watson and Miller (1973) studied five affected families and discussed the possible dominant inheritance and variable expressivity of this disorder. Alagille et al. (1975) reported that 3 of 15 patients had sibs with neonatal cholestasis. LaBreque et al. (1982) reported a four-generation family in which 15 of 24 individuals demonstrated at least one of the characteristics of AGS, although only 3 had jaundice in the neonatal period. Throughout all of the reports, transmission was consistent with an autosomal dominant pattern of inheritance, but the penetrance of the disorder was clearly reduced and expressivity was quite variable (Shulman et al., 1984; Dhorne-Pollet et al., 1994; Spinner et al., 1994).

The finding of multiple AGS patients with a cytogenetically visible deletion or translocation of chromosome 20 led to the assignment of AGS to 20p12 (Byrne et al., 1986; Anad et al., 1990; Spinner et al., 1994). While the percentage of patients with a chromosomal deletion or rearrangement was found to be quite low (<7%) (Krantz et al., 1997), these patients were instrumental in establishing the precise localization of the genomic region containing the disease gene. In 1997, two groups were able to demonstrate that *JAG1* was physically located within the commonly deleted region on the short arm of chromosome 20 and that mutations in *JAG1* were found in patients with AGS (Li et al., 1997; Oda et al., 1997).

JAG1 Protein Structure

JAG1 is a cell surface protein with a single-pass transmembrane domain; it is one of a family of ligands for the Notch transmembrane receptors. In humans, there are four Notch receptors: Notch1, 2, 3, and 4. JAG1 and the Notch receptors are components of the highly conserved Notch signaling pathway. As noted in Chapter 39, this pathway has been primarily studied in the fruit fly *Drosophila melano-gaster* and the nematode *Caenorhabditis elegans* and functions in many different cell types throughout development to regulate cell fate decisions (Artavanis-Tsakonas et al., 1999; Weinmaster, 2000). Homozygous mutations of Notch are lethal in flies, with affected flies demonstrating hypertrophy of the nervous system, thereby indicating the inability for appropriate cells to adopt an alternative cell fate (Artavanis-Tsakonas et al., 1999). The finding that mutations in *JAG1* cause AGS indicates that Notch signaling is important in the normal development of the organ systems affected—the liver, heart, skeleton, eye, face, kidney, and others.

Table 40–1. Therapeutic Modalities in Alagille Syndrome

Symptom	Pharmacologic Therapy	Dietary and Other Therapies
Fat malabsorption	Medium-chain tryglicerides (added to diet)	Optimize carbohydrate and protein intake
Fat-soluble vitamin deficiency (vitamin D, E, and A levels should be routinely monitored, and PT/PTT should be monitored as an indicator of vitamin K deficiency); inability to correct coagulopathy in some patients may indicate severe synthetic liver dysfunction	Vitamin K (oral/intramuscular); vitamin D (oral/intramuscular—absorption of vitamin D may be enhanced by administration of D-α-tocopheryl polyethylene glycol-1000 succinate [TPGS]); vitamin E (oral) (TPGS-soluble preparation); vitamin A (oral/intramuscular—not usually indicated and not readily available; monitor for liver toxicity)	
Pruritus	Ursodeoxycholic acid (choleretic; paradoxically appears to exacerbate pruritus in some patients); antihistamines; rifampin (inhibits uptake of bile acids into hepatocytes); cholestyramine (binds bile salts and prevents reabsorption—some children develop severe acidosis on this therapy); naltrexone (opioid antagonist); phenobarbitol (?efficacy)	Hydrate skin with emollients; trim fingernails; ultraviolet therapy (?efficacy)
Decreased bone density, osteoporosis	Calcium supplements	Routinely monitor bone density with DEXA scans

Source: Adapted from Piccoli and Witzleben, 2000.

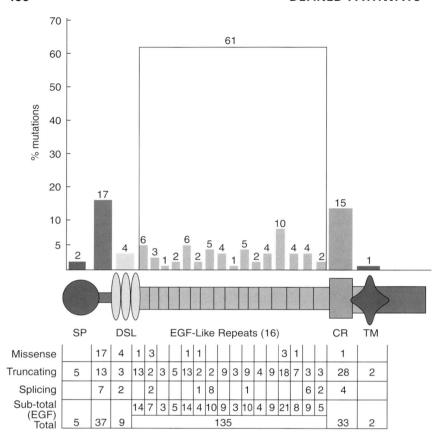

Figure 40–3. Representation of the domains of the Jagged1 protein. SP, signal peptide; DSL, highly conserved region among all Notch ligands named for Delta, Serrate, and Lag-2 (ligands from *Drosophila* [Delta and Serrate] and *C. elegans* [Lag-2]). Graph represents the distribution of different types of mutations—missense, protein truncating (frameshift, nonsense), and splicing—across the different regions and the percentage contribution to the total of reported mutations. Numbers of mutations seen in a published review of 230 patients are indicated below the figure. (From Spinner et al., 2001.)

	SP	DSL		E1	E2	E3	E4	E5	E6	E7	E8	E9	E10	E11	E12	E13	E14	E15	E16	CR	TM
Missense		17	4	1	3			1	1							3	1			1	
Truncating	5	13	3	13	2	3	5	13	2	2	9	3	9	4	9	18	7	3	3	28	2
Splicing		7	2		2				1	8			1					6	2	4	
Sub-total (EGF)				14	7	3	5	14	4	10	9	3	10	4	9	21	8	9	5		
Total	5	37	9	135 (EGF-Like Repeats)																33	2

JAG1 shares structural similarity with all of the Notch ligands identified to date (*Delta* and *Serrate* in *D. melanogaster*; *LAG2* in *C. elegans*; Jagged2, Delta-like 2, Delta-like 3, and Delta like-4 in vertebrates). All ligands contain a large extracellular domain, a transmembrane domain, and a small intracellular portion (Figure 40–3). The extracellular domains of the protein include a 21 amino acid signal peptide, a 40 amino acid DSL region that is highly conserved among all Notch ligands (DSL is named for Delta, Serrate and Lag-2), 16 epidermal growth factor (EGF)–like regions and a cysteine-rich region. The EGF-like repeats consist of 40 to 50 amino acids and are found in a large number of extracellular proteins with diverse functions. They invariably contain six conserved cysteine residues that form three disulfide bonds, which are believed to be important for protein stabilization and protein–protein interaction (Campbell and Bork, 1993). A subset of the EGF-like repeats in human JAG1 are calcium binding, and the presence of calcium has been shown to be essential for mouse Jagged1–Notch interaction (Shimizu et al., 1999). JAG1 contains a 24 amino acid insertion that interrupts the tenth EGF repeat.

Expression of JAG1

The timing and specificity of the Notch receptor–ligand interactions are not completely understood at this time. However, expression studies indicate that this is most likely a dynamic process, and any given ligand may interact with different Notch receptors, depending on the tissue type and developmental stage. This is borne out by studies demonstrating that mouse JAG1 interacts with Notch 1, 2, and 3. These interactions minimally require the DSL region, which is important for ligand–receptor binding, while the EGF-like domains modulate the signaling activity (Shimizu et al., 1999). The expression patterns of *JAG1*, as well as of the Notch receptors, have been studied in detail in a variety of species and tissues during development. Overall, the expression pattern of JAG1 correlates with the clinical features seen in AGS. Expression studies in mice, rats, and humans have implicated JAG1 in the development of the central nervous system, heart, lung, liver, skeletal system, kidney, gallbladder, limb bud, testis, and teeth

(Lindsell et al., 1997; Mitsiadis et al., 1997; Loomes et al., 1999; Crosnier et al., 2000a; Jones et al., 2000). In adults, *JAG1* is expressed at high levels in the heart, skeletal muscle, pancreas, placenta, lung, and kidney (Mitsiadis et al., 1997; Loomes et al., 1999).

Molecular Biology of and Mutations in *JAG1*

The *JAG1* gene is located on human chromosome 20, within band p12. The *JAG1* cDNA (GenBank accession # 4557678) is 6 kb with a coding region of 3657 nucleotides (Oda et al., 1997). At the genomic level, *JAG1* occupies 36,000 bp of DNA sequence and is encoded within 26 exons. The overall DNA sequence homology of human *JAG1* to the rat is 88.8%, with 96.7% identity in the coding region (Oda et al., 1997).

To date, over 300 AGS probands have been studied molecularly, and *JAG1* mutations have been demonstrated in ~70% (Krantz et al., 1998; Yuan et al., 1998; Crosnier et al., 1999; Spinner et al., 2001). Most of the reported studies have utilized cytogenetics and fluorescence in situ hybridization (FISH) to screen for deletions, and single-strand conformation polymorphism (SSCP) analysis to screen for intragenic mutations. Across all studies, total gene deletions have been identified in 3% to 7% of patients. The other 65% of mutations are intragenic, and 72% of these are protein truncating (frameshift and nonsense). Some 9% of patients have splicing mutations, and 9% have missense mutations. The mutations are distributed across the entire coding region of the *JAG1* gene (Fig. 40–3). *JAG1* mutations have been found to be de novo in 56% to 70% of cases (Krantz et al., 1998; Crosnier et al., 1999). In some cases, mosaicism has been identified in a parent with no clinically evident signs of AGS, complicating carrier identification and genetic diagnosis (Giannakudis et al., 2001; Laufer-Cahana et al., 2002).

Missense mutations are of particular interest because they provide clues as to which portions of the JAG1 protein are crucial to normal functioning. Functional studies of a small set of JAG1 missense mutations have revealed that several of these lead to functional haploinsufficiency, due to the improper modification of the newly translated protein, which is therefore not properly targeted to the cell surface (Morrissette et al., 2001). This has been shown for the L37S and R184H missense mutations (Morrissette et al., 2001) and recently for the P810L mutation (Lu et al., 2002). Another missense mutation (G274D) leads to a partial phenotype of cardiac defects and the absence of liver involvement (Eldadah et al., 2001).

Mutations in *JAG1* could cause AGS, either by inducing haploinsufficiency of the JAG1 protein or by causing a dominant–negative effect. Under a model of haploinsufficiency, an alteration in one of the *JAG1* genes leads to a complete lack of product or a severely defective product, resulting in insufficient protein. Genes showing haploinsufficiency code for products that are needed in specific tissues in large quantity, such that having only one functional copy does not allow enough of the protein product to be made. Alternatively, the quantity of the gene product may be tightly regulated because it interacts in precise amounts with another protein, and excess of the other protein may be toxic to the cell. The fact that large deletions of 20p12, including the entire *JAG1* gene cause AGS is good evidence that some cases of AGS are caused by haploinsufficiency for *JAG1*. A dominant–negative effect is also a potential mechanism for a dominant disorder. In this case, the mutant protein antagonizes the activity of the remaining wild-type protein, so that normal function of the gene is obliterated. Interestingly, in *Drosophila*, there have been *Delta* and *Serrate* mutants reported that appear similar to the *JAG1* mutations seen in AGS, and these have been shown to function in a dominant–negative fashion (Sidow et al., 1997). In humans, there are currently no data supporting dominant–negative JAG1 mutations in AGS. However, a non-transmembrane form of Jagged-1 has been studied. This secreted form of JAG1 was found to be biologically active in a cell culture system designed to study the differentiation of endothelial cells (Wong et al., 2000). It is possible that these types of *JAG1* mutations might result in a phenotype that is different from AGS, and new strategies will be required to identify these.

Phenotypic Variability and Modifiers

The AGS phenotype demonstrates variable expressivity with clinical effects ranging from subclinical to life threatening. The only reliable indicator of mortality has been found to be the presence of complex heart disease. In newborns with AGS and hepatic involvement, it is not possible to predict which patients will progress to end-stage liver disease (Emerick et al., 1999). Although it had been hoped that genetic studies would reveal a correlation between the genetic mutation and phenotype to explain the clinical variability, this has not been the case.

Even within families segregating a single mutation, the expressivity of the disorder has been found to range from mild to severe (Shulman et al., 1984; Spinner, et al., 1994, Li et al., 1997). An exception to this seems to be a family described by Eldadah et al. (2001). In this large, multigeneration family, a missense mutation (G274D) was found to be segregating with apparently isolated cardiac disease. The cardiac disease in this family consisted of tetralogy of Fallot (5 of 14 individuals), ventricular septal defect with aortic dextroposition (1 of 14 individual), peripheral pulmonic stenosis (6 of 14 individuals), and unspecified cardiac disease (2 of 14 individuals). These cardiac abnormalities are consistent with those seen in AGS. This missense mutation has not been seen in any of the over 200 patients studied with AGS.

Expression and functional studies of this mutant have demonstrated that it is "leaky"—that is, some of the G274D protein molecules are normally processed and transported to the cell surface where they function appropriately, while some of them are incorrectly processed and transported. These results suggest that while haploinsufficiency for JAG1 is associated with the well-characterized phenotype of AGS, the "leaky" G274D mutant, which allows more JAG1 protein to reach the cell surface, is associated with a cardiac-specific phenotype (Lu et al., 2003). Therefore, cardiac development appears to be more sensitive to JAG1 dosage than is liver development. This is the first *JAG1* mutation identified with a phenotypic correlation.

The lack of consistent phenotypes both within and between families with the same *JAG1* mutations suggests that there are modifiers of the AGS phenotype. These modifiers could be genetic or environ-

mental. Some support for the presence of potential genetic modifiers comes from work in the mouse. A mouse knockout of the Jag1 gene has been reported (Xue et al., 1999). Homozygotes for the Jag1 null allele die by 11.5 days post conception (dpc) from vascular defects, and therefore only limited developmental analysis is possible due to the lethality before any key steps in organogenesis. The Jag1 mutant heterozygotic mice exhibit eye defects but do not demonstrate the liver, cardiac, or other common abnormalities seen in human patients with AGS. Recent evidence has demonstrated that mice that are doubly heterozygous for *Jag1* and *Notch2* mutations are an excellent model for AGS (McCright et al., 2002). These mice are jaundiced and have bile duct, heart, eye, and kidney abnormalities that are similar to those seen in AGS patients. This work points to *Notch2* as a potential genetic modifier of the effect of a *JAG1* mutation in humans.

Genetic studies will expand our knowledge of the clinical manifestations of a *JAG1* mutation. In families in which there is a *JAG1* mutation segregating, only about 25% of those carrying the mutation meet the clinical criteria for AGS. Therefore, it can be anticipated that individuals who do not meet the complete criteria, and who do not have a family member with AGS, may also be found to have mutations in *JAG1*. Some individuals with cardiac findings in the absence of liver abnormalities have been found to have *JAG1* mutations (Krantz et al., 1999b; Eldadah et al., 2001).

The identification of *JAG1* as the disease gene for AGS links a critical developmental pathway to a multisystem congenital disorder in humans. Two other Notch signaling pathway genes involved in human disease are Notch3 (mutations in which cause CADASIL) and DLL3 (mutations in which cause spondylocostal dysostosis) (Joutel et al., 1996; Bulman et al., 2000). It is anticipated that mutations in other members of the Notch signaling pathway will be found to cause other human disorders, contributing further insight into the molecular basis of both human disease and normal and abnormal development.

GENETIC COUNSELING

At this time, diagnosis of AGS is made on a clinical basis. JAG1 mutations are found in only 70% of clinically defined probands, and molecular testing is not readily available. FISH analysis can be carried out using a probe that contains *JAG1*, which will show a deletion in 3% to 7% of patients (Krantz et al., 1997).

Genetic counseling for AGS can be complicated. While the disorder is known to be autosomal dominant, the expressivity is highly variable. It may be difficult to correctly identify a carrier parent if clinical features of AGS are not evident. In order to evaluate parents as potential carriers of a *JAG1* mutation, clinical evaluation—including analysis of liver function, cardiac evaluation, radiograph of the spine, ophthalmologic examination, and evaluation of facial features—by a clinical geneticist should be carried out. Approximately 50% to 70% of cases of AGS result from a de novo *JAG1* mutation (Crosnier et al., 1999; Spinner et al., 2001). If parents do not carry a mutation or deletion identified in a child with AGS, then their risk of recurrence is very low, as germline mosaicism remains a possibility but has not been documented in AGS to date. Individuals without clinical manifestations of AGS have been identified, however, who were found to be mosaic for point mutations and deletions (Giannakudis et al., 2001, Laufer-Cahana et al., 2002). This makes recurrence risk counseling based solely on a thorough clinical exam of the parents inaccurate.

Prenatal diagnosis can be carried out if a *JAG1* mutation can be detected in an affected member of the family. However, it should be considered that even if the presence of a *JAG1* mutation is confirmed prenatally, there is no way to predict the severity of the clinical features, which may range from mild to severe.

REFERENCES

Alagille D, Habib EC, Thomassin N (1969). L'atresie des voies biliaires intrahepatiques avec voies biliaires extrahepatiques permeables chez l'enfant. *J Par Pediatr* 301–318.

Alagille D, Odievre M, Gautier M, Dommergues JP (1975). Hepatic ductular hypoplasia associated with characteristic facies, vertebral malformations, retarded physical, mental, and sexual development, and cardiac murmur. *J Pediatr* 86: 63–71.

Alagille D, Estrada A, Hadchouel M, Gautier M, Odievre M, Dommergues JP (1987). Syndromic paucity of interlobular bile ducts. *J Pediatr* 110: 195–200.

Anad F, Burn J, Matthews D, Cross I, Davison BCC, Mueller R, Sands M, Lillington DM, Eastham E (1990). Alagille syndrome and deletion of 20p. *J Med Genet* 27: 729–737.

Artavanis-Tsakonas S, Rand MD, Lake RJ (1999). Notch signaling: cell fate control and signal intergration in development. *Science* 284: 770–776.

Berard E, Sarles J, Triolo V, Gagnadoux MF, Wernert F, Hadchouel M, Niaudet P (1998). Renovascular hypertension and vascular anomalies in Alagille syndrome. *Pediatr Nephrol* 12: 121–124.

Brodsky MC, Cunniff C (1993). Ocular anomalies in the Alagille syndrome (arteriohepatic dysplasia). *Ophthalmology* 100: 1767–1774.

Bulman MP, Kusumi K, Frayling TM, McKeown C, Garrett C, Lander ES, Krumlauf R, Hattersley AT, Ellard S, Turnpenny PD (2000). Mutations in the human delta homologue, DLL3, cause axial skeletal defects in spondylocostal dysostosis. *Nat Genet* 24: 438–441.

Byrne JLB, Harrod MJE, Friedman JM, Howard-Peebles PN (1986). Del(20p) with manifestations of arteriohepatic dysplasia. *Am J Med Genet* 24: 673–678.

Campbell ID, Bork P (1993). Epidermal growth factor-like modules. *Curr Opin Struct Biol* 3: 385–392.

Cardona J, Houssin D, Gauthier F, Devictor D, Losay J, Hadchouel M, Bernard O (1995). Liver transplantation in children with Alagille syndrome: a study of twelve cases. *Transplantation* 60: 339–342.

Chong SKF, Lindridge J, Moniz C, Mowat AP (1989). Exocrine pancreatic insufficiency in syndromic paucity of interlobular bile ducts. *J Pediatr Gastroeneterol Nutr* 9: 445–449.

Collins DM, Shannon FT, Campbell CB (1981). Bile acid metabolism in mild arteriohepatic dysplasia. *Aust N Z J Med* 11: 48–51.

Crosnier C, Driancourt C, Raynaud N, Dhorne-Pollet S, Pollet N, Bernard O, Hadchouel M, Meunier-Rotival M (1999). Mutations in JAGGED1 gene are predominantly sporadic in Alagille syndrome. *Gastroenterology* 116: 1141–1148.

Crosnier C, Attie-Bitach T, Encha-Razavi F, Audollent S, Soudy F, Hadchouel M, Meunier-Rotival M, Vekemans M (2000a). JAGGED1 gene expression during human embryogenesis elucidates the wide phenotypic spectrum of Alagille syndrome. *Hepatology* 32: 574–581.

Crosnier C, Lyavieris P, Neunier-Rotival M, Hadchouel M (2000b). Alagille syndrome: the widening spectrum of arteriohepatic dysplasia. *Clin Liver Dis* 4: 765–768.

Danks DM, Campbell PE, Jack I, Rogers J, Smith AL (1977). Studies of the aetiology of neonatal hepatitis and biliary atresia. *Arch Dis Child* 52: 360–367.

Deprettere A, Portmann B, Mowat AP (1987). Syndromic paucity of the intrahepatic bile ducts: diagnostic difficulty; severe morbidity throughout early childhood. *J Pediatr Gastroenteral Nutr* 6: 865–871.

Desmaze C, Deleuze JF, Dutrillaux AM, Thomas G, Hadchouel M, Aurias A (1992). Screening of microdeletions of chromosome 20 in patients with Alagille syndrome. *J Med Genet* 29: 233–235.

Dhorne-Pollet S, Deleuze J-F, Hadchouel M, Bonaiti-Pellie C (1994). Segregation analysis of Alagille syndrome. *J Med Genet* 31: 453–457.

Eldadah ZA, Hamosh A, Biery NJ, Montgomery RA, Duke M, Elkins R, Dietz HC (2001). Familial tetralogy of Fallot caused by mutation in the jagged1 gene. *Hum Mol Genet* 10: 163–169.

Emerick KM, Rand EB, Goldmuntz E, Krantz ID, Spinner NB, Piccoli DA (1999). Features of Alagille syndrome in 92 patients: frequency and relation to prognosis. *Hepatology* 29: 822–829.

Giannakudis J, Ropke A, Kujat A, Krajewska-Walasek M, Hughes H, Fryns JP, Bankier A, More D, Schlicker M, Hansmann IP (2001). Parental mosaicism of JAG1 mutations in families with Alagille syndrome. *Eur J Hum Genet* 9: 209–216.

Greenwood RD, Rosenthal A, Crocker AC, Nadas AS (1976). Syndrome of intrahepatic biliary dysgenesis and cardiovascular malformations. *Pediatrics* 58: 243–247.

Gurkan A, Emre Su, Fishbein TM, Brady L, Millis M, Birnbaum A, Kim-Schluger L, Sheiner PA (1999). Unsuspected bile duct paucity in donors for living-related liver transplation: two case reports. *Transplantation* 67: 416–418.

Habib R, Dommergues JP, Gubler MC, Hadchouel M, Gautier M, Odievre M, Alagille D (1987). Glomerular mesangiolipidosis in Alagille syndrome (arteriohepatic dysplasia). *Pediatr Nephrol* 1: 455–464.

Henriksen NT, Langmark F, Sorland SJ, Fausa O, Landaas S, Aagenaes O (1977). Hereditary cholestasis combined with peripheral plumonary stenosis and other anomalies. *Acta Paediatr Scand* 66: 7–15.

Heubi JE, Higgins JV, Argao EA, Sierra RI, Specker BL (1997). The role of magnesium in the pathogenesis of bone disease in childhood cholestatic liver disease: a preliminary report. *J Pediatr Gastroenterol Nutr* 25: 301–306.

Hingorani M, Nischal KK, Davies A, Bentley C, Vivian A, Baker AJ, Mieli-Vergani G, Bird AC, Aclimandos WA (1999) Ocular abnormalities in Alagille syndrome. *Ophthalmology* 106: 330–337.

Hoffenberg EJ, Narkewicz MR, Sondheimer JM, Smith DJ, Silverman A, Sokol RJ (1995). Outcome of syndromic paucity of interlobular bile ducts (Alagille syndrome) with onset of cholestasis in infancy. *J Pedsiatr* 127: 220–224.

Hyams JS, Berman MM, Davis BH (1983). Tubulointerstitial nephropathy associated with arteriohepatic dysplasia. *Gastroenterology* 85: 430–434.

Johnson BL (1990). Ocular pathologic features of arteriohepatic dysplasia (Alagille syndrome). *Am J Ophthalmol* 110: 504–512.

Jones EA, Clement-Jones M, Wilson DI (2000). JAGGED1 expression in human embryos: correlation with the Alagille syndrome phenotype. *J Med Genet* 37: 663–668.

Joutel A, Corpechot C, Ducros A, Vahedi K, Chabriat H, Mouton P, Alamowitch S, Domenga V, Cecillion M, Marechal E, et al. (1996). Notch3 mutations in CADASIL, a hereditary adult-onset condition causing stroke and dementia. *Nature* 383: 707–710.

Kamath BM, Loomes KM, Oakey RJ, Emerick KE, Conversano T, Spinner NB, Piccoli DA, Krantz ID (2002a). Facial features in Alagille syndrome: specific or cholestasis facies? *Am J Med Genet* 112: 163–170.

Kamath BM, Loomes KM, Oakey RJ, Krantz ID (2002b). Supernumerary digital flexion

creases; an additional clinical manifestation of Alagille syndrome. *Am J Med Genet* 112: 171–175.

Kamath BM, Stolle C, Bason L, Colliton RP, Piccoli DA, Spinner NB, Krantz ID (2002c). Craniosynostosis in Alagille syndrome. *Am J Med Genet* 112: 176–180.

Krantz ID, Rand EB, Genin A, Hunt P, Jones M, Louis AA, Graham JM Jr, Bhatt S, Piccoli DA, Spinner NB (1997). Deletions of 20p12 in Alagille syndrome: frequency and molecular characterization. *Am J Med Genet* 70: 80–86.

Krantz, ID, Colliton RP, Genin A, Rand EB, Li L, Piccoli DA, Spinner NB (1998). Spectrum and frequency of Jagged1 (JAG1) mutations in Alagille syndrome patients and their families. *Am J Hum Genet* 62: 1361–1369.

Krantz ID, Piccoli DA, Spinner NB (1999a). Clinical and molecular genetics of Alagille syndrome. *Curr Opin Pediatr* 11: 558–564.

Krantz ID, Smith R, Colliton RP, Tinkel H, Zackai EH, Piccoli DA, Goldmuntz E, Spinner NB (1999b). *Jagged1* mutations in patients ascertained with isolated congenital heart defects. *Am J Med Genet* 84: 56–60.

LaBrecque DR, Mitros FA, Nathan RJ, Romanchuk KG, Judisch GF, El-Khoury GH (1982). Four generations of arteriohepatic dysplasia. *Hepatology* 2: 467–474.

Laufer-Cahana A, Krantz ID, Bason LD, Lu FM, Piccoli DA, Spinner NB (2002). Alagille syndrome inherited from a phenotypically normal mother with a mosaic 20p microdeletion. *Am J Med Genet* 112: 190–193.

Li L, Krantz ID, Den Y, Genin A, Banta AB, Collins CC, Qi M, Trask BJ, Kuo WL, Cochran J, et al. (1997). Alagille syndrome is caused by mutations in human *Jagged1*, which encodes a ligand for Notch1. *Nat Genet* 16: 243–251.

Lindsell CE, Shawber CJ, Boulter J, Weinmaster G (1995). Jagged: a mammalian ligand that activates Notch1. *Cell* 80: 909–917.

Lindsell CE, Boulter J, DiSibio G, Gossler A, Weinmaster G (1997). Expression patterns of Jagged, Delta1, Notch1, Notch2 and Notch3 genes identify ligand–receptor pairs that may function in neural development. *Mol Cell Neurosci* 8: 14–27.

Loomes KM, Underkoffler LA, Morabito J, Gottlieb S, Piccoli DA, Spinner NB, Baldwin HS, Oakey RJ (1999). The expression of Jagged1 in the developing mammalian heart correlates with cardiovascular disease in Alagille syndrome. *Hum Mol Genet* 8: 2443–2449.

Lu F, Morrisette JJ, Spinner NB (2003). Conditional JAG1 mutation shows the developing heart is more sensitive than developing liver to JAG1 dosage. *Am J Hum Gen* 72: 1065–1070.

Martin SR, Garel L, Alvarez F (1996). Alagille's syndrome associated with cystic renal disease. *Arch Dis Child* 74: 232–235.

McCright B, Lozier J, Gridley T (2002). A mouse model of Alagille syndrome: Notch2 as a genetic modifier of Jag1 haploinsufficiency. *Development* 129: 1075–1082.

McDonald-McGinn DM, Kirschner R, Goldmuntz E, Sullivan K, Eicher P, Gerdes M, Moss E, Solot C, Wang P, Jacobs I, et al. (1999). The Philadelphia story: the 22q11.2 deletion—report on 250 patients. *Genet Couns* 10: 11–24.

Mitsiadis TA, Henrique D, Thesleff I, Lendahl U (1997). Mouse Serrate-1 (Jagged-1): expression in the developing tooth is regulated by epithelial–mesenchymal interactions and fibroblast growth factor-4. *Development* 124: 1473–1483.

Morrissette JJD, Colliton RP, Spinner NB (2001). Defective intracellular transport and processing of JAG1 missense mutation in Alagille syndrome. *Hum Mol Genet* 10: 405–413.

Nischal KK, Hingorani M, Bentley CR, Vivian AJ, Bird AC, Baker AJ, Mowat AP, Mieli-Vergani G, Aclimandos WA (1997). Ocular ultrasound in Alagille syndrome. *Ophthalmology* 104: 79–85.

Novotny NM, Zetterman RK, Antonson DL, Vanderhoof JA (1981). Variation in liver histology in Alagille's syndrome. *Am J Gastroenterol* 75: 449–450.

Oda T, Elkahloun AG, Pike BL, Okajima K, Krantz ID, Genin A, Piccoli DA, Meltzer PS, Spinner NB, Collins FS, Chandrasekharappa SC (1997). Mutations in the human Jagged1 gene (JAGL1) are responsible for Alagille syndrome. *Nat Genet* 16: 235–242.

Piccoli DA, Spinner NB (2001). Alagille syndrome and the Jagged1 gene. *Semin Liver Dis* 21: 525–534.

Piccoli DA, Witzleben CL (2000). Disorders of the intrahepatic bile ducts. In: *Pediatric Gastrointestinal Disease: Clinical Manifestations and Management, 4th Edition*. Walker DA, Durie PR, Hamilton JR, et al. (eds.) B. C. Decker, Philadelphia, pp. 1362–1384.

Puklin JE, Riely CA, Simon RM, Cotlier E (1981). Anterior segment and retinal pigmentary abnormalities in arteriohepatic dysplasia. *Ophthalmology* 88: 337–347.

Quiros-Tejeira RE, Ament ME, Heyman MB, Martin MG, Rosenthal P, Hall TR, McDiarmid SV, Vargas JH (1999). Variable morbidity in Alagille syndrome: a review of 43 cases. *J Pediatr Gastroenterol Nutr* 29: 431–437.

Rachmel A, Zeharia A, Neuman-Levin M, Weitz R, Shamir R, Dinari G (1989). Alagille syndrome associated with Moyamoya disease. *Am J Med Genet* 33: 89–91.

Romanchuk KG, Judisch GF, LaBrecque DR (1981). Ocular findings in arteriohepatic dysplasia (Alagille's syndrome). *Can J Ophthalmol* 16: 94–99.

Rosenfield NS, Kelley MJ, Jensen PS, Cotlier E, Rosenfield AT, Riely CA (1980). Arteriohepatic dysplasia: radiologic features of a new syndrome. *Am J Roentgenol* 135: 1217–1223.

Russo PA, Ellis D, Hashida Y (1987). Renal histopathology in Alagille's syndrome. *Pediatr Pathol* 7: 557–568.

Schonck M, Hoorntje S, van Hooff J (1998). Renal transplantation in Alagille syndrome. *Nephrol Dial Transplant* 13: 197–199.

Shefler AG, Chan MKH, Ostman-Smith IO (1997). Middle aortic syndrome in a boy with arteriohepatic dysplasia (Alagille syndrome). *Pediatr Cardiol* 18: 232–234.

Shimizu K, Chiba S, Kumano K, Hosoya N, Takahashi T, Kanda Y, Hamada Y, Yazaki Y, Hirai H (1999). Mouse jagged1 physicially interacts with notch2 and other notch receptors: assessment by quantitative methods. *J Biol Chem* 274: 32961–32969.

Shulman SA, Hyams JS, Gunta R, Greenstein RM, Cassidy SB (1984). Arteriohepatic dysplasia (Alagille syndrome): extreme variability among affected family members. *Am J Med Genet* 19: 325–332.

Sidow A, Bulotsky MS, Kerrebrock AW, Bronson RT, Daly MJ, Reeve MP, Hawkins TL, Birren BW, Jaenisch R, Lander ES (1997). Serrate2 is disrupted in the mouse limb-development mutant syndactylism. *Nature* 389: 722–725.

Silberbach M, Lashley D, Reller MD, Kinn WF, Terry A, Sunderland CO (1994): Arteriohepatic dysplasia and cardiovascular malformations. *Am Heart J* 127: 695–699.

Smith R, Goldmuntz E, Shin J, Kranyz ID, Spinner NB (1998). Human Jagged1 mutations in patients presenting with tetralogy of Fallot. *Am J Hum Genet* 63: A2.

Sokol RJ, Heubi JE, Balistreri WF (1983). Intrahepatic "cholestasis facies": is it specific for Alagille syndrome? *J Pediatr* 103: 205–208.

Spinner NB, Rand EB, Fortina P, Genin A, Taub R, Semeraro A, Piccoli DA (1994). Cytologically balanced t(2;20) in a two-generation family with Alagille syndrome: cytogenetic and molecular studies. *Am J Hum Genet* 55: 238–243.

Spinner NB, Colliton RP, Crosnier C, Krantz ID, Hadchouel M, Meunier-Rotival M (2001). Mutation update: Jagged1 mutations in Alagille syndrome. *Hum Mutat* 17: 18–33.

Tolia V, Dubois RS, Watts FB, Perrin E (1987). Renal abnormalities in paucity of interlobular bile ducts. *J Ped Gastroenterol Nutr* 6: 971–976.

Tzakis AG, Reyes J, Tepetes K, Tzoracoleftherakis V, Todo S, Starzl TE (1993). Liver transplantation for Alagille's syndrome. *Arch Surg* 128: 337–339.

Vobecky SJ, Williams WG, Trusler GA, Coles JG, Rebeyka IM, Smallhorn J, Burrows P, Gow R, Freedom RM (1993). Survival analysis of infants under age 18 months presenting with tetralogy of Fallot. *Ann Thorac Surg* 56: 944–949.

Waring GO, Rodrigues MM, Laibson PR (1975). Anterior chamber cleavage syndrome: a stepladder classification. *Surv Ophthalmol* 20: 3–27.

Watson GH, Miller V (1973). Arteriohepatic dysplasia, familial pulmonary arterial stenosis with neonatal liver disease. *Arch Dis Child* 48: 459–466.

Weinmaster G (2000). Notch signal transduction: a real Rip and more. *Curr Opin Genet Dev* 10: 363–369.

Wells KK, Pulido JS, Judisch GF, Ossoinig KC, Fisher TC, LaBrecque DR (1993). Ophthalmic features of Alagille syndrome (arteriohepatic dysplasia). *J Pediatr Ophthalmol Strabismus* 30: 130–135.

Wong MKK, Prudovsky I, Vary C, Booth C, Liaw L, Mousa S, Small D Maciag T (2000). A non-transmembrane form of Jagged-1 regulates the formation of matrix dependent chord-like structures. *Biochem Biophys Res Comm* 268: 853–859.

Woolfenden AR, Albers GW, Steinberg GK, Hahn JS, Johnston DC, Farrell K (1999). Moyamoya syndrome in children with Alagille syndrome: additional evidence of a vasculopathy. *Pediatrics* 103: 505–508.

Xue Y, Gao X, Lindsell CE, Norton CR, Chang B, Hicks C, Gendron-Maguire M, Rand EB, Weinmaster G, Gridley T (1999). Embryonic lethality and vascular defects in mice lacking the notch ligand Jagged1. *Hum Mol Genet* 8: 723–730.

Yuan ZR, Zohsaka T, Ikegaya T, Suzuki T, Okano S, Abe J, Kobayashi N, Yamade M (1998). Mutational analysis of the *Jagged1* gene in Alagille syndrome families. *Hum Mol Genet* 7: 1363–1369.

41 | *DLL3* and Spondylocostal Dysostosis

PETER D. TURNPENNY AND KENRO KUSUMI

The delta-like 3 (*DLL3*) gene, which maps to chromosome 19q13.1 in humans, has a significant developmental role in somitogenesis, particularly in patterning events of sclerotomal tissues, from which the axial skeleton and ribs are derived. *DLL3* encodes a ligand for the Notch family of receptors and shows spatially restricted patterns of expression during somite formation. It is presumed to have a key role in the cell-signaling processes that give rise to somite boundary formation, which proceeds in a rostral–caudal direction with a precise temporal periodicity driven by an internal oscillator, or molecular "segmentation clock." Mutated *DLL3* results in abnormal vertebral segmentation throughout the entire spine, usually with rib fusions, and these features define spondylocostal dysostosis (SCD)—a short-trunk, short-stature condition with nonprogressive kyphoscoliosis, usually without additional abnormalities. To date, *DLL3* mutations have been found in autosomal recessive (AR) SCD, and this is characterized by a consistent radiological phenotype, where the vertebral bodies in childhood have smooth outlines—for which we coin the term "pebble beach sign." Furthermore, we designate this form of SCD, due to mutated *DLL3*, as type 1. At least one form of non-*DLL3* SCD occurs, apparently with AR inheritance and sometimes associated with other anomalies, where the vertebral bodies have more angular radiological outlines, which we designate SCD type 2. These forms of SCD are distinct from the very severe truncal shortening condition, spondylothoracic dysplasia (STD), also demonstrating AR inheritance, in which the ribs fan out with a crab-like appearance on X-ray. Most frequently documented in Puerto Ricans, this condition has been mapped to chromosome 2q32. Abnormal vertebral segmentation is a common developmental defect, but the radiological phenotypes are very diverse, and cases demonstrating clear mendelian inheritance are relatively rare. The identification of *DLL3* makes it possible to start building a classification based on genotype–phenotype correlation.

ROLE IN THE NOTCH SIGNALING DEVELOPMENTAL PATHWAY

Somitogenesis in Normal Development

A critical function of the notch pathway is in the embryonic formation of somites. Somites are paired blocks of paraxial mesoderm that are patterned from the presomitic mesoderm, in a sequential process called somitogenesis (reviewed in detail in Chapter 10). Somitogenesis takes place between 20 and 35 days of human embryonic development (Fig. 41–1). In this process the somites are laid down in a rostro–caudal direction, first forming the most rostral somites and progressively laying down more caudal somites (Fig. 41–2). In the chick and mouse a pair of somites are formed with precise periodicity every 90 and 120 minutes, respectively (Fig. 41–3). Somites ultimately give rise to three substructures: sclerotome, which forms the axial skeleton and ribs; dermotome, which forms the dermis; and myotome, which forms the axial musculature.

In normal development, differentiation of the somite leads to the ventral sections that form the sclerotome, while the dorsolateral part forms the dermomyotome (Keynes and Stern, 1988). Early somites are also partitioned into rostral and caudal compartments, and embryonic studies of notch pathway genes such as *Dll3* show compartment-specific expression. The vertebrae are formed from the caudal part of one somite and the adjacent rostral part of the next, a phe-

nomenon that is known as "resegmentation" (Fig. 41–4), while the axial muscle groups connecting the vertebrae result from the rostral–caudal segments within one somite. The so-called resegmentation phenomenon was proposed a century and a half ago on the basis of histological studies of embryos (Remak, 1850). Although this hypothesis was challenged (Verbout, 1985), several embryological experiments have upheld it (Bagnall et al, 1989; Ewan and Everett, 1992; Goldstein and Kalcheim, 1992), and recently the *Mesp2* gene has been shown to be required for the rostral–caudal compartmentalization of somites (Saga et al., 1997), acting through regulation of the notch pathway (Takahashi et al., 2000).

Notch Signaling Pathway and Delta-like 3

The notch signaling pathway has diverse functional roles in human embryonic development. This pathway is named for the *Notch* receptor, identified in *Drosophila* as the first characterized developmental mutation (Poulson, 1937). Subsequent studies have revealed a Notch signaling pathway in *Drosophila* and other organisms, including *C. elegans*, zebrafish, chick, mouse, rat, and humans (Fig. 41–5; reviewed in Mumm and Kopan, 2000, and in Chapter 39 of this book). Notch receptors are activated by serrate/jagged and delta classes of ligand, and delta-like 3 (*DLL3*) is one of three identified mammalian delta molecules. The ability of notch receptors to be activated by ligand is modulated by members of the *fringe* gene family (Evrard et al., 1998; Zhang and Gridley, 1998; Bruckner et al., 2000; Moloney et al., 2000). Upon activation by ligand, the notch receptor undergoes a cleavage by presenilin, to release the intracellular signaling domain (notch-ic). Notch-ic then moves to the nucleus and converts suppressors of hairless/CSL from repressors to activators of the *hairy-enhancer of split* (*HES*) genes. *HES* genes regulate the *achaete-scute/ASCL* genes.

In somitogenesis, the main role for both murine *Dll3* and its human homolog *DLL3* appears to lie in the initial formation of somite segments. Loss of *Dll3* function, due to gene truncation or deletion, results in severe disruption of normal somite patterning. This was first identified in the pudgy mouse (Fig. 41–6), an X-ray-induced mutant (Grüneberg, 1961) that is homozygous for a severe *Dll3* truncation mutation (Kusumi et al., 1998). Targeted deletion of *Dll3* displays defects similar to, but slightly more severe than, the pudgy mouse (Dunwoodie et al., 2002). The phenotype due to mutated human *DLL3* is strikingly similar (Fig. 41–7) (Turnpenny et al., 1991, 1999, 2003; Bulman et al., 2000), with multiple vertebral segmentation defects and rib fusions, which define the entity spondylocostal dysostosis.

CLINICAL DESCRIPTION OF THE SYNDROME

Nomenclature

At present, evidence from genotype–phenotype studies suggests that mutated *DLL3* is associated with a consistent pattern of abnormal vertebral segmentation, inherited as an autosomal recessive condition (Turnpenny et al., 2003). However, the term "spondylocostal dysostosis" (SCD) has been applied widely to a variety of radiological phenotypes, and it is therefore necessary to review the use of terminology.

Spondylocostal Dysostosis/Dysplasia

In both the medical literature and current clinical practice there is considerable confusion surrounding the term *spondylocostal dysostosis*.

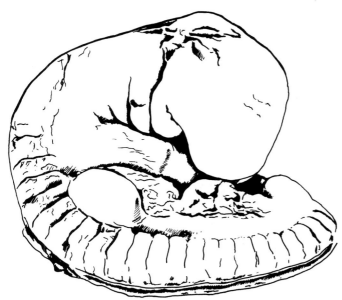

Figure 41–1. Line drawing of a human embryo at 35 days, showing the segmentation of tissues lateral to the neural tube into multiple, regular somites.

Not only has it been used, and continues to be used, for a variety of different radiological phenotypes, but a number of alternative terms are frequently applied interchangeably. Thus, the term is often applied to any radiograph of the spine and thoracic cage that includes multiple vertebral segmentation defects (even if the defects are restricted to a few vertebrae) in combination with abnormal rib alignment, with or without points of fusion between adjacent ribs. It is also frequently used when there is marked asymmetry of the thoracic cage with a significant reduction in rib number on one side (or sometimes both sides), often in association with scoliosis (Fig. 41–8) and including, of course, abnormal vertebral segmentation. Although different scoliotic and kyphotic curves are frequently present in these disorders, the group of conditions must be defined by the segmentation defect or defects rather than by spinal curvature.

The key radiological feature is the presence of irregularly shaped vertebrae that do not conform to their normal pattern. Excluded, therefore, are the various forms of severe platyspondyly conditions which are part of a generalized skeletal *dysplasia*, as well as a large number of rare but reasonably well delineated syndromes that include limited forms of abnormal vertebral segmentation, as listed in Table 41–1. Rather, SCD and associated conditions with multiple vertebral segmentation defects are truly developmental malformations and are properly designated *dysostoses*.

Costovertebral Dysplasia

In the older literature the term *costovertebral dysplasia* can be found (Norum and McKusick, 1969; Cantú et al., 1971; Bartsocas et al., 1974; David and Glass, 1983), but it is seldom used today. It is less appropriate than SCD, not only because these are not primarily dysplasias but also because the term diverts attention from the primary developmental defect having occurred in the formation of vertebrae.

Jarcho-Levin Syndrome

Many clinicians continue to use the eponymous *Jarcho-Levin syndrome* (JLS) across the spectrum of radiological phenotypes that include abnormal vertebral segmentation and rib alignment. In 1938 two siblings with severe segmentation defects of the entire vertebral column, though most severe in the thoracic region, and with fusion of several ribs were reported (Jarcho and Levin, 1938). Both siblings died in infancy of respiratory failure, and the firstborn may also have had dextrocardia. With fusion of many vertebral bodies, there were overlapping features with Klippel-Feil syndrome.

Spondylothoracic Dysplasia

The term *spondylothoracic dysplasia* is best reserved for the distinctive autosomal recessive condition, most commonly reported in Puerto Ricans, which is characterized by severe truncal shortening and a radiological appearance of the ribs fanning out from their vertebrocostal origin in a "crab-like" fashion (Fig. 41–9). Fusion of the ribs is present posteriorly at their vertebral origin, and otherwise they are usually neatly aligned and packed tightly together. The thoracic vertebrae appear most severely affected and "telescoped" together, and this condition has a distinctive phenotype that has been well characterized in recent studies (Cornier et al., 2000).

Infant mortality is approximately 50% due to restrictive respiratory insufficiency, and the widespread axial skeletal effects justify designation as a dysplasia. The term *spondylothoracic dysostosis/dysplasia* (STD) was first proposed by Moseley and Bonforte (1969), and genetic mapping studies have suggested the locus is within chromosome band 2q32 (Santiago-Cornier et al., 2001). Studies of the ultrastructure in JLS at necropsy are scarce. However, one report (Solomon et al., 1978) comments on an increased ratio between cartilage and bone on parasagittal sections of the vertebral bodies, with persistence of cartilage about the midline. The ossification centers were disorganized and varied in size and distribution, and in the lateral portion of some vertebral bodies longitudinal clefts of cartilage separated anterior and posterior ossification centers. Although the modeling of the vertebral bodies was severely disorganized, microscopic bone formation and structure were not disturbed.

A number of cases in the literature demonstrating this typical STD phenotype, predominantly in Puerto Ricans, are reported as examples of JLS (Lavy et al., 1966; Moseley and Bonforte, 1969; Pochaczevsky et al., 1971; Pérez-Comas and García-Castro, 1974; Gellis and Feingold, 1976; Trindade and de Nóbrega, 1977; Solomon et al., 1978; Tolmie et al., 1987; Schulman et al., 1993; McCall et al., 1994; Mortier et al., 1996), but it appears that Jarcho and Levin described a different condition which is closer to STD type 2 (see page 477) rather than STD. Certain other case reports designated as "JLS" are neither very similar to those described by Jarcho and Levin nor consistent with STD (Poor et al., 1983; Karnes et al., 1991; Simpson et al., 1995; Aurora et al., 1996; Eliyahu et al., 1997; Rastogi et al., 2002). Once a gene for STD in the Puerto Rican cohort is characterized, it will be possible to undertake genotype–phenotype studies that will further facilitate classification of this group of disorders.

Sporadically Occurring Abnormal Vertebral Segmentation

In clinical practice sporadically occurring cases of abnormal vertebral segmentation are far more common than those which are familial and apparently demonstrating mendelian inheritance. These sporadic cases

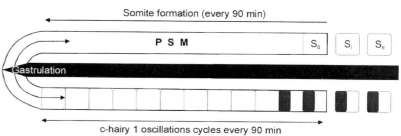

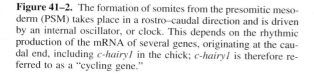

Figure 41–2. The formation of somites from the presomitic mesoderm (PSM) takes place in a rostro–caudal direction and is driven by an internal oscillator, or clock. This depends on the rhythmic production of the mRNA of several genes, originating at the caudal end, including *c-hairy1* in the chick; *c-hairy1* is therefore referred to as a "cycling gene."

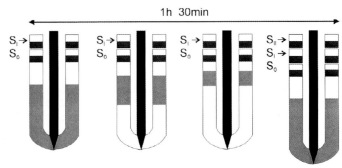

Figure 41–3. The internal oscillator, or clock, is determined by the expression of cycling genes that appear as a wave with their origin at the caudal end of the PSM. This wave sweeps across the PSM once during each somite formation and narrows as it proceeds in a caudal direction. It does not result from cell displacement but, instead, appears to reflect intrinsically coordinated pulses of mRNA expression.

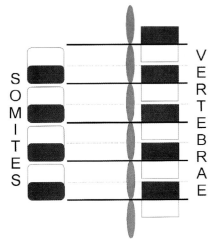

Figure 41–4. The early somites show internal differentiation into rostral and caudal compartments. Ultimately, in development, the vertebrae are formed from the caudal part of one somite and the adjacent rostral part of the next, a process known as "resegmentation."

are more likely to be associated with additional anomalies and are discussed in this section.

Association with Neural Tube Defects

A relatively common association with severely disorganized vertebrae, and rib alignment and number, is neural tube defect (NTD). This often gives rise to the most severely disrupted radiological phenotypes within this group (Fig. 41–10), but there is no evidence at present that *DLL3* is implicated in the causation. In our view it is debatable whether this NTD-associated group should be classified as part of the spondylocostal dysostoses. The primary developmental pathology presumably lies in the processes that determine neural tube closure rather than vertebral segmentation, with the latter causally linked as a consequential effect or sequence. The association of NTD with abnormal vertebral segmentation has been well documented (Wynne-Davies, 1975; Eller and Morton, 1970; McLennan, 1976; Naik et al., 1978; Lendon et al., 1981; Kozlowski, 1984; Giacoia and Say, 1991; Martínez-Frías et al., 1994; Sharma and Phadke, 1994), and the point has been made previously that classification should be based on the basic cause rather than on the radiological features (Martínez-Frías, 1996). Similarly, an association between either spina bifida occulta or diastematomyelia (or both) and costovertebral anomalies has been well reported (Poor et al., 1983; Aymé and Preus, 1986; Herold et al., 1988; Reyes et al., 1989), thus strongly suggesting a causal link or sequence, though the mechanisms remain to be elucidated.

Association with Multiple Congenital Abnormalities

As with NTD, multiple congenital abnormalities (MCA) occur relatively commonly in association with multiple vertebral segmentation defects, and such cases are far more likely to be sporadic rather than familial.

Epidemiological studies have highlighted the wide heterogeneity of this group (Martínez-Frías and Urioste, 1994), and the literature has been well reviewed by Mortier et al. (1996). Anal and urogenital anomalies are the most frequently occurring (Eller and Morton., 1970; Pochaczevsky et al., 1971; Bonaime et al., 1978; Devos et al., 1978; Poor et al., 1983; Kozlowski, 1984; Tolmie et al., 1987; Roberts et al., 1988; Gaicoia and Say, 1991; Karnes et al., 1991; Murr et al., 1992; Lin and Harster, 1993; Mortier et al., 1996), followed by a variety of congenital heart disease conditions (Delgoffe et al., 1982; Kozlowski, 1984; Ohzeki et al., 1990; Aurora et al., 1996; Mortier et al., 1996).

Limb abnormalities occur but are generally of a minor nature; they include talipes and oligodactyly or polydactyly (Karnes et al., 1991; Mortier et al., 1996). Infrequently, diaphragmatic hernia is a feature (Martínez-Frías et al., 1994; Lam et al., 1999). As a minor anomaly, inguinal and abdominal hernias are frequently reported in association with multiple vertebral segmentation defects. It is not clear at present whether these are part of the primary developmental abnormality complex or secondary to increased intra-abdominal pressure as a result of having a shortened spine and trunk. Many case reports could reasonably be assigned a diagnosis of the VATER (vertebral defects, anal atresia, tracheoesophageal fistula, radial defects, and renal anomalies) or VACTERL (vertebral defects, anal atresia, cardiac defects, tracheo-esophageal fistula, radial defects, and renal anomalies, non-radial limb defects) associations (Kozlowski, 1984), and this would appear to be a very heterogeneous group with few clues regarding causation at the present time.

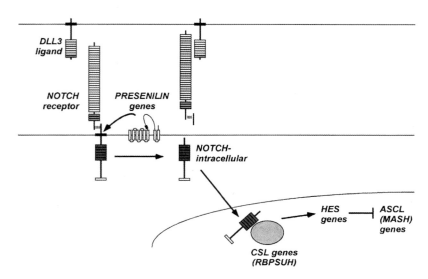

Figure 41–5. Notch is a large transmembrane receptor able to recognize two sets of transmembrane ligands, Delta and Serrate. Upon ligand binding, Notch undergoes a proteolytic cleavage by *presenilin* at membrane level, leading to the translocation of its intracytoplasmic domain (notch-ic) into the nucleus where it converts suppressors of hairless/CSL from repressors to activators of the *hairy* and *enhancer of split family*—which are the cycling genes exhibiting a rhythmic pattern of expression across the PSM.

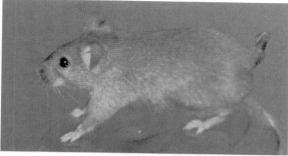

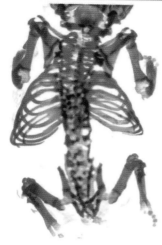

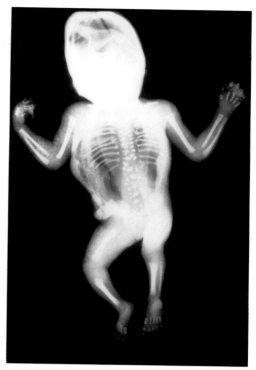

Figure 41–6. The pudgy mouse, an X-ray–induced mutant (Grüneberg, 1961), shown to be homozygous for a severe *Dll3* truncation mutation (Kusumi et al., 1998). Staining of the skeleton (*bottom*) reveals multiple vertebral segmentation defects and irregularly aligned ribs with points of fusion.

Association with Abnormal Karyotypes
It is important to include among the sporadic cases those in which a chromosomal abnormality has been found. Such cases are relatively rare, but seldom is investigation for tissue mosaicism undertaken (for example, by skin biopsy), so underdiagnosis of this group is possible. Apart from trisomy 8 mosaicism (Riccardi, 1977), there is no obvious pattern to the group with chromosome abnormalities. Deletions affecting both 18q (Dowton et al., 1997) and 18p (Nakano et al., 1977) have been reported, in addition to a supernumerary dicentric 15q marker (Crow et al., 1997) and an apparently balanced translocation between chromosomes 14 and 15 (De Grouchy et al., 1963) in the earliest period of investigative cytogenetics. In addition, one author (P.D.T.) is personally aware of a patient with a minor degree of segmentation abnormality who is mosaic for Klinefelter's syndrome. One can obviously postulate that haploinsufficiency may be unmasking a new mendelian locus for SCD, but the paucity and diversity of these cases may indicate that the resulting SCD in association with MCA represents a common pathway of complex pleiotropic developmental mechanisms that are sensitive to a range of unbalanced karyotypes.

Familial Abnormal Vertebral Segmentation
Monogenic forms of multiple vertebral segmentation defects, whether in "pure" form or "syndromic," are relatively rare compared to sporadically occurring cases. The phenotype defining autosomal recessive (AR) STD has been described above. In addition, there is a milder phenotype for which AR inheritance is either clear-cut or very likely (Norum and McKusick, 1969; Cantú et al., 1971; Castroviejo et al., 1973; Bartsocas et al., 1974; Silengo et al., 1978; Beighton and Horan, 1981; David and Glass, 1983; Poor et al., 1983; Young and Moore, 1984; Roberts et al., 1988; Turnpenny et al., 1991, 1999; Satar et al., 1992; Bulman et al., 2000). These cases are pure, nonsyndromic, forms of SCD and are characterized by multiple hemivertebrae throughout the entire spine (Figs. 41–7, 41–11). The trunk is shortened to a variable degree, the abdomen is protruberant (Fig. 41–12), and life-threatening complications are rare,

Figure 41–7. A fetus with vertebral segmentation defects throughout the spine and abnormally aligned ribs with points of fusion. This fetus was homozygous for *DLL3* mutations and is classified as having SCD type 1.

though one of the affected cases in the family reported by Turnpenny et al. (1991) succumbed at age 7 months with a large patent ductus arteriosus and a hypoplastic diaphragm at necropsy. Some other reports have also highlighted persistent foramen ovale. However, in general, this is a relatively mild and generally pure SCD phenotype and is the one in which *DLL3* mutations have been identified. As with JLS, inguinal hernias in males has been reported (Bonaime et al., 1978; Turnpenny et al., 1991), and mental retardation is not a feature. Published work on the ultra-

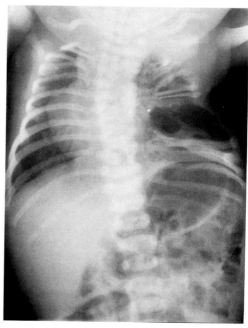

Figure 41–8. Multiple vertebral segmentation defects predominantly affect the thoracic spine and demonstrate marked asymmetry of rib formation. No *DLL3* mutations were identified.

Table 41–1. Some Syndromes and Conditions That Include Abnormal Vertebral Segmentation

Acrofacial dysostosis
Aicardi
Alagille
Anhalt
Atelosteogenesis III
Axial mesodermal dysplasia
Casamassima
Caudal regression
CHARGE association
Chromosomal abnormalities
Covesdem
Currarino
De la Chapelle
DiGeorge/Sedláčková
Dysspondylochondromatosis
Femoral hypoplasia–unusual facies
Fibrodysplasia ossificans progressiva
Frontonasal dysplasia
Fryns-Moerman
Goldenhar/Facio-auriculo-vertebral spectrum
Holmes-Schimke
Incontinentia pigmenti
Jarcho-Levin
Kabuki
Kaufman-McKusick
Klippel-Feil
Larsen
Maternal diabetes
MURCS association
Multiple pterygium syndrome
Pascual-Castroviejo
PHAVER
RAPADILINO
Robinow
Rokitansky sequence
Rolland-Desbuquois
Silverman
Simpson-Golabi-Behmel
Sirenomelia
Spondylocarpotarsal dysostosis
Spondylocostal dysostosis
Thakker-Donnai
Toriello
Urioste
VATER/VACTERL associations
Verhove-Vanhorick
Zimmer

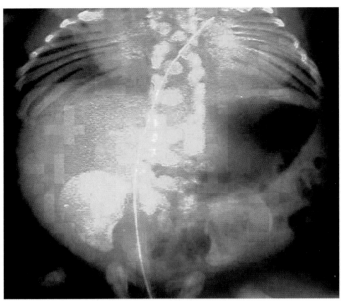

Figure 41–9. Spondylothoracic dysplasia. Radiologically this is characterized by severe truncal shortening, and the ribs fan out in a "crab-like" fashion. Fusion of the ribs is essentially at their vertebrocostal origin and, unlike SCD, seldom do the ribs show abnormal alignment with points of fusion along their length. (Image supplied courtesy of Alberto Santiago-Cornier, Ponce School of Medicine, Ponce, Puerto Rico.)

consistent within families and not dissimilar to that observed in *DLL3*-linked cases, with involvement of all vertebrae. Indeed, we have shown (Floor et al., 1989) that SCD is due to homozygously mutated *DLL3*, and the inheritance is pseudo-dominant (unpublished). This raises the question whether AD SCD families exist.

Summary

In this section we have discussed the different SCD phenotypes. There is marked heterogeneity and delineation is problematic. It is our view that

structure features of SCD is lacking; however, one author (P.D.T.) is personally aware of recent studies undertaken on one case and, although modeling of the vertebral bodies was disorganized, microscopic bone formation and structure were not disturbed.

Several families apparently demonstrating AR SCD, but with syndromic associations, have been reported. These include SCD with anal and urogenital anomalies (Casamassima et al., 1981), two affected siblings where one had hexadactyly of the left foot while the other had tetralogy of Fallot (Franceschini et al., 1974), and two siblings with congenital heart disease (Simpson et al., 1995). In all of these families, the spinal radiological phenotype is different from the *DLL3*-linked cases. The family described by Wadia et al. (1978), the so-called COVESDEM syndrome, is most likely AR Robinow syndrome.

A small number of SCD families demonstrating vertical transmission, and therefore probable autosomal dominant (AD) inheritance, have been reported (Van der Sar, 1952; Rütt and Degenhardt, 1959; Peralta et al., 1967; Rimoin et al., 1968; Kubryk and Borde, 1981; Temple et al., 1988; Floor et al., 1989; Lorenz and Rupprecht, 1990). These are generally mild, nonsyndromic cases. The radiological phenotype of the spine is very variable in one family (Temple et al., 1988), with restrictive pulmonary failure in the most severely affected adult but very limited spinal involvement in the mildest case. In four of the other families (Van der Sar, 1952; Rimoin et al., 1968; Floor et al., 1989; Lorenz and Rupprecht, 1990) the radiological phenotype is more

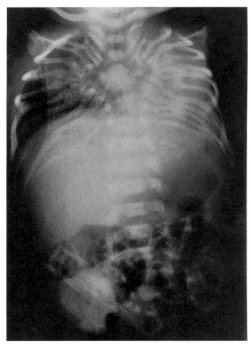

Figure 41–10. Severe mid-thoracic abnormal vertebral segmentation in association with neural tube defect. Apart from the region involved, segmentation is normal.

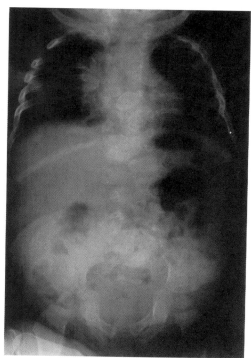

Figure 41–11. Spondylocostal dysostosis due to mutated *DLL3* type 1. Note the smooth vertebral body borders throughout the spine—the "pebble beach" sign.

the term "spondylocostal dysostosis" should be reserved for cases of multiple vertebral segmentation defects that affect the entire spine, usually combined with abnormally aligned ribs, frequently showing points of fusion. STD is a separate, distinct phenotype, and JLS (i.e., the condition described by Jarcho and Levin in 1938) appears different again and should

not be used indiscriminately. As we discuss further below ("SCD in Clinical Practice"), mutation analysis on different forms of SCD suggests a significant phenotype–genotype correlation, making it possible to delineate SCD type 1 (due to mutated *DLL3*) and at least one other form, for which we suggest, at present, the designation SCD type 2. In due course, it may transpire that several further subtypes can be delineated.

MOLECULAR GENETICS OF THE *DLL3* LOCUS AND DISEASE-CAUSING MUTATIONS

Genetic mapping by standard homozygosity of descent techniques (Lander and Botstein, 1987; Turnpenny et al., 1999) was used to identify a locus for AR SCD at chromosome 19q13.1 between markers D19S570 and D19S412, which included the extensive Arab-Israeli kindred first reported by Turnpenny et al. (1991). This region shares syntenic conservation with the murine chromosome 7 region that harbors the *Dll3* gene (Giampetro et al., 1999), which is truncated in the pudgy mouse (Kusumi et al., 1998). With the axial skeletal phenotype of pudgy demonstrating striking similarity to our AR SCD families, we hypothesized that a human *Dll3* ortholog would be a candidate gene for the SCD locus. This proved to be so in three consanguineous families (Bulman et al., 2000). The organization of human *DLL3* is shown in Figure 41–13. The reading frame of the gene spans 1.9 kb and consists of 9 exons. The exon–intron junctions within the predicted amino acid sequence are identical to those of mouse *Dll3*, except for the terminal exon, which corresponds to a fusion of mouse exons 9 and 10, resulting in a human protein of 32 additional amino acids. There is variability in the size of the mouse and human introns. The gene is sequentially ordered with a delta-serrate-lag (DSL) domain, six highly conserved epidermal growth factor (EGF) repeats, and the transmembrane (TM) region.

Autosomal Recessive SCD

A total of 17 *DLL3* mutations have now been published (Bultman et al., 2000; Sparrow et al., 2002; Bonafé et al., 2003; Turnpenny et al., 2003), and these are listed in Table 41–2. Those mutation data have been derived from a total of 18 families, 13 of whom are consanguineous.

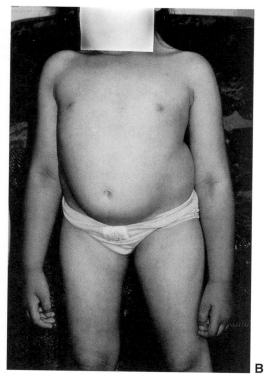

A   **B**

Figure 41–12. Clinical appearance of a child with SCD type 1 due to mutated *DLL3*. Note the shortened spine in relation to the limbs (*A*) and a thoracic lordosis. The shortened trunk can be appreciated in the frontal view, as well as the abdominal protrusion (*B*).

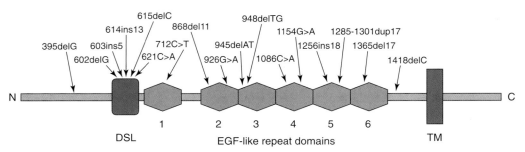

Figure 41–13. Organization of the *DLL3* gene. DSL, delta-serrate-lag domain; EGF, epidermal growth factor domain(s); TM, transmembrane domain.

Three mutations have been identified in more than one family. The 945delAT (T315C316del2) mutation has been found in two ethnic Pakistani kindreds originating from Kashmir, and analysis of DNA markers flanking the *DLL3* locus has identified a common haplotype, supporting the likelihood that these two kindreds have a common ancestry. Similarly, the 614insGTCCGGGACTGCG (R205ins13) mutation is found in two families, both consanguineous—one ethnic Lebanese Arabs and the other ethnic Turks. Haplotype analysis supports the likelihood of a common ancestry for these two Levant kindreds of the Middle East. The 593insGCGGT (S198ins5) mutation is present in the Arab-Israeli kindred, homozygous in those affected; in the Spanish family, the affected child is heterozygous for the same mutation. Haplotype analysis on these two pedigrees does *not* support a common ancestry, and the 593insGCGGT mutation is therefore believed to be recurrent, occurring as it does within a region of the gene with multiple repeat GCGGT sequences. Slipped mispairing during DNA replication probably explains the generation of this insertion mutation.

All the mutations identified in these AR SCD cases are clustered in exons 4–8 and are therefore located in the extracellular domain. Five of these are sited in the highly conserved EGF repeat domains. Fourteen mutations predict either a stop codon (three mutations) or a downstream protein truncation (eleven mutations). There are two missense mutations, one of which (G385D) results in the substitution of a highly conserved charged polar residue, glycine, for a nonpolar residue, aspartic acid, in the fifth EGF. The conservation of this residue

extends from *Drosophila melanogaster* through to humans, and substitution is therefore likely to disrupt conformation of the DLL3 protein, perhaps altering its ligand properties with notch or modification by the oscillator, or segmental clock, mediated by *lunatic fringe*. This mutation was found in a Pakistani family originating from Rawalpindi and was not found in a total of 72 controls—39 ethnic Pakistanis and 33 Arab-Israelis (Bulman et al., 2000). In addition, there is one donor splice site mutation (868del11) in exon 6. All of these mutations demonstrate that the membrane anchoring and correctly folded EGF-like repeats of DLL3 are essential for normal somitogenesis.

These mutations which cause AR SCD give rise to a consistent radiological and clinical phenotype (Turnpenny et al., 2003). Multiple vertebral segmentation defects (hemivertebrae) are present throughout the spine, and there is consistency in the abnormal form and shape of the vertebrae in the different regions from cervical to lumbar. As discussed below ("SCD in Clinical Practice"), the radiological appearances in childhood are of vertebrae which are circular or ovoid on anteroposterior projection, and they have smooth outlines.

One family from this cohort manifests abnormal clinical features in addition to the pure SCD that characterizes the rest of them. The affected siblings homozygous for the exon 8 mutation 1365del-CGCTCCCGGCTACATGG have manifested a form of distal arthrogryposis in keeping with a fetal akinesia sequence, and both succumbed in early childhood, though the exact reasons are unclear (C. McKeown, personal communication). There is multiple inbreeding in this particular family, and it is possible that a separate AR condition

Table 41–2. Mutations Identified within the *DLL3* Gene

Exon	Nucleotide	Amino Acid	Predicted Protein Alteration	Mutation Status	Ethnic Origin
4	395delG	G132del1	Frameshift—83 new amino acids and premature truncation	Heterozygous	Jewish—Ashkenazi (plus one Sephardic in family background)
5	603insGCGGT*	S198ins5	Frameshift—39 new amino acids and premature truncation	Homozygous	Arab-Israeli‡
				Heterozygous	Spanish‡
5	602delG	G201del1	Frameshift—39 new amino acids and premature truncation	Homozygous	Northern European
5	614insGTCCGGGACTGCG	R205ins13	Frameshift—15 new amino acids and premature truncation	Homozygous	Turkish†
				Homozygous	Arab-Lebanese†
5	615delC	R205del1	Frameshift	Heterozygous	European (Swiss)
5	621C > A	C207X	TGC > TGA (stop)	Heterozygous	Mixed European
6	712C > T	R238X	Stop	Heterozygous	European (Swiss)
6	868del11		Donor splice site deleted	Homozygous	Pakistani
7	926G > A	C309Y	Missense	Homozygous	Palestinian Arab
7	945delAT*	T315C316del2	Frameshift—16 new amino acids and premature truncation	Homozygous	Pakistani (Kashmir)†
					Pakistani (Kashmir)†
7	948delTG	A317del1	Frameshift—114 new amino acids and premature truncation	Heterozygous	English
7	1086C > A	C362X	Stop	Homozygous	Turkish
8	1285–1301dupCGCGCGGACCCGTGCGC	P437dup17	Frameshift	Homozygous	European (Swiss)
8	1154G > A	G385D	Gly > Asp in EGF5	Homozygous	Pakistani (Rawalpindi)
8	1256ins18		Fameshift	Heterozygous	Southern European
8	1365delCGCTCCCGGCTACATGG	C655M660del17	Frameshift—4 new amino acids and premature truncation	Homozygous	Pakistani
8	1418delC	A473del1	Frameshift—74 new amino acids and premature truncation	Heterozygous	Mixed European

*The nomenclature for these mutations has been modified slightly from that originally published (Bulman et al., 2000).
†Haplotype analysis supports the possibility of a common ancestry in these families with the same mutation.
‡Haplotype analysis does not support the probability of a common ancestry in these families with the same mutation.

is segregating coincidentally to SCD; the parents have one normal child, and thus far SCD has cosegregated with the abnormal neurological features.

Autosomal Dominant SCD

Thus far in AR SCD, no mutations have been identified that affect either the transmembrane (TM) or intracellular domains (ICD) of the DLL3 protein. However, we are aware of a patient with a de novo heterozygous ICD mutation consisting of a single nucleotide change—C1562T (S521F) in exon 8. The affected child has abnormal vertebral segmentation of a similar form to the AR cases, but, unlike the latter, it is very limited in its extent to a few vertebrae in the mid-thoracic region (S. Dunwoodie and R. Savarirayan, personal communication). At present, the pathogenicity of this S521F mutation is not established, but as a truncation of the intracellular domain of Delta or Serrate it may produce a dominant–negative phenotype. It has recently been shown that delta ligand activation of notch signaling requires endocytosis (Parks et al., 2000). It would be instructive to determine if the S521F type of mutation in delta ICD could potentially alter ligand conformation to disrupt normal endocytosis. Further studies are needed to establish whether *DLL3* mutations affecting the ICD consistently give rise to abnormal vertebral segmentation—that is, a form of SCD.

SCD IN CLINICAL PRACTICE

Establishing the Diagnosis: SCD Type 1

Clinically, SCD is a radiological diagnosis, and the variety of phenotypes seen in practice, and reported in the literature, has been discussed here. Minor forms of abnormal vertebral segmentation may only be diagnosed incidentally as a result of radiographs undertaken for unrelated reasons, but severe forms are usually diagnosed in the newborn period because truncal shortening is evident, with a short neck and protruberant abdomen. The presence or absence of additional anomalies is potentially significant in terms of a possible syndrome diagnosis, and standard karyotyping should be undertaken. In the face of a normal standard karyotype from peripheral blood lymphocytes, investigation for possible chromosomal mosaicism by skin biopsy is justified if suggestive features, such as asymmetry and neurodevelopmental delay, are present. This may be important for genetic counseling. Additional conventional investigations worth considering are renal ultrasound and echocardiography. If appropriate, the presence of neurological features should prompt magnetic resonance imaging of the spine in view of the occasional association with anomalies such as diastematomyelia.

It has already been mentioned that AR SCD due to mutated *DLL3* has a characteristic and consistent radiological phenotype (Figs. 41–7, 41–11). All vertebrae are involved, with no region preferentially affected, and the kyphoscoliotic curves are mild. These spinal curvatures are nonprogressive and on current experience a spine with abnormal segmentation that manifests progressive scoliotic deformity is unlikely to be due to mutated *DLL3*. Abnormal alignment of the ribs is likely to be a clear radiological feature, usually with points of fusion posteriorly or close to the costovertebral origin of the ribs. Occasionally rib number is reduced in *DLL3*-linked SCD. Many sporadic cases of abnormal vertebral segmentation, which will frequently be diagnosed as cases of SCD, have limited involvement of the vertebral column, and rib number may be both significantly reduced and asymmetrical (Fig. 41–8).

The form of the misshapen vertebrae in AR SCD due to mutated *DLL3* is emerging as characteristic and consistent (Turnpenny et al., 2003). These are circular or ovoid radiologically on anteroposterior projection and lack angular features (Figs. 41–7, 41–11). They have the appearance of smooth, eroded stones on a pebble beach, and we therefore suggest a new sign in skeletal radiology—the "pebble beach" sign. Furthermore, we suggest this strong phenotype–genotype correlation should be designated "SCD type 1," based on the characteristic and consistent phenotype for which the molecular genetic defect is now established. Confirmation of SCD type 1 is now possible by direct sequencing of *DLL3* or by appropriate mutation detection methods.

Establishing the Diagnosis: SCD Type 2

At least one other form of SCD occurs, based on a definition of SCD that combines the features of all vertebrae showing features of abnormal segmentation and the ribs being abnormally aligned but essentially symmetrical in number. In several cases of this kind, we have not found mutations in *DLL3*. In one consanguineous family, it has been possible to exclude linkage to *DLL3*. These cases differ in a subtle way from SCD type 1. The form of the misshapen vertebrae tends to be more angular than circular or ovoid, and there is more variability of form throughout the spinal column. An example is shown in Figure 41–14. In some cases, the lumbar vertebrae are distinct in form from the thoracic, demonstrating less segmentation disruption and a degree of platyspondyly. It is justified to include these cases as SCD given their clinical similarity to SCD type 1, and we therefore suggest the designation "SCD type 2." However, the mode of inheritance is not clear in all cases, and within this group there may well be heterogeneity. One such case in our cohort, for example, is an isolated case in the family who has cardiac situs inversus. The involvement of the entire spinal column in SCD type 2 suggests the likelihood of a disorder, or disorders, following mendelian inheritance, but the molecular basis remains to be elucidated. Progress is hampered by the apparent unavailability of any large affected kindred to facilitate genetic mapping studies.

Prenatal Diagnosis

Experience indicates that some couples at risk of having children with SCD choose prenatal diagnosis (PND) and termination of pregnancy, whereas others can accept and absorb the condition into their family, continuing to have children despite the genetic risk. The general absence of additional malformations or mental retardation in SCD type 1 should be mentioned in counseling before PND, and within an affected family these aspects may already be appreciated. If, following the birth (or termination) of an affected offspring, the molecular defect(s) in *DLL3* have been identified, early PND by chorionic villus sampling (CVS) is possible, taking the usual precautions to ensure that the DNA analyzed has contributions from both parents. To date there

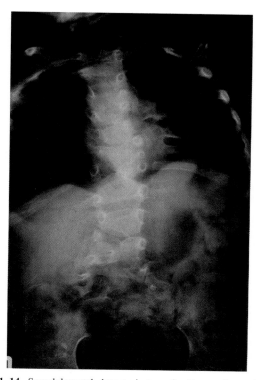

Figure 41–14. Spondylocostal dysostosis type 2. Abnormal vertebral segmentation throughout the spine with abnormal rib alignment and relatively "angular" contours to the vertebrae, but no mutations identified in *DLL3*. This is similar to, but distinct from, the radiological appearance of SCD type 1.

has been one report of PND using molecular genetic testing in a family with two affected offspring homozygous for a *DLL3* mutation (Whittock, et al., 2003)

PND has been achieved using imaging techniques. The first such diagnosis was made in 1979 using standard radiographs in the third trimester (Pérez-Comas and García-Castro). Naturally, the advent of ultrasonographic examination has transformed the ability to detect this condition prenatally. This has been reported several times (Apuzzio et al., 1987; Tolmie et al., 1987; Romero et al., 1988; Marks et al., 1989; Eliyahu et al., 1997; Lawson et al., 1997; Wong and Levine, 1998; Hull et al., 2001). All these case reports refer to the PND of "JLS" rather than SCD. However, the phenotype reported by Eliyahu is clearly SCD rather than JLS/STD, and the subjects are members of the same family reported by Turnpenny et al. (1991, 1999), whose *DLL3* mutation is established (Bulman et al., 2000). In the majority of these cases the diagnosis was made in the mid trimester between 16 and 23 weeks, based on the findings of a shortened spine, disorganization of the vertebral bodies, posterior fusion of the ribs, reduced chest diameter, protruberant abdomen, and normal long bone measurements. Apuzzio et al. (1987) discuss the difficulties in making an ultrasonographic diagnosis of JLS, but technical advances in image resolution are facilitating earlier diagnosis. Indeed, there have been two reports of first trimester diagnosis at 12 weeks using this modality (Eliyahu et al., 1997; Hull et al., 2001) in patients known to be at risk and therefore followed from early pregnancy. No misdiagnoses occurred. In the most recent of these cases (Hull et al., 2001) three-dimensional ultrasound was used to confirm a totally disorganized spine. Other accompanying features have included cystic hygroma and mild polyhydramnios.

Apart from the family reported by Eliyahu et al. (1997), one of us (P.D.T.) is aware that other SCD type 1 cases have been diagnosed prenatally on a number of occasions, generally in the early part of the second trimester. With ever-improving imaging technologies, it is likely that ultrasonography will have a far greater role in the prenatal diagnosis of SCD and JLS than CVS and mutation analysis. Not only is it becoming rapidly possible to make a diagnosis by ultrasound as early as CVS, but it avoids subjecting the fetus to the risk of an invasive procedure.

A potential dilemma arises when a disorganized spine (without NTD) is unexpectedly detected by routine ultrasound. In the absence of a positive family history or parental consanguinity, the precise type of abnormal vertebral segmentation present and the pattern of inheritance are likely to be in doubt. The offer of fetal karyotyping is fully justified with counseling provision appropriate to the outcome. Detailed ultrasonography looking for additional anomalies should be undertaken. The presence of multiple congenital abnormalities increases the likelihood of a sporadically occurring case, as well as the possibility of neurodevelopmental delay. Serial assessment of thoracic volume may give an indication of the risk of respiratory failure in infancy or early childhood, although no study addressing this specific question in this group of disorders has been undertaken. Interpretation of the findings must therefore follow the general principles with which an experienced ultrasonographer will be familiar.

Management and Treatment

SCD due to mutated *DLL3* tends to be a mild condition in medical terms. The spinal malformation is radiologically dramatic but does not cause a progressive kyphoscoliosis; neurological complications are not reported. Surgical interference of the spine is therefore unlikely to be necessary. This is not necessarily true of other forms of SCD that are not *DLL3*-linked. Some cases demonstrate progressive spinal curvature, and the presence of diastematomyelia may give rise to neurological complications. In doubtful cases, therefore, serial radiological assessment at intervals through childhood is indicated, accompanied by detailed clinical, especially neurological, evaluation. As mentioned already in this section, renal and cardiac imaging is indicated and should be undertaken in infancy.

The presence of either inguinal or abdominal hernias (or both) will be evident on clinical examination and will require surgical intervention according to normal principles. The most serious potential com-

plication, however, is the threat of respiratory failure due to restricted chest size and reduced thoracic cage and lung volume, which may be exacerbated in some forms of SCD by progressive and marked scoliosis. This is only a small threat in AR SCD due to mutated *DLL3*, but it may be life-threatening in STD and other severe, sporadic forms of abnormal vertebral segmentation. Approximately 50% of children with the classic STD phenotype succumb to respiratory failure in early childhood. The effect of long-term intensive care in severe cases remains to be evaluated. It is these cases which are at most theoretical risk of abdominal wall herniation and the consequences of nonintervention; however, morbidity due to strangulated hernias has not, to our knowledge, been reported.

Some individuals with SCD type 1 have significant short stature, and this is also true of survivors with STD. The possible psychological impact in these cases has not been evaluated but may be significant in some cases. Additionally, the stigmatization of having a birth defect may, in some ethnic communities, greatly reduce marriage prospects for affected females.

Counseling

Familial forms of SCD following mendelian inheritance are more commonly AR than AD. This is true so far for SCD type 1, due to mutated *DLL3*, STD, and some other forms of SCD (designated type 2 at present) that are distinct from the *DLL3* phenotype. When normal parents have had more than one affected child—preferably confirmed by normal spinal radiology in the parents—counseling for AR inheritance is straightforward. However, multiple consanguinity is common in some ethnic communities, and the possibility of pseudodominance must be considered where there is parent–child transmission. Although some intrafamilial variability may occur (Cantú et al., 1971; Franceschini et al., 1974; Trindade and de Nóbrega, 1977; Turnpenny et al., 1991), the phenotype and severity is reasonably consistent, and for SCD type 1 we have shown this to be largely true between affected families (Turnpenny et al., 2003).

Families demonstrating clear AD inheritance appear to be rare, but when this pattern is present, especially in the absence of consanguinity, counseling is again straightforward, with the cautionary note that variability may be a feature (Temple et al., 1988). As noted previously, we have observed pseudodominance (unpublished) in a family previously reported as AD SCD (Floor et al., 1989).

Genetic counseling may be difficult, however, when the clinician is faced with an isolated case where the precise classification is uncertain. The presence of additional organ system anomalies makes it more likely that the case is sporadic (Mortier et al., 1996), but this is not an absolute principle (Casamassima et al., 1981). When accompanied by open spina bifida, risk counseling is probably the most appropriate, although the dilemmas presented by this situation have been discussed (Sharma and Phadke, 1994). There do not appear to be any truly familial cases of SCD or STD incorporating open myelomeningocele, though several reports interpret the presence of open neural arches of the vertebrae as "spina bifida" (Moseley and Bonforte, 1969; Pochaczevsky et al., 1971; Solomon et al., 1978) in cases that otherwise bear the features of STD. We presume the primary pathology in these cases is abnormal vertebral segmentation rather than failure of neural tube closure. In a study of a heterogeneous group of patients with "congenital scoliosis" with more than one abnormally degmented vertebrae (not single isolated vertebral defects), Wynne-Davies (1975) found a sibling recurrence risk of 2–3%.

At present, it appears that abnormal segmentation throughout the entire spine is more likely to be due to single gene damage than cases where abnormal segmentation is restricted to a region such as the thoracic spine. However, there are apparent exceptions to this rule, as highlighted by the case of monozygotic twins discordant for SCD (Van Thienen and Van der Auwera, 1994), and AR Robinow syndrome is also a notable exception. Where the entire spine is involved, and the case is isolated, it is not possible to be confident of the pattern of inheritance, for this could be AR or AD. It is possible with experience, however, to be reasonably confident of SCD type 1 on the basis of the entire spine being involved, and with the presence of the pebble beach sign. In many cases doubt will remain, but in due course it will hopefully be possible to offer more comprehensive genetic testing to resolve the causation, and with further epidemiological analysis to develop more accurate risk assessment based on a combination of the phenotype and the outcome of mutation screening.

DELTA-LIKE MUTATIONS IN MODEL SYSTEMS

Delta (*Dl*) and *Notch* are among the first characterized developmental mutations in the *Drosophila* model system (Poulson, 1937). *Dl* is required for numerous embryonic processes, including determination of neurogenic and muscle cell fates, as well as antennal, leg, retinal, wing, and bristle development (Muskavitch, 1994). Up to 288 mutation alleles have been recorded for *Dl*, with many displaying both dominantly inherited visible phenotypes and recessive embryonic lethality (Flybase). Mutation analysis in *Dl* has demonstrated the functional role of the delta-serrate-lag2 conserved (DSL) domain and 9 EGF-like domains of this notch ligand. Cell aggregation assays have been used to show that these *Dl* domains interact with EGF repeats 11 and 12 of the *Notch* receptor. Secreted extracellular forms of *Dl* exhibit antagonistic effects for transmembrane *Dl* ligand signaling.

Vertebrate homologs of *Dl* have been identified in numerous model systems. In the mouse, targeted mutations of delta-like 1 (*Dll1*) have been reported, with recessive embryonic lethality due to defects in vascular formation and somitogenesis (Hrabé de Angelis et al., 1997). Human defects of *DLL1* have not yet been identified. Two mutation alleles have been reported for *Dll3* that both severely disrupt somite segmentation—the *Dll3^pu* (*pudgy*) 4 bp deletion and a targeted deletion (Kusumi et al., 1998; Dunwoodie et al., 2002). *Dll3* somite malformations were recessively inherited, but abnormal expression of *Dll3* itself was noted in paraxial mesoderm of heterozygous *Dll3^pu* embryos, suggesting autoregulation. Furthermore, transgenic insertion of genomic clones containing *Dll3* did not result in skeletal defects, possibly due to regulatory compensation of extra *Dll3* transgenic copies. Delta-like 4 (*Dll4*) has been cloned in mouse and humans and was found to be expressed in arterial epithelium (Shutter et al., 2000), but mutations have not been reported.

In zebrafish, four homologs (*deltaA, deltaB, deltaC,* and *deltaD*) have been cloned, and the *after eight* spontaneous mutation in *deltaD* disrupts segmentation in somitogenesis (Haddon et al., 1998; Holley et al., 2000). X-Delta-2 has been cloned in the frog *Xenopus laevis*, and overexpression of truncated, extracellular-only forms of the ligand disrupted normal somitogenesis (Jen et al., 1997). Due to divergent gene duplication events in vertebrate evolution between mammals and fish/amphibians, it is not possible to define exact orthologs for the delta-like genes. Confusingly, the EGF repeat-containing gene, delta homolog-like 1 (*DLK1*), has been described, but it is divergent in sequence from the *DLL* genes. To avoid confusion, the mammalian homologs have been given the nomenclature *DLL1, DLL3,* and *DLL4*. Overall, mutation analysis from model systems has demonstrated that the *DLL* genes play roles in multiple developmental events, particularly in somitogenesis for vertebrate genes.

DEVELOPMENTAL PATHOGENESIS IN SPONDYLOCOSTAL DYSOSTOSIS

Recent developmental and genetic studies have contributed greatly to our understanding of somite segmentation. Biological theorists have long speculated on the mechanism that underlies the repatterning of homogeneous mesoderm during somitogenesis into discrete, regularly-sized somite segments. Somitogenesis is the basis for regular patterning of the vertebrae, discs, and spinal nerves that comprise the adult spine. One popular model invokes an oscillator or clock (Fig. 41–3), which regulates the patterning of somites (reviewed in Palmeirim et al., 1997; Pourquié and Kusumi, 2001). Physical evidence for such an oscillator was provided by observations that notch pathway genes display dynamic expression, including lunatic fringe (*Lfng*), hairy/enhancer of split homologs-1 and 7 (*Hes1, Hes7*) in the mouse, and c-*hairy-1*, c-*hairy-2,* and c-*hey-2* in the chick (Forsberg et al., 1998; McGrew et al., 1998; Aulehla and Johnson, 1999; Jiang et al., 2000; Jouve et al., 2000; Leimeister et al., 2000; Bessho et al., 2001). Ex-

pression of these genes was observed to oscillate toward the rostral margin of the unsegmented, presomitic mesoderm, in synchrony with each somite cycle. Mutations of noncycling genes in the notch pathway, including *Dll3*, have been found to disrupt these oscillations, providing a developmental mechanism for the segmentation defects of spondylocostal dysostosis (Kusumi et al., 1998). The function of these oscillations is currently being debated, but one model proposes that the "somite clock" is responsible for synchronizing cohorts of cells within the presomitic mesoderm, to refine to prospective somite borders (Jiang et al., 2000). In a second model, the oscillations are thought to regulate rostral versus caudal somite cell identity and patterning of boundaries. In addition, the determination of somite boundaries has been found to be regulated by the molecule FGF8 in the chick (Dubrulle et al., 2001). FGF8 was found to maintain presomitic mesodermal cells in an immature state; moreover, the proposective boundary cells were transiently determined at a FGF8 threshold boundary, approximately four somite-widths caudal to the PSM border. Existence of both FGF8 and oscillatory genes of the notch pathway were essential for determining these prospective borders.

Intriguingly, genes of the notch signaling pathway including *Dll3* have been found to be expressed during dynamic patterning of the central nervous system (Kusumi et al., 2001), and defects have been reported in *Dll3^pu* neuroventricles (Kusumi et al., 1998; Dunwoodie et al., 2002). Work is ongoing in the chick, mouse, and zebrafish model systems to determine the role of the notch pathway genes, including *Dll3*, in these other patterning mechanisms. Our further understanding of delta-like 3 and other genes of the notch signaling pathway in model systems will facilitate the unraveling of this developmental pathway in humans, thus providing the opportunity to study candidate genes in different phenotypes where the dominant feature is abnormal vertebral segmentation.

REFERENCES

Apuzzio JJ, Diamond N, Ganesh V, Desposito F (1987). Difficulties in the prenatal diagnosis of Jarcho-Levin syndrome. *Am J Obstet Gynecol* 156: 916–918.

Aulehla A, Johnson RL (1999). Dynamic expression of lunatic fringe suggests a link between notch signaling and an autonomous cellular oscillator driving somite segmentation. *Dev Biol* 207: 49–61.

Aurora P, Wallis CE, Winter RM (1996). The Jarcho-Levin syndrome (spondylocostal dysplasia) and complex congenital heart disease: a case report. *Clin Dysmorphol* 5: 165–169.

Aymé S, Preus M (1986). Spondylocostal/spondylothoracic dysostosis: the clinical basis for prognosticating and genetic counselling. *Am J Med Genet* 24: 599–606.

Bagnall KM, Higgins SJ, Sanders EJ (1989). The contribution made by cells from a single somite to tissues within a body segment and assessment of their integration with similar cells from adjacent segments. *Development* 107: 931–943.

Bartsocas CS, Kiossoglou KA, Papas CV, Xanthou-Tsingoglou M, Anagnostakis DE, Daskalopoulou HD (1974). Costovertebral dysplasia. *Birth Defects OAS* 10(9): 221–226.

Beighton P, Horan FT (1981). Spondylocostal dysostosis in South African sisters. *Clin Genet* 19: 23–25.

Bessho Y, Miyoshi G, Sakata R, Kageyama R (2001). Hes7: a bHLH-type repressor gene regulated by Notch and expressed in the presomitic mesoderm. *Genes Cells* 6: 175–185.

Bonafé L, Giunta C, Gassner M, Steinmann M, Superti-Furga A (2003). A cluster of autosomal recessive spondylocostal dysostosis caused by three newly identified *DLL3* mutations segregating in a small village. *Clin Genet* 64: 28–35.

Bonaime JL, Bonne B, Joannard A, Guerard L, Guilhot J, Cotton B, Butel J, et al. (1978). Le syndrome de dysostose spondylothoracique ou spondylocostale. *Pédiatrie* 33: 173–188.

Bruckner K, Perez L, Clausen H, Cohen S (2000). Glycosyl transferase activity of Fringe modulates Notch–Delta interactions. *Nature* 406: 411–415.

Bulman MP, Kusumi K, Frayling TM, McKeown C, Garrett C, Lander ES, Krumlauf R, Hattersley AT, Ellard S, Turnpenny PD (2000). Mutations in the human *Delta* homologue, *DLL3*, cause axial skeletal defects in spondylocostal dysostosis. *Nat Genet* 24: 438–441.

Cantú JM, Urrusti J, Rosales G, Rojas A (1971). Evidence for autosomal recessive inheritance of costovertebral dysplasia. *Clin Genet* 2: 149–154.

Casamassima AC, Morton CC, Nance WE, Kodroff M, Caldwell R, Kelly T, Wolf B (1981). Spondylocostal dysostosis associated with anal and urogenital anomalies in a Mennonite sibship. *Am J Med Genet* 8: 117–127.

Castroviejo P, Rodriguez-Costa T, Castillo F (1973). Spondylo-thoracic dysplasia in three sisters. *Dev Med Child Neurol* 15: 348–354.

Cornier AS, Ramrez-Lluch N, Arroyo S, Marquez A, Acevedo J, Warman M (2000). Natural history of Jarcho-Levin syndrome. *Am J Hum Genet* 67(4)(Suppl.2): 56(A238). (Abstract).

Crow YJ, Tolmie JL, Rippard K, Nairn L, Wilkinson AG, Turner T (1997). Spondylocostal dysostosis associated with a 46,XX, +15,dic(6;15)(q25;q11.2) translocation. *Clin Dysmorphol* 6: 347–350.

David TJ, Glass A (1983). Hereditary costovertebral dysplasia with malignant cerebral tumour. *J Med Genet* 20: 441–444.

De Grouchy J, Mlynarski JC, Maroteaux P, Lamy M, Deshaies G, Benichou C, Salmon C (1963). Syndrome polydysspondylique par translocation 14–15 et dyschondrostéose chez un même sujet: ségrégation familiale. *C R Acad Sci [D] Paris* 256: 1614–1616.

Delgoffe C, Hoeffel JC, Worms AM, Bretagne MC, Pernot C, Pierson M (1982). Dysostoses spondylocostales et cardiopathies congénitales. *Ann Pédiatr* 29: 135–139.

Devos EA, Leroy JG, Braeckman JJ, Vanden Bulcke L-J, Langer LO (1978). Spondylocostal dysostosis and urinary tract anomaly: definition and review of an entity. *Eur J Pediatr* 128: 7–15.

Dowton SB, Hing AV, Sheen-Kaniecki V, Watson MS (1997). Chromosome 18q22.2–qter deletion and a congenital anomaly syndrome with multiple vertebral segmentation defects. *J Med Genet* 34: 414–417.

Dubrulle J, McGrew MJ, Pourquié O (2001). FGF signaling controls somite boundary position and regulates segmentation clock control of spatiotemporal Hox gene activation. *Cell* 106: 219–232.

Dunwoodie SL, Clements M, Sa X, Conlon R, Beddington RSP (2002) Axial skeletal defects caused by mutation in the spondylocostal dysostosis/pudgy gene *Dll3* are associated with disruption of the segmentation clock within the presomitic mesoderm. *Development* 129: 1795–1806.

Eliyahu S, Weiner E, Lahav D, Shalev E (1997). Early sonographic diagnosis of Jarcho-Levin syndrome: a prospective screening program in one family. *Ultrasound Obstet Gynecol* 9: 314–318.

Eller JL, Morton JM (1970). Bizarre deformities in offspring of user of lysergic acid diethylamide. *N Engl J Med* 283: 395–397.

Evrard YA, Lun Y, Aulehla A, Gan L, Johnson RL (1998). *lunatic fringe* is an essential mediator of somite segmentation and patterning. *Nature* 394: 377–381.

Ewan KB, Everett AW (1992). Evidence for resegmentation in the formation of the vertebral column using the novel approach of retroviral-mediated gene transfer. *Exp Cell Res* 198: 315–320.

Floor E, De Jong RO, Fryns JP, Smulders C, Vles JSH (1989). Spondylocostal dysostosis: an example of autosomal dominant inheritance in a large family. *Clin Genet* 36: 236–241.

Forsberg H, Crozet F, Brown NA (1998). Waves of mouse Lunatic fringe expression, in four-hour cycles at two-hour intervals, precede somite boundary formation. *Curr Biol* 8: 1027–1030.

Franceschini P, Grassi E, Fabris C, Bogetti G, Randaccio M (1974). The autosomal recessive form of spondylocostal dysostosis. *Radiology* 112: 673–675.

Gellis SS, Feingold M (1976). Picture of the month: spondylothoracic dysplasia. *Am J Dis Child* 130: 513–514.

Giacoia GP, Say B (1991). Spondylocostal dysplasia and neural tube defects. *J Med Genet* 28: 51–53.

Giampietro PF, Raggio CL, Blank RD (1999). Synteny-defined candidate genes for congenital and idiopathic scoliosis. *Am J Med Genet* 83: 164–177.

Goldstein RS, Kalcheim C (1992). Determination of epithelial half-somites in skeletal morphogenesis. *Development* 116: 441–445.

Grüneberg H (1961). Genetical studies on the skeleton of the mouse. *Genet Res Camb* 2: 384–393.

Haddon C, Smithers L, Schneider-Maunoury S, Coche T, Henrique D, Lewis J (1998). Multiple delta genes and lateral inhibition in zebrafish primary neurogenesis. *Development* 125(3): 359–370.

Herold HZ, Edlitz M, Barochin A (1988). Spondylothoracic dysplasia. *Spine* 13: 478–481.

Holley SA, Geisler R, Nusslein-Volhard C (2000). Control of her1 expression during zebrafish somitogenesis by a delta-dependent oscillator and an independent wave-front activity. *Genes Dev* 14(13): 1678–1690.

Hrabé de Angelis M, McIntyre J, Gossler A (1997). Maintenance of somite borders in mice requires the Delta homologue Dll1. *Nature* 386: 717–721.

Hull AD, James G, Pretorius DH (2001). Detection of Jarcho-Levin syndrome at 12 weeks by nuchal translucency screening and three-dimensional ultrasound. *Prenat Diagn* 21: 390–394.

Jarcho S, Levin PM (1938). Hereditary malformation of the vertebral bodies. *Bull Johns Hopkins Hosp* 62: 216–226.

Jen W-C, Wettstein D, Turner D, Chitnis A, Kintner C (1997). The Notch ligand, X-Delta-2, mediates segmentation of the paraxial mesoderm in Xenopus embryos. *Development* 124: 1169–1178.

Jiang YJ, Aerne BL, Smithers L, Haddon C, Ish-Horowicz D, Lewis J (2000). Notch signalling and the synchronization of the somite segmentation clock. *Nature* 408(6811): 475–479.

Jouve C, Palmeirim I, Henrique D, Beckers J, Gossler A, Ish-Horowicz D, Pourquié O (2000). Notch signalling is required for cyclic expression of the hairy-like gene HES1 in the presomitic mesoderm. *Development* 127: 1421–1429.

Karnes PS, Day D, Barry SA, Pierpoint MEM (1991). Jarcho-Levin syndrome: four new cases and classification of subtypes. *Am J Med Genet* 40: 264–270.

Keynes RJ, Stern, CD (1988). Mechanisms of vertebrate segmentation. *Development* 103: 413–429.

Kozlowski K (1984). Spondylo-costal dysplasia. *Fortschr Röntgenstr* 140: 204–209.

Kubryk N, Borde M (1981). La dysostose spondylocostale. *Pédiatrie* 17: 137–146.

Kusumi K, Sun ES, Kerrebrock AW, Bronson RT, Chi D-C, Bulotsky MS, Spencer JB, Birren BW, Frankel WN, Lander ES (1998). The mouse pudgy mutation disrupts *Delta* homologue Dll3 and initiation of early somite boundaries. *Nat Genet* 19: 274–278.

Kusumi K, Dunwoodie SL, Krumlauf R (2001). Dynamic expression patterns of the pudgy/spondylocostal dysostosis gene *DLL3* in the developing nervous system. *Mech Dev* 100: 141–144.

Lam YH, Eik-Nes SH, Tang MHY, Lee CP, Nicholls JM (1999). Prenatal sonographic features of spondylocostal dysostosis and diaphragmatic hernia in the first trimester. *Ultrasound Obstet Gynecol* 13: 213–215.

Lander ES, Botstein D (1987). Homozygosity mapping: a way to map human recessive traits with the DNA of inbred children. *Science* 236: 1567–1570.

Lavy NW, Palmer CG, Merritt AD (1966). A syndrome of bizarre vertebral anomalies. *J Pediatr* 69: 1121–1125.

Lawson ME, Share J, Benacerraf B, Krauss CM. (1997). Jarcho-Levin syndrome: prenatal diagnosis, perinatal care and followup of siblings. *J Perinatol* 17: 407–409.

Leimeister C, Dale K, Fischer A, Klamt B, Hrabé de Angelis M, Radtke F, McGrew MJ, Pourquié O, Gessler M (2000). Oscillating expression of c-hey2 in the presomitic mesoderm suggests that the segmentation clock may use combinatorial signaling through multiple interacting bHLH factors. *Dev Biol* 227: 91–103.

Lendon RG, Wynne-Davies R, Lendon M (1981). Are congenital vertebral anomalies and spina bifida cystica aetiologically related? *J Med Genet* 18: 424–427.

Lin AE, Harster GA (1993). Another case of spondylocostal dyplasia and severe anomalies. *Am J Med Genet* 46: 476–477. (Letter).

Lorenz P, Rupprecht E (1990). Spondylocostal dysostosis: dominant type. *Am J Med Genet* 35: 219–221.

Marks F, Hernanz-Schulman M, Horii S, Greenland VC, Lustig I, Snyder J, Young BK, Greco MA, Subramanyam B, Genieser NB (1989). Spondylothoracic dysplasia: clinical and sonographic diagnosis. *J Ultrasound Med* 8: 1–5.

Martínez-Frías ML (1996). Multiple vertebral segmentation defects and rib anomalies. *Am J Med Genet* 66: 91.

Martínez-Frías ML, Urioste M (1994). Segmentation anomalies of the vertebrae and ribs: a developmental field defect—epidemiologic evidence. *Am J Med Genet* 49: 36–44.

Martínez-Frías ML, Bermejo E, Paisán L, Martín M, Egüés J, López JA, Martínez S, Orbea C, et al. (1994). Severe spondylocostal dysostosis associated with other congenital anomalies: a clinical/epidemiological analysis and description of ten cases from the Spanish Registry. *Am J Med Genet* 51: 203–212.

McCall CP, Hudgins L, Cloutier M, Greenstein RM, Cassidy SB (1994). Jarcho-Levin syndrome: unusual survival in a classical case. *Am J Med Genet* 49: 328–332.

McGrew MJ, Dale JK, Fraboulet S, Pourquié O (1998). The lunatic fringe gene is a target of the molecular clock linked to somite segmentation in avian embryos. *Curr Biol* 8: 979–982.

McLennan JE (1976). Rib anomalies in myelodysplasia. *Biol Neonate* 29: 129–141.

Moloney DJ, Panin VM, Johnston SH, Chen J, Shao L, Wilson R, Wang Y, Stanley P, Irvine KD, Haltiwanger RS, et al. (2000). Fringe is a glycosyltransferase that modifies Notch. *Nature* 406: 360–375.

Mortier GR, Lachman RS, Bocian M, Rimoin DL (1996). Multiple vertebral segmentation defects: analysis of 26 new patients and review of the literature. *Am J Med Genet* 61: 310–319.

Moseley JE, Bonforte RJ (1969). Spondylothoracic dysplasia: a syndrome of congenital anomalies. *Am J Roentgenol* 106: 166–169.

Mumm JS, Kopan R (2000). Notch signaling: from the outside in. *Dev Biol* 228: 151–165.

Murr MM, Waziri MH, Schelper RL, Abu-Youself M (1992). Case of multiple vertebral anomalies, cloacal dysgenesis, and other anomalies presenting prenatally as cystic kidneys. *Am J Med Genet* 42: 761–765.

Muskavitch MAT (1994). Delta-notch signaling and *Drosophila* cell fate choice. *Dev Biol* 166: 415–430.

Naik PR, Lendon RG, Barson AJ (1978). A radiological study of vertebral and rib malformations in children with myelomeningocele. *Clin Radiol* 29: 427–430.

Nakano S, Okuno T, Hojo H, Misawa S, Abe T (1977). 18p-syndrome associated with hemivertebrae, fused ribs and micropenis. *Jpn J Hum Genet* 22: 27–32.

Norum RA, McKusick VA (1969). Costovertebral anomalies with apparent recessive inheritance. *Birth Defects OAS* 18: 326–329.

Ohzeki T, Shiraishi M, Matsumoto Y, Takagi J, Motozumi H, Hanaki K (1990). Sporadic occurrence of spondylocostal dysplasia and mesocardia in a Japanese girl. *Am J Med Genet* 37: 427–428.

Palmeirim I, Henrique D, Ish-Horowicz D, Pourquié O (1997). Avian hairy gene expression identifies a molecular clock linked to vertebrate segmentation and somitogenesis. *Cell* 91: 639–648.

Parks AL, Klueg KM, Stout JR, Muskavitch MA (2000). Ligand endocytosis drives receptor dissociation and activation in the Notch pathway. *Development* 127: 1373–1385.

Peralta A, Lopez C, Gracia R, Crespo LM (1967). Polidispondilia familiar. *Rev Pediatr Obstet Gynecol [Pediatr]* 7: 93–96.

Pérez-Comas A, García-Castro JM (1974). Occipito-facial-cervico-thoracic-abdomino-digital dysplasia: Jarcho-Levin syndrome of vertebral anomalies. *J Pediatr* 85: 388–391.

Pérez-Comas A, García-Castro JM (1979). Prenatal diagnosis of OFCTAD dysplasia or Jarcho-Levin syndrome. New York: Alan R. Liss for the National Foundation, March of Dimes. *Birth Defects: OAS* 14(5A): 39–44.

Pochaczevsky R, Ratner H, Perles D, Kassner G, Naysan P (1971). Spondylothoracic dysplasia. *Radiology* 98: 53–58.

Poor MA, Alberti A, Griscom T, Driscoll SG, Holmes LB (1983). Nonskeletal malformations in one of three siblings with Jarcho-Levin syndrome of vertebral anomalies. *J Pediatr* 103: 270–272.

Poulson DF (1937). Chromosomal deficiencies and embryonic development of *Drosophila melanogaster*. *Proc Natl Acad Sci USA* 23: 133–137.

Pourquié O, Kusumi K (2001). When body segmentation goes wrong. *Clin Genet* 60: 409–416.

Rastogi D, Rosenzweig EB, Koumbourlis A (2002). Pulmonary hypertension in Jarcho-Levin syndrome. *Am J Med Genet* 107: 250–252.

Remak R (1850). *Untersuchungen über die Entwicklung der Wirbeltiere*. Reimer, Berlin.

Reyes MC, Morales A, Harris V, Barreta TM, Goldbarg H (1989). Neural defects in Jarcho-Levin syndrome. *J Child Neurol* 4: 51–54.

Riccardi VM (1977). Trisomy 8: an international study of 70 patients. *Birth Defects OAS* 13(3C): 171–184.

Rimoin DL, Fletcher BD, McKusick VA (1968). Spondylocostal dysplasia. *Am J Med Genet* 45: 948–953.

Roberts AP, Conner AN, Tolmie JL, Connor JM (1988). Spondylothoracic and spondylocostal dysostosis. *J Bone Joint Surg Br* 70B: 123–126.

Romero R, Ghidini A, Eswara MS, Seashore MR, Hobbins JC (1988). Prenatal findings in a case of spondylocostal dysplasia type I (Jarcho-Levin syndrome). *Obstet Gynecol* 71: 988–991.

Rütt A, Degenhardt KH (1959). Beitrag zur Ätiologie und Pathogenese von Wirbelsäulenmißbildungen. *Arch Orthop Unfallchir* 51: 120–139.

Saga Y, Hata N, Koseki H, Taketo MM (1997). Mesp2: a novel mouse gene expressed in the presegmented mesoderm and essential for segmentation initiation. *Genes Dev* 11: 1827–1839.

Santiago-Cornier A, Ramirez N, Franceschini V, Acevedo J, Roman H, Rosado E, Garcia L, Torres J (2001). Mapping of spondylothoracic dysplasia (Jarcho-Levin syndrome) to chromosome 2q32.1 in Puerto Rican population. *Am J Hum Genet* 69(4)(Suppl): 514(A1946). (Abstract).

Satar M, Kozanoglu MN, Atilla E (1992). Identical twins with an autosomal recessive form of spondylocostal dysostosis. *Clin Genet* 41: 290–292.

Schulman M, Gonzalez MT, Bye MR (1993). Airway abnormalities in Jarcho-Levin syndrome: a report of two cases. *J Med Genet* 30: 875–876.

Sharma AK, Phadke SR (1994). Another case of spondylocostal dysplasia and severe anomalies: a diagnostic and counseling dilemma. *Am J Med Genet* 50: 383–384.

Shutter JR, Scully S, Fan W, Richards WG, Kitajewski J, Deblandre GA, Kintner C, Stark KL (2000). *Dll4*, a novel Notch ligand expressed in arterial endothelium. *Genes Dev* 14: 1313–1318.

Silengo MC, Cavallaro S, Franceschini P (1978). Recessive spondylocostal dysostosis: two new cases. *Clin Genet* 13: 289–294.

Simpson JM, Cook A, Fagg NLK, MacLachlan NA, Sharland GK (1995). Congenital heart disease in spondylothoracic dysostosis: two familial cases. *J Med Genet* 32: 633–635.

Solomon L, Jimenez B, Reiner L (1978). Spondylothoracic dysostosis. *Arch Pathol Lab Med* 102: 201–205.

Sparrow DB, Clements M, Withington SL, Scott AN, Novotny J, Sillence D, Kusumi K, Beddington RSP, Dunwoodie SL (2002). Diverse requirements for Notch signalling in mammals. *Int J Dev Biol* 46: 365–374.

Takahashi Y, Koizumi K, Takagi A, Kitajima S, Inoue T, Koseki H, Saga Y (2000). Mesp2 initiates somite segmentation through the Notch signalling pathway. *Nat Genet* 25: 390–396.

Temple IK, Thomas TG, Baraitser M (1988). Congenital spinal deformity in a three generation family. *J Med Genet* 25: 831–834.

Tolmie JL, Whittle MJ, McNay MB, Gibson AAM, Connor JM (1987). Second trimester prenatal diagnosis of the Jarcho-Levin syndrome. *Prenat Diagn* 7: 129–134.

Trindade CEP, de Nóbrega FJ (1977). Spondylothoracic dysplasia in two siblings. *Clin Pediatr* 16: 1097–1099.

Turnpenny PD, Thwaites RJ, Boulos FN (1991). Evidence for variable gene expression in a large inbred kindred with autosomal recessive spondylocostal dysostosis. *J Med Genet* 28: 27–33.

Turnpenny PD, Bulman MP, Frayling TM, Abu-Nasra TK, Garrett C, Hattersley AT, Ellard S (1999). A gene for autosomal recessive spondylocostal dysostosis maps to 19q13.1–q13.3. *Am J Hum Genet* 65: 175–182.

Turnpenny PD, Whittock NV, Duncan J, Dunwoodie S, Kusumi K, Ellard S (2003). Novel mutations in *DLL3*, a somitogenesis gene encoding a ligand for the Notch signalling pathway, cause a consistent pattern of abnormal vertebral segmentation in spondylocostal dysostosis. *J Med Genet* 40: 333–339.

Van der Sar A (1952). Hereditary multiple hemivertebrae. *Docum Med Geographica Tropica* 4: 23–28.

Van Thienen M-N, Van der Auwera BJ (1994). Monozygotic twins discordant for spondylocostal dysostosis. *Am J Med Genet* 52: 483–486.

Verbout AJ (1985). The development of the vertebral column. *Adv Anat Embryol Cell Biol* 90: 1–122.

Wadia RS, Shirole DB, Dikshit MS (1978). Recessively inherited costovertebral segmentation defect with mesomelia and peculiar facies (Covesdem syndrome). *J Med Genet* 15: 123–127.

Whittock NV, Turnpenny PD, Tuerlings J, Ellard S (2003). Molecular genetic prenatal diagnosis for a case of autosomal recessive spondylocostal dysostosis. *Prenat Diagn* (in press).

Wong G, Levine D (1998). Jarcho-Levin syndrome: two consecutive pregnancies in a Puerto Rican couple. *Ultrasound Obstet Gynecol* 12: 70–73.

Wynne-Davies R (1975). Congenital vertebral anomalies: aetiology and relationship to spina bifida cystica. *J Med Genet* 12: 280–288.

Young ID, Moore JR (1984). Spondylocostal dysostosis. *J Med Genet* 21: 68–69.

Zhang N, Gridley T (1998). Defects in somite formation in *lunatic fringe*-deficient mice. *Nature* 394: 374–377.

Part I.
The Sex Determination Pathway

42 | Introduction to the Sex Determination Pathway: Mutations in Many Genes Lead to Sexual Ambiguity and Reversal

ROBERT P. ERICKSON

Sexual differentiation is a dynamic process that is subject to a sequential program. This program is so ordered that it can be carried to completion in consecutive stages, often described in the literature as (*1*) the establishment of chromosomal sex at fertilization, (*2*) the development of gonadal sex, and (*3*) the development of the secondary sexual characteristics, collectively called the sexual phenotype. However, recent research has shown that sex differences are present immediately after fertilization, thus suggesting that sexual development should be considered to include a stage of pregonadal sexual dimorphism. This paradigm of a developmental cascade constitutes the central dogma of sexual differentiation, formulated in principle by A. Jost at the end of the 1940s to explain the results of his experiments on fetal castration in rabbits. He observed that the extirpation of the gonads (ovaries or testes) before sexual differentiation had occurred invariably resulted in the development of the fetuses in a female-type pattern (Jost, 1953).

In considering the pathway of genetic expression for sex determination, *SRY* (sex-determining region, Y chromosome) is usually placed "at the top." However, SOX9 has now clearly been implicated as one of the major downstream regulators of male sexual determination, and *SRY* may be its antirepressor in the gonad. Haploinsufficiency of SOX9 has long been known to have a major effect on human sexual determination, as seen in the sex reversal or sexual ambiguity that is frequently found in campomelic dysplasia. The discovery that increased dosage of SOX9 could masculinize the fetus (Huang et al., 1999) and substitute for *Sry* in mice (Vidal et al., 2001) has strongly demonstrated its major role. Because *Sox9* expression in mice is not detected until embryonic day 9 (Wright et al., 1995) while *SRY/Sry* is expressed in the preimplantation embryo (Zwingman et al., 1993; Ao et al., 1994), I start the description of the cascade with *SRY*.

SRY AND Y-CHROMOSOMAL SEX DETERMINATION

SRY Is *TDF*

In 1959 four reports demonstrated the crucial role of the Y chromosome in sex determination in mammals: Welshons and Russell (1959) showed that XO mice are female; Jacobs and Strong (1959) showed the karyotype 47,XXY as a male with Klinefelter's syndrome; Ford and colleagues (1959b) reported the 45,XO karyotype in a woman with Turner's syndrome; and Ford and colleagues (1959a) described two supernumerary chromosomes (an X and a 21, giving the karyotype 48,XXY,+21) in a male with Klinefelter's and Down syndromes. These observations demonstrated that the presence of a Y chromosome, independent of the number of X chromosomes, resulted in the development of a mammalian embryo as a male, whereas in the absence of the Y chromosome, it developed as a female. Thus, the Y chromosome appeared to possess a gene or genes whose presence or absence determined the destiny of the bipotential gonad as a testis or ovary, respectively. Once the choice was made, gonadal hormones would control the development of the dimorphic secondary sex characteristics (Jost et al., 1973). In the human, the hypothetical Y-chromosomal gene(s) was named *TDF* (testis-determining factor), and in mice *tdy* (testis-determining gene on the Y).

The next major question was whether *TDF* is one gene and, if so, where on the Y chromosome it is located. The discovery that 46,XX males usually have translocations of Yp to one of their Xps was a major breakthrough in the ability to map a single *TDF* on the Y chromosome (Evans et al., 1979; Magenis et al., 1982). The X and Y pair at meiosis in homologous segments located at the termini of their arms. Because of the high rate of genetic exchange between the X and Y chromosomes in these regions, genes located in them appear to be neither X-linked nor Y-linked, and thus these portions of the sex chromosomes are called "pseudoautosomal." The occurrence of crossovers centromeric to the Y_p pseudoautosomal region can result in the transfer of *TDF* to the X chromosome. Such translocations involve an illegitimate recombination during paternal meiosis due to crossing over between unpaired segments (Gueallaen et al., 1984; Stalvey et al., 1989). Molecular analyses of the different fragments of Y chromosome present in such patients permitted the construction of a deletion map of the Y chromosome (Vergnaud et al., 1986; Nakahori et al., 1991). Such mapping demonstrated that the terminal region of Yp, adjacent to the pseudoautosomal region (and including it, but with the knowledge that the pseudoautosomal region was shared with females), is essential for testicular differentiation. Finer mapping continued, and since translocation breakpoints may contain multiple small rearrangements, one candidate gene was mistakenly identified because of such complexity: Page et al. (1987) found a highly conserved sequence that seemed to map with a male-determining Y fragment, and they named it zinc finger Y, *ZFY*. They also found that one of their XX males did not have *ZFY*, and later the finding of more such patients suggested that *ZFY* could not be *TDF* (Palmer et al., 1989; Verga and Erickson, 1989).

The resumed search for *TDF* was targeted on 35 kb of DNA between the proximal limit of the pseudoautosomal region of the Y chromosome and the breakpoint in XX,*ZFY*-negative males. The subclones generated from this target were hybridized with DNA from males of various mammals. One subclone detected sex-specific sequences in multiple mammals (Sinclair et al., 1990). The nucleotide sequence of this subclone encoded a protein that contained a segment of 80 amino acids homologous to the mating-type protein of the *mat-3M* gene in *Schizosaccharomyces pombe* and to a conserved 80 amino acid DNA-binding motif present in the HMG1 and HMG1 (high mobility group) proteins (Sinclair et al., 1990) and in other transcription-regulating proteins (Jantzen et al., 1990). Northern analyses of a variety of tissues disclosed a transcript of 1.1 kb only in the testes. This gene, designated *SRY* (sex-determining region, Y chromosome) was suggested to be *TDF* (Sinclair et al., 1990). Soon thereafter, mutations in *SRY* were found in some cases of XY, or pure gonadal dysgenesis (Berta et al., 1990; Jäger et al., 1990; Hawkins et al., 1992; Affara et al., 1993).

The mouse *Sry* gene was cloned at the same time as *SRY* by homology (Gubbay et al., 1990). Mice transgenic for a 14 kb fragment containing *Sry* showed 40,XX sex-reversal—that is, mice otherwise destined to be female had a normal male appearance, although they were sterile (Koopman et al., 1991). Testes of these mice were histologically similar to those of human XX males. Sex reversal did not always occur, however, even with a particular transgenic insertion. This incomplete penetrance seems unrelated to variation in number of *Sry* transgenes, although it may be related to the influence of genetic background on *Sry* transgene expression (Hacker et al., 1995). It will be of interest to determine whether variations in genetic modifiers are also the explanation for the various phenotypes of particular mutations in *SRY*. In this context, it is relevant to point out that *SRY* did not cause sex reversal in transgenic mice; therefore, it is not nearly as conserved in function as some human genes that can work even in *Drosophila*. However, the HMG box can be "swapped" between Sox3, Sox9, and Sry and still function normally in sex determination (Bergstrom et al., 2000).

The *SRY* gene has a simple structure, with only one exon and no introns. The 5′ flanking sequence does not contain TATA or CAAT boxes; it is GC rich and contains two tandem Sp1 recognition sites, a sequence known to potentiate transcription (Vilain et al., 1992). The region transcribed consists of 841 bp, resulting in a transcript of 1.1 kb, while the translated region consists of 612 bp, producing a protein of 204 amino acids with a molecular weight of 23.9 kDa. The *SRY* gene is flanked by two regions rich in adenine and thymidine (AT)–containing inverted repeat sequences, suggesting that this gene has its origin in the retroposition of the transcript of some other gene during human evolution. The region that codes for the HMG box is located practically in the center of the *SRY* gene, at amino acids 57–137 of the protein (Su and Lau, 1993).

The HMG boxes of SRY and Sry correspond to generalized HMG boxes (Bianchi et al., 1992) and contain two nuclear localization signals (Sudbeck and Scherer, 1997). The SRY HMG box binds to synthetic DNA fragments of the sequence AACAAAG (Nasrin et al., 1991); however, it also binds to cruciform DNA structures independent of their sequence (Ferrari et al., 1992). This ambiguity about the basis of DNA binding is apparently resolved by structural studies showing that the consensus sequence and the cruciform structure adopt a similar confirmation in solution (King and Weiss, 1993). The resolution of the solution structure of the SRY-octamer DNA complex indicates that a concave surface, made of several amino acids, binds to the minor groove, thus inducing a large conformational change in the DNA (Werner et al., 1995). The solution structure also aids the interpretation of the effects of mutations in *SRY*. Several mutations showing variable penetrance cause defects that would be expected to destabilize the protein, presumably leading to more rapid degradation. Other mutations in the HMG box alter the confirmation of DNA-contact sites in a way that precludes the usual deformation of the DNA (Werner et al., 1995; Murphy et al., 2001). In addition to the HMG box, *Sry* contains a large glutamine repeat region that is important for function in *Mus musculus musculus* but not in other species of mice (Dubin and Ostrer, 1994; Bowles et al., 1999). *SRY* can be phosphorylated in vitro, and the phosphorylated form binds DNA more tightly but the relevance of this phosphorylation has not been shown in vivo (Desclozeaux et al. 1998). SRY and other SOX proteins have also been shown to be involved in pre-mRNA splicing, but the importance of this role is not yet clear (Ohe et al., 2002).

What Regulates *SRY* and What Are Its Targets?

Initial studies on the expression of *Sry* did not disclose expression until day 11.5. The evidence that this expression was in presumptive Sertoli cells came from the use of a mutation that prevents germ cell migration into the gonadal ridge (Koopman et al., 1990). This late expression raises the question of what controls *Sry* expression. Perhaps a clue to the control of *Sry* expression comes from the finding of much earlier expression in preimplantation embryos. A pathway to include this observation and the probable role of SRY in the regulation of other genes is depicted in Figure 42–1. PCR studies of mouse embryos from embryonic days 1.5 to 4.5 found abundant evidence for transcription of *Sry* (and *Zfy*) from two-cell to blastocyst stages (Zwingman et al., 1993), and this result was confirmed in human embryos (Ao et al., 1994). Quantitation disclosed that there are approximately 40 to 100 copies per cell in a male blastocyst (Cao et al., 1995). As in adult mouse testes (Capel at al, 1993; Zwingman et al., 1994), both circular (nontranslated) and linear (potentially translatable) *Sry* RNAs are found (Boyer and Erickson, 1993). The functional importance of circular transcripts of *Sry* is unclear; they are not made by *SRY*. The difference is explained by the finding that *Sry* is located in the middle of a large inverted repeat, whereas *SRY* is not. The mouse urogenital ridge transcript is linear and contains 3.5 kb of 3′ UTR (Hacker et al., 1995).

A potential SRY-binding sequence AACAAAG has been identified at positions −3 to +4 relative to the site of transcription initiation of the *SRY* gene (or at −15 − −9 from the second transcriptional site;

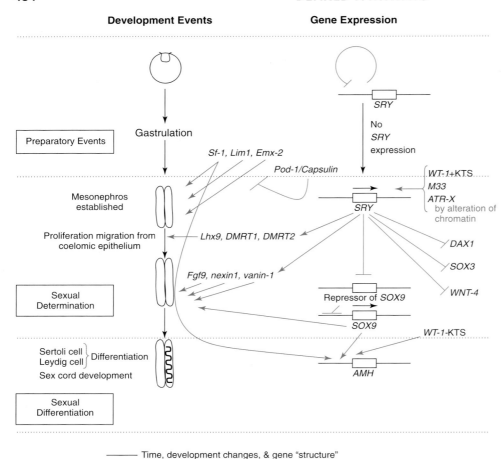

Figure 42–1. The role of *SRY* in testis determination. A hypothetical autoinhibitory role for the preimplantation expression of *SRY* is indicated with "release" by chromatin-altering proteins (middle right) at the time of sex-specific gonadal differentiation. The possible role of many other genes is also indicated. Inhibitory pathways in red, stimulatory pathways in green.

Margarit et al., 1998). Thus, a possible autoregulatory role has been suggested (Vilain et al., 1992), and the early expression of *SRY/Sry* might be autoinhibitory. This inhibition might be released by chromatin changes or other alterations later in development. This potential self-binding site is well conserved in higher primates (Margarit et al., 1998).

Several genes are involved in chromatin structure, and their mutations cause partial or complete sex reversal. The knockout of *M33*, the mouse homolog of *Drosophila Polycomb* which regulates chromatin structure, shows hermaphroditism with intersex genitalia or complete male-to-female sex reversal (Katoh-Fukui et al., 1998). In these mutants with a disrupted C-terminal domain, the primordial gonad failed to grow at the normal time of *Sry* expression, suggesting that M33 may be upstream of *Sry*. Another gene implicated in sex determination is *XH2* (X-linked helicase 2, also known as *ATR-X*), and it might also have a role in the chromatin changes that alter the expression of *SRY*. This gene is mutated in ATR-X—a syndrome of α-thalassemia (sometimes), mental *r*etardation, and mapping to the *X*—which also can show sexual ambiguity (Gibbons et al., 1995). This helicase-related protein interacts with E2H2 heterochromatin proteins (Cardoso et al., 1998) and alters DNA methylation (Gibbons et al., 2000). Intriguingly, marsupials have X and Y copies, and their Y (*ATRY*) copy is only expressed in testes (Pask et al., 2000). Pask et al. (2000) suggest that *ATRY* may be a more ancestral sex-determining gene than *SRY*. If this is so, chromatin changes could be the initial stage in sex determination, possibly "releasing" *SRY* from its autoinhibition and preventing reinhibition. Non-chromatin altering gene products which may alter *Sry* expression are Gata4 and its partner, FogZ (Tevosian et al., 2002).

It has been proposed, with much circumstantial evidence, that SRY counteracts a negative regulator of sex determination. According to

this hypothesis, the HMG domain of SRY binds to regulatory DNA sequences of a hypothetical gene "Z," which is considered to be a negative regulator of male sex determination (McElreavey et al., 1993). This interaction of SRY with the "Z" gene is postulated to inhibit its transcription and, thus, its regulatory effect, resulting in a male phenotype. Graves (1998) has suggested that *SRY*'s inhibitory target is *SOX3*. *SOX3* is not required for male differentiation (Stevanovic et al., 1993) and is more abundantly expressed in female than in male genital ridges (Collignon et al., 1996). Thus, *Sox3*, which is most abundantly expressed in the embryonic nervous system, may be a master regulator for ovarian development that is inhibited by *Sry*. Since *Sry* binds to the same DNA sequence as *Sox3*, but with higher affinity (Collignon et al., 1996), the inhibition could be a simple, nonproductive displacement of *Sox3* at a binding site.

The original "Z" gene was thought to be located on Xp21 (McElreavey et al., 1993). A number of 46,XY individuals with sex reversal have partial duplications of Xp and an intact *SRY* gene. They usually have normal female external and internal genitalia with partial gonadal dysgenesis (Bardoni et al., 1994). Bernstein and colleagues (1980) presented two cases and concluded that "testis-determining genes of the Y chromosome may be suppressed by regulatory elements of the X." When the X-homolog of *ZFY*, *ZFX*, was discovered and found to be in the duplicated Xp region, it was suggested as the negative regulator (Scherer et al., 1989). If this is the cause of the sex reversal, however, subjects with a 46,XXY karyotype should not develop testes because *ZFX* escapes inactivation. Thus, whatever the locus (or loci) on Xp is, it should be X-inactivated, or XXY would not develop as males under this hypothesis. Indeed, some XXY triploids have shown sexual ambiguity (Graham et al., 1989), and lack of X-inactivation in the triploids may be the cause (Petit et al., 1992).

Ogata and coworkers (Ogata et al., 1992; Ogata and Matsuo, 1994) further defined the critical region for Xp duplication with sex reversal, and Bardoni and colleagues (1994) narrowed it to a 160 kb span. The latter hypothesized a single gene in the region and named it DSS (*dosage sensitive sex reversal*). This region includes *DAX1* (*dosage sensitive sex reversal–adrenal hypoplasia congenita gene on the X chromosome gene 1*), a gene whose defects cause adrenal hypoplasia congenita (Muscatelli et al., 1994; Zanaria et al., 1994). DAX1 (and WT1) are discussed in Chapter 45, "DAX1 and X-Linked Adrenal Hypoplasia Congenita and XY Sex Reversal." *DAX1* is a candidate for DSS. *DAX1* is an orphan member of the nuclear hormone receptor family, meaning that its ligand is unknown.

DAX1 is related to *SF1*, which is involved in gonad development (see later in this chapter). Capel (1995) has argued that *DAX1* may be involved in the fetal response to maternal hormones in such a manner that an increased dosage of *DAX1* would override the *SRY* signal for testis development. This hypothesis is supported by the fact that *DAX1* is normally down-regulated in the developing testis while its expression persists in the developing ovary (Swain et al., 1996), and overexpression in *Dax1* transgenics delays testicular development and can result in sex reversal in the presence of weak-functioning (hypomorphic) *Sry* (Swain et al., 1998). If *DAX1* is DSS, it indicates that DSS is not necessary for male differentiation, because absence of *Dax1* function does not impair phenotypic male or female development (Yu et al., 1998). In fact, *Dax1*-deficient 40,XY mice are males with small testes and infertility due to abnormal proliferation and differentiation of Leydig and Sertoli cells (Jeffs et al., 2001). New data on *DAX1*'s role in peritubular myoid cell differentiation in early testis development is reviewed in Chapter 45. *DAX1* is autosomal in marsupials, suggesting that its X location is not critical for its potential role in sexual differentiation (Pask et al., 1997). Thus, if *SRY* inhibits *DAX1* expression (an inhibition which can be overridden with excess dosage of *DAX1*), the inhibition would be one of a female program of development—that is, as in the case of the postulated role of *SOX3*, *SRY*s interaction would be inhibitory to ovarian development rather than stimulatory to male development.

Another gene involved in dosage-dependent 46,XY sex reversal is *WNT-4*, which maps to distal 1p; duplications of this gene sometimes cause male pseudohermaphroditism (Garcia-Heras et al., 1999). The *Wnt-4* knockout doesn't affect male sexual development, but the females are masculinized (Vainio et al., 1999). Interestingly, *WNT-4*'s overexpression (in transfection experiments with cultured Sertoli and Leydig cells) appears to result in up-regulation of *DAX-1*, linking these two dosage-dependent, female sexual development program-enhancing, pathways (Jordan et al., 2001).

Fibroblast growth factor 9 (Fgf9) may be an important mediator of *SRY* action (Colvin et al., 2001). The *Fgf9* knockout shows deficient mesonephric cell migration into the gonad, deficient mesenchymal proliferation, decreased function of Sertoli cells, and frequent sex reversal. Other candidates for a role in the regulation or function of *Sry* have emerged from microarray experiments. A search for genes expressed differentially between the two sexes after overt gonad differentiation led to the discovery of two—*nexin*-1 and *vanin*-1—that show male-specific expression before this differentiation (Grimmond et al., 2000). Of the two, only *nexin*-1, a serine protease inhibitor with a binding site for WT-1 (see below) in its promoter (Erno et al., 1996), is possibly expressed in time (at embryonic day 11.25) to influence *Sry* (onset at day 10.5 by the most sensitive techniques [Hacker et al., 1995]). However, it seems more likely that *nexin-1* is downstream of *Sry* and involved in the rapid proliferation of the male coelomic epithelium seen at this time (Schmahl et al., 2000). HMG domain proteins appear to gain their DNA-binding specificity from protein cofactors (reviewed in Kamachi et al., 2000). A candidate for a co-regulator protein for SRY, SIP-1, has been identified by a yeast two-hybrid screen (Poulat et al., 1997), but its role in sex determination is not yet known.

Is *SRY* Essential and Can *SOX9* Substitute for It?

In addition to the question of what regulates *SRY*—since it does not seem to be continuously expressed from preimplantation development to the time of gonadal sex differentiation—is the question of the essentiality of *SRY*. It clearly is not essential in all mammals. The males of several species of voles (Just et al., 1995) and spinous country-rats

(Sutou et al., 2001) develop appropriately without it. This evolutionary evidence is supported by clinical data. Molecular investigations into the XX true hermaphrodites more frequently seen among South African Bantus have also not detected Y chromosomal sequences (Ramsay et al., 1988). Extensive studies in this group show no evidence of *SRY* in ovarian or testicular biopsy tissue (Spurdle et al., 1995). Thus, mammalian male sex determination can certainly occur in the absence of *SRY*. Campomelic dysplasia, due to haploinsufficiency of SOX9, is discussed fully in Chapter 43, "SOX9 and Campomelic Dysplasia and Sex Reversal." As already mentioned, activation of *SOX9* is clearly one method by which an *SRY*-negative individual can develop such a male phenotype. *Sox9* transgenics develop a normal male appearance in the absence of *Sry* (Vidal et al., 2001), and increased dosage of SOX9, due to a chromosomal duplication, strongly masculinized a fetus (Huang et al., 1999).

Further evidence for the important role of *Sox9*, at least in mouse sexual differentiation, comes from a new dominant insertional mutation, *Odsex* (Bishop et al., 2000). *Odsex* represents a 150 kb deletion that maps about 1 million bp upstream of *Sox9*. Mice that are 40,XX, lack *Sry*, and carry this deletion up-regulate *Sox9* expression in fetal gonads and develop as phenotypic males (Bishop et al., 2000). In addition, it has been shown that in the human testes, the time of activation of the targets of *SOX9* transcription corresponds to a time when SOX9 is found in the nucleus instead of the cytoplasm (de Santa Barbara et al., 2000). *SOX9*, and its role in development, seems more widely conserved than does *SRY*.

SRY is thus postulated to be the deinhibitor of a yet to be identified inhibitor (possibly the "Z" gene) of *SOX9* since no evidence for a role of SRY in *SOX9* expression has come to light. However, the role that is being elucidated is probably most essential in mammals: although *SOX9* is found to be expressed in avian (Morais da Silva et al., 1996) and reptilian testes; in a careful study of temperature-dependent sex determination in the American alligator, SOX9 is only detected after testes formation had started—that is, after sex determination (Western et al., 1999). In addition, in birds, SOX9 expression follows the expression of antimüllerian hormone (AMH), even though AMH is a presumptive target of *SOX9* regulation in mammals (Oreal et al., 1998). Although it would simplify explanations of sex determination if *SOX9* were linked to sex determination in *SRY*-negative mammals, genetic segregation of allelic variants with gender was not found in an *SRY*-negative species of vole (Baumstark et al., 2001). Evolutionary conservation of sex chromosomes is strong, and one can hypothesize that some Y-chromosomal gene other than *SRY* now controls *SOX9* in such species.

The downstream targets of *SOX9* are now being elucidated. *SOX9* has been found to have a major effect on AMH transcription, whereas SF1 has only a minor effect in vivo (Arango et al., 1999). GATA-4 also plays a major role in stimulating transcription of AMH (Viger et al., 1998) and could be downstream, as well as upstream (see above), of *SOX9* (Fig. 42–1). Although SF1 has earlier roles in gonadal development (see below), it is believed that SF1 is a key coactivator of AMH expression by SOX9. Both SOX9 and SF1 coassociate and, although their binding sites are 40 bp apart on the DNA, it has been proposed that the local bending of the DNA by SOX9 could contribute to stabilization of a transcriptional regulator form of SF1 (de Santa Barbara et al., 1998). Thus, SF1 may be the specific gonadal coactivator for SOX9 (as discussed above in regard to SRY and SIP-1), while some other coactivator—possibly including phosphorylation by protein kinase A (Huang et al., 2000)—is involved in promoting COL-IIα1 expression, the relevant target in bone. AMH and the testosterone production by Leydig cells become the major downstream regulators of the male phenotype.

Jost's experiments (Jost et al., 1973), already described, established that although sex-determining genes are responsible for directing the development of the gonad, secondary sexual differentiation of external genitalia and internal duct systems is under hormonal control in humans and other eutherian mammals. Indifferent (bipotential) external structures are initially present in males and females. The testis produces androgens, which masculinize the labioscrotal folds (to form a scrotum) and the genital tubercle (to form the penis). In the absence of the testis, and, thus, of high levels of androgen molecules, the labio-scrotal folds fail to fuse and form labia, and the genital tubercle becomes the clitoris. Internally, the mesonephric (wolffian) and para-mesonephric (müllerian) ducts develop into male or female structures, respectively. Testicular androgen promotes development of the wolffian ducts (WD) into epididymides, vasa deferentia, and seminal vesicles, and absence of androgens leads to WD degeneration. Also produced in the testis is AMH, which causes degeneration of the müllerian duct (MD). In the female, in absence of AMH, the MD becomes the uterine tubes, uterus, and upper part of the vagina. Mutations in *AMH* and its receptor are fully discussed in Chapter 44, "AMH/MIS and Its Receptors and Sexual Ambiguity and Persistent Müllerian Derivatives." Prostaglandin D2 may also provide an important paracrine role in male gonadal differentiation, especially in the presence of germ cells (Adams and McLaren, 2002). Obviously, many different genes are involved in realizing this program, and some of them are discussed in the next section.

GENE ACTION IN THE GONADAL RIDGE PRIOR TO SEX-SPECIFIC GONADAL DIFFERENTIATION

This description of gene action during sex determination and differentiation begins with the time of expression of *SRY*, since it is testes-determining factor. However, a number of other genes are expressed in the gonadal ridge before *SRY* is expressed, and they are essential for sexual development; in fact, absence of some of these genes leads to sex reversal. Again, their putative interactions are depicted in Fig. 42–1 while the time of expression of many of these genes is in Figure 42–2.

Emx2, Lhx1, and Sf-1

The absence of certain genes causes a lack of any visible gonadal development, and some of these genes are also implicated in renal development. For example, knockouts (KOs) for *Emx2* do not have kidneys, ureters, gonads, or genital tracts (Miyamoto et al., 1997). Although *WT1* (see below) and other genes that are normally expressed in the metanephric mesenchyme were initially expressed normally in this KO, subsequent expression was greatly reduced, and degeneration and apoptosis occurred (Miyamoto et al., 1997). Kidneys and gonads are also missing in *Lhx1* KOs (Shawlot and Behringer, 1995). This is not surprising, given the very early role of *Lhx1* in gastrulation.

Another gene whose absence prevents gonad formation is *Sf-1*, or steroidogenic factor-1. SF-1 is homologous to the *Drosophila* gene *Fushi tarazu* 1 factor and sometimes is referred to as *Ftz F*1; it is an orphan nuclear receptor that has been shown to be a key regulator of steroidogenic enzymes in adrenocortical cells (see above; Lala et al., 1992). Developmental studies demonstrated that Sf-1 is expressed in

the urogenital ridge at embryonic day 9 to 9.5 in the mouse. This is at an early stage of organogenesis of the developing gonads and before *Sry* is expressed (Ikeda et al. 1994); the same result has been confirmed in humans (de Santa Barbara et al., 2000). The knockout of *Sf-1* resulted in mice that died 8 days after birth (Luo et al., 1994; Sadovsky et al., 1995). The KO mice lacked adrenal glands and gonads and had a resulting deficiency in corticosterone that was the likely cause of death. More recent expression studies (Hatano et al., 1994; Shen et al., 1994) have demonstrated a sexually dimorphic expression pattern of *Sf-1* with persistence in males and a discontinuation of expression in females, which was hypothesized to link the expression of *Sry* to that of the AMH. SF1 was shown to regulate AMH expression in vitro (Shen et al., 1994) and in vivo (Giuli et al., 1997), but another in vitro study could not demonstrate that SF-1 could mediate between *SRY* and AMH (Haqq et al., 1994 as discussed in the preceeding section). Dramatic costimulation of the AMH promoter by Wt-1 (isoforms lacking lys-thr-ser between the third and fourth zinc finger [-KTS] as further discussed in what follows) with SF-1 has been demonstrated (Nachtigal et al., 1998) and can be antagonized by Dax1; transcription of the Leydig insulin-like gene is also mediated (Zimmerman et al., 1998).

We predicted that human mutations in SF-1 would lead to "a phenotype associated with predominantly female appearance and severe neonatal problems due to lack of steroid hormones" (Pinsky et al., 1999). Such a patient has now been described. A 46,XY female with adrenal failure at 2 weeks of life was found to have a 2 bp mutation at exon 3, resulting in a mutated glycine, which is an essential part of the zinc finger and is important for DNA binding (Achermann et al., 1999). The region of 9q33 to which *SF-1* maps (Taketo et el, 1995) has not yet been associated with cytogenetic abnormalities and problems of sexual differentiation.

Other Genes Expressed before Sry with a Role in Sex Determination

Several genes that are expressed in mouse gonadal ridge at day 9.5, before sexual determination becomes evident, may have a role in preparing the gonad for sexual differentiation (Fig. 41–1). These include *Sf-1* and *Lhx-1* (already discussed), *Dmrt-1* and -2, *Pod-1/Capsulin*, and *Wt-1*.

Dmrt-1 maps to distal 9p, and it has long been known that deletions on distal 9p are frequently associated with 46,XY sex reversal. These are reviewed, and the essential chromosomal region is better defined, in Flejter et al. (1998). Surprisingly, a mammalian homolog of a gene shared by *C. elegans* and *Drosophila*, which is involved in the sex differentiation cascade, was found to have a mammalian homolog that mapped to this region (Raymond et al., 1998). This is particularly intriguing since conservation of sex determination pathways

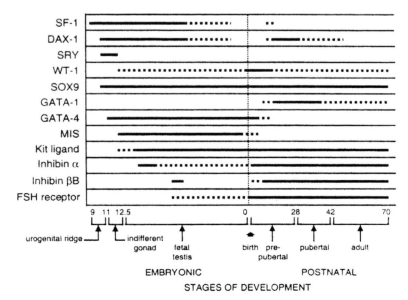

Figure 42–2. The time of expression of many genes in Sertoli cells. (Reproduced from Viger et al., *Development* 125: 2665 (1998), by permission of the authors and The Company of Biologists, Cambridge, UK.)

has been an exception, not a rule. While mutations in this highly conserved *DMRT-1* gene are infrequent in 46,XY males, the most recent deletional mapping of the critical region on 9p includes both *DMRT-1* and a homologous gene, *DMRT-2* (Raymond et al., 1999b). Thus, haploinsufficiency of both genes may contribute to 46,XY sex reversal. Expression studies of *Dmrt-1* have shown that it is expressed in the genital ridge at day 9.5 (Raymond et al., 1999a). Initially, expression is equal in genital ridges of both sexes, but gradually expression is limited to the male gonad (Moniot et al., 2000). *Dmrt-1* is also expressed in the genital ridge and in the wolffian duct before sexual differentiation in the avian embryo, which is not true of *SRY* (Raymond et al., 1999a). *DMRT-1* is appropriately temperature-controlled in the turtle gonad before sexual differentiation (Kettlewell et al., 2000) and is expressed during gonadal development and spermatogenesis even in fish (Marchand et al., 2000). Thus, as might be expected for a gene with homology to a *C. elegans* and *Drosophila* gene involved in sex determination, *DMRT-1* may have a more conserved role in sexual determination in vertebrates than does *SRY*.

Members of the *Lhx* family may be near the "top" of the cascade. *Lhx* refers to the LIM homeobox family, a gene family of nongrouped homeobox-containing transcription factors (Hobert and Westphal, 2000). As mentioned, *Lhx1* absence prevents kidney and gonad development. *Lhx-1* and *Lhx-9* transcripts are present in the urogenital ridges of mice at embryonic day 9.5 (Birk et al., 2000). The KO of *Lhx-9* fails to form a gonad because somatic cells of the genital ridge fail to proliferate despite normal germ cell migration (Birk et al., 2000). 40,XY mice with the KO were phenotypically female and had no gonads. Presumably, cell migration from the mesonephros, an important source of cells in the developing gonad (Tilmann and Capel, 1999), also did not occur. Importantly, evidence was also provided that *Sf-1* expression was markedly decreased (Birk et al., 2000).

Another gene possibly involved in *Sf-1* expression is *Pod-1/Capsulin*. This gene was found by differential cDNA screening of embryonic day 13.5 male versus female gonads (Tamura et al., 2001). Its time course of expression is similar to that of *Sf-1*, but the two do not colocalize. Importantly, co-transfection of *Pod-1* with *Sf-1* resulted in repression of *Sf-1* expression (Tamura et al., 2001).

The association between the Wilms' tumor 1 (*WT1*) gene and testis development was recognized from investigations into the Denys-Drash syndrome and the WAGR syndrome; WAGR consists of Wilms' tumor, *a*niridia, *g*enitourinary anomalies, and mental *r*etardation and is caused by deletions of 11p13 and hemizygosity in this region. Further, the phenotype of the deletions suggested that there was a tumor suppressor in this region related to Wilms tumor (for review, see Hastie, 2001). In Denys-Drash syndrome, there is a complex nephropathy and sexual ambiguity. Patients with the WAGR syndrome may have undescended testes and hypospadias, whereas male patients with Denys-Drash syndrome may have female or ambiguous external genitalia with dysgenic gonads.

When the *WT1* gene was cloned, it was found to code for a DNA-binding, zinc-finger transcription factor with several isoforms due to alternative splicing. Expression studies show that high levels of *WT1* are expressed in the developing kidney, especially in glomeruli and mesangial cells that are involved in the above-mentioned nephropathy. High levels were also found in the indifferent gonads, in Sertoli cells, and in granulosa cells. It has been suggested that the *WT1* gene is involved in mesenchymal–epithelial interactions (van Heyningen and Hastie, 1992)—for example, between Sertoli cells and Leydig cells. Such interactions are crucial in both the developing kidney and gonad. Analysis of the defects of kidney development in *Wt-1* knockout mice strongly support the notion that Wt-1 is involved in the urogenital mesenchyme-to-epithelial transition (Sainio et al., 1997). It is probable that defects in these interactions disrupt testicular development so that Leydig cell function and testosterone production are inadequate. This could explain the pseudohermaphroditism sometimes seen in Denys-Drash syndrome.

Recent work has focused on the important role of two different isoforms of *WT-1*. Although *WT-1* has at least 24 different isoforms, alternative splice donor sites at the end of exon 9, leading to the insertion or omission of three amino acids (KTS), lead to a variation in isoforms which is extremely conserved in evolution (Kent et al., 1995).

Children with Frasier syndrome, a variant of Denys-Drash, with late-onset glomerular nephropathy are mostly mutant for this splice site which creates the KTS insertion and, thus, have a deficiency of the KTS positive isoform (Little et al., 1999). This was confirmed in mice which were designed to express only the KTS positive or KTS negative isoforms. The heterozygous mice, with a reduction of the *Wt-1* KTS positive isoform as predicted from the patients, created a model for Frasier syndrome (Hammes et al., 2001). Homozygous mice deficient for either isoform died at birth due to kidney defects. The homozygous mice lacking the *Wt-1* KTS positive isoforms also showed a complete XY sex reversal because of a dramatic reduction of *Sry* expression (Hammes et al., 2001). Since the −KTS isoform has been shown to be a transcriptional regulator of *Dax-1*, one method by which the KTS-deficient positive isoform *Wt-1* mice could be sex reversed would be by up-regulation of *Dax-1* from the unopposed action of the KTS minus isoform (Kim et al., 1999). Hammes et al. (2001) suggest that *WT-1* KTS positive isoform may be an important activator of *SRY* in the developing gonad. Hossein and Saunders (2001), however, have shown that *WT-1* KTS minus isoform but not *WT-1* KTS positive isoform, could activate *SRY*. To make things more complex, *WT-1* has been shown to be a target gene of *SRY* in vitro but not in vivo (Toyooka et al., 1998). Thus, interactions between *Sry* and *Wt-1* in the developing mouse gonad are important, but it is not yet clear what is the precise pathway or the mechanism of control of their interaction in sexual determination.

Hastie (2001) has argued that the frequent, but also frequently not complete, 46X,Y sex reversal seen in Frasier patients (where the level of *WT-1* −KTS isoforms are increased 50%) makes an increase in the KTS minus isoform unlikely to be the cause of the phenotype of the KTS positive isoform knockout. In fact, since the WT-1 −KTS isoform has been shown to have a potential role in the regulation of AMH, one might anticipate less sexual ambiguity with increased expression of the WT-1 −KTS isoform (Shimamura et al., 1997). However, as previously discussed, Sox9 seems to be the most crucial transcriptional activator of AMH gene expression (Arango et al., 1999).

Finally, Hammes et al. (2001) explored the possible role of increased expression of *Dax-1* in the *Wt-1* −KTS isoform knockout mice and did not find an increase. Since the *WT-1* KTS positive isoform has been thought to be less involved in transcriptional activation and more involved in RNA processing (Davies et al., 1998; Little et al., 1999), it is possible that the *Wt-1* KTS positive isoform effect on *Sry* expression could be more involved with alterations in chromatin structure, which could lead to the above-hypothesized release of a previous autoinhibition of *Sry* expression.

SEXUAL DIFFERENTIATION

Female Pseudohermaphroditism with Normal Female Internal Structures

While it is apparent that antimüllerian hormone and testosterone are the major regulators of external male differentiation secreted by the testes, the nature and action of the genes involved are the subject of much current research. Other gene products are also involved, as indicated by the short anogenital distance in the hypertestosterone XX*Sxr*, sex-reversed mouse (Atkinson and Blecher, 1994). Human patients again give a hint as to the complexities of gene regulation of sexual differentiation. While it is well known that a number of karyotypic abnormalities are associated with sexual ambiguity, such as 9p and 10q deletions, 1p and X duplications, and others (many of them mentioned in this chapter), a group of patients with female pseudohermaphroditism with caudal dysplasia hint at the activation of genes involved in sexual differentiation (these clinical entities are not covered further elsewhere in this volume).

Female pseudohermaphroditism (FPH) may be defined as an apparent male or an individual with an ambiguous external genital appearance accompanying a normal female karyotype. Following the report by Perloff et al. (1953), several publications have described a distinct form of FPH that is associated with malformations of the internal genital, urinary, and gastrointestinal tracts (Carpentier and Potter, 1959; Lubinsky, 1980; Hokamp and Muller, 1983; Robinson and Tross, 1984). These defects include atresia or duplication of the uterus and vagina, fistulas between the urinary and gastrointestinal and genital tracts, urethral stenosis or atresia, and various skeletal anomalies including vertebral and radial defects. They may occur in the apparent absence of testosterone or *SRY* (Erickson et al., 1997).

The disorder is likely to have heterogeneous causes, some of them genetic. Lubinsky (1980) suggested that this spectrum of defects could be explained as a disturbance of a specific caudal developmental field (a single morphogenetically reactive unit in the embryo), with female pseudohermaphroditism serving as a relatively rare marker of this process that occurs in the absence of testosterone. Robinson and Tross (1984) hypothesized a primary defect in the cloacal membrane and emphasized the absence of a median perineal raphe in their five cases (one male); some, or all, of their cases may differ from others because of clustering or doxylamine succinate exposure (or both). Escobar et al. (1987) have proposed that this combination of defects reflects the failure of migration or of the urorectal septum to fuse with the cloacal membrane. When this interaction does not occur, the cloacal membrane does not divide. Since the raphe of the male scrotum reflects the re-fusion of these folds, those cases of FPH with caudal anomalies in which there is no raphe may represent this mechanism. Failure of division in the posterior, anal portion may persist as imperforate anus, also a possible distinguishing feature of two causes. The failure of the cloacal membrane to separate could also reflect an excess of local mesoderm. Such an excess might contribute to enlargement of the phallus in such cases, even in the absence of testosterone. It may also be relevant to cases of penoscrotal transposition in which overlapping birth defects occur (MacKenzie et al., 1994; Parida et al., 1995). In the case of penoscrotal transposition, the "excess" mesoderm would be more posterior (and augmented by testosterone in these 46,XY cases).

What might be the cause of this failure of the cloacal membrane to divide? Patients ascertained because of other defects—for example, prune belly sequence or bilateral renal agenesis—have a similar pattern of caudal malformations (Carpentier and Potter, 1959; Reinberg et al., 1991). Furthermore, this pattern of dysmorphism, but without FPH, is found in the VACTERL (*v*ertebral-*a*nal-*c*ardiac-*TE* fistula *r*adial [or *r*enal]-other *l*imb), and MURCS (*mü*llerian duct aplasia-*r*enal aplasia, *c*ervicothoracic *s*omite dysplasia) associations, and Rokitansky, caudal dysplasia, and exstrophy of the bladder and cloaca sequences. These three conditions usually occur sporadically in families. The effects of maternal diabetes have been implicated in both the VACTERL association and the caudal dysplasia sequence, but in most

cases, the cause is unknown. Autosomal dominant inheritance of multiple caudal anomalies has also been described (Erickson et al., 1990). The search for genes involved is more easily performed in mice.

Some Genes Involved in External Sexual Differentiation

The role of growth factors in the differentiation of the genital tubercle (GT) has been explored in mice. The possible roles of many of these genes are depicted in Figure 42–3. While *Fgf9* is implicated in gonadal differentiation, *Fgf8* and *10* are implicated in external sexual differentiation and the knockout of *Fgf10* has quite marked sexual ambiguity (Haraguchi et al., 2000). The interaction of a number of these factors, in a pathway initiated by Sonic hedgehog (Shh), has been studied in organ cultures of murine genital tubercles (Haraguchi et al., 2001). Genital tubercles explants were treated with beads soaked in Shh, and gene expression was studied by in situ hybridization. Bone morphogenetic protein 4, Fgf10, Gli1, Hoxd13, and Ptch1 all showed increased expression in the Shh-treated outgrowths (Haraguchi et al., 2001). Antibodies to Shh and the *Shh* knockout were also studied. $Shh^{-/-}$ embryos showed no external genitalia at 12.5 days gestation and showed down-regulation of *Fgf8*. Cultured GT explants treated with antibody to Shh also showed marked down-regulation of *Fgf10*. Shh is known to influence three Gli transcription factors. Haraguchi et al. (2001) studied *Gli2* knockout mice which exhibited ventral malformations of the GT.

These findings are also relevant to the hypospadias seen in Smith-Lemli-Opitz syndrome. As has been frequently discussed, part of the developmental defects seen in this cholesterol synthesis deficiency may be due to altered Shh signaling because of possible absence of the cholesterol moiety normally found at the C terminus. This is a controversial subject because many effects of Shh do not depend on the cholesterol moiety (see Chapter 16, "An Introduction to Sonic Hedgehog Signaling") and holoprosencephaly (a birth defect sometimes seen in Smith-Lemli-Opitz syndrome) occurs with Shh haploinsufficiency while hypospadias does not (see Note Added in Proof). Shh is also required for prostate development (Podlasek et al., 1999). In contrast, Desert hedgehog is required to maintain germ cells in the testis (Bitgood et al., 1996).

While *Wnt4* is implicated in gonadal differentiation, *Wnt5a* has also been implicated in genital tubercle development (Yamaguchi et al., 1999). Also, the role of AMH in development seems quite dependent on the signaling molecule *Wnt-7a*. The knockout for *Wnt-7a* has

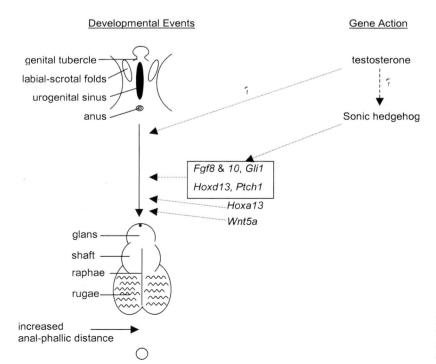

Figure 42–3. Possible role of various genes in development of the external male genitalia. Many genes have been implicated in masculine development of the genital tubercle, and most of them are depicted here. Stimulatory pathways shown by dotted lines.

postaxial hemimelia but otherwise is fully viable, although sterile (Parr and McMahon, 1995). Studies on this mutant (Miller and Sassoon, 1998; Parr and McMahon, 1998), as well as on the spontaneous mutant in *Wnt-7a* that is identified by the similar phenotype (Parr et al., 1998), led to the recognition that males failed to undergo regression of the müllerian duct while females show abnormal oviduct and uterine development. It was found that the antimüllerian hormone receptor was not being expressed in the males (Parr and McMahon, 1998); thus, *Wnt-7a* is essential for AMH function. In addition, *Hoxa-10* and *Hoxa-11* expression was abnormal postnatally in the female oviduct and uterus of these mutants (Miller and Sassoon, 1998), indicating that *Wnt-7a* is important for maintaining their expression.

Multiple *Hox* genes are involved in sexual differentiation. Hypodactyly is a semidominant mutation in mice due to deficiency of *Hoxa-13* (Mortlock et al., 1996). The homozygous embryos rarely survive to adulthood, but when they do, they are infertile. Altered expression of multiple *Hoxd* genes occurs in the mouse mutation *Ulnaless* and is associated with abnormalities of the penile bone (Peichel et al., 1997). The *Hoxd-13* homozygous knockouts are infertile and have an altered penile bone (Dollé et al., 1993). The compound double homozygous deficiency of *Hoxa-13* and *Hoxd-13* showed a complete absence of external genitalia (Kondo et al., 1997). Haploinsufficiency of the *Hoxa* cluster was associated with some genital abnormalities (unilateral cryptorchidism and a ventral-bowed penis), as well as with several other abnormalities, possibly due to the deletion of other genes in the karyotypically visible deletion (Devriendt et al., 1999). Patients with haploinsufficiency of the *HOXD* complex had genital anomalies of a small phallus and no palpable testes in one case, and penoscrotal transposition with micropenis in a second case, as well as several limb and other abnormalities (Del Campo et al., 1999) while hand-foot-genital syndrome with male cryptorchidism and hypospadias is due to mutations in *HOXA13* (Mortlock and Innis, 1997; see Chapter 48, "HOXA13 and the Hand-Foot-Genital and Guttmacher Syndromes").

NOTE ADDED IN PROOF

Recent data suggest that sterol deficiency inhibits *smoothened* transduction of *Shh* signalling (Cooper et al., 2003).

CONCLUSION

The sex determination pathway, like most developmental pathways, has a strong tendency to maintain its function—that is, it is homeostatic. Thus, haploinsufficiency of SOX9—in the human condition, campomelic dysplasia—only results in sexual reversal a portion of the time, while sexual ambiguity and a normal-appearing male phenotype in these $SOX9^{+/-}$, 46,XY individuals are nearly equally frequent outcomes. In a similar manner, a low number of mice that are nulls for fibroblast growth factor 9 manage to develop as normal males (Colvin et al., 2001). Redundancy in pathways, as already discussed, is part of the mechanism by which the homeostatic continuation of male sexual development occurs. One can surmise that a number of genes in the pathway might be up- or down-regulated to compensate for deficiencies in other members of the pathway. We know that the degree of homeostasis is altered by modifying genes; a good example is the Y^{dom} effect on the C57BL6/J background versus that on the *Mus poschiavanus* background (Washburn et al., 2001). Thus, further understanding of the sex determination pathway will come from studies of altered gene expression in deficient states and the location and identification of modifier genes that alter the pathway.

REFERENCES

Achermann JC, Ito M, Hindmarsh PC, Jameson JL (1999). A mutation in the gene encoding steroidogenic factor-1 causes XY sex reversal and adrenal failure in humans. *Nat Genet* 22: 125–126.

Adams IA, McLaren A (2002). Sexually dimorphic development of mouse primordial germ cells: switching from oogenesis to spermatogenesis. *Development* 129: 1155–1164.

Affara NA, Chalmers IJ, Ferguson-Smith MA (1993). Analysis of SRY in 22 sex-reversed XY females identifies four new point mutations in the conserved DNA binding domain. *Hum Mol Genet* 2: 785–789.

Ao A, Erickson RP, Winston RM, Handyside AH (1994). Transcription of paternal Y-linked genes in the human zygote as early as the pronucleate stage. *Zygote* 2: 281–287.

Arango NA, Lovell-Badge R, Behringer RR (1999). Targeted mutagenesis of the endogenous mouse *Mis* gene promoter: in vivo definition of genetic pathways of vertebrate sexual development. *Cell* 99: 409–419.

Atkinson TG, Blecher SR (1994). Aberrant anogenital distance in XXSxr ("sex-reversed") mice. *J Zool* 233: 581–589.

Bardoni B, Zabaria E, Guioli S, Floridia G, Worley KC, Tonini G, Ferrante E, Chiumello G, McCabe ERB, Fraccaro M, et al. (1994). A dosage sensitive locus at chromosome Xp21 is involved in male to female sex reversal. *Nat Genet* 7: 497–501.

Baumstark A, Akhverdyan M, Schulze A, Reisert I, Vogel W, Just W (2001). Exclusion of SOX9 as the testis determining factor in *Ellobius lutescens*: evidence for another testis determining gene besides SRY and SOX9. *Mol Genet Metab* 72: 61–66.

Bergstrom DE, Young M, Albrecht KH, Eicher E (2000). Related function of mouse SOX3, SOX9 and SRY HMG domains assayed by male sex determination. *Genesis* 29: 111–124.

Bernstein R, Jenkins T, Dawson B, Wagner J, Dewald G, Koo GC, Wachtel SS (1980). Female phenotype and multiple abnormalities in sibs with a Y chromosome and partial X chromosome duplication: H-Y antigen and Xg blood group findings. *J Med Genet* 17: 291–300.

Berta P, Hawkins JR, Sinclair AH, Taylor A, Griffiths BL, Goodfellow PN, Fellous M (1990). Genetic evidence equating *SRY* and the testis-determining factor. *Nature* 348: 448–450.

Bianchi ME, Falciola L, Ferrari S, Lilley DMJ (1992). The DNA binding site of HMG1 protein is composed of two similar segments (HMG boxes), both of which have counterparts in other eukaryotic regulatory proteins. *EMBO J* 11: 1055–1063.

Birk OS, Casiano DE, Wassif CA, Cogliati T, Zhao L, Zhao Y, Grinberg A, Huang S, Kreidberg JA, Parker KL, et al. (2000). The LIM homeobox gene *Lhx9* is essential for mouse gonad formation. *Nature* 403: 909–913.

Bishop CE, Whitworth DJ, Qin Y, Agoulnik AI, Agoulnik IU, Harrison WR, Behringer RR, Overbeek PA (2000). A transgenic insertion upstream of *Sox9* is associated with dominant XX sex reversal in the mouse. *Nat Genet* 26: 490–494.

Bitgood MJ, Shen L, McMahon AP (1996). Sertoli cell signaling by Desert hedgehog regulates the male germline. *Curr Biol* 6: 298–304.

Bowles J, Cooper L, Berkman J, Koopman P (1999). *Sry* requires a CAG repeat domain for male sex determination in *Mus muculus*. *Nat Genet* 22: 405–408.

Boyer T, Erickson RP (1993). Detection of circular and linear transcripts of *Sry* in preimplantation mouse embryos: differences in requirement for reverse transcriptase. *Biochem Biophys Res Commun* 198: 492–496.

Cao QP, Gaudette MF, Robinson DH, Crain WR (1995). Expression of the mouse testis-determining gene *Sry* in male preimplantation embryos. *Mol Reprod Dev* 40: 196–204.

Capel B (1995). New bedfellows in the mammalian sex-determination affair. *Trends Genet* 11: 161–163.

Capel B, Swain A, Nicolis S, Hacker A, Walter M, Koopman P, Goodfellow P, Lovell-Badge R (1993). Circular transcripts of the testis-determining gene *Sry* in adult mouse testis. *Cell* 73: 1019–1030.

Cardoso C, Timsit S, Villard L, Khrestchatisky M, Fontes M, Colleaux L (1998). Specific interaction between the *XNP/ATR-X* gene product and the SET domain of the human EZH2 protein. *Hum Mol Genet* 7: 679–684.

Carpentier PJ, Potter EL (1959). Nuclear sex and genital malformation in 48 cases of renal agenesis, with special reference to non-specific female pseudohermaphroditism. *Am J Obstet Gynecol* 78: 235–258.

Collignon J, Sockanathan S, Hacker A, Cohen-Tannoudji M, Norris D, Rastan S, Stevanovic M, Goodfellow PN, Lovell-Badge R (1996). A comparison of the properties of *Sox-3* with *Sry* and two related genes, *Sox-1* and *Sox-2*. *Development* 122: 509–520.

Colvin JS, Green RP, Schmahl J, Capel B, Ornitz DM (2001). Male-to-female sex reversal in mice lacking fibroblast growth factor 9. *Cell* 104: 875–889.

Cooper MK, Wassif CA, Krakowiak PA, Taipale J, Gong R, Kelley RI, Porter FD, Beachy PA (2003). A defective response to Hedgehog signalling in disorders of cholesterol synthesis. *Nature Genetics* 33: 508–513.

Davies RC, Calvo C, Bratt E, Larsson S, Lamond AI, Hastie ND (1998). WT1 interacts with the splicing factor U2AF65 in an isoform-dependent manner and can be incorporated into spliceosomes. *Genes Dev* 12: 3217–3225.

Del Campo M, Jones MC, Veraksa AN, Curry CJ, Jones KL, Mascarello JT, Ali-Kahn-Catts Z, Drumheller T, McGinnis W (1999). Monodactylous limbs and abnormal genitalia are associated with hemizygosity for the human 2q31 region that includes the *HOXD* cluster. *Am J Hum Genet* 65: 104–110.

de Santa Barbara P, Bonneaud N, Boizet B, Desclozeaux M, Moniot B, Sudbeck P, Scherer G, Poulat F, Berta P (1998). Direct interaction of SRY-related protein SOX9 and steroidogenic factor 1 regulates transcription of the human anti-müllerian hormone gene. *Mol Cell Biol* 18: 6653–6665.

de Santa Barbara P, Moniot B, Poulat F, Berta P (2000). Expression and subcellular localization of SF-1, SOX9, WT1, and AMH proteins during early human testicular development. *Dev Dyn* 217: 293–298.

Desclozeaux M, Poulat F, de Santa Barbara P, Capony J-P, Turowski P, Jay P, Méjean C, Moniot B, Boizet B, Berta P (1998). Phosphorylation of an N-terminal motif enhances DNA-binding activity of the human SRY protein. *J Bio Chem* 273: 7988–7995.

Devriendt K, Jaeken J, Matthijs G, Van Esch H, Debeer P, Gewillig M, Fryns J-P (1999). Haploinsufficiency of the HOXA gene cluster, in a patient with hand-foot-genital syndrome, velopharyngeal insufficiency, and persistent patent ductus botalli. *Am J Hum Genet* 65: 249–251.

Dollé P, Dierich A, LeMeur M, Schimmang T, Schuhbaur B, Chambon P, Duboule D (1993). Disruption of the *Hoxd-13* gene induces localized heterochrony leading to mice with neotenic limbs. *Cell* 75: 431–441.

Dubin RA, Ostrer H (1994). Sry is a transcriptional activator. *Mol Endocrinol* 8: 1182–1192.

Erickson RP, Verga V, Dasouki M (1990). Use of a probe for the putative sex determining gene, Zinc finger Y, in the study of patients with ambiguous genitalia and XY gonadal dysgenesis. *Am J Med Genet* 36: 232–236.

Erickson RP, Stone JF, McNoe LA, Eccles MR (1997). Molecular and clinical studies of three cases of female pseudohermaphroditism with caudal dysplasia suggest multiple etiologies. *Clin Genet* 51: 331–337.

Erno H, Kury P, Botteri FM, Monard D (1996). A Krox binding site regulates protease nexin-1 promoter activity in embryonic heart, cartilage and parts of the nervous system. *Mech Dev* 60: 139–150.

Escobar LF, Weaver DD, Bixler D, Hodes MR, Mitchell M (1987). Urorectal septum malformation sequence. *Am J Dis Child* 141: 1021–1024.

Evans HS, Buckton KE, Spowart G, Carothers AD (1979). Heteromorphic X chromosomes in 46,XX males: evidence for the involvement of X–Y interchange. *Hum Genet* 49: 11–31.

Ferrari S, Harley VR, Pontiggia A, Goodfellow PN, Lovell-Badge R, Bianchi ME (1992). *SRY* like HMG1, recognizes sharp angles in DNA. *EMBO J* 11: 4497–4506.

Flejter WL, Fergestad J, Gorski J, Varvill T, Chandrasekharappa S (1998). A gene involved in XY sex reversal is located on chromosome 9, distal to marker D9S1779. *Am J Hum Genet* 63: 794–802.

Ford CE, Jones KW, Miller OJ, Mittwoch U, Penrose LS, Ridler M, Shapiro A (1959a). The chromosomes in a patient showing both mongolism and the Klinefelter syndrome. *Lancet* 1: 709–710.

Ford CE, Jones KW, Polani PE, De Almedia JC, Briggs JH (1959b). A sex chromosome anomaly in a case of gonadal dysgenesis (Turner's syndrome). *Lancet* 1: 711.

Garcia-Heras J, Corley N, Garcia MF, Kukolich MK, Smith KG, Day DW (1999). De novo partial duplications 1p: report of two new cases and review. *Am J Med Genet* 82: 261–264.

Gibbons RJ, Picketss DJ, Villard L, Higgs DR (1995). Mutations in a putative global transcriptional regulators cause X-linked mental retardation with α-thalassemia (ATR-X syndrome). *Cell* 80: 837–845.

Gibbons RJ, McDowell TL, Raman S, O'Rourke DM, Garrick D, Ayyub H, Higgs DR (2000). Mutations in ATRX, encoding a SWI/SNF-like protein, cause diverse changes in the pattern of DNA methylation. *Nat Genet* 24: 368–371.

Giuli G, Shen W-H, Ingraham HA (1997). The nuclear receptor SF-1 mediates sexually dimorphic expression of müllerian inhibiting substance, in vivo. *Development* 124: 1799–1807.

Graham JM Jr, Rawnsley AF, Simmons GM, Wurster-Hills DH, Park JP, Parin-Padilla M, Crow HC (1989). Triploidy: pregnancy complications and clinical findings in seven cases. *Prenat Diagn* 9: 409–419.

Graves JA (1998). Interactions between *SRY* and *SOX* genes in mammalian sex determination. *Bioessays* 20: 264–269.

Grimmond S, Van Hataren N, Siggers P, Arkell R, Larder R, Bento Soares M, de Fatima Bonaldo M, Smith L, Tymowska-Lalanne Z, Wells C, Greenfield A (2000). Sexually dimorphic expression of protease nexin-1 and vanin-1 in the developing mouse gonad prior to overt differentiation suggests a role in mammalian sexual development. *Hum Mol Genet* 9: 1553–1560.

Gubbay J, Collignon J, Koopman P, Capel B, Aconomou A, Münsterberg A, Vivian N, Goodfellow P, Lovell-Badge R (1990). A gene mapping to the sex-determining region of the mouse Y chromosome is a member of a novel family of embryonically expressed genes. *Nature* 346: 245–250.

Gueallaen G, Casanova M, Bishop C, Geldwerth D, Andre G, Fellous M, Weissenboch J (1984). Human XX males with Y single-copy DNA fragments. *Nature* 307: 172–173.

Hacker A, Capel B, Goodfellow P, Lovell-Badge R (1995). Expression of *Sry*, the mouse sex-determining region gene. *Development* 121: 1603–1614.

Hammes A, Guo J-K, Lutch G, Leheste J-R, Landrock D, Ziegler U, Gubler M-C, Schedl A (2001). Two splice variants of the Wilms' tumor 1 gene have distinct functions during sex determination and nephron formation. *Cell* 106: 319–329.

Haqq CM, King C-Y, Donahoe PK, Weiss MA (1994). Molecular basis of mammalian sexual determination: activation of müllerian inhibiting substance gene expression *SRY*. *Science* 266: 1494–1500.

Haraguchi R, Suzuki K, Murakami R, Sakai M, Kamikawa M, Kengaku M, Sekine K, Kawano H, Kato S, Ueno N, Yamada G (2000). Molecular analysis of external genitalia formation: the role of fibroblast growth factor (Fgf) genes during genital tubercle formation. *Development* 127: 2471–2479.

Haraguchi R, Mo R, Hui CC, Motoyama J, Makino S, Shiroishi T, Gaffield W, Yamada G (2001). Unique functions of Sonic hedgehog signaling during external genitalia development. *Development* 128: 4241–4250.

Hastie ND (2001). Life, sex, and WT1 isoforms: three amino acids can make all the difference. *Cell* 106: 391–394.

Hatano O, Takayama K, Imai T, Waterman MR, Takakusu A, Omura T, Morohasi K-I (1994). Sex-dependent expression of a transcription factor, Ad4BP, regulating steroidogenic P-450 genes in the gonads during prenatal and postnatal rat development. *Development* 20: 2787–2797.

Hawkins JR, Taylor A, Goodfellow PN, Migeon CJ, Smith KD, Berkovitz GD (1992). Evidence for increased prevalence of *SRY* mutations in XY females with complete rather than partial gonadal dysgenesis. *Am J Hum Genet* 51: 979–984.

Hobert O, Westphal H (2000). Functions of LIM-homeobox genes. *Trends Genet* 16: 75–83.

Hokamp HG, Muller KM (1983). Prune belly syndrome and female pseudohermaphroditism. *Pathol Res Pract* 117: 76–83.

Hossain A, Saunders GF (2001). The human sex-determining gene *SRY* is a direct target of *WT1*. *J Biol Chem* 276: 16817–16823.

Huang B, Wang S, Ning Y, Lamb AN, Bartley J (1999). Autosomal XX sex reversal caused by duplication of *SOX9*. *Am J Med Genet* 87: 349–353.

Huang W, Zhou X, Lefebvre V, de Crombrugghe B (2000). Phosphorylation of SOX9 by cyclic AMP-dependent protein kinase A enhances SOX9's ability to transactivate a *Col2a1* chondrocyte-specific enhancer. *Mol Cell Biol* 20: 4149–4158.

Ikeda Y, Shen W-H, Ingraham HA, Parker KL (1994). Developmental expression mouse steroidogenic factor 1, an essential regulator of the steroid hydrolaxes. *Mol Endocrinol* 8: 654–662.

Jacobs PA, Strong JA (1959). A case of human intersexuality having a possible XXY sex-determining mechanism. *Nature* 183: 302.

Jäger RJ, Anvret M, Hall K, Scherer G (1990). A human XY female with a frame shift mutation in the candidate testis-determining gene *SRY*. *Nature* 348: 452–454.

Jantzen H-M, Admon A, Bell SP, Tjian R (1990). Nucleolar transcription factor hUBf contains a DNA-binding motif with homology to HMG proteins. *Nature* 344: 830–836.

Jeffs B, Meeks JJ, Ito M, Martinson FA, Matzuk MM, Jameson JL, Russell LD (2001). Blockage of the rete testis and efferent ductules by ectopic Sertoli and Leydig cells causes infertility in dax1-deficient male mice. *Endocrinology* 142: 4486–4495.

Jordan BK, Mohammed M, Saunders TC, Délot E, Chen X-N, Dewing P, Swain A, Rao PN, Elejakde BR, Vilain E (2001). Up-regulation of WNT-4 signaling and dosage-sensitive sex reversal in humans. *Am J Hum Genet* 68: 1102–1109.

Jost A (1953). Problems of fetal endocrinology: the gonadal and hypophyseal hormones. *Recent Prog Horm Res* 8: 379.

Jost A, Vigier B, Prepin J, Perchellet JP (1973). Studies on sex differentiation in mammals. *Recent Prog Horm Res* 29: 1–41.

Just W, Rau W, Vogel W, Akhverdian M, Fredga K, Graves JA, Lyapunova E (1995). Absence of *Sry* in species of the role *Ellobius*. *Nat Genet* 11: 117–118.

Kamachi Y, Uchikawa M, Kondoh H (2000). Pairing SOX off with partners in the regulation of embryonic development. *Trends Genet* 16: 182–187.

Katoh-Fukui Y, Tsuchiya R, Shiroishi T, Nakahara Y, Hashimoto N, Noguchi K, Higashinakagawa T (1998). Male-to-female sex reversal in *M33* mutant mice. *Nature* 393: 688–692.

Kent J, Coriat AM, Sharpe PT, Hastie ND, van Heyningen V (1995). The evolution of WT1 sequence and expression pattern in the vertebrates. *Oncogene* 11: 1781–1792.

Kettlewell JR, Raymond CS, Zarkower D (2000). Temperature-dependent expression of turtle Dmrt1 prior to sexual differentiation. *Genesis* 26: 174–178.

Kim J, Prawitt D, Bardeesy N, Torban E, Vicaner C, Goodyer P, Zabel B, Pelletier J (1999). The Wilms' tumor suppressor gene (wt1) product regulates *Dax-1* gene expression during gonadal differentiation. *Mol Cell Biol* 19: 2289–2299.

King C-Y, Weiss MA (1993). The SRY high-mobility-group box recognizes DNA by partial intercalation in the minor groove: a topological mechanism of sequence specificity. *Proc Natl Acad Sci USA* 90: 11990–11994.

Kondo T, Zákány J, Innis JW, Duboule D (1997). Of fingers, toes and penises. *Nature* 390: 29.

Koopman P, Münsterberg A, Capel B, Vivian N, Lovell-Badge R (1990). Expression of a candidate sex-determining gene during mouse testis differentiation. *Nature* 348: 450–452.

Koopman P, Gubbay J, Vivan N, Goodfellow P, Lovell-Badge R (1991). Male development of chromosomally female mice transgenic for *Sry*. *Nature* 351: 117–121.

Lala DS, Rice DA, Parker KL (1992). Steroidogenic factor 1, a key regulator of steroidogenic enzyme expression, is the mouse homolog of fushi tarazu factor 1. *Mol Endocrinol* 6: 1249–1258.

Little M, Holmes G, Walsh P (1999). WT1: what has the last decade told us? *Bioessays* 21: 191–202.

Lubinsky MS (1980). Female pseudohermaphroditism and associated anomalies. *Am J Med Genet* 6: 123–136.

Luo X, Ikeda Y, Parker KL (1994). A cell-specific nuclear receptor is essential for adrenal and gonadal development and sexual differentiation. *Cell* 77: 481–490.

MacKenzie J, Chitayat D, McLorie G, Balfe JW, Pandit PB, Blecher SR (1994). Penoscrotal transposition: a case report and review. *Am J Med Genet* 49: 103–107.

Magenis RE, Webb MJ, McKean RS, Tomar D, Allen LJ, Kammer H, VanDyke DL, Louvien E (1982). Translocation (X;Y)(p22.33;p11.2) in XX males: etiology of male phenotype. *Hum Genet* 62: 271–276.

Marchand O, Govoroun M, D'Cotta H, McMeel O, Lareyre J, Bernot A, Laudet V, Guiguen Y (2000). DMRT1 expression during gonadal differentiation and spermatogenesis in the rainbow trout, *Oncorhynchus mykiss*. *Biochim Biophys Acta* 1493: 180–187.

Margarit E, Guillén A, Rebordosa C, Vidal-Taboada J, Sánchez M, Ballesta F, Oliva R (1998). Identification of conserved potentially regulatory sequences of the SRY gene from 10 different species of mammals. *Biochem Biophys Res Commun* 245: 370–377.

McElreavey K, Vilain E, Abbas N, Herskowitz I, Fellous M (1993). A regulatory cascade hypothesis for mammalian sex determination: *SRY* represses a negative regulator of male development. *Proc Natl Acad Sci USA* 90: 3368–3372.

Miller C, Sassoon DA (1998). Wnt-7a maintains appropriate uterine patterning during the development of the mouse female reproductive tract. *Development* 125: 3201–3211.

Miyamoto N, Yoshida M, Kuratani S, Matsuo I, Aizawa S (1997). Defects of urogenital development in mice lacking *Emx2*. *Development* 124: 1653–1664.

Moniot B, Berta P, Sherer G, Sudbeck P, Poulat F (2000). Male specific expression suggests role of DMRT1 in human sex determination. *Mech Dev* 91: 323–325.

Morais da Silva S, Hacker A, Harley V, Goodfellow P, Swain A, Lovell-Badge R (1996). *SOX9* expression during gonadal development implies a conserved role for the gene is testis differentiation in mammals and birds. *Nat Genet* 14: 62–68.

Mortlock DP, Innis JW (1997). Mutation of *HOXA-13* in hand-foot-genital syndrome. *Nat Genet* 15: 179–180.

Mortlock DP, Post LC, Innis JW (1996). The molecular basis of hypodactyly (*Hd*): a deletion in *Hoxa13* leads to arrest of digital arch formation. *Nat Genet* 13: 284–289.

Murphy EC, Zhurkin VB, Louis JM, Cornilescu G, Clore GM (2001). Structural basis for SRY-dependent 46-X,Y sex reversal: modulation of DNA bending by a naturally occurring point mutation. *J Mol Biol* 312: 481–499.

Muscatelli F, Strom TM, Walker AP, Zanaria E, Récan D, Meindl A, Bardoni B, Guioli S, Zehetner G, Rabl W, et al. (1994). Mutations in the *DAX-1* gene give rise to both X-linked adrenal hypoplasia congenita and hypogonadotropic hypogonadism. *Nature* 372: 672–676.

Nachtigal MW, Hirokawa Y, Enyeart-VanHouten DL, Flanagan JN, Hammer GD, Ingraham HA (1998). Wilms' tumor 1 and Dax-1 modulate the orphan nuclear receptor SF-1 in sex-specific gene expression. *Cell* 93: 445–454.

Nakahori Y, Tamua T, Nagafuchi S, Fujieda K, Minowada S, Fukutani K, Fuse H, Hayashi K, Kuroki Y, Fukushima Y, et al. (1991). Molecular cloning and mapping of 10 new probes on the human Y chromosome. *Genomics* 9: 765–769.

Nasrin N, Buggs C, Kong XF, Carnazza J, Goebl M, Alexander-Bridges M (1991). DNA-binding properties of the product of the testis-determining gene and a related protein. *Nature* 354: 317–320.

Ogata T, Matsuo N (1994). Testis determining gene(s) on the X chromosome short arm: chromosomal localization and possible role in testis determination. *J Med Genet* 31: 349–350.

Ogata T, Hawkins JR, Taylor A, Matsuo N, Hata J, Goodfellow PN (1992). Sex reversal in a child with a 46,X,Yp+ karyotype: support for the existence of a gene(s), located in distal Xp, involved in testis formation. *J Med Genet* 29: 226–230.

Ohe K, Lalli E, Sassone-Corsi P (2002). A direct role of SRY and SOX proteins in pre-mRNA splicing. *Proc Natl Acad Sci USA* 99: 1146–1151.

Oreal E, Lieau C, Mattel MG, Josso N, Picard JY, Carre-Eusebe D, Magre S (1998). Early expression of AMH in chicken embryonic gonads precedes testicular SOX9 expression. *Dev Dyn* 212: 522–532.

Page DC, Mosher R, Simpson EM, Fisher EMC, Mardon G, Pollack J, McGillivray B, de la Chappele A, Brown LG (1987). The sex-determining region or the human Y chromosome encodes a finger protein. *Cell* 51: 1091–1104.

Palmer MS, Sinclair AH, Berta P, Ellis NA, Goodfellow PN, Abbas NE, Fellous M (1989). Genetic evidence that *ZFY* is not the testis-determining factor. *Nature* 342: 937–939.

Parida SK, Hall BD, Barton L, Fujimoto A (1995). Penoscrotal transposition and associated anomalies: report of five new cases and review of the literature. *Am J Med Genet* 59: 69–75.

Parr BA, McMahon AP (1995). Dorsalizing signal Wnt-7a required for normal polarity of D–V and A–P axes of mouse limb. *Nature* 374: 350–353.

Parr BA, McMahon AP (1998). Sexually dimorphic development of the mammalian reproductive tract requires *Wnt-7a. Nature* 395: 707–710.

Parr BA, Avery EJ, Cygan JA, McMahon AP (1998). The classical mouse mutant postaxial hemimelia results from a mutation in the *Wnt 7*a gene. *Dev Biol* 202: 228–234.

Pask A, Toder R, Wilcox SA, Camerino G, Graves JA (1997). The candidate sex-reversing *DAX1* gene is autosomal in marsupials: implications for the evolution of sex determination in mammals. *Genomics* 41: 422–426.

Pask A, Renfree MB, Marshall Graves JA (2000). The human sex-reversing ATRX gene has a homologue on the marsupial Y chromosome, ATRY: implications for the evolution of mammalian sex determination. *Proc Natl Acad Sci USA* 97: 13198–13202.

Peichel CL, Prabhakaran B, Vogt TF (1997). The mouse *Ulnaless* mutation deregulates posterior *HoxD* gene expression and alters appendicular patterning. *Development* 124: 3481–3492.

Perloff WH, Conger KB, Ley L (1953). Female pseudohermaphroditism: a description of two unusual cases. *J Clin Endocrinol* 13: 783–790.

Petit P, Moerman PH, Fryns JP (1992). Full 69,XXY triploidy and sex-reversal: a further example of true hermaphrodism associated with multiple malformations. *Clin Genet* 41: 175–177.

Pinsky L, Erickson RP, Schimke RN (1999). *Genetic Disorders of Human Sexual Development.* Oxford University Press, New York, pp. 11–38.

Podlasek CA, Barnett DH, Clemens JQ, Bak PM, Bushman W (1999). Prostate development requires Sonic hedgehog expressed by the urogenital sinus epithelium. *Dev Biol* 209: 28–39.

Poulat F, de Santa Barbara P, Desclozeaux M, Soullier S, Moniot B, Bonneaud N, Boizet B, Berta P (1997). The human testis determining factor *SRY* binds a nuclear factor containing PDZ protein interaction domains. *J Biol Chem* 272: 7167–7172.

Ramsay M, Berstein R, Zwane E, Page DC, Jenkins T (1988). XX true hermaphroditism in southern African blacks: an enigma of primary sexual differentiation. *Am J Hum Genet* 43: 4–13.

Raymond CS, Shamu CE, Shen MM, Seifert KJ, Hirsch B, Hodgkin J, Zarkower D (1998). Evidence for evolutionary conservation of sex-determining genes. *Nature* 391: 691–695.

Raymond CS, Kettlewell JR, Hirsch B, Bardwell VJ, Zarkower D (1999a). Expression of *Dmrt1* in the genital ridge of mouse and chicken embryos suggests a role in vertebrate sexual development. *Dev Biol* 215: 208–220.

Raymond CS, Parker ED, Kettlewell JR, Brown LG, Page DC, Kusz K, Jaruzelska J, Reinberg Y, Flejter WL, Bardwell VJ, et al. (1999a) A region of human chromosome 9p required for testis development contains two genes related to known sexual regulators. *Hum Mol Genet* 8: 989–996.

Reinberg Y, Shapiro E, Manivel JC, Manley CB, Pettinato G, Gonzales R (1991). Prune belly syndrome in females: a triad of abdominal muscular deficiency and anomalies of the urinary and genital systems. *J Pediatr* 118: 395–398.

Robinson Jr HB, Tross K (1984). Agenesis of the cloacal membrane: a possible teratogenic anomaly. *Perspect Pediatr Pathol* 8: 79–96.

Sadovsky Y, Crawford PA, Woodson KG, Polish JA, Clements MA, Tourtellotte L M, Simburger K, Milbrandt J (1995). Mice deficient in the orphan receptor steroidogenic factor 1 lack adrenal glands and gonads but express P450 side-chain-cleavage enzyme in the placenta and have normal embryonic serum levels of corticosteroids. *Proc Natl Acad Sci USA* 92: 10939–10943.

Sainio K, Hellstedt P, Kreidberg JA, Saxen L, Sariola H (1997). Differential regulation of two sets of mesonephric tubules by WT-1. *Development* 124: 1293–1299.

Scherer G, Schempp W, Baccichetti C, Lensini E, Bricarelli FD, Carbone LD, Wolf U (1989). Duplication of an Xp segment that includes the ZFX locus causes sex inversion in man. *Hum Genet* 81: 291–294.

Schmahl J, Eicher EM, Washburn LL, Capel B (2000). *Sry* induces cell proliferation in the mouse gonad. *Development* 127: 65–73.

Shawlot W, Behringer RR (1995). Requirement for *Lim1* in head-organizer function. *Nature* 374: 425–430.

Shen W-H, Moore CCD, Ikeda Y, Parker KL, Ingraham HA (1994). Nuclear receptor steroidogenic factor 1 regulates the müllerian inhibiting substance gene: a link to the sex determination pathway. *Cell* 77: 651–661.

Shimamura R, Fraizer GC, Trapman J, Lau YfC, Saunders GF (1997). The Wilms' tumor gene WT1 can regulate genes involved in sex determination and differentiation: SRY, müllerian-inhibiting substance, and the androgen receptor. *Clin Cancer Res* 3: 2571–2580.

Sinclair AH, Berta P, Palmer MS, Hawkins JR, Griffiths BL, Smith MJ, Foster JW, Frischauf A-M, Lovell-Badge R, Goodfellow PN (1990). A gene from the human sex-determining region encodes a protein with homology to a conserved DNA-binding motif. *Nature* 346: 240–244.

Spurdle AB, Shankman S, Ramsay M (1995). XX true hermaphroditism in southern African blacks: exclusion of SRY sequences and uniparental disomy of the X chromosome. *Am J Hum Genet* 55: 53–56.

Stalvey JRD, Durbin EJ, Erickson RP (1989). Sex vesicle "entrapment": translocation or nonhomologous recombination of misaligned Yp and Xp as alternative mechanisms for abnormal inheritance of the sex-determining region. *Am J Med Genet* 32: 546–572.

Stevanovic M, Lovell Badge R, Collignon J, Goodfellow PN (1993). SOX3 is an X-linked gene related to SRY. *Hum Mol Genet* 2: 2007–2012.

Su H, Lau YC (1993). Identification of the transcriptional unit, structural organization, and promoter sequence of the human sex-determining region Y (*SRY*) gene, using a reverse genetic approach. *Am J Hum Genet* 52: 24–38.

Sudbeck P, Scherer G (1997). Two independent nuclear localization signals are present in the DNA-binding high mobility group domains of SRY and SOX9. *J Biol Chem* 272: 27848–27852.

Sutou S, Mitsui Y, Tsuchiya K (2001). Sex determination without the Y chromosome in two Japanese rodents *Tokudaia osimensis osimensis* and *Tokudaia osimensis* spp. *Mamm Genome* 12: 17–21.

Swain A, Zanaria E, Hacker A, Lovell-Badge R, Camerino G (1996). Mouse *Dax1* expression is consistent with a role in sex determination as well as in adrenal and hypothalamus function. *Nat Genet* 12: 404–409.

Swain A, Narvaez V, Burgoyne P, Camerino G, Lovell-Badge R (1998). *Dax1* antagonizes *Sry* action in mammalian sex determination. *Nature* 391: 761–767.

Taketo M, Parker KL, Howard TA, Tsukiyama T, Wong M, Niwa O, Morton CC, Miron PM, Seldin MF (1995). Homologs of *Drosophila* Fushi-Tarazu factor 1 map to mouse chromosome 2 and human chromosome 9q33. *Genomics* 25: 565–567.

Tamura M, Kanno Y, Chuma S, Saito T, Nakatsuji N (2001). *Pod-1/Capsulin* shows a sex- and stage-dependent expression pattern in the mouse gonad development and represses expression of Ad4BP/SF-1. *Mech Dev* 102: 135–144.

Tevosian SG, Albrecht KH, Crispino JD, Fujiwara Y, Eicher EM, Orkin SH (2002). Gonadal differentiation, sex determination and normal *Sry* expression in mice require direct interaction between transcription factors GATA4 and FOG2. *Development* 129: 4627–4634.

Tilmann C, Capel B (1999). Mesonephric cell migration induces testis cord formation and Sertoli cell differentiation in the mammalian gonad. *Development* 126: 2883–2890.

Toyooka Y, Tanaka SS, Hirota O, Tanaka S, Takagi N, Yamanouchi K, Tojo H, Tachi C (1998). Wilms' tumor suppressor gene (*WT1*) as a target gene of SRY function in a mouse ES cell line transfected with SRY. *Int J Dev Biol* 42: 1143–1151.

Vainio S, Heikkila M, Kispert A, Chin N, McMahon AP (1999). Female development in mammals is regulated by Wnt-4. *Nature* 397: 405–409.

van Heyningen V, Hastie ND (1992). Wilms' tumor: reconciling genetics and biology. *Trends Genet* 8: 16–21.

Verga V, Erickson RP (1989). An extended long-range restriction map of the human sex-determining region on Yp, including *ZFY*, finds marked homology on XP and no detectable Y sequences in an XX male. *Am J Hum Genet* 44: 756–765.

Vergnaud G, Page DC, Simmler MC, Brown L, Rouyer F, Noel B, Botstein D, de la Chapelle A, Weissenbach J (1986). A deletion map of the human Y chromosome based on DNA hybridization. *Am J Hum Genet* 38: 109–124.

Vidal VPI, Chaboissier M-C, de Rooij DG, Schedl A (2001). *Sox9* induces testis development in XX transgenic mice. *Nat Genet* 28: 216–217.

Viger RS, Mertineit C, Trasier JM, Nemer M (1998). Transcription factor GATA-4 is expressed in a sexually dimorphic pattern during mouse gonadal development and is a potent activator of the müllerian inhibiting substance promoter. *Development* 125: 2665–2675.

Vilain E, Fellous M, McElreavey K (1992). Characterization and sequence of the 5' flanking region of the human testis-determining factor *SRY. Methods Mol Cell Biol* 3: 128–134.

Washburn LL, Albrecht KH, Eicher EM (2001). C57BL/6J-*T*-associated sex reversal in mice is caused by reduced expression of a *Mus domesticus Sry* allele. *Genetics* 158: 1675–1681.

Welshons WJ, Russell LB (1959). The Y-chromosome as the bearer of male determining factors in the mouse. *Proc Natl Acad Sci USA* 45: 560.

Werner MH, Huth JR, Gronenborn AV, Clore GM (1995). Molecular basis of human 46,XY sex reversal revealed from the three-dimensional solutions structure of the human *SRY*-DNA complex. *Cell* 81: 705–714.

Western PS, Harry JL, Graves JAM, Sinclair AH (1999). Temperature-dependent sex determination: upregulation of *SOX9* expression after commitment to male development. *Dev Dyn* 214: 171–177.

Wright E, Hargrave MR, Christiansen J, Cooper L, Kun J, Evans T, Gangadharan U, Greefield A, Koopman P (1995). The *Sry*-related gene *Sox9* is expressed during chondrogenesis in mouse embryos. *Nat Genet* 9: 15–20.

Yamaguchi TP, Bradley A, McMahon AP, Jones S (1999). A Wnt5a pathway underlies outgrowth of multiple structures in the vertebrate embryo. *Development* 126: 1211–1223.

Yu RN, Ito M, Saunders TL, Camper SA, Jameson JL (1998). Role of *Ahch* in gonadal development and gametogenesis. *Nat Genet* 20: 353–357.

Zanaria E, Muscatelli F, Bardoni B, Strom TM, Guioli S, Guo W, Lalli E, Moser C, Walker AP, McCabe ERB, et al. (1994). An unusual member of the nuclear hormone receptor superfamily responsible for X-linked adrenal hypoplasia congenita. *Nature* 372: 635–641.

Zimmerman S, Schwärzler A, Buth S, Engel W, Adham IM (1998). Transcription of the Leydig insulin-like gene is mediated by steroidogenic factor-1. *Mol Endocrinol* 12: 706–713.

Zwingman T, Erickson RP, Boyer T, Ao A (1993). Transcription of the sex determining region genes *Sry* and *Zfy* in the mouse preimplantation embryo. *Proc Natl Acad Sci USA* 90: 814–817.

Zwingman T, Fujimoto H, Lai L-W, Boyer T, Ao A, Stalvey JRD, Blecher SR, Erickson RP (1994). Transcription of circular and noncircular forms of *Sry* in mouse testes. *Mol Reprod Dev* 37: 370–381.

43 | *SOX9* and Campomelic Dysplasia and Sex Reversal

SAHAR MANSOUR

Campomelic dysplasia (CMD) is a rare, usually lethal skeletal dysplasia. Unlike other forms of skeletal dysplasia, it is frequently associated with XY sex reversal. The gene for this condition, *SOX9*, was identified in 1994. As suggested by the phenotype in CMD, *SOX9* is an important gene, not only in the sex determination pathway but also in chondrogenesis. In this chapter I discuss *SOX9* and its role in both the sex determination pathway and the cartilage and collagen pathway. The clinical and radiological features of CMD are described, including the phenotype and complications in survivors with this condition.

LOCUS AND DEVELOPMENTAL PATHWAYS

SOX9 and CMD

A few case reports were published that described CMD with chromosomal translocations involving chromosome 17q (Young et al., 1992; Tommerup et al., 1993). This led to the hypothesis that the gene for CMD is located at or near the breakpoint of these translocations. The murine *Sox9* had been localized to mouse chromosome 11 in an area that is homologous to distal chromosome 17q. Although the human *SOX9* gene was not at the translocation breakpoint, it was within an 88 kb region. Because the mouse *Sox9* gene is expressed in skeletal tissue during mouse embryogenesis, it was regarded as a strong candidate gene for CMD (Wright et al., 1995). *SOX9* was first cloned in 1994 (Foster et al., 1994; Wagner et al., 1994).

Heterozygous mutations in *SOX9* were identified in six of nine patients with CMD. These were all either de novo mutations or not present in 100 controls. All of these mutations were predicted to cause protein truncation and therefore loss of function of the protein. The predicted loss of function of these mutants and the absence of mutations in both alleles suggest that this is an autosomal dominant condition due to haploinsufficiency of the gene.

Sox9 and Collagen Development

Because campomelic dysplasia is a skeletal dysplasia, it is clear that *SOX9* has an important role in the development of bone and cartilage. The mechanism, however, is still not fully understood. During chondrogenesis in the mouse, *Sox9* is expressed with *Col2a1*, the gene that encodes a major cartilage matrix protein, type II collagen. The first intron of the type II collagen gene contains regulatory sequences that are required for chondrocyte-specific expression of this gene. It has been shown that the SOX9 protein binds specifically to sequences in the first intron of *COL2A1* (Bell et al., 1997). In transgenic mice, mutations of these sequences abolish Sox9 binding and therefore expression of a *Col2a1*-driven reporter gene (col2a1 lacZ). Ectopic expression of Sox9 transactivates *Col2a1* and the *Col2a1*-driven reporter gene in some tissues. This activation demonstrates that *COL2A1* expression is directly regulated by the SOX9 protein. Abnormal expression of collagen II results in the skeletal changes seen in CMD.

SOX9 and Sex Determination

SOX9 has a major role in the vertebrate sex determination pathway. Although the mechanism is still not completely understood, recent studies are providing some clues. These studies have been thoroughly reviewed in Chapter 42.

Heterozygous levels of *SOX9* are close to a threshold for gonadal development. Below this threshold, the Sertoli's cells fail to be either initiated or maintained. A dosage effect is further suggested by the report of a single case of XX sex reversal due to a 17q23–24 duplication (the region containing *SOX9*)(Huang et al., 1999).

Gonadal development depends on the expression of a subgroup of genes, including *WT1, GATA4,* and *SF1,* as well as *LIM1* and *LHX9.* These genes are probably transcriptional activators. There is strong evidence that SF1, WT1, and GATA4 participate with SOX9 in the activation of antimüllerian hormone (*AMH*). The regulation of *AMH* is complex; protein–protein interactions exist between SOX9 and SF1, SF1 and GATA4, and SF1 and WT1. Although the *AMH* promotor has binding sites for SOX9, SF1, and GATA4, it appears that SOX9 has a pivotal role in *AMH* activation. Mutations in the SOX9-binding site of *AMH* in mice leads to complete absence of *AMH* transcription and therefore to the persistence of müllerian ducts in transgenic mice (whereas mutations in the SF1 binding site cause the müllerian ducts to only partially regress (Arango et al., 1999)). Therefore, SF1 may be the specific gonadal coactivator for *SOX9*, while other coactivators are required for promoting expression of *COL2A1.*

CLINICAL DESCRIPTION

Campomelic dysplasia (CMD) was first described by Maroteaux et al. in 1971. The name is derived from the Greek *campo,* meaning "bowed" (or *campto* meaning "bent") and *melia* meaning "limb."

CMD was initially thought to be an autosomal recessive condition because of recurrences in siblings. It is now believed to be an autosomal dominant condition with a high incidence of sporadic new dominant mutations because of the degree of lethality. Evidence to support this includes segregation analysis, which demonstrates a ratio of 0.05 (Mansour et al., 1995), and identification of heterozygous mutations in *SOX9* (Foster et al., 1994). Recurrences of CMD in siblings have been reported, and these may be explained by gonadal (or somatic) mosaicism in one parent. The recurrence risk is approximately 2% to 5%. The clinical and radiological features of this condition are now well defined and characteristic (Mansour et al., 1995).

Clinical Features

Neonates with this condition are born with disproportionate short stature (Fig. 43–1). The limbs appear shorter than the trunk. There is usually bowing of the lower limbs (91%), frequently with pre-tibial dimpling (88%). The face is dysmorphic, with relative macrocephaly (87%), lowset ears (88%), hypertelorism, a depressed nasal bridge (90%), long philtrum, and micrognathia (93%). Two-thirds of affected cases have a midline posterior cleft palate. There is often bilateral talipes equinovarus (94%), with or without a "sandal gap" between the hallux and the second toe. Congenital dislocation of the hips is a common finding (82%). Congenital heart disease (22%) is also a feature but is usually minor (ventricular septal defects or atrial septal defects). Renal abnormalities also occurred; they were mainly hydronephrosis (23%)(Mansour et al., 1995).

The most unusual feature of this rare skeletal dysplasia is the presence of sex reversal in males. The ratio of chromosomal male to female affected patients approximated 1:1, supporting an autosomal mode of inheritance; however, there appeared to be a preponderance of female infants (72%) (another 17% had ambiguous genitalia [Fig. 43–1]). This is because almost three-quarters of infants with a male

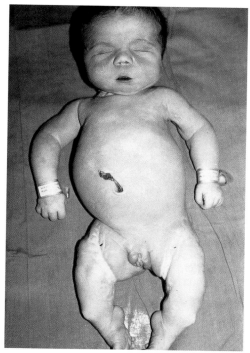

Figure 43–1. A neonate with campomelic dysplasia with micrognathia, depressed nasal bridge, relative macrocephaly, ambiguous genitalia and bowed long bones.

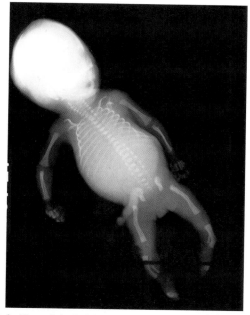

Figure 43–2. The radiological features of a fetus with campomelic dysplasia, showing hypoplastic scapulae, non-mineralization of the thoracic pedicles, 11 pairs of ribs, bowed femora, bowed tibiae, and vertical narrow iliac wings. (Reproduced with permission from *Journal of Medical Genetics*, Mansour et al. 1995, 32: 415–420.)

karyotype (46,XY) had female or ambiguous genitalia. This varied from a bifid scrotum with hypospadius to complete female genitalia with an enlarged clitoris. Histopathology of the gonads in affected males with sex reversal also varied from ovotestes to normal ovarian tissue.

There did not appear to be any correlation between sex reversal and prognosis for survival. Respiratory distress was a consistent feature and was due to the presence of a small thorax and a degree of tracheomalacia. In the vast majority of cases, the respiratory distress led to lethality in the neonatal period or infancy (90%). In a few cases, the patients survived the first year of life and developed further complications (described below).

Radiological Findings

The diagnosis of CMD is made by the characteristic radiological features (Fig. 43–2). Radiological diagnostic criteria do exist, but only as an aid to diagnosis, and they mainly apply to the neonatal period. These include hypoplastic scapulae, bowed femora, bowed tibiae, vertical narrow iliac wings, and nonmineralization of the thoracic pedicles. Probably the most important feature is hypoplasia of the scapulae, which was present in 92% of cases. Despite the name of the condition, only 80% to 90% had bowing of the long bones, and there have been a number of patients described with "acampomelic" campomelic dysplasia.

Other important radiological features include small thorax with slender ribs and 11 pairs of ribs. X-rays of the spine show hypoplastic vertebral bodies, abnormal cervical vertebrae, and kyphoscoliosis. The pelvic changes are fairly distinctive, with vertically narrow iliac bones, abnormal ischial bones, and no ossification of the pubic bones. Dislocation of the hips may also be seen radiologically. In the lower limbs—apart from the bowing of the long bones, as previously mentioned—there is delayed ossification of the distal femoral and proximal tibial epiphyses and hypoplasia of the fibulae. The talus may be absent. The long bones of the upper limbs may also be bowed, and most cases have a short first metacarpal bone. There is frequently dislocation of the radial head (Mansour et al., 1995).

Recently, the radiological features of five survivors of campomelic dysplasia have been reviewed (Offiah et al., 2002; Mansour et al.,

2002). These five people also have additional characteristic radiological features. There is still bowing of the long bones, hypoplastic scapulae, 11 pairs of ribs, and short metacarpals, but in addition, the pelvis shows narrow iliac bones with defective ischiopubic ossification, hypoplastic lesser trochanters, and elongated femoral necks (Fig. 43–3: patient 4 from Mansour et al., 2002). The patellae are hypoplastic or absent. Progressive kyphoscoliosis is seen with dysraphism usually of the cervical or lumbar spine (Fig. 43–4: patient 5 from Mansour et al., 2002).The pelvic features overlap with a rare autosomal dominant condition, ischiopubic-patella (IPP) syndrome, and it is believed that some published case reports of IPP may actually be survivors of CMD (Offiah et al., 2002).

Prenatal Diagnosis

Features on prenatal ultrasound include short and bowed long bones (especially femora). This can be confused with other skeletal dysplasias (e.g., osteogenesis imperfecta type II or III). The differential

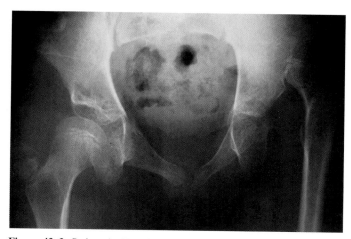

Figure 43–3. Patient 4: AP pelvis (aged 9 years) showing short ischia, defective ossification of the inferior pubic rami, dislocated left hip, narrow vertical iliac wings, and slender superior pubic rami. (Reproduced with permission from *Journal of Medical Genetics*, Mansour et al. 2002.)

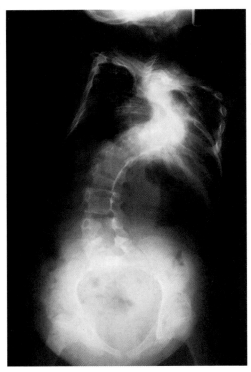

Figure 43–4. Patient 5: AP thoracolumbar spine (aged 11 years) showing significant scoliosis, cervical and lumbar dysraphism, defective ischiopubic ossification, and "drumstick" proximal femora. (Reproduced with permission from *Journal of Medical Genetics*, Mansour et al. 2002.)

diagnosis can be narrowed if there is the presence of ambiguous genitalia or sex reversal. Other ultrasonic markers include cystic hygroma (11 to 20 weeks) or polyhydramnios in the third trimester. Obviously, there is a much higher chance of detecting this condition antenatally if there has been a previously affected sibling.

Chromosomal Translocations

A number of reports of campomelic dysplasia indicate de novo chromosomal translocations involving chromosome 17q. Some of the individuals described have also had XY sex reversal. These reports led to the identification of *SOX9* (Tommerup et al., 1993; Foster et al., 1994).

There are a number of interesting points about this group of patients. For example, although the breakpoints were all on chromosome 17q, they were not at the same location, and none of the breakpoints actually disrupted the gene itself. The possible mechanisms for this are discussed later in this chapter. Of the seven reported cases of CMD with a translocation (Tommerup et al., 1993; Mansour et al., 1995) (excluding termination of pregnancy) five survived the first year of life and were still alive at the time of publication. It may be that this subgroup of cases of campomelic dysplasia is more likely to survive the neonatal period and have a less severe phenotype. They have less respiratory distress in the neonatal period and are less likely to have bowing of the long bones.

Survivors of CMD

Increasingly, it is recognized that a small number of affected individuals survive the first year of life. We recently reported five patients with CMD who were between 7 and 20 years old (Mansour et al., 2002). All of them had genetic or cytogenetic evidence of CMD: two had a chromosomal translocation involving the long arm of chromosome 17; the other three had mutations in *SOX9*. Of these five, one had asymmetrical involvement and was much less severely affected than the other four; she also had a daughter with classical CMD who died in the neonatal period. It was therefore likely that this individual had a somatic mosaic mutation in *SOX9*.

There were consistent clinical and radiological features in this group

and similar complications. The dysmorphic facies was distinctive and has already been described. Complications included respiratory and orthopedic problems. Four had respiratory problems, including neonatal respiratory distress, recurrent apneas, and chest infections and stridor. One boy required a tracheostomy for the first 6 years of life. The respiratory problems were worse in infancy (especially the neonatal period) but improved in later childhood. These same four individuals, however, developed a marked and progressive kyphoscoliosis, which compromised respiratory function. All five were very short, with heights significantly below the third centile. The body proportions changed with age, however, so that at birth the limbs were disproportionately short, but with the increasing kyphoscoliosis (and therefore short trunk), the limbs appeared relatively long (Fig. 43–5: patient 5 from Mansour et al., 2002). There was mild to moderate global developmental delay, but this was much more marked in the gross motor skills (probably because of the presence of hypotonia and respiratory problems) and less marked in the social skills. Most of these patients had significant conductive hearing loss. Myopia was present in the older patients, and dental caries with irregular teeth were also a problem. Apart from the progressive kyphoscoliosis, there were a number of other orthopedic complications, including talipes equinovarus, congenital subluxation or dislocation of the hips and dislocation of the radial heads, which caused limited supination. Sex reversal was only present in one of these cases and was associated with a paracentric inversion of chromosome 17q; there was one male with normal genitalia.

A number of explanations for survival in this condition are possible. The first explanation, as mentioned, is somatic mosaicism of the *SOX9* mutation. This is often difficult to prove at a molecular level but is suggested if there is either a milder phenotype in association with asymmetry or the birth of a more severely affected offspring. Also as mentioned, CMD with a chromosomal translocation may have a milder phenotype, but the mechanism for this is not yet understood. Alternatively, a milder mutation in *SOX9* may result in survival of the affected individual. The lack of genotype–phenotype correlation is discussed later in this chapter, and it may be that affected babies are more likely to survive because of improvements in neonatal care. It is possible that there are more survivors of this condition who have not been diagnosed as it is considered to be a lethal condition. A recent study reviewed cases of ischiopubic-patella syndrome. Some of these patients had other radiological features suggestive of CMD. Two of the

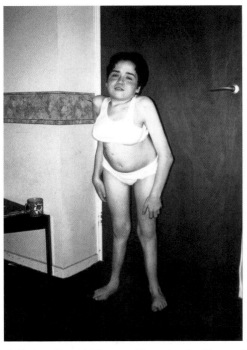

Figure 43–5. Patient 5, aged 21 years. (Reproduced with permission from *Journal of Medical Genetics*, Mansour et al. 2002.)

patients described here as survivors of CMD were originally thought to have IPP but were then found to have mutations in *SOX9*. It may be that there are other patients with this condition who also have mutations in *SOX9*.

SOX9 GENE AND ITS MUTATIONAL SPECTRUM

The *SRY* (*sex-determining region Y*) gene has a highly conserved 80 amino acid motif, called the "high mobility group" (HMG) domain. This HMG domain is conserved in other transcription factors with DNA-binding properties. A subgroup of genes share more than 60% homology with the HMG domain and were therefore named *SOX/Sox* (*Sry-related box*) genes. Because of the degree of homology, it is assumed that this subgroup are also transcription factors.

The *SOX9* gene encodes a 509 amino acid polypeptide containing an *SRY* homology domain. The homeobox domain has 71% homology with the *SRY* HMG domain (76% homology at the amino acid level). It is the only *SOX* gene to include introns and has three exons (all the other SOX genes are single exons). The HMG domain is encoded by exon 1.

Function of *SOX9*

A strong sequence conservation of *SOX9* throughout mammalian evolution suggests that this gene is an important regulatory factor. In the fetus, expression of *SOX9* has been demonstrated in the testes, chondrocytes, perichondrium, brain, liver, and kidney. In adults, expression of *SOX9* has been demonstrated in adult testes, heart, brain kidney, pancreas, and prostate (Foster et al., 1994; Wagner et al., 1994).

The HMG domain is important for DNA binding. This domain can bind to a minor groove of the DNA and cause the double helix to bend and unwind, thus causing an angulation of the DNA that is characteristic of SOX proteins. This action is thought to be important for the initiation of transcription. Unwinding of the DNA double helix may allow the gene promotors to be in a more open conformation and therefore enhance transcriptional activation (Marshall and Harley, 2000).

The PQS domain at the *SOX9* C terminus is rich in proline, glutamines, and serines and comprises 108 residues. This is the major transcriptional activation domain. The PQA domain comprises 41 residues; is rich in prolines, glutamines, and alanines; and is required for maximal activation of target genes (McDowall et al., 1999). This domain is only conserved in mammals and, therefore, may be involved in the mammalian sex-determining mechanism.

SOX9 has a preference for particular binding sites, but interaction between SOX9 and other proteins must play an important part in determining tissue-specific gene regulation. For example, although SOX9 is involved in sex determination and collagen formation, collagen genes are not transcribed in the testes, and the antimüllerian hormone (AMH), is not transcribed by chondrocytes.

Genotype–Phenotype Correlation

Meyer et al. (1997) looked at the distribution and nature of *SOX9* mutations, including 10 novel mutations. The mutations were evenly distributed in the three exons. There were missense mutations, nonsense mutations, and frameshift and splice site mutations. The nonsense mutation Q117X was associated with removal of 80% of the protein, but the patient was still alive at the age of 12. Other mutations, which left most of the protein intact, were found in patients who died in the neonatal period. One mutation, Y440X, was associated with prolonged survival. The two patients with this mutation were still alive at 4 and 9 years of age. This mutation occurred in exon 3, the PQS domain, and retained some residual activity of the SOX9 protein. Apart from this mutation, there did not appear to be any correlation between the location or nature of the mutation and the severity of the condition.

One frameshift mutation, a single A insertion in codon 368, was found in an XY male and in an XY sex-reversed female. This suggests that the sex reversal may be due to variable penetrance. Sex reversal was associated with mutations in all three exons, and there was again no correlation with the nature of the mutations. Meyer et al. (1997) also looked for *SOX9* mutations in 18 female patients with XY gonadal dysgenesis, but they did not find any mutations. This sug-

gests that *SOX9* mutations do not usually result in XY sex reversal without the skeletal malformations.

Chromosomal 17q Rearrangements and Effect on *SOX9*

A total of 14 patients have been reported with chromosomal translocations and inversions associated with campomelic dysplasia but with breakpoints outside the coding region of *SOX9*. One group (Pfeifer et al., 1999) mapped six breakpoints to an interval that was 140 to 950 kb proximal to *SOX9*. Genomic sequencing of the region up to 1063 kb from the *SOX9* 5′ flanking region was determined and analyzed by the gene prediction program, GENSCAN, and by searching of dbEST. No genes or transcripts were identified.

The mutational mechanism in these cases remains speculative. It may be due to disruption of alternative transcripts from one or more upstream promotors, but because of the distribution of breakpoints over such a long distance, this would imply a very long intron. Alternative suggestions are position effects, altering *SOX9* expression by translocation of the gene into a heterochromatic environment, and disruption of a second CMD-causing gene in 17q. No genes appear to exist in this region, however.

The most likely explanation is that the breakpoint causes removal of one or more *cis*-regulating elements from an extended *SOX9* control region. There are probably multiple *cis*-acting elements scattered over a region more than 350 kb upstream of *SOX9*. These may be regulators of *SOX9* which interact with the distant *SOX9* through a looping mechanism. Loss of a regulator may result in inadequate, reduced expression of *SOX9* but possibly not absence of the gene product.

GENETIC COUNSELING AND MANAGEMENT

CMD is a sporadic condition with a very high rate of new dominant mutations, but there is a small but significant risk of gonadal mosaicism or even somatic mosaicism. It is worth examining the parents of the affected individual and measuring their heights. If they are of normal stature and have no significant skeletal abnormalities, the recurrence risk is approximately 2% to 5%. This risk is based on previous reported studies, but because the numbers are small, the figure is an estimated risk of recurrence due to gonadal mosaicism.

In theory, prenatal diagnosis can be offered if a *SOX9* mutation has been identified, but few diagnostic laboratories currently offer this service. Therefore, prenatal diagnosis can be offered by detailed fetal scans. Ultrasound at 12 weeks could pick up cystic hygromas and possibly short, bowed or bent long bones. The karyotype of the fetus may be useful to exclude or confirm sex reversal or chromosomal rearrangements (although the fetal sex cannot be determined on ultrasound before 16 weeks).

The prognosis of CMD is usually poor, with the majority dying in the neonatal period or infancy. As discussed here, there is a small chance of survival, but survival would be accompanied by a number of respiratory and orthopaedic complications. The respiratory complications after the neonatal period include recurrent apneas and chest infections. One of the surviving patients mentioned required a tracheostomy for 6 years. The apneas are life threatening but become less frequent as the child becomes older. However, the progressive kyphoscoliosis can result in increasingly poor respiratory function.

The orthopedic complications are numerous. The major problem is the progressive kyphoscoliosis, which can be very severe and difficult to manage. Three of the survivors had several operations, but they failed to stop the deterioration of the back. Other orthopedic complications include congenital dislocation or subluxation of the hips, dislocation of the radial heads, and bilateral metatarsus varus. The bowing of the long bones in the survivors was not very marked and therefore did not appear to cause complications.

Survivors of this condition should have regular checks for the other associated features, which include myopia, conductive hearing loss, and dental caries (with irregular teeth). There are usually mild to moderate learning difficulties, and these patients should be assessed carefully for any special educational or physical needs they may have at school (Mansour et al., 2002).

MUTANTS IN ORTHOLOGOUS GENES

The mouse homolog has already been discussed in the beginning of this chapter. *SOX9* appears to have a male-specific role in mammals, birds, and reptiles. In the chicken embryo and alligator, expression of *SOX9* occurs much later and follows expression of *AMH*—that is, after sex determination. *SOX9* may therefore be required in different stages of testis development in different vertebrates, and only some of these functions have been conserved through evolution, see Chapter 42. Consequently, it may be that *SOX9* is required for later testis-specific functions (Morais da Silva et al., 1996).

DEVELOPMENTAL PATHOGENESIS

Chondrogenesis

Studies using mouse *Sox9* knockout chimeras showed that mesenchymal cells that did not contain *Sox9* did not differentiate into chondrocytes and were not present in cartilage tissue. Also, teratomas derived from *Sox9* knockout embryonic stem cells showed no cartilage formation (Bi et al., 1999). This suggests that *Sox9* is the first transcription factor that is essential for chondrocyte differentiation and cartilage formation. There is some suggestion that *L-SOX5* and *SOX6* are also involved in expression of *COL2A1*. *L-Sox5* and *Sox6* are coexpressed with *Sox9* in all chondrogenic sites in the mouse. The 48 bp chondrocyte-specific enhancer region in the first intron of *Col2a1* binds all three of these Sox proteins and is cooperatively activated by these proteins (Lefebvre et al., 1998).

Another collagen gene, *Col11a2*, encoding collagen type XI, is also important for the formation of collagen fibril formation and skeletal morphogenesis. This gene contains a 60 bp region in intron 1 that acts as a promotor region for the gene. Within this region there is a 7 bp sequence that binds to the Sox9 protein. Mutations in this sequence result in complete loss of the enhancer activity. This suggests that this 7 bp sequence within intron 1 plays a critical role in the cartilage-specific enhancer of *Col11a2* through Sox9-mediated transcriptional activity (Liu et al., 2000). Sox9 is probably involved at a very early stage of chondrogenesis and may be the major transcription factor in controlling chrondrogenesis.

Sex Determination Pathway

There is already some evidence that although *Sry* is expressed first in the genital ridge, it is closely followed by expression of *Sox9*. By 11.5 dpc, *Sox9* is clearly expressed in the developing XY gonads but is absent in XX gonads. Although *Sox9* stays on, however, *Sry* is switched off after a very short time. There is, as yet, no evidence for a direct role of Sry in expression of *Sox9*, but there is some evidence that Sry prevents inhibition of *Sox9* by its action on another gene, possibly *Sox3*. This is covered in more detail in Chapter 42.

Other investigations have suggested that ectopic expression of *Sox9* in XX gonads is sufficient to initiate male development; therefore, all downstream events in testis determination are initiated by *Sox9* (Vidal et al., 2001). The *Odsex* mouse provides further evidence that *Sox9* is crucial for male sex determination. This mouse is the result of a new dominant insertion of a mutation upstream of *Sox9*, leading to an activation of *Sox9* in both XX and XY gonads. This results in male development of all mutant XX mice. The nature of this mutation is not un-

derstood. It may cause a loss of negative regulatory elements of *Sox9*, or it may have a direct effect on enhancer elements (Bishop et al., 2000). *Sox9* may be the only crucial gene downstream of *Sry* for the initiation and maintenance of Sertoli cell differentiation (Lovell-Badge, 2002).

References

Arango NA, Lovell-Badge R, Behringer RR (1999). Targeted mutagenesis of the endogenous mouse Mis gene promoter: in vivo definition of genetic pathways of vertebrate sexual development. *Cell* 99: 409–419.

Bell DM, Leung KK, Wheatley SC, Ng LI, Zhou S, Ling KW, Sham MH, Koopman P, Tam PP, Cheah KS (1997). SOX9 directly regulates the type II collagen gene. *Nat Genet* 16: 174–178.

Bi W, Deng JM, Zhang Z, Behringer RR, de Crombrugghe (1999). Sox9 is required for cartilage formation. *Nat Genet* 22(1): 85–89.

Bishop CE, Whitworth DJ, Qin Y, Agoulnik AI, Agoulnik IU, Harrison WR, Behringer RR, Overbeek PA (2000). A transgenic insertion upstream of *Sox9* is associated with dominant XX sex reversal in the mouse. *Nat Genet* 26: 490–494.

Foster JW, Dominguez-Steglich MA, Guioli S, Kwok C, Weller PA, Stevanovic M, Weissenbach J, et al. (1994). Campomelic dysplasia and autosomal sex reversal caused by mutations in an *SRY*-related gene. *Nature* 372: 525–530.

Huang B, Wang S, Ning Y, Lamb AN, Bartley J (1999). Autosomal XX sex reversal caused by duplication of SOX9. *Am J Med Genet* 87: 349–353.

Lefebvre V, Li P, de Crombrugghe B (1998). A new long form of Sox5 (L-Sox5), Sox6 and Sox9 are coexpressed in chondrogenesis and cooperatively activate the type II collagen gene. *EMBO J* 17: 5718–5733.

Liu Y, Li H, Tanaka K, Tsumaki N, Yamada Y (2000). Identification of an enhancer sequence within the first intron required for cartilage-specific transcription of the α2 (XI) collagen gene. *J Biol Chem* 275: 12712–12718.

Lovell-Badge R, Canning C, Sekido R (2002). *Sex-Determining Genes in Mice: Building Pathways—The Genetics and Biology of Sex Determination*. Novartis Foundation Symposium 244. Wiley, New York.

Mansour S, Hall CM, Pembury ME, Young ID (1995). A clinical and genetic study of campomelic dysplasia. *J Med Genet* 32: 415–420.

Mansour S, Offiah AC, McDowall S, Sim P, Tolmie J, Hall CM (2002). The phenotype of survivors of campomelic dysplasia. *J Med Genet* 39: 597–602.

Maroteaux P, Spranger J, Opitz JM, Kucera J, Lowry RB, Schimke RN, Kagan SM (1971). Le syndrome campomelique. *Presse Med* 79: 1157–1162.

Marshall OJ, Harley VR (2000). Molecular mechanisms of SOX9 action. *Mol Genet Metab* 71: 455–462.

McDowall S, Argentaro A, Ranganathan S, Weller P, Mertin S, Mansour S, Tolmie J, Harley V (1999). Functional and structural studies of wild type SOX9 and mutations causing campomelic dysplasia. *J Biol Chem* 274: 24023–24030.

Meyer J, Sudbeck P, Held M, Wagner T, Schmitz ML, Bricarelli FI, Eggermont E, Freidrich U, Haas OA, Kobelt A, et al. (1997). Mutational analysis of the SOX9 gene in campomelic dysplasia and autosomal sex reversal: lack of genotype/phenotype correlations. *Hum Mol Genet* 6(1): 91–8.

Morais da Silva S, Hacker A, Harley V, Goodfellow P, Swain A, Lovell-Badge R (1996). Sox9 expression during gonadal development implies a conserved role for the gene in testis differentiation in mammals and birds. *Nat Genet* 14: 62–68.

Offiah AC, Mansour S, McDowall S, Tolmie J, Sim P, Hall CM (2002). Surviving campomelic dysplasia has the radiological features of the previously reported ischio-pubic-patella syndrome. *J Med Genet* 39: e50.

Pfeifer D, Kist R, Dewar K, Devon K, Lander ES, Birren B, Korniszewski L, Back E, Scherer G (1999). Campomelic dysplasia translocation breakpoints are scattered over a 1 Mb proximal to SOX9: evidence for an extended control region. *Am J Hum Genet* 65: 111–124.

Tommerup N, Schempp W, Meincke P, et al. (1993). Assignment of an autosomal sex reversal locus (SRA1) and campomelic dysplasia (CMPD1) to 17q24.3 to q25.1. *Nat Genet* 4: 170–174.

Vidal VPI, Chaboissier M-C, de Rooij DG, Schedl A (2001). Sox9 induces testis development in XX transgenic mice. *Nat Genet* 28: 216–217.

Wagner T, Wirth J, Meyer J, Zabel B, Held M, Zimmer J, Pasantes J, Bricarelli FD, Keutel J, Hustert F, et al. (1994). Autosomal sex reversal and campomelic dysplasia are caused by mutations in and around the SRY-related gene SOX9. *Cell* 79: 1111–1120.

Wright E, Hargrave MR, Christiansen J, Cooper L, Kun J, Evans T, Gangadharan U, et al. (1995). The *Sry*-related gene Sox-9 is expressed during chondrogenesis in mouse embryos. *Nat Genet* 9: 15–20.

Young ID, Zuccollo J, Maltby EL, Broderick NJ (1992). Campomelic dysplasia associated with a de novo 2q;17q reciprocal translocation. *J Med Genet* 29: 251–252.

44 | *AMH/MIS* and Its Receptors and Sexual Ambiguity and Persistent Müllerian Derivatives

JEAN-YVES PICARD

Antimüllerian hormone (AMH), also called müllerian inhibiting substance (MIS), is a member of the transforming growth factor β (TGF-β) family, produced exclusively by the gonads, that plays an important role in sex differentiation and gonadal function.

The primary role of AMH is to induce regression of the müllerian ducts, which otherwise would develop into uterus, fallopian tubes, and upper vagina. Fetal Sertoli cells begin to produce AMH immediately after testicular sex is determined; it follows that müllerian regression is the first sign of male sex differentiation, beginning at 8 fetal weeks in the human fetus and 13–14 dpc in the fetal rat. Regression proceeds rapidly in a cranio–caudal direction, provided the müllerian ducts have been exposed to the hormone before the end of a critical "window" of sensitivity, ending at 8 weeks in the human fetus (Josso et al., 1977) and 16 dpc in the rat (Picon, 1969). Androgens, produced by fetal Leydig cells, masculinize the external genitalia and urogenital sinus and promote the differentiation of wolffian ducts into male efferent ducts and accessory organs but fail to influence the fate of müllerian ducts.

AMH plays other roles in the reproductive tract. In freemartins, when female fetuses are exposed to testicular secretions of a male twin, it represses ovarian growth, kills germ cells, and may even produce masculinization (Jost et al., 1972). A similar picture is observed in female transgenic mice that express the human AMH gene under the control of the metallothionein promoter (Behringer et al., 1990). In the adult female ovary, AMH represses follicular maturation by inhibiting aromatase synthesis, expression of the LH receptor (di Clemente et al., 1994a), and epidermal growth factor–induced proliferation and function of human granulosa cells (Kim et al., 1992). AMH also affects Leydig cell development and function (Racine et al., 1998; Teixeira et al., 1999; Trbovich et al., 2001). It inhibits Leydig cell differentiation and decreases the expression of steroidogenic enzymes, thus leading to a decrease in testicular testosterone secretion.

AMH is a 560 amino acid glycoprotein formed by two 70 kDa monomers linked by disulfide bonds. The hormone is cleaved at a proteolytic site 109 amino acids upstream of the C terminus, yielding a short bioactive C-terminal domain with homology to members of the TGF-β family and a long N terminus with no bioactivity of its own but which enhances the bioactivity of the C terminus (Wilson et al., 1993). AMH is synthesized by Sertoli cells immediately after testis determination and is produced at high levels up to puberty, at which time it is repressed by testicular androgens (al-Attar et al., 1997). AMH is also produced from birth onward in the female by ovarian granulosa cells (Münsterberg and Lovell-Badge, 1991). AMH does not appear to play a major physiological role after birth, but it has been used as a marker of gonadal function/tumorigenesis in both sexes. An assay kit is now commercially available (from Immunotech Coulters) for measuring AMH in human serum.

The human AMH gene was cloned by Cate et al. (1986). It is located on the tip of the short arm of chromosome 19, band p13.3 (Cohen-Haguenauer et al., 1987). Only 2.75 kbp in length, it contains 5 exons; the 3′ end of the fifth one is particularly GC-rich and codes for the bioactive C-terminal domain. The minimal promoter is only 200 bp (Giuili et al., 1997) and is flanked by a household gene coding for spliceosome SAP 62 (Dresser et al., 1995). This AMH promoter contains binding sites for three transcription factors, the most potent of which are SOX9, modulated by SF-1, and GATA-4 (Arango et al., 1999).

AMH TRANSDUCTION CASCADE

Members of the TGF-β family signal through two distinct membrane-bound serine/threonine kinase receptors. Receptor type II binds to the ligand, and the type II/ligand complex recruits receptor type I, which acts as a signal transducer by binding to and activating specific Smad molecules (Massagué and Chen, 2000). The gene for the AMH type II receptor (AMHR-II), located on chromosome 12 q13, is 8 kbp long and divided into 11 exons (Imbeaud et al., 1995a). Exons 1–3 code for the signal sequence and extracellular domain, exon 4 for most of the transmembrane domain, and exons 5–11 for the intracellular serine/threonine kinase domains. Exon 2 undergoes alternative splicing in rabbit (di Clemente et al., 1994b) and dog (Messika-Zeitoun, unpublished data) but not in man (Imbeaud et al., 1995a) or rat (Baarends et al., 1994). AMHR-II is expressed in the mesenchymal cells that surround the müllerian duct, and also in gonads on Sertoli, Leydig and granulosa cells. The mature form of the human receptor is expressed at the cell surface and has a mass of 82 kDa (Faure et al., 1996).

The identity of the AMH type I receptor remains controversial. Binding of the ligand to the extracellular domain of AMHR-II successively triggers interaction with a bone morphogenetic protein (BMP) type I receptor, BMPR-IB/ALK6, phosphorylation of Smad1 and its entry into the nucleus (Gouédard et al., 2000). BMPR-IB is duly expressed in developing müllerian ducts, but up to now there is no evidence to show that its presence is required for AMH-mediated müllerian regression, which follows a β-catenin-dependent pathway (Allard et al., 2000). Smad 1 could be activated by different type I receptors in different tissues; indeed, evidence has been presented for the involvement of other BMP type I receptors such as ActR-I/ALK2 (Clarke et al., 2001; Visser et al., 2001) and BMPR-IA/ALK3 (Jamin et al., 2002) in AMH action. The latter appears particularly important for müllerian regression, since conditional inactivation of the gene leads to persistence of müllerian derivatives in mice. All the candidate type I receptors for AMH use Smads 1, 5, and 8 as intracellular effectors. A suggested transduction pathway for AMH is shown in Figure 44–1.

CLINICAL DESCRIPTION OF PERSISTENT MÜLLERIAN DUCTS SYNDROME

Since regression of müllerian ducts is the major role played by AMH in development, it is not surprising that persistence of müllerian derivatives is the hallmark of AMH and AMH receptor mutations. Affected subjects are, by definition, genotypic (46, XY) and phenotypic (external genitalia normally virilized) males, frequently with cryptorchidism that is sometimes associated with inguinal hernia. The hernia may appear incarcerated, in spite of the lack of symptoms of intestinal obstruction, but this discrepancy is usually not correctly interpreted. Sonography could be useful but is rarely performed unless an older sibling has been diagnosed with the condition.

The presence of müllerian derivatives is usually discovered at surgery. Two anatomical forms of persistent müllerian duct syndrome (PMDS) have been described. The most common one is characterized by the association of unilateral cryptorchidism and controlateral hernia. One testis has descended into the scrotum, and the ipsilateral uterus and fallopian tube have either entered the inguinal canal—a condition known as hernia uteri inguinalis—or, alternatively, can be

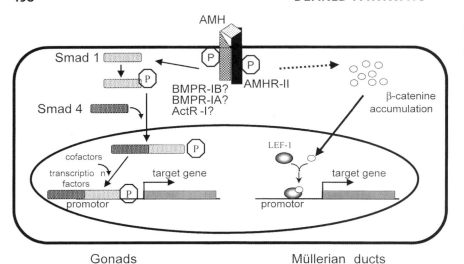

Figure 44–1. The antimüllerian hormone (AMH) signaling cascade. (Adapted from Massagué and Weis-Garcia, 1996.)

dragged into it by gentle traction, pulling the controlateral testis and fallopian tube in their wake. Often, no traction is necessary because the controlateral testis is already in the hernial sac. Tranverse testicular ectopia, as this condition is called, is extremely frequent in PMDS (Thompson et al., 1994). More rarely, PMDS presents as bilateral cryptorchidism, the uterus is fixed in the pelvis, and both testes are embedded in the broad ligament (Fig. 44–2). These clinical variants are not genetically determined and may occur within the same sibship (Guerrier et al., 1989).

In PMDS, the testes are abnormally mobile because they are not anchored to the bottom of the processus vaginalis by a normal male gubernaculum but are connected instead to elongated, thin, round ligaments (Hutson et al., 1994). This hypermobility could favor testicular torsion and subsequent testicular degeneration, and a high incidence of such degeneration has been reported in PMDS (Imbeaud et al., 1995b).

Testes are normally differentiated and, in the absence of long-standing cryptorchidism, usually contain germ cells, but often they are not properly connected to male excretory ducts due to aplasia of the epi-

didymis and the upper part of the vas deferens (Imbeaud et al., 1996). It is usually difficult to bring the testes down to a normal position; even after careful dissection, the free segment of the spermatic cord is very short because the vasa deferentia are embedded in the mesosalpynx, lateral uterine wall, and cervix.

Few associated clinical abnormalities have been described, apart from testicular tumors (Nishioka et al., 1992; Snow et al., 1995) and colon adenocarcinoma and medullary thyroid cancer, which developed in one patient at age 77 (Imbeaud et al., 1996). Associated defects are more frequent in patients with unexplained PMDS. Except in patients with testicular degeneration, serum testosterone and response to chorionic gonadotropin are normal. In contrast, the level of circulating AMH is extremely variable and depends on the molecular basis of the condition (Fig. 44–3). Female relatives of AMH-resistant patients who share their genetic background are phenotypically normal and fertile.

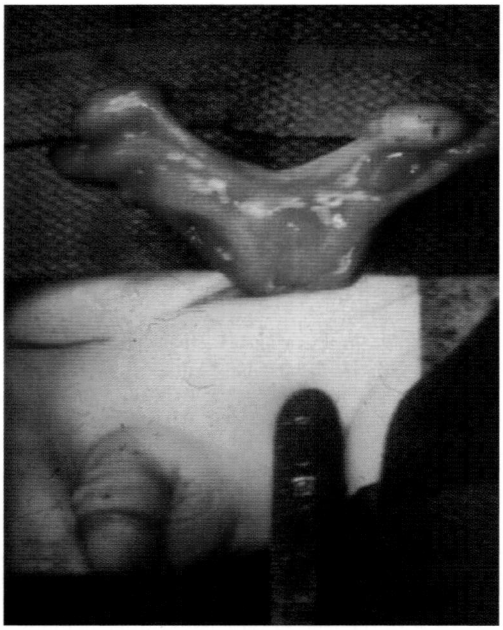

Figure 44–2. Operative view of patient with persistent müllerian duct syndrome (PMDS): the testes are tightly attached to the müllerian derivatives. (From Carré-Eusèbe et al., 1992, with permission.)

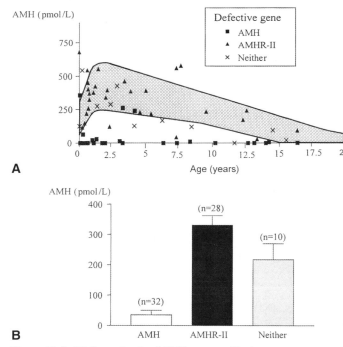

Figure 44–3. (*A*) Serum levels of AMH, measured by immunoassay, according to genotype. Normal range is shaded. (*B*) Mean and standard error of the mean (SEM) of serum AMH levels. Only patients under the age of 15 are included, because serum AMH is not informative in older subjects. (From Belville et al., 1999, with permission.)

MUTATIONS

Isolated persistence of müllerian derivatives can be ascribed either to lack of production of AMH, usually because of mutations of the AMH gene, or to resistance of target organs, which is a consequence of mutations of the components of the AMH transduction cascade. Our own experience is based on 76 families who were screened for mutations of the AMH or AMHR-II gene from 1988 to 2002. Transmission is according to an autosomal recessive pattern.

AMH Gene Mutations

AMH gene mutations, detected in 47% of PMDS families, are present across the length of the gene, except exon 4, and are particularly frequent in exon 1 and in the 3' end of exon 5, which codes the bioactive C terminus (Fig. 44–4A). Most mutations are different: only 9 out of 35 were recurrent, in exon 1 and in the 3' end of exon 5, representing, respectively, 43% and 28% of total mutations. As usual (Cooper and Krawczak, 1993), transitions were more frequent than transversions. No mutations were detected in the proximal promoter.

In most cases of AMH gene mutations, serum levels of AMH are very low or undetectable. This is of diagnostic importance in children, but not after puberty when AMH production by Sertoli cells is normally repressed. In rare cases, AMH gene mutations were found in patients with no müllerian derivatives. One patient presented with transverse testicular ectopia, practically never seen in the absence of PMDS (Thompson et al., 1994), and another had a brother with classical PMDS. Possibly, the müllerian derivatives degenerated in late fetal life.

AMH Type II Receptor Mutations

In contrast to AMH gene mutations, serum levels of AMH are normal in these patients. AMHR-II mutations were present in 38% of PMDS families; 52% of these were compound heterozygous (Fig. 44–5). Serum AMH concentration was normal for the patients' ages. Some 25 different mutations of AMHR-II were spread over the length of the gene (Fig. 44–4B); most are missense, transitions being more frequent than transversions. Six mutations were recurrent (Fig. 44–4B). The most frequent, d6331–6357, a deletion of 27 bp in exon 10 (Imbeaud et al., 1996), was present in 45% of families of this group, either in the homozygous state or coupled with missense mutations. An interesting mutation truncates the protein immediately after the transmembrane domain. This type of mutation is usually dominant-negative in other members of the TGF-β family, but in the PMDS family there was no phenotype in heterozygotes. PMDS was present only in subjects who bore a mutation on the other AMHR-II allele (Messika-Zeitoun et al., 2001).

Genetic Transmission

Both AMH and AMHR-II mutations are transmitted as autosomal recessive conditions due to mutations on both alleles of the affected gene. Some 61% of AMH mutations were homozygous, due to a high proportion of patients from Arab or Mediterranean countries who are characterized by a high rate of consanguinity. The ethnic origin of homozygous patients with AMHR-II mutations clearly differed from that of patients with AMH mutations, with a lower proportion of Arab and Mediterranean patients and a higher proportion of Asians, both Turkish and Pakistani. In contrast, the ethnic origin of AMH and AMHR-II compound heterozygotes was very similar, with a high proportion of French and northern European subjects (Fig. 44–5).

In exceptional cases, however, extensive searches yielded mutations on only one allele. Possibly, the other allele bears a splicing mutation, which went undetected because testicular RNA was unavailable. Dominant-negative activity of receptor type II mutations is unlikely. In one patient, d6331–6357 was found: this is a very common mutation that does not produce a phenotype in other heterozygous males. The other case is a deletion in the signal peptide; the resultant protein could not be inserted into the plasma membrane and thus could not bind to the wild-type protein to impair its activity.

(A) AMH gene

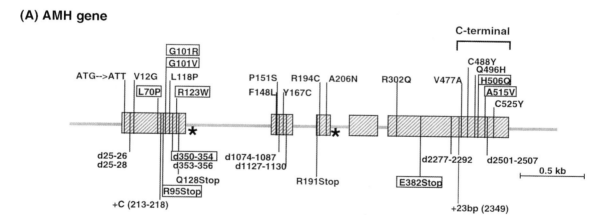

(B) AMHR-II gene

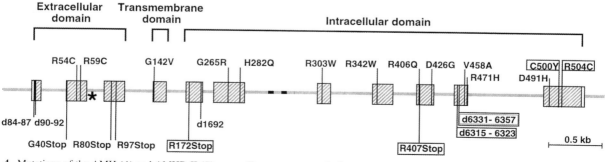

Figure 44–4. Mutations of the AMH (*A*) and AMHR-II (*B*) genes. Exons are shaded. Recurrent mutations are boxed, the very frequent mutation d6331–6357 is surrounded by a double box. Asterisks represent splice mutations. The 3' end of exon 5 codes for the C-terminal, bioactive domain of the AMH protein. (Completed from Belville et al., 1999, with permission.)

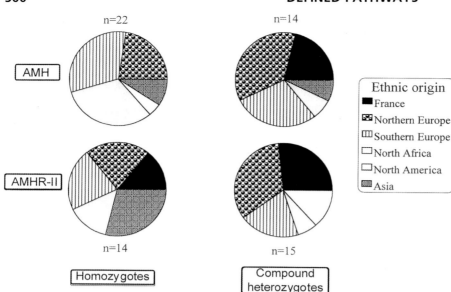

n=22   n=14

AMH

AMHR-II

n=14   n=15

Homozygotes   Compound
                     heterozygotes

Ethnic origin
■ France
▨ Northern Europe
▥ Southern Europe
□ North Africa
□ North America
▨ Asia

Figure 44–5. Ethnic origin and allelic status of patients with AMH or AMHR-II mutations. The five patients in whom a mutation was detected on a single allele are included; *n* represents the number of families in each group. (From Josso et al., 2002, with permission.)

Mutations in Other Genes

In 11 families representing 15% of the total number, no mutation of either the AMH or the AMHR-II genes was detectable. No large DNA rearrangements were seen by Southern blotting. Unexplained PMDS may reflect mutations in components downstream of the type II receptor in the AMH transduction cascade, especially the type I receptor(s) or Smad molecules. The knockout phenotype (Baur et al., 2000; Yi et al., 2000) of BMPR-IB/ALK6, a candidate type I receptor for AMH (Gouédard et al., 2000), is characterized by severe chondrodystrophies, whereas cartilage defects have not been described in PMDS. Smad molecules are probably not involved, either, because their mutations are usually associated with a high incidence of cancer, which is not observed in PMDS. Unexplained persistence of müllerian derivatives is often associated with other malformations and may not be due to mutations of elements of the AMH signaling cascade.

MANAGEMENT OF PMDS PATIENTS

Surgical Treatment

Correct surgical management of PMDS requires recognition of the condition by the surgeon and confirmation with testicular biopsies and chromosomal studies. PMDS is usually discovered incidentally during surgery for undescended testis or inguinal hernia. Sonography could be useful but is rarely performed unless an older sibling has been diagnosed with the condition. The initial procedure includes testicular biopsies, herniorraphy, and replacement of the gonads within the scrotum. The presence and duration of cryptorchidism will affect otherwise normal testicular histology. After confirmation of the diagnosis of PMDS and of integrity of the testes, definitive surgery should be performed to remove the corpus of the uterus and fallopian tubes, enabling fixation of the testes in the scrotum.

Preservation of the müllerian derivatives is incompatible with successful orchidopexies because the testes and vasa deferentia are tethered to the uterus. Furthermore, with sexual maturation, the uterus may hypertrophy and cause discomfort. The preferred operation includes proximal salpingectomies, leaving the fimbriae with the epididymes, thus releasing the testes (Fig. 44–6A,B). The vasa deferentia are then dissected from the lateral uterine walls and left intact with pedicles of myometrium, and a corporeal hysterectomy is performed, with or without removal of the vestigial cervix (Fig. 44–6C) (Loeff et al., 1994).

Fertility of the Patient

Lack of proper communication between the testis and excretory ducts and difficulties at orchidopexy probably contribute to explain the rarity

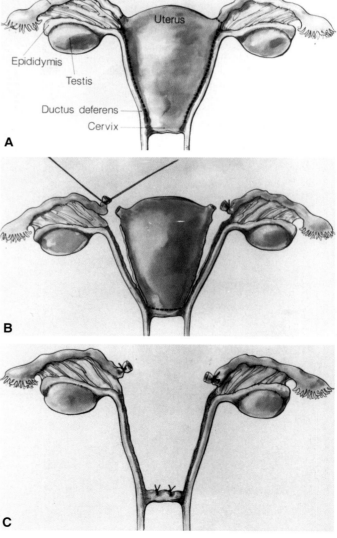

Figure 44–6. Definitive surgical management of persistent müllerian duct syndrome (PMDS). (From Loeff et al., 1994, with permission.)

of fertility in PMDS patients—only 11%, according to a Kuwait study (Farag, 1993). Perhaps early correction of cryptorchidism, preventing testicular alteration or degeneration, and better information made available to surgeons on this rare condition will improve fertility.

GENETIC COUNSELING

PMDS syndrome is not as rare as once thought. Cases observed in France lead to an estimation of its prevalence in a range greater than 1 male birth in 100,000. PMDS is not severe enough for systematic prenatal diagnosis, with eventual subsequent decision to abort. Early discovery and treatment could prevent risks of degeneration and malignancy of the testes, with no impediment for normal sexuality. The question of fertility of the treated patients remains more controversial.

Up to now the identified mutations responsible for PMDS are recessive, and each parent of an affected boy is generally heterozygous for the mutations. The risk for another boy to be affected is 1 in 4.

The physiological role in females of AMH secreted by granulosa cells remains unclear. But taking into account our observation of an affected PMDS boy's mother homozygous for the same mutation, AMH, even if it is involved in ovarian development and function, appears to be a dispensable factor. Thus parents could probably be reassured concerning the fate of their female offspring.

REFERENCES

Allard S, Adin P, Gouédard L, di Clemente N, Josso N, Orgebin-Crist MC, Picard JY, Xavier F (2000). Molecular mechanisms of hormone-mediated müllerian duct regression: involvement of β-catenin. *Development* 127: 3349–3360.

Arango NA, Lovell-Badge R, Behringer RR (1999). Targeted mutagenesis of the endogenous mouse Mis gene promoter: in vivo definition of genetic pathways of vertebrate sexual development. *Cell* 99: 409–419.

al-Attar L, Noël K, Dutertre M, Belville C, Forest MG, Burgoyne PS, Josso N, Rey R (1997). Hormonal and cellular regulation of Sertoli cell anti-müllerian hormone production in the postnatal mouse. *J Clin Invest* 100: 1335–1343.

Baarends WM, van Helmond MJL, Post M, van der Schoot PCJM, Hoogerbrugge JW, de Winter JP, Uilenbroek JTJ, Karels B, Wilming LG, Meijers JHC, et al. (1994). A novel member of the transmembrane serine/threonine kinase receptor family is specifically expressed in the gonads and in mesenchymal cells adjacent to the müllerian duct. *Development* 120: 189–197.

Baur ST, Mai JJ, Dymecki SM (2000). Combinatorial signaling through BMP receptor IB and GDF5: shaping of the distal mouse limb and the genetics of distal limb diversity. *Development* 127: 605–619.

Behringer RR, Cate RL, Froelick GJ, Palmiter RD, Brinster RL (1990). Abnormal sexual development in transgenic mice chronically expressing müllerian inhibiting substance. *Nature* 345: 167–170.

Belville C, Josso N, Picard JY (1999). Persistence of müllerian derivatives in males. *Am J Med Genet* 89: 218–223.

Carré-Eusèbe D, Imbeaud S, Harbison M, New M I, Josso N, Picard J Y (1992). Variants of the anti-müllerian hormone gene in a compound heterozygote with the persistent müllerian duct syndrome and his family. *Hum Genet* 90: 389–394.

Cate RL, Mattaliano RJ, Hession C, Tizard R, Farber NM, Cheung A, Ninfa EG, Frey AZ, Gash DJ, Chow EP, et al. (1986). Isolation of the bovine and human genes for müllerian inhibiting substance and expression of the human gene in animal cells. *Cell* 45: 685–698.

Clarke TR, Hoshiya Y, Yi SE, Liu XH, Lyons KM, Donahoe PK (2001). Müllerian inhibiting substance signaling uses a bone morphogenetic protein (BMP)–like pathway mediated by ALK2 and induces Smad6 expression. *Mol Endocrinol* 15: 946–959.

Cohen-Haguenauer O, Picard JY, Mattei MG, Serero S, Nguyen VC, de Tand MF, Guerrier D, Hors-Cayla MC, Josso N, Frézal J (1987). Mapping of the gene for anti-müllerian hormone to the short arm of human chromosome 19. *Cytogenet Cell Genet* 44: 2–6.

Cooper DN, Krawczak M (1993). *Human Gene Mutations*. Bios Science Publishers, Eynsham, U.K.

di Clemente N, Goxe B, Remy JJ, Cate RL, Josso N, Vigier B, Salesse R (1994a). Inhibitory effect of AMH upon the expression of aromatase and LH receptors by cultured granulosa cells of rat and porcine immature ovaries. *Endocrine* 2: 553–558.

di Clemente N, Wilson CA, Faure E, Boussin L, Carmillo P, Tizard R, Picard JY, Vigier B, Josso N, Cate RL (1994b). Cloning, expression and alternative splicing of the receptor for anti-müllerian hormone. *Mol Endocrinol* 8: 1006–1020.

Dresser DW, Hacker A, Lovell-Badge R, Guerrier D (1995). The genes for a spliceosome protein (SAP62) and the anti-müllerian hormone (AMH) are contiguous. *Hum Mol Genet* 4: 1613–1618.

Farag TI (1993). Familial persistent müllerian duct syndrome in Kuwait and neighboring populations. *Am J Med Genet* 47: 432–434.

Faure E, Gouédard L, Imbeaud S, Cate RL, Picard JY, Josso N, di Clemente N (1996). Mutant isoforms of the anti-müllerian hormone type II receptor are not expressed at the cell membrane. *J Biol Chem* 271: 30571–30575.

Giuili G, Shen WH, Ingraham HA (1997). The nuclear receptor SF-1 mediates sexually dimorphic expression of müllerian inhibiting substance, in vivo. *Development* 124: 1799–1807.

Gouédard L, Chen YG, Thevenet L, Racine C, Borie S, Lamarre I, Josso N, Massagué J, di Clemente N (2000). Engagement of bone morphogenetic protein type IB receptor and Smad1 signaling by anti-müllerian hormone and its type II receptor. *J Biol Chem* 275: 27973–27978.

Guerrier D, Tran D, van der Winden JM, Hideux S, Van Outryve L, Legeai L, Bouchard M, van Vliet G, de Laet MH, Picard JY, et al. (1989). The persistent müllerian duct syndrome: a molecular approach. *J Clin Endocrinol Metab* 68: 46–52.

Hutson JM, Davidson PM, Reece L, Baker ML, Zhou B (1994). Failure of gubernacular development in the persistent müllerian duct syndrome allows herniation of the testes. *Pediatr Surg Int* 9: 544–546.

Imbeaud S, Faure E, Lamarre I, Mattei MG, di Clemente N, Tizard R, Carré-Eusèbe D, Belville C, Tragethon L, Tonkin C, et al. (1995a). Insensitivity to anti-müllerian hormone due to a spontaneous mutation in the human anti-müllerian hormone receptor. *Nat Genet* 11: 382–388.

Imbeaud S, Rey R, Berta P, Chaussain JL, Wit JM, Lustig RH, De Vroede MAM, Picard JY, Josso N (1995b). Progressive testicular degeneration in the persistent müllerian duct syndrome. *Eur J Pediatr* 154: 187–190.

Imbeaud S, Belville C, Messika-Zeitoun L, Rey R, di Clemente N, Josso N, Picard JY (1996). A 27 base-pair deletion of the anti-müllerian type II receptor gene is the most common cause of the persistent müllerian duct syndrome. *Hum Mol Genet* 5: 1269–1279.

Jamin SP, Arango NA, Mishina Y, Behringer RR (2002). Genetic studies of MIS signalling in sexual development. In: *The Genetics and Biology of Sex Determination*. Chadwick D & Goode J (eds.) Novartis Foundation, Wiley, New York, pp. 157–168.

Josso N, Picard JY, Tran D (1977). The anti-müllerian hormone. *Recent Prog Horm Res* 33: 117–160.

Josso N, Belville C, Picard JY (2002). Persistence of müllerian derivatives in males. In: *Reproductive Medicine: Molecular, Cellular and Genetic Fundamentals*. 2nd Ed. Fauser BCJM (ed.) New York City: Parthenon Publishing.

Jost A, Cressent M, Dupouy JP, Magre S, Perchellet JP, Perlman S, Prepin J, Vigier B (1972). Becoming a male. *Adv Biosci* 10: 3–13.

Kim JH, Seibel MM, MacLaughlin DT, Donahoe PK, Ransil BJ, Hametz PA, Richards CJ (1992). The inhibitory effects of müllerian-inhibiting substance on epidermal growth factor induced proliferation and progesterone production of human granulosa-luteal cells. *J Clin Endocrinol Metab* 75: 911–917.

Loeff DS, Imbeaud S, Reyes HM, Meller JL, Rosenthal IM (1994). Surgical and genetic aspects of persistent müllerian duct syndrome. *J Pediatr Surg* 29: 61–65.

Massagué J, Chen YG (2000). Controlling TGF-β signaling. *Gene Dev* 14: 627–644.

Massagué J, Weis-Garcia F (1996). Serine/threonine kinase receptors: mediators of transforming growth factor β family signals. *Cancer Surv* 27: 41–64.

Messika-Zeitoun L, Gouédard L, Belville C, Dutertre M, Lins L, Imbeaud S, Hughes IA, Picard JY, Josso N, di Clemente N (2001). Autosomal recessive segregation of a truncating mutation of anti-müllerian hormone type II receptor in a family affected by the persistent müllerian duct syndrome contrasts with its dominant negative activity in vitro. *J Clin Endocrinol Metab* 86: 4390–4397.

Münsterberg A, Lovell-Badge R (1991). Expression of the mouse anti-müllerian hormone gene suggests a role in both male and female sex differentiation. *Development* 113: 613–624.

Nishioka T, Kadowaki T, Miki T, Hanai J (1992). Persistent müllerian duct syndrome. *Hinyokika Kiyo* 38: 89–92.

Picon R (1969). Action du testicule foetal sur le développement in vitro des canaux de Müller chez le rat. *Arch Anat Microsc Morphol Exp* 58: 1–19.

Racine C, Rey R, Forest MG, Louis F, Ferré A, Huhtaniemi I, Josso N, di Clemente N (1998). Receptors for anti-müllerian hormone on Leydig cells are responsible for its effects on steroidogenesis and cell differentiation. *Proc Natl Acad Sci USA* 95: 594–599.

Snow BW, Rowland RG, Seal GM, Williams SD (1985). Testicular tumor in patient with persistent müllerian duct syndrome. *Urology* 26: 495–497.

Teixeira J, Fynn-Thompson E, Payne A, Donahoe PK (1999). Müllerian-inhibiting substance regulates androgen synthesis at the transcriptional level. *Endocrinology* 140: 4732–4738.

Thompson ST, Grillis MA, Wolkoff LH, Katzin WE (1994). Transverse testicular ectopia in a man with persistent müllerian duct syndrome. *Arch Pathol Lab Med* 118: 752–755.

Trbovich AM, Sluss PM, Laurich VM, ONeill FH, NacLaughlin DT, Donahoe PK, Teixeira J (2001). Müllerian inhibiting substance lowers testosterone in luteinizing hormone-stimulated rodents. *Proc Natl Acad Sci USA* 98: 3393–3397.

Visser JA, Olaso R, Verhoef-Post M, Kramer P, Themmen APN, Ingraham HA (2001). The serine/threonine transmembrane receptor ALK2 mediates müllerian inhibiting substance signaling. *Mol Endocrinol* 15: 936–945.

Wilson CA, di Clemente N, Ehrenfels C, Pepinsky RB, Josso N, Vigier B, Cate RL (1993). müllerian inhibiting substance requires its N-terminal domain for maintenance of biological activity, a novel finding within the TGF-β superfamily. *Mol Endocrinol* 7: 247–257.

Yi SE, Daluiski A, Pederson R, Rosen V, Lyons KM (2000). The type I BMP receptor BMPRIB is required for chondrogenesis in the mouse limb. *Development* 127: 621–630.

45 | *DAX1* and X-Linked Adrenal Hypoplasia Congenita and XY Sex Reversal

ERIC VILAIN AND EDWARD R. B. MCCABE

DAX1 (dosage-sensitive sex reversal, adrenal hypoplasia congenita critical region on the X chromosome, gene 1) is the nuclear receptor protein encoded by the gene *NR0B1*, which maps to Xp21 (McCabe, 2001a; Phelan and McCabe, 2001). It is an unusual member of the nuclear receptor superfamily. DAX1 is similar in sequence in its C-terminal portion to that of the typical ligand-binding domain (LBD) of other members of the superfamily (Zanaria et al., 1994; Guo et al., 1995b; Burris et al., 1996). The N-terminal portion of DAX1 is composed of 3.5 amino acid repeats and is similar to only one other superfamily member, SHP, encoded by *NR0B2*, which contains only one of these repeats (Seol et al., 1996; Nuclear Receptor Nomenclature Committee, 1999; McCabe, 2001a).

DAX1 is expressed at all levels of the steroidogenic axis, which is composed of the hypothalamus, pituitary, adrenal cortex, and gonads (McCabe, 2001a). Investigations of patients and mice with alterations in DAX1 expression indicate that this protein is critical for normal development of each of the tissues within the hypothalamic-pituitary-adrenal/gonadal axis.

As indicated by its somewhat cumbersome name (Zanaria et al, 1994), genetic alterations in DAX1 expression are associated with dosage-sensitive sex reversal (DSS) and adrenal hypoplasia congenita (AHC) (McCabe, 2001a). The X-linked cytomegalic form of AHC is caused by intragenic loss-of-function mutations in or complete deletion of *NR0B1* (Muscatelli et al., 1994; Zanaria et al., 1994; Guo et al., 1995; Zhang et al., 1998; Phelan and McCabe, 2001). Affected males with AHC have hypogonadotropic hypogonadism (HH) that becomes clinically evident at adolescence. Duplication of the 160 kb critical region that contains the *NR0B1* locus results in female or ambiguous external genitalia in an XY genotypic individual, a developmental disorder known as DSS (Arn et al., 1994; Bardoni et al., 1994; Baumstark et al., 1996).

ROLE OF DAX1 IN DEVELOPMENT

Adrenal Development

The adrenal cortex and the medulla, though housed within the same capsule, represent two distinct tissues with very different embryologic origins (McCabe, 2001a). The adrenal cortical anlagen are mesodermal and develop from the posterior abdominal wall mesenchyme that is close to the cephalic portion of the mesonephros. The adrenal medulla primordia derive from neural crest cells and originate in the paraaortic sympathetic ganglia.

The development of the adrenal cortex involves two distinct waves of coelomic epithelial cell migration, one at approximately 32 and the other at 37 days postfertilization in humans (McCabe, 2001a). In addition, the mesonephric glomerular medial wall epithelium gives rise to the cells that become the cortical capsule and structural elements. The adult (permanent or definitive) cortex develops in the subcapsular region, and the fetal (provisional) cortex develops more deeply. The migrating adrenal medullary neural complexes pass through the developing cortices from approximately 7 to 14 weeks postfertilization. Disorganization of these tissues results in neuroblastic nodules that are normal developmental arrests within the fetal adrenal cortex and must be distinguished from early malignant neuroblastomas (Lack and Kozakewich 1990a, 1990b).

In the human fetus, the adrenal gland is a prominent organ, achieving a size larger than the kidney in the second trimester (McCabe, 2001a). Within the adrenal gland of the fetus, the size of the outer adult zone is exceeded in size by the inner fetal zone, the latter representing up to 80% of the adrenal cortex at birth. There is a rapid reduction in the fetal zone following birth: by 2 months of age it represents only 25% of the cortex, and by 1 year it can no longer be identified. While apoptosis may contribute to the loss of the fetal zone (McCabe, 2001a), there is also evidence that the inner fasciculata and reticularis derive from fetal zone cells (Sucheston and Cannon, 1968; Lack and Kozakewich, 1990b).

Stem cells in the capsule or immediate subcapsular region appear to be responsible for the maintenance of the adrenal cortex (McCabe, 2001a). Adrenal cortical tissue has been reported to regenerate from transplanted capsular fragments (Skelton, 1959; Belloni et al., 1990). Centripetal movement of adrenal cortical cells has been observed, with cell division more frequent in the glomerulosa and cell death more common in the reticularis (Zajicek et al., 1986; Vinson et al., 1992). A mechanism that involves replenishment of the adrenal cortex from stem cells in the cortical capsular region, centripetal migration through the cortex, and programmed cell death at the corticomedullary junction is consistent with the available data (McCabe, 2001a).

Role of DAX1 and SF1 in Adrenal Development

DAX1 loss-of-function mutations result in the X-linked cytomegalic form of AHC (McCabe, 2001a; Phelan and McCabe, 2001). Affected patients usually have adrenal cortical tissue present, though it is hypoplastic. Occasionally, however, no adrenal tissue can be identified despite a careful and thorough search, and this is consistent with adrenal aplasia (Stempfel and Engel, 1960; Sperling et al., 1973; Pakravan et al., 1974; Wittenberg, 1981; McCabe, 2001a). The adrenal cortical tissue in the cytomegalic form of AHC shows characteristic histopathological changes (Uttley, 1968; Seltzer et al., 1985; Lack and Kozakewich, 1990b; McCabe, 2001a). The definitive adult zone is absent or nearly absent. The hypoplastic cortex has a disorganized appearance, with micronodules that contain eosinophilic cells. It is assumed that this residual cortex represents tissue with persistence of fetal zone characteristics that may continue past the age when the fetal cortex typically disappears (Seltzer et al., 1985).

DAX1 and steroidogenic factor 1 (SF1) are nuclear receptors that are involved in the normal development of the steroidogenic axis (Achermann et al, 2000; McCabe, 2001a, 2002). mRNAs for SF1 and DAX1, and for their murine orthologs Ftzf1 and Ahch, are expressed throughout the steroidogenic axis (Ikeda et al., 1994, 1996; Zanaria et al., 1994; Guo et al., 1995a; Bae et al., 1996). Developmental expression of *DAX1/Ahch* occurs throughout the hypothalamic-pituitary-adrenal/gonadal axis at the same time or slightly later than *SF1/Ftzf1* (Tables 45–1 to 45–3). *Ahch* and *Ftzf1* are expressed in the murine adrenal primordia at 11 dpc (Table 45–4). *Ahch* is also expressed in embryonic stem (ES) cells, and its expression appears to be critical for ES cell survival, since unconditional ES cell knockout of *Ahch* has not been observed (Yu et al., 1998b; Achermann et al., 2000; Clipsham et al., 2001).

DAX1 and SF1 are components in an extremely complex network involved in transcriptional regulation during development (McCabe, 2002). The *DAX1* and *Ahch* promoters contain sequences in positions similar to the SF1 response element (RE) consensus sequence (Burris et al., 1995; Bae et al., 1996; Guo et al., 1996). The human RE

Table 45–1. SF1/Ftzf1 and DAX1 Expression in the Developing Mammalian Central Nervous System

	Pituitary		Hypothalamus	
	Ftzf1 (SF1)	Dax1 (DAX1)	Ftzf1 (SF1)	Dax1 (DAX1)
MOUSE (DPC)				
9.5		1st ↑ protein (p) Rathke's pouch, dorsal region (Ikeda et al., 2001)	1st ↑ p proencephalon/diencephalons (Ikeda et al., 2001)	1st ↑ p proencephalon/diencephalons (Ikeda et al., 2001)
11.0			1st ↑ r hypothalamic primordium (Dellovade et al., 2000) (Sf-1 earliest marker for cells that form VMH)	
11.5	1st ↑ RNA (r) in developing anterior pituitary (Ikeda et al., 1994)	1st ↑ RNA (r) Rathke's pouch, limited to dorsal side (Ikeda et al., 1996)	↑ r hypothalamic primordium (Ikeda et al., 1994)	1st apparent ↑ r hypothalamic primordium (Ikeda et al., 1996; Swain et al., 1996)
12.5	←→ r	↓↓ p in dorsal Rathke (Ikeda et al., 2001)	↑ p (Dellovade et al., 2000)	
13.5	1st ↑ protein (p) in Rathke's pouch, at ventralmost side (Ikeda et al., 2001)	↓↓ p in dorsal Rathke, but still some detected (Ikeda et al., 2001)	↑ p (Dellovade et al., 2000) (VMH cells now immuno-histochem.ically distinct)	
14.5	←→ r, ←→ p limited to anterior lobe (Ikeda et al., 2001)	1st ↑ p in anterior pituitary, likely gonadotropes (Ikeda et al., 1996, 2001; Swain et al., 1996; (co-loc. Kawabe et al., 1999) w/ Sf-1 [Kawabe et al., 1999; Ikeda et al., 2001;])	↑ p (Kawabe et al., 1999)	↑ p anterior hypothalamus (Kawabe et al., 1999)
18.5			↑ p (Dellovade et al., 2000) (VMH histologically distinct)	
P0	↑ p in gonadotropes (Kawabe et al., 1999)		←→ p VMH (Kawabe et al., 1999)	1999) p variable stain VMH (Kawabe et al., 1999)
P5		↑ p in gonadotropes of rat (Ikeda et al., 2001)		
P21		↓↓ p in Dax-1+/Sf-1− cells (very rarely found) (Ikeda et al. 2001)		
ADULT	Anterior pituitary gonadotropes (Ingraham et al., 1994; Ikeda et al., 1995; Swain et al., 1996)	Anterior pituitary gonadotropes (Kawabe et al., 1999)	←→ p VMH (Ingraham et al., 1994; Ikeda et al., 1995)	←→ p VMH (Kawabe et al., 1999; Swain et al., 1996)
HUMAN				
ADULT	Anterior pituitary gonadotroph (Aylwin et al., 2001)	Anterior pituitary gonadotroph (Aylwin et al., 2001)	?	←→ p (Guo et al., 1995a)

Human genes in parentheses.

dpc, days postcoitum (mouse); p, protein expression; r, RNA expression; ←→, persists; ↑, appears or increases slightly; ↓↓ decreases strongly; VMH, ventromedial hypothalamus.

binds SF1 specifically (Burris et al.,1995), and SF1/Ftzf1 enhances DAX1/Ahch expression (Vilain et al., 1997; Yu et al., 1998a; Kawabe et al., 1999). Numerous potential gene targets for SF1 have been identified, suggesting involvement in sex determination, sexual differentiation, steroidogenesis, and lipid metabolism (Achermann et al., 2000). The Ftzf1 and Wt1 proteins interact directly to promote synergistically müllerian inhibiting substance (MIS) expression (Nactigal et al., 1998). Ahch antagonizes the synergy, most likely through heterodimerization between Ftzf1 and Ahch. A similar mechanism appears to be involved in the regulation of expression of the high-density lipoprotein receptor (Hdlr) (Lopez et al., 2001). Sterol regulatory element-binding protein-1a (Srebp1a) and Ftzf1 positively regulate transcription of Hdlr. Ahch inhibits the activities of both Srebp1 and Ftzf1, though apparently through different mechanisms. The involvement of these genes, Ahch and Ftzf1, which are more typically considered to be regulators of sex determination/sexual differentiation, with Hdlr and Srebp1, suggests a molecular basis through this system for at least some of the gender-specific aspects of fat metabolism.

Based on these observations of a positive influence of Ftzf1 and a negative effect of Ahch on the regulation of expression of these two different gene products, Wt1 and Hdlr, it is likely that additional systems will show counterregulatory activating and inhibiting influences of the paired transcription factors, SF1/Ftzf1 and DAX1/Ahch. Mangelsdorf (2001) has noted that there is an evolutionary relationship between the paralogous pairs of genes, SF1 and luteinizing hormone re-

leasing hormone 1 (LRH1), and DAX1 and short heterodimer partner (SHP). Just as SF1 and DAX1 are positive and negative regulators, respectively, of the pathways that are involved in sex determination and sexual differentiation, their respective paralogs, LRH1 and SHP, have the same counterregulatory relationship in bile acid metabolism.

These counterbalancing influences, positive for Ftzf1 and negative for Ahch, on adrenal cortical cellular proliferation and steroidogenic function have been confirmed in vivo in murine knockout models (Babu et al., 2002). Homozygosity for targeted disruption of $Ftzf1^{-/-}$ in mice results in adrenal aplasia (Luo et al., 1994), and heterozygotes (+/−) evidence adrenal hypoplasia (Babu et al., 2002), indicating the importance of Ftzf1 in early adrenal development. Ftzf1 also plays a role in maintenance of adult adrenal cortical cell proliferation potential following unilateral adrenalectomy, as demonstrated in experiments with Ftzf1 heterozygotes (Beuschlein et al., 2002). Hemizygous males (*/−) after conditional Ahch-targeted disruption show normal initial development of the adrenal cortex, but the normal fetal X-zone regression is lacking with sexual maturation (Yu et al., 1998b; Achermann et al., 2000). Compound Ftzf1 heterozygotes (+/−) : Ahch hemizygotes (*/−) showed neither the reduced adrenal weight nor the reduced steroidogenesis in response to stress characteristic of the Ftzf1 heterozygotes (Babu et al, 2001). These results were interpreted to support an in vivo model in which Ahch antagonizes the positive actions of Ftzf1 on adult adrenal cortical cell proliferation and steroidogenesis.

Table 45–2. Expression of SF1/Ftzf1 and DAX1 during Development of the Adrenal Cortex

P (dpc)	Mouse		CS (dpo)	Human	
	Ftzf1	Dax1		SF1	DAX1
9.0	1st ↑ RNA (r) adrenogonadal primordium (Ikeda et al., 1994)	1st ↑ r adrenogonadal primordium (Swain et al., 1996)	32/14	1st ↑ p rotein (p) adrenogonadal primordium (in cells under genital ridge medial to mesonephros) (Hanley et al., 1999, 2001)	
11.0	↑ r throughout adrenal primordium (Ikeda et al., 1994; Hatano et al., 1996; Swain et al., 1996) (after gonads and adrenals separate)	↑ r adrenal primordium (Swain et al., 1996)	33/15	1st ↑ r adrenal primordium (Hanley et al., 2001); ↑ p (Hanley et al., 1999); (cortex begin distinction) (Hanley et al., 1999)	1st ↑ r adrenal primordium (Hanley et al., 2000, 2001)
13.5	↑ ↑ r in adrenal cortex only (Ikeda et al., 1994; Swain et al., 1996)	↑ r in adrenal cortex mostly (Swain et al., 1996)			
17.5	⟷ r adrenocortical zones (Ikeda et al., 1994; Swain, et al., 1996)	⟷ r adrenocortical zones (Ikeda et al., 1994; Swain et al., 1996)	52/21	↑ r throughout cortex (fetal zone apparent) (Hanley et al., 2001)	↑ r low throughout cortex (Hanley et al., 2000, 2001)
P0 P21	↓ r overall in rat (Hatano et al., 1994)		3 weeks	⟷ r adrenocortical zones (Hanley et al., 2001) low r in fetal zone (Hanley et al., 2001)	⟷ r adrenocortical zones (Hanley et al., 2001) low r in fetal zone (Hanley et al., 2001)
Adult	Adrenal cortex (Honda et al., 1993; Morohashi et al., 1994); zona glomerulosa, z. fasciculata, z. reticularis, none in medulla	Adrenal cortex (Kawabe et al., 1999): zona glomerulosa, z. fasciculata, z. reticularis, none in medulla	Adult	Adrenal cortex (Shibata et al., 2001); zona glomerulosa, z. fasciculata, z. reticularis, none in medulla	Adrenal cortex (Shibata et al., 2001); zona glomerulosa, z. fasciculata, z. reticularis, none in medulla

P, postnatal day (mouse); dpc, days postcoitum (mouse); CS, carnegie stage (human); dpo, days postovulation (human); r, RNA expression; p, protein expression: ⟷, persists; ↓, decreases slightly; ↑, appears or increases slightly; ↑ ↑, increases strongly.

Role of DAX1 and SF1 in Hypothalamic and Pituitary Development

DAX1/Ahch is expressed in the human and murine hypothalamus and pituitary (Zanaria et al., 1994; Guo et al., 1995a; Bae et al., 1996; Ikeda et al., 1996) (Table 45–1). In the mouse, Ahch expression is observed at E9.5 in the proencephalon, followed by the ventromedial hypothalamus (VMH) and the anterior pituitary gonadotropes (Ikeda et al., 1996, 2001). In addition to this pattern of expression being consistent with the hypogonadotropic hypogonadism observed among patients with *DAX1* mutations, male murine *Ahch* hemizygotes (*/−) have hypogonadism (Jeffs et al., 2001a).

Ftzf1 is expressed in the murine ventral proencephalon at E9.5, the same stage that Ahch is expressed in the proencephalon (Ikeda et al., 2001) (Table 45–1). *Ftzf1* is also expressed subsequently in the ventral medial hypothalamus, the anterior pituitary, and the gonadotropes (Ikeda et al., 1994, 1996; Ingraham et al., 1994; Roselli et al., 1997). Ftzf1 is critical for normal formation and function of the CNS portion of the steroidogenic axis, since development of the ventromedial nucleus (VMN) and the gonadotropes is disrupted after targeted disruption of *Ftzf1−/−* in the mouse (Ikeda et al., 1995; Shinoda et al., 1995). When a Cre-loxP construct was used to generate mice with specific inactivation of *Ftzf1* in the anterior pituitary, the resulting animals exhibited hypogonadotropic hypogonadism (HH) (Zhao et al., 2001).

Role of DAX1 in Sex Determination and Gonadal Development

Dax1 is one of the still relatively small number of genes known to be involved in mammalian sex determination. In mammals, sex determination refers to the developmental decision that orients the undifferentiated and bipotential gonad into a testis or an ovary. In males, this process is triggered by SRY, an HMG-related transcription factor that is encoded on the Y chromosome (Sinclair et al., 1990). Sry is expressed in the developing testis between 10.5 and 12.5 dpc in the mouse (Koopman et al., 1990). In females, *SRY* is not present and testes do not develop. Mutations in *SRY* result in the early arrest of testicular development, leading in humans to an XY female phenotype with gonadal dysgenesis (Vilain and McCabe, 1998; see Chapter 42).

The molecular events downstream of SRY are poorly understood. Only a small number of genes are known to be responsible for the oc-

currence of XY females with gonadal dysgenesis (see Table 45–4). *DAX1*, when duplicated and presumably overexpressed in an XY individual, is responsible for a female phenotype (Arn et al., 1994; Bardoni et al., 1994; Baumstark et al., 1996). In addition, Ahch was shown to antagonize Sry action in a transgenic mouse model (Swain et al., 1998). DAX1 is expressed in the genital ridge at 11.5 dpc in both sexes, but at 13.5 dpc it is turned down in male gonads while it remains on in female gonads (Table 45–3). These data have resulted in the concept that DAX1 acts as an "anti-testis" gene, preventing normal male differentiation of the embryonic gonad (Goodfellow and Camerino, 1999). When SRY is present, this "anti-testis" action would be antagonized, and the testes would develop normally. When DAX1 is duplicated, it would overcome SRY "pro-male" action, and testicular tissue would not develop. Recent analysis of Ahch knockout shows that DAX1 may also be important for testis determination (Meeks et al., 2003).

DAX1 belongs to the emerging category of sex-determining genes (along with *WNT4*) that antagonize male development. They are expressed in both male and female gonads until about E12, at which point they are turned off in males and continue to be expressed in females (Swain et al., 1996; Vainio et al., 1999). Therefore, they are also potential promoters of ovarian development. The other categories of genes involved in sex determination are promoters of testicular development (such as *SRY* and *SOX9*) and transcription factors (e.g., *SF1* and *WT1*), which are involved in both early gonadal development and throughout the differentiation of sex-specific cell types. The roles for *DAX1* and other sex determination genes are depicted in Figure 45–1; see also Chapter 42.

X-LINKED ADRENAL HYPOPLASIA CONGENITA AND HYPOGONADOTROPIC HYPOGONADISM

Clinical Description

X-linked inheritance of the cytomegalic form of AHC is well documented (McCabe, 2001a). Patients with a contiguous gene syndrome involving the deletion of the AHC locus, along with the loci for glycerol kinase (GK) and Duchenne muscular dystrophy (DMD), permitted the mapping of AHC to Xp21 before a detailed physical map was available in this region (Guggenheim et al., 1980; Hammond et al., 1985; Patil et al., 1985; Bartley et al., 1986; Clarke et al., 1986; Dunger

Table 45–3. Expression Profile of SF-1/Ftzf1 and DAX-1 in Mouse and Human Gonads

Developmental stage (dpc or postnatal for mouse)	RNA		Protein		Site of Expression	
	M	F	M	F	M	F
Ftzf1 EXPRESSION PROFILE, MOUSE GONADS*						
E9.5	+	+	+	+	Indifferent gonads (presumptive gonad in urogenital ridge)	
E10.5	+	+	+	+	Indifferent gonads	
E11.5	+	+	+	+	Indifferent gonads	
E12	+	+	+	+	Indifferent gonads	
E12.5	++	+	++	++	Highest in interstitial region (Leydig cells); testicular cords, seminiferous tubules	Primordial ovary
E13.5	++	+	++	++	Interstitial region (Leydig cells)	
E14.5	++	+	++	++	Increasing expression	
E15.5	++	+	++	++	Increasing expression	
E16.5	++	+	++	+	Increasing expression	
E17.5	++	+	++	+		
E18.5	+	+	++	+		Follicles?
P0			++		Sertoli/Leydig cells	Granulosa/interstitial cells (higher in interstitial cells)
P5			++		Sertoli/Leydig cells (decreasing expression in Sertoli cells)	
P7			++		Sertoli/Leydig cells (decreasing expression in Sertoli cells)	
P15	+		++		Sertoli/Leydig cells (much lower in Sertoli cells)	
P21			++		Sertoli/Leydig cells (much lower in Sertoli cells)	
Adult	+	+	++	+	Leydig cells	Stromal/granulosa cells of primordial, primary, and preantral follicles; strong expression in granulosa/theca and internal cells of antral/atretic follicles
SF-1 EXPRESSION PROFILE, HUMAN GONADS†						
32/14	+	+			Indifferent gonad (medial to mesonephros)	
33/15	+	+			Indifferent gonad	
41/17	+	+			Indifferent gonad (absent from primordial germ cells)	
44/18	+	+			Developing testes	
52/21	+	+			Interstitial region (Leydig cells); higher in sex cords	Developing ovary (diffuse expression)
18 week	+	+			Higher in interstitial region; sex coreds	Developing ovary (coelomic epithelium)
Adult						
DAX-1 EXPRESSION PROFILE, MOUSE GONADS‡						
E9.5	−	−	−	−		
E10.5	−	−	−	−	Somatic cells of genital ridge	
E11.5	++	++	++	++	Somatic cells of genital ridge (coelomic epithelium)	
E12	+	++	+	++		Cells proximal to mesonephros
E12.5	+	++	+	++	+ in cells at gonad/mesonephros junction Sertoli/Leydig cells	Primordial ovary
E13.5	+	++	+	++	Sertoli/Leydig cells	Coelomic epithelium
E14.5	+	++	+	++	Sertoli/Leydig cells; interstitial cells	Coelomic epithelium
E15.5	+	++	+	+	Sertoli/Leydig cells	
E16.5	+	+	+	+	Sertoli/Leydig cells	
E17.5	+	+	+	+	Sertoli/Leydig cells	Coelomic epithelium
E18.5			++	+		
P0			++	+		
P5	+	+	++	+	Sertoli cells	Developing follicle
P7	+		+		Sertoli cells	
P14	+	+	+		Sertoli cells	Granulosa/interstitial cells
P21	++	+	+		Sertoli cells	Granulosa/interstitial cells
Adult	+	+	+	+	Leydig cells (low expression in Sertoli cells)	Stromal (theca/granulosa) cells (absent from follicle cells and luteinizing cells of graffian follicles)
DAX-1 EXPRESSION PROFILE, HUMAN GONADS§						
32/14	−	−				
33/15	+	+			Indifferent gonadal ridge	
41/17	+	+			Indifferent gonadal ridge	
44/18	+	+			Indifferent gonadal ridge	
52/21	+	+			RNA mainly detected in developing sex cords	
18 week	+	+			Fetal testis	Fetal ovary
Adult						

Sources
*Ikeda et al., 1993, 1994, 1996, 2001; Bakke et al., 2001a.
†Takeyama et al., 1995; Ramayya et al., 1997; Hanley et al., 1999; Bakke et al., 2001a,b.
‡Ikeda et al., 1996, 2001; Swain et al., 1996; Nachtigal et al., 1998; Kawabe et al., 1999.
§Hanley et al., 2000.

Table 45–4. Genes of Human Sex Determination

Gene	Function	Localization	Phenotype	
			Mutation/Deletion	Duplication
SRY	Transcription factor	Yp11.3	XY female	Normal
DAX1	Transcription factor	Xp21.3	AHC	XY female
SOX9	Transcription factor	17q24	XY female, CD	XX male
DMRT1	Transcription factor	9p24.3	(XY female)	?
SF1	Transcription factor	9q33	XY female, AHC	?
WT1	Transcription factor	11p13	XY female, DDS	?
Wnt-4	Signaling molecule	1p35	?	XY female

AHC, adrenal hypoplasia congenita; CD, campomelic dysplasia; DDS, dosage-sensitive sex reversal.

et al., 1986; McCabe 2001a, 2001b). The involvement of these additional genes in a contiguous gene syndrome will be evidenced by elevated circulating creatine kinase with DMD, and with "pseudohypertriglyceridemia" (Goussalt et al., 1982) due to elevated blood glycerol and glyceroluria with GKD, as well as increased circulating corticotropin with AHC (McCabe, 2001a).

X-linked isolated AHC associated with HH is caused by intragenic mutations in *DAX1* (Muscatelli et al., 1994; Zanaria et al., 1994; Guo et al., 1995b).

Presentation with signs and symptoms of adrenal insufficiency, including life-threatening clinical and metabolic decompensation, occurs most typically early in life. In a series of 17 patients who presented clinically, the median age for initial symptoms was 3 weeks, with a range of 1 week to 3 years (Peter et al., 1998). Two brothers in this series with deletion of *DAX1* and *GK* illustrate the variability in expressivity that is associated with *DAX1* mutations: one had his first salt wasting episode at 1 month of age, and the other was diagnosed with a similar episode at 3 years of age. The two brothers we described originally (McCabe et al., 1977)—with what is now recognized as a contiguous gene syndrome involving complete deletion of *DAX1* (Worley et al., 1993; Guo et al., 1995) associated with breakpoints in telomeric *IL1RAPL1* and centromeric *DMD* genes (Niakan et al., 2001)—presented initially at 33 months and 6 years of age (Guggenheim et al., 1980). Occasionally, adrenal insufficiency may not present acutely until 10 years of age (Meakin et al., 1959; Golden et al., 1977), and in one family, not until 17 to 32 years of age (Brochner-Mortensen, 1956). While these families are consistent with

X-linked inheritance, it must be noted that *DAX1* mutations have not been demonstrated in these latter three families. Delayed onset in some patients presumably represents interindividual variability in the duration of residual adrenal cortical function and differences in environmental stress exposures. Variability in expressivity will be due to the influence of modifier genes (see below).

There is not only variability in expressivity but also variability in penetrance of AHC among individuals with *DAX1* mutations. A family with X-linked inheritance of a *DAX1* nonsense mutation included a homozygous female who appeared to be the product of a gene conversion event and exhibited HH but not adrenal insufficiency (Merke et al., 1999). Males hemizygous for this nonsense mutation included two brothers, who presented with adrenal insufficiency at 14 and 16 days of age and manifested HH in adolescence, and their maternal grandfather who was unaffected. Another family has been reported in which the proband is heterozygous for a missense mutation, C200W, and has AHC (unpublished manuscript). However, the proband's heterozygous sister and hemizygous father are both unaffected. Variability in penetrance is influenced by modifier genes. At least for the C200W mutation, intrinsic properties of the mutant protein also influence penetrance.

The adrenal insufficiency of AHC has been misdiagnosed as congenital adrenal hyperplasia (Peter et al, 1998; McCabe et al., 2001a). In a series of 18 patients with AHC from 16 families, the most typical presentation (16 individuals) was with salt wasting; one presented with a hypoglycemic seizure, and another was diagnosed prenatally and treated presymptomatically (Peter et al., 1998). Wheezing has been attributed to adrenal insufficiency in AHC (Sakura et al., 1991). Since proopiomelanocortin (POMC) is the precursor protein from which the melanocyte-stimulating hormones (γ_3-MSH and α-MSH), as well as corticotropin, and other peptides, are produced by posttranslational processing, patients with AHC and elevated corticotropin may have hyperpigmentation that may be quite prominent with coal-black skin coloration (Jones et al., 1995).

The X-linked form of AHC is associated typically with HH (McCabe, 2001a). The HH in these patients results from combined hypothalamic and pituitary defects (Habiby et al., 1996), which is consistent with the normal expression of *DAX1* in both the hypothalamus and the pituitary (Guo et al., 1995a). The possibility of delayed puberty in female carriers of *DAX1* mutations (Seminara et al., 1999) is consistent with the role of dosage in *DAX1* function. Interestingly, despite the fact that HH that is clinically evident in affected individuals during adolescence, the "mini-puberty of infancy" is normal in these individuals (Takahashi et al., 1997; Kaiserman et al., 1998; Peter et al., 1998). This clinical observation suggests differences in regulation of the hypothalamus-pituitary-gonadal axis between infancy and adolescence, or erosion of axis function with age in affected males. X-linked AHC has been associated in one family with androgenic precocity (Wittenberg, 1981).

Molecular Genetics

The majority of patients in whom mutations have been identified have had involvement of DAX1 (Phelan and McCabe, 2001). In this recent compendium of 85 DAX1 mutations, the most common were frameshifts (49%), followed by nonsense mutations (28%), missense mutations (20%), and in-frame codon deletions (2%) (Fig. 45–2). The frameshift and nonsense mutations are distributed throughout the two exons of the *DAX1* coding sequence. Six of the missense mutations

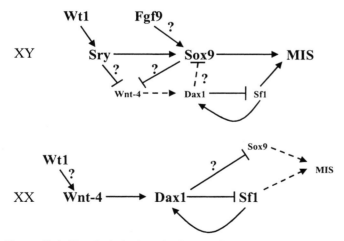

Figure 45–1. Hypothetical schematic diagram of the human sex determination pathway. In XY individuals, expression of SRY may inhibit the action of WNT-4 and, consequently, of DAX1. Low levels of DAX1 cannot fully inhibit the male pathway composed of the activation of Sox9 and MIS. Expression of müllerian inhibiting substance (MIS) is the first indication of testicular formation. In XX individuals, WNT4 up-regulates the expression of DAX1. Then, DAX1 expression antagonizes the male pathway and MIS is turned off. Genes in large print are "on." Genes in small print are "off." The interaction of genes that are on is shown in solid lines. The interaction of genes that are off is shown in dashed lines.

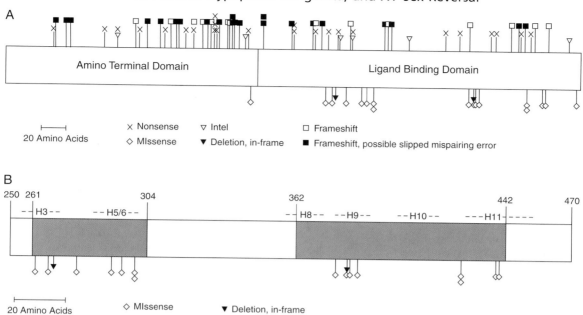

Figure 45–2. (*A*) Mutations in DAX1 including nonsense (X); missense (open diamond); insertion/deletion (open triangle); in-frame deletion (closed triangle); frameshift (open square); and frameshift, possible slipped mispairing error (closed square). (*B*) Amino-acid-altering mutations localize preferentially to the structural subdomain of the ligand-binding domain (LBD). (From Phelan and McCabe, Mutations in *NROB1* (DAX1) and *NR5A1* (SF1) responsible for adrenal hypoplasia congenita, *Human Mutation*, 2001, Wiley-Liss, Inc., a subsidiary of John Wiley and Sons, Inc.)

had previously been shown to map to the C-terminal half of the DAX1 protein, within the structural subdomain of the ligand-binding domain (LBD) (Zhang et al., 1998). Among the 17 missense mutations in the more recent report, these six plus nine additional ones map to this same domain, as well as the two in-frame codon deletions (Phelan and McCabe, 2001). The two exceptions are C200W, which is predicted to map to the hinge region of the protein (unpublished manuscript), and L466R, which is predicted to map to the ligand-binding subdomain of the LBD in a region that corresponds to the activation function-2 (AF2) site in other nuclear receptor proteins (Phelan and McCabe, 2001).

Three patients have been described with mutations in *SF1* (*NR5A1*) associated with AHC, two in the DNA-binding domain (DBD) and one in the hinge region (Achermann et al., 1999b, 2002; Biason-Lauber and Schoenle, 2000; Phelan and McCabe, 2001; Ozisik et al., 2002). The G35E mutation in the P-box of the DBD was observed in a 46,XY sex-reversed female who presented with signs of adrenal insufficiency in the first month of life (Achermann et al., 1999b). The individual was heterozygous for this de novo missense mutation that exhibited loss of function with respect to SF1-response-element binding and target-gene transactivation (Achermann et al., 1999b; Ito et al., 2000). The other mutation in the SF1 DBD is R92Q in the A-box (involved in stabilization of SF1 monomeric binding to DNA through interaction with the minor groove) (Achermann et al., 2002) This patient also exhibited early onset of adrenal insufficiency and 46,XY sex reversal. However, the affected individual was homozygous for the R92Q allele, and heterozygotes had no significant phenotypic abnormalities. Consistent with these clinical observations, the R92Q mutation had less of an effect on DNA binding and transaction than did G35E. The de novo mutation in a conserved residue in the hinge region, R255L, was observed in a heterozygous prepubertal 46,XX female with apparently normal ovarian function and AHC (Biasson-Lauber and Schoenle, 2000). The R255L mutant SF1 protein was transcriptionally inactive.

The phenotypic differences between humans with *SF1* and mice with *Ftzf1* mutations clearly show species differences. Whereas the human 45,XX prepubertal patient has apparently intact ovarian function (Biason-Lauber and Schoenle, 2000), female mice with targeted mutation of *Ftzf1* have gonadal agenesis. The 46,XY humans and the mice with *SF1/Ftzf1* mutations have XY sex reversal with streaklike dysgenetic gonads in the humans and gonadal agenesis in the mice,

though the humans are heterozygotes and the mice are homozygotes (Luo et al., 1994; Sadovsky et al., 1995; Achermann et al., 1999b, 2002). Although AHC may be observed in humans heterozygous for *SF1* mutations, and homozygous mice have adrenal aplasia, heterozygous mice do exhibit a mild adrenal phenotype (Bland et al., 2000).

Diagnosis

The diagnosis of *DAX1* haploinsufficiency should be suspected in males with AHC, particularly when there is an X-linked pattern of inheritance and an association with hypogonadotropic hypogonadism (McCabe, 2001a). *DAX1* mutations also have been rarely observed in females with AHC (Bartley et al., 1982; unpublished manuscript). If a *DAX1* mutation is not identified in a patient with AHC, then a mutation in *SF1* should be considered. The possibility of an *SF1* mutation is particularly compelling in an individual with XY sex reversal and AHC (Achermann et al., 1999b, 2002). In an individual with XY sex reversal and normal adrenal function, DSS with a genomic duplication of the Xp21 region that contains *DAX1* should be considered in the differential diagnosis (McCabe, 2001a). Identification of *DAX1* and *SF1* mutations should rely on genomic sequencing (Wong et al., 1996; Zhang et al., 1998, 2001; Phelan and McCabe, 2001; Ozicik et al., 2002).

Management

Treatment involves glucocorticoid and mineralocorticoid replacement for management of AHC and testosterone supplementation at puberty for HH (Grumbach and Styne, 1992; McCabe, 2001a). If ambiguous genitalia are present, then appropriate consideration and decision-making should occur (see following discussion at "Management").

XY SEX REVERSAL

Clinical Description

Duplication of the dosage-sensitive, sex reversal (DSS) locus, located on Xp21.3 and including the *DAX1* gene, leads to XY gonadal dysgenesis (Arn et al., 1994; Bardoni et al., 1994; Baumstark et al., 1996). Gonadal dysgenesis is a defect in normal development, in which the gonads fail to differentiate into testes in XY individuals. The gonads become small and fibrous, with no oocytes, and are termed "streak" gonads. XY female patients with gonadal dysgenesis are sometimes referred to as "XY sex-reversed" patients or individuals with "XY sex reversal" (Simpson and Martin, 1981). Although widely used, this terminology is somewhat vague as it does not distinguish XY females with gonadal dysgenesis from XY females with androgen resistance. The nomenclature of XY gonadal dysgenesis is essentially based on pathological and cytogenetic findings (Berkovitz and Seeherunvong, 1998). Pure gonadal dysgenesis refers to gonads that are composed of fibrous tissue only, without evidence of testicular tissue. The phenotype of the external genitalia is female without ambiguity. Mixed gonadal dysgenesis is characterized by asymmetric gonadal development, typically with a streak gonad on one side and a testis, generally cryptorchid, on the other side. Because of the presence of some testicular tissue, the external genitalia are ambiguous, with frequent asymmetry of the labioscrotal folds, which are more masculinized on the testis side. The internal genitalia may also be asymmetric, with one fallopian tube on the streak gonad side. These patients have a mosaic chromosomal constitution that frequently includes a 45,X cell line.

Partial gonadal dysgenesis refers to streak gonads that contain some functional testicular tissue. As a consequence, the external genitalia are partially masculinized, and the sexual phenotype is ambiguous. Partial gonadal dysgeneses are thought to be the consequence of molecular defects downstream from that of pure gonadal dysgenesis. Mutations of SRY, the primary trigger of the sex determination pathway, are almost always responsible for pure gonadal dysgenesis. Partial gonadal dysgeneses are almost never explained by mutations in SRY. One exception is a deletion 3' of the SRY open reading frame that leads to partial gonadal dysgenesis (McElreavey et al., 1996). Another is a missense mutation in the 5' non-HMG box region of SRY (Domenice et al., 1998).

Duplication of the DSS locus leads, in most individuals, to XY females with pure gonadal dysgenesis, and, occasionally, to XY intersex individuals, presumably with XY partial gonadal dysgenesis. This complete defect of gonadal development has several associated biological and clinical phenomena. The absence of testicular development results in two major endocrine consequences: a low level of androgens (leading to feminization of the external genitalia, with normal clitoris and labia) and the absence of secretion of MIS by the Sertoli cells, resulting in the persistence of the müllerian structures (uterus, fallopian tubes, and upper part of the vagina). The latter characteristic is essential in the differential diagnosis of XY females with androgen resistance, who do not have remaining müllerian structures because of the normal secretion of MIS. Individuals with pure gonadal dysgenesis are typically not recognized at birth, as they appear as normally developed girls. They usually present around 14 years of age for delayed puberty and primary amenorrhea. They are generally taller than average (review in Vilain, 2000). Laboratory evaluation shows elevated serum gonadotropins (LH and FSH). Patients with XY pure gonadal dysgenesis have an increased risk of gonadoblastoma, a tumor composed of germ cell nests, sex cord cells, and calcifications. Gonadoblastomas develop in 10% to 30% of patients with streak gonads and a Y chromosome (Rutgers, 1991).

Molecular Genetics

Duplication of DSS, a 160 kb critical locus on Xp21.3 that includes DAX1, results in XY individuals with female or ambiguous genitalia (Arn et al., 1994; Bardoni et al., 1994; Baumstark et al., 1996). DAX1 is a good candidate for the DSS phenotype because of its localization within the critical region and because it encodes a putative transcription factor that is expressed in the developing gonads, adrenals, hypothalamus, and pituitary (Swain et al., 1996). A mouse transgenic model overexpressing Ahch results in XY mice that are phenotypically female, suggesting that DAX1 is the gene primarily responsible for DSS (Swain et al., 1998).

Diagnosis

When the diagnosis of gonadal dysgenesis is suspected, a blood karyotype should be requested. This may reveal a cytogenetically visible deletion of Xp21.3, which contains DAX1. If the patient is an XY fe-

male with gonadal dysgenesis and no visible chromosomal abnormality, the first molecular diagnostic test to be performed should be evaluation for an SRY mutation. If no mutation is found in SRY, the search for a small duplication within DSS, including DAX1, can be undertaken. This is usually performed by Southern blot of the patient's DNA hybridized with a DAX1 probe. This test is typically difficult to interpret, as it measures the genic dose of DAX1 and aims to differentiate between one copy (normal XY male) and two copies (XY female with duplication of DSS). In order to increase accuracy, it is advised to run, in addition to the patient's sample, DNA from a normal male (one dose), a normal female (two doses), and, if available, from cell lines with 47,XXX (three doses) and 49,XXXXY (four doses). In addition, the blot should be rehybridized with an autosomal probe to normalize the results for the amount of DNA loaded. Rarely is the breakpoint of the duplication close enough to the probe to produce a Southern blot pattern that is different from normal and that has a junction fragment.

An alternative test for duplication is fluorescence in situ hybridization (FISH). The main advantage of FISH is to avoid the difficult interpretation of a Southern blot and to provide clearer pictures of duplications. The main drawback is the lack of sensitivity, since if the duplication is too small and contiguous to the normal locus, then only one spot will be seen. Because patients with XY gonadal dysgenesis are not fertile, the issue of prenatal diagnosis is typically not relevant. However, with the increased frequency of pregnancies after age 35, the prenatal discovery of sex reversal (XX male or XY female)—or the misattribution of phenotypic sex based on chromosomal analysis without visualization of the genitalia—has increased. If the prenatal karyotype is 46,XY and the ultrasound shows female fetal genitalia, additional molecular tests may clarify the diagnosis. Androgen resistance should first be ruled out because of its higher incidence. An important diagnostic clue to androgen resistance is a positive family history for XY females, primary amenorrhea, sexual ambiguity, or even male infertility consistent with an X-linked pattern of inheritance. A second clue is the absence of a uterus. However, presence or absence of a uterus is hard to evaluate prenatally.

Most duplications of DSS result in pure gonadal dysgenesis in XY individuals. Typically, they present at adolescence for delayed puberty and primary amenorrhea. Diagnosis is initially based on the clinical observation of normal females with eunuchoid proportions and small or absent breast development. There are likely to be no associated malformations or dysmorphic features. Their stature is normal or tall. The absence of congenital anomalies and the normal height differentiates the clinical presentations of XY pure gonadal dysgenesis from Turner syndrome (45,X). External genitalia are often normal but occasionally appear hypoplastic. The laboratory results show high levels of LH and FSH that demonstrate a primary gonadal insufficiency. Blood karyotype may reveal a cytogenetically visible rearrangement of Xp. Because of the risk of gonadoblastoma, bilateral gonadectomy is recommended and may be performed by laparoscopy. Careful examination, including histological examination of the gonads, allows physicians to establish the final diagnosis by demonstrating the presence of a uterus (typically infantile), fallopian tubes, and elongated, thin, rudimentary streak gonads that are composed of fibrous ovarian-like stroma (Sohval, 1965).

Management

Management of XY females with pure gonadal dysgenesis—whether caused by duplication of DSS, mutation of SRY, or any other genetic mechanism—is similar to the management of delayed puberty and primary amenorrhea. Estrogen replacement therapy is best started with physiological doses of estradiol to allow patients to achieve their genetic growth potential. Estradiol intramuscularly (IM) at 0.25 mg per month to start, with a dosage increase of 0.25 mg every 6 months up to 1.0 to 1.5 mg per month, is recommended. An oral alternative would be 5 μg of ethinyl estradiol daily, 3 out of 4 weeks, increased progressively to the adult dose of 20 μg (Sperling et al., 1973). Progestin is usually added 2 years after menarche—for example, medroxyprogesterone acetate, 5 to 10 mg at bedtime for 7 to 14 days, during the second and third week of estrogens. Eventually, once optimal height has been achieved, treatment with birth control pills is the most convenient form of therapy. In the case of a patient born with an intersex condition, a specialized team composed of a pediatric endocrinologist, a pediatric urologist, a geneticist, and a psychologist should rapidly evaluate, discuss, and explain options of management to the parents. Gender (male or female) should be assigned based on the knowledge of the diagnoses, the clinical outcome studies, and the combined opinions of the specialized team and the parents. Performing early genital surgery, or delaying it until the patient consents, should be presented to the parents as options. Communicating with patient support groups is also recommended.

ANIMAL MODELS

Transgenic Mice

Involvement of DAX1 in mammalian sex determination has initially been inferred from the identification of a 160 kb critical region responsible, when duplicated, for XY sex reversal in humans (Arn et al., 1994; Bardoni et al., 1994; Baumstark et al., 1996). This 160 kb DSS locus contains the *DAX1* gene, as well as other expressed sequence tags or genes such as the *MAGE* genes. Although *DAX1* is the best candidate gene to be involved in sex determination because of its pattern of developmental expression and sexually dimorphic gonadal expression, other sex-determining genes within DSS cannot be ruled out by the positional mapping of human Xp21 duplication. The evidence that *DAX1* is directly involved in sex determination should come from transgenic experiments, showing that extra copies of *DAX1/Ahch* alone result in an XY female phenotype. Such an animal model was generated by Swain and colleagues (1998). An 11 kb fragment of *Ahch* promoter drove its gonadal expression identically to the endogenous *Ahch* expression. The mouse *Ahch* cDNA was then inserted downstream of the previously identified 11 kb *Ahch* promoter. Even in the four mouse lines that displayed levels of exogenous *Ahch* expression higher than the endogenous *Ahch* (up to five times the normal level), no XY sex reversal was observed. At the adult stage, these transgenic mice did not show a phenotype similar to XY humans with a duplicated DSS. However, testicular differentiation (evaluated by the presence of testicular cords and *Mis* expression) was significantly delayed at E12.5, but was normal at E13.5. In addition, in mice homozygous for the *Ahch* transgene, XY males displayed infertility with a block in spermatogenesis.

XY sex reversal was only observed when the *Mus musculus* transgenic mice were bred with mice carrying a *Mus domesticus poschiavinus* strain Y chromosome, Y^{pos} (Swain et al., 1998). Y^{pos} is known to be associated with sex reversal on a C57BL/6 background (Eicher et al., 1982). On a mixed genetic background, Y^{pos} is associated with a 14 hour delay of testis cord formation (Palmer and Burgoyne, 1991), due to low levels of *Sry* expression. Since the *Ahch* transgenic mice have a mixed background, the occurrence of XY sex reversal can be attributed to the overexpression of *Ahch*. In the context of a low level of expressed Sry, *Ahch* transgenic mice mimic the phenotype observed in DSS patients.

It can be concluded that Dax1 acts antagonistically to Sry and that the mechanisms of mammalian sex determination are highly sensitive to the relative dosage of these two genes. The observation of sex reversal only if there is a low level of *Sry* expression in *Ahch* transgenic mice may reflect differences between human and murine sex determination, such as differences in expression and sequence of *SRY/Sry*. In fact, rapid evolution of *SRY* and *DAX1* has been demonstrated among mammals (Whitfield et al., 1993; Patel et al., 2001).

A less likely possibility, but one that remains open to speculation, is the presence of additional genes within the DSS locus that code for proteins that may act synergistically with DAX1.

Knockout Mice

To better understand the physiological function of DAX1/Ahch in adrenal and gonadal development, a knockout mouse model was generated (Yu et al., 1998b). The Ahch profile of expression (turned off in male gonads after E12.5), as well as its antagonistic action to SRY/Sry,

suggests an "anti-testis" role during development. The Ahch expression profile in the developing ovary also raises the possibility of a role in ovarian development. If this is the case, XX mice deleted for *Ahch* should not have normal ovaries.

Attempts to delete the first exon of Ahch using a standard gene-targeting strategy failed to generate viable targeted embryonic stem (ES) cells (Yu et al., 1998b). As *Ahch* was shown to be expressed in ES cells, this suggests a role of Ahch for the survival of ES cells (Clipsham et al., 2001). Using a Cre-mediated disruption of Ahch exon 2 (with the CMV promoter driving Cre expression), a murine model for AHC was generated (Yu et al., 1998b).

Heterozygous females for the *Ahch* deletion showed no phenotype. Males who have only a single *Ahch*-deleted allele were normal in terms of viability and size. However, the fetal adrenal X-zone did not regress as it normally should after puberty (Dunn, 1970). As in humans with X-linked AHC, the adrenal cortex of the male knockout mice contained X-zone (similar to human fetal) cells, but unlike the humans, there was a normal adult zone (glomerulosa and fasciculata) and normal secretion of corticosteroids. External and internal genitalia of male knockout mice were phenotypically normal, but testes were smaller and showed a progressive loss of germ cells throughout postnatal maturation, with complete loss at 14 weeks. These observations suggest that Ahch is important for the maintenance of spermatogenesis. Unlike in humans with AHC, the knockout mice did not display hypo-gonadotropic hypogonadism, thus suggesting that the spermatogenetic defect was not caused by low secretion of GnRH, LH, and FSH but by a primary testicular failure. Further analysis revealed that *Ahch*-deficient mice displayed a blockage of the rete testis and efferent ductules by ectopic Sertoli and Leydig cells, causing infertility (Jeffs et al., 2001a). On a Y^{pos} background, XY knockout mice are female, suggesting, in this genetic context, a role for DAX1 in testis determination (Meeks et al., 2003).

Females homozygous for the deletion of *Ahch* exon 2 showed normal ovarian structure and fertility (Yu et al., 1998b). The only significant change from wild-type females was the presence, in some follicles, of multiple oocytes. These results suggest that Ahch may not be involved in ovarian formation. However, only exon 2 was deleted and an abnormal transcript was observed (RN Yu, personal communication). Together with the absence of adrenal, hypothalamic, and pituitary dysfunction, as observed in humans mutated for *Dax1*, these mice may represent a hypomorphic phenotype from which no definite conclusion could be drawn in terms of involvement of Ahch in ovarian development. Alternatively, the detailed mechanisms of development and the roles of partners in these complex developmental networks undoubtly differ between species. Nevertheless, the *Ahch* knockout mice provide a good model for studying certain aspects of Ahch function. For instance, it was thought that Ahch repressed all the Ftzf1-activated targets using in vitro transfection studies; however, in vivo analysis of the *Ahch* knockout mice revealed that aromatase (cyp19) is the main physiological target of *Ahch* in Leydig's cells (Wang et al., 2001). The Ahch-deficient mice also provided information about the roles of Ahch in various gonadal cell types. When rescued by a *Mis*-promoter-driven Ahch transgene, the Ahch-deficient male mice showed a Sertoli cell–specific rescue of fertility, but the testicular morphology remained abnormal (Jeffs et al., 2001b). This suggested that Ahch plays a crucial role not only in Sertoli cells but also in Leydig cell development and function.

DEVELOPMENTAL PATHOGENESIS

Summary

The clinical findings among humans and mice with mutations in *DAX1/Ahch* very clearly show the importance of this orphan nuclear receptor in the development of the hypothalamic-pituitary-adrenal/gonadal axis. The developmental profiles of *DAX1/Ahch* and *SF1/Ftzf1*, as well as the pathogenesis among those with mutations in these genes, suggest the interaction of DAX1/Ahch with SF1/Ftzf1 in the normal development of the steroidogenic axis. The precise nature of the interaction(s) of these transcription factors in normal development remains to be clarified (McCabe, 2001a).

An SF1 RE is conserved in the human and murine *DAX1* promoters (Burris et al., 1995; Bae et al., 1996; Guo et al., 1996). This RE binds SF1 specifically (Burris et al., 1995) and is used by SF1 to increase DAX1 expression in a human adrenal cortical carcinoma all line NCI H295 (Vilain et al., 1997).

DAX1 appears to be a transcriptional repressor, but the mechanism of this repression is still under examination. DAX1 binds to hairpin DNA structural motifs to decrease target gene expression (Zazopoulos et al., 1997). Ahch may heterodimerize with Ftzf1 to block the interaction of Ftzf1 with Wt1 to stimulate MIS expression (Nachtigal et al., 1998) and with Srebp1a to stimulate Hdlr expression (Lopez et al., 2001). In addition, DAX1 contains putative transcriptional silencing domains, one of which in the carboxy terminus suggests similarity with the AF2 region of other nuclear receptors (Ito et al., 1997; Lalli et al., 1997; Achermann et al., 2000).

DAX1 mutations interfere with transcriptional silencing (Achermann et al., 2000; McCabe, 2001a). Since the majority of the *DAX* mutations are frameshift or nonsense changes and since the AF2-like domain is at the carboxy terminus, then these mutations would eliminate this putative silencing domain (Achermann et al., 2000). Naturally occurring mutations, including single amino acid changes, interfere with transcriptional silencing (Ito et al., 1997; Lalli et al., 1997). N-CoR is a co-regulator recruited by DAX1 to SF1 (Crawford et al., 1998). Since these factors vary in abundance with different cell types, they could contribute to variability in silencing by cell type and promoter (Lalli et al., 1997).

Consequences of Complexity

The complexity of the DAX1 and SF1 transcriptional regulatory networks contributes to the stability of these critical developmental networks and also helps explain their vulnerability (McCabe, 2002). These networks have the hub-and-spoke structure that is typical of scale-free networks (Albert et al., 2000; Tu, 2000; Dipple et al., 2001; Clipsham et al., 2002). The highly robust character of scale-free networks is important for systems that are essential for steroidogenic axis development and sex determination (McCabe, 2002). In general, these developmental processes proceed, normally, despite significant variation and even component failure imposed by genetic and environmental causes (Dipple et al., 2001).

Examination of the structural features that provide these scale-free networks with their functional robustness also provides clues to their vulnerability (Dipple et al., 2001; Clipsham et al., 2002). Compromise of highly connected nodes or nonredundant "trunk lines" begin to fragment the system. In the past, a mutation in a component like *DAX1* has frequently been considered to be an interruption of a transcriptional pathway or cascade. *DAX1*, however, is a highly connected node in this scale-free system, and mutation of *DAX1* removes an entire network segment (Clipsham et al., 2002).

The complexity of the transcriptional regulatory networks involved in steroidogenic axis development and sex determination also provides insight into why a patient's genotype rarely predicts their phenotype (Dipple and McCabe, 2000a, 2000b; Dipple et al., 2001; McCabe, 2002). Modifying influences—whether genetic or environmental—are capable of altering flux through the network, thereby altering the individual's phenotype. This concept is supported by the field of metabolic control analysis, which has shown that for most pathways there is no rate-limiting step (Dipple and McCabe, 2000b). Also consistent with this concept are the clinical observations were categorized as "synergistic heterozygosity" when Vockley et al., 2000 observed a number of individuals who initially were recognized to be heterozygous for a mutation in only a single enzyme in a pathway. Subsequent molecular genetic analysis showed, however, that these patients were heterozygotes for at least one additional enzyme in the same pathway. In accord with metabolic control analysis, if there is not a single rate-limiting step in a pathway, then heterozygosity for two steps may be equivalent in phenotypic consequences to homozygosity for a single step. We would argue that, on the basis of network complexity, those nodes susceptible to synergistic heterozygosity would be those that are the more highly connected and more vulnerable nodes, or they would represent nonredundant trunk lines between such nodes (Dip-

ple et al., 2001). Such patients also demonstrate that patients' phenotypes are the consequences of network flux, so that variations in more than one step will influence flux and therefore phenotype.

Our understanding of complex systems, like those in which DAX1 is engaged, remains quite primitive (Koshland, 1998). We must begin to understand and model protein networks using concepts from engineering, electronics, and computer design (Biay, 1995; Hartwell et al., 1999). Recent design and construction of an oscillatory network composed of transcriptional regulators and referred to as a "repressilator" clearly has conceptual appeal in molecular developmental endocrinology (Elowitz and Leibler, 2000). Further study is required to fully understand such complex genetic circuits (Judd et al., 2000).

References

Achermann JC, Gu W-X, Kotlar TJ, Meeks JJ, Sabacan LP, Seminara SB, Habiby RL, Hindmarsh PC, Bick DP, Sherins RJ, et al. (1999a). Mutational analysis of *DAX1* in patients with hypogonadotropic or pubertal delay. *J Clin Endocrinol Metab* 84: 4497–4500.

Achermann JC, Ito M, Ito M, Hindmarsh PC, Jameson JL (1999b). A mutation in the gene encoding steroidogenic factor-1 causes XY sex reversal and adrenal failure in humans. *Nat Genet* 22: 125–126.

Achermann JC, Baxter J, Jameson JL (2000). SF-1 and DAX-1 in adrenal development and pathology. In: *Adrenal Disease in Childhood*, vol. 2. Hughes JA, Clark AJ (eds.) Karger, pp. 1–23.

Achermann JC, Ozisik G, Ito M, Orun UA, Harmanci K, Gurakan B, Jameson JL (2002). Gonadal determination and adrenal development are regulated by the orphan nuclear receptor, steroidogenic factor-1, in a dose-dependent manner. *J Clin Endocrinol Metab* 87: 1829–1833.

Albert R, Jeong H, Barbasi A-L (2000). Error and attack tolerance of complex networks. *Nature* 406: 378–382.

Arn P, Chen H, Tuck Muller CM, Mankinen C, Wachtel G, Li S, Shen CC, Wachtel SS (1994). SRVX, a sex-reversing locus in Xp21.2 to p22.11. *Hum Genet* 93: 389–393.

Aylwin SJ, Welch JP, Davey CL, Geddes JF, Wood DF, Besser GM, Grossman AB, Monson JP, Burrin JM (2001). The relationship between steroidogenic factor 1 and DAX-1 expression and in vitro gonadotropin secretion in human pituitary adenomas. *J Clin Endocrinol Metab* 86: 2476–2483.

Babu PS, Bavers DL, Beuschlein F, Shah S, Jeffs B, Jameson JL, Hammer GD (2002). Interaction between Dax-1 and steroidogenic factor-1 in vivo: increased adrenal responsiveness to ACTH in the absence of Dax-1. *Endocrinology* 143: 665–673.

Bae DS, Schaefer ML, Partan BW, Muglia L (1996). Characterization of the mouse DAX1 gene reveals evolutionary conservation of a unique amino-terminal motif and widespread expression in mouse tissue. *Endocrinology* 137: 3921–3927.

Bakke M, Zhao L, Parker KL (2001a). Approaches to define the role of SF-1 at different levels of the hypothalamic-pituitary-steroidogenic organ axis. *Mol Cell Endocrinol* 179: 33–37.

Bakke M, Zhao L, Hanley NA, Parker KL (2001b). SF-1: a critical mediator of steroidogenesis. *Mol Cell Endocrinol* 171: 5–7.

Bardoni B, Zanaria E, Guioli S, Floridia G, Worley KC, Tonini G, Ferrante E, Chiumello S, McCabe ERB, Fraccaro M, et al. (1994). A dosage sensitive locus at chromosome Xp21 is involved in male to female sex reversal. *Nat Genet* 7: 497–501.

Bartley JA, Miller DK, Hayford JT, McCabe ERB (1982). The concordance of X-linked glycerol kinase deficiency with X-linked adrenal hypoplasia in two families. *Lancet* 2: 733–736.

Bartley JA, Patil S, Davenport S, Goldstein D, Pickens J (1986). Duchenne muscular dystrophy, glycerol kinase deficiency, and adrenal insufficiency associated with Xp21 interstitial deletion. *J Pediatr* 108: 189–192.

Baumstark A, Barbi G, Djalali M, Geerkens C, Mitulla B, Mattfeldt T, Cabra del Almeida JC, Vargas FR, Llerna JC (1996). Xp-duplications with and without sex reversal. *Hum Genet* 97: 79–86.

Belloni AS, Neri G, Musajo FG, Andreis PA, Boscaro M, D'Agostino D, Rebuffat P, Boshier DP, Gottardo E, Mazzocchi G, Nussdorfer GG (1990). Investigations on the morphology and function of adrenocortical tissue regenerated from gland capsular fragments autotransplanted in the musculus gracilis of the rat. *Endocrinology* 126: 3251–3262.

Berkovitz GD, Seeherunvong T (1998). Abnormalities of gonadal differentiation. *Baillieres Clin Endocrinol Metab* 12: 133–142.

Beuschlein F, Mutch C, Bauers DL, Ulrich-Lai YM, Engeland WC, Keegan C, Hamma GD (2002). Steroidogenic factor-1 is essential for compensatory adrenal growth following unilateral adrenalectomy. *Endocrinology* 148: 3122–3135.

Biason-Lauber A, Schoenle EJ (2000). Apparently normal ovarian differentiation in a prepubertal girl with transcriptionally inactive steroidogenic factor1 (NR5A/SF1) and adrenocortical insufficiency. *Am J Hum Genet* 67: 1563–1568.

Biay D (1995). Protein molecules as computational elements in living cells. *Nature* 376: 307–312.

Bland ML, Jamieson CA, Akana SF, Bornstein SR, Eisenhofer G, Dallman MF, Ingraham HA (2000). Haploinsufficiency of steroidogenic factor-1 in mice disrupts adrenal development leading to an impaired stress response. *Proc Natl Acad Sci USA* 97: 14488–14493.

Brochner-Mortensen K (1956). Familial occurrence of Addison's disease. *Acta Med Scand* 156: 205–290.

Burris TP, Guo W, Le T, McCabe ERB (1995). Identification of a putative steroidogenic factor-1 response element in the DAX-1 promoter. *Biochem Biophys Res Commun* 214: 576–581.

Burris TP, Guo W, McCabe ERB (1996). The gene responsible for adrenal hypoplasia congenital, DAX1, encodes a nuclear hormone receptor that defines a new class within the superfamily. In: *Recent Progress in Hormone Research*. Conn PM (ed.) Endocrine Society, Bethesda, Md., pp. 241–260.

Clarke A, Roberts SH, Thomas NST, Whitfield A, Williams J, Harper PS (1986). Duchenne muscular dystrophy with adrenal insufficiency and glycerol kinase deficiency: high resolution cytogenetic analysis with molecular, biochemical and clinical studies. *J Med Genet* 23: 501–508.

Clipsham RC, Zhang Y-H, Huang B-L, McCabe ERB (2001). *Ahch* expression in murine embryonic stem cells: a model system for investigating the role of *Ahch* in early ontogeny. In: *Proceedings of the 83rd Annual Meeting of the Endocrine Society, Denver, Colorado*. A585. The Endocrine Society Press, Bethesda, MD.

Clipsham R, Zhang Y-H, Huang B-L, McCabe ERB (2002). Genetic network identification by high density, multiplexed reversed transcriptional (HD-MRT) analysis in steroidogenic axis model cell lines *Mol Genet Metab* 77: 159.

Crawford PA, Dorn C, Sadovsky Y, Milbrandt J (1998). Nuclear receptor DAX-1 recruits nuclear receptor corepressor N-CoR to steroidogenic factor. *Mol Cell Biol* 18: 2949–2956.

Dellovade TL, Young M, Ross EP, Henderson R, Caron K, Parker K, Tobet SA (2000). Disruption of the gene encoding SF-1 alters the distribution of hypothalamic neuronal phenotypes. *J Comp Neurol* 423: 579–589.

Dipple KM, McCabe ERB (2000a). Modifier genes convert "simple" mendelian disorders to complex traits. *Mol Genet Metab* 71: 43–50.

Dipple KM, McCabe ERB (2000b). Phenotypes of patients with "simple" mendelian disorders are complex traits: thresholds, modifiers, and system dynamics. *Am J Hum Genet* 66: 1729–1735.

Dipple KM, Phelan JK, McCabe ERB (2001). Consequences of complexity within biological networks: robustness and health, or vulnerability and disease. *Mol Genet Metab* 74: 45–50.

Domenice S, Yumie Nishi M, Correia Billbeck AE, Latronico AC, Aparecida Medeiros M, Russel AJ, Vass K, Marino Carvalho F, Costa Frade EM, Prado Arnhold IJ, Bilharinho Mendonca B (1998). A novel missense mutation (S18N) in the 5′ non-HMG box region of the SRY gene in a patient with partial gonadal dysgenesis and his normal male relatives. *Hum Genet* 102: 213–215.

Dunger DB, Davies KE, Pembrey M, Lake B, Pearson P, Williams D, Whitfield A, Dillon MJ (1986). Deletion of the X chromosome detected by direct DNA analysis in one of two unrelated boys with glycerol kinase deficiency, adrenal hypoplasia and Duchenne muscular dystrophy. *Lancet* 1: 585–587.

Dunn TB (1970). Normal and pathologic anatomy of the adrenal gland of the mouse, including neoplasms. *J Natl Cancer Inst* 44: 1323–1389.

Eicher EM, Washburn LL, Whitney JB 3rd, Morrow KE (1982). *Mus poschiavinus* Y chromosome in the C57BL/6J murine genome causes sex reversal. *Science* 217: 535–537.

Elowitz MB, Leibler S (2000). A synthetic oscillatory network of transcriptional regulators. *Nature* 403: 335–338.

Golden MP, Lippe BM, Kaplan SA (1977). Congenital adrenal hypoplasia and hypogonadotropic hypogonadism. *Am J Dis Child* 131: 1117–1118.

Goodfellow PN, Camerino G (1999). Dax-1, an "antitestis" gene. *Cell Mol Life Sci* 55: 857–863.

Goussault Y, Turpin E, Neel D, Dreux C, Chann B, Bakir R, Rouffy J (1982). "Pseduo-hypertriglyceridemia" caused by hyperglycerolemia due to congenital enzyme deficiency. *Clin Chem Acta* 123: 269–274.

Grumbach MM, Styne DM (1992). Puberty: ontogamy neuroendocrinology, physiology and disorders. In: *Williams Textbook of Endocrinology*. Williams JD, Foster BW (eds.) W. B. Saunders, Philadelphia, 1139–1221.

Guggenheim MA, McCabe ERB, Roig M, Goodman SI, Lum GM, Bullen WW, Ringel SP (1980). Glycerol kinase deficiency with neuromuscular, skeletal and adrenal abnormalities. *Ann Neurol* 7: 441–449.

Guo W, Burris TP, McCabe ERB (1995a). Expression of DAX-1, the gene responsible for X-linked adrenal hypoplasia congenital and hypogonadotropic hypogonadism in the hypothalamic-pituitary/gonadal axis. *Biochem Mol Med* 56: 8–13.

Guo W, Mason JS, Stone CG, Morgan SA, Madu SI, Baldini A, Lindsay EA, Biesecker LG, Copeland KC, Horlick MNB, et al. (1995b). Diagnosis of X-linked adrenal hypoplasia congenital by mutation analysis of DAX-1 gene. *JAMA* 274: 324–330.

Guo W, Burris TP, Zhang Y-H, Huang B-L, Mason J, Copeland KC, Kupfer SR, Pagon RA, McCabe ERB (1996). Genomic sequence of the DAX1 gene: an orphan nuclear receptor responsible for X-linked adrenal hypolplasia congenital and hypogonadotropic hypogonadism. *J Clin Endocrinol Metab* 82: 2481–2486.

Habiby RL, Boepple P, Nachtigall L, Sluss PM, Crowley WF Jr, Jameson JL (1996). Adrenal hypoplasia congenital with hypogonadotropic hypogonadism: evidence that DAX1 mutations lead to combined hypothalamic and pituitary defects in gonadotropin production. *J Clin Invest* 98: 1055–1062.

Hammond J, Howard NJ, Brookwell R, Purvis-Smith S, Wilcken B, Hoogenraad N (1985). Proposed assignment of loci for X-linked adrenal hypoplasia and glycerol kinase genes. *Lancet* 1: 54.

Hanley NA, Ball SG, Clement-Jones M, Hagan DM, Strachan T, Lindsay S, Robson S, Ostrer H, Parker KL, Wilson DI (1999). Expression of steroidogenic factor 1 and Wilms' tumour 1 during early human gonadal development and sex determination. *Mech Dev* 87: 175–180.

Hanley NA, Hagan DM, Clement-Jones M, Ball SG, Strachan T, Salas-Cortes L, McElreavey K, Lindsay S, Robson S, Bullen P, et al. (2000). SRY, SOX9, and DAX1 expression patterns during human sex determination and gonadal development. *Mech Dev* 91: 403–407.

Hanley NA, Rainey WE, Wilson DI, Ball SG, Parker KL (2001). Expression profiles of SF-1, DAX1 and CYP17 in the human fetal adrenal gland: Potential interactions in gene regulation. *Mol Endocrinol* 15: 57–68.

Hartwell L, Hopfield JJ, Leibler S, Murray AW (1999). From molecular to modular cell biology. *Nature* 402: C47–C52.

Hatano O, Takayama K, Imai T, Waterman MR, Takakusu A, Omura T, Morohashi K (1994). Sex-dependent expression of a transcription factor, Ad4BP, regulating steroidogenic P-450 genes in the gonads during prenatal and postnatal rat development. *Development* 120: 2787–2797.

Hatano O, Takakusu A, Nomura M, Morohashi K (1996). Identical origin of adrenal cortex and gonad revealed by expression profiles of Ad4BP/SF-1. *Genes Cells* 1: 663–671.

Honda S, Morohashi K, Nomura M, Takeya H, Kitajima M, Omura T (1993). Ad4BP regulating steroidogenic P-450 gene is a member of steroid hormone receptor superfamily. *J Biol Chem* 268: 7494–7502.

Ikeda Y, Lala DS, Luo X, Kim E, Moisan MP, Parker KL (1993). Characterization of the mouse FTZ-F1 gene, which encodes a key regulator of steroid hydroxylase gene expression. *Mol Endocrinol* 7: 852–860.

Ikeda Y, Shen W-H, Ingraham HA, Nilson JH, Parker KL (1994). Developmental expression of mouse steroidogenic factor-1, an essential regulator of the steroid hydroxylases. *Mol Endocrinol* 8: 654–662.

Ikeda Y, Luo X, Addub R, Nilson JH, Parker KL (1995). The nuclear receptor steroidogenic factor 1 is essential for the formation of the ventromedial hypothalamic nucleus. *Mol Endocrinol* 9: 478–486.

Ikeda Y, Shen WH, Ingraham HA, Parker KL (1994). Developmental expression of mouse steroidogenic factor-1, an essential regulator of the steroid hydroxylases. *Mol Endocrinol* 8: 654–662.

Ikeda Y, Swain A, Weber TJ, Hentges KE, Zanaria E, Lalli E, Tamai KT, Sassone-Corsi P, Lovell-Badge R, Camerino G, Parker KL (1996). Steroidogenic factor 1 and Dax-1 colocalize in multiple cell lineages: potential links in endocrine development. *Mol Endocrinol* 10: 1261–1272.

Ikeda Y, Takeda Y, Shikayama T, Mukai T, Hisano S, Morohashi K-I (2001). Comparative localization of Dax-1 and Ad4BP/SF-1 during development of the hypothalamic-pituitary-gonadal axis suggests their closely related and distinct functions. *Dev Dyn* 220: 363–376.

Ingraham HA, Lala DS, Ikeda Y, Luo K, Shen WH, Nachtigal MW, Abbud R, Nilson JH, Parker KL (1994). The nuclear receptor steroidogenic factor 1 acts at multiple levels of the reproductive axis. *Genes Dev* 8: 2302–2312.

Ito M, Yu R, Jameson JL (1997). DAX-1 inhibits SF-1-mediated transactivation via a carboxy-terminal domain that is deleted in adrenal hypoplasia congenital. *Mol Cell Biol* 17: 1476–1483.

Ito M, Achermann JC, Jameson JL (2000). A naturally occurring steroidogenic factor-1 mutation exhibits differential bindings and activation of target genes. *J Biol Chem* 275: 31708–31714.

Jeffs B, Meeks JJ, Ito M, Martinson FA, Matzuk MM, Jameson JL, Russell LD (2001a). Blockage of the rete testis and efferent ductules by ectopic Sertoli and Leydig cells causes infertility in Dax1-deficient male mice. *Endocrinology* 142: 4486–4495.

Jeffs B, Ito M, Yu RN, Martinson FA, Wang ZJ, Doglio LT, Jameson JL (2001b). Sertoli cell-specific rescue of fertility, but not testicular pathology in *Dax1* (*Ahch*)-deficient male mice. *Endocrinology* 142: 2481–2488.

Jones D, Kay M, Craigen W, McCabe ERB, Hawkins H, Dominey A (1995). Coal-black hyperpigmentation at birth in a child with congenital adrenal hypoplasia. *J Am Acad Dermatol* 33: 323–326.

Judd EM, Laub MT, McAdams HH (2000). Toggles and oscillators: new generic circuit designs. *Bioessays* 22: 507–509.

Kaiserman KB, Nakamoto JM, Geffner ME, McCabe ERB (1998). Minipuberty of infancy and adolescent pubertal function in adrenal hypoplasia congenital. *J Pediatr* 133: 300–302.

Kawabe K, Shikayama T, Tsuboi H, Oka S, Oba K, Yanase T, Nawata H, Morohashi K (1999). Dax-1 as one of the target genes of Ad4BP/SF-1. *Mol Endocrinol* 13: 1267–1284.

Koopman P, Munserberg A, Capel B, Vivian N, Lovell-Badge R (1990). Expression of a candidate sex-determining gene during mouse testis differentiation. *Nature* 348: 450–452.

Koshland DE Jr. (1998). The era of pathway quantification. *Science* 280: 852–853.

Lack EE, Kozakewich HPW (1990a). Adrenal neuroblastoma, ganglioneuroblastoma, and related tumors. In: *Pathology of the Adrenal Glands*. Lack EE (ed.) Churchill Livingstone, New York, pp. 277–309.

Lack EE, Kozakewich HPW (1990b). Embryology, developmental anatomy, and selected aspects on non-neoplastic pathology. In: *Pathology of the Adrenal Glands*. Lack EE (ed.) Churchill Livingstone, New York, pp. 1–74.

Lalli E, Bardoni B, Zazopoulos E, Wurtz JM, Strom TM, Moras D, Sassone-Corsi P (1997). A transcriptional silencing domain in DAX-1 whose mutation causes adrenal hypoplasia congenital. *Mol Endocrinol* 11: 1950–1960.

Lopez D, Shea-Eaton W, Sanchez MD, McLean MP (2001). DAX-1 represses the high-density lipoprotein receptor through interaction with positive regulators sterol regulatory element-binding protein-1a and steroidogenic factor-1. *Endocrinology* 142: 5097–5106.

Luo X, Ikeda Y, Parker KL (1994). A cell-specific nuclear receptor is essential for adrenal and gonadal development and sexual differentiation. *Cell* 77: 481–490.

Mangelsdorf DJ (2001). Regulation of sterol homeostasis by nuclear receptors. In: *Proceedings of the 83rd Annual Meeting of the Endocrine Society, Denver, Colorado*. L4-2: 19. The Endocrine Society Press, Bethesda, MD.

McCabe ERB (2001a). Adrenal hypoplasias and aplasias. In: *The Metabolic and Molecular Bases of Inherited Diseases, 8th Edition*. Scriver CR, Beaudet AL, Sly WS, Valle D, Childs B, Vogelstein B (eds.) McGraw-Hill, New York, pp. 4263–4274.

McCabe ERB (2001b). Disorders of glycerol metabolism. In: *The Metabolic and Molecular Bases of Inherited Diseases, 8th Edition*. Scriver CR, Beaudet AL, Sly SW, Valle D, Childs B, Vogelstein B (eds.) McGraw-Hill, New York, pp. 2217–2237.

McCabe ERB (2002). Vulnerability within a robust complex system: DAX-1 mutations and steroidogenic axis development. *J Clin Endocrinol Metab* 87: 41–43.

McCabe ERB, Phelan J (2001). Mutations in *NR0B1* (DAX1) and *NR5A1* (SF1) responsible for adrenal hypoplasia congenita. *Hum Mut* 18: 472–487.

McCabe ERB, Fennessey PV, Guggenheim MA, Miles BS, Bullen WW, Sceats DJ, Goodman SI (1997). Human glycerol kinase deficiency with hyperglycerolemia and glyceroluria. *Biochem Biophys Res Commun* 78: 1327–1333.

McElreavey K, Vilain E, Barbaux S, Fuqua JS, Fechner PY, Souleyreau N, Doco-Fenzy M, Gabriel R, Quereux C, Fellous M, Berkovitz GD (1996). Loss of sequences 3′ to the testis-determining gene, SRY, including the Y pseudoautosomal boundary associated with partial testicular determination. *Proc Natl Acad Sci USA* 93: 8590–8594.

Meakin JW, Nelson DH, Thron GW (1959). Addison's disease in two brothers. *J Clin Endocrinol Metab* 19: 726–731.

Meeks JJ, Weiss J, Jameson JL (2003). Dax1 is required for testis determination. *Nature Genet* 34: 32–33.

Merke DP, Tajima T, Baron J, Cutler GB (1999). Hypogonadotropic hypogonadism in a female caused by an X-linked recessive mutation in the DAX1 gene. *N Engl J Med* 340: 1248–1252.

Morohashi K, Iida H, Nomura M, Hatano O, Honda S, Tsukiyama T, Niwa O, Hara T,

Takakusu A, Shibata Y (1994). Functional difference between Ad4BP and ELP, and their distributions in steroidogenic tissues. *Mol Endocrinol* 8: 643–653.

Muscatelli F, Strom TM, Walker AP, Zanaria E, Recan D, Meindl A, Bardoni B, Guillo S, Zehetner G, Robl W, et al. (1994). Mutations in the DAX-1 gene give rise to both X-linked adrenal hypoplasia congenital and hypogonadotropic hypogonadism. *Nature* 372: 672–676.

Nachtigal MW Hirokawa Y, Enyeart-VanHouten DL, Flanagan JN, Hammer GD, Ingraham HA (1998). Wilms' tumor 1 and Dax–1 modulate the orphan nuclear receptor SF-1 in sex-specific gene expression. *Cell* 93: 445–454.

Niakan WW, Zhang Y-H, Huang B-L, McCabe ERB (2001). Complex glycerol kinase deficiency: defining the deletional breakpoints in the original patient described with this contiguous gene syndrome. *Am J Hum Genet* 69: 2654A.

Nuclear Receptor Nomenclature Committee (1999). A unified nomenclature system for the nuclear receptor superfamily. *Cell* 97: 161–163.

Ozisik G, Achermann JC, Jameson JL (2002). The role of SF1 in adrenal and reproductive function: insight from naturally occurring mutations in humans. *Mol Genet Metab* 76: 85–91.

Pakravan P, Kenny FM, Depp R, Allen AC (1974). Familial congenital absence of the adrenal glands: evaluation of the glucocorticoid, mineralocorticoid and estrogen metabolism in the perinatal period. *J Pediatr* 84: 74–78.

Palmer JS, Burgoyne PS (1991). The *Mus musculus domesticus* Tdy allele acts later than the *Mus musculus* Tdy allele: a basis for XY sex-reversal in C56BL/6-YPOS mice. *Development* 113: 709–714.

Patel M, Dorman KS, Zhang Y-H, Huang B-L, Arnold AP, Sinsheimer JS, Vilain E, McCabe ERB (2001). Primate DAX1, SRY, and SOX9: evolutionary stratification of sex-determination pathway. *Am J Hum Genet* 68: 275–280.

Patil SR, Bartley JA, Murray JC, Ionasescu VV, Pearson PL (1985). X-linked glycerol kinase, adrenal hypoplasia and myopathy map at Xp21. *Cytogenet Cell Genet* 40: 720–721.

Peter M, Viemann M, Partsch C-J, Sippell WG (1998). Congenital adrenal hypoplasia: clinical spectrum, experience with hormonal diagnosis, and report on new point mutations of the DAX-1 gene. *J Clin Endocrinol Metab* 83: 2666–2674.

Phelan JK, McCabe ERB (2001). Mutations in *NR0B1* (DAX1) and *NR5A1* (SF1) responsible for adrenal hypoplasia congenital. *Hum Mutat* 18: 472–487.

Ramayya MS, Zhou J, Kino T, Segars JH, Bondy CA, Chrousos GP (1997). Steroidogenic factor 1 messenger ribonucleic acid expression in steroidogenic and nonsteroidogenic human tissues: Northern blot and in situ hybridization studies. *J Clin Endocrinol Metab* 82: 1799–1806.

Roselli CE, Jorgensen EZ, Doyle MW, Ronnekleiv OK (1997). Expression of the orphan receptor steroidogenic factor-1 mRNA in the rat medial basal hypothalamus. *Brain Res Mol Brain Res* 44: 66–72.

Rutgers JL (1991). Advances in the pathology of intersexed conditions. *Hum Pathol* 22: 884–891.

Sadovsky Y, Crawford PA, Woodson KG, Polish JA, Clements MA, Tourtellotte LM, Simburger K, Millbrandt J (1995). Mice deficient in the orphan receptor steroidogenic factor 1 lack adrenal glands and gonads but express P450 side-chain-cleavage enzyme in the placenta and have normal embryonic serum levels of corticosteroids. *Proc Natl Acad Sci USA* 92: 10939–10943.

Sakura N, Nishimura S, Kawahara N, Komazawa Y, Yamaguchi S (1991). Asthma as the first presenting symptom of complex glycerol kinase deficiency. *Acta Paediatr Scand* 80: 723–725.

Seltzer WK, Firminger H, Klein J, Pike A, Fennessey P, McCabe ERB (1985). Adrenal dysfunction in glycerol kinase deficiency. *Biochem Med* 33: 189–199.

Seminara SB, Achermann JC, Genel M, Jameson JL, Crowley WF Jr. (1999). X-linked adrenal hypoplasia congenita: a mutation in *DAX1* expands the phenotypic spectrum in males and females. *J Clin Endocrinol Metab* 84: 4501–4509.

Seol W, Choi H-S, Moore DD (1996). An orphan nuclear hormone receptor that lacks a DNA binding domain and heterodimerizes with other receptors. *Science* 272: 1336–1339.

Shibata H, Ikeda Y, Mukai T, Morohashi K, Kurihara I, Ando T, Suzuki T, Kobayashi S, Murai M, Saito I, Saruta T (2001). Expression profiles of COUP-TF, DAX-1 and SF-1 in the human adrenal gland and adrnocortical tumors: possible implications in steroidogenesis. *Mol Genet Metab* 74: 206–216.

Shinoda K, Lei H, Yoshii H, Nomura M, Nagano M, Shiba H, Sasaki H, Osawa Y, Ninomiya Y, Niwa O, et al. (1995). Developmental defects of the ventromedial hypothalamus nucleus and pituitary gonadotroph in the Ftz-F1 disrupted mice. *Dev Dyn* 204: 22–29.

Simpson JL, Martin AO (1981). Gonadal dysgenesis: genetic heterogeneity based upon observation, H-Y antigen status, and segregation analysis. *Hum Genet* 58: 91–97.

Sinclair AH, Berta P, Palmer MS, Hawkin JR, Griffiths BL, Smith MJ, Foster JM, Frischauf AM, Lovell-Badge R, Goodfellow PN (1990). A gene from the human sex-determining region encodes a protein with homology to a conserved DNA binding motif. *Nature* 346: 240–244.

Skelton FR (1959). Adrenal regeneration and adrenal regeneration hypertension. *Physiol Rev* 39: 162–182.

Sohval AR (1965). Pure gonadal dysgenesis. *Am J Med* 38: 615–625.

Sperling MA, Wolfsen AR, Fisher DA (1973). Congenital adrenal hypoplasia: an isolated defect of organogenesis. *J Pediatr* 82: 444–449.

Stempfel RS Jr., Engel FL (1960). A congenital, familial syndrome of adrenocortical insufficiency without hypoaldosteronism. *J Pediatr* 57: 443–451.

Sucheston ME, Cannon MS (1968). Development of zonular patterns in the human adrenal gland. *J Morphol* 126: 477–491.

Swain A, Zanaria E, Hacker A, Lovell-Badge R, Camerino G (1996). Mouse Dax1 expression is consistent with a role in sex determination as well as in adrenal and hypothalamus function. *Nat Genet* 12: 404–409.

Swain A, Narvaez V, Burgoyne P, Camerino G, Lovell-Badge R (1998). Dax1 antagonizes Sry action in mammalian sex determination. *Nature* 391: 761–767.

Takahashi T, Shoji Y, Haraguchi N, Takahashi I, Takada G (1997). Active hypothalamic-pituitary-gonadal axis in an infant with X-linked adrenal hypoplasia congenital. *J Pediatr* 130: 485–488.

Takayama K, Sasano H, Fukaya T, Morohashi K, Suzuki T, Tamura M, Costa MJ, Yajima A (1995). Immunohistochemical localization of Ad4-binding protein with correlation to steroidogenic enzyme expression in cycling human ovaries and sex cord stromal tumors. *J Clin Endocrinol Metab* 80: 2815–2821.

Tu Y (2000). How robust is the internet? *Nature* 406: 353–354.

Uttley WS (1968). Familial congenital adrenal hypoplasia. *Arch Dis Child* 43: 724–730.

Vainio S, Heikkila M, Kispert A, Chin N, McMahon AP (1999). Female development in mammals is regulated by Wnt-4 signalling. *Nature* 397: 405–409.

Vilain E (2000). Genetics of sexual development. *Annu Rev Sex Res* 11: 1–25.

Vilain E, McCabe ERB (1998). Mammalian sex determination from gonads to brain. *Mol Genet Metab* 65: 74–84.

Vilain E, Guo W, Zhang Y-H, McCabe ERB (1997). DAX1 gene expression upregulated by steroidogenic factor 1 in an adrenocortical carcinoma cell line. *Biochem Mol Med* 61: 1–8.

Vinson GP, Whitehouse B, Hinson J (1992). *The Adrenal Cortex*. Prentice Hall, Englewood Cliffs, N.J.

Vockley J, Rinaldo P, Bennett MJ, Matern D, Vladutiu GD (2000). Synergistic heterozygosity: disease resulting from multiple partial defects in one or more metabolic pathways. *Mol Genet Metab* 71: 10–18.

Wang ZJ, Jeffs B, Ito M, Achermann JC, Yu RN, Hales DB, Jameson JL (2001). Aromatase (CYP19) expression is up-regulated by targeted disruption of Dax1. *Proc Natl Acad Sci USA* 98: 7988–7993.

Whitfield LS, Lovell-Badge R, Goodfellow PN (1993). Rapid sequence evolution of the mammalian sex-determining gene SRY. *Nature* 364: 713–715.

Wittenberg DF (1981). Familial X-linked adrenocortical hypoplasia association with androgenic precocity. *Arch Dis Child* 56: 633–636.

Wong M, Ramayya MS, Chrousos GP, Driggers PH, Parker KL (1996). Cloning and sequence analysis of the human gene encoding steroidogenic factor 1. *J Mol Endocrinol* 17: 139–147.

Worley KC, Ellison KA, Zhang Y-H, Wang D-F, Mason J, Roth EJ, Adams V, Fogt DD, Zhu X-M, Towbin JA, et al. (1993). Yeast artificial chromosome cloning in the glycerol kinase and adrenal hypoplasia congenita region of Xp21. *Genomics* 16: 407–416.

Yu RN, Ito M, Jameson JL (1998a). The murine Dax-1 promoter is stimulated by SF-1 (steroidogenic factor-1) and inhibited by COUP-TF (chicken ovalbumin upstream promoter-transcription factor) via a composite nuclear receptor-regulatory element. *Mol Endocrinol* 12: 1010–1022.

Yu RN, Ito M, Saunders TL, Camper SA, Jameson JL (1998b). Role of Ahch in gonadal development and gametogenesis. *Nat Genet* 20: 353–357.

Zajicek G, Ariel I, Arber N (1986). The streaming adrenal cortex: direct evidence of centripetal migration of adenocytes by estimation of cell turnover rate. *J Endocrinol* 111: 477–482.

Zanaria E, Muscatelli F, Bardoni B, Strom TM, Guioli S, Guo W, Lalli E, Moser C, Walker AP, McCabe ERB, et al. (1994). A novel and unusual member of the nuclear hormone receptor superfamily is responsible for X-linked adrenal hypoplasia congenita. *Nature* 372: 635–641.

Zazopoulos E, Lalli E, Stocco DM, Sassone-Corsi P (1997). DNA binding and transcriptional repression by DAX-1 blocks steroidogenesis. *Nature* 390: 311–315.

Zhang Y-H, Guo W, Wagner RL, Huang B-L, McCabe L, Vilain E, Burris TP, Anyane-Yeboa K, Burghes AHM, Chitayat D, et al. (1998). DAX1 mutations map to putative structural domains in a deduced three-dimensional model. *Am J Hum Genet* 62: 855–864.

Zhang Y-H, Huang B-L, Anyane-Yeboa K, Carvalho JA, Clemons RD, Cole T, De Figueiredo BC, Lubinsky M, Metzger DL, Quadrelli R, et al. (2001). Nine novel mutations in *NROB1* (DAX1) causing adrenal hypoplasia congenita. *Hum Mutat* 18: 547.

Zhao L, Bakke M, Parker KL (2001). Pituitary-specific knockout of steroidogenic factor 1. *Mol Cell Endocrinol* 185: 27–32.

IV

GENE FAMILIES NOT YET IN PATHWAYS

Part A.
The Homeobox Gene Family

46 | The Role of *Hox* and *Dlx* Gene Clusters in Evolution and Development

FRANK H. RUDDLE

The genetic basis of development was significantly advanced in the early 1980s with the elucidation of the molecular structure of the homeotic genes. These genes constituted a large family characterized by a conserved 183 nt domain termed the "homeobox" (Gehring, 1998). The homeobox encodes a 61 amino acid helix–turn–helix configuration that serves as a DNA-binding domain. The gene products of the homeotic genes serve as transcription factors and have been shown to regulate a variety of developmental processes, particularly in early development but at other stages in the life cycle as well.

In this chapter, I restrict attention to members of the mammalian homeobox gene family that are organized as multigene clusters. These constitute two distinct genetic systems: the *Hox* and the distalless (*Dlx*) cluster systems. The two systems together regulate pattern formation in vertebrates over the entire rostral–caudal body axis; in addition, they contribute significantly to limb pattern formation. I examine the structure and function of these multigene ensembles, as well as their evolutionary origins and contributions to phylogenetic diversity. I also explore the special developmental genetic properties of multigene clusters and their unique role in development and evolution.

STRUCTURE

There are 39 *Hox* genes in man and mouse; these genes are organized into four clusters, each of which contains between 9 and 11 genes. The clusters map to loci on four different chromosomes. There are six

Dlx genes organized into three clusters of two genes each. Interestingly, the *Dlx* bigene clusters are physically linked to the *Hox* clusters over a distance of approximately 1 Mb. The linkage relationships are as follows: *Hoxa* (human chromosome 7p15–p14) to *Dlx5–6*; *Hoxb* (17q21–22) to *Dlx3–7*; and *Hoxd* (2q31–32) to *Dlx1–2*. *Hoxc* (12q13) has not been shown to possess a *Dlx* partner (Fig. 46–1).

The *Hox* and *Dlx* clusters show interesting nucleotide sequence colinear relationships because of their duplication histories. The *Hox* genes between clusters can be aligned by nucleotide and amino acid similarities in the coding regions (Bailey et al., 1997). A total of 13 cognate or paralogous groups can be defined that show an ancestral relation. On this basis, one would expect a total of 52 genes, but gene loss during the duplication process has reduced gene number to the observed 39. Paralogy groups 4,9, and 13 have four members; 2, 7, and 12 have but two; and the rest have three. The *Dlx* genes can be similarly arranged into paralog groups, but this is not reflected in their terminology (Stock et al., 1996). It can be shown, by sequence comparisons, that *Dlx 1, 6,* and *7* constitute one cognate group, and *Dlx 2, 3,* and *5* make up the other. The human and mouse *Hox* gene clusters measure about 120 kb in length, and the *Hox* genes are spaced at approximately 10 kb intervals. The *Dlx* bigene clusters measure between 20 and 30 kb overall, and the genes within a cluster are separated by 10 to 20 kb of noncoding DNA (Sumiyama et al., 2002b).

Two homeotic even-skipped genes, *Evx-1* and *Evx-2*, are closely linked with Hox clusters *Hoxa* and *Hoxd*, respectively. *Evx-1* maps 44

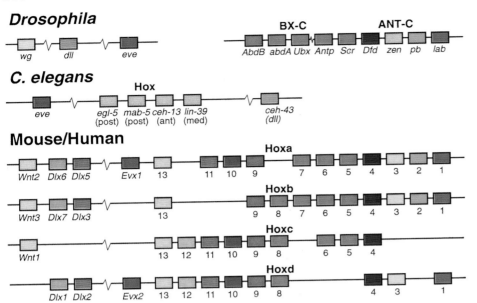

Figure 46–1. *Hox* and *Dlx* clusters showing physical colinearity. Identical colors within species indicate vertical paralogy groups, and different colors indicate laterally arranged paralogous genes, with the exception of *Hox* genes 5 through 8 that take the same blue color, because of their sequence similarity in the homeodomain. Identical colors between genes in different species indicate an orthologous relationship. Other aspects of this figure are discussed in the text.

kb upstream of *Hoxa-13*, and its paralog maps 12 kb upstream of Hoxd-13. The *Evx* genes are divergently transcribed with respect to the *Hox* genes. The intervals separating the *Evx* genes and the *Hox* clusters contain many lines, sines, and other repetitive elements, suggesting a degree of functional isolation between the *Hox* clusters and the *Evx* genes. However, genetic experiments have been reported that indicate a degree of functional interaction between *Evx-2* and *Hoxd-13*. The functional relationship between the *Evx* genes and the *Hox* clusters remains to be defined fully. Numerous additional genes of developmental significance map in the vicinity of the *Hox–Dlx* clusters (Ruddle et al., 1994). Many are members of multigene families whose paralogs map in the vicinity of several clusters. For example, members of the *Wnt* gene family—*Wnt-1, -2,* and *-3*—map in the vicinity of *Hoxc, a,* and *b* respectively.

Recently, in part in conjunction with the various genome-sequencing projects, it has been possible to obtain full nucleotide sequence maps for a number of Hox clusters. Interestingly, the first full sequence was reported for the horn shark (*Heterodontus francisci*) (Kim et al., 2000). The horn shark *Hoxa* sequence was found to be surprisingly similar in a number of respects to that of the human Hoxa sequence, but especially so in terms of gene spacing in spite of the 300 million year difference in the origins of the two species (Fig. 46–2). More recently, comparisons of gene spacing between different mammalian species confirm the conservation of gene spacing within orthologous clusters. This feature is consistent with the emerging view that the clusters are highly integrated in a functional sense and that conservation of noncoding domains is necessary for normal function.

GENERAL PATTERNS OF GENE EXPRESSION

The *Hox* paralogous groups show a fascinating spatial colinear relationship with the developing anterior/posterior (A/P) axis. The 3′ termini of the clusters that contain paralogous group 1 are expressed at or near the midbrain/hindbrain junction. Progressively higher-order

paralog groups are expressed in more posterior regions. The 5′ termini contains paralog group 13 and is expressed in the most posterior region of the axis. Thus, the expression patterns of the *Hox* genes are deployed over the A/P axis in a spatially colinear pattern, corresponding to their physical order in the gene cluster (McGinnis and Krumlauf, 1992). The *Dlx* gene expression domain overlaps that of the *Hox* genes in the pharyngeal and hindbrain regions. They also express in the midbrain and forebrain regions. Thus, together, the *Hox* and *Dlx* systems influence pattern formation over the entire rostrocaudal axis. Moreover, the expression of the *Hox* genes progress in a temporal sense from the 3′ end of the cluster to the 5′ terminus in concert with morphogenetic modifications that take place in an early to late time frame and progress from rostral to caudal positions. This correlation between *Hox* expression and anterior to the posterior developmental process is termed "temporal colinearity."

The *Hox* and *Dlx* genes also control patterning in the developing limb. Proximal and distal identities are controlled by the deployment of *Hox* paralog group 9 proximally and, again progressively, *Hox 10, 11, 12,* and *13* more distally. Interestingly, the *Hoxd* cluster shows major involvement (Spitz et al., 2001). The *Dlx* genes are also expressed in the developing limb buds, but their developmental role is not yet clearly understood. The 5′ genes of the *Hoxd* cluster also have an important role in the patterning of the urogenital system (Duboule, 1995).

Spatial colinearity is a striking feature of the Hox cluster system that has not yet been explained satisfactorily in functional or evolutionary terms. Functionally, one can speculate that the cluster is highly integrated in the sense of a supergene. Support for this notion comes from several sources. We have shown that the clusters are devoid of long interspersed elements (LINES) and short interspersed elements (SINES) that are known to interfere with normal gene expression by interference with endogenous *cis* controls (Kim et al., 2000). Gene spacing within clusters is highly conserved, as described above. Evi-

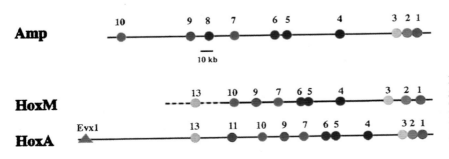

Figure 46–2. Similar gene spacing in *Hox* clusters. Relative gene spacing within *Hox* clusters based on contig mapping (Amp) and complete nucleotide sequencing (HoxM and HoxA). Amp is the amphioxus cluster, HoxM cluster is the horn shark Hox A ortholog, and HoxA is the human HoxA cluster.

dence has been presented supporting enhancer-sharing indicative of integration of gene transcription by *cis* regulatory mechanisms. Experiments have shown that gene reporters taken from one region of a cluster and transplanted to a different site assume the regulatory patterns of expression that are typical of the latter location (Kmita et al., 2000). One might predict that such a system would be adaptive in the sense that mutations occurring at one site would be required to be adaptive to adjacent regions as well, assuring developmental integration along the axis.

Evolutionarily, a gene complex might arise from a single homeotic gene that initially exerted identity control over the entire A/P axis. Lateral gene duplication could then lead subsequently to a two-gene cluster in which the two genes assumed identity control over anterior and posterior domains, respectively. Subsequent lateral gene duplications would continue to subdivide the cluster into domains colinear with the A/P axis. Any gene duplication inconsistent with spatial colinearity would be eliminated as nonadaptive.

EVOLUTION

It is important to consider the evolution for the Hox and Dlx clusters, since an understanding of their evolutionary history contributes to our comprehension of their genetic and developmental roles in extant forms. We can gain insight into the formation of the human clusters by the phylogenetic examination of a broad spectrum of extant species. The homeotic gene clusters were first described in *Drosophila*, and largely for this reason the *Drosophila* cluster has served as a prototype (Lewis, 1992). It consists of nine genes divided into two subclusters (termed the *Antennapedia* and the *Bithorax* clusters), separated by a 1 Mb insert. Eight *Drosophila* genes show a clear orthologous relationship with corresponding human *Hox* cluster genes (paralog groups 1–9), as shown in Figure 46–1. The *Drosophila* and human genes occur in the same serial order, showing a precise physical colinear relationship.

This property is observed in all species examined to date, with the exception of *Caenorhabditis*, in which several of the genes are inverted in comparison with other clusters. The *Drosophila* orthologs of *Wnt*, *Dlx*, and *Evx*—namely, *wg*, *dll*, and *eve*—are not tightly linked to the *Drosophila* cluster mapping elsewhere in the *Drosophila* genome. The subcluster organization of the *Drosophila* cluster is considered a derived trait, since more primitive insects possess a single contiguous cluster. Apart from the minor differences between *Drosophila* and human *Hox* clusters, there is a remarkable overall conservation in the clusters, considering the 1-billion-year time divergence in the evolution of the two species. Functional conservation is also indicated by similar patterns of spatial colinearity in the two species.

The invertebrate species examined to date have a single *Hox* cluster. The evolution of the clusters observed in a variety of invertebrate species is believed to have arisen as a singular event, since all clusters show strong orthologous relationships. Presumably, a one-cluster *Hox* system can adequately support the relatively simple and small body plans of the invertebrates. Expansion of the *Hox* gene system is observed in the deuterostomes. The echinoderms possess a one-cluster system, but we see here for the first time evidence of a 5′ serial extension of genes arising from the group 9 gene (Martinez et al., 1999). This extends the basal 9-gene cluster to a 13-gene cluster, as seen in the human and mouse clusters.

Amphioxus, a cephalochordate, has recently been shown to have a 14-gene cluster. This would suggest that in vertebrates there has been a deletion of paralog group 14 (Shimeld and Holland, 2000). The 5′ extension represents a signal event in the evolution of the vertebrates, since in higher forms these genes have been coopted into the patterning of fins, limbs, and the urogenital system—all unique body plan innovations found only in the vertebrates.

Sequence comparisons among the human and mouse paralogy groups suggest an increase of gene number by lateral gene duplication, by processes similar to unequal crossing over. Three related groups of genes have been defined as arising from a primordial cluster of three genes. One group, consisting of paralog groups 1–3, shows anterior expression. A second, consisting of paralog groups 4–8, shows

mid-body expression. A third, consisting of paralog groups 9–13, shows expression over the posterior axis. One might predict that these units might comprise functional subdomains within the clusters.

The vertebrates are notable in that they are unique among multicellular animals in having several *Hox* clusters. It is generally believed that cluster duplication occurred in the context of whole genome duplications (Ruddle et al., 1999). It is estimated that at least two, possibly three, genome duplication events occurred in the evolution of the basal vertebrates, based largely on the chromosome map positions of gene family paralogs. Many *Hox* gene clusters have been observed in all of the major vertebrate groups, but the precise number of clusters has not been determined unequivocally in all groups. For example, in the jawless fishes we have evidence for three or possibly four *Hox* clusters for the lamprey (*Petromyzon marinus*). In the horn shark there is good evidence for two clusters, and in recent unpublished findings, we have obtained additional evidence for a total of four. In the mammals there is excellent evidence for four *Hox* clusters, but this number is primarily based on only two species—humans and mouse.

The ray-finned fishes represent a totally unexpected situation. Here it has been shown only recently that these species have experienced an additional duplication, giving rise to species such as the zebrafish and the pufferfish with 7 to 8 Hox clusters (Amores et al., 1998; Meyer and Schartl, 1999). It will be of great interest to pinpoint the time of this additional *Hox* cluster duplication in the basal actinopterygian fishes. The *Hox* cluster duplication in the ray-finned fishes is the most recent duplication event known. The duplication is accompanied by an enormous radiation in body forms, represented by an estimated 25,000 species, and it invades all freshwater and saltwater environments. As such, ray-finned fishes provide a singular opportunity to study the evolutionary mechanism and consequence of Hox cluster duplication.

The process of *Hox* cluster duplication is becoming clearer as more species are studied with respect to *Hox* cluster number, especially by using full-sequence analysis. The phylogenetic relationship between the four *Hox* clusters in humans and mouse has become somewhat clear through sequence comparisons between the clusters (Bailey et al., 1997). To date this has been restricted to the homeobox sequences or the sequences of closely linked paralogs such as the collagen genes. There is general agreement that the duplication events leading to the higher vertebrates occurred as distinct events that were separated by a significantly long period of time. We have taken the position that the *Hoxa* and *Hoxd* clusters group together and are more primitive. This is consistent with gene spacing similarity between the *Hoxa* cluster seen in amphioxus, horn shark, and humans. It is also consistent with respect to the linkage relationships between the *Hox* and *Dlx* clusters. The phylogenetically more primitive *Dlx* clusters are *Dlx1–2* and *Dlx5–6* are linked to the *Hoxd* and *Hoxa* clusters, respectively. The most recent *Dlx* cluster is *Dlx3–7*, which maps with the *Hoxb* cluster. The *Hoxb* and *Hoxc* clusters are believed to be more recent, and these clusters show a significantly greater number of linked paralogs such than wnt than would be expected. While a good case can be made for a *Hoxa* : *Hoxd* :: *Hoxb* : *Hoxc* topology, it must be recognized that other topologies have been put forward and the topology issue is not as yet definitively resolved.

It is becoming clear that *Hox* cluster duplication is biologically important beyond the simple increase in cluster number. If one compares the sequence of the Hoxa cluster between the horn shark and humans, one observes a high degree of sequence similarity in both coding and noncoding regions, in spite of the 300 million years difference in the origins of the two species. However, if one extends the comparison to the duplicated *Hoxaa* and *Hoxab* clusters in the zebrafish (*Danio rerio*), then one sees a dramatic modification in cluster architecture and patterns of sequence similarity. The duplicated zebrafish clusters are significantly shorter, and many of the noncoding motifs that are conserved between horn shark and humans are absent. Moreover, while some coding elements are present in both daughter clusters, others are retained in only one cluster, whereas several are lost altogether. Thus it appears that Hox cluster duplication can be associated with dramatic alterations in cluster organization and, presumably, in cluster function.

The reduction in cluster size associated with duplication is interesting with respect to observed differences in *Hox* cluster size in the deuterosomes. The sea urchin has an overall size of about 400 kb, amphioxus 200 kb, horn shark–man–mouse 120 kb, and zebrafish 40 to 80 kb. One might speculate that each reduction in size was associated with a gene duplication event. This would imply duplication and cluster loss in the transition from the echinoderms to the protochordates. These early events, taking place presumably in the Cambrian period some 500 million years ago, may only be susceptible to speculation. However, the more recent duplication in the ray-finned fishes offers an opportunity to study a duplication event at first hand in both structural and functional terms.

Ohno (1970) introduced an important concept regarding the way genetic diversity might arise and mediate the evolutionary process. He postulated that gene duplication followed by gene diversification could be a significant source of genetic and concomitant phenotypic diversity. This concept is particularly relevant to the duplication of the *Hox* and *Dlx* clusters that play major developmental and evolutionary roles in patterning the rostral–caudal and appendicular axes. Ohno conceived two basic possibilities. In the first, the gene of interest would duplicate, and both daughter derivatives would diverge. In the second, following duplication, one daughter would maintain the configuration of the parent, while the other would undergo divergence. The latter scenario can be termed the semiconservative duplication model.

A priori, the semiconservative model would seem appropriate to *Hox* cluster duplication if we assume that the cluster is a highly complex genetic entity and that normal developmental patterning depends on this cluster. Thus, according to this view, in the transition from a single cluster to multiclusters, one cluster would be mainly conserved, whereas the others would diverge, thus supporting newly acquired features. We have speculated that the *Hoxa* cluster may represent such a conserved cluster (Kim et al., 2000). This speculation is based on the following considerations. First, the Hoxa cluster resembles the amphioxus cluster to a greater degree than the other clusters because of the retention of genes and their spacing. Second, sequence comparisons among the clusters, together with outgroup comparisons, suggest that the Hoxa cluster—together with the *Hoxd* cluster—is primitive. Admittedly, these considerations are shallow and certainly not definitive. It is hoped that greater understanding will come as we analyze the *Hox* cluster sequences of additional species and better understand their individual functional attributes.

DEVELOPMENTAL EXPRESSION AND FUNCTION

The expression of the *Hox* genes can be divided into two temporally distinct modes: activation and maintenance. Activation occurs in the mouse around 7.0 to 7.5 dpc. The genes are expressed initially in the tail bud and the adjoining allantois. Gene expression then extends anteriorly in a staggered array, with the more 3′ genes establishing anterior boundaries in more rostral positions and the more 5′ genes forming anterior boundaries in more posterior positions in serial correspondence with the physical order of the genes in the cluster. Once the anterior positions of gene expression are set, gene expression drops first in posterior positions, and loss of expression extends anteriorly to establish a distinct posterior boundary of expression for each gene. Thus, the rostro/caudal axis is divided into a number of distinct zones of expression extending from the midbrain/hindbrain junction to the tail bud.

Hox gene expression on the A/P axis is different in the mesodermal and ectodermal anlagen. The anterior limit of expression for a particular *Hox* gene is uniformly offset posteriorly by about six somites in the mesoderm anlage in relation to the ectodermal anlage. Thus, the zones of mesodermal and ectodermal expression for individual *Hox* genes do not overlap to any appreciable extent along the rostro/caudal axis. The offset between expression in mesodermal and ectodermal anlagen may be adaptive since it precludes the simultaneous effect of *Hox* gene mutation on mesodermal and ectodermal derivatives within the same zone.

Activation represents a mensuration activity in which the ante-rior/posterior axis is divided into a number of anatomically specific zones. Mutations in *Hox* genes specifically affect the body plan anatomy in zones where they are expressed, as discussed below. Activation is complete by 9.5 to 10 dpc. The zonal patterns are then maintained throughout morphogenesis. There is growing evidence that the transcriptional regulation of the *Hox* genes during activation and maintenance is governed by different mechanisms, and there is growing evidence that the *Polycomb* and *Trithorax* group genes play a critical part in maintaining *Hox* gene expression, although the mechanism of expression maintenance has not yet been elucidated (Hanson et al., 1999).

Moreover, expression of the *Hox* genes is not limited to the embryonic phase of development. For example, *Hoxb-8* has been shown to express in the adult brain (Greer and Capecchi, 2002), and numerous *Hox* genes have essential roles in differentiating the formed elements of the blood (Takeshita et al., 1993). The *Dlx7* gene has been shown to regulate hemoglobin expression in the differentiation of red cells (Chase et al., 2002). The role of *Hox* genes in the adult is probably underappreciated, since adult tissues have not yet been systematically surveyed for *Hox* gene expression.

Hox gene mutations affect the body plan in the zone of *Hox* gene expression. For example, the zone of expression of *Hoxc-8* in the mouse in the mesodermal anlage ranges from an anterior position in somite 15 to a posterior position in somite 23. This interval spans the posterior portion of the thorax (thoracic vertebrae 4–13) and the anterior domain of the lumbar region (lumbar vertebrae 1–2). A *Hoxc-8* loss-of-function mutation produced by gene targeting in embryonic stem cells results in homeotic transformation (anteriorization) of the first lumbar vertebra into a thoracic vertebra bearing a rib. Not all mutations produce a homeotic phenotype. *Hoxc-8* loss-of-function mutation results in a nonhomeotic phenotypic defect in limb development and is characterized by a congenital prehension defect of the forepaws (clenched fist), resulting from a faulty nerve/muscle interconnection. Gain-of-function mutations have also been produced and show a variety of developmental abnormalities. However, these mutations are more difficult to interpret mechanistically, since the developmental basis of their action is frequently obscure.

Loss-of-function *Hox* mutations have been shown in a number of instances to produce only a mild effect or, in some instances, no observable effect on phenotype. This has been shown to be due to redundancy effects mediated by paralogous isoforms that substitute for the absent gene. Redundancy effects have been well demonstrated for the paralogous genes *Hoxa-3*, *Hoxb-3*, and *Hoxd-3* (Greer et al., 2000). It has been shown for murine *Hox3* that the progressive addition of loss-of-function mutations within its paralog group correlates with progressive severity of phenotype. For example, animals homozygously deficient for *Hoxd-3* have a mild defect in the structure of the first vertebra (atlas), while the addition of deficiency mutations in the paralogous genes *Hoxa-3* and *Hoxb-3* progressively increases the malformation of the atlas.

It is of particular interest that the coding regions of the *Hox3* paralogs are similar, sharing approximately 50% identity in their protein-coding sequences (Greer et al., 2000). It has been shown in gene-swapping experiments that an exchange of coding sequence between clusters results in normal expression and development. Using stem cell gene-targeting methodologies, the coding region of the *Hoxa-3* gene was placed into the *Hoxd-3* locus, maintaining proper relationships between donor coding and recipient noncoding domains. Similarly, the *Hoxd-3* gene was inserted into the *Hoxa-3* position. The experiment is revealing, since it demonstrates that the coding regions are sufficiently similar that they can substitute for one another functionally. Importantly, the experiment also shows that the control domains among the *Hox3* paralogs have diverged and perform different patterns of the regulation that is essential for normal development. These results underscore the growing realization that both temporal and spatial regulation of expression are critical for pattern formation. These findings also support the notion that modification of noncoding control sequences may represent a significant mechanism for the generation of evolutionary diversity.

Considerable progress has been made in understanding *Hox* gene transcriptional regulation in *Drosophila*. Progress has been slower in the mouse, but useful information has been obtained in a few systems, notably for *Hoxc-8*. To discover enhancer elements, the upstream ~10 kb was inserted upstream of LacZ driven by a minimal promoter to produce a reporter construct that could be introduced into mice transgenically (Shashikant and Ruddle, 1996). Embryos were examined for expression at 10.5 days in mesodermal and ectodermal locations that had been predicted by previously established *Hoxc-8* endogenous expression studies. Appropriate expression patterns were found to be mediated by a small, 200 nt, element that mapped 3 kb of the *Hoxc-8* promoter. This element is presently termed the early enhancer (EE), since it regulates early expression associated with gene activation. Gel retardation experiments showed that at least five protein binding sites of 8 to 10 nt length mapped into this site. These motifs were designated from 3′ to 5′ as A through E. A and D are presumed caudal binding sites, based on motif sequence and binding studies. The B, C, and E sites may respond to forkhead, hox, and high-mobility-type proteins based on motif sequence signatures, respectively. The motifs were shown to have enhancer properties by mutational analysis in the context of transgene experiments. Moreover, the upstream noncoding region of *Hoxc-8* has been examined by sequence comparisons between humans and mouse. These studies showed an average sequence similarity of approximately 65%. In the enhancer region, however, sequence conservation averages 90%, and the protein sites show absolute identity. Mutational analysis involving combinations of mutations and their effects on reporter expression indicate that the binding sites are interactive combinatorially in the sense of an enhanceosome. The current experimental results suggest that the early enhancer is highly integrated in structure and function. This view is consistent with the high degree of sequence conservation for the EE demonstrated among the principal orders of mammals and extending to the representatives of birds and bony fish with some reduction in sequence similarity, especially in the fishes.

We have recently carried out mutational analysis of the endogenous *Hoxc-8* early enhancer. In the first experiment, the 200 nt EE was deleted by homologous recombination in primary stem cells. Derived mice, homozygous for the deletion, show a series of skeletal modifications that involve the cervical, thoracic, and lumbar regions, a number of which are homeotic in character. Unexpectedly, the EE deletion does not eliminate *Hoxc-8* expression. It delays the onset of expression and results in weak expression in early embryos. Mutant animals show normal expression of *Hoxc-8* from day 11 on. The result is in agreement with our designation of EE as governing early expression and the activation of Hoxc-8 expression. The data also implicate additional noncoding motifs as necessary for *Hoxc-8* expression, especially in the context of late expression and maintenance. Subsequent experiments will focus on the modification of the EE. We previously replaced the mouse EE with the chick EE in reporter-transgene experiments. The expression of *Hoxc-8* was posteriorized in a manner consistent with *Hoxc-8* rostro–caudal expression in the chick (Belting et al., 1998). This experiment shows that avian EE can respond to murine signals, but, interestingly, the EE influences *Hoxc-8* expression consistent with avian expression. It will be of interest to replace the endogenous mouse EE with that of the chick to determine if the body plan might be modified in the direction of the chick.

Distalless (*Dlx*) transcriptional control is beginning to yield to analysis. As described above, there are six *Dlx* genes arranged as three bigene clusters. The genes in each cluster are transcribed convergently so that they have a common 3′ domain. The *Dlx3–7* gene is of interest because phylogenetically it is more diverged than the other two and controls the development of more recently acquired vertebrate features such as placentation and the regulation of hemoglobin expression in erythrocyte differentiation (Sumiyama et al., 2002). *Dlx 3–7* is expressed in early development in the limb bud and in the first and second visceral arches, but unlike the other two *Dlx* bigene clusters, *Dlx 3–7* is not expressed in the central nervous system.

Recently, we compared the intermediate noncoding 3′ sequence shared by *Dlx3* and *Dlx7* in humans and mouse. Five putative control elements of high-sequence similarity were located (Sumiyama et al., 2002). Sequence similarity ranged from 86% to 90% in elements of 183 to 358 nt. The entire bigene cluster was isolated, and a LacZ reporter was inserted in frame by homologous recombination into the first exon of *Dlx3*. This construct, measuring ~80 kb, essentially reconstituted the endogenous pattern of Dlx3 when inserted in transgenic mice. Ablation and isolation of the putative control elements in a series of transgenic experiments verified their capacity to regulate *Dlx3* expression in limb bud and visceral arches. Evidence was also adduced to support the view that these control elements may simultaneously regulate both the *Dlx7* and *Dlx3* genes, a property previously termed "enhancer sharing." Enhancer sharing was first reported for the *Hox* clusters and may be a common property of gene clusters, contributing to coordination of gene expression within the cluster.

Sequence comparisons combined with transgenic functional analysis of gene expression is beginning to yield information on regulatory links between the *Dlx* bigene clusters. Previously, it was established that the Dlx2 protein could bind specifically with an element in the intermediate domain of the *Dlx5–6* cluster. *Dlx2* is expressed before *Dlx5–6* expression, and it was shown that *Dlx5–6* activation depends on *Dlx2* expression. Our recent studies on *Dlx3–7* have revealed a motif that is highly similar to the *Dlx5–6* sequence response to Dlx2. This element is located within one of the *Dlx3–7* enhancer elements. Thus, we can postulate the coordinate activation of both the *Dlx5–6* and *Dlx3–7* clusters by the early expression of *Dlx2*. These findings represent one of the first clear-cut examples of regulation between paralogous clusters located on different chromosomes.

CONCLUSION AND SPECULATION

The *Hox* and *Dlx* systems are remarkable in that they accomplish two seemingly opposite processes: stable developmental control and evolutionary plasticity. I take the view that these systems in their intrinsic design are, in fact, adapted to these capabilities. As indicated in this chapter, the clusters are both highly integrated in terms of *cis* control elements and highly redundant. Small nucleotide substitutions in *cis* control elements can make substantive modifications in the developmental plan, but these alterations are generally subtle and buffered by semiredundant clusters. Thus, genetic modifications in the developmental process can be readily introduced that carry a negligible genetic load and can spread through a population rapidly as neutral or slightly adaptive traits. Under the appropriate environmental conditions this can lead to the accumulation, interaction, and accommodation of successive mini-mutations that, together, modify the body plan in adaptive directions. According to this scenario, adaptive body plan modifications could occur rapidly over a relatively short time span. This epigenetic system is itself adaptive and is optimized by selection. Elsewhere, I have referred to the *Hox/Dlx* system as an "evo/devo (evolution and development) machine."

The current prevalent view is that the *Hox/Dlx* systems are highly conserved and that there is little genetic variation. Indeed, there are a number of instances of extremely highly conserved elements that show little change over hundreds of million years. These conserved elements impress us, and surely must be functionally significant, but I submit they are not representative of the overall system.

I predict on the basis of what I have said in this chapter that if we look carefully, we will find sequence variants in the *Hox* and *Dlx* clusters that represent recent adaptations to the body plan, as well as variants very much like polymorphisms that are neutral in character, but may well be adaptive under certain future environmental circumstances. It will be of interest to search for such characters among various representatives of the mammals—primates, inbred lines of mice, and racial and ethnic groups of humans—then within such populations. It will be important to relate these variants to corresponding body plan features and possible risk of developmental aberration. Particular variants may carry development risk under certain environmental conditions such as exposure to pollutants, diet, and medication.

Possibly one can look forward to a new branch of pediatrics that focuses on such problems and which surveys the evo/devo machine for risk factors and offers means for either avoidance or prevention (or both)—a new field, that we might term *epigenetic medicine*.

ACKNOWLEDGMENTS

This work is supported by the National Institutes of Health (GM09966 and NS 43525), National Science Foundation (IBN-9905403), and Department of Energy (DOE-DE-FG02-01ER63274). I thank Drs. Chris Amemiya, Aster Juan, Kenta Sumiyama, and Gunter Wagner for their critical reading of the manuscript and helpful discussions. It gives me great pleasure to dedicate this article to Ms. Alexis (Lexi) Henley Shohet on the occasion of her first birthday—1 September 2002.

REFERENCES

Amores A, Force A, Yan Y-L, Joly L, Amemiya CT, Fritz A, Ho R, Langeland J, Prince V, Wang Y-L, et al. (1998). Zebrafish Hox clusters and vertebrate genome evolution. *Science* 282: 1711–1714.

Bailey WJ, Kim J, Wagner GP, Ruddle FH (1997). Phylogenetic reconstruction of vertebrate Hox cluster duplications. *Mol Biol Evol* 14: 843–853.

Belting HG, Shashikant CS, Ruddle FH (1998). Modification of expression and *cis*-regulation of *Hoxc8* in the evolution of diverged axial morphology. *Proc Natl Acad Sci USA* 95: 2355–2360.

Chase M, Fu S, Haga S, Davenport G, Stevenson H, Do K, Morgan D, Mah A, Berg P (2002). BP1, a homeodomain-containing isoform of Dlx4, represses the β-globin gene. *Mol Cell Biol* 22: 2505–2514.

Duboule D (1995). Vertebrate *Hox* genes and proliferation: an alternative pathway to homeosis? *Curr Opin Genet Dev* 5: 525–528.

Gehring WJ (1998). *Master Control Genes in Development and Evolution.* Yale University Press, New Haven.

Greer JM, Capecchi MR (2002). *Hoxb8* is required for normal grooming behavior in mice. *Neuron* 33: 23–34.

Greer JM, Puetz J, Thomas KR, Capecchi MR (2000). Maintenance of functional equivalence during paralogous *Hox* gene evolution. *Nature* 403: 661–664.

Hanson RD, Hess JL, Yu BD, Ernst P, Lohuizen MV, Berns A, Lugt NMTvd (1999). Mammalian *Trithorax* and *Polycomb*-group homologues are antagonistic regulators of homeotic development. *Proc Natl Acad Sci USA* 96: 14372–14377.

Kim CB, Amemiya CT, Bailey W, Kawasaki K, Mezey J, Miller W, Minoshima S, Shimiza N, Wagner G, Ruddle FH (2000). Hox cluster genomics in the horn shark, *Heterodontus francisci. Proc Natl Acad Sci USA* 97: 1655–1660.

Kmita M, van der Hoeven F, Zakany J, Krumlauf R, Duboule D (2000). Mechanisms of *Hox* gene colinearity: transposition of the anterior *Hoxb1* gene into the posterior HoxD complex. *Genes Dev* 14: 198–211.

Lewis EB (1992). Clusters of master control genes regulate the development of higher organisms. *JAMA* 267: 287–289.

Martinez P, Rast JP, Arenas-Mena C, Davidson EH (1999). Organization of an echinoderm *Hox* gene cluster. *Proc Natl Acad Sci USA* 96: 1469–1474.

McGinnis W, Krumlauf R (1992). Homeobox genes and axial patterning. *Cell* 68: 283–302.

Meyer A, Schartl M (1999). Gene and genome duplications in vertebrates: the one-to-four (-to-eight in fish) rule and the evolution of novel gene functions. *Curr Opin Cell Biol* 11: 699–704.

Ohno S (1970). *Evolution by Gene Duplication.* Springer Verlag, New York.

Ruddle FH, Bentley KL, Murtha MT, Risch N (1994). Gene loss and gain in the evolution of the vertebrates. *Dev Suppl* 155–161.

Ruddle FH, Amemiya CT, Carr JL, Kim CB, Ledje C, Shashikant CS, Wagner G (1999). Evolution of chordate Hox gene clusters. *Ann NY Acad Sci* 870: 238–248.

Shashikant CS, Ruddle FH (1996). Combinations of closely situated *cis*-acting elements determine tissue-specific patterns and anterior extent of early *Hoxc8* expression. *Proc Natl Acad Sci USA* 93: 12364–12369.

Shimeld SM, Holland PWH (2000). Vertebrate innovations. *Proc Natl Acad Sci USA* 97: 4449–4452.

Spitz F, Gonzalez F, Peichel C, Vogt T, Duboule D, Zakany J (2001). Large scale transgenic and cluster deletion analysis of the HoxD complex separate an ancestral regulatory module from evolutionary innovations. *Genes Dev* 15: 2209–2214.

Stock DW, Ellies DL, Zhao Z, Ekker M, Ruddle FH, Weiss KM (1996). The evolution of the vertebrate Dlx gene family. *Proc Natl Acad Sci USA* 93: 10858–10863.

Sumiyama K, Irvine S, Stock D, Weiss K, Kawasaki K, Shimizu N, Shashikant CS, Miller W, Ruddle FH (2002). Genomic structure and functional control of the Dlx 3–7 bigene cluster. *Proc Natl Acad Sci USA* 99: 780–785.

Takeshita K, Bollekens JA, Hijiya N, Ratajczak M, Ruddle FH (1993). A homeobox gene of the Antennapedia class is required for human adult erythropoiesis. *Proc Natl Acad Sci USA* 90: 3535–3538.

47 | *HOXD13* and Synpolydactyly

FRANCES R. GOODMAN AND PETER J. SCAMBLER

HOXD13, the most 5′ member of the *HOXD* gene cluster, encodes a highly conserved transcription factor which plays a crucial role in the development of the autopod; but the molecular pathway in which it acts is poorly understood. Little is known about how its expression is regulated, and none of its target genes or transcriptional cofactors has yet been identified. Synpolydactyly (SPD), the first human birth defect found to be caused by mutations in a *HOX* gene, is a rare, dominantly inherited malformation of the hands and feet, characterized by soft tissue syndactyly between the third and fourth fingers and between the fourth and fifth toes, with variable digit duplication in the syndactylous web. Most cases result from different-sized expansions of a polyalanine tract in HOXD13's N-terminal region, and both penetrance and phenotypic severity have been shown to correlate positively with expansion size. The mutant protein appears to interfere functionally with both the remaining wild-type HOXD13 and other 5′ HOXD proteins expressed in the developing autopod, acting as a "super" dominant-negative. A milder atypical form of SPD, characterized by a distinctive foot phenotype, results from a variety of other *HOXD13* mutations, all of which are likely to cause functional haploinsufficiency. In addition, two unusual forms of brachydactyly distinct from SPD but exhibiting overlap with brachydactyly types D and E, result from specific missense mutations in the HOXD13 homeodomain, which alter rather than abolish DNA binding. The abnormalities in these conditions appear to reflect disturbances of patterning and growth both at the early stage of autopod development in undifferentiated mesenchyme and at a later stage in the chondrogenic cells of cartilaginous bone models. These observations suggest that HOXD13's downstream targets are likely to include genes with important roles in cell sorting/boundary formation and cell cycle control.

DEVELOPMENTAL PATHWAY

Hox genes encode a highly conserved family of transcription factors which play fundamental roles in morphogenesis during embryonic development (McGinnis and Krumlauf, 1992; Krumlauf, 1994; Mark et al., 1997). Most vertebrates (including humans) have 39 *Hox* genes grouped into four clusters, named *HoxA*, *HoxB*, *HoxC*, and *HoxD*, each located on a different chromosome and containing 9–11 genes (see Chapter 46). In general, the order in which these genes are arranged within each cluster corresponds to their temporal and spatial expression patterns during development, a phenomenon known as *temporal and spatial colinearity*. Thus, genes at the 3′ end of each cluster are expressed early, in anterior and proximal regions, whereas genes at the 5′ end of each cluster are expressed later, in more posterior and distal regions (Krumlauf, 1994). While all *Hox* genes help pattern the vertebrate embryo along the primary body axis (head-to-tail), the most 5′ members of the *HoxA* and *HoxD* clusters also play an important part in patterning the secondary body axes (limbs and external genitalia).

Hoxd13 in Development

Hoxd13, the most 5′ member of the *HoxD* cluster, is expressed in three distinct regions during vertebrate development: the trunk, the limb buds, and the genital tubercle (Dollé et al., 1991a,b). Along the trunk, its expression is restricted to the most posterior neural tube and somites (future tail region) and the most distal gut and urogenital tract (future rectum, lower ureters and bladder, lower vas deferens and accessory sex glands in males, and lower uterus and vagina in females) (Dollé et al., 1991b; Kondo et al., 1996; Podlasek et al., 1997). In the limb

buds, its expression is also posteriorly and distally restricted but occurs in two distinct phases (Nelson et al., 1996). During the first phase, which corresponds to the specification of the zeugopod (lower arm/leg), the five most 5′ *Hoxd* genes (*Hoxd9–Hoxd13*) are expressed as a concentric nested set centered around the posterior/distal margin of the limb. *Hoxd13* is the last member of the cluster to be expressed and has the smallest expression domain. During the second phase, which corresponds to the specification of the autopod (hand/foot), the four most 5′ *Hoxd* genes (*Hoxd10–Hoxd13*) are expressed in similar domains across the distal end of the limb. *Hoxa13*, the only *Hoxa* gene expressed in the autopod, also occupies a similar domain. Interestingly, studies in chick have shown that *Hoxd13* is the first member of its cluster to be activated in this second phase and that its expression domain is slightly larger than those of the other 5′ *Hoxd* genes, extending right up to the anterior margin of the limb (Nelson et al., 1996). This unusual reversal of the principles of temporal and spatial colinearity points to a dominant role for *Hoxd13* in autopod development.

Although *Hox* genes help specify segment identity along the primary body axis, their role in patterning the developing limbs is rather different (Mark et al., 1997). Contrary to previous expectations, they do not appear to specify upper, as opposed to lower, limb identity or the identities of the different digits. Targeted mutagenesis and overexpression of individual and multiple 5′ *Hoxd* and *Hoxa* genes, including *Hoxd13*, in mouse and chick, result not in homeotic transformations of the limbs but in alterations in the size, shape, and number of particular bones associated with delays in chondrification and ossification (Dollé et al., 1993; Favier and Dollé, 1997). These findings indicate that the 5′ *Hoxd* and *Hoxa* genes help determine region-specific growth and differentiation in the skeletal elements of the limb. Different *Hox* genes expressed in the same region appear to have both unique and overlapping roles. Thus, homozygous *Hoxd13* and *Hoxa13* knockout mice exhibit quite distinct autopod defects, indicating that the two genes are not functionally equivalent; but *Hoxd13*/*Hoxa13* double mutants have more severe defects than single mutants, revealing that the two genes can also partially compensate for each other (Fromental-Ramain et al., 1996). In mutants lacking both copies of both genes, the limbs are truncated at the level of the distal zeugopod, showing that autopod growth and patterning is dependent on *Hox13* gene function.

Regulation and Targets

The 5′ *Hoxd* and *Hoxa* genes are downstream effectors of signals from the two organizing regions, the zone of polarizing activity (ZPA) and the apical ectodermal ridge (AER), which together pattern the anteroposterior and proximodistal axes of the limb bud (Johnson and Tabin, 1997; Tickle, 2000). In the 5′ *Hoxd* genes, the early phase of posteriorly nested expression in the zeugopod described above appears to be activated in direct response to *Sonic hedgehog* (*Shh*) signaling (see Chapter 16) from the ZPA. Signaling from the AER is also required for initiation of this phase, although not for its maintenance (Laufer et al., 1994; Nelson et al., 1996). The late phase of distal expression in the autopod is likely regulated by downstream mediators of *Shh* signaling, especially bone morphogenetic protein-2 (*Bmp-2*; see Chapter 24) in the mesoderm and fibroblast growth factor 4 (*Fgf-4*; see Chapter 32) from the AER (Duprez et al., 1996). *Shh* signaling also appears to regulate 5′ *Hoxd* gene expression in the developing gut and genital tubercle (Roberts et al., 1998; Haraguchi et al., 2001).

As suggested by the phenomenon of temporal and spatial colinearity mentioned above, the expression of each *Hox* cluster as a whole is likely to be coordinated by complex regulatory mechanisms (van der Hoeven et al., 1996). The initial activation of the entire mouse *HoxD* cluster, for instance, appears to be subject to repression by a regulatory element upstream of the cluster, which is later sequentially relieved in a 3′ to 5′ direction (Kondo and Duboule, 1999). Within the cluster, expression of multiple neighboring genes is probably regulated by global enhancer sequences, such as the "digit enhancer" thought to control expression of the four most 5′ *Hoxd* genes and the adjacent *Evx2* gene in the autopod and genital tubercle (Hérault et al., 1999). Individual 5′ *Hoxd* genes are also subject to cross-regulatory and autoregulatory controls (Zappavigna et al., 1991). Nevertheless, no transcription factor that directly regulates the expression of any of the 5′ *Hoxd* genes, including *Hoxd13*, has yet been identified. One possible candidate is the POZ/zinc-finger transcription factor Plzf (Barna et al., 2000).

Although Hox proteins have long been recognized to act as transcriptional activators and repressors, very few of their target genes are currently known. In particular, no direct target of Hoxd13 has yet been identified. These targets are nevertheless likely to be genes of fundamental interest since they are expected to encode proteins with roles in basic cellular processes, such as proliferation, differentiation, migration, and survival (Graba et al., 1997).

Most, if not all, Hox proteins are now thought to interact with specific DNA-binding partners, forming multimeric protein complexes that direct transcription of their targets (Mann and Affolter, 1998). Known partners of the 3′ Hox proteins include members of the Pbx and Meis/Prep1 families of homeodomain proteins. There is little evidence that these proteins can bind DNA cooperatively with the 5′ Hox proteins even in vitro, however (Shen et al., 1997a,b); and in vivo their nuclear expression is sharply restricted to the proximal portion of the limb bud, indicating that they cannot interact with the 5′ Hoxd and Hoxa13 proteins during autopod development (Mercader et al., 1999; Capdevila et al., 1999). Thus, the DNA-binding partners and transcriptional cofactors of Hoxd13 also remain to be identified.

PHENOTYPE

SPD is a rare, dominantly inherited distal limb malformation, characterized, as its name indicates, by a combination of syndactyly (joined digits) and polydactyly (extra digits). It was first described over a century ago as an incidental finding in one of the earliest reported patients with Fabry disease (Anderson, 1898), and that description is still a good one:

> Both hands are contracted at the middle and distal joints, and the middle and distal phalanges of the fourth finger on each hand are duplicated, the two digits being enclosed in one cutaneous investment. His mother and sister, and three out of four of his children, have congenital deformities like his own.

Typical SPD

These digital abnormalities typically occur in a highly specific distribution, which differs in the hands and feet (Fig. 47–1). Thus, there is soft tissue syndactyly between the third and fourth fingers and between the fourth and fifth toes, with a supernumerary digit in the syndactylous web. Incomplete penetrance and variable expression are common, however; and involvement is often strikingly asymmetrical (Thomsen, 1927; Cross et al., 1967; Merlob and Grunebaum, 1986; Sayli et al., 1995). From one to all four limbs can be affected, and severity ranges from just partial or complete soft tissue syndactyly, without an extra digit (Fig. 47–1*A,E*), through duplication of just the distal or the distal and middle phalanges (Fig. 47–1*C*) to duplication of all three phalanges, with a bifid or extra central metacarpal/metatarsal (Fig. 47–1*B,D,F*). In the hands, contractures at the interphalangeal joints often cause the webbed fingers to be held in fixed flexion. As syndactyly can occur without polydactyly but polydactyly does not occur without syndactyly, SPD has been classified as one of the syndactylies (syndactyly type II) (Temtamy and McKusick, 1978).

In addition, there is often clinodactyly, camptodactyly, and/or brachydactyly of the fifth fingers, due to hypoplasia of the fifth middle phalanges (Fig. 47–1*B–D*), and brachydactyly of the second to fifth toes,

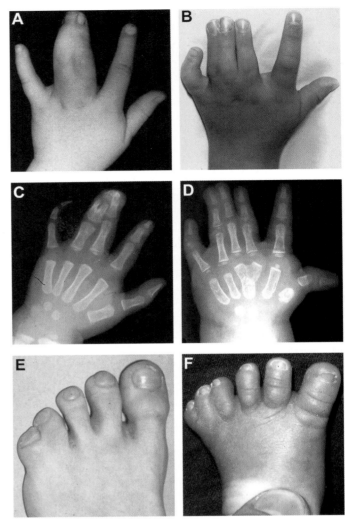

Figure 47–1. Typical synpolydactyly phenotype caused by polyalanine tract expansions in HOXD13. (*A*) Syndactyly between the third and fourth fingers in a girl heterozygous for a seven-residue expansion. (*B*) Syndactyly between the third and fourth fingers, a complete extra digit in the syndactylous web, and clinodactyly of the fifth finger in a boy heterozygous for a 14-residue expansion. (*C*) Duplicated fourth distal and middle phalanges, broad fourth proximal phalanx, and hypoplastic fifth middle phalanx in a boy heterozygous for a seven-residue expansion. (*D*) Duplicated third distal, middle, and proximal phalanges; Y-shaped third metacarpal; hypoplastic fifth middle phalanx; and radially deviated thumb with short first metacarpal in a boy heterozygous for a 14-residue expansion. (*E*) Syndactyly between the fourth and fifth toes in a boy heterozygous for a seven-residue expansion. (*F*) Syndactyly between the fourth and fifth toes, with an extra toe in the syndactylous web, in a boy heterozygous for a nine-residue expansion.

due to hypoplasia or absence of the second to fifth middle phalanges (Camera et al., 1995). Other minor foot abnormalities, such as syndactyly between the second and third toes or an overriding fourth or fifth toe, may also occur and may even be the only clinical manifestation in very mildly affected individuals (Goodman et al., 1997). Although abnormalities do not usually extend as far anteriorly as the first digits or as far proximally as the carpals/tarsals, individuals from one severely affected family demonstrated broad radially deviated, proximally placed thumbs with short first metacarpals (Fig. 47–1*B,D*), broad halluces, and enlarged capitate bones (third distal carpals) (Goodman et al., 1997).

Atypical SPD

An atypical form of SPD, characterized by a novel foot phenotype, has recently been identified in five unrelated families (Goodman et al., 1998; Calabrese et al., 2000; Debeer et al., 2002; Kan et al., 2003). Although the external appearance of the feet is often unremarkable, on radiological examination all affected individuals in these families share a distinctive set of bilateral, symmetrical abnormalities (Fig. 47–2A). First, there are small spurs of bone in the first web spaces, representing partial duplication of the bases of the second metatarsals and sometimes also similar spurs in the fourth web spaces, representing partial duplication of the fourth metatarsals. Second, the bones of the first digital ray (the distal and proximal phalanges of the hallux and the first metatarsal) are unusually broad. Third, there is hypoplasia of the middle phalanges and/or symphalangism of the middle and distal phalanges in the second to fifth toes. Typical SPD of the third/fourth fingers and the fourth/fifth toes occurs only at low penetrance in these families and is usually unilateral and mild (just soft tissue syndactyly or duplication of a distal phalanx). Bilateral fifth finger clinodactyly, however, is present in almost all affected individuals.

Homozygous SPD

Only eight patients with a homozygous form of SPD have been reported (Akarsu et al., 1995; Muragaki et al., 1996). All have extremely small hands and feet. One, from a consanguineous American SPD

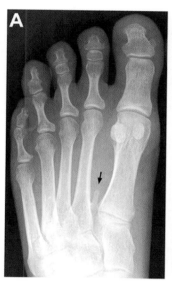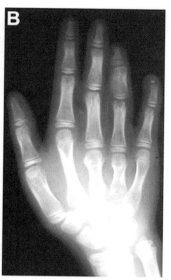

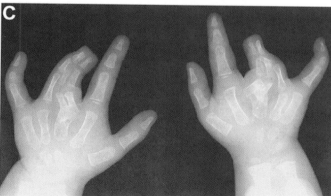

Figure 47–2. Phenotypes caused by other *HOXD13* mutations. (*A*) Partial duplication of the bases of the second metatarsal in the first web space (arrowed), broadening of the hallux and first metatarsal, and hypoplasia or symphalangism of the second to fifth middle phalanges in a woman with a missense mutation in exon 2 (892C>T [R31W] in Fig. 47–3). (*B*) Widening of the fourth middle phalanx (representing attempted duplication), hypoplasia of the fifth distal phalanx, and marked shortening of the third, fourth, and fifth metacarpals (a feature of brachydactyly type E) in a girl with a missense mutation in exon 2 (940A>C [I47L] in Fig. 47–3). (*C*) Complete cutaneous syndactyly between the third and fourth fingers, duplication of all three phalanges of the third fingers, broad third metacarpals, and hypoplastic fifth middle phalanges in a girl heterozygous for a 117 kb microdeletion that removes *HOXD9-HOXD13* and *EVX2*.

family, has duplication of the distal phalanges of the thumbs, short fingers with hypoplastic middle phalanges, syndactyly between the third to fifth fingers, small rounded metacarpals, and two extra distal carpals. In the feet, she has only three very short toes, with a relatively normal first metatarsal, a short second metatarsal, and a single small bone replacing the third to fifth metatarsals (Muragaki et al., 1996). The remaining seven patients, from the same consanguineous Turkish SPD family, have still more severe abnormalities. In the hands, there is complete soft tissue syndactyly, hypoplasia or absence of the nails, and brachydactyly and camptodactyly of the fingers, resulting in a "paw-like" appearance. Radiographs reveal between six and eight rudimentary digits, with small and malformed phalanges, metacarpals, and distal carpals. In the feet, there is also complete soft tissue syndactyly but no polydactyly. Radiographs reveal deformity, fusion, or absence of most of the phalanges, metatarsals, and distal tarsals (Akarsu et al., 1995). The severe limb malformations in these homozygotes indicate that SPD is a semidominant condition.

Abnormalities Outside the Autopod

Interestingly, one of the two SPD homozygotes for whom radiographs of the entire spine have been obtained shows total coccygeal agenesis (Akarsu et al., 1996). This is the only reported instance of skeletal involvement outside the distal limb in SPD. In the severely affected SPD family mentioned above, male heterozygotes were born with mid-penile hypospadias (Goodman et al., 1997). This is the only reported instance of extraskeletal involvement in SPD.

MUTATIONS IN *HOXD13*

The clue to the molecular basis of SPD came from linkage studies of the remarkable Turkish family mentioned above, which included 182 living affected individuals and in which the condition could be traced back over seven generations, spanning at least 140 years (Sayli et al., 1995). These studies mapped the SPD locus to chromosome 2q31, where the *HOXD* cluster is located (Sarfarazi et al., 1995); and mutations in *HOXD13* were soon after identified in four unrelated SPD families (Muragaki et al., 1996; Akarsu et al., 1996), making SPD the first human malformation syndrome shown to be caused by mutations in a *HOX* gene.

The genomic structure of *HOXD13* is depicted in Figure 47–3. It comprises just two exons, separated by an 808 bp intron and encoding a protein of 335 amino acids. Exon 1, which contains bases 1–757 of the coding sequence, includes a 45 bp imperfect trinucleotide repeat encoding a 15-residue polyalanine tract in the protein's N-terminal region. Exon 2, which contains bases 757–1008 of the coding sequence, includes the 180 bp homeobox, a highly conserved sequence element found in all *Hox* genes, encoding the 60–amino acid homeodomain, a DNA-binding motif in the protein's C-terminal region. The only polymorphism in the coding sequence reported to date is a G/A single nucleotide polymorphism at base 180, in the codon for alanine 12 of the polyalanine tract, which does not change the amino acid (Goodman et al., 1997).

Polyalanine Tract Expansions

Most cases of SPD are now known to be caused by different-sized insertions in the trinucleotide repeat in exon 1, resulting in an expanded polyalanine tract containing between 7 and 14 extra alanine residues. Such expansions have been reported in 26 unrelated SPD families (Muragaki et al., 1996; Akarsu et al., 1996; Goodman et al., 1997; Baffico et al., 1997; Kjaer et al., 2002). They have been shown to be meiotically stable over at least six generations in one family (Goodman et al., 1997) and over at least seven generations in another (Akarsu et al., 1996), and meiotic instability has never been observed. The expansions in HOXD13 thus differ sharply from the "dynamic" expansions underlying conditions such as Huntington's disease, fragile X syndrome, and myotonic dystrophy, which exhibit marked meiotic instability, and usually increase in size on transmission, causing increasingly severe disease in successive generations. In the dynamic expansions, there are long stretches of perfect trinucleotide repeats, which predispose to strand slippage on replication (Ashley and War-

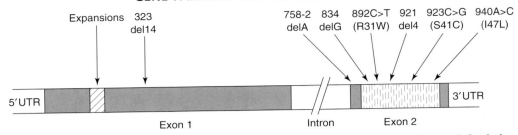

Figure 47–3. Genomic structure of *HOXD13*, showing the imperfect trinucleotide repeat in exon 1 (hatched box), the homeobox in exon 2 (stippled box), and the sites of all intragenic mutations identified to date.

ren, 1995). The repeat encoding the HOXD13 polyalanine tract, however, is imperfect, due to the use of four alternative codons for alanine (GCA, GCC, GCG, and GCT). Such cryptic interruptions are thought to prevent strand slippage. Instead, the polyalanine tract expansions in HOXD13 probably represent small duplications, caused by unequal crossing over between two normal alleles that have become misaligned during replication (Warren, 1997).

A study of 20 typical SPD families with different-sized expansions has found that both penetrance and severity of phenotype correlate with expansion size (Goodman et al., 1997). All 17 nonpenetrant mutation carriers identified in the study harbored a seven-alanine expansion, the shortest expansion known to be pathological; and in two large, fully ascertained pedigrees harboring seven-alanine and nine-alanine expansions, the penetrance was 86% and 97%, respectively (Akarsu et al., 1996; Goodman et al., 1997). An analysis of the number of limbs affected shows a statistically highly significant trend toward increasing involvement of both the hands and the feet with increasing expansion size ($P = 0.012$ for hands and $P < 0.00005$ for feet). There is also a strong trend toward more complete digit duplication with increasing expansion size. This genotype–phenotype correlation culminates in the only known family with a 14-alanine expansion, the longest so far identified. This is the severely affected family mentioned above, in which affected individuals have the most extensive limb abnormalities, including malformations of the thumbs, halluces, and distal carpals, and in which affected males have hypospadias (Goodman et al., 1997). The same correlation is also evident in SPD homozygotes. Thus, the American patient with the milder limb phenotype is homozygous for a seven-alanine expansion (Muragaki et al., 1996), whereas the seven Turkish patients with the more severe limb phenotype are homozygous for a nine-alanine expansion (Akarsu et al., 1996).

Other *HOXD13* Mutations

Three different intragenic deletions in *HOXD13* have been reported in three unrelated families. The first, a six-generation Italian family, harbors a 14 bp deletion in exon 1 (323 del14 in Fig. 47–3), which removes bases 323–336 of the coding sequence, creating a frameshift leading to a premature stop codon at bases 681–683 (Goodman et al., 1998). This deletion is predicted to result in a truncated protein containing only the first 107 amino acids of the wild-type protein, followed by 115 amino acids with no counterpart in the wild-type protein and lacking the entire homeodomain. The second, a five-generation Scottish family, harbors a deletion of a single G residue in exon 2 (834 delG in Fig. 47–3), which removes base 834 of the coding sequence, creating a frameshift leading to a premature stop codon at bases 935–937 (Goodman et al., 1998). This deletion is predicted to result in a truncated protein containing the first 278 amino acids of the wild-type protein, followed by 33 amino acids with no counterpart in the wild-type protein and lacking the last 49 amino acids of the homeodomain, including the entire recognition helix. The third, a two-generation Italian family, harbors a 4 bp deletion in exon 2 (921 del4 in Fig. 47–3), which removes bases 921–924 of the coding sequence, creating a frameshift again leading to a premature stop codon at bases 935–937 (Calabrese et al., 2000). This deletion is predicted to result in a truncated protein containing the first 307 amino acids of the wild-type protein, followed by 3 amino acids with no counterpart in the wild-type protein and lacking the last 20 amino acids of the homeodomain, again including the entire recognition helix. All mutation carriers in all three families have the atypical SPD phenotype described above.

Exactly the same atypical phenotype has also been observed in two further families. One, a three-generation English family, harbors a deletion of a single A residue 2 bases upstream of the start of exon 2 (758 −2 delA in Fig. 47–3) (Kan et al., 2003). The other, a four-generation Belgian family, harbors a C-to-T transition in exon 2, at position 892 of the coding sequence, which changes amino acid 298 (residue 31 of the homeodomain) from arginine to tryptophan (892C>T [R31W] in Fig. 47–3) (Debeer et al., 2002). The foot abnormalities in one member of this family are illustrated in Fig. 47–2*A*.

A very similar phenotype has also been reported in a father and daughter who share a 117 kb microdeletion at the 5′ end of the *HOXD* cluster (Goodman et al., 2002). Although the daughter has severe bilateral SPD in the hands (Fig. 47–2*C*), the father has only bilateral partial cutaneous syndactyly between the third and fourth fingers. Both patients, however, have virtually the same foot abnormalities as those seen in the atypical form of SPD. The microdeletion, whose extent has been defined precisely, removes just *HOXD9–HOXD13* and *EVX2* and extends only 85 kb upstream of *HOXD13*.

Two further missense mutations in exon 2 of *HOXD13* have recently been reported, both associated with limb phenotypes that are distinct from SPD. In three English families who are probably related through a common affected ancestor, a novel dominantly-inherited combination of polydactyly and brachydactyly, exhibiting overlap with brachydactyly type E (illustrated in Fig. 47–2*B*), segregates with an A-to-C transversion at position 940 of the coding sequence (Caronia et al., 2003; Johnson et al., 2003). This changes amino acid 314 (residue 47 of the homeodomain) from isoleucine to leucine (940A>C [I47L] in Fig. 47–3). In another English family, a dominantly-inherited brachydactyly exhibiting overlap with brachydactyly types D and E segregates with a C-to-G transition at position 923 of the coding sequence (Johnson et al., 2003). This changes amino acid 308 (residue 41 of the homeodomain) from serine to cysteine (923C>G [S41C] in Fig. 47–3).

DIAGNOSIS AND MANAGEMENT

The diagnosis of SPD is based on careful clinical and radiological assessment of the patient's hands and feet, followed by sequence analysis of *HOXD13* to identify the causative mutation. If a mutation is not detected, cytogenetic and/or haplotype analysis should be undertaken to search for a deletion affecting the 5′ end of the *HOXD* cluster. Most patients will require surgery of the hands and feet, to release the syndactyly and remove the extra digits, partly to improve function and partly for cosmetic reasons. Patients should be advised that any child born to a mutation carrier has a 50% chance of also carrying the mutation.

ANIMAL MODELS

The *spdh* Mouse

The best animal model for SPD is the synpolydactyly homolog (*spdh*) mouse, a spontaneous mutant carrying a seven-residue expansion in the N-terminal polyalanine tract of mouse Hoxd13, which, like that of human HOXD13, is normally 15 residues long (Johnson et al., 1998; Bruneau et al., 2001). Only 30% of *spdh* heterozygotes have limb defects, and these consist only of slight shortening of the second and fifth middle phalanges, with occasional carpal fusions. *spdh* homozygotes, however, have marked shortening, malformation, and occasional bony fusion of the digits in all four limbs, with partially penetrant central poly-dactyly in the hindlimbs. Homozygous males also have agenesis of the preputial glands and abnormalities of the seminal vesicles and are infer-tile. The limb defects in *spdh* heterozygotes are much milder than those in most humans heterozygous for a seven-alanine expansion, and those in *spdh* homozygotes are similar but not identical to those in the only known human homozygous for a seven-alanine expansion, who actually has oligodactyly in the feet (Muragaki et al., 1996). This may reflect a species difference in the effects of the mutation. Even in human het-erozygotes, however, seven-alanine expansions are associated with the lowest penetrance and the mildest and most variable phenotype.

Abnormalities of autopod development in *spdh* homozygotes have been observed at two distinct stages (Johnson et al., 1998; Bruneau et al., 2001). First, the early precartilaginous digital condensations are short-ened and abnormally spaced, with a wide gap between the third and fourth condensations in the hindlimb, leading to the formation of a su-pernumerary central condensation. Second, chondrification and ossifica-tion of the phalanges and metacarpals/tarsals are markedly delayed, with loss of the normal regular pattern of ossification centers. This appears to be due to a delayed transition from proliferative to hypertrophic chon-drocytes in the growth plates. A more recent study has additionally shown that phalangeal joint formation is impaired (Albrecht et al., 2002).

The *Del3* Mouse

A second model for SPD is provided by mice carrying a targeted dele-tion of the three most 5' *Hoxd* genes, *Hoxd11*, *Hoxd12*, and *Hoxd13* (*Del3*) (Zákány and Duboule, 1996). *Del3* heterozygotes have hy-poplastic second and fifth middle phalanges, but *Del3* homozygotes have shortening, webbing, and fusion of the digits, with central poly-dactyly, especially in the hindlimbs, and malformations and fusions of the carpals/tarsals. These abnormalities are again similar, although not identical, to those seen in SPD heterozygotes and homozygotes. In *Del3* homozygotes, as in *spdh* homozygotes, the precartilaginous digital condensations are abnormally small, extra condensations de-velop, and both chondrification and ossification are delayed. Ho-mozygous males also have a reduction in the size of the penis and penian bone (Zákány et al., 1997).

The *Hoxd13* Knockout Mouse

Mice with targeted disruptions of the homeobox of *Hoxd13* have also been generated by two different groups, with virtually identical results (Dollé et al., 1993; Davis and Capecchi, 1996). Only 36%–50% of het-erozygotes have any abnormalities, and these consist of a small extra postaxial bony element, usually in the forelimbs only, sometimes ac-companied by minor defects of the metacarpals and distal carpals (Davis and Capecchi, 1996; Kondo et al., 1996). Homozygotes have more marked limb abnormalities, particularly in the forelimbs, including short-ening of all the digits, especially digits two and five, due mainly to hypoplasia/absence of the middle phalanges and, in about 50%, a rudi-mentary extra postaxial digit. There are also fusions of the metacar-pophalangeal joints, shortening and thickening of the metatarsals (espe-cially the first metatarsals, which have an unusual anterior protrusion), and minor malformations of the distal carpals/tarsals. During autopod development, the precartilaginous digital condensations are reduced in width and length and there is often a large field of uncondensed cells posteriorly, in which an extra condensation forms. Both chondrification and ossification of almost all the skeletal elements are strikingly delayed.

Homozygous *Hoxd13* knockout mice also have abnormalities of the lowest (fourth) sacral vertebra (Dollé et al., 1993). In addition, males are infertile, with shortening and deformity of the proximal part of the penian bone (normally a site of strong *Hoxd13* expression), agenesis of the bulbourethral glands, and abnormalities of the seminal vesicles and prostate (Podlasek et al., 1997). They also exhibit disorganization of the internal anal sphincter, leading in 30% to anal prolapse (Kondo et al., 1996).

Hoxd13 Misexpression in Chick

Ectopic overexpression of *Hoxd13* in the developing chick limb pro-duces shortening of the long bones of the stylopod and zeugopod, es-pecially the tibia (Goff and Tabin, 1997). This is first apparent at a rel-atively late stage, during growth of the cartilaginous models, and is as-sociated with decreased chondrocyte proliferation in the growth plates.

DEVELOPMENTAL PATHOGENESIS

Polyalanine Expansions

The polyalanine tract expansions in HOXD13 that cause typical SPD have proved to be the first instance of a novel class of mutation. Simi-lar expansions have now been identified in HOXA13, causing hand-foot-genital syndrome (Goodman et al., 2000; Debeer et al., 2002), as well as in two other homeodomain transcription factors: ARX, causing men-tal retardation and epilepsy (Stromme et al., 2002) and PHOX2B, caus-ing congenital central hypoventilation syndrome (Amiel et al., 2003); and four nonhomeodomain transcription factors: CBFA1, causing clei-docranial dysplasia (Mundlos et al., 1997), ZIC2 (see Chapter 18), caus-ing holoprosencephaly (Brown et al., 1998), FOXL2 (see Chapter 85), causing blepharophimosis-ptosis-epicanthus inversus syndrome (Crisponi et al., 2001) and SOX3, causing mental retardation and growth hormone deficiency (Laumonnier et al., 2002). Interestingly, the length of the expanded tract that causes disease is similar in all eight proteins (20–29 residues), suggesting a common underlying mechanism.

Although polyalanine tracts are a frequent motif in transcription fac-tors, their normal function is not known. They may act as flexible spacer elements between other domains (Karlin and Burge, 1996), or they may bind proteins with which the transcription factors interact, such as DNA-binding partners or transcriptional cofactors (Han and Manley, 1993; Licht et al., 1994). The effects of expanding such tracts are also not yet understood. In the case of HOXD13, at least, even a 14-residue expan-sion does not affect the mutant protein's stability or nuclear localization (Goodman, unpublished data). Moreover, the increase in penetrance and phenotypic severity observed in SPD patients with increasingly large ex-pansions is consistent with a progressive gain of function.

The similarity between the limb abnormalities in homozygous *Del3* mice and those in SPD patients has led to the suggestion that mutant HOXD13 protein carrying an expanded polyalanine tract may exert a dominant-negative effect over the remaining wild-type HOXD13 and over HOXD11, HOXD12, and possibly the other HOX proteins (HOXD10 and HOXA13) expressed in the developing autopod (Zákány and Duboule, 1996). This hypothesis is supported by recent studies in *spdh* mice (Bruneau et al., 2001). The mutant Hoxd13 is produced at the same time and in the same distribution as wild-type Hoxd13 and at virtually the same levels. Unlike mutant proteins car-rying large polyglutamine tract expansions, it does not induce in-creased apoptosis. It also has no effect on the expression of other *Hox* genes in the autopod. Genetic complementation experiments, however, indicate that it not only has lost its own normal function but also in-terferes with the functions of both wild-type Hoxd13 and other 5' Hoxd proteins (although probably not with Hoxa13).

While polyalanine tract expansions should not affect HOXD13's ability to bind DNA, they may well disrupt interactions between the N-terminal region of HOXD13 and other proteins, whether by steric hindrance or by altering the orientation of adjacent N-terminal do-mains. Alternatively, they may allow abnormal protein–protein inter-actions to occur, perhaps by directly binding another protein. What-ever the exact molecular mechanism, the result is evidently to perturb some or all of HOXD13's normal functions. The mutant protein can nevertheless interfere functionally with the remaining wild-type HOXD13 as well as with other 5' HOXD proteins in the developing autopod, probably by competing for binding-site occupancy, thus act-ing as a "super" dominant-negative.

Loss-of-Function Mutations

Five of the other *HOXD13* mutations described above produce virtu-ally the same atypical form of SPD, suggesting that they act by a very similar mechanism, which differs subtly from the mechanism by which the polyalanine tract expansions act. The most likely explanation is that all five mutations result in functional haploinsufficiency for *HOXD13*. The three frameshifting deletions (323 del14, 834 delG, and 921 del4) are predicted to result in truncated proteins lacking all or most of the homeodomain and, therefore, unable to bind DNA. Preliminary findings indicate that these mutant proteins are stable but completely inactive both *in vitro* and *in vivo* (Goodman, unpublished data). The 758 −2 delA mutation disrupts the consensus AG splice acceptor site of exon 2, and is likely to cause a failure of normal splicing, abolishing the production of functional protein from the mutant allele (Kan et al., 2003). The 892C>T missense mutation alters a highly-conserved arginine residue in helix II of the homeodomain, which is thought to form salt bridges with both a phosphate group in the DNA backbone and with a highly-conserved glutamate residue in helix III, and is predicted to destabilize the homeodomain–DNA complex (Debeer et al., 2002). The similarity between the phenotype caused by these five loss-of-function mutations and that observed in the father and daughter with the microdeletion at the 5′ end of the *HOXD* cluster suggests that the chief cause of the abnormalities in these two patients is probably also haploinsufficiency for *HOXD13*, although in their case haploinsufficiency for *HOXD10–HOXD12* and *EVX2* may be an additional factor (Goodman et al., 2002).

The limb abnormalities in carriers of all five mutations differ in a number of ways, however, from those in *Hoxd13* knockout mice. In particular, neither the fully penetrant atypical foot phenotype nor the partially penetrant central SPD in the hands characteristic of these patients occurs in heterozygous or homozygous *Hoxd13* knock-outs. There are several possible explanations for these phenotypic differences. The consequences of haploinsufficiency for *HOXD13* may differ in humans and mice, either because of differences between the two species in sensitivity to reduced *HOXD13* gene dosage or because of subtle differences in the role played by *HOXD13* during early human and murine autopod development. Alternatively, the targeted mouse mutations may not have resulted in a straightforward loss of Hoxd13 function, perhaps because insertion of a selectable marker cassette has disrupted the expression of neighboring genes in the *HoxD* cluster (Olson et al., 1996).

Specific Substitutions in the Homeodomain

The I47L (940A>C) and S41C (923C>G) missense mutations in the homeodomain both produce novel phenotypes, and are likely to act through distinct mechanisms. The former affects a highly-conserved residue in the recognition helix which directly contacts target DNA, but represents a conservative substitution, suggesting that it may perturb rather than abolish HOXD13's DNA-binding capacity. Interestingly, this mutation has recently been shown to impair DNA binding at some but not all sites bound by the wild-type protein (Caronia et al., 2003; Johnson et al., 2003), resulting in a selective rather than a generalised loss of HOXD13 function both in vitro and in vivo (Caronia et al., 2003). The latter affects a less conserved residue between helices II and III, but again appears to subtly alter rather than abolish DNA binding (Johnson et al., 2003).

Distribution of Abnormalities

As described above, the limb abnormalities in SPD most commonly involve the central and postaxial digits but can extend as far anteriorly as the first digits and as far proximally as the distal carpals in both heterozygotes and homozygotes. This distribution corresponds closely to the second of the two phases of *Hoxd13* expression in the developing mouse and chick limb, during specification of the autopod (Dollé et al., 1991a; Nelson et al., 1996). Interestingly, in both the typical and atypical forms of SPD, there are striking and consistent differences between the pattern of abnormalities in the upper and lower limbs. In the hands, the digital webbing and duplication are always central, never preaxial or postaxial. Indeed, syndactyly between the third and fourth fingers, with or without an extra digit in the syndactylous web, has been reported in at least one member of virtually every family carrying a heterozygous *HOXD13* mutation, suggesting that this abnormality is a hallmark of disturbed *HOXD13* function. In the feet, however, the digital webbing and duplication are always postaxial, never preaxial or central. Moreover, the distinctive features of the atypical form of SPD are confined to the feet alone. These observations imply that, in humans at least, *HOXD13* plays different roles in the developing hands and feet, perhaps contributing to the significant morphological differences between them.

The limb abnormalities in SPD also vary markedly in severity not only between and within affected families but also within one affected individual. Much of the interfamilial and intrafamilial variation can be explained by differences in the underlying mutations. Thus, as explained above, the highest penetrance and most severe phenotypes are associated with the longest polyalanine tract expansions, while the lowest penetrance and mildest phenotypes are associated with loss-of-function mutations. The greatest interfamilial and intrafamilial variation in penetrance and severity occurs in families carrying the smallest expansions, perhaps reflecting the greater relative influence of other genetic factors in these cases (Goodman et al., 1997).

The strikingly asymmetrical limb involvement common in individual SPD patients, however, has occurred against a uniform genetic background, suggesting that the underlying mechanism may be stochastic. Interestingly, there is increasing evidence that both the initiation and maintenance of gene expression are stochastic processes. A study modeling such processes mathematically has shown that loss of one copy of a gene increases both stochastic delays in gene activation and stochastic reductions in gene expression levels, particularly if the gene in question is positively autoregulated (Cook et al., 1998). The dominant-negative and loss-of-function mutations in *HOXD13* described above could well cause these kinds of stochastic disturbance of expression from the remaining wild-type *HOXD13* allele. These in turn could lead to asymmetrical limb abnormalities if, as seems likely, the correct timing and level of *HOXD13* expression in a small field of mesenchymal precursor cells are crucial for normal autopod development (Nelson et al., 1996).

The total coccygeal agenesis reported in one SPD homozygote (Akarsu et al., 1996) and the hypospadias reported in male SPD heterozygotes carrying the longest known polyalanine tract expansion (Goodman et al., 1997) are consistent with the observed expression of mouse *Hoxd13* in the most posterior part of the developing trunk and urogenital tract (Dollé et al., 1991a). In particular, hypospadias is thought to result from failure of the urogenital folds to fuse during urethral development, and mouse *Hoxd13* has been shown to be expressed in the most distal epithelium of the urogenital sinus, which gives rise to the urogenital folds (Dollé et al., 1991b). Genital abnormalities and infertility are also common in male mice homozygous for spontaneous and targeted mutations in *Hoxd13*, as described above, and hypospadias is a frequent malformation in male patients heterozygous for mutations in the closely related paralogous gene *HOXA13* (Mortlock and Innis, 1997; Goodman et al., 2000).

Disturbed Autopod Patterning and Growth

The abnormalities in SPD are not morphological transformations of the autopod segment of the limb or alterations of digit identity but, rather, changes in the number, separation, size, and shape of specific skeletal elements. The same is true of the limb abnormalities in the corresponding mouse mutants. As described earlier, they appear to arise at two distinct stages of autopod development, first during the growth and patterning of undifferentiated mesenchymal cells in the limb bud core and later during the growth and differentiation of chondrogenic cells in the cartilaginous bone models. This is consistent with the tissue-specific expression of *Hoxd13* within the mouse autopod, which (like that of *Hoxd10–12* and *Hoxa13*) initially comprises the entire mesenchymal core but is then restricted first to the precartilaginous condensations and later to the perichondrium and proliferating chondrocytes of the cartilaginous models (Dollé et al., 1991a; Zákány and Duboule, 1996).

Insight into the molecular basis of some of these effects has been provided by studies of a mouse *Hoxa13* knockout (see Chapter 48) generated by targeted insertion of the *GFP* gene (Stadler et al., 2001), which, like previous *Hoxa13* knockouts (Fromental-Ramain et al., 1996), exhibits absence of the first digits and central syndactyly. Homozygous *Hoxa13^GFP*-expressing mesenchymal cells form fewer and smaller precartilaginous aggregates than wild-type cells *in vitro*, and the mesenchyme in mutant autopods is disorganized. Moreover, at the stage when cells expressing wild-type *Hoxa13* become restricted to the digital condensations, *Hoxa13^GFP*-expressing cells remain in the interdigital zones, where they appear unable to respond to normal apoptotic signals. Underlying these defects is a disturbance of the ephrin(Eph)/Eph-receptor signaling system, which is known to play a crucial role in cell sorting and boundary formation (Frisén et al., 1999). Several 3′ *HoxA* and *HoxB* genes have previously been shown to regulate EphA receptors involved in hindbrain rhombomere boundary formation and axon guidance (Studer et al., 1998). In *Hoxa13^GFP* mutants, expression of the EphA7 receptor is markedly reduced and expression of one of its ligands, EphA3, persists throughout the cartilaginous condensations and interdigital zones along with *Hoxa13^GFP* instead of becoming restricted to the perichondrium. These findings suggest that Hoxa13 directly regulates the expression of *EphA7* (and possibly of other *EphA* receptors). Hoxd13 has been proposed to play a similar role (Stadler et al., 2001), and indeed overexpression of wild-type human HOXD13 in the developing chick autopod has recently been shown to produce a marked increase in the expression levels of *EphA7* in the perichondrium of the digital condensations (Caronia et al., 2003).

Both the syndactyly and the polydactyly caused by *HOXD13* mutations could readily be explained by perturbations of this kind in cell sorting and cell adhesion. Ectopic expression of *Hoxd* genes in the interdigital zones has previously been associated with reduced apoptosis leading to persistent interdigital webbing (Morgan et al., 1992; Barna et al., 2000). Moreover, overexpression of *Hoxa13* in chick limb buds causes increased mesenchymal cell adhesiveness, leading to ectopic cartilage formation in the zeugopod and preaxial polydactyly in the autopod (Yokouchi et al., 1995).

The shortening or absence of skeletal elements, however, is more likely to reflect impaired cell proliferation. As described above, the middle phalanges of the fifth fingers and second to fifth toes are frequently hypoplastic in SPD heterozygotes. Similar hypoplasia/aplasia of the middle phalanges, especially of the second and fifth digits, is common in mice carrying mutations in individual 5′ *Hoxd* genes, including *Hoxd13*, and in *Hoxa13* as well as in compound mutants (Davis and Capecchi, 1996; Fromental-Ramain et al., 1996). The second and fifth digital rays are the last to condense, and the middle phalanges are the last digital segments to form; thus, this particular defect may result from a reduction in the number of precursor cells in the undifferentiated mesenchyme (Davis and Capecchi, 1996). Similarly, the more extensive hypoplasia/aplasia of skeletal elements found in SPD homozygotes could result from reduced cell division both at this early stage and later in the chondrogenic cells of the growth plates. If so, the HOXD13 targets may well include genes with key functions in cell cycle control.

At present, we understand very little about HOXD13's role at the cellular or molecular level. Identification of the pathways in which it acts and the genes it regulates should shed important light both on the pathogenesis of SPD and other limb malformations and on the development of the autopod, its evolutionary origins, and its diversity.

REFERENCES

Akarsu AN, Akhan O, Sayli BS, Sayli U, Baskaya G, Sarfarazi M (1995). A large Turkish kindred with syndactyly type II (synpolydactyly). 2. Homozygous phenotype? *J Med Genet* 32: 435–441.

Akarsu AN, Stoilov I, Yilmaz E, Sayli BS, Sarfarazi M (1996). Genomic structure of *HOXD13* gene: a nine polyalanine duplication causes synpolydactyly in two unrelated families. *Hum Mol Genet* 5: 945–952.

Albrecht AN, Schwabe GC, Stricker S, Boddrich A, Wanker EE, Mundlos S (2002). The synpolydactyly homolog (spdh) mutation in the mouse—a defect in patterning and growth of limb cartilage elements. *Mech Dev* 112: 53–67.

Amiel J, Laudier B, Attie-Bitach T, Trang H, de Pontual L, Gener B, Trochet D, Etchevers H, Ray P, Simmoneau M, Vekemans M, Munnich A, Gaultier C, Lyonnet S (2003). Polyalanine expansion and frameshift mutations of the paired-like homeobox gene PHOX2B in congenital central hypoventilation syndrome. *Nat Genet* 10: 459–460.

Anderson W (1898). A case of "angeio-keratoma." *Br J Dermatol* 10: 113–117.

Ashley CT, Warren ST (1995). Trinucleotide repeat expansion and human disease. *Annu Rev Genet* 29: 703–728.

Baffico M, Baldi M, Cassan PD, Costa M, Mantero R, Garani P, Camera G (1997). Synpolydactyly: clinical and molecular studies on four Italian families. *Eur J Hum Genet* 5(Suppl 1): A142.

Barna M, Hawe N, Niswander L, Pandolfi PP (2000). Plzf regulates limb and axial skeletal patterning. *Nat Genet* 25: 166–172.

Brown SA, Warburton D, Brown LY, Yu C, Roeder ER, Stengel-Rutkowski S, Hennekam RCM, et al. (1998). Holoprosencephaly due to mutations in ZIC2, a homologue of *Drosophila odd-paired*. *Nat Genet* 20: 180–183.

Bruneau S, Johnson K R, Yamamoto M, Kuroiwa A, Duboule D (2001). The mouse *Hoxd13^spdh* mutation, a polyalanine expansion similar to human type II synpolydactyly (SPD), disrupts the function but not the expression of other *Hoxd* genes. *Dev Biol* 237: 345–353.

Calabrese O, Bigoni S, Gualandi F, Trabanelli C, Camera G, Calzolari E (2000). A new

mutation in *HOXD13* associated with foot pre-postaxial polydactyly. *Eur J Hum Genet* 8(Suppl 1): 140.

Camera G, Camera A, Pozzolo S, Costa M, Mantero R (1995). Synpolydactyly (type II syndactyly) with aplasia/hypoplasia of the middle phalanges of the toes: report on a family with eight affected members in four generations. *Am J Med Genet* 55: 244–246.

Capdevila J, Tsukui T, Rodríguez Esteban C, Zappavigna V, Izpisúa Belmonte JC (1999). Control of vertebrate limb outgrowth by the proximal factor *Meis2* and distal antagonism of BMPs by Gremlin. *Mol Cells* 4: 839–849.

Caronia G, Goodman FR, McKeown CME, Scambler PJ, Zappavigna V (2003). An I47L substitution in the HOXD13 homeodomain causes a novel human limb malformation by producing a selective loss of function. *Development* 130: 1701–1712.

Cook DL, Gerber AN, Tapscott SJ (1998). Modeling stochastic gene expression: implications for haploinsufficiency. *Proc Natl Acad Sci USA* 95: 15641–15646.

Crisponi L, Deiana M, Loi A, Chiappe F, Uda M, Amati P, Bisceglia L, Zelante L, Nagaraja R, Porcu S, et al. (2001). The putative forkhead transcription factor FOXL2 is mutated in blepharophimosis/ptosis/epicanthus inversus syndrome. *Nat Genet* 27: 159–166.

Cross HE, Lerberg DB, McKusick VA (1967). Type II syndactyly. *Am J Hum Genet* 20: 368–380.

Davis AP, Capecchi MR (1996). A mutational analysis of the 5′ *HoxD* genes: dissection of genetic interactions during limb development. *Development* 122:1175–1185.

Debeer P, Bacchelli C, Scambler PJ, De Smet L, Fryns JP, Goodman FR (2002). Severe digital abnormalities in a patient heterozygous for both a novel missense mutation in HOXD13 and a polyalanine tract expansion in HOXA13. *J Med Genet* 39: 852–856.

Dollé P, Izpisúa-Belmonte JC, Boncinelli E, Duboule D (1991a). The *Hox4.8* gene is localized at the 5′ extremity of the *Hox4* complex and is expressed in the most posterior parts of the body during development. *Mech Dev* 36: 3–13.

Dollé P, Izpisúa-Belmonte J C, Brown J M, Tickle C, Duboule D (1991b). *HOX4* genes and the morphogenesis of mammalian genitalia. *Genes Dev* 5: 1767–1767.

Dollé P, Dierich A, LeMeur M, Schimmang T, Schuhbaur B, Chambon P, Duboule D (1993). Disruption of the *Hoxd13* gene induces localized heterochrony leading to mice with neotenic limbs. *Cell* 75: 431–441.

Duprez DM, Kostakopoulou K, Francis-West PH, Tickle C, Brickell PM (1996). Activation of *Fgf-4* and *HoxD* gene expression by *BMP-2* expressing cells in the developing chick limb. *Development* 122: 1821–1828.

Favier B, Dollé P (1997). Developmental functions of mammalian *Hox* genes. *Mol Hum Reprod* 3: 115–131.

Frisén J, Holmberg J, Barbacid M (1999). Ephrins and their Eph receptors: multitalented directors of embryonic development. *EMBO J* 18: 5159–5165.

Fromental-Ramain C, Warot X, Messadecq N, LeMeur M, Dollé P, Chambon P (1996). *Hoxa13* and *Hoxd13* play a crucial role in the patterning of the limb autopod. *Development* 122: 2997–3011.

Goff DJ, Tabin CJ (1997). Analysis of *Hoxd13* and *Hoxd11* misexpression in chick limb buds reveals that *Hox* genes affect both bone condensation and growth. *Development* 124: 627–636.

Goodman FR, Mundlos S, Muragaki Y, Donnai D, Giovannucci-Uzielli ML, Lapi E, Majewski F, McGaughran J, McKeown C, Reardon W, et al. (1997). Synpolydactyly phenotypes correlate with size of expansions in HOXD13 polyalanine tract. *Proc Natl Acad Sci USA* 94: 7458–7463.

Goodman FR, Giovannucci-Uzielli ML, Hall C, Reardon W, Winter R, Scambler P (1998). Deletions in *HOXD13* segregate with an identical, novel foot malformation in two unrelated families. *Am J Hum Genet* 63: 992–1000.

Goodman FR, Bacchelli C, Brady AF, Brueton LA, Fryns JP, Mortlock DP, Innis JW, Holmes LB, Donnenfeld AE, Feingold M, et al. (2000). Novel *HOXA13* mutations and the phenotypic spectrum of hand-foot-genital syndrome. *Am J Hum Genet* 67: 197–202.

Goodman FR, Majewski F, Collins AL, Scambler PJ (2002). A 117-kb microdeletion removing *HOXD9-HOXD13* and *EVX2* causes synpolydactyly. *Am J Hum Genet* 70: 547–555.

Graba Y, Aragnol D, Pradel J (1997). *Drosophila* Hox complex downstream targets and the function of homeotic genes. *Bioessays* 19: 379–388.

Han K, Manley JL (1993). Transcriptional repression by the *Drosophila* Even-skipped protein: definition of a minimal repression domain. *Genes Dev* 7: 491–503.

Haraguchi R, Mo R, Hui C, Motoyama J, Makino S, Shiroishi T, Gaffield W, Yamada G (2001). Unique functions of Sonic hedgehog signaling during external genitalia development. *Development* 128: 4241–4250.

Hérault Y, Beckers J, Gerard M, Duboule D (1999). *Hox* gene expression in limbs: colinearity by opposite regulatory controls. *Dev Biol* 208: 157–165.

Johnson D, Kan SH, Oldridge M, Trembath RC, Roche P, Esnouf RM, Giele H, Wilkie AOM (2003). Missense mutations in the homeodomain of HOXD13 are associated with brachydactyly types D and E. *Am J Hum Genet* 72: 984–997.

Johnson KR, Sweet HO, Donahue LR, Ward-Bailey P, Bronson RT, Davisson MT (1998). A new spontaneous mouse mutation of *Hoxd13* with a polyalanine expansion and phenotype similar to human synpolydactyly. *Hum Mol Genet* 7: 1033–1038.

Johnson RL, Tabin CJ (1997). Molecular models for vertebrate limb development. *Cell* 90: 979–990.

Kan SH, Johnson D, Giele H, Wilkie AOM (2003). An acceptor splice site mutation in *HOXD13* results in variable hand, but consistent foot malformations. *Am J Med Genet* (in press).

Karlin S, Burge C (1996). Trinucleotide repeats and long homopeptides in genes and proteins associated with nervous system disease and development. *Proc Natl Acad Sci USA* 93: 1560–1565.

Kjaer KW, Hedeboe J, Bugge M, Hansen C, Friis-Henriksen K, Vestergaard MB, Tommerup N, Opitz JM (2002). HOXD13 polyalanine tract expansion in classical synpolydactyly type Vordingborg. *Am J Med Genet* 110: 116–121.

Kondo T, Duboule D (1999). Breaking colinearity in the mouse HoxD complex. *Cell* 97: 407–417.

Kondo T, Dollé P, Zákány J, Duboule D (1996). Function of posterior *HoxD* genes in the morphogenesis of the anal sphincter. *Development* 122: 2651–2659.

Krumlauf R (1994). *Hox* genes in vertebrate development. *Cell* 78: 191–201.

Laufer E, Nelson CE, Johnson RL, Morgan BA, Tabin C (1994). Sonic hedgehog and Fgf-4 act through a signaling cascade and feedback loop to integrate growth and patterning of the developing limb bud. *Cell* 79: 993–1003.

Laumonnier F, Ronce N, Hamel BCJ, Thomas P, Lespinasse J, Raynaud M, Paringaux C, van Bokhoven H, Kalscheuer V, Fryns JP, Chelly J, Moraine C, Briault S (2002). Transcription factor SOX3 is involved in X-linked mental-retardation with growth hormone deficiency. *Am J Hum Genet* 71: 1450–1455.

Licht JD, Hanna-Rose W, Reddy JC, English MA, Ro M, Grossel M, Shaknovich R, Hansen U (1994). Mapping and mutagenesis of the amino-terminal transcriptional repression domain of the *Drosophila* Kruppel protein. *Mol Cell Biol* 14: 4057–4066.

Mann RS, Affolter M (1998). Hox proteins meet more partners. *Curr Opin Genet Dev* 8: 423–429.

Mark M, Rijli FM, Chambon P (1997). Homeobox genes in embryogenesis and pathogenesis. *Pediatr Res* 42: 421–429.

McGinnis W, Krumlauf R (1992). Homeobox genes and axial patterning. *Cell* 68: 283–302.

Mercader N, Leonardo E, Azpiazu N, Serrano A, Morata G, Martínez-AC, Torres M (1999). Conserved regulation of proximodistal limb axis development by Meis1/Hth. *Nature* 402: 425–429.

Merlob P, Grunebaum M (1986). Type II syndactyly or synpolydactyly. *J Med Genet* 23: 237–241.

Morgan BA, Izpisúa-Belmonte JC, Duboule D, Tabin CJ (1992). Targeted misexpression of *Hox4.6* in the avian limb bud causes apparent homeotic transformations. *Nature* 358: 236–239.

Mortlock DP, Innis JW (1997). Mutation of *HOXA13* in hand-foot-genital syndrome. *Nat Genet* 15: 179–180.

Mundlos S, Otto F, Mundlos C, Mulliken JB, Aylsworth AS, Albright S, Lindhout D, Cole WG, Henn W, Knoll JHM, et al. (1997). Mutations involving the transcription factor CBFA1 cause cleidocranial dysplasia. *Cell* 89: 773–779.

Muragaki Y, Mundlos S, Upton J, Olsen BR (1996). Altered growth and branching patterns in synpolydactyly caused by mutations in *HOXD13*. *Science* 272: 548–551.

Nelson CE, Morgan BA, Burke AC, Laufer E, DiMambro E, Murtaugh LC, Gonzales E, Tessarollo L, Parada LF, Tabin C (1996). Analysis of *Hox* gene expression in the chick limb bud. *Development* 122: 1449–1466.

Olson EN, Arnold HH, Rigby PW, Wold BJ (1996). Know your neighbors: three phenotypes in null mutants of the myogenic bHLH gene *MRF4*. *Cell* 85: 1–4.

Podlasek CA, Duboule D, Bushman W (1997). Male accessory sex organ morphogenesis is altered by loss of function of *Hoxd13*. *Dev Dyn* 208: 454–465.

Roberts DJ, Smith DM, Goff DJ, Tabin CJ (1998). Epithelial-mesenchymal signaling during the regionalization of the chick gut. *Development* 125: 2791–2801.

Sarfarazi M, Akarsu AN, Sayli BS (1995). Localization of the syndactyly type II (synpolydactyly) locus to 2q31 region and identification of tight linkage to *HOXD8* intragenic marker. *Hum Mol Genet* 4: 1453–1458.

Sayli BS, Akarsu AN, Sayli U, Akhan O, Ceylaner S, Sarfarazi M (1995). A large Turkish kindred with syndactyly type II (synpolydactyly). 1. Field investigation, clinical and pedigree data. *J Med Genet* 32: 421–434.

Shen WF, Rozenfeld S, Lawrence HJ, Largman C (1997a). The Abd-B-like Hox homeodomain proteins can be subdivided by the ability to form complexes with Pbx1a on a novel DNA target. *J Biol Chem* 272: 8198–8206.

Shen WF, Montgomery JC, Rozenfeld S, Moskow JJ, Lawrence HJ, Buchberg AM, Largman C (1997b). AbdB-like Hox proteins stabilize DNA binding by the Meis1 homeodomain proteins. *Mol Cell Biol* 17: 6448–6458.

Stadler HS, Higgins KM, Capecchi MR (2001). Loss of *Eph-receptor* expression correlates with loss of cell adhesion and chondrogenic capacity in *Hoxa13* mutant limbs. *Development* 128: 4177–4188.

Stromme P, Mangelsdorf ME, Shaw MA, Lower KM, Lewis SME, Bruyere H, Lutcherath V, Gedeon AK, Wallace RH, Scheffer IE, Turner G, Partington M, Frints SGM, Fryns JP, Sutherland GR, Mulley JC, Gecz J (2002). Mutations in the human ortholog of aristaless cause X-linked mental retardation and epilepsy. *Nat Genet* 30: 441–445.

Studer M, Gavalas A, Marshall H, Ariza-McNaughton L, Rijli FM, Chambon P, Krumlauf R (1998). Genetic interactions between *Hoxa1* and *Hoxb1* reveal new roles in regulation of early hindbrain patterning. *Development* 125: 1025–1036.

Temtamy SA, McKusick VA (1978). Syndactyly as an isolated malformation. In: *The Genetics of Hand Malformations*. Birth Defects Original Article Series, Volume XIV. Bergsma D (ed.) Alan R. Liss, New York, pp. 301–322.

Thomsen O (1927). Einige Eigentümlichkeiten der erblichen Poly-und Syndaktylie bei Menschen. *Acta Med Scand* 65: 609–644.

Tickle C (2000). Limb development: an international model for vertebrate pattern formation. *Int J Dev Biol* 44: 101–108.

van der Hoeven F, Zákány J, Duboule D (1996). Gene transpositions in the *HoxD* complex reveal a hierarchy of regulatory controls. *Cell* 85: 1025–1035.

Warren S T (1997). Polyalanine expansion in synpolydactyly might result from unequal crossing-over of *HOXD13*. *Science* 275: 408–409.

Yokouchi Y, Nakazato S, Yamamoto M, Goto Y, Kameda T, Iba H, Kuroiwa A (1995). Misexpression of *Hoxa13* induces cartilage homeotic transformation and changes cell adhesiveness in chick limb buds. *Genes Dev* 9: 2509–2522.

Zákány J, Duboule D (1996). Synpolydactyly in mice with a targeted deficiency in the *HoxD* complex. *Nature* 384: 69–71.

Zákány J, Fromental-Ramain C, Warot X, Duboule D (1997). Regulation of number and size of digits by posterior *Hox* genes: a dose-dependent mechanism with potential evolutionary implications. *Proc Natl Acad Sci USA* 94: 13695–13700.

Zappavigna V, Renucci A, Izpisúa-Belmonte JC, Urier G, Peschle C, Duboule D (1991). *HOX4* genes encode transcription factors with potential auto- and cross-regulatory capacities. *EMBO J* 10: 4177–4187.

48 | *HOXA13* and the Hand-Foot-Genital and Guttmacher Syndromes

JEFFREY W. INNIS

*H*OX gene mutations in humans associated with specific morphological defects have been described for only three of the 39 known genes (see Chapter 46): *HOXD13* (see Chapter 47), *HOXA13*, and *HOXA11*. Except for the newly described mutation in human *HOXA11* (Thompson and Nguyen, 2000), this subject has been reviewed (Innis, 1997; Veraksa et al., 2000; Goodman and Scambler, 2001). All of these human syndromes are associated with heterozygous *HOX* mutations that are inherited in an autosomal dominant pattern with almost complete penetrance. Heterozygous premature chain termination as well as missense and alanine expansion mutations in *HOXA13* cause distal limb and genitourinary (GU) malformations in humans. Haploinsufficiency for HOXA13 in humans causes hand-foot-genital syndrome (HFGS), which is characterized by symmetrical preaxial deficiency of the hands and feet, fifth digit clinodactyly, and frequent but incompletely penetrant GU defects including incomplete müllerian fusion in females and hypospadias in males. Mutations that code for in-frame alanine expansions in the largest of three, long polyalanine tracts also result in typical HFGS features. However, missense mutations in the HOXA13 homeodomain may act dominantly to cause a more severe HFGS-like phenotype or the Guttmacher syndrome of preaxial deficiency, postaxial polydactyly, and hypospadias. Mouse models of *Hoxa13* deficiency have revealed similar malformations, illustrating the conservation of Hox function and the utility of mouse models for understanding the cellular consequences of *HOX* mutations in humans.

ROLE OF THE LOCUS IN THE DEVELOPMENTAL PATHWAY

HOXA13 is a member of the *AbdB*-like paralogue group of HOX transcription factor proteins that are transcribed early in development. *HOXA13* is the last gene of the *Hoxa* cluster to be activated, and it is expressed in distal structures of the limb and trunk during development. *Hoxa13* is also active in the adult in additional tissues, although its role is not known. Paralogous and nonparalogous compound *Hox* gene mutants exhibit nonallelic noncomplementation, illustrating genetic cooperation in growth and differentiation. *Hox* paralogue group 13 genes, *Hoxa13* and *Hoxd13*, are critical in autopod growth and patterning; development of posterior axial structures, including the distal digestive, urinary, and reproductive tracts; and mesenchymal/endothelial organization in the umbilical artery during embryogenesis. *Hoxa13* and *Hoxd13* expression patterns overlap but are not identical, in abundance or in distribution, in tissues where they are both expressed. Despite the differences, the effects of combined mutations illustrate the cooperative, quantitative nature of their genetic input. In the developing limb, one function of HOXA13 is to promote the growth of mesenchyme, particularly the preaxial tissues that will give rise to the thumbs or great toes, as well as aggregation, cell adhesion, and perichondrial boundary formation in the autopod through regulation of the ephrin A7 (*EphA7*) receptor and EphA3 ligand expression. In the vascular walls of the umbilical arteries, HOXA13 deficiency reduces *EphA7* and *EphA4* expression and there is a failure of cell sorting between the endothelium and the vascular mesenchyme. *Hoxa13* is also expressed early along the length of the müllerian ducts and subsequently restricted in expression to the cervix and vagina. Thus, the role of *Hoxa13* in embryogenesis is both promotion of growth and organization of mesenchymal condensations in the limbs, cellular stratification within the umbilical arteries, as well as definition of tissue boundaries of male and female reproductive organs.

CLINICAL DESCRIPTION

There are two human syndromes associated with mutations in *HOXA13*, HFGS and Guttmacher syndrome. Inherited and sporadic cases of HFGS have been described. Guttmacher syndrome is similar to HFGS but distinct in its expression of postaxial polydactyly and uniphalangeal second toes with nail hypoplasia and has been reported in one family.

HFGS

The first clinical reports of HFGS (OMIM 140000) appeared in 1970 (Stern et al., 1970; Poznanski et al., 1970). Several additional families or cases have since been described and updated (Poznanski et al., 1975; Giedion and Prader, 1976; Elias et al., 1978; Goeminne et al., 1981; Verp et al., 1983; Halal, 1988; Verp, 1989; Cleveland and Holmes, 1990; Donnenfeld et al., 1992; Fryns et al., 1993; Devriendt et al., 1999; Goodman et al., 2000). The clinical manifestations of HFGS are limited to the upper and lower distal limb structures and the urogenital tract. The hallmark in the skeletal system is bilateral thumb and great toe hypoplasia, primarily due to shortening of the distal phalanx and/or the first metacarpal or metatarsal (Fig. 48–1). Shortening is often mild but may be more severe in selected cases (Goodman et al., 2000). There may be limited metacarpophalangeal flexion of the thumb or inability to oppose the thumb and fifth finger. Often, the thenar eminences are hypoplastic. There is very often fifth finger clinodactyly, which is secondary to a shortened middle phalanx. Altered dermatoglyphics of the hands (Stern et al., 1970; Giedion and Prader, 1976; Halal, 1988) have been reported and primarily involve distal placement of the axial triradius, lack of thenar or hypothenar patterning, low arches on the thumbs, thin ulnar loops (deficiency of radial loops and whorls), and a greatly reduced ridge count on fingers. The feet are often short. The great toe may be medially deviated (hallux varus) and is a useful diagnostic clue when present (Cleveland and Holmes, 1990). The nail on the great toe and the size of the calcaneus may be small.

Radiographic findings and a characteristic metacarpophalangeal profile have been described (Poznanski et al., 1970, 1975; see also Giedion and Prader, 1976; Halal, 1988) and include hypoplasia of distal phalanx and first metacarpal of the thumbs and great toes, pointed distal phalanges of the thumb, and the great toes often lack normal tufts. There are selected fusions of the tarsals or carpals; shortening of the calcaneus; occasional bony fusions of the middle and distal phalanges of the second, third, fourth, or fifth toes; and retardation of carpal or tarsal maturation. The metacarpophalangeal profile reflects shortening of the first metacarpal and first and second phalanges, as well as the second phalanx of the second and fifth digits.

There is some minor variation in the severity of the limb defects between individuals; however, the defects are usually very similar bilaterally. Radius/ulna, humerus, tibia/fibula, and femur segments are normal. Ambulation is not affected, although one report described an adult who had difficulty with balance standing upright. Abnormalities of muscle other than thenar hypoplasia have not been reported. The skeletal manifestations within families appear to be the most penetrant, whereas there is variability in the penetrance and/or severity of genital anomalies.

GU problems in females include vesicoureteral reflux secondary to ureteric incompetence, hypospadiac urethra, ectopic ureteral orifices, subsymphyseal epispadias, urinary incontinence, patulous urethra,

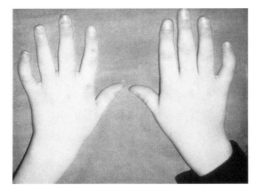

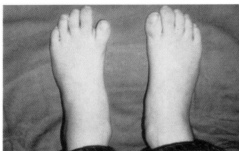

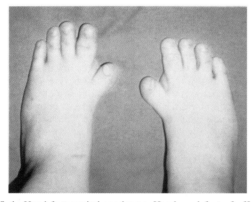

Figure 48–1. Hand-foot-genital syndrome. Hands and feet of affected individuals. Note short thumbs and clinodactyly of the fifth fingers, as well as hypoplastic nails, medial deviation, and shortening of the great toes. (From Mortlock and Innis, 1997, with permission.)

trigonal hypoplasia, and small hymenal opening (Poznanski et al., 1975; Halal, 1988; Verp, 1989; Donnenfeld et al., 1992). Various degrees of incomplete müllerian fusion with or without two cervices or a longitudinal vaginal septum have been reported. Miscarriage or premature labor may occur. The consequences of vesicoureteral reflux or obstruction may include recurrent urinary tract infections and chronic pyelonephritis. Recurrent urinary tract infections may begin in infancy. Renal insufficiency leading to renal transplant was reported in one female individual (Halal, 1988). Surgical correction of ureter placement and bladder outlet as well as removal of longitudinal vaginal septae or hymenectomy for tight constriction ring has been reported. Menstruation is usually of normal onset. The increased risk for premature labor, premature birth, fetal loss, or stillborns is well known in females with varying degrees of incomplete müllerian fusion.

Males may have hypospadias of variable severity with or without chordee. While many are glandular (Giedion and Prader, 1976), two males with grades II and III (Donnenfeld et al., 1992) and one with grade IV (Fryns et al., 1993) hypospadias have been reported.

Of all reports of HFGS-affected males, only one has had a documented history of urinary tract infection (UTI) (Donnenfeld et al., 1992). In this same family, the two affected boys had hypospadias (grades II and III), one had bilateral vesicoureteral reflux (with UTI

history), and the other had uteropelvic junction (UPJ) obstruction. This is the same family reported by Verp et al. (1983, family 1) and updated by Donnenfeld et al. (1992). The extent to which males have had thorough urological evaluations is unknown.

Affected males are not at increased risk for cryptorchidism and are fertile, while HFGS females may have difficulties with premature labor or early pregnancy loss, presumably secondary to uterine structural abnormalities. No anomalies of the prostate or seminal vesicles have been described, although specific examinations of these structures have not been reported.

Other rare reported abnormalities, which may be unrelated to the gene defect, include strabismus (Elias et al., 1978), ventriculoseptal defect (propositus of Stern et al., 1970), inguinal hernia, epididymal cyst, short stature, cervical ribs, supernumerary nipple, late enuresis, lower limit of functioning, onychodysplasia (Halal, 1988), sacral dimple (Fryns et al., 1993), and psychomotor retardation, microcephaly, and hypertelorism (in one of four affected members of a family) (Fryns et al., 1993). External ears are normal in patients with HFGS.

Chromosome analysis of HFGS patients is usually normal. There is one report of a chromosomal deletion involving the entire *HOXA* cluster on chromosome 7p14-15 (Devriendt et al., 1999). In this report, the findings were typical for HFGS but additional anomalies were present, presumably secondary to deletion of the other genes in the *HOXA* cluster or adjacent genes. In reports in which the condition affects multiple family members, HFGS follows an autosomal-dominant pattern of inheritance with complete penetrance, with variability in expression of the urogenital phenotype. Sporadic, new mutation cases have been reported. Only one report (Giedion and Prader, 1976) has described three affected boys of apparently unaffected parents, suggesting the possibility of gonadal mosaicism, a rare autosomal-recessive form, or incomplete penetrance.

Genetic mapping performed on the original family to be described with this disorder localized the mutation near the *HOXA* cluster of genes on 7p14-p15, and a mutation was subsequently identified in the *HOXA13* gene (Mortlock and Innis, 1997). This family had a G-to-A transition leading to the substitution of an invariant tryptophan residue with a premature stop codon (W369X) in the critical DNA-binding homeodomain (Table 48–1). Since the original report, additional mutations have been described in *HOXA13*, including nonsense, missense, and alanine expansion mutations (Goodman et al., 2000; Innis et al., 2002).

Guttmacher Syndrome

Guttmacher syndrome (OMIM 176305) is a dominantly inherited combination of preaxial deficiency, postaxial polydactyly of the hands only, and hypospadias. It was first reported in 1993 in three individuals from a single family (Guttmacher, 1993). Acquisition of developmental milestones, like HFGS, is normal. There are no other known cases.

The skeletal features of affected patients are very similar to those of HFGS (Fig. 48–2), including hypoplastic thumbs and halluces, fifth finger clinobrachydactyly, and hypospadias. However, two of its features, unilateral or bilateral postaxial polydactyly of the hands and short or uniphalangeal second toes with absent nails, are unique and not seen in HFGS patients. Limited range of motion at the interphalangeal joints of the thumbs and uniphalangeal halluces were described. The two affected males had glandular hypospadias. The single female in the family apparently had a normal urinary tract by ultrasound examination, although she had one UTI. Whether or not more common abnormalities of the ureters, as described in HFGS, occur is unknown. Transmission is autosomal-dominant. Two mutations in one allele of *HOXA13* were found in this family (Innis et al., 2002) (Table 48–1).

MOLECULAR GENETICS OF THE LOCUS

Hox genes are members of a highly conserved set of transcription factor genes that were first discovered in *Drosophila* through work on classical mutants, such as Antennapedia (Scott, 1992; Carroll, 1995, and references therein). *Hox* genes are found in all animal species and

Table 48–1. Human *HOXA13* Gene Mutations

Mutation	Exon	nt*;DNA alteration	Protein	Region	Reference
Nonsense-inherited	2	1107;TGG_TGA	W369X	Homeodomain (W48X)#	Mortlock and Innis (1997)
Nonsense-inherited	2	1093;CAG_TAG	Q365X	Homeodomain (Q44X)	Goodman et al. (2000)
Nonsense-de novo	1	407;TCG_TAG‖	S136X		Goodman et al. (2000)
Nonsense-inherited	1	586;CAG_TAG	Q196X		Goodman et al. (2000)
Missense-de novo	2	1114;AAC_CAC	N372H	Homeodomain (N51H)	Goodman et al. (2000)
Missense-inherited†	2	1112;CAG_CTG	Q371L	Homeodomain (Q50L)	Innis et al. (2002)
Deletion-inherited†		-78/-79;del GC	—	Promoter	Innis et al. (2002)
Expansion-inherited	1	ins 18 bases	+6 alanines	Polyalanine 18**	Utsch et al. (2002)
Expansion-inherited	1	387;ins 24 bases	+8 alanines	Polyalanine 18	Goodman et al. (2002)
Expansion-inherited‡	1	ins 27 bases	+9 alanines	Polyalanine 18	
Expansion-inherited§	1	ins 30 bases	+10 alanines	Polyalanine 18	

*nt, nucleotide number of the cDNA beginning with the A of the start codon = +1.
†Guttmacher syndrome (MIM 176305), both mutations on the same allele (Innis et al., 2002).
‡F. Goodman (personal communication).
§T. Williams and J.W. Innis (unpublished).
‖Mistakenly reported originally as an A_C substitution (Goodman et al., 2000).
#With homeodomain residues numbered 1–60.
**This is the largest of three alanine repeats at 18 residues and, like the other two, is encoded by an imperfect trinucleotide repeat (Fig. 48–3).

are united by several distinctive features (see Chapter 46). They are (*1*) related to the *Drosophila* homeotic selector genes, (*2*) arranged in clusters, and (*3*) expressed along the body axis in precise domains that correlate with their relative gene order in the complexes, a feature termed *colinearity* (Duboule and Morata, 1994). Colinearity exhibits both spatial and temporal components. Subsequent to gastrulation and embryonic development, *Hox* genes may be expressed in many organs, even in adults. Examples include *Hoxc13* in the skin (Godwin and Capecchi, 1998; see also Duboule, 1998) and mouse *Hox9* paralogue expression in the adult breast (Chen and Capecchi, 1999). All *Hox* genes contain a 183 bp homeobox that codes for a 60–amino acid helix-turn-helix protein motif called a *homeodomain*, which is capable of binding to DNA (Gehring et al., 1994a,b). In mammals, there are four clusters of *HOX* genes, thought to have arisen through two duplication events from a single ancestral *HOX* cluster composed of

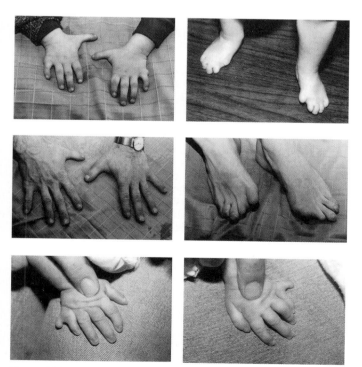

Figure 48–2. Guttmacher syndrome. Phenotype of the hands and feet of individuals with preaxial deficiency, postaxial polydactyly, and hypospadias. Upper left, after excision of extra postaxial digit. Middle left, after excision of right unilateral postaxial digit. Bottom panels, feet not shown. (Reprinted from Guttmacher, 1993, with permission.)

13 genes (Ruddle et al., 1994). The initial duplication of the *HOX* clusters, followed by selective gene loss within individual duplicate clusters, has led to the current arrangement of *HOX* genes in modern mammals. Extant *HOX* genes can be classified by homology as belonging to one of 13 ancestral paralogous groups (Scott, 1992). Of these, HOX paralogue groups 9–13 are most similar to the *Drosophila Abdominal-B* (*AbdB*) gene.

HOX proteins are composed of a 60–amino acid homeodomain (positioned near the C terminus of each protein) and substantial N-terminal amino acid sequences. Binding and functional specificity are regulated by the homeodomain and by cofactor associations with the homeodomain and its N-terminal arm or other parts of the protein (Mann and Chan, 1996; Mann and Affolter, 1998). The amino acid sequences of the homeodomains are highly conserved. Residues that are characteristic of paralogous groups within and around the homeodomains have been identified (Sharkey et al., 1997). Interestingly, the nonhomeodomain regions of HOX protein paralogues diverge greatly and may comprise as much as 80% of the protein. *AbdB*-like HOX proteins interact and stabilize DNA binding by MEIS1 protein, a TALE-class homeodomain-containing transcription factor (Shen et al., 1997; Bürglin, 1997).

Human (*HOXA13*, OMIM 142959) and mouse (*Hoxa13*) genes have two exons (Mortlock et al., 1996; Mortlock and Innis, 1997) (Fig. 48–3). Transcription-initiation sites have been mapped in mouse limb bud (−62 relative to the A residue of the translation-initiation codon) and placental mRNA (Mortlock et al., 1996; Post and Innis, 1999a,b). Northern blot analysis of 11.5-day normal mouse embryonic mRNA revealed the presence of two distinct transcripts of approximately 2.4 and 3.8 kb when hybridized with *Hoxa13*-specific probes. Heterogeneity of transcript size is due to usage of two different AAUAAA polyadenylation signals in the 3′-untranslated region (Mortlock et al., 1996). The first exon is highly GC-rich and is approximately 1 kb in length. The intron is composed of about 700 bp; and the second exon, which encodes the homeodomain, is either 1.4 or 2.8 kb, depending on polyadenylation signal usage. The mRNA splicing position within the coding sequence is identical between the mouse and human genes.

Conceptual translation of the mouse mRNA codes for a 386–amino acid protein of approximately 39 kDa, whereas the human mRNA codes for a protein of 388 amino acids. In vitro transcription/translation assays with mouse *Hoxa13* gene sequences showed initiation of translation at two in-frame methionines, which are separated by 15 amino acids. HOXA13 protein synthesis initiating at the first methionine is expressed in mouse limb buds and in vitro (Post et al., 2000). Whether or not initiation occurs at the second in-frame methionine in vivo is not known; however, initiation at the second methionine would omit a highly conserved protein domain at the amino terminus (Mortlock et al., 2000).

For HOXA13, and like most HOX proteins, the 60–amino acid homeodomain is encoded by the second exon and translation contin-

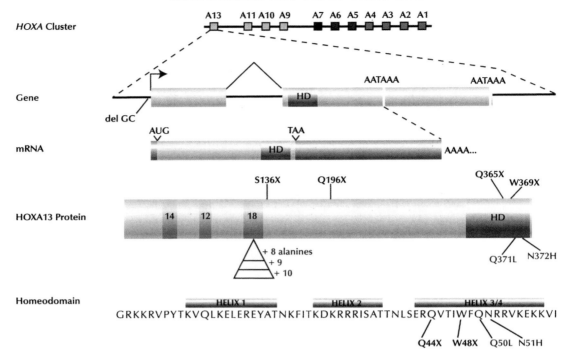

Figure 48–3. Molecular genetics of *HOXA13*. *HOXA13* is located on chromosome 7p14 at the 5′ end of the *HOXA* cluster of genes. See text for additional details. Mutations are indicated. Del GC refers to the 2 bp deletion that is found in the same *HOXA13* allele as the Q50L missense mutation in the homeodomain in Guttmacher syndrome.

ues for seven amino acids after the end of the core homeodomain sequence. The HOXA13 60–amino acid homeodomain sequences of human, mouse, chicken, and axolotl proteins are identical; but they differ slightly from zebrafish HOXA13a and HOXA13b orthologues at positions 2 and 3, respectively (Gardiner et al., 1995; Mortlock et al., 1996; Mortlock and Innis, 1997; A. Kuroiwa, personal communication). Residues immediately amino-terminal to the homeodomain are also very highly conserved, as are selected residues or motifs encoded by the first exon.

HOXA13 protein has three large polyalanine repeats (Mortlock et al., 1996, 2000) of 14, 12, and 18 residues encoded by imperfect trinucleotide repeats in the first exon. Other, shorter alanine repeats are also present in the amino-terminal portion of the protein. Mortlock et al. (2000) amplified N-terminal *Hoxa13* coding sequences from fish, amphibian, reptile, chicken, and marsupial and eutherian mammal genomic DNA. Compared with fish HOXA13, the mammalian protein is larger by 35% owing to accumulation of polyalanine repeats and flanking segments rich in proline, glycine, or serine within the first 215 amino acids. Certain residues and amino acid motifs are strongly conserved, and numerous HOXA13 N-terminal domains were also shared in the paralogous HOXB13, HOXC13, and HOXD13 proteins. Some conserved regions are unique to HOXA13. Two domains highly conserved in HOXA13 orthologues are shared with *Drosophila* AbdB and other vertebrate *AbdB*-like proteins. Marsupial and eutherian mammal HOXA13 proteins have three, large homopolymeric alanine repeats of 14, 12, and 17–18 residues that are absent in reptiles, birds, and fish. Therefore, the repeats arose after the divergence of reptiles from the lineage that gave rise to mammals. In contrast other, short homopolymeric alanine repeats in mammalian HOXA13 have remained virtually the same length, suggesting that forces driving or limiting repeat expansion are context-dependent. Consecutive stretches of identical third-base usage in alanine codons within the large repeats were found, supporting replication slippage as a mechanism for their generation. However, numerous species-specific base substitutions affecting third-base alanine repeat codon positions were observed, particularly in the largest repeat. Since the large alanine repeats were likely present prior to eutherian mammal development, as suggested by the opossum data, a dynamic process of recurring replication slippage (or unequal crossing over) and point mutation within alanine repeat codons could reconcile these observations. Moreover, this process could also account for the numerous proline-, serine-, and glycine-rich codons flanking the largest repeat.

HOXA13 MUTATIONS IN HFGS AND GUTTMACHER SYNDROME

Table 48–1 lists the known mutations in human *HOXA13* relative to the nucleotide sequence and domain structure, and Figure 48–3 depicts the gene position of the mutations, particularly those in the homeodomain in relation to the three α helices. Nonsense, missense, and alanine expansion mutations have been identified in the protein-coding regions of the gene in HFGS patients. In addition, a large chromosomal deletion has been described, which was shown to delete the entire human *HOXA* cluster (Devriendt et al., 1999). Nonsense mutations in the first or second exon have been described, and one missense mutation (N51H) located in the homeodomain was found in one HFGS patient. All mutations in the homeodomain have been confined to the third helix, which is critical for DNA binding.

All of the HFGS in-frame polyalanine expansions (+6, +8, +9, and +10 alanines) identified so far have been localized to the third large repeat (normal length 18), and all are meiotically stable through many generations, unlike typical trinucleotide repeat disorders such as fragile X syndrome. These polyalanine expansions may occur through unequal crossing over (Warren, 1997) or replication slippage. Variations in the length of this largest repeat have been found only in affected HFGS patients and not in controls.

No reported cases of homozygosity for *HOXA13* mutations have been reported. However, a double heterozygote carrying a HOXA13 polyalanine expansion (nine residues) allele and a HOXD13 missense mutation in the homeodomain has been identified (Goodman et al., personal communication).

In Guttmacher syndrome, affected individuals are heterozygous for a novel missense mutation (Q50L) in the HOXA13 homeodomain, which arose on an allele already carrying a 2 bp deletion (del GC −78/−79) (Figs. 48–2, 48–3) in the gene's highly conserved promoter region (Innis et al., 2002). This deletion produces no detectable abnormalities on its own as two individuals carry the promoter mutation without apparent phenotypic abnormalities. The missense mutation, which alters a key residue in the recognition helix of the homeodomain, is likely to perturb HOXA13's DNA-binding properties and appears to have both a loss and a specific gain of function.

GENOTYPE–PHENOTYPE CORRELATIONS

The number of patients with HFGS for whom mutations in HOXA13 have been identified is small. Nonetheless, the HFGS limb phenotype in patients with the four heterozygous nonsense mutations in either exon 1 or 2 as well as the polyalanine expansions are very similar to those described for the patient with cytogenetic deletion of the *HOXA* cluster. Therefore, the typical HFGS features appear to result from HOXA13 haploinsufficiency. Minor differences may be attributable to effects of other genetic loci or stochastic variables.

The two missense mutations (N51H and Q50L) are instructive. The patient with N51H had a more severe HFGS phenotype, and the Guttmacher syndrome family with the Q50L mutation exhibited entirely different features, including postaxial polydactyly in the upper limbs only and uniphalangeal second toes with absent nails. The effects of these mutations on DNA binding have not been examined. However, generally speaking, it appears that *HOXA13* missense mutations may produce more severe HFGS features or unusual digital malformations.

Hypospadias does not always occur in affected males. When it does, it is most often glandular, although there is variability in severity even in males with the same mutation. It appears that females are more likely to have more severe problems in the GU tract than males (Poznanski et al., 1975). Further conclusions are limited by the available information in only a few families.

The variables that determine whether or not a *HOXA13* mutation carrier will develop GU problems are not clear. It is the author's experience, however, that male or female carriers of alanine tract expansions may have increased penetrance and severity of urinary problems. This is not to say that patients with other mutations should not be evaluated thoroughly for GU problems. This tentative observation is supported by the fact that the only reported HFGS males with UTIs, reflux, or UPJ obstruction are those of Donnenfeld et al. (1992), which is the family with the eight-alanine expansion. Females in this same family also stand out in terms of the severity of their GU tract problems (Verp et al., 1983; Donnenfeld et al., 1992).

Similarly, in the family with the 10-residue alanine expansion, there are nine affected females, all of whom have GU problems (Innis, unpublished observations): seven have had recurrent UTIs, incontinence, ureteral reflux, or misplaced urethra and two have had only a longitudinal vaginal septum. Eight have had surgery including hymenectomy, laparoscopy, cystoscopy, intravenous pyelography (IVP), urethral size reduction, and uterine surgery for incomplete müllerian fusion. In this family, there are 15 affected males. Of the four for whom medical information is available, three have glandular hypospadias.

In a German HFGS family (Becker et al., 2002; Utsch et al., 2002), a six-alanine repeat expansion was described. The affected male proband had glandular hypospadias, and both his affected mother and grandmother had uterus bicornus unicollis with double cervix. The mother also had a longitudinal vaginal septum. Unfortunately, no information could be obtained regarding the urinary tract in the affected individuals.

Therefore, while the proposed correlation between alanine repeat mutations and severity of urinary tract problems in general is tentative and needs to be examined more rigorously with other families, it may be that carriers of a polyalanine expansion are more likely to have urinary tract problems, particularly if they are females.

ESTABLISHING THE DIAGNOSIS

A thorough examination must be performed including the hands, feet, and genitalia. The characteristic hand abnormalities, primarily small thumbs and fifth finger clinodactyly, along with small great toes, possibly with hallus varus, should prompt suspicion of HFGS. Radiographs of the skeleton are very helpful as skeletal defects are 100% penetrant and the diagnosis can be made from these films (Poznanski et al., 1970). Ears are normal in HFGS and in Guttmacher syndrome,

and major anomalies in other systems are usually not seen in HFGS. Familial involvement with autosomal-dominant inheritance is supportive of the diagnosis. GU defects are the most variable and should be examined for in every patient suspected of HFGS. However, since the hand and foot anomalies can be mild, patients with HFGS may present for medical evaluation of recurrent miscarriage, UTI, incontinence, ureteral reflux, or hypospadias. Women found to have incomplete müllerian fusion of any degree should have a thorough evaluation of their hands and feet, as well as assessment of bladder/ureter function and urethral competence. Males with hypospadias, while commonly observed in isolation or in combination with other syndromes, should have a thorough evaluation of their hands and feet. Numerous disorders with aplastic or hypoplastic thumbs, often with other anomalies, are known that should be considered in the differential diagnosis of HFGS.

Perhaps the most similar syndromes in the differential diagnosis include those affecting both the thumbs/hallaces and the müllerian derivatives. Pinsky (1974) described a community of acral/genital or distal limb/müllerian malformation syndromes. These include camptobrachydactyly (Edwards and Gale, 1972), vaginal atresia/polydactyly (McKusick et al., 1964), HFGS, and three additional syndromes that also had external and/or middle ear anomalies. Several additional reports of individuals with similar clinical findings affecting the digits and reproductive tract have been described since. Hennekam (1989) reported a family with moderately shortened hallaces, incomplete müllerian fusion, and small, thickened, dysplastic helices but without hand anomalies or the typical HFGS metacarpophalangeal profile. No detectable mutation in *HOXA13* could be identified in this patient (Goodman et al., 2000). A report by Halal (1986) described a unique family with müllerian duct anomalies and upper limb hypoplasia of varying severity, and Michels and Caskey (1979) described two cases of müllerian aplasia and hypoplastic thumbs. Whether or not these are the result of mutations in *HOX* genes is unknown. Analysis of *HOX* gene structure in such candidate syndromes should be facilitated by the availability of primer sets recently described for all *HOX* genes (Kosaki et al., 2002).

Prenatal ultrasound visualization of short thumbs or great toes may suggest the diagnosis, but its accuracy is unknown. Prenatal *HOXA13* DNA mutation analysis has not been reported.

KNOWN THERAPIES

Serious clinical consequences of *HOXA13* mutations relate primarily to the GU and reproductive systems, which may require medical therapy or surgery. Ureteral reflux has been documented in both sexes. Individuals with clinical findings compatible with HFGS should have formal urological evaluation including renal imaging and IVP and/or voiding cystourethrogram to examine for vesicoureteral reflux. Recurrent UTI may be improved by prophylactic antibiotic therapy. Knowledge of the anatomy of the uterus in affected individuals is helpful prospectively in the management of pregnancy and delivery.

COUNSELING AND PROGNOSIS

Autosomal-dominant inheritance with 100% penetrance and variable expression has been observed. Skeletal severity may vary slightly within a family and is not often associated with fine motor problems. Urogenital defects are variable. Intelligence and life span are normal. Medical problems primarily revolve around GU reflux and complications, incontinence, and pregnancy loss or premature labor. Surgery may be required to reimplant ureters or correct hypo- or epispadias, incontinence, or other urological complications. Longitudinal vaginal septum and other forms of incomplete müllerian fusion should have formal obstetric evaluation. Renal transplant has been reported in one patient.

NATURAL AND ENGINEERED MUTATIONS IN ORTHOLOGOUS GENES

A considerable understanding of the consequences of *HOXA13* mutation has been derived from studies in mice. Early expression studies followed by careful phenotypic characterization of spontaneous and targeted null alleles in mice, as well as mouse and chick misexpression experiments, have shown important quantitative and qualitative roles for HOXA13 in development. In the following discussion, segments of the developing limb are referred to as the *autopod* (hand or foot), *zeugopod* (radius/ulna or tibia/fibula), or *stylopod* (humerus or femur).

Expression

The mouse *Hoxa13* gene is expressed in the developing limb buds, urogenital structures, distal gastrointestinal tract, umbilical arteries, and isolated placenta (Haack and Gruss, 1993; Mortlock et al., 1996; Fromental-Ramain et al., 1996a; Warot et al., 1997; Stadler et al., 2001). *Hoxa13* expression begins at embryonic day (e) 10.5 in the forelimb in wild-type mice, and mutant mice show visible effects of *Hoxa13* deficiency approximately 24 (*Hypodactyly*) to 48 (targeted mutants) hours later.

Human and mouse *AbdB*-like *HOXA* gene expression has also been evaluated in the female reproductive tract by *in situ* hybridization (Taylor et al., 1997; Ma et al., 1998; Post and Innis, 1999b). Using probes to *Hoxa9*, *-a10*, *-a11*, and *-a13*, expression was demonstrated for all genes along the length of the developing paramesonephric duct in the embryonic mouse. From as early as e16.5 to 2 weeks of age, spatial restriction of the anterior and posterior extents of expression of the *Hoxa* genes becomes apparent: *Hoxa9* in the oviduct, *Hoxa10* and *Hoxa11* in the uterus, *Hoxa11* and *Hoxa13* in the uterine cervix, and only *Hoxa13* in the vagina. Expression in these structures continues into adult life with the same spatial tissue restriction. Adult human tissues showed the same spatial expression pattern along the length of the müllerian derivatives. *HOXA13* is strongly expressed in the cervix and the vaginal epithelium below the keratin as they are in the mouse. Therefore, there is strong conservation of the *Hoxa* expression domains from mice to humans, which persists postnatally even though the mouse has a bicornuate uterus and humans have a unicornuate uterus. Therefore, early HOX expression may promote growth of the müllerian duct, but later spatial restriction in both humans and mice is associated with definition of the identities of sections of the reproductive tract rather than the overall plan or shape of the müllerian derivatives.

At e12.5, mouse *Hoxa13* is expressed in the mesenchyme of the developing genital tubercle, the mesenchyme around the urogenital sinus, and the sinus epithelium. At e14.5, expression is observed also in the distal portions of the müllerian and wolffian (mesonephric) ducts, the wall of the developing urinary bladder, as well as the walls of the umbilical arteries (Warot et al., 1997; Stadler et al., 2001). Newborn males also exhibit expression in the prostate, seminal vesicles, and bulbourethral gland. *Hoxa13* is believed to play an important role in prostate ductal morphogenesis and clefting in the seminal vesicle (Warot et al., 1997; Podlasek et al., 1999, 2002). Females show abundant expression in the developing cervix and vagina (Warot et al., 1997; Post and Innis, 1999b), the urethral mesenchyme and epithelia, and, importantly, the points of entrance of the ureters into the bladder. *Hoxa13* is also expressed in the epithelia, not the muscular layer, of the hindgut and rectum.

Reverse transcription PCR studies also show expression of *Hoxa13* in mouse skeletal muscle, lung, bladder, ascending and descending colon, appendix, and placenta (Mouse Genome Informatics Database, www.informatics.jax.org). Weaker signals have been detected in whole brain, heart, long bones, paw, ileum, and cervix.

The expression and function of *Hoxa13* have also been explored in the chick. *Hoxa13* is expressed in the developing chick limb bud beginning at stage 22. After spreading across the entire autopod, *Hoxa13* expression begins to be excluded from areas of mesenchymal condensation except for the perichondrium (Yokouchi et al., 1991; Nelson et al., 1996). Therefore, cells actively condensing to form cartilage downregulate the mRNA abundance for *Hoxa13*.

In addition, HOXA13 protein is expressed within limb myoblasts restricted to the posterior part of the dorsal/ventral muscle masses in chick wings and legs (Yamamoto et al., 1998). Expression of HOXA13 protein is the first indication of the segregation of myogenic cells into dorsal and ventral muscle masses. HOXA13 expression in chick au-

topodal mesenchyme requires the apical ectodermal ridge (AER), not the zone of polarizing activity (ZPA), whereas posterior myogenic cell HOXA13 expression is dependent on the ZPA and not the AER. Bone morphogenetic protein 2 (BMP2) is capable of inducing, and NOGGIN/CHORDIN of downregulating, the expression of HOXA13 from the posterior muscle masses, implying that the ZPA may mediate the positive induction of HOXA13 via BMP2. Thus, HOXA13 expression in muscle precursors requires signals distinct from the nonmuscle mesenchyme of the developing limb bud.

The axolotl is a urodele amphibian (*Ambystoma mexicanum*) that has been a model system for experimental regeneration of amputated limbs (Gardiner et al., 1995). Axolotl *Hoxa13* is expressed during limb development and upregulated very early during regeneration of limbs in the mesenchyme. Subsequent to blastema formation, *Hoxa13* becomes distally restricted, whereas *Hoxa9* is expressed throughout the blastema, expression patterns more akin to the developmental "nested" expression pattern. Thus, axolotl limbs are capable of reactivating expression of *Hox* genes during regeneration, and *Hoxa13* expression is one of the earliest markers for this intriguing process.

Mouse Mutants

A natural, spontaneous mutation and several targeted gene disruptions of mouse *Hoxa13* have been described. All *Hoxa13* mutants exhibit defects of the limbs, GU tract, and, as homozygotes, embryonic lethality. *Hypodactyly* (*Hoxa13^Hd*) is a mutation in *Hoxa13* that arose spontaneously (Hummel, 1970). Heterozygous mutants have shortening of the first digit on all four feet (Fig. 48–4), and this phenotype was the clue that led to the identification of *HOXA13* mutation in human HFGS (Mortlock and Innis, 1997). Mice homozygous for *Hoxa13^Hd* have only a single digit on each paw (Hummel, 1970; Mortlock et al., 1996). Heterozygous *Hoxa13^Hd/+* mouse skeletal defects are 100% penetrant and identifiable without molecular typing. Targeted mutants have been constructed by homologous recombination in embryonic stem cells (Fromental-Ramain et al., 1996a; Stadler et al., 2001). Targeted

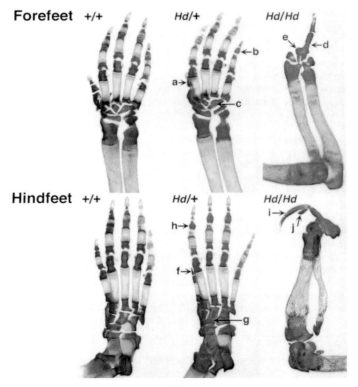

Figure 48–4. Hypodactyly (*Hoxa13^Hd*) forelimbs and hindlimbs. See text for details. Arrows: *a* and *f*, hypoplastic digit 1; *b* and *h*, delayed ossification phalanx 2; *c* and *g*, carpal or tarsal fusions; *d* and *e*, incompletely formed digit and carpal; *i* and *j*, one digit with rudimentary anterior metatarsal. (Reprinted from Mortlock et al., 1996, with permission.)

Hoxa13+/− heterozygous mouse mutants have a subtler, incompletely penetrant phenotype, with no alteration of the first metatarsal or proximal phalanx, whereas *Hoxa13Hd/+* heterozygotes frequently exhibit such shortening. Homozygous mutants of both mutations are more severely affected than the heterozygote, and *Hoxa13Hd/Hd* mutants have considerably more severe limb abnormalities than the targeted homozygous mutants. In addition, *in utero* (e11.5–e15.5) lethality is uniform in targeted mutants; however, rare, liveborn male and female *Hoxa13Hd/Hd* mice, many of which grow to adulthood, have been described (Mortlock et al., 1996; Robertson et al., 1996, 1997; Post and Innis, 1999a,b). *Hoxa13* homozygous mutant mice die in utero secondary to umbilical artery stenosis (Warot et al., 1997), not from an effect of lack of expression in the placenta as mutants have no placental phenotype (Mortlock et al., 1996; Warot et al., 1997). Alterations in the terminal structures of the GU and digestive tracts in both males and females of both natural and targeted mutations have been described (Warot et al., 1997; Post and Innis, 1999b). Despite documented expression of the *Hoxa13* gene in other tissues of the mouse, abnormalities in structures other than the limbs and GU tracts have not been described.

Hypodactyly (*Hoxa13Hd*)

Limbs. *Hoxa13Hd/Hd* embryos begin to show a slight reduction in the amount of anterior limb bud tissue in the developing autopod beginning at approximately e11.5–e12 (Mortlock et al., 1996; Robertson et al., 1996, 1997; Post and Innis, 1999a). Whole-mount in situ hybridization with antisense *Hoxa13* RNA probes has shown that the expression pattern of the mutant mRNA is normally distributed in the autopod, although its abundance appears increased (Post and Innis, 1999a). In heterozygous mutant forelimbs and hindlimbs, complete penetrance of digit 1 reduction is observed. Reduction varies from shortening of the nail to loss of the terminal phalanx or of two phalanges. Incomplete penetrance was observed for alterations in the timing of ossification events in specific cartilaginous elements of the autopod, and fusions of carpals or tarsals also were observed. Specifically, in the forelimb, there are often delays in metacarpal ossification and digit 5 second phalanx ossification as well as abnormal d1-d2-c carpal fusion and d4 carpal ossification (Mortlock et al., 1996). In the hindlimbs, there are delays in the ossification of the second phalanges of digits 2 and 5 and inappropriate cuneiforme3-naviculare tarsal fusion. Limb malformations are symmetrical in individual *Hoxa13Hd/+* and *Hoxa13Hd/Hd* animals, and radius/ulna and tibia/fibula elements are normal.

Robertson et al. (1996) showed that *Hoxa13Hd/Hd* limb buds exhibit increased cell death and that the AER persists longer than expected. *Hoxa13Hd/Hd* cells formed fewer cartilage nodules in micromass cultures compared to wild-type or heterozygous mutant cells. This effect was cell-autonomous and not secondary to an inhibitory factor secreted into the medium by mutant cells. This was hypothesized to be a defect in aggregation or in cartilage differentiation, leading to delay or abnormal patterning of the mutant limb buds.

Post and Innis (1999a) showed not only increased cell death but also that cell death and narrowing of the *Hoxd13* RNA expression domain in the autopods of *Hoxa13Hd/Hd* mice distinguish them from targeted *Hoxa13−/−* mice. Through alternate strain crosses, genetic background was excluded as the basis for the phenotypic differences between *Hoxa13Hd/Hd* and targeted mutants. In addition, compound heterozygotes (*Hoxa13−/Hd*) exhibit a phenotype intermediate to either homozygote, suggesting a unique, negative role of the *Hoxa13Hd* allele during limb development.

Urogenital Structures. Heterozygous *Hoxa13Hd/+* mice are normal in all respects in terms of apparent reproductive and urinary function. Heterozygous mutant males have abnormalities of the accessory sex organs (Podlasek et al., 1999). The seminal vesicles are derivatives of the wolffian ducts, sites of *Hoxa13* expression. Of *Hoxa13Hd/+* mutants, 86% had smaller seminal vesicles with an abnormal semicircular shape and markedly reduced secondary and tertiary branching. Other wolffian duct derivatives, including the epididymis, ductus deferens, and ampullary gland, were normal. Of the GU sinus deriv-

atives, the coagulating gland showed fewer than two main ducts per lobe in 29% of heterozygotes but normal numbers of duct tips. The dorsolateral prostate and ventral prostate gland showed size reductions in half of the mutants examined, with a significant reduction in the number of duct tips. Despite these abnormalities, heterozygous *Hoxa13Hd/+* males are fertile, and mendelian ratios are observed for normal and mutant offspring of heterozygous males and females (Post and Innis, 1999b). Heterozygous *Hoxa13Hd/+* females exhibit anterior transformation of cervical tissue to a uterine stromal phenotype, which is accentuated in the homozygote and occasionally includes uterus-specific glands in the transformed cervical region. The columnar-to-squamosal epithelial transition that characterizes mature cervical–vaginal tissue is positioned within uterus-like stroma rather than cervical tissue in these mutants, suggesting that this postnatal developmental transition occurs independently of the underlying stromal characteristics (Post and Innis, 1999b).

Hoxa13Hd/Hd mice of both sexes usually die *in utero*, although a few survive and 25 (7 males and 18 females) have been evaluated (Post and Innis, 1999b). *Hoxa13Hd/Hd* females survive more frequently to birth than males. Surviving adult *Hoxa13Hd/Hd* homozygotes of both sexes are infertile. *Hoxa13Hd/Hd* adult females produce apparently functional germ cells as determined by superovulation and ovarian histology but exhibit profound hypoplasia of the cervix and vaginal cavity and a marked reduction of the anovaginal distance. *Hoxa13* expression is localized to the cervical and vaginal tissues, consistent with the observed defects. Adult *Hoxa13Hd/Hd* males have a severely hypoplastic and misshapen penian bone and are incapable of copulating. The penian bone develops by a combination of endochondral and intramembranous ossification, but the defects observed in *Hoxa13Hd/Hd* males are limited to the region of endochondral bone formation. Thus, infertility in *Hoxa13Hd/Hd* homozygous mutants is related to hypoplasia of the vaginal cavity and cervix in females and deficiency of the os penis in males. Mutants also occasionally exhibit vesicouterine fistula and hydronephrosis (Mortlock et al., 1996), similar to *Hoxa13−/+/Hoxd13−/−* mutants (Warot et al., 1997). These findings suggest that the *Hoxa13Hd* mutation has negative effects beyond simple *Hoxa13* loss in GU development, like the limb, perhaps through cell death or inhibition of *Hoxd* function. The defects in *Hoxa13Hd/Hd* mutants have many similarities to those of targeted *Hoxa13−/−/Hoxd13−/−* double-mutants.

Molecular Genetics. *Hoxa13Hd* is a 50 bp deletion within the coding sequences of the first exon of *Hoxa13* (Mortlock et al., 1996). The *Hoxa13Hd* deletion does not interfere with steady-state mRNA levels. The *Hoxa13Hd* deletion is a simultaneous loss- and gain-of-function allele of *Hoxa13*. Post et al. (2000) showed that the *Hoxa13Hd* deletion results in a translational frameshift that leads to the loss of wild-type HOXA13 protein and the simultaneous production of a novel, stable protein in the limb buds of mutant mice. The mutant protein was shown to consist of the first 25 amino acids of the wild-type HOXA13 sequence, followed by 275 amino acids of a novel arginine- and lysine-rich sequence, and the protein lacks the homeodomain. Like wild-type HOXA13, the mutant protein is localized to the nucleus in transfected COS-7 cells, perhaps mediated by the arginine- and lysine-rich peptide sequences encoded by the mRNA after the translational frameshift. Misexpression of the mutant mRNA throughout the developing limb bud in transgenic mice led to reduction or absence of proximal and distal (autopod) limb structures. It was proposed that production of the mutant protein leads to profound loss of digits in the autopod of *Hoxa13Hd/Hd* mice, making them more severely affected compared with targeted mutants. The existence of the novel protein in GU structures has not been examined.

Targeted *Hoxa13* Mutant Mice

Fromental-Ramain et al. (1996a) created two different targeted *Hoxa13* gene disruptions using embryonic stem cell technology. In the first, a neomycin resistance cassette (Neo^r) was inserted into the EcoRV site of the homeobox, disrupting the HOXA13 protein sequence in the middle of the second α helix of the homeodomain (Fig. 48–2). In the second, a 2.8 kb deletion encompassing the first exon, intron, and coding portion of the second exon was constructed. The phenotypes of mice with the Neo^r cassette insertion in the homeodomain and the gene deletion were identical.

Stadler et al. (2001) reported the phenotype of two *Hoxa13* loss-of-function alleles created by insertion of a *GFPneo* gene into the *Hoxa13* homeodomain also using homologous recombination in embryonic stem cells. Neo^r was removed in one strain by Cre-mediated recombination of flanking lox sites, leaving only the *GFP* gene inframe with the *Hoxa13* coding sequences. Both mice had similar phenotypes in heterozygous and homozygous form and were similar to those of Fromental-Ramain et al. (1996a).

Limbs. The four targeted null alleles of *Hoxa13* exhibit limb phenotypes in heterozygous or homozygous mutant mice that are very similar to each other. However, other than for in utero death, the limb phenotypes are milder compared to *Hypodactyly* mice, as described above. In contrast to the *Hypodactyly* mouse mutant, targeted *Hoxa13*$^{-/-}$ mutants can be analyzed only up until e15.5 when in utero death prevents further examination. Targeted heterozygotes (*Hoxa13*$^{+/-}$) show incomplete penetrance for a missing or shortened digit 1 in the forelimbs and an altered terminal phalanx in the hindlimbs. Incomplete penetrance of the soft tissue syndactyly of digits 2 and 3 is observed in the hindlimbs. Homozygote forelimbs and hindlimbs exhibit fully penetrant loss of digit 1, lack of second phalanges in digits 2 and 5, webbing between digits 2 and 3, and significantly delayed carpal condensations. Digit 5 condensation is delayed in mutant forelimbs and very small in the hindlimbs. Digits 2, 3, and 5 of the forelimbs and hindlimbs are smaller, yet the second phalangeal elements of digits 2 and 5 are absent in the forelimbs while those elements of all hindlimb digits are missing at e15.5. The distal radius/ulna and tibia/fibula zeugopod segments are normal. Mice homozygous for a null allele of *Hoxa13* (*Hoxa13*$^{-/-}$) have four digits on each paw but no digit 1. Neither heterozygous nor homozygous *Hoxa13* mutant mice exhibit polydactyly.

Urogenital Structures. Targeted heterozygous *Hoxa13*$^{+/-}$ mutants have apparently normal GU structures. Since targeted *Hoxa13* null homozygotes die in utero between e11.5 and e15.5, examination of the GU phenotypes in embryos at e13.5 and e14.5 was performed by Warot et al. (1997). At these stages in normal embryos, the wolffian and müllerian ducts are closely apposed to the GU sinus. However, *Hoxa13*$^{-/-}$ mutant ducts at this stage are far away and the GU sinuses of *Hoxa13*$^{-/-}$ mutants are hypoplastic. The caudal segments of the developing müllerian ducts are small or nonexistent at e14.5 in mutants; thus, absence or delay in their growth results from HOXA13 deficiency. Ureter development, beginning with sprouting from the wolffian/mesonephric ducts, is not appropriate in *Hoxa13*$^{-/-}$ mutants either in that proximity to the GU sinus is too far rostral to be appropriately incorporated into the bladder. *Hoxa13*$^{-/-}$ mutant bladder development is also severely impaired and noticeable by poor development of the rostral extension of the GU sinus. Thus, the poor placement of the ureters relative to the developing bladder in mouse mutants may offer an explanation for the abnormal positioning of the ureters and ureteral reflux in humans with *HOXA13* mutations.

A synergistic effect of *Hoxa13* and *Hoxd13* in GU development is also observed (Warot et al., 1997; Kondo et al., 1997).

DEVELOPMENTAL PATHOGENESIS

Skeletal Phenotype of HFGS and Guttmacher Syndrome

Haploinsufficiency for HOXA13 in humans appears to be the underlying mechanism for most cases of HFGS. This is supported by comparison of individuals with nonsense point mutations with the patient carrying the chromosomal *HOXA* cluster deletion and by analysis of the phenotypes of engineered and natural mouse mutants.

All *HOXA13* in-frame polyalanine expansions appear to create null alleles since patients with these mutations have a phenotype compatible with haploinsufficiency. It is unknown whether this results from downregulation of mutant allele transcription, mutant mRNA instability, reduced translation, protein mislocalization or degradation, or

normal protein quantity with reduced transcriptional activity. These *HOXA13* alanine expansion mutations stand in contrast with *HOXD13* polyalanine expansions in human and mouse synpolydactyly, wherein a dominant effect of the mutant allele increases with increasing length of the expansion and is associated with impairment of function, but not expression, of other *Hoxd* genes (Goodman et al., 1997; Bruneau et al., 2001; Albrecht et al., 2002).

The two reported missense mutations (N51H, Q50L) may lead to more severe outcomes or unique phenotypes; however, firm conclusions cannot be made given the small number of patients. Nonetheless, it is instructive to consider how such phenotypes may occur and how gain-of-function effects may be exerted.

The Q50L missense mutation in the homeobox is critical in the Guttmacher syndrome phenotype. Residue 50 lies in the recognition helix of the homeodomain, with the glutamine side chain positioned within the major groove of the DNA. A glutamine residue is present at this position in all invertebrate and vertebrate HOX proteins; however, other homeodomain-containing transcription factors have a variety of different amino acids at this position, including lysine, serine, histidine, cysteine, alanine, glycine, and isoleucine (Gehring et al., 1994a; Bürglin, 1997). Residue 50 was shown to be a key determinant of the DNA-binding specificity of different homeodomains (Hanes and Brent, 1989; Treisman et al., 1989; Schier and Gehring, 1992). More recent structural studies have confirmed this observation but have added that its contribution to binding affinity and specificity depends on the identity of the amino acid occupying the position (Tucker-Kellogg et al., 1997; Fraenkel and Pabo, 1998; Grant et al., 2000). The type of interaction, whether by hydrogen bonding or van der Waals' forces, is dependent on the identity of the amino acid at this position. These forces affect binding affinity and may affect in vivo functional characteristics. For example, an engineered Q50A substitution in the engrailed homeodomain results in only a twofold reduction in DNA-binding affinity at a TAA**TTA** engrailed consensus binding site, but a Q50K substitution changes the binding site preference to TAAT**CC**, with significantly increased affinity (Ades and Sauer, 1994). The only naturally occurring missense mutation previously reported at this position is Q50P in the HLXB9 homeodomain (Hagan et al., 2000), which is predicted to result in complete loss of function due to disruption of the α-helical structure of the recognition helix (see Chapter 46). The Q50L mutation may not affect protein stability in this way, yet it almost certainly changes HOXA13's DNA-binding properties.

Several features of Guttmacher syndrome suggest that the Q50L mutation leads to loss of normal HOXA13 activity. The combination of hypoplastic thumbs and halluces, fifth finger clinobrachydactyly, and hypospadias is typical in HFGS caused by different nonsense mutations in *HOXA13*. Loss of HOXA13 activity in Guttmacher syndrome probably results from altered DNA binding by the HOXA13^{Q50L} mutant protein at normal HOXA13 target sites or at least a subset of these sites.

However, haploinsufficiency cannot explain the two additional features that distinguish Guttmacher syndrome from HFGS: postaxial polydactyly of the hands and uniphalangeal second toes with absent nails (Fig. 48–3). These features do not occur in any of the patients or mouse mutants described above with mutations only in *Hoxa13* and cannot therefore be attributed to loss of HOXA13 activity. Their presence suggests that the Q50L mutation also produces a specific gain of function. This could result from altered DNA binding or transcriptional activity by the HOXA13^{Q50L} mutant protein at a subset of normal HOXA13 target sites and/or at novel target sites, especially sites normally bound by other homeodomain proteins. Interestingly, 6%, 30%, and 50% of *Hoxd12*$^{+/-}$, *Hoxd13*$^{+/-}$, and *Hoxd13*$^{-/-}$ mice, respectively, have a rudimentary extra postaxial digit in the forelimbs, as do 80%–86% of *Hoxd12*$^{+/-}$/*Hoxd13*$^{+/-}$ *trans*-heterozygotes (Dollé et al., 1993; Davis and Capecchi, 1996; Kondo et al., 1996). Moreover, compound *Hoxd13*$^{-/-}$ *Hoxa13*$^{+/-}$ mutants have as many as seven digits in the forelimbs, as do mice homozygous for a deletion that removes *Hoxd11*, *Hoxd12*, and *Hoxd13* (Fromental-Ramain et al., 1996a; Zákány et al., 1997). Similarly, patients heterozygous for specific mutations in *HOXD13* have postaxial polydactyly of the feet (Muragaki et al., 1996; Goodman et al., 1998; see Chapter 47), and patients homozygous for a polyalanine tract expansion in HOXD13 can have up to eight rudimentary digits in the hands (Akarsu et al., 1995). The postaxial polydactyly in Guttmacher syndrome might therefore stem from functional interference by the HOXA13^{Q50L} mutant protein with one or more of the posterior HOXD proteins expressed in the developing forelimb autopod. This possibility is even more compelling considering that the Q50L mutation also leads to some loss of HOXA13 function. The two additional digital abnormalities in Guttmacher syndrome differ in the hands (an extra sixth digit) and feet (a hypoplastic second digit), whereas the digital abnormalities in patients with typical HFGS are always analogous in all four limbs. This suggests that the gain of function exerted by the HOXA13^{Q50L} mutant protein may involve different target genes or different target gene effects in the upper as opposed to the lower limbs.

The other reported missense mutation in *HOXA13*, a *de novo* N51H substitution in the homeodomain (Goodman et al., 2000), causes severely hypoplastic thumbs, absent halluces, rudimentary first metatarsals, and short second to fifth digits due to middle phalanx hypoplasia, with neither postaxial polydactyly nor terminal phalangeal involvement of the second toes. Two amino acid substitutions affecting adjacent residues in the HOXA13 recognition helix, which might be expected to have similar functional consequences, thus give rise to quite distinct limb phenotypes, suggesting that each perturbs DNA binding or transcriptional activity in a specific, different way. It will be interesting to explore these differences further once bona fide target genes and relevant binding sequences have been identified.

HOXA13 and GU Development

The effects of the *HOXA13* mutations on GU development suggest that there have been significant constraints on the structure and expression of HOXA13 during evolution because HOXA13 alterations could have had deleterious consequences on the development of the genitalia and, thus, reproductive fitness. However, mice heterozygous for *Hoxa13* null mutations exhibit minor features of the skeleton and no GU phenotype, whereas humans have very similar skeletal malformations yet often serious GU defects, particularly in females. This could result from fundamental differences in the way that HOXA13 is utilized in the GU tracts of mice and humans or, once again, differences in expression or paralogue group functional redundancy.

Evaluation of the patterns of *Hoxa* gene expression in mouse and human müllerian derivatives shows conservation of spatial expression patterns and persistence of expression throughout adults. This observation in both bicornuate (mice) and unicornuate (humans) müllerian derivatives suggests that the mechanisms that determine the ultimate shape of the uterus may not be dependent on *Hoxa* expression. Instead, incomplete müllerian fusion in humans in HOXA13 deficiency appears to be secondary to a defect in distal müllerian duct proliferation.

The work of Zhao and Potter (2001) also supports the view that one role of *Hox* genes in the müllerian duct is to define qualitative features. *Hoxa13* homeodomain swapping for that of *Hoxa11* results in differentiation of the reproductive tract in areas of endogenous *Hoxa11* expression to cervix/vagina identity. Therefore, the various forms of incomplete müllerian fusion, especially those without limb anomalies suggestive of *HOXA13* mutation, may more likely be secondary to non-*HOX* gene defects. In addition, cases of müllerian hypoplasia or aplasia present in the human population may more likely represent individual *HOX* mutations or perhaps simultaneous knockout of expression of multiple *HOXA* genes due to disruption of a müllerian-duct specific *cis*-acting element or enhancer protein.

Function of HOXA13 in Limb Morphogenesis

Much of our understanding of *Hox* gene function in mammals derives from studies in which the genes have been disrupted by targeted homologous recombination in mouse embryonic stem cells. The human mutations that have been described also extend our knowledge of conservation of *HOX* gene functions as well as our understanding of the effects of novel mutations on phenotype.

Evaluation of the phenotypes of mice with single- and double-mutants has shown that HOX genes function in areas of autopodal expression in redundant, quantitative ways and in qualitative ways to promote morphological development in vertebrates. The concept of cooperation and redundancy of function of Hox paralogues and non-paralogues in limb morphogenesis has been reviewed (Rijli and Chambon, 1997).

The phenotypic consequences of single *Hox* gene loss often differ between paralogues, even those expressed in identical distributions. Such differences at the single-gene level have been interpreted to mean that the genes may have redundant or common functional targets as well as functions unique to each. Combined loss of paralogous genes, however, results in loss of structures, demonstrating strong genetic interactions of both genes in controlling growth and patterning of these structures. However, until recently, the distinctions between single-mutants could not be conclusively proven to be due to special attributes of each protein or other causes. Greer et al. (2000) showed that mouse *Hoxd3* and *Hoxa3* can fully substitute for one another, giving rise to a normal phenotype, suggesting that they are equivalent functionally even when expressed from the other allele. Such equivalence may not mean that each gene in its own context is expressed the same as the other paralogue(s) in each cell type but that apparent qualitative differences observed in single gene mutants may reflect quantitative variation in individual protein expression in specific cell types. This model would imply that there is a common set of target genes capable of sensing minor differences in levels of expression. Where differences in timing or expression domains of paralogues exist, the potential for unique functions increases. In this model, variation in the total amount of paralogue mRNA, the rate of mRNA translation, and protein posttranslational modifications could be levels of control over the output of HOX activity.

In the limb, similar quantitative involvement has been proven by nonallelic non-complementation exhibited by mice deleted for several *Hox* genes; however, important differences exist. For example, *Hoxa11/Hoxd11* double-mutants lack almost all of the radius and ulna. Paralogous *Hoxa9* and *Hoxd9* single-mutants also show unique phenotypes, though clearly nonequivalent functions in stylopod development were found in double-mutants (Fromental-Ramain et al., 1996b). In this pair, *Hoxa9* loss in the stylopod is fully compensated by *Hoxd9*, whereas the reverse is not true.

Hoxa13 and *Hoxd13* single-mutants or combined double/single-mutants of each combination show distinct phenotypes (Fromental-Ramain et al., 1996a). Human HOXA13 haploinsufficiency alone causes similar defects to heterozygous null *Hoxa13* mouse mutants, implying a conserved role for HOXA13 in mice and humans. In *Hoxa13* mouse mutants, there is no primary digit 1 condensation in the forelimbs or hindlimbs, suggesting that the contribution of *Hoxa13* to digit 1 development is early. In these situations, wild-type *Hoxd13* (or other Hox expression in the autopod) gene dosage is insufficient to rescue loss of *Hoxa13*. Additional loss of *Hoxd13* results in loss of separate autopodal structures, as would be expected if group 13 gene dosage were critical for autopod development. However, the thumbs and great toes in mice and humans are unique and dependent on HOXA13 alone for growth. This may be partly explained by the patterns of expression of *Hoxd13* and *Hoxa13*. *Hoxa13* appears to reach more anteriorly and proximally within the autopod, particularly early in development (Nelson et al., 1996; Post and Innis, 1999a). Differences in the abundance and distribution of *Hoxa13* and *Hoxd13* expression are very evident in the developing GU tract as well (Warot et al., 1997). Therefore, HOXA13 dosage is critical, by itself, in the preaxial region of the developing autopod early, and heterozygous effects in humans and mice carrying null alleles are expected and observed. Interestingly, adding additional Hox dosage to the thumb or great toe region might be expected to change the growth outcome of those mesenchymal condensations. Transgenic overexpression of HOXA13 in chick limbs occasionally induces an extra anterior digit in the wings and legs (Yokouchi et al., 1995). In addition, transgenic overexpression of *Hoxd12* in the developing autopod induces triphalangeal thumbs or preaxial mirror-image duplications secondary to ectopic anterior Sonic hedgehog (Shh) expression (Knezevic et al., 1997).

Therefore, the emerging picture is that after the duplications of the ancestral Hox cluster, apparent divergence in paralogue function has come about by changes in the domains of expression, timing, and expression level for individual members in cells, rather than by variation in the properties of each paralogue. Such regulatory changes are likely to be important in the phenotypic differences between species, and mutations in the *cis*-acting regulatory sequences are candidates in certain forms of congenital malformation. To date, no regulatory mutations have been identified in human *HOX* genes, although a promoter mutation in the human *HOXA13* gene, without apparent phenotypic effect by itself, has been described in Guttmacher syndrome (Innis et al., 2002). A predictable consequence of a dysregulated posterior *Hox* gene in developing human limbs might be phocomelia or other segmental deficiencies or perhaps polydactyly depending on which gene was expressed and what domain was involved. Identification of enhancer and insulator elements for *Hox* gene limb expression may facilitate exploration for mutations in conditions hypothesized to be secondary to altered human *HOX* gene regulation.

Regulatory Targets of *HOX* Genes

The role of *HOX* gene expression is to regulate the expression of genes to promote selective growth and differentiation of developing or developed structures. In *Drosophila*, expression of many genes is affected in HOM/Hox mutants, suggesting that many, if not all, genes are regulated directly or indirectly by HOX proteins (Liang and Biggin, 1998) and that regulation occurs at many levels of the hierarchy of genetic networks (Weatherbee et al., 1998). If, as expected, this occurs with vertebrate HOX proteins, it remains to be determined what genes in what hierarchies are influenced to what magnitude to influence morphogenetic outcomes in tissues. Clearly, HOX paralogue protein dosage is critical to morphogenetic outcome, as revealed by non-allelic noncomplementation, and has been interpreted to indicate that HOX proteins have common regulatory targets. So far, it appears that some targets of *Hox* gene regulation in the limbs include the *Hox* genes themselves and cell adhesion molecule receptors or ligands.

HOX proteins regulate each other, and there are important qualitative differences between individual gene products. This conclusion is derived from studies showing strong qualitative effects of HOX proteins ectopically expressed in regions more anterior or proximal than usual. In such natural or experimental situations, it has been observed that more posterior *HOX* proteins generally exert functional dominance over other (normally more anterior) HOX gene products, giving rise to malformations or "posterior" transformations of axial or limb structures. This interesting aspect of HOX function, noted initially in *Drosophila* (termed *phenotypic suppression*) and subsequently in mice (*posterior prevalence*), is poorly understood at the molecular level (reviewed by Botas, 1993; Duboule and Morata, 1994).

In the mouse mutant *Ulnaless*, for example, the expression domains of *Hoxd12* and *Hoxd13* in the limb bud are expanded anteriorly and proximally and *Hoxd12* expression is reduced in the autopod. Mutants also show *Hoxd11* reduction of expression in the autopod as well as the zeugopod. The unlinked *Hoxa11* gene is also reduced in expression. This suggested that the reduction in size of the radius and ulna, like the absence of *Hoxd11* and *Hoxa11* in targeted mutants, is secondary to downregulation of expression by the posterior *Hoxd13* and *Hoxd12* gene products (Peichel et al., 1997; Hérault et al., 1997). Similar reductions in zeugopod size were also observed in cases of *Hoxd13* misexpression in chickens and as a consequence of certain targeted mutants in mice (van der Hoeven et al., 1996; Goff and Tabin, 1997). *Hoxa13* misexpression as described in the chick was also associated with reduction of growth of zeugopodal elements, presumably secondary to downregulation of expression of more proximal genes (Yokouchi et al., 1995).

Furthermore, the closely related *AbdB*-like orthologues *Hoxa13* and *Hoxa11* are not functionally equal. In the experiments described above by Zhao and Potter (2001), who replaced the endogenous *Hoxa13* homeobox with that encoded by the *Hoxa11* sequence, the forelimbs of mutants demonstrated shortening of the radius and ulna and the histology of the mutant uterus revealed a homeotic transformation to a cervical/vaginal histology. Interestingly, the mutant kidney, male reproductive tract, and axial skeleton were normal. The effects of *Hoxa11*^{a13HD} expression on uterine and limb development indicate that the *Hoxa13* and the *Hoxa11* homeoboxes, despite being very

closely related, are not functionally equivalent and point to important qualitative differences in morphological outcome promoted by individual HOX proteins.

HOXA13 also controls morphogenesis by regulating cell adhesion and aggregation. A role for *Hoxa13* in promoting cell adhesion was suggested by early data with chicken models and in *Hypodactyly* mutant mice (Yokouchi et al., 1995; Robertson et al., 1996). In the chick, HOXA13 misexpression promoted shortening of proximal skeletal elements and HOXA13-expressing cells harvested from infected limbs self-associated in mixed limb bud cultures. Thus, HOXA13 was felt to induce the capacity for limb bud mesenchyme to associate and form aggregations akin to prechondrogenic condensations.

Impaired cell adhesion in limb buds would help to explain the delay in condensation of precartilaginous autopodal elements in *Hoxa13* mutant mice. New data confirm a role for HOXA13 in promoting cell adhesion and mesenchymal aggregation in the developing limb bud mesenchyme, as well as organization of the mesenchymal–endothelial cell boundary of the umbilical arteries through regulation of ephrin receptor/ligand expression (Stadler et al., 2001).

REFERENCES

Ades SE, Sauer RT (1994). Differential DNA-binding specificity of the engrailed homeodomain: the role of residue 50. *Biochemistry* 33: 9187–9194.

Akarsu AN, Akhan O, Sayli BS, Sayli U, Baskaya G, Sarfarazi M (1995). A large Turkish kindred with syndactyly type II (synpolydactyly). 2. Homozygous phenotype? *J Med Gen* 32: 435–441.

Albrecht AN, Schwabe GC, Stricker S, Boddrich A, Wanker EE, Mundlos S (2002). The synpolydactyly homolog (spdh) mutation in the mouse—a defect in patterning and growth of limb cartilage elements. *Mech Dev* 112: 53–67.

Becker K, Brock D, Ludwig M, Bidlingmaier F, Albers N, Lentze MJ, Utsch B (2002). Das dominant vererbte Hand-Fuβ-Genital-Syndrom: Malformationen der distalen Extremitäten mit Fehlbildungen des Urogenitaltraktes. *Monatsschr Kinderh* (in press).

Botas J (1993). Control of morphogenesis and differentiation by HOM/Hox genes. *Curr Opin Cell Biol* 5: 1015–1022.

Bruneau S, Johnson KR, Yamamoto M, Kuroiwa A, Duboule D (2001). The mouse *Hoxd13*^{spdh} mutation, a polyalanine expansion similar to human type II synpolydactyly (SPD), disrupts the function but not the expression of other *Hoxd* genes. *Dev Biol* 237: 345–353.

Bürglin TR (1997). Analysis of TALE superclass homeobox genes (*MEIS, PBC, KNOX, Iroquois, TGIF*) reveals a novel domain conserved between plants and animals. *Nucleic Acids Res* 25: 4173–4180.

Carroll SB (1995). Homeotic genes and the evolution of arthropods and chordates. *Nature* 376: 479–485.

Chen F, Capecchi MR (1999). Paralogous mouse *Hox* genes, *Hoxa9, Hoxb9*, and *Hoxd9*, function together to control development of the mammary gland in response to pregnancy. *Proc Natl Acad Sci USA* 96: 541–546.

Cleveland RH, Holmes LB (1990). Hand-foot-genital syndrome: the importance of hallux varus. *Pediatr Radiol* 20: 339–343.

Davis AP, Capecchi MR (1996). A mutational analysis of the 5′ HoxD genes: dissection of genetic interactions during limb development in the mouse. *Development* 122: 1175–1185.

Devriendt K, Jaeken J, Matthijs G, Van Esch H, Debeer P, Gewillig M, Fryns J-P (1999). Haploinsufficiency of the *HOXA* gene cluster in a patient with hand-foot-genital syndrome, velopharyngeal insufficiency, and persistent patent ductus Botalli. *Am J Hum Genet* 65: 249–251.

Dollé P, Dierich A, LeMeur M, Schimmang T, Schuhbaur B, Chambon P, Duboule D (1993). Disruption of the *Hoxd-13* gene induces localized heterochrony leading to mice with neotenic limbs. *Cell* 75: 431–441.

Donnenfeld AE, Schrager DS, Corson SL (1992). Update on a family with hand-foot-genital syndrome: hypospadias and urinary tract abnormalities in two boys from the fourth generation. *Am J Med Genet* 44: 482–484.

Duboule D (1998). *Hox* is in the hair: a break in colinearity? *Genes Dev* 12: 1–4.

Duboule D, Morata G (1994). Colinearity and functional hierarchy among genes of the homeotic complexes. *Trends Genet* 10: 358–364.

Edwards JA, Gale RP (1972). Camptobrachydactyly: a new autosomal dominant trait with two probable homozygotes. *Am J Hum Genet* 24: 464–474.

Elias S, Simpson JL, Feingold M, Sarto G (1978). The hand-foot-uterus syndrome: a rare autosomal dominant disorder. *Fertil Steril* 29: 239–240.

Fraenkel E, Pabo CO (1998). Comparison of X-ray and NMR structures for the Antennapedia homeodomain–DNA complex. *Nat Struct Biol* 5: 692–697.

Fromental-Ramain C, Warot X, Messadecq N, LeMeur M, Dolle P, Chambon P (1996a). *Hoxa-13* and *Hoxd-13* play a crucial role in the patterning of the limb autopod. *Development* 122: 2997–3011.

Fromental-Ramain C, Warot X, Lakkaraju S, Favier B, Haack H, Birling C, Dierich A, Dolle P, Chambon P (1996b). Specific and redundant functions of the paralogous *Hoxa-9* and *Hoxd-9* genes in forelimb and axial skeleton patterning. *Development* 122: 461–472.

Fryns JP, Vogels A, Decock P, van den Berghe H (1993). The hand-foot-genital syndrome: on the variable expression in affected males. *Clin Genet* 43: 232–234.

Gardiner DM, Blumberg B, Komine Y, Bryant SV (1995). Regulation of HoxA expression in developing and regenerating axolotl limbs. *Development* 121: 1731–1741.

Gehring WJ, Affolter M, Bürglin T (1994a). Homeodomain proteins. *Annu Rev Biochem* 63: 487–526.

Gehring WJ, Qian YQ, Billeter M, Furukubo-Tokunaga K, Schier AF, Resendez-Perez D, Affolter M, Otting G, Wuthrich K (1994b). Homeodomain-DNA recognition. *Cell* 78: 211–223.
Giedion A, Prader A (1976). Hand-foot-uterus (HFU) syndrome with hypospadias: the hand-foot-genital (HFG) syndrome. *Pediatr Radiol* 4: 96–102.
Godwin AR, Capecchi MR (1998). *Hoxc13* mutant mice lack external hair. *Genes Dev* 12: 11–20.
Goeminne L (1981). Syndroom van Poznanski-Stern. *Tijdschr Geneeskunde* 37: 1461–1465.
Goff DJ, Tabin CJ (1997). Analysis of Hoxd-13 and Hoxd-11 misexpression in chick limb buds reveals that *Hox* genes affect both bone condensation and growth. *Development* 124: 627–636.
Goodman F, Scambler P (2001). Human *HOX* gene mutations. *Clin Genet* 59: 1–11.
Goodman FR, Mundlos S, Muragaki Y, Donnai D, Giovannuci-Uzielli ML, Lapi E, Majewski F, McGaughran J, McKeown C, Reardon W, et al. (1997). Synpolydactyly phenotypes correlate with size of expansions in *HOXD13* polyalanine tract. *Proc Natl Acad Sci* USA 94: 7458–7463.
Goodman FR, Giovannucci-Uzielli ML, Hall C, Reardon W, Winter R, Scambler P (1998). Deletions in *HOXD13* segregate with an identical, novel foot malformation in two unrelated families. *Am J Hum Genet* 63: 992–1000.
Goodman FR, Bacchelli C, Brady AF, Brueton LA, Fryns J-P, Mortlock DP, Innis JW, Holmes LB, Donnenfeld AE, Feingold M, et al. (2000). Novel *HOXA13* mutations and the phenotypic spectrum of hand-foot-genital syndrome. *Am J Hum Genet* 67: 197–202.
Grant RA, Rould MA, Klemm JD, Pabo CO (2000). Exploring the role of glutamine 50 in the homeodomain–DNA interface: crystal structure of engrailed (Gln50 → Ala) complex at 2.0 Å. *Biochemistry* 39: 8187–8192.
Greer JM, Puetz J, Thomas KR, Capecchi MR (2000). Maintenance of functional equivalence during paralogous *Hox* gene evolution. *Nature* 403: 661–665.
Guttmacher AE (1993). Autosomal dominant preaxial deficiency, postaxial polydactyly, and hypospadias. *Am J Med Genet* 46: 219–222.
Haack H, Gruss P (1993). The establishment of murine Hox-1 expression domains during patterning of the limb. *Dev Biol* 157: 410–422.
Hagan DM, Ross AJ, Strachan T, Lynch SA, Ruiz-Perez V, Wang YM, Scambler P, Custard E, Reardon W, Hassan S, et al. (2000). Mutation analysis and embryonic expression of the *HLXB9* Currarino syndrome gene. *Am J Hum Genet* 66: 1504–1515.
Halal F (1986). A new syndrome of severe upper limb hypoplasia and müllerian duct anomalies. *Am J Med Genet* 24: 119–126.
Halal F (1988). The hand-foot-genital (hand-foot-uterus) syndrome: family report and update. *Am J Med Genet* 30: 793–803.
Hanes S, Brent R (1989). DNA specificity of the bicoid activator protein is determined by homeodomain recognition helix residue 9. *Cell* 57: 1275–1283.
Hennekam RCM (1989). Acral-genital anomalies combined with ear anomalies. *Am J Med Genet* 33: 454–455.
Herault Y, Fraudeau N, Zakany J, Duboule D (1997). *Ulnaless* (*Ul*), a regulatory mutation inducing both loss-of-function and gain-of-function of posterior *Hoxd* genes. *Development* 124: 3493–3500.
Hummel K (1970). *Hypodactyly*, a semidominant lethal mutation in mice. *J Hered* 61: 219–220.
Innis JW (1997). Role of *HOX* genes in human development. *Curr Opin Pediatr* 9: 617–622.
Innis JW, Goodman FR, Bacchelli C, Williams TM, Mortlock DP, Sateesh P, Scambler PJ, McKinnon W, Guttmacher AE (2002). A *HOXA13* allele with a missense mutation in the homeobox and a dinucleotide deletion in the promoter underlies Guttmacher syndrome. *Hum Mutat* 19: 573–574.
Knezevic V, Santo RD, Schughart K, Huffstadt U, Chiang C, Mahon KA, Mackem S (1997). *Hoxd-12* differentially affects preaxial and postaxial chondrogenic branches in the limb and regulates *Sonic hedgehog* in a positive feedback loop. *Development* 124: 4523–4536.
Kondo T, Dollé P, Zákány J, Duboule D (1996). Function of posterior *HoxD* genes in the morphogenesis of the anal sphincter. *Development* 122:2651–2659.
Kondo T, Zakany J, Innis JW, Duboule D (1997). Of fingers, toes and penises. *Nature* 390:29.
Kosaki K, Kosaki R, Suzuki T, Yoshihashi H, Sasaki K, Tomita M, McGinnis W, Matsuo N (2002). A complete mutation analysis panel of the 39 human *HOX* genes. *Teratology* 65: 47–49.
Liang Z, Biggin MD (1998). Eve and ftz regulate a wide array of genes in blastoderm embryos: the selector homeoproteins directly or indirectly regulate most genes in *Drosophila*. *Development* 125: 4471–4482.
Ma L, Benson G, Hyunjung L, Dey S, Maas R (1998). *Abdominal B* (*AbdB*) Hoxa genes: regulation in adult uterus by estrogen and progesterone and repression in müllerian duct by the synthetic estrogen diethylstilbestrol (DES). *Dev Biol* 197: 141–154.
Mann RS, Affolter M (1998). Hox proteins meet more partners. *Curr Opin Genet Dev* 8: 423–429.
Mann RS, Chan S-K (1996). Extra specificity from extradenticle: the partnership between HOX and PBX/EXD homeodomain proteins. *Trends Genet* 12: 258–262.
McKusick VA, Bauer RL, Koop CE, Scott RB (1964). Hydrometrocolpos as a simply inherited malformation. *J Amer Med Assoc* 189: 813–816.
Michels V, Caskey CT (1979). Müllerian aplasia with hypoplastic thumbs: two case reports. *Int J Gynaecol Obstet* 17: 6–10.
Mortlock DP, Innis JW (1997). Mutation of *HOXA13* in hand-foot-genital syndrome. *Nat Genet* 15: 179–180.
Mortlock DP, Post LC, Innis JW (1996). The molecular basis of Hypodactyly (*Hd*): a deletion in *Hoxa13* leads to arrest of digital arch formation. *Nat Genet* 13: 284–289.
Mortlock DP, Sateesh P, Innis JW (2000). Evolution of N-terminal sequences of the vertebrate HOXA13 protein. *Mamm Genome* 11: 151–158.
Muragaki Y, Mundalos S, Upton J, Olsen BR (1996). Altered growth and branching patterns in synpolydactyly caused by mutations in HOXD13. *Science* 222: 548–551.
Nelson CE, Morgan BA, Burke AC, Laufer E, DiMambro E, Murtaugh LC, Gonzales E, Tessarollo L, Parada LF, Tabin C (1996). Analysis of *Hox* gene expression in the chick limb bud. *Development* 122: 1449–1466.
Peichel CL, Prabhakaran B, Vogt TF (1997). The mouse *Ulnaless* mutation deregulates posterior *HoxD* gene expression and alters appendicular patterning. *Development* 124: 3481–3492.
Pinsky L (1974). A community of human malformation syndromes involving the müllerian ducts, distal extremities, urinary tract, and ears. *Teratology* 9: 65–80.
Podlasek CA, Clemens JQ, Bushman W (1999). *Hoxa-13* gene mutation results in abnormal seminal vesicle and prostate development. *J Urol* 161: 1655–1661.
Podlasek C, Houston J, McKenna KE, McVary KT (2002). Posterior *Hox* gene expression in developing genitalia. *Evol Dev* 4: 142–163.
Post LC, Innis JW (1999a). Altered Hox expression and increased cell death distinguish *Hypodactyly* from *Hoxa13* null mice. *Int J Dev Biol* 43: 287–294.
Post LC, Innis JW (1999b). Infertility in adult *Hypodactyly* mice is associated with hypoplasia of distal reproductive structures. *Biol Reprod* 61: 1402–1408.
Post LC, Margulies EH, Kuo A, Innis JW (2000). Severe limb defects in *Hypodactyly* mice result from expression of a novel, mutant HOXA13 protein. *Dev Biol* 217: 290–300.
Poznanski AK, Stern AS, Gall JC (1970). Radiographic findings in the hand-foot-uterus syndrome (HFUS). *Radiology* 95: 129–134.
Poznanski AK, Kuhns LR, Lapides J, Stern AM (1975). A new family with the hand-foot-genital syndrome—a wider spectrum of the hand-foot-uterus syndrome. *Birth Defects* 11: 127–135.
Rijli FM, Chambon P (1997). Genetic interactions of *Hox* genes in limb development: learning from compound mutants. *Curr Opin Genet Dev* 7: 481–487.
Robertson KE, Chapman MH, Adams A, Tickle C, Darling SM (1996). Cellular analysis of limb development in the mouse mutant *Hypodactyly*. *Dev Genet* 19: 9–25.
Robertson KE, Tickle C, Darling SM (1997). *Shh*, *Fgf4* and *Hoxd* gene expression in the mouse limb mutant hypodactyly. *Int J Dev Biol* 41: 733–736.
Ruddle FH, Bartels JL, Bentley KL, Kappen C, Murtha MT, Pendleton JW (1994). Evolution of *HOX* genes. *Annu Rev Genet* 28: 423–442.
Schier AF, Gehring W (1992). Direct homeodomain–DNA interaction in the regulation of the *fushi-tarazu* gene. *Nature* 356: 804–807.
Scott MP (1992). Vertebrate homeobox gene nomenclature. *Cell* 71: 551–553.
Sharkey M, Graba Y, Scott MP (1997). *Hox* genes in evolution: protein surfaces and paralog groups. *Trends Genet* 13: 145–151.
Shen W-F, Montgomery JC, Rozenfeld S, Moskow JJ, Lawrence HJ, Buchberg AM, Largman C (1997). AbdB-like Hox proteins stabilize DNA binding by the Meis1 homeodomain proteins. *Mol Cell Biol* 17: 6448–6458.
Stadler HS, Higgins KM, Capecchi MR (2001). Loss of *Eph-receptor* expression correlates with loss of cell adhesion and chondrogenic capacity in *Hoxa13* mutant limbs. *Development* 128: 4177–4188.
Stern AM, Gall JC, Perry BL, Stimson CW, Weitkamp LR, Poznanski AK (1970). The hand-foot-uterus syndrome. *J Pediatr* 77: 109–116.
Taylor HS, Vanden Heuvel GB, Igarashi P (1997). A conserved *Hox* axis in the mouse and human female reproductive system: late establishment and persistent adult expression of the *Hoxa* cluster genes. *Biol Reprod* 57: 1338–1345.
Thompson A, Nguyen L (2000). Amegakaryocytic thrombocytopenia and radio-ulnar synostosis are associated with *HOXA11* mutation. *Nat Genet* 26: 397–398.
Treisman J, Gonczy P, Vashishtha M, Harris E, Desplan C (1989). A single amino acid can determine the DNA binding specificity of homeodomain proteins. *Cell* 59: 553–562.
Tucker-Kellogg L, Rould MA, Chambers KA, Ades SE, Sauer RT, Pabo CO (1997). Engrailed (Gln50 → Lys) homeodomain–DNA complex at 1.9 Å resolution: structural basis for enhanced affinity and altered specificity. *Structure* 5: 1047–1054.
Utsch B, Becker K, Brock D, Lentze M, Bidlingmaier F, Ludwig M (2002). A novel stable polyalanine [poly(A)] expansion in the HOXA13 gene associated with hand-foot-genital syndrome: proper function of poly(A)-harbouring transcription factors depends on a critical repeat length? *Hum Genet* 110: 488–494.
van der Hoeven F, Zakany J, Duboule D (1996). Gene transpositions in the *HOXD* complex reveal a hierarchy of regulatory controls. *Cell* 85: 1025–1035.
Veraksa A, Del Campo M, McGinnis W (2000). Developmental patterning genes and their conserved functions: from model organisms to humans. *Mol Genet and Metab* 69: 85–100.
Verp MS (1989). Urinary tract abnormalities in hand-foot-genital syndrome. *Am J Med Genet* 32: 555.
Verp MS, Simpson JL, Elias S, Carson S, Sarto G, Feingold M (1983). Heritable aspects of uterine anomalies. I. Three familial aggregates with müllerian fusion anomalies. *Fertil Steril* 40: 80–85.
Warot X, Fromental-Ramain C, Fraulob V, Chambon P, Dolle P (1997). Gene dosage-dependent effects of the *Hoxa-13* and *Hoxd-13* mutations on morphogenesis of the terminal parts of the digestive and urogenital tracts. *Development* 124: 4781–4791.
Warren ST (1997). Polyalanine expansion in synpolydactyly might result from unequal crossing over of *HOXD13*. *Science* 275: 408–409.
Weatherbee SD, Halder G, Kim J, Hudson A, Carroll S (1998). Ultrabithorax regulates genes at several levels of the wing-patterning hierarchy to shape the development of the *Drosophila* haltere. *Genes Dev* 12: 1474–1482.
Yamamoto M, Gotoh Y, Tamura K, Tanaka M, Kawakami A, Ide H, Kuroiwa A (1998). Coordinated expression of *Hoxa-11* and *Hoxa-13* during limb muscle patterning. *Development* 125: 1325–1335.
Yokouchi Y, Sasaki H, Kuroiwa A (1991). Homeobox gene expression correlated with the bifurcation process of limb cartilage development. *Nature* 353: 443–445.
Yokouchi Y, Nakazato S, Yamamoto M, Goto Y, Kameda T, Iba H, Kuroiwa A (1995). Misexpression of *Hoxa-13* induces cartilage homeotic transformation and changes cell adhesiveness in chick limb buds. *Genes Dev* 9: 2509–2522.
Zákány J, Fromental-Ramain C, Warot X, Duboule D (1997). Regulation of number and size of digits by posterior *Hox* genes: a dose-dependent mechanism with potential evolutionary implications. *Proc Natl Acad Sci USA* 94: 13695–13700.
Zhao Y, Potter SS (2001). Functional specificity of the *Hoxa13* homeobox. *Development* 128: 3197–3207.

49 | Transcription Factors Involved in Disorders of Forebrain and Pituitary Development

KATHRYN WOODS AND MEHUL T. DATTANI

The pituitary gland is a central regulator of growth, reproduction, and homeostasis. During embryogenesis, complex molecular pathways are established to define the development of the pituitary. Given the close anatomical and developmental relationship between the forebrain and anterior pituitary any aberration in this process will impinge not only on the development of the anterior pituitary, but also on the development of other structures, particularly other forebrain structures, the developing eye, and the cerebellum. This suggestion has been borne out by descriptions of the genetic basis of syndromes affecting the pituitary, such as septo-optic dysplasia (SOD). Elucidation of the molecular basis of disorders affecting solely the pituitary and syndromes in which the pituitary is but one component can lead to a better understanding of the complex genetic pathways that result in normal patterning of the forebrain and structures such as the anterior pituitary.

DEVELOPMENT OF THE PITUITARY GLAND

The pituitary gland is a central regulator of growth, metabolism, and development in children. Its complex functions are mediated via hormone-signaling pathways that regulate the finely balanced homeostatic control in vertebrates. These hormone-signaling pathways coordinate signals from the hypothalamus to the peripheral endocrine organs, such as the thyroid, adrenal gland, and gonads. The pituitary gland consists of two main lobes, the anterior and posterior lobes, with a smaller intermediate lobe. The anterior and intermediate lobes are derived from the oral ectoderm, while the posterior lobe is derived from the neural ectoderm (Schwind, 1928; Kaufman et al., 1992).

Development of this gland follows a similar pattern in a number of different species but has been best studied in rodents such as the mouse and rat. In the mouse, anterior pituitary development occurs in four distinct stages: pituitary placode formation, development of the rudimentary Rathke's pouch, formation of the definitive pouch, and terminal differentiation of the various cell types in a temporally and spatially regulated manner (Simmons et al., 1990; Japon et al., 1994).

The onset of pituitary organogenesis coincides with a thickening of the oral ectoderm on embryonic day (E) 8.0 in mice. It has been postulated that a signal from the neural ectoderm induces this thickening of the underlying oral ectoderm, with subsequent formation of Rathke's pouch. Molecules such as fibroblast growth factor 8 (FGF8), bone morphogenetic protein 4 (BMP4), and Nkx2.1 (Lazzaro et al., 1991; Ericson et al., 1998; Takuma et al., 1998), which are expressed in the neural ectoderm and not in Rathke's pouch, are thought to play a significant role in normal anterior pituitary development, as illustrated by the phenotype of mouse mutants that are either null or hypomorphic for these alleles. Following induction of the pituitary placode, this then invaginates on E8.5 to form the rudimentary Rathke's pouch, from which the anterior and intermediate lobes derive.

Rathke's pouch develops in a two-step process that requires at least two sequential inductive signals from the diencephalon. First, the induction and formation of the pouch rudiment are dependent on BMP4. Second, FGF8, which is also present in the hypothalamus and not in Rathke's pouch, activates the key regulatory genes LIM homeobox 3 (*Lhx3*) and *Lhx4*, which are essential for subsequent development of the pouch rudiment into a definitive pouch (Takuma et al., 1998).

During the second stage of pituitary development, the oral ectodermal epithelial pouch continues to bud upward, while the posterior part of the diencephalon evaginates downward to form the infundibulum. The pouch makes direct cell–cell contact with the neuroepithelium of the nascent diencephalon at E8.5–9.0 (Jacobsen et al., 1979). This apposition of Rathke's pouch and the diencephalon is maintained throughout the early stages of pituitary organogenesis, with no inward movement and proliferation of mesodermal cells at this stage; and this close relationship together with various animal experimental manipulations has long suggested that inductive tissue interactions are involved in the process (Takuma et al., 1998).

From E9.5 onward, mesodermal cells migrate into this area and proliferate, thus ensuring separation of the brain and oral cavities. The fact that the oral and neural ectodermal tissues maintain contact during this structural rearrangement implies that direct contact and signaling between these two structures is still essential for this stage of pituitary organogenesis. Formation of the definitive pouch occurs between E10.5 and E12.0. The pouch epithelium continues to proliferate as it closes and separates from the underlying oral ectoderm, forming the definitive Rathke's pouch abutting the neurally derived infundibulum. The pouch is still connected to the oral cavity via an epithelial stalk; however, continued growth upward of the pouch leads to thinning of this stalk, with eventual loss of the connection.

The final stage of pituitary gland development entails the terminal differentiation of the progenitor cells into the distinct cell types found within the mature pituitary gland. To facilitate the correct cell specification, a morphogenetic code must be established so that at any point within the pituitary a cell can maintain its identity. This polarization of the pituitary gland is initiated by genes for extrinsic factors such as *Fgf8*, *Bmp2*, and *Bmp4*, which emanate from the surrounding tissues, namely, the infundibulum and the juxtapituitary mesenchyme. The effect of the signaling molecules on the anterior pituitary gland is to establish gradients of transcription factors intrinsically with *Lhx3*, *Six3*, *Prophet of Pit1* (*Prop1*), and *Nkx3.1* being expressed dorsoventrally and *Islet-1* (*Isl1*), *Lhx4*, *Six1*, *Brain-4* (*Brn4*), and *Pituitary–forkhead* (*P-frk*) being expressed ventrodorsally (Sheng et al., 1997; Treier et al., 1998; Sheng and Westphal, 1999). These genetic gradients lead to a wave of cell differentiation along the ventrodorsal axis, with ventral thyrotrope and corticotrope cells being the first to differentiate, followed by somatotrope, dorsal thyrotrope, gonadotrope, and lactotrope cell differentiation in a precise temporal and spatial pattern. The progenitors of the hormone-secreting cell types proliferate ventrally from the pouch between E12.5 and E15.5 to populate what will form the anterior lobe. The mature anterior pituitary gland is populated by five neuroendocrine cell types, each defined by the hormone produced: corticotropes (corticotropin), thyrotropes (thyrotrophin), gonadotropes (luteinizing hormone [LH], follicle-stimulating hormone [FSH]), somatotropes (growth hormone [GH]), and lactotropes (prolactin [PRL]) (for review see Dasen and Rosenfeld, 1999). The remnants of the dorsal portion of the pouch form the intermediate lobe, containing the melanotrope cell type that produces the hormone proopiomelanocortin (POMC), the precursor protein to the melanocyte-stimulating hormone (MSH), and endorphins. Each of the five anterior pituitary cell types differentiates in a temporally and spatially regulated manner (Simmons et al., 1990; Japon et al., 1994), and this process is dependent on a number of transcription factors. A tissue-specific POU domain factor, POU1F1 (PIT1), is required for the terminal differentiation, growth, and survival of somatotropes, lactotropes, and thyrotropes (Li et al., 1990; Aarskog et al., 1997), while

Figure 49–1. Schematic of pituitary development, highlighting the numerous genes known to be important.

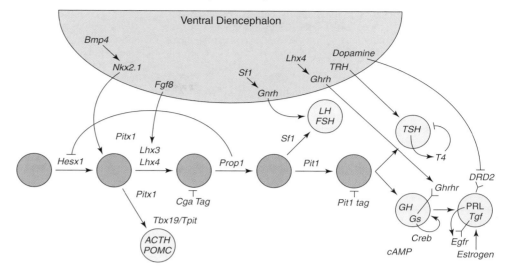

the nuclear receptor steroidogenic factor-1 (Sf1) is expressed later in the nascent gonadotrope lineage (Ingraham et al., 1994). The paired-domain transcription factor Prop1 appears to be essential for the determination of the gonadotrope lineage as well as the Pou1f1-dependent lineage in humans (Li et al., 1990).

Hence, a number of transcription factors and signaling molecules are implicated in the various stages of pituitary gland development (Figs. 49–1, 49–2). The current understanding of the complex interactions that occur during the development of the pituitary is shown in Figure 49–1, including the various genes implicated in the formation of a normal pituitary gland. At the far left, the cells within the primordium of the pituitary are competent to differentiate into all cell types. Following expression of the earliest markers of pituitary gland development (e.g., *Hesx1*), further signaling pathways are established, whereby signals emanate from within the pituitary gland proper and from the ventral diencephalon and then direct these cells toward terminal differentiation of the cell types of the pituitary. Figure 49–2 indicates the time of expression of some of the important molecules implicated in pituitary development. The genes that are expressed early are implicated initially in organ commitment but may also be involved in the downstream regulation of genes that have specific roles in directing the cells toward a particular fate.

In comparison with the rodent, little is known about pituitary de-

velopment in humans. However, it appears that the embryological development of the human pituitary mirrors that seen in the rodent. Spontaneous or artificially induced mutations in the mouse have led to significant insights into human pituitary disease, and identification of mutations associated with human pituitary disease have in turn been invaluable in defining the genetic cascade responsible for the development of this embryological tissue.

MUTATIONS LEADING TO PITUITARY DISEASE IN HUMANS

For some time now, the significance of genes expressed as the pituitary cells commit to a particular cell fate has been known, and mutations within genes such as *GH-1* and *GH-releasing hormone receptor* (*GHRHR*) have been extensively documented (Procter et al., 1998; Lin-Su and Wajnrajch, 2002). Only recently have mutations been described within the genes expressed earlier in the developmental pathway. In humans, developmental defects of the pituitary are rare and characterized by a highly variable phenotype, even between affected individuals within the same family. Patients usually present with deficiencies in one or more of the hormones secreted by the anterior pituitary and are classified as having either an isolated hormone deficiency, e.g., GH deficiency (GHD), or combined pituitary hormone

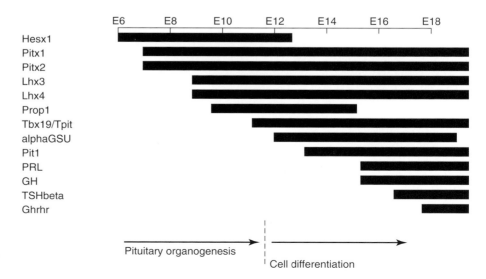

Figure 49–2. Onset and length of expression of various pituitary genes.

deficiency (CPHD). These hormonal deficits can also be described as part of a syndrome, with patients manifesting abnormalities in extrapituitary structures, usually in structures sharing an embryological origin, such as the eye and forebrain in SOD.

HESX1 and SOD

Extrapolation from murine studies has implicated the *HESX1* gene in the etiology of SOD. *Hesx1* is a member of the *paired-like* class of homeobox genes, which is first expressed in the midline anterior visceral endoderm as gastrulation commences in the mouse. Expression is then induced in the adjacent ectoderm in a region fated to form the forebrain. Subsequently, *Hesx1* is expressed at the anterior extreme of the rostral neural folds, finally becoming restricted to the ventral diencephalon by E9.0. Concurrently, *Hesx1* is also expressed in the thickened layer of oral ectoderm that will evaginate to form Rathke's pouch. *Hesx1* continues to be expressed within the developing anterior pituitary until E11.5, when expression becomes downregulated in a specific spatiotemporal pattern correlating with progressive pituitary cell differentiation. By E15.5, expression is undetectable (Dattani et al., 1998; Martinez-Barbera et al., 2000).

SOD: Clinical Description

SOD, also known as de Morsier's syndrome, is a rare condition originally described in 1941 (Reeves, 1941) in a 7-month-old baby with absence of the septum pellucidum and optic nerve anomalies. It is a highly heterogeneous syndrome characterized by the classical triad of optic nerve hypoplasia; midline neuroradiological abnormalities, such as agenesis of the corpus callosum and absence of the septum pellucidum; and pituitary hypoplasia with consequent pituitary hormone deficiency. Neurological deficit is common, ranging from global retardation to focal deficits such as epilepsy or hemiparesis (Kuriyama et al., 1988; Miller et al., 2000). Neuroradiological abnormalities are present in up to 75%–80% of patients with optic nerve hypoplasia, which in turn may be unilateral or bilateral, and may be the first presenting feature, with later onset of endocrine dysfunction (Izenberg et al., 1984; Arslanian et al., 1984; Shammas et al., 1993; Willnow et al., 1996). Bilateral optic nerve hypoplasia is commoner (88% compared with 12% unilateral cases), and other ophthalmological deficits include anophthalmia or microphthalmia. Pituitary hypoplasia may manifest as endocrine deficits varying from isolated GHD to panhypopituitarism. A decrease in growth rate due to GHD is the commonest presenting feature, with hypoglycemia, polyuria, and polydipsia be-

ing less common. Either sexual precocity or failure to develop in puberty may occur, and abnormal hypothalamic neuroanatomy or function may be a feature, as may diabetes insipidus. The endocrinopathy may evolve with a progressive loss of endocrine function over time. The commonest endocrinopathy is GHD, followed by thyrotropin and corticotropin deficiency. Gonadotropin secretion may be retained in the face of other pituitary hormone deficiencies.

Several etiologies have been postulated to account for the sporadic occurrence of SOD, such as viral infections, environmental teratogens, and vascular or degenerative damage. It appears that the developmental anomaly takes place during a critical period of embryogenesis between 3 and 6 weeks of gestation in humans. Two significant developments take place at this stage. First, the telencephalic and optic vesicles and the retinal ganglion cells differentiate. Second, the lamina terminalis thickens, and its subsequent differentiation results in formation of the corpus callosum, anterior commissure, and fornix. Any insult that occurs at this stage has the potential to produce failure of ganglion cell formation with subsequent hypoplasia of optic nerves and chiasm in the first instance and lack of commissural or septal formation in the second instance. Familial cases of SOD are rare and may be associated with either an autosomal-dominant or an autosomal-recessive inheritance (Blethen and Weldon, 1985; Benner et al., 1990; Wales and Quarrell, 1996).

Molecular Genetics of SOD

Initially, a homozygous missense mutation within the homeobox of *HESX1* was identified in two siblings with SOD (Dattani et al., 1998). These children were born within a highly consanguineous pedigree and presented in the newborn period with hypoglycemia secondary to cortisol deficiency. Subsequent testing confirmed panhypopituitarism. Neuroradiological imaging revealed agenesis of the corpus callosum, optic nerve hypoplasia, a hypoplastic anterior pituitary gland, and an ectopic/undescended posterior pituitary gland. The mutation resulted in the substitution of an arginine residue by cysteine at position 160 of the coding region (position 53 of the *HESX1* homeodomain).

A large number of patients with sporadic SOD and its milder variants were screened for heterozygous *HESX1* mutations. To date, three novel heterozygous mutations have been published: Q6H, S170L, and T181A (Thomas et al., 2001) (Fig. 49–3). All three mutations are associated with a milder phenotype than the homozygous R160C substitution, invariably leading to isolated GHD with or without an ectopic/undescended posterior pituitary. The S170L substitution is lo-

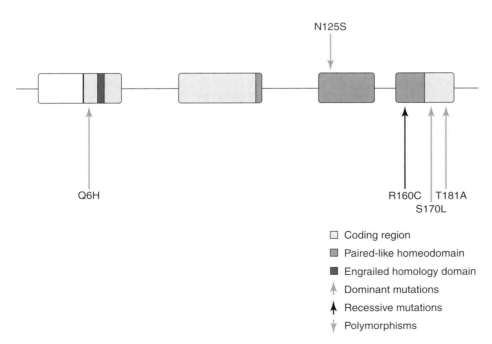

N125S

Q6H

R160C   T181A
S170L

☐ Coding region

▦ Paired-like homeodomain

■ Engrailed homology domain

↑ Dominant mutations

↟ Recessive mutations

↓ Polymorphisms

Figure 49–3. Diagram showing the position of mutations and polymorphisms within *HESX1*.

cated three residues downstream of the carboxy terminus of the homeodomain in a highly conserved region of *HESX1* and was first described in two siblings with isolated GHD, one of whom also had optic nerve hypoplasia. Subsequently, the same mutation was found in a child with isolated GHD with an ectopic/undescended posterior pituitary. The mutation was not found in 140 control chromosomes. The Q6H substitution occurs at a highly conserved residue at the N terminus in a patient who presented with GH and thyrotropin deficiency and an ectopic/undescended posterior pituitary. The T181A change is located at the carboxy terminus of the protein and was observed in an individual with GHD and absence of the posterior pituitary bright spot. Once again, neither of these changes was found in 140 control chromosomes. Compound heterozygosity within *HESX1* was excluded by performing haplotype analysis (Thomas et al., 2001).

Establishing the Diagnosis

The phenotype of SOD is highly variable, and a diagnosis is made on the basis of a combination of any two of the three cardinal features described above. Only 30% of SOD cases demonstrate all three features, 62% manifesting hypopituitarism and 60% showing an absent septum pellucidum (Morishima and Aranoff, 1986). Acers (1983) reported that of 45 individuals with optic nerve hypoplasia, 12 had associated midline brain defects, with six of these individuals also demonstrating hypopituitarism. The condition is thought to be more frequent in children born to younger mothers (mean maternal age 22 years), although this has been disputed. In some studies, there is a preponderance of primigravida mothers.

The diagnosis is usually made at an early stage, although careful investigation is essential to make a diagnosis. The patient usually presents either with early endocrinopathy in the form of central (hypothalamo-pituitary) hypothyroidism and hypoglycemia due to hypocortisolism or with visual impairment, which may itself be variable. Later on, growth failure may mark a diagnosis of GHD. Gonadotropin secretion is variable, with the majority of children who manifest an endocrinopathy being gonadotropin-deficient. These patients may present with genital abnormalities in the form of a micropenis associated with cryptorchidism. A small proportion of children may actually show signs of early or precocious puberty. Diabetes insipidus may also be a feature. The diagnosis of an endocrinopathy is made by performing tests of cortisol secretion, such as an insulin tolerance test or a glucagon test, assessment of the concentrations of insulin-like growth factor-1 (IGF-1) and its binding protein (IGFBP3), an LH-releasing hormone (LHRH) test (to assess gonadotropin secretion), and a thyrotropin-releasing hormone (TRH) test to assess secretion of thyrotropin. A water-deprivation test may be indicated if a diagnosis of diabetes insipidus needs to be excluded.

A complete ophthalmological assessment should include fundoscopy, visual evoked potentials, and an electroretinogram. Neuroradiological imaging will reveal the full extent of the syndrome and may show signs of optic nerve hypoplasia, other midline defects such as agenesis of the corpus callosum and absence of the septum pellucidum, anterior pituitary hypoplasia, an ectopic/undescended posterior pituitary, and other associated abnormalities such as schizencephaly.

Given the variability of the phenotype, prenatal genetic diagnosis would be limited to those pedigrees in which homozygous mutations of *HESX1* have been identified. The severity of the SOD phenotype may justify a prenatal diagnosis, particularly in families in which blindness and developmental delay form predominant features of the syndrome. However, to date, only one homozygous mutation of *HESX1* has been described in the literature, so caution needs to be exercised in the use of prenatal diagnosis, particularly in view of the variably penetrant nature of the condition. Prenatal diagnosis in the dominant forms should be actively discouraged given the variable penetrance with typically milder phenotypes.

Management

SOD is a complex disorder, the management of which requires a multidisciplinary approach. Given the visual impairment, careful assessment by a visual developmental team is required. Psychological input may be necessary given the association between behavioral difficulties and SOD. The child may also manifest a seizure disorder and require input from a neurologist, particularly with respect to anticonvulsant therapy.

The mainstay of treatment remains endocrine. Hormone replacement will be required depending on the endocrinopathy present. Hormonal agents used will include glucocorticoids such as hydrocortisone, thyroxine, and sex steroids such as ethinylestradiol and testosterone, with progestagens to ensure regular menstrual cycles in girls. All of these can be administered orally. Many of these children are GH-deficient and will therefore require treatment with recombinant human GH, which is administered subcutaneously on a daily basis. Diabetes insipidus may be a feature, necessitating deamino-8-D-arginine vasopressin (DDAVP, desmopressin) treatment, which may be administered orally or intranasally. The combination of DDAVP and hydrocortisone treatment needs to be carefully managed, particularly at times of intercurrent illness. Occasionally, children with SOD may enter puberty at an early age, when treatment with a gonadotropin hormone–releasing hormone agonist may be required. In the long term, the condition needs to be carefully monitored, particularly as the endocrinopathy may evolve. Hence, all children should have their growth and puberty monitored carefully.

Genetic counseling should be approached cautiously in these individuals. Homozygous mutations within *HESX1* can be predicted to lead to a phenotype. However, heterozygous mutations are variably penetrant, and the risks of recurrence cannot be accurately assessed in these individuals. Additionally, the role of other genetic and environmental factors modifying the phenotype needs to be taken into account when assessing risks of recurrence. It is, however, becoming increasingly clear that some forms of SOD will have an underlying genetic basis and that our understanding of the etiology is at present rudimentary.

Mutations in Orthologous Genes

Targeted disruption of this gene in mice gave rise to a highly variable phenotype in which homozygous mice showed a combination of the following phenotypic features: a reduction in the prospective forebrain tissue, decreased head size, absence of the developing optic vesicles, severe microphthalmia, and craniofacial dysplasia. All homozygous mice showed an abnormal but variable phenotype at birth, while a small percentage (1%) of the heterozygous pups also showed a morphologically abnormal phenotype. Detailed analysis of the affected animals demonstrated abnormalities of the septum pellucidum and the corpus callosum, absence of the optic cups and the olfactory placodes, hypothalamic abnormalities, and a dysplastic or absent Rathke's pouch. In the majority of *Hesx1* mutants, pituitary development proceeded beyond the formation of Rathke's pouch; however, 5% of the *Hesx1* null mutants demonstrated aplasia of the anterior pituitary (Dattani et al., 1998; Dasen et al., 2001). At E12.5, multiple oral invaginations led to the formation of multiple pituitary glands, with cellular overproliferation. The terminal differentiation of hormone-producing cell types was normal by E16.5, with expression of α-*GSU*, *TSHβ*, *GH*, *POMC*, and *Pou1f1*. The expression domains of *Lhx3* and *Prop1* were expanded and extended into the more anterior region of oral ectoderm. The expression domains of *Fgf8* and *Fgf10* in the infundibulum were expanded more rostrally, and these data therefore suggest that *Hesx1* is required for the maintenance of proper FGF expression domains. *Fgf8* in turn regulates *Hesx1* expression since expression of *Fgf8* under the control of the *Pitx1* promoter led to complete loss of *Hesx1* expression (Dasen et al., 2001). These in vivo data are consistent with the function of *Hesx1* as a repressor.

Developmental Pathogenesis of SOD

The identification of mutations within *HESX1* and the study of the functional consequences of these mutations have contributed to a greater understanding of the role of the gene in normal and abnormal brain development.

Studies carried out by us and others are elucidating the various functions of *HESX1* during development. The repressor function of *Hesx1* can be attributed to the presence of a highly conserved repressor domain, eh1, so called because a similar repressor domain has been described in engrailed (En) and Goosecoid (Gsc), both of which act as repressors within the developing brain. Additionally, Hesx1 has a second repressor domain within the homeodomain (Dasen et al., 2001). The protein interacts with the mammalian Groucho homologue transducer of split enhancer-like 1 (TLE1) via eh1 and with the nuclear receptor corepressor 1 (NCoR1) via the homeodomain (Xu et al., 1999). In keeping with these data, expression of GRO/TLE1 overlaps with that of *Hesx1* between E9.5 and E12.0 in Rathke's pouch (Dasen et al., 2001). Using *in vitro* transfection studies, we have demonstrated that HESX1 is a transcriptional repressor that is promoter-specific (Brickman et al., 2001). The protein represses at the SV40 promoter but not the E4 promoter, suggesting that it requires interaction with other homeodomain partners to achieve its repressor effect since the SV40 promoter contains binding sites for other homeodomain proteins and E4 does not. The repressor function of HESX1 resides in 37 amino acids at the N terminus of the HESX1 protein (the repressor domain containing the eh1 domain). Additionally, using a mammalian two-hybrid system, we have demonstrated that the repressor domain is implicated in homo- and heterodimerization of HESX1 with partner proteins (Brickman et al., 2001).

Functional analysis of the R160C mutation was based on knowledge of the functions of homeodomain proteins. This arginine residue is highly conserved in the majority of homeodomain proteins and implicated in the binding of target DNA by the homeodomain. In particular, Arg^{53} makes contact with the phosphate backbone within the major groove of DNA. Functional analysis of this mutation showed that the mutant protein failed to bind the consensus P3 sequence to which paired-like homeodomain proteins can bind as dimers. The wild-type protein had a high affinity for the P3 site (K_d 10 nM), whereas the mutant protein failed to bind even at 1000-fold higher concentrations. Intriguingly, when increasing concentrations of R160C HESX1 were added to the wild-type protein, the mutant protein resulted in loss of DNA binding by the wild-type protein (Brickman et al., 2001). This in vitro dominant-negative effect was recapitulated in transfection studies (Brickman et al., 2001). Additionally, it was shown that the dominant-negative effect was the result of the formation of inactive dimers of wild-type and R160C HESX1. The dimerization was mediated by the eh1 domain (Brickman et al., 2001). In spite of these findings, obligate heterozygous carriers within the highly consanguineous pedigree were phenotypically normal. Two possibilities could account for this phenomenon: (*1*) as with the mutant mice, the penetrance of heterozygous mutations may be variable and only a small proportion of heterozygous individuals manifest a phenotype and (*2*) only a small proportion of HESX1 homodimers is sufficient to prevent the manifestation of a phenotype.

The mechanisms by which the heterozygous mutations lead to a phenotype are, at present, poorly understood. The S170L substitution leads to a four- to sevenfold reduction in the binding of HESX1 to P3 (Thomas et al., 2001). It is unlikely that this change on its own is responsible for the phenotype observed in patients since more profound functional changes in the R160C protein are not associated with a heterozygous phenotype. One possible mechanism may lie in the interaction of HESX1 with other as yet unidentified partner proteins. Functional analysis of the latter two mutations is currently under way. The presence of heterozygous *HESX1* mutations in association with a milder, variably penetrant phenotype is similar to the murine model, where heterozygous *Hesx1* null mice can also variably demonstrate a phenotype. The association of a phenotype with heterozygous mutations within a condition in which homozygous mutations have been described and where obligate carriers manifest no phenotype would indicate that the inheritance of this disorder is complex and may involve a number of genes and/or environmental factors.

Mutations within *HESX1* have been associated with SOD and milder pituitary phenotypes (Dattani et al., 1998; Thomas et al., 2001). Nevertheless, the majority of patients screened in our studies show no mutation of *HESX1*. There may be several explanations for this. Variable phenotypes may actually reflect the heterogeneity of multiple conditions, with different pathways affecting forebrain/midbrain development. Alternatively, the variability could theoretically reflect a single SOD phenotype with the same genetic defect (e.g., *HESX1*) but which

is variably penetrant, in which case alterations in regulatory regions may also contribute to the etiology of this condition. For instance, forebrain and pituitary-specific regulatory regions may account for the temporal pattern of expression of *HESX1* within these regions, and mutations in one or the other region may lead to a principally forebrain or pituitary phenotype. Additionally, like holoprosencephaly (Wallis and Muenke, 2000), SOD may have a multigenic basis, and mutations in as yet unidentified genes could contribute to some cases. To date, the targets and partners of *HESX1* remain unknown. These may shed further light on the molecular basis of not only SOD but of various other pituitary disorders. Elucidation of the functional significance of the *HESX1* mutations in our SOD patients will lead to a detailed understanding of the function of this homeodomain protein in the development of the forebrain and pituitary.

LHX3 AND *LHX4* AND COMPLEX PITUITARY PHENOTYPES

LHX3/LHX4

Lhx3 (*P-Lim/Lim-3*) is a LIM-containing homeobox gene (Seidah et al., 1994; Bach et al., 1995). It contains two LIM domains that mediate protein–protein interactions and *trans*-activation functions and a DNA-binding homeodomain. Expression of *Lhx3* is initially observed throughout the developing brain and spinal cord but, by E9.5 in the mouse embryo, is restricted to the invaginating Rathke's pouch (Zhadanov et al., 1995). *Lhx4* is a second LIM homeobox gene closely related to *Lhx3*, with a very similar expression pattern in the developing pituitary. While the expression pattern of *Lhx3* is relatively broad within the pituitary during development, *Lhx4* expression is observed in a restricted pattern within the *Lhx3* expression domain. At E9.5, *Lhx4* transcripts are observed throughout the developing pituitary gland; by E12.5, *Lhx4* expression is restricted to the future anterior lobe of the pituitary; and by E15.5, *Lhx4* expression is down-regulated throughout the anterior pituitary (Sheng et al., 1997; Yamashita et al., 1997).

Clinical Description of Syndromes Associated with *LHX3/LHX4* Mutations

The affected patients harboring a mutation within the *LHX3* gene had severe growth retardation and were deficient in all but one of the anterior pituitary hormones (corticotropin). Additionally, they presented with a phenotype characterized by elevated and anteverted shoulders, leading to the clinical appearance of a short and stubby neck associated with a severe restriction of the rotation of the cervical spine, resulting in limited head rotation. Magnetic resonance imagining (MRI) of the neck revealed an abnormally steep cervical spine. One of the affected patients also demonstrated an enlarged pituitary on MRI scanning (Netchine et al., 2000).

The proband within the family carrying an *LHX4* mutation presented with GH, thyrotropin, and corticotropin deficiency (Machinis et al., 2001). The probands were too young for assessment of their gonadotropin secretion. Neuroimaging of the affected individuals revealed the presence of a small sella turcica, a persistent craniopharyngeal canal, a hypoplastic anterior pituitary lobe, and an ectopic/undescended posterior pituitary. Additionally, the cerebellar tonsils were abnormal.

Molecular Genetics of Syndromes Associated with *LHX3/LHX4* Mutations

Mutations within the *LHX3* gene were reported in two unrelated consanguineous pedigrees (Netchine et al., 2000). In the first family, a homozygous missense mutation led to substitution of an invariant tyrosine residue by cysteine, Y116C. In the second, the mutation was a homozygous 23 bp deletion predicted to result in a severely truncated protein lacking the entire homeodomain. Both parents were heterozygous for this deletion and manifested no phenotype, suggesting an autosomal-recessive phenotype.

Mutations within the *LHX4* gene were described in a large consanguineous family (Machinis et al., 2001). The mutation within this family was a heterozygous G>C transversion at the 3′ end of intron

4. This splice site change affects the invariant AG dinucleotide of the splice acceptor site and leads to the generation of two alternatively spliced isoforms.

Establishing the Diagnosis

The diagnosis of anterior pituitary hormone deficiency is usually considered if a patient presents with short stature and poor growth velocity. Other features alerting the clinician include central hypothyroidism, often presenting in the newborn period with failure to thrive and prolonged jaundice, and genital abnormalities in the form of a micropenis with cryptorchidism, suggesting gonadotropin deficiency. Mutations within *LHX4*, but not *LHX3*, appear to be associated with corticotropin deficiency, and these patients may therefore present with neonatal hypoglycemia and convulsions (Netchine et al., 2000; Machinis et al., 2001). Combined pituitary hormone testing in the form of a GH provocation test, TRH test, and LHRH test may be indicated. Neuroimaging is mandatory and may reveal anterior pituitary hypoplasia. Cerebellar abnormalities may be observed in children with *LHX4* mutations. MRI of the cervical spine may reveal abnormalities in children with *LHX3* mutations.

Genetic prenatal diagnosis remains a possibility for these syndromes; however, neither syndrome is associated with severely disabling features. Only two pedigrees with *LHX3* mutations and one with *LHX4* mutations have been described. Hence, at present, given the lack of extensive knowledge regarding penetrance and phenotypes associated with mutations within these genes and given that both syndromes are treatable, prenatal diagnosis cannot be recommended.

Management

The mainstay of management remains endocrine, with replacement of the appropriate hormones. Hence, in the case of *LHX3* deficiency, treatment would need to be instituted with recombinant hGH, thyroxine, and sex steroids, while with *LHX4* mutations, treatment with recombinant hGH, thyroxine, hydrocortisone, and possibly sex steroids would need to be instituted. Mutations within these genes may be associated with other, as yet unidentified phenotypes. Given the association of extrapituitary abnormalities, the role of other disciplines, such as neurology, may need to be considered.

Genetic counseling may be possible in the case of both *LHX3* and *LHX4* mutations; but given that the conditions are not life-threatening and are amenable to treatment, its role remains questionable.

Mutations in Orthologous Genes

In targeted murine *Lhx3* null mutants, initiation of Rathke's pouch is normal but further development of the rudimentary pouch is not seen. The cells within the anterior pituitary are unable to proliferate and commit to a cellular differentiation pathway so that with the exception of a small number of corticotropes, no anterior pituitary cells are present. Homozygous pups either are stillborn or die early in the neonatal period (Sheng et al., 1996). Targeted mutagenesis of the *Lhx4* gene revealed a much milder phenotype than that observed with the *Lhx3*$^{-/-}$ mouse. Homozygous pups displayed mild hypopituitarism with a reduction in the number of somatotropes and lactotropes and consequent GH, PRL, and LH deficiency (Sheng et al., 1997). The cell lineages in this null mouse are specified normally but then fail to expand. This is thought to be the result of a wave of precursor cell death (Raetzman et al., 2002). There was no obvious heterozygous phenotype (Sheng et al., 1997). The phenotype of the *Lhx3*$^{-/-}$, *Lhx4*$^{-/-}$ double-mutant is much more severe than that of either null mutant on its own (Sheng et al., 1997). Development of the pituitary is arrested at the rudimentary stage, suggesting that there is, to some degree, functional redundancy between these two LIM homeobox genes. *Lhx4* is essential for the early expression of *Lhx3*, but there is a second phase of *Lhx3* expression which is independent of *Lhx4* (Raetzman et al., 2002).

Developmental Pathogenesis of Syndromes Associated with *LHX3/LHX4* Mutations

LHX3 mutations appear to be recessively inherited and are associated with a defined phenotype. The mechanism underlying the cervical spine abnormality remains unknown. The Y116C substitution is within the second LIM domain of the protein, a region involved in forming the zinc finger–binding motif. This motif is implicated in protein–protein interactions; and consequently, a mutation within this region would be predicted to disrupt the function of this protein. Transient transfection studies demonstrated that the two published mutations failed to activate the α-GSU promoter (Sloop et al., 2001), which is expressed in the pituitary at an early developmental stage. Additionally, the truncated protein lacking the homeodomain was unable to bind a consensus high-affinity LHX3-binding site, whereas the Y116C missense mutation showed no effect on DNA binding (Sloop et al., 2001). The two LIM domains are important for interactions with partner proteins such as C-LIM (Bach, 2000), POU1F1 (Bach et al., 1995), MRGI (Glenn and Maurer, 1999), and Selective LIM-binding factor (SLB) (Howard and Maurer, 2000). The ability of the mutated protein Y116C to interact with these putative partners was investigated in in vitro binding assays; it was shown that while the ability of LHX3(Y116C) to interact with Pou1f1 was retained, the binding affinity was reduced (Sloop et al., 2001).

The mutation identified within the *LHX4* gene would be predicted to interfere with the normal splicing of this gene. Transfection studies revealed that the mutation led to splicing defects whereby mutant isoforms of the protein were generated, due to utilization of two cryptic splice acceptor sites present within exon 5. Both of these variant *LHX4* isoforms led to disruption of the homeodomain of this gene (Machinis et al., 2001). A heterozygous mutation of this gene appears to be sufficient to result in a disease phenotype, whereas heterozygous changes within *LHX3* do not result in a clinical phenotype, even though on analysis of murine null mutants, homozygous disruption of *Lhx3* led to a more severe phenotype than that observed with *Lhx4* (Sheng et al., 1997).

POU1F1 AND *PROP1* AND *CPHD*

POU1F1/PROP1

POU1F1 (*PIT1*) is a member of the POU family of transcription factors, characterized by the presence of a highly conserved bipartite DNA-binding domain, comprising the POU-specific domain (POU-S) and the POU homeodomain (POU-HD) (Herr et al., 1988). *Pou1f1* is expressed relatively late during anterior pituitary development (see Fig. 49–2); transcripts are first observed at E14.5 and then continue to be specifically expressed in the anterior pituitary throughout adulthood. Expression is restricted to the thyrotrope, somatotrope, and lactotrope cell lineages, consistent with functional studies of this protein, which show that expression of the *GH*, *PRL*, *TSH-β* subunit, and *GHRHR* genes is regulated by POU1F1. Pou1f1 binds to its own proximal promoter and upregulate its own expression (Delhase et al., 1996).

PROP1 is a pituitary-specific homeodomain transcription factor of the *paired-like* class. Expression is first observed in the dorsal region of Rathke's pouch at E10.5, peaks at E12.0, and is completely undetectable by E15.5. Expression of *Prop1* is observed specifically in those cells that will later express *Pou1f1* (Andersen et al., 1995; Sornson et al., 1996), although the role of *Prop1* in gonadotrope development remains unclear.

Clinical Description of CPHD Phenotypes Associated with *POU1F1* and *PROP1* Mutations

The first human mutations in *POU1F1* were reported in a child with combined GH and PRL deficiency with severe central hypothyroidism (Tatsumi et al., 1992). The patient was homozygous for a nonsense mutation in *POU1F1*. Further mutations were described in two Dutch families with GH, PRL, and thyrotropin deficiencies (Pfaffle et al., 1992). Within the first family, affected individuals had mild central hypothyroidism and normal-sized anterior pituitary glands on MRI with normal serum thyroxine levels before commencing GH treatment. In the second family, the children had more severe central hypothyroidism and small anterior pituitaries. Since the original description of *POU1F1* mutations in humans, 14 different mutations in at least

19 families have been described in *POU1F1* (see Fig. 49–4). The mutations are present mainly in the POU-S and POU-HD regions. In affected individuals, the phenotype is characterized by severe GH and PRL deficiencies, with variable thyrotropin deficiency. The variability in the size of the anterior pituitary is a feature of *POU1F1* mutations in humans, with some individuals showing anterior pituitary hypoplasia and others showing a normal pituitary gland on MRI. The posterior pituitary and pituitary stalk are of normal size and position.

Given the rarity of *POU1F1* mutations within the phenotype of CPHD, it became clear that other genes were implicated. Patients with a phenotype similar to that of patients with *POU1F1* mutations were originally screened for mutations in *PROP1*, with no success. It was not until patients with a more severe CPHD phenotype (GH, PRL, and TSH deficiency with additional LH and FSH deficiency) were screened that human mutations within this gene were identified (Wu et al., 1998). Patients with *PROP1* mutations were unable to enter puberty, or puberty was arrested due to gonadotropin deficiency. Evolving cortisol deficiency has also been described in a small number of patients (Deladoey et al., 1999; Mendonca et al., 1999; Asteria et al., 2000). These data suggest a role for *PROP1* in the differentiation of somatotropes, lactotropes, caudomedial thyrotropes, and gonadotropes in humans. To date, 14 different recessive mutations have been documented in a total of 61 different families with CPHD, making *PROP1* the most commonly implicated gene in CPHD (Cogan et al., 1998) (see Fig. 49–5). In a study of 73 patients with CPHD, 35 were found to have mutations of *PROP1*, with marked phenotypic variability (Deladoey et al., 1999). Additionally, pituitary enlargement with subsequent involution has also been reported in patients with *PROP1* mutations (Fofanova et al., 1998; Mendonca et al., 1999; Rosenbloom et al., 1999). The mechanism underlying this phenomenon remains unknown.

Molecular Genetics of CPHD

The mutation first identified in the *POU1F1* gene was a nonsense homozygous mutation within the POU-S domain, leading to a severely truncated protein lacking 171 amino acids, including half of the POU-S and all of the POU-HD regions. Such a protein would be unable to bind to downstream targets such as the GH, PRL, and thyrotropin promoters (Tatsumi et al., 1992). In the first Dutch family, the mutation was a homozygous substitution A158P in the POU-S domain of the gene. In the second family, affected children were compound heterozygotes for the A158P substitution from their father and a deletion of the entire *POU1F1* gene from their mother (Pfaffle et al., 1992). In addition to these recessive mutations, a number of dominant mutations have been described, the R271W substitution in the carboxy terminus of the homeodomain of *POU1F1* being the most frequent (Radovick et al., 1992; Ohta et al., 1992).

Four families with CPHD were associated with homozygosity or compound heterozygosity for inactivating mutations of the *PROP1* gene (Wu et al., 1998). So far, all *PROP1* mutations are inherited in an autosomal-recessive manner. Two of the described mutations, microdeletions within exon 2, occur at a high frequency within *PROP1* families: a 2 bp ΔGA 301/302 deletion (Wu et al., 1998) and a ΔGA 149/150 or ΔA 150 (Fofanova et al., 1998).

Establishing the Diagnosis of CPHD

The diagnosis of CPHD is based on the documentation of low growth velocity in conjunction with GHD on provocative testing, thyrotropin deficiency characterized by a low thyrotropin in conjunction with a low thyroxine level, and a suboptimal thyrotropin response to TRH, PRL deficiency in response to TRH stimulation, and, in the case of *PROP1* mutations, gonadotropin deficiency in response to gonadotropin-releasing hormone and probable cortisol deficiency in response to provocation with either hypoglycemia or synacthen. Additionally, an MRI scan of the pituitary will reveal a normal, hypoplastic, or enlarged pituitary gland with no other midline defects. The posterior pituitary is usually eutopic.

There is at present no need for prenatal diagnosis given that the condition is eminently treatable. However, the thyroxine level should be checked postnatally in order to diagnose the condition as quickly as possible and thereby institute treatment rapidly with a view to preventing brain damage. Since the condition is treatable, antenatal diagnosis should certainly not be considered. Early genetic testing may be important for the early diagnosis of these disorders so that hypothyroidism and GHD may be diagnosed quickly with the rapid commencement of treatment.

Management of CPHD

Growth should be carefully monitored, and if the growth velocity is poor and GHD confirmed on provocative testing, then treatment with recombinant hGH should be commenced. Thyroxine should be commenced if the free or total thyroxine concentration is low. Sex steroids in the form of estrogen or testosterone should be commenced if gonadotropin deficiency is confirmed. Hydrocortisone should be commenced if cortisol secretion is impaired. If a mutation within *PROP1* is documented and cortisol secretion is normal, then cortisol secretion should be assessed at regular intervals as it may be impaired at a later date. If a pituitary mass is present, serial MRI scans are indicated to monitor the size of the mass.

Counseling may be available for both *POU1F1* and *PROP1* mutations. Although genetic counseling is possible in CPHD due to recessive *POU1F1* and *PROP1* mutations, it can be difficult in patients with dominant mutations since the penetrance can be variable (Radovick et al., 1992; Ohta et al., 1992).

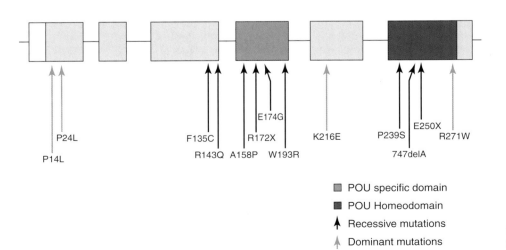

P14L   P24L   F135C   R143Q   A158P   R172X   E174G   W193R   K216E   P239S   747delA   E250X   R271W

■ POU specific domain
■ POU Homeodomain
↟ Recessive mutations
↟ Dominant mutations

Figure 49–4. Diagram showing the position of mutations within *POU1F1*.

Mutations in Orthologous Genes

Two spontaneously occurring mouse mutants of *Pou1f1*, the Snell (*Pit1*^{dw}) and Jackson (*Pit1*^{dwj}) mice, have been described (Duquesnoy, 1975). Homozygous mutant mice showed pituitary hypoplasia with absence of somatotropes, lactotropes, and thyrotropes. Both of these phenotypes result from mutations within the *Pou1f1* gene (Li et al., 1990). The Snell dwarf mouse results from the substitution of a tryptophan residue by cysteine (W261C) within the POU-HD. The Jackson phenotype is the result of either an insertion or an inversion of a 4 kb fragment within the gene, which would be predicted to disrupt protein function.

PROP1 was positionally cloned using the Ames dwarf mouse (*Prop1*^{df}) (Duquesnoy, 1975). This spontaneously occurring mouse mutant had a phenotype somewhat similar to those of the Snell (*Pit1*^{dw}) and Jackson (*Pit1*^{dwj}) mice, except that in addition to the lack of thyrotrope, somatotrope, and lactotrope cells, there was a reduction in the number of gonadotrope cells (Li et al., 1990). The genetic basis for this phenotype was the result of a mutation in the *Prop1* gene, a homozygous point mutation within the first α helix of the *Prop1* homeodomain leading to substitution of a serine residue with proline (S38P), with consequent reduction in the binding of Prop1 to its target DNA (Sornson et al., 1996).

More detailed analysis of *Prop1*^{df} mutant mice has revealed a hypocellular anterior pituitary at E14.5 with an abnormally expanded Rathke's pouch, though in contrast to the hypocellularity seen in the *Lhx4*$^{-/-}$ mouse, this does not appear to be the result of increased cell death (Raetzman et al., 2002). Analysis of *Prop1*$^{df/df}$ *Lhx4*$^{-/-}$ double-mutants has suggested a genetic interaction between Prop1 and Lhx4. Such interactions may explain some of the phenotypic heterogeneity observed in humans with *PROP1* mutations. Premature expression of *Prop1* during early murine pituitary gland development led to complete absence of the anterior pituitary gland (Dasen et al., 2001).

Developmental Pathogenesis of the Condition

So far, 14 mutations have been described in the *POU1F1* gene (Fig. 49–4). Only a few of the *POU1F1* mutations have been studied in any detail. The mutations inherited recessively affect the structure of the POU-S and POU-HD regions, whereas the dominant mutations are generally found outside the DNA-binding domains (Tatsumi et al., 1992; Pfaffle et al., 1992; Radovick et al., 1992; Ohta et al., 1992). The A158P mutated protein can bind to target promoters but cannot activate transcription from either the GH or PRL promoters (Pfaffle et al., 1992). In transfection studies, the R271W mutation acts as a dominant-negative and prevents transcriptional activation by the wild-type protein (Radovick et al., 1992; Ohta et al., 1992).

The 2 bp ΔGA 301/302 deletion (Wu et al., 1998) and the ΔGA 149/150 or ΔA 150 (Fofanova et al., 1998) frameshift mutation within *PROP1* introduce premature stop codons within the open reading frame of this gene, leading to truncated protein products that lack the DNA-binding domain. The ΔGA 301/302 mutation is the most commonly reported; it has been reported as a *de novo* mutation and in all ethnic populations studied. The mutation lies within a GA repeat sequence, suggesting that this is a mutational hot spot. All other mutations so far reported affect the highly conserved homeodomain. Mutations are either missense within this region; nonsense, leading to a truncated protein lacking a functional homeodomain; or splicing, again leading to a disrupted homeodomain. As *PROP1* mutations are always inherited in a recessive manner, the consequences of the mutations are the result of loss of a functional protein as opposed to a dominant-negative effect. Of note is the enlarged sella turcica observed in association with *PROP1* mutations (Mendonca et al., 1999). The exact mechanism underlying the pituitary enlargement remains unclear, and biopsy of the mass in a single patient revealed amorphous tissue with occasional fibroblastic cells but no identifiable anterior pituitary cell types (Parks et al., 1998). This enlargement of the sella turcica is also observed with *LHX3* mutations. There is no clear genotype–phenotype correlation; the cortisol deficiency in particular appears to be unpredictable, and the mechanism remains poorly understood.

TBX19/TPIT AND ISOLATED CORTICOTROPIN DEFICIENCY

TBX19/TPIT

T-box genes are a family of transcription factors that play critical roles during embryonic development (Papaioannou and Silver, 1998). The characteristic feature of this family of genes is a DNA-binding domain spanning 180 bp, the T-box. The first member of this family to be identified was the mouse *Brachyury* (*T*) gene, which was positionally cloned in 1990 (Wilkinson et al., 1990). Twelve human T-box genes have been identified to date (Yi et al., 1999). Limited expression data in humans suggest that the homologues are expressed in a similar manner to their murine counterparts, with distinct temporal and spatial expression patterns during development (Chapman et al., 1996; Smith 1997). Members of this family play a role in human genetic disorders (Bamshad et al., 1997; Basson et al., 1997; Li et al., 1997).

Previous studies have shown an interaction between Pitx1 and Tbx4 in the developing hindlimb (Logan and Tabin, 1999). The transcription factor Pitx1 was originally identified as a result of its cell-specific transcription of the *POMC* gene, and originally it was thought to be a corticotrope-specific factor (Lamonerie et al., 1996). Subsequently, expression of *Pitx1* has been shown in all anterior pituitary

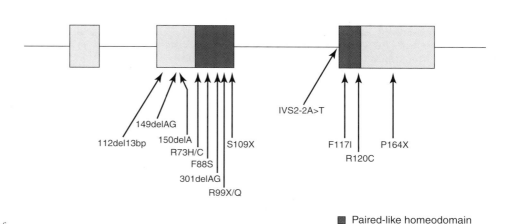

149delAG

112del13bp   150delA   S109X

R73H/C

F88S

301delAG

R99X/Q

IVS2-2A>T

F117I   P164X

R120C

■ Paired-like homeodomain

↑ Recessive mutations

Figure 49–5. Diagram showing the position of mutations within *PROP1*.

cell types (Lanctot et al., 1999). Therefore, it is not possible to explain the corticotrope-specific expression of *POMC* as being solely due to regulation by Pitx1; interaction with some other factor must be involved. The identification of the T-box gene *TBX19/TPIT*, present within the POMC-expressing cell lineage, was therefore of obvious interest (Lamolet et al., 2001). Expression of this gene is first observed at E11.5 within the caudoventral aspect of the developing anterior pituitary gland. By E12.5, the expression of *Tbx19/Tpit* is restricted to those cells that will subsequently become the POMC-expressing cells of the anterior pituitary, suggesting that *TBX19/TPIT* is required for corticotrope cell differentiation and activation of POMC transcription (Lamolet et al., 2001; Liu et al., 2001).

Clinical Description

Mutations within *TBX19/TPIT* were identified in two patients who presented with very similar symptoms, namely isolated corticotropin deficiency (Lamolet et al., 2001). Specifically, a very low basal plasma cortisol level was seen with no corticotropin response to corticotropin-releasing hormone (CRH). However, a cortisol response to corticotropin administration was maintained.

Molecular Genetics

The patient from the first family was found to carry a homozygous nonsense mutation within *TBX19/TPIT*, leading to a premature termination codon, resulting in a truncated protein lacking most of the carboxy terminus (R286X) (Lamolet et al., 2001). The mutation within the second family (Delcros et al., 1988) was a heterozygous point mutation within the T-box, resulting in substitution of a serine residue by phenylalanine at a highly conserved residue (S128F) (Lamolet et al., 2001).

Establishing the Diagnosis

Patients usually present with symptoms of cortisol deficiency, namely, early-onset hypoglycemia, adrenal insufficiency and collapse with intercurrent illness, and recurrent infections. Later on, fatigue may be a major feature. Investigations should include a 24-hour plasma cortisol profile, synacthen tests (physiological or standard), plasma corticotropin and a CRH test. The concentration of cortisol in the plasma will be low, as will the corticotropin concentration. CRH will lead to a sub-optimal elevation in corticotropin concentration. The cortisol response to synacthen (exogenous corticotropin) will either be normal or suboptimal. Prenatal diagnosis is not indicated in isolated corticotropin deficiency

Management

The condition is eminently treatable, necessitating the use of glucocorticoids in the form of either hydrocortisone or prednisolone. Maintenance doses should be used. The dose should be doubled at times of intercurrent illness or stress, e.g., surgery or injury. The disease can be perfectly controlled using glucocorticoids.

Developmental Pathogenesis of the Condition

Experimental data have shown that in transfection experiments a strong synergistic effect is observed between Tbx19/Tpit and Pitx1 on the POMC promoter (Lamolet et al., 2001; Liu et al., 2001). The specific expression of *Tbx19/Tpit* in pituitary POMC-expressing cells and its obvious involvement in regulation of the *POMC* gene support the hypothesis that mutations within this gene would result in an isolated deficiency of pituitary POMC/corticotropin. This indeed was the case. Functional analysis of the mutations has not been performed. The phenotype seen in the patient harboring a homozygous mutation resulting in a truncated protein is undoubtedly due to a loss of function. However, the heterozygous point mutation within the T box could result in a phenotype either due to a dominant-negative effect or due to haploinsufficiency as described for other mutations within T-box genes (Basson et al., 1999; Cross et al., 2000).

EMX2 AND SCHIZENCEPHALY

EMX2 is a homeobox gene (Simeone et al., 1992) and one of two homologues of the *Drosophila* gap gene *empty spiracles* (*ems*) (Dalton et al., 1989). Extensive research into the role of this gene within the developing forebrain has established it as one of the earliest markers of cerebral cortex. Expression begins at E8.5 in the developing forebrain, specifically within the anterior dorsal neuroectodermal regions of the embryo. By E9.5, the expression domain is defined by an anterior boundary overlapping that of *Emx1* and a posterior boundary within the roof of the presumptive diencephalon. By E12.5, there is a distinct gradient of expression of *Emx2*, specifically within the neuroepithelium. Within the posterior dorsal telencephalon, there is a greater intensity of signal, which then decreases toward the anterior boundary (Simeone et al., 1992). This posterior–anterior gradient may be due to a gradient of maturing neuroblasts during corticogenesis, with mature cells being seen earlier in more anterior regions (Cecchi et al., 1999). The specific expression pattern observed with *Emx2* suggests that this homeobox gene plays a significant role in early forebrain development.

Clinical Description

Schizencephaly is a rare human disorder normally classified as a cell-migration disorder. It has a highly variable phenotype that can encompass normal intelligence, seizures, and severe neurological defects. Neuroradiological examination of affected individuals shows a full-thickness cleft within the cerebral hemispheres. This cleft is characterized by an infolding of gray matter from the cerebral cortex into the ventricle, termed the *pial-ependymal seam*. Within the cleft, the cortical pia and the ventricular ependyma are fused (Barkovich et al., 1989; Barkovich and Kjos, 1992).

Molecular Genetics

To date, 13 individuals have been shown to harbor heterozygous mutations within *EMX2* (Brunelli et al., 1996; Faiella et al., 1997). The first mutations were described in three families. The first proband, who manifested severe cortical defects, harbored an insertion within the homeobox of *EMX2*. Analysis of the parents of this individual showed that this must be a *de novo* mutation (Brunelli et al., 1996). The next two patients had somewhat milder phenotypes, and both had a single-base substitution at the 3' splice site of intron 1 (at positions -1 and -4 respectively).

Establishing the Diagnosis and Management

The diagnosis is revealed on MRI. An electroencephalogram may be indicated if seizures form part of the clinical picture. Management involves treatment of the various clinical features such as convulsions with, e.g., anticonvulsants.

Mutations in Orthologous Genes

Mice homozygous for a targeted deletion in the *Emx2* locus (*Emx2*$^{-/-}$) are unable to survive past the neonatal period, the phenotype including absence of kidneys and other urogenital defects such as absence of the gonads and genital tracts (Pellegrini et al., 1996; Miyamoto et al., 1997; Yoshida et al., 1997). A role for *Emx2* in patterning the proximal structures of the developing limb, namely, the scapula and ilium, has also been described (Pellegrini et al., 2001). Homozygous pups show altered patterning of the hippocampus, reduced olfactory bulbs and absence of the dentate gyrus (Pellegrini et al., 1996; Miyamoto et al., 1997; Yoshida et al., 1997). More detailed analysis of the cells within the cortical plate showed that the neurons displayed abnormal migration patterns, similar to those seen in the *Reeler* mouse mutant phenotype. Indeed, *reelin* expression was absent in the forebrain of the *Emx2*$^{-/-}$ mice, in regions that would normally be expected to express this transcript (Mallamaci et al., 2000).

Developmental Pathogenesis

The mutation resulting in a frameshift led to the production of a missense protein with an altered carboxy terminus, specifically affecting the recognition helix of the homeodomain with presumably consequent loss of function. Both the splice site mutations affect normal splicing of the gene, and RNase protection analysis of the cytoplasm of cells transfected with the mutant forms of this gene failed to detect any correctly spliced product (Brunelli et al., 1996). On the basis of the small population of patients with schizencephaly due to *EMX2* mutations, tentative genotype–phenotype correlations can be made. More severe mutations affecting splicing or causing frameshifts seem to be associated with a more severe bilateral phenotype, while missense mutations are more likely to be associated with a milder phenotype. While schizencephaly has no direct endocrine or pituitary involvement per se, there have been a number of reports in which SOD is associated with schizencephaly (Barkovich et al., 1989; De Smedt et al., 2000; Miller et al., 2000). It has been proposed that schizencephaly may be a further dysmorphic manifestation of this highly variable disorder (Kuban et al., 1989; Nuri Sener, 1996; Ramos Fernandez et al., 1996). However, the association between these two disorders may reflect a mutation in an as yet unknown gene important for normal forebrain development.

CONCLUSIONS

Normal development of the forebrain and pituitary gland is the result of a complex cascade of developmental genes. The many components of this increasingly complex genetic cascade form a coordinated pathway of signaling molecules, transcription factors, and downstream target genes. However, elucidation of the intricate relationships between the numerous genes expressed during the development of these structures is still at an early stage. Our understanding of the molecular basis of forebrain and pituitary disorders in human is still in its infancy and to date has been mainly dependent on the identification of spontaneous mutations or artificially targeted mutations in mice. The phenotype of these mutant mice can then be extrapolated to human conditions and the homologous candidate gene screened for mutations in the appropriate cohort of patients. This approach has proved highly successful, with mutations in *POU1F1* and *PROP1* accounting for a proportion of CPHD cases. The genes *HESX1*, *LHX3*, and *LHX4* were chosen for mutation screening on the basis of the phenotype of mice with targeted deletions of the relevant gene; again, this approach proved to be successful, although mutations within these three genes appear to be less frequent. Although this approach of identifying candidate genes based on mouse phenotypes has proved successful, it should nevertheless be approached with caution. Significant differences between the expression patterns of these developmental genes and the phenotypes arising as a result of targeted mutagenesis are apparent. This is best exemplified by *LHX4*, whereby a phenotype in the mouse is observed only in homozygous murine null mutants and a phenotype in humans has been described in association with heterozygous mutations.

The considerable phenotypic variability within and between families is a feature of mutations within *HESX1*, *PROP1*, and, to a lesser extent, *POU1F1*. In the case of *HESX1* and *POU1F1*, both dominant and recessive forms of inheritance have been described. With the identification of heterozygous mutations in families in which obligate carriers show no disease phenotype, the penetrance of many of these mutations appears to be incomplete. The variability of phenotype and penetrance may indeed be indicative of an interaction with environmental modifiers or with other genes, as has been described in Bardet-Biedl syndrome (Katsanis et al., 2001).

The literature suggests an association of SOD with various environmental factors, e.g., drugs and alcohol. These factors may modify an underlying genetic predisposition to the disorder. The hypothesis that genetic interactions may be important in the etiology of these disorders opens up exciting possibilities, given the large number of genes implicated in forebrain and pituitary development. We have already identified a number of polymorphisms within both introns and exons of a number of important developmental genes, including *HESX1*. Some of these may be functionally relevant (Brickman et al., 2001) but unable to generate a phenotype in isolation. However, a particular combination of polymorphisms in different developmental genes could account for the variability in both phenotype and inheritance that is observed within these disorders.

Finally, only coding regions of various genes have been screened for mutations. Little is known about the identity and role of various promoters and enhancers. With the fruition of the Human Genome Project, it is now possible to identify both promoter and enhancer re-

gions for the genes in question. Embryogenesis is a highly complex process, and one could speculate that subtle differences in the expression of various genes and, hence, proteins could result in abnormal phenotypes. Promoter or enhancer regions may differentially regulate the temporal and spatial patterns of expression of various genes. Mutations within these regions could potentially explain the phenotypic variations observed in a condition such as SOD. Recognition of such regions will be made possible through identification of conserved genomic regions between different species. It is possible that a number of genetic variations in non-coding regions may actually alter the expression of these critical developmental genes. Hence, one could predict that the identification of polymorphisms within these regions may be as important as functional amino acid substitutions arising as a result of mutations within the coding regions of various genes.

The identification of genetic mutations in rare human disorders leads to a greater understanding of normal human development. The identification of mutations in novel candidate genes, the possible interaction with other genes and/or environmental factors, and the identification of sequence changes in putative promoters/enhancers will add a further layer to the complexity of disorders such as CPHD and SOD. The sequencing of the human genome is making this task ever more accessible and will enable us to understand the complex and intricate relationships within the genetic cascade that ultimately lead to the normal development of structures such as the forebrain and pituitary gland.

REFERENCES

Aarskog D, Eiken HG, Bjerknes R, Myking OL (1997). Pituitary dwarfism in the R271W *Pit-1* gene mutation. *Eur J Pediatr* 156: 829–834.

Acers TE (1983). Optic nerve hypoplasia and visual function (a quantitative correlation). *J Okla State Med Assoc* 76: 409–413.

Andersen B, Pearse RV, Jenne K, Sornson M, Lin SC, Bartke A, Rosenfeld MG (1995). The *Ames dwarf* gene is required for *Pit-1* gene activation. *Dev Biol* 172: 495–503.

Arslanian SA, Rothfus WE, Foley-TP J, Becker DJ (1984). Hormonal, metabolic, and neuroradiologic abnormalities associated with septo-optic dysplasia. *Acta Endocrinol Copenh* 107: 282–288.

Asteria C, Oliveira JH, Abucham J, Beck-Peccoz P (2000). Central hypocortisolism as part of combined pituitary hormone deficiency due to mutations of *PROP-1* gene. *Eur J Endocrinol* 143: 347–352.

Bach I (2000). The LIM domain: regulation by association. *Mech Dev* 91: 5–17.

Bach I, Rhodes SJ, Pearse RV, Heinzel T, Gloss B, Scully KM, Sawchenko PE, Rosenfeld MG (1995). P-Lim, a LIM homeodomain factor, is expressed during pituitary organ and cell commitment and synergizes with Pit-1. *Proc Natl Acad Sci USA* 92: 2720–2724.

Bamshad M, Lin RC, Law DJ, Watkins WC, Krakowiak PA, Moore ME, Franceschini P, Lala R, Holmes LB, Gebuhr TC, et al. (1997). Mutations in human *TBX3* alter limb, apocrine and genital development in ulnar-mammary syndrome. *Nat Genet* 16: 311–315.

Barkovich AJ, Kjos BO (1992). Schizencephaly: correlation of clinical findings with MR characteristics. *AJNR Am J Neuroradiol* 13: 85–94.

Barkovich AJ, Fram EK, Norman D (1989). Septo-optic dysplasia: MR imaging. *Radiology* 171: 189–192.

Basson CT, Bachinsky DR, Lin RC, Levi T, Elkins JA, Soults J, Grayzel D, Kroumpouzou E, Traill TA, Leblanc-Straceski J, et al. (1997). Mutations in human *TBX5* [corrected] cause limb and cardiac malformation in Holt-Oram syndrome. *Nat Genet* 15: 30–35.

Basson CT, Huang T, Lin RC, Bachinsky DR, Weremowicz S, Vaglio A, Bruzzone R, Quadrelli R, Lerone M, Romeo G, et al. (1999). Different *TBX5* interactions in heart and limb defined by Holt-Oram syndrome mutations. *Proc Natl Acad Sci USA* 96: 2919–2924.

Benner JD, Preslan MW, Gratz E, Joslyn J, Schwartz M, Kelman S (1990). Septo-optic dysplasia in two siblings. *Am J Ophthalmol* 109: 632–637.

Blethen SL, Weldon VV (1985). Hypopituitarism and septooptic "dysplasia" in first cousins. *Am J Med Genet* 21: 123–129.

Brickman JM, Clements M, Tyrell R, McNay D, Woods K, Warner J, Stewart A, Beddington RS, Dattani M (2001). Molecular effects of novel mutations in *Hesx1/HESX1* associated with human pituitary disorders. *Development* 128: 5189–5199.

Brunelli S, Faiella A, Capra V, Nigro V, Simeone A, Cama A, Boncinelli E (1996). Germline mutations in the homeobox gene *EMX2* in patients with severe schizencephaly. *Nat Genet* 12: 94–96.

Cecchi C, Mallamaci A, Boncinelli E (1999). Mouse forebrain development. The role of *Emx2* homeobox gene. *C R Acad Sci III* 322: 837–842.

Chapman DL, Garvey N, Hancock S, Alexiou M, Agulnik SI, Gibson-Brown JJ, Cebra-Thomas J, Bollag RJ, Silver LM, Papaioannon VE (1996). Expression of T-box family genes Tbx1–Tbx5 during early mouse development. *Dev Dyn* 206: 379–390.

Cogan JD, Wu W, Phillips JA, Arnhold IJ, Agapito A, Fofanova OV, Osorio MG, Bircan I, Moreno A, Mendonca BB (1998). The *PROP1* 2-base pair deletion is a common cause of combined pituitary hormone deficiency. *J Clin Endocrinol Metab* 83: 3346–3349.

Cross SJ, Ching YH, Li QY, Armstrong-Buisseret L, Spranger S, Lyonnet S, Bonnet D, Penttinen M, Jonveaux P, Leheup B, et al. (2000). The mutation spectrum in Holt-Oram syndrome. *J Med Genet* 37: 785–787.

Dalton D, Chadwick R, McGinnis W (1989). Expression and embryonic function of empty spiracles: a *Drosophila* homeo box gene with two patterning functions on the anterior–posterior axis of the embryo. *Genes Dev* 3: 1940–1956.

Dasen JS, Rosenfeld MG (1999). Signaling mechanisms in pituitary morphogenesis and cell fate determination. *Curr Opin Cell Biol* 11: 669–677.

Dasen JS, Barbera JP, Herman TS, Connell SO, Olson L, Ju B, Tollkuhn J, Baek SH, Rose DW, Rosenfeld MG (2001). Temporal regulation of a paired-like homeodomain repressor/TLE corepressor complex and a related activator is required for pituitary organogenesis. *Genes Dev* 15: 3193–3207.

Dattani MT, Martinez Barbera JP, Thomas PQ, Brickman JM, Gupta R, Martensson IL, Toresson H, Fox M, Wales JK, Hindmarsh PC, et al. (1998). Mutations in the homeobox gene *HESX1/Hesx1* associated with septo-optic dysplasia in human and mouse. *Nat Genet* 19: 125–133.

Deladoey J, Fluck C, Buyukgebiz A, Kuhlmann BV, Eble A, Hindmarsh PC, Wu W, Mullis PE (1999). "Hot spot" in the *PROP1* gene responsible for combined pituitary hormone deficiency. *J Clin Endocrinol Metab* 84: 1645–1650.

Delcros B, Campagne D, Bratos M, Vanlieferinghen P, Demeocq F, Malpeuch G (1988). Growth hormone deficiency and primary empty sella turcica in children [in French]. *Ann Pediatr (Paris)* 35: 123–128.

Delhase M, Castrillo JL, De-La-Hoya M, Rajas F, Hooghe PE (1996). AP-1 and Oct-1 transcription factors down-regulate the expression of the human *PIT1/GHF1* gene. *J Biol Chem* 271: 32349–32358.

De Smedt S, Demaerel P, Casaer P, Casteels I (2000). Septo-optic dysplasia in combination with a pigmented skin lesion: a case report with nosological discussion. *Eur J Paediatr Neurol* 4: 189–193.

Duquesnoy RJ (1975). The pituitary dwarf mouse: a model for study of endocrine immunodeficiency disease. *Birth Defects* 11: 536–543.

Ericson J, Norlin S, Jessell TM, Edlund T (1998). Integrated FGF and BMP signaling controls the progression of progenitor cell differentiation and the emergence of pattern in the embryonic anterior pituitary. *Development* 125: 1005–1015.

Faiella A, Brunelli S, Granata T, D'Incerti L, Cardini R, Lenti C, Battaglia G, Boncinelli E (1997). A number of schizencephaly patients including 2 brothers are heterozygous for germline mutations in the homeobox gene *EMX2*. *Eur J Hum Genet* 5: 186–190.

Fofanova OV, Takamura N, Kinoshita E, Parks JS, Brown MR, Peterkova VA, Evgrafov OV, Goncharov NP, Bulatov AA, Dedov II, et al. (1998). A mutational hot spot in the *Prop-1* gene in Russian children with combined pituitary hormone deficiency. *Pituitary* 1: 45–49.

Glenn DJ, Maurer RA (1999). MRG1 binds to the LIM domain of Lhx2 and may function as a coactivator to stimulate glycoprotein hormone alpha-subunit gene expression. *J Biol Chem* 274: 36159–36167.

Herr W, Sturm RA, Clerc RG, Corcoran LM, Baltimore D, Sharp PA, Ingraham HA, Rosenfeld MG, Finney M, Ruvkun G, et al. (1988). The POU domain: a large conserved region in the mammalian *pit-1, oct-1, oct-2*, and *Caenorhabditis elegans unc-86* gene products. *Genes Dev* 2: 1513–1516.

Howard PW, Maurer RA (2000). Identification of a conserved protein that interacts with specific LIM homeodomain transcription factors. *J Biol Chem* 275: 13336–13342.

Ingraham HA, Lala DS, Ikeda Y, Luo X, Shen WH, Nachtigal MW, Abbud R, Nilson JH, Parker KL (1994). The nuclear receptor steroidogenic factor 1 acts at multiple levels of the reproductive axis. *Genes Dev* 8: 2302–2312.

Izenberg N, Rosenblum M, Parks JS (1984). The endocrine spectrum of septo-optic dysplasia. *Clin Pediatr (Phila)* 23: 632–636.

Jacobsen AG, Miyamoto DM, Mai SH (1979). Rathke's pouch morphogenesis in the chick embryo. *J Exp Zool* 207: 351–366.

Japon MA, Rubinstein M, Low MJ (1994). In situ hybridization analysis of anterior pituitary hormone gene expression during fetal mouse development. *J Histochem Cytochem* 42: 1117–1125.

Katsanis N, Ansley SJ, Badano JL, Eichers ER, Lewis RA, Hoskins BE, Scambler PJ, Davidson WS, Beales PL, Lupski JR (2001). Triallelic inheritance in Bardet-Biedl syndrome, a mendelian recessive disorder. *Science* 293: 2256–2259.

Kaufman MH (1992). *An Atlas of Mouse Development*. Academic Press, New York.

Kuban KC, Teele RL, Wallman J (1989). Septo-optic-dysplasia-schizencephaly. Radiographic and clinical features. *Pediatr Radiol* 19: 145–150.

Kuriyama M, Shigematsu Y, Konishi K, Konishi Y, Sudo M, Haruki S, Ito H (1988). Septo-optic dysplasia with infantile spasms. *Pediatr Neurol* 4: 62–65.

Lamolet B, Pulichino A, Lamonerie T, Gauthier Y, Brue T, Enjalbert A, Drouin J (2001). A pituitary cell–restricted T box factor, Tpit, activates POMC transcription in cooperation with Pitx homeoproteins. *Cell* 104: 849–859.

Lamonerie T, Tremblay JJ, Lanctot C, Therrien M, Gauthier Y, Drouin J (1996). Ptx1, a bicoid-related homeo box transcription factor involved in transcription of the proopiomelanocortin gene. *Genes Dev* 10(10): 1284–1295.

Lanctot C, Gautheir Y, Drouin J (1999). *Pituitary homeobox 1 (Ptx1)* is differentially expressed during pituitary development. *Endocrinology* 140(3): 1416–1422.

Lazzaro D, Price M, de Felice M, Di Lauro R (1991). The transcription factor *TTF-1* is expressed at the onset of thyroid and lung morphogenesis and in restricted regions of the foetal brain. *Development* 113: 1093–1104.

Li S, Crenshaw EB, Rawson EJ, Simmons DM, Swanson LW, Rosenfeld MG (1990). Dwarf locus mutants lacking three pituitary cell types result from mutations in the POU-domain gene *pit-1*. *Nature* 347: 528–533.

Li QY, Newbury-Ecob RA, Terrett JA, Wilson DI, Curtis AR, Yi CH, Gebuhr T, Bullen PJ, Robson SC, Strachan T, et al. (1997). Holt-Oram syndrome is caused by mutations in *TBX5*, a member of the *Brachyury (T)* gene family. *Nat Genet* 15: 21–29.

Lin-Su K, Wajnrajch MP (2002). Growth hormone releasing hormone (GHRH) and the GHRH receptor. *Rev Endocrinol Metab Disord* 3: 313–323.

Liu J, Lin C, Gleiberman A, Ohgi KA, Herman T, Huang HP, Tsai MJ, Rosenfeld MG (2001). Tbx19, a tissue-selective regulator of POMC gene expression. *Proc Natl Acad Sci USA* 98: 8674–8679.

Logan M, Tabin CJ (1999). Role of Pitx1 upstream of Tbx4 in specification of hindlimb identity. *Science* 283: 1736–1739.

Machinis K, Pantel J, Netchine I, Leger J, Camand OJ, Sobrier ML, Moal FD, Duquesnoy P, Abitbol M, Czernichow P, et al. (2001). Syndromic short stature in patients with a germline mutation in the lim homeobox *lhx4*. *Am J Hum Genet* 69: 961–968.

Mallamaci A, Mercurio S, Muzio L, Cecchi C, Pardini CL, Gruss P, Boncinelli E (2000). The lack of *Emx2* causes impairment of Reelin signaling and defects of neuronal migration in the developing cerebral cortex. *J Neurosci* 20: 1109–1118.

Martinez-Barbera JP, Rodriguez TA, Beddington RS (2000). The homeobox gene *Hesx1* is required in the anterior neural ectoderm for normal forebrain formation. *Dev Biol* 223: 422–430.

Mendonca BB, Osorio MG, Latronico AC, Estefan V, Lo LS, Arnhold IJ (1999). Longitudinal hormonal and pituitary imaging changes in two females with combined pituitary hormone deficiency due to deletion of A301,G302 in the *PROP1* gene. *J Clin Endocrinol Metab* 84: 942–945.

Miller SP, Shevell MI, Patenaude Y, Poulin C, O'Gorman AM (2000). Septo-optic dysplasia plus: a spectrum of malformations of cortical development. *Neurology* 54: 1701–1703.

Miyamoto N, Yoshida M, Kuratani S, Matsuo I, Aizawa S (1997). Defects of urogenital development in mice lacking *Emx2*. *Development* 124: 1653–1664.

Morishima A, Aranoff GS (1986). Syndrome of septo-optic-pituitary dysplasia: the clinical spectrum. *Brain Dev* 8: 233–239.

Netchine I, Sobrier ML, Krude H, Schnabel D, Maghnie M, Marcos E, Duriez B, Cacheux V, Moers A, Goossens M, et al. (2000). Mutations in *LHX3* result in a new syndrome revealed by combined pituitary hormone deficiency. *Nat Genet* 25: 182–186.

Nuri Sener R (1996). Septo-optic dysplasia associated with cerebral cortical dysplasia (cortico-septo-optic dysplasia). *J Neuroradiol* 23: 245–247.

Ohta K, Nobukuni Y, Mitsubuchi H, Fujimoto S, Matsuo N, Inagaki H, Endo F, Matsuda I (1992). Mutations in the *Pit-1* gene in children with combined pituitary hormone deficiency. *Biochem Biophys Res Commun* 189: 851–855.

Papaioannou VE, Silver LM (1998). The T-box gene family. *Bioessays* 20: 9–19.

Parks JS, Brown MR, Baumbach L, Sanchez JC, Stanley CA, Gianella-Neto D, Wu W, Oyesiku N (1998). Natural history and molecular mechansims of hypopituitarism with large sella turcica. Presented at the American Endocrine Society Meeting. New Orleans, June 24–27, 1998 Abstract no. P3-409 pg 470.

Pellegrini M, Mansouri A, Simeone A, Boncinelli E, Gruss P (1996). Dentate gyrus formation requires *Emx2*. *Development* 122: 3893–3898.

Pellegrini M, Pantano S, Fumi MP, Lucchini F, Forabosco A (2001). Agenesis of the scapula in *Emx2* homozygous mutants. *Dev Biol* 232: 149–156.

Pfaffle RW, DiMattia GE, Parks JS, Brown MR, Wit JM, Jansen M, Van-der-Nat H, Van-den-Brande JL, Rosenfeld MG, Ingraham HA (1992). Mutation of the POU-specific domain of Pit-1 and hypopituitarism without pituitary hypoplasia. *Science* 257: 1118–1121.

Procter AM, Phillips JA, Cooper DN (1998). The molecular genetics of growth hormone deficiency. *Hum Genet* 103: 255–272.

Radovick S, Nations M, Du Y, Berg LA, Weintraub BD, Wondisford FE (1992). A mutation in the POU-homeodomain of *Pit-1* responsible for combined pituitary hormone deficiency. *Science* 257(5073): 1115–1118.

Raetzman LT, Ward R, Camper SA (2002). *Lhx4* and *Prop1* are required for cell survival and expansion of the pituitary primordia. *Development* 129: 4229–4239.

Ramos Fernandez JM, Martinez San Millan J, Barrio Castellano R, Yturriaga Matarranz R, Lorenzo Sanz G, Aparicio Meix JM (1996). Septo-optic dysplasia: report of 6 patients studied with MR and discussion on its pathogenesis [in Spanish]. *An Esp Pediatr* 45: 614–618.

Reeves DL (1941). Congenital absence of septum pellucidum. *Bull Johns Hopkins Hosp* 69: 61–71.

Rosenbloom AL, Almonte AS, Brown MR, Fisher DA, Baumbach L, Parks JS (1999). Clinical and biochemical phenotype of familial anterior hypopituitarism from mutation of the *PROP1* gene. *J Clin Endocrinol Metab* 84: 50–57.

Schwind JL (1928). The development of the hypophysis cerebri of the albino rat. *Am J Anat* 41: 295–315.

Seidah NG, Barale JC, Marcinkiewicz M, Mattei MG, Day R, Chretien M (1994). The mouse homeoprotein mLIM-3 is expressed early in cells derived from the neuroepithelium and persists in adult pituitary. *DNA Cell Biol* 13: 1163–1180.

Shammas NW, Brown JD, Foreman BW, Marutani DR, Maddela D, Tonner D (1993). Septo-optic dysplasia associated with polyendocrine dysfunction. *J Med* 24: 67–74.

Sheng HZ, Westphal H (1999). Early steps in pituitary organogenesis. *Trends Genet* 15: 236–240.

Sheng HZ, Zhadanov AB, Mosinger B, Fujii T, Bertuzzi S, Grinberg A, Lee EJ, Huang SP, Mahon KA, Westphal H (1996). Specification of pituitary cell lineages by the LIM homeobox gene *Lhx3*. *Science* 272: 1004–1007.

Sheng HZ, Moriyama K, Yamashita T, Li H, Potter SS, Mahon KA, Westphal H (1997). Multistep control of pituitary organogenesis. *Science* 278: 1809–1812.

Simeone A, Acampora D, Gulisano M, Stornaiuolo A, Boncinelli E (1992). Nested expression domains of four homeobox genes in developing rostral brain. *Nature* 358: 687–690.

Simmons DM, Voss JW, Ingraham HA, Holloway JM, Broide RS, Rosenfeld MG, Swanson LW (1990). Pituitary cell phenotypes involve cell-specific Pit-1 mRNA translation and synergistic interactions with other classes of transcription factors. *Genes Dev* 4: 695–711.

Sloop KW, Parker GE, Hanna KR, Wright HA, Rhodes SJ (2001). LHX3 transcription factor mutations associated with combined pituitary hormone deficiency impair the activation of pituitary target genes. *Gene* 265: 61–69.

Smith J (1997). *Brachyury* and *T-box* genes. *Curr Opin Gen Dev* 7: 474–479.

Sornson MW, Wu W, Dasen JS, Flynn SE, Norman DJ, O'Connell SM, Gukovsky I, Carriere C, Ryan AK, Miller AP, et al. (1996). Pituitary lineage determination by the Prophet of Pit-1 homeodomain factor defective in Ames dwarfism. *Nature* 384: 327–333.

Takuma N, Sheng HZ, Furuta Y, Ward JM, Sharma K, Hogan LM, Pfaff SL, Westphal H, Kimura S, Mahon KA (1998). Formation of Rathke's pouch requires dual induction from the diencephalon. *Development* 125: 4835–4840.

Tatsumi K, Miyai K, Notomi T, Kaibe K, Amino N, Mizuno Y, Kohno H (1992). Cretinism with combined hormone deficiency caused by a mutation in the *PIT1* gene. *Nat Genet* 1: 56–58.

Thomas PQ, Dattani MT, Brickman JM, McNay D, Warne G, Zacharin M, Cameron F, Hurst J, Woods K, Dunger D, et al. (2001). Heterozygous *HESX1* mutations associated with isolated congenital pituitary hypoplasia and septo-optic dysplasia. *Hum Mol Genet* 10: 39–45.

Treier M, Gleiberman AS, O'Connell SM, Szeto DP, McMahon JA, McMahon AP, Rosenfeld MG (1998). Multistep signaling requirements for pituitary organogenesis in vivo. *Genes Dev* 12: 1691–1704.

Wales JK, Quarrell OW (1996). Evidence for possible mendelian inheritance of septo-optic dysplasia. *Acta Paediatr* 85: 391–392.

Wallis D, Muenke M (2000). Mutations in holoprosencephaly. *Hum Mutat* 16: 99–108.

Wilkinson DG, Bhatt S, Herrmann BG (1990). Expression pattern of the mouse *T* gene and its role in mesoderm formation. *Nature* 343: 657–659.

Willnow S, Kiess W, Butenandt O, Dorr HG, Enders A, Strasser Vogel B, Egger J, Schwarz HP (1996). Endocrine disorders in septo-optic dysplasia (De Morsier syndrome)—evaluation and follow up of 18 patients. *Eur J Pediatr* 155: 179–184.

Wu W, Cogan JD, Pfaffle RW, Dasen JS, Frisch H, O'Connell SM, Flynn SE, Brown MR, Mullis PE, Parks JS, et al. (1998). Mutations in *PROP1* cause familial combined pituitary hormone deficiency. *Nat Genet* 18: 147–149.

Xu L, Glass CK, Rosenfeld MG (1999). Coactivator and corepressor complexes in nuclear receptor function. *Curr Opin Genet Dev* 9: 140–147.

Yamashita T, Moriyama K, Sheng HZ, Westphal H (1997). *Lhx4*, a LIM homeobox gene. *Genomics* 44: 144–146.

Yi CH, Terrett JA, Li QY, Ellington K, Packham EA, Armstrong-Buisseret L, McClure P, Slingsby T, Brook JD (1999). Identification, mapping, and phylogenomic analysis of four new human members of the T-box gene family: *EOMES, TBX6, TBX18,* and *TBX19*. *Genomics* 55: 10–20.

Yoshida M, Suda Y, Matsuo I, Miyamoto N, Takeda N, Kuratani S, Aizawa S (1997). *Emx1* and *Emx2* functions in development of dorsal telencephalon. *Development* 124: 101–111.

Zhadanov AB, Bertuzzi S, Taira M, Dawid IB, Westphal H (1995). Expression pattern of the murine LIM class homeobox gene *Lhx3* in subsets of neural and neuroendocrine tissues. *Dev Dyn* 202: 354–364.

50 | *IDX1* and Pancreatic Agenesis and Type 2 Diabetes

MELISSA K. THOMAS AND JOEL F. HABENER

Islet duodenum homeobox-1 (IDX1) is a pancreas-specific home-odomain transcription factor that regulates embryonic pancreatic development, the expression of genes essential for glucose sensing and metabolism, and the differentiation and function of insulin-producing beta cells in the endocrine pancreas. Expression of IDX1 is confined primarily to the developing embryonic pancreas and the adult pancreas, and IDX1 function is essential for the proper development of both the exocrine and endocrine pancreas. Mutations in the *IDX1* gene are associated with multiple metabolic phenotypes in humans.

IDX1 AND THE DEVELOPMENT OF THE PANCREAS

IDX1 (Miller et al., 1994) was cloned in multiple laboratories and is known in the literature by several names, including IPF-1 (Ohlsson et al., 1993), STF-1 (Leonard et al., 1993), GSF (Marshak et al., 1996), and PDX-1 (Offield et al., 1996). The human gene, known as *IPF-1*, consists of two exons located at chromosome 13q12.1 (Stoffel et al., 1995; Inoue et al., 1996).

IDX1 contains a conserved homeodomain DNA-binding domain, which is related to *Antennapedia* in *Drosophila melanogaster* (Fig. 50–1). The amino acid sequences of IDX1 orthologs are highly conserved in a wide variety of species, including zebrafish (Milewski et al., 1998) and frogs (Wright et al., 1989). The *IDX1* gene is located within a parahox cluster that includes genes for the transcription factors *GSX* and *CDX* (Brooke et al., 1998). Amino-terminal sequences within the protein comprise transcriptional activation domains and contain regions that interact with coactivators including cAMP response element–binding protein–binding protein (CBP) and p300 (Asahara et al., 1999; Qiu et al., 2002) and homeodomain proteins including pbx (Peers et al., 1995; Swift et al., 1998).

Expression of IDX1 is confined largely to the developing embryonic pancreas and the adult pancreas, although limited expression occurs in the CNS (Guz et al., 1995; Schwartz et al., 2000). In mouse embryos, IDX1 expression is first detected at embryonic day (e)8.5 in a small segment of patterned foregut endoderm that is destined to become the pancreas (Fig. 50–2). During the early stages of pancreatic development in the mouse, IDX1 is expressed throughout the dorsal and ventral buds of the pancreas, with subsequent restriction of expression to the developing ductal tree as it undergoes branching morphogenesis and to the associated cells of the endocrine pancreas embedded in the ducts. At the time of birth, IDX1 is expressed in the insulin-producing beta cells within the islets of Langerhans and in a small subset of somatostatin-expressing delta cells (Guz et al., 1995). Studies in transgenic mice show that a 4.6 kb segment of the mouse *Idx1* promoter contains all of the regulatory sequences that are needed to specify the embryonic and adult pancreatic expression patterns of the homeoprotein (Stoffers et al., 1999; Gannon et al., 2001).

IDX1 function is essential for the proper development of both the exocrine and endocrine pancreas. Homozygous disruption of IDX1 expression (*Idx1* gene knockout) in mice results in pancreatic agenesis because of a failure of the ventral and dorsal pancreatic buds to develop (Jonsson et al., 1994; Offield et al., 1996). In *Idx1* knockout mice, the pancreatic epithelium is unable to appropriately signal to the pancreatic mesenchyme and pancreatic development is arrested at the formation of the initial rudimentary dorsal pancreatic bud (Ahlgren et al., 1996; Offield et al., 1996). Lineage tracing studies in mouse models demonstrate that embryonic progenitor cells that express IDX1 dif-ferentiate into pancreatic endocrine, exocrine, and ductal cell types (Herrera, 2000; Gu et al., 2002). During embryonic development of the pancreas, IDX1 facilitates the budding of the endoderm epithelium and participates in the specification of the endocrine and exocrine compartments of the pancreas. Electroporation experiments in chick embryos indicate that IDX1 expression in and of itself is sufficient to induce epithelial budding (Grapin-Botton et al., 2001). Furthermore, ectopic expression of IDX1 in the exocrine compartment late in embryonic development disrupts normal development of the exocrine pancreas (Heller et al., 2001). IDX1 is required in the later stages of pancreatic development for expansion of the pancreatic cell mass, and this function is dependent on interactions with pbx homeoproteins (Dutta et al., 2001).

Multiple signaling cascades and transcription factors converge to regulate IDX1 expression during embryonic development of the pancreas as well as in adult pancreatic beta cells. Conserved regions among the mouse, human, and chick *Idx1* promoters mediate pancreatic beta cell–specific expression and are regulated by the transcription factor hepatocyte nuclear factor-3β (HNF-3β) (Wu et al., 1997; Gerrish et al., 2000; Marshak et al., 2000; Ben-Shushan et al., 2001; Gannon et al., 2001). In experimental animal and cell culture model systems, *idx1* expression is regulated by the transcription factors HNF-1α and HNF-1β, which are implicated in human forms of monogenic diabetes and maturity-onset diabetes of the young (MODY), and by upstream stimulatory factor (USF), promoter-specific factors SP1, and SP3 (Sharma et al., 1996; Qian et al., 1999; Ben-Shushan et al., 2001; Gerrish et al., 2001; Shih et al., 2001; Sun and Hopkins, 2001). The activin/transforming growth factor-β (TGF-β) and hedgehog signaling pathways regulate IDX1 expression levels in the developing and adult pancreas (Hebrok et al., 1998, 2000; Thomas, 2002; Thomas et al., 2001b).

IDX1 IN THE REGULATION OF GLUCOSE HOMEOSTASIS

IDX1 was identified first as a regulator of insulin and somatostatin gene expression (Leonard et al., 1993; Ohlsson et al., 1993; Miller et al., 1994). Extensive studies in several laboratories established that IDX1 is a central component in the regulation of glucose-responsive enhancers that are conserved in rat and human insulin promoters. IDX1 binds to A boxes (encoding conserved nucleotide sequences GTAATC) in the promoters and acts in concert with basic helix-loop-helix transcription factors that bind adjacent E boxes (encoding conserved nucleotide sequences CANNTG), such as Beta2/NeuroD, E12, and E47, to provide both basal and glucose-stimulated transcriptional activation of the insulin promoters. This synergistic transcriptional activation is mediated in part through protein–protein interactions (Ohneda et al., 2000) and the interactions of IDX1 with the coactivators CBP and p300, which stabilize transcriptional enhanceasome multiprotein complexes on the insulin promoter (Asahara et al., 1999; Qiu et al., 2002).

IDX1 also regulates glucose sensing by the insulin-producing pancreatic beta cells within the endocrine pancreas by way of regulating the promoters of the glucose transporter-2 (Glut-2) and glucokinase genes (Waeber et al., 1996; Watada et al., 1996). Additional targets of IDX1 regulation include islet amyloid polypeptide (IAPP) (Serup et al., 1996; Carty et al., 1997), heparin-binding epidermal growth fac-

Figure 50–1. Schematic diagram of IDX1 protein structure. Amino acid positions are designated by number. Transcriptional activation and DNA-binding domains are depicted. Positions of known mutations are designated.

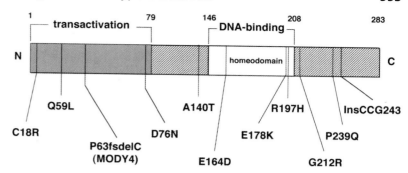

tor-like growth factor (HB-EGF) (Kaneto et al., 1997), and fibroblast growth factor receptor-1 signaling in the developing pancreas (Hart et al., 2000). The functional significance of the regulation of somatostatin expression by IDX1 remains to be elucidated.

Heterozygous disruption of *Idx1* expression in mice (haploinsufficiency) leads to impaired glucose tolerance (Ahlgren et al., 1998; Dutta et al., 1998) and defective glucose-stimulated insulin secretion (Brissova et al., 2002). Pancreas-specific extinction of *Idx1* expression after the pancreas develops in a rat insulin promoter-cre/lox mouse model results in a diabetes phenotype that is accompanied by reduced expression levels of Glut-2 and disorganized increased numbers of glucagon-producing alpha cells within the pancreatic islets (Ahlgren et al., 1998). Inducible suppression of IDX1 mRNA expression increases fasting glucose levels and decreases insulin-to-glucose ratios in older, but not in younger, transgenic mice (Thomas et al., 2001a). Expression levels of the IDX1 protein are tightly regulated in normal pancreatic beta cells, in part by autoregulation of *Idx1* gene expression at the level of the promoter (Thomas et al., 2001a). The reduction of *Idx1* gene dosage accelerates the development of fasting hyperglycemia in mouse models of inducible suppression of *Idx1* expression (Thomas et al., 2002). Metabolic phenotypes associated with IDX1 deficiency likely reflect dysregulation of a combination of glucose sensing, insulin gene expression, and insulin secretion.

IDX1 functions as a metabolic sensor because extracellular glucose levels regulate its phosphorylation (Macfarlane et al., 1994, 1997), nuclear translocation (Rafiq et al., 1998; Macfarlane et al., 1999b), DNA-binding activity (Melloul et al., 1993; Macfarlane et al., 1994), and transcriptional activation potency (Petersen et al., 1998; Shushan et al., 1999). Analyses of insulin receptor substrate-2 (IRS-2) knockout mouse models indicate that IDX1 functions downstream of the insulin-signaling pathway in the regulation of pancreatic beta cell mass (With-

ers et al., 1999; Kushner et al., 2002). IDX1 can "rescue" the development of diabetes in mice lacking the gene encoding IRS-2 (Kushner et al., 2002). The IRS-2 branch of the insulin/insulin-like growth factor signaling system mediates peripheral insulin action and pancreatic beta cell growth and function. Both IDX1 levels and beta cell mass are reduced in the islets from IRS-2 knockout mice. The transgene expression of IDX1 in IRS-2 knockout mice restores beta cell mass and function and promotes normal glucose tolerance throughout life without the development of diabetes (Kushner et al., 2002). Pathophysiologic conditions such as hyperglycemia, hyperlipidemia, and excess glucocorticoids suppress *Idx1* expression (Olson et al., 1995; Sharma et al., 1995; Gremlich et al., 1997; Sharma et al., 1997; Zangen et al., 1997).

Increasing evidence implicates IDX1 as an essential protein required for the differentiation of new beta cells from stem/progenitor cells within the adult pancreas. Mice heterozygous for *Idx1* disruption demonstrate a trend toward reduced pancreatic beta cell mass (Dutta et al., 1998). Expression of IDX1 is associated with cellular proliferation in several model systems. In cultured cells derived from human islets, IDX1-expressing cells proliferate *ex vivo* (Beattie et al., 1999). In experimental systems for endocrine pancreatic differentiation of mouse or human embryonic stem cells, expression of IDX1 is induced (Gerrish et al., 2000; Schuldiner et al., 2000; Assady et al., 2001; Lumelsky et al., 2001). Differentiation of adult pancreas-derived stem/progenitor cells also is associated with induction of nuclear IDX1 expression (Bonner-Weir et al., 2000; Zulewski et al., 2001).

Agents that induce pancreatic beta cell neogenesis (defined as differentiation of new pancreatic beta cells from progenitor cells), such as glucagon-like-peptide-1 (GLP-1) or its agonist exendin-4, induce *IDX1* expression in cellular models of pancreatic beta cell progenitors

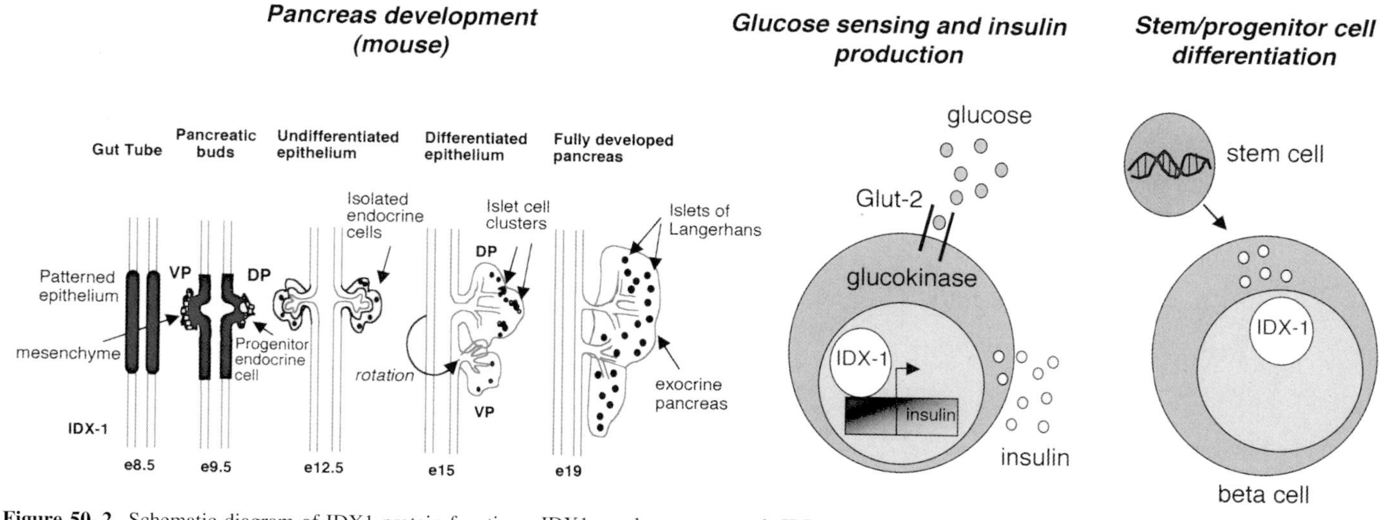

Figure 50–2. Schematic diagram of IDX1 protein functions. IDX1 regulates pancreatic development (*left*). IDX1 expression patterns in the developing mouse pancreas are depicted as black regions, with approximate embryonic ages (in days) designated for each developmental stage. (Adapted from Thomas and Habener, 2002.) Ventral (VP) and dorsal (DP) pancreatic buds are designated. IDX1 regulates glucose-sensing and insulin production in pancreatic beta cells (*middle*). IDX1 regulatory targets glucose transporter-2 (Glut-2), glucokinase, and insulin are depicted. IDX1 expression is a critical step in the differentiation of new pancreatic beta cells from stem/progenitor cells (*right*).

(Zhou et al., 1999; Abraham et al., 2002) and *in vivo* (Stoffers et al., 2000). Regenerating pancreatic beta cells express IDX1 in models of pancreatic injury. In response to administration of the beta cell toxin streptozotocin, a population of somatostatin- and IDX1-coexpressing cells appear in islets and are proposed to represent islet progenitors (Fernandes et al., 1997). Similarly, IDX1 expression increases in both the ductal epithelium from which new pancreatic beta cells arise and islets of the regenerating pancreas in a partial pancreatectomy model (Sharma et al., 1999). Overexpression of IDX1 in the liver induces insulin gene expression in a subpopulation of cells, demonstrating that IDX1 can "reprogram" extrapancreatic (liver) cells into pancreatic beta cell phenotypes (Ferber et al., 2000). Collectively, these studies imply that the induction of IDX1 expression is a critical step in the differentiation of new pancreatic beta cells from stem/progenitor cells.

CLINICAL CONSEQUENCES OF *IDX1* MUTATIONS

Mutations in the *IDX1* gene are associated with multiple metabolic phenotypes in humans. Homozygous disruption of the *Idx1* gene (nullizygosity) results in pancreatic agenesis (Stoffers et al., 1997a), heterozygosity for an inactivating mutation is associated with heritable autosomal-dominant MODY4 (Stoffers et al., 1997b), and heterozygous carriers of missense mutations exhibit a predisposition to the development of adult-onset diabetes (Hani et al., 1999; Macfarlane et al., 1999a) (Table 50–1). Studies of IDX1 function provide striking examples of bi-directional translational research in which mutant phenotypes in humans and mice are highly concordant.

MOLECULAR GENETICS

The first identified mutation in the human *IDX1 (IPF1)* gene was in a patient with pancreatic agenesis. A female Caucasian infant was diagnosed with pancreatic agenesis shortly after birth (Wright et al., 1993). The combined clinical presentation of neonatal diabetes mellitus and pancreatic exocrine insufficiency suggested the absence of a pancreas. The diagnosis was confirmed by abdominal ultrasound. Replacement therapy with insulin and pancreatic enzymes allowed the child to grow and develop normally. Genotyping of the child identified homozygosity for a single cytosine nucleotide deletion within codon 63 in exon 1 of the transcriptional activation domain of the *Idx1* gene (Pro63fsdelC) (Stoffers et al., 1997a). This inactivating deletion mutation shifted the reading frame of the protein with the translation of 59 new codons and terminated the transcript upstream of the conserved homeodomain DNA-binding domain. The extended family of the child with pancreatic agenesis has a high prevalence of early-onset diabetes, with an average age at onset of 35 years and autosomal-dominant inheritance across six generations (Stoffers et al., 1997b). No mutations in the known MODY genes coding for *HNF-4α*, *HNF-1α*, or *glucokinase* were identified in the family members. The Pro63fsdelC *IDX1* mutation segregated with early-onset diabetes in this extended family with a two-point lod score of 3.43. Accordingly, *IDX1* was designated MODY4. Of the six genes with identified mutations linked to MODY syndromes, five are transcription factors implicated in insulin gene regulation and/or pancreatic development (Fajans et al., 2001). Most of the MODY4 family members with dia-

betes were managed with diet or oral hypoglycemic agents without signs of ketosis or severe insulin deficiency. Careful clinical phenotyping of individuals with the Pro63fsdelC mutation by five-step hyperglycemic clamp testing demonstrated that the mutation is associated with a higher fasting glucose level, decreased insulin-to-glucose ratio, and loss of the first-phase insulin secretory response to glucose stimulation (Clocquet et al., 2000). Of note, individuals with the Pro63fsdelC mutation demonstrated increased insulin sensitivity compared to family member control subjects without the mutation.

Functional studies revealed that two isoforms of IDX1 protein are generated by the Pro63fsdelC *IDX1* mutation: a truncated form, which encodes the transcriptional activation domain with novel carboxy-terminal sequences, and a second isoform generated by internal translation, which lacks the transcriptional activation domain but contains the homeodomain DNA-binding domain and the carboxy-terminal sequences of native IDX1 (Stoffers et al., 1998). Because the second IDX1 protein isoform inhibits the transcriptional activation functions of wild-type IDX1, a dominant-negative function of the mutant proteins was proposed to contribute to the molecular mechanism that leads to the observed phenotype.

A child born with severe permanent neonatal diabetes was shown to have pancreatic hypoplasia and compound heterozygous mutations (E164D and E178K) in the homeodomain (exon 2) of IDX1 (Schwitzgebel et al., 2002). In studies in vitro, the mutated IDX1 protein has a shorter half-life and diminished interactions with E47 and Beta2/NeuroD.

Several missense mutations in *IDX1* are associated with a predisposition to the development of Type 2 diabetes, with a later age at onset than MODY4. Two single amino acid substitutions (Q59L and D76N) and one in-frame proline insertion (InsCCG243) were identified in a French population (Hani et al., 1999). The InsCCG243 *IDX1* mutation was linked to an autosomal-dominant late-onset diabetes with progressive impairment of insulin secretion. The Q59L and D76N *IDX1* mutations were less penetrant and conferred a relative risk of 12.6 for the development of diabetes. These missense mutations were associated with a reduction in glucose-stimulated insulin secretion. Plasma insulin-to-glucose ratios were reduced substantially in carriers of the D76N *Idx1* mutation in response to oral glucose tolerance tests. Missense *IDX1* mutations with the amino acid substitutions (C18R, D76N, and R197H) were identified in patients with adult-onset diabetes in a Caucasian population from the United Kingdom (Macfarlane et al., 1999a). In a Danish population, the D76N *IDX1* mutation was identified but did not segregate with the diabetes phenotype; however, a MODY patient was identified with a novel A140T *IDX1* mutation (Hansen et al., 2000).

Several cosegregations of *IDX1* mutations with MODY3 mutations (in *HNF-1α*) were noted in Scandinavian patients (Weng et al., 2001). The P239Q *IDX1* mutation cosegregated with a MODY3 mutation (R272C in *HNF-1α*) in one MODY family and was observed independently in three families with Type 2 diabetes. The D76N *IDX1* mutation also cosegregated with a MODY3 mutation (S315fsinsA in *HNF-1α*) and was observed in two Scandinavian families with adult-onset diabetes. An additional G212R *IDX1* mutation was identified in a Scandinavian family with early-onset diabetes (defined as less than 40 years of age). Glucose tolerance testing of Scandinavian nondia-

Table 50–1. Known Mutations in the *IDX1* (*IPF1*) Gene Associated with the Development of Type 2 Diabetes Mellitus

Mutation	Population	Phenotype	References
C18R	UK	Early-late-onset DM	Macfarlane et al., 1999a
Q59L	France	Early-late-onset DM	Hani et al., 1999; Waeber et al., 2000
P63fsdelC	USA	MODY4, pancreatic agenesis	Stoffers et al., 1997a,b
D76N	France, UK, Denmark	Early/late-onset DM	Hani et al., 1999; Macfarlane et al., 1999a; Hansen et al., 2000
A140T	Denmark	Early-onset DM	Hansen et al., 2000
E164D	Switzerland	Permanent neonatal DM	Schwitzgebel et al., 2002
E178K	Switzerland	Permanent neonatal DM	Schwitzgebel et al., 2002
R197H	UK	Late-onset DM	Macfarlane et al., 1999a
G212R	Sweden	No cosegregation	Weng et al., 2001
P239Q	Sweden	Early-late-onset DM, gestational DM	Weng et al., 2001, 2002
InsCCG243	France	Late-onset DM	Hani et al., 1999

DM, diabetes mellitus; MODY, maturity-onset diabetes of youth.

betic carriers of the *IDX1* mutations revealed increased glucose levels and reduced insulin-to-glucose ratios compared to noncarrier family member controls (Weng et al., 2001). A complex mouse model with a double heterozygous disruption of the *IDX1* and *HNF-1α* genes developed progressive impaired glucose tolerance, diminished glucose-stimulated insulin secretion, and abnormalities in islet cell architecture (Shih et al., 2002). A French family was identified in which the cosegregation of the Q59L *IDX1* mutation with a missense mutation (S59N) in the islet-brain-1 (*IBL*) gene resulted in the development of insulin-dependent diabetes (Waeber et al., 2000). Most of the functional studies of *IDX1* mutations demonstrate decreased transcriptional activation of insulin promoter–reporter constructs *in vitro* (Hani et al., 1999; Macfarlane et al., 1999a; Hansen et al., 2000; Weng et al., 2001).

In a group of Swedish women with gestational diabetes mellitus and a family history of diabetes, mutations in the MODY2, MODY3, and MODY4 genes were found (Weng et al., 2002). One patient with gestational diabetes mellitus carried the P239Q *IDX1* mutation. She required supplemental insulin therapy during her pregnancy; however, her glucose tolerance was normal a year after delivery. This phenotype suggests that in the presence of the P239Q *IDX1* missense mutation the pancreatic beta cells could not compensate for the increased insulin resistance and insulin requirements of pregnancy. Screening of additional women with gestational diabetes and of children and adolescents with impaired glucose tolerance or diabetes for *IDX1* and other MODY gene mutations will be important in the setting of the epidemic increase in obesity and the metabolic syndrome in younger populations.

MANAGEMENT: THERAPEUTIC AND PROGNOSTIC IMPLICATIONS

The prevalence of *IDX1* mutations in patients with Type 2 diabetes is unknown, but estimates from population-based studies range from 1% to 6% (Reis et al., 2000). Furthermore, the predictive value of genetic screening for *IDX1* mutations is not yet established (Hattersley, 1998). Studies in mouse models suggest that IDX1 deficiency from the transient suppression of *Idx1* expression, in the absence of mutations in the *Idx1* gene, is sufficient to induce fasting hyperglycemia in older mice (Thomas et al., 2001a). Thus, therapeutic approaches to restore normal IDX1 expression levels and function in pancreatic beta cells may have broad application for individuals with Type 2 diabetes. GLP-1 agonists and inhibitors of GLP-1 cleavage by dipeptidyl peptidase IV are in clinical trials for the treatment of diabetes. These agents function, at least in part, to increase the expression and activation of IDX1. Studies of the regulation of IDX1 expression are likely to identify additional signaling pathways that merit consideration for therapeutic development for cell-based or small molecule treatments of diabetes (Thomas et al., 2001b).

MUTATIONS IN ORTHOLOGOUS GENES

Engineered *Idx1* mutations in the mouse are discussed in earlier sections.

DEVELOPMENTAL PATHOGENESIS

The mechanisms by which IDX1 mutations result in pancreatic agenesis and diabetes are discussed in earlier sections.

REFERENCES

Abraham EJ, Leech CA, Lin J, Zulewski H, Habener JF (2002). Insulinotropic hormone glucagon-like peptide-1 differentiation of human pancreatic islet–derived progenitor cells into insulin-producing cells. *Endocrinology* 143: 3152–3161.
Ahlgren U, Jonsson J, Edlund H (1996). The morphogenesis of the pancreatic mesenchyme is uncoupled from that of the pancreatic epithelium in IPF1/PDX1-deficient mice. *Development* 122: 1409–1416.
Ahlgren U, Jonsson J, Jonsson L, Simu K, Edlund H (1998). β-cell-specific inactivation of the mouse *Ipf1/Pdx1* gene results in loss of the β-cell phenotype and maturity onset diabetes. *Genes Dev* 12: 1763–1768.
Asahara H, Dutta S, Kao HY, Evans RM, Montminy M (1999). Pbx–Hox heterodimers recruit coactivator–corepressor complexes in an isoform-specific manner. *Mol Cell Biol* 19: 8219–8225.

Assady S, Maor G, Amit M, Itskovitz-Eldor J, Skorecki KL, Tzukerman M (2001). Insulin production by human embryonic stem cells. *Diabetes* 50: 1691–1697.
Beattie GM, Itkin-Ansari P, Cirulli V, Leibowitz G, Lopez AD, Bossie S, Mally MI, Levine F, Hayek A (1999). Sustained proliferation of PDX-1+ cells derived from human islets. *Diabetes* 48: 1013–1019.
Ben-Shushan E, Marshak S, Shoshkes M, Cerasi E, Melloul D (2001). A pancreatic beta-cell-specific enhancer in the human *PDX-1* gene is regulated by hepatocyte nuclear factor 3beta (HNF-3beta), HNF-1alpha, and SPs transcription factors. *J Biol Chem* 276: 17533–17540.
Bonner-Weir S, Taneja M, Weir GC, Tatarkiewicz K, Song KH, Sharma A, O'Neil JJ (2000). In vitro cultivation of human islets from expanded ductal tissue. *Proc Natl Acad Sci USA* 97: 7999–8004.
Brissova M, Shiota M, Nicholson WE, Gannon M, Knobel SM, Piston DW, Wright CV, Powers AC (2002). Reduction in pancreatic transcription factor PDX-1 impairs glucose-stimulated insulin secretion. *J Biol Chem* 277: 11225–11232.
Brooke NM, Garcia-Fernandez J, Holland PWH (1998). The *ParaHox* gene cluster is an evolutionary sister of the *Hox* gene cluster. *Nature* 392: 920–922.
Carty MD, Lillquist JS, Peshavaria M, Stein R, Soeller WC (1997). Identification of *cis*- and *trans*-active factors regulating human islet amyloid polypeptide gene expression in pancreatic beta-cells. *J Biol Chem* 272: 11986–11993.
Clocquet AR, Egan JM, Stoffers DA, Muller DC, Wideman L, Chin GA, Clarke WL, Hanks JB, Habener JF, Elahi D (2000). Impaired insulin secretion and increased insulin sensitivity in familial maturity-onset diabetes of the young 4 (insulin promoter factor 1 gene). *Diabetes* 49: 1856–1864.
Dutta S, Bonner-Weir S, Montminy M, Wright C (1998). Regulatory factor linked to late-onset diabetes? *Nature* 392: 560.
Dutta S, Gannon M, Peers B, Wright C, Bonner-Weir S, Montminy M (2001). PDX: PBX complexes are required for normal proliferation of pancreatic cells during development. *Proc Natl Acad Sci USA* 98: 1065–1070.
Fajans SS, Bell GI, Polonsky KS (2001). Molecular mechanisms and clinical pathophysiology of maturity-onset diabetes of the young. *N Engl J Med* 345: 971–980.
Ferber S, Halkin A, Cohen H, Ber I, Einav Y, Goldberg I, Barshack I, Seijffers R, Kopolovic J, Kaiser N, et al. (2000). Pancreatic and duodenal homeobox gene 1 induces expression of insulin genes in liver and ameliorates streptozotocin-induced hyperglycemia. *Nat Med* 6: 568–572.
Fernandes A, King LC, Guz Y, Stein R, Wright CVE (1997). Differentiation of new insulin-producing cells is induced by injury in adult pancreatic islets. *Endocrinology* 138: 1750–1762.
Gannon M, Gamer LW, Wright CV (2001). Regulatory regions driving developmental and tissue-specific expression of the essential pancreatic gene *pdx1*. *Dev Biol* 238: 185–201.
Gerrish K, Gannon M, Shih D, Henderson E, Stoffel M, Wright CV, Stein R (2000). Pancreatic beta cell-specific transcription of the *pdx-1* gene. The role of conserved upstream control regions and their hepatic nuclear factor 3beta sites. *J Biol Chem* 275: 3485–3492.
Gerrish KE, Cissell MA, Stein R (2001). The role of hepatic nuclear factor 1α and PDX-1 in transcriptional regulation of the pdx-1 gene. *J Biol Chem* 276: 47775–47784.
Grapin-Botton A, Majithia AR, Melton DA (2001). Key events of pancreas formation are triggered in gut endoderm by ectopic expression of pancreatic regulatory genes. *Genes Dev* 15: 444–454.
Gremlich S, Bonny C, Waeber G, Thorens B (1997). Fatty acids decrease IDX-1 expression in rat pancreatic islets and reduce GLUT2, glucokinase, insulin, and somatostatin levels. *J Biol Chem* 272: 30261–30269.
Gu G, Dubauskaite J, Melton DA (2002). Direct evidence for the pancreatic lineage: NGN3+ cells are distinct from duct progenitors. *Development* 129: 2447–2457.
Guz Y, Montminy MR, Stein R, Leonard J, Gamer LW, Wright CVE, Teitelman G (1995). Expression of murine STF-1, a putative insulin gene transcription factor, in β cells of pancreas, duodenal epithelium and pancreatic exocrine and endocrine progenitors during ontogeny. *Development* 121: 11–18.
Hani EH, Stoffers DA, Chevre JC, Durand E, Stanojevic V, Dina C, Habener JF, Froguel P (1999). Defective mutations in the insulin promoter factor-1 (IPF-1) gene in late-onset Type 2 diabetes mellitus. *J Clin Invest* 104: R41–48.
Hansen L, Urioste S, Petersen HV, Jensen JN, Eiberg H, Barbetti F, Serup P, Hansen T, Pedersen O (2000). Missense mutations in the human insulin promoter factor-1 gene and their relation to maturity-onset diabetes of the young and late-onset Type 2 diabetes mellitus in Caucasians. *J Clin Endocrinol Metab* 85: 1323–1326.
Hart AW, Baeza N, Apelqvist A, Edlund H (2000). Attenuation of FGF signalling in mouse beta-cells leads to diabetes. *Nature* 408: 864–868.
Hattersley AT (1998). Maturity-onset diabetes of the young: clinical heterogeneity explained by genetic heterogeneity. *Diabetes Med* 15: 15–24.
Hebrok M, Kim SK, Melton DA (1998). Notochord repression of endodermal sonic hedgehog permits pancreas development. *Genes Dev* 12: 1705–1713.
Hebrok M, Kim SK, St Jacques B, McMahon AP, Melton DA (2000). Regulation of pancreas development by hedgehog signaling. *Development* 127: 4905–4913.
Heller RS, Stoffers DA, Bock T, Svenstrup K, Jensen J, Horn T, Miller CP, Habener JF, Madsen OD, Serup P (2001). Improved glucose tolerance and acinar dysmorphogenesis by targeted expression of transcription factor PDX-1 to the exocrine pancreas. *Diabetes* 50: 1553–1561.
Herrera PL (2000). Adult insulin- and pancreas-producing cells differentiate from two independent cell lineages. *Development* 127: 2317–2322.
Inoue H, Riggs AC, Tanizawa Y, Ueda K, Kuwano A, Liu L, Donis-Keller H, Permutt MA (1996). Isolation, characterization, and chromosomal mapping of the human insulin promoter factor 1 (*IPF-1*) gene. *Diabetes* 45: 789–794.
Jonsson J, Carlsson L, Edlund T, Edlund H (1994). Insulin-promoter-factor 1 is required for pancreas development in mice. *Nature* 371: 606–609.
Kaneto H, Miyagawa J, Kajimoto Y, Yamamoto K, Watada H, Umayahara Y, Hanafusa T, Matsuzawa Y, Yamasaki Y, Higashiyama S, et al. (1997). Expression of heparin-binding epidermal growth factor-like factor during pancreas development. A potential role of PDX-1 in transcriptional activation. *J Biol Chem* 272: 29137–29143.

Kushner JA, Ye J, Schubert M, Burks DJ, Dow MA, Flint CL, Dutta S, Wright CV, Montminy MR, White MF (2002). Pdx1 restores beta cell function in Irs2 knockout mice. *J Clin Invest* 109: 1193–1201.

Leonard J, Peers B, Johnson T, Ferreri K, Lee S, Montminy MR (1993). Characterization of somatostatin transactivating factor-1, a novel homeobox factor that stimulates somatostatin expression in pancreatic islet cells. *Mol Endocrinol* 7: 1275–1283.

Lumelsky N, Blondel O, Laeng P, Velasco I, Ravin R, McKay R (2001). Differentiation of embryonic stem cells to insulin-secreting structures similar to pancreatic islets. *Science* 292: 1389–1394.

Macfarlane WM, Read ML, Gilligan M, Bujalska I, Docherty K (1994). Glucose modulates the binding activity of the β cell transcription factor IUF-1 in a phosphorylation-dependent manner. *Biochem J* 303: 625–631.

Macfarlane WM, Smith SB, James RF, Clifton AD, Doza YN, Cohen P, Docherty K (1997). The p38/reactivating kinase mitogen-activated protein kinase cascade mediates the activation of the transcription factor insulin upstream factor 1 and insulin gene transcription by high glucose in pancreatic beta-cells. *J Biol Chem* 272: 20936–20944.

Macfarlane WM, Frayling TM, Ellard S, Evans JC, Allen LI, Bulman MP, Ayres S, Shepherd M, Clark P, Millward A, Demaine A, et al. (1999a). Missense mutations in the insulin promoter factor-1 gene predispose to Type 2 diabetes. *J Clin Invest* 104: R33–R39.

Macfarlane WM, McKinnon CM, Felton-Edkins ZA, Cragg H, James RF, Docherty K (1999b). Glucose stimulates translocation of the homeodomain transcription factor PDX1 from the cytoplasm to the nucleus in pancreatic beta-cells. *J Biol Chem* 274: 1011–1016.

Marshak S, Totary H, Cerasi E, Melloul D (1996). Purification of the beta-cell glucose-sensitive factor that transactivates the insulin gene differentially in normal and transformed islet cells. *Proc Natl Acad Sci USA* 93: 15057–15062.

Marshak S, Benshushan E, Shoshkes M, Havin L, Cerasi E, Melloul D (2000). Functional conservation of regulatory elements in the *pdx-1* gene: PDX-1 and hepatocyte nuclear factor 3β transcription factors mediate β-cell-specific expression. *Mol Cell Biol* 20: 7583–7590.

Melloul D, Ben-Neriah Y, Cerasi E (1993). Glucose modulates the binding of an islet-specific factor to a conserved sequence within the rat I and the human insulin promoters. *Proc Natl Acad Sci USA* 90: 3865–3869.

Milewski WM, Duguay SJ, Chan SJ, Steiner DF (1998). Conservation of PDX-1 structure, function, and expression in zebrafish. *Endocrinology* 139: 1440–1449.

Miller CP, McGehee RE, Habener JF (1994). IDX1: a new homeodomain transcription factor expressed in rat pancreatic islets and duodenum that transactivates the somatostatin gene. *EMBO J* 13: 1145–1156.

Offield MF, Jetton TL, Labosky PA, Ray M, Stein RW, Magnuson MA, Hogan BLM, Wright CVE (1996). PDX-1 is required for pancreatic outgrowth and differentiation of the rostral duodenum. *Development* 122: 983–995.

Ohlsson H, Karlsson K, Edlund T (1993). IPF1, a homeodomain-containing transactivator of the insulin gene. *EMBO J* 12: 4251–4259.

Ohneda K, Mirmira RG, Wang J, Johnson JD, German MS (2000). The homeodomain of PDX-1 mediates multiple protein–protein interactions in the formation of a transcriptional activation complex on the insulin promoter. *Mol Cell Biol* 20: 900–911.

Olson LK, Sharma A, Peshavaria M, Wright VE, Towle HC, Robertson RP, Stein R (1995). Reduction of insulin gene transcription in HIT-T15 β cells chronically exposed to a supraphysiologic glucose concentration is associated with loss of STF-1 transcription factor expression. *Proc Natl Acad Sci USA* 92: 9127–9131.

Peers B, Sharma S, Johnson T, Kamps M, Montminy M (1995). The pancreatic islet factor STF-1 binds cooperatively with Pbx to a regulatory element in the somatostatin promoter: importance of the FPWMK motif and of the homeodomain. *Mol Cell Biol* 15: 7091–7097.

Petersen HV, Peshavaria M, Pedersen AA, Philippe J, Stein R, Madsen OD, Serup P (1998). Glucose stimulates the activation domain potential of the PDX-1 homeodomain transcription factor. *FEBS Lett* 431: 362–366.

Qian J, Kaytor EN, Towle HC, Olson LK (1999). Upstream stimulatory factor regulates *Pdx-1* gene expression in differentiated pancreatic beta-cells. *Biochem J* 341: 315–322.

Qiu Y, Guo M, Huang S, Stein R (2002). Insulin gene transcription is mediated by interactions between the p300 coactivator and PDX-1, BETA2, and E47. *Mol Cell Biol* 22: 412–420.

Rafiq I, Kennedy HJ, Rutter GA (1998). Glucose-dependent translocation of insulin promoter factor-1 (IPF-1) between the nuclear periphery and the nucleoplasm of single MIN6 β-cells. *J Biol Chem* 273: 23241–23247.

Reis AF, Ye WZ, Dubois-Laforgue D, Bellanne-Chantelot C, Timsit J, Velho G (2000). Mutations in the insulin promoter factor-1 gene in late-onset Type 2 diabetes mellitus. *Eur J Endocrinol* 143: 511–513.

Schuldiner M, Yanuka O, Itskovitz-Eldor J, Melton DA, Benvenisty N (2000). From the cover: effects of eight growth factors on the differentiation of cells derived from human embryonic stem cells. *Proc Natl Acad Sci USA* 97: 11307–11312.

Schwartz PT, Perez-Vellamil B, Rivera A, Moratalla R, Vallejo M (2000). Pancreatic homeodomain transcription factor IDX1/IPF1 expressed in developing brain regulates somatostatin gene transcription in embryonic neural cells. *J Biol Chem* 275: 19106–19114.

Schwitzgebel VM, Mamin A, Brun T, Ritz-Laser B, Zaiko M, Maret A, Theintz GE, Philippe J (2002). Decreased IPF1 level due to compound heterozygous mutation leads to agenesis of human pancreas. Endocrine Society. Annual Meeting Program, June 19–22, San Francisco, California. Abstract nr. PI-26.

Serup P, Jensen J, Andersen FG, Jørgensen MC, Blume N, Holst JJ, Madsen OD (1996). Induction of insulin and islet amyloid polypeptide production in pancreatic islet glucagonoma cells by insulin promoter factor 1. *Proc Natl Acad Sci USA* 93: 9015–9020.

Sharma A, Olson LK, Robertson RP, Stein R (1995). The reduction of insulin gene transcription in HIT-T15 β cells chronically exposed to high glucose concentration is associated with the loss of RIPE3b1 and STF-1 transcription factor expression. *Mol Endocrinol* 9: 1127–1134.

Sharma S, Leonard J, Lee S, Chapman HD, Leiter EH, Montminy MR (1996). Pancreatic islet expression of the homeobox factor STF-1 relies on an E-box motif that binds USF. *J Biol Chem* 271: 2294–2299.

Sharma S, Jhala US, Johnson T, Ferreri K, Leonary J, Montminy M (1997). Hormonal regulation of an islet-specific enhancer in the pancreatic homeobox gene *STF-1*. *Mol Cell Biol* 17: 2598–2604.

Sharma A, Zangen DH, Reitz P, Taneja M, Lissauer ME, Miller CP, Weir GC, Habener JF, Bonner-Weir S (1999). The homeodomain protein IDX1 increases after an early burst of proliferation during pancreatic regeneration. *Diabetes* 48: 507–513.

Shih DQ, Screenan S, Munoz KN, Philipson L, Pontoglio M, Yaniv M, Polonsky KS, Stoffel M (2001). Loss of HNF-1alpha function in mice leads to abnormal expression of genes involved in pancreatic islet development and metabolism. *Diabetes* 50: 2472–2480.

Shih DQ, Heimesaat M, Kuwajima S, Stein R, Wright CV, Stoffel M (2002). Profound defects in pancreatic beta-cell function in mice with combined heterozygous mutations in Pdx-1, Hnf-1alpha, and Hnf-3beta. *Proc Natl Acad Sci USA* 99: 3818–3823.

Shushan EB, Cerasi E, Melloul D (1999). Regulation of the insulin gene by glucose: stimulation of *trans*-activation potency of human PDX-1 N-terminal domain. *DNA Cell Biol* 18: 471–479.

Stoffel M, Stein R, Wright CV, Espinosa R 3rd, Le Beau MM, Bell GI (1995). Localization of human homeodomain transcription factor insulin promoter factor 1 (IPF1) to chromosome band 13q12.1. *Genomics* 28: 125–126.

Stoffers DA, Zinkin NT, Stanojevic V, Clarke WL, Habener JF (1997a). Pancreatic agenesis attributable to a single nucleotide deletion in the human *IPF1* coding region. *Nat Genet* 15: 106–110.

Stoffers DA, Ferrer J, Clarke WL, Habener JF (1997b). Early-onset type-II diabetes mellitus (MODY4) linked to *IPF-1*. *Nat Genet* 17: 138–139.

Stoffers DA, Stanojevic V, Habener JF (1998). Insulin promoter factor-1 gene mutation linked to early-onset type 2 diabetes mellitus directs expression of a dominant negative isoprotein. *J Clin Invest* 102: 232–241.

Stoffers DA, Heller RS, Miller CP, Habener JF (1999). Developmental expression of the homeodomain protein IDX1 in mice transgenic for an IDX1 promoter/lacZ transcriptional reporter. *Endocrinology* 140: 5374–5381.

Stoffers DA, Kieffer TJ, Hussain MA, Drucker DJ, Bonner-Weir S, Habener JF, Egan JM (2000). Insulinotropic glucagon-like peptide 1 agonists stimulate expression of homeodomain protein IDX1 and increase islet size in mouse pancreas. *Diabetes* 49: 741–748.

Sun Z, Hopkins N (2001). *vhnf1*, the MODY5 and familial GCKD-associated gene, regulates regional specification of the zebrafish gut, pronephros, and hindbrain. *Genes Dev* 15: 3217–3229.

Swift GH, Liu Y, Rose SD, Bischof LJ, Steelman S, Buchberg AM, Wright CVE, MacDonald RJ (1998). An endocrine–exocrine switch in the activity of the pancreatic homeodomain protein PDX1 through formation of a trimeric complex with PBX1b and MRG1 (MEIS2). *Mol Cell Biol* 18: 5109–5120.

Thomas MK (2002). Hedgehog signaling in pancreas development and the regulation of insulin production. *Curr Opin Endocrinol Diabetes* 9: 168–173.

Thomas MK, Habener JF (2002). Pancreas development. In: *Immunologically Mediated Endocrine Diseases.* Gill GR (ed.) Lippincott Williams & Wilkins, Philadelphia, pp. 141–166.

Thomas MK, Devon ON, Lee JH, Peter A, Schlosser DA, Tenser MS, Habener JF (2001a). Development of diabetes mellitus in aging transgenic mice following suppression of pancreatic homeoprotein IDX1. *J Clin Invest* 108: 319–329.

Thomas MK, Lee JH, Rastalsky N, Habener JF (2001b). Hedgehog signaling regulation of homeodomain protein islet duodenum homeobox-1 expression in pancreatic beta-cells. *Endocrinology* 142: 1033–1040.

Thomas MK, Devon ON, Gannon M, Wright C, Habener JF (2002). Age- and gene dose-dependent diabetes as a result of inducible suppression of pdx-1 expression. Endocrine Society. Annual Meeting Program, June 19–22, 2002, San Francisco, California. Abstract nr. PI-24.

Waeber G, Thompson N, Nicod P, Bonny C (1996). Transcriptional activation of the *GLUT2* gene by the IPF-1/STF-1/IDX1 homeobox factor. *Mol Endocrinol* 10: 1327–1334.

Waeber G, Delplanque J, Bonny C, Mooser V, Steinmann M, Widmann C, Miklossy J, Dina C, Hani EH, Vionnet N, et al. (2000). The gene *MAPK8IP1*, encoding islet-brain-1, is a candidate for Type 2 diabetes. *Nat Genet* 24: 291–295.

Watada H, Kajimoto Y, Umayahara Y, Matsuoka T, Kaneto H, Fujitani Y, Kamada T, Kawamori R, Yamasaki Y (1996). The human glucokinase gene beta-cell-type promoter: an essential role of insulin promoter factor 1/PDX-1 in its activation in HIT-T15 cells. *Diabetes* 45: 1478–1488.

Weng J, Macfarlane WM, Lehto M, Gu HF, Shepherd LM, Ivarsson SA, Wibell L, Smith T, Groop LC (2001). Functional consequences of mutations in the MODY4 gene (*IPF1*) and coexistence with MODY3 mutations. *Diabetologia* 44: 249–258.

Weng J, Ekelund M, Lehto M, Li H, Ekberg G, Frid A, Aberg A, Groop LC, Berntorp K (2002). Screening for MODY mutations, GAD antibodies, and Type 1 diabetes–associated HLA genotypes in women with gestational diabetes mellitus. *Diabetes Care* 25: 68–71.

Withers DJ, Burks DJ, Towery HH, Altamuro SL, Flint CL, White MF (1999). Irs-2 coordinates Igf-1 receptor-mediated beta-cell development and peripheral insulin signalling. *Nat Genet* 23: 32–40.

Wright CV, Schnegelsberg P, De Robertis EM (1989). XlHbox 8: a novel *Xenopus* homeo protein restricted to a narrow band of endoderm. *Development* 105: 787–794.

Wright NM, Metzger DL, Borowitz SM, Clarke WL (1993). Permanent neonatal diabetes mellitus and pancreatic exocrine insufficiency resulting from congenital pancreatic agenesis. *Am J Dis Child* 147: 607–609.

Wu J-L, Gannon M, Peshavaria M, Offield MF, Henderson E, Ray M, Marks A, Gamer LW, Wright CVE, Stein R (1997). Hepatocyte nuclear factor 3β is involved in pancreatic β-cell-specific transcription of the *pdx-1* gene. *Mol Cell Biol* 17: 6002–6013.

Zangen DH, Bonner-Weir S, Lee CH, Latimer JB, Miller CP, Habener JF (1997). Reduced insulin, GLUT2, and IDX1 in β-cells after partial pancreatectomy. *Diabetes* 46: 258–264.

Zhou J, Wang X, Pineyro MA, Egan JM (1999). Glucagon-like peptide 1 and exendin-4 convert pancreatic AR42J cells into glucagon- and insulin-producing cells. *Diabetes* 48: 2358–2366.

Zulewski H, Abraham EJ, Gerlach MJ, Daniel PB, Moritz W, Muller B, Vallejo M, Thomas MK, Habener JF (2001). Multipotential nestin-positive stem cells isolated from adult pancreatic islets differentiate *ex vivo* into pancreatic endocrine, exocrine, and hepatic phenotypes. *Diabetes* 50: 521–533.

51 | *MSX1* and Partial Anodontia, Orofacial Clefting, and the Witkop Syndrome

MARIE-JOSÉ H. VAN DEN BOOGAARD

Msx1, isolated by homology to the Drosophila muscle-segment homeobox (msh) gene, is highly conserved; it plays an important role in inductive epithelial–mesenchymal interactions, leading to vertebrate organogenesis, and is involved in cell differentiation. During embryonic development, *Msx1* is intensely expressed in the facial primordium and in a variety of embryonic tissues requiring epithelial–mesenchymal interactions for their morphogenesis, such as limb buds and tooth buds.

Msx1 knockout mice exhibit craniofacial defects including cleft palate, abnormalities of the middle ear, defective nail plate, and absent tooth development.

MSX1 mutations in humans are associated with similar phenotypes: partial anodontia, nonsyndromic clefting, and Witkop syndrome (tooth–nail syndrome, OMIM 189500).

The *MSX* genes of vertebrates comprise a small family of homeobox-containing genes. The *msh/msx* gene family is one of the most evolutionarily highly conserved families of homeobox-containing genes and is represented in different species (Table 51–1) (Holland, 1991; reviewed by Davidson, 1995; Bendall and Abate-Shen, 2000).

Three subclasses can be identified in vertebrates based on a few differences in the homeodomain and neighboring regions of the proteins: Msx1, Msx2 (formerly Hox 7.1 and Hox 8, respectively; for new nomenclature, see Scott, 1992), and Msx3. These genes encode closely related homeodomains.

The observation that *Msx* genes are highly conserved, the specific expression pattern of *Msx1*, its involvement in epithelial–mesenchymal interaction, and the role of *Msx1* in the regulation of cellular differentiation by transcriptional repression suggest that *Msx1* plays an essential role in vertebrate development (Davidson, 1995; Bendall and Abate-Shen, 2000). This is supported by the observation that mutations in *Msx1* result in congenital anomalies in both mice and humans.

ROLE OF MSX1 IN DEVELOPMENT

Expression Pattern of *Msx1*

Msx1 is broadly expressed during embryogenesis and organogenesis, and extensive studies of its expression in mouse embryos have been performed (Hill et al., 1989; Robert et al., 1989; MacKenzie et al., 1991a,b; reviewed by Davidson and Hill, 1991; Davidson, 1995; Sadler and Potts, 1997; Houzelstein et al., 1997, 1999, 2000; Bendall and Abate-Shen, 2000). During embryonic development, *Msx1* is expressed in a variety of tissues in a dynamic manner. The earliest expression in the mouse embryo is detectable in the primitive streak, followed by expression in the neural crest and in cells derived from the neural crest before, during, and after their migration.

Striking expression is seen in craniofacial structures, like the nasal and maxillary processes and mandibular arch, and later in the mouth structures that develop from the arch (Fig. 51–1 shows 11.5 days postconception [dpc]). *Msx1* is expressed in the dental papilla and surrounding mesenchymal tissue (Fig. 51–2 shows 13.5 dpc).

The developing limb bud is another major site of *Msx1* expression (Fig. 51–1). During development, the transcripts become restricted to the distal portion of the developing limb bud, which is essential for limb morphogenesis (Hill et al., 1989; Robert et al., 1989; MacKenzie et al., 1991b; reviewed in Cohn and Tickle, 1996; Houzelstein et al., 1997; Johnson and Tabin, 1997; Bendall and Abate-Shen, 2000).

Expression of *Msx1* has also been reported in the lateral dermomyotome of brachial and thoracic somites, in limb muscle precursor cells migrating to the forelimb, and in a subset of dermal progenitor cells originating from the somites (Houzelstein et al., 1999, 2000). In addition, *Msx1* is expressed in specific organs such as the heart (Robert et al., 1989; Chan-Thomas et al., 1993) and eye (Monaghan et al., 1991).

Postnatal expression of *Msx1* was found in the epidermis (Noveen et al., 1995; Stelnicki et al., 1997), uterus (Pavlova et al., 1994), mammary gland (Friedmann and Daniel, 1996; Phippard et al., 1996), and sutural and bone tissue (Kim et al., 1998; Orestes-Cardoso et al., 2001).

The expression pattern of *Msx1* suggests that it plays an important role in growth, morphogenesis, and organ development, characterized by coordinated growth and cell differentiation in the epithelium and mesenchyme cells (Davidson, 1995; Thesleff et al., 1995). In these processes, there must be a finely regulated balance between proliferation and differentiation. Programmed cell death also contributes to this fine balance (Bendall and Abate-Shen, 2000).

Role of *Msx1* in Apoptosis

The observation of overlapping expression of *Msx1* and *Msx2* (Fig. 51–3) preceding programmed cell death, during embryogenesis, as well as in cell studies suggests that *Msx1* may also participate in apoptosis (Marazzi et al., 1997). For example, both *Msx1* and *Msx2* are both expressed in the neural crest and at the interdigital necrotic zones in the distal limbs (reviewed by Davidson, 1995; Bendall and Abate-Shen, 2000).

Studies performed in a cellular model system provided evidence that *Msx2* is a key regulator of cell death in the bone morphogenetic protein (Bmp)–mediated pathway of apoptosis (Marazzi et al., 1997). In vivo, forced expression of *Msx2* also leads to apoptosis (Takahashi et al., 1998).

Although *Msx1* is required for *Bmp4* expression in dental mesenchyme and *Bmp4* induces expression of *p21* and *Msx2* (Jernvall et al., 1998; reviewed in Peters and Balling, 1999) (Fig. 51–4), both of which are associated with programmed cell death, it is not clear if *Msx1* is directly involved in programmed cell death.

Msx1 in Epithelial–Mesenchyme Signaling and Pattern Formation

In the mandibular arch and limb processes, *Msx1* transcripts accumulate in zones of ectodermal–mesodermal cell contact; this leads to the hypothesis that *Msx1* is involved with epithelial–mesenchymal interaction (Robert et al., 1989; Davidson and Hill, 1991). Grafting and tissue recombination studies show that this epithelium–mesenchyme interaction is important in the outgrowth of the limb (Davidson et al., 1991; Robert et al., 1991), outgrowth of facial processes, and correct skeletogenesis in the mandibular arch (Wedden, 1987; Wedden et al., 1988; Richman and Tickle, 1989; Brown et al., 1993; Mina et al., 1995; Francis-West et al., 1998; Bendall and Abate-Shen, 2000; Mina 2001a,b). Observations in mutant animals also support the hypothesis that *Msx1* is involved in this interaction (Davidson, 1995). Chick mutants showed that signals emanating from the overlying ectoderm control mesenchymal expression of *Msx1* at the distal tip of the limb bud. In the limbless chick mutant, which lacks an apical ectodermal ridge, mesenchymal expression of *Msx1* is reduced but can be restored to normal levels by grafting an apical ridge from a normal embryo

Table 51–1. *Msx/Msh* Genes in Different Species

Species	*Msh*-like Gene	References
Human	*MSX1, MSX2*	Ivens et al., 1990; Hewitt et al., 1991; Jabs et al., 1993; Vastardis et al., 1996; Van den Boogaard et al., 2000; Wilkie et al., 2000; Jumlongras et al., 2001
Mouse	*Msx1, Msx2, Msx3*	Hill et al., 1989; Robert et al., 1989; Monaghan et al., 1991; Bell et al., 1993; Shimeld et al., 1996; Wang et al., 1996
Chicken/quail	*Msx1, Msx2*	Takahashi and Le Douarin, 1990;* Coelho et al., 1991a; Yokouchi et al., 1991; Suzuki et al, 1991; Nohno et al., 1992
Frog (*Xenopus*)	*Msx1, Msx2*	Su et al., 1991
Zebrafish	*MsxA-MsxD*	Ekker et al., 1992; Akimenko et al., 1995
Newt/axolotl	*NvMsx1, AmMsx1, AmMsx2*	Crews et al., 1995; Carlson et al., 1998; Koshiba et al., 1998
Ascidian	*msh*	Holland, 1991
Drosophila	*msh*	Robert et al., 1989
Honeybee	*msh*	Walldorf et al., 1989
Hydra	*msh*	Schummer et al., 1992

*Quail *Msx2* was initially thought to be orthologous to murine *Msx1/Hox7* and therefore designated as *Quox7* in the reference. In later publications, it was renamed *Quox8*.
Source: Davidson (1995), Bendall and Abate-Shen (2000).

(Coelho et al., 1991b). Furthermore, experimental removal of the apical ectodermal ridge in developing chick limb buds showed that the apical ectodermal ridge is a source of instructive signals for *Msx1* expression (Robert et al., 1991).

Tooth Development and *Msx1*

Tooth development is also regulated by reciprocal interaction between epithelium and mesenchyme (Mina and Kollar, 1987; Lumsden, 1988; Jowett et al., 1993; reviewed in Thesleff et al., 1995; Maas and Bei, 1997; Stock et al., 1997; Thesleff and Sharpe, 1997; Peters and Balling, 1999). Grafting and tissue recombination studies showed that the dental epithelium contains instructive signals for tooth formation and that *Msx1* is expressed in the mesenchyme in response to signals from the overlying epithelium (Mina and Kollar, 1987; Lumdsen, 1988; Jowett et al., 1993; Wang et al., 1998).

For example, expression of *Bmp4* and fibroblast growth factor 8 (*Fgf8*) in the epithelium induces mesenchymal expression of *Msx1*.

MSX1 subsequently induces *Bmp4* expression in the dental mesenchyme and is also involved in the maintenance of BMP4 (Fig. 51–4).

Mesenchymal BMP4 signaling is involved in the induction of the enamel knot: the transition from the bud to the cap stage. This is an important step in tooth development.

Furthermore, *Msx1* is required for expression of *Fgf3* in the dental mesenchyme. FGFs control mesenchymal cell proliferation, which is also an important process in tooth development. After the cap stage, tooth development becomes independent of *Msx1* (Bei et al., 2000).

Of course, many other genes are also involved in tooth development. *Msx1* interacts with several of these genes (Fig. 51–4) (Jowett et al., 1993; Vainio et al., 1993; Chen et al., 1996; reviewed in Thesleff and Sharpe, 1997; Bei and Maas, 1998; Tucker et al, 1998; reviewed in Peters and Balling, 1999; Zhang et al., 1999, 2000; Bei et al., 2000; Bendall and Abate-Shen, 2000).

Msx1 Is Involved in Cellular Differentiation and Proliferation

While *Msx1* is correlated with inductive–epithelial interaction, where coordinated growth and cell differentiation in the epithelium and mesenchyme cell occur, it has been suggested that *Msx1* could also be involved in cell proliferation and cell differentiation (Davidson, 1995). Indeed, the *Msx1* gene is expressed in mesodermal progenitor cells migrating from the primitive streak, where inhibition of cellular differentiation is important (Bendall et al., 1999; Houzelstein et al., 1999).

At a later stage, *Msx1* is associated with specific proliferative zones. For example, in the developing mouse limb bud, there is striking ex-

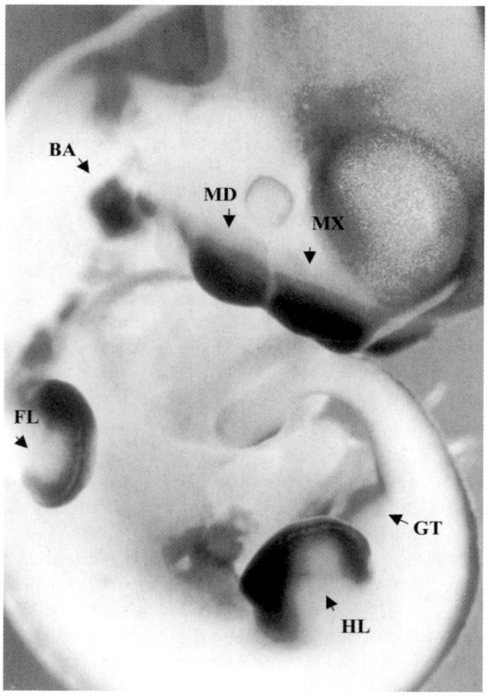

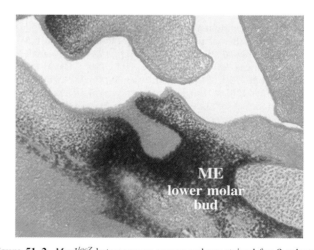

Figure 51–1. Whole-mount heterozygous *Msx1*^lacZ mouse embryo stained for β-galactosidase. Stage 11.5 days postcoitum. BA, branchial arch; MD, mandibular process; MX, maxillary process; FL, forelimb bud; HL, hindlimb bud; GT, genital tubercle. (With thanks to D. Houzelstein and B. Robert.)

Figure 51–2. *Msx1*^lacZ heterozygous mouse embryo stained for β-galactosidase. Stage 13.5 days postcoitum. Magnification of the lower tooth bud. ME, mesectoderm. (With thanks to D. Houzelstein, A. Bach, and B. Robert.)

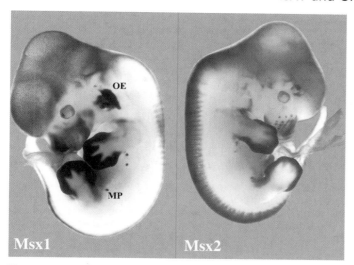

Figure 51–3. Whole-mount heterozygous mouse embryos for *Msx1*ˡᵃᶜᶻ and *Msx2*ˡᵃᶜᶻ stained for β-galactosidase. Stage 12.5 days postcoitum. OE, outer ear; MP, mammary primordium. (With thanks to M.A. Nicola, A. Bach, and B. Robert.)

pression of *Msx1* in the proliferative and undifferentiated cells of the progress zone. During limb development, *Msx1* is downregulated in cells that leave the progress zone and differentiate (Hill et al., 1989; Robert et al., 1989; reviewed in Bendall and Abate-Shen, 2000; Hu et al., 2001). Thus, expression demarcates the boundary between undifferentiated cells expressing *Msx1* and differentiated cells not expressing *Msx1* (Odelberg et al., 2000).

Msx1 can also be reinduced during regeneration and is then probably involved in redifferentiation (Davidson, 1995; Bendall and Abate-Shen, 2000). *Msx1* expression was observed in fetal and neonatal mice when limb regeneration was induced by amputation of distal digit structures (Reginelli et al., 1995). After amputation of the fin of adult zebrafish, in which *msx* transcripts are normally undetectable, *msx* genes are reinduced during regeneration (Akimenko et al., 1995). Urodele amphibians show a striking plasticity in cellular differentiation and are capable of regenerating several anatomic structures (Odelberg et al., 2000). Froglet blastema expresses *Msx1* (Endo et al., 2000). The blastema is a pool of proliferating progenitor cells, which are formed during regeneration by cell dedifferentiation. In limb regeneration in adult urodele amphibians, *Msx1* reactivation accompanies the dedifferentiation of the mesenchyme (Crews et al., 1995; Simon et al., 1995; Koshiba et al., 1998).

The hypothesis that *Msx1* plays a crucial role in cell differentiation can be supported by cell culture data (Hu et al., 2001). Forced expression of *Msx1* in myogenic precursors blocked myogenic terminal differentiation, repressing the expression of lineage-specific genes, like *MyoD*. This resulted in a highly proliferative transformed phenotype (Song et al., 1992; Woloshin et al., 1995). A similar ability to inhibit differentiation was observed in adipocytes, chondrocytes, and osteoblasts (Hu et al., 2001).

There is also evidence that terminally differentiated murine myotubes can be induced to de-differentiate to proliferating mononucleated cells by MSX1. These cells were capable of redifferentiating into different cell types, expressing characteristic markers of chondrogenesis, adipogenesis, myogenesis, and osteogenesis (Odelberg et al., 2000). In addition, ectopic expression of *Msx1* during chicken embryogenesis showed inhibition of the development of limb musculature and repression of MyoD in vivo (Bendall et al., 1999).

Msx1 and Proliferative Capacity in Adulthood

Msx1 expression also appears to correlate with the maintenance of proliferative capacity of tissues that are capable of renewal in adulthood (Bendall and Abate-Shen, 2000). In adulthood, *Msx1* is expressed in stem cells of uterine epithelium (Pavlova et al., 1994), mammary

epithelium (Friedmann and Daniel, 1996; Phippard et al., 1996), and basal epithelium of the dermis (Noveen et al., 1995). *Msx1* is also expressed in bone tissue. In bone, progenitor as well as differentiating and differentiated cells of osteoblastic, chondroblastic, osteoclastic, and chondroclastic lineages could express *Msx1* (Kim et al., 1998; Orestes-Cardosa et al., 2001). *Msx1* downregulated *Cbfa1*, a master gene of skeletal cell differentiation (Blin-Wakkach et al., 2001). Orestes-Cardosa et al. (2001) proposed that *Msx1* might determine local pools of bone cells in the osteoprogenitor compartment. This could be a result of inhibition of terminal differentiation and enhancement of cell proliferation, which is important for bone growth and homeostasis (Kim et al., 1998).

In summary, the expression patterns of *Msx* genes are consistent with a role as general inhibitors of cell differentiation during embryogenesis and maintenance of proliferative capacity of tissues in adulthood, which is important in morphogenesis and growth (Davidson, 1995; Bendall and Abate-Shen, 2000; Hu et al., 2001).

Msx1 Is Involved in the Cell Cycle

Inhibition of cell differentiation due to *Msx1* is correlated with upregulation of *cyclin D1* and *Cdk4* activity (Hu et al., 2001). *Cyclin D1* inhibits differentiation of multiple cell lineages. Inhibition by *cyclin D1* is the result of its ability to block the cell from exiting from the cell cycle and undergoing terminal differentiation.

A model was proposed for the mechanism by which the *Msx1* gene inhibits cellular differentiation, in which the primary function of Msx1 is to maintain cyclin D1 expression in the progenitor population during development. In this model, Msx1 sustains cells in a proliferative state, without actively promoting proliferation. Hu et al. (2001) proposed that loss of Msx1 function would cause premature exit of a cell from the cell cycle and result in differentiation and decreased proliferation, thus impairing growth and morphogenesis.

While upregulation of cyclin D1 is often found in breast carcinoma and Msx1 has the potential to upregulate cyclin D1, Hu et al. (2001) suggested that Msx1 may play a role in breast cancer. This hypothesis deserves further study. However, Park et al. (2001) observed overexpression of Msx1 in human ovarian cancer cell lines, which suppressed cell proliferation; they considered that this could be due to Msx1 repressing cell cycle progression. These reports support the notion that Msx1 is involved in tumorigenesis, but its precise biological function in cancer cells remains unclear.

MSX1 Protein Is a Potent Transcriptional Repressor

As already discussed, an important function of Msx1 is to inhibit cellular differentiation. Probable mechanisms are downregulation of master genes (like *Cbfa1*) and upregulation of genes (like *cyclin D1*) involved in cell differentiation (Blin-Wakkach et al., 2001; Hu et al., 2001).

The biological function of the homeobox gene *Msx1* was at first described as transcriptional regulation, by DNA binding to specific DNA sequences (Catron et al., 1993). The DNA-binding specificity of MSX1 results from the cumulative action of residues in the N-terminal arm and helices I, II, and III of the homeodomain (Isaac et al., 1995; Zhang et al., 1997; Bendall et al., 1998, 1999; Bendall and Abate-Shen, 2000).

Transcription studies revealed that Msx proteins are mainly potent transcriptional repressors (Catron et al., 1995, 1996; Zhang et al., 1996, 1997; reviewed in Bendall and Abate-Shen, 2000). Although the MSX1 homeodomain binds with high affinity to a specific DNA site (containing the TAAT sequence), the homeodomain DNA-binding activity is not required for this transcriptional repression by Msx1 (Catron et al., 1996). Msx1 appears to repress transcription through protein–protein interactions, mediated by the homeodomain (Zhang et al., 1996). Several models of repression have been discussed by Zhang et al. (1996, 1997) and Bendall and Abate-Shen (2000).

In their review, Bendall and Abate-Shen (2000) proposed that the repression could be a result of direct interaction with the preinitiation complex, blocking the basal transcription machinery by preventing interaction with transcriptional activators. It was demonstrated that

Msx1 proteins could interact with the TATA-binding protein (TBP). TBP is a core component of the basal transcription machinery, which mediates activation (Zhang et al., 1996, 1997; reviewed in Lee and Young, 1998; Bendall and Abate-Shen, 2000). Also, the presence of Msx1 in a multiprotein transcriptional complex containing a basal transcription factor (TBP), a sequence–specific activator (Sp1), and a coactivator (cAMP response element–binding protein–binding protein/p300) was demonstrated by Shetty et al. (1999).

However, the repression may also be due to interaction of the Msx1 protein with the DNA-bound activator, thereby blocking its function of activating the transcription (Bendall and Abate-Shen, 2000).

Another suggested mode of repression is the interaction of Msx1 with other homeoproteins, preventing them from DNA binding and thereby inhibiting transcriptional activation (Zhang et al., 1997; Bendall and Abate-Shen, 2000). Heterodimer formation between the homeoproteins Msx and Dlx (a transcriptional activator) results in functional antagonism (Zhang et al., 1997). Furthermore, heterodimer formation between Msx1 and genes coding for members of the LIM and Pax families prevents DNA binding of Msx1 and the other protein involved (Zhang et al., 1997; Bendall et al., 1998, 1999; Bendall and Abate-Shen, 2000).

Interestingly, the *Lhx2* LIM-homeobox gene (functionally interchangeable with the *ap* gene in *Drosophila*) and Msx1 expression patterns in the mouse are complementary in most tissues. However, in the developing limb, they are coexpressed (Lu et al., 2000). In *Drosophila*, this spatial relationship of expression patterns for *ap* and *msh* was also recognized. The expression patterns of both genes in the mouse and *Drosophila* suggest that the regulation of these genes has been conserved during evolution (Lu et al., 2000). In *Drosophila*, the *msh* gene acts downstream of *ap* and is involved in dorsal identity specification in wing development (Milan et al., 2001).

In vivo, complex formation between Msx1 and Pax3 may prevent premature activation of myogenic genes (*MyoD*) in migratory limb muscle precursor cells during their migration (Bendall et al., 1999).

Regulation of *Msx1* Expression

A finely tuned regulation of *Msx1* is important for balanced cell growth and differentiation, and *Msx1* appears to be involved in the regulation of its own transcription. The *Msx1* promotor may itself be subject to *Msx1*-mediated transcriptional repression. Thus, *Msx1* has an autoinhibitory activity (Shetty et al., 1999).

Another mechanism is the presence of antisense (AS) RNA. Involvement of endogenous AS RNAs in the regulation of gene expression has been documented for various genes. In most cases, regulation occurs at the translational level. The AS transcript hybridizes to the sense transcript and blocks access of the translation machinery

to the sense transcript. This leads to reduced levels of protein synthesis (reviewed in Inouye, 1988; Kumar and Carmichael, 1998). The presence of endogenous *Msx1* AS RNA (*Msx1*-AS RNA) has been demonstrated in mice, rats, and humans (Blin-Wakkach et al., 2001). The *Msx1*-AS cDNA is complementary to the region extending from the 3′ end of exon 2 to the middle of intron 1 of the genomic *Msx1* DNA sequence. In vivo data showed that the balance between the levels of *Msx1* RNA and *Msx1*-AS RNA is related to expression of the *Msx1* protein (Blin-Wakkach et al., 2001).

CLINICAL FEATURES ASSOCIATED WITH MSX1 MUTATIONS IN HUMANS

MSX1 mutations are associated with three clinically related phenotypes: partial anodontia, orofacial clefting, and Witkop syndrome. So far, three human *MSX1* mutations have been documented. The mutations were identified in three unrelated families with familial tooth agenesis (Vastardis et al., 1996; van den Boogaard et al., 2000; Jumlongras et al., 2001) (see Table 51–3).

The first family had an autosomal-dominant form of hypodontia [OMIM 106600] caused by an R196P missense mutation in *MSX1* (Vastardis et al., 1996). Affected individuals most frequently showed agenesis of the maxillary and mandibular second premolars; some affected individuals missed the maxillary first premolars and mandibular first molars. Skull X-rays showed loss of proper tooth inclination in relation to the jaws. The maxilla was also slightly shorter than the mandibula, although both were within normal limits. Affected individuals showed no craniofacial abnormalities, nor were nail or limb defects mentioned.

In the second family, another *MSX1* mutation (S105X) was associated with familial tooth agenesis and various combinations of cleft lip and cleft lip/palate (nonsyndromic cleft lip with or without cleft palate [OMIM 119530]/isolate cleft palate [OMIM 119540]) (van den Boogaard et al., 2000). There were 12 affected members in the second family (Fig. 51–5). Four males had a cleft. The 5-year-old proband (IV-1) and a maternal uncle (III-3) had a cleft palate. II-3 had a cleft alveolar ridge, and III-9 had a cleft lip and palate. Eleven family members lacked some permanent teeth (Table 51–2). The pattern of tooth agenesis was almost identical to that of the first family described with an *MSX1* mutation. Most affected individuals were missing both mandibular and maxillary second premolars. The third molar was also frequently absent. In most cases, the pattern of dental agenesis was bilaterally symmetrical. As far as we know, the affected family members showed no nail defects.

The third *MSX1* mutation (S202X) was identified in a three-generation family with familial tooth agenesis in combination with dysplastic toenails and/or fingernails, diagnosed as tooth-and-nail syn-

Table 51–2. Pattern of Tooth Agenesis in a Dutch Family with S105X *MSX1* Mutation Associated with Clefting and Tooth Agenesis

Pedigree ID	Dental Arch	Missing Permanent Teeth															
		Right								Left							
		8	7	6	5	4	3	2	1	1	2	3	4	5	6	7	8
II-1	Maxillary													*			
	Mandibular			*				*		*							
II-4	Maxillary	*			*									*			*
	Mandibular	*			*									*			*
II-5	Maxillary	*			*	*								*			*
	Mandibular	*			*									*		*	*
III-1	Maxillary	*			*	*							*	*			*
	Mandibular	*			*									*			*
III-4	Maxillary				*									*			
	Mandibular				*									*			
III-8	Maxillary				*	*		*			*		*	*			
	Mandibular																
III-9	Maxillary				*	*		*					*	*			
	Mandibular	*			*									*			*
III-13	Maxillary	*	*		*			*			*			*		*	*
	Mandibular	*	*		*								*	*	*	*	*

*Missing tooth; 1, central incisor; 2, lateral incisor; 3, canine; 4 and 5, first and second premolars, respectively; 6, 7, and 8, first, second, and third molars, respectively.

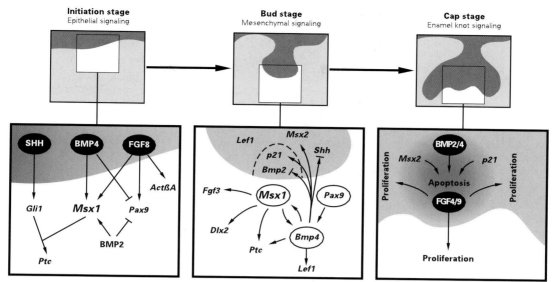

Figure 51–4. Schematic representation of reciprocal signaling between the epithelium and mesenchyme during the early phases of tooth development; initiation stage, bud stage, and cap stage. (Adapted from Peters and Balling, 1999, and Cohen, 2000, with additional data from Zhang et al., 1999, 2000.)

drome, also known as Witkop syndrome or nail dysgenesis and hypodontia (Jumlongras et al., 2001).

No orofacial cleft or any other craniofacial abnormalities were present in affected members of this family. However, affected individuals had a large number of congenitally missing permanent teeth (11–28), which showed a specific pattern. The premolars, first molars, and third molars were predominantly absent. In a few cases, other teeth, like incisors and canines, were also missing. The permanent teeth that were present appeared smaller in the mesiodistal dimension and had shorter root lengths than normal. The primary dentition was normal, except in one affected individual in whom the mandibular right primary central and lateral incisor was fused. Affected members had a prominent maxillar frenulun, and frenectomy was required to accommodate dental prostheses.

In most cases, nail dysplasia was present. The toenails were more severely affected, especially the fifth toenail. The skin, sweat glands, and hair were normal.

Partial Anodontia

The tooth phenotype in families with an *MSX1* mutation is different from common hypodontia. The reported frequencies of hypodontia in the general population lie within the range 1.6%–10.1%. This figure excludes the absence of third molars, which occurs in 20% of the population (Graber, 1978; Schalk-van der Weide, 1992; Cohen, 2000). The most commonly missing permanent teeth are premolars and maxillary lateral incisors (Symons et al., 1993), for which *MSX1* and *MSX2* have been excluded as candidate genes (Nieminen et al., 1995).

Interestingly, the reported *MSX1* mutations seem to affect predominantly the second premolars and the first and third molars. Several authors have discussed the possible cause of this selective tooth agenesis (Vastardis et al., 1996; Thesleff, 1996; Peters and Balling, 1999; Jumlongras et al., 2001).

The basic genetic mechanisms of tooth development are conserved between different tooth classes. The teeth within a class evolve as a unit. Several models have been proposed to explain the differences in shape between tooth classes. One model presumes a prespecification of neural crest cells, which determine the identity of each individual tooth. Another model suggests that different tooth types develop from initially identical tissue and that the differences in development are due to influences from the molecular environment. There can be positional differences between the gradients and presence of other homeoproteins, resulting in different tooth types (Stock et al., 1997; Peters and Balling, 1999). Indeed, ectopic expression of *Barx1* in the distal presumptive incisor mesenchyme, due to inhibition of BMP4 signal-

ing, results in transformation of tooth identity from incisor to molar (Tucker et al., 1998). These findings support the idea that homeobox genes are involved in the determination of different tooth types.

It was suggested that the timing of *MSX1* expression and the presence or absence of possible redundancy from other genes could be critical for the development of specific teeth (Thesleff, 1996; Jumlongras et al., 2001) and could explain the specific pattern of tooth agenesis associated with *MSX1* mutation.

Furthermore, the missing teeth are the last to develop from each tooth class and might therefore be more susceptible to defects during development than the other elements (Thesleff, 1996).

Orofacial Clefting

In one family with an *MSX1* mutation, we found four affected individuals with an orofacial cleft (van den Boogaard et al., 2000). In general, the prevalence of orofacial cleft at birth varies from 1 in 500 to 1 in 2500, depending on ethnic background, geographic origin and socioeconomic status. The etiology of orofacial clefting is complex, and several genetic and environmental factors are involved (Schutte and Murray, 1999; Spritz, 2001; Murray, 2002).

Genetic epidemiological studies suggest that several interacting loci, including a major gene, are involved in the etiology of orofacial clefting and may account for approximately half of the familial occurrences (FitzPatrick and Farral, 1993; Christensen and Mitchell, 1996). Several candidate genes (e.g., *MTHFR, TGFA, BCL3, DLX2, MSX1,* and *TGFB3*) have been screened for linkage disequilibrium with clefting. Significant linkage disequilibrium was found between cleft lip (with or without cleft palate) and isolated cleft palate and *MSX1* (Lidral et al., 1998; Beaty et al., 2001). A Danish study provided further evidence that the risk of isolated cleft palate may be influenced by variation at the locus for *MSX1*. This could not be confirmed for cleft lip with or without cleft palate (Mitchell et al., 2001). A study performed in a Chilean population also showed association between *MSX1* and nonsyndromic cleft lip/palate. This was more pronounced for males (Blanco et al., 2001). Another study using a case-parent trio design confirmed that the candidate *MSX1* plays an etiological role in isolated nonsyndromic oral clefting (Beaty et al., 2002). Detection of an *MSX1* mutation in individuals with orofacial clefting confirmed *MSX1* as a candidate gene for orofacial clefting (van den Boogaard et al., 2000).

Previous studies suggested an etiological distinction between isolated cleft palate and cleft lip with or without cleft palate (Fraser, 1955, 1970). However, cases of cleft palate only and of cleft lip and cleft palate were seen in the second *MSX1* family. This mixed clefting phenotype is also noted in families affected with the syndromic forms of orofacial clefting Van der Woude's syndrome and ectrodactyly–ectodermal dysplasia–clefting. These syndromes are caused by mutations in the *IRF6* and *TP63* genes, respectively (Celli et al., 1999; McGrath et al., 2001; Kondo et al., 2002). Interestingly, Kondo et al. (2002) suggested that both these genes and *MSX1* are involved in common genetic pathways.

In humans, tooth agenesis is noted in about 35% of individuals with isolated cleft palate, despite the fact that the cleft does not directly involve the tooth-bearing area (Ranta, 1986). This suggests that odontogenesis and palate formation are developmentally related events and that a single gene could be involved in both processes. Since *MSX1* is associated with both tooth agenesis and orofacial clefting, it might be such a single gene.

Witkop Syndrome (Tooth-and-Nail Syndrome)

In one family, the *MSX1* mutation is associated with features of Witkop syndrome. This family was first described in 1997 by Stimson et al.

Witkop (1965) described autosomal-dominant hypoplasia of the nails with hypodontia. This combination of symptoms was common in the Dutch Mennonites of Canada (Chitty et al., 1996). The combination of hypodontia with dysplastic nails was first reported by Weech (1929), though more fully by Witkop (1965) and Witkop et al. (1975) (see Murdoch-Kinch et al., 1993). The incidence has been estimated to be approximately 1 to 2:10,000 (Witkop, 1990). Since the original communication, several other families and cases with Witkop syndrome have been reported (Redpath and Winter, 1969; Giansanti et al., 1974; Hudson and Witkop, 1975; Murdoch-Kinch et al., 1993; reviewed by Chitty et al., 1996; Garzon and Paller, 1996; Stimson et al., 1997; Zabawski and Cohen, 1999; Hodges and Harley, 1999; Jumlongras et al., 2001).

The main features of Witkop syndrome are a variable number and variable types of congenitally missing permanent teeth. The teeth may be widely spaced. Anodontia is rare in this disorder but has been reported (Giansanti et al., 1974). The deciduous teeth may be normal, but there are some reports of congenitally missing deciduous teeth (Chitty et al., 1996). Tooth shape may also be conical.

The nails are generally thin, slow-growing, brittle, and spoon-shaped. In most cases, the toenails are more severely affected than the fingernails.

The phenotypic expression, including tooth and nail defects, seems, however, to be highly variable. In some instances, the only features are marked longitudinal ridges and pitting (Giansanti et al., 1974). The nail defects improve with age, so these may not be detectable in adulthood. Older children and adults frequently have normal fingernails but small, spoon-shaped toenails.

The hair has a normal distribution, but it may be fine and slow-growing. Sparse eyebrows have been described in a few affected individuals (Chitty et al., 1996).

Affected individuals have no typical facial phenotype. However, there may be a small jaw, eversion of the lower lip as a result of the tooth agenesis, and maxillary hypoplasia.

One family with only one affected individual with a cleft palate has been reported (Chitty et al., 1996). We can speculate whether this is part of the phenotypic expression of a probable *MSX1* mutation in this family. In this case, the phenotypes between the three MSX1 families show more overlap and are less distinguishable (see Table 51–3). Also, because the deciduous teeth may be normal and the nail abnormalities may be very mild in Witkop syndrome and since these symptoms

could have been missed in the other two *MSX1* families, the overlap in phenotypes might be more obvious than previously suggested (Jumlongras et al., 2001).

Other Symptoms of the Spectrum

Because there are only a few families in which an *MSX1* mutation has been identified and since they were selected on the presence of tooth agenesis, we cannot exclude that *MSX1* is involved in a range of other phenotypes. *MSX1* mutations may result in abnormalities of other structures or tissues where *MSX1* is expressed and may be associated with less prominent abnormalities in tooth development. For example, during development, Msx1 is expressed in the CNS, and *MSX1* mutation may be related to abnormal morphology of specific brain structures, although this has not been established.

In addition, it is well known that a different pathogenic effect of mutations can result in a different phenotype. Genotype–phenotype studies of the *MSX2* gene provide an example of this: loss-of-function mutation in *MSX2* results in defective cranial osteogenesis and enlarged parietal foraminae, while a gain of function results in premature cranial suture differentiation, ossification, and hence craniosynostosis (Ferguson, 2000; Cohen, 2000). To date, no gain-of-function mutations in *MSX1* have been reported.

However, it has been suggested that overexpression of *MSX1* may also play a role in mammary carcinoma and ovarian cancer (Hu et al., 2001; Park et al., 2001). Thus, the recognized phenotype of *MSX1* mutations could be a result of selection bias. To elucidate the possible phenotypic expression of *MSX1* mutations, it is necessary to identify more families with *MSX1* mutations and to study other congenital abnormalities that could be related to MSX1.

MOLECULAR GENETICS OF *MSX1*

Structure of *Msx1*

The murine homologue of *Msh*, *Msx1* (formerly *Hox7*), was characterized and mapped to mouse chromosome 5 (Hill et al., 1989; Robert et al., 1989). In 1990, the human locus was mapped to chromosome 4 (4p16.1), a region thought to be involved in Wolf-Hirschhorn syndrome (Ivens et al., 1990). Subsequently, the structure and sequence of the human homeobox gene *MSX1* were reported by Hewitt et al. (1991). The homeodomain of 60 amino acids is highly conserved, consisting of an N-terminal arm and helices I, II, and III. Human and murine *Msx1* show 94% identity in the homeodomain at the DNA level. Homology at the nucleotide coding level was 80% (Hewitt et al., 1991; Padanilam et al., 1992).

Sequence analysis of the human *MSX1* gene showed that it has two exons separated by an intron of approximately 1.6 kb. The intron is located 40 bp upstream of the homeobox, a position comparable to that in other homeobox genes (Hewitt et al., 1991). Exon 2 contains the homeobox.

The gene is approximately 4 kb. The human *Msx1* cDNA is 1719 bp long. The gene encodes a protein of 297 amino acids, and the homeodomain extends from residues 165 through 225. *MSX1* has a putative GC-rich promotor region. The 5′ upstream region does not contain a TATA box, although an AT-rich region is present with a CCAAT box upstream. There are several GC boxes.

Comparing the *Msx1* cDNA sequence from five species revealed a strictly conserved, 66 bp region at the 3′ noncoding end that contains a consensus TATA box, identified as the initiation site of Msx1-AS RNA transcription (Blin-Wakkach et al., 2001). *Msx1* codes for a DNA-binding protein, which functions as a transcriptional repressor through its interaction with general transcription factors and other homeoproteins. The homeodomain is essential for these functions and important for protein stability (Hu et al., 1998).

MSX1 Mutations in Humans

Three mutations have been reported in three unrelated families (Table 51–3, Fig. 51–6) (Vastardis et al., 1996; van den Boogaard et al., 2000; Jumlongras et al., 2001). In these families, affected individuals are heterozygous for an autosomal-dominant mutation.

Table 51–3. Published *MSX1* Mutations in Humans

Reference	Mutation	Type of Mutation	Phenotype		
			Tooth Agenesis	Oral Clefting	Nail Defect
Vastardis et al., 1996	R196P	Missense	+	−	−
Van den Boogaard et al., 2000	S105X	Nonsense	+	+	−
Jumlongras et al., 2001	S202X	Nonsense	+	−	+

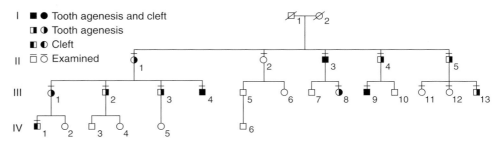

Figure 51–5. Pedigree and symptoms of the Dutch family with the S105X *MSX1* mutation.

The first mutation was detected in a family with autosomal-dominant agenesis of the second premolars and third molars (Vastardis et al., 1996). An arg196-to-pro (R196P) missense mutation in the homeodomain of the *MSX1* gene was identified.

The second reported mutation is a heterozygous C→A transversion, creating a stop codon in exon 1 (S105X) (van den Boogaard et al., 2000). This mutation is associated with autosomal-dominant tooth agenesis combined with oral clefting. The stop mutation is proximal to the homeodomain in exon 2.

The third *MSX1* mutation concerns a heterozygous C→A transversion resulting in replacement of serine codon 202 by a stop codon in exon 2 (S202X) (Jumlongras et al., 2001). This mutation causes Witkop syndrome.

Both R196P and S202X mutations are located in the homeobox coding region in exon 2 and occur within helix II. This helix, like the N-terminal arm and helix I, is important for protein stability. Helix II, however, does not contribute to DNA binding, transcriptional repression, or protein interaction (Shang et al., 1994; Isaac et al., 1995; Zhang et al., 1996, 1997; Hu et al., 1998).

R196P is located at a position that plays a crucial role in protein structure and stability (Hu et al., 1998). The truncated S202X protein lacks a part of helix II, helix III, and the entire C-terminal region. Helix III contributes to DNA binding and protein interaction, including heterodimerization with Dlx (Jumlongras et al., 2001).

Phenotype–Genotype Correlation

The *MSX1* mutations show overlapping and nonoverlapping phenotypes. All three mutations (S105X, R196P, S202X) are responsible for autosomal-dominant selective tooth agenesis of especially the premolars, first molars, and third molars. However, the *MSX1* mutations S105X and S202X are also associated with combinations of tooth agenesis with oral clefting and tooth agenesis with nail defects (Witkop syndrome), respectively. Because of the varying degree of nail abnormalities or even the absence of nail abnormalities in Witkop syndrome, this additional symptom could have been missed or simply not present in the other families described.

The presence or absence of nail defects or orofacial clefting might be related to the type of mutation and other possible modifying factors (sense/AS, molecular environment, genetic background, environmental factors). The phenotype of *MSX1* mutation probably represents only one spectrum of symptoms, including selective tooth agenesis, orofacial clefting, and nail abnormalities.

Haploinsufficiency

Haploinsufficiency is the probable cause for the phenotype of all three mutations. The effect of the MSX1 (R196P) mutation was studied by biochemical and functional analyses (Hu et al., 1998). MSX1 (R196P) has a perturbed structure and reduced thermostability compared with wild-type MSX1, resulting in severe impairment of biochemical activities. There is little or no ability to interact with DNA or other protein factors, and MSX1 (R196P) does not have the ability to act as a transcription repressor. MSX1 (R196P) is inactive in vivo. The effect of MSX1 (R196P) was examined in developing chicken limb buds but not in developing teeth. Biochemical studies demonstrated that MSX1 (R196P) has no apparent novel activities. Since MSX1 (R196P) appears to be inactive, haploinsufficiency is the most likely pathogenic mechanism for the tooth agenesis in the family with the R196P mutation (Hu et al., 1998).

S105X is a stop mutation proximal to the homeodomain in exon 2, which probably also leads to haploinsufficiency (van den Boogaard et al., 2000).

The S202X mutation leads to a truncated protein, missing part of the homeodomain and the C-terminal end. This protein is probably not properly folded, is unstable, or is unable to bind to DNA (Jumlongras et al., 2001). However, we can hypothesize that S202X is stable and the N-terminal arm of the homeodomain still has some function.

Although Msx1 has been well studied and haploinsufficiency is most likely to be the pathogenic mechanism, there remains much to be discovered about its mode of action (Bendall and Abate-Shen, 2000).

We cannot exclude that the different mutations may have diverging effects on pathways still to be elucidated. This could explain the different phenotypes of the mutations seen between the families, especially the presence of orofacial clefting in the family with S105X and the absence of clefting in the families with R196P and S202X. It is interesting that both R196P and S202X families have a mutation in helix II of the homeodomain in exon 2 and that the mutation associated with clefting is located in exon 1. In addition, R196P, which is associated with selective tooth agenesis and no other features, is a missense mutation. In contrast, the mutations (S105X and S202X) associated with tooth agenesis in combination with orofacial clefting and nail abnormalities, respectively, are both nonsense mutations.

Sense–AS

Msx1 expression can be regulated by the balance between the levels of *Msx1* RNA and *Msx1*-AS RNA. The ratio of both *Msx1* RNAs appears to be a key factor for cell differentiation and phenotypic expression in mineralized tissues (Blin-Wakkach et al., 2001). However, what effect do mutations in *Msx1* have on the balance of the two *Msx1* RNAs and expression of the *Msx1* protein? When mutations can interfere in this mode of gene regulation, the sense/AS mechanism could be an important element of the pathogenic mechanism and could explain the gradational effects seen in different mutations. We can speculate if the position of the mutation, in exon 1 versus exon 2, plays a role in its effect on the ratio of both *Msx1* RNAs. A nonsense mutation in the 5' site of the gene might be associated with absent mRNA, which could influence the ratio of *Msx1* RNA and *Msx1*-AS RNA. Further studies are needed to evaluate these possible mechanisms.

Variable Expression

We see great intrafamilial and interfamilial clinical variability in families carrying an *MSX1* mutation. This clinical variability could be explained by other genes acting in the same or in different developmental pathways, possibly as modifiers on the effect of the Msx1 mutation.

The biological function of the MSX1 protein might also be context-dependent and influenced by the molecular environment of the tissue in which it is expressed (Bendall and Abate-Shen, 2000). Many cell adhesion molecules, extracellular matrix components, and cell surface matrix receptors have been associated with morphogenesis (Thesleff et al., 1995). Differences in genetic background might also be responsible for the phenotypic differences. The families originate from different countries. Msx1 may also be involved in sex-dependent susceptibility to orofacial clefting (Blanco et al., 2001).

In addition to potential modifier genes, molecular environment, and genetic background, environmental factors may modulate the clinical expression. Smoking and alcohol consumption during pregnancy appeared to be associated with an increased risk for cleft palate and cleft lip with or without cleft palate, respectively, if the infant had an allelic variant of the MSX1 site (Romitti et al., 1999). Another study provided evidence for an interaction between infants' *MSX1* genotype and maternal smoking (Beaty et al., 2002).

DIAGNOSIS

The main features of the phenotypes associated with *MSX1* mutation are selective tooth agenesis, probably in combination with nail abnormalities or orofacial clefting. Since the tooth abnormalities may not be present in childhood and the nail defects improve with age, it may be difficult to recognize these symptoms as part of the phenotypic spectrum of the *MSX1* phenotype. Furthermore, nail and tooth abnormalities are common symptoms of several forms of ectodermal dysplasia, a heterogeneous group of disorders characterized by defects in at least two ectodermally derived organs, such as teeth, nails, hair, and sweat glands (Slavkin et al., 1998).

However, the *MSX1* mutation phenotype can be distinguished from several forms of ectodermal dysplasia by the presence of only teeth and/or nail abnormalities, and the features do not meet the criteria of specific ectodermal dysplasias. In addition, *MSX1* mutation seems to affect only specific types of permanent teeth: premolars, first molars, and third molars. When clefting is present, other causes or syndromes have to be excluded since clefting is a feature of more than 400 syndromes. A careful family history must be obtained to confirm an autosomal-dominant pattern for this disorder because of its variable expression.

MANAGEMENT

Abnormal dentition seems to be the most common feature of the *MSX1* mutation. Affected individuals have a variable number and variable types of congenitally absent permanent teeth. Early correction of dental abnormalities is essential in the management of this disorder. Surgical repairs for various clefts of the lip and palate may also be indicated.

Another aspect of patient care is counseling of affected individuals and family members because the inheritance is autosomal-dominant. Since there may be considerable variation in expression, gene carriers may have only minimal signs, but they can be identified by mutation analysis once a pathogenic mutation has been identified in the family.

KNOCKOUT MOUSE

To determine the phenotypic consequences of deficiency of *Msx1*, two homozygous *Msx1*[−/−] mice were created (Satokata and Maas, 1994; Houzelstein et al., 1997). In the first knockout, a PMC1*neo* gene was introduced into helix III of the homeodomain, truncating the gene 3' in the homeodomain (Satokata and Maas, 1994). In the second knockout, a reporter *nlacZ* gene, containing a nuclear localization signal (n), was introduced at the same restriction site where the PMC1*neo* gene

was introduced in the first knockout. While the mutated gene forms an Msx1–β-galactosidase fusion protein, *Msx1* expression could be studied by β-galactosidase histoenzymology (Houzelstein et al., 1997).

Homozygous mice died a few hours after birth and exhibited marked congenital abnormalities. They failed to form teeth and had craniofacial defects, with absence of the alveolar bones in the mandible and maxilla and lesser abnormalities in the parietal, frontal, and nasal membrane bones; cleft of the secondary palate; and abnormalities of the malleus in the middle ear. They also exhibited defective nail plates (Jumlongras et al., 2001).

It was striking that most other sites where *Msx1* is strongly expressed appeared to be normal, and several possible explanations have been suggested (Satokata and Maas, 1994; Davidson, 1995; Thesleff et al., 1995; Catron et al., 1996; Houzelstein et al., 1997).

Firstly, the phenotype reported may not represent the real null mutation. In the knockouts, the mutation truncates the gene 3' in the homeodomain. Thus, the N-terminal arm of the homeodomain is still present, which might leave residual activity of the protein (Davidson, 1995). However, the mutations may nevertheless be null because of the disturbance of the three-dimensional structure of the mutant protein (Houzelstein et al., 1997).

Secondly, expression in the unaffected tissues in the knockout mice may be superfluous (Thesleff et al., 1995). *Msx1* may have no function at all in these tissues (Houzelstein et al., 1997). In this respect, expression of AS *Msx1* may play a role.

Thirdly, other cofactors are necessary for the proper functioning of Msx1, and Msx1 is nonfunctional in sites where the cofactor is not expressed or absent (Houzelstein et al., 1997).

Several authors have suggested that the absence of phenotypic alterations in tissues expressing Msx1 could be explained by functional redundancy of Msx1 and Msx2 (Satokata and Maas, 1994; Catron et al., 1996; Houzelstein et al., 1997). Msx1 and Msx2 are expressed in overlapping patterns, although there are discrete differences (Fig. 51–3) (Catron et al., 1996; Houzelstein et al., 1997; Sadler and Potts, 1997; M.-A. Nicola, unpublished data). Msx2 expression in the frontonasal process is much more restricted than expression of Msx1. With respect to tooth development, Msx2 is preferentially expressed in dental ectoderm and Msx1 is expressed in dental mesenchyme (MacKenzie et al., 1991a,b, 1992; Chen et al., 1996; Maas et al., 1996; Houzelstein et al., 1997; Thesleff and Sharpe, 1997). With respect to early limb development, the expression pattern shows considerable overlap, although the exact level of expression of Msx1 and Msx2 differs (Hill et al., 1989; Coelho et al., 1991a,b; Robert et al., 1991; Yokouchi et al., 1991; Nohno et al., 1992; Catron et al., 1996; Houzelstein et al., 1997; Bendall and Abate-Shen, 2000).

In the limbs, expression of Msx1 and Msx2 seems sufficiently similar to permit Msx2 to compensate for Msx1, but in the facial region and the teeth, this is not the case. It is proposed that the redundancy may be achieved through different mechanisms, which have similar functional outcomes (Catron et al., 1996; Houzelstein et al., 1997).

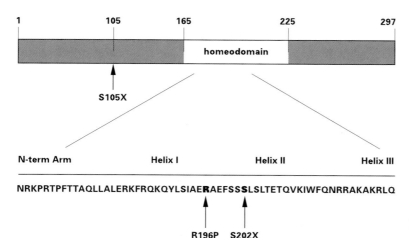

Figure 51–6. Simple schematic diagram of Msx1 showing the published human *MSX1* mutation.

Analyses show that Msx1 and Msx2 have similar DNA-binding and transcriptional properties but that these functions are modulated differently by their nonconserved N-terminal regions.

For some pathways, other proteins with similar functions may compensate for Msx1. The regulation of expression of proteins where Msx1 is involved might be subject to additional mechanisms, which compensate for the absence of Msx1.

DEVELOPMENTAL PATHOGENESIS OF THE CONDITION

To date, *MSX1* mutations have been identified in three unrelated families (Vastardis et al., 1996; van den Boogaard et al., 2000, Jumlongras et al., 2001) (Table 51–3, Fig. 51–6). The mutations in *MSX1* are associated with selective tooth agenesis and selective tooth agenesis in combination with nonsyndromic orofacial clefting and nail abnormalities (Witkop syndrome), respectively (Fig. 51–5, Fig. 51–6, Table 51–2).

The homeobox gene *Msx1* is highly conserved and therefore expected to play an important role in embryonic development. *Msx1* has been found in regions of cephalic neural crest migration and differentiation, as well as in the derived mesenchyme cells (Hill et al., 1989; Robert et al., 1989; MacKenzie et al., 1991a,b; reviewed by Davidson and Hill, 1991; Davidson 1995; Sadler and Potts, 1997; Houzelstein et al., 1997, 1999, 2000; Bendall and Abate-Shen, 2000).

Msx1 is also involved in epithelial–mesenchymal interaction by mediating and controlling the expression of inductive signals transmitted between the epithelial and mesenchymal layers during tooth development and development of the mandibular arch and limb buds (Davidson, 1995; Thesleff and Sharpe, 1997; Francis-West et al., 1998; reviewed in Peters and Balling, 1999; Zhang et al., 1999; Bei et al., 2000; reviewed in Bendall and Abate-Shen, 2000; Mina, 2001a,b). The main function of *Msx1* is to maintain the proliferative capacity of precursor cells of the mesenchyme by preventing their differentiation. Premature differentiation results in decreased proliferation and, thus, impaired outgrowth and morphogenesis. In addition, *Msx1* might be indirectly involved in programmed cell death, which also contributes to morphogenesis (Marazzi et al., 1997).

Msx1 regulates cellular differentiation by transcriptional repression and protein–protein interaction (Zhang et al., 1997, 1999; Bendall and Abate-Shen, 2000). Msx1 could suppress terminal differentiation in myoblasts and osteoblasts by repression of MyoD and Cbfa1 expression, respectively. Protein complex formation between Msx and Pax3 may prevent premature activation of myogenic genes in migratory limb muscle precursor cells during their migration (Houzelstein et al., 1999; Bendall et al., 1999; Orestes-Cardosa et al., 2001). Hu et al. (2001) proposed that *Msx1* gene expression also maintains cyclin D1 expression and prevents cells from exiting the cell cycle, thereby inhibiting terminal differentiation of precursor cells.

During embryogenesis, Msx1 is broadly expressed. There was obvious expression in the craniofacial structures, including facial processes, tooth buds, and limb buds. Thus, mutations in Msx1 were expected to be associated with abnormal morphogenesis of these structures (Hill et al., 1989; Robert et al., 1989; MacKenzie et al., 1991a,b; reviewed by Davidson and Hill, 1991; Davidson 1995; Sadler and Potts, 1997; Houzelstein et al., 1997, 1999; Bendall and Abate-Shen, 2000).

The phenotypic consequences of lacking *Msx1* function were examined in homozygous *Msx1*$^{-/-}$ mice. All *Msx1*$^{-/-}$ mice exhibit cleft secondary palate, deficiency of alveolar mandible and maxilla, and failure of tooth development. Additionally, they manifest abnormalities of the skull, malleus, nasal bones, conchae, and nail plates (Satokata and Maas, 1994; Houzelstein et al., 1997; Jumlongras et al., 2001). Several authors have suggested that the apparent absence of abnormalities in other tissues expressing Msx1 could be an effect of functional redundancy of Msx2 (Satokata and Maas, 1994; Catron et al., 1996; Houzelstein et al., 1997). The expression patterns of Msx1 and Msx2 overlap considerably, although they are not identical. Likewise, the functions of Msx1 and Msx2 are similar but not equal (Catron et al., 1996). Another possibility is that Msx1 has no function in any of the tissues where it is expressed (Houzelstein et al., 1997).

The phenotypic spectrum in the families with an *MSX1* mutation shows a clear resemblance to the phenotype seen in knockout mice. The phenotype in the families is probably due to haploinsufficiency. All three mutations will affect the homeodomain, which is essential for DNA binding, transcriptional repression, protein–protein interaction, and protein stability of Msx1. Msx1 regulates cellular differentiation with these mechanisms.

The mutation (R196P) in the family with autosomal-dominant selective tooth agenesis is located in exon 2 in the coding region for helix II of the homeodomain, at a position that is important for protein stability. Biochemical and functional analyses show that the mutant protein exhibits little or no activity (Hu et al., 1998). The mutation (S202X), associated with Witkop syndrome, is also located in helix II in exon 2 and results in a truncated protein, which lacks helix III and the total C-terminal region. The mutation (S105X), associated with tooth agenesis and orofacial clefting, is located in exon 1 proximal to the homeodomain. The effect of both mutations, S202X and S105X, probably also leads to haploinsufficiency.

However, we cannot rule out that other mechanisms may be at work in addition to, or instead of, haploinsufficiency in causing the different phenotypes seen in humans with an *MSX1* mutation. Until the function of the Msx1 protein and regulation of the gene expression have been investigated and the effects of the mutations better understood, we cannot determine a definite pathogenetic mechanism for the deformities so far associated with these mutations.

ACKNOWLEDGMENTS

We thank D. Lindhout, J.K. Ploos van Amstel, F.A. Beemer, F. Meijlink, and J. Senior for reading the manuscript and M.J.H.M. van den Boogaard for creating Figure 51–4. Dr. Robert, Pasteur Institute, Paris, kindly provided Figures 51–1, 51–2, and 51–3.

REFERENCES

Akimenko MA, Johnson SL, Westerfield M, Ekker M (1995). Differential induction of four *msx* homeobox genes during fin development and regeneration in zebra fish. *Development* 121: 347–357.

Beaty TH, Wang H, Hetmanski JB, Fan YT, Zeiger JS, Liang KY, Chiu YF, Vanderkolk CA, Seifert KC, Wulfsberg EA, et al. (2001). A case-control study of nonsyndromic oral clefts in Maryland. *Ann Epidemiol* 11: 434–442.

Beaty TH, Hetmanski JB, Zeiger JS, Fan YT, Liang KY, Vanderkolk CA, McIntosh I (2002). Testing candidate genes for non-syndromic oral clefts using a case-parent trio design. *Genet Epidemiol* 22: 1–11.

Bei M, Maas R (1998). FGFs and BMP4 induce both *Msx1*-independent and *Msx1*-dependent signaling pathways in early tooth development. *Development* 125: 4325–4333.

Bei M, Kratochwil K, Maas RL (2000). BMP4 rescues a non-cell-autonomous function of *Msx1* in tooth development. *Development* 127: 4711–4718.

Bell JR, Noveen A, Liu YH, Ma L, Dobias S, Kundu R, Luo W, Xia Y, Lusis AJ, Snead ML (1993). Genomic structure, chromosomal location, and evolution of the mouse *Hox8* gene. *Genomics* 17: 800.

Bendall AJ, Abate-Shen C (2000). Roles for Msx and Dlx homeoproteins in vertebrate development. *Gene* 247: 17–31.

Bendall AJ, Rincon-Limas DE, Botas J, Abate-Shen C (1998). Protein complex formation between *Msx1* and Lhx2 homeoproteins is incompatible with DNA binding activity. *Differentiation* 63: 151–157.

Bendall AJ, Ding J, Hu G, Shen MM, Abate-Shen C (1999). *Msx1* antagonizes the myogenic activity of Pax3 in migrating limb muscle precursors. *Development* 126: 4965–4976.

Blanco R, Chakraborty R, Barton SA, Carreno H, Paredes M, Jara L, Palomino H, Schull WJ (2001). Evidence of a sex-dependent association between the *Msx1* locus and nonsyndromic cleft lip with or without cleft palate in the Chilean population. *Hum Biol* 73: 81–89.

Blin-Wakkach C, Lezot F, Ghoul-Mazgar S, Hotton D, Monteiro S, Teillaud C, Pibouin L, Orestes-Cardoso S, Papagerakis P, Macdougall M, et al. (2001). Endogenous *Msx1* antisense transcript: in vivo and in vitro evidences, structure, and potential involvement in skeleton development in mammals. *Proc Natl Acad Sci USA* 98: 7336–7341.

Brown JM, Wedden SE, Millburn GH, Robson LG, Hill RE, Davidson DR, Tickle C (1993). Experimental analysis of the control of expression of the homeobox-gene *Msx-1* in the developing limb and face. *Development* 119: 41–48.

Carlson MR, Bryant SV, Gardiner DM (1998). Expression of Msx-2 during development, regeneration, and wound healing in axolotl limbs. *J Exp Zool* 282: 715–723.

Catron KM, Iler N, Abate C (1993). Nucleotides flanking a conserved TAAT core dictate the DNA binding specificity of three murine homeodomain proteins. *Mol Cell Biol* 13: 2354–2365.

Catron KM, Zhang H, Marshall SC, Inostroza JA, Wilson JM, Abate C (1995). Transcriptional repression by Msx-1 does not require homeodomain DNA-binding sites. *Mol Cell Biol* 15: 861–871.

Catron KM, Wang H, Hu G, Shen MM, Abate-Shen C (1996). Comparison of MSX-1 and MSX-2 suggests a molecular basis for functional redundancy. *Mech Dev* 55: 185–199.

Celli J, Duijf P, Hamel BC, Bamshad M, Kramer B, Smits AP, Newbury-Ecob R, Hennekam RC, Van Buggenhout G, Van Haeringen A, et al. (1999). Heterozygous germline mutations in the p53 homolog p63 are the cause of EEC syndrome. *Cell* 99: 143–153

Chan-Thomas PS, Thompson RP, Robert B, Yacoub MH, Barton PJ (1993). Expression of homeobox genes *Msx-1* (*Hox-7*) and *Msx-2* (*Hox-8*) during cardiac development in the chick. *Dev Dyn* 197: 203–216.

Chen Y, Bei M, Woo I, Satokata I, Maas R (1996). *Msx1* controls inductive signaling in mammalian tooth morphogenesis. *Development* 122: 3035–3044.

Chitty LS, Dennis N, Baraitser M (1996). Hidrotic ectodermal dysplasia of hair, teeth, and nails: case reports and review. *J Med Genet* 33: 707–710.

Christensen K, Mitchell LE (1996). Familial recurrence-pattern analysis of nonsyndromic isolated cleft palate—a Danish Registry study. *Am J Hum Genet* 58: 182–190.

Coelho CN, Sumoy L, Rodgers BJ, Davidson DR, Hill RE, Upholt WB, Kosher RA (1991a). Expression of the chicken homeobox-containing gene *GHox-8* during embryonic chick limb development. *Mech Dev* 34: 143–154.

Coelho CN, Krabbenhoft KM, Upholt WB, Fallon JF, Kosher RA (1991b). Altered expression of the chicken homeobox-containing genes *GHox-7* and *GHox-8* in the limb buds of limbless mutant chick embryos. *Development* 113: 1487–1493.

Cohen MM Jr (2000). Craniofacial disorders caused by mutations in homeobox genes *MSX1* and *MSX2*. *J Craniofac Genet Dev Biol* 20: 19–25.

Cohn MJ, Tickle C (1996). Limbs: a model for pattern formation within the vertebrate body plan. *Trends Genet* 12: 253–257.

Crews L, Gates PB, Brown R, Joliot A, Foley C, Brockes JP, Gann AA (1995). Expression and activity of the newt *Msx-1* gene in relation to limb regeneration. *Proc R Soc Lond B Biol Sci* 259: 161–171.

Davidson D (1995). The function and evolution of *Msx* genes: pointers and paradoxes. *Trends Genet* 11: 405–411.

Davidson DR, Hill RE (1991). *Msh*-like genes: family of homeobox genes with wide-ranging expression during vertebrate development. *Semin Dev Biol* 2: 405–412.

Davidson DR, Crawley A, Hill RE, Tickle C (1991). Position-dependent expression of two related homeobox genes in developing vertebrate limbs. *Nature* 352: 429–431.

Ekker M, Akimenko MA, Bremiller R, Westerfield M (1992). Regional expression of three homeobox transcripts in the inner ear of zebra fish embryos. *Neuron* 9: 27–35.

Endo T, Tamura K, Ide H (2000). Analysis of gene expressions during *Xenopus* forelimb regeneration. *Dev Biol* 220: 296–306.

Ferguson MW (2000). A hole in the head. *Nat Genet* 24: 330–331.

FitzPatrick D, Farrall M (1993). An estimation of the number of susceptibility loci for isolated cleft palate. *J Craniofac Genet Dev Biol* 13: 230–235.

Francis-West P, Ladher R, Barlow A, Graveson A (1998). Signalling interactions during facial development. *Mech Dev* 75: 3–28.

Fraser FC (1955). Thoughts on the etiology of clefts of the palate and lip. *Acta Genet* 5: 358–369.

Fraser FC (1970). The genetics of cleft lip and cleft palate. *Am J Hum Genet* 22: 336–352.

Friedmann Y, Daniel CW (1996). Regulated expression of homeobox genes *Msx-1* and *Msx-2* in mouse mammary gland development suggests a role in hormone action and epithelial–stromal interactions. *Dev Biol* 177: 347–355.

Garzon MC, Paller AS (1996). What syndrome is this? Witkop tooth and nail syndrome. *Pediatr Dermatol* 13: 63–64.

Giansanti JS, Long SM, Rankin JL (1974). The "tooth and nail" type of autosomal dominant ectodermal dysplasia. *Oral Surg Oral Med Oral Pathol* 37: 576–582.

Graber LW (1978). Congenital absence of teeth: a review with emphasis on inheritance patterns. *J Am Dent Assoc* 96: 266–275.

Hewitt JE, Clark LN, Ivens A, Williamson R (1991). Structure and sequence of the human homeobox gene *HOX7*. *Genomics* 11: 670–678.

Hill RE, Jones PF, Rees AR, Sime CM, Justice MJ, Copeland NG, Jenkins NA, Graham E, Davidson DR (1989). A new family of mouse homeo box-containing genes: molecular structure, chromosomal location, and developmental expression of Hox-7.1. *Genes Dev* 3: 26–37.

Hodges SJ, Harley KE (1999). Witkop tooth and nail syndrome: report of two cases in a family. *Int J Paediatr Dent* 9: 207–211.

Holland PW (1991). Cloning and evolutionary analysis of *msh*-like homeobox genes from mouse, zebrafish and ascidian. *Gene* 98: 253–257.

Houzelstein D, Cohen A, Buckingham ME, Robert B (1997). Insertional mutation of the mouse *Msx1* homeobox gene by an *nlacZ* reporter gene. *Mech Dev* 65: 123–133.

Houzelstein D, Auda-Boucher G, Cheraud Y, Rouaud T, Blanc I, Tajbakhsh S, Buckingham ME, Fontaine-Perus J, Robert B (1999). The homeobox gene *Msx1* is expressed in a subset of somites, and in muscle progenitor cells migrating into the forelimb. *Development* 126: 2689–2701.

Houzelstein D, Cheraud Y, Auda-Boucher G, Fontaine-Perus J, Robert B (2000). The expression of the homeobox gene *Msx1* reveals two populations of dermal progenitor cells originating from the somites. *Development* 127: 2155–2164.

Hu G, Vastardis H, Bendall AJ, Wang Z, Logan M, Zhang H, Nelson C, Stein S, Greenfield N, Seidman CE, et al. (1998). Haploinsufficiency of *Msx1*: a mechanism for selective tooth agenesis. *Mol Cell Biol* 18: 6044–6051.

Hu G, Lee H, Price SM, Shen MM, Abate-Shen C (2001). *Msx* homeobox genes inhibit differentiation through upregulation of cyclin D1. *Development* 128: 2373–2384.

Hudson CD, Witkop CJ (1975). Autosomal dominant hypodontia with nail dysgenesis. Report of twenty-nine cases in six families. *Oral Surg Oral Med Oral Pathol* 39: 409–423.

Inouye M (1988). Antisense RNA: its functions and applications in gene regulation—a review. *Gene* 72: 25–34.

Isaac VE, Sciavolino P, Abate C (1995). Multiple amino acids determine the DNA binding specificity of the Msx-1 homeodomain. *Biochemistry* 34: 7127–7134.

Ivens A, Flavin N, Williamson R, Dixon M, Bates G, Buckingham M, Robert B (1990). The human homeobox gene *HOX7* maps to chromosome 4p16.1 and may be implicated in Wolf-Hirschhorn syndrome. *Hum Genet* 84: 473–476.

Jabs EW, Muller U, Li X, Ma L, Luo W, Haworth IS, Klisak I, Sparkes R, Warman ML, Mulliken JB (1993). A mutation in the homeodomain of the human *MSX2* gene in a family affected with autosomal dominant craniosynostosis. *Cell* 75: 443–450.

Jernvall J, Aberg T, Kettunen P, Keranen S, Thesleff I (1998). The life history of an embryonic signaling center: BMP-4 induces p21 and is associated with apoptosis in the mouse tooth enamel knot. *Development* 125: 161–169.

Johnson RL, Tabin CJ (1997). Molecular models for vertebrate limb development. *Cell* 90: 979–990.

Jowett AK, Vainio S, Ferguson MW, Sharpe PT, Thesleff I (1993). Epithelial-mesenchymal interactions are required for *msx 1* and *msx 2* gene expression in the developing murine molar tooth. *Development* 117: 461–470.

Jumlongras D, Bei M, Stimson JM, Wang WF, DePalma SR, Seidman CE, Felbor U, Maas R, Seidman JG, Olsen BR (2001). A nonsense mutation in *MSX1* causes Witkop syndrome. *Am J Hum Genet* 69: 67–74.

Kim HJ, Rice DP, Kettunen PJ, Thesleff I (1998). FGF-, BMP- and Shh-mediated signalling pathways in the regulation of cranial suture morphogenesis and calvarial bone development. *Development* 125: 1241–1251.

Kondo S, Schutte B, Richardson R, Bjork B, Knight A, Watanabe Y, Howard E, Ferreira de Lima R, Daack-Hirsch S, Sander A, et al. (2002). Mutations in *IRF6* cause Van der Woude and popliteal pterygium syndromes. *Nat Genet* 32: 285–289.

Koshiba K, Kuroiwa A, Yamamoto H, Tamura K, Ide H (1998). Expression of *Msx* genes in regenerating and developing limbs of axolotl. *J Exp Zool* 282: 703–714.

Kumar M, Carmichael GG (1998). Antisense RNA: function and fate of duplex RNA in cells of higher eukaryotes. *Microbiol Mol Biol Rev* 62: 1415–1434.

Lee TI, Young RA (1998). Regulation of gene expression by TBP-associated proteins. *Genes Dev* 12: 1398–1408.

Lidral AC, Romitti PA, Basart AM, Doetschman T, Leysens NJ, Daack-Hirsch S, Semina EV, Johnson LR, Machida J, Burds A, et al. (1998). Association of *Msx1* and TGFB3 with nonsyndromic clefting in humans. *Am J Hum Genet* 63: 557–568.

Lu CH, Rincon-Limas DE, Botas J (2000). Conserved overlapping and reciprocal expression of msh/Msx1 and apterous/Lhx2 in *Drosophila* and mice. *Mech Dev* 99:177–181.

Lumsden AG (1988). Spatial organization of the epithelium and the role of neural crest cells in the initiation of the mammalian tooth germ. *Development* 103(Suppl): 155–169.

Lyons GE, Houzelstein D, Sassoon D, Robert B, Buckingham ME (1992). Multiple sites of Hox-7 expression during mouse embryogenesis: comparison with retinoic acid receptor mRNA localization. *Mol Reprod Dev* 32: 303–314.

Maas R, Bei M (1997). The genetic control of early tooth development. *Crit Rev Oral Biol Med* 8: 4–39.

Maas R, Chen YP, Bei M, Woo I, Satokata I (1996). The role of *Msx* genes in mammalian development. *Ann NY Acad Sci* 785: 171–181.

MacKenzie A, Ferguson MW, Sharpe PT (1991a). Hox-7 expression during murine craniofacial development. *Development* 113: 601–611.

MacKenzie A, Leeming GL, Jowett AK, Ferguson MW, Sharpe PT (1991b). The homeobox gene *Hox 7.1* has specific regional and temporal expression patterns during early murine craniofacial embryogenesis, especially tooth development in vivo and in vitro. *Development* 111: 269–285.

MacKenzie A, Ferguson MW, Sharpe PT (1992). Expression patterns of the homeobox gene, *Hox-8*, in the mouse embryo suggest a role in specifying tooth initiation and shape. *Development* 115: 403–420.

Marazzi G, Wang Y, Sassoon D (1997). Msx2 is a transcriptional regulator in the BMP4-mediated programmed cell death pathway. *Dev Biol* 186: 127–138.

McGrath JA, Duijf PHG, Doetsch V, Irvine AD, De Waal R, Vanmolkot KRJ, Kelly A, Atherton DJ, Griffiths AD, Orlow SJ, et al. (2001). Hay-Wells syndrome is caused by heterozygous missense mutations in the SAM domain of p63. *Hum Mol Genet* 10: 221–229.

Milan M, Weihe U, Tiong S, Bender W, Cohen SM (2001). msh specifies dorsal cell fate in the *Drosophila* wing. *Development* 128: 3263–3268.

Mina M (2001a). Morphogenesis of the medial region of the developing mandible is regulated by multiple signaling pathways. *Cells Tissues Organs* 169: 295–301.

Mina M (2001b). Regulation of mandibular growth and morphogenesis. *Crit Rev Oral Biol Med* 12: 276–300.

Mina M, Kollar EJ (1987). The induction of odontogenesis in non-dental mesenchyme combined with early murine mandibular arch epithelium. *Arch Oral Biol* 32: 123–127.

Mina M, Gluhak J, Upholt WB, Kollar EG, Rogers B (1995). Experimental analysis of *Msx1* and *Msx2* gene expression during chick mandibular morphogenesis. *Dev Dyn* 202: 195–214.

Mitchell LE, Murray JC, O'Brien S, Christensen K (2001). Evaluation of two putative susceptibility loci for oral clefts in the Danish population. *Am J Epidemiol* 153: 1007–1015.

Monaghan AP, Davidson DR, Sime C, Graham E, Baldock R, Bhattacharya SS, Hill RE (1991). The *Msh*-like homeobox genes define domains in the developing vertebrate eye. *Development* 112: 1053–1061.

Murdoch-Kinch CA, Miles DA, Poon CK (1993). Hypodontia and nail dysplasia syndrome. Report of a case. *Oral Surg Oral Med Oral Pathol* 75: 403–406.

Murray JC (2002). Gene/environment causes of cleft lip and/or palate. *Clin Genet* 61: 248–256.

Nieminen P, Arte S, Pirinen S, Peltonen L, Thesleff I (1995). Gene defect in hypodontia: exclusion of *MSX1* and *MSX2* as candidate genes. *Hum Genet* 96: 305–308.

Nohno T, Noji S, Koyama E, Nishikawa K, Myokai F, Saito T, Taniguchi S (1992). Differential expression of two *msh*-related homeobox genes *Chox-7* and Chox-8 during chick limb development. *Biochem Biophys Res Commun* 182: 121–128.

Noveen A, Jiang TX, Ting-Berreth SA, Chuong CM (1995). Homeobox genes *Msx-1* and *Msx-2* are associated with induction and growth of skin appendages. *J Invest Dermatol* 104: 711–719.

Odelberg SJ, Kollhoff A, Keating MT (2000). Dedifferentiation of mammalian myotubes induced by msx1. *Cell* 103: 1099–1109.

Orestes-Cardoso SM, Nefussi JR, Hotton D, Mesbah M, Orestes-Cardoso MD, Robert B, Berdal A (2001). Postnatal *Msx1* expression pattern in craniofacial, axial, and appendicular skeleton of transgenic mice from the first week until the second year. *Dev Dyn* 221: 1–13.

Padanilam BJ, Stadler HS, Mills KA, McLeod LB, Solursh M, Lee B, Ramirez F, Buetow KH, Murray JC (1992). Characterization of the human HOX 7 cDNA and identification of polymorphic markers. *Hum Mol Genet* 1: 407–410.

Park J, Park K, Kim S, Lee JH (2001). *Msx1* gene overexpression induces G₁ phase cell arrest in human ovarian cancer cell line OVCAR3. *Biochem Biophys Res Commun* 281: 1234–1240.

Pavlova A, Boutin E, Cunha G, Sassoon D (1994). Msx1 (Hox-7.1) in the adult mouse uterus: cellular interactions underlying regulation of expression. *Development* 120: 335–345.

Peters H, Balling R (1999). Teeth. Where and how to make them. *Trends Genet* 15: 59–65.

Phippard DJ, Weber-Hall SJ, Sharpe PT, Naylor MS, Jayatalake H, Maas R, Woo I, Roberts-Clark D, Francis-West PH, Liu YH, et al. (1996). Regulation of Msx-1, Msx-2, Bmp-2 and Bmp-4 during foetal and postnatal mammary gland development. *Development* 122: 2729–2737.

Ranta R (1986). A review of tooth formation in children with cleft lip/palate. *Am J Orthod Dentofacial Orthop* 90: 11–18.

Redpath TH, Winter GB (1969). Autosomal dominant ectodermal dysplasia with significant dental defects. *Br Dent J* 126: 123–128.

Reginelli AD, Wang YQ, Sassoon D, Muneoka K (1995). Digit tip regeneration correlates with regions of *Msx1* (Hox 7) expression in fetal and newborn mice. *Development* 121: 1065–1076.

Richman JM, Tickle C (1989). Epithelia are interchangeable between facial primordial of chick embryos and morphogenesis is controlled in the mesenchyme. *Dev Biol* 136: 201–210

Robert B, Sassoon D, Jacq B, Gehring W, Buckingham M (1989). *Hox-7*, a mouse homeobox gene with a novel pattern of expression during embryogenesis. *EMBO J* 8: 91–100.

Robert B, Lyons G, Simandl BK, Kuroiwa A, Buckingham M (1991). The apical ectodermal ridge regulates *Hox-7* and *Hox-8* gene expression in developing chick limb buds. *Genes Dev* 5: 2363–2374.

Romitti PA, Lidral AC, Munger RG, Daack-Hirsch S, Burns TL, Murray JC (1999). Candidate genes for nonsyndromic cleft lip and palate and maternal cigarette smoking and alcohol consumption: evaluation of genotype-environment interactions from a population-based case-control study of orofacial clefts. *Teratology* 59: 39–50.

Sadler TW, Potts LF (1997). Making sense with anti-sense; determining the role of *Msx* genes in mouse whole embryo culture. In: *Studies in Somatology and Craniofacial Biology.* Cohen MM Jr, Baum BJ (eds.) IOS Press, Amsterdam, pp. 59–66.

Satokata I, Maas R (1994). *Msx1* deficient mice exhibit cleft palate and abnormalities of craniofacial and tooth development. *Nat Genet* 6: 348–356.

Schalk-van der Weide Y (1992). Oligodontia: A Clinical, Radiographic and Genetic Evaluation. University of Utrecht, Utrecht, the Netherlands. Dissertation.

Schummer M, Scheurlen I, Schaller C, Galliot B (1992). *HOM/HOX* homeobox genes are present in hydra (*Chlorohydra viridissima*) and are differentially expressed during regeneration. *EMBO J* 11: 1815–1823.

Schutte BC, Murray JC (1999). The many faces and factors of orofacial clefts. *Hum Mol Genet* 8: 1853–1859.

Scott MP (1992). Vertebrate homeobox gene nomenclature. *Cell* 71: 551–553.

Shang Z, Isaac VE, Li H, Patel L, Catron KM, Curran T, Montelione GT, Abate C (1994). Design of a "minimal" homeodomain: the N-terminal arm modulates DNA binding affinity and stabilizes homeodomain structure. *Proc Natl Acad Sci USA* 91: 8373–8377.

Shetty S, Takahashi T, Matsui H, Ayengar R, Raghow R (1999). Transcriptional autorepression of *Msx1* gene is mediated by interactions of *Msx1* protein with a multi-protein transcriptional complex containing TATA-binding protein, Sp1 and cAMP-response-element-binding protein-binding protein (CBP/p300). *Biochem J* 339(Pt 3): 751–758.

Shimeld SM, McKay IJ, Sharpe PT (1996). The murine homeobox gene *Msx-3* shows highly restricted expression in the developing neural tube. *Mech Dev* 55: 201–210.

Simon H-G, Nelson C, Goff D, Laufer E, Morgan BA, Tabin C (1995). Differential Expression of myogenic regulatory genes and *Msx-1* during dedifferentiation and redifferentiation of regenerating amphibian limbs. *Dev Dyn* 202: 1–12.

Slavkin HC, Shum L, Nuckolls GH (1998). Ectodermal dysplasia: a synthesis between evolutionary, developmental, and molecular biology and human clinical genetics. In: *Molecular Basis of Epithelial Appendage Morphogenesis: Molecular Biology Intelligence Unit.* Chuong C-M (ed.) RG Landes, Austin, pp. 15–37.

Song K, Wang Y, Sassoon D (1992). Expression of Hox-7.1 in myoblasts inhibits terminal differentiation and induces cell transformation. *Nature* 360: 477–481.

Spritz RA (2001). The genetics and epigenetics of orofacial clefts. *Curr Opin Pediatr* 13: 556–560.

Stelnicki EJ, Komuves LG, Holmes D, Clavin W, Harrison MR, Adzick NS, Largman C (1997). The human homeobox genes *MSX-1, MSX-2,* and *MOX-1* are differentially expressed in the dermis and epidermis in fetal and adult skin. *Differentiation* 62: 33–41.

Stimson JM, Sivers JE, Hlava GL (1997). Features of oligodontia in three generations. *J Clin Pediatr Dent* 21: 269–275.

Stock DW, Weiss KM, Zhao Z (1997). Patterning of the mammalian dentition in development and evolution. *Bioessays* 19: 481–490.

Su MW, Suzuki HR, Solursh M, Ramirez F (1991). Progressively restricted expression of a new homeobox-containing gene during *Xenopus laevis* embryogenesis. *Development* 111: 1179–1187.

Suzuki HR, Padanilam BJ, Vitale E, Ramirez F, Solursh M (1991). Repeating developmental expression of *G-Hox 7*, a novel homeobox-containing gene in the chicken. *Dev Biol* 148: 375–388.

Symons AL, Stritzel F, Stamation J (1993). Anomalies associated with hypodontia of the permanent lateral incisor and second premolar. *J Clin Pediatr Dent* 17: 109–111.

Takahashi Y, Le Douarin N (1990). cDNA cloning of a quail homeobox gene and its expression in neural crest–derived mesenchyme and lateral plate mesoderm. *Proc Natl Acad Sci USA* 87: 7482–7486.

Takahashi K, Nuckolls GH, Tanaka O, Semba I, Takahashi I, Dashner R, Shum L, Slavkin HC (1998). Adenovirus-mediated ectopic expression of Msx2 in even-numbered rhombomeres induces apoptotic elimination of cranial neural crest cells in ovo. *Development* 125: 1627–1635.

Thesleff I (1996). Two genes for missing teeth. *Nat Genet* 13: 379–380.

Thesleff I, Sharpe P (1997). Signalling networks regulating dental development. *Mech Dev* 67: 111–123.

Thesleff I, Vaahtokari A, Partanen AM (1995). Regulation of organogenesis. Common molecular mechanisms regulating the development of teeth and other organs. *Int J Dev Biol* 39: 35–50.

Tucker AS, Matthews KL, Sharpe PT (1998). Transformation of tooth type induced by inhibition of BMP signaling. *Science* 282: 1136–1138.

Vainio S, Karavanova I, Jowett A, Thesleff I (1993). Identification of BMP-4 as a signal mediating secondary induction between epithelial and mesenchymal tissues during early tooth development. *Cell* 75: 45–58.

Van den Boogaard MJ, Dorland M, Beemer FA, Ploos van Amstel HK (2000). *Msx1* mutation is associated with orofacial clefting and tooth agenesis in humans. *Nat Genet* 24: 342–343.

Vastardis H, Karimbux N, Guthua S W, Seidman JG, Seidman CE (1996). A human *Msx1* homeodomain missense mutation causes selective tooth agenesis. *Nat Genet* 13: 417–421.

Walldorf U, Fleig R, Gehring WJ (1989). Comparison of homeobox-containing genes of the honeybee and *Drosophila*. *Proc Natl Acad Sci USA* 86: 9971–9975.

Wang W, Chen X, Xu H, Lufkin T (1996). *Msx3*: a novel murine homologue of the *Drosophila msh* homeobox gene restricted to the dorsal embryonic central nervous system. *Mech Dev* 58: 203–215.

Wang YH, Upholt WB, Sharpe PT, Kollar EJ, Mina M (1998). Odontogenic epithelium induces similar molecular responses in chick and mouse mandibular mesenchyme. *Dev Dyn* 213: 386–397.

Wedden SE (1987). Epithelial–mesenchymal interactions in the development of chick facial primordia and the target of retinoid action. *Development* 99: 341–351.

Wedden SE, Ralphs JR, Tickle C (1988). Pattern formation in the facial primordia. *Development* 103(Suppl): 31–40.

Weech AA (1929). Hereditary ectodermal dysplasia (congenital ectodermal defect). *Am J Dis Child* 37: 766–790.

Wilkie AOM, Tang Z, Elanko N, Walsh S, Twigg SRF, Hurst JA, Wall SA, Chrzanowska, Maxson RE Jr (2000). Functional haploinsufficiency of the human homeobox gene *MSX2* casuses defects in skull ossification. *Nat Genet* 24: 387–390.

Witkop CJ Jr (1965). Genetic diseases of the oral cavity. In: *Oral pathology.* Tiecke RW (ed.) McGraw-Hill, New York, pp. 812–813.

Witkop CJ Jr (1990). Hypodontia-nail dysgenesis. In: *Birth Defect Encyclopedia: The Comprehensive, Systematic, Illustrated Reference Source for the Diagnosis, Delineation, Etiology, Biodynamics, Occurrence, Prevention, and Treatment of Human Anomalies of Clinical Relevance.* Buyse ML (ed.) Center for Birth Defects Information Services, Dover, MA, p. 920.

Witkop CJ Jr, Brearley LJ, Gentry WC (1975). Hypoplastic enamel, onycholysis, and hypohidrosis inherited as an autosomal dominant trait: a review of ectodermal dysplasia syndromes. *Oral Surg Oral Med Oral Pathol* 30: 71–86.

Woloshin P, Song K, Degnin C, Killary AM, Goldhamer DJ, Sassoon D, Thayer MJ (1995). MSX1 inhibits myoD expression in fibroblast × 10T1/2 cell hybrids. *Cell* 82: 611–620.

Yokouchi Y, Ohsugi K, Sasaki H, Kuroiwa A (1991). Chicken homeobox gene *Msx-1*: structure, expression in limb buds and effect of retinoic acid. *Development* 113: 431–444.

Zabawski EJ Jr, Cohen JB (1999). Hereditary hypodontia and onychorrhexis of the fingernails and toenail koilonychia: Witkop tooth- and nail syndrome. *Dermatol Online J* 5: 3.

Zhang H, Catron KM, Abate-Shen C (1996). A role for the Msx-1 homeodomain in transcriptional regulation: residues in the N-terminal arm mediate TATA binding protein interaction and transcriptional repression. *Proc Natl Acad Sci USA* 93: 1764–1769.

Zhang H, Hu G, Wang H, Sciavolino P, Iler N, Shen MM, Abate-Shen C (1997). Heterodimerization of Msx and Dlx homeoproteins results in functional antagonism. *Mol Cell Biol* 17: 2920–2932.

Zhang Y, Zhao X, Hu Y, St Amand T, Zhang M, Ramamurthy R, Qiu M, Chen Y (1999). *Msx1* is required for the induction of Patched by Sonic hedgehog in the mammalian tooth germ. *Dev Dyn* 215: 45–53.

Zhang Y, Zhang Z, Zhao X, Yu X, Hu Y, Geronimo B, Fromm SH, Chen YP (2000). A new function of BMP4: dual role for BMP4 in regulation of Sonic hedgehog expression in the mouse tooth germ. *Development* 127: 1431–1443.

52 | *MSX2* and *ALX4* and Craniosynostosis and Defects in Skull Ossification

ULRICH MÜLLER

Mutations in the homeobox gene *MSX2* can result in both craniosynostosis (the premature fusion of the calvarial sutures) and its opposite, parietal foramina (the delayed ossification along the sagittal sutures). The one *MSX2* mutation (Pro148His) described in craniosynostosis to date results in a gain of gene fuction due to increased binding to the consensus MSX binding site and the subsequent overstimulation of *MSX2* target genes. Conversely, haploinsufficiency of *MSX2* is the cause of parietal foramina. Haploinsufficiency of another homeobox gene, *ALX4*, can also underlie parietal foramina. No mutation has yet been discovered in this gene in craniosynostosis.

Normal differentiation of the skull involves ossification and growth of the cranial plates and their fusion along the calvarial sutures. This process is finely tuned and well coordinated with the growth of the developing brain. Numerous polypeptides including bone morphogenetic proteins (BMPs), fibroblast growth factors (FGFs; see Chapter 32) and their receptors (FGFRs; see Chapter 33), and transcription factors control these developmental processes. In principle, disturbances in the function of any one of these polypeptides can result in malformations of the head and can interfere with normal development and operation of the brain. In this chapter I focus on the role of the homeotic genes *MSX2* and *ALX4* in abnormal differentiation of the skull, specifically in craniosynostosis and parietal foramina.

CRANIOSYNOSTOSIS AND PARIETAL FORAMINA

Craniosynostosis, the premature fusion of the calvarial sutures, is a particularly common malformation of the skull. It occurs in about 1 in 2500 newborns (Lajeunie et al., 1995, 1996) and has been described in over 100 syndromes (Winter and Baraitser, 1996). Several forms of craniosynostosis are inherited as autosomal dominant traits, with craniosynostosis as the sole or predominant finding. Depending on which suture is involved, the cranial manifestation may be turribrachycephaly (coronal suture), scaphocephaly (sagittal suture), plagiocephaly (coronal or lambdoid suture), or combinations thereof (reviewed by Müller et al., 1997). Secondary neurological and ophthalmological complications can occur and include epileptic seizures, headaches, mental retardation, optic atrophy due to increased intracranial pressure, and hydrocephalus due to Arnold-Chiari malformation. In a few rare instances, agenesis of the corpus callosum has been observed (reviewed by Wilkie, 1997; Jones, 1988).

While craniosynostosis is caused by abnormally accelerated differentiation of the bones of the skull, a delay in this developmental process can result in parietal foramina (PFM), also referred to as foramina parietalia permagna (FPP) (reviewed by Cohen, 2000). PFM are oval, symmetrical defects in the parietal bones located along the sagittal sutures. Their size decreases with time, and they are usually clinically insignificant. Occasionally, however, PFM are associated with headaches or structural or vascular malformations of the brain, or they may be so large as to require neurosurgical intervention (Pang and Lin, 1982; Preis et al., 1995).

MSX2 AND *ALX4*

Human *MSX2* is a member of the vertebrate *Msx* family of homeobox genes that were isolated based on their homology to *Drosophila* gene *Msh* (muscle segment homeobox gene). There are three murine *Msx* genes, *Msx1* (see Chapter 51), *Msx2* (this chapter), and *Msx3*. Unlike the *Hox* (homeobox-containing) genes (see Chapter 46), the *Msx* genes are not clustered on chromosomes. The human ortholog of *Msx2* was assigned to the distal long arm of chromosome 5 (5q34–q35) (Jabs et al., 1993) and positioned between the genes *CSX* (cardiac homeobox gene) proximally and *DRD1* (dopamin receptor D1) distally on a yeast artificial chromosome (YAC) contig of 5q35.1 (Kostrzewa et al., 1998). *MSX2* is composed of two exons separated by a large intron. The gene encodes a 267 amino acid protein with a homeobox domain of 60 amino acids. Overall identity to the mouse ortholog is 92%, with the homeobox domains being 100% identical in both species (Bell et al., 1993; Jabs et al., 1993).

While *Msx3* is primarily expressed in the central nervous system (Shimeld et al., 1996; Wang et al., 1996), *Msx2* and closely related *Msx1* are expressed in multiple tissues at many stages of development, including eyes, ears, and tooth buds; the nasal, maxillary, and mandibular processes; and the bones of the skull (Monaghan et al., 1991; MacKenzie et al., 1992; Jabs et al., 1993; Jowett et al., 1993). *Msx2* is also highly expressed in cells at the extreme ends of the osteogenic fronts of the calvarial sutures (Jabs et al., 1993).

MSX1 and 2, together with a wealth of additional genes, are regulated by Wnt protein (Wnt-3A; Willert et al., 2002) (see Chapter 22). Bone morphogenetic protein-4 (BMP-4) is also an important upstream regulator of MSX2/Msx2 expression (e.g., Graham et al., 1994). In a cell system, BMP-4 and Wnt-3A were found to act synergistically on the expression levels of *Msx1* and 2 among other genes. However, BMP-4 exerts its effects as early as at 30 minutes, while Wnt acts only after 2 hours (Willert et al., 2002). YY1, a transcription factor with four zinc finger domains, is another BMP-4 independent upstream regulator of *Msx2* that might be required to maintain optimal *Msx2* gene expression. Binding of YY1 to the promoter region of *Msx2* results in activation of this gene (Tan et al., 2002).

Downstream genes regulated by *Msx2* include *Runx2*, which codes for a runt domain transcription factor (Ito, 1999; see Chapter 29). *Runx2* plays an important role in ossification by the regulation of osteoblast-specific genes, such as osteocalcin. Using a cell system, Shirakabe et al. (2001) showed that the homeobox protein *Msx2* can interfere with *Runx2* activity. Interaction of *Msx2* and *Runx2* represses the ability of *Runx2* to regulate expression of downstream genes. Another homeobox protein, Dlx5 (homolog of the *Drosophila* distalless, Dll, gene) interferes with the Runx2–Msx2 interaction, thus reversing the repression of *Runx2* activity by *Msx2*.

Human *ALX4* (aristaless-like homeobox gene) is related to the *Drosophila* gene *aristaless* and to a group of vertebrate genes, including *Alx3*, *Prx1*, *Prx2*, and *Cart1* (Opstelten et al., 1991; Cserjesi et al., 1992,; Zhao et al., 1993; Rudnick et al., 1994; Qu et al., 1997a, 1997b). *Aristaless* refers to absent or reduced aristae (sense organs at the tip of the antennae) that—among other features—are found in flies with mutations of this homeobox gene. Human *ALX4* is located in the proximal short arm of chromosome 11 (11p11.2) in close proximity to the gene *EXT2*, mutations of which cause multiple exostoses. *ALX4* is composed of at least four exons coding for a paired-type homeodomain protein of 411 amino acids. Overall identity to the mouse ortholog is 92.5%, with the homeobox region being 100% identical in both species (Wuyts al al., 2000a).

In the mouse, *Alx4* is expressed in osteoblast precursors of most bones, in addition to various tissues such as the dermal papillae of hair and whisker follicles, the dental papillae of teeth, and a subset of mesenchymal cells in pubescent mammary glands (Hudson et al., 1998). Whole-mount in situ experiments during development demonstrated expression of *Alx4* in both the craniofacial region and the anterior aspect of the developing limb buds (Qu et al., 1997b). Based on this finding, Qu et al. (1997b) suggest that *Alx4* has a role in the patterning of structures derived from craniofacial mesenchyme, the first branchial arch, and the limb bud.

Both *Alx4* and *Alx3* are downstream targets of Twist, which is required for normal limb and craniofacial development (Loebel et al., 2002; see Chapter 34). Furthermore, *Alx4* interacts with lymphoid enhancer-binding factor (LEF-1) in mesenchymal cells of developing bones, limbs, hair, whiskers, teeth, and mammary tissues. LEF-1 and *Alx4* appear to interact through a specific proline-rich domain in the N-terminal region of *Alx4* and in the DNA-binding domain (HMG-box) of LEF-1. Specific binding of LEF-1 and *Alx4* to the promoter of neural cell adhesion molecule (N-CAM) modulates its activity (Boras and Hamel, 2002).

CRANIOSYNOSTOSIS, BOSTON TYPE (TYPE 2) AND *MSX2*

A mutation in *MSX2* was shown to be the underlying cause of craniosynostosis in a large family. In this family, craniosynostosis is inherited as an autosomal dominant trait. The phenotype of affected individuals varies greatly and ranges from clinically insignificant forehead recession (Fig. 52–1a), via turribrachycephaly (Fig. 52–1b) and frontal bossing (Fig. 52–1c), to kleeblattschädel anomaly (cloverleaf skull, Fig. 52–1d). Because this family was studied by researchers at Children's Hospital in Boston (Müller et al., 1993; Warman et al., 1993) the craniosynostosis in this family is referred to as "craniosynostosis, Boston type." A better term, suggested by Victor McKusick, might be craniosynostosis, type 2 (OMIM 604757). Linkage analysis in this family located the craniosyostosis locus in the distal long arm

of chromosome 5 (Müller et al., 1993), in the same general region to which *MSX2* had been assigned (Jabs et al., 1993). *MSX2* was therefore studied as a candidate gene for craniosynostosis in the Boston family.

Linkage analysis using a short tandem repeat polymorphism (STRP) marker in the large intron of *MSX2* gave a high LOD score ($Z_{max} = 4.8$ at $\theta \rightarrow 0$), and subsequent sequencing of the gene in patients revealed a C→A transversion at nucleotide 64 of exon 2. This results in an amino acid change from Pro (CCC) to His (CAC) at position 7 of the homeodomain of *MSX2* (Pro148His; Table 52–1). The proline in the homeodomain of Msx2 has been highly conserved during vertebrate evolution. This, together with the high expression of *Msx2* in the calvarial sutures argues for a causative role of the mutation in diseases of the skull.

Expression of the murine counterpart of the human Pro148His *MSX2* mutation in mice and the induction of craniosynostosis in the transgenic animals has proved beyond doubt the causative nosologic role of the mutation (Liu et al., 1995). The Pro → His mutation at position 7 of the homeodomain results in a gain of function of Msx2 by increasing and stabilizing binding of the homeodomain to DNA without altering nucleotide sequence binding preferences. Using gel shift analysis, Ma et al. (1996) showed that the binding affinity of Pro148His Msx2 to a sequence that contains the consensus Msx binding site, TAATTG, is dramatically increased as compared to wild-type Msx2.

Furthermore, binding site selection analyses demonstrated that the mutation has virtually no effect on site specificity of Msx2 binding. The experiments suggest that craniosynostosis in Pro148His Msx2 results from overstimulation of the Msx2 target sequences. This is consistent with findings in mice overexpressing wild-type human MSX2 which also develop craniosynostosis (Liu et al., 1999). In addition, overexpression of Msx2 in cultured chick calvarial osteoblasts prevents osteoblast differentiation but enhances growth of undifferenti-

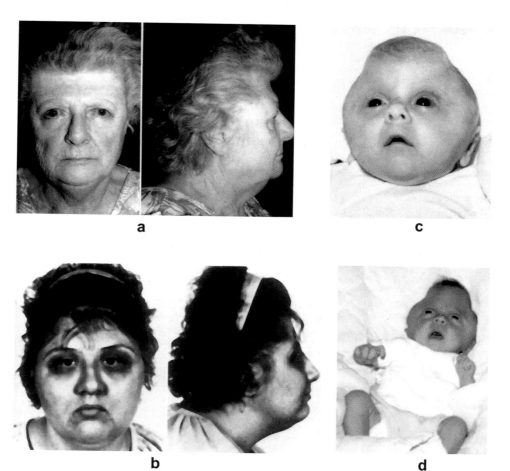

Figure 52–1. Different manifestations of craniosynostosis, Boston type. All individuals carry the P148H mutation in *MSX2*. (*a*) Recession of forehead; (*b*) turribrachycephaly; (*c*) frontal bossing; (*d*) kleeblattschädel anomaly.

Table 52–1. Mutation in *MSX2*

Mutation (Amino Acid Substitution)	Location in Gene	Phenotype*	Reference
P148H	Exon 2	Craniosynostosis	Jabs et al., 1993
A89X	Exon 1	PFM	Wuyts et al., 2000b
W115X	Exon 1	PFM	Wuyts et al., 2000b
L154P	Exon 2	PFM	Wuyts et al., 2000b
RK159–160del	Exon 2	PFM	Wilkie et al., 2000
R172H	Exon 2	PFM	Wilkie et al., 2000; Wuyts et al., 2000b
206 kb deletion	Deletion of entire gene	PFM	Wilkie et al., 2000

*PFM, parietal foramina.

ated osteoblasts (Dodig et al., 1999). Taken together, these findings suggest that both overexpression of MSX2 and the Pro148His mutation accelerate suture formation by prevention of calvarial osteoblast differentiation and enhancement of growth.

To date, affected members of the Boston family are the only reported cases with craniosynostosis and a mutation in *MSX2*.

PARIETAL FORAMINA AND *MSX2*

Parietal foramina (PFM) (or foramina parietalia permagna; FPP) (OMIM 168500) and craniosynostosis may be considered the opposite extremes of a spectrum of abnormal ossification processes of the skull. As discussed in this chapter, *Msx2* overexpression in cultured osteoblasts and in transgenic mice inhibits calvarial osteoblast differentiation and stimulates both proliferation of undifferentiated osteoblasts and premature closure of the calvarial sutures. Conversely, inhibition of *Msx2* expression stimulates osteoblast differentiation and may delay proliferation of osteoblasts and suture closure (Dodig et al., 1999). This was proven in *Msx2*-deficient mice that have defects of skull ossification, notably of the frontal bone, and persistent calvarial foramina (Satokata et al., 2000).

Given the effects observed after down-regulation of *Msx2* in cultured chick osteoblasts and in mice, a deficiency of *MSX2* might also cause related effects in humans. To date, two groups of investigators have reported a total of six different mutations in both exons of *MSX2* in patients with PFM (Wilkie et al., 2000; Wuyts et al., 2000b; Table 52–1). One of these mutations was a deletion of 206 kb in the distal long arm of chromosome 5, including the entire *MSX2* gene (Wilkie et al., 2000). Obviously, haploinsufficiency of *MSX2* accounts for PFM in the deletion case. Analysis of the remaining mutations in both exons 1 and 2 suggests that these DNA alterations result in haploinsufficiency of *MSX2* as well. In addition, two nonsense mutations in exon 1 (Table 52–1) result in truncation of MSX2 and loss of the homeodomain. The L154P, RK159–160 del, and R172H mutations (Table 52–1) occurred in the homeodomain at positions necessary for DNA binding and appear to interrupt critical contacts of MSX2 with its target sequences.

Although deficiency of Msx2 has similar effects in mice and humans, there are important differences. Unlike in humans, heterozygous deletions of *Msx2* in mice *(Msx+/−)* do not have a phenotypic effect. The abnormal findings in ossification are only observed in homozygous *(Msx2−/−)* mice that show a central defect of the frontal bone, in contrast to humans in whom the parietal bones are affected. These findings may be ascribed to differences in *Msx2* dosage sensitivity between the two species.

PARIETAL FORAMINA AND *ALX4*

PFM can also be caused by mutations in the homeobox gene *ALX4*. Evidence of involvement of *ALX4* in the formation of PFM came from findings in the 11p11.2 contiguous gene-deletion syndrome, also referred to as Potocki-Shaffer syndrome (PSS) (OMIM #601224). Monosomy of 11p11.2 in PSS results in biparietal foramina, multiple exostoses, dysmorphic features, and mental retardation. Wu et al. (2000) argued that haploinsufficiency of a homolog of *MSX2* could cause PFM in the 11p11.2 contiguous gene-deletion syndrome. They performed a BLASTN homology search of the complete coding sequence of *MSX2* against the genome-sequence database and identified a bacterial artificial chromosome (BAC) derived from chromosome 11 that displayed 26 bp of 100% sequence identity to parts of the homeodomain of *MSX2*. In situ hybridization of this BAC to chromosomes from patients assigned it to the critical interval of the PSS. A homology search of the sequences flanking the homeobox of the gene revealed a high degree of homology to mouse *Alx4*. Based on its location, its bone-specific expression, and its function in the development of skull and limb bones of the mouse, the authors postulated that haploinsufficiency of *ALX4* is the cause of PFM in the 11p11.2 contiguous gene-deletion syndrome.

Applying a similar approach, Wuyts et al. (2000a) identified an *Alx4* homolog in the deleted interval of the PSS. After characterization of the genomic structure of human *ALX4*, they performed mutation analysis in patients with isolated, autosomal dominant PFM (OMIM #168500) in whom a mutation in *MSX2* had been previously excluded. They found two different mutations in two out of six families tested (Table 52–2): one mutation resulted in a frameshift and premature termination of the polypeptide (S168fs); the other one was a missense mutation (R272P). Both mutations are consistent with the assumption that haploinsufficiency of *ALX4* results in PFM. While the polypeptide is truncated in the frameshift mutation, a highly evolutionarily conserved arginine in the homeobox domain was exchanged by a proline. This probably resulted in disruption of DNA binding and a loss of ALX4 function. An additional three loss-of-function mutations of *ALX4* in PFM were described by Mavrogiannis et al. (2001) (Table 52–2). Two of these were nonsense mutations and resulted in complete or partial elimination of the DNA-binding homeodomain of ALX4. The third mutation occurred at the highly conserved arginine at position 218. Exchange of this arginine by a glutamine probably interferes with DNA contact of the amino-terminal arm of the homeodomain. Interestingly, in the mouse, the identical mutation underlies the Strong's luxoid allele that abolishes DNA binding of Alx4 and subsequent transcriptional activation (Qu et al., 1998).

Table 52–2. Mutations in *ALX4*

Mutation (Amino Acid Substitution)	Location in Gene*	Phenotype†	Reference
Q140X	C418T exon 1	PFM	Mavrogiannis et al., 2001
S168fs	504delT exon 2	PFM	Wuyts et al., 2000a
R218Q	G653A exon 2	PFM	Mavrogiannis et al., 2001
Q246X	C736T exon 2	PFM	Mavrogiannis et al., 2001
R272P	G815C exon 3	PFM	Wuyts et al, 2000a

*Sizes of the four exons are 466, 311, 129, and 330 bp, respectively.
†PFM, parietal foramina.

DEVELOPMENTAL PATHOGENESIS AND CONCLUSIONS

Both *Msx2* and *Alx4* have important roles in osteogenesis. Upstream regulators of *Msx2* include BMP-4 and Wnt. Furthermore, the YY1 transcription factor is required for fine tuning of *Msx2* expression. YY1 action is independent of the BMP-4 signal transduction pathway. Downstream genes of *Msx2* include *Runx2*, which is a significant regulator of osteoblast-specific genes. A gain-of-function mutation in *MSX2* (Pro148His) results in craniosynostosis by increasing binding to the consensus *Msx*-binding site, thus overstimulating *Msx2* target genes. The mutation does not appear to affect interaction of *Msx2* and *Runx2* or the resulting repression of *Runx2* activity; however, regulation of *Msx2* (Pro148His) by Dlx5 appears to be abolished (Shirakabe et al., 2001). Loss-of-function mutations of *Msx2* result in PFM. It can be postulated that the reduced repression of *Runx2* by *Msx2* and the resulting increased action of Dlx5 on *Runx2* interfere with normal regulation of osteoblast-specific genes and thus with osteogenesis. Exact mechanisms, however, are not yet known.

Alx4 is regulated by the transcription factor TWIST that is mutated in Saethre-Chotzen syndrome, which is characterized by craniosynostosis and abnormal limb development (see Chapter 34). Known mutations in *Alx4* result in a loss of gene function by abolishing DNA binding and subsequent regulation of downstream genes and giving rise to PFM. PFMs caused by mutations in either *MSX2* or *ALX4* are phenotypically indistinguishable. It is presently not clear, however, whether *MSX2* and *ALX4* act in the same or in related (perhaps parallel) pathways.

REFERENCES

Bell JR, Noveen A, Liu YH, Ma L, Dobias S, Kundu R, Luo W, Xia Y, Lusis AJ, Snead ML, Maxson R (1993). Genomic structure, chromosomal location, and evolution of the mouse Hox8 gene. *Genomics* 16: 123–131.

Boras K, Hamel PA (2002). Alx4 binding to LEF-1 regulates N-CAM promoter activity. *J Biol Chem* 277: 1120–1127.

Cohen MM Jr. (2000). Craniofacial disorders caused by mutations in homeobox genes MSX1 and MSX2. *J Craniofac Genet Dev Biol* 20: 19–25.

Cserjesi P, Lilly B, Bryson L, Wang Y, Sassoon DA, Olson EN (1992). Mhox: a mesodermally restricted homeodomain protein that binds an essential site in the muscle creatine kinase enhancer. *Development* 115: 1087–1101.

Dodig M, Tadic T, Kronenberg MS, Dacic S, Liu Y-H, Maxson R, Rowe DW, Lichtler AC (1999). Ectopic Msx2 overexpression inhibits and Msx2 antisense stimulates calvarial osteoblast differentiation. *Dev Biol* 209: 298–307.

Graham A, Francis-West P, Brickell P, Lumsden A (1994). The signalling molecule BMP4 mediates apoptosis in the rhombencephalic neural crest. *Nature* 372: 684–686.

Hudson R, Taniguchi-Sidle A, Boras K, Wiggan O, Hamel PA (1998). Alx-4, a transcriptional activator whose expression is restricted to sites of epithelial–mesenchymal interactions. *Dev Dyn* 213: 159–169.

Ito Y (1999). Molecular basis of tissue-specific gene expression mediated by the Runt domain transcription factor PEBP2/CBF. *Genes Cells* 4: 685–696.

Jabs EW, Müller U, Li X, Ma L, Luo W, Haworth IS, Klisak I, Sparkes R, Warman ML, Mulliken JB, et al. (1993). A mutation in the homeodomain of the human *MSX2* gene in a family affected with autosomal dominant craniosynostosis. *Cell* 75: 443–450.

Jones KL (1988). *Smith's Recognizable Patterns of Human Malformation*. W. B. Saunders Company, Philadelphia.

Jowett AK, Vainio S, Ferguson MWJ, Sharpe PT, Thesleff I (1993). Epithelial–mesenchymal interactions are required for msx1 and msx2 gene expression in the developing murine molar tooth. *Development* 117: 461–470.

Kostrzewa M, Krings BW, Dixon MJ, Eppelt K, K`hler A, Grady DL, Steinberger D, Fairweather ND, Moyzis RK, Monaco AP, Müller U (1998). Integrated physical and transcript map of 5q31.3–qter. *Eur J Hum Genet* 6: 266–274.

Lajeunie E, Le Merrer M, Bonaiti-Pellie C, Marchac D, Renier D (1995). Genetic study of nonsyndromic coronal craniosynostosis. *Am J Med Genet* 55: 500–504.

Lajeunie E, Le Merrer M, Bonaiti-Pellie C, Marchac D, Renier D (1996). Genetic study of scaphocephalie. *Am J Med Genet* 62: 282–285.

Liu YH, Kundu R, Wu L, Luo W, Ignelzi MA Jr., Snead ML, Maxson RE Jr. (1995). Premature suture closure and ectopic cranial bone in mice expressing Msx2 transgenes in the developing skull. *Proc Natl Acad Sci USA* 92: 6137–6141.

Liu YH, Tang Z, Kundu RK, Wu L, Luo W, Zhu D, Sangiorgi F, Snead ML, Maxson RE

(1999). Msx2 gene dosage influences the number of proliferative osteogenic cells in growth centers of the developing murine skull: a possible mechanism for MSX2-mediated craniosynostosis in humans. *Dev Biol* 205: 260–274.

Loebel DAF, O'Rourke MP, Steiner KA, Banyer J, Tam PPL (2002). Isolation of differentially expressed genes from wild-type and Twist mutant mouse limb buds. *Genesis* 33: 103–113.

Ma L, Golden S, Wu L, Maxson R (1996). The molecular basis of Boston-type craniosynostosis: the Pro148 → His mutation in the N-terminal arm of the MSX2 homeodomain stabilizes DNA binding without altering nucleotide sequence preferences. *Hum Mol Genet* 5: 915–920.

MacKenzie A, Ferguson MWJ, Sharpe PT (1992). Expression patterns of the homeobox gene, Hox—8, in the mouse embryo suggest a role in specifying tooth initiation and shape. *Development* 115: 403–420.

Mavrogiannis LA, Antonopoulou I, Baxova A, Kutilek S, Kim CA, Sugayama SM, Salamanca A, Wall SA, Morris-Kay GM, Wilkie AOM (2001). Haploinsufficiency of the human homeobox gene *ALX4* causes skull ossification defects. *Nat Genet* 27: 17–18.

Monaghan AP, Davidson DR, Sime C, Graham E, Baldock R, Bhattacharya SS, Hill RE (1991). The Msh-like homeobox genes define domains in the developing vertebrate eye. *Development* 112: 1053–1061.

Müller U, Warman ML, Mulliken JB, Weber JL (1993). Assignment of a gene locus involved in craniosynostosis to chromosome 5qter. *Hum Mol Genet* 2: 119–122.

Müller U, Steinberger D, Kunze S (1997). Molecular genetics of craniosynostotic syndromes. *Graefe's Arch Clin Exp Ophthalmol* 235: 545–550.

Opstelten D-JE, Vogels R, Robert B, Kalkhoven E, Zwartkruis F, de Laaf L, Destrée OH, Deschamps J, Lawson KA, Meijlink F (1991). The mouse homeobox gene, S8, is expressed during embryogenesis predominantly in mesenchyme. *Mech Dev* 34: 29–41.

Pang D, Lin A (1982). Symptomatic large parietal foramina. *Neurosurgery* 11: 33–37.

Preis S, Engelbrecht V, Lenard HG (1995). Aplasia cutis congenita and enlarged parietal foramina (Catlin marks) in a family. *Acta Paediatr* 84: 701–702.

Qu S, Li LY, Wisdom R (1997a). Alx-4: cDNA cloning and characterization of a novel paired-type homeodomain protein. *Gene* 203: 217–223.

Qu S, Niswender KD, Ji Q, Van der Meer R, Keeney D, Magnuson MA, Wisdom R (1997b). Polydactyly and ectopic ZPA formation in Alx-4 mutant mice. *Development* 124: 3999–4008.

Qu S, Tucker SC, Ehrlich JS, Levorse JM, Flaherty LA, Wisdom R, Vogt TF (1998). Mutations in mouse *Aristaless-like 4* cause *Strong's luxoid* polydactly. *Development* 125: 2711–2721.

Rudnick A, Ling TY, Odagiri H, Rutter WJ, German MS (1994). Pancreatic β cells express a diverse set of homeobox genes. *Proc Natl Acad Sci USA* 91: 12203–12207.

Satokata I, Ma L, Ohshima H, Bei M, Woo I, Nishizawa K, Maeda T, Takano Y, Uchiyama M, Heaney S, et al. (2000). Msx2 deficiency in mice causes pleiotropic defects in bone growth and ectodermal organ formation. *Nat Genet* 24: 391–395.

Shimeld S, McKay IJ, Sharpe PT (1996). The murine homeobox gene Msx-3 shows highly restricted expression in the developing neural tube. *Mech Dev* 55: 201–210.

Shirakabe K, Terasawa K, Miyama K, Shibuya H, Nishida E (2001). Regulation of the activity of the transcription factor Runx2 by two homeobox proteins, Msx2 and Dlx5. *Genes Cells* 6: 851–856.

Tan DP, Nonaka K, Nuckolls GH, Liu YH, Maxson RE, Slavkin HC, Shum L (2002). YY1 activates Msx2 gene independent of bone morphogenetic protein signalling. *Nucleic Acids Res* 30: 1213–1223.

Wang W, Chen X, Xu H, Lufkin T (1996). Msx3: a novel murine homologue of the *Drosophila* msh homeobox gene restricted to the dorsal embryonic central nervous system. *Mech Dev* 58: 203–215.

Warman ML, Mulliken JB, Hayward P, Müller U (1993). Newly recognized autosomal dominant disorder with craniosynostosis. *Am J Med Genet* 46: 444–449.

Wilkie AOM (1997). Craniosynostosis: genes and mechanisms. *Hum Mol Genet* 6: 1647–1656.

Wilkie AOM, Tang Z, Elanko N, Walsh S, Twigg SRF, Hurst JA, Wall SA, Chrzanowska KH, Maxson RE (2000). Functional haploinsufficiency of the human homeobox gene *MSX2* causes defects in skull ossification. *Nat Genet* 24: 387–390.

Willert J, Epping M, Pollack JR, Brown PO, Nusse R (2002). A transcriptional response to Wnt protein in human embryonic carcinoma cells. *BMC Dev Biol* 2: 8.

Winter RM, Baraitser M (1996). *The London Dysmorphology Database*. Oxford University Press, Oxford.

Wu Y-Q, Badano JL, McCaskill C, Vogel H, Potocki L, Shaffer LG (2000). Haploinsufficiency of *ALX4* as a potential cause of parietal foramina in the 11p11.2 contiguous gene-deletion syndrome. *Am J Hum Genet* 67: 1327–1332.

Wuyts W, Cleiren E, Homfray T, Rasore-Quartino A, Vanhoenacker F, Van Hul W (2000a). The *ALX4* homeobox gene is mutated in patients with ossification defects of the skull (foramina parietalia permagna, OMIM 168500). *J Med Genet* 37: 916–920.

Wuyts W, Reardon W, Preis S, Homfray T, Rasore-Quartino A, Christians H, Willems PJ, Van Hul W (2000b). Identification of mutations in the *MSX2* homeobox gene in families affected with foramina parietalia permagna. *Hum Mol Genet* 9: 1251–1255.

Zhao G-Q, Zhou X, Eberspaecher H, Solursh M, De Crombrugghe B (1993). Cartilage homeoprotein 1, a homeoprotein selectively expressed in chondrocytes. *Proc Natl Acad Sci USA* 90: 8633–8637.

53 | *SHOX* and Dyschondrosteosis and the Turner Syndrome

JAY W. ELLISON

The story of the *SHOX* gene is an example of how observations of different clinical disorders can eventually converge on a single gene. The disorders in this case are dyschondrosteosis, a skeletal dysplasia; Turner syndrome, an aneuploid condition resulting from a missing sex chromosome; and idiopathic short stature (ISS). *SHOX* is implicated in each of these conditions, although its contribution to the phenotypes varies with respect to both level of involvement and level of experimental proof. The predicted nature of the gene product (as a DNA-binding transcriptional regulator), its abundant expression in bone, and the skeletal phenotypes of patients all point to the placement of *SHOX* in a developmental pathway of bone development. The details of this pathway are at present largely lacking; studies of *SHOX* have thus far largely been confined to defining the spectrum of clinical phenotypes associated with mutations in the gene. It is expected that close attention to clinical features combined with basic cell biology studies will eventually reveal details of the role of *SHOX* in growth and bone development.

CLINICAL DISORDERS

The beginnings of the mapping of an X-chromosomal stature locus can be traced to the report of a male with a terminal deletion of Xp who was affected by multiple clinical phenotypes including X-linked ichthyosis, chondrodysplasia punctata, mental retardation, and growth delay (Curry et al., 1984). The patient's mother, who was a carrier of the deletion, exhibited short stature. Additional studies of individuals with Xp deletions led to the assignment of a short stature locus to distal Xp, encompassing the pseudoautosomal region (PAR) (Ballabio et al., 1989). Further narrowing of the critical region to the distal 700 kb of the PAR was accomplished largely by Ogata and coworkers (1992, 1995), who detected submicroscopic pseudoautosomal deletions in patients exhibiting short stature as their only phenotypic abnormality. The hypothesis accompanying these observations was that haploinsufficiency for a gene or genes in the critical deleted region was responsible for the short stature phenotype. A search for genes in this critical region led to the cloning of the *SHOX* gene, as described below. At the end of this section, we will further discuss the evidence for the role of SHOX in ISS.

Turner syndrome is characterized clinically by four cardinal features: (*1*) short stature, (*2*) ovarian failure due to dysgenesis and accelerated oocyte loss, (*3*) a variety of major and minor malformations, and (*4*) a high rate (>95%) of embryonic lethality (Lippe, 1991). There is great variability in the frequency of observed malformations, which may include cardiovascular, renal, and skeletal anomalies. A number of physical features often associated with Turner syndrome, such as webbing of the neck, dysmorphic ears, low posterior hairline, and hyperconvexity of the nails, are believed to be secondary to fetal lymphedema, which is mostly resolved by the time of birth. These latter features are probably more properly referred to, in the parlance of clinical genetics, as "deformations."

Short stature and ovarian failure are the most consistent features seen in Turner syndrome. Turner girls are generally below average in length at birth, and their growth rate is reduced significantly in childhood, leading to moderate short stature during this period (−2 S.D.) (Ranke et al., 1983; Even et al., 2000). Lack of the pubertal growth spurt results in a final adult average height of Turner females of about

4'8"–4'9" (Lyon et al., 1985; Rosenfeld et al., 1998). The growth failure in Turner syndrome is often fairly proportionate, although there is some shortening of the lower extremities. Frank mesomelia of the arms is sometimes present, and Madelung deformity is seen occasionally (Lippe, 1991). Furthermore, well-known features of Turner syndrome are cubitus valgus (an increased "carrying angle"), short fourth metacarpals, and occasionally a short neck (Lippe, 1991). Thus, skeletal abnormalities do occur in Turner females, albeit with much less consistency than an overall decrease in linear growth.

In 1965, not long after Turner syndrome was found to be caused by partial or complete monosomy for the X chromosome, it was hypothesized that the genes involved in the disorder escaped the process of X-chromosome inactivation and had functional homologs on the Y chromosome (Ferguson-Smith, 1965). It was proposed that a single, rather than the normal double, dose of such genes led to the phenotypic abnormalities seen in Turner females. This was a remarkably prescient inference at a time when no genes that escaped X inactivation had yet been identified. Phenotype–karyotype correlations made at that time and in subsequent years using cases of partial X monosomy enabled workers to narrow the location of the culpable genes to the short arm of the X chromosome. The identification of pseudoautosomal genes, beginning with the cloning of *MIC2* (Buckle et al., 1985), provided a set of candidate genes fulfilling the gene dosage requirements for the (anti-Turner) genes proposed by Ferguson-Smith (1965). Additional X/Y homologous (but nonpseudoautosomal) gene pairs, such as *ZFX/ZFY* (Page et al., 1987; Schneider-Gadicke et al., 1989) and *RPS4X/RPS4Y* (Fisher et al., 1990), added to the list of candidates; but evidence for their role in Turner syndrome remained elusive. The identification of *SHOX* within the Xp/Yp PAR demonstrated escape from X-chromosome inactivation, and the correlation of its deletion with short stature in the patients noted above immediately made *SHOX* a strong candidate for contributing to the short stature seen in Turner syndrome (Rao et al., 1997; Ellison et al., 1997). Direct proof of this role is difficult to come by, as it is for any single gene that is part of an aneuploid condition. The evidence consists primarily of a correlation between short stature and a single copy of *SHOX* in both Turner patients and patients with *SHOX* deletions and inactivating mutations. The case for the involvement of *SHOX* in the occasional skeletal abnormalities seen in Turner syndrome rests on the known role of *SHOX* in skeletal malformations in another set of patients (see below).

Quite apart from investigations of Turner syndrome and Xp microdeletion patients was the description of an inherited skeletal dysplasia called *dyschondrosteosis*. This term was introduced in the description of a young woman with short stature associated with mesomelic shortening of both upper and lower extremities (Leri and Weill, 1929). Radiologic findings included bowing of the radius and dorsal subluxation of the distal ulna. An individual with dyschondrosteosis is shown in Figure 53–1, demonstrating the mesomelic shortening. Subsequent reports noted the familial nature of the syndrome and its clinical variability and refined the radiologic criteria. An autosomal-dominant mode of transmission was observed, with a preponderance of affected females over males (Langer, 1965; Herdman et al., 1966). Severity was generally greater in females, which may have provided an ascertainment bias. The radius was often more severely affected than the ulna, often leading to a clinically obvious

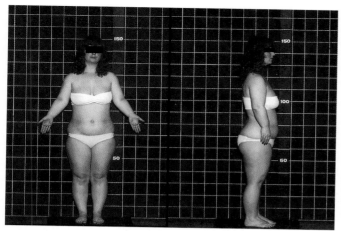

Figure 53–1. A patient with Leri-Weill dyschondrosteosis. Note the short stature and mesomelic shortening of the upper and lower extremities.

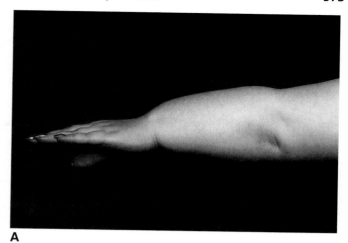

A

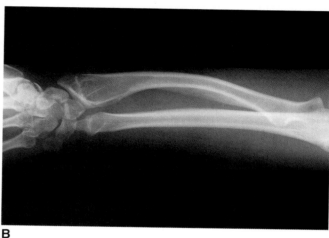

B

Figure 53–2. (*A*) The forearm is of the individual in Figure 53–1, showing a Madelung deformity. Note the prominence of the subluxed ulna. (*B*) X-ray of a different patient with dyschondrosteosis and Madelung deformity. Evident are the bowed radius with an angulated distal epiphysis, proximal displacement and slight triangulation of the carpal bones, and lack of articulation of the distal ulna.

sign known as Madelung deformity. This latter entity had been first described in 1878 as a dorsal subluxation of the hand with prominence of the distal ulna (Madelung, 1878). Madelung deformity in the patient depicted in Figure 53–1 is shown more clearly in Figure 53–2*A*, where prominence of the subluxed ulna is evident. The initial description predated X-ray studies, and in subsequent years, further reports noted the frequent familial nature of the condition and outlined its radiographic features. Madelung deformity can be unilateral and can have both nongenetic and genetic causes, and it was not appreciated until after the report by Langer (1965) that a sizable proportion of Madelung deformity cases likely represent a manifestation of dyschondrosteosis (Herdman et al., 1966). Besides shortening of the forearm bones in dyschondrosteosis, there is premature fusion of the medial portion of the distal radial epiphysis, leading to an angulated growth plate and bowing of the radius. There is an increased spacing between radius and ulna, and disproportionate growth of the ulna leads to its lack of articulation with the wrist bones, with resulting dorsal subluxation. In addition, there is proximal placement and triangulation of the carpal bones, which often become wedged between the ulna and the angulated distal radius. These radiologic signs are demonstrated in Figure 53–2*B*, which shows a case of Madelung deformity associated with dyschondrosteosis.

Incomplete penetrance and variable expressivity are often observed in families with dyschondrosteosis (Dawe et al., 1982). The lower extremities are less often affected than the upper, but there can be shortening of both the tibia and fibula. There can also be tibiofibular disproportion leading to tibia varum. Normal stature is not infrequently observed due to the lack of lower extremity involvement (Langer, 1965; Dawe et al., 1982). Males are less frequently, and in general less severely, affected.

Proof that *SHOX* is the causative gene in dyschondrosteosis quickly followed its cloning. Two groups performed linkage analysis on families with dyschondrosteosis and found significant linkage to the Xp/Yp PAR (Belin et al., 1998; Shears et al., 1998). The expression pattern of *SHOX* and its implication in short stature made it an attractive candidate gene, and both groups demonstrated *SHOX* deletions or mutations in affected members of a number of families (Belin et al., 1998; Shears et al., 1998).

A more severe form of mesomelic dwarfism has been observed in offspring when both parents have dyschondrosteosis. This entity, Langer mesomelic dwarfism, is characterized by severe shortening of both forearm and lower leg bones and can involve the mandible (Langer, 1967). It was hypothesized that the severely affected individuals described by Langer represented the homozygous manifestation of the genetic defect found in dyschondrosteosis (Espiritu et al., 1975; Fryns and Van Den Berghe, 1979). For some time, this proposal was debated, but its validity was confirmed following identifi-

cation of the *SHOX* gene as the causal factor in dyschondrosteosis (Belin et al., 1998). More recently, direct proof of homozygous *SHOX* deficiency has been reported in patients with Langer mesomelic dwarfism (Robertson et al., 2000; Shears et al., 2002; Zinn et al., 2002).

It is instructive to consider the roles of *SHOX* in Turner syndrome and ISS relative to its contribution to the phenotype in dyschondrosteosis. *SHOX* mutations are clearly causal in the latter condition, although there is variable expressivity and reduced penetrance for both skeletal malformations and stature (Dawe et al., 1982). The similarity of the occasional skeletal abnormalities seen in Turner syndrome with those seen in dyschondrosteosis make it perfectly reasonable to conclude that haploinsufficiency of *SHOX* contributes to the abnormal skeletal features in Turner syndrome. It has been speculated that ovarian failure in Turner patients, by resulting in reduced estrogen levels, is protective against the deforming influence of *SHOX* deficiency (Kosho et al., 1999), which is why most Turner patients do not show frank skeletal deformity. The quantitative contribution of *SHOX* hemizygosity to the short stature in Turner syndrome has been estimated at two-thirds by one group; i.e., two-thirds of the growth deficit is due to having a single copy of *SHOX* (Ross et al., 2001). This figure was derived by comparing heights of females with dyschondrosteosis to heights in Turner females. Such an extrapolation should be viewed with caution. Growth patterns in Turner syndrome are no doubt influenced by dosage inequity of other X-linked or pseudoautosomal genes, and occur in the context of steroid hormone insufficiency. In addition, growth rates are different in Turner patients compared to patients with Leri-Weill syndrome. The latter grow at a rate that is parallel to the normal growth curve but displaced downward by about 2 S.D. (Kosho et al., 1999). Turner patients, however, grow at a slower rate during childhood and a still slower rate during puberty (Lyon et al., 1985; Even et al., 2000). Furthermore, some dyschondrosteosis patients are of normal stature, while short stature is virtually universal in Turner syndrome. Thus, it seems somewhat overly simplistic to assign a quantitative contribution of *SHOX* haploinsufficiency to the growth retardation in Turner syndrome.

Another question that remains unresolved is the role of *SHOX* in isolated ISS, i.e., short stature (defined as stature greater than 2 S.D. below ethnic norms) that is not accompanied by other syndromic features or by skeletal features reminiscent of dyschondrosteosis. In the original paper describing the cloning of *SHOX*, 91 patients (primarily Japanese) were screened for *SHOX* mutations by single-strand conformation polymorphism (SSCP) analysis followed by DNA sequencing, and a nonsense mutation was found in a single patient (Rao et al., 1997). Musebeck et al. (2001) looked for *SHOX* deletions in 35 patients with ISS and found none. Binder et al. (2000) carried out a similar analysis on 68 ISS patients and found a single case of a *SHOX* deletion. In the largest study to date, Rappold et al. (2002) studied 750 ISS patients by SSCP screening and 150 patients by fluorescence in situ hybridization (FISH) analysis. They found three mutations in each group and concluded that *SHOX* mutations account for 2.4% of ISS cases, thus making it a quantitatively significant cause of short stature. The clear implication was that *SHOX* analysis should be part of a routine work-up of short stature, much as karyotyping of short females and growth hormone studies currently are. However, a closer look at the data of Rappold et al. (2002) calls their conclusions into question. Firstly, the authors derived their 2.4% figure by extrapolating the detection rates of each of the two techniques to patients not investigated by that method. Such extrapolations with small numbers of positive patients seems risky, especially after one looks closely at the patients themselves. Two of the six patients with *SHOX* abnormalities had other conditions plausibly related to their short stature (growth hormone deficiency and hypogonadism), two more had mothers with Madelung deformity and either scoliosis or short limbs, and another patient developed Madelung deformity with the onset of puberty. Thus, these five patients should have been excluded from the analysis either because of associated conditions or because they reflect the variable expressivity of dyschondrosteosis. This leaves a single ISS patient (who was prepubertal) with a *SHOX* mutation among 900 patients in that study. Regarding the other cited studies, the patient representing the single *SHOX* mutation in the original report is the same patient in the Rappold et al. (2002) study who later developed Madelung deformity. Furthermore, the single patient detected by Binder et al. (2000) was noted to have mild mesomelia and mild triangulation of the carpal bones, findings that could be considered mild versions of what is observed in Madelung deformity. The reasonable conclusion from all these studies is that, if one obtains a careful family history (including an examination of family members) and excludes skeletal dysplasia and other preexisting syndromic conditions, the yield of *SHOX* mutations in the work-up of patients with ISS will be exceedingly low, if not virtually zero. The flip side of that conclusion is that a detailed examination of short patients for mild skeletal manifestations of dyschondrosteosis may identify a subset of patients in whom *SHOX* testing is worthwhile.

MOLECULAR GENETICS

The *SHOX* gene was independently cloned by two groups through a traditional positional cloning approach. Cloned genomic DNA from the 700 kb critical deleted region defined by Ogata and colleagues (1992) (see above) was subjected to standard gene identification methods (Rao et al., 1997; Ellison et al., 1997). The former group further narrowed the critical region to a 140 kb area by analyzing a deletion in an additional short stature patient, and *SHOX* was found to reside in this critical region. There were some differences in the findings of the two groups who isolated the gene: Rao et al. (1997) described two

patterns of alternative mRNA splicing, leading to two isoforms that differed in the length and composition of their C-terminal ends; while Ellison et al. (1997) detected an additional 5′ noncoding exon. These features are diagrammed in Figure 53–3. The predicted protein encoded by *SHOX* contains a homeodomain and thus is presumed to be a DNA-binding transcription factor. Although very low levels of *SHOX* expression are found in a variety cell lines and tissues (Rao et al., 1997; Ellison et al., 1997), the highest levels of expression have been found in bone marrow–derived stem cells and in cultured trabecular bone cells, which have an osteoblast-like phenotype. The 5′ exon was found in mRNA from these latter cells (Ellison, unpublished) and has not been observed in other cell types in which *SHOX* is expressed (Rappold, personal communication). Thus, this may be a unique transcription-start site in more differential bone cells. As expected from its pseudoautosomal location, *SHOX* escapes the process of X-chromosome inactivation (Rao et al., 1997).

Reports of patients with chromosomal abnormalities involving deletion of distal Xp, including X;Y translocations (Youlton et al., 1985; Guichet et al., 1997), established deletions as one mutational mechanism leading to dyschondrosteosis. The patients of Ogata et al. (1992, 1995) and Rao et al. (1997) in whom the critical *SHOX* deleted region was defined showed that submicroscopic microdeletions were another mutational mechanism. What was not expected was that deletions would continue to be the predominant mechanism in patients with dyschondrosteosis. In the first two reports describing the association of *SHOX* mutations in the disorder, 15 families were reported, and gene deletions were present in affected individuals in 13 of these families (Belin et al., 1998; Shears et al., 1998). Subsequent reports have continued to show a high incidence of deletions, in the range of 40%–80% of patients (Schiller et al., 2000; Musebeck et al., 2001; Grigelioniene et al., 2001; Ross et al., 2001; Cormier-Daire et al., 2001; Falcinelli et al., 2002). The sizes of the deletions were generally not determined, although one group reported a range of 0.1-9 megabases (Schiller et al., 2000). It is interesting to speculate that the high rate of deletion may be related to the enhanced rate of recombination in the PAR in male meiosis. To date, however, no evidence for a recurrent deletional mechanism has been described. A number of examples of contiguous gene deletion syndromes have been found in which deletion of neighboring genes causes additional phenotypes such as mental retardation, chondrodysplasia punctata, or ichthyosis (Seidel et al., 2001; Vassal et al., 2001).

The preponderance of deletions in dyschondrosteosis patients clearly establishes haploinsufficiency as the mechanism leading to the phenotype. A summary of the nondeletion *SHOX* mutations reported to date is given in Table 53–1. These intragenic mutations show an interesting pattern. About half of the mutations lead to protein truncation. Nine are missense mutations, and all but one of these are located within the homeobox (coding for amino acid residues 117–177, see Table 53–1). Thus, haploinsufficiency of the *SHOX* protein appears to be the exclusive, or at least overwhelmingly major, mechanism leading to the short stature and dyschondrosteosis phenotypes.

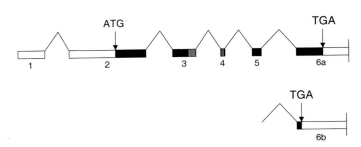

Figure 53–3. Exon and coding sequence organization of the *SHOX* gene. Exon lengths are drawn to scale except for the sixth exons. Exons 1 and 2 are as determined by Ellison et al. (1997). Both alternatively spliced sixth exons demonstrated by Rao et al. (1997) are shown. Exon 6b lies about 13 kb 3′ of 6a in genomic DNA. The 6a and 6b exons have been truncated for this figure. Introns are not drawn to scale. Untranslated regions are white, coding sequence is black or gray, and the homeobox sequence is gray.

Table 53–1. Summary of *SHOX* Intragenic Mutations

DNA Change	Coding Change	Mutation Type	References
del 197-198GC	—	Frameshift	Huber et al., 2001
del 222-232	—	Frameshift	Grigelioniene et al., 2001
G272T	E61X	Nonsense	Rappold et al., 2002
del 272G	—	Frameshift	Grigelioniene et al., 2000
C425T	Q112X	Nonsense	Huber et al., 2001
del 449A	—	Frameshift	Ross et al., 2001
del 465C	—	Frameshift	Falcinelli et al., 2002
A474T	Q128L (2 cases)	Missense	Grigelioniene et al., 2001; Ross et al., 2001
C485G	L132V	Missense	Grigelioniene et al., 2000
T497C	F136L	Missense	Falcinelli et al., 2002
G536T	E149X	Nonsense	Huber et al., 2001
C548G	R153G	Missense	Falcinelli et al., 2002
G549T	R153L	Missense	Grigelioniene et al., 2000
T552C	L154P	Missense	Ross et al., 2001
ins 5726T	—	Frameshift	Huber et al., 2001
C593T	R168W	Missense	Ogata et al., 2002
C608T	R173C (2 cases)	Missense	Huber et al., 2001; Shears et al., 2002
C674T	R195X (7 casers)	Nonsense	Rao et al., 1997; Belin et al., 1998; Clement-Jones et al., 2000; Rappold et al., 2002; Grigelioniene et al., 2001; Ross et al., 2001
C688G	Y199X	Nonsense	Shears et al., 1998
G761A	A224T	Missense	Rappold et al., 2002
del 776-787	del H229-L232	Deletion	Rappold et al., 2002

Specific nucleotide changes are designated using the numbering system of Genbank entry Y11535. Mutations are listed top to bottom beginning with the 5'-most mutation. Multiple independent occurrences of mutations are indicated.

There have been no reports of any correlation between mutation type and phenotype.

ESTABLISHING THE DIAGNOSIS

SHOX mutations have been demonstrated in various ways. FISH analysis with cosmid probes has been the usual method of detecting gene deletions. Another method used to detect deletions has been the use of highly informative polymorphic markers surrounding the gene (Binder et al., 2000; Falcinelli et al., 2002). When parental DNA is available and the parents contain different alleles, the observation of hemizygosity in an affected individual allows one to infer the existence of a *SHOX* deletion. Screening for point mutations has been accomplished by direct DNA sequencing, with or without prior screening of PCR products by SSCP analysis. Using these methods, several groups have reported mutation detection rates for *SHOX* of about 60%–80% in patients with dyschondrosteosis (Schiller et al., 2000; Grigelioniene et al., 2001; Falcinelli et al., 2002). The failure to detect *SHOX* mutations in a significant number of dyschondrosteosis patients has led some to conclude that there is locus heterogeneity for the disorder (Schiller et al., 2000). A similar conclusion was recorded by one group based on limited linkage studies in two families (Cormier-Daire et al., 2001). Ross et al. (2001) detected *SHOX* mutations in 100% of 21 dyschondrosteosis families that they studied. These authors used a combination of FISH to look for deletions and denaturing high-performance liquid chromatography (DHPLC) to look for point mutations. It is not immediately clear from this work whether the greater detection rate reflects a greater sensitivity of DHPLC or a more careful selection of patients (or both). Nonetheless, there does not appear to be any firm evidence for locus heterogeneity in Leri-Weill dyschondrosteosis.

In contrast to dyschondrosteosis, isolated Madelung deformity (defined as Madelung deformity with normal stature) appears to be heterogenous. Grigelioniene et al. (2001) investigated 28 dyschondrosteosis families and seven sporadic cases of isolated Madelung deformity for *SHOX* mutations by a variety of methods, including FISH, Southern blotting, direct sequencing, flanking polymorphism analysis, and fiber-FISH analysis. These workers found *SHOX* mutations in 22 dyschondrosteosis cases but in none of the sporadic isolated Madelung deformity cases, although interestingly a tandem duplication of *SHOX* was found in one case of isolated Madelung deformity.

TREATMENT AND COUNSELING

The efficacy of growth hormone supplementation in girls with Turner syndrome (Rosenfeld et al., 1998) immediately suggests a treatment option for patients with short stature associated with *SHOX* deficiency. Large-scale studies of growth hormone treatment of patients with dyschondrosteosis or *SHOX*-associated short stature are just beginning, but reports are available of such treatment in a few cases. Shanske et al. (1999) reported an increase in height velocity from 2.8 to 9.4 cm/year in a prepubertal boy following a 12-month period of growth hormone treatment. This boy had a Y;13 translocation that resulted in deletion of the Yp PAR, including *SHOX*. Binder et al. (2000) treated two siblings with a nonsense *SHOX* mutation for 12 months with growth hormone and observed increases in height velocity that were virtually identical to that observed by Shanske et al. (1999). They noted, however, that the increase in growth of the lower extremities was less than that observed in the trunk and arms. Ogata et al. (2001) treated three patients with *SHOX*-associated short stature. A prepubertal boy with a Y-chromosome microdeletion that included *SHOX* showed a significant increase in height velocity. A prepubertal girl with the same nonsense mutations as the patients of Binder et al. (2000) was treated for several years with growth hormone and achieved a moderate increase in height velocity. The third patient treated by Ogata et al. (2001) had an apparently unbalanced X;2 translocation, which resulted in a derivative X chromosome that was deleted for distal Xp (including *SHOX*) and trisomic for distal 2p. There was evidence of selective inactivation of the derivative X such that the extra 2p sequences were also inactivated. Thus, it was presumed that there was no functional chromosomal imbalance other than for the distal Xp sequences. This girl showed no increase in height velocity during her period of growth hormone treatment, which was from age 6 to age 14 years. Thus, the experience with these patients showed a variable response of growth to supplemental growth hormone therapy.

The two female patients of Ogata et al. (2001) were also treated briefly with gonadotropin-releasing hormone (GnRH). The rationale for this treatment is that by suppressing gonadal estrogen production with GnRH, epiphyseal closure could be delayed and, thus, a longer period of growth before puberty would be offered. In addition, because estrogen may contribute to the skeletal deformities seen in dyschondrosteosis and some girls with Turner syndrome, it was hoped that GnRH therapy would prevent the deformities in the treated girls. The second case (the girl who showed a moderate response to growth hormone therapy) showed mild curvature of the radius at 10 years and

10 months of age, 14 months after GnRH was begun. The third case, who had not responded to growth hormone, went on to develop a full-blown Madelung deformity. Because of her partial aneuploidy, the latter patient may not be the best patient from whom to draw general conclusions. Nonetheless, the data are insufficient to allow us to determine whether growth hormone therapy (with or without GnRH) will be universally successful in treating patients with SHOX deficiency. It seems that special caution should be applied in treating females with normal gonadal function since there may be a risk of asymmetric growth and consequent exacerbation of skeletal deformities.

Counseling of patients with deletions or mutations of the SHOX gene is at once straightforward, and yet also fraught with some uncertainty. There is a 50% chance of an affected parent transmitting the altered gene to an offspring. The gene lies in the PAR of the X and Y chromosomes, so counseling for transmission of an altered allele is generally done as for autosomal-dominant disorders. The distal location of SHOX within the PAR dictates that the obligatory crossover within this region will be proximal to the gene in the great majority of meioses. Therefore, inheritance of SHOX alleles in a sex-linked pattern is expected to occur only slightly more than half the time.

More problematic is the counseling regarding what to expect in the phenotype of a SHOX heterozygote. The variability seen both within and among families reflects a wide range of clinical phenotypes, from normal or only mildly proportionate short stature to rather marked mesomelia and skeletal deformity. The risk of the more severe clinical features is substantially greater in females than in males. Advice on supplemental hormone therapy would probably need to be individualized, based on early growth patterns and close skeletal examination.

HOMOLOGOUS GENES IN OTHER SPECIES

Rovescalli et al. (1996) described the cloning of a mouse homeobox-containing gene that they called Og-12. When SHOX was subsequently isolated, a comparison of the two genes showed extensive similarity over much of the predicted protein sequence, including an identical homeodomain as well as conserved exon–intron junctions (Rao et al., 1997; Ellison et al., 1997). Despite extensive divergence in the region upstream of the homeodomain, it seemed reasonable at the time to assume that Og-12 was the mouse ortholog of SHOX, especially given the documented divergence of other human pseudoautosomal genes from their mouse counterparts (Ellison et al., 1996). However, the cloning and characterization of the human gene OG12X (Semina et al., 1998) showed that SHOX2 is the ortholog of Og-12. The proteins encoded by the two genes are identical, and they map to respective chromosomal regions that exhibit conserved synteny (Semina et al., 1998). Repeated attempts to clone the SHOX ortholog in the mouse have failed (J. Ellison, unpublished, and G. Rappold, personal communication), and the latest draft of the mouse genome sequence shows no gene more closely related to SHOX than Og-12. Homologous genes have been reported in other species, but these genes are clearly orthologs of OG12X (Joly et al., 1997). Thus, it appears that OG12X (also called SHOX2) represents the ancestral gene and that human SHOX is the product of a more recent gene duplication. Both mouse Og-12 and human OG12X/SHOX2 are expressed in a variety of tissues during embryonic development (Semina et al., 1998; Clement-Jones et al., 2000), while SHOX expression is limited, being mainly expressed in the limbs and pharyngeal arches (Clement-Jones et al., 2000) as well as the cultured bone-derived cells noted earlier (Ellison et al., 1997). It is not clear if SHOX and SHOX2 are expressed in the same cells in humans. Therefore, SHOX may have evolved a specialized function in humans that is served in the mouse by Og-12/Shox2. At any rate, the lack of a mouse ortholog has prevented the generation of an animal model for studying SHOX function. An Og-12 knock-out mouse, which has not been reported, would seem at best to be a model for a combined SHOX plus SHOX2 deficiency. Given the widespread expression of SHOX2, this may create problems in correlating phenotypic features to a particular human gene. Perhaps a tissue-specific (i.e., bone) knockout would provide an opportunity for learning about SHOX function in an experimental animal.

DEVELOPMENTAL PATHOGENESIS

The finding of a homeodomain in a predicted protein encoded by SHOX leads to the assumption that it acts as a DNA-binding transcriptional regulator. The pathogenesis of the abnormalities seen in patients with SHOX mutations is thus presumed to be the dysregulated expression of the target genes of SHOX. Haploinsufficiency of a transcription factor leading to developmental abnormalities is a commonly observed phenomenon. The finding of high levels of expression in cultured bone-derived cells (Ellison et al., 1997) and a causative role in skeletal dysplasia imply a primary role in the developing skeleton. The significance of the low level of expression (detectable only by reverse-transcription PCR) in a wide variety of cultured cells is not clear. In situ hybridization studies in human embryos showed SHOX expression in developing limb and in the mesenchymal core of the first and second pharyngeal arches (Clement-Jones et al., 2000). The pharyngeal arch expression presumably explains the mandibular abnormalities seen in some patients with Langer mesomelic dwarfism, who carry homozygous SHOX mutations. It also may explain the micrognathia occasionally seen in females with Turner syndrome. Beyond this correlation of SHOX expression with phenotypic features, there are scant data regarding the cellular or molecular details of the developmental pathway in which SHOX operates. A SHOX expression plasmid was cotransformed with a reporter gene that was downstream of a consensus homeodomain binding sequence (Rao et al., 2001). When bone-derived cells (from an osteosarcoma) were used in these experiments, cotransformation resulted in increased expression of the reporter gene. This study implies that SHOX acts by stimulating transcription of genes in bone cells, but it does not really give us more information than already inferred on the basis of its expression pattern and its homeodomain (other than perhaps that it does not act strictly as a repressor of transcription). There are currently no published reports that identify target genes of SHOX or proteins with which it interacts. Perhaps a fruitful strategy would be to incorporate studies of patients with phenotypes similar to that seen in SHOX-deficient patients. The lack of SHOX mutations in the families with isolated Madelung deformity reported by Grigelionione et al. (2001) implies the possible existence of a distinct locus for this inherited disorder. Other cases of familial mesomelic shortening (Fasanelli et al., 1983; Fujimoto et al., 1998) might lead to the discovery of other genes that act in the same developmental pathway as SHOX. Such genes would become candidates for encoded upstream SHOX regulators, downstream targets, or proteins that interact with the SHOX protein.

Observations of cellular processes accompanying bone morphogenesis may help to provide clues about the physiologic role of SHOX in skeletal development. In dyschondrosteosis, there is dysplasia at the ulnar aspect of the distal radial growth plate, which leads to narrowing and premature fusion at this site. Continued growth of other parts of the growth plates leads to asymmetric growth and bowing of the radius. Munns et al. (2001) examined the growth plate morphology in resected specimens from patients with dyschondrosteosis. They found disruption of the normal cellular architecture with loss of the normal columnar stacking pattern of chondrocytes. Instead, nests of chondrocytes were found with juxtaposed cells of different maturational stages. There was expansion of the hypertrophic layer of chondrocytes and a concomitant reduction in the proliferative layer. In addition, microscopic islands of cartilage were found in the osteoid matrix adjacent to the growth plate. These observations suggest that defects in chondrocyte maturational processes are associated with the growth plate abnormalities. Whether these processes are directly or indirectly related to SHOX function remains to be answered.

NOTE ADDED IN PROOF

A SHOX mutation database has been established (Niesler et al., 2002). The URL is http://www.shox.uni-hd.de.

A recent report by Stuppia et al. (2003) suggests that the frequency of SHOX mutations in idopathic short stature may be higher than previously estimated. In their Italian group of patients, they found not only a higher frequency of deletions (7% of all patients), but also three (of 56) patients with an identical missense mutation, bringing the total in this group to 12.4% of ISS patients with *SHOX* mutations. Although a greater methodologic sensitivity with direct DNA sequencing may partially explain the higher frequency, one must also question the possibility of patient selection bias or a founder effect in this Italian population. Certainly more large-scale studies with better methods are needed to address the question of SHOX's role in ISS.

REFERENCES

Ballabio A, Bardoni B, Carrozzo R, Andria G, Bick D, Campbell L, Hamel B, Ferguson-Smith MA, Gimelli G, Fraccaro M, et al. (1989). Contiguous gene syndromes due to deletions in the distal short arm of the human X chromosome. *Proc Natl Acad Sci USA* 86(24): 10001–10005.

Belin V, Cusin V, Viot G, Girlich D, Toutain A, Moncla A, Vekemans M, Le Merrer M, Munnich A, Cormier-Daire V (1998). *SHOX* mutations in dyschondrosteosis (Leri-Weill syndrome). *Nat Genet* 19(1): 67–69.

Binder G, Schwarze CP, Ranke MB (2000). Identification of short stature caused by *SHOX* defects and therapeutic effect of recombinant human growth hormone. *J Clin Endocrinol Metab* 85(1): 245–249.

Buckle V, Mondello C, Darling S, Craig IW, Goodfellow PN (1985). Homologous expressed genes in the human sex chromosome pairing region. *Nature* 317(6039): 739–741.

Clement-Jones M, Schiller S, Rao E, Blaschke RJ, Zuniga A, Zeller R, Robson S C, Binder G, Glass I, Strachan T, et al. (2000). The short stature homeobox gene *SHOX* is involved in skeletal abnormalities in Turner syndrome. *Hum Mol Genet* 9(5): 695–702.

Cormier-Daire V, Huber C, Munnich A (2001). Allelic and nonallelic heterogeneity in dyschondrosteosis (Leri-Weill syndrome). *Am J Med Genet* 106(4): 272–274.

Curry CJ, Magenis RE, Brown M, Lanman JT Jr, Tsai J, O'Lague P, Goodfellow P, Mohandas T, Bergner EA, Shapiro LJ (1984). Inherited chondrodysplasia punctata due to a deletion of the terminal short arm of an X chromosome. *N Engl J Med* 311(16): 1010–1015.

Dawe C, Wynne-Davies R, Fulford GE (1982). Clinical variation in dyschondrosteosis. A report on 13 individuals in 8 families. *J Bone Joint Surg Br* 64(3): 377–381.

Ellison J, Li X, Francke U, Shapiro LJ (1996). Rapid evolution of human pseudoautosomal genes and their mouse homologs. *Mamm Genome* 7: 25–30.

Ellison JW, Wardak Z, Young MF, Gehron Robey P, Laig-Webster M, Chiong W (1997). *PHOG*, a candidate gene for involvement in the short stature of Turner syndrome. *Hum Mol Genet* 6(8): 1341–1347.

Espiritu C, Chen H, Woolley PV Jr (1975). Mesomelic dwarfism as the homozygous expression of dyschondrosteosis. *Am J Dis Child* 129(3): 375–377.

Even L, Cohen A, Marbach N, Brand M, Kauli R, Sippell W, Hochberg Z (2000). Longitudinal analysis of growth over the first 3 years of life in Turner syndrome. *J Pediatr* 137(4): 460–464.

Falcinelli C, Iughetti L, Percesepe A, Calabrese G, Chiarelli F, Cisternino M, De Sanctis L, Pucarelli I, Radetti G, Wasniewska M, et al. (2002). *SHOX* point mutations and deletions in Leri-Weill dyschondrosteosis. *J Med Genet* 39(6): E33.

Fasanelli S, Iannaccone G, Bellussi A (1983). A possibly new form of familial bone dysplasia resembling dyschondrosteosis. *Pediatr Radiol* 13(1): 25–31.

Ferguson-Smith MA (1965). Karyotype-phenotype correlations in gonadal dysgenesis and their bearing on pathogenesis of malformations. *J Med Genet* 2: 142–155.

Fisher EM, Beer-Romero P, Brown LG, Ridley A, McNeil JA, Lawrence JB, Willard HF, Bieber FR, Page DC (1990). Homologous ribosomal protein genes on the human X and Y chromosomes: escape from X inactivation and possible implications for Turner syndrome. *Cell* 63(6): 1205–1218.

Fryns JP, Van Den Berghe H (1979). Langer type of mesomelic dwarfism as the possible homozygous expression of dyschondrosteosis. *Hum Genet* 46(1): 21–27.

Fujimoto M, Kantaputra PN, Ikegawa S, Fukushima Y, Sonta S, Matsuo M, Ishida T, Matsumoto T, Kondo S, Tomita H, et al. (1998). The gene for mesomelic dysplasia Kantaputra type is mapped to chromosome 2q24-q32. *J Hum Genet* 43: 32–36.

Grigelioniene G, Eklof O, Ivarsson SA, Westphal O, Neumeyer L, Kedra D, Dumanski J, Hagenas L (2000). Mutations in short stature homoebox containing gene (SHOX) in dyschondrosteosis but not in hypochondroplasia. *Hum Genet* 107: 145–149.

Grigelioniene G, Schoumans J, Neumeyer L, Ivarsson A, Eklof O, Enkvist O, Tordai P, Fosdal I, Myhre A G, Westphal O, et al. (2001). Analysis of short stature homeobox-containing gene (*SHOX*) and auxological phenotype in dyschondrosteosis and isolated Madelung deformity. *Hum Genet* 109(5): 551–558.

Guichet A, Briault S, Le Merrer M, Moraine C (1997). Are t(X;Y) (p22;q11) translocations in females frequently associated with Madelung deformity? *Clin Dysmorphol* 6(4): 341–345.

Herdman RC, Langer LO, Good RA (1966). Dyschondrosteosis. The most common cause of Madelung's deformity. *J Pediatr* 68(3): 432–441.

Huber C, Cusin V, Le Merrer M, Mathieu M, Sulmont V, Dagoneau N, Munnich A, Cormier-Daire V (2001). SHOX point mutations in dyschondrosteosis. *J Med Genet* 38: 323.

Joly JS, Bourrat F, Nguyen V, Chourrout D (1997). *Ol-Prx 3*, a member of an additional class of homeobox genes, is unimodally expressed in several domains of the developing and adult central nervous system of the medaka (*Oryzias latipes*). *Proc Natl Acad Sci USA* 94(24): 12987–12992.

Kosho T, Muroya K, Nagai T, Fujimoto M, Yokoya S, Sakamoto H, Hirano T, Terasaki H, Ohashi H, Nishimura G, et al. (1999). Skeletal features and growth patterns in 14 patients with haploinsufficiency of *SHOX*: implications for the development of Turner syndrome. *J Clin Endocrinol Metab* 84(12): 4613–4621.

Langer LO (1965). Dyschondrosteosis, a heritable bone dysplasia with characteristic roentgenograqhic features. *AJR Am J Roentgenol* 95: 178–188.

Langer LO Jr (1967). Mesomelic dwarfism of the hypoplastic ulna, fibula, mandible type. *Radiology* 89(4): 654–660.

Leri A, Weill J (1929). Une affection congenitale et symetrique du development osseux: la dyschondrosteoste. *Bull Mem Soc Med Hop Paris* 53: 1491–1494.

Lippe B (1991). Turner syndrome. *Endocrinol Metab Clin North Am* 20(1): 121–152.

Lyon AJ, Preece MA, Grant DB (1985). Growth curve for girls with Turner syndrome. *Arch Dis Child* 60(10): 932–935.

Madelung O (1878). Die spontane subluxation der hand nach norne. *Arch Klin Chir* 23: 395–412.

Munns CF, Glass IA, LaBrom R, Hayes M, Flanagan S, Berry M, Hyland VJ, Batch JA, Philips GE, Vickers D (2001). Histopathological analysis of Leri-Weill dyschondrosteosis: disordered growth plate. *Hand Surg* 6(1): 13–23.

Musebeck J, Mohnike K, Beye P, Tonnies H, Neitzel H, Schnabel D, Gruters A, Wieacker PF, Stumm M (2001). Short stature homeobox-containing gene deletion screening by fluorescence in situ hybridisation in patients with short stature. *Eur J Pediatr* 160(9): 561–565.

Niesler B, Fischer C, Rappold GA (2002). The human SHOX mutation database. *Hum Mutat* 20(5): 338–341.

Ogata T, Goodfellow P, Petit C, Aya M, Matsuo N (1992). Short stature in a girl with a terminal Xp deletion distal to DXYS15: localisation of a growth gene(s) in the pseudoautosomal region. *J Med Genet* 29(7): 455–459.

Ogata T, Yoshizawa A, Muroya K, Matsuo N, Fukushima Y, Rappold G, Yokoya S (1995). Short stature in a girl with partial monosomy of the pseudoautosomal region distal to DXYS15: further evidence for the assignment of the critical region for a pseudoautosomal growth gene(s). *J Med Genet* 32(10): 831–834.

Ogata T, Onigata K, Hotsubo T, Matsuo N, Rappold G (2001). Growth hormone and gonadotropin-releasing hormone analog therapy in haploinsufficiency of *SHOX*. *Endocr J* 48(3): 317–322.

Ogata T, Muroya K, Sasaki G, Nishimura G, Kitoh H, Hattori T (2002). SHOX nullizgosity and haploinsufficiency in a Japanese family: implication for the development of Turner skeletal features. *J Clin Endocrinol Metab* 87: 1390–1394.

Page DC, Mosher R, Simpson EM, Fisher EM, Mardon G, Pollack J, McGillivray B, de la Chapelle A, Brown LG (1987). The sex-determining region of the human Y chromosome encodes a finger protein. *Cell* 51(6): 1091–1104.

Ranke MB, Pfluger H, Rosendahl W, Stubbe P, Enders H, Bierich JR, Majewski F (1983). Turner syndrome: spontaneous growth in 150 cases and review of the literature. *Eur J Pediatr* 141(2): 81–88.

Rao E, Weiss B, Fukami M, Rump A, Niesler B, Mertz A, Muroya K, Binder G, Kirsch S, Winkelmann M, et al. (1997). Pseudoautosomal deletions encompassing a novel homeobox gene cause growth failure in idiopathic short stature and Turner syndrome. *Nat Genet* 16(1): 54–63.

Rao E, Blaschke RJ, Marchini A, Niesler B, Burnett M, Rappold GA (2001). The Leri-Weill and Turner syndrome homeobox gene *SHOX* encodes a cell-type specific transcriptional activator. *Hum Mol Genet* 10(26): 3083–3091.

Rappold GA, Fukami M, Niesler B, Schiller S, Zumkeller W, Bettendorf M, Heinrich U, Vlachopapadoupoulou E, Reinehr T, Onigata K, et al. (2002). Deletions of the homeobox gene *SHOX* (short stature homeobox) are an important cause of growth failure in children with short stature. *J Clin Endocrinol Metab* 87(3): 1402–1406.

Robertson SP, Shears DJ, Oei P, Winter RM, Scambler PJ, Aftimos S, Savarirayan R (2000). Homozygous deletion of *SHOX* in a mentally retarded male with Langer mesomelic dysplasia. *J Med Genet* 37(12): 959–964.

Rosenfeld RG, Attie KM, Frane J, Brasel JA, Burstein S, Cara JF, Chernausek S, Gotlin RW, Kuntze J, Lippe BM, et al. (1998). Growth hormone therapy of Turner syndrome: beneficial effect on adult height. *J Pediatr* 132(2): 319–324.

Ross JL, Scott C Jr, Marttila P, Kowal K, Nass A, Papenhausen P, Abboudi J, Osterman L, Kushner H, Carter P, et al. (2001). Phenotypes associated with *SHOX* deficiency. *J Clin Endocrinol Metab* 86(12): 5674–5680.

Rovescalli AC, Asoh S, Nirenberg M (1996). Cloning and characterization of four murine homeobox genes. *Proc Natl Acad Sci USA* 93(20): 10691–10696.

Schiller S, Spranger S, Schechinger B, Fukami M, Merker S, Drop SL, Troger J, Knoblauch H, Kunze J, Seidel J, et al. (2000). Phenotypic variation and genetic heterogeneity in Leri-Weill syndrome. *Eur J Hum Genet* 8(1): 54–62.

Schneider-Gadicke A, Beer-Romero P, Brown L G, Nussbaum R, Page D C (1989). *ZFX* has a gene structure similar to *ZFY*, the putative human sex determinant, and escapes X inactivation. *Cell* 57(7): 1247–1258.

Seidel J, Schiller S, Kelbova C, Beensen V, Orth U, Vogt S, Claussen U, Zintl F, Rappold GA (2001). Brachytelephalangic dwarfism due to the loss of ARSE and *SHOX* genes resulting from an X;Y translocation. *Clin Genet* 59(2): 115–121.

Semina EV, Reiter RS, Murray JC (1998). A new human homeobox gene *OGI2X* is a member of the most conserved homeobox gene family and is expressed during heart development in mouse. *Hum Mol Genet* 7(3): 415–422.

Shanske A, Ellison J, Vuguin P, Dowling P, Wasserman E, Heinrich J, Saenger P (1999). Deletion of the pseudoautosomal region in a male with a unique Y;13 translocation and short stature. *Am J Med Genet* 82(1): 34–39.

Shears DJ, Vassal HJ, Goodman FR, Palmer RW, Reardon W, Superti-Furga A, Scambler PJ, Winter RM (1998). Mutation and deletion of the pseudoautosomal gene *SHOX* cause Leri-Weill dyschondrosteosis. *Nat Genet* 19(1): 70–73.

Shears DJ, Guillen-Navarro E, Sempere-Miralles M, Domingo-Jimenez R, Scambler PJ, Winter RM (2002). Pseudodominant inheritance of Langer mesomelic dysplasia caused by a *SHOX* homeobox missense mutation. *Am J Med Genet* 110(2): 153–157.

Stuppia L, Calabrese G, Gatta V, Pintor S, Morizio E, Fantasia D, Guanciali Franchi P, Rinaldi MM, Scarano G, Concolino D, Giannotti A, Petreschi F, Anzellotti MT, Pomilio M, Chiarelli F, Tumini S, Palka G. SHOX mutations detected by FISH and direct sequencing in patients with short stature. *J Med Genet* 40: E11.

Vassal H, Medeira A, Cordeiro I, Santos HG, Castedo S, Saraiva C, da Silva PM, Monteiro C (2001). Terminal deletion of Xp22.3 associated with contiguous gene syndrome: Leri-Weill dyschondrosteosis, developmental delay, and ichthyosis. *Am J Med Genet* 99(4): 331–334.

Youlton R, Castillo S, Be C (1985). XY translocation in a woman with dyschondrosteosis and sterility. *Rev Med Chil* 113(3): 228–230.

Zinn AR, Wei F, Zhang L, Elder FF, Scott CI Jr, Marttila P, Ross JL (2002). Complete *SHOX* deficiency causes Langer mesomelic dysplasia. *Am J Med Genet* 110(2): 158–163.

54 | *HLXB9* and Sacral Agenesis and the Currarino Syndrome

STEPHEN SCHERER, GIUSEPPE MARTUCCIELLO, ELENA BELLONI, AND MICHELE TORRE

Agenesis of the sacrum is a defect that involves the spinal column, with varying degrees of severity. It is usually sporadic in origin and associated with maternal diabetes. There are also familial forms, such as the Currarino syndrome, in which the defects are transmitted through entire pedigrees, with reduced penetrance in some cases.

The genetics underlying sacral agenesis remained unknown for many years, although various genes were tested as candidates for the disease. In 1995, there was still no association with any specific autosome. This is probably because a clear distinction among the various forms in which a disease manifests itself is necessary to understand the genetic cause(s). It can now be said that a disease called *sacral agenesis* proper does not exist as a single entity; rather, it is a morphologic anomaly that is part of a very complex spectrum of developmental malformations, with each driven by the anomalous functioning of one or more genes or gene pathways.

In 1998, molecular genetic studies demonstrated the involvement of the *HLXB9* (also called *HB9*, *SCRA1*, or *HOXHB9*) gene in families affected by agenesis of the terminal part of the spinal column. A closer clinical analysis of the cases described, along with further studies, demonstrated that the gene was directly linked to a specific form of sacral agenesis, the Currarino syndrome (CS). A second study that analyzed both families and sporadic cases with other symptoms affecting the caudal region confirmed that defects of *HLXB9* are specific to CS and likely not involved in other malformations.

Given these findings, it becomes evident that a complete description of the embryology of the sacral region, and of the different anomalies that affect it, is necessary to fully understand the molecular genetics of this complex condition.

CLINICAL MANIFESTATIONS AFFECTING THE SACRAL REGION, EMBRYOLOGY, AND DEVELOPMENT

Development of the spinal column begins in embryonic life and ends in the third decade of life (Tortori Donati et al., 2000; Diel et al., 2001). The first stage is mesenchymal: the major steps are gastrulation (weeks 2–3) and primary neurulation (weeks 3–4). Gastrulation (see Chapter 5) is the process by which the bilaminar disc is converted into a trilaminar disc, when, on day 14–15, the mesoblast (future mesoderm) migrates between the two existing layers. No mesodermal cells migrate along the midline. Subsequently, they join medially to form the notochord (gestational day 17), which induces the ectoderm to form the neural plate; the plate then folds to become the neural tube (primary neurulation). During neurulation, ectodermal cells progressively disconnecting from the lateral walls of the neural folds differentiate into the neural crest. The lateral mesoderm thickens to become the paraxial mesoderm, and from this structure, by the end of gestational week 5, 42 to 44 somites arise.

The second stage is chondrification (see Chapter 11), which starts in gestational week 5 and results in cartilagineous vertebral column. In weeks 5 to 6, another important phenomenon begins: secondary neurulation and retrogressive differentiation. With this process, the remaining sacrococcygeal metameres, distal to the caudal end of the neural plate (located at S3–S5 level), are formed. This process continues until gestational day 48. The third stage, primary ossification, occurs in three ossification centers: costal, neural, and central. In the sacrum, the costal centers produce on both sides the lateral mass and

the sacral alae (Fig. 54–1). The neural centers contribute to the neural arch and the posterolateral vertebral body. The central ossification center forms the mid-portion of the vertebral body. The last stage is secondary ossification, with an accessory ossification center on each sacral vertebral body, and the fusion of discs, lasting until the third decade.

At birth, three ossification centers for each vertebra are present: one for the body and one for each half of the posterior vertebral arch. The costal element may be visible on each side of S1–S3 (Denton, 1982). The arch and the body fuse at the age of 7 years, and the laminae fuse posteriorly at the age of 7 to 10 years. The coccyx may or may not be ossified at birth. The appearance of the ossification center of the coccyx starts at birth (for the first coccygeal vertebra) and lasts more than 14 years (Belot and Lepennetier, 1969). The knowledge of these processes is important for the correct interpretation of sacrum imaging in infancy and childhood. The following is a description of the congenital lesions, arising from defects in one or more stages of the sacral development.

TRANSITIONAL VERTEBRA

This anomaly is very common (20% of the general population) and can be characterized by the "sacralization" of L5 vertebra or "lumbarization" of S1 (Diel et al., 2001). In the first case, L5 is incorporated into the sacrum; in the second case, S1 is positioned above the superior margin of the sacrum. This anomaly is asymptomatic, but it is important to be aware of it to avoid potential mistakes in the count of sacral vertebrae.

SIRENOMELIA

Known in ancient Greece, sirenomelia is characterized essentially by the fusion of the lower limbs at varying degrees, with the absence of normal rotation (apodia, monopodia, and dipodia), associated anorectal malformations (ARMs), absent or arrested genital development, absent or cystic kidneys, pelvic alterations, preaxial defects of upper limbs, intestinal malformations, persistent cloaca, cardiopathies, and vertebral, vertebrocostal, and lumbosacral defects (Lerone et al., 1997). Because of bilateral renal dysgenesis or agenesis, sirenomelia is not compatible with life. The incidence is 1:60,000 live births, with a male/female ratio of 2:7, and presents a low risk of recurrence (Kallen and Winberg, 1974). The defects observed in this sequence are thought to be due to an early alteration of vascular development (Stevenson et al., 1986).

SACRAL AGENESIS AND CAUDAL REGRESSION SYNDROME

The caudal regression syndrome (CRS) is a heterogeneous constellation of caudal anomalies that include varying degrees of agenesis of the spinal column, ARMs, genitourinary anomalies, and pulmonary hypoplasia (Duhamel, 1961). This syndrome presents some typical features (Cama et al., 1996): (1) cutaneous signs (lumbosacral agenesis with flattening of the buttock and shortening of the intergluteal cleft), (2) total or partial sacrococcygeal agenesis, (3) vertebral or skeletal dysmorphia (scoliosis, kyphoscoliosis, rib anomalies, hip dislocation, and lower limb deformities such as clubfoot), (4) cardiac

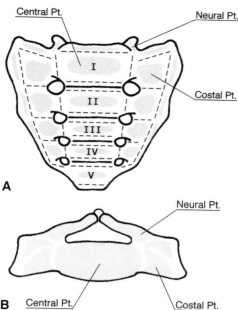

Figure 54–1. Two views of the three ossification centers (costal, neural, and central) in the primary ossification of the sacrum.

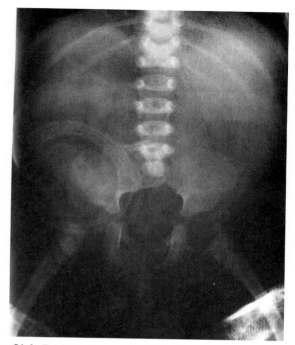

Figure 54–2. Total sacral agenesis with involvement of lumbar vertebra 5 (sacral agenesis type 1).

malformations (tetralogy of Fallot), (5) ARMs, (6) genitourinary disorders (renal unilateral or bilateral aplasia or dysplasia, vesicoureteral reflux, ureterocele, hypospadias, and malformed external genitalia), and (7) pulmonary hypoplasia.

The incidence of CRS is approximately 1:7500 births, but some authors report an incidence varying from 1:200 to 1000 (Wilmshurst et al., 1999) to 1:10,000 to 20,000 (Diel et al., 2001). CRS may be found in multisystemic malformations such as omphalocele, cloacal extrophy imperforate anus, and spinal deformities (OEIS), and vertebral, anorectal, cardiac, tracheoesophageal, renal, and limb anomalies (VACTERL syndrome). A well-known risk factor is maternal diabetes: 8% to 16% of CRS patients have a diabetic mother. The risk that a diabetic pregnant woman has an affected child is thought to be 1% (Passarge and Lenz, 1966). Others report a lower incidence of 1.27:1000 (Lenz and Kucera, 1967, Kalter, 1993).

It is possible to diagnose CRS antenatally or at birth. Some cases of sacral agenesis are diagnosed later, with the child usually presenting with urologic problems or constipation. A review of the literature (Wilmshurst et al., 1999) showed that the age range at presentation is wide; in only one study was the diagnosis made for half of the cases in the newborn period. The most common complaint in cases diagnosed later was urinary incontinence.

The degree of spine involvement can vary. Different classifications for sacral agenesis have been proposed. Renshaw (1978) suggested four classifications: type 1, total or partial unilateral sacral agenesis; type 2, partial sacral agenesis with a partial but bilaterally symmetric defect and a stable articulation between the ilia and a normal or hypoplastic S1; type 3, variable lumbar and total sacral agenesis with the ilia articulating with the sides of the lowest vertebra present; and type 4, variable lumbar and total sacral agenesis, with the caudal endplate of the lowest vertebra resting above either fused ilia or an iliac amphiarthrosis.

Another classification was proposed by Kalitzki (1965) and adopted with minor modifications by Pang (1993) and Cama et al. (1996). The classification proposed by Cama et al. involves five specific categories: type 1, total sacral agenesis with normal or short transverse pelvic diameter and involvement of some lumbar vertebrae (Fig. 54–2); type 2, total sacral agenesis without involvement of lumbar vertebrae; type 3, subtotal sacral agenesis or sacral hypodevelopment (with S1 present) (Fig. 54–3); type 4, hemisacrum (Fig. 54–4); and type 5, coccygeal agenesis.

Central nervous system involvement is present in almost all cases

and can lead to neurologic clinical deficit or, when occult, can be discovered with ultrasonographic or magnetic resonance studies.

In severe forms, with total sacral agenesis (types 1 and 2 of Cama et al.'s classification) or subtotal sacral agenesis (type 3), the corresponding metameres of the spinal cord are also absent and the spinal cord terminates abruptly and is often club shaped. The higher the termination of the cord, the more severe is the malformation, with more

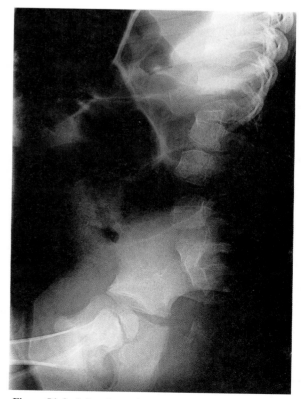

Figure 54–3. Subtotal sacral agenesis (sacral agenesis type 3).

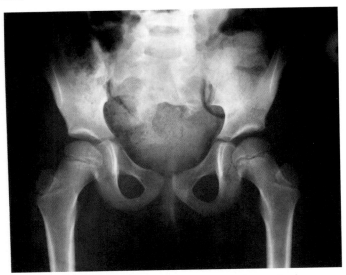

Figure 54–4. Hemisacrum (sacral agenesis type 4).

absent vertebrae. In the most severe cases described (Blery et al., 1983; Mihmanli et al., 2001), the spinal cord terminated at the mid-portion of the thoracic tract, and vertebrae caudal to this level were absent. Some malformations of cauda equina and/or anterior meningocele can be associated.

In other less severe forms, S2 or more caudal sacral vertebrae are present; only metameres developed with secondary neurulation are absent. The conus medullaris is elongated and stretched caudally and is tethered by a tight filum terminale, intradural lipoma, terminal myelocystocele, or lypomyelomeningocele (Naidich et al., 1966). In some rare cases, the cord is not tethered, and the only characteristic is a conus medullaris without tip. When tethered cord is associated with CRS, the conus medullaris is abnormally low (below L3 vertebral level). The clinical signs are related to tethering of the spinal cord or filum terminale to the surrounding tissues and include motor and sensory dysfunction of the legs, muscle atrophy or hypoplasia, decreased or hyperactive reflexes, urinary incontinence, and orthopedic deformities (Tortoti Donati et al., 2000).

ARMs are frequently associated with CRS. Seven of 26 CRS patients (27%) presented with ARMs in the series of Cama et al. (1996), and 48% presented in the series of Renshaw (1978). ARMs encompass a large spectrum of diseases, including mild and severe forms. The modern classification of ARMs was proposed by Peña in 1995 and is based in both sexes on the presence and site of rectal fistulas. In males, the categories are ARM with rectovesical fistula, ARM with rectoprostatic fistula, ARM with rectobulbar fistula, ARM with rectoperineal fistula, and other cases (ARM without fistula or rectal stenosis). In females, the categories are ARM with rectocloacal fistula (persistent cloaca), ARM with rectovestibular fistula, ARM with rectoperineal fistula, and other cases (ARM without fistula or rectal stenosis).

Bowel function is frequently impaired in children with CRS. The neurogenic bowel is characterized by severe constipation and/or fecal incontinence. In a series of 23 cases (Renshaw, 1978), these symptoms were present in 19 (83%) patients.

Genitourinary anomalies are also very common in children affected by CRS. Neurogenic bladder is present in 80% to 100% of cases (Cama et al., 1996; Renshaw, 1978; Wilmshurst et al., 1999). A bladder motility disorder can be clinically evident or be discovered after urodynamic evaluation. Vesicoureteral reflux was present in 19% (Cama et al., 1996) to 45% (Wilmshurst et al., 1999) of children. Renal aplasia or dysplasia should be investigated in these patients. In 22 patients presenting with sacral agenesis (Wilmshurst et al., 1999), 7 (32%) presented with renal scarring and 3 (14%) presented with chronic renal failure at diagnosis. Orthopedic disorders were present in 24 of 26 patients (92%) studied by Cama et al. (1996) and in 14 of 22 patients (64%) studied by Wilmshurst et al. (1999). The most common anomaly was clubfoot; other frequent disorders were hip dislocation and scoliosis.

Other possible malformations that are less frequently associated with CRS are cardiac and pulmonary anomalies. Six of 26 children (23%) (Cama et al., 1996) had cardiac malformations.

From these data, it is clear that CRS is a multisystem syndrome; for this reason, a multidisciplinary approach is essential. The medical and surgical treatment of CRS has the following goals (Cama et al., 1996): (1) surgical treatment of malformations associated with sacral agenesis; (2) preservation and/or improvement of renal, cardiac, and gastrointestinal function; (3) prevention of early and late complications (neurologic worsening, spinal deformities, and infections); and (4) achievement of essential functions, including walking and urinary and fecal continence.

The number of sacral vertebrae is an important prognostic factor in children affected by CRS, but it is not always easy to determine it on the basis of sacral radiographs. In 1995, Alberto Peña proposed the "sacral ratio" (SR) as an objective and reliable tool to evaluate sacral development. He proposed SR as a prognostic factor for children affected by ARMs. Anteroposterior (AP) and lateral (L) radiographs of the sacrum make it possible to calculate AP- and L-SR (Peña, 1995). SR is obtained through the division between two distances (Fig. 54–5), with the first from the lowest point of the sacrum (or of the coccyx, if present) to the segment joining the two posterior iliac spines (BC in Fig. 54–5) and the second from this segment to that joining the upper points of the iliac crests (AB in Fig. 54–5). The ratio of BC to AB

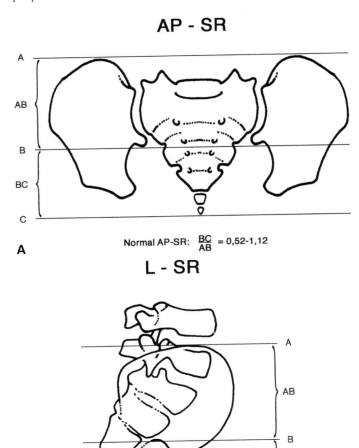

Figure 54–5. The sacral ratio (SR) is calculated by dividing BC by AB. (*A*) Anteroposterior (AP)-SR. (*B*) Lateral (L)-SR. The normal values in the general population are shown.

is the SR, which is a good parameter of sacral development. A low SR is an index of sacral hypoplasia, and this implies a worse functional prognosis, according to Peña (1995). In 100 normal children, the average AP-SR calculated by Peña (1995) was 0.74, and L-SR was 0.77.

In a study by Torre et al. (2001), SR in the normal population was evaluated in 147 children of different ages to assess the normal range of variability. SR was measured in 59 children with ARMs to verify whether it is a clinically reliable prognostic factor in these patients. The values obtained were correlated with associated medullary anomalies, intestinal innervation, and functional prognosis, in terms of fecal and urinary continence.

Finally, in 25 cases (15 patients with ARMs and 10 control subjects), multiple measurements of SR were obtained at different ages in the same subject to verify whether SR could change with growth. The average AP-SR was 0.74. In children more than 5 years, AP-SR increased to an average of 0.82. The AP-SR values observed in this normal population ranged from 0.52 to 1.12. The average L-SR was 0.75. In children older than 5 years, L-SR increased to 0.91. The range of L-SR values was from 0.52 to 1.18. The correlation between SR and medullary anomalies in patients with ARMs was statistically significant. The correlation between SR and intestinal innervation was not significant; however, in children with a low SR, the presence of innervation anomalies were more frequent than it was in those with a normal SR (75% versus 60%).

Follow-up data on fecal and urinary continence revealed a correlation between SR and fecal and urinary continence in these patients.

In 25 cases, SR was calculated at different ages. In 8 of 10 control subjects, the authors observed an increase in SR values with growth; in the remaining 2 subjects, SR decreased with growth. In 15 patients with ARMs, SR decreased over time in 14. This study by Torre et al. (2001) led to the following conclusions. (1) In the normal population, the average values of AP-SR and L-SR are very similar to those reported in the literature (Peña, 1995). However, SR proved to have a wide range of values in the normal population: 0.52 to 1.12 (AP-SR) and 0.52 to 1.18 (L-SR). This result led the authors to consider AP-SR and L-SR values to be pathologic only if they were lower than 0.52. (2) An SR value of lower than 0.52 is well correlated with a higher risk of medullary anomalies and with a poor functional prognosis in terms of fecal and urinary continence. (3) Age seems to be a possible variability factor of SR. In fact, SR tends to increase in the normal population with growth, whereas it tends to decrease in patients with ARMs. The increased SR values in older children among the normal population could be explained in part by the progressive development of coccygeal ossification nuclei, appearing at birth and lasting for more than 14 years. In patients with ARM, SR values decrease with age. A possible explanation is that the sacrum in these patients is congenitally involved and cannot grow proportionally with the child and his or her pelvic bones; therefore, congenital sacral involvement becomes more evident at older ages, with a decrease in SR values.

CURRARINO SYNDROME

Currarino syndrome (CS) is a particular form of CRS. In this entity, sacral anomaly is type IV of the Cama et al. (1996) classification and consists of a pathognomonic hemisacrum, with the preservation of S1 (see Fig. 54–4). This syndrome was first described as a triad of anorectal anomaly, hemisacrum, and presacral mass (Currarino et al., 1981). Other reports described the syndrome as "ASP" (anal atresia, sacral anomalies, and presacral mass). Belloni et al. (2000) called the disorder Currarino syndrome; and this is the most appropriate name because there often are features present other than just the triad of hemisacrum, presacral mass, and ARM (Lynch et al., 2000). This affection can be sporadic or familial, with an autosomal dominant transmission. An important clinical sign in these patients is severe constipation, which can be the earliest symptom. In some cases, the syndrome is incomplete, presenting with only one or two malformations. The hemisacrum or bifid sacrum is present in every case. Every type of ARM (see the classification earlier) can be present but ARM

with perineal fistula is the most common. The presacral mass can be a presacral teratoma, an anterior meningocele, an enteric cyst, or a complex of more than one. Some cases of malignancy have been described in the literature (Norum et al., 1991; Tander et al., 1999).

In the largest series from a review of the literature (Lynch et al., 2000) the female/male ratio was 1.7:1. The greater number of females can be explained by the associated gynecologic and urinary tract problems seen in women. In these patients, there was a broad range of clinical signs and symptoms associated with CS (constipation, bowel obstruction, perianal sepsis, urinary and gynaecologic problems, spinal cord tethering, meningitis, anterior meningocele, and presacral mass), but 33% of cases were asymptomatic. Prenatal diagnosis is very rare (Friedmann et al., 1997), with only three cases described so far, but it is possible if there is a presacral mass. Current prenatal diagnosis can be based on molecular genetic analysis.

MOLECULAR GENETIC STUDIES REGARDING THE SR: INVOLVEMENT OF THE *HLXB9* GENE IN CS

Several cytogenetic defects have been associated with sacral malformations, including deletions of the long arm of chromosome 7 (7q). In 1995, Linch et al. (1995) showed for the first time, in an analysis of two families, genetic linkage with the q36 region of human chromosome 7 through the use of a fully penetrant dominant inheritance model. Figure 54–6 shows the results obtained for the most informative pedigree presented in this first study, indicating that the affected gene was located between the D7S396 marker and the chromosome 7 telomere. The clinical description of the family members showed that some, but not all, of the affected individuals were characterized by the presence of a presacral mass and/or an ARM. These traits are typical of the CS, and it could be demonstrated that in each case there was a defect in the sacral bones, which the authors reported as sacral agenesis, presumably indicating the presence of a hemisacrum. This specific defect is the most distinctive of the syndrome, being always present in the patients, whereas the lack of the other anomalies of the triad was not difficult to see in many of the affected individuals.

The 7q36 region had been involved in different developmental abnormalities, such as holoprosencephaly and triphalangeal thumb, giving rise to the hypothesis that various genes that play a role in some developmental step may be located in this area (Belloni et al., 1996). The construction of a detailed physical map of the long arm of chromosome 7, and of q36 in particular, allowed positioning of several genes in the region. Refined mapping of the cytogenetic anomalies associated with the different phenotypes observed in other patients helped to further refine the region. These studies lead to the identification of *Sonic Hedgehog* (*SHH*) as the causative gene for holoprosencephaly (Belloni et al., 1996; Rossler et al., 1996) and to the precise localization of two homeobox genes known to have a role in early development, *EN2* and *HLXB9*, near the interval defined by Lynch et al. in 1995. An exhaustive analysis of the *SHH* gene and promoter sequence was performed in two studies (Vargas et al., 1998; Seri et al., 1999) with an aim to evaluate its involvement in sacral anomalies and CS. This gene is expressed in the spinal cord, as demonstrated by studies performed on normal and *Shh*$^{-/-}$ transgenic mice (Chiang et al., 1996), supporting the hypothesis of its possible involvement in anomalies that affect the sacral region. The resulting absence of sequence anomalies in the studied patients showed that *SHH* likely did not contribute to abnormalities that affect the sacrum. Moreover, linkage analysis on additional families affected by sacral agenesis confirmed the involvement of the terminal end of 7q (Ross et el., 1998; Seri et al., 1999) and allowed a more refined positioning of the causative gene distal to the D7S559 marker, confirming the exclusion of the *SHH* gene, which had been mapped centromerically. At the same time, these results lead to the conclusion that *EN2* could not be considered a candidate because it was located upstream of *SHH* (Figs. 54–7 and 54–8).

HLXB9, the third candidate gene, however, was located precisely within the interval defined by the linkage analysis, between the D7S559 and D7S2423 markers. Cloned in 1994 (Harrison et al., 1994), *HLXB9* was initially found to be expressed exclusively in pancreatic and lymphoid tissues, as shown by Northern blot experiments per-

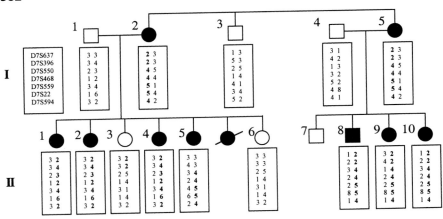

Figure 54–6. Linkage analysis in the pedigree described by Lynch et al. in 1995. The disease-associated haplotypes are indicated in bold. Individuals II-3 and II-5 are those defining the locus location between D7S396 and the chromosome 7 telomere. (From Lynch et al., 1995.)

formed on a variety of human tissues. Nevertheless, later studies carried out in *Xenopus laevis* (Saha et al., 1997) demonstrated that the homologous gene *xHB9* was expressed in the spinal cord, (more precisely, at the level of the tailbud), raising the possibility of a role of the human gene in sacral development. To understand the role of *HLXB9* in early development, Ross et al. (1998) analyzed its expression in human embryos, finding that at Carnegie stage 19 (48 postovulatory days), gene expression was found in the anterior horn regions of the spinal cord.

Based on these functional data, the gene was tested for direct involvement in sacral malformations by searching for mutations in the gene sequence of affected individuals and families. The *HLXB9* gene contains three exons. A combination of DGGE, single-strand conformation polymorphism, and direct DNA sequencing experiments, as described in three successive studies (Ross et al., 1998; Belloni et al., 2000; Hagan et al., 2000), demonstrated the presence of mutations in

the gene coding sequence, as well as intron-exon boundaries, in both sporadic and familial cases, proving a causative role of *HLXB9* in sacral abnormalities.

Table 54–1 summarizes the *HLXB9* mutations found to date, as well their localization within the gene sequence. For each mutation, a similar change was not observed in any of at least 100 normal chromosomes examined. As also indicated in Figure 54–9, all of the missense mutations cluster in the portion of the gene coding for the homeodomain, with each resulting in nonconservative amino acid substitutions. A comparison of the mutated human residues with those in the mouse, chicken, *X. laevis*, and sea urchin homologue genes revealed that they are highly conserved residues throughout evolution (Fig. 54–10). This suggests that an amino acid change in the homeobox would severely affect the normal functioning of the protein. In a similar way, the splicing mutations detected in three of the affected cases hit nucleotides either in the acceptor or in the donor splicing sites, which are 100% conserved, indicating that an abnormal protein will be obtained. All of the frameshift mutations, as well as those leading to the change of a residue into a stop codon, give rise to a truncated product. In a few cases, hemizygous microdeletion of *HLXB9* could be observed: this was shown either by means of microsatellite analysis, within the D7S637–D7S594 interval, or by assessing the status of the intragenic polymorphic alanine stretch, as determined by the presence of a CGC repeat in this region.

In conclusion, a total of nine missense, two nonsense, seven frameshift, and two splicing mutations, along with six hemizygous microdeletions, have been published to date. Because haploinsufficiency of *HLXB9* has been considered the pathogenic event in those cases carrying deletions of the 7q35-tel region on one allele and given the autosomal dominant inheritance of the disease, it can be inferred that all of the mutations found in the studied patients represent loss-of-function alleles.

The presence of a poly-alanine tract has been described in other homeobox gene sequences (see Chapters 63 and 64). In some cases, variation in the length of the triplet repeat is associated with disease conditions such as synpolydactyly, oculopharyngeal muscular dystrophy, and cleidocranial dysplasia (Mundlos et al., 1997; Goodman et al., 1997; Brais et al., 1998). A similar condition was not determined in the patients affected by sacral anomalies, because all of the alleles observed in the patients could also be detected in normal control subjects. In the study performed by Belloni et al. 2000, CGC_{11} was determined to be the most common allele in the general population, accounting for 90.23% of the chromosomes analyzed. Other alleles observed were CGC_{12} (1.7%), CGC_9 (7.47%), and CGC_8 (0.6%). These were all determined to be heterozygous changes. In only one sample among the affected patients and the control subjects was it

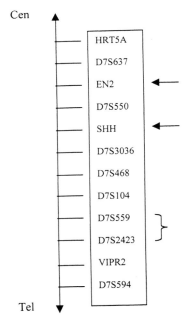

Figure 54–7. Marker and gene order (7cen-qter) within the 7q36 region involved in sacral abnormalities. The positions of *SHH* and *EN2* are indicated, as well as the interval containing *HLXB9*, as defined by linkage analysis (data derived from the chromosome 7 database: http://www.chr7.org/).

Figure 54–8. Linkage analysis in the pedigree described by Ross et al. in 1998. The disease-associated haplotypes are indicated in bold. Individuals II-4, III-5, and III-6 are those defining the locus location between D7S559 and the chromosome 7 telomere. A second pedigree from the same study helped in the further definition of the locus, between D7S559 and D7S2423. (From Ross et al., 1998.)

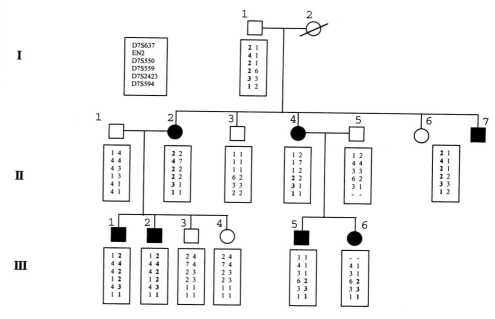

possible to reveal a homozygous change in the poly-alanine tract, giving rise to the CGC_9/CGC_9 allelic combination. This sample came from the control collection (a total of 100 normal chromosomes were included in the study): nevertheless, a closer clinical investigation showed that the individual lacked fusion of the posterior arch of the vertebrae, with scoliosis on the left side. In any case, no association between the repeat length and the presence of a sacral condition in this individuals, as well as in other affected or normal individuals, could be established because the alleles observed in the patients were also detected in control subjects. In addition to patient-specific mutations, HLXB9 analysis revealed the presence of sequence polymorphism (Table 54–2).

In some of the familial cases, individuals carrying a familial mutation are asymptomatic, and no sacral abnormality could be shown after radiographic analysis. This was shown, for instance, in the families carrying 48insC, 859-2A → G, and T248S (Ross et al., 1998; Belloni et al., 2000), leading to the conclusion that the disease phenotype is transmitted with reduced penetrance.

Table 54–1. Identified *HLXB9* Mutations

	Mutation cDNA (Genomic)	Mutation Position	Mutation Type	Comments
1	*48insC (*125insC)	Exon 1	Frameshift	Familial
2	234delG (307delG)	Exon 1	Frameshift	Sporadic
3	331delG (408delG)	Exon 1	Frameshift	Familial
4	337delC (414delC)	Exon 1	Frameshift	Familial
5	del14nt406-419 (del14nt483-496)	Exon 1	Frameshift	Familial
6	409delG (486delG)	Exon 1	Frameshift	Familial
7	Y166X	Exon 1	Nonsense	Sporadic
8	*575delA (*652delA)	Exon 1	Frameshift	Familial
9	R247G	Exon 2	Missense	Familial
10	R247H	Exon 2	Missense	Familial
11	T248S	Exon 2	Missense	Familial
12	Q261X	Exon 2	Nonsense	Familial
13	858+1G → A (4291G → A)	Intron 2	Splicing	Familial
14	859-2A → G (4889A → G)	Intron 2	Splicing	Familial
15	*W290G	Exon 3	Missense	Familial
16	W290L	Exon 3	Missense	Familial
17	Q292P	Exon 3	Missense	Familial
18	R294W	Exon 3	Missense	Familial
19	R295W	Exon 3	Missense	Sporadic
20	R295Q	Exon 3	Missense	Familial
21	Hemizygous deletion of *HLXB9*	—	—	Familial
22	Hemizygous deletion of *HLXB9*	—	—	Familial
23	Hemizygous deletion of *HLXB9*	—	—	Sporadic
24	Hemizygous deletion of *HLXB9*	—	—	Familial
25	Hemizygous deletion of *HLXB9*	—	—	Sporadic
26	Hemizygous deletion of *HLXB9*	—	—	Sporadic

*The mutation has been identified in two independent cases (Ross et al., 1998; Belloni et al., 2000; Hagan et al., 2000).

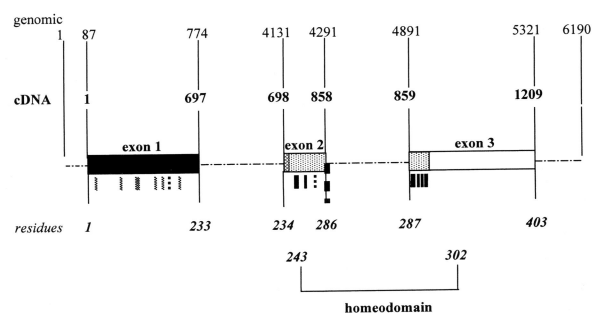

Figure 54–9. Structure of the *HLXB9* gene. Numbers in black indicate the nucleotide numeration according to the genomic sequence; numbers in bold indicate the nucleotide numeration according to the cDNA sequence; and numbers in gray indicate the residue numeration. The shaded regions within exons 2 and 3 represent the homeodomain. The position of the mutations in indicated by the vertical bars: gray, frameshift; dotted black, nonsense; black, missense; and dotted gray, splicing mutations.

As pointed out in the clinical description, the spectrum of ARMs is very broad, and only 29% of cases have been described in association with sacral anomalies, giving rise to various CRS phenotypes. Consequently, to reach a complete understanding of the genetic causes of CRS, it is reasonable to separately address the different aspects of this pathologic condition, considering each subgrouping of patients to be a different clinical entity. This was accomplished, after the description of the involvement of *HLXB9* in sacral agenesis (Ross et al., 1998), in the study by Belloni et al. (2000), which aimed to provide a more refined definition of the genetic role of *HLXB9* in the different cases of ARM associated with sacral abnormalities. The patients who were analyzed are reported in Table 54–3, and their clinical conditions are given, defining the three categories into which they have been classified. *HLXB9* mutations have been identified only in those individuals diagnosed with CS. The observation was consistent with what was presented in the original report (Ross et al., 1998), which described the identification of six different mutations in unrelated individuals collectively grouped as having dominantly inherited sacral agenesis. Closer examination of the clinical data revealed the presence of either CS or partial characteristics reminiscent of CS. Instead, the results obtained refined the involvement of this homeogene in spe-cific anorectal and sacral anomalies, showing that it is possible to exclude a role for *HLXB9* in caudal regression categories 3 and 5, as well as total sacral agenesis (categories 1 and 2). This was confirmed in the study by Hagan et al. (2000), with the finding of 13 additional mutations (all reported in Table 54–1), all in CS families or sporadic patients. This study included the analysis of an additional 32 patients with partial, atypical, or related phenotypes (ARMs, total sacral agenesis, sacrococcygeal teratomas, and spina bifida occulta). Mutations were not detected in this additional cohort of patients, confirming that the CS phenotype is specifically linked to anomalies involving only the *HLXB9* gene. Although it is possible that a mutation or DNA sequence variation in the noncoding region of *HLXB9* could be present in these individuals, a more likely possibility is that other genes are important in the pathogenesis of these malformations.

No *HLXB9* mutations have been detected in some of the familial and sporadic cases analyzed. This suggests that there could be genetic heterogeneity for this syndrome or that some nongenetic determinants should be taken into consideration, at least for the sporadic cases. In this regard, Hagan et al. (1995) tested other candidate genes, based not on their chromosomal location but instead on their potential functional relationship with *HLXB9*. In particular, a gene known to be in-

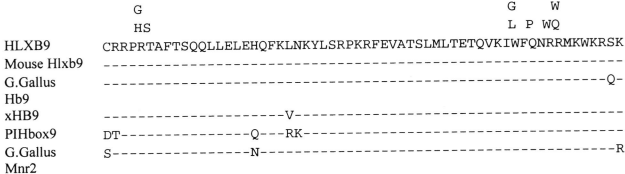

Figure 54–10. Comparison of the human, mouse, chicken, *Xenopus*, and sea urchin *HLXB9* homologues at the homeodomain. The high homology with the chicken *Mnr2* homeobox is also shown. The position of the nine missense mutations detected in patients with Curranno syndrome is indicated. (From Hagan et al., 1999.)

Table 54–2. Described *HLXB9* Sequence Polymorphisms

Sequence Polymorphisms (cDNA)
-519delC
-293C $\rightarrow$ G
$858+92$A $\rightarrow$ G
$859-131$T $\rightarrow$ C
Sequence variation in intron 2
433 (P119P)

Source: Belloni et al., 2000; Hagan et al., 2000.

volved in the same pathway, *ISL1*, was screened by SSCP analysis for the presence of mutations in five sporadic CS patients, who do not carry *HLXB9* sequence abnormalities; no pathogenic DNA sequence changes were detected, (Riggs et al., 1995).

To date, no gene other than *HLXB9* has been shown to be involved in sacral malformations, and its specific role in CS supports the hypothesis that the various conditions affecting the normal sacral and anorectal development depend on the abnormal functioning of different genes. Further linkage studies are therefore necessary to determine the genetic association existing with other anomalies, such as total sacral agenesis. In consideration of all of the mutations discovered in CS patients and families, no obvious genotype–phenotype correlation has been observed. The only relevant observation is that patients carrying large deletions at 7q have a more complex phenotype, which can often include developmental delay.

The identification of *HLXB9* as the causative gene for CS has important diagnostic value because it can allow the assessment of the disease status not only in affected but also in individuals who are asymptomatic heterozygotes. As pointed out earlier, CS is an autosomal dominant disorder with variable expression and reduced penetrance, meaning that molecular genetic analysis becomes relevant in detecting those individuals who do not clearly show the disease phenotype. Moreover, the hereditary nature of the disorder prompts genetic counseling to be offered to the members of CS families, in such a way that the identification of asymptomatic carriers could lead to a reduction in morbidity. Moreover, the identification of at-risk subjects could allow careful planning of pregnancies and the appropriate treatment of affected children at birth.

In this regard, it has been shown that prenatal ultrasonography is not a completely accurate method of investigation, because it identifies only the presence of a presacral mass, but not in all cases, making molecular analysis the most reliable diagnostic approach (reviewed in Lynch et al., 2000). In familial cases, all first-degree relatives should be offered genetic testing, in combination with a pelvic radiograph, which remains the clinical investigation of choice, allowing also the recognition of subtle abnormalities. Individuals with an abnormal radiograph should then be examined with further and more detailed investigations, such as pelvic MRI or CT scanning, to completely characterize the anomalies.

HLXB9 AND SACRAL DEVELOPMENT: THE ANIMAL MODELS

The ablation of *Hlxb9* expression was studied in two murine knockout models, generated either by homologous recombination in ES cells (Li et al., 1999) or by deletion of exon 3, which contains the terminal part of the homeodomain (Harrison et al., 1999). Heterozygous mice had no apparent abnormalities, but the homozygous mutants *Hlxb9*$^{-/-}$ were not viable. Analysis of the embryos from interrupted pregnancies revealed that they had no obvious morphologic abnormality, except for the fact that they were smaller than their normal littermates and showed a curled body. Despite these anomalies, the skeletal development appeared to be normal: differential staining of the cartilage and bones, as well as radiographic examination, did not reveal any sacral abnormalities in the mutant mice. As described at the time of its cloning, *HLXB9* expression was evidenced only in pancreatic and lymphoid tissues; although early B- and T-lymphocyte development in the knockout mice appeared intact, defects were described in the development of the pancreas. The first anomaly was observed in the dorsal part of the devel-

oping pancreas, where the correspondent epithelial bud was absent. On the other side, the ventral bud was present, but further analysis showed that at this location, spatial organization of the endocrine cells in the deriving islets of Langerhans seemed to be affected. Contrary to the typical structure of maturing islets, where α-cells are located at the periphery surrounding a core of β-cells, the mouse homozygous mutants failed to reach this level of organization. Taken altogether, these data showed that *Hlxb9* is selectively required in the initial stages of dorsal pancreatic development, allowing the evagination and subsequent development of the dorsal bud. On the ventral side, its function is not required for the generation of endocrine and exocrine cells, which are independent of this homeogene, whereas it is necessary for the differentiation and maturation steps, leading to the formation of functional islets. Human *HLXB9* expression during embryogenesis was examined by Hagan et al. (2000), revealing that the gene can be detected again in the dorsal and ventral regions of the pancreas, although there is not the same variation in the levels of expression seen in mouse. There also are differences in the timing of the gene expression between human and mouse, suggesting that pancreas development might follow different steps. Despite these observations, pancreatic malformation or malfunction has never been observed in CS patients. Interestingly, Kalter (1993) reported the association between maternal diabetes and caudal dysplasia, whereas the teratogenic effects of insulin have been reported in animals affected by caudal malformations. Because the spectrum of defects that characterize caudal dysplasia is broad and includes anomalies of the sacral region, the study performed by Hagan et al. (2000) put forth the hypothesis of an involvement of *HLXB9* in this disease condition. This will require mutation analysis in affected cases (study in progress).

Based on the fact that a primary notochordal defect in the tail bud has been proposed as the pathogenic mechanism leading to CS, *HLXB9* expression in human embryos was also examined in this location. The gene expression could not be detected in the tail bud nothocord or even in more anterior regions of the nothocord, starting from Carnegie stage 12 (CS12). This might reflect the low sensitivity of standard in situ hybridization techniques, leaving open the possibility that the most significant expression at this embryonic location occurs in the very first developmental stages and then lowers to undetectable levels. This hypothesis finds support in the studies by Harrison et al. (1999) and Li et al. (1999), describing *Hlxb9* expression in mice. In this case, the gene can be detected at high levels in the notochord and the tail bud only before E10, which corresponds to CS12 in humans. This suggests that *HLXB9* might affect early notochordal development, whereas other genes downstream in the *HLXB9* pathway might act in later stages, when the formation of the vertebrae is completed. Human HLXB9 expression was also found during the development of the foregut, including the pharynx, esophagus, and stomach. The situation in mouse is quite different, because the gene is detectable in also the midgut or the hindgut, sites not identified in the human expression pattern, even after a very detailed examination. These differences have also been pointed out in other studies (Yamaguchi et al., 1999; Fougerousse et al., 2000) and they might be important in the understanding of the phenotypic features seen in the *Hlxb9* knockout mice compared with what is observed in humans.

Finally, the analysis of the *Hlxb9*$^{-/-}$ mice demonstrated defects affecting the motor neurons (Arber et al., 1999; Thaler et al., 1999), a defect never described in patients (but *HLXB9* expression has been seen in human motor neurons during the development of the spinal cord). It is important to point out that the affected neurons in the mutant mice are not restricted to the sacral region but instead involve the spinal cord at all levels. It seems that the use of *Hlxb9* mouse models to study the human disease might be somewhat limited, given the differences in the phenotypes derived by the lack of *HLXB9* expression, in particular for those defects affecting the sacral region. Similar examples with other genes and the corresponding human diseases have already been described (e.g., with the *Shh* knockout mice in holoprosencephaly). This means that although the differences in the expression and consequent function of the mouse compared with those of the human gene might be relevant in understanding all the aspects of the disease, the role of *HLXB9* in human development might be

Table 54–3. Patients in Three Groups According to Their Sacral Phenotype, Analyzed for the Presence of Mutations Affecting *HLXB9*

Patient	Sacral Phenotype (Category 4)	HB9 Associated Anomalies	HB9 Mutation
GROUP 1: CURRARINO SYNDROME			
1	Hemisacrum	ARM with rectoperineal fistula, anterior meningocele, tethered cord, presacral teratoma	HB9 del
2	Hemisacrum	ARM with rectoperineal fistula, anterior meningocele	384delG exon 1
11	Hemisacrum	ARM with rectoperineal fistula, anterior meningocele, tethered cord, hydromyelia	R295W exon 3/a
15	Hemisacrum	ARM with rectoperineal fistula, anterior meningocele	None
19	Hemisacrum	ARM without fistula, hypospadia, Down syndrome	None
59	Hemisacrum	ARM with rectoperineal fistula, little bladder capacity	$858+1G \rightarrow A$ exon 2
60	Hemisacrum	ARM with rectoperineal fistula	T248S exon 2
66	Hemisacrum	ARM with rectoperineal fistula, presacral teratoma	None
69	Hemisacrum	ARM, presacral mass, tethered cord, rectal duplication, bifid clitoris, lipoma of conus, holoprosencephaly	HB9 del
70	Hemisacrum	ARM, presacral mass	HB9 del

Patient	Sacral Phenotype (Category 3)	Associated Anomalies	HB9 Mutation
GROUP 2: CAUDAL REGRESSION SYNDROME (CRS) + ARM + SACRAL HYPODEVELOPMENT			
3	CRS; agenesis of coccix and one sacral vertebra, SR = 0.43	ARM with rectobulbar fistula, lipoma of filum, hydromyelia, vertebral anomalies (L3-L4), syndactyly of 2°-3° toes	None
4	CRS, agenesis of coccix and one sacral vertebra, SR = 0.70	ARM with rectobulbar fistula, bilateral vescicoureteral reflux, vertebral anomalies (L2-L5)	None
	CRS, SR = 0.55	ARM with rectoprostatic fistula, lipoma of terminal filum, hydromielia, tethered cord, intraatrial defect, pulmonary artery stenosis, syndactyly of 3°-4° fingers	None
14	CRS, SR = 0.45	ARM with rectovesical fistula	None
16	CRS, agenesis of coccix and one sacral vertebra, SR = 0.35	ARM with rectocloacal fistula, duplicity of uterus and vagina	None
18	CRS	ARM with rectobulbar fistula, posterior meningocele	None
24	CRS, SR = 0.24	ARM with rectocloacal fistula, lipoma of terminal filum, tethered cord, right ureterocele, bilateral congenital club foot, intraabdominal testis	None
25	CRS, agenesis of coccix and one sacral vertebra, SR = 0.54	ARM with rectobulbar fistula, intraventricular defect	None
29	CRS, agenesis of coccix and three sacral vertebrae, SR = 0.33	ARM with rectoperineal fistula, high medullary cone (D11), vertebral fusion (L4-L5), annular pancreas, inferior limb arthrogryposis, bilateral congenital clubfoot	None
30	CRS, agenesis of coccix and one sacral vertebra, SR = 0.58	ARM with rectocloacal fistula, tethered cord, L5 schisis, bicornate uterus	None
31	CRS, SR = 0.54	ARM with rectovestibular fistula, macrocrania	None
33	CRS, SR = 0.55	ARM with rectovestibular fistula, thickened filum terminale, tethered cord, hemangiomatosis	None
35	CRS, SR = 0.56	ARM with rectoperineal fistula, mild atrophy of cerebral cortex, hypoparathyroidism	None
36	CRS, agenesis of coccix, SR = 0.54	ARM with rectobulbar fistula, low medullary cone (L4), open foramen ovale, right hydronephrosis, anomalies of cervical spine and 1° right rib	None
68	CRS, SR = 0.27	ARM with rectocloacal fistula, monolateral renal dysgenesis	None

Patient	Sacral Phenotype (Categories 1 and 2)	Associated Anomalies	HB9 Mutation
GROUP 3: TOTAL SACRAL AGENESIS + ARM			
9	CRS, complete sacral agenesis	ARM with rectoprostatic fistula, high medullary cone (D11), hydromyelia, right multicystic kidney, left megaureter, right hernia and undescended testis	None
20	CRS, agenesis of sacral vertebrae and one lumbar vertebra	ARM with rectobulbar fistula, bilateral congenital clubfoot, monolateral renal dysplasia, hypospadia	None

ARM, anorectal malformation.

more complex than what is observed in the animal model. A more complete understanding of the pathway in which *HLXB9* directly interacts will be the most accurate way to unravel its role in the pathogenesis of CS and in human sacral development.

REFERENCES

Arber S, Han B, Mendelsohn M, Smith M, Jessell TM, Sockanathan S (1999). Requirement for the homeobox gene Hb9 in the consolidation of motor neuron identity. *Neuron* 23: 659–674.

Belloni E, Martucciello G, Verderio D, Ponti E, Seri M, Jasonni V, Torre M, Ferrari M, Tsui LC, Scherer SW (2000). Involvement of the HLXB9 homeobox gene in Currarino syndrome. *Am J Hum Genet* 66:312–319.

Belloni E, Muenke M, Roessler E, Traverso G, Siegel-Bartelt J, Frumkin A, Mitchell HF, Donis-Keller H, Helms C, Hing AV, et al. (1996). Identification of Sonic hedgehog as a candidate gene responsible for holoprosencephaly. *Nat Genet* 14: 353–356.

Belot J, Lepennetier F (1969). *Anatomie Radiographique du squelette normal.* Atlas. Amédée Legrand & C. Editeurs, Paris.

Blery M, Chagnon S, Pennecot GF, Philippe JF (1983). Dorsolumbosacral agenesis. A propos of 2 cases. Review of the literature. *J Radiol* 64: 171–176.

Brais B, Bouchard J-P, Xie X-G, Rochefort DL, Chretien N, Tome FMS, Lafreniere FMS, Rommens JM, Uyama E, Nohira O, et al. (1998). Short GCG expansion in the PABP2 gene cause oculopharingeal muscular dystrophy. *Nat Genet* 18: 164–167.

Cama A, Palmieri A, Capra V, Piatelli GL, Ravegnani M, Fondelli P (1996). Multidisciplinary management of caudal regression syndrome (26 cases). *Eur J Pediatr Surg* 6 S1:44–45.

Chiang C, Litingtung Y, Lee E, Young KE, Corden JL, Westphal H, Beachy PA (1996). Cyclopia and defective axial patterning in mice lacking Sonic hedgehog gene function. *Nature* 383: 407–413.

Currarino G, Coln D, Votteler T (1981). Triad of anorectal, sacral, and presacral anomalies. *AJR Am J Roentgenol* 137: 395–398.

Denton JR (1982). The association of congenital spinal anomalies with imperforate anus. *Clin Orthop Relat Res* 162: 91–98.

Diel J, Ortiz O, Losada RA, Price DB, Hayt MW, Katz DS (2001). The sacrum: pathologic spectrum, multi-modality imaging, and subspeciality approach. *Radiographics* 21: 83–104.

Duhamel B (1961). From the mermaid to anal imperforation: the syndrome of caudal regression. *Arch Dis Child* 36: 152–155.

Fougerousse F, Bullen PJ, Herasse M, Lindsay S, Richard I, Wilson D, Suel L, Durand M, Robson S, Abitbol M, et al. (2000). Human-mouse differences in the embryonic expression patterns of developmental control genes and disease genes. *Hum Mol Genet* 9: 165–173.

Friedmann W, Henrich W, Dimer JS, Bassir C, Kunze J, Dudenhausen JW (1997). Prenatal diagnosis of Currarino triad. *Eur J Ultrasound* 6: 191–196.

Goodman FR, Mundlos S, Muragaki Y, Donnai D, Giovannucci-Uzielli ML, Lapi E, Majewski F, McGaughran J, McKeown C, Reardon W, et al. (1997). Synpolydactyly phenotypes correlate with size of expansion in HOXD13 poly-alanine tract. *PNAS* 94: 7458–7463.

Hagan DM, Ross AJ, Strachan T, Lynch SA, Ruiz-Perez V, Wang YM, Scambler P, Custard E, Reardon W, Hassan S, et al. (2000). Mutation analysis and embryonic expression of the HLXB9 Currarino syndrome gene. *Am J Hum Genet* 66: 1504–1515.

Harrison KA, Druey KM, Deguchi Y, Tuscano JM, Kehrl JH (1994). A novel human homeobox gene distantly related to proboscipedia is expressed in lymphoid and pancreatic tissues. *J Biol Chem* 269: 19968–19975.

Harrison KA, Thaler J, Pfaff SL, Gu H, Kehrl JH (1999). Pancreas dorsal lobe agenesis and abnormal islets of Langerhans in Hlxb9-deficient mice. *Nat Genet* 23: 71–75.

Kalitzki M (1965). Congenital malformations and diabetes. *Lancet* 2: 641–642.

Kallen B, Winberg I (1974). Caudal mesoderm pattern of anomalies: from renal agenesis to sirenomelia. *Teratology* 9: 99–112.

Kalter H (1993). Case reports of malformations associated with maternal diabetes: history and critique. *Clin Genet* 43: 174–179.

Lenz W, Kucera J (1967). L'étiologie de la régression caudale (agénésie du sacrum). *Med Hyg* 25: 241–243.

Lerone M, Bolino A, Martucciello G (1997). The genetics of anorectal malformations: a complex matter. *Semin Pediatr Surg* 6: 1–11.

Li H, Arber S, Jessel TM, Edlund H (1999). Selective agenesis of the dorsal pancreas in mice lacking homeobox gene Hlxb9. *Nat Genet* 23: 67–70.

Lynch SA, Wang Y, Strachan T, Burn J, Lindsay S (2000). Autosomal dominant sacral agenesis: Currarino syndrome. *J Med Genet* 37: 561–566.

Lynch SA, Bond PM, Copp AJ, Kirwan WO, Nour S, Balling R, Mariman E, Burn J, Strachan T (1995). A gene for autosomal dominant sacral agenesis maps to the holoprosencephaly region at 7q36. *Nat Genet* 11: 93–95.

Mihmanli I, Kurugoglu S, Kantarci F, Kanberoglu K (2001). Dorsolumbosacral agenesis. *Pediatr Radiol* 31: 286–288.

Mundlos S, Otto F, Mundlos C, Mulliken JB, Aylsworth AS, Albright S, Lindhout D, Cole WG, Henn W, Knoll JH, et al. (1997). Mutations involving the transcription factor CBFA1 cause cleidocranial dysplasia. *Cell* 89: 773–779.

Naidich TP, Zimmerman RA, McLone DG, Raybaud CA, Altman NR, Braffman BH (1996). Congenital anomalies of the spine and spinal cord. In: *Magnetic Resonance Imaging of the Brain and Spine, 2nd Edition*. Atlas SW (ed.) Lippincott-Raven, Philadelphia, pp. 1265–1337.

Norum J, Wist E, Bostad L (1991). Incomplete Currarino syndrome with a presacral leiomyosarcoma. *Acta Oncol* 30: 987–988.

Pang D (1993). Sacral agenesis and caudal spinal cord malformations. *Neurosurgery* 32: 755–779.

Passarge E, Lenz W (1966). Syndrome of caudal regression in infants of diabetic mothers: observations of further cases. *Pediatrics* 37: 672–675.

Pena A (1995). Anorectal malformations. *Semin Pediatr Surg* 4: 35–47.

Renshaw TS (1978). Sacral agenesis. *J Bone Joint Surg* 60-A: 373–383.

Riggs AC, Tanizawa Y, Aoki M, Wasson J, Ferrer J, Rabin DU, Vaxillaire M, Froguel P, Gough S, Liu L, et al. (1995). Characterization of the LIM/homeodomain gene islet-1 and single nucleotide screening in NIDDM. *Diabetes* 44: 689–694.

Ross AJ, Ruiz-Perez V, Wang Y, Hagan DM, Scherer SW, Lynch SA, Lindsay S, Custard E, Belloni E, Wilson DI, et al. (1998). A homeobox gene, HLXB9, is the major locus for dominantly inherited sacral agenesis. *Nat Genet* 20: 358–361.

Saha MS, Miles RR, Grainger RM (1997). Dorsal-ventral patterning during neural induction in Xenopus: assessment of spinal cord regionalization with xHB9, a marker for the motor neuron region. *Dev Biol* 187: 209–223.

Seri M, Martucciello G, Paleari L, Bolino A, Priolo M, Salemi G, Forabosco P, Caroli F, Silengo M, Zelante L, et al. (1999). Exclusion of the Sonic Hedgehog gene as responsible for Currarino syndrome and anorectal malformations with sacral hypodevelopment. *Hum Genet* 104: 108–110.

Stevenson RE, Jones KL, Paelan MC (1986). Vascular steal: the pathogenetic mechanism producing sirenomelia and associated defects of the viscera and soft tissues. *Pediatrics* 78: 451–457.

Tander B, Baskin D, Bulut M (1999). A case of incomplete Currarino triad with malignant transformation. *Pediatr Surg Int* 15: 409–410.

Thaler J, Harrison K, Sharma K, Lettieri K, Kehrl J, Pfaff SL (1999). Active suppression of interneuron programs within developing motor neurons revealed by analysis of homeodomain factor Hb9. *Neuron* 23: 675–687.

Torre M, Martucciello G, Jasonni V (2001). Sacral development in anorectal malformations and in normal population. *Pediatr Radiol* 31: 858–862.

Tortoti Donati P, Rossi A, Cama A (2000). Spinal dysraphism: a review of neuroradiological features with embryological correlations and proposal for a new classification. *Neuroradiology* 42: 471–491.

Vargas FR, Roessler E, Gaudenz K, Belloni E, Whitehead AS, Kirke PN, Mills JL, Hooper G, Stevenson RE, Cordeiro I, et al. (1998). *Hum Genet* 102: 387–392.

Wilmshurst JM, Kelly R, Borzyskowski M (1999). Presentation and outcome of sacral agenesis: 20 years' experience. *Dev Med Child Neurol* 41: 806–812.

Yamaguchi TP, Bradley A, McMahon AP, Jones S (1999). A Wnt5a pathway underlies outgrowth of multiple structures in the vertebrate embryo. *Development* 126: 1211–1223.

55 | *EYA1* and the Branchio-Oto-Renal Syndrome

ROBERT T. MOY AND RICHARD L. MAAS

Mutation of *EYA1* is an established cause of branchio-oto-renal (BOR) syndrome (OMIM 113650). This gene, which belongs to a highly conserved family of transcriptional coactivators, is thought to function through its recruitment to specific enhancers by members of the Six family of homeoproteins. Thus, *EYA1* heterozygosity is currently thought to underlie the BOR phenotype through an inability to activate transcription from Six-responsive elements to appropriate levels. The resultant phenotype typically includes deafness with associated otic, renal, and branchial abnormalities, though highly variable expressivity often means that all three BOR characteristics are rarely found in a single patient.

BOR syndrome is an autosomal-dominant developmental disorder typically characterized by branchial clefts, hearing loss, and renal abnormalities. Although incomplete penetrance and variable expressivity have made it difficult to establish its true prevalence, BOR syndrome is thought to be rare, with an approximate incidence of 1:40,000. Furthermore, BOR syndrome was implicated as the cause of deafness in approximately 2% of congenitally deaf children (Fraser et al., 1980). First characterized by Melnick and colleagues in 1976, BOR syndrome has been known by a variety of names, including *Melnick-Fraser syndrome, branchio-oto (BO) syndrome, branchio-oto-ureteral (BOU) syndrome, preauricular pit cervical fistula hearing loss syndrome, and earpits-deafness syndrome.* Of these, *BOR* and *BO* are the most commonly used terms, with BOR relating to cases in which renal anomalies occur in at least some family members and BO to cases in which renal anomalies are not present. However, while it is certain that some cases of BO are variants of BOR syndrome, others are genetically distinct. Another related syndrome, BOU, is often regarded as a form of BOR, although it is unknown whether BOU maps to the BOR locus. Indeed, BOR syndrome may be genetically heterogeneous: while a preponderance of BO and BOR syndrome cases are associated with mutations in the *EYA1* locus at 8q13.3, others resembling BOR syndrome are not.

Loss-of-function mutations and deletions of the *EYA1* gene, a homolog of the *Drosophila eyes absent (eya)* gene, are an established cause of BOR syndrome, and *Eya1*$^{+/-}$ mutant mice display a phenotype which highly resembles that expressed in BOR syndrome patients. Hence, BOR syndrome is an autosomal-dominant disorder that results from haploinsufficiency for *EYA1*. *EYA1* encodes a putative transcriptional cofactor and is part of a family of genes whose members have been found in organisms ranging from humans to plants. Structurally, Eya proteins consist of two conserved domains, a relatively divergent N-terminal proline-, serine-, and threonine-rich (PST) domain and a highly conserved C-terminal Eya domain. These domains appear to encode a transcriptional activation module and a protein–protein interaction module, respectively. Eya proteins are thus thought to act as transcriptional coactivators, with other DNA-binding transcription factors recruiting the transcriptional activation activity of the PST domain through interactions with the Eya domain. In this chapter, we review the phenotypic features of BOR syndrome and explore how *EYA1* mutations may cause the BOR phenotype, drawing on information from both human genetic studies and developmental investigations in *Eya1*-deficient model organisms, such as the mouse and fly.

STRUCTURE AND FUNCTION OF *EYA1*

eyes absent (eya), named after its mutant phenotype in *Drosophila*, was first discovered by positional cloning (Bonini et al., 1993). In contrast to the single *eya* gene in *Drosophila*, four *Eya* family members, designated *Eya1–4*, are known to exist in the mouse and human. There are single known family members in *Caenorhabditis elegans, Xenopus*, zebrafish, *Fugu*, squid, rice, and *Arabidopsis*, though additional family members probably exist in *Xenopus*, zebrafish, and *Fugu* (Sahly et al., 1999; Borsani et al., 1999; Takeda et al., 1999; David et al., 2001). Three members exist in chick (Borsani et al., 1999). Eya family members are frequently expressed in tissues undergoing differentiation, making it plausible that Eya expression subserves similar functions in disparate organisms.

EYA1 Encodes Several Splice Variants with Different Coding Potentials

The human *EYA1* gene is located at 8q13.3 and consists of 16 exons spaced over 156 kb, with introns ranging in size from 0.1 to 27.5 kb (Abdelhak et al., 1997a). Three *EYA1* splice isoforms, *EYA1A, EYA1B*, and *EYA1C*, have been identified which differ in their 5′ ends. *EYA1A* is 3.8 kb and has at least two distinct 3′ untranslated regions (UTRs) (Abdelhak et al., 1997a). *EYA1B* differs from *EYA1A* in that it contains a 128 bp insertion that creates a stop codon just after the proposed start codon for *EYA1A*. Thus, it has been proposed that an alternative start codon exists for *EYA1B*. *EYA1C* is similar to *EYA1B* but has an additional 584 bp replacement of the 5′ UTR. Thus, EYA1B and EYA1C share the same coding potential, while the N terminus of *EYA1A* differs from that of the other isoforms (Abdelhak et al., 1997b). Little is known about how these isoforms differ in function or how their expression is controlled, although their existence implies that EYA1 function may be partly regulated at the level of alternative splicing (Fig. 55–1).

The Structure of EYA1 Suggests a Function as a Transcriptional Coactivator

EYA1A is a 559–amino acid protein with a mass of 61.2 kDa. Sequence analysis reveals five potential *N*-glycosylation sites, four potential protein kinase C sites, and a single potential site for cAMP-dependent protein kinase C phosphorylation (Abdelhak et al., 1997a). There are also two mitogen-activated protein kinase (MAPK) sites, which modulate Eya function in the fly (Hsiao et al., 2001). Structurally, Eya family members have two distinct domains, a PST domain and a highly conserved Eya domain. The functional conservation of at least two of these isoforms is demonstrated by the ability of murine *Eya2* to functionally restore eyes in an *eya* mutant background (Bonini et al., 1997) (Fig. 55–2).

The Eya Domain Mediates Protein–Protein Interactions

Although Eya proteins contain no previously identified motifs, the identity between Eya family members is especially high (70%–88%) within the 271–amino acid C-terminal Eya domain. The highly conserved nature of the Eya domain over a variety of species suggests a conserved role, probably as a region of protein–protein interactions. A potential structural homology between this domain and the haloacid dehalogenase-like hydrolase family of proteins exists (PFAM Swiss prot: Q99502, http://pfam.wustl.edu/cgi-bin/getswisspfam?key=Q99502), though the significance of this is unknown.

The Eya domain acts as a site of protein–protein interactions in vertebrates and invertebrates. Proteins encoded by the *Six* and *Dach* gene families as well as the Gα$_i$ and Gα$_z$ G-protein subunits bind this domain in yeast two-hybrid and glutathione-*S*-transferase (GST) pull-

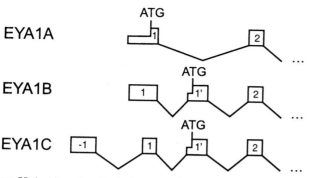

Figure 55–1. Alternate splice isoforms of *EYA1*. The N terminus of the protein encoded by *EYA1A* consists of exons 1 and 2, with a start codon located in exon 1. The protein encoded by *EYA1B* utilizes exons 1 and 2, along with exon 1′. Exon 1′ results in a frameshift from the start codon located in exon 1. It is hypothesized that an alternate start sequence, located in exon 1′, is utilized in *EYA1B* and *EYA1C*. The N terminus of the protein encoded by *EYA1C* consists of exons 1′ and 2 and a shortened region of exon 1. Additionally, an exon, denoted −1, is utilized in this isoform.

down assays (Chen et al., 1997; Pignoni et al., 1997; Fan et al., 2000). While Six and Dach proteins bind to Eya domains of diverse Eya family members, the Gα subunits have thus far been examined only for interactions with Eya2. Whether these proteins can bind Eya1 simultaneously is unknown, though the size of the Eya domain suggests this possibility. The importance of the Eya domain and its interactions in vivo is demonstrated by missense mutations in this region, which are associated with BOR syndrome (Abdelhak et al., 1997b). Recent data have demonstrated that these missense mutations interfere with Six1 and Six2 binding and produce a loss-of-function phenotype (Buller et al., 2001). Further highlighting the importance of Eya protein complexes, coexpression of either *dac* or *so* with *eya* results in a synergistic enhancement in the ability of Eya to induce ectopic eye formation in flies (Chen et al., 1997; Pignoni et al., 1997).

The PST Domain Is a Transcriptional Activation Domain
Despite their relatively high content of proline, serine, and threonine, the PST domains of Eya family members are not highly conserved. While The PST domains of Eya1 and -2 act as transcriptional activators, the PST domain of Eya3 activates transcription less efficiently (Xu et al., 1997b). These differences may provide a mechanism of selective transcriptional control through the divergent abilities of the

PST domains of different Eya family members to activate transcription in different contexts. Consistent with this model, differences in the ability of Eya1, -2, and -3 to synergize with Six family members in the activation of transcription from a Six-responsive reporter construct have been reported (Ohto et al., 1999). Although it has been suggested that the PST domain forms β-pleated sheets similar to those found in the yeast acidic activators GAL4 and GCN4, the exact nature of transcriptional activation by the PST domain is unknown (Leuther et al., 1993; Van Hoy et al., 1993).

The Pattern of *Eya1* Expression Suggests Its Importance in Multiple Developmental Processes

Eya1 Expression in the Mouse and Human
The mouse has served as the major source of information concerning mammalian *Eya1* expression during embryogenesis. In the mouse, *Eya1* expression is found in the brain, cranial placodes (lens, otic, nasal, Rathke's pouch, trigeminal, and all other ectodermal placodes and their derivatives), and areas of inductive tissue interactions, including the kidney primordium, presomitic mesoderm, branchial arches, gut, genital tubercle, tendon, dorsal root ganglia, dorsal neural tube, floorplate, vomeronasal organ, tooth germ, and whisker follicle (Xu et al., 1997a). Consistent with current models of Eya function, *Eya1* expression overlaps with that of *Pax* and *Six* family members.

As in the mouse, human *EYA1* is expressed in the fetal brain and kidney, the latter consistent with a role in kidney formation. Adult expression of *EYA1* is found in heart, brain, and skeletal muscle but not lung, kidney, or pancreas (Abdelhak et al., 1997a). The role of EYA1 in the adult human is currently unknown, and our understanding of *EYA1* expression in humans is incomplete. However, the developmental expression of *Eya1* in the mouse is sufficient to explain the constellation of affected organs in BOR syndrome.

EYA1: Function

The combination of a large, highly conserved protein-binding domain with a transcriptional activation domain suggests that Eya1 functions as a transcriptional coactivator. In such a model, a DNA-binding protein recruits the PST activation domain of Eya into proximity with DNA via interactions with the Eya domain. The synergistic increase in the ability of the DNA-binding, homeodomain-containing protein So to form ectopic eyes when coexpressed with Eya supports the *in vivo* functional relevance of this model for modular transcriptional activation. Further support for an Eya1 coactivator function derives from the finding that Eya1, -2, and -3 can dramatically increase the activa-

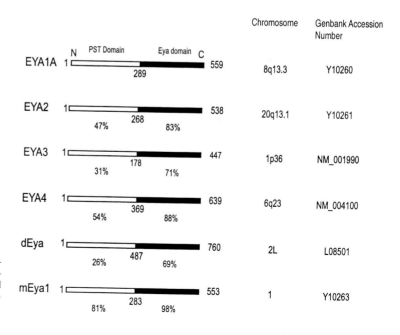

Figure 55–2. EYA1A is a member of a highly conserved family of proteins and consists of two domains: a loosely conserved N-terminal PST domain, which can act as a transcriptional activator, and a highly conserved Eya domain, which can act as a site of protein–protein interactions. Identity between the Eya and PST domains was calculated using BLAST2.

tion of gene expression by Six1, -2, -4, and -5 (Ohto et al., 1999; Fan et al., 2000). Since four known *Eya* genes exist in mouse and human, a combinatorial model of transcriptional activation by Six and Eya family members is possible. In this combinatorial model, different DNA-binding proteins could bind a variety of Eya proteins, with each combination subserving a separate function. This model would provide an elegant mechanism for the activation of selective sets of genes in a highly regulatable manner by a small number of proteins.

Control of Eya Function at the Protein Level

Nuclear Localization. Unlike *Drosophila* Eya, mammalian Eya family members appear to lack nuclear localization signals. Thus, Eya1 may be cytoplasmic, though nuclear translocation can be induced by cotransfection with Six family members (Ohto et al., 1999). As might therefore be expected, both nuclear and cytoplasmic Eya1 are found in developing tissues (Purcell, 2001). Six-mediated nuclear translocation can be blocked by activated $G\alpha_z$ and $G\alpha_i$ G-protein subunits, which bind and thus sequester Eya2 in the cytoplasm (Fan et al., 2000). Thus, several systems may control the nuclear translocation of Eya and modulate Eya function. It is not known whether EYA1 function is controlled in a similar manner, but the high degree of similarity between human and murine Eya1 suggests that this is likely.

Eya Function Is Regulated Through Phosphorylation. Phosphorylation is a common form of regulation at the protein level. Eya contains two MAPK sites, which are located just N-terminal to the Eya domain. These sites are conserved in *Drosophila*, human, and mouse Eya1. In *Drosophila*, these MAPK sites can modulate Eya function as SαA mutations that destroy the MAPK consensus sites and decrease the ability of Eya to induce ectopic eyes. Conversely, S→E or S→D mutations, which mimic phosphorylation, increase the rate of induction of eyes by Eya. This phosphorylation can be mediated by extracellular signal–regulated kinase (ERK), Janus kinase (JNK), p38a, or p38b (Hsiao et al., 2001). The mechanism by which phosphorylation leads to increased eye induction is currently unknown, as is whether this regulation applies to human EYA1. Nonetheless, the conservation of the MAPK sites through mouse and human suggests that phosphorylation by MAPK may be a general mechanism of Eya regulation.

EYA1 Function Is Dependant on Protein–Protein Interactions

As a transcriptional cofactor, the function of EYA1 is determined by the proteins with which it interacts. Several families of EYA1-interacting proteins are known. These interacting proteins are of importance to BOR syndrome as they define the function of EYA1 in vivo and, and in principle, their respective genes are likely to represent potential genetic modifiers of the BOR phenotype.

sine oculis (so)/Six: Interacting Proteins Which Can Direct EYA1 to Promoter Sequences. There are currently six known Six family members in the mouse and three known members in the fly. *Six* genes encode DNA-binding proteins containing two conserved regions, a Six domain and a Six homeodomain. Six family members can interact with the Eya domain through the Six domain (Pignoni et al., 1997; Ohto et al., 1999). The Six homeodomain binds DNA and potentially directs Six-associated Eya family members to specific promoter sequences. Consistent with a hypothesized role as an Eya-interacting protein, Six family members have expression patterns which overlap with Eya expression (Xu et al., 1997b; Ohto et al., 1998, 1999). Mice null for *Six4* and *Six5* have been made. While *Six4* mutant mice have no detectable phenotype, *Six5* mutant mice display cataracts (Sarkar et al., 2000; Klesert et al., 2000; Ozaki et al., 2001). Six3 is believed to function during oculogenesis and neural development as expression of *Six3* can lead to the formation of ectopic lenses and ectopic optic vesicle-like structures in *Medaka* and mouse, respectively (Oliver et al., 1996; Loosli et al., 1999; Lagutin et al., 2001). In humans, mutations in the homeodomain of SIX3 are associated with holoprosencephaly at the HPE2 locus at 2p21 (Wallis et al., 1999). *SIX1* and *SIX2* are the most relevant *Six* genes to BOR syndrome as they are expressed in the developing ear and kidney.

dachshund (dac)/Dach: The Possibility of Multiple Coactivators in EYA1 Protein Complexes. There are currently two known *dac* homologs in mice and one in humans (Hammond et al., 1998; Kozmik et al., 1999; Caubit et al., 1999; Davis et al., 1999, 2001b). Like Eya family members, Dach contains no known DNA-binding domains or specific DNA-binding activity, though they share a region of homology with the ski/sno family of transcriptional cofactors. Thus, Dach family members are also thought to function as transcriptional cofactors. In vertebrates, *Dach1* is expressed in the eye, limb, and CNS, including the otic vesicle (Caubit et al., 1999; Davis et al., 1999). *Dach1* mutant mice are perinatal-lethal due to a failure to suckle and exhibit cyanosis and respiratory distress, though no anatomical abnormalities have been found (Davis et al., 2001a). The proteins encoded by the *Drosophila* homologs of *Dach1* and *Eya1*, *dac* and *eya*, interact in directed yeast two-hybrid and GST pulldown assays. Functionally, coexpression of *eya* and *dac* leads to a synergistic increase in the induction of ectopic eyes relative to that produced by *eya* or *dac* overexpression alone (Shen and Mardon, 1997).

$G\alpha_z$ and $G\alpha_i$ G-Protein Subunits: A Possible Mechanism for the Cytoplasmic Sequestration of EYA1. Mechanisms which regulate the function of other Eya family members are probably also utilized to control EYA1 function. Recently, Eya2 was found to interact with the $G\alpha_z$ and $G\alpha_i$ G-protein subunits. $G\alpha_z$ and $G\alpha_i$ subunits, which mimic activated $G\alpha_z$ and $G\alpha_i$ but not wild-type $G\alpha_z$ and $G\alpha_i$, can bind and sequester Eya2 in the cytoplasm, blocking the ability of Eya2 to act as a transcriptional cofactor (Fan et al., 2000). Thus, G-protein signaling may modulate Eya2 signaling. Although whether EYA1 can bind the α subunits of activated G proteins is currently unknown, $G\alpha_z$ plays roles in neurotransmission and platelet activation while $G\alpha_i$ plays roles in multiple systems (for review, see Ho and Wong, 2001).

EYA1 FUNCTIONS IN AN EVOLUTIONARILY CONSERVED GENETIC PATHWAY THAT CONTROLS THE DEVELOPMENT OF MULTIPLE ORGANS

EYA1 Functions as Part of a Highly Conserved Genetic Network

The nonlethal eye phenotype of *eyes absent* flies as well as the ability of ectopic *eya* expression to induce ectopic eyes have allowed for powerful epistasis analyses of the pathway in which *eya* functions. *Pax6* (see Chapter 62) and one of its two *Drosophila* homologs, *eyeless* (*ey*), are conserved genes acting during early mammalian and insect eye formation. Evidence that these genes act near the top of the genetic pathway controlling eye formation is provided by experiments demonstrating that misexpression of *Pax6* results in the formation of ectopic eyes in *Drosophila* and *Xenopus* (Halder et al., 1995; Chow et al., 1999). Furthermore, signaling upstream of *ey/Pax6* is conserved and the two murine *Pax6* promoters can partially reproduce the expression induced by the *ey* promoter in the fly (Xu et al., 1999a). Thus, *Pax6* exists in a pathway which is highly conserved in organisms across metazoa, from fly to human.

In *Drosophila*, *eya* mutations can phenocopy mutations in *eyeless*, resulting in apoptotic loss of eye imaginal disc cells (Bonini et al., 1993). Several lines of evidence demonstrate that Eya family members function downstream of Pax family members. First, *ey* is expressed before *eya* and *so* (Halder et al., 1998). Second, *ey* can induce *eya* and *so* independently during the formation of ectopic eyes, and *eyeless* does not elicit the formation of ectopic eyes in *eya* and *so* mutant lines (Halder et al., 1998; Chen et al., 1999). Finally, *so* and *eya* are not expressed in *ey* mutant flies, while *eyeless* is expressed in both *eya* and *so* mutant lines (Halder et al., 1998). These results lead to a model in which *eya* and *so* function together downstream of *ey* to mediate critical functions in eye formation.

A role for a *Drosophila* bone morphogenetic protein (BMP) homolog (see Chapter 24), *decapentaplegic* (*dpp*), in the control of *eya* expression was first noticed when it was found that *ey* can only induce *so* and *eya* in portions of the imaginal disc which express *dpp*.

This was further demonstrated by overexpression of *dpp*, which increases the area of *so*, *dac*, and *eya* expression (Chen et al., 1999). Thus, *ey* and *dpp* function upstream of *eya*. The highly conserved nature of Pax signaling suggests that Pax family members and BMP family members act upstream of *EYA1* to regulate *EYA1* expression. Consistent with the *Drosophila* data, *Pax6* mutant *Small eye* (*Sey/Sey*) mice show reduced *Eya1* expression in the lens, nasal placodes, and the pituitary anlage Rathke's pouch (Xu et al., 1997a).

The *Pax-Eya-Six* Network Has Been Recruited for Use in the Development of Several Tissues

The Six-Eya system is utilized by other *Pax* genes (see Chapter 59). For example, in the ear and kidney, instead of *Pax6*, *Pax2* is required for organogenesis (Torres et al., 1995). Consistent with a role upstream of *Eya1*, *Pax2* expression is unchanged in *Eya1* mutant animals. Similarly, otic expression of both *Pax8* and *Pax2* is unaffected in an *Eya1* null background (Xu et al., 1999b). The *Pax-Eya-Six* genetic network is also conserved in the chick, where Eya2 can synergize with Six1 or Dach2 under Pax3 in the expression of myogenic genes (Heanue et al., 1999).

Genes Acting Downstream of *EYA1*

While the function of EYA1 suggests multiple downstream targets, currently, *Dach1* and *-2*, *Six1* and *-2*, and glia-derived neurotrophic factor (*GDNF*; see Chapter 35) are the best candidates for genes whose expression, and hence function, reside downstream of Eya family members (Xu et al., 1999b). These genes do not form linear genetic cascades but integrated networks of action. In *Drosophila*, *dac* is downstream of the So-Eya cassette but forms a positive feedback loop to regulate these genes (Chen et al., 1997). In vertebrates, *Dach2* can induce *Pax3* expression (Heanue et al., 1999). Surprisingly, *Dach1* expression is not decreased in the otic or optic structures of the *Eya1* mutant mouse (Heanue et al., 2002). Likewise, *dac*, *so*, and *eya* can also feedback to positively regulate *ey* expression (Chen et al., 1997; Pignoni et al., 1997) (Fig. 55–3).

CLINICAL DESCRIPTION OF BOR SYNDROME

The major diagnostic criteria for BOR syndrome are preauricular pits, branchial fistulas, hearing loss, and renal hypoplasia. Coincident occurrence of all of these anomalies in an individual is relatively rare, so the coincidence of these characteristics among family members is often sufficient for the BOR syndrome diagnosis. In addition, several other tissues may be affected. The cranial nerves, especially the facial nerve, are often abnormal. Skeletal, thyroid, and parathyroid anomalies are rare but relevant as the mouse model displays these abnormalities. Variable expressivity can result in not only different organs being affected but also asymmetrical severity within affected systems.

Prevalence of BOR Syndrome

BOR syndrome is a rare disorder whose phenotypic variance hinders attempts to quantify its prevalence in the general population. Using

the presence of preauricular pits as a diagnostic sign of BO and BOR, 19 of 421 profoundly deaf, white schoolchildren in Montreal were determined to have BO or BOR (Fraser et al., 1980). Assuming that half of these children have renal anomalies and that profound deafness occurs at a rate of 1:1000 in the general population, a prevalence of 1:40,000 was extrapolated for BOR syndrome. This number is a broad estimate as only 16% of BOR patients display profound deafness (Chen et al., 1995). Furthermore, this number was generated from a single racial category in a small geographic area. In fact, the prevalence of preauricular pits varies widely between ethnic groups. In blacks, preauricular pits occur at a rate of 5.2% compared to under 1% for whites and 0.1% for Asian Indians (Bergsma, 1979). Whether these differing rates of preauricular pits are manifestations of a higher rate of BOR syndrome in certain populations is unknown. Preauricular pits are also more common in newborn females than in males (2:1), though there is no difference between the sexes in the incidence of BOR syndrome (Buyse, 1990). Thus, while the best available estimates place the incidence of BOR syndrome at 1:40,000, the actual number may be very different.

Penetrance and Expressivity of BOR Syndrome

Although the expression of certain phenotypic manifestations of BOR syndrome varies, the overall penetrance of BOR syndrome is high (99%), with almost all known carriers showing some characteristic of the disorder (Fraser et al., 1980). Expressivity, though, can vary greatly. This results in a variety of organs being affected with differing severity and a range of phenotypes from outwardly normal to lethal, due to bilateral renal agenesis or severe renal dysplasia. Furthermore, many organs can appear to be completely unaffected only to have severe disorders in the bilateral partner or to be severely abnormal in the next generation (Fig. 55–4).

The highly variable expression of the BOR syndrome phenotype could be caused by several mechanisms. If Eya function is dependent on multiple interacting proteins, these might correspond to distinct genetic modifier loci and could underlie phenotypic variation. This is supported by the *Eya1* null mouse, where genetic background influences cleft secondary palate formation (Xu et al., 1999b). Thus, variability occurs within BOR families, which presumably share the same mutation.

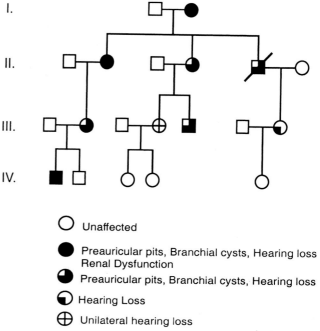

Figure 55–4. A typical brachio-oto-renal syndrome family pedigree. Note the high penetrance and variable expressivity (Modified with permission of Wiley-Liss Inc., from Kumar et al., 1998b.)

○ Unaffected

● Preauricular pits, Branchial cysts, Hearing loss Renal Dysfunction

◗ Preauricular pits, Branchial cysts, Hearing loss

◔ Hearing Loss

⊕ Unilateral hearing loss

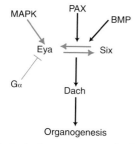

Figure 55–3. A hypothetical scheme to account for the role of Eya1 in mammalian organogenesis. Red arrows denote protein–protein interactions leading to positive regulation of Eya function. Red line indicates a protein–protein interaction leading to a potential negative regulation of Eya function. Black arrows denote genetic interactions. MAPK, mitogen-activated protein kinase; BMP, bone morphogenetic protein.

Several other mechanisms may explain interfamilial variation of the BOR syndrome phenotype. As the *Eya1* phenotype in mouse is extremely sensitive to *Eya1* gene dosage, small changes in the ability of Eya to function may cause significant changes in phenotype. This is demonstrated by anomalies such as the absence of the thymus and parathyroids, which are present in homozygous, but not heterozygous, *Eya1* mutant mice (Xu et al., 1999b). Another possible, but less likely, cause of phenotypic variability may be deregulated expression of *EYA1* splice variants. Altered expression or changes in the ratio of splice isoforms can cause variable phenotypic expressivity. In addition, mutation of specific enhancer regions could decrease or abolish *Eya1* expression in specific tissues while leaving others untouched. Finally, the variety of mutations within *EYA1* may lead to proteins of differing function. These mechanisms need not be exclusive, and it is likely that many may contribute to the variability found in BOR syndrome.

Characteristics of BOR Syndrome

Branchial Anomalies in BOR Syndrome
Branchial anomalies in BOR syndrome include preauricular pits and branchial cleft fistulas (Fig. 55–5). These occur commonly, with frequencies of 77% and 63%, respectively (Fraser et al., 1980). Preauricular pits are typically shallow, pinhead-sized depressions in the helix of the ear near its upper attachment. These occur rarely in the general population but more commonly in certain ethnic groups.

Branchial cleft fistulas are usually inconspicuous openings which occur in the lower third of the neck, usually on the median border of the sternomastoid muscle. These fistulas are often noted if they ooze or become infected. Preauricular tags are also a relatively common characteristic of BOR syndrome, being found in 13% of patients (Chen et al., 1995).

Abnormalities of the palate affect around 7% of BOR patients (Chen et al., 1995). Cleft palate and short or constricted palate make up the majority of these anomalies (Cremers and Fikkers-van Noord, 1980; Chen et al., 1995; Konig et al., 1994). Facial characteristics of BOR syndrome include long and narrow facies and deep overbite. In addition, agnathia occurs in 4% of the BOR population (Chen et al., 1995). BOR patients with hypodontia have also been described (Weber and Kousseff, 1999). Based on the expression of *Eya1* in some of these tissues, it is likely that the presence of some of these ancillary phenotypic manifestations reflects the intrinsic activity of *EYA1*, influenced by the presence of specific modifier loci in different genetic backgrounds.

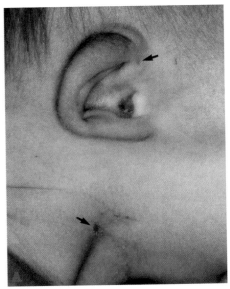

Figure 55–5. Typical characteristics of branchio-oto-renal syndrome. Note the preauricular pit (upper arrow) and the branchial fistula (lower arrow). Also note the small, cup-shaped pinna. (Reprinted with permission of Wiley-Liss, Inc., from Kumar et al., 1998b.)

The number of branchial anomalies correlates with the occurrence of deafness. Thus, while BOR patients with two or fewer branchial anomalies have an 81% chance of being deaf, those with three or more anomalies are deaf 97% of the time. In contrast, no correlation was found between the number or combination of BOR syndrome characteristics (pits, fistulas, and deafness) and renal abnormalities (Fraser et al., 1980).

Otic and Vestibular Anomalies in BOR Syndrome
Hearing loss is the most common symptom of BOR syndrome, occurring in 98% of patients. Though common, the severity and causes of this hearing loss vary (Chen et al., 1995). Onset of deafness can range from birth to adulthood (Buyse, 1990). Regarding deafness in BOR patients, 30% has been attributed to conductive hearing loss, 22% to sensorineural causes, and 48% to a combination of conductive and sensorineural causes (Fraser et al., 1980). The severity of the hearing loss also varies. In one study, 16% of BOR patients exhibited profound hearing loss, with 33% having severe, 22% moderate, and 27% mild hearing loss (Chen et al., 1995). Although most cases of BOR-related hearing loss are congenital, progressive hearing loss has also been described on several occasions and may connote a maintenance requirement for EYA1 function in the adult ear (Fraser et al., 1978; Stuckens et al., 2001; Kemperman et al., 2001).

Middle Ear Anomalies in BOR Syndrome.
Middle ear anomalies often result in conductive deafness, which affects 30% of BOR syndrome patients (Fraser et al., 1980). Most cases of conductive deafness in BOR syndrome are caused by ossicle malformation or fusion. Like many other tissues affected in BOR syndrome, the ossicle phenotype is highly variable and often asymmetrical. Affected ossicles in BOR syndrome patients can range from hypoplastic to absent and can display a wide range and variety of malformations (Fraser et al., 1980; Heimler and Lieber, 1986; Ng et al., 1989). Malpositioned ossicles are fairly common, occurring in 50% of BOR patient ears. Ossicle malformation is also relatively common, occurring at a rate of 33%. Less common are ossicle–ossicle fusions, resulting in lateral chain fixation (25%) and ossicle dislocation (17%) (Chen et al., 1995). Even when the ossicles are functional, auditory signals may not be transmitted to the cochlea as the oval window may be absent or fused to the ossicles (Ostri et al., 1991; Graham and Allanson, 1999). Several other middle ear anomalies are also known to occur in BOR patients. For example, the middle ear cavity may be reduced or expanded in size (Greenberg et al., 1988; Ostri et al., 1991). Additionally, there have been several accounts of *cholesteatomas*, which are masses of keratinized skin in the middle ear (Lipkin et al., 1986; Konig et al., 1994; Graham and Allanson, 1999; Worley et al., 1999).

Outer Ear Anomalies in BOR Syndrome.
Pinnae deformities are common in BOR patients (36%) and typically range from crumpled or hypoplastic helices to cup-shaped, anteverted pinnae (Chen et al., 1995). Additionally, the auditory canal can be severely affected. Auditory canal atresia is found in 12.5% of BOR patients, and auditory canal stenosis is present in 21% (Chen et al., 1995). Atresic auditory canals may lead to conductive deafness. Less common outer ear anomalies include low-set ears and microtia (Fraser et al., 1983; Rollnick and Kaye, 1985; Heimler and Lieber, 1986; Ostri et al., 1991; Worley et al., 1999).

Inner Ear Anomalies in BOR Syndrome.
Inner ear anomalies are commonly found in BOR patients and underlie sensorineural hearing loss. Typically, these anomalies are represented by hypoplastic or dysplastic cochlea, which occur in 62.5% and 33% of BOR patients, respectively. There are also multiple accounts of complete absence of the cochlea and of Mondini-type cochlear defects (1.5 instead of 2.5 turns) (Fitch et al., 1976; Melnick et al., 1976; Fraser et al., 1980; Cremers and Fikkers-van Noord, 1980; Ng et al., 1989; Chen et al., 1995; Worley et al., 1999). These defects can result in fewer cochlear neurons (Fitch et al., 1976) and a hypoplastic cochlear nerve.

Given the high rate of cochlear anomalies, the temporal and developmental similarities between cochlear and vestibular formation, and the early developmental role of *EYA1*, it is not surprising that the vestibular system is often affected in BOR syndrome. Among BOR patients, 12.5% display absent or abnormal semicircular canals and 46%, an enlarged vestibular aqueduct (Chen et al., 1995). In addition, the labyrinths may display reduced or absent irritability, even when present.

Renal Anomalies in BOR Syndrome

Renal anomalies in BOR syndrome can range from clinically insignificant to bilateral agenesis, with a range of hypodysplasia, either uni- or bilaterally (Melnick et al., 1978; Carmi et al., 1983). In an extreme case demonstrating the wide variation that can occur within families, a patient with chronic renal failure received a transplant from his affected mother, who had no evidence of kidney abnormalities (Ni et al., 1994). The prevalence of renal anomalies varies greatly between diagnostic methods and research groups. In a study in which excretory urography was used to identify renal anomalies, 16/16 BOR patients were found to have renal anomalies (Van Widdershoven et al., 1983). Thus, while most BOR patients probably have renal anomalies, only 33% show disturbed glomerular filtration and only 10%–25% have medically severe renal problems (Cremers and Fikkers-van Noord, 1980). Therefore, mild renal abnormalities with no significant clinical sequelae represent the majority of renal anomalies in BOR patients.

Chen et al. (1995) used intravenous pyelography (IVP) to demonstrate that 62% of BOR patients (*n* = 21) have renal anomalies. These anomalies were delineated further into renal agenesis, hypoplasia, and dysplasia, which occurred at rates of 29%, 19%, and 14%, respectively. It is important to bear in mind that the reported incidence of severe kidney abnormalities may be low as a result of perinatal lethality. Kidney ectopias have also been reported on three separate occasions and polycystic kidneys are relatively common (Carmi et al., 1983; Rollnick and Kaye, 1985; Daggilas et al., 1992). Though most renal symptoms in BOR syndrome are not progressive, BOR-associated progressive renal failure has been reported on several occasions (Misra and Nolph, 1998; Rodriguez-Soriano et al., 2001).

The renal pelvis and ureter are also sites of malformation in BOR syndrome patients. Abnormalities of the renal pelvis include bifid renal pelvis and extra renal pelvis (Fraser et al., 1980; Heimler and Lieber, 1986; Konig et al., 1994). Ureteral malformations include megaureter, ureter duplications, and ureteropelvic junction obstructions (Fraser et al., 1983; Heimler and Lieber, 1986). These anomalies can lead to vesicoureteral reflux (Heimler and Lieber, 1986; Weber and Kousseff, 1999; Bellini et al., 2001). A single case of ureter agenesis has been reported (Melnick et al., 1978). Thus, BOR syndrome can result in multiple types of ureteral malformation, which could account for the ureteral findings in BOU syndrome. This is consistent with our current understanding of the role of *Eya1* in murine kidney development.

Cranial Nerve Anomalies in BOR Syndrome

Cranial nerve problems occur commonly in BOR syndrome, with 21% of patients expressing anomalies of the facial nerve (Chen et al., 1995). This can result in facial paralysis, which occurs in about 4% of BOR patients (Cremers and Fikkers-van Noord, 1980). Similarly, facial nerve hypoplasia and misguided course have also been demonstrated (Chitayat et al., 1992; Chen et al., 1995). As in the case of the ureters, duplication as well as agenesis can occur. Duplication of the facial nerve occurs in 8% of BOR patients (Chen et al., 1995). Other cranial nerves can also be affected in BOR syndrome, and congenital vocal cord paresis, possibly due to facial nerve error, has been reported (Weber and Kousseff, 1999).

Lacrimation is often affected in BOR syndrome as lacrimal duct aplasia and stenosis can occur; these were included as diagnostic signs of BOR syndrome in many early papers (Melnick et al., 1976; Fraser et al., 1978; Konig et al., 1994; Chen et al., 1995). Control of both lacrimation and salivation is mediated by the facial nerve. Gustatory lacrimation, or "crocodile tears," a rare disorder resulting in tear formation upon salivation, has been described in BOR syndrome patients, including the only known case of familial gustatory lacrimation (Preisch et al., 1985; Chen et al, 1995; Weber and Kousseff, 1999;

Graham and Allanson, 1999). Gustatory lacrimation could be caused by errors of cranial nerve pathfinding resulting from misrouting of facial nerve fibers such that axons normally destined for the submandibular ganglion, which controls salivation, enter the major superficial petrosal nerve, enervating the pterygopalatine ganglion, which controls lacrimation. These pathfinding errors may result from errors in neuronal identity specification.

Rare BOR Phenotypes Associated with *EYA1* Mutation

Several other clinical findings have been associated with BOR syndrome but are seen only rarely. Thus, it is unknown whether these represent true manifestations of the BOR syndrome phenotype. An advantage of the mouse model of BOR syndrome is that the homozygous *Eya1* mutant mouse carries a complete null mutation and, thus, represents the strongest possible phenotype. Thus, the presence of certain anomalies in the mouse model strongly suggests that their incidental association in BOR syndrome is also due to *EYA1* mutation.

Though rare, thyroid and parathyroid anomalies in BOR syndrome patients have been reported. Reports of thyroid and parathyroid anomalies consist of euthyroid goiter and absent parathyroids (Heimler and Lieber, 1986; Chen et al., 1995; Weber and Kousseff, 1999). Homozygous *Eya1* mutant mice lack parathyroids and have hypoplastic thyroids (Xu et al., 1999b). Thus, it is likely that these anomalies are associated with a strong loss of *EYA1* function at these loci during development.

In addition, rib, skull, hip, and vertebral skeletal anomalies have been found in BOR patients. These findings are consistent with the *Eya1* mutant mouse in which rib, skull, hip, and neck anomalies occur (Xu et al., 1999b). These anomalies correspond to *Eya1* expression in cartilaginous condensations and strongly suggest that *Eya1* plays a role in skeletogenesis (Xu et al., 1999b). Skeletal anomalies in BOR patients vary, and there are only single accounts of each anomaly listed except hip dysplasia, which has been reported twice. When considered as a whole with the mouse data, it is apparent that skeletal anomalies can be manifestations of BOR syndrome. A full list of skeletal anomalies found in BOR syndrome patients includes congenital hip dysplasia, osteosclerosis, excess ribs, microcephaly, shoulder abnormalities, rachensis, incomplete closure of the left palpebral fissure, cervical and spinal anomalies, lumbar meningomyelocele, and a variety of hand and foot anomalies (Fraser et al., 1980; Carmi et al., 1983; Pennie and Marres, 1992; Konig et al., 1994; Torres-Peris, 1994; Chen et al., 1995; Weber and Kousseff, 1999; Graham and Allanson, 1999).

Considering that the genetic pathways governing eye formation are highly conserved between fly and human and that *eya* is necessary for fly eye development, the lack of a prevalent, early eye phenotype in BOR syndrome is quite surprising. Three families with eye disorders (congenital cataracts, Peter's anomaly, persistence of pupillary membrane) were demonstrated to have missense mutations in the Eya domain of *EYA1*, although two of these families did not display BOR syndrome (Azuma et al., 2000). These may be cases where BOR characteristics either are not apparent due to penetrance and expressivity issues or a gain-of-function mutation or may be unrelated to the apparent *EYA1* mutation. Arguing for the significance of these ocular phenotypes, however, is their resemblance to phenotypes found in aniridia patients, who are haploinsufficient for *PAX6*, a putative upstream regulator of *EYA1* function in early eye development.

EYA1 MUTATIONS CAN CAUSE BOR SYNDROME

In 1997, a human ortholog of the *Drosophila eya* gene was identified as a cause of BOR syndrome by positional cloning (Abdelhak et al., 1997a). Soon afterward, *EYA1* mutations were demonstrated to underlie BO syndrome as well, though they are not the sole cause (Cremers and Fikkers-van Noord, 1980; Vincent et al., 1997; Kumar et al., 1998a). To date, nearly 30 distinct *EYA1* mutations have been isolated (summarized in Table 55–1). These range from cytogenetic scale deletions of the gene or larger to individual point mutations, which change the identity of single amino acids.

Interestingly, many of these mutations affect the highly conserved Eya domain, and all known phenotype-related missense mutations oc-

Table 55–1. Known Phenotype-Inducing Mutations of *EYA1*

Mutation	Result	Phenotype	Reference
297del	Frameshift	BOR syndrome	Vincent et al., 1997
387insT	Frameshift	BOR syndrome	Rickard et al., 2000
Y244X	Stop codon	BOR syndrome	Rickard et al., 2000
755insC	Frameshift	BOR syndrome	Abdelhak et al., 1997a,b
R264X	Stop codon	BOR syndrome	Fukada et al., 2001
R265X	Stop codon	BOR syndrome	Rickard et al., 2000
W275X	Stop codon	BOR syndrome	Abdelhak et al., 1997a,b
868-1G → A	Splicing error	BOR syndrome	Rickard et al., 2000
870insGT	Frameshift	BOR syndrome	Vincent et al., 1997
E330K	Missense mutation	Bilateral persistence of the pupillary membrane	Azuma et al., 2000
1041G → T	Splicing error	BOR syndrome	Rickard et al., 2000
1042-13 23 bp inversion	Splicing error	BOR syndrome	Rickard et al., 2000
G393S	Missense mutation	BOR syndrome, nystagmus, and congenital cataracts	Azuma et al., 2000
R407Q	Missense mutation	BOR syndrome	Kumar et al., 1998a
1251T → CC	Frameshift	BOR syndrome	Abdelhak et al., 1997a,b
1359insC	Frameshift	BOR syndrome	Abdelhak et al., 1997b
S454P	Missense mutation	BOR syndrome	Abdelhak et al., 1997b
1372T → AGAGC	Frameshift	BOR syndrome	Abdelhak et al., 1997a,b
L472R	Missense mutation	BOR syndrome	Abdelhak et al., 1997b
1498+2T → G	Splicing error	BOR syndrome	Abdelhak et al., 1997a,b
R514G	Missense mutation	Congenital cataracts, Peter's anomaly	Azuma et al., 2000
1501del4	Frameshift	BOR syndrome	Kumar et al., 1998a
1555ins4	Frameshift	BOR syndrome	Abdelhak et al., 1997b
1592delC	Frameshift	BOR syndrome	Kumar et al., 1998a
1599+5G → C	Slicing error	BOR syndrome	Abdelhak et al., 1997b
1599+1G → A	Splicing error	BOR syndrome	Rodriguez-Soriano et al., 2001
L547P	Missense mutation	BOR syndrome	Rickard et al., 2000
X559Y	Stop codon error	BOR syndrome	Rickard et al., 2000

cur in this region (Abdelhak et al., 1997b; Kumar et al., 1998a; Azuma et al., 2000; Rickard et al., 2000). Since these missense mutations in the Eya domain typically result in a phenotype similar to that associated with *EYA1* deletions, it can be concluded that these represent loss-of-function mutations. Hence, the Eya domain is critical for EYA1 function. Though many of the mutations associated with phenotypes are found in the EYA domain, these mutations are relatively evenly spread throughout this domain and there are no mutational hot spots. This suggests that the Eya domain functions as a single large, well-ordered domain rather than as a series of small subdomains. The lack of BOR-associated missense mutations in the PST domain may reflect a lack of critical residues due to the flexible structure postulated for PST domains (Fig. 55–6).

BOR vs. BO Syndrome

Whether BOR and BO syndromes are separate entities has been the subject of debate. Nonetheless, it is certain that many cases of BO have minor renal anomalies and are thus truly cases of BOR syndrome. Additionally, cases of BO syndrome have been genetically mapped to the *EYA1* locus at 8q13 (Cremers and Fikkers-van Noord, 1980; Vincent et al., 1997), and a frameshift within *EYA1* was even found in

one case (Vincent et al., 1997). Thus, *EYA1* mutations can underlie both BO and BOR syndromes.

The high degree of phenotypic variance in BOR and BO syndrome patients has led some to invoke genetic heterogeneity as a cause. In support of this, 60% of BOR families tested did not have identifiable mutations within the *EYA1* gene (Kumar et al., 1998a). Furthermore, cases of BO which do not localize to the 8q region have also been noted (Kumar et al., 1998b; Stratakis et al., 1998). A second locus for BO syndrome was discovered at 1q31 (Kumar et al., 2000), although the BO-associated gene at this locus has yet to be identified. It will be interesting to see what relation exists between this gene and *EYA1*. Like *EYA1*-mediated BOR syndrome, this BO syndrome segregates in an autosomal-dominant fashion and gives rise to conductive or mixed hearing loss and preauricular sinuses. Though families in this pedigree differ from BOR families in having commissural lip pits, the lip pits do not cosegregate with the 1q31 locus (Kumar et al., 2000). It is also unknown whether renal anomalies can be associated with mutations at this locus. In sum, although *EYA1* mutations can cause both BO and BOR syndromes, there are likely to be additional genes whose mutations also underlie these syndromes.

BOU syndrome consists of the branchial and otic characteristics of

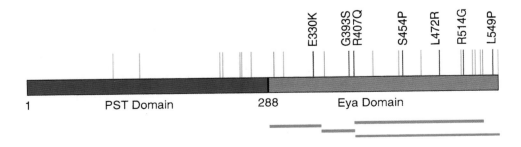

1   PST Domain   288   Eya Domain

■ Genomic deletion
▨ Frameshift or Termination
▩ Splicing error
■ Missense mutation

Figure 55–6. Distribution of phenotype-associated mutations of *EYA1*. Note the clustering of mutations in the Eya domain. All known phenotype-associated mutations affect the Eya domain.

BO and BOR syndrome along with uretal abnormalities, duplication of the ureters, or bifid renal pelvis (Fraser et al., 1983). BOU is thought to be a variant of BOR syndrome as a range of phenotypes can be found which span from BOU to BOR syndrome (Konig et al., 1994). However, BOU syndrome has not yet been associated with mutations at the *EYA1* locus.

Genotype–Phenotype Correlations

The variable expressivity of *EYA1* mutations, especially the asymmetrical phenotypic manifestations and intrafamily variability, make genotype to phenotype correlations difficult. No correlation between phenotype and genotype has been reported thus far.

ESTABLISHING A BOR DIAGNOSIS

The highly variable nature of BOR syndrome complicates its diagnosis. Thus, while preauricular pits and deafness are fairly common in BOR syndrome patients, renal abnormalities often go undetected. Generally, the presence of a branchial, otic, or renal phenotype in a first-degree relative is used to establish the diagnosis. The differential diagnosis includes Treacher-Collins syndrome, hemifacial microsomia, and other BO syndromes, including BO and BOU.

MANAGEMENT OF BOR SYNDROME

Therapies

Treatment of BOR syndrome is largely symptomatic. Hearing aids may be used for patients with hearing loss. Operation on the ossicles is possible but difficult. Operation can also be used to correct external auricular malformations, cleft palate, and branchial sinuses and cysts. Renal transplantation may be indicated for patients with severe renal abnormalities.

Genetic Counseling

Commercial testing for BOR syndrome is not available. Given the reported 40% rate of finding mutations within *EYA1* in BOR syndrome patients (Kumar et al., 1998a), such testing would currently be of potential value only in cases where the parental mutation is known and readily detectable. The high penetrance and autosomal-dominant nature of BOR syndrome mean that approximately 50% of offspring from an affected parent should display some characteristics of BOR syndrome. Thus, it is suggested that all family members of BOR syndrome patients be tested for hearing and renal anomalies. The concurrence of branchial with renal anomalies also suggests that patients who display preauricular pits or branchial fistulas with hearing loss should be tested for renal problems. Prenatal ultrasound may also be used to track kidney formation during the development of potential affected fetuses.

Future Prospects

Near-term prospects for BOR syndrome include more accurate testing, through the localization of additional BOR loci; a more complete definition of the *EYA1* locus; and a better understanding of EYA1 regulation and function. In the future, studies into the nature of the phenotypic variability observed in BOR syndrome could lead to the ability to predict or alleviate symptoms through the identification and modulation of factors which affect expressivity. Furthermore, as cases of progressive hearing loss and renal failure have been described, future studies may lead to the ability to stop or slow the progression of these disorders.

ANIMAL MODELS OF BOR SYNDROME

Drosophila

The *eya* fly mutant was isolated because of its eponymous *eyes absent* phenotype, which is caused by cell death anterior to the morphogenetic furrow in the fly eye (Bonini et al., 1993). It was later demonstrated that *eya* is necessary for both the initiation and pro-gression of the morphogenetic furrow (Pignoni et al., 1997). Though mutations in *eya* can result in loss of the eyes, most *eya* mutations are embryonic-lethal (Leiserson et al., 1998). Non-eye abnormalities include reduced or absent ocelli (*Drosophila* photoreceptive organs), abnormal brain morphology, female sterility, abnormal gonad formation, and abnormal head involution (Nusslein-Volhard et al., 1984, cited in Bonini et al., 1997). Though the phenotypes of *eya* mutant flies and humans are divergent, the highly conserved nature of the *Pax-Eya-Six* signaling pathway makes *Drosophila* an attractive model for the study of many aspects of *EYA1* function.

Mouse

Heterozygous *Eya1* Mutant Mice Express a BOR Syndrome-Like Phenotype

Eya1$^{+/-}$ mice display a phenotype similar to BOR syndrome (Xu et al., 1999b). All *Eya1$^{+/-}$* mice have some degree of hearing loss, and a small percentage display renal abnormalities, including renal hypoplasia and unilateral renal agenesis (Xu et al., 1999b). These findings were independently confirmed by a spontaneous, weaker loss-of-function mutation in the *Eya1^{BOR}* mouse, where insertion of an intracisternal A particle into exon 7 of *Eya1* results in a recessive BOR-like phenotype (Johnson et al., 1999).

As would be expected if Eya1 function is dependent on a number of factors, genetic background of the mouse (129/SV or Balb/C vs. C57BL6/6J) markedly influences cleft secondary palate phenotype. While all 129/SV and Balb/C *Eya1$^{-/-}$* mice displayed cleft secondary palate, all C57BL/6J mice displayed abnormal fusion of the palatal shelves with the nasal septum. Anomalies in these mice which also exist in human BOR patients include hearing loss, cochlear nerve misrouting, malformed ossicles, atrophy of the spiral ganglion, vestibular labyrinth anomalies, and renal defects (Xu et al., 1999b). The high degree of phenotypic similarity between BOR syndrome patients and *Eya1$^{+/-}$* mice makes these mice an attractive model to study the developmental basis for BOR syndrome associated defects.

Eya1$^{-/-}$ Mice Die Perinatally and Display Multiple Abnormalities

Homozygous mutant animals express more severe versions of the heterozygous phenotype in addition to displaying other abnormalities not present in heterozygotes. These animals display complete renal agenesis with 100% penetrance, which is sufficient to explain their perinatal demise. Furthermore, the external ears and the ossicles of the middle ear are absent or malformed, inner ear structures such as the cochlea never form, and the auditory canal is atretic. The functional requirement for the observed placodal expression of *Eya1* during embryogenesis manifests itself as an absence of the facioacoustic (VII–VIII) and petrosal ganglia (IX). Axon misrouting has been noted for the cochlear and vagus nerves, suggesting a role in pathfinding or ganglion identity specification. As noted earlier, other similarities between these mice and BOR syndrome patients include craniofacial and skeletal defects, parathyroid abnormalities, and cleft palate (Xu et al., 1999b).

DEVELOPMENTAL MECHANISMS UNDERLYING BOR SYNDROME PATHOGENESIS

While it is hypothesized that EYA1 functions with other proteins to specify organ identity, the pathogenic mechanisms responsible for BOR syndrome are currently only partly understood. However, data on Eya family members in a variety of organisms have provided some insight into the possible developmental mechanisms responsible for BOR syndrome pathogenesis. In particular, the *Eya1* mutant mouse has been used to determine the earliest stages at which anatomical defects are present and can serve as a valuable model to test hypotheses about how *Eya1* mutations lead to the BOR phenotype.

Possible Mechanisms Leading to Kidney Anomalies in BOR Syndrome

Mammalian kidney formation is dependent on inductive interactions between the ureteric bud and the metanephric mesenchyme (see Chapter 13). The expression profile of *Eya1* in the developing murine kidney suggests a model by which EYA1 may function in early kidney formation. *Eya1* is initially expressed in the nephrogenic cord and the uninduced metanephric mesenchyme. Upon induction of the metanephric mesenchyme by the ureteric bud, *Eya1* expression becomes restricted to the induced metanephric mesenchyme (Xu et al., 1999b). Thus, Eya1 function may be required in the metanephric mesenchyme for proper early induction of the kidney. This finding has been greatly strengthened by findings in the *Eya1* null mouse. In this mouse, the ureteric bud never forms and the metanephric mesenchyme undergoes apoptosis. This suggests that metanephric *Eya1* expression is necessary for ureteric bud outgrowth and for subsequent inductive interactions that underlie the early stages of kidney formation.

The *Pax-Eya-Six* pathway, which was determined through epistasis analysis in *Drosophila*, appears to be conserved during mammalian kidney formation. *Pax2* (see Chapter 60) is necessary for kidney formation and appears to function upstream of *Eya1* (Torres et al., 1995; Xu et al., 1999b). Six family members are also expressed in the developing kidney, suggesting that Six–Eya1 interactions may underlie Eya1 function in the kidney. Six1 is expressed in nephrogenic cord, while *Six2* is also expressed in the metanephric mesenchyme but not the ureteric bud (Oliver et al., 1995; Xu et al., 1999b).

Kidney formation has been well studied, and several extracellular molecules have been hypothesized to act as signals for ureteric bud outgrowth. Of these, the most compelling is GDNF (see Chapter 35). GDNF is expressed in the metanephric mesenchyme, while its receptor, c-ret (see Chapter 36) receptor tyrosine kinase (RTK), is expressed in the mesonephric duct, becoming restricted to the ureteric bud upon bud induction (Pachnis et al., 1993). As in *Eya1*, mice mutant for *GDNF*, *c-ret*, or a GDNF coreceptor, *GDNFR-α*, display kidney agenesis (Sanchez et al., 1996; Pichel et al., 1996; Moore et al., 1996; Durbec et al., 1996; Jing et al., 1996). Moreover, GDNF expression is undetectable in the *Eya1* null mouse, suggesting that Eya1 may regulate *GDNF*. A loss of GDNF function would be sufficient to provide a mechanism by which the kidney agenesis phenotype occurs in *Eya1*$^{-/-}$ mice (Xu et al., 1999b).

These studies on the *Eya1* null mouse are formally relevant only to the homozygous condition. Errors in EYA1 function may occur at many levels which are not identified in the *Eya1* null mouse because they occur subsequent to ureteric bud outgrowth. Thus, *Eya1* continues to be expressed in the developing kidney after ureteric bud outgrowth. Specifically, *Eya1* is expressed in the condensing mesenchyme which surrounds new ureteric branches (Kalatzis et al., 1998). *Eya1* expression in the kidney decreases during development and is not detectable in the mature kidney (Abdelhak et al., 1997a). Nonetheless, it is also possible that the haploid levels of EYA1, as found in most BOR syndrome patients, may cause an intermediate lack of ureteric bud outgrowth, which could help to explain the disparate renal phenotypes seen in BOR patients.

Possible Mechanisms Leading to Otic and Vestibular Anomalies in BOR Syndrome

The mammalian ear is formed by a complex set of tissue interactions. The ear of the *Eya1* null mouse is characterized by a series of abnormalities, each of which may have a different origin. *Eya1* null mice lack inner ear structures, such as the cochlea. This correlates well with *Eya1* expression in the developing otic structures. *Eya1* is selectively expressed in the ventromedial wall of the otic vesicle, the portion where the sensory epithelia of the inner ear will form (Kalatzis et al., 1998). The inner ear phenotype in the *Eya1* null mouse is caused by a failure of otic vesicle development, which is associated with widespread apoptotic cell death within the otic vesicle (Xu et al., 1999b). Absent or hypoplastic cochlea are sometimes found in BOR syndrome patients. This is likely caused by either a failure of otic vesicle development or a diminished otic vesicle due to increased apoptosis.

Later in development, *Eya1* expression continues in a variety of inner ear structures which may be malformed in BOR syndrome patients. These include the neuroepithelium of the floor of the cochlear duct and spiral ganglion, which go on to form hair cells and the organ of Corti. *Eya1* expression continues through the maturation of the inner ear structures. *Eya1* expression is also found in the developing sensory epithelium of the vestibular components of the inner ear (Kalatzis et al., 1998). Thus, heterozygosity may cause dose-dependent phenotypes in the ear. Alternately, the various ear phenotypes found in BOR syndrome may be the result of different processes. Of note, *Six1* is expressed in the otic vesicle; thus, Six1 and Eya1 may interact in the otic vesicle during otic development (Oliver et al., 1995).

The middle ear is formed by derivatives of the first and second branchial arches. Though expressed in the branchial arches, *Eya1* does not seem to be expressed in the dorsal first or second branchial arches, regions that will form the ossicles. Thus, in cases where the ossicles are missing, *Eya1* mutation may lead to a phenotype through indirect, potentially inductive interactions with the dorsal first and second branchial arches (Kalatzis et al., 1998). *Eya1* is also expressed in developing endochondral structures and may cause ossicle fusion by interfering with their separation from each other (Xu et al., 1997b). Although BOR syndrome is often characterized by misshapen pinnae, *Eya1* is expressed adjacent to, but not within, the epithelium of the first branchial arch and its surrounding mesenchyme, tissues which will form the external ear (Kalatzis et al., 1998).

Possible Mechanisms Leading to Branchial Anomalies in BOR Syndrome

Eya1 is expressed in the developing branchial arches and clefts and may thus cause the branchial anomalies found in BOR syndrome. Branchial cleft expression in particular may lead to the formation of branchial fistulas. Though little is known about the formation of preauricular pits and branchial fistulas, preauricular pits are thought to be caused by incomplete fusion of the first branchial cleft. Incomplete fusion of the second branchial cleft is thought to underlie branchial fistulas.

CONCLUSION

BOR syndrome is a rare disorder which results in a highly variable phenotype which affects branchial structures, the otic system, and renal structures. A suitable mouse model for this disorder has been made, and investigations on the mechanism of how *EYA1* dysfunction leads to the BOR phenotype have resulted in substantial progress. Future progress will involve a better understanding of the *EYA1* locus, how its gene product functions, and how the relevant developmental processes may be manipulated to ameliorate the pathological and clinical features of BOR syndrome.

REFERENCES

Abdelhak S, Kalatzis V, Heilig R, Compain S, Samson D, Vincent C, Weil D, Cruaud C, Sahly I, Leibovici M, et al. (1997a). A human homologue of the *Drosophila eyes absent* gene underlies branchio-oto-renal (BOR) syndrome and identifies a novel gene family. *Nat Genet* 15: 157–164.

Abdelhak S, Kalatzis V, Heilig R, Compain S, Samson D, Vincent C, Levi-Acobas F, Cruaud C, Le Merrer M, Mathieu M, et al. (1997b). Clustering of mutations responsible for branchio-oto-renal (BOR) syndrome in the eya homologous region (eyaHR) of *EYA1*. *Hum Mol Genet* 6: 2247–2255.

Azuma N, Hirakiyama A, Inoue T, Asaka A, Yamada M (2000). Mutations of a human homologue of the *Drosophila eyes absent* gene (*EYA1*) detected in patients with congenital cataracts and ocular anterior segment anomalies. *Hum Mol Genet* 9: 363–366.

Bellini C, Piaggio G, Massocco D, Perfumo F, Bertini I, Gusmano R, Serra G (2001). Branchio-oto-renal syndrome: a report on nine family groups. *Am J Kidney Dis* 37: 505–509.

Bergsma D (ed.) (1979). *Birth Defects Compendium*, 2nd Edition. Alan R. Liss, New York.

Bonini NM, Leiserson WM, Benzer S (1993). The *eyes absent* gene: genetic control of cell survival and differentiation in the developing *Drosophila* eye. *Cell* 72: 379–395.

Bonini NM, Bui QT, Gray-Board GL, Warrick JM (1997). The *Drosophila eyes absent* gene directs ectopic eye formation in a pathway conserved between flies and vertebrates. *Development* 124: 4819–4826.

Borsani G, DeGrandi A, Ballabio A, Bulfone A, Bernard L, Banfi S, Gattuso C, Mariani M, Dixon M, Donnai D, et al. (1999). *EYA4*, a novel vertebrate gene related to *Drosophila eyes absent*. *Hum Mol Genet* 8: 11–23.

Buller C, Xu X, Marquis V, Schwanke R, Xu PX (2001). Molecular effects of Eya1 domain mutations causing organ defects in BOR syndrome. *Hum Mol Genet* 10: 2775–2781.

Buyse ML (ed.) (1990). *Birth Defects Encyclopedia : The Comprehensive, Systematic, Illustrated Reference Source for the Diagnosis, Delineation, Etiology, Biodynamics, Occurrence, Prevention, and Treatment of Human Anomalies of Clinical Relevance*. Blackwell, Dover, MA, pp. 243–244.

Carmi R, Binshtock D, Abeliovich D, Bar-Ziv J (1983). The branchio-oto-renal (BOR) syndrome: report of bilateral renal agenesis in three sibs. *Am J Med Genet* 14: 625–627.
Caubit X, Thangarajah R, Theil T, Wirth J, Nothwang HG, Ruther U, Krauss S (1999). Mouse Dac, a novel nuclear factor with homology to *Drosophila* dachshund shows a dynamic expression in the neural crest, the eye, the neocortex, and the limb bud. *Dev Dyn* 214: 66–80.
Chen A, Francis M, Ni L, Cremers CW, Kimberling WJ, Sato Y, Phelps PD, Bellman SC, Wagner MJ, Pembrey M, et al. (1995). Phenotypic manifestations of branchio-oto-renal syndrome. *Am J Med Genet* 58: 365–370.
Chen R, Amoui M, Zhang Z, Mardon G (1997). Dachshund and eyes absent proteins form a complex and function synergistically to induce ectopic eye development in *Drosophila*. *Cell* 91: 893–903.
Chen R, Halder G, Zhang Z, Mardon G (1999). Signaling by the TGF-β homologue *decapentaplegic* functions reiteratively within the network of genes controlling retinal cell fate determination in *Drosophila*. *Development* 126: 935–943.
Chitayat D, Hodgkinson KA, Chen MF, Haber GD, Nakishima S, Sando I (1992). Branchio-oto-renal syndrome: further delineation of an underdiagnosed syndrome. *Am J Med Genet* 43: 970–975.
Chow RL, Altmann CR, Lang RA, Hemmati-Brivanlou A (1999). Pax6 induces ectopic eyes in a vertebrate. *Development* 126: 4213–4222.
Cremers CWRJ, Fikkers-van Noord M (1980). The earpits-deafness syndrome: clinical and genetic aspects. *Int J Pediatr Otorhinolaryngol* 2: 309–322.
Daggilas A, Antoniades K, Palasis S, Aidonis A (1992). Branchio-oto-renal dysplasia associated with tetralogy of Fallot. *Head Neck* 14: 139–142.
David R, Ahrens K, Wedlich D, Schlosser G (2001). *Xenopus Eya1* demarcates all neurogenic placodes as well as migrating hypaxial muscle precursors. *Mech Dev* 103: 189–192.
Davis RJ, Shen W, Heanue TA, Mardon G (1999). Mouse *Dach*, a homologue of *Drosophila dachshund*, is expressed in the developing retina, brain and limbs. *Dev Genes Evol* 209: 526–536.
Davis RJ, Shen W, Sandler YI, Amoui M, Purcell P, Maas R, Ou CN, Vogel H, Beaudet AL, Mardon G (2001a). *Dach1* mutant mice bear no gross abnormalities in eye, limb, and brain development and exhibit postnatal lethality. *Mol Cell Biol* 21: 1484–1490.
Davis RJ, Shen W, Sandler YI, Heanue TA, Mardon G (2001b). Characterization of mouse *Dach2*, a homologue of *Drosophila dachshund*. *Mech Dev* 102: 169–179.
Durbec P, Marcos-Gutierrez CV, Kilkenny C, Grigoriou M, Wartiowaara K, Suvanto P, Smith D, Ponder B, Constantini F, Saarma M (1996). GDNF signaling through the Ret receptor tyrosine kinase. *Nature* 381: 789–793.
Fan X, Brass LF, Poncz M, Spitz F, Maire P, Manning DR (2000). The alpha subunits of G_z and G_i interact with the eyes absent transcription cofactor Eya2, preventing its interaction with the six class of homeodomain-containing proteins. *J Biol Chem* 275: 32129–32134.
Fitch N, Lindsay J, Srolovitz H (1976). Severe renal dysgenesis produced by a dominant gene. *Am J Dis Child* 130: 1356–1357.
Fraser FC, Ling D, Clogg D, Nogrady B (1978). Genetic aspects of the BOR syndrome—branchial fistulas, ear pits, hearing loss, and renal anomalies. *Am J Med Genet* 2: 241–252.
Fraser FC, Sproule JR, Halal F (1980). Frequency of the branchio-oto-renal (BOR) syndrome in children with profound hearing loss. *Am J Med Genet* 7: 341–349.
Fraser FC, Ayme S, Halal F, Sproule J (1983). Autosomal dominant duplication of the renal collecting system, hearing loss, and external ear anomalies: a new syndrome? *Am J Med Genet* 14: 473–478.
Fukada S, Kuroda T, Chida E, Shimizu R, Usami S, Koda E, Abe S, Namba A, Kitamura K, Inuyama Y (2001). A family affected by branchio-oto syndrome with EYA1 mutations. *Auris Nasus Larynx* 28(Suppl): S7–S11.
Graham GE, Allanson JE (1999). Congenital cholesteatoma and malformations of the facial nerve: rare manifestations of the BOR syndrome. *Am J Med Genet* 86: 20–26.
Greenberg CR, Trevenen C, Evans JA (1988). The BOR syndrome and renal agenesis—prenatal diagnosis and further clinical delineation. *Prenat Diagn* 8: 103–108.
Halder G, Callaerts P, Gehring WJ (1995). Induction of ectopic eyes by targeted expression of the *eyeless* gene in *Drosophila*. *Science* 267: 1788–1792.
Halder G, Callaerts P, Flister S, Walldorf U, Kloter U, Gehring WJ (1998). *Eyeless* initiates the expression of both *sine oculis* and *eyes absent* during *Drosophila* development. *Development* 125: 2181–2191.
Hammond KL, Hanson IM, Brown AG, Lettice LA, Hill RE (1998). Mammalian and *Drosophila dachshund* genes are related to the *Ski* proto-oncogene and are expressed in eye and limb. *Mech Dev* 74: 121–131.
Heanue TA, Reshef R, Davis RJ, Mardon G, Oliver G, Tomarev S, Lassar AB, Tabin CJ (1999). Synergistic regulation of vertebrate muscle development by *Dach2, Eya2,* and *Six1,* homologs of genes required for *Drosophila* eye formation. *Genes Dev* 13: 3231–3243.
Heanue TA, Davis RJ, Rowitch DH, Kispert A, McMahon AP, Mardon G, Tabin CJ (2002). *Dach1*, a vertebrate homologue of *Drosophila dachshund*, is expressed in the developing eye and ear of both chick and mouse and is regulated independently of *Pax* and *Eya* genes. *Mech Dev* 111: 75–87.
Heimler A, Lieber E (1986). Branchio-oto-renal syndrome: reduced penetrance and variable expressivity in four generations of a large kindred. *Am J Med Genet* 25: 15–27.
Ho MKC, Wong YH (2001). G_z signaling: emerging divergence from G_i signaling. *Oncogene* 20: 1615–1625.
Hsiao FC, Williams A, Davies EL, Rebay I (2001). Eyes absent mediates cross-talk between retinal determination genes and the receptor tyrosine kinase signaling pathway. *Dev Cell* 1: 51–61.
Jing S, Wen D, Yu Y, Holst PL, Luo Y, Fang M, Tamir R, Antonio L, Hu Z, Cupples R, et al. (1996). GDNF-induced activation of the rat protein tyrosine kinase is mediated by GDNFR-alpha, a novel receptor for GDNF. *Cell* 85: 1113–1124.
Johnson KR, Cook SA, Erway LC, Matthews AN, Sanford LP, Paradies NE, Friedman RA (1999). Inner ear and kidney anomalies caused by IAP insertion in an intron of the *Eya 1* gene in a mouse model of BOR syndrome. *Hum Mol Genet* 8: 645–653.
Kalatzis V, Sahly I, El-Amraoui A, Petit C (1998). *Eya1* expression in the developing ear and kidney: towards the understanding of the pathogenesis of branchio-oto-renal (BOR) syndrome. *Dev Dyn* 213: 486–499.
Kemperman MH, Stinckens C, Kumar S, Huygen PL, Joosten FB, Cremers CW (2001). Progressive fluctuant hearing loss, enlarged vestibular aqueduct, and cochlear hypoplasia in branchio-oto-renal syndrome. *Otol Neurotol* 22: 637–643.
Klesert TR, Cho DH, Clark JI, Maylie J, Adelman J, Snider L, Yuen EC, Soriano P, Tapscott SJ (2000). Mice deficient in Six5 develop cataracts: implications for myotonic dystrophy. *Nat Genet* 25: 105–109.
Konig R, Fuchs S, Dukiet C (1994). Branchio-oto-renal (BOR) syndrome: variable expressivity in a five-generation pedigree. *Eur J Pediatr* 153: 446–450.
Kozmik Z, Pfeffer P, Kralova J, Paces J, Paces V, Kalousova A, Cvekl A (1999). Molecular cloning and expression of the human and mouse homologues of the *Drosophila dachshund* gene. *Dev Genes Evol* 209: 537–545.
Kumar S, Kimberling WJ, Weston MD, Schaefer BG, Berg MA, Marres HAM, Cremers CWRJ (1998a). Identification of three novel mutations in human EYA1 protein associated with branchi-oto-renal syndrome. *Hum Mutat* 11: 443–449.
Kumar S, Marres HAM, Cremers CWRJ, Kimberling WJ (1998b). Autosomal-dominant branchio-otic (BO) syndrome is not allelic to the branchio-oto-renal (BOR) gene at 8q13. *Am J Med Genet* 76: 395–401.
Kumar S, Deffenbacher K, Marres HAM, Cremers CWRJ, Kimberling WJ (2000). Genomewide search and genetic localization of a second gene associated with autosomal dominant branchio-oto-renal syndrome: clinical and genetic implications. *Am J Hum Genet* 66: 1715–1720.
Lagutin O, Zhu CC, Furuta Y, Rowitch DH, McMahon AP, Oliver G (2001). *Six3* promotes the formation of ectopic optic vesicle-like structures in mouse embryos. *Dev Dyn* 221: 342–349.
Leiserson WM, Benzer S, Bonini NM (1998). Dual functions of the *Drosophila eyes absent* gene in the eye and embryo. *Mech Dev* 73: 193–202.
Leuther KK, Salmeron JM, Johnston SA (1993). Genetic evidence that an activation domain of GAL4 does not require acidity and may form a beta sheet. *Cell* 72: 575–585.
Lipkin DF, Coker NJ, Jenkins HA (1986). Hereditary cholesteatoma. A variant of branchio-oto-renal dysplasia. *Arch Otolaryngol Head Neck Surg* 112: 1097–1100.
Loosli F, Winkler S, Wittbrodt J (1999). *Six3* overexpression initiates the formation of ectopic retina. *Genes Dev* 13: 649–654.
Melnick M, Bixler D, Nance WE, Silk K, Yune H (1976). Familial branchio-oto-renal dysplasia: a new addition to the branchial arch syndromes. *Clin Genet* 9: 25–34.
Melnick M, Hodes ME, Nance WE, Yune H, Sweeney A (1978). Branchio-oto-renal dysplasia and branchio-oto dysplasia: two distinct autosomal dominant disorders. *Clin Genet* 13: 425–442
Misra M, Nolph KD (1998). Renal failure and deafness: branchio-oto-renal syndrome. *Am J Kidney Dis* 32: 334–337.
Moore MW, Klein RD, Farinas I, Sauer H, Armanini M, Phillips H, Reichardt LF, Ryan AM, Carver-Moore K, Rosenthal A (1996). Renal and neuronal abnormalities in mice lacking GDNF. *Nature* 382: 76–79.
Ng YY, Bellman S, Phelps PD (1989). Computed tomography of earpits-deafness syndrome. *Br J Radiol* 62: 947–949.
Ni L, Wagner MJ, Kimberling WJ, Pembrey ME, Grundfast KM, Kumar S (1994). Refined localization of the branchiootorenal syndrome by linkage and haplotype analysis. *Am J Med Genet* 51: 176–184.
Ohto H, Takizawa T, Saito T, Kobayashi M, Ikeda K, Kawakami K (1998). Tissue and developmental distribution of *Six* family gene products. *Int J Dev Biol* 42: 141–148.
Ohto H, Kamada S, Tago K, Tominaga S-H, Ozaki H, Sato S, Kawakami K (1999). Cooperation of Six and Eya in activation of their target genes through nuclear translocation of Eya. *Mol Cell Biol* 19: 6815–6824.
Oliver G, Wehr R, Jenkins NA, Copeland NG, Cheyette BN, Hartenstein V, Zipursky SL, Gruss P (1995). Homeobox genes and connecting tissue patterning. *Development* 121: 693–705.
Oliver G, Loosli F, Koster R, Wittbrodt J, Gruss P (1996). Ectopic lens induction in fish in response to the murine homeobox gene *Six3*. *Mech Dev* 60: 233–239.
Ostri B, Johnsen T, Bergmann I (1991). Temporal bone findings in a family with branchio-oroto-renal syndrome (BOR). *Clin Otolaryngol* 100: 928–932.
Ozaki H, Watanabe Y, Takahashi K, Kitamura K, Tanaka A, Urase K, Momoi T, Sudo Ksakagami J, Asano M, Iwakura Y, et al. (2001). *Six4*, a putative myogenin gene regulator, is not essential for mouse embryonic development. *Mol Cell Biol* 21: 3343–3350.
Pachnis V, Mankoo B, Costantini F (1993). Expression of the c-*Ret* proto-oncogene during mouse embryogenesis. *Development* 119: 1005–1017.
Pennie BH, Marres HAM (1992). Shoulder abnormalities in association with the branchio-oto-renal dysplasia in a patient who also has familial joint laxity. *Int J Pediatr Otorhinolaryngol* 23: 269–273.
Pichel JG, Shen L, Sheng HZ, Gramholm AC, Drago J, Grinberg A, Lee EJ, Huang SP, Saarma M, Hoffer BJ, et al. (1996). Defects in enteric innervation and kidney development in mice lacking GDNF. *Nature* 382: 73–76.
Pignoni F, Hu B, Zavitz KH, Xiao J, Garrity PA, Zipursky SL (1997). The eye-specification proteins So and Eya form a complex and regulate multiple steps in *Drosophila* eye development. *Cell* 91: 881–891.
Preisch JW, Bixler D, Ellis FD (1985). Gustatory lacrimation in association with the brachio-oto-renal syndrome. *Clin Genet* 27: 506–509.
Purcell P (2001). Genes involved in early development of mouse cranial sensory placodes. PhD thesis, Harvard University, Boston, MA.
Rickard S, Boxer M, Trompeter R, Bitner-Glindzicz M (2000). Importance of clinical evaluation and molecular testing in the branchio-oto-renal (BOR) syndrome and overlapping phenotypes. *J Med Genet* 37: 623–627.
Rodriguez-Soriano J, Vallo A, Bilboa JR, Castano L (2001). Branchio-oto-renal syndrome: identification of a novel mutation in the *EYA1* gene. *Pediatr Nephrol* 16: 550–553.
Rollnick BR, Kaye CI (1985). Hemifacial microsomia and the branchio-oto-renal syndrome. *J Craniofac Genet Dev Biol Suppl* 1(Suppl): 287–295.

Sahly I, Andermann P, Petit C (1999). The zebrafish *eya1* gene and its expression pattern during embryogenesis. *Dev Genes Evol* 209: 399–410.

Sanchez MP, Silos-Santiago I, Frisen J, He B, Lira SA, Barbacid M (1996). Renal agenesis and the absence of enteric neurons in mice lacking GDNF. *Nature* 382: 70–73.

Sarkar PS, Appukuttan B, Han J, Ito Y, Ai C, Tsai W, Chai Y, Stout JT, Reddy S (2000). Heterozygous loss of *Six5* in mice is sufficient to cause ocular cataracts. *Nat Genet* 25: 110–114.

Shen W, Mardon G (1997). Ectopic eye development in *Drosophila* induced by directed *dac* expression. *Development* 124: 45–52.

Stratakis CA, Lin J-P, Rennert OM (1998). Description of a large kindred with autosomal dominant inheritance of branchial arch anomalies, hearing loss and ear pits, and exclution of the branchio-oto-renal (BOR) syndrome gene locus (chromasome 8q13.3). *Am J Med Genet* 79: 209–214.

Stuckens C, Standaert L, Casselman JW, Huygen PL, Kumar S, Van de Wallen J, Cremers CW (2001). The presence of a widened vestibular aqueduct and progressive sensorineural hearing loss in the branchio-oto-renal syndrome. A family study. *Int J Pediatr Otorhinolaryngol* 59: 163–172.

Takeda Y, Hatano S, Sentoku N, Matsuoka M (1999). Homologs of animal eyes absent (*eya*) genes are found in higher plants. *Mol Gen Genet* 262: 131–138.

Torres M, Gomez-Pardo E, Dressler GR, Gruss P (1995). *Pax2* controls multiple steps of urogenital development. *Development* 121: 4057–4065.

Torres-Peris V, Jorda E, Ramon D, Peiro J, Revert A, Torres-Larrosa T (1994). Melnick-Fraser syndrome. *Dermatology* 189: 103–104.

Van Hoy M, Leuther KK, Kodadek T, Johnston SA (1993). The acidic activation domains of the GCN4 and GAL4 proteins are not alpha helical but form beta sheets. *Cell* 72:587–594.

Van Widdershoven J, Monnens L, Assmann K, Cremers C (1983). Renal disorders in the branchio-oto-renal syndrome. *Helv Paedeatr Acta* 38: 513–522.

Vincent C, Kalatzis V, Abdelhak S, Chaib H, Compain S, Helias J, Vaneecloo FM, Petit C (1997). BOR and BO syndromes are allelic defects of EYA1. *Eur J Hum Genet* 5: 242–246.

Wallis DE, Roessler E, Hehr U, Nanni L, Wiltshire T, Richieri-Costa A, Gillessen-Kaesbach G, Zackai EH, Rommens J, Muenke M (1999). Mutations in the homeodomain of the human *SIX3* gene cause holoprosencephaly. *Nat Genet* 22: 196–198.

Weber KM, Kousseff BG (1999). "New" manifestations of BOR syndrome. *Clin Genet* 56: 306–312.

Worley GA, Vats A, Harcourt J, Albert DM (1999). Bilateral cholesteatoma in branchio-oto-renal syndrome. *J Laryngol Otol* 113: 841–843.

Xu PX, Woo I, Her H, Beier DR, Maas RL (1997a). Mouse *Eya* homologues of the *Drosophila eyes absent* gene require *Pax6* for expression in lens and nasal placode. *Development* 124: 219–231.

Xu PX, Cheng J, Epstein JA, Maas RL (1997b). Mouse *Eya* genes are expressed during limb tendon development and encode a transcriptional activation function. *Proc Natl Acad Sci USA* 94: 11974–11979.

Xu PX, Zhang X, Heaney S, Yoon A, Michelson AM, Maas RL (1999a). Regulation of Pax6 expression is conserved between mice and flies. *Development* 126: 383–395.

Xu PX, Adams J, Peters H, Brown MC, Heaney S, Maas R (1999b). *Eya1* deficient mice lack ears and kidneys and exhibit abnormal apoptosis of organ primordia. *Nat Genet* 23: 113–117.

56 | *PITX2* and *PITX3* and the Axenfeld-Rieger Syndrome, Iridogoniodysgenesis and Iris Hypoplasia, Peters Anomaly, and Anterior Segment Ocular Dysgenesis

ELENA V. SEMINA

*P*ITX2 and *PITX3* genes represent members of the family of homeobox-containing transcription factor genes, PITX, that plays an important role in embryonic development in different species. Humans with mutations in the *PITX* genes exhibit a variety of developmental defects, including such debilitating ocular conditions as glaucoma, cataracts, and corneal opacities. Moreover, the *PITX2* gene is a critical factor in the regulation of left-right asymmetry in embryogenesis and is likely to play a role in hematopoietic stem cell biology, GABAergic neuron differentiation, and tumorigenesis. The *PITX3* gene, in addition to its role in ocular development, appears to be involved in governing the development of the mesencephalic dopaminergic system that has been implicated in some psychiatric disorders. Therefore, the *PITX* genes represent important components of the network of genes directing the development of multiple organs in different species. Studies of the *PITX* roles in embryogenesis and cell fate decisions will lead to further exploration of the disorders associated with alterations in these genes. This should provide insight into the mechanisms of normal embryonic development, allow the identification of other disease genes, and lead to the better diagnosis and treatment of the associated conditions.

THE *PITX* GENE FAMILY

The human *PITX2* gene (originally called *RIEG/Rieg*) was first identified by positional cloning of the gene responsible for 4q25-linked cases of Rieger syndrome (now called Axenfeld-Rieger syndrome [ARS]; see later) (Semina et al., 1996b). The positional cloning steps included linkage mapping of the ARS gene to the 4q25 region (Murray et al., 1992), fine mapping of the two independent translocation breakpoints that occurred in unrelated ARS patients and involved the 4q25 region (Datson et al., 1996; Semina et al., 1996a), construction of the DNA contig encompassing the critical interval, and, finally, identification and analysis of genes located within the interval. The *PITX2* gene was shown to (1) map to the critical region known to contain the ARS gene, (2) be in close proximity to the two ARS breakpoints, and (3) contain multiple mutations in ARS patients and not in healthy control individuals. In addition, mouse *Pitx2* gene was isolated and showed remarkable homology with the human gene at both the nucleotide and protein levels. By in situ hybridization on whole mount embryos and sections, the *Pitx2* mRNA was detected in the mesenchyme around the developing eye and in the epithelium and mesenchyme of the maxilla and mandible, dental lamina, umbilical region, pituitary, midbrain region, and limbs (Semina et al. 1996b) (Fig. 56–1). The ocular, dental, and umbilical sites of *Pitx2* expression were consistent with the human disease phenotype.

The mouse *Pitx2* gene was also identified independently by researchers who study genes expressed in pituitary (*Ptx2*, Gage and Camper, 1997) and brain (*Otlx2*, Mucchielli et al., 1996; *Brx1*, Kitamura et al., 1997). The human *PITX2* was later isolated by another group as a target of *All1* (Arakawa et al., 1998). The *All1* gene is frequently altered in human acute leukemias that results in a loss of All1 function and missing expression of *Pitx2*, which suggests a role for *PITX2* in tumorigenesis. Degar et al. (2001) report an identification of *Pitx2* in a search for genes that are preferentially expressed in hematopoietic stem/progenitor cells and not in their differentiated progeny, suggesting a role for *Pitx2* in hematopoietic stem cell biology. Westmoreland et al. (2001) proposed that *Pitx2* is also involved in controlling GABAergic neuron differentiation.

The *PITX2* gene was shown to express up to three different mRNA isoforms in different species (Gage and Camper, 1997; Arakawa et al., 1998; Essner et al., 2000; Schweickert et al., 2000). The specific role of each of the isoforms has not yet been fully clarified, although differences in an expression pattern and a phenotypic effect have been noted (Essner et al., 2000; Schweickert et al., 2000; Liu et al., 2001).

The *PITX2* gene became the second member of the PITX family. The first gene, *Pitx1* (originally called *P-OTX* or *Ptx1*), was identified as a pituitary factor (Lamonerie et al., 1996; Szeto et al., 1996). The PITX family at this time consists of three genes, *PITX1* through *PITX-3*, that show overlapping expression patterns (see Fig. 56–1 reviewed in Gage et al., 1999b).

The human and mouse *PITX3/Pitx3* genes were identified in a search for additional members of the PITX family (Semina et al., 1997, 1998). The *PITX3/Pitx3* showed 100% identity to *PITX2/Pitx2* in the homeodomain (HD) region with overall identity at the protein level being at 78%. The earliest expression of the mouse *Pitx3* gene was detected in the lens at the placode stage, where it continued to be expressed until birth (Semina et al., 1997) (see Fig. 56–1). The murine *Pitx3* gene was localized to the distal region of chromosome 19 (Semina et al., 1997), and the human *PITX3* gene was mapped to 10q25. Expression pattern of the mouse *Pitx3* gene suggested that it might be involved in ocular phenotypes, particularly the ones that include abnormal lens development. Therefore, after the placement of the *PITX3* gene to the 10q25 region, we examined several ocular pedigrees for linkage to the *PITX3* locus. A six-generation family affected with anterior segment ocular dysgenesis with cataracts (ASOD) (Hittner et al., 1982) exhibited linkage to 10q24-25 with an lod score of 4.8 at $\theta = 0$ with the marker D10S192. Subsequent analysis of the *PITX3* gene sequence in DNA from affected members of this pedigree identified causative mutation in the gene. Screening of other ocular families identified another mutation in an isolated cataract patient (Semina et al., 1998) (Fig. 56–2, see also later).

The rat *Pitx3* gene was also independently identified; it was shown to be involved in the development of the mesencephalic dopaminergic system that controls behavior and movement and has been implicated in psychiatric and affective disorders (Smidt et al., 1997; Cazorla et al., 2000; Lebel et al., 2001).

ARS, ASOD, AND OTHER DISORDERS OF THE ANTERIOR SEGMENT ASSOCIATED WITH MUTATIONS IN *PITX* GENES

The human disorders associated with mutations in the *PITX2* and *PITX3* genes are summarized in Table 56–1.

The *PITX2* gene was originally discovered as the first causative gene for Rieger syndrome, which is now termed Axenfeld-Rieger syndrome (OMIM 180500) (Alward et al., 2000). ARS is an autosomal dominant disorder with specific ocular, dental, and umbilical anomalies (see Fig. 56–3) (Axenfeld, 1920; Berg, 1932; Rieger, 1934, 1935; Alward, 2000). ARS is characterized by complete penetrance, but variable expressivity was recorded in families. Classic ARS manifestations include specific ocular, dental, and umbilical anomalies; glaucoma, which is present in about 8% of patients at birth, 50% by the second decade, and 60% thereafter, seems to be the most debilitating feature of this condition. Specific ARS ocular anomalies include a prominent annular white line near the limbus at the level of Desce-

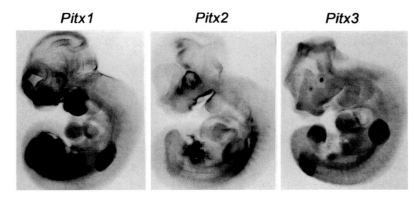

Pitx1   *Pitx2*   *Pitx3*

Figure 56–1. Whole-mount in situ hybridization on mouse day-11 embryos with antisense digoxigenin-labeled riboprobes derived from the mouse *Pitx1*, *Pitx2*, and *Pitx3* cDNAs as indicated. Bars, 0.55 mm.

ment membrane (posterior embryotoxon), hypoplastic iris, iridocorneal adhesions, and glaucoma (Shields, 1983; Shields et al., 1985; Ritch et al., 1996). The condition was first noted by Axenfeld, who described posterior embryotoxon in 1920 (Axenfeld, 1920). Later, Rieger reported a patient with posterior embryotoxon, iris hypoplasia, and pupillary defects. Rieger (1934, 1935) also noted the nonocular developmental defects such as craniofacial dysmorphism, dental hypoplasia, and redundant periumbilical skin. In 1932, Berg described a similar condition that included iris hypoplasia and iridocorneal adhesions but lacked posterior embryotoxon; he named it iridogoniodysgenesis (IGD). The patients with IGD were reported to occasionally have the same nonocular defects; therefore, the diagnosis of Axenfeld/Rieger/iridogoniodysgenesis anomaly was suggested when the corresponding ocular defect appeared to be the only clinical finding in the family, whereas when the ocular features were accompanied by systemic anomalies, it was regarded as a respective syndrome. All of these conditions were found to be caused by mutations in the same genes (Table 56–2; also see later); therefore, the term Axenfeld-Rieger syndrome was proposed to consolidate all of these overlapping phenotypes to eliminate confusing subclassification and to allow easier communication between investigators (Alward, 2000).

Dental defects in ARS vary from small teeth to complete anodontia. Missing lateral mandibular incisors are described as the most common feature. Umbilical anomalies range from isolated redundant umbilical skin to severe hernias or omphalocele. Other anomalies include maxillary hypoplasia, dysplastic ears, hearing loss, pituitary and cardiac anomalies, short stature, hydrocephalus, hypospadius, and limb defects (Fitch and Kaback, 1978; Brooks et al. 1989; Tsai and Grajewski, 1994; Mammi et al., 1998).

Peters' anomaly (OMIM 604229 and 603807) is a rare condition characterized by central corneal leukoma, absence of the posterior corneal stroma and Descemet membrane, varying degree of iris and lenticular attachments to the central aspect of the posterior cornea, and cataracts in some cases (Peters, 1906). Peters' anomaly is often associated with other systemic anomalies (Peters' plus syndrome; OMIM 261540). It is usually transmitted as an autosomal recessive trait; many sporadic cases are reported as well.

ASOD (OMIM 107250) is the collective term that refers to congenital disease that results from abnormally developed structures lining the anterior segment, including the anterior chamber angle, iris, cornea, and lens. Some of these conditions can be categorized as specific anomalies such as Axenfeld-Rieger anomaly or Peters' anomaly. ASOD consists of a highly variable and heterogeneous group of conditions and can be associated with a variety of systemic abnormalities.

THE MOLECULAR GENETICS OF ANTERIOR SEGMENT DISORDERS ASSOCIATED WITH *PITX* MUTATIONS

Frequency and Spectrum of *PITX* Mutations in Human Disorders

Ocular expression of the *PITX2* mutations shows broad variability, both between and within families. The reported phenotypes include Rieger and Axenfeld anomaly, iris hypoplasia, IGD, Peters' anomaly, and partial aniridia (see Table 56–1). The umbilical and dental anomalies are

highly penetrant; only about 9% of patients with *PITX2* mutations display isolated ocular defects. In classic ARS patients, the frequency of the *PITX2* mutations is about 40% (Semina et al., 1996; Perveen et al., 2000). Among other anomalies associated with *PITX2* mutations, Meckel's diverticulum and severe omphalocele are the most common.

The spectrum of *PITX3* mutations is not well defined yet because of the small number of etiologic mutations so far identified. The *PITX3* gene was found to be affected in two unrelated families characterized by cataracts with or without anterior segment anomalies. The first family is a six-generation pedigree with 15 living affected members who were diagnosed with ASOD (Hittner et al., 1982). All of the affected members were characterized by corneal opacities with or without iris adhesions and cataracts; optic nerve abnormalities were seen in 20% of individuals with the disorder (Fig. 56–2). The phenotype was highly variable and ranged from posterior embryotoxon with mild cataract to severe corneal opacity with moderate cataract; the visual acuity varied from 20/20 in at least one eye to hand motion only. The proband underwent corneal transplantation and an extracapsular cataract extraction in one eye at the age of 6 weeks. Microscopic studies of the proband's cornea showed no evidence of Descemet's layer or resid-

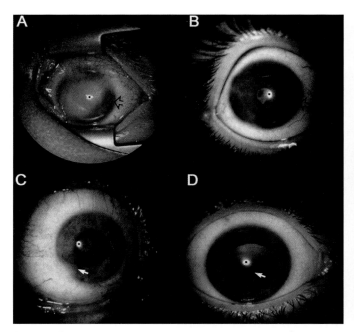

Figure 56–2. Variable expressivity in family with anterior segment ocular dysgenesis. (*A*) A dense central corneal leucoma with an iris adhesion obscures a small central cataractous lens. (*B*) A dense central cataractous lens overshadows a translucent central corneal leucoma. (*C*) A dense central cataractous lens overshadows a dense peripheral corneal leucoma with an iris adhesion. (*D*) Both a small corneal opacity and a small lens opacity might easily escape detection without both a family history and a slit lamp examination. Open arrowhead indicates Schwalbe's ring; white arrow, corneal opacity (leucoma); black arrow, lens opacity (cataract). The white dot with black center is an artifact. (From *Nat Genet* [1998] 19: 167–170.)

Table 56–1. Summary of *PITX2* and *PITX3* Mutations

Gene	No.	Mutation/Position*	Predicted Effect/Location*	Ocular Phenotype/Other Features	Reference
PITX2	1	T744A	L54Q/HD	ARA/dental and umbilical defects	Semina et al., 1996
	2	A785C	T68P/HD	ARA/dental and umbilical defects	Semina et al., 1996
	3	G789A	R69H/HD	Iridogoniodysgenesis/dental and umbilical defects	Kulak et al., 1998
	9	G830C	V83L/HD	ARA/dental and umbilical defects	Priston et al., 2001
	4	C833T	R84W/HD	Iris hypoplasia/dental and umbilical s defects in 1 of 15 studied patients	Alward et al., 1997
	5	G to C/exon 3, 3'ss (+5)	Aberrant splicing/exon 4 (affects part of HD and C-term)	ARA/dental and umbilical defects, severe omphalocele	Semina et al., 1996
	6	A to G/exon 4, 5'ss (-11)	Aberrant splicing/exon 4 (affects part of HD and C-term)	ARA/dental and umbilical defects	Semina et al., 1996
	7	G855C	R91P/HD	ARA/dental and umbilical defects (2), Meckel's diverticulum	Semina et al., 1996; Priston et al., 2001
	8	G982A	W135STOP/C-term	ARA/dental and umbilical defects, severe omphalocele, Meckel's diverticulum	Semina et al., 1996
	10	Duplication of 21 bp 713-733	Duplication of T54 through Q50/HD	ARA/maxillary hypoplasia, normal teeth and umbilicus	Priston et al., 2001
	11	A to T/exon 4, 5'ss (-2)	Aberrant splicing/exon 4 (affects part of HD and C-term)	ARA, Peters' anomaly, cataract/dental and umbilical defects	Perveen et al., 2000; Doward et al., 1999
	12	1083_ins C	Frameshift P167_/C-term	ARA, Peters' anomaly/dental defects	Perveen et al., 2000
	13	G to C/exon 3, 5'ss (-1)	Aberrant splicing/exon 3 (affects part of N-term, HD, C-term)	ARA, partial aniridia/dental and umbilical defects, joint hypermobility, anteriorly placed anus	Perveen et al., 2000
	14	A939_del	Frameshift Q119_/C-term	ARA/dental and umbilical defects	Perveen et al., 2000
	15	TA1235-1236_AAG	Frameshift T218_/C-term	ARA/dental and umbilical defects, Meckel's diverticulum	Perveen et al., 2000
	16	A845G	K88E/HD	ARA, bilateral corneal opacity, partial aniridia/dental and umbilical defects, hyperflexible joints	Saadi et al., 2001
	17	AA868-869_ del	Frameshift R95_/HD and C-term	ARA/dental and umbilical defects, imperforate anus, pectus deformity, finger pulp defect	Perveen et al., 2000
	18	C851T	R90C/HD	ARA/dental and umbilical defects, cleft palate, cleft uvula, learning difficulties, edentulos	Perveen et al., 2000
	19	Breakpoint t(4:16)/5–15 kb upstream	Loss of expression	ARA/dental and umbilical defects	Semina et al., 1996
	20	Breakpoint t(4:11)/55–65 kb upstream	Loss of expression	ARA/dental and umbilical defects, polydactyly, developmental delay	Semina et al., 1996
	21	Breakpoint t(4:12)/90 kb upstream	Loss of expression	ARA/dental and umbilical defects	Flomen et al., 1998
	22	Deletion (4) (q24q26)	Deletion of *PITX2* gene	ARA, microphthalmia/dysplastic ears, narrow palate, VSD, mental retardation and other MCA	Schinzel et al., 1997
	23	Deletion (4)(q25q27)	Deletion of *PITX2* gene	ARA/dental anomalies, dyscrania, dysplastic ears	Flomen et al., 1998
PITX3	1	Insertion of 17 bp at 660	Frameshift/G219_ C-term	Anterior segment ocular dysgenesis	Semina et al., 1998
	2	G41A	S13N/N-term	Cataract	Semina et al., 1998

*Position/location is shown according to Semina et al. (1996).
ARA, Axelfeld-Rieger anomaly; VSD, ventricular septal defect; HD, homeodomain.

ual endothelial cells even in the far periphery of the corneal button and thickening of the acellular Bowman's layer. The cataractous changes appeared to be cortical, suggesting that only the last-forming fibers were affected. The second family represents a single pedigree consisting of unaffected father and a mother and a child who were affected with an isolated autosomal dominant congenital cataract (ADCC).

Molecular Genetics and Functional Analysis of Pitx2 and Pitx3 Normal and Mutant Proteins

The *PITX2* and *PITX3* genes encode HD-containing transcription factors that regulate the expression of other genes during embryogenesis. The HD transcription factors function to specifically bind DNA in the regulatory regions of their downstream genes to control their activities; the HD region plays a major role in the DNA binding, whereas the other regions of the proteins can moderate the specificity of this contact.

The HD regions of the proteins encoded by *PITX2* or *PITX3* are identical and show the strongest similarity to the *paired-like* and the *bicoid-like* HD (Semina et al., 1996, 1997, 1998; Amendt et al., 1998).

The *bicoid*-related proteins share a lysine residue at position 9 of the third helix of the HD, which has been shown to determine the specificity of binding to 3'CC dinucleotide following the TAAT core (Gehring et al., 1994). Consistent with this prediction, it was demonstrated that both PITX2 and PITX3 can strongly bind to the DNA sequence 5'-TAATCC-3' and to other *bicoid* sequences and to transactivate promoters containing these sequences (Amendt et al., 1998; Cazorla et al., 2000; Lebel et al., 2001). These identical DNA-binding specificities of PITX2 and PITX3 proteins are not surprising because their HD sequences are the same. Similar phenomena were reported for other transcription factors, and either such proteins could be functionally redundant or their specificity will reside in functions other than DNA binding (Hellqvist et al., 1998).

Protein–protein interactions play important roles in the modulation of HD protein binding and transcriptional activity (Treisman et al., 1992; Bendall et al., 1998; Carroll and Vize, 1999; Perrone et al., 1999). This combinatorial control of regulation is thought to enable the formation of more complex networks (multiprotein complexes) involved in regulation of gene expression in eukaryotic organisms (Wolberger, 1998).

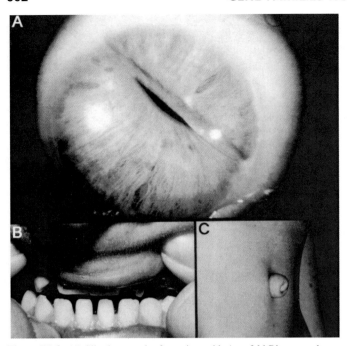

Figure 56–3. (*A*) Slit photograph of a patient with Axenfeld-Rieger syndrome. The hypoplastic iris allows the pupillary sphincter muscle to be seen as a band around the pupil. The pupil is distorted (corectopia). The distinct white line in the periphery of the cornea is termed "posterior embryotoxon" and represents a prominent and anteriorly displaced Schwalbe's line of trabecular meshwork, which is not normally visible. (*B*) This patient has both oligodontia, as evident by missing maxillary lateral incisors (canines are in the lateral incisor position), and microdontia, as present in the mandibular central incisors. (*C*) Photograph of the abdominal area showing characteristic umbilical abnormalities due to failure of the periumbilical skin to involute. (From *Nat Genet* [1996] 14: 392–399.)

For the Pitx2 protein, it was shown that the C-terminal tail, which is deleted in some ARS patients, regulates Pitx2 activity through interactions with other proteins (Amendt et al., 1998, 1999, 2000). In fact, the Pitx2 protein may not be fully activated until expression of the appropriate cofactor (Amendt et al., 1999). Another PITX family member, Pitx1, was shown to be involved in interactions with Pit-1, Clim1,Clim2, and bHLH transcription factors, which result in synergistic transcriptional activation of genes in pituitary cells (Szeto et al. 1996; Bach et al., 1998; Poulin et al., 2000). The C-terminal tails of Pitx proteins contain a 14–amino acid motif that is shared by many *paired-like* HD proteins expressed in ocular tissues (Semina et al., 1996; Furukawa et al., 1997; Mathers et al., 1997) and may represent an interacting site with a common family of proteins as has been shown, for example, for EXD/PBX and HOX protein families (Shanmugam et al., 1997).

The majority of the *PITX2* mutations are located in the homeobox region of the gene encoding the HD. These mutations are most likely to generate a null allele, which was shown to be true in several cases (Amendt et al., 1998; Kozlowski and Walter, 2000; Priston et al., 2001). These findings, supported by reports of large deletions that encompass the whole *PITX2* gene in some ARS patients (Schinzel et al., 1997; Flomen et al., 1998), strongly suggest haploinsufficiency as an etiologic mechanism of ARS. Several translocation breakpoints were localized at about 5 to about 90 kb upstream of the *PITX2* gene (Semina et al., 1996; Flomen et al., 1998). The phenomenon, when development of a disease is caused by chromosomal rearrangements outside the transcription and promoter regions, is recognized as "position effect" and was described for a number of transcription factor genes (Kleinjan and van Heyningen, 1998). There are a number of mechanisms that can explain this phenomenon, such as removal of locus-specific enhancer elements or a chromatin-organizing region from the gene that results in reduction in its expression.

There have been several reports that connected phenotypic spectrum of the anterior segment features in ARS with residual activity of the mutant PITX2 protein. In Kozlowski and Walter (2000) and Priston et al. (2001) tested the activity of different mutant PITX2 proteins

Table 56–2. Current Genetic Data for Anterior Segment Disorders and Cataracts, with Ocular Component of the Phenotype Shown in Parentheses for Syndromes

Disorder	Location	Gene	Function
Aniridia, Peters' anomaly, iris hypoplasia, foveal hypoplasia, cataract, keratitis, ARS	11p13	*PAX6*	Paired-box transcription factor
ARS, iris hypoplasia, Peters' and Rieger anomalies, IGD	4q25	*PITX2*	HD-transcription factor
Alagille syndrome (posterior embryotoxon)	20p12	*JAG1*	Ligand for a Notch receptor
ARA, IGD, anterior segment dysgenesis, ARS	6p25	*FOXC1*	Fork-head transcription factor
Anterior segment dysgenesis, cataracts	10q24-25	*PITX3*	HD-transcription factor
Nail-patella syndrome (open angle glaucoma)	9q34	*LMX1B*	LIM-HD transcription factor
Microphthalmia, cataracts, iris anomalies	14q24	*CHX10*	HD-transcription factor
Anterior segment dysgenesis, cataracts	8q13.3	*EYA1*	Transcription factor
Anterior segment dysgenesis, cataracts	1p32	*FOXE3*	Fork-head transcr. factor
Craniosynostosis with anterior segment dysgenesis	10q26	*FGFR2*	Fibroblast growth factor receptor
Anterior segment dysgenesis and cataract	16q23.2	*MAF*	Basic leucine zipper (bZIP) transcription factor
Primary open-angle glaucoma (GLC1A)	1q24-25	*MYOC*	Unknown
Primary congenital glaucoma (GLC3A), Peters' anomaly	2p22-21	*CYP1B1*	Cytochrome
Primary congenital glaucoma (GLC3B)	1p36	—	—
Primary open-angle glaucoma (GLC1B, GLC1C, GLC1D, GLC1E, GLC1F)	2q; 3q; 8q; 10p; 7q35	—	—
AD-nanophthalmos (NNO1) with hyperopia and glaucoma	11	—	—
Pigment dispersion syndrome	7q35-36	—	—
ARS	13q14	—	—
ARS	16q24	—	—
Cataract (autosomal dominant and recessive)	1q; 22q; 21q; 13q; 11q; 12q; 2q; 17q; multiple other loci	*GJA8, CRYBB2, CRYAA, GJA3, CRYAB, MIP, CRYGD, CRY-GC, CRYBA1*	Gap-junction connexin and crystallin proteins, major intrinsic protein

ARS, Axenfeld-Rieger syndrome; IGD, iridogoniodysgenesis; ARA, Axenfeld-Rieger anomaly; AD, autosomal dominant.
Source: Pax6 (Glaser et al., 1992; Jordan et al., 1992); PITX2 (Semina et al., 1996b); JAG1 (Li et al., 1997); FOXC1 (Kume et al., 1998; Mears et al., 1998; Nishimura et al., 1998; Mirzayans et al., 1999); PITX3 (Semina et al., 1998a); LMX1B (Chen et al., 1998; Vollrath et al., 1998); CHX10 (Persin et al., 2000); EYA1 (Abdelhak et al., 1997; Azuma et al., 2000); FOXE3 (Semina et al., 2001); FGFR2 (Okajima et al., 1999); MAF (Jamieson et al., 2002); MYOC (Stone et al., 1997); CYP1B1 (Stoilov et al., 1997; Vincent et al., 2001); GJA8 (Shiels et al., 1998), CRYBB2 (Litt et al., 1997), CRYAA (Litt et al., 1998), GJA3 (Mackay et al., 1999), CRYAB (Vicart et al., 1998; Berry et al., 2000), MIP (Berry et al., 2000; Sidjanin et al., 2001), CRYGD (Heon et al., 1999; Stephan et al., 1999), CRYGC (Heon et al., 1999; Ren et al., 2000), CRYBA1 (Kannabiran et al., 1998), GLC3B (Akarsu et al., 1996); GLC1B, GLC1C, GLC1D, GLC1E, GLC1F (Stoilova et al., 1996; Wirtz et al., 1997, 1999; Sarfarazi et al., 1998; Trifan et al., 1998); NNO1 (Othman et al., 1998); ARS at 13q (Phillips et al., 1996); pigment dispersion syndrome (Andersen et al., 1997), ARS at 16q (Nishimura et al., 2000).

through DNA-binding shifts and transactivation studies. These studies demonstrated that there is a positive correlation between the severity of ARS ocular phenotype and the loss of activity by corresponding mutant PITX2 protein: the mutant protein associated with iris hypoplasia (Alward et al., 1998) showed the most retained activity, followed by the IGD mutant (Kulak et al., 1998) and, finally, mutant proteins associated with the Axenfeld-Rieger ocular defects (posterior embryotoxon, iridocorneal adhesions, iris hypoplasia, glaucoma) that were proved to be nonfunctional. In line with these reports, Saadi et al. (2001) presented identification of the first dominant negative mutation in the PITX2 HD in an ARS patient with pronounced ocular findings (partial aniridia in addition to ARA). This mutation disrupted the critical *bicoid*-specific lysine residue at position 9 of the third (recognition) helix of the HD and changed it into glutamic acid. This resulted not only in the creation of a nonfunctional mutant allele but also in suppression of the wild-type protein activity. Priston et al. (2001) also presented the first phenomenon of increased transactivation activity by the mutant PITX2 protein associated with ARS, suggesting that elevated activity of the one PITX2 allele may be as physiologically disruptive as a null allele.

The *PITX3* mutations demonstrate a different distribution in comparison to *PITX2*: of two mutations identified to date, one is located in the region that encodes the N-terminal region of the protein, and the other encodes the C-terminal region; no mutations in the homeobox region, where the *PITX2* mutations are clustered, have been identified. The first mutation that was found in ASOD individuals (see earlier) is a 17-bp insertion carrying an extra copy of an 11-bp repeat present in the normal sequence of the gene (Semina et al., 1998). The insertion results in a frame shift in the 3′ end of the coding region, so that the mutant protein is predicted to contain an intact HD sequence but to lack 82 C-terminal amino acids, including the conserved 14–amino acid motif. The second mutation that was identified in ADCC individuals is a G-to-A nucleotide substitution, resulting in a serine-to-asparagine change in the N-terminal region of the translated protein. The exact mechanism of either ASOD or ADCC mutation in the *PITX3* gene is yet unknown; however, because the HD region is intact in both mutant proteins, they are likely to retain their DNA-binding activity but to be defective in carrying out other functions. Such defects in protein function could produce a dominant negative effect. Identification of additional mutations in the *PITX3* gene is critical for further characterization of the primary phenotypes associated with alterations in this gene and for establishment of the phenotype–genotype correlations.

ESTABLISHING THE DIAGNOSIS

ARS and Axenfeld-Rieger anomaly, anterior segment dysgenesis, and other related anomalies are diagnosed on the basis of clinical findings. The main characteristic feature of the Axenfeld-Rieger disorder is abnormal development of the anterior segment of the eye (see earlier), which is usually easily detectable at birth but may require a detailed ophthalmologic examination in some mildly affected patients. Individuals who present with umbilical hernias, redundant periumbilical skin, or omphalocele at birth or dental anomalies later in life should be evaluated by an ophthalmologist for Axenfeld-Rieger ocular anomalies to verify the diagnosis. This is important because patients with Axenfeld-Rieger disorders are at high risk for the development of glaucoma and should be carefully monitored.

MANAGEMENT, SPECIFIC TREATMENT, AND COUNSELING

The dental defects associated with ARS usually require orthodontic and prosthodontic treatment as a result of malocclusion associated with multiple missing teeth. The redundant periumbilical skin does not usually cause any medical problems and is a cosmetic defect, but umbilical hernias and omphalocele require surgical interference in severe cases. The most challenging therapeutic efforts in the Axenfeld-Rieger spectrum and other anterior segment disorders involve the treatment of glaucoma when present (Petersen and Boger, 2002). If the diagnosis of Axenfeld-Rieger disorder is suspected, the intraocular pressure should be examined and followed up. Unfortunately, Axenfeld-Rieger–associated glau-

coma is very difficult to manage with medication, and surgery (filtration surgery, cryoablation, or a tube shunt) is also often unsuccessful. For patients with bilateral visually disabling corneal opacity (Peters' anomaly, ASOD), penetrating keratoplasty is recommended. This is a corneal transplant procedure that may restore vision to otherwise blind eyes. In case of congenital cataracts that are causing a severe reduction in vision, a cataract extraction procedure (lensectomy, lens aspiration) is recommended, with the aim to remove the natural lens of the eye that has become cloudy. In general, pediatric disorders such as congenital glaucoma, cataract, and corneal opacities are treatable but treatment is problematic, and they remain the most common causes of childhood blindness. The complex nature and severity of developmental anomalies, intense inflammation, amblyopia, problems with tissue repair, regeneration, and scarring play roles in the failure of treatment.

Several genes associated with anterior segment disorders have been identified that can be tested in affected pedigrees on a research basis to provide better counseling for families (see Table 56–2; see also later). Analyses of the disease-associated genes will provide insight into the mechanisms of normal development of these structures and the disease pathogenesis and therefore may eventually provide a better treatment for these debilitating conditions.

ANIMAL PHENOTYPES ASSOCIATED WITH *Pitx2* AND *Pitx3* ALTERATIONS

The *Pitx2* gene has been shown to play a crucial role in heart development and determination of left/right patterning of visceral organs in vertebrates (Harvey et al., 1998; Logan et al., 1998; Piedra et al., 1998; Ryan et al., 1998; Yoshioka et al., 1998). The *Pitx2*$^{-/-}$ homozygous mice demonstrate multiple defects in abdominal wall, heart, lung, brain, ocular, and pituitary development that lead to their death around embryonic days 9.25 to 15 (Gage et al., 1999a; Kitamura et al., 1999; Lin et al., 1999; Lu et al., 1999; Liu et al., 2002). Ocular defects in the *Pitx2*$^{-/-}$ mice include dysgenesis of the extraocular muscle and thickening of the mesothelial layer of the cornea resulting in enophthalmos. In contrast to the multiple anomalies identified in mice homozygous for the *Pitx2* null allele, ARS patients with known *PITX2* mutations do not demonstrate any visible heart, lung, brain, or pituitary anomalies, which may be explained by the dominant nature of this disorder as one normal copy of the *PITX2* gene is present in these individuals. Mutations in both copies of the *PITX2* gene may be associated with a more severe phenotype that is still to be determined or results in embryonic death.

The roles of different human *PITX2* isoforms have yet to be elucidated. The *pitx2a* and *pitx2b* isoforms were found to have different expression patterns and distinct genetic pathways upstream and downstream of each isoform in zebrafish and frog (Essner et al., 2000; Schweickert et al., 2000). Their functions may also be different as, for example, ectopic expression of isoforms *a* and *b* in a frog shows that both isoforms can alter left-right development, but *pitx2a* has a slightly stronger effect on the laterality of a heart (Essner et al., 2000). All of the *PITX2*-ARS mutations that have been identified to date are located in the last two *PITX2* exons encoding the HD and C-terminal regions, which are common for all of the isoforms. The isoform-specific mutations may be responsible for a different phenotype or phenotypes that have yet to be discovered.

The mouse *Pitx3* gene was mapped to the region of chromosome 19 where the mutant recessive phenotype *aphakia* (*ak*) had been previously mapped (Varnum and Stevens, 1968, 1975). Affected mice demonstrate abnormal lens development that leads to the reduced eye size and overall ocular disorganization. Detailed examination of the *aphakia* embryos detected that the first abnormalities in lens development are seen slightly before closure of the lens cup at day 10.5–11 dpc: there is a progressive accumulation of cells, released by the lens epithelium, in the lumen of the lens cup, so that by the time of lens vesicle formation the lumen is entirely obliterated (Varnum and Stevens, 1968; Zwaan et al., 1975). After 11 days pc, no further organization of the lens takes place: the lens vesicle does not detach from the ectoderm, the anterior segment is not formed, and the cells at the posterior wall never elongate to become lens fibers.

By in situ hybridization, we detected no expression in the lens placode and lens pit or later in the lens remnants in the *ak/ak* animals (Semina et al., 2000). Rieger et al. (2001) used the quantitative PCR approach to show that expression of the *Pitx3* transcript is diminished to 5% of its normal amount in cDNA derived from heads of days 11.5–15.5 *ak/ak* and wild-type embryos. When the *Pitx3* promoter region was studied, two deletions in the *ak/ak* genomic DNA were identified: of 652 nucleotides (Δ652) residing at a distance of 2.5 kb from the start of the *Pitx3* cDNA and of 1432 nucleotides (Δ1432) surrounding noncoding exon 1 (Semina et al., 2000; Rieger et al., 2001). Although *aphakia* mice seem to retain some *Pitx3* expression, it is suggested that severe reduction of this expression or complete loss of it during certain stages of ocular development is responsible for the ocular anomalies in these animals. The creation of *Pitx3*$^{-/-}$ knockout mice, which was initiated at several laboratories, will show whether the complete loss of *Pitx3* expression results in a phenotype that differs from *aphakia*.

THE DEVELOPMENTAL PATHOGENESIS OF THE DISORDERS ASSOCIATED WITH *PITX* MUTATIONS

Anomalies associated with ARS seem to result from arrest in development as originally suggested by Shields (1983). In human ocular development, the arrest was proposed to occur at the late stages and to result in retention of the primordial corneal endothelial layer over portions of iris and the anterior chamber. This leads to a variety of iris anomalies and compression and/or incomplete development of trabecular meshwork and Schlemm's canal, structures that control the flow of aqueous humor from the eye into the venous system. In normal eyes, the primordial corneal endothelial layer creates a closed cavity to form the anterior chamber and then later progressively disappears, with some remaining cells establishing the endothelial lining of the trabecular meshwork. The corneal endothelial layer is produced by mesenchymal cells of neural crest origin that populate many other anterior segment structures as well as the pituitary gland, bones, and cartilage of the upper face and the dental papillae. Therefore, developmental arrest involving neural crest could also explain the ocular, facial, and tooth anomalies that are characteristic of this condition (Shields, 1983; Shields et al., 1985).

Studies of mice with complete loss of *Pitx2* function (see also earlier) demonstrated arrest of ocular development at the stage when lens vesicle separates from corneal ectoderm. This separation is thought to be facilitated by differentiation of corneal endothelium and is normally followed by the formation of anterior segment structures in the opening space (Reneker et al., 2000). *Pitx2*$^{-/-}$ mice demonstrate displaced irregular pupil and a lack of anterior chamber, extraocular muscles, and differentiated cornea (specifically corneal endothelium), whereas the mesothelial layer of the cornea is increased 5- to 10-fold at some stages (Gage et al., 1999b; Kitamura et al., 1999; Li et al., 1999; Lu et al., 1999). These findings indicate the importance of *Pitx2* for proper migration and/or differentiation of neural crest–derived mesenchymal cells, suggesting that the same process is likely to be disturbed in patients with Axenfeld-Rieger disorders.

Ocular defects in humans with mutations in the *PITX3* gene and *aphakia* mice are likely to also be due to arrest at the late stages of ocular development. In *aphakia* mice, the ocular development is arrested at the same stage as in the *Pitx2*$^{-/-}$ mice—the lens vesicle separation from the corneal ectoderm (see also earlier). The primary defect seem to be abnormal development of the lens, which is consistent with the *Pitx3* expression in mouse embryos. Defects in cellular adhesion, migration, and differentiation of neural crest cells have been suggested to occur in *aphakia* eye development, and it must be determined which of them represents a primary or secondary defect. It has been demonstrated that removal or replacement of the lens leads to arrest in anterior segment development, as no recognizable corneal endothelium, corneal stroma, iris stroma, or anterior chamber was found in lens-less eyes. Instead, there was a disorganized aggregate of mesenchymal cells beneath the corneal epithelium (Beebe and Coats, 2000). Therefore, PITX factors appear to be involved in a complex crosstalk between different developing tissues during anterior segment development that guides the proper formation of these structures.

Haploinsufficiency seems to be the main underlying mechanism of

ARS produced by *PITX2* mutations, whereas the dominant negative effect is likely to be the cause of anterior segment dysgenesis and cataract in patients with *PITX3* mutations (see earlier). Both the *PITX2* and *PITX3* mutations demonstrate significant interfamilial and intrafamilial differences in phenotype, indicating that individual variations in multiple other factors affect expressivity of the disorder. This phenomenon has been reported for many "single-gene" diseases (Quinn et al., 1997; Griep et al., 1998; Chang et al., 1999; Farley et al., 1999; Gong et al., 1999; Hong et al., 1999; Ireda et al., 1999). Identification and examination of genes involved in PITX pathways, analyses of genes with similar expression and/or associated disease phenotype, and studies of environmental factors should help to reveal the nature of this phenotypic variability and to provide a basis for studies of the related complex ocular disorders.

Genes responsible for conditions similar to those caused by PITX mutations could be involved in PITX pathways and therefore provide insight into the mechanisms of these pathologies. Heterogeneity of ARS was originally proposed because of the identification of different chromosomal anomalies in patients with the syndrome and was later confirmed through linkage and gene identification studies. The majority of reported cytogenetic abnormalities include deletions/translocations affecting 4q, 13q, and 6p and trisomy/monosomy 9, 16, 18, 20, and 21, where anomalies of 4, 13, and 6 chromosomes were associated with syndromic features, while the other cases were mostly characterized with only ocular findings (reviewed in Rogers, 1988). Five genetic loci and three causative genes for ARS are identified to date. In addition to the *PITX2* gene at the 4q25, which is described here, these loci include *FOXC1* at 6p25 (Mirzayans et al., 2000), *PAX6* at 11p13 (Riise et al., 2001), and unknown genes at 13q14 (Phillips et al., 1996) and 16q24 (Nishimura et al., 2000). The same as *PITX2*, *FOXC1* and *PAX6* were shown to be involved in a variety of overlapping phenotypes: aniridia, Peters' anomaly, iris hypoplasia, Rieger anomaly, and ARS for *PAX6* and ARS and Axenfeld-Rieger and anomaly, IGD, iris hypoplasia, and anterior segment dysgenesis for *FOXC1* (see Table 56–2 and references therein). Similar conditions are caused by mutations in *JAG1* (posterior embryotoxon in Alagille syndrome; Li et al., 1997), *LIMX1B* (open-angle glaucoma in nail-patella syndrome; Chen et al., 1998; Vollrath et al., 1998), and a variety of glaucoma genes (see Table 56–2). Anterior segment dysgenesis with and without cataracts or nonocular features is an extremely heterogeneous condition. In addition to the above-mentioned genes that are involved in the Axenfeld-Rieger spectrum, causes include mutations in *EYA1* (anterior segment dysgenesis; Azuma et al., 2000), *FGFR2* (craniosynostosis syndrome with anterior segment dysgenesis; Okajima et al., 1999), *FOXE3* (cataract and anterior segment dysgenesis; Semina et al., 2001), and *MAF* (cataract, anterior segment dysgenesis and coloboma; Jamieson et al., 2002). A variety of cataract-causing genes have also been reported (see Table 56–2). Most of the genes identified to date that are involved in the Axenfeld-Rieger spectrum and other anterior segment disorders are transcription factors that regulate the expression of other genes during development. Identification of their downstream targets is of high priority to better understand the mechanisms of normal development and associated abnormalities and to identify future therapeutic strategies.

ACKNOWLEDGMENTS

I am grateful to Dr. Jeffrey C. Murray for introducing me to studies of Axenfeld-Rieger syndrome and for his guidance, friendship, and support over the years of my postdoctoral training and in the following years. I am also thankful to Drs. Andy Russo, Brad Amendt, and Tord Hjalt for their support and collaboration on studies of PITX2 protein. I give many thanks to Rebecca Reiter, Dee Even, Carrie Funkhauser, Bonnie Ludwig, and Gretchen Mondt, who helped me with numerous aspects of this study. This study would not have been possible without support from many physicians and their patients who contributed samples for analysis, in particular, Drs. W. Lee Alward, Pierre Bitoun and Helen Mintz-Hittner. The study was supported by funds from the National Eye Institute, National Institutes of Health.

REFERENCES

Abdelhak S, Kalatzis V, Heilig R, Compain S, Samson D, et al. (1997). A human homologue of the Drosophila eyes absent gene underlies branchio-oto-renal (BOR) syndrome and identifies a novel gene family. *Nat Genet* 15(2): 157–164.

Akarsu AN, Turacli ME, Aktan SG, Barsoum-Homsy M, Chevrette L, Sayli BS, Sarfarazi M (1996). A second locus (GLC3B) for primary congenital glaucoma (Buphthalmos) maps to the 1p36 region. *Hum Mol Genet* 5(8): 1199–1203.

Alward WL (2000). Axenfeld-Rieger syndrome in the age of molecular genetics. *Am J Ophthalmol* 130(1): 107–115.

Alward WL, Semina EV, Kalenak JW, Heon E, Sheth BP, Stone EM, Murray JC (1998). Autosomal dominant iris hypoplasia is caused by a mutation in the Rieger syndrome (RIEG/PITX2) gene. *Am J Ophthalmol* 125(1): 98–100.

Amendt BA, Semina EV, Alward WL (2000). Rieger syndrome: a clinical, molecular, and biochemical analysis. *Cell Mol Life Sci* 57(11): 1652–1666.

Amendt BA, Sutherland LB, Russo AF (1999). Multifunctional role of the Pitx2 homeodomain protein C-terminal tail. *Mol Cell Biol* 19(10): 7001–7010.

Amendt BA, Sutherland LB, Semina EV, Russo AF (1998). The molecular basis of Rieger syndrome. Analysis of Pitx2 homeodomain protein activities. *J Biol Chem* 273(32): 20066–20072.

Andersen JS, Pralea AM, DelBono EA, Haines JL, Gorin MB, Schuman JS, Mattox CG, Wiggs JL (1997). A gene responsible for the pigment dispersion syndrome maps to chromosome 7q35-q36. *Arch Ophthalmol* 115(3): 384–388.

Arakawa H, Nakamura T, Zhadanov AB, Fidanza V, Yano T, Bullrich F, Shimizu M, Blechman J, Mazo A, Canaani E, et al. (1998). Identification and characterization of the ARP1 gene, a target for the human acute leukemia ALL1 gene. *Proc Natl Acad Sci USA* 95(8): 4573–4578.

Axenfeld T (1920). Embryotoxon corneae posteris. *Ber Dtsch Ophthalmol Ges* 42: 381–382.

Azuma N, Hirakiyama A, Inoue T, Asaka A, Yamada M (2000). Mutations of a human homologue of the Drosophila eyes absent gene (EYA1) detected in patients with congenital cataracts and ocular anterior segment anomalies. *Hum Mol Genet* 9(3): 363–366.

Bach I, Carriere C, Ostendorff HP, Andersen B, Rosenfeld MG (1997). A family of LIM domain-associated cofactors confer transcriptional synergism between LIM and Otx homeodomain proteins. *Genes Dev* 11(11): 1370–1380.

Beebe DC, Coats JM (2000). The lens organizes the anterior segment: specification of neural crest cell differentiation in the avian eye. *Dev Biol* 220(2): 424–431.

Bendall AJ, Rincon-Limas DE, Botas J, Abate-Shen C (1998). Protein complex formation between Msx1 and Lhx2 homeoproteins is incompatible with DNA binding activity. *Differentiation* 63(3): 151–157.

Berg F (1932). Erbliches jugendliches glaukom. *Acta Ophthalmol* 10: 568–587.

Berry V, Francis P, Kaushal S, Moore A, Bhattacharya S (2000). Missense mutations in MIP underlie autosomal dominant 'polymorphic' and lamellar cataracts linked to 12q. *Nat Genet* 25(1): 15–17.

Berry V, Francis P, Reddy MA, Collyer D, Vithana E, et al. (2001). Alpha-b crystallin gene (cryab) mutation causes dominant congenital posterior polar cataract in humans. *Am J Hum Genet* 69(5): 1141–1145.

Brooks JK, Coccaro PJ Jr, Zarbin MA (1989). The Rieger anomaly concomitant with multiple dental, craniofacial, and somatic midline anomalies and short stature. *Oral Surg Oral Med Oral Pathol* 68(6): 717–724.

Carroll TJ, Vize PD (1999). Synergism between Pax-8 and lim-1 in embryonic kidney development. *Dev Biol* 214(1): 46–59.

Cazorla P, Smidt MP, O'Malley KL, Burbach JP (2000). A response element for the homeodomain transcription factor Ptx3 in the tyrosine hydroxylase gene promoter. *J Neurochem* 74(5): 1829–1837.

Chang B, Smith RS, Hawes NL, Anderson MG, Zabaleta A, Savinova O, Roderick TH, Heckenlively JR, Davisson MT, John SW (1999). Interacting loci cause severe iris atrophy and glaucoma in DBA/2J mice. *Nat Genet* 21(4): 405–409.

Chen H, Lun Y, Ovchinnikov D, Kokubo H, Oberg KC, Pepicelli CV, Gan L, Lee B, Johnson RL (1998). Limb and kidney defects in Lmx1b mutant mice suggest an involvement of LMX1B in human nail patella syndrome. *Nat Genet* 19(1): 51–55.

Datson NA, Semina E, van Staalduinen AA, Dauwerse HG, Meershoek EJ, Heus JJ, Frants RR, den Dunnen JT, Murray JC, van Ommen GJ (1996). Closing in on the Rieger syndrome gene on 4q25: mapping translocation breakpoints within a 50-kb region. *Am J Hum Genet* 59(6): 1297–1305.

Degar BA, Baskaran N, Hulspas R, Quesenberry PJ, Weissman SM, Forget BG (2001). The homeodomain gene Pitx2 is expressed in primitive hematopoietic stem/progenitor cells but not in their differentiated progeny. *Exp Hematol* 29(7): 894–902.

Doward W, Perveen R, Lloyd IC, Ridgway AE, Wilson L, Black GC (1999). A mutation in the RIEG1 gene associated with Peters' anomaly. *J Med Genet* 36(2): 152–155.

Essner JJ, Branford WW, Zhang J, Yost HJ (2000). Mesendoderm and left-right brain, heart and gut development are differentially regulated by pitx2 isoforms. *Development* 127(5): 1081–1093.

Farley FA, Lichter PR, Downs CA, McIntosh I, Vollrath D, Richards JE (1999). An orthopaedic scoring system for nail-patella syndrome and application to a kindred with variable expressivity and glaucoma. *J Pediatr Orthop* 19(5): 624–631.

Fitch N, Kaback M (1978). The Axenfeld syndrome and the Rieger syndrome. *J Med Genet* 15(1): 30–34.

Flomen RH, Vatcheva R, Gorman PA, Baptista PR, Groet J, Barisic I, Ligutic I, Nizetic D (1998). Construction and analysis of a sequence-ready map in 4q25: Rieger syndrome can be caused by haploinsufficiency of RIEG, but also by chromosome breaks approximately 90 kb upstream of this gene. *Genomics* 47(3): 409–413.

Furukawa T, Kozak CA, Cepko CL (1997). rax, a novel paired-type homeobox gene, shows expression in the anterior neural fold and developing retina. *Proc Natl Acad Sci USA* 94(7): 3088–3093.

Gage PJ, Camper SA (1997). Pituitary homeobox 2, a novel member of the bicoid-related family of homeobox genes, is a potential regulator of anterior structure formation. *Hum Mol Genet* 6(3): 457–464.

Gage PJ, Suh H, Camper SA (1999a). Dosage requirement of Pitx2 for development of multiple organs. *Development* 126(20): 4643–4651.

Gage PJ, Suh H, Camper SA (1999b). The bicoid-related Pitx gene family in development. *Mamm Genome* 10(2): 197–200.

Gehring WJ, Qian YQ, Billeter M, Furukubo-Tokunaga K, Schier AF, et al. (1994). Homeodomain-DNA recognition. *Cell* 78(2): 211–223.

Glaser T, Walton DS, Maas RL (1992). Genomic structure, evolutionary conservation and aniridia mutations in the human PAX6 gene. *Nat Genet* 2(3): 232–239.

Gong X, Agopian K, Kumar NM, Gilula NB (1999). Genetic factors influence cataract formation in alpha 3 connexin knockout mice. *Dev Genet* 24(1-2): 27–32.

Griep AE, Krawcek J, Lee D, Liem A, Albert DM, Carabeo R, Drinkwater N, McCall M, Sattler C, Lasudry JG, et al. (1998). Multiple genetic loci modify risk for retinoblastoma in transgenic mice. *Invest Ophthalmol Vis Sci* 39(13): 2723–2732.

Hellqvist M, Mahlapuu M, Blixt A, Enerback S, Carlsson P (1998). The human forkhead protein FREAC-2 contains two functionally redundant activation domains and interacts with TBP and TFIIB. *J Biol Chem* 273(36): 23335–23343.

Heon E, Priston M, Schorderet DF, Billingsley GD, Girard PO, et al. (1999). The gamma-crystallins and human cataracts: a puzzle made clearer. *Am J Hum Genet* 65: 1261–1267.

Hittner HM, Kretzer FL, Antoszyk JH, Ferrell RE, Mehta RS (1982). Variable expressivity of autosomal dominant anterior segment mesenchymal dysgenesis in six generations. *Am J Ophthalmol* 93(1): 57–70.

Hjalt TA, Amendt BA, Murray JC (2001). PITX2 regulates procollagen lysyl hydroxylase (PLOD) gene expression: implications for the pathology of Rieger syndrome. *J Cell Biol* 152(3): 545–552.

Hjalt TA, Semina EV, Amendt BA, Murray JC (2000). The Pitx2 protein in mouse development. *Dev Dyn* 218(1): 195–200.

Jamieson RV, Perveen R, Kerr B, Carette M, Yardley J, Heon E, Wirth MG, van Heyningen V, Donnai D, Munier F, et al. (2002). Domain disruption and mutation of the bZIP transcription factor, MAF, associated with cataract, ocular anterior segment dysgenesis and coloboma. *Hum Mol Genet* 11(1): 33–42.

Jordan T, Hanson I, Zaletayev D, Hodgson S, Prosser J, Seawright A, Hastie N, van Heyningen V (1992). The human PAX6 gene is mutated in two patients with aniridia. *Nat Genet* 1(5): 328–332.

Kannabiran C, Rogan PK, Olmos L, Basti S, Rao GN, Kaiser-Kupfer M, Hejtmancik JF (1998). Autosomal dominant zonular cataract with sutural opacities is associated with a splice mutation in the betaA3/A1-crystallin gene. *Mol Vis* 23(4): 21.

Kitamura K, Miura H, Yanazawa M, Miyashita T, Kato K (1997). Expression patterns of Brx1 (Rieg gene), Sonic hedgehog, Nkx2.2, Dlx1 and Arx during zona limitans intrathalamica and embryonic ventral lateral geniculate nuclear formation. *Mech Dev* 67(1): 83–96.

Kitamura K, Miura H, Miyagawa-Tomita S, Yanazawa M, Katoh-Fukui Y, Suzuki R, Ohuchi H, Suehiro A, Motegi Y, Nakahara Y, et al. (1999). Mouse Pitx2 deficiency leads to anomalies of the ventral body wall, heart, extra- and periocular mesoderm and right pulmonary isomerism. *Development* 126(24): 5749–5758.

Kleinjan DJ, van Heyningen V (1998). Position effect in human genetic disease. *Hum Mol Genet* 7(10): 1611–1618.

Kozlowski K, Walter MA (2000). Variation in residual PITX2 activity underlies the phenotypic spectrum of anterior segment developmental disorders. *Hum Mol Genet* 9(14): 2131–2139.

Kulak SC, Kozlowski K, Semina EV, Pearce WG, Walter MA (1998). Mutation in the RIEG1 gene in patients with iridogoniodysgenesis syndrome. *Hum Mol Genet* 7(7): 1113–1117.

Kume T, Deng KY, Winfrey V, Gould DB, Walter MA, Hogan BL (1998). The forkhead/winged helix gene Mf1 is disrupted in the pleiotropic mouse mutation congenital hydrocephalus. *Cell* 93(6): 985–996.

Lamonerie T, Tremblay JJ, Lanctot C, Therrien M, Gauthier Y, Drouin J (1996). Ptx1, a bicoid-related homeo box transcription factor involved in transcription of the pro-opiomelanocortin gene. *Genes Dev* 10(10): 1284–1295.

Lebel M, Gauthier Y, Moreau A, Drouin J (2001). Pitx3 activates mouse tyrosine hydroxylase promoter via a high-affinity binding site. *J Neurochem* 77(2): 558–567.

Li L, Krantz ID, Deng Y, Genin A, Banta AB, Collins CC, Qi M, Trask BJ, Kuo WL, Cochran J, et al. (1997). Alagille syndrome is caused by mutations in human Jagged1, which encodes a ligand for Notch1. *Nat Genet* 16(3): 243–251.

Lin CR, Kioussi C, O'Connell S, Briata P, Szeto D, Liu F, Izpisua-Belmonte JC, Rosenfeld MG (1999). Pitx2 regulates lung asymmetry, cardiac positioning and pituitary and tooth morphogenesis. *Nature* 401: 279–282.

Litt M, Carrero-Valenzuela R, LaMorticella DM, Schultz DW, Mitchell TN, et al. (1997). Autosomal dominant cerulean cataract is associated with a chain termination mutation in the human beta-crystallin gene CRYBB2. *Hum Mol Genet* 6: 665–668.

Litt M, Kramer P, LaMorticella DM, Murphey W, Lovrien EW, Weleber RG (1998). Autosomal dominant congenital cataract associated with a missense mutation in the human alpha crystallin gene CRYAA. *Hum Mol Genet* 7(3): 471–474.

Liu C, Liu W, Lu MF, Brown NA, Martin JF (2001). Regulation of left-right asymmetry by thresholds of Pitx2c activity. *Development* 128(11): 2039–2048.

Logan M, Pagan-Westphal SM, Smith DM, Paganessi L, Tabin CJ (1998). The transcription factor Pitx2 mediates situs-specific morphogenesis in response to left-right asymmetric signals. *Cell* 94(3): 307–317.

Lu MF, Pressman C, Dyer R, Johnson RL, Martin JF (1999). Function of Rieger syndrome gene in left-right asymmetry and craniofacial development. *Nature* 401: 276–278.

Mackay D, Ionides A, Kibar Z, Rouleau G, Berry V, Moore A, Shiels A, Bhattacharya S (1999). Connexin46 mutations in autosomal dominant congenital cataract. *Am J Hum Genet* 64(5): 1357–1364.

Mammi I, De Giorgio P, Clementi M, Tenconi R (1998). Cardiovascular anomaly in Rieger Syndrome: heterogeneity or contiguity? *Acta Ophthalmol Scand* 76(4): 509–512.

Mathers PH, Grinberg A, Mahon KA, Jamrich M (1997). The Rx homeobox gene is essential for vertebrate eye development. *Nature* 387:603–607.

Mears AJ, Jordan T, Mirzayans F, Dubois S, Kume T, et al. (1998). Mutations of the forkhead/winged-helix gene, FKHL7, in patients with Axenfeld-Rieger anomaly. *Am J Hum Genet* 63(5): 1316–1328.

Mirzayans F, Gould DB, Heon E, Billingsley GD, Cheung JC, Mears AJ, Walter MA (2000). Axenfeld-Rieger syndrome resulting from mutation of the FKHL7 gene on chromosome 6p25. *Eur J Hum Genet* 8(1): 71–74.

Mucchielli ML, Mitsiadis TA, Raffo S, Brunet JF, Proust JP, Goridis C (1997). Mouse Otlx2/RIEG expression in the odontogenic epithelium precedes tooth initiation and requires mesenchyme-derived signals for its maintenance. *Dev Biol* 189(2): 275–284.

Murray JC, Bennett SR, Kwitek AE, Small KW, Schinzel A, Alward WL, Weber JL, Bell GI, Buetow KH (1992). Linkage of Rieger syndrome to the region of the epidermal growth factor gene on chromosome 4. *Nat Genet* 2(1): 46–49.

Nishimura DY, Searby CC, Borges AS, Carani JCE, Betinjane AJ, Stone EM, Susanna R, Alward WLM, Sheffield VC (2000). Identification of a fourth Rieger syndrome locus at 16q24. ASHG meeting, Philadelphia.

Nishimura DY, Swiderski RE, Alward WL, Searby CC, Patil SR, Bennet SR, Kanis AB, Gastier JM, Stone EM, Sheffield VC (1998). The forkhead transcription factor gene FKHL7 is responsible for glaucoma phenotypes which map to 6p25. *Nat Genet* 19(2): 140–147.

Okajima K, Robinson LK, Hart MA, Abuelo DN, Cowan LS, Hasegawa T, Maumenee IH, Wang Jabs E (1999). Ocular anterior chamber dysgenesis in craniosynostosis syndromes with a fibroblast growth factor receptor 2 mutation. *Am J Med Genet* 85(2): 160–170.

Othman MI, Sullivan SA, Skuta GL, Cockrell DA, Stringham HM, Downs CA, Fornes A, Mick A, Boehnke M, Vollrath D, et al. (1998). Autosomal dominant nanophthalmos (NNO1) with high hyperopia and angle-closure glaucoma maps to chromosome 11. *Am J Hum Genet* 63(5): 1411–1418.

Percin FE, Ploder LA, Yu JJ, Arici K, Horsford JD, et al. (2000). Human microphthalmia associated with mutations in the retinal homeobox gene CHX10. *Nat Genet* 25(4): 397–401.

Perrone L, Tell G, Di Lauro R (1999). Calreticulin enhances the transcriptional activity of thyroid transcription factor-1 by binding to its homeodomain. *J Biol Chem* 274(8): 4640–4645.

Perveen R, Lloyd IC, Clayton-Smith J, Churchill A, van Heyningen V, Hanson I, Taylor D, McKeown C, Super M, Kerr B, et al. (2000). Phenotypic variability and asymmetry of Rieger syndrome associated with PITX2 mutations. *Invest Ophthalmol Vis Sci* 41(9): 2456–2460.

Peters A (1906). Ueber angeborene Defektbildung der Descemetschen Membran. *Klin Mbl Augenheilk* 44: 27–40, 105–119.

Petersen RA, Boger WP III (2002). Pediatric ophthalmology. In: *Manual of Ocular Diagnosis and Therapy*. Pavan-Langston D (ed.) Lippincott Williams and Wilkins, Philadelphia, chap. 11.

Phillips JC, del Bono EA, Haines JL, Pralea AM, Cohen JS, Greff LJ, Wiggs JL (1996). A second locus for Rieger syndrome maps to 13q14. *Am J Hum Genet* 59(3): 613–619.

Piedra ME, Icardo JM, Albajar M, Rodriguez-Rey JC, Ros MA (1998). Pitx2 participates in the late phase of the pathway controlling left-right asymmetry. *Cell* 94(3): 319–324.

Poulin G, Lebel M, Chamberland M, Paradis FW, Drouin J (2000). Specific protein-protein interaction between basic helix-loop-helix transcription factors and homeoproteins of the Pitx family. *Mol Cell Biol* 20(13): 4826–4837.

Priston M, Kozlowski K, Gill D, Letwin K, Buys Y, Levin AV, Walter MA, Heon E (2001). Functional analyses of two newly identified PITX2 mutants reveal a novel molecular mechanism for Axenfeld-Rieger syndrome. *Hum Mol Genet* 10(16): 1631–1638.

Reneker LW, Silversides DW, Xu L, Overbeek PA (2000). Formation of corneal endothelium is essential for anterior segment development—a transgenic mouse model of anterior segment dysgenesis. *Development* 127(3): 533–542.

Rieger H (1934). Verlagerung und schitzform der pupille mit hypopasie des irisvordblattes. *Z Augenheilk* 84: 98–99.

Rieger H (1935). Beitraege zur kenntnis seltener und entrundung der pupille. *Albrecht von Graefes Arch Klin Exp Ophthalmol* 133: 602–635.

Rieger DK, Reichenberger E, McLean W, Sidow A, Olsen BR (2001). A double-deletion mutation in the Pitx3 gene causes arrested lens development in aphakia mice. *Genomics* 72(1): 61–72.

Riise R, Storhaug K, Brondum-Nielsen K (2001). Rieger syndrome is associated with PAX6 deletion. *Acta Ophthalmol Scand* 79(2): 201–203.

Ritch R, Shields MB, Krupin T (1996). *The Glaucomas*. Mosby, St. Louis, pp. 717–725, 875.

Ryan AK, Blumberg B, Rodriguez-Esteban C, Yonei-Tamura S, Tamura K, Tsukui T, de la Pena J, Sabbagh W, Greenwald J, Choe S, et al. (1998). Pitx2 determines left-right asymmetry of internal organs in vertebrates. *Nature* 394: 545–551.

Saadi I, Semina EV, Amendt BA, Harris DJ, Murphy KP, Murray JC, Russo AF (2001). Identification of a dominant negative homeodomain mutation in Rieger syndrome. *J Biol Chem* 276(25): 23034–23041.

Sarfarazi M, Child A, Stoilova D, Brice G, Desai T, Trifan OC, Poinoosawmy D, Crick RP (1998). Localization of the fourth locus (GLC1E) for adult-onset primary open-angle glaucoma to the 10p15-p14 region. *Am J Hum Genet* 62(3): 641–652.

Schinzel A, Brecevic L, Dutly F, Baumer A, Binkert F, Largo RH (1997). Multiple congenital anomalies including the Rieger eye malformation in a boy with interstitial deletion of (4) (q25 → q27) secondary to a balanced insertion in his normal father: evidence for haplotype insufficiency causing the Rieger malformation. *J Med Genet* 34(12): 1012–1014.

Schweickert A, Campione1 M, Steinbeisser H, Blum M (2000). Pitx2 isoforms: involvement of Pitx2c but not Pitx2a or Pitx2b in vertebrate left-right asymmetry. *Mech Dev* 90(1): 41–51.

Semina EV, Reiter RS, Murray JC (1997). Isolation of a new homeobox gene belonging to the Pitx/Rieg family: expression during lens development and mapping to the aphakia region on mouse chromosome 19. *Hum Mol Genet* 6(12): 2109–2116.

Semina EV, Brownell I, Mintz-Hittner HA, Murray JC, Jamrich M (2001). Mutations in the human fork-head transcription factor gene *FOXE3* cause anterior segment ocular dysgenesis and cataracts. *Hum Mol Genet* 10(3): 231–236.

Semina EV, Murray JC, Reiter R, Hrstka RF, Graw J (2000). Deletion in the promoter region and altered expression of Pitx3 homeobox gene in aphakia mice. *Hum Mol Genet* 9(11): 1575–1585.

Semina EV, Ferrell RE, Mintz-Hittner HA, Bitoun P, Alward WL, Reiter RS, Funkhauser C, Daack-Hirsch S, Murray JC (1998). A novel homeobox gene PITX3 is mutated in families with autosomal-dominant cataracts and ASMD. *Nat Genet* 19(2): 167–170.

Semina EV, Datson NA, Leysens NJ, Zabel BU, Carey JC, Bell GI, Bitoun P, Lindgren C, Stevenson T, Frants RR, et al. (1996a). Exclusion of epidermal growth factor and high-resolution physical mapping across the Rieger syndrome locus. *Am J Hum Genet* 59(6): 1288–1296.

Semina EV, Reiter R, Leysens NJ, Alward WL, Small KW, Datson NA, Siegel-Bartelt J, Bierke-Nelson D, Bitoun P, Zabel BU, et al. (1996b). Cloning and characterization of a novel bicoid-related homeobox transcription factor gene, RIEG, involved in Rieger syndrome. *Nat Genet* 14(4): 392–399.

Shanmugam K, Featherstone MS, Saragovi HU (1997). Residues flanking the HOX YPWM motif contribute to cooperative interactions with PBX. *J Biol Chem* 272(30): 19081–19087.

Shields MB (1983). Axenfeld-Rieger syndrome: a theory of mechanism and distinctions from the iridocorneal endothelial syndrome. *Trans Am Ophthalmol Soc* 81: 736–784.

Shields MB, Buckley E, Klintworth GK, Thresher R (1985). Axenfeld-Rieger syndrome. A spectrum of developmental disorders. *Surv Ophthalmol* 29(6): 387–409.

Shiels A, Mackay D, Ionides A, Berry V, Moore A, Bhattacharya S (1998). A missense mutation in the human connexin50 gene (GJA8) underlies autosomal dominant "zonular pulverulent" cataract, on chromosome 1q. *Am J Hum Genet* 62(3): 526–532.

Sidjanin DJ, Parker-Wilson DM, Neuhauser-Klaus A, Pretsch W, Favor J, Deen PM, et al. (2001). A 76-bp deletion in the Mip gene causes autosomal dominant cataract in Hfi mice. *Genomics* 74(3): 313–319.

Smidt MP, van Schaick HS, Lanctot C, Tremblay JJ, Cox JJ, van der Kleij AA, Wolterink G, Drouin J, Burbach JP (1997). A homeodomain gene Ptx3 has highly restricted brain expression in mesencephalic dopaminergic neurons. *Proc Natl Acad Sci USA* 94(24): 13305–13310.

St. Amand TR, Ra J, Zhang Y, Hu Y, Baber SI, Qiu M, Chen Y (1998). Cloning and expression pattern of chicken Pitx2: a new component in the SHH signaling pathway controlling embryonic heart looping. *Biochem Biophys Res Commun* 247(1): 100–105.

Stephan DA, Gillanders E, Vanderveen D, Freas-Lutz D, Wistow G, Baxevanis AD, Robbins CM, VanAuken A, Quesenberry MI, Bailey-Wilson J, et al. (1999). Progressive juvenile-onset punctate cataracts caused by mutation of the gammaD-crystallin gene. *Proc Natl Acad Sci USA* 96(3): 1008–1012.

Stoilov I, Akarsu AN, Sarfarazi M (1997). Identification of three different truncating mutations in cytochrome P4501B1 (CYP1B1) as the principal cause of primary congenital glaucoma (buphthalmos) in families linked to the GLC3A locus on chromosome 2p21. *Hum Mol Genet* 6(4): 641–647.

Stoilova D, Child A, Trifan OC, Crick RP, Coakes RL, Sarfarazi M (1996). Localization of a locus (GLC1B) for adult-onset primary open angle glaucoma to the 2cen-q13 region. *Genomics* 36(1): 142–150.

Stone EM, Fingert JH, Alward WLM, Nguyen TD, Polansky JR, Sunden SLF, Nishimura D, Clark AF, Nystuen A, Nichols BE, et al. (1997). Identification of a gene that causes primary open angle glaucoma. *Science* 275: 668–670.

Szeto DP, Ryan AK, O'Connell SM, Rosenfeld MG (1996). P-OTX: a PIT-1-interacting homeodomain factor expressed during anterior pituitary gland development. *Proc Natl Acad Sci USA* 93(15): 7706–7710.

Treisman J, Harris E, Wilson D, Desplan C (1992). The homeodomain: a new face for the helix-turn-helix? *Bioessays* 14(3): 145–150.

Trifan OC, Traboulsi EI, Stoilova D, Alozie I, Nguyen R, Raja S, Sarfarazi M (1998). A third locus (GLC1D) for adult-onset primary open-angle glaucoma maps to the 8q23 region. *Am J Ophthalmol* 126(1): 17–28.

Tsai JC, Grajewski AL (1994). Cardiac valvular disease and Axenfeld-Rieger syndrome. *Am J Ophthalmol* 118(2): 255–256.

Varnum DS, Stevens LC (1968). Aphakia, a new mutation in the mouse. *J Hered* 59(2): 147–150.

Varnum DS, Stevens LC (1975). Aphakia linked with brachymorphic. *Mouse News Lett* 53: 35.

Vicart P, Caron A, Guicheney P, Li Z, Prevost MC, et al. (1998). A missense mutation in the alphaB-crystallin chaperone gene causes a desmin-related myopathy. *Nat Genet* 20(1): 92–95.

Vincent A, Billingsley G, Priston M, Williams-Lyn D, Sutherland J, Glaser T, Oliver E, Walter MA, Heathcote G, Levin A, et al. (2001). Phenotypic heterogeneity of CYP1B1 mutations in a patient with Peters' anomaly. *J Med Genet* 38: 324–326.

Vollrath D, Jaramillo-Babb VL, Clough MV, McIntosh I, Scott KM, Lichter PR, Richards JE (1998). Loss-of-function mutations in the LIM-homeodomain gene, LMX1B, in nail-patella syndrome. *Hum Mol Genet* 7(7): 1091–1098.

Westmoreland JJ, McEwen J, Moore BA, Jin Y, Condie BG (2001). Conserved function of Caenorhabditis elegans UNC-30 and mouse Pitx2 in controlling GABAergic neuron differentiation. *J Neurosci* 21(17): 6810–6819.

Wirtz MK, Samples JR, Kramer PL, Rust K, Topinka JR, Yount J, Koler RD, Acott TS (1997). Mapping a gene for adult-onset primary open-angle glaucoma to chromosome 3q. *Am J Hum Genet* 60(2): 296–304.

Wirtz MK, Samples JR, Rust K, Lie J, Nordling L, Schilling K, Acott TS, Kramer PL (1999). GLC1F, a new primary open-angle glaucoma locus, maps to 7q35-q36. *Arch Ophthalmol* 117(2): 237–241.

Wolberger C (1998). Combinatorial transcription factors. *Curr Opin Genet Dev* 8(5): 552–559.

Yoshioka H, Meno C, Koshiba K, Sugihara M, Itoh H, Ishimaru Y, Inoue T, Ohuchi H, Semina EV, Murray JC, et al. (1998). Pitx2, a bicoid-type homeobox gene, is involved in a lefty-signaling pathway in determination of left-right asymmetry. *Cell* 94(3): 299–305.

Zwaan J (1975). Immunofluorescent studies on aphakia, a mutation of a gene involved in the control of lens differentiation in the mouse embryo. *Dev Biol* 44(2): 306–312.

57 | *CSX/NKX2-5* and Congenital Heart Disease

PATRICK Y. JAY, ANDREW J. POWELL, MEGAN C. SHERWOOD, AND SEIGO IZUMO

Nkx2-5 is a homeodomain-containing transcription factor that is required for normal embryonic cardiac development. Loss of the homologous gene *tinman* in *Drosophila* results in absence of the dorsal vessel, the fly equivalent of the heart. A homozygous null mutation of Nkx2-5 in mouse causes arrest of cardiac development during looping of the heart tube and embryonic lethality. The heterozygous null mutation in mice replicates some of the defects observed in humans. The first reported patients had a familial syndrome of atrial septal defect (ASD) and atrioventricular (AV) conduction block. Additional mutations have been discovered in a wide range of congenital heart defects, including ASD and ventricular septal defect (VSD), tetralogy of Fallot, and Ebstein's malformation of the tricuspid valve. Mutations of Nkx2-5 are also associated with deleterious effects on cardiac rhythm and function in some patients. The diagnosis and management of such patients are discussed. Finally, mouse models and biochemical experiments suggest that developmental pathogenesis involves numerous molecular interactions between Nkx2-5, other transcription factors, and gene-regulatory sequences. The many interactions and subtle hemodynamic variables likely influence the spectrum of cardiac phenotypes associated with Nkx2-5 mutations.

ROLE OF THE SPECIFIC LOCUS AND DEVELOPMENTAL SYSTEM

Drosophila tinman and the vertebrate homologue *Nkx2-5* play essential roles in cardiac development. Similarities of cardiac morphogenesis in *Drosophila* and the early vertebrate embryo through the linear heart tube stage suggest an evolutionarily conserved genetic program (see Chapter 9). In *Drosophila* and vertebrate embryos, the heart forms in the midline by fusion of cardiac primordia from the left and right lateral mesoderm. The heart of the fruit fly and early vertebrate embryo is a linear vessel, which pumps by peristalsis. Components of the ancient program were then adapted to construct the four-chambered heart that separates the pulmonary and systemic circulations of air-breathing vertebrates. The heart tube loops to the right, chambers develop, and valves form. In air-breathing animals, the left (systemic) and right (pulmonary) circulations are separated by septation of the atria, ventricles, and great arteries. The expression patterns and analysis of mutant animals indicate that *tinman* and *Nkx2-5* play important roles throughout cardiac development. In the literature, *tinman* has previously been referred to as *NK4* (Kim and Nirenberg, 1989) and *msh-2* (Bodmer et al., 1990). *Nkx2-5* is also known as *Csx* (for cardiac-specific homeobox [Komuro and Izumo, 1993]) and *Nkx2.5*.

Nkx2-5 and *tinman* are the first expressed genes to delineate the precardiac mesoderm and developing heart (Harvey, 1996). *tinman* is initially expressed in the primordial mesoderm of the blastoderm prior to gastrulation and the entire mesoderm as it spreads dorsally on the right and left sides of the embryo. *tinman* expression becomes restricted to the dorsal mesoderm and is present at later stages only in the heart tube (Bodmer et al., 1990). Loss of *tinman* results in absence of the heart, gut muscle, and some somatic muscles, tissues that are derived from the dorsal mesoderm (Azpiazu and Frasch, 1993; Bodmer, 1993). Ubiquitous expression of *tinman* driven by a heat shock promoter rescues loss of these tissues but does not cause formation of ectopic myocardium (Bodmer, 1993). Therefore, *tinman* is necessary but not sufficient to specify cardiac and other tissues derived from the dorsal mesoderm.

The role of *tinman* in cardiac specification motivated the search for a murine homologue. In contrast to early *tinman* expression in the primordial mesoderm, *Nkx2-5* is first expressed in the left and right anterolateral plate mesoderm and subjacent endoderm and continues to be expressed in the heart at all stages of development (Komuro and Izumo, 1993; Lints et al., 1993). Nkx2-5 protein is present in other embryonic, but not postnatal, tissues, including the tongue, some cranial muscles, pylorus, spleen, and scattered cells in the liver (Kasahara et al., 1998). Ectopic expression of Nkx2-5 in the embryonic chick gut causes morphologic transformation of the gizzard epithelium to that of the pylorus. Conversely, inhibition of Nkx2-5 in the pylorus causes the epithelium to be coated with a keratin-like substance normally present in the gizzard, suggesting a role in pyloric sphincter specification (Smith et al., 2000). In general, however, the function of Nkx2-5 in noncardiac tissues is unknown.

A homozygous null mutation in mouse of Nkx2-5 is lethal at embryonic day 9–10. Unlike *tinman*, *Nkx2-5* is not essential for specification of cardiac tissue because a heart tube forms in null mutant embryos. In the normal mouse at embryonic day 9–10, the looping heart tube has four discernible chambers, a narrow AV canal, and a formed outflow tract but no septa or valves. The null mutant heart tube loops partially before the embryo dies of cardiac insufficiency. The atrial and ventricular chambers lack distinct left and right components. The AV canal is wide, and the outflow tract is stenotic. The ventricular trabeculae and endocardial cushions are absent. The null mutant embryo shows signs of heart failure, including severe growth retardation, pericardial effusion, and diminished arterial and yolk sac vessel development (Lyons et al., 1995; Tanaka et al., 1999a). The term *heart failure* can be misleading if interpreted from the perspective of postnatal physiology because specific etiologies may be unique to the embryonic heart. Inadequate cardiac output may also result from developmental abnormalities of the outflow tract or AV canal (Ishiwata, Yamasaki, and Izumo, unpublished observations), myocardial growth, force generation, or some combination.

Close inspection of heterozygous null mutant mice has revealed abnormalities similar to those seen in human patients. The first observed defect was in the atrial septum. In the fetus, physiologic right-to-left shunting occurs through the foramen ovale and ductus arteriosus. The foramen ovale is a hole in the atrial septum secundum, which is covered on the left atrial side by the septum primum. The septum primum acts as a flap valve, which closes after birth when the pressure of the left atrium exceeds that of the right atrium. Usually, formation of fibrous adhesions between the septa primum and secundum closes the potential communication. The process is incomplete, however, in approximately 27% of individuals (Hagen et al., 1984), resulting in a patent foramen ovale (PFO) that may permit the passage of paradoxical emboli that cause stroke. Secundum ASDs result from an insufficiency of the septum primum to cover the foramen. Tanaka et al. (unpublished data) found that 20% of heterozygous null mutant mice had a secundum ASD, as determined by echocardiography and gross pathologic examination. No wild-type mice had an ASD. The absence of right atrial or ventricular dilation suggested that the shunt flow across the ASD was not physiologically significant. In contrast, Biben et al. (2000) found that only 5 of 425 heterozygous mutants and 0 of 415 wild-type mice had an ASD. They noted a PFO in 66% of the heterozygous mutant mice, a 2.5- to 3.5-fold higher incidence than that in wild-type. PFOs were associated with aneurysms in the septum primum, which may result from increased flow through the PFO. The size of the defect may be affected by modifier genes as the size of the atrial septum seems to depend on the particular mouse strain. The varied results of the two groups could result from the different genetic backgrounds of the mice studied or differences in the interpretation of a quantitative trait, namely, the size of an ASD, which both groups found with higher prevalence in Nkx2-5 heterozygous mice.

Haploinsufficiency of Nkx2-5 in mice also causes an increased incidence of bicuspid aortic valve, in which one of the three leaflet commissures is fused. In humans, bicuspid aortic valves, the associated aortic stenosis, and other left-heart obstructive lesions are heritable (Ferencz et al., 1989; Huntington et al., 1997), but there are no reports of human Nkx2-5 mutations in these diseases. Wild-type mice have a low incidence of bicuspid aortic valve, 0.5%–1.4% depending on the strain. Heterozygous mutant Nkx2-5 mice have a 4- to 7.8-fold increased incidence (Biben et al., 2000).

Heterozygous null mutant mice have defects in cardiac conduction. Biben et al. (2000) discovered prolongation of the P–R interval in female heterozygous mice of the C57Bl/6 background. Tanaka et al. (unpublished data) found prolongation of the P–R and QRS intervals by ambulatory telemetry and surface electrocardiogram in mice of both sexes, probably because of finer time resolution in the measurements. In vivo intracardiac electrophysiologic studies reveal a prolonged *A–H interval*, the time required for a signal to travel from the sinus node to the His bundle. Either slow conduction through the atrial myocardium or an increased delay in the AV node may prolong the A–H interval. Abnormalities in AV node function detected by rapid atrial

pacing suggest that abnormal prolongation of the A–H interval occurs in the AV node.

Nkx2-5 activates the expression of genes that affect cardiac development and function, as inferred from the mutant phenotypes. Few transcriptional targets are known that can clearly explain the cardiac abnormalities associated with Nkx2-5 mutation. Target genes have generally been identified either by examination of in situ expression in null mutant embryos or in cell culture by co-transfection of Nkx2-5 and a candidate gene promoter construct. In the latter experiment, a promoter for the gene of interest, which should contain one or more Nkx2-5-binding sites (Chen and Schwartz, 1995), is fused to a reporter such as β-galactosidase or luciferase. Transcriptional activation of the construct by co-transfected Nkx2-5 increases reporter enzyme activity. Results of the in vitro assay, however, may not reproduce the in vivo gene expression pattern if other factors regulate transcription in situ (Lints et al., 1993; Chen and Schwartz, 1996; Tanaka et al., 1999a). Transgenic mice that have the promoter–reporter gene construct may also be crossed with Nkx2-5 knockout mice to examine *in vivo* regulation (Zou et al., 1997).

CLINICAL DESCRIPTION OF SYNDROME AND ANATOMIC PATHOLOGY

Mutations of Nkx2-5 in humans are associated with a wide range of cardiac anatomic malformations, AV conduction defects, and less commonly reported abnormalities of myocardial function. The inheritance pattern is autosomal-dominant with variable penetrance. No extracardiac defects have been described in humans with isolated Nkx2-

Table 57–1. Classification of Structural and Functional Heart Defects and Their Association with *Nkx2-5* Mutation in Human and Mouse Based on a Schema from the Baltimore–Washington Infant Study

Mechanism	Diagnostic Type	Human	Mouse
Lateralization and looping	Laterality disturbances, complex defects, and corrected (L) transposition		
Malformations of the ventricular outlets and arterial trunks			
I. Mesenchymal cell migration	Normally related (spiral) great arteries		
	Tetralogy of Fallot	X	
	Double outlet right ventricle	X	
	Common arterial trunk		
	VSD, supracristal type		
	Aorticopulmonary window		
	Interrupted aortic arch		
II. Complete transposition	Transposed (parallel) great arteries		
	With intact ventricular septum		
	With VSD		
	With double outlet right ventricle		
	With pulmonary/tricuspid atresia		
Extracellular matrix defects	AV septal defects		
	Complete and partial types		
	VSD type		
Hemodynamic (flow) defects	Left-sided obstructive lesions		
	Hypoplastic left heart syndrome		
	Coarctation of the aorta		
	Aortic valve stenosis		X
	Bicuspid aortic valve		X
	Right-sided obstructive lesions		
	Pulmonic valve stenosis		
	Pulmonary atresia with intact ventricular septum		
	Tricuspid atresia (hypoplasia)	X	
	Septation defects and patent duct		
	VSD, membranous type	X	
	ASD	X	X
	Patent arterial duct		
Cell death	VSD, muscular type	X	
	Ebstein anomaly	X	
Targeted growth	Total and partial anomalous pulmonary venous return		
Contraction, growth, and rhythm	Ventricular dysfunction	X	
	Ventricular hypertrophy	X	
	Ventricular non-compaction	X	
	Arrhythmia	X	X
	AV conduction block	X	X

Anatomic defects and functional disorders are divided into hypothetical developmental pathways and physiologic function. Published associations of *Nkx2-5* mutation with specific cardiac defects or disease in human or mouse are noted. VSD, ventricular septal defect; ASD, atrial septal defect; AV, atrioventricular.

5 mutations. Humans who have chromosomal deletions that include the Nkx2-5 locus do have cardiac and noncardiac defects (Pauli et al., 1999; Schafer et al., 2001). Schott et al. (1998) first mapped mutations of Nkx2-5 to chromosome 5q35 in families with ASDs and AV conduction defects. Members of the same families who were not genotyped had other congenital heart defects, including VSDs, tetralogy of Fallot, subvalvar aortic stenosis, and mitral valve fenestration. Subsequent family studies confirmed that Nkx2-5 affects the development of multiple cardiac structures (Table 57–1) (Benson et al., 1999). A few examples of some of the defects associated with Nkx2-5 mutations are shown (Fig. 57–1).

Nkx2-5 mutations also affect cardiac function. First, AV conduction defects were described in the originally identified families. Many of these patients received pacemakers. The phenotype is usually interpreted as demonstrating a role for Nkx2-5 in the maintenance of the postnatal conduction system, but a congenital defect may also be

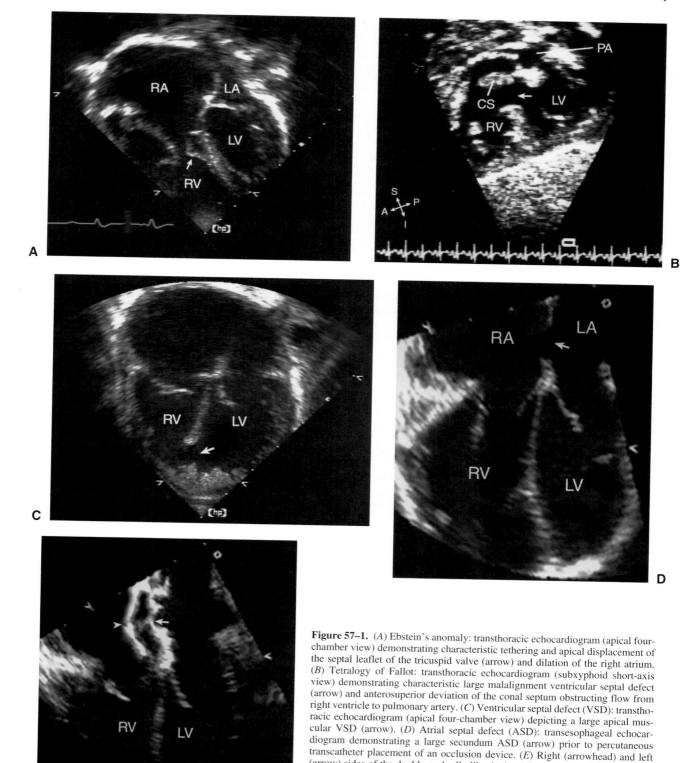

Figure 57–1. (*A*) Ebstein's anomaly: transthoracic echocardiogram (apical four-chamber view) demonstrating characteristic tethering and apical displacement of the septal leaflet of the tricuspid valve (arrow) and dilation of the right atrium. (*B*) Tetralogy of Fallot: transthoracic echocardiogram (subxyphoid short-axis view) demonstrating characteristic large malalignment ventricular septal defect (arrow) and anterosuperior deviation of the conal septum obstructing flow from right ventricle to pulmonary artery. (*C*) Ventricular septal defect (VSD): transthoracic echocardiogram (apical four-chamber view) depicting a large apical muscular VSD (arrow). (*D*) Atrial septal defect (ASD): transesophageal echocardiogram demonstrating a large secundum ASD (arrow) prior to percutaneous transcatheter placement of an occlusion device. (*E*) Right (arrowhead) and left (arrow) sides of the double-umbrella-like device grip each side of the atrial septum to close the ASD. RA, right atrium; LA, left atrium; RV, right ventricle; LV, left ventricle; CS, conal septum; PA, pulmonary artery.

present since Nkx2-5 is expressed at higher levels in the embryonic conduction system than in the surrounding myocardium (Thomas et al., 2001). Members of families in which conduction defects have been identified seem to have an increased risk of sudden death; whether death was due to a primary arrhythmic event or secondary to untreated complete heart block was not reported (Benson et al., 1998, 1999).

Second, left ventricular hypertrophy and heart failure have been noted in a few families. Left ventricular hypertrophy for which no obvious cause was identified occurred with low penetrance (Schott et al., 1998; Benson et al., 1999). Members of one family were diagnosed with a familial cardiomyopathy because of echocardiographic evidence of ventricular dysfunction and arrhythmias (Benson et al., 1999). Ventricular non-compaction, a rare disorder in which the myocardium is spongy with dense trabeculations, has also been described (Pauli et al., 1999). These infrequent observations suggest that Nkx2-5 plays an unexplored role in myocardial growth and function.

MOLECULAR GENETICS OF THE LOCUS, MUTATIONS, AND PHENOTYPE–GENOTYPE CORRELATIONS

The NK family of transcription factors, which includes *tinman* and *Nkx2-5*, was discovered in a *Drosophila* genomic DNA library screen for the conserved DNA-binding sequences of homeobox proteins (Kim and Nirenberg, 1989). The family is divided into two groups, NK-1 and NK-2. A conserved tyrosine residue at position 54 of the homeodomain distinguishes the NK-2 subgroup. Most NK-2 proteins have two conserved peptide domains, TN and NK2-SD. *Nkx2-5* contains both domains, but *tinman* lacks the NK2-SD domain (Fig. 57–2). The function of the domains is unknown.

Correlations of a specific Nkx2-5 mutation with a phenotype are difficult because of the small number of patients studied so far, but some patterns are emerging. Homeodomain and some nonsense mutations diminish or abolish DNA binding (Kasahara et al., 2000). Each of these DNA-binding mutations in familial and sporadic cases is associated with a high incidence of AV block. No conduction defect has been observed in the small number of patients with mutations that do not affect DNA binding (Benson et al., 1999; Goldmuntz et al., 2001). The similarity to the loss-of-function phenotype in the mouse suggests that the association is real.

There are few reported cases of mutations that are not expected to, or do not, affect DNA binding. Four missense mutations were described in 6 of 114 tetralogy of Fallot patients who did not have a chromosome 22q11 deletion (Goldmuntz et al., 2001). Three of the mutations were in the conserved TN or NK2-SD domain. None of these patients had a conduction defect.

The incidence of Nkx2-5 mutation in most forms of congenital heart disease is unknown. In two studies of patients who had tetralogy of Fallot but not the chromosome 22q11 deletion, 7 of a combined population of 124 carried an Nkx2-5 mutation in the coding sequence, suggesting a 5% incidence (Benson et al., 1999; Goldmuntz et al., 2001). In a small survey of idiopathic second- or third-degree AV

block, 1 of 10 patients carried a mutation; his father, who had an unknown genotype, died suddenly at age 29 (Benson et al., 1999).

DIAGNOSIS IN THE INDIVIDUAL AND FETUS

No diagnostic test for Nkx2-5 mutations exists for routine clinical use, but a family history of nonsyndromic congenital heart disease or association of AV block and heart defect would suggest the presence of a mutation. Therefore, the two practical diagnostic questions are as follows: (*1*) Does the patient or fetus have a congenital heart defect, AV block, or cardiac dysfunction? (*2*) Is the cardiac diagnosis part of a familial pattern that suggests a genetic cause? These questions, albeit mundane, should be considered to guide optimal management and counseling. For more complete descriptions of the diagnosis and management of specific cardiac defects and diseases, the reader is referred to any of several pediatric cardiology texts (Fyler, 1992; Garson et al., 1997; Allen et al., 2000).

The clinical presentation of a patient with an Nkx2-5 mutation depends on the cardiac phenotype. Structural malformations are usually first suspected after an abnormal physical examination, which prompts diagnostic imaging by echocardiography or cardiac catheterization (Fyler and Nadas, 1992; Pelech, 1998). The defects that have been described in human Nkx2-5 mutation may be detected at any age from the fetus to adult. In the newborn, cyanotic or duct-dependent lesions that have been described include Ebstein's anomaly and tetralogy of Fallot with either pulmonic stenosis or pulmonary atresia. In the infant, large VSDs and, rarely, ASDs permit a left-to-right shunt that causes pulmonary overcirculation and signs of tachypnea and failure to thrive. At any age, septal and valvular defects may manifest as wide, fixed splitting of the second heart sound (ASD), murmurs (ASD, VSD, valvar stenosis, or regurgitation), and clicks (aortic or pulmonic stenosis). The clinical findings are more easily detected after the newborn period, when right ventricular pressure has dropped and the heart rate is slower.

A cardiac conduction defect is not easily diagnosed by physical examination unless there is bradycardia or an irregular rhythm, signs of second- or third-degree AV block. Patients with second- or third-degree block may have syncope. First-degree AV block can be diagnosed only by electrocardiogram (EKG) (Walsh and Saul, 1992). Cardiomyopathy may be diagnosed by history or physical examination when the disease is moderate or severe but may be subclinical in mild cases. Echocardiogaphy or cardiac catheterization is useful to assess the disease (Colan et al., 1992).

Most major cardiac defects, some rhythm abnormalities, and dysfunction may also be diagnosed prenatally by ultrasound (Cohen, 2001). Routine obstetric ultrasound may reveal an anatomic abnormality. Fetal bradycardia may suggest AV block, evident as AV dissociation by echocardiography. Referral to a pediatric cardiologist with expertise in fetal echocardiography is valuable for diagnosis, counseling, and planning of perinatal and subsequent cardiac care. Fetal diagnosis by a pediatric cardiologist may be more accurate

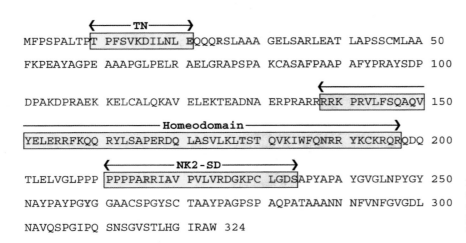

```
                 ← ——— TN ——— →
MFPSPALTPT PFSVKDILNL EQQQRSLAAA GELSARLEAT LAPSSCMLAA  50

FKPEAYAGPE AAAPGLPELR AELGRAPSPA KCASAFPAAP AFYPRAYSDP 100

                                     ←———————————————
DPAKDPRAEK KELCALQKAV ELEKTEADNA ERPRARRRK PRVLFSQAQV 150

 ———————————————— Homeodomain ————————————————→
YELERRFKQQ RYLSAPERDQ LASVLKLTST QVKIWFQNRR YKCKRQRQDQ 200

            ←——————— NK2-SD ———————→
TLELVGLPPP PPPPARRIAV PVLVRDGKPC LGDSAPYAPA YGVGLNPYGY 250

NAYPAYPGYG GAACSPGYSC TAAYPAGPSP AQPATAAANN NFVNFGVGDL 300

NAVQSPGIPQ SNSGVSTLHG IRAW 324
```

Figure 57–2. Human Nkx2-5 amino acid sequence. Conserved subdomains are indicated in boxes. Reported nonsense (blue) and missense (red) mutations discovered in patients with congenital heart disease are indicated in boldface.

(Berghella et al., 2001; Meyer-Wittkopf et al., 2001), but this depends on local practice patterns. A "normal" fetal echocardiographic diagnosis, however, cannot rule out certain postnatal heart defects, such as ASD, smaller VSDs, patent ductus arteriosus, aortic coarctation, or minor valve abnormalities. Fetal physiology and current imaging resolution can make these defects challenging to diagnose.

Most cases of congenital heart disease are sporadic, which does not exclude a genetic cause; but many careful studies prove that there is an increased incidence of congenital heart disease within families of an affected proband. If a parent has a congenital heart defect, the percentage of concordantly affected children ranges approximately 1%–12%, which is severalfold higher than the fractional percentage risk for the specific lesion in the general population (Nora, 1994). Inclusion of discordant lesions raises the relative risk further. If a child has congenital heart disease, approximately 4% of siblings were found to have a defect compared to 1% in a matched control population in the Baltimore–Washington Infant Study (Ferencz et al., 1989). It is therefore always appropriate to elicit a family history even if one cannot identify the genetic mutation. Given the varied presentations of Nkx2-5 mutation reported within the same family, one should inquire about diagnosed congenital heart defects, arrhythmias or asymptomatic EKG abnormalities, and cardiomyopathies. Questions should be asked about sudden, unexpected death or syncope suggestive of unrecognized arrhythmia and infant or childhood deaths suggestive of unrepaired lesions. Such information should heighten clinical suspicion for the presence of heart disease in relatives and future children. Early recognition of defects such as ASDs and aortic stenosis can prevent the late sequelae of arrhythmia and heart failure. As the natural history of patients with specific gene mutations becomes known, specific prognostic information may be offered.

MANAGEMENT, TREATMENT, AND COUNSELING

Similar to the diagnostic approach outlined above, management is directed toward the patient's cardiac condition and genetic counseling. No current approach is tailored for the patient with a known or suspected Nkx2-5 mutation, but the clinician may have a higher index of suspicion for AV block, arrhythmias, and ventricular dysfunction, which may arise even after the congenital heart defect is repaired or palliated. The details of the management of the many forms of cardiac disease associated with Nkx2-5 mutation are beyond the scope of this chapter, but a discussion of general principles may be useful for the noncardiologist.

First, is intervention required, or is observation sufficient? The spectrum of disease reported with Nkx2-5 mutation ranges from minor to severe. Heart defects or dysfunctions that do or will cause symptoms if untreated require intervention, e.g., tetralogy of Fallot or large ASDs. In contrast, small ASDs or VSDs do not impose a deleterious shunt volume and can close spontaneously. Similarly, isolated first-degree AV block or mild valvular stenosis generally causes no symptoms. Minor defects thus do not warrant the risk of intervention but should be followed for the potential development of complications, e.g., aortic regurgitation caused by prolapse of the right coronary cusp into a membranous VSD. Subacute bacterial endocarditis prophylaxis is recommended for certain defects during dental and certain surgical procedures involving the respiratory, gastrointestinal, and genitourinary mucosa (Dajani et al., 1997).

If treatment of a defect is necessary, the goal is to normalize the mechanical work of the heart through surgery or interventional cardiac catheterization (Fig. 57–1). For example, defects that impose a large volume overload require closing the holes (ASDs, VSDs) or repair or replacement of regurgitant valves. Pressure-overload lesions, e.g., aortic valve stenosis, may be relieved by percutaneous balloon dilation, surgical valvotomy, or valve replacement. If the patient has only one functional ventricle, as in hypoplastic left-heart syndrome or tricuspid atresia, a series of palliative operations are performed (Forbess et al., 1997; Bove, 1998). Each successive step decreases the volume load on the ventricle. The final stage, the Fontan procedure, separates the pulmonary and systemic circulations, placing them in series, and the single ventricle is the systemic pump. In addition, other

lesions that increase the work of the heart are addressed by interventional catheterization or surgery at each stage.

The goal of management of the functional abnormalities associated with Nkx2-5 mutation is to maintain as normal as possible cardiac rhythm and contractile function. AV conduction defects that cause symptoms or increase the risk of sudden death require placement of a cardiac pacemaker. Arrhythmias are treated with medications, pacing, interventional cardiac electrophysiology, or a combination to minimize their occurrence. An automatic implanted cardiac defibrillator may be placed for life-threatening rhythms. Current therapy for heart failure is aimed at inhibiting the neurohormonal response in the adrenergic and renin-angiotensin-aldosterone systems, which slows the progression of disease, and minimizing symptoms and potential sequelae, e.g., anticoagulation to prevent thromboembolism (Hunt et al., 2001). Cardiac transplantation is a last management option in end-stage heart failure.

Management of the unborn fetus is a rapidly changing field that has exciting therapeutic potential. Current practice focuses on fetal echocardiographic diagnosis and parental counseling. An abnormal obstetric ultrasound examination is a clear indication for fetal echocardiography. Another indication is a family history of congenital heart disease, especially if a parent is affected (Cohen, 2001). An accurate diagnosis aids counseling, which can be reassuring or helpful for decision making regarding continuation of the pregnancy. Clinicians can help prepare the parents emotionally and practically for choices regarding pre- and postnatal management. Although it is unclear whether fetal diagnosis affects postnatal or operative mortality, it can reduce the morbidity resulting from shock and acidosis in the newborn with an undiagnosed duct-dependent lesion (Bonnet et al., 1999; Kumar et al., 1999; Tworetzky et al., 2001). Some evidence indicates that prenatal diagnosis improves neurologic outcomes (Mahle et al., 2001).

Awareness of the increased familial risk for congenital heart disease and the ability to make accurate fetal diagnoses will be especially important if therapeutic *in utero* intervention becomes an effective option. Serial fetal echocardiographic examinations demonstrate that the severity of defects can progress during gestation. Obstruction of left ventricular blood flow from aortic or mitral stenosis, for example, can be associated with progression to severe left-heart obstruction or hypoplasia (Hornberger et al., 1995a; Simpson and Sharland, 1997; Yagel et al., 1997; Agnoleti et al., 1999). Progression has also been reported for right-sided lesions such as Ebstein's malformation and tetralogy of Fallot (Hornberger et al., 1991, 1995b). These observations have prompted interventional cardiologists to attempt balloon dilation of fetal valvular aortic stenosis. Initial results in a very small group have been poor but should improve as technical problems are solved (Kohl et al., 2000).

Finally, genetic counseling can be as important to patients and families as interventional therapy. Unfortunately, variable penetrance and the absence of diagnostic tests for Nkx2-5 mutation preclude precise predictions regarding recurrence or prognosis. Estimates of the relative risk of recurrence from epidemiologic studies cannot be extrapolated to individual families. Given this caveat, the clinician should consider the specific circumstances of the family. Some reassurance may be given in sporadic cases of nonsyndromic congenital heart disease. Although future offspring or siblings have a severalfold higher risk of a heart defect, the absolute risk is generally less than 15% (Boughman et al., 1987; Nora, 1994). A conscientious cardiac physical examination and evaluation for abnormal results should suffice for relatives of sporadic cases. Fetal echocardiography should be obtained if the need for reassurance is great or the proband's defect is particularly severe. When the family history suggests a mendelian inheritance pattern, it seems prudent to elicit a careful cardiac history and physical examination for all relatives, to obtain an EKG or echocardiogram if there is a suspicion for abnormality, and to obtain a fetal echocardiogram for each pregnancy.

DEVELOPMENTAL PATHOGENESIS

The heart form is the culmination of multiple, complex morphogenetic processes beginning before the embryonic heart tube develops. A genetic blueprint directs the processes, but mechanical forces also mold the heart through blood flow. Nkx2-5 regulates gene expression before the heart tube has formed and throughout development. Thus, a congenital heart defect could result from a direct effect of Nkx2-5 on the development of the affected structure or an indirect effect that perturbs the normal flow of blood.

Genes that affect cardiac morphogenesis may be divided into two categories: (1) effector genes that directly affect tissue shape or function, e.g., cytoskeletal or extracellular matrix proteins or components of the excitation–contraction mechanism, and (2) patterning genes that regulate the expression of effector or other patterning genes, e.g., transcription factors and signaling pathway molecules. *Nkx2-5* is in the latter group. For example, complete loss of *Nkx2-5* leads to absence of eHAND expression, a basic helix-loop-helix transcription factor that is normally expressed in the murine left ventricle and precardiac mesoderm (Tanaka et al., 1999a; Yamagishi et al., 2001). A double knockout of *Nkx2-5* and dHAND, a basic helix-loop-helix transcription factor expressed in the murine right ventricle, causes the ventricular chamber not to develop in the embryonic heart tube, although a small group of cells that express ventricular genes is present (Yamagishi et al., 2001). Most of the few known downstream targets of *Nkx2-5* have been identified by in situ analysis of null mutant embryos at or before the looped heart tube stage. The *Nkx2-5* regulated genes that effect subsequent cardiac development probably have only subtle, but significant, quantitative differences from the normal level, localization, or timing of expression of target genes in heterozygous mutants. Identification of the genes is a major challenge.

In contrast, the molecular interactions that involve *Nkx2-5* in cardiac gene transcription are better understood. First, in vitro cotransfection experiments demonstrate clearly that combinations of cardiac transcription factors act together to regulate the expression of target genes. The atrial natriuretic factor (ANF) promoter is the best-studied model (Fig. 57–3). The ANF promoter contains multiple binding sites for Nkx2-5, Tbx2 or Tbx5, GATA4, and serum response factor (SRF). Nkx2-5 can physically associate with itself (Kasahara et al., 2001), GATA4 (Durocher et al., 1997; Lee et al., 1998), or Tbx5 (Bruneau et al., 2001; Hiroi et al., 2001) to activate ANF gene expression synergistically. (A GATA4–SRF complex also activates gene expression [Belaguli et al., 2000].) Nkx2-5 and Tbx5 similarly activate Connexin40 expression (Bruneau et al., 2001). Interestingly, Tbx2 appears to compete with Tbx5 for the same binding site; a complex composed of Tbx2 and Nkx2-5 represses ANF gene transcription (Habets et al., 2002). Many other transcription factors are expressed in specific chambers or cells of the heart (Bruneau, 2002). Thus, the intersecting expression patterns of cardiac transcription factors can govern the spatiotemporal regulation of gene expression.

Second, modulation of the stoichiometric relationships between the concentration of Nkx2-5, the number of available binding sites in a promoter, and the binding affinity is another key regulatory mechanism. The haploinsufficient mutant phenotype proves the relevance of the concentration of Nkx2-5. In vitro, cotransfection of a dominant-negative Nkx2-5 mutant isoform that dimerizes with wild-type Nkx2-5 but does not bind DNA reduces transcription from the ANF pro-

moter (Kasahara et al., 2001). The ANF promoter contains at least three Nkx2-5 consensus binding sites, two of which are adjacent to each other and associated with Nkx2-5 dimerization (Chen and Schwartz, 1995; Lee et al., 1998; Kasahara et al., 2000). Deletion of individual binding sites decreases Nkx2-5-activated transcription (Lee et al., 1998; Bruneau et al., 2001). Other transcription factors, such as COUP-TF1, can block Nkx2-5-binding sites to prevent transcription (Guo et al., 2001). Furthermore, the binding sites may be entirely inaccessible when repressor elements in the regulatory sequence mediate the recruitment of deacetylated histones (Kuwahara et al., 2001). Finally, phosphorylation of Nkx2-5, which occurs *in vivo*, increases its affinity for consensus binding sequences (Kasahara and Izumo, 1999).

Sophisticated variations on the simple stoichiometric model probably exist but have not been explored in detail. For instance, multiple enhancers drive developmental stage- and chamber-specific expression of Nkx2-5 (Lien et al., 1999; Reecy et al., 1999; Schwartz and Olson, 1999; Tanaka et al., 1999b). Two groups that examined mutations of regulatory sequences that might cause localized deficiencies of Nkx2-5 focused on expression in early embryonic stages but not potential effects on cardiac development (Liberatore et al., 2002; Lien et al., 2002).

Most research has focused on the molecular biology and genetics of Nkx2-5 mutation, with little attention to the influence of hemodynamics in shaping the heart. Experimental perturbation of blood flow in embryonic chick hearts, however, produces defects resembling hypoplastic left-heart syndrome, semilunar valve abnormalities, pharyngeal arch artery anomalies, and VSDs (Hogers et al., 1999; Sedmera et al., 1999). A clear genetic example comes from mice with a double heterozygous mutation of Jag1 and Notch2, a model for Alagille syndrome. Jag1 and Notch2 are ligand and receptor, respectively, involved in intercellular signaling, cell fate specification, and embryonic patterning (see Chapters 39 and 40). Jag1 is expressed in the pulmonary trunk and aorta and Notch2, in the pulmonary trunk, aorta, ventricle, and atrial wall. Double-mutant mice have a hypoplastic pulmonary artery, VSD, and aorta overriding the right ventricle, which resembles tetralogy of Fallot and fits the expression pattern of both genes. However, they also have ASDs, even though neither Jag1 nor Notch2 is expressed in the atrial septum (McCright et al., 2002). The ASDs probably result from increased right-to-left shunting at the atrial level in the embryo secondary to the right ventricular outflow tract obstruction. Similarly, Nkx2-5 mutation may subtly affect the development or function of an early structure that perturbs blood flow and causes abnormal development of other, later structures.

Given the many molecular, genetic, and hemodynamic interactions involved in cardiac development, it becomes clearer why heterozygous mutations of *Nkx2-5* can cause congenital and postnatal heart disease with variable penetrance and presentation. The heart is the product of multiple serial and parallel processes, each of which has a different dependence on Nkx2-5 dosage and other variables for normal completion. Less than normal levels of Nkx2-5 lead to decreased, but not absent, expression of certain cardiac genes, which increases the probability of, but does not commit the heart to, a defect. Polymorphisms of interacting transcription factors, regulatory sequences, or downstream effectors and chaotic perturbations of blood flow alter the probability of any given patient (or mouse) developing a malformation. Furthermore, normal development of various cardiac structures or functions must have a different dependence on Nkx2-5 interactions with DNA or proteins. For example, almost all reported patients with DNA-binding mutations develop AV block but few develop tetralogy of Fallot. In contrast, mutations of conserved Nkx2-5 subdomains, which presumably mediate protein–protein interactions, have been associated with tetralogy of Fallot but not AV block.

To clarify the developmental processes that Nkx2-5 may affect, it would be useful to organize the phenotypes reported in mice and humans into a conceptual framework. Table 57–1 classifies the cardiac abnormalities according to the schema adopted by the Baltimore–Washington Infant Study. The goal of this population-based study was to identify genetic and environmental etiologies for congenital heart disease. The investigators classified defects according to presumed

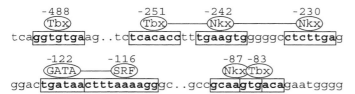

Figure 57–3. Multiple cardiac transcription factors bind to sequences in the atrial natriuretic factor promoter to regulate gene expression. Transcription factor binding sites demonstrated in vivo or in vitro are shown. Lines connect transcription factors that form hetero- or homodimeric protein–DNA complexes, which activate or repress transcription. The binding sites at positions −87 and −83 for the Nkx2-5 and Tbx transcription factors overlap, but the functional significance is unknown. Bases are numbered with respect to the transcription-start site (Argentin et al., 1985; GenBank accession number K02062). GATA, GATA4; Nkx, Nkx2-5; SRF, serum response factor; Tbx, Tbx2 or -5.

embryologic timing of the affected structure and by developmental mechanisms (Ferencz, 1997). The schema, albeit oversimplified and imperfect, should help clinicians and scientists think about what processes Nkx2-5 may regulate.

SUMMARY

A mysterious mix of environmental and genetic factors was once thought to cause congenital heart disease, but discoveries in the past decade have significantly revised this perception. Cardiac transcription factors, like *tinman* and *Nkx2-5*, play essential roles in cardiac development in fly and mouse. The presence of heterozygous mutations in patients with congenital heart disease proved the clinical relevance and has motivated intense scrutiny of the heterozygous mouse phenotype and molecular biology of Nkx2-5. This basic research has illuminated the potential mechanisms that underlie variable penetrance and pleiomorphic phenotypes in Nkx2-5 mutation. The early scientific advances have not altered the therapeutic management or counseling of patients with Nkx2-5 mutation. This will undoubtedly change as knowledge grows regarding Nkx2-5-regulated pathways and the incidence and natural history of Nkx2-5 mutation in humans.

REFERENCES

Agnoleti G, Annecchino F, Preda L, Borghi A (1999). Persistence of the left superior caval vein: can it potentiate obstructive lesions of the left ventricle? *Cardiol Young* 9: 285–290.

Allen HD, Gutgesell HP, Clark EB, Driscoll DJ (2000). *Moss and Adams' Heart Disease in Infants, Children, and Adolescents, Including the Fetus and Young Adult.* Lippincott Williams & Wilkins, Philadelphia.

Argentin S, Nemer M, Drouin J, Scott GK, Kennedy BP, Davies PL (1985). The gene for rat atrial natriuretic factor. *J Biol Chem* 260: 4568–4571.

Azpiazu N, Frasch M (1993). *Tinman* and *Bagpipe*: two homeo box genes that determine cell fates in the dorsal mesoderm of *Drosophila. Genes Dev* 7: 1325–1340.

Belaguli NS, Sepulveda JL, Nigam V, Charron F, Nemer M, Schwartz RJ (2000). Cardiac tissue enriched factors serum response factor and GATA-4 are mutual coregulators. *Mol Cell Biol* 20: 7550–7558.

Benson DW, Sharkey A, Fatkin D, Lang P, Basson CT, McDonough B, Strauss AW, Seidman JG, Seidman CE (1998). Reduced penetrance, variable expressivity, and genetic heterogeneity of familial atrial septal defects. *Circulation* 97: 2043–2048.

Benson DW, Silberbach GM, Kavanaugh-McHugh A, Cottrill C, Zhang Y, Riggs S, Smalls O, Johnson MC, Watson MS, Seidman JG, et al. (1999). Mutations in the cardiac transcription factor NKX2.5 affect diverse cardiac developmental pathways. *J Clin Invest* 104: 1567–1573.

Berghella V, Pagotto L, Kaufman M, Huhta JC, Wapner RJ (2001). Accuracy of prenatal diagnosis of congenital heart defects. *Fetal Diagn Ther* 16: 407–412.

Biben C, Weber R, Kesteven S, Stanley E, McDonald L, Elliott DA, Barnett L, Koentgen F, Robb L, Feneley M, et al. (2000). Cardiac septal and valvular dysmorphogenesis in mice heterozygous for mutations in the homeobox gene *Nkx2-5. Circ Res* 87: 888–895.

Bodmer R (1993). The gene *Tinman* is required for specification of the heart and visceral muscles in *Drosophila. Development* 118: 719–729.

Bodmer R, Jan LY, Jan YN (1990). A new homeobox-containing gene, *Msh-2*, is transiently expressed early during mesoderm formation of *Drosophila. Development* 110: 661–669.

Bonnet D, Coltri A, Butera G, Fermont L, Le Bidois J, Kachaner J, Sidi D (1999). Detection of transposition of the great arteries in fetuses reduces neonatal morbidity and mortality. *Circulation* 99: 916–918.

Boughman JA, Berg KA, Astemborski JA, Clark EB, McCarter RJ, Rubin JD, Ferencz C (1987). Familial risks of congenital heart defect assessed in a population-based epidemiologic study. *Am J Med Genet* 26: 839–849.

Bove EL (1998). Current status of staged reconstruction for hypoplastic left heart syndrome. *Pediatr Cardiol* 19: 308–315.

Bruneau BG (2002). Transcriptional regulation of vertebrate cardiac morphogenesis. *Circ Res* 90: 509–519.

Bruneau BG, Nemer G, Schmitt JP, Charron F, Robitaille L, Caron S, Conner DA, Gessler M, Nemer M, Seidman CE, et al. (2001). A murine model of Holt-Oram syndrome defines roles of the T-box transcription factor Tbx5 in cardiogenesis and disease. *Cell* 106: 709–721.

Chen CY, Schwartz RJ (1995). Identification of novel DNA binding targets and regulatory domains of a murine Tinman homeodomain factor, Nkx-2.5. *J Biol Chem* 270: 15628–15633.

Chen CY, Schwartz RJ (1996). Recruitment of the Tinman homolog Nkx-2.5 by serum response factor activates cardiac alpha-actin gene transcription. *Mol Cell Biol* 16: 6372–6384.

Cohen MS (2001). Fetal diagnosis and management of congenital heart disease. *Clin Perinatol* 28: ii–vi.

Colan SD, Spevak PJ, Parness IA, Nadas AS (1992). Cardiomyopathies. In: *Nadas' Pediatric Cardiology.* Fyler DC (ed.) Hanley & Belfus, Philadelphia, pp. 329–361.

Dajani AS, Taubert KA, Wilson W, Bolger AF, Bayer A, Ferrieri P, Gewitz MH, Shulman ST, Nouri S, Newburger JW, et al. (1997). Prevention of bacterial endocarditis. Recommendations by the American Heart Association. *JAMA* 277: 1794–1801.

Durocher D, Charron F, Warren R, Schwartz RJ, Nemer M (1997). The cardiac transcription factors Nkx2-5 and GATA-4 are mutual cofactors. *EMBO J* 16: 5687–5696.

Ferencz C (1997). Categorization of cardiovascular malformations for risk factor analysis. In: *Genetic and Environmental Risk Factors of Major Cardiovascular Malformations: The Baltimore-Washington Infant Study 1981–1989.* Ferencz C, Loffredo CA, Correa-Villasenor A, Wilson PD (eds.) Futura, Armonk, NY, pp. 13–28.

Ferencz C, Boughman JA, Neill CA, Brenner JI, Perry LW (1989). Congenital cardiovascular malformations: questions on inheritance. Baltimore–Washington Infant Study Group. *J Am Coll Cardiol* 14: 756–763.

Forbess JM, Cook N, Serraf A, Burke RP, Mayer JE Jr, Jonas RA (1997). An institutional experience with second- and third-stage palliative procedures for hypoplastic left heart syndrome: the impact of the bidirectional cavopulmonary shunt. *J Am Coll Cardiol* 29: 665–670.

Fyler DC (ed.) (1992). *Nadas' Pediatric Cardiology.* Hanley & Belfus, Philadelphia.

Fyler DC, Nadas AS (1992). History, physical examination and laboratory tests. In: *Nadas' Pediatric Cardiology.* Fyler DC (ed.) Hanley & Belfus, Philadelphia, pp. 101–116.

Garson A, Bricker JT, Fisher DJ, Neish SR (1997). *The Science and Practice of Pediatric Cardiology.* Lippincott Williams & Wilkins, Philadelphia.

Goldmuntz E, Geiger E, Benson DW (2001). NKX2.5 mutations in patients with tetralogy of Fallot. *Circulation* 104: 2565–2568.

Guo L, Lynch J, Nakamura K, Fliegel L, Kasahara H, Izumo S, Komuro I, Agellon LB, Michalak M (2001). COUP-TF1 antagonizes Nkx2.5-mediated activation of the calreticulin gene during cardiac development. *J Biol Chem* 276: 2797–2801.

Habets PEMH, Moorman AFM, Clout DEW, van Roon MA, Lingbeek M, van Lohuizen M, Campione M, Christoffels VM (2002). Cooperative action of Tbx2 and Nkx2.5 inhibits ANF expression in the atrioventricular canal: implications for cardiac chamber formation. *Genes Dev* 16: 1234–1246.

Hagen PT, Scholz DG, Edwards WD (1984). Incidence and size of patent foramen ovale during the first 10 decades of life: an autopsy study of 965 normal hearts. *Mayo Clin Proc* 59: 17–20.

Harvey RP (1996). NK-2 homeobox genes and heart development. *Dev Biol* 178: 203–216.

Hiroi Y, Kudoh S, Monzen K, Ikeda Y, Yazaki Y, Nagai R, Komuro I (2001). Tbx5 associates with Nkx2-5 and synergistically promotes cardiomyocyte differentiation. *Nat Genet* 28: 276–280.

Hogers B, DeRuiter MC, Gittenberger-de Groot AC, Poelmann RE (1999). Extraembryonic venous obstructions lead to cardiovascular malformations and can be embryolethal. *Cardiovasc Res* 41: 87–99.

Hornberger LK, Sahn DJ, Kleinman CS, Copel JA, Reed KL (1991). Tricuspid valve disease with significant tricuspid insufficiency in the fetus: diagnosis and outcome. *J Am Coll Cardiol* 17: 167–173.

Hornberger LK, Sanders SP, Rein AJ, Spevak PJ, Parness IA, Colan SD (1995a). Left heart obstructive lesions and left ventricular growth in the midtrimester fetus. A longitudinal study. *Circulation* 92: 1531–1538.

Hornberger LK, Sanders SP, Sahn DJ, Rice MJ, Spevak PJ, Benacerraf BR, McDonald RW, Colan SD (1995b). In utero pulmonary artery and aortic growth and potential for progression of pulmonary outflow tract obstruction in tetralogy of Fallot. *J Am Coll Cardiol* 25: 739–745.

Hunt HA, Baker DW, Chin MH, Cinquegrani MP, Feldmanmd AM, Francis GS, Ganiats TG, Goldstein S, Gregoratos G, Jessup ML, et al. (2001). ACC/AHA guidelines for the evaluation and management of chronic heart failure in the adult: executive summary. A report of the American College of Cardiology/American Heart Association Task Force on Practice Guidelines (Committee to Revise the 1995 Guidelines for the Evaluation and Management of Heart Failure): Developed in Collaboration with the International Society for Heart and Lung Transplantation, Endorsed by the Heart Failure Society of America. *Circulation* 104: 2996–3007.

Huntington K, Hunter AG, Chan KL (1997). A prospective study to assess the frequency of familial clustering of congenital bicuspid aortic valve. *J Am Coll Cardiol* 30: 1809–1812.

Kasahara H, Izumo S (1999). Identification of the in vivo casein kinase II phosphorylation site within the homeodomain of the cardiac tissue-specifying homeobox gene product Csx/Nkx2.5. *Mol Cell Biol* 19: 526–536.

Kasahara H, Bartunkova S, Schinke M, Tanaka M, Izumo S (1998). Cardiac and extracardiac expression of Csx/Nkx2.5 homeodomain protein. *Circ Res* 82: 936–946.

Kasahara H, Lee B, Schott JJ, Benson DW, Seidman JG, Izumo S (2000). Loss of function and inhibitory effects of human CSX/NKX2.5 homeoprotein mutations associated with congenital heart disease. *J Clin Invest* 106: 299–308.

Kasahara H, Usheva A, Ueyama T, Aoki H, Horikoshi N, Izumo S (2001). Characterization of homo- and heterodimerization of cardiac Csx/Nkx2.5 Homeoprotein. *J Biol Chem* 276: 4570–4580.

Kim Y, Nirenberg M (1989). *Drosophila* NK-homeobox genes. *Proc Natl Acad Sci USA* 86: 7716–7720.

Kohl T, Sharland G, Allan LD, Gembruch U, Chaoui R, Lopes LM, Zielinsky P, Huhta J, Silverman NH (2000). World experience of percutaneous ultrasound-guided balloon valvuloplasty in human fetuses with severe aortic valve obstruction. *Am J Cardiol* 85: 1230–1233.

Komuro I, Izumo S (1993). Csx: a murine homeobox-containing gene specifically expressed in the developing heart. *Proc Natl Acad Sci USA* 90: 8145–8149.

Kumar RK, Newburger JW, Gauvreau K, Kamenir SA, Hornberger LK (1999). Comparison of outcome when hypoplastic left heart syndrome and transposition of the great arteries are diagnosed prenatally versus when diagnosis of these two conditions is made only postnatally. *Am J Cardiol* 83: 1649–1653.

Kuwahara K, Saito Y, Ogawa E, Takahashi N, Nakagawa Y, Naruse Y, Harada M, Hamanaka I, Izumi T, Miyamoto Y, et al. (2001). The neuron-restrictive silencer element–neuron-restrictive silencer factor system regulates basal and endothelin 1-inducible atrial natriuretic peptide gene expression in ventricular myocytes. *Mol Cell Biol* 21: 2085–2097.

Lee Y, Shioi T, Kasahara H, Jobe SM, Wiese RJ, Markham BE, Izumo S (1998). The cardiac tissue–restricted homeobox protein Csx/Nkx2.5 physically associates with the zinc finger protein GATA4 and cooperatively activates atrial natriuretic factor gene expression. *Mol Cell Biol* 18: 3120–3129.

Liberatore CM, Searcy-Schrick RD, Vincent EB, Yutzey KE (2002). *Nkx-2.5* gene induction in mice is mediated by a smad consensus regulatory region. *Dev Biol* 244: 243–256.

Lien CL, Wu C, Mercer B, Webb R, Richardson JA, Olson EN (1999). Control of early cardiac-specific transcription of Nkx2-5 by a GATA-dependent enhancer. *Development* 126: 75–84.

Lien CL, McAnally J, Richardson JA, Olson EN (2002). Cardiac-specific activity of an *Nkx2-5* enhancer requires an evolutionarily conserved Smad binding site. *Dev Biol* 244: 257–266.

Lints TJ, Parsons LM, Hartley L, Lyons I, Harvey RP (1993). Nkx-2.5: a novel murine homeobox gene expressed in early heart progenitor cells and their myogenic descendants. *Development* 119: 419–431.

Lyons I, Parsons LM, Hartley L, Li R, Andrews JE, Robb L, Harvey RP (1995). Myogenic and morphogenetic defects in the heart tubes of murine embryos lacking the homeo box gene Nkx2-5. *Genes Dev* 9: 1654–1666.

Mahle WT, Clancy RR, McGaurn SP, Goin JE, Clark BJ (2001). Impact of prenatal diagnosis on survival and early neurologic morbidity in neonates with the hypoplastic left heart syndrome. *Pediatrics* 107: 1277–1282.

McCright B, Lozier J, Gridley T (2002). A mouse model of Alagille syndrome: Notch2 as a genetic modifier of Jag1 haploinsufficiency. *Development* 129: 1075–1082.

Meyer-Wittkopf M, Cooper S, Sholler G (2001). Correlation between fetal cardiac diagnosis by obstetric and pediatric cardiologist sonographers and comparison with postnatal findings. *Ultrasound Obstet Gynecol* 17: 392–397.

Nora JJ (1994). From generational studies to a multilevel genetic–environmental interaction. *J Am Coll Cardiol* 23: 1468–1471.

Pauli RM, Scheib-Wixted S, Cripe L, Izumo S, Sekhon GS (1999). Ventricular noncompaction and distal chromosome 5q deletion. *Am J Med Genet* 85: 419–423.

Pelech AN (1998). The cardiac murmur. When to refer? *Pediatr Clin North Am* 45: 107–122.

Reecy JM, Li X, Yamada M, DeMayo FJ, Newman CS, Harvey RP, Schwartz RJ (1999). Identification of upstream regulatory regions in the heart-expressed homeobox gene *Nkx2-5*. *Development* 126: 839–849.

Schafer IA, Robin NH, Posch JJ, Clark BA, Izumo S, Schwartz S (2001). Distal 5q deletion syndrome: phenotypic correlations. *Am J Med Genet* 103: 63–68.

Schott JJ, Benson DW, Basson CT, Pease W, Silberbach GM, Moak JP, Maron BJ, Seidman CE, Seidman JG (1998). Congenital heart disease caused by mutations in the transcription factor NKX2-5. *Science* 281: 108–111.

Schwartz RJ, Olson EN (1999). Building the heart piece by piece: modularity of *cis*-elements regulating Nkx2-5 transcription. *Development* 126: 4187–4192.

Sedmera D, Pexieder T, Rychterova V, Hu N, Clark EB (1999). Remodeling of chick embryonic ventricular myoarchitecture under experimentally changed loading conditions. *Anat Rec* 254: 238–252.

Simpson JM, Sharland GK (1997). Natural history and outcome of aortic stenosis diagnosed prenatally. *Heart* 77: 205–210.

Smith DM, Nielsen C, Tabin CJ, Roberts DJ (2000). Roles of BMP signaling and Nkx2.5 in patterning at the chick midgut–foregut boundary. *Development* 127: 3671–3681.

Tanaka M, Chen Z, Bartunkova S, Yamasaki N, Izumo S (1999a). The cardiac homeobox gene *Csx/Nkx2.5* lies genetically upstream of multiple genes essential for heart development. *Development* 126: 1269–1280.

Tanaka M, Wechsler SB, Lee IW, Yamasaki N, Lawitts JA, Izumo S (1999b). Complex modular *cis*-acting elements regulate expression of the cardiac specifying homeobox gene *Csx/Nkx2.5*. *Development* 126: 1439–1450.

Thomas PS, Kasahara H, Edmonson AM, Izumo S, Yacoub MH, Barton PJ, Gourdie RG (2001). Elevated expression of Nkx-2.5 in developing myocardial conduction cells. *Anat Rec* 263: 307–313.

Tworetzky W, McElhinney DB, Reddy VM, Brook MM, Hanley FL, Silverman NH (2001). Improved surgical outcome after fetal diagnosis of hypoplastic left heart syndrome. *Circulation* 103: 1269–1273.

Walsh EP, Saul JP (1992). Cardiac arrhythmias. In: *Nadas' Pediatric Cardiology*. Fyler DC (ed.) Hanley & Belfus, Philadelphia, pp. 377–433.

Yagel S, Weissman A, Rotstein Z, Manor M, Hegesh J, Anteby E, Lipitz S, Achiron R (1997). Congenital heart defects: natural course and in utero development. *Circulation* 96: 550–555.

Yamagishi H, Yamagishi C, Nakagawa O, Harvey RP, Olson EN, Srivastava D (2001). The combinatorial activities of Nkx2.5 and dHAND are essential for cardiac ventricle formation. *Dev Biol* 239: 190–203.

Zou Y, Evans S, Chen J, Kuo HC, Harvey RP, Chien KR (1997). CARP, a cardiac ankyrin repeat protein, is downstream in the Nkx2-5 homeobox gene pathway. *Development* 124: 793–804.

58 | *LMX1B* and the Nail Patella Syndrome

BRENDAN LEE AND ROY MORELLO

Nail patella syndrome (NPS) is a dominantly inherited skeletal malformation syndrome. Patients have characteristic features including nail and patella hypoplasia, elbow and knee deformities, nephropathy, and ocular defects. The condition is characterized by high penetrance, variable expressivity, and significant intrafamilial variability. Diagnosis is based on clinical criteria. Morbidity is associated with functional limitations caused by joint abnormalities, risk of developing nephrotic syndrome (which may progress to end-stage renal disease), and risk of developing glaucoma and ocular hypertension. NPS is caused by loss-of-function mutations in the LIM homeodomain (LHX) transcription factor *LMX1B*. *LMX1B* specifies a transcriptional network important in pattern formation of the limb as well as cell maturation and differentiation in both the kidney and CNS. In the limb, *LMX1B* is a unique mesenchymal determinant of dorsal cell fate. In the kidney, it regulates podocyte-specific expression of glomerular basement membrane type IV collagen. Moreover, it specifies morphogenesis of secondary foot processes and directs the expression of unique components of a specialized cell–cell adhesion complex, the slit diaphragm. Finally, it has emerging roles in the survival of mesencephalic dopaminergic neurons, the regulation of dorsoventral projections of motor axons in the vertebrate limb, and the differentiation of periocular mesenchyme. The pathogenesis of NPS reflects a loss of dorsal specification of soft tissues of the limb and disrupted proliferation of anterior relative to posterior skeletal elements. The nephropathy arises in part due to an architectural defect in a primary component of the filtration barrier of the kidney, the glomerular basement membrane (GBM). Glaucoma is likely secondary to anterior segment dysgenesis in the eye. How the function of *LMX1B* in other developmental programs impacts the pathogenesis of the NPS phenotype is still unclear.

LMX1B: HISTORY AND PLEIOTROPIC ROLE DURING LIMB PATTERN FORMATION

Lmx1b is a homeobox-containing transcription factor belonging to the subfamily of LHX transcription factors (Hobert and Westphal, 2000). These molecules, in addition to containing a homeodomain, are characterized by the presence of two cysteine- and histidine-rich zinc finger-like motifs, called LIM domains, at the amino-terminal region of the protein (Sanchez-Garcia and Rabbitts, 1994; Dawid et al., 1998). The LIM domain name derived from its original description in the three genes *Lin11*, *Isl1*, and *Mec3*. These conserved domains are thought to mediate protein–protein interactions. Hence, they help to specify the context-dependent action of LHX transcription factors (German et al., 1992; Ostendorff et al., 2000). Based on the conserved features and similarities among their homeodomains, the LHX transcription factors have been divided into six subgroups: the Apterous group, the Lhx6/7 group, the Islet group, the Lmx group, the Lim-3 group, and the Lin-11 group. Each subgroup contains several genes that have been identified in both vertebrates and invertebrates (for review, see Hobert and Westphal, 2000). The LHX transcription factors have important functions in several developmental processes, including cell fate specification, pattern formation, promotion of cell survival, and cell differentiation (Taira et al., 1994; Pfaff et al., 1996; Porter et al., 1997; Sheng et al., 1997; Benveniste et al., 1998; Rodriguez-Esteban et al., 1998; Sagasti et al., 1999).

The *Lmx1b* ortholog was originally isolated in the chick (*C-Lmx1*)

(Riddle et al., 1995; Vogel et al., 1995). It was first thought to be the avian ortholog of the hamster gene *Lmx1* (German et al., 1992). Later, Iannotti et al. (1997) isolated a novel human *LMX1* gene, distinct from the human ortholog of the hamster gene (*LMX1.1 or LMX1A*) and termed it *LMX1.2*. Sequence analysis demonstrated that *LMX1.2* (later renamed *LMX1B*) was the true human ortholog of the *C-Lmx1* gene, thus revealing that mammals possess at least two *Lmx1* homologs with different functions.

C-Lmx1 misexpression experiments using the avian retrovirus system elucidated its function and importance in determining dorsal cell fate during limb bud development (Riddle et al., 1995; Vogel et al., 1995). Vertebrate limb bud development is a highly organized process and represents a paradigm for developmental biology studies (see Chapter 12). The prospective limb bud cells originate in the lateral plate mesoderm. To develop an anatomical and well-defined functional structure, limb bud cells need to be specified along three spatial axes: proximal/distal (P/D), anterior/posterior (A/P), and dorsal/ventral (D/V). Mesenchymal–ectodermal interactions are critical in this process. Fibroblast growth factors (*Fgfs*, see Chapter 32) are secreted factors in the apical ectodermal ridge that help to specify the outgrowth of the limb along the P/D axis, while sonic hedgehog (*Shh*; see Chapter 16) signaling, originating from the posterior mesoderm (zone of polarizing activity), is responsible for determination of the A/P axis. Finally, several signaling molecules (*Wnt7a* [see Chapter 22], *Radical Fringe, En-1*) contribute to the establishment of the D/V axis in part by specifying the position of the apical ectodermal ridge. These three processes are intimately interconnected (for review of limb development, see Capdevila and Izpisua Belmonte, 2001, and Chapter 12). *Wnt7a* in the dorsal ectoderm and *En-1* in the ventral ectoderm are the molecular cues that direct cells in the mesoderm to adopt a D/V polarity (Wurst et al., 1994; Parr and McMahon, 1995; Logan et al., 1997; Loomis et al., 1998). Experiments performed on the chicken have demonstrated that *Wnt7a* is able to induce *C-Lmx1* expression in the dorsal mesenchyme of the limb bud (Riddle et al., 1995; Vogel et al., 1995). At least in the zeugopod and autopod, *C-Lmx1* is necessary and sufficient to establish dorsal cell fate commitment. In addition, *Wnt7a* mis-expression in the ventral ectoderm induces ectopic *C-Lmx1* expression in the ventral mesoderm of the limb bud and converts these cells from a ventral to a dorsal fate.

Lmx1b inactivation in the mouse confirmed the chick studies and demonstrated that *Lmx1b* is a unique determinant of mesenchymal dorsal structures during limb bud development. *Lmx1b*$^{-/-}$ mice are born live but die within 24 hours with multiple defects (Chen et al., 1998a). The most striking affect is in the limbs, which show complete ventralization of the dorsal mesoderm-derived tissues at the zeugopodal and autopodal levels. In addition to absent patella development (typically derived from the dorsal patellar tendon), the distal duplication of the ventral pattern involves muscles, tendons, and sesamoid bones, with apparent absence of nails (Chen et al., 1998a). Other skeletal defects are present, including the absence of distal ulna, small scapulae, misoriented clavicles, and iliac anomalies. In situ hybridization studies in wild-type mice demonstrated that *Lmx1b* is expressed in the limb bud as early as embryonic day (E) 8.5 through E16.5 (Cygan et al., 1997). Moreover, its limb expression is temporally and spatially restricted with a P/D and an A/P gradient of expression starting at E12.5 and extinguishing by E16.5 (Fig. 58–1) (Dreyer et al., 2000). Comparative studies between *Wnt7a* null mice and *Lmx1b* null mice

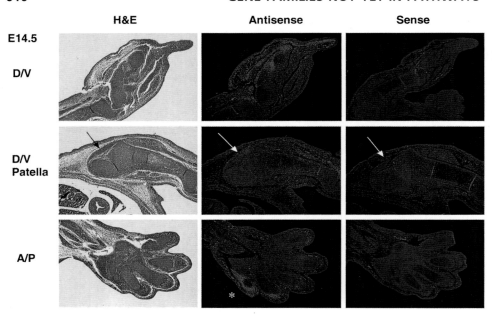

E14.5

D/V

D/V
Patella

A/P

H&E   Antisense   Sense

Figure 58–1. RNA in situ hybridization of embryonic day 14.5 (E14.5) mouse limb sections using *Lmx1b* probe. *Top row*: Forelimb dorsal/ventral (D/V) sections showing expression in dorsal mesenchyme (presumptive muscle, tendon, ligaments). *Middle row*: Hindlimb D/V section with arrow pointing to patella showing similar patterns of expression. *Bottom row*: Forelimb anterior/posterior (A/P) section showing graded expression (*) from anterior to posterior digits. (Reprinted from Dreyer et al., *Hum Mol Genet* 9: 1067–1074, 2000.)

suggest that the dorsalization of the proximal limb bud is still dependent on *Lmx1b*, even if its expression in this region might be independent of *Wnt7a* and rather induced by some other yet unknown factor (Chen and Johnson, 1999).

The *Lmx1b* gene contains eight exons and encodes for an approximately 6 kb mRNA and a 379–amino acid protein (Fig. 58–2). It contains, from the N-terminal to the C-terminal region, four recognizable functional domains: a LIM-A and a LIM-B domain (for protein in-

teraction), a homeodomain (for DNA binding), and a glutamine-rich and serine-rich domain (with putative transcriptional activation function). *Lmx1b*, like its homolog *Lmx1a*, likely exerts its function via a transcriptional activation complex that is specified by interactions with other transcriptional factors or cofactors via the LIM domains (German et al., 1992; Johnson et al., 1997; Dreyer et al., 2000). Some interacting proteins have been described to either positively or negatively regulate LHX transactivation of target genes. These interactors

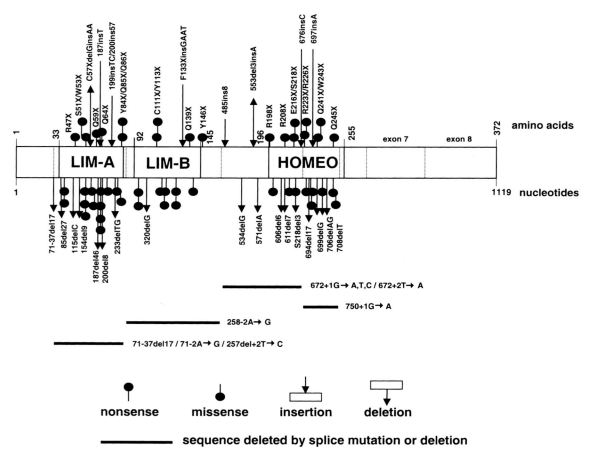

Figure 58–2. Schematic of *LMX1B* gene. Respective exons are delineated by thin lines. Functional domains are listed within boxes. Mutations are shown above and below as per schema.

Figure 58–3. Two-year-old nail patella syndrome patient's hands. Arrows: dysplastic first and second digits in the *left panel* and thumb in the *right panel.*

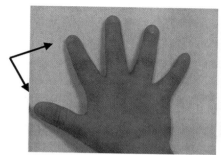
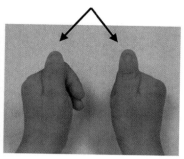

include *Ldb1* (Agulnick et al., 1996), *RLIM* (Bach et al., 1999), *E47* (German et al., 1992), *Chip* (van Meyel et al., 1999), and LIM-only (*LMO*) proteins (Milan et al., 1998; Milan and Cohen, 1999). The cofactor RLIM is able to ubiquitinate cofactors bound to LHX proteins, thus leading to their degradation via the 26S proteasome pathway (Ostendorff et al., 2002).

NPS: CLINICAL FEATURES AND NATURAL HISTORY

NPS is a dominantly inherited pleiotropic skeletal malformation syndrome exhibiting high penetrance and significant variable expressivity (Jones, 1997). Because multiple organ systems are affected, it is likely that the underlying gene function in multiple developmental pathways. The clinical features include abnormal nails and skeleton, especially involving the knees and elbows. Familial associations of defective elbows, knees, and nails had been made in several reports dating back to the 1800s (Little, 1897). Since then, the association has been given multiple names, including *hereditary osteo-onychodysplasia* and *Fong disease* (Fong, 1946; Roekerath, 1951). The ocular finding of a cloverleaf appearance of the iris and the unique radiographic association of iliac horns to NPS were made in the mid-1900s (Flickinger and Spivey, 1969). The cosegregation of primary open angle glaucoma (POAG) was made much later (Lichter et al., 1997). Nephropathy, which accounts for significant morbidity in NPS, was described in the mid-1900s (Brixey and Burke, 1950; Hawkings and Smith, 1950). Many more excellent studies have since documented the incidence of multiple features of this disease (Bongers et al., 2002). The main conclusion that can be drawn is that, while many of the unique features are found in a majority of patients, there is great intrafamilial variability for the severity of each feature. This makes presymptomatic counseling especially difficult.

The nail dysplasia is often noticeable at birth and can be seen as nail hypoplasia, anonychia, longitudinal ridging, splitting, and spooning of the nail (Stratigos and Baden, 2001; Fistarol and Itin, 2002). Interestingly, the nails of the anterior digits of the upper limb are usually more affected, with a gradation of severity from the anterior (thumb side) to the posterior (fifth digit) sides of the hand (Fig. 58–3). For example, patients often have affected first and second digits. The toenails are often not involved. In the literature review of Bongers et al. (2002) 95% of NPS patients had nail abnormalities. A characteristic feature is the presence of triangular-appearing lunulae of the nails (Mellotte and Eastwood, 1995). Although a cosmetic problem, the nail dysplasia does not cause significant long-term morbidity. Another classical feature found in NPS is patellar abnormalities ranging from hypoplasia to aplasia. It is found in over 90% of patients and may lead to recurrent dislocation or subluxation, leg extension lag, and significant knee pain (Guidera et al., 1991; Bongers et al., 2002).

Ocular findings including pigmentation of the inner margin of the iris (Lester's line) and iris processes have few functional implications (Flickinger and Spivey, 1969). However, POAG is a variable feature of NPS (Lichter et al., 1997; Craig and Mackey, 1999). In an ocular investigation of NPS patients, ocular hypertension and glaucoma were found in 7% and 10% of cases, respectively. In a minority of cases, other ocular complications, such as cataracts and microcornea, have been reported (Sweeney et al., 2001).

Multiple skeletal features are found in NPS. The most characteristic ones affect the pelvis, the elbows, the knees, and the feet (Guidera et al., 1991). A pathognomonic feature found in NPS is triangular dorsolateral projections off the ilia (Fong, 1946; Hawkings and Smith, 1950; Sartoris and Resnick, 1987). These are termed *iliac horns* and are found in 70%–80% of NPS patients (Fig. 58–4). Iliac horns do not affect gait or other function (Bongers et al., 2002). Relevant for skele-

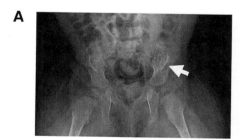
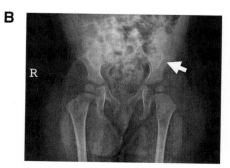
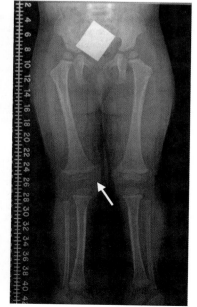

Figure 58–4. Pelvic radiographs of nail patella syndrome. (*A*) Seven-month-old girl: arrow points to iliac horns. (*B*) Fourteen-month-old girl: arrow points to iliac horns. (*C*) Eighteen-month-old girl: arrow points to mild prominence of medial femoral condyle and genu varum.

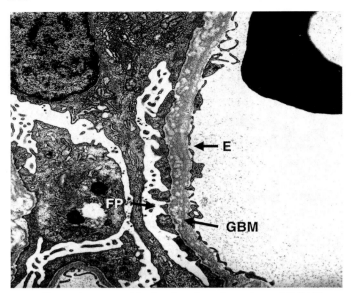

Figure 58–5. Ultrastructural findings in nail patella syndrome (NPS) kidneys. Transmission electron micrograph of kidney biopsy from NPS patient shows thickened, moth-eaten appearance of glomerular basement membrane (GBM). Podocyte foot processes (FP) and endothelial fenestrations (E) appear intact. (Reprinted from Morello and Lee, *Pediatr Res* 51: 551–558, 2002.)

tal function are the findings of elbow dysplasia, often with radial head subluxation or dislocation, as well as foot deformities, including talipes equinovarus (Hogh and Macnicol, 1985; Fiedler et al., 1987). The former can be found in up to 90% of patients and will prevent full extension, pronation, or supination while leaving the patient with flexion contractures. A clinical scoring system has been proposed to grade the severity of orthopedic findings (Farley et al., 1999). Muscle aplasia has also been described (Jones, 1997). When involving the pectoralis, biceps, and triceps muscles, shoulder instability may develop.

The clinical complication having the greatest impact on long-term morbidity in NPS is nephropathy (Mihatsch and Zollinger, 1980). This often begins as microalbuminuria and progresses to frank proteinuria. It is less commonly associated with hematuria, though in a proportion of cases frank end-stage renal failure can develop. In two separate studies, 25% and 62% of patients had renal involvement; end-stage renal disease (ESRD) developed in 2% and 15%, respectively (Sweeney et al., 2001; Bongers et al., 2002). While light microscopic alterations on renal biopsy may not be apparent in all cases, it is likely that all NPS patients have alterations on the ultrastructural level (Gubler et al., 1980; Taguchi et al., 1988; Drut et al., 1992). These have been well documented in fetal and adult cases. Characteristic changes include diffuse and irregular thickening of the GBM with lucencies that give it a "moth-eaten" appearance (Fig. 58–5). In addition, there is often deposition of fibrillar collagen bundles within the GBM. Podocyte foot processes may also be irregular, though this may

be due to effacement with progression of the nephropathy. Because some of the ultrastructural findings are reminiscent of those seen in Alport's syndrome, the type IV collagen genes were initially considered good candidates for this condition. However, the multisystemic involvement made this less likely. Unfortunately, there are no good clinical predictors of progression to ESRD or of whether a patient will develop clinical nephropathy.

There have been other rare associations reported with NPS, including mental retardation, psychosis, and cleft lip/palate. There are also several reports of additional clinical conditions coincident with NPS in the same patient, e.g., achondroplasia, IgA nephropathy, and sensorineural hearing loss (Hussain and Hope, 1994; Chuah et al., 1999; Wright et al., 2000; Gao et al., 2001). These are likely to be incidental findings and not associated with common pathogenetic mechanisms.

Patients often present with minor skeletal problems, e.g., involving the feet, when seen by orthopedic surgeons. Nephropathy is often not diagnosed until the third decade of life, unless presymptomatic monitoring has been initiated due to another affected family member (Sweeney et al., 2001). If there is progression to ESRD, it rarely occurs prior to the fourth decade. Limitation of joint mobility at the elbow due to dislocation, flexion contractures, or pterygia and hyperextension of the knee may ultimately limit function (Guidera et al., 1991). This may also put the patient at risk for early-onset arthritis. Ultimately, because glaucoma can develop in a subset of patients from birth until well into adulthood, monitoring is also indicated at the time of diagnosis. Unfortunately, there are no good clinical or molecular markers to predict progression on these fronts, and prospective monitoring is indicated as part of the health-care maintenance program of patients.

MOLECULAR GENETICS OF *LMX1B* MUTATIONS IN NPS

NPS was one of the first human genetic conditions successfully studied by linkage. It was linked to the ABO blood group locus and the adenylate kinase 1 gene (Renwick and Lawler, 1955; Schleutermann et al., 1969). Subsequently, multiple family studies further refined the region to chromosome 9q34 (Campeau et al., 1995; McIntosh et al., 1997). *LMX1B* was ultimately identified as the gene mutated in this condition by comparative phenotypic analysis with the mouse model and synteny with the NPS locus (Chen et al., 1998a; Dreyer et al., 1998). Since the original description of the first mutations in the *LMX1B* gene, at least 90 different mutations in more than 150 unrelated families have been described (Table 58–1) (Bongers et al., 2002). Included are missense, nonsense, and splice mutations as well as microinsertions and deletions. The mutations described to date have been localized to either exon 2, 3, 4, or 5, while none has been identified in exon 1, 6, 7, or 8 (Vollrath et al., 1998; Clough et al., 1999; Seri et al., 1999; Hamlington et al., 2000, 2001; Sweeney et al., 2001). The majority of mutations affect the LIM domains (especially the LIM-A domain) or the homeodomain, while no mutations have yet been described in the glutamine- and serine-rich carboxy-terminal domain (Table 58–1, Fig. 58–2). The microinsertions and deletions as well as the splice and nonsense mutations cause a frameshift or exon skip-

Table 58–1. *LMX1B* Mutations in Nail Patella Syndrome

Location	Mutation	Type	Comment	References
LIM-A domain	71-37del17	D	Loss of exon 2, frameshift, PTC	Hamlington et al., 2000
	71-2A → G	S	Loss of exon 2, frameshift, PTC	Clough et al., 1999
	71-1G → A	S	Frameshift, PTC	McIntosh et al., 1998
	85del27	D	Disrupt Zn finger	Clough et al., 1999
	C36R	M	Disrupt Zn finger	Clough et al., 1999
	C36S	M	Disrupt Zn finger	Clough et al., 1999
	115delC	D	Frameshift, PTC	Hamlington et al., 2001
	R47X	N	PTC	Hamlington et al., 2001
	S51X	N	PTC	Hamlington et al., 2001
	154del9	D	Disrupt Zn finger	Clough et al., 1999
	W53X	N	PTC	Clough et al., 1999
	H54N	M	Disrupt Zn finger	Hamlington et al., 2001
	H54Y	M	Disrupt Zn finger	Clough et al., 1999

(*continued*)

Table 58–1. *Continued*

Location	Mutation	Type	Comment	References
	H54Q	M	Disrupt Zn finger	Clough et al., 1999
	C57R	M	Disrupt Zn finger	Clough et al., 1999
	C57X(delGinsAA)	D/I	PTC	Hamlington et al., 2001
	L58W	M	Disrupt Zn finger	Hamlington et al., 2001
	Q59X	N	PTC	Vollrath et al., 1998
	C60G	M	Disrupt Zn finger	Clough et al., 1999
	C60R	M	Disrupt Zn finger	Hamlington et al., 2001
	C60Y	M	Disrupt Zn finger	Clough et al., 1999
	C60F	M	Disrupt Zn finger	Hamlington et al., 2001
	187insT	I	Frameshift, PTC	Clough et al., 1999
	187del46	D	Frameshift, PTC	Clough et al., 1999
	C63R	M	Disrupt Zn finger	Clough et al., 1999
	Q64X	N	PTC	Clough et al., 1999
	199insTC	I	Frameshift, PTC	Clough et al., 1999
	200del8	D	Frameshift, PTC	Clough et al., 1999
	200ins57	I	Disrupt Zn finger	Hamlington et al., 2001
	233delTG	D	Frameshift, PTC	Vollrath et al., 1998
	C80W	M	Disrupt Zn finger	Hamlington et al., 2001
	D83G	M	Disrupt Zn finger	Clough et al., 1999
	Y84X	N	PTC	Clough et al., 1999
	Q85X	N	PTC	Hamlington et al., 2001
	Q86X	N	PTC	Hamlington et al., 2001
	257del+2T → C	S	Loss of exon 2, frameshift, PTC	McIntosh et al., 1998
LIM-B domain	258-2A → G	S	Loss of exon3, frameshift, PTC	Clough et al., 1999
	C95Y	M	Disrupt Zn finger	Clough et al., 1999
	C95F	M	Disrupt Zn finger	Vollrath et al., 1998
	320delG	D	Frameshift, PTC	McIntosh et al., 1998
	C111X	N	PTC	Clough et al., 1999
	Y113X	N	PTC	Clough et al., 1999
	H114Y	M	Disrupt Zn finger	Hamlington et al., 2001
	C117Y	M	Disrupt Zn finger	Hamlington et al., 2001
	C120S	M	Disrupt Zn finger	Clough et al., 1999
	C123Y	M	Disrupt Zn finger	Clough et al., 1999
	C123F	M	Disrupt Zn finger	Clough et al., 1999
	F133X(insGAAT)	I	PTC	Clough et al., 1999
	Q139X	N	PTC	Clough et al., 1999
	C142W	M	Disrupt Zn finger	McIntosh et al., 1998
	Y146X	N	PTC	McIntosh et al., 1998
Linker	485ins8	I	Frameshift, PTC	McIntosh et al., 1998
	534delG	D	Frameshift, PTC	McIntosh et al., 1998
	553del3insA	D/I	Frameshift, PTC	Hamlington et al., 2001
	571delA	D	Frameshift, PTC	Hamlington et al., 2001
Homeodomain	R198X	N	PTC	Dreyer et al., 1998
	R200Q	M	Affect DNA binding	McIntosh et al., 1998
	606del6	D	Affect DNA binding	Hamlington et al., 2001
	611del7	D	Frameshift, PTC	McIntosh et al., 1998
	R208X	N	PTC	Vollrath et al., 1998
	A213P	M	Affect DNA binding	McIntosh et al., 1998
	E216X	N	PTC	McIntosh et al., 1998
	S218del3	D	Affect DNA binding	Hamlington et al., 2001
	S218P	M	Affect DNA binding	McIntosh et al., 1998
	S218X	N	PTC	Clough et al., 1999
	R223X	N	PTC	McIntosh et al., 1998
	672+1G → A	S	Loss of exon 4, frameshift, PTC	McIntosh et al., 1998
	672+1G → T	S	Loss of exon 4, frameshift, PTC	McIntosh et al., 1998
	672+1G → C	S	Loss of exon 4, frameshift, PTC	Hamlington et al., 2001
	672+2T → A	S	Loss of exon 4, frameshift, PTC	Clough et al., 1999
	R226X	N	PTC	McIntosh et al., 1998
	676insC	I	Frameshift, PTC	Hamlington et al., 2001
	R226P	M	Affect DNA binding	McIntosh et al., 1998
	L229P	M	Affect DNA binding	Clough et al., 1999
	A230V	M	Affect DNA binding	McIntosh et al., 1998
	694del17	D	Frameshift, PTC	Hamlington et al., 2001
	697insA	I	Frameshift, PTC	Dreyer et al., 1998
	699delG	D	Frameshift, PTC	Seri et al., 1999
	706delAG	D	Frameshift, PTC	Seri et al., 1999
	708delT	D	Frameshift, PTC	Clough et al., 1999
	Q241X	N	PTC	Clough et al., 1999
	W243X	N	PTC	McIntosh et al., 1998
	W243C	M	Affect DNA binding	Hamlington et al., 2001
	Q245X	N	PTC	McIntosh et al., 1998
	N246K	M	Affect DNA binding	Dreyer et al., 1998
	A249P	M	Affect DNA binding	Knoers et al., 2000
	750+1G → A	S	Loss of exon 5	McIntosh et al., 1998

D, deletion mutation; N, nonsense mutation; M, missense mutation; S, splice mutation; I, insertion mutation.

ping, thereby generating a premature termination codon in the open reading frame. The predicted truncated transcripts have never actually been observed in vivo. It is likely that nonsense-mediated RNA decay prevents the production of a truncated protein. These data have supported a model of haploinsufficiency in the pathogenesis of NPS. Missense mutations within the LIM domains, however, invariably affect conserved residues and are predicted to disrupt the regionally encoded zinc-finger structure. Mutations affecting the homeodomain interfere with or abolish DNA binding in vitro (Dreyer et al., 1998; McIntosh et al., 1998). These in vitro binding assays were performed utilizing as a probe the *FLAT* element. This was described previously as part of the insulin mini-enhancer complex. It serves as a target of the *Lmx1a* gene, a homolog of *Lmx1b* that shares an identical homeodomain on the sequence level (German et al., 1992). Large deletions encompassing the *LMX1B* locus have yet to be described, but the underlying mechanism of NPS is still thought to be haploinsufficiency. All currently described mutations are predicted to cause loss of a functional allele. A dominant-negative effect is unlikely, especially with the description of a balanced translocation with one of the breakpoints involving the *LMX1B* gene (Duba et al., 1998).

Unfortunately, because of disease heterogeneity within and among families, it has not been possible to establish a genotype–phenotype correlation. An identical mutation affecting multiple families may cause nephropathy in some, but not all, members (Knoers et al., 2000). The same situation is true for the association of open angle glaucoma with NPS. The absence of mutations affecting the carboxy-terminal region of *LMX1B* is interesting and raises important questions. It is possible that such mutations may not have an effect on limb development and that this function is dependent only on the LIM or the homeodomain (Clough et al., 1999).

ESTABLISHING THE NPS DIAGNOSIS

While NPS exhibits high penetrance, significant variable expressivity may make diagnosis difficult, especially in mild cases. The diagnosis is straightforward when the classic tetrad of abnormal nails, elbows, knees, and iliac horns is found on physical exam. Nail dystrophy, patellar abnormalities, and elbow dysplasia are most prevalent. However, because many patients present with minor skeletal complaints, especially involving the feet, the multi-systemic nature of the underlying condition may not always be appreciated.

Nail dysplasia is easily diagnosed and usually found at birth. Because patella ossify over a wide range of ages in childhood and depending on sex, radiographic studies may miss hypoplasia. However, direct physical examination in conjunction with ultrasonography can be used in younger children (Miller et al., 1998). In older children, radiographic studies are adequate. Other imaging technologies, such as magnetic resonance imaging, can also detect the presence of patella hypoplasia. Iliac horns, while not present in all NPS patients, are quite specific and can be identified by plane radiographs of infants and young children. A complete list of radiographic features in NPS including more subtle ones (that may help to solidify a clinical diagnosis) is given in Table 58–2. While not required for diagnosis, the finding of ocular abnormalities and/or nephropathy would also confirm the clinical suspicion of NPS. A formal ophthalmologic evaluation to detect ocular hypertension would also be helpful. Urine analysis and/or 24-hour urine collection for protein can detect nephropathy.

DNA testing is not available on a clinical basis. However, testing can be arranged on a research basis. Since mutations are not found in all cases, presymptomatic or prenatal testing can be performed on a research basis by undertaking linkage analysis. Prenatal diagnosis has also been reported, using ultrasonography to detect skeletal alterations including iliac horns, absent patellae, and lower extremity alterations (Feingold et al., 1998; McIntosh et al., 1999; Pinette et al., 1999). Because the ultrastructural alterations of the kidney in NPS occur even prenatally, diagnosis via prenatal renal biopsy could also be considered, though there would be significant risks (Gubler and Levy, 1993).

The differential diagnosis may include several conditions that have in common some of the skeletal features of NPS. For example, patella aplasia-hypoplasia syndrome is dominantly inherited and has been

Table 58–2. Radiographic Findings in Nail Patella Syndrome

Hypoplastic or aplastic patella
Iliac horn
Elongated radius with hypoplasia of radial head
Hypoplasia of the capitellum
Flaring of the iliac wing with small iliac angle
Prominence of the medial femoral condyle
Other less common findings:
  Joint asymmetry
  Clinodactyly
  Camptodactyly
  Symphalangism
  Calcaneovalgus deformity
  Subluxation of the tarsal–metatarsal joint
  Small acromion with hypoplastic scapula

mapped to chromosome 17q21-22 (Bernhang and Levine, 1973; Mangino et al., 1999). These patients do not have the ocular, renal, nail, or other skeletal findings of NPS. Like NPS, Meier-Gorlin syndrome is characterized by patellar hypoplasia and elbow dislocation (Bongers et al., 2001a; Cohen et al., 2002). However, it is recessively inherited and characterized by failure to thrive and dysmorphic features, i.e., micrognathia and microtia. Sequence analysis of *LMX1B* in these patients failed to identify mutations. Finally, ischiopatellar syndrome or small patella syndrome is a dominantly inherited condition characterized by patella hypoplasia (Scott and Taor, 1979; Bongers et al., 2001b). However, patients also have upper femur abnormalities and pelvic abnormalities including ischial hypoplasia and delayed ossification of the ischiopubic junction. Allelism with NPS was excluded, but the analysis was not informative for the patella aplasia locus. Radial head dislocation has also been reported to be inherited in a dominant fashion as an isolated finding; its relation with *LMX1B* is unclear (Reichenbach et al., 1995).

When glaucoma is the primary ascertainment criteria, the diagnosis of various forms of juvenile-onset POAG should be differentiated (Craig and Mackey, 1999). Some of these conditions also present with pigmentary alterations of the irides. However, the distinction from NPS should be straightforward based on the skeletal findings in NPS. Finally, the diagnosis may in rare cases be first raised by histopathologic findings on renal biopsy for evaluation of steroid-resistant nephrotic syndrome. In this case, the histopathologic features bear some similarities to Alport's syndrome and to collagen type III glomerulopathy (Noel et al., 1989; Imbasciati et al., 1991; Gubler et al., 1993; Bodziak et al., 1994). In either case, the skeletal findings in NPS help to make the distinction relatively straightforward. Ultimately, the finding of multiorgan system involvement helps to distinguish it from other genetic entities that primarily affect the skeleton, eyes, or kidneys in an isolated fashion.

MANAGEMENT, TREATMENT, AND COUNSELING

Patients at diagnosis should have full orthopedic, ophthalmologic, and nephrologic evaluations. Acute and long-term morbidity is usually associated with orthopedic problems. Foot abnormalities are a chief complaint (Hogh and Macnicol, 1985; Fiedler et al., 1987). Knee and elbow complaints also cause chronic problems (Guidera et al., 1991). In general, a conservative approach should be taken and surgery considered when functional limitations outweigh risks in each situation. Operations to correct foot and ankle deformities were most common in one study of 44 patients (Guidera et al., 1991). Knee extensor operations and foot posteromedial releases produced good results. Interestingly, elbow reconstructive procedures were rarely indicated. In another report, radial head resection relieved minor pain but did not improve elbow motion (Yakish and Fu, 1983). The Stanisavljevic procedure has been used to correct permanent patella dislocation and improve extension lag at the knee (Marumo et al., 1999). Surgical interventions should be considered, especially when gait is markedly affected.

Few studies have addressed the efficacy of different treatment options for patients who suffer from glaucoma. Hence, a traditional oph-

Figure 58–6. Expression of *Lmx1b* in embryonic mouse kidneys. *Left panel*: Hematoxylin and eosin (H&E) stain of embryonic day 14.5 (E14.5) mouse kidney in transverse section. *Right panel*: RNA in situ hybridization of E14.5 kidney section with *Lmx1b* showing glomerular-specific expression (arrow). (Reprinted from Morello et al., *Nat Genet* 27: 205–208, 2001.)

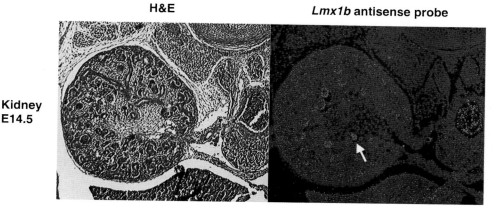

thalmologic approach should be taken. Mouse studies point to a possible dysgenesis of the anterior chamber as an underlying defect (Chen et al., 1998b). In all patients, prospective monitoring for development of ocular hypertension is indicated, given the variability of this feature in NPS.

Similarly, long-term morbidity arises from the development of nephropathy. While this usually does not become clinically significant until later in life, prospective monitoring should be instituted in order to identify microalbuminuria and proteinuria. Initially in childhood, routine urinanalysis is sufficient for this purpose. However, for follow-up of clinical nephropathy, 24-hour urine collections to calculate proteinuria and creatinine clearance are indicated, as well as a full nephrology evaluation. Since the nephropathy in this condition is not immunologically related, it is likely to be steroid-resistant. Ultimately, for ESRD, kidney transplantation is curative because of the cell-autonomous nature of the underlying kidney defect (Uranga et al., 1973; Verdich, 1980; Chan et al., 1988; Bodziak et al., 1994).

Patients and their families should be counseled on the dominant pattern of inheritance and the associated recurrence risk. Parents of newly diagnosed patients should be evaluated for subtle signs of NPS since this would directly affect recurrence for future offspring. No clear cases of germinal mosaicism have been reported, though this remains a formal possibility. Counseling should also stress the significant intrafamilial variability and lack of adequate genotype–phenotype correlations or clinical indices to predict the development of either glaucoma or nephropathy.

MOUSE MODELS OF *Lmx1b* FUNCTION AND ITS EMERGING ROLE IN CELLULAR DIFFERENTIATION

The only existing mouse model for study of *Lmx1b* function has been created by a targeted deletion of exons 3–7 of the *Lmx1b* gene in mouse embryonic stem cells with the subsequent generation of heterozygous and homozygous knockout mice (Chen et al., 1998a). Mutant *Lmx1b* mice are born live with multiple defects but die within 24 hours for reasons that remain to be determined. As expected, they showed dorsal-to-ventral conversion of mesenchymal tissues in both fore- and hindlimbs, especially at the zeugopodal and autopodal levels, confirming previous studies describing the importance of *Lmx1b* for the determination of dorsal structures during chick limb development (Riddle et al., 1995; Vogel et al., 1995). The correlation of *LMX1B* mutations with NPS pointed to the previously unappreciated function of this transcription factor in kidney development.

Lmx1b null mice also exhibit kidney defects (see Chapter 13 for review), characterized by accumulation of glycoproteins in the distal collecting tubules as well as an abnormal GBM upon ultrastructural examination (Chen et al., 1998a). This is highly reminiscent of the features observed in NPS kidney biopsies. *Lmx1b* is indeed expressed at all levels of glomerular maturation, beginning with the S-shaped bodies and continuing to the mature glomeruli following birth (Fig. 58-6). *Lmx1b* expression and its importance during metanephric kidney development is correlated with the nephropathy observed in NPS

patients. Interestingly, the mutant phenotype in the limb and kidney is apparent in null mice, while the clinical features are apparent in heterozygous states in humans. This may point to differences in dosage sensitivity of these developmental pathways in mice vs. humans.

The mutant mice have proven extremely useful in elucidating the underlying molecular defects in *Lmx1b$^{-/-}$* kidney. *Lmx1b$^{-/-}$* mice have a strongly decreased level of expression of α4(IV) and α3(IV) collagen subunits in the GBM. This likely contributes to the architectural alteration of the GBM as well as the proteinuria observed in both mutant mice and NPS patients (Morello et al., 2001). This downregulation is due to loss of direct transactivation of the *Col4a3/Col4a4* gene locus by *Lmx1b*. LMX1B was found to be capable of binding an enhancer-like element in the first intron of *Col4a4*, which regulates the expression of both *Col4a4* and *Col4a3* (Morello et al., 2001); hence, these molecules are the first identified downstream targets of *Lmx1b* to be activated during metanephric kidney development. More recent studies have suggested that *Lmx1b* also directly regulates the expression of two other genes, *Cd2ap* and *Nphs2* (Podocin) (Miner et al., 2002; Rohr et al., 2002). These proteins are podocyte differentiation markers and contribute to the formation of the slit diaphragm between podocyte foot processes. Moreover, mutations in these genes have been implicated in genetic forms of nephrotic syndrome (Shih et al., 1999; Boute et al., 2000). *Lmx1b$^{-/-}$* podocytes show developmental arrest, with immature foot processes and abnormal slit diaphragm formation. Hence, these results highlighted the importance of *Lmx1b* for proper podocyte maturation and terminal differentiation, especially foot process formation on both the molecular and phenotypic levels (Morello and Lee, 2002).

The association between NPS and POAG has prompted investigations of the potential role played by *Lmx1b* during eye formation and development. *Lmx1b$^{-/-}$* mouse embryos show ocular abnormalities at E15.5 and develop iris and ciliary body hypoplasia and corneal stromal defects at the newborn stage. Therefore, *Lmx1b* is an important regulator of murine eye anterior segment morphogenesis and patterning (Pressman et al., 2000). These findings suggest a potential developmental origin of POAG in NPS patients.

Chen et al. (1998b) documented *Lmx1b* expression in the progenitors of some calvarial bones and in the neuroepithelium underlying the calvarial region. The finding of multiple calvarial defects and suture abnormalities in *Lmx1b$^{-/-}$* mice suggests another role for this transcription factor in the patterning and morphogenesis of the cranial vault.

Studies in the chicken have reported a role of *Lmx1b* during anterior CNS development. Its expression was detected in the ventral and dorsal midline, in a population of dorsal interneurons of the developing spinal cord, and in the rostral domain of the isthmus (Adams et al., 2000). Evidence suggested that in the isthmus organizer *Lmx1b* is an effector of *Fgf8* and is able to regulate *Wnt1* expression. It can also play a role in the formation of the mesencephalic/metencephalic boundary (Adams et al., 2000). Further experiments in mice and humans showed *Lmx1b* expression in developing mesencephalic dopamine neurons, which was maintained throughout adult life (Smidt et al., 2000). Interestingly, *Lmx1b*$^{-/-}$ mesencephalic dopamine neurons did not activate the expression of a mesencephalic dopamine neuron-specific homeodomain gene, *Ptx3*; and these cells were eventually lost during development (Smidt et al., 2000). Finally, the elegant work of Kania et al. (2000) showed the important function played by *Lmx1b* in the dorsal mesenchymal limb bud cells for providing axon guidance to the motor neuron projections originating from the lateral motor column of the spinal cord and in the establishment of a distinct dorsal and ventral trajectory. Together, these studies show a diverse role for *Lmx1b* in the regulation of cellular maturation in neurons and podocytes. However, how it specifies dorsal position in developing limb mesenchyme is still unclear.

PATHOGENESIS OF NPS AND IMPORTANT QUESTIONS

The NPS phenotype is caused by dysregulation of a complex transcriptional network specified by *LMX1B* (Hermanns and Lee, 2001). The outcome of this dysregulation is complex on the cellular level, but phenotypically it relates to defects in cellular maturation and pattern specification. Unfortunately, especially in the latter case, none of the direct target genes is known. The soft tissue and skeletal defects (patella) in NPS reflect a deficiency of dorsal specification of the developing limb during a very restricted time in embryonic development (Dreyer et al., 2000). Both nails and patella are derived from dorsal mesenchyme. At the same time, the elbow abnormalities (radial head dislocation with elongated radius, asymmetric joints, medial vs. lateral femoral condylar prominence, etc.) are likely a reflection of dysregulated A/P patterning and the gradient of *Lmx1b* expression along that axis (Dreyer et al., 2000). The null mouse model clearly demonstrates the loss of dorsalization of the limb with conversion of muscle, tendon, and ligaments from a dorsal to a ventral pattern. Similarly, a proliferation defect of anterior relative to posterior skeletal elements is evident in both humans and mice. NPS patients have an elongated radius, while *Lmx1b*$^{-/-}$ mice have ulnar hypoplasia (Chen et al., 1998a).

In contrast to the limb-patterning defect, the nephropathy arises from a defect in cellular maturation and differentiation (Morello and Lee, 2002). *Lmx1b* is expressed in both embryonic and adult kidney glomeruli. The defective GBM in NPS is likely due in part to dysregulated production of glomeruli-specific α4(IV) and α3(IV) collagen by podocytes (Morello et al., 2001). However, null mice have a more severe phenotype and show arrested podocyte differentiation with decreased expression of podocin and Cd2ap and paucity of foot processes (Miner et al., 2002; Rohr et al., 2002). How this translates to the NPS phenotype given only haploinsufficiency of LMX1B is unclear. Ultrastructural studies in humans have not demonstrated a clear defect in slit diaphragm formation. Another clinical question is the etiology of fibrillar collagen deposition in NPS patient GBM. This, however, is not prevalent in *Lmx1b*$^{-/-}$ mouse GBM. From these studies, it is clear that the basic architectural defect in GBM of NPS patients is due to *Lmx1b* dysregulation of key matrix components.

The ocular defects in NPS reflect the function of *Lmx1b* in anterior chamber morphogenesis. It is expressed in periocular mesenchyme, which gives rise to sclera, cornea, ciliary body, iris, and trabeculae; and null mice have abnormal cornea, ciliary body, and iris (Pressman et al., 2000). Since its expression persists into adulthood, it is unclear whether the glaucoma observed in NPS is due to dysgenesis of these anterior chamber components during development and/or to loss of some maintenance function in adulthood. Since null mice die in the perinatal period, no studies are available at later time points. At the same time, no histopathologic studies of NPS anterior chamber structure have been reported. The expression and function of *Lmx1b* in the CNS is intriguing and raises the question of whether some of the psychiatric associations reported in NPS may be related to dysregulation of dopaminergic neurons (Smidt et al., 2000). Another interesting clinical question is the etiology of muscle hypoplasia. This may be secondary to axonal innervation defects due to the role of *Lmx1b* in D/V projection of motor axons (Kania et al., 2000). Finally, it is intriguing that no mutations have been found in the carboxy-terminal domain. This raises the question of whether a different phenotype might result from alterations in this portion of the molecule.

There are important basic questions that remain to be addressed. For example, there are still no other mesenchymal determinants of dorsal pattern in the developing limb. In fact, our understanding of the molecular determinants of D/V pattern formation in the limb is dwarfed in comparison to the data on A/P pattern specification. Identifying downstream targets of *Lmx1b* in limb development may help in this regard. Full delineation of the *Lmx1b* transcriptional network may be critical for elucidating the molecular mechanisms that control cell process formation. *Lmx1b* mutant podocytes do not form secondary foot processes. Given the similarities of podocytes and neurons, such studies may lend insight into cellular processes such as cytoskeletal reorganization. Clearly, comparative analysis of the mouse model and the NPS phenotype will help to answer these clinical questions.

ACKNOWLEDGMENTS

The authors thank O. Hernandez for administrative assistance, S. Carter, R.N., for clinical assistance, and T. Bertin for review of the manuscript. Portions of this work were supported by the National Institutes of Health, March of Dimes, the Arthritis Foundation, and the Baylor College of Medicine Child Health Research Center and Mental Retardation Research Center. R.M. is supported by a fellowship from the Italian Telethon Foundation.

REFERENCES

Adams KA, Maida JM, Golden JA, Riddle RD (2000). The transcription factor Lmx1b maintains Wnt1 expression within the isthmic organizer. *Development* 127: 1857–1867.

Agulnick AD, Taira M, Breen JJ, Tanaka T, Dawid IB, Westphal H (1996). Interactions of the LIM-domain-binding factor Ldb1 with LIM homeodomain proteins. *Nature* 384: 270–272.

Bach I, Rodriguez-Esteban C, Carriere C, Bhushan A, Krones A, Rose DW, Glass CK, et al. (1999). RLIM inhibits functional activity of LIM homeodomain transcription factors via recruitment of the histone deacetylase complex. *Nat Genet* 22: 394–399.

Benveniste RJ, Thor S, Thomas JB, Taghert PH (1998). Cell type-specific regulation of the *Drosophila* FMRF-NH2 neuropeptide gene by Apterous, a LIM homeodomain transcription factor. *Development* 125: 4757–4765.

Bernhang AM, Levine SA (1973). Familial absence of the patella. *J Bone Joint Surg A* 55: 1088–1090.

Bodziak KA, Hammond WS, Molitoris BA (1994). Inherited diseases of the glomerular basement membrane. *Am J Kidney Dis* 23: 605–618.

Bongers EM, Opitz JM, Fryer A, Sarda P, Hennekam RC, Hall BD, Superneau DW, et al. (2001a). Meier-Gorlin syndrome: report of eight additional cases and review. *Am J Med Genet* 102: 115–24.

Bongers EM, Van Bokhoven H, Van Thienen MN, Kooyman MA, Van Beersum SE, Boetes C, Knoers NV, et al. (2001b). The small patella syndrome: description of five cases from three families and examination of possible allelism with familial patella aplasia-hypoplasia and nail-patella syndrome. *J Med Genet* 38: 209–214.

Bongers EM, Gubler MC, Knoers NV (2002). Nail-patella syndrome. Overview on clinical and molecular findings. *Pediatr Nephrol* 17: 703–712.

Boute N, Gribouval O, Roselli S, Benessy F, Lee H, Fuchshuber A, Dahan K, et al. (2000). NPHS2, encoding the glomerular protein podocin, is mutated in autosomal recessive steroid-resistant nephrotic syndrome. *Nat Genet* 24: 349–354.

Brixey AM, Burke RM (1950). Arthro-onychodysplasia. *Am J Med* 8: 738–744.

Campeau E, Watkins D, Rouleau GA, Babul R, Buchanan JA, Meschino W, Der Kaloustian VM (1995). Linkage analysis of the nail-patella syndrome. *Am J Hum Genet* 56: 243–247.

Capdevila J, Izpisua Belmonte JC (2001). Patterning mechanisms controlling vertebrate limb development. *Annu Rev Cell Dev Biol* 17: 87–132.

Chan PC, Chan KW, Cheng IK, Chan MK (1988). Living-related renal transplantation in a patient with nail-patella syndrome. *Nephron* 50: 164–166.

Chen H, Johnson RL (1999). Dorsoventral patterning of the vertebrate limb: a process governed by multiple events. *Cell Tissue Res* 296: 67–73.

Chen H, Lun Y, Ovchinnikov D, Kokubo H, Oberg KC, Pepicelli CV, Gan L, et al. (1998a). Limb and kidney defects in Lmx1b mutant mice suggest an involvement of LMX1B in human nail patella syndrome. *Nat Genet* 19: 51–55.

Chen H, Ovchinnikov D, Pressman CL, Aulehla A, Lun Y, Johnson RL (1998b). Multiple calvarial defects in lmx1b mutant mice. *Dev Genet* 22: 314–320.

Chuah KL, Tan PH, Choong HL, Lai D, Chiang C (1999). Nail-patella syndrome and IgA nephropathy in a Chinese woman. *Pathology* 31: 345–349.

Clough MV, Hamlington JD, McIntosh I (1999). Restricted distribution of loss-of-function mutations within the *LMX1B* genes of nail-patella syndrome patients. *Hum Mutat* 14: 459–465.

Cohen A, Mulas R, Seri M, Gaiero A, Fichera G, Marini M, Baffico M, et al. (2002). Meier-Gorlin syndrome (ear-patella-short stature syndrome) in an Italian patient: clinical evaluation and analysis of possible candidate genes. *Am J Med Genet* 107: 48–51.

Craig JE, Mackey DA (1999). Glaucoma genetics: where are we? Where do we go? *Curr Opin Ophthalmol* 10: 126–134.

Cygan JA, Johnson RL, McMahon AP (1997). Novel regulatory interactions revealed by studies of murine limb pattern in Wnt-7a and En-1 mutants. *Development* 124: 5021–5032.

Dawid IB, Breen JJ, Toyama R (1998). LIM domains—multiple roles as adapters and functional modifiers in protein interactions. *Trends Genet* 14: 156–162.

Dreyer SD, Zhou G, Baldini A, Winterpacht A, Zabel B, Cole W, Johnson RL, et al. (1998). Mutations in LMX1B cause abnormal skeletal patterning and renal dysplasia in nail patella syndrome. *Nat Genet* 19: 47–50.

Dreyer SD, Morello R, German MS, Zabel B, Winterpacht A, Lunstrum GP, Horton WA, et al. (2000). LMX1B transactivation and expression in nail-patella syndrome. *Hum Mol Genet* 9: 1067–1074.

Drut RM, Chandra S, Latorraca R, Gilbert-Barness E (1992). Nail-patella syndrome in a spontaneously aborted 18-week fetus: ultrastructural and immunofluorescent study of the kidneys. *Am J Med Genet* 43: 693–696.

Duba HC, Erdel M, Loffler J, Wirth J, Utermann B, Utermann G (1998). Nail patella syndrome in a cytogenetically balanced t(9;17)(q34.1;q25) carrier. *Eur J Hum Genet* 6: 75–79.

Farley FA, Lichter PR, Downs CA, McIntosh I, Vollrath D, Richards JE (1999). An orthopaedic scoring system for nail-patella syndrome and application to a kindred with variable expressivity and glaucoma. *J Pediatr Orthop* 19: 624–631.

Feingold M, Itzchak Y, Goodman RM (1998). Ultrasound prenatal diagnosis of the nail-patella syndrome. *Prenat Diagn* 18: 854–856.

Fiedler BS, De Smet AA, Kling TF Jr, Fisher DR (1987). Foot deformity in hereditary onycho-osteodysplasia. *Can Assoc Radiol J* 38: 305–308.

Fistarol SK, Itin PH (2002). Nail changes in genodermatoses. *Eur J Dermatol* 12: 119–128.

Flickinger RR Jr, Spivey BE (1969). Lester's line in hereditary osteo-onychoysplasia. *Arch Ophthalmol* 82: 700–703.

Fong EE (1946). Iliac horns (symmetrical bilateral central posterior iliac processes): a case report. *Radiology* 47: 517–518.

Gao X, Miyai T, Tahara T, Mae H, Takai T, Kawaguchi S, Sugihara K, et al. (2001). IgA nephropathy associated with nail-patella syndrome in a 7-year-old girl. *Pediatr Int* 43: 434–436.

German MS, Wang J, Chadwick RB, Rutter WJ (1992). Synergistic activation of the insulin gene by a LIM-homeo domain protein and a basic helix-loop-helix protein: building a functional insulin minienhancer complex. *Genes Dev* 6: 2165–2176.

Gubler MC, Levy M (1993). Prenatal diagnosis of nail-patella syndrome by intrauterine kidney biopsy. *Am J Med Genet* 47: 122–124.

Gubler MC, Levy M, Naizot C, Habib R (1980). Glomerular basement membrane changes in hereditary glomerular diseases. *Renal Physiol* 3: 405–413.

Gubler MC, Dommergues JP, Foulard M, Bensman A, Leroy JP, Broyer M, Habib R (1993). Collagen type III glomerulopathy: a new type of hereditary nephropathy. *Pediatr Nephrol* 7: 354–360.

Guidera KJ, Satterwhite Y, Ogden JA, Pugh L, Ganey T (1991). Nail patella syndrome: a review of 44 orthopaedic patients. *J Pediatr Orthop* 11: 737–742.

Hamlington JD, Clough MV, Dunston JA, McIntosh I (2000). Deletion of a branch-point consensus sequence in the *LMX1B* gene causes exon skipping in a family with nail patella syndrome. *Eur J Hum Genet* 8: 311–314.

Hamlington JD, Jones C, McIntosh I (2001). Twenty-two novel LMX1B mutations identified in nail patella syndrome (NPS) patients. *Hum Mutat* 18: 458.

Hawkings CF, Smith OE (1950). Renal dysplasia in a family with multiple hereditary abnormalities including iliac horns. *Lancet* I: 803–808.

Hermanns P, Lee B (2001). Transcriptional dysregulation in skeletal malformation syndromes. *Am J Med Genet* 106: 258–271.

Hobert O, Westphal H (2000). Functions of LIM-homeobox genes. *Trends Genet* 16: 75–83.

Hogh J, Macnicol MF (1985). Foot deformities associated with onycho-osteodysplasia. A familial study and a review of associated features. *Int Orthop* 9: 135–138.

Hussain SS, Hope GA (1994). Sensorineural hearing loss and nail patella syndrome. *Arch Otolaryngol Head Neck Surg* 120: 674–675.

Iannotti CA, Inoue H, Bernal E, Aoki M, Liu L, Donis-Keller H, German MS, et al. (1997). Identification of a human *LMX1* (*LMX1.1*)-related gene, *LMX1.2*: tissue-specific expression and linkage mapping on chromosome 9. *Genomics* 46: 520–524.

Imbasciati E, Gherardi G, Morozumi K, Gudat F, Epper R, Basler V, Mihatsch MJ (1991). Collagen type III glomerulopathy: a new idiopathic glomerular disease. *Am J Nephrol* 11: 422–429.

Johnson JD, Zhang W, Rudnick A, Rutter WJ, German MS (1997). Transcriptional synergy between LIM-homeodomain proteins and basic helix-loop-helix proteins: the LIM2 domain determines specificity. *Mol Cell Biol* 17: 3488–3496.

Jones KL (1997). Nail-patella syndrome. In: *Smith's Recognizable Patterns of Human Malformation*. Saunders, Philadelphia, pp. 438–439.

Kania A, Johnson RL, Jessell TM (2000). Coordinate roles for LIM homeobox genes in directing the dorsoventral trajectory of motor axons in the vertebrate limb. *Cell* 102: 161–173.

Knoers NV, Bongers EM, van Beersum SE, Lommen EJ, van Bokhoven H, Hol FA (2000). Nail-patella syndrome: identification of mutations in the *LMX1B* gene in Dutch families. *J Am Soc Nephrol* 11: 1762–1766.

Lichter PR, Richards JE, Downs CA, Stringham HM, Boehnke M, Farley FA (1997). Cosegregation of open-angle glaucoma and the nail-patella syndrome. *Am J Ophthalmol* 124: 506–515.

Little EM (1897). Congenital absence or delayed development of the patella. *Lancet* II: 781–784.

Logan C, Hornbruch A, Campbell I, Lumsden A (1997). The role of Engrailed in establishing the dorsoventral axis of the chick limb. *Development* 124: 2317–2324.

Loomis CA, Kimmel RA, Tong CX, Michaud J, Joyner AL (1998). Analysis of the genetic pathway leading to formation of ectopic apical ectodermal ridges in mouse Engrailed-1 mutant limbs. *Development* 125: 1137–1148.

Mangino M, Sanchez O, Torrente I, De Luca A, Capon F, Novelli G, Dallapiccola B (1999). Localization of a gene for familial patella aplasia-hypoplasia (PTLAH) to chromosome 17q21-22. *Am J Hum Genet* 65: 441–447.

Marumo K, Fujii K, Tanaka T, Takeuchi H, Saito H, Koyano Y (1999). Surgical management of congenital permanent dislocation of the patella in nail patella syndrome by Stanisavljevic procedure. *J Orthop Sci* 4: 446–449.

McIntosh I, Clough MV, Schaffer AA, Puffenberger EG, Horton VK, Peters K, Abbott MH, et al. (1997). Fine mapping of the nail-patella syndrome locus at 9q34. *Am J Hum Genet* 60: 133–142.

McIntosh I, Dreyer SD, Clough MV, Dunston JA, Eyaid W, Roig CM, Montgomery T, et al. (1998). Mutation analysis of *LMX1B* gene in nail-patella syndrome patients. *Am J Hum Genet* 63: 1651–1658.

McIntosh I, Clough MV, Gak E, Frydman M (1999). Prenatal diagnosis of nail-patella syndrome. *Prenat Diagn* 19: 287–288.

Mellotte GJ, Eastwood JB (1995). Pathognomonic sign of triangular lunulae in the nail-patella syndrome. *Nephrol Dial Transplant* 10: 300–301.

Mihatsch MJ, Zollinger HU (1980). Kidney disease. *Pathol Res Pract* 167: 88–117.

Milan M, Cohen SM (1999). Regulation of LIM homeodomain activity in vivo: a tetramer of dLDB and apterous confers activity and capacity for regulation by dLMO. *Mol Cells* 4: 267–273.

Milan M, Diaz-Benjumea FJ, Cohen SM (1998). Beadex encodes an LMO protein that regulates Apterous LIM-homeodomain activity in *Drosophila* wing development: a model for *LMO* oncogene function. *Genes Dev* 12: 2912–2920.

Miller TT, Shapiro MA, Schultz E, Crider R, Paley D (1998). Sonography of patellar abnormalities in children. *AJR Am J Roentgenol* 171: 739–742.

Miner JH, Morello R, Andrews KL, Li C, Antignac C, Shaw AS, Lee B (2002). Transcriptional induction of slit diaphragm genes by Lmx1b is required in podocyte differentiation. *J Clin Invest* 109: 1065–1072.

Morello R, Lee B (2002). Insight into podocyte differentiation from the study of human genetic disease: nail-patella syndrome and transcriptional regulation in podocytes. *Pediatr Res* 51: 551–558.

Morello R, Zhou G, Dreyer SD, Harvey SJ, Ninomiya Y, Thorner PS, Miner JH, et al. (2001). Regulation of glomerular basement membrane collagen expression by LMX1B contributes to renal disease in nail patella syndrome. *Nat Genet* 27: 205–208.

Noel LH, Gubler MC, Bobrie G, Savage CO, Lockwood CM, Grunfeld JP (1989). Inherited defects of renal basement membranes. *Adv Nephrol Necker Hosp* 18: 77–94.

Ostendorff HP, Bossenz M, Mincheva A, Copeland NG, Gilbert DJ, Jenkins NA, Lichter P, et al. (2000). Functional characterization of the gene encoding RLIM, the corepressor of LIM homeodomain factors. *Genomics* 69: 120–130.

Ostendorff HP, Peirano RI, Peters MA, Schluter A, Bossenz M, Scheffner M, Bach I (2002). Ubiquitination-dependent cofactor exchange on LIM homeodomain transcription factors. *Nature* 416: 99–103.

Parr BA, McMahon AP (1995). Dorsalizing signal Wnt-7a required for normal polarity of D–V and A–P axes of mouse limb. *Nature* 374: 350–353.

Pfaff SL, Mendelsohn M, Stewart CL, Edlund T, Jessell TM (1996). Requirement for LIM homeobox gene Isl1 in motor neuron generation reveals a motor neuron-dependent step in interneuron differentiation. *Cell* 84: 309–320.

Pinette MG, Ukleja M, Blackstone J (1999). Early prenatal diagnosis of nail-patella syndrome by ultrasonography. *J Ultrasound Med* 18: 387–389.

Porter FD, Drago J, Xu Y, Cheema SS, Wassif C, Huang SP, Lee E, et al. (1997). *Lhx2*, a LIM homeobox gene, is required for eye, forebrain, and definitive erythrocyte development. *Development* 124: 2935–2944.

Pressman CL, Chen H, Johnson RL (2000). LMX1B, a LIM homeodomain class transcription factor, is necessary for normal development of multiple tissues in the anterior segment of the murine eye. *Genesis* 26: 15–25.

Reichenbach H, Hormann D, Theile H (1995). Hereditary congenital posterior dislocation of radial heads. *Am J Med Genet* 55: 101–104.

Renwick JH, Lawler SD (1955). Genetical linkage between the ABO and nail-patella loci. *Ann Hum Genet* 19: 312–331.

Riddle RD, Ensini M, Nelson C, Tsuchida T, Jessell TM, Tabin C (1995). Induction of the LIM homeobox gene Lmx1 by WNT7a establishes dorsoventral pattern in the vertebrate limb. *Cell* 83: 631–640.

Rodriguez-Esteban C, Schwabe JW, Pena JD, Rincon-Limas DE, Magallon J, Botas J, Belmonte JC (1998). Lhx2, a vertebrate homologue of apterous, regulates vertebrate limb outgrowth. *Development* 125: 3925–3934.

Roekerath W (1951). Hereditaire osteo-onycho-dysplasie. *Fortschr Roentgenstr* 75: 700–712.

Rohr C, Prestel J, Heidet L, Hosser H, Kriz W, Johnson RL, Antignac C, et al. (2002). The LIM-homeodomain transcription factor Lmx1b plays a crucial role in podocytes. *J Clin Invest* 109: 1073–1082.

Sagasti A, Hobert O, Troemel ER, Ruvkun G, Bargmann CI (1999). Alternative olfactory neuron fates are specified by the LIM homeobox gene lim-4. *Genes Dev* 13: 1794–1806.

Sanchez-Garcia I, Rabbitts TH (1994). The LIM domain: a new structural motif found in zinc-finger-like proteins. *Trends Genet* 10: 315–320.

Sartoris DJ, Resnick D (1987). The horn: a pathognomonic feature of paediatric bone dysplasias. *Aust Paediatr J* 23: 347–349.

Schleutermann DA, Bias WB, Murdoch JL, McKusick VA (1969). Linkage of the loci for the nail-patella syndrome and adenylate kinase. *Am J Hum Genet* 21: 606–630.

Scott JE, Taor WS (1979). The "small patella" syndrome. *J Bone Joint Surg B* 61: 172–175.

Seri M, Melchionda S, Dreyer S, Marini M, Carella M, Cusano R, Piemontese MR, et al. (1999). Identification of *LMX1B* gene point mutations in Italian patients affected with nail-patella syndrome. *Int J Mol Med* 4: 285–290.

Sheng HZ, Moriyama K, Yamashita T, Li H, Potter SS, Mahon KA, Westphal H (1997). Multistep control of pituitary organogenesis. *Science* 278: 1809–1812.

Shih NY, Li J, Karpitskii V, Nguyen A, Dustin ML, Kanagawa O, Miner JH, et al. (1999). Congenital nephrotic syndrome in mice lacking CD2-associated protein. *Science* 286: 312–315.

Smidt MP, Asbreuk CH, Cox JJ, Chen H, Johnson RL, Burbach JP (2000). A second independent pathway for development of mesencephalic dopaminergic neurons requires Lmx1b. *Nat Neurosci* 3: 337–341.

Stratigos AJ, Baden HP (2001). Unraveling the molecular mechanisms of hair and nail genodermatoses. *Arch Dermatol* 137: 1465–1471.

Sweeney E, Fryer AE, Mountford RC, Green AJ, McIntosh I (2001). Nail patella syndrome: a study of 123 patients from 43 British families and detection of 16 novel mutations of LMX1B. *Am J Hum Genet* 69: A72.

Taguchi T, Takebayashi S, Nishimura M, Tsuru N (1988). Nephropathy of nail-patella syndrome. *Ultrastruct Pathol* 12: 175–183.

Taira M, Otani H, Jamrich M, Dawid IB (1994). Expression of the LIM class homeobox gene *Xlim-1* in pronephros and CNS cell lineages of *Xenopus* embryos is affected by retinoic acid and exogastrulation. *Development* 120: 1525–1536.

Uranga VM, Simmons RL, Hoyer JR, Kjellstrand CM, Buselmeier TJ, Najarian JS (1973). Renal transplantation for the nail patella syndrome. *Am J Surg* 125: 777–779.

van Meyel DJ, O'Keefe DD, Jurata LW, Thor S, Gill GN, Thomas JB (1999). Chip and apterous physically interact to form a functional complex during *Drosophila* development. *Mol Cells* 4: 259–265.

Verdich J (1980). Nail-patella syndrome associated with renal failure requiring transplantation. *Acta Derm Venereol* 60: 440–443.

Vogel A, Rodriguez C, Warnken W, Izpisua Belmonte JC (1995). Dorsal cell fate specified by chick Lmx1 during vertebrate limb development [erratum appears in *Nature* 1996;379(6568). 848]. *Nature* 378: 716–720.

Vollrath D, Jaramillo-Babb VL, Clough MV, McIntosh I, Scott KM, Lichter PR, Richards JE (1998). Loss-of-function mutations in the LIM-homeodomain gene, *LMX1B*, in nail-patella syndrome. *Hum Mol Genet* 7: 1091–1098.

Wright MJ, Ain MC, Clough MV, Bellus GA, Hurko O, McIntosh I (2000). Achondroplasia and nail-patella syndrome: the compound phenotype. *J Med Genet* 37: E25.

Wurst W, Auerbach AB, Joyner AL (1994). Multiple developmental defects in Engrailed-1 mutant mice: an early mid-hindbrain deletion and patterning defects in forelimbs and sternum. *Development* 120: 2065–2075.

Yakish SD, Fu FH (1983). Long-term follow-up of the treatment of a family with nail-patella syndrome. *J Pediatr Orthop* 3: 360–363.

Part B.
The Paired-Box (PAX) Gene Pathway

59 | Introduction to Paired-Box Genes

PETROS PETROU AND PETER GRUSS

The paired box–containing (*Pax*) genes are a family of highly conserved transcriptional regulators that play essential roles in diverse processes of early animal development and cell-fate specification. The discovery of their characteristic feature, the paired box, had its origin in the extensive systematic mutagenesis screen performed in the fruit fly *Drosophila melanogaster* (Nüsslein-Volhard and Wieschaus, 1980). The isolation and subsequent cloning of the genes affected in the mutants with defects in primary body patterning and segmentation revealed that many of them encode transcriptional regulators which share common amino acid motifs. The paired box was named after the segmentation gene *paired* and identified as a common sequence motif shared by *paired* and the two genes of the *gooseberry* locus of *Drosophila*, *gooseberry-proximal* (*gsb-p*) and *gooseberry-distal* (*gsb-d*) (Bopp et al., 1986). The same genes shared a second sequence domain of about 180 bp, which was identified in the genes underlying homeotic transformations in the fly and therefore termed the *homeobox* (McGinnis et al., 1984; Scott and Weiner, 1984). Two additional genes, *Pox-meso* and *Pox-neuro*, were subsequently identified in *Drosophila* as paired box–containing genes that, in contrast to *paired*, did not contain a homeobox (Bopp et al., 1989). The discovery of the paired box in *Drosophila* was followed by an extensive search for *Pax* genes in the genomes of other species. Based on their sequence similarity to the *Drosophila* genes, paired box–containing genes were sub-

sequently identified in a variety of organisms. Nine paired box–containing genes (*Pax1*–*Pax9*) have so far been identified in the mouse and human (reviewed in Dahl et al., 1997; Mansouri et al., 1999; Underhill, 2000; Chi and Epstein, 2002), which, in contrast to *Hox* genes (Kessel and Gruss, 1990), are not organized in chromosome clusters. Paired box–containing genes have also been identified in the genomes of other metazoans, such as nematodes and arthropods, as well as in more primitive organisms like hydrozoa, porifera, and anthozoa (Sun et al., 1997; Hoshiyama et al., 1998; Groger et al., 2000). The current scenario for the evolution of the paired domain (PD) suggests that it is derived from an ancestral transposase which was fused to a homeodomain (HD) shortly after the emergence of metazoans (Breitling and Gerber, 2000). Thus, the *Pax* family is comprised of genes that arose very early in evolution and are highly conserved throughout phyla.

STRUCTURE AND ORGANIZATION OF MAMMALIAN *Pax* GENES

The defining feature of all Pax proteins is the presence of the PD. This is often associated with additional structural motifs like an HD and/or a short sequence with the consensus (H/Y)S(I/V)(N/S)G(I/L)LG, which is termed the *octapeptide*. Similar to the protein paired of

Pax subclass	Structure				Chromosome		Embryonic expression	Mutants	
	PD	OP	HD	PST	Mouse	Human		Mouse	Human
Pax3					1	2q35	brain, dorsal neural tube, neural crest, dermomyotome, limb bud	*Splotch*	Waardenburg
Pax7					4	1p36.2	brain, dorsal neural tube, neural crest, dermomyotome (onset later than *Pax3*)		
Pax4					6	7q32	endocrine pancreas, neural tube		Diabetes Type II
Pax6					2	11p13	brain, ventral neural tube, eye and nasal structures, pituitary, endocrine pancreas	*Small eye*	Aniridia
Pax2					19	10q25	isthmus, ear, eye, excretory system, specific neural tubes cell types	*Krd, 1^{neu}*	renal coloboma
Pax5					4	9p13	isthmus, neural tube, B lymphocytes		congenital hypothyroidism
Pax8					2	2q12-14	isthmus, neural tube, thyroid		
Pax1					2	20p11	sclerotome, pharyngeal pouches, thymus	*Undulated*	
Pax9					12	14q12-13	sclerotome, developing tooth mesenchyme		oligodontia

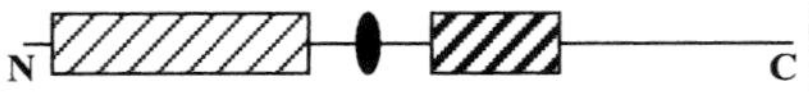

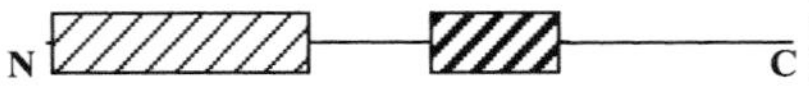

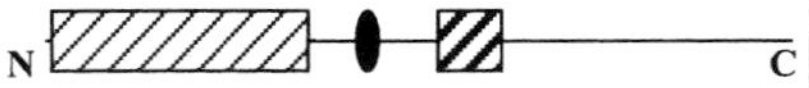

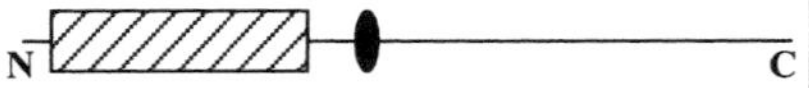

Figure 59–1. Overview of the mammalian Pax protein family. The nine Pax proteins are classified into four paralogous groups. Within individual groups, Pax proteins share a high degree of sequence identity in the paired domain and exhibit similar protein architecture as well as overlapping expression patterns of the corresponding genes. Mouse mutants and human syndromes that result from *Pax* gene mutations are indicated (references provided in text). PD, paired domain; OP, octapeptide; HD, paired-type homeodomain; PST, proline-, serine-, and threonine-rich region.

Drosophila, the mammalian Pax3, Pax4, Pax6, and Pax7 proteins contain an additional HD, which is referred to as "paired-type" HD. The octapeptide is conserved in all Pax proteins with the exception of Pax4 and Pax6, while Pax2, Pax5, and Pax8 contain only a remnant of the HD, which includes the amino-terminal α-helix. Based on the specific assembly of these structural motifs as well as on their genomic organization, the nine mammalian *Pax* genes have been classified into four paralogous groups (Fig. 59–1). *Pax* genes belonging to the same subclass share high sequence identity within the PD and similar expression patterns during embryonic development. All murine *Pax* genes exhibit specific spatial and temporal expression patterns during embryogenesis, and all, with the exception of *Pax1* and *Pax9*, are expressed in the developing central nervous system (Stoykova and Gruss, 1994). Their expression in the mouse starts between days 8 and 9.5 of embryonic development.

Pax GENE MUTATIONS AND DEVELOPMENTAL ABNORMALITIES

The elucidation of the role of *Pax* genes, including their classification into molecular pathways, is of enormous interest not only for the field of developmental biology but also for clinical research. The essential role of *Pax* genes in development and organogenesis is exemplified by the fact that the majority of them have mutations that underlie congenital abnormalities in the mouse and human. An interesting feature common to several *Pax* genes is that heterozygous mutations give rise to semidominant phenotypes. These mutations affect only a subset of the cell types in which the corresponding gene is expressed. Although haploinsufficiency is not a common feature shared by the majority of the vertebrate transcription factors (Engelkamp and van Heyningen, 1996), the dependence of proper development on the maintenance of a permissive *Pax* gene dosage is remarkable. The molecular basis of the occurrence of haploinsufficient syndromes upon reduction of functional *Pax* gene dosage remains unresolved.

Pax MUTATION PHENOTYPES

A frameshift mutation in one *Pax1* allele leading to a single amino acid exchange gives rise to the semidominant *Undulated* (*Un*) phenotype in mice, which is characterized by a kinky-tail phenotype. Homozygous mutants exhibit defects in the vertebral axis that originate from defective patterning of the sclerotome in which *Pax1* is expressed (Balling et al., 1988). No human congenital syndrome has so far been correlated with mutations in the *PAX1* gene.

Naturally occurring heterozygous mutations in the *PAX2* gene un-

derlie the renal-coloboma syndrome, an autosomal-dominant disorder characterized by renal hypoplasia and optic nerve colobomas (Sanyanusin et al., 1995; reviewed in Eccles and Schimmenti, 1999; see Chapter 60). This phenotype is consistent in the mouse (Favor et al., 1996) and results in both species from the same insertion of a single base pair that leads to a frameshift within the paired box. Gene-targeting studies have established an essential role for Pax2 in kidney, eye, and inner ear development (Torres et al., 1995), while Pax2 activity in the isthmic organizer is necessary for the proper development of the midbrain and cerebellum (Urbànek et al., 1997).

A further naturally occurring mutation that leads to a semidominant disorder, the mouse *Splotch* (*Sp*) mutation (Auerbach, 1954) and the corresponding Waardenburg's syndrome (WS) in humans, result from heterozygous mutations in *Pax3/PAX3* (Epstein et al., 1991; Baldwin et al., 1992; Tassabehji et al., 1992; see Chapter 61). Patients with WS are primarily characterized by pigmentation defects and deafness. Consistent with this phenotypic alteration, *Sp* mice exhibit coat color abnormalities. These disorders are caused by defects in the development of derivatives of the neural crest as a consequence of *Pax3* haploinsufficiency. Homozygous *Sp* embryos exhibit extensive neural crest deficiencies, such as heart defects, which finally cause embryonic lethality (Conway et al., 1997a, b), dysgenesis or absence of numerous peripheral ganglia (Lang et al., 2000), and neural tube defects. In addition to the function of Pax3 in neural crest cells and their derivatives and consistent with its expression in the dermomyotome of developing somites, functional Pax3 is required for the formation of some types of skeletal muscle.

In the case of *Pax4*, targeted ablation of the gene in the mouse genome revealed its crucial function in the development of an endodermally derived organ, the pancreas. In the absence of functional Pax4, the insulin producing beta cells and the somatostatin-producing delta cells of the endocrine pancreas fail to differentiate from precursor cells (Sosa-Pineda et al., 1997). Interestingly, the function of *Pax* genes in the specification of pancreatic cell types is not exclusively restricted to *Pax4* since the activity of a second *Pax* gene, *Pax6*, is required for the development of the glucagon-producing alpha cells (St-Onge et al., 1997). Moreover, a role for Pax2 in the regulation of the glucagon promoter has also been proposed (Ritz-Laser et al., 2000). Two recent studies implicate impaired *PAX* gene function in the pathogenesis of human diabetes. A missense mutation in the *PAX4* paired box was shown to correlate with Type 2 diabetes (Shimajiri et al., 2001), whereas different *PAX6* gene mutations were linked with glucose intolerance in Japanese patients (Yasuda et al., 2002).

The role of *Pax5* during embryonic development has been assessed by the generation of a null allele by homologous recombination. In homozygous mutants, differentiation of the B cells from lymphoid precursors is arrested at the pro-B-cell stage (Urbánek et al., 1994). Similar to *Pax2*, *Pax5* is expressed at the mid–hindbrain boundary and is required for the proper patterning of the posterior midbrain (Urbánek et al., 1994).

The *Pax6* gene holds an outstanding position within the *Pax* gene family. It is the gene that most impressively reflects the major features of this family, such as the high evolutionary conservation, the ability to direct organ formation, as well as the high degree of dosage sensitivity (see Chapter 62). *Pax6* function is tightly correlated with the development of the visual system in both vertebrates and invertebrates. The remarkable ability of *Pax6* to direct organ formation has been demonstrated in *Drosopeyhila*, in which targeted expression of both the fly *Pax6* ortholog *eyeless(ey)* as well as the mouse *Pax6* resulted in the formation of ectopic compound eyes (Halder et al., 1995). *Pax6*-like genes from other species were also shown to induce ectopic eyes in *Drosophila* (Glardon et al., 1997; Tomarev et al., 1997; Nornes et al., 1998). These findings established *Pax6* as a "master control gene" of organogenesis and led to substantial reconsideration of the assumption that different eye types have arisen independently during evolution. Heterozygous mutations in *Pax6* give rise to the semidominant *small eye* (*sey*) phenotype in mice and rats (Hill et al., 1991) and lead to a variety of ocular defects in humans, such as aniridia, cataracts, and optic nerve colobomas (Jordan et al., 1992; Glaser et al., 1994). The occurrence of ocular abnormalities upon overexpression of *PAX6* in transgenic mice further demonstrates the need for a permissive threshold of *Pax6* gene dosage for normal eye development (Schedl et al., 1996). Outside the eye, Pax6 is expressed in the prosencephalon, where it defines the di–mesencephalic boundary (Matsunaga et al., 2000) and is involved in the patterning of the neocortex (Bishop et al., 2000). Pax6 activity is furthermore required for the proper development of nasal structures, for the differentiation of pancreatic endocrine precursors (see above), and for the specification of regional neuronal identity in the neural tube (Ericson et al., 1997; Briscoe et al., 2000).

Targeted disruption of *Pax7* affected the emigration of cephalic neural crest cells, resulting in craniofacial abnormalities (Mansouri et al., 1996). Furthermore, the absence of myogenic satellite cells in adult skeletal muscle of *Pax7*-deficient mice demonstrates the absolute requirement of Pax7 for the specification of this cell lineage (Seale et al., 2000). Gene-targeting studies in mice (Mansouri et al., 1998) as well as the identification of heterozygous mutations in *PAX8* in patients with congenital hypothyroidism (Macchia et al., 1998) established a role for *Pax8/PAX8* in the development of the thyroid gland.

Finally, inactivation of *Pax9* in mice revealed its importance for the development of derivatives of the third and fourth pharyngeal pouches and resulted in additional craniofacial abnormalities (Peters et al., 1998). Mutations affecting *PAX9* gene function have been discovered in cases of human oligodontia (Stockton et al., 2000) and are consistent with the lack of teeth in *Pax9*-deficient mice (Peters et al., 1998; see Chapter 63). Thus, mammalian *Pax* genes play a pivotal role in organ formation and the specification of cell types during embryonic development.

Pax GENES IN REGULATORY HIERARCHIES

The phenotypic alterations resulting from mutations in the different *Pax* genes suggest that they occupy high positions in the respective genetic hierarchies that underlie organogenesis. The best example that demonstrates the capacity of a *Pax* gene to initiate the complete cascade of events that lead to organ formation is the ability of *ey/Pax6* to induce ectopic eyes in *Drosophila* (Halder et al., 1995). *Ey* is upstream of several other identified genes involved in compound eye formation, including *sine oculis* (*so*), *eyes absent* (*eya*), and *dachshund* (*dac*) (Bonini et al., 1993; Cheyette et al., 1994; Mardon et al., 1994). Interestingly, this master regulatory function of *ey/Pax6* is not restricted to the fly but is also conserved in vertebrates and involves the same players (Chow et al., 1999). Data from *Drosophila* argue, however, against a linear arrangement of these factors in the regulatory hierarchy that controls eye development and suggest the existence

of more complicated interwoven feedback loops that are utilized to sustain *ey* expression (Halder et al., 1998). Studies in *Drosophila* identify the epidermal growth factor receptor (Egfr) and Notch signaling pathways as potential upstream regulators of *ey* activity (Kumar and Moses, 2001). Whether *Pax6* is under the control of the same signaling pathways during mammalian eye development remains to be shown. The ability of *Pax6* to direct de novo organ formation does not seem to apply to structures outside the eye, suggesting that *Pax6* acts more downstream in the corresponding genetic programs. In many of these instances, *Pax6* function is mainly required for the assignment of positional information or the specification of cell fate, whereas its precise position within regulatory pathways remains to be defined. In the retina, conditional inactivation of *Pax6* just after the formation of retinal progenitor cells revealed its function upstream of basic helix-loop-helix (bHLH) factors that control the differentiation of these progenitors to the different retinal cell types (Marquardt et al., 2001). Additional *in vitro* studies have implicated Pax6 in the regulation of the activity of a number of other different genes. In the pancreas, Pax6 seems to directly regulate expression of the glucagon gene (Hussain and Habener, 1999). Also, the activity of the crystallin genes in the lens fiber compartment is very likely under the direct control of Pax6 (reviewed in Cvekl and Piatigorsky, 1996). Moreover, several studies implicate Pax6 function in the regulation of cell adhesion molecules (Stoykova et al., 1997; Meech et al., 1999). The finding that Pax8 induces a transcriptional response from the promoter of the neural cell adhesion molecule *in vitro* (Holst et al., 1994) suggests that regulation of cell adhesion molecule gene expression is probably a more general feature of Pax protein function.

Pax3 is crucial for the development of some types of skeletal muscle and upon ectopic expression is able to activate the myogenic program in embryonic mesoderm and neural tissue (Maroto et al., 1997). This enabled the placement of *Pax3* upstream of *Myf5* and the myogenic regulator *MyoD*. Several parallels can be drawn between *Pax6* and *Pax3* concerning their function in genetic hierarchies. First, both genes are able to redirect cell fate and trigger a specific genetic pathway when expressed ectopically with Pax6, having the striking effect to lead to the formation of a complete organ. Second, although Pax6 and Pax3 specify different developmental programs, they seem to cooperate with similar factors. As in the case of *Pax6* in the eye (see above), mouse orthologs of *so*, *eya*, and *dac* (*Six1*, *Eya2*, and *Dach2*) function together with *Pax3* during myogenesis (Heanue et al., 1999; Relaix and Buckingham, 1999). *In vitro* studies verified the capacity of Pax3 to initiate the myogenic program in pluripotent cells and to induce the expression of *Six1* and *Eya2* prior to the induction of *MyoD* (Ridgeway and Skerjanc, 2001). Furthermore, Pax3 directly controls expression of the tyrosine kinase receptor c-Met (Epstein et al., 1996), which is essential for the migration of hypaxial muscle precursors from the somites toward the limb buds (Bladt et al., 1995). Little information exists concerning the classification of the rest of the *Pax* genes in regulatory networks. For the induction of *Pax1* expression in the sclerotome, the secreted factor from the notochord, Sonic hedgehog (Shh), was shown to be necessary, thus positioning *Pax1* downstream of the *Shh* signaling pathway (Fan and Tessier-Lavigne, 1994; Fan et al., 1995). Pax9, which is expressed in the sclerotome in a similar but not identical manner to Pax1 (Neubüser et al., 1995), acts downstream of the *Uncx4.1* homeobox gene in the caudolateral sclerotome (Mansouri et al., 2000). In the developing kidney, Pax2 plays a crucial role during the interaction between the ureteric bud and the surrounding mesenchyme, which gives rise to the formation of the metanephros. Pax2 directly induces expression of the *Wilms' tumor gene 1* (*WT1*) in the metanephric mesenchyme (Dehbi et al., 1996), while subsequently *Pax2* gene activity is repressed by WT1, thus allowing terminal differentiation of the kidney epithelial structures (Ryan et al., 1995). Pax5 was originally identified to be the B cell-specific activator protein that was able to regulate expression of the *CD19* gene (Adams et al., 1992). Binding sites for Pax5 have been identified in a number of additional genes in the B-cell lineage, such as *LEF-1*, *N-myc*, and *PD-1* (Nutt et al., 1998), as well as in the promoter of the *mb-1* gene that encodes for the Ig α chain (Fitzsimmons et al., 1996). Consistent with the essential function of Pax8 in the development of the thyroid gland, thyroid-specific genes were found to be directly regulated by Pax8 (Zannini et al., 1992).

FUNCTIONAL REDUNDANCY WITHIN THE *Pax* FAMILY

The high sequence conservation of the PD in addition to the overlapping expression pattern of the murine *Pax* genes that belong to the same subclass raises the question of the existence of redundant functions. Indeed, functional redundancy involving several paralogous *Pax* genes could be demonstrated with the generation of compound mutants. *Pax1* single mutants exhibit distinct malformations of the vertebral column, which are not encountered upon loss of function of the paralogous gene *Pax9*. Absence of functional *Pax9* in the *Pax1* mutant background, however, gives rise to more severe vertebral column defects (Peters et al., 1999). *Pax2* and *Pax5* are coexpressed in the isthmic organizer, with *Pax2* being expressed earlier than *Pax5*. Both the existence of a more severe phenotype in the *Pax2/Pax5* compound mutant (Urbànek et al., 1997; Schwarz et al., 1997) as well as the ability of *Pax5* to completely rescue the *Pax2* phenotype in the brain (Bouchard et al., 2000) demonstrate the functional equivalence of *Pax2* and *Pax5*. Redundant functions have also been proposed for *Pax3* and *Pax7* in the dorsal neural tube (Mansouri and Gruss, 1998).

Pax GENES AND ONCOGENESIS

Increased *Pax* transcriptional activity has been strongly implicated in oncogenesis (Maulbecker and Gruss, 1993). Although it is not yet clear whether increased *Pax* gene expression is sufficient for cellular transformation, several *Pax* genes are persistently expressed in tumor-derived cell lines. *PAX2* and *PAX8* are expressed in Wilms' tumor (Dressler and Douglass, 1992; Poleev et al., 1992). Pax5 has been associated with regulation of the *p53* tumor-suppressor gene (Stuart et al., 1995), while PAX8 has been implicated in the activation of the *BCl2* apoptosis-suppressor gene (Hewitt et al., 1997). Additionally, several chromosomal translocations involving *PAX* genes have been correlated with various types of cancer (reviewed in Barr, 1997). Alveolar rhabdomyosarcoma is a pediatric smooth muscle cancer that can result from a t(2;13) chromosomal translocation, leading to fusion of the PAX3 DNA-binding domains to the transactivation domain of the forkhead family factor *FKHR* (Barr et al., 1993; Galili et al., 1993). An analogous translocation, t(1;13), resulting in a PAX7–FKHR fusion protein, has also been reported (Davis et al., 1994). These translocations give rise to gene products that are more potent activators than the wild-type proteins (Fredericks et al., 1995) and that exhibit distinct DNA-binding and regulatory properties (Bennicelli et al., 1996). Translocations involving *PAX5* or *PAX8* can result in large cell lymphoma (Busslinger et al., 1996) and thyroid carcinoma (Kroll et al., 2000), respectively. The correlation between oncogenesis and *PAX* gene dysfunction suggests a role for *PAX* genes in the regulation of the cell cycle and proliferation.

BIOCHEMICAL PROPERTIES OF Pax PROTEINS

The paired box is the defining sequence motif of all *Pax* genes. It encodes a domain of 128 amino acids in length, which is always located at the N-terminal end and represents the longest structural domain of Pax proteins. Relatively late after its discovery, the PD was defined as a sequence-specific DNA-binding activity through studies with the *Drosophila* protein paired and the promoter of the *even skipped* gene (Treisman et al., 1991). Subsequent studies demonstrated the capacity of most of the other Pax proteins to interact with the *even skipped* promoter and established the members of the Pax protein family as sequence-specific DNA-binding proteins. Toward an understanding of the genetic pathways that are controlled by Pax proteins, a substantial amount of effort has been invested in the identification of Pax target genes. This was facilitated by the identification of binding sites for the PD of different Pax proteins in vitro by binding-site selection (Epstein et al., 1994a; Chalepakis and Gruss, 1995). The attempt, however, to identify Pax target promoters on the basis of their sequence

similarity to the *in vitro* derived consensus sequences has been successful only in limited instances. This was mainly due to the fact that natural binding sites significantly differ from the optimal PD recognition sites that were obtained in vitro and shown to be highly related among the PDs of different Pax proteins. Thus, the ability of the various Pax proteins to participate in different developmental pathways despite the capacity of their PDs to bind to similar sequences was a paradox for a long time. Today, it is clear that DNA recognition by Pax proteins is much more complex than originally assumed and that biological diversity within the Pax protein family is achieved both at the level of DNA binding as well as through interactions with other proteins that confer novel properties to Pax proteins.

Studies on Pax5 first demonstrated that the PD consists of two subdomains with distinct DNA-binding capacities (Czerny et al., 1993). The two subdomains were thereafter termed the PAI and RED domains, for the N-terminal and the C-terminal subdomains, respectively (PAI + RED = PAIRED) (Jun and Desplan, 1996). Hence, the bipartite nature of the PD that would allow the combinatorial or selective use of the two subdomains can significantly contribute to the expansion of the PD recognition repertoire. Indeed, several lines of evidence support this model. First, individual Pax proteins make distinct use of the PAI and RED subdomains for their DNA binding. For example, the sequence which was selected in vitro by the *Drosophila* protein paired was only 14 bp long (Jun and Desplan, 1996), in contrast to the longer ones selected by Pax5 (Czerny et al., 1993) and Pax6 (Epstein et al., 1994a), suggesting that the RED domain does not significantly contribute to the overall protein binding. The absolute requirement of the PAI domain for paired function was further underscored by the finding that the RED domain of paired is dispensable for the rescue of *paired* mutants in *Drosophila* (Bertuccioli et al., 1996). Second, in several cases, the binding activity of the individual subdomains seems to be regulated *in vivo* by alternative splicing. Alternative splicing results, in the case of *Pax6* and *Pax8*, in isoforms that contain additional amino acids, which impair the DNA-binding activity of the PAI domain. These isoforms exclusively interact with DNA through the RED domain (Epstein et al., 1994b; Kozmik et al., 1997). Interestingly, the protein Lune, which is the product of the gene *eye gone* of *Drosophila*, turned out to be unique within the *Pax* family since it contains a partial PD that consists only of the RED domain (Jun et al., 1998). Lune, which is involved in eye development, shares DNA-binding properties with the alternatively spliced Pax6 isoform.

The solution of the crystal structure of the PD of the *Drosophila paired* (Xu et al., 1995) and PAX6 (Xu et al., 1999) provided insights into the bipartite nature of the PD and the contributions of the individual subdomains to the overall binding. The crystallographic data confirmed the minor contribution of the RED domain of paired in PD DNA recognition. Moreover, significant information concerning the role of the RED domain in DNA binding came from the solution of the PAX6 DNA crystal structure. Both the PAI and the RED subdomains were folded in a classical helix-turn-helix motif reminiscent of the archetypal structure with which various procaryotic proteins interact with DNA. The recognition helix of each subdomain makes significant contacts in the major groove of the DNA in a way that the two subdomains are related by a twofold symmetry axis (Fig. 59–2). Furthermore, the linker region between the two subdomains represents a flexible β-hairpin structure that makes minor groove contacts (Xu et al., 1999). The importance of the linker region in PD DNA binding is exemplified by the existence of Pax3 isoforms that differ in their ability to utilize the linker region and the RED domain in sequence recognition (Vogan and Gros, 1997). Adoption of the modular structure by the PD described above seems to be induced upon DNA binding. Based on circular dichroism spectroscopy data of the Pax6 PD in solution, it has been proposed that it is largely structureless, whereas upon binding on the consensus DNA-recognition site, the PD was shown to exhibit a high content of α-helical structure (Epstein et al., 1994a). The apparent ability of the PD to change its conformation depending on whether it is bound on DNA or not might reflect regulatory mechanisms of Pax protein function.

Four of the nine mammalian Pax proteins possess, in addition to the PD, a second DNA-binding motif, the paired-type homeodomain

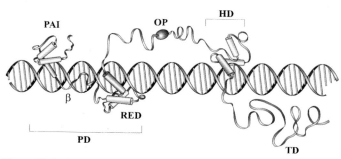

Figure 59–2. Structure and binding mode of Pax proteins on DNA target sites. The two subdomains (PAI and RED) of the paired domain (PD) and the paired-type homeodomain (HD) exhibit helix-turn-helix folding. The recognition helix of each individual binding motif contacts the major groove of DNA. The two subdomains of the PD are separated by a β-hairpin structure (β), which contributes to the overall binding. In some Pax proteins, a conserved octapeptide (OP) is located between the PD and the HD. A transactivation domain is usually located at the C terminus. (Reproduced from Chi N, Epstein JA *Trends Genet* 2002; 18:43, with the permission of Elsevier.)

(HD). Hence, in addition to the bipartite PD, Pax3, Pax7, Pax4 and Pax6 contain a total of three DNA-interacting modules. This suggests that the use of the HD either exclusively or in combination with the PAI and/or the RED domain could provide a much higher degree of specificity in target site recognition. Indeed, cooperativity between the PD and the HD in binding site recognition could be demonstrated *in vitro* (Jun and Desplan, 1996). *In vivo*, however, Pax proteins seem to differ in the extent of the HD contribution to the overall protein function. While for the rescue of *paired* mutants in *Drosophila* the HD of paired is absolutely required (Bertuccioli et al., 1996; Miskiewicz et al., 1996), the HD of eyeless seems to be dispensable for protein function *in vivo*. This is supported by the finding that an *ey* variant without the HD maintains the potential to rescue the mutant *ey* phenotype and, furthermore, to induce the formation of eyes upon ectopic expression (Punzo et al., 2001). The DNA-binding properties of the isolated HD have been assessed in vitro. Paired-type HDs can cooperatively dimerize on palindromic sites of the type 5′-TAAT(N)$_{2-3}$ATTA-3′ (Wilson et al., 1993). In vivo, however, there is no evidence for a PD-independent function of the HD. In vitro data rather support the notion that the HD in Pax proteins does not function independently and that its activity in terms of DNA binding is modulated by the PD (Underhill and Gros, 1997; Singh et al., 2000).

Pax PROTEINS AS TRANSCRIPTIONAL MODIFIERS

The current view on the function of Pax proteins implies sequence-specific binding on enhancer DNA sequences of target genes and subsequent modification of transcriptional activity. The function of Pax proteins as transcriptional modifiers is accomplished at two levels: first, through their intrinsic transcriptional stimulatory or repressor potential and, second, through DNA-dependent and –independent interactions with other proteins. Pax proteins are characterized by the presence of a high content of the amino acids **p**roline, **s**erine, and **t**hreonine in the C-terminal end, which is thus termed the *PST* region. The necessity for an intact PST domain for normal Pax protein function became evident from the finding that a nonsense mutation leading to a truncated PST region in the *PAX6* gene correlated with ocular defects and aniridia (Glaser et al., 1994). The same mutation was further shown to give rise to a protein variant with significantly reduced transactivation properties compared to wild-type PAX6. In the case of Pax6, it has been proposed that the activity of the PST region is probably regulated by phosphorylation through mitogen-activated protein kinases (Mikkola et al., 1999). Further studies on Pax6 and the regulation of the activity of the *crystallin* genes in the murine lens revealed an additional function of Pax6 as a repressor. In contrast to its activator function in the transcription of the *α-Crystallins* (reviewed in Cvekl and Piatigorsky, 1996), Pax6 exerts a negative effect on the activity of the *β-Crystallin* genes (Duncan et al., 1998). Functional dis-

section studies assigned repressor functions to other Pax proteins and identified specific protein segments as repressor domains. In the case of Pax3, fusion of different segments of the protein to a heterologous DNA-binding domain identified the region composed of the first 90 N-terminal amino acids, which extends into the PD to exhibit transcription-inhibitory activity (Chalepakis et al., 1994). As in the case of Pax6, the transactivation properties of Pax3 were conferred by the C terminus. A similar study on Pax2 further supported the general function of the C terminus of Pax proteins as an activation domain (Lechner and Dressler, 1996). Moreover, the same study identified the conserved octapeptide present in Pax2, Pax5, and Pax8 as capable of downmodulating the transcriptional activity of the C terminus. A function as a repressor of the promoters of the *glucagon* and *insulin* genes during early pancreatic development has been assigned to PAX4 (Smith et al., 1999). The repressor function of PAX4 is thought to be important for differentiation of the beta cell lineage and the suppression of alpha cell fate in the endocrine pancreas.

Pax PROTEINS AND COFACTORS

Evidence accumulating during the past few years supports the idea that Pax proteins undergo physical interactions with other proteins. This mechanism provides a simple and economical way to create new properties that enable proteins to perform additional functions. Association of Pax with other partners serves either to modify the effect of Pax proteins on the transcriptional activity of target genes or to inactivate the DNA-binding properties of specific Pax protein domains. Interestingly, the data reported so far implicate all structural motifs of the Pax proteins in interactions with other proteins. Using two-hybrid technology, members of the Groucho family of transcriptional corepressors were identified as interacting partners of Pax5 (Eberhard et al., 2000). Association with Groucho proteins is mediated by the conserved octapeptide and the C terminus of Pax5. Thus, the function of Pax5 as transcriptional repressor is thought to involve a complex assembly with Groucho proteins. Additionally, Pax5 forms protein complexes with the TATA box–binding protein (TBP) and the retinoblastoma (Rb) protein (Eberhard and Busslinger, 1999). The partial HD of Pax5 functions in this case as an interacting motif. HD-mediated interactions with TBP and Rb were also reported for Pax6 (Cvekl et al., 1999). The above data suggest that Pax proteins establish direct contacts with components of the basal transcription machinery and imply a link between Pax activity and the cell cycle. Physical association between Pax6 and numerous homeoproteins, like Chx10, Six3, Lhx2, En1, Prep1, Prox1, and HoxB1, were reported in vitro (Mikkola et al., 2001). In some of these cases, binding of Pax6 to the above proteins resulted in an increase of the transcription activation potential. The Pax3 HD is directly involved in the interaction between Pax3 and the HIRA corepressor (Magnaghi et al., 1998), Rb family proteins (Wiggan et al., 1998), and the Daxx repressor (Hollenbach et al., 1999). The interaction between Pax3 and HIRA is of particular interest since *HIRA* maps to the critical region (22q11) responsible for the human DiGeorge syndrome (DGS) (Lamour et al., 1995), which is characterized by defects in neural crest–derived organs. The types of cardiac defect seen in humans with DGS reflect those observed in *Splotch* mice, raising the possibility that genes downstream of Pax3 are affected in DGS. Since HIRA exerts its repressor function by local remodeling of chromatin structure, its interaction with Pax3 implies the involvement of chromatin modifications in the process of *Pax*-mediated repression. Moreover, the complex formation between HIRA and Pax3 might play a role in the pathogenesis of DGS. Among the reported interactions between Pax and other proteins, several are directly mediated through the PD. Two types of PD-mediated interaction involving Pax proteins can be distinguished, DNA-dependent and –independent. The demonstration of an interaction between Pax5 and members of the Ets family of transcription factors was the first report of a DNA-dependent interaction involving a Pax protein (Fitzsimmons et al., 1996). The interaction between Pax5 and a subset of Ets proteins plays a role in the regulation of the β cell-specific expression of the *mb-1* gene. DNA-bound Pax5 results in the recruitment of Ets proteins to a binding site on the *mb-1* promoter, for which the Ets proteins on their own have low intrinsic affinity. Insight into the molecular details of the cooperative association between Ets and Pax proteins was provided by the solution of the crystal structure of a ternary complex containing the PD of Pax5 and the Ets domain of Ets1 bound to DNA (Garvie et al., 2001). Pax5 alters the DNA contacts made by Ets-1, allowing the protein to form more favorable interactions with the low-affinity binding site. A comparison with the crystal structure of DNA-bound Pax6 (Xu et al., 1999) revealed, furthermore, that the majority of the residues used for DNA binding are conserved between Pax5 and Pax6. Similar to Pax5 and Ets, Pax6 and Sox2 are involved in a cooperative, DNA-dependent interaction that plays a role in the regulation of the δ-crystallin gene (Kamachi et al., 2001). The complex assembly between Pax6 and Sox2 enables the strong binding of Pax6 to an otherwise nonoptimal binding site. Cooperation between Pax and Sox proteins in different developmental programs seems to be a more general mechanism within the Pax protein family that also applies to other members. The combined function of Pax3 and Sox10 seems to play a role in the development of neural crest–derived structures. Adjacent binding sites for Pax3 and Sox10 were identified in the promoter of the c-RET gene, which is often mutated in cases of Hirschsprung's syndrome (Lang et al., 2000). In addition, Pax3 and Sox10 are involved in the synergistic activation of the promoter of the MITF gene, which is required for melanocyte maturation (Potterf et al., 2000). Further reports implicate additional DNA-dependent interactions between Pax6 and other proteins that are involved in target gene regulation. For the regulation of the glucagon promoter, it is thought that Pax6 functions as a complex with p300 and Cdx2. The interaction between Pax6 and Cdx2 is directly mediated by the PD (Ritz-Laser et al., 1999), whereas the assembly of the above ternary complex on the glucagon promoter results in increased transcriptional activity (Hussain and Habener, 1999).

DNA-independent interactions in which the PD is directly involved mostly result in the inhibition of the DNA-binding activity of the PD. Id proteins belong to the family of HLH proteins and function as inhibitors of cellular differentiation through association with other family members and inhibition of their binding on DNA target sites (reviewed in Norton et al., 1998; Norton, 2000). Through complex assembly with Pax2, Pax5, and Pax8, Id proteins were shown to function as antagonists of Pax activity by inhibiting the DNA binding of the PD (Roberts et al., 2001). Similar interactions that impair the binding activity of the Pax6 PD were reported with the quail Engrailed1 (En1) (Plaza et al., 1997) and the Mitf transcription factor (Planque et al., 2001a). In the latter case, the RED subdomain of Pax6 functions as a protein–protein interaction motif.

Besides its function as a transactivation domain, the C-terminal PST region of Pax6 directly binds Maf members of the bZip family of transcription factors (Planque et al., 2001b). This interaction was implicated in the regulation of the glucagon promoter, leading to enhanced transcriptional activity.

Despite the numerous reports implicating Pax proteins in interactions with other factors, the biological function of the resulting complexes could be elucidated in only very few cases. Extensive research in this field is required to shed light on the significance of complexes in vivo in which Pax proteins are involved.

CONCLUDING REMARKS

Since the discovery of Pax genes, their function and regulation have been the subject of intensive investigation. Pax genes have been established as crucial regulators of development and organogenesis in different species, which reflects the evolutionary conservation of specific developmental programs. The gradual understanding of their function at the molecular level reveals the mechanisms that contribute to the diversity within the Pax family. These mechanisms include the selective or combinatorial use of the distinct motifs for DNA binding, the intrinsic potential of Pax proteins to modify transcription of target genes, as well as their ability to fine-tune these activities by undergoing interactions with other proteins. The remarkable ability of Pax genes to maintain or direct pluripotent cell populations toward a specific fate opens new, challenging perspectives for their use in the treatment of disease.

REFERENCES

Adams B, Dörfler P, Aguzzi A, Kozmik Z, Urbánek P, Maurer-Fogy I, Busslinger M (1992). Pax-5 encodes the transcription factor BSAP and is expressed in B lymphocytes, the developing CNS, and adult testis. Genes Dev 6: 1589–1607.

Auerbach R (1954). Analysis of the developmental effects of a lethal mutation in the house mouse. J Exp Zool 127: 305–329.

Baldwin CT, Hoth CF, Amos JA, da-Silva EO, Milunski A (1992). An exonic mutation in the HuP2 paired domain gene causes Waardenburg's syndrome. Nature 355: 637–638.

Balling R, Deutsch U, Gruss P (1988). Undulated, a mutation affecting the development of the mouse skeleton, has a point mutation in the paired box of Pax-1. Cell 55: 531–535.

Barr FG (1997). Chromosomal translocations involving paired box transcription factors in human cancer. Int J Biochem Cell Biol 29: 1449–1461.

Barr FG, Galili N, Holick J, Biegel JA, Rovera G, Emanuel BS (1993). Rearrangement of the PAX3 paired box gene in the pediatric solid tumor alveolar rhabdomyosarcoma. Nat Genet 3: 113–117.

Bennicelli JL, Edwards RH, Barr FG (1996). Mechanism for transcriptional gain of function resulting from chromosomal translocation in alveolar rhabdomyosarcoma. Proc Natl Acad Sci USA 93: 5455–5459.

Bertuccioli C, Fasano L, Jun S, Wang S, Sheng G, Desplan C (1996). In vivo requirement for the paired domain and homeodomain of the paired segmentation gene product. Development 122: 2673–2685.

Bishop KM, Goudreau G, O'Leary DD (2000). Regulation of area identity in the mammalian neocortex by Emx2 and Pax6. Science 288: 344–349.

Bladt F, Riethmacher D, Isenmann S, Aguzzi A, Birchmeier C (1995). Essential role for the c-met receptor in migration of myogenic precursor cells into the limb bud. Nature 376: 768–771.

Bonini NM, Leiserson WM, Benzer S (1993). The eyes absent gene: genetic control of cell survival and differentiation in the developing eye. Cell 72: 379–395.

Bopp D, Burri M, Baumgartner S, Frigerio G, Noll M (1986). Conservation of a large protein domain in the segmentation gene paired and in functionally related genes of Drosophila. Cell 47: 1033–1040.

Bopp D, Jamet E, Baumgartner S, Burri M, Noll M (1989). Isolation of two tissue-specific Drosophila paired box genes, Pox meso and Pox neuro. EMBO J 8: 3447–3457.

Bouchard M, Pfeffer P, Busslinger M (2000). Functional equivalence of the transcription factors Pax2 and Pax5 in mouse development. Development 127: 3703–3713.

Breitling R, Gerber J-K (2000). Origin of the paired domain. Dev Genes Evol 210: 644–650.

Briscoe J, Pierani A, Jessel TM, Ericson J (2000). A homeodomain protein code specifies progenitor cell identity and neuronal fate in the ventral neural tube. Cell 101: 435–445.

Busslinger M, Klix N, Pfeffer P, Graninger PG, Kozmik Z (1996). Deregulation of PAX-5 by translocation of the Eμ enhancer of the IgH locus adjacent to two alternative PAX-5 promoters in a diffuse large-cell lymphoma. Proc Natl Acad Sci USA 93: 6129–6134.

Chalepakis G, Gruss P (1995). Identification of DNA recognition sequences for the Pax3 paired domain. Gene 162: 267–270.

Chalepakis G, Jones FS, Edelman GM, Gruss P (1994). Pax-3 contains domains for transcription activation and transcription inhibition. Proc Natl Acad Sci USA 91: 12745–12749.

Cheyette BNR, Green PJ, Martin K, Garren H, Hartenstein V, Zipursky SL (1994). The Drosophila sine oculis locus encodes a homeodomain-containing protein required for the development of the entire visual system. Neuron 12: 977–996.

Chi N, Epstein JA (2002). Getting your Pax straight: Pax proteins in development and disease. Trends Genet 18: 41–47.

Chow RL, Altmann CR, Lang RA, Hemmati-Brivanlou A (1999). Pax6 induces ectopic eyes in a vertebrate. Development 126: 4213–4222.

Conway SJ, Henderson DJ, Copp AJ (1997a). Pax3 is required for cardiac neural crest migration in the mouse: evidence from the splotch (Sp2H) mutant. Development 124: 505–514.

Conway SJ, Henderson DJ, Kirby ML, Anderson RH, Copp AJ (1997b). Development of a lethal congenital heart defect in the splotch (Pax3) mutant mouse. Cardiovasc Res 36: 163–173.

Cvekl A, Piatigorsky J (1996). Lens development and crystallin gene expression: many roles for Pax-6. Bioessays 18: 621–630.

Cvekl A, Kashanchi F, Brady JN, Piatigorsky J (1999). Pax-6 interactions with TATA-box-binding protein and retinoblastoma protein. Invest Opthalmol Vis Sci 40: 1343–1350.

Czerny T, Schaffner G, Busslinger M (1993). DNA sequence recognition by Pax proteins: bipartite structure of the paired domain and its binding site. Genes Dev 7: 2048–2061.

Dahl E, Koseki H, Balling R (1997). Pax genes and organogenesis. Bioessays 19: 755–765.

Davis RJ, D'Cruz CM, Lovell MA, Biegel JA, Barr FG (1994). Fusion of PAX7 to FKHR by the variant t(1;13)(p36;q14) translocation in alveolar rhabdomyosarcoma. Cancer Res 54: 2869–2872.

Dehbi M, Ghahremani M, Lechner M, Dressler G, Pelletier J (1996). The paired box transcription factor PAX2 positively modulates expression of the Wilms tumor supressor gene (WT1). Oncogene 13: 447–453.

Dressler GR, Douglass EC (1992). Pax-2 is a DNA-binding protein expressed in embryonic kidney and Wilms tumor. Proc Natl Acad Sci USA 89: 1179–1183.

Duncan MK, Haynes JI2nd, Cvekl A, Piatigorski J (1998). Dual roles for Pax-6: a transcriptional repressor of lens fiber cell-specific beta-crystallin genes. Mol Cell Biol 18: 5579–5586.

Eberhard D, Busslinger M (1999). The partial homeodomain of the transcription factor Pax-5 (BSAP) is an interaction motif for the retinoblastoma and TATA-binding proteins. Cancer Res 59(Suppl 7): 1716S–1724S.

Eberhard D, Jimenez G, Heavey B, Busslinger M (2000). Transcriptional repression by Pax5 (BSAP) through interaction with corepressors of the Goucho family. *EMBO J* 19: 2292–2303.

Eccles MR, Schimmenti LA (1999). Renal-coloboma syndrome: a multi-system developmental disorder caused by PAX2 mutations. *Clin Genet* 56: 1–9.

Engelkamp D, van Heyningen V (1996). Transcription factors in disease. *Curr Opin Genet Dev* 6: 334–342.

Epstein DJ, Malo D, Vekemans M, Gros P (1991). Molecular characterisation of a deletion encompassing the Splotch mutation on mouse chromosome 1. *Genomics* 10: 89–93.

Epstein J, Cai J, Glaser T, Jepeal L, Maas R (1994a). Identification of a *Pax* paired domain recognition sequence and evidence for DNA-dependent conformational changes. *J Biol Chem* 269: 8355–8361.

Epstein JA, Glaser T, Cai J, Jepeal L, Walton DS, Maas RL (1994b). Two independent and interactive DNA-binding subdomains of the Pax6 paired domain are regulated by alternative splicing. *Genes Dev* 8: 2022–2034.

Epstein JA, Shapiro DN, Cheng J, Lam PY, Maas RL (1996). Pax3 modulates expression of the c-Met receptor during limb muscle development. *Proc Natl Acad Sci USA* 93: 4213–4218.

Ericson J, Rashbass P, Schedl A, Brenner-Morton S, Kawakami A, van Heyningen V, Jessel TM, Briscoe J (1997). Pax6 controls progenitor cell identity and neuronal fate in response to graded Shh signaling. *Cell* 90: 169–180.

Fan CM, Tessier-Lavigne M (1994). Patterning of mammalian somites by surface ectoderm and notochord: evidence for sclerotome induction by a *hedgehog* homolog. *Cell* 79: 1175–1186.

Fan CM, Porter JA, Chiang C, Chang DT, Beachy PA, Tessier-Lavigne M (1995). Long-range sclerotome induction by *sonic hedgehog*—direct role of the amino-terminal cleavage product and modulation by the cyclic AMP signaling pathway. *Cell* 81: 457–465.

Favor J, Sandulache R, Neuhauser-Klaus A, Pretsch W, Chatterjee B, Senft E, Wurst W, Blanquet V, Grimes P, Sporle R, et al. (1996). The mouse $Pax2^{1Neu}$ mutation is identical to a human *PAX2* mutation in a family with renal-coloboma syndrome and results in developmental defects of the brain, ear, eye and kidney. *Proc Natl Acad Sci USA* 93: 13870–13875.

Fitzsimmons D, Hodsdon W, Wheat W, Maira S-M, Wasylyk B, Hagman J (1996). Pax-5 (BSAP) recruits *Ets* proto-oncogene family proteins to form functional ternary complexes on a B-cell-specific promoter. *Genes Dev* 10: 2198–2211.

Fredericks WJ, Galili N, Mukhopadhyay S, Rovera G, Bennicelli J, Barr FG, Rauscher FJ (1995). The PAX3-FKHR fusion protein created by the t(2;13) translocation in alveolar rhabdomyosarcoma is a more potent transcriptional activator than PAX3. *Mol Cel Biol* 15: 1522–1535.

Galili N, Davis RJ, Fredericks WJ, Mukhopadhyay S, Rauscher FR, Emanuel BS, Rovera G, Barr FG (1993). Fusion of a fork head domain gene to *PAX3* in the solid tumour alveolar rhabdomyosarcoma. *Nat Genet* 5: 230–235.

Garvie CW, Hagman J, Wolberger C (2001). Structural studies of Ets-1/Pax5 complex formation on DNA. *Mol Cells* 8: 1267–1276.

Glardon S, Callaerts P, Halder G, Gehring WJ (1997). Conservation of *Pax-6* in a lower chordate, the ascidian *Phallusia mammilata*. *Development* 124: 817–825.

Glaser T, Jepeal L, Edwards JG, Young SR, Favor J, Maas RL (1994). *PAX6* gene dosage effect in a family with congenital cataracts, aniridia, anophthalamia and central nervous system defects. *Nat Genet* 7: 463–471.

Groger H, Callaerts P, Gehring WJ, Schmid V (2000). Characterization and expression analysis of an ancestor-type *Pax* gene in the hydrozoan jellyfish *Podocoryne carnea*. *Mech Dev* 94: 157–169.

Halder G, Callaerts P, Gehring WJ (1995). Induction of ectopic eyes by targeted expression of the *eyeless* gene in *Drosophila*. *Science* 267: 1788–1792.

Halder G, Callaerts P, Flister S, Walldorf U, Kloter U, Gehring WJ (1998). Eyeless initiates the expression of both *sine oculis* and *eyes absent* during *Drosophila* compound eye development. *Development* 125: 2181–2191.

Heanue TA, Reshef R, Davis RJ, Mardon G, Oliver G, Tomarev S, Lassar AB, Tabin CJ (1999). Synergistic regulation of vertebrate muscle development by Dach2, Eya2 and Six1, homologs of genes required for *Drosophila* eye formation. *Genes Dev* 13: 3231–3243.

Hewitt SM, Hamada S, Monarres A, Kottical LV, Saunders GF, McDonnell TJ (1997). Transcriptional activation of the bcl-2 apoptosis suppressor gene by the paired box transcription factor PAX8. *Anticancer Res* 17: 3211–3215.

Hill RE, Favor J, Hogan BLM, Ton CCT, Saunders GF, Hanson IM, Prosser J, Jordan T, Hastie ND, van Heyningen V (1991). Mouse *Small eye* results from mutations in a paired-like homeobox-containing gene. *Nature* 354: 522–525.

Hollenbach AD, Sublett JE, McPherson CJ, Grosveld G (1999). The Pax3-FKHR oncoprotein is unresponsive to the Pax3-associated repressor hDaxx. *EMBO J* 18: 3702–3711.

Holst BD, Goomer RS, Wood IC, Edelman GM, Jones FS (1994). Binding and activation of the promoter for the neural cell adhesion molecule by Pax-8. *J Biol Chem* 269: 22245–22252.

Hoshiyama D, Suga H, Iwabe N, Koyanagi M, Nikoh N, Kuma K, Matsuda F, Honjo T, Miyata T (1998). Sponge Pax cDNA related to Pax-2/5/8 and ancient gene duplication in the Pax family. *J Mol Evol* 47: 640–648.

Hussain MA, Habener JF (1999). Glucagon gene transcription activation mediated by synergistic interactions of Pax-6 and cdx-2 with the p300 co-activator. *J Biol Chem* 274: 28950–28957.

Jordan T, Hanson I, Zaletayev D, Hodgson S, Prosser J, Seawright A, Hastie N, van Heyningen V (1992). The human *PAX6* gene is mutated in two patients with aniridia. *Nat Genet* 1: 328–332.

Jun S, Desplan C (1996). Cooperative interactions between paired domain and homeodomain. *Development* 122: 2639–2650.

Jun S, Wallen VR, Goriely A, Kalionis B, Desplan C (1998). Lune/eye gone, a Pax-like protein, uses a partial paired domain and a homeodomain for DNA recognition. *Proc Natl Acad Sci USA* 95: 13720–13725.

Kamachi Y, Uchikawa M, Tanouchi A, Sekido R, Kondoh H (2001). Pax6 and Sox2 form a co-DNA-binding partner complex that regulates initiation of lens development. *Genes Dev* 15: 1272–1286.

Kessel M, Gruss P (1990). Murine developmental control genes. *Science* 249: 374–379.

Kozmik Z, Czerny T, Busslinger M (1997). Alternatively spliced insertions in the paired domain restrict the DNA sequence specificity of Pax6 and Pax8. *EMBO J* 16: 6793–6803.

Kroll TG, Sarraf P, Pecciarini L, Chen CJ, Mueller E, Spiegelman BM, Fletcher JA (2000). PAX8-PPARgamma1 fusion oncogene in human thyroid carcinoma. *Science* 289: 1357–1360.

Kumar J, Moses K (2001). EGF receptor and Notch signaling act upstream of Eyeless/Pax6 to control eye specification. *Cell* 104: 687–697.

Lamour V, Lecluse Y, Desmaze C, Spector M, Bodescot M, Aurias A, Osley MA, Lipinski M (1995). A human homolog of the *S. cerevisiae* HIR1 and HIR2 transcriptional repressors cloned from the DiGeorge syndrome critical region. *Hum Mol Genet* 4: 791–799.

Lang D, Chen F, Milewski R, Li J, Lu MM, Epstein JA (2000). Pax3 is required for enteric ganglia formation and functions with Sox10 to modulate expression of c-ret. *J Clin Invest* 106: 963–971.

Lechner MS, Dressler GR (1996). Mapping of Pax-2 transcription activation domains. *J Biol Chem* 271: 21088–21093.

Macchia PE, Lapi P, Krude H, Pirro MT, Missero C, Chiovato L, Souabni A, Baserga M, Tassi V, Pinchera A, et al. (1998). Pax8 mutations associated with congenital hypothyroidism caused by thyroid dysgenesis. *Nat Genet* 19: 83–86.

Magnaghi P, Roberts C, Lorain S, Lipinski M, Scambler PJ (1998). HIRA, a mammalian homologue of *Saccharomyces cerevisiae* transcriptional co-repressors, interacts with Pax3. *Nat Genet* 20: 74–77.

Mansouri A, Gruss P (1998). *Pax3* and *Pax7* are expressed in commissural neurons and restrict ventral neuronal identity in the spinal cord. *Mech Dev* 78: 171–178.

Mansouri A, Stoykova A, Torres M, Gruss P (1996). Dysgenesis of cephalic neural crest derivatives in $Pax7^{-/-}$ mutant mice. *Development* 122: 831–838.

Mansouri A, Chowdhury K, Gruss P (1998). Follicular cells of the thyroid gland require *Pax8* gene function. *Nat Genet* 19: 87–90.

Mansouri A, Goudreau G, Gruss P (1999). *Pax* genes and their role in organogenesis. *Cancer Res* 59: 1707–1709.

Mansouri A, Voss AK, Thomas T, Yokota Y, Gruss P (2000). *Uncx4.1* is required for the formation of the pedicles and proximal ribs and acts upstream of *Pax9*. *Development* 127: 2251–2258.

Mardon G, Solomon NM, Rubin GM (1994). *dachshund* encodes a nuclear protein required for normal eye and leg development in *Drosophila*. *Development* 120: 3473–3486.

Maroto M, Reshef R, Munsterberg AE, Koester S, Goulding M, Lassar AB (1997). Ectopic *Pax-3* activates *MyoD* and *Myf-5* expression in embryonic mesoderm and neural tissue. *Cell* 89: 139–148.

Marquardt T, Ashery-Padan R, Andrejewski N, Scardigli R, Guillemot F, Gruss P (2001). Pax6 is required for the multipotent state of retinal progenitor cells. *Cell* 105: 43–55.

Matsunaga E, Araki I, Nakamura H (2000). *Pax6* defines the di-mesencephalic boundary by repressing *En1* and *Pax2*. *Development* 127: 2357–2365.

Maulbecker CC, Gruss P (1993). The oncogenic potential of *Pax* genes. *EMBO J* 12: 2361–2367.

McGinnis W, Levine MS, Hafen E, Kuroiwa A, Gehring WJ (1984). A conserved DNA sequence in homoeotic genes of the *Drosophila antennapedia* and *bithorax* complexes. *Nature* 308: 428–433.

Meech R, Kallunki P, Edelman GM, Jones FS (1999). A binding site for homeodomain and Pax proteins is necessary for L1 cell adhesion molecule gene expression by Pax-6 and bone morphogenetic proteins. *Proc Natl Acad Sci USA* 96: 2420–2425.

Mikkola I, Bruun J-A, Bjorkoy G, Holm T, Johansen T (1999). Phosphorylation of the transactivation domain of Pax6 by extracellular signal–regulated kinase and p38 mitogen-activated protein kinase. *J Biol Chem* 274: 15115–15126.

Mikkola I, Bruun J-A, Holm T, Johansen T (2001). Superactivation of Pax6-mediated transactivation from paired domain–binding sites by DNA-independent recruitment of different homeodomain proteins. *J Biol Chem* 276: 4109–4118.

Miskiewicz P, Morissey D, Lan Y, Raj L, Kessler S, Fujoka M, Goto T, Weir M (1996). Both the paired domain and homeodomain are required for *in vivo* function of *Drosophila* paired. *Development* 122: 2709–2718.

Neubüser A, Koseki H, Balling R (1995). Characterization and developmental expression of *Pax9*, a paired box containing gene related to *Pax1*. *Dev Biol* 170: 701–716.

Nornes S, Clarkson M, Mikkola I, Pedersen M, Bardsley A, Martinez JP, Krauss S, Johansen T (1998). Zebrafish contains two *pax6* genes involved in eye development. *Mech Dev* 77: 185–196.

Norton JD (2000). Id helix-loop-helix in cell growth, differentiation and tumourigenesis. *J Cell Sci* 113(Pt 2): 3897–3905.

Norton JD, Deed RW, Craggs G, Sablitzky F (1998). Id helix-loop-helix proteins in cell growth and differentiation. *Trends Cell Biol* 8: 58–65.

Nüsslein-Volhard C, Wieschaus E (1980). Mutations affecting segment number and polarity in *Drosophila*. *Nature* 287: 795–801.

Nutt SL, Morrison AM, Dorfler P, Rolink A, Busslinger M (1998). Identification of BSAP (Pax-5) target genes in early B-cell development by loss- and gain-of-function experiments. *EMBO J* 17: 2319–2333.

Peters H, Neubüser A, Kratochwil K, Balling R (1998). *Pax9* deficient mice lack pharyngeal pouch derivatives and teeth and exhibit craniofacial and limb abnormalities. *Genes Dev* 12: 2735–2747.

Peters H, Wilm B, Sakai N, Imai K, Maas R, Balling R (1999). Pax1 and Pax9 synergistically regulate vertebral column development. *Development* 126: 5399–5408.

Planque N, Leconte L, Conquell MF, Martin P, Saule S (2001a). Specific Pax-6/microphthalmia transcription factor interactions involve their DNA-binding domains and inhibit transcriptional properties of both proteins. *J Biol Chem* 276: 29330–29337.

Planque N, Leconte L, Coquelle MF, Benkhelifa S, Martin P, Felder-Schmittbuhl M-P,

Saule S (2001b). Interaction of Maf transcription factors with Pax-6 results in synrgistic activation of the glucagon promoter. *J Biol Chem* 276: 35751–35760.

Plaza S, Langlois M-C, Turque N, LeCornet S, Bailly M, Bègue A, Quatannens B, Dozier C, Saule S (1997). The homeobox-containing engrailed-1 (En-1) product down-regulates the expression of *Pax-6* through a DNA binding-independent mechanism. *Cell Growth Differ* 8: 1115–1125.

Poleev A, Fickenscher H, Mundlos S, Winterpacht A, Zabel B, Fidler A, Gruss P, Plachov D (1992). *PAX8*, a human paired box gene: isolation and expression in developing thyroid, kidney and Wilms' tumor. *Development* 116: 611–623.

Potterf SB, Furumura M, Dunn KJ, Arnheiter H, Pavan WJ (2000). Transcription factor hierarchy in Waardenburg syndrome: regulation of MITF expression by SOX10 and PAX3. *Hum Genet* 107: 1–6.

Punzo C, Kurata S, Gehring W (2001). The *eyeless* homeodomain is dispensable for eye development in *Drosophila*. *Genes Dev* 15: 1716–1723.

Relaix F, Buckingham M (1999). From insect eye to vertebrate muscle: redeployment of a regulatory network. *Genes Dev* 13: 3171–3178.

Ridgeway AG, Skerjanc IS (2001). Pax3 is essential for skeletal myogenesis and the expression of Six1 and Eya2. *J Biol Chem* 276: 19033–19039.

Ritz-Laser B, Estreicher A, Klages N, Saule S, Philippe J (1999). Pax-6 and Cdx-2/3 interact to activate glucagon gene expression on the G1 element. *J Biol Chem* 274: 4124–4132.

Ritz-Laser B, Estreicher A, Gauthier B, Philippe J (2000). The paired homeodomain transcription factor Pax-2 is expressed in the endocrine pancreas and transactivates the glucagon gene promoter. *J Biol Chem* 275: 32708–32715.

Roberts EC, Deed WR, Inoue T, Norton JD, Sharrocks A (2001). Id helix-loop-helix proteins antagonize Pax transcription factor activity by inhibiting DNA binding. *Mol Cell Biol* 21: 524–533.

Ryan G, Steele-Perkins V, Morris JF, Rauscher FJ III, Dressler GR (1995). Repression of *Pax-2* by *WT1* during normal kidney development. *Development* 121: 867–886.

Sanyanusin P, Schimmenti LA, McNoe LA, Ward TA, Pierpont MEM, Sullivan MJ, Dobyns WB, Eccles MR (1995). Mutation of the *PAX2* gene in a family with optic nerve colobomas, renal anomalies and vesicoureteral reflux. *Nat Genet* 9: 358–363.

Schedl A, Ross A, Lee M, Engelkamp D, Rashbass P, van Heyningen V, Hastie N (1996). Influence of *PAX6* gene dosage on development: overexpression causes severe eye abnormalities. *Cell* 86: 71–82.

Schwarz M, Alvarez-Bolado G, Urbanek P, Busslinger M, Gruss P (1997). Conserved biological function between *Pax-2* and *Pax-5* in midbrain and cerebellum development: evidence from targeted mutations. *Proc Natl Acad Sci USA* 94: 14518–14523.

Scott MP, Weiner AJ (1984). Structural relationships among genes that control development: sequence homology between the *antennapedia, ultrabithorax* and *fushi tarazu* loci of *Drosophila. Proc Natl Acad Sci USA* 81: 4115–4119.

Seale P, Sabourin LA, Girgis-Gabardo A, Mansouri A, Gruss P, Rudnicki MA (2000). Pax7 is required for the specification of myogenic satellite cells. *Cell* 102: 777–786.

Shimajiri Y, Sanke T, Furuta H, Hanabusa T, Nakagawa T, Fujitani Y, Kajimoto Y, Takasu N, Nanjo K (2001). A missense mutation of *PAX4* gene (R121W) is associated with type 2 diabetes in Japanese. *Diabetes* 50: 2864–2869.

Singh S, Stellrecht CM, Tang HK, Saunders GF (2000). Modulation of PAX6 homeodomain function by the paired domain. *J Biol Chem* 275: 17306–17313.

Smith SB, Ee HC, Conners JR, German MS (1999). Paired-homeodomain transcription factor PAX4 acts as a transcriptional repressor in early pancreatic development. *Mol Cell Biol* 19: 8272–8280.

Sosa-Pineda B, Chowdhury K, Torres M, Oliver G, Gruss P (1997). The *Pax4* gene is essential for differentiation of insulin-producing beta cells in the mammalian pancreas. *Nature* 386: 399–402.

Stockton DW, Das P, Goldenberg M, D'Souza RN, Patel PI (2000). Mutation of *Pax9* is associated with oligodontia. *Nat Genet* 24: 18–19.

St-Onge L, Sosa-Pineda B, Chowdhury K, Mansouri A, Gruss P (1997). *Pax6* is required for differentiation of glucagon-producing α-cells in mouse pancreas. *Nature* 387: 406–409.

Stoykova A, Gruss P (1994). Roles of *Pax*-genes in developing and adult brain as suggested by expression patterns. *J Neurosci* 14: 1395–1412.

Stoykova A, Götz M, Gruss P, Price J (1997). *Pax6*-dependent regulation of adhesive patterning, *R-cadherin* expression and boundary formation in developing forebrain. *Development* 124: 3765–3777.

Stuart ET, Haffner R, Oren M, Gruss P (1995). Loss of p53 function through Pax-mediated transcriptional repression. *EMBO J* 14: 5638–5645.

Sun H, Rodin A, Zhou Y, Dickinson DP, Harper DE, Hewett-Emmett D, Li WH (1997). Evolution of paired domains: isolation and sequencing of jellyfish and hydra *Pax* genes related to *Pax-5* and *Pax-6*. *Proc Natl Acad Sci USA* 94: 5156–5161.

Tassabehji M, Read AP, Newton VE, Harris R, Balling R, Gruss P, Strachan T (1992). Waardenburg's syndrome patients have mutations in the human homologue of the *Pax-3* paired box gene. *Nature* 355: 635–636.

Tomarev SI, Callaerts P, Kos L, Zinovieva R, Halder G, Gehring W, Piatigorsky J (1997). Squid Pax-6 and eye development. *Proc Natl Acad Sci USA* 94: 2098–2100.

Torres M, Gomez-Pardo E, Dressler GR, Gruss P (1995). *Pax-2* controls multiple steps of urogenital development. *Development* 4057–4065.

Treisman J, Harris E, Desplan C (1991). The paired box encodes a second DNA-binding domain in the Paired homeo domain protein. *Genes Dev* 5: 594–604.

Underhill AD (2000). Genetic and biochemical diversity in the *Pax* gene family. *Biochem Cell Biol* 78: 629–638.

Underhill DA, Gros P (1997). The paired-domain regulates DNA binding by the homeodomain within the intact Pax-3 protein. *J Biol Chem* 272: 14175–141812.

Urbánek P, Wang Z-Q, Fetka I, Wagner EF, Busslinger M (1994). Complete block of early B cell differentiation and altered patterning of the posterior midbrain in mice lacking Pax5/BSAP. *Cell* 79: 901–912.

Urbànek P, Fetka I, Meisler MH, Busslinger M (1997). Cooperation of *Pax2* and *Pax5* in midbrain and cerebellum development. *Proc Natl Acad Sci USA* 94: 5703–5708.

Vogan KJ, Gros P (1997). The C-terminal subdomain makes an important contribution to the DNA binding activity of the Pax-3 paired domain. *J Biol Chem* 272: 28289–28295.

Wiggan O, Taniguchi-Sidle A, Hamel PA (1998). Interaction of the pRb-family proteins with factors containing paired-like homeodomains. *Oncogene* 16: 227–236.

Wilson D, Sheng G, Lecuit T, Dostatni N, Desplan C (1993). Cooperative dimerization of paired class homeo domains on DNA. *Genes Dev* 7: 2120–2134.

Xu W, Rould MA, Jun S, Desplan C, Pabo CO (1995). Crystal structure of a paired domain-DNA complex at 2.5 Å resolution reveals structural basis for Pax developmental mutations. *Cell* 80: 639–650.

Xu HE, Rould MA, Xu W, Epstein JA, Maas RL, Pabo CO (1999). Crystal structure of the human Pax6 paired domain–DNA complex reveals specific roles for the linker region and carboxy-terminal subdomain in DNA binding. *Genes Dev* 13: 1263–1275.

Yasuda T, Kajimoto Y, Fujitani Y, Watada H, Yamamoto S, Watarai T, Umayahara Y, Matsuhisa M, Gorogawa S, Kuwayama Y, et al. (2002). *PAX6* mutation as a genetic factor common to aniridia and glucose intolerance. *Diabetes* 51: 224–230.

Zannini M, Francis-Lang H, Plachov D, Di Lauro R (1992). Pax-8, a paired domain-containing protein, binds to a sequence overlapping the recognition site of a homeodomain and activates transcription from two thyroid-specific promoters. *Mol Cell Biol* 12: 4230–4241.

60 | *PAX2* and the Renal-Coloboma Syndrome

MICHAEL R. ECCLES

THE *PAX2* LOCUS AND DEVELOPMENTAL PATHWAY

PAX2, the second member of the *PAX* gene family, is located in a gene-rich region of human chromosome 10, near the boundary of bands q24 and q25 (Eccles et al., 1992; Stapleton et al., 1993; Narahara et al., 1997). Unlike the *PAX3* and *PAX6* genes, which led to the mapped locations of the disease loci for Waardenburg's syndrome and aniridia, respectively (Strachan and Read, 1994), the identification and mapping of the *PAX2* gene did not immediately suggest the existence of a known disease locus. Ultimately, it was the expression pattern of *PAX2* that provided clues leading to the association of *PAX2* mutations with renal-coloboma syndrome (Sanyanusin et al., 1995b). *PAX2* is expressed in fetal brain, spinal cord, eye, ear, urogenital tract, and kidney (Dressler et al., 1990; Nornes et al., 1990; Eccles et al., 1992; Terzic et al., 1998; Tellier et al., 2000). Following birth, *PAX2* expression declines in many tissues (Dressler and Douglass, 1992; Eccles et al., 1992) but remains in parts of the urogenital tract.

Expression of *Pax2* in Brain Development

PAX2 plays an important role in formation of the mid–hindbrain boundary, a process involving segmentation of the neural tube into midbrain and hindbrain vesicles (Favor et al., 1996). In mice, *Pax2* is initially expressed widely in the neural tube, in regions destined to become the forebrain to the prospective anterior hindbrain (Nornes et al., 1990). This expression occurs during the late primitive streak stage, before somitogenesis (Rowitch and McMahon, 1995). Later, *Pax2* is detected in the embryonic midbrain in an overlapping pattern at the boundary between the midbrain and hindbrain, concurrently with expression of *Pax5* and *Pax6* (Nornes et al., 1990). *Pax5* expression is dependent on *Pax2* expression (Pfeffer et al., 2000), and expression of both genes is necessary to establish the mid–hindbrain boundary (Schwarz et al., 1999). In addition to the mid–hindbrain boundary, *Pax2* is expressed in fetal spinal interneurons in the ventricular zone (Nornes et al., 1990; Burrill et al., 1997), and in certain GABAergic interneurons in the cerebellum (Maricich and Herrup, 1999).

Expression of *Pax2* in Eye Development

Correct development of the eye, including the optic nerve and optic chiasm, depends on the appropriate level and timing of *PAX2* expression (Torres et al., 1996). The eye develops from the optic vesicle, which invaginates to form the optic cup and closes along the ventral surface at the optic fissure. *Pax2* is expressed initially in the distal portions of the optic vesicle (Nornes et al., 1990) and later in the ventral half of the optic cup and stalk, the optic fissure, the early retinal tissue surrounding the fissure, and the ventral half of the optic stalk. After closure of the optic fissure, expression of *Pax2* subsides, except for the optic stalk, where *Pax2* is essential for establishing the correct axonal trajectories from the eye to the diencephalon (forebrain) and for the formation of the optic chiasm (Nornes et al., 1990; Torres et al., 1996). As the optic stalk develops and becomes the optic nerve, expression of *Pax2* is continuous between the optic nerve and the neuroepithelium of the ventral forebrain (Macdonald et al., 1997), later becoming restricted to the optic nerve (Nornes et al., 1990).

Expression of *Pax2* in Ear Development

Expression of *Pax2* is required for inner ear development, following invagination of the ectodermal placodes adjacent to the hindbrain region to form the otic vesicle (Torres et al., 1996). *Pax2* is expressed in the neurogenic tissues of the inner ear that later form the saccula and cochlea (Nornes et al., 1990). Initially, *Pax2* is expressed throughout the otic vesicle, but at later stages expression is restricted to regions flanking the neural tube and then to the more ventral parts of the otic vesicle (Torres and Giraldez, 1998; Groves and Bronner-Fraser, 2000).

Expression of *Pax2* in Kidney and Urogenital Tract Development

Pax2 plays an important role both in the initial stages of urogenital tract development and later during kidney growth and development (Sanyanusin et al., 1995b; Torres et al., 1995; see Chapter 13). The first stage of kidney development involves the formation of a transient kidney called the *mesonephros* in the rostral portions of the mesonephric duct. *Pax2* is expressed in the mesonephric nephrons and the mesonephric duct (Dressler et al., 1990). Following caudal extension of the mesonephric duct, also called the *wolffian duct*, the ureteric bud sprouts and branches toward the nephrogenic mesenchyme. *Pax2* is expressed in the ureteric bud as it invades the nephrogenic mesenchyme, inducing epithelial differentiation of the mesenchyme (Fig. 60–1) (Dressler et al., 1990). Concomitantly, *Pax2* expression is induced in the nephrogenic mesenchyme, although this expression rapidly abates as the epithelial cells begin to form S-shaped bodies, glomeruli, and tubules comprising the proximal end of the nephron (Dressler et al., 1990; Eccles et al., 1992).

Pax2 is not expressed in mature glomeruli or in proximal or distal tubules. Throughout formation of the metanephros, *Pax2* is continually expressed in the branching ureteric bud, which eventually forms the urothelium of the ureter, renal pelvis, and collecting ducts (Dressler et al., 1990; Eccles et al., 1992), and in newly induced mesenchyme. The ureteric bud undergoes repeated cycles of arborization and extension upon contact with the mesenchyme. Reciprocal signals from the mesenchyme and the ureteric bud promote guidance and differentiation of the ureteric bud and mesenchymal cells. The process of branching of the ureteric bud, then induction and differentiation to form new nephrons, followed by ureteric bud branching is reiterated throughout fetal life until the full complement of nephrons has been generated. *Pax2* is expressed at low levels in the collecting ducts of adult kidneys and at higher levels in certain kidney diseases or during kidney regeneration (Eccles et al., 1992; Winyard et al., 1996; Imgrund et al., 1999).

In males, the wolffian duct is derived from the mesonephric duct, while the paramesonephric duct degenerates. Several structures of the male genital tract derive from the wolffian duct, including the vas deferens, epididymis, and ductuli efferentes. Formation of these structures is dependent on the expression of *Pax2* in the wolffian duct (Torres et al., 1995), and *Pax2* continues to be expressed in the vas deferens, epididymis, and ductuli efferentes in adult males (Fickenscher et al., 1993; Oefelein et al., 1996).

In females, the mullerian duct is derived from the paramesonephric duct, which develops in parallel to the mesonephric duct and goes on to form several structures of the female genital tract, including the oviducts and uterus, while the mesonephric duct degenerates. Formation of these structures is dependent on expression of *Pax2* in the paramesonephric duct (Torres et al., 1995), and *Pax2* continues to be expressed in the oviducts of adult females (Fickenscher et al., 1993; Oefelein et al., 1996).

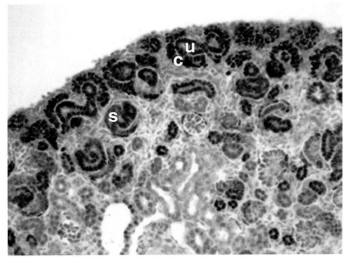

Figure 60–1. Pax2 expression pattern in fetal kidney. The photo shows Pax2 protein expressed in ureteric buds (U), condensing mesenchyme (C), and S-shaped bodies (S) in mouse fetal kidney at embryonic day 19. Pax2 protein was detected using a polyclonal anti-Pax2 antibody and diaminobenzidine staining. Magnification is ×200.

CLINICAL DESCRIPTION OF RENAL-COLOBOMA SYNDROME

Mutations in *PAX2* result in a rare, dominantly inherited, autosomal disorder of the eyes and kidneys, renal-coloboma syndrome (RCS). RCS was first reported by Reiger (1977). However, it was only in 1995 that a causal association with heterozygous mutations in the *PAX2* gene was established (Sanyanusin et al., 1995b). RCS is known by several different names in the literature, including *papillorenal syndrome* (Bron et al., 1988), *morning glory syndrome* (Karcher, 1979), *coloboma-ureteral-renal syndrome* (Schimmenti et al., 1995), and *optic nerve coloboma with renal disease* (Weaver et al., 1988; Narahara et al., 1997). Some uncertainty has been expressed as to whether RCS is the right name for this syndrome as it is clear that not all patients have optic nerve colobomas (Devriendt et al., 1998; Parsa et al., 2001). Indeed, a range of ocular abnormalities, including optic disc dysplasia and morning glory disc anomaly, are associated with renal disease in RCS. Nevertheless, colobomas of the optic nerve appear to be the most frequent eye abnormality occurring in association with renal disease in RCS (Tables 60–1, 60–2).

General Features and Incidence

Ocular and kidney abnormalities are the main presenting features in RCS, while vesicoureteral reflux (VUR), hearing loss, and CNS ab-

Table 60–1. Percent Penetrance of Clinical Features of Renal-Coloboma Syndrome

Clinical Phenotype	Percent Penetrance of Phenotype (*n* = 60)	Percent of Patients with Ocular Abnormalities or Renal Hypoplasia and the Clinical Phenotype
Ocular abnormality	87%	100%*
Reduced visual acuity	50%	58%*
Isolated ocular abnormality	13%	15%*
Renal hypoplasia	70%	100%†
Renal disease	65%	97%†
Renal transplant	38%	60%†
Isolated renal hypoplasia	5%	10%†
Vesicoureteral reflux	17%	12%†
Hearing loss	3%	—
CNS abnormalities	2%	—

*Ocular abnormality.
†Renal hypoplasia.

Table 60–2. Ocular Abnormalities in Renal-Coloboma Syndrome Patients

Eye or Fundus Abnormality (*n* = 118 Eyes)	No. Eyes with Phenotype	No. Eyes with Reduced Visual Acuity
Optic nerve coloboma	50	38
Optic disc pit	22	4
Optic disc dysplasia	20	9
Morning glory disc anomaly	2	2
Optic disc hypoplasia	3	2
Microphthalmia	2	2
Orbital cyst	1	1
Redundant fibroglial tissue	6	2
Retinal detachment	2	2
Myopia	20	14
Nystagmus	10	4
Strabismus	4	2
Amblyopia	4	4

normalities are less frequently observed (Table 60–1). The incidence of RCS in the population is unknown, and it may be under-diagnosed. This may in part be due to insufficient knowledge and experience in recognizing RCS as a specific disease entity as it is easy to miss subtle signs of dysplastic changes in the fundus during an ophthalmic examination.

Ocular Abnormalities and Visual Acuity

Clinical Presentation

Fifty percent of RCS patients present with a reduction in visual acuity of one or both eyes, sometimes with considerable variation between them (see Table 60–1). Myopia (25%), nystagmus (10%), strabismus (5%), and cataracts have also been reported in RCS patients (Table 60–2), while amblyopia and esotropia are also frequent. Limitation of visual acuity to light and color perception only, detection of hand movements, or counting of fingers held at arm's length is relatively infrequent. Often, the deficit in visual acuity is progressive, although the severity and nature of the ocular lesions correlate with loss of visual acuity (Dureau et al., 2001).

Abnormalities of the Fundus and Globe

Defects of the fundus are present in approximately 90% of RCS patients (Table 60–1), including optic nerve colobomas (Fig. 60–2). Defects involving the entire globe and/or retro-orbital structures are un-

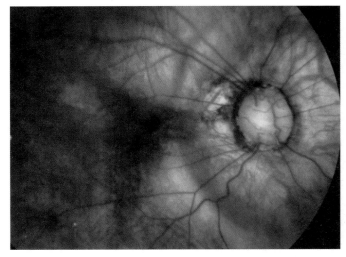

Figure 60–2. Fundus of a patient with renal-coloboma syndrome showing an optic nerve coloboma. Note the tortuosity of blood vessels emanating from the optic nerve coloboma and the pallor of the surrounding retina, indicative of retinal thinning.

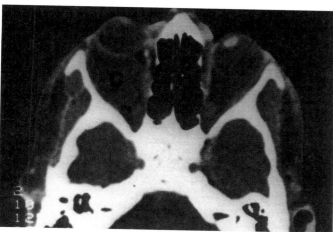

Figure 60–3. Computed tomographic scan of the head of a patient with renal-coloboma syndrome showing a retro-orbital cyst (C) immediately behind the microphthalmic eye. (Reproduced from Schimmenti et al., 1997, *Am J Hum Genet* 60: 872, University of Chicago Press.)

common; in one patient, a CT scan of the head revealed a retro-orbital cyst in one eye, which was also microphthalmic (Fig. 60–3).

Included in the spectrum of ocular defects in RCS patients are optic disc dysplasia, morning glory disc anomaly with radial emergence of the retinal vessels, abnormal patterns of the cilioretinal arteries, excavation of the optic nerve, partial coloboma of the optic nerve including optic nerve pits, large temporal pits, and peripapillary choroiditis. Around the rim of the optic nerve, the fundus often shows thinning of the retinal epithelium and alterations in the pigmentation of the retina or macula. Associated anomalies include macula colobomas and/or redundant fibroglial tissue. A proportion of patients have altered retinal vessel patterns and optic disc anomalies (Table 60–2) with no measurable defect in visual acuity.

Physiological Eye Abnormalities
Reduced optic nerve conduction in some RCS patients is suggested by an increased latency and decreased amplitude in visual evoked potentials (VEPs) (Sanyanusin et al., 1995a). Intraocular pressure and retinal thickness may also sometimes be abnormal, as detailed in a recent ophthalmological study of several RCS patients (Parsa et al., 2001).

Developmental Origin of Eye Abnormalities
As with sporadic or autosomal-dominant ocular colobomas (Pagon, 1981; Pagon et al., 1981), the eye defects in RCS are thought to arise from defective closure of the optic fissure during eye development. Failure of embryonic optic fissure closure is associated with a spectrum of anomalies, including optic nerve or disc colobomas, retro-orbital cysts, and colobomas of the eyelid, iris, lens, or choroid.

Urological Abnormalities

The Kidneys and Renal Failure
Clinical Presentation. Abnormal kidney morphogenesis and function is the second most frequent feature characterizing RCS, with mild or severe renal disease occurring in approximately 65% of patients and renal hypoplasia (small kidneys) in 70% (Table 60–1). Nonspecific markers of renal disease that are elevated in RCS patients include blood pressure, serum creatinine, and blood urea nitrogen.

Renal hypoplasia is usually bilateral, although marked variability in the severity of renal abnormalities and the degree of renal hypoplasia occurs (Devriendt et al., 1998; Porteous et al., 2000; Gus et al., 2001). Unilateral renal agenesis is also observed occasionally. Cystic kidneys, reflux nephropathy due to VUR (see below), and dysplastic changes occur in approximately 10% of RCS patients, with or without renal hypoplasia. A quarter of RCS patients have no renal abnormalities.

Primary Renal Hypoplasia in the Absence of Ocular Anomalies.
Sporadic cases of isolated renal hypoplasia have been identified as part of the spectrum of RCS, involving patients with isolated renal hypoplasia and normal eyes upon ophthalmological examination who have *PAX2* mutations (Dureau et al., 2001; Nishimoto et al., 2001; Salomon et al., 2001). *PAX2* mutations were not identified in the majority of patients with isolated renal hypoplasia, although subtle abnormalities of the eyes were identified in up to 37% of patients with isolated renal hypoplasia upon reexamination (Salomon et al., 2001; Dureau et al., 2001; Nishimoto et al., 2001). Oligomeganephronia is a variant of renal hypoplasia, characterized by a reduced number of nephrons, overall smaller kidney size, and hypertrophied nephrons (Royer et al., 1967), in which *PAX2* mutations have also recently been identified (Salomon et al., 2001). Isolated renal hypoplasia is a major cause of end-stage renal failure in children (Woolf, 1998); all patients with isolated renal hypoplasia should have an eye examination to determine whether they have RCS.

Histopathological Abnormalities of the Kidneys.
In gross appearance, the kidneys of RCS patients often have thinner cortical regions and hypoplastic papillae, containing fewer collecting ducts than normal (Weaver et al., 1988; Devriendt et al., 1998). Histological sections from renal cortical biopsies of patients with RCS and chronic renal failure reveal decreased numbers of glomeruli, mesangial fibrosis, glomerulosclerosis, involuting glomeruli, and hyalinization of glomeruli. Tubular atrophy may be evident in a portion of the tubules, while the remaining tubules appear to be hypertrophied (Fig. 60–4) (Weaver et al., 1988; Schimmenti et al., 1995; Devriendt et al., 1998).

Clinical Course of Renal Abnormalities.
Figure 60–5 shows the left and right kidney lengths in 11 patients with RCS, expressed as a percentage of normal kidney length for age and sex. On average, the length of kidneys with renal hypoplasia is 60% of normal. The renal disease in RCS is progressive, culminating in end-stage renal failure in 33% of patients with *PAX2* mutations. Eight percent of RCS patients had end-stage renal failure before the age of 10, while 17% had developed end-stage renal disease by age 20. Interestingly, end-stage renal failure occurred in 97% of RCS patients who had renal hypoplasia (Table 60–1), suggesting that there is a strong correlation between kidney size and susceptibility to renal disease. The renal abnormalities are not reversible, and the renal disease bears little relationship to the type of mutation, except that renal failure was less severe in patients with nontruncating rather than truncating mutations of *PAX2* (Table 60–3).

Vesicoureteral Reflux
Clinical Presentation. Seventeen percent of patients with RCS were reported to have VUR, due to a malformation of the vesi-

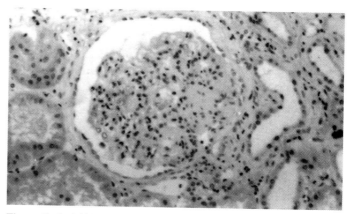

Figure 60–4. A kidney section prepared from the renal biopsy of an 18-year-old patient with renal-coloboma syndrome, prior to renal transplant. Hematoxylin and eosin stain. Note the glomerulosclerosis of the glomerulus. (Reproduced from Schimmenti et al., 1997, *Am J Hum Genet* 60: 873, University of Chicago Press.)

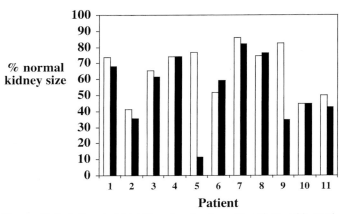

Figure 60–5. Left and right kidney lengths from 11 patients with renal-coloboma syndrome who have renal hypoplasia. Left (white) and right (black) kidney lengths, as measured by ultrasound, are shown as a percentage of normal kidney length for age and sex. (Reproduced with modifications from Porteous et al., 2000, *Hum Mol Genet* 9: 6, Oxford University Press.)

coureteral junction of the ureter (Table 60–1) (Eccles et al., 1996). VUR involves the regurgitation of urine from the bladder via the ureter into/toward the kidney (Eccles et al., 1996; Eccles and Jacobs, 2000). While not all patients with RCS have VUR, the incidence of VUR among RCS patients may be underestimated because VUR tends to be asymptomatic and often resolves spontaneously in early childhood (Bailey and Rolleston, 1997).

Usually, the initial presentation of VUR is pyelonephritis, resulting from an ascending urinary tract infection, or renal failure, resulting from scar formation and loss of renal function, called *reflux nephropathy* (Bailey and Rolleston, 1997). VUR is detected by micturating cystourethrogram, while the extent of renal damage is determined using a dimethyl succinic acid scan.

Clinical Course of VUR.

High-grade VUR (VUR of grades III or IV) in RCS patients is expected to contribute to the progression of renal failure and may require surgical reimplantation of the ureters to correct the reflux. Histopathological changes in renal tissue of patients with VUR include interstitial fibrosis, glomerulosclerosis, and tubular atrophy, which are relatively nonspecific changes. Lower grades of VUR are usually of lesser clinical consequence.

Developmental Abnormalities Associated with VUR.

The shape and position of the ureteric orifice in the bladder wall are abnormal in patients with VUR (Eccles and Jacobs, 2000). This may be due to altered timing of branching of the ureteric bud from the wolffian duct.

Inner Ear Abnormalities

Approximately 5% of RCS patients have hearing loss in the high-frequency range (Sanyanusin et al., 1995b; Schimmenti et al., 1997; Porteous et al., 2000). The exact anatomical nature of this deficit is unknown, but it is presumed to be due to abnormal development of the neurogenic portion of the inner ear.

CNS Abnormalities

One patient with a *PAX2* mutation presented with renal anomalies, optic nerve colobomas, hydrocephalus together with platybasia, and severe Chiari malformation type 1 (Schimmenti et al., 1999). The relatively low frequency of this phenotype in patients with *PAX2* mutation may be because the tissues of the mid-/hindbrain are not as sensitive to dosage levels of PAX2 protein as the eyes and kidneys during development.

Other Abnormalities

Soft skin and joint laxity have been reported in some RCS patients (Sanyanusin et al., 1995b; Schimmenti et al., 1997, 1999). The *PAX2* gene is not expressed in skin or in limb formation, and the reason for

these anomalies in RCS is not known. Bilateral cryptorchidism was reported in one patient with renal hypoplasia and optic nerve colobomas (Porteous et al., 2000). Even though *PAX2* is expressed in the epididymis and vas deferens, this abnormality could be just a sporadic occurrence because of the relatively high incidence of cryptorchidism in general. Febrile and clonic seizures have been reported in several RCS patients (Sanyanusin et al., 1995b; Schimmenti et al., 1997). Again, whether seizures are caused by *PAX2* mutations is not known.

Variable Expression of the RCS Phenotype

Expression of the RCS phenotype is extremely variable (Table 60–3), whether patients are unrelated with different mutations or from the same family with identical mutations, as illustrated in Figure 60–6. Variability in the phenotypic expression of RCS is notable even in different tissues in the same individual. For instance, the severity of ocular disease does not correlate with that of the kidneys, and between one affected eye or kidney and the contralateral organ, there may be considerable variation. The same sort of variability is evident in inbred *Pax2* mutant mice (Favor et al., 1996). These findings suggest that stochastic, rather than genetic, background effects play a role in the variability of the phenotype.

MUTATIONS IN *PAX2* CAUSING RCS AND STRUCTURE/FUNCTION RELATIONSHIPS

The *PAX2* gene comprises 12 exons spanning approximately 80 kb of genomic DNA (Sanyanusin et al., 1996) and encodes a 48–50 kDa protein containing an octapeptide domain and a partial homeodomain in addition to the paired box (Dressler and Douglass, 1992; Eccles et al., 1992).

The majority of the 13 reported *PAX2* mutations occur within the paired box domain (Fig. 60–7). This domain is composed of two helix-turn-helix motifs, forming two distinct subdomains, referred to as the *PAI* (N-terminal) and *RED* (C-terminal) *domains* (see Chapter 59) (Epstein et al., 1994; Kozmik et al., 1997; Xu et al., 1999). The PAI subdomain of PAX2 is thought to make most of the DNA contacts (Xu et al., 1999). Seven mutations (mutations 2, 4–7, 12, 13) in PAX2 have been identified in the PAI subdomain, many of which are frameshift mutations, resulting in protein truncation (Fig. 60–7). A highly ordered linker region, which also makes extensive DNA contacts, is contained between the the two DNA-binding subdomains and immediately adjacent to two in-frame mutations (mutations 6 and 7) in the *PAX2* gene (Fig. 60–7). The precise effect of the two missense mutations is unknown, but they may disturb the structure of this part of the protein or alter amino acids with a direct role in protein–DNA interactions (Devriendt et al., 1998). A frameshift mutation (mutation 11) has been identified in exon 3 of *PAX2* in the RED subdomain (Dureau et al., 2001).

The occurrence of frameshift or nonsense mutations in the PAI subdomain is predicted to result in extremely truncated PAX2 proteins with a short region encoding part of the paired box DNA-binding domain, followed by a stretch of abnormal reading frame and a premature stop codon. These polypeptides, if expressed, would possess little or no DNA-binding ability.

In addition to the paired box domain, mutations have been reported in the octapeptide domain, partial homeodomain, and transactivation domain of *PAX2* (mutations 1 and 8–10). The octapeptide domain represses transcriptional activation of target genes, while the partial homeodomain interacts with the retinoblastoma 1 (RB1) and TATA-binding proteins (Eberhard et al., 2000). The truncating frameshift and nonsense mutations affecting these domains in *PAX2* probably destroy PAX2 activity by removing the transactivation domain in the carboxyl terminus, which is essential for the transcriptional activation of target genes (Dorfler and Busslinger, 1996). If truncated proteins resulting from these mutations are expressed, it is likely that they would bind DNA but not transactivate target genes; therefore, the DNA-binding ability of these proteins potentially could act in a dominant-negative fashion. The transactivation domain contains a conserved 55–amino acid sequence rich in proline, serine, and threonine (PST), characteristic of transcription factors involved in intracellular signaling (Dor-

Table 60–3. Summary of *PAX2* Mutations Documented in the Literature

Site and Nature of Mutation	First Amino Acid Affected	Domain Affected	Consequences of Mutation	No. Patients with Mutation	Recurrent	Percent Carrying Mutation with Ocular Anomalies	Percent Carrying Mutation with Renal Anomalies or VUR	Reference
1 Exon 5 - delC1104	188	Octapeptide domain	Reading frameshift, PTT	4	No	100%	75%	Sanyanusin et al., 1995a
2 Exon 2 - insG619	26	Paired box domain	Reading frameshift, PTT	23	+13X	91%	78%	Sanyanusin et al., 1995b; Schimmenti et al., 1997; Amiel et al., 2000; Porteous et al., 2000; Dureau et al., 2001; Ford et al., 2001; Salomon et al., 2001
2a Exon 2 - delG619	26	Paired box domain	Reading frameshift, PTT	2	No	100%	100%	Schimmenti et al., 1999
2b Exon 2 - insertion of 2Gs at position 619	26	Paired box domain	Reading frameshift, PTT	1	No	100%	100%	Amiel et al., 2000
3 Translocation (10; 13) (q24;q12.3)	—	Paired box domain	Chromosome translocation within intron 3 or 4	1	No	100%	100%	Narahara et al., 1997
4 Exon 2 - del674-695	43	Paired box domain	Reading frameshift, PTT	1	No	100%	100%	Schimmenti et al., 1997
5 Exon 2 - delT611	23	Paired box domain	Reading frameshift, PTT	1	No	100%	100%	Cunliffe et al., 1998
6 Exon 3 - G769A	74	Paired box domain	Reading frameshift, PTT	6	No	100%	100%	Devriendt et al., 1998
7 Exon 3 -duplication of positions 763–768	76	Paired box domain	Reading frameshift, PTT	1	No	100%	100%	Devriendt et al., 1998
8 Exon 7 - C1289T	251	Partial homeodomain	Insertion of a stop codon, PTT	9	No	100%	56%	Porteous et al., 2000
9 Exon 9 -C1566A	344	Transactivation domain	Insertion of a stop codon, PTT	2	No	0%	100%	Nishimoto et al., 2001
10 Exon 7 - C1318T	261	Transactivation domain	Insertion of a stop codon, PTT	1	No	100%	100%	Nishimoto et al., 2001
11 Exon 3 - delG832	97	Paired box domain	Reading frameshift, PTT	2	No	100%	100%	Dureau et al., 2001
12 Exon 2 - del658-663	38	Paired box domain	Reading frameshift, PTT	1	No	100%	100%	Dureau et al., 2001
13 Exon 2 - delT602	20	Paired box domain	Reading frameshift, PTT	1	No	100%	100%	Chung et al., 2001

PTT, premature termination of translation.

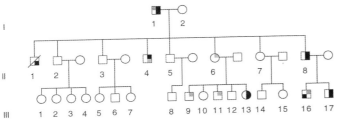

Figure 60–6. Pedigree of a family with renal-coloboma syndrome showing marked variability in ocular and renal disease in different individuals. Individuals in three generations of the pedigree (I, II, and III) are shown, as previously reported (Porteous et al., 2000). Square symbols denote males, while circles denote females. The first quadrant in each symbol depicts ocular disease. Gray denotes fundus abnormalities only, and black denotes fundus abnormalities with reduced visual acuity. The second quadrant depicts renal disease. Gray in the second quadrant denotes renal hypolasia without renal failure, and black denotes renal hypoplasia and renal failure. The third quadrant depicts vesicoureteral reflux. The fourth quadrant depicts sensorineural hearing loss. Gray denotes mild hearing loss. (Reproduced with modifications from Porteous et al., 2000, *Hum Mol Genet* 9: 3, Oxford University Press.)

fler and Busslinger, 1996). A mutation (mutation 9) in *PAX2* has been reported in exon 9, inside the transactivation domain (Nishimoto et al., 2001).

In addition to the mutations above, a balanced chromosomal translocation involving the *PAX2* locus, between chromosomes 10 and 13, t(10;13), was identified in one patient with RCS (Narahara et al., 1997). Table 60–3 summarizes all *PAX2* mutations and polymorphisms that have been documented. The identification of mutations spanning from the paired box to the transactivation domain indicates that mutations occurring anywhere throughout the *PAX2* gene can result in RCS. The reader is directed to the Human *PAX2* Allelic Variant Database (http://www.hgu.mrc.ac.uk/Softdata/PAX2/) for further information.

The pattern of inheritance of *PAX2* mutations is similar to that of other human PAX syndromes, such as *PAX3* in Waardenburg's syndrome types I and III and *PAX6* in aniridia (Epstein, 1995). The *PAX2*, *PAX3*, and *PAX6* genes have an interesting characteristic in that a dominant phenotype is observed for a heterozygous mutation, indicating haploinsufficiency of *PAX* gene products (Fisher and Scrambler, 1994; Epstein, 1995; Sanyanusin et al., 1995b). For mutations in *Pax2*, the phenotype is more severe in homozygous *Pax2* mutant mice than in heterozygous *Pax2* mutants. Null *Pax2* alleles generated by homologous recombination in mice (Torres et al., 1995) provide evidence that RCS is associated with sensitivity to reduced *Pax2* gene

dosage. Although monoallelic expression, as described for the stochastically expressed *Pax5* gene (Nutt and Busslinger, 1999), may be one way to explain haploinsufficiency of Pax gene products, *Pax2* is biallelically expressed in fetal mouse kidneys between 12 days postcoitum and 1 day postnatal (Porteous et al., 2000).

A Frequent *PAX2* Mutation

A recurrent G-insertion (or G-deletion) mutation in a guanosine homonucleotide tract (G619insertion/deletion) in exon 2 of *PAX2* has been identified 14 times independently in unrelated families (Table 60–3). Remarkably, ocular and renal defects in *Pax2*[1Neu] mice (see below) are associated with an identical G-insertion mutation in the mouse *Pax2* gene (Favor et al., 1996). The most likely explanation for the high frequency of the G619insertion mutation in comparison to other *PAX2* mutations is that the DNA in this region is "slippery," leading to forward or backward skipping by the DNA polymerase. This would result in insertion or deletion of nucleotides during replication and, as a consequence, expansion or contraction of the homoguanosine tract.

Phenotype–Genotype Correlations

Although data on 60 patients with *PAX2* mutations are available, there is little to indicate that the location or the type of mutation in *PAX2* can influence the phenotypic expression of RCS. Indeed, the variability of phenotype in individuals with an identical mutation is greater than differences associated with different mutations. For instance, the G619 mutation has been identified in patients with very severe ocular and renal abnormalities as well as in patients who are only mildly affected or who have isolated renal hypoplasia (Table 60–3). Two mutations, a missense mutation and an in-frame codon insertion in exon 3 of *PAX2*, appear to result in slightly milder phenotypes than average for *PAX2* mutations (Devriendt et al., 1998). However, it is not possible to make any conclusions from these data as the number of mutations is too small (Table 60–3).

Diagnosis of RCS

Patients with RCS usually present with ocular and renal abnormalities. A tentative diagnosis of RCS may be made based on the presence of either an optic nerve or optic disc abnormality together with one or more of the following kidney abnormalities: renal hypoplasia of one or both kidneys, renal agenesis, renal disease, or VUR. Such patients should be examined for *PAX2* mutations. While some patients who have these abnormalities may not yield *PAX2* mutations, it is clear that these patients have classic features of RCS, indistinguishable from those patients who do have *PAX2* mutations.

Some additional features have been observed in several patients with RCS and *PAX2* mutation, including cryptorchidism, microcephaly, and nephrolithiasis. However, these abnormalities are sporadic and not generally considered part of the syndrome. Patients with additional features, such as clubfoot, polydactyly, etc., have not been found to have *PAX2* mutations.

Genetic Heterogeneity

More than 10 patients have been described who have classic RCS based on the criteria described above but who do not have a *PAX2* mutation (Dureau et al., 2001; Salomon et al., 2001). Indeed, approximately 40% of RCS patients do not appear to have *PAX2* mutations. This means either that the *PAX2* mutation screening is not sensitive enough, that mutations occur in another domain of *PAX2* such as the promoter region, or that there is genetic heterogeneity of RCS.

Related Conditions

One condition that may be a variant of RCS is dominantly inherited isolated optic nerve colobomas, although molecular analyses of DNA from a large cohort of patients presenting with sporadic or hereditary isolated optic nerve colobomas and related eye abnormalities revealed a *PAX2* mutation in only one patient with an associated renal malformation (Cunliffe et al., 1998).

Primary isolated VUR is another condition that like RCS is dominantly inherited. However, *PAX2* mutations were absent in several

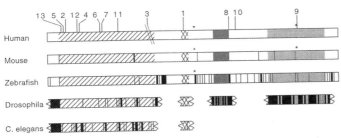

Figure 60–7. Structural features and mutations within PAX2. *Top bar* shows the human PAX2 protein, and the numbers above the bar refer to the mutations identified in PAX2 (see Table 60–3). The bar is divided into several domains as follows: hatching represents the paired box domain; cross-hatching represents the octapeptide domain; dark gray box represents the partial homeodomain; light gray box represents the transactivation domain. Asterisks denote the positions of alternatively spliced exons. Also shown are the mouse, zebrafish, *Drosophila, and C. elegans* Pax2 proteins. Vertical lines drawn on these bars denote positions at which the amino acids vary from the human PAX2 protein. Proteins and the positions of the mutations are drawn to scale. Broken bars of the *Drosophila* and *C. elegans* proteins indicate that the proteins are larger than shown and only the homologous domains are represented. The *C. elegans* protein contains no partial homeodomain or transactivation domain homology.

families with primary isolated VUR (Choi et al., 1998). Furthermore, dominantly inherited VUR in several families was not linked to the *PAX2* locus (Choi et al., 1998; Feather et al., 2000).

THERAPIES, GENETIC COUNSELING, AND PROGNOSTIC INFORMATION

There is no known therapy for RCS. Treatment for end-stage renal failure requires renal dialysis and ultimately renal transplant. Eye abnormalities in RCS patients often lead to reduced visual acuity and can lead to complications such as retinal detachment unless appropriate ocular follow-up is done.

In counseling patients and families with RCS, it is important to remember the considerable phenotypic variability. Correct diagnosis and genetic counseling are important as mildly affected parents may have severely affected offspring.

ANIMAL MODELS OF RCS AND MUTATIONS IN ORTHOLOGOUS *Pax2* GENES

Mutations in *Pax2* orthologues have been described in several species, including mice, zebrafish, *Drosophila* and *Caenorhabditis elegans*. In each species, *Pax2* mutations cause disrupted development, although the tissues affected are variable. Mice provide an excellent animal model of RCS; and as described below, three different *Pax2* mutations affect predominantly eye and kidney development in a dominant fashion, strikingly similar to the situation in humans. Zebrafish *Pax2* mutants also have eye and kidney abnormalities, although kidney development in fish does not exactly mimic that in mice and humans. *Drosophila Pax2* mutants have abnormalities affecting the development of eye and sensory organ precursor cells, while *C. elegans Pax2* mutants have developmental abnormalities of the uterus and male tail.

In spite of similarities in the *Pax2* gene between species (Fig. 60–7), very distantly related species have rather more differences in *Pax2* structure than similarities, which is reflected in both *Pax2* expression patterns and putative roles in organogenesis. It is encouraging, however, that analogous organs are affected by *Pax2* mutations in fish and humans, suggesting that it is reasonable to extrapolate from *Pax2* mutations in other vertebrate systems to putative effects in humans.

Mouse *Pax2* Mutants as Models of RCS

Mice have a single *Pax2* gene on chromosome 19, showing very high conservation with human *PAX2* (98.5% at the amino acid level) (Fig. 60–7). *Pax2* mutations in mice include *Krd* (Keller et al., 1994), *Pax2*[1Neu] (Favor et al., 1996), and a targeted disruption of the *Pax2* gene (Torres et al., 1995).

Krd heterozygous mutant mice exhibit **k**idney and **r**etinal **d**efects and were generated by transgene insertional mutagenesis. Insertion of the transgene on mouse chromosome 19 induced a chromosomal deletion of approximately 7 Mb of DNA, involving the entire *Pax2* gene and flanking regions (Keller et al., 1994). Homozygous *Krd* mutant embryos are preimplantation-lethal, probably due to the deletion of essential genes in this interval.

Heterozygous mutant *Krd* mice have reduced cell numbers in the inner cell and ganglion cell layers of the retina as well as abnormalities in electroretinogram recordings, which suggest alterations in photoreceptor and bipolar cell function (Keller et al., 1994). Movements of epithelial cells expressing *Pax2* in the posterior optic cup and optic stalk of the developing eye are also altered in *Krd* mutant mice. Consequently, this leads to improper formation of the optic fissure (Otteson et al., 1998).

Renal abnormalities in heterozygous *Krd* mutant mice include small kidneys with fewer glomeruli and less well-developed medulla and cortical regions than in wild-type mice. The kidney phenotype is highly variable, ranging from severe renal hypoplasia to normal size. Often, one kidney is small and the other within the normal range. Complete absence of a kidney, hydroureter, or cystic kidney abnormalities are observed on occasion (Keller et al., 1994).

The *Pax2*[1Neu] mutation was identified through mutagenesis experiments undertaken to identify genetic determinants of eye disease. The mutation is a G-nucleotide insertion in exon 2 of the *Pax2* gene, which occurs in a homonucleotide tract of seven Gs and is identical to the G619 insertion mutation in humans (Favor et al., 1996).

The *Pax2*[1Neu] mutation is semidominant, having both heterozygous and homozygous phenotypes. Homozygous *Pax2*[1Neu] mutant mice have a number of defects in organ development, but fetuses survive until birth and die perinatally. Abnormalities include agenesis of the urogenital tract, exencephaly, and abnormalities of the inner ear, optic nerves, and optic chiasm (Favor et al., 1996).

The wolffian duct in homozygous *Pax2*[1Neu] mutant mice appears normal at 9–10 days postcoitum, but the caudal wolffian duct degenerates after that. As a result, at embryonic day 12.5, the ureteric bud does not appear, causing renal agenesis. Structures such as the vas deferens and epididymis, which also develop from the wolffian duct, are unable to form in *Pax2*[1Neu−/−] mutants.

In *Pax2*[1Neu] homozygous mutant mice, the mullerian duct also degenerates, leading to absence of the oviducts, uterus, and vagina in females. Both wolffian and müllerian ducts express *Pax2* during development and are derived from the intermediate mesoderm. While endoderm-derived structures such as the urethra, bladder, and prostate glands are normal in *Pax2*[1Neu−/−] mutant mice, these are surrounded by blunt-ended remnants of the genital ridge (Favor et al., 1996). The same pattern of abnormalities in the urogenital tract occurs in mice harboring a targeted disruption of *Pax2*, as described below (Torres et al., 1995).

Heterozygous *Pax2*[1Neu] mutant mice show predominantly kidney and eye defects, analogous to the eye and kidney abnormalities in humans with *PAX2* mutations and similar to those observed in *Krd* mutant mice. The genital tracts in the *Pax2*[1Neu] heterozygotes appear normal (Favor et al., 1996).

In contrast to the *Pax2*[1Neu] allele, the targeted mutation in *Pax2* knockout mice was generated by homologous recombination using a targeting vector containing a neomycin cassette. In this mutation, part of *Pax2* exons 1 and 2 as well as the intron sequence in between were replaced, resulting in a truncated Pax2 protein (Torres et al., 1995). *Pax2* knockout mice show essentially identical urogenital features to *Pax2*[1Neu] mice, with similar CNS and ocular phenotypes, although exencephaly does not occur as frequently as in *Pax2*[1Neu] mice, possibly because of differences in the genetic backgrounds of the two strains (Torres et al., 1996). Ear defects include an enlarged chamber in the inner ear, abnormal organs of Corti, and lack of cochlear innervation. The eye abnormalities are consistent with failure of optic fissure closure. In addition, axons of the optic nerve are reduced in number and unable to form a chiasm, projecting only ipsilaterally (Torres et al., 1996).

Pax2 Mutations in Zebrafish, *Drosophila*, and *C. elegans*

Zebrafish

The zebrafish genome has been partially duplicated, resulting in two *Pax2* genes, *Pax2.1* and *Pax2.2* (Pfeffer et al., 1998). Despite genome duplication, mutagenesis of the zebrafish genome resulted in identification of zebrafish *no isthmus* (*noi*) alleles of the *Pax2.1* gene (Brand et al., 1996; Lun and Brand, 1998). As the name suggests, the mid–hindbrain boundary (isthmus) does not form in *noi* homozygous mutants, and development of the optic stalk of the zebrafish eye is also affected (Pfeffer et al., 1998). In addition, *Noi* mutants have twice the number of hair cells in the inner ear as *Pax2.1* is epistatic to both Delta and Notch signaling pathways (Riley et al., 1999).

Pax2.1 expression in the zebrafish pronephros assumes a pattern that is similar in many respects to mammalian *Pax8* in the fetal kidney (Drummond, 2000). However, *Pax2.1* mutations cause disrupted development of the pronephros (Majumdar et al., 2000), while in contrast, *Pax8* mutations do not affect the mammalian kidney (Macchia et al., 1998; Mansouri et al., 1998). In this regard, the zebrafish pronephros is less complex than the mammalian metanephros, and the *noi* phenotype does not resemble renal abnormalities in *Pax2* mutant mice as *noi* mutants lack pronephric tubules (Majumdar et al., 2000). Nevertheless, while *Pax2.1* and *Pax8* appear to have swapped roles in zebrafish, there is evolutionary conservation of coordinate regulation between the *Pax2*, *Pax5*, and *Pax8* genes in fish and mammals, with Pax2 at the top of the regulatory cascade (Noll, 1993; Pfeffer et al., 1998, 2002, 2002).

Drosophila

Among invertebrates, the *Drosophila melanogaster Pax2* gene is the most studied (D-*Pax2*). Two mutations, *Sparkling* and *Shaven,* in D-*Pax2* enhancer elements have been identified (Fu et al., 1998). *Sparkling* mutants (*Spa*) have a rough eye phenotype due to disruption of the hexagonal lattice of ommatidia, indicating that D-*Pax2* expression is required for the specification of cone and primary pigment cells of the eye discs in the late larval and pupal stages (Fu and Noll, 1997). *Shaven* (*Sv*) mutations cause elimination of shaft and glial cells, which are important for the development of the mechanosensory bristles in adult flies (Fu et al., 1998). Again, Notch signaling pathways are thought to play a role in *Sv* expression (Kavaler et al., 1999).

C. elegans

Pax2 orthologues have been identified in jellyfish (Sun, 1997; Groger et al., 2000), sponges (Hoshiyama et al., 1998), and the nematode *C. elegans* (Chamberlin et al., 1997). The *C. elegans Pax2* gene, *egl-38*, is required for the hermaphrodite egg-laying apparatus and development of the male tail (Chamberlin et al., 1997).

DEVELOPMENTAL PATHOGENESIS OF RCS

How do *PAX2* mutations result in RCS? The information gleaned from structure/function relationships of *Pax2* presented above does not suggest a mechanism. Recently, however, new clues have been obtained from animal models. Loss-of-function *PAX2* mutations are predicted to lead to either delayed, inhibited, or altered development of the affected tissues. Renal hypoplasia is frequent in heterozygous *Pax2*[1Neu+/−] mutant mice and associated with excessive amounts of apoptosis during development (Porteous et al., 2000; Torban et al., 2000). The highest levels of apoptosis occurred at embryonic day 16, in mutant collecting ducts (Fig. 60–8). In contrast, very little difference was observed in the number of dividing cells in fetal kidneys between mutant and wild-type mice (Porteous et al., 2000; Torban et al., 2000). Assuming that kidney growth is a balance between the increase of cell numbers by cell division and reduction of cell numbers by attrition through apoptosis, these results suggest that renal hypo-

plasia in *Pax2*[1Neu] mice involves excessive cell death in the developing kidneys.

While apoptotic cell death conveniently fits with the notion that cell loss may lead to small kidneys, cell death is a relatively nonspecific outcome and does not necessarily explain the reduction in ureteric bud branching and the presence of fewer nephrons in *Pax2*[1Neu] mutant kidneys. How could apoptosis cause this phenotype? A related question is whether apoptosis is the primary outcome of the *PAX2* mutation in the ureteric bud. Some researchers consider apoptosis to be a default mechanism by which the body eliminates cells that fail to fulfill the correct developmental program. Therefore, the finding of elevated apoptosis in *PAX2* mutant kidneys does not necessarily mean that the function of *PAX2* is to promote cell survival during development. Indeed, *PAX2* may well have other primary functions, and apoptosis may simply be a nonspecific outcome of failed development in *Pax2* mutant mice.

To address the question of whether apoptosis plays a primary role in the survival of renal medullary collecting duct cells, expression of *Pax2* was studied in the mouse inner medullary collecting duct cell line mIMCD-3. These cells express high levels of endogenous *Pax2*. Following transfection of an antisense *Pax2* expression construct into mIMCD-3 cells, endogenous *Pax2* dropped to an undetectable level. Concomitantly, a sharp increase in apoptotic cell death was observed (Torban et al., 2000). In contrast, *Pax2* expression protected HEK293 human fetal kidney cells from apoptosis induced with the proapoptotic gene *caspase-2* (Torban et al., 2000). Taken together, these data suggest that *Pax2* does have a primary role in the survival of medullary collecting duct cells during development.

Assuming that *Pax2* does play a role in facilitating cell survival during development, the question of how apoptosis in the medullary collecting duct cells leads to renal hypoplasia still needs to be answered. In *Pax2* mutant mice, one of the effects of the *Pax2* mutation was a decreased rate of new nephron induction since the total number of early epithelial structures (at the tips of ureteric buds) and glomeruli (representing more advanced nephrons) was strikingly reduced in the mutant kidneys. These nephrons, although reduced in number, appeared to have normal morphology (Porteous et al., 2000). Reduced rates of new nephron induction could be caused by excessive apoptosis in the ureteric bud. It might be envisaged, for example, that the branching of the ureteric bud is severely reduced by apoptosis. A model of inhibition of branching as a result of excessive apoptosis has been proposed to explain how apoptosis could cause renal hypoplasia in RCS (Torban et al., 2000). Whether similar involvement of apoptosis is responsible for the ocular phenotype in RCS has yet to be determined.

Another question arising from the studies described above is the mechanism by which *Pax2* facilitates cell survival. It may be that the transcriptional targets of *Pax2* are important in promoting cell survival (Stuart et al., 1995; Pfeffer et al., 2000). However, little is known about the transcriptional targets of Pax2. Likewise, there is little known in this regard about factors that regulate the *Pax2* gene, although the human and mouse *Pax2* promoters have been isolated and characterized in some detail (Ryan et al., 1995; Stayner et al., 1998; Kuschert et al., 2001). Clearly, much work still needs to be done to dissect the molecular pathways involving *Pax2* and to fully characterize the pathogenic mechanisms involved in RCS.

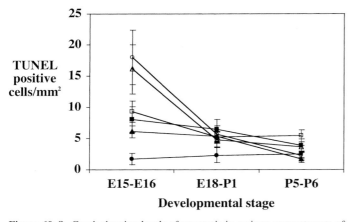

Figure 60–8. Graph showing levels of apoptosis in various compartments of the kidney at different stages of development in *Pax2* mutant mice. Apoptosis was measured as the number of terminal deoxynucleotidyl transferase–mediated dUTP nick end labeling (TUNEL)-positive cells per unit area of the kidney section, as reported previously (Porteous et al., 2000). TUNEL-positive cells were counted at embryonic day 15–16 (E15–E16), embryonic day 18 to postnatal day 1 (E18–P1), and postnatal day 5–6 (P5–P6). Circles show apoptosis in either mutant (open symbols) or wild-type littermate collecting ducts (filled symbols). Triangles show apoptosis in mutant (open) or wild-type littermate renal cortex (filled). Squares show apoptosis in mutant (open) or wild-type littermate glomeruli (filled). Each point represents the analysis of at least nine kidneys.

REFERENCES

Amiel J, Audollent S, Joly D, Dureau P, Salomon R, Tellier AL, Auge J, Bouissou F, Antignac C, Gubler MC, et al. (2000). PAX2 mutations in renal-coloboma syndrome: mutational hotspot and germline mosaicism. *Eur J Hum Genet* 8: 820–826.

Bailey RR, Rolleston GL (1997). Vesicoureteric reflux and reflux nephropathy: the Christchurch contribution. *N Z Med J* 25: 266–269.

Brand M, Heisenberg CP, Jiang YJ, Beuchle D, Lun K, Furutani-Seiki M, Granato M, Haffter P, Hammerschmidt M, Kane DA, et al. (1996). Mutations in zebrafish genes affecting the formation of the boundary between midbrain and hindbrain. *Development* 123: 179–190.

Bron AJ, Burgess SEP, Awdry PN, Oliver D, Arden G (1988). An inherited association of optic disc dysplasia and renal disease. Report and review of the literature. *Ophthalmic Paediatrics* 10: 185–198.

Burrill JD, Moran L, Goulding MD, Sauerssig H (1997). PAX2 is expressed in multiple spinal cord interneurons, including a population of EN1+ interneurons that require PAX6 for their development. *Development* 124: 4493–4503.

Chamberlin HM, Palmer RE, Newman AP, Sternberg PW, Baillie DL, Thomas JH (1997). The *PAX* gene *egl-38* mediates developmental patterning in *Caenorhabditis elegans*. *Development* 124: 3919–3928.

Choi K-L, McNoe LA, French MC, Guilford PJ, Eccles MR (1998). Absence of *PAX2* gene mutations in patients with primary familial vesicoureteric reflux. *J Med Genet* 35: 338–339.

Chung GW, Edwards AO, Schimmenti LA, Manligas GS, Zhang YH, Ritter R, 3rd (2001). Renal-coloboma syndrome: report of a novel *PAX2* gene mutation. *Am J Ophthalmol* 132: 910–914.

Cunliffe HE, McNoe LA, Ward TA, Devriendt K, Brunner HG, Eccles MR (1998). The prevalence of *PAX2* mutation in patients with isolated colobomas or colobomas associated with urogenital anomalies. *J Med Genet* 35: 806–812.

Devriendt K, Matthijs G, Damme BV, Caesbroeck DV, Eccles M, Vanrenterghem Y, Fryns J-P, Leys A (1998). Missense mutation and hexanucleotide duplication in the *PAX2* gene in two unrelated families with renal-coloboma syndrome (MIM 120330). *Hum Genet* 103: 149–153.

Dorfler P, Busslinger M (1996). C-terminal activating and inhibitory domains determine the transactivation potential of BSAP (Pax-5), Pax-2 and Pax-8. *EMBO J* 15: 1971–1982.

Dressler GR, Douglass EC (1992). Pax-2 is a DNA-binding protein expressed in embryonic kidney and Wilms tumor. *Proc Natl Acad Sci USA* 89: 1179–1183.

Dressler GR, Deutsch U, Chowdhury K, Nornes HO, Gruss P (1990). *Pax2*, a new murine paired-box containing gene and its expression in the developing excretory system. *Development* 109: 787–795.

Drummond IA (2000). The zebrafish pronephros: a genetic system for studies of kidney development. *Pediatr Nephrol* 14: 428–435.

Dureau P, Attie-Bitach T, Salomon R, Bettembourg O, Amiel J, Uteza Y, Dufier JL (2001). Renal coloboma syndrome. *Ophthalmology* 108: 1912–1916.

Eberhard D, Jimenez G, Heavey B, Busslinger M (2000). Transcriptional repression by Pax5 (BSAP) through interaction with corepressors of the Groucho family. *EMBO J* 19: 2292–2303.

Eccles MR, Jacobs GH (2000). The genetics of primary vesico-ureteric reflux. *Ann Acad Med Singapore* 29: 337–345.

Eccles MR, Wallis LJ, Fidler AE, Spurr NK, Goodfellow PJ, Reeve AE (1992). Expression of the *PAX2* gene in human fetal kidney and Wilms tumour. *Cell Growth Differ* 3: 279–289.

Eccles MR, Bailey RR, Abbott GD, Sullivan MJ (1996). Unravelling the genetics of vesicoureteric reflux: a common familial disorder. *Hum Mol Genet* 5: 1425–1429.

Epstein CJ (1995). The new dysmorphology: application of insights from basic developmental biology to the understanding of human birth defects. *Proc Natl Acad Sci USA* 92: 8566–8573.

Epstein JA, Glaser T, Cai J, Jepal L, Walton DS, Maas RL (1994). Two independent and interactive DNA-binding subdomains of the Pax6 paired domain are regulated by alternative splicing. *Genes Dev* 8: 2022–2034.

Favor J, Sandulache R, Neuhauser-Klaus A, Pretsch W, Chatterjee B, Senft E, Wurst W, Blanquet V, Grimes P, Sporle R, et al. (1996). The mouse Pax2 1Neu mutation is identical to a human PAX2 mutation in a family with renal-coloboma syndrome and results in developmental defects of the brain, ear, eye, and kidney. *Proc Natl Acad Sci USA* 93: 13870–13875.

Feather SA, Malcolm S, Woolf AS, Wright V, Blaydon D, Reid CJ, Flinter FA, Proesmans W, Devriendt K, Carter J, et al. (2000). Primary, nonsyndromic vesicoureteric reflux and its nephropathy is genetically heterogeneous, with a locus on chromosome 1. *Am J Hum Genet* 66: 1420–1425.

Fickenscher HR, Chalepakis G, Gruss P (1993). Murine Pax-2 protein is a sequence-specific trans-activator with expression in the genital system. *DNA Cell Biol* 12: 381–391.

Fisher E, Scrambler P (1994). Human haploinsufficiency—one for sorrow, two for joy. *Nat Genet* 7: 5–7.

Ford B, Rupps R, Lirenman D, Van Allen MI, Farquharson D, Lyons C, Friedman JM (2001). Renal-coloboma syndrome: prenatal detection and clinical spectrum in a large family. *Am J Med Genet* 99: 137–141.

Fu W, Noll M (1997). The Pax2 homolog sparkling is required for development of cone and pigment cells in the *Drosophila* eye. *Genes Dev* 2066–2077.

Fu W, Duan H, Frei E, Noll M (1998). shaven and sparkling are mutations in separate enhancers of the *Drosophila* Pax2 homolog. *Development* 125: 2943–2950.

Groger H, Callaerts P, Gehring WJ, Schmid V (2000). Characterization and expression analysis of an ancestor-type *pax* gene in the hydrozoan jellyfish *Podocoryne carnea*. *Mech Dev* 94: 157–169.

Groves AK, Bronner-Fraser M (2000). Competence, specification and commitment in otic placode induction. *Development* 127: 3489–3499.

Gus PI, de Souza CF, Porteous S, Eccles M, Giugliani R (2001). Renal-coloboma syndrome in a Brazilian family. *Arch Ophthalmol* 119: 1563–1565.

Hoshiyama D, Suga H, Iwabe N, Koyanagi M, Nikoh N, Kuma K, Matsuda F, Honjo T, Miyata T (1998). Sponge Pax cDNA related to Pax-2/5/8 and ancient gene duplications in the Pax family. *J Mol Evol* 47: 640–648.

Imgrund M, Grone E, Grone HJ, Kretzler M, Holzman L, Schlondorff D, Rothenpieler UW (1999). Re-expression of the developmental gene Pax-2 during experimental acute tubular necrosis in mice 1. *Kidney Int* 56: 1423–1431.

Karcher H (1979). Zum Morning Glory Syndrome. *Klin Monatsbl Augenheilkd* 175: 835–840.

Kavaler J, Fu W, Duan H, Noll M, Posakony JW (1999). An essential role for the *Drosophila* Pax2 homolog in the differentiation of adult sensory organs. *Development* 126: 2261–2272.

Keller SA, Jones JM, Boyle A, Barrow LL, Kilen PD, Green DG, Kapousta NV, Hitchcock PF, Swank RT, Meisler MH (1994). Kidney and retinal defects (Krd), a transgene induced mutation with a deletion of mouse chromosome 19 that includes the Pax-2 locus. *Genomics* 23: 309–320.

Kozmik Z, Czerny T, Busslinger M (1997). Alternatively spliced insertions in the paired domain restrict the DNA sequence specificity of Pax6 and Pax8. *EMBO J* 16: 6793–6803.

Kuschert S, Rowitch DH, Haenig B, McMahon AP, Kispert A (2001). Characterization of Pax-2 regulatory sequences that direct transgene expression in the wolffian duct and its derivatives. *Dev Biol* 229: 128–140.

Lun K, Brand M (1998). A series of *no isthmus (noi)* alleles of the zebrafish *pax2.1* gene reveals multiple signaling events in development of the midbrain–hindbrain boundary. *Development* 125: 3049–3062.

Macchia PE, Lapi P, Krude H, Pirro MT, Missero C, Chiovato L, Souabni A, Baserga M, Tassi V, Phichera A, et al. (1998). *PAX8* mutations associated with congenital hypothyroidism caused by thyroid dysgenesis. *Nat Genet* 19: 83–86.

Macdonald R, Scholes J, Strähle U, Brennan C, Holder N, Brand M, Wilson SW (1997). The Pax protein Noi is required for commissural axon pathway formation in the rostral forebrain. *Development* 124: 2397–2408.

Majumdar A, Lun K, Brand M, Drummond IA (2000). Zebrafish no isthmus reveals a role for pax2.1 in tubule differentiation and patterning events in the pronephric primordia. *Development* 127: 2089–2098.

Mansouri A, Chowdhury K, Gruss P (1998). Follicular cells of the thyroid gland require *Pax8* gene function. *Nat Genet* 19: 87–90.

Maricich SM, Herrup K (1999). Pax-2 expression defines a subset of GABAergic interneurons and their precursors in the developing murine cerebellum. *J Neurobiol* 41: 281–294.

Narahara K, Baker E, Ito S, Yokoyama Y, Yu S, Hewitt D, Sutherland GR, Eccles MR, Richards RI (1997). Localisation of a 10q breakpoint within the *PAX2* gene in a patient with a de novo t(10:13) translocation and optic nerve coloboma-renal disease. *J Med Genet* 34: 213–216.

Nishimoto K, Iijima K, Shirakawa T, Kitagawa K, Satomura K, Nakamura H, Yoshikawa N (2001). *PAX2* gene mutation in a family with isolated renal hypoplasia. *J Am Soc Nephrol* 12: 1769–1772.

Noll M (1993). Evolution and role of *Pax* genes. *Curr Opin Genet Dev* 3: 595–605.

Nornes HO, Dressler GR, Knapik EW, Deutsch U, Gruss P (1990). Spatially and temporally restricted expression of Pax2 during murine neurogenesis. *Development* 109: 797–809.

Nutt SL, Busslinger M (1999). Monoallelic expression of *Pax5*: a paradigm for the haploinsufficiency of mammalian *Pax* genes? *Biol Chem* 380: 601–611.

Oefelein M, Grapey D, Schaeffer T, Chin-Chance C, Bushman W (1996). *Pax-2*: a developmental gene constitutively expressed in the mouse epididymis and ductus deferens. *J Urol* 156: 1204–1207.

Otteson DC, Shelden E, Jones JM, Kameoka J, Hitchcock PF (1998). Pax2 expression and retinal morphogenesis in the normal and Krd mouse. *Dev Biol* 193: 209–224.

Pagon RA (1981). Ocular coloboma. *Surv Ophthalmol* 25: 223–236.

Pagon RA, Graham JM, Zonana J, Yong S-L (1981). Coloboma, congenital heart disease, and choanal atresia with multiple anomalies: CHARGE association. *J Pediatr* 99: 223–227.

Parsa CF, Silva ED, Sundin OH, Goldberg MF, De Jong MR, Sunness JS, Zeimer R, Hunter DG (2001). Redefining papillorenal syndrome: an underdiagnosed cause of ocular and renal morbidity. *Ophthalmology* 108: 738–749.

Pfeffer PL, Gerster T, Lun K, Brand M, Busslinger M (1998). Characterization of three novel members of the zebrafish Pax2/5/8 family: dependency of Pax5 and Pax8 expression on the Pax2.1 (noi) function. *Development* 125: 3063–3074.

Pfeffer PL, Bouchard M, Busslinger M (2000). Pax2 and homeodomain proteins cooperatively regulate a 435 bp enhancer of the mouse *Pax5* gene at the midbrain–hindbrain boundary. *Development* 127: 1017–1028.

Pfeffer PL, Payer B, Reim G, di Magliano MP, Busslinger M (2002). The activation and maintenance of Pax2 expression at the mid–hindbrain boundary is controlled by separate enhancers. *Development* 129: 307–318.

Porteous S, Torban E, Cho NP, Cunliffe H, Chua L, McNoe L, Ward T, Souza C, Gus P, Giugliani R, et al. (2000). Primary renal hypoplasia in humans and mice with PAX2 mutations: evidence of increased apoptosis in fetal kidneys of Pax2(1Neu)$^{+/-}$ mutant mice. *Hum Mol Genet* 9: 1–11.

Reiger G (1977). krankheitsbil der Handmannschen sehnervenanomalie: windenbluten-(Morning Glory) syndrom? *Klin Monatsbl Augenheilkd* 170: 697–706.

Riley BB, Chiang M, Farmer L, Heck R (1999). The *deltaA* gene of zebrafish mediates lateral inhibition of hair cells in the inner ear and is regulated by pax2.1. *Development* 126: 5669–5678.

Rowitch DH, McMahon AP (1995). Pax-2 expression in the murine neural plate precedes and encompasses the expression domains of Wnt-1 and En-1. *Mech Dev* 52: 3–8.

Royer P, Habib R, Courtecuisse V, Leclerc F (1967). Bilateral renal hypoplasia with oligonephronia. *Arch Fr Pediatr* 24: 249–268.

Ryan G, Steele-Perkins C, Morris JF III, FJR, Dressler GR (1995). Repression of Pax-2 by WT1 during normal kidney development. *Development* 121: 867–875.

Salomon R, Tellier AL, Attie-Bitach T, Amiel J, Vekemans M, Lyonnet S, Dureau P, Niaudet P, Gubler MC, Broyer M (2001). PAX2 mutations in oligomeganephronia. *Kidney Int* 59: 457–462.

Sanyanusin P, McNoe LA, Sullivan MJ, Weaver RG, Eccles MR (1995a). Mutation of PAX2 in two siblings with renal-coloboma syndrome. *Hum Mol Genet* 4: 2183–2184.

Sanyanusin P, Schimmenti LA, McNoe LA, Ward TA, Pierpont MEM, Sullivan MJ, Dobyns WB, Eccles MR (1995b). Mutation of the *PAX2* gene in a family with optic nerve colobomas, renal anomalies and vesicoureteral reflux. *Nat Genet* 9: 358–363.

Sanyanusin P, Norrish JH, Ward TA, Nebel A, McNoe LA, Eccles MR (1996). Genomic structure of the human PAX2 gene. *Genomics* 35: 258–261.

Schimmenti LA, Pierpont ME, Carpenter BLM, Kashtan CE, Johnson MR, Dobyns WB (1995). Autosomal dominant optic nerve colobomas, vesicoureteral reflux, and renal anomalies. *Am J Med Genet* 59: 204–208.

Schimmenti LA, Cunliffe HE, McNoe LA, Ward TA, French MC, Shim HH, Zhang Y-H, Proesmans W, Leys A, Byerly KA, et al. (1997). Further delineation of renal-coloboma syndrome in patients with extreme variability of phenotype and identical PAX2 mutations. *Am J Hum Genet* 60: 869–878.

Schimmenti LA, Shim HH, Wirtschafter JD, Panzarino VA, Kashtan CE, Kirkpatrick SJ, Wargowski DS, France TD, Michel E, Dobyns WB (1999). Homonucleotide expansion and contraction mutations of PAX2 and inclusion of Chiari 1 malformation as part of renal-coloboma syndrome. *Hum Mutat* 14: 369–376.

Schwarz M, Alvarez-Bolado G, Dressler G, Urbanek P, Busslinger M, Gruss P (1999). Pax2/5 and Pax6 subdivide the early neural tube into three domains. *Mech Dev* 82: 29–39.

Stapleton P, Weith A, Urbánek P, Kozmik Z, Busslinger M (1993). Chromosomal localization of seven *PAX* genes and cloning of a novel family member, *PAX-9*. *Nat Genet* 3: 292–298.

Stayner CK, Cunliffe HE, Ward TA, Eccles MR (1998). Cloning and characterization of the human PAX2 promoter. *J Biol Chem* 273: 25472–25479.

Strachan T, Read AP (1994). *PAX* genes. *Curr Opin Genet Dev* 4: 427–438.

Stuart ET, Haffner R, Oren M, Gruss P (1995). Loss of p53 function through PAX-mediated transcriptional repression. *EMBO J* 14: 5638–5645.

Sun H (1997). Evolution of paired domains: isolation and sequencing of jellyfish and hydra *Pax* genes related to Pax-5 and Pax-6. *Proc Natl Acad Sci* 94: 5156–5161.

Tellier AL, Amiel J, Delezoide AL, Audollent S, Auge J, Esnault D, Encha-Razavi F, Munnich A, Lyonnet S, Vekemans M, et al. (2000). Expression of the *PAX2* gene in human embryos and exclusion in the CHARGE syndrome. *Am J Med Genet* 93: 85–88.

Terzic J, Muller C, Gajovic S, Saraga-Babic M (1998). Expression of *PAX2* gene during human development. *Int J Dev Biol* 42: 701–707.

Torban E, Eccles M, Favor J, Goodyer P (2000). PAX2 suppresses apoptosis in renal collecting duct cells. *Am J Pathol* 157: 833–842.

Torres M, Giraldez F (1998). The development of the vertebrate inner ear. *Mech Dev* 71: 5–21.

Torres M, Gomez-Pardo E, Dressler GR, Gruss P (1995). Pax-2 controls multiple steps of urogenital development. *Development* 121: 4057–4065.

Torres M, Gomez-Pardo E, Gruss P (1996). Pax2 contributes to inner ear patterning and optic nerve trajectory. *Development* 122: 3381–3391.

Weaver RG, Cashwell LF, Lorentz W, Whiteman D, Geisinger KR, Ball M (1988). Optic nerve coloboma associated with renal disease. *Am J Med Genet* 29: 597–605.

Winyard PJD, Risdon RA, Sams VR, Dressler GR, Woolf AS (1996). The PAX2 transcription factor is expressed in cystic and hyperproliferative dysplastic epithelia in human kidney malformations. *J Clin Invest* 98: 451–459.

Woolf AS (1998). Emerging roles of obstruction and mutations in renal malformations. *Pediatr Nephrol* 12: 690–694.

Xu HE, Rould MA, Xu W, Epstein JA, Maas RL, Pabo CO (1999). Crystal structure of the human Pax6 paired domain–DNA complex reveals specific roles for the linker region and carboxy-terminal subdomain in DNA binding. *Genes Dev* 13: 1263–1275.

61 | *PAX3* and the Waardenburg Syndrome Type 1

ANDREW READ

PAX3 is one of the nine human genes of the PAX family of transcription factors (see Chapter 59; Chi and Epstein, 2002). PAX genes are defined by the presence of a paired box, encoding a 128– or 129–amino acid DNA-binding paired domain (PD). Like several others of the family, *PAX3* also encodes a second DNA-binding domain, a paired-type homeodomain (HD). PAX family members are dispersed around the human genome, with *PAX3* being located on the distal long arm of chromosome 2 at 2q35-q36.

PAX3 GENE STRUCTURE AND TRANSCRIPTION

The *PAX3* gene comprises 10 exons covering 99 kb of genomic DNA (Table 61–1). Exons 2–4 encode the PD and exons 5–6 the HD. Several splice variants have been reported (Fig. 61–1) (Barber et al., 1999). Most importantly, the use of two alternative splice acceptors separated by three nucleotides at the start of exon 3 produces forms with (+Q) or without (−Q) glutamine at amino acid 108. These variants have shown differential patterns of transcriptional activation in an in vitro assay (Vogan et al., 1996). A splice donor at nucleotide 248 of exon 8 is ignored in some transcripts, in which case translation proceeds for six codons (SKPWTF) into intron 8 before hitting a stop (isoform C). When intron 8 is spliced out, the C terminus, encoded by exon 9, is AFHYLKPDIA (isoform D). The intron 9 donor splice site is not seen in mouse or quail (Barber et al., 1999), so exon 10 is probably specific to certain human transcripts. If exon 10 is used, it would encode a further 21 amino acids and a 3′ untranslated region (UTR) of about 1300 nucleotides (isoform E). Reverse-transcriptase PCR experiments on human muscle RNA produced products containing exons 8, 9, and 10 without introns 8 and 9 (Barber et al., 1999). Additionally, 3′ rapid amplification of cDNA ends (RACE) extension of RNA from human adult cerebellum suggested the existence of messengers truncated at exon 4 (isoforms A, B), which if translated would encode proteins lacking the HD (Tsukamoto et al., 1994).

PAX3 EXPRESSION DURING DEVELOPMENT

PAX3 expression has been studied mainly in the mouse. In mouse embryos studied by in situ hybridization (Stuart et al., 1994, and references therein), expression is seen in the dorsal part of the neural tube, including the neural crest, starting at embryonic day (E) 8–8.5. In human embryos, *PAX3* is expressed in the CNS during the period of neural tube closure and later in the somites (Gérard et al., 1995). Neural crest cells migrate throughout the embryo; differentiate into many cell types including melanocytes, enteric and peripheral ganglia, and Schwann cells; and populate tissues including some facial bones and parts of the cardiac outflow tract. Pax3-expressing cells in mouse embryos migrate from the dermomyotome into the limb buds around E9.5, where they induce formation of limb muscles. In the future, global studies of gene expression by microarrays or serial analysis of gene expression (SAGE) may also help to define the patterns of *PAX3* expression in normal and abnormal cells.

DEFINING THE DOWNSTREAM TARGETS OF *PAX3*

As with all transcription factors, defining the downstream targets of *PAX3* has proved difficult. Possible approaches include comparisons of genes expressed in normal and *PAX3* mutant cells, genetic studies of animal models to detect epistatic and hypostatic effects, studies of *in vitro* DNA binding, chromatin immunoprecipitation, and studies of the changes in gene-expression patterns when *PAX3* is transfected into a suitable recipient cell. The main animal model is the *Splotch* (*Sp*) mouse, described below. Chromatin immunoprecipitation and targeted expression microarray studies have not been reported for *Pax3*; therefore, the main investigations at the molecular level have been into DNA binding.

DNA Targets of PAX3

DNA-binding studies using PCR selection have defined oligonucleotide sequences to which the PD and HD of PAX3 or related proteins separately show the strongest binding (Wilson et al., 1993; Chalepakis and Gruss, 1995). However, the biological relevance of these findings is open to some doubt. First, there is good evidence that when a Pax protein binds DNA, the various domains do not act independently. PDs themselves comprise two linked helix-turn-helix (HTH) motifs (Xu et al., 1999; Garvie et al., 2002), each rather analogous to the HD HTH and able to bind DNA. Different DNA sequences are recognized depending on whether the N-terminal or C-terminal HTH predominates in the overall PD DNA binding (Czerny et al., 1993; Epstein et al., 1994). On top of this, the PD influences DNA binding by the HD (Underhill and Gros, 1997), as do C-terminal parts of the protein (Vogan and Gros, 1997). A second limitation on the relevance of the selection procedure comes from the likelihood that biologically relevant targets may well not show the strongest binding. The most interesting developmental events involve divergence of a previously homogeneous cell population into distinct subpopulations with different developmental destinies, and these switches most likely involve finely balanced and rather weak interactions so that only a proportion of targets respond. Testimony to this is the way that many developmental defects, including type 1 Waardenburg syndrome (WS1), are dominantly inherited because of haploinsufficiency of a transcription factor. Finally, transcription factors typically act in a combinatorial way, with combinations of proteins binding in a highly specific way to targets that are relatively weak and nonspecific for the individual proteins. This mechanism has been well described for PAX5 (Garvie et al., 2002) and is likely to apply equally to PAX3.

For all of these reasons, we still know relatively little about the downstream targets of PAX3 during development. However, several have been identified, including *MITF* (Watanebe et al., 1998), *MET* (Epstein et al., 1996), *RET* (Lang et al., 2000), and (perhaps indirectly) *MyoD* and/or *Myf5* (Tajbakhsh et al., 1997); and each of these helps to explain features of Waardenburg syndrome.

Other Interactions of PAX3

Protein–protein interactions are just as important as DNA binding in explaining how PAX3 affects expression of a target gene. The C-terminal part of the PAX3 protein includes a typical serine- and threonine-rich transactivation domain, but *in vitro* DNA-binding studies have shown that PAX3 can have both stimulatory and inhibitory effects on transcription. Identified protein partners include the Sox10 transcription factor and two likely corepressors, HIRA (Magnaghi et al., 1998) and hDaxx (Hollenbach et al., 1999).

CLINICAL FEATURES OF WS1

WS1 is defined by a variable combination of hearing loss, patchy depigmentation, and dystopia canthorum (Table 61–2). Many other oc-

Table 61–1. Structure of the Human *PAX3* Gene

Unit	Start Position (nt)	End Position (nt)	Length (nt)	Amino Acids	Note
Exon 1	1	263	263	1–29	
Intron 1	264	1580	1317		
Exon 2	1581	1816	236	29–107	Paired domain: amino acids 34–162
Intron 2	1817	3136	1320		
Exon 3	3137	3266	130	108–151	−Q form uses splice acceptor 3 nt downstream, lacks Q108
Intron 3	3267	4489	1223		
Exon 4	4490	4262	133	151–196	Isoform A reads through splice donor, adds 19 extra residues, then STOP
Intron 4	4263	66,510	62,248		
Exon 4A	4866	4988	124	[196–206]	Isoform B uses normal intron 4 donor splice site, splices onto exon 4A, adding 10 extra residues, then STOP
Exon 5	66,511	66,718	208	196–264	Homeodomain: amino acids 219–278
Intron 5	66,719	77,406	10,688		
Exon 6	77,407	77,573	167	265–320	
Intron 6	77,574	78,439	866		
Exon 7	78,440	78,654	215	320–391	
Intron 7	78,655	96,603	17,949		
Exon 8	96,604	96,850	247	392–474	Isoform C reads through splice donor, adds 6 extra residues (SKPWTF), then STOP
Intron 8	96,851	97,347	497		
Exon 9	97,348	97,378	31	474–483	Isoform D reads through splice donor to STOP 1 nt downstream
Intron 9	97,377	97,457	171		Donor splice site not conserved in mouse
Exon 10	97,458	98,916	1369	483–503	Human-specific? 1305 nt 3′ untranslated region

casional complications have been reported, though, as discussed below, it is doubtful whether most of these are truly related to WS1.

Hearing Loss

Hearing loss is congenital, nonprogressive, and sensorineural. Liu et al. (1995) noted hearing loss in 35/60 personally examined cases (58%), a figure very similar to the 57% obtained in a literature search (Table 61–2). This is rather lower than the figure of 77% for WS2, but that probably just reflects the greater difficulty of making a diagnosis of WS2 without hearing loss as a pointer. The degree of loss can vary even within families. In the 35 affected WS1 patients, the loss was unilateral in 9 and bilateral in 24; in 21 of the latter, it was symmetrical and usually profound. Various audiogram shapes have been reported (Newton, 1990), including configurations associated with a profound bilateral or unilateral impairment, U-shaped audiograms in one or both ears, unilateral and bilateral low-frequency impairments, profound loss in one ear and moderate U-shaped or low-frequency loss in the other, and audiometric dips.

Few studies have been made of the temporal bones of WS1 patients. Fisch (1959) described atrophy of the stria vascularis, absence of hair cells, and a severe decrease of spiral ganglion cells in the cochlea of a 3-year-old girl with profound hearing loss and probable WS1. Merchant et al. (2001) reported findings in a woman with unambiguous WS1 (*PAX3* mutation S201X). She had unilateral low-frequency sensorineural hearing loss, which correlated precisely with absence of melanocytes, absence of the stria vascularis, and missing hair cells in

just the apical part of the affected cochlea; the contralateral cochlea was normal. This shows very clearly that absence of melanocytes is the primary cause of the hearing loss.

Pigmentary Changes

Pigmentary anomalies affect the hair, eyes, and skin. In the hair, a white forelock is the commonest feature. Locks of other colors or at other positions on the head have been described, but it is not clear that any of those cases have definite WS1. The forelock may be present at birth or may appear later, in which case it is often the precursor of general graying that can start as early as the teens. The early graying of WS typically starts in the midline, rather than around the temples. A white forelock may be present at birth and then disappear, only to return later. Table 61–2 shows that about half of all subjects currently or previously had a white forelock, which could vary in size from a few hairs to an impressive blaze. Women in particular often disguise a forelock by dyeing, so it is necessary to ask specifically.

In the eyes, typical findings include complete heterochromia (one blue eye and one brown) or segmental heterochromia (two colors within one iris, usually as sharply demarcated radial segments). Frills of a rather different color around the pupil are a normal variant and not associated with WS. Table 61–2 shows that 15%–18% of subjects had both irides brilliant blue with hypoplastic stroma. These "Waardenburg blue eyes" are particularly noticeable when they occur in a person from an ethnic group where most people have brown eyes. Small patches of hypopigmented skin are common in people with

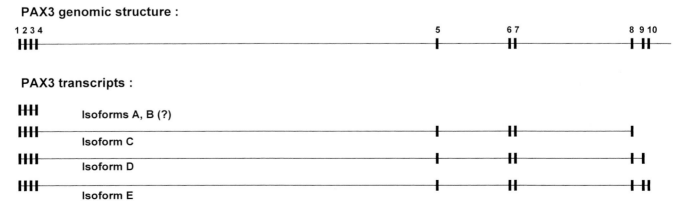

Figure 61–1. Structure of the *PAX3* gene and its transcripts. The sequence normally quoted is for isoform C. It is not clear whether isoforms A, B, and E are genuine functional transcripts. See Table 61–1 for +Q and −Q isoforms.

Table 61–2. Frequencies of Clinical Features in Subjects with Type 1 Waardenburg Syndrome

Feature	% of Personally Examined Series (n = 60)	% of Literature Series (n = 210)
Sensorineural hearing loss >25 dB	58	57
Heterochromia (two different-colored eyes or two colors within one eye)	15	31
Hypoplastic blue eyes	15	18
White forelock (now or reported)	48	43
Early graying (age <30 years)	38	23
Hypo- or hyper-pigmented skin patches	37	30

Source: Liu et al., 1995.

WS1. The extent of depigmentation is usually quite minor, unlike in piebaldism (see below).

Dystopia Canthorum

Arias (1971) was the first to point out that families with WS could be divided into those where all affected people had dystopia canthorum (type 1) and those where nobody had dystopia (type 2). *Dystopia* is an outward displacement of the inner canthi only, which is different from the outward displacement of the entire globe seen in hypertelorism (but, confusingly, many WS1 patients also have hypertelorism). Dystopia is associated with fusion of the eyelids medially and opening of the inferior lacrimal puncta opposite the iris rather than the sclera. Dystopia is difficult to diagnose reliably just by clinical impression and should be determined by measuring the eyes and calculating the W index (see below). If the two Waardenburg Consortium papers (Farrer et al., 1992, 1995) are compared, it can be seen that the first paper suggests that only a proportion of WS1 families are linked to 2q, while the second paper reports complete concordance. The first paper relied on clinical judgment of dystopia (by experienced clinicians); the second substituted the W index. Dystopia is seen in 98%–99% of WS1 subjects and is much the most reliable hallmark of WS1. Together with dystopia, there is often a characteristic facial build, with a broad high nasal root, hypoplastic alae nasi, and eyebrows that flare medially or tend to grow together (*synophrys*).

Many other abnormalities have been reported in subjects with WS, and these are considered in the discussion of counseling below.

MOLECULAR GENETICS OF WS1

WS1 is currently unique among human auditory-pigmentary syndromes in being apparently genetically homogeneous. No doubt, exceptions will be found sooner or later, but at present no case of unambiguous WS1 has been shown to be caused by mutation in any gene other than *PAX3* (although *PAX3* mutations are involved in conditions other than WS1, see below). *PAX3* mutations have not been found in all WS1 patients tested, but the main reason for this is probably the imperfect sensitivity of current mutation-scanning technologies.

Many different *PAX3* mutations have been described, including whole gene deletions, single nucleotide substitutions causing missense or nonsense mutations, frameshifting and frame-neutral small insertion/deletion mutations, and splice-site changes (see, e.g., Tassabehji et al., 1995). Missense mutations show a very good correlation with codons for amino acids known to make crucial protein–DNA contacts (Xu et al., 1995), while nonsense and frameshifting mutations are scattered through exons 2–6 of the gene (Fig. 61–2).

Such mutational diversity is typical of diseases caused by loss of function. Since WS1 is a dominant condition and affected people are heterozygous, this indicates that haploinsufficiency is the pathogenic mechanism. This again is typical of transcription factors, where a finely balanced action may be required to divert a subset of cells down a certain developmental route.

As often happens with conditions caused by haploinsufficiency, WS1 is almost as variable within families as between families. No genotype–phenotype correlations are strong enough to be usefully predictive for individuals. However, careful statistical studies of a large series (DeStefano et al., 1998) showed that a cohort of people with mutations that introduced a premature termination codon upstream of the HD had a significantly increased risk of each type of pigmentary anomaly compared to a cohort with point mutations causing amino acid substitutions in the HD. Nonsense-mediated mRNA decay (NMD) (Frischmeyer and Dietz, 1999) makes it likely that the former class of alleles produced no PAX3 protein. No correlations were found between type of mutation and risk of hearing loss.

The only notable genotype–phenotype correlation may be with mutation of asparagine-47. Two families have been described with different missense mutations affecting this amino acid. Hoth et al. (1993) showed that the mutation N47H was the cause of the only known example of a family in which "type 3 WS" was transmitted as a dominant condition. Later, Asher et al. (1996a) showed that the mutation N47K caused a unique syndrome, craniofacial-deafness-hand syndrome (MIM 122880), in a single family. Interestingly, the N47H mutation (numbered N14H by the authors) conferred unique DNA-binding behavior in vitro (Fortin et al., 1997).

A curious feature of the molecular pathology is the lack of mutations in the 3′ part of the gene. Routine mutation screening has normally covered exons 1–8, corresponding to isoform C in Figure 61–1; many patients have also been screened for mutations in exons 9 and 10, yet almost no mutations have been found downstream of the HD. The lack of missense mutations might suggest that no single amino acid in the C-terminal part of the protein is necessary for its presumed function in transactivation; the almost complete lack of premature termination mutations is harder to understand. Premature termination codons normally trigger NMD, so no functional mRNA is produced from such alleles. However, premature termination codons in the final exon of a gene or within about 50 nucleotides of the splice site of the penultimate exon usually escape NMD (Frischmeyer and Dietz, 1999). If so, such mutant alleles might produce a protein containing the PD and HD, but lacking all or part of the C-terminal sequence. PAX3 protein with a changed or truncated C terminus may be lethal or may produce a syndrome that is different from WS, and

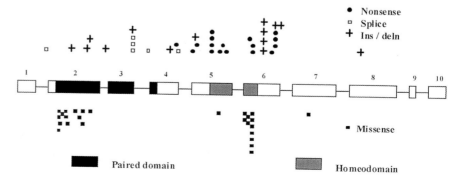

Figure 61–2. *PAX3* mutations in types 1 and 3 Waardenburg syndrome. The figure shows a typical selection of mutations (Tassabehji et al., 1995; Tassabehji et al., unpublished data). Missense mutations are concentrated in the N-terminal helix-turn-helix portion of the paired domain and the recognition helix (third helix) of the homeodomain; mutations of any type are seldom found downstream of the homeodomain.

the relevant patients have not yet been tested. Whatever the explanation, this is very different from *PAX6*, where mutations are found in all parts of the gene.

A final interesting finding in the molecular pathology of *PAX3* was the discovery of gain-of-function mutations in the tumor alveolar rhabdomyosarcoma. A chromosomal translocation characteristic of these tumors, t(2;13)(q35;q14), creates a novel chimeric gene comprising exons 1–7 of *PAX3* followed by exons of *FKHR*, a transcription factor gene of the forkhead family (Galili et al., 1993). This encodes a protein that binds to PAX3 targets but is overactive, not responding to the repressor hDaxx (Hollenbach et al., 1999). As well as having neoplastic growth properties, the cells take on some properties of striated muscle cells, no doubt reflecting the role of PAX3 in the formation of limb muscles.

ESTABLISHING THE DIAGNOSIS OF WS1

Clinical diagnostic criteria for WS have been set by the Waardenburg Consortium (Table 61–3) (Farrar et al., 1992). For WS1, the ultimate criterion is demonstration of a *PAX3* mutation; however, this service is not widely available and sensitivity is not 100%, so diagnosis is normally made on clinical grounds. Other types of WS are not discrete genetic entities; thus, their diagnostic criteria are much more arbitrary. If we had better insight into the genetic bases of WS2, we might write different criteria.

The presenting symptom is almost always hearing loss, normally in a baby or child. Standard audiological examination will reveal a sensorineural loss, but as described above, the severity, audiogram shape, and symmetry (unilateral or bilateral) are quite variable and do not help establish the diagnosis. Progressive loss is very unusual and a strong pointer to alternative diagnoses. The loss in WS (of all types) is normally congenital and nonprogressive.

Occasionally, patients present because of pigmentary features, usually patchy skin depigmentation. Pronounced depigmentation is unusual in WS and, if present, suggests a diagnosis of piebaldism (MIM 172800). Hearing loss is unusual but not unknown in piebaldism, and there tends to be a characteristic distribution of the depigmentation. A diagnosis of piebaldism would be confirmed by finding a mutation in the *KIT* gene.

Dystopia canthorum is the key indicator of WS1. The inner canthal, interpupillary, and outer canthal distances (*a*, *b*, *c* respectively) should be measured in millimeters with a rigid ruler placed against the forehead and the W index then calculated using the formula (Arias and Mota, 1978) $W = X + Y + (a/b)$, where $X = \{2a - 0.2119c - 3.909\}/c$ and $Y = \{2a - 0.2497b - 3.909\}/b$. The formula (derived

from a discriminant analysis) can easily be set up on a spreadsheet and is supposed to be applicable to patients of any age or ethnic group. Dystopia is present if the value of W is 1.95 or greater.

Originally, the threshold was set at $W = 2.07$ (Arias and Mota, 1978), but it was moved to 1.95 in light of the results of Farrar et al. (1995). In that study, 67 families with WS (type 1 or 2) were tested for linkage to 2q35. All families showing linkage had a W value, averaged across all affected members tested, of 1.95 or more, and no unlinked families had $W > 1.95$. Using the older threshold of 2.07, one family was misclassified and had been previously reported as an example of a WS2 family with a *PAX3* mutation (Tassabehji et al., 1993). Individuals vary, and inevitably the occasional person will be found who has WS1 (proved by *PAX3* mutation analysis) but whose W value falls below the 1.95 threshold; conversely, dystopia as defined here is not an infallible indicator of WS1.

Prenatal diagnosis is possible where there is a proven *PAX3* mutation, but the procedure can tell only whether or not the fetus carries the mutation. It is not possible to say how severely affected it would be; in particular, it is not possible to predict the presence or degree of hearing loss. Variability within families is not substantially less than that between families. Understandably, very few couples request prenatal diagnosis.

MANAGEMENT, TREATMENT, AND COUNSELING OF WAARDENBURG SYNDROME

There is no special management or treatment for WS. The hearing loss is normally nonprogressive and is treated symptomatically (including consideration of cochlear implant), just as for any other hearing loss. Occasional patients request cosmetic surgery for the dystopia. Because of the small risk of neural tube defects (see below), it would seem prudent for women pregnant with a fetus at risk of WS1 to use periconceptional folate supplements.

If the diagnosis of WS1 is firm, the risk of a child carrying the *PAX3* mutation is 1 in 2. Because of reduced penetrance, the risk of the child being clinically affected is lower and can be estimated from the figures in Table 61–2 (Liu et al., 1995). Counseling might largely focus on the risk of any of the very large number of reported rare complications (summarized by Da Silva, 1991). The difficulty here is that most of those case reports were not of patients with proven *PAX3* mutations or even, in most cases, dystopia canthorum. Almost certainly, the literature is heavily contaminated with patients who had other illdefined neurocristopathies, rather than WS1. Hirschsprung disease, for example, certainly occurs in combination with auditory-pigmentary symptoms (Shah-Waardenburg syndrome, see Chapter 38) but is not a feature of WS1.

Abnormalities truly associated with WS1 probably include neural tube defects, limb contractures, and maybe Sprengel's shoulder.

- Neural tube defects occur in most or all homozygous *Splotch* mouse embryos (depending on the particular mutation) and in one of the three reported cases of human homozygotes (Aymé and Philip 1995). Spina bifida occurs rarely but at greater than background frequency in WS1 patients (Kromberg and Krause, 1993), and *PAX3* mutations are found at a low but significant level in patients with spina bifida (Hol et al., 1995). One family where WS1 seemed particularly associated with spina bifida (Kromberg and Krause, 1993) turned out to have exactly the same *PAX3* mutation as another large family where none of seven affected people had spina bifida (A.P. Read, upublished data); thus, there is no evident predictor of the risk.
- Limb contractures define Klein-Waardenburg syndrome or WS3 (MIM 148820), a condition also caused by *PAX3* mutations. However, WS3 patients are a mixture of rare, very severely affected homozygotes and more mildly affected heterozygotes. Affected relatives of heterozygous WS3 patients typically have WS1 (e.g., family WS.105 in Tassabehji et al., 1995). With the possible exception of mutation at asparagine-47 (see above), there is no evidence that any genotype is at particularly high risk.

Table 61–3. Diagnostic Criteria for Type 1 Waardenburg Syndrome (WS1)

Major criteria:
- Sensorineural hearing loss >25 dB for at least two frequencies between 250 and 4000 Hz, without evidence of middle ear effusion and without evidence to suggest that presbyacusis or another factor accounts for the elevated hearing threshold
- Iris pigmentary abnormality: two eyes of different color, or iris bicolor/segmental heterochromia, or characteristic brilliant blue (sapphire) iris ("Waardenburg blue eye")
- Hair hypopigmentation: white forelock or white hairs within eyebrow, eyelashes, or other locations
- Dystopia canthorum: W index >1.95
- First-degree relative previously diagnosed with WS1

Minor criteria:
- Congenital leukoderma: several areas of hypopigmented skin
- Synophrys or medial eyebrow flaring
- Broad high nasal root
- Hypoplasia of alae nasi
- Premature graying: predominance of white scalp hairs before age 30

To be classified as affected, an individual must have either two major or one major and two minor criteria. Experience subsequent to publication of these criteria suggests that dystopia canthorum plus one other major sign is a suitable minimal criterion.
Source: Farrer et al., 1992.

• We have noted Sprengel's shoulder more frequently than expected in our own series of WS1 patients.

ANIMAL MODELS OF WS

The *PAX* gene family was first identified through homology to the *paired* mutant of *Drosophila melanogaster*, and *prd* has been used as the archetypal PAX protein in many of the studies of *in vitro* DNA binding. However, the only good animal model of WS1 is the *Splotch* mouse. Several alleles are known. The original spontaneous *Sp* mutant has a change, TCTCCAG to CGTGTG that abolishes the splice acceptor (underlined) at the end of intron 3. *Splotch-retarded* (*Sp*^{r}), the most severe allele, has a large chromosomal deletion. *Sp*^{2H} has a 32-base deletion in the HD, and *Sp*^{d}, the mildest allele, has a missense mutation, G42R, within the PD. Heterozygous *Splotch* mice (all alleles) have a white belly spot but normal hearing (Steel and Smith, 1992). *Sp*^{r} heterozygotes are also growth-retarded (interestingly, so was a boy with WS1 caused by a 7 Mb chromosomal deletion [Tassabehji et al., 1994]). Homozygotes have lethal neural tube defects; 60% die at E13.5–14.5 from heart defects. Homozygosity for *Sp*^{r} causes preimplantation lethality, possibly due to lack of other genes encompassed by the deletion.

DEVELOPMENTAL PATHOGENESIS OF WS

The varying penetrance of the different features of WS1 may reflect the sensitivity of different developmental processes to reduced PAX3 protein dosage. Dystopia canthorum, being the most highly penetrant feature, must result from the most dosage-sensitive process. Curiously, *Splotch* mice do not have very evident dystopia, although cranial morphology does depend subtly on the genetic background (Asher et al., 1996b). At the other end of the scale, limb defects and neural tube defects are only very occasionally seen in heterozygotes. Patients with these features may be especially sensitive because of their genotype at other loci that interact with *PAX3* or control the same developmental processes; alternatively, there may be a role for random chance in these events.

WS1 is the only clearly defined genetic entity in the large group of human auditory-pigmentary syndromes. Toriello (1995) described 18 syndromes that involve sensorineural hearing loss and abnormal pigmentation. Some of these (e.g., types 2 and 4 WS) are known to be genetically heterogeneous. Thus, upward of two dozen human conditions combine sensorineural hearing loss with abnormal pigmentation (normally patchy depigmentation) of the skin, hair, and/or irides.

Many other mammalian species show a similar combination of deafness and white spotting or white coat (Steel and Bock, 1983). The common feature is a patchy absence of melanocytes. The hearing loss arises from an absence of intermediate cells in the stria vascularis of the cochlea. These cells are a specialized set of melanocytes, and they are required to maintain the unusual ionic composition of the cochlear endolymph. In their absence, there is no hearing (Steel and Barkway 1989; Merchant et al., 2001). Melanocytes are physically absent from the affected areas; this is in contrast to albinism, where melanocytes are present but cannot make melanin because of an inborn error of metabolism, usually absence of tyrosinase. Albinos have grossly normal hearing. All melanocytes, except those of the retinal pigmented epithelium, arise from the embryonic neural crest, which is where *PAX3* is expressed (see above). Thus, the main features of WS1 are explicable in terms of a neurocristopathy, and the bewildering variety of other human auditory-pigmentary anomalies is only to be expected, given the very complicated genetic programs controlling neural crest differentiation.

REFERENCES

Arias S (1971). Genetic heterogeneity in the Waardenburg syndrome. *Birth Defects* 7: 87–101.
Arias S, Mota M (1978). Apparent non-penetrance for dystopia in Waardenburg syndrome type I, with some hints on the diagnosis of dystopia canthorum. *J Genet Hum* 26: 103–131.
Asher JH Jr, Sommer A, Morrell R, Friedman TB (1996a). Missense mutation in the paired domain of *PAX3* causes craniofacial-deafness-hand syndrome. *Hum Mutat* 7: 30–35.

Asher JH Jr, Harrison RW, Morell R, Carey ML, Friedman TB (1996b). Effects of *PAX3* modifier genes on craniofacial morphology, pigmentation and viability: a murine model of Waardenburg syndrome variation. *Genomics* 34: 285–298.
Aymé S, Philip N (1995). Possible homozygous Waardenburg syndrome in a fetus with exencephaly. *Am J Med Genet* 59: 263–265.
Barber TD, Barber MC, Cloutier TE, Friedman TB (1999). *PAX3* gene structure, alternative splicing and evolution. *Gene* 237: 311–319.
Chalepakis G, Gruss P (1995). Identification of DNA recognition sequences for the Pax3 paired domain. *Gene* 162: 267–270.
Chi N, Epstein JA (2002). Getting your Pax straight: *Pax* genes in development and disease. *Trends Genet* 18: 41–47.
Czerny T, Schaffner G, Büsslinger M (1993). DNA sequence recognition by Pax proteins: bipartite structure of the paired domain and its binding site. *Genes Dev* 7: 2048–2061.
Da-Silva EO (1991). Waardenburg I syndrome: a clinical and genetic study of two large Brazilian kindreds, and literature review. *Am J Med Genet* 40: 65–74.
DeStefano AL, Cupples A, Arnos KS, et al. (1998). Correlation between Waardenburg syndrome phenotype and genotype in a population of individuals with identified *PAX3* mutations. *Hum Genet* 102: 499–506.
Epstein JA, Glaser T, Cai J, Jepeal L, Walton DS, Maas RL (1994). Two independent and interactive DNA binding subdomains of the *PAX6* paired domain are regulated by alternative splicing. *Genes Dev* 8: 2022–2034.
Epstein JA, Shapiro DN, Cheng J, Lam PY, Maas RL (1996). *Pax3* modulates expression of the c-Met receptor during limb muscle development. *Proc Natl Acad Sci USA* 93: 4213–4218.
Farrer L, Grundfast KM, Amos J, et al. (1992). Waardenburg syndrome is caused by defects at multiple loci, one of which is between *ALPP* and *FN1* on chromosome 2: first report of the Waardenburg consortium. *Am J Hum Genet* 50: 902–913.
Farrer L, Arnos KS, Asher J, et al. (1995). Locus heterogeneity for Waardenburg syndrome is predictive of clinical subtypes. *Am J Hum Genet* 55: 728–737.
Fisch L (1959). Deafness as part of an hereditary syndrome. *J Layngol Otol* 73: 355–382.
Fortin AS, Underhill DA, Gros P (1997). Reciprocal effect of Waardenburg syndrome mutations on DNA binding by the *Pax-3* paired domain and homeodomain. *Hum Mol Genet* 6: 1781–1790.
Frischmeyer PA, Dietz HC (1999). Nonsense-mediated mRNA decay in health and disease. *Hum Mol Genet* 8: 1893–1900.
Galili N, Davis RJ, Fredericks WJ, Mukhopadhyay S, Rauscher FJ, Emanuel BS, Rovera G, Barr FG (1993). Fusion of a fork head domain gene to *PAX3* in the solid tumour alveolar rhabdomyosarcoma. *Nat Genet* 5: 230–235.
Garvie CW, Hagman J, Wolberger C (2002). Structural studies of Ets-1/Pax5 complex formation in DNA. *Mol Cell* 8: 1267–1276.
Gérard M, Abitol M, Delezoide A-L, Dufier J-L, Mallet J, Vekemans M (1995). *PAX* genes expression during human embryonic development, a preliminary report. *C R Acad Sci Paris* 318: 57–66.
Hol FA, Hamel BC, Geurds MP, Mullaart RA, Barr FG, Macina RA, Mariman EC (1995). A frameshift mutation in the gene for *PAX3* in a girl with spina bifida and mild signs of Waardenburg syndrome. *J Med Genet* 32: 52–56.
Hollenbach AD, Sublett JE, McPherson CJ, Grosveld G (1999). The Pax3-FKHR oncoprotein is unresponsive to the Pax3-associated repressor hDaxx. *EMBO J* 18: 3702–3711.
Hoth CF, Milunsky A, Lipsky N, Sheffer R, Clarren SK, Baldwin CT (1993). Mutations in the paired domain of the human *PAX3* gene cause Klein-Waardenburg syndrome (WS-III) as well as Waardenburg syndrome type 1 (WS-1). *Am J Hum Genet* 52: 455–462.
Kromberg JGR, Krause A (1993). Waardenburg syndrome and spina bifida. *Am J Med Genet* 45: 536–537.
Lang D, Chen F, Milewski R, Li J, Lu MM, Epstein JA (2000). *Pax3* is required for enteric ganglia formation and functions with *Sox10* to modulate expression of c-ret. *J Clin Invest* 106: 963–971.
Liu XZ, Newton VE, Read AP (1995). Waardenburg syndrome type II: phenotypic findings and diagnostic criteria. *Am J Med Genet* 55: 95–100.
Magnaghi P, Roberts C, Lorain S, Lipinski M, Scambler PJ (1998). *HIRA*, a mammalian homologue of *Saccharomyces cerevisiae* transcriptional co-repressors, interacts with *Pax3*. *Nat Genet* 20: 74–77.
Merchant SN, McKenna MJ, Baldwin CT, Milunsky A, Nadol JB (2001). Otopathology in a case of type 1 Waardenburg's syndrome. *Ann Otol Rhinol Laryngol* 110: 875–882.
Newton VE (1990). Hearing loss and Waardenburg syndrome: implications for genetic counselling. *J Laryngol Otol* 104: 97–103.
Steel KP, Barkway C (1989). Another role for melanocytes: their importance for normal stria vascularis development in the mammalian inner ear. *Development* 107: 453–463.
Steel KP, Bock GR (1983). Hereditary inner-ear abnormalities in animals. *Arch Otolaryngol* 109: 22–29.
Steel KP, Smith RJH (1992). Normal hearing in *Splotch* (Spl/+), the mouse homologue of Waardenburg syndrome type 1. *Nat Genet* 2: 75–79.
Stuart ET, Kioussi C, Gruss P (1994). Mammalian *PAX* genes. *Annu Rev Genet* 28: 219–236.
Tajbakhsh S, Rocancourt D, Cossu G, Buckingham M (1997). Redefining the genetic hierarchies controlling skeletal myogenesis: *Pax-3* and *Myf-5* act upstream of *MyoD*. *Cell* 89: 127–138.
Tassabehji M, Read AP, Newton VE, Gruss P, Harris R, Strachan T (1993). Mutations in the *PAX3* gene causing Waardenburg syndrome type 1 and type 2. *Nat Genet* 3: 26–30.
Tassabehji M, Newton VE, Leverton K, et al. (1994). *PAX3* gene structure and mutations: close analogies between Waardenburg syndrome and the Splotch mouse. *Hum Mol Genet* 3: 1069–1074.
Tassabehji M, Newton VE, Liu XZ, et al. (1995). The mutational spectrum in Waardenburg syndrome. *Hum Mol Genet* 4: 2131–2137.
Toriello HV (1995). Genetic hearing loss associated with integumentary disorders. In: Gorlin RJ, Toriello HV, Cohen MM (eds) *Hereditary Hearing Loss and Its Syndromes.* Oxford University Press, Oxford, pp. 368–412.

Tsukamoto K, Nakamura Y, Niikawa N (1994). Isolation of two isoforms of the *PAX3* gene transcripts and their tissue-specific alternative expression in human adult tissues. *Hum Genet* 93: 270–274.

Underhill DA, Gros P (1997). The paired domain regulates DNA binding by the homeodomain within the intact *Pax-3* protein. *J Biol Chem* 272: 14175–14182.

Vogan KJ, Gros P (1997). The C-terminal subdomain makes an important contribution to the DNA binding activity of the *Pax-3* paired domain. *J Biol Chem* 282: 89–95.

Vogan KJ, Underhill DA, Gros P (1996). An alternative splicing event in the *Pax-3* paired domain identifies the linker region as a key determinant of paired domain DNA-binding activity. *Mol Cell Biol* 16: 6677–6686.

Watanebe A, Takeda K, Ploplis B, Tachibana M (1998). Epistatic relationship between Waardenburg syndrome genes *MITF* and *PAX3*. *Nat Genet* 18: 283–286.

Wilson D, Sheng G, Lecuit T, Dostatni N, Desplan C (1993). Cooperative dimerization of paired class homeo domains on DNA. *Genes Dev* 7: 2120–2134.

Xu W, Rould MA, Jun S, Desplan C, Pabo CO (1995). Crystal structure of a paired domain–DNA complex at 2.5 Å resolution reveals structural basis for Pax developmental mutations. *Cell* 80: 639–650.

Xu HE, Rould MA, Xu W, Epstein JA, Maas RL, Pabo CO (1999). Crystal structure of the human *PAX6* paired domain with a 26 base pair DNA: new perspectives on paired domain–DNA interactions. *Genes Dev* 13: 1263–1275.

62 | *PAX6* and Aniridia and Related Phenotypes

VERONICA VAN HEYNINGEN AND KATHLEEN WILLIAMSON

LOCUS AND DEVELOPMENTAL PATHWAY: IDENTIFICATION OF *PAX6* AS THE GENE MUTATED IN ANIRIDIA

Positional Cloning

The *PAX6* gene on chromosome 11p13 was isolated by positional cloning (Ton et al., 1991) as a strong candidate gene for the human eye anomaly aniridia (OMIM 106210) (Fig. 62–1). The gene was identified within the aniridia subregion of the Wilms' tumor, aniridia, genitourinary abnormalities, and mental retardation (WAGR, OMIM 194072) contiguous deletion site. Its expression pattern, assessed by RNA in situ hybridization in human and mouse development, is consistent with a role for *PAX6* in developmental eye disease, although it is broader than the spectrum of tissues affected in aniridia.

Sequence analysis revealed that the *PAX6* gene is a predicted transcriptional regulator, highly conserved across many phyla (see below).

Validation of the Disease Association

Following the positional cloning, intragenic mutations were defined in a high proportion of aniridia cases, confirming that *PAX6* is the major, perhaps even the sole, gene implicated in this anomaly (Jordan et al., 1992; Glaser et al., 1992; Axton et al., 1997; Gronskov et al., 2001). Most mutations associated with classical aniridia are clear loss-of-function changes (Hanson and van Heyningen, 1995; Prosser and van Heyningen, 1998), suggesting that this is another developmental anomaly resulting from haploinsufficiency of a transcriptional regulator (Seidman and Seidman, 2002).

PAX6 EXPRESSION DURING DEVELOPMENT

Eye Development

Although early eye expression was initially studied in a 49-day-gestation human embryo (Fig. 62–2) (Ton et al., 1991), much of the normal expression data for *Pax6* come from in situ hybridization and immunohistochemical analyses in the mouse, where these studies are more readily carried out at all stages of development. Further information has been gained from phenotypic analysis of the semidominant Small eye (*Sey*) mouse model for aniridia (Hill et al., 1991). There are several *Sey Pax6* alleles, including a targeted loss-of-function mutant where *lacZ* expression is driven by the endogenous *Pax6* regulatory system (St Onge et al., 1997) and some ethyl nitrosourea (ENU)-induced mutants (Favor et al., 2001; Thaung et al., 2002). Heterozygous mutant mice provide a good model overall for human aniridia. The effect of homozygous loss of Pax6 function can also be studied during mouse gestation since *Pax6* null mice survive to birth and die neonatally (Hill et al., 1991). The lethal phenotype (*anophthalmia*, no olfactory structures and severe brain abnormalities) is very similar to the only reported clearly defined *PAX6* null human infant (Glaser et al., 1994a).

Pax6 is expressed from mouse embryonic day 8 (E8) onward, at the early stages of eye development, in both neural and surface ectoderm (Grindley et al., 1995; Cvekl and Piatigorsky, 1996). Neuroectoderm evaginates to give rise to the optic vesicle, which, following obligatory but transient contact with the surface ectoderm, invaginates to produce the double-layered optic cup that differentiates into the pigmented and neural layers of the retina. Following contact with the op-

tic vesicle, the surface ectoderm thickens to produce the lens placode. The placodal surface ectoderm then invaginates and pinches off to form the lens primordium; the rejoined surface ectoderm becomes the cornea. All layers of the developing eye therefore express *Pax6*. The retinal epithelial layer ceases to express *Pax6* before the pigment cells migrate in, but the neural retina continues to require *Pax6* expression following its initial specification. If *Pax6* expression is abrogated after the retinal progenitor cells have populated the developing retina but before differentiation into distinct cell types, only amacrine cells are produced (Marquardt et al., 2001; Marquardt and Gruss, 2002). A series of helix-loop-helix (HLH) genes are Pax6 targets and regulate retinal cell type identity.

The iris, initially an extension of the retina to which neural crest and mesenchymal cells later migrate, also expresses *Pax6* during development.

Correct development of the eye requires *Pax6* expression in the surface ectoderm both before and after contact with the optic vesicle (Grindley et al., 1995; Ashery-Padan et al., 2000; Dimanlig et al., 2001). If lens development is disturbed by turning off the late surface ectoderm expression of *Pax6*, then retinal development is also disrupted, demonstrating once more the interdependent development of the two components (Ashery-Padan et al., 2000). Lens epithelial cells and corneal limbal cells continue to express *Pax6* in the adult, where Pax6 may play a role in tissue maintenance. The role of *Pax6* in eye development is highly conserved throughout evolution (Gehring and Ikeo, 1999).

Olfactory System

Pax6 expression is required in the developing nasal placode and continues in the periglomerular and granular cell layers of the adult olfactory bulb and in the olfactory epithelium (Stoykova and Gruss, 1994; Davis and Reed, 1996; Dellovade et al., 1998). One of the well-established sites of continuing adult neural cell generation is the Pax6-positive rostral migratory stream, which continues to populate the olfactory system in rodents.

Brain and Neural Tube

A complex spatiotemporal expression pattern has been defined in the developing brain and neural tube for *Pax6*, as well as many other developmental regulators. Strong expression is seen in the cortical layers of the telencephalon and diencephalon (Stoykova and Gruss, 1994), where Pax6 plays a role in the specification of cellular (Gotz et al., 1998) and regional (Bishop et al., 2000) identity.

There is a clear boundary at the midbrain, where expression stops (Matsunaga et al., 2000). *Pax6* is also expressed in the thalamus (Stoykova and Gruss, 1994), pineal (Estivill-Torrus et al., 2001), and pituitary (Walther and Gruss, 1991; Bentley et al., 1999). In *Pax6* null mice, development of the corticothalamic and thalamocortical axes is severely disrupted (Pratt et al., 2000). In the hindbrain, the rhombic lip, precerebellar nuclei, and cerebellar external granular layer express Pax6 (Engelkamp et al., 1999). Expression persists into adulthood in many of these structures (Stoykova and Gruss, 1994). At the cellular level, the role of Pax6 is complex; it is generally confined to dividing cells, but in some cases expression persists in postmitotic cells (Estivill-Torrus et al., 2002). Expression in the spinal cord is confined to the ventral region, where Pax6 plays a key role in the development of motor neurons (Ericson et al., 1997). Reciprocal regulation between

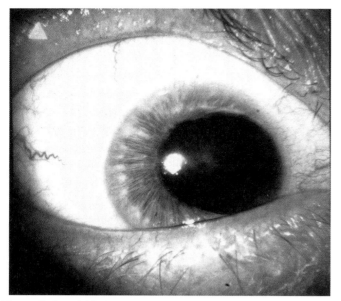

Figure 62–1. Aniridia in an adult eye, illustrating the variable iris hypoplasia. The pupil is enlarged and eccentric, with abnormal thin iris structure on the left and virtually no iris remnant on the right.

Pax6 and the HLH gene *Neurogenin2* has been demonstrated in this region (Scardigli et al., 2001), and further investigation may reveal parallels in the retina.

Pancreas

Outside the CNS, the endocrine cells of the developing and mature pancreas are another site of *Pax6* expression (St Onge et al., 1997). Interestingly, although pancreatic beta cells share with neurons the expression of several markers that otherwise seem neuron-specific, there is emerging evidence that there is no neuronal lineage contribution to the endocrine pancreas (Edlund, 2002).

Expression Studies in Human Tissues

Information on gene expression in humans is more limited, although PAX6 expression was observed in the developing eye at 6–22 weeks' gestation by immunohistochemical staining (Nishina et al., 1999) and at 7 weeks by in situ hybridization (Ton et al., 1991) (Fig. 62–2). Northern blot analysis on 17- to 22-week human fetal RNA was also reported (Ton et al., 1991). A series of human (and mouse) cell lines that express PAX6 at high levels have been useful for functional studies.

Spatiotemporal and Quantitative Control of Expression

How the correct expression of a complex developmental regulator like *PAX6* is controlled is not understood. There is some evidence for control of the timing, site, and level of gene expression through multiple

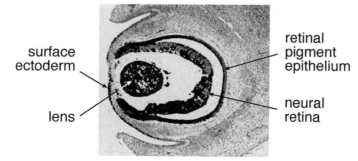

Figure 62–2. *PAX6* expression by radioactive *in situ* hybridization on the developing human eye. Section of 7-week-gestation human fetal eye showing the expression pattern of *PAX6* in the double-layered retina, the developing lens, and the surface ectoderm, which will form the cornea.

upstream (Williams et al., 1998; Kammandel et al., 1999; Dimanlig et al., 2001), intragenic (Plaza et al., 1995a; Marquardt et al., 2001), and downstream (Kleinjan et al., 2001; Griffin et al., 2002) regulatory elements (see below, Gene Structure and Genomic Organization).

CLINICAL PHENOTYPES ASSOCIATED WITH *PAX6* MUTATIONS

Aniridia and Related Eye Anomalies

Despite the broad expression of *Pax6* in the developing CNS, haploinsufficiency and the heterozygous *PAX6* missense mutations observed so far have been associated predominantly with aniridia and related eye phenotypes in humans and rodents.

Aniridia OMIM 106210 is a relatively rare (~1:60,000) developmental eye anomaly. Although often described as an anterior segment malformation, it is more correctly classified as a panocular abnormality, in line with the broad ocular expression pattern of *PAX6*. An autosomal-dominant segregation pattern is clearly observed in large families. The phenotype is variable, even within kindreds (Hittner et al., 1980); but careful clinical study confirms a high degree of penetrance (Mintz-Hittner et al., 1992).

The most obvious phenotypic feature of aniridia is iris hypoplasia of variable extent (Fig. 62–1), from almost complete absence of the iris to cryptic thinning of the iris stroma recognizable only under iris *trans*-illumination. Other iris defects include persistent iris strands, vascular loops and pupillary margin irregularities, and abnormal collarette (Mintz-Hittner et al., 1992). Variant aniridia phenotypes, with abnormal but not absent iris tissue, are more often associated with *PAX6* missense mutations (Hanson et al., 1999; van Heyningen and Williamson, 2002). Some *PAX6* mutations have been associated with congenital or early-onset cataracts (Epstein et al., 1994; Hanson et al., 1999).

Virtually all aniridia cases have foveal hypoplasia (OMIM 136520), a major cause of reduction in visual acuity (Azuma et al., 1996; Hanson et al., 1999). Its consistent presence from birth is thought to lead to the development of nystagmus in a high proportion of cases (Hanson et al., 1999; Sonoda et al., 2000).

Cataracts and glaucoma are frequently associated with aniridia (Khaw, 2002), occasionally congenitally but more often as later components of disease progression. Subluxation of the lens can be a feature (Day, 1990). Defects of the anterior chamber angle and ciliary body are implicated in abnormalities of the aqueous circulation. The anterior chamber may also be disrupted by the presence of persistent iris strands, synechiae, and lens–iris or lens–corneal adhesions. Some cases of Peters' anomaly result from *PAX6* mutations (Hanson et al., 1994; van Heyningen and Williamson, 2002). The lens–corneal adhesion phenotype is frequently seen in the original Edinburgh *Sey* mice (with a stop codon mutation in the linker region of the gene). However, most cases of Peters' anomaly are not associated with *PAX6* intragenic mutations (Churchill et al., 1998). Other associated abnormalities include corneal defects, such as keratitis (Mirzayans et al., 1995), opacification, pannus, and microcornea. In addition, limbal stem cell deficiency has been documented in aniridia (Dua et al., 2000; Daniels et al., 2001), and this is thought to make patients particularly susceptible to adverse effects of surgery for cataract, trabeculectomy, or corneal problems (Khaw, 2002). Comparison of human corneal features with those in the more accessible developing and mature cornea in heterozygous Small eye mice suggests that the rodent model is similar to human and may provide an experimental system for improving surgery outcomes (Ramaesh et al., 2003).

Possible Nonocular Effects of *PAX6* Mutation

Surprisingly, in view of the *PAX6* expression pattern in the developing telencephalon, diencephalon, rhombomeres, and cerebellum, there have been no consistent reports of any neurological involvement in aniridia cases. Nonocular abnormalities have, however, been reported in a few cases with established *PAX6* point mutations. Behavioral problems were described in two aniridia families (Heyman et al., 1999; Malandrini et al., 2001). Structural brain abnormalities (absence of anterior commissure) and anosmia/hyposmia (in some accompanied by olfactory bulb hypoplasia) were found in 12 cases where structural magnetic resonance imaging (MRI) was carried out and the Pennsylvania University Smell Test administered to 14 adult aniridia patients, each with identified *PAX6* mutations (Sisodiya et al., 2001). Anosmia had previously been mentioned in an aniridia case with a defined *PAX6* mutation (Martha et al., 1995). There was an increased incidence of epilepsy in the cohort studied by MRI, including both familial and sporadic instances, although the sample was too small for clear statistical analysis. Further MRI analysis, looking at an enlarged cohort, revealed the absence or hypoplasia of the pineal in 20/24 subjects, whose circadian activities now need to be assessed (Mitchell et al., 2003).

One study suggested a link between *PAX6* pancreatic expression and glucose intolerance in four aniridia individuals with known *PAX6* mutations (Yasuda et al., 2002).

Deletion-Associated Syndromic Aniridia

A proportion of aniridia cases are syndromic, primarily as a component of the WAGR deletion syndrome. Deletions virtually always arise *de novo*, except in rare cases where a parent carries a balanced insertional translocation (Lavedan et al., 1989). The severity of the phenotype is generally correlated with the size of the deletion: large deletions are frequently associated with developmental delay, mental retardation, and a variety of anomalies, including vertebral malformations and cardiac abnormalities (van Heyningen et al., 1985).

Of major concern, however, is whether the deletion encompasses the *WT1* Wilms' tumor predisposition gene or its control region. *WT1* lies about 700 kb centromeric to the *PAX6* gene, so submicroscopic deletions which delete *WT1* may be present in some sporadic and a few very rare familial *PAX6* deletion cases. In XY individuals, deletion of *WT1* is often heralded by genitourinary abnormalities such as cryptorchidism and hypospadias or occasionally complete sex reversal which may be associated with the presence of abnormal gonadal remnants that may themselves pose a risk of gonadoblastoma (van Heyningen et al., 1990; see Chapter 42). Gonadal abnormalities are much rarer and more difficult to identify in XX individuals with *WT1* deletion. Glomerular sclerosis may also be present from an early stage, or it may develop later, sometimes leading to end-stage renal failure (Breslow et al., 2000). However, when one copy of the *WT1* gene is deleted, the main risk requiring regular follow-up is that of Wilms' tumor (Fantes et al., 1992; Drechsler et al., 1994; Crolla et al., 1997; Gronskov et al., 2001; Muto et al., 2002; Crolla and van Heyningen, 2002).

Aniridia-like Phenotypes not Related to PAX6

Rare cases of aniridia associated with cerebellar ataxia and mild mental retardation (Gillespie's syndrome) have been reported (Crawfurd et al., 1979; Nevin and Lim, 1990). No *PAX6* mutations have been identified in Gillespie's syndrome (Glaser et al., 1994b), and it is likely that a different gene underlies this form of aniridia, which has also been reported to be distinct in terms of eye phenotype. One case was a child with an

apparently balanced de novo translocation, which may give clues to the identification of a Gillespie's syndrome gene (Dollfus et al., 1998).

MOLECULAR GENETICS OF THE *PAX6* LOCUS AND MUTATION SPECTRUM

Motifs and Function Prediction

The 422–amino acid PAX6 protein is a proposed tissue-specific transcriptional regulator with two DNA-binding domains: a paired domain, with homology to the *Drosophila* segmentation gene *paired* (Burri et al., 1989), and a paired-type homeodomain (Galliot et al., 1999). The two DNA-binding domains are separated by a linker region, and at the C terminus there is a proline-, serine-, and threonine-rich (PST) transactivation domain (Fig. 62–3A).

Evolutionary Conservation

PAX6 shows 100% amino acid identity and 95% nucleotide identity over the full sequence between mouse and human homologues, with a single amino acid difference in the alternatively spliced exon 5a. The paired and homeodomains are about 90% amino acid-identical to the *Drosophila* pax6 orthologue, at the *eyeless* locus, and >80% identical to the *Caenorhabditis elegans* pax6 orthologue at the *vab3* locus (Chisholm and Horvitz, 1995).

Gene Structure and Genomic Organization

The *PAX6* transcription unit, producing a 2.7 kb message, consists of 14 exons and spans a 22 kb genomic stretch (Glaser et al., 1992; Miles et al., 1998) (Fig. 62–3A,B). An alternatively spliced exon 5a is present, the inclusion of which is seen in most tissues to produce a minor isoform containing 14 additional amino acids in the paired domain, altering its conformation and DNA-binding specificity (Epstein et al., 1994). Two alternative promoters (Plaza et al., 1995b) and upstream (Kammandel et al., 1999) as well as intragenic (Plaza et al., 1995a) regulatory elements have been identified (Fig. 62–3B). Aniridia-associated chromosomal translocation and inversion breakpoints distal to the *PAX6* transcription unit (Fantes et al., 1995) suggested the presence of downstream long-range control elements, extending the genomic region covered by the functional gene to >180 kb (Fig. 62–3B). With this idea in mind, yeast artificial chromosome (YAC) transgenic mice were produced using a large human YAC containing the *PAX6* gene with 200 kb of genomic sequence flanking the gene on each side. This large YAC could fully correct the heterozygous and homozygous (lethal) phenotypes of the mouse *Sey* mutant (Schedl et al., 1996). A smaller YAC stretching almost to the distal patient breakpoint could not correct the *Sey* phenotypes (Kleinjan et al., 2001). It was also shown coincidentally that Pax6 dosage is critical for eye development as mice with five copies of the larger YAC transgene in

Figure 62–3. (*A*) Exonic organization of the *PAX6* gene. Schematic diagram illustrating the motif structure of PAX6, with the position of the exons marked along the top and the numbering of the motif-boundary amino acid residues marked along the bottom. UTR, untranslated region; PD, paired domain; HD, homeodomain; PST, proline-, threonine-, and serine-rich transactivation domain. (*B*) Genomic environment of the *PAX6* gene and its regulatory elements. Exons are shown in black; neighboring *ELP4* gene exons are shown in gray. The diagram is not to scale. EE is the upstream ectodermal enhancer (see, e.g., Dimanlig et al., 2001). P0 and P1 are the two alternative *PAX6* promoters (Plaza et al., 1995b). NRE is the neural retina-specific enhancer (see Marquardt et al., 2001, and references therein). The most distal breakpoint associated with aniridia is marked, as is the end of the YAC, which is able to correct the mouse *Small eye* phenotype. Downstream enhancer function has been defined (Kleinjan et al., 2001; Griffin et al., 2002).

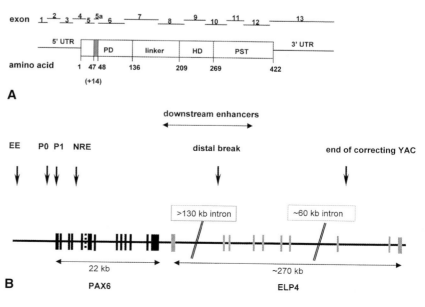

addition to their own endogenous two copies of *Pax6* showed a microphthalmic phenotype distinct from the haploinsufficient phenotype (Schedl et al., 1996). Following this demonstration of phenotypic correction with a large fragment of genomic DNA covering the regions up to and beyond the most distal patient breakpoint (Fantes et al., 1995) (Fig. 62–3*B*), the region was functionally dissected using a number of approaches. Sequence comparisons between species over the whole region revealed a high degree of conservation that extends far beyond the transcription unit (Plaza et al., 1995a; Miles et al., 1998) and contains identifiable elements with *PAX6*-related regulatory function (Kammandel et al., 1999; Lauderdale et al., 2000; Kleinjan et al., 2001; Dimanlig et al., 2001; Griffin et al., 2002).

WAGR region sequence analysis revealed that much of the downstream control region for *PAX6* is within a ubiquitously expressed neighboring gene, now identified as elongation protein 4 (*ELP4*), part of a complex with RNA polymerase 2 (Kleinjan et al., 2002). This association presumably underlies, at least in part, the existence of the large conserved WAGR synteny region in vertebrates (Glaser et al., 1990; Miles et al., 1998). Sequences were obtained from a human phage artificial chromosome (PAC) contig (Niederfuhr et al., 1998; http://www.sanger.ac.uk/cgi-bin), and mouse and *Fugu rubripes* bacterial artificial chromosomes (BACs) (Miles et al., 1998). Phylogenetic sequence comparison led to the identification of conserved, and therefore probably functionally significant, noncoding regions, some of which are being assessed (Kleinjan et al., 2001, 2002; Griffin et al., 2002).

Spectrum of *PAX6* Mutations Causing Disease

The published intragenic mutations in *PAX6* are collected in a regularly curated online database (http://pax6.hgu.mrc.ac.uk). In general, nucleotide changes are found throughout the gene, with the 223 changes in the database distributed as follows: 41% in the paired domain, 13% in the linker region, 15% in the homeodomain, and 18% in the PST region. The documented changes in the paired domain and homeodomain are shown graphically (Fig. 62–4*A,B*). Only four different polymorphic changes are reported, a surprisingly low number which emphasizes the incredibly high level of sequence conservation in *PAX6*.

Premature Protein Termination

An exceptionally high proportion of the aniridia-associated changes lead to predicted premature protein truncation (Hanson and van Heyningen, 1995; Prosser and van Heyningen, 1998). This is perhaps in line with haploinsufficiency as the mutational mechanism responsible for the aniridia phenotype. The dearth of missense mutations was, nevertheless, unexpected because missense changes may also be expected to lead to loss of function, particularly in such a highly conserved gene (see above). Perhaps heterozygous absence of a PAX6 protein or RNA product is required for the classical aniridia phenotype.

The most frequently recurring mutations are C40X (3×), R67X (3×), R203X (9×), and R240X (15×), with the last two involving CpG dinucleotide changes.

Splicing Mutations

The only other recurrent change is a splice donor mutation in the +1 position of intron 6 (×7), where a G residue is replaced by each of the other three nucleotides. This splice mutation was first observed with, and can be verified by, nested reverse-transcription with RNA prepared from nonexpressing lymphoblastoid cell lines, showing that this change results in an in-frame deletion of 36 amino acids from the paired domain as a weak cryptic splice site in exon 6 is utilized instead of the mutated donor site. Other intronic donor and acceptor sites carry occasional mutations. A unique and interesting splice mutation reported is at the splice acceptor site of intron 5a, which is suggested to increase the ratio of +5a to −5a isoforms of *PAX6* (Epstein et al., 1994). The phenotype is juvenile-onset cataracts, glaucoma, and nystagmus but with relatively normal irides. Since the role of exonic splice enhancers has been described, a number of missense changes in various genes have been reclassified as splicing mutations (Cartegni et al., 2002). Some of

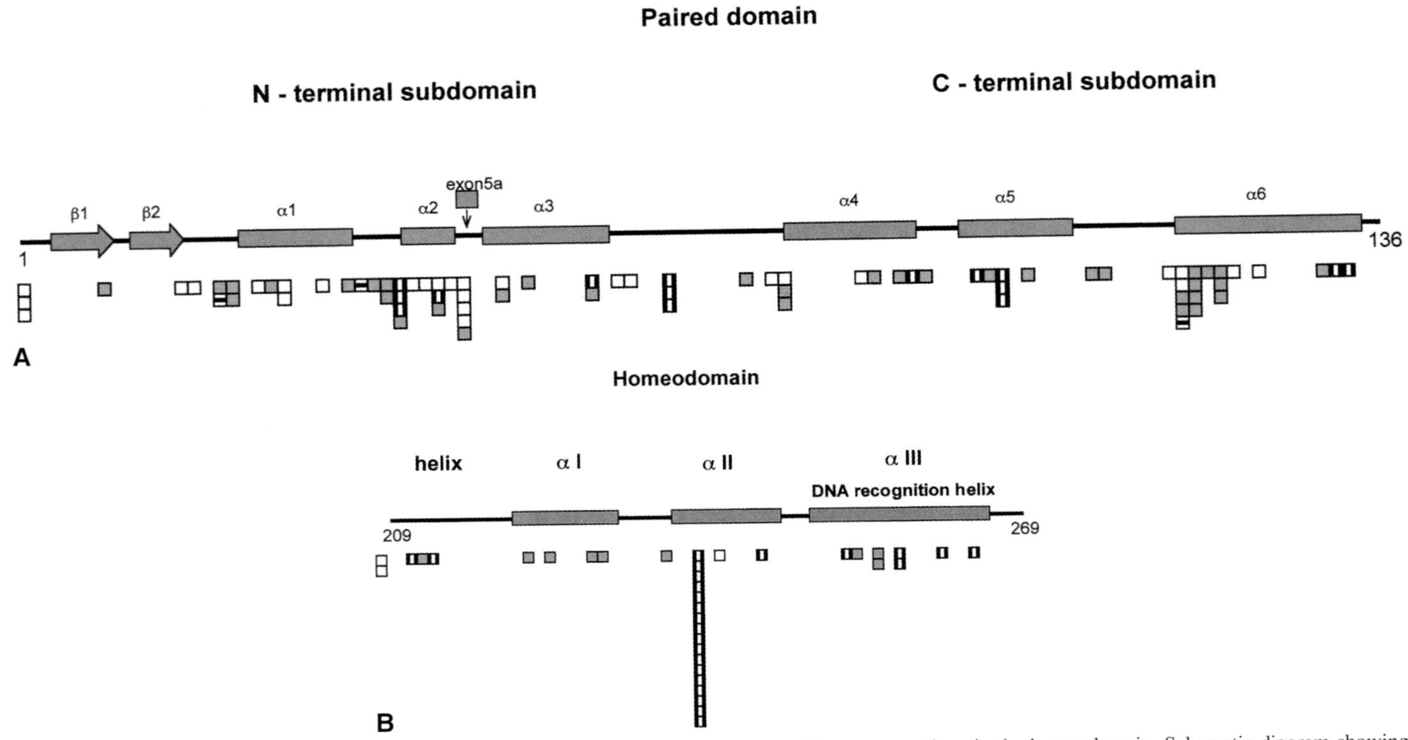

Figure 62–4. (*A*) Documented human mutations in the paired domain (PD). Schematic diagram showing the organization of the PD protein structure. The N- and C-terminal subdomains are marked, with β sheets and α helices detailed. Open boxes, missense mutations (see Table 62–1 for specific details); shaded boxes, frameshift mutations; horizontal filled boxes, in-frame deletions; vertical filled boxes, nonsense mutations (http://pax6.hgu.mrc.ac.uk). (*B*) Documented human mutations in the homeodomain. Schematic diagram showing the protein structure of the homeodomain. The α-helical regions are detailed. Open boxes, missense mutations (see Table 62–1 for specific details); shaded boxes, frameshift mutations; vertical filled boxes, nonsense mutations.

the missense changes described below may in reality be splicing mutations (see Table 62–1). It may be particularly interesting to assess this with the four independently arising identical changes (V7D) reported to cause microphthalmia with congenital cataract and anterior segment defects (Axenfeldt's and Peters' anomalies) (Azuma et al., 1999).

Missense Mutation

A missense mutation was first identified in a family with variant anterior segment abnormalities including bilateral Peters' anomaly with lens–corneal adhesions resulting in central corneal leukoma in one child (Hanson et al., 1994). Although most cases of Peters' anomaly are not caused by *PAX6* mutations (Churchill et al. 1998), two further cases with missense changes in the N-terminal portion of the paired domain have been identified (Wolf et al., 1998) close to the first Peters' anomaly mutation. A carefully selected set of so-called variant aniridias are caused by missense mutations, most of which are confined to the paired domain (Hanson et al. 1999; van Heyningen and Williamson, 2002) (Table 62–1). The phenotypes described in these cases include isolated foveal hypoplasia: hypocellular macular region in the retina with apparently normal irides, in two cases with an R128C change (Azuma et al., 1996; van Heyningen and Williamson, 2002). Familial cataracts, in some cases associated with partial iris hypoplasia, have been associated with several paired domain missense changes (van Heyningen and Williamson, 2002) (Table 62–1).

A deficit of missense mutations remains in regions of the protein outside the paired domain. The homeodomain in particular shows a very low frequency of missense changes. Just N-terminal to the home-

odomain, R208W (Hanson et al., 1993) and R208Q (Gronskov et al., 1999) have been reported; but the latter change was present together with A79E on the other allele of the individual with familial aniridia, the R208Q allele was present in her unaffected mother, and A79E was inherited from her affected father. Similarly, R242T was found in a boy with unilateral iris coloboma without any visual problems (Morrison et al., 2002), and the mutation was also present in his unaffected mother. Both R208 and R242 are highly conserved arginine residues that are expected to be functionally critical. However, there has been some suggestion from work in *Drosophila* that an intact pax6 homeodomain is not required for visual system development (Punzo et al., 2001).

A few putative missense changes in the linker region or in the PST-rich transactivation domain are described in Table 62–1. The Q422R mutation, in the final codon before termination, was described in a case with the unusual phenotype of uveal ectropion (misalignment of different iris layers), corneal abnormalities, and posterior embryotoxon (prominent Schwalbe line) (Azuma and Yamada, 1998). A second report of the same amino acid change had the features of aniridia (Singh et al., 2001). Recently several missense mutations, predominately on the transactivating domain, but also one in the paired and one in the homeodomain, were reported in association with optic nerve malformations (Azuma et al., 2003).

Predicted C-Terminal Extension

A category of changes that may have distinct associated subphenotypes includes mutations at the C terminus, where a short stretch of five to seven amino acids shows high sequence conservation between

Table 62–1. *PAX6* **Missense Mutations and Associated Phenotypes**

PAX6 Mutation*	Inheritance	Phenotype/Comments
M1Q	n/a†	Aniridia
M1V	Sporadic	Aniridia
M1K	Familial	Aniridia, late cataract, lens ectopia, glaucoma
N17S (2 mutns)	Sporadic	Aniridia, cataract (N17S is on the same allele as I29V)
G18W	Familial	Peters' anomaly, congenital cataract
G18R	Familial	Peters' anomaly, bilateral
R26G	Familial	Peters' anomaly
I29V (2 mutns)	Sporadic	Aniridia, cataract (I29V is on the same allele as N17S)
I29S	Sporadic	Aniridia
A33P	Familial	Partial aniridia with significant iris remnants, congenital cataract
I42S	Familial	Aniridia, congenital cataract
S43P	Familial	Aniridia, cataract, microcornea with vascularization
R44Q	Sporadic	Aniridia, cataract
Q47R	Sporadic	Aniridia (mutation may cause aberrant splicing)
V7D‡ (exon 5a)	Familial	Peters' anomaly, microphthalmia, congenital cataract
V7D‡ (exon 5a)	n/a	Axenfeldt's anomaly, microcornea
V7D‡ (exon 5a)	n/a	Peters' anomaly, cataract, microcornea, brain abnormality
V7D‡ (exon 5a)	Sporadic	Microphthalmia, congenital cataract
V53L	Familial	Aniridia
T63P	Familial	Aniridia, cataract, glaucoma
G64V	Familial	Peripheral corneal epithelium abnormality, congenital cataract
V78A	Familial	Foveal hypoplasia, nystagmus
A79E	Familial	Aniridia, cataract (carried by affected father and by viable compound heterozygote
I87R	Sporadic	Aniridia
P118R	Familial	Aniridia
S119R	Sporadic	Aniridia
S119R	Familial	Aniridia, ptosis, mild mental retardation, behavioral abnormalities
V126D	Familial (germline mosaic)	Ectopia pupillae, optic nerve hypoplasia, keratitis
R128C ×2	Familial	Isolated foveal hypoplasia
Q178H	Familial	Aniridia, optic nerve hypoplasia, cataract
R208W	Familial	Aniridia
R208Q	Familial	No phenotype (allele carried by unaffected mother and by viable compound heterozygous daughter with A79E)
R242T	Familial	Mild partial aniridia, also carried by unaffected mother
Q255H	Sporadic	Aniridia (mutation may cause aberrant splicing)
S353A	Familial	Aniridia
P375Q	n/a	Aniridia
G387D	Familial	Aniridia, but mutation comes from unaffected father
Q422R	Sporadic	Uveal ectropion, corneal epithelium abnormality, posterior embryotoxon
Q422R	n/a	Aniridia, cataract, mild lens subluxation

*Original references for mutations can be found at http://pax6.hgu.mrc.ac.uk
†n/a, not assessed.
‡The exon 5a alternative splice is numbered separately.

vertebrates and invertebrates, suggesting that this region may be involved in functional interactions. Several cases of X423L (Baum et al., 1999; Sisodiya et al., 2001; Singh et al., 2001) and one of X423Y (Gronskov et al., 2001) have been reported. A progressive retinal dystrophy phenotype with relatively well-preserved iris and epilepsy in three affected individuals was seen in two unrelated families with X423L (Sisodiya et al., 2001; Sisodiya and Moore, unpublished data). In common with many of the remaining cohort of patients who had MRI (mostly typical PAX6-haploinsufficient aniridia cases), the X423L individual showed severe hyposmia and absent anterior commissure (Sisodiya et al., 2001).

C-terminal extensions are predicted in one of the three possible reading frames, not only for X423 mutations but also for some out-of-frame insertions and deletions near the C terminus. In each frame, a string of seven or eight lysines is present as the human PAX6 termination codon, UAA, is followed by 23 adenines. A 10 bp deletion seven amino acids before the stop codon results in a predicted C-terminal extension of 35 amino acids in a family where aniridia cosegregates with behavioral problems and significant frontal lobe dysfunction (Heyman et al., 1999).

Chromosomal Rearrangements

The haploinsufficiency phenotype of aniridia was suggested by the early identification of chromosomal deletions (Hittner et al., 1979) when the contiguous deletion syndrome of WAGR was first defined. The nature of the associated anomalies depends on the extent of the deletion. Wilms tumor predisposition is one of the most frequent associations that needs to be identified, to monitor for the earliest signs of tumor (Fantes et al., 1992; Crolla et al., 1997; Gronskov et al., 2001; Muto et al., 2002; Crolla and van Heyningen, 2002). The nature and extent of other associated anomalies depend on the loci included in the deletion (Bruns et al., 1991; McGaughran et al., 1995). The gene(s) implicated in the mental retardation phenotype has been a subject to controversy (Schwartz et al., 1995; Guillemot et al., 1999).

Submicroscopic deletions and other rearrangements leading to aniridia can be assessed most readily using a panel of fluorescence in situ hybridization (FISH) probes for chromosomal analysis (Fantes et al., 1992; Crolla et al., 1997; Gronskov et al., 2001; Muto et al., 2002; Crolla and van Heyningen, 2002). Cryptic deletions of the PAX6 downstream regulator region (Lauderdale et al., 2000) may be more frequent than previously suspected and require the availability of a cosmid contig for routine FISH analysis of the whole region (Crolla and van Heyningen, unpublished data). The aniridia phenotype in these microdeletion cases is indistinguishable from loss-of-function intragenic mutations. Some very small deletions or other genomic rearrangements that disrupt tissue-specific regulators may lead to phenotypes other than aniridia, although the nature of the phenotypes to be expected is difficult to predict and this area could require help from analysis of targeted mouse deletions. Not all PAX6 regulatory elements have been defined. No upstream (centromeric) chromosomal breakpoints disrupting PAX6 function have been identified. Rare cases of duplication of the region may be seen. One case with a strabismus phenotype and mild developmental delay at the time of diagnosis has been described (Aalfs et al., 1997).

Establishing the Diagnosis

In most cases, aniridia is identified soon after birth, when the infant fails to respond normally to light and to visual stimuli. It is frequently first noticed by the mother. Classical aniridia with extensive reduction in iris tissue should be readily identifiable. Some of the variant aniridia phenotypes may be more difficult to diagnose. Foveal hypoplasia is one of the key features of eye abnormalities resulting from PAX6 mutation. This can be readily identified using fluoresceine angiography (Hittner et al., 1980). When the iris is more or less intact, iris trans-illumination will help to identify mild anomalies. Early diagnosis of de novo sporadic aniridia cases is important because microdeletions, which may include the WT1 gene and are usually not associated with other phenotypic features, should be identified quickly so that screening can begin for Wilms' tumor and possible renal anomalies (Fantes et al., 1992; Crolla et al., 1997). Diagnosis of the eye phenotype may help prevent some of the progressive features of aniridia, such as glaucoma.

Ophthalmologists suggest that prenatal diagnostic testing for aniridia is rarely requested, unless there is a badly affected parent who wishes to prevent the birth of a similarly affected child. Very occasionally, both members of a couple are affected with aniridia, giving a 25% risk of a pregnancy with a PAX6 homozygous (or compound heterozygous), neonatally lethal fetus. In such cases, if the parental mutations are known, chorionic villus sampling or amniocentesis can provide tissue samples for prenatal diagnosis.

MANAGEMENT, TREATMENT, AND COUNSELING

Although aniridia is a progressive eye disease, with frequent development of glaucoma and cataracts, it has been proposed that preventive gonioscopy (Chen and Walton, 1999) can help to preserve sight.

As discussed above, de novo cases of sporadic aniridia should be studied for the presence of a deletion that may extend to the Wilms' tumor predisposition locus. Cases with WT1 deleted must be monitored regularly for the development of Wilms' tumor and for possible symptoms of renal failure which would require urgent treatment. Genital and gonadal anomalies may also be present if WT1 is deleted, particularly in XY individuals. Sexual ambiguity or sex reversal may mask the presence of streak gonads, which are generally best removed to prevent gonadoblastoma.

Counseling for aniridia would cover the phenotypic heterogeneity and the progressive nature of the disease, including the degree of visual impairment.

PAX6 IN MODEL ORGANISMS

The Pax6 gene has become a paradigm for the investigation of gene function through a wide spectrum of model systems. This is in large measure because of the highly conserved role of Pax6 genes in eye development. There has been considerable controversy over whether the evolution of eyes is truly monophyletic, as suggested by the universal involvement of Pax6 orthologues as key regulators of eye development (Pennisi, 2002; Pichaud and Desplan, 2002). Major model systems for dissecting Pax6 function have come from both vertebrates and invertebrates. The availability of different model systems is an incredible bonus for a wide-ranging and rounded approach to understanding gene function in normal development and in disease (van Heyningen, 1997).

Vertebrates

The Sey mouse was identified as a likely model for aniridia on the basis of the homologous map position of the Small eye locus and the human eye anomaly. The point mutation in two different mouse alleles was identified even before the first human intragenic mutation (Hill et al., 1991). Subsequently, several other ENU mutagenesis–derived alleles have been defined (Favor and Neuhauser-Klaus, 2000; Favor et al., 2001; Thaung et al., 2002). A rat Pax6 mutant has also been described (Matsuo et al., 1993).

The spectrum of mutations in the mouse is similar to that in humans. However, the phenotypic variation, though quite broad for each allele studied, does not seem to correlate with the distinctions seen in the human cohort. This may be due in part to the fact that the mouse eye is differently organized in some ways. For example, no fovea is present in the retina as mice are nocturnal. Therefore, it is not surprising that the R128C mutation, which is associated with isolated foveal hypoplasia in the two human cases where it has been seen, does not show the same phenotype in mice (Thaung et al., 2002). Reduced eye size seen in mice is not echoed in human aniridia, where eye size is normal. However, mouse eyes in general, and the lens in particular, are proportionately much larger than their human counterparts. The mouse Pax6 phenotype almost invariably includes cataract (in fact, much of the ENU screening that has revealed new Pax6 alleles was initially looking for cataracts (Favor and Neuhauser-Klaus, 2000; Favor et al., 2001). The original Edinburgh Sey mouse (Roberts, 1967) presents with the Peters' anomaly phenotype at high frequency (Hanson et al., 1994).

In the mouse, a lacZ reporter targeted mutation has also been produced with complete truncation of the Pax6 gene, showing a phenotype indistinguishable from other, later terminating predicted protein truncations (St Onge et al., 1997). The *Sey* mouse model has been very widely used to investigate the role of Pax6 in the development of the CNS (Caric et al., 1997; Osumi et al., 1997; Ericson et al., 1997; Gotz et al., 1998; Engelkamp et al., 1999; Stoykova et al., 2000; Vitalis et al., 2000; Takahashi and Osumi, 2002). Informative conditional knockouts for lens development (Ashery-Padan et al., 2000) and retinal differentiation (Marquardt et al., 2001) have been described. Mouse deletion models for WAGR syndrome have also been studied (Glaser et al., 1990; Cattanach et al., 1996; Kent et al., 1997). Interestingly, heterozygous mice do not present with kidney tumors.

Using the various mouse models, a vast amount of work has been done on the role of *Pax6* in the development of the eye, brain, spinal cord, olfactory system, and pancreas. Many of these studies have used homozygous *Pax6* null mice to study Pax6 function throughout gestation, but clearly adult phenotypes cannot be assessed.

The mouse model system has also been useful in defining the interactions of the *Pax6* gene at the protein and DNA levels with other genes in eye development, for example, interactions with other major regulators of eye development, such as Six3 (Ashery-Padan et al., 2000), where mutual regulation of *Pax6* and *Six3* may be a critical mechanism in the heterozygous lens phenotype seen in mice (Goudreau et al., 2002). Interaction both at the protein level and through promoter regulation is found with some interactors, such as Sox2 (Kamachi et al., 2001) and MAF (Sakai et al., 2001; Planque et al., 2001). Some unknown downstream targets of Pax6 have begun to be defined (Bernier et al., 2001).

Much of the dissection of the *PAX6* regulatory elements was carried out using mouse transgenesis (see above, Gene Structure and Genomic Organization). Some studies have used cell culture and transfection systems (Xu and Saunders, 1998; Zheng et al., 2001). Analysis of PAX6 functional domains (Tang et al., 1997, 1998; Xu and Saunders, 1998; Singh et al., 2000) and of mutant alleles (Tang et al., 1998; Singh et al., 1998, 2001) was carried out using in vitro assays and cultured cell studies in a variety of systems, including quail (Plaza et al., 1993; Turque et al., 1994; Plaza et al. 1995a,b).

Other vertebrates have been widely used to study Pax6 function in different ways. An example to single out here is the use of *Xenopus* to show that ectopic expression of *Pax6* can induce the formation of eye primordia (Chow et al., 1999).

Invertebrates

The highly conserved ancestral role of *Pax6* in eye development across many phyla was first noted when the remarkable homology of the dipteran and mammalian mutant phenotypes was discovered (Quiring et al., 1994). Astonishingly, *Pax6* genes from several different sources were shown to be capable of inducing the development of eyes at foreign sites when ectopically expressed in the *Drosophila* leg, wing, and antennal imaginal discs (Halder et al., 1995). There is a wide-ranging literature on the role of *Pax6* in eye development across different phyla (Gehring and Ikeo, 1999).

Other, nonocular conserved functions for *Pax6* are seen in CNS development, reflected to some extent in both *Drosophila* (Kurusu et al., 2000; Callaerts et al., 2001) and the *C. elegans vab3* mutations (Chisholm and Horvitz, 1995). Interestingly, several of the *C. elegans pax6* mutant alleles reported are identical to human aniridia-associated mutations. *C. elegans* also has a second phenotype associated with its *pax6* locus: *mab18*, which has abnormal male mating behavior and sensory mutations. The *pax6* gene is implicated, as a different transcriptional isoform, where the paired domain is absent through alternative promoter usage and splicing (Zhang and Emmons, 1995). Suggestions for the existence of a homologous vertebrate transcript with no paired domain have been made for the quail (Turque et al., 1994).

SUMMARIZING THE DEVELOPMENTAL PATHOGENESIS OF *PAX6*

PAX6/Pax6 plays several major roles at different stages in eye development. It is expressed at different times in different sites, almost certainly under distinct but overlapping control from other interacting genes. Pax6 is a DNA-binding transcription factor that regulates a large array of downstream genes, genes acting in parallel pathways such as *Six3*, and even itself (autoregulation). It shows a very high degree of evolutionary conservation at the level of both sequence and function. This has made possible the use of many different model organisms, suitable for different experimental approaches, in the analysis of function. Of course, there are differences as well as similarities in the role of even highly conserved genes in different systems. For example, *Pax6* shows strong dosage sensitivity in mammals but not in *Drosophila*. However, even in humans and mice, haploinsufficiency affects only some developmental systems; so far, the eye is most obviously affected; but with more careful analysis of phenotypes (suggested by knowledge of the expression pattern and the homozygous phenotype in the mouse model system), olfactory system abnormalities are emerging, as well as possible brain malformations (Sisodiya et al., 2001). The similarities and differences between different model systems can in themselves be instructive; for example, *Drosophila* pax6 regulates the expression of *rhodopsin*, but this level of regulation is lost in vertebrates, where regulation of *crystallin* expression is seen (Cvekl and Piatigorsky, 1996) and Pax6 plays a major role in the control of lens development as well as retinal development and differentiation. Given this diversity of roles, it is not surprising that aniridia is now recognized as a panocular disease and that other associated anomalies, mostly not of great clinical significance, are also emerging.

Naturally occurring mutations in the human population have revealed a broad spectrum of different changes. Most mutations are unique or seen only occasionally. However, despite this wealth of different mutations, there are still some "missing" mutations, for example, missense changes in the homeodomain. It is almost certain that such mutations do arise as a result of random nucleotide changes. In view of the high degree of *PAX6* sequence conservation, it seems likely that missense changes in this region would have adverse effects. Why do we not see these mutations? It has been surprising that the one or two homeodomain missense mutations seen are associated with very mild, weakly penetrant phenotypes. They might not be revealed by phenotypes in the heterozygous state, and since humans are outbred, the chance of seeing them in the homozygous state may be very low. The most likely explanation, however, may be that in looking mainly at eye anomalies we are practising ascertainment bias. The missing mutations may be associated with a very different neurological, olfactory, or pancreatic phenotype, which we have not yet deciphered as relevant to PAX6 function. One way to decide what to look for would be to create some of these mutations specifically in the mouse.

Other phenotypes may also be associated with mutations at some of the emerging regulatory element sites. These regions may also be implicated in cases of aniridia-like and related eye development phenotypes where *PAX6* intragenic mutations have not been identified. The difficulty with identifying such changes unequivocally is to demonstrate their effect convincingly.

PAX6 has been a splendid paradigm that continues to yield insight into disease mechanisms, normal development, and evolution.

REFERENCES

Aalfs CM, et al. (1997). Tandem duplication of 11p12-p13 in a child with borderline development delay and eye abnormalities: dose effect of the *PAX6* gene product? *Am J Med Genet* 73: 267–271.

Ashery-Padan R, et al. (2000). Pax6 activity in the lens primordium is required for lens formation and for correct placement of a single retina in the eye. *Genes Dev* 14(21): 2701–2711.

Axton R, et al. (1997). The incidence of PAX6 mutation in patients with simple aniridia: an evaluation of mutation detection in 12 cases. *J Med Genet* 34(4): 279–286.

Azuma N, Yamada M (1998). Missense mutation at the C terminus of the *PAX6* gene in ocular anterior segment anomalies. *Invest Ophthalmol Vis Sci* 39(5): 828–830.

Azuma N, et al. (1996). PAX6 missense mutation in isolated foveal hypoplasia. *Nat Genet* 13(2): 141–142.

Azuma N, et al. (1999). Missense mutation in the alternative splice region of the *PAX6* gene in eye anomalies. *Am J Hum Genet* 65(3): 656–663.

Azuma N, Yamaguchi Y, Handa H, Tadokoro K, Asaka A, Kawase E, Yamada M (2003). Mutations of the PAX6 gene detected in patients with a variety of optic-nerve malformations. *Am J Hum Genet* 72: 1565–1570.

Baum L, et al. (1999). Run-on mutation and three novel nonsense mutations identified in the *PAX6* gene in patients with aniridia. *Hum Mutat* 14(3): 272–273.

Bentley CA, et al. (1999). Pax6 is implicated in murine pituitary endocrine function. *Endocrine* 10(2): 171–177.

Bernier G, et al. (2001). Isolation and characterization of a downstream target of Pax6 in the mammalian retinal primordium. *Development* 128(20): 3987–3994.

Bishop KM, Goudreau G, O'Leary DD (2000). Regulation of area identity in the mammalian neocortex by Emx2 and Pax6. *Science* 288 (5464): 344–349.

Breslow NE, et al. (2000). Renal failure in the Denys-Drash and Wilms' tumor-aniridia syndromes. *Cancer Res* 60(15): 4030–4032.

Bruns G, et al. (1991). A gene and breakpoint anchored map of the WAGR deletion region of human chromosome-11p. *Cytogenet Cell Genet* 58: 1956.

Burri M, et al. (1989). Conservation of the paired domain in metazoans and its structure in three isolated human genes. *EMBO J* 8(4): 1183–1190.

Callaerts P, et al. (2001). *Drosophila* Pax-6/eyeless is essential for normal adult brain structure and function. *J Neurobiol* 46(2): 73–88.

Caric D, et al. (1997). Determination of the migratory capacity of embryonic cortical cells lacking the transcription factor Pax-6. *Development* 124(24): 5087–5096.

Cartegni L, Chew SL, Krainer AR (2002). Listening to silence and understanding nonsense: exonic mutations that affect splicing 1. *Nat Rev Genet* 3(4): 285–298.

Cattanach BM, et al. (1996). Two Sey (Pax6) mutants. *Mouse Genome* 94: 678.

Chen TC, Walton DS (1999). Goniosurgery for prevention of aniridic glaucoma 1. *Arch Ophthalmol* 117(9): 1144–1148.

Chisholm AD, Horvitz HR (1995). Patterning of the *Caenorhabditis elegans* head region by the Pax-6 family member vab-3. *Nature* 377 (6544): 52–55.

Chow RL, et al. (1999). Pax6 induces ectopic eyes in a vertebrate. *Development* 126 (19): 4213–4222.

Churchill AJ, et al. (1998). PAX6 is normal in most cases of Peters' anomaly. *Eye* 12(Pt 2): 299–303.

Crawfurd MD, Harcourt RB, Shaw PA (1979). Non-progressive cerebellar ataxia, aplasia of pupillary zone of iris, and mental subnormality (Gillespie's syndrome) affecting 3 members of a non-consanguineous family in 2 generations. *J Med Genet* 16(5): 373–378.

Crolla JA, et al. (1997). A FISH approach to defining the extent and possible clinical significance of deletions at the WAGR locus. *J Med Genet* 34(3): 207–212.

Crolla JA, van Heyningen V (2002). Frequent chromosome aberrations revealed by molecular cytogenetic studies in referred aniridia cases. *Am J Hum Genet* 71: 1138–1149.

Cvekl A, Piatigorsky J (1996). Lens development and crystallin gene expression: many roles for Pax-6. *Bioessays* 18(8): 621–630.

Daniels JT, et al. (2001). Corneal stem cells in review. *Wound Repair Regen* 9(6): 483–494.

Davis JA, Reed RR (1996). Role of Olf-1 and Pax-6 transcription factors in neurodevelopment. *J Neurosci* 16(16): 5082–5094.

Day S, Narita A (1997). Uveal tract. In: *Pediatric Ophthalmology, 2nd Edition.* Taylor D (ed.) Blackwell Scientific, Oxford, Chap. 38, pp. 410–444.

Dellovade TL, Pfaff DW, Schwanzel-Fukuda M (1998). Olfactory bulb development is altered in small-eye (Sey) mice. *J Comp Neurol* 402(3): 402–418.

Dimanlig PV, et al. (2001). The upstream ectoderm enhancer in Pax6 has an important role in lens induction. *Development* 128(22): 4415–4424.

Dollfus H, et al. (1998). Gillespie syndrome phenotype with a t(X;11)(p22.32;p12) de novo translocation. *Am J Ophthalmol* 125(3): 397–399.

Drechsler M, et al. (1994). Molecular analysis of aniridia patients for deletions involving the Wilms-tumor gene. *Hum Genet* 94: 331–338.

Dua HS, et al. (2000). Limbal stem cell deficiency: concept, aetiology, clinical presentation, diagnosis and management. *Indian J Ophthalmol* 48(2): 83–92.

Edlund H (2002). Organogenesis: pancreatic organogenesis, developmental mechanisms and implications for therapy. *Nat Rev Genet* 3(7): 524–532.

Engelkamp D, et al. (1999). Role of Pax6 in development of the cerebellar system. *Development* 126(16): 3585–3596.

Epstein JA, et al. (1994). Two independent and interactive DNA-binding subdomains of the Pax6 paired domain are regulated by alternative splicing. *Genes Dev* 8(17): 2022–2034.

Ericson J, et al. (1997). Graded sonic hedgehog signaling and the specification of cell fate in the ventral neural tube. *Cold Spring Harb Symp Quant Biol* 62: 451–466.

Estivill-Torrus G, et al. (2001). The transcription factor Pax6 is required for development of the diencephalic dorsal midline secretory radial glia that form the subcommissural organ. *Mech Dev* 109(2): 215–224.

Estivill-Torrus G, et al. (2002). Pax6 is required to regulate the cell cycle and the rate of progression from symmetrical to asymmetrical division in mammalian cortical progenitors. *Development* 129(2): 455–466.

Fantes JA, et al. (1992). Submicroscopic deletions at the WAGR locus, revealed by nonradioactive in situ hybridization. *Am J Hum Genet* 51: 1286–1294.

Fantes J, et al. (1995). Aniridia-associated cytogenetic rearrangements suggest that a position effect may cause the mutant phenotype. *Hum Mol Genet* 4: 415–422.

Favor J, Neuhauser-Klaus A (2000). Saturation mutagenesis for dominant eye morphological defects in the mouse *Mus musculus*. *Mamm Genome* 11(7): 520–525.

Favor J, et al. (2001). Molecular characterization of Pax6(2Neu) through Pax6(10Neu). An extension of the Pax6 allelic series and the identification of two possible hypomorph alleles in the mouse *Mus musculus*. *Genetics* 159(4): 1689–1700.

Galliot B, de Vargas C, Miller D (1999). Evolution of homeobox genes: Q50 Paired-like genes founded the Paired class. *Dev Genes Evol* 209(3): 186–197.

Gehring WJ, Ikeo K (1999). Pax6: mastering eye morphogenesis and eye evolution. *Trends Genet* 15(9): 371–377.

Glaser T, Lane J, Housman D (1990). A mouse model of the aniridia-Wilms tumor deletion syndrome. *Science* 250(4982): 823–827.

Glaser T, Walton DS, Maas RL (1992). Genomic structure, evolutionary conservation and aniridia mutations in the human *PAX6* gene. *Nat Genet* 2: 232–239.

Glaser T, et al. (1994a). *PAX6* gene dosage effect in a family with congenital cataracts, aniridia, anophthalmia and central nervous system defects. *Nat Genet* 7(4): 463–471.

Glaser T, et al. (1994b). Absence of *PAX6* gene mutations in Gillespie syndrome (partial aniridia, cerebellar ataxia, and mental retardation). *Genomics* 19(1): 145–148.

Gotz M, Stoykova A, Gruss P (1998). Pax6 controls radial glia differentiation in the cerebral cortex. *Neuron* 21(5): 1031–1044.

Goudreau G, et al. (2002). Mutually regulated expression of Pax6 and Six3 and its implications for the Pax6 haploinsufficient lens phenotype. *Proc Natl Acad Sci USA* 99(13): 8719–8724.

Griffin C, et al. (2002). New 3′ elements control Pax6 expression in the developing pretectum, neural retina and olfactory region. *Mech Dev* 112(1–2): 89–100.

Grindley JC, Davidson DR, Hill RE (1995). The role of Pax-6 in eye and nasal development. *Development* 121(5): 1433–1442.

Gronskov K, et al. (1999). Mutational analysis of PAX6: 16 novel mutations including 5 missense mutations with a mild aniridia phenotype. *Eur J Hum Genet* 7(3): 274–286.

Gronskov K, et al. (2001). Population-based risk estimates of Wilms tumor in sporadic aniridia. A comprehensive mutation screening procedure of PAX6 identifies 80% of mutations in aniridia. *Hum Genet* 109(1): 11–18.

Guillemot F, Auffray C, Devignes MD (1999). Detailed transcript map of a 810-kb region at 11p14 involving identification of 10 novel human 3′ exons. *Eur J Hum Genet* 7(4): 487–495.

Halder G, Callaerts P, Gehring WJ (1995). Induction of ectopic eyes by targeted expression of the eyeless gene in Drosophila. *Science* 267(5205): 1788–1792.

Hanson I, van Heyningen V (1995). Pax6: more than meets the eye. *Trends Genet* 11(7): 268–272.

Hanson IM, et al. (1993). PAX6 mutations in aniridia. *Hum Mol Genet* 2(7): 915–920.

Hanson IM, et al. (1994). Mutations at the PAX6 locus are found in heterogeneous anterior segment malformations including Peters' anomaly. *Nat Genet* 6(2): 168–173.

Hanson I, et al. (1999). Missense mutations in the most ancient residues of the PAX6 paired domain underlie a spectrum of human congenital eye malformations. *Hum Mol Genet* 8(2): 165–172.

Heyman I, et al. (1999). Psychiatric disorder and cognitive function in a family with an inherited novel mutation of the developmental control gene PAX6. *Psychiatr Genet* 9(2): 85–90.

Hill RE, et al. (1991). Mouse small eye results from mutations in a paired-like homeobox-containing gene. *Nature* 354(6354): 522–525.

Hittner HM, Riccardi VM, Francke U (1979). Aniridia caused by a heritable chromosome 11 deletion. *Ophthalmology* 86(6): 1173–1183.

Hittner HM, et al. (1980). Variable expressivity in autosomal dominant aniridia by clinical, electrophysiologic, and angiographic criteria. *Am J Ophthalmol* 89(4): 531–539.

Jordan T, et al. (1992). The human *PAX6* gene is mutated in two patients with aniridia. *Nat Genet* 1: 328–332.

Kamachi Y, et al. (2001). Pax6 and SOX2 form a co-DNA-binding partner complex that regulates initiation of lens development. *Genes Dev* 15(10): 1272–1286.

Kammandel B, et al. (1999). Distinct *cis*-essential modules direct the time–space pattern of the *Pax6* gene activity. *Dev Biol* 205(1): 79–97.

Kent J, et al. (1997). The reticulocalbin gene maps to the WAGR region in human and to the small eye Harwell deletion in mouse. *Genomics* 42: 260–267.

Khaw PT (2002). Aniridia. *J Glaucoma* 11(2): 164–168.

Kleinjan DA, et al. (2001). Aniridia-associated translocations, DNase hypersensitivity, sequence comparison and transgenic analysis redefine the functional domain of PAX6. *Hum Mol Genet* 10(19): 2049–2059.

Kleinjan DA, et al. (2002). Characterization of a novel gene adjacent to *PAX6*, revealing synteny conservation with functional significance. *Mamm Genome* 13(2): 102–107.

Kurusu M, et al. (2000). Genetic control of development of the mushroom bodies, the associative learning centers in the *Drosophila* brain, by the eyeless, twin of eyeless, and Dachshund genes. *Proc Natl Acad Sci USA* 97(5): 2140–2144.

Lauderdale JD, et al. (2000). 3′ Deletions cause aniridia by preventing *PAX6* gene expression. *Proc Natl Acad Sci USA* 97(25): 13755–13759.

Lavedan C, et al. (1989). Molecular definition of de novo and genetically transmitted WAGR-associated rearrangements of 11p13. *Cytogenet Cell Genet* 50(2–3): 70–74.

Malandrini A, et al. (2001). PAX6 mutation in a family with aniridia, congenital ptosis, and mental retardation. *Clin Genet* 60(2): 151–154.

Marquardt T, Gruss P (2002). Generating neuronal diversity in the retina: one for nearly all. *Trends Neurosci* 25(1): 32–38.

Marquardt T, et al. (2001). Pax6 is required for the multipotent state of retinal progenitor cells. *Cell* 105(1): 43–55.

Martha A, et al. (1995). Three novel aniridia mutations in the human *PAX6* gene. *Hum Mutat* 6(1): 44–49.

Matsunaga E, Araki I, Nakamura H (2000). Pax6 defines the di–mesencephalic boundary by repressing En1 and Pax2. *Development* 127(11): 2357–2365.

Matsuo T, et al. (1993). A mutation in the *Pax-6* gene in rat small eye is associated with impaired migration of midbrain crest cells. *Nat Genet* 3(4): 299–304.

McGaughran JM, Ward HB, Evans DR (1995). WAGR syndrome and multiple exostoses in a patient with del(11)(p11.2-p14.2). *J Med Genet* 32: 823–824.

Miles C, et al. (1998). Complete sequencing of the Fugu WAGR region from WT1 to PAX6: dramatic compaction and conservation of synteny with human chromosome 11p13. *Proc Natl Acad Sci USA* 95: 13068–13072.

Mintz-Hittner HA, et al. (1992). Criteria to detect minimal expressivity within families with autosomal dominant aniridia. *Am J Ophthalmol* 114(6): 700–707.

Mirzayans F, et al. (1995). Mutation of the *PAX6* gene in patients with autosomal dominant keratitis. *Am J Hum Genet* 57(3): 539–548.

Mitchell TN, Free SL, Williamson KA, Stevens JM, Churchill AJ, Hanson IM, Shorvon SD, Moore AT, Van Heyningen V, Sisodiya SM (2003). Polymicrogyria and abscence of pineal gland due to PAX6 mutation. *Ann Neurol* 53: 658–663.

Morrison D, et al. (2002). National study of microphthalmia, anophthalmia, and coloboma (MAC) in Scotland: investigation of genetic aetiology. *J Med Genet* 39(1): 16–22.

Muto R, et al. (2002). Prediction by FISH analysis of the occurrence of Wilms tumor in aniridia patients. *Am J Med Genet* 108(4): 285–289.

Nevin NC, Lim JH (1990). Syndrome of partial aniridia, cerebellar ataxia, and mental retardation—Gillespie syndrome. *Am J Med Genet* 35(4): 468–469.

Niederfuhr A, et al. (1998). A sequence-ready 3-Mb PAC contig covering 16 breakpoints of the Wilms tumor aniridia region of human chromosome 11p13. *Genomics* 53: 155–163.

Nishina S, et al. (1999). PAX6 expression in the developing human eye. *Br J Ophthalmol* 83(6): 723–727.

Osumi N, et al. (1997). Pax-6 is involved in the specification of hindbrain motor neuron subtype. *Development* 124(15): 2961–2972.

Pennisi E (2002). Evolution of developmental diversity. Evo-devo devotees eye ocular origins and more. *Science* 296(5570): 1010–1011.

Pichaud F, Desplan C (2002). *Pax* genes and eye organogenesis. *Curr Opin Genet Dev* 12(4): 430–434.

Planque N, et al. (2001). Interaction of Maf transcription factors with Pax-6 results in synergistic activation of the glucagon promoter. *J Biol Chem* 276(38): 35751–35760.

Plaza S, Dozier C, Saule S (1993). Quail Pax-6 (Pax-QNR) encodes a transcription factor able to bind and trans-activate its own promoter. *Cell Growth Differ* 4(12): 1041–1050.

Plaza S, et al. (1995a). Identification and characterization of a neuroretina-specific enhancer element in the quail *Pax-6 (Pax-QNR)* gene. *Mol Cell Biol* 15(2): 892–903.

Plaza S, et al. (1995b). Quail Pax-6 (Pax-QNR) mRNAs are expressed from two promoters used differentially during retina development and neuronal differentiation. *Mol Cell Biol* 15(6): 3344–3353.

Pratt T, et al. (2000). A role for Pax6 in the normal development of dorsal thalamus and its cortical connections. *Development* 127(23): 5167–5178.

Prosser J, van Heyningen V (1998). PAX6 mutations reviewed. *Hum Mutat* 11(2): 93–108.

Punzo C, Kurata S, and Gehring WJ (2001). The eyeless homeodomain is dispensable for eye development in *Drosophila*. *Genes Dev* 15(13): 1716–1723.

Quiring R, et al. (1994). Homology of the eyeless gene of *Drosophila* to the Small eye gene in mice and aniridia in humans. *Science* 265(5173): 785–789.

Ramaesh T, Collinson JM, Ramaesh K, Kaufman MH, West JD, Dhillon B (2003). Corneal abnormalities in Pax6+/− small eye mice mimic human aniridia-related keratopathy. *Invest Ophthalmol Vis Sci* 44: 1871–1878.

Roberts RC (1967). Small eyes—a new dominant mutation in the mouse. *Genet Res* 9: 121–122.

Sakai M, et al. (2001). Regulation of c-*maf* gene expression by Pax6 in cultured cells. *Nucleic Acids Res* 29 (5): 1228–1237.

Scardigli R, et al. (2001). Crossregulation between Neurogenin2 and pathways specifying neuronal identity in the spinal cord. *Neuron* 31(2): 203–217.

Schedl A, et al. (1996). Influence of *PAX6* gene dosage on development: overexpression causes severe eye abnormalities. *Cell* 86(1): 71–82.

Schwartz F, et al. (1995). cDNA sequence, genomic organization, and evolutionary conservation of a novel gene from the WAGR region. *Genomics* 29: 526–532.

Seidman JG, Seidman C (2002). Transcription factor haploinsufficiency: when half a loaf is not enough. *J Clin Invest* 109(4): 451–455.

Singh S (1998). Truncation mutations in the transactivation region of PAX6 result in dominant-negative mutants. *J Biol Chem* 273(34): 21531–21541.

Singh S, et al. (2000). Modulation of PAX6 homeodomain function by the paired domain. *J Biol Chem* 275(23): 17306–17313.

Singh S, et al. (2001). Missense mutation at the C-terminus of PAX6 negatively modulates homeodomain function. *Hum Mol Genet* 10(9): 911–918.

Sisodiya SM, et al. (2001). PAX6 haploinsufficiency causes cerebral malformation and olfactory dysfunction in humans. *Nat Genet* 28(3): 214–216.

Sonoda S, et al. (2000). A novel *PAX6* gene mutation (P118R) in a family with congen-ital nystagmus associated with a variant form of aniridia. *Graefes Arch Clin Exp Ophthalmol* 238(7): 552–558.

St Onge L, et al. (1997). Pax6 is required for differentiation of glucagon-producing alpha-cells in mouse pancreas. *Nature* 387(6631): 406–409.

Stoykova A, Gruss P (1994). Roles of *Pax* genes in developing and adult brain as suggested by expression patterns. *J Neurosci* 14(3 Pt 2): 1395–1412.

Stoykova A, et al. (2000). Pax6 modulates the dorsoventral patterning of the mammalian telencephalon. *J Neurosci* 20(21): 8042–8050.

Takahashi M, Osumi N (2002). Pax6 regulates specification of ventral neurone subtypes in the hindbrain by establishing progenitor domains. *Development* 129(6): 1327–1338.

Tang HK, Chao LY, Saunders GF (1997). Functional analysis of paired box missense mutations in the *PAX6* gene. *Hum Mol Genet* 6(3): 381–386.

Tang HK, Singh S, Saunders GF (1998). Dissection of the transactivation function of the transcription factor encoded by the eye developmental gene *PAX6*. *J Biol Chem* 273(13): 7210–7221.

Thaung C, et al. (2002). Novel ENU-induced eye mutations in the mouse: models for human eye disease. *Hum Mol Genet* 11(7): 755–767.

Ton CC, et al. (1991). Positional cloning and characterization of a paired box– and home-obox-containing gene from the aniridia region. *Cell* 67(6): 1059–1074.

Turque N, et al. (1994). *Pax-QNR/Pax-6*, a paired box– and homeobox-containing gene expressed in neurons, is also expressed in pancreatic endocrine cells. *Mol Endocrinol* 8(7): 929–938.

van Heyningen V (1997). Model organisms illuminate human genetics and disease. *Mol Med* 3(4): 231–237.

van Heyningen V, Williamson KA (2002). PAX6 in sensory development. *Hum Mol Genet* 11(10): 1161–1167.

van Heyningen V, et al. (1985). Molecular analysis of chromosome 11 deletions in aniridia-Wilms tumor syndrome. *Proc Natl Acad Sci USA* 82(24): 8592–8596.

van Heyningen V, et al. (1990). Role for the Wilms tumor gene in genital development? *Proc Natl Acad Sci USA* 87(14): 5383–5386.

Vitalis T, et al. (2000). Defect of tyrosine hydroxylase-immunoreactive neurons in the brains of mice lacking the transcription factor Pax6. *J Neurosci* 20(17): 6501–6516.

Walther C, Gruss P (1991). *Pax-6*, a murine paired box gene, is expressed in the developing CNS. *Development* 113(4): 1435–1449.

Williams SC, et al. (1998). A highly conserved lens transcriptional control element from the *Pax-6* gene. *Mech Dev* 73(2): 225–229.

Wolf MT, et al. (1998). Ten novel mutations found in aniridia. *Hum Mutat* 12(5): 304–313.

Xu ZP, Saunders GF (1998). PAX6 intronic sequence targets expression to the spinal cord. *Dev Genet* 23(4): 259–263.

Yasuda T, et al. (2002). PAX6 mutation as a genetic factor common to aniridia and glucose intolerance. *Diabetes* 51(1): 224–230.

Zhang Y, Emmons SW (1995). Specification of sense-organ identity by a *Caenorhabditis elegans* Pax-6 homologue. *Nature* 377(6544): 55–59.

Zheng JB, et al. (2001). Activation of the human *PAX6* gene through the exon 1 enhancer by transcription factors SEF and Sp1. *Nucleic Acids Res* 29(19): 4070–4078.

63 | *PAX9* and Hypodontia

PRAGNA I. PATEL AND DONALD T. BROWN

The most common abnormality affecting the formation of the dentition is deviation from the usual number of the human permanent dentition (a total of 32 teeth in both jaws) or the deciduous dentition (20 total teeth in both jaws). When the number of teeth is less than the normal complement of dentition, the condition is known as *hypodontia*. Other anomalies seen in association with hypodontia include small tooth size (*microdontia*) and anomalies in tooth shape, most commonly tapering or "peg-shaped" teeth (McKeown et al., 2001; Brook et al., 2002). Frameshift, nonsense, and missense mutations in the human *PAX9* gene have been associated with hypodontia involving primarily posterior teeth. Severe hypodontia associated with a submicroscopic deletion involving loss of the entire gene in one family supports a model implicating haploinsufficiency of *PAX9* as the primary cause for hypodontia involving molar teeth. Both primary and permanent dentition are affected, with the effects being more prominent in the case of permanent teeth. PAX9 is a member of a family of transcription factors characterized by a common DNA-binding domain called the paired domain. It is highly homologous to PAX1, with which it shares an overlapping pattern of expression. PAX9 is a 342–amino acid protein encoded by a single gene mapping to human chromosome 14q21. Homozygous *Pax9* mutant mice die shortly following birth. They lack a thymus, parathyroid glands, and ultimobranchial bodies. Mutant mice have a cleft secondary palate at birth, and tooth development is arrested at the bud stage, resulting in the absence of all teeth. Heterozygous mutants display no discernible defects.

LOCUS AND DEVELOPMENTAL PATHWAY

As discussed in Chapter 59, *PAX9* is the ninth member of the paired domain–containing family of genes and encodes a 342–amino acid protein encoded by a single gene mapping to human chromosome 14q21 and to mouse chromosome 12 (Stapleton et al., 1993; Wallin et al., 1993). The paired domain constitutes 125 amino acids at the amino-terminal end of the protein, followed by a highly hydrophilic 76-residue region rich in proline, serine and glutamine residues. This is followed by a conserved octapeptide sequence and then the carboxy-terminal portion of the protein (Fig. 63–1). *PAX9* is highly homologous to *PAX1*, particularly within the paired box domain, and belongs to one of four *PAX* gene subfamilies whose members lack a paired-type homeodomain. The *Pax9* gene has been identified in several vertebrates, including zebrafish (Nornes et al., 1996), chick (Muller et al., 1996), mouse (Wallin et al., 1993), and human (Stapleton et al., 1993). In zebrafish, two putative proteins, Pax9a and Pax9b, have been implicated that are identical for 212 amino acids from the N terminus, including the 125–amino acid paired domain and the conserved octapeptide sequence, but differ in the C-terminal sequences downstream of the octapeptide (Nornes et al., 1996) (Fig. 63–1). Examination of the murine *Pax9* genomic sequence suggests that expression of a Pax9b protein is feasible by skipping exon 3, akin to the situation described in zebrafish (Nornes et al., 1996). Zebrafish Pax9 has a DNA-binding specificity that is distinct from Pax6 but similar to that for Pax1 and –2 (Nornes et al., 1996). A Pax9-specific target DNA sequence has not been identified.

PAX9 expression displays a spatially and temporally restricted pattern during development, suggesting a critical role in morphogenesis (Neubuser et al., 1995). As well, *Pax9* and *Pax1* expression follows an overlapping but not identical pattern during murine development

(Neubuser et al., 1995). In the developing vertebral column, *Pax9* expression is first evident around embryonic day 8.5 in the epithelium of the foregut. By E9.5, it is expressed in the pharyngeal pouches, the caudal half of each sclerotome, the hindgut, and the underlying mesenchyme. Beginning at E11.5, in addition to expression in these structures, high levels of *Pax9* expression are evident in the limb buds and in multiple locations within the nonneural parts of the head, including the nasal mesenchyme, the mandibulary and maxillary components of the first branchial arch, and the tongue. The complex expression pattern of *Pax9* during murine development suggests that it plays a crucial role in organogenesis. Indeed, disruption of the *Pax9* gene in the mouse results in severe developmental anomalies, including lack of a thymus, parathyroid glands, and ultimobranchial bodies as well as complete absence of teeth (Peters et al., 1998a). Deformities of all limbs, the craniofacial region, and visceral skeleton also result from complete *Pax9* deficiency. In humans, mutations in *PAX9* result in the congenital absence of predominantly posterior teeth, particularly molar teeth (Stockton et al., 2000).

Pax9 and *Pax1* are two members of the PAX family of genes that are most closely related with an overall protein sequence similarity of 79% (Neubuser et al., 1995). The sequences of the carboxy termini of the proteins are, however, completely divergent. The genes display an overlapping yet distinct pattern of expression in the sclerotomes, which represent the ventromedial compartment of the somites that form the vertebral column. They also display an overlapping pattern of expression in the endodermally derived epithelium of the pharyngeal pouches, which gives rise to the thymus, parathyroid glands, ultimobranchial bodies, Eustachian tube, and tonsils. Expression of *Pax9* and *Pax1* is observed in adjacent, nonoverlapping, mesenchymal domains of the limbs. Notably, however, while wide expression of *Pax9* is seen in the neural crest–derived mesenchyme that develops into craniofacial structures including teeth, *Pax1* expression is not observed in these regions. Furthermore, *Pax9* expression is independent of *Pax1* expression, as demonstrated by normal *Pax9* expression in *Pax1* mutant embryos (Neubuser et al., 1995).

Pax9 AND TOOTH DEVELOPMENT

Tooth development is a result of complex, reciprocal interactions between the dental epithelium and mesenchyme, with a shift of odontogenic potential to and fro between these tissues (see Chapter 15). Odontogenesis is initiated in the dental epithelium between E9.0 and E11.5, with the first morphological sign being the appearance of the dental lamina. The latter then grows into the underlying mesenchyme of the first branchial arch to form an epithelial bud (bud stage, E13.5). Mesenchymal cells then collect around the bud forming the dental papilla, the precursor to the tooth pulp and dentin-secreting odontoblasts. This is followed by additional soft tissue phases, including the cap stage (E14.5), during which odontoblasts are formed, and the bell stage (E15.5), when the enamel-depositing ameloblasts are formed.

Several transcription factors, growth factors, signaling molecules, and extracellular matrix molecules are expressed in a spatially and temporally restricted pattern in the epithelium and mesenchyme during the odontogenic process (see Chapter 15). The ability to perform tissue-recombination experiments to combine oral epithelium with non-dental neural crest–derived mesenchyme and aboral epithelium with dental mesenchyme has advanced our understanding of the hier-

Figure 63–1. Schematic diagram of the *PAX9* gene and location of mutations in hypodontia patients. (*A*) Top diagram shows human exons and introns. *Pax9a* and *Pax9b* represent the alternatively spliced isoforms described in zebrafish. (*B*) The PAX9 protein, showing the paired domain and conserved octapeptide. Locations of mutations described in hypodontia patients are indicated above the protein.

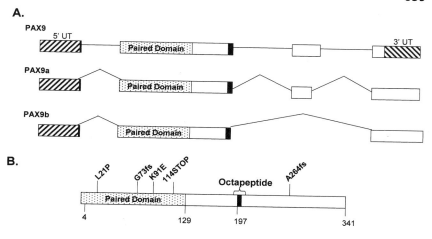

archy and role of the various factors in the odontogenic process (Mina and Kollar, 1987; Lumsden, 1988). *Pax9* is key among these factors, and its expression is noted at prospective sites of all teeth before there are any morphological signs of odontogenesis (Neubuser et al., 1997). Thus, *Pax9* expression can be seen in the mesenchyme of the mandibular arch at the prospective site of the molar from E10.0 onward, followed by expression at the prospective sites of the incisors; and expression is seen until E16.5. Expression of *Pax9* in the mandibular arch is induced by diffusible factors present in the oral epithelium, and candidates for these are Fgf8 and Fgf9, members of the fibroblast growth factor family (Neubuser et al., 1997). *Fgf8* is, however, expressed widely in the oral epithelium, thereby raising the question as to the mechanism underlying the restricted pattern of expression of *Pax9* only in prospective sites of tooth formation. Bone morphogenetic protein 4 (Bmp4) and Bmp2, members of the transforming growth factor β family, are candidates for molecules that antagonize the *Pax9*-inducing activity of Fgf8, and this has been proven by studies using in vitro explants (Neubuser et al. 1997). As well, the patterns of expression of *Bmp2* and *Bmp4* are in agreement with this hypothesis.

At E11.5, the odontogenic potential shifts from the epithelium to the mesenchyme concomitantly with a shift in *Bmp4* expression to the dental mesenchyme from the epithelium. At this stage, the bud stage, both *Pax9* and *Msx1* are expressed in the mesenchyme and their expression is key to the maintenance of the odontogenic potential of the dental mesenchyme. *Pax9* expression now becomes independent of activating epithelial signals as well as the inhibitory effects of BMPs (Neubuser et al., 1997). As well, Pax9 and Msx1 play a regulatory role in the maintenance of *Bmp4* expression and signaling, which is important in the induction of the transient enamel knot, which guides the next stage of tooth development. Interestingly, tooth development in both *Pax9* and *Msx1* mutant mice is arrested at the bud stage (Satokata and Maas, 1994; Peters et al., 1998b), thus suggesting their similar and nonredundant roles in signaling progression to the cap stage of tooth development.

CLINICAL FEATURES OF HYPODONTIA

Hypodontia is the most common abnormality affecting the formation of the dentition. Hypodontia of the primary dentition is uncommon, with a prevalence rate of <0.5%, and has no significant sex distribution difference (Tavajohi-Kermani et al., 2002). It is often followed by hypodontia in the same region of the permanent dentition. The prevalence of hypodontia in the permanent dentition, excluding third molars, ranges between 2.3% and 10% (Rose, 1966). Typically, a third of the hypodontia patients surveyed have one or more affected first-degree relative (Brook, 1984). The prevalence of hypodontia in relation to severity has been studied quite extensively. Most hypodontia cases, ranging from 80% to 85% in different studies, involve the absence of one or two teeth (Muller et al., 1970). Agenesis of six or more missing teeth, classified as severe hypodontia or oligodontia, is much less prevalent and occurs in roughly 0.5% of the population (Hobkirk and Brook, 1980). The tooth most commonly missing is the

third molar (or wisdom tooth) in as much as 20% of the population (Lavelle et al., 1970; Shapiro and Farrington, 1983). The second most commonly missing tooth is reported to be the maxillary lateral incisor by some investigators (Brekhus et al., 1944; Muller et al., 1970) and the mandibular second premolar by others (Dolder, 1937; Grahnen, 1956). The lowest incidence of tooth agenesis occurs in the lower central and lateral permanent incisors. Agenesis of maxillary permanent central incisors, maxillary permanent cuspids, and maxillary permanent first molars is rare (Tavajohi-Kermani et al., 2002).

Hypodontia can be found as an independent congenital oral trait (nonsyndromic) or with a generalized syndrome, or it can be acquired. It is an associated finding in at least 49 syndromes listed in the Online Mendelian Inheritance in Man database (http://www.nlbi.nlm. nih.gov/omim). The nonsyndromic form of hypodontia can be sporadic or familial. There have been reports of hypodontia inherited in an autosomal-dominant, autosomal-recessive, or X-linked fashion. The autosomal-dominant pattern of single gene inheritance has been suggested most frequently for hypodontia. The autosomal-dominant form displays phenotypic heterogeneity, as measured by the nature of the missing teeth and other alterations in the teeth. This is related to genetic heterogeneity illustrated by positional cloning of two underlying genes, *MSX1* (Vastardis et al., 1996) (see Chapter 51) and *PAX9* (Stockton et al., 2000) an unknown gene on chromosome 10 (Liu et al., 2001), and possibly another gene(s) (Vastardis, 1996; Arte et al., 2001). Hypodontia has also been attributed to polygenic inheritance (Suarez and Spence, 1974).

The permanent dentition of a typical patient with a *PAX9* mutation reveals a consistent pattern of severe hypodontia involving the majority of molar teeth. The primary dentition in these individuals varies from being apparently normal to missing one or more primary molar teeth. Craniofacial symmetry is normal, although the absence of posterior teeth results in a noticeable reduction in the vertical dimensions of the face. Decreased maxillary jaw size is also a common finding. Intraoral examination typically reveals multiple missing teeth in all four quadrants accompanied by atrophy of maxillary and mandibular alveolar ridges. Those teeth present are spaced apart but are of healthy periodontal status, as indicated from normal probing depths. All erupted permanent teeth typically show reduced mesiodistal dimensions when compared to unaffected siblings or relatives. In addition, the permanent maxillary lateral incisors appear peg-like. In cases where succedaneous teeth are missing, i.e., second premolars and lower central incisors, the primary predecessors are commonly retained in the arches.

Figure 63–2 shows the intraoral cavities of a pair of identical twins bearing an insertion mutation within the *PAX9* gene. While the overall pattern of missing teeth is similar, differences in the identities of some of the missing teeth are interesting to note, suggesting that nongenetic environmental or unknown stochastic factors can influence the clinical phenotype in patients. Likewise, Figure 63–3 shows a panoramic radiograph of an 11-year-old girl and her mother, demonstrating a similar variation in the identity of the teeth missing. Figure

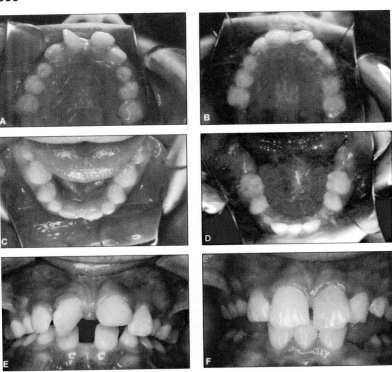

Figure 63–2. Intraoral photographs of 10-year-old identical twins with 288 bp insertion within the second exon of the *PAX9* gene. Twin A is shown in panels *A*, *C*, and *E* and twin B is shown in panels *B*, *D*, and *F*. Twin A is missing all maxillary second premolars and molars, the right mandibular central incisor, and all right and left mandibular first and third molars. Twin B is missing all maxillary second premolars and molars, the mandibular central incisors, and the mandibular second and third molars.

63–4 shows a schematic representation of the pattern of missing teeth in 9 members of a family we studied within which a missense mutation in *PAX9* was found to be segregating (Das et al., 2002a). There is variable expressivity of the phenotype since different members of the same sibship (III:9, III:10; V:5, V:6) and extended members of the family have a similar, but not identical, pattern of missing teeth. This is likely due to the effect of unknown modifying genes and other nongenetic stochastic factors.

Figure 63–5 shows an analysis of data published on the permanent dentition of 43 hypodontia patients with a *PAX9* mutation (Goldenberg et al., 2000; Nieminen et al., 2001; Frazier-Bowers et al., 2002; Das et al., 2002a,b). When including third molars, patients were missing an average of 14 teeth. With the exception of one patient who was

missing only two third molars (Das et al., 2002b), all other patients did not bear any third molars. Similarly, except for one patient who retained her second molars (Das et al., 2002b), all other patients were missing at least one second molar, with >74.4% missing all of their second molars. Over 9.3% of patients retained all of their first molars, while roughly a third of patients were missing all of their first molars. Thus, overall these data are consistent with a *PAX9* mutation being typically associated with the absence of all second and third molars and at least two first molars. Some patients were missing other classes of teeth as well, particularly second premolars, central incisors, and/or lateral incisors: 84% of patients were missing one or more second pre-

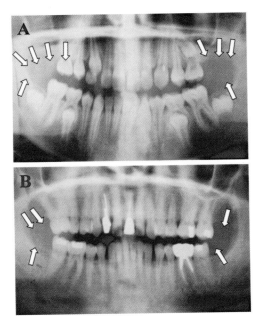

Figure 63–3. Panoramic radiographs illustrating hypodontia in an 11-year-old girl (*A*) and her mother (*B*) caused by a missense mutation in *PAX9*.

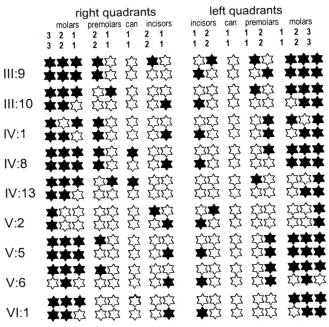

Figure 63–4. Schematic representation of the hypodontia phenotype in members of a family segregating a missense mutation in *PAX9*. Filled and open stars indicate missing teeth and teeth present, respectively. can, canines.

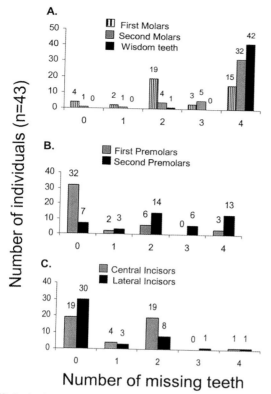

Figure 63–5. Analysis of data on hypodontia of permanent dentition of 43 individuals bearing mutations in the *PAX9* gene. The actual number of individuals missing each class of tooth is indicated above each bar.

molars, while 56% and 30% of patients were missing central and lateral incisors, respectively. It remains to be seen whether the absence of incisor teeth is truly associated with modifier gene effects on the *PAX9* mutation or if these effects are attributable to distinct mutations in another gene(s) also segregating within the same families.

MUTATIONS IN *PAX9* ASSOCIATED WITH HYPODONTIA

Our laboratory first reported the association of a mutation in *PAX9* with oligodontia (Stockton et al., 2000). We studied a large family segregating autosomal dominant oligodontia involving primarily molars (Goldenberg et al., 2000; Stockton et al., 2000). The proband and his two affected brothers had several developmentally absent permanent teeth. The most severely affected family member lacked 18 permanent teeth, including all maxillary and mandibular first, second, and third molars; second premolars; as well as mandibular central incisors. In the least affected member, all maxillary and mandibular second and third molars, maxillary first molars, first premolars, as well as mandibular central incisors were absent. Forty-three members of the family were sampled, of whom 19 were affected. To identify the locus responsible for the molar hypodontia, a genomewide search was performed, which localized the gene to a 25 cM interval in chromosome 14 q21. *PAX9* had been previously mapped to this region by fluorescence in situ hybridization, and this map location was confirmed using a radiation hybrid panel. Sequencing of exon 2 of *PAX9* revealed an insertion of a G residue at nucleotide 218 (+1 = A of ATG codon) (Stockton et al., 2000). The mutation results in an abnormal amino acid sequence starting at amino acid 73, which is in a highly conserved region 70 amino acids into the paired domain and between the N-terminal and C-terminal DNA-binding domains. A premature stop codon is created 243 amino acids after the insertion, reducing the size of the protein by 25 amino acid residues. A frameshift mutation resulting from insertion of a G residue at nucleotide +793 and premature truncation at amino acid 315 was recently reported (Frazier-

Bowers et al., 2002). Several other categories of mutations within *PAX9* have been reported in families with hypodontia. Nieminen et al. (2001) reported a nonsense mutation at amino acid residue 114 within the paired domain. We found missense mutations in two large families that resulted in substitution of glutamic acid for lysine at residue 91 and proline for leucine at residue 21, both within the paired domain of PAX9 (Das et al., 2002b). In addition to these single-base mutations, we recently reported a 288 bp insertion within exon 2 that resulted in a frameshift at residue 58 and premature truncation of the protein at residue 177 (Das et al., 2002b). As well, we reported a submicroscopic deletion of >57 kb involving the *PAX9* gene in a small nuclear family affected with severe hypodontia of the primary and permanent dentition (Das et al., 2002a). Two genes map within the deletion interval in the latter family: *PAX9*, the only odontogenic gene within the interval, and *SLC25A21*, encoding a mitochondrial oxodicarboxylate carrier. The latter suggested that human *PAX9* is a dosage-sensitive gene, with haploinsufficiency resulting in hypodontia.

The mode of action of the submicroscopic deletion involving *PAX9* is quite obviously due to haploinsufficiency for *PAX9* (Das et al., 2002a). The functional effects of the other categories of mutations are less obvious; but given the phenotypic similarities between the patients with the large deletion and those with the other types of mutation, it may be reasonable to assume that an insufficient level of PAX9 or functionally inactive PAX9 results in hypodontia of posterior teeth. The frameshift, nonsense, and insertion mutations are predicted to result in proteins lacking part or all of the paired domain and might therefore be expected to cause loss of function. We have recently identified two missense mutations resulting in amino acid substitutions within the paired domain. It is possible that these proteins, whose synthesis and stability are likely not affected, fail to recognize the target DNA sequence, resulting in functional haploinsufficiency. The other possibility is that they may recognize new targets, resulting in a novel gain of function. Given the overall phenotypic similarities of these patients to those bearing the other classes of mutations, the former possibility is most likely the mechanism of action of the missense mutations. While patients with *PAX9* mutations typically lack at least six or more molar teeth, there is considerable intrafamilial variability in the identity of the teeth missing among affected members of the families within which various *PAX9* mutations are reported to segregate, and the molecular basis of this is largely unknown.

DIAGNOSTIC CONSIDERATIONS

Normal development of permanent teeth implies the presence of tooth buds for all permanent teeth by the preteen years and significant crown formation by the early teens. The exception to this may be the third molar teeth, which may have delayed development, not showing calcification until the late teen years. The congenital absence of a tooth cannot be established accurately unless one knows the dental age of the patient and the approximate timing of onset of calcification of the crowns of the teeth under normal circumstances. The dental age will determine if a tooth is missing or if there is delayed development of a tooth bud that has not begun to calcify. When hypodontia is suspected, the full extent of the condition may be diagnosed in patients of 8 years or older. Healthy premolars are unlikely to develop after age 8 years (Proffit, 1986). A detailed medical history and examination allows exclusion of (*1*) ectodermal dysplasia (associated with sparse hair and absence of sweating) and (*2*) specific syndromes where hypodontia is an associated feature, such as cleft lip and palate, Down syndrome, and Rieger's syndrome. A detailed medical and dental history, a detailed clinical dental examination, and radiographic studies (typically a panoramic radiograph, which gives a simultaneous view of the right and left sides of both upper and lower jaws on one film and will include any unerupted permanent teeth) are necessary. In conjunction with noting the patient's dental history and any supplementary information they may provide to rule out possible causes of tooth loss; tooth agenesis is then confirmed. Thus, phenocopies arising from events such as traumatic tooth loss, tooth decay, or extraction are greatly minimized. Anomalies such as ectopic canines, peg-shaped laterals, taurodontism, and rotated premolars, which have been noted in hypodontia families (Arte et al., 2001), are recorded. Dental transposition is an anomaly involving the positional interchange of two teeth and most commonly involves the maxillary canine and first premolar teeth. Peg-shaped or congenitally missing permanent lateral incisors frequently are associated with tooth transposition (Talbot and Hill, 2002). Tooth dimensions may be recorded on patient study models using image analysis techniques. All fully erupted, permanent, unrestored teeth on study models are measured (McKeown et al., 2001). Tooth dimensions include mesiodistal and buccolingual diameters as well as perimeter, area, and measures of tooth shape (taper). Dental records are evaluated to determine overlap with previously described forms of tooth anomaly. In each case/family, the consistent absence of several molar teeth would suggest that the patient(s) may bear a mutation in the *PAX9* gene, which could be tested by mutation analysis of *PAX9*. The absence of other classes of teeth in families with a *PAX9* mutation may be due to variable expressivity or to mutations in another gene(s).

MANAGEMENT OF HYPODONTIA

Therapeutic options include retaining the primary tooth, orthodontic treatment to close the edentulous spaces, dental surgical implants, and fixed or removable dental prosthetic appliances. The decision to close the space via orthodontic therapy is complex and determined by a number of issues. It is usually best if the space is closed and a natural tooth substituted for the missing one. The two treatment options available for treating missing maxillary permanent lateral incisors are (*1*) to open the space and prosthetically replace the missing tooth and (*2*) to close the space and use the permanent cuspid as the lateral incisor. The cuspid can be reshaped to obtain the best esthetics (Kokich, 2002). Retaining the primary tooth can be an option in an ideal occlusion. The lower primary second molars may be left in place and have been reported to be retained as long as the fourth to the sixth decade of life and usually remain useful at least until the early twenties. Some mesiodistal width reduction of these teeth may be necessary to achieve the best compromise of dental interdigitation.

Long-term retention of the maxillary primary lateral incisors is usually unacceptable due to the frequent resorption of their root structure by the erupting permanent cuspids. Many times, the erupting cuspid will spontaneously substitute for the maxillary permanent lateral incisors. In that case, the primary cuspid has no successor and the permanent bicuspid frequently must be moved into that position after removal of the primary cuspid (Proffit, 1986). If permanent teeth are absent and there is crowding of the existing dentition, extraction of the primary teeth and orthodontic treatment to close the space is often the best choice.

Early removal of retained primary second molar teeth with no successor at age 7–9 years will usually reduce the overall orthodontic treatment time, with mesial drift of the lower first molars occurring prior to the onset of comprehensive treatment in the teen years (Proffit, 1986).

Autotransplantation of the other natural teeth in the patient's mouth is a good alternative to the other treatments discussed if conditions permit. Unerupted teeth are the best candidates because their root apices are not fully formed and will have higher success rates. Tooth transplantation success rates have been 79% when studied 17–41 years posttreatment. Autotransplantation of developing premolars is becoming an attractive consideration because of their capacity for functional adaptation and preservation of the alveolar bony ridge (Czochrowska et al., 2002). Premolars and third molars are the best choices for autogenous transplantation because of their root contour, relative dispensability, and the late age at which they remain viable (Northway, 2002). Unerupted third molars that may be typically used for this purpose are unfortunately not available in the vast majority of patients with hypodontia due to *PAX9* mutations.

MUTATIONS IN ORTHOLOGOUS GENES

Much of what is known about vertebrate tooth development has been gleaned from studies in the mouse, aided by expression analyses of key genes in the developing mouse tooth organ, as well as by functional in vivo and in vitro tooth recombinations and bead implanta-

tion assays. In addition, dental anomalies apparent upon targeted inactivation of various genes have unearthed new molecular players, enabled delineation of the in vivo functions of these molecules, and provided strong candidates for human genetic conditions involving tooth anomalies. This is clearly illustrated by studies on the *Pax9* orthologue in the mouse. *Pax9*-deficient mice were generated in the Balling laboratory by insertion of a promoterless *Escherichia coli* ATG-*lacZ*-poly(A) cassette and the *PGK-neo* gene (Peters et al., 1998b). Heterozygous *Pax9^{lacZ}* mice are viable and fertile and do not display any discernible defects, suggesting that, in contrast to humans, *Pax9* is apparently not dosage-sensitive in mice. Homozygous *Pax9*-deficient mice die soon after birth and display numerous developmental anomalies. They lack a thymus, parathyroid glands, and ultimobranchial bodies, all of which are derivatives of the pharyngeal pouches. Examination of mutant embryos revealed that at E10.0 the pharyngeal pouches appeared normal. At E11.5, the development of the third and fourth pharyngeal pouches is retarded and the derivative organs, including the thymus and parathyroid lands, do not develop. Mutant mice have a cleft secondary palate at birth, and this is likely the cause of the respiratory difficulties in the pups that result in early mortality. The palatal shelves appear elevated and seem normal at E12.0 but begin to reveal an abnormal broad shape at E13.5. Pax9 is thus critical for regulation of the shape of palatal shelves but is apparently not required for their elevation. All teeth are also absent in homozygous animals. Histological analysis during development revealed that up to E12.5, normal and mutant mice showed no differences. However, at E13.5, there was a discernible difference in the extent of condensation of mesenchymal cells surrounding the bud, and at E14.5, only a rudimentary bud was evident in the mutant mice. These studies clearly illustrated that Pax9 is required for tooth development before or at the bud stage.

Pax9 is also required for skeletal development of the skull and larynx. Mutant animals had specific skeletal defects of craniofacial development. Malformations of the tympanic ring, Reichert's cartilage, hyoid bone, thyroid cartilage, and cricoid cartilage occurred, and these correlated with the embryonic expression of *Pax9* in these regions, with the exception of the laryngeal cartilages. Deformities in the latter are likely due to failure to interact with the pharyngeal endoderm. Homozygous *Pax9^{lacZ}* mice develop preaxial digit duplications in both forelimbs and hindlimbs. A small supernumerary toe is formed in the hindlimb, with a milder effect in the forelimb, where the supernumerary digit does not separate from the thumb.

The pleiotropic effects of *Pax9* deficiency suggest that Pax9 plays a key role in regulating organogenesis in widely differing anatomical parts of the developing mouse. These regulatory functions are neither cell-specific nor restricted to a particular germ cell layer. The common denominator is the apparent existence of PAX9-binding sequences in the regulatory domains of genes that play a critical role in the development of the various organs in which *Pax9* is expressed and that are affected in deficient animals. Not all organs revealing *Pax9* expression during development are affected, however, in the mutants. These include the salivary glands, epithelia lining the upper digestive tract, tail, elbow, knee, tongue, and brain. It is plausible that the early death of mutant mice precludes analysis of the effect of Pax9 deficiency on these organs and structures and may require examination in conditional knockout mice (Peters et al., 1998a).

DEVELOPMENTAL PATHOGENESIS

The prospective sites of tooth development are marked by *Pax9* expression well before there are any physical signs of tooth morphogenesis. In *Pax9*-deficient mice, there is a failure of the mesenchyme to condense around the epithelial bud, thus arresting tooth development at the bud stage (Peters et al., 1998b). *Msx1*-deficient mice show the same phenotype (Satokata and Maas, 1994). Moreover, *Pax9* and *Msx1* show overlapping patterns of expression, thus supporting the hypothesis that they act in the same developmental pathway. Expression of *Msx1* and *Bmp4* is thought to be maintained in the dental mesenchyme via a positive feedback loop and may be essential to allow progression from the bud to the cap stage.

Peters et al. (1998a) investigated whether *Pax9*-deficient embryos had lost their potential for epithelial morphogenesis, by conducting tissue recombination experiments. The combination of *Pax9*-deficient E13.5 mesenchyme and normal epithelium failed to form teeth, while the combination of normal mesenchyme and *Pax9*-deficient epithelium yielded at least one tooth per graft. Thus, these studies show that the effects of *Pax9* deficiency on epithelial development can be overcome by normal mesenchyme from the bud stage.

Molecular changes in dental mesenchyme are affected by a number of molecules, including Bmp4, Msx1, lymphoid enhancer-binding factor 1 (Lef1), and Pax9. Analysis of the expression of these genes in *Pax9*-deficient mice determined that, while at E12.0 the expression of *Bmp4*, *Msx1*, and *Lef1* was normal, by E13.5 mesenchymal *Bmp4* expression was very low, as was that of *Msx1* and *Lef1* (Peters et al., 1998a). Bmp4 induces expression of *Msx1* and *Lef1*; thus, it appears that Pax9 is required to maintain *Bmp4* expression in the dental mesenchyme, and its downregulation has a direct impact on *Msx1* and *Lef1* expression. Maintenance of the expression of *Bmp4*, shown to be involved in enamel knot induction in the next stage of odontogenesis, may require *Pax9* expression. Thus, at a critical stage of tooth development, Pax9 may act upstream of Bmp4, Msx1, and Lef1. Supporting this hypothesis is the observation that *Pax9* expression is apparently unaltered in homozygous *Msx1* and *Lef1* embryos.

Heterozygous dominant mutations in *MSX1* (Vastardis et al. 1996) and *PAX9* (Stockton et al., 2000) each affect the third molars, or "wisdom teeth," with the majority of patients displaying agenesis of these teeth. In addition to the absence of third molars, *PAX9* mutations affect formation of the first and second molars and occasionally the maxillary second premolars, while *MSX1* mutations are characterized by absence of the second premolars. Direct comparisons with the mouse are impeded by the simpler dentition in mice, with the presence of only incisors and molar teeth. However, these observations in human tooth anomalies suggest that, while *MSX1* and *PAX9* may act in the same developmental pathway, their unique spatially restricted expression pattern may signal the specification of different shapes of teeth. This is in keeping with the theory of an overlapping odontogenic homeobox code, first proposed by Sharpe (1995), wherein he suggested that overlapping domains of several homeobox genes in mandibular mesenchyme might determine the shape of teeth that develop at a particular position. *PAX9* likely represents the odontogenic code for the development of molars in humans, given the dramatic deleterious effect of *PAX9* mutations on the development of permanent human molars. Opposing or synergistic effects of a modifier gene(s) may play a role in the variable expressivity of a mutation in *PAX9*, resulting in different overall patterns of hypodontia in individual patients within a family.

ACKNOWLEDGMENTS

We thank A. Rohr, P. Das and T. Bowerman for assistance with graphics. We are grateful to the families who shared clinical data for this chapter and their dentists for providing it. The authors acknowledge support from NIH grant DE14102 and grants from the Texas Applied Technology Program and the American Association of Orthodontists Foundation.

REFERENCES

Arte S, Nieminen P, Apajalahti S, Haavikko K, Thesleff I, Pirinen S (2001). Characteristics of incisor-premolar hypodontia in families. *J Dent Res* 80: 1445–1450.

Brekhus P, Oliver C, Montelius G (1944). A study of the pattern and combination of congenitally missing teeth in man. *J Dent Res* 23: 117–131.

Brook AH (1984). A unifying aetiological explanation for anomalies of human tooth number and size. *Arch Oral Biol* 29: 373–378.

Brook AH, Elcock C, Al-Sharood MH, McKeown HF, Khalaf K, Smith RN (2002). Further studies of a model for the aetiology of anomlies of tooth number and size in humans. *Connect Tiss Res* 43: 289–295.

Czochrowska EM, Stenvik A, Bjercke B, Zachrisson BU (2002). Outcome of tooth transplantation: survival and success rates 17–41 years posttreatment. *Am J Orthod Dentofacial Orthop* 121: 110–119.

Das P, Stockton DW, Bauer C, Shaffer LG, D'Souza RN, Wright JT, Patel PI (2002a).

Haploinsufficiency of *PAX9* is associated with autosomal dominant hypodontia. *Hum Genet* 110: 371–376.

Das P, Hai M, Elcock C, Leal S, Brown DT, Brook AH, Patel PI (2003). Novel missense mutations and a 288-bp exonic insertion in the *PAX9* gene in families with autosomal dominant hypodontia. *Am J Med Genet* 118A: 35–42.

Dolder E (1937). Deficient dentition. *Dent Pract Dent Rec* 57: 142.

Frazier-Bowers SA, Guo DC, Cavender A, Xue L, Evans B, King T, Milewicz D, D'Souza RN (2002). A novel mutation in human *PAX9* causes molar oligodontia. *J Dent Res* 81: 129–133.

Goldenberg M, Das P, Messersmith M, Stockton DW, Patel PI, D'Souza RN (2000). Clinical, radiographic and genetic evaluation of a novel form of autosomal dominant oligodontia. *J Dent Res* 79: 1469–1475.

Grahnen HJ (1956). Hypodontia in the permanent dentition. *Odontologisk Revy* 7: 1.

Hobkirk JA, Brook AH (1980). The management of patients with severe hypodontia. *J Oral Rehabil* 7: 289–298.

Kokich VO Jr (2002). Congenitally missing teeth: orthodontic management in the adolescent patient. *Am J Orthod Dentofacial Orthop* 121: 594–595.

Lavelle CL, Ashton EH, Flinn RM (1970). Cusp pattern, tooth size and third molar agenesis in the human mandibular dentition. *Arch Oral Biol* 15: 227–237.

Liu W, Wang H, Zhao S, Zhao W, Bai S, Zhao Y, Xu S, Wu C, Huang W, Chen Z, et al. (2001). The novel gene locus for agenesis of permanent teeth (He-Zhao deficiency) maps to chromosome 10q11.2. *J Dent Res* 80: 1716–1720.

Lumsden AG (1988). Spatial organization of the epithelium and the role of neural crest cells in the initiation of the mammalian tooth germ. *Development* 103(Suppl): 155–169.

McKeown HF, Robinson DL, Elcock C, Brook AH (2001). Tooth dimensions in hypodontia patients, their unaffected relatives and a control group measured by a new image analysis system. *Eur J Orthod* 24: 131–141.

Mina M, Kollar EJ (1987). The induction of odontogenesis in non-dental mesenchyme combined with early murine mandibular arch epithelium. *Arch Oral Biol* 32: 123–127.

Muller TP, Hill IN, Peterson AC, Blayney JR (1970). A survey of congenitally missing permanent teeth. *J Am Dent Assoc* 81: 101–107.

Muller TS, Ebensperger C, Neubuser A, Koseki H, Balling R, Christ B, Wilting J (1996). Expression of avian Pax1 and Pax9 is intrinsically regulated in the pharyngeal endoderm, but depends on environmental influences in the paraxial mesoderm. *Dev Biol* 178: 403–417.

Neubuser A, Koseki H, Balling R (1995). Characterization and developmental expression of *Pax9*, a paired-box-containing gene related to *Pax1*. *Dev Biol* 170: 701–716.

Neubuser A, Peters H, Balling R, Martin GR (1997). Antagonistic interactions between FGF and BMP signaling pathways: a mechanism for positioning the sites of tooth formation. *Cell* 90: 247–255.

Nieminen P, Arte S, Tanner D, Paulin L, Alaluusua S, Thesleff I, Pirinen S (2001). Identification of a nonsense mutation in the *PAX9* gene in molar oligodontia. *Eur J Hum Genet* 9: 743–746.

Nornes S, Mikkola I, Krauss S, Delghandi M, Perander M, Johansen T (1996). Zebrafish Pax9 encodes two proteins with distinct C-terminal transactivating domains of different potency negatively regulated by adjacent N-terminal sequences. *J Biol Chem* 271: 26914–26923.

Northway W (2002). Autogenic dental transplants. *Am J Orthod Dentofacial Orthop* 121: 592–593.

Peters H, Neubuser A, Kratochwil K, Balling R (1998a). *Pax-9* deficient mice lack pharyngeal pouch derivatives and teeth and exhibit craniofacial and limb abnormalities. *Genes Dev* 12: 2735–2747.

Peters H, Neubuser A, Kratochwil K, Balling R (1998b). Pax9-deficient mice lack pharyngeal pouch derivatives and teeth and exhibit craniofacial and limb abnormalities. *Genes Dev* 12: 2735–2747.

Proffit WR (1986). Treatment of non-skeletal problems in preadolescent children. In: *Contemporary Orthodontics*. C.V. Mosby, St. Louis, pp. 312–353.

Rose JS (1966). A survey of congenitally missing teeth, excluding third molars, in 6000 orthodontic patients. *Dent Pract Dent Rec* 17: 107–114.

Satokata I, Maas R (1994). Msx1 deficient mice exhibit cleft palate and abnormalities of craniofacial and tooth development. *Nat Genet* 6: 348–356.

Shapiro SD, Farrington FH (1983). A potpourri of syndromes with anomalies of dentition. *Birth Defects* 19: 129–140.

Sharpe PT (1995). Homeobox genes and orofacial development. *Connect Tissue Res* 32: 17–25.

Stapleton P, Weith A, Urbanek P, Kozmik Z, Busslinger M (1993). Chromosomal localization of seven *PAX* genes and cloning of a novel family member, *PAX-9*. *Nat Genet* 3: 292–298.

Stockton DW, Das P, Goldenberg M, D'Souza RN, Patel PI (2000). Mutation of PAX9 is associated with oligodontia. *Nat Genet* 24: 18–19.

Suarez BK, Spence MA (1974). The genetics of hypodontia. *J Dent Res* 53: 781–785.

Talbot TQ, Hill AJ (2002). Transposed and impacted maxillary canine with ipsilateral congenitally missing lateral incisor. *Am J Orthod Dentofacial Orthop* 121: 316–323.

Tavajohi-Kermani H, Kapur R, Sciote JJ (2002). Tooth agenesis and craniofacial morphology in an orthodontic population. *Am J Orthod Dentofacial Orthop* 122: 39–47.

Vastardis H (1996). Genetic approaches to understanding tooth development: a human *MSX1* homeodomain missense mutation causes selective tooth agenesis (dissertation). Boston, MA: Harvard University.

Vastardis H, Karimbux N, Guthua SW, Seidman IG, Seidman CE (1996). A human MSX 1 homeodomain missense mutation causes selective tooth agenesis. *Nat Genet* 13: 417–421.

Wallin J, Mizutani Y, Imai K, Miyashita N, Moriwaki K, Taniguchi M, Koseki H, Balling R (1993). A new Pax gene, *Pax-9*, maps to mouse chromosome 12. *Mamm Genome* 4: 354–358.

Part C.
The Forkhead Gene Family

64 | Introduction to Forkhead Genes

NAOYUKI MIURA, TAO WANG, AND TOMOKI TAMAKOSHI

HISTORY OF FORKHEAD (WINGED HELIX) GENES

Among the genes that determine development, cell fate, and differentiation in higher organisms, transcription factors play key roles in morphogenesis. Forkhead (winged helix) is one of these transcription factors. A *Drosophila* mutant was found and named *fork head* (*fkh*) (Weigel et al., 1989). *Fkh* mutations cause homeotic transformation of ectodermal portions of the gut: foregut and hindgut are replaced by ectopic head structures in *fkh* mutant embryos. A year later, a second transcription factor, named hepatocyte nuclear factor-3α (*HNF-3α*), a hepatocyte-enriched gene in the rat (Lai et al., 1990), was biochemically purified and cloned. In November 1990, in a letter to the editor of *Cell*, Weigel and Jackle (1990) reported a 100-amino acid conservation between *Drosophila* fkh and rat HNF-3α and named it the *forkhead domain*. Several laboratories started cloning the new family of genes with a forkhead domain. In 1993, the three-dimensional structure of HNF-3γ, a subfamily member of HNF-3α, was determined. The forkhead domain is comprised of the structure helix(H_1)-turn-helix(H_2)-turn-helix(H_3)-β sheet-loop(W_1)-β sheet-loop(W_2). It is characterized by two unique loops connected to the helix-turn-helix and thus was called *winged helix* (Clark et al. 1993). These authors showed that the domain contacts a target DNA mainly with the third helix and second loop as a monomer. Thus, *winged helix* is the same as *forkhead*; *winged helix* is a name for the three-dimensional structure and *forkhead* is a name for the amino acid con-

servation. More than 100 *forkhead* genes have now been cloned, about 30 of them in the mouse (Kaufman and Knochel, 1996).

In different species, these genes have been given such names as *MFH-1*, *Lun*, *Mf1–3*, *Bf1–2*, *fkh1–6*, *HFH1–8*, and *FREAC1–7*. In some cases, a partial cDNA and similar but distinct genes have been cloned. Researchers determined the expression pattern of the cloned gene and suggested its role in development. Gene knockout technology has been used to uncover the developmental roles of cloned genes in mice. The phenotypes of knockout mice were sometimes expected, sometimes unexpected.

As the number of *forkhead*/winged helix genes in higher organisms increased, confusion arose: one gene had several names, and two genes had similar names. To avoid such complexity and introduce a common language, a nomenclature conference was held at La Jolla in November 1998, and the participants agreed that we would call the *forkhead*/winged helix genes by a unified, systematic name, *Fox* (Forkhead box). Fox proteins were assigned to individual subclasses based on phylogenetic analysis. Subclasses were designated by a letter, and within each subclass proteins were given an Arabic numeral. Therefore, the current name of any Fox protein is "Fox, subclass N, member X," or, for example, "Foxc2." Abbreviations for chordate Fox proteins are upper-case letters for humans (e.g., FOXC2); only the first letter is capitalized for mice (e.g., Foxc2); and the first and subclass letters are capitalized for all other chordates (e.g., FoxC2) (Kaestner et al., 2000). Current assignments for the chordate Fox proteins are listed at the Fox

Table 64–1. New Nomenclature for *Fox* Genes*

Subclass Member	Subclass 1	2	3	4
A or a	HNF3α	HNF3β	HNF3γ	
B or b	Mf3/fkh5/TWH	fkh4		
C or c	Mf1/FKHL7	MFH1/FKHL14		
D or d	Bf2/FREAC4	Mf2	HFH2/genesis	HFH6/fkh2
E or e	TTF2/FKHL15	HFKH4	HKH7/FREAC8	
F or f	HFH8/FREAC1	Lun/FREAC2		
G or g	Bf1			
H or h	FAST			
I or i	HFH3/FREAC6/FRH10			
J or j	HFH4			
K or k	MNF			
L or l	fkh6/FREAC7			
M or m	HFH11/Trident			
N or n	WHN	HTLF	CHES1	
O or o	FKHR	AF6q21	FKHRL1	AFX
P or p	QRF		scurfin	
Q or q	HFH1L			

*Original names are placed across the columns (in rows) for each subclass (column headings) and subclass member (first column). For example, Foxc2 is the new systematic name of MFH-1, Foxf2 is that of Lun, Foxg1 is that of Bf1, and so on. Only frequently used names are shown.

Source: http://www.biology.pomona.edu/foxbyclass.html

nomenclature web site (http://www.biology.pomona.edu/fox.html). Systematic and original names are summarized in Table 64–1.

FORKHEAD FORMS SUBFAMILIES OF TRANSCRIPTION FACTORS

The forkhead domain is a DNA-binding domain. Conservation of the amino acid sequence in the forkhead domain among members varies from 95% to 30%. The family can be divided into subclasses depending on the degree of conservation of the forkhead domain. Subclass A consists of homologues of *fork head*. Subclass B is most similar to subclass A, subclass C is the next most similar, and so on. Subclass P means a lesser similarity to subclass A. Examples of amino acid sequences of Foxa, Foxc, Foxf, and Foxp proteins are listed in Figures 64–1 through 64–4, respectively. The HNF-3β identity of subclasses A, C, F, and P are about 95%, 70%, 55%, and 30%, respectively.

TARGET GENES OF FORKHEAD GENES

A transcription factor binds to a target DNA site and acts as a transcriptional activator or repressor. The amino acid sequences of the forkhead domain in Foxf1 and Foxf2 proteins are completely identi-

```
Foxa1    1  MLGTVKMEGHESNDWNSYYADTQEAYSSVPVSNMNSGLGSMNSMNTYMTMNTMTTSG--N    58
Foxa2    1  MLGAVKMEGLEPSDWSSYYAEPEG-YSSVS--NMNAGLG-MNGMNTYMSMSAAAMGGGSG    56
Foxa3    1  -----------------------------------------------------MLGSVK     6

Foxa1   59  -MTPASFNMS-YANT-GLGAGLSPGAVAGMPGAS--AGAMN-SMTAAGVTAMGTALSPGG   112
Foxa2   57  NMSAGSMNMSSYVGA-GMSPSLAGMSP-GAGAMA---GM-SGSAGAAGVAGMGPHLSPS-   109
Foxa3    7  -MEAHDLAEWSYYPEAGEVYSPVNPVP-TMAPLNSYMTLNPLSSPYPPGGLQASPLPTGP    64

Foxa1  113  MGSMGAQPATSMNGLGPYAAAMNPCMSPMAYAPSNLGRSRAGGGGDAKTFKRSYPHAKPP   172
Foxa2  110  LSPLGGQAAGAMGGLAPYANM-NS-MSPM-YGQAGLSRAR-----DPKTYRRSYTHAKPP   161
Foxa3   65  LAPPAPTAPLGPT-FPSLGTGGSTGGSASGYVAPGPGLVHGKEMA--KGYRRPLAHAKPP   121

Foxa1  173  YSYISLITMAIQQAPSKMLTLSEIYQWIMDLFPYYRQNQQRWQNSIRHSLSFNDCFVKVA   232
Foxa2  162  YSYISLITMAIQQSPNKMLTLSEIYQWIMDLFPFYRQNQQRWQNSIRHSLSFNDCFLKVP   221
Foxa3  122  YSYISLITMAIQQAPGKMLTLSEIYQWIMDLFPYYRENQQRWQNSIRHSLSFNDCFVKVA   181

Foxa1  233  RSPDKPGKGSYWTLHPDSGNMFENGCYLRRQKRFKCEKQPGAGGGSGGGGSKGGPESRKD   292
Foxa2  222  RSPDKPGKGSFWTLHPDSGNMFENGCYLRRQKRFKCEKQLALKEAAGAASSGGK----KT   277
Foxa3  182  RSPDKPGKGSYWALHPSSGNMFENGCYLRRQKRFKLEEKAKKGNSATSASRNGTAGSATS   241

Foxa1  293  -PSG-PGNPSAESPLHRGVHGKASQLE-GAPAPGPAASP-QTLDHSGATATGGASE--LK   346
Foxa2  278  AP-GSQA---SQAQLGEAAGSA-SETPAGTESPHSSASPCQEHKRGGLSELKGAPASALS   332
Foxa3  242  ATTTAATA------VTSP----------AQ--PQPT--PSEPEAQSGDDVGG------LD   275

Foxa1  347  SPASSSAPPISSGPGA-LASVPPSHPAHGLAPHESQLHLKGDPRYSFNHPFSINNLMSSS   405
Foxa2  333  PPEPAPSPGQQQQAAAHLLG-PPHHP--GLPPEA-H--LKPEHHYAFNHPFSINNLMSSE   386
Foxa3  276  CASP---PSSTPYFSG-LE----------LPGE-----LKLDAPYNFNHPFSINNLMSE-   315

Foxa1  406  EQQH----------KLDFKAYEQALQYSP-YGATLPASLPLGSASVATRSPIEPSALEP--   453
Foxa2  387  QQHHHSHHHHQPHKMDLKAYEQVMHYPGGYGSPMPGSLAMGPV--TNKAGLDASPLAADT   444
Foxa3  316  -QTST------PSKLDVG-FGG-------YGAES------GEPGV---------------   339

Foxa1  454  AYYQGVYSRPVLNTS   468
Foxa2  445  SYYQGVYSRPIMNSS   459
Foxa3  340  -YYQSLYSRSLLNAS   353
```

Figure 64–1. Amino acid sequences of *forkhead* orthologue, class A Fox proteins. Identical amino acids are boxed.

```
Foxc1    1  MQARYSVSSPNSLGVVPYLGGEQSYYRAAAAAAGGGMTAMPAPMSVYSHPAHAEQYPGSM   60
Foxc2    1  MQARYSVSDPNV-GVVPYLSEQN-YYRAAG-----SMGGMASPMGVYSG--HPEQYGAGM   51

Foxc1   61  ARAMGPYTPQPQP-KDMVKPPYSYIALITMAIQNAPDKKITLNGIYQFIMDRFPFYRDNK  119
Foxc2   52  GRSMAPYHHQHAAPKDLVKPPYSYIALITMAIQNAPEKKITLNGIYQFIMDRFPFYRENK  111

Foxc1  120  QGWQNSIRHNLSLNECFVKVPRDDKKPGKGSYWTLDPDSYNMFENGSFLRRRRRFKKKDA  179
Foxc2  112  QGWQNSIRHNLSLNECFVKVPRDDKKPGKGSYWTLDPDSYNMFENGSFLRRRRRFKKKDV  171

Foxc1  180  VKDKEEKGRLHLQEPPPPQAGRQPAPAPPEQAEGSAPGPQPPPVRIQDIKTENGTCPSPP  239
Foxc2  172  PKDKEERAHLK--EPPSTTAKGAPTGTPVAD--G----PKEAEKKVVV-KSEAASPALPV  222

Foxc1  240  QPLSPAAALGSGSAATVPKIESPDSSSSLSSGSSPPGSLPSARPLSLDAAEPAPPPQPA  299
Foxc2  223  ITKVE--TLSPEGALQAS----PRSASSTPA-GSPD-GSLPEHHAAAPNGL---------  265

Foxc1  300  PPPHHSQGFSVDNIMTSLRGSPQGSAAELGSGLLASAAASSRAGIAP-PLALGAYSPGQS  358
Foxc2  266  P------GFSVETIMT-LRTSPPGG--DLSPAA-----A--RAGLVVPPLALP-YAAAPP  308

Foxc1  359  SLMSSPCSQSSSAGSSGGGGGGGGGGGGSSSAAGVTGGAATYHCNLQAMSLYAAGERGGHL  418
Foxc2  309  AAMTQPCAQGLEAAGSAGYQCSMRAMSLYT---GAERPAHV-CVPPALDEALSDHPSGPG  364

Foxc1  419  QGPAGGAGSAAVDDP-LPDYSLPPATSSSSSSLSHGGGGQEASHHPASHQ-GRLTS-WYL  475
Foxc2  365  S-PLGALNLAAGQEGALGASGHHHQHH---GHLHPQAPPPAP-QPEPAPQPATQATSWYL  419

Foxc1  476  NQAGGDLGHLASAAAAAAAAAAYPGQQQNFHSVREMFESQRIGLNNSPVNGNS--S--CQM  531
Foxc2  420  NHGG-DLSHLPGH-------TFATQQQTEPNVREMFNSHRLGLDNSSLGESQVSNASCQL  471

Foxc1  532  AFPASQSLYRTSGAFVYDCSKF                                       553
Foxc2  472  PYRATPSLYRHAAPYSYDCTKY                                       493
```

Figure 64–2. Amino acid sequences of class C Fox proteins.

cal (Fig. 64–3), and those in Foxc1 and Foxc2 proteins are identical except for two amino acids (they are only aspartic acid to glutamic acid changes) (Fig. 64–2). In these cases, one can expect that Foxf1 and Foxf2 proteins bind to the same target gene(s) and that Foxc1 and Foxc2 proteins also bind to the same but another target(s). The target genes of each forkhead gene are important to determine. However, except for several genes that FoxA proteins regulate, only a few target genes have been identified. Theoretically, regulatory DNAs, called *enhancers* and *promoters*, are composed of multiple *cis* elements, to which each transcription factor can bind as a monomer or multimer. Transcriptional activity is determined by the synergistic action of these elements. Furthermore, a transcription factor can bind to a sequence slightly different from the consensus binding site. In this case, a neighboring transcription factor can efficiently help (or sometimes inhibit) the binding of the Fox protein to a weak binding site. The multiple combinations of *cis* elements and cooperative actions of transcription factors govern the mystery of transcriptional regulation. Identifying the target genes that each Fox protein regulates represents a barrier to surmount.

STRUCTURE AND CHROMOSOMAL LOCALIZATION OF FORKHEAD GENES

The structure of forkhead genes is variable. *Foxc1*, *Foxc2*, and *Foxg1* genes are devoid of introns. *Foxa1–3*, *Foxf1*, and *Foxf2* genes have one intron. In contrast, *Foxp1*, *Foxp2*, and *Foxp3* genes have more than 10 introns (Fig. 64–4). It is well known that *Hox* genes are clustered in four chromosomes in mouse and human. Unlike *Hox*, *Fox* genes are located on various chromosomes. *Foxa1*, *Foxa2*, *Foxa3*, *Foxc1*, and *Foxc2* genes are located on mouse chromosomes 12, 7, 2, 13, and 8, respectively. As partially discussed in Chapters 66 and 65, *FOXF1*, *FOXC2*, and *FOXL1* genes are located on human chromo-

```
Foxf1    1  ------------------------------------------------------------    1
Foxf2    1  MSTEGGPPPPPPRPPPAPLRRACSPAPGALQAALMSPPPAATLESTSSSSSSSSSASCASS   60

Foxf1    1  ----------------M-DPAAAGPTKAKKTNAGVRRPEKPPYSYIALIVMAIQSSPSK   42
Foxf2   61  SSNSVSASAGACKSAASSGG-AGAGSGGTKKATSGLRRPEKPPYSYIALIVMAIQSSPSK  119

Foxf1   43  RLTLSEIYQFLQARFPFFRGAYQGWKNSVRHNLSLNECFIKLPKGLGRPGKGHYWTIDPA  102
Foxf2  120  RLTLSEIYQFLQARFPFFRGAYQGWKNSVRHNLSLNECFIKLPKGLGRPGKGHYWTIDPA  179

Foxf1  103  SEFMFEEGSFRRRPRGFRRKCQALKPVMSMVN-GLGFNH-L-PDTYGFQGSGG--LSCAP  157
Foxf2  180  SEFMFEEGSFRRRPRGFRRKCQALKPMYHRMVSGLGFGASLLPQGFDFQAPPSAPLGCHG  239

Foxf1  158  NSLALEGGLGMMNGHLAGNVDGM--ALPS----HSVPHLPSNGGHSYMGGCGGSAA----  207
Foxf2  240  QGG-YGG-LDMMPAGYDTGAGAPGHAHPQHLHHHHVPHMSPNPGSTYMASCPVPAGPAGV  297

Foxf1  208  ---------G-EMPHHDSSVPASPLLPAGAGGVMEPHAVMSSSAAAWPPAASAALNSGAS  257
Foxf2  298  GAAAGGGGGGGDYGPDSSSSPVPSSPAMAS-AIEC-HSPYTSPAAHWSSPGASP------  349

Foxf1  258  MIKQQP-LSPCNPAAN-P-LSGSISTHSLEQPYLHQNSHNGPAELQGIPRYHSQSPSMCD  314
Foxf2  350  MLKQPPALTPSSNPAASAGLHPSMSSYSLEQSYLHQNAREDLSV--GLPRYQHHSTPVCD  407

Foxf1  315  RKEFVFSFNAMASSSMHTTGGGSYYHQQVT--YQDIKPCVM                     353
Foxf2  408  RKDFVLNFNGISS--FHPSASGSYYHHHQSVCQDIKPCVM                      446
```

Figure 64–3. Amino acid sequences of class F Fox proteins.

```
Foxp1a    1  MMQESGSETKSNGSAIQNGSSGGN-HLLECGALRDTRSNGEAPAVDLGAADLAHVQQQQQ       59
Foxp1b    1  MMQESGSETKSNGSAIQNGSSGGN-HLLECGALRDTRSNGEAPAVDLGAADLAHVQQQQQ       59
Foxp1c    1  -----------------------------------------------------------       1
Foxp2     1  MMQESVTETISNSSMNDNGMSTLSSQ-LDAGS-RDGRSSGDTSSE-VSTVELLHLQQQ-      56
Foxp3     1  -----------------------------------------------------------       1

Foxp1a   60  QALQVARQLLLQQQQQQQQQQQQQQQQQQQQQQQQQQQQQQQQQQQQQVSGLKSPKRNDK      119
Foxp1b   60  QALQVARQLLLQQQQQQQQQQQQQQQQQQQQQQQQQQQQQQQQQQQQQVSGLKSPKRNDK      119
Foxp1c    1  -----------------------------------------------------------       1
Foxp2    57  -ALQAARQLLLQQ----------------------------------QTSGLKSPKSSEK       81
Foxp3     1  -----------------------------------------------------------       1

Foxp1a  120  QPALQVPVSVAMMTPQVITPQQMQQILQQQVLSPQQLQVLLQQQQALMLQQQ-LQEFYKK      178
Foxp1b  120  QPALQVPVSVAMMTPQVITPQQMQQILQQQVLSPQQLQVLLQQQQALMLQQQ-LQEFYKK      178
Foxp1c    1  -----------------------------------------------------------       1
Foxp2    82  QRPLQVPVSVAMMTPQVITPQQMQQILQQQVLSPQQLQALLQQQQAVMLQQQQLQEFYKK      141
Foxp3     1  -----------------------------------------------------------       1

Foxp1a  179  QQEQLQLQLLQQQH--------------------------------AGKQPKEQ        200
Foxp1b  179  QQEQLQLQLLQQQH--------------------------------AGKQPKEQ        200
Foxp1c    1  -----------------------------------------------------        1
Foxp2   142  QQEQLHLQLLQQQQQQQQQQQQQQQQQQQQQQQQQQQQQQQQQQQQQQQQQQH-PGKQAKEQ  200
Foxp3     1  -----------MPNPRPAKPMAPSLALGPSPGVLPSWKTAPKGS----ELLGTRGSGG     43

Foxp1a  201  Q-------VATQQLAFQQQLLQMQQLQQQHL-LSLQRQGLLTIQPGQPALFLQ-PLAQGM      251
Foxp1b  201  Q-------VATQQLAFQQQLLQMQQLQQQHL-LSLQRQGLLTIQPGQPALFLQ-PLAQGM      251
Foxp1c    1  -----------------------------------------------------------M        1
Foxp2   201  QQQQQQQLAAQQLVFQQQLLQMQQLQQQHLLSLQRQGLISIPPGQAALPVQ-SLPQAG      259
Foxp3    44  PFQGRDLRSGAHTSSSLNPLPPSQ-L--Q-----LPTVPLVMVAPSGARLGPSPHLQALL       95

Foxp1a  252  II-PTELQQ-LWKEVTSAHTAEETTSSNHS-S--LDLTSTCVSSSAP---SKSSLIMNPHA      303
Foxp1b  252  II-PTELQQ-LWKEVTSAHTAEETTSSNHS-S--LDLTSTCVSSSAP---SKSSLIMNPHA      303
Foxp1c    2  II-PTELQQ-LWKEVTSAHTAEETTSSNHS-S--LDLTSTCVSSSAP---SKSSLIMNPHA       53
Foxp2   260  LSPAEIQQ-LWKEVTGVHSMEDNGIKHG--G--LDLTTNNSSTTSSTTSKASPPITHHS      314
Foxp3    96  QDRPHFMHQLST-MDAHAQTPVLQVRPLDNPAMISLPPPSAATGVFSLKARPGLPPGINV      154

Foxp1a  304  STNG---QLS--VHTPKRESLSHEEHPHSH---PLY---GHGVCKWPGCEAVCDDFPAFL      352
Foxp1b  304  STNG---QLS--VHTPKRESLSHEEHPHSH---PLY---GHGVCKWPGCEAVCDDFPAFL      352
Foxp1c   54  STNG---QLS--VHTPKRESLSHEEHPHSH---PLY---GHGVCKWPGCEAVCDDFPAFL      102
Foxp2   315  IVNG---QSS--MLNARRDSSSHEETGASH---TLY---GHGVCKWPGCESICEDFGQFL      363
Foxp3   155  ASLEWVSREPALLCTIFPRSGTPRKDSNLLAAPQGSMPLLANGVCKWPGCEKVFEEPEEFL      214

Foxp1a  353  KHLNSEHALDDRSTAQCRVQMQVVQQLELQLAKDKERLQAMMTHLHVKSTEPKAAPQPLN      412
Foxp1b  353  KHLNSEHALDDRSTAQCRVQMQVVQQLELQLAKDKERLQAMMTHLHVKSTEPKAAPQPLN      412
Foxp1c  103  KHLNSEHALDDRSTAQCRVQMQVVQQLELQLAKDKERLQAMMTHLHVKSTEPKAAPQPLN      162
Foxp2   364  KHLNNEHALDDRSTAQCRVQMQVVQQLEIQLSKERERLQAMMTHLHMRPSEPKPSEKPLN      423
Foxp3   215  KHCQADHLLDEKGKAQCLLQREVVQSLEQQLELEKEKLGAMQAHLAGKMALAKAPSVAS-      273

Foxp1a  413  LVSSVTLSKSASEASPQSLPHTPTTPAPLTPVTQGPSVITTTSMHTVGPIRRRYSDKYN      472
Foxp1b  413  LVSSVTLSKSASEASPQSLPHTPTTPAPLTPVTQGPSVITTTSMHTVGPIRRRYSDKYN      472
Foxp1c  163  LVSSVTLSKSASEASPQSLPHTPTTPAPLTPVTQGPSVITTTSMHTVGPIRRRYSDKYN      222
Foxp2   424  LVSSVTMSKNMLETSPQSLPQTPTTPTAPVTPITQGPSVITPASVPNVGAIRRRHSDKYN      483
Foxp3   274  MDKSSCCIVATSTQGSV-LPAWSAPREW--------HDG----GLFA---VRRHLWGSHG      317

Foxp1a  473  VPISSADIAQNQEFYKNAEVRPPFTYASLIRQAILESPEKQLTLNEIYNWFTRMFAYFRR      532
Foxp1b  473  VPISSADIAQNQEFYKNAEVRPPFTYASLIRQAILESPEKQLTLNEIYNWFTRMFAYFRR      532
Foxp1c  223  VPISSADIAQNQEFYKNAEVRPPFTYASLIRQAILESPEKQLTLNEIYNWFTRMFAYFRR      282
Foxp2   484  IPMSSE-IAPNYEFYKNADVRPPFTYATLIRQAIMESSDRQLTLNEIYSWFTRTFAYFRR      542
Foxp3   318  NSSFPEFFHNM-DYFKYHNMRPPFTYATLIRWAILEAPERQRTLNEIYHWFTRMFAYFRN      376

Foxp1a  533  NAATWKNAVRHNLSLHKCFVRVENVKGAVWTVDEVEFQKRRPQKISGNPSLIKNMQSSHA      592
Foxp1b  533  NAATWKAS--------------------------------------------------      540
Foxp1c  283  NAATWKNAVRHNLSLHKCFVRVENVKGAVWTVDEVEFQKRRPQKISGNPSLIKNMQSSHA      342
Foxp2   543  SAATWKNAVRHNLSLHKCFVRVENVKGAVWTVDEVEYQKRRSQKITGSPTLVKNIPTSLG      602
Foxp3   377  HPATWKNAIRHNLSLHKCFVRVESEKGAVWTVDEFEFRKKRSQR---------------      420

Foxp1a  593  YCTPLNAALQASMAENSIPLYTTASMGNPTLGSLASAIREELNGAMEHTNSNESDSSPGR      652
Foxp1b  541  -----------MAENSIPLYTTASMGNPTLGSLASAIREELNGAMEHTNSNESDSSPGR      588
Foxp1c  343  YCTPLNAALQASMAENSIPLYTTASMGNPTLGSLASAIREELNGAMEHTNSNESDSSPGR      402
Foxp2   603  YGAALNASLQAALAESSLPLLSNPGLINNASSGLLQAVHEDLNGSLDHIDSNGNSS-PGC      661
Foxp3   421  -----------------------------------------------------------      421

Foxp1a  653  SPMQAVHPIHVKEEPLDPEEAEGPLSLVTTANHSPDFDHDRDYEDEPVNEDME          705
Foxp1b  589  SPMQAVHPIHVKEEPLDPEEAEGPLSLVTTANHSPDFDHDRDYEDEPVNEDME          641
Foxp1c  403  SPMQAVHPIHVKEEPLDPEEAEGPLSLVTTANHSPDFDHDRDYEDEPVNEDME          455
Foxp2   662  SPQPHIHSIHVKEEPVIAEDEDCPMSLVTTANHSPELEDDREIEEEPLSEDLE          714
Foxp3   421  --------------------PNKCS----N--PCP----          429
```

Figure 64–4. Amino acid sequences of class P Fox proteins. Three alternative splicing forms are identified in the *Foxp1* gene (*Foxp1a*, *Foxp1b*, and *Foxp1c*). It is known that the *Foxp3* gene is mutated in *scurfy* mutant mice.

667

some 16 and *FOXC1*, *FOXF2*, and *FOXQ1* genes are on human chromosome 6. These facts are interesting from the viewpoints of gene evolution and geographical gene expression.

INTRACELLULAR LOCALIZATION AND SIGNALING PATHWAY OF FOX PROTEINS

Most transcription factor proteins are localized in the nucleus. Consistent with this rule, most Fox proteins are present in the nucleus. Deletional analysis of the Foxa2 protein revealed that the nuclear localization signal is within the forkhead domain (Qian and Costa, 1995). The FOXC1 protein has two separate nuclear localization signals in the forkhead domain, one rich in basic amino acid residues and a second highly conserved among FOX proteins (Berry et al., 2002). Exceptionally, FoxO proteins are translocated between the cytoplasm and nucleus. FOXO proteins are in the cytoplasm when their unique serine/threonine residues are phosphorylated; unphosphoylated proteins are in the nucleus (described later).

EACH TYPE OF KNOCKOUT MOUSE SHOWS DISTINCT PLEIOTROPIC PHENOTYPES

Like their random genomic organization, there appear to be no simple rules governing the spatial and temporal expression pattern of *Fox* genes, unlike patterns shown by *Hox* genes. Rather, it appears that several members of *Fox* may direct cell proliferation, cell fate determination, and cell differentiation in many different or divided regions. For example, after *Foxg1*, *Foxd1*, and *Foxb1* genes are expressed in the neural tube, *Foxg1* is expressed in the telencephalon and nasal retina, *Foxd1* is expressed in the diencephalon and temporal retina, and *Foxb1* is expressed in the hypothalamus and spinal cord. *Foxc2* and *Foxc1* genes are expressed in the presomitic mesoderm at an early stage, but some regions of expression overlap and others do not at later stages (Kaestner et al., 1996; Iida et al., 1997; Kume et al., 1998). Several *Fox* genes are expressed in the developing lung and several different ones in the developing kidney. In summary, each member has a microscopically distinct expression pattern in various regions of any organ, and several members constitute a team directing morphogenesis of the organ or the tissue.

To clarify the developmental roles of each *Fox* gene in this complex family, many laboratories have made knockout mice deficient in one gene function. The phenotypes of some knockout mice are summarized in Table 64–2. It has also been discovered that *Foxc1*, *Foxe3*, *Foxn1*, *Foxp3*, and *Foxq1* genes are mutated in *congenital hydrocephalus* (*ch*), *dysgenetic lens* (*dyl*), *nude*, *scurfy*, and *satin* mutant mice (Nehls et al., 1994; Kume et al., 1998; Blixt et al., 2000; Brunkow et al., 2001 ; Hong et al., 2001). These natural and artificial mutant mice are the best model animals for understanding human congenital diseases and their underlying molecular mechanisms.

OTHER FUNCTIONS OF FOX PROTEINS

As Fox proteins have diverse domain sequences and complex expression patterns, they might play different roles in various regions of the body. We certainly cannot describe all roles of Fox proteins in de-

tail. Rather, we will describe some special functions that have been extensively analyzed.

Foxj1 is expressed in the developing respiratory and reproductive epithelium (Hackett et al., 1995) and choroid plexus epithelium (Lim et al., 1997). A detailed analysis showed that *Foxj1* is expressed in ciliated epithelial cells in the developing mouse lung (Tichelaar et al., 1999a,b; Blatt et al., 1999); that is, *foxj1* is expressed in ciliated tissues found in proximal respiratory epithelium, oviduct, haploid sperm, and choroid plexus. *Foxj1* knockout mice show complete absence of cilia (or flagella in the case of sperm) and random left–right asymmetry (Chen et al., 1998; Brody et al., 2000). Consistently, transgenic mice in which the *Foxj1* gene is ectopically expressed under the surfactant protein C promoter display distal respiratory epithelial cell differentiation and morphology. The presence of the Foxj1 protein inhibits markers of nonciliated cells and induces those of ciliated cells (Tichelaar et al., 1999a,b). These data support the strict role of the Foxj1 protein in ciliogenesis.

The FoxH protein was initially identified in the activin signaling pathway. When activin binds to the cell surface activin receptor, the Smad2, Smad4, and FoxH proteins form a complex and bind to the target gene, *Mix1* (Chen et al., 1996). They are also involved in transforming growthfactor-β signaling and nodal signaling (Labbe et al., 1998; Zhou et al., 1998; Liu et al., 1999; Saijoh et al., 2000) (see Chapter 24). *Foxh1* knockout mice show abnormal anterior–posterior patterning and failure to form the node and its derivatives (Yamamoto et al., 2001; Hoodless et al., 2001).

Like DAF-16 in *Caenorhabditis elegans*, which is involved in longevity (Ogg et al., 1997; Lin et al., 1997), the FoxO subfamily (Foxo1, Foxo3, Foxo4) (Anderson et al., 1998) is involved in regulating the cell cycle and apoptosis. The unique feature of this subfamily is the cytoplasmic-nuclear relocalization of the Fox protein (Takaishi et al., 1999; Kops et al., 2002). The most convincingly demonstrated substrates for protein kinase B/Akt are the FoxO subfamily of forkhead transcription factors (Biggs et al., 1999; Kops et al., 1999). Phosphorylation of FoxO proteins results in their binding to 14-3-3 proteins and then expulsion from the nucleus, causing loss of transcriptional activity and decreased expression of proteins that promote cell death and cell cycle arrest (Brunet et al., 1999; Downward and Leevers, 2001). Mammalian Foxo3 functions at the G_2 to M checkpoint in the cell cycle, triggering the repair of damaged DNA. Overall, FoxO proteins regulate the resistance of cells to stress and may affect organism life span (Tran et al., 2002).

LESSONS FROM MUTANT ANALYSES

After the discovery of the forkhead family, many knockout mice have been developed to uncover the functions of the members of this family. Also, positional cloning makes it possible to identify the causative genes for inherited human and rodent disorders. Based on the experimental results and findings in our laboratory and in others, we will discuss several implications.

Members of the Subfamily May Play Compensatory Roles

Foxc2 and Foxc1 have a practically identical forkhead domain (only two D–E changes) with similar flanking protein structures (Miura et

Table 64–2. Phenotypes of *Fox* Gene Knockout Mice

Gene	Phenotype	References
Foxa2	Defects in node and notochord	Ang and Rossant, 1994; Weinstein et al., 1994
Foxg1	Small cerebral hemispheres	Xuan et al., 1995
Foxd1	Defect in transformation in renal tubular epithelium, abnormality in collecting ducts	Hatini et al., 1996
Foxn1	Nude mice, athymus	Nehls et al., 1996
Foxb1	Growth retardation, defect in milk ejection reflex, motor weakness	Labosky et al., 1997; Dou et al., 1997
Foxc2	Interruption of aortic arch, defects in skeletogenesis	Iida et al., 1997; Winnier et al., 1997
Foxi1	Abnormalities in stomach and jejunum	Kaestner et al. 1997; Fukamachi et al., 2001
Foxc1	Glaucoma, hydrocephalus, defects in skeletogenesis	Kume et al., 1998
Foxe1	Cleft palate, thyroid agenesis	DeFelice et al., 1998
Foxi1	Defects in inner ear	Hulander et al., 1998
Foxj1	Situs inversus, defective ciliogenesis, hydrocephalus	Chen et al., 1998; Brody et al., 2000
Foxk1	Abnormal muscle regeneration	Garry et al., 2000
Foxh1	Abnormal A–P patterning, defects in node and notochord	Yamamoto et al., 2001; Hoodless et al., 2001

al., 1993, 1997; Kume et al., 1998) (Fig. 64–2) and may have similar functions. *Foxc2* knockout mice show interruption of the aortic arch, ventral septal defect, and abnormalities in skeletogenesis (Iida et al., 1997). *Foxc1* knockout mice have hydrocephalus, glaucoma, and abnormalities of the skeleton, kidney, and ureter (Kume et al., 1998). Interestingly, double heterozygotes (*Foxc2*[+/−], *Foxc1*[+/−]) die prenatally and have cardiovascular abnormalities (Winnier et al., 1999). *Foxc1*[+/−] mice and *Foxc2*[+/−] mice show aberrant ocular development. Iris and corneal abnormalities are seen more in *Foxc1*[+/−] mice and less often in *Foxc2*[+/−] mice (Smith et al., 2000). Kidney abnormalities were observed frequently in *Foxc1*[−/−] mice and rarely in *Foxc2*[−/−] mice. Furthermore, double homozygotes (*Foxc2*[−/−], *Foxc1*[−/−]) have no somites or segmented paraxial mesoderm (Kume et al., 2001). This indicates that *Foxc2* and *Foxc1* cooperate in somitogenesis and that one gene can compensate for the other in single homozygotes (Iida et al., 1997; Winnier et al., 1997). Foxc2 and Foxc1 might play similar but distinct roles in various tissues, for example, the outflow tract of heart, eyes, kidneys, and somites. Overall, it seems that Foxc2 contributes more to cardiovascular formation and Foxc1 contributes more to eye and kidney formation (see Chapter 66).

Forkhead Genes as Causative Genes for Inherited Disorders

Positional cloning is a powerful method to identify the causative gene for inherited disorders. Mutations have now been found in several *FOX* genes. Some patients with hereditary lymphedema distichiasis (LD) syndrome have mutations in the *FOXC2* gene (Fang et al., 2000; Erickson et al., 2001; Bell et al., 2001) (see Chapter 66), those with congenital glaucoma have mutations in the *FOXC1* gene (Nishimura et al., 1998, 2001; Lehmann et al., 2000; Saleem et al., 2001) (see Chapter 65), those with the blepharophimosis/ptosis/epicanthus inversus syndrome (BPES) have mutations in the *FOXL2* gene (Crisponi et al., 2001; DeBaere et al., 2001; Yamada et al., 2001) (see Chapter 65), and those with anterior segment ocular dysgenesis and cataracts have mutations in the *FOXE3* gene (Semina et al., 2001). These four diseases are transmitted as dominant traits. In recessive traits, mutations in *FOXE1*, *FOXN1*, and *FOXP3* genes are found in patients with thyroid agenesis, those with alopecia universalis, and those with immune dysregulation,polyendocrinopathy, enteropathy, X-linked syndrome, respectively (Clifton-Bligh et al., 1998; Ahmad et al., 1998; Chatila et al., 2000; Wildin et al., 2001; Bennett et al., 2001). In 5 years, the number of *FOX* genes found to be involved in hereditary diseases will surely increase.

Forkhead Genes: Dominant Trait and Gene Dosage Effect

As in cases of *TBX5* in Holt-Oram syndrome, *TBX3* in ulnar-mammary syndrome, and *TBX1* in DiGeorge syndrome, *FOXC2* in LD, *FOXC1* in glaucoma, and *FOXL2* in BPES are dominant traits. It is common that heterozygotes of transcription factor genes show symptoms (Seidman and Seidman, 2002). Typically, two cases are possible: one is a dominant-negative type and the other is a haploinsufficiency type. Several lines of evidence favor the second possibility in the case of the dominant trait of *FOX* genes. The exact molecular mechanism in which the half-dose of transcription factor is not enough for maintaining normal function is not known. Speculation focuses on multiple target motifs in the regulatory regions and synergistic actions of transcription factors; that is, the target gene expression may depend on the concentration of a key transcription factor. Therefore, we think that gene dosage is an important point in determining the ultimate function of the transcription factor. A half-dose may not be sufficient for function, and a double dose may exert abnormal function. The complexity and pleiotropicity of symptoms in human patients and knockout mice make it difficult for researchers to better understand the causes and symptoms. Sometimes phenotypes of knockout mice appear different from those of humans. One important point is that experimental mice have a limited genetic background but humans have a mixed genetic background. It is necessary to carefully consider the whole picture of inherited diseases from multiple viewpoints.

PERSPECTIVES

From a fertilized egg, the cell continues proliferation, cell fate determination, and body formation in a uterus. Developmental gene programs and cell–cell interactions make the organism what it is. During the complex developmental processes, several gene families are involved. One key family is the *Fox* genes. In organogenesis, dozens or hundreds of genes act coordinately to make an organ. It is like an orchestra playing a symphony. The first violins (*Foxc2*) and second violins (*Foxc1*) may play harmonic sounds with distinct tones. They play with the other string instruments as well as other types of instrument to produce the symphony. Without any one member, the music is incomplete, whether such incompleteness is recognized or not. We expect that mutations in dozens of genes may result in a similar phenotype. For better understanding, the collection of more cases with inherited diseases and the development of more sophisticated methods to analyze phenotypes of knockout mice are needed. We have come halfway but now have plenty of questions to be answered. We realize that Fox proteins act as pleiotropically as does a fox.

ACKNOWLEDGMENTS

N.M. thanks Reiko Miura for continuous support. We acknowledge Yukie Nishizawa and Mayumi Hara for secretarial assistance and Rikako Katsu for technical assistance.

REFERENCES

Ahmad W, Haque MF, Brancolini V, Tsou HC, Haque S, Lim H, Aita VM, Owen J, deBlaquiere M, Frank J, et al. (1998). Alopecia universalis associated with a mutation in the human hairless gene. *Science* 279: 720–724.

Anderson MJ, Viars CS, Czekay S, Cavenee WK, Arden KC (1998). Cloning and characteriztion of three human forkhead genes that comprise an FKHR-like gene subfamily. *Genomics* 47: 187–199.

Ang SL, Rossant J (1994). HNF-3β is essential for node and notochord formation in mouse development. *Cell* 78: 561–574.

Bell R, Brice G, Child AH, Murday VA, Mansour S, Sandy CJ, Collin JRO, Brady AF, Callen DF, Burnand K, et al. (2001). Analysis of lymphoedema-distichiasis families for FOXC2 mutations reveals small insertions and deletions throughout the gene. *Hum Genet* 108: 546–551.

Bennett CL, Christie J, Ramsdell F, Brunkow ME, Ferguson PJ, Whitesell L, Kelly TE, Saulsbury FT, Chance PF, Ochs HD (2001). The immune dysregulation, polyendocrinopathy, enteropathy, X-linked syndrome (IPEX) is caused by mutations of FOXP3. *Nat Genet* 27: 20–21.

Berry FB, Saleem RA, Walter MA (2002). FOXC1 transcriptional regulation is mediated by N- and C-terminal activation domains and contains a phosphorylated transcriptional inhibitory domain. *J Biol Chem* 277: 10292–10297.

Biggs WH, Meisenhelder J, Hunter T, Cavenee WK, Arden KC (1999). Protein kinase B/Akt-mediated phosphorylation promotes nuclear exclusion of the winged helix transcription factor FKHR1. *Proc Natl Acad Sci USA* 96: 7421–7426.

Blatt EN, Yan XH, Wuerffel MK, Hamilos DL, Brody SL (1999). Forkhead transcription factor HFH-4 expression is temporally related to ciliogenesis. *Am J Respir Cell Mol Biol* 21: 168–176.

Blixt A, Mahlapuu M, Aitola M, Pelto-Huikko M, Enerback S, Carlsson P (2000). A forkhead gene, FoxE3, is essential for lens epithelial proliferation and closure of the lens vesicle. *Genes Dev* 14: 245–254.

Brody SL, Yan XH, Wuerffel MK, Song SK, Shapiro SD (2000). Ciliogenesis and leftright axis defects in forkhead factor HFH-4-null mice. *Am J Respir Cell Mol Biol* 23: 45–51.

Brunet A, Bonni A, Zigmond MJ, Lin MZ, Juo P, Hu LS, Aderson MJ, Arden KC, Blenis J, Greenberg ME (1999). Akt promotes cell survival by phosphorylating and inhibiting forkhead transcription factor. *Cell* 96: 857–868.

Brunkow ME, Jeffery EW, Hjerrild KA, Paeper B, Clark LB, Yasayko S-A, Wilkinson JE, Galas D, Ziegler SF, Ramsdell F (2001). Disruption of a new forkhead/winged-helix protein, scurfin, results in the fatal lymphoproliferative disorder of the scurfy mouse. *Nat Genet* 27: 68–73.

Chatila TA, Blaeser F, Ho N, Lederman HM, Voulgaropoulos C, Helms C, Bowcock AM (2000). JM2, encoding a fork head-related protein, is mutated in X-linked autoimmunity-allergic disregulation syndrome. *J Clin Invest* 106: R75–R81.

Chen X, Rubock MJ, Whitman M (1996). A transcriptional partner for MAD proteins in TGF-β signalling. *Nature* 383: 691–696.

Chen J, Knowles HJ, Hebert JL, Hackett BP (1998). Mutation of the mouse heptocyte nuclear factor/forkhead homologue 4 gene results in an absence of cilia and random left–right asymmetry. *J Clin Invest* 102: 1077–1082.

Clark KL, Halay ED, Lai E, Burley SK (1993). Co-crystal structure of the HNF-3/fork head DNA-recognition motif resembles histone H5. *Nature* 364: 412–420.

Clifton-Bligh R, Wentworth JM, Heinz P, Crisp MS, John R, Lazrus JH, Ludgate M, Chatterjee VK (1998). Mutation of gene encoding human TTF-2 associated with thyroid agenesis, cleft palate and choanal atresia. *Nat Genet* 19: 399–401.

Crisponi L, Deiana M, Loi A, Chiappe F, Uda M, Amati P, Bisceglia L, Zelante L, Nagaraja R, Porcu S, et al. (2001). The putative forkhead transcription factor FOXL2 is mutated in blepharophimosis/ptosis/epicanthus inversus syndrome. *Nat Genet* 27: 159–166.

De Baere E, Dixon MJ, Small KW, Jabs EW, Leroy BP, Devriendt K, Gillerot Y, Mortier G, Meire F, Maldergem LV, et al. (2001). Spectrum of FOXL2 gene mutations in blepharophimosis-ptosis-epicanthus inversus (BPES) families demonstrates a genotype–phenotype correlation. *Hum Mol Genet* 10: 1591–1600.

De Felice M, Ovitt C, Biffali E, Rodriguez-Mallon A, Arra C, Anastassiadis K, Macchia PE, Mattei M, Mariano A, Scholer H, et al. (1998). A mouse model for hereditary thyroid dysgenesis and cleft palate. *Nat Genet* 19: 395–398.

Dou C, Ye X, Stewart C, Lai SC (1997). TWH regulates the development of subsets of spinal cord neurons. *Neuron* 18: 539–551.

Downward J, Leevers SJ (2001). Trachealess—a new transcription factor target for PKB/Akt. *Dev Cell* 1: 726–728.

Erickson RP, Dagenais SL, Caulder MS, Downs CA, Herman G, Jones MC, Kerstjens-Frederikse WS, Lidral AC, McDonald M, Nelson CC, et al. (2001). Clinical heterogeneity in lymphoedema-distichiasis with FOXC2 truncating mutations. *J Med Genet* 38: 761–766.

Fang J, Dagenais SL, Erickson RP, Arlt MF, Glynn MW, Gorski JL, Seaver LH, Glover TW (2000). Mutations in FOXC2 (MFH-1), a forkhead faily transcription factor, are responsible for the hereditary lymphedema-distichiasis syndrome. *Am J Hum Genet* 67: 1382–1388.

Fukamachi H, Fukuda K, Suzuki M, Furumoto Y, Ichinose M, Shimizu S, Tsuchiya S, Horie S, Suzuki Y, Saito Y, et al. (2001). Mesenchymal transcription factor Fkh6 is essential for the development and differentiation of parietal cells. *Biochem Biophys Res Commun* 280: 1069–1076.

Garry DJ, Meeson A, Elterman J, Zhao Y, Yang P, Bassel-Duby R, Williams RS (2000). Myogenic stem cell function is impaired in mice lacking the forkhead/winged helix protein MNF. *Proc Natl Acid Sci USA* 97: 5416–5421.

Hackett BP, Brody SL, Liang M, Zeitz IZ, Bruns LA, Gitlin JD (1995). Primary structure of hepatocyte nuclear factor/forkhead homologue 4 and characterizaton of gene expression in the developing respiratory and reproductive epithelium. *Proc Natl Acad Sci USA* 92: 4249–4253.

Hatini V, Huh SO, Herzlinger D, Soares VC, Lai E (1996). Essential role of stromal mesenchyme in kidney morphogenesis revealed by targeted disruption of winged helix transcription factor BF-2. *Genes Dev* 10: 1467–1478.

Hong H-K, Noveroske JK, Headon DJ, Liu T, Sy M-S, Justice MJ, Chakravarti A (2001). The winged helix/forkhead transcription factor foxq1 regulates differentiation of hair in satin mice. *Genesis* 29: 163–171.

Hoodless PA, Pye M, Chazaud C, Labbe E, Attisano L, Rossant J, Wrana J (2001). FoxH1 (Fast) functions to specify the anterior primitive streak in the mouse. *Genes Dev* 15: 1257–1271.

Hulander M, Wurst W, Carlsson P, Enerback S (1998). The winged helix transcription factor Fkh10 is required for normal development of the inner ear. *Nat Genet* 20: 374–376.

Iida K, Koseki H, Kakinuma H, Kato N, Mizutani-Koseki Y, Ohuchi H, Yoshioka H, Noji S, Kawamira K, Kataoka Y, et al. (1997). Essential roles of the winged helix transcription factor MFH-1 in aortic arch patterning and skeletogenesis. *Development* 124: 4627–4638.

Kaestner KH, Bleckmann SC, Monaghan AP, Schlondorff J, Mincheva A, Lichter P, Schutz G (1996). Clustered arrangement of winged helix genes fkh-6 and MFH-1: possible implications for mesoderm development. *Development* 122: 1751–1758.

Kaestner KH, Silberg DG, Traber PG, Schutz G (1997). The mesenchymal winged helix transcription factor Fkh6 is required for the control of gastrointestinal proliferation and differentiation. *Genes Dev* 11: 1583–1595.

Kaestner KH, Knochel W, Martinez DE (2000). Unified nomenclature for the winged helix/forkhead transcription factors. *Genes Dev* 14: 142–146.

Kaufmann E, Knochel W (1996). Five years on the wings of fork head. *Mech Dev* 57: 3–20.

Kops GJPL, de Ruiter ND, De Vries-Smith AMM, Powell DR, Bos JL, Burgering BMT (1999). Direct control of the forkhead transcription factor AFX by protein kinase B. *Nature* 398: 630–634.

Kops GJPL, Medema RH, Glassford J, Essers MAG, Dijkers PF, Coffer PJ, Lam EW-F, Burgering BMT (2002). Control of cell cycle exit and entry by protein kinase B-regulated forkhead transcription factors. *Mol Cell Biol* 22: 2025–2036.

Kume T, Deng K-Y, Winfrey V, Gould DB, Walter MA, Hogan BLM (1998). The forkhead/winged helix gene Mf1 is disrupted in the pleiotropic mouse mutation congenital hydrocephalus. *Cell* 93: 985–996.

Kume T, Jiang H, Topczewska JM, Hogan BLM (2001). The murine winged helix transcription factors, Foxc1 and Foxc2, are both required for cardiovascular development and somitogenesis. *Genes Dev* 15: 2470–2482.

Labbe E, Silvestri C, Hoodless PA, Wrana JL, Attisano L (1998). Smad2 and Smad3 positively and negatively regulate TGFβ-dependent transcription through the forkhead DNA-binding protein FAST2. *Mol Cells* 2: 109–120.

Labosky PA, Winnier GE, Jetton TL, Hargett L, Ryan AK, Rosenfeld MG, Parlow AF, Hogan BLM (1997). The winged helix gene, Mf3, is required for normal development of the diencephalom and midbrain, postnatanl growth and the milk-ejection reflex. *Development* 124: 1263–1274.

Lai E, Prezioso VR, Smith E, Litvin O, Costa RH, Darnell JE Jr (1990). HNF-3A, a hepatocyte-enriched transcription factor of novel structure is regulated transcriptionally. *Genes Dev* 4: 1427–1436.

Lehmann OJ, Ebenezer ND, Jordan T, Fox M, Ocaka L, Payne A, Leroy B, Clark BJ, Hitchings RA, Povey S, et al. (2000). Chromosomal duplication involving the forkhead transcription factor gene *FOXC1* causes iris hypoplasia and glaucoma. *Am J Hum Genet* 67: 1129–1135.

Lim L, Zhou H, Coata RH (1997). The winged helix transcription factor HFH-4 is expressed during choroid plexus epithelial development in the mouse embryo. *Proc Natl Acad Sci USA* 94: 3094–3099.

Lin K, Dorman JB, Rodan A, Kenyon C (1997). daf-16: an HNF-3/forkhead family member that can fnction to double the life-span of *Caenorhabditis elegans*. *Science* 278: 1319–1323.

Liu B, Dou C-L, Prabhu L, Lai E (1999). FAST-2 is mammalian winged-helix protein which mediates transforming growth factor β signals. *Mol Cell Biol* 19: 424–430.

Miura N, Wanaka A, Tohyama M, Tanaka K (1993). MFH-1, a new member of the fork head domain family, is expressed in developing mesenchyme. *FEBS Lett* 326: 171–176.

Miura N, Iida K, Kakinuma H, Yang X-L, Sugiyama T (1997). Isolation of the mouse (MFH-1) and human (FKHL14) mesenchyme fork head-1 genes reveals conservation of their gene and protein structures. *Genomics* 41: 489–492.

Nehls M, Pfeifer D, Schorpp M, Hedrich H, Boehm T (1994). New member of the winged-helix protein family disrupted in mouse and rat nude mutations. *Nature* 372: 103–107.

Nehls M, Kyewski B, Messerle M, Waldschutz R, Schuddekopf K, Smith AJH, Boehm T (1996). Two genetically separable steps in the differentiation of thymic epithelium. *Science* 272: 886–889.

Nishimura DY, Swiderski RE, Alward WLM, Searby CC, Patil SR, Bennet SR, Kanis AB, Gastier JM, Stone EM, Sheffield VC (1998). The forkhead transcription factor gene *FKHL7* is responsible for glaucoma phenotypes which map to 6p25. *Nat Genet* 19: 140–147.

Nishimura DY, Searby CC, Alward WL, Walton D, Craig JE, Mackey DA, Kawase K, Kanis AB, Patil SR, Stone EM, et al. (2001). A spectrum of FOXC1 mutations suggests gene dosage as a mechanism for developmental defects of the anterior chamber of the eye. *Am J Genet* 68: 364–372.

Ogg S, Paradis S, Gottlieb S, Patterson G, Lee L, Tissenbaum HA, Ruvkun G (1997). The fork head transcription factor DAF-16 transduces insulin-like metabolic and longevity signals in *C. elegans*. *Nature* 389: 994–999.

Qian X, Costa RH (1995). Analysis of hepatocyte nuclear factor-3β protein domains required for transcriptional activation and nuclear targeting. *Nucleic Acids Res* 23: 1184–1191.

Saijoh Y, Adachi H, Sakuma R, Yeo CY, Yashiro K, Watamabe M, Hashiguchi H, Mochida M, Ohishi S, Kawabata M, et al. (2000). Left–right asymmetric expression of lefty2 and nodal is induced by a signaling pathway that includes the transcription factor FAST2. *Mol Cells* 5: 35–47.

Saleem RA, Banerjee-Basu S, Berry FB, Baxevanis AD, Walter MA (2001). Analyses of the effects that disease-causing missense mutations have on the structure and function of the winged-helix protein FOXC1. *Am J Hum Genet* 68: 627–641.

Seidman JG, Seidman C (2002). Transcription factor haploinsufficiency: when half a loaf is not enough. *J Clin Invest* 109: 451–455.

Semina EV, Brownell I, Mintz-Hittner HA, Murray JC, Jamrich M (2001). Mutations in the human forkhead transcription factor FOXE3 associated with anterior segment ocular dysgenesis and cataracts. *Hum Mol Genet* 10: 231–236.

Smith RS, Zabaleta A, Kume T, Savinova OV, Kidson SH, Martin JE, Nishimura DY, Alward WLM, Hogan BLH, John SWM. (2000). Haploinsufficiency of the transcription factors FOXC1 and FOXC2 results in aberrant ocular development. *Hum Mol Genet* 9: 1021–1032.

Takaishi H, Konishi H, Masuzaki H, Ono Y, Saito N, Kitamura T, Ogawa W, Kasuga M, Kikkawa U, Nishizuka Y (1999). Regulation of nuclear transcription of forkhead transcription factor AFX by protein kinase B. *Proc Natl Acad Sci USA* 96: 11836–11841.

Tichelaar JW, Lim L, Costa RH, Whitsett JA (1999a). HNF-3/Forkhead homologue-4 influences lung morphogenesis and respiratory epithelial cell differentiation in vivo. *Dev Biol* 213: 405–417.

Tichelaar JW, Wert SE, Costa RH, Kimura S, Whitsett JA (1999b). HNF-3/Forkhead homologue-4 (HFH-4) is expressed in ciliated epithelial cells in the developing mouse lung. *J Histochem Cytochem* 47: 823–831.

Tran H, Brunet A, Grenier JM, Datta SR, Fornace AJ Jr, DiStefano PS, Chiang LW, Greenberg ME (2002). DNA repair pathway stimulated by the forkhead transcription factor FOXO3a though the Gadd45 protein. *Science* 296: 530–534.

Weigel D, Jackle H (1990). The fork head domain: a novel DNA binding motif of eukaryotic transcription factors? *Cell* 63: 455–456.

Weigel D, Jurgens G, Kuttner F, Seifert E, Jackle H (1989). The homeotic gene fork head encodes a nuclear protein and is expressed in the terminal regions of the *Drosophila* embryo. *Cell* 57: 645–658.

Weinstein DC, Altaba AR, Chen WS, Hoodless P, Prezioso VR, Jessell TM, Darnell JE (1994). The winged-helix transcription factor HNF-3β is required for notochord development in the mouse embryo. *Cell* 78: 575–588.

Wildin RS, Ramsdell F, Peake J, Faravelli F, Casanova J-L, Mazzella M, Goulet O, Perroni L, Bricarelli FD, Byrne G, et al. (2001). X-linked neonatal diabetes mellitus, enteropathy and endocrinopathy syndrome is the human equivalent of mouse scurfy. *Nat Genet* 27: 18–20.

Winnier GE, Hargett L, Hogan BLM (1997). The winged helix transcription factor MFH1 is required for proliferation and patterning of paraxial mesoderm in the mouse embryo. *Genes Dev* 11: 926–940.

Winnier GE, Kume T, Deng K, Rogers R, Bundy J, Raines C, Walter MA, Hogan BLM, Conway SJ (1999). Roles for the winged helix transcription factors MF1 and MFH1 in cardiovascular development revealed by nonallelic noncomplementation of null alleles. *Dev Biol* 213: 418–431.

Xuan S, Baptista CA, Balas G, Tao W, Soares VC, Lai E (1995). Winged helix transcription factor BF-1 is essential for the development of the cerebral hemispheres. *Neuron* 14: 1141–1152.

Yamada T, Hayasaka S, Matsumoto M, Esa T, Hayasaka Y, Endo M (2001). Heterozygous 17-bp deletion in the forkhead transcription factor gene, *FOXL2*, in a Japanese family with blepharomosis-epicanthus inversus syndrome. *J Hum Genet* 46: 733–736.

Yamamoto M, Meno C, Sakai Y, Shiratori H, Mochida K, Ikawa Y, Saijoh Y, Hamada H (2001). The transcription factor FoxH1 (FAST) mediates nodal signaling during anterior-posterior patterning and node formation in the mouse. *Genes Dev* 15: 1242–1256.

Zhou S, Zawel L, Lengauer C, Kinzler KW, Vogelstein B (1998). Characterization of human FAST-1, a TGFβ and activin signal transducer. *Mol Cells* 2: 121–127.

65 | *FOXC1* and *FOXL2* and the Axenfeld-Rieger Malformations and the Blepharophomisis, Ptosis, and Epicanthus Inversus Syndrome

RAMSEY A. SALEEM, FRED B. BERRY, AND MICHAEL A. WALTER

The complex process of embryogenesis proceeds through molecular signaling and regulation by developmentally important transcription factors. Of the regulatory molecules known, members of the ever-growing Forkhead family of transcription factors are recognized to play key roles in the development of a wide range of organisms (Kaufmann and Knochel, 1996). Forkhead transcription factors are characterized by the presence of a conserved 110–amino acid DNA-binding domain, the forkhead domain (FHD) (Fig. 65–1). This DNA-binding motif is a variant of the helix-turn-helix motif, consisting of one minor and three major α helices, two β sheets, and two large loops that form "wing-like" structures. As a result, FHDs are often referred to as "winged-helix domains." Increasingly, winged-helix or *FOX* (Forkhead Box) genes have been implicated in human heritable disorders. *FOXC1* and *FOXL2* are two of four FOX genes known to be involved in diseases with ocular manifestations. *FOXC1* mutations underlie ocular anterior segment dysgenesis with an increased risk of glaucoma and systemic defects, while *FOXL2* mutations cause blepharophimosis, ptosis, and epicanthus inversus syndrome (BPES), an autosomal-dominant disorder affecting the eyelids and tissues surrounding the eye. In this chapter, we will discuss the involvement of *FOXC1* and *FOXL2* in development as well as the pathology that results when these genes are altered.

FOXC1

Axenfeld-Rieger malformations cause a spectrum of ocular anterior segment defects and increase the risk of glaucoma in patients by 50%. Genetically heterogeneous, Axenfeld-Rieger malformations are transmitted in an autosomal-dominant manner and are highly penetrant. Mutations in *FOXC1* underlie Axenfeld-Rieger malformations, mapping to 6p25. *FOXC1* mutations can reduce the levels of FOXC1 protein, inhibit DNA binding of FOXC1, and/or reduce levels of FOXC1 transactivation. Although the missense mutations studied thus far have not shown a strong genotype–phenotype correlation, patients with *FOXC1* duplications appear to have a higher incidence of glaucoma. Animal studies have shown that *Foxc1* is a key regulator of somitogenesis, interacting with several genes, including components of the Notch signaling pathway. These studies have also shown that *Foxc1* plays critical roles in the normal development of the ocular, skeletal, cardiac, and urogenital systems.

Locus and Developmental Pathway

FOXC1 is located at 6p25 in the human genome and is a single-exon gene. The 1659 bp open reading frame encodes a protein, 553 amino acids in length, that localizes to the nucleus and contains several functional domains (Saleem et al., 2001; Berry et al., 2002) (Fig. 65–1). The FOXC1 FHD binds a consensus DNA sequence (RTAAAYA) (Pierrou et al., 1994) and contains amino acid regions necessary for correct nuclear targeting (Berry et al., 2002). Amino acid residues 168–176 in the C-terminal portion of the FHD are required for the nuclear localization of FOXC1 and, when fused to a green fluorescent protein (GFP) reporter, are able to target the GFP reporter to the nucleus. These sequences thus represent a bona fide nuclear localization signal. At the N terminus of the FHD, amino acid residues 78–93 constitute a required accessory domain for efficient targeting of FOXC1 to the nucleus but are not sufficient for the nuclear localization of a GFP reporter.

FOXC1 is able to transactivate gene expression of a reporter construct (Saleem et al., 2001; Berry et al., 2002), an activity mediated by N- and C-terminal activation domains (Berry et al., 2002) (Fig. 65–1). The N-terminal activation domain is located within amino acid residues 1–51, while the C-terminal activation domain is located within amino acid residues 435–553. FOXC1 constructs lacking these domains are unable to transactivate gene expression, while fusion of these activation domains to a GAL4 DNA-binding domain increases transcriptional activation of a GAL4 reporter gene. Interestingly, the C-terminal activation domain–GAL4 DNA-binding domain fusion protein is able to transactivate gene expression at levels 10 times that of full-length FOXC1–GAL4 DNA-binding domain chimeric proteins. The comparatively lower transactivation ability of full-length FOXC1 may be due to the presence of an inhibitory domain located within amino acid residues 215–365 (Berry et al., 2002) (Fig. 65–1). The FOXC1 inhibitory domain is not able to independently repress transcription but instead inhibits the transcriptional potential of activation domains. Additionally, amino acid residues 215 and 366 are phosphorylated, thus altering the protein conformation of FOXC1, and can be dephosphorylated by treatment with calf intestinal phosphatase (Berry et al., 2002).

FOXC1 is expressed in multiple fetal and adult tissues, as determined by Northern blot analysis (Pierrou et al., 1994; Mears et al., 1998; Nishimura et al., 1998). A 3.9–4.5 kb mRNA is detected, with the highest expression in adult kidney, heart, peripheral blood leukocytes, and prostate and in fetal kidney. An alternative transcript, 3.4–4.0 kb in size, is found in fetal kidney, likely generated by differential polyadenylation (Pierrou et al., 1994; Mears et al., 1998; Nishimura et al, 1998). PCR analysis detects *FOXC1* in human fetal craniofacial RNA and in human adult iris (Mears et al., 1998).

Foxc1 (formerly *Mf1* and *Fhk1*) is the murine homologue of human *FOXC1*. At the amino acid level, the FHD of human FOXC1 and murine Foxc1 are identical, and outside the FHD the proteins are 92% identical. Adult expression of murine *Foxc1* is present in multiple tissues, with the exception of liver (Hiemisch et al., 1998; Nishimura et al., 1998). The highest expression of mouse *Foxc1* is found in heart, kidney, adrenal glands, and brain, as determined by RNase protection assays (Hiemisch et al., 1998). Embryonically, *Foxc1* expression has been studied extensively. A significant advance in these studies was the generation of a mouse in which *Foxc1* is replaced by the *LacZ* gene (*Foxc1^lacZ*), allowing analysis of *Foxc1* promoter activity by staining for β-galactosidase (Kume et al., 1998).

Expression of *Foxc1* in the Somites and Presomitic Mesoderm

Embryonic expression of *Foxc1* is detected throughout the mesoderm, with the exception of the notochord (Sasaki and Hogan, 1993). Between 7.5 and 9.0 days post coitum (dpc), *Foxc1* is first expressed in the developing embryo in the presomitic mesoderm (PSM) and somites (Sasaki and Hogan, 1993; Hiemisch et al., 1998). Interestingly, immunohistochemistry experiments show that by 9.5 dpc Foxc1 protein forms a gradient from low levels in the posterior PSM to high levels in the anterior PSM (Kume et al., 2001). Transverse sections at the PSM level also detect the highest levels of *Foxc1* mRNA closest to the neural tube, forming a dorsal/ventral gradient (Kume et al., 2000). The zebrafish *FOXC1* homologue, *foxc1a*, is expressed in the developing somites (Topczewska et al., 2001). As somitogenesis proceeds, it becomes evident that Foxc1 is also involved in skeletal development,

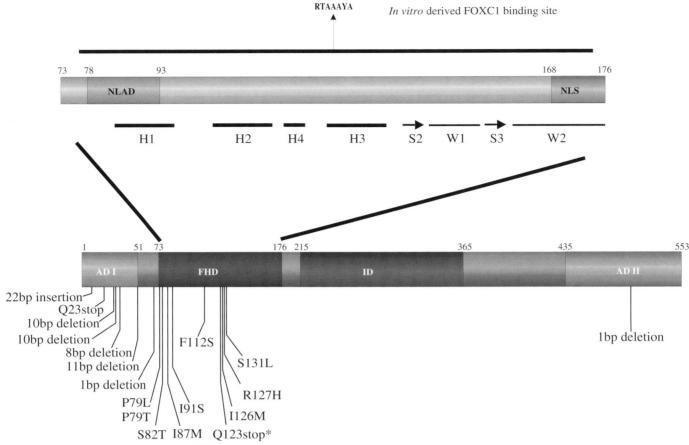

Figure 65–1. Schematic representation of FOXC1 domains and *FOXC1* mutations. AD I, activation domain 1 (N terminus); FHD, forkhead domain; ID, inhibitory domain; AD II, activation domain 2 (C terminus); NLAD, nuclear localization accessory factor; NLS, nuclear localization signal. *Congenital hydrocephalus mutation identified in mouse.

where it is expressed by 11.5–12.5 dpc in the condensing mesenchyme of the vertebrae and forelimbs (Hiemisch et al., 1998; Kume et al., 1998).

Cardiac Expression of *Foxc1*

Foxc1 is involved in early cardiac development. Between 7.5 and 9.0 dpc, *Foxc1* is first seen in the developing embryo in the first branchial arches (Sasaki and Hogan, 1993; Hiemisch et al., 1998). *Foxc1* is also weakly expressed during early embryogenesis in the endocardium, the dorsal portion of the pericardial peritoneal canal (Swiderski et al., 1999), the pharyngeal arch system, and the endothelium of the heart (Winnier et al., 1999). There is clear expression of *Foxc1* in the heart at 10.5–11.5 dpc as the valves and septae form, with expression in the mesenchyme and endothelium of the aortic arches at 10.5 dpc (Winnier et al., 1999). By 11.5–13 dpc, *Foxc1* is expressed in the mesenchyme surrounding all arterial vessels, the mesenchyme of each leaflet of the semilunar valves, the future spiral septum outflow tract, the future atrial septum, the endocardial cushion tissue of the heart, and the semilunar, tricuspid, and mitral valves. *Foxc1* is also expressed uniformly throughout the smooth muscle of the pulmonary trunk (Swiderski et al., 1999; Winnier et al., 1999). Swiderski et al. (1999) also found expression of *Foxc1* in the trabeculated region of the ventricular wall, the aortic and pulmonary valves, and the septum primum. By 15 dpc, there is a general decrease in *Foxc1* expression but a persistence of signal in the atrial septum and the mitral, tricuspid, aortic, and pulmonary valves (Swiderski et al., 1999). *Foxc1* expression is still present in adult mouse cardiac tissue in the aorta, the pulmonary trunk, the endocardium, and the smooth muscle and endothelium of the coronary vessels (Winnier et al., 1999).

Urogenital Expression of *Foxc1*

Expression of *Foxc1* is also observed in the presumptive intermediate mesoderm, which will give rise to the urogenital system (Kume et al., 2000). At 9.5 dpc, there is urogenital expression in the mesonephric mesenchyme alongside the Wolffian duct (Kume et al., 2000). *Foxc1* is expressed weakly in the Wolffian duct itself, though by 11.5–12.5 dpc no expression in the Wolffian duct can be seen. As development of the urogenital system proceeds, Foxc1 becomes expressed in the metanephric mesenchyme.

Ocular Expression of *Foxc1*

Expression of *Foxc1* is also seen in the cells that will give rise to the ocular tissues. From days 10.5 to 11.5 dpc, *Foxc1* is highly expressed in the head mesenchyme and by 11.5–12.5 dpc the specific ocular tissues expressing *Foxc1* can be identified. *Foxc1* is expressed in the mesenchymal cells of the optic cup between the lens and the retina, the periocular mesenchyme, the cornea, the prospective trabecular meshwork, the sclera, the ectoderm of the future inner eyelids, and the future conjunctival epithelium (Kidson et al., 1999). *Foxc1* expression persists in the prospective trabecular meshwork, the sclera, and the conjunctival epithelium at 16.5 dpc (Kidson et al., 1999).

Expression of *Foxc1* throughout embryogenesis in the PSM, somites, and the developing cardiovascular and urogenital systems and the prevalence of *Foxc1* in the forming ocular tissues suggest that *Foxc1* plays an important role in embryogenesis. In particular, the prevalent ocular expression of *Foxc1* is consistent with *Foxc1* being a major eye development locus. The discovery of *FOXC1* mutations in Axenfeld-Rieger malformation patients confirms this idea.

Clinical Description

Axenfeld-Rieger malformations are a group of genetically and phenotypically heterogeneous disorders leading to aberrant development of the eye (Fig. 65–2) as well as other tissues. Axenfeld-Rieger malformations have been mapped to three chromosomal loci: 4q25, 6p25, and 13q14. While the gene at 13q14 has yet to be identified, it is known that mutations in *PITX2* cause Axenfeld-Rieger malformations mapping to 4q25 (Semina et al., 1996). Mutations in *FOXC1* underlie Axenfeld-Rieger malformations mapping to 6p25 (Mears et al., 1998; Nishimura et al., 1998). Axenfeld-Rieger malformations are transmitted in an autosomal-dominant manner and are highly penetrant but vary greatly in expressivity. Patients with Axenfeld-Rieger malformations typically have a 50% higher incidence of glaucoma.

Historically, Axenfeld-Rieger malformations have been classified as Axenfeld's anomaly, Rieger's anomaly, or Rieger's syndrome, a group of related conditions. Patients were considered to have Axenfeld's anomaly when they presented with iris strands connecting the iridocorneal angle to the trabecular meshwork and a prominent, anteriorly displaced Schwalbe's line. If a patient presented with iris hypoplasia, corectopia (abnormal situation of the pupil), or polycoria, he or she was considered to have Rieger's anomaly. When these findings were concurrent with systemic defects, patients were considered to have Rieger's syndrome. Systemic findings associated with *FOXC1* mutations include maxillary hypoplasia, telecanthus, hypertelorism, a broad and flat nasal bridge, hypodontia, hypospadism, and a protruding umbilicus. Cardiac anomalies such as atrial septal defects, mitral valve defects, and tricuspid valve defects have been found in patients with *FOXC1* mutations, although evidence of *FOXC1* underlying cardiac defects in humans is still anecdotal (Mears et al., 1998; Winnier et al., 1999; Swiderski et al., 1999).

The overlap of ocular and nonocular defects in patients with Axenfeld's anomaly, Rieger's anomaly, and Rieger's syndrome makes this classification scheme somewhat arbitrary, leading to the proposal that these defects be classified as Axenfeld-Rieger anomaly for patients presenting with ocular defects only and Axenfeld-Rieger syndrome for patients presenting with ocular and systemic defects (Shields, 1983). In light of recent molecular data showing that mutations to a single gene can cause both the anomalous and syndromic forms of Axenfeld-Rieger, we propose that the term *Axenfeld-Rieger malformations* be used to describe these defects (Lines et al., 2002).

Identification of the Gene and Mutational Spectrum

The terminal end of chromosome 6 was known to contain a locus important for ocular development from clinical and cytogenetic analyses of patients with distal deletions of 6p or ring chromosome 6 (Zurcher et al., 1990; Palmer et al., 1991; Plaja et al., 1994). Patients with 6p terminal deletions presented with various ocular defects, such as iris hypoplasia and glaucoma; nonocular defects, including facial and dental anomalies; and cardiac defects. Linkage analysis in two families presenting with iris hypoplasia, goniodysgenesis, and a high frequency of juvenile glaucoma demonstrated the presence of an important ocular development locus at 6p25 and identified *FOXC1* as a candidate gene (Mears et al., 1996). Subsequent linkage analysis in a family diagnosed with Axenfeld-Rieger anomaly demonstrated that this disease phenotype also mapped to a critical region located at 6p25 (Gould et al., 1997). Identification of this important ocular locus led to direct analysis of candidate genes within the 6p25 critical region. These analyses allowed two groups to independently identify mutations in *FOXC1* within families diagnosed with Axenfeld-Rieger malformations (Mears et al., 1998; Nishimura et al., 1998). Concurrent with the findings in humans, *Foxc1* was identified as the gene underlying the mouse *congenital hydrocephalus* phenotype (Kume et al., 1998; Hong et al., 1999). Interestingly, some patients with deletions of 6p25 also present with hydrocephalus (Kume et al., 1998).

Mutations reported thus far in *FOXC1* have been largely frameshift mutations upstream of the FHD that result in truncated proteins and missense mutations within the FHD itself (see Table 65–1 and Fig. 65–1). One exception is a single base pair deletion found downstream

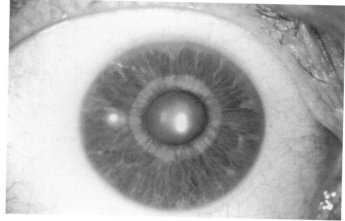

Figure 65–2. Photograph showing Axenfeld-Rieger malformations in a patient eye. Note the iris hypoplasia, prominent iris sphincter muscle (white ring around pupil), and corectopia.

of the FHD that removes only the last 49 amino acids of *FOXC1* (Nishimura et al., 2001), possibly inactivating the potent C-terminal transactivation domain (Berry et al., 2002). Interestingly, the *FOXC1* F112S mutation corresponds to the same position as an F98S mutation in *Foxe3* found in the mouse mutant *dysgenic lens* (Blixt et al., 2000). Similarly, the R127H mutation in *FOXC1* corresponds to the R127H mutation in *FOXP2*, a gene involved in speech capacity (Lai et al., 2001). The occurrence of analogous missense mutations in different *FOX* genes is likely indicative of a low tolerance for change and a high degree of conservation of key residues within the FHD.

Biochemical analysis of five of the *FOXC1* missense mutations (S82T, I87M, F112S, I126M, S131L) located within the FHD demonstrated that these mutations perturb FOXC1 activity (Saleem et al., 2001). The I87M mutation markedly reduces levels of FOXC1 protein, either by reducing the ability of cells to translate *FOXC1* mRNA or by reducing the stability of the FOXC1 protein. FOXC1 harboring the S82T and S131L mutations shows reduced binding to a synthetic FOXC1-binding site, while FOXC1 F112S or I126M mutants bind the FOXC1-binding site at near wild-type levels. The I126M mutation was also found to have altered binding specificity. All of the mutants of FOXC1 tested showed reduced ability to transactivate luciferase reporter assays, although to different extents. The S82T mutation shows almost 60% of wild-type FOXC1 transactivation ability, while the S131L mutation shows no transactivation ability. Based on the above data, it is likely that the net effect of these *FOXC1* mutations is to reduce the expression of FOXC1 target genes and that they represent loss-of-function mutations.

While the above data indicate that loss-of-function mutations in *FOXC1* underlie Axenfeld-Rieger malformations, recent data suggest that increased *FOXC1* gene dosage may also be deleterious (Lehmann et al., 2000; Nishimura et al., 2001). Specifically, patients with *FOXC1* duplications may have up to 150% of wild type FOXC1 activity (three active alleles), while patients carrying the S82T FOXC1 mutation may retain 78% of normal FOXC1 activity (the activity of FOXC1 S82T and the wild-type allele). The evidence that either loss-of-function mutations or increased gene dosages induce Axenfeld-Rieger malformations suggests that normal development is quite sensitive to *FOXC1* levels, reflecting stringent upper and lower critical thresholds for *FOXC1* activity. Additionally, the missense mutations do not appear to have strong genotype–phenotype correlations in *FOXC1* pathogenesis, though this may reflect the activity of modifier loci. Patients carrying the S82T *FOXC1* allele, which has a high amount of residual activity, can have a more severe phenotype than patients with an S131L *FOXC1* allele, which has no activity (Saleem et al., 2001). Lehmann et al. (2000) noted, however, that patients with duplications of *FOXC1* appear to have a higher incidence of glaucoma, suggesting that an increase in *FOXC1* dosage may have a more deleterious effect than reduction in *FOXC1* dosage.

Table 65–1. Summary of Human Mutations Reported in *FOXC1*

Mutation	Position	Clinical Features	Reference
P79L	236	NL	Nishimura et al., 2001
P79T	235	Early-onset glaucoma, posterior embryotoxon, iris hypoplasia, iris strands, scrotum defects, persistence of pupillary membrane, atrial septal defects	Suzuki et al., 2001
S82T	245	Glaucoma, corectopia, goniodysgenesis, iris hypoplasia, iris strands, posterior embryotoxon, atrial septal defects, hearing loss	Mears et al., 1998
I87M	261	Glaucoma, iris strands, goniodysgenesis, posterior embryotoxon	Mears et al., 1998
I91S	273	Severe early-onset glaucoma, iris hypoplasia	Kawase et al., 2001
F112S	335	A spectrum of anterior segment defects, mitral valve defects, mitral and tricuspid valve defects	Nishimura et al., 1998; Swiderski et al., 1999
I126M	378	Glaucoma, severe Axenfeld's anomaly	Nishimura et al., 2001
R127H	381	Severe early-onset glaucoma, iris hypoplasia	Kawase et al., 2001
S131L	392	Glaucoma, classic Rieger's anomaly, Axenfeld's anomaly	Nishimura et al., 1998, 2001
Q23Stop	67	Iris hypoplasia, corectopia, posterior embryotoxon, iris strands, flat midface, microdontia, umbilical anomalies, cardiac defects, hearing loss	Mirzayans et al., 2000
10 bp deletion	93–102	Glaucoma, iris hypoplasia, goniodysgenesis	Mears et al., 1998
11 bp deletion	153–162	Glaucoma, Rieger's anomaly, iris hypoplasia	Nishimura et al., 1998
22 bp insertion	26–47	NL	Nishimura et al., 2001; Kawase et al., 2001
10 bp deletion	99–108	NL	Nishimura et al., 2001
8 bp deletion	116–123	NL	Nishimura et al., 2001
1 bp deletion	210	Ocular findings not listed, atrial septal defects	Swiderski et al., 1999
1 bp insertion	262–265	NL	Nishimura et al., 2001
1 bp insertion	286	Congenital glaucoma, posterior embryotoxon, iris hypoplasia, hypertelorism	Kawase et al., 2001
1 bp deletion	1512	NL	Nishimura et al., 2001
6p25 duplication	NA	Glaucoma, iris hypoplasia, iris strands, goniodysgenesis	Lehmann et al., 2000
6p25 duplication	NA	Iris hypoplasia	Nishimura et al., 2001
6p25 duplication	NA	NL	Nishimura et al., 2001

NA, not applicable; NL, not listed.

Management and Counseling

The most severe consequence of Axenfeld-Rieger malformations is the increased risk of developing glaucoma. The glaucoma that Axenfeld-Rieger patients develop is managed with a variety of pharmacologic and surgical treatments (Shields, 1989). In adult cases, a medical course of treatment is initially recommended. These treatments include the use of β-blocking agents and carbonic anhydrase inhibitors to reduce the production of aqueous humor. Surgery is recommended in cases where medical treatment does not help and in infantile cases. Surgical treatments include goniotomy, trabeculotomy, and trabeculectomy. The latter surgical procedure is the most common treatment used for patients with Axenfeld-Rieger-associated glaucoma.

Animal Models and Mutations in Orthologous Genes
The *Congenital Hydrocephalus* Mouse
A point mutation in *Foxc1*, generating a truncated protein that lacks the FHD, underlies the spontaneous mouse mutation *congenital hydrocephalus (ch)*, described by Gruneberg (1943; Kume et al., 1998; Hong et al., 1999). The phenotype of homozygous *Foxc1^lacZ^* null mutants is identical to the *ch* phenotype (Kume et al., 1998).

*Foxc1^lacZ^* and *ch* Homozygous Nulls Have Severe Developmental Defects
ch (Foxc1^lacZ^) homozygous null mice have massively enlarged cerebral hemispheres that are hemorrhagic, with a dark purplish blue color. All *ch* homozygous mice die pre- or perinatally as a result of respiratory failure, showing an absence of expanded alveoli (Hong et al., 1999; Winnier et al., 1999). At 14.5 dpc, *ch (Foxc1^lacZ^)* homozygous mutant embryos can be clearly distinguished from their wild-type littermates by frontal bulging of the head and a striking lack of the cranial vault, due to absence of the calvarial bones, giving the top of the head a flat appearance. *ch (Foxc1^lacZ^)* homozygous null embryos show a reduction in size of the basio-occipital, exo-occipital, and hyoid bones. The superoccipital bone is severely malformed, while the mandible, squamous, and zygomatic bones are misshapen and massively ossified. Additionally, the nasal septum is reduced, leading to the characteristic short snout appearance. In the axial skeleton, the dorsal neural arches of the vertebral, including the axis and atlas, fail to fuse along the length of the whole vertebral column, with a reduction of the lateral arches and vertebral bodies (Kume et al., 1998; Hong et al., 1999). The rib cage and ribs in *ch (Foxc1^lacZ^)* homozygous null embryos are reduced and fragile, showing an absence of the sternum ossification centers except in the manubrium, a weak attachment of the right and left costal cartilage, and a misshapen and fragmented xiphoid process (Kume et al., 1998; Hong et al., 1999). The severe skeletal defects in homozygotes, particularly with respect to facial bone development, are reminiscent of the syndromic features in patients with Axenfeld-Rieger malformations.

The development of other systems is also affected in *ch (Foxc1^lacZ^)* homozygous null embryos. Sections of fixed 16.5 dpc embryos show disruptions to some blood vessels in the brain (Kume et al., 1998). Ocular findings include open eyelids, failure of the anterior chamber to form, iris hypoplasia, attachment of the lens to the cornea, thickening of the corneal epithelium, absence of the corneal endothelium, and disorganized corneal stroma (Kume et al., 1998; Kidson et al., 1999). Interestingly, the thickened corneal epithelium shows expansion of *Foxc1^lacZ^* expression, raising the possibility of a self-regulating mechanism (Kidson et al., 1999). In addition to the other corneal anomalies, there is absence of organized zonular occludens junctions in *ch (Foxc1^lacZ^)* homozygous null corneal mesenchyme cells, indicating that *Foxc1* may play a role in regulating extracellular matrix components (Kidson et al., 1999). Evidence from mouse expression data, the ocular defects in the *ch* mouse, and the ocular defects found in humans with *FOXC1* mutations demonstrate the importance of *FOXC1* in ocular development.

ch (Foxc1^lacZ^) homozygous null embryos also show malformations of the cardiovascular and urogenital systems. Cardiovascular defects include type B interruptions, a clear coarctation, or a narrowing of the aortic arch (Winnier et al., 1999). Additional cardiac defects of *ch (Foxc1^lacZ^)* homozygous nulls include infundibular hypertrophy, ventricular septal defects, and aortic and pulmonary valve dysplasia. The pulmonary and aortic valve leaflets of homozygous mutant mice are thickened and partially fused at the commissures. Urogenital defects in *ch (Foxc1^lacZ^)* homozygous mice include duplex kidneys connected to double ureters and fluid-filled enlargement of the kidney and ureter (Green, 1970; Kume et al., 2000). Only one of the ureters is fluid-filled and dilated; the other ureter is normal (Kume et al., 2000). An ectopic ureteric bud forms in *ch* (*Foxc1^lacZ*) homozygous mutants by 11 dpc anteriorly to the normal ureteric bud, the wolffian duct is kinked and displaced medially, and the normal ureteric bud is much broader than in wild-type mice. It is thought that reciprocal interactions between the ectopic bud and the nephrogenic mesenchyme induce formation of an ectopic kidney, which fuses with the normal kidney (Green, 1970; Kume et al., 2000). Both sexes (males 75% and females 100%) of *ch* (*Foxc1^lacZ*) homozygous mutants show anteriorly displaced gonads compared to wild-type mice (Green 1970; Kume et al., 2000). The range of defects found in *ch* (*Foxc1^lacZ*) homozygous mutants demonstrates that *Foxc1* is an important regulator of skeletal, ocular, cardiac, and urogenital development.

The penetrance of many of these developmental anomalies can vary depending on the genetic background of the *ch* (*Foxc1^lacZ*) homozygous mutant (Hong et al., 1999; Winnier et al., 1999; Kume et al., 2000; Smith et al., 2000). *Foxc1* malformations tend to show greater penetrance on CHMU/Le × C57BL/6 backgrounds in comparison to other backgrounds, such as 129 × black Swiss or CAST. Interestingly, *ch* (*Foxc1^lacZ*) homozygous cardiac anomalies are still highly penetrant on a 129 × black Swiss background (Winnier et al., 1999). The differential effects of background on penetrance are likely due to modifier genes that modulate the effect of *Foxc1* deficiencies. The identities of any modifier genes are unknown.

Foxc1^lacZ and *ch* Heterozygotes Have Ocular Defects Similar to Axenfeld-Rieger Malformations

Heterozygous *ch* (*Foxc1^lacZ*) mice have numerous ocular anterior segment malformations, although there is a range of expressivity (Hong et al., 1999; Smith et al., 2000). Slit-lamp analysis revealed anterior segment malformations of heterozygous *ch* (*Foxc1^lacZ*) that included progressive corectopia (abnormal situation of the pupil), irregularly shaped pupils, iridocorneal adhesions and iris tears, a progressively thinning iris, posterior embryotoxon, scleralization of the peripheral cornea, and corneal opacities. Older heterozygous *ch* mice have a high incidence of corneal opacification, neovascularization, and cataracts.

Interestingly, histologic analysis determined that anterior segment defects occur in *Foxc1^lacZ* heterozygotes regardless of the background (Smith et al., 2000). The severity of the specific defect varies greatly between eyes and within individual eyes. The majority of eyes analyzed have varying degrees of abnormality in the iridocorneal angles. Abnormalities of the iridocorneal angle include a reduced or absent Schlemm's canal, enlarged blood vessels, iris strands, and a hypoplastic, compressed, or absent trabecular meshwork (TM). Cells resembling TM mesenchymal precursor cells sometimes occupy areas lacking a TM. Interestingly, some *ch* heterozygotes on a CHUM/Le background presented with hypoplastic ciliary bodies and short, thin ciliary processes, while no ciliary body defects were found in *Foxc1^lacZ* heterozygotes on any of the backgrounds tested (Smith et al., 2000).

The TM is normally composed of spaced trabecular beams and organized collagen and elastic tissue, allowing drainage of the aqueous humour from the eye. Electron microscopy of the TM in *Foxc1^lacZ* mice shows regional affected areas with disruptions of the extracellular matrix (Smith et al., 2000). Affected regions sometimes contain cells that resemble TM precursor cells, or in other areas, the TM cells have a normal appearance but are densely packed and continuous. Schlemm's canal contains giant vacuoles or is absent in some areas with abnormal TM cells. That the ocular findings in mouse *Foxc1* heterozygotes recapitulate the ocular phenotypes of *FOXC1* insufficiencies in humans shows that there is likely a high degree of conservation in FOXC1 function between mouse and human.

Developmental Pathogenesis

While the upstream regulators and downstream targets of FOXC1 remain unknown, there is a significant amount of data revealing genes that show altered expression on *Foxc1^-/-* single homozygous and *Foxc1^-/-*/Foxc2^-/- compound homozygous backgrounds (see Table 65–2). In *Foxc1^-/-* homozygotes, two genes regulating urogenital development, *Gdnf* and *Eya1*, show expression that is anteriorly expanded (Kume et al., 2000). *Gdnf* is expressed in the mesenchyme of the developing urogenital system, and both *Gdnf* and *Eya1* are required for ureteric bud formation (Moore et al., 1996; Abdelhak et al., 1997). Homozygous nulls of either *Gdnf* or *Eya1* do not form ureteric buds. *Eya1* homozygous nulls do not express *Gdnf* in the nephrogenic mesenchyme, suggesting that *Eya1* acts upstream of *Gdnf* to regulate *Gdnf* expression.

Experiments using micromass cultures of the sternum primordium from *Foxc1^-/-* homozygotes indicate that *Foxc1* mediates bone morphogenetic protein 2 (BMP2) and transforming growth factor β1 (TGF-β1) signaling (Kume et al., 1998). Wild-type cultures will show enhanced chondrogenesis in response to BMP2 or TGF-β1, but this response is drastically reduced in *Foxc1^-/-* homozygote micromass cultures, indicating that *Foxc1* is required for cartilage development. It is also possible that Foxc1 regulates its own expression. As mentioned above, in *Foxc1^lacZ* homozygous mutants, *Foxc1^lacZ* expression persists in the presumptive corneal mesenchyme, whereas in normal embryos *Foxc1* is downregulated as the endothelial cells differentiate (Kidson et al., 1999).

Many genetic and systemic defects are observed only on compound *Foxc1^-/-*/Foxc2^-/- homozygous backgrounds (see above), demonstrating that, to some extent, *Foxc1* and *Foxc2* can complement each other. Compound homozygotes do not express *paraxis* in the somites and anterior PSM, the normal sites of *paraxis* expression, while *Foxc1^-/-* and *Foxc2^-/-* single homozygotes show no *paraxis* defect (Burgess et al., 1995; Kume et al., 2001). Interestingly, the mesodermal cells are correctly specified as paraxial mesoderm, as indicated by *Mox1* and *pMesogenin1* expression, but show a significant differentiation defect, as indicated by an absence of *Pax1* and *MyoD* expression (Kume et al., 2001) (Table 65–2). In zebrafish, *foxc1a* regulates the expression of *paraxis* (Topczewska et al., 2001). *Foxc1^-/-*/Foxc2^-/- compound homozygotes also have defects in Notch signaling in the anterior PSM (Kume et al., 2001). Notch sig-

Table 65–2. Summary of Genes Affected in *Foxc1^-/-* Single Homozygotes

Gene	Function/Expression	Defect	Reference
Foxc1	Downregulated in the corneal endothelium as the presumptive corneal mesenchyme differentiates	Endothelial cells do not differentiate, and *Foxc1^lacZ* expression persists	Kidson et al., 1999
Gdnf	Essential for ureteric bud formation	Anterior and medial expansion of Gndf expression	Kume et al., 2000
Eya1	Expression overlaps with *Gdnf*, essential for ureteric bud formation, likely upstream of *Gdnf*	Anterior expansion of *Eya1* expression	Kume et al., 2000
BMP2	Wild-type micromass cultures of sternal primordium undergo enhanced chondrogenesis in the presence of BMP2	Micromass cultures of sternal primordium from *Foxc1^-/-* cells have significantly reduced response to BMP2	Kume et al., 1998
TGFβ1	Wild-type micromass cultures of sternal primordium undergo enhanced chondrogenesis in the presence of TGF-β1	Micromass cultures of sternal primordium from *Foxc1^-/-* cells have significantly reduced response to TGF-β1	Kume et al., 1998
zo1	Major component of bands of occluding junctions between wild-type endothelial cells	Absent in mutant *Foxc1^-/-* cells, punctate expression seen in mesenchyme adjacent to lens of eye	Kidson et al., 1999

Table 65–3. Summary of Genes Affected in *Foxc1*$^{-/-}$/*Foxc2*$^{-/-}$ Compound Homozygotes

Gene	Function/Expression	Defect
Paraxis	Normally expressed in somites, anterior PSM	No expression, very low levels anteriorly near neural tube
Tbx18	Normally expressed in anterior portion of somite	No expression, expression normal in single *Foxc1*$^{-/-}$ and *Foxc2*$^{-/-}$ homozygotes
Uncx4.1	Normally expressed in posterior portion of somite	No expression, expression normal in single *Foxc1*$^{-/-}$ and *Foxc2*$^{-/-}$ homozygotes
Pax1	Normally expressed in somites	No expression in somites
MyoD	Normally expressed in somites	No expression in somites
ephrinB2	ephrin/Eph pathway involved in formation of boundary between S0 and S1 somites	*ephrinB2* is expressed but expression is downregulated and diffuse
Notch1	Expressed in anterior PSM with highest levels in S2 somite	Strongly downregulated, only very faint bands in presumptive S1 and S2 somites
Mesp2	A bHLH transcription factor expressed in anterior portion of S2 somite, may function to specify anterior cell fate	Strongly downregulated
Mesp1	Closely related to *Mesp2*	Strongly downregulated
Lunatic Fringe	Encodes a modulator of Notch receptor activity	Reduced expression with diffuse expression pattern
Dll1	Encodes a Notch ligand, expressed throughout PSM and posterior half of S1 somite	Anterior boundary diffuse, expression in somite region diffuse
Hes5	A target of the Notch signaling pathway, expressed in two stripes of the anterior PSM	Pattern of expression diffuse and downregulated, expression normal in neural tube

PSM, presomitic mesoerm; bHLH, basic helix-loop-helix.
Source: Kume et al., 2001.

naling, in conjunction with *Mesp2*-mediated downregulation of *Dll1* in the anterior somite, is thought to be required for the establishment of anterior and posterior cell fates within the anterior portion of the PSM (Takahashi et al., 2000). Compound null homozygotes of *Notch1* and *Notch4* (*Notch1*$^{-/-}$/*Notch4*$^{-/-}$) or the Notch signaling genes *presenilin1* and *presenilin2* (*presenilin1*$^{-/-}$/*presenilin2*$^{-/-}$) have cardiovascular and somite formation defects similar to *Foxc1*$^{-/-}$/*Foxc2*$^{-/-}$ compound homozygous nulls (Donoviel et al., 1999; Krebs et al., 2000). *Notch1*, normally expressed in the anterior PSM, with highest expression in somite S2, is strongly downregulated in *Foxc1*$^{-/-}$/*Foxc2*$^{-/-}$ compound homozygous nulls, as are other genes in Notch signaling pathways (*Mesp2, Mesp1, Lunatic fringe, Dll1, Hes5*; see Table 65–3). There is thought to be a regulatory loop between *Mesp2, Notch1*, and *Dll1* in the anterior PSM (Takahashi et al., 2000). In *Dll1* homozygous mutants, *Foxc1* is expressed at lower levels in the somites and PSM compared to wild-type embryos (Kume et al., 2001). Additionally, there is ectopic expression of *Foxc1* throughout the neural tube of the *Dll1* homozygous null embryo. Given that *Foxc1* is expressed, although at lower levels, in the *Dll1* null mouse, Foxc1 is not thought to be an obligatory component of the Mesp2–Notch1–Dll1 regulatory loop (Kume et al., 2001).

Zebrafish appear to recapitulate, to some extent, the function of *foxc1a* in the genetic regulation of somitogenesis. Expression of *mesp-b* is absent, while *notch6* and *notch5* are strongly downregulated in foxc1a "knock down" fish (Topczewska et al., 2001) (Table 65–4). Similar to *Foxc1*$^{-/-}$/*Foxc2*$^{-/-}$ compound homozygous mice, *foxc1a* knockdown zebrafish show strong downregulation of *ephrinB3* and *ephrinA4*, genes required to establish intersomitic boundaries (see Tables 65–3 and 65–4).

Clearly, FOXC1 is important for the normal development of ocular, skeletal, cardiovascular, and urogenital systems. Defects such as Axenfeld-Rieger anomalies are thought to arise from a defect in migration and differentiation of neural crest mesenchyme involved in the formation of the eye (Mears et al., 1996). FOXC1 is likely to

play a role in signaling cascades that lead to differentiation of the neural crest mesenchyme or in regulating the cell fates of the developing ocular tissues. The fact that the extracellular matrix component *zo1* is not expressed properly raises the possibility that FOXC1 regulates the expression or function of proteins involved in cell–cell adhesion (Kidson et al., 1999). Smith et al. (2000) also found deficiencies in the ocular extracellular matrix of *Foxc1* heterozygotes. Similarly, the failure of *Foxc1*$^{-/-}$ sternum primordial cells to condense and differentiate into cartilage in response to BMP2 and TGF-β1 may indicate abnormal cell–cell adhesion (Kume et al, 1998; Kidson et al., 1999).

Foxc1 may interact with factors in the Notch signaling pathway to regulate gene expression and may also interact with other *Fox* genes that are expressed in the axial, nonaxial, and lateral plate mesoderm (Kume et al., 2001). Expression of both *Foxc1* and *Foxc2* overlaps with that of Foxb1 and Foxd2 (Kume et al., 2001). Alternatively, it has been proposed that Foxc1 may remodel the chromatin structure, and thus regulate transcription, of genes involved in mesodermal development, similar to models proposed for *Foxa2* (Kume et al., 1998; Cirillo and Zaret, 1999; Kume et al., 2001). Given the wide expression of *FOXC1* and its involvement in a variety of developmental systems, it may be found that FOXC1 has diverse functions that change in different tissues at specific times. Whatever the normal roles are, FOXC1 is undeniably an important regulator of embryogenesis.

FOXL2

BPES (OMIM 110100) is an autosomal-dominant disorder affecting the eyelids and tissues surrounding the eye. It is also commonly associated with infertility in females resulting from premature ovarian failure. This disorder is classified into two forms (Zlotogora et al., 1983): BPES type I, in which the eyelid malformations are associated with ovarian failure and female infertility, and BPES type II, where only the eyelid abnormalities are observed. Both types of this disorder have

Table 65–4. Summary of Genes Affected in Zebrafish *foxc1a* Knockdowns

Gene	Function/Expression	Defect
paraxis	Normally expressed in somites, anterior PSM	No expression
mesp-b	A bHLH transcription factor expressed in anterior portion of S2 somite, may function to specify anterior cell fate	No expression
ephrinB2	ephrin/Eph pathway involved in formation of boundary between S0 and S1 somites	Strongly downregulated
notch5	Highly expressed in developing somites	Strongly downregulated
notch6	Highly expressed in developing somites	Strongly downregulated, boundaries expanded
ephA4	ephrin/Eph pathway involved in formation of boundary between S0 and S1 somites	Strongly downregulated

PSM, presomitic mesoderm; bHLH, basic helix-loop-helix.
Source: Topczewska et al., 2001.

been linked to the same chromosomal location, 3q23; and recently, mutations in patients with BPES types I and II have been identified in the *FOXL2* gene, which lies in 3q23 (Crisponi et al., 2001; De Baere et al., 2001; Yamada et al., 2001). The *FOXL2* mutations identified in patients with both forms of BPES are varied and include nonsense mutations, missense mutations, and insertions and deletions resulting in frameshift mutations. Genotype–phenotype correlations associated with these mutations may provide insight into the form of BPES that affects a given individual. Mutations resulting in BPES type I are predicted to create a truncated form of FOXL2, whereas mutations that are predicted to extend the FOXL2 protein are found in patients with BPES type II (Crisponi et al., 2001; De Baere et al., 2001; Yamada et al., 2001). How both forms of BPES differentially arise from such *FOXL2* mutations is not known.

Locus and Developmental Pathway

FOXL2 is also a member of the growing family of forkhead/winged helix transcription factors implicated in a number of human heritable diseases (reviewed in more detail in Chapter 64). *FOXL2* has been mapped to chromosome 3q23 and encodes a 2.7 kb mRNA transcript (Crisponi et al., 2001). Like many *FOX* genes, *FOXL2* contains a single coding exon. The predicted protein encoded by the *FOXL2* gene is composed of 376 amino acids and contains the evolutionarily conserved 110–amino acid FHD. Downstream of the FHD lies an alanine-rich region, which may be involved in transcriptional regulation (Tjian and Maniatis, 1994; Shim et al., 2000). Apart from these two domains, FOXL2 bears little similarity to any other protein functional domain. The consensus DNA-binding sites and targets for FOXL2 transcriptional regulation have yet to be identified.

Expression studies of *FOXL2* in mice reveal a restricted pattern of expression and suggest a role in the formation of the pituitary gland and the eyelid and maintenance of the ovary. In the pituitary, *FOXL2* displays a highly restricted expression pattern at 10.5 dpc in the ventralmost portion of Rathke's pouch (Treier et al., 1998). Its spatially restricted expression pattern suggests that it may act in establishing a gradient of transcription factors involved in pituitary cell lineage determination (Treier et al., 1998). At 13.5–15.5 dpc, *FOXL2* is highly expressed in the margins of the eyelid forming outside of the cornea, in the mesenchyme around the optic cup, and in the protruding ridges of the developing eyelid (Crisponi et al., 2001). Formation of the mouse eyelid is initiated by 15.5 dpc, consistent with *FOXL2* expression in the periocular mesenchyme (Findlater et al., 1993). The eyelids develop from the surface ectodermal folds arising from the frontonasal and maxillary processes. Proliferation of the underlying mesenchyme causes the eyelid fold to lengthen and cover the surface of the cornea. The eyelids will then fuse and remain closed until birth. In the adult mouse ovary, *FOXL2* mRNA is predominantly localized to the follicle cells surrounding the oocyte but absent from the oocyte itself (Crisponi et al., 2001). Northern blot data reveal an exclusive expression pattern of *FOXL2* in the adult human ovary. Expression of *FOXL2* in follicular cells but not in the oocyte proper suggests a role in the maintenance of the ovary (Crisponi et al., 2001). The expression patterns presented for *FOXL2* foretell a role for *FOXL2* in the etiology of BPES.

Clinical Description

BPES is an autosomal-dominant disorder that was first described by Vignes (1889) as dysplasia of the eyelids. It is characterized by a reduction of the width of the palpebral fissure (blepharophimosis), drooping of the upper eyelid (ptosis), and formation of a small skin fold arising from the lower eyelid and running up to the nasal bridge (epicanthus inversus) (Fig. 65–3). Ultimately, the effect of these malformations is a reduction of the size of the palpebral aperture, and patients often display a characteristic posture, with brow furrowed and the head tilted back to compensate for the reduced eyelid opening. Acquisition of this posture as an infant can impair the development of sitting and walking as the child will often topple over backward to see from the lowered eyelids (Oley and Baraitser, 1988). In addition to these characteristic eyelid anomalies, patients may present a spectrum of nonocular features, including a flat and low nasal bridge, an

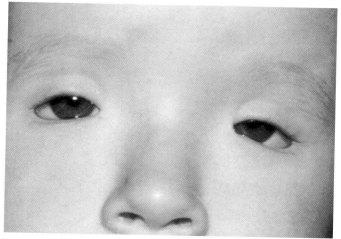

Figure 65–3. Eyelid and facial features of a blepharophomisis, ptosis, and epicanthus inversus syndrome–affected child.

increase in the vertical height of the eyebrows, protruding cup-shaped ears, as well as cardiac defects (Beauchamp, 1980). Rare cases of learning difficulties have been detected in BPES, although these are unusual and may represent an extreme phenotype (Harrar et al., 1995) or comorbidity.

Additional features commonly associated with BPES are menstrual irregularities (primary or secondary amenorrhea), primary ovarian failure, and female infertility. BPES females afflicted with primary ovarian failure display normal secondary sexual characteristics; however, they present with elevated gonadotropin levels and decreased estradiol and progesterone levels and ultimately cease menses (Townes and Muechler, 1979; Fraser et al., 1988; Prueitt and Zinn, 2001). Males with BPES are fertile, and in many pedigrees, BPES is transmitted only through males.

Identification of the Gene and Mutational Spectrum

The identification of BPES patients with balanced translocations or deletions involving chromosome 3q23 instigated the search for the responsible gene within this region. Physical mapping and positional cloning had also placed the locus responsible for BPES at 3q23. De Baere et al. (2001) identified *BPES1* as a candidate gene for BPES; it was disrupted by a balanced translocation t(3;4)(q23;p15.2). However, upon screening of BPES patients, no disease-causing mutations were found in *BPES1*. Crisponi et al. (2001) mapped a t(3;7) breakpoint and identified two novel genes at this interval: *c3orf5* and *FOXL2*. No disease-causing mutations were found in *c3orf5*; however, five distinct *FOXL2* mutations were discovered in patients with BPES type I or II. Since then a spectrum of BPES-causing mutations have been assigned to *FOXL2* (Crisponi et al., 2001; De Baere et al., 2001; Yamada et al., 2001) (Fig. 65–4).

BPES types I and II result from distinct types of mutation in the *FOXL2* gene. The disease-causing mutations ascribed to *FOXL2* include missense mutations, nonsense mutations, and insertions and deletions resulting in frameshift mutations (Fig. 65–4). These mutations in the predicted protein can lie upstream of the FHD, within the FHD, or downstream of the FHD. It is hypothesized that the differentiation of the two forms of BPES is not determined by the type or location of the *FOXL2* mutation but, rather, is the effect of the mutation on the position of the predicted termination codon. Mutations found in BPES type I patients are predicted to create a premature stop codon in the *FOXL2* open reading frame. This stop codon may result from nonsense mutations or from deletions and duplications resulting in frameshift mutations (Crisponi et al., 2001; De Baere et al., 2001). Mutations resulting in BPES type II are predicted to extend the *FOXL2* open reading frame from 5 to 156 amino acids. The type of mutations include in-frame duplications of residues in the poly-Ala region (Crisponi et al., 2001; De Baere et al., 2001), an in-frame deletion and duplication that is also predicted to extend the poly-Ala region (De

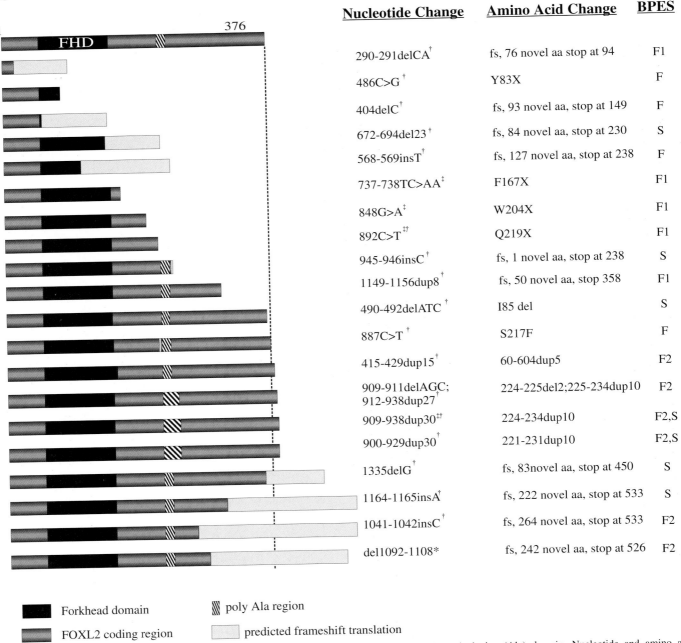

Nucleotide Change	Amino Acid Change	BPES
290-291delCA[†]	fs, 76 novel aa stop at 94	F1
486C>G[†]	Y83X	F
404delC[†]	fs, 93 novel aa, stop at 149	F
672-694del23[†]	fs, 84 novel aa, stop at 230	S
568-569insT[†]	fs, 127 novel aa, stop at 238	F
737-738TC>AA[‡]	F167X	F1
848G>A[‡]	W204X	F1
892C>T[‡‡]	Q219X	F1
945-946insC[†]	fs, 1 novel aa, stop at 238	S
1149-1156dup8[†]	fs, 50 novel aa, stop 358	F1
490-492delATC[†]	I85 del	S
887C>T[†]	S217F	F
415-429dup15[†]	60-604dup5	F2
909-911delAGC; 912-938dup27[†]	224-225del2;225-234dup10	F2
909-938dup30[‡‡]	224-234dup10	F2,S
900-929dup30[†]	221-231dup10	F2,S
1335delG[†]	fs, 83novel aa, stop at 450	S
1164-1165insA[†]	fs, 222 novel aa, stop at 533	S
1041-1042insC[†]	fs, 264 novel aa, stop at 533	F2
del1092-1108*	fs, 242 novel aa, stop at 526	F2

Legend:
- Forkhead domain
- poly Ala region
- FOXL2 coding region
- predicted frameshift translation

Figure 65–4. Summary of *FOXL2* mutations in blepharophomisis, ptosis, and epicanthus inversus syndrome (BPES) patients. Schematic representation of the *FOXL2* mutations on the predicted amino acid sequence is presented on the left. Gray bar represents the FOXL2 protein sequence, while the light box represents the predicted change in translation resulting from frameshift (fs) mutations. The Forkhead domain (FHD) is denoted by a black rectangle. Hatched box represents the polyalanine (Ala) domain. Nucleotide and amino acid changes are presented in first and second columns, respectively. The form of BPES is indicated in the third column: F1, familial BPES type I; F2, familial BPES type II; F, familial BPES of undetermined form; S, sporadic BPES. (From †De Baere et al., 2001; ‡Crisponi et al., 2001; *Yamada et al., 2001.)

Baere et al., 2001), a 17 bp deletion downstream of the predicted FHD (Yamada et al., 2001), as well as single-nucleotide insertions that shift the reading frame to extend the termination codon (De Baere et al., 2001). However, a number of *FOXL2* mutations were identified in families in which the form of BPES could not be determined because the pedigrees contained only either affected males or affected, pre-pubescent females. Additionally, a number of *FOXL2* mutations were found in sporadic cases (De Baere et al., 2001). Until the reproductive status of affected females can be determined, such genotype–phenotype correlations must remain speculative.

The breakpoint in BPES patients with cytogenetic abnormalities lies several hundred kilobases upstream of the *FOXL2* gene (Crisponi et al., 2001). It is thought that the effect of these mutations results from deletion of a distal enhancer that may disrupt *FOXL2* expression

(Crisponi et al., 2001; De Baere et al., 2001). Typically, BPES patients with translocations or microdeletions involving 3q23 present a broader spectrum and more severe features, such as learning and developmental delays, microcephaly, microphthalmia, and joint abnormalities (Williamson et al., 1981; Fujita et al., 1992; Cabral de Almeida et al., 1993; Fryns et al., 1993; Jewett et al., 1993; Boccone et al., 1994; Ishikiryama and Goto, 1994; Small et al., 1995; Warburg et al., 1995).

Management and Counseling

BPES is treated by surgical means to repair the ptosis and to improve the cosmetic appearance of the affected individual. Surgery is often initiated between the ages of 3 and 5 years. Counseling of BPES patients may be problematic as determination of the form of BPES may prove to be difficult in sporadic cases or in cases where little family history is known. BPES is a congenital disorder, and the eyelid malformations will be identified quite early in life. However, in female patients, infertility will not be diagnosed until later. The psychologic burden of the facial abnormalities and female infertility can greatly affect the quality of life of BPES patients. BPES males are fertile, yet there is a risk of transmitting the BPES type II mutation to female offspring. If the family history presents with affected females who are fertile, then it is likely that the patients are BPES type I and that affected female patients will be fertile. However, some affected BPES type II females present with menstrual and endocrine abnormalities. Mutational screening of *FOXL2* may permit a more accurate and reliable diagnosis of the particular form of BPES.

Animal Models and Mutations in Orthologous Genes

To date, targeted deletions of the mouse *Foxl2* gene have yet to be reported. However, the polled/intersex syndrome (PIS) in goats has been suggested to be an animal model for primary ovarian failure associated with BPES type II (Crisponi et al., 2001; Vaiman et al., 1999). This syndrome results in the absence of horn and sex reversal in females. The mutation afflicting the PIS goat maps to 1q31 (Vaiman et al., 1999), a region with conserved synteny to human 3q23; thus, *FOXL2* was considered an attractive candidate gene for PIS. Furthermore, Pailhoux and colleagues (2001) have determined that the PIS mutation is a deletion of a 11.7 kb element in the critical PIS region that affects transcription of *FOXL2* and *PISRT1*, a 1.5 kb mRNA devoid of an open reading frame. *FOXL2* expression was dramatically reduced in the developing gonads of PIS goats. Expression of *FOXL2* in the eyelid was not affected, consistent with the absence of eyelid malformations in PIS goats. This PIS deletion is located 200 kb upstream of the *FOXL2* gene and is believed to delete an enhancer essential for ovarian expression of *FOXL2* (Pailhoux et al., 2001). A similar position effect may also be responsible for the BPES phenotype in patients with 3;7 and 3;4 balanced translocations as the breakpoint regions in these patients lie 180 kb 5′ to the *FOXL2* locus (Crisponi et al., 2001). Such a cytogenetic rearrangement may disrupt the function of an enhancer region and alter the expression of *FOXL2* (Crisponi et al., 2001; De Baere et al., 2001; Pailhoux et al., 2001).

Developmental Pathogenesis

How do mutations in *FOXL2* differentially give rise to BPES types I vs. II? It is possible that the BPES type I mutations predicted to produce a truncated protein containing a partial or complete FHD may act in a dominant-negative manner by competing with wild-type FOXL2 for DNA-binding sites. The similarity of BPES phenotypes in patients with truncating *FOXL2* mutations to those patients carrying balanced translocations suggests that haploinsufficiency of a *FOXL2* null allele may underlie the effects of the *FOXL2* mutations. One possibility is that the introduction of the premature stop codon renders the mutant mRNA susceptible to mRNA surveillance and leads to its degradation through nonsense-mediated decay pathways (Frischmeyer and Dietz, 1999). Thus, only a single copy of *FOXL2* would be present. In type II BPES mutations, these alterations may reduce the activity of *FOXL2* to levels that are low enough to impair proper eyelid formation yet not affect ovarian maintenance. The reduction in activity may also stem from decreased protein stability rather than formation of a less active FOXL2. As in the case of FOXC1, decreased transcriptional activation of FOXL2 below a critical threshold level may initiate progression of the disease phenotype. Further molecular examination of the effects of BPES disease-causing mutations on the function of FOXL2 will be required to understand the role of FOXL2 in the manifestation of type I vs. type II BPES.

Transcriptional targets for FOXL2 have yet to be identified, and their determination will aid in the understanding of how FOXL2 contributes to the pathogenesis of BPES. At present, the role of FOXL2 in eyelid development and ovarian maintenance remains unknown. *FOXL2* is expressed in periocular mesenchyme, which contributes to the formation of eyelids. As FOXC1 is integral in the differentiation of mesenchyme cells (Kume et al., 1998), so too may be FOXL2 in the differentiation of periocular mesenchyme. The failure of eyelid fusion in mice has been associated with mutations in a number of genes,

including *TGF-α* (Carroll et al., 1998), MEK kinase 1 (Yujiri et al., 2000), the epidermal growth factor receptor (Chen et al., 2000), and the retinoid X receptor-α (Mascrez et al., 2001). Targeted deletion of the activin/inhibin-β B subunit (*Inhbb*) gene in mice produced a compound phenotype consisting of eyelid abnormalities as well as female reproductive deficiencies (Vassalli et al., 1994). The similarities between the *Inhbb* knockout mouse and BPES type II patients suggests that FOXL2 may participate in some aspect of the inhibin–TGF-β signaling pathways (Crisponi et al., 2001). One may speculate that the FOXL2 controls transcription of some of these genes required in the cascade of events essential for proper eyelid formation during development and ovarian maintenance in adult life.

CONCLUSION

FOXC1 and FOXL2 are distantly related members of the forkhead family of transcription factors that share a common DNA-binding motif yet have little similarity in the remainder of the encoded protein. Mutations in both genes result in autosomal-dominant disorders presenting ocular and craniofacial findings. Haploinsufficiency of *FOXC1* and *FOXL2* leads to the progression of Axenfeld-Rieger malformations and BPES, respectively, demonstrating the exquisite sensitivity of the development of the eye to even slight alterations in gene function. Interestingly, *ch* (*Foxc1^lacZ*) homozygous null embryos are born with open eyelids, suggesting that FOXC1 and FOXL2 may play opposing roles in eyelid formation (Kume et al., 1998). Eyelid malformations in BPES type II patients are thought to arise from *FOXL2* mutations producing a hypomorphic allele (Crisponi et al., 2001; De Baere et al., 2001). However, such mutations do not appear to affect ovarian maintenance, suggesting that the eyelids are more sensitive to FOXL2 activity than are the ovaries. In the case of FOXC1, stringent threshold levels of FOXC1 activity exist and deviations above and below such critical levels may underlie Axenfeld-Rieger malformations and other ocular anomalies (Lehmann et al., 2000; Saleem et al., 2001). The identification of target genes regulated by FOXC1 and FOXL2 as well as the determination of proteins interacting with these molecules will aid in elucidating the biologic roles of both FOXC1 and FOXL2.

NOTE ADDED IN PROOF

De Baere et al. (2003) describe 21 new *FOXL2* mutations in BPES patients leading to a revision of the genotype-phenotype correlation. Specifically, *FOXL2* mutations predicted to extend the protein while retaining an intact FHD and poly Ala tract were detected in patients with either BPES type I or II.

REFERENCES

Abdelhak S, Kalatzis V, Heilig R, Compain S, Samson D, Vincent C, Weil D, Cruaud C, Sahly I, Leibovici M, et al. (1997). A human homologue of the *Drosophila eyes absent* gene underlies branchio-oto-renal (BOR) syndrome and identifies a novel gene family. *Nat Genet* 15: 157–164.

Beauchamp GR (1980). Blepharophimosis and cardiopathy. *J Pediatr Ophthalmol Strabismus* 17: 227–228.

Berry FB, Saleem RA, Walter MA (2002). FOXC1 transcriptional regulation is mediated by N-and C-terminal activation domains and contains a phosphorylated transcriptional inhibitory domain. *J Biol Chem* 277: 10292–10297.

Blixt A, Mahlapuu M, Aitola M, Pelto Huikko M, Enerback S, Carlsson P (2000). A forkhead gene, *FoxE3*, is essential for lens epithelial proliferation and closure of the lens vesicle. *Genes Dev* 14: 245–254.

Boccone L, Meloni A, Falchi AM, Usai V, Cao A (1994). Blepharophimosis, ptosis, epicanthus inversus syndrome, a new case associated with de novo balanced autosomal translocation [46,XY,t(3;7)(q23;q32)]. *Am J Med Genet* 51: 258–259.

Burgess R, Cserjesi P, Ligon KL, Olson EN (1995). Paraxis: a basic helix-loop-helix protein expressed in paraxial mesoderm and developing somites. *Dev Biol* 168: 296–306.

Cabral de Almeida JC, Llerena JC, Neto JBG, Jung M, Martins RR (1993). Another example favouring the location of BPES at 3q2. *J Med Genet* 30: 86.

Carroll JM, Luetteke NC, Lee DC, Watt FM (1998). Role of integrins in mouse eyelid development: studies in normal embryos and embryos in which there is a failure of eyelid fusion. *Mech Dev* 78: 37–45.

Chen B, Bronson RT, Klaman LD, Hampton TG, Wang JF, Green PJ, Magnuson T, Douglas PS, Morgan JP, Neel BG (2000). Mice mutant for Egfr and Shp2 have defective cardiac semilunar valvulogenesis. *Nat Genet* 24: 296–299.

Cirillo LA, Zaret KS (1999). An early developmental transcription factor complex that is more stable on nucleosome core particles than on free DNA. *Mol Cells* 4: 961–969.

Crisponi L, Deiana M, Loi A, Chiappe F, Uda M, Amati P, Bisceglia L, Zelante L, Nagaraja R, Porcu S, et al. (2001). The putative forkhead transcription factor FOXL2 is mutated in blepharophimosis/ptosis/epicanthus inversus syndrome. *Nat Genet* 27: 159–166.

De Baere E, Dixon MJ, Small KW, Jabs EW, Leroy BP, Devriendt K, Gillerot Y, Mortier G, Meire F, Van Maldergem L, et al. (2001). Spectrum of *FOXL2* gene mutations in blepharophimosis-ptosis-epicanthus inversus (BPES) families demonstrates a genotype–phenotype correlation. *Hum Mol Genet* 10: 1591–1600.

DeBaere E, Beysen D, Oley C, Lorenz B, Cocquet J, De Sutter P, Devriendt K, Dixon M, Fellous M, Fryns J-P, et al. (2003). FOXL2 and BPES: mutational hotspots, phenotypic variability, and revision of the genotype-phenotype correlation. *Am J Hum Genet* 72: 478–487.

Donoviel DB, Hadjantonakis AK, Ikeda M, Zheng H, Hyslop PS, Bernstein A (1999). Mice lacking both presenilin genes exhibit early embryonic patterning defects. *Genes Dev* 13: 2801–2810.

Findlater GS, McDougall RD, Kaufman MH (1993). Eyelid development, fusion and subsequent reopening in the mouse. *J Anat* 183: 121–129.

Fraser IS, Shearman RP, Smith A, Russell P (1988). An association among blepharophimosis, resistant ovary syndrome, and true premature menopause. *Fertil Steril* 50: 747–751.

Frischmeyer PA, Dietz HC (1999). Nonsense-mediated mRNA decay in health and disease. *Hum Mol Genet* 8: 1893–1900.

Fryns JP, Stromme P, van den Berghe H (1993). Further evidence for the location of the blepharophimosis syndrome (BPES) at 3q22.3-q23. *Clin Genet* 44: 149–151.

Fujita H, Meng J, Kawamura M, Tozuka N, Ishii F, Tanaka N (1992). Boy with a chromosome del(3)(q12q23) and blepharophimosis syndrome. *Am J Med Genet* 44: 434–436.

Gould DB, Mears AJ, Pearce WG, Walter MA (1997). Autosomal dominant Axenfeld-Rieger anomaly maps to 6p25. *Am J Hum Genet* 61: 765–768.

Green MC (1970). The developmental effects of congenital hydrocephalus (ch) in the mouse. *Dev Biol* 23: 585–608.

Gruneberg H (1943). Congenital hydrocephalus in the mouse, a case of spurious pleiotropism. *J Genet* 45: 1–21.

Harrar HS, Jeffery S, Patton MA (1995). Linkage analysis in blepharophimosis-ptosis syndrome confirms localisation to 3q21-24. *J Med Genet* 32: 774–777.

Hiemisch H, Monaghan AP, Schutz G, Kaestner KH (1998). Expression of the mouse *Fkh1/Mf1* and *Mfh1* genes in late gestation embryos is restricted to mesoderm derivatives. *Mech Dev* 73: 129–132.

Hong HK, Lass JH, Chakravarti A (1999). Pleiotropic skeletal and ocular phenotypes of the mouse mutation congenital hydrocephalus (ch/Mf1) arise from a winged helix/forkhead transcriptionfactor gene. *Hum Mol Genet* 8: 625–637.

Ishikiryama S, Goto M (1994). Blepharophimosis, ptosis, epicanthus inversus syndrome (BPES) and microcephaly. *Am J Med Genet* 52: 245.

Jewett T, Rao PN, Weaver RG, Stewart W, Thomas IT, Pettenati MJ (1993). Blepharophimosis, ptosis, and epicanthus inversus syndrome (BPES) associated with interstitial deletion of band 3q22: review and gene assignment to the interface of band 3q22.3 and 3q23. *Am J Med Genet* 47: 1147–1150.

Kaufmann E, Knochel W (1996). Five years on the wings of fork head. *Mech Dev* 57: 3–20.

Kawase C, Kawase K, Taniguchi T, Sugiyama K, Yamamoto T, Kitazawa Y, Alward WL, Stone EM, Nishimura DY, Sheffield VC (2001). Screening for mutations of Axenfeld-Rieger syndrome caused by *FOXC1* gene in Japanese patients. *J Glaucoma* 10: 477–482.

Kidson SH, Kume T, Deng K, Winfrey V, Hogan BL (1999). The forkhead/winged-helix gene, *Mf1*, is necessary for the normal development of the cornea and formation of the anterior chamber in the mouse eye. *Dev Biol* 211: 306–322.

Krebs LT, Xue Y, Norton CR, Shutter JR, Maguire M, Sundberg JP, Gallahan D, Closson V, Kitajewski J, Callahan R, et al. (2000). Notch signaling is essential for vascular morphogenesis in mice. *Genes Dev* 14: 1343–1352.

Kume T, Deng KY, Winfrey V, Gould DB, Walter MA, Hogan BL (1998). The forkhead/winged helix gene *Mf1* is disrupted in the pleiotropic mouse mutation congenital hydrocephalus. *Cell* 93: 985–996.

Kume T, Deng K, Hogan BL (2000). Murine forkhead/winged helix genes *Foxc1* (*Mf1*) and *Foxc2* (*Mfh1*) are required for the early organogenesis of the kidney and urinary tract. *Development* 127: 1387–1395.

Kume T, Jiang H, Topczewska JM, Hogan BLM (2001). The murine winged helix transcription factors, Foxc1 and Foxc2, are both required for cardiovascular development and somitogenesis. *Genes Dev* 15: 2470–2482.

Lai CS, Fisher SE, Hurst JA, Vargha Khadem F, Monaco AP (2001). A forkhead-domain gene is mutated in a severe speech and language disorder. *Nature* 413: 519–523.

Lehmann OJ, Ebenezer ND, Jordan T, Fox M, Ocaka L, Payne A, Leroy BP, Clark BJ, Hitchings RA, Povey S, et al. (2000). Chromosomal duplication involving the forkhead transcription factor gene *FOXC1* causes iris hypoplasia and glaucoma. *Am J Hum Genet* 67: 1129–1135.

Lines MA, Kozlowski K, Walter MA (2002). Molecular genetics of Axenfeld-Rieger malformations. *Hum Mol Genet* 11: 1177–1187.

Mascrez B, Mark M, Krezel W, Dupe V, LeMeur M, Ghyselinck NB, Chambon P (2001). Differential contributions of AF-1 and AF-2 activities to the developmental functions of RXRα. *Development* 128: 2049–2062.

Mears AJ, Mirzayans F, Gould DB, Pearce WG, Walter MA (1996). Autosomal dominant iridogoniodysgenesis anomaly maps to 6p25. *Am J Hum Genet* 59: 1321–1327.

Mears AJ, Jordan T, Mirzayans F, Dubois S, Kume T, Parlee M, Ritch R, Koop B, Kuo WL, Collins C, et al. (1998). Mutations of the forkhead/winged-helix gene, *FKHL7*, in patients with Axenfeld-Rieger anomaly. *Am J Hum Genet* 63: 1316–1328.

Mirzayans F, Gould DB, Heon E, Billingsley GD, Cheung JC, Mears AJ, Walter MA (2000). Axenfeld-Rieger syndrome resulting from mutation of the FKHL7 gene on chromosome 6p25. *Eur J Hum Genet* 8: 71–74.

Moore MW, Klein RD, Farinas I, Sauer H, Armanini M, Phillips H, Reichardt LF, Ryan AM, Carver-Moore K, Rosenthal A (1996). Renal and neuronal abnormalities in mice lacking GDNF. *Nature* 382: 76–79.

Nishimura DY, Swiderski RE, Alward WL, Searby CC, Patil SR, Bennet SR, Kanis AB, Gastier JM, Stone EM, Sheffield VC (1998). The forkhead transcription factor gene *FKHL7* is responsible for glaucoma phenotypes which map to 6p25. *Nat Genet* 19: 140–147.

Nishimura DY, Searby CC, Alward WL, Walton D, Craig JE, Mackey DA, Kawase K, Kanis AB, Patil SR, Stone EM, et al. (2001). A spectrum of *FOXC1* mutations suggests gene dosage as a mechanism for developmental defects of the anterior chamber of the eye. *Am J Hum Genet* 68: 364–372.

Oley C, Baraitser M (1988). Blepharophimosis, ptosis, epicanthus inversus syndrome (BPES syndrome). *J Med Genet* 25: 47–51.

Pailhoux E, Vigier B, Chaffaux S, Servel N, Taourit S, Furet JP, Fellous M, Grosclaude F, Cribiu EP, Cotinot C, et al. (2001). A 11.7-kb deletion triggers intersexuality and polledness in goats. *Nat Genet* 29: 453–458.

Palmer CG, Bader P, Slovak ML, Comings DE, Pettenati MJ (1991). Partial deletion of chromosome 6p: delineation of the syndrome. *Am J Med Genet* 39: 155–160.

Pierrou S, Hellqvist M, Samuelsson L, Enerback S, Carlsson P (1994). Cloning and characterization of seven human forkhead proteins: binding site specificity and DNA bending. *EMBO J* 13: 5002–5012.

Plaja A, Vidal R, Soriano D, Bou X, Vendrell T, Mediano C, Pueyo JM, Labrana X, Sarret E (1994). Terminal deletion of 6p: report of a new case. *Ann Genet* 37: 196–199.

Prueitt RL, Zinn AR (2001). A fork in the road to fertility. *Nat Genet* 27: 132–134.

Saleem RA, Banerjee-Basu S, Berry FB, Baxevanis AD, Walter MA (2001). Analyses of the effects that disease-causing missense mutations have on the structure and function of the winged-helix protein FOXC1. *Am J Hum Genet* 68: 627–641.

Sasaki H, Hogan BL (1993). Differential expression of multiple fork head related genes during gastrulation and axial pattern formation in the mouse embryo. *Development* 118: 47–59.

Semina EV, Reiter R, Leysens NJ, Alward WL, Small KW, Datson NA, Siegel-Bartelt J, Bierke-Nelson D, Bitoun P, Zabel BU, et al. (1996). Cloning and characterization of a novel bicoid-related homeobox transcription factor gene, *RIEG*, involved in Rieger syndrome. *Nat Genet* 14: 392–399.

Shields MB (1983). Axenfeld-Rieger syndrome: a theory of mechanism and distinctions from the iridocorneal endothelial syndrome. *Trans Am Ophthalmol Soc* 81: 736–784.

Shields MB (1989). Axenfeld-Rieger syndrome. In: *The Glaucomas*. Ritch R, Shields MB, Krupin T (eds.) CV Mosby, St. Louis, pp. 885–896.

Shim YS, Jang YK, Lim MS, Lee JS, Seong RH, Hong SH, Park SD (2000). Rdp1, a novel zinc finger protein, regulates the DNA damage response of rhp51(+) from *Schizosaccharomyces pombe*. *Mol Cell Biol* 20: 8958–8968.

Small KW, Stalvey M, Fisher L, Mullen L, Dickel C, Beadles K, Reimer R, Lessner A, Lewis K, Pericak-Vance MA (1995). Blepharophimosis syndrome is linked to chromosome 3q. *Hum Mol Genet* 4: 443–448.

Smith RS, Zabaleta A, Kume T, Savinova OV, Kidson SH, Martin JE, Nishimura DY, Alward WL, Hogan BL, John SW (2000). Haploinsufficiency of the transcription factors FOXC1 and FOXC2 results in aberrant ocular development. *Hum Mol Genet* 9: 1021–1032.

Suzuki T, Takahashi K, Kuwahara S, Wada Y, Abe T, Tamai M (2001). A novel (Pro79Thr) mutation in the FKHL7 gene in a Japanese family with Axenfeld-Rieger syndrome. *Am J Ophthalmol* 132: 572–575.

Swiderski RE, Reiter RS, Nishimura DY, Alward WL, Kalenak JW, Searby CS, Stone EM, Sheffield VC, Lin JJ (1999). Expression of the *Mf1* gene in developing mouse hearts: implication in the development of human congenital heart defects. *Dev Dyn* 216: 16–27.

Takahashi Y, Koizumi K, Takagi A, Kitajima S, Inoue T, Koseki H, Saga Y (2000). Mesp2 initiates somite segmentation through the Notch signalling pathway. *Nat Genet* 25: 390–396.

Tjian R, Maniatis T (1994). Transcriptional activation: a complex puzzle with few easy pieces. *Cell* 77: 5–8.

Topczewska JM, Topczewski J, Shostak A, Kume T, Solnica-Krezel L, Hogan BL (2001). The winged helix transcription factor Foxc1a is essential for somitogenesis in zebrafish. *Genes Dev* 15: 2483–2493.

Townes PL, Muechler EK (1979). Blepharophimosis, ptosis, epicanthus inversus, and primary amenorrhea. A dominant trait. *Arch Ophthalmol* 97: 1664–1666.

Treier M, Gleiberman AS, O'Connell SM, Szeto DP, McMahon JA, McMahon AP, Rosenfeld MG (1998). Multistep signaling requirements for pituitary organogenesis in vivo. *Genes Dev* 12: 1691–1704.

Vaiman D, Schibler L, Oustry-Vaiman A, Pailhoux E, Goldammer T, Stevanovic M, Furet JP, Schwerin M, Cotinot C, Fellous M, et al. (1999). High-resolution human/goat comparative map of the goat polled/intersex syndrome (PIS): the human homologue is contained in a human YAC from HSA3q23. *Genomics* 56: 31–39.

Vassalli A, Matzuk MM, Gardner HA, Lee KF, Jaenisch R (1994). Activin/inhibin beta B subunit gene disruption leads to defects in eyelid development and female reproduction. *Genes Dev* 8: 414–427.

Vignes A (1889). Epicanthus heredetaire. *Rev Gen Ophtalmol (Paris)* 8: 438–439.

Warburg M, Bugge M, Brondum-Nielsen K (1995). Cytogenetic findings indicate heterogeneity in patients with blepharophimosis, epicanthus inversus, and developmental delay. *J Med Genet* 32: 19–24.

Williamson RA, Donlan MA, Dolan CR, Thuline HC, Harrison MT, Hall JG (1981). Familial insertional translocation of a portion of 3q into 11q resulting in duplication and deletion of region 3q22.1 leads to q24 in different offspring. *Am J Med Genet* 9: 105–111.

Winnier GE, Kume T, Deng K, Rogers R, Bundy J, Raines C, Walter MA, Hogan BL, Conway SJ (1999). Roles for the winged helix transcription factors MF1 and MFH1 in cardiovascular development revealed by nonallelic noncomplementation of null alleles. *Dev Biol* 213: 418–431.

Yamada T, Hayasaka S, Matsumoto M, Budu Esa T, Hayasaka Y, Endo M (2001). Heterozygous 17-bp deletion in the forkhead transcription factor gene, *FOXL2*, in a Japanese family with blepharophimosis-ptosis-epicanthus inversus syndrome. *J Hum Genet* 46: 733–736.

Yujiri T, Ware M, Widmann C, Oyer R, Russell D, Chan E, Zaitsu Y, Clarke P, Tyler K, Oka Y, Fanger GR, Henson P, Johnson GL (2000). MEK kinase 1 gene disruption alters cell migration and c-Jun NH2-terminal kinase regulation but does not cause a measurable defect in NF-kappaB activation. *Proc Natl Acad Sci USA* 97: 7272–7277.

Zlotogora J, Sagi M, Cohen T (1983). The blepharophimosis, ptosis, and epicanthus inversus syndrome: delineation of two types. *Am J Hum Genet* 35: 1020–1027.

Zurcher VL, Golden WL, Zinn AB (1990). Distal deletion of the short arm of chromosome 6. *Am J Med Genet* 35: 261–265.

66 | *FOXC2* and Lymphedema Distichiasis

ROBERT P. ERICKSON

Lymphedema distichiasis (LD) is a dominantly inherited syndrome of high penetrance and extremely variable expression. Its most constant feature is distichiasis, a double row of eyelashes due to secondary eyelashes growing from the meibomian glands. Lymphedema is typically of adolescent onset but can be so severe as to cause hydrops fetalis and may not appear at all. LD results from heterozygosity for null mutations at *FOXC2*. *FOXC2* is a member of the forkhead transcription factor family. This gene family codes for transcription factors with both positive and negative effects on transcription. The pattern of embryonic expression of *Foxc2* and the phenotype of homozygous nulls predict the extra clinical features seen in LD: cleft palate, cardiac abnormalities, extradural spinal cysts, and ptosis. To date, only 2 of 42 published mutations have been missense, strongly suggesting that it is haplodeficiency which results in the phenotype. Thus, the great clinical variability is likely to result from the effects of modifier genes.

LOCUS AND DEVELOPMENTAL PATHWAY

As discussed in Chapter 64, forkhead transcription factors have multiple roles in development. *FOXC2* maps to 16q24.3 and lies in a cluster of three forkhead genes (Fig. 66–1). It produces a 2.2 kb transcript with a 1.5 kb single exon coding region that is highly (~70%) GC-rich (Kaestner et al., 1996). The FOXC2 protein contains 501 amino acids. The one known domain in the gene is the forkhead domain. Its promoter and regulatory sequences have not been characterized. One functional Foxc2 consensus forkhead domain-binding site has been defined in a reporter assay system (Miura et al., 1997). However, binding specificity in vivo is thought to involve both the conserved forkhead domain and flanking sequences (Miura et al., 1997). There are currently no known gene targets for this transcription factor.

The role of *Foxc2* was initially explored by expression studies during early mouse embryogenesis (Kaestner et al., 1996). In situ hybridizations showed expression in the embryonic mesoderm of day 7.5 embryos, both anterior and posterior to the node but not including the extra-embryonic mesoderm. As development continued, *Foxc2* transcripts were detected in somites, mesoderm, head, and endocardium at embryonic day 8.25. By embryonic day 10.5, expression was very strong in the somites and dorsal aorta (Kaestner et al., 1996). *Foxc2* expression in the head region was particularly prominent in the cartilaginous condensation around the optic vesicle and the skull underlying the midbrain and hindbrain (Iida et al., 1997). This mesenchyme gives rise to palatal processes and the outer layer of the optic vesicle. The mandibular component of the first branchial arch also showed strong expression of *Foxc2*. At day 11.5, *Foxc2* expression was prominent surrounding the optic cup, including the prospective sclerotic coat of the eyeball (Iida et al., 1997).

The requirement for *Foxc2* expression in these various regions in normal development was explored by creating knockouts for the gene. Some *Foxc2* homozygous embryos died in utero (40%) and others at birth (60%) with heart defects (Iida et al., 1997). Almost all of the homozygous knockout embryos had interruptions, coarctation, or tubular hypoplasia of the aortic arch. All newborns had complete cleft secondary palate. There were abnormalities of the skull, including abnormal formation of the optic canal, absence of the posterior wall of the foramen ovale, and fusion of the malleus and incus, primarily defects of neural crest origin (Iida et al., 1997). Axial skeletal anomalies with short vertebral bodies, spina bifida, and spina bifida occulta were found.

Foxc2 interacts with Foxc1 (see Chapter 65) in cardiac, renal, and ocular development. The Foxc1 DNA-binding domain has 97% identity and 99% similarity to that of Foxc2 (Kume et al., 2000), and the two genes show very similar expression patterns. The interactions of Foxc2 and Foxc1 in cardiac development were shown by creating double heterozygotes for the two knockouts (Winnier et al., 1999). These compound heterozygotes showed interruptions and coarctation of the aortic arch, dysgenesis of pulmonary and aortic valves, ventricular septal defect, and other cardiac abnormalities. They died before birth. Because single heterozygotes were thought to be completely recessive (without detectable abnormalities), the finding of such severe cardiac abnormalities in double heterozygotes strongly implicated an important interaction between Foxc1 and Foxc2. The importance of this interaction was further demonstrated by the phenotype of the compound homozygous deficiency (Kume et al., 2001). The $Foxc1^{-/-}$, $Foxc2^{-/-}$ embryos die earlier (day 9.5) with more severe cardiac and vascular abnormalities, an absent second branchial arch, a complete lack of somites, and usually an open neural tube.

In the kidney, *Foxc1* was initially transcribed at higher levels than *Foxc2*, particularly on embryonic day 10.5 in the mesonephric mesenchyme, while *Foxc2* transcripts were higher around the ureter bud (Kume et al., 2000). Homozygous *Foxc1* knockout mice had hydronephrosis and hydroureter on some genetic backgrounds; other genetic backgrounds showed very low penetrance with only 2% of homozygotes showing kidney abnormalities. Taking advantage of these differences in genetic backgrounds, Kume et al. (2000) made the double compound heterozygote $Foxc1^{+/-}$, $Foxc2^{+/-}$ on the genetic background with a low frequency of kidney defects for $Foxc1^{-/-}$ mice. Interaction of the two genes was shown, with one-third of the compound heterozygotes showing hypoplastic kidneys and two-thirds having a single hydroureter.

Minor ocular anterior chamber abnormalities were noted in *Foxc2* knockout heterozygotes (Smith et al., 2000). While the *Foxc1* homozygous knockout was characterized by severe abnormalities of the eye with absence of the anterior chamber (Kidson et al., 1999), eye defects in heterozygous *Foxc1* deficiency were also seen on some genetic backgrounds (Hong et al., 1999). The double heterozygote $Foxc1^{+/-}$, $Foxc2^{+/-}$ had a similar range of ocular abnormalities to that seen in the $Foxc2^{+/-}$ alone but a more severe deficiency of mesenchyme-derived iris stroma (Smith et al., 2000).

Given these observations, one might have predicted that the human *FOXC2* mutation would result in a syndrome of cardiac, ocular, and renal findings with cleft palate. The route to discovering that *FOXC2* mutations caused LD was an indirect one, and ocular (predictable) and lymphatic abnormalities (not predictable) turned out to be the major features.

CLINICAL FEATURES

Although co-occurrence of distichiasis and lymphedema was reported over a century ago (Kuhnt, 1899), familial LD was first reported by Campbell (1945) and subsequently in Neel and Schull's (1954) early textbook of human genetics as an example of the co-inheritance of two apparently unrelated traits. A full report of an apparently different family (both described by colleagues in Ann Arbor, Michigan, but

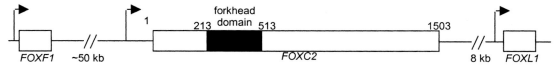

Figure 66–1. Genomic structure of *FOXC2* and surrounding region.

the publications used different University of Michigan pedigree numbers and the pedigrees did not look congruent) described it as an autosomal-dominant disorder presenting in a large pedigree as lymphedema of the limbs with variable age at onset, double rows of eyelashes (distichiasis), and variable expression of photophobia, ectropion, and webbing of the neck (Falls and Kertesz, 1964). Later reports added other variable features, including cardiac defects, cleft palate, and spinal extradural cysts (Robinow et al., 1970; Schwartz et al., 1980; Corbett et al., 1982; Goldstein et al., 1985) which suggested a defect in a gene with pleiotropic effects acting during development. Young patients with distichiasis and cleft palate (Bartley and Jackson, 1989) probably represent the syndrome and would later develop lymphedema. Families with cleft palate and lymphedema in which no mention of distichiasis is made (Figueroa et al., 1983) may also have LD but with mild distichiasis.

Clinical findings in many case reports are summarized in Table 66–1. There may be some duplication as some patients may be included in more than one report. *FOXC2* mutations are highly penetrant, the excess seen in Table 66–1 presumably being due to ascertainment bias. Lymphedema and distichiasis were equally common, but lymphedema occurred in all families with age dependence. Lymphedema occurs most often by puberty; however, in our family 5, the 26-year-old mother does not yet have lymphedema, and in our family 3, there are three adults over 19 years of age with no clinical lymphedema (Erickson et al., 2001). Brice et al. (2002) present sex-dependent cumulative penetrance rates, with 50% of males affected by age 12 and 50% of females by age 22. Even when lymphedema is not apparent, an underlying lymphangiodysplasia and lymphatic insufficiency may, nonetheless, be present and visible on imaging studies. However, lymphedema has sometimes been so great as to result in therapeutic abortion for hydrops fetalis: the hydrops fetalis was so severe that it was thought to be due to Turner's syndrome in our family 1 (Fang et al., 2000). (The karyotype was normal in one of the hydropic fetuses [Seaver, 2001].) Distichiasis is the most constant finding in the affected individuals we studied, with high penetrance (Erickson et al., 2001). Cleft palate has been quite frequent in the af-

fected members of families, and tetralogy of Fallot has been the most common congenital heart anomaly (see Table 66–1 for summary of findings), both occurring in approximately 10% of the affected individuals we have studied.

Thus, heterozygosity for *FOXC2* mutations leads to a variably expressed, multiple malformation syndrome in which we find distichiasis to be the most common feature. Finegold et al. (2001), Bell et al. (2001), and Brice et al. (2002) have also presented recent mutational analyses of LD families. Our results are in general agreement with their findings. However, there are some differences with the results of Finegold et al. (2001) in which lymphedema, rather than distichiasis, was the constant feature in families. These authors reported one family in which only lymphedema, and not distichiasis, was found. This led Finegold et al. (2001) to implicate *FOXC2* mutations in a large number of lymphedema syndromes and to emphasize the heterogeneity of previously separated lymphedema syndromes. However, this was one small family of the 11 studied by the authors and of the 42 total with *FOXC2* mutations from the combined studies and is, thus, not typical. This discrepancy may represent the method of ascertainment in that our families were ascertained for lymphedema and distichiasis, while lymphedema alone was the main criterion in the study by Finegold and colleagues. However, mild cases of distichiasis may be detected only by an ophthalmologist.

The lymphatic abnormalities in LD have not been extensively studied. Kinmonth (1972) performed lymphangiograms in several patients with probable LD and found an increased number and slight broadening of the lymphatics (Fig. 66–2). Dale (1987) reported bilateral hyperplasia to be consistently associated with lymphedema in LD. Rosbotham et al. (2000) performed lymphoscintigraphy in a number of individuals from a large pedigree. They found delayed arrival to the inguinal nodes of the ^{99}Tc-antimony sulfide colloid injected into the first web space of the foot to be a useful classification tool. Several members of the family who denied lymphedema had abnormally slow transport.

One would not have predicted lymphatic abnormalities in humans haplodeficient for *FOXC2* on the basis of the knockout phenotype (see above). However, genes frequently have different roles at different

Table 66–1. Penetrance and Clinical Findings in Lymphedema Distichiasis

Reference	No. Affected*/ No. at Risk	Lymphedema	Distichiasis	Cleft Palate	Heart Defect	Other†
Neel and Schull, 1954	6/10	7	7	0	0	0
Falls and Kertesz, 1964	9/17	8	9	0	0	6
Goldstein et al., 1985	4/4	3	5	0	3	4
Robinow et al., 1970	2/6	2	3	0	0	2
Jester, 1977	1/1	1	1	0	0	0
Shammas et al., 1979	7/18	5	9	0	0	6
Pap et al., 1980	10/26	10	5	0	0	5
Schwartz et al., 1980	2/2	2	3	0	0	3
Dale, 1987	10/18	8	4	0	0	0
Temple and Collin, 1994	1/1	2	2	1	0	2
Chen et al., 1996	1/2	1	1	0	1	0
Mangion et al., 1999	23/37	20	19	1	3	4
Rosbotham et al., 2000	20/32	18	13	0	1	3
Fang et al., 2000	8/11	6	8	1	1	0
Bell et al., 2001	21/36‡	32	32	?	?	?
Finegold et al., 2001	—	48	33	3	4	10
Erickson et al., 2001§	10/17	16	30	2	3	2
Total	135/238	189	184	8	16	47

*When data (e.g., pedigree) allow this to be determined.
†Spinal extradural cysts, ptosis, webbed neck, extropion.
‡Two unaffected but carrying mutation identified.
§Cases not reported in first publication from same group.

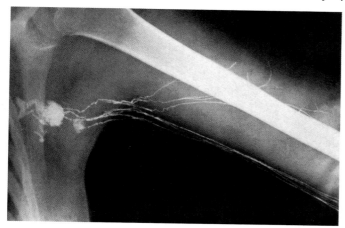

Figure 66–2. Axillary lymphangiogram of female patient with presumed lymphedema distichiasis (cleft palate and lymphedema with onset at 9 years). Note hyperplastic lymphatic vessels with accessory ones filled by retrograde flow. (From Kinmonth [1982]. *The Lymphatics: Surgery, Lymphography and Diseases of the Chyle and Lymph Systems.* London: Edward Arnold, p. 113.)

stages of development, and the homozygous null reveals early gene action. The story is reminiscent of the developmental program elucidated for vascular endothelial growth factor C (VEGF-C) and its receptor, VEGFR-3 (Lymboussaki et al., 1999) (see Chapter 101). The knockout for VEGFR-3 died at embryonic day 9.5 secondary to cardiac failure with enlarged blood vessels which had defective lumens (Dumont et al., 1998). However, a role in later lymphatic development was suggested by the pattern of expression of VEGF-C and VEGFR-3 (Kukk et al., 1996) and confirmed by overexpression of VEGF-C in adult mice (Jelsch et al., 1997). A different, later developmental role is also suggested by the divergent pattern of expression of VEGF-C from the other VEGFs at later stages. Thus, FOXC2 may play an important role in lymphatic development which has yet to be elucidated, or there may be important species differences between its role in mice and humans. The primary defect in distichiasis is in the meibomian glands, which can be small or absent and can have the accessory cilia emerging from their orifices (Fig. 66–3). It has varied markedly in severity among our patients: from a few fine accessory eyelashes, noted only by the physician, to such severe corneal abrasions that surgical removal of the eyelid margin was performed. The mouse heterozygote for the *Foxc2* knockout can have a short Schlemm's canal, aberrantly developed trabecular network, and iris hypoplasia; but no abnormalities of eyelids were originally described (Smith et al., 2000). The iris hypoplasia noted in mice suggests that

photophobia in some *FOXC2* mutant patients could be secondary to light transmission through the iris instead of secondary to corneal irritation by aberrant eyelashes. The influence of other genes, e.g., *Foxc1* deficiency (see above), on this part of the phenotype warrants further study.

IDENTIFICATION OF GENE AND MUTATIONAL SPECTRUM

A gene for LD was mapped to 16q24.3 (Mangion et al., 1999). Several years earlier, we had reported neonatal lymphedema similar to that in Turner syndrome associated with a Y:16 translocation (Erickson et al., 1995). We searched for an "anti-Turner" gene that could be involved in preventing lymphedema on the Y chromosome side of the translocation because of the known association of Xp with preventing lymphedema in Turner's syndrome and the Y chromosome with preventing lymphedema in males (Drury et al., 1998). However, we were not able to find a candidate gene in this portion of the Y chromosome. With the report of LD linking to 16q near our chromosomal breakpoint, we searched the chromosome 16 side of the translocation and found *FOXC2,* mutations of which cause LD (Fang et al., 2000).

We initially reported mutations in the *FOXC2* gene in two families and a probable position effect in the original Y:16 translocation patient. Our and other analyses of *FOXC2* mutations in additional families with LD found that truncating mutations can be associated with a variety of phenotypes (see Table 66–1). A variety of mutations were found in these families, including nonsense mutations, single nucleotide insertions and deletions, and some insertion/deletions. All insertions and deletions led to frameshifts, and all mutations are predicted to truncate the FOXC2 protein. There was no apparent correlation of phenotype with mutant alleles. These results are consistent with our earlier interpretation that haploinsufficiency for *FOXC2* is responsible for the phenotype (Fang et al., 2000). Only two missense mutations in *FOXC2* have been reported (Fang et al., 2000; Bell et al., 2001; Finegold et al., 2001; Erickson et al., 2001; Brice et al., 2002) among 42 LD families, a marked contrast to the findings with *FOXC1* mutations and Axenfeld-Rieger anomaly (Saleem et al., 2001).

COUNSELING AND TREATMENT

Counseling issues in LD are not simple. While it is dominantly inherited with quite high penetrance, the variable expressivity is extreme. As already mentioned, the lymphedema can be so severe that hydrops fetalis is diagnosed, and this has led to *in utero* termination (Seaver, 2001). Tetralogy of Fallot and cleft palate, of course, are usually repairable but are, nonetheless, severe birth defects. The less frequent complication of extradural spinal cysts can also lead to major surgical procedures. The distichiasis is usually more readily controlled. Thus, genetic counseling is a 50% risk per pregnancy to an affected individual but with great variability in the "risk for what."

Although there are operative procedures for lymphedema, they remain very controversial, whereas physical manipulative treatments involving external compression and massage are well established (Földi, 1983; Ko et al., 1998). Physiotherapy consisting of compression bandaging and gentle lymphatic massage provides a mainstay of treatment. Meticulous skin care, wearing of low-stretch compression garments, and raising the affected extremities are also strongly recommended (International Society of Lymphology Executive Committee, 1995). These approaches can result in about a 50% decrease in lymphedema volume and prevent the development of hardened skin and subcutaneous tissues. Thus, although there is no treatment which will completely eliminate the lymphedema, these treatments will make it much more manageable.

MUTATIONS IN ORTHOLOGOUS GENES

At the beginning of this chapter, we discussed the homozygous *Foxc2* knockout, to indicate its role in early development and its relationship to associated birth defects. We and our associates have now studied

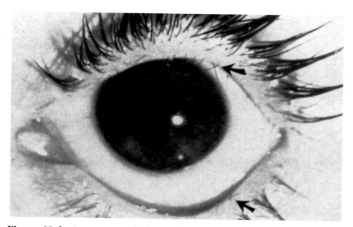

Figure 66–3. Accessory eyelashes at the site of meibomian gland openings (arrows) in patient with lymphedema distichiasis. (From Stammos et al. [1979]. Distichiasis of the lids and lymphedema of the lower extremities: a report of ten cases. *J Pediatr Ophthalmol Strabismus* 16: 130; by permission of author and publisher.)

Foxc2 heterozygous knockouts for features related to LD (Krieder-man et al., 2003). In contrast to the claim that heterozygotes were normal, a notion already found erroneous in regard to the anterior chamber of the eye, features of LD were found. Young *Foxc2*$^{+/-}$ mice demonstrated prompt but distinctively abnormal dynamic visual lymphangiograms under high-power dissecting microscopy following intradermal administration of Evans blue dye in the hindpaws, forepaws, and snout. Compared to control +/+ mice, there was rapid visualization of an increased number and/or diameter of lymphatic truncal collectors in the limbs and centrally, including the thoracic duct, and increased number and size of regional lymph nodes draining each injection site. In addition, Evans blue–stained lymph refluxed promptly retrograde from the cisterna chyli into dilated lymphatic channels in the hepatic hilum, mesentery, mesenteric lymph nodes, and intestinal wall through visible yet apparently incompetent interlymphangion valves. Rhythmic contractions were noted in the larger excised popliteal, axillary, jugular, and mesenteric lymph nodes. The enlarged Evans blue–stained thoracic duct was patent to its termination in the left subclavian vein without evidence of obstruction. Except for lymphatic system abnormalities, no other gross anatomic abnormalities or organ pathology, including of the cardiovascular system, were found, and neither peripheral lymphedema nor chylous or nonchylous effusion was observed. This abnormal phenotype was much less detectable in aged mice.

These distinctive visual lymphangiograms conform closely to those few reported images generated in LD patients by Kinmonth (1972) using lipid contrast conventional lymphography, namely, generalized increase in number and size of peripheral and central lymphatic collecting trunks (termed *bilateral lymphatic hyperplasia*) and lymph nodes combined with retrograde truncal lymph reflux (Fig. 66–2). This LD dynamic lymphatic imaging pattern is in direct contrast to the typical findings in most patients with congenital hereditary lymphedema (Milroy type) of delayed lymph transport and hypoplasia or aplasia of the lower and occasionally upper limb deep lymphatic system associated with lymph node hypoplasia and lymph reflux into the superficial valveless dermal lymphatic apparatus.

DEVELOPMENTAL PATHOGENESIS

Increased FOXC2 expression in mouse adipocytes results in an insulin-sensitive phenotype in both white and brown adipose tissue (Cederberg et al., 2001). Overexpression of FOXC2 mostly led to elevated levels of a variety of mRNAs which increase the sensitivity of the β-adrenergic–cAMP–protein kinase A signaling pathway. In contrast, given our recent findings of increased lymphatics and lymph nodes in young *Foxc2* heterozygotes, a negative effect of FOXC2 on lymphangiogenic factors seems more plausible than upregulation of gene activity. Forkhead family transcription factors have been implicated in both transactivation and repression of target genes (Kaufmann and Knochel, 1996). Therefore, downregulation could occur by direct repression or by activation of other genes (e.g., other transcription factors) that repress transcription. Factors known to be involved in lymphatic development (see Chapters 101 and 102) include VEGF-C, VEGF-D, VEGFR-3, PROX1, and ANG2. Knockouts of *Vegfr-3*, the receptor for Vegf-C and Vegf-D, show vascular defects (Dumont et al., 1998) and do not survive to the age of lymphatic development, while overexpression of Vegf-C and Vegf-D in the skin of transgenic mice produces hyperplasia and overgrowth of lymphatic tissues (Jelsch et al., 1997), a finding similar to that seen in patients with LD. Experimental analyses in mice should allow substantiation of this hypothesis.

The search for modifying genes would certainly include *FOXC1*. As already discussed, there is a large overlap in the pattern of expression and interaction with *FOXC2* in a variety of phenotypes. This is especially apparent in the double *Foxc1, Foxc2* knockout. The pattern of gene expression in these compound homozygotes implicates an interaction of *Foxc1/2* with the Notch signaling pathway (Kume et al., 2001). Of course, variation in hypothetical target genes (e.g., *VEGF-C, VEGF-D, VEGFR-3, PROX1,* and *ANG2*) could also explain the marked variability in patients for severity of lymphedema and associated malformations.

REFERENCES

Bartley GB, Jackson IT (1989). Distichiasis and cleft palate. *Plast Reconstr Surg* 84: 129–132.

Bell R, Brice G, Child AH, Murday VA, Mansour S, Sandy CJ, Collin JRO, Brady AF, Callen DF, Burnand K, et al. (2001). Analysis of lymphoedema-distichiasis families for *FOXC2* mutations reveals small insertions and deletions throughout the gene. *Hum Genet* 108: 546–511.

Brice G, Mansour S, Bell R, Collin JRO, Child AH, Brady AF, Sarfarazi M, Burnand KG, Jeffery S, Mortimer P, et al. (2002). Analysis of the phenotypic abnormalities in lymphoedema distichiasis syndrome in 74 patients with *FOXC2* mutations or linkage to 16q24. *J Med Genet* 39: 478–483.

Campbell KN (1945). Milroy's disease: chronic hereditary edema. Univ Hosp Bull Univ Mich 11: 69–70.

Cederberg A, Grønning I M, Ahren B, Taskén K, Carlsson P, Enerbäk S (2001). *FOXC2* is a winged helix gene that counteracts obesity, hypertriglyceridemia, and diet-induced insulin resistance. *Cell* 6: 563–573.

Chen E, Larabell SK, Daniels JM, Goldstein S (1996). Distichiasis–lymphedema syndrome: tetralogy of Fallot, chylothorax, and neonatal death. *Am J Med Genet* 66: 273–75.

Corbett CRR, Dale RF, Coltart DJ, Kinmonth JB (1982). Congenital heart disease in patients with primary lymphoedemas. *Lymphology* 15: 85–90.

Dale RF (1987). Primary lymphoedema when found with distichiasis of the type defined as bilateral hyperplasia by lymphology. *J Med Genet* 24: 170–171.

Drury SS, Erickson RP, Glover TW (1998). Y:16 translocation breakpoint associated with a partial Turner phenotype identifies a foamy virus insertion. *Cytogenet Cell Genet* 80: 199–203.

Dumont DJ, Jussila L, Taipale J, Lymboussaki A, Mustonen T, Pajusola K, Breitman M, Alitalo K (1998). Cardiovascular failure in mouse embryos deficient in VEGF receptor-3. *Science* 282: 946–949.

Erickson RP, Hudgins L, Stone JF, Schmidt S, Wilke C, Glover TW (1995). A "balanced" Y: 16 translocation associated with Turner-like neonatal lymphedema suggests the location of a potential anti-Turner gene on the Y chromosome. *Cytogenet Cell Genet* 71: 163–167.

Erickson RP, Dagenais SL, Caulder MS, Downs CA, Herman G, Jones MC, Kerst Jens-Frederikse WS, Lidral AC, McDonald M, Nelson CC, et al. (2001). Clinical heterogeneity in lymphedema-distichiasis with *FOXC2* truncating mutations. *J Med Genet* 38: 761–766.

Falls HF, Kertesz ED (1964). A new syndrome combining pterygium colli with developmental anomalies of the eyelids and lymphatics of the lower extremities. *Trans Am Ophthalmol Soc* 62: 248–275.

Fang JM, Dagenais SL, Erickson RP, Arlt MF, Glynn MW, Gorski JL, Seaver LH, Glover TW (2000). Mutations in *FOXC2 (MFH-1)*, a forkhead family transcription factor, are responsible for the hereditary lymphedema-distichiasis syndrome. *Am J Hum Genet* 67: 1382–1388.

Figueroa AA, Pruzansky S, Rollnick SR (1983). Meige disease (familial lymphedema praecox) and cleft palate: report of a family and review of the literature. *Cleft Palate J* 20: 151–157.

Finegold DN, Kimak MA, Lawrence EC, Levinson KL, Cherniske EM, Poser SNR, Dunlap JW, Ferrell RE (2001). Truncating mutations in *FOXC2* cause multiple lymphedema syndromes. *Hum Mol Genet* 10: 1185–1189.

Földi M (1983). Lymphoedema. In: *Lymphangiology*. Foldi M, Casley-Smith JR (eds). Shattauer-Verlag, Stuttgart, p. 666–706.

Goldstein S, Qazi QH, Fitzgerald J, Goldstein L, Friedman AP, Sawyer P (1985). Distichiasis, congenital heart defects and mixed peripheral vascular anomalies. *Am J Med Genet* 20: 283–294.

Hong H-K, Lazz JH, Chakravarti A (1999). Pleiotropic skeletal and ocular phenotypes of the mouse mutation congenital hydrocephalus (ch/Mfl) arise from a winged helix-forkhead transcription factor gene. *Hum Mol Genet* 8: 625–637.

Iida K, Koseki H, Kakinuma H, Kato N, Mizutani-Koseki Y, Ohuchi H, Yoshioka H, Noji S, Kawamura K, Kataoka Y, et al. (1997). Essential roles of the winged helix transcription factor MFH-1 in aortic arch patterning and skeletogenesis. *Development* 124: 4627–4638.

International Society of Lymphology Executive Committee (1995). The diagnosis and treatment of peripheral lymphedema. Consensus document of the International Society of Lymphology Executive Committee. *Lymphology* 28: 113–117.

Jelsch M, Kaipainen A, Joukov V, Meng X, Lakso M, Rauvala H, Swartz M, Fukumura D, Jain R, Alitalo K (1997). Hyperplasia of lymphatic vessels in VEGF-C transgenic mice. *Science* 276: 1423–1425.

Jester HG (1977). Lymphedema-distichiasis. A rare hereditary syndrome. *Hum Genet* 39: 113–116.

Kaestner KH, Bleckmann SC, Monaghan AP, Schlondorff J, Mincheva A, Lichter P, Schutz G (1996). Clustered arrangement of winged helix genes *fkh-6* and *MFH-1*; possible implications for mesoderm development. *Development* 122: 1751–1758.

Kaufmann E, Knochel W (1996). Five years on the wings of fork head. *Mech Dev* 57: 3–20.

Kidson SH, Kume T, Deng K, Winfrey V, Hogan BLM (1999). The forehead/winged helix gene, *MF1*, is necessary for the normal development of the cornea and formation of the anterior chamber in the mouse eye. *Dev Biol* 211: 306–322.

Kinmonth JB (1972). *The Lymphatics: Surgery, Lymphography and Diseases of the Chyle and Lymph Systems*. Edward Arnold, London, pp. 116–127.

Ko D, Lerner R, Klose G, Cosimi A (1998). Effective treatment of lymphedema of the extremities. *Arch Surg* 133: 452–458.

Kriederman B, Myloyde T, Witte M, Dagenais SL, Witte C, Rennels M, Bernas M, Erickson R, Caulden MS, Miura N, Jackson D, Brooks B, Glover TW (2003). *FOXC2*$^{+/-}$ mice are a model for autosomal dominant lymphedema-distichiasis syndrome. *Hum Molec Genet*, in press.

Kuhnt H (1899). Ueber distichiasis (congenita) vera. *Z Augenh* 2: 46–57.

Kukk E, Lymboussaki A, Taira S, Kaipainen A, Jeltsch M, Joukov V, Alitalo K (1996). VEGF-C receptor binding and pattern of expression with VEGFR-3 suggests a role in lymphatic vascular development. *Development* 122: 3829–3837.

Kume T, Deng K, Hogan BLM (2000). Murine forkhead/winged helix genes *Foxc1 (Mf1)* and *Foxc2 (mfh1)* are required for the early organogenesis of the kidney and urinary tract. *Development* 127: 1387–1395.

Kume T, Jiang HY, Topczewska JM, Hogan BLM (2001). The murine winged helix transcription factors, Foxc1 and Foxc2, are both required for cardiovascular development and somatogenesis. *Genes Dev* 15: 2470–2482.

Lymboussaki A, Olofsson B, Eriksson U, Alitalo K (1999). Vascular endothelial growth factor (VEGF) and VEGF-C show overlapping binding sites in embryonic endothelial and distinct sites in differentiated adult endothelia. *Circ Res* 85: 999.

Mangion J, Rahman N, Mansour S, Brice G, Rosbotham J, Child A H, Murday V A, Mortimer P S, Barfoot R, Sigurdsson A, et al. (1999). A gene for lymphedema-distichiasis maps to 16q24.3. *Am J Hum Genet* 65: 427–432.

Miura N, Iida K, Kakinuma H, Yang X L, Sugiyama T (1997). Isolations of the mouse *(MFH-1)* and human *(FKHL-14)* mesenchyme fork head-1 genes reveals conservation of their gene and protein structures. *Genomics* 41: 489–492.

Neel JV, Schull WJ (1954). *Human Heredity.* University of Chicago Press, Chicago, pp. 50–51.

Pap Z, Bíró T, Szabó L, Papp Z (1980). Syndrome of lymphoedema and distichiasis. *Hum Genet* 53: 309–310.

Robinow M, Johnson GF, Verhagen AD (1970). Distichiasis-lymphoedema. A hereditary syndrome of multiple congenital defects. *Am J Dis Child* 119: 343–347.

Rosbotham JL, Brice GW, Child AH, Nunan TO, Mortimer PS, Burnand KG (2000). Distichiasis-lymphoedema: clinical features, venous function and lymphoscintigraphy. *J Dermatol* 142: 148–152.

Saleem RA, Banerjee-Basu S, Berry FB, Baxevania AD, Walter MA (2001). Analyses of the effects that disease-causing missense mutations have on the structure and function of the winged-helix protein FOXC1. *Am J Hum Genet* 68: 27–41.

Schwartz JF, O'Brien MS, Hoffman JS Jr (1980). Hereditary spinal arachnoid cysts, distichiasis, and lymphedema. *Ann Neurol* 7: 340–343.

Seaver LH (2001). Non-immune hydrops and cystic hygroma in the lymphedema-distichiasis syndrome. *Proc Greenwood Genet Center* 20: 5–8.

Shammas HJF, Tabbara KF, Der Kaloustian VM (1979). Distichiasis of the lids and lymphedema of the lower extremities: a report of ten cases. *J Pediatr Ophthalmol Strabismus* 16: 129–132.

Smith RS, Zabaleta A, Kume T, Savinova OV, Kidson SH, Martin JE, Nishimura DY, Alward WL, Hogan BLM, John SWM (2000). Haploinsufficiency of the transcription factors FOXC1 and FOXC2 results in aberrant ocular development. *Hum Mol Genet* 9: 1021–1032.

Stammos et al. (1979). Distichiasis of the lids and lymphedema of the lower extremities: a report of ten cases. *J Pediatr Ophthalmol Strabismus* 16:130; by permission of author and publisher.

Temple IK, Collin JRO (1994). Distichiasis-lymphoedema syndrome: a family report. *Clin Dysmorphol* 3: 139–142.

Winnier GE, Kume T, Deng K, Rogers R, Bundy J, Raines C, Walter MA, Hogan BLM, Conway SJ (1999). Roles for the winged helix transcription factors MF1 and MFH1 in cardiovascular development revealed by non-allelic non-complementation of null alleles. *Dev Biol* 213: 418–431.

Part D.
The T-Box Gene Family

67 | Introduction to the *T-Box* Genes and Their Roles in Developmental Signaling Pathways

VIRGINIA E. PAPAIOANNOU AND SARAH N. GOLDIN

The history of the T-box gene family began with the 1927 discovery of a semidominant mutation in mice, named *Brachyury* (short tail), or simply *T*, for tail. The mutation affects both embryonic viability in homozygotes and tail development in heterozygotes (Dobrovolskaïa-Zavadskaïa, 1927). In the following decades, the embryological defects caused by the *T* mutation were exhaustively studied. Finally, in 1990, the *T* gene was cloned (Herrmann et al., 1990). At the same time, Pflugfelder et al. (1990) were analyzing the *Drosophila melanogaster optomotor blind* (*omb*) mutant, characterized by the absence of giant neurons in the lobular plate of the optic lobe of the adult fly. Upon cloning the *omb* gene, they recognized that *omb* and *T* share a domain of homology and demonstrated that this domain possesses a general DNA-binding affinity (Pflugfelder et al., 1992). Subsequently, the *omb*-homologous domain of T was shown to bind specifically to DNA, and its preferred in vitro target sequence was identified (Kispert and Herrmann, 1993). Then in 1995 it was shown that *T* encodes a transcription factor capable of regulating expression of a reporter via the identified target sequence (Kispert, 1995). Based on the limited number of DNA-binding motifs and the observation that gene families are the norm for transcription factors, it seemed likely that *T* and *omb* represented just two members of a larger gene family. This prediction was born out by Bollag et al. (1994), who demonstrated the existence of a family of *T*-related genes in the mouse genome, which was christened the T-box gene family after the region of homology that encodes most of the DNA-binding domain. Thus, the defining feature of the T-box gene family is a conserved sequence encoding a polypeptide domain that extends across a region of 180–200 amino acid residues and is called the T-box domain or T domain (Kispert and Herrmann, 1993; Bollag et al., 1994).

Since 1994, new members of the family have been discovered in an ever-widening circle of species so that today the family contains over 100 genes (Papaioannou, 2001). The evolutionary relationships between the various members of the gene family are being elucidated by phylogenetic analysis. Support has been found for the hypothesis that DNA-binding activity is conserved among all proteins containing the T-box domain. The discovery of a consensus binding motif and determination of the structure of the *Xbra* T domain bound to DNA have opened the way to a better understanding of the interaction of T-box genes with DNA. Subsequently, potential downstream targets of many different T-box genes have been identified by a variety of direct and indirect in vivo and in vitro techniques. T-box genes have been implicated as players in many of the signaling pathways used throughout development. Interest in the functional role of individual family members has been heightened by the dramatic phenotypes of T-box gene mutations in diverse species including *Drosophila*, zebrafish, mouse, and human, which have profound developmental consequences.

686

EVOLUTION OF THE *T-BOX* GENE FAMILY

Phylogenetic analysis has indicated that the T-box family is ancient, with members present in species from hydra to humans. The family's initial expansion from a single progenitor sequence appears to have occurred at the outset of metazoan evolution (Agulnik et al., 1996). Comprehesive phylogenetic analyses (Ruvinsky et al., 2000b; Papaioannou, 2001) indicate that the genomes of most animal species will have at least five T-box genes (corresponding to the five subfamilies shown in Fig. 67–1 and Table 67–1) and that all chordates could have eight or more.

Phylogenetic analysis allows the identification of likely orthologs across different species as well as paralogs within a species. Orthologous genes are defined as direct descendents from a single ancestral gene present in a common ancestral species or, in other words, separation by speciation. Paralogous genes are defined as genes descendent from a single ancestral gene separated by gene duplication within a species. The relative time of duplication, whether by speciation or gene duplication, can be inferred from the phylogentic tree (Fig. 67–1). For example, orthologs of the first cloned T-box gene, mouse *T*, have been identified in many vertebrate and invertebrate species and are found in the T subfamily. A duplication event appears to have occurred in an ancestor of the vertebrate lineage to generate the paralogous genes *T* and *Tbx19*. Similarly, a *Xenopus*-specific gene duplication appears to have generated the paralogous gene pair *Xbra* and *Xbra3*.

In comparisons between closely related species, such as mouse and human, it is generally possible to recognize orthologous genes. However, with more distantly related species, the distinction between true orthologs and subfamily members can sometimes be more difficult to make. For example, when mouse *Tbr1* was first identified, it was thought to be the ortholog of *Xenopus Eomesodermin* (*Eomes*) (Bulfone et al., 1995). Later, mouse *Eomes* was cloned and recognized as the true ortholog, due to its much greater degree of sequence identity to *Eomes* (Wattler et al., 1998) (Fig. 67–1). Orthology is defined purely on the basis of evolutionary heritage, as deduced from sequence identity, chromosomal location, and intron/exon structure. Orthologs are likely to perform related functions in different species such that they may be expressed at comparable times in comparable tissues and/or may exert related genetic and biochemical effects. However, conserved functional attributes cannot be used as evidence for orthology. The Tbx6 subfamily is particularly instructive on this point. The zebrafish gene *tbx6* was so named largely because of its apparent functional similarity to the mouse gene *Tbx6*, as deduced from a similar expression pattern in nascent mesoderm at gastrulation and in paraxial mesoderm at tail bud stages (Chapman et al., 1996a; Hug et al., 1997). Phylogenetic analysis, however, indicates that the two genes are not true orthologs as they likely diverged prior to the speciation event that separated the bony fish and tetrapod lineages (see Fig. 67–1) (Ruvinsky et al., 2000b). In fact, the original naming of the Tbx6 subfamily was erroneously based more on the conserved expression patterns of most of its members than on an understanding of their evolutionary relationships. Even today, except for the human/mouse/*Xenopus TBX6/Tbx6* and human/mouse *MGA/Mga* orthologous groups, the relationships between members of the subfamily, both across and within species, are largely unclear. Perhaps there are still undiscovered T-box genes that will help to clarify the issue. Alternatively, these genes may have diverged beyond easy understanding of orthology despite a common heritage, or the subfamily may be the result of combinations of lineage-specific gene losses and duplications such that orthologs will never be found in all species.

Analysis of the genomic structure of a number of T-box genes has provided independent support for the phylogenetic tree based on amino acid sequences (Wattler et al., 1998), and differences in intron position or number brought about by intron deletion, sliding, or insertion are features that can further clarify relationships between subfamily members. The *MGA/Mga* gene is highly unusual in this respect. It codes for a dual-specificity protein that contains both a T-box and a Myc-like basic-helix-loop-helix-leucine zipper (bHLHZ) domain. Genomic sequencing showed that the T-box domain is encoded by a single-unit exon, unlike all other T-box genes, which show general conservation of intron/exon structure with the T-box encoded by three to five exons. Thus, *MGA/Mga* could be the product of the retrotransposition of a *T-box* gene into a gene coding for a Max-interacting bHLHZ protein (Hurlin et al., 1999). *MGA/Mga* falls within the Tbx6 subfamily and is the probable ortholog of a newt gene, *CpUbiqT* (Papaioannou, 2001). It will be very interesting to discover if this gene shares the unusual genomic structure of *MGA/Mga* and whether it also encodes for a dual-specificity transcription factor.

The power of phylogenetic analysis in reconstructing the evolution of groups of related genes is shown by the *Tbx2* subfamily. The phylogenetic tree indicates that *Tbx2* and *Tbx3* form a paralogous gene pair, as do *Tbx4* and *Tbx5*. Genomic mapping of the genes in both mice and humans showed that *Tbx2* and *Tbx4* exist as a linked pair, as do *Tbx3* and *Tbx5*. Thus, we have proposed a model for the evolution of this subfamily, hypothesizing an initial tandem duplication of a single ancestral gene by unequal crossing over to form a two-gene cluster that later duplicated and was dispersed to different chromosomal locations (Fig. 67–2) (Agulnik et al., 1996). Estimates of the timing of this duplication and dispersal event place it before the separation of the bony fish and tetrapod lineages, suggesting that the genomic arrangement of these two T-box clusters should be similar in all vertebrates (Ruvinsky et al., 2000a).

With the complete sequence of the human genome available, the full complement of T-box genes present in *Homo sapiens* has likely been identified. There are 18 T-box genes in the human genome. Mouse orthologs have been identified for all but one of these genes, *TBX23* (Table 67–1). *TBX23* is most likely a non-functional pseudogene as its putative open reading frame contains several stop codons. Thus, this gene may represent a human genome-specific duplication, perhaps of *TBX19*, which is also located on chromosome 1, or its cognate pseudogene may have been lost from the mouse genome. Conversely, human orthologs have been identified for all murine T-box genes discovered to date. Surprisingly, the human genome does not appear to contain a Tbx6 subfamily ortholog to *Xenopus VegT* and zebrafish *tbx16*, nor has such a gene been identified in mouse. This absence may indicate loss of a *VegT*-like gene in the mammalian lineage. Similarly, human *TBX6* and mouse *Tbx6* orthologs have not been identified in nonmammalian lineages apart from *Xenopus* (Uchiyama et al., 2001).

The phylogenetic tree presented in Figure 67–1 is based on comparisons of the T-box domain amino acid sequence of each gene. In general, T-box genes do not show marked conservation outside of the T-box, with specific instructive exceptions. Orthologs of the same T-box gene across species generally show conservation both within the T-box and across the entire open reading frame (Fig. 67–3A). Consider, for example, the canonical *T*, or *Brachyury*, gene. The T-box domain amino acid sequences of zebrafish (*Danio rerio*) *T*, *Xenopus Xbra*, chicken *T*, and human *T* are, respectively, 88%, 93%, 97%, and 97% identical to that of mouse *T*. Additionally, these orthologs are highly related across the entire open reading frame with *D. rerio T* 63%, *Xenopus Xbra* 75%, chicken *T* 80%, and human *T* 90% identical to mouse *T*. In fact, this comparison of sequence across the entire open reading frame can often be used to clarify issues of confused orthology.

Due to their common evolutionary heritage, orthologs often show conservation of nonexonic transcriptional regulatory elements as well and, thus, may be regulated by similar upstream factors. Therefore, it is highly likely that orthologs will function in related molecular pathways across different species. For example, *Xenopus VegT* expression in the dorsal marginal zone and blastopore lip at mid- to late gastrulation is dependent on fibroblast growth factor (FGF) signaling (Lustig et al., 1996). Similarly, expression of the zebrafish ortholog *tbx16/spadetail* (*spt*) in the germ ring at mid-gastrulation is maintained by FGF signaling (Griffin et al., 1998).

Paralogous gene pairs within a species may also show conservation of non-T-box amino acid sequences and of transcriptional regulatory elements. Consider the case of the paralogous mouse genes *Tbx4* and *Tbx5*. In addition to being 94% identical across their T-box amino acid sequences, the C-terminal domain of *Tbx5* is approximately 38% iden-

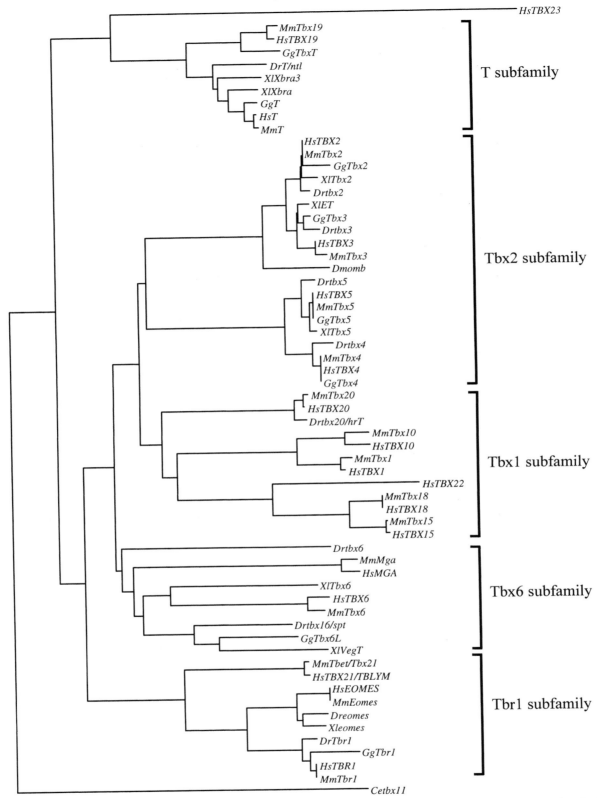

Figure 67–1. Phylogenetic tree of T-box genes of zebrafish, *Xenopus*, chicken, mouse, and human. The T-box domain amino acid sequences of T-box genes identified in *Homo sapiens* (*Hs*), *Mus Musculus* (*Mm*), *Xenopus laevis* (*Xl*), *Gallus gallus* (*Gg*), and *Danio rerio* (*Dr*); of the *Drosophila melanogaster* gene *omb*; and of *Caenorhabditis elegans tbx11* were used to generate a phylogenetic tree. The five subfamilies are delineated by brackets to the right. Phylogenetic analysis was conducted using the ClustalW software package (http://www.ebi.ac.uk/clustalw/) accessed via the European Bioinformatics Institute (EBI) (http://www.ebi.ac.uk/). Sequences were aligned with ClustalW and then subjected to Phylip analysis in the same EBI interface (no distance correction, gapped areas included). Phylip outputs were interpreted using the tree-drawing program NJplot (Perrier and Gouy, 1996) obtained from Pôle Bio-Informatique Lyonnais (http://pbil.univ-lyonl.fr/). *Cetbx11* was outgrouped to root the tree. The following sequences were excluded from the tree due to insufficient sequence data: *Drtbax*, *XlTbx4*, and *GgTbr2*.

Table 67–1. _T-Box_ Gene Orthologs in Mouse and Human, Grouped by Subfamily

Mouse Gene*	Chromosome Location	Mutations	Reference	Human Gene*	Chromosome Location	Human Syndrome	Reference
T	17.4	T, T^{2J}, T^{or4}, T^{orl}, T^{hp}, T^{kt1}, T^{137}, T^{wis}, T^{c}, T^{c-2H}	Herrmann, 1992; Papaioannou, 2001	T	6q27	Spina bifida (candidate)	Edwards et al., 1996
Tbx19 (Tpit)	1.86	—	Lamolet et al., 2001; Liu et al., 2001	TBX19 (TPIT)	1q23-q24	Isolated deficiency of pituitary pro-opiomelanocortin-derived corticotropin	Yi et al., 1999; Lamolet et al., 2001
	—		—	TBX23 (pseudogene)	1	—	Ruvinsky et al., 2000b
Tbx1	16.6	$Tbx1^{tm1Pa}$	Bollag et al., 1994; Jerome et al., 2001	TBX1	22q11	DiGeorge (candidate)	Chieffo et al., 1997
Tbx10	19.2	—	Agulnik et al., 1998; Wattler et al., 1998; Law et al., 1998	TBX10	11q13	—	Law et al., 1998
Tbx15	3.49	—	Agulnik et al., 1998; Wattler et al., 1998	TBX15	1p13	Acromegaloid facial appearance (candidate)	Agulnik et al., 1998
Tbx18	9	—	Kraus et al., 2001	TBX18	6q14-q15	—	Yi et al., 1999
Tbx20	9	—	Carson et al., 2000; Meins et al., 2000	TBX20	7p15.1-p13	—	Ruvinsky et al., 2000b; Meins et al., 2000
Tbx22		—	Herr, et al., 2003	TBX22	Xq13.1-21.1	Cleft palate with ankyloglossia	Ruvinsky et al., 2000a; Laugier-Anfossi et al., 2000
Tbx2	11.46		Bollag et al., 1994	TBX2	17q23	—	Campbell et al., 1995; Law et al., 1995
Tbx3	5.67	$Tbx3^{tm1Pa}$	Bollag et al., 1994; Davenport et al., 2003	TBX3	12q23-q24	Ulnar-mammary	Li et al., 1997; Bamshad et al., 1997
Tbx4	11.46	$Tbx4^{tm1Pa}$	Agulnik et al., 1996; Naiche and Papaioannou, 2003	TBX4	17q2-q22	—	Yi et al., 2000
Tbx5	5.67	$Tbx5^{del}$	Agulnik et al., 1996; Bruneau et al., 2001	TBX5	12q23-q24	Holt-Oram	Li et al., 1997; Basson et al., 1997
Tbx6	7.6	$Tbx6^{tm1Pa}$	Agulnik et al., 1996; Chapman et al., 1998, 1996a	TBX6	16p12-q12	—	Papapetrou et al., 1999; Yi et al., 1999
Mga	2.67	—	Hurlin et al., 1999	MGA	15q14	—	Hurlin et al., 1999 (GenBank clone RP1110756, accession AC073657)
Tbr1	2.33	$Tbr1^{-}$ Eo^{lacZ}	Bulfone et al., 1995, 1998	TBR1	—	—	Bulfone et al., 1995
Eomes (Tbr2)	9.64	—	Wattler et al., 1998; Hancock et al., 1999; Russ et al., 2000	Eomes (TBR2)	3p21.3-p21.2	—	Campbell et al., 1998; Yi et al., 1999
Tbx21 (Tbet)	11	$Tbet^{-}$	Zhang et al., 2000, 2002	TBX21 (TBLYM)	17	Asthma (candidate)	Ruvinsky et al., 2000b; Zhang and Yang, 2000; Finnotto et al., 2002

*Names in parentheses are aliases.

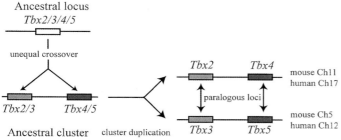

Figure 67–2. Model for the evolution of the Tbx2 subfamily in vertebrates, which hypothesizes an initial tandem duplication of a single ancestral gene by unequal crossing over to form a two-gene cluster that later duplicated and was dispersed to different chromosomal locations (Agulnik et al., 1996). Chromosomal locations for the mouse and human genes are indicated.

tical to that of *Tbx4*. An interspecific comparison of the complete protein sequence of *Tbx4* and *Tbx5* orthologs shows that several short amino acid stretches are invariantly conserved in the C-terminal domains of both proteins (Fig. 67–3*B*) (A.L. Naiche, personal communication).

In some cases, nonorthologous members of a subfamily in different species show amino acid conservation outside of the T box. Consider, for example, the Tbr1 subfamily (Fig. 67–3*C*). Within the T box, the amino acid sequence of *Xenopus Eomes* is 93% identical to that of mouse *Eomes* and 84% identical to that of mouse *Tbr1*. The C-terminal protein domain of *Xenopus Eomes* is 72% identical to that of its ortholog mouse *Eomes* but 45% identical to that of the nonorthologous subfamily member mouse *Tbr1*, with the identity concentrated in four major stretches. The conservation of non-T-box sequences between family members can help us gain insight into the proteins' biochemistry and mode of action. If a specific function of one family member (e.g., interaction with an accessory protein) has been localized to a region of the protein that is conserved in another T-box protein, it is possible that the two proteins will share that function.

EVIDENCE FOR *T-BOX* GENES AS TRANSCRIPTION FACTORS

DNA Binding and Identification of Specific Binding Sequences

With the discovery of a conserved region of homology between *Drosophila omb* and mouse *Brachyury*, the DNA-binding property of the T-box proteins and their potential role as transcription factors were recognized. Nonspecific binding of *in vitro* synthesized Omb to calf thymus DNA was the first evidence for DNA binding. This activity was shown to reside in the domain conserved between Omb and T (Pflugfelder et al., 1992), which became known as the T-box domain or T domain (Kispert and Herrmann, 1993; Bollag et al., 1994). Specific target DNA sequences recognized by the T-box domain were first identified by binding site selection using *in vitro* synthesized mouse T protein and a mixture of random oligonucleotides. From these studies, a 20-base, nearly palindromic binding site (TG/CACACCT//AGGTGTGAAATT) was defined as the consensus T-box domain–binding sequence. The T protein binds this inverted repeat as a monomer and can bind to variously spaced and oriented half-sites (AGGTGTGAAA) (Kispert and Herrmann, 1993).

The architecture of the T-box domain sequence-specific DNA recognition was revealed by solving the X-ray crystallographic structure of the *Xenopus* Xbra DNA-binding domain in complex with a 24-nucleotide palindromic DNA duplex (Fig. 67–4) (Muller and Herrmann, 1997). The X-ray structure reveals that the T domain can bind as a dimer, although the protein is in solution as a monomer, and that it contacts the DNA in both the major and minor grooves. There is a novel protein–DNA interaction in which a C-terminal helix is embedded into an enlarged minor groove of DNA without bending the DNA. The dimer interface lies above the minor groove such that the dimer forms a large arc spanning the DNA, allowing it to contact the 20 bp DNA-recognition sequence via the minor groove. This configuration results in a large hole between the dimer interface and the contact regions of each monomer with its DNA half-site (Muller and Herrmann, 1997).

A. T orthologs

	% identity	
	T-box	ORF
Danio rerio T/ntl	88	63
Xenopus Xbra	93	75
chicken T	97	80
human T	97	90
mouse T		

B. Paralogs

	% identity	
	T-box	C term
mouse Tbx5	94	38
mouse Tbx4		

C. Tbr1 subfamily

	% identity	
	T-box	C term
Xenopus Eomes	93	72
mouse Eomes	84	45
mouse Tbr1		

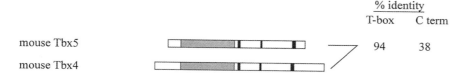

Figure 67–3. Examples of similarities and differences in amino acid sequence among orthologs, paralogs, and subfamily members in the T-box gene family. Boxes represent open reading frames (ORFs), drawn to scale. T-box domains are shaded gray. *C-term* refers to all protein sequences from the end of the T-box domain to the C-terminal end of the protein. (*A*) Comparison of T orthologs from different species. Percent identities of T-box domains and entire ORFs to those of mouse T are indicated. (*B*) Comparison of murine T-box gene paralogs Tbx4 and Tbx5. Percent identities of Tbx5 T-box and C terminus to those of Tbx4 are indicated. Black boxes represent three peptide sequences in the C-terminal domain that are invariantly conserved across all known Tbx4 and Tbx5 orthologs. (*C*) Comparison of Tbr1 subfamily members. *Xenopus* Eomes and mouse Eomes are orthologs. *Xenopus* Eomes and mouse Tbr1 are nonorthologous, nonparalogous subfamily members. Percent identities of *Xenopus* Eomes T-box and C-terminal end to those of mouse Eomes and Tbr1 are indicated.

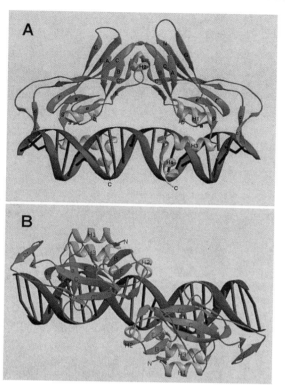

Figure 67–4. Ribbon diagram of the *Xenopus Brachyury* T-domain dimer bound to DNA. Depicted are residues 39–221 of both monomers and the 24 mer DNA duplex. (*A*) View perpendicular to the DNA axis with the dyad vertical. (*B*) Rotated by 90 degrees around the DNA axis with respect to *A*. (Reprinted with permission from Muller and Herrmann, 1997.)

Since these early studies, proteins from *Brachyury* orthologs in other species, as well as several other T-box genes, namely, mouse *Tbx3, Tbx6,* and *Tbr1*; human *TBX5*; and *Xenopus Eomes* and *VegT*, have been found to demonstrate sequence-specific DNA binding to the T consensus or very similar sequences (Kispert and Herrmann, 1993; Holland et al., 1995; Papapetrou et al., 1999; Hsueh et al., 2000; Conlon et al., 1996, 2001; Ghosh et al., 2001; Carlson et al., 2001). Furthermore, similar sequences, referred to as "T-binding elements" (TBEs), have been found in the promoters of a number of potential downstream target genes (reviewed by Papaioannou, 2001) (Table 67–2). All metazoan species appear to have multiple T-box genes; and although they are expressed in highly specific patterns during development, there are many areas of expression overlap. Because of the high degree of conservation of the T-box sequences, it is likely that all T-box proteins will have similar DNA-binding specificity and could potentially heterodimerize with other T-box proteins during DNA binding. Additionally, whether or not there is heterodimerization, different T-box proteins may compete for binding sites in tissues in which they are coexpressed due to different affinity for specific sequences or specific spacing/orientation of TBEs.

Although the potential for interactions and/or competition between different T-box proteins is considerable, relatively few studies have investigated the role of heterodimerization and/or competitive binding. In vitro synthesized mouse Tbx6 was found to bind efficiently to the T consensus target sequence, forming two complexes of different mobilities, representing monomeric and dimeric forms of the protein bound to DNA. However, no evidence for binding of Tbx6/T heterodimers was found when the two proteins were combined in the same binding assay reaction (Papapetrou et al., 1999). The consensus binding site for human TBX5 is contained within the consensus binding site for T, but T does not bind the TBX5 site, possibly indicating more stringent binding requirements for T (Ghosh et al., 2001). In *Xenopus*, several T-box genes have overlapping expression in the early embryo. As will be discussed later, genes of a novel family of paired-

Table 67–2. Putative Downstream Target Genes of Vertebrate T-Box Transcription Factors, Grouped by Subfamily, with the Nature of the Evidence that They Are Direct Downstream Target Genes*

T-Box Transcription Factor	Downstream Target Gene	Nature of Target Protein	Transcriptional Activity	Nature of Evidence that Gene Is a Downstream Target
Xenopus Xbra	*eFGF*	Growth factor	Activation	2 half-sites in promoter, reporter assay
	Bix4	Homeobox transcription factor	Activation	3 half-sites in promoter, rapid induction by Xbra, transcription assay
	Xwnt11	Ligand	Activation	Rapid induction by Xbra, coexpression
Mouse T	*fgf4*	Growth factor	Activation	Binding site in promoter
Human T	*FGF4*	Growth factor	Activation	Binding site in promoter
Mouse Tbx19	*pro-opiomelano-cortin (POMC)*	Hormone	Activation	Binding site in promoter, expression, transcription assay, mutant phenotype
Mouse/human Tbx2	*pleiotrophin (osf-1)*	Heparin-binding protein	Activation	Binding site in promoter, expression unregulated
	Cdkn2a (p19^{ARF})	Cyclin-dependent kinase inhibitor	Repression	Functional screen, transcription assay
	tyrosinase-related protein-1 (trp-1)	Melanin synthesis enzyme	Repression	2 half-sites in promoter, binding and transcription assay
Mouse/human Tbx5	*connexin 40 (cx40)*	Gap junction subunit	Activation	Lower expression in *Tbx5* mutants, *Tbx5* mutant phenotype, 5 binding sites in promoter, binding and transcription assays
	atrial natriuretic factor (ANF, Nppa)	Peptide hormone	Activation	Lower expression in *Tbx5* mutants, *Tbx5* mutant phenotype, 3 half-sites in promoter, binding and transcription assays
Xenopus VegT	*Xnr1*	Transforming growth factor-β growth factor	Activation	Binding sites in promoter, transcription assay
	Bix1	Homeobox transcription factor	Activation	Rapid induction by Xbra, timing of expression
	Bix4	Homeobox transcription factor	Activation	3 half-sites in promoter, binding and transcription assays
	Paraxial protocadherin (PAPC)	Transmembrane, cell adhesion	Activation	Transcription assay, ectopic expression
Zebrafish tbx16	*paraxial protocadherin*	Transmembrane, cell adhesion	Activation	Expression, mutant analysis
Mouse Tbx21 (Tbet)	*IL-2*	Cytokine	Repression	Binding sites in promoter, expression, transcription assay, *Tbet* mutant phenotype
	INF-γ	Antiviral	Activation	Binding sites in promoter, expression, transcription assay, *Tbet* mutant phenotype
Mouse Tbr1	*reelin*	Extracellular matrix glycoprotein	Activation	Binding sites in promoter, transcription assay, *Tbr1* mutant phenotype

*See text for references.

type homeobox genes, the *Bix* genes, are induced in *Xenopus* by both Xbra and VegT. While *Bix1* is induced equally strongly by either Xbra or VegT, *Bix4* is more efficiently activated by VegT (Casey et al., 1999). The *Bix4* regulatory region contains two 10 bp T-box domain–binding sites within 70 bp of the transcription-start site and a third related site 15 bp upstream. Xbra and VegT bind to the middle site, while Xbra binds strongly and VegT very weakly to the proximal site. The middle site is necessary for *Bix4* expression in the endoderm, while all three sites are required for correct spatial expression at the early gastrula stage. Binding site selection experiments show that Xbra, VegT, and Eomesodermin bind the same core sequence but select paired sites that differ in their orientation and spacing (Tada et al., 1998; Casey et al., 1999; Conlon et al., 2001). Taken together, these studies indicate that regulation of downstream genes by T-box proteins is likely to be complex, especially in areas where two or more T-box genes have overlapping expression.

Evidence for Transcriptional Regulatory Activity

Determining the transcriptional regulatory activity of a DNA-binding protein and identifying direct downstream target genes are not simple matters. There are several levels of evidence to consider. In vitro assays that make use of target DNA-binding sequences fused to reporter genes provide indirect evidence for regulatory activity of DNA-binding proteins and can also be used to test the role of particular protein domains. These assays, however, are removed from a biological context and indicate what a protein is capable of doing, not necessarily what it normally does. Gene-expression patterns consistent with activation or repression can be examined in in vitro assays or within tissues in vivo. Coexpression of a putative transcription factor and a potential target in the same cells is indirect evidence for transcriptional activation or repression, provided the transcription factor expression temporally precedes target gene expression or extinction of expression, respectively. Rapid induction of gene expression in in vivo assays, such as the animal cap assay in *Xenopus* embryos, identifies potential downstream targets for activation; and conversely, rapid loss of expression of genes following expression of the transcription factor can identify potential targets for repression. Gene-expression patterns in animals that are mutant for putative transcription factors can provide further evidence for regulatory relationships. These various functional and expression assays become more powerful and more direct when combined with evidence from genomic sequence analysis that T-box domain–binding sites actually exist in the regulatory regions of the potential target genes and, further, that these target sites mediate gene expression. The more complete the evidence is, the greater the confidence that a specific gene is a biologically meaningful downstream target of T-box genes (Table 67–2).

Evidence for transcriptional activity of T-box proteins was first demonstrated for mouse T in in vitro transcription assays. The T-box domain resides in the N-terminal domain, whereas the C-terminal region has a complex domain structure with two activation domains and two domains that block activation. The regulatory activity of the protein in transcriptional assays is affected by the number and spacing of TBEs in target DNA (Kispert and Herrmann, 1993; Kispert et al., 1995). It thus seems possible that T protein in vivo, and by extension other T-box proteins, may interact with half-sites of particular spacing and orientation and that selection of the binding sites could be influenced by factors interacting with the T-box protein and/or the TBEs. There is circumstantial evidence for the involvement of accessory proteins that might form a bridge between two T proteins bound to neighboring target sites, stabilize DNA–T protein complexes, or determine whether the protein acts as a repressor or activator (Kispert and Herrmann, 1993; Kispert et al., 1995).

Two T orthologs, zebrafish T and *Xenopus* Xbra, as well as *Xenopus* VegT and Eomes, act as transcriptional activators in yeast and mammalian cell culture transcription assay systems, with the activation domain residing in the C-terminal domain (Conlon et al., 1996, 2001). *Xenopus* ET, however, represses both basal and activated transcription in assays in human cell lines and *Xenopus* embryos. A domain found to be necessary and sufficient for repression is highly conserved in the human ortholog, *TBX3*, and in the closely related *TBX2*.

These human genes and their mouse orthologs can act as transcriptional repressors (Carreira et al., 1998; He et al., 1999, Carlson et al., 2001).

Mga is an unusual T-box gene in that it codes for a protein containing both a T-box domain and a bHLHZ domain and is thus thought to function as a dual-specificity transcription factor capable of regulating the expression of both Max-network and T-box domain target genes. The transcriptional activity of bHLHZ proteins is mediated by heterodimerization with the small bHLHZ protein Max, required for specific DNA binding to E-box sequences. The mouse gene *Mga* was discovered through a yeast two-hybrid screen for Max-interacting proteins. In vitro binding and transcription assays indicate that Mga is capable of regulating transcription from promoters containing either TBE or Myc/Max-binding sites and that cellular Max levels dictate whether it functions as a repressor or an activator (Hurlin et al., 1999).

Identification of Downstream Target Genes

A Variety of T-Box Targets in a Variety of Species and Tissues

Table 67–2 lists potential downstream target genes of vertebrate T-box proteins for which fairly convincing evidence of a direct transcriptional regulatory link exists. These genes encode a variety of different types of protein and undoubtedly represent only a small subset of the genes regulated by T-box proteins. Many more direct and indirect downstream target genes are likely to emerge as T-box genes come under greater scrutiny.

Several genes were identified in a screen for *Brachyury*-inducible genes in *Xenopus*. One of these genes codes for the ligand *Xwnt11* and another is *Bix4* (*Brachyury*-inducible homeobox-containing gene-4), both of which are implicated in regulating the movements of gastrulation in the early embryo (Tada et al., 1998; Tada and Smith, 2000; Saka et al., 2000). Additional experiments with candidates isolated in this screen illustrate just how complicated the correct identification of downstream target genes can be. Both *Bix4* and *Bix1* were induced by Xbra in the assay and *Bix4* has TBEs in its promoter; however, they can both also be activated by another T-box protein, VegT. Which is the real inducer? It is quite possible that both Xbra and VegT regulate or coregulate these *Bix* genes in vitro, but the timing of expression of *Bix1* makes it a more attractive candidate as a direct target of VegT (Tada et al., 1998). Thus, the promiscuous binding of different T-box proteins to the target DNA-binding sequence and the overlapping expression patterns of different T-box genes must be considered in determining the biological relevance of particular candidate target genes identified in induction assays.

Other potential downstream targets of VegT in *Xenopus* embryos include the transforming growth factor-β (TGF-β) growth factor *Xnr1*, the promoter of which contains two potential VegT-binding sites that will activate a reporter gene in the presence of VegT (Hyde and Old, 2000), and *paraxial protocadherin* (*PAPC*), which is ectopically expressed in response to *VegT* mRNA injection into embryos (Kim et al., 1998). *PAPC* encodes a transmembrane cell adhesion molecule and is a potential target of the zebrafish *VegT* ortholog *tbx16* or *spt*, although it is not known whether it is a direct or an indirect target. During gastrulation, *PAPC* expression is closely correlated with that of *tbx16*, although later it is expressed independently of *tbx16* in somites. Concordantly, zebrafish *papc* expression is greatly reduced in *spt* mutants at gastrulation but reappears at the time of tail somite formation. Furthermore, a dominant-negative form of *papc* mRNA disrupts the convergence movements of gastrulating embryos in a manner reminiscent of the *spt* mutation (Yamamoto et al., 1998), suggesting that they are in the same pathway.

Tbx5 is one of several T-box genes expressed in the developing heart of vertebrates and is implicated by its mutant effects in humans and mice in the control of heart development (Basson et al., 1997; Li et al., 1997; Bruneau et al., 2001; see Chapter 69). Based on alterations of gene-expression patterns in the hearts of mutant mice, *connexin 40* (*cx40*) and *atrial natriuretic factor* (*ANF*, also called *Nppa*), which are both required for normal heart development, were identified as potential direct targets of Tbx5. Both of these genes satisfy virtually all of the criteria of direct targets: their expression patterns overlap with *Tbx5* in the developing heart, their expression is diminished in heterozygous *Tbx5* mutant hearts and absent in homozygous hearts, they are activated by Tbx5, and they contain TBEs in their promoters that are necessary and sufficient for activation by Tbx5 (Bruneau et al., 2001; Ghosh et al., 2001). *cx40* is one of several gap junction subunit genes expressed in cardiac cells and is important in the conduction system of the heart. *ANF* is a peptide hormone produced in the heart in response to atrial stretch and other stimuli and is regionally expressed in the developing heart tube.

Tbx21 (also known as *Tbet* in mouse and *TBLYM* in human) is restricted in its expression to T-helper (T$_H$) cells of the immune system. Potential T-box domain binding sites have been detected in the promoters of the T-cell specific genes *IL-2* and *INF-γ*, and transcription reporter assays indicate that *Tbx21* represses *IL-2*, *IL-4*, and *IL-5* and activates *INF-γ* expression in CD4, but not CD8, T cells. *Tbx21* controls the differentiation of the T$_H$1 cell lineage from naive helper cells by initiating the T$_H$1 genetic program and repressing the opposing T$_H$2 program (Szeto et al., 1999; Szabo et al., 2002). In mice with a mutation in *Tbx21*, CD4 cells express lower levels of *INF-γ*, providing additional evidence that it is a direct target (Szabo et al., 2002).

Mouse *Tbx2* is widely expressed in a variety of cell and tissue types during development, including chondrocyte/osteoblast cell types (Chapman et al., 1996b; Chen et al., 2001). A microarray analysis of *Tbx2*-expressing and -nonexpressing cell lines identified a variety of potential downstream targets, including cell cycle control genes and genes involved in the chrondrocyte/osteoblast cell differentiation pathways. Support that at least some of these *Tbx2*-regulated genes are direct targets comes from the recognition of TBEs in the regulatory region of human pleiotrophin (*osf-1*), a secreted heparin-binding protein in fetal cartilage (Chen et al., 2001).

In a study of the regulation of mouse *tyrosinase-related protein-1* (*trp-1*), which corresponds to the *brown* coat color locus, two melanocyte-specific regulatory elements in the promoter were found to contain a sequence similar to a half-site of the Brachyury consensus binding site. Tbx2, which is thought to be the only T-box gene expressed in melanoblasts and melanocytes, is capable of binding to these half-sites and repressing transcription in melanocyte and melanoma cell lines. This suggests that Tbx2 may regulate *trp-1* expression during melanocyte development in vivo and points to an important role for Tbx2 in the melanoblast survival and differentiation pathway (Carreira et al., 1998).

Human TBX2 and TBX3 were both identified in functional screens as negative regulators of the cell cycle control gene *Cdkn2a* (also called *p19^{ARF}* in mouse and *p14^{ARF}* in humans). The importance of repression of a cell cycle regulator is emphasized by the observation that *TBX2* is amplified in certain types of breast cancer (Jacobs et al., 2000; Brummelkamp et al., 2001). It first appeared that both the mouse and human genes were directly repressed by TBX2 through an interaction with the promoter that did not involve a consensus T-box domain binding site. However, a variant T-site was later identified in the initiator that binds both Tbx2 and Tbx3 (Lingbeek et al., 2002).

T-Box Genes as Targets of T-Box Genes

There are a few examples of T-box genes regulating other T-box genes. The regulatory pathways of three *Xenopus* genes, *Eomes*, *VegT*, and *Xbra*, that are expressed in response to early mesoderm inducers have been investigated using the animal cap assay (reviewed in Papaioannou and Silver, 1998). This assay, which measures the induction of genes in response to injection of mRNA into the isolated animal pole of an embryo, provides evidence for autoregulation of these genes and for regulatory networks linking all three genes. However, making the distinction between direct and indirect regulation will require additional evidence.

There is evidence for autoregulation of *T* from several other species. In the ascidian *Halocynthia roretzi*, a TBE has been identified in the *T* promoter that is responsible for expression in reporter assays, indicating direct control (Takahashi et al., 1999). In *Xenopus*, there is ev-

idence for indirect autoregulation of the *T* ortholog *Xbra*, requiring the intermediary of FGF signaling (Tada et al., 1997). Thus, *eFGF* is a potential target of Xbra and is induced as a cell-autonomous, immediate-early response to *Xbra* expression. Two potential TBEs have been found in the *Xenopus eFGF* upstream regulatory region. Xbra can bind to one of these half-sites and activate transcription in a reporter gene assay, but full induction requires both half-sites. One of these binding sites is conserved in mouse and human *FGF4* regulatory regions, possibly indicating that FGF is downstream of *T* in these species as well (Casey et al., 1998). However, a reporter transgene assay was used in *Brachyury* null cells in combination with normal cells in mouse chimeras to study the regulation of *T*, and it was found that *T* promoter activity is maintained in *T/T* cells through midgestation. Thus, unlike *Xenopus*, there is no evidence that the T protein is required for the maintenance of *T* expression in the primitive streak of mice. *Fgf4* (an ortholog of Xenopus *eFGF*) is also expressed in *T/T* cells in these chimeras, indicating that this gene does not depend on T in a regulatory loop, as has been postulated for *Xenopus* (Schmidt et al., 1997).

Transcriptional Regulation through Interactions with Other Proteins

T-box proteins have the potential to homodimerize and/or heterodimerize with one another to effect transcriptional regulation, although this has not been demonstrated in vivo. In addition, a few cases of interactions with other proteins have been found to be important in specific contexts, and it is likely that additional interacting proteins will be discovered that are accessory or obligatory partners in DNA binding and transcriptional regulation. For example, Tbx5 was isolated in a yeast two-hybrid screen using the cardiac homeodomain transcription factor Nkx2-5 as bait. Although TBEs in the promoters of *ANF* and *cx40* are necessary and sufficient for activation by Tbx5 in cardiac cells, as described above, the existence of binding sites for Nkx2-5 near the TBEs in both of these genes prompted the investigation of possible cooperation of these two transcription factors. It was found that Tbx5 and Nkx2-5 physically interact, synergistically activating *ANF* and *cx40*. The overlapping expression of these factors makes it highly likely that this interaction is biologically meaningful (Bruneau et al., 2001; Hiroi et al., 2001).

Another homeodomain transcription factor, Pitx1, is an obligate partner of Tbx19 (also called Tpit) for the activation of *pro-opiomelanocortin* (*POMC*) transcription in pituitary melanotrophs and corticotrophs through binding to adjacent binding sites in the promoter. *Tbx19* is expressed only in these two pituitary cell types and, together with Pitx1, is responsible for the tissue-specific expression of *POMC*. Interestingly, Tbx1, which is in a different T-box subfamily and is the only other T-box protein expressed in these cells, does not synergize with Tpit (Lamolet et al., 2001; Liu et al., 2001).

A different type of protein–protein interaction is seen with mouse Tbr1. This protein interacts with the membrane-associated guanylate kinase CASK/LIN-2 in neural cells. Tbr1 binds the guanylate kinase domain of CASK and then redistributes to the nucleus. Although Tbr1 is capable by itself of binding to T-box domain binding sequences and activating expression, activity is greatly enhanced when Tbr1 is associated with CASK. Two TBEs have been found in the regulatory region of the *reelin* gene, and Tbr1-CASK induces expression of *reelin* in a transcription reporter assay. Additional evidence that *reelin* is a genuine downstream target of Tbr1-CASK comes from the neurological phenotype of mice with mutations in *reelin*, which is similar to mice with a *Tbr1* mutation (Bulfone et al., 1998; Hsueh et al., 2000).

T-BOX GENE INVOLVEMENT IN SIGNALING PATHWAYS

T-box transcription factors are involved in at least six of the main developmental signaling pathways (Table 67–3). In the following sections, we present examples of the most direct evidence for T-box genes as downstream targets or upstream effectors in signaling pathways in vertebrates, with a few examples from invertebrates. Because research

Table 67–3. *T-Box* **Gene Participation in Signaling Pathways***

Signaling Pathway	Signaling Pathway Component	Role	*T-Box* Gene	Tissue Affected
Wnt	Wingless signaling molecule	Activator/repressor	*Drosophila H15* and *omb*	Wing and leg imaginal discs
	Wnt3a signaling molecule (via TCF/β-catenin/LEF1)	Activator	Mouse *T*	Primitive streak
TGF-β	Decapentaplegic (BMP2/4) signaling molecule	Activator/repressor	*Drosophila omb* and *H15*	Wing and leg imaginal discs
	Activin signaling molecule	Activator	*Xenopus Xbra*, *VegT*, and *Eomes*; chicken *Tbx6L*	Early embryo
	BMP2 signaling molecule	Activator	Chicken *Tbx2*	Heart
	BMP4 signaling molecule	Activator	Chicken *Tbx5*	Eye
	oep intracellular protein	Interacting protein	Zebrafish *ntl*	Mesoderm
	SIP1 interacting protein	Repressor	*Xenopus Xbra*	Early embryo
	Xnf1 transcription factor	Target	*Xenopus VegT*	Early embryo
Hedgehog	shh signaling molecule	Activator	Mouse and chick *Tbx1*	Pharyngeal region
	shh signaling molecule	Activator	Mouse and chick *Tbx2*	Limb
FGF	bFGF signaling molecule	Activator	*Xenopus Xbra* and *VegT*	Early embryo
	FGF4 signaling molecule	Activator	Chicken *Tbx6L*	Early embryo
	FGF4 signaling molecule	Activator	Mouse *Eomes*	Trophectoderm
	FGFR1 receptor	Activator	Mouse *T* and *Tbx6*	Nascent paraxial mesoderm
Notch	Suppressor of hairless (SuH) binding protein	Activator	Ascidian *CiBra*	Notochord
	Su(H)2 binding protein	Activator	Human *TBX19*	Unknown
Receptor guanylate cyclase	*ANF* peptide hormone	Target	Mouse *Tbx5*	Heart

*The examples shown are only those cases where direct evidence exists for *T-box* gene involvement in specific tissues (see text for references) and do not represent the full range of *T-box* gene involvement in each pathway nor the full range of signaling pathways in which *T-box* genes may function.

TGF, transforming growth factor; TCF, T-cell factor; LEF, lymphoid enhancer factor; BMP, bone morphogenetic protein; shh, sonic hedgehog; bFGF, basic fibroblast growth factor; oep, one-eyed pinhead; SIP, Smad interacting protein.

into the T-box gene family is still in its infancy, this survey does not represent the full range of T-box gene involvement in each pathway or the full range of signaling pathways in which T-box genes may function. Many additional studies provide indirect evidence of involvement in various tissues and in intersecting regulatory pathways. The studies reviewed here offer a tantalizing, if incomplete, glimpse of the complexity of T-box gene involvement in developmental pathways and point the way to further investigation.

Wnt Signaling Pathway

The Wnts comprise a large family of ligands with several receptors of the Frizzled family (see Chapter 22). Evidence from mouse mutants implicates *Wnt* in the regulation of maintenance (but not initiation) of *T* expression, at least in the primitive streak. *Wnt3a* null mutants have a phenotype strikingly similar to *T/T* mutant embryos, including the formation of ectopic neural tubes ventral to the primitive streak, as do double-mutants for *Lef1* and *Tcf1*, downstream effectors of Wnt signaling (Yamaguchi et al., 1999; Galceran et al., 1999). Although expression of *T* in the node and notochord is unaffected in *Wnt3a* mutant embryos, *T* is downregulated in the primitive streak prior to the onset of the mutant phenotype. Examination of *T* regulatory sequences reveals two canonical T-cell transcription factor (TCF)-binding sites to which β-catenin/lymphoid enhancer factor-1 (LEF-1) specifically binds and which, when mutated, abolish binding and reporter gene expression both in vivo and in vitro. Furthermore, *Wnt3a* mutants can be rescued by an activated form of LEF-1 (Galceran et al., 2001). The TCF-binding sites are conserved in the regulatory region of *Xenopus Xbra*. The distal TCF site alone (or both TCF sites together) is required for activity (Clements et al., 1996; Latinkic et al., 1997; Yamaguchi et al., 1999; Arnold et al., 2000). *Brachyury* expression is induced in embryonic stem cells cocultured with Wnt3a-producing fibroblasts, a clear demonstration that *Brachyury* expression can be induced by Wnt3a (Arnold et al., 2000).

Drosophila is particularly amenable for elucidating signaling pathways and has been a fruitful source for information about T-box genes. Expression of the Tbx2 subfamily gene *omb* in the wing, leg, and genital imaginal discs is under the control of the diffusible factors *wingless* (*wg*) (Wnt signaling pathway) and *decapentaplegic* (*dpp*) (receptor serine/threonine kinase TGF-β pathway), which in turn are downstream of *hedgehog* (*hh*) signaling (Lecuit et al., 1996; Nellen et al., 1996). *Omb* along with another T-box gene, *H15*, from the Tbx1 subfamily, appears to have a role in establishing dorsal/ventral polar-

ity in the leg. In response to *hh* signaling from the posterior cells of the leg disc, *dpp* and *wg* are induced in the dorsal and ventral anterior cells, respectively, and in turn specify dorsal and ventral identity through mutual repression and activation of the region-specific target genes *omb* and *H15* (Brook and Cohen, 1996). This interaction provides an example of the intersection of three different signaling pathways, Wnt, Hedgehog and TGF-β, controlling two different T-box genes, *omb* and *H15*, to establish complex developmental patterning.

TGF-β Signaling Pathway

The TGF-β signaling pathway is characterized by multiple ligands of the bone morphogenetic protein (BMP) family, including activin and nodal, and multiple receptors affecting transcription via the Smad proteins (see Chapter 24). In *Xenopus*, *Xbra* expression and consequently mesoderm formation are induced in equatorial cells of the blastula under the influence of growth factor-like signals from the vegetal hemisphere. Candidates for the mesoderm-inducing signals include members of the FGF family (see below) and the TGF-β family (activin and Vg1). The timing of *Xbra* induction and the lack of inhibition by a protein synthesis inhibitor indicate that *Xbra* expression is an immediate-early response at least to activin and basic FGF and that the gene is thus a direct target of mesoderm induction. Although overexpression of constitutively active activin receptors or Smad proteins strongly induces expression of *Xbra*, it is not known whether Smad proteins bind directly to *Xbra* regulatory sequences (Smith et al., 1991, 1997). The novel Smad-interacting protein-1 (SIP1), a zinc finger/homeodomain repressor, was found to interact with Smad proteins and to bind to sequences in the *Xbra* promoter. Overexpression of SIP1 represses *Xbra*, which raises the possibility that activation of *T* by activin may be a release from repression (Verschueren et al., 1999; Lerchner et al., 2000).

There is good evidence that the zebrafish gene *one-eyed pinhead* (*oep*), which codes for an epidermal growth factor–CFC family extracellular ligand, is a cofactor for nodal signaling (Gritsman et al., 1999). This gene is essential for the formation of anterior axial structures and shows a genetic interaction with the *T* ortholog *ntl*, which affects posterior somites. In *oep;ntl* double-mutant fish, the phenotype is more severe than expected on the basis of additive effects and all but the most anterior somites are disrupted, revealing a partially overlapping requirement for *oep* and *ntl* in mesoderm formation. This interaction links *ntl* with the TGF-β pathway, although *oep* is not required for the regulation of *ntl* expression (Schier et al., 1997).

In addition to the evidence for T-box genes being downstream of this signaling pathway, evidence has been presented that the TGF-β growth factor Xnr1 is a direct downstream target of *Xenopus* VegT (Table 67–2). The initiation of endoderm-specific gene expression by VegT in *Xenopus* embryos is dependent on the TGF-β factors Xnr1, -2, and -4 (Xanthos et al., 2001). Other evidence for involvement of T-box genes in the TGF-β pathway is indirect. In chick, *Tbx2* appears to be downstream of Bmp2 in the heart (Yamada et al., 2000), *Tbx6L* may be downstream of activin (Knezevic et al., 1997), and *Tbx5* appears to be downstream of Bmp4 in the ventral eye (Koshiba-Takeuchi et al., 2000).

Hedgehog Signaling Pathway

There are several hedgehog ligands and receptors that are widely used in early development (see Chapter 16). In the mouse, *Tbx1* expression is dependent on Sonic hedgehog (Shh) signaling during pharyngeal arch development. Expression is decreased in *shh* mutant mice in the mesodermal core of arches and is not present in the pharyngeal endoderm, although expression is not affected elsewhere in the embryo. Similarly, in the chick, Shh can induce *Tbx1* expression in the pharyngeal region (Garg et al., 2001). *Tbx2* can also be induced in the developing limb of the chick in response to exogenous Shh (Gibson-Brown et al., 1998).

FGF Signaling Pathway

The FGF signaling pathway includes many mitogens and growth factor ligands, such as FGF, and frequently involves cross-talk with other signaling pathways (see Chapter 32). As discussed earlier, members of the FGF family are candidate inducers of *Xbra* in *Xenopus* embryos. FGF exerts its effects through the mitogen-activated protein kinase pathway, although nothing is known about how this signal-transduction pathway interacts with the *Xbra* promoter (reviewed by Smith et al., 1995, 1997). FGF4 (and activin, as mentioned above) induces chicken *Tbx6L* in primary cultures of dispersed blastoderm cells, and induction is dependent on protein synthesis (Knezevic et al., 1997). In the primitive streak of mouse embryos, both *T* and *Tbx6* are downregulated in FGFR1 mutant cells, specifically in the precursors of the paraxial mesoderm. Furthermore, it has been postulated that FGFR1 indirectly modulates Wnt signaling, which in turn activates *T*, indicating a probable interconnection between these two pathways in the morphogenesis and patterning of mesoderm at gastrulation (Ciruna and Rossant, 2001).

Mouse *Eomes* is expressed in the trophoblast layer of the blastocyst and in trophectoderm stem cells in vitro, which are maintained as stem cells with FGF4. Upon removal of FGF4, *Eomes* is rapidly downregulated and the cells differentiate, indicating that *Eomes* is downstream of FGF signaling. It has been proposed that FGF4/FGFR2 and Eomes are part of the signaling pathway required for the maintenance of the proliferative undifferentiated state of the extraembryonic ectoderm (Tanaka et al., 1998).

Notch Signaling Pathway

Evidence that T-box genes are targets of Notch signaling comes from the ascidian *Ciona intestinalis* (see Chapter 39). The regulatory region of the ascidian *T* ortholog, *CiBra*, which is responsible for notochord-specific expression, contains a specific binding element and is activated by the Suppressor of Hairless [Su(H)] protein of the Notch signaling pathway. This observation suggests that the notochord-specific pattern of *T* may be downstream of Notch signaling, at least in this species (Corbo et al., 1998). Evidence from mice with mutations in components of the Notch signaling pathway, however, does not support a role for the Notch pathway in *T* regulation in this species as the notochord appears to be unaffected (Kusumi et al., 1998). The promoter of human *TBX19*, which is in the same subfamily, bears similarity to the promoter region of *Ciona* in that it contains Su(H)2-binding sites (Yi et al., 1999); but no functional or regulatory information is available for this gene. These observations illustrate the limitations and dangers inherent in extrapolation between species where gene regulation may have evolved differently.

Receptor Guanylate Cyclase Pathway

As previously described, mouse Tbx5 activates *ANF*, a peptide ligand of the receptor guanylate cyclase pathway (Table 67–2). This factor is regionally expressed in the heart and may play a role in region-specific differentiation.

T-BOX GENES AND DEVELOPMENTAL DISORDERS

As will be discussed more fully in the following chapters dealing with specific human syndromes, mutations of T-box genes are responsible for several human developmental disorders and are suspected of playing a role in several others (Table 67–1). Mutations in *TBX3* and *TBX5* (see Chapter 69) are causative in the ulnar-mammary and Holt-Oram syndromes, respectively (Bamshad et al., 1997; Basson et al., 1997; Li et al., 1997). *TBX1* is located within the critical deletion region mapped for DiGeorge syndrome (Chieffo et al., 1997), and the phenotype of *Tbx1* mutant mice (see below) further indicates a causative role for *TBX1* mutations in DiGeorge syndrome (Jerome and Papaioannou, 2001; see Chapter 68). Isolated deficiency of pituitary corticotropin can be caused by mutations in the *TBX19/TPIT* gene (Lamolet et al., 2001), X-linked cleft plate with ankyloglossia is caused by mutations in *TBX22* (Braybrook et al., 2001), and *TBX21/TBLYM* is implicated in asthma (Finnotto et al., 2002).

T-box gene mutations likewise have profound developmental consequences in animals such as mouse and zebrafish. Animal models are amenable to genetic and developmental analyses and, therefore, represent an invaluable resource for investigating the causal relationships between gene alterations and developmental abnormalities. In addition to the spontaneously occurring T-box gene mutations that have been identified in mouse and zebrafish, custom-made mutations are being engineered in mice using gene-targeting techniques. The capacity of animal models to provide insight into the clinical etiology of human disorders is powerfully illustrated by the examples of mouse *Tbx1*, *Tbx3*, and *Tbx5*. The developmental expression patterns and the chromosomal locations of these genes were used to predict their human orthologs' roles in the DiGeorge, ulnar-mammary, and Holt-Oram syndromes long before the human orthologs were cloned (Bollag et al., 1994; Agulnik et al., 1996; Chapman et al., 1996b). The availability of mouse models for human developmental disorders, such as the mouse *Tbx1* mutant model for DiGeorge, will allow for a deeper understanding of the molecular, cellular, and morphogenetic mechanisms by which complex developmental anomalies arise.

Trunk and Tail: *T* and *Tbx6* Subfamily Genes

Many mouse mutant alleles are available for the canonical *T* gene (Beddington et al., 1992). The *T* deletion allele first reported (Dobrovolskaïa-Zavadskaïa, 1927) has been well characterized (Gluecksohn-Schonheimer, 1944; Gruneberg, 1958; Yanagisawa et al., 1981; Herrmann et al., 1990; Wilkinson et al., 1990; Rashbass et al., 1991; Herrmann, 1992). At embryonic day (e) 8.5, homozygous mutant embryos exhibit an enlarged and bulky primitive streak due to an increase in posterior primitive streak cell number. Despite normal rates of cell proliferation, these embryos show insufficient mesoderm production and a concomitant irregular increase in the ectodermal cell population. This mesoderm insufficiency most severely affects the chordamesoderm such that the notochordal plate forms but fails to differentiate into the notochord and eventually degenerates. In the absence of a notochord, the neural tube becomes kinked and somite formation is disrupted. In these embryos, the head appears normal but axial elongation ceases as mesodermal defects become apparent. The degree of abnormality increases along the anterior/posterior axis such that the posterior region is entirely missing in later stages of development. Homozygous mutant embryos eventually die at around e10.5 due to developmental failure of the allantois, a posterior mesoderm-derived tissue. Heterozygous mutant mice are born with shortened tails and one or more malformed and/or fused sacral vertebrae.

The zebrafish *ntl* homozygous recessive lethal mutant phenotype is caused by a mutation in the *T* ortholog. Homozygous *ntl/ntl* embryos fail to form differentiated notochord, lack posterior embryonic structures, and have abnormally shaped anterior somites (Schulte-Merker, 1995). Similarly, a missense mutation in the T-box of canine *T* leads to the heterozygous short tail, or bobtail, phenotype of the Welsh Corgi breed. This missense mutation was shown to abrogate *in vitro* DNA-binding activity of canine T (Haworth, 2001). These defects in zebrafish and dog are analogous to those observed in mouse *T* homozygous and heterozygous mutants, respectively, indicating a conserved developmental role for the three orthologs. In humans, an allele association test was used to show evidence for a significant association between transmission of the $TIVS_7$-2 allele of human *T* and spina bifida, although a causal relationship has not been established (Morrison et al., 1996).

In 1998, the zebrafish homozygous recessive lethal *spt* phenotype was shown to be caused by mutation of the ortholog of *Xenopus VegT*, known as *tbx16* (Griffin et al., 1998; Ruvinsky et al., 1998). Homozygous *spt/spt* embryos have major trunk mesoderm deficiencies but relatively normal notochord and tail development. Tail bud stage mutant embryos show depleted paraxial mesoderm such that there are no trunk somites, only scattered mesenchymal cells, and a few clusters of cells adjacent to the notochord. The notochord and spinal cord form normally in the trunk but then develop bends and kinks. Anterior head and neural development is normal, as are tail somite segmentation and differentiation (Kimmel et al., 1989).

Mice carrying a targeted mutation of the *Tbx6* locus were generated by Chapman and Papaioannou (1998). Mice heterozygous for the targeted allele are normal, while homozygous mutant embryos show a striking phenotype in which the tail bud enlarges and the trunk paraxial mesoderm differentiates inappropriately as neural tubes in place of somites. Mutants die at mid-gestation from vascular failure, which may be secondary to the lack of paraxial mesoderm and somites. This phenotype indicates that neural differentiation is a default pathway for mesoderm cells exiting the primitive streak and that *Tbx6* normally either inhibits neural fate or imposes mesodermal fate.

Tbx1 and the DiGeorge Syndrome

Targeted mutations designed to generate a null allele of mouse *Tbx1* have been made by several laboratories (Merscher et al., 2001; Lindsay et al., 2001; Jerome and Papaioannou, 2001). Mice heterozygous for a *Tbx1* mutation have a high incidence of cardiac outflow tract anomalies, while homozygous mutant embryos display a wide range of developmental anomalies, including thymic and parathyroid hypoplasia, cardiac outflow tract abnormalities, abnormal facial structures, low-set and abnormally folded or absent external ears, abnormal vertebrae, and cleft palate. The human DiGeorge/velocardiofacial syndrome is a dominant developmental disorder commonly associated with a deletion of chromosomal region 22q11. The deletion usually, but not always, includes *TBX1* along with many other genes; and because of the wide spectrum of abnormalities, multiple gene involvement has been postulated. However, based on the array of phenotypes seen in *Tbx1* mutant mice, which closely matches that seen in human DiGeorge/velocardiofacial patients, *Tbx1* was identified as a key gene in the etiology of the disorder (Jerome and Papaioannou, 2001). These *Tbx1* mutant mice provide the best animal model to date for human DiGeorge/velocardiofacial syndrome.

Tbx3: A Mouse Model for Ulnar-Mammary Syndrome

Mutations in *TBX3* in humans are responsible for the developmental disorder ulnar-mammary syndrome. This syndrome is characterized primarily by deficiencies or duplications in the posterior part of the forelimb and apocrine/mammary gland hypoplasia (see Chapter 69). Among mice carrying a targeted mutation in *Tbx3*, heterozygotes are apparently normal, whereas the homozygous phenotype recapitulates the predominant features of ulnar-mammary syndrome in limb and mammary gland development and reveals novel roles for *Tbx3* (Davenport et al., unpublished data). Homozygous mice lack mammary gland primordia, and the forelimbs show variable lack of development of the posterior elements (digits and ulna). However, unlike in human patients, the hindlimb is even more severely affected than the forelimb, with truncated development of the posterior and distal elements. The endoderm layer of the yolk sac of homozygous embryos degen-

erates at mid-gestation and the embryos die. This defect could not be predicted from the human heterozygous phenotype but corresponds to embryonic expression of *Tbx3* in the precursors of the yolk sac (Chapman et al., 1996b).

Tbx5: A Mouse Model for Holt-Oram Syndrome

The Holt-Oram syndrome in humans, which is caused by mutations in *TBX5*, is characterized by hand and heart malformations, including septal defects and abnormal cardiac electrophysiology (see Chapter 69). A mutation was created in mouse *Tbx5*, and the resultant mutant animals provide a good model for the human syndrome. Heterozygous mice have forelimb defects and reduced viability, which can be attributed to atrial and ventricular septal defects and conduction system disease. Homozygous mutant mice are more severely affected and show arrested cardiac development during gestation (Bruneau et al., 2001). Several downstream target genes of *Tbx5* were identified in this study, illustrating the usefulness of mouse models for the molecular analysis of human syndromes.

Tbx21/Tbet: An Asthma Model

Szabo et al. (2002) and Finotto et al. (2002) described the effects of a targeted mutation of *Tbet* in mice. Homozygous mutant mice are viable and appear grossly normal. However, homozygous mutant CD4 T cells and natural killer (NK) cells show a marked decrease in INF-γ synthesis during primary stimulation, while heterozygous CD4 T cells and NK cells show a milder defect in INF-γ production. In the absence of *Tbet*, CD4 T cells fail to differentiate into the T_H1 lineage and default to the T_H2 state, while NK cells show diminished cytolytic function. These alterations in immune system function correlate with the appearance of asthmatic inflammatory symptoms in both heterozygous and homozygous mutant mice. A connection with asthma in humans is strongly indicated by the reduced expression of *Tbet* in asthma patients and by the position of *Tbet* in a chromosomal region linked to asthma (Finotto et al., 2002).

Mutants in Search of a Syndrome

Several other mutations have been reported in mouse T-box genes that do not correlate with any known human syndromes. Nonetheless, these mutant mice provide models for the investigation of certain developmental processes and may eventually be associated with human disease. Like other T-box gene mutations, a targeted mutation in *Tbx4* results in a phenotype that is predicted by its developmental expression pattern in the allantois and the hindlimb (Chapman et al., 1996b; Naiche and Papaioannou, 2003). Heterozygous embryos are normal, whereas homozygous mutant embryos die at mid-gestation due to a failure of the allantois to establish a placental connnection. Hindlimb development is severely compromised, with little outgrowth of the limb bud.

Russ et al. (2000) reported the generation of mice carrying a targeted allele of *Eomes*. While mice heterozygous for the mutant allele are healthy and fertile, homozygous mutant embryos arrest at the blastocyst stage. Mutant embryos implant into the uterine wall but arrest shortly thereafter and fail to form organized embryonic or extraembryonic structures. In in vitro blastocyst culture, mutant trophectoderm fails to differentiate into trophoblast. Analysis of aggregation chimeras between homozygous mutant embryonic stem cells and tetraploid host embryos, in which all embryonic tissue is embryonic stem cell–derived, revealed a requirement for *Eomes* at gastrulation. Chimeric embryos at e7.5 show thickening of the epiblast with morphological signs of epithelial-to-mesenchymal transition but no emergence of embryonic or extraembryonic mesoderm. Marker analysis suggests that this defect results from a failure of migration toward the primitive streak rather than a loss of axis specification or mesoderm induction per se.

Mice carrying a targeted mutation of *Tbr1* were created by Bulfone et al. (1998). Mice heterozygous for the targeted allele are indistinguishable from wild-type littermates, while homozygous mutants do not nurse and die shortly after birth. The mutants' brains are smaller than those of wild-type littermates, and their cortical neuron laminar organization is disrupted. The number of preplate cells is reduced, with a concomitant deficiency in their derivatives. The olfactory bulb of mutants is small due to a reduction in total cell number. Specifically, the mitral cell layer is absent such that there are no identifiable mitral or tufted projection neurons.

CONCLUSIONS

Mutations in *T-box* genes have unequivocally demonstrated the importance of this gene family in a wide spectrum of developmental processes and pointed to their causative role in the etiology of specific human disorders. Studies linking specific *T-box* genes to specific signaling pathways are accumulating. Although these studies only scratch the surface, T-box genes have been intimately involved in all pathways examined so far and will no doubt prove to be key elements in the normal development of many tissues and organs.

ACKNOWLEDGMENTS

This chapter is based on work supported by National Institutes of Health grants RO1 HD33082 and RO1 GM60561 and National Science Foundation grant IBN 9985953. We thank the members of our laboratory for support and helpful discussions.

REFERENCES

Agulnik SI, Garvey N, Hancock S, Ruvinsky I, Chapman DL, Agulnik I, Bollag R, Papaioannou V, Silver LM (1996). Evolution of mouse *T-box* genes by tandem duplication and cluster dispersion. *Genetics* 144: 249–254.

Agulnik SI, Papaioannou VE, Silver LM (1998). Cloning, mapping and expression analysis of *TBX15*, a new member of the T-box gene family. *Genomics* 51: 68–75.

Arnold SJ, Stappert J, Bauer A, Kispert A, Herrmann BG, Kemler R (2000). *Brachyury* is a target gene of the Wnt/β-catenin signaling pathway. *Mech Dev* 91: 249–258.

Bamshad M, Lin RC, Law DJ, Watkins WS, Krakowiak PA, Moore ME, Franceschini B, Lala R, Holmes LB, Gebuhr TC, et al. (1997). Mutations in human *TBX3* alter limb, apocrine and genital development in ulnar-mammary syndrome. *Nature Genet.* 16: 311–315.

Basson CT, Bachinsky DR, Lin RC, Levi T, Elkins J, Soults J, Grayzel D, Kroumpousou K, Traill TA, Leblanc-Straceski J, et al. (1997). Mutations in human cause limb and cardiac malformations in Holt-Oram syndrome. *Nat Genet* 15: 30–35.

Beddington RSP, Rashbass P, Wilson V (1992). *Brachyury*—a gene affecting mouse gastrulation and early organogenesis. *Dev Suppl* 157–165.

Bollag RJ, Siegfried Z, Cebra-Thomas JA, Garvey N, Davison EM, Silver LM (1994). An ancient family of embryonically expressed mouse genes sharing a conserved protein motif with the T locus. *Nat Genet* 7: 383–389.

Braybrook C, Doudney K, Marcano ACB, Arnason A, Bjornsson A, Patton MA, Goodfellow PJ, Moore GE, Stanier P (2001). The T-box transcription factor gene *TBX22* is mutated in X-linked cleft palate and ankyloglossia. *Nat Genet* 29: 179–183.

Brook WJ, Cohen SM (1996). Antagonistic interactions between wingless and decapentaplegic responsible for dorsal–ventral pattern in the *Drosophila* leg. *Science* 273: 1373–1377.

Brummelkamp TR, Kortlever RM, Lingbeek M, Trettel F, MacDonald ME, van Lohuizen M, Bernards R (2001). *TBX-3*, the gene mutated in ulnar-mammary syndrome, is a negatvie regulator of *p19ARF* and inhibits senescence. *J Cell Biol* 277: 6567–6572.

Bruneau BG, Nemer G, Schmitt JP, Charron F, Robitaille L, Caron S, Conner DA, Gessler M, Nemer M, Seidman CE, et al. (2001). A murine model of Holt-Oram syndrome defines roles of the T-box transcription factor Tbx5 in cardiogenesis and disease. *Cell* 106: 709–721.

Bulfone A, Smiga SM, Shimamura K, Peterson A, Puelles L, Rubenstein JLR (1995). *T-brain-1*: a homolog of *Brachyury* whose expression defines molecularly distinct domains within the cerebral cortex. *Neuron* 15: 63–78.

Bulfone A, Wang F, Hevner R, Anderson S, Cutforth T, Chen S, Meneses J, Pedersen R, Axel R, Rubenstein JLR (1998). An olfactory sensory map develops in the absence of normal projection neurons or GABAergic interneurons. *Neuron* 21: 1273–1282.

Campbell C, Goodrich K, Casey G, Beatty B (1995). Cloning and mapping of a human gene (*TBX2*) sharing a highly conserved protein motif with the *Drosophila omb* gene. *Genomics* 28: 255–260.

Campbell CE, Casey G, Goodrich K (1998). Genomic structure of *TBX2* indicates conservation with distantly related T-box genes. *Mamm Genome* 9: 70–73.

Carlson H, Ota S, Campbell CE, Hurlin PJ (2001). A dominant repression domain in Tbx3 mediates transcriptional repression and cell immortalization: relevance to mutations in Tbx3 that cause ulnar-mammary syndrome. *Hum Mol Genet* 10: 2403–2413.

Carreira S, Dexter TJ, Yavuzer U, Easty DJ, Goding CR (1998). Brachyury-related transcription factor Tbx2 and repression of the melanocyte-specific TRP-1 promoter. *Mol Cell Biol* 18: 5099–5108.

Carson CT, Kinzler ER, Parr BA (2000). *Tbx12*, a novel T-box gene, is expressed during early stages of heart and retinal development. *Mech Dev* 96: 137–140.

Casey ES, O'Reilly M-AJ, Conlon FL, Smith JC (1998). The T-box transcription factor Brachyury regulates expression of *eFGF* through binding to a non-palindromic response element. *Development* 125: 3887–3894.

Casey ES, Tada M, Fairclough L, Wylie CC, Heasman J, Smith JC (1999). Bix4 is activated directly by VegT and mediates endoderm formation in *Xenopus* development. *Development* 126: 4193–4200.

Chapman DL, Papaioannou VE (1998). Three neural tubes in mouse embryos with mutations in the T-box gene, *Tbx6*. *Nature* 391: 695–697.

Chapman DL, Agulnik I, Hancock S, Silver LM, Papaioannou VE (1996a). Tbx6, a mouse T-box gene implicated in paraxial mesoderm formation at gastrulation. *Dev Biol* 180: 534–542.

Chapman DL, Garvey N, Hancock S, Alexiou M, Agulnik S, Gibson Brown JJ, Cebra-Thomas J, Bollag RJ, Silver LM, Papaioannou VE (1996b). Expression of the T-box family genes, *Tbx1–Tbx5*, during early mouse development. *Dev Dynam* 206: 379–390.

Chen J-R, Zhong Q, Wang J, Cameron RS, Borke JL, Isales CM, Bollag RJ (2001). Microarray analysis of *Tbx2*-directed gene expression: a possible role in osteogenesis. *Mol Cell Endocrinol* 177: 43–54.

Chieffo C, Garvey N, Roe B, Zhang G, Silver L, Emanuel BS, Budarf ML (1997). Isolation and characterization of a gene from the DiGeorge chromosomal region (DGCR) homologous to the mouse *Tbx1* gene. *Genomics* 43: 267–277.

Ciruna B, Rossant J (2001). FGF signaling regulates mesoderm cell fate specification and morphogenetic movement at the primitive streak. *Dev Cell* 1: 37–49.

Clements D, Taylor HC, Herrmann BG, Stott D (1996). Distinct regulatory control of the *Brachyury* gene in axial and non-axial mesoderm suggests separation of mesodermal lineages early in mouse gastrulation. *Mech Dev* 56: 139–149.

Conlon FL, Sedgwick SG, Weston KM, Smith JC (1996). Inhibition of Xbra transcription activation causes defects in mesodermal patterning and reveals autoregulation of Xbra in dorsal mesoderm. *Development* 122: 2427–2435.

Conlon FL, Fairclough L, Price BMJ, Casey ES, Smith JC (2001). Determinants of T box protein specificity. *Development* 128: 3749–3758.

Corbo JC, Fujiwara S, Levine M, Di Gregorio A (1998). Suppressor of hairless activates *Brachyury* expression in the *Ciona* embryo. *Dev Biol* 203: 358–368.

Davenport TG, Jerome-Majewska LA, Papaioannou VE (2003). Mammary gland, limb, and yolk sac defects in mice lacking *Tbx3*, the gene mutated in human ulnar mammary syndrome. *Development* 130: 2263–2273.

Dobrovolskaïa-Zavadskaïa N (1927). Sur la mortification spontanée de la queue che la souris nouveau-née et sur l'existence d'un caractère (facteur) héréditaire "non viable." *C R Seances Soc Biol* 97: 114–116.

Edwards YH, Putt W, Lekoape KM, Stott D, Fox M, Hopkinson DA, Sowden J (1996). The human homolog *T* of the mouse *T* (*Brachyury*) gene; structure, cDNA sequence, and assignment to chromosome 6q27. *Genome Res* 6: 226–233.

Finnotto S, Neurath MF, Glickman JN, Qin S, Lehr HA, Green FHY, Ackerman K, Haley K, Galle PR, Szabo SJ, et al. (2002). Development of spontaneous airway changes consistent with human asthma in mice lacking T-bet. *Science* 295: 336–338.

Galceran J, Farinas I, Depew MJ, Clevers H, Grosschedl R (1999). *Wnt3a*−/−-like phenotype and limb deficiency in Lef1−/− Tcf1−/− mice. *Genes Dev* 13: 709–717.

Galceran J, Hsu S-C, Grosschedl R (2001). Rescue of *Wnt* mutation by an activated form of LEF-1: regulation of maintenance but not initiation of *Brachyury* expression. *Proc Natl Acad Sci USA* 98: 8668–8673.

Garg V, Yamagishi C, Hu T, Kathiriya IS, Yamagishi H, Srivastava D (2001). *Tbx1*, a DiGeorge syndrome candidate gene, is regulated by sonic hedgehog during pharyngeal arch development. *Dev Biol* 235: 62–73.

Ghosh TK, Packham EA, Bonser AJ, Robinson TE, Cross SJ, Brook JD (2001). Characterization of the TBX5 binding site and analysis of mutations that cause Holt-Oram syndrome. *Hum Molec Genet* 10: 1983–1994.

Gibson-Brown JJ, Agulnik SI, Silver LM, Niswander L, Papaioannou VE (1998). Involvement of T-box genes *Tbx2–Tbx5* in vertebrate limb specification and development. *Development* 125: 2499–2509.

Glueksohn-Schonheimer S (1944). The development of normal and homozygous Brachy (*T/T*) mouse embryos in the extraembryonic coelom of the chick. *Proc Natl Acad Sci USA* 30: 134–140.

Griffin KJP, Amacher SL, Kimmel CB, Kimelman D (1998). Molecular identification of *spadetail*: regulation of zebrafish trunk and tail mesoderm formation by T-box genes. *Development* 125: 3379–3388.

Gritsman K, Zhang J, Cheng S, Heckscher E, Talbot WS, Schier AF (1999). The EGF-CFC protein one-eyed pinhead is essential for nodal signaling. *Cell* 97: 121–132.

Gruneberg H (1958). Genetical studies on the skeleton of the mouse XXIII. The development of brachyury and Anury. *J Embryol Exp Morphol* 6: 424–443.

Hancock SN, Agulnik SI, Silver LM, Papaioannou VE (1999). Mapping and expression analysis the mouse ortholog of *Xenopus Eomesodermin*. *Mech Dev* 81: 205–208.

Haworth K, Putt W, Cattanach B, Breen M, Binns M, Lingaas F, Edwards YH (2001). Canine homolog of the T-box transcription factor T; failure of the protein to bind to its DNA target leads to a short-tail phenotype. *Mamm Genome* 12: 212–218.

He M-L, Wen L, Campbell CE, Wu JY, Rao Y (1999). Transcription repression by *Xenopus* ET and its human ortholog *TBX3*, a gene involved in ulnar-mammary syndrome. *Proc Natl Acad Sci USA* 96: 10212–10217.

Herr A, Meunier D, Muller I, Rump A, Fundele R, Ropers HH, Nuber UA (2003). Expression of mouse Tbx22 supports its role in palatogenesis and glossogenesis. *Dev Dyn* 226: 579–586.

Herrmann BG (1992). Action of the *Brachyury* gene in mouse embryogenesis. *Ciba Found Symp* 165: 78–91.

Herrmann BG, Labiet S, Poustka A, King T, Lehrach H (1990). Cloning of the *T* gene required in mesoderm formation in the mouse. *Nature* 343: 617–622.

Hiroi Y, Kudoh S, Monzen K, Ikeda Y, Yazaki Y, Nagai R, Komuro I (2001). Tbx5 associates with Nkx2-5 and synergistically promotes cardiomyocyte differentiation. *Nature Genet.* 28: 276–280.

Holland PWH, Koschorz B, Holland LZ, Herrmann BG (1995). Conservation of *Brachyury* (*T*) genes in amphioxus and vertebrates: developmental and evolutionary implications. *Development* 121: 4283–4291.

Hsueh Y-P, Wang T-F, Yang F-C, Sheng M (2000). Nuclear translocation and transcription regulation by the membrane-associated guanylate kinase CASK/LIN-2. *Nature* 404: 298–302.

Hug B, Walter V, Grunwald DJ (1997). *tbx6*, a *Brachyury*-related gene expressed by ventral mesendodermal precursors in the zebrafish embryo. *Dev Biol* 183: 61–73.

Hurlin PJ, Steingrimsson E, Copeland NG, Jenkins NA, Eisenman RN (1999). Mga, a dual-specificity transcription factor that interacts with Max and contains a T-domain DNA-binding motif. *EMBO J* 18: 7019–7028.

Hyde CE, Old RW (2000). Regulation of the early expression of *Xenopus nodal-related 1* gene, Xnr1. *Development* 127: 1221–1229.

Jacobs JJL, Robanus-Maandag E, Kristel P, Lingbeek M, Nederlof PM, van Welsem T, van de Vijver MJ, Koh EY, Daley GQ, van Lohuizen M (2000). Senescence bypass screen identifies *TBX2*, which represses *Cdkn2a* (*p19ARF*) and is amplified in a subset of human breast cancers. *Nat Genet* 26: 291–299.

Jerome LA, Papaioannou VE (2001). DiGeorge syndrome phenotype in mice mutant for the T-box gene, *Tbx1*. *Nat Genet* 27: 286–291.

Kim S-H, Yamamoto A, Bouwmeester T, Agius E, De Robertis EM (1998). The role of Paraxial Protocadherin in selective adhesion and cell movements of the mesoderm during *Xenopus* gastrulation. *Development* 125: 4681–4691.

Kimmel CB, Kane DA, Walker C, Warga RM, Rothman MB (1989). A mutation that changes cell movement and cell fate in the zebrafish embryo. *Nature* 337: 358–362.

Kispert A (1995). The Brachyury protein: a T-domain transcription factor. *Semin Dev Biol* 6: 395–403.

Kispert A, Herrmann BG (1993). The *Brachyury* gene encodes a novel DNA binding protein. *EMBO J* 12: 3211–3220.

Kispert A, Koschorz B, Herrmann, BG (1995). The T protein encoded by *Brachyury* is a tissue-specific transcription factor. *EMBO J* 14: 4763–4772.

Knezevic V, De Santo R, Mackem S (1997). Two novel chick T-box genes related to mouse *Brachyury* are expressed in different, non-overlapping mesodermal domains during gastrulation. *Development* 124: 411–419.

Koshiba-Takeuchi K, Takeuchi JK, Matsumoto K, Momose T, Uno K, Hoepker V, Ogura K, Takahashi N, Nakamura H, Yasuda K, et al. (2000). Tbx5 and the retinotectum projection. *Science* 287: 134–137.

Kraus F, Haenig B, Kispert A (2001). Cloning and expression analysis of the mouse T-box gene *Tbx18*. *Mech Dev* 100: 83–86.

Kusumi K, Sun E, Kerrebrock AW, Bronson RT, Chi D-C, Bulotsky M, Spencer JB, Birren BW, Frankel WN, Lander ES (1998). The mouse pudgy mutation disrupts *Delta* homologue *Dll3* and initiation of early somite boundaries. *Nat Genet* 19: 274–278.

Lamolet B, Pulichino A-M, Lamonerie T, Gauthier Y, Brue T, Enjalbert A, Drouin J (2001). A pituitary cell-restricted T box factor, Tpit, activates POMC transcription in cooperation with Pitx homeoproteins. *Cell* 104: 849–859.

Latinkic BV, Umbhaure M, Neal KA, Lerchner W, Smith JC, Cunliffe V (1997). The *Xenopus Brachyury* promoter is activated by FGF and low concentrations of activin and suppressed by high concentrations of activin and by paired-type homeodomain proteins. *Genes Dev* 11: 3265–3276.

Laugier-Anfossi F, Villard L (2000). Molecular characterization of a new human T-box gene (*TBX22*) located in Xq21.1 encoding a protein containing a truncated T-domain. *Gene* 255: 289–296.

Law DJ, Gebuhr T, Garvey N, Agulnik SI, Silver LM (1995). Identification, characterization and localization to chromosome 17q21-22 of the human TBX2 homolog, member of a conserved developmental gene family. *Mamm Genome* 6: 793–797.

Law DJ, Garvey N, Agulnik SI, Perlroth V, Hahn OM, Rhinehart RE, Gubuhr TC, Silver LM (1998). TBX10, a member of the *Tbx1*-subfamily of conserved developmental genes, is located at human chromosome 11q13 and proximal mouse chromosome 19. *Mamm Genome* 9: 397–399.

Lecuit T, Brook WJ, Ng M, Calleja M, Sun H, Cohen SM (1996). Two distinct mechanisms for long-range patterning by Decapentaplegic in the *Drosophila* wing. *Nature* 381: 387–393.

Lerchner W, Latinkic BV, Remacle JE, Huylebroeck D, Smith JC (2000). Region-specific activation of the *Xenopus Brachyury* promoter involves active repression in ectoderm and endoderm: a study using transgenic frog embryos. *Development* 127: 2729–2739.

Li QY, Newbury-Ecob RA, Terrett JA, Wilson DI, Curtis ARJ, Yi CH, Gebuhr T, Bullen PJ, Robson SC, Strachan T, et al. (1997). Holt-Oram syndrome is caused by mutations in *TBX5*, a member of the *Brachyury (T)* gene family. *Nat Genet* 15: 21–29.

Lindsay EA, Vitelli F, Su H, Morishima M, Huynh T, Pramparo T, Jurecic V, Ogunfinu G, Sutherland HF, Scambler PJ, et al. (2001). *Tbx1* haploinsufficiency in the DiGeorge syndrome region causes aortic arch defects in mice. *Nature* 410: 97–101.

Lingbeek ME, Jacobs JJL, van Lohuizen M (2002). The T-box repressors *TBX2* and *TBX3* specifically regulate the tumor-suppressor $p14^{ARF}$ via a variant T-site in the initiator. *J Biol Chem* 277: 26120–26127.

Liu J, Lin C, Gleiberman A, Ohgi KA, Herman T, Huang H-P, Tsai M-J, Rosenfeld MG (2001). *Tbx19*, a tissue-selective regulator of POMC gene expression. *Proc Natl Acad Sci USA* 98: 8674–8679.

Lustig KD, Kroll KL, Sun EE, Kirschner MW (1996). Expression cloning of a *Xenopus* T-related gene (*Xombi*) involved in mesodermal patterning and blastopore lip formation. *Development* 122: 4001–4012.

Meins M, Henderson DJ, Bhattacharya SS, Sowden JC (2000). Characterization of the human *TBX20* gene, a new member of the T-box gene family closely related to the *Drosophila H15* gene. *Genomics* 67: 317–332.

Merscher S, Funke B, Epstein JA, Heyer J, Puech A, Lu MM, Xavier RJ, Demay MB, Russell RG, Factor S, et al. (2001). *TBX1* is responsible for cardiovascular defects in velo-cardio-facial/DiGeorge syndrome. *Cell* 104: 619–629.

Morrison K, Papapetrou C, Attwood J, Hol F, Lynch SA, Sampath A, Hamel B, Burn J, Sowden J, Stott D, et al. (1996). Genetic mapping of the human homologue (*T*) of mouse *T* (*Brachyury*) and a search for allele association between human *T* and spina bifida. *Hum Mol Genet* 5: 669–674.

Muller CW, Herrmann BG (1997). Crystallographic structure of the T domain-DNA complex of the *Brachyury* transcription factor. *Nature* 389: 884–888.

Naiche LA, Papaioannou VE (2003). Loss of *Tbx4* blocks hindlimb development and affects vascularization and fusion of the allantois. *Development* 130: 2681–2693.

Nellen D, Burke R, Struhl G, Basler K (1996). Direct and long-range action of a DPP morphogen gradient. *Cell* 85: 357–368.

Papaioannou VE (2001). T-box genes in development: from hydra to humans. *Int Rev Cytol* 207: 1–70.

Papaioannou VE, Silver LM (1998). The T-box gene family. *Bioessays* 20: 9–19.

Papapetrou C, Putt W, Fox M, Edwards YH (1999). The human *TBX6* gene: cloning and assignment to chromosome 16p11.2. *Genomics* 55: 238–241.

Perriere G, Gouy M (1996). WWW-Query: an on-line retrievel system for biological sequence banks. *Biochimie* 78: 364–369.

Pflugfelder GO, Schwarz H, Roth H, Poeck B, Sigl A, Kerscher S, Jonschker B, Pak WL, Heisenberg M (1990). Genetic and molecular characterization of the *optomoter-blind* gene locus in *Drosophila melanogaster*. *Genetics* 126: 91–104.

Pflugfelder GO, Roth H, Poeck B (1992). A homology domain shared between *Drosophila optomotor-blind* and mouse *Brachyury* is involved in DNA binding. *Biochem Biophys Res Commun* 186: 918–925.

Rashbass P, Cooke LA, Herrmann BG, Beddington RSP (1991). A cell autonomous function of *Brachyury* in *T/T* embryonic stem cell chimaeras. *Nature* 353: 348–351.

Russ AP, Wattler S, Colledge WH, Aparicio SAJR, Carlton MBL, Pearce JJ, Barton SC, Surani MA, Ryan K, Nehls MC, et al. (2000). *Eomesodermin* is required for mouse trophoblast development and mesoderm formation. *Nature* 404: 95–98.

Ruvinsky I, Silver L, Ho R (1998). Characterization of the zebrafish *tbx16* gene and evolution of the vertebrate T-box family. *Dev Genes Evol* 208: 94–99.

Ruvinsky I, Oates AC, Silver LM (2000a). The evolution of paired appendages in vertebrates: T-box genes in the zebrafish. *Dev Genes Evol* 210: 82–91.

Ruvinsky I, Silver LM, Gibson-Brown JJ (2000b). Phylogenetic analysis of T-box genes demonstrates the importance of amphioxus for understanding evolution of the vertebrate genome. *Genetics* 156: 1249–1257.

Saka Y, Tada M, Smith JC (2000). A screen for targets of the *Xenopus* T-box gene *Xbra*. *Mech Dev* 93: 27–39.

Schier AF, Neuhauss SCF, Helde KA, Talbot WS (1997). The *one-eyed pinhead* gene functions in mesoderm and endoderm formation in zebrafish and interacts with *no tail*. *Development* 124: 327–342.

Schmidt C, Wilson V, Stott D, Beddington RSP (1997). *T* promoter activity in the absence of functional T protein during axis formation and elongation in the mouse. *Dev Biol* 189: 161–173.

Schulte-Merker S (1995). The zebrafish *no tail* gene. *Semin Dev Biol* 6: 411–416.

Smith JC, Price BMJ, Green JBA, Weigel D, Herrmann BG (1991). Expression of a Xenopus homolog of *Brachyury* (*T*) is an immediate-early response to mesoderm induction. *Cell* 67: 79–87.

Smith JC, Cunliffe V, O'Reilly M-AJ, Schulte-Merker S, Umbhauer M (1995). *Xenopus Brachyury*. *Semin Dev Biol* 6: 405–410.

Smith JC, Armes NA, Conlon FL, Tada M, Umbhauer M, Weston KM (1997). Upstream and downstream from *Brachyury*, a gene required for vertebrate mesoderm formation. *Cold Spring Harb Symp Quant Biol* LXII: 337–346.

Szabo SJ, Kim ST, Costa GL, Zhang X, Fathman CG, Glimcher LH (2002). A novel transcription factor, T-bet, directs Th1 lineage commitment. *Cell* 100: 655–669.

Szabo SJ, Sullivan BM, Stemmann C, Satoskar AR, Sleckman BP, Glimcher LH (2002). Distinct effects of T-bet in TH1 lineage commitment and IFN-gamma production in CD4 and CD8 T cells. *Science* 295: 338–342.

Szeto DP, Rodriguez-Esteban C, Ryan AK, O'Connell SM, Liu F, Kioussi C, Gleiberman AS, Izpisua-Belmonte JC, Rosenfeld MG (1999). Role of the Bicoid-related homeodomain factor Pitx1 in specifying hindlimb morphogenesis and pituitary development. *Genes Dev* 13: 484–494.

Tada M, Smith JC (2000). *Xwnt11* is a target of *Xenopus* Brachyury: regulation of gastrulation movements via Dishevelled, but not through the canonical Wnt pathway. *Development* 127: 2227–2238.

Tada M, O'Reilly M-AJ, Smith, JC (1997). Analysis of competence and of *Brachyury* autoinduction by use of hormone-inducible *Xbra*. *Development* 124: 2225–2234.

Tada M, Casey ES, Fairclough L, Smith JC (1998). *Bix1*, a direct target of *Xenopus* T-box genes, causes formation of ventral mesoderm and endoderm. *Development* 125: 3997–4006.

Takahashi H, Mitani Y, Satoh G, Satoh N (1999). Evolutionary alterations of the minimal promoter for notochord-specific *Brachyury* expresssion in ascidian embryos. *Development* 126: 3725–3734.

Tanaka S, Kunath T, Hadjantonakis A-K, Nagy A, Rossant J (1998). Promotion of trophoblast stem cell proliferation by FGF4. *Science* 282: 2072–2075.

Uchiyama H, Kobayashi T, Yamashita A, Ohno S, Yabe S (2001). Cloning and characterization of the T-box gene *Tbx6* in *Xenopus laevis*. *Dev Growth Differ* 43: 657–669.

Verschueren K, Remacle JE, Collart C, Kraft H, Baker BS, Tylzanowski P, Nelles L, Wuytens G, Su M-T, Bodmer R, et al. (1999). SIP1, a novel zinc finger/homeodomain repressor, interacts with Smad proteins and binds to 5′-CACCT sequences in candidate target genes. *J Biol Chem* 274: 20489–20498.

Wattler S, Russ A, Evans M, Nehls M (1998). A combined analysis of genomic and primary protein structure defines the phylogenetic relationship of new members of the T-box family. *Genomics* 48: 24–33.

Wilkinson DG, Bhatt S, Herrmann BG (1990). Expression pattern of the mouse *T* gene and its role in mesoderm formation. *Nature* 343: 657–659.

Xanthos JB, Kofron M, Wylie C, Heasman J (2001). Maternal VegT is the initiator of a molecular nework specifying endoderm in *Xenopus laevis*. *Development* 128: 167–180.

Yamada M, Revelli J-P, Eichele G, Barron M, Schwartz RJ (2000). Expression of chick *Tbx-2*, *Tbx-3*, and *Tbx-5* genes during early heart development: evidence for BMP2 induction of *Tbx2*. *Dev Biol* 228: 95–105.

Yamaguchi TP, Takada S, Yoshikawa Y, Wu N, McMahon AP (1999). *T* (Brachyury) is a direct target of Wnt3a during paraxial mesoderm specification. *Genes Dev* 13: 3185–3190.

Yamamoto A, Amacher SL, Kim S-H, Geissert D, Kimmel CB, De Robertis EM (1998). Zebrafish *paraxial protocadherin* is a downstream target of *spadetail* involved in morphogenesis of gastrula mesoderm. *Development* 125: 3389–3397.

Yanagisawa KO, Fujimoto H, Urushihara H (1981). Effects of the Brachyury (*T*) mutation on morphogenetic movement in the mouse embryo. *Dev Biol* 87: 242–248.

Yi C-H, Terrett JA, Li Q-Y, Ellington K, Packham EA, Armstrong-Buisseret L, McClure P, Slingsby T, Brook JD (1999). Identification, mapping, and phylogenomic analysis of four new human members of the T-box gene family: *EOMES*, *TBX6*, *TBX18*, and *TBX19*. *Genomics* 55: 10–20.

Yi C-H, Russ A, Brook JD (2000). Virtual cloning and physical mapping of a human T-box gene, *TBX4*. *Genomics* 67: 92–95.

Zhang W-X, Yang SY (2000). Cloning and characterization of a new member of the T-box gene family. *Genomics* 70: 41–48.

68 | *TBX1* and the DiGeorge Syndrome Critical Region

SCOTT E. KLEWER, RAYMOND B. RUNYAN, AND ROBERT P. ERICKSON

Congenital cardiovascular malformation is the most common class of birth defects and one of the three most common causes of death in the first year of life (Rubin et al., 1985). Abnormal gene dosage is the best understood genetic cause of congenital heart defects (CHDs). The most common genetic cause of CHDs is trisomy-21 (Down syndrome), which affects approximately 1 in 1000 fetuses and is associated with a 40% incidence of cardiac defects (Adams et al., 1981). Inappropriate gene dosage caused by gene deletions is also associated with congenital heart disease. Children with DiGeorge syndrome or sequence (DGS) who display a recognizable spectrum of craniofacial anomalies, abnormal morphogenesis of the cardiac outflow tract and great vessels (aorta, subclavian, pulmonary arteries), and thymic and parathyroid defects often have microdeletions of chromosome 22q11 (Driscoll et al., 1993). Identical chromosome 22q11 deletions have been identified in patients with velocardiofacial syndrome (VCFS), conotruncal anomaly face syndrome (CAFS), and isolated CHDs (Goldmuntz et al., 1998). Deletion of this region on chromosome 22, called the "DiGeorge critical region" (DGCR), is the second most common known genetic cause of congenital heart disease (Goodship et al., 1998). The heterogeneous clinical manifestations of these 22q11 deletion syndromes have captured the interest and attention of clinical and molecular geneticists hoping to dissect the genetic basis of this human chromosomal haploinsufficiency.

LOCUS AND DEVELOPMENTAL PATHWAY

The characteristic organs affected in DGS include the face and palate, the parathyroid and thymus, the cardiac outflow tract, and the great vessels. Typically, CGS patients suffer varying degrees of underdevelopment of these organs, each of which forms from the embryonic pharyngeal pouches (Robinson, 1975; Rohn et al., 1984). Thus, the developmental pathogenesis of DGS and other 22q11 deletion syndromes has been attributed to abnormal morphogenesis of the pharyngeal pouches. Disruption of the molecular pathways that direct development of the pharyngeal pouch primordia, its vascular supply, or the cells that migrate through the region has been implicated in causing the 22q11 deletion syndrome phenotypes (Epstein, 2001; Vitelli et al., 2002).

The DGCR on human chromosome 22q11 contains at least 35–40 genes, including *Tbx1* (Fig. 68–1) (Chieffo et al., 1997; Dunham et al., 1999). As discussed later in this chapter (Mutants in Orthologues), animal models strongly implicate *Tbx1* as the gene responsible for the abnormal cardiovascular patterning observed in mouse models of human 22q11 deletion syndromes. *Tbx1* shares a common DNA-binding domain with other *T-box* gene members and is phylogenetically similar to the *Drosophila omb* gene and the mouse *brachyury*, gene, symbol *T* from tailless, from which it gets its name (Pflugfelder et al., 1992). During mouse development, *Tbx1* is strongly expressed in the pharyngeal endoderm and present in the mesodermal core of the pharyngeal pouches (Jerome and Papaioannou, 2001; Merscher et al., 2001; Paylor et al., 2001). Vitelli and colleagues (2002) generated a transgenic mouse carrying a *Tbx1-lacZ* reporter gene to characterize the developmental fate of *Tbx1*-expressing cells. These studies demonstrate that *Tbx1* displays both anterior/posterior and medial/lateral gradients in the developing pharyngeal regions. During the critical period of pharyngeal morphogenesis in the mouse (embryonic day [E] 9.5–E11.5), *Tbx1* expression is most pronounced in the most recently formed pharyngeal pouch. *Tbx1* is expressed by mesenchymal cells in the pharyngeal arch surrounding the developing aortic arch arteries, which are destined to become the future great vessels (subclavians, carotids, transverse aorta, and ductus arteriosus). Within the developing heart tube, *Tbx1* is expressed by cells within the inner curvature of the heart following cardiac looping. As heart development proceeds, *Tbx1*-expressing cells expand into the primitive cardiac outflow tract and eventually are found along the entire length of the pulmonary artery and aorta, including the septum of the truncus arteriosus (Fig. 68–2). These expression data demonstrate that *Tbx1* is expressed within the cardiovascular regions that are most frequently affected in chromosome 22q11 deletion syndromes. In addition, the dynamic expression patterns of *Tbx1* in the developing pharyngeal regions suggest that it is involved in the normal growth process of the embryonic pharyngeal pouches.

CLINICAL DESCRIPTION

At least three distinct clinical entities have been associated with 22q11 deletions. They all share cardiac defects and atypical facies. Because one of them, DGS, also has thymic hypoplasia and hypoparathyroidism while another, VCFS, has frequent oral-facial clefting, the acronym *CATCH 22* (**c**ardiac defects, **a**typical facies, **t**hymic hypoplasia, **c**lefting, and **h**ypoparathyroidism) was used to categorize this group of defects. Given the literary connotation of the acronym, *22q11 deletion syndrome* has become a more accepted term to describe this group of disorders (Goldmuntz et al., 1998).

DGS has also been called the III–IV pharyngeal pouch complex defect. Commonly accepted features of DGS include absence or hypoplasia of the thymus and/or parathyroid glands (DiGeorge, 1965). The fuller spectrum of the sequence includes cardiovascular anomalies, among which interrupted aortic arch and truncus arteriosus are common, and craniofacial anomalies, among which micrognathia, ear abnormalities, blunted nose, and hypertelorism are most common. Cleft palate or bifid uvula sometimes occur (Carey, 1980).

Molecular genetic and refined cytogenetic approaches helped to define the basis of DGS. Scambler et al. (1991), used probes from 22q11-pter to show that a subset of markers is hemizygous in DGS patients (i.e., there were microdeletions not visible at the cytogenetic level). High-resolution karyotypes disclosed visible deletions in one-third of cases (Wilson et al., 1992), while a careful study of 35 patients disclosed deletions in 33 when molecular probes were used (Carey et al., 1992). As more probes from 22q11 were identified, it was eventually found that almost all patients are deleted in this region. For instance, D22S75 and D22S259 were deleted in 14 of 14 patients (Driscoll et al., 1992). However, genetic heterogeneity is clearly present with a number of other chromosomal regions sometimes implicated, particularly 10p (Bartsch et al., 1999; Dasouki et al., 1997; Greenberg et al., 1987; Koenig et al., 1987; Schuffenhauer et al., 1998). With current fluorescence in situ hybridization (FISH) assays, microdeletion of 22q11 can be detected in 90% of people with the full DGS phenotype (Driscoll et al., 1993).

An exciting extension of 22q11 deletion research was the finding of similar deletions in two other distinct clinical syndromes. Driscoll et al. (1992) identified 22q11 deletions for the same two probes (D22S259 and D22S75) that are consistently deleted in DGS in 14 of 15 patients with VCFS. This was initially surprising since there was

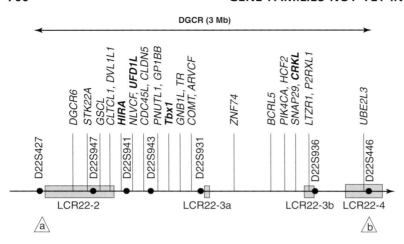

Figure 68–1. Schematic diagram of the DiGeorge critical region (DGCR) associated with 22q11 deletion syndromes. The DGCR is flanked by markers D22S427 (*a*), located 2.5 Mb from the centromere, and D22S446 (*b*), located 5.5 Mb from the centromere. The 3 Mb DGCR, the typically deleted region, is flanked by two low copy repeats (LCRs, gray boxes). Two additional LCR regions are located within the DGCR and may be responsible for the less common 22q11 deletions (Shaikh et al., 2000). Genes listed are only those with a designated Human Genome Organization gene name and are ordered (left to right) from centromere to telomere. Genes with demonstrated roles in cardiac development are in bold. Gene data, marker data, and chromosomal location are extracted from National Center of Biotechnology Information sequence data (contigs NT_011519 and NT_011520) and referenced with the chromosome 22 gene list (http://www.sanger.ac.uk).

minimal apparent overlap reported between DGS and VCFS. What we now call VCFS was first described by Shprintzen et al. (1978) as a combination of an unusual "pear-shaped" nose and other facial anomalies, including a retruded mandible, frequent heart defects, cleft palate, and learning disabilities. An earlier report emphasized the cardiac defects (Stern et al., 1977). Delayed development is frequently associated with microcephaly. In addition to the unusual nose, the face is long with relative malar flatness. The micrognathia is severe enough that about 15% of patients exhibit Robin's sequence (Arvystas and Shprintzen, 1984). Reviews of large numbers of cases have shown that about 10% have cleft palate and 35% have velum insufficiency (Ryan et al., 1997). Also, this survey found hypocalcemia in 60%, reflecting the overlap with DGS (Ryan et al., 1997). The frequency of psychiatric disorders, including bipolar and delusional disorders, is very high (Carlson et al., 1997a,b), with a large amount of attention-deficit hyperactivity disorder as well (Moss et al., 1999). Importantly, some children diagnosed with DGS at birth develop a typical VCFS appearance in later childhood (Stevens et al., 1990). Geneticists now report that 70% of people with VCFS features carry a 22q11 microdeletion (Driscoll et al., 1993).

During the period that U.S. and European dysmorphologists were characterizing DGS and VCFS, pediatric cardiologists were defining a combination of CHDs involving abnormal outflow tract formation and peculiar facial characteristics in the Asian population (Takao et al., 1980; Shimizu et al., 1984). Individuals with this syndrome, CAFS, display a typical facies and cleft palate but no thymic or parathyroid hypoplasia. Similar to DGS and VCFS patients, molecular genetic studies have shown that chromosome 22q11 deletions are common in subjects with CAFS (Scambler et al., 1992; Burn et al., 1993; Seaver et al., 1994).

Meanwhile, and independently in the United States, several children with a conotruncal cardiac malformation, pulmonary atresia with ventricular septal defect (PA/VSD), were noted to have a similar craniofacial appearance. A study by dysmorphologist examiners unaware of the cardiac lesion was designed to evaluate the possibility that a recognizable phenotype was associated with PA/VSD. Nearly half of 14 children with cyanotic heart lesions were considered to have similar craniofacial appearances, which were most similar to CAFS. The distinctive facial appearance included hypertelorism and an unusual nose with deeply grooved nasal alae, creating a prominent nasal tip that was quite different from the VCFS nose. Dental caries, minor ear anomalies, and long and slender fingers were also common. All cases with the identified phenotype had 22q11 deletions. Interestingly, all deletions were maternal in origin, suggesting a parent of origin effect in CAFS (Seaver et al., 1994).

The finding of 22q11 deletions has been demonstrated once in yet another distinctive but rare cardiac facial syndrome, Kenny-Caffey syndrome (Sabry et al., 1998). Kenny-Caffey syndrome has both dominant and recessive forms. Growth retardation, hypoparathyroidism, and cortical thickening of the long bones with medullary stenosis are the most constant features. Importantly, the recessive form maps to 1q42-43 (Diaz et al., 1998). Most geneticists consider the identification of 22q11 deletions in Kenny-Caffey syndrome to probably be the result of phenotypic overlap with VCFS in one family.

Cardiac defects are a well-recognized abnormality of the 22q11 deletion syndromes, affecting approximately 75% of all patients who demonstrate hemizygosity for the 22q11 locus. Although most patients

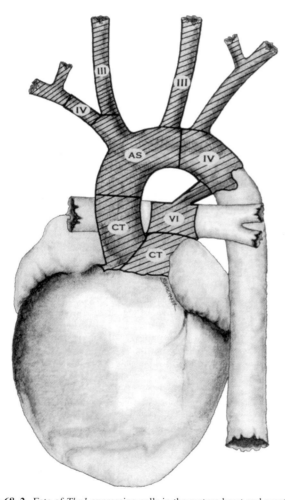

Figure 68–2. Fate of *Tbx1*-expressing cells in the mature heart and great vessels. The mature cardiac outflow tract, including the ascending aorta and main pulmonary artery, develops from the conotruncus (CT) and the aortic sac (AS). The right and left carotid and subclavian arteries develop from pharyngeal arch arteries III and IV, respectively. Left pharyngeal arch artery IV also forms the distal transverse aorta, and pharyngeal arch artery VI forms the ductus arteriosus. Right artery VI normally involutes. *Tbx1*-expressing cells (hatched area) can be localized in all vascular structures derived from the cardiac outflow tract and pharyngeal arch arteries.

Table 68–1. Congenital Heart Disease in 22q11 Deletion Syndromes and Isolated Cases*

Type	DGS	VCFS	CAFS	22q11 Deletion in Isolated CHD†
Tetralogy of Fallot	20%	4%	73%	15%
Truncus Arteriosus	26%	0	2%	35%
VSD/malaligned VSD	12%	37%	12%	33%
Interrupted aortic arch	38%	0	4%	50%
Aortic arch anomaly	14%	11%	5%	—
DORV	0	0	2%	5%
TGA	6%	0	1%	0

*Percent incidence of congenital heart defect (CHD) type in DiGeorge syndrome (DGS) (Van Mierop and Kutsche, 1986), velocardiofacial syndrome (VCFS) (Young et al., 1980), and conotruncal anomaly face syndrome (CAFS) (Momma and Takao, 1989). VSD, ventricular septal defect; DORV, double outlet right ventricle; TGA, transposition of the great arteries.

†Percentage of isolated CHD found to carry 22q11 deletion (Goldmuntz et al., 1998).

share a similar deletion of chromosome 22q11, a wide variety of cardiac phenotypes are observed (Table 68–1). The explanation for the distinctiveness in some cases and overlap in others remains to be defined. The nature of most CHDs in 22q11.2 microdeletions can be classified as "conotruncal," or cardiac outflow tract defects, often complicated by abnormalities of the major vascular structures that arise from the pharyngeal arch arteries (Fig. 68–2).

Because of the well-recognized association between 22q11 hemizygosity and cardiac defects in DGS, VCFS, and CAFS, investigators began assaying children with isolated CHDs for the presence of 22q11 deletions. In these nonsyndromic individuals, 22q11 deletions were detected in 15% of patients with tetralogy of Fallot, 35% with truncus arteriosus, and 50% with interrupted aortic arch type B (Goldmuntz et al., 1998). The likelihood of a 22q11 deletion appears greater for non-syndromic children with cardiac outflow tract defects plus abnormal aortic arch anatomy (right aortic arch or cervical aortic arch) and/or abnormal pulmonary artery branching (discontinuous or hypoplastic).

One common CHD involving abnormal cardiac outflow tract and great vessel development is transposition of the great arteries (TGA). TGA was initially reported to occur in 13% of children hemizygous for the DGCR when assessed by Southern blotting (Melchionda et al., 1995), but this was not confirmed with contemporary FISH analysis (Marino et al., 2001). Most contemporary pediatric cardiologists do not consider TGA to be a cardiac defect that is associated with 22q11 deletion syndromes.

IDENTIFICATION OF THE GENE AND MUTATIONAL SPECTRUM

De la Chapelle and colleagues (1981) identified a DGS family with a chromosome 20;22 translocation and suggested that the DGS was due to either a chromosome 22 deletion or a chromosome 20 duplication. Chromosome 22q11 hemizygosity was confirmed as being responsible for some DGS cases by identifying affected patients with 22q11 translocations to other chromosomes (Kelley et al., 1982). Microdeletions of a 2–3 Mb region on chromosome 22q11 have been detected in 90% of DGS patients, 70% of those with VCFS, and 15% of people with isolated conotruncal cardiac defects (Driscoll et al., 1993; Goldmuntz et al., 1998).

Substantial research efforts have been focused on dissecting the commonly deleted chromosome 22q11 region in DGS, VCFS, and CAFS. Initial efforts attempted to narrow the DGCR by characterizing the overlapping regions for different 22q11 deletion patients. Using this approach, a common, large 3 Mb interstitial deletion was discovered that accurately identifies nearly 90% of DGS patients (Kerstjens-Frederikse et al., 1999; Lindsay et al., 2001). This chromosome 22q11 deletion, termed the *typically deleted region* (TDR), is flanked by markers *D22S427* and *D22S801* (LN80) (Fig. 68–1). Subsequent investigations have further refined the DGCR to a 1.5 Mb region in a smaller percentage of patients (Lindsay et al., 1995; Shaikh et al., 2000). Alternatively, some patients carry 22q11 deletions that have no overlap with the TDR (Shaikh et al., 2000).

Knowledge of the complete DNA sequence of chromosome 22 has greatly facilitated definition of the DGCR (Dunham et al., 1999). Approximately 35–40 genes have been localized to the DGCR TDR (Fig. 68–1). The dramatic clinical variability of identical TDR deletions has complicated definition of the genes responsible for the various "pharyngeal" phenotypes that are associated with 22q11 deletion syndromes, but candidate genes for the observed cardiovascular phenotypes include the transcription factors *TBX1* (Lindsay et al., 2001) and *HIRA* (Farrell et al., 1999), the ubiquitin processing gene *UFD1L* (Yamagishi et al., 1999), and the adapter protein CRKL (Guris et al., 2001). The apparent redundancy of developmental expression of these genes combined with the lack of identified single gene mutations in patients with cardiac outflow tract abnormalities has led many to speculate that the cardiovascular sequelae of 22q11 deletions are the result of several contiguous chromosome 22 genes (Goodship and Burn, 2000; Schinke and Izumo, 2001).

Multiple low copy DNA repeat (LCR) elements have been identified on chromosome 22. LCR recombination is a well-characterized mechanism of chromosomal rearrangement (Shaikh et al., 2000). Interestingly, four LCRs are located in the chromosome 22q11 region. Abnormal recombination between these elements has been proposed as a mechanism for the observed instability of the DGCR (Halford et al., 1993; Lindsay et al., 1993; Collins et al., 1997). Haploinsufficiency of multiple genes, resulting from abnormal recombination of LCRs flanking the DGCR, is consistent with the molecular genetic observations in 22q11 deletion syndrome patients (Kerstjens-Frederikse et al., 1999). Some of the clinical features of 22q11 deletion syndromes are reminiscent of those in patients exposed in utero to the teratogen isotretinoin (Lammer et al., 1985). It therefore appears that 22q11 deletion syndromes may represent a contiguous gene haploinsufficiency syndrome influenced by environmental challenges/exposures.

COUNSELING AND TREATMENT

The overall birth prevalence of 22q11 deletions is reported to be at least 1 in 4000 (Goodship et al., 1998). Identification of many of the classic facial features of 22q11 deletion syndromes can be rather subjective, and some important features of 22q11 deletion syndromes, including speech and learning disorders and psychological issues, may not be present until later childhood or adolescence. In addition, the associated vascular anomalies, such as isolated right aortic arch, cervical aortic arch, aberrant subclavian artery, aorticopulmonary collaterals, and discontinuous branch pulmonary arteries, may be silent and undetected by routine pediatric management. Therefore, the true incidence of 22q11 deletions in the population is not known, but current estimates are likely to be low.

Patients with 22q11 deletions may present with diverse clinical symptoms, including palatal abnormalities, craniofacial dysmorphism, absent thymus, or hypocalcemia. Typically, cardiac defects are the usual focus of initial clinical management of neonates with 22q11 deletion syndromes. Early neonatal echocardiography is essential for any child with clinical features of abnormal pharyngeal development for suspected congenital heart disease.

The initial treatment of neonates with 22q11 deletion syndromes is dictated by the type of cardiac defect diagnosed by noninvasive or invasive testing, including echocardiography, magnetic resonance imaging, and occasionally cardiac catheterization. Infants with interrupted aortic arch, critical coarctation of the aorta, or severe pulmonary outflow tract obstruction typically require stabilization with continuous prostaglandin E_1 infusion to maintain patency of the ductus arteriosus in preparation for palliative or complete repair before discharge from the nursery. Repair of these abnormalities may carry mortality risks greater than 50% (Klewer et al., 1998). Most 22q11 deletion syndrome infants with cardiac outflow tract abnormalities, including persistent truncus arteriosus, tetralogy of Fallot, or malaligned outflow tract VSD, undergo complete surgical repair within the first year of life. For many of these patients, subsequent cardiac surgical interventions are required to resolve morbidity related to early surgical repairs (e.g., conduit replacement, valvuloplasty). Minor great vessel abnormalities, including aberrant subclavian artery or right aortic arch, are typically silent and require no intervention. Occasionally, however, malposition of the great vessels can affect normal pulmonary or esophageal function.

The relationship between 22q11 deletion syndromes and significant abnormalities of cardiac outflow tract morphogenesis or great vessel development is well recognized. Because of the high frequency of 22q11 deletions in liveborns and the occurrence of other clinically relevant abnormalities in facial structure and thymic function, patients with these types of CHD should be examined by a geneticist for the presence of noncardiac pharyngeal abnormalities, which may aide in identifying those patients likely to have a 22q11 deletion.

An important consideration is whether FISH analysis for 22q11 deletions is warranted in families that have a child born with an isolated CHD. Goodship and colleagues (1998) performed FISH analysis for 22q11 deletions in 170 infants with significant cardiac defects requiring early intervention, who were identified from 69,129 live births. The incidence of 22q11 deletions was only 3% for infants with any type of significant congenital heart disease, which led the authors to not recommend routine FISH analysis for 22q11 deletions for all children with significant CHDs. In contrast, Goldmuntz and colleagues (1998) analyzed patients with isolated cardiac outflow tract or great vessel abnormalities and identified 22q11 deletions in 15%–50% of these patients, depending on the cardiac lesion. Their results suggest that it is reasonable to perform FISH analysis for 22q11 deletions on patients with isolated cardiac outflow tract defects. Many pediatric centers have embraced this philosophy and routinely perform FISH analysis for 22q11 deletions prior to any surgical intervention for infants with cardiac outflow tract defects.

Ongoing long-term follow-up studies will assist in developing appropriate recommendations for which pediatric cardiology patients should be tested for a chromosome 22q11 deletion. Ultimately, this genetic information can identify patients who might benefit from multispecialty programs with cardiology, immunology, speech and development, and psychology specialists to limit the morbidities of abnormal pharyngeal development caused by 22q11 deletions.

MUTANTS IN ORTHOLOGUES

Important questions surrounding 22q11 deletion syndromes have yet to be resolved by human molecular genetics, including accounting for the observed clinical heterogeneity of this uniform chromosomal deletion and understanding the mechanism of how abnormal dosage of chromosome 22q11 genes affects pharyngeal development. To gain insight into the role of genes located in the DGCR, developmental biology researchers have begun utilizing genetic engineering in mice to examine the functional role of these factors during development.

The mouse is an ideal model to study DGCR genes because human chromosome 22q11 is highly conserved on mouse chromosome 16 (Sutherland et al., 1998). As a proof of that principle, Lindsay and colleagues (1999) used homologous recombination to create *Df1* mice, which lacked 18 genes contained within the human DGCR. Heterozygous *Df1/+* mice had a high incidence of cardiac defects attributed to abnormal fourth pharyngeal arch artery development. Importantly, the *Df1/+* cardiac defects could be "rescued" by mating with transgenic mice harboring a duplication of the deleted *Df1* region. This study demonstrated that reduced dosage of these 18 genes within the mouse equivalent of the human DGCR is necessary and sufficient for the observed cardiovascular phenotypes. There were no craniofacial, thyroid, parathyroid, or thymic abnormalities observed in *Df1/+* mice. Using similar approaches, Kimber et al. (1999) generated mice lacking at least seven DGCR genes that displayed completely normal cardiovascular development, and Puech et al. (2000) generated a mouse model lacking 16 DGCR genes that also were without cardiovascular abnormalities. Alignment of the regions deleted in these mouse equivalents of human 22q11 deletion syndromes narrowed the list of candidate genes for cardiac phenotypes in the mouse to only six. One of the remaining candidate genes was *Tbx1*.

The role of *Tbx1* in pharyngeal arch artery development was confirmed in subsequent mouse studies. Cardiac defects in *Df1/+* mice were completely rescued by mating with transgenic mice carrying a

Tbx1 PI Artificial Chromosomes (PAC) (Lindsay et al., 2001). In addition, cardiac outflow tract defects in mice hemizygous for a 1.5 Mb region corresponding to 22q11 were partially rescued by mating with transgenic mice carrying a human *Tbx1* Bacterial Artificial Chromosome (BAC) (Merscher et al., 2001). These studies demonstrate that *Tbx1* haploinsufficiency is responsible for the cardiac phenotypes observed in the mouse equivalent of human 22q11 deletion syndromes.

The requirements of *Tbx1* in pharyngeal development have also been examined directly in a knockout mouse model. Jerome and Papaioannou (2001) generated *Tbx1*$^{-/-}$ mice, which displayed a spectrum of developmental anomalies reminiscent of human DGS. Abnormal facial development, cleft palate, thymic and parathyroid hypoplasia, cardiac outflow tract malalignment, and disrupted aortic arch arteries were observed in *Tbx1*$^{-/-}$ mice. *Tbx1*$^{+/-}$ heterozygous mice lived but displayed a high incidence of small or absent fourth aortic arch arteries during development.

Although *Tbx1* appears to be the major candidate gene responsible for the cardiac phenotype in mouse models of human 22q11 deletion syndromes, existing human molecular genetic data suggest that 22q11 deletion syndromes are most likely a contiguous gene deletion syndrome. With respect to other genes in the DGCR, the requirement of *CRKL* has been examined in the mouse. Ablation of the murine equivalent of this gene, *Crkol*, results in a pharyngeal phenotype (Guris et al., 2001). *Crkol*$^{-/-}$ mice are embryonic-lethal and display abnormal aortic arch development and cardiac outflow tract defects. However, *Crkol*$^{+/-}$ heterozygous mice do not display a cardiac phenotype. Although deletion of *UFD1L* was suggested to be causative for interrupted aortic arch type B in a child (Yamagishi et al., 1999), isolated disruption of *UFD1L*, which occurred in the genetic engineering that created the *Df1* mouse, did not result in cardiac defects (Lindsay et al., 1999; Goodship and Burn, 2000). Finally, decreasing the expression of *Hira* (formerly *Tuple1*) with antisense oligonucleotides in cardiac neural crest cells resulted in a high incidence of truncus arteriosus in an avian model (Farrell et al., 1999). In the mouse, ablation of *Hira* by homologous recombination resulted in defective gastrulation and early embryonic lethality. *Hira*$^{+/-}$ heterozygous mice, however, did not display any cardiovascular phenotype (Roberts et al., 2002).

T box–mediated gene transcription is obviously important in cardiovascular development (as evident by this chapter and Chapter 69). The pathways affected directly or indirectly by *Tbx1* remain to be defined. Through the use of animal models of cardiovascular development, the upstream and downstream targets of the *Tbx1* pathway are being investigated. In zebrafish, a mutant named van Gogh (*vgo*) lacks pharyngeal arches (Piotrowski and Northcutt, 1996; Schilling et al., 1996). Identification of the gene responsible for the *vgo* phenotype may shed important insight into pharyngeal patterning. Other reports implicate *Hira* and members of the fibroblast growth factor (Fgf) family in pharyngeal arch development. It remains to be determined how *Tbx1*, *Hira*, and Fgf family members might interact genetically during aortic arch and pharyngeal development. It is clear that animal models will greatly contribute to our understanding of the interactions between *Tbx1* and other genes within the DGCR and elsewhere in the genome. Ultimately, genetically engineered animal models might facilitate understanding of the nature of the phenotypic heterogeneity of DGCR haploinsufficiency and may aide in determining whether 22q11 deletion syndromes are single-gene or contiguous gene deletion syndromes.

DEVELOPMENTAL PATHOGENESIS

In considering the developmental pathogenesis of the 22q11 deletions, the analysis is complex due to the variety of genes and activities found within the deletion region. The obvious involvement of pharyngeal arches, facial dysmorphogenesis, and outflow tract anomalies argues for a role of the neural crest population. However, gene expression data suggest that the developmental pathogenesis is more complex than simply direct loss of the neural crest cell population.

Briefly, craniofacial morphogenesis is characterized by the interactions and activities of several cell populations. The jaw and anterior cervical region of the developing embryo are distinguished by a bilateral series of five pharyngeal arches, numbered I–IV and VI (Fig.

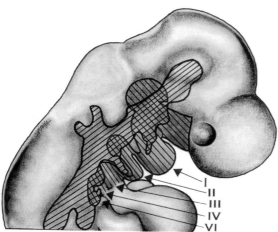

Figure 68–3. Comparison of *Tbx1* expression and neural crest cell migration in the developing pharyngeal region of embryonic day 10.5. mouse. *Tbx1* is expressed by cells in the pharyngeal mesenchyme (▨). The course of cranial neural crest cell migration into the pharyngeal region (▧) demonstrates overlap with *Tbx1* expression. These expression data are supportive of potential cell-nonautonomous interactions between neural crest cells and pharyngeal primordia/tissues. Expression data adopted from *Tbx1* and neural crest fate mapping mouse models (Jiang et al., 2000; Vitelli et al., 2002).

68–3). Each pharyngeal arch has an external covering of ectoderm, an internal lining of endoderm (facing the developing gut tube), and a central population of neural crest cells and mesoderm (Sadler, 2000). The core of each pharyngeal arch is mesodermal in origin and contains mesenchymal cells that will contribute to skeletal muscle elements and an aortic arch vessel. Surrounding the core of each arch is a population of neural crest cells (Graham and Smith, 2001). While neural crest cells are the source of the connective tissue elements of the anterior face and cervical region, they also play a significant role in tissue interactions required for normal morphogenesis. For example, thymic and thyroid cells are derived from endoderm in the clefts between pharyngeal arches III and IV and between IV and VI. Neurocristopathies are often associated with defects in the thymus and thyroid (Bolande, 1997). These are likely to be caused by a failure of signaling between neural crest cells and endoderm. One example of such an interaction can be seen in the *hoxa-3* mutant mouse (Manly and Capecchi, 1995). In this case, thymic and thyroid maldevelopment appear to be caused by failure of the neural crest to provide appropriate developmental cues to the pharyngeal primordia.

The structures most commonly affected in 22q11 deletions, including the face and palate, thymus gland, parathyroid gland, cardiac outflow tract, and great vessels, are derived from the embryonic pharyngeal regions. The hypothesis that the pharyngeal phenotype of DGS is due to abnormal neural crest cell development is supported by several lines of experimental evidence in animal models. In the avian system, neural crest cells migrate into the pharyngeal arches and cardiac outflow tract and are required for normal heart and great vessel development. Ablation of the neural crest cell population causes cardiac defects that include truncus arteriosus in manipulated chick embryos (Kirby and Waldo, 1995). Partial neural crest cell ablation causes less severe cardiac defects in chick embryos, including VSD and/or great vessel misalignment and abnormal great vessel patterning (Nishibatake et al., 1987).

Although these experiments show defects due to a lack of neural crest cells, they do not distinguish between defects due to direct loss of the cell population or loss of signaling either to or from the neural crest cell population. The recent work by Vitelli and colleagues (2002) showing expression of Tbx1 in cells adjacent to the neural crest suggests that the role of the neural crest in pharyngeal arch development may be mediated, in part, by reciprocal interactions between the neural crest and the adjacent endoderm. Interruption of this tissue interaction in either direction may be related to the dysmorphogenesis seen in DGS.

It has been speculated that *Tbx1* has multiple roles in pharyngeal development, including an early cell-autonomous role in endoderm growth and patterning and a later cell-non-autonomous function, supporting the development of pharyngeal arch and pouch derivatives. The latter role may be mediated through signaling to neural crest–derived cells. An understanding of the mechanisms of action of *Tbx1* and identification of its genetic pathways will ultimately be required to understand normal and abnormal pharyngeal development.

ACKNOWLEDGMENTS

We thank Ms. Shannon Shoemaker for her artistic expertise, utilized for the diagrams included in this chapter.

REFERENCES

Adams MM, Erickson JD, Layde PM, Oakley GP (1981). Down's syndrome. Recent trends in the United States. *JAMA* 246: 758–760.
Arvystas M, Shprintzen RJ (1984). Craniofacial morphology in the velocardiofacial syndrome. *J Craniofac Genet Dev Biol* 4: 39–46.
Bartsch O, Wagner A, Hinkel GK, Lichtner P, Murken J, Schuffenhauer S (1999). No evidence for chromosomal microdeletions at the second DiGeorge syndrome locus on 10p near D10S585. *Am J Med Genet* 83: 425–426.
Bolande RP (1997). Neurocristopathy: its growth and development in 20 years. *Pediatr Pathol Lab Med* 17: 1–25.
Burn J, Takao A, Wilson D, Cross I, Momma K, Wadey R, Scambler P, Goodship J (1993). Conotruncal anomaly face syndrome is associated with a deletion within chromosome 22q11. *J Med Genet* 30: 822–824.
Carey AH, Kelley D, Halford S, Wadey R, Wilson D, Goodship J, Burn J, Paul T, Sharkey A, Dumanski J, Nordenskjold M, Williamson R, Scambler PJ (1992). Molecular genetic study of the frequency of monosomy 22q 11 in DiGeorge syndrome. *Am J Hum Genet* 51: 964–970.
Carey JC (1980). Spectrum of the DiGeorge "syndrome." *J Peds* 96: 955–956.
Carlson C, Sirotkin H, Pandita R, Goldberg R, McKie J, Wadey R, Patanjali SR, Weissman SM, Anyane-Yeboa K, Warburton D, et al. (1997a). Molecular definition of 22q11 deletions in 151 Velo-Cardio-Facial syndrome patients. *Am J Hum Genet* 61: 620–629.
Carlson C, Papolos D, Pandita RK, Faedda GL, Veit S, Goldberg R, Shprintzen R, Kucherlapati R, Morrow B (1997b). Molecular analysis of velo-cardio-facial syndrome patients with psychiatric disorders. *Am J Hum Genet* 60: 851–859.
Chieffo C, Garvey N, Gong W, Roe B, Zhang G, Silver L, Emanuel BS, Budarf ML (1997). Isolation and characterization of a gene from the DiGeorge chromosomal region homologous to the mouse *Tbx1* gene. *Genomics* 43: 267–277.
Collins JE, Mungall AJ, Badcock KL, Fay JM, Dunham I (1997). The organization of the gamma-glutamyl transferase genes and other low copy repeats in human chromosome 22q11. [erratum appears in *Genome Res* 1997;7(9):942]. *Genome Res* 7: 522–531.
Dasouki M, Jurecic V, Phillips JA III, Whitlock JA, Baldini A (1997). DiGeorge anomaly and chromosome 10p deletions: One or two loci? *Am J Med Genet* 73: 72–75.
de la Chapelle A, Herva R, Koivisto M, Aula P (1981). A deletion in chromosome 22 can cause DiGeorge syndrome. *Hum Genet* 57: 253–256.
Diaz GA, Khan KT, Gelb BD (1998). The autosomal recessive Kenny-Caffey syndrome locus maps to chromosome 1q42-q43. *Genomics* 54: 13–18.
DiGeorge AM (1965). Discussion of a new concept of the cellular basis of immunology. *J Peds* 67: 907.
Driscoll DA, Budarf ML, Emanuel BS (1992). A genetic etiology for DiGeorge syndrome: Consistent deletions and microdeletions of 22q11. *Am J Hum Genet* 50: 924–933.
Driscoll DA, Salvin J, Sellinger B, Budarf ML, McDonald-McGinn DM, Zackai EH, Emanuel BS (1993). Prevalence of 22q11 microdeletions in DiGeorge and velocardiofacial syndromes: implications for genetic counselling and prenatal diagnosis. *J Med Genet* 30: 813–817.
Dunham I, Shimizu N, Roe BA, Chissoe S, Hunt AR, Collins JE, Bruskiewich R, Beare DM, Clamp M, Smink LJ, et al. (1999). The DNA sequence of human chromosome 22. [erratum appears in *Nature* 2000;404(6780):904]. *Nature* 402: 489–495.
Epstein JA (2001). Developing models of DiGeorge syndrome. *Trends Genet* 17: S13–S17.
Farrell MJ, Stadt H, Wallis KT, Scambler P, Hixon RL, Wolfe R, Leatherbury L, Kirby ML (1999). *HIRA*, a DiGeorge syndrome candidate gene, is required for cardiac outflow tract septation. *Circ Res* 84: 127–135.
Goldmuntz E, Clark BJ, Mitchell LE, Jawad AF, Cuneo BF, Reed L, McDonald-McGinn D, Chien P, Feuer J, Zackai EH, et al. (1998). Frequency of 22q11 deletions in patients with conotruncal defects. *J Am Coll Cardiol* 32: 492–498.
Goodship JA, Burn J (2000). UFD1L is not the monogenic basis for heart defects associated with the CATCH phenotype. *Mol Med Today* 6: 14.
Goodship J, Cross I, LiLing J, Wren C (1998). A population study of chromosome 22q11 deletions in infancy. *Arch Dis Child* 79: 348–351.
Graham A, Smith A (2001). Patterning the pharyngeal arches. *Bioessays* 23: 54–61.
Greenberg et al. (1987). Hypoparathyroidism and T cell immune defect in a patient with 10p deletion syndrome. *J Pediatr* 109: 489–492.
Guris DL, Fantes J, Tara D, Druker BJ, Imamoto A (2001). Mice lacking the homologue of the human 22q11.2 gene *CRKL* phenocopy neurocristopathies of DiGeorge syndrome. *Nat Genet* 27: 293–298.
Halford S, Lindsay E, Nayudu M, Carey AH, Baldini A, Scambler PJ (1993). Low-copy-number repeat sequences flank the DiGeorge/velo-cardio-facial syndrome loci at 22q11. *Hum Mol Genet* 2: 191–196.
Jerome LA, Papaioannou VE (2001). DiGeorge syndrome phenotype in mice mutant for the T-box gene, *Tbx1*. *Nat Genet* 27: 286–291.
Jiang X, Rowitch DH, Soriano P, McMahon AP, Sucov HM (2000). Fate of the mammalian cardiac neural crest. *Dev Suppl* 127: 1607–1616.

Kelley RI, Zackai EH, Emanuel BS, Kistenmacher M, Greenberg F, Punnett HH (1982). The association of the DiGeorge anomalad with partial monosomy of chromosome 22. *J Pediatr* 101: 197–200.

Kerstjens-Frederikse WS, Kurahashi H, Driscoll DA, Budarf ML, Emanuel BS, Beatty B, Scheidl T, Siegel-Bartelt J, Henderson K, Cytrynbaum C, et al. (1999). Microdeletion 22q11.2: clinical data and deletion size. *J Med Genet* 36: 721–723.

Kimber WL, Hsieh P, Hirotsune S, Yuva-Paylor L, Sutherland HF, Chen A, Ruiz-Lozano P, Hoogstraten-Miller SL, Chien KR, Paylor R, et al. (1999). Deletion of 150 kb in the minimal DiGeorge/velocardiofacial syndrome critical region in mouse. *Hum Mol Genet* 8: 2229–2237.

Kirby ML, Waldo KL (1995). Neural crest and cardiovascular patterning. *Circ Res* 77: 211–215.

Klewer SE, Behrednt DM, Atkins DL (1998). Truncus arteriosus. In: *Perspectives in Pediatric Cardiology*, volume 6. Moller JH (ed.) Futura, Armonk, NY, pp. 271–286.

Koenig R et al. (1987). Hypoparathyroidism with partial monosomy 10p. *J Pediatr* 111: 310.

Lammer EJ, Chen DT, Hoar RM, Agnish ND, Benke PJ, Braun JT, Curry CJ, Fernhoff PM, Grix AW Jr, Lott IT (1985). Retinoic acid embryopathy. *N Engl J Med* 313: 837–841.

Lindsay EA, Halford S, Wadey R, Scambler PJ, Baldini A (1993). Molecular cytogenetic characterization of the DiGeorge syndrome region using fluorescence in situ hybridization. *Genomics* 17: 403–407.

Lindsay EA, Greenberg F, Shaffer LG, Shapira SK, Scambler PJ, Baldini A (1995). Submicroscopic deletions at 22q11.2: variability of the clinical picture and delineation of a commonly deleted region. *Am J Med Genet* 56: 191–197.

Lindsay EA, Botta A, Jurecic V, Carattini-Rivera S, Cheah YC, Rosenblatt HM, Bradley A, Baldini A (1999). Congenital heart disease in mice deficient for the DiGeorge syndrome region. *Nature* 401: 379–383.

Lindsay EA, Vitelli F, Su H, Morishima M, Huynh T, Pramparo T, Jurecic V, Ogunrinu G, Sutherland HF, Scambler PJ, et al. (2001). *Tbx1* haploinsufficieny in the DiGeorge syndrome region causes aortic arch defects in mice. *Nature* 410: 97–101.

Manley NR, Capecchi MR (1995). The role of Hoxa-3 in mouse thymus and thyroid development. *Development* 121: 1989–2003.

Marino B, Digilio MC, Toscano A, Anaclerio S, Giannotti A, Feltri C, de Ioris MA, Angioni A, Dallapiccola B (2001). Anatomic patterns of conotruncal defects associated with deletion 22q11. *Genet Med* 3: 45–48.

Melchionda S, Digilio MC, Mingarelli R, Novelli G, Scambler P, Marino B, Dallapiccola B (1995). Transposition of the great arteries associated with deletion of chromosome 22q11. *Am J Cardiol* 75: 95–98.

Merscher S, Funke B, Epstein JA, Heyer J, Puech A, Lu MM, Xavier RJ, Demay MB, Russell RG, Factor S, et al. (2001). TBX1 is responsible for cardiovascular defects in velo-cardio-facial/DiGeorge syndrome. *Cell* 104: 619–629.

Momma K, Takao A (1989). Right ventricular concentric hypertrophy and left ventricular dilation by ductal constriction in fetal rats. *Circ Res* 64: 1137–1146.

Moss EM, Batshaw ML, Solot CB, Gerdes M, McDonald-McGinn DM, Driscoll DA, Emanuel BS, Zackai EH, Wang PP (1999). Psychoeducational profile of the 22q11.2 microdeletion: A complex pattern. *J Pediatr* 134: 193–198.

Nishibatake M, Kirby ML, Van Mierop LH (1987). Pathogenesis of persistent truncus arteriosus and dextroposed aorta in the chick embryo after neural crest ablation. *Circulation* 75: 255–264.

Paylor R, McIlwain KL, McAninch R, Nellis A, Yuva-Paylor LA, Baldini A, Lindsay EA (2001). Mice deleted for the DiGeorge/velocardiofacial syndrome region show abnormal sensorimotor gating and learning and memory impairments. *Hum Mol Genet* 10: 2645–2650.

Pflugfelder GO, Roth H, Poeck B (1992). A homology domain shared between *Drosophila* optomotor-blind and mouse Brachyury is involved in DNA binding. *Biochem Biophys Res Commun* 186: 918–925.

Piotrowski T, Northcutt RG (1996). The cranial nerves of the Senegal bichir, *Polypterus senegalus* [osteichthyes: actinopterygii: cladistia]. *Brain Behav Evol* 47: 55–102.

Puech A, Saint-Jore B, Merscher S, Russell RG, Cherif D, Sirotkin H, Xu H, Factor S, Kucherlapati R, Skoultchi AI (2000). Normal cardiovascular development in mice deficient for 16 genes in 550 kb of the velocardiofacial/DiGeorge syndrome region. *Proc Natl Acad Sci USA* 97: 10090–10095.

Roberts C, Sutherland HF, Farmer H, Kimber W, Halford S, Carey A, Brickman JM, Wynshaw-Boris A, Scambler PJ (2002). Targeted mutagenesis of the *Hira* gene results in gastrulation defects and patterning abnormalities of mesoendodermal derivatives prior to early embryonic lethality. *Mol Cell Biol* 22: 2318–2328.

Robinson HB Jr. (1975). DiGeorge's or the III–IV pharyngeal pouch syndrome: pathology and a theory of pathogenesis. *Perspect Pediatr Pathol* 2: 173–206.

Rohn RD, Leffell MS, Leadem P, Johnson D, Rubio T, Emanuel BS (1984). Familial third–fourth pharyngeal pouch syndrome with apparent autosomal dominant transmission. *J Pediatr* 105: 47–51.

Rubin JD, Ferencz C, McCarter RJ, Wilson PD, Boughman JA, Brenner JI, Neill CA, Perry LW, Hepner SI, Downing JW (1985). Congenital cardiovascular malformations in the Baltimore-Washington area. *Md Med J* 34: 1079–1083.

Ryan AK, Goodship JA, Wilson DI, Philip N, Levy A, Seidel H, Schuffenhauer S, Oechsler H, Belohradsky B, Prieur M, et al. (1997). Spectrum of clinical features associated with interstitial chromosome 22q11 deletions: a European collaborative study. *J Med Genet* 34: 798–804.

Sabry MA, Zaki M, Abul Hassan SJ, Ramadan DG, Abdel Rasool MA, al Awadi SA, al Saleh Q (1998). Kenny-Caffey syndrome is part of the CATCH 22 haploinsufficiency cluster. *J Med Genet* 35: 31–36.

Sadler TW (2000). *Langman's Medical Embryology*, 8th Edition. Lippincott Williams & Wilkins, Baltimore.

Scambler PJ, Kelly D, Lindsay E, Williamson R, Goldberg R, Shprintzen R, Wilson DI, Goodship JA, Cross IE, Burn J (1992). Velo-cardio-facial syndrome associated with chromosome 22 deletions encompassing the DiGeorge locus. *Lancet* 339: 1138–1139.

Schilling TF, Piotrowski T, Grandel H, Brand M, Heisenberg CP, Jiang YJ, Beuchle D, Hammerschmidt M, Kane DA, Mullins MC, et al. (1996). Jaw and branchial arch mutants in zebrafish. I: Branchial arches. *Dev Suppl* 123: 329–344.

Schinke M, Izumo S (2001). Deconstructing DiGeorge syndrome. *Nat Genet* 27: 238–240.

Schuffenhauer S, Lichtner P, Peykar-Derakhshandeh P, Murken J, Haas OA, Back E, Wolff G, Zabel B, Barisic I, Rauch A, Borochowitz Z, Dallapiccola B, Ross M, Meitinger T (1998). Deletion mapping on chromosome 10p and definition of a critical region for the second DiGeorge syndrome locus (DGS2). *Eur J Hum Genet* 6: 213–225.

Seaver LH, Pierpont JW, Erickson RP, Donnerstein RL, Cassidy SB (1994). Pulmonary atresia associated with maternal 22q11.2 deletion: possible parent of origin effect in the conotruncal anomaly face syndrome. *J Med Genet* 31: 830–834.

Shaikh TH, Kurahashi H, Saitta SC, O'Hare AM, Hu P, Roe BA, Driscoll DA, McDonald-McGinn DM, Zackai EH, Budarf ML, et al. (2000). Chromosome 22-specific low copy repeats and the 22q11.2 deletion syndrome: genomic organization and deletion endpoint analysis. *Hum Mol Genet* 9: 489–501.

Shimizu T, Takao A, Ando M, Hirayama A (1984). Conotruncal face syndrome: its heterogeneity and association with thymus involution. In: *Congenital Heart Disease: Causes and Processes*, Nora JJ, Takao A (eds.) Futura, Mount Kisco, NY, pp. 29–41.

Shprintzen RJ, Goldberg RB, Lewin ML, Sidoti EJ, Berkman MD, Argamaso RV, Young D (1978). A new syndrome involving cleft palate, cardiac anomalies, typical facies, and learning disabilities: velo-cardio-facial syndrome. *Cleft Palate J* 15: 56–62.

Stern AM et al. (1977). An association of aorticotruncoconal abnormalities, velopalative incompetence and unusual spine fusion. *Birth Defects* 13: 259.

Stevens CA, Carey JC, Shigeoka AO (1990). DiGeorge anomaly and velocardialfacial syndrome. *Peds* 85: 526–530.

Sutherland HF, Kim UJ, Scambler PJ (1998). Cloning and comparative mapping of the DiGeorge syndrome critical region in the mouse. *Genomics* 52: 37–43.

Takao A, Ando M, Cho K, Kinouchi A, Murakami Y (1980). Etiologic categorization of common congenital heart disease. In: *Etiology and Morphogenesis of Congenital Heart Disease*. Van Praagh R, Takao A (eds.) Futura, Mount Kisco, NY, pp. 253–269.

Van Mierop LH, Kutsche LM (1986). Cardiovascular anomalies in DiGeorge syndrome and importance of neural crest as a possible pathogenetic factor. *Am J Cardiol* 58: 133–137.

Vitelli F, Morishima M, Taddei I, Lindsay EA, Baldini A (2002). *Tbx1* mutation causes multiple cardiovascular defects and disrupts neural crest and cranial nerve migratory pathways. *Hum Mol Genet* 11: 915–922.

Wilson DJ, Cross JE, Goodship JA, Brown J, Scambler PJ, Bain HH, Taylor JFN, Walsh K, Bankier A, Burn J, Wolstenholme J (1992). A prospective cytogenetic study of 36 cases of DiGeorge syndrome. *Am J Human Genet* 51: 957–963.

Yamagishi H, Garg V, Matsuoka R, Thomas T, Srivastava D (1999). A molecular pathway revealing a genetic basis for human cardiac and craniofacial defects. *Science* 283: 1158–1161.

Young D, Shprintzen RJ, Goldberg RB (1980). Cardiac malformations in the velocardiofacial syndrome. *Am J Cardiol* 46: 643–648.

TBX3 and *TBX5* and the Ulnar-Mammary and Holt-Oram Syndromes

MICHAEL J. BAMSHAD AND LYNN B. JORDE

Ulnar-mammary syndrome (UMS) and Holt-Oram syndrome (HOS) are rare, autosomal-dominant, multiple-malformation disorders. UMS is characterized by apocrine abnormalities including breast defects and malformations of the posterior elements of the upper limb. In contrast, HOS is typified by heart malformations, most commonly an atrial septal defect (ASD) or ventricular septal defect (VSD), conduction abnormalities, and defects of the anterior elements of the upper limb. UMS and HOS are caused by myriad different mutations in *TBX3* and *TBX5*, respectively, two members of the T-box gene family linked together on chromosome 12q24. For both conditions, there is little evidence to support a genotype-phenotype correlation. The long-term care of patients with UMS or HOS can be challenging, but in general, most patients do well. In the heart, TBX5 physically interacts with Nkx2-5 to transactivate *atrial natriuretic factor* (*ANF*) and connexin-40 (*cx40*). In the limb, Tbx5 appears to activate *fibroblast growth factor-10* (*Fgf10*) directly to initiate forelimb bud outgrowth and determine, in part, forelimb identity. Tbx3 acts as a negative repressor of *p19^{ARF}* and *p53* and interferes with apoptosis. In vitro studies demonstrate that substitutions in the DNA-binding domain of TBX3 and TBX5 or proteins with truncations in the C terminus of TBX3 and TBX5 fail to bind DNA and lose their transcriptional properties. Loss of Tbx3 repressor activity may promote a pro-apoptotic path that results in a diminished number of mesodermal cells in the developing limb and breast. Loss of Tbx5 activity appears to result in the downregulation of several genes critical for normal heart development. Mice haploinsufficient for *Tbx3* or lacking functional *Tbx5* exhibit malformations that recapitulate UMS and HOS, respectively.

T-box genes are members of a highly conserved family of transcription factors that share a region of homology to the DNA-binding domain (T box) of the mouse *Brachyury* (or *T*) gene product (Herrmann et al., 1990; Bollag et al., 1994). The spatial and temporal expression patterns of T-box genes are tightly regulated, underscoring the critical roles that they play in morphogenesis and organogenesis (see Chapter 67). To date, more than 20 different T-box genes have been found in humans; based on their phylogenetic relationships, they can be classified into several different subgroups. One subgroup consists of the four T-box genes *TBX2*, *TBX3*, *TBX4*, and *TBX5*. These T-box genes are thought to have arisen from a common ancestor (*TBX2/3/4/5*) that underwent unequal crossover to create the genes *Tbx2/3* and *Tbx4/5* (Fig. 69–1). This was followed by a duplication event that produced the cognate pairs *TBX2/TBX3* and *TBX4/TBX5* and the linked pairs *TBX3/TBX5* and *TBX2/TBX4* (Agulnik et al., 1996; Ruvinsky et al., 2000). The role of T-box genes in human disease was brought to focus when mutations in *TBX3* and *TBX5* were found to cause the multiple malformations in UMS (OMIM 181450) (Bamshad et al., 1995, 1997) and HOS (OMIM 142900) (Terrett et al., 1994; Basson et al., 1994, 1997; Li et al., 1997).

TBX3 and *TBX5* are located on chromosome 12q24.1, with *TBX5* mapping approximately 265 kb centromeric of *TBX3*. *TBX3* is composed of eight exons that encode at least four different transcripts (Fig. 69–2) (Bamshad et al., 1999). The most common full-length transcript is 5.2 kb and has an open reading frame of 2172 bp that encodes a protein with 723 amino acid residues. One alternative transcript of *TBX3* contains 60 bp inserted between exons 2 and 3 encoded by an alternatively spliced exon 2a (Fig. 69–2). The region of *TBX3* into which exon 2a is spliced encodes the highly conserved DNA-binding

domain of the TBX3 protein. Insertion of these 20–amino acid residues into the middle of the T box is likely to alter its DNA-binding properties, although this has yet to be fully characterized. Another alternative transcript of *TBX3* splices the 5′ sequence of exon 1 to exon 7 in-frame and eliminates the T box. This is analogous to transcripts lacking a homeobox, which have been reported for several *Hox* genes (Chariot et al., 1995).

The T-box domain of human *TBX3* is composed of 180 amino acid residues between residues 105 and 285. Sequence conservation is high, being 98% identical to the T-box domain of mouse and chick Tbx3 and about 95% identical to the T-box domain of human TBX2. The T-box domain of TBX3 shares 62% identical residues with the T-box domain of human TBX5 and about 50% identical residues with the T-box domain of mouse T. *TBX5* is composed of at least nine exons that encode several alternatively spliced transcripts (Fig. 69–3). The major transcript encodes a product of 518 amino acid residues, which is 97% homologous to mouse Tbx5 (Li et al., 1997; Basson et al., 1997, 1999). Like other T-box genes, the T-box domain of TBX5 is composed of ~184 amino acid residues (~62–246), and it is 99% identical to the T-box domain of mouse and chick Tbx5 (Bruneau et al., 1999). Conservation among homologues of *TBX5* is substantially reduced preceding and immediately following the T-box domain.

In vitro PCR-based binding selection experiments led to the identification of a 22-nucleotide palindromic DNA-binding site for mouse T (Kispert and Herrmann, 1993). The crystal structure of its homolgoue in *Xenopus* (i.e., Xbra) bound to DNA demonstrated binding of a T-box dimer to this site (Müller and Herrmann, 1997). In this structure, each monomer contacted one half-site and monomers interacted with each other via a hydrophobic interface. Electrophoretic mobility shift assays (EMSAs) using the T-box domain of human T and the full-length T showed a similar pattern of binding (Papapetrou et al., 1997). The structure of the T-box domain (residues 101–291) of TBX3 bound to human DNA at a resolution of 1.7 Å has been solved (Coll et al., 2002). The T-box domain consists of a seven-stranded β-barrel domain belonging to the s-type immunoglobulin domain class. The β barrel is composed of two β-pleated sheets and two smaller sheets that close the β barrel toward the DNA. Loops extending from one of the β-barrel domains and a C-terminal extension contact the major and minor grooves of DNA, respectively. In contrast to T, two TBX3 monomers bind independently to the palindromic DNA duplex used for cocrystallization without stabilizing the monomer–monomer interaction. This suggests that TBX3 binds as a monomer to single sites, consistent with the observation that all targets of T-box proteins identified to date contain only single sites. TBX5 binds to a core eight nucleotides, which are part of the *Brachyury* consensus half-site, and to the full-length *Brachyury* site (Ghosh et al., 2001). The former sequence is present in the upstream region of several important genes that are expressed in the developing heart (e.g., cardiac α-actin, cardiac myosin heavy chain α, cardiac myosin heavy chain β, myosin light chain 1A, myosin light chain 1B, and cardiac-specific homeobox [i.e., Nkx2-5]).

Deletion mutants of mouse *T* have shown that the C-terminal region following the T-box domain has two transactivating and two repressing regions (Kispert et al., 1995). However, there is little sequence conservation outside of the T-box domain of different T-box proteins, so inferences of function among the T-box genes should be interpreted with caution. Although the regions preceding and follow-

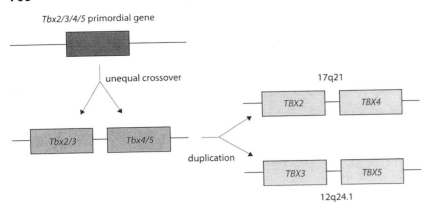

Figure 69–1. Schematic of the evolution of the two gene clusters containing *Tbx2* and *Tbx5* by unequal crossover of a primordial gene (*Tbx2/3/4/5*) followed by cluster duplication to produce the linked gene pairs *TBX3/TBX5* and *TBX2/TBX4* on human chromosomes 12q24.1 and 17q21, respectively.

ing the T-box domain vary in length and primary sequence even among *TBX3* orthologues, there is experimental evidence that some functional characteristics are conserved. Transcriptional assays using C-terminal truncation mutants have demonstrated that the C-terminal region of human *TBX3* contains several regions which either activate or repress transcription (He et al., 1999; Carlson et al., 2001). One particular region that included amino acid residues 567–623 repressed transcription levels to near that of the wild-type protein and showed a dominant repression activity (Carlson et al., 2001).

MALFORMATION SYNDROMES CAUSED BY MUTATIONS IN *TBX3* AND *TBX5*

UMS

Mutations in *TBX3* cause the rare multiple-malformation disorder UMS. It was originally reported in the 19th century in a woman with mammary hypoplasia, inability to lactate, and absence of digits 3, 4, and 5 as well as the ulna (Gilly, 1882). However, it was not until the late 20th century that its mode of inheritance and phenotypic characteristics were more fully characterized (Pallister et al., 1976; Schinzel et al., 1987). By the mid-1990s, approximately 10 families with UMS had been reported (Gonzales et al., 1976; Hecht and Scott, 1984; Meinecke et al., 1989; Franceschini et al., 1992), though more than half of all affected individuals belong to a single kindred (Bamshad et al., 1996). After the discovery that mutations in *TBX3* cause UMS, about 10 additional families with UMS have been identified (Bamshad, unpublished data).

The most salient features of UMS are upper limb malformations, apocrine gland/mammary hypoplasia and/or dysfunction, and genital anomalies. Most affected individuals have posterior (i.e., postaxial or ulnar) upper limb deficiencies (Fig. 69–4). These defects range from mild hypoplasia of the terminal phalanx of the fifth digit, which can be detected only radiographically, to absence of the third, fourth, and

fifth digits of the hand and absence of the ulna accompanied by hypoplasia of the upper arm. The appearance of either of these defects is quite characteristic, though not pathognomonic. Complete absence of the hand and deficiencies of more anterior parts of the upper limb (e.g., fourth digit) in the presence of normal posterior elements (e.g., fifth digit) are very rare and should raise suspicion about the diagnosis. Accordingly, the most posterior elements of the upper limb are almost always more severely affected than the anterior parts. Nevertheless, an individual with UMS having a typical split hand/foot malformation and a mutation in *TBX3* has been reported (Franceschini et al., 1992). Phocomelia is not a characteristic of UMS.

In contrast to limb deficiencies, some individuals with UMS have duplications of the fifth digit (i.e., posterior polydactyly). Several individuals have demonstrated posterior polydactyly of one limb and absence of the posterior elements of the contralateral limb (Bamshad et al., 1996). UMS is also one of several conditions characterized by defects of dorsal/ventral patterning characterized by partial duplication of the nail on the ventral surface of the fifth digit (Fig. 69–5). This is sometimes accompanied by a dorsalization of the skin of the fifth digit. Thus, the proximal/distal, anterior/posterior, and dorsal/ventral axes of the developing upper limb can be affected in individuals with UMS. Alternatively, some individuals with UMS have normal upper limbs (Meinecke et al., 1989; Bamshad et al., 1996). The lower limbs of individuals with UMS can also be affected, although this is less frequent. To date, these malformations have been limited to syndactyly of the posterior digits, hypoplasia of the fifth digit, and unilateral posterior polydactyly (Schinzel et al., 1987; Bamshad et al., 1996, 1999).

Apocrine abnormalities in UMS range from minimally diminished axillary hair and perspiration accompanied by normal breast development and lactation to complete absence of the breasts and no axillary hair or perspiration. Individuals often have moderately reduced axillary hair and perspiration, absence of hair on the anterior chest wall, along with hypoplasia of the areola and/or breast. The abnormalities

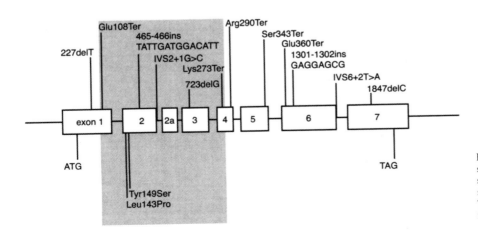

Figure 69–2. Schematic illustration of the genomic structure of *TBX3* (not to scale) with the nature and position of each mutation identified. Individual exons are shown as numbered boxes, and the region encoding the T box is shaded. Only a single mutation (227delT) is found in more than one proband.

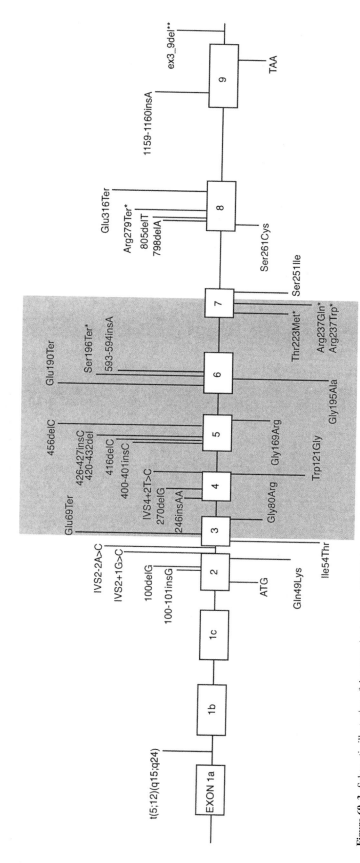

Figure 69–3. Schematic illustration of the genomic structure of *TBX5* (not to scale) with the nature and position of each mutation identified. Individual exons are shown as numbered boxes, and the region encoding the T box is shaded. Mutations found in more than one proband are denoted by an asterisk. A mutation that results in the deletion of exons 3–9 is indicated by a pair of asterisks.

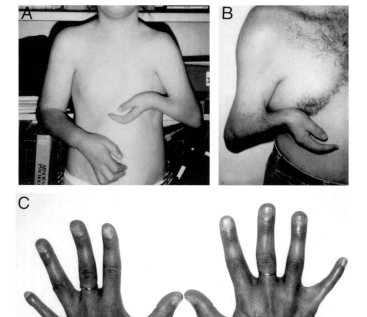

Figure 69–4. Typical limb malformations found in ulnar-mammary syndrome. (*A* and *B*) Absence of digits 3, 4, and 5 and ulna accompanied by hypoplasia of the radius and humerus. Note in *B* the mild webbing across the anterior axillary fold, a circumscribed patch of the anterior chest lacking hair, and hypoplasia of the nipple. (*C*) Bilateral hypoplasia of the second and third phalanges of the fifth digit. Note the slightly bulbous tip of the left fifth digit accompanied by hypoplasia of the nail, resulting in a very characteristic appearance.

of perspiration tend to be more apparent in males than females, while the breast abnormalities are more noticeable in females. Some women have morphologically normal breasts but are unable to produce breast milk. Individuals with either unilateral or bilateral supernumerary nipples have also been reported (Bamshad et al., 1996).

Myriad low-frequency malformations have been observed in individuals with UMS. Genital anomalies such as micropenis, hypospa-

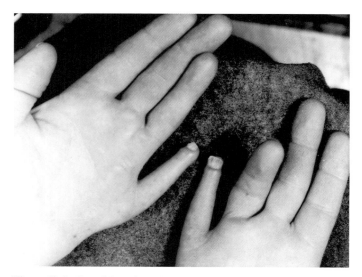

Figure 69–5. One of the unique abnormalities in individuals with ulnar-mammary syndrome is dorsalization of the posterior edge of the upper limb manifest by duplication of the nailbed and epidermal structures (i.e., hair and pigmentation pattern) on the palmar surface of the hands.

dias, cryptorchidism, and shawl scrotum have been observed in males (Schinzel et al., 1987; Bamshad et al., 1996; Sasaki et al., 2002). In females, imperforate hymen, small uterus, and bicornate uterus have been reported. Males commonly experience delayed pubertal development, though it has been reported in both sexes. Dental abnormalities include ectopic, hypoplastic, or absent canine teeth. Obesity was originally emphasized as a major feature of UMS (Schinzel, 1987), although it is probably only a low-frequency finding.

Expression of UMS is highly variable within and between families, and several obligate carriers, apparently nonpenetrant, have been reported (Bamshad et al., 1996). Although, the sample size of independent cases of UMS is relatively small, there does not appear to be any correlation between the severity of limb and nonlimb defects. The severity of defects appears to be similar between males and females, and no parent-of-origin effects have been noted.

HOS

A significant association between the frequency of congenital heart defects and abnormalities of the radius was noted more than 50 years ago (Birch-Jensen, 1949; Temtamy and McKusick, 1978), including observations of families in whom the transmission of limb and heart defects was consistent with autosomal-dominant inheritance. A report of a family with similar abnormalities in 1960 built upon these observations and led to the widespread acknowledgment that these findings were, in many cases, a specific syndrome (Holt and Oram, 1960). This disorder subsequently became known as Holt-Oram syndrome and was shown to be caused by mutations in *TBX5* (Basson et al., 1997; Li et al., 1997). To date, several hundred putative cases of HOS have been reported (Gall et al., 1966; Temtamy and McKusick, 1978; Newbury et al., 1996).

HOS is characterized by abnormalities of the anterior (i.e., preaxial or radial) elements of the upper limbs accompanied by cardiac malformations. The limb malformations in individuals with HOS are typically bilateral and asymmetric, with the left side often more severely affected than the right side (Gall et al., 1966; Newbury et al., 1996). The limb malformations in HOS are markedly variable within and between families. The mildest malformations of the limb are, arguably, abnormalities of the size, shape, and number of carpal bones as manifest by hypoplasia/fusion or accessory carpals (Poznanski et al., 1970). Mild thenar hypoplasia may similarly be the only limb abnormality observed in an affected individual. Functionally, the most minor abnormalities noted are limited opposability of the thumb or limited supination, either of which may be present in the absence of skeletal defects. Clinodactyly of the fifth digit and brachydactyly caused by hypoplasia of the middle phalanges are also relatively minor manifestations of HOS. The most common limb malformations reported involve abnormalities of the thumb. These include a triphalangeal thumb, digitalized thumb with two phalanges, hypoplasia or absence of the thumb, and combinations thereof (Fig. 69–6). More than 50% of individuals have abnormalities of the forearm, most commonly hypoplasia or absence of the radius (Fig. 69–6). This is often accompanied by hypoplasia of the ulna, though it is usually affected to a lesser degree. Abnormalities of the posterior skeletal elements of the upper limb are never found in the absence of defects of the anterior elements.

Malformations of the upper arm and shoulder girdle are more common than is often appreciated, hypoplasia of the humerus causing shortening of the upper arm in approximately 50% of cases. The head of the humerus is commonly hypoplastic, though this can be a subtle finding. The clavicles are normal in only a minority of individuals with HOS. More often, they are hypoplastic, though the acromioclavicular joint is frequently described as prominent on external exam. In combination with hypoplasia of the pectoralis major and/or deltoids, these abnormalities underlie the characteristic appearance of sloping shoulders in individuals with HOS. The most severe limb malformation reported in individuals with HOS is bilateral phocomelia (Temtamy and McKusick, 1978). Complete transverse defects and absence of an entire arm are rarely, if ever, manifestations of HOS.

More than 95% of individuals with HOS have detectable cardiac involvement, although this estimate is dependent on the ascertainment

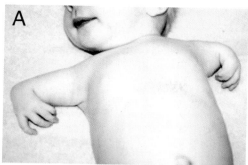

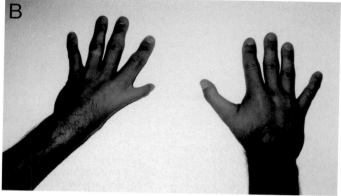

Figure 69–6. (*A*) Bilateral absence of the first digit, radius, ulna, and severe hypoplasia of the humerus. (*B*) Bilateral hypoplasia of the first digit. Note that the left side is more severely affected than the right side in both *A* and *B*.

criteria (Newbury et al., 1996; Sletten and Pierpont, 1996). Most individuals have structural heart disease, the most common being a secundum ASD. This often results in a common atrium syndrome with or without anomalous pulmonary venous return. The second most frequent heart malformation is VSD. Typically, only a single septal defect is present, though some patients have both. Myriad other cardiac malformations have been reported, including patent ductus arteriosus, endocardial cushion defect, mitral valve prolapse, aortic stenosis, and hypoplastic left heart (Newbury et al., 1996; Sletten and Pierpont, 1996). Ventricular outflow tract abnormalities have been reported but are very uncommon.

Conduction abnormalities are common and may be present in the absence of structural heart disease. More frequently, however, conduction abnormalities occur together with a structural heart defect. The most common electrocardiographic (ECG) finding is a prolonged P–R interval. Less frequent ECG abnormalities include sinus bradycardia, progressive atrioventricular block, atrial fibrillation, and left bundle branch block.

DIAGNOSIS

Diagnostic Criteria

The variable expressivity of UMS and HOS can make the assignment of a definitive diagnosis challenging, particularly in a sporadic case. As a consequence, specific criteria have been proposed to facilitate the diagnostic process.

Some combinations of defects (e.g., posterior limb deficiencies in the absence of axillary hair or sweating) are virtually pathognomonic of UMS. However, the diagnosis of UMS is often challenging, particularly in sporadic cases if only the limb defects are present and/or prepubertal children because many of the abnormalities are not detectable until puberty (e.g., the presence of axillary hair). In addition to a family history of a posterior limb duplication and/or deficiency, the presence of two or more of the following diagnostic criteria is required to diagnose UMS: hypoplasia or absence of the posterior elements of the upper limb, posterior polydactyly, dorsalization of the

ventral surface of the fifth digit including isolated duplication of the nail, mammary hypoplasia/aplasia, decreased ability to lactate, supernumerary nipples, diminished axillary sweating and reduced body odor, sparse or absent axillary hair, and delayed puberty. In some cases, definitive diagnosis may not be possible in the absence of genetic testing.

Several factors make the definitive diagnosis of HOS more challenging than that of UMS. The number of organs and body areas affected in individuals with HOS is more limited compared to UMS, but the spectrum of limb and heart malformations appears to be broader. The congenital heart defects in HOS are more common than the malformations observed in individuals with UMS; thus, their cooccurrence with limb abnormalities is anticipated to be more frequent. Furthermore, heart and hand malformations are commonly found in syndromes and associations that may be difficult to distinguish from HOS (see below, Differential). Lastly, none of the abnormalities observed in individuals with HOS is pathognomonic. As a consequence, even the strictest clinical criteria may not define a genetically homogeneous set of individuals.

Given these qualifications, commonly used clinical diagnostic criteria for HOS include the presence of an affected family member, bilateral anterior upper limb defects, and an ASD or characteristic conduction abnormality. Families in which two or more individuals have only limb or only heart malformations would not meet the criteria for HOS. Diagnosis of HOS is also based, in part, on the absence of malformations that are not usually observed in individuals with HOS (e.g., malformations of the lower limb) or a suitable alternative diagnosis (e.g., trisomy 18).

Differential

The alternative diagnoses that should be considered in an individual suspected of having UMS are limited. Foremost, it should be remembered that UMS is very rare. Thus, even though posterior polydactyly is a feature of UMS, it occurs much more frequently as an isolated malformation. Most often, the diagnosis of UMS is entertained in a child presenting with a posterior limb deficiency. While this malformation is uncommon, even most children with this defect do not have UMS.

Conditions characterized by limb deficiencies similar to those observed in UMS include Brachmannn-De Lange syndrome, Poland's anomaly, split hand/foot malformation (SHFM) syndrome (see Chapter 105), hand-foot-uterus syndrome (HFUS, OMIM 140000; see Chapter 48), and scalp-ear-nipple syndrome (SENS, OMIM 181270). Most children with Brachmann-De Lange syndrome have facial characteristics and a spectrum of additional malformations that make them easily distinguishable from children with UMS. Although there are rare reports of bilateral Poland's anomaly (Karnak et al., 1998), the overwhelming majority of children with Poland's anomaly have unilateral and ipsilateral malformations of the limb and chest wall, whereas the defects in UMS are usually bilateral. Although hypoplasia of the breast is observed in both conditions, the pectoralis muscles are usually normal in UMS. An individual with UMS and absence of the fourth digit resembling a typical SHFM has been reported (Franceschini et al., 1992), but normal posterior elements of the hand in the presence of defects of more anterior structures (e.g., a "split hand") are very rare in UMS. SHFM accompanied by ectodermal findings is common in individuals with ectrodactyly and ectodermal dysplasia with cleft lip and/or palate (EEC) syndrome (OMIM 604292, see Chapter 105), but the palate, skin, scalp hair, nails, lacrimal glands, and lacrimal ducts of individuals with UMS are usually normal. Manifestations of HFUS that are similar to UMS include digital hypoplasia, supernumerary nipples, and genital anomalies (Rogers and Anderson, 1995), although abnormalities of axillary hair and perspiration are not observed in HFUS. SENS is characterized by breast hypoplasia, diminished axillary perspiration, dental anomalies, abnormally shaped ears, and limb defects (Edwards et al., 1994). However, the most common limb defect in SENS is syndactyly, not a deficiency or duplication of the upper limb.

The diagnostic possibilities for individuals who present with limb and heart defects is moderately large, but only a few of these conditions are relatively common. The most frequent diagnoses that are characterized by a pattern of malformations similar to HOS are VATER/VACTERL (includes vertebral, anal, cardiac, tracheal, esophageal, radial, renal, and limb anomalies) association, thrombocytopenia and absent radius (TAR) syndrome (OMIM 274000), Fanconi's anemia, Okihiro's syndrome (OMIM 126800), and several hand-heart syndromes. Diagnosis of either VATER or VACTERL association requires more than the presence of only structural heart and anterior upper limb defects (Botto et al., 1997). However, renal dysplasia, tracheoesophageal fistula with esophageal atresia, and vertebral anomalies are relatively common defects and may be found coincidentally in some individuals with HOS. Similarly, Fanconi's anemia can present with malformations resembling HOS or the VATER/VACTERL associations, making it difficult to differentiate among these diagnoses. Abnormalities of the shoulder girdle and chest wall, however, are much more common in individuals with HOS. TAR syndrome can be distinguished from HOS by the presence of a normal or slightly hypoplastic thumb accompanied by severe hypoplasia or aplasia of the radius (Hall et al., 1969).

Several different hand-heart syndromes that are transmitted in an autosomal-dominant pattern have been described. Okihiro's syndrome is characterized by anterior upper limb malformations and structural defects that can be indistinguishable from HOS (Okihiro et al., 1977). The radial defects can range from hypoplasia of the thenar eminence with or without thumb abduction and apposition weakness, hypoplasia or absence of the thumb, and hypoplasia or absence of the radius and ulna. In addition, however, individuals with Okihiro's syndrome have ocular defects consistent with Duane's anomaly, which is an inability to abduct the globe, reduced ability to adduct the globe, retraction of the globe and narrowing of the palpebral fissure upon adduction, and abnormal convergence. Duane's anomaly can be unilateral or bilateral. The locus for Okihiro's syndrome has been identified recently; it is caused by mutations in *SALL4* (Kohlhase et al., 2002). The hand-heart syndromes that are commonly included in the differential diagnosis of HOS are heart-hand syndrome II (Tabatznik's syndrome) and III (OMIM 140450), both of which are very rare. Moreover, the phenotypes of neither of these are very similar to common presentations of HOS. Tabatznik's syndrome is characterized by brachydactyly type D (i.e., a short and broad terminal phalanx of the thumb) or mild thumb hypoplasia accompanied by supraventricular tachycardia (Temtamy and McKusick, 1978; Silengo et al., 1990). A hand malformation resembling brachydactyly type C (shortening of the proximal and middle phalanges of the second and third digits sometimes accompanied by carpal fusion) and sick-sinus syndrome occur together in hand-heart syndrome III (Ruiz De La Fuente and Prieto, 1980). In contrast to HOS, however, the feet are also affected in this condition, albeit to a lesser degree.

SPECTRUM OF MUTATIONS IN *TBX3* AND *TBX5*

To date, 14 different mutations in *TBX3* have been found in 15 kindreds with UMS (Fig. 69–2), including missense, nonsense, frameshift, and splice-site mutations (Bamshad et al., 1997, 1999; Sasaki et al., 2002; Bamshad, unpublished data). With the exception of 227delT, each mutation has been found in only one family. Two missense mutations in exon 2 (Leu^{143}Pro and Tyr^{149}Ser) produce nonconservative amino acid substitutions in the T box. Both of these substitutions are predicted to disturb the β barrel of TBX3 and reduce the stability of the DNA-binding domain (Coll et al., 2002), and both disrupt normal TBX3 function (Brummelkamp et al., 2002). Six mutations in *TBX3* disrupt the T box and produce a protein fragment that has reduced, if any, DNA-binding activity. Six mutations in *TBX3* are located 3′ of the region encoding the T box. These mutant alleles are transcribed and translated, but the truncated TXB3 proteins exhibit diminished or complete loss of transcriptional repression activity (Carlson et al., 2001). Taken together with the observation that TBX3 binds as a monomer, these data suggest that UMS results from functional haploinsufficiency of TBX3 protein, a conclusion that is consistent with lack of genotype–phenotype correlation in UMS (Bamshad et al., 1999).

The allelic spectrum of HOS is more complex than that of UMS (Fig. 69–3), with ~35 different mutations discovered to date (Brassington et al., 2003; Li et al., 1997; Basson et al., 1997, 1999; Cross et al., 2000; Yang et al., 2000; Akrami et al., 2001). In addition to missense, nonsense, frameshift, and splice-site mutations, a deletion encompassing exons 3–9 (Akrami et al., 2001) and a translocation that putatively disrupts *TBX5* (Basson et al., 1997) have been reported. In contrast to mutations in *TBX3*, many of the mutations in *TBX5* have been found in more than one family. Three of these are missense mutations (Thr^{223}Met, Arg^{237}Gln, and Arg^{237}Trp), and two are nonsense mutations (Ser^{196}Ter and Arg^{279}Ter). These five mutations account for about 50% of all cases of HOS found to be caused by mutations in *TBX5*. The Arg^{279}Ter mutation, found in a total of six familial and sporadic cases of HOS, is a caused by a C-to-T transition of 1500 bp. The cytosine is part of a CG doublet that may represent a mutation hot spot in *TBX5*.

While mutations have been found in virtually every family meeting the diagnostic criteria for UMS, *TBX5* mutations have been found in only ~30%–35% of cases meeting the diagnostic criteria for HOS (Brassington et al., 2003; Cross et al., 2000). There are several possible explanations. First, many cases diagnosed as HOS could be phenocopies, particularly because all of the sporadic cases and many of the HOS families are too small to be informative for linkage analysis. This is consistent with a higher mutation detection rate in familial vs. sporadic cases (Brassington et al., 2003). Second, in most studies, *TBX5* is screened for mutations by sequencing only the regions that will be translated. Thus, large deletions or mutations in untranslated regions that could disrupt normal TBX5 function would not be detected. However, a search for large deletions in 20 cases of HOS in which no mutations in *TBX5* had been found yielded only one new mutation (Akrami et al., 2001). Similarly, screening the untranslated regions of *TBX5* in ~30 patients with HOS, who did not have mutations in the translated portion of *TBX5*, did not increase the detection rate (Brassington et al., 2003). Third, HOS may be a genetically heterogeneous disorder. This is consistent with the observation that HOS does not map to 12q24 in some kindreds (Terrett et al., 1994), although no additional loci have been identified. Finally, there may be regulatory regions important for normal *TBX5* function that have not yet been identified and may harbor mutations causing HOS. These explanations are not mutually exclusive, and each is likely to be responsible, in part, for the low rate of detection of mutations in *TBX5* causing HOS.

MANAGEMENT

The management of an individual with a multiple malformation syndrome caused by a mutation in *TBX3* or *TBX5* often requires a multidisciplinary approach. Specialties that often participate include genetics, orthopedics, plastic surgery, cardiology, and endocrinology. Early diagnosis affords important information about natural history. This allows an opportunity to implement preventive measures and institute screening to facilitate early diagnosis and intervention.

Initial Evaluation

The initial assessment of an individual suspected of having UMS, HOS, or a related disorder should be focused on the broad collection of phenotypic data. Data to be collected include detailed obstetrical, medical, developmental, and family histories and a comprehensive physical examination. Documentation of at least a three-generation pedigree is also recommended. It is also often helpful to examine photographs of the parents taken when they were children, siblings, and extended family members. This is especially useful when determining whether a particular physical characteristic is a diagnostic clue or part of the phenotypic background of the family or both (i.e., when a parent or relative is unknowingly affected as well).

In addition to general inquiries about medical history, more detailed questions should be asked about the organ systems and body areas typically affected. For example, for postpubertal individuals suspected of having UMS it is important to inquire about the presence of axillary hair and sweating; the need to shave the axilla and/or use deodorant; the presence of supernumerary teeth; the presence of breast hypoplasia or marked breast asymmetry; the ability to lactate (e.g., engorgement, milk expression); and the onset of puberty, including the pitch of the voice. Limb abnormalities in suspected cases of UMS are usually the ascertaining feature, though the clinician may need to inquire about the inability to completely flex the fifth digit and the presence of a partial nail on the ventral surface of the fifth digit. Most of the features of HOS are notable on physical exam or will be detected via imaging studies of the chest, upper limbs, and heart. Ancillary information that may be helpful includes the presence of a symptomatic arrhythmia (e.g., syncope, palpitations), limited supination of the forearm, diminished range of motion of the thumb or wrist, increased rang of motion of the shoulder (due to hypoplasia of the clavicles), and weakness of the shoulder caused by muscular hypoplasia.

The physical exam should include a detailed survey of the individual and overall morphological characteristics of the hands, wrists, forearms, upper arms, and chest. The general relationships among the parts of the hands (e.g., length of digits, spacing between digits) should be observed, and subsequently each part should be examined individually. The thumb is a particularly complex body part, and skill is required to differentiate between normal variations and abnormal findings. Sloping shoulders are most easily detected by examination from the rear.

Individuals provisionally diagnosed with UMS need not be referred to any other specialists if their limb malformations are not severe. Aside from the limb defects, the most disturbing feature of UMS is delayed puberty in boys and breast hypoplasia in girls. Testosterone therapy in males with delayed puberty has been variably effective (Schinzel et al., 1987; Sasaki et al., 2002). For women with moderate to severe breast hypoplasia, referral to a plastic surgeon for counseling about reconstruction or augmentation is appropriate. All individuals suspected of having HOS should be referred to a cardiologist for further evaluation, including an ECG and echocardiogram. For UMS, imaging of the limbs to better define the underlying skeletal structure is of interest but usually not necessary for diagnostic purposes. In contrast, imaging studies of the limb are commonly needed to confirm the diagnosis of HOS in an individual as carpal defects may otherwise go undetected (Poznanski et al., 1970). An anterior/posterior radiograph of the chest should also be performed to detect subtle abnormalities of the clavicles. Prior to surgical palliation or correction of a limb malformation, the skeletal structures of the affected limb(s) should be imaged by standard radiography or magnetic resonance imaging.

Repair of Malformations

Many of the abnormalities found in individuals with UMS or HOS require surgical palliation or correction. Most individuals with HOS have either an ASD or a VSD, and if these do not close spontaneously, they can be surgically repaired with a very high rate of success. Thus, the first surgical procedure that many individuals with HOS undergo is repair of a structural cardiac defect. The age at which this is done is of course dependent on the type and severity of the underlying cardiac malformation. Repair of more severe and/or complex heart defects is often associated with substantially higher morbidity, and for some rare abnormalities (e.g., hypoplastic left heart) the treatment options are limited to palliative repair or transplant (Sletten and Pierpont, 1996).

The need for surgical intervention to treat the limb defects found in individuals with mutations in *TBX3* or *TBX5* is highly variable. The overwhelming principle to keep in mind is that the function of the limbs should be optimized, and sometimes this means that no surgical procedure is indicated. In some cases of HOS, it is necessary to reconstruct the thumb or create an equivalent digit from another finger. Limb defects that result in truncations of the arm or leg may necessitate amputation if it is likely to improve the fit of a prosthesis.

Long-Term Care and Prognosis

The long-term care of individuals with UMS or HOS does not commonly require ongoing medical intervention. The physical impairments caused by limb and heart malformations are usually the most salient problems at birth and often the most difficult to manage. Once these malformations have been treated, if necessary, most individuals do very well. The exception is children with HOS who have a complex heart malformation; they tend to do more poorly. Children with limb malformations that result in little functional impairment may require no intervention; thus, seek the advice of a specialist only as needed. Even children with severe limb malformations are remarkably adaptive, though they may need more services before and after surgical palliation or correction.

For males with UMS, a notable concern as they get older is hypogonadism accompanied by delayed puberty. Often, they do not undergo pubertal changes and develop secondary sexual characteristics until their late teens or early twenties. However, pubertal development inevitably does take place, leading to normal secondary sexual characteristics and, apparently, function. Several males with UMS have demonstrated low levels of testosterone; low to low-normal responses of luteinizing hormone and follicle-stimulating hormone to gonadotropin-releasing hormone stimulation tests; and normal testosterone response to human gonadotropin-stimulation tests (Sasaki et al., 2002). These findings are consistent with the suggestion that males with UMS suffer from a mild gonadotropin deficiency (Schinzel et al., 1987; Meinecke et al., 1989). Treatment with testosterone has led to increases in penile length (Schinzel et al., 1987; Sasaki et al., 2002).

Women with UMS and, less frequently, HOS may have breast hypoplasia that may be severe enough for them to seek reconstruction or augmentation. In UMS, the morphology of the breast may be normal, despite an inability or reduced ability to lactate. The etiology of this functional defect is unknown, though the histological appearance of the glandular breast tissue of several women with UMS and reduced lactation was normal (Bamshad, unpublished data). Males with UMS may develop gynecomastia that is symptomatic enough to warrant treatment, although this is usually because of its cosmetic significance.

The overall prognosis for individuals with UMS or HOS is quite good, and many, if not most, individuals with UMS or HOS do not require specialized medical care throughout life. As awareness has increased among health professionals, the practical management of cases has improved. Likewise, among the general public, there is growing acceptance of individuals with medical disabilities. It is not clear that this has diminished the psychological impact of these disorders on affected individuals, though the perception of isolation felt by some patients may have been lessened.

A variety of different advocacy groups for people with only limb defects, only heart malformations, and HOS exist. These groups concentrate on disseminating accurate information to health-care providers and families of affected individuals, promoting the exchange of information among patients and their families, advocating for issues directly pertinent to the perceived needs of their community, and, to a limited extent, supporting clinical research.

Recurrence Risk

UMS and HOS are transmitted in an autosomal-dominant pattern. Accordingly, once a diagnosis is established, the recurrence risk for each disorder is 50%. However, atypical and nonpenetrant cases can diminish the accuracy of estimates of the recurrence risk in individual cases. Thus, the empirical recurrence risk may be less than 50% in sporadic cases putatively diagnosed as HOS in which a mutation in *TBX5* is not identified. However, no such empirical risks have been estimated. Mutation testing for UMS and HOS is available on a research basis.

MODELS OF DISEASE

The most common birth defects observed in humans are those of the limbs and the heart, congenital heart defects being the most common cause of infant mortality in the United States. Knowledge of the pathogenesis of these defects has increased rapidly over the last decade, in part because identification of the molecular basis of human malformation syndromes such as UMS and HOS has often hastened the creation of a model of the condition in an organism such as a mouse or chick. These models can subsequently be studied and manipulated in ways that are neither ethically appropriate nor technically feasible in humans.

The malformations observed in patients with UMS and HOS were hypothesized to be caused by functional haploinsufficiency of *TBX3* and *TBX5*. Thus, one strategy used to clarify their roles in normal development was to create loss-of-function murine mutants (i.e., knockout mice). In practice, this has proved to be challenging, and to date only one group has published the results of their attempts to create knockout mice, specifically mice lacking functional *Tbx5* (Bruneau et al., 2001). To create a Tbx5 null mutant, a mutant allele of *Tbx5* in which exon 3 was flanked by loxP sequences was engineered. Mice bearing this allele were bred to transgenic mice constitutively expressing Cre recombinase. In the presence of Cre, a new *Tbx5* allele was created that lacked exon 3, leading to aberrant splicing of exons 2 and 4 and an allele that, if translated, would consist of only 53 amino acid residues. Presumably, this peptide was inactive.

Mice bearing one nonfunctional allele of Tbx5 (i.e., *Tbx5*$^{+/-}$) recapitulated many of the phenotypic characteristics of HOS, although the severity of the phenotype varied depending on the strain of mouse (Bruneau et al., 2001). This observation is consistent with the variable expression of limb and heart malformations found in many HOS families, further supporting the existence of modifier genes. Only 10% of crosses between 129SvJ Ella-Cre mice and 129SvEv *Tbx5*$^{+/lox}$ mice yielded live pups, the remaining 90% having complex cardiac defects that caused death in utero. In contrast, crosses between 129SvJ Ella-Cre and *Tbx5*$^{+/lox}$ black Swiss mice produced viable and fertile mice with relatively mild heart and limb malformations, through approximately 40% of these *Tbx5*$^{+/-}$ embryos died in utero as well. The mice surviving to 8 weeks of age had dilated atria and large ASDs, whereas the *Tbx5*$^{+/-}$ embryos harvested at day 16.5 were found to have large ASDs and either membranous or muscular VSDs. Conduction abnormalities in surviving mice included first- and second-degree atrioventricular block as well as sinoatrial pauses. The forelimbs of these mice exhibited elongated phalanges of the first digit and a hypoplastic falciformis. No conduction abnormalities were found in the absence of structural heart defects, and the size of the ASD did not correlate with the presence of conduction defects (Bruneau, personal communication).

Development in mice with two nonfunctional alleles of *Tbx5* (i.e., *Tbx5*$^{-/-}$ mice) appeared to be arrested at embryonic day 9.5, and all mice died before embryonic day 10.5 (Bruneau et al., 2001). The primitive inflow tract, atria, and left ventricle were severely hypoplastic; and as a consequence, the right ventricle and outflow tract were markedly distorted. Markers that demarcate particular cardiac cell lineages were variably affected in *Tbx5*$^{-/-}$ mice. *eHand* transcripts that identify the primitive left ventricle were present, *Nkx2-5* expression was reduced, and expression of *ANF* and *cx40* transcripts was absent. The promoters of *ANF* and *cx40* were subsequently found to contain two and five T box–binding elements, respectively, that are homologous to half of the *Brachyury* consensus site. In EMSAs, the *ANF* and *cx40* promoters competed for endogenous T-box proteins from atrial cardiomyocyte nuclear extracts and interacted with recombinant Tbx5. It was further shown that Tbx5 physically interacts with Nkx2-5 to synergistically transactivate *ANF* and *cx40* (Bruneau et al., 2001; Hiroi et al., 2001).

Creation of a murine model of UMS has proven to be more difficult than anticipated, although it has been accomplished (Davenport et al., 2003). Mice heterozygous for a targeted mutation in *Tbx3* appear normal, while homozygotes lack mammary glands, the ulna, and the posterior digits (see Chapter 67). Other strategies to model UMS have attempted to create conditional mutants in which *Tbx3* expression in specific spatial (e.g., forelimb) and temporal (e.g., limb initiation) intervals is eliminated (Moon and Bamshad, unpublished data).

DEVELOPMENTAL PATHOGENESIS

T-box genes are highly conserved among chordates and exhibit tightly regulated spatial and temporal expression patterns during embryogenesis, suggesting that they play important roles in development. This inference was underscored by the discovery that mutations in *TBX3*

and *TBX5* cause multiple-malformation syndromes in humans. As a consequence, understanding the roles of *TBX3* and *TBX5* in normal development has been a major area of investigation over the last several years.

Tbx3/TBX3 is expressed in a wide variety of areas in mouse (Chapman et al., 1996), chick (Gibson-Brown et al., 1996), and human (Bamshad et al., 1999), although most of the tissues and organs in which it is expressed are normal in individuals with UMS. Thus, *TBX3* is likely to play myriad roles in development, although normal levels of TBX3 protein are not necessary for the normal development of many of the tissues in which it is expressed. In contrast, two of the three tissues/areas in which *Tbx5/TBX5* is expressed (i.e., heart and forelimb) are abnormal in individuals with HOS, suggesting that these tissues may be more sensitive to changes in *TBX5* dosage. In addition to the heart and limb, *Tbx5* is expressed in the dorsal side of the developing eye in chick and appears to be involved in determination of the dorsal/ventral axis and the projection of axons between the retina and the tectum (Koshiba-Takeuchi et al., 2000; Uemonsa et al., 2002). *Tbx2* and *Tbx3* are also expressed in the neural retina and have been suggested to provide positional information and differentiation of distinct cell types across the laminar axis of the retina (Sowden et al., 2001).

Expression of *Tbx5* in the developing heart has been widely reported in mice (Chapman et al., 1996; Li et al., 1997; Bruneau et al., 1999, 2001; Liberatore et al., 2000), chick (Gibson-Brown et al., 1996; Bruneau et al., 1999; Liberatore et al., 2000), frog (Horb and Thomsen, 1999), and human (Li et al., 1997; Hatcher et al., 2000). Early in murine embryogenesis, *Tbx5* is expressed uniformly throughout the cardiac crescent, but it is not required for formation of the cardiac crescent (Bruneau et al., 1999, 2001). In the linear heart tube, *Tbx5* expression is greater at the posterior end than the anterior end. Upon looping, *Tbx5* is expressed in the presumptive left ventricle but not in the presumptive right ventricle or outflow tract. In contrast, in human embryos, it is expressed in both ventricles (Li et al., 1997; Hatcher et al., 2000). *Tbx5* is also expressed in the atrial part of the atrioventricular valves and the left side of the ventricular septum. Thus, the pattern of expression provides an embryological basis for the malformations observed in mice lacking one or two functional copies of Tbx5 and in individuals with HOS.

Tbx5 is expressed in heart tissues that are not typically affected in individuals with HOS. For example, although Tbx5 is expressed in the developing atrioventricular valves, these valves are rarely abnormal in individuals with HOS. Studies of the expression pattern of TBX5 protein in human embryonic patterns have reconciled these differences. In a 10-week human heart, TBX5 is present in the walls and septa of all four cardiac chambers, but its expression is higher in the atria than in the ventricles (Hatcher et al., 2000). This may explain, in part, the observation that ASDs are more common than VSDs in individuals with HOS. TBX5 is not expressed in the developing atrioventricular valves or the outflow tract. Interestingly, expression of TBX5 was found to be graded within the myocardium (i.e., higher in the epicardium and lower in the endocardium) of the left-sided, but not right-sided, chambers of the heart. Lastly, TBX5 is also expressed in the adult heart, although the functional significance of this observation remains unknown.

TBX5 is expressed in the atrioventricular node, and this may account for the progressive atrioventricular block observed in individuals with HOS. *Tbx5* also directly activates the transcription of *cx40*, which encodes a component of the gap junctions present at the appositions between Purkinje fibers. Normal levels of *cx40* are necessary to form gap junctions to facilitate the rapid conduction of impulses in the His-Purkinje system. Mice lacking *cx40* have conduction defects (e.g., atrioventricular block) similar to those found in individuals with HOS, although they do not exhibit septal defects (Simon et al., 1998). However, *cx40* is not expressed in the atrioventricular node. This suggests that the conduction defects observed in individuals with HOS may be caused by one or more mechanisms.

The role of T-box genes in limb development has been a popular area of investigation for several reasons. First, the limb has long been considered an excellent model for studying pattern formation and the regulation of growth. Second, in the mid-1990s, studies in mice revealed that the expression patterns of T-box genes in the limb are highly restricted. *Tbx5* is expressed throughout the forelimb, whereas expression of *Tbx4* is limited to the hindlimb (Chapman et al., 1996; Gibson-Brown et al., 1996, 1998). This suggested that *Tbx5* and *Tbx4* might play important roles in determining forelimb and hindlimb identity, respectively. Third, the limb malformations observed in humans with UMS and HOS preferentially affect either the posterior or anterior elements of the upper limb, respectively. This indicates that *TBX3* and *TBX5* might play complementary roles in patterning the anterior/posterior axis of the upper limb (Bamshad et al., 1997).

Over the last few years, a substantial body of experimental data has established that *Tbx5* and *Tbx4* are early markers of the forelimb/wing and hindlimb/leg fields, respectively, in mouse (Chapman et al., 1996; Gibson-Brown et al., 1998), chick (Gibson-Brown et al., 1996; Isaac et al., 1998; Logan et al., 1998; Ohuchi et al., 1998; Rodriguez-Esteban et al., 1999; Saito et al., 2002), and frog (Takabatake et al., 2000). This pattern is conserved in zebrafish as well, with *Tbx5* and *Tbx4* controlling the pattern of pectoral and pelvic fin formation, respectively (Tamura et al., 1999; Begemann and Ingham, 2000; Ahn et al., 2002). While a similar expression pattern is observed in regenerating newt limbs (Simon et al., 1998), *Tbx4* and *Tbx5* appear to be coexpressed in the developing newt limbs (Khan et al., 2002). The mechanism by which limb identity is established in the presence of both Tbx4 and Tbx5 is unknown. The roles of most of the genes that are differentially expressed between the forelimb and hindlimb are unknown. In the hindlimb, the homeobox transcription factor *Pitx1* acts upstream of *Tbx4*, and its expression is necessary for normal hindlimb patterning (Logan et al., 1998; Lanctot et al., 1999; Logan and Tabin, 1999; Szeto et al., 1999).

Misexpression experiments in chick confirm that Tbx4 and Tbx5 also regulate, in part, limb identity (Logan and Tabin, 1999; Rodriguez-Esteban et al., 1999; Takeuchi et al., 1999). For example, misexpression of *Tbx5* in the leg bud induces wing-like skeletal elements and epithelial structures (e.g., feathers instead of scales), while *Tbx4* misexpression in the wing bud results in the formation of a wing with a leg-like appearance, including digits with claws (Takeuchi et al., 1999). FGF-induced ectopic limbs in the flank have wing- or leg-like characteristics depending on the expression patterns of *Tbx5* and *Tbx4*, respectively (Ohuchi et al., 1998; Takeuchi et al., 1999). Limb-specific expression of *Hoxc* genes is also perturbed by misexpressing *Tbx4* and *Tbx5*, suggesting that some *Hox* genes are downstream targets of Tbx4 and Tbx5 in chick limb buds.

Tbx5 misexpression in the leg bud was originally shown to repress *Tbx4* expression, suggesting that one role of *Tbx5* was to repress *Tbx4* expression (Takeuchi et al., 1999). However, *Tbx4* is not expressed in the forelimb field of *Tbx5* null mutants (Agarwal et al., 2002), and conditional deletion of *Tbx5* in the limb at embryonic day 9.5 does not result in the conversion of forelimb to hindlimb identity. These results suggest that T-box genes are not the sole determinants of limb identity. While the forelimb field of *Tbx5*$^{-/-}$ embryos forms, these embryos do not form forelimb buds, and FGF and Wnt regulatory loops are not established. Moreover, *Fgf10* is not expressed in the lateral plate mesoderm of *Tbx5*$^{-/-}$ embryos, and *Tbx5* directly activates *Fgf10* in early limb bud mesenchyme. This suggests that the primary role of *Tbx5* may be to initiate forelimb bud outgrowth from the lateral plate mesoderm (Agarwal et al., 2002).

Similar to the action of *Tbx5* in cardiogenesis, normal development of the limb also appears to be dosage-sensitive. This implies that the varied severity of upper limb truncation defects observed in individuals with HOS may be related to *TBX5* dosage. However, different individuals with the same *TBX5* mutation, including parent–offspring pairs, commonly exhibit upper limb truncations that range from mild to severe. This variability could be due to the effects of modifier genes influencing *TBX5* dosage. If so, one prediction is that the degree of severity of limb defects should be correlated with the degree of relatedness between affected members of the same kindred. This has yet to be formally tested in a large sample of HOS families confirmed to have mutations in *TBX5*. Dosage sensitivity of normal limb development also suggests that mutations that affect the transcriptional efficiency of *TBX5* may cause HOS. This is particularly intriguing because mutations in the coding region account for only 35% of mutations found in probands with HOS. However, no such mutations have been reported.

The role of *Tbx3* in development has been studied less extensively compared to *Tbx5*. The expression pattern in the developing forelimb is complex. In chick and mouse, *Tbx3* is expressed along the anterior and posterior margins of the forelimb separated by a stripe of cells that do not express *Tbx3* (Chapman et al., 1996; Gibson-Brown et al., 1998; Tümpel et al., 2002). Expression along the posterior edge extends into the hand and foot plates to the very tip of the autopod. According to fate maps of stage 20 chick limb buds, these cells along the posterior margin expressing *Tbx3* will give rise to the ulna and posterior digits. In contrast, cells along the anterior margin expressing *Tbx3* contribute little, if anything, to the limb (Vargesson et al., 1997). This is consistent with the observation that limb malformations in individuals with UMS always affect the posterior structures of the upper limb. *Tbx3* is also expressed in the apical ectodermal ridge, a region of specialized epithelium overlying the distal tip of the limb bud that coordinates, in part, outgrowth and pattern formation and the interdigital areas, although expression is eventually limited to the edges of the digital rays.

Characterization of the molecular and cellular processes disrupted by mutations in *TBX5* and *TBX3* is beginning to provide additional insight into the pathogenesis of HOS and UMS, respectively. Basson et al., (1999) reported a correlation between the locations of missense mutations in *TBX5* and the severity of heart and limb malformations in individuals with HOS. Specifically, an amino acid substitution in the N-terminal end of the T-box (Gly^{80}Arg) was found to cause severe heart malformations and mild limb defects in a single large kindred. In contrast, amino acid substitutions in the C-terminal end of the T-box (Arg^{237}Gln, Arg^{237}Trp) were found to cause mild cardiac abnormalities and severe limb defects. Transactivation studies using a native promoter of ANF demonstrated that Tbx5 mutants with a Gly^{80}Arg substitution failed to activate ANF, whereas Tbx5 mutants with a Arg^{237}Gln substitution activated ANF to a level similar to wild-type Tbx5 (Hiroi et al., 2001). Thus, this result might explain the more severe heart malformations caused by the Gly^{80}Arg substitution. However, this conclusion will have to be reconciled with subsequent binding studies of mutant Tbx5 proteins with the same amino acid substitutions, which demonstrated that both Tbx5 mutants failed to bind to a preferred target DNA sequence identified via an in vitro selection procedure (Ghosh et al., 2001). Multiple missense mutations that disrupt the C terminus of the T box have been found in individuals with either mild limb or severe heart limb malformations and no evidence of a genotype–phenotype correlation (Brassington et al., 2003). In contrast to the loss of DNA-binding activity caused by Gly^{80}Arg and Arg^{237}Gln substitutions, binding activity is retained in TBX5 proteins with both the Ser^{252}Ile and Gly^{169}Arg substitutions (Ghosh et al., 2001). A mutant TBX5 protein (Arg^{279}Ter) missing part of the C-terminal domain also retains strong binding activity, although it is unknown whether it is biologically active.

The mouse mutant *Brachyury* is caused by a 200 kb deletion that removes the entire *T* gene and effectively produces a null mutation, and the observed defects in *Brachyury* are thought to result from haploinsufficiency of T protein. In contrast, other *T* alleles (e.g., T^{wis}, T^c, T^{c-2H}) are due to insertions and deletions that cause frameshifts and truncated T proteins (Herrmann, 1991). These alleles retain their DNA-binding activity *in vitro* and produce more severe developmental defects than observed in *T* null mutants. Thus, it has been suggested that they act as dominant-negative mutations (Herrmann, 1991).

Wild-type Tbx3 binds to the canonical *Brachyury*-binding site as a monomer and represses transcription (He et al., 1999; Carlson et al., 2001). However, several regions within Tbx3 have repression, and at least one region has activation activity, though only when isolated from other regions of Tbx3. A key repression domain (amino acids 567–623) resides in the C terminus and is dominant over the activity of transcriptional activators (Carlson et al., 2001). Mutations in *TBX3* that disrupt the DNA-binding domain are predicted to create null alleles, while mutations causing C-terminal truncations could produce null alleles or have a dominant-negative effect. In vitro transcriptional assays have demonstrated that mutations in *TBX3* that cause substitutions in the DNA-binding domain as well as those predicted to encode truncated Tbx3 proteins exhibit either diminished (Tbx3-433 and Tbx3-605) or no (Tbx3-300, Tbx-343, Tbx360) repressor activity (Carlson et al., 2002). Tbx3-652 repressed transcription at a level similar to wild-type Tbx3. These data demonstrate that UMS is caused by haploinsufficiency.

In cell culture, Tbx3 is capable of immortalizing mouse embryo fibroblasts by acting as a negative repressor of p19^{ARF} and p53 and, thus, interferes with apoptosis (Brummelkamp et al., 2002; Carlson et al., 2002). Both missense mutations in *TBX3* (Leu^{143}Pro and Y^{149}Ser) as well as C-terminal truncation mutants fail to repress p19^{ARF} and lose the ability to inhibit apoptotic activity. Thus, the malformations observed in individuals with UMS may be caused by a failure to protect progenitor populations of mesodermal cells from apoptosis. This is similar to effects of mutations in *TP63* that result in a reduction in progenitor cell populations and cause limb and ectodermal defects in EEC syndrome (see Chapter 105) and confirms the hypothesis that EEC syndrome and UMS have a common pathogenetic mechanism (Bamshad et al., 1997).

TBX3 is widely expressed in a variety of tissue and organs that are not affected in individuals with UMS (Bamshad et al., 1999). In other words, development of most tissues in which *TBX3* is expressed is normal in individuals with UMS. This suggests that different tissues may require quantitatively different levels of normal TBX3 protein. Alternatively, other genes, including T-box genes, with expression domains overlapping *TBX3* (e.g., *TBX2*), may be able to compensate for reduced levels of normal TBX3 protein in certain tissues and organs. Such functional redundancy is also observed for other families of transcription factors that play prominent roles in limb development and cause human birth defect syndromes (e.g., *HOX* genes).

Defects of the apocrine glands, teeth, and external genitalia are common in individuals with UMS (Bamshad et al., 1996). This is consistent with the observation that *Tbx3* is expressed in mammary buds, jaw mesenchyme, and genital tubercle (Chapman et al., 1996). Mammary buds are epithelial structures derived from the surface ectoderm. The mammary buds interact with a thickened ridge of underlying mesenchyme (i.e., the milk ridge) to form the branching duct system of the breast (Hennighausen and Robinson, 1998). Similarly, tooth development is initiated by the inductive effect of the oral epithelium on the underlying mesenchyme (Thesleff and Sharpe, 1997), and the epithelium of the genital tubercle has an inductive effect on the underlying mesenchyme that will eventually form the external genitalia (Dolle et al., 1991). Although the apical ectodermal ridge of the limb bud is organized differently, the mammary buds, the oral epithelium, and the epithelium of the genital tubercle each exhibit a similar inductive effect of epithelium on mesenchyme or vice versa.

TBX3 is widely expressed in adult tissues, although the role of *TBX3* beyond organogenesis is largely unexplored. Because delayed puberty is a consistent feature of individuals with UMS, it has been suggested that *TBX3* might participate in the transcriptional control system of the hypothalamic–pituitary–adrenal axis (Bamshad et al., 1996). This is consistent with the observation that *TBX3* is expressed in the adult pituitary and adrenal glands. Moreover, another T-box gene, Tbx19, is essential for the differentiation of pro-opiomelanocortin cells, and mutations in TBX19 cause isolated deficiency of adrenocorticotropin (Lamolet et al., 2001).

REFERENCES

Agarwal P, Wylie JN, Galceran J, Arkhitko O, Li C, Deng C, Grosschedl R, Bruneau BG (2003). Tbx5 is essential for forelimb bud initiation following patterning of the limb field in the mouse embryo. *Development* 130: 623–633.

Agulnik SI, Garvey N, Hancock S, Ruvinsky I, Chapman DL, Agulnik I, Bollag R, Papaioannou V, Silver LM (1996). Evolution of mouse T-box genes by tandem duplication and cluster dispersion. *Genetics* 144: 249–254.

Ahn D, Kourakis MJ, Rohde LA, Silver LM, Ho RK (2002). T-box gene *tbx5* is essential for formation of the pectoral limb bud. *Nature* 417: 754–758.

Akrami SM, Winter RM, Brook JD, Armour JAL (2001). Detectioin of a large tbx5 deletion in a family with Holt-Oram syndrome. *J Med Genet* 38: E44.

Bamshad M, Krakowiak PA, Watkins WS, Root S, Carey JC, Jorde LB (1995). A gene for ulnar-mammary syndrome maps to 12q23-q24.1. *Hum Mol Genet* 4: 1973–1977.

Bamshad M, Root S, Carey JC (1996). Clinical analysis of a large kindred with the Pallister ulnar-mammary syndrome. *Am J Med Genet* 65: 325–331.

Bamshad M, Lin RC, Law DJ, Watkins WS, Krakowiak PA, Moore ME, Franceschini P, Lala R, Holmes LB, Gebuhr TC, et al. (1997). Mutations in human TBX3 alter limb, apocrine and genital development in ulnar-mammary syndrome. *Nat Genet* 16: 311–315.

Bamshad M, Le T, Watkins WS, Dixon ME, Kramer BE, Roeder AD, Carey JC, Root S, Schinzel A, Van Maldergem L, et al. (1999). The spectrum of mutations in TBX3 genotype/phenotype relationship in ulnar-mammary syndrome. *Am J Hum Genet* 64: 1550–1562.

Basson CT, Cowley GS, Solomon SD, Weissman B, Poznanski AK, Traill TA, Seidman JG, Seidman CE (1994). The clinical and genetic spectrum of the Holt-Oram syndrome (heart-hand syndrome). *N Engl J Med* 330: 885–891.

Basson CT, Bachinsky DR, Lin RC, Levi T, Elkins JA, Soults J, Grayzel D, Kroumpouzou E, Traill TA, Leblanc-Straceski J, et al. (1997). Mutations in human [TBX3] cause limb and cardiac malformation in Holt-Oram syndrome. *Nat Genet* 15: 30–35.

Basson CT, Huang T, Lin RC, Bachinsky DR, Weremowicz S, Vaglio A, Bruzzone R, Quadrelli R, Lerone M, Romeo G, et al. (1999). Different tbx5 interactions in heart and limb defined by Holt-Oram syndrome mutations. *Proc Natl Acad Sci USA* 96: 2919–2924.

Begemann G, Ingham PW (2000). Developmental regulation of Tbx5 in zebrafish embryogenesis. *Mech Dev* 90: 299–304.

Birch-Jensen A (1949). Congenital Deformities of the Upper Extremities. Copenhagen: Ejnar Munksgaard.

Bollag RJ, Siegfried RJ, Cebra-Thomas JA, Garvey N, Davison EM, Silver LM (1994). An ancient family of embryonically expressed mouse genes sharing a conserved protein motif with the T locus. *Nat Genet* 7: 383–389.

Botto LD, Khoury MJ, Mastroiacovo P, Castilla EE, Moore CA, Skjaerven R, Mutchinick OM, Borman B, Cocchi G, Czeizel AE, et al. (1997). The spectrum of congenital anomalies of the VATER association: an international study. *Am J Med Genet* 71: 8–15.

Brassington AE, Sung SS, Toydemir RM, Le T, Roeder AD, Rutherford AE, Whitby FG, Jorde LB, Bamshad MJ (2003). Expressivity of Holt-Oram syndrome is not predicted by *TBX5* genotype. *Am J Hum Genet* (in press).

Brummelkamp TR, Kortlever RM, Lingbeek M, Trettel F, MacDonald ME, Lohuizen MV, Bernards R (2002). *Tbx-3*, the gene mutated in ulnar-mammary syndrome, is a negative regulator of p19^{ARF} and inhibits senescence. *J Biol Chem* 277: 6567–6572.

Bruneau BG, Logan M, Davis N, Levi T, Tabin CJ, Seidman JG, Seidman CE (1999). Chamber-specific cardiac expression of tbx5 and heart defects in Holt-Oram syndrome. *Dev Biol* 211: 100–108.

Bruneau BG, Nemer G, Schmitt JP, Charron F, Robitaille L, Caron S, Conner DA, Gessler M, Nemer M, Seidman CE, et al. (2001). A murine model of Holt-Oram syndrome defines roles of the T-box transcription factor tbx5 in cardiogenesis and disease. *Cell* 106: 709–721.

Carlson H, Ota S, Campbell C, Hurlin PJ (2001). A dominant repression domain in tbx3 mediates transcriptional repression and cell immortalization: relevance to mutations in tbx3 that cause ulnar-mammary syndrome. *Hum Mol Genet* 10: 2403–2413.

Carlson H, Ota S, Song Y, Chen Y, Hurlin PJ (2002). Tbx3 impinges on the p53 pathway to suppress apoptosis, facilitate cell transformation and block myogenic differentiation. *Oncogene* 21: 3827–3835.

Chapman DL, Garvey N, Hancock S, Alexiou M, Agulnik SI, Gibson-Brown JJ, Cebra-Thomas J, Bollag RJ, Silver LM, Papaioannou VE (1996). Expression of the T-box family genes, *Tbx1–Tbx5*, during early mouse development. *Dev Dyn* 206: 379–390.

Chariot A, Moreau L, Senterre G, Sobel ME, Castronovo V (1995). Retinoic acid induces three newly cloned HOXA1 transcripts in MCF7 breast cancer cells. *Biochem Biophys Res Commun* 215: 713–720.

Coll M, Seidman JG, Müller CW (2002). Structure of the DNA-bound T-box domain of human tbx3, a transcription factor responsible for ulnar-mammary syndrome. *Structure* 10: 343–356.

Cross SJ, Ching Y, Li QY, Armstrong-Buisseret L, Spranger S, Lyonnet S, Bonnet D, Penttinen M, Jonveaux P, Leheup B, et al. (2000). The mutations spectrum in Holt-Oram syndrome. *J Med Genet* 37: 785–787.

Davenport TG, Jerome-Majewska LA, Papaioannou VE (2003). Mammary gland, limb and yolk sac defects in mice lacking tbx3, the gene mutated in human ulnar mammary syndrome. *Development* 130: 2263–2273.

Dolle P, Izpisua-Belmonte JC, Brown JM, Tickle C, Duboule D (1991). *Hox-4* genes and the morphogenesis of mammalian genitalia. *Genes Dev* 5: 1767–1776.

Edwards MJ, McDonald D, Moore P, Rae J (1994). Scalp-ear-nipple syndrome: additional manifestations. *Am J Med Genet* 50: 247–250.

Franceschini P, Vardeu MP, Dalforno L, Signorile F, Franceschini D, Lala R, Matarazzo P (1992). Possible relationship between ulnar-mammary syndrome and split hand with aplasia of the ulna syndrome. *Am J Med Genet* 44: 807–812.

Gall JC, Stern AM, Cohen MM, Adams MS, Davidson RT (1966). Holt-Oram syndrome: clinical and genetic study of a large family. *Am J Hum Genet* 18: 187–199.

Ghosh TK, Packman EA, Bonser AJ, Robinson TE, Cross SJ, Brook SJ (2001). Characterization of the TBX5 binding site and analysis of mutations that cause Holt-Oram syndrome. *Hum Mol Genet* 10: 1983–1994.

Gibson-Brown JJ, Agulnik SI, Chapman DL, Alexious M, Garvey N, Silver LM, Papaioannou VE (1996). Evidence of a role for T-box genes in the evolution of limb morphogenesis and the specification of forelimb/hindlimb identity. *Mech Dev* 56: 93–101.

Gibson-Brown JJ, Agulnik SI, Silver LM, Niswander L, Papaioannou VE (1998). Involvement of T-box genes *Tbx2–Tbx5* in vertebrate limb specification and development. *Development* 125: 2499–2509.

Gilly E (1882). Absence complète des mamelles chez une femme mère: atropie du membre superieur droit. *Courrier Med* 32: 27–28.

Gonzalez CH, Herrmann J, Opitz JM (1976). Mother and son affected with the ulnar-mammary syndrome type Pallister. *Eur J Pediatr* 123: 225–235.

Hall JG, Levin J, Kuhn JP, Ottenheimer EJ, Van Berkum KAP, McKusick VA (1969). Thrombocytopenia with absent radius (TAR). *Medicine* 48: 411–439.

Hatcher CJ, Goldstein MM, Mah CS, Delia S, Basson CT (2000). Identification and localization of tbx5 transcription factor during human cardiac morphogenesis. *Dev Dyn* 219: 90–95.

He M, Wen L, Campbell CE, Wu JY, Rao Y (1999). Transcription repression by *Xenopus ET* and its human ortholog *tbx3*, a gene involved in ulnar-mammary syndrome. *Proc Natl Acad Sci USA* 96: 10212–10217.

Hecht JT, Scott CI Jr (1984). The Schinzel syndrome in a mother and daughter. *Clin Genet* 25: 63–67.

Hennighausen L, Robinson GW (1998). Think globally, act locally: the making of a mouse mammary gland. *Genes Dev* 12: 449–455.

Herrmann BG (1991). Expression pattern of the *Brachyury* gene in whole-mount Twis/Twis mutant embryos. *Development* 113: 913–917.

Herrmann BG, Labeit S, Poustka A, King TR, Lehrach H (1990). Cloning of the T gene required in mesoderm formation in mouse. *Nature* 343: 617–622.

Hiroi Y, Kudoh S, Monzen K, Ikeda Y, Yazaki Y, Nagai R, Komuro I (2001). Tbx5 associates with Nkx2-5 and synergistically promotes cardiomyocyte differentiation. *Nat Genet* 28: 276–280.

Holt M, Oram S (1960). Familial heart disease with skeletal malformation. *Br Heart J* 22: 236–242.

Horb ME, Thomsen GH (1999). Tbx5 is essential for heart development. *Development* 126: 1739–1751.

Isaac A, Rodriguez-Esteban C, Ryan A, Altabef M, Tsukui T, Patel K, Tickle C, Izpisua-Belmonte JC (1998). *Tbx* genes and limb identity in chick embryo development. *Development* 125: 1867–1875.

Karnak I, Tanyel FC, Tunçbilek E, Unsal M, Büyükpamukçu N (1998). Bilateral Poland anomaly. *Am J Med Genet* 75: 505–507.

Khan P, Linkhart B, Simon H (2002). Different regulation of T-box genes *Tbx4* and *Tbx5* during limb development and limb regeneration. *Dev Biol* 250: 383–392.

Kispert A, Herrmann BG (1993). The *Brachyury* gene encodes a novel DNA binding protein. *EMBO J* 12: 3211–3220.

Kispert A, Koschorz B, Herrmann BG (1995). The T protein encoded by Brachyury is a tissue-specific transcription factor. *EMBO J* 14: 4763–4772.

Kohlhase J, Heinrich M, Shubert L, Liebers M, Kispert A, Laccone F, Turnpenny P, Winter RM, Reardon W (2002). Okihiro syndrome is caused by SALL4 mutations. *Hum Mol Genet* 11: 2979–2987.

Koshiba-Takeuchi K, Takeuchi JK, Matsumoto K, Momose T, Uno K, Hoepker V, Ogura K, Takahashi N, Nakamura H, Yusuda K, et al. (2000). Tbx5 and the retinotectum projection. *Science* 287: 134–137.

Lamolet B, Pulichino AM, Lamonerie T, Gauthier Y, Brue T, Enjalbert A, Drouin J (2001). Pituitary cell-restricted T box facdtdor, Tpit, activates POMC transcription in cooperation with Pitx homeoprotein. *Cell* 104: 849–859.

Lanctot C, Moreau A, Chamberland M, Tremblay ML, Drouin J (1999). Hindlimb patterning and mandible development require the Ptx1 gene. *Development* 126: 1805–1810.

Li QY, Newbury-Ecob RA, Terrett JA, Wilson DI, Curtis ARJ, Yi CH, Gebuhr T, Bullen PJ, Robson SC, Strachan T, et al. (1997). Holt-Oram syndrome is caused by mutations in *TBX5*, a member of the *Brachyury* (T) gene family. *Nat Genet* 15: 21–29.

Liberatore CM, Searcy-Schrick RD, Yutzey KE (2000). Ventricular expression of the tbx5 inhibits normal heart chamber development. *Dev Biol* 223: 169–180.

Logan M, Tabin CJ (1999). Role of pitx1 upstream of tbx4 in specification of hindlimb identity. *Science* 283: 1736–1739.

Logan M, Simon HG, Tabin C (1998). Differential regulation of T-box and homeobox transcription factors suggests roles in controlling chick limb-type identity. *Development* 125: 2825–2835.

Meinecke P, Stier U, Blunck W (1989). Normal hands and feet in the ulnary-mammary syndrome. *Dysmorphol Clin Genet* 3: 61–64.

Müller CW, Herrmann BG (1997). Crystallographic structure of the T domain–DNA complex of the Brachyury transcription factor. *Nature* 389: 884–888.

Newbury RA, Leanage R, Raeburn JA, Yound ID (1996). Holt-Oram syndrome: a clinical genetic study. *J Med Genet* 33: 300–307.

Ohuchi H, Takeuchi J, Yoshioka H, Ishimaru Y, Ogura K, Takahashi N, Ogura T, Noji S (1998). Correlation of wing-leg identity in ectopic FGF-induced chimeric limbs with the differential expression of chick tbx5 and tbx4. *Development* 125: 51–60.

Okihiro MM, Tasaki T, Nakano KK, Bennett BK (1977). Duane syndrome and congenital upper-limb anomalies: a familial occurrence. *Arch Neurol* 34: 174–179.

Pallister PD, Herrmann J, Opitz JM (1976). Studies of malformation syndromes in man XXXXII: a pleiotropic dominant mutation affecting skeletal, sexual and apocrine-mammary development. *Birth Defects* 12: 247–254.

Papapetrou C, Edwards YH, Sowden JC (1997). The T transcription factor functions as a dimer and exhibits a common human polymorphism Gly-177-Asp in the conserved DNA-binding domain. *FEBS Lett* 409: 201–206.

Poznanski AK, Gall JC Jr., Stern AM (1970). Skeletal manifestations of the Holt-Oram syndrome. *Radiology* 94: 45–54.

Rodriguez-Esteban C, Tsukui T, Yonei S, Magallon J, Tamura T, Belmonte JCI (1999). The T-box genes *tbx4* and *tbx5* regulate limb outgrowth and identity. *Nature* 398: 814–818.

Rogers C, Anderson G (1995). Hand-foot-uterus syndrome in a patient with overlapping phenotypic features. *Proc Greenwood Genet Center* 14: 17–20.

Ruiz de la Fuente S, Prieto F (1980). Heart-hand syndrome. III. A new syndrome in three generations. *Hum Genet* 55: 43–47.

Ruvinsky I, Gibson-Brown JJ (2000). Genetic and developmental bases of serial homology in vertebrate limb evolution. *Development* 127: 5233–5244.

Saito D, Yonei-Tamura S, Kano K, Ide H, Tamura K (2002). Specification and determination of limb identity: evidence for inhibitory regulation of *Tbx* gene expression. *Development* 129: 211–220.

Sasaki G, Ogata T, Ishii T, Hasegawa T, Sata S, Matsuo N (2002). Novel mutation of tbx3 in a Japanese family with ulnar-mammary syndrome: implication for impaired sex development. *Am J Med Genet* 110: 365–369.

Schinzel A (1987). Ulnar-mammary syndrome. *J Med Genet* 24: 778–781.

Schinzel A, Illig R, Prader A (1987). The ulnar-mammary syndrome: an autosomal dominant pleiotropic gene. *Clin Genet* 32: 160–168.

Silengo MC, Biagioli M, Guala A, Lopez-Bell G, Lala R (1990). Heart-hand syndrome II. A report of Tabatznik syndrome with new findings. *Clin Genet* 38: 105–113.

Simon AM, Goodenoug DA, Paul DL (1998). Mice lacking connexin40 have cardiac conduction abnormalities characteristic of atrioventricular block and bundle branch block. *Curr Biol* 8: 295–298.

Sletten LJ, Pierpont ME (1996). Variation in severity of cardiac disease in Holt-Oram syndrome. *Am J Med Genet* 65: 128–132.

Sowden JC, Holt JKL, Meins M, Smith HK, Bhattacharya SS (2001). Expression of *Drosophila* omb-related T-box genes in the developing human and mouse neural retina. *Invest Ophthalmol Vis Sci* 42: 3095–3102.

Szeto DP, Rodriguez-Esteban C, Ryan AK, O'Connell SM, Lui F, Kioussi C, Gleiberman AS, Izpisua-Belmonte JC, Rosenfeld MG (1999). Role of the Bicoid-related homeodomain factor Pitx1 in specifying hindlimb morphogenesis and pituitary development. *Gene Dev* 13: 484–494.

Takabatake Y, Takabatake T, Takeshima K (2000). Conserved and divergent expression of T-box genes *Tbx2–Tbx5* in *Xenopus*. *Mech Dev* 91: 433–437.

Takeuchi JK, Koshiba-Takeuchi K, Matsumoto K, Vogel-Hopker A, Naitoh-Matsuo M, Ogura K, Takahashi N, Yasuda K, Ogura T (1999). *Tbx5* and *Tbx4* genes determine the wing/leg identity of limb buds. *Nature* 398: 810–814.

Tamura K, Yonei-Tamura S, Belmonte JCI (1999). Differential expression of tbx4 and tbx5 in zebrafish fin buds. *Mech Dev* 87: 181–184.

Temtamy SA, McKusick VA (1978). *The Genetics of Hand Malformations*. Alan R. Liss, New York, pp. 117–133.

Terrett JA, Newbury-Ecob R, Cross GS, Fenton I, Raeburn JA, Young ID, Brook JD (1994). Holt-Oram syndrome is a genetically heterogeneous disease with one locus mapping to human chromosome 12q. *Nat Genet* 6: 401–404.

Thesleff I, Sharpe P (1997). Signalling networks regulating dental development. *Mech Dev* 67: 111–123.

Tümpel S, Sanz-Ezquerro JJ, Isaac A, Eblaghie MC, Dobson J, Tickle C (2002). Regulation of *Tbx3* expression by anteroposterior signalling in vertebrate limb development. *Dev Biol* 250: 251–262.

Uemonsa T, Sakagami K, Yasuda K, Araki M (2002). Development of dorsal–ventral polarity in the optic vesicle and its presumptive role in eye morphogenesis as shown by embryonic transplantation and in ovo explant culturing. *Dev Biol* 248: 319–330.

Vargesson N, Clarke JD, Vincent K, Coles C, Wolpert L, Tickle C (1997). Cell fate in the chick limb bud and relationship to gene expression. *Development* 124: 1909–1918.

Yang J, Hu D, Xia J, Yang Y, Ying B, Hu J, Zhou X (2000). Three novel TBX5 mutations in Chinese patients with Holt-Oram syndrome. *Am J Med Genet* 92: 237–240.

V
PROCESSES

Part A.
Regulation of Chromatin Structure and Gene Expression

70 | Mechanisms of Regulated Gene Transcription

MICHAEL G. ROSENFELD, KRISTEN JEPSEN, OLA HERMANSON, AND CHRISTOPHER K. GLASS

Precisely regulated patterns of gene expression underlie the development and homeostatic control of all metazoan organisms. In turn, regulation occurs at the level of gene transcription, RNA processing, export, mRNA stability, and translation, and complex machinery that serves to regulate gene transcription affords highly gene-specific patterns of regulation.

Studies of the molecular basis for gene transcription have linked the processes of transcription initiation, elongation of nascent transcripts, mRNA splicing, termination, and polyadenylation, as well as the control of RNA stability (reviewed in Maniatis and Reed, 2002). Coupling between transcription and RNA splicing is well-documented (Bentley, 1999; Hirose and Manley, 2000; Proudfoot et al., 2000; Shatkin and Manley, 2000; Cramer et al., 2001). The control of transcription involves DNA-bound transcription factors, which can function as either activators or repressors, and factors that act without binding DNA, resulting in "*trans*"-activation or repression events. Transcription requires the actions of families of complexes essential for the function of RNA polymerase II (Pol II), including TFIIA, TFIIB, TFIID, TFIIE, TFIIF, and TFIIH (Conaway and Conaway, 1993; Orphanidus et al., 1996; Roeder, 1996; Lemon and Tjian 2000; Butler and Kadonaga, 2002). Indeed, various combinations of the TATA box, TFIIB recognition element, initiator (Inr), and downstream core promoter element serve to provide specific complex enhancers (Butler and Kadonaga, 2002). The "general" transcription factors position and orient Pol II on the canonic elements, determining the initiation site. DNA binding transcription factors, which constitute a significant percentage of the mammalian genome, are generally divided into families based on shared properties of their DNA-binding domains, such as nuclear receptors, homeodomain proteins, the winged helix family, the Cys·His zinc finger family, β-helix-loop-helix factors, CCATT binding factors, and others. These DNA-binding transcription factors, however, appear to require the recruitment of multiple complexes, containing regulating molecules referred to as co-activators or co-repressors, that serve as a functional linkage between DNA bound transcription factors and the core machinery (reviewed in Kingston and Narlikar, 1999; Glass and Rosenfeld, 2000), which includes factors that bind at the core, such as TAFs, TFIIA, NC2, and PC4, and with Pol II (mediator SMCC/Srb) (Myers and Kornberg, 2000). Together, these factors constitute the preinitiation complex, with cofactors that are recruited by DNA-bound transcription factors at promoters or enhancers, serving to alter chromatin structure and impinge on core machinery, regulating gene expression. Co-activator complexes contain factors with a series of enzymatic activities, including histone factor acetyltransferase, protein methyltranserase, DNA methylase, ADP ribosyltransferase, and protein kinase activity, and that act as remodeling complexes (e.g., SWI/SNF, ISWF-ATPases) (reviewed in Lemon and Tjian, 2000), which are recruited to DNA-bound transcription factors. Positioning of the promoter is achieved under control of TFIIE and the helicase functions of TFIIH, with Pol II disengagement required for RNA elongation. The transcriptional machinery required can be considered as those components required for transcription from a naked DNA template and those factors required to permit transcription from a chromatinized template. The DNA-binding transcription factors communicate with the core machinery via recruitment of complexes referred to as co-activators or co-repressors. Literally, hundreds of such cofactors have been identified. The balance of co-activator and co-repressor complexes serves to regulate not only activation or repression events but also the level of specific gene expression.

The complexity of regulatory machinery is expanded by the presence of the alternative splice forms of many components, their covalent modification, and specific temporal and spatial expression of gene families and the spatial regulation of their expression. Further, many co-activators and co-repressors have been identified as present in multiple complexes. For example, more than 70 "co-activators" have been demonstrated for nuclear receptors (reviewed in Hermanson et al., 2002).

Activation of events in the context of dynamically regulated chromatinized templates requires a factor-mediated transition between compact heterochromatinized regions and derepressed regions capable of activation. This is a critical process in developmental and cell-type specification events.

The complexity imposed by the large number of co-regulatory complexes provides a potential molecular basis for cell-type and promoter-specific patterns of gene expression and the ability to integrate multiple signaling pathways to achieve selective patterns of gene expression at the level of the nucleus. Further, the potential specificity of the regulating machinery provides an opportunity to intervene in a gene-selective or even a gene-specific manner to modify the pattern of gene expression. The principle of transcriptional regulation, which underlies many diseases of development, homeostasis, and tumor formation, is exemplified by the regulation of gene expression by nuclear receptors.

TRANSCRIPTIONAL CO-ACTIVATORS IN NUCLEAR RECEPTOR FUNCTION

Members of the nuclear receptor superfamily can directly activate or repress target genes by binding to hormone response elements (HREs) in promoter or enhancer regions. Alternatively, these factors can bind to other DNA sequence-specific activators and can either enhance or inhibit the transcriptional activities of other classes of transcription factors, referred to as *transrepression* (Fig. 70–1). Nuclear receptor DNA response elements recruit specific receptor homodimers on heterodimers based on the orientation and spacing of the core binding motifs. When these are present as direct repeats, asymmetry is provided to the response element (Glass and Rosenfeld, 2000). Nuclear receptor functions are directed by specific activation domains—one in the N terminus, referred to as *activation function 1* (AF1), and a second in the C-terminal ligand binding domain (LBD), referred to as *activation function 2* (AF2) (Bourguet et al., 2000). Most evidence supports a model in which ligand-dependent exchange of co-repressors for co-activators serves as the basic mechanism for switching gene re-

pression to activation and indicates the level of their activity. It appears that co-regulatory complexes are differentially used in both a cell- and promoter-specific manner to activate or repress gene transcription. Because the co-regulatory components recruited to the nuclear receptors are themselves targets of regulation by diverse intracellular signaling pathways, this provides a combinatorial code for tissue- and gene-specific responses. These factors use both their specific enzymatic and platform assembly functions to mediate nuclear receptor genetic programs critical for developmental and homeostatic processes in metazoans.

A diverse group of proteins have emerged as potential co-activators for nuclear receptors (Fig. 70–2). Ligand-dependent recruitment of co-activators is dependent on AF2, which consists of a short conserved helical sequence within the C terminus of the LBD (Bourguet et al., 2000). A large number of factors interact with nuclear receptors, in either a ligand-independent or a ligand-dependent manner, and are often components of large, multiprotein complexes, most of these factors interact with the LBD, but a distinct set of co-activators are associated with the N-terminal domain. Because interaction helices with a core LXXLL that interact with a single nuclear receptor C-terminal hydrophobic pocket are used by so many co-activators, a major conceptual problem is that the number of potential co-regulators clearly exceeds the capacity for direct interaction by a single receptor (Rosenfeld and Glass, 2001; McKenna et al., 2002). The most plausible hypothesis for why the number of potential co-regulators exceeds the capacity for direct interaction by a single receptor is that transcriptional activation by nuclear receptors involves the actions and possible interactions of multiple factors. These factors could act in either a sequential and/or a combinatorial manner to reorganize chromatin templates and to modify and recruit basal factors and RNA polymerase II (Wu, 1997; Wade and Wolffe, 1999). It is likely that these co-activator complexes provide specific enzymatic functions required to remodel chromatin and to alter properties of DNA binding factors, as well as the function of platforms that are required for interactions with components of the core machinery.

Several insights into the mechanisms by which co-activator complexes are recruited to nuclear receptors in a ligand-dependent manner have been provided by the identification of one group of co-activators, the p160 family of nuclear receptor co-activators, referred to as SRC1/NCOA1, TIF2/GRIP1, and P/CIP/A1B-1/ACTR/RAC/TRAM-1 (Glass and Rosenfeld, 2000; McKenna et al., 1999). The p160 factors consist of three members that exhibit a common domain structure. A central conserved domain mediates ligand-dependent interactions with the nuclear receptor LBD, whereas the conserved C-terminal transcriptional activation domains mediate interactions with either CBP/p300 or with protein arginine methyltransferase (Chen et al., 1999; Koh et al., 2001), respectively, thereby recruiting additional complexes to promoter-bound nuclear receptors in a ligand-dependent manner (Torchia et al., 1997; Kurokawa et al., 1998). Biochemical studies have also demonstrated strong, ligand-dependent interactions between nuclear receptors and p140 factors, probably representing the co-regulator RIP140, which results in a reproductive defect in female mice on gene deletion (White et al., 2000) but which can serve as a negative regulator of specific p160-dependent activation events.

One way of considering the requirement for the numerous complexes that mediate nuclear receptor–dependent transcription is that distinct protein complexes are required to act sequentially, combinatorially, or in parallel to mediate specific required events. For example, one group of recruited proteins that disrupts chromatin formation, such as the BRG-1 complex, functioning analogous to the yeast SWI/SNF complex, may be responsible for chromatin remodeling. Factors such as CBP, p300, and pCAF/GCN5L have acetyltransferase activity (Yang et al., 1996; Grant et al., 1997). Biochemical studies and protein–protein interaction screens suggest that many of these proteins function as components of large, multiprotein complexes and that additional enzymatic activities may be important for their function. For example, p160 co-activator proteins, such as GRIP-1, can associate with arginine methyltransferase 1 (CARM1), which potentiates ligand-dependent transcription by several nuclear receptors (Chen et al.,

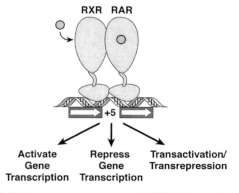

Figure 70–1. Nuclear receptors, such as the REX.RAR heterodimer, can either activate or repress gene transcription or act in *trans* with other DNA-binding factors to initiate or repress gene expression.

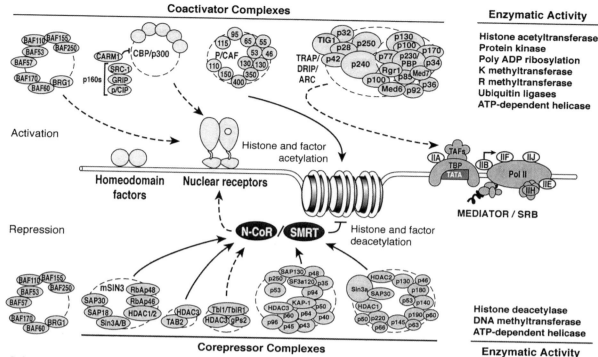

Figure 70–2. Cofactor complexes regulate gene expression. Alternative recruitment of multiple coactivator complexes (a few are schematically) or corepressor complexes (only N-CoR/SMRT complexes are shown) lead to gene activation of repression. In each case, numerous enzymatic activities contribute to the activation or repression events.

1999). PRMTI, a second arginine methyltransferase related to CARM1, also functions independently as a nuclear receptor co-activator (Koh et al., 2001). The CBP/P300 co-activators can recruit additional factors with HAT activity, such as the p/CAF/Gcn5L complexes (Ogryzko et al., 1996; Kurokawa et al., 1998). The number of subunits and their varying contents and conformations of the recruited complexes may explain why distinct acetyltransferases are required by different DNA-bound transcription factors on specific gene targets (Korzus et al., 1998).

In addition to co-activator complexes that harbor nucleosome remodeling or histone acetyltransferase, a series of other co-activator complexes have been identified. The most well characterized of these is the TRAP/DRIP/ARC complex, which enhances the transcriptional activities of nuclear receptors and other signal-dependent transcription factors in vitro (Rachez et al., 1998; Fondell et al., 1999; Näär et al., 1999). The TRAP/DRIP/ARC complex is recruited to nuclear receptors in a ligand-dependent manner via a 220-kDa component referred to as PBP/TRAP220/DRIP205 (Lee et al., 1995b; Zhu et al., 1997). Disruption of the *TRAP/220/DRIP205/PBP* gene in the mouse results in early embryonic lethality (E11.5), and initial studies in mouse embryo fibroblasts (MEFs) have suggested a defect in ligand-dependent thyroid hormone and peroxisome proliferator-activated receptor-γ (PPARγ) function (Lee et al., 1995b; Näär et al., 1999). Other classes of transcription factors appear to remain competent to activate transcription in these cells, consistent with the model that distinct components interact with different DNA-binding transcription factors. The TRAP/DRIP/ARC complex consists of more than a dozen polypeptides, a subset of which appears to constitute modules that are components of other activator complexes, including CRSP, NAT, SMCC, and mouse Srb mediator, none of which have known HAT activity (Fondell et al., 1999; Ito et al., 1999; Naar et al., 1999) but which may interact with additional complexes. Although the TRAP/DRIP/ARC complex is not stably associated with RNA polymerase II, it can be co-immunoprecipitated in the presence of ligand-activated vitamin D receptor (Rachez et al., 1999). Thus, either conformational changes and/or recruitment of additional components permits a stable interaction with RNA polymerase II complexes.

Complexes that contain factors similar or homologous to factors in the yeast mediator complex (i.e., TRAP-SMCC-DRIP-ARC) have been isolated by co-precipitation of different transcription factors.

Many of the proteins in the TRAP-SMSCC-DRIP-ARC complex are present in more than one complex and might be involved in bridging the RNA polymerase II complex with basal transcription factors, although additional functions for these factors must also be considered. Related complexes include CRSP and PC2 (Ryu and Tjian, 1999), ARC/DRIP/TRAP (Yuan et al., 1998; Näär et al., 1999; Rachez et al., 1999) and NAP/SMCC/Srb (Sun et al., 1998; Gu et al., 1999).

Many or most co-activator complexes can act in synergy or antagonistically to other complexes. For example, ASC2 is a complex that interacts not only with nuclear receptors but also with CBP/p300 or the DRIP130/CRSP130/Sur2 component of TRAP/DRIP/ARC, via a domain in its C terminus (Lee et al., 1999), as well as with factors of the basal transcription complex (Yao et al., 1998).

Consistent with their functions, diverse phenotypes are observed in mice deleted or mutated for genes encoding these coactivators. Mice lacking CBP or p300 die early in embryogenesis, with severe defects in hematopoiesis and neural development (Yao et al., 1998; Oike et al., 1999); defects include impairment in retinoic acid receptor signaling (Yao et al., 1998) and evidence that p300 regulates proliferation. Animals lacking PBP/TRIP2/TRAP220/DRIP205/RB18A, a co-activator component of the mediator complex, also show embryonic lethality and impaired transcription by thyroid receptor and PPAR (Ito et al., 2000; Zhu et al., 2000). Mice lacking p160 factors, such as NCoA1/SRC1/p160, are viable and grossly normal, probably because of functional redundancy among the three class members (Xu et al., 1998), but exhibit defects of steroid and thyroid hormone action (Xu et al., 1998; Weiss et al., 1999; Wang et al., 2000). Levels of the nuclear receptor co-activator pCIP/ACTR/AIB1/SRC3 (Torchia et al., 1997) are increased in certain epithelial breast cancers (Anzick et al., 1997). Chromosomal rearrangements leading to either constitutively active or disrupted function of CBP or p300 have been demonstrated in certain leukemias such as acute myeloid leukemia (AML) (Ida et al., 1997; Darimont et al., 1998). Conversely, co-repressors such as N-CoR and SMRT have also been linked to AML, in addition to PML, via translocations to generate ETO and retinoic acid receptor fusions, respectively (Puigsever et al., 1998; Stromberg et al., 1999).

The fact that many co-regulators exhibit temporal and/or tissue-specific differences in expression, with levels often varying dramatically among tissues and specific cell types (Monsalve et al., 2000), provides one explanation for differential gene regulation in distinct cell types (Moilanen et al., 1999). For example, the dramatic increase in the levels of PGC1 in brown fat provides a cell- and tissue-specific mechanism for transcriptional regulation by PPARγ. Functionally, PGC1 also regulates RNA processing when bound to a promoter (Wang et al., 2000). Many co-regulators, such as PGC1, are present in different protein–protein complexes at different times in the same cell. In other cases, the intracellular partitioning of cofactors in nucleus and cytoplasm provides a regulated step in the control of gene expression (Glass and Rosenfeld, 2000).

In summary, biochemical and genetic studies suggest that co-regulatory complexes are differentially used in both a cell- and promoter-specific manner to activate or repress gene transcription. These co-regulatory components are themselves targets of diverse intracellular signaling pathways and provide a combinatorial code for tissue- and gene-specific responses, using both enzymatic and platform assembly functions to mediate the actions of nuclear receptor genetic programs critical for developmental and homeostatic processes in metazoan organisms.

The direct evidence of the roles of multiple complexes has been fortified by chromatin immunoprecipitation assays. For example, a number of complexes are "simultaneously" bound to estrogen receptor target genes in response to hormone (Shang et al., 2000). Whether these complexes indeed simultaneously contact each estrogen receptor is not yet established through this technique, especially in light of evidence of rapid turnover of DNA-bound receptors (McNally et al., 2000). A rapid turnover of receptors has been reported on response elements of hormonally induced genes, based on the turnover of fluorescent-labeled glucocorticoid receptors in a cell line containing a multimerized integrate of mouse mammary tumor virus (MMTV) promoter/transcription units (McNally et al., 2000). Because this rapid exchange involves receptors particularly associated with different co-activator complexes, one could speculate that this would provide a mechanism for combinatorial regulation of gene expression. Alternatively, multiple complexes may be components of a "super" activation complex, but with variation in the primary contact or contacts with DNA-bound transcription factors.

COFACTOR REGULATION

Many co-regulators shuttle between intracellular compartments, often by associating with a DNA-binding transcription factor or cofactors (Korzus et al., 1998; McInerney et al., 1998; Heery et al., 2001). Indeed, specific classes of transcription factors, including nuclear receptors, translocate between cytoplasm and nucleus, and their appear to serve as co-regulators for actions of other classes of transcription factors, such as nuclear factor-κB and certain Smads.

Protein kinases such as MEKK1 and CASK/LIN2 can translocate to the nucleus and exert roles in derepression and activation of specific transcription factors (Rachez et al., 1998; Baek et al., 2002). Another putative mechanism for modulating cellular co-regulator levels and function is regulated proteolysis. Regulated proteolysis of DNA-binding transcription factors has previously been implicated in cell cycle regulation (Näär et al., 1999).

Several proteins involved in proteolysis have been suggested as nuclear receptor co-regulators. Three of the TRAP/DRIP/Arc proteins are involved in proteolysis (Lee et al., 1995a). Studies have demonstrated ligand-induced ubiquitination and proteosome-dependent degradation of nuclear receptors, such as thyroid hormone receptor (Ito et al., 1999), but it is not known which factors regulate such degradation events. Proteolysis is a suggested regulatory mechanism for specific nuclear receptor–mediated transcription (McKenna et al., 2002), and such mechanisms have been suggested to play a role in neurodegenerative diseases, such as Alzheimer's disease (Alves-Rodrigues et al., 1998).

The activities of many co-regulators, including CBP, p300, and the p160 factors, are modulated by protein kinases, including those involved in the regulation of cell cycle progression (Ait-Si-Ali et al.,

1998), but the full in vivo functional significance remains to be determined (McKinsey et al., 2000; Zhou et al., 2000). Modulation of co-regulators through a crosstalk of phosphorylation and acetylation events may mediate signal-specific gene regulation events (Boyes et al., 1998; Deckert and Struhl, 2001). Conversely, regulation of histone deacetylase activity and subcellular localization by CaM kinases and mitogen-activated protein (MAP) kinases have been reported (Imhof et al. 1997; Munshi et al. 1998).

ACETYLATION AND METHYLATION OF TRANSCRIPTION FACTORS

Many co-regulators, including CBP, p300, p/CAF, and GCN5, contain acetyltransferase activity–modifying histones, transcription factors, and other co-regulators in function. These factors acetylate specific lysines in the N termini of histone tails. Hyperacetylation of histones H3 and H4 is associated with increased transcriptional activity on many promoters (Perissi et al., 1999). A histone "code" has been described in which the multiple modifications of each of the histone cores, including acetylation, methylation, phosphorylation, ADP ribosylation effecting histones H3, H4, H2A, and H2B, acts as "marks" of gene activation or repression events. Different combinations of modifications have distinct regulatory consequences (Jenuwein and Allis, 2001). Acetylation can alter the activity of DNA-binding transcription factors (Bannister et al., 2000; Soutoglou et al., 2000) and basal transcription factors (Chen et al., 1999). An example is HMG 17, which can interact with the thyroid hormone receptor (Ito et al., 1999; Rachez et al., 1999; Koh et al., 2001). A functional role for the acetylation of co-regulators has been suggested, such as modulation of their interactions (Xu et al., 2001).

Both DNA and protein methylation are regulators of gene transcription. One nuclear receptor coactivator, CARM1, is an arginine methyltransferase that is recruited to other co-activators, such as SRC-1/NCoA-1/p160 (Chen et al., 1999). A second arginine methyltransferase has also been shown to interact with p160 cofactors and to increase the transcriptional activity of nuclear receptors (Lanz et al., 1999). Consistent with the increasing evidence of links between methylation and acetylation, there is a reciprocal modulation of histone phosphorylation–acetylation events by methylation (Jenuwein and Allis, 2001). Several RNA processing factors are also modulated by methylation (Shi et al., 2001), and a small RNA (SRA) has been suggested to serve as a co-activator for steroid receptors (Lanz et al., 2002), interacting with multiple nuclear receptor–associated co-regulators (Shi et al., 2001; Watanabe et al., 2001). It is likely that there may be many small RNAs and RNA-binding factors that will be specifically linked to gene transcription and methylation events and also modulate cellular localization events. For example, nuclear translocalization of STAT1 and its association with PIAS1/GBP is regulated by the methyltransferase PRMT1 (Mowen et al., 2001). Thus, numerous enzymatic activities that include methylation, phosphorylation, acetylation, and ADP ribosylation are suggested to serve important functions in the modulation of transcriptional activation, acting at the level of both chromatin and the transcription apparatus.

TRANSCRIPTIONAL REPRESSION

Transcriptional repression plays as equally a fundamental role as does activation in developmental and homeostatic regulation. Repression has been demonstrated to occur via several distinct mechanisms, including competition for DNA binding with activators, sequestering or relocalizing of activators, interactions with core transcriptional machinery, DNA methylation, and the recruitment of complexes with histone deacetylase activity. Even recruitment of a loss of effective DNA binding activation or co-activator can reduce gene expression and constitute a "repressive" event.

The knowledge that the thyroid hormone and retinoic acid receptors (T₃R and RAR) actively repress transcription in the absence of their cognate ligands via transferable repression domains (Baniahmad et al., 1992; Xu et al., 1996) led to the identification of a 270-kDa protein associated with unliganded T₃R/RXR heterodimers and the cloning of the nuclear receptor co-repressor (N-CoR) (Hörlein et al., 1995) and a homologous protein termed silencing mediator of retinoic acid and thyroid hormone receptors (SMRTs) (Chen and Evans, 1995; Ordentlich et al., 1999; Park et al., 1999).

N-CoR and SMRT both contain conserved bipartite nuclear receptor interaction domains (Seol et al., 1996; Zamir et al., 1996; Li et al., 1997a), with each containing a critical L-X-X-X-I-X-X-X-I/L motif, which included the L/I-X-X-I/V-I motif termed the CoRNR box (Hu and Lazar, 1999; Nagy et al., 1999; Perissi et al., 1999). This motif is similar to the L-X-X-L-L recognition motif present in nuclear receptor co-activators (Heery et al., 1997; Torchia et al., 1997). N-CoR and MSRT contain four independent repressor domains that are capable of transferring active repression to a heterologous DNA-binding domain (Chen and Evans, 1995; Hörlein et al., 1995; Ordentlich et al., 1999; Park et al., 1999). Further analysis of the nuclear receptor interaction domains revealed that each is predicted to form an extended alpha helix one helical turn longer than the co-activator motif. Preferences of RAR for SMRT and T_3R for N-CoR (Cohen et al., 2000) are due to specific sequences in the L-X-X-X-I-X-X-X-I/L motif (Hu et al., 2001) with a thyroid hormone receptor (T_3R)-specific interaction domain present in N-CoR but not in SMRT (Cohen et al., 2001).

Deletion of the murine *N-CoR* locus relieves nuclear receptor–mediated repression of specific genes and altered patterns of transcription in *N-CoR$^{-/-}$* cells result in blocks at specific points in erythrocyte, thymocyte and neural development. These data indicate that N-CoR is a required component of short-term active repression by nuclear receptors and other factors. N-CoR also appears to be required for a specific subset of long-term repression events (Jepsen et al., 2000). Available data suggest that specific combinations of co-repressors and histone deacetylases mediate the gene-specific actions of DNA-bound repressors on development of multiple organ systems.

IDENTIFICATION OF HISTONE DEACETYLASE PROTEINS

The observation that acetylation of specific lysines in the amino termini of histones correlates with increased transcription, while heterochromatic regions are generally hypoacetylated (Grunstein, 1990; Turner, 1993), led to efforts to isolate and characterize the role of histone deacetylases (HDACs) in transcriptional repression. Experiments in yeast identified two complexes with HDAC activity, HDA and HDB (Rundlett et al., 1996), that contained two closely related HDACs: Hda-1 and RPD3 (Vidal and Gaber, 1991; Rundlett et al., 1996). Subsequently, large families of HDAC proteins were classified on the basis of their homology to RPD3 or Hda-1 as class I or class II HDACs, respectively (for a review, see Gray and Ekstrom, 2001). N-CoR and SMRT were found to be associated with the mammalian homologues of the yeast proteins RPD3/HDAC1 and Sin3 (Heinzel et al., 1997; Nagy et al., 1997).

RPD3 is linked via epistasis to Sin3 (RPD1) (Bowdish and Mitchell, 1993; McKenzie et al., 1993; Vidal and Gaber, 1991), which was initially identified in genetic screens for reverting mutations allowing expression of HO in the absence of *Swi5* (Nasmyth et al., 1987), linking them to chromatin remodeling events (Winston and Carlson, 1992). RPD3 is required to achieve full repression and full activation of transcription of several target genes in yeast (Vidal and Gaber, 1991; Vannier et al., 1996), providing genetic proof of the role of specific histone deacetylation events in the regulation of gene repression.

Experiments that purified recombinant *Drosophila* HDAC1 in in vitro transcription assays on chromatinized templates (Huang and Kadonaga, 2001) demonstrate that HDAC1 alone can mediate histone deacetylation, and a Gal4-dHDAC1 fusion protein could repress transcription on chromatinized templates but not on naked DNA templates, suggesting that HDAC actions block at the initiation step of transcription. Some system HDAC proteins appear to require association with N-CoR or SMRT for full enzymatic activity (Wen et al., 2000; Guenther et al., 2001).

In addition to the related class I and class II HDAC families, the silent information regulator 2 (SIR2)-like proteins constitute a third class of HDAC activity (class III HDACs) (for review, see Gottschling, 2000).

Initial genetic data suggested that Sir2p may have a role in histone deacetylation modulating silenced regions of the yeast genome (Rine et al., 1979; Nasmyth, 1982; Braunstein et al., 1993). The human Sir2p homologue was shown to possess nicotinamide adenine dinucleotide (NAD)-dependent ADP-ribosyltransferase activity (Tsang and Escalante-Semerena, 1998), and Sir2p is an NAD-dependent histone deacetylase (Imai et al., 2000; Landry et al., 2000; Smith et al., 2000). Despite the linkage of histone deacetylation to gene regulation, it is intriguing that expression of just 2% of cellular genes is changed with TSA treatment, despite the expected increase in core histone acetylation (Van Lint et al., 1996). Further, Rpd3-deleted strains in yeast have defects in both transcriptional repression and activation (Vidal et al., 1991; Gray and Levine, 1996; Rundlett et al., 1996) and in fact show increased repression at telomeric heterochromatin (Rundlett et al., 1996). Thus, co-repressor and co-activator actions reflect promoter-specific use of co-regulatory factors, whereas different transcriptional activators confer distinct patterns of histone acetylation, which are not fully correlated with transcriptional activation, actions of Sin3a and Rpd3, cause decreased acetylation of histones (Deckert and Struhl, 2001).

In turn, the histone deacetylases are associated with a series of distinct repression complexes. For example, HDACs 1 and 2 have been found in several complexes, including the Sin associated protein complex (Zhang et al., 1997, 1998a), and the NURD (nucleosome remodeling and histone deacetylation) (Tong et al., 1998; Xue et al., 1998; Zhang et al., 1998c, 1999) complexes. The NURD complex has ATP-dependent chromatin remodeling activity (reviewed in Knoepfler and Eisenman, 1999). Both complexes also contain retinoblastoma protein (Rb)-associated proteins RbAp-46 and -48, along with complex-specific components, including DNA methyl-binding protein. One possibility is that a core HDAC complex can differentially recruit additional proteins, imparting distinct functional roles. Complexes purified using either anti-HDAC1 or 2 antibodies overlap significantly with the NURD complex, including the presence of MTA 2, the ATPase Mi-2, RbAp-46 and -48, and methyl-CpG–binding domain proteins (MBD) 2 and/or 3 (Xu et al., 1998; Humphrey et al., 2001). This links proteins involved in binding methylated CpG dinucleotides and gene silencing to histone deacetylases, consistent with interactions of the methyl-CpG–binding protein, MeCP2, Sin3A, and HDACs (Jones et al., 1998; Nan et al., 1998). Indeed, whereas MeCP2 has not been identified in complexes with N-CoR or SMRT, it does interact specifically with N-CoR (Kokura et al., 2001). Thus, analogous to events in gene activation, transcriptional repression involves actions of ATP-dependent chromatin remodeling complexes, histone deacetylation, and DNA methylation and their interactions.

Conversely, a single co-repressor, such as N-CoR, can interact with different HDACs, including HDAC1, 2, and 3 (Guenther et al., 2000; Li et al., 2000; Underhill et al., 2000; Wen et al., 2000; Jones et al., 2001). In N-CoR complexes containing HDAC1 and 2, Sin3a was also present, which is consistent with the SAP complex (Zhang et al., 1997; Zhang et al., 1998a). Biochemical purification of complexes using anti–N-CoR or anti-HDAC3 antibodies also revealed a distinct complex containing HDAC3, N-CoR or SMRT, and transducin beta-like protein 1 (TBL-1) (Guenther et al., 2000; Li et al., 2000; Underhill et al., 2000; Wen et al., 2000). TBL-1 has six WD-40 repeats (Bassi et al., 1999), a motif also present in the Tup1 and Groucho corepressors, and is homologous to the *Drosophila* protein ebi, which is involved in epidermal growth factor receptor signaling pathways (Dong et al., 1999). An additional component of the N-CoR/Tbl1/Tbl1R/HDAC3 complex, Gps2, has been identified (Zhang et al., 2000). N-CoR/SMRT/HDAC3 complexes may also contain Krab-associated protein 1 (KAP-1), which interacts with members of the heterochromatin protein 1 (HP1) family and several members of the Swi/Snf ATP-dependent chromatin remodeling complex, analogous to other dependent chromatin remodeling proteins (Underhill et al., 2000). In addition to the biochemical copurification of N-CoR or SMRT with HDACs, several groups have also shown the third repressor domain of N-CoR or SMRT can directly interact with HDAC4, 5, and 7 in vitro (Huang et al., 2000; Kao et al., 2000).

HDAC 1 and 2 have also been identified as part of a complex containing CoREST and a novel protein homologous to a diverse group of oxidases and dehydrogenases (Humphrey et al., 2001; You et al., 2001), which was also present in one version of the NURD complex (Tong et al., 1998). This binding protein suggests a potential regulated enzymatic activity, analogous to the C-terminal binding proteins (CtBP), which have homology to dehydrogenase enzymes (Nibu et al., 1998; Schaeper et al., 1998), and X-ray crystallography confirms a structural similarity (Kumar et al., 2002).

OTHER TRANSCRIPTION FACTOR PARTNERS

N-CoR or SMRT can serve as co-repressors for several members of the nuclear receptor superfamily, including v-ErbA (Chen and Evans, 1995; Busch et al., 2000) RevErb (Zamir et al., 1996), COUP-transcription factors (Shibata et al., 1997), PPARγ (Dowell et al., 1999), and DAX1 (Crawford et al., 1998). Although steroid hormone receptors do not appear to interact with N-CoR or SMRT in the absence of ligand (Chen and Evans, 1995; Hörlein et al., 1995), both the estrogen receptor (ER) and progesterone receptor (PR) can interact with these co-repressors in the presence of their respective antagonists to repress transcription (Xu et al., 1996; Jackson et al., 1997; Smith et al., 1997; Lavinsky et al., 1998). In chromatin immunoprecipitation (ChIP) assays performed in the breast tumor–derived cell line MCF-7, N-CoR and SMRT were present on the estrogen-responsive cathepsin D and pS2 promoters in the presence of the antagonist tamoxifen but not estrogen (Shang et al., 2000). Together, the data suggest a role for N-CoR and SMRT in mediating the antagonist-associated effects of steroid hormone receptors (Chen and Evans, 1995; Hörlein et al., 1995).

In addition to their interactions with members of the nuclear receptor family, N-CoR and SMRT have been implicated as co-repressors for a variety of unrelated transcription factors that regulate diverse cellular processes. SMRT can be recruited to repress transcription by serum response factor (SRF), activating protein-1 (AP-1), and nuclear factor-κB (NFκB), transcription factors that are involved in the stimulation of cellular proliferation processes (Lee et al., 2000). N-CoR and SMRT have both been implicated as involved in abrogating transcription by the evolution-related POU homeodomain factors Pit-1 (Xu et al., 1998) and Oct-1 (Kakizawa et al., 2001), which have important developmental roles, and by the homeobox factor PBX (Asahara et al., 1999; Shanmugam et al., 1999), which is an important determiner of cell fate and segment identity. These co-repressors also interact with the Poz/zinc finger transcription factor BCL-6, which may influence apoptosis (Dhordain et al., 1998; Huynh and Bardwell, 1998; Wong and Privalsky, 1998), with the bHLH proteins MAD (Heinzel et al., 1997), MyoD (Bailey et al., 1999), and HES-related repressor proteins (Iso et al., 2001), to suppress proliferation or induce terminal differentiation, and with the Notch-activated adapter protein Su(H)/RBP-J/CBF1 (Kao et al., 1998), which influences differentiation, proliferation, and apoptosis in many developmental systems.

REGULATION OF N-CoR/SMRT

The actions of N-CoR and SMRT are analogous to most co-repressors and are regulated at multiple levels. The N-terminus of N-CoR interacts with mSiah2, the mammalian homologue of *Drosophila Seven in absentia* (Zhang et al., 1998b), mSiah2 has been implicated in regulating proteasomal degradation of proteins (Hu et al., 1997; Li et al., 1997b; Tang et al., 1997). Co-expression of N-CoR and mSiah2 resulted in a dramatic decrease of N-CoR protein levels, an effect that can be blocked by proteasome inhibitors (Zhang et al., 1998b).

Although their association with nuclear receptors is clearly controlled at the hormone binding level, there have also been several systems in which cell-signaling events seem capable of regulating the association with and thus activity of N-CoR or SMRT. Treatment of treated MCF-7 or HeLa cells with forskolin, which stimulates the PKA pathway, or EGF, which stimulates the MAPK and PKC pathways, results in decreased association of N-CoR and ER in the presence of the antagonist tamoxifen (Lavinsky et al., 1998) and could convert tamoxifen from an antagonist to an agonist of ER-mediated transcription (Lavinsky et al.,

1998). Activation of the mitogen-activated protein kinase (MAPK) pathway by L-throxine (T_4) results in serine phosphorylation of TRβ1 and dissociation of SMRT in a hormone-independent manner. Similarly, phosphorylation of SMRT by MAPK-extracellular signal–regulated kinase 1 (MEK-1) and MEK-1 kinase (MEKK) can inhibit interactions between SMRT and nuclear receptors or PLZF (Hong and Privalsky, 2000). In contrast, phosphorylation of SMRT by the protein kinase casein kinase II (CK2) stabilizes the SMRT–nuclear receptor interaction (Zhou et al., 2001). Thus, different cell signaling pathways can effect different transcriptional outcomes.

In addition to their role in imposing protein–protein interaction changes, cell-signaling pathways have also been shown to cause changes in subcellular distribution, presumably to restrict the access of transcription factors to co-repressors. CamKIV-dependent phosphorylation of the NFκB p65 subunit result can not only in an exchange of SMRT for CBP but also in translocation of SMRT to the cytoplasm (Jang et al., 2001). Akt1, MEK-1, and MEKK-1 signaling also result in a redistribution of SMRT and N-CoR from the nucleus to the perinucleus or cytoplasm (Hong and Privalsky, 2000; Baek et al., 2002; Hermanson et al., 2002). Interestingly, co-repressors may themselves shuttle associated proteins to the nucleus, as appears to be the case for both Su(H)/RBP-J/CBF1 (Zhou and Hayward, 2001) and certain HDAC proteins (Wu et al., 2001). Intracellular signaling events are also thought to influence the subcellular distribution of HDAC proteins (Grozinger and Schreiber, 2000; McKinsey et al., 2000a, 2000b) and thus may be a general mechanism by which corepressor proteins are regulated.

Although negative regulation of co-repressor function is achieved by protein degradation and by altering protein–protein interactions or subcellular localization, there also are examples of regulation of the specificity of co-repressor function at the level of association with other co-repressor molecules to form distinct co-repressor complexes. The Ski proto-oncogene family, which includes the proteins Ski and Sno, have been found to complex with N-CoR, SMRT, HDACs, and Sin3 to regulate transcriptional repression by MAD and TRβ (Nomura et al., 1999). A co-repressor complex containing N-CoR and Ski or Sno has also been implicated as a negative regulator of the TGFβ signaling pathway (Luo et al., 1999; Stroschein et al., 1999). Ski or Sno, together with N-CoR, forms complexes with the SMAD proteins that positively regulate TGFβ signaling, resulting in repression of TGFβ-activated transcription (Luo et al., 1999; Stroschein et al., 1999). A Ski-related factor, Dach, can also act as a co-repressor, by interacting with homeodomain regulators, the six genes (Li et al., 2002). As the data collected increase, there will doubtlessly prove to be additional mechanisms by which both the regulation and specificity of N-CoR and SMRT activity are controlled.

Thus, the numerous complexes that compete for interactions with DNA binding proteins serve to set the precise level of gene activation or repression and are themselves the objects of dynamic regulation by numerous posttranslational modifications regulating subcellular localization and degradation, function, and binding. In concert with a similar intricate regulation of core machinery, promoter-specific and cell type–specific patterns of regulated gene expression are observed.

REFERENCES

Ait-Si-Ali S, Ramirez S, Barre FX, Dkhissi F, Magnaghi-Jaulin L, Girault JA, Robin P, Knibiehler M, Pritchard LL, Ducommun B, et al. (1998). Histone acetyltransferase activity of CBP is controlled by cycle-dependent kinases and oncoprotein E1A. *Nature* 396: 184–186.

Alves-Rodrigues A, Gregori L, Figueiredo-Pereira ME (1998). Ubiquitin, cellular inclusions and their role in neurodegeneration. *Trends Neurosci* 21: 516–520.

Anzick SL, Kononen J, Walker RL, Azorsa DO, Tanner MM, Guan XY, Sauter G, Kallioniemi OP, Trent JM, Meltzer PS (1997). AIB1, a steroid receptor coactivator amplified in breast and ovarian cancer. *Science* 277: 965–968.

Asahara H, Dutta S, Kao HY, Evans RM, Montminy M (1999). Pbx-Hox heterodimers recruit coactivator-corepressor complexes in an isoform-specific manner. *Mol Cell Biol* 19: 8219–8225.

Baek SH, Kioussi C, Briata P, Wang D, Nguyen HD, Ohgi KA, Glass CK, Wynshaw-Boris A, Rose DW, Rosenfeld MG (2003). Regulated subset of G1 growth-control genes in response to derepression by the Wnt pathway. *Proc Natl Acad Sci USA* 100: 3245–3250.

Bailey P, Downes M, Lau P, Harris J, Chen SL, Hamamori Y, Sartorelli V, Muscat GE (1999). The nuclear receptor corepressor N-CoR regulates differentiation: N-CoR directly interacts with MyoD. *Mol Endocrinol* 13: 1155–1168.

Baniahmad A, Kohne AC, Renkawitz R (1992). A transferable silencing domain is present in the thyroid hormone receptor, in the v-erbA oncogene product and in the retinoic acid receptor. *EMBO J* 11: 1015–1023.
Bannister AJ, Miska EA, Gorlich D, Kouzarides T (2000). Acetylation of import in-alpha nuclear import factors by CBP/p300. *Curr Biol* 10: 467–470.
Bassi MT, Ramesar RS, Caciotti B, Winship IM, De Grandi A, Riboni M, Townes PL, Beighton P, Ballabio A, Borsani G (1999). X-linked late-onset sensorineural deafness caused by a deletion involving OA1 and a novel gene containing WD-40 repeats. *Am J Hum Genet* 64: 1604–1616.
Bentley D (1999). Coupling RNA polymerase II transcription with pre-mRNA processing. *Curr Opin Cell Biol* 11: 347–351.
Bourguet W, Germain P, Gronemeyer H (2000). Nuclear receptor ligand-binding domains: three-dimensional structures, molecular interactions and pharmacological implications. *Trends Pharm Sci* 21: 381–388.
Bowdish KS, Mitchell AP (1993). Bipartite structure of an early meiotic upstream activation sequence from Saccharomyces cerevisiae. *Mol Cell Biol* 13: 2172–2181.
Boyes J, Byfield P, Nakatani Y, Ogryzko V (1998). Regulation of activity of the transcription factor GATA-1 by acetylation. *Nature* 396: 594–598.
Braunstein M, Rose AB, Holmes SG, Allis CD, Broach JR (1993). Transcriptional silencing in yeast is associated with reduced nucleosome acetylation. *Genes Dev* 7: 592–604.
Busch K, Martin B, Baniahmad A, Martial JA, Renkawitz R, Muller M (2000). Silencing subdomains of v-ErbA interact cooperatively with corepressors: involvement of helices 5/6. *Mol Endocrinol* 14: 201–211.
Butler JE, Kadonaga JT (2002). The RNA polymerase II core promoter: a key component in the regulation of gene expression. *Genes Dev* 16: 2583–2592.
Chen JD, Evans RM (1995). A transcriptional co-repressor that interacts with nuclear hormone receptors. *Nature* 377: 454–457.
Chen D, Ma H, Hong H, Koh SS, Huang S-M, Schurter BT, Aswad DW, Stallcup MR (1999). Regulation of transcription by a protein methyltransferase. *Science* 284: 2174–2176.
Cohen RN, Putney A, Wondisford FE, Hollenberg AN (2000). The nuclear corepressors recognize distinct nuclear receptor complexes. *Mol Endocrinol* 14: 900–914.
Cohen RN, Brzostek S, Kim B, Chorev M, Wondisford FE, Hollenberg AN (2001). The specificity of interactions between nuclear hormone receptors and corepressors is mediated by distinct amino acid sequences within the interacting domains. *Mol Endocrinol* 15: 1049–1061.
Conaway RC, Conaway JW (1993). General initiation factors for RNA polymerase II. *Annu Rev Biochem* 62: 161–190.
Crawford PA, Dorn C, Sadovsky Y, Milbrandt J (1998). Nuclear receptor DAX-1 recruits nuclear receptor corepressor N-CoR to steroidogenic factor 1. *Mol Cell Biol* 18: 2949–2956.
Darimont BD, Wagner RL, Apriletti JW, Stallcup MR, Kushner PJ, Baxter JD, Fletterick RJ, Yamamoto KR (1998). Structure and specificity of nuclear receptor-coactivator interactions. *Genes Dev* 12: 3343–3356.
Deckert J, Struhl K (2001). Histone acetylation at promoters is differentially affected by specific activators and repressors. *Mol Cell Biol* 21: 2726–2735.
Dhordain P, Lin RJ, Quief S, Lantoine D, Kerckaert JP, Evans RM, Albagli O (1998). The LAZ3(BCL-6) oncoprotein recruits a SMRT/mSIN3A/histone deacetylase containing complex to mediate transcriptional repression. *Nucleic Acids Res* 26: 4645–4651.
Dong X, Tsuda L, Zavitz KH, Lin M, Li S, Carthew RW, Zipursky SL (1999). ebi regulates epidermal growth factor receptor signaling pathways in Drosophila. *Genes Dev* 13: 954–965.
Dowell P, Ishmael JE, Avram D, Peterson VJ, Nevrivy DJ, Leid M (1999). Identification of nuclear receptor corepressor as a peroxisome proliferator-activated receptor alpha interacting protein. *J Biol Chem* 1274: 15901–15907.
Fondell JD, Guermah M, Malik S, Roeder RG (1999). Thyroid hormone receptor-associated proteins and general positive cofactors mediate thyroid hormone receptor function in the absence of the TATA box-binding protein-associated factors of TFIID. *Proc Natl Acad Sci USA* 96: 1959–1964.
Glass CK, Rosenfeld MG (2000). The coregulator exchange in transcriptional functions of nuclear receptors. *Genes Dev* 14: 121–141.
Gottschling DE (2000). Gene silencing: two faces of SIR2. *Curr Biol* 10: R708–R711.
Grant PA, Duggan L, Cote J, Roberts SM, Brownell JE, Candau R, Ohba R, Owen-Hughes T, Allis CD, Winston F, et al. (1997). Yeast Gcn5 functions in two multisubunit complexes to acetylate nucleosomal histones: characterization of an Ada complex and the SAGA (Spt/Ada) complex. *Genes Dev* 11: 1640–1650.
Gray SG, Ekstrom TJ (2001). The human histone deacetylase family. *Exp Cell Res* 262: 75–83.
Gray S, Levine M (1996). Transcriptional repression in development. *Curr Opin Cell Biol* 8: 358–364.
Grunstein M (1990). Histone function in transcription. *Annu Rev Cell Biol* 6: 643–678.
Guenther MG, Barak O, Lazar MA (2001). The SMRT and N-CoR corepressors are activating cofactors for histone deacetylase 3. *Mol Cell Biol* 21: 6091–6101.
Guenther MG, Lane WS, Fischle W, Verdin E, Lazar MA, Shiekhattar R (2000). A core SMRT corepressor complex containing HDAC3 and TBL1, a WD40-repeat protein linked to deafness. *Genes Dev* 14: 1048–1057.
Heery DM, Kalkhoven E, Hoare S, Parker MG (1997). A signature motif in transcriptional co-activators mediates binding to nuclear receptors. *Nature* 387: 733–736.
Heinzel T, Lavinsky RM, Mullen TM, Soderstrom M, Laherty CD, Torchia J, Yang WM, Brard G, Ngo SD, Davie JR, et al. (1997). A complex containing N-CoR, mSin3 and histone deacetylase mediates transcriptional repression. *Nature* 387: 43–48.
Hermanson O, Jepsen K, Rosenfeld MG (2002). N-CoR controls differentiation of neural stem cells into astrocytes. *Nature* 419: 934–939.
Hirose Y, Manley JL (2000). RNA polymerase II and the integration of nuclear events. *Genes Dev* 14: 1415–1429.
Hong SH, Privalsky ML (2000). The SMRT corepressor is regulated by a MEK-1 kinase pathway: inhibition of corepressor function is associated with SMRT phosphorylation and nuclear export. *Mol Cell Biol* 20: 6612–6625.
Hörlein AJ, Naar AM, Heinzel T, Torchia J, Gloss B, Kurokawa R, Ryan A, Kamei Y, Soderstrom M, Glass CK, et al. (1995). Ligand-independent repression by the thyroid hormone receptor mediated by a nuclear receptor co-repressor. *Nature* 377: 397–404.
Hu X, Lazar MA (1999). The CoRNR motif contains the recruitment of corepressors by nuclear hormone receptors. *Nature* 402: 93–96.
Hu I, Lazar MA (2000). Transcriptional repression by nuclear hormone receptors. *Trends Endocrinol Metab* 11: 6–10.
Hu X, Li Y, Lazar MA (2001). Determinants of CoRNR-dependent repression complex assembly on nuclear hormone receptors. *Mol Cell Biol* 221: 1747–1758.
Hu G, Chung YL, Glover T, Valentine V, Look AT, Fearon ER (1997). Characterization of human homologs of the Drosophila seven in absentia (sina) gene. *Genomics* 46: 103–111.
Huang X, Kadonaga JT (2001). Biochemical analysis of transcriptional repression by Drosophila histone deacetylase 1. *J Biol Chem* 276: 12497–12500.
Huang EY, Zhang J, Miska EA, Guenther MG, Kouzarides T, Lazar MA (2000). Nuclear receptor corepressors partner with class II histone deacetylases in a Sin3-independent repression pathway. *Genes Dev* 14: 45–54.
Humphrey GW, Wang Y, Russanova VR, Hirai T, Qin J, Nakatani Y, Howard BH (2001). Stable histone deacetylase complexes distinguished by the presence of SANT domain proteins CoREST/kiaa0071 and Mta-L1. *J Biol Chem* 276: 6817–6824.
Huynh KD, Bardwell VJ (1998). The BCL-6 POZ domain and other POZ domains interact with the co-repressors N-CoR and SMRT. *Oncogene* 17: 2473–2484.
Ida K, Kitabayashi I, Taki T, Taniwaki M, Noro K, Yamamoto M, Ohki M, Hayashi Y (1997). Adenoviral E1A-associated protein p300 is involved in acute myeloid leukemia with t(11;22)(q23;q13). *Blood* 90: 4699–4704.
Imai S, Armstrong CM, Kaeberlein M, Guarente L (2000). Transcriptional silencing and longevity protein Sir2 is an NAD-dependent histone deacetylase. *Nature* 403: 795–800.
Imhof A, Yang XJ, Ogryzko VV, Nakatani Y, Wolffe AP, Ge H (1997). Acetylation of general transcription factors by histone acetyltransferases. *Curr Biol* 7: 689–692.
Iso T, Sartorelli V, Poizat C, Iezzi S, Wu HY, Chung G, Kedes L, Hamamori Y (2001). HERP, a novel heterodimer partner of HES/E(spl) in Notch signaling. *Mol Cell Biol* 21: 6080–6089.
Ito M, Yuan CX, Okano HJ, Darnell RB, Roeder RG (2000). Involvement of the TRAP220 component of the TRAP/SMCC coactivator complex in embryonic development and thyroid hormone action. *Mol Cell* 5: 683–693.
Ito M, Yuan CX, Malik S, Gu W, Fondell JD, Yamamura S, Fu ZY, Zhang X, Qin J, Roeder RG (1999). Identity between TRAP and SMCC complexes indicates novel pathways for the function of nuclear receptors and diverse mammalian activators. *Mol Cell* 3: 361–370.
Jackson TA, Richer JK, Bain DL, Takimoto GS, Tung L, Horwitz KB (1997). The partial agonist activity of antagonist-occupied steroid receptors in controlled by a novel hinge domain-binding coactivator L7/SPA and the corepressors N-CoR or SMRT. *Mol Endocrinol* 11: 693–705.
Jenuwein T, Allis CD (2001). Translating the histone code. *Science*. 293: 1074–1080.
Jepsen K, Hermanson O, Onami TM, Gleiberman AS, Lunyak V, McEvilly RJ, Kurokawa R, Kuman V, Liu F, Seto E, et al. (2000). Combinatorial roles of the nuclear receptor corepressor in transcription and development. *Cell* 102: 753–763.
Jones PL, Veenstra GJ, Wade PA, Vermaak D, Kass SU, Landsberger N, Strouboulis J, Wolffe AP (1998). Methylated DNA and MeCP2 recruit histone deacetylase to repress transcription. *Nat Genet* 19: 187–191.
Kakizawa T, Miyamoto T, Ichikawa K, Takeda T, Suzuki S, Mori J, Kumagai M, Yamashita K, Hashizume K (2001). Silencing mediator for retinoid and thyroid hormone receptors interacts with octamer transcription factor-1 and acts as a transcriptional repressor. *J Biol Chem* 276: 9720–9725.
Kao HY, Downes M, Ordentlich P, Evans RM (2000). Isolation of a novel histone deacetylase reveals that class I and class II deacetylases promote SMRT-mediated repression. *Genes Dev* 14: 55–66.
Kingston RE, Narlikar GJ (1999). ATP-dependent remodeling and acetylation as regulators of chromatin fluidity. *Genes Dev* 13: 2339–2352.
Knoepfler PS, Eisenman RN (1999). Sin meets NuRD and other tails of repression. *Cell* 99: 447–450.
Koh SS, Chen D, Lee YH, Stallcup MR (2001). Synergistic enhancement of nuclear receptor function by p160 coactivators and two coactivators with protein methyltransferase activities. *J Biol Chem* 276: 1089–1098.
Koh S, Chen D, Lee Y, Stallcup M (2001). Synergistic enhancement of nuclear receptor function by p160 coactivators and two coactivators with protein methyltransferase activities. *J Biol Chem* 276: 1089–1098.
Korzus E, Torchia J, Rose DW, Xu L, Kurokawa R, McInerney EM, Mullen TM, Glass CK, Rosenfeld MG (1998). Transcription factor-specific requirements for coactivators and their acetyltransferase functions. *Science* 279: 703–707.
Kumar V, Carlson JE, Ohgi KA, Edwards TA, Rose DW, Escalante CR, Rosenfeld MG, Aggarwal AK (2002). Transcription corepressor CtBP is an NAD(+)-regulated dehydrogenase. *Mol Cell* 10: 857–869.
Kurokawa R, Kalafus D, Ogliastro MH, Kioussi C, Xu L, Torchia J, Rosenfeld MG, Glass CK (1998). Differential use of CREB binding protein-coactivator complexes. *Science* 279: 700–703.
Landry J, Slama JT, Sternglanz R (2000). Role of NAD(+) in the deacetylase activity of the SIR2-like proteins. *Biochem Biophys Res Commun* 278: 685–690.
Lanz RB, McKenna NJ, Onate SA, Albrecht U, Wong J, Tsai SY, Tsai MJ, O'Malley BW (1999). A steroid receptor coactivator, SRA, functions as an RNA and is present in an SRC-1 complex. *Cell* 97: 17–27.
Lee JW, Choi HS, Gyuris J, Brent R, Moore DD (1995a). Two classes of proteins dependent on either the presence or absence of thyroid hormone for interaction with the thyroid hormone receptor. *Mol Endocrinol* 9: 243–254.
Lee JW, Ryan F, Swaffield JC, Johnston SA, Moore DD (1995b). Interaction of thyroid-hormone receptor with a conserved transcriptional mediator. *Nature* 374: 91–94.

Lee SK, Anzick SL, Choi JE, Bubendorf L, Guan XY, Jung YK, Kallioniemi OP, Kononen J, Trent JM, Azorsa D, et al. (1999). A nuclear factor, ASC-2, as a cancer-amplified transcriptional coactivator essential for ligand-dependent transactivation by nuclear receptors in vivo. *J Biol Chem* 274: 34283–34293.
Lemon B, Tjian R (2000). Orchestrated response: a symphony of transcription factors for gene control. *Genes Dev* 14: 2551–2569.
Li H, Leo C, Schroen DJ, Chen JD (1997a). Characterization of receptor interaction and transcriptional repression by the corepressor SMRT. *Mol Endocrinol* 11: 2025–2037.
Li S, Li Y, Carthew RW, Lai ZC. (1997b). Photoreceptor cell differentiation requires regulated proteolysis of the transcriptional repressor Tramtrack. *Cell* 90: 469–478.
Li J, Wang J, Nawaz Z, Liu J, Qin J, Wong J (2000). Both corepressor proteins SMRT and N-CoR exist in large protein complexes containing HDAC3. *EMBO J* 19: 4342–4350.
McInerney EM, Rose DW, Flynn SE, Westin S, Mullen TM, Krones A, Inostroza J, Torchia J, Nolte RT, Assa-Munt N, et al. (1998). Determinants of coactivator LXXLL motif specificity in nuclear receptor transcriptional activation. *Genes Dev* 12: 3357–3368.
McKenna NJ, Lanz RB, O'Malley BW. (1999). Nuclear receptor coregulators: cellular and molecular biology. *Endocr Rev* 20: 321–344.
McKinsey TA, Zhang CL, Lu J, Olson EN (2000). Signal-dependent nuclear export of a histone deacetylase regulates muscle differentiation. *Nature* 408: 106–111.
McNally JG, Muller WG, Walker D, Wolford R, Hager GL (2000). The glucocorticoid receptor: rapid exchange with regulatory sites in living cells. *Science* 287: 1262–1265.
Moilanen AM, Karvonen U, Poukka H, Yan W, Toppari J, Janne OA, Palvimo JJ (1999). A testis-specific androgen receptor coregulator that belongs to a novel family of nuclear proteins. *J Biol Chem* 274: 3700–3704.
Monsalve M, Wu Z, Adelmant G, Puigserver P, Fan M, Spiegelman BM (2000). Direct coupling of transcription and mRNA processing through the thermogenic coactivator PGC-1. *Mol Cell* 6: 307–316.
Mowen KA, Tang J, Zhu W, Schurter BT, Shuai K, Herschman HR, David M (2001). Arginine methylation of STAT1 modulates IFNalpha/beta-induced transcription. *Cell* 2104: 731–741.
Munshi N, Merika M, Yie J, Senger K, Chen G, Thanos D (1998). Acetylation of HMG I(Y) by CBP turns off IFN beta expression by disrupting the enhanceosome. *Mol Cell* 2: 457–467.
Myers LC, Kornberg RD (2000). Mediator of transcriptional regulation. *Annu Rev Biochem* 69: 729–749.
Näär AM, Beaurang PA, Zhou S, Abraham S, Solomon W, Tijian R (1999). Composite coactivator ARC mediates chromatin-directed transcriptional activation. *Nature* 398: 828–832.
Nagy L, Kao H, Love J, Li C, Banayo E, Gooch J, Krishna V, Chatterjee K, Evans R, Schwabe J (1999). Mechanism of corepressor binding and release from nuclear hormone receptors. *Genes Dev* 13: 3209–3216.
Nan X, Ng HH, Johnson CA, Laherty CD, Turner BM, Eisenman RN, Bird A (1998). Transcriptional repression by the methyl-CpG-binding protein MeCP2 involves a histone deacetylase complex. *Nature* 393: 386–389.
Nasmyth K, Seddon A, Ammerer G (1987). Cell cycle regulation of SW15 is required for mother-cell-specific HO transcription in yeast. *Cell* 49: 549–558.
Nibu Y, Zhang H, Levine M (1998). Interaction of short-range repressors with Drosophila CtBP in the embryo. *Science* 280: 101–104.
Ogryzko VV, Schiltz RL, Russanova V, Howard BH, Nakatani Y (1996). The transcriptional coactivators p300 and CBP are histone acetyltransferases. *Cell* 87: 953–959.
Oike Y, Takakura N, Hata A, Kaname T, Akizuki M, Yamaguchi Y, Yasue H, Araki K, Yamamura K, Suda T (1999). Mice homozygous for a truncated form of CREB-binding protein exhibit defects in hematopoiesis and vasculo-angiogenesis. *Blood* 93: 2771–2779.
Ordentlich P, Downes M, Xie W, Genin A, Spinner NB, Evans RM (1999). Unique forms of human and mouse nuclear receptor corepressor SMRT. *Proc Natl Acad Sci USA* 96: 2639–2644.
Orphanidus G, Lagrange T, Reinberg D (1996). The general transcription factors of RNA polymerase II. *Genes Dev* 10: 2657–2683.
Park EJ, Schroen DJ, Yang M, Li H, Li L, Chen JD (1999). SMRTe, a silencing mediator for retinoid and thyroid hormone receptors extended isoform that is more related to the nuclear receptor corepressor. *Proc Natl Acad Sci USA* 96: 3519–3524.
Perissi V, Staszewski LM, McInerney EM, Kurokawa R, Krones A, Rose DW, Milburn MV, Glass CK, Rosenfeld MG (1999). Molecular determinants of nuclear receptor-corepressor interaction. *Genes Dev* 13: 3198–3208.
Proudfoot N (2000). Connecting transcription to messenger RNA processing. *Trends Biochem Sci* 25: 290–293.
Puigserver P, Wu Z, Park CW, Graves R, Wright M, Spiegelman BM (1998). A cold-inducible coactivator of nuclear receptors linked to adaptive thermogenesis. *Cell* 92: 829–839.
Rachez C, Suldan Z, Ward J, Chang CPB, Burakov D, Erdjument-Bromage H, Tempst P, Freedman LP (1998). Ligand-dependent transcription activation by nuclear receptors requires the DRIP complex. *Genes Dev* 12: 1787–1800.
Rine J, Strathern JN, Hicks JB, Herskowitz I (1979). A suppressor of mating-type locus mutations in Saccharomyces cerevisiae: evidence for and identification of cryptic mating-type loci. *Genetics* 93: 877–901.
Roeder RG (1996). The role of general initiation factors in transcription by RNA polymerase II. *Trends Biochem Sci* 21: 327–335.
Rundlett SE, Carmen AA, Kobayashi R, Bavykin S, Turner BM, Grunstein M (1996). HDA1 and RPD3 are members of distinct yeast histone deacetylase complexes that regulate silencing andtranscription. *Proc Natl Acad Sci USA* 93: 14503–14508.
Ryu S, Tjian R (1999). Purification of transcription cofactor complex CRSP. *Proc Natl Acad Sci USA* 96: 7137–7142.
Schaeper U, Subramanian T, Lim L, Boyd JM, Chinnadurai G (1998). Interaction between a cellular protein that binds to the C-terminal region of adenovirus E1A (CtBP) and a novel cellular protein is disrupted by E1A through a conserved PLDLS motif. *J Biol Chem* 273: 8549–8552.
Seol W, Mahon MJ, Lee YK, Moore DD (1996). Two receptor interacting domains in the nuclear hormone receptor corepressor RIP13/N-CoR. *Mol Endocrinol* 10: 1646–1655.
Shang Y, Hu X, DiRenzo J, Lazar MA, Brown M (2000). Cofactor dynamics and sufficiency in estrogen receptor-regulated transcription. *Cell* 103: 843–852.
Shanmugam K, Green NC, Rambaldi I, Saragovi HU, Featherstone MS (1999). PBX and MEIS as non-DNA-binding partners in trimeric complexes with HOX proteins. *Mol Cell Biol* 19: 7577–7588.
Shi Y, Downes M, Xie W, Kao HY, Ordentlich P, Tsai CC, Hon M, Evans RM (2001). Sharp, an inducible cofactor that integrates nuclear receptor repression and activation. *Genes Dev* 15: 1140–1151.
Shibata H, Nawaz Z, Tsai SY, O'Malley BW, Tsai MJ (1997). Gene silencing by chicken ovalbumin upstream promoter-transcription factor I (COUP-TFI) is mediated by transcriptional corepressors, nuclear receptor-corepressor (N-CoR) and silencing mediator for retinoic acid receptor and thyroid hormone receptor (SMRT). *Mol Endocrinol* 11: 714–724.
Smith CL, Nawaz Z, O'Malley BW (1997). Coactivator and corepressor regulation of the agonist/antagonist activity of the mixed antiestrogen, 4-hydroxytamoxifen. *Mol Endocrinol* 11: 657–666.
Smith JS, Brachmann CB, Celic I, Kenna MA, Muhammad S, Starai VJ, Avalos JL, Escalante-Semerena JC, Grubmeyer C, Wolberger C, et al. (2000). A phylogenetically conserved NAD+-dependent protein deacetylase activity in the Sir2 protein family. *Proc Natl Acad Sci USA* 97: 6658–6663.
Soutoglou E, Katrakili N, Talianidis I (2000). Acetylation regulates transcription factor activity at multiple levels. *Mol Cell* 5: 745–751.
Stromberg H, Svensson SP, Hermanson O (1999). Distribution of CREB-binding protein immunoreactivity in the adult rat brain. *Brain Res* 818: 510–514.
Tong JK, Hassig CA, Schnitzler GR, Kingston RE, Schreiber SL (1998). Chromatin deacetylation by an ATP-dependent nucleosome remodelling complex. *Nature* 395: 917–921.
Torchia J, Rose DW, Inostroza J, Kamei Y, Westin S, Glass CK, Rosenfeld MG (1997). The transcriptional co-activator p/CIP binds CBP and mediates nuclear-receptor function. *Nature* 387: 677–684.
Tsang AW, Escalante-Semerena JC (1998). CobB, a new member of the SIR2 family of eucaryotic regulatory proteins, is required to compensate for the lack of nicotinate mononucleotide: 5,6-dimethylbenzimidazole phosphoribosyltransferase activity in cobT mutants during cobalamin biosynthesis in Salmonella typhimurium LT2. *J Biol Chem* 273: 31788–31794.
Turner BM (1993). Decoding the nucleosome (review). *Cell* 75: 5–8.
Underhill C, Qutob MS, Yee SP, Torchia J (2000). A novel nuclear receptor corepressor complex, N-CoR, contains components of the mammalian SWI/SNF complex and the corepressor KAP-1. *J Biol Chem* 275: 40463–40470.
Van Lint C, Emiliani S, Verdin E (1996). The expression of a small fraction of cellular genes is changed in response to histone hyperacetylation. *Gene Exp* 5: 245–253.
Vannier D, Balderes D, Shore D (1996). Evidence that the transcriptional regulators SIN3 and RPD3, and a novel gene (SDS3) with similar functions, are involved in transcriptional silencing in S. cerevisiae. *Genetics* 144: 1343–1353.
Vidal M, Gaber RF (1991). RPD3 encodes a second factor required to achieve maximum positive and negative transcriptional states in Saccharomyces cerevisiae. *Mol Cell Biol* 11: 6317–6327.
Wade PA, Wolffe AP (1999). Transcriptional regulation: SWItching circuitry. *Curr Biol* 9: R221–R224.
Wang Z, Rose DW, Hermanson O, Liu F, Herman T, Wu W, Szeto D, Gleiberman A, Krones A, Pratt K, et al. (2000). Regulation of somatic growth by the p160 coactivator p/CIP. *Proc Natl Acad Sci USA* 97: 13549–13554.
Watanabe M, Yanagisawa J, Kitagawa H, Takeyama K, Ogawa S, Arao Y, Suzawa M, Kobayashi Y, Yano T, Yoshikawa H, et al. (2001). A subfamily of RNA-binding DEAD-box proteins acts as an estrogen receptor alpha coactivator through the N-terminal activation domain (AF-1) with an RNA coactivator, SRA. *EMBO J* 20: 1341–1352.
Weiss RE, Xu J, Ning G, Pohlenz J, O'Malley BW, Refetoff S (1999). Mice deficient in the steroid receptor co-activator 1 (SRC-1) are resistant to thyroid hormone. *EMBO J* 18: 1900–1904.
Wen YD, Perissi V, Staszewski LM, Yang WM, Krones A, Glass CK, Rosenfeld MG, Seto E (2000). The histone deacetylase-3 complex contains nuclear receptor corepressors. *Proc Natl Acad Sci USA* 97: 7202–7207.
White R, Leonardsson G, Rosewell I, Ann Jacobs M, Milligan S, Parker M (2000). The nuclear receptor co-repressor nrip1 (RIP140) is essential for female fertility. *Nat Med* 6: 1368–1374.
Winston F, Carlson M (1992). Yeast SNF/SWI transcriptional activators and the SPT/SIN chromatin connection. *Trends Genet* 8: 387–391.
Wong CW, Privalsky ML (1998). Transcriptional repression by the SMRT-mSin3 corepressor: multiple interactions, multiple mechanisms, and a potential role for TFIIB. *Mol Cell Biol* 18: 5500–5510.
Wu C (1997). Chromatin remodeling and the control of gene expression. *J Biol Chem* 272: 28171–28174.
Wu X, Li H, Park EJ, Chen JD (2001). SMRTE inhibits MEF2C transcriptional activation by targeting HDAC4 and 5 to nuclear domains. *J Biol Chem* 276: 24177–24185.
Xu J, Nawaz Z, Tsai SY, Tsai MJ, O'Malley BW (1996). The extreme C terminus of progesterone receptor contains a transcriptional repressor domain that functions through a putative corepressor. *Proc Natl Acad Sci USA* 93: 12195–12199.
Xu J, Qiu Y, DeMayo FJ, Tsai SY, Tsai MJ, O'Malley BW (1998). Partial hormone resistance in mice with disruption of the steroid receptor coactivator-1 (SRC-1) gene. *Science* 279: 1922–1925.
Xu W, Chen H, Du K, Asahara H, Tini M, Emerson BM, Montminy M, Evans RM (2001). A transcriptional switch mediated by cofactor methylation. *Science* 294: 2507–2511.
Xue Y, Wong J, Moreno GT, Young MK, Cote J, Wang W (1998). NURD, a novel complex with both ATP-dependent chromatin-remodeling and histone deacetylase activities. *Mol Cell* 2: 851–861.
Yang XJ, Ogryzko VV, Nishikawa J, Howard BH, Nakatani Y (1996). A p300/CBP-associated factor that competes with the adenoviral oncoprotein E1A. *Nature* 382: 319–324.
Yao TP, Oh SP, Fuchs M, Zhou ND, Ch'ng LE, Newsome D, Bronson RT, Li E, Liv-

ingston DM, Eckner R (1998). Gene dosage-dependent embryonic development and proliferation defects in mice lacking the transcriptional integrator p300. *Cell* 93: 361–372.

You A, Tong JK, Grozinger CM, Schreiber SL (2001). CoREST is an integral component of the CoREST-human histone deacetylase complex. *Proc Natl Acad Sci USA* 98: 1454–1458.

Yuan CX, Ito M, Fondell JD, Fu ZY, Roeder RG (1998). The TRAP220 component of a thyroid hormone receptor-associated protein (TRAP) coactivator complex interacts directly with nuclear receptors in a ligand-dependent fashion. *Proc Natl Acad Sci USA* 95: 14584.

Zamir I, Harding HP, Atkins GB, Horlein A, Glass CK, Rosenfeld MG, Lazar MA (1996). A nuclear hormone receptor corepressor mediates transcriptional silencing by receptors with distinct repression domains. *Mol Cell Biol* 16: 5458–5465.

Zhang J, Kalkum M, Chait BT, Roeder RG (2002). The N-CoR-HDAC3 nuclear receptor corepressor complex inhibits the JNK pathway through the integral subunit GPS2. *Mol Cell* 9: 611–623.

Zhang J, Guenther MG, Carthew RW, Lazar MA (1998b). Proteasomal regulation of nuclear receptor corepressor-mediated repression. *Genes Dev* 12: 1775–1780.

Zhang Y, Iratni R, Erdjument-Bromage H, Tempst P, Reinberg D. (1997). Histone deacetylases and SAP18, a novel polypeptide, are components of a human Sin3 complex. *Cell* 89: 357–364.

Zhang Y, LeRoy G, Seelig HP, Lane WS, Reinberg D (1998c). The dermatomyositis-specific autoantigen Mi2 is a component of a complex containing histone deacetylase and nucleosome remodeling activities. *Cell* 95: 279–289.

Zhang Y, Ng HH, Erdjument-Bromage H, Tempst P, Bird A, Reinberg D (1999). Analysis of the NuRD subunits reveals a histone deacetylase core complex and a connection with DNA methylation. *Genes Dev* 13: 1924–1935.

Zhang Y, Sun ZW, Iratni R, Erdjument-Bromage H, Tempst P, Hampsey M, Reinberg D (1998a). SAP30, a novel protein conserved between human and yeast, is a component of a histone deacetylase complex *Mol Cell* 1: 1021–1031.

Zhou S, Hayward SD (2001). Nuclear localization of cbf1 is regulated by interactions with the SMRT corepressor complex. *Mol Cell Biol* 21: 6222–6232.

Zhou Y, Gross W, Hong SH, Privalsky ML (2001). The SMRT corepressor is a target of phosphorylation by protein kinase CK2 (casein kinase II). *Mol Cell Biochem* 220: 1–13.

Zhou X, Richon VM, Wang AH, Yang XJ, Rifkind RA, Marks PA (2000). Histone deacetylase 4 associates with extracellular signal-regulated kinases 1 and 2, and its cellular localization is regulated by oncogenic Ras. *Proc Natl Acad Sci USA* 97: 14329–14333.

Zhu Y, Qi C, Jain S, Rao MS, Reddy JK (1997). Isolation and characterization of PBP, a protein that interacts with peroxisome proliferator-activated receptor. *J Biol Chem* 272: 25500–25506.

71 | *CBP* and the Rubinstein-Taybi Syndrome

FRED PETRIJ, MARTIJN H. BREUNING, RAOUL C.M. HENNEKAM,
AND RACHEL H. GILES

The Rubinstein-Taybi syndrome (RTS, OMIM 180849) is caused by de novo occurring heterozygous constitutional mutations of the cAMP response element–binding protein (CREB)–binding protein gene (*CREBBP* or *CBP*) gene (OMIM 600140). These mutations are presumed to lead to haploinsufficiency of the CBP protein. The main clinical features of the syndrome are abnormalities of the face, thumbs, and big toes as well as growth and mental retardation.

The CBP protein functions as a transcriptional cofactor by forming a physical bridge between the different components of the transcription machinery. It also functions as a potent histone acetyltransferase (HAT), making the DNA accessible to transcription factors. It is a mediator of different signaling pathways and participates in basic cellular functions. CBP and its close relative p300 play a key role as downstream effectors in the hedgehog, decapentaplegic, wingless (WNT), and Toll developmental pathways.

The human *CBP* gene is located on chromosome band 16p13.3 and has 31 translated exons that are spread over 154 kb of genomic DNA. The CBP protein consists of 2442 amino acids (265 kDa). The *CBP* gene is highly conserved: several *CBP* othologs have been cloned, such as the *Mus musculus Cbp*, the *Drosophila melanogaster dCBP*, and the *Caenorhabditis elegans cbp-1*. CBP does not appear to have a yeast ortholog, however. *Cbp* knockout mice show a phenotype similar to the RTS phenotype in humans. Although much can be learned from the orthologous mutations engineered to date, ultimately the only way to dissect CBP's role in development will be through the use of further genetic approaches in model organisms.

DEVELOPMENTAL SYSTEM

As reviewed in Chapter 70, almost all developmental pathways culminate in interactions that require CBP and its close relative p300. These cofactors harbor intrinsic HAT enzymatic activity (Bannister and Kouzarides, 1996; Ogryzko et al., 1996), which seems to be essential to the key role they play as downstream effectors in the hedgehog, decapentaplegic, wingless (WNT), and Toll developmental pathways. CBP and p300 bind and regulate the activity of dozens of DNA-binding transcription factors (Fig. 71–1). CBP and p300 closely resemble each other biochemically; however, in vivo studies have shown relevant biological differences. Although mutations in *p300* have been reported in primary tumors, no germline mutations of *p300* have been associated with human disease. In this chapter, we discuss how heterozygous constitutional mutations of the *CBP* gene cause the congenital malformation syndrome RTS. We conclude that a 50% reduction in CBP protein levels during one or more critical stage(s) in fetal development is sufficient to cause the range of symptoms that collectively form RTS.

CLINICAL DESCRIPTION

In 1957, three Greek orthopedic surgeons described a 7-year-old boy in the French orthopedic journal *Revue d'Orthopédie* as "a new case of congenital malformations of the thumbs absolutely symmetrical" (Michail et al., 1957). Other characteristics were "mental deficiency and physical underdevelopment, conical face with long Cyrano-type nose, muscular hypotonia with platypodia, funnel chest, cryptorchidism and spindle-legs slightly turgid." In that same year, the pediatrician Jack Rubinstein investigated a 3.5-year-old girl with similar findings in his newly opened Cincinnati Center for Developmental Disorders (Rubinstein, 1990). In the next few years, he was able to collect 6 other cases with similar features. In 1963, he and the pediatric radiologist Hooshang Taybi from Oklahoma reported on these 7 children in the *American Journal of Diseases of Children* as a possible new mental retardation syndrome (Rubinstein and Taybi, 1963), being unaware of the French paper. Later, Rubinstein assigned the "bibliographic certificate of birth" of the syndrome to his Greek colleagues (Rubinstein, 1974). Warkany (1974) ended the discussion about the entity's name by calling it the Rubinstein-Taybi syndrome (RTS), a term already used in 1964 by Coffin (1964) and Job et al. (1964).

RTS is a well-defined syndrome with a characteristic face, broad thumbs, broad big toes, and mental retardation as major clinical hallmarks. RTS is generally a de novo occurring autosomal-dominant trait. The empiric recurrence risk for a couple with a previous child with RTS is as low as 0.1%. If, however, a person with RTS is able to reproduce, the recurrence risk could be as high as 50%. Birth prevalence is 1 in 100,000–125,000. RTS has been described in populations of many different ancestries; however, the number of reports on non-Caucasian patients is low (Petrij et al., 2001).

Three cases are described in the literature in which women likely to be affected with RTS have had a child with the syndrome (Hennekam et al., 1989; Marion et al., 1993; Petrij et al., 2000a). In all three cases, the children clearly had more pronounced dysmorphic features and were more mentally retarded than their mothers. The diagnosis in the mothers would have been difficult without the more pronounced phenotype of their children. The fact that all three mothers were able to reproduce is probably related to their relatively mild phenotypes. The mild phenotype can be explained by the variability of the syndrome or a somatic mosaicism. Molecular analyses on mother and child were not performed in two cases (Hennekam et al., 1989; Marion et al., 1993) and were inconclusive in the third (Petrij et al., 2000a). All three mothers had at least one unaffected child (Hennekam et al., 1989; RW Marion, personal communication, 1996; J.J. van der Smagt, personal communication, 2001). Two unpublished affected parent–child pairs are known to one of us (R.C.M.H.): in one, both mother and child are severely affected; in the other, the mother is more severely affected than the child. Molecular studies in these cases are pending.

Because different clinical features play a different role during the life of an RTS patient, we will partition the clinical history of these patients into three age groups: 0–2 years, 2–12 years, and 12 years and older.

Clinical Features

The main clinical features of the syndrome are abnormalities of the face, thumbs, and big toes as well as growth and mental retardation. The facial appearance is striking: microcephaly, downslanting palpebral fissures, broad nasal bridge, beaked nose with the nasal septum extending below the alae, highly arched palate, and mild micrognathia (Fig. 71–2A,B). Broad thumbs and broad big toes are present in almost all cases (Fig. 71–3). Terminal broadening of the phalanges of the fingers, persistent fetal pads, clinodactyly of the fifth finger, overlapping of the toes, and angulation deformities of the thumbs and halluces can also be present. There is marked growth retardation with poor weight gain during infancy, often replaced by overweight in later childhood

Figure 71–1. CBP/p300 molecular organization and interactions. Interacting proteins are shown at the *top* of the figure; functional domains are depicted *below*. Many known interactions are not included due to space limitations. (Modified from Goodman and Smolik, 2000, reprinted from *Genes Dev* with permission from Cold Spring Harbor Laboratory Press.)

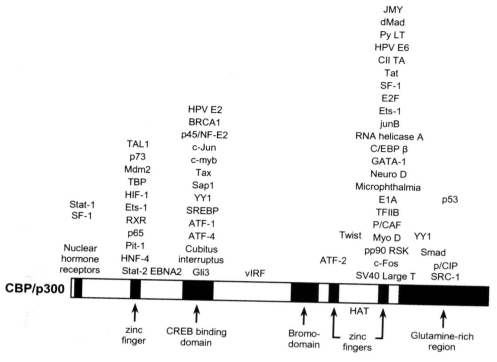

(Fig. 71–4). Global mental deficiency is characteristic, with an average IQ between 35 and 50. Behavior is characterized by short attention span, poor coordination, and sudden mood changes. Other findings may include eye anomalies (nasolacrimal duct obstruction, ptosis of eyelids, congenital or juvenile glaucoma, and refractive errors), specific dental anomalies (talon cusps of the permanent incisors), a variety of congenital heart defects, and skin anomalies (supernumerary nipples, nevus flammeus, hirsutism, and keloid formation). The clinical history often shows feeding problems and recurrent conjunctivitis in the neonatal period, respiratory problems in the first decade, and lifelong constipation. An inventory of the major features of RTS and their frequency is given in Table 71–1. In general, RTS patients are in good health. Although an increased risk for different types of tumor is known, life expectancy seems to be normal (Petrij et al., 2001).

0–2 Years

Length, weight, and occipitofrontal circumference (OFC) at birth are between the 25th and 50th percentiles, except for the OFC of males, which is at the 2nd percentile (Rubinstein, 1990; Stevens et al., 1990b). Average birth length is 49 cm (range 43.9–53.3 cm), and average birth weight is 3.1 kg (range 2.05–4.28 kg). Mean OFC is 34.2 cm (males) and 32.2 cm (females) (range 29–38 cm) (Stevens et al., 1990b). Poor weight gain during infancy is usual (Stevens et al., 1990b). In the first few months, all growth curves decline: length to the 5th percentile, weight below the 5th percentile, and head OFC to the 2nd percentile, leading to microcephaly. In the first year of life, 80% of children with RTS have feeding problems, which are mainly caused by general hypotonia, gastroesophageal reflux (GER), and recurrent upper respiratory infections. As long as the weight percentile keeps up with the length percentile, no direct intervention is necessary. Most feeding problems resolve after a period of 1 year (Grunow, 1982; Hennekam et al., 1990b). Constipation is a frequent (71%) and persistent problem in RTS patients, starting in babies and toddlers. It is a primary problem, not secondary to the feeding problems. Constipation should be treated by diet or laxative medication, also because it can play a role in vesicoureteral reflux and urinary tract infections.

General psychomotor development is delayed. Eye contact is delayed as well, but as soon eye contact is established, RTS babies make contact easily. Most parents describe them as easy-going and loving babies. Table 71–2 gives an overview of the general developmental milestones (Hennekam et al., 1992).

Upper respiratory infections, (aspiration) pneumonias, and middle ear infections are frequent in children with RTS (51%). Aberrant craniofacial anatomy and GER are the main causes. If GER seems to be the major cause of the upper respiratory infections and (aspiration) pneumonias, it should be treated with medication. Patients with recurrent ear infections should be referred to a pediatric otolaryngologist as middle ear disease is more common (50%) and more severe in children with RTS.

Children with RTS frequently have lacrimal duct obstructions (43% bilateral, 7% unilateral), which often lead to recurrent conjunctivitis. Surgical intervention may be necessary if the problems do not resolve. In some cases, placement of glass tear ducts is required, but this is usually performed only when the patient has reached adulthood. Other frequent ocular problems are ptosis (45%), strabismus (58%), and refractive errors (41%). Cataract, glaucoma, and coloboma occur less frequently (<10%). In some RTS patients, surgery is required to correct a ptosis or strabismus. During the first 2 years of life, correction of refractive errors is seldom needed. Because of the high frequency of eye problems in RTS, it is important to refer a child with a probable diagnosis of RTS to a pediatric ophthalmologist within the first few weeks of life (van Genderen et al., 2000).

The average age at which a congenital heart malformation is diagnosed in RTS patients is 6.4 months (range first day to 12 years). Of RTS patients, 32% have a congenital heart malformation, 65% of whom have a single defect (posterior descending artery, ventral or atrial septal defects, coarctation, or pulmonic stenosis) and 35% two or more defects or a complex malformation (Table 71–1). In half of the cases with a single defect, surgery is needed compared to 80% of the more complex cases.

Almost all boys with RTS have incomplete or delayed descent of the testicles. Surgery is needed before the age of 2 years in almost all cases because spontaneous full descent is not to be expected. Hypospadias is seen in 11% of boys with RTS. Surgery should be considered only if the hypospadias is severe or in cases with recurrent infections. All RTS children who have had one or more urinary tract infections should undergo an ultrasound examination because 52% have kidney anomalies. If a child with RTS has a neurogenic bladder or a change in bowel or bladder function, an evaluation for tethered cord, by magnetic resonance imaging of the lower spinal cord, should be performed.

The main nondental oral aspects of RTS are a thin upper lip (40%), small oral opening (56%), pouting lower lip (38%), retro/micrognathia

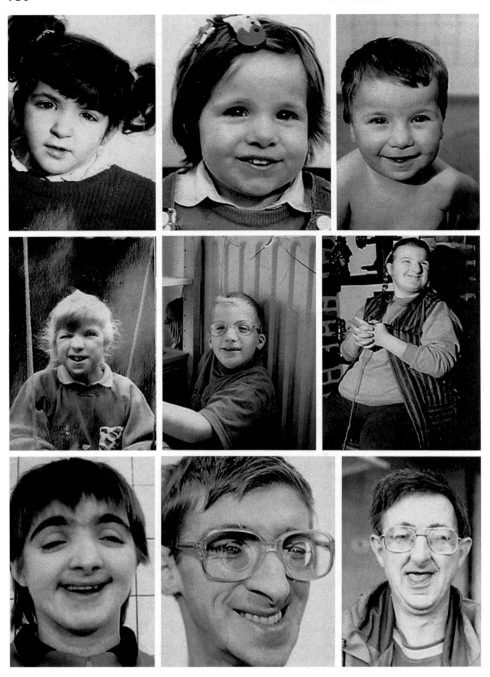

Figure 71–2A. Variability of facial dysmorphism as seen in nine Rubinstein-Taybi syndrome patients at different ages. *Top row*: 3.1 years, 2.0 years, and 2.2 years. *Middle row*: 13.4 years, 10.3 years, and 18.7 years. *Bottom row*: 20.1 years, 34.4 years, and 45.3 years. Note the relatively mild phenotype of the three children in the top row. The top left girl has a deletion of the entire *CBP* gene (see Fig. 71–7, patient RT2906).

(56%), and highly arched narrow palate (93%). Cleft uvula, cleft palate, or (more rarely), cleft lip can be part of the syndrome. Timing of the eruption of deciduous and permanent dentition is normal. The malpositioned and crowded teeth (62%) often have marked caries (36%), which is possibly caused by problems in dental care due to the small opening of the mouth, malpositioning and malformation of the teeth, and noncooperation of the patients. Hypodontia, hyperdontia, and natal teeth can be manifestations of the syndrome. The most important dental feature in RTS is the very high incidence of talon cusps in the permanent dentition (92%). They can be present in the deciduous dentition (9%) or sometimes can be detected in the jaws by orthopanthomogram. Talon cusps are accessory cusp-like structures on the lingual side, mostly of the incisors (Fig. 71–5). Two or more talon cusps are rarely found in the normal population or in other syndromes. Therefore, this finding strongly supports the diagnosis of RTS (Hennekam and Van Doorne, 1990).

Children with significant angulation of the thumbs should be considered for surgical repair prior to the age of 2 years because these angulations can have serious consequences for the functional ability of the hands (Wood and Rubinstein, 1987). Surgery of angulated great toes is performed only when they hinder walking or wearing footwear. Hypermobility of the joints is seldom a problem at this early age.

RTS children can be difficult to intubate because of the easy collapsibility of the laryngeal wall. In RTS children, an anesthesiologist comfortable with complex pediatric airway problems should perform the general anesthesia if needed. Because of these problems, RTS children should be intubated earlier and extubated later than other children. The flaccid larynx may also cause significant sleep apnea at this age.

2–12 Years

The constipation, eye problems, swallowing problems, aspirations, anesthetic problems, and upper respiratory infections will remain pres-

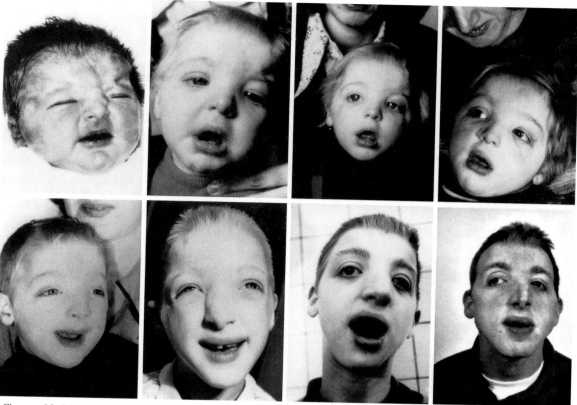

Figure 71–2B. Change of facial characteristics with age in one individual. *Top row*: 1 week, 1.2 years, 2.2 years, and 3.4 years. *Bottom row*: 5.3 years, 10.1 years, 15.5 years, and 29.1 years. Note the difference in slanting of the palpebral fissures and the position of the nasal septum.

ent during childhood. The upper respiratory infections gradually subside: 26% before the age of 6 years and 61% before the age of 12 years (Grunow, 1982; Hennekam et al., 1990b). The majority of the RTS children will become continent for urine and feces.

In the first few months of life, average length falls from the 50th to the 5th percentile. During the preschool and early school years, height keeps following these centiles. Figure 71–4 shows that the height curves for males and females are very similar. Growth velocity is below the mean but within the normal range until early adolescence (Stevens et al., 1990b). In males and females, average weight is at the 50th percentile at birth but falls below the 5th percentile in the first few months. Males gain weight mainly during the preschool and school years. Their average weight is in the 5th–50th percentile, but by the time adolescence emerges it drops below the 5th percentile again. As seen in Figure 71–4, males are overweight for their age during childhood. The overweight in females starts somewhat later (early adolescence) but can remain a problem throughout life (Hennekam et al., 1990b). Dietary measures are often required for boys during childhood and for girls from early adolescence onward.

The mean age at which RTS children start to walk is 35 months (range 18–54). In cases with angulated great toes, orthopedic intervention is sometimes needed.

The first few words will be spoken around the second year. Two- or three-word sentences will take as long as 4 years and sometimes even 7 years, so there is a large spread in speech development. Despite the oral anatomical abnormalities, the "speech mechanism" seems to be intact. Some children display a nasal type of speech. Although the vocabulary is limited (corresponding to the IQ), the communicative abilities of RTS children are often relatively good. However, some individuals are nonverbal and use sign language or other systems to communicate. Children in this age group are in general friendly, happy, and easy-going. Nevertheless, 25% of the parents of RTS children in this age group report behavioral problems, often characterized by short attention span, stubbornness, lack of perseverance,

claiming behavior, and sudden mood changes (Hennekam et al., 1992). Most children with RTS need some degree of individualized programming, whether in specialized or inclusive settings. They often need speech therapy, physical therapy, and pedagogic guidance.

Refractive errors are present in 41% of RTS children. The majority have myopia, but hypermetropia and astigmatism also occur (van Genderen et al., 2000). In this age group, correction of these refractive errors becomes important. Many children are photophobic (50%). At this age, retinal dysfunction does not play an important role in the quality of vision (see below).

The majority of the dental problems are described above (see 0–2 Years). However, talon cusps are a feature of the permanent dentition (92%) and much less so of the deciduous dentition (9%). Talon cusps can give rise to caries by accumulation of food remains behind them. It is possible to grind off the tips or fill up the space between the cusps and the teeth. Malpositioned and crowded teeth could make surgical intervention sometimes necessary. The person who carries out any dental procedure should be familiar with the anesthetic problems of RTS patients (see above) (Hennekam and Van Doorne, 1990).

Because RTS patients start to walk within this age range (on average at 35 months), general hypotonia and hyperextensibility of the joints due to lax ligaments (82%) can become more problematic. If there is a weight problem as well, the overweight should certainly be addressed. The gait is commonly stiff and sometimes waddling. Children with RTS have an increased risk for dislocation of the radial head and the patella. Patellar dislocation can be particularly burdensome (Hennekam et al., 1990b; Moran et al., 1993; Stevens, 1997) and can have great consequences for the mobility of the patient. If not treated in time, patellar dislocation can lead to complications such as genua valga, tibial torsion, and flexion contracture. Around 10 years of age, children with RTS can start developing a kyphosis, lordosis, and scoliosis. Other skeletal anomalies include sternal abnormalities, rib defects, spina bifida, flat acetabular angles, slipped capital femoral epi-

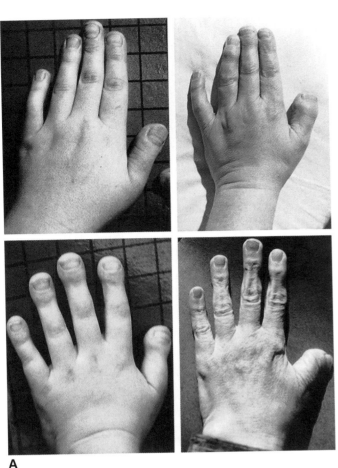

A

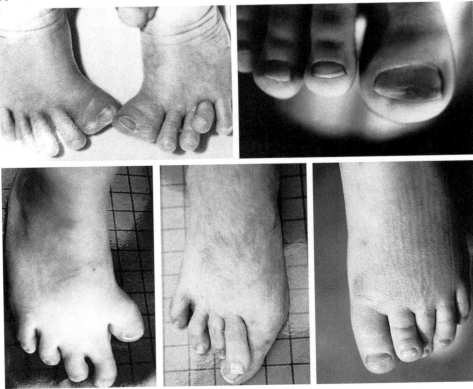

B

Figure 71–3. (*A*) Hands of four Rubinstein-Taybi syndrome (RTS) patients. Thumbs are broad (87%), sometimes showing signs of duplication of the distal phalanges (although genuine preaxial polydactyly does not occur). Angulation deformities of the thumbs occur in 33% of cases (22% bilateral, 11% unilateral). Terminal broadening of the other phalanges can be seen in 64% of RTS patients (appearing mushroom-shaped on X-ray). (*B*) Feet of five RTS patients. Halluces are always broad (100%), showing no or just minimal signs of duplication, or have real duplications of the distal phalanges (11%). Angulation deformities can be present in the varus (7%) or valgus (17%) position (*bottom left* and *bottom middle*, respectively). Varus deformities sometimes require surgery.

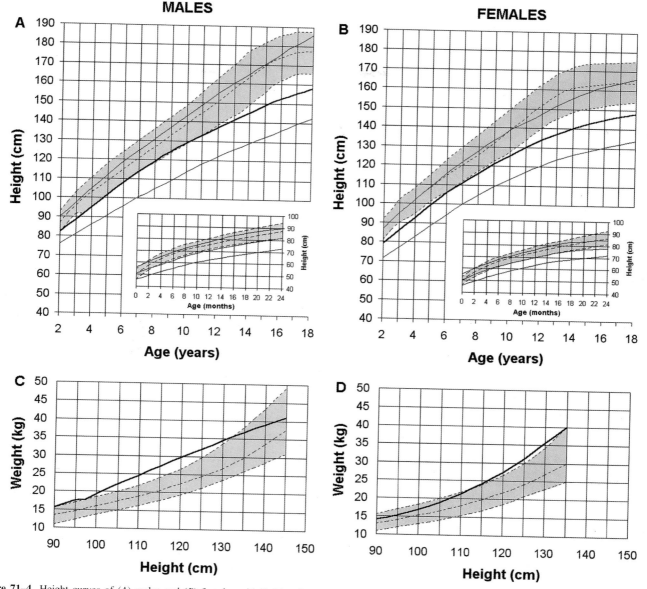

Figure 71–4. Height curves of (*A*) males and (*B*) females with Rubinstein-Taybi syndrome (RTS) (mean ± 2 S.D., solid lines) compared to normal individuals (dashed lines) and average weight-for-height of (*C*) males and (*D*) females with RTS (solid line) compared to 5th, 50th, and 95th percentiles in normal individuals (dashed lines). (Modified from Stevens et al., 1990, reprinted from *Am J Med Genet* with permission from John Wiley & Sons, Inc.)

physis (Bonioli et al., 1993), flaring of ilia, notched ischia, and increased risk of fractures (Hennekam et al., 1990b; Rubinstein, 1990). Various other low-frequency anomalies have been discussed by Rubinstein (1990), Robson et al. (1980), and Hennekam et al. (1990b).

Obstructive sleep apnea syndrome is often (11%) a considerable problem (Hennekam et al., 1990b; Zucconi et al., 1993). It may be caused by the combination of a narrow palate, micrognathia, hypotonia, obesity, and easy collapsibility of the laryngeal walls (Hennekam et al., 1990b). In one patient, these complaints necessitated a tracheostomy. Indicative for obstructive sleep apnea syndrome are snoring, particular sleeping posture (often, the children sleep with the head between the knees), superficial sleep in the night, and excessive sleepiness during the daytime. Continuous positive airway pressure may elevate the problem but is often not accepted by RTS patients. Sleeping

in an optimal posture seems to be the most simple solution (Hennekam et al., 1990b; Zucconi et al., 1993).

An increased tumor risk has been recognized (Miller and Rubinstein, 1995). The reported tumors include nasopharyngeal rhabdomyosarcoma (Sobel and Woerner, 1981), intraspinal neurilemmoma (Russell et al., 1971), pheochromocytoma (Bonioli and Bellini, 1992), meningioma (Bilir et al., 1990; Hennekam et al., 1990b), other brain tumors (Hennekam et al., 1990a; Lannering et al., 1990; D'Cruz et al., 1993; Evans et al., 1993; Skousen et al., 1996), pilomatrixoma (Cambiaghi et al., 1994; Masuno et al., 1998), and acute leukemia (Jonas et al., 1978). About half of the tumors are malignant. The majority of tumors are neural tube derivatives. Treatment is like in other individuals. In 86% of cases, the diagnosis has been made before the age of 15 years (Miller and Rubinstein, 1995).

Table 71–1. Medical Problems of the Rubinstein-Taybi Syndrome

Feature	Percentage ($n = 95$)
Pregnancy	
Gestational length	39.9 (range 32–44) weeks
Polyhydramnios	30
Infancy history	
Respiratory problems	51
Feeding problems	80
Constipation	71
Poor weight gain	80
Medical history	
Visual problems	84
Strabismus	58
Refractive error	41
Astigmatism	18
Other	4
Cataracts	7
Glaucoma	8
Coloboma	5
Tear duct obstruction	39
Ptosis	45
Hearing loss	24
Frequent middle ear infections	60
Congenital heart defects	32
PDA	13
VSD	12
ASD	10
Coarctation	3
Pulmonic stenosis	2
Urinary tract infection	22
Keloids or hypertrophic scarring	25
Severe constipation	44
Epilepsy	23

PDA, posterior descending artery; VSD, ventricular septal defect; ASD, atrial septal defect.
Source: Gorlin et al., 2001; Petrij et al., 2001.

12 Years and Older

The constipation, eye problems, malignancies, obstructive sleep apneas, and anesthetic problems (see above) remain present during adolescence and adulthood. In general, RTS patients remain the friendly, loving personalities they were during childhood, although sudden mood changes can occur. If they are not allowed to indulge their increased need for daytime sleep, then mood changes, excitability, and irritability can occur. The need for daytime sleep can be caused by obstructive sleep apneas during night. Long-term obstructed respiration can lead to pulmonary hypertension, which in its turn can cause right ventricle hypertrophia and ultimately decompensatio cordis. Treatment of pulmonary hypertension is necessary.

Neither boys nor girls will experience a pubertal growth spurt, which contributes to their short stature as adults (Fig. 71–4). Values for final height and mean OFC at adulthood are 153.1 cm and 54.7 cm for males and 146.7 cm and 52.4 cm for females, respectively. Average adult height is about 3 S.D. below the mean. The average OFC of males is smaller at birth (2nd percentile) and throughout childhood (−4 S.D.) than that of females (almost at the 50th percentile and below the 2nd percentile), but at adulthood the mean OFC of males is around the 25th percentile and that of females around the 5th percentile. School-age boys and adolescent girls tend to be overweight

Table 71–2. Developmental Milestones of Rubinstein-Taybi Syndrome (RTS) Children Compared to Normal Children

Milestone	Average Age (Months)		Range (Months)	
	RTS	Normal	RTS	Normal
Laughing	2.5	2	2–6	2
Roll over	10	6	4–18	5–7
Sit	16	7	9–24	6–8
Crawl	19	9	12–36	8–10
Stand	29	9	11–80	8–10
Walk	35	14	18–54	12–15

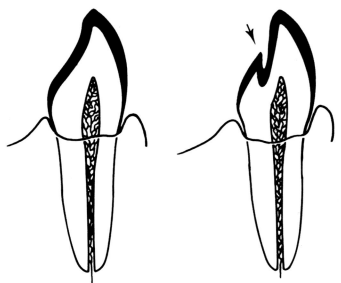

Figure 71–5. Schematic drawing of a talon cusp (arrow) compared with a normal incisor. The talon cusp may also contain a pulp chamber. They are rarely found in the normal population or other syndromes. Two or more talon cusps strongly support the Rubinstein-Taybi syndrome diagnosis (Hennekam and Van Doorne, 1990).

for height (Fig. 71–4). Several patients have vigorous appetites in late childhood or early adolescence (Stevens et al., 1990b).

Puberty starts at normal age. Girls often have hypermenorrhagia or metrorrhagia. The contraceptive pill can often resolve this problem. Contraindications of this treatment are not described. Because some of the adolescents and adults are sexually active, males as well as females, this issue needs to be addressed.

Keloids (22%) or hypertrophic scarring (16%) have been described in 25% of cases (Rohlfing et al., 1971; Goodfellow et al., 1980; Selmanowitz and Stiller, 1981; Sammartino et al., 1986; Hennekam et al., 1990b; Stevens et al., 1990a; Gorlin et al., 2001; Petrij et al., 2001). They can cause pain and extreme itchiness. The localization of keloid formation is unremarkable, i.e., the upper part of the back, chest, shoulders, and upper arms. Sometimes only minimal trauma, such as a bee sting or rubbing clothes, can instigate the keloid formation. Keloids are very therapy-resistant; local corticosteroids, oral antihistamines, or laser therapy are often ineffective and sometimes even cause more damage than good. Avoiding skin trauma is the only preventive measure that can be taken.

Malignancies, should they occur, will generally manifest before the age of 15 years (86%) (Miller and Rubinstein, 1995). However, meningiomas are more likely to occur around 40 years of age.

Van Genderen et al. (2000) described a high frequency of retinal dysfunction (78%) in RTS patients. Electroretinographic investigations showed cone or cone–rod dysfunction in 58%, and visual evoked potentials (VEPs) showed an abnormal waveform in 63% of 24 investigated patients. With age, retinal as well as electrophysiological abnormalities occurred more frequently. In the age group below 15 years, only minor abnormalities were found. Because of the high frequency of ocular abnormalities, visual function tests and electrophysiological investigations should be performed in every RTS patient at regular intervals. Retinal dysfunction cannot be treated, but it is important to know this at an early stage, to make proper adjustments to the natural environment of the patient.

Several pubertal patients have severe and prolonged aseptic hip joint inflammations (Perthes like). In general, this problem resolves without intervention, but symptomatic treatment might be necessary because of the pain (Gorlin et al., 2001). Tethered cord has been described in RTS (Rosenbaum et al., 1990) but remains uncommon. Change in bowel or bladder habits or change in gait could indicate that a tethered cord is evolving. Slipped capital femoral epiphysis, which occurs preferably in adolescence, can become a major problem. Initially, it is often silent; but if there are symptoms, the radiographic progress is often already severe. Pain or a change in gait should always be carefully evaluated in RTS.

MOLECULAR GENETICS

The Human RTS Locus Is Positioned on Chromosome Band 16p13.3

Imaizumi and Kuroki (1991) and shortly thereafter Tommerup et al. (1992) described RTS patients with a de novo reciprocal translocation that was consistent for one of the breakpoints, a t(2;16)(p13.3;p13.3) and a t(7;16)(q34;p13.3). All previously reported chromosomal rearrangements, reviewed by Hennekam et al. (1990a), had been inconsistent with regard to their breakpoints. Lacombe et al. (1992) confirmed the assignment of RTS to 16p13.3 by reporting a de novo pericentric inversion, inv(16)(p13.3q13).

Breuning et al. (1993) reported another t(16;20) and investigated the 16p13.3 region using two-color fluorescence in situ hybridization (FISH). The rank order of approximately 80 chromosome 16p cosmids was determined. The breakpoints of the t(2;16) and the t(7;16) mapped between the cosmids N2 (D16S138) and RT1 (D16S237). In the years that followed, four additional gross chromosomal rearrangements involving 16p13.3 were discovered (Table 71–3).

Breuning et al. (1993) analyzed 24 RTS patients by FISH using the N2 and RT1 probes and found that the RT1 signal was missing from one chromosome 16 in six patients (25%). For five of these patients, the parents were available for FISH studies; none showed an RT1 microdeletion, indicating a de novo rearrangement. Using molecular markers, Hennekam et al. (1993) found a copy of chromosome 16 from both parents in all 19 RTS patients studied, excluding uniparental disomy as a causative mechanism for RTS. The initial estimation of 25% microdeletions may have been an overestimation due to small numbers. An inventory of all RTS microdeletions published so far (Breuning et al., 1993; Masuno et al., 1994; Petrij et al., 1995, 2000a; McGaughran et al., 1996; Wallerstein et al., 1997; Taine et al., 1998; Bartsch et al., 1999; Blough et al., 2000; Murata et al., 2001) shows that the actual 16p microdeletion frequency in RTS is around 10% (Table 71–4). Clinical features were essentially the same in patients with or without detectable deletions, with the possible exception of microcephaly, angulation of thumbs and halluces, and partial duplication of halluces (Hennekam et al., 1993).

Cloning the RTS Gene Region

Breuning et al. (1993) demonstrated not only that the chromosomal breakpoints leading to RTS map to the area between N2 and RT1 but that this area is also home to somatic chromosomal rearrangements leading to leukemia (Petrij et al., 1995; Giles et al., 1995, 1997b). These authors embarked upon cloning the gene for the RTS and the gene for acute myeloid leukemia (AML) associated with the translocation t(8;16)(p11;p13.3) (Wessels et al., 1991). t(8;16) is a somatic rearrangement associated with AML subtype M4/M5. AML patients observed with this translocation often exhibit erythrophagocytosis and generally have a poor prognosis (reviewed in Velloso et al., 1996). Cosmids N2 and RT1 were used as starting points for a classical positional cloning effort. In this way, a genomic map of 1.2 Mb was constructed (Giles et al., 1997a).

Table 71–3. Translocations and Pericentric Inversions Reported in Rubinstein-Taybi Syndrome

Chromosomal Rearrangement		References
t(2;16)[JAP]	(p13.3;p13.3)	Imaizumi and Kuroki, 1991
t(7;16)	(q34;p13.3)	Tommerup et al., 1992
inv(16)[FRA]	(p13.3q13)	Lacombe et al., 1992
inv(16)[NOR]	Unknown	Breuning et al., 1993; Petrij et al., 1995
t(16;20)	(p;q)	Petrij et al., 1995
t(2;16)[NL]	(q36.3;p13.3)	Petrij et al. 1995; Petrij et al., 2000b
t(1;16)	(p34.1;p13.2)	Wallerstein et al., 1997
t(16;Y)	Unknown	Blough, personal communication, 1998

Cloning of the CBP Gene

A subclone from cosmid RT1 showed conservation with DNA from several species (zoo-blot). This subclone was used to screen a human fetal brain cDNA library. This method resulted in a cDNA clone which contained an open reading frame of 573 bp and a poly-A tail. The open reading frame of this cDNA showed 92% DNA homology with murine Cbp (Chrivia et al., 1993; Petrij et al., 1995; Giles et al., 1997a).

CBP was characterized in 1993 in the mouse by Chrivia et al. (1993) as a transcriptional co-activator. The protein was named after its interaction with the CREB protein (Kwok et al., 1994). Although officially the gene is named CREBBP, it is generally referred to by its shorter acronym CBP. CBP and its chromosome 22 homolog p300 (Eckner et al., 1994; Lundblad et al., 1995) have been found not just to function as transcriptional coactivators by forming a physical bridge between the different components of the transcription machinery but also as potent HATs by making the DNA accessible to transcription factors. They are mediators of different signaling pathways and participants in basic cellular functions such as DNA repair, cell growth, cell differentiation, apoptosis, and tumor suppression (see below and Chapter 70). In other words, CBP and p300 are at the center of multiple signal-transduction pathways and thereby regulate the expression of many genes (reviewed by Goodman and Smolik, 2000).

Twelve of the 13 known RTS and t(8;16)-AML breakpoints are restricted to a 15–20 kb area (Fig. 71–6). However, the RTS t(2;16)[NL] breakpoint maps approximately 100 kb more telomeric than this breakpoint cluster, which indicated that the RTS gene is spread over quite a stretch of genomic DNA (>100 kb) (Petrij et al., 1995; Giles et al., 1997a). A part of the breakpoint region, the area just telomeric of cosmid RT166, is unstable in cosmids and yeast artificial chromosomes (YACs). Multiple attempts to isolate this DNA fragment in cosmid, fosmid, PAC, or bacterial artificial chromosome (BAC) libraries initially failed. Large-scale chromosome 16 sequence analysis performed at the Los Alamos National Laboratory identified a 165 kb BAC clone (GenBank accession AC007151) containing the 5′ end of the CBP gene (including exons 1–3) (Coupry et al., 2002). Sequence analysis revealed the exact size of intron 2 (39,517 bp) and the distance between cosmids RT203 and RT166 (11,173 bp). A NIX analysis of the unstable region of CBP indicated the presence of 57% interspersed repeats (27.7% of SINEs, 17.8% of LINEs, 0.8% of long terminal repeat elements, and 10.7% of MER elements). In comparison, two other cosmids covering the 3′ part of the CBP gene (i.e., RT191 and RT102) presented a total of 28.6% and 35.3% interspersed repeats, respectively (Coupry et al., 2002). The high density of repeat elements observed in

Table 71–4. Reported Rubinstein-Taybi Syndrome Microdeletion Frequency

Authors	Patients Studied	Microdeletions	Non-RT1/RT100 (5 Cosmids Tested)	%
Breuning et al., 1993	24	6	—	25
Masuno et al., 1994	25	1	—	4
McGaughran et al., 1996	16	2	—	13
Wallerstein et al., 1997	64	7	—	11
Taine et al., 1998	30	3	—	10
Bartsch et al., 1999	45	4	—	9
Blough et al., 2000	66	5	—	8
Petrij et al., 2000a	105	9	2/66	9
Murata et al., 2001	16	1	2/23	6
Total	391	38	4	10

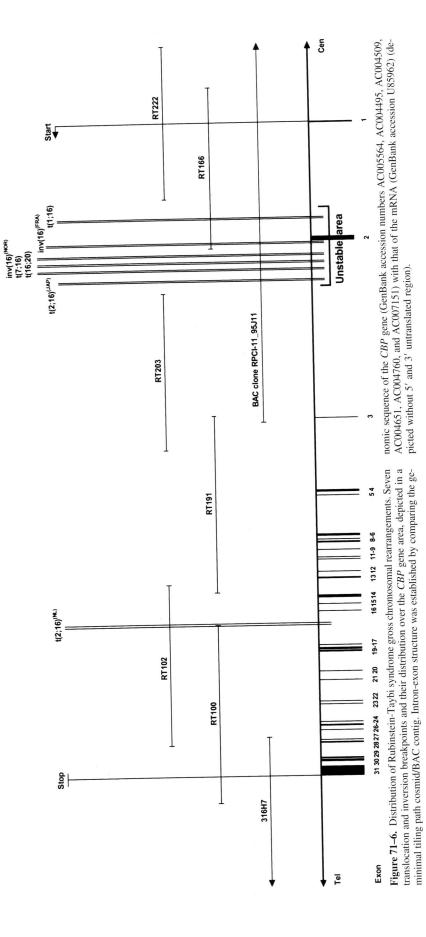

Figure 71–6. Distribution of Rubinstein-Taybi syndrome gross chromosomal rearrangements. Seven translocation and inversion breakpoints and their distribution over the *CBP* gene area, depicted in a minimal tiling path cosmid/BAC contig. Intron-exon structure was established by comparing the genomic sequence of the *CBP* gene (GenBank accession numbers AC005564, AC004495, AC004509, AC004651, AC004760, and AC007151) with that of the mRNA (GenBank accession U85962) (depicted without 5′ and 3′ untranslated region).

the 5′ region of the *CBP* gene could be responsible for the observed instability leading to numerous chromosomal rearrangements.

The human *CBP* cDNA measures 9068 bp in length, of which 7329 bp are translated into 2442 amino acids (GenBank accession 85962). The protein is 265 kDa. The human *CBP* gene (154 kb) consists of 31 exons (Petrij, 2000; Petrij et al., 2000a) and is transcriptionally oriented from centromere to telomere (Giles et al., 1997a) (see Fig. 71–6 and Table 71–5).

CBP Mutation Analysis in RTS Patients

RTS diagnostics start with careful clinical evaluation, which was and still is the hallmark of diagnostics. Although translocations and inversions form the minority of *CBP* mutations in RTS, the diagnostic procedure should be followed by karyotyping. To date, eight gross chromosomal rearrangements involving chromosome band 16p13.3 have been reported (see Table 71–3). The positions of seven of these eight known RTS translocations and inversions were determined by FISH, fiber FISH, and Southern analysis (Fig. 71–6).

Initially, cosmid RT1 and later RT100 were used in FISH experiments for RTS microdeletion detection. Because these two cosmids cover only the 3′ end of the human *CBP* gene, 5′ microdeletions would not be detected using them alone. Ideally, five cosmids (RT100,

RT102, RT191, RT203, and RT166) should be used to detect all submicroscopic deletions in patients with a clinical picture of RTS (Blough et al., 2000; Petrij et al., 2000a, 2001). Cosmids were used from the physical mapping effort as probes for FISH experiments on material from 21 RTS patients with microdeletions. In a nondeletion individual, each cosmid tested gives two distinct signals, one from each chromosome 16. However, when the genomic area corresponding to one or more of these cosmids is deleted, only one signal, from the unaffected chromosome 16, will be observed. Using this method, Petrij et al. (2000a) measured the deleted areas in 21 RTS patients. All deletions affected at least some part of the *CBP* gene, which ranged from 50 to >650 kb (Fig. 71–7). Coupry et al. (2002) found suitable polymorphic repeats in intron 1 (MS1) and in the large intron 2 (MS2 and MS4) and located the already known marker D16S3065 in intron 13 of the *CBP* gene. Assuming obligate heterozygosity (parental DNA should be available), these four intragenic markers can be used in RTS deletion detection as well. Because the four markers do not cover the 3′ end of the *CBP* gene, 3′ cosmids (e.g., RT100 and RT102) used in FISH experiments remain necessary to guarantee full coverage. MS1, MS2, and MS4 have been submitted to dbSTS with the accession numbers G72365, G72366, and G72367, respectively.

Translocations, inversions, and microdeletions certainly indicated

Table 71–5. Intron–Exon Boundaries of Human *CBP*

Exon	*CBP* (nt from ATG)	GenBank U85962 (nt)	Exon Size (nt)	LANL Cosmid	GenBank Accession	Exon (Cosmid/BAC Position)	Intron (Cosmid/BAC Position)	Intron Size (nt)
1	1–85	819–903	85	RT166	AC005564	8013–8097	8098–36910*	28,813
				BAC	AC007151	69479–69563	40657–69478*	
2	86–798	904–1616	713	RT166	AC005564	36911–37623	37624–37930†	
				BAC	AC007151	39944–40656	427–39943	39,517
3	799–975	1617–1793	177	RT203	AC004495	28034–28210	28211–35528†	
				RT191	AC004509	467–643	644–17619	16,976
				BAC	AC007151	250–426	1–249†	
4	976–1216	1794–2034	241	RT191	AC004509	17620–17860	17861–19151	1291
5	1217–1330	2035–2148	114	RT191	AC004509	19152–19265	19266–28319	9054
6	1331–1573	2149–2391	243	RT191	AC004509	28320–28562	28563–29939	1377
7	1574–1676	2392–2494	103	RT191	AC004509	29940–30042	30043–30367	325
8	1677–1823	2495–2641	147	RT191	AC004509	30368–30514	30515–32428	1914
9	1824–1941	2642–2759	118	RT191	AC004509	32429–32546	32547–33063	517
10	1942–2113	2760–2931	172	RT191	AC004509	33064–33235	33236–33588	353
11	2114–2158	2932–2976	45	RT191	AC004509	33589–33633	33634–36552	2919
12	2159–2283	2977–3101	125	RT191	AC004509	36553–36677	36678–37315	638
13	2284–2463	3102–3281	180	RT191	AC004509	37316–37495	37496–39595†	+2100
				RT102	AC004651		1–2492	+2492
							overlap	−1828
14	2464–2880	3282–3698	417	RT102	AC004651	2493–2909	2910–4125	2764
15	2881–3060	3699–3878	180	RT102	AC004651	4126–4305	4306–5569	1216
16	3061–3250	3879–4068	190	RT102	AC004651	5570–5759	5760–14506	1264
17	3251–3369	4069–4187	119	RT102	AC004651	14507–14625	14626–15430	8747
18	3370–3609	4188–4427	240	RT102	AC004651	15431–15670	15671–16102	805
19	3610–3698	4428–4516	89	RT102	AC004651	16103–16191	16192–21672	432
20	3699–3779	4517–4597	81	RT102	AC004651	21673–21753	21754–23795	5481
21	3780–3836	4598–4654	57	RT102	AC004651	23796–23852	23853–28124	2042
22	3837–3914	4655–4732	78	RT102	AC004651	28125–28202	28203–28517	4272
23	3915–3982	4733–4800	68	RT102	AC004651	28518–28585	28586–32929	315
24	3983–4133	4801–4951	151	RT102	AC004651	32930–33080	33081–33754	4344
25	4134–4280	4952–5098	147	RT102	AC004651	33755–33901	33902–34806	674
26	4281–4394	5099–5212	114	RT102	AC004651	34807–34920	34921–36663	905
27	4395–4560	5213–5378	166	RT102	AC004651	36664–36829	36830–37275	1743
				316H7	AC004760	710–875	876–1321	
28	4561–4728	5379–5546	168	RT102	AC004651	37276–37443	37444–41541	446
				316H7	AC004760	1322–1489	1490–5587	
29	4729–4890	5547–5708	162	RT102	AC004651	41542–41703	41704–42016†	4098
				316H7	AC004760	5588–5749	5750–6051	
30	4891–5172	5709–5990	282	316H7	AC004760	6052–6333	6334–7650	302
31	5173–7329	5991–8147	2157	316H7	AC004760	7651–9807		1317
CBP translated sequence			7329					
5′UTR			818				Σ introns	144,861
3′UTR			921		U85962			
CBP transcript			9068		U89355			

*Difference in intron 1 size between cosmid RT166 and the bacterial artificial chromosome (BAC) clone is due to polymorphic di- and trinucleotide repeats.
†End of the cosmid or beginning of the BAC clone (which was sequenced in reversed orientation).

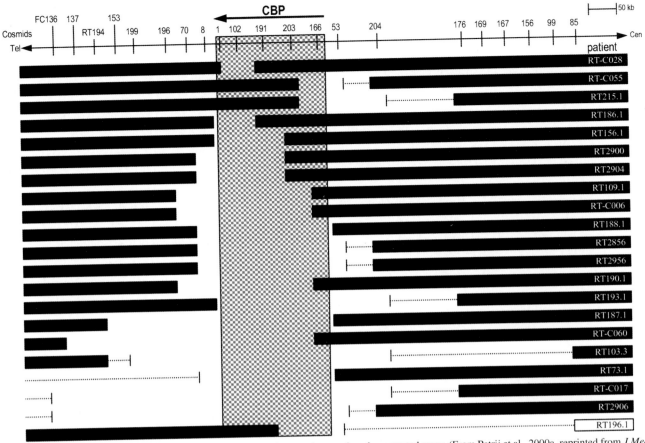

Figure 71-7. Schematic representation of 21 Rubinstein-Taybi microdeletions. Black bars represent undeleted DNA; dashed lines represent uncloned or untested areas. (From Petrij et al., 2000a, reprinted from *J Med Genet* with permission from the BMJ Publishing Group.)

that the *CBP* gene was disrupted in these RTS patients. However, a second gene, contained within *CBP*'s introns, could still be involved. Petrij et al. (1995) used the protein truncation test (PTT) (Roest et al., 1993) to look for translation-terminating *CBP* mutations in RTS patients without rearrangements. Two of 16 patients showed mutations resulting in a truncated protein product (Fig. 71–8). Sequence analyses confirmed these results. In both patients, a codon for glutamine was changed into a stop codon by a C-to-T substitution (at nt 406 and nt 1069, respectively). Both patients had classical RTS phenotypes. In one of these cases, the mutation destroyed a *Pvu*II restriction site. This site was present in both chromosomes of the parents, indicating

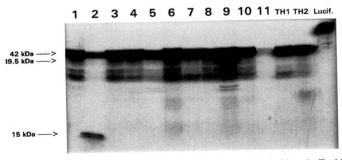

Figure 71-8. Truncated CBP proteins in two patients with Rubinstein-Taybi syndrome. Protein truncation test was performed on the first 1.2 kb of the human *CBP* cDNA. Patient samples 2 and 9 show a truncated protein of 15 and 39.5 kDa, respectively (normal is 42 kDa). On this autoradiogram, 11 patients are depicted. TH, control individuals; luciferase lane contains a control for the translation reaction. Samples of five additional patients were analyzed on another gel but did not reveal truncated proteins (Petrij et al., 1995, reprinted from *Nature* with permission from Macmillan Magazines Limited.)

a *de novo* mutation. In a series of 21 additional RTS patients analyzed by the same technique, Petrij et al. (2000a) found one 11 bp deletion and one mutation affecting the splicing of the second exon. Thus, using the PTT technique, about 11% (4/37) of truncating mutations could be discovered.

Coupry et al. (2002) analyzed 63 RTS patients. Three microdeletions were detected by RT100 FISH analysis. The remaining group of 60 patients was analyzed by various techniques, and 27 mutations were identified: two microdeletions by microsatellite analysis, one intronic rearrangement by Southern blot, one truncated RNA by Northern blot, one small intragenic deletion by reverse-transcription PCR, and 22 point mutations resulting in either stop codons (13/22), amino acid substitutions (4/22), or abnormal splicing of the *CBP* RNA (5/22) by direct sequencing. These results showed that a combination of various techniques is able to identify a CBP mutation in 47.6% (30/63) of RTS cases.

Petrij et al. (2000b) set up a Western blot approach to gain more insight into whether this approach could be used for diagnostic purposes or as a prescreening method of RTS patients. In preliminary experiments with SDS-PAGE gels of a higher percentage (10%, 12.5%, 15%, and 20%) separating smaller proteins, they found that two known RTS point mutations (Petrij et al., 1995) which should result in relatively small truncated CBP proteins did not give clear signals in Western blot experiments with polyclonal antibody A-22 raised against the N terminus of CBP, whereas for another (inv[16]^NOR) case a truncated fragment could be detected. These data indicate that the truncated mRNAs are not always stable, perhaps due to nonsense-mediated decay. In agreement with the haploinsufficiency hypothesis, they observed in some cases, including the t(2;16)^NL case (see below), lower levels of full-length CBP compared to control persons as well as loading controls for each lane. Western blotting can thus be used for diagnostic purposes only as an ancillary approach. However, if protein extracts are made directly from blood, Western blotting is relatively simple, fast, and inexpensive and may therefore be valuable for prescreening suspected RTS cases in research settings to select samples for further analysis. Particularly those cases which display a truncated band and/or lower levels of the CBP protein may be of interest for further analysis at the DNA level.

Murata et al. (2001) suggested that RTS could be caused by loss of CBP's HAT activity since all previously reported RTS mutations were lacking all or part of the HAT domain. They also reported the first missense mutation found in an RTS patient. This mutation is located within the HAT domain of *CBP*: a G → C mutation at nucleotide 4951 that changed amino acid 1378 from arginine (CGG) to proline (CCG). Murata et al. (2001) introduced the identical missense mutation into the recombinant mouse *Cbp*. It abolished the HAT activity of CBP and the ability of CBP to transactivate CREB in HAT assays and in microinjection experiments. Kalkhoven et al. (2003) showed mutations in two RTS patients (one missense and one exon 22 splice site mutation) affecting the plant homeodomain CPHDS-type zinc finger which forms a part of the CBP HAT domain.

The Western blot analysis which Petrij et al. (2000b) performed on an RTS t(2;16)(q36.3;p13.3) concurred with this HAT hypothesis. All RTS translocations and inversions, except for t(2;16)[NL], could theoretically produce only proteins containing a very small part of the N terminus of CBP (266 amino acids or less). In (2;16)[NL], a stable truncated protein of half the normal length in addition to expression of the wild-type allele (Fig. 71–9) resulted in a child with characteristics of RTS. Because the protein observed from the Western analysis (slightly larger than 112 kDa) corresponds with the predicted protein size (119 kDa) generated by this translocation, we do not expect that the translocation results in fusion of CBP with another protein. It is unknown whether N-terminal functions are affected, for instance, by aberrant folding of the truncated protein. However, one intriguing possibility is that the C terminus of CBP is necessary for normal development. The truncated t(2;16)[NL] CBP protein lacks, in any event, various functional domains, including its HAT domain and the binding domain for the HAT P/CAF, which probably results in total loss of CBP function in chromatin remodeling. However, other regions binding to transcriptional regulators or cell cycle proteins have also been lost, such as the E1A-binding domain that also binds the basal transcription factor IIB and the region binding the transcription factor SRC1. Identification of this patient expressing a C-terminally truncated but stable CBP protein has delineated potential candidate domains.

However, Coupry et al. (2002) found three missense mutations (exon 31) and one nonsense mutation (exon 30) by direct sequencing. These mutations are positioned 3′ of CBP's HAT domain. Furthermore, they described a fourth missense mutatation positioned 5′ of the HAT domain (exon 15). It was not shown whether these mutations lead to stable proteins or have intact HAT activity. Nevertheless, these data may indicate that mutations in domains not necessarily affecting the HAT function of CBP could also lead to RTS (e.g., mutations in the E1A-binding domain or the C-terminal glutamine-rich region). More work should be done on how CBP mutations lead to the RTS phenotype.

About half of RTS cases remain unexplained. Other mechanisms that could lead to reduced CBP production, such as splice site muta-

tions, promoter mutations, mutations within a possible locus control region, or mutations leading to defective protein processing, cannot be excluded as causative mechanisms for RTS.

CBP Mutations in Leukemia

Shortly after the discovery of *CBP* disruption in several RTS cases, Giles et al. (1995) demonstrated that the *CBP* gene was also disrupted in three t(8;16)-AML patients. Later, Borrow et al. (1996) reported the fusion of *CBP* with the *MOZ* (monocytic leukemia zinc finger) gene on chromosome 8. Another leukemia-associated somatic translocation has been described: t(11;16). Unlike t(8;16)-AML, t(11;16) is not confined to AML but has also been observed in chronic myeloid leukemia and myelodysplastic syndrome and is almost never de novo but arises after anticancer treatment. In this case, the *MLL* (mixed lineage leukemia) gene is the fusion partner of *CBP* (Rowley et al., 1997; Sobulo et al., 1997; Taki et al., 1997). CBP is thus implicated in leukemia as well as embryonic development (Giles et al., 1998b).

Haploinsufficiency

The occurrence of point mutations in a single gene implies that RTS is not caused by a contiguous gene syndrome, in which the deletion of several adjacent genes causes a composite set of abnormalities, as had been previously proposed. Several of the microdeletions remove the entire *CBP* gene (Fig. 71–7), which makes a dominant-negative model unlikely as well. A haploinsufficiency model, in which two functional copies of the gene are required to produce sufficient product for normal development, seems to be a more likely explanation for the RTS phenotype (Petrij et al., 1996).

In agreement with the haploinsufficiency hypothesis, Petrij et al. (2000b) observed in some cases, including the t(2;16)[NL] case (see above), lower levels of full-length CBP compared to control persons as well as loading controls for each lane (Fig. 71–9). Accordingly, mouse knockout experiments showed that loss of one *Cbp* allele is indeed sufficient to cause skeletal malformations (Tanaka et al., 1997).

Levels of CBP may be particularly crucial at certain stages of embryonic development, explaining the RTS phenotype. Although there are several postnatal problems in RTS patients, such as an increased predisposition for neoplasia, keloid formation, aseptic hip joint inflammations, and growth retardation, it remains uncertain whether haploinsufficiency of CBP has direct pathophysiological consequences after birth. Haploinsufficiency of CBP does not necessarily lead to leukemia. CBP's oncogenic role in AML is due to its participation in a fusion transcript. Preliminary data indicate (see below) that the neoplasia and keloid formation in RTS are caused by biallelic *CBP* mutations rather than haploinsufficiency of CBP.

ESTABLISHING THE DIAGNOSIS

The diagnosis is based on the clinical presentation (see above, Clinical Description). Combined cytogenetic and molecular investigations of the *CBP* gene area on chromosome 16p13.3 can confirm the diagnosis in 50% of cases. Gross chromosomal rearrangements such as translocations and inversions are rarely found, whereas microdeletions occur in approximately 10% of cases (Table 71–4). Nonsense, missense, and splicing mutations are reported as well (Petrij et al., 1995, 2000a; Murata et al., 2001; Coupry et al., 2002). Heterogeneity remains possible, but no reports on involvement of other genes have been published.

MANAGEMENT, TREATMENT, AND COUNSELING

Counseling

The needs of parents, sibs, and other family members of a child with RTS should not be underestimated. They have great needs for definitive diagnosis; understanding; genetic counseling, including estimation of recurrence risk; and especially adequate information and help for providing optimal guidance and care to their child. Furthermore, proper molecular diagnostic tools should be available because they are invaluable in differentiating RTS from other inherited diseases with often much higher recurrence risks (Petrij et al., 2001).

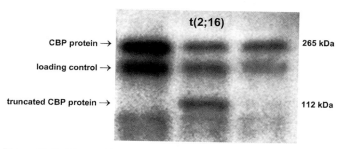

Figure 71–9. Western blot analysis of Rubinstein-Taybi syndrome t(2;16)[NL] (*middle*) and two controls (*left* and *right*) showing a truncated CBP protein in the translocation case. Lower levels of full-length CBP compared to control persons as well as loading controls for each lane can be seen. (Modified from Petrij et al., 2000b, reprinted from *Am J Med Genet* with permission from John Wiley & Sons, Inc.)

Management

Early diagnosis of RTS is critical, particularly because certain symptoms can be relieved. For example, many RTS children have nutritional deficiencies that, if recognized early on, can be addressed and corrected. Undescended testes in males can be surgically corrected. Complete cardiac and pulmonary examinations should be performed in newly diagnosed patients, allowing early treatment and/or surgery. If surgery or anesthetic is required, doctors should be aware that RTS patients are susceptible to tracheal collapse, cardiac arrhythmias, or reflux. Furthermore, RTS patients run a higher risk of contracting cancer. Regular check-ups allow early recognition of developing malignancies and thus increase the chances of successful intervention (Petrij, 2000; Petrij et al., 2001).

Health-watch programs specifically for persons with RTS have been developed in the United States and the Netherlands. Health-watch programs act as guides of methods to deal with the specific medical problems of an entity. They indicate problems that need extra medical attention, require treatment, or regular monitoring and evaluation over time. A summary of such a program is given in the clinical part of this chapter and in Table 71–6. The quality of life for RTS patients, as well as their parents, can only benefit from proper diagnosis, counseling, and guidance.

Treatment

Research will clarify the pathways in which CBP is involved and to what extent mutations in *CBP* lead to derailment of these pathways and to the developmental problems in RTS. A thorough understanding of the pathophysiology of RTS would stimulate the design of therapeutic approaches for some of the RTS-related medical problems, such as keloid formation or treatment or prevention of malignancies (Petrij et al., 2001). Inborn errors of development such as angulation deformities of the thumbs and halluces or congenital heart defects require standard practices of symptom relief. Until the in vivo functionality of CBP is better defined, there is no available treatment for RTS.

MUTATIONS IN ORTHOLOGOUS GENES

Advances in the understanding of CBP *in vivo* function have largely stemmed from the use of animal models. CBP does not appear to have an ortholog in yeast, although three CBP orthologs were reported in the *C. elegans* genome (Lundblad et al., 1995). The *Drosophila* ortholog of CBP (dCBP) possesses all of the protein-interaction motifs and appears to function in a fashion similar to its human counterpart (Akimaru et al., 1997a,b).

CBP and p300 seem to be expressed in almost identical patterns in the developing mouse embryo (Partanen et al., 1999), explaining why these proteins are highly redundant. Targeted disruption of the *Cbp* gene in mice has revealed interesting parallels with RTS. Firstly, mice lacking a single *Cbp* allele manifest various skeletal abnormalities, including delayed ossification (33%), a large anterior fontanel (67%),

and abnormal ossification of the sternum, xiphoid process, and axial bone (29%) (Tanaka et al., 1997) (Fig. 71–10). In another study, mice heterozygous for a truncated Cbp (Oike et al., 1999) demonstrate mental deficiency, growth retardation (100%), poor locomotor activity (100%), retarded osseous maturation (100%), large anterior fontanel (100%), hypoplastic maxilla with narrow palate (100%), cardiac abnormalities (17%), skeletal abnormalities (7%), and reduced weight of white adipose tissue (Yamauchi et al., 2002). However, broad digits were not observed in any of the mice. A third mouse model hemizygous for Cbp (Fig. 71–11) confirmed the previous findings and uncovered an increased risk for developing neoplasia (Kung et al., 2000). These manifestations resemble many of those seen in human RTS patients (Hennekam et al., 1990b; Tanaka et al., 1997; Oike et al., 1999). When *Cbp* is homozygously knocked out, the mice do not survive past 9–11 days of gestation (Tanaka et al., 1997; Yao et al., 1998). Examination of these embryos reveals that they have abnormal neural tube closure defects (Yao et al., 1998). Heterozygous p300 inactivation has no visible effect in the mutant mice that survive birth; however, up to 55% of the heterozygous mice die in utero, depending on the genetic background. Mice homozygous for p300 inactivating mutations strongly resemble *Cbp* knockout mice: they die after 9–11 days of gestation, displaying defects in neural tube closure, cell proliferation, and cardiac development (Yao et al., 1998). Remarkably, crossing the *Cbp* and *p300* heterozygous mutants produced double-heterozygous *Cbp/p300* mutant embryos, which died *in utero* and otherwise shared phenotypic similarities to both *Cbp* and *p300* homozygous mutants. These results suggest that CBP and p300 exert common embryonal survival functions and that the combined dose of CBP and p300 is critical for mouse embryonic development (see Table 71–7).

Oike *et al.* (1999) described defects in primitive hematopoiesis and vasculogenesis in mice homozygous for a truncated *Cbp* allele. Kung

Table 71–6. Rubinstein-Taybi Syndrome Health Watch Program

	Age group (years)		
	0–2	2–12	>12
Evaluations should be performed every	3 months	1–2 years	3–5 years
Developmental problems	+	+	+
Growth retardation	+	+	+
Feeding problems	+	+	+/−
Constipation	+	+	+
Upper respiratory infections	+	+	+/−
Eye problems	+	+	+
Heart malformations	+	+/−	+/−
Genitourinary tract problems	+	+/−	+/−
Oral problems	+	+	+/−
Orthopedic problems	+	+	+/−
Anesthetic problems	+	+	+
Obstructive sleep apnea syndrome	~	+	+
Tumors	~	~	+
Keloids	~	~	+

+, evaluation necessary; +/−, if symptoms are present; ~, rare.

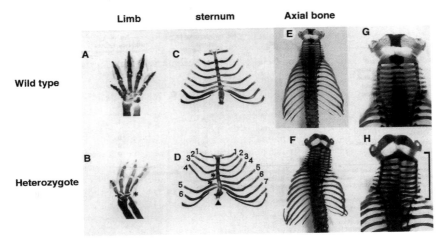

Limb   sternum   Axial bone

Wild type

Heterozygote

Figure 71–10. Severe abnormalities in *Cbp* heterozygous mice. Bone and cartilage stained specimens of (*A,B*) the right forelimbs and (*C,D*) sternums of a wild-type (*A,C*) and a *Cbp* heterozygous mouse (*B,D*). *Oligodactyly and misalignment of rib pairs can be observed. Only six ribs can be seen on the right side. Dorsal view of the vertebrae of (*E,G*) a wild-type and (*F,H*) a heterozygote. In the heterozygote, 10 ribs on the right side, 14 ribs on the left side, asymmetric cervical vertebrae, extra split thoracic vertebrae, and scoliosis were observed. (From Tanaka et al., 1997, reprinted from *Proc Natl Acad Sci USA* with permission from the National Academy of Sciences USA.)

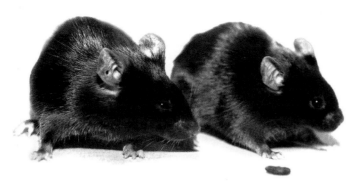

Figure 71–11. Normal littermate (*left*), *Cbp* hemizygous mouse (*right*), and normal mouse feces (*middle*). *Cbp* hemizygous mice are smaller than their littermates and have beaked noses and various other skeletal abnormalities that make them easy to distinguish (photo kindly provided by T.P. Yao).

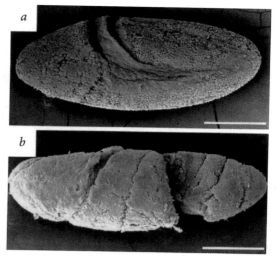

Figure 71–12. *Drosophila* CBP mutation experiments. (*a*) Stage 9 wild-type control embryo. (*b*) Late-stage 10 hemizygous CBP mutant embryo. (From Akimuru et al., 1997b, reprinted with permission from *Nat Genet* of the Nature Publishing Group.)

et al. (2000) documented multilineage defects in hematopoietic differentiation; *Cbp* hemizygous mice and, as the mice age, a high incidence of hematopoietic malignancies. Some of these malignancies are characterized by a loss of heterozygosity of the second *Cbp* allele, supplying the first direct evidence for CBP's role as a tumor-suppressor protein. RTS patients do not have a particular tendency to develop hematological malignancies, and there is only preliminary evidence suggesting the somatic inactivation of the second *CBP* allele in RTS patient tumors (Giles, unpublished data; Petrij, 2000). However, CBP's participation in fusion proteins created by somatic rearrangements in AML does reflect an important role for CBP in human myeloid development.

As in RTS patients, it is not possible to directly link the murine *Cbp* mutant phenotypes to one or more particular pathways. One study suggests that the cardiac abnormalities in homozygous $Cbp^{-/-}$ mice might result from defective MEF-2 signaling (Yao et al., 1998), a transcription factor that regulates the expression of muscle-specific genes. Another study (Bamforth et al., 2001) compared this phenotype to knockout mice lacking the transcription factor Cited2 (CBP/p300-interacting transactivator with ED-rich tail), which recapitulate some aspects of the cranio-facial and cardiac abnormalities seen in RTS patients. It has been suggested that CBP's tumor-suppressor activity lies in its negative control of the Wnt signaling pathway (Waltzer and Bienz, 1999; Kung et al., 2000), although by blocking differentiation, Cbp heterozygosity places a pool of immature cells at increased risk for accumulating additional genetic changes that contribute to neoplastic transformation. To summarize the murine data, p300 is essential for normal cardiac and neural development, whereas CBP is essential for neurulation, hematopoietic differentiation, angiogenesis, and skeletal and cardiac development (Yao et al., 1998; Oike et al., 1999; Kung et al., 2000).

Drosophila CBP (dCBP) seems to be required for multiple developmental processes as well. Embryos lacking dCBP have severe phenotypes, lacking head, thorax, and both the dorsal and ventricular cuticle structures (Akimaru et al., 1997a). Maternal dCBP can partially rescue embryos that lack dCBP, producing embryos with a twisted germ band in which both mesoderm and ectoderm cells are missing (Fig. 71–12), loss of naked cuticle, and reduction in the hairs and bristles in the denticle belt. Two-hybrid screens identified dCBP as a co-

factor for the transcription factor cubitus interruptus (ci), the downstream effector in the hedgehog (HH) signaling pathway (Akimaru et al., 1997a). Many lines of evidence suggest that dCBP is required for the ci-mediated expression of wg, the ortholog of the mammalian Wnt signalling pathway. ci is a member of the GLI family of zinc finger proteins. Interaction between human CBP and GLI3 has been confirmed, and specific interaction domains have been mapped (Dai et al., 1999). Interestingly, truncating mutations in different domains of GLI3 have been identified in patients with the Greig's cephalosyndactyly syndrome, Pallister-Hall syndrome, postaxial polydactyly type A, autosomal-dominant preaxial polydactyly type IV, and postaxial polydactyly type A/B (Vortkamp et al., 1991; Kang et al., 1997; Radhakrishna et al., 1997; Wild et al., 1997; Kalff-Suske et al., 1999; Villavicencio et al., 2000), five syndromes with distinct and overlapping features, all including limb dysmorphisms (Fig. 71–13). During embryogenesis Sonic Hedgehog–Patched–GLI (*SHH–PTCH–GLI*) pathway genes induce cell proliferation in a tissue-specific manner, leading to a number of human birth defects when mutated. If the SHH–PTCH–GLI pathway (see Fig. 71–13A and Chapter 16) is aberrantly activated during adult life, the resulting cellular proliferation manifests as cancer. Studying these types of pathway is essential for understanding the mechanisms of human birth defects and cancer simultaneously (Villavicencio et al., 2000).

In the same dCBP mutants, as described above, the twisted germband phenotype (Fig. 71–12) suggested that dCBP might mediate the dorsal-dependent expression of the *twist* gene (see Chapter 34). Indeed, dCBP is also a cofactor for the transcription factor dorsal (Akimaru et al., 1997b). By analogy, CBP, which interacts with the human ortholog of dorsal, nuclear factor (NF)-κB (RelA subunit), probably affects expression of the human *TWIST* gene. Haploinsufficiency for human TWIST has been reported to be responsible for the Saethre-Chotzen syndrome, a disease strongly resembling RTS, particularly in digit (compare Figs. 71–3, 71–13B) and craniofacial dysmorphisms (Howard et al., 1997). The syndromes are similar enough

Table 71–7. Combined Dose of Cbp/p300 Is Critical for Mouse Development

Cbp	p300	Phenotype	Reference
++	++	Normal	—
+−	++	Skeletal abnormalities, growth and mental retardation, predisposition to hematologic cancers, reduced white adipose tissue	Tanaka et al., 1997; Oike et al., 1999; Kung et al., 2000; Yamauchi et al., 2002
−−	++	Embryonic-lethal (E9–11)	Yao et al., 1998; Kung et al., 2000; Tanaka et al., 2000
++	+−	Reduced pre- and postnatal viability but otherwise normal	Yao et al., 1998
++	−−	Embryonic-lethal (E9–11)	Yao et al., 1998
+−	+−	Embryonic-lethal (E9–11)	Yao et al., 1998

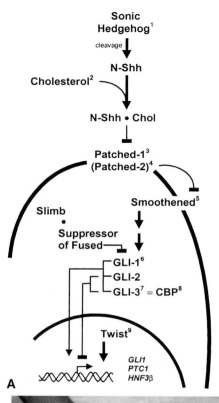

Sonic Hedgehog[1]

↓ cleavage

N-Shh

Cholesterol[2]

N-Shh • Chol

⊣

Patched-1[3]
(Patched-2)[4]

Smoothened[5]

Slimb •
Suppressor of Fused ⊣

GLI-1[6]
GLI-2
GLI-3[7] = CBP[8]

Twist[9]

GLI1
PTC1
HNF3β

A

1. Holoprosencephaly

2. Smith-Lemli-Opitz

3. Gorlin Syndrome
   Basal Cell Carcinoma
   Medulloblastoma
   Trichoepithelioma
   Esophageal Squamous Cell Carcinoma
   Bladder Transitional Cell Carcinoma

4. Basal Cell Carcinoma
   Medulloblastoma

5. Basal Cell Carcinoma
   Medulloblastoma

6. Basal Cell Carcinoma
   Glioblastoma
   Rhabdomyosarcoma
   Osteosarcoma
   Predicts Sarcoma Grade

7. Greig Syndrome
   Pallister-Hall Syndrome
   Postaxial Polydactyly A
   Preaxial Polydactyly IV
   Postaxial Polydactyly A/B

8. Rubinstein-Taybi

9. Saethre-Chotzen

Figure 71–13. (*A*) The Sonic Hedgehog (SHH)–Patched (PTCH)–GLI pathway (*left*) and its links to human diseases (*right*) (see also Chapters 16–20). (Modified from Villavicencio et al., 2000, reprinted from *Am J Hum Genet* with permission from the University of Chicago Press.) (*B*) Examples of the possible effects of mutations in some of the *SHH-PTCH-GLI* pathway genes: cutaneous syndactyly of first to fourth fingers of a patient with Gorlin's syndrome, preaxial polydactyly of the feet of a patient with Greig's syndrome, and mild broadening of the thumb of a patient with Saethre-Chotzen syndrome. Compare these limb dysmorphisms with those of Rubinstein-Taybi patients as shown in Figure 71–3.

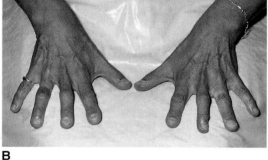
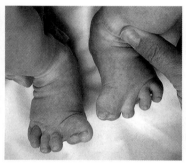
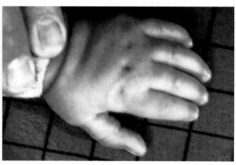

B

phenotypically to warrant confusion in at least some cases. Lowry (1990) reported a patient in which the clinical diagnosis was changed from RTS to Saethre-Chotzen. Mouse knockouts of *Cbp*, *p300*, and *Twist* also result in similar phenotypes (Chen and Behringer, 1995). Abrogation of NF-κB in the developing chick limb bud, normally activated in response to the Toll signal-transduction pathway, first identified in studies of dorsoventral polarity formation of *Drosophila* embryo (Drier and Steward, 1997), resulted in reduced *TWIST* expression (Bushdid et al., 1998; Kanegae et al., 1998). Interestingly, TWIST has been proposed to inhibit myogenesis in epithelial tissues by inhibiting the acetyltransferase activity of CBP/p300 (Hamamori et al., 1999). This negative feedback regulatory mechanism suggests that the similar Saethre-Chotzen and RTS phenotypes result from reduced *TWIST* expression combined with hyperacetylation activity of CBP and p300 (Fig. 71–14). In Saethre-Chotzen patients, reduced levels of TWIST will not adequately regulate CBP/p300 HAT activity, resulting in hyperacetylation of target histones and cellular proteins. Alternatively, reduced CBP levels in RTS patients are insufficient to support normal levels of *TWIST* expression, which is then unable to inhibit CBP acetyltransferase activity. Thus, although CBP levels are low in RTS patients, the acetyltransferase activity of CBP could be disproportionally high and, combined with reduced *TWIST* expression, capable of generating a Saethre-Chotzen-like phenotype (Fig. 71–14).

Shi and Mello (1998) investigated the developmental role of the *C. elegans* ortholog of CBP, cbp-1. When cbp-1 function was blocked by RNA interference (RNAi), embryos were produced lacking all

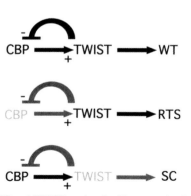

Figure 71–14. CBP and TWIST are involved in a negative feedback loop that may explain the similarities observed in Rubinstein-Taybi syndrome (RTS) and Saethre-Chotzen syndrome (SC) patients. In a wildtype (WT) cell (*upper cartoon*), CBP is required for expression of the *TWIST* gene. TWIST in turn inhibits CBP's histone acetyltransferase (HAT) activity. In RTS patients (*middle cartoon*), half the level of CBP (light gray) results in lower TWIST expression, which is then less efficient (gray) at regulating HAT activity of the CBP that is present. SC patients (*lower cartoon*) are haploinsufficient for TWIST (light gray), which will also only partially regulate CBP HAT activity (gray). Haploinsufficiency for either CBP or TWIST disturbs this negative feedback loop and results in the hyperacetylation of CBP substrates. It follows that the phenotypic overlap seen between patients with these two syndromes might be explained by reduced levels of TWIST coupled with increased CBP HAT activity.

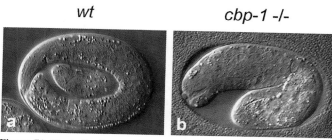

wt   *cbp-1 -/-*

Figure 71–15. A *C. elegans cbp-1* deletion mutant displays an embryonic-lethal phenotype. Animals homozygous for the *cbp-1* deletion die at the 1.5- to 2-fold stage of embryonic development. Normarski images of (*A*) a wild-type (wt) and (*B*) a homozygous mutant (−/−) animal are shown. The wild-type embryo is at the pretzel stage, while the *cbp-1* mutant embryo is at the 1.5- to 2-fold stage. (From Victor et al., 2002, reprinted from *EMBO Rep* with permission from Oxford University Press.)

mesodermal, endodermal, and hypodermal cells. Strikingly, in the absence of functional cbp-1, many of the cell lineages undergo extra cell divisions and all embryos exhibit neuronal differentiation. These data suggest that cbp-1 might be a component of all nonneuronal developmental pathways. By simultaneously suppressing the function of the *C. elegans* othologs of the histone deacetylases HDAC1 and RBBP4, endoderm differentiation is largely restored. More recent studies (Calvo et al., 2001; Victor et al., 2002) detail the requirement of cbp-1 for endoderm differentiation (Fig. 71–15) and show that this process is dependent on cbp-1's HAT activity. The fact that cbp-1 normally promotes differentiation and development in *C. elegans* by antagonizing the activities of histone deacetylases demonstrates the importance of interplay between acetyltransferases and deacetylases in the regulation of cell fate–determining genes during development. These data support the hypothesis that RTS is caused by a compromising mutation to CBP's HAT activity (Murata et al., 2001). However, cbp-1 RNAi would disturb multiple transcriptional pathways important for development, making it difficult to draw definitive conclusions about the HAT function of cbp-1 in development specifically. Alternative genetic approaches in *C. elegans* should be taken to address this very relevant question.

DEVELOPMENTAL PATHOGENESIS

Because large deletions of the *CBP* gene have been identified in RTS patients as well as point mutations resulting in a premature truncation of the protein, it is generally believed that haploinsufficiency for CBP is responsible for RTS. At birth, RTS patients have several developmental problems, described above, suggesting that at certain stages of fetal development high CBP levels are critical for normal organogenesis. RTS is a syndrome with a highly variable phenotype. This variability could be caused by different mutations in *CBP*, genetic heterogeneity (mutations in different genes), or genes modifying the effect of the germline mutation (genetic background). The constellation of symptoms seen in RTS can be explained by CBP's role as a transcriptional coactivator. Because CBP is involved in the regulation of many other genes, the polymorphic nature of these genes could amplify the variability of clinical manifestations as seen in RTS. By elucidating the mutation spectrum, it would be possible to identify which signal-transduction pathways are disturbed by specific *CBP* mutations. Several domains are particularly interesting to screen for missense mutations, such as those involved in interactions with transcription factor GLI3 or NF-κB (RelA subunit).

Oike et al. (1999) proposed a dominant-negative mechanism, in which a truncated CBP hampers the function of the full-length protein. The hypothesis was based on comparison of two different mouse models. One *Cbp*[+/−] mutant mouse model, in which amino acids 29–265 were replaced by a targeting vector, exhibited a few features of RTS but did not have any detectable heart abnormalities (Tanaka et al., 1997). The other, *Cbp*[+/−], where the one *Cbp* allele was truncated at residue 1085, showed many characteristics of RTS including cardiac anomalies (Oike et al., 1999). By chance, this position in the

mouse exactly corresponds to amino acid 1084 in humans and is thereby a perfect model for the t(2;16)[NL] RTS patient (Petrij et al., 2000b). This patient does not have a significantly more severe phenotype than other RTS patients. Moreover, compared to three patients with defined hemizygous deletions affecting the entire *CBP* gene (Breuning et al., 1993; Hennekam et al., 1993; Petrij et al., 1995), no significant differences in phenotype were observed. We therefore cannot reach the same conclusions as Oike et al. (1999). Whether a dominant-negative effect of certain CBP mutations exists remains unanswered. Genetic background plays a critical role in RTS phenotype, and extrapolation of results from mouse experiments to the human situation is always imperfect.

If CBP and p300 are so similar, can inactivating germline mutations of p300 cause RTS? While the biochemical overlap between these two proteins makes p300 mutations in RTS a possibility, two lines of evidence suggest that this is rarely, if ever, the case. Firstly, chromosomal rearrangements in confirmed RTS patients have always involved the *CBP* locus on chromosomal band 16p13.3, whereas no rearrangements at the *p300* locus at 22q13 have been reported (Giles et al., 1998a). Secondly, targeted disruption of *Cbp* and *p300* genes in mice reveals that heterozygous *Cbp* mutants display skeletal abnormalities resembling many of those seen in human RTS patients. Normal levels of p300 are unable to compensate for the reduced CBP levels, either because of different temporal and/or spatial expression patterns or because of as yet unknown differences in physiological function. Heterozygous *p300* inactivation, however, has no visible effect on mutant mice that survive birth; but up to 55% of heterozygous p300 mice die *in utero*. Interestingly, mice heterozygous for both *Cbp* and *p300* null mutations exhibit the same phenotype as either *Cbp* or *p300* homozygous mutant mice (Yao et al., 1998). One could postulate a "triploinsufficiency" model in which losing one of the four *CBP/p300* alleles leads to major health problems and losing two alleles leads to embryonal death (Giles, 1998) (see Table 71–7). Concordantly, Partanen *et al.* (1999) described an extensively, but not fully, overlapping expression pattern of *Cbp* and *p300* during development, suggesting common as well as distinct biochemical functions. Although interpretation is somewhat complicated because of differences in genetic background, the mouse data suggest that *p300* may be less appropriate as a candidate gene for RTS.

Genetic background almost certainly plays a role in the severity of the disease. Three documented RTS mothers produced RTS children with a more severe phenotype than they had themselves. Presumably, the children have the same *CBP* mutation as the mothers; thus, it would be reasonable to expect a similar phenotype. However, the mild phenotype in the mothers might be due to their favorable (epi)genetic background or a somatic mosaicism.

Although RTS patients do not exhibit neurodegeneration, some insight into their neurogenic phenotype can be derived from Huntington's disease. Huntington's disease (OMIM 143100) is a slowly progressive autosomal-dominant neurodegenerative disease, characterized by gradually evolving involuntary movements (chorea), progressive dementia, and psychiatric disturbances, especially mood disorder and personality changes. Huntington's disease is caused by the presence of expanded poly-Q in mutant huntingtin, which leads to its abnormal proteolytic cleavage with liberation of toxic N-terminal fragments that tend to aggregate. Subsequent nuclear translocation of the cleaved mutant huntingtin is associated with formation of intranuclear protein aggregates and neurotoxicity. Mutant huntingtin sequesters CBP (not p300) in these aggregates, thereby resulting in neuronal death (Steffan et al., 2000; Nucifora et al., 2001). Overexpression of CBP rescues neurons expressing huntingtin with an expanded glutamine repeat, and treatment of these cells with histone deacetylase inhibitors can reduce the toxicity caused by polyglutamine aggregates (Steffan et al., 2000; McCampbell et al., 2000, 2001; McCampbell and Fishbeck 2001a). It is interesting to speculate that a reduction in cellular CBP levels is toxic to neurons and could be responsible for some of the neuronal phenotype seen in RTS patients, such as the cone–rod dysfunction and the abnormal VEPs.

Another feature of RTS is the somewhat increased predisposition to certain types of cancer (Miller and Rubinstein, 1995). Keloids (22%) and hypertrophic scarring (16%) also have been described in RTS

(Hennekam et al., 1990b). The higher prevalence of cancer in RTS patients fits the "two-hit" model for tumor-suppressor proteins proposed by Knudson (1971). Preliminary data (obtained by Southern analyses) indicate that a somatic loss of heterozygosity of CBP indeed took place in, respectively, a meningioma and a keloid of two different RTS patients (Giles, unpublished; Petrij, 2000). Cbp is biallelically mutated in plasmacytomas of hemizygous *Cbp* knock-out mice (Kung et al., 2000). To elucidate its role as a tumor suppressor in human hematopoietic cancers and to differentiate between a simple gain of function by forming fusion proteins or by combining this with a loss of heterozygosity, leukemic cells with translocations affecting one *CBP* allele should be examined for mutations in their second *CBP* allele. Waltzer and Bienz (1999) showed that by acetylating the transcription factor dTCF, dCBP negatively regulated the wingless (wg) pathway in Drosophila. It follows that ablating CBP would allow unbridled activation of wingless target genes, including oncogenes such as c-*MYC*. Inappropriate WNT signaling is present in virtually all colorectal cancers and common in breast carcinomas and pilomatrixomas (reviewed in Bienz and Clevers, 2000). Determining the presence of nuclear β-catenin, which binds T-cell transcription factor to activate transcription and is the hallmark of active WNT signaling, or documenting overexpression of WNT target genes would establish whether tumors in RTS patients are products of aberrant WNT signalling.

Evidence suggests that levels of CBP are limiting in cells. The fact that CBP interacts with several proteins, each with a different affinity, suggests that reduced levels of CBP will affect certain interactions, while other interactions/pathways will be affected less. How crosstalk between different developmental pathways occurs is an emerging field in itself. Of particular interest is the potential interplay between acetylase and methylase in maintaining the dynamic balance of gene activation and silencing. CBP and p300 are methylation substrates for the methyltransferase CARM1 (Xu et al., 2001). Methylation of a specific arginine residue in the KIX domain (CREB-binding domain) inhibits CREB signaling (and presumably all transactivation by proteins that associate with the KIX domain) while selectively enhancing nuclear hormone receptor–mediated transcription. It has been suggested that methylation-directed cofactor switching can provide a simple way of crosstalk between two potentially competing signaling pathways.

The ability of CBP to serve as a mediator of both cell proliferation and growth arrest pathways remains a paradox. One hypothesis for how this homeostasis is maintained places tumor-suppressor proteins p53 and BRCA1 at center stage. Acetylation of p53 by CBP/p300 affects the strength of p53 binding to a promoter region; this acetylation switches the affinity for particular promoters, perhaps due to a change in conformation. Cellular stress will disrupt the MDM2–p53 interaction through phosphorylation of specific residues (Prives, 1998). This results in stabilization and activation of the p53 protein. This is sufficient for activation of target genes regulated by high-affinity binding sites, such as p21, resulting in cell-cycle arrest. However, if an apoptotic response is needed, p53 will bind to the first half of BRCA1. CBP/p300, which is also bound to BRCA1, can subsequently acetylate the C terminus of p53. After this, p53 can be released again, and the acetylation of its C terminus results in a switch in affinity. The low-affinity sites (like the *BAX* promoter) are now bound with high affinity, and a new class of target genes is activated. One could speculate that reduced cellular levels of CBP would drive p53's choice of promoter toward those with a high affinity, resulting in cell-cycle arrest. Mouse embryonic fibroblasts derived from Cbp homozygous mice have impaired proliferation, supporting this hypothesis (Yao et al., 1998).

Compellingly, phenotypic overlap between RTS and other diseases with identified mutations has been documented. As discussed above, evidence from *Drosophila* and humans suggests a link between the pathophysiology of the Saethre-Chotzen syndrome and RTS. Similarities between RTS and Greig's cephalosyndactyly syndrome in limb and craniofacial dysmorphisms have also been noted. Greig's cephalosyndactyly syndrome is caused by truncating mutations of the *GLI3* gene (see Chapter 20). GLI is the human ortholog of the *Drosophila* CI, a protein that is regulated by dCBP in the hedgehog

signaling pathway. The interaction coupled with the phenotypic similarity suggests that mutations in CBP may impair some of GLI3's activity in activating downstream hedgehog target genes, resulting in overlapping etiologies between RTS and Greig's cephalosyndactyly syndrome.

Because CBP is so prevalent in developmental pathways, linking RTS phenotypic characteristics to a specific developmental process seems impossible. Clinicians and molecular biologists must team up better to examine and make use of the naturally occurring CBP mutant, RTS patients. Phenotype–genotype correlations should be detailed. Questions concerning the role of HAT activity during development, subcellular localization of CBP during development, whether WNT signaling initiates RTS tumors after loss of the second allele, and the role of CBP in neural, myeloid, bone, and cardiac development can be addressed. Ultimately, the only way to dissect CBP's role in development will be through use of further genetic approaches in model organisms. Although CBP seems to be well conserved throughout evolution, much of the work in model organisms has yet to have confirmed functional consequences in humans.

ACKNOWLEDGMENTS

The authors thank Drs. L.M. Soors d'Ancona, S. Wiley, and J.H. Rubinstein for sharing data on the development of a health-watch program for RTS children; Dr. J.H. Roelfsema for critical reading; V. Petrij-Brückmann for the layout of Figures 71–1 through 71–4, 71–6, 71–7, and 71–13, and Drs. T.P. Yao, J.H. Roelfsema, and Y. Shi for contributing Figures 71–11, 71–14, and 71–15, respectively.

REFERENCES

Akimaru H, Chen Y, Dai P, Hou DX, Nonaka M, Smolik SM, Armstrong S, Goodman RH, Ishii S (1997a). *Drosophila* CBP is a co-activator of cubitus interruptus in hedgehog signalling. *Nature* 386: 735–738.

Akimaru H, Hou DX, Ishii S (1997b). *Drosophila* CBP is required for dorsal-dependent *twist* gene expression. *Nat Genet* 17: 211–214.

Bamforth SD, Braganca J, Eloranta JJ, Murdoch JN, Marques FI, Kranc KR, Farza H, Henderson DJ, Hurst HC, Bhattacharya S (2001). Cardiac malformations, adrenal agenesis, neural crest defects and exencephaly in mice lacking Cited2, a new Tfap2 co-activator. *Nat Genet* 29: 469–474.

Bannister AJ, Kouzarides T (1996). The CBP co-activator is a histone acetyltransferase. *Nature* 384: 641–643.

Bartsch O, Wagner A, Hinkel GK, Krebs P, Stumm M, Schmalenberger B, Bohm S, Balci S, Majewski F (1999). FISH studies in 45 patients with Rubinstein-Taybi syndrome: deletions associated with polysplenia, hypoplastic left heart and death in infancy. *Eur J Hum Genet* 7: 748–756.

Bienz M, Clevers H (2000). Linking colorectal cancer to Wnt signaling. *Cell* 103: 311–320.

Bilir BM, Bilir N, Wilson GN (1990). Intracranial angioblastic meningioma and an aged appearance in a woman with Rubinstein-Taybi syndrome. *Am J Med Genet Suppl* 6: 69–72.

Blough RI, Petrij F, Dauwerse JG, Milatovich-Cherry A, Weiss L, Saal HM, Rubinstein JH (2000). Variation in microdeletions of the cyclic AMP-responsive element–binding protein gene at chromosome band 16p13.3 in the Rubinstein-Taybi syndrome. *Am J Med Genet* 90: 29–34.

Bonioli E, Bellini C (1992). Rubinstein-Taybi syndrome and pheochromocytoma. *Am J Med Genet* 44: 386.

Bonioli E, Bellini C, Senes FM, Palmieri A, Di Stadio M, Pinelli G (1993). Slipped capital femoral epiphysis associated with Rubinstein-Taybi syndrome. *Clin Genet* 44: 79–81.

Borrow J, Stanton VP Jr, Andresen JM, Becher R, Behm FG, Chaganti RSK, Civin CI, Disteche C, Dubé I, Frischauf AM, et al. (1996). The translocation t(8;16)(p11;p13) of acute myeloid leukemia fuses a putative acetyl transferase to the CREB-binding protein. *Nat Genet* 14: 33–41.

Breuning MH, Dauwerse JG, Fugazza G, Saris JJ, Spruit L, Wijnen H, Tommerup N, van der Hagen CB, Imaizumi K, Kuroki Y, et al. (1993). Rubinstein-Taybi syndrome caused by submicroscopic deletions within 16p13.3. *Am J Hum Genet* 52: 249–254.

Bushdid PB, Brantley DM, Yull FE, Blaeuer GL, Hoffman LH, Niswander L, Kerr LD (1998). Inhibition of NF-kappaB activity results in disruption of the apical ectodermal ridge and aberrant limb morphogenesis. *Nature* 392: 615–618.

Calvo D, Victor M, Gay F, Sui G, Luke MP, Dufourcq P, Wen G, Maduro M, Rothman J, Shi Y (2001). A POP-1 repressor complex restricts inappropriate cell type-specific gene transcription during Caenorhabditis elegans embryogenesis. *EMBO J* 20: 7197–7208.

Cambiaghi S, Ermacora E, Brusasco A, Canzi L, Caputo R (1994). Multiple pilomatricomas in Rubinstein-Taybi syndrome: a case report. *Pediatr Dermatol* 11: 21–25.

Chen ZF, Behringer RR (1995). Twist is required in head mesenchyme for cranial neural tube morphogenesis. *Genes Dev* 9: 686–699.

Chrivia JC, Kwok RPS, Lamb N, Haglwara M, Montimny MR, Goodman RH (1993). Phosphorylated CREB binds specifically to the nuclear protein CBP. *Nature* 365: 855–859.

Coffin GS (1964). Brachydactyly, peculiar faces and mental retardation. *Am J Dis Child* 108: 351–359.

Coupry I, Roudaut C, Stef M, Deirue MA, Marshe E, Burgelin I, Taine L, Lacombe D,

Benoît A (2002). Molecular analysis of the *CREBBP* gene in 60 patients with Rubinstein-Taybi syndrome. *J Med Genet* (in press).
Dai P, Akimaru H, Tanaka Y, Maekawa T, Nakafuku M, Ishii S (1999). Sonic Hedgehog–induced activation of the Gli1 promoter is mediated by GLI3. *J Biol Chem* 274: 8143–8152.
D'Cruz CA, Karmizin N, Johal JS, Halligan G, Faerber EN (1993). Malignant neoplasms in patients with the Rubinstein-Taybi syndrome. *Pediatr Pathol* 13: 102.
Drier EA, Steward R (1997). The dorsoventral signal transduction pathway and the Rel-like transcription factors in Drosophila. *Semin Cancer Biol* 8: 83–92.
Eckner R, Ewen ME, Newsome D, Gerdes M, DeCaprio JA, Lawrence JB, Livingston DM (1994). Molecular cloning and functional analysis of the adenovirus E1A-associated 300-kD protein (p300) reveals a protein with properties of a transcriptional adaptor. *Genes Dev* 8: 869–884.
Evans G, Burnell L, Campbell R, Gattamaneni HR, Birch J (1993). Congenital anomalies and genetic syndromes in 173 cases of medulloblastoma. *Med Pediatr Oncol* 21: 433–434.
Giles RH (1998). CBP/p300 transgenic mice. *Trends Genet* 14: 214.
Giles RH, Petrij F, Dauwerse JG, van der Reijden BA, Beverstock GC, Hagemeijer A, Breuning MH (1995). The translocation t(8;16) in ANLL M4/M5 disrupts the *CBP* gene on chromosome 16. *Blood* 86: 35a.
Giles RH, Petrij F, Dauwerse HG, den Hollander AI, Lushnikova T, van Ommen GJ, Goodman RH, Deaven LL, Doggett NA, Peters DJ, et al. (1997a). Construction of a 1.2-Mb contig surrounding, and molecular analysis of, the human CREB-binding protein (*CBP/CREBBP*) gene on chromosome 16p13.3. *Genomics* 42: 96–114.
Giles RH, Dauwerse JG, Higgins C, Petrij F, Wessels JW, Beverstock GC, Döhner H, Jotterand-Bellomo M, Falkenburg JHF, Slater RM, et al. (1997b). Detection of *CBP* rearrangements in acute myelogenous leukemia with t(8;16). *Leukemia* 11: 2087–2096.
Giles RH, Dauwerse JG, van Ommen GJB, Breuning MH (1998a). Do chromosomal bands 16p13 and 22q11-13 share ancestral origins? *Am J Hum Genet* 63: 1240–1242.
Giles RH, Peters DJM, Breuning MH (1998b). Conjunction dysfunction: CBP/p300 in human disease. *Trends Genet* 14: 178–183.
Goodfellow A, Emmerson RW, Calvert HT (1980). Rubinstein-Taybi syndrome and spontaneous keloids. *Clin Exp Dermatol* 5: 369–370.
Goodman RH, Smolik S (2000). CBP/p300 in cell growth, transformation, and development. *Genes Dev* 14: 1553–1577.
Gorlin RJ, Cohen MM, Hennekam RCM (2001). Rubinstein-Taybi syndrome. *Syndromes of the Head and Neck.* Oxford University Press, New York, pp. 382–387.
Grunow JE (1982). Gastroesophageal reflux in Rubinstein-Taybi syndrome. *J Pediatr Gastroenterol Nutr* 1: 273–274.
Hamamori Y, Sartorelli V, Ogryzko V, Puri PL, Wu HY, Wang JY, Nakatani Y, Kedes L (1999). Regulation of histone acetyltransferases p300 and PCAF by the bHLH protein twist and adenoviral oncoprotein E1A. *Cell* 96: 405–413.
Hennekam RCM, Van Doorne JM (1990). Oral aspects of Rubinstein-Taybi syndrome. *Am J Med Genet Suppl* 6: 42–47.
Hennekam RCM, Lommen EJ, Strengers JL, Van Spijker HG, Jansen-Kokx TM (1989). Rubinstein-Taybi syndrome in a mother and son. *Eur J Pediatr* 148: 439–441.
Hennekam RCM, Stevens CA, Van de Kamp JJ (1990a). Etiology and recurrence risk in Rubinstein-Taybi syndrome. *Am J Med Genet Suppl* 6: 56–64.
Hennekam RCM, Van Den Boogaard MJ, Sibbles BJ, Van Spijker HG (1990b). Rubinstein-Taybi syndrome in the Netherlands. *Am J Med Genet Suppl* 6: 17–29.
Hennekam RCM, Baselier AC, Beyaert E, Bos A, Blok JB, Jansma HB, Thorbecke-Nilsen VV, Veerman H (1992). Psychological and speech studies in Rubinstein-Taybi syndrome. *Am J Ment Retard* 96: 645–660.
Hennekam RCM, Tilanus M, Hamel BC, Voshart-van Heeren H, Mariman EC, van Beersum SE, van den Boogaard MJ, Breuning MH (1993). Deletion at chromosome 16p13.3 as a cause of Rubinstein-Taybi syndrome: clinical aspects. *Am J Hum Genet* 52: 255–262.
Howard TD, Paznekas WA, Green ED, Chiang LC, Ma N, Ortiz De Luna RI, Garcia Delgado C, Gonzalez-Ramos M, Kline AD, Wang Jabs E (1997). Mutations in *TWIST*, a basic helix-loop-helix transcription factor, in Saethre-Chotzen syndrome. *Nat Genet* 15: 36–41.
Imaizumi K, Kuroki Y (1991). Rubinstein-Taybi syndrome with de novo reciprocal translocation t(2;16)(p13.3;p13.3). *Am J Med Genet* 38: 636–639.
Job JC, Rossier A, de Grandprey J (1964). Etudes sur les nanismes constitutionnels. II. Le syndrome de Rubinstein et Taybi. *Ann Pediatr* 11: 646.
Jonas DM, Heilbron DC, Ablin AR (1978). Rubinstein-Taybi syndrome and acute leukemia. *J Pediatr* 92: 851–852.
Kalff-Suske M, Wild A, Topp J, Wessling M, Jacobsen EM, Bornholdt D, Engel H, Heuer H, Aalfs CM, Ausems MG, et al. (1999). Point mutations throughout the *GLI3* gene cause Greig cephalopolysyndactyly syndrome. *Hum Mol Genet* 8: 1769–1777.
Kalkhoven E, Roelfsema JH, Teynissen H, Den Boor A, Ariyurck Y, Zantema A, Breuning MH, Hennekan RCM, Peters DJM (2003). Loss of CBP acetyltransferase activity by PHD finger mutations in Rubenstein-Taybi syndrome. *Hum Mol Genet* 12: 441–450.
Kanegae Y, Tavares AT, Izpisua Belmonte JC, Verma IM (1998). Role of Rel/NF-kappaB transcription factors during the outgrowth of the vertebrate limb. *Nature* 392: 611–614.
Kang S, Graham JM Jr, Olney AH, Biesecker LG (1997). GLI3 frameshift mutations cause autosomal dominant Pallister-Hall syndrome. *Nat Genet* 15: 266–268.
Knudson AG (1971). Mutation and cancer: statistical study of retinoblastoma. *Proc Natl Acad Sci USA* 68: 820–823.
Kung AL, Rebel VI, Bronson RT, Ch'ng LE, Sieff CA, Livingston DM, Yao TP (2000). Gene dose-dependent control of hematopoiesis and hematologic tumor suppression by CBP. *Genes Dev* 14: 272–277.
Kwok RPS, Lundblad JR, Chrivia JC, Richards JP, Bächinger HP, Brennan RG, Roberts SGE, Green MR, Goodman RH (1994). Nuclear protein CBP is a coactivator for the transcription factor CREB. *Nature* 370: 223–226.
Lacombe D, Saura R, Taine L, Battin J (1992). Confirmation of assignment of a locus for Rubinstein-Taybi syndrome gene to 16p13.3. *Am J Med Genet* 44: 126–128.
Lannering B, Marky I, Nordborg C (1990). Brain tumors in childhood and adolescence in west Sweden 1970–1984. Epidemiology and survival. *Cancer* 66: 604–609.
Lowry RB (1990). Overlap between Rubinstein-Taybi and Saethre-Chotzen syndrome: a case report. *Am J Med Genet* 6: 73–76.
Lundblad JR, Kwok RPS, Laurance ME, Harter ML, Goodman RH (1995). Adenoviral E1A-associated protein p300 as a functional homologue of the transcriptional co-activator CBP. *Nature* 374: 85–88.
Marion RW, Garcia DM, Karasik JB (1993). Apparent dominant transmission of the Rubinstein-Taybi syndrome. *Am J Med Genet* 46: 284–287.
Masuno M, Imaizumi K, Kurosawa K, Makita Y, Petrij F, Dauwerse H G, Breuning MH, Kuroki Y (1994). Submicroscopic deletion of chromosome region 16p13.3 in a Japanese patient with Rubinstein-Taybi syndrome. *Am J Med Genet* 53: 352–354.
Masuno M, Imaizumi K, Ishii T, Kuroki Y, Baba N, Tanaka Y (1998). Pilomatrixomas in Rubinstein-Taybi syndrome. *Am J Med Genet* 77: 81–82.
McCampbell A, Fischbeck KH (2001). Polyglutamine and CBP: fatal attraction? *Nat Med* 7: 528–530.
McCampbell A, Taylor JP, Taye AA, Robitschek J, Li M, Walcott J, Merry D, Chai Y, Paulson H, Sobue G, et al. (2000). CREB-binding protein sequestration by expanded polyglutamine. *Hum Mol Genet* 9: 2197–2202.
McCampbell A, Taye AA, Whitty L, Penney E, Steffan JS, Fischbeck KH (2001). Histone deacetylase inhibitors reduce polyglutamine toxicity. *Proc Natl Acad Sci USA* 98: 15179–15184.
McGaughran JM, Gaunt L, Dore J, Petrij F, Dauwerse HG, Donnai D (1996). Rubinstein-Taybi syndrome with deletions of FISH probe RT1 at 16p13.3: two UK patients. *J Med Genet* 33: 82–83.
Michail J, Matsoukas J, Theodorou S (1957). Pouce bot arque enforte abductions extension et autres symptomes concimants. *Rev Chir Orthop* 43: 142–146.
Miller RW, Rubinstein JH (1995). Tumors in Rubinstein-Taybi syndrome. *Am J Med Genet* 56: 112–115.
Moran R, Calthorpe D, McGoldrick F, Fogarty E, Dowling F (1993). Congenital dislocation of the patella in Rubinstein Taybi syndrome. *Ir Med J* 86: 34–35.
Murata T, Kurokawa R, Krones A, Tatsumi K, Ishii M, Taki T, Masuno M, Ohashi H, Yanagisawa M, Rosenfeld MG, et al. (2001). Defect of histone acetyltransferase activity of the nuclear transcriptional coactivator CBP in Rubinstein-Taybi syndrome. *Hum Mol Genet* 10: 1071–1076.
Nucifora FC Jr, Sasaki M, Peters MF, Huang H, Cooper JK, Yamada M, Takahashi H, Tsuji S, Troncoso J, Dawson VL, et al. (2001). Interference by huntingtin and atrophin-1 with cbp-mediated transcription leading to cellular toxicity. *Science* 291: 2423–2428.
Ogryzko VV, Schiltz RL, Russanova V, Howard BH, Nakatani Y (1996). The transcriptional coactivators p300 and CBP are histone acetyltransferases. *Cell* 87: 953–959.
Oike Y, Hata A, Mamiya T, Kaname T, Noda Y, Suzuki M, Yasue H, Nabeshima T, Araki K, Yamamura K (1999). Truncated CBP protein leads to classical Rubinstein-Taybi syndrome phenotypes in mice: implications for a dominant-negative mechanism. *Hum Mol Genet* 8: 387–396.
Partanen A, Motoyama J, Hui CC (1999). Developmentally regulated expression of the transcriptional cofactors/histone acetyltransferases CBP and p300 during mouse embryogenesis. *Int J Dev Biol* 43: 487–494.
Petrij F (2000). Molecular Analysis of the Rubinstein-Taybi Syndrome. Leiden University, Leiden.
Petrij F, Giles RH, Dauwerse JG, Saris JJ, Hennekam RCM, Masuno M, Tommerup N, van Ommen GJB, Goodman RH, Peters DJM, et al. (1995). Rubinstein-Taybi syndrome is caused by mutations in the transcriptional co-activator CBP. *Nature* 376: 348–351.
Petrij F, Giles RH, Dorsman JC, Dauwerse JG, van Ommen GJB, Peters DJM, Breuning MH (1996). Haploinsufficiency of CBP leads to the Rubinstein-Taybi syndrome. *Am J Hum Genet* 59(Suppl): A142.
Petrij F, Dauwerse HG, Blough RI, Giles RH, van der Smagt JJ, Wallerstein R, Maaswinkel-Mooy PD, van Karnebeek CD, van Ommen GJ, van Haeringen A, et al. (2000a). Diagnostic analysis of the Rubinstein-Taybi syndrome: five cosmids should be used for microdeletion detection and low number of protein truncating mutations. *J Med Genet* 37: 168–176.
Petrij F, Dorsman JC, Dauwerse HG, Giles RH, Peeters T, Hennekam RC, Breuning MH, Peters DJ (2000b). Rubinstein-Taybi syndrome caused by a de novo reciprocal translocation t(2;16)(q36.3;p13.3). *Am J Med Genet* 92: 47–52.
Petrij F, Giles RH, Breuning MH, Hennekam RCM (2001). Rubinstein-Taybi syndrome. In: *The Metabolic and Molecular Bases of Inherited Disease*. Scriver CR, Beaudet AL, Sly WS, Valle D, Childs B, Vogelstein B (eds.) McGraw-Hill, New York, pp. 6167–6182.
Prives C (1998). Signaling to p53: breaking the MDM2-p53 circuit. *Cell* 95: 5–8.
Radhakrishna U, Wild A, Grzeschik KH, Antonarakis SE (1997). Mutation in GLI3 in postaxial polydactyly type A. *Nat Genet* 17: 269–271.
Robson MJ, Brown LM, Sharrard WJ (1980). Cervical spondylolisthesis and other skeletal abnormalities in Rubinstein-Taybi syndrome. *J Bone Joint Surg Br* 62: 297–299.
Roest PAM, Roberts RG, Sugino S, van Ommen GJB, den Dunnen JT (1993). Protein truncation test (PTT) for rapid detection of translation-terminating mutations. *Hum Mol Genet* 2: 1719–1721.
Rohlfing B, Lewis K, Singleton EB (1971). Rubinstein-Taybi syndrome. Report of an unusual case. *Am J Dis Child* 121: 71–74.
Rosenbaum KN, Johnson DL, Fitz CR, McCullogh DC (1990). Tethered cord in Rubinstein-Taybi syndrome. *Am J Hum Genet Suppl* 47: A75.
Rowley JD, Reshmi S, Sobulo O, Musvee T, Anastasi J, Raimondi S, Schneider NR, Barredo JC, Cantu ES, Schlegelberger B, et al. (1997). All patients with the t(11;16)(q23;p13.3) that involves MLL and CBP have treatment-related hematologic disorders. *Blood* 90: 535–541.
Rubinstein JH (1974). Fatherhood of the so-called Rubinstein-Taybi syndrome. *Am J Dis Child* 128: 424.
Rubinstein JH (1990). Broad thumb-hallux (Rubinstein-Taybi) syndrome 1957–1988. *Am J Med Genet Suppl* 6: 3–16.
Rubinstein JH, Taybi H (1963). Broad thumbs and toes and facial abnormalities. *Am J Dis Child* 105: 588–608.
Russell NA, Hoffman HJ, Bain HW (1971). Intraspinal neurilemoma in association with the Rubinstein-Taybi syndrome. *Pediatrics* 47: 444–447.

Sammartino A, Cerbella R, Lembo G, Federico A, Loffredo L (1986). Rubinstein-Taybi syndrome with multiple keloids. *J Fr Ophtalmol* 9: 725–729.

Selmanowitz VJ, Stiller MJ (1981). Rubinstein-Taybi syndrome. Cutaneous manifestations and colossal keloids. *Arch Dermatol* 117: 504–506.

Shi Y, Mello C (1998). A CBP/p300 homolog specifies multiple differentiation pathways in *Caenorhabditis elegans*. *Genes Dev* 12: 943–955.

Skousen GJ, Wardinsky T, Chenaille P (1996). Medulloblastoma in patient with Rubinstein-Taybi syndrome. *Am J Med Genet* 66: 367.

Sobel RA, Woerner S (1981). Rubinstein-Taybi syndrome and nasopharyngeal rhabdomyosarcoma. *J Pediatr* 99: 1000–1001.

Sobulo OM, Borrow J, Tomek R, Reshmi S, Harden A, Schlegelberger B, Housman D, Doggett NA, Rowley JD, Zeleznik-Le NJ (1997). MLL is fused to CBP, a histone acetyltransferase, in therapy-related acute myeloid leukemia with a t(11;16)(q23;p13.3). *Proc Natl Acad Sci USA* 94: 8732–8737.

Steffan JS, Kazantsev A, Spasic-Boskovic O, Greenwald M, Zhu YZ, Gohler H, Wanker EE, Bates GP, Housman DE, Thompson LM (2000). The Huntington's disease protein interacts with p53 and CREB-binding protein and represses transcription. *Proc Natl Acad Sci USA* 97: 6763–6768.

Stevens CA (1997). Patellar dislocation in Rubenstein-Taybi syndrome. *Am J Med Genet* 72: 188–190.

Stevens CA, Carey JC, Blackburn BL (1990a). Rubinstein-Taybi syndrome: a natural history study. *Am J Med Genet Suppl* 6: 30–37.

Stevens CA, Hennekam RC, Blackburn BL (1990b). Growth in the Rubinstein-Taybi syndrome. *Am J Med Genet Suppl* 6: 51–55.

Taine L, Goizet C, Wen ZQ, Petrij F, Breuning MH, Ayme S, Saura R, Arveiler B, Lacombe D (1998). Submicroscopic deletion of chromosome 16p13.3 in patients with Rubinstein-Taybi syndrome. *Am J Med Genet* 78: 267–270.

Taki T, Sako M, Tsuchida M, Hayashi Y (1997). The t(11;16)(q23;p13) translocation in myelodysplastic syndrome fuses the *MLL* gene to the *CBP* gene. *Blood* 89: 3945–3950.

Tanaka Y, Naruse I, Maekawa T, Masuya H, Shiroishi T, Ishii S (1997). Abnormal skeletal patterning in embryos lacking a single Cbp allele: a partial similarity with Rubinstein-Taybi syndrome. *Proc Natl Acad Sci USA* 94: 10215–10220.

Tanaka Y, Naruse I, Hongo T, Xu M, Nakahata T, Maekawa T, Ishii S (2000). Extensive brain hemorrhage and embryonic lethality in a mouse null mutant of CREB-binding protein. *Mech Dev* 95: 133–145.

Tommerup N, van der Hagen CB, Heiberg A (1992). Tentative assignment of a locus for Rubinstein-Taybi syndrome to 16p13.3 by a de novo reciprocal translocation, t(7;16)(q34;p13.3). *Am J Med Genet* 44: 237–241.

van Genderen MM, Kinds GF, Riemslag FC, Hennekam RC (2000). Ocular features in Rubinstein-Taybi syndrome: investigation of 24 patients and review of the literature. *Br J Ophthalmol* 84: 1177–1184.

Velloso ERP, Mecucci C, Michaux L, van Orshoven A, Stul M, Boogaerts M, Bosly A, Cassiman J-J, van den Berghe H (1996). Translocation t(8;16)(p11;p13) in acute nonlymphocytic leukemia: report on two new cases and review of the literature. *Leuk Lymphoma* 21: 137–142.

Victor M, Bei Y, Gay F, Calvo D, MelloC, Shi Y (2002). HAT activity is essential for CBP-1 dependent transcription and differentiation in *Caenorhabditis elegans*. *EMBO Rep* 3: 50–55.

Villavicencio EH, Walterhouse DO, Iannaccone PM (2000). The sonic hedgehog-patched-Gli pathway in human development and disease. *Am J Hum Genet* 67: 1047–1054.

Vortkamp A, Gessler M, Grzeschik K-H (1991). GLI3 zinc-finger gene interrupted by translocations in Grieg syndrome families. *Nature* 352: 539–540.

Wallerstein R, Anderson CE, Hay B, Gupta P, Gibas L, Ansari K, Cowchock FS, Weinblatt V, Reid C, Levitas A, et al. (1997). Submicroscopic deletions at 16p13.3 in Rubinstein-Taybi syndrome: frequency and clinical manifestations in a North American population. *J Med Genet* 34: 203–206.

Waltzer L, Bienz M (1999). A function of CBP as a transcriptional co-activator during Dpp signalling. *EMBO J* 18: 1630–1641.

Warkany J (1974). Difficulties of classification and terminology of syndromes of multiple congenital anomalies. *Am J Dis Child* 128: 424–425.

Wessels JW, Mollevanger P, Dauwerse JG, Cluitmans FH, Breuning MH, Beverstock GC (1991). Two distinct loci on the short arm of chromosome 16 are involved in myeloid leukemia. *Blood* 77: 1555–1559.

Wild A, Kalff-Suske M, Vortkamp A, Bornholdt D, Konig R, Grzeschik KH (1997). Point mutations in human GLI3 cause Greig syndrome. *Hum Mol Genet* 6: 1979–1984.

Wood VE, Rubinstein JH (1987). Surgical treatment of the thumb in the Rubinstein-Taybi syndrome. *J Hand Surg [Br]* 12: 166–172.

Xu W, Chen H, Du K, Asahara H, Tini M, Emerson BM, Montminy M, Evans RM (2001). A transcriptional switch mediated by cofactor methylation. *Science* 294: 2507–2511.

Yamauchi T, Oike Y, Kamon J, Waki H, Komeda K, Tsuchida A, Date Y, Li MX, Miki H, Akanuma Y, et al. (2002). Increased insulin sensitivity despite lipodystrophy in Crebbp heterozygous mice. *Nat Genet* 30: 221–226.

Yao TP, Oh SP, Fuchs M, Zhou ND, Ch'ng LE, Newsome D, Bronson RD, Livingston DM, Eckner R (1998). Gene dosage-dependent embryonic development and proliferation defects in mice lacking the transcriptional integrator p300. *Cell* 93: 361–372.

Zucconi M, Ferini-Strambi L, Erminio C, Pestalozza G, Smirne S (1993). Obstructive sleep apnea in the Rubinstein-Taybi syndrome. *Respiration* 60: 127–132.

72 | *ATRX* and X-Linked *α*-Thalassemia Mental Retardation Syndrome

RICHARD J. GIBBONS AND TAKAHITO WADA

The rare association of *α*-thalassemia and mental retardation (MR) was recognized 20 years ago by Weatherall and colleagues (1981). It was known that *α*-thalassemia arises when there is a defect in the synthesis of the *α*-globin chains of adult hemoglobin (HbA, $\alpha_2\beta_2$). When these authors encountered three mentally retarded children with *α*-thalassemia and a variety of developmental abnormalities, their interest was stimulated by the unusual nature of the *α*-thalassemia. The children were of northern European origin, where *α*-thalassemia is uncommon; and although one would have expected to find clear signs of this inherited anemia in their parents, it appeared to have arisen de novo in the affected offspring. It was thought that the combination of *α*-thalassemia, MR (ATR), and the associated developmental abnormalities represented a new syndrome and that a common genetic defect might be responsible for the diverse clinical manifestations. This conjecture has been confirmed, and what has emerged is the identification of two quite distinct syndromes: ATR-16, a contiguous gene syndrome, and ATR-X, which results from mutation of a putative chromatin remodeling factor.

In ATR-16, there are large (1–2 Mb) chromosomal rearrangements that delete many genes, including the *α*-globin genes from the tip of the short arm of chromosome 16 (Wilkie et al., 1990a). MR is in the mild to moderate range, and there is considerable variation in the phenotype, which has been ascribed in part to differences in the size of the 16p deletion. In many cases, the deletion has resulted from an unbalanced chromosomal translocation. Hence, aneuploidy of a second chromosome is present and probably contributes to the clinical picture.

In the second syndrome, initially called nondeletional *α*-thalassemia/MR syndrome and subsequently ATR-X (McKusick 300032), Wilkie et al. (1990b) demonstrated that there were no structural abnormalities in the *α*-globin cluster. This group of patients presented with a much more uniform phenotype and a recognizable facial dysmorphism (see below). Recognition of characteristic facial features from previously published case reports of X-linked MR suggested that this syndrome results from mutations in an X-encoded factor that is a putative regulator of gene expression.

ATRX FUNCTION

ATRX Locus

The five original "nondeletion" cases described by Wilkie et al. (1990b) were sporadic in nature, and apart from all being male, there were no immediate clues to the genetic etiology. Somatic cell hybrids composed of a mouse erythroleukemia cell line containing chromosome 16 (wherein the *α*-globin gene lies) derived from an affected boy produced human *α*-globin in a manner indistinguishable from a similar hybrid containing chromosome 16 from a normal individual. It seemed likely that the defect in globin synthesis lay *in trans* to the globin cluster. This was confirmed in a family with four affected sibs in whom the condition segregated independently of the *α*-globin cluster. In more extended families, affected individuals were always related via the female line, suggesting an X-linked pattern of inheritance. Consistent with this was the normal phenotype of obligate female carriers associated with a highly skewed pattern of X inactivation (Gibbons et al., 1992).

Linkage analysis in 16 families mapped the disease interval to Xq13.1-q21.1. A candidate gene approach was undertaken, which cap-italized on advances in gene trap techniques. Fontés and colleagues developed a strategy for isolating cDNA fragments by hybridization to cloned DNA from Xq13.3 (Gecz et al., 1994). A number of these cDNA fragments were hybridized to DNA from a group of affected individuals. An absent hybridization signal was noted in one patient when an 84 bp cDNA fragment, E4, was used. E4 was shown to be part of a gene known as *XH2/XNP* (Gibbons et al., 1995b). Subsequently, a 2 kb genomic deletion was demonstrated in this individual.

We now know that the *ATRX* gene spans about 300 kb of genomic DNA and contains 36 exons (Picketts et al., 1996). It encodes at least two alternatively spliced, ~10.5 kb mRNA transcripts which differ at their 5′ ends and are predicted to give rise to slightly different proteins of 265 and 280 kDa.

Within the N-terminal region lies a complex cysteine-rich segment (ADD, Fig. 72–1). The ADD comprises a PHD-like zinc finger and an additional putative zinc-binding C_2C_2 motif just upstream (Gibbons et al., 1997). The PHD finger is a zinc-binding domain (Cys_4-His-Cys_3), 50–80 amino acids in length, that has been identified in an increasing number of proteins, many of which are thought to be involved in chromatin-mediated transcriptional regulation (Aasland et al., 1995). The solution structure of the PHD motif has been determined for two proteins, the human William-Beuren syndrome transcription factor (WSTF) (Pascual et al., 2000) and the transcriptional corepressor KAP1 (Capili et al., 2001). This shows it to be an interleaved zinc finger. In terms of charge and topology, there are no structural features typical of a nucleic acid–binding protein, which suggests that the PHD zinc finger is unlikely to be a DNA-binding domain. The functional significance of the ADD segment is demonstrated by the high degree of conservation between human and mouse (97 of 98 amino acids) and the fact that it represents a major site of mutations in patients with ATR-X syndrome, containing over 60% of all mutations (Fig. 72–1 and see below).

The central and C-terminal regions show the greatest conservation between murine and human sequences (94%) (Picketts et al., 1998). The central portion of the molecule contains motifs that identify ATRX as a novel member of the SNF2 subgroup of a superfamily of proteins. This group of proteins is characterized by the presence of seven highly conserved co-linear helicase motifs. Other members of the SNF2 subfamily are involved in a wide variety of cellular functions, including regulation of transcription (SNF2, MOT1, and brahma), control of the cell cycle (NPS1), DNA repair (RAD16, RAD54, and ERCC6), and mitotic chromosomal segregation (lodestar). An interaction with chromatin has been shown for SNF2 and brahma and may be a common theme for all members of this group (reviewed in Carlson and Laurent, 1994). The ATRX protein, although showing marginally higher sequence homology to RAD54 than other members of this group, does not obviously fall into a particular functional category by virtue of homology in these flanking segments. There is no clinical evidence of ultraviolet sensitivity or the premature development of malignancy in the ATR-X syndrome, which might point to this being a defect in DNA repair. Furthermore, cytogenetic analysis has not demonstrated any evidence of abnormal chromosome breakage or segregation. Rather, the consistent association of ATR-X with *α*-thalassemia suggests that the protein normally exerts its effect at one or more of the many stages involved in gene expression.

The extreme C terminus of ATRX encodes two additional domains of potential functional importance which are highly conserved in

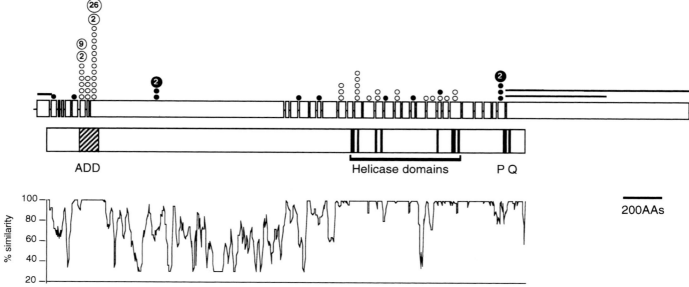

Figure 72–1. Schematic diagram of the complete *ATRX* cDNA: boxes represent the 35 exons (excluding the alternatively spliced exon 7); thin horizontal lines represent introns (not to scale). The largest open reading frame is shown as an open box. The principal domains, the zinc finger motif (ADD), and the highly conserved helicase motif are indicated, as are the P box (P) and a glutamine-rich region (Q). In the lower part of the figure is a graphical representation of the amino acid similarity between human and mouse ATRX proteins.

In the upper part of the figure, 60 different *ATRX* mutations from Table 72–2 are illustrated. The positions of the mutations are shown by circles: filled circles represent mutations (nonsense or leading to a frameshift) that would cause protein truncation; open circles represent missense mutations; deletions are indicated by horizontal dashed lines. Recurrent mutations are illustrated by larger circles, and the number of independent families is indicated.

mouse. The P box (Fig. 72–1) is an element conserved among other SNF2-like family members involved in transcriptional regulation, and a stretch of glutamine residues (Q box) represents a potential protein-interaction domain.

Studies of ATRX Function

Expression Studies

In the human adult, ATRX mRNA has a widespread pattern of expression, with particularly high expression in the brain, heart, and skeletal muscle (Stayton et al., 1994). *Mxnp* (the mouse homologue) is expressed very early in development. At the earliest stage examined, the early primitive streak stage (7.0 days postcoitum [dpc]), a diffuse signal was detected, with a stronger signal present at the posterior amniotic fold, which later gives rise to the chorion. In middle-gestation (11.5 dpc) embryo, Mxnp expression is generalized. With time, the intensity of the signal in the trunk decreases and there is a changing pattern of signal in the CNS, which by birth becomes restricted to a limited number of sites in which active cell proliferation occurs (Stayton et al., 1994).

Cellular Localization

A panel of antibodies has been developed against the ATRX protein, and by Western blot analysis in normal individuals, all of these detect a fragment of ~280 kDa, consistent with the predicted size of the ATRX protein (McDowell et al., 1999). Immunocytochemical analysis and indirect immunolocalization demonstrate that ATRX is a nuclear protein with a punctate staining pattern. In mouse cells at interphase, >90% ATRX protein colocalizes with 4′,6-diamidino-2-phenylindole bright regions of the nucleus, which represent pericentromeric heterochromatin, and this association is maintained in metaphase. In human cells at interphase, the pattern of staining is similarly punctate but the relationship to pericentromeric heterochromatin is less clear-cut. In unsynchronized HeLa cells, there is a considerable variation from cell to cell in the proportion of ATRX co-localizing with centromeric signals. Berube et al. (2000) used sequential extraction of HeLa and 293 cells to demonstrate that, during interphase, the majority of ATRX is tightly associated with the nuclear matrix. During metaphase, ATRX is associated with the centromeres, and this is

concomitant with phosphorylation of ATRX. As a consequence, it is possible that the distribution of ATRX during the cell cycle in human cells is phosphorylation-dependent. One additional striking finding in human metaphase preparations is that ATRX antibodies consistently localize to the short arms of acrocentric chromosomes and colocalize with a transcription factor (upstream binding factor) that is known to bind the rDNA arrays in nucleolar organizer regions.

Functional Consequences of Mutations

The effects of ATRX mutations on the chromatin structure of the rDNA arrays located in these regions have been studied. Although no gross changes in DNAase1, micrococcal nuclease, or endonuclease accessibility were detected, striking differences were noted in the pattern of rDNA methylation between normal controls and patients with ATR-X syndrome (Gibbons et al., 2000). In normal individuals, approximately 20% of the transcribed units were methylated, whereas in ATR-X patients, rDNA genes were substantially unmethylated. The hypomethylated regions in ATR-X individuals localized within the CpG-rich region of the rDNA repeat, which contains the transcribed 28S, 18S, and 5.8S genes and resembles a large CpG island.

Since ATRX is also associated with heterochromatin, which contains a substantial proportion of the highly repetitive DNA in mammalian genomes, these methylation studies were extended to other repetitive sequences containing CpG dinucleotides known to be epigenetically modified by methylation. In this way, two additional sequences were identified that were abnormally methylated in ATR-X patients. Y-specific repeats (DYZ2) were almost all methylated in ATR-X patients, while ~6% were unmethylated in peripheral blood of normal individuals. Subtle changes in the pattern of methylation were also observed in the TelBam3.4 family of repeats, which are mainly found in the subtelomeric regions. To date, no change in the pattern of methylation has been detected in the α-globin gene cluster, which might explain the reduced expression of the α-globin genes compared with expression of the β-globin genes. However, the subtle changes in methylation seen in the repetitive sequences of rDNA and DYZ2 are probably below the level of detection at single-copy loci.

These findings are most clearly related to the effects of mutations of the *DDM1* gene of *Arabidopsis thaliana*, which, like ATRX, encodes a SWI/SNF protein (Jeddeloh et al., 1999). Mutations of *DDM1* display a number of developmental defects and are hypomethylated at a variety of CpG-rich repetitive elements, including rDNA, centromeric repeats, and telomere-associated sequences (Vongs et al., 1993; Kakutani et al., 1995; Jacobsen, 1999). These observations raise the possibility that ATRX in mammalian cells and DDM1 in plants provide the ATPase-dependent chromatin-remodeling activity to a complex involved in the establishment or maintenance of DNA methylation.

Interestingly, the ADD of ATRX is most closely related to that found in the recently characterized human DNMT3 family of de novo methyltransferases, providing one possible link between ATRX and the methylation machinery (Xie et al., 1999). Putative ATRX orthologues in *Caenorhabditis elegans* and *Drosophila melanogaster*, organisms which do not have DNA methylation, are lacking the ADD motif seen in mammalian ATRX protein and in a putative plant orthologue (Villard et al., 1999b). One possibility is that ATRX protein and the DNMT3 methyltransferases interact with similar proteins via this motif.

Protein Interactions

Like other members of the SNF2 family, ATRX appears to to be part of a multiprotein complex. Preliminary experiments show that ATRX fractionates as a very large complex (>1 Md) by Superose 6 gel filtration. One of the proteins with which ATRX has been shown to interact is the heterochromatin protein HP1. Analysis of ATRX in a yeast two-hybrid screen has shown that it interacts with a murine homologue (mHP1α) of the *Drosophila* heterochromatic protein HP1; the N-terminal region (326–1196) of ATRX (which lies outside the ADD) interacts with the shadow chromodomain of mHP1α (Le Douarin et al., 1996). This region of ATRX is relatively poorly conserved between mouse and human but includes a pentapeptide segment highly similar to an HP1-binding domain (Smothers and Henikoff, 2000) as well as the coiled-coil motif, which could mediate the interaction. Further evidence comes from indirect immunoflourescence, where it has been shown in mouse cells that the ATRX protein colocalizes with mHP1α at pericentromeric heterochromatin during interphase and mitosis (McDowell, et al., 1999). Finally ATRX and HP1 coimmunoprecipitate using either anti-ATRX or anti-HP1 antibodies (Berube et al., 2000).

Recent evidence suggests that HP1, a known chromatin-binding protein implicated in both gene silencing and supranucleosomal chromatin structure, is a structural adapter, whose role is to assemble macromolecular complexes in chromatin. It appears to be targeted by binding, via its chromodomain, to methylated lysine-9 of histone H3 (Bannister et al., 2001; Lachner et al., 2001). This modification of the histone tail is catalyzed by a methyltransferase activity of the protein SUV39H1 (Rea et al., 2000). An interaction between ATRX and HP1 may be sufficient to colocalize ATRX within heterochromatin via a protein–protein interaction.

In a more directed use of the yeast two-hybrid system, Cardoso et al. (1998) investigated the interaction of ATRX with a variety of heterochromatin-associated proteins. An interaction was demonstrated between ATRX (475–734) and the SET domain of polycomb group protein EZH2.

The ADD domain of ATRX is another potential site for protein interaction. The ADD domain of Dnmt3a interacts with the histone deacetylase HDAC1 (Fuks et al., 2001). Interestingly, the PHD motif of Mi2β also binds HDAC1, and it is possible that this component of the ADD domain is responsible for binding HDAC. In addition, the ADD domain of Dnmt3 binds to the sequence-specific DNA-binding protein RP58. A similar interaction between ATRX and other sequence-specific DNA-binding proteins may be responsible for targeting ATRX to specific loci or alternatively recruiting specific loci to repressive heterochromatin.

CLINICAL AND HEMATOLOGICAL FINDINGS IN ATR-X SYNDROME

Since the identification of the *ATRX* gene, numerous other forms of syndromal X-linked MR (often representing single family reports) have been identified as resulting from ATRX mutations: Juberg-Mar-

Table 72–1. Clinical Findings in 168 ATR-X Syndrome Patients

Clinical Finding	Total*	%
Profound mental retardation	160/167†	96
Characteristic face	138/147	94
Skeletal abnormalities	128/142	90
HbH inclusions	130/147	88
Neonatal hypotonia	88/105	84
Genital abnormalities	119/150	79
Microcephaly	103/134	77
Gut dysmotility	89/117	76
Short stature	73/112	65
Seizures	53/154	34
Cardiac defects	32/149	21
Renal/urinary abnormalities	23/151	15

*Total represents the number of patients on whom appropriate information is available and includes patients who do not have α-thalassemia but in whom *ATRX* mutations have been identified.

†One patient too young (<1 year) to assess degree of mental retardation.

sidi (Villard et al., 1996a), X-linked MR with spastic paraplegia (Lossi et al., 1999), Carpenter-Waziri (Abidi et al., 1999), Holmes-Gang (Stevenson et al., 2000a), and Smith-Fineman-Myers (Villard et al., 2000) syndromes. As will be discussed, there is little rationale for separating these into distinct disorders. For the purpose of this chapter, these conditions have been amalgamated under the term *ATR-X syndrome*. A total of 168 cases of ATR-X syndrome from over 100 families have now been characterized, and a definite phenotype is emerging (Table 72–1).

Neonatal Period

Pregnancy is usually uneventful and proceeds to term, and in 90% of cases birth weight is normal. Affected neonates usually have marked hypotonia and associated feeding difficulties. Poor temperature control, hypoglycemia, apneic episodes, abnormal movements, and seizures have also been noted on a number of occasions.

Psychomotor Retardation and the CNS

In early childhood, all milestones are delayed. Many patients do not walk until later in childhood, and some never ambulate. Most have no speech, although there are several cases in which individuals are limited to a handful of words or signs. They frequently have only situational understanding and are dependent for almost all activities of daily living. More recent reports, however, point to a wider spectrum of intellectual handicap than previously thought. A mutation in the *ATRX* gene has been identified in a family originally described by Carpenter and colleagues (1999). All affected males have moderate MR and exhibit expressive language delay, though no psychometric evaluation is available. Guerrini and colleagues (2000) reported a mutation in an Italian family with four affected male cousins: one has profound MR, whereas the others have IQs of 41, 56, and 58. The basis for this marked variation is unknown. Generally, affected individuals continue to acquire new skills, though a brief period of neurological deterioration has been reported in three cases. In one report, electroencephalographic (EEG) changes were consistent with encephalitis (Donnai et al., 1991). The family originally reported by Holmes and Gang (1984) was subsequently shown to have an *ATRX* mutation (Stevenson, et al., 2000a). All three affected males from this family died in childhood, and the death of one was attributed to encephalitis.

As affected individuals age, there is often a tendency toward spasticity. A recent report described a family with an *ATRX* mutation in which affected members had spastic paraplegia from birth (Lossi et al., 1999).

Seizures occur in approximately one-third of cases, and most frequently are clonic/tonic or myoclonic in nature. A number of parents have reported jerking movements which are not associated with epileptiform activity on EEG.

Assessment of vision and hearing is difficult. Vision usually appears normal, although two cases have been reported as blind. Optic atrophy or pale discs are commonly noted, as are refractive errors (especially myopia). Sensorineural deafness has previously been considered a feature that distinguishes ATR-X syndrome from the allelic condition Juberg-Marsidi syndrome (Saugier-Veber et al., 1995). However, of the 13 cases with a documented sensorineural hearing deficit, seven have ATR-X syndrome, i.e., presence of α-thalassemia.

Although head circumference is usually normal at birth, post-natal microcephaly usually develops. Macrocephaly has not been reported.

Computed tomography or magnetic resonance brain imaging are generally unremarkable, although mild cerebral atrophy may be seen. In two cases, partial or complete agenesis of the corpus callosum has been reported. There have been autopsy reports in only three cases. The brain was small in each; in two the morphology was normal, and in one the temporal gyri on the right were indistinct, with hypoplasia of the cerebral white matter.

Behavioral Phenotype

No systematic study of behavior has been carried out in ATR-X syndrome. Consequently, most reports of behavioral characteristics are anecdotal, and ascertainment has been limited. Nevertheless, a thumbnail sketch of the mannerisms of this condition is slowly emerging (Kurosawa et al., 1996; Wada et al., 1998), and this may be diagnostic.

Subjects are usually described by their parents as content and of a happy disposition. Affected individuals exhibit a wide range of emotions that are usually appropriate to their circumstances. There have been reports, however, of unprovoked emotional outbursts with sustained laughing or crying. There may be emotional fluctuation, with sudden switches between almost manic-like excitement or agitation to withdrawal and depression. In several instances, episodes of crying have been thought to be associated with pain, possibly of a gastrointestinal origin (see below).

Whereas many individuals are affectionate to their caregivers and appreciate physical contact, some cases exhibit autistic-like behavior: patients appear to be in a world of their own, show little interest or even recognition of those around them, and avoid eye contact. The latter behavior may be associated with an unusual and persistent posture, such as sitting with the head tilted, gazing upward.

Affected persons may be restless, exhibiting choreoathetoid movements. Frequently, they put their hands into their mouths and may induce vomiting. Sometimes, they engage in self-injurious behavior, biting or hitting themselves. They may hit, push, or squeeze their necks with their hands to the point of cyanosis, a state they may also achieve through breath-holding. Repetitive stereotypic movements may be manifest, and these may vary from pill-rolling or hand-flapping to spinning around on one spot while gazing into a light. These characteristic behaviors are reminiscent of Angelman's syndrome and may lead to diagnostic confusion.

Autism occurs more often in some genetic abnormalities producing MR (e.g., fragile X syndrome, Rett syndrome, and tuberous sclerosis) than in others (e.g., Down syndrome or Prader-Willi syndrome) (Dykens and Volkmar, 1997). It is possible that some neurobiological mechanisms that produce MR are more likely to lead to autism than others, and ATRX may have a role in such a pathway.

Facial Anomalies

Distinctive facial traits are most readily recognized in early childhood and the gestalt is probably secondary to facial hypotonia (Fig. 72–2a,b). The frontal hair is often upswept and there is telecanthus, epicanthic folds, flat nasal bridge, mid-face hypoplasia, and a small triangular upturned nose with the alae nasi extending below the columella and septum. The upper lip is tented and the lower lip full and everted, giving the mouth a "carp-like" appearance. The frontal incisors are frequently widely spaced, the tongue protrudes, and there is prodigious dribbling. The ears may be simple, slightly low-set, and posteriorly rotated.

Genital Abnormalities

Genital abnormalities are seen in 80% of children. These may be very mild, e.g., undescended testes or deficient prepuce; but the spectrum of abnormality extends through hypospadias to micropenis (Fig. 72–3a) to ambiguous or external female genitalia (Fig. 72–3b). The most severely affected children, who are clinically defined as male pseudohermaphrodites, are usually raised as females. In such cases, there are no mullerian structures present and dysgenetic testes or streak gonads have been found intra-abdominally (Wilkie, et al., 1990b; Ion et al., 1996). Of particular interest is the finding that these abnormalities breed true within families (McPherson et al., 1995). Puberty is frequently delayed and in a few cases appears to be arrested. Curiously, premature adrenarche has been noted in two children.

Skeletal Abnormalities

A wide range of relatively mild skeletal abnormalities have been noted, some of which are probably secondary to hypotonia and immobility (Gibbons et al., 1995a). Fixed flexion deformities, particularly of the fingers, are common. Other abnormalities of the fingers and toes that have been observed are clinodactyly, brachydactyly, tapering of the fingers, drum stick phalanges, cutaneous syndactyly, overlapping of the digits, and a single case with a bifid thumb. Foot deformities occur in 29% and include pes planus, talipes equinovarus, and talipes calcaneovalgus. Almost a third of cases have kyphosis and/or scoliosis, and chest wall deformity has been seen in 10 cases. Sacral dimples were present in three cases, radiological spina bifida in two, and other abnormalities of the vertebrae in five. Only a few of the cases have had thorough radiological investigation. In those who have, the most common findings were delayed bone age and coxa valga. Short stature was seen in two-thirds of cases. Longitudinal data are available in only a few cases. As has been noted previously, in some patients growth retardation is apparent throughout life, whereas in others it manifests at a later stage, e.g., at the time of the pubertal growth spurt.

Miscellaneous Abnormalities

Recurrent vomiting, regurgitation, or gastroesophageal reflux, particularly in early childhood, is a common finding and seems likely to be a

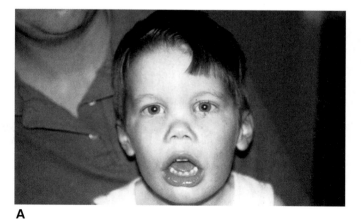

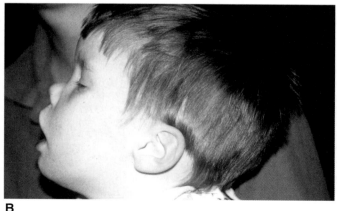

A   **B**

Figure 72–2. Four-year-old male with ATR-X syndrome showing (*A*) typical facial appearance and (*B*) mid-face hypoplasia. (From Gibbons et al., 1995a.)

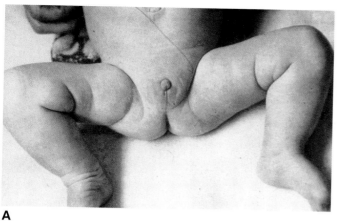
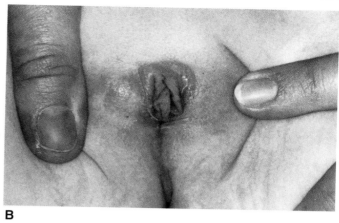

Figure 72–3. (*A*) Micropenis in a subject with ATR-X syndrome. (Taken from Gibbons et al., 1995a.) (*B*) External genitalia in ATR-X subject with male pseudohermaphroditism. (Taken from Wilkie et al., 1990b.)

manifestation of a more generalized dysmotility of the gut. In severe cases, surgical treatment by fundoplication has been undertaken, as has feeding gastrostomy. An apparent reluctance to swallow has been reported by several parents and probably reflects the dyscoordinated swallowing that has been observed radiologically in two well-studied cases. The tendency to aspiration is commonly implicated as a cause of death in early childhood. Excessive drooling is very common, as is frequent eructation. Constipation occurs often and in some individuals is a major management problem. Hospital admissions for recurrent ileus have been reported in two cases, and reduced intestinal mobility has been observed radiologically in four cases. Two patients required partial resection of the ileum after developing ischemia of the small bowel, which in one case was attributed to a volvulus. Volvulus has been reported in an additional case. One child required a right hemicolectomy following an episode of necrotizing enterocolitis at 13 days of age.

There is evidence to suggest that affected individuals are susceptible to peptic ulceration. Esophagitis, esophageal stricture, and peptic ulcer have been observed endoscopically in single cases. In five cases, there has been evidence of an upper gastrointestinal bleed, one of

which required transfusion (hemoglobin 5 g/dl). Pain resulting from peptic ulceration is one possible explanation for the episodes of persistent crying and food refusal reported by a number of parents.

A wide range of cardiac abnormalities have been noted: septal defects (10 cases), patent ductus arteriosus (6 cases), pulmonary stenosis (3 cases), aortic stenosis (2 cases), tetralogy of Fallot (2 cases), and single cases of transposition of the great arteries, dextracardia with situs solitus, and aortic regurgitation.

Renal abnormalities (hydronephrosis, renal hypoplasia or agenesis, polycystic kidney, vesicoureteric reflux) may present with recurrent urinary tract infections.

Hematology

Although initially the presence of α-thalassemia was one of the defining elements of the syndrome, it is clear that there is considerable variation in the hematological manifestations associated with *ATRX* mutations. A number of families have been identified in which some or all of the affected members have no signs of α-thalassemia (Villard et al., 1996b,c) (Table 72–2). Nevertheless, the test for α-thalassemia

Table 72–2. Summary of *ATRX* Mutations

No.	Exon/intron*	Mutation†	De Novo Mutation‡	No. of Peds	No. of Cases	M R§	Genital Abnormality‖	HbH Cells**	Reference
1	1	EX1_2del		1	2		+ to ++	0	(Gibbons and Higgs, 2000)
2	2	109C>T; R37X		1	4	Mild-profound	n to ++	0 to 0.006	(Guerrini et al., 2000)
3	6	413_414delAA; K138fs		1	1		+	0	(Gibbons and Higgs, 2000)
4	8	524G>A; G175E		1	1		+	0	(Villard et al., 1999)
5	8	528_529insCAA; 176_177insQ		1	3		+	0.003 to 0.12	(Gibbons et al., 1997)
6	8	536A>G; S c532-594del; V178_K198del	+	9	10		n to +++	0 to 1.5	(Picketts et al., 1996); (Gibbons et al., 1997); (Villard et al., 1999); (Wada et al., 2000); (Gibbons and Higgs, 2000)
7	8	568C>G; P190A		1	1		++	4.8	(Gibbons et al., 1997)
8	8	568C>T; P190S		2	2		n	+ to 5	(Gibbons and Higgs, 2000); (Villard et al., 1999)
9	8	569C>T; P190L	+	1	1		+	+	(Wada et al., 2000)
10	8	576G>C; L192F		1	1		n	<0.01	(Gibbons et al., 1997)
11	8	580G>A; V194I		1	1		+	11.6	(Wada et al., 2000)
12	9	599G>C; C200S	+	1	1		++	31.5	(Gibbons et al., 1997)
13	9	656A>C; Q219P		1	1		n	+	(Villard et al., 1999)
14	9	658T>C; C220R		1	1		++	0.01	(Gibbons et al., 1997)
15	9	659G>A; C220Y		1	3		n	nd	(Stevenson et al., 2000)
16	10	665G>C; W222S		1	1		++	0.003	(Gibbons et al., 1997)
17	10	666G>T; W222C		1	1		++	4	unpublished
18	10	717C>A; F239L		1	1		U	2	(Gibbons and Higgs, 2000)
19	10	719G>T; C240F	+	1	1		++	6	(Gibbons et al., 1997)
20	10	731T>A; I244N	+	1	1		+	16	(Gibbons and Higgs, 2000)

(*continued*)

Table 72–2. Summary of *ATRX* Mutations *Continued*

No.	Exon/intron*	Mutation†	De Novo Mutation‡	No. of Peds	No. of Cases	MR§	Genital Abnormality‖	HbH Cells**	Reference
21	10	736C>T; R246C	+	26	32		n to ++++	0 to 14	(Gibbons et al., 1997); (Gibbons and Higgs, 2000); (Wada et al., 2000); unpublished
22	10	737G>T; R246L		2	2		n to +	+ to 1.0	(Fichera et al., 1998); (Villard et al., 1999)
23	10	739A>G; N247D		1	1		++	+	(Gibbons and Higgs, 2000)
24	10	745G>T; G249C	+	1	1		+	+	(Villard et al., 1999)
25	10	746G>A; G249D	+	1	2		++	2.5 to 3.9	(Gibbons et al., 1997)
26	10	787T>C; W263R		1	1		n	0.4	(Gibbons and Higgs, 2000)
27	10	797A>G; Y266C		1	1		++	10	(Gibbons and Higgs, 2000)
28	10	1725delA; K575fs		1	1		++	2.8	unpublished
29	10	1727C>A; S576X		2	6		n to +++	1.4 to 10	(Gibbons and Higgs, 2000)
30	10	1748delC; T583fs		1	1		n	0	(Gibbons and Higgs, 2000)
31	int12	3944-2A>G; S insertion 86bp (fs)		1	1		++	3.7	(Fichera et al., 1998)
32	15	4317G>A; S insertion 53bp (fs)		1	2		++ to +++	0.9 to 3.6	(Picketts et al., 1996)
33	17	4613T>G; V1538G		1	1		+++	11	(Picketts et al., 1996)
34	17	4617_4622del; 1540_1541delDE		1	2		n to +++	0.9 to 1.0	(Gibbons and Higgs, 2000)
35	17	4654G>T; V1552F		1	2		+ to +++	41 to 56	(Wada et al., 2000)
36	19	4826A>G; H1609R		1	1		+++	1.6	(Gibbons et al., 1995)
37	19	4840T>C; C1614R		1	1		+++++	>5	(Gibbons et al., 1995)
38	19	4864G>A; A1622T	+	1	1		++	18.2	(Gibbons and Higgs, 2000)
39	19	4934T>C; L1645S		1	1		n	0.2	(Wada et al., 2000)
40	19	4950G>T; K1650N		1	2		n	0.4 to 0.6	(Gibbons et al., 1995)
41	20	5039T>C; I1680T		1	1		+++++	+	(Gibbons and Higgs, 2000)
42	21	5137C>T; P1713S		1	1		n	0	(Villard et al., 1996)
43	21	5225G>A; R1742K	+	1	3	Moderate	++	3	(Lossi et al., 1999)
44	int 21	5273-10T>A; S c5273_5448del; Y1758X		1	3		n to +++	<0.001 to 30	(Villard et al., 1996)
45	23	5498A>G; Y1833C		1	1		++	0.2	(Gibbons and Higgs, 2000)
46	23	5540A>G; Y1847C		1	1		+	+	(Wada et al., 2000)
47	25	5721G>A; S c5698_5786del; G1900fs		1	1		+++	+	unpublished
48	int 26	5957-2A>G; S c5957_6022del; p1986_2007del	+	1	1		+	+	(Gibbons and Higgs, 2000)
49	27	6104A>T; D2035V		1	2		+++	7 to 27	(Gibbons et al., 1995)
50	28	6149T>C; I2050T		1	4		n	U	(Abidi et al., 1999)
51	int 28	6218-12574G>A; S insertion 124bp (fs)	+	1	1		++	1.4	(Picketts et al., 1996)
52	29	6250T>C; Y2084H		1	1		++	>5	(Gibbons et al., 1995)
53	30	6392G>A; R2131Q		1	3		+++	U	(Villard et al., 1996)
54	30	6488A>G; Y2163C	+	1	1		+	12	(Gibbons et al., 1995)
55	35	7156C>T; R2386X	+	2	3		++++ to +++++	v.rare to 0.02	(Gibbons et al., 1995) (Gibbons and Higgs, 2000)
56	35	7162G>T; E2388X		1	2		+++++	0.03	(Gibbons et al., 1995)
57	int 35	7201-2A>G; S c7201_7208del; L2401fs		1	2		++	0	(Villard et al., 2000)
58	int 35	7201-2delCTAA; S c7201_7208del; L2401fs		1	5		+++++	0***	(Ion et al., 1996)
59	36	IVS35_8789del		1	3		+++++	0.03 to 1.1	(Gibbons et al., 1995)
60	36	EX36del		1	2		+++++	6.5	(Gibbons and Higgs, 2000)

*Exon or intron in which mutation lies; numbering based on a total of 36 exons with exon 7 spliced out (accession U72937).

†Nomenclature of mutations as recommended by Dunnen and Antonarakis (2000). For base substitutions, the DNA mutation is followed by the amino acid change; for splicing abnormalities (S), the resulting principal cDNA is given (preceded by *c*); mutations leading to frameshift are indicated by *fs* and, where appropriate, the first affected amino acid is given; where the precise extent of a deletion is not determined, the deleted exons are indicated. All amino acid substitutions occur at residues conserved in the predicted human and mouse protein sequences.

‡+ indicates that this mutation arises de novo in a member of the family.

§Unless shown otherwise, mental retardation (MR) was profound (severity as defined in ICD-10 [1992] classification.)

‖For a given mutation, the range of genital abnormalities present is shown: n, normal; +, very mild, e.g., high-lying testes; ++, cryptorchidism; +++, hypospadias; ++++, micropenis; +++++, ambiguous genitalia or male pseudohermaphrodite.

**For a given mutation, the proportion of cells with HbH inclusions is shown. Where values from more than one individual are available, a range is shown. + indicates when inclusions were observed but not quantified.

***0/5000 red cells had HbH inclusions but α/β-globin chain ratio = 0.85, 15% below control samples. U, undetermined.

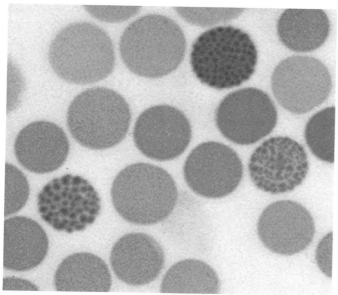

Figure 72–4. Photomicrograph of the peripheral blood of a case with ATR-X syndrome, showing three cells containing HbH inclusions.

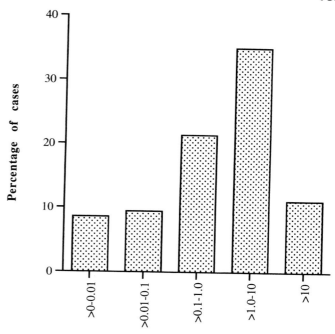

Percentage cells with HbH inclusions

Figure 72–5. Percentage of cells with HbH inclusions in cases in which the presence of inclusions has been demonstrated and quantified ($n = 103$).

is simple and, when positive, quickly establishes the diagnosis. The most sensitive test uses light microscopy to detect red cells containing HbH inclusions (Fig. 72–4) after incubation, at room temperature, of venous blood with 1% brilliant cresyl blue for 4–24 hours. HbH is unstable, and cells with inclusions may be more difficult to find in older blood samples. When the family history and phenotype are strongly suspect, a careful search for inclusions should be made in all affected individuals and repeated if necessary as they may be very infrequent (Fig. 72–5). In most cases of ATR-X, there is insufficient HbH to be detected by electrophoresis. The hematology is often surprisingly normal considering the presence of α-thalassemia (Fig. 72–6 and 72–7). Neither the hemoglobin concentration nor the mean cell hemoglobin is as severely affected as in the classical forms of α-thalassemia, which are associated with *cis*-acting mutations in the α-globin complex (Fig. 72–7), and this probably reflects the different pathophysiology of the conditions.

Life Expectancy

Of the 168 patients described, there have been 25 deaths. The cause was established in just over half, of which there were six cases of pneumonia and four of aspiration of vomitus. Cases appear to be particularly vulnerable in early childhood, with 19 of the deaths occur-

ring under the age of 5 years; this may be associated with the fact that gastroesophageal reflux and vomiting are often more severe in the early years. There are no long-term longitudinal data in this relatively newly described syndrome, but a number of affected individuals are fit and well in their 30s and 40s.

Phenotype of Carriers

Female carriers are intellectually normal, and no consistent physical manifestations have been observed. There is no increase in the rate of miscarriage for them. Rare cells with HbH inclusions may be found in about a quarter of obligate carriers (Gibbons et al., 1995a). Studies of the pattern of X inactivation in carriers of ATR-X syndrome show that, in most females, the abnormal X chromosome is predominantly inactivated in cells from a variety of tissues. This would explain the scarcity of cells with HbH inclusions in these individuals (Gibbons et al., 1992) and why no abnormality in rDNA methylation is observed in female carriers (Gibbons and Higgs, unpublished observation).

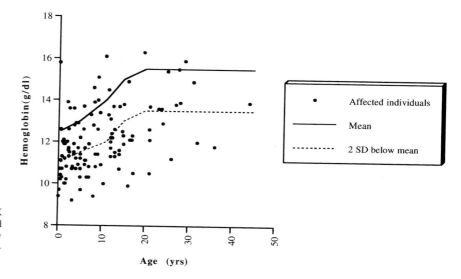

Figure 72–6. Hemoglobin levels in subjects with ATR-X syndrome at various ages. Solid line indicates the mean and dashed line, 2 SD below the mean (Dallman, 1977). For any given subject, only one result within each consecutive 5-year period is given.

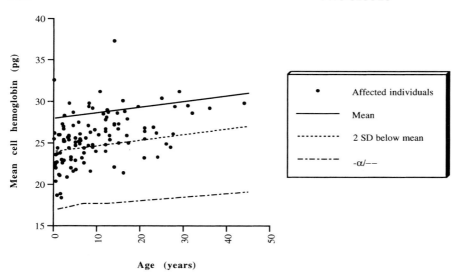

Figure 72–7. Mean cell hemoglobin levels in subjects with ATR-X syndrome at various ages. Mean values for individuals with α-thalassemia resulting from a −α/−− genotype are shown.

MUTATIONS OF THE *ATRX* GENE AND THEIR ASSOCIATED PHENOTYPE

Allelic Conditions

Since its identification in 1995, the *ATRX* gene has emerged as the disease gene for numerous forms of syndromal X-linked MR: X-linked α-thalassemia/MR or ATR-X (Gibbons et al., 1995b), Carpenter-Waziri syndrome (Abidi et al., 1999), Holmes-Gang syndrome (Stevenson et al., 2000a), Juberg-Marsidi syndrome (Villard et al., 1996a), and Smith-Fineman-Myers syndrome (Villard et al., 2000). It is also the disease gene for X-linked MR with spastic paraplegia (Lossi et al., 1999). It has been estimated that approximately 10% of named X-linked MR syndromes are candidates for allelism based on phenotypic findings. These include XLMR-arch fingerprints-hypotonia, Brooks, Chudley-Lowry, Miles-Carpenter, Proud, Vasquez, Young-Hughes, and XLMR-psoriasis syndromes (Stevenson et al., 2000b). It is now important to establish the full range of disease-causing mutations, to facilitate genetic counseling and to elucidate functionally important aspects of the protein.

Distribution of Mutations

To date, 60 different mutations have been documented in 97 separate families (Table 72–2 and Fig. 72–1). The missense mutations, in particular, are clustered in two regions, the ADD domain and the helicase domain. Analysis of the mutations and their resulting phenotypes allows important conclusions to be drawn.

Mutations of ATRX Probably Cause Reduced Function

A number of mutations predicted to cause protein truncation are scattered throughout the gene (Table 72–2). Such mutations would be expected to result in loss of function if critical domains are removed. It is clear, however, that these mutations are not lethal. Furthermore, the resulting phenotype is similar to that seen in other mutations. Using monoclonal antibodies against ATRX and Western blot analysis, it has been possible to look at the ATRX protein in patients with mutations predicted to cause protein truncations. A curious observation is that not only is the predicted truncated product observed but a small amount of full-length product is also observed (McDowell et al., 1999). The reason for full-length product is as yet unexplained, though alternate splicing has been excluded. It is possible that complete absence of ATRX, a true null, may be lethal; but a comprehensive analysis of ATRX protein in many different patients will be needed to address this issue.

Levels of ATRX protein were substantially reduced in a number of patients with missense mutations involving the ADD domain (McDowell, et al., 1999; Cardoso et al., 2000). The recent determination of the structure of two PHD zinc fingers casts light on how mutations might affect protein structure and stability (Pascual et al., 2000; Capili et al., 2001). By comparing the equivalent residues of ATRX with those for KAP-1, the naturally occurring mutations fall into four groups (Fig. 72–8): loss of zinc-binding cysteine residues, which would affect protein folding; introduction of additional potentially

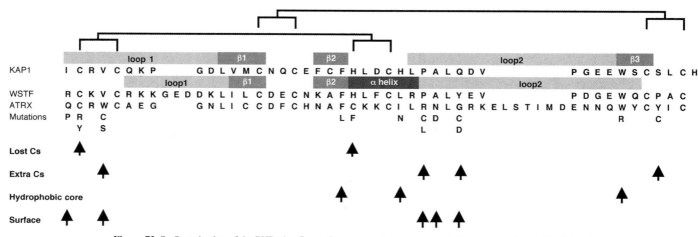

Figure 72–8. Organization of the PHD zinc finger. Sequence and structural motif alignment for KAP-1, WSTF, and ATRX and a schematic depicting zinc ligation. Positions of ATRX mutations are shown and classified (see text).

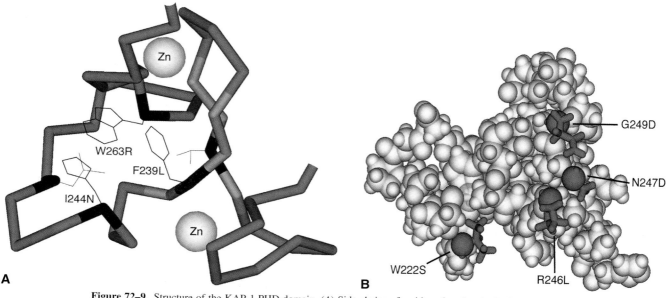

Figure 72–9. Structure of the KAP-1 PHD domain. (*A*) Side chains of residues forming the hydrophobic core are shown in wire form. Mutations of the analogous ATRX residues are highlighted and labeled. (*B*) Four of the five surface residues that are mutated in ATRX are shown.

zinc-binding cysteines, which are likely to cause incorrect folding by competing for the zinc atoms; mutations affecting the tightly packed hydrophobic core (Fig. 72–9*a*), which experimentally are as debilitating as mutations in zinc-binding cysteines; mutations affecting residues predicted to be exposed on the surface of the protein (Fig. 72–9*b*). In this last class, Capili et al. (2001) suggested mutations at these residues may interfere with specific protein–protein interactions. It is intriguing that three of these residues (Fig. 72–9*b*; R246L, N247D, and G249D) are clustered and may disrupt a particular interaction.

All of the helicase mutations so far described are located adjacent to, rather than within, the seven highly conserved motifs that characterize the SNF2 helicase/ATPase proteins. In other SNF2 proteins, mutations that fall in the motifs completely abolish activity. It is possible that the ATRX mutations alter, rather than abolish, the protein activity. These findings are consistent with the view that the common final pathway of ATRX mutations is a decrease, rather than abolition, of ATRX activity.

Genotype–Phenotype Correlations

Since the discovery of the *ATRX* gene, most new cases have been defined on the basis of severe MR, with the typical facial appearance associated with a mutation in the *ATRX* gene. This allows a less biased evaluation of the effect of *ATRX* mutations on the commonly associated clinical manifestations. The severity of three aspects of the phenotype (MR, genital abnormality, and α-thalassemia) are quantifiable to some degree.

The greatest variation in intellectual handicap is associated with a truncating mutation at the N terminus of the protein (Guerrini et al., 2000). Analysis of the RNA derived from patient cell lines showed no alternate splicing that might be associated with skipping of the mutation and degrees of phenotypic rescue. As discussed above, protein analysis by Western blotting has shown small amounts of full-length protein for each patient. This may be associated with inefficient recognition of the premature stop codon or possibly the use of an alternative, downstream translational initiation codon. Nevertheless, there is no correlation between the degree of retardation and the amount of full-length protein.

There are now eight different mutations associated with the most severe urogenital abnormalities (Table 72–2). In five, the protein is truncated, resulting in loss of the C-terminal domain, including a conserved element (P in Fig. 72–1) and polyglutamine tract (Q in Fig. 72–1). From the available data, it appears that, in the absence of the C-terminal domain, severe urogenital abnormalities are likely (though not inevitable as one mutation in this region was associated with cryptorchidism), suggesting that this region may play a specific role in

urogenital development. Consistent with this, in families with such mutations, severe urogenital abnormalities breed true (McPherson et al., 1995; Ion et al., 1996), and a nonsense mutation (55, Table 72–2) gives rise to a similar phenotype in two unrelated families. At other sites, however, there is no obvious link between phenotype and genotype, and there is considerable variation in the degree of abnormality seen in individuals with identical mutations.

The relationship between ATRX mutations and α-thalassemia is unclear. Since the presence of excess β chains (HbH inclusions) was originally used to define the ATR-X syndrome, current observations are inevitably biased. Nevertheless, there is considerable variability in the degree to which α-globin synthesis is affected by these mutations, as judged by the frequency of cells with HbH inclusions. Some patients do not have HbH inclusions (Villard et al., 1996a–c), although this does not rule out downregulation of α-globin expression since inclusions may not appear until there is 30%–40% reduction in α-chain synthesis (Higgs et al., 1989). It is interesting that patients with identical mutations may have very different, albeit stable, degrees of α-thalassemia, suggesting that the effect of the ATRX protein on α-globin expression may be modified by other genetic factors. This is most clearly illustrated by comparing the hematology of cases with identical mutations (Table 72–2). In the 5′ splicing mutation (6, Table 72–2), there are 10 affected individuals from nine different families, and the frequency of cells with HbH inclusions varies from 0% to 1.5%. Furthermore, comparison of the 32 cases from 26 pedigrees with the common 736C>T mutation (21, Table 72–2) shows an even greater variation in the frequency of HbH inclusions (0%–14%). This may be analogous to mutations of other members of the SNF2 family, whose effects are modified by a variation in many genes encoding proteins that interact with SNF2-like proteins (Hirschhorn et al., 1992; Carlson and Laurent, 1994).

In conclusion, there is a broad phenotypic spectrum associated not only with different *ATRX* mutations but also with identical mutations. In different reports, the presence or absence of certain findings has been emphasized, but the case for phenotype splitting is not persuasive. Systematic mutation analysis of a broad population of patients with learning difficulties should help to determine the extent of the phenotypic spectrum associated with *ATRX* mutations and their prevalence.

DIAGNOSIS AND COUNSELING

Diagnosis

For the clinician and the family of a mentally retarded male, the important consideration is accurate and speedy diagnosis. Research over the last 5 years has provided an array of useful findings for the identification of ATR-X syndrome and its clinical variants. A search for HbH inclusions is an easy and rapid first-line test that will confirm the diagnosis in many cases. The observation of methylation abnormalities in ATR-X patients potentially adds a new valuable and complementary screening test for diagnosis. If these tests are negative and where the index of suspicion is high, it may be worth proceeding to mutation analysis or checking for reduced levels of ATRX protein to confirm the diagnosis.

Differential Diagnosis

The diagnosis of ATR-X syndrome is relatively straightforward in patients who present with typical clinical features and HbH inclusions. However, where the hematology has not been checked or HbH inclusions are absent, diagnostic difficulty may arise. Coffin-Lowry syndrome may be confused with ATR-X syndrome, particularly in early childhood. Distinguishing features are the downslanting palpebral fissures, broad nose, pudgy and tapering digits, absence of genital abnormalities, and the frequent presence of carrier manifestations in Coffin-Lowry syndrome. There is phenotypic overlap with Angelman's syndrome (profound MR with absent speech and walking, seizures, happy disposition, emotional lability) and Smith-Lemli-Opitz (facial dysmorphism, skeletal and genital abnormalities). Diagnostic testing or mutational analysis should allow these conditions to be excluded in most cases.

Mutation Analysis

The gene is large, and comprehensive mutation analysis, even of the coding region, is a time-consuming and expensive enterprise. Given that the missense mutations are clustered in the ADD and helicase domains, it is sensible to commence with these segments. Analysis of the ATRX protein may show a truncation in affected individuals, which allows more directed sequencing.

Identification and Counseling of Female Carriers

ATR-X syndrome is a recessive X-linked condition. Female carriers are phenotypically and intellectually normal; therefore, additional tests are required to determine a female's genotype. In the past, skewed X inactivation has been utilized as a marker for carriers of the ATRX mutation. However, 5%–10% of normal females have skewed X inactivation, and occasional female carriers have a balanced pattern (Gibbons et al., 1992); therefore, this method should be used with caution. Of obligate female carriers, 25% exhibit rare cells with HbH inclusions, but obviously a negative result does not exclude carriage of a mutation. Since the identification of the ATRX gene, mutation detection has become the mainstay of carrier identification. In families in which the causative mutation has not been identified, linked markers may be used to identify whether descendants of an obligate carrier have inherited the disease-associated haplotype.

For the female who has been identified as a carrier, there is a 50% risk of passing on the disease allele; but since only males are clinically affected, the risk of having an affected child is 25% for each pregnancy. Prenatal diagnosis for such at-risk females is feasible.

The principal issue when counseling is determining the risk of recurrence for families with a sporadic case of ATR-X. One small study showed that 17/20 mothers of sporadic cases were carriers (Bachoo and Gibbons, 1999). Therefore, in families where the mutation has not been identified, 85% of the mothers of sporadic cases would be expected to be carriers.

Another important consideration concerns the possibility of germline mosaicism. This has been reported in ATR-X syndrome and means that, despite a negative mutation test, a mother of an ATR-X case may still be at risk of further affected offspring (Bachoo and Gibbons, 1999). It is advisable to offer all mothers of affected children prenatal diagnosis even if they are negative for the ATRX mutation.

MUTATIONS IN ORTHOLOGOUS GENES

There are no published animal models for ATR-X syndrome.

DEVELOPMENTAL PATHOGENESIS

On the basis of "guilt by association," it would seem most likely that ATRX, as a heterochromatic protein, is involved in repression of gene expression. How then might mutations of ATRX cause reduced expression of the α-globin genes compared with the β-globin genes? The first question is whether α-globin expression is reduced or β-globin expression is increased. Indirect evidence supports a model with reduced α-globin expression. Unfortunately, there are no reports of individuals with three copies of the β-globin genes in whom the effect of increased β-globin expression might be observed. However, individuals with an increase in the number of α- or γ-globin genes do not have anemia or hypochromic microcytic red cells (Higgs et al., 1980; Fei et al., 1989), whereas those with reduced numbers of α-, β-, or γ-globin genes do. Therefore, it seems most likely that the hypochromic microcytic anemia observed in ATR-X syndrome is due to reduced α-globin gene expression.

It is not clear how loss-of-function mutations (see below) in a protein associated with repressive heterochromatin might lead to reduced expression of a target gene. One possibility is that it is a neutral chromatin remodeling protein that may be involved in activation or repression, depending on its location in euchromatin or heterochromatin, respectively. Other possibilities are that it acts to prevent the repressive effects of heterochromatin on neighboring euchromatic genes or indirectly as a repressor of another gene repressor. The changes in DNA methylation observed in patients with ATRX mutations have been seen only in heterochromatic loci; no changes in methylation have yet been observed in genes whose expression is perturbed in ATR-X syndrome.

Features of the phenotype, for example, the presence and severity of α-thalassemia, are variable even for a given mutation; and it seems likely that modifying genes are involved. Obvious candidates are genes encoding for other protein components of heterochromatin.

In future, a considerable amount of work will be necessary to integrate the phenotype of ATR-X syndrome with the molecular mechanisms responsible. Important research areas will be identification of target genes whose expression is directly influenced by ATRX, determination of how ATRX is directed within the nucleus to its target sites, characterization of the multiprotein complex of which ATRX is a component, analysis of the biochemical properties of ATRX, and resolution of the direct and indirect consequences of ATRX mutations.

REFERENCES

Aasland R, Gibson TJ, Stewart AF (1995). The PHD finger: implications for chromatin-mediated transcriptional regulation. *Trends Biochem Sci* 20: 56–59.

Abidi F, Schwartz CE, Carpenter NJ, Villard L, Fontes M, Curtis M (1999). Carpenter-Waziri syndrome results from a mutation in XNP. *Am J Med Genet* 85: 249–251.

Bachoo S, Gibbons RJ (1999). Germline and gonosomal mosaicism in the ATR-X syndrome. *Eur J Hum Genet* 7: 933–936.

Bannister AJ, Zegerman P, Partridge JF, Miska EA, Thomas JO, Allshire RC, Kouzarides T (2001). Selective recognition of methylated lysine 9 on histone H3 by the HP1 chromo domain. *Nature* 410: 120–124.

Berube NG, Smeenk CA, Picketts DJ (2000). Cell cycle–dependent phosphorylation of the ATRX protein correlates with changes in nuclear matrix and chromatin association. *Hum Mol Genet* 9: 539–547.

Capili AD, Schultz DC, Rauscher IF, Borden KL (2001). Solution structure of the PHD domain from the KAP-1 corepressor: structural determinants for PHD, RING and LIM zinc-binding domains. *EMBO J* 20: 165–177.

Cardoso C, Timsit S, Villard L, Khrestchatisky M, Fontès M, Colleaux L (1998). Specific interaction between the XNP/ATR-X gene product and the SET domain of the human EZH2 protein. *Hum Mol Genet* 7: 679–684.

Cardoso C, Lutz Y, Mignon C, Compe E, Depetris D, Mattei MG, Fontes M, Colleaux L (2000). ATR-X mutations cause impaired nuclear location and altered DNA binding properties of the XNP/ATR-X protein. *J Med Genet* 37: 746–751.

Carlson M, Laurent BC (1994). The SNF/SWI family of global transcriptional activators. *Curr Opin Cell Biol* 6: 396–402.

Carpenter NJ, Qu Y, Curtis M, Patil SR (1999). X-linked mental retardation syndrome with characteristic "coarse" facial appearance, brachydactyly, and short stature maps to proximal Xq. *Am J Med Genet* 85: 230–235.

Dallman PR (1977). The red cell. In: *Blood and Blood-Forming Tissues*. Dallman PR (ed.) Appleton-Century-Crofts, New York, pp. 1109–1113.

Donnai D, Clayton-Smith J, Gibbons RJ, Higgs DR (1991). The non-deletion α thalassaemia/mental retardation syndrome. Further support for X linkage. *J Med Genet* 28: 742–745.

Dunnen JT, Antonarakis SE (2000). Mutation nomenclature extensions and suggestions to describe complex mutations: a discussion. *Hum Mutat* 15: 7–12.

Dykens EM, Volkmar FR (1997). Medical conditions associated with autism. In: *Handbook of *Autism and Pervasive Developmental Disorders.* Cohen DJ, Volkmar FR (eds.) Wiley, New York, pp. 388–410.

Fei YJ, Kutlar F, Harris HF, Wilson MM, Milana A, Sciacca P, Schiliro G, Masala B, Manca L, Altay Ç, et al. (1989). A search for anomalies in the ζ, α, β, and γ globin gene arrangements in normal black, Italian, Turkish and Spanish newborns. *Hemoglobin* 13: 45–65.

Fuks F, Burgers WA, Godin N, Kasai M, Kouzarides T (2001). Dnmt3a binds deacetylases and is recruited by a sequence-specific repressor to silence transcription. *EMBO J* 20: 2536–2544.

Gecz J, Pollard H, Consalez G, Villard L, Stayton C, Millasseau P, Krestchatisky M, Fontes M (1994). Cloning and expression of the murine homologue of a putative human X-linked nuclear protein gene closely linked to PGk1 in Xq13.3. *Hum Mol Genet* 3: 39–44.

Gibbons RJ, Higgs DR (2000). The molecular-clinical spectrum of the ATR-X xyndrome. *Am J Med Genet* 97: 204–212.

Gibbons RJ, Suthers GK, Wilkie AOM, Buckle VJ, Higgs DR (1992). X-linked α thalassemia/mental retardation (ATR-X) syndrome: localisation to Xq12-21.31 by X-inactivation and linkage analysis. *Am J Hum Genet* 51: 1136–1149.

Gibbons RJ, Brueton L, Buckle VJ, Burn J, Clayton-Smith J, Davison BCC, Gardner RJM, Homfray T, Kearney L, Kingston HM, et al. (1995a). The clinical and hematological features of the X-linked α thalassemia/mental retardation syndrome (ATR-X). *Am J Med Genet* 55: 288–299.

Gibbons RJ, Picketts DJ, Villard L, Higgs DR (1995b). Mutations in a putative global transcriptional regulator cause X-linked mental retardation with α-thalassemia (ATR-X syndrome). *Cell* 80: 837–845.

Gibbons RJ, Bachoo S, Picketts DJ, Aftimos S, Asenbauer B, Bergoffen J, Berry SA, Dahl N, Fryer A, Keppler K, et al. (1997). Mutations in a transcriptional regulator (hATRX) establish the functional significance of a PHD-like domain. *Nat Genet* 17: 146–148.

Gibbons RJ, McDowell TL, Raman S, O'Rourke DM, Garrick D, Ayyub H, Higgs DR (2000). Mutations in ATRX, encoding a SWI/SNF-like protein, cause diverse changes in the pattern of DNA methylation. *Nat Genet* 24: 368–371.

Guerrini R, Shanahan JL, Carrozzo R, Bonanni P, Higgs DR, Gibbons RJ (2000). A nonsense mutation of the *ATRX* gene causing mild mental retardation and epilepsy. *Ann Neurol* 47: 117–121.

Higgs DR, Old JM, Pressley L, Clegg JB, Weatherall DJ (1980). A novel α-globin gene arrangement in man. *Nature* 284: 632–635.

Higgs DR, Vickers MA, Wilkie AOM, Pretorius I-M, Jarman AP, Weatherall DJ (1989). A review of the molecular genetics of the human α-globin gene cluster. *Blood* 73: 1081–1104.

Hirschhorn JN, Brown SA, Clark CD, Winston F (1992). Evidence that SNF2/SWI2 and SNF5 activate transcription in yeast by altering chromatin structure. *Genes Dev* 6: 2288–2298.

Holmes LB, Gang DL (1984). Brief clinical report: an X-linked mental retardation syndrome with craniofacial abnormalities, microcephaly and club foot. *Am J Med Genet* 17: 375–382.

ICD-10 (1992). *The ICD-10 Classification of Mental and Behavioural Disorders. Clinical Description and Diagnostic Guidelines.* WHO, Geneva.

Ion A, Telvi L, Chaussain JL, Galacteros F, Valayer J, Fellous M, McElreavey K (1996). A novel mutation in the putative DNA helicase XH2 is responsible for male-to-female sex reversal associated with an atypical form of the ATR-X syndrome. *Am J Hum Genet* 58: 1185–1191.

Jacobsen SE (1999). Gene silencing: maintaining methylation patterns. *Curr Biol* 9: R617–R619.

Jeddeloh JA, Stokes TL, Richards EJ (1999). Maintenance of genomic methylation requires a SWI2/SNF2-like protein. *Nat Genet* 22: 94–97.

Kakutani T, Jeddeloh JA, Richards EJ (1995). Characterization of an Arabidopsis thaliana DNA hypomethylation mutant. *Nucleic Acids Res* 23: 130–137.

Kurosawa K, Akatsuka A, Ochiai Y, Ikeda J, Maekawa K (1996). Self-induced vomiting in X-linked α-thalassemia/mental retardation syndrome. *Am J Med Genet* 63: 505–506.

Lachner M, O'Carroll D, Rea S, Mechtler K, Jenuwein T (2001). Methylation of histone H3 lysine 9 creates a binding site for HP1 proteins. *Nature* 410: 116–120.

Le Douarin B, Nielsen AL, Garnier J-M, Ichinose H, Jeanmougin F, Losson R, Chambon P (1996). A possible involvement of TIF1α and TIF1β in the epigenetic control of transcription by nuclear receptors. *EMBO J* 15: 6701–6715.

Lossi AM, Millan JM, Villard L, Orellana C, Cardoso C, Prieto F, Fontes M, Martinez F (1999). Mutation of the *XNP/ATR-X* gene in a family with severe mental retardation.

spastic paraplegia and skewed pattern of X inactivation: demonstration that the mutation is involved in the inactivation bias. *Am J Hum Genet* 65: 558–562.

McDowell TL, Gibbons RJ, Sutherland H, O'Rourke DM, Bickmore WA, Pombo A, Turley H, Gatter K, Picketts DJ, Buckle VJ, et al. (1999). Localization of a putative transcriptional regulator (ATRX) at pericentromeric heterochromatin and the short arms of acrocentric chromosomes. *Proc Natl Acad Sci USA* 96: 13983–13988.

McPherson E, Clemens M, Gibbons RJ, Higgs DR (1995). X-linked alpha thalassemia/mental retardation (ATR-X) syndrome. A new kindred with severe genital anomalies and mild hematologic expression. *Am J Med Genet* 55: 302–306.

Pascual J, Martinez-Yamout M, Dyson HJ, Wright PE (2000). Structure of the PHD zinc finger from human Williams-Beuren syndrome transcription factor. *J Mol Biol* 304: 723–729.

Picketts DJ, Higgs DR, Bachoo S, Blake DJ, Quarrell OWJ, Gibbons RJ (1996). *ATRX* encodes a novel member of the SNF2 family of proteins: a common mechanism underlying the ATR-X syndrome. *Hum Mol Genet* 5: 1899–1907.

Picketts DJ, Tastan AO, Higgs DR, Gibbons RJ (1998). Comparison of the human and murine *ATRX* gene identifies highly conserved, functionally important domains. *Mamm Genome* 9: 400–403.

Rea S, Eisenhaber F, O'Carroll D, Strahl BD, Sun ZW, Schmid M, Opravil S, Mechtler K, Ponting CP, Allis CD, et al. (2000). Regulation of chromatin structure by site-specific histone H3 methyltransferases. *Nature* 406: 593–599.

Saugier-Veber P, Munnich A, Lyonnet S, Toutain A, Moraine C, Piussan C, Mathieu M, Gibbons RJ (1995). Letter to the Editor: Lumping Juberg-Marsidi syndrome and X-linked α-thalassemia/mental retardation syndrome? *Am J Med Genet* 55: 300–301.

Smothers JF, Henikoff S (2000). The HP1 chromo shadow domain binds a consensus peptide pentamer. *Curr Biol* 10: 27–30.

Stayton CL, Dabovic B, Gulisano M, Gecz J, Broccoli V, Giovanazzi S, Bossolasco M, Monaco L, Rastan S, Boncinelli E, et al. (1994). Cloning and characterisation of a new human Xq13 gene, encoding a putative helicase. *Hum Mol Genet* 3: 1957–1964.

Stevenson RE, Abidi F, Schwartz CE, Lubs HA, Holmes LB (2000a). Holmes-Gang syndrome is allelic with XLMR-hypotonic face syndrome. *Am J Med Genet* 94: 383–385.

Stevenson RE, Schwartz CE, Schroer RJ (2000b). *X-Linked Mental Retardation.* Oxford University Press, New York.

Villard L, Gecz J, Mattéi JF, Fontés M, Saugier-Veber P, Munnich A, Lyonnet S (1996a). XNP mutation in a large family with Juberg-Marsidi syndrome. *Nat Genet* 12: 359–360.

Villard L, Lacombe D, Fontés M (1996b). A point mutation in the *XNP* gene, associated with an ATR-X phenotype without α-thalassemia. *Eur J Hum Genet* 4: 316–320.

Villard L, Toutain A, Lossi A-M, Gecz J, Houdayer C, Moraine C, Fontès M (1996c). Splicing mutation in the *ATR-X* gene can lead to a dysmorphic mental retardation phenotype without α-thalassemia. *Am J Hum Genet* 58: 499–505.

Villard L, Bonino MC, Abidi F, Ragusa A, Belougne J, Lossi AM, Seaver L, Bonnefont JP, Romano C, Fichera M, et al. (1999a). Evaluation of a mutation screening strategy for sporadic cases of ATR-X syndrome. *J Med Genet* 36: 183–186.

Villard L, Fontes M, Ewbank JJ (1999b). Characterization of xnp-1, a *Caenorhabditis elegans* gene similar to the human *XNP/ATR-X* gene. *Gene* 236: 13–19.

Villard L, Fontes M, Ades LC, Gecz J (2000). Identification of a mutation in the *XNP/ATR-X* gene in a family reported as Smith-Fineman-Myers syndrome. *Am J Med Genet* 91: 83–85.

Vongs A, Kakutani T, Martienssen RA, Richards EJ (1993). *Arabidopsis thaliana* DNA methylation mutants. *Science* 260: 1926–1928.

Wada T, Nakamura M, Matsushita Y, Yamada M, Yamashita S, Iwamoto H, Masuno M, Imaizumi K, Kuroki Y (1998). Three Japanese children with X-linked alpha-thalassemia/mental retardation syndrome (ATR-X) [in Japanese]. *No To Hattatsu* 30: 283–289.

Weatherall DJ, Higgs DR, Bunch C, Old JM, Hunt DM, Pressley L, Clegg JB, Bethlenfalvay NC, Sjolin S, Koler RD, et al. (1981). Hemoglobin H disease and mental retardation. A new syndrome or a remarkable coincidence? *N Engl J Med* 305: 607–612.

Wilkie AOM, Buckle VJ, Harris PC, Lamb J, Barton NJ, Reeders ST, Lindenbaum RH, Nicholls RD, Barrow M, Bethlenfalvay NC, et al. (1990a). Clinical features and molecular analysis of the α_thalassaemia/mental retardation syndromes. I. Cases due to deletions involving chromosome band 16p13.3. *Am J Hum Genet* 46: 1112–1126.

Wilkie AOM, Zeitlin HC, Lindenbaum RH, Buckle VJ, Fischel-Ghodsian N, Chui DHK, Gardner-Medwin D, MacGillivray MH, Weatherall DJ, Higgs DR (1990b). Clinical features and molecular analysis of the α thalassemia/mental retardation syndromes. II. Cases without detectable abnormality of the α globin complex. *Am J Hum Genet* 46: 1127–1140.

Xie S, Wang Z, Okano M, Nogami M, Li Y, He WW, Okumura K, Li E (1999). Cloning, expression and chromosome locations of the human *DNMT3* gene family. *Gene* 236: 87–95.

73 | *IGF2, H19, p57*^{KIP2}, and *LIT1* and the Beckwith-Wiedemann Syndrome

MICHAEL R. DEBAUN AND ANDREW P. FEINBERG

Beckwith-Wiedemann syndrome (BWS) (OMIM 130650) is a syndrome of prenatal overgrowth, birth defects, and predisposition to cancer and therefore of great interest in understanding embryogenesis and malignancy. BWS is also a paradigm to evaluate the role of epigenetics, that is, heritable information not within the DNA sequence itself, because it involves both imprinted genes and altered DNA methylation. Through its molecular characterization, it has been possible to define the first epigenotype–phenotype relationship in human genetics: several genes in an imprinted genomic domain of 11p15 are involved in the disorder, with *IGF2* and *H19* linked to cancer risk and *p57*^{KIP2} and *LIT1*, an antisense RNA, linked to overgrowth and midline abdominal wall defects. There also are likely additional genes involved in the pathogenesis of BWS.

ROLE OF THE SPECIFIC LOCUS

The BWS locus on 11p15 coincides with an approximately 1-Mb domain of imprinted genes, those that show preferential expression of the maternal or paternal allele. This domain is itself divided into two imprinted subdomains, and BWS patients show genetic or epigenetic alterations in one or both of these domains, specifically the following. (1) paternal uniparental disomy (UPD) of 11p15, in which the maternal copy is replaced with a duplicated paternal copy; UPD affects all or most of these genes. (2) loss of imprinting (LOI) of insulin-like growth factor II (*IGF2*), involving activation of the normally silent maternally inherited allele of *IGF2*; IGF2 is an autocrine growth factor, and the effective doubling of its dose by LOI likely leads to premalignant lesions termed *nephrogenic rests* (NRs), as well as cancer. (3) Abnormal methylation of the normally unmethylated maternal allele of a "differentially methylated region" (DMR) upstream of H19; this aberrant methylation is the likely mechanism of LOI of *IGF2* (see 2 above). *IGF2* and *H19* are within the more telomeric imprinted subdomain. *H19* itself has no known function, except that the DMR regulates *IGF2* expression. (4) Mutations of *p57*^{KIP2}, a cyclin-dependent kinase inhibitor that causes G₁/S cell cycle arrest; *p57*^{KIP2} is an imprinted gene normally expressed from the maternal allele. (5) LOI of *LIT1*, which codes for an untranslated RNA within the voltage-gated potassium channel gene *KvLQT1*; LOI of *LIT1* involves biallelic expression and loss of methylation of the normally methylated maternal allele of a DMR upstream of *LIT1*. Like *H19*, *LIT1* has no known intrinsic function other than to regulate the expression of other genes in *cis*, and *p57*^{KIP2} is a likely target. *LIT1* and *p57*^{KIP2} are within the more centromeric imprinted subdomain. (6) Germline chromosomal rearrangements, either balanced rearrangements interrupting the *KvLQT1* gene, or a second gene, *ZnF215*, which codes for a zinc finger protein of unknown function, located several megabases centromeric to *KvLQT1*. In addition, some patients show unbalanced duplications of the 11p15 region. The chromosomal rearrangements are hypothesized to separate *p57*^{KIP2}, and possibly other maternally expressed genes, from its enhancer.

CLINICAL DESCRIPTION

BWS is one of the most commonly recognized overgrowth syndromes, with an estimated incidence of 1:14,000 births. The syndrome was independently described by J. B. Beckwith at the annual meeting of the Western Society for Pediatric Research in 1963 (Beckwith, 1963) and H. R. Wiedemann in 1964 (Wiedemann, 1964) and was initially referred to as the EMG syndrome for its original distinguishing features: exomphalos, macroglossia, and gigantism. Infants with BWS present with a distinctive craniofacial phenotype and may have multiple congenital anomalies (Table 73–1). The most common five features identified at birth are macroglossia, macrosomia, birth weight and length greater than the 90th percentile, midline abdominal wall defects (omphalocele, diastasis recti, and umbilical hernia), ear pits or creases, and neonatal hypoglycemia.

To better define the natural history of BWS and to provide a large epidemiologic database and biological repository for genotype–phenotype analyses, a BWS registry was established in 1994 at the Genetic Epidemiology Branch of the National Cancer Institute (NCI). For those families who agreed to participate, a comprehensive questionnaire was completed. Informed consent and medical information release documents were obtained. Definition of BWS was based on a physician's diagnosis of BWS and phenotypic manifestations of at least two of the five most common features associated with BWS, given earlier. The clinical definition used for BWS is limited because no standard diagnostic criteria exist that have been independently verified with patients who have either genetic or epigenetic mutations. When molecular analyses were completed in children who met the NCI diagnostic criteria for BWS, only 7 of 10 children had genetic or epigenetic mutations (DeBaun et al., 2002). Further, among the children who met the definition of BWS, no obvious clinical differences where present when comparing children with and without genetic or epigenetic mutations. These findings suggest that other genetic or epigenetic mutations not yet identified are responsible for disease in approximately one third of children with BWS.

In the BWS registry, only 13% of the children had all five of the most common features associated with BWS. Based on the data from the BWS registry, the most common clinical or laboratory features associated with BWS are macroglossia (94%), abdominal wall defects (umbilical hernia/omphalocele or diastasis recti) (74%), ear pits ear grooves (68%), hemangiomas (typically nevus flammeus on the forehead and back of the neck) (63%), and neonatal hypoglycemia at birth (52%). In addition, 12% of the children had a documented hearing loss. Characterization of the hearing loss is incomplete. However, conduction hearing loss resulting from stapedial fixation (Paulsen, 1973; Daugbjerg and Everberg, 1984; Takahashi et al., 1996) has been reported. Finally, genitourinary anomalies include undescended testes (44%), hypospadias (8%), and cliteromegaly (9%).

Both direct and indirect evidence points to hyperinsulinemia as the cause of hypoglycemia in this population. Initial support for excessive insulin release was based on Beckwith's original observation that two of six patients had an enlarged pancreas ranging from 2.5 to 3.5 times the normal weight and all six had islet cell hyperplasia. Indirect support for hyperinsulinemia includes the requirement of more than 10 to 12 mg of glucose/kg/min to barely maintain euglycemia, circulating insulin levels that are either high or not appropriately suppressed, urinary or plasma ketones that are low, and an exaggerated response to exogenous glucagon.

A greater than expected number of infants were born prematurely (<37 weeks' gestation), and the pregnancies were associated with other complications. Fifty percent of the infants with BWS were born prematurely, and polyhydramnios was reported as a complication in 43% of the pregnancies. Polyhydramnios was previously reported to occur in greater than expected frequency by Weng et al. (1995).

Table 73–1. Clinical Features Associated with Documented Children with Either Genetic or Epigenetic Mutations Occurring in BWS

Commonly present
  Prenatal overgrowth
    Weight greater than 90th percentile
  Craniofacial
    Macroglossia
    Ear pits/creases
    Prominent occiput
    Wide and flat nasal bridge
    Nevus flammeus
  Genitourinary malformations
    Hydronephrosis
    Undescended testicle
    Cliteromegaly
    Hypospadias
  Abdominal wall defects
    Diastasis recti
    Umbilical hernia
    Omphalocele
  Musculoskeletal
    Asymmetry of the limbs
    Joint laxity
    Thoracic cage abnormalities
      Pectus carinatum or excavatum
  Hearing impairment
    Eighth nerve deficit
    Bone conduction defect
Occasional
  Cleft lip/palate
  Hemangiomas

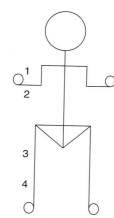

Figure 73–1. Musculoskeletal evaluation in children with Beckwith-Wiedemann syndrome. Limb measurements. Limb lengths were measured from (1) acromioclavicular joint to olecranon, (2) olecranon to ulnar styloid, (3) anterior superior iliac spine to superior patellar border, and (4) superior patellar border to medial malleolus. Limb girths were measured at the midportion of the quadriceps and midportion of the gastrocnemius.

The craniofacial features of children with BWS are distinctive and include prominent occiput, maxillary hypoplasia with a broad nasal bridge, and facial nevus flammeus typically seen at birth with decreasing intensity over time. Premature infants with BWS have been initially thought to have normal facial features but later develop macroglossia and other facial features associated with BWS (Motokura et al., 1991). Ear creases are located on the anterior or posterior portion of the earlobe (Fishman et al., 1983). In addition, ear pits are located on the anterior or posterior portion of the helix (Fishman et al., 1983). Various combinations of posterior and anterior creases and pits can occur with no clinical significance. Children with BWS may have cleft lips and palates, although a full description of the types and frequency of cleft lips and palates is lacking.

Children with BWS can have asymmetry of the limbs or face, as well as joint laxity, scoliosis, and thoracic cage abnormalities. In the only systematic assessment of the musculoskeletal children with BWS, 55 children were examined by physiatrists (Gerber, 2001). Definitions for the various musculoskeletal manifestations were determined based on assessment of patients with BWS. Asymmetry of length or girth was defined as greater than 10% discrepancy between the right and left sides. Scoliosis was identified as present or absent by inspection of the thoracolumbar vertebral alignment and scapular prominence in standing and forward flexion. Ligamentous laxity was considered present if the thumb reached the ventral forearm, the knees or elbows achieved greater than 5-degree hyperextension, or the calcaneus was everted more than 10 degrees and the medial arch was flattened. Thoracic cage asymmetry was noted if nipples were discordant in height. An approach to evaluate the musculoskeletal system in children is described in Figure 73–1. In addition to the measurements of the lower extremities, an anterior posterior radiograph of the lower extremities with a ruler may be the most objective measure to assess as well as to follow leg length discrepancy. Joint laxity, the most common clinical feature, occurred in 70% of the children; 65% had thoracic cage asymmetry, including 25% with either pectus carinatum or excavatum, and 16% had scoliosis. Asymmetry of the girth or length of a limb occurred in at least 10%.

Children with BWS can have both malignant and nonmalignant manifestations of renal disease (Fig. 73–2, Table 73–2). Wilms tumor and nephroblastomatosis are the malignant and premalignant mani-

festations of renal disease in children with BWS. Nonmalignant renal disease in children with BWS is very important to identify because these abnormalities can be confused with Wilms tumor and/or nephroblastomatosis. These nonmalignant abnormalities include multiple caliceal cysts or diverticulae, hydronephrosis, and medullary cysts resulting from dilated collecting ducts with decreased numbers of Henle loops in the medulla (renal medullary dysplasia). The dilated ducts may affect some or all of the medullary pyramids. If severe and widespread, it can evolve into medullary sponge kidney, manifested by severe collecting duct dilatation with microcalcifications, and predisposition to recurrent pyelonephritis. In 152 patients with BWS, 45 nonmalignant renal abnormalities were identified: medullary cysts (13%), caliceal diverticulae (1%), hydronephrosis (12%), and nephrolithiasis (6.4%) (Choyke et al., 1998). The majority of the patients were asymptomatic. Clinical manifestations of the patients who were symptomatic included urinary tract infections, flank pain due to nephrolithiasis, and progressive renal disease requiring dialysis (Choyke et al., 1998). The incidence of these nonmalignant renal conditions is unknown.

Children with BWS have a particular propensity for congenital NRs, which are also referred to as nephroblastomatosis. NRs represent the abnormal persistence of fetal embryonal cells or their derivatives. Two patterns of NRs exist: perilobar and intralobar. Perilobar NRs are primarily located in the periphery of the renal lobe, sharply demarcated from the normal renal tissue, and in their active growth phase, they consist of blastemal or embryonal epithelial cell types. Intralobar NRs occur throughout the kidney and are characterized by multiple cell types, including immature or mature stroma. The lesions appear to be normal nephrons without a distinct border. The intralobar NRs occur less frequently. Occasionally, severe neonatal nephromegaly due to excessive proliferation of nephrons, and not nephroblastomatosis, during late intrauterine life (hyperplastic nephromegaly) is noted.

The clinical features of BWS in the BWS registry are summarized in Table 73–1. Neither gender nor ethnicity was associated with BWS.

THE GENETICS OF BWS

BWS has attracted great interest from both molecular biologists and clinical geneticists because it serves as a model for understanding the epigenetics of cancer. *Epigenetics* is the stable transmission of genetic information that does not involve the sequence itself. The type of epigenetic change critical to BWS is genomic imprinting, which involves the silencing of a specific parentally inherited allele. Imprinting challenges conventional mendelian dogma, in that for imprinted genes, traits do not segregate or assort independently: for a paternally expressed gene, only the paternal "trait" is transmitted to progeny,

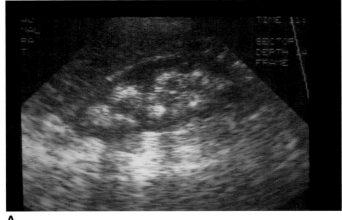

A

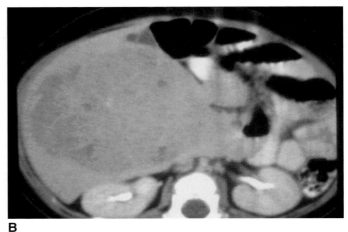

B

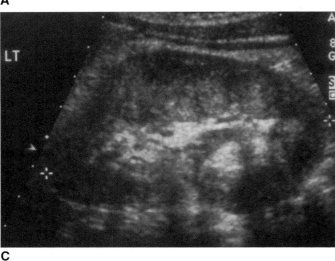

C

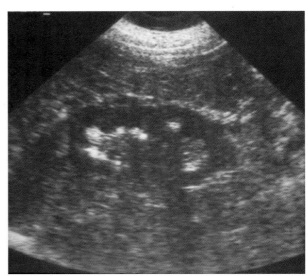

D

Figure 73–2. (*A*) Renal sonogram demonstrating echogenic renal pyramids typical of medullary sponge kidney in a child with Beckwith-Wiedemann syndrome (BWS). (*B*) Computed tomography scan with intravenous contrast demonstrating a large hepatoblastoma in a child with BWS. (*C*) A 2-year-old child with BWS and nephromegaly. The kidney measures 9 cm (99th percentile) in length. (*D*) Renal sonogram demonstrating multiple stones (echogenic foci with shadowing) in the renal medulla in a teenager with BWS.

whereas the maternal trait, silent in one generation when passed from mother to son, reappears in the next.

Rarely, patients with BWS provided initial clues that imprinting was a basis for the etiology of BWS when two separate chromosomal rearrangements involving 11p15 were identified: (1) balanced re-arrangements always with a breakpoint within 11p15 and (2) unbal-anced duplications always including 11p15 within the duplicated seg-ment, although the region of duplication can include most of the short arm of chromosome 11 (Hoovers et al., 1995). In addition, it was ob-served that all of the balanced rearrangements involved the maternal 11p15, and that all of the unbalanced duplications involved the pa-ternal 11p15 (Mannens et al., 1995). These observations suggested that BWS could involve an imprinted gene, that is, a gene showing

Table 73–2. Nonmalignant Renal Abnormalities in Patients with Beckwith-Wiedemann Syndrome

Renal Abnormality	Patients (%) (n = 152)	Median Age (yr)	Range at Time of Diagnosis
Medullary renal cysts	13	6	2 days to 23 years
Caliceal diverticula	1.3	1.5	1 to 2 years
Hydronephrosis	12	1	5 months to 30 years
Nephrolithiasis	4	16	3 months to 30 years
Total	25	1.4	2 days to 30 years

parent of origin-specific allele silencing. In this case, there is no sim-ple model that would best fit the chromosomal data, because the bal-anced rearrangements suggest truncation of a maternally expressed gene and the unbalanced duplications suggest duplication of a pater-nally expressed gene. Confirmation of a role for genomic imprinting came from the observation of paternal UPD in a larger but still mi-nority proportion of patients (Henry et al., 1993).

The first resolution of the BWS imprinting dilemma came from the discovery of human imprinted genes, specifically *IGF2*, the gene on 11p15 for insulin-like growth factor II an important autocrine growth factor in cancer (Ogawa et al., 1993; Rainier et al., 1993). Moreover, *IGF2* was found to undergo LOI in embryonal tumors, specifically those that affect BWS patients (Ogawa et al., 1993; Rainier et al., 1993). LOI involves activation of the normally silent maternal allele of *IGF2* and silencing of the normally expressed maternal allele of a nearby untranslated RNA termed H19. As expected, normal cells of BWS also exhibited LOI of *IGF2* but only in a minority of patients (Weksberg et al., 1993). LOI of *IGF2* could account for UPD and un-balanced paternal duplications, as all would yield a double dose of *IGF2* and, presumably, overgrowth, but it would not account for the maternal balanced rearrangements. Insight into the role of these re-arrangements came from the discovery that virtually all of them in-terrupt a 350-kb gene encoding the voltage-gated potassium channel gene *K$_V$LQT1*, which is imprinted and expressed from the maternal allele prenatally but not is not imprinted in the heart (Lee et al., 1997b). This was the first known example of tissue-specific imprinting. The mechanism whereby disruption of K_VLQT1 causes BWS is not, however, because of its effect on the gene itself, as deletional mutagenesis of the gene in the mouse causes a model of Jervell-Lange-Nielsen syndrome (hereditary deafness and arrhythmia) but not BWS (Lee et al., 2000). Rather, disruption of BWS acts by its effect on imprinting of one or more nearby genes, also on 11p15, but more than 500 kb removed from *IGF2* and *H19*. One target of the rearrangements appears to be the cyclin-dependent kinase inhibitor gene *p57*^{KIP2}, because this gene is mutated in the germline in approximately 5% of BWS patients (Hatada et al., 1996; Lee et al., 1997a; O'Keefe et al., 1997).

A better understanding of the mechanism of epigenetic alterations in BWS came from the discovery of a 60-kb untranslated RNA, antisense in orientation and within K_VLQT1, but expressed oppositely to K_VLQT1 and to *p57*^{KIP2}, that is, from the paternal allele. This RNA, termed *LIT1*, for long intronic transcript 1, undergoes LOI in approximately half of BWS children. In this case, LOI involves activation of the normally silent maternal allele of *LIT1* (Lee et al., 1999). *LIT1* likely serves as a transcriptional repressor of *p57*^{KIP2} and other maternally expressed genes on 11p15, and LOI of *LIT1* leads to complete or nearly complete loss of expression of the transcripts that it regulates.

The mechanism of LOI, both of *IGF2* and of *LIT1*, involves DNA methylation, a covalent modification of the nucleotide cytosine (Moulton et al., 1994; Steenman et al., 1994). For both genes, a DMR is normally methylated on one parental allele and is unmethylated on the other. In the case of *IGF2*, methylation on the paternal allele of a DMR between *IGF2* and *H19*, and located just upstream of *H19*, causes the paternal allele to be activated by an enhancer shared between *IGF2* and *H19*. On the maternal allele, the unmethylated DMR binds the insulator protein CTCF and likely other chromatin proteins as well, blocking access of the shared enhancer to the maternal allele of *IGF2*, leading to silencing of that copy (Cui et al., 2001). LOI of *IGF2* in BWS and in embryonal tumors, both in BWS patients and occurring sporadically in the general pediatric population, involves aberrant methylation of the maternal *H19* DMR, silencing of the maternal *H19* allele, and activation of the maternal *IGF2* allele (Feinberg, 2001, 2002).

The mechanism of LOI of *LIT1* also involves DNA methylation, but in contrast to *IGF2*, it involves *hypomethylation* rather than *hypermethylation*. Here, a DMR upstream of *LIT1* is normally methylated on the *maternal* allele and unmethylated on the *paternal* allele.

The unmethylated paternal allele allows expression of *LIT1* and repression of *p57*^{KIP2} and other genes, and LOI of *LIT1* in BWS involves biallelic activation of *LIT1* and thus biallelic repression of *p57*^{KIP2} (Lee et al., 1999; Feinberg, 2002).

Although the genetics of BWS is complex, it is easier to visualize in the context of the present understanding that 11p15 contains a cluster of imprinted genes distributed over 1 Mb, with two imprinted domains under independent imprinting regulation (Fig. 73–3). One domain includes the genes *p57*^{KIP2}, *LIT1*, and K_VLQT1, and the candidate tumor suppressor genes *TSSC3* and *TSSC5*. The second domain includes *IGF2* and *H19*. Within these domains, a delicate balance of growth promotion and growth inhibition has arisen through evolution, with *H19* antagonizing *IGF2* and *LIT1* antagonizing *p57*^{KIP2}. Alterations of either domain can lead to the features of BWS, presumably because of activation of common final targets for cell growth. Thus, LOI of *IGF2* involves epigenetic disruption of the *IGF2-H19* domain, with biallelic activation of *IGF2* and biallelic silencing of *H19*. LOI of *LIT1* involves epigenetic disruption of the *p57*^{KIP2}-*LIT1*-K_VLQT1 domain, with biallelic activation of *LIT1* and biallelic silencing of *p57*^{KIP2}. Mutations in *p57*^{KIP2} simply silence this gene directly. The balanced chromosomal rearrangements are predicted to separate *p57*^{KIP2} from its enhancer, and UPD has the equivalent effect of LOI of both domains (i.e., switching from a maternal to a paternal epigenotype).

An important prediction of the two-domain hypothesis is that the phenotype of BWS will depend on which domain or domains is involved in a given patient. For example, LOI of *IGF2* occurs commonly in sporadically occurring tumors, but LOI of *LIT1* is not found in these tumors (Lee et al., 1999). Thus, one would predict that LOI involving the *IGF2-H19* domain predisposes to cancer in BWS patients with this alteration. A test of this hypothesis required a systematic analysis of epigenotype and phenotype together in a single cohort of patients.

The first epigenotype–phenotype analysis in human disease was performed in a defined population of BWS patients. The BWS registry systematically examined a cohort of 92 patients with BWS and molecular analysis of both *H19* and *LIT1*. The study cohort had the same frequency of clinical features as the larger cohort of 187 children in the registry but without biological specimens. This study reached three major conclusions (DeBaun et al., 2002): (1) LOI of *H19-IGF2* confers a significant increased risk of cancer, 41% versus 10%, with an odds ratio of 6.2 (95% confidence interval [CI], 1.7 to 19.8); (2) LOI of *LIT1* was significantly associated with birth defects; and (3) UPD was significantly associated with hypoglycemia (DeBaun et al., 2002).

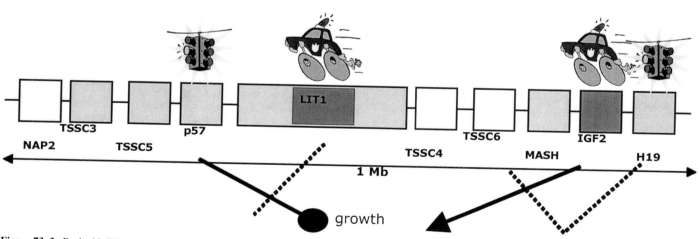

Figure 73–3. Beckwith-Wiedemann syndrome (BWS) can be viewed as a disorder affecting an imprinted gene domain of 11p15, in which two imprinted subdomains independently contribute to growth regulation, and disturbances in either of which can lead to manifestations of BWS. The more centromeric subdomain, including *p57*^{KIP2} and *LIT1*, is more closely related to prenatal growth and midline closure, and the more telomeric subdomain, including *H19* and insulin-like growth factor II gene (*IGF2*) is more closely related to growth of the kidney and liver and to embryonal tumors. *IGF2* is regulated by *H19* imprinting, and *p57*^{KIP2} is regulated by *LIT1* imprinting. In common with all of the potential genetic and epigenetic abnormalities (described in detail in the text) is a switch from maternal to paternal epigenotype, in the case of imprinting disturbances, or a switch from maternal to paternal genotype, in the case of uniparental disomy. Growth promoting genes are depicted by a speeding car and growth inhibitory genes by a traffic light.

Bliek et al. (2001) also observed an association between aberrant methylation of H19 and cancer. The phenotypes associated with epigenetic alterations of the two domains differed significantly, in each case with $P < 0.01$, but they did overlap. The implication is the two domains have a converging but nonidentical effect on gene expression and phenotype. The results support Haig's hypothesis that imprinted genes have evolved to develop counteracting roles in growth regulation between maternally and paternally expressed genes, when the genes are linked (Haig and Graham, 1991). They also offer a powerful clinical opportunity to assess risk of specific phenotypes depending on the epigenetic alteration. Finally, the result showing a specific association of UPD with hypoglycemia, but no such association with LOI of either domain alone, implies that the gene for hypoglycemia is not IGF2, H19, LIT1, or p57^{KIP2} but instead another gene within 11p15 that becomes duplicated in the paternal allele. One possibility is the insulin gene itself, suggesting that it might be imprinted in the developing pancreas.

ESTABLISHING THE DIAGNOSIS

The diagnosis of BWS is based on a constellation of clinical findings commonly recognized at birth but may be more readily identified after a few months of age (particularly for premature infants). Two suggested diagnostic criteria have been described for BWS. The first, by DeBaun et al. (2002), was for research classification only, and includes a clinical diagnosis of BWS plus two of the five most common features: (1) macroglossia, (2) birth weight and length greater than 90th percentile, (3) hypoglycemia in the first month of life, (4) ear creases or ear pits, and (5) midline abdominal wall defects (omphalocele, diastasis recti, and umbilical hernia). The second, by Elliot et al. (1994), includes the presence of either three major features (anterior abdominal wall defect, macroglossia, or prepostnatal overgrowth) or two major plus three minor findings (ear pits, nevus flammeus, neonatal hypoglycemia, nephromegaly, or hemihyperplasia). The minimum number of major or minor features required to make the diagnosis of BWS has not been determined, and we do not think that will be possible in the absence of more complete genotypic understanding. Although molecular diagnosis of BWS is now available, only about two thirds of the children with a clinical diagnosis of BWS will have a recognized genetic or epigenetic mutation. The absence of a mutation in a child with clinical findings suggestive of BWS should not preclude a diagnosis of BWS.

Given the protean presentation of BWS and the observation that a minority of children will have all of the five most common features associated of BWS, a high index of suspicion is required to make the diagnosis. Any infant presenting with macrosomia and hypoglycemia who is not an infant of diabetic mother should be evaluated for BWS. Similarly, a geneticist should evaluate an infant presenting with omphalocele or macroglossia, with or without other BWS features. The most common overgrowth syndrome that should be considered in the differential diagnosis of an infant with suspected BWS is the Simpson-Golabi-Behmel syndrome (SGB) (see Chapter 96). SBG is an X-linked disorder with a phenotype similar to BWS, including macrosomia, macroglossia, and renal anomalies. There also appears to be a predisposition to Wilms tumor in individuals with SGB. However, these two disorders can usually be distinguished from one another based on the different craniofacial features, including macrocephaly in SGB patients. Other overgrowth syndromes that do not share visceral abnormalities with BWS include the Sotos, Weaver, and Marshall-Smith syndromes. These disorders are all characterized by early overgrowth and advanced bone age, hypotonia, and neurodevelopmental impairment.

BWS remains a clinical diagnosis. Nevertheless, molecular diagnostic testing is a new useful adjunct to the history and physical examination, and it offers the promise of improved genetic counseling. Although most BWS patients presenting to geneticists have undergone karyotyping, the yield is low, less than 1%. It still can be useful, however, particularly if there are other congenital malformations or mental retardation, suggesting chromosomal duplication, or a history of multiple spontaneous abortions in the mother, suggesting a balanced chromosomal rearrangement. UPD testing is widely offered, and here,

too, the yield is low, approximately 10%. However, the advantage of UPD testing is that its presence suggests a theoretically zero recurrence risk, because all known cases involve somatic mosaicism, a postzygotic event.

The most robust molecular testing is done for imprinting abnormalities, focused on the DMRs of LIT1 and H19, because they do not depend on the presence of a transcribed polymorphism with LIT1 or IGF2 for an RT-PCR test. We know of only one CLIA-certified laboratory that offers methylation testing (Washington University), although this test will likely become more common. It is particularly important to be able to detect partial LOI. Thus, "MSP," or methylation-specific PCR, is not a suitable test because it is nonquantitative and can fail to detect mosaicism in Prader-Willi syndrome. Methylation testing must be done by either quantitative Southern blot hybridization or one of the newer quantitative methylation assays, such as Methyl-light. Finally, mutational analysis for p57^{KIP2} can be performed to identify the 5% of patients with mutations in this gene, although it is not currently offered in a CLIA setting.

MANAGEMENT, TREATMENT, AND COUNSELING

The recognition of hypoglycemia in the first few hours of life is important and a common feature in infants with BWS, occurring in approximately 50% of children surveyed (DeBaun et al., 2000). The prevalence of hypoglycemia remains to be defined because of the lack of prospective studies, the lack of consensus for definition of hypoglycemia, and failure to recognize BWS. One prospective study addressing hypoglycemia evaluated 39 infants younger than 1 year with BWS. The authors defined hypoglycemia based on the criteria by Cornblath and Schwartz (1993): glucose levels less than 30 mg/dl in full term or less than 20 mg/dl in preterm. In this group, 12 of 35 infants had hypoglycemia. The majority of infants with hypoglycemia are asymptomatic and become normoglycemic within the first 3 days of life. The presence of persistent hypoglycemia beyond the neonatal period has become recognized. In the BWS registry, 4% of the children were evaluated and treated for hypoglycemia beyond the neonatal period (DeBaun et al., 2002). A variety of therapeutic interventions were used in the group who had persistent hypoglycemia, including tube feedings, oral hyperglycemic agents, and, for a few patients, partial pancreatectomy (DeBaun et al., 2000).

The majority of infants with BWS and hypoglycemia can be managed with frequent feedings and/or intravenous or enteral infusions of glucose. In persistent hypoglycemia, blood obtained at the time of hypoglycemia with accurate glucose measurement and an assessment of insulin, ketone bodies (β-hydroxybuturate and/or acetoacetate), lactate, cortisol, growth hormone, and urine glucose measurements are important. Table 73–3 represents a suggested evaluation for a child with suspected BWS who has persistent hypoglycemia.

Macroglossia is often a major cause of cosmetic concern. This may cause poor self-esteem in patients with BWS. The tongue size may vary considerably. No definitive approach to managing macroglossia has been developed; however, some craniofacial teams advocate partial glossectomy before primary teeth eruption to prevent malocclusion of the teeth. The most common surgical technique is the anterior three-dimensional "W" technique performed by the craniofacial team at St. Louis Children Hospital, Washington University School of Medicine. This team has evaluated well over 100 children with BWS and

Table 73–3. Evaluation for Hypoglycemia in Beckwith-Wiedemann Syndrome

Test	Result	Interpretation
Insulin level	High	Consistent with hyperinsulinemia
Ketone bodies (β-hydroxybutyrate and/or acetoacetate)	Present	Metabolic disease
Urinalysis for ketones	Low	Consistent with hyperinsulinemia
Growth hormone	Low	Hypopituitarism
Cortisol	Low	Adrenal insufficiency
Lactate	High	Metabolic disease

performed lingual reduction in at least 75 infants. After "W" lingual reduction, typically normal feeding patterns were resumed within 1 month for infants and within 2 months for toddlers, and normal sleep pattern was commonly reestablished within 2 weeks. Longitudinal data determining beneficial effects of lingual reduction are lacking and require a systematic evaluation.

Patients, parents, and clinicians should be aware of these musculoskeletal abnormalities and the need for monitoring over time to assess their functional impact and the possible need for treatment, because several of the findings such as subluxation of the joints or asymmetry of the lower extremities may require intervention. Unfortunately, the optimal strategy for assessment and management of these clinical manifestations has not been determined.

Actively growing nephrogenic rests may result in multiple renal masses that are grossly identical to Wilms tumor. Newly appearing renal lesions can result in confusion when clinical management decisions must be made, because radiographic imaging and surgical inspection frequently cannot distinguish between Wilms tumor and NRs. A renal biopsy may not clear up the ambiguity, because the histologic appearances of Wilms tumor and NRs are quite similar. When a biopsy of a renal mass is performed and histologic review occurs, a margin of normal and abnormal tissue should be selected to help distinguish between NRs and Wilms tumor. Subtle findings associated with Wilms tumor include the elliptically shaped nephroblastoma cells circumscribed by fibrosis as opposed to a circular shape of nephroblastoma cells without fibrosis band.

Cancer occurs at least 600 times more frequently in children with BWS than in children without BWS (DeBaun and Tucker, 1998). The incidence of cancer is age related, with the highest risk occurring in children younger than 4 years, but with substantial risk continuing up to approximately 10 years of age. No reports have indicated that teenagers or adults with BWS have an increased risk of cancer. In the BWS registry, the only registry that followed children with BWS longitudinally, the average annual incidence of cancer in the first 4 years of life was 0.027 case of cancer per person-year, and at between 4 and 10 years of age, the incidence was 0.002 case of cancer per person-year. If 100 children with BWS were followed from birth until 10 years of age, approximately 10 cases of cancers would be expected before 4 years of age, and 1 case of cancer would be expected at between 4 and 10 years of age. In the first 4 years of life, the relative risk (RR) of Wilms tumor (RR = 816; 95% CI, 359 to 1156), neuroblastoma (RR = 197; 95% CI, 22 to 711), and hepatoblastoma (RR = 2280; 95% CI, 928 to 11,656) is high (DeBaun and Tucker, 1998). Other cancers that occur with an increased frequency in this population include rhabdomyosarcoma and adrenal cortical carcinoma.

The usefulness of cancer screening in children with BWS has been demonstrated in retrospective and anecdotal studies. Although limited due to small numbers and study design, these studies have provided a compelling rationale to use renal sonography to screen for Wilms tumor in an interval of 4 months or less and alpha-fetoprotein (AFP) to screen for hepatoblastoma at intervals of 6 to 12 weeks.

The liver, spleen, pancreas, kidneys, and adrenal glands should be systematically examined, and the renal length should be determined. The size of the kidney is important to determine because the presence of persistent nephromegaly throughout the early infant period is associated with Wilms tumor. Because the risk of tumor and other nonmalignant conditions is high in this population, a low clinical threshold should be maintained to obtain additional imaging studies of the kidneys. There is no clear clinical advantage of magnetic resonance imaging studies over computed tomography scans of the kidney.

The evidence to support screening with Wilms tumor is primarily based on the large international case-control study where patients with either BWS or idiopathic hemihypertrophy (IH) were screened at intervals of at least every 4 months. Controls were patients with either BWS or IH that were not effectively screened, either screened at intervals greater than 4 months or not screened at all. In this study, none of the patients that were effectively screened (*n* = 15) with renal sonography had late-stage Wilms tumor (stage III and IV), whereas 42% (*n* = 59) of the patients who were never screened developed late-

stage Wilms tumor. Identifying children with Wilms tumor at an early stage (stage I and II) results in less toxic chemotherapy and no irradiation, thus providing a clearcut benefit for early detection of Wilms tumor (Choyke et al., 1999). When a renal lesion is identified on sonographic examination, we recommend that an enhanced computed tomography or magnetic resonance imaging examination with 5-mm-thick sections be performed before surgery.

Further supporting evidence for screening for Wilms tumor includes the size of the Wilms tumor in children who are screened versus that in the nonscreened population. In the case series of children who are screened at intervals of 4 months or less, the average Wilms tumor diameter was 3.4 cm (Choyke et al., 1999). However, in two series of patients with sporadic Wilms tumor, the average diameter was 11 and 13 cm, respectively (Fishman et al., 1983; Hugosson et al., 1995). In addition to regularly scheduled abdominal sonographic examinations for detection of Wilms tumor, an assessment of AFP for the detection of hepatoblastoma is of clinical use. In a small case series of 5 children with BWS or IH for whom serial serum AFP screening, usually in combination with abdominal ultrasonography, led to the early detection of hepatoblastoma, all five hepatoblastomas were stage I as opposed to the general hepatoblastoma population, in whom two of three were stages III/IV at diagnosis (Clericuzio, 2002). For children with BWS or IH, we recommend serum AFP screening every 6 to 12 weeks until 4 years of age. The age at which screening ceases for either Wilms tumor or hepatoblastoma should be based on the age of the patient, the age-specific incidence of the cancer, and the added value that each parent has for knowing the results of the screening test. For Wilms tumor, the age that screening should stop is unclear, but approximately 90% of the Wilms tumors in children with BWS occur before 8 years of age (Beckwith, 1998). Sonographic screening evaluations generally stop by 8 years of age; screening beyond 8 years of age may provide reassurance to the parents and may have some minimum clinical usefulness. These perceived benefits must be balanced by the increased rate of false-positive test results that may result in unnecessary diagnostic imaging and surgery. In a retrospective analysis, two patients underwent inappropriate complete nephrectomies based on lesions believed to be Wilms tumor as a result of imaging studies. Subsequently, these lesions were determined to be a complicated renal cyst and NR after pathologic evaluation, respectively (Choyke et al., 1999).

A similar rationale applies for stopping AFP measurements for screening for hepatoblastoma. Approximately 90% of all hepatoblastomas occur before 3 years of age (Ross and Gurney, 1998). Screening beyond this age carries diminishing rates of true-positive results, while increasing the risk of false-positive results.

To identify the potential use of a screening intervention trial, a cost-benefit analysis of screening for Wilms tumor and hepatoblastoma was conducted. Based on data from the BWS registry at the NCI, the National Wilms Tumor Study (NWTS), and large published series, two hypothetical cohorts of 1000 infants born with BWS were modeled to demonstrate a benefit of screening for Wilms tumor or hepatoblastoma. When variables such as cost of screening examination, discount rate, and effectiveness of screening were varied based on high and low estimates, the incremental cost per life-year saved for screening up until the age of 4 years remained comparable to acceptable population-based cancer screening ranges (<$50,000 per life-year saved). Until a formal screening trial is undertaken, the quarterly abdominal sonographic examinations in children with BWS represent a reasonable strategy for cancer screening (Mcneil et al., 2001).

Counseling for recurrence has been limited by the absence of adequate molecular tools. However, the presence of a defined molecular abnormality can be useful in estimating recurrence risk and the risk of transmitting BWS to offspring. A chromosomal rearrangement should be approached in the same manner as other chromosomal rearrangements; that is, the parents should be tested, and in this case prenatal testing could be offered. Mutations in *p57*KIP2, if found, can be most helpful in counseling. When transmitted through the father, the phenotype is null or minimal, and the penetrance of BWS when transmitted through the mother is high, although there are no series providing precise numbers. A potential issue for *p57*KIP2 mutational testing is that a positive result is clear if there is a nonsense mutation, but missense mutations might or might not be significant and therefore the genetic testing must be performed on multiple family members and related to the phenotype in the family. UPD, when present, suggests a zero recurrence risk, because all known cases involve somatic mosaicism. However, in the absence of a very large series, a recurrence risk of less than 5% should be reported. Testing for LOI will be informative in the largest number of BWS patients, is positive in over half of patients, and can involve *LIT1*, *H19*, or, rarely, both. Indeed, UPD testing could be reserved for those patients in whom methylation assays are positive for both *LIT1* and *H19*, similar to the sequence of testing often used for PWS. This approach would, however, miss UPD limited to one gene, although that has not yet been described. Counseling for patients with methylation abnormalities is limited, at this point, to confirmation of the diagnosis, albeit an important consideration. Although the type of abnormality does stratify risk of cancer, we believe that patients with *LIT1* abnormalities alone should be subjected to the same screening program as those with *H19* abnormalities, until other confirming epigenotype–phenotype studies are available. The recurrence risk for methylation abnormalities and the risk of transmission are at the present unknown but under intense investigation by the authors and others. In the absence of those data, we do not recommend prenatal diagnosis by methylation testing at this time.

ANIMAL MODELS

An animal model for *p57*KIP2 knockout involves deletional mutagenesis of the gene. It is an embryonic lethal when transmitted from the mother, and the phenotype involves midline abdominal wall defects and cleft palate, reinforcing the notion that this gene is involved developmentally in midline closure and consistent with the epigenotype–phenotype analysis of BWS patients (Zhang et al., 1997). However, the mice do not show overgrowth, and clearly mutation of *p57*KIP2 is not lethal in humans. Several animal models exist for deletion of the *H19* DMR, which has a similar effect as its methylation. Mice show biallelic expression of *IGF2* and prenatal overgrowth but no other developmental abnormality and no cancer phenotype (Leighton et al., 1995; Ripoche et al., 1997; Thorvaldsen et al., 1998). A combined mutational model involving a cross between both loci shows both phenotypes described here, as well as macroglossia, suggesting a cooperative role between the two loci (Caspary et al., 1999). An engineered translocation of mouse chromosome 7, involving the orthologous region to human 11p15, shows inactivation of *p57*KIP2 (Cleary et al., 2001), confirming the hypothesis advanced by Lee et al. (1999) that the balanced chromosomal rearrangements separate this gene from its enhancer.

DEVELOPMENTAL PATHOGENESIS

BWS has served as a model of the epigenetics of disease and of cancer in particular. The greatest insight has come in understanding the developmental pathogenesis of cancer, because of parallel studies performed on the epigenetics of embryonal tumors, to which BWS patients are at increased risk. The original discovery of LOI was of Wilms tumors (WT) in more than half of sporadic cases, and this finding was later extended to BWS. LOI involves biallelic expression of *IGF2* (i.e., aberrant activation of the normally silent maternal allele of *IGF2*) as well as silencing of the maternal *H19*. The molecular mechanism in embryonal tumors is methylation of the *H19* ICR, which blocks access of the insulator protein CTCF, allowing a shared enhancer to activate the maternal *IGF2* allele (Cui et al., 1999). The developmental pathogenesis of tumors has been a conundrum until recently, however, as another WT locus on chromosome 11, *WT1*, was identified earlier and involves a classic knudsonian two-hit kinetics of inactivation of a tumor suppressor gene. Furthermore, germline mutations in *WT1* lead to the Denys-Drash syndrome of genitourinary malformations, renal dysplasia, and tumors.

An advance in understanding the developmental pathogenesis was made by Ravenel et al. (2001). These authors found that WT with LOI of *IGF2* are of a pathologic subtype distinct from those with LOH and

mutations of *WT1*. LOI pathology reflects a developmental stage of nephrogenesis corresponding to committed nephroblasts, whereas tumors with normal imprinting and/or LOH reflect an earlier stage of renal development in which the nephroblasts are immature and pluripotent, capable of differentiating into heterotypic elements such as muscle and cartilage. Furthermore, Ravenel et al. (2001) found that tumors with LOI show a specific increase in IGF2 expression, without alterations of other imprinted genes in the same 11p15 domain. These results are consistent with studies showing that IGF2 is a mitogen expressed specifically in proliferative kidney, relatively late in development (Hedborg et al., 1994). Thus, LOI leads to overexpression of IGF2 and increased mitogenesis. Two predictions of this model are that tumors in BWS patients or sporadic tumors with LOI occur in the periphery of the developmental renal lobe, that is, at greater distance from the collecting system than tumors in Denys-Drash syndrome or with sporadically occurring *WT1* mutations; and that LOI is also present in premalignant NRs, as they are the developmental precursor of WT. Both predictions were borne out. Furthermore, LOI was found to explain the bimodal age distribution of WT (Ravenel et al., 2001). Thus, late-arising tumors, accounting for about half of sporadic cases, do not involve two hits of a tumor suppressor gene, as the Knudson model predicts, but instead involve epigenetic alterations of *IGF2*. This result is consistent with the later developmental role of IGF2 in nephrogenic proliferation, compared with the earlier developmental role of WT1 in kidney formation. A developmental model of the epigenetics of WT and BWS is shown in Figure 73–4. These results would also explain why BWS patients with epigenetic alterations of *H19* and *IGF2* are at a substantially greater risk of cancer, specifically the type that involves LOI of *IGF2*.

The developmental pathogenesis of birth defects in BWS is less clear, although the mouse models suggest a critical role for *p57*KIP2 in midline closure, presumably by inhibiting cell cycle progression on detection of the appropriate signals for midline apposition. Overgrowth itself is still puzzling, as that was more specifically associated with imprinting abnormalities in the *LIT1-p57*KIP2 domain, yet mice with *p57*KIP2 mutations do not show overgrowth. A clue to developmental mechanism comes from a study by Grandjean et al. (2000), who found that IGF2 can itself serve as a negative regulator of *p57*KIP2 expression, implying a common signaling pathway. It is likely that

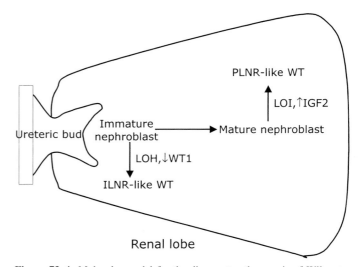

Figure 73–4. Molecular model for the divergent pathogenesis of Wilms tumor (WT). Immature nephroblasts develop in proximity to the ureteric bud and migrate to the periphery of the developing renal lobe as they mature. *WT1* mutations, decreased *WT1* expression, and 11p loss of heterozygosity (LOH) interfere with maturation and lead to intralobar nephrogenic rest (ILNR)-like Wilms tumor derived from pluripotent nephroblasts, accounting for the presence of heterotypic elements, such as muscle and cartilage. In contrast, loss of imprinting of the insulin-like growth factor II (*IGF2*) gene in mature nephroblasts leads to increased *IGF2* expression, a failure of proliferation arrest, and the development of perilobar nephrogenic rest (PLNR)-like tumors at the periphery of the renal lobe. (Reprinted with permission from Raven et al. [2001].)

IGF2 and *p57*^{KIP2} have overlapping functions within the cell that are developmentally defined.

REFERENCES

Beckwith JB (1963). Extreme cytomegaly of the adrenal fetal cortex omphalocele, hyperplasia of kidneys and pancreas, and Leydig cell hyperplasia-another syndrome? Annual Meeting of the Western Society for Pediatric Research, Los Angeles, CA.

Beckwith JB (1998). Children at increased risk for Wilms tumor: monitoring issues. *J Pediatr* 132: 377–379.

Bliek J, Maas SM, Ruijter JM, Hennekam RC, Alders M, Westerveld A, Mannens MM (2001). Increased tumour risk for BWS patients correlates with aberrant H19 and not KCNQ1OT1 methylation: occurrence of KCNQ1OT1 hypomethylation in familial cases of BWS. *Hum Mol Genet* 10: 467–476.

Caspary T, Cleary MA, Perlman EJ, Zhang P, Elledge SJ, Tilghman SM (1999). Oppositely imprinted genes p57Kip2 and Igf2 interact in a mouse model for Beckwith-Wiedemann syndrome. *Genes Dev* 13: 3115–3125.

Choyke PL, Siegel MJ, Craft AW, Green DM, DeBaun MR (1999). Screening for Wilms tumor in children with Beckwith-Wiedemann syndrome or idiopathic hemihypertrophy. *Med Pediatr Oncol* 32: 196–200.

Choyke PL, Siegel MJ, Oz O, Sotelo-Avila C, DeBaun MR (1998). Nonmalignant renal disease in pediatric patients with Beckwith-Wiedemann syndrome. *AJR Am J Roentgenol* 171: 733–737.

Cleary MA, van Raamsdonk CD, Levorse J, Zheng BH, Bradley A, Tilghman SM (2001). Disruption of an imprinted gene cluster by a targeted chromosomal translocation in mice. *Nat Genet* 29: 78–82.

Clericuzio C (2002). Serum alpha-fetoprotein screening for hepatoblastoma in children with high-risk phenotypes. Proceedings of the Greenwood Genetic Center.

Cornblath M, Schwartz R (1993). Hypoglycemia in the neonate. *J Pediatr Endocrinol* 6: 113–129.

Cui H, Niemitz EL, Ravenel JD, Onyango P, Brandenburg SA, Lobanenkov VV, Feinberg AP (2001). Loss of imprinting of insulin-like growth factor-II in Wilms' tumor commonly involves altered methylation but not mutations of CTCF or its binding site. *Cancer Res* 61: 4947–4950.

Daugbjerg P, Everberg G (1984). A case of Beckwith-Wiedemann syndrome with conductive hearing loss. *Acta Paediatr Scand* 73: 408–410.

DeBaun MR, Tucker MA (1998). Risk of cancer during the first four years of life in children from the Beckwith-Wiedemann Syndrome Registry. *J Pediatr* 132: 398–400.

DeBaun MR, King AA, White N (2000). Hypoglycemia in Beckwith-Wiedemann syndrome. *Semin Perinatol* 24: 164–171.

DeBaun MR, Niemitz EL, McNeil DE, Brandenburg SA, Lee MP, Feinberg AP (2002). Epigenetic alterations of H19 and LIT1 distinguish patients with Beckwith-Wiedemann syndrome with cancer and birth defects. *Am J Hum Genet* 70: 604–611.

Elias ER, DeBaun MR, Feinberg AP (1998). Beckwith-Wiedemann syndrome. In: *Principles of Molecular Medicine.* Jameson JL (ed.) Humana Press, Cambridge.

Elliott M, Bayly R, Cole T, Temple IK, Maher ER (1994). Clinical features and natural history of Beckwith-Wiedemann syndrome: presentation of 74 new cases. *Clin Genet* 46: 168–174.

Feinberg AP (2001). Genomic Imprinting and cancer. In: *The Metabolic and Molecular Bases of Inherited Disease.* Scriver CR, Beaudet AL, Sly WS, Valle D (eds.) McGraw-Hill, New York, pp. 525–537.

Feinberg A (2002). Genetic and epigenetic contributions to tumour evolution. In: *Seminars in Cancer Biology.* Klein G (ed.) Academic Press Ltd., in press.

Fishman EK, Hartman DS, Goldman SM, Siegelman SS (1983). The CT appearance of Wilms tumor. *J Comput Assist Tomogr* 7: 659–665.

Grandjean V, Smith J, Schofield PN, Ferguson-Smith AC (2000). Increased IGF-II protein affects p57KIP2 expression in vivo and in vitro: implications for Beckwith-Wiedemann syndrome. *Proc Natl Acad Sci USA* 97: 5279–5284.

Haig D, Graham C (1991). Genomic imprinting and the strange case of the insulin-like growth factor II receptor. *Cell* 64: 1045–1046.

Hatada H, Ohashi Y, Fukushima Y, Kaneko M, Inoue Y, Komoto A, Okada S, Ohishi A, Nabetani H, Morisaki M, et al. (1996). An imprinted gene p57KIP2 is mutated in Beckwith-Wiedemann syndrome. *Nat Genet* 14: 171–173.

Henry I, Bonaiti-Pellie C, Chehensse V, Beldjord C, Schwartz C, Utermann G, Junien C (1991). Uniparental paternal disomy in a genetic cancer-predisposing syndrome. *Nature* 351: 665–667.

Hoovers JMN, Kalikin LM, Johnson LA, Alders M, Redeker B, Law DJ, Bliek J, Steenman M, Benedict M, Wiegant J, et al. (1995). Multiple genetic loci within 11p15 defined by Beckwith-Wiedemann syndrome rearrangement breakpoints and subchromosomal transferable fragments. *Proc Natl Acad Sci USA* 92: 12456–12460.

Hugosson C, Nyman R, Jacobsson B, Jorulf H, Sackey K, McDonald P (1995). Imaging of solid kidney tumours in children. *Acta Radiol* 36: 254–260.

Lee MP, Hu RJ, Johnson LA, Feinberg AP (1997b). Human KVLQT1 gene shows tissue-specific imprinting and encompasses Beckwith-Wiedemann syndrome chromosomal rearrangements. *Nat Genet* 15: 181–185.

Lee MP, DeBaun M, Randhawa GS, Reichard BA, Feinberg AP (1997a). Low frequency of p57KIP2 mutation in Beckwith-Wiedemann syndrome. *Am J Hum Genet* 61: 304–309.

Lee MP, DeBaun MR, Mitsuya K, Galonek HL, Brandenburg S, Oshimura M, Feinberg AP (1999). Loss of imprinting of a paternally expressed transcript, with antisense orientation to KVLQT1, occurs frequently in Beckwith-Wiedemann syndrome and is independent of insulin-like growth factor II imprinting. *Proc Natl Acad Sci USA* 96: 5203–5208.

Lee MP, Ravenel JD, Hu RJ, Lustig LR, Tomaselli G, Berger RD, Brandenburg SA, Litzi TJ, Bunton TE, Limb C, et al. (2000). Targeted disruption of the Kvlqt1 gene causes deafness and gastric hyperplasia in mice. *J Clin Invest* 106: 1447–1455.

Leighton PA, Ingram RS, Eggenschwiler J, Efstratiadis A, Tilghman SM (1995). Disruption of imprinting caused by deletion of the H19 gene region in mice. *Nature* 375: 34–39.

Mannens M, Hoovers JMN, Redeker E, Verjaal M, Feinberg AP, Little P, Boavida M, Coad N, Steenman M, Bliek J, et al. Parental imprinting of human chromosome region 11p15.4-pter involved in the Beckwith-Wiedemann syndrome and various human neoplasia. *Eur J Hum Genet* 2: 3–23.

McNeil DE, Brown M, Ching A, DeBaun MR (2001). Screening for Wilms tumor and hepatoblastoma in children with Beckwith-Wiedemann syndromes: a cost-effective model. *Med Ped Oncol* 37: 349–356.

Motokura T, Bloom T, Kim HG, Juppner H, Ruderman JV, Kronenberg HM, Arnold A (1991). A novel cyclin encoded by a bcl1-linked candidate oncogene. *Nature* 350: 512–515.

O'Keefe D, Dao D, Zhao L, Sanderson R, Warburton D, Weiss L, Anyane-Yeboa K, Tycko B (1997). Coding mutations in p57KIP2 are present in some cases of Beckwith-Wiedemann syndrome but are rare or absent in Wilms tumors. *Am J Hum Genet* 61: 295–303.

Ogawa O, Eccles MR, Szeto J, McNoe LA, Yun K, Maw MA, Smith PJ, Reeve AE (1993). Relaxation of insulin-like growth factor II gene imprinting implicated in Wilms' tumour. *Nature* 362: 749–751.

Onyango P, Miller W, Lehoczky J, Leung C, Birren B, Wheelan S, Dewar K, Feinberg A (2000). Sequence and comparative analysis of the mouse 1 megabase region orthologous to the human 11p15 imprinted domain. *Genome Res* 10: 1697–1710.

Paulsen K (1973). Otological features in exomphalos-macro-glossia-gigantism syndrome (Wiedemann's syndrome). *Z Laryngol Rhinol Otol* 52: 793–798.

Rainier S, Johnson LA, Dobry CJ, Ping AJ, Grundy PE, Feinberg AP (1993). Relaxation of imprinted genes in human cancer. *Nature* 362: 747–749.

Ravenel JD, Broman KW, Perlman EJ, Niemitz EL, Jayawardena TM, Bell DW, Haber DA, Uejima H, Feinberg AP (2001). Loss of imprinting of insulin-like growth factor-II (IGF2) gene in distinguishing specific biological subtypes of Wilms tumor. *J Natl Cancer Inst* 93: 1698–703.

Ripoche MA, Kress C, Poirier F, Dandolo L (1997). Deletion of the H19 transcription unit reveals the existence of a putative imprinting control element. *Genes Dev* 11: 1596–1604.

Ross JA, Gurney JG (1998). Hepatoblastoma incidence in the United States from 1973 to 1992. *Med Pediatr Oncol* 30: 141–142.

Steenman MJ, Rainier S, Dobry CJ, Grundy P, Horon IL, Feinberg AP (1994). Loss of imprinting of IGF2 is linked to reduced expression and abnormal methylation of H19 in Wilms' tumour. *Nat Genet* 7: 433–439.

Takahashi S, Shinoda H, Nakano Y (1996). Congenital stapedial fixation associated with Beckwith-Wiedemann syndrome: two cases of a woman and her brother. *Am J Otol* 17: 111–114.

Thorvaldsen JL, Duran KL, Bartolomei MS (1998). Deletion of the H19 differentially methylated domain results in loss of imprinted expression of H19 and Igf2. *Genes Dev* 12: 3693–3702.

Weksberg R, Shen DR, Fei YL, Song QL, Squire J (1993). Disruption of insulin-like growth factor 2 imprinting in Beckwith-Wiedemann syndrome. *Nat Genet* 5: 143–150.

Weng EY, Moeschler JB, Graham JM Jr (1995). Longitudinal observations on 15 children with Wiedemann-Beckwith syndrome. *Am J Med Genet* 56: 366–373.

Wiedemann HR (1964). Complexe malformatif familial avec hernie ombilicale et macroglossie: un "syndrome nouveau?" *J Genet Hum* 13: 223–232.

Zhang P, Liegeois NJ, Wong C, Finegold M, Hou H, Thompson JC, Silverman A, Harper JW, DePinho RA, Elledge SJ (1997). Altered cell differentiation and proliferation in mice lacking p57KIP2 indicates a role in Beckwith-Wiedemann syndrome. *Nature* 387: 151–158.

74 | 15q11-13 and the Prader-Willi Syndrome

SHAWN E. MCCANDLESS AND SUZANNE B. CASSIDY

Prader-Willi syndrome (PWS [OMIM 176270]) is a multisystem disorder with a recognizable pattern of dysmorphic features and major neurologic, cognitive, endocrine, and behavioral abnormalities, all of which are referable to a characteristic pattern of CNS maldevelopment. Newborns have profound hypotonia, feeding difficulties, and poor weight gain. Later, they develop hyperphagia leading to obesity, short stature, characteristic physical appearance, and a characteristic pattern of behavior problems that includes obsessive-compulsive traits. Management centers on control of food intake to avoid obesity, medical treatment of endocrine abnormalities, and behavior management techniques. Diagnosis is based on clinical findings, confirmed by demonstration of lack of biparental expression of the genes in the region.

PWS was the first recognized human disorder related to genomic imprinting and the first shown to be due to uniparental disomy (UPD). It is caused by failure of expression of paternally expressed genes in the PWS region of chromosome 15. This can be due to deletion of paternally contributed chromosome 15, maternal UPD, or disruption or deletion of the imprinting center responsible for altering the paternal imprint. Maternally imprinted genes in the region include *SNURF-SNRPN*; two *MAGE* family genes, *MAGEL2* and *NECDIN*; *MKRN3*; *IPW*; and several clusters of tandemly duplicated small nucleolar RNAs (snoRNAs). The specific relationship between the failure of gene expression and the physical and behavioral phenotype is not known; the mechanism of action of the imprinting switch also is not known. A variety of mouse models have been developed. Several have a phenotype with perinatal failure to thrive and lethality. None have survived long enough for it to be determined whether they will recapitulate the hyperphagic obesity phenotype.

DEVELOPMENTAL PATHWAY

PWS is an example of a genomic disorder (Lupski, 1998; Ji et al., 2000; Nicholls and Knepper, 2001) that results from lack of the typical expression of one or more imprinted genes. The phenotype is not the direct result of a DNA sequence change, as is a traditional genetic disorder. Instead, it is due to changes that affect the genomic structure and epigenetic phenomena that lead to differential expression of alleles from parents of a particular sex (imprinting), recurrent rearrangements due to the presence of low-copy repeats (duplicons), and correction of meiotic errors (trisomy rescue). It was one of the first human disorders of this type to be delineated. The genomic structure of the region has been reviewed in detail (Nicholls and Knepper, 2001).

The basic defect in PWS is the lack of expression of the genes from either allele in a region of DNA located at chromosome 15q11-13 (Nicholls, 1989; Nicholls and Knepper, 2001). In the normal situation, several genes in this region display genomic imprinting, which means that they are differentially expressed based on the sex of the parent from whom the chromosome on which they lie was inherited. In the case of PWS, there is a lack of expression of one or more genes on 15q11-13 that are normally expressed only from the paternally inherited chromosome (Nicholls, 1989; Nicholls and Knepper, 2001). Angelman syndrome is a clinically distinct disorder thought to be due to the lack of expression of a gene or genes within the same chromosome region that is normally expressed in the brain only from the maternally inherited chromosome (Kishino et al., 1997; Rougeulle et al., 1997; Vu and Hoffman, 1997).

CLINICAL DESCRIPTION

The first identification that the features of PWS represented a recurrent and recognizable pattern was made by Prader, Labhart, and Willi in 1956 (Prader et al., 1956). The clinical characteristics and natural history have been described in detail in a number of clinical series and reviews (Zellweger and Schneider, 1968; Hall and Smith, 1972; Holm and Laurnen, 1981; Bray et al., 1983; Butler et al., 1986; Cassidy and Ledbetter, 1989; Butler, 1990; Cassidy, 1997). The findings that have the greatest impact on health and quality of life are the predisposition to morbid obesity and the cognitive and behavioral characteristics.

Although PWS is considered to be a dysmorphic syndrome, the dysmorphic findings are fairly subtle. They consist of dolichocephaly, narrow bifrontal diameter, "almond-shaped" and sometimes upslanting palpebral fissures, narrow nasal bridge, and downturned mouth (Fig. 74–1). In addition, the hands and feet are short, the hands are narrow with absent hypothenar bulge, and the fingers are often tapered. Puffy/fatty dorsa of the hands and fingers, as well as of the feet, are frequent. Treatment with growth hormone from an early age may make these features less evident (based on personal experience), and there are data to suggest that the facial phenotype is less striking when the disorder results from UPD rather than deletion (Cassidy et al., 1997).

Hypotonia

Central hypotonia is a hallmark of PWS, and there is no convincing case of a patient with the disorder who lacks this feature. Although it persists throughout life, the most profound consequence occurs during the perinatal period and early infancy. It is associated with decreased fetal movement, abnormal fetal position, and difficulty at the time of delivery, often necessitating cesarean section. The hypotonia at birth is of varying severity but often is profound. A state of hypoarousal is present, with little spontaneous movement and a very weak cry. The child sleeps excessively and does not awaken to feed. Reflexes may be decreased or absent. Almost invariably, the suck is poor, causing significant feeding problems; consequent failure to thrive is common. Breastfeeding is rarely possible; almost always the child must be fed with a special nipple or, more often, gavage. Infantile lethargy, with decreased arousal and weak cry, is also a prominent finding. When neuromuscular electrophysiological and muscle biopsy studies are conducted as part of a diagnostic evaluation, the results are normal or nonspecific. The hypotonia, poor suck, and lethargy gradually improve with time, although muscle tone is never completely normal. There often is a period of normal feeding after a varying number of weeks or months. Motor milestones are delayed. The average age of sitting is 12 months; that of walking is 24 months. Adults remain mildly hypotonic with decreased muscle bulk and tone. The muscle hypotonia likely contributes to the characteristic poorly articulated, and often hypernasal, speech, as well as to the facial appearance, scoliosis/kyphosis, osteoporosis, and poor coordination. Hypotonia is such a characteristic finding that it is recommended that all newborns with persistent hypotonia be tested for PWS (Miller et al., 1999; Gunay-Aygun et al., 2001).

Hyperphagia and Obesity

At some time in the first 5 or 6 years of life, the child with PWS has the sudden onset of hyperphagia. Hyperphagia appears to be related

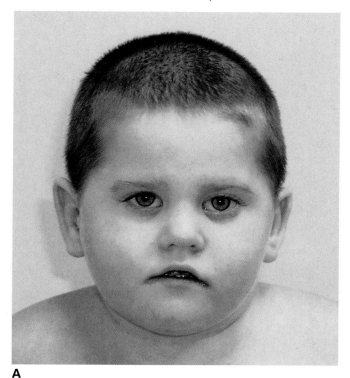

A

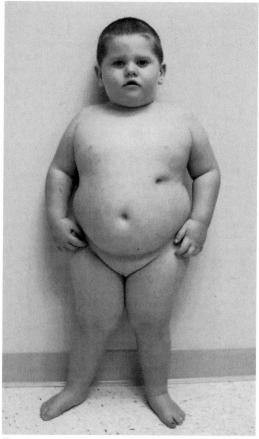

B

Figure 74–1. Typical physical manifestations in a male with Prader-Willi syndrome. (*A*) Note the bifrontal narrowing, almond-shaped palpebral fissures, and down-turned corners of mouth with dried saliva. (*B*) Truncal obesity (with scar from gastrostomy), hypogenitalism, and small hands and feet.

to a hypothalamic abnormality resulting in a lack of sense of satiety (Zipf and Berntson, 1987; Holland et al., 1993, 1995). Food-seeking behavior is common and includes hoarding or foraging for food, eating of unappealing substances such as garbage, pet food, and frozen food, and stealing of food or money to buy food. A high threshold for vomiting may complicate bingeing on spoiled food from the garbage or such items as boxes of sugar or frozen uncooked meat. Toxicity from emetics that fail to induce vomiting has occurred.

The obesity of PWS is not present at birth or during the early period of severe hypotonia but generally begins between the ages of 1 and 6 years. Obesity is nearly always present after age 6 years unless it is actively avoided, and the proportion of fat mass to lean body mass is high even in thin infants with PWS (Butler, 1990). The obesity is centrally distributed, with relative sparing of the distal extremities; even individuals who are not overweight tend to deposit fat on the abdomen, buttocks, and thighs.

Avoidance of obesity is one of the most difficult management problems, and obesity is generally believed to be the major cause of morbidity and mortality in this disorder. Longevity may be nearly normal if appropriate weight is maintained (Greenswag, 1987; Cassidy et al., 1994). Cardiopulmonary compromise (pickwickian syndrome) results from excessive obesity, as do type II diabetes mellitus, hypertension, thrombophlebitis, and chronic leg edema. Sleep apnea occurs at increased frequency, but there are other sleep disturbances seen in PWS, such as hypoventilation and altered sleep architecture, that appear to be unrelated to obesity (Hertz et al., 1995). Aberrant levels of oxytocin have been identified and may be associated with the impaired satiety response characteristic of the syndrome (Martin et al., 1998).

Cognition and Behavior

The cognitive and behavioral issues in PWS have a major impact on quality of life. Mild global developmental delay is present in most affected individuals. There is a wide range of cognitive function, with

an average IQ of approximately 65 to 70. A synthesis of IQ data from 575 subjects in 57 published studies found that 34% had mild mental retardation, 27% had moderate delays, and 6% had severe to profound levels of impairment (Curfs and Fryns, 1992). A surprisingly large percentage, 32%, exhibited IQ scores above 70, the established cutoff for mental retardation.

Commonly, affected individuals can read, write, and perform simple arithmetic. Adaptive behavior is rarely commensurate with IQ scores (Dykens and Cassidy, 2002). Many people with PWS have relative strengths in tasks assessing visuospatial processing and long-term memory and relative weakness in arithmetic, sequential tasks, and short-term memory (Curfs and Fryns, 1992; Taylor, 1988; Curfs, 2002; Dykens and Cassidy, 2002). Interestingly, many people with PWS have shown a true cognitive strength in working jigsaw puzzles (Dykens, 2002) and word-find puzzles (based on personal observation).

Although verbal skills are often a relative strength in many people with PWS, speech is generally poorly articulated and frankly apraxic. Studies have identified high-pitched nasal speech qualities, errors with certain speech sounds and complex syntax, poor narrative retelling abilities, and reduced vocabulary skills relative to age expectations in up to 85% to 90% of affected individuals (Kleppe et al., 1990; Akefeldt et al., 1997; Lewis, 2002). Speech and articulation difficulties are likely related to oral muscular hypotonia, and perhaps to the characteristic thick, viscous saliva (Kleppe et al., 1990).

As many as 85% of people with PWS exhibit significant maladaptive behavior (Dykens and Cassidy, 1995, 1999, 2002; Clarke et al., 1996; Dykens and Kasari, 1997). Indeed, behavioral problems constitute one of the major diagnostic criteria (Holm et al., 1993), and the behavioral phenotype is often quite characteristic (Dykens and Cassidy, 1995; Clarke et al., 1996; Dykens and Kasari, 1997; Cassidy and Morris, 2002). In general, problem behaviors can be food-related, impulse control, obsessive-compulsive, or other affective disorders (Dykens and Cassidy, 2002). Other behaviors include high rates of tantrums, impulsivity, stubbornness, arguing with others, disobedience, lability, skin picking, compulsions, withdrawal, and anxiety (Dykens and Cassidy, 1995; Dykens et al., 1996; State et al., 1999). Parents often complain about repetitive question asking, excessive talking, and verbal perseveration (Dykens, 1996). Behavioral issues frequently jeopardize home life, group home placements, and school and employment situations (based on personal experience).

Obsessive-compulsive symptoms occur in about 70% of patients (Dykens et al., 1996). This is particularly interesting in light of findings that people with PWS have high levels of serotonin in the cerebrospinal fluid (Martin et al., 1998) and that brains taken at autopsy from people with PWS have decreased numbers and size of oxytocin-secreting cells in the paraventricular nucleus of the hypothalamus (Swaab, 1997; Goldstone et al., 2002). Oxytocin is involved in serotonin metabolism (Dykens and Cassidy, 2002).

A number of reports have demonstrated that psychosis develops in a small but significant proportion of people with PWS, generally in late adolescence or early adulthood. In addition to several case reports, two studies in larger numbers of individuals found that 6% to 12% showed psychotic symptoms and visual or auditory hallucinations (Stein et al., 1994; Beardsmore et al., 1998; Clarke, 1998; Clarke et al., 1998; Boer et al., 2002). These rates are high relative to those for other people with mental retardation. A specific type, cycloid psychosis, has been noted in a number of those with psychiatric symptoms. Although many individuals responded well to standard therapy, several showed disorganized thinking or behavior that persisted over the years.

Other Clinical Findings

Hypogonadism and short stature are sufficiently frequent to be included among the major diagnostic criteria (Holm et al., 1993). There are several other findings that are typically seen in people with PWS, including a number of autonomic nervous system abnormalities, high pain threshold, sleep abnormalities, scoliosis, and vision impairment.

Hypogonadism

Hypogonadism is present in most individuals with PWS and is of prenatal onset. It is hypothalamic in origin, and in general, gonadotropins, estrogen, and testosterone are deficient. External genitalia are initially small and remain relatively small throughout life unless sex hormone replacement therapy is used. Hypogonadism is manifested in males as unilateral or bilateral cryptorchidism (in 80%), scrotal hypoplasia (small, hypopigmented, and poorly rugated), and, often, a small penis. In females, there is hypoplasia of the labia minora and clitoris (Cassidy, 1984). Hypogonadism is also manifested as abnormal pubertal development in both sexes (Kauli et al., 1978; Vanelli et al., 1984; Stein et al., 1994; Beardsmore et al., 1998; Clarke, 1998; Clarke et al., 1998; Linnemann et al., 1999; Schmidt and Schwarz, 2001; Boer et al., 2002). Although pubic and axillary hair may develop early (premature adrenarche) or normally, the remainder of pubertal development is usually delayed and incomplete. True precocious puberty has been described rarely. Adult males only occasionally have a voice change, male body habitus, or substantial facial or body hair. In females, breast development generally begins at a normal age, although it is difficult to differentiate from the pseudogynecomastia due to fat accumulation that occurs in both sexes. Menarche may occur as late as the 30s, particularly in association with significant weight loss in obese individuals, but there usually is amenorrhea or oligomenorrhea. In both males and females, sexual activity is rare. Two women with molecularly confirmed PWS (one with deletion and one with uniparental disomy) have brought pregnancies to term (Akefeldt et al., 1999; Eiholzer et al., 2001; Schulze et al., 2001), however, so although most affected individuals are infertile, this should not be presumed. Systematic studies of gonadal structure and function are lacking, particularly in the prenatal and neonatal period. Testosterone and estrogen are generally low for age in males and females, respectively, as is follicle-stimulating hormone and usually luteinizing hormone in both sexes, although the range is wide (Jeffcoate et al., 1980; Bray et al., 1983; Cassidy, 1984; Lee, 1995; Burman et al., 2001). Because the pituitary gland and gonads are normal but understimulated, treatment with pituitary or gonadal hormones can improve secondary sex characteristics.

Short Stature

Most individuals with PWS are short for their family. There are many data indicating reduced growth hormone secretion in PWS, as has been documented in at least 15 studies involving more than 300 affected children (reviewed in Burman et al., 2001). In contrast to normal individuals with obesity, who may show blunted growth hormone response to stimulation, those with PWS have shown low levels of insulin-like growth factor I and insulin-like growth factor–binding protein 3 (Radetti et al., 1998; Park et al., 1999; Scacchi et al., 1999; Corrias et al., 2000). Growth hormone deficiency can account for the altered body composition with a high fat-to-lean body mass ratio, reduced muscle mass, osteopenia, central distribution of obesity, and delayed bone age seen in some patients. Growth hormone treatment corrects the characteristic small hands and feet.

EPIDEMIOLOGY OF PWS

PWS has been described in a wide variety of ethnic and racial backgrounds, with no recognized predilection. The prevalence is variously quoted as 1:10,000 to 1:25,000 (Burd et al., 1990), although no population-based screening studies have been reported. Most cases occur sporadically, although carriers of balanced translocations may have multiple affected children. The sons of a woman with an imprinting defect may have multiple affected children, leading to the suggestion of a "grandmatrilineal" inheritance pattern (Ming et al., 2000).

MOLECULAR GENETICS

There are several ways that the paternally inherited genes in 15q11-13 may fail to be expressed, causing PWS. Approximately 70% result from an interstitial deletion of the PWS region on the paternally inherited chromosome 15. There are two common proximal breakpoints in the region and one common breakpoint at the distal end of the region (Christian et al., 1995; Robinson et al., 1998; Amos-Landgraf et al., 1999). More than 95% of studied individuals with deletions have these common breakpoints spanning a 4-Mb region. Work suggests that this recurrent common deletion is due to the presence of multiple copies of repeated sequences flanking the deleted region (Buiting et al., 1992, 1998; Amos-Landgraf et al., 1999; Ji et al., 1999). These sequences, derived from a recurrently duplicated ancestral gene (HERC2), are referred to as the "END repeat" (Amos-Landgraf et al., 1999; Ji et al., 2000). These so-called "duplicons" (Christian et al., 1999; Ji et al., 2000) may result in aberrant recombination leading to deletion or, in other cases, duplication of the intervening sequence.

About 15% of cases result from the absence of paternally contributed alleles due to maternal UPD. This term describes the situation in which both copies of chromosome 15 are inherited from a single parent—the mother in the case of PWS (Nicholls et al., 1989). A two-step process explains most cases of maternal UPD. First, there is a maternal nondysjunction event that leads to an ovum disomic for chromosome 15. After fertilization with a normal sperm, the blastocyst with trisomy 15 is destined for spontaneous abortion unless a second event, usually thought to be anaphase lag, produces a daughter cell that has lost one of the three chromosomes 15. This process, referred to as "trisomy rescue," has been documented based on the presence of a trisomic cell line in the placenta with UPD in the embryo (Cassidy et al., 1992; Purvis-Smith et al., 1992; Roberts et al., 1997; European Collaborative Research on Mosaicism in CVS [EUCROMIC], 1999).

A third cause of PWS is the presence of a chromosome 15 from each parent (biparental inheritance), both of which are maternally imprinted. This "imprinting defect" is the result of a failure to erase the paternal grandmother's chromosome 15 imprint and apply the male-appropriate imprint in the father's germ line. When the father passes on the chromosome 15 that he inherited from his mother, the maternal imprint of that chromosome must be switched to the paternal imprint in the father's germ line. In the case of the PWS region of chro-

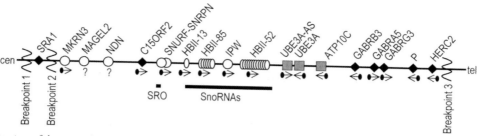

Figure 74–2. Genomic structure of the approximately 4-Mb Prader-Willi syndrome region of chromosome 15q11-13. White circles represent maternally imprinted genes (expressed only from paternally inherited chromosomes), gray rectangles represent paternally imprinted genes, and black diamonds represent genes that are expressed biparentally. *SRA1* is not imprinted (Nicholls and Knepper, 2001), and *C15ORF2* is expressed only in testis and biparentally (Nicholls and Knepper, 2001). *UBE3A-AS* is an antisense transcript of *UBE3A* (Rougeulle, 1998). The small bar labeled SRO is the smallest region of overlap of microdeletions and defines the region containing the imprinting center. Small arrows show the orientation of transcription. See text for a discussion of other features.

mosome 15, the maternal imprint is characterized by hypermethylation of a series of CpG islands in the promoter regions of the imprinted genes (Driscoll et al., 1992; Glenn et al., 1993). This in turn alters the histone acetylation pattern and interferes with the translational process, presumably by leading to an unfavorable genomic structure for the binding of transcription factors and the translational machinery (Saitoh and Wada, 2000). Imprinting defects in PWS cause persistence of the hypermethylation on the chromosome 15 passed from the father.

Two types of imprinting defects have been found to cause PWS (Nicholls, 1998; Ohta et al., 1999). One is associated with a microdeletion of a small region that includes the PWS imprinting center. The specific sequence and the mechanism of action of the imprinting center are not known. The smallest region of overlap among individuals with these microdeletions of the imprinting center is about 4 kb, located at the 5′ end of the *SNURF-SNRPN* gene (see later) within 15q11-13 (Fig. 74–2). In a second group of imprinting defects, no deletion or mutation is found. These are presumed to have occurred sporadically, suggesting the possiblity of a random failure to properly initiate or complete the imprint switching process. Together, these two types of imprinting defects account for fewer than 5% of affected individuals.

Last, there are several reports of individuals with balanced translocations of chromosome 15 who have the PWS phenotype. The breakpoints of these translocations are either associated with cryptic deletions or disrupt the imprinting center (Bray et al., 1983; Sun et al., 1996; Kuslich et al., 1999; Butler and Thompson, 2000; Wirth et al., 2001).

Importantly, there have been no well-documented cases of clinically typical PWS in individuals who do not have one of these mechanisms leading to the lack of expression of the paternally inherited genes. The lack of cases with mutations in single genes in the region suggests that PWS likely represents a true multigene disorder.

Maternally Imprinted Genes in the Region

Figure 74–2 shows the genomic structure of the PWS/AS region of chromosome 15. This region contains several paternally active genes, two maternally active genes (*UBE3A* and *ATP10C*), and several nonimprinted genes. The nonimprinted genes are not likely candidates for the various abnormalities seen in patients with PWS. These include a family of γ-aminobutyric acid (GABA) receptors (GABRB1, GABRB2, and GABRB3) and the *P* gene, or mouse pink-eye dilution locus (Nicholls and Knepper, 2001). The *P* gene has been shown to be the gene involved in oculocutaneous albinism type II (Ramsay et al., 1992; Rinchik et al., 1993; Lee et al., 1994), an autosomal recessive disorder. Therefore, although haploinsufficiency for the *P* gene is not strictly implicated in PWS, it may explain the relative hypopigmentation seen in some individuals with PWS due to 15q deletion (Wiesner et al., 1987; Butler, 1989; King et al., 1993; Lee et al., 1994; Cassidy et al., 1997).

Maternally imprinted genes in the region, that is, those expressed only from the paternally inherited allele, must all be considered potential candidate genes for phenotypic features of PWS. They include the previously noted *SNURF-SNRPN*, *NDN* (protein, NECDIN), *MAGEL2*, *MKRN3* (previously called *ZNF127* because of its zinc finger domain), *IPW*, and three families of snoRNA clusters *HBII-13*, *HBII-85*, and *HBII-52* (Nicholls and Knepper, 2001). The functions of *MKRN3* and *IPW* are unknown. A *Zpf127* (mouse homologue of *MKRN3*) knockout mouse is said to be fertile and not obese, although behavioral evaluation has not been reported (Jong et al., 1999). Similarly, a radiation-induced deletion including *Ipw* in a mouse does not appear to be associated with the PWS phenotype when passed from a male (Johnson et al., 1995). This suggests that *IPW* is not directly responsible for the PWS phenotype.

The *SNURF-SNRPN* locus has received the most attention, in part because the 5′ end of this gene contains the PWS imprinting center (Ohta et al., 1999; Bielinska et al., 2000; Nicholls and Knepper, 2001). This fascinating gene has been shown to have a polycistronic structure, similar in some ways to genes typically seen in microbes (Gray, 1999a). In addition to the functional control of the imprinting process, this sequence codes for two different proteins and an snoRNA (Gray et al., 1999a; Cavaille et al., 2000; Nicholls and Knepper, 2001; Runte et al., 2001). The initially described functional protein was SmN, thought to function in RNA splicing in the brain (Ozcelik et al., 1992; Gray et al., 1999b). *SNURF* (*SNRPN* Upstream Reading Frame) contains the putative PWS imprinting center, suggesting a probable role in PWS (Gray et al., 1999a; Runte et al., 2001). The small protein transcribed from this reading frame has also been proposed to have a role in the regulation of SmN expression (Gray et al., 1999b; Nicholls and Knepper, 2001). The snoRNA *HBII-13* is contained in intron 12 of the *SNURF-SNRPN* gene (Wirth et al., 2001), although no specific function has been identified.

NDN (NECDIN) (Jay et al., 1997; MacDonald and Wevrick, 1997; Maruyama et al., 1991; Sutcliffe et al., 1997) and *MAGEL2* (Boccaccio et al., 1999; Lee et al., 2000), two members of the *MAGE* (melanoma antigen E) family of genes, map to the PWS region and are maternally imprinted. These proteins are thought to be involved in cell cycle control and apoptosis by linking cell surface receptors to regulatory pathways (Barker and Salehi, 2002). *Magel2* has been shown to be highly expressed in the hypothalamus of the mouse embryo (Boccaccio et al., 1999; Lee et al., 2000), a brain structure that is the source of a variety of clinical findings in PWS, including hypogonadism and appetite control abnormalities. Little else is known about the function or significance of *MAGEL2* (Nicholls and Knepper, 2001). Another MAGE family protein, NECDIN (Neurally differentiated Embryonal Carcinoma–Derived prote*IN*; Maruyama et al., 1991), is also maternally imprinted (Jay et al., 1997; MacDonald and Wevrick, 1997; Sutcliffe et al., 1997). NECDIN has been shown to bind to a variety of transcription factors and can interfere with postmitotic cell proliferation (Barker and Salehi, 2002).

The snoRNA genes, *HBII-13* (present in a single copy) and the tandemly repeated, multicopy *HBII-52*, and *HBII-85* are maternally imprinted and clustered within the PWS region and are expressed in the brain (Barker and Salehi, 2002; Cavaille et al., 2000; de los Santos et al., 2000). *HBII-52* contains sequence complimentary to a region of the serotonin receptor 2C mRNA, suggesting a possible RNA target (Cavaille et al., 2000; Barker and Salehi, 2002). The functions and targets of the other snoRNAs are not known (Nicholls and Knepper, 2001). The role, if any, of these genes in PWS has not been elucidated.

Additional, as yet unidentified, genes may also be present within the 4-Mb PWS/AS region.

Genotype–Phenotype Correlation

Several studies have attempted to correlate the molecular cause of PWS with the clinical findings (Gillessen-Kaesbach et al., 1995; Mitchell et al., 1996; Cassidy et al., 1997; Gunay-Aygun et al., 1997). The rarity of individuals with imprinting defects has limited this to comparing individuals with deletions with those with UPD. Subtle differences have been found. Patients with deletions are more likely to have hypopigmentation (Butler, 1989; Gillessen-Kaesbach et al., 1995; Mitchell et al., 1996; Cassidy et al., 1997), although this does not appear to correlate with the haplotype in the region of the *P* gene in the undeleted chromosome (Spritz et al., 1997). A variety of behavior problems, including skin picking (Dykens et al., 1999; Symons et al., 1999), maladaptive behaviors, and distress related to compulsive symptoms (Dykens et al., 1999), appear to be more severe in individuals with deletions.

Individuals with UPD have increased maternal age (Gillessen-Kaesbach et al., 1995), which is not surprising in light of the presumed mechanism of trisomy rescue. Different studies have drawn different conclusions as to differences in birthweight and early feeding difficulties (Gillessen-Kaesbach et al., 1995; Mitchell et al., 1996; Gunay-Aygun et al., 1997). Possibly because of the somewhat milder phenotype, individuals with UPD tend to be diagnosed later than do individuals with deletions (Gunay-Aygun et al., 1997). This difference may disappear as physicians become more familiar with PWS and the diagnostic strategies available. Verbal IQ (Roof et al., 2000) and overall IQ (Cassidy et al., 2000) have been shown to be slightly higher in individuals with UPD than in those with a deletion.

ESTABLISHING THE DIAGNOSIS OF PWS

Diagnostic criteria for PWS have been developed (Holm et al., 1993) and updated in light of the development of unambiguous molecular tests that show reduced sensitivity of clinical criteria for diagnosing PWS (Gunay-Aygun et al., 2001). Clinical criteria may be used to identify people for whom further testing is indicated, but definitive diagnosis requires the documentation of a lack of paternally contributed genes in the PWS region. The initial test generally performed for the purpose of diagnosing PWS is a methylation-sensitive analysis by Southern blotting using methylation-sensitive restriction enzymes (Kubota et al., 1996b, 1996a) or a methylation-sensitive PCR-based approach (Zeschnig et al., 1997; Muralidhar and Butler 1998). Both approaches have been shown to be very effective. An approach that avoids methylation analysis has been proposed using RT-PCR to document the lack of expression of a maternally imprinted gene in the region, *SNRPN* (Kubota et al., 1996a, 1996b; Wevrick and Francke, 1996; Chotai and Payne, 1998).

Many practitioners order high-resolution chromosome analysis simultaneously with the methylation study in recognition that the chromosome analysis will be needed regardless of the result of the more specific test. If the methylation analysis is normal, chromosome analysis is needed because among people referred for PWS testing, another, unexpected, chromosomal rearrangement is frequently found. If the methylation test result is positive, chromosome analysis is needed to identify the molecular cause of the abnormal methylation. If a deletion is not seen on routine chromosome analysis, fluorescence in situ hybridization (FISH) using the *SNRPN* probe should be performed to rule out deletions. *SNRPN* is the best probe for FISH studies because it includes the PWS imprinting center, of which small deletions may lead to the PWS phenotype (Buiting et al., 1995; Saitoh et al., 1997; Nicholls et al., 1998; Ohta et al., 1999). Last, if no deletion is found, microsatellite studies to rule out UPD should be performed (Shaffer et al., 2001). If no deletion or UPD is found to explain an abnormal pattern of methylation, an error of the imprinting center is presumed.

This is significant because the recurrence risk is higher, as great as 50% with each pregnancy, in imprinting defects.

FISH, microsatellite studies for UPD, and methylation analysis have all been validated for prenatal diagnosis in amniocytes or chorionic villi (Kubota et al., 1996a; Glenn et al., 2000), and all three are available clinically. Further testing to confirm the cause of the imprinting defect is available only on a research basis.

MANAGEMENT

As with most chronic diseases, the treatment of PWS centers on the management of its manifestations. The management changes with age, focusing in infancy on feeding and muscle tone issues. Later, the focus changes to control of eating and weight, education, and behavior management. In adult life, the added issues of dealing with secondary complications, activities of daily living, and mental health concerns take on increasing importance. Several thorough discussions of management issues have been previously published (Greenswag and Alexander, 1995; Cassidy, 2001).

In the newborn with PWS, feeding via gavage is often required for up to 6 months. Feeding with systems designed for infants with cleft palate, such as the Haberman™ nipple or Pigeon feeder, may be useful. Nasogastric tubes are generally well tolerated; gastrostomy placement is usually avoidable. Nutritional management during infancy should involve the use of concentrated formulas to minimize volume requirements. Caloric requirements at this stage are similar to or greater than those for neonates without PWS. Weight and length should be closely monitored to avoid poor growth related to the increased work of feeding.

Cryptorchidism in males is common and often requires surgical intervention. Because fertility has not been observed in males with PWS, early surgical intervention is less urgent and may be best delayed until the early feeding problems are resolved. Injections of human chorionic gonadotropin (hCG) may help bring the testes farther down the inguinal canal and enlarge the scrotum and, occasionally, can obviate the need for surgical intervention.

Management issues in childhood center on nutrition, behavior, and education. Nutritional counseling for the family should begin in infancy to ensure the child develops appropriate food preferences from an early age. It is important to ensure that the family is not restricting fats excessively in infancy for fear of the later development of obesity. Fats are essential for brain growth, and there is no evidence to suggest that restriction of fats in infancy will improve weight management later in life. Because the muscle mass is disproportionately low for any given body size, caloric requirements for older children with PWS are often as low as 60% of those for normally proportioned children of the same body weight (Holm and Pipes, 1976). It is critical to monitor growth and to record measurements on a standard growth curve regularly so that excess weight gain can be identified and dealt with early. Vitamin and mineral (especially calcium and vitamin D) intake must be monitored, and supplements should be given as needed.

The feeling of hunger is never completely relieved in individuals with PWS, even after eating a large meal. Sight, smell, or discussion of food will make the child with PWS uncomfortable. Their tendency to obsessive thinking can make it difficult for them to concentrate on anything else if there is food visible in the room; this is an important fact for school workers. Likewise, individuals with PWS are not well equipped to help with food preparation and cleanup, and these tasks should be avoided. All caretakers need to understand these factors, including grandparents and extended family members, neighbors, friends, and church and school providers.

Behavior management also should begin early because it clearly is easier to avoid the development of problem behaviors than it is to treat them. Affected children in general respond well to routine, regular schedules, and advance notice of transitions in activities. Parents should be instructed on the importance of setting limits and reinforcing them consistently and strongly. Redirection, positive reinforcement, and nonfood reward systems often work well. Most experts believe that giving or withholding food should not be used as a reward or a punishment for a person with PWS.

Pharmacologic interventions are frequently helpful, particularly in dealing with anxiety disorders and obsessive-compulsive behaviors. In one report from a rehabilitation hospital with expertise in caring for patients with PWS, as many as 75% of individuals admitted for crisis management of PWS required some type of psychotropic medication to adequately manage behavior or psychiatric symptoms (Brice, 2000). The same review of the experience of a single unit (Brice, 2000) found that the medications most commonly used are the selective serotonin reuptake inhibitors, which are helpful with both anxiety and obsessive symptoms. For individuals with aggression or severe mood instability, mood stabilizers such as sodium valproate or lithium may be helpful. Less commonly, these problems may require treatment with an antipsychotic agent, a therapy that may also be indicated for older teens and adults with psychotic symptoms. Individuals with PWS tend to be sensitive to medications, and it is prudent to start new drugs at the low end of the dosage range. Pharmacologic agents directed at reducing appetite have been ineffective in PWS (Zipf and Berntson, 1987; Fieldstone et al., 1998; Yaryura-Tobias et al., 1998; Ming et al., 2000). Several case reports of surgical attempts to limit obesity have had mixed results (Touquet et al., 1983; Miyata et al., 1990; Dousei et al., 1992; Antal and Levin, 1996; Grugni et al., 2000), likely due to the inability to affect the lack of sense of satiety.

There are three randomized controlled trials of growth hormone replacement therapy in PWS, all of which have demonstrated improved linear growth velocity (Fig. 74–3), body composition, muscle function, and level of activity (Hauffa, 1997; Lindgren et al., 1997, 1998; Eiholzer et al., 1998, 2000; Carrel et al., 1999, 2001; Lindgren and Ritzen, 1999; Eiholzer and l'Allemand, 2000). Body composition changes include increased lean muscle mass and decreased fat mass (Figs. 74–4 and 74–5) There also is an associated increase in energy level and willingness to partake in physical activity (Hauffa, 1997; Eiholzer et al., 1998). Further, there is evidence of improvement in the decreased respiratory drive in response to increased CO_2 concentrations (Lindgren et al., 1999). Linear growth increases markedly in the first year and then settles into a slower, but higher than baseline, rate in the second year. These benefits continued through 4 years of continuous therapy at doses of 1 to 1.5 mg/M^2/day but not with low-dose therapy (0.3 mg/M^2/day) (Carrel et al., 2001). Side effects of human growth hormone therapy appear to be rare but include pedal edema, worsening of scoliosis, and risk of pseudotumor cerebri.

Approval for use of human growth hormone therapy is for children older than 3 years of age, as neither infants nor adults were included in the original studies. A small clinical trial of growth hormone in infants with PWS suggests benefit (Eiholzer et al., 2001). Similarly, growth hormone may be beneficial in maintaining muscle bulk and body composition in adults (Mogul et al., 2000). Further studies in both age groups are under way.

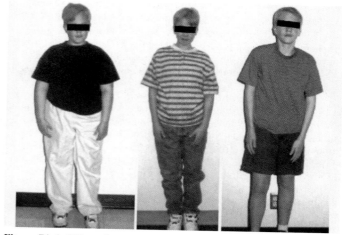

Figure 74–4. Effect of growth hormone on body composition showing the same individual at (A) initiation of therapy with recombinant human growth hormone, (B) after 12 months of therapy, and (C) after 24 months of therapy. Note the striking changes in body habitus. (Photograph courtesy of Aaron L. Carrel, MD, published with permission of Lippincott, Williams & Wilkins, Philadelphia.)

Because of the relative intensity of living with an individual with PWS families are often ready for the child with PWS, to leave home on becoming an adult. Often, a group home setting, especially those specifically designated for individuals with PWS, can significantly reduce the burden of exposure to food.

MOUSE MODELS

The human PWS region of chromosome 15q11-13 is syntenic to the central region of mouse chromosome 7 with similar genomic structure and organization, including imprinting patterns (Nicholls and Knepper, 2001). On the other hand, the imprinting mechanisms may have diverged as suggested by a transgenic mouse whose *Snrpn* sequence, including the purported IC region, was replaced with human *SNRPN* sequence, causing biallelic expression of the genes in the region (Blaydes et al., 1999).

There are mouse models for the common deletion (Gabriel et al., 1999), for maternal UPD for the relevant region (Cattanach et al., 1992), and for an imprinting mutation (Yang et al., 1998; Blaydes et al., 1999; Bielinska et al., 2000). In addition, there are knock-out mod-

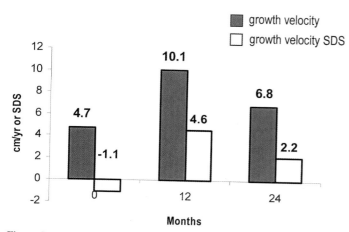

Figure 74–3. Effect of treatment with recombinant human growth hormone on growth velocity. Mean growth velocity in cm/yr and standard deviations (SDS) are shown at start of therapy and after 12 and 24 months of therapy. (Data from Carrel et al., 1999.)

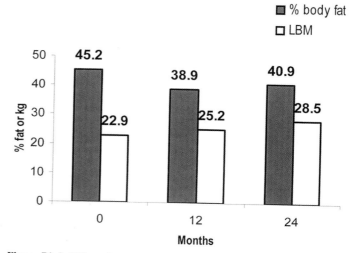

Figure 74–5. Effect of treatment with recombinant human growth hormone on percent body fat and lean body mass (LBM) at start of therapy and after 12 and 24 months of therapy. (Data from Carrel et al., 1999.)

els for *NECDIN* (Gerard et al., 1999; Tsai et al., 1999a; Muscatelli et al., 2000) and *SNRPN* (Tsai et al., 1999b). A variety of abnormalities have been described in these mice, yet none completely recapitulates the clinical findings and course of human PWS (Cattanach et al., 1992; Blaydes et al., 1999; Gabriel et al., 1999; Gerard et al., 1999; Tsai et al., 1999a, 1999b; Bielinska et al., 2000; Lee et al., 2000; Muscatelli et al., 2000).

A targeted deletion of mouse chromosome 7 from exon 2 of *Snrpn* to *Ube3a* leads to a phenotype similar to the newborn presentation of PWS when paternally inherited—hypotonia and growth retardation—and high mortality rates by the time of weaning (Tsai et al., 1999b). Surviving mice were fertile and did not become obese. Genes outside the region of the deletion (e.g., *Necdin*) were normally expressed, confirming that the imprinting center is upstream of exon 2 of *Snrpn*.

Similarly, a transgenic mouse with a deletion of the entire PWS region has a perinatal lethal phenotype with low muscle activity when inherited paternally (Gabriel et al., 1999). There was no obvious phenotype in maternally inherited deletions in either case. When *Snrpn* was deleted but the imprinting center was left intact, all offspring were phenotypically normal regardless of whether the deletion was inherited paternally or maternally (Yang et al., 1998). A slightly larger *Snrpn* deletion that included the imprinting center caused a phenotype similar to the mice described earlier with deletions of the larger PWS region (Yang et al., 1998). Thus, there are reasonable mouse models for the neonatal phenotype caused by both deletion and imprinting defects. Interestingly, mice chimeric for an imprinting center deletion show evidence of loss of the paternal imprint in somatic cells, suggesting that the imprinting center is necessary not only for initiation of the paternal imprint but also for its maintenance (Bielinska et al., 2000).

Three different mouse strains have been created with targeted disruption of the *Necdin* gene (Gerard et al., 1999; Tsai et al., 1999a; Muscatelli et al., 2000). One line showed no identifiable phenotype when the *Necdin* deletion was passed by either parent (Tsai et al., 1999a), but the background strain was not reported, nor was the breeding strategy described. The other two *Necdin* knockout models, both expressed on a C57Bl6/J background, had different phenotypes. One had significant perinatal lethality associated with respiratory distress and cyanosis (Gerard et al., 1999). Further crosses on a hybrid background lead to reduction, and even normalization, of the neonatal lethal phenotype, suggesting a strong background effect for this particular characteristic. Those surviving the neonatal period had normal fertility and did not become obese. Expression studies staining with X-gal showed no evidence of the inserted *LacZ*-containing maternally inherited allele in many areas of the brain, including the hypothalamus.

The remaining *Necdin*-deficient mouse model (Muscatelli et al., 2000) also showed a significant postnatal mortality rate that was decreased by further outcrosses. Additional phenotyping of these mice showed increased skin-scraping behavior in the knockout, a behavior possibly comparable to skin picking in people with PWS. They did have better than normal function in spatial learning and memory, suggesting a possible connection with the visuospatial strength shown in individuals with PWS (e.g., skill with jigsaw puzzles; Dykens et al., 2002). They also observed reduced numbers of hypothalamic oxytocin- and leutinizing hormone–releasing hormone–producing neurons, possibly reflecting part of the appetite control defect and hypogonadotropic hypogonadism seen in PWS.

The differences in the three *Necdin* knockout models may be due to minor differences in the approach used to produce the knockout, but more likely they reflect the presence of modifier genes and epigenetic differences based on the genetic background (Nicholls, 1999).

PATHOGENESIS

Despite the large body of literature describing the genomic structure of the PWS region of chromosome 15, very little is known about the specific mechanisms by which failure of expression of the genes involved leads to failure of normal development. The primary phenotypic findings in PWS appear to be secondary to abnormal CNS development. The genes in the region are expressed in the brain and, by homology to other genes, are suggested to have a regulatory function in other pathways. These pathways have not been elucidated. *SNRPN* appears to function as a subunit of the spliceosome in the CNS and therefore may affect transcription of genes involved in a variety of aspects of neurodevelopment. snoRNAs in the region may also have a role in RNA processing in the CNS. *NECDIN* may be involved in postmitotic cell proliferation, and *MAGEL2* may have a role in apoptosis, suggesting a possible role for both in the development of nuclei in the hypothalmus disordered in PWS. Deletion of the *P* gene has an obvious role in pigmentation in patients with deletions. We believe that most, if not all, of the dysmorphic characteristics are secondary to hypotonia and endocrine dysfunction and that they become significantly less obvious during growth hormone therapy.

CONCLUSION

PWS is complex in terms of molecular basis, clinical manifestations, and management. Little is understood about the pathogenesis despite a dramatic increase in research on genetics and genotype–phenotype correlation. It is anticipated that mouse models, which exist for all three causes of PWS, will be of great benefit in understanding the fundamental processes that have gone awry in affected individuals. It is also hoped that these studies will lead to innovative treatments, such as reversal of imprinting, that may improve understanding of the control of gene expression but also benefit the lives of the families who live with this condition.

ACKNOWLEDGMENTS

The authors wish to thank Dr. Robert Nicholls for his helpful input.

REFERENCES

Greenswag LR, Alexander RC (1995). *Management of Prader-Willi syndrome, 2nd edition.* Springer-Verlag, New York.

Akefeldt A, Akefeldt B, Gillberg C (1997). Voice, speech and language characteristics of children with Prader-Willi syndrome. *J Intellect Disabil Res* 41(Pt 4): 302–311.

Akefeldt A, Tornhage CJ, Gillberg C (1999). A woman with Prader-Willi syndrome gives birth to a healthy baby girl. *Dev Med Child Neurol* 41: 789–790.

Amos-Landgraf JM, Ji Y, Gottlieb W, Depinet T, Wandstrat AE, Cassidy SB, Driscoll DJ, Rogan PK, Schwartz S, Nicholls RD (1999). Chromosome breakage in the Prader-Willi and Angelman syndromes involves recombination between large, transcribed repeats at proximal and distal breakpoints. *Am J Hum Genet* 65: 370–386.

Antal S, Levin H (1996). Biliopancreatic diversion in Prader-Willi syndrome associated with obesity. *Obes Surg* 6: 58–62.

Barker PA, Salehi A (2002). The MAGE proteins: Emerging roles in cell cycle progression, apoptosis, and neurogenetic disease. *J Neurosci Res* 67: 705–712.

Beardsmore A, Dorman T, Cooper SA, Webb T (1998). Affective psychosis and Prader-Willi syndrome. *J Intellect Disabil Res* 42(Pt 6): 463–471.

Bielinska B, Blaydes SM, Buiting K, Yang T, Krajewska-Walasek M, Horsthemke B, Brannan CI (2000). De novo deletions of *SNRPN* exon 1 in early human and mouse embryos result in a paternal imprint switch. *Nat Genet* 25: 74–78.

Blaydes SM, Elmore M, Yang T, Brannan CI (1999). Analysis of murine *Snrpn* and human *SNRPN* gene imprinting in transgenic mice. *Mamm Genome* 10: 549–555.

Boccaccio I, Glatt-Deeley H, Watrin F, Roeckel N, Lalande M, Muscatelli F (1999). The human *MAGEL2* gene and its mouse homologue are paternally expressed and mapped to the Prader-Willi region. *Hum Mol Genet* 8: 2497–2505.

Boer H, Holland A, Whittington J, Butler J, Webb T, Clarke D (2002). Psychotic illness in people with Prader Willi syndrome due to chromosome 15 maternal uniparental disomy. *Lancet* 359: 135–136.

Bray GA, Dahms WT, Swerdloff RS, Fiser RH, Atkinson RL, Carrel RE (1983). The Prader-Willi syndrome: a study of 40 patients and a review of the literature. *Medicine (Balt)* 62: 59–80.

Brice J (2000). Behaviorial and psychotropic interventions in persons with Prader-Willi syndrome. *Endocrinologist* 10: 27S–30S.

Buiting K, Gross S, Ji Y, Senger G, Nicholls RD, Horsthemke B (1998). Expressed copies of the *MN7 (D15F37)* gene family map close to the common deletion breakpoints in the Prader-Willi/Angelman syndromes. *Cytogenet Cell Genet* 81: 247–253.

Buiting K, Saitoh S, Gross S, Dittrich B, Schwartz S, Nicholls RD, Horsthemke B (1995). Inherited microdeletions in the Angelman and Prader-Willi syndromes define an imprinting centre on human chromosome 15. *Nat Genet* 9: 395–400.

Buiting K, Greger V, Brownstein BH, Mohr RM, Voiculescu I, Winterpacht A, Zabel B, Horsthemke B (1992). A putative gene family in 15q11-13 and 16p11.2: possible implications for Prader-Willi and Angelman syndromes. *Proc Natl Acad Sci USA* 89: 5457–5461.

Burd L, Vesely B, Martsolf J, Kerbeshian J (1990). Prevalence study of Prader-Willi syndrome in North Dakota. *Am J Med Genet* 37: 97–99.

Burman P, Ritzen EM, Lindgren AC (2001). Endocrine dysfunction in Prader-Willi syndrome: a review with special reference to GH. *Endocr Rev* 22: 787–799.

Butler MG (1989). Hypopigmentation: a common feature of Prader-Labhart-Willi syndrome. *Am J Hum Genet* 45: 140–146.

Butler MG (1990). Prader-Willi syndrome: current understanding of cause and diagnosis. *Am J Med Genet* 35: 319–332.

Butler MG, Thompson T (2000). Prader-Willi syndrome: Clinical and genetic findings. *Endocrinologist* 10: 3S–16S.

Butler MG, Meaney FJ, and Palmer CG (1986). Clinical and cytogenetic survey of 39 individuals with Prader-Labhart-Willi syndrome. *Am J Med Genet* 23: 793–809.

Carrel AL, Myers SE, Whitman BY, Allen DB (1999). Growth hormone improves body composition, fat utilization, physical strength and agility, and growth in Prader-Willi syndrome: A controlled study. *J Pediatr* 134: 215–221.

Carrel AL, Myers SE, Whitman BY, Allen DB (2001). Sustained benefits of growth hormone on body composition, fat utilization, physical strength and agility, and growth in Prader-Willi syndrome are dose-dependent. *J Pediatr Endocrinol Metab* 14: 1097–1105.

Cassidy SB (1984). Prader-Willi syndrome. *Curr Prob Pediatr* 14(1): 1–55.

Cassidy SB (1997). Prader-Willi syndrome. *J Med Genet* 34: 917–923.

Cassidy SB (2001). Prader-Willi syndrome. In: *Management of Genetic Syndromes.* Cassidy SB, Allanson JE (eds.) Wiley-Liss, New York, pp. 301–322.

Cassidy SB, Ledbetter DH (1989). Prader-Willi syndrome. *Neurol Clin* 7: 37–54.

Cassidy SB, Morris CL (2002). Behavioral phenotypes. *Adv Pediatr* 49: 59–86.

Cassidy SB, Devi A, Mukaida C (1994). Aging in Prader-Willi syndrome: 22 patients over age 30 years. *Proc Greenwood Genet Center* 13: 102–103.

Cassidy SB, Dykens E, Williams CA (2000). Prader-Willi and Angelman syndromes: sister imprinted disorders. *Am J Med Genet* 97: 136–146.

Cassidy SB, Lai LW, Erickson RP, Magnuson L, Thomas E, Gendron R, Herrmann J (1992). Trisomy 15 with loss of the paternal 15 as a cause of Prader-Willi syndrome due to maternal disomy. *Am J Hum Genet* 51: 701–708.

Cassidy SB, Forsythe M, Heeger S, Nicholls RD, Schork N, Benn P, Schwartz S (1997). Comparison of phenotype between patients with Prader-Willi syndrome due to deletion 15q and uniparental disomy 15. *Am J Med Genet* 68: 433–440.

Cattanach BM, Barr JA, Evans EP, Burtenshaw M, Beechey CV, Leff SE, Brannan CI, Copeland NG, Jenkins NA, Jones J (1992). A candidate mouse model for Prader-Willi syndrome which shows an absence of *Snrpn* expression. *Nat Genet* 2: 270–274.

Cavaille J, Buiting K, Kiefmann M, Lalande M, Brannan CI, Horsthemke B, Bachellerie JP, Brosius J, Huttenhofer A (2000). Identification of brain-specific and imprinted small nucleolar RNA genes exhibiting an unusual genomic organization. *Proc Natl Acad Sci USA* 97: 14311–14316.

Chotai KA, Payne SJ (1998). A rapid, PCR based test for differential molecular diagnosis of Prader-Willi and Angelman syndromes. *J Med Genet* 35: 472–475.

Christian SL, Fantes JA, Mewborn SK, Huang B, Ledbetter DH (1999). Large genomic duplicons map to sites of instability in the Prader-Willi/Angelman syndrome chromosome region (15q11-q13). *Hum Mol Genet* 8: 1025–1037.

Christian SL, Robinson WP, Huang B, Mutirangura A, Line MR, Nakao M, Surti U, Chakravarti A, Ledbetter DH (1995). Molecular characterization of two proximal deletion breakpoint regions in both Prader-Willi and Angelman syndrome patients. *Am J Hum Genet* 57: 40–48.

Clarke D (1998). Prader-Willi syndrome and psychotic symptoms: 2. a preliminary study of prevalence using the Psychopathology Assessment Schedule for Adults with Developmental Disability checklist. *J Intellect Disabil Res* 42(Pt 6): 451–454.

Clarke DJ, Boer H, Chung MC, Sturmey P, Webb T (1996). Maladaptive behaviour in Prader-Willi syndrome in adult life. *J Intellect Disabil Res* 40(Pt 2): 159–165.

Clarke D, Boer H, Webb T, Scott P, Frazer S, Vogels A, Borghgraef M, Curfs LM (1998). Prader-Willi syndrome and psychotic symptoms: 1. case descriptions and genetic studies. *J Intellect Disabil Res* 42(Pt 6): 440–450.

Corrias A, Bellone J, Beccaria L, Bosio L, Trifiro G, Livieri C, Ragusa L, Salvatoni A, Andreo M, Ciampalini P, et al. (2000). GH/IGF-I axis in Prader-Willi syndrome: evaluation of IGF-I levels and of the somatotroph responsiveness to various provocative stimuli. Genetic Obesity Study Group of Italian Society of Pediatric Endocrinology and Diabetology. *J Endocrinol Invest* 23: 84–89.

Curfs LMG (2002). Psychological profile and behavioral characteristics in Prader-Willi syndrome. In: *Prader-Willi Syndrome and Other 15q Deletion Disorders.* Edited by: Cassidy SB (ed.). Springer-Verlag, Berlin, pp. 211–222.

Curfs LM, Fryns JP (1992). Prader-Willi syndrome: a review with special attention to the cognitive and behavioral profile. *Birth Defects Orig Artic Ser* 28: 99–104.

de los Santos T, Schweizer J, Rees CA, Francke U (2000). Small evolutionarily conserved RNA, resembling C/D box small nucleolar RNA, is transcribed from *PWCR1*, a novel imprinted gene in the Prader-Willi deletion region, which is highly expressed in brain. *Am J Hum Genet* 67: 1067–1082.

Dousei T, Miyata M, Izukura M, Harada T, Kitagawa T, Matsuda H (1992). Long-term follow-up of gastroplasty in a patient with Prader-Willi syndrome. *Obes Surg* 2: 189–193.

Driscoll DJ, Waters MF, Williams CA, Zori RT, Glenn CC, Avidano KM, Nicholls RD (1992). A DNA methylation imprint, determined by the sex of the parent, distinguishes the Angelman and PWS syndromes. *Genomics* 13: 917–924.

Dykens EM (2002). Are jigsaw puzzle skills 'spared' in persons with Prader-Willi syndrome? *J Child Psychol Psychiatry* 43: 343–352.

Dykens EM, Cassidy SB (1995). Correlates of maladaptive behavior in children and adults with Prader-Willi syndrome. *Am J Med Genet* 60: 546–549.

Dykens EM, Cassidy SB (1999). PWS. In: *Handbook of Neurodevelopmental and Genetic Disorders in Children.* Goldstein S, Reynolds CR (eds.) Guilford Press, New York, pp. 525–554.

Dykens EM, Cassidy SB (2002). Prader-Willi and Angelman syndrome: cognitive and behavioral phenotypes. In: *Genetics and Neurobehavioral Disorders.* Fisch GS (ed.) Humana Press, Totowa, NJ.

Dykens EM, Kasari C (1997). Maladaptive behavior in children with Prader-Willi syndrome, Down syndrome, and nonspecific mental retardation. *Am J Ment Retard* 102: 228–237.

Dykens EM, Cassidy SB, King BH (1999). Maladaptive behavior differences in Prader-Willi syndrome due to paternal deletion versus maternal uniparental disomy. *Am J Ment Retard* 104: 67–77.

Dykens EM, Leckman JF, Cassidy SB (1996). Obsessions and compulsions in Prader-Willi syndrome. *J Child Psychol Psychiatry* 37: 995–1002.

Eiholzer U, l'Allemand D (2000). Growth hormone normalises height, prediction of final height and hand length in children with Prader-Willi syndrome after 4 years of therapy. *Horm Res* 53: 185–192.

Eiholzer U, l'Allemand D, van der Sluis I, Steinert H, Gasser T, Ellis K (2000). Body composition abnormalities in children with Prader-Willi syndrome and long-term effects of growth hormone therapy. *Horm Res* 53: 200–206.

Eiholzer U, Schlumpf M, Nordmann Y, l'Allemand D (2001). Early manifestations of Prader-Willi syndrome: influence of growth hormone. *J Pediatr Endocrinol Metab* 14(suppl 6): 1441–1444.

Eiholzer U, Gisin R, Weinmann C, Kriemler S, Steinert H, Torresani T, Zachmann M, Prader A (1998). Treatment with human growth hormone in patients with Prader-Labhart-Willi syndrome reduces body fat and increases muscle mass and physical performance. *Eur J Pediatr* 157: 368–377.

European Collaborative Research on Mosaicism in CVS (EUCROMIC) (1999). Trisomy 15 CPM: probable origins, pregnancy outcome and risk of fetal UPD. *Prenat Diagn* 19: 29–35.

Fieldstone A, Zipf WB, Sarter MF, Berntson GG (1998). Food intake in Prader-Willi syndrome and controls with obesity after administration of a benzodiazepine receptor agonist. *Obes Res* 6: 29–33.

Gabriel JM, Merchant M, Ohta T, Ji Y, Caldwell RG, Ramsey MJ, Tucker JD, Longnecker R, Nicholls RD (1999). A transgene insertion creating a heritable chromosome deletion mouse model of Prader-Willi and Angelman syndromes. *Proc Natl Acad Sci USA* 96: 9258–9263.

Gerard M, Hernandez L, Wevrick R, Stewart CL (1999). Disruption of the mouse *necdin* gene results in early post-natal lethality. *Nat Genet* 23: 199–202.

Gillessen-Kaesbach G, Robinson W, Lohmann D, Kaya-Westerloh S, Passarge E, Horsthemke B (1995). Genotype-phenotype correlation in a series of 167 deletion and non-deletion patients with Prader-Willi syndrome. *Hum Genet* 96: 638–643.

Glenn CC, Deng G, Michaelis RC, Tarleton J, Phelan MC, Surh L, Yang TP, Driscoll DJ (2000). DNA methylation analysis with respect to prenatal diagnosis of the Angelman and Prader-Willi syndromes and imprinting. *Prenat Diagn* 20: 300–306.

Glenn CC, Nicholls RD, Robinson WP, Saitoh S, Niikawa N, Schinzel A, Horsthemke B, Driscoll DJ (1993). Modification of 15q11-q13 DNA methylation imprints in unique Angelman and Prader-Willi patients. *Hum Mol Genet* 2: 1377–1382.

Goldstone AP, Unmehopa UA, Bloom SR, Swaab DF (2002). Hypothalamic NPY and agouti-related protein are increased in human illness but not in Prader-Willi syndrome and other obese subjects. *J Clin Endocrinol Metab* 87: 927–937.

Gray TA, Saitoh S, Nicholls RD (1999a). An imprinted, mammalian bicistronic transcript encodes two independent proteins. *Proc Natl Acad Sci USA* 96: 5616–5621.

Gray TA, Smithwick MJ, Schaldach MA, Martone DL, Graves JA, McCarrey JR, Nicholls RD (1999b). Concerted regulation and molecular evolution of the duplicated *SNRPB'/B* and *SNRPN* loci. *Nucleic Acids Res* 27: 4577–4584.

Greenswag LR (1987). Adults with Prader-Willi syndrome: a survey of 232 cases. *Dev Med Child Neurol* 29: 145–152.

Grugni G, Guzzaloni G, Morabito F (2000). Failure of biliopancreatic diversion in Prader-Willi syndrome. *Obes Surg* 10: 179–181.

Gunay-Aygun M, Heeger S, Schwartz S, Cassidy SB (1997). Delayed diagnosis in patients with Prader-Willi syndrome due to maternal uniparental disomy 15. *Am J Med Genet* 71: 106–110.

Gunay-Aygun M, Schwartz S, Heeger S, O'Riordan MA, Cassidy SB (2001). The changing purpose of Prader-Willi syndrome clinical diagnostic criteria and proposed revised criteria. *Pediatrics* 108: E92.

Hall BD, Smith DW (1972). Prader-Willi syndrome. A resume of 32 cases including an instance of affected first cousins, one of whom is of normal stature and intelligence. *J Pediatr* 81: 286–293.

Hauffa BP (1997). One-year results of growth hormone treatment of short stature in Prader-Willi syndrome. *Acta Paediatr Suppl* 423: 63–65.

Hertz G, Cataletto M, Feinsilver SH, Angulo M (1995). Developmental trends of sleep-disordered breathing in Prader-Willi syndrome: the role of obesity. *Am J Med Genet* 56: 188–190.

Holland AJ, Treasure J, Coskeran P, Dallow J (1995). Characteristics of the eating disorder in Prader-Willi syndrome: implications for treatment. *J Intellect Disabil Res* 39(Pt 5): 373–381.

Holland AJ, Treasure J, Coskeran P, Dallow J, Milton N, Hillhouse E (1993). Measurement of excessive appetite and metabolic changes in Prader-Willi syndrome. *Int J Obes Relat Metab Disord* 17: 527–532.

Holm VA, Laurnen EL (1981). Prader-Willi syndrome and scoliosis. *Dev Med Child Neurol* 23: 192–201.

Holm VA, Pipes PL (1976). Food and children with Prader-Willi syndrome. *Am J Dis Child* 130: 1063–1067.

Holm VA, Cassidy SB, Butler MG, Hanchett JM, Greenswag LR, Whitman BY, Greenberg F (1993). Prader-Willi syndrome: consensus diagnostic criteria. *Pediatrics* 91: 398–402.

Jay P, Rougeulle C, Massacrier A, Moncla A, Mattei MG, Malzac P, Roeckel N, Taviaux S, Lefranc JL, Cau P, et al. (1997). The human necdin gene, *NDN*, is maternally imprinted and located in the Prader-Willi syndrome chromosomal region. *Nat Genet* 17: 357–361.

Jeffcoate WJ, Laurance BM, Edwards CR, Besser GM (1980). Endocrine function in the Prader-Willi syndrome. *Clin Endocrinol (Oxf)* 12: 81–89.

Ji Y, Eichler EE, Schwartz S, Nicholls RD (2000). Structure of chromosomal duplicons and their role in mediating human genomic disorders. *Genome Res* 10: 597–610.

Ji Y, Walkowicz MJ, Buiting K, Johnson DK, Tarvin RE, Rinchik EM, Horsthemke B, Stubbs L, Nicholls RD (1999). The ancestral gene for transcribed, low-copy repeats in the Prader-Willi/Angelman region encodes a large protein implicated in protein trafficking, which is deficient in mice with neuromuscular and spermiogenic abnormalities. *Hum Mol Genet* 8: 533–542.

Johnson DK, Stubbs LJ, Culiat CT, Montgomery CS, Russell LB, Rinchik EM (1995).

Molecular analysis of 36 mutations at the mouse pink-eyed dilution (*p*) locus. *Genetics* 141: 1563–1571.
Jong MT, Gray TA, Ji Y, Glenn CC, Saitoh S, Driscoll DJ, Nicholls RD (1999). A novel imprinted gene, encoding a RING zinc-finger protein, and overlapping antisense transcript in the Prader-Willi syndrome critical region. *Hum Mol Genet* 8: 783–793.
Kauli R, Prager-Lewin R, Laron Z (1978). Pubertal development in the Prader-Labhart-Willi syndrome. *Acta Paediatr Scand* 67: 763–767.
King RA, Wiesner GL, Townsend D, White JG (1993). Hypopigmentation in Angelman syndrome. *Am J Med Genet* 46: 40–44.
Kishino T, Lalande M, Wagstaff J (1997). *UBE3A/E6-AP* mutations cause Angelman syndrome. *Nat Genet* 15: 70–73.
Kleppe SA, Katayama KM, Shipley KG, Foushee DR (1990). The speech and language characteristics of children with Prader-Willi syndrome. *J Speech Hear Disord* 55: 300–309.
Kubota T, Aradhya S, Macha M, Smith AC, Surh LC, Satish J, Verp MS, Nee HL, Johnson A, Christan SL, et al. (1996a). Analysis of parent of origin specific DNA methylation at *SNRPN* and *PW71* in tissues: implication for prenatal diagnosis. *J Med Genet* 33: 1011–1014.
Kubota T, Sutcliffe JS, Aradhya S, Gillessen-Kaesbach G, Christian SL, Horsthemke B, Beaudet AL, Ledbetter DH (1996b). Validation studies of *SNRPN* methylation as a diagnostic test for Prader-Willi syndrome. *Am J Med Genet* 66: 77–80.
Kuslich CD, Kobori JA, Mohapatra G, Gregorio-King C, Donlon TA (1999). Prader-Willi syndrome is caused by disruption of the *SNRPN* gene. *Am J Hum Genet* 64: 70–76.
Lee PDK (1995). Endocrine and metabolic aspects of Prader-Willi syndrome. In: *Management of Prader-Willi syndrome*. Greenswag LR, Alexander RC (eds.) Springer-Verlag, New York, pp. 32–57.
Lee S, Kozlov S, Hernandez L, Chamberlain SJ, Brannan CI, Stewart CL, Wevrick R (2000). Expression and imprinting of *MAGEL2* suggest a role in Prader-Willi syndrome and the homologous murine imprinting phenotype. *Hum Mol Genet* 9: 1813–1819.
Lee ST, Nicholls RD, Bundey S, Laxova R, Musarella M, Spritz RA (1994). Mutations of the *P* gene in oculocutaneous albinism, ocular albinism, and Prader-Willi syndrome plus albinism. *N Engl J Med* 330: 529–534.
Lewis B, Lewis B, Freebairn L, Heeger S, Cassidy S (2002). Speech and Language Skills of Individuals with Prader-Willi syndrome. *Am J Speech-Language Pathol* 11: 1–10.
Lindgren AC, Ritzen EM (1999). Five years of growth hormone treatment in children with Prader-Willi syndrome. Swedish National Growth Hormone Advisory Group. *Acta Paediatr Suppl* 88: 109–111.
Lindgren AC, Hellstrom LG, Ritzen EM, Milerad J (1999). Growth hormone treatment increases CO_2 response, ventilation and central inspiratory drive in children with Prader-Willi syndrome. *Eur J Pediatr* 158: 936–940.
Lindgren AC, Hagenas L, Muller J, Blichfeldt S, Rosenborg M, Brismar T, Ritzen EM (1997). Effects of growth hormone treatment on growth and body composition in Prader-Willi syndrome: a preliminary report. The Swedish National Growth Hormone Advisory Group. *Acta Paediatr Suppl* 423: 60–62.
Lindgren AC, Hagenas L, Muller J, Blichfeldt S, Rosenborg M, Brismar T, Ritzen EM (1998). Growth hormone treatment of children with Prader-Willi syndrome affects linear growth and body composition favourably. *Acta Paediatr* 87: 28–31.
Linnemann K, Schroder C, Mix M, Kruger G, Fusch C (1999). Prader-Labhart-Willi syndrome with central precocious puberty and empty sella syndrome. *Acta Paediatr* 88: 1295–1297.
Lupski JR (1998). Genomic disorders: structural features of the genome can lead to DNA rearrangements and human disease traits. *Trends Genet* 14: 417–422.
MacDonald HR, Wevrick R (1997). The *necdin* gene is deleted in Prader-Willi syndrome and is imprinted in human and mouse. *Hum Mol Genet* 6: 1873–1878.
Martin A, State M, Anderson GM, Kaye WM, Hanchett JM, McConaha CW, North WG, Leckman JF (1998). Cerebrospinal fluid levels of oxytocin in Prader-Willi syndrome: a preliminary report. *Biol Psychiatry* 44: 1349–1352.
Maruyama K, Usami M, Aizawa T, Yoshikawa K (1991). A novel brain-specific mRNA encoding nuclear protein (necdin) expressed in neurally differentiated embryonal carcinoma cells. *Biochem Biophys Res Commun* 178: 291–296.
Miller SP, Riley P, Shevell MI (1999). The neonatal presentation of Prader-Willi syndrome revisited. *J Pediatr* 134: 226–228.
Ming JE, Blagowidow N, Knoll JH, Rollings L, Fortina P, McDonald-McGinn DM, Spinner NB, Zackai EH (2000). Submicroscopic deletion in cousins with Prader-Willi syndrome causes a grandmatrilineal inheritance pattern: effects of imprinting. *Am J Med Genet* 92: 19–24.
Mitchell J, Schinzel A, Langlois S, Gillessen-Kaesbach G, Schuffenhauer S, Michaelis R, Abeliovich D, Lerer I, Christian S, Guitart M, et al. (1996). Comparison of phenotype in uniparental disomy and deletion Prader-Willi syndrome: sex specific differences. *Am J Med Genet* 65: 133–136.
Miyata M, Dousei T, Harada T, Aono T, Kitagawa T, Nose O, Kawashima Y (1990). Metabolic changes following gastroplasty in Prader-Willi syndrome—a case report. *Jpn J Surg* 20: 359–364.
Mogul HR, Medhi M, Zhang S, Southren AL (2000). Prader-Willi syndrome in adults. *Endocrinologist* 10: 65S–70S.
Muralidhar B, Butler MG (1998). Methylation PCR analysis of Prader-Willi syndrome, Angelman syndrome, and control subjects. *Am J Med Genet* 80: 263–265.
Muscatelli F, Abrous DN, Massacrier A, Boccaccio I, Le Moal M, Cau P, Cremer H (2000). Disruption of the mouse *Necdin* gene results in hypothalamic and behavioral alterations reminiscent of the human Prader-Willi syndrome. *Hum Mol Genet* 9: 3101–3110.
Nicholls RD (1999). Incriminating gene suspects, Prader-Willi style. *Nat Genet* 23: 132–134.
Nicholls RD, Knepper JL (2001). Genome organization, function, and imprinting in Prader-Willi and Angelman syndromes. *Annu Rev Genomics Hum Genet* 2: 153–175.
Nicholls RD, Saitoh S, Horsthemke B (1998). Imprinting in Prader-Willi and Angelman syndromes. *Trends Genet* 14: 194–200.
Nicholls RD, Knoll JH, Butler MG, Karam S, Lalande M (1989). Genetic imprinting suggested by maternal heterodisomy in nondeletion Prader-Willi syndrome. *Nature* 342: 281–285.
Ohta T, Gray TA, Rogan PK, Buiting K, Gabriel JM, Saitoh S, Muralidhar B, Bilienska B, Krajewska-Walasek M, Driscoll DJ, et al. (1999). Imprinting-mutation mechanisms in Prader-Willi syndrome. *Am J Hum Genet* 64: 397–413.
Ozcelik T, Leff S, Robinson W, Donlon T, Lalande M, Sanjines E, Schinzel A, Francke U (1992). Small nuclear ribonucleoprotein polypeptide N (*SNRPN*), an expressed gene in the Prader-Willi syndrome critical region. *Nat Genet* 2: 265–269.
Park MJ, Kim HS, Kang JH, Kim DH, Chung CY (1999). Serum levels of insulin-like growth factor (IGF)-I, free IGF-I, IGF binding protein (IGFBP)-1, IGFBP-3 and insulin in obese children. *J Pediatr Endocrinol Metab* 12: 139–144.
Prader A, Labhart A, Willi A (1956). Ein syndrom von adipositas, kleinwuchs, kryptorchismus und oligophrenie nach myotonieartigem zustand im neugeborenenalter. *Schweiz Med Wochen* 86: 1260–1261.
Purvis-Smith SG, Saville T, Manass S, Yip MY, Lam-Po-Tang PR, Duffy B, Johnston H, Leigh D, McDonald B (1992). Uniparental disomy 15 resulting from "correction" of an initial trisomy 15. *Am J Hum Genet* 50: 1348–1350.
Radetti G, Bozzola M, Pasquino B, Paganini C, Aglialoro A, Livieri C, Barreca A (1998). Growth hormone bioactivity, insulin-like growth factors (IGFs), and IGF binding proteins in obese children. *Metabolism* 47: 1490–1493.
Ramsay M, Colman MA, Stevens G, Zwane E, Kromberg J, Farrall M, Jenkins T (1992). The tyrosinase-positive oculocutaneous albinism locus maps to chromosome 15q11.2-q12. *Am J Hum Genet* 51: 879–884.
Rinchik EM, Bultman SJ, Horsthemke B, Lee ST, Strunk KM, Spritz RA, Avidano KM, Jong MT, Nicholls RD (1993). A gene for the mouse pink-eyed dilution locus and for human type II oculocutaneous albinism. *Nature* 361: 72–76.
Roberts E, Stevenson K, Cole T, Redford DH, Davison EV (1997). Prospective prenatal diagnosis of Prader-Willi syndrome due to maternal disomy for chromosome 15 following trisomic zygote rescue. *Prenat Diagn* 17: 780–783.
Robinson WP, Dutly F, Nicholls RD, Bernasconi F, Penaherrera M, Michaelis RC, Abeliovich D, Schinzel AA (1998). The mechanisms involved in formation of deletions and duplications of 15q11-q13. *J Med Genet* 35: 130–136.
Roof E, Stone W, MacLean W, Feurer ID, Thompson T, Butler MG (2000). Intellectual characteristics of Prader-Willi syndrome: comparison of genetic subtypes. *J Intellect Disabil Res* 44(Pt 1): 25–30.
Rougeulle C, Glatt H, Lalande M (1997). The Angelman syndrome candidate gene, *UBE3A/E6-AP*, is imprinted in brain. *Nat Genet* 17: 14–15.
Runte M, Huttenhofer A, Gross S, Kiefmann M, Horsthemke B, Buiting K (2001). The IC-SNURF-SNRPN transcript serves as a host for multiple small nucleolar RNA species and as an antisense RNA for *UBE3A*. *Hum Mol Genet* 10: 2687–2700.
Saitoh S, Wada T (2000). Parent-of-origin specific histone acetylation and reactivation of a key imprinted gene locus in Prader-Willi syndrome. *Am J Hum Genet* 66: 1958–1962.
Saitoh S, Buiting K, Cassidy SB, Conroy JM, Driscoll DJ, Gabriel JM, Gillessen-Kaesbach G, Glenn CC, Greenswag LR, Horsthemke B, et al. (1997). Clinical spectrum and molecular diagnosis of Angelman and Prader-Willi syndrome patients with an imprinting mutation. *Am J Med Genet* 68: 195–206.
Scacchi M, Pincelli AI, Cavagnini F (1999). Growth hormone in obesity. *Int J Obes Relat Metab Disord* 23: 260–271.
Schmidt H, Schwarz HP (2001). Premature adrenarche, increased growth velocity and accelerated bone age in male patients with Prader-Labhart-Willi syndrome. *Eur J Pediatr* 160: 69–70.
Schulze A, Mogensen H, Hamborg-Petersen B, Graem N, Ostergaard JR, Brondum-Nielsen K (2001). Fertility in Prader-Willi syndrome: a case report with Angelman syndrome in the offspring. *Acta Paediatr* 90: 455–459.
Shaffer LG, Agan N, Goldberg JD, Ledbetter DH, Longshore JW, Cassidy SB (2001). American College of Medical Genetics statement on diagnostic testing for uniparental disomy. *Genet Med* 3: 206–211.
Spritz RA, Bailin T, Nicholls RD, Lee ST, Park SK, Mascari MJ, Butler MG (1997). Hypopigmentation in the Prader-Willi syndrome correlates with *P* gene deletion but not with haplotype of the hemizygous *P* allele. *Am J Med Genet* 71: 57–62.
State M, Dykens EM, Rosner B, Martin A, King BH (1999). Obsessive-compulsive symptoms in Prader-Willi and "Prader-Willi-like" patients. *J Am Acad Child Adolesc Psychiatry* 38: 329–334.
Stein DJ, Keating J, Zar HJ, Hollander E (1994). A survey of the phenomenology and pharmacotherapy of compulsive and impulsive-aggressive symptoms in Prader-Willi syndrome. *J Neuropsychiatry Clin Neurosci* 6: 23–29.
Sun Y, Nicholls RD, Butler MG, Saitoh S, Hainline BE, Palmer CG (1996). Breakage in the *SNRPN* locus in a balanced 46,XY,t(15;19) Prader-Willi syndrome patient. *Hum Mol Genet* 5: 517–524.
Sutcliffe JS, Han M, Christian SL, Ledbetter DH (1997). Neuronally-expressed *necdin* gene: an imprinted candidate gene in Prader-Willi syndrome. *Lancet* 350: 1520–1521.
Swaab DF (1997). Prader-Willi syndrome and the hypothalamus. *Acta Paediatr Suppl* 423: 50–54.
Symons FJ, Butler MG, Sanders MD, Feurer ID, Thompson T (1999). Self-injurious behavior and Prader-Willi syndrome: behavioral forms and body locations. *Am J Ment Retard* 104: 260–269.
Taylor RL (1988). Cognitive and behavioral features. In: *Prader-Willi syndrome: Selected Research and Management Issues* Caldwell ML, Taylor RL (eds.) Springer-Verlag, New York, pp. 29–42.
Touquet VL, Ward MW, Clark CG (1983). Obesity surgery in a patient with the Prader-Willi syndrome. *Br J Surg* 70: 180–181.
Tsai TF, Armstrong D, Beaudet AL (1999a). *Necdin*-deficient mice do not show lethality or the obesity and infertility of Prader-Willi syndrome. *Nat Genet* 22: 15–16.
Tsai TF, Jiang YH, Bressler J, Armstrong D, Beaudet AL (1999b). Paternal deletion from *Snrpn* to *Ube3a* in the mouse causes hypotonia, growth retardation and partial lethality and provides evidence for a gene contributing to Prader-Willi syndrome. *Hum Mol Genet* 8: 1357–1364.

Vanelli M, Bernasconi S, Caronna N, Virdis R, Terzi C, Giovannelli G (1984). Precocious puberty in a male with Prader-Labhart-Willi syndrome. *Helv Paediatr Acta* 39: 373–377.

Vu TH, Hoffman AR (1997). Imprinting of the Angelman syndrome gene, *UBE3A*, is restricted to brain. *Nat Genet* 17: 12–13.

Wevrick R, Francke U (1996). Diagnostic test for the Prader-Willi syndrome by *SNRPN* expression in blood. *Lancet* 348: 1068–1069.

Wiesner GL, Bendel CM, Olds DP, White JG, Arthur DC, Ball DW, King RA (1987). Hypopigmentation in the Prader-Willi syndrome. *Am J Hum Genet* 40: 431–442.

Wirth J, Back E, Huttenhofer A, Nothwang HG, Lich C, Gross S, Menzel C, Schinzel A, Kioschis P, Tommerup N, et al. (2001). A translocation breakpoint cluster disrupts the newly defined 3′ end of the *SNURF-SNRPN* transcription unit on chromosome 15. *Hum Mol Genet* 10: 201–210.

Yang T, Adamson TE, Resnick JL, Leff S, Wevrick R, Francke U, Jenkins NA, Copeland NG, Brannan CI (1998). A mouse model for Prader-Willi syndrome imprinting-centre mutations. *Nat Genet* 19: 25–31.

Yaryura-Tobias JA, Grunes MS, Bayles ME, Neziroglu F (1998). Hyperphagia and self-mutilation in Prader-Willi syndrome: psychopharmacological issues. *Eat Weight Disord* 3: 163–167.

Zellweger H, Schneider HJ (1968). Syndrome of hypotonia-hypomentia-hypogonadism-obesity (HHHO) or Prader-Willi syndrome. *Am J Dis Child* 115: 588–598.

Zeschnigk M, Lich C, Buiting K, Doerfler W, Horsthemke B (1997). A single-tube PCR test for the diagnosis of Angelman and Prader-Willi syndrome based on allelic methylation differences at the *SNRPN* locus. *Eur J Hum Genet* 5: 94–98.

Zipf WB, Berntson GG (1987). Characteristics of abnormal food-intake patterns in children with Prader-Willi syndrome and study of effects of naloxone. *Am J Clin Nutr* 46: 277–281.

DNMT3B and the Immunodeficiency-Centromeric Instability-Facial Anomalies Syndrome

DEBORAH BOURC'HIS, FRANÇOISE LEDEIST, AND EVANI VIEGAS-PÉQUIGNOT

ICF syndrome (OMIM 242860) is a rare recessive autosomal disease characterized by variable combined immunodeficiency (I), centromeric instability (C) and facial anomalies (F) (Hultén, 1978; Tiepolo et al., 1978, 1979). The dysmorphic facial features include hypertelorism, low-set ears, micrognathia, a flat nasal bridge, and an epicanthus. The unusually decondensed and juxtacentromeric heterochromatin of chromosomes 1 and 16 and, less frequently, chromosome 9 is abnormally hypomethylated in all ICF tissues. The hypomethylated classical satellite 2 is the preferential breakpoint for the deletions and duplications of chromosome arms observed in the lymphocyte cells of patients with ICF. This syndrome can be diagnosed on the basis of these characteristic chromosome abnormalities and the variable immunodeficiency associated with life-threatening infections. The ICF locus has been mapped to 20q11-13, and mutations have been observed in the *DNMT3B* gene in several patients. The *DNMT3B* (ICF) gene is required for de novo methylation and normal development.

ICF syndrome is the first known human disease directly related to a constitutive DNA methylation defect. This methylation effect primarily affects classical satellite repeats (Jeanpierre et al., 1993; Miniou et al., 1994). Most of the cases of ICF described (about 35 patients) were found in Europe, although some families from North Africa have also been described. Only two patients from the United States and two families from Japan have been reported (Fryns et al., 1981; Howard et al., 1985; Carpenter et al., 1987; Valkova et al., 1987; Maraschio et al., 1988; Turleau et al., 1989; Fasth et al., 1990; Bauld et al., 1991; Tüküm et al., 1992; Gimelli et al., 1993; Jeanpierre et al., 1993; Smeets et al., 1994; Brown et al., 1995; Franceschini et al., 1995; Sawyer et al., 1995; Schuffenhauer et al., 1995; and unpublished observations). The frequency of ICF is probably underestimated because karyotype analysis, which is the most reliable means of diagnosis, is not systematically recommended in case of severe combined immunodeficiency.

Homozygosity mapping in consanguineous families showed that the ICF locus maps to 20q11-q13 (Wijmenga et al., 1998). Direct mutation screening then showed that *DNMT3B* was the gene responsible for ICF syndrome (Hansen et al., 1999; Okano et al., 1999; Xu et al., 1999). *DNMT3B* belongs to the family of DNA methyltransferases that contain specific catalytic domains responsible for the methylation of cytosines in CpG dinucleotides in mammals (Bestor and Verdine, 1994; Okano et al., 1998; Bestor, 2000). DNA methylation may modify gene expression and helps to maintain chromatin in a repressive state (Wolffe and Matzke, 1999). In mammals, methylation patterns are shaped by methyltransferases with different biochemical properties: Dnmt1 is involved in the maintenance of methylation patterns by methylating the hemimethylated DNA created after each replication cycle, whereas Dnmt3a and 3b are thought to be involved in de novo methylation given their ability to methylate unmethylated DNA. *Dnmt3a* and *3b* are expressed at high levels in embryonic stem (ES) cells (Okano et al., 1999). They reset methylation patterns during the gastrula stage, after the massive wave of demethylation that occurs during preimplantation development (Howlett and Reik, 1991; Rougier et al., 1998; Mayer et al., 2000). Dnmt3b is essential for development, as shown by the early embryonic lethal phenotype of knockout mice carrying a total loss-of-function *Dnmt3b* mutation (Okano et al., 1999). ICF patients and *Dnmt3b*$^{-/-}$ mice display altered juxta/pericentromeric DNA methylation in classical satellite and minor satellite sequences, respectively, suggesting that Dnmt3b has a specialized function in heterochromatin methylation. It has been hypothesized that the loss of classical satellite methylation in ICF patients interferes with specific gene silencing processes in *trans*, causing immunodeficiency and facial dysmorphism (Xu et al., 1999).

CLINICAL DESCRIPTION OF THE SYNDROME

The clinical manifestations of ICF syndrome are facial abnormalities, mental retardation, and failure to thrive. However, these clinical features are clearly variable. Facial abnormalities consist mainly of hypertelorism, a flat nasal bridge, a protruding tongue, epicanthal folds, low-set ears, and micrognathia (Figure 75–1). However, manifestations such as hyper-pigmented skin spots (Tiepolo et al., 1979) and telangiectasis are observed in a small number of patients. Bipartite nipples have been reported in two cases (Franceschini et al., 1995). Growth retardation, due at least in part to malabsorption, is usually seen during infancy, and in some cases it is detected at birth (Fasth et al., 1990; Smeets et al., 1994; Brown et al., 1995). Growth retardation can be associated with a small head circumference (Fasth et al., 1990; Brown et al., 1995). Psychomotor development is slow and sometimes is associated with an ataxic gait, choreoathetoid tremors, and neurological degeneration (Tiepolo et al., 1979). Mild mental retardation has been described in about 45% of patients, but only a few cases of severe mental retardation have been reported. However, all of these features vary, in terms of association and intensity, from one patient to another one. Some patients present with no typical clinical features, as seen in a brother of one proband (Gimelli et al., 1993) who presented immunologic and cytogenetic features but no clinical manifestations. Clinical progress is marked by recurrent infections related to the immunodeficiency, consisting essentially of pneumonia and diarrhea. However, we cannot rule out the possibility of a primary intestinal mucosal defect (Turleau et al., 1989). The small number of analyzed patients all underwent puberty normally.

The extent of the immunodeficiency is also variable, ranging from a severe combined immunodeficiency to nearly normal immunity. The most common feature is hypogammaglobulinemia. The humoral defect usually involves all the immunoglobulin isotypes (IgG, IgA, IgM, and IgE), at varying levels. However, in some cases, the levels of only one or two immunoglobulin isotypes are low, usually IgM and IgE (Gimelli et al., 1993), IgA and IgE (Tiepolo et al., 1979), or IgA alone. Complete agammaglobulinemia is rare (Brown et al., 1995). In some cases, cellular immunity is also impaired (Tiepolo et al., 1979). In these cases, the cellular defect consists of T-cell lymphopenia (Fasth et al., 1990), particularly involving the CD4 T-cell population, associated with functional failures that include poor response to mitogens and to recall antigens (Turleau et al., 1989). Most patients with ICF receive regular infusions of immunoglobulins, but they frequently die during childhood or adolescence. Despite the combined immunodeficiency observed in some ICF patients, no malignancy, such as lymphoma or another type of tumor, has been observed so far.

KARYOTYPE ABNORMALITIES AND MOLECULAR DEFECTS IN PATIENTS WITH ICF

The first relationship between ICF syndrome and DNA methylation was the indication that the chromosomal abnormalities found in PHA-stimulated lymphocytes (T cells) of ICF patients mimic those observed in normal lymphocytes treated with the demethylating agent, 5-aza-

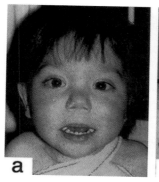
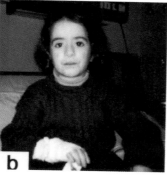

Figure 75–1. Front view of two immunodeficiency-centromeric instability-facial anomalies (ICF) syndrome patients with several of the facial abnormalities. (From Turleau et al., 1989 and Miniou et al., 1994.)

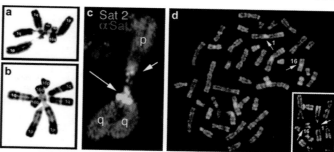

Figure 75–2. Chromosomes from ICF patients with immunodeficiency-centromeric instability-facial anomalies (ICF) syndrome. Typical figures of ICF patients after Giemsa staining (*a*) and R-banding (*b*) (Xu et al., 1999) showing associations and decondensations of constitutive heterochromatin from chromosomes 1 and 16 (p, short arm; q, long arm). (*c*) In situ hybridization using classical satellite 2 (*large arrow* on the *left*) and alpha satellite (*small arrow* on the *right*) probes on chromosome 1 of an ICF patient showing the duplication of the chromosome arms (p, short arm; q, long arm) (Xu et al., 1999). The breakpoint of the chromosomal rearrangement is located on classical satellite 2. (*d*) Indirect immunofluorescence with 5-methylcytosine monoclonal antibody in control cells showing the methylated state of the constitutive heterochromatin of chromosomes 1 and 16. *Left* (*inset*): chromosomes from an ICF patient showing the undermethylation of the constitutive heterochromatin.

cytidine (Jeanpierre et al., 1993). In both cases, constitutive heterochromatin, mainly located in the vicinity of centromeres, was abnormally decondensed and formed associations, leading to typical multiradiate configurations (Figure 75–2, a and b). The syndrome can be diagnosed on the basis of these abnormalities and the presence of a variable combined immunodeficiency. The frequency of rearrangements in lymphocytes ranges from 20% to 80% among patients (Miniou et al., 1994).

These rearrangements mainly involve the constitutive heterochromatin of chromosomes 1 and 16 and include whole arm deletions, duplications, and isochromosomes. The heterochromatin of chromosomes 9 and Y may be stretched, but in general, these chromosomes do not participate in the multiradiate configurations. Rearrangements involving two chromosomes, such as translocations, are rare, but when they do occur, chromosome 1 or 16 or both are involved. Chromosome nondisjunction and chromosome pulverization have been described occasionally. In fibroblast and bone marrow cells, these typical configurations are absent or present at a low frequency (Howard et al., 1985; Carpenter et al., 1987; Fasth et al., 1990; Gimelli et al., 1993). ICF patients have a increased frequency of micronuclei, in accordance with their genome instability (Miniou et al., 1994; Stacey et al., 1995). Multiradiate configurations have been detected in ICF lymphoblast cell lines (B cells) (Ji et al., 1997), but the significance of these observations is unclear because heterochromatin can be decondensed and display low levels of methylation even in normal lymphoblast cultures (Vilain et al., 2000).

The constitutive heterochromatin methylation defect was confirmed by use of a specific 5-methylcytosine antibody on chromosomes (Figure 75–2d) and nuclei and by Southern blot analysis using satellite-specific probes. ICF methylation profiles are comparable to those observed in normal extraembryonic tissues (Jeanpierre et al., 1993; Miniou et al., 1994). In humans, constitutive heterochromatin is mainly composed of classical and alpha satellites. Classical satellite 2 is mostly located in the juxtacentromeric region of chromosomes 1 and 16. Classical satellite 3 is found in the juxtacentromeric region of chromosome 9 and in the long arm of chromosome Y. Finally, classical satellite 1 is located in the long arm of Y chromosome. Alpha satellites are present in all chromosomes. They are specific for each chromosome and map to the centromeric regions (Jeanpierre, 1994; Miniou et al., 1994; Schueler et al., 2001).

Classical satellite 2 sequences are systematically demethylated in ICF patients, and they are the preferential breakpoint for the chromosome rearrangements characteristic of this syndrome (Figure 75–2, a–c). Interestingly, the association between satellite 2 hypomethylation and chromosome instability has also been observed in solid tumors, lymphomas, and leukemia (Narayan et al., 1998). In contrast, alpha satellites are heterogeneously demethylated in ICF patients, suggesting that the methylation of the two components of human constitutive heterochromatin is differentially regulated (Jeanpierre et al., 1993; Miniou et al., 1994, 1997b).

Facultative heterochromatin, represented by the inactive X chromosome (Xi) in females, is globally undermethylated in ICF patients,

as shown by immunofluorescence studies with 5-methylcytosine antibodies (Miniou et al., 1994; Bourc'his et al., 1999) (Figure 75–3a). In normal females, this antibody revealed that the Xi is equally as methylated as the active X chromosome and as all of the other chromosomes. At the molecular level, in normal females, the methylation of CpG islands in X-linked inactivated genes is associated with the repressive state of Xi. This profile may change in female ICF patients, depending on the patient and the gene considered (Figure 75–3b). RT-PCR (Hansen et al., 2000) and enzymatic dosage (Bourc'his et al., 1999), revealed that three of the nine X-linked genes tested were subject to biallelic expression in three patients with demethylated CpG islands. Although the replication timing of the ICF undermethylated Xi was found to be normal at the chromosome level, replication was found to occur slightly early for two loci showing reactivation. No differences between normal and ICF females have been found for other parameters related to X inactivation, such as Barr body formation at interphase, XIST expression, and the typical distribution of XIST RNA

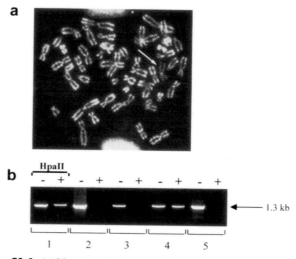

Figure 75–3. (*a*) Metaphase from an immunodeficiency-centromeric instability-facial anomalies (ICF) syndrome female patient after indirect immunofluorescence with 5-methylcytosine antibody. The arrow indicates the undermethylated inactive X chromosome. (*b*) Methylation status of CpG islands of the X-linked *MAOA* gene analyzed by a PCR-based assay using uncut (−) and *Hpa*II-cut (+) DNA. *Lane 1*, female control leukocytes; *lane 2*, male control leukocytes; *lane 3*, patient ICF 1 fibroblasts; *lane 4*, patient ICF 1 leukocytes; *lane 5*, patient ICF 2 leukocytes (from Bourc'his et al., 1999).

on Xi. Similarly, no phenotypic or clinical differences have been observed between male and female ICF patients.

Other repeated DNA sequences are also affected by the ICF methylation defect. These include young Alu sequences (Miniou et al., 1997a) and D4Z4 and NBL2 repeats (Kondo et al., 2000). The methylation patterns of some imprinted loci such as H19, PW71, and D15S9 (P32 probe) are modified in some, but not in all, studied patients (Schuffenhauer et al., 1995; Xu et al., 1999). Finally, 7% of the total decrease in genome methylation is detected in brain cells in ICF patients (Tuck-Muller et al., 2000), illustrating that the ICF methylation defect is targeted to specific loci.

To gain insight into the functional consequences of the ICF methylation defect, cDNA microarrays were used to analyze more than 5000 genes in four patients (Ehrlich et al., 2001). This revealed that several genes were dysregulated. Most of these dysregulated genes are involved in immune function. No change in methylation status was observed in the promoter regions of these underexpressed or overexpressed genes, suggesting that the methylation defect does not directly affect these sequences but instead affects their expression in an indirect or a *trans* manner. However, this study was performed in lymphoblast cell lines, which present variable methylation patterns and are prone to culture effects even when derived from normal individuals (Vilain et al., 2000). More information is needed about RNA changes in other tissues and about protein expression before we can draw conclusions about the biologic relevance of this lymphogenesis-associated gene dysregulation in ICF syndrome.

In conclusion, several DNA repeated sequences or genes may be demethylated in ICF patients. The methylation of classical satellite DNA is systematically altered. However, the methylation of other loci is highly variable. The methylation status of classical satellites in ICF patients was originally thought to be identical to that of extraembryonic tissues, which escape the wave of de novo methylation after implantation and remain undermethylated compared with the embryo itself. The hypothesis that ICF syndrome results from the failure to establish accurate methylation patterns during the gastrula stage was finally confirmed after the identification of mutations in the de novo methyltransferase DNMT3B in ICF patients. In agreement with this specific developmental function, *DNMT3B* is highly expressed in ES cells and very early postimplantation embryos but is down-regulated in differentiated cells.

MUTATIONS IN PATIENTS WITH ICF

DNMT3B, a gene involved in the de novo methylation of DNA, has been found to be mutated in unrelated ICF patients (Hansen et al., 1999; Xu et al., 1999). This gene spans about 47 kb and contains 24 exons, of which 6 are subject to alternative splicing. Two alternative 5′ exons have been found. The human mRNA is 4.3 kb long and is mainly expressed in the thymus and testis in adults (Hansen et al., 1999; Xu et al., 1999). *DNMT3B* transcripts are abundant in undifferentiated mouse ES cells and early embryos, which is consistent with it having de novo methylation activity. The carboxyl-terminal domain includes five of the most conserved DNA methyltransferase motifs. The amino-terminal region of *DNMT3B* contains a cysteine-rich domain that is related to a region of the putative DNA helicase, ATRX, which is mutated in patients affected by alpha-thalassemia–mental retardation (ATRX) syndrome (Gibbons et al., 2000). A PWWP domain is located to the amino terminus of DNMT3B. This PWWP domain has the ability to bind DNA in vitro (Qiu et al., 2002).

This diversity of reported mutations is remarkable for such a rare disease and may exclude some founder effects and mutational hotspots. Patients are homozygous or compound heterozygous for exonic mutations that are mostly concentrated in the catalytic domain of *DNMT3B*. Parents of patients have been found to be heterozygous for the mutant allele. One case of de novo mutation was reported, but paternity was not determined (Hansen et al., 1999; Okano et al., 1999). Mutations generally correspond to a single base substitution, and most affect invariant positions in *DNMT3B* and *3A*. Two groups of mutations have been found, missense and splice-site mutations, which do not completely abolish enzymatic activity, and nonsense mutations,

which can lead to a lack of functional protein (Wijmenga et al., 2000). Functional analysis using a stable episomal system showed that the D809G mutation, located on motif X of the catalytic domain, reduces the DNA methytransferase activity (Xu et al., 1999). No patients are homozygous for mutations that remove amino-terminal sequences. All of the patients carrying nonsense mutations have a missense mutation in the other allele, illustrating that total loss of function is probably not compatible with life. A large region of the catalytic domain, involving the highly conserved motifs IV and VI, has been deleted in *Dnmt3b* mutant mice (Okano et al., 1999) and is indeed associated with an early embryonic lethal phenotype.

Twenty-seven patients have been studied in total. No *DNMT3B* exonic mutations were detected in about 37% of the cases (Wijmenga et al., 2000; unpublished cases). Exonic mutations in the closely related *DNMT3A* gene (mapped in 2p23), which also has a de novo methyltransferase activity, were not found in these patients. The lack of mutations in the catalytic domain of *DNMT3B* suggests that another gene is involved in ICF syndrome or that mutations are located in regulatory sequences in this class of patients. The hypothesis of genetic heterogeneity is reinforced by the fact that some ICF patients from consanguineous families are not homozygous-by-descent in the *DNMT3B* region (Wijmenga et al., 2000). Genotype–phenotype correlations in ICF patients cannot be performed yet, because of the incomplete clinical information for some patients and families, the rarity of the syndrome, the extreme variability of phenotypic features and methylation defects, and the potential genetic heterogeneity of the disease.

GENETIC COUNSELING AND PROGNOSTIC INFORMATION

ICF syndrome can accurately be diagnosed by performing karyotype analysis or Southern blot analysis with classical satellite 2–specific probes on blood samples from fetuses in week 18 or 19 of gestation (Miniou et al., 1997b). The results of other prenatal diagnosis methods that can be performed earlier during the gestation period, such chorionic villous sampling (CVS; week 13) and amniotic fluid analysis (week 11), are not reliable. Heterochromatin decondensation and hypomethylation on chromosomes 1, 9, 16, and Y may be found in both amniocytes and chorionic villi without having any pathologic relevance (Kokalj-Vokac et al., 1998). The diagnostic method based only on the detection of mutations in the catalytic domain of *DNMT3B* is not always informative, as shown by the fact that exonic mutations are not detected in the catalytic domain of about 37% of the patients. Genetic counseling, with a favorable outcome, was given with a probability of greater than 90% that the fetus will be unaffected. In fact, a diagnostic method combining linkage and CVS karyotype analysis was used during a pregnancy conceived by a consanguineous couple in a family with an affected child from a previous pregnancy. The D20S850 marker, which is closely linked to the *DNMT3B* gene (20q11-q13), was informative and indicated that the fetus was heterozygous for the critical region. Postnatal analysis of peripheral blood confirmed that the child was unaffected (Bjorck et al., 2000).

The evolution of the disease is variable. Patients generally die during infancy or adolescence; only patients with less severe immunologic defects survive. Death is often associated with severe bacterial or viral infections, leading to pulmonary and gastrointestinal problems. No tumors have been reported in patients with ICF despite the methylation defect. However, this syndrome is generally associated with a poor prognosis.

DEVELOPMENTAL PATHOGENESIS

The gene responsible for ICF, *DNMT3B*, is required for the establishment of DNA methylation patterns during early development. DNA methylation is one of the major epigenetic marks of the human genome and is involved in gene repression (Zaret and Wolffe, 2001). This situation makes it difficult to evaluate the relationship between genetic and developmental abnormalities in ICF syndrome.

In ES cells and early mouse embryos, Dnmt3b is responsible for the methylation of pericentromeric heterochromatin (Okano et al.,

1999). In accordance, all ICF patients display hypomethylation of classical satellite 2, a main component of human constitutive heterochromatin (Miniou et al., 1994). Several lines of evidence indicate that heterochromatin may be directly or indirectly involved in gene silencing (Gasser, 2001). For instance, during mouse lymphocyte differentiation, silenced genes and other components of the repressive machinery co-localize with heterochromatin foci (Brown et al., 1997). Thus, the loss of methylation of constitutive heterochromatin in ICF patients may interfere with lymphocyte transcriptional repression and generate the characteristic immunodeficiency (Xu et al., 1999). Efforts to understand the basis of epigenetic regulation in mammals may help to elucidate the relationship between genetic and developmental abnormalities in ICF syndrome.

ACKNOWLEDGMENTS

We are grateful for support from the Association pour la Recherche sur le Cancer (ARC) and the Ligue Contre le Cancer, Comité de Paris.

REFERENCES

Bauld R, Grace E, Richards N, Ellis PM (1991). The ICF syndrome: a rare chromosome instability syndrome. *J Med Genet* 28: 63.

Bestor TH (2000). The DNA methyltransferases of mammals. *Hum Mol Genet* 9: 2395–2402.

Bestor TH, Verdine GL (1994). DNA methyltransferases. *Curr Opin Cell Biol* 6: 380–389.

Bjorck EJ, Bui TH, Wijmenga C, Grandell U, Nordenskjold M (2000). Early prenatal diagnosis of the ICF syndrome. *Prenat Diagn* 20: 828–831.

Bourc'his D, Miniou P, Jeanpierre M, Molina-Gomes D, Dupont JM, De Saint-Basile G, Maraschio P, Tiepolo L, Viegas-Péquignot E (1999). Abnormal methylation does not prevent X inactivation in ICF patients. *Cytogenet Cell Genet* 84: 245–252.

Brown DC, Grace E, Sumner AT, Edmunds AT, Ellis PM (1995). ICF syndrome (immunodeficiency, centromeric instability and facial anomalies): investigation of heterochromatin abnormalities and review of clinical outcome. *Hum Genet* 96: 411–416.

Brown KE, Guest SS, Smale ST, Hahm K, Merkenschlager M, Fisher AG (1997). Association of transcriptionally silent genes with Ikaros complexes at centromeric heterochromatin. *Cell* 91: 845–854.

Carpenter NJ, Filipovich A, Blaese RM, Carey TL, Berkel AI (1987). Variable immunodeficiency with abnormal condensation of the heterochromatin of chromosomes 1, 9 and 16. *J Pediatr* 112: 757–760.

Ehrlich M, Buchanan KL, Tsien F, Jiang G, Sun B, Uicker W, Weemaes CM, Smeets D, Sperling K, Belohradsky BH, et al. (2001). DNA methyltransferase 3B mutations linked to the ICF syndrome cause dysregulation of lymphogenesis genes. *Hum Mol Genet* 10: 2917–2931.

Fasth A, Forestier E, Holmberg E, Holmgren G, Nordenson I, Söderström T, Wahlström J (1990). Fragility of the centromeric region of chromosome 1 associated with combined immunodeficiency in siblings. *Acta Paediatr Scand* 79: 605–612.

Franceschini P, Martino S, Ciocchini M, Ciuti E, Vardeu MP, Guala A, Signorile F, Camerano P, Franceschini D, Tovo PA (1995). Variability of clinical and immunological phenotype in immunodeficiency-centromeric instability-facial anomalies syndrome. Report of two new patients and review of the literature. *Eur J Pediatr* 154: 840–846.

Fryns JP, Azou M, Eggermont E, Pedersen JC, Van den Berghe H (1981). Centromeric instability of chromosomes 1, 9 and 16 associated with combined immunodeficiency. *Hum Genet* 57: 108–110.

Gasser SM (2001). Positions of potential: nuclear organization and gene expression. *Cell* 104: 639–642.

Gibbons RJ, McDowell TL, Raman S, M. ORD, Garrick D, Ayyub H, Higgs DR (2000). Mutations in ATRX, encoding a SWI/SNF-like protein, cause diverse change in the pattern of DNA methylation. *Nat Genet* 24: 368–371.

Gimelli G, Varone P, Pezzolo A, Lerone M, Pistoia V (1993). ICF syndrome with variable expression in sibs. *J Med Genet* 30: 429–432.

Hansen RS, Stoger R, Wijmenga C, Stanek AM, Canfield TK, Luo P, Matarazzo MR, D'Esposito M, Feil R, Gimelli G, et al. (2000). Escape from gene silencing in ICF syndrome: evidence for advanced replication time as a major determinant. *Hum Mol Genet* 9: 2575–2587.

Hansen RS, Wijmenga C, Luo P, Stanek AM, Canfield TK, Weemaes CMR, Gartler SM (1999). The DNMT3B DNA methyltransferase gene is mutated in the ICF immunodeficiency syndrome. *Proc Natl Acad Sci USA* 96: 14412–14417.

Howard PJ, Lewis IJ, Harris F, Walker S (1985). Centromeric instability of chromosomes 1 and 16 with variable immune deficiency: a new syndrome. *Clin Genet* 27: 501–505.

Howlett SK, Reik W (1991). Methylation levels of maternal and paternal genomes during preimplantation development. *Development* 113: 119–127.

Hultén M (1978). Selective somatic pairing and fragility at 1q12 in a boy with common variable immunodeficiency: a new syndrome. *Clin Genet* 14: 294–295.

Jeanpierre M (1994). Human satellites 2 and 3. *Ann Génét* 37: 163–171.

Jeanpierre M, Turleau C, Aurias A, Prieur M, Ledeist F, Fischer A, Viegas-Péquignot E (1993). An embryonic-like methylation pattern of classical satellite DNA is observed in ICF syndrome. *Hum Mol Genet* 2: 731–735.

Ji W, Hernandez R, Zhang XY, Qu GZ, Frady A, Varela M, Ehrlich M (1997). DNA demethylation and pericentromeric rearrangements of chromosome 1. *Mutat Res* 379: 33–41.

Kokalj-Vokac N, Zagorac A, Pristovnik M, Bourgeois C, Dutrillaux B (1998). DNA methylation of the extraembryonic tissues: an in situ study on human metaphase chromosomes. *Chrom Res* 6: 161–166.

Kondo T, Bobek MP, Kuick R, Lamb B, Zhu X, Narayan A, Bourc'his D, Viegas-Péquignot E, Ehrlich M, Hanash SM (2000). Whole-genome methylation scan in ICF syndrome: hypomethylation of non-satellite DNA repeats D4Z4 and NBL2. *Hum Mol Genet* 9: 597–604.

Maraschio P, Zuffardi O, Dalla FT, Tiepolo L (1988). Immunodeficiency, centromeric heterochromatin instability of chromosomes 1, 9, and 16, and facial anomalies: the ICF syndrome. *J Med Genet* 25: 173–180.

Mayer W, Niveleau A, Walter J, Fundele R, T. H (2000). Demethylation of the zygotic paternal genome. *Nature* 403: 501–502.

Miniou P, Bourc'his D, Molina Gomes D, Jeanpierre M, Viegas-Péquignot E (1997a). Undermethylation of Alu sequences in ICF syndrome: molecular and in situ analysis. *Cytogenet Cell Genet* 77: 308–313.

Miniou P, Jeanpierre M, Blanquet V, Sibella V, Bonneau D, Herbelin C, Fischer A, Niveleau A, Viegas-Péquignot E (1994). Abnormal methylation pattern in constitutive and facultative (X inactive chromosome) heterochromatin of ICF patients. *Hum Mol Genet* 3: 2093–2102.

Miniou P, Jeanpierre M, Bourc'his D, Coutinho Barbisa AC, Blanquet V, Viegas-Péquignot E (1997b). Alpha-satellite DNA methylation in normal individuals and in ICF patients: heterogeneous methylation of constitutive heterochromatin in adult and fetal samples. *Hum Genet* 99: 738–745.

Narayan A, Ji W, Zhang XY, Marrogi A, Graff JR, Baylin SB, Ehrlich M (1998). Hypomethylation of pericentromeric DNA in breast adenocarcinomas. *Int J Cancer* 77: 833–838.

Okano M, Bell DW, Haber DA, Li E (1999). DNA methyltransferases Dnmt3a and Dnmt3b are essential for de novo methylation and mammalian development. *Cell* 99: 247–257.

Okano M, Xie S, Li E (1998). Cloning and characterization of a family of novel mammalian DNA (cytosine-5) methyltransferases. *Nat Genet* 19: 219–220.

Qiu C, Sawada K, Zhang X, Cheng X (2002). The PWWP domain of mammalian DNA methyltransferase Dnmt3b defines a new family of DNA-binding folds. *Nat Struct Biol* 9: 217–224.

Rougier N, Bourc'his D, Molina Gomes D, Niveleau A, Plachot M, Pàldi A, Viegas-Péquignot E (1998). Chromosome methylation patterns during mammalian preimplantation development. *Genes Dev* 12: 2108–2113.

Sawyer JR, Swanson CM, Wheeler G, Cunniff C (1995). Chromosome instability in ICF syndrome: formation of micronuclei from multibranched chromosomes 1 demonstrated by fluorescence in situ hybridization. *Am J Med Genet* 56: 203–209.

Schueler MG, Higgins AW, Rudd MK, Gustashaw K, Willard HF Genomic and genetic definition of a functional human centromere. *Science* 294: 109–115.

Schuffenhauer S, Bartsch O, Stumm M, Buchholz T, Petropoulou T, Kraft S, Belohradsky B, Hinkel GK, Meitinger T, Wegner RD (1995). DNA, FISH and complementation studies in ICF syndrome: DNA hypomethylation of repetitive and single copy loci and evidence for a trans acting factor. *Hum Genet* 96: 562–571.

Smeets DF, Moog U, Weemaes CM, Vaes PG, Merkx GF, Niehof JP, Hamers G (1994). ICF syndrome: a new case and review of the literature. *Hum Genet* 94: 240–246.

Stacey M, Bennett MS, Hulten M (1995). FISH analysis on spontaneously arising micronuclei in the ICF syndrome. *J Med Genet* 32: 502–508.

Tiepolo L, Maraschio P, Gimelli G, Cuoco C, Gargani GF, Romano C (1978). Concurrent instability at specific sites of chromosomes 1, 9 and 16 resulting in multi-branched structures. *Clin Genet* 14: 313–314.

Tiepolo L, Maraschio P, Gimelli G, Cuoco C, Gargani GF, Romano C (1979). Multibranched chromosomes 1, 9 and 16 in a patient with combined IgA and IgE deficiency. *Hum Genet* 51: 127–137.

Tuck-Muller CM, Narayan A, Tsien F, Smeets DF, Sawyer J, Fiala ES, Sohn OS, Ehrlich M (2000). DNA hypomethylation and unusual chromosome instability in cell lines from ICF syndrome patients. *Cytogenet Cell Genet* 89: 121–128.

Tükün A, Bökesoy I, Gürsel T, Tümer L, Tunaoglu S, Uluoglu O (1992). Two siblings with ICF syndrome: case reports and review. *Dysmorph Clin Genet* 6: 135–140.

Turleau C, Cabanis MO, Girault D, Ledeist F, Mettey R, Puissant H, Prieur M, de Grouchy J (1989). Multibranched chromosomes in the ICF syndrome: immunodeficiency, centromeric instability, and facial anomalies. *Am J Med Genet* 32: 420–424.

Valkova G, Ghenev E, Tzancheva M (1987). Centromeric instability of chromosomes 1, 9 and 16 with variable immune deficiency. Support of a new syndrome. *Clin Genet* 31: 119–124.

Vilain A, Bernardino J, Gerbault-Seureau M, Vogt N, Niveleau A, Lefrançois D, Malfoy B, Dutrillaux B (2000). DNA methylation and chromosome instability in lymphoblastoid cell lines. *Cytogenet Cell Genet* 90: 93–101.

Wijmenga C, Hansen RS, Gimelli G, Bjorck EJ, Davies EG, Valentine D, Belohradsky BH, van Dongen JJ, Smeets DF, van den Heuvel LP, et al. (2000). Genetic variation in ICF syndrome: evidence for genetic heterogeneity. *Hum Mutat* 16: 509–517.

Wijmenga C, van den Heuvel LP, Strengman E, Luyten JA, van der Burgt IJ, de Groot R, Smeets DF, Draaisma JM, van Dongen JJ, De Abreu RA, et al. (1998). Localization of the ICF syndrome to chromosome 20 by homozygosity mapping. *Am J Hum Genet* 63: 803–809.

Wolffe AP, Matzke MA (1999). Epigenetics: regulation through repression. *Science* 286: 481–486.

Xu G-L, Bestor TH, Bourc'his D, Hsieh C-L, Tommerup N, Bugge M, Hulten M, Qu X, Russo JJ, Viegas-Péquignot E (1999). Chromosome instability and immunodeficiency syndrome caused by mutations in a DNA methyltransferase gene. *Nature* 402: 187–191.

Zaret K, Wolffe AP (2001). Chromosomes and expression mechanisms. *Curr Opin Genet Dev* 11: 111–227.

MARIA ZENIOU, SYLVIE JACQUOT, JEAN-PIERRE DELAUNOY, AND ANDRÉ HANAUER

Loss-of-function mutations in the gene encoding the protein kinase ribosomal S6 serine/threonine kinase 2 (RSK2) are responsible for Coffin-Lowry syndrome (CLS; OMIM 303600), a syndromic form of X-linked mental retardation. Cardinal features of CLS are growth and psychomotor retardation, characteristic facial and digital abnormalities, and progressive skeletal deformations.

RSK2 belongs to the 90 kDa RSK family, which includes four highly related members in humans, RSK1 through -4, which are derived from four independent genes. RSKs act at the distal end of the Ras/mitogen-activated protein kinase (MAPK) signaling pathway, phosphorylate, and activate a variety of nuclear and cytoplasmic proteins in response to a broad range of cellular perturbations, including stimulation with growth factors and neurotransmitters, and UV irradiation. RSKs have been implicated in several important cellular events, including proliferation and differentiation, response to stress, and apoptosis. It is still unclear whether distinct physiological functions are regulated by the four proteins or whether their functions are in large part overlapping. However, two specific physiological substrates have been definitively identified for RSK2; the transcription factor cAMP response element binding (CREB) protein and histone H3, a modulator of chromatin and gene expression. Therefore, at least some of the CLS phenotypic features may be caused by perturbations in intracellular signaling pathways that link mitogen-induced signals to CREB protein–regulated gene expression. Particularly, the involvement of CREB protein in learning and memory processes may explain the mental impairment observed in RSK2-deficient patients. An RSK2-deficient mouse has been created that exhibits growth retardation and impaired learning. It represents a powerful tool to elucidate the molecular mechanisms that generate the CLS phenotype.

RSK2 mutations in patients with CLS are extremely heterogeneous and lead to premature termination of translation and/or to loss of phosphotransferase activity. No obvious correlation is observed between the position or type of the *RSK2* mutations and the severity or particular clinical features of CLS. However, significantly milder disease was noted in a few cases with missense mutations, leaving a residual RSK2 kinase activity.

THE RSK FAMILY OF SERINE/THREONINE KINASES

MAPK Signaling Pathways

Cells in multicellular organisms must communicate with each other to control their growth, regulate their development, and coordinate their functions. External signals involved in these processes are received at transmembrane receptors and relayed to cytosolic or nuclear effectors through signal transduction cascades. The activities of the many enzymes that compose these cascades are regulated by their phosphorylation state (Karim and Hunter, 1995). Among the signaling cascades involved in the response to many extracellular signals in eukaryotic organisms are those that activate the MAPK family of kinases. The members of this family of kinases are characterized by their activation by MAPK kinases (MEKs) through dual phosphorylation of threonine and tyrosine residues in the activation loop and by their substrate specificity, which is proline-directed phosphorylation of ser-

ine or threonine. Three major MAPK families have been identified in mammalian cells, including the extracellular signal-regulated kinase (ERK) pathway and the stress-activated p38 and Jun kinase (JNK) pathways (Cano and Mahadevan, 1995; Karin and Hunter, 1995). The ERK pathway is strongly activated by growth factors via the *Ras* protooncogene and is involved in proliferation, differentiation, and transformation. This pathway is also activated through signaling molecules like protein kinase C, phosphoinositol 3-kinase, cytosolic calcium, or cAMP and by many peptide hormones and neurotransmitters. Stress-activated MAPKs respond to stress factors (UV radiation, heat shock, oxidative and osmotic stress) or cytokines, which leads to cell death, survival, or defense. Various cytosolic and nuclear substrates for MAPKs have been identified, including several transcription factors (Karim and Hunter, 1995). A subset of MAPK targets is itself composed of protein kinases. The gene encoding RSK2 is a member of a family of such kinases (known as p90^{rsk} or the RSK or MAPKAP-K1 family) targeted by the MAPK/ERK pathway. RSKs have been implicated in several important cellular events, including proliferation and differentiation, response to stress, and apoptosis (Blenis, 1993).

Structure and Role of RSKs in Signal Transduction

The first ribosomal S6 kinase protein was identified in 1985 in *Xenopus laevis* through cellular fractionation, and it was initially characterized as a 90-kDa protein capable of phosphorylating the 40S ribosomal subunit protein S6 (Erikson and Maller, 1985). Therefore, RSKs were initially thought to play a role in cell growth through the regulation of translation. However, although the ribosomal S6 protein is a good substrate in vitro, it was shown that it is not a substrate in vivo (von Manteuffel et al., 1997). RSK family members have subsequently been identified in many other species, including *Caenorhabditis elegans, Drosophila melanogaster*, chicken, mouse, and humans (Grove et al., 1993; Wassarman et al., 1994; Zhao et al., 1995). In *Drosophila*, only one RSK protein is known, whereas in mammals, four members have been characterized so far. The four human RSK proteins—RSK1, RSK2, RSK3, and RSK4—are very similar in length (735, 740, 733, and 745 amino acid residues, respectively) and show 75% to 80% amino acid identity. They are encoded by four distinct genes mapping to chromosomes 3 (*RSK1*), Xp22.2 (*RSK2*), 6q27 (*RSK3*), and Xq21 (*RSK4*). Only the genomic structure of the human *RSK2* gene has been completely determined, and its coding sequence is split into 22 exons (Jacquot et al., 1998a). RSK proteins are composed of two functional kinase catalytic domains, linked together by a regulatory linker region (Fig. 76–1). Each domain is related to a different class of protein kinases (Bjorbaek et al., 1995).

Although widely distributed, the four mammalian RSK proteins show varying tissue expression: RSK1 is most abundantly expressed in hematopoietic cells, intestine, and liver; RSK2, heart, pancreas, and skeletal muscle; RSK3, lung and skeletal muscle; and RSK4, kidney and brain (Moller et al., 1994; Zhao et al., 1995; Yntema et al., 1999).

A considerable body of evidence has accumulated showing that RSKs are downstream components of the Ras/MEK/ERK signaling pathway. The activation of ERKs leads to the activation of RSKs in essentially all cases in which both kinase activities have been measured. RSKs, like ERKs, are activated by mitogens such as growth factors, phorbol esters, neurotransmitters, and hormones (Frödin and

Figure 76–1. Structure of ribosomal S6 serine/threonine kinase (RSK) proteins. Amino acid numbering refers to human RSK2. PDK1, 3-phosphoinositide–dependent protein kinase-1; ERK, extracellular signal-regulated kinase.

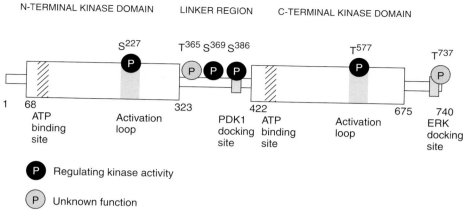

Gammeltoft, 1999) (Fig. 76–2). ERKs phosphorylate and directly activate the carboxyl-terminal kinase domain of RSK (Zhao et al., 1996) in response to an extracellular mitogenic stimulation. It has, however, become apparent that the role of RSKs is not restricted to the mitogenic response and that they can integrate the effect of various other signals and pathways (Tan et al., 1999; Bertolotto et al., 2000; Mérienne et al., 2000).

Regulation of RSK Enzymatic Activity

It is well established that the N-terminal kinase domain is responsible for phosphotransferase activity toward substrates, whereas the C-terminal kinase domain is necessary for enzymatic activation of the N-terminal kinase domain (Zhao et al., 1995; Fisher and Blenis, 1996). RSK phosphotransferase activity is accompanied by the phosphorylation of at least six residues, of which four have been shown to modulate kinase activity (one threonine and three serines) (Dalby et al., 1998; Fig. 76–3). On stimulation, ERK binds to a docking site located at the extreme C terminus of RSK (Smith et al., 1999) and phosphorylates Ser369 (using human RSK2 numbering) in the linker region and Thr577 in the activation loop of the C-terminal kinase domain (Fig. 76–3A). These events lead to activation of the C-terminal catalytic domain, which then enhances the N-terminal kinase activity via a mechanism involving autophosphorylation of an additional serine residue (Ser386 in human

RSK2) in the linker region (Fisher and Blenis, 1996; Dalby et al., 1998; Fig. 76–3B). Recent studies have shown that the 3-phosphoinositide–dependent protein kinase-1 (PDK1) is involved in the activation of the N-terminal kinase domain by phosphorylating a serine residue within the activation loop of this domain (Ser227 in human RSK2). How PDK1 and ERK cooperate to activate the N-terminal domain of RSK has also been unraveled. PDK1 is recruited to RSK at a docking site, encompassing Ser386 (human RSK2) in the linker region and in an Ser386 phospho–dependent manner (Fig. 76–3B). Recruitment of PDK1 results in phosphorylation and activation of PDK1 itself (Fig. 76–3C). Activated PDK1 phosphorylates Ser227 and thereby activates the N-terminal catalytic domain (Fig. 76–3C) (Frödin et al., 2000). Thus, RSK enzymatic activity results from the synergistic action of at least two signaling pathways: the ERK pathway and the PDK1 pathway. The activated N-terminal domain phosphorylates substrates on threonine and serine residues within the basophilic consensus motif Arg/Lys-X-Arg-X-X-Ser/Thr or Arg-Arg-X-Ser/Thr (Leigton et al., 1995).

RSK Functions

An Important Role in Transcriptional Regulation

In nonstimulated cells, RSK proteins are present in both the cytoplasmic and nuclear compartments (Chen et al., 1992). In response to

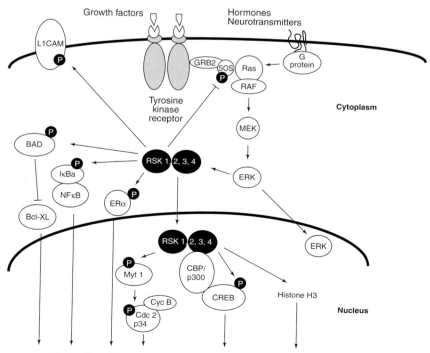

Figure 76–2. The ribosomal S6 serine/threonine kinase (RSK) signaling pathway. L1CAM, L1 cell adhesion molecule; GRB2, growth factor receptor–bound protein 2; SOS, Son-of-Sevenless; MEK, mitogen-activated protein kinase kinase; ERK, extracellular signal-regulated kinase; BAD, BCL2 antagonist of cell death; NK-κB, nuclear factor-κB; ERα, estrogen nuclear alpha receptor; CBP, CREB-binding protein; CREB, cAMP response element binding protein.

a

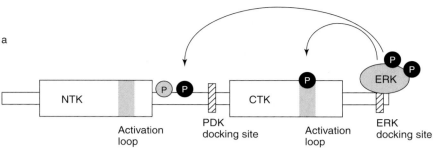

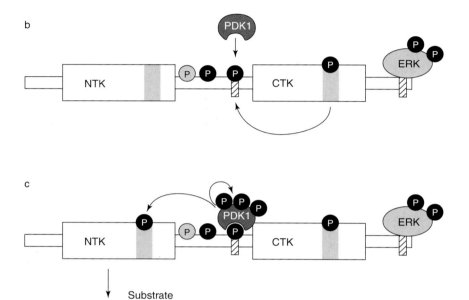

Figure 76–3. Events leading to ribosomal serine/threonine kinase (RSK) phosphotransferase activity. Activation of RSKs in vivo is associated with increased phosphorylation at six sites, of which four modulate kinase activity. The various putative or established RSK nuclear (NTK) and cytosolic (CTK) substrates are represented. PDK, 3-phosphoinositide–dependent protein kinase; ERK, extracellular signal-regulated kinase.

a mitogenic stimulation, both cytoplasmic and nuclear RSKs are activated and an increase in the nuclear pool is observed, suggesting a function in the nucleus (Zhao et al., 1995). The finding that RSKs efficiently phosphorylate transcription factors such as c-Fos, c-Jun, Nur77, or SRF in vitro supports a role for RSKs in the transcriptional control of gene expression (Blenis, 1993). In vivo studies have subsequently confirmed most of these substrates (Swanson et al., 1999; Brüning et al., 2000). Additional transcription factors, including the estrogen nuclear alpha receptor (ERα) (Joel et al., 1998) and CREB protein (Xing et al., 1996), have been identified as in vivo targets of RSKs. CREB protein, an important regulator of immediate-early gene expression, is implicated in various functions such as cell proliferation (Barton et al. 1996) and survival (Bonni et al, 1999). Ca^{2+}, cAMP, growth factors, and stress activate CREB protein through phosphorylation at Ser133 (Xing et al., 1996; De Cesare et al., 1998), indicating that CREB protein is an effector of multiple signaling pathways. Phosphorylation of CREB protein at Ser133 leads to the recruitment of the transcriptional coactivator CREB-binding protein (CBP) or p300 and induction of genes containing the cAMP response element (CRE) in the promoter. Growth factor-mediated CREB activation is Ras/ERK dependent (Ginty et al., 1994), and RSK2 has been shown to specifically phosphorylate CREB at Ser133 in cells stimulated with endothelium growth factor (EGF) (Xing et al., 1996). This result was confirmed in fibroblasts lacking functional RSK2 (De Cesare et al., 1998). Furthermore, lack of EGF-induced CREB phosphorylation in these cells correlated with a drastic reduction in c-*fos* induction, an immediate-early gene whose expression is regulated by CREB protein. Coffin-Lowry fibroblasts expressed normal levels of RSK1 and RSK3, indicating that they cannot replace RSK2 in EGF-induced activation of CREB protein in fibroblasts. By using mouse RSK2-defi-

cient cell lines, Brüning et al. (1997) confirmed that RSK2 is required for growth factor–stimulated expression of c-Fos.

RSK1 was shown to phosphorylate ERα at Ser167 in response to growth factor stimulation and thus to enhance its transcriptional activity (Joel et al., 1998).

RSKs were also demonstrated to associate with CBP and p300 in response to growth factor signaling. CBP and p300 are nuclear proteins that function as transcriptional coactivators of many transcription factors by creating a physical bridge between the transcription factor and the basal transcriptional machinery and by altering the chromatin structure (Montminy, 1997). The increasing variety of transcription factors that associate with CBP and p300, including CREB protein, c-Fos, c-Jun, STAT, MyoD, nuclear factor-κB (NF-κB), and steroid receptors, suggests that multiple cellular events may be coordinated by these proteins. Formation of the RSK–CBP complex was shown to repress cAMP-inducible transcription by CREB protein while allowing Ras-responsive transcription to be induced (Nakajima et al., 1996).

In addition to phosphorylating transcription factors, RSKs may be implicated in eliciting targeted alterations in the chromatin environment encompassing specific genes through the phosphorylation of nucleosomal and chromatin proteins. It has been known for a long time that histones are in vitro substrates of RSKs (Chen et al., 1992). Recent results have indicated that phosphorylation of histone H3 (at Ser10) is dramatically impaired in fibroblasts and in ES cells lacking RSK2 activity (Sassone-Corsi et al., 1999). Phosphorylation of Ser10 of histone H3 is believed to facilitate acetylation of Lys14 and thereby favor chromatin decondensation and transcription. Thus, in response to growth factor stimulation, CREB protein and histone H3 activities may be coordinately regulated through phosphorylation by RSK2, leading to the synergistic transcriptional activation of CREB-regulated genes.

In addition to a role in the nucleus, RSKs have been shown to phosphorylate IκBα, a cytosolic inhibitor of the transcription factor NF-κB (Schouten et al., 1997). NF-κB regulates the expression of various genes involved in inflammatory processes, proliferation, and apoptosis in response to a broad range of stimuli, including interleukin 1, the tumor necrosis factor α, and phorbol ester (Verma et al., 1995). NF-κB is present in an active form in the cytoplasm, bound to the inhibitory protein IκBα. On phosphorylation, IκBα is rapidly degradated, freeing NF-κB to translocate to the nucleus and to activate the expression of its target genes. A study identified two cytokine-responsive kinases that can phosphorylate IκBα (Zandi et al., 1997). However, coexpression studies have subsequently indicated that in phorbol ester–induced cells, RSK may also phosphorylate IκBα and stimulate NF-κB activation (Schouten et al., 1997). Thus, mitogenic stimulation of RSK may promote cell survival through indirect activation of genes responsive to NF-κB.

Other Cellular Actions

Son of sevenless (SOS) is an important guanine nucleotide exchange factor for Ras that becomes phosphorylated on serine and threonine residues after stimulation of the cells with growth factors. These phosphorylations are mediated in part by RSK2 and play a role in the negative feedback of Ras stimulation (Douville and Downward, 1997). Thus, RSK2 plays a role in the down-regulation of its own pathway.

Cytokines and growth factors promote cell survival in part through phosphorylation of the pro-apoptotic BCL2 antagonist of cell death (BAD) protein at two critical sites: Ser112 and Ser136. BAD phosphorylated at either of these sites binds to the cytosolic 14.3.3 protein, which prevents its dimerization with the anti-apoptotic BclX protein and, thus, apoptosis (Bertolotto et al., 2000). Although Ser136 is phosphorylated by protein kinase B, RSKs have been implicated in the phosphorylation of BAD at Ser112 (Bonni et al., 1999). Depending on the inducer, RSK-mediated phosphorylation of BAD Ser112 is ERK (Bonni et al., 1999) or protein kinase C dependent (Bertolotto et al., 2000). Thus, RSK may also promote cell survival through direct phosphorylation of BAD.

Finally, RSKs have been shown to associate with the L1 cell adhesion molecule, L1CAM, at the membrane and to phosphorylate it at a serine residue. L1CAM is involved in neuronal cell migration and axon growth during embryogenesis as well as in synaptic plasticity. This phosphorylation may regulate the interaction of L1CAM and intracellular signaling cascades or cytoskeletal elements involved in neurite outgrowth (Schaefer et al., 1999).

Although reported studies have considerably extended understanding of RSKs, many questions still remain. The respective contributions of each RSK family member to the in vivo activation of most known substrates are not well defined. Only two specific physiological substrates have, for example, been definitively identified for RSK2, the kinase that is inactivated in patients with CLS; CREB protein (De Cesare et al., 1998) and histone H3 (Sassone-Corsi et al., 1999). Another point that has not yet been addressed is whether various external stimuli preferentially lead to activation of a particular RSK protein in cell lines or tissues or whether their functions are in large part redundant. More important, although it is clearly established that the RSK signaling pathway plays an important role in cellular events such as growth and differentiation, the relevance of these events to the normal development and functioning of the whole organism is unknown. The identification of the CLS caused by inactivation of human RSK2 has shown that although RSK2 is widely expressed, it appears unnecessary for most aspects of normal growth and differentiation; most tissues and organs develop quite normally. The CLS phenotype also reveals that RSK2 has a unique role in cognitive function and skeletal development.

CLINICAL PHENOTYPE OF CLS

CLS is a syndromic form of X-linked mental retardation characterized in male patients by psychomotor retardation, growth retardation, and various skeletal anomalies. Typical facial changes and specific clinical and radiological hand aspects exhibited by patients are essential clues for diagnosis. CLS has been reported in families of European, Asian, and African origin (see references in Young, 1988). The incidence is unknown but is probably 1 to 2:100,000 males.

Inheritance

Coffin et al. (1966), Lowry et al. (1971), Procopis and Turner (1972), and Temtamy et al. (1975) suspected X-linked inheritance, and partial expression in a substantial proportion of female carriers led to the proposition of a semidominant mode of X-linked transmission. Genetic mapping studies definitively assigned the CLS locus to the X chromosome (Hanauer et al., 1988; Biancalana et al., 1992). Although no genetic heterogeneity has been detected, it cannot be completely excluded, based on the large number of patients referred to our diagnostic laboratory with a CLS phenotype but without detectable mutation in the *RSK2* gene (see later). An interstitial deletion on chromosome 10q was detected in a mentally retarded patient reported as being "CLS-like" (McCandless et al., 2000).

Clinical Features

The diagnosis is based on clinical examination. In adult male patients, the disease has a well-defined phenotype and can in most cases be diagnosed by professionals who are trained in genetic disorders. However, its clinical presentation may markedly vary both in severity and in the expression of uncommonly associated features, leading occasionally to diagnostic difficulties. In addition, in infancy the physical characteristics are usually very mild and CLS may be confused with other syndromes.

Skeletal Abnormalities

Intrauterine growth is often slow, but the birth weight is usually in the normal range. Growth retardation becomes apparent after the first months of life. Final adult height is usually below the third centile. Nevertheless, a normal stature should not exclude the diagnosis of CLS.

Facial features include a prominent forehead and supraorbital ridges with hypertelorism and downslanting of the palpebral fissures. The nose is bulbous with a thick septum and anteverted nares as well as thick alae. The mouth is wide and often open with full everted lips and small, irregular or missing teeth. Early loss of teeth is frequently noticed. The tongue tends to protrude and typically shows a deep median furrow. The ears, although of normal length, are often prominent or low set. Both microcephaly and macrocephaly have been reported but only in a small proportion of patients.

Limb abnormalities are relatively minor but characteristic of CLS. The hands are large with soft, lax skin and short, tapered, and puffy fingers with small nails (Fig. 76–4). The finger joints are frequently hyperextensible. Dermatoglyphic studies consistently reveal an unusual transversal hypothenar crease. Because of the presence of increased subcutaneous fat, forearm fullness is sometimes noticeable and may serve as an early aid in diagnosis (Hersh et al., 1984). Flat feet are frequent in patients with CLS.

Other frequent skeletal changes are spinal kyphosis and scoliosis with dysplasia of the vertebral bodies at the thoracolumbar junction. Kyphosis and scoliosis may be caused by the associated ligamentous laxity and changes in the intervertebral discs. Less constant skeletal features include pectus carinatum or excavatum and cervical ribs, narrow iliac wings, and shortening of the long bones of the lower limbs. Skeletal changes show progressive deterioration, and the spinal deformations often require surgical correction. The age of onset of puberty is usually normal or slightly late.

Radiological Findings

Radiological findings may include large frontal sinuses, calvarial hyperostosis, anterior wedging of the vertebral bodies, narrow intervertebral spaces, short sternum with failure of longitudinal fusion of the paired sternal segments, and ligamentum flava calcification. Some patients have a delayed bone age and a relative osteopenia. Most characteristic are the short metacarpals and phalanges, with tufting of the extremities of the distal phalanges. These changes, which may show

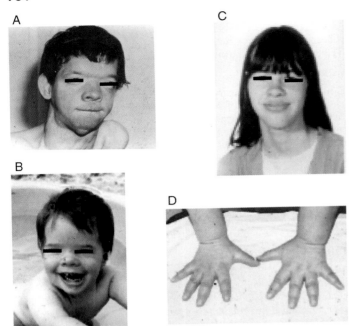

Figure 76–4. Patients with Coffin-Lowry syndrome (CLS). (*A*) Typical facial gestalt in a male. (*B*) The face of this 2-year-old boy is already peculiar, and most of the typical facial aspects of CLS are emerging: hypertelorism, frontal bossing with prominent supraorbital ridges, round nasal tip, full lips, and teeth anomalies. (*C*) Mild facial features in a female patient. (*D*) Characteristic hands with tapering fingers in a young boy.

progressive deterioration, are not pathognomonic but sufficiently distinctive to provide a good clue to the diagnosis. Brain anomalies such as hydrocephalus and corpus callosum agenesis have been occasionally described (Coffin et al., 1966; Lowry et al., 1971; Tentamy et al., 1975; Hunter et al., 1982; Ozden et al., 1994; Soekarman and Fryns, 1994).

Psychomotor Development and Behavior

The cognitive deficit in males with CLS is significant, with IQ scores ranging from 15 to 60 but clustering in the severe range. Partington et al. (1988) found no evidence for intellectual deterioration with age, although this had previously been reported (Coffin et al., 1966, Procopis et al., 1972). Development of speech is always involved but to varying degrees. Motor development is also delayed and marked in infancy by hypotonia. The mean age of walking is 3 years. Difficulties in ambulation may persist with a clumsy gait or resume during childhood.

Affected individuals tend to be loving, friendly, and easy to get along with. Their temperament often remains friendly throughout life. Despite their limited verbal abilities, their communication skills are good.

Other Clinical Features

Sensorineural hearing deficit has been described in numerous patients (Wilson et al., 1981; Hunter et al., 1982; Collacott et al., 1987; Hartsfield et al., 1993). Significant deafness concerns approximately one third of patients with CLS. The deficit is bilateral and may be highly variable in severity. In addition, there might be intrafamilial variability (Hartsfield et al., 1993). Regular hearing checks are recommended because late-onset deafness has been described (Rosanowski et al., 1998).

Seizures have been described in approximately one third of patients with CLS (Lowry et al., 1971; Fryns et al., 1977; Partington et al., 1988). Seizures do not appear to be of a specific type and are not particularly resistant to antiepileptic drugs.

Fryns et al. (1977) described the frequent occurrence of episodes of sudden, nonepileptic collapses with atonia in two CLS-affected brothers. These drop attacks were generally induced by a loud noise,

a surprise, or excitement, and their severity and frequency worsened with age. Subsequently, these authors observed the same sudden collapse phenomenon in an additional male of 20 patients with CLS whom they examined (Fryns and Smeets, 1998). Crow et al. (1998) reported the same nonepileptic collapses with atonia, which they described as a cataplexy-like phenomenon, in two males and one female. Electroencephalography, MRI, and brain and cerebral angiography results were normal in these patients. Caraballo et al. (2000) stated that these drop episodes are an unusual form of exaggerated startle response, differing from hypereplexia. The origin of the drop episodes remains unclear. Benzodiazepine administration reduced the frequency of drop episodes in one patient (Nakamura et al., 1998).

Cardiac involvement has been noted since the first description of the syndrome (Coffin et al., 1966). There are scanty reports mentioning various cardiac problems, namely, mitral valve regurgitation, heart murmur, myocardiopathy, and endomyocardial fibroelastosis (Tentamy et al., 1975; Hunter et al., 1982; Della Cella et al., 1987; Machin et al., 1987; Charles et al., 1988; Gilgenkrantz et al., 1988; Plomp et al., 1995; Massin et al., 1999). Thus, a myocardial disorder seems to be part of CLS and requires specific cardiac follow-up.

Diagnosis in Infancy

The clinical features of CLS are not evident at birth or even in infancy. Pregnancy is often uneventful, but an excess of amniotic fluid together with a reduction in fetal movements has been noted before delivery. Affected newborn boys usually show only hypotonia and hyperlaxity of joints. Retardation of growth and psychomotor development become gradually evident after the first months of life. Facial coarsening is mild and usually hard to recognize in infancy, becoming progressively pronounced and characteristic only in late childhood. Similarly, a delayed closure of the anterior fontanel beyond the age of 2 years has been reported in several cases. However, in infancy, a prominent forehead with a large anterior fontanel, hypertelorism, bulbous nose with anteverted nares, full upper lip, fullness of the forearms, transverse hypothenar crease, and tapered fingers are notable. Other possible early signs are sensorineural hearing deficit and microcephaly (Harsfield et al., 1993). Sternal malformations have been described in a few boys at birth (Tentamy et al., 1975); however, skeletal deformities usually become apparent only after the age of 2 years.

Clinical Expression in Female Patients

Some of the physical features seen in males may also be found in females, but they are neither as prominent nor as constant. The most consistent features are large and soft fleshy hands with distal tapering fingers and a tendency to obesity. Hand radiographs show similar findings as those in male patients. Less frequently, a short stature, a coarse face with prominent brow, hypertelorism, pouting lips, and thick nasal tissues are seen (see Fig. 76–4). Cognitive function of female carriers may be mildly impaired or normal. Frequently, they are reported to have learning difficulties at school. Epilepsy may develop (Partington et al., 1988; Plomp et al., 1995). Psychiatric illness (depression, psychotic behavior, and schizophrenia) has been described in a few female patients (Haspeslagh et al., 1984; Collacott et al., 1987).

Differential Diagnosis

In very young male patients, the mild physical characteristics of CLS may be confused with other syndromes. Among these are most notably alpha-thalassemia with mental retardation syndrome (ATR-X, OMIM 300032), fragile X syndrome (OMIM 309550), Sotos syndrome (OMIM 117550), Williams syndrome (OMIM 194050), lysosomal storage disease (Plomp et al., 1995), and some chromosomal anomalies, as previously discussed (McCandless et al., 2000).

THE MOLECULAR BASIS OF CLS

Spectrum of Mutations

By screening 250 unrelated individuals with clinical features suggestive of CLS, more than 75 distinct disease-associated *RSK2* mutations

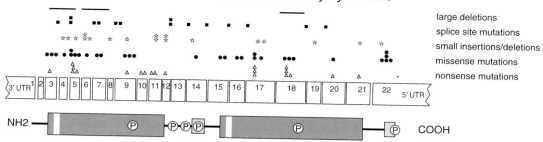

Figure 76–5. Mutation spectrum of the ribosomal S6 serine/threonine kinase-2 (*RSK2*) gene. Mutations so far detected are shown above the schematic representation of the RSK2 transcript and protein.

were identified in 85 of the patients (Fig. 76–5) (Trivier et al., 1996; Jacquot et al., 1998a; Abidi et al., 1999; Delaunoy et al., 2001). Approximately 40% of these mutations were missense mutations, 20% were nonsense mutations, 20% were splicing errors, and 20% were short deletion or insertion events. Only three large deletions, two involving two exons and the third involving only one exon, have been found so far. Mutations have occurred throughout all exons, except exons 1 and 2, and only 11 mutations have been found in more than one family: the most prevalent alterations are three nonsense mutations (three occurrences each) and a missense mutation (three occurrences) (Fig. 76–5). It is intriguing that a high rate of new mutations was observed. Indeed, in a total of 41 families for which samples were available from the mothers of the probands, two thirds (27 of 41) of the mutations arose de novo in the proband. This high proportion of de novo mutation is very unusual in X-linked disorders and has received no explanation as yet. Evidence for germinal mosaicism was clearly demonstrated in two families (Jacquot et al., 1998b; Horn et al., 2001) (Fig. 76–6), and strong suggestion was provided by a few additional families. Ten mutations have been identified in young fe-male probands who had learning disability and mild but suggestive physical phenotype but who had no affected male relatives (Delaunoy et al., 2001).

Two thirds of *RSK2* mutations result in premature translation termination, of which the vast majority has been shown or can be predicted to cause complete loss of function of the mutant allele. One third of *RSK2* mutations exert their effects by substituting one amino acid for another. A number of these missense mutations alter known phosphorylation sites (or surrounding amino acids belonging to their recognition motifs) critical for RSK2 catalytic function, ATP-binding sites, or the ERK docking site, and their detrimental effect is obvious. The mechanism by which the remaining missense mutations exert their effects is less evident, but in most cases the secondary structure of the kinase domains is likely to be disrupted.

Genotype–Phenotype Relationship

No consistent relationship has been observed between specific mutations and the severity of the disease or the expression of particular features. The extent of protein truncations shows no correlation with the disease severity. This makes genetic counseling difficult because an estimation of the severity of involvement cannot be given to parents. It is interesting, however, that significantly milder disease was noted in some cases carrying missense mutations compared with the vast majority of those with truncating mutations. For instance, the I189K mutation, which results in a mutant protein retaining 10% of residual enzymatic activity, was identified in two slightly retarded male siblings with a very mild form of CLS (Manouvrier-Hanu et al., 1999). The less severely affected male of our cohort of patients expressed a mutant protein retaining 20% of residual kinase activity (Merienne et al., 1999). The patient bearing this mutation and his affected male relatives were only mildly mentally retarded. This family was previously reported as a nonsyndromic X-linked mental retardation family (Donnelly et al., 1994), and these patients cannot be formally classified as CLS patients because they do not exhibit any physical feature of the syndrome. Thus, the tendency in some patients carrying a missense mutation to be less affected suggests a pivotal role of residual enzyme activity in determining the severity of symptoms. It is, however, difficult to extend this observation to all known missense mutations because detailed clinical data and cell lines, which are necessary for assessing the kinase activity, of a high proportion of patients have not been available. In addition, patients have been examined by different clinicians, and there was no common definition of severity. Nevertheless, investigation in a few families with multiple affected members revealed that there may be intrafamilial variability for severity or for expression of uncommonly associated features. Thus, current data suggest that the genotype of the mutation is not the only determinant in the phenotypic expression. Environmental factors or other components that contribute to the same physiological function as the RSK2 protein may also influence the presentation of the disease. Modifying genes could be those encoding other RSK members or the closely related mitogen- and stress-activated protein kinases (MSKs) (see the review by Frödin and Gammeltoft, 1999) or genes that encode proteins that participate in the same pathway.

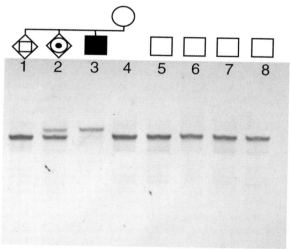

Figure 76–6. Single-strand conformation polymorphism (SSCP) analysis of exon 5 and flanking intron boundaries in five sporadic cases showing clinical features highly suggestive of Coffin-Lowry syndrome (lanes 3 and 5–8). Primers and conditions used for RT-PCR amplification and SSCP analysis have been described previously (Jacquot et al., 1998a). A band shift caused by a C-to-T transition at nucleotide 328 was found in the first male patient (lane 3). The mutation resulted in the creation of a premature stop codon (R110X). His unaffected mother did not carry the mutation (lane 4), demonstrating the occurrence of a de novo event. Two prenatal diagnoses were performed. A female fetus (lane 2) was found to be heterozygous for the band shift, and thus a carrier, whereas a subsequent male fetus (lane 1) carried a normal allele. These results, confirmed by direct sequencing of the PCR products, provided evidence for gonadal mosaicism. Four additional and unrelated males (lanes 5–8) showed normal bands.

MOLECULAR DIAGNOSIS FOR CLS

In the series of 250 patients clinically diagnosed with CLS and referred to our laboratory for mutation screening, a mutation was identified in only 34%. As stated previously, most clinical features are nonspecific and clinical examination may not always distinguish CLS from other mental retardation syndromes, in particular, in very young children. In addition, most cases (around 80%) of CLS are sporadic. Thus, it is very likely that misdiagnosis played the most important role in the failure to detect more mutations in our series of patients. Therefore, screening for RSK2 mutations appears essential to firmly establish the diagnosis of CLS in the majority of patients and to establish molecular prenatal or carrier diagnosis to families.

Mutation Screening

Mutation screening of the RSK2 gene is performed in our laboratory by single-strand conformation polymorphism analysis of PCR-amplified exons from genomic DNA (see Fig. 76–6), followed by sequencing of products exhibiting variants (Jacquot et al., 1998a; Delaunoy et al., 2001). Although no "hot spot" for mutations is apparent, some clustering can be observed. A larger number of mutations are localized within exon 5 (13%), exon 17 (10%), and exons 9 and 18 (each 9%). It is thus relevant to screen mutations starting from these exons.

Functional Assays

Given the complex structure of the *RSK2* gene and the diversity of mutations, a systematic search for mutations can be a time-consuming and expensive process. Therefore, Western blot and kinase assay tests have been set up that are of great value in the differential diagnosis of CLS (Merienne et al., 1998). Based on current knowledge of the nature of mutations in *RSK2*, it can be estimated that Western blot analysis of RSK2 allows the detection of up to 70% of the mutated RSK2 proteins. Western blot analysis can be performed on lymphocyte protein extracts prepared directly from fresh (less than 24 hours) blood samples or from a lymphoblast or a fibroblast cell line (Fig. 76–7). The remaining RSK2 mutations are missense changes that have for the most part been shown to result in partial or complete loss of RSK2 phosphotransferase activity. Thus, an in vitro kinase assay was also developed. This latter assay would be the diagnostic method of choice because it has the potential to detect all classes of mutations and to provide information on a possible residual enzyme activity. However, it can be used only on a fibroblast cell line. Both Western blot and kinase assays can be used for prenatal diagnosis because the RSK2 protein is readily detectable in cultured amniocytes (Fig. 76–7). Unfortunately, female carrier detection is not feasible with Western blot analysis or kinase assay because of random X inactivation.

TREATMENT

There is no specific treatment for CLS. Current effective management of patients focuses on supportive and symtomatic therapy. In particular, sensorineural hearing deficit should be addressed very early to improve the development and quality of life of the patients. Progressive spine deformation (scoliosis/kyphosis) may require surgery in adulthood.

ANIMAL MODEL

A mouse model for CLS, obtained through homologous recombination and carrying targeted mutations at the *Rsk2* locus, was described (Dufresne et al., 2001). Mutant mice show no obvious skeletal abnormality but weigh 10% less and are 14% shorter than wild-type littermates. Glycogen metabolism in skeletal muscle is slightly altered. Treatment with either insulin or exercise resulted in an elevated and prolonged activation of ERK1 and ERK2 phosphorylation in the muscle of mutant mice, suggesting that RSK2 plays an important functional role in feedback inhibition of ERK signaling in vivo. The mice also exhibit impaired learning and poor coordination, providing evidence that RSK2 has similar roles in mental functioning in both mice and humans. Thus, these mice could provide a valuable model for the study of CLS and a powerful tool to examine in greater detail the role of RSK2 in brain development, cognitive function, and bone formation. A more profound understanding of the physiological roles of RSK2 and the pathophysiology is the prerequisite for the suggestion of possible therapeutical approaches.

POSSIBLE PATHOGENIC MECHANISMS

The nature of the anatomical and physiological defects in CLS patients in relation to *RSK2* mutations is still poorly understood. However, the fact that cognitive impairment is a prominent feature indicates an important role of RSKs in development and/or function of the central nervous system. At a macroscopic level, no reproducible pathological abnormalities have been reported, suggesting that RSK2 is not required for major aspects of brain development. The possibility that RSKs are involved in more subtle processes like neuronal plasticity has begun to receive attention. The ERK-MAPK signaling cascade is required for both long-term memory formation and synaptic plasticity (Atkins et al., 1998; Silva et al., 1998; Blum et al., 1999). A defect in CREB phosphorylation is also a potential cause of the cognitive impairment because cells derived from patients with CLS are deficient in EGF-stimulated CREB phosphorylation (De Cesare et al., 1998). A growing body of evidence documents CREB activation as an essential step in the process of learning and long-term memory formation (Yin et al., 1994; Gass et al., 1998). Long-term potentiation, a long-lasting increase in the efficacy of synaptic transmission, is postulated to be a model for cellular mechanisms underlying learning and memory acquisition (Bliss et al., 1993). Long-term potentiation requires the synthesis of proteins, and activation of the transcription factor CREB represents one step in the cascade of events leading to this protein synthesis. Interestingly, Harum et al. (2001) demonstrated a direct relationship between the magnitude of in vitro RSK2-mediated CREB phosphorylation and intelligence level in patients with CLS. This result supports the hypothesis that the Ras-MAPK pathway signaling through RSK2 to CREB plays a prominent role in cognitive dysfunction in patients with CLS. Genes anticipated to have altered regulation due to impaired CREB activation are those with a CREB binding site within their promoter region. In addition to several immediate-early genes and transcription factors regulated by CREB, there are numbers of other genes with promoters that include a CRE sequence whose products are involved in learning. These latter genes include those encoding the brain-derived neurotrophic factor (BDNF), the transcription factor C/EBP, and the extracellular protease tissue plasminogen activator (tPA). Perturbation in the transcriptional regulation of these genes, and others, are hypothesized to underlie at least some aspects of the CLS phenotype.

RSK2 has also been identified in *N*-methyl-D-aspartate (NMDA) receptor multiprotein complexes isolated from mouse brain (Husi et al., 2000). The NMDA receptor has been implicated in the induction of synaptic plasticity through activation of second-messenger pathways.

It is noteworthy that two putative substrates of RSK2—CBP and L1CAM—have also been implicated in brain function and mental retardation. Mutations in the gene encoding CBP were found to cause

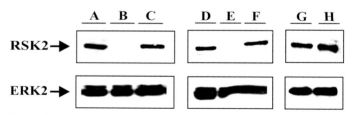

Figure 76–7. Western blot analysis of the ribosomal S6 serine/threonine kinase-2 (RSK2) (*top*) and extracellular signal-regulated kinase-2 (ERK1) (*bottom*) proteins (control for protein amount) in lymphoblast (*left*) and fibroblast (*middle*) cell lines and cultured amniocytes (*right*). Lanes A, C, D, and F represent normal control males, and lanes B and E are Coffin-Lowry syndrome–affected male patients carrying truncating RSK2 mutations. Lanes G and H are from normal male fetuses.

Rubinstein-Taybi syndrome (RTS; OMIM 180849) (Petrij et al., 1995; see Chapter 71). RTS is an autosomal dominant disorder characterized by retarded growth and mental function and various skeletal abnormalities. Indeed, some similarities exist between the phenotypes of patients with RTS and patients with mutations in RSK2, suggesting that a defect in CBP transcriptional regulation could contribute to the CLS phenotype. Formation of the CBP–RSK complex was proposed to contribute to the ability of nerve growth factor to induce neuronal differentiation (Nakajima et al., 1996). Mutations in the L1CAM gene are responsible for an X-linked neurological disorder that has been described as CRASH syndrome (OMIM 303350). One of the most consistent features in affected boys is mental retardation. Phosphorylation of L1CAM by RSK may regulate the interaction of L1CAM and intracellular signaling cascades or cytoskeletal elements involved in neurite outgrowth (Schaefer et al., 1999). Critical aims of current studies are to verify whether these candidate RSK effectors actually serve as physiologically relevant effectors of RSK2 function and to define their precise contribution to RSK2 signaling in cognitive function.

It is unclear how mutations in *RSK2* give rise to skeletal defects in CLS. However, studies with a fibroblast cell line derived from a patient with CLS have indicated that the cells are defective in c-*fos* gene expression induced by EGF (De Cesare et al., 1998). Various studies have established a unique role for the nuclear transcription factor c-*fos* in regulating the differentiation and activity of specific bone cell populations during development. It is interesting that phenotypic manifestations of mice lacking c-*fos* include growth retardation and deficiencies in bone remodeling and tooth eruption, highly reminiscent of those expressed by patients with CLS (Wang et al., 1992). Thus, it can be hypothesized that the loss of c-*fos* regulation in patients with CLS is responsible, at least in part, for skeletal changes and teeth abnormalities. Moreover, the mild behavioral abnormalities shown by the c-*fos* knockout mice further strengthens the similarity with the CLS phenotype.

The mouse model that has been reported will be important to obtain further insight into the molecular mechanisms that lead to CLS.

NOTE ADDED IN PROOF

One of the most provocative recent observations in BWS is that there may be an excess of assisted reproductive technology (ART) among IVF patients. DeBaun et al. (2003) found that ART was approximately 6-fold more common among BWS patients than in the general population. This difference was not specific to the mode of ART, as it included both in vitro fertilization and intracytoplasmic sperm injection. However, almost all of the patients showed a hypomethylation defect involving imprinting of *LIT1*. Maher et al. (2003) also found a fourfold excess of ART among IVF patients, also with a hypomethylation imprinting defect. Since overgrowth is a common feature of in vitro culture of ruminants, with imprinting defects, it is reasonable that in vitro culture can lead to imprinting and overgrowth defects in humans. It is most important that careful outcomes measures be put in place for ART to look for this phenomenon, since it may be avoidable, and it may also provide clues to prenatal epigenetic causes of birth defects in non-ART and non-BWS population.

ACKNOWLEDGMENTS

We are deeply indebted to the many CLS families and clinicians around the world who made possible the CLS study. We gratefully acknowledge Prof. J. L. Mandel, all of the members of our research group, and collaborators, past and present, for their enduring contribution.

REFERENCES

Abidi F, Jacquot S, Lassiter C, Trivier E, Hanauer A, Schwartz CE (1999). Novel mutations in Rsk-2, the gene for Coffin-Lowry syndrome (CLS). *Eur J Hum Genet* 7: 20–26.

Atkins CM, Selcher JC, Petraitis JJ, Trzaskos JM, Sweatt JD (1998). The MAPK cascade is required for mammalian associative learning. *Nat Neurosci* 1: 602–609.

Barton WW, Wilcoxen SE, Christensen PJ, Paine R (1996). Association of ICAM-1 with the cytoskeleton in rat alveolar epithelial cells in primary culture. *Am J Physiol* 271: L707–L718.

Bertolotto C, Maulon L, Filippa N, Baier G, Auberger P (2000). Protein kinase C theta and epsilon promote T-cell survival by a rsk-dependent phosphorylation and inactivation of BAD. *J Biol Chem* 275: 37246–37250.

Biancalana V, Briard ML, David A, Gilgenkrantz S, Kaplan J, Mathieu M, Piussan C, Poncin J, Schintzel A, Oudet C, et al. (1992). Confirmation and refinement of the genetic localization of the Coffin-Lowry syndrome locus in Xp22.1-p22.2. *Am J Hum Genet* 50: 981–987.

Bjorbaek C, Vik TA, Echwald SM, Yang PY, Vestergaard H, Wang JP, Webb GC, Richmond K, Hansen T, Erikson RL, et al. (1995). Cloning of a human insulin-stimulated protein kinase (ISPK-1) gene and analysis of coding regions and mRNA levels of the ISPK-1 and the protein phosphatase-1 genes in muscle from NIDDM patients. *Diabetes* 44: 90–97.

Blenis J (1993). Signal transduction via the MAP kinases; proceed at your own RSK. *Proc Natl Acad Sci* USA 90: 5889–5892.

Bliss TVP, Collingridge GL (1993). A synaptic model of memory: long-term potentiation in the hippocampus. *Nature* 361: 31–39.

Blum S, Moore AN, Adams F, Dash PK (1999). A mitogen-activated protein cascade in the CA1/CA2 subfield of the dorsal hippocampus is essential for long-term spatial memory. *J Neurosci* 19: 3535–3544.

Bonni A, Brunet A, West AE, Datta SR, Takasu MA, Greenberg ME (1999). Cell survival promoted by the Ras-MAPK signaling pathway by transcription-dependent and –independent mechanisms. *Science* 286: 358–362.

Bruning JC, Gillette JA, Zhao Y, Bjorbaeck C, Kotzka J, Knebel B, Avci H, Hanstein B, Lingohr P, Moller DE, et al. (2000). Ribosomal subunit kinase-2 is required for growth factor-stimulated transcription of the c-Fos gene. *Proc Natl Acad Sci USA* 97: 2462–2467.

Cano E, Mahadevan LC (1995). Parallel signal processing among mammalian MAPKs. *Trends Biochem Sci* 20: 117–122.

Caraballo R, Tesi Rocha A, Medina C, Fejerman N (2000). Drop episodes in Coffin-Lowry syndrome: an unusual type of startle response. *Epileptic Disord* 2: 173–1766.

Charles S, Passuti N, Rogez JM, David A (1988). Fatal cardiac complications in a child operated on for severe scoliosis with a Coffin-Lowry syndrome. A propos of a case. *Chir Pediatr* 29: 36–38.

Chen RH, Sarnecki C, Blenis J (1992). Nuclear localization and regulation of erk- and rsk-encoded protein kinases. *Mol Cell Biol* 12: 915–927.

Coffin GS, Siris E, Wegienka LC (1966). Mental retardation with osteocartilaginous anomalies. *Am J Dis Child* 112: 205–213.

Collacott RA, Warrington JS, Young ID (1987). Coffin-Lowry syndrome and schizophrenia: a family report. *J Ment Defic Res* 31: 1999–1207.

Crow YJ, Zuberi SM, McWilliam R, Tolmie JL, Hollman A, Pohl K, Stephenson JB (1998). "Cataplexy" and muscle ultrasound abnormalities in Coffin-Lowry syndrome. *J Med Genet* 35: 94–98.

Dalby KN, Morrice N, Caudwell FB, Avruch J, Cohen P 1998). Identification of regulatory phosphorylation sites in mitogen-activated protein kinase (MAPK)-activated protein kinase-1a/p90rsk that are inducible by MAPK. *J Biol Chem* 273: 1496–1505.

DeBaun MR, Niemitz EL, Feinberg AP. Association of in vitro fertilization with Beckwith-Wiedemann syndrome and epigenetic alternations of LIT1 and H19 (2003). *Am J Hum Genet* 72: 156–160.

Delaunoy JP, Abidi F, Zeniou M, Jacquot S, Merienne K, Pannetier S, Schmitt M, Schwartz CE, Hanauer A (2001). Mutations in the X-linked RSK2 gene (RPS6KA3) in patients with Coffin-Lowry syndrome. *Hum Mut* 17: 103–116.

De Cesare D, Jacquot S, Hanauer A, Sassone-Corsi P (1998). Rsk-2 activity is necessary for epidermal growth factor-induced phosphorylation of CREB protein and transcription of c-fos gene. *Proc Natl Acad Sci USA* 95: 12202–12207.

Della Cella G, Stagnaro MG, Beluschi C, Forni GL (1987). Coffin-Lowry syndrome. Description of 2 cases associated with cardiovascular anomalies. *Pediatr Med Chir* 9: 229–232.

Donnelly AJ, Choo KH, Kozman HM, Gedeon AK, Danks DM, Mulley JC (1994). Regional localisation of a non-specific X-linked mental retardation gene (MRX19) to Xp22. *Am J Med Genet* 51: 581–585.

Douville E, Downward J (1997). EGF induced SOS phosphorylation in PC12 cells involves P90 RSK-2. *Oncogene* 15: 373–383.

Dufresne SD, Bjorbaek C, El-Haschimi K, Zhao Y, Aschenbach WG, Moller DE, Goodyear LJ (2001). Altered extracellular signal-regulated kinase signaling and glycogen metabolism in skeletal muscle from p90 ribosomal S6 kinase 2 knockout mice. *Mol Cell Biol* 21: 81–87.

Erikson E, Maller JL (1985). A protein kinase from Xenopus eggs specific for ribosomal protein S6. *Proc Natl Acad Sci USA* 82: 742–746.

Fisher TL, Blenis J (1996). Evidence for two catalytically active kinase domains in pp90rsk. *Mol Cell Biol* 16: 1212–1219.

Frödin M, Gammeltoft S (1999). Role and regulation of 90 kDa ribosomal S6 kinase (RSK) in signal transduction. *Mol Cell Endocrinol* 25: 65–77.

Frödin M, Jensen CJ, Merienne K, Gammeltoft S (2000). A phosphoserine-regulated docking site in the protein kinase RSK2 that recruits and activates PDK1. *EMBO J* 19: 2924–2934.

Fryns JP, Smeets E. (1998) "Cataplexy" in Coffin-Lowry syndrome. *J Med Genet* 35: 702.

Fryns JP, Vinken L, Van den Berghe P (1977). The Coffin syndrome. *Hum Genet* 10: 271–306.

Gass P, Wolfer DP, Balschun D, Rudolph D, Frey U, Lipp HP, Schutz G (1998). Deficits in memory tasks of mice with CREB mutations depend on gene dosage. *Learn Mem* 5: 274–288.

Ginty DD, Bonni A, Greenberg ME (1994). Nerve growth factor activates a Ras-dependent protein kinase that stimulates c-fos transcription via phosphorylation of CREB. *Cell* 77: 713–725.

Gilgenkrantz S, Mujica P, Gruet P, Tridon P, Schweitzer F, Nivelon-Chevallier A, Nivelon JL (1988). Coffin-Lowry syndrome: a multicenter study. *Clin Genet* 34: 230–245.

Grove JR, Price DJ, Banerjee P, Balasubramanyam A, Ahmad MF, Avruch J (1993). Protein Regulation of an epitope-tagged recombinant Rsk-1 S6 kinase by phorbol ester and ERK/MAP kinase. *Biochemistry* 32: 7727–7738.

Hanauer A, Alembik Y, Gilgenkrantz S, Mujica P, Nivelon-Chevallier A, Pembrey ME,

Young ID, Mandel JL (1988). Probable localisation of the Coffin-Lowry locus in Xp22.2-p22.1 by multipoint linkage analysis. *Am J Med Genet* 30: 523–530.

Hartsfield JK Jr, Hall BD, Grix AW, Kousseff BG, Salazar JF, Haufe SM (1993). Pleiotropy in Coffin-Lowry syndrome: sensorineural hearing deficit and premature tooth loss as early manifestations. *Am J Med Genet* 45: 552–557.

Harum KH, Alemi L, Johnston MV (2001). Cognitive impairment in Coffin-Lowry syndrome correlates with reduced RSK2 activation. *Neurology* 56: 207–214.

Haspeslagh M, Fryns JP, Beusen L, Van Dessel F, Vinken L, Moens E, Van den Berghe H (1984). The Coffin-Lowry syndrome. A study of two new index patients and their families. *Eur J Pediatr* 143: 82–86.

Hersh JH, Weisskopf B, DeCoster C (1984). Forearm fullness in Coffin-Lowry syndrome: a misleading yet possible early diagnostic clue. *Am J Med Genet* 18: 195–199.

Horn D, Delaunoy JP, Kunze J (2001). Prenatal diagnosis in Coffin-Lowry syndrome demonstrates germinal mosaicism confirmed by mutation analysis. *Prenat Diag* 21: 881–884.

Hunter AG, Partington MW, Evans JA (1982) The Coffin-Lowry syndrome. Experience from four centres. *Clin Genet* 21: 321–335.

Husi H, Ward MA, Choudhary JS, Blackstock WP, Grant SG (2000). Proteomic analysis of NMDA receptor-adhesion protein signaling complexes. *Nat Neurosci* 3: 661–669.

Impey S, Smith DM, Obrietan K, Donahue R, Wade C, Storm DR (1998). Stimulation of cAMP response element (CRE)-mediated transcription during contextual learning. *Nat Neurosci* 1: 595–601.

Jacquot S, Merienne K, Pannetier S, Blumenfeld S, Schinzel A, Hanauer A (1998b). Germline mosaicism in Coffin-Lowry syndrome. *Eur J Hum Genet* 6: 578–582.

Jacquot S, Merienne K, De Cesare D, Pannetier S, Mandel JL, Sassone-Corsi P, Hanauer A (1998a). Mutation analysis of the RSK2 gene in Coffin-Lowry patients: extensive allelic heterogeneity and a high rate of de novo mutations. *Am J Hum Genet* 63: 1631–1640.

Joel PB, Smith J, Sturgill TW, Fisher TL, Blenis J and Lannigan DA (1998). pp90rsk1 regulates estrogen receptor-mediated transcription through phosphorylation of Ser-167. *Mol Cell Biol* 18: 1978–1984.

Karin M, Hunter T (1995). Transcriptional control by protein phosphorylation: signal transmission from the cell surface to the nucleus. *Curr Biol* 5: 747–757.

Leighton IA, Dalby KN, Caudwell FB, Cohen PT, Cohen P 1995). Comparison of the specificities of p70 S6 kinase and MAPKAP kinase-1 identifies a relatively specific substrate for p70 S6 kinase: the N-terminal kinase domain of MAPKAP kinase-1 is essential for peptide phosphorylation. *FEBS Lett* 375: 289–293.

Lowry B, Miller JR, Fraser FC (1971). A new dominant gene mental retardation syndrome. Association with small stature, tapering fingers, characteristic facies, and possible hydrocephalus. *Am J Dis Child* 121: 496–500.

Machin GA, Walther GL, Fraser VM (1987). Autopsy findings in two adult siblings with Coffin-Lowry syndrome. *Am J Med Genet* 3(Suppl): 303–309.

Maher ER, Brueton LA, Bowdin SC, Lutharia A, Cooper W, Cole TR, Macdonald F, Sampson JR, Barratt CL, Reik W, Hawkins MM (2003). Beckwith-Wiedemann syndrome and assisted reproduction technology (ART). *J Med Genet* 40: 62–64.

McCandless SE, Schwartz S, Morrison S, Garlapati K, Robin NH (2000) Adult with an interstitial deletion of chromosome 10 [del(10)(q25.1q25.3)]: overlap with Coffin-Lowry syndrome. *Am J Med Genet* 13: 93–98.

Manouvrier-Hanu S, Amiel J, Jacquot S, Merienne K, Moerman A, Coeslier A, VallÇe L, Croquette MF, Hanauer A (1999). Unreported RSK2 missense mutation in two male siblings with an unusually mild form of Coffin-Lowry syndrome. *J Med Genet* 36: 775–778.

Massin MM, Radermecker MA, Verloes A, Jacquot S, Grenade T (1999). Cardiac involvement in Coffin-Lowry syndrome. *Acta Paediatr* 88: 468–470.

Merienne K, Jacquot S, Zeniou M, Pannetier S, Sassone-Corsi P, Hanauer A (2000). Activation of RSK by UV-light: phosphorylation dynamics and involvement of the MAPK pathway. *Oncogene* 19: 4221–4229.

Merienne K, Jacquot S, Trivier E, Pannetier S, Rossi A, Schinzel A, Castellan C, Kress W, Hanauer A (1998). Rapid immunoblot and kinase assay tests for a syndromal form of X-linked mental retardation: Coffin-Lowry syndrome. *J Med Genet* 35: 890–894.

Merienne K, Jacquot S, Pannetier S, Zeniou M, Bankier A, Gecz J, Mandel JL, Mulley J, Sassone-Corsi P, Hanauer A (1999). A missense mutation in RPS6KA3 (RSK2) responsible for non-specific mental retardation. *Nat Genet* 22: 13–14.

Moller DE, Xia CH, Tang T, Zhu A, Jakubowsky M (1994). Human rsk isoforms: cloning and characterization of tissue-specific expression. *Am J Physiol* 266: C351–C359.

Montminy M (1997). Transcriptional activation. Something new to hang your HAT on. *Nature* 387: 654–655.

Nakajima T, Fukamizu A, Takahashi J, Gage FH, Fisher T, Blenis J, Montminy MR (1996). The signal-dependent coactivator CBP is a nuclear target for pp90RSK. *Cell* 86: 465–474.

Nakamura M, Yamagata T, Momoi MY, Yamazaki T (1998). Drop episodes in Coffin-Lowry syndrome: exaggerated startle responses treated with clonazepam. *Pediatr Neurol* 19: 148–150.

Ozden A, Dirik E, Emel A, Sevinc N (1994). Callosal dysgenesis in a patient with Coffin-Lowry syndrome. *Indian J Pediatr* 61: 101–103.

Partington MW, Mulley JC, Sutherland GR, Thode A, Turner G (1988). A family with the Coffin Lowry syndrome revisited: localization of CLS to Xp21-pter. *Am J Med Genet* 30: 509–521.

Petrij F, Giles RH, Dauwerse HG, Saris JJ, Hennekam RC, Masuno M, Tommerup N, van Ommen GJ, Goodman RH, Peters DJ (1995). Rubinstein-Taybi syndrome caused by mutations in the transcriptional co-activator CBP. *Nature* 376: 348–351.

Plomp AS, De Die-Smulders CEM, Meinecke P, Ypma-Verhulst JM, Lissone DA, Fryns JP (1995). Coffin-Lowry syndrome: clinical aspects at different ages and symptoms in female carriers. *Gen Counsel* 6: 259–268.

Procopis PG, Turner B (1972). Mental retardation, abnormal fingers, and skeletal anomalies: Coffin's syndrome. *Am J Dis Child* 124: 258–261.

Rosanowski F, Hoppe U, Proschel U, Eysholdt U (1998). Late-onset sensorineural hearing loss in Coffin-Lowry syndrome. *ORL J Otorhinolaryngol Relat* 60: 224–226.

Sassone-Corsi P, Mizzen CA, Cheung P, Crosio C, Monaco L, Jacquot S, Hanauer A, Allis CD (1999). Requirement of Rsk-2 for epidermal growth factor-activated phosphorylation of histone H3. *Science* 285: 886–890.

Schaefer AW, Kamiguchi H, Wong EV, Beach CM, Landreth G, Lemmon V (1999). Activation of the MAPK signal cascade by the neural cell adhesion molecule L1 requires L1 internalization. *J Biol Chem* 274: 37965–37973.

Schouten GJ, Vertegaal AC, Whiteside ST, Israel A, Toebes M, Dorsman JC, van der Eb AJ, Zantema A (1997). IkappaB alpha is a target for the mitogen-activated 90 kDa ribosomal S6 kinase. *EMBO J* 16: 3133–3144.

Silva AJ, Kogan JH, Frankland PW, Kida S (1998). CREB and memory. *Annu Rev Neurosci* 21: 127–148.

Smith JA, Poteet-Smith CE, Malarkey K, Sturgill TW (1999). Identification of an extracellular signal-regulated kinase (ERK) docking site in ribosomal S6 kinase, a sequence critical for activation by ERK in vivo. *J Biol Chem* 274: 2893–2898.

Soekarman D, Fryns JP (1994). Corpus callosum agenesis in Coffin-Lowry syndrome. *Genet Couns* 5: 77–80.

Swanson KD, Taylor LK, Haung L, Burlingame AL and Landreth GE. (1999). Transcription factor phosphorylation by pp90(rsk2). Identification of Fos kinase and NGFI-B kinase I as pp90(rsk2). *J Biol Chem* 274: 3385–3395.

Tan Y, Ruan H, Demeter MR, Comb MJ (1999). p90(RSK) blocks bad-mediated cell death via a protein kinase C-dependent pathway. *J Biol Chem* 274: 34859–34867.

Tentamy SA, Miller JD, Hussels-Maumenee I (1975). The Coffin-Lowry syndrome: an inherited facio-digital mental retardation syndrome. *J Pediatr* 86: 724–731.

Trivier E, De Cesare D, Jacquot S, Pannetier S, Zackai E, Young I, Mandel JL, Sassone-Corsi P, Hanauer A (1996). Mutations in the kinase Rsk-2 associated with Coffin-Lowry syndrome. *Nature* 384: 567–570.

Verma IM, Stevenson JK, Schwarz EM, Van Antwerp D, Miyamoto S (1995). Rel/NF-kappa B/I kappa B family: intimate tales of association and dissociation. *Genes Dev* 9: 2723–2735.

von Manteuffel SR, Dennis PB, Pullen N, Gingras AC, Sonenberg N, Thomas G (1997). The insulin-induced signalling pathway leading to S6 and initiation factor 4E binding protein 1 phosphorylation bifurcates at a rapamycin-sensitive point immediately upstream of p70s6k. *Mol Cell* 17: 5426–5436.

Wassarman DA, Solomon NM. Rubin GM (1994). The Drosophila melanogaster ribosomal S6 kinase II-encoding sequence. *Gene* 144: 309–310.

Wilson WG, Kelly TE (1981). Brief clinical report: early recognition of the Coffin-Lowry syndrome. *Am J Med Genet* 8: 215–220.

Wang ZQ, Ovitt C, Grigoriadis AE, Mohle-Steinlein U, Ruther U, Wagner EF (1992). Bone and haematopoietic defects in mice lacking c-fos. *Nature* 360: 741–745.

Xing J, Ginty DD, Greenberg ME (1996). Coupling of the RAS-MAPK pathway to gene activation by RSK2, a growth factor-regulated CREB kinase. *Science* 273: 959–963.

Yin JC, Wallach JS, Del Vecchio M, Wilder EL, Zhou H, Quinn WG, Tully T (1994). Induction of a dominant negative CREB transgene specifically blocks long-term memory in Drosophila. *Cell* 79: 49–55.

Yntema HG, van den Helm B, Kissing J, van Duijnhoven G, Poppelaars F, Chelly J, Moraine C, Fryns JP, Hamel BC, Heilbronner H, et al. (1999). A novel ribosomal S6-kinase (RSK4; RPS6KA6) is commonly deleted in patients with complex X-linked mental retardation. *Genomics* 15: 332–343.

Young ID (1988). The Coffin-Lowry syndrome. *J Med Genet* 25: 344–348.

Zandi E, Rothwarf DM, Delhase M, Hayakawa M, Karin M (1997). The IkappaB kinase complex (IKK) contains two kinase subunits, IKKalpha and IKKbeta, necessary for IkappaB phosphorylation and NF-kappaB activation. *Cell* 91: 243–252.

Zhao Y, Bjorbaek C, Moller DE (1996). Regulation and interaction of pp90(rsk) isoforms with mitogen-activated protein kinases. *J Biol Chem* 271: 29773–29779.

Zhao Y, Bjorbaek C, Weremowicz S, Morton CC, Moller DE (1995). RSK3 encodes a novel pp90rsk isoform with a unique N-terminal sequence: growth factor-stimulated kinase function and nuclear translocation. *Mol Cell Biol* 15: 4353–4363.

Part B.
Transcription Factors

77 | *MITF* and the Waardenburg Type II and Albinism-Deafness (Tietz) Syndromes

MASAYOSHI TACHIBANA

Waardenburg syndrome type II (WS2) is an auditory-pigmentary syndrome whose symptoms (hearing loss and iris/skin pigmentary disturbance) may be attributable to physical absence of melanocytes in the cochlea, eyes, and skin. Molecular analysis of mutant mice with a phenotype resembling WS2 led to the cloning of a transcriptional factor gene, *MITF* (**mi**crophthalmia-associated **t**ranscription **f**actor). MITF is a transcription factor with a basic helix-loop-helix leucine zipper (bHLHZip) that differentiates cells into melanocytes and transactivating genes specific to melanocytes. Loss-of-function mutations of the *MITF* gene have been found in WS2 individuals, and gain-of-function mutations of this gene have been found in individuals with Tietz syndrome, another auditory-pigmentary syndrome.

CLONING AND FUNCTION OF *MITF*

Mouse Model of WS2

The transgenic mouse mutant *VGA-9* displays white coat color, small eyes, and deafness. Due to its phenotypic resemblance, it was found to be allelic with the natural mouse mutant *microphthalmia* (*mi*) and proposed as an animal model for WS2 (OMIM 193510). These mice lack melanocytes in the skin and eyes, and the cochleae display pro-

gressive degeneration (Tachibana et al., 1992). The form of degeneration was consistent with the cochleo-saccular type that is observed in various mice with pigmentation anomalies (Steel et al., 1987). *VGA-9* mice initially respond to sound, but the startle response is lost as the mice reach the age of 1 month. The stria vascularis lacks intermediate cells and is highly atrophic, and the scala media collapses with age. The hair cells of the organ of Corti form normally, but with age the outer hair cells degenerate and the inner hair cells remain relatively intact (Tachibana et al., 1992). Strial intermediate cells are neural crest–derived melanocytes and are essential for normal development and function of the cochlea (reviewed in Tachibana, 1999). Thus, all phenotypes of *VGA-9* mice, i.e., white coat color, small eyes, and deafness, may be related to the physical absence of pigment cells.

Cloning of *MITF* and Its Isoforms

The gene responsible for the *VGA-9* mouse phenotype and its human homolog, termed *MITF*, has been cloned (Hodgkinson et al., 1993; Tachibana et al., 1994). *MITF* encodes a bHLHZip protein and was assigned to human chromosome 3p14.1-p12.3 (Tachibana et al., 1994). Depending on the length of the first exon, four isoforms of MITF, termed MITF-A, -C, -H and -M, have been cloned (reviewed in Shibahara et al., 2001). The shortest isoform, MITF-M, is expressed selectively and abundantly in neural crest–derived melanocyte lineage cells, which also express MITF-A and MITF-H. MITF-C is expressed in many cell types, including retinal pigment epithelium, but is undetectable in cells of the melanocyte lineage (Fuse et al., 1999).

Function of *MITF*

Expression of MITF-M induces characteristics of melanocytes (Tachibana et al., 1996) and activates many melanocyte-specific genes (reviewed in Tachibana, 2000), which include genes for tyrosinase; tyrosine-related protein-1 (TRP-1); a melanosomal protein, QNR-71; and a receptor for α-melanocyte-stimulating hormone, *MC1R* (Moro et al., 1999; Adachi et al., 2000). Considering this, MITF may also be read as **m**elanocyte-**i**nducible **t**ranscription **f**actor.

Clinical Features of WS2

WS represents a group of human auditory-pigmentary syndromes first described by a Dutch ophthalmologist and geneticist (Waardenburg, 1951). This syndrome is now subcategorized into four types according to clinical features (reviewed in Read and Newton, 1997). All types of WS have skin/hair/iris pigmentation anomalies and hearing loss, i.e., auditory-pigmentary symptoms, which may be explained by the physical absence of pigment cells in the skin, hair, iris, and cochlea. WS2 is notable only for these auditory-pigmentary symptoms, while the other types of WS are associated with additional symptoms: WS1 (OMIM 193510) is associated with lateral displacement of the inner canthi of eyes (dystopia canthorum); WS3 (also known as Klein-Waardenburg syndrome, OMIM 148820), with hypoplasia of the upper limb muscles; and WS4 (also known as Waardenburg-Shah syndrome, OMIM 277580), with Hirschsprung disease. While WS1, WS2, and WS3 are inherited in an autosomal dominant fashion, WS4 is inherited as both autosomal dominant and recessive forms.

Diagnostic criteria for WS2 have been proposed as follows. Individuals fulfilling two of these criteria should be counted as affected (Liu et al., 1995) and should not be associated with other symptoms, such as dystopia canthorum, limb deformity, or Hirschsprung disease:
1. Congenital sensorineural hearing loss
2. Pigmentary disturbance of iris
   a. Complete heterochromia irides (two eyes of different color)
   b. Partial or segmental heterochromia (segments of blue or brown pigmentation in one or both eyes)
   c. Hypoplastic blue eyes (characteristic brilliant blue in both eyes)
3. Pigmentary disturbance of the hair
   a. White forelock from birth or in teens
   b. Premature graying before age 30 years
4. A first- or second-degree relative with two or more of criteria 1–3

The case shown in Figure 77–1 has profound congenital sensorineural hearing loss, complete heterochromia irides, and white forelock but no dystopia canthorum, limb deformity, Hirschsprung disease, or WS relatives. Therefore, this individual was diagnosed as a *de novo* case of WS2.

A survey of 124 cases of WS2 and 270 cases of WS1 revealed considerable differences of phenotypic penetrance (Liu et al., 1995): congenital senorineural hearing loss occurred in 77% and 57%; heterochromia irides in 48% and 27%; hypoplastic blue eye in 9% and 17%; white forelock in 9% and 17%; early graying in 23% and 26%; and white skin patches in 6% and 31%, respectively. The higher incidence of hearing loss in WS2 may be due to the difficulty of diagnosing WS2 in individuals without hearing loss. The hearing loss is congenital, sensorineural, and non-progressive, showing marked variation between and within families: 84% are reported to have bilateral loss and 40%, profound loss.

In the skin and hair of WS individuals, the affection is usually patchy and appears as a white spot (leukoderma) and early white forelock. The white forelock usually appears before age 30 years; it may appear at birth and persist or disappear (sometimes reappear). In the eyes, absence of melanocytes of the iris produces heterochromia irides (two different-colored eyes or two different colors within a single eye); and in the inner ear, absence of melanocytes of the stria vascularis (strial intermediate cells) results in sensorineural hearing loss.

MUTATIONS OF *MITF*

Mutations in WS2

A linkage analysis of WS2 families mapped the responsible gene to the *MITF* locus (Hughes et al., 1994), and indeed, mutations have been found in WS2 families (Tassabehji et al., 1994): to date, nine types of mutation have been found in the coding region of the *MITF* gene (Fig. 77–2) (Read and Newton, 1997). The change R203K seems to be neutral since it was found in a proband but did not track with WS. Curiously, *MITF* mutations account for only a minor portion (~15%) of WS2 cases (Read and Newton, 1997), and a mutational search in important portions of the *MITF* promoter failed to find any mutation in WS2 families (Jacquemin et al., 2001).

Haploinsufficiency vs. Dominant-Negative Model

WS2 is an autosomal dominant disorder. Several molecular mechanisms for such a dominant mutation have been proposed (reviewed in Wilkie, 1994), notably haploinsufficiency (reduced gene dosage, expression, or protein activity) and dominant-negative effects. Function analysis of two mutations (R214Stop and R259Stop) has revealed that mutant MITF proteins do not have any apparent dominant-negative effect (Nobukuni et al., 1996). Including these two, most of the known *MITF* mutations in WS2 compromise the HLHZip region (Fig. 77–2), making dimerization of mutant MITF with wild-type MITF difficult and dominant-negative effects unlikely. In these mutations, haploinsufficiency due to loss of function probably is the mutational mechanism responsible for WS2.

A gain-of-function *MITF* mutation involving dominant-negative function seems to cause a different autosomal dominant auditory-pigmentary syndrome. An in-frame deletion mutation (DelR217) has been found in two families of albinism-deafness (Tietz) syndrome (MIM 103500). Individuals with this syndrome have generalized skin/ocu-

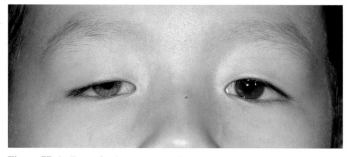

Figure 77–1. Face of a de novo case of Waardenburg syndrome (WS) type II (courtesy of Dr. Norio Sakai, Department of Developmental Medicine [Pediatrics], Osaka University Graduate School of Medicine, Osaka, Japan). Note complete hetrochromia irides of eyes but absence of dystopia canthorum. This 4-year-old boy also has profound congenital sensorineural hearing loss and some white hairs at the forelock, but no leukoderma was apparent. No relatives, including parents, showed WS symptoms.

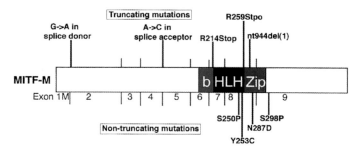

Figure 77–2. Mutations of the *MITF* gene in Waardenburg syndrome type II (WS2). Note that, except for the S298P mutation, all mutations compromise the basic helix-loop-helix (bHLH) Zip region. Splice donor and R214Stop mutations were found in two separate WS2 families. (For references on each mutation, see Read and Newton, 1997.)

lar albinism and constant profound hearing loss, symptoms similar to, but more severe than, those of WS2. DelR217 compromises the DNA-binding basic domain of MITF but retains the dimerization HLHZip domain. Therefore, it is likely that, in heterozygous Tietz syndrome individuals, DelR217-MITF binds with wild-type MITF and interferes with the dimer's DNA binding, a dominant-negative effect. Indeed, the identical mutation in mice, causing a semi-dominant phenotype in vivo, was shown to have a dominant-negative effect in vitro (Hemesath et al., 1994). Although S298P also does not compromise the dimerization domain, this mutation was found in WS2 and thus probably does not have a dominant-negative effect. Ser^{298} is a phosphorylation site: mutation at this site reduced DNA binding and transactivating activity in vitro (Takeda et al., 2000).

EPISTATIC RELATIONSHIPS BETWEEN WS GENES

The genes responsible for each type of WS have been cloned. While practically all cases of WS1 and WS3 show mutated *PAX3*, WS4 individuals are either homozygously mutated in *EDN3* (the endothelin-3 gene) or *EDNRB* (the endothelin receptor B gene) or heterozygously mutated in *SOX10*. In addition to *MITF*, it was recently found that *SLUG*, a transcription factor gene, was mutated in WS2 individuals (Sánchez-Martin et al., 2002).

An epistatic relationship between *PAX3* or *SOX10* and *MITF* has been elucidated. PAX3 and SOX10, as a transcription factor, synergically transactivate *MITF*, and mutations of *PAX3* and *SOX10* in WS cause auditory-pigmentary symptoms, probably through failure of *MITF* transactivation (Watanabe et al., 1998; Bondurand et al., 2000). It was recently shown that MITF transcriptionally transactivates *SLUG* (Sánchez-Martin et al., 2002). EDN3–EDNRB interaction probably activates MITF at the protein and promoter levels through the cytoplasmic signaling pathway (reviewed in Tachibana, 2000). We recently found that one type of homozyous *Ednrb* mutation in mice causes auditory-pigmentary symptoms but not Hirshsprung's disease (unpublished data). These findings suggest that some types of mutation in *PAX3*, *SOX10*, *EDN3*, or *EDNRB* cause auditory-pigmentary symptoms but not other symptoms and thus constitute WS2.

REFERENCES

Adachi S, Morii E, Kim D, Ogihara H, Jippo T, Ito A, Lee Y-M, Kitamaura Y (2000). Involvement of *mi*-transcription factor in expression of α-melanocyte-stimulating hormone receptor in cultured mast cells of mice. *J Immunol* 164: 855–860.

Bondurand N, Pingaut V, Goerich DE, Lemort N, Sock E, Caignec CL, Wegner M, Goossens M (2000). Interaction among *SOX10*, *PAX3* and *MITF*, three genes altered in Waardenburg syndrome. *Hum Mol Genet* 9: 1907–1917.

Fuse N, Yasumoto K, Takeda K, Amae S, Yoshizawa M, Udono T, Takahashi K, Tamai M, Tomita Y, Tachibana M, et al. (1999). Molecular cloning of cDNA encoding a novel microphthalmia-associated transcription factor isoform with a distinct amino-terminus. *J Biochem* 126: 1043–1051.

Hemesath TJ, Steingrímsson E, McGill G, Hansen MJ, Yaught J, Hodgkinson CA, Arnheiter H, Copeland NG, Jenkins NA, Fisher DE (1994). *microphthalmia*, a critical factor in melanocyte development defines a discrete transcription factor family. *Gene Dev* 8: 2770–2780.

Hodgkinson CA, Moore KJ, Nakayama A, Steingrímsson E, Copeland NG, Jenkins NA, Arnheiter H (1993). Mutations at the mouse microphthalmia locus are associated with defects in a gene encoding a novel basic-helix-loop-helix-zipper protein. *Cell* 74: 395–404.

Hughes AE, Nwton VE, Liu XZ, Read AP (1994). A gene for Waardenburg type 2 maps close to the human homologue of the microphthalmia gene at chromosome 3p12-p14.1. *Nat Genet* 7: 509–512.

Jacquemin P, Lannoy VJ, O'Sullivan J, Read A, Lemaigre FP, Rousseau GG (2001). The transcription factor Onecut-2 controls the *Microphthalmia*-associated transcription factor gene. *Biochem Biophys Res Commun* 285: 1200–1205.

Liu X-Z, Newton VE, Read AP (1995). Waardenburg syndrome type II: phenotypic findings and diagnostic criteria. *Am J Med Genet* 55: 95–100.

Moro O, Ideta R, Ifuku O (1999). Characterization of the promoter region of the human melanocortin-1 receptor (*MC1R*) gene. *Biochem Biophys Res Commun* 262: 452–460.

Nobukuni Y, Watanabe A, Takeda K, Skarka H, Tachibana M (1996). Analyses of loss-of-function mutations of the *MITF* gene suggest that haploinsufficiency is a cause of Waardenburg syndrome type 2A. *Am J Hum Genet* 59: 76–83.

Read AP, Newton VE (1997). Waardenburg syndrome. *J Med Genet* 34: 656–665.

Sánchez-Martin M, Rodoriquez-Garcia A, Perez-Losada J, Sagrera A, Read AP, Sánchez-Garcia I (2002). *SLUG* (*SNAI2*) deletions in patients with Waardenburg disease. *Hum Mol Genet* 11: 3231–3236.

Shibahara S, Takeda K, Yasumoto K, Udono T, Watanabe K, Saito H, Takahashi K (2001). Microphthalmia-associated transcription factor (MITF): multiplicity in structure, function, and regulation. *J Invest Dermatol Symp Proc* 6: 99–104.

Steel KP, Barkway C, Bock GR (1987). Strial dysfunction in mice with cochleo-saccular abnormalities. *Hear Res* 27: 11–26.

Tachibana M (1999). Sound needs sound melanocytes to be heard. *Pigment Cell Res* 12: 344–354.

Tachibana M (2000). MITF: a stream flowing for pigment cells. *Pigment Cell Res* 12: 230–240.

Tachibana M, Hara Y, Vyas D, Hodgkinson C, Fex J, Grundfast K, Arnheiter H (1992). Cochlear disorder associated with melanocyte anomaly in mice with a transgenic insertional mutation. *Mol Cell Neurosci* 3: 433–445.

Tachibana M, Perez-Jurado LA, Nakayama A, Hodgkinson CA, Li X, Schneider M, Miki T, Fex J, Francke U, Arnheiter H (1994). Cloning of *MITF*, the human homolog of the mouse microphthalmia gene and assignment to chromosome 3p14.1-p12.3. *Hum Mol Genet* 3: 553–557.

Tachibana M, Takeda K, Nobukuni Y, Urabe K, Long JE, Meyers KA, Aaronson SA, Miki T (1996). Ectopic expression of *MITF*, a gene for Waardenburg syndrome type 2, converts fibroblasts to cells with melanocyte characteristics. *Nat Genet* 14: 50–54.

Takeda K, Takemoto C, Kobayashi I, Watanabe A, Nobukuni Y, Fisher DE, Tachibana M (2000). Ser298 of MITF, a mutation site in Waardenburg syndrome type 2, is a phosphorylation site with functional significance. *Hum Mol Genet* 9: 125–132.

Tassabehji M, Newton VE, Read AP (1994). Waardenburg syndrome type 2 caused by mutations in the human microphthalmia (*MITF*) gene. *Nat Genet* 8: 251–255.

Waardenburg PJ (1951). A new syndrome combining developmental anomalies of the eyelids, eyebrows and nose root with pigmentary defects of the iris and head hair and with congenital deafness. *Am J Hum Genet* 3: 195–253.

Watanabe A, Takeda K, Ploplis B, Tachibana M (1998). Epistatic relationship between Waardenburg syndrome genes *MITF* and *PAX3*. *Nat Genet* 18: 283–286.

Wilkie AOM (1994). The molecular basis of genetic dominance. *J Med Genet* 31: 89–98.

FRANS P. M. CREMERS AND COR W. R. J. CREMERS

THE POU PROTEIN FAMILY: FLEXIBLE TRANSCRIPTION FACTORS

POU3F4 belongs to a superfamily of POU domain transcription factors that are characterized by two evolutionary conserved subdomains: a POU-specific domain and a POU homeodomain. The POU domain was first identified 14 years ago and takes its name after the first four transcription factors in which it was found: mammalian Pit-1, Oct-1, Oct-2, and *Caenorhabditis elegans* Unc86 (Clerc et al., 1988; Herr et al., 1988; Ingraham et al., 1988; Sturm et al., 1988; Finney and Ruvkun, 1990). The POU subdomains are connected through a variable and flexible linker, and together they partially encircle defined DNA sequences in the promoter region of a variety of genes. Several POU domain members, including POU3F4, bind to octamer sequence elements.

The POU domain for which there is most structural data is derived from Oct-1. Crystallographic and biochemical studies have shown that the bipartite POU domain can assume a variety of conformations, depending on the DNA element. Some POU proteins (e.g., Oct-1) act as monomers; others (e.g., Pit-1) cooperatively form dimers. The binary complex(es) provide distinct platforms for the recruitment of specific regulators to control transcription, by either stimulation or repression.

More than 150 POU-domain proteins are currently known (Schultz et al., 2000). POU proteins regulate many fundamental developmental and homeostatic processes. They have been grouped into seven distinct classes according to linker length and composition (Spaniol et al., 1996). The neuronally expressed Pit proteins define class I. The ubiquitously expressed Oct-1 (POU2F1) and tissue-specific Oct-2 (POU2F2) are representatives of class II. Brn-1 (POU3F3), Brn-2 (POU3F2), Brn-4 (POU3F4), and Tst-1 (POU3F1), which are involved in neural development, comprise class III. The Brn3 (Pou4f) proteins and Unc86 are involved in embryonic development and comprise class IV. Class V POU proteins generally are involved in early embryogenesis and class VI POU proteins are expressed in the central nervous system. Class VII POU proteins are critical for early developmental stages (Spaniol et al., 1996; Ryan and Rosenfeld, 1997).

Several POU proteins are important for inner ear development. The POU transcription factor Pou4f1 (Brn3c) regulates soma size, target field innervation, and axon pathfinding of inner ear sensory neurons. Absence of Pou4f1 results in the down-regulation of the neurotrophin receptor TrkC and a selective loss of TrkC neurons in the spiral ganglion (Huang et al., 2001). This innervation defect is similar to that of TrkC$^{-/-}$ mice. Inactivation of *Pou4f3* (also named *Brn-3c* or *Brn-3.1*) leads to sensorineural deafness and vestibular impairment (Erkman et al., 1996). Mutations in *POU4F3* were found to be associated with a progressive autosomal dominant form of nonsyndromic sensorineural hearing loss in humans (DFNA15) (Vahava et al., 1998). The role of POU3F4 in inner ear development is outlined in detail next.

DIVERSE ROLES OF POU3F4 IN MAMMALIAN EMBRYONIC DEVELOPMENT AND HOMEOSTASIS

Spatiotemporal Expression of POU3F4

POU3F4 orthologs have been identified in mouse (*Brn-4/Pou3f4*), rat (*RHS2*), and amphibian *X. laevis* (*XLPOU2*), but not in zebrafish (Hara et al., 1992; le Moine and Young, 1992; Mathis et al., 1992; Witta et al., 1995; Spaniol et al., 1996). The high evolutionary conservation of POU3F4 is illustrated by the fact that *X. laevis* XLPOU2 shows 92% identity with human POU3F4 at the amino acid level (Witta et al., 1995). The nomenclature indicated above is not used consistently. *Brn-4* is mostly used to designate the mouse ortholog of *POU3F4*, while *Pou3f4* is the officially approved mouse gene symbol. In one rat study, *Brn-4* is used instead of *RSH2* (Alvarez-Bolado et al., 1995).

Because of its homology to POU-domain proteins from classes III and IV, which play important roles in brain development, most studies concentrated on the *Brn-4/RSH2* expression pattern in the developing brain of mice and rats (Hara et al., 1992; le Moine and Young, 1992; Mathis et al., 1992; Okazawa et al., 1996). The diverse roles of the four intronless class III POU-domain proteins—Brn-1, Brn-2, Brn-4, and Tst-1—in the developing rat brain were extensively studied by Alvarez-Bolado and coworkers (1995). In situ hybridization analysis indicates that in the ventricular, subventricular, and mantle layer of the forebrain neural tube, class III POU proteins display a unique expression pattern. Within each particular region, or layer within a region, none to four of the mRNAs may be detected, and this pattern changes during development. Expression of *Brn-4* is initially broad throughout the neural tube and becomes much more restricted in the adult, where its expression is confined to the striatum (telencephalon), the medial habenula, the paraventricular and supraoptic nuclei, and the subcommissural organ.

POU3F4 expression outside the developing central nervous system was found in human fetal kidney, the rat and mouse otic vesicle, the mouse fetal muscle, and the *X. laevis* prenephros (le Moine and Young, 1992; Witta et al., 1995; Dominov and Miller, 1996). Surprisingly, *Pou3f4* was also found to be expressed in pancreatic α-cells of adult mice (Hussain et al., 1997). Although formal proof for *POU3F4* expression in these tissues in humans has not been established, it seems clear that this gene has a large functional repertoire.

Phippard et al. (1998) investigated the subcellular expression of Brn-4 in the ontogeny of the mouse ear. Employing immunohistochemistry, Brn-4 was localized in the nucleus of ventral mesenchymal cells in the earliest developmental stages of otic capsule (10.5–11.5 days postcoitus), correlating with the onset of mesenchymal condensation. Subsequent events in formation of the bony labyrinth require extensive remodeling of mesenchyme to form openings in the temporal bone. Strikingly, during the further differentiation of the otic capsule, the subcellular localization of Brn-4 changes. The Brn-4 protein remains nuclear in those regions of the otic capsule that give rise to the cellular regions of the mature bony labyrinth, while it shifts to perinuclear/cytoplasmic in those regions of the otic capsule that will cavitate to form acellular regions in the temporal bone, such as the scala tympani, the scala vestibuli, and the IAC.

Transcriptional Regulation of the *POU3F4* gene

Malik and coworkers (1996) identified the 5′-CAATATGCTAAT-3′ sequence as the preferred DNA-binding site of Brn-4. By using DNase I footprinting analysis, they also revealed that recombinant Brn-4 was able to protect five sites between −457 and +22 of its own promoter, suggesting autoregulation. Autoregulation was previously observed for Pit-1 (McCormick et al., 1988; Rhodes et al., 1993). Analysis of the *Pou3f4* promoter using transgenic mice containing a *LacZ* reporter gene that was driven by different portions of a 6 kb DNA sequence containing its promoter revealed at least two positive *cis*-acting elements that direct expression to the developing neural tube but not to the inner ear (Heydemann et al., 2001). One enhancer was situated between −3.3 and −1.2 kb upstream; another was located within −0.6 kb. Transgenic expression is restricted to cells of ectodermal origin in regions that broadly overlap with other members of the POU-domain gene family (He et al., 1989).

In early *X. laevis* development, the POU3F4 ortholog XLPOU2 is induced by noggin (Witta et al., 1995). Noggin is a polypeptide secreted by Spemann's organizer in amphibians (Smith and Harland, 1992), a region that produces signals which induce the formation of neural tissue from the overlying dorsal ectoderm (Lamb et al., 1993). Thus, XLPOU2 is an early response gene of the endogenous neural inducer noggin. In the mouse E14 striatum, Pou3f4 is expressed predominantly in the subventricular zone (le Moine and Young, 1992; Mathis et al., 1992; Alvarez-Bolado et al., 1995). Immunohistochemical analyes show that Pou3f4-expressing cells are neuronal precursors.

Pou3f4 expression could be upregulated in postmitotic neuronal precursor cells using either insulin-like growth factor-I (IGF-1) or brain-derived neurotrophic factor (BDNF) (Shimazaki et al., 1999). Other POU class III genes, such as *Pou3f2* and *Pou3f3*, did not exhibit this upregulation. These findings suggest that, in part, Pou3f4 mediates the actions of epigenetic signals that induce striatal neuron-precursor differentiation.

In the developing mouse skeletal muscle, myogenin-dependent *Brn-4* expression was observed. *Brn-4* was expressed together with other POU genes, including *Emb* and *Oct-1*, but, contrary to *Brn-4*, the latter two genes are also expressed in postnatal and adult muscle (Dominov and Miller, 1996).

Downstream Target Genes of POU3F4

So far, three different target genes of POU3F4 have been identified: the preglucagon, the D_{1A} dopamine receptor, and the involucrin genes. The proglucagon gene is specifically expressed in the α-cells of the islets of Langerhans, the intestines, selected ganglia of the brain stem, and the hypothalamus. Its promoter contains several AT-rich motifs, which prompted Hussain and coworkers to test the possibility whether POU-domain genes are expressed in pancreatic α-cells. By means of RT-PCR, *Brn-4* mRNA could be readily identified. Reporter gene studies showed Brn-4-dependent activation of proglucagon transcription (Hussain et al., 1997). Okazawa and coworkers (1996) reported the regulation of striatal D_{1A} dopamine receptor gene transcription by Brn-4 and found two Brn-4 binding sites in the intron of this gene. In situ hybridization revealed colocalization of Brn-4 and D_{1A} mRNA at the level of a single neuron in the rat striatum where this dopamine receptor is most abundantly expressed. Human involucrin, a precursor of the keratinocyte cornified envelope, is specifically expressed in the suprabasal epidermal layers. Welter et al. (1996) demonstrated that several POU-homeodomain transcription factors, including Brn-4/Pou3f4, suppress transcription of human involucrin in an octamer binding site–independent manner. Probably, POU proteins interact with other proteins in the vicinity of the TATA-box.

CLINICAL FEATURES OF DFN3

X-linked deafness type 3 (DFN3) is the most frequent X-linked form of inherited deafness. In most cases, patients show a mixed type of deafness, including fixation of the stapes. After the stapedial footplate has been surgically opened to replace the fixed stapes, a heavy flow (previously often denoted as a perilymphatic gusher) of cerebrospinal fluid is observed (Nance et al., 1971). Cerebrospinal fluid can enter the vestibule as a result of the lateral widening of the bony internal auditory canal (IAC) (Glasscock, 1973; Cremers et al., 1985; Michel et al., 1991; Phelps et al., 1991; Talbot and Wilson, 1994; Tang and Parnes, 1994) (see Fig. 78–1). High-resolution computer-assisted tomography reveals the temporal bone defects. Stapes gusher is a dreaded complication because it can cause dizziness in the patient and increase the level of hearing loss (Glasscock, 1973; Cremers et al., 1983).

Two family studies have presented detailed audiometric findings in

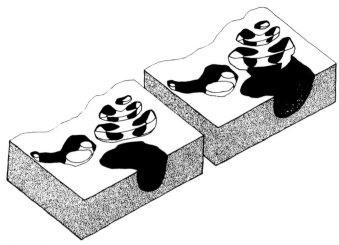

Figure 78–1. Three-dimensional picture of part of the normal temporal bone (left side) and a temporal bone observed in a typical patient with X-linked deafness type 3 (DFN3; right side). In the patient with DFN3, both the inner ear canal and its connection to the inner ear are substantially widened. (Adapted with permission from Cremers et al., 2000.)

affected males (Nance et al., 1971; Cremers, 1985; Cremers et al., 1985) and in female carriers (Nance et al., 1971; Cremers and Huygen, 1983). The hearing loss in the affected males has a conductive and a sensorineural component. In case there is a large conductive component of over 30 to 40 dB, this could be the result of a stapes fixation. Smaller conductive losses are considered to be the result of a widened vestibule, leading to a loss of energy of fluid waves on their way to the cochlea. The sensorineural component is progressive; affected males will become profoundly deaf. It is assumed that changing cerebrospinal fluid pressures will be conducted along the induced IAC, and this will effectively damage the inner ear. Traumas to the head are supposed to accelerate the progress of the hearing loss. In one report, DFN3 was diagnosed in two sisters with the full-blown clinical picture described above (Papadaki et al., 1998). The expression of an X-linked recessive gene defect in carrier females might be due to preferential inactivation of the X chromosome, which carries the normal *POU3F4* allele as observed in other instances (Naumova et al., 1996, 1998; Plenge et al., 1997; Parolini et al., 1998). Alternatively, both females carry a dominant *POU3F4* mutation.

MOLECULAR GENETICS OF DFN3

Mutations Affecting the *POU3F4* Gene Directly

The DFN3 gene was mapped to the proximal part of the long arm of the X chromosome by genetic linkage analyses of large families (Brunner et al., 1988; Wallis et al., 1988) and by the identification of microscopically visible Xq21 deletions that are associated with complex phenotypes consisting of choroideremia, nonspecific mental retardation, and DFN3 (Tabor et al., 1983; Nussbaum et al., 1987; Cremers et al., 1988, 1989). Subsequently, smaller-sized deletions were found in patients with classic DFN3 (Bach et al., 1992; Huber et al., 1994; Piussan et al., 1995), and the underlying gene *POU3F4* could be identified by using a positional candidate gene cloning approach (de Kok et al., 1995b). The absence of the *POU3F4* gene in three patients with DFN3, as well as the identification of point mutations in DFN3 patients without detectable chromosomal abnormalities, clearly established the pathologic role of this gene.

Mutation analysis of the *POU3F4* gene can be efficiently performed by sequence analysis of five overlapping polymerase chain reaction (PCR) fragments spanning the 1083 bp open reading frame (ORF) (de Kok et al., 1995b). Mutation analysis in 33 patients revealed 15 small mutations in the *POU3F4* gene (Fig. 78–2), 5 of which result in premature termination of translation, 9 of which result in amino acid substitutions, and 1 of which results in a deletion of two amino acids at

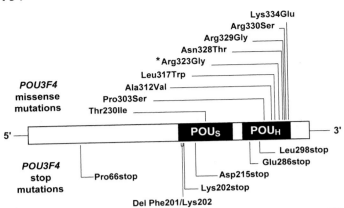

Figure 78–2. Fifteen small mutations identified in the *POU3F4* gene. The POU domains and the positions of the mutations are drawn to scale. The missense mutations are clustered in the POU homeodomain (POU_H). The stop mutations are in the POU-specific domain (POU_S). The asterisk marks a mosaic de novo mutation. Here, 50% of this patients' peripheral blood cell DNA carried the Arg323Gly mutation, and 50% contained the normal sequence (de Kok et al., 1997). (Adapted with permission from Cremers et al., 2000.)

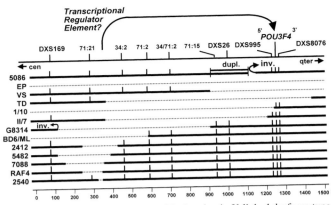

Figure 78–3. Genomic map of the critical region in X-linked deafness type 3 (DFN3) and chromosomal abnormalities associated with classic DFN3. Except for the deletion observed in patient II/7, deletions either span the *POU3F4* gene or overlap 900 kb proximal to the *POU3F4* gene. Patient 5086 carries a paracentric inversion (q21.1–q21.3) associated with a 150 kb duplication (de Kok et al., 1995a). Deletions are indicated by dotted lines. (Adapted with permission from Cremers et al., 2000.)

the beginning of the POU-specific domain (Bitner-Glindzicz et al., 1995; de Kok et al., 1995b, 1997; Friedman et al., 1997; Hagiwara et al., 1998; Y. J. M. de Kok and F. P. M. Cremers, unpublished results). As expected, the protein-truncating mutations were found throughout the ORF. In contrast, the missense mutations are clustered in the α3-helix of the POU homeodomain. According to nuclear magnetic resonance and crystallographic studies of Oct-1, the mutated amino acid residues at positions 230 (located in the α3-helix POU-specific domain), 328, 330, and 334 (all located in the α3-helix of the POU homeodomain) contact the major groove or backbone of the octamer binding sequence (Klemm et al., 1994). Pro303, Ala312, and Arg323 are strictly conserved residues among members of the six classes of the POU domain superfamily (Okamoto et al., 1993). Additional evidence for pathogenicity of the Asn328Thr and Arg330Ser mutations is provided by Liang and coworkers (1995), who show that mutations at homologous positions in Pit-1 result in reduction of DNA binding and transcriptional activation. Leu317 and Arg329 are conserved in at least four of the six classes of POU proteins (Okamoto et al., 1993), indicating that most if not all missense mutations have a severe effect on the proper binding of POU3F4 to its target sequence(s).

The Arg323Gly missense mutation was found in a sporadic DFN3 patient who was proven to be mosaic for this mutation. Some 50% of his peripheral blood cell DNA carried the missense mutation, and 50% carried the wild-type DNA sequence (de Kok et al., 1997).

Deletions, Inversions, and Duplications Proximal to *POU3F4*

Upon cloning of the *POU3F4* gene, we initially identified three DFN3-associated deletions that span the *POU3F4* gene, and at least three that were located upstream of the gene (Fig. 78–3). The largest deletion (patient EP) is estimated to span 5 Mb of Xq21.1. By constructing a 1500 kb cosmid contig, a detailed physical map of the proximal region was generated. Figure 78–3 shows the most important DNA markers in the map, as well as all deletions, inversions, and duplications thus far identified in patients with the classic DFN3 phenotype. At the telomeric side, these deletions do not extend farther than approximately 200 kb distal to the *POU3F4* gene, thereby forming the proximal margin of the critical interval for a gene involved in nonspecific mental retardation (Yntema et al., 1999).

Remarkably, eight proximal deletions, one of which is associated with a paracentric inversion (G8314; inv(q13q21.2); Bitner-Glindzicz et al., 1994), overlap in a small chromosomal segment 900 kb proximal to *POU3F4*. The smallest of these deletions comprises 8 kb and was identified in a male patient (number 2540) belonging to one of the two DFN3 families that were previously used for the genetic linkage mapping of the gene defect (Brunner et al., 1988). In one patient

(patient GL), six microdeletions had been reported, but reexamination with the restriction enzyme *Taq*I did not confirm this original finding. Thus, all proximal deletions observed so far, except deletion II/7, overlap the 8 kb segment deleted in patient 2540. The deletion observed in patient II/7 is situated between the *POU3F4* gene and the proximal 8 kb segment, indicating that other *POU3F4*-regulatory elements might be residing in this region.

Southern blot analyses of the critical 8 kb region in human, mouse, hamster, and bovine revealed significant evolutionary conservation. Sequence analysis of the 8 kb DNA segment in humans and mouse revealed a stretch of at least 2 kb of sequence that was 80% identical between these species (F. P. M. Cremers and Y. J. M. de Kok, unpublished data). Extensive cDNA library screening and database comparisons, however, did not reveal any transcribed sequences.

In one DFN3 patient, a paracentric inversion (q21.1–q21.31) associated with a 150 kb duplication (patient 5086), dislocated the *POU3F4* gene approximately 3 to 5 Mb away from the proximal DNA element (de Kok et al., 1995a).

Clustering of Missense Mutations in *POU3F4*

Missense mutations in the *POU3F4* gene are conspicuously clustered in the POU homeodomain (Fig. 78–2). Possibly, missense mutations outside the POU domains lead to a completely different phenotype or, alternatively, are embryonic lethal. Based on the octamer site-independent suppression activity of POU3F4 in human involucrin transcription, it can be hypothesized that POU3F4 segments outside the POU domains not only function as transactivation domains but also are implicated in POU protein heterodimerization or interactions with other transcriptional regulators. Missense mutations may have a dominant negative effect on the proper function of other (POU-domain) proteins that play important roles in embryonic development.

ESTABLISHING THE DIAGNOSIS AND MANAGEMENT OF PATIENTS

When a mixed type of deafness is found in a male patient, a detailed CT scan should be performed to trace the typical radiologic features of this disease. X-linked inheritance in some cases might be supported by family data. It is of crucial importance to diagnose this disease before deciding to perform an exploratory tympanotomy and to open the footplate. The audiometric configuration is also specific, showing large conductive components for the low frequencies and almost no conductive hearing loss for the high frequencies. In case DFN3 is suspected, a molecular diagnosis can be established in more than 80% of the cases by sequence analysis of the intronless *POU3F4* gene and deletion analysis of the critical 8 kb segment situated 900 kb proximal to *POU3F4*. When no mutation is found, and the family is large enough, linkage analysis with DNA markers residing in Xq21.2 can be employed to investigate whether the gene defect is positioned in the DFN3 critical region. Genetic counseling is helpful to protect family members from eventful ear surgery. Hearing aids are needed for revalidation.

MOUSE MODELS FOR DFN3

Three mouse models for DFN3 were generated, two via targeted mutagenesis (Minowa et al., 1999; Phippard et al., 1999) and one in a random mutagenesis program (Phippard et al., 2000). Via homologous recombination in embryonic stem cells, Minowa and colleagues (1999) deleted the entire coding sequence of the mouse *Pou3f4* gene. The *Pou3f4*$^{-/Y}$ male mice exhibited profound deafness. However, no gross morphological changes in the conductive ossicles or cochlea were detected, although there was a dramatic reduction in endocochlear potential. Electron microscopy revealed severe ultrastructural alterations in cochlear spiral ligament fibrocytes which are located beneath the stria vascularis. The number of fibrocytes was reduced; they showed cell shape abnormalities and had few mitochondria. Fibrocytes are mesenchymal in origin and probably play a critical role in potassium ion homeostasis. In a parallel study, Phippard and coworkers replaced the endogenous *Pou3f4* gene by a *LacZ* reporter gene (Phippard et al., 1999). Male mice with a mutant *Pou3f4* locus demonstrated vertical head bobbing, changes in gait, reduced whisker mobility, and hearing loss.

One of the major malformations contributing to hearing loss in human patients with mutations in the human *Pou3f4* ortholog is stapes fixation, which compromises sound conduction through the middle ear ossicular system. Pou3f4-deficient mice have a normal incus and malleus but a generally thinner and abnormally formed stapes. The stapes footplate lies in the oval window, and the morphology and area of the footplate effects the efficiency with which sound energy is transmitted into the cochlear fluids. The normal footplate displays a convex surface, whereas the surface of the mutant footplate is flattened. The sole of the normal footplate is ovoid shaped; the mutant footplate displays a polygonal morphology. The cochlea show overall hypoplasia, most obvious in the basal turn due to the fact that the scala tympani adopt a more flattened elliptical shape with an apparent reduction in volume. In addition, the mutant cochlea on average consists of only one and one-half turn compared to a one and three-quarter turn in the normal cochlea. The spiral limbus, a supporting structure of the organ of Corti, shows a reduction in size. Also, in the study of Minowa et al. (1999), fibrocytes of the spiral ligament are thinner and less adherent than in the wild-type mouse, resulting in acellular spaces in the regions where fibrocytes normally underlie the stria vascularis.

As in humans with DFN3, the temporal bone of Pou3f4 knockout mice show severe abnormalities. All three foramina of the IAC, through which the auditory and facial nerves are conveyed through the temporal bone to the brain stem, are enlarged. In addition, the superior semicircular canal is constricted, possibly explaining the head bobbing of mutant mice and the compromised vestibular function. In addition, other temporal bone structures are thinner than normal, in accordance with the hypothesis that the *Pou3f4* gene may be necessary for the survival of mesenchymal cells during the remodeling in the development of the otic capsule (Phippard et al., 1998).

A mouse mutant that arose in a radiation mutagenesis experiment, *sex-linked fidget (slf)*, carries an inversion that abolishes *Pou3f4* gene expression in the embryonic inner ear, but not in the neural tube, corroborating the existence of an inner ear–specific regulatory DNA element located far upstream of the mouse and human *POU3F4* genes (Phippard et al., 2000). As a result of functional deficits in the auditory and vestibular systems, *slf* mice, and *Pou3f4*$^{-/-}$ female or *Pou3f4*$^{-/Y}$ male mice generated through targeted mutagenesis, display behavioral anomalies including vertical head bobbing and hearing loss. Anatomic and histologic abnormalities include a reduction in the coiling of the cochlea and hypoplasia of otic mesenchyme-derived cochlear structures such as the spiral limbus, the scala tympani, and strial fibrocytes. Apparently, *POU3F4* enhances the survival of mesodermal cells during the mesenchymal remodeling that forms the ma-

ture bony labyrinth and regulates inductive signaling mechanisms in the otic mesenchyme.

DEVELOPMENTAL PATHOGENESIS OF DFN3

The compact genomic structure of the *POU3F4* gene and the identification of deletions and inversions far upstream of the gene enabled the detection of 28 mutations in 33 unrelated DFN3 patients. *POU3F4* point mutations or small deletions were found in 15 patients; deletions encompassing the entire *POU3F4* gene were found in 3; and deletions, a deletion/inversion, and a duplication/inversion involving sequences proximal to *POU3F4* were found in 10 patients. In 5 patients, no mutations were found, but not all patients were investigated for inversions and deletions outside the *POU3F4* gene and for deletions of the 8 kb proximal DNA element. The deletion observed in patient II/7 resides between the *POU3F4* gene and the proximal hotspot for deletions (Fig. 78–3), indicating that other important sequences are disrupted. Why and how proximal deletions and inversions give rise to the DFN3 phenotype remains to be elucidated.

Several human genetic diseases have been found to be associated with structural rearrangements outside the transcription units and are generally referred to as "position effect mutations" (Kleinjan and van Heyningen, 1998, and references therein). Most of these genes, such as *POU3F4*, display tissue-specific fetal expression patterns, thus rendering the analysis of transcriptional activity very difficult. The distance between the *POU3F4* gene and its putative control region as defined by small deletions located 900 kb upstream is the largest reported thus far (Kleinjan and van Heyningen, 1998). Strikingly, an inversion/duplication with a breakpoint 170 kb proximal to *POU3F4* is also associated with full-blown DFN3. The relatively small size of some of the proximal deletions, as well as the absence of structural rearrangements distal to *POU3F4*, argue against a role for position-effect variegation, like heterochromatin spreading from nearby chromosomal regions. More likely, a specific transcriptional regulator element, maybe a so-called locus control region, is situated in the proximal region. It will be of interest to study the presence of DNAse I hypersensitive sites in this region and to investigate the effect of disruption of the orthologous region in the mouse.

Mutations that inactivate mouse *Pou3f4* lead to developmental abnormalities in the middle ear ossicles, a reduction in the coiling of the cochlea, and hypoplasia of mesenchyme-derived cochlear structures. Also, there is a bulbous dilatation of the lateral portion of the internal auditory canal with incomplete separation from the cochlea and widening of the first part of the facial nerve. The lack of overt abnormalities outside the temporal bone suggests that in other tissues the absence of POU3F4 can be compensated for by other POU-domain proteins, most likely members of the class III (POU3F1, POU3F2, POU3F3) and class IV (e.g., POU4F1, POU4F3, POU4F2) POU proteins.

Since all DFN3 patients display the hallmarks of the disease, a genotype–phenotype correlation cannot be made. Apart from DFN3, one patient (TD) also shows hypogonadism. Although this feature was also observed in affected relatives of TD, it is not clear whether hypogonadism is related to the absence of *POU3F4* in these patients (Myhre et al., 1982).

None of the genes described in this chapter that are thought to be regulated by POU3F4 are likely to be involved in temporal bone modeling during otogenesis. More than 50 genes have been reported to be expressed in the inner ear (Torres and Giraldez, 1998), and it is likely that this list will continue to grow. To unravel the precise role of POU3F4 in inner ear development it will be necessary to identify the proteins that act upstream or downstream of POU3F4.

REFERENCES

Alvarez-Bolado G, Rosenfeld MG, Swanson LW (1995). Model of forebrain regionalization based on spatiotemporal patterns of POU-III homeobox gene expression, birthdates, and morphological features. *J Comp Neurol* 355: 237–295.

Bach I, Brunner HG, Beighton P, Ruvalcaba RHA, Reardon W, Pembrey ME, van der Velde-Visser SD, Bruns GAP, Cremers CWRJ, Cremers FPM, Ropers H-H (1992). Microdeletions in patients with gusher-associated, X-linked mixed deafness (DFN3). *Am J Hum Genet* 50: 38–44.

Bitner-Glindzicz M, de Kok Y, Summers D, Huber I, Cremers FPM, Ropers H-H, Reardon W, Pembrey ME, Malcolm S (1994). Close linkage of a gene for X linked deafness to three microsatellite repeats at Xq21 in radiologically normal and abnormal families. *J Med Genet* 31: 916–921.

Bitner-Glindzicz M, Turnpenny P, Höglund P, Kääriäinen H, Sankila E-M, van der Maarel SM, de Kok YJM, Ropers H-H, Cremers FPM, Pembrey M, Malcolm S (1995). Further mutations in *Brain 4* (POU3F4) clarify the phenotype in the X-linked deafness, DFN3. *Hum Mol Genet* 4: 1467–1469.

Brunner HG, van Bennekom CA, Lambermon EMM, Oei TL, Cremers CWRJ, Wieringa B, Ropers H-H (1988). The gene for X-linked progressive mixed deafness with perilymphatic gusher during stapes surgery (DFN3) is linked to PGK. *Hum Genet* 80: 337–340.

Clerc RG, Corcoran LM, LeBowitz JH, Baltimore D, Sharp PA (1988). The B-cell-specific Oct-2 protein contains POU box- and homeo box-type domains. *Genes Dev* 2: 1570–1581.

Cremers CWRJ (1985). Audiological features of the X-linked progressive mixed deafness syndrome with perilymphatic gusher during stapes surgery. *Am J Otol* 6: 243–246.

Cremers CWRJ, Huygen PLM (1983). Clinical features of female heterozygotes in the X-linked mixed deafness syndrome (with perilymphatic gusher during stapes surgery). *J Pediatr Otorhinolaryng* 6: 179–185.

Cremers CWRJ, Hombergen GCJH, Wentges RThR (1983). Perilymphatic gusher and stapes surgery: a predictable complication? *Clin Otolaryngol* 8: 235–240.

Cremers CWRJ, Hombergen GCHJ, Scaf JJ, Huygen PLM, Volkers WS, Pinckers AJLG (1985). X-linked progressive mixed deafness with perilymphatic gusher during stapes surgery. *Arch Otolaryngol* 111: 249–254.

Cremers FPM, van de Pol TJR, Wieringa B, Hofker MH, Pearson PL, Pfeiffer RA, Mikkelsen M, Tabor A, Ropers H-H (1988). Molecular analysis of male-viable deletions and duplications allows ordering of 52 DNA probes on proximal Xq. *Am J Hum Genet* 43: 452–461.

Cremers FPM, van de Pol TJR, Diergaarde PJ, Wieringa B, Nussbaum RL, Schwartz M, Ropers H-H (1989). Physical fine mapping of the choroideremia locus using Xq21 deletions associated with complex syndromes. *Genomics* 4: 41–46.

Cremers, Cremers CWRJ, Ropers H-H (2000). The ins and outs of X-linked deafness type 3. In: *Genetics in Oto-Rhino-Laryngology*. Kitamura K, Steel KP (eds.) S. Karger AG, Basel, pp. 184–195.

de Kok YJM, Merkx GFM, van der Maarel SM, Huber I, Malcolm S, Ropers H-H, Cremers FPM (1995a). A duplication/paracentric inversion associated with familial X-linked deafness (DFN3) suggests the presence of a regulatory element more than 400 kb upstream of the *POU3F4* gene. *Hum Mol Genet* 4: 2145–2150.

de Kok YJM, van der Maarel SM, Bitner-Glindzicz M, Huber I, Monaco AP, Malcolm S, Pembrey ME, Ropers H-H, Cremers FPM (1995b). Association between X-linked mixed deafness and mutations in the POU domain gene *POU3F4*. *Science* 267: 685–688.

de Kok YJM, Cremers CWRJ, Ropers H-H, Cremers FPM (1997). The molecular basis of X-linked deafness type 3 (DFN3) in two sporadic cases: identification of a somatic mosaicism for a *POU3F4* missense mutation. *Hum Mutation* 10: 207–211.

Dominov JA, Miller JB (1996). POU homeodomain genes and myogenesis. *Dev Genet* 19: 108–118.

Erkman L, McEvilly RJ, Luo L, Ryan AK, Hooshmand F, O'Connell SM, Keithley EM, Rapaport DH, Ryan AF, Rosenfeld MG (1996). Role of transcription factors Brn-3.1 and Brn-3.2 in auditory and visual system development. *Nature* 381: 603–606.

Finney M, Ruvkun G (1990). The unc-86 gene product couples cell lineage and cell identity in *C. elegans*. *Cell* 63: 895–905.

Friedman RA, Bykhovskaya Y, Tu G, Talbot JM, Wilson DF, Parnes LS, Fischel-Ghodsian N (1997). Molecular analysis of the *POU3F4* gene in patients with clinical and radiographic evidence of X-linked mixed deafness with perilymphatic gusher. *Ann Otol Rhinol Laryngol* 106: 320–325.

Glasscock ME (1973). The stapes gusher. *Arch Otolaryngol* 98: 82–91.

Hagiwara H, Tamagawa Y, Kitamura K, Kodera K (1998). A new mutation in the *POU3F4* gene in a Japanese family with X-linked mixed deafness (DFN3). *Laryngoscope* 108: 1544–1547.

Hara Y, Rovescalli AC, Kim Y, Nirenberg M (1992). Structure and evolution of four POU domain genes expressed in mouse brain. *Proc Natl Acad Sci USA* 89: 3280–3284.

He X, Treacy MN, Simmons DM, Ingraham HA, Swanson LW, Rosenfeld MG (1989). Expression of a large family of POU-domain regulatory genes in mammalian brain development. *Nature* 340: 35–41.

Herr W, Sturm RA, Clerc RG, Corcoran LM, Baltimore D, Sharp PA, Ingraham HA, Rosenfeld MG, Finney M, Ruvkun G (1988). The POU domain: a large conserved region in the mammalian pit-1, oct-1, oct-2, and *Caenorhabditis elegans* unc-86 gene products. *Genes Dev* 2: 1513–1516.

Heydemann A, Nguyen LC, Crenshaw EB, III (2001). Regulatory regions from the Brn4 promoter direct LACZ expression to the developing forebrain and neural tube. *Brain Res Dev Brain Res* 128: 83–90.

Huang EJ, Liu W, Fritzsch B, Bianchi LM, Reichardt LF, Xiang M (2001). Brn3a is a transcriptional regulator of soma size, target field innervation and axon pathfinding of inner ear sensory neurons. *Development* 128: 2421–2432.

Huber I, Bitner-Glindzicz M, de Kok YJM, van der Maarel SM, Ishikawa-Brush Y, Monaco AP, Robinson D, Malcolm S, Pembrey ME, Brunner HG, et al. (1994). X-linked mixed deafness (DFN3): cloning and characterization of the critical region allows the identification of novel microdeletions. *Hum Mol Genet* 3: 1151–1154.

Hussain MA, Lee J, Miller CP, Habener JF (1997). POU domain transcription factor brain 4 confers pancreatic α-cell-specific expression of the proglucagon gene through interaction with a novel proximal promoter G1 element. *Mol Cell Biol* 17: 7186–7194.

Ingraham HA, Chen RP, Mangalam HJ, Elsholtz HP, Flynn SE, Lin CR, Simmons DM, Swanson L, Rosenfeld MG (1988). A tissue-specific transcription factor containing a homeodomain specifies a pituitary phenotype. *Cell* 55: 519–529.

Kleinjan D-J, van Heyningen V (1998). Position effect in human genetic disease. *Hum Mol Genet* 7: 1611–1618.

Klemm JD, Rould MA, Aurora R, Herr W, Pabo CO (1994). Crystal structure of the Oct-1 POU domain bound to an octamer site: DNA recognition with tethered DNA-binding modules. *Cell* 77: 21–32.

Lamb TM, Knecht AK, Smith WC, Stachel SE, Economides AN, Stahl N, Yancopolous GD, Harland RM (1993). Neural induction by the secreted polypeptide noggin. *Science* 262: 713–718.

le Moine C, Young WS III (1992). *RHS2*, a POU domain-containing gene, and its expression in developing and adult rat. *Proc Natl Acad Sci USA* 89: 3285–3289.

Liang J, Moye-Rowley S, Maurer RA (1995). In vivo mutational analysis of the DNA binding domain of the tissue-specific transcription factor, Pit-1. *J Biol Chem* 270: 25520–25525.

Malik KF, Kim J, Hartman AL, Kim P, Scott Young III W (1996). Binding preferences of the POU domain protein Brain-4: implications for autoregulation. *Mol Brain Res* 38: 209–221.

Mathis JM, Simmons DM, He X, Swanson LW, Rosenfeld MG (1992). Brain 4: a novel mammalian POU domain transcription factor exhibiting restricted brain-specific expression. *EMBO J* 11: 2551–2561.

McCormick A, Wu D, Casatrillo JL, Dana S, Strobl J, Thompson EB, Karin M (1988). Extinction of growth hormone expression in somatic cell hybrids involves repression of the specific *trans*-activator GHF-1. *Cell* 55: 379–389.

Michel O, Breunsbach J, Matthias R (1991). Das angeborene Liquordrucklabyrinth. *HNO* 39: 486–490.

Minowa O, Ikeda K, Sugitani Y, Oshima T, Nakai S, Katori Y, Suzuki M, Furukawa M, Kawase T, Zheng Y, et al. (1999). Altered cochlear fibrocytes in a mouse model of DFN3 nonsyndromic deafness. *Science* 285: 1408–1411.

Myhre SA, Ruvalcaba RHA, Kelley VC (1982). Congenital deafness and hypogonadism: a new X-linked recessive disorder. *Clin Genet* 22: 299–307.

Nance WE, Setleff R, McLeod A, Sweeney A, Cooper C, McConnell F (1971). X-linked mixed deafness with congenital fixation of the stapedial footplate and perilymphatic gusher. *Birth Defects, Orig Artic Ser* 7: 64–69.

Naumova AK, Plenge RM, Bird LM, Leppert M, Morgan K, Willard HF, Sapienza C (1996). Heritability of X chromosome: inactivation phenotype in a large family. *Am J Hum Genet* 58: 1111–1119.

Naumova AK, Olien L, Bird LM, Smith M, Verner AE, Leppert M, Morgan K, Sapienza C (1998). Genetic mapping of X-linked loci involved in skewing of X chromosome inactivation in the human. *Eur J Hum Genet* 6: 552–562.

Nussbaum RL, Lesko JG, Lewis RA, Ledbetter SA, Ledbetter DH (1987). Isolation of anonymous DNA sequences from within a submicroscopic X chromosomal deletion in a patient with choroideremia, deafness, and mental retardation. *Proc Natl Acad Sci USA* 84: 6521–6525.

Okamoto K, Wakamiya M, Noji S, Koyama E, Taniguchi S, Takemura R, Copeland NG, Gilbert DJ, Jenkins NA, Muramatsu M, Hamada H (1993). A novel class of murine POU gene predominantly expressed in central nervous system. *J Biol Chem* 268: 7449–7457.

Okazawa H, Imafuku I, Minowa MT, Kanazawa I, Hamada H, Mouradian MM (1996). Regulation of striatal D1A dopamine receptor gene transcription by Brn-4. *Proc Natl Acad Sci USA* 93: 11933–11938.

Papadaki E, Prassopoulos P, Bizakis J, Karampekios S, Papadakis H, Gourtsoyiannis N (1998). X-linked deafness with stapes gusher in females. *Eur J Radiol* 29: 71–75.

Parolini O, Ressmann G, Haas OA, Pawlowsky J, Gadner H, Knapp W, Holter W (1998). X-linked Wiskott-Aldrich syndrome in a girl. *N Engl J Med* 338: 291–295.

Phelps PD, Reardon W, Pembrey M, Bellman S, Luxon L (1991). X-linked deafness, stapes gushers and a distinctive defect of the inner ear. *Neuroradiology* 33: 326–330.

Phippard D, Heydeman A, Lechner M, Lu L, Lee D, Kyin T, Grenshaw EB III (1998). Changes in the subcellular localization of the *Brn4* gene product precede mesenchymal remodeling of the otic capsule. *Hearing Res* 120: 77–85.

Phippard D, Lu L, Lee D, Saunders JC, Crenshaw EB III (1999). Targeted mutagenesis of the POU-domain gene Brn4/Pou3f4 causes developmental defects in the inner ear. *J Neurosci* 19: 5980–5989.

Phippard D, Boyd Y, Reed V, Fisher G, Masson WK, Evans EP, Saunders JC, Crenshaw EB III (2000). The sex-linked fidget mutation abolishes Brn4/Pou3f4 gene expression in the embryonic inner ear. *Hum Mol Genet* 9: 79–85.

Piussan C, Hanauer A, Dahl N, Mathieu M, Kolski C, Biancalana V, Heyberger S, Strunski V (1995). X-linked progressive mixed deafness: a new microdeletion that involves a more proximal region in Xq21. *Am J Hum Genet* 56: 224–230.

Plenge RM, Hendrich BD, Schwartz C, Arena JF, Naumova A, Sapienza C, Winter RM, Willard HF (1997). A promoter mutation in the XIST gene in two unrelated families with skewed X-chromosome inactivation. *Nat Genet* 17: 353–356.

Rhodes SJ, Chen R, DiMattia GE, Scully KM, Kalla KA, Lin S-C, Yu VC, Rosenfeld MG (1993). A tissue-specific enhancer confers Pit-1-dependent morphogen inducibility and autoregulation on the *Pit-1* gene. *Genes Dev* 7: 913–932.

Ryan AK, Rosenfeld MG (1997). POU domain family values: flexibility, partnerships, and developmental codes. *Genes Dev* 11: 1207–1225.

Schultz J, Copley RR, Doerks T, Ponting CP, Bork P (2000). SMART: a web-based tool for the study of genetically mobile domains. *Nucleic Acids Res* 28: 231–234.

Shimazaki T, Arsenijevic Y, Ryan AK, Rosenfeld MG, Weiss S (1999). A role for the POU-III transcription factor Brn-4 in the regulation of striatal neuron precursor differentiation. *EMBO J* 18: 444–456.

Smith WC, Harland RM (1992). Expression cloning of noggin, a new dorsalizing factor localized to the Spemann organizer in *Xenopus* embryos. *Cell* 70: 829–840.

Spaniol P, Bornmann C, Hauptmann G, Gerster T (1996). Class III POU genes of zebrafish are predominantly expressed in the central nervous system. *Nucleic Acids Res* 24: 4874–4881.

Sturm RA, Das G, Herr W (1988). The ubiquitous octamer-binding protein Oct-1 contains a POU domain with a homeo box subdomain. *Genes Dev* 2: 1582–1599.

Tabor A, Andersen O, Lundsteen C, Niebuhr E, Sardemann H (1983). Interstitial deletion in the "critical region" of the long arm of the X chromosome in a mentally retarded boy and his normal mother. *Hum Genet* 64: 196–199.

Talbot JM, Wilson DF (1994). Computed tomographic diagnosis of X-linked congenital mixed deafness, fixation of the stapedial footplate, and perilymphatic gusher. *Am J Otol* 15: 177–182.

Tang A, Parnes LS (1994). X-linked progressive mixed hearing loss: computed tomography findings. *Ann Otol Rhinol Laryngol* 103: 655–657.

Torres M, Giraldez F (1998). The development of the vertebrate inner ear. *Mech Dev* 71: 5–21.

Vahava O, Morell R, Lynch ED, Weiss S, Kagan ME, Ahituv N, Morrow JE, Lee MK, Skvorak AB, Morton CC, et al. (1998). Mutation in transcription factor *POU4F3* associated with inherited progressive hearing loss in humans. *Science* 279: 1950–1954.

Wallis C, Ballo R, Wallis G, Beighton P, Goldblatt J (1988). X-linked mixed deafness with stapes fixation in a Mauritian kindred: linkage to Xq probe pDP34. *Genomics* 3: 299–301.

Welter JF, Gali H, Crish JF, Eckert RL (1996). Regulation of human involucrin promoter activity by POU domain proteins. *J Biol Chem* 271: 14727–14733.

Witta SE, Agarwal VR, Sato SM (1995). *XLPOU 2*, a noggin-inducible gene, has direct neuralizing activity. *Development* 121: 721–730.

Yntema HG, van den HB, Kissing J, van Duijnhoven G, Poppelaars F, Chelly J, Moraine C, Fryns JP, Hamel BC, Heilbronner H, et al. (1999). A novel ribosomal S6-kinase (RSK4; RPS6KA6) is commonly deleted in patients with complex X-linked mental retardation. *Genomics* 62: 332–343.

79 | *TFAP2B* and the Char Syndrome

MASAHIKO SATODA AND BRUCE D. GELB

Char syndrome, a disorder affecting cardiovascular, craniofacial, and limb development, results from altered activity of the transcription factor, TFAP2B. Mutant TFAP2B alleles act in a dominant negative fashion. Homo- and heterodimers containing mutant TFAP2B molecules either do not bind target gene sequences or fail to transactivate gene expression properly.

The disorder is transmitted as an autosomal dominant trait by the gene that encodes TFAP2B, localized to chromosomal region 6p12. The human *TFAP2B* cDNA and genomic sequences have been isolated, characterized, and used to analyze the mutations causing Char syndrome. The six identified defects have been point mutations in the coding region, with all but one affecting the basic domain that is critical for DNA binding.

Clinical manifestations include a typical dysmorphic appearance, patent ductus arteriosus (PDA), and aplasia or hypoplasia of the middle phalanx of the fifth finger. Other features observed with lower frequency include muscular ventricular septal defects and complex heart disease, hypodontia, foot anomalies, polythelia, and developmental delay, as well as visual and hearing abnormalities. Lifespan is normal with minimal morbidity related to the disorder.

Diagnosis is usually made by clinical examination. Demonstration of *TFAP2B* defects confirm the diagnosis, but no coding changes are identifiable in approximately 50% of patients. Prenatal diagnosis of Char syndrome might be attempted with ultrasonography but could be technically challenging.

Therapy is directed at discovering and treating PDA and other cardiac disease. Preventive pediatric care is appropriate for developmental, visual, and hearing issues.

CLINICAL DESCRIPTION AND HISTORICAL ASPECTS

Florence Char, an American geneticist, described a novel syndrome in 1978, based on her observations with a four-generation Arkansas family (Char, 1978). The principal features that she noted were facial dysmorphia consisting of a short philtrum, patulous lips, ptosis, and low-set ears (Fig. 79–1A), aplasia of a phalanx in the fifth fingers (Fig. 79–1B), and PDA. Dr. Char noted that the mode of inheritance of this disorder was autosomal dominant and that expression of the trait was variable.

Since that description of the trait that is now referred to eponymously, a limited number of additional publications have described additional families inheriting Char syndrome (Temple, 1992; Davidson, 1993; Sletten and Pierpont, 1995; Slavotinek et al., 1997; Bertola et al., 2000; Sweeney et al., 2000; Zannolli et al., 2000). In addition, the original kindred described by Char was reevaluated 30 years later, by which time a number of additional affected individuals were available (Satoda et al., 1999). Clinical descriptions of the affected individuals in those families expanded the range of abnormalities associated with Char syndrome (Table 79–1). Most of these features have varied significantly between and within families inheriting Char syndrome. The exception is the dysmorphia, which has been present in all patients although it is less marked among affected individuals in one family (Sletten and Pierpont, 1995). The variability of the expression of the Char syndrome phenotype was compared between two large kindreds with 19 and 14 affected individuals (the original Char and Sletten kindreds, respectively) (Satoda et al., 1999). PDA prevalence was 21% in the former and 71% in the latter, while the prevalence of fifth-finger abnormalities was 89%

and 0%, respectively. In all families with several affected individuals, the pattern of inheritance is autosomal dominant with complete penetrance.

There are no data about the anatomy or histology of the ductus arteriosus or other affected structures in Char syndrome.

THE MOLECULAR GENETICS OF *TFAP2B*

Gene Assignment

The locus for human *TFAP2B* was assigned to chromosomal band 6p12 using fluorescence in situ hybridization (FISH), as well as with physical mapping. Williamson and coworkers (1996) fluorescently labeled a human genomic P1 clone–derived artificial chromosome (PAC) clone containing the *TFAP2B* gene and showed that it hybridized to 6p12 on human metaphase chromosome preparations. *TFAP2B* was mapped physically using radiation hybrid and yeast artificial chromosome (YAC) mapping techniques. As part of the Human Genome Project, sequence-tagged site (STS) SGC31053, which corresponds to sequence from intron 1 of the *TFAP2B* gene, was mapped with radiation hybrid clone panels into the region that contains several genes which had been mapped to 6p12. Satoda and coworkers (2000) also amplified this STS from CEPH megaYAC clones 849b3, 754a3, 858b11, 771c3, and 921c5, colocalizing it with the Char syndrome critical region and several genes assigned to 6p12.

The *TFAP2B* cDNA

Moser and coworkers (1995) cloned the mouse *Tfap2b* cDNA using its homology to *Tfap2a*. First, a human genomic bacteriophage library was screened with a portion of the human *TFAP2A* cDNA. This resulted in the isolation of two weakly hybridizing phage clones that contained sequences homologous to exons 2–6. This, in turn, led to a screening of a mouse fetal cDNA phage library and the isolation of cDNAs with the entire coding region. Williamson and coworkers (1996) isolated the orthologous human cDNA from a breast cancer–derived cell line. The 1391 bp human cDNA has 5′ and 3′ untranslated regions of 32 and 9 bp, respectively. The open reading frame (ORF) of 1350 bp encodes a 450-residue polypeptide with a predicted unglycosylated $M_r = 49,266$. The predicted protein sequence has the typical organization of AP-2 transcription factors: an N-terminal transactivation domain, a basic domain, and a C-terminal helix–span–helix (HSH) domain (Fig. 79–2A). The sequence of the basic and HSH domain are highly conserved with the other three human AP-2 proteins (Fig. 79–2B), as well as those in other organisms such as mouse, chicken, frog, and fly (e.g., *Drosophila* AP-2 and human TFAP2A are 68% identical). The transactivation domains are far more divergent among the AP-2 proteins (e.g., *Drosophila* AP-2 and human TFAP2A are only 28% identical). The TFAP2B transactivation domain, like those of most of the AP-2 proteins, contains a PY motif (XPPXY) and certain other conserved residues, which are critical for transactivating gene expression (Wankhade et al., 2000).

The expression pattern of *Tfap2b* has been studied during mouse embryogenesis (Moser et al., 1997b). At the earliest stage examined, 8 days postcoitus (d.p.c.), *Tfap2b* expression is observed in the lateral head mesenchyme, the neural fold, and the extraembryonic trophoblast. At 10 d.p.c., *Tfap2b* is expressed in the mid- and hindbrain, the spinal cord, the dorsal root ganglia, the facial mesenchyme, the

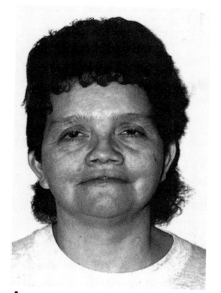

A

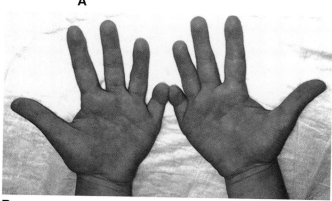

B

Figure 79–1. (*A*) Typical facial features of Char syndrome in an affected 46-year-old woman from the Arkansas family. The short philtrum, prominent lips, flat nasal bridge with upturned nares, midface hypoplasia, and ptosis are evident. (*B*) Hands of the same individual with Char syndrome. The fifth middle phalanges are absent, and the fifth proximal and distal phalanges are hypoplastic.

first branchial arch, and the surface ectoderm. Later, during organogenesis, *Tfap2b* continues to be expressed in the midbrain and the facial mesenchyme and is expressed in the kidney and the corneal epithelium. This tissue-specific expression pattern has overlap with other AP-2 genes in some structures at certain time points, but is unique overall.

The *TFAP2B* Gene

The *TFAP2B* gene spans approximately 24.5 kb and is divided into eight exons (Fig. 79–3). Exon 1 contains the 5′ untranslated region, the translation initiation ATG, and several additional codons. Exon 2 is an alternative exon with nine codons and appears to be skipped in most transcripts. Exon 3, at 459 bp, is relatively long for an internal exon. Exon 8 contains the stop codon. This exonic organization is well conserved among the genes in the AP-2 family. Other features of the *TFAP2B* gene, such as identification of the transcription initiation site and the critical enhancer elements, have not been delineated.

MOLECULAR PATHOLOGY OF CHAR SYNDROME

TFAP2B Gene Defects

Satoda and coworkers (1999) identified *TFAP2B* as the Char syndrome disease gene using a positional candidacy approach. Initially, two

Table 79–1. Clinical Features of Char Syndrome

Dysmorphia
  Broad forehead
  Hypertelorism
  Ptosis
  Flat nasal bridge
  Flat nasal tip
  Short philtrum
  Patulous lips
  Low set pinnae
Cardiovascular
  Patent ductus arteriosus
  Muscular ventricular septal defect
  Complex defects
Skeletal
  Clinodactyly of the fifth fingers
  Hypoplasia or aplasia of middle phalanx of the fifth fingers
  Polydactyly of the toes
  Partial syndactyly of the toes
  Abnormal fifth toes (broad, externally rotated)
Ophthalmalogic
  Strabismus
  Myopia
Polythelia
Dental/oral
  Hypodontia of permanent teeth
  High arched palate
Developmental delay, mild

multigenerational kindred, the original family discovered by Florence Char (1978) and a second kindred identified by Sletten and Pierpont (1995), were used to perform linkage analysis (Satoda et al., 1999). Significant linkage was found with several polymorphic DNA markers mapping to chromosome 6p12–p21. The maximal two-point LOD score was 8.39, achieved with marker *D6S1638*. Both families contributed positively to the LOD scores obtained with markers from that region and independently provided evidence for linkage. Haplotype analysis identified recombinant events that defined the Char syndrome locus with high probability to a 3.1 cM region between *D6S459/ D6S1632/D6S1541* and *D6S1024*. While genetic heterogeneity is suspected for Char syndrome (discussed below), no proof of that has been reported using linkage exclusion mapping.

Next, Satoda and coworkers (2000) discovered that missense mu-

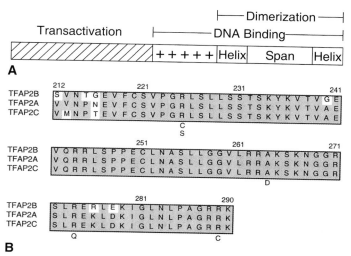

Figure 79–2. (*A*) Domain arrangement of a prototypical AP-2 protein. Slashes are the N terminus, plus signs are the basic domain, and the rest is the C terminus. (*B*) Clustal W alignment of the basic and helix–span–helix (HSH) regions of the human TFAP2 protein sequences with five Char syndrome mutations. Identical amino acid residues are shaded in gray. The basic region of TFAP2B extends from residue 212 to residue 287, and the first helix of the HSH motif extends from residue 288 to residue 315. (From Williams and Tjian, 1991.)

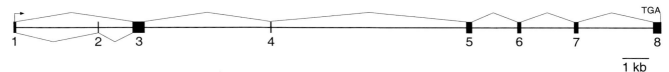

Figure 79–3. Genomic organization of the human *TFAP2B* gene. The eight exons are indicated, including exon 2, which is not present in most *TFAP2B* transcripts. The translation initiation ATG in exon 1 and the TGA stop codon in exon 8 are shown. The scale in kilobases is shown.

tations in *TFAP2B* cause Char syndrome. As discussed, they physically mapped *TFAP2B* into the critical region for Char syndrome and then performed mutation analysis with the original Char kindred and a modest Scottish family (Davidson, 1993). Both families were inheriting exon 5 missense mutations, which were, respectively, a C-to-A transversion at nucleotide 791 that predicted the substitution of an alanine by an aspartic acid residue at codon 264 (A264D) and a C-to-T transition at nucleotide 865 that predicted the substitution of an arginine by a cysteine at codon 289 (R289C). Subsequently, this research group genotyped an additional eight unrelated patients and families with Char syndrome (Zhao et al., 2001). They identified four additional missense mutations (Table 79–2). No mutation was found in four individuals with Char syndrome. While the mutation analysis scanned only the coding exons and their intron boundaries, the dominant negative effects of the mutations that were identified suggested that changes in regulatory regions of the *TFAP2B* gene would be unlikely to cause Char syndrome. Thus, Char syndrome may prove to be genetically heterogeneous.

Several features of the six Char syndrome mutations that have been identified to date are noteworthy. First, they are all missense mutations. This makes it less likely that they cause haploinsufficiency, a notion bolstered by the mutant protein characterization studies described in this chapter. Second, five of the six *TFAP2B* gene defects affect residues in the basic or HSH domain (Fig. 79–2B). Since those domains are critical for DNA binding, it seems that the pathogenic mechanism underlying Char syndrome relates to perturbed binding of AP-2 dimers that contain mutant TFAP2B to their target gene regulatory sites. Third, four of the six Char syndrome mutations alter arginine residues. As discussed by Zhao et al., the disproportion of arginine missense mutations observed in *TFAP2B* and other transcription factors (Basson et al., 1999; International Agency for Research on Cancer, 2001) can be attributed to synergism between fundamental genetic and structural mechanisms. A genetic mechanism is invoked because four of the six codons coding for arginine contain CpG dinucleotides, which are susceptible to mutagenesis (Holliday and Grigg, 1993). In fact, all four *TFAP2B* arginine residues that are mutated are encoded by CGX codons. The structural mechanism relates to that fact that arginine residues are known to play critical functions in the binding of transcription factors to their target sequences (Pabo and Sauer, 1992). Specifically, they can form hydrogen bonds with bases, as well as with phosphate groups in the DNA backbone.

The effects of the six TFAP2B mutant proteins have been characterized in vitro and in cell culture (Satoda et al., 2000; Zhao et al., 2001). Electromobility shift assays (EMSAs) were used to assess the ability of mutant TFAP2B proteins to bind TFAP2 target DNA sequence. Wild-type and mutant proteins were translated in vitro and incubated with the palindromic TFAP2 recognition sequence from position −180 of the human metallothionein-2A gene (*MT2A*-180). The P62R proteins, which have normal basic and HSH sequences, engen-

dered a normal shift (Fig. 79–4A). Among the mutants that affect the basic or HSH domains, the R274Q protein weakly bound the sequence while the other four mutants did not. When these mutants were co-expressed with a truncated TFAP2A protein that retains its dimerization and DNA-binding functions, it was observed that heterodimers containing R225S, R274Q, and P62R did bind target sequence, while R225C heterodimers were not able to do so (Fig. 79–4B). Protein crosslinking documented that R225C protein dimerizes, establishing its deficit as a failure of DNA binding per se.

The six TFAP2B mutants have been expressed transiently in NIH3T3 cells, either alone or with wild type TFAP2B, and their ability to transactivate a chloramphenicol acetyl transferase (CAT) reporter gene was assessed (Satoda et al., 2000; Zhao et al., 2001). When expressed singly, all mutants engendered significantly less CAT expression than the wild type did (Fig. 79–5A). When co-expressed with wild-type TFAP2B, all mutants significantly reduced the CAT expression expected from the wild-type protein (Fig. 79–5B). This documented that the mutant wild-type heterodimers were not transactivating efficiently, clear evidence that the mutants have dominant

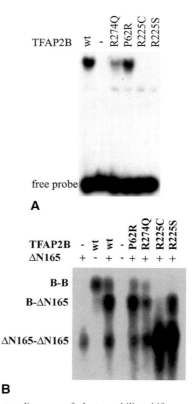

B

Figure 79–4. Autoradiograms of electromobility shift assays (EMSAs) performed using recombinant TFAP2B proteins. (*A*) EMSAs performed with singly translated recombinant TFAP2B proteins that had been incubated with ^{32}P-labeled DNA with the consensus TFAP2 binding sequence. The free probe is shown. (*B*) EMSA performed with co-translated TFAP2B and truncated TFAP2A proteins. Truncated TFAP2A (N165), which retains dimerization and DNA-binding properties, was co-translated with wild-type and mutant TFAP2B. TFAP2 proteins were incubated with ^{32}P-labeled DNA with the consensus TFAP2 binding sequence and electrophoresed. The two homodimer species (upper and lower shifted complexes) and the heterodimer (intermediate shifted complex) are shown.

Table 79–2. TFAP2B Mutations Causing Char Syndrome

Family	Nucleotide substitution	Exon	Amino acid substitution	Functional domain
Minnesota	C185 > G	2	P62R	Transaction
Palestine	C673 > T	4	R225C	Basic
England	C673 > A	4	R225S	Basic
Arkansas	C791 > A	5	A264D	Basic
Australia	G821 > A	5	R274Q	Basic
Scotland	C865 > T	5	R289C	Helix–span–helix

Source: Zhao et al., 2001.

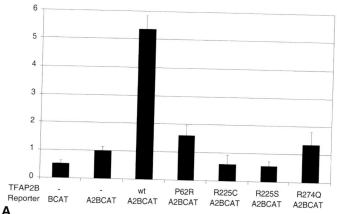

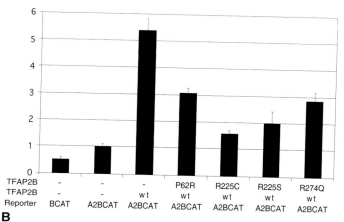

Figure 79–5. Transactivation assays with wild-type and mutant TFAP2B in NIH3T3 cells. (*A*) Cells were transfected transiently with 1.5 μg of the chloramphenicol acetyl transferase (CAT) reporter construct (A2BCAT) with three copies of TFAP2-binding sequence or an equivalent amount of the CAT-only construct (BCAT). To test for transactivation, 0.3 μg wild-type (wt) or mutant *TFAP2B* construct was co-transfected with A2BCAT. After 48 hours, cells were lysed and the CAT concentrations in the lysates were determined. To normalize for transfection efficiency, 0.5 μg of pQB125 was co-transfected, and GFP fluorescence was measured. The bars indicate the mean and standard errors from three independent transfections. Units are arbitrary and the mean from the condition with only A2BCAT was set at 1.0. (*B*) Transient co-expression of wild and mutant *TFAP2B* genes in NIH3T3 cells. Co-transfections and analysis were performed as described in A. Total DNA used during the transfection was made equivalent for all conditions with an unrelated plasmid.

negative effects. There were some significant differences among the mutants, with the R225C and A264D (see Table 79–2 and Satoda et al., 2000) proteins having the most negative effects.

Genotype–Phenotype Correlation

As documented in the preceding section, five of the six *TFAP2B* mutations have affected DNA binding, while one mutation, P62R, affected the transactivation domain. While the functional profile of P62R was similar to that of R274Q and R289C, the phenotype associated with P62R was strikingly different. The facial dymorphia originally described by Florence Char has been consistent among affected individuals with relatively little intra- or interfamilial variation. The family bearing the P62R mutation consistently had a much milder facial dysmorphism, such that the original assignment of affectation status for some individuals in that kindred without PDA was in error. In addition, other families with multiple affected individuals have revealed some persons with abnormalities of the hands, ranging from aplasia of the middle phalanx of the fifth digit to clinodactyly. None of the 14 affected members of the family inheriting the P62R mutation had such hand defects.

Despite the mild facial and hand phenotype, the prevalence of PDA and other cardiovascular defects in the family inheriting P62R was high. This discrepancy between the effects of P62R on cardiac development versus those on craniofacial and hand development requires explanation, particularly since two other mutants with comparable dominant negative effects are associated with the typical Char syndrome phenotype. One potential basis for this phenomenon would depend on the expression patterns of TFAP2 coactivators. The PY motif has been shown to mediate interactions between transcription factors and coactivators (Yagi et al., 1999). Thus, adverse effects of P62R could be more marked in certain tissues, in which coactivators interacting with the PY motif play a greater role in modulating transcriptional activation. Testing of this hypothesis, particularly with respect to cardiovascular development, must await identification of the relevant TFAP2B coactivators.

DIAGNOSIS

Clinical Evaluation

The diagnosis of Char syndrome depends on the clinical features and an awareness of the condition. Since all affected individuals have dysmorphia, which is usually striking and distinctive, an examination of the facial features will usually prompt the proper diagnosis. The other major features—abnormal fifth fingers and PDA—are variably present. In the experience at our center, two unrelated patients were found to have Char syndrome after intervention for a PDA, which is a disproportionate occurrence compared to the worldwide experience. This suggests that this condition is less rare than might be inferred from the literature and that it is underdiagnosed due to the unfamiliarity of most physicians with it. When suspected, examination by a clinical geneticist should result in an accurate diagnosis. Cardiologic evaluation with echocardiography and roentgenography of the hands may assist the clinician in making this diagnosis.

Prenatal Diagnosis

There are no reports of prenatal diagnosis of Char syndrome. Such efforts would appear to be difficult for at-risk fetuses and nearly impossible for de novo cases. The ductus arteriosus is normally open during fetal life so that this cardinal feature cannot be determined in utero. No attempt at detecting the dysmorphic features using fetal ultrasound has been described, but this is likely to be technically challenging in most instances. If present, aplasia of the middle phalanx of one or both fifth fingers could be detected when the diagnosis of Char syndrome is suspected.

TREATMENT

Clinical Management

The major focus for managing patients with Char syndrome concerns the cardiovascular involvement. Infants and children suspected of having Char syndrome need a careful cardiac evaluation, usually including an echocardiogram. Evaluation in the newborn nursery may not be completely informative since the ductus arteriosus may remain open for several days in any neonate. Management of PDA after the immediate newborn period is determined by the degree of shunting. No information is available concerning the likelihood of spontaneous closure of a patent duct after the first weeks of life in patients with Char syndrome, but it is likely to be rather low. Standard care with surgical ligation or ductal occlusion at catheterization can be offered to patients with Char syndrome and a PDA.

Mothers carrying fetuses at risk for Char syndrome—that is, offspring of affected mothers or fathers—should have fetal echocardiography at about 18 to 20 weeks after gestation to rule out complex congenital heart disease (CHD). If CHD is present, such findings might alter the management of the infant at birth, as well as suggest a need to change the delivery site to a center that is able to provide urgent interventions for complex heart defects.

Children with Char syndrome need careful pediatric attention during infancy and childhood. Although certain medical problems such as hearing loss, visual problems, and developmental delay are relatively infrequent among affected children, their prevalence is greater than in the general population. Since those difficulties can be ameliorated through early intervention, preventive pediatric care is appropriate. The most striking external aspects of Char syndrome—namely, the dysmorphia and hand anomalies—require no special care early in life. The dysmorphic features do become important as patients go through childhood and adolescence because of their stigmatizing effects. No data are available about the success of plastic surgical intervention for the facial features in Char syndrome.

Genetic Counseling

Genetic counseling for Char syndrome is relatively straightforward since this trait is autosomal dominant with complete penetrance. Emphasis is necessary on the variability of the phenotype within families, particularly when an affected family member has experienced severe cardiac or neurodevelopmental problems. The recurrence risk for couples with a prior child with an apparently de novo case of Char syndrome is quite low since the disorder is fully penetrant, mitigated by the possibility of gonadal mosaicism. Clinical DNA diagnostics are not available for this disorder and are not anticipated soon because of the rarity of the condition and the apparent genetic heterogeneity.

MUTATIONS IN ORTHOLOGOUS GENES

Moser and coworkers (1997a) generated a mouse model with complete deficiency of Tfap2b using targeted gene disruption in embryonic stem cells. Mice that were heterozygous for the $Tfap2b^-$ allele were phenotypically normal, while homozygotes died in the newborn period. It was shown that $Tfap2b^{-/-}$ mice have polycystic kidneys with cysts in the collecting ducts and distal tubules. These renal changes occurred relatively late in kidney development and were due to excessive apoptosis in the affected regions that was accompanied by down-regulation of anti-apoptotic genes. These investigators did not note any malformations in structures comparable to those affected in Char syndrome.

The genome of the fruit fly, *Drosophila melanogaster*, contains a single AP-2 gene (*dAP-2*). The gene has been cloned (Bauer et al., 1998; Monge and Mitchell, 1998), and several mutant alleles have been generated (Kerber et al., 2001; Monge et al., 2001). Flies with null mutations die as adults or late pupae. They have an abnormal phenotype that includes severely shortened legs with absent tarsal joints, as well as reduced proboscis. While embryonic brain development is normal, defects do exist in the central complex of the protocerebrum. Hypomorphic *dAP-2* alleles have less severe effects on leg shortening. Interestingly, these mutations result in ectopic growth in the eye territory, including supernumerary antennae, potentially through a developmental mechanism that might be relevant for the polythelia observed in some individuals with Char syndrome.

One particularly interesting *Drosophila dAP-2* mutation is R243C (Monge et al., 2001), which alters the arginine residue corresponding to the one mutated in the Char syndrome allele, R225C. In flies, R243C is a null mutant associated with a severe phenotype comparable to that observed with CRIM-negative mutants. When paired with hypomorphic mutations, the R243C allele caused a more severe phenotype, evidence of a dominant negative effect. These results provided confirmation in vivo of the dominant negative effects that were documented in vitro and in cell culture with the TFAP2B R225C mutant protein.

Developmental Pathogenesis of Char Syndrome

The phenotype of Char syndrome includes developmental defects in craniofacial, limb, and cardiovascular development. The pathogenesis of the disorder must result from perturbations in the gene-expression programs induced by TFAP2B in relevant cells and tissues during organogenesis, but the present state of our knowledge is, in several respects, inadequate to provide a meaningful understanding of those issues. First, understanding the specific mechanisms by which the dominant negative *TFAP2B* mutations result in the specific developmental abnormalities observed in Char syndrome would require a thorough elucidation of the upstream regulators and downstream effectors for TFAP2B. Second, the importance of the TFAP2B dimerization

partners (about which little is known except that they appear to be limited to other AP-2 transcription factors) is strongly suggested by the completely discrepant phenotypes in patients with Char syndrome and Tfap2b-deficient mice. Third, an incisive assessment of disease pathogenesis is further hindered by the fact that Tfap2b expression pattern in mice, as published, does not correlate with certain aspects of the phenotype (e.g., no expression was noted in developing mouse limbs, but ulnar ray derivatives are affected in individuals with Char syndrome). Despite those limitations, certain inferences about the developmental pathogenesis of Char syndrome can be drawn from studies of the AP-2 gene family.

While the upstream regulators of the AP-2 genes generally and TFAP2B specifically have not been delineated in a thorough way, Stephen Cohen's group recently identified Notch signaling as an upstream regulator of *dAP-2* (Kerber et al., 2001). They documented that Notch signaling is necessary to induce *dAP-2* and that a constitutively active form of Notch causes ectopic *dAP-2* expression. They also showed that dAP-2 is necessary but not sufficient for inducing leg joints in flies: that is, dAP-2 is not the only mediator of Notch signaling required for joint formation. Finally, this group showed that dAP-2 is necessary for the survival of interjoint cells but is not expressed in them; it acts in a non-cell-autonomous manner. While the relevance of these observations to mammalian development remains to be established, the apoptosis of distinct renal cellular components observed in Tfap2b-deficient mice may be a correlate.

AP-2 proteins have been implicated in the regulation of a large number of genes. This includes some for which functionality has been documented and a much greater number for which AP-2 consensus-binding elements have been identified in gene promoters and enhancers. The regulation of AP-2-responsive genes can be positive (e.g., transforming growth factor-α and cyclin-dependent kinase inhibitor 1A) or negative (e.g., c/EBP-α and c-*myc*). The members of the AP-2 transcription factor family are generally viewed as interchangeable in transactivating gene expression, but this is not always the case. For example, TFAP2B transactivates expression from the c-erbB-2 promoter less potently than does TFAP2A or C (Bosher et al., 1996).

One AP-2-regulated gene with potential relevance for the Char syndrome phenotype is *Hoxa2* (Maconochie et al., 1999). *Hoxa2* is expressed in cranial neural crest cells that migrate into the second branchial arch, a structure that contributes to craniofacial development. The *Hoxa2* gene contains an enhancer with a functional AP-2 binding site that positively regulates expression in the branchial arch (but is not required for expression in the hindbrain) (Maconochie et al., 1999). Loss of Tfap2a does not alter *Hoxa2* expression in the second branchial arch, suggesting that either other AP-2 proteins are relevant or that overall AP-2 levels are critical for induction of *Hoxa2* expression. Proof of the latter concept exists: when either *Tfap2a* or *Tfap2c* is overexpressed in developing mice, the *Hoxa2* promoter is activated in the first branchial arch (as assessed with a reporter gene) where the gene is not normally expressed. Of note, *Hoxa2* activation did not occur ubiquitously or even in all tissues where the *Ap-2* genes are ordinarily expressed at high level (e.g., the frontonasal mesenchyme).

These findings with *Hoxa2* bear directly on the pathogenesis of Char syndrome, particularly to the rather specific pattern of developmental abnormalities. Since the *TFAP2B* mutations associated with this disorder act in a dominant-negative manner, it seems that reduced total AP-2 activity, an integration of all available AP-2 proteins expressed in a given cell, has adverse affects on the regulation of critical downstream genes. The specificity in affected tissues results from two factors. Since half of the TFAP2B molecules are not functional, tissues in which TFAP2B constitutes a large percentage of total AP-2 protein are more likely to be adversely affected. Second, genes for which the normal integrated AP-2 level is marginally adequate to result in their expression or repression are at greater risk for misregulation when TFAP2B mutant proteins reduce total AP-2 activity. Thus, there could be cells or tissues in which *TFAP2B* is expressed robustly, but the presence of a mutant allele has minimal or no adverse effects due to the overall abundance of AP-2 activity. Conversely, there can be tissues with relatively modest levels of TFAP2B where the dominant-negative effects of the mutant allele can result in dramatic abnormalities in proliferation or differentiation. These disparate outcomes are even more understandable if one considers that the relative potencies of the AP-2 proteins, presumptively including heterodimers, are not equivalent for the regulation of individual genes. These factors may explain apparent inconsistencies such as why craniofacial development is normal in mice lacking both *Tfap2b* alleles but the presence of one dominant-negative *TFAP2B* allele results in distinct facial dysmorphia in humans.

One striking feature of Char syndrome is PDA, a relatively common form of congenital heart disease for which *TFAP2B* is the first human disease gene to be identified. While no direct information about the pathogenesis of PDA in Char syndrome is available, recent work by Henry Sucov's group concerning cardiac developmental defects in *Tfap2a*$^{-/-}$ mice provides important insights (Brewer et al., 2002). While previous investigators had established a wide range of development abnormalities in *Tfap2a*$^{-/-}$ mice, Sucov's group documented that they had conotruncal cardiac defects, with double-outlet right ventricle being most prevalent. Using a *LacZ* reporter allele knocked into the *Tfap2a* locus, they showed expression in neural crest cells during their migration into the cardiac outflow tract. Expression was not detected later during outflow tract development (e.g., aortopulmonary septation). This is most likely due to down-regulation of *Tfap2a* rather than loss of that subset of cells, although fate mapping studies are required to establish this formally. When the knock-in allele was present in homozygosity, the same range of cardiac defects was observed as found in *Tfap2a*$^{-/-}$ mice but the migration pattern of the positively stained cardiac neural crest cells was normal. This documented that Tfap2a is not necessary for cardiac neural crest cell migration and that cardiac defects attributable to Tfap2a deficiency appear to arise through perturbations of cardiac outflow tract development per se. Since the ductus arteriosus develops from the left sixth aortic arch artery and receives an important contribution from migrating neural crest cells (Waldo et al., 1999), an analogous situation may hold for mutant TFAP2B and Char syndrome. That is, the pathogenesis of PDA in Char syndrome is predicted to arise not from a failure of neural crest cells to migrate properly to the sixth arch but, rather, from perturbed development of smooth muscle cells in the developing ductus arteriosus.

ACKNOWLEDGMENTS

This work was supported in part from awards from the National Institutes of Health (HD38018 to BDG and A59998 to JDL) and the March of Dimes (FY00-246 to BDG).

REFERENCES

Basson CT, Huang T, Lin RC, Bachinsky DR, Weremowicz S, Vaglio A, Bruzzone R, Quadrelli R, Lerone M, Romeo G, et al. (1999). Different TBX5 interactions in heart and limb defined by Holt-Oram syndrome mutations. *Proc Natl Acad Sci USA* 96: 2919–2924.

Bauer R, McGuffin ME, Mattox W, Tainsky MA (1998). Cloning and characterization of the *Drosophila* homologue of the AP-2 transcription factor. *Oncogene* 17: 1911–1922.

Bertola DR, Kim CA, Sugayama SM, Utagawa CY, Albano LM, Gonzalez CH (2000). Further delineation of Char syndrome. *Pediatr Int* 42: 85–88.

Bosher JM, Totty NF, Hsuan JJ, Williams T, Hurst HC (1996). A family of AP-2 proteins regulates c-erbB-2 expression in mammary carcinoma. *Oncogene* 13: 1701–1707.

Brewer S, Jiang X, Donaldson S, Williams T, Sucov HM (2002). Requirement for AP-2α in cardiac outflow tract morphogenesis. *Mech Dev* 110: 139–149.

Char F (1978). Peculiar facies with short philtrum, duck-bill lips, ptosis and low-set ears: a new syndrome? *Birth Defects Orig Artic Ser* 14: 303–305.

Davidson HR (1993). A large family with patent ductus arteriosus and unusual face. *J Med Genet* 30: 503–505.

Holliday R, Grigg GW (1993). DNA methylation and mutation. *Mutat Res* 285: 61–67.

International Agency for Research on Cancer (2001). IARC PT53 mutation database, http://www.iarc.fr/p53/Index.html.

Kerber B, Monge I, Mueller M, Mitchell PJ, Cohen SM (2001). The AP-2 transcription factor is required for joint formation and cell survival in *Drosophila* leg development. *Development* 128: 1231–1238.

Maconochie M, Krishnamurthy R, Nonchev S, Meier P, Manzanares M, Mitchell PJ, Krumlauf R (1999). Regulation of Hoxa2 in cranial neural crest cells involves members of the AP-2 family. *Development* 126: 1483–1494.

Monge I, Mitchell PJ (1998). DAP-2, the *Drosophila* homolog of transcription factor AP-2. *Mech Dev* 76: 191–195.

Monge I, Krishnamurthy R, Sims D, Hirth F, Spengler M, Kammermeier L, Reichert H, Mitchell PJ (2001). *Drosophila* transcription factor AP-2 in proboscis, leg and brain central complex development. *Development* 128: 1239–1252.

Moser M, Imhof A, Pscherer A, Bauer R, Amselgruber W, Sinowatz F, Hofstadter F, Schule R, Buettner R (1995). Cloning and characterization of a second AP-2 transcription factor: AP-2 β. *Development* 121: 2779–2788.

Moser M, Pscherer A, Roth C, Becker J, Mucher G, Zerres K, Dixkens C, Weis J, Guay-Woodford L, Buettner R, Fassler R (1997a). Enhanced apoptotic cell death of renal epithelial cells in mice lacking transcription factor AP-2β. *Genes Dev* 11: 1938–1948.

Moser M, Ruschoff J, Buettner R (1997b). Comparative analysis of AP-2α and AP-2β gene expression during murine embryogenesis. *Dev Dyn* 208: 115–124.

Pabo CO, Sauer RT (1992). Transcription factors: structural families and principles of DNA recognition. *Annu Rev Biochem* 61: 1053–1095.

Satoda M, Pierpont ME, Diaz GA, Bornemeier RA, Gelb BD (1999). Char syndrome, an inherited disorder with patent ductus arteriosus, maps to chromosome 6p12–p21. *Circulation* 99: 3036–3042.

Satoda M, Zhao F, Diaz GA, Burn J, Goodship J, Davidson HR, Pierpont ME, Gelb BD (2000). Mutations in TFAP2B cause Char syndrome, a familial form of patent ductus arteriosus. *Nat Genet* 25: 42–46.

Slavotinek A, Clayton-Smith J, Super M (1997). Familial patent ductus arteriosus: a further case of CHAR syndrome. *Am J Med Genet* 71: 229–232.

Sletten LJ, Pierpont ME (1995). Familial occurrence of patent ductus arteriosus. *Am J Med Genet* 57: 27–30.

Sweeney E, Fryer A, Walters M (2000). Char syndrome: a new family and review of the literature emphasising the presence of symphalangism and the variable phenotype. *Clin Dysmorphol* 9: 177–182.

Temple IK (1992). Char syndrome (unusual mouth, patent ductus arteriosus, phalangeal anomalies). *Clin Dysmorphol* 1: 17–21.

Waldo KL, Lo CW, Kirby ML (1999). Connexin 43 expression reflects neural crest patterns during cardiovascular development. *Dev Biol* 208: 307–323.

Wankhade S, Yu Y, Weinberg J, Tainsky MA, Kannan P (2000). Characterization of the activation domains of AP-2 family transcription factors. *J Biol Chem* 275: 29701–29708.

Williams T, Tjian R (1991). Characterization of a dimerization motif in AP-2 and its function in heterologous DNA-binding proteins. *Science* 251: 1067–1071.

Williamson JA, Bosher JM, Skinner A, Sheer D, Williams T, Hurst HC (1996). Chromosomal mapping of the human and mouse homologues of two new members of the AP-2 family of transcription factors. *Genomics* 35: 262–264.

Yagi R, Chen LF, Shigesada K, Murakami Y, Ito Y (1999). A WW domain-containing yes-associated protein (YAP) is a novel transcriptional co-activator. *EMBO J* 18: 2551–2562.

Zannolli R, Mostardini R, Matera M, Pucci L, Gelb BD, Morgese G (2000). Char syndrome: an additional family with polythelia, a new finding. *Am J Med Genet* 95: 201–203.

Zhao F, Weismann CG, Satoda M, Pierpont ME, Sweeney E, Thompson EM, Gelb BD (2001). Novel TFAP2B mutations that cause Char syndrome provide a genotype–phenotype correlation. *Am J Hum Genet* 69: 695–703.

Part C.
Posttranslational Control and Ubiquination

80 | An Introduction to Posttranslational Control by Ubiquitin-Dependent Proteolysis

PETER K. JACKSON

Posttranslational modification of proteins allows an expansion of the side chain chemistry of the standard translationally encoded amino acids to expand the range of protein activities. The ability to reversibly modify proteins at specific times provides a flexible means for regulating protein function on a wide range of time scales. A selective list of posttranslational modifications is provided in Table 80–1. To create this broad repertoire, a large number of protein-modifying enzymes and cofactors evolved to catalyze these alterations, typically on specific consensus sites within target proteins. For a given posttranslational mechanism to function, both the *trans*-acting modifying enzymes and the *cis*-acting sites of modification on protein targets must be intact. A broad range of human genetic diseases has already been found to involve deficiencies in both the modifying enzymes and their recognition sites on protein targets, and more examples are likely on the way.

Among the most highly studied posttranslational mechanisms is the addition of the 76 amino acid protein ubiquitin to other proteins, a modification used (*1*) to tag proteins for proteolytic destruction by a pathway to be described here and (*2*) to more directly modify the activity of proteins (although here the mechanisms are more poorly understood). The degradation of a protein by the ubiquitin pathway requires (*1*) tagging of the substrate protein by covalently attaching multiple ubiquitin molecules, typically to create polyubiquitin chains,

and (*2*) degradation of the tagged protein by the 26S proteasome, a large protease complex, generating peptides from the target protein and recycling the ubiquitin molecules. Degradation of intracellular proteins by the ubiquitination–proteasome pathway is highly selective, which can potentially account for the wide range of protein half-lives from minutes (e.g., the tumor-suppressor protein p53) to days (e.g., many cytoskeletal proteins).

The conjugation of ubiquitin to proteins requires a series of ubiquitination enzymes, including the E1 (ubiquitin-activating), E2 (ubiquitin-conjugating), and E3 (ubiquitin-ligase) enzymes (see the Glossary to this chapter for definitions of each). These form a ubiquitin enzyme shuttle to activate ubiquitin and assemble ubiquitin chains onto target proteins (Fig. 80–1). Of these, the largest group are the E3 ubiquitin ligases, which typically bind to substrates and direct ubiquitin chain addition onto those targets. There are possibly several hundred E3 enzymes of various classes. For comparison, measurements of the number of ubiquitinated proteins suggest that as many as 30% to 40% of all proteins may be ubiquitinated in mammalian cells (Schubert et al., 2000). The consequences of ubiquitination for this vast range of proteins is in many cases to regulate the specific protein's stability, but in some cases it alters the protein's activity. The control of protein stability can range from the "switch-like" destruction of regulatory proteins—as seen in the control of mitosis—to the homeosta-

Table 80–1. List of Posttranslational Modifications

Additions to hydroxyl groups (S/T/Y)
  Phosphorylation
  Sulfation
Sulfhydral modification
  Disulfide bond
  Oxidation
  Cysteinylation
  Glutathionylation
Amine modification: lysine side chain or N-terminus
  Methylation
  Formylation
  Acetylation
  Lipoic acid addition
  Farnesylation
  Myristoylation
  Palmitoylation
  Biotinylation
  Stearoylation
  Farnesylation
  Geranylgeranylation
Additions to acids and amides: (E/D/Q/N)
  Pyroglutamic acid (Q)
  Deamidation (Q/N)
  Carboxylation (E/D)
Carbohydrate addition (S/T/N)
  Pentoses
  Deoxyhexoses
  Hexosamines
  Hexoses
  N-acetylhexosamines
  Sialic acid
Other additions
  Prolyl or asparaginyl hydroxylation
  Tyrosination

tic or "thermostat-like" balancing of protein levels in response to metabolic stimuli.

Whether used as a switch or a thermostat, the misregulation of ubiquitination enzymes or the altered access of ubiquitination pathways to specific protein targets can lead to distinct human pathologies. At this time, a small number of human genetic diseases have been linked to misregulation of protein ubiquitination, exemplified by the chapters on Angelman syndrome (Chapter 81) by Joseph Wagstaff and on von Hippel-Lindau disease (Chapter 82) by Eamonn Maher. But the molecular identification of families of ubiquitin ligases is very recent, and a limited number of pathways have been described. Many more connections are likely to follow.

In this chapter I discuss the basic mechanisms of ubiquitination and destruction by the proteasome and then provide examples of how

adapter proteins and ancillary factors allow the coupling of the basic ubiquitination machines to specific biological systems.

BIOCHEMISTRY OF UBIQUITINATION AND FUNCTION OF UBIQUITIN LIGASES

The ubiquitination–proteasome system is thought to be the major pathway for proteolysis outside the lysosome. Ubiquitination and proteasome–dependent degradation can occur in the cytosol and nucleus, and, indeed, the proteasome is present in both locations (Peters et al., 1994). The pathway does not appear to operate within membrane-bounded organelles, where the proteasome is excluded. Protein targets can include soluble proteins, components of protein complexes, integral membrane proteins, and even proteins that have undergone retrograde transport from the ER.

In addition to specific triggering of the destruction of regulatory proteins in signaling pathways, ubiquitination is used to rid the cell of abnormal proteins including misfolded or unassembled proteins in both normal conditions and under cellular stress (Wickner et al., 1999; Hohfeld et al., 2001). There appears to be a strong coupling between cellular chaperone systems and ubiquitination. A reasonable model is that unfolded proteins are acted on by the chaperone system to facilitate rapid folding, but proteins that persist in an unfolded state have the opportunity to be modified by the slower ubiquitination pathway. Indeed, the proteasome has a series of associated chaperone activities, which are certainly important for delivering the ubiquitinated target through a channel into the central cavity of the proteasome (Wang et al., 1999b; Baumeister et al., 2000). But it may be that these or other chaperone activities act on ubiquitinated proteins as a second mechanism to facilitate protein folding (see, for example, Hohfeld et al., 2001).

Even though a large percentage of cellular proteins are ubiquitinated, the ubiquitination system is very selective and uses specific targeting signals, often coupled to specific posttranslational modifications such as phosphorylation. The use of reversible posttranslational modifications allows the protein to be targeted for destruction at a specific time distinct from when the protein is produced and used.

PRODUCTION OF UBIQUITIN, UBIQUITIN CHAINS, AND UBIQUITIN-LIKE MOLECULES

Ubiquitin is a 76 amino acid protein encoded by a series of different genes, including polyubiquitin genes that encode polypeptides with tandemly repeated ubiquitin monomers (Pickart, 1998). These can be proteolytically processed into ubiquitin monomers by ubiquitin-specific proteases. In the simplest case, this processing event removes a short C-terminal extension to create the C-terminal diglycine, found in the mature ubiquitin protein. The C-terminal glycine forms isopeptide bonds with ϵ-amino groups of lysine side chains of either target proteins or—in the case of polyubiquitin chains—side chain lysines of ubiquitin itself. This C-terminal glycine is also the site activated by the E1 enzyme to form thiolesters first with the E1, which activates the ubiquitin to be transferred to form a thiolester with an E2 enzyme.

There are multiple lysines on ubiquitin, but Lys48 is most commonly used to assemble polyubiquitin chains destined for destruction by the proteasome. Other side chain lysines are known to be or are implicated in distinct cellular processes. For example, Lys63-linked ubiquitin is required for DNA damage checkpoint signaling and for signaling IκB destruction in the NFκB transcriptional pathway (discussed below under UEV proteins). Additional examples are known and have been reviewed by Pickart (1998).

When added as a monomer, ubiquitin can play an important role in noncatabolic processes that range from histone regulation and endocytosis to virus budding (reviewed in Hicke, 2001). Recently, a number of ubiquitin-like molecules (Ubls), including the protein SUMO (small ubiquitin-related modifier, also called sentrin), Nedd8/Rub1, and several even more exotic Ubls (Hochstrasser, 1998, 2001; Jackson, 2001; Ohsumi, 2001) have been found added to target proteins through isopeptide bonds to lysine side chains. Here, monoubiquitin and monoaddition of its Ubl cousins appear to function as posttranslational modifiers of protein function and likely reflect a more ances-

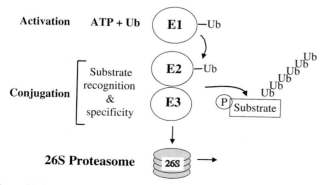

Figure 80–1. The ubiquitin proteasome pathway. A cascade of ubiquitin enzymes (E1, E2, E3) identify the site of ubiquitin chain addition and direct proteins to the 26S proteasome source for degradation. E1, ubiquitin-activating enzymes; E2, ubiquitin-conjugative enzymes; E3, ubiquitin-ligase enzymes.

tral role for the ubiquitin structural fold in regulating protein activity. The biological roles of Ubl modification range even more broadly. Notably, modification by SUMO can play critical roles in several nuclear and cytoplasmic processes, including nuclear transport, the regulation of transcription, the targeting of transcriptional regulators to subnuclear domains, and the regulation of mitosis. These Ubls have their own E1, E2, and (in the case of SUMO) even their own E3 enzymes. The implication is that this family of Ubl modifications and their enzymes may regulate a variety of cellular responses by altering protein activity and localization.

PROTEASOME

The proteasome is the cellular protease complex that directs destruction of both ubiquitinated proteins and some non-ubiquitinated proteins (Rechsteiner, 1998). The complex is also important for peptide processing, at least for antigen presentation by the immune system. A detailed discussion of the proteasome is beyond the context of the current chapter, and the role of the proteasome in human disease has not been explored in detail. A brief description for the purposes of understanding ubiquitin-dependent proteolysis follows.

The proteasome is a 26S complex composed of a core 20S particle containing the protease activity and two 19S regulatory particles that cap the core particle. The 20S core is composed of four stacked rings of seven subunits each. The inner rings contain β-subunits, which are threonine proteases. The outer rings are regulatory α-subunits and contain sequences that gate protein entry into the protease core. The 19S regulatory caps contain ATPase chaperones and several isopeptidase functions (see under isopeptidases) that allow ubiquitinated proteins to be unfolded and deubiquitinated before destruction.

The proteasome is thus a very general cellular regulator, but many questions remain about the diversity of its composition, biochemical activities, and function. It has attracted attention recently as a therapeutic target for cancer (Goldberg and Rock, 2002).

ENZYMOLOGY OF UBIQUITIN CHAIN ADDITION

Ubiquitination of a substrate requires a ubiquitin enzyme shuttle using E1, E2, and E3 enzymes to direct the formation of ubiquitin chains on specific substrates (Fig. 80–1). Among these enzymes, the E3 ubiquitin ligases appear to bind substrates and recruit the ubiquitin-charged E2, thereby stimulating the formation of polyubiquitin chains on particular protein targets. Although only a few detailed examples exist, it appears likely that E3 binding to substrate is the rate-limiting step for at least some ubiquitination reactions, and that ubiquitin-charged E2s can be created independently of E3-substrate binding.

E1 Enzymes

To activate the 76 amino acid ubiquitin protein, one active site within the E1 enzyme uses ATP to create a ubiquitin-adenylate (plus pyrophosphate) coupled to the C-terminal Gly76 of ubiquitin. This activated form is transferred to a cysteine within the active site of the E1 enzyme to form a thiolester linked to the ubiquitin C terminus. In both yeast and mammals, there appears to be one major E1 gene (Scheffner et al., 1998). In humans, the E1 gene is located on the short arm of the X chromosome (Xp11.23) and exhibits X-inactivation. This locus appears to be highly mutable because a number of mammalian cell lines have been found with mutations in the E1 (Finley et al., 1984). Lesions in the E1 locus are very likely to be lethal.

The E1 enzymes for the Ubls, including SUMO and NEDD8, have been described (Hochstrasser, 2000a, 2000b) and are discussed in the following section. Of interest is that the E1 proteins for SUMO and NEDD8, although highly conserved, are encoded by two polypeptides that separate the N-terminal adenylate binding function and the C-terminal thiolester function. For the ubiquitin E1, in both yeast and mammals, these enzymatic functions are combined in a single polypeptide.

E2 Enzymes

Once the E1 has been "charged" with ubiquitin through the thiolester bond, the E1 is competent to transfer ubiquitin via transesterification to an active site cysteine of an E2 enzyme. The E2, or ubiquitin-conjugating (UBC), enzymes are a highly conserved family with at least 13 E2s in yeast and over 30 members in humans. Although several of the better-studied E2s—such as UBC3/Cdc34, UBC4, UBC5, and UBC7—appear to function broadly with a large number of E3 and ubiquitin targets, some of the UBCs are distinct in their functional properties and localization (Scheffner et al., 1998). Most UBCs exhibit a core domain of ~16 kDa, but a number have specific C-terminal extensions or a short N-terminal extension, or both. Critical to the function of the E2s is the active site cysteine. The crystal structures of various E2 enzymes suggest a relatively flat structure where the cysteine sits in a shallow cleft between a four α-helix domain and a four-stranded β-sheet (Scheffner et al., 1998).

Among the E2 enzymes, at least two are known to be the critical E2s for the ubiquitin-like molecules SUMO and NEDD8, called Ubc9 and Ubc12, respectively. The selectivity of these E2s for their ubiquitin variants has been demonstrated (see Hochstrasser, 2002), although the chemical and structural basis for this selectivity is still being investigated. Addition of SUMO, NEDD8, and other Ubls is thought to occur primarily as monomers, and the addition of these proteins does not direct proteins to the proteasome. The addition of SUMO is thought to change both the localization and activity of proteins. NEDD8 addition is also thought to regulate the activity of proteins, and the best-characterized molecular target to date is a subunit of the SCF ubiquitin ligases (described below). The addition of these and other related Ubls has been previously reviewed (Hochstrasser, 2000a, 2001, 2002; Hicke, 2001; Jackson, 2001).

UEV Proteins

In addition to canonical E2 proteins, a small family of closely related proteins that lack the essential thiolester-forming cysteine are called Ub-conjugating enzyme variants (UEVs). UEVs have a central domain similar to true Ubcs. The best-characterized UEV is the yeast MMS2 gene, which is important for RAD6-dependent postreplication DNA repair (Broomfield et al., 1998; Hofmann and Pickart, 1999). The Mms2 protein was found to form a complex with a conventional E2, called Ubc13, and an E3 ubiquitin ligase, Rad6. Both biochemical and genetic studies support that this complex stimulates addition of ubiquitin to Lys63 (as opposed to the conventional Lys48 addition) to a yet unidentified target. Recently, a crystal structure revealed that Mms2 and Ubc13 can form a dimeric complex that may suggest how two ubiquitin monomers are brought into proximity for ubiquitination (VanDemark et al., 2001), although little is understood biochemically. These UEV proteins have been implicated in DNA repair in yeast and in cytokine signaling through the TNF/NFκB pathway in mammals, the cell cycle, and other pathways (Deng et al., 2000). These proteins constitute a distinct subfamily with the E2 enzymes, and at least two genes (one on 20q13.2) encode possibly four or more variants (Franko et al., 2001; Ashley et al., 2002). Although the role of these genes in DNA damage and in cytokine signaling suggest their importance in human physiology, little is known about the function of these genes in human disease.

E3 Ubiquitin Ligases

The ability of E3 enzymes to stimulate ubiquitination of specific targets remained somewhat mysterious until the molecular identification of their constituents in the mid to late 1990s and through the biochemical and structural studies revealing their function that is still in progress. The E3 ubiquitin ligases function either enzymatically or as a scaffold for the E2 enzymes to facilitate transfer of ubiquitin to substrates and the assembly of a ubiquitin chain. The molecular composition of E3s range from a single multidomain polypeptide to large, multicomponent complexes. Typically, the E3s contain a domain important for catalysis and a separate domain important for substrate binding (Jackson et al., 2000). Indeed, characterizing the substrate-binding domains for specific ubiquitin ligases has led to the identification of substrates that participate in many different pathways. Many steps are poorly understood, including how the overall complex is organized to transfer ubiquitin to substrates, how ubiquitin chains are formed, how these complexes are assembled, and how they are regulated by a growing list of ancillary factors.

To date, there are two major structural classes of E3 ubiquitin ligases, the HECT (homologous to E6-AP C terminus) domain and RING (Really Interesting New Gene) finger ubiquitin ligases, although newer studies suggest additional structures called PHD and UBA domains may possess E3 or enhance activity (Hatakeyama et al., 2001; Jiang et al., 2001; Lu et al., 2002; Patterson, 2002)

The HECT-domain proteins are a modest-sized family of proteins with connections to several important biological functions, including the human disease Angelman syndrome (see Chapter 81) and the ability of human papillomaviruses to inactivate the tumor suppressor p53. In the largest class of E3 ubiquitin ligases, the so-called RING finger proteins use a zinc-binding function to stimulate catalysis of ubiquitin chain formation and may combine substrate binding and catalytic domains within a single polypeptide. Alternatively, a smaller RING finger polypeptide can be associated within the context of a multiprotein complex with separate polypeptides containing (1) the RING finger and associated catalytic polypeptides and (2) substrate binding (or "adapter") functions.

HECT-Domain E3 Ubiquitin Ligases

HECT-domain proteins are found broadly in eukaryotes and are defined by a 350 amino acid C-terminal HECT homology domain, originally identified in E6-AP (Scheffner, 1998). A current estimate is that there are at least 28 HECT-domain proteins in humans (Scarafia et al., 2000).

The first identified HECT-domain protein and indeed one of the first E3 defined was E6-AP, identified by the Howley group (Huibregtse et al., 1993; Scheffner et al., 1993). E6-AP (for E6-associated protein) was identified as the E3 recruited by the human papillomavirus E6 oncoprotein to induce degradation of the p53 tumor suppressor, a critical function for the virus to evade DNA damage responses. Within the HECT domain of E6-AP, a conserved cysteine forms a thiolester with ubiquitin (Scheffner et al., 1995). The ubiquitinated E3 can then directly catalyze ubiquitin transfer to the target protein. Other ubiquitin ligases are not thought to form thiolester bonds with ubiquitin, but possibly form transient associations with activated ubiquitin moieties to catalyze transfer to substrates. Outside the catalytic domain, HECT-domain proteins are often large proteins (90 to 200 kDa) with extensive N-terminal domains. In this class of ubiquitin ligases, it appears that the N terminus confers the ability to bind substrate, and the C-terminal HECT domain serves to directly transfer ubiquitin from a thiolester linkage to the substrate.

A growing number of HECT-domain proteins have now been linked to interesting physiological processes, and in a few cases target proteins or candidate targets have been identified. In the human Nedd4 protein and its budding yeast homolog, Rsp5, the N terminus contains several "WW domains" (Sudol, 1998; Wang et al., 1999a), which direct binding to proteins containing proline-rich PPXY motifs (Rotin, 1998).

In the human NEDD4 ubiquitin ligase, the N terminus allows an interaction with the amiloride-sensitive epithelial sodium channel (EnaC) and in yeast Rsp5, the WW motifs are critical for interaction with its target, the large subunit of RNA polymerase (Wang et al., 1999a). A NEDD4-like subfamily of the HECT-domain proteins has been reviewed (Harvey and Kumar, 1999). In the case of human NEDD4, its binding with EnaC appears to require proline-rich sequences in EnaC's β- and γ-chains, a site for mutations in patients with Liddle syndrome (Staub et al., 2000). Here, the inability of EnaC to bind NEDD4 corresponds to an inability of the channel to be ubiquitinated and destroyed, and patients with Liddle syndrome appear to accumulate EnaC. By increasing the amount of active channel, the result is an increase in the levels of sodium (and water) retained, thus leading to hypertension. The role that other pathways controlling hypertension might play in this pathway are also being explored (Kamynina and Staub, 2002). The yeast *Rsp5* gene has a variety of other roles, including control of permeases and endocytosis.

Recently, a novel HECT domain E3, Xsmurf1, was shown to bind, ubiquitinate, and regulate the stability of the Smad1 regulator of BMP signaling (Zhu et al., 1999). BMPs (bone morphogenetic proteins) are members of the TGF-β growth factor family (see Chapter 24). A num-

ber of Smurf-related genes have been implicated in signaling pathways in humans and flies (see, for example, Kavsak et al., 2000; Arora and Warrior, 2001; Bonni et al., 2001). Other interesting HECT-domain proteins include the fission yeast Pub1 gene, which controls ubiquitin-dependent destruction of the cell cycle regulatory phosphatase Cdc25 (Nefsky and Beach, 1996), and the mouse *Itchy* gene, which is involved in inflammatory responses, as suggested by the name associated with the gene deficiency (Perry et al., 1998; Fang et al., 2002). With the number of uncharacterized human HECT-domain proteins, it appears likely that many more physiologically interesting processes will be linked to this class of E3 enzymes in years to come.

RING Finger E3 Ubiquitin Ligases

The largest number of ubiquitin ligases contain a RING finger, a domain central to catalysis. Indeed, reconstitution studies show that fusions between GST and many (and possibly most) RING finger proteins will stimulate ubiquitin chain formation in the presence of purified ubiquitin, E1, and E2 components and ATP (Lorick et al., 1999). Thus, the RING finger plus an E2 enzyme appear to form the catalytic core necessary for ubiquitin chain formation. If the E3 protein or complex contains both a RING and a specific substrate-binding domain, a simple model is that these two functions cooperate to attach a ubiquitin chain to a specific substrate (Jackson et al., 2000). Whereas additional functions with the E3 enzyme likely remain to be defined, the simplified model can help explain how substrate recognition is coupled to substrate ubiquitination. I begin with the SCF complexes; then consider RING finger complexes, including the APC, VHL, and other cullin complexes; and then conclude with single polypeptide RING finger E3 proteins.

SCF (Skp1, Cullin, F-box) Complexes. The SCF class of ubiquitin ligases form complexes that contain at least four proteins: Skp1, the cullin protein Cul1, the RING finger protein Rbx1, and an F-box protein, a substrate-binding protein (see Fig. 80–2). Other proteins associated with SCF ubiquitin ligases are still being defined, but biochemical reconstitution of these four components plus E1 and E2 enzymes is sufficient for ubiquitin chain formation on an appropriately modified substrate.

SCF substrates are bound directly by the F-box proteins, which contain a ~45 amino acid motif called an F-box and serve as adapter proteins by binding to substrates through several different protein–protein interaction domains (Jackson et al., 2000, discussed below). The F-box is required for binding to Skp1, which, in turn, associates with Cul1. A recent crystal structure of a partial SCF complex reveals that the cullin protein acts as a scaffold, bringing the E2 ubiquitin-conjugating enzyme into close proximity with the rest of the complex (Zheng et al., 2002). There are at least six human cullins, including Cul1-5 and Apc2. Cul1, Cul2, and Apc2 functions in known E3 complexes (discussed below). The remaining cullins are likely to organize ubiquitin ligase complexes similar to SCF and Cul1. Human Roc1/Rbx1/Hrt1, a protein containing a RING-H2 finger domain, appears to promote association of the cullin protein with the E2 enzyme and to enhance ubiquitin ligase activity (Kamura et al., 1999; Ohta et al., 1999; Skowyra et al., 1999; Tan et al., 1999). The RING-H2 is one of a class of RING finger domains containing an octet of Zn^{2+}-binding cysteine and histidine residues that may participate in E2 binding and catalysis.

The F-box adapter proteins direct ubiquitination of diverse substrates. There are 16 F-box proteins in *S. cerevisiae*, ~100 in the complete *C. elegans* genome, and more than 50 in vertebrates (Jackson et al., 2000). In the highly studied SCF^{Cdc4}, SCF^{Skp2}, and SCF$^{\beta-TrCP}$ complexes, substrate phosphorylation is required for binding to the F-box protein. In the budding yeast SCF^{Cdc4} complex, the WD40-repeat domain of Cdc4 binds each of its known substrates (Sic1p, Cdc6p, and Gcn4p) in a phosphorylation-dependent fashion (see Jackson et al., 2000 and references therein). The SCF$^{\beta-TrCP}$ complex recognizes a specific phosphoserine motif (DSGφXS) found in the regulatory proteins IκBα and β-catenin. Skp2, a leucine-rich repeat containing F-box protein, also recognizes only the phosphorylated form of the Cdk regulator p27^{Kip1}. Although phosphorylation is clearly required for the

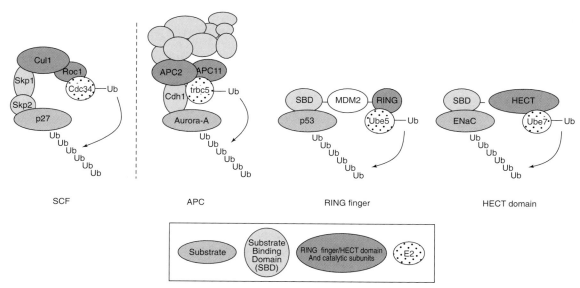

Figure 80–2. The architecture of known ubiquitin ligases.

binding of specific substrates to their F-box adapter, it not clear whether phosphorylation merely serves to improve the affinity of substrate to the F-box protein, or has additional roles.

Among the 70 or more F-boxes, many fall into specific groups (Cenciarelli et al., 1999; Regan-Reimann et al., 1999; Winston et al., 1999). The largest group, exemplified by Skp2 (also called Fbl1), contain C-terminal leucine-rich repeats (LRRs), where a variable number of α/β leucine-rich repeats can form a structure like a segment of a doughnut, to interact with target proteins. There are at least 18 of these so-called Fbl (F-box LRR domain) proteins. A second large group, exemplified by the protein β-TrCP (or Fbw1) has C-terminal WD40 domains, which typically form a 7-fold symmetric β-propeller, again implicated in protein–protein interaction. There are at least 11 Fbw (F-box WD40 repeat) proteins. The remaining F-box proteins are a more diverse group and have simply been called Fbx. Among this group, several of the F-box proteins may not function as adapters for SCF complexes, but may use the F-box to bind Skp1 for some more general function. Examples exist in yeast proteins involved in endocytosis (Galan et al., 2001), kinetochore assembly (Connelly and Hieter, 1996; Kaplan et al., 1997; Stemmann et al., 2002), the vacuolar ATPase (Galan et al., 2001); and in human cell cycle control proteins including the regulators cyclin F (Bai et al., 1996) and Emi1 (Reimann et al., 2001).

In each of the better-understood cases described above, where phosphorylation of the target protein is essential for F-box binding, the phosphorylation of the substrate is highly regulated by ancillary factors. Further, in many cases, the rate-limiting step for destruction of the target is the phosphorylation event. Thus, posttranslational modifications like phosphorylation can function as the trigger for protein destruction.

The Anaphase-Promoting Complex (APC).

The APC was the first multicomponent ubiquitin ligase described and is required for the degradation of substrates that control the metaphase-to-anaphase transition and for the destruction of cyclin B to allow exit from mitosis. Like the SCF complex, the APC contains a cullin homolog, Apc2, and a RING-H2 finger protein similar to Rbx1 called Apc11. Reconstitution studies show that these two proteins form the catalytic core of the APC and are sufficient for ubiquitin chain assembly in vitro (Gmachl et al., 2000; Tang et al., 2001)

The APC associates with two WD repeat–containing adapter proteins, Cdc20/Fizzy and Cdh1/Hct1/Fizzy-related. Both bind the APC and have recently been shown to be important for substrate binding (Burton and Solomon, 2000; Hilioti et al., 2001; Pfleger et al., 2001a; Schwab et al., 2001), although the specific determinants of binding remain unclear. The APC also contains other components (at least 11

polypeptides in total), but the role of these additional components and the possible heterogeneity of APC composition are not understood. Two general destruction signals have been identified in substrates targeted for destruction by the APC—the destruction box (or D-box) and the KEN box (Pfleger and Kirschner, 2000). The D-box motif is found in all the known APC^{Cdc20} substrates, but also in some APC^{Cdh1} substrates, whereas the KEN box appears to target substrates specifically to only APC^{Cdh1}. Thus, Cdh1 can target ubiquitination of both D-box- and KEN-box-containing substrates. Although the D-box and KEN-box motifs appear to be necessary for Cdc20- and Cdh1-activated substrate ubiquitination, it is not clear whether either Cdc20 or Cdh1 is sufficient for direct binding of these recognition sequences or whether additional sequences or factors can contribute to adapter binding.

Ubiquitination of APC substrates is regulated both by phosphorylation of the APC core components and by phosphorylation of at least the Cdh1 adapter protein (Kramer et al., 2000). The APC is also controlled by inhibitory proteins that bind to the Cdc20 and Cdh1 adapter proteins. These include the spindle assembly checkpoint protein Mad2, which binds Cdc20 and inhibits APC activity following spindle damage (Shah and Cleveland, 2000); a closely related protein, called Mad2B, which binds and inhibits Cdh1 (Chen and Fang, 2001; Pfleger et al., 2001b), and the Emi1 protein (Reimann et al., 2001; Hsu et al., 2002), which binds both Cdc20 and Cdh1 to inhibit their activity during interphase.

A growing number of APC substrates has begun to implicate this complex in controlling more than mitosis, a topic that has been recently reviewed (Harper et al., 2002; Peters, 2002).

Von Hippel-Lindau and Other Cullin-Based E3 Ligases.

Another E3 ligase complex that was discovered in the mid- to late 90s was the von Hippel-Lindau (VHL) complex, named for its association with the genetic disease VHL, a familial cancer syndrome. The von Hippel-Lindau (VHL)/ElonginC/ElonginB (or VBC) ubiquitin ligase contains the VHL tumor suppressor, which is inactivated in von Hippel-Lindau disease and in over 80% of sporadic renal cell carcinomas (recently reviewed in Kamura et al., 2002 and discussed in Chapter 82 by Eamon Maher). The VBC ubiquitin ligase is structurally similar to the SCF E3 complex. It contains ROC1, Cul2 protein, a protein homologous to Skp1 called elongin C, and VHL, an adapter protein that binds to Elongin C through a special motif, the BC-box. This motif is found in a number of proteins, including VHL, Elongin A, and members of the suppressor of cytokine signaling (SOCS) family, where it is embedded within an "SOCS-box" domain. The BC motif is necessary and sufficient for VHL, Socs1, and Socs3 to bind elongin C (Stebbins et al., 1999; Zhang et al., 1999). The BC-box–elongin C interaction may strongly parallel the F-box–Skp1 interaction, and the number of SOCS boxes appears to be at least 26 (W. Harper, personal communication). Interestingly, elongin B is homologous to ubiquitin, although its role is unclear. The topic will be covered in detail in Chapter 82 by Eamonn Maher.

VHL down-regulates hypoxia-inducible mRNAs (Kaelin and Maher, 1998), in large part by controlling proteolysis of hypoxia-regulated transcription factors Hif1α and Hif2α (Maxwell et al., 1999). The VHL ubiquitin ligase binds Hif1α and Hif2α and regulates their destruction (Maxwell et al., 1999; Ohh et al., 2000). The recent crystal structure of the VHL/ElonginC/ElonginB complex reveals one face of the VHL molecule where Elongin C binds and another region that appears to be important for binding substrate. Both substrate-binding and elongin C–binding regions are frequently mutated in distinct classes of VHL disease (Stebbins et al., 1999).

An important development in the VHL story came from the study of how the VHL adapter protein recognizes its substrate Hif1α in the presence of oxygen, thus triggering ubiquitin-dependent destruction. A critical posttranslational modification of Hif1α is the creation of a hydroxylproline group (Ivan et al., 2001), an alteration that requires a specific prolyl hydroxylase, described in the worm and called egl9 (Epstein et al., 2001). Thus, by recognizing a modification requiring an oxygen cofactor, the VHL adapter becomes a critical oxygen sensor. Recent studies suggest that even more modifications may participate in this sensing mechanism (Bruick and McKnight, 2001, 2002; Lando et al., 2002). The fascinating implication for other adapter proteins is that a broad range of posttranslationally modified proteins can be recognized by as yet undiscovered adapter functions. Indeed, a recent F-box protein Fbx2 has been demonstrated to target glycosylated proteins for destruction (Yoshida et al., 2002).

VHL is the best-studied Cul2/SOCS-box complex, but a growing number of provocative stories of SOCS-box protein have been described (see a recent review by Kile et al., 2002). A large number of these proteins have other protein–protein interaction domains, including a number that have SH2 domains and participate in tyrosine kinase signaling pathways.

The strong similarities between the SCF complex and the Cul2/SOCS-box complexes suggests that the other cullins (Cul3, Cul4, and Cul5) are likely to organize similar adapter complexes. In the case of Cul3, this protein appears to be important for the regulation of cyclin E levels (Singer et al., 1999), but the remaining components of the complex are not yet known. Nonetheless, the strong similarities among these complexes and the fairly detailed knowledge of which domains mediate association between cullins and their partners should provide a rough roadmap for future molecular identifications. Whether each cullin will have a close homolog of Skp1 and a specific class of adapter proteins like the F-boxes and SOCS-boxes, or whether some of these proteins are reused in multiple complexes, remains to be investigated. Indeed, recent data suggest that Cul5 may associate with some of the same accessory proteins that Cul2 does (Kamura et al., 2001).

Single Polypeptide RING Finger E3 Proteins.

A growing number of E3 ubiquitin ligases have been found to contain an N-terminal substrate-binding domain and a C-terminal RING finger within the same polypeptide. One estimate of the number of such genes in the human genome is ~210 (Human Genome Consortium, 2001), making this the 15th largest gene family, although another reference suggests over 460 such genes (Patterson, 2002). This large number of RING finger proteins may account for the destruction of a much larger number of proteins. Together with over 70 F-boxes, 26 SOCS-box proteins, 28 HECT-domain proteins, and several U-box- and PHD-domain ligases (see below), we may count over 340 (or even 590!) likely E3 ubiquitin ligases! Moreover, several individual E3s are known to ubiquitinate many different substrates, using a variety of ancillary factors. Thus, a vast number of specific proteins can be recognized for ubiquitination.

Within the single polypeptide RING finger proteins, a number of classes have begun to emerge. Because would be difficult to comprehensively cover RING finger E3 proteins here, I briefly discuss several of the best understood examples, especially those with relevance to human physiology.

1. *Cbl and Cbl family members.* In one of the better understood examples, Cbl, an adapter protein containing both SH2 and C3HC4 RING finger domains, functions as a ubiquitin ligase that recognizes tyrosine-phosphorylated substrates through its SH2 domain (Joazeiro et al., 1999). Cbl-mediated ubiquitination of active receptor protein-tyrosine kinases serves a regulatory role in receptor desensitization (Levkowitz et al., 1999). Mutations in the Cbl RING finger at Trp408—a conserved residue in several RING finger–containing proteins including Apc11, Roc1, and Roc2—render Cbl unable to promote degradation. C-terminal to the Cbl RING finger, there is a DOC domain, a motif found in APC10, cullins, and HECT-domain proteins and thought to be important for ubiquitination (Grossberger et al., 1999). Oncogenic versions of Cbl contain deletions or point mutations in the RING domain, suggesting that Cbl becomes transforming by losing the activity of the RING finger (i.e., ubiquitin-ligase activity), thus causing hyperactivation of tyrosine kinase signaling. There is now a small family of Cbl ligases that appear to function in a variety of contexts to dampen or shape tyrosine kinase signaling responses (Rao et al., 2002).

2. *Mdm2.* In another highly studied example, the p53 regulator Mdm2 uses an N-terminal p53 binding function and a C-terminal RING-H2 finger to direct the ubiquitination of the tumor suppressor p53 (Fang et al., 2000; Honda and Yasuda, 2000). The ubiquitin ligase activity of the p53 regulator Mdm2 is RING finger–dependent for both p53 ubiquitination and Mdm2 autoubiquitination. The observation that E3s are capable of autoubiquitination suggests one mechanism by which the E3s, many of which are unstable, may self-regulate their own function. Replacement of the Mdm2 RING finger domain with the RING finger from a heterologous RING protein rescued the autoubiquitination and degradation of Mdm2 but was not able to facilitate ubiquitination of p53, suggesting that the RING domain is required to impart some degree of specificity in recognition of heterologous substrates (Fang et al., 2000). However, RING finger mutations do not disrupt binding between Mdm2 and p53, indicating that RINGs are not necessarily involved in substrate binding. MdmX, a structurally related protein to Mdm2, has been shown to regulate both Mdm2 and p53 levels through its RING finger domain (Sharp et al., 1999). The Mdm2 and MdmX RING finger domains interact, and such an interaction appears to be important for MdmX-mediated stabilization of Mdm2 and of p53. Thus, some RING finger proteins may regulate others by direct interaction of their RING domains.

3. *IAP (Inhibitors of Apoptosis).* A fascinating class of RING finger proteins are the inhibitors of apoptosis, or IAPs. This class of proteins is conserved from worms and flies to mammals and participates in the regulation of apoptosis (and likely other processes) by inhibiting the activity of caspases, the cellular proteases that serve as both regulators and effectors of apoptosis (Salvesen and Duckett, 2002). The ability of caspases to cleave proteins during programmed cell death is inhibited by the IAPs through a characteristic protein–protein interaction domain found in the IAP proteins, called the BIR (baculovirus IAP repeats) motif. In addition to these domains, many IAP proteins also contain RING finger domains (Martin, 2002; Salvesen and Duckett, 2002), and recent evidence shows that they can be triggered to undergo autoubiquitination in response to signals that trigger programmed cell death (PCD). The current model is that this autoubiquitination would cause the IAP to be destroyed, thereby allowing caspase activation and PCD (Salvesen and Duckett, 2002), although additional possibilities remain to be explored. A biochemical pathway regulating IAP autoubiquitination is currently being explored both in *Drosophila* and in human cells (Martin, 2002), but additional insight into more general mechanisms controlling RING finger proteins may appear in this context.

4. *BRCA1.* BRCA1 is a well-known tumor-suppressor gene involved in hereditary cancers of the breast and ovary (Deng and Brodie, 2000; Deng and Scott, 2000). More recently, a heterodimeric complex of BRCA1 and BARD1 has been shown to possess ubiquitin ligase activity through the RING domains of each protein (reviewed

in Baer and Ludwig, 2002). Strikingly, cancer-predisposing mutations have been identified in the RING domain of BRCA1 that abolish not only BRCA1's ubiquitin ligase activity but also its function in the G2/M checkpoint (Ruffner et al., 2001). BRCA1 associates with the centrosome during mitosis through a γ-tubulin-binding domain (Hsu and White, 1998; Hsu et al., 2001). Mouse embryonic fibroblasts harboring a deletion of exon 11 of BRCA1, which contains the γ-tubulin-binding domain, exhibit a defective G2/M checkpoint, centrosome amplification, and aneuploidy (Xu et al., 1999; Brodie and Deng, 2001), hinting that the mitotic localization of BRCA1 to the centrosome is critical for accurate cell division and genomic stability. Exon 11 also includes a nuclear localization sequence (NLS), but NLS-deficient BRCA1 is still capable of nuclear import and formation of DNA damage–induced nuclear foci through association with BARD1 (Fabbro et al., 2002). Moreover, overexpression of the BRCA1 γ-tubulin-binding domain causes centrosome amplification and spindle abnormalities, presumably by preventing endogenous, full-length BRCA1 from associating with mitotic centrosomes (Hsu et al., 2001). Whether the ubiquitin ligase activity of BRCA1 is required at the centrosome for genomic stability is an important question that remains to be addressed.

5. *TRIADs, Including Parkin and Dorfin.* Another rapidly expanding area is the effect of E3 ubiquitin ligases in the nervous system, both in signaling pathways (some of which are pathways common to development) and most strikingly in neurodegenerative disease. In neurodegeneration, a simple model is that persistent downregulation of a specific ubiquitin ligase or enzyme that processes ubiquitinated proteins causes an abnormal accumulation of these proteins. This deficiency may be accelerated by the accumulation of unfolded proteins (in the case where such accumulation exceeds the capacity of the ubiquitination-destruction system). The net result is that homeostasis fails, and the accumulation of some protein leads to neuronal dysfunction and pathology, typically cell death. In one example, the accumulation of the presynaptic protein α-synuclein is associated with a variety of diseases called "α-synucleinopathies," which include both Parkinson disease and Lewy-body-associated dementias (see Giasson and Lee, 2001, for a review). In a small number of cases, dominant mutations in α-synuclein (A53T) appear to result in Lewy pathology.

In autosomal recessive juvenile parkinsonism (AR-JP), mutations in the *parkin* gene are strongly associated with the disease. AR-JP is characterized by clinical indications characteristic of Parkinson (including tremor and dyskinesia) plus histological features typical of Parkinson disease, including neuronal loss and gliosis. The mutations in the *parkin* gene (6q25.2–q27) include missense mutations, small deletions, exon deletions, nonsense mutations, and frameshift mutations (Kitada et al., 1998; Lucking et al., 2001). Generally in patients with AR-JP, both alleles show coding-region mutations that cause inactivation of the parkin protein. Parkin has an N-terminal ubiquitin-like domain and an unusual C-terminal structure where two RING finger domains are separated by a specialized cysteine-rich motif that is similar to a RING domain called an in-between region (IBR). Together, this unusual tripartite sequence has been called a TRIAD (van der Reijden et al., 1999; Rankin et al., 2001), and recent data suggest that the TRIAD domain of parkin associates with the E2 UbcH7 and has E3 ubiquitin ligase activity (Shimura et al., 2000; Zhang et al., 2000). Many of the mutations have been found to be or would be predicted to be deficient in E3 activity (Giasson and Lee, 2001).

The implication is that mutations in parkin cause the accumulation of specific substrates that lead to neuronal defects. Indeed, parkin has been shown to ubiquitinate α-synuclein (Chung et al., 2001), but the cellular defects seen with patients with parkin deficiencies do not uniformly show Lewy pathology, so α-synuclein may not be the only parkin target. Indeed, parkin appears to bind and ubiquitinate (*1*) a synaptic vesicle protein, CDCre11 (Zhang et al., 2000), (*2*) synphilin-1, an α-synuclein interacting protein (Chung et al., 2001), and (*3*) a special glycosylated form of α-synuclein (Giasson and Lee, 2001). The function of parkin in normal physiology is also being investigated,

and there is some evidence to suggest that it may be involved in the response to unfolded proteins (Imai et al., 2001, 2002).

In addition to the fascinating physiology of parkin, the structure of TRIAD domains is intriguing. Some structure-function analysis has shown that at least the first RING finger domain of parkin is important for E3 activity, although the biochemical function of the dual RING fingers and the IBR is not clear. There are at least 22 proteins that have a TRIAD structure, including another E3 ubiquitin ligase implicated in neurogenerative disease, called Dorfin (Niwa et al., 2001, 2002), and a small family of proteins implicated in development, related to the *Drosophila* gene Ariadne (Moynihan et al., 1999; Aguilera et al., 2000; Tan et al., 2000; Ardley et al., 2001). Of considerable interest is that a small number of genes contain only an IBR region exclusive of RING domains (discussed below), including the mitotic regulator Emi1, which regulates another E3 ubiquitin ligase, the APC (Reimann et al., 2001).

Other Single Ring Finger Polypeptide Ubiquitin Ligases (SRFP).

There are a number of other highly studied RING finger ubiquitin ligases, including those that participate in the N-end rule (Varshavsky, 2000), a pathway critical for protein processing in all eukaryotes and the SIAH (seven-in-absentia) regulators of cell growth and morphology (Polekhina et al., 2002). These and other new families of SRFPs will be important to explore for their connections to human physiology and disease.

New Classes of E3 Ubiquitin Ligases.

1. *U-Boxes.* Recent data show that proteins containing a U-box are important for ubiquitin-dependent protein degradation (see review in Patterson, 2002). The U-box was first identified in the yeast ubiquitination factor UFD2 (ubiquitin fusion degradation protein 2) (Koegl et al., 1999) and has been found in a number of proteins implicated in ubiquitination processes (Patterson, 2002). The U-box is a 75 amino acid domain similar in structure to a RING finger, but lacking the canonical cysteines for coordinating Zn^{2+} (Aravind and Koonin, 2000). Recent biochemical data support that U-box domains are indeed ubiquitin ligases (Alberti et al., 2001; Hatakeyama et al., 2001; Jiang et al., 2001). A small number of U-boxes have been characterized in detail (Patterson, 2002), but UFD2 was originally characterized as an "E4," an activity thought to regulate the formation of longer ubiquitin chains. However, the ability of such a domain to have E3 activity suggests that there may be distinct kinds of E3s that promote the assembly of chains of different lengths. In one model, some E3s might initiate chains and then "switch" to another E3 to promote the assembly of longer chains. It is also possible that these types of activities are not really qualitatively different, but that quantitative differences show varying in vitro activities. Little is known about the role of these genes in human physiology, but UFD2 has been implicated in neurodegeneration in mice (Conforti et al., 2000) and in the unfolded protein response (Patterson, 2002).

2. *PHD Fingers.* Among the other new protein domains that function as E3 ubiquitin ligases, the PHD domain within the protein kinase MEKK1 appears to function to cause the degradation of the Erk1 and 2 protein kinases, a phosphorylation target of MEKK1 (Lu et al., 2002). The PHD or (plant homeodomain), also called the LAP (or leukemia-associated protein) domain, shows similarity to the RING finger domain and contains the familiar octet of cysteines and histidines for metal binding. PHDs have been found in many proteins involved in chromatin-mediated transcription (Aasland et al., 1995), but their biochemical activity is unclear. Whether each of these proteins is involved in ubiquitination or whether the same domain can have an additional chromatin-associated function is not clear. There has been evidence that ubiquitination processes can be organized directly on chromatin (Furstenthal et al., 2001) and may also regulate transcription (Kaiser et al., 2000; Kuras et al., 2002), so there may be a connection between the two functions.

3. *SUMO Ligases.* The ability of the U-box domain to serve as an E3 without the benefit of the Zn^{2+} binding cysteines suggests that variations on a conserved structure may allow a conserved enzymatic

function to be functionally altered for specific reactions. Indeed, the zinc-binding function within the IBR of a TRIAD might suggest that a C6HC structure modulates the E3 functions in a yet undefined fashion.

Recently, a modified form of the RING finger, called the Siz/PIAS-RING, or SP-RING, has been shown to be important for the function of E3 ligases that promote the addition of the ubiquitin-like protein SUMO to substrate proteins (Johnson and Gupta, 2001). These SUMO ligases appear to stimulate the addition of SUMO to specific target proteins that regulate a variety of processes, including mitotic progression, nuclear transport, and transcriptional repression, a topic that has been reviewed recently (Hochstrasser, 2001; Jackson, 2001). In humans, there is a family of at least four PIAS proteins, which may each be SUMO ligases regulating a variety of responses, including transcriptional responses in well-known signaling pathways and nuclear localization (Jackson, 2001). Whether additional E3 ligases function to promote the addition of other ubiquitin-like molecules, such as NEDD8, remains to be seen.

UBIQUITIN ISOPEPTIDASES

The formation of ubiquitin chains is reversible, and once ubiquitin chains have been formed, a series of deubiquitinating enzymes (or DUBs) can hydrolyze them. There are currently three known classes of deubiquitinating enzymes, two of which have been reviewed (Wilkinson and Hochstrasser, 1998), although others will certainly be described. A brief description of the enzymatic function, gene families, and potential physiological roles of each follows.

UCH Genes

Ubiquitin genes are encoded as fusion proteins (Pickart, 1998); this includes the polyubiquitin genes believed to encode the majority of cellular ubiquitin. These linear peptides must be processed (like a "cookie cutter") to generate ubiquitin monomers using a peptidase activity described as a ubiquitin C-terminal hydrolase (UCH). The UCH genes encode thiol proteases that cleave ubiquitin after Gly76 to reveal the C-terminal end. A modest number of human UCH genes have been described (Larsen et al., 1998). At this point, few specific UCHs have been linked to human physiology or disease, although a recent connection of a UCH gene to Parkinson disease has been described (Leroy et al., 1998).

UBP Genes

Once ubiquitin chains have been formed, there are a number of possibilities for deubiquitinating enzymes to process or recycle these proteins. Because ubiquitin chains are formed through isopeptide bonds to the Lys48 of the proximal ubiquitin (or less often to other lysine side chains), these DUBs are called isopeptidases, or ubiquitin-processing peptidases (UBPs) The UBPs are a much larger gene family, ranging from 50 to 250 kDa, with at least 16 UBPs in yeast and an even larger number in humans. These proteins are also thiol proteases and sensitive to thiol reagents, but not to inhibitors of serine proteases. There are a number of potential biochemical roles for UBPs, including the recycling of ubiquitin monomers, proofreading of misformed or trapped ubiquitin chains, the regulation of ubiquitination and degradation, and possibly the generation of dynamic ubiquitin chains (Wilkinson and Hochstrasser, 1998). The physiology of UBPs remains poorly understood.

UBPs have been implicated in a number of physiological processes including growth control, development, and the metabolism of degradation intermediates (Wilkinson and Hochstrasser, 1998). In one example, a UBP called tre-2 (Papa and Hochstrasser, 1993) has been shown to function as an oncogene when an inactivated mutant is overexpressed. Given the diversity of enzymes in the UBP family, these genes are quite likely to have roles in human physiology and disease.

JAMM Domain Genes

Very recently, a new family of metalloprotease domains was discovered that function as isopeptidases for ubiquitin and potentially a number of ubiquitin-like molecules (Cope et al., 2002; Verma et al., 2002).

In many fungi, animals, and plants, a protein complex called the signalosome is a conserved multiprotein complex (~8 subunits) that has several subunits that share homology with the regulatory lid complex from the proteasome. The signalosome plays regulatory roles in the function of SCF ubiquitin ligases and a number of physiological processes in eukaryotes. Recent evidence shows that the signalosome contains an activity that can hydrolyze the isopeptide linkage of the ubiquitin-like molecule NEDD8 from target proteins including cullins (the scaffold protein for SCF complexes), where the NEDD8 modification is required for SCF activity. One subunit of the signalosome, called Jab1 or Csn5, is essential for the isopeptidase activity and contains a highly conserved metalloisopeptidase domain, called the Jab1/MPN domain–associated metallopeptidase (JAMM). Mutations of the essential $EX_nHXHX_{10}D$ motif abolished the isopeptidase activity of the signalosome. As a result, the activity of representative SCF complexes were altered, as reflected in the loss of NEDD8 modification.

A similar JAMM domain was observed in the RPN11 subunit of the proteasome lid in a conserved site (Verma et al., 2002). Here, mutation of the JAMM domain showed that these proteasomes were defective in destroying ubiquitinated substrates. Thus, it appears that deubiquitination is critical for a protein to be processed by the proteasome, suggesting that the critical functions of the proteasome lid (regulatory particle) include not only recognition of ubiquitinated substrates but also the deubiquitination of these substrates, thereby releasing them into the protease core of the proteasome.

Remaining JAMM-domain proteins have yet to be explored, but a reasonable possibility is that they function as isopeptidases for other ubiquitin-like molecules. Again, connections to human physiology and pathology will be of great interest.

UBIQUITIN-DEPENDENT PROTEOLYSIS: CONTROL BY ANCILLARY FACTORS

Although the core components of the ubiquitination pathways are becoming better defined, the coupling of the ubiquitination machinery to specific cellular responses appears to be dominated by ancillary factors that gate the ubiquitination process. The requirement for phosphorylation of specific F-box targets is a prime example. In the case of the Wnt-signaling pathway (see Chapter 22), phosphorylation of the transcription factor β-catenin is mediated by a kinase complex that includes the Wnt regulatory factors Axin, the APC (adenomatous polyposis coli) tumor suppressor, and the kinase GSK3. In the absence of Wnt signaling, the Axin/APC complex directs GSK3 phosphorylation on β-catenin. In turn, the $SCF^{\beta-TrCP}$ ubiquitin ligase binds and triggers the ubiquitin-dependent destruction of β-catenin (for reviews, see Wodarz and Nusse, 1998; Huelsken and Birchmeier, 2001; Moon et al., 2002). When Wnt signals are present, the Axin/APC/GSK3 complex no longer phosphorylates β-catenin, so the protein accumulates and translocates to the nucleus to promote transcription of Wnt targets. Here, the elaborate regulatory complex that controls β-catenin phosphorylation is more the rule than the exception.

In another example, destruction of the $p27^{Kip1}$ inhibitor of cyclin E/Cdk2—a kinase complex that regulates DNA replication—is mediated by the SCF^{Skp2} complex. In mammalian cells, the ability of p27 to be phosphorylated on a conserved site and recognized by the SCF complex requires not only the phosphorylation but also the physical presence of the cyclin E/Cdk2 complex and the Cdk-associated protein Cks1 (Montagnoli et al., 1999; Ganoth et al., 2001; Harper, 2001). In the early *Xenopus* embryo, a detailed assembly pathway coupled to the formation of a replication initiation complex is essential for recruiting a related cyclin E/Cdk2/inhibitor complex to origins of DNA replication and then only triggering destruction of the inhibitor (and thus activation of the kinase) when the assembly pathway is successfully completed (Furstenthal et al., 2001).

The importance of these examples is that the destruction of regulatory proteins may be tightly coupled to other regulatory or structural changes in the cell, thus making destruction contingent on specific events. As more examples are examined, more general regulatory themes may appear. But simply enough, if destruction of a regulatory protein serves as a trigger to inactivate an inhibitor to initiate a process or destroy a positive regulator to conclude a process, then ubiquitination enzymes can be physically coupled to these processes to ensure both spatial and temporal accuracy.

Other posttranslational modifications such as the modification of Hif1-α by proline hydroxylation and its recognition by the VHL adapter protein hint at the broad possibilities for triggering protein destruction of very specific pools of protein modified for regulatory purposes. Moreover, having a broad array of adapter molecules in the genome and having the core ubiquitination machinery be modular, evolutionary forces can create new recognition functions without altering the core components.

TARGETS OF UBIQUITINATION: DISCOVERING THEIR BIOLOGY

Although genetics and molecular biology have now provided multiple examples of ubiquitin ligases that are associated with specific targets, probably the most important question is what are the consequences of ubiquitination and destruction of these specific protein targets? Typically this means identifying the specific cis-acting sequences within the protein recognized by the E3 ubiquitin ligase, making mutations that block binding of the ligase, establishing that these mutations indeed stabilize the target protein, and then characterizing the phenotypic and biochemical consequences of having a "nondestructable" version of the protein.

The specific experimental manipulations accompanying this kind of characterization are straightforward (although not necessarily simple) applications of molecular biology and having a nondestructable regulator of a specific process can be an invaluable tool. The creation of a nondestructable mitotic cyclin B (Murray et al., 1989) provided a powerful reagent for inducing a stable mitotic state in *Xenopus* egg extracts, cultured cells, yeast, and *Drosophila* embryos. The ability to freeze a mitotic state, normally only transiently occurring, provided a biochemical and genetic setting to discover how a host of mitotically regulated mechanisms (spindle assembly, nuclear envelope breakdown, chromosome condensation, to name a few) functioned.

However, there are cautions to be exercised when using a nondestructable mutant to characterize the role of a particular destruction pathway. It is quite possible either that a physiological block is created by such a mutant, but that cells or organisms can proceed via an alternative or adaptive pathway, or that the block is firm but pathological consequences ensue. Kinetic analysis should help determine what the immediate consequences of blocking destruction are. Alternatively, inactivating the critical ubiquitination enzymes, generally the E3 ligase or the specific adapter (F-box) subunit, by siRNA or dominant negative techniques should stabilize the target protein and may show an interpretable phenotype. Here, the major difficulty is that many E3s will have multiple substrates and functions, so it may be difficult to sort out which stabilized target is giving the phenotype.

Even with these cautions, these types of studies have been very telling and continue to introduce an expanding range of new cellular pathways. An obvious analogy is the stunning progress made over the past decades in understanding how transcriptional control regulates a wide variety of cellular pathways. In the case of transcription, the relative slowness of transcriptional responses limits the kinds of processes under this level of control. Studying the more rapid processes amenable to proteolytic control will allow interrogation of a much broader range of cellular pathways and should open up many new areas of physiology in the years to come.

GLOSSARY OF UBIQUITINATION ENZYMES

Ubiquitin-dependent proteolysis occurs following the covalent addition of a polyubiquitin chain to a specific target protein. Polyubiquitination targets proteins to the 26S proteasome, an ATP- and ubiquitin-dependent protease complex. The cascade of E1, E2, and E3 enzymes activate the ubiquitin and facilitate the assembly of the multiubiquitin chain. Generally, the E3s are the most diverse group.

Ubiquitin (Ub): A 76 amino acid protein with the C-terminal glycine (Gly76) residue capable of forming an isopeptide bond with a side chain lysine on a target protein or one of the side chain lysines of ubiquitin itself (notably Lys48). There are a number of ubiquitin-like molecules (Ubls), such as SUMO-1 and NEDD8/Rub1, that are added as monomers to side chain lysines.

E1, a ubiquitin-activating enzyme: Ubiquitin is activated by the E1 enzyme and ATP to form a thiolester linkage between the C-terminal glycine 76 and a conserved active site cysteine. Uba1 is the major form of this enzyme in yeast and humans.

E2, a ubiquitin-conjugating enzyme: After activation by the E1, ubiquitin is transesterified to a conserved cysteine of an E2 enzyme. There are 13 E2s in yeast and approximately 30–50 in vertebrates. The genetic name for these enzymes includes the three-letter code "Ubc." Except for Ubc9 (a SUMO-conjugating enzyme) and Ubc12 (a NEDD8/Rub1-conjugating enzyme), the Ubcs have varying genetically defined functions in ubiquitination, but some overlapping roles. Ubc3 is also known as Cdc34, a crucial E2 enzyme in the SCF ubiquitin ligase.

E3, a ubiquitin ligase: The E3 ubiquitin ligases couple with the E2s to bind substrate and assemble a multiubiquitin chain on the substrate. For the HECT-domain E3s, the E3 itself forms a thiolester with ubiquitin and presumably participates in transferring the ubiquitin directly to the substrate. For the E3 complexes containing cullins or RING finger proteins, no direct thiolester between E3 and ubiquitin has been identified. In these E3 classes, the ubiquitin ligase might function to facilitate the interaction between substrate and E2 enzyme (see main text for further discussion).

E4, a multiubiquitin chain assembly factor: The budding yeast UFD2 has been called an E4 protein. The protein binds to multiubiquitin chains and may facilitate part of the ubiquitin-dependent proteolysis pathway following ubiquitin chain assembly.

The 26S proteasome: The proteasome is an abundant protease complex comprising a 20S core particle (CP) flanked by two 19S regulatory particles (RP). The CP is cylindrical, with narrow channels feeding a central cavity with multiple protease sites. The RPs regulate substrate access at both ends of the core. The RP itself contains a base, which contains ATPase subunits thought to unfold substrates for access to the core, and a lid, which contains subunits for binding multiubiquitin chains and ubiquitin-deconjugating enzymes (isopeptidases).

Ubiquitin hydrolases (isopeptidases) or deubiquitinating enzymes (DUBs): A diverse group of enzymes that hydrolyze isopeptide bonds in a multiubiquitin chain. These enzymes might provide regulatory and proofreading functions for assembly of ubiquitin chains and also allow recycling of ubiquitin monomers.

REFERENCES

Aasland R, Gibson TJ, Stewart AF (1995). The PHD finger: implications for chromatin-mediated transcriptional regulation. *Trends Biochem Sci* 20: 56–59.

Aguilera M, Oliveros M, Martinez-Padron M, Barbas JA, Ferrus A (2000). Ariadne-1: a vital *Drosophila* gene is required in development and defines a new conserved family of ring-finger proteins. *Genetics* 155: 1231–1244.

Alberti S, Patterson C, Hohfeld J, Demand J (2001). Cooperation of a ubiquitin domain protein and an E3 ubiquitin ligase during chaperone/proteasome coupling. *Curr Biol* 11: 1569–1577.

Aravind L, Koonin EV (2000). The U box is a modified RING finger: a common domain in ubiquitination. *Curr Biol* 10: R132–R134.

Ardley HC, Tan NG, Rose SA, Markham AF, Robinson PA (2001). Features of the parkin/ariadne-like ubiquitin ligase, HHARI, that regulate its interaction with the ubiquitin-conjugating enzyme, Ubch7. *J Biol Chem* 276: 19640–19647.

Arora K, Warrior R (2001). A new Smurf in the village. *Dev Cell* 1: 441–442.

Ashley C, Pastushok L, McKenna S, Ellison MJ, Xiao W (2002). Roles of mouse UBC13 in DNA postreplication repair and Lys63-linked ubiquitination. *Gene* 285: 183–191.

Baer R, Ludwig T (2002). The BRCA1/BARD1 heterodimer, a tumor suppressor complex with ubiquitin E3 ligase activity. *Curr Opin Genet Dev* 12: 86–91.

Bai C, Sen P, Hofmann K, Ma L, Goebl M, Harper JW, Elledge SJ (1996). SKP1 connects cell cycle regulators to the ubiquitin proteolysis machinery through a novel motif, the F-box. *Cell* 86: 263–274.

Baumeister W, Steven A, Zwickl P (2000). The proteasome: a supramolecular assembly designed for controlled proteolysis. *Curr Opin Struct Biol* 10: 242–250.

Bonni S, Wang HR, Causing CG, Kavsak P, Stroschein SL, Luo K, Wrana JL (2001). TGF-β induces assembly of a Smad2-Smurf2 ubiquitin ligase complex that targets SnoN for degradation. *Nat Cell Biol* 3: 587–595.

Brodie SG, Deng CX (2001). BRCA1-associated tumorigenesis: what have we learned from knockout mice? *Trends Genet* 17: S18–22.

Broomfield S, Chow BL, Xiao W (1998). MMS2, encoding a ubiquitin-conjugating-enzyme-like protein, is a member of the yeast error-free postreplication repair pathway. *Proc Natl Acad Sci USA* 95: 5678–5683.

Bruick RK, McKnight SL (2001). A conserved family of prolyl-4-hydroxylases that modify HIF. *Science* 294: 1337–1340.
Bruick RK, McKnight SL (2002). Transcription: oxygen sensing gets a second wind. *Science* 295: 807–808.
Burton JL, Solomon MJ (2000). Hs11p, a Swe1p inhibitor, is degraded via the anaphase-promoting complex. *Mol Cell Biol* 20: 4614–4625.
Cenciarelli C, Chiaur DS, Guardavaccaro D, Parks W, Vidal M, Pagano M (1999). Identification of a family of human F-box proteins. *Curr Biol* 9: 1177–1179.
Chen J, Fang G (2001). MAD2B is an inhibitor of the anaphase-promoting complex. *Genes Dev* 15: 1765–1770.
Chung KK, Zhang Y, Lim KL, Tanaka Y, Huang H, Gao J, Ross CA, Dawson VL, Dawson TM (2001). Parkin ubiquitinates the α-synuclein-interacting protein, synphilin-1: implications for Lewy-body formation in Parkinson disease. *Nat Med* 7: 1144–1150.
Conforti L, Tarlton A, Mack TG, Mi W, Buckmaster EA, Wagner D, Perry VH, Coleman MP (2000). A Ufd2/D4Cole1e chimeric protein and overexpression of Rbp7 in the slow Wallerian degeneration (WldS) mouse. *Proc Natl Acad Sci USA* 97: 11377–11382.
Connelly C, Hieter P (1996). Budding yeast SKP1 encodes an evolutionarily conserved kinetochore protein required for cell cycle progression. *Cell* 86: 275–285.
Cope GA, Suh GS, Aravind L, Schwarz SE, Zipursky SL, Koonin EV, Deshaies RJ (2002). Role of predicted metalloprotease motif of Jab1/Csn5 in cleavage of NEDD8 from CUL1. *Science* 15: 15.
Deng CX, Brodie SG (2000). Roles of BRCA1 and its interacting proteins. *Bioessays* 22: 728–737.
Deng CX, Scott F (2000). Role of the tumor suppressor gene Brca1 in genetic stability and mammary gland tumor formation. *Oncogene* 19: 1059–1064.
Deng L, Wang C, Spencer E, Yang L, Braun A, You J, Slaughter C, Pickart C, Chen ZJ (2000). Activation of the IκB kinase complex by TRAF6 requires a dimeric ubiquitin-conjugating enzyme complex and a unique polyubiquitin chain. *Cell* 103: 351–361.
Epstein AC, Gleadle JM, McNeill LA, Hewitson KS, O'Rourke J, Mole DR, Mukherji M, Metzen E, Wilson MI, Dhanda A, et al. (2001). *C. elegans* EGL-9 and mammalian homologs define a family of dioxygenases that regulate HIF by prolyl hydroxylation. *Cell* 107: 43–54.
Fabbro M, Rodriguez JA, Baer R, Henderson BR (2002). BARD1 induces BRCA1 intranuclear foci formation by increasing RING-dependent BRCA1 nuclear import and inhibiting BRCA1 nuclear export. *J Biol Chem* 277: 21315–21324.
Fang D, Elly C, Gao B, Fang N, Altman YC, Joazeiro CA, Hunter T, Copeland N, Jenkins N, Liu YC (2002). Dysregulation of T lymphocyte function in itchy mice: a role for Itch in TH2 differentiation. *Nat Immunol* 3: 281–287.
Fang S, Jensen JP, Ludwig RL, Vousden KH, Weissman AM (2000). Mdm2 is a RING finger–dependent ubiquitin protein ligase for itself and p53. *J Biol Chem* 275: 8945–8951.
Finley D, Ciechanover A, Varshavsky A (1984). Thermolability of ubiquitin-activating enzyme from the mammalian cell cycle mutant ts85. *Cell* 37: 43–55.
Franko J, Ashley C, Xiao W (2001). Molecular cloning and functional characterization of two murine cDNAs which encode Ubc variants involved in DNA repair and mutagenesis. *Biochim Biophys Acta* 1519: 70–77.
Furstenthal L, Swanson C, Kaiser BK, Eldridge AG, Jackson PK (2001). Triggering ubiquitination of a CDK inhibitor at origins of DNA replication. *Nat Cell Biol* 3: 715–722.
Galan JM, Wiederkehr A, Seol JH, Haguenauer-Tsapis R, Deshaies RJ, Riezman H, Peter M (2001). Skp1p and the F-box protein Rcy1p form a non-SCF complex involved in recycling of the SNARE Snc1p in yeast. *Mol Cell Biol* 21: 3105–3117.
Ganoth D, Bornstein G, Ko TK, Larsen B, Tyers M, Pagano M, Hershko A (2001). The cell-cycle regulatory protein Cks1 is required for SCF(Skp2)-mediated ubiquitinylation of p27. *Nat Cell Biol* 3: 321–324.
Giasson BI, Lee VM (2001). Parkin and the molecular pathways of Parkinson's disease. *Neuron* 31: 885–888.
Gmachl M, Gieffers C, Podtelejnikov AV, Mann M, Peters JM (2000). The RING-H2 finger protein APC11 and the E2 enzyme UBC4 are sufficient to ubiquitinate substrates of the anaphase-promoting complex. *Proc Natl Acad Sci USA* 97: 8973–8978.
Goldberg AL, Rock K (2002). Not just research tools: proteasome inhibitors offer therapeutic promise. *Nat Med* 8: 338–340.
Grossberger R, Gieffers C, Zachariae W, Podtelejnikov AV, Schleiffer A, Nasmyth K, Mann M, Peters JM (1999). Characterization of the DOC1/APC10 subunit of the yeast and the human anaphase-promoting complex. *J Biol Chem* 274: 14500–14507.
Harper JW (2001). Protein destruction: adapting roles for Cks proteins. *Curr Biol* 11: R431–R435.
Harper JW, Burton JL, Solomon MJ (2002). The anaphase-promoting complex: it's not just for mitosis any more. *Genes Dev* 16: 2179–2206.
Harvey KF, Kumar S (1999). Nedd4-like proteins: an emerging family of ubiquitin-protein ligases implicated in diverse cellular functions. *Trends Cell Biol* 9: 166–169.
Hatakeyama S, Yada M, Matsumoto M, Ishida N, Nakayama KI (2001). U box proteins as a new family of ubiquitin-protein ligases. *J Biol Chem* 276: 33111–33120.
Hicke L (2001). Protein regulation by monoubiquitin. *Nat Rev Mol Cell Biol* 2: 195–201.
Hilioti Z, Chung YS, Mochizuki Y, Hardy CF, Cohen-Fix O (2001). The anaphase inhibitor Pds1 binds to the APC/C-associated protein Cdc20 in a destruction box-dependent manner. *Curr Biol* 11: 1347–1352.
Hochstrasser M (1998). There's the rub: a novel ubiquitin-like modification linked to cell cycle regulation. *Genes Devel* 12: 901–907.
Hochstrasser M (2000). Biochemistry: all in the ubiquitin family. *Science* 289: 563–564.
Hochstrasser M (2001). SP-RING for SUMO: new functions bloom for a ubiquitin-like protein. *Cell* 107: 5–8.
Hochstrasser M (2002). New structural clues to substrate specificity in the "ubiquitin system." *Mol Cell* 9: 453–454.
Hofmann RM, Pickart CM (1999). Noncanonical MMS2-encoded ubiquitin-conjugating enzyme functions in assembly of novel polyubiquitin chains for DNA repair. *Cell* 96: 645–653.
Hohfeld J, Cyr DM, Patterson C (2001). From the cradle to the grave: molecular chaperones that may choose between folding and degradation. *EMBO Rep* 2: 885–90.
Honda R, Yasuda H (2000). Activity of MDM2, a ubiquitin ligase, toward p53 or itself is dependent on the RING finger domain of the ligase. *Oncogene* 19: 1473–1476.
Hsu LC, White RL (1998). BRCA1 is associated with the centrosome during mitosis. *Proc Natl Acad Sci USA* 95: 12983–12988.
Hsu LC, Doan TP, White RL (2001). Identification of a γ-tubulin-binding domain in BRCA1. *Cancer Res* 61: 7713–7718.
Hsu JY, Reimann JD, Sorensen CS, Lukas J, Jackson PK (2002). E2F-dependent accumulation of hEmi1 regulates S phase entry by inhibiting APCCdh1. *Nat Cell Biol* 22: 22.
Huelsken J, Birchmeier W (2001). New aspects of Wnt signaling pathways in higher vertebrates. *Curr Opin Genet Dev* 11: 547–553.
Huibregtse JM, Scheffner M, Howley PM (1993). Cloning and expression of the cDNA for E6-AP, a protein that mediates the interaction of the human papillomavirus E6 oncoprotein with p53. *Mol Cell Biol* 13: 775–784.
Human Genome Consortium (2001). Initial sequencing and analysis of the human genome. *Nature* 409: 860–921.
Imai Y, Soda M, Inoue H, Hattori N, Mizuno Y, Takahashi R (2001). An unfolded putative transmembrane polypeptide, which can lead to endoplasmic reticulum stress, is a substrate of Parkin. *Cell* 105: 891–902.
Imai Y, Soda M, Hatakeyama S, Akagi T, Hashikawa T, Nakayama KI, Takahashi R (2002). CHIP is associated with Parkin, a gene responsible for familial Parkinson's disease, and enhances its ubiquitin ligase activity. *Mol Cell* 10: 55–67.
Ivan M, Kondo K, Yang H, Kim W, Valiando J, Ohh M, Salic A, Asara JM, Lane WS, Kaelin WG Jr. (2001). HIFα targeted for VHL-mediated destruction by proline hydroxylation: implications for O2 sensing. *Science* 292: 464–468.
Jackson PK (2001). A new RING for SUMO: wrestling transcriptional responses into nuclear bodies with PIAS family E3 SUMO ligases. *Genes Dev* 15: 3088–3103.
Jackson PK, Eldridge AG, Freed E, Furstenthal L, Hsu JY, Kaiser BK, Reimann JD (2000). The lore of the RINGs: substrate recognition and catalysis by ubiquitin ligases. *Trends Cell Biol* 10: 429–439.
Jiang J, Ballinger CA, Wu Y, Dai Q, Cyr DM, Hohfeld J, Patterson C (2001). CHIP is a U-box-dependent E3 ubiquitin ligase: identification of Hsc70 as a target for ubiquitylation. *J Biol Chem* 276: 42938–42944.
Joazeiro CA, Wing SS, Huang H, Leverson JD, Hunter T, Liu YC (1999). The tyrosine kinase negative regulator c-Cbl as a RING-type, E2-dependent ubiquitin-protein ligase. *Science* 286: 309–312.
Johnson ES, Gupta AA (2001). An E3-like factor that promotes SUMO conjugation to the yeast septins. *Cell* 106: 735–744.
Kaelin WG Jr, Maher ER (1998). The VHL tumour-suppressor gene paradigm. *Trends Genet* 14: 423–426.
Kaiser P, Flick K, Wittenberg C, Reed SI (2000). Regulation of transcription by ubiquitination without proteolysis: Cdc34/SCF(Met30)-mediated inactivation of the transcription factor Met4. *Cell* 102: 303–314.
Kamura T, Koepp DM, Conrad MN, Skowyra D, Moreland RJ, Iliopoulos O, Lane WS, Kaelin WG Jr, Elledge SJ, Conaway RC, et al. (1999). Rbx1, a component of the VHL tumor suppressor complex and SCF ubiquitin ligase. *Science* 284: 657–661.
Kamura T, Burian D, Yan Q, Schmidt SL, Lane WS, Querido E, Branton PE, Shilatifard A, Conaway RC, Conaway JW (2001). Muf1, a novel Elongin BC-interacting leucine-rich repeat protein that can assemble with Cul5 and Rbx1 to reconstitute a ubiquitin ligase. *J Biol Chem* 276: 29748–29753.
Kamura T, Conaway JW, Conaway RC (2002). Roles of SCF and VHL ubiquitin ligases in regulation of cell growth. *Prog Mol Subcell Biol* 29: 1–15.
Kamynina E, Staub O (2002). Concerted action of ENaC, Nedd4-2, and Sgk1 in transepithelial Na^+ transport. *Am J Physiol Renal Physiol* 283: F377–387.
Kaplan KB, Hyman AA, Sorger PK (1997). Regulating the yeast kinetochore by ubiquitin-dependent degradation and Skp1p-mediated phosphorylation. *Cell* 91: 491–500.
Kavsak P, Rasmussen RK, Causing CG, Bonni S, Zhu H, Thomsen GH, Wrana JL (2000). Smad7 binds to Smurf2 to form an E3 ubiquitin ligase that targets the TGFβ-receptor for degradation. *Mol Cell* 6: 1365–1375.
Kile BT, Schulman BA, Alexander WS, Nicola NA, Martin HM, Hilton DJ (2002). The SOCS box: a tale of destruction and degradation. *Trends Biochem Sci* 27: 235–241.
Kitada T, Asakawa S, Hattori N, Matsumine H, Yamamura Y, Minoshima S, Yokochi M, Mizuno Y, Shimizu N (1998). Mutations in the parkin gene cause autosomal recessive juvenile parkinsonism. *Nature* 392: 605–608.
Koegl M, Hoppe T, Schlenker S, Ulrich HD, Mayer TU, Jentsch S (1999). A novel ubiquitination factor, E4, is involved in multiubiquitin chain assembly. *Cell* 96: 635–644.
Kuras L, Rouillon A, Lee T, Barbey R, Tyers M, Thomas D (2002). Dual regulation of the met4 transcription factor by ubiquitin-dependent degradation and inhibition of promoter recruitment. *Mol Cell* 10: 69–80.
Lando D, Peet DJ, Whelan DA, Gorman JJ, Whitelaw ML (2002). Asparagine hydroxylation of the HIF transactivation domain a hypoxic switch. *Science* 295: 858–861.
Larsen CN, Krantz BA, Wilkinson KD (1998). Substrate specificity of deubiquitinating enzymes: ubiquitin C-terminal hydrolases. *Biochemistry* 37: 3358–3368.
Leroy E, Boyer R, Auburger G, Leube B, Ulm G, Mezey E, Harta G, Brownstein MJ, Jonnalagada S, Chernova T, et al. (1998). The ubiquitin pathway in Parkinson's disease. *Nature* 395: 451–452.
Levkowitz G, Waterman H, Ettenberg SA, Katz M, Tsygankov AY, Alroy I, Lavi S, Iwai K, Reiss Y, Ciechanover A, et al. (1999). Ubiquitin ligase activity and tyrosine phosphorylation underlie suppression of growth factor signaling by c-Cbl/Sli-1. *Mol Cell* 4: 1029–1040.
Lorick KL, Jensen JP, Fang S, Ong AM, Hatakeyama S, Weissman AM (1999). RING fingers mediate ubiquitin-conjugating enzyme (E2)-dependent ubiquitination. *Proc Natl Acad Sci USA* 96: 11364–11369.
Lu Z, Xu S, Joazeiro C, Cobb MH, Hunter T (2002). The PHD domain of MEKK1 acts as an E3 ubiquitin ligase and mediates ubiquitination and degradation of ERK1/2. *Mol Cell* 9: 945–956.
Lucking CB, Bonifati V, Periquet M, Vanacore N, Brice A, Meco G (2001). Pseudo-dom-

inant inheritance and exon 2 triplication in a family with parkin gene mutations. *Neurology* 57: 924–927.

Martin SJ (2002). Destabilizing influences in apoptosis: sowing the seeds of IAP destruction. *Cell* 109: 793–796.

Maxwell PH, Wiesener MS, Chang GW, Clifford SC, Vaux EC, Cockman ME, Wykoff CC, Pugh CW, Maher ER, Ratcliffe PJ (1999). The tumour suppressor protein VHL targets hypoxia-inducible factors for oxygen-dependent proteolysis. *Nature* 399: 271–275.

Montagnoli A, Fiore F, Eytan E, Carrano AC, Draetta GF, Hershko A, Pagano M (1999). Ubiquitination of p27 is regulated by Cdk-dependent phosphorylation and trimeric complex formation. *Genes Dev* 13: 1181–1189.

Moon RT, Bowerman B, Boutros M, Perrimon N (2002). The promise and perils of Wnt signaling through β-catenin. *Science* 296: 1644–1646.

Moynihan TP, Ardley HC, Nuber U, Rose SA, Jones PF, Markham AF, Scheffner M, Robinson PA (1999). The ubiquitin-conjugating enzymes UbcH7 and UbcH8 interact with RING finger/IBR motif-containing domains of HHARI and H7-AP1. *J Biol Chem* 274: 30963–30968.

Murray AW, Solomon MJ, Kirschner MW (1989). The role of cyclin synthesis and degradation in the control of maturation promoting factor activity. *Nature* 339: 280–286.

Nefsky B, Beach D (1996). Pub1 acts as an E6-AP-like protein ubiquitiin ligase in the degradation of cdc25. *EMBO J* 15: 1301–1312.

Niwa J, Ishigaki S, Doyu M, Suzuki T, Tanaka K, Sobue G (2001). A novel centrosomal ring-finger protein, dorfin, mediates ubiquitin ligase activity. *Biochem Biophys Res Commun* 281: 706–713.

Niwa JI, Ishigaki S, Hishikawa N, Yamamoto M, Doyu M, Murata S, Tanaka K, Taniguchi N, Sobue G (2002). Dorfin ubiquitylates mutant SOD1 and prevents mutant SOD1-mediated neurotoxicity. *J Biol Chem* 26: 26.

Ohh M, Park C, Ivan M, Hofman MA, Kim T, Huang LE, Pavletich N, Chau V, Kaelin WG (2000). Ubiquitination of hypoxia-inducible factor requires direct binding of the β-domain of the von Hippel-Lindau protein. *Nat Cell Biol* 2: 423–427.

Ohsumi Y (2001). Molecular dissection of autophagy: two ubiquitin-like systems. *Nat Rev Mol Cell Biol* 2: 211–216.

Ohta T, Michel JJ, Schottelius AJ, Xiong Y (1999). ROC1, a homolog of APC11, represents a family of cullin partners with an associated ubiquitin ligase activity. *Mol Cell* 3: 535–541.

Papa FR, Hochstrasser M (1993). The yeast DOA4 gene encodes a deubiquitinating enzyme related to a product of the human tre-2 oncogene. *Nature* 366: 313–319.

Patterson C (2002). A new gun in town: the U box is a ubiquitin ligase domain. *Science's STKE [Electronic Resource]: Signal Transduction Knowledge Environment* 2002: E4.

Perry W, Hustad C, Swing D, O'Sullivan T, Jenkins N, Copeland N (1998). The itchy locus encodes a novel ubiquitin protein ligase that is disrupted in a18H mice. *Nat Genet* 18(2): 143–146.

Peters J (2002). The anaphase-promoting complex: proteolysis in mitosis and beyond. *Mol Cell* 9: 931–943.

Peters JM, Franke WW, Kleinschmidt JA (1994). Distinct 19 S and 20 S subcomplexes of the 26 S proteasome and their distribution in the nucleus and the cytoplasm. *J Biol Chem* 269: 7709–7718.

Pfleger CM, Kirschner MW (2000). The KEN box: an APC recognition signal distinct from the D box targeted by Cdh1. *Genes Dev* 14: 655–665.

Pfleger CM, Lee E, Kirschner MW (2001a). Substrate recognition by the Cdc20 and Cdh1 components of the anaphase-promoting complex. *Genes Dev* 15: 2396–2407.

Pfleger CM, Salic A, Lee E, Kirschner MW (2001b). Inhibition of Cdh1-APC by the MAD2-related protein MAD2L2: a novel mechanism for regulating Cdh1. *Genes Dev* 15: 1759–1764.

Pickart CM (1998). *Polyubiquitin Chains in Ubiquitin and the Biology of the Cell.* Plenum Press, New York.

Polekhina G, House CM, Traficante N, Mackay JP, Relaix F, Sassoon DA, Parker MW, Bowtell DD (2002). Siah ubiquitin ligase is structurally related to TRAF and modulates TNF-α signaling. *Nat Struct Biol* 9: 68–75.

Rankin CA, Joazeiro CA, Floor E, Hunter T (2001). E3 ubiquitin-protein ligase activity of Parkin is dependent on cooperative interaction of RING finger (TRIAD) elements. *J Biomed Sci* 8: 421–429.

Rao N, Dodge I, Band H (2002). The Cbl family of ubiquitin ligases: critical negative regulators of tyrosine kinase signaling in the immune system. *J Leukoc Biol* 71: 753–763.

Rechsteiner M (1998). *The 26S Proteasome in Ubiquitin and the Biology of the Cell.* Plenum Press, New York.

Regan-Reimann JD, Duong QV, Jackson PK (1999). Identification of novel F-box proteins in *Xenopus laevis. Curr Biol* 9: R762–763.

Reimann JD, Freed E, Hsu JY, Kramer ER, Peters JM, Jackson PK (2001). Emi1 is a mitotic regulator that interacts with Cdc20 and inhibits the anaphase promoting complex. *Cell* 105: 645–655.

Rotin D (1998). WW (WWP) domains: from structure to function. *Curr Top Microbiol Immunol* 228: 115–133.

Ruffner H, Joazeiro CA, Hemmati D, Hunter T, Verma IM (2001). Cancer-predisposing mutations within the RING domain of BRCA1: loss of ubiquitin protein ligase activity and protection from radiation hypersensitivity. *Proc Natl Acad Sci USA* 98: 5134–5139.

Salvesen GS, Duckett CS (2002). IAP proteins: blocking the road to death's door. *Nat Rev Mol Cell Biol* 3: 401–410.

Scarafia LE, Winter A, Swinney DC (2000). Quantitative expression analysis of the cellular specificity of HECT-domain ubiquitin E3 ligases. *Physiol Genomics* 4: 147–153.

Scheffner M, Huibregtse JM, Vierstra RD, Howley PM (1993). The HPV-16 E6 and E6-AP complex functions as a ubiquitin-protein ligase in the ubiquitination of p53. *Cell* 75: 495–505.

Scheffner M, Nuber U, Huibregtse JM (1995). Protein ubiquitination involving an E1-E2-E3 enzyme ubiquitin thioester cascade. *Nature* 373: 81–83.

Scheffner M, Smith S, Jentsch S (1998). *The Ubiquitin-Conjugation System in Ubiquitin and the Biology of the Cell.* Plenum Press, New York.

Schubert U, Anton LC, Gibbs J, Norbury CC, Yewdell JW, Bennink JR (2000). Rapid degradation of a large fraction of newly synthesized proteins by proteasomes. *Nature* 404: 770–774.

Schwab M, Neutzner M, Mocker D, Seufert W (2001). Yeast Hct1 recognizes the mitotic cyclin Clb2 and other substrates of the ubiquitin ligase APC. *EMBO J* 20: 5165–5175.

Shah JV, Cleveland DW (2000). Waiting for anaphase: Mad2 and the spindle assembly checkpoint. *Cell* 103: 997–1000.

Sharp DA, Kratowicz SA, Sank MJ, George DL (1999). Stabilization of the MDM2 oncoprotein by interaction with the structurally related MDMX protein. *J Biol Chem* 274: 38189–38196.

Shimura H, Hattori N, Kubo S, Mizuno Y, Asakawa S, Minoshima S, Shimizu N, Iwai K, Chiba T, Tanaka K, Suzuki T (2000). Familial Parkinson disease gene product, parkin, is a ubiquitin-protein ligase. *Nat Genet* 25: 302–305.

Singer JD, Gurian-West M, Clurman B, Roberts JM (1999). Cullin-3 targets cyclin E for ubiquitination and controls S phase in mammalian cells. *Genes Dev* 13: 2375–2387.

Skowyra D, Koepp DM, Kamura T, Conrad MN, Conaway RC, Conaway JW, Elledge SJ, Harper JW (1999). Reconstitution of G1 cyclin ubiquitination with complexes containing SCFGrr1 and Rbx1. *Science* 284: 662–665.

Staub O, Abriel H, Plant P, Ishikawa T, Kanelis V, Saleki R, Horisberger JD, Schild L, Rotin D (2000). Regulation of the epithelial Na+ channel by Nedd4 and ubiquitination. *Kidney Int* 57: 809–815.

Stebbins CE, Kaelin WG Jr, Pavletich NP (1999). Structure of the VHL-ElonginC-ElonginB complex: implications for VHL tumor suppressor function. *Science* 284: 455–461.

Stemmann O, Neidig A, Kocher T, Wilm M, Lechner J (2002). Hsp90 enables Ctf13p/Skp1p to nucleate the budding yeast kinetochore. *Proc Natl Acad Sci USA* 99: 8585–8590.

Sudol M (1998). From Src homology domains to other signaling modules: proposal of the "protein recognition code." *Oncogene* 17: 1469–1474.

Tan NG, Ardley HC, Rose SA, Leek JP, Markham AF, Robinson PA (2000). Characterisation of the human and mouse orthologues of the *Drosophila* ariadne gene. *Cytogenet Cell Genet* 90: 242–245.

Tan P, Fuchs SY, Chen A, Wu K, Gomez C, Ronai Z, Pan ZQ (1999). Recruitment of a ROC1-CUL1 ubiquitin ligase by Skp1 and HOS to catalyze the ubiquitination of I-κ B-α. *Mol Cell* 3: 527–533.

Tang Z, Li B, Bharadwaj R, Zhu H, Ozkan E, Hakala K, Deisenhofer J, Yu H (2001). APC2 Cullin protein and APC11 RING protein comprise the minimal ubiquitin ligase module of the anaphase-promoting complex. *Mol Biol Cell* 12: 3839–3851.

VanDemark AP, Hofmann RM, Tsui C, Pickart CM, Wolberger C (2001). Molecular insights into polyubiquitin chain assembly: crystal structure of the Mms2/Ubc13 heterodimer. *Cell* 105: 711–720.

van der Reijden BA, Erpelinck-Verschueren CA, Lowenberg B, Jansen JH (1999). TRIADs: a new class of proteins with a novel cysteine-rich signature. *Protein Sci* 8: 1557–1561.

Verma R, Aravind L, Oania R, McDonald WH, Yates IJ, Koonin EV, Deshaies RJ (2002). Role of Rpn11 metalloprotease in deubiquitination and degradation by the 26S proteasome. *Science* 15: 15.

Wang G, Yang J, Huibregtse JM (1999a). Functional domains of the Rsp5 ubiquitin-protein ligase. *Mol Cell Biol* 19: 342–352.

Wang HR, Nederlof P, Baumeister W, Zwickl P (1999b). The proteasome: a macromolecular assembly designed for controlled proteolysis. *Biol Chem* 380: 1183–1192.

Wickner S, Maurizi MR, Gottesman S (1999). Posttranslational quality control: folding, refolding, and degrading proteins. *Science* 286: 1888–1893.

Wilkinson KD, Hochstrasser M (1998). *The Deubiquitinating Enzymes in Ubiquitin and the Biology of the Cell.* Plenum Press, New York.

Winston JT, Koepp DM, Zhu C, Elledge SJ, Harper JW (1999). A family of mammalian F-box proteins. *Curr Biol* 9: 1180–1182.

Wodarz A, Nusse R (1998). Mechanisms of Wnt signaling in development. *Annu Rev Cell Dev Biol* 14: 59–88.

Xu X, Weaver Z, Linke SP, Li C, Gotay J, Wang XW, Harris CC, Ried T, Deng CX (1999). Centrosome amplification and a defective G2-M cell cycle checkpoint induce genetic instability in BRCA1 exon 11 isoform-deficient cells. *Mol Cell* 3: 389–395.

Yoshida Y, Chiba T, Tokunaga F, Kawasaki H, Iwai K, Suzuki T, Ito Y, Matsuoka K, Yoshida M, Tanaka K, Tai T (2002). E3 ubiquitin ligase that recognizes sugar chains. *Nature* 418: 438–442.

Zhang JG, Farley A, Nicholson SE, Willson TA, Zugaro LM, Simpson RJ, Moritz RL, Cary D, Richardson R, Hausmann G, et al. (1999). The conserved SOCS box motif in suppressors of cytokine signaling binds to elongins B and C and may couple bound proteins to proteasomal degradation. *Proc Natl Acad Sci USA* 96: 2071–2076.

Zhang Y, Gao J, Chung KK, Huang H, Dawson VL, Dawson TM (2000). Parkin functions as an E2-dependent ubiquitin-protein ligase and promotes the degradation of the synaptic vesicle-associated protein, CDCrel-1. *Proc Natl Acad Sci USA* 97: 13354–13359.

Zheng N, Schulman B, Song L, Miller J, Jeffrey P, Wang P, Chu C, Koepp D, Elledge S, Pagano M, et al. (2002). Structure of the Cul1-Rbx1-Skp1-F box-Skp2 SCF ubiquitin ligase complex. *Nature* 416: 703–709.

Zhu H, Kavsak P, Abdollah S, Wrana JL, Thomsen GH (1999). A SMAD ubiquitin ligase targets the BMP pathway and affects embryonic pattern formation. *Nature* 400: 687–693.

81 | *UBE3A* and the Angelman Syndrome

JOSEPH WAGSTAFF

Angelman syndrome (AS) is a neurodevelopmental disorder caused by deficiency of the ubiquitin-protein ligase UBE3A in the brain. The genetic pathogenesis of AS is complex, because the *UBE3A* gene shows parent-specific differential expression, or imprinting, limited to the brain. In most tissues, the maternal and paternal alleles of *UBE3A* are expressed equally; in some brain regions, however, the maternal allele is expressed at a much higher level than the paternal allele. Therefore, any genetic mechanism leading to absence of a functional allele of *UBE3A* inherited from the mother causes AS; absence of a functional paternal allele of *UBE3A* causes no phenotypic effects. UBE3A was first identified as a ubiquitin protein ligase that, in the presence of E6 proteins from high-risk human papillomaviruses (HPVs), ubiquitinates the p53 tumor suppressor, thereby targeting it for degradation by the proteasome. The p53 protein does not appear to be a UBE3A substrate in normal human tissues. The substrate(s) of UBE3A that fail to be ubiquitinated in the brains of AS patients, and that lead to the neurological manifestations of AS, remain to be identified.

ROLE OF UBE3A AND UBIQUITIN PATHWAY

The protein product of *UBE3A*, also known as E6-AP (E6-associated protein), was first identified by Huibregtse et al. (1991, 1993) as a cellular protein that interacts with the E6 proteins of high-risk tumorigenic HPVs. Cervical cancer cells (such as HeLa cells) infected with high-risk HPVs contain very low levels of the tumor suppressor p53. Huibregtse et al. demonstrated that the UBE3A/E6 complex acts as an E3 ubiquitin-protein ligase with p53 as substrate. Multiubiquitination renders p53 a substrate for degradation by the proteasome, thus accounting for the low p53 levels in cells infected with high-risk HPVs.

UBE3A contains a C-terminal domain conserved in ubiquitin-protein ligases from yeast to human, referred to as the HECT (homologous to E6-AP C terminus) domain (Huibregtse et al., 1995). Unlike other E3s, UBE3A and other HECT-domain proteins form a thioester bond with ubiquitin before ubiquitin is transferred to substrates. Transfer of ubiquitin to substrates by UBE3A requires (*1*) binding of an E2-ubiquitin conjugate to the HECT domain of UBE3A; (*2*) transfer of ubiquitin from the E2 to the catalytic cysteine of UBE3A, with formation of a thioester linkage; and (*3*) transfer of ubiquitin from UBE3A to substrate. In vitro, UBE3A can accept ubiquitin from at least two E2 enzymes, UBCH7 and UBCH8 (Kumar et al., 1997). Huang et al. (1999) have determined the crystal structure of the UBE3A HECT domain that is bound to UBCH7.

The role of UBE3A in the pathogenesis of AS is clearly not catalysis of p53 ubiquitination, because this reaction depends on E6 proteins from high-risk HPVs, and no E6 proteins or E6 homologs are present in normal human tissues. Therefore, it is reasonable to assume that other UBE3A substrates exist for which ubiquitination does not require HPV E6. Only a small number of E6-independent UBE3A substrates have been identified, all by P. Howley's group using a two-hybrid approach. These substrates are HHR23A and HHR23B, human homologs of the yeast Rad23 DNA repair protein (Kumar et al., 1999), and active BLK, a B-lymphocyte-specific Src-family kinase (Oda et al., 1999).

The possibility that UBE3A has functions other than its ubiquitin-protein ligase activity was raised by Nawaz et al. (1999), who recovered UBE3A in a two-hybrid screen using the ligand-binding domain of human progesterone receptor as bait. They showed, using an in vitro assay, that UBE3A coactivates the transcriptional activity of the progesterone receptor in a hormone-dependent manner. They also showed that missense mutant forms of UBE3A that cause AS are not defective in this coactivation function.

CLINICAL DESCRIPTION OF AS

Major clinical features of AS include severe mental retardation with lack of speech, easily provoked smiling and laughter, seizure disorder, distinctive gait with widely separated feet and raised arms flexed at the elbows and wrists, tremulous movements, and sleep disorder (Williams et al., 1995b) (Fig. 81–1). Dysmorphic features are not striking in young children with AS; however, as AS individuals age, characteristic facial features may become apparent, such as prognathism, wide mouth, and widely spaced teeth. Clayton-Smith (1993) has suggested that these changes probably are caused by constant tongue thrusting. Many AS individuals show normal head circumference at birth, with a decline in the head circumference percentile with age; however, true microcephaly (head circumference <2nd percentile) is absent in a substantial fraction of AS individuals. The natural history of the mental impairment in AS is generally static, with slow attainment of new skills and no developmental regression; exceptions to this generalization usually involve poorly controlled seizures with consequent loss of developmental milestones.

MOLECULAR GENETICS OF AS AND GENOTYPE–PHENOTYPE CORRELATIONS

Genetic Etiologies of AS

Most cases of AS are sporadic; however, a significant number of cases of familial AS in siblings or in more distant relatives have been reported. Although AS was first described as a clinical entity in 1965 (Angelman, 1965), no genetic correlate was found until 1987, when two groups reported deletions of 15q11–q13 in AS individuals (Kaplan et al., 1987; Magenis et al., 1987). The deletions were indistinguishable cytogenetically from those reported in individuals with Prader-Willi syndrome (PWS) by Ledbetter et al. (1981). Knoll et al. (1989) reported that, whereas PWS deletions involve de novo loss from the paternal chromosome 15, AS deletions involve loss from the maternal chromosome 15. The fact that identical deletions on the maternal and paternal copies of chromosome 15 lead to two completely distinct clinical syndromes led to the suggestion that gene expression in this region is different on the maternal and paternal homologs—that is, that 15q11–q13 is affected by genetic imprinting (see later in this chapter). Detection of deletions of 15q11–q13 by standard cytogenetic techniques is subject to a high frequency of false-positive and false-negative determinations (Delach et al., 1994). More accurate deletion detection in this region has been facilitated by fluorescence in situ hybridization (FISH) assays. FISH has shown that approximately 70% of individuals clinically diagnosed with AS have 15q11–q13 deletions. The size of these deletions has been estimated to be ~4 Mb (Christian et al., 1998), with limited heterogeneity of breakpoints flanking the commonly deleted region. With only one known exception (Kokkonen and Leisti, 2000), these deletions always

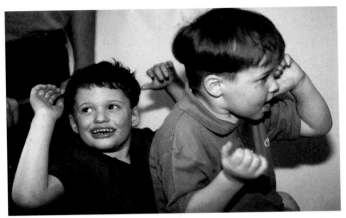

Figure 81–1. Photograph of two brothers with Angelman syndrome caused by a *UBE3A* missense mutation. Note smiling, widely spaced teeth, and flexion at elbows and wrists. (Photo courtesy of Roberta Pagon, M.D.)

occur de novo, presumably during oogenesis, and cause sporadic cases of AS.

Three other common molecular genetic causes of AS are known: point mutations within the *UBE3A* gene, imprinting defects, and paternal uniparental disomy (UPD) for chromosome 15. *UBE3A* spans 100 kb within 15q11–q13 and contains 16 exons (Kishino and Wagstaff, 1998). A balanced 15q inversion that causes AS when transmitted maternally has a breakpoint within intron 1 of *UBE3A* (Kishino et al., 1997). To date, almost 60 distinct point mutations of *UBE3A* have been identified (Fig. 81–2). Maternal transmission of *UBE3A* mutations causes AS; paternal transmission has no detectable phenotypic effect (see Fig. 81–3 for a representative pedigree). This unusual behavior is the result of brain-specific imprinting of *UBE3A* (Albrecht et al., 1997; Rougeulle et al., 1997; Vu and Hoffman, 1997; Jiang et al., 1998): the maternal allele of *UBE3A* is transcribed at a much higher level in brain than is the paternal allele, with the consequence that only mutations of the maternal allele of *UBE3A* or deletions of maternal 15q11–q13 lead to significant brain deficiency of UBE3A protein.

Among the *UBE3A* mutations shown in Fig. 81–2, 63% are frameshifts, 14% are nonsense mutations, 10% are missense mutations, 9% are in-frame additions or deletions, 3% are splice site mutations, and one mutation deletes the stop codon and is predicted to cause an elongated protein. Exon 9 mutations account for 45% of the point mutations in Fig. 81–2, a higher frequency than for any other single exon; however, this frequency of mutations is not dispropor-

tionate to exon size, because exon 9 constitutes 49% of the *UBE3A* coding region. Exons 15 and 16, by contrast, contain 29% of the point mutations, whereas they only constitute 10% of the *UBE3A* coding region. Although exons 15 and 16 encode part of the HECT domain that includes the catalytic cysteine of UBE3A, it is unlikely that the higher-than-expected frequency of mutations in this region is related to its functional importance; the frequency of chain-terminating mutations (frameshifts and nonsense mutations) among exon 15 and 16 mutations is 61%, which is not significantly different from the frequency within the gene as a whole. More likely, DNA sequence features of these exons contribute to the higher-than-expected mutation frequency.

Most *UBE3A* mutations in unrelated AS individuals are unique; among the 58 point mutations shown in Figure 81–2, 50 have been reported in only one individual or pedigree; 6 have been reported twice; 1 has been reported three times; and 1 has been reported in four AS individuals.

A third major cause of AS is "imprinting defects," which are found in 3% to 5% of AS individuals. This category has been referred to in some earlier publications as "imprinting mutations." AS imprinting-defect individuals show abnormal cytosine methylation at several diagnostic sites in the AS/PWS region without having either typical ~4 Mb maternal deletions in 15q11–q13 or paternal UPD 15. Normal human somatic cell DNA is cytosine-methylated on the maternal copy of the *SNRPN* promoter region, with almost complete lack of cytosine methylation on the paternal copy of the same region (Sutcliffe et al., 1994; Glenn et al., 1996); similar maternal-specific cytosine methylation is present at locus *D15S63* (Dittrich et al., 1993) and at the promoters of the *NDN* (Jay et al., 1997) and *ZNF127* (Driscoll et al., 1992) loci. In imprinting-defect AS individuals, the maternal copies of these regions lack cytosine methylation, as do the paternal copies (Buiting et al., 1998). Therefore, it is believed that both the maternal and paternal *UBE3A* alleles in these individuals have the paternal pattern of expression (i.e., hypoactive) in brain cells. A major step in understanding the mechanistic basis of imprinting defects came with the description in 1995 of small deletions >20 kb upstream of the *SNRPN* promoter in two families with AS imprinting defects (Buiting et al., 1995). Since that time, seven additional deletions have been described in patients with AS imprinting defects (Buiting et al., 1999; Ohta et al., 1999), and these deletions define an 880 bp smallest region of overlap (SRO) ~35 kb upstream of *SNRPN*, referred to as the AS-IC (Fig. 81–4). The relationship between these deletions and AS imprinting defects is intriguing: only ~20% of AS imprinting defect patients have AS-IC deletions (Buiting et al., 1999), and in the remaining ~80%, sequencing of the AS-IC has shown no evidence of point mutation or other sequence alteration.

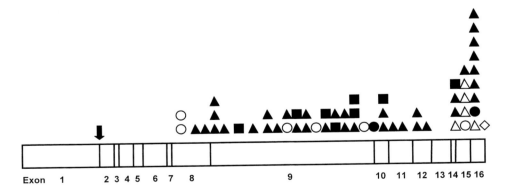

Exon   1   2 3 4 5 6 7 8   9   10 11 12 13 14 15 16

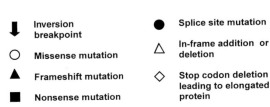

Figure 81–2. *UBE3A* mutations in individuals with Angelman syndrome. Mutations shown are from published sources (Kishino et al., 1997; Fung et al., 1998; Malzac et al., 1998; Baumer et al., 1999; Fang et al., 1999; Russo et al., 2000; Lossie et al., 2001), as well as unpublished mutations from the author's laboratory. Each symbol represents a unique mutation; repeated occurrences of the same mutation are not shown.

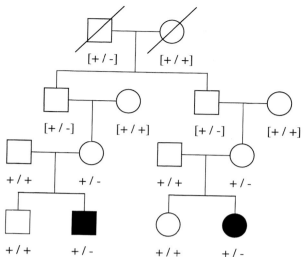

Figure 81–3. Pedigree of family in which two second cousins are affected by Angelman syndrome caused by the same *UBE3A* frameshift mutation (Malzac et al., 1998). The AS phenotype is shown by the filled symbols. Genotypes are either heterozygous for the *UBE3A* mutation (+/−) or homozygous wild type (+/+). Genotypes of the grandparents and great grandparents are inferred and are enclosed by brackets. Paternal transmission of the *UBE3A* mutation from the grandfathers, who are brothers, to their daughters, has no phenotypic effect; maternal transmission of the mutation causes AS.

all polymorphic genetic loci), and paternal UPD 15 is associated with both advanced maternal age and advanced paternal age (Robinson et al., 2000). One hypothesis consistent with both the high frequency of isodisomy in paternal UPD 15 and the advanced maternal age is that these individuals arise from fertilization of a chromosome 15 nullisomic egg by a normal sperm; the resulting zygote will be monosomic for chromosome 15, and there will be strong selection for duplication of the single paternal chromosome 15, yielding paternal isodisomy for chromosome 15. A small fraction of paternal UPD 15 individuals have two distinct paternal copies of chromosome 15, presumably as a result of a paternal meiotic error followed by loss of the maternal chromosome 15 during early development.

Between 10% and 20% of individuals with a clinical diagnosis of AS show no evidence of large deletions, *UBE3A* mutation, imprinting defect, or UPD. Whether these individuals actually show defective UBE3A enzyme activity in brain cells, which is inferred to be the common pathogenetic feature of the known etiologic categories of AS, is unknown. Some of these individuals may have distinct disorders that mimic AS phenotypically, while some may have genetic or epigenetic abnormalities of *UBE3A* that are not detected by current clinical laboratory tests (i.e., single-exon or multiexon deletions of *UBE3A*, *UBE3A* promoter mutations, or imprinting defects limited to *UBE3A*).

Genotype/Phenotype Correlations in AS

AS individuals with large deletions, *UBE3A* mutations, imprinting defects, and UPD share certain clinical features that lead to clinical suspicion of AS and subsequent laboratory confirmation. However, severity of the clinical features of AS shows some correlation with etiologic category. Many individuals with large-deletion AS show hypopigmentation (compared to familial background) of skin, hair, and eyes, which is much rarer in other categories of AS; this hypopigmentation is thought to reflect heterozygous deletion of the *OCA2* (*p*) locus, which is homozygously mutated in type II oculocutaneous albinism. Several reports have shown that both imprinting defect and UPD AS individuals, on average, show less severe motor and speech delay, as well as a lower incidence of microcephaly and severe seizures, than do individuals with large-deletion AS (Moncla et al., 1999; Lossie et al., 2001). *UBE3A* mutation individuals tend to show phenotypic severity intermediate between the severe large-deletion phenotype and the milder imprinting defect/UPD phenotype. For instance, Lossie et al. (2001) showed that the incidence of significant seizures (grand mal seizures requiring administration of at least one anticonvulsant) was 90% in the large-deletion group, 53% in the *UBE3A* mutation group, and 14% in both the imprinting-defect and UPD groups. There is significant phenotypic variability within each etiologic category, so that for most quantifiable features, there is substantial overlap between the ranges for the four etiologic categories.

A simple model to explain the genotype–phenotype correlations in AS posits that the clinically recognizable AS phenotype is produced by absence of a *UBE3A* allele with the high level of expression in brain cells that is characteristic of a normal maternal allele. Therefore, an individual with a maternally transmitted *UBE3A* mutation would

Many of the deletion-positive imprinting defects show familial recurrence: maternal transmission of these AS-IC deletions causes AS, while paternal transmission has no phenotypic effect. On the other hand, recurrence has never been reported in families with a deletion-negative AS imprinting defect patient. These observations have led to the proposal that deletion-negative AS imprinting defects result from a random, low-probability failure to establish the maternal imprint on a genetically normal maternal chromosome 15, whereas a chromosome with a deleted AS-IC is blocked from establishing the maternal imprint for the AS/PWS region after maternal transmission, but can establish the paternal imprint normally after paternal transmission (Buiting et al., 1998). The mechanism by which the AS-IC regulates either imprint establishment or maintenance (or both) over the ~2 Mb region in 15q11–q13 that contains imprinted genes is not known. The AS-IC contains upstream exon 5 of *SNRPN* (exon U5) (Buiting et al., 1999), which is present in a small fraction of somatic *SNRPN* transcripts; the significance of this observation is not clear.

The fourth main etiology of AS is paternal uniparental disomy (UPD) of chromosome 15, observed in 2% to 3% of AS individuals. As with large-deletion AS, AS individuals with paternal UPD 15 lack a maternal copy of 15q11–q13; unlike large-deletion AS, these individuals have two paternal copies of 15q11–q13. Most paternal UPD 15 is isodisomy (i.e., the two paternal chromosomes are identical for

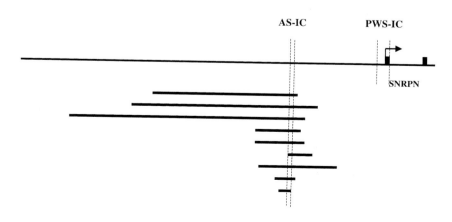

Figure 81–4. Imprinting-defect deletions and the region of deletion overlap in Angelman syndrome. Schematic, not drawn to scale, adapted from Buiting et al. (1999) and Ohta et al. (1999), shows that the overlap of nine AS imprinting-defect deletions defines an 880 bp region of deletion overlap, designated here as AS-IC. This region lies ~35 kb centromeric from the major promoter of *SNRPN*, which lies within the Prader-Willi syndrome imprinting center (PWS-IC).

have the core AS phenotype. This phenotype can be modified by other genetic abnormalities found in the other etiologic categories. Individuals with large deletions lack maternal copies of at least 10 genes in addition to *UBE3A* (Nicholls et al., 1998); some of these genes are expressed exclusively from the paternal chromosome (e.g., *SNRPN*), so their deletion should be inconsequential. Others are expressed from both chromosomes, and the effects of heterozygous deletion of those genes may interact with the effects of lack of a maternal *UBE3A* allele in brain cells to exacerbate the phenotype. Large AS deletions include a cluster of three GABA$_A$-receptor subunit genes, and deletion of one of these, *GABRB3*, has been proposed as a modifying factor that increases the severity of deletion AS compared to *UBE3A* mutation AS (Minassian et al., 1998). In contrast, AS individuals with imprinting defects or UPD, while lacking a 15q11–q13 region that functions as a normal maternal region, have an extra copy of a functionally paternal region. Studies of *UBE3A* expression in mouse and human brains have shown that, while the paternal allele is hypoactive compared to the maternal allele, it does have some transcriptional activity (Albrecht et al., 1997; Rougeulle et al., 1997; Vu and Hoffman, 1997), which is variable in different brain regions. The presence of a hypoactive paternal *UBE3A* allele may therefore act as a positive modifier, reducing the severity of the imprinting defect and UPD phenotypes. It should be noted that there is no evidence that extra copies of active paternal alleles of imprinted 15q11–q13 genes such as *SNRPN* have any deleterious effect on the phenotype of imprinting defect and UPD AS individuals.

Within the *UBE3A* mutation category, no studies have been reported that show correlations between mutation type or location and phenotypic severity. Also, there have been no reports correlating enzymatic activity of mutant UBE3A proteins with phenotype. Nawaz et al. (1999) determined both ubiquitin-protein ligase activity (with HHR23A as substrate) and transcriptional coactivator activity of five UBE3A proteins with mutations found in AS individuals. All five mutant proteins showed normal coactivation activity, but four of the mutant proteins showed absent or severely decreased ubiquitin-protein ligase activity. (One mutant protein, I804K, showed normal activity in both assays.) Their results indicate that the AS phenotype is almost certainly due to lack of the ubiquitin-protein ligase activity of UBE3A, rather than the transcriptional coactivator function.

ESTABLISHING THE DIAGNOSIS

Clinical suspicion of AS is based on the presence of characteristic neurological and developmental problems, as well as typical features of easily provoked laughter and smiling. A guide to clinical diagnosis of AS was published in 1995 (Table 81–1) (Williams et al., 1995a). No clinical scoring system has been devised that is able to distinguish AS from non-AS individuals reliably. Until laboratory diagnostic testing reveals a molecular abnormality in the 10% to 20% of individuals who appear clinically to have AS but have no correlated laboratory testing abnormality, the clinical diagnosis of AS will continue to have aspects of art as well as science.

Laboratory testing for AS usually involves conventional G-banded chromosome analysis followed by either FISH or methylation testing, or both (Table 81–2). Probes from 15q11–q13 commonly used for AS FISH contain either locus *D15S10* (very close to *UBE3A*) or *SNRPN* (>500 kb proximal to UBE3A). Almost all AS deletions include both of these loci, so probes for these two loci are equally sensitive in deletion detection. Commercially available probes for these loci are often combined with a probe for distal 15q to identify chromosome 15, and

Table 81–1. Clinical Diagnostic Criteria in Angelman Syndrome

Consistent features (100%)
  Developmental delay, functionally severe
  Speech impairment, none or minimal use of words; receptive and nonverbal communication skills higher than verbal ones
  Movement or balance disorder, usually ataxia of gait and/or tremulous movement of limbs
  Behavioral uniqueness: any combination of frequent laughter/smiling; apparent happy demeanor; easily excitable personality, often with hand flapping movements; hypermotoric behavior; short attention span
Frequent features (more than 80%)
  Delayed growth in head circumference, sometimes resulting in microcephaly by age 2
  Seizures, onset <3 years of age
  Abnormal EEG, characteristic pattern with large amplitude slow-spike waves (usually 2–3/sec), facilitated by eye closure
Associated features (20%–80%)
  Flat occiput
  Occipital groove
  Protruding tongue
  Tongue thrusting; suck/swallowing disorders
  Feeding problems during infancy
  Prognathism
  Wide mouth, widely spaced teeth
  Frequent drooling
  Excessive chewing/mouthing behaviors
  Strabismus
  Hypopigmented skin, light hair and eye color (compared to family)
  Hyperactive lower limb deep tendon reflexes
  Uplifted, flexed arm position, especially during ambulation
  Increased sensitivity to heat
  Sleep disturbance
  Attraction to or fascination with water

Source: Williams et al., 1995a.

with a chromosome 15–specific α-satellite probe to detect rare cryptic translocations involving chromosome 15 and another acrocentric chromosome.

Two probes have been widely used for methylation analysis in AS: a probe from the *SNRPN* promoter region (Glenn et al., 1996), and a probe from the *D15S63* locus (Dittrich et al., 1993). Either of these probes can be hybridized to Southern blots of DNA digested with a methylation-sensitive restriction enzyme to determine whether a methylated (maternal) or nonmethylated (paternal) copy of the region is present. Kubota et al. (1996) have shown that *D15S63* is normally methylated in lymphocyte DNA but not in amniocytes or chorionic villi, while *SNRPN* is normally methylated in both prenatal tissues and can therefore be used for prenatal diagnostic testing. Several groups (Kubota et al., 1997; Zeschnigk et al., 1997) have also described methylation-specific PCR assays for sodium bisulfite–treated DNA that can be used to determine the presence of DNA with either the maternal or paternal methylation pattern at the *SNRPN* locus.

The sensitivity of FISH in AS is approximately 70%, while the sensitivity of methylation testing is approximately 75%. Although this might appear to favor methylation analysis as the initial test for AS, a positive FISH test establishes both the diagnosis and the etiologic category (deletion) with a single test, while a positive (i.e., paternal-only) methylation test may be found in an AS individual with either deletion, imprinting defect, or UPD. Presence of hypopigmentation relative to family background in an AS individual increases the likelihood of a deletion, so FISH may be the most reasonable first test in this situation. If an individual has a positive FISH test and a clinical

Table 81–2. Genetic Etiologies and Diagnostic Test Results in Angelman Syndrome

Etiologic Category	Occurrence (% of AS)	Recurrence Risk (%)	FISH	Methylation	Polymorphism Analysis	*UBE3A* Mutation Analysis
Deletion	70	<1	Deletion	Paternal only		
UBE3A mutation	5–10	<1–50	No deletion	Biparental	Biparental	Mutation present
Imprinting defect	3–5	<1–50	No deletion	Paternal only	Biparental	
Paternal UPD	2–3	<1	No deletion	Paternal only	Paternal only	

picture consistent with AS, then the diagnosis of deletion AS is almost certain. If there is a negative FISH test and a positive methylation test, then the individual may have either an imprinting defect or paternal UPD 15. The possibility of paternal UPD is usually tested by analysis of several microsatellite loci on 15q, both within the AS-deletion region and outside, in DNA from the AS individual and both parents; lack of a maternal contribution for one or more loci outside of the AS-deletion region establishes the diagnosis of UPD. If UPD is not present, with negative FISH testing and paternal-only methylation testing, the individual is then categorized as having an imprinting defect. Testing for small deletions near *SNRPN* in imprinting-defect individuals is not available on a clinical basis but is available through a small number of research laboratories.

If methylation testing (with or without FISH) is negative and the clinical suspicion of AS is high, the next step in diagnostic evaluation is *UBE3A* mutation analysis. Clinical UBE3A mutation analysis in most cases is based on genomic DNA and is restricted to the coding exons (7–16) of *UBE3A*. Several strategies have been used for *UBE3A* mutation analysis, including direct sequencing, single-strand conformation polymorphism (SSCP) analysis, and denaturing high-performance liquid chromatography (DHPLC) analysis. The incidence of *UBE3A* mutations among individuals with a clinical diagnosis of AS, negative methylation analysis, and negative FISH, has ranged from 5% to 50% (Malzac et al., 1998; Baumer et al., 1999; Fang et al., 1999) and clearly reflects differing criteria for clinical diagnosis in different centers. All studies have noted that the frequency of *UBE3A* mutations in familial cases is higher than that in sporadic cases. It is important for those performing and interpreting *UBE3A* mutation results to note the presence of two highly conserved processed pseudogenes of *UBE3A* on chromosomes 2 and 21 (Kishino and Wagstaff, 1998), which may be amplified by some exon primers.

MANAGEMENT AND COUNSELING

Counseling regarding recurrence risk of deletion AS is straightforward: only one instance of familial recurrence of deletion AS has been reported (Kokkonen and Leisti, 2000), and the recurrence risk is generally thought to be less than 1%. In spite of this very low recurrence risk, many couples choose to have prenatal diagnosis by FISH for reassurance after the birth of a previous child with deletion AS. Standard prenatal cytogenetic analysis is generally not sufficiently sensitive to detect AS deletions. As with deletion AS, AS caused by UPD usually has a low recurrence risk. There has been only one report of AS UPD in the offspring of a father with a Robertsonian translocation involving chromosome 15 (Zackai et al., 1995); such a paternal chromosome translocation might cause an increased recurrence risk.

Counseling after having a child with an imprinting defect is more complex. Counseling in these cases is facilitated by determination of AS-IC deletion status, which is currently performed only in a small number of laboratories. If an AS child has an IC deletion, then parental DNA should be tested for the deletion. If the mother is heterozygous for the same IC deletion present in the child, then the risk of recurrence of AS in subsequent children of the mother is 50% (regardless of the father's genetic contribution). Prenatal diagnosis in such cases could be performed either by methylation testing using the *SNRPN* probe or by direct DNA analysis of the IC deletion. If the mother is not detectably heterozygous or mosaic for the same IC deletion as the child, then the risk of AS in a subsequent child is significantly less than 50%. However, the possibility of undetected mosaicism in the mother, possibly limited to the germ line, makes it worthwhile to consider prenatal methylation analysis or IC deletion DNA analysis in these cases. If an AS child with imprinting defect has no detectable AS-IC deletion, the recurrence risk of AS in subsequent pregnancies appears to be much lower than 50% (Buiting et al., 1998); in fact, no recurrences have been reported in families with IC-deletion negative-imprinting defects. However, the numbers of patients studied so far is small, and it is probably worth discussing the possibility of prenatal methylation analysis with parents in these circumstances.

Counseling after detection of a *UBE3A* mutation in a child with AS requires testing of the mother to determine whether the mutation was inherited or occurred de novo. If the mother is heterozygous for the mutation, then the risk of AS in each of her subsequent pregnancies will be 50%. Testing of the mother's parents and siblings is advisable under these circumstances. Direct detection of the mutation can be performed for prenatal diagnosis. If the mother is not heterozygous for the mutation, the mutation is probably a de novo occurrence with a low risk of recurrence. However, several clinically normal mothers of *UBE3A*-mutation AS children have shown low-level mosaicism for the child's *UBE3A* mutation in lymphocyte DNA (Malzac et al., 1998), so that lack of clear evidence that the mother is a heterozygote does not necessarily imply a near-zero recurrence risk.

A difficult counseling situation arises when a child whose clinical phenotype is consistent with AS shows no abnormality in FISH, methylation, or *UBE3A* mutation testing (Stalker and Williams, 1998). We and others have found familial AS cases in which all diagnostic testing is negative, so that the chance of recurrence in the situation of negative testing is clearly appreciable. A first step in this situation is to review the clinical findings in the child to determine if another diagnosis, such as Rett syndrome, ATR-X (see Chapter 72), or chromosome 22q distal deletion, might be compatible with the clinical phenotype (Williams et al., 2001). If the phenotype is clearly that of AS, one possible avenue to prenatal diagnosis, based on the assumption that the AS child has a genetic lesion in the vicinity of *UBE3A* that has not been detected, is haplotype analysis. The affected child, mother, father, and siblings can be tested for polymorphic microsatellite markers in the AS deletion region, including markers that flank *UBE3A*. The AS child's maternal haplotype is then provisionally the AS haplotype. If there are unaffected siblings who have inherited the other maternal haplotype, this would be consistent with the hypothesis that the mother is heterozygous for an AS mutation in the region. If unaffected siblings share the maternal haplotype with the AS child, this indicates that either (*1*) the AS mutation has occurred de novo in the child or is mosaic in the mother or (*2*) the child's AS phenotype is not caused by a sequence alteration in the AS deletion region.

Prenatal diagnosis based on haplotyping could be carried out if the AS child's maternal haplotype is not present in any unaffected siblings. However, there are numerous possible pitfalls to this approach, including misidentification of a normal fetus as affected if the mother is not a mutation heterozygote, as well as misidentification of an affected fetus as normal if the AS child's phenotype is not caused by sequence alteration in 15q11–q13. We have studied a family with six children, three of whom have AS, that illustrates the complexities of haplotype analysis in this condition. Two of the three AS children have the same maternal haplotype, and the third has a crossover within the AS region; two of the unaffected children have the opposite maternal haplotype from the two AS children, but one unaffected child has the same maternal haplotype as the two AS children. This puzzling situation was clarified when it was found that the three AS children have the same *UBE3A* missense mutation, and their mother is a low-level mosaic for the same mutation, so that she can transmit either the normal or the mutant allele on the same haplotype (Malzac et al., 1998).

Management of AS usually involves a team of caregivers, including the primary physician, clinical geneticist, neurologist, teachers, and therapists. Major goals of management in AS should be optimization of function, enhancement of communication, prevention of morbidity due to seizures or injury, and support of parents who are often dealing with very severe behavioral problems and sleep disorders in their AS children. Major medical issues in AS include the following:

1. *Seizure disorder.* Most AS individuals have seizures at some time during their lives, and almost all seizure types can be seen. The age of onset of AS seizures is usually before 3 years, and a typical EEG pattern is seen in some AS individuals (Boyd et al., 1988). The most commonly used medications for AS seizures are valproic acid and clonazepam (Williams et al., 1995b), although some AS patients are successfully treated with other medications such as ethosuximide and topiramate. There are some reports of exacerbation of AS seizures by carbamazepine and vigabatrin (Kuenzle et al., 1998; Ruggieri and McShane, 1998).

2. *Sleep disorder.* Sleep disturbance is another common finding in AS individuals. The relationship between sleep disorder and seizure disorder is not clear: many parents report that their AS child's sleep disorder began at the same time as her seizure disorder, and parents also often report that long periods of sleep disturbance appear to precede periods of seizure activity. Sleep problems in the AS child often lead to sleep problems for the entire family, with consequent disruption of family relationships, school, and work. Medications that have been used to treat AS sleep disorder include diphenhydramine, clonidine, chloral hydrate, clonazepam, and melatonin.

3. *Feeding problems.* Feeding problems—involving tongue thrusting, incoordination of sucking and swallowing, and gastroesophageal reflux—are common in infants with AS but tend to improve with age. If such problems persist and are associated with poor weight gain, consultation with a pediatric gastroenterologist is recommended. Occasional AS children have sufficiently severe gastroesophageal reflux to require gastrostomy with fundoplication.

4. *Scoliosis.* Scoliosis occurs in some adolescents with AS, especially in those who are nonambulatory. This may require bracing or surgical correction.

Often the major nonmedical concern of parents of AS children is communication therapy for their nonverbal child. Because of the variability in cognitive levels and communication skills among AS individuals, some of which is correlated with diagnostic category, communication therapy must be tailored to individual strengths and weaknesses. For most AS children, speech is unlikely ever to progress past one or two words, so nonverbal means of communication should be emphasized. These means may involve photograph displays for choosing, or more stylized symbol displays; some individuals with AS are able to use sign language. Receptive language skills should also be an emphasis of communication therapy.

Most children with AS eventually become ambulatory, and because of their high activity level, muscle strength, curiosity, and fascination with water, they are at high risk of injuring themselves. Most of these children require constant supervision, and many parents have designed "safe rooms" for their AS child to sleep in or to play in without supervision. However, some AS children have injured themselves severely in supposedly "safe" rooms, so that parents need to be cautious about any unsupervised activity of their AS child.

Families with AS children often are coping with severe sleep problems in the child and in the rest of the family, along with severe behavioral problems in the AS child and with medical issues such as seizure control and feeding difficulties. Many parents who have found it difficult to face these situations in isolation have found significant benefit from AS parent support groups, including the Angelman Syndrome Foundation (ASF) (http://www.angelman.org) in the United States and the International Angelman Syndrome Organization (IASO) (http://www.asclepius.com/iaso). These organizations have helped AS parents make contact with other AS parents through online listservs and through regional meetings, as well as to bring families into contact with professionals who have expertise in medical and developmental issues of AS individuals.

MUTATIONS IN ANIMAL MODELS

Targeted mutations of *Ube3a* have been produced in two mouse models. The first mouse knockout was reported by Jiang et al. (1998), and was constructed by replacing exon 2 (homologous to human exon 8) with a Neo^R cassette. Mice that inherited the mutant allele either maternally or paternally were viable, as were homozygotes, although their viability was reduced compared to heterozygotes. Maternal allele–deficient mice, but not paternal allele–deficient mice, were shown to have defects in motor coordination and in context-dependent fear conditioning. Maternal allele–deficient mice also had defective hippocampal long-term potentiation and showed audiogenic seizure activity that was modulated by genetic background. Jiang et al. presented evidence for increased levels of cytoplasmic p53 in Purkinje cells and in hippocampal neurons of maternal allele–deficient mice, compared to wild-type controls.

Miura et al. (2002) produced a different knockout mouse model, with deletion of the portion of *Ube3a* encoding the C-terminal 87 amino acids, including the catalytic cysteine; this deleted region was replaced by an internal ribosome entry site linked to a Neo^R-lacZ fusion protein, so that transcription of the knockout allele leads to β-galactosidase expression. Mice that inherited this knockout allele maternally showed motor deficits and context-dependent fear conditioning deficits similar to those observed by Jiang et al.; they also were defective in the hidden-platform phase of the Morris water maze task, which tests hippocampal function. None of the mice showed spontaneous motor seizures, but most of the maternal allele–deficient mice showed hippocampal EEG abnormalities with episodes of high-amplitude spikes (two to four per second), accompanied by lack of movement. The EEG abnormalities resolved quickly after administration of either valproic acid or ethosuximide. These maternal allele–deficient mice showed no evidence of increased p53 levels in either the cerebellum or the hippocampus. LacZ staining showed maternal-specific expression in many cortical regions including the hippocampus, with biparental expression in the choroid plexus. There was also maternal-specific lacZ staining in cerebellar cells near the Purkinje cell layer, but not in the Purkinje cells themselves.

Both of these maternal *Ube3a*–deficient mouse models mimic some important aspects of AS, including motor abnormalities, learning deficits, and EEG abnormalities. Neither mouse model shows any detectable structural abnormality of brain cells, although in both models, maternal *Ube3a*–deficient mice have reduced brain size postnatally. The differences between the two models in some aspects, such as presence of spontaneous motor seizures and accumulation of p53 in neurons, may be due to different strain backgrounds or to differences between the gene targeting strategies employed.

DEVELOPMENTAL PATHOGENESIS

AS is caused by lack of a functional maternal allele of *UBE3A*, which encodes a ubiquitin-protein ligase. The two major questions to be answered about the developmental pathogenesis of AS are, first, what are the mechanisms that lead to brain-specific partial silencing of the paternal allele of *UBE3A* and activation of the maternal allele, and, second, how does deficiency of the UBE3A ubiquitin-protein ligase protein in brain cells, caused by lack of a maternal *UBE3A* allele, cause the clinical manifestations that we recognize as AS?

Evidence for brain-specific imprinting of *UBE3A* has come from in situ hybridization to brains of mice lacking maternal *Ube3a* alleles (Albrecht et al., 1997; Jiang et al., 1998) and from RNA analysis of brain tissue from AS-deletion individuals (Rougeulle et al., 1997). Albrecht et al. (1997) used mice with paternal UPD for the region of chromosome 7 containing *Ube3a* to demonstrate that the maternal allele of *Ube3a* is expressed preferentially in hippocampal neurons and Purkinje cells. Jiang et al. (1998) tested expression in *Ube3a* maternal-knockout and paternal-knockout mice by in situ hybridization; they found absence of detectable expression of *Ube3a* from the paternal allele in Purkinje cells and hippocampal neurons; however, in some brain regions, such as pyriform cortex, they found equal expression of maternal and paternal alleles of *Ube3a*. Rougeulle et al. (1998) analyzed postmortem samples of frontal cortex from AS deletion, PWS deletion, and control individuals and showed that deletion of the maternal *UBE3A* allele reduced *UBE3A* expression to approximately 10% of control levels.

Understanding brain-specific imprinting of *UBE3A* will require an understanding of the mechanisms that regulate imprinted gene expression in 15q11–q13. We know that establishment of the maternal pattern of gene expression in the AS/PWS region requires the AS-IC, located ~35 kb proximal to *SNRPN* and >500 kb proximal to *UBE3A*, unless the PWS-IC, which overlaps the *SNRPN* promoter, is absent. The molecular function of the AS-IC is not known, other than the fact that it contains upstream exon U5 of *SNRPN*. The maternal pattern of gene expression is correlated with cytosine methylation of the PWS-IC, which is unmethylated on the paternal chromosome. It is clear in humans that this PWS-IC cytosine methylation is not the gametic imprint for the AS/PWS region, because (in contrast to mouse) this region is not cytosine-methylated in human oocytes (El-Maarri et al.,

2001). Brannan and Bartolomei (1999) have proposed that the function of the AS-IC is to prevent establishment of the paternal pattern of gene expression, which depends on the PWS-IC. Evidence for paternal-specific transcription in the antisense orientation to *UBE3A* has been presented in humans (Rougeulle et al., 1998; Runte et al., 2001) and mouse (Chamberlain and Brannan, 2001). Runte et al. (2001) have shown evidence for paternal-specific transcription spanning the >500 kb between the PWS-IC and *UBE3A*, in antisense orientation to *UBE3A*. They have hypothesized that this transcript may function to repress *UBE3A* sense-strand expression from the paternal allele. However, it is still not clear whether there is a cause-and-effect relationship between the antisense transcript and repression of *UBE3A* expression, and it is not clear if there is a continuous antisense transcript extending from the PWS-IC to *UBE3A*.

Other possible long-range mechanisms by which the AS-IC and/or PWS-IC may interact with *UBE3A* include chromatin looping, sliding of one or more proteins along the chromosome, or spreading of protein complexes from a nucleation site, such as the AS-IC, to the target, in this case *UBE3A*. No parent-specific epigenetic modifications of the *UBE3A* promoter region have been reported; Lossie et al. (2001) have examined cytosine methylation of this region in human lymphocyte, brain, and germ cell DNA and have found no evidence of differential cytosine methylation between maternal and paternal alleles. We (T. Kishino and J. Wagstaff, unpublished data) have found similar lack of differential methylation in human lymphocyte DNA and mouse brain DNA; we also have found no evidence for parent-specific differential histone acetylation or differential histone methylation near the *UBE3A* promoter in human lymphocyte chromatin.

Mutation or absence of the maternal allele of *UBE3A* results in deficiency, but not complete absence, of UBE3A protein in brain, due to silencing of the paternal allele. How deficiency of UBE3A protein in brain leads to the clinical manifestations of AS is as poorly understood as the mechanism of brain-specific imprinting. We know of three substrates for UBE3A-mediated ubiquitin-protein ligase activity: p53, which is an E6-dependent substrate, and HHR23A/HHR23B, as well as active BLK kinase, which are E6-independent substrates. The p53 protein is unlikely to play a role in pathogenesis of AS, because all in vitro and in vivo data (other than the results of Jiang et al., 1998) indicate that p53 is a UBE3A substrate only in the presence of E6 protein from high-risk HPVs. HHR23A and HHR23B are E6-independent substrates. Kumar et al. (1999) found that these proteins undergo UBE3A-dependent degradation only during S phase, so it is unlikely that levels of this protein would be significantly altered in postmitotic neurons. However, there have been no published reports of the abundance of HHR23A or HHR23B in AS or *Ube3a*$^{m-/p+}$ brains, so the possibility of an involvement of these proteins in AS pathogenesis cannot be excluded. Finally, BLK is a B-lymphocyte-specific protein and therefore it probably is not involved in AS pathogenesis.

A major goal for future AS research will be to identify additional UBE3A substrates and to devise methods to assess the roles of these substrates in AS pathogenesis. Although most investigators have assumed that ubiquitination of proteins by UBE3A always targets them for proteolysis, it is worth bearing in mind that some ubiquitinations serve to alter protein function, without altering protein stability (Finley, 2001). Therefore, protocols that screen for accumulated proteins in AS (or AS mouse model) brains may miss important substrates. Previous screening for UBE3A substrates has primarily involved two-hybrid hunts for proteins that interact with catalytically inactivated UBE3A mutants; future directions may involve direct screening of in vitro translated proteins or protein pools for modification by UBE3A. After additional substrates have been identified, assessment of their roles in AS will involve measurement of protein levels in AS vs. wild-type brains and determination of the effects of ubiquitination on substrate function and stability. An important functional assay for roles of a candidate substrate in AS pathogenesis will be to introduce a form of the protein that is resistant to UBE3A modification into transgenic mice, and to assay the mice for aspects of the AS mouse phenotype.

ACKNOWLEDGMENTS

I would like to thank Carolyn Ohle for valuable comments on the manuscript.

REFERENCES

Albrecht U, Sutcliffe JS, Cattanach BM, Beechey CV, Armstrong D, Eichele G, Beaudet AL (1997). Imprinted expression of the murine Angelman syndrome gene, Ube3a, in hippocampal and Purkinje neurons. *Nat Genet* 17: 75–78.

Angelman H (1965). "Puppet" children: a report on three cases. *Dev Med Child Neurol* 7: 681–688.

Baumer A, Balmer D, Schinzel A (1999). Screening for UBE3A mutations in a group of Angelman syndrome patients selected according to non-stringent clinical criteria. *Hum Genet* 105: 598–602.

Boyd S, Harden A, Patton M (1988). The EEG in early diagnosis of the Angelman (happy puppet) syndrome. *Eur J Pediatr* 147: 508–513.

Brannan CI, Bartolomei MS (1999). Mechanisms of genomic imprinting. *Curr Opinion Genet Devel* 9: 164–170.

Buiting K, Saitoh S, Gross S, Dittrich B, Schwartz S, Nicholls RD, Horsthemke B (1995). Inherited microdeletions in the Angelman and Prader-Willi syndromes define an imprinting centre on human chromosome 15. *Nat Genet* 9: 395–400.

Buiting K, Dittrich B, Gross S, Lich C, Farber C, Buchholz T, Smith E, Reis A, Burger J, Nothen MM, et al. (1998). Sporadic imprinting defects in Prader-Willi syndrome and Angelman syndrome: implications for imprint-switch models, genetic counseling, and prenatal diagnosis. *Am J Hum Genet* 63: 170–180.

Buiting K, Lich C, Cottrell S, Barnicoat A, Horsthemke B (1999). A 5-kb imprinting center deletion in a family with Angelman syndrome reduces the shortest region of deletion overlap to 880 bp. *Hum Genet* 105: 665–666.

Chamberlain S, Brannan CI (2001). The Prader-Willi syndrome imprinting center activates the paternally expressed murine Ube3a antisense transcript but represses paternal Ube3a. *Genomics* 73: 316–322.

Christian S, Bhatt N, Martin S, Sutcliffe J, Kubota T, Huang B, Mutirangura A, Chinault A, Beaudet AL, Ledbetter D (1998). Integrated YAC contig map of the Prader-Willi/Angelman region on chromosome 15q11–q13 with average STS spacing of 35 kb. *Genome Res* 8: 146–157.

Clayton-Smith J (1993). Clinical research on Angelman syndrome in the United Kingdom: observations on 82 affected individuals. *Am J Med Genet* 46: 12–15.

Delach J, Rosengren S, Kaplan L, Greenstein R, Cassidy S, Benn P (1994). Comparison of high resolution chromosome banding and fluorescence in situ hybridization (FISH) for the laboratory evaluation of Prader-Willi syndrome and Angelman syndrome. *Am J Med Genet* 52: 85–91.

Dittrich B, Buiting K, Gross S, Horsthemke B (1993). Characterization of a methylation imprint in the Prader-Willi syndrome chromosome region. *Hum Mol Genet* 2: 1995–1999.

Driscoll DJ, Waters M, Wiliams C, Zori R, Glenn C, Avidano K, Nicholls RD (1992). A DNA methylation imprint, determined by the sex of the parent, distinguishes the Angelman and Prader-Willi syndromes. *Genomics* 13: 917–924.

El-Maarri O, Buiting K, Peery E, Kroise P, Balaban B, Wagner K, Urman B, Heyd J, Lich C, Brannan C, et al. (2001). Methylation imprints on human chromosome 15 are established during or after fertilization. *Nat Genet* 27: 341–344.

Fang P, Lev-Lehman E, Tsai T-F, Matsuura T, Benton CS, Sutcliffe JS, Christian SL, Kubota T, Halley DJ, Meijers-Heijboer H, et al. (1999). The spectrum of mutations in UBE3A causing Angelman syndrome. *Hum Mol Genet* 8: 129–135.

Finley D (2001). Signal transduction: an alternative to destruction. *Nature* 412: 283–286.

Fung DCY, Yu B, Cheong KF, Smith A, Trent RJ (1998). UBE3A "mutations" in two unrelated and phenotypically different Angelman syndrome patients. *Hum Genet* 102: 487–492.

Glenn C, Saitoh S, Jong M, Filbrandt M, Surti U, Driscoll DJ, Nicholls RD (1996). Gene structure, DNA methylation, and imprinted expression of the human SNRPN gene. *Am J Hum Genet* 58: 335–346.

Huang L, Kinnucan E, Wang G, Beaudenon S, Howley PM, Huibregtse JM, Pavletich NP (1999). Structure of an E6AP-UbcH7 complex: insights into the ubiquitin-protein ligase/ubiquitin-conjugating enzyme cascade. *Science* 286: 1321–1326.

Huibregtse JM, Scheffner M, Howly PM (1991). A cellular protein mediates association of p53 with the E6 oncoprotein of human papillomavirus types 16 or 18. *EMBO J* 10: 4129–4135.

Huibregtse JM, Scheffner M, Howley PM (1993). Cloning and expression of the cDNA for E6-AP, a protein that mediates the interaction of the human papillomavirus E6 oncoprotein with p53. *Mol Cell Biol* 13: 775–784.

Huibregtse JM, Scheffner M, Beaudenon S, Howley PM (1995). A family of proteins structurally and functionally related to the E6-AP ubiquitin-protein ligase. *Proc Natl Acad Sci USA* 92: 2563–2567.

Jay P, Rougeulle C, Massacrier A, Moncla A, Mattei M-G, Malzac P, Roeckel N, Taviaux S, Lefranc J-L, Cau P, et al. (1997). The human necdin gene, NDN, is maternally imprinted and located in the Prader-Willi syndrome chromosomal region. *Nat Genet* 17: 357–361.

Jiang Y, Armstrong D, Albrecht U, Atkins CM, Noebels JL, Eichele G, Sweatt JD, Beaudet AL (1998). Mutation of the Angelman ubiquitin ligase in mice causes increased cytoplasmic p53 and deficits of contextual learning and long-term potentiation. *Neuron* 21: 799–811.

Kaplan L, Wharton R, Elias E, Mandell F, Donlon T, Latt S (1987). Cinical heterogeneity associated with deletions in the long arm of chromosome 15: report of three new cases and their possible genetic significance. *Am J Med Genet* 28: 45–53.

Kishino T, Wagstaff J (1998). Genomic organization of the UBE3A/E6-AP gene and related pseudogenes. *Genomics* 47: 101–107.

Kishino T, Lalande M, Wagstaff J (1997). UBE3A/E6-AP mutations cause Angelman syndrome. *Nat Genet* 15: 70–73.

Knoll JHM, Nicholls RD, Magenis RE, Graham JM Jr, Lalande M, Latt SA (1989). Angelman and Prader-Willi syndromes share a common chromosome 15 deletion but differ in parental origin of the deletion. *Am J Med Genet* 32: 285–290.

Kokkonen H, Leisti J (2000). An unexpected recurrence of Angelman syndrome suggestive of maternal germ-line mosaicism of del(15)(q11q13) in a Finnish family. *Hum Genet* 107: 83–85.

Kubota T, Aradhya S, Macha M, Smith A, Surh L, Satish J, Verp M, Nee H, Johnson A, Christian S, et al. (1996). Analysis of parent of origin specific DNA methylation at SNRPN and PW71 in tissues: implication for prenatal diagnosis. *J Med Genet* 33: 1011–1014.

Kubota T, Das S, Christian S, Baylin S, Herman J, Ledbetter D (1997). Methylation-specific PCR simplifies imprinting analysis. *Nat Genet* 16: 16–17.

Kuenzle C, Steinlin M, Wohlrab G, Boltshauser E, Schmitt, B (1998). Adverse effects of vigabatrin in Angelman syndrome. *Epilepsia* 39: 1213–1215.

Kumar S, Kao WH, Howley PM (1997). Physical interaction between specific E2 and Hect E3 enzymes determines functional cooperativity. *J Biol Chem* 272: 13548–13554.

Kumar S, Talis AL, Howley PM (1999). Identification of HHR23A as a substrate for E6-associated protein-mediated ubiquitination. *J Biol Chem* 274: 18785–18792.

Ledbetter DH, Ricciardi VM, Airhart SD, Strobel RJ, Keenan BS, Crawford JD (1981). Deletions of chromosome 15 as a cause of the Prader-Willi syndrome. *N Engl J Med* 304: 325–329.

Lossie A, Whitney M, Amidon D, Dong H, Chen P, Theriaque D, Hutson A, Nicholls R, Zori R, Wiliams C, et al. (2001). Distinct phenotypes distinguish the molecular classes of Angelman syndrome. *J Med Genet* 38: 834–845.

Magenis R, Brown M, Lacy D, Budden S, LaFranchi S (1987). Is Angelman syndrome an alternate result of del(15)(q11q13)? *Am J Med Genet* 28: 829–838.

Malzac P, Webber H, Moncla A, Graham JM Jr, Kukolich M, Williams C, Pagon RA, Ramsdell LA, Kishino T, Wagstaff J (1998). Mutation analysis of UBE3A in Angelman syndrome patients. *Am J Hum Genet* 62: 1353–1360.

Minassian B, DeLorey T, Olsen R, Philippart M, Bronstein Y, Zhang Q, Guerrini R, Van Ness P, Livet M, Delgado-Escueta AV (1998). Angelman syndrome: correlations between epilepsy phenotypes and genotypes. *Ann Neurol* 43: 485–493.

Miura K, Kishino T, Li E, Webber H, Dikkes P, Holmes G, Wagstaff J (2002). Neurobehavioral and electroencephalographic abnormalities in Ube3a maternal-deficient mice. *Neurobiol Dis* 9:149–159.

Moncla A, Malzac P, Voelckel M-A, Auquier P, Girardot L, Mattei M-G, Philip N, Mattei J-F, Lalande M, Livet M-O (1999). Phenotype-genotype correlation in 20 deletion and 20 non-deletion Angelman syndrome patients. *Eur J Hum Genet* 7: 131–139.

Nawaz Z, Lonard D, Smith C, Lev-Lehman E, Tsai S, Tsai M-J, O'Malley B (1999). The Angelman syndrome-associated protein, E6-AP, is a coactivator for the nuclear hormone receptor superfamily. *Mol Cell Biol* 19: 1182–1189.

Nicholls RD, Saitoh S, Horsthemke B (1998). Imprinting in Prader-Willi and Angelman syndromes. *Trends Genet* 14: 194–200.

Oda H, Kumar S, Howley PM (1999). Regulation of the Src family tyrosine kinase Blk through E6AP-mediated ubiquitination. *Proc Natl Acad Sci USA* 96: 9557–9562.

Ohta T, Buiting K, Kokkonen H, McCandless S, Heeger S, Leisti H, Driscoll DJ, Cassidy SB, Horsthemke B, Nicholls RD (1999). Molecular mechanism of Angelman syndrome in two large families involves an imprinting mutation. *Am J Hum Genet* 64: 385–396.

Robinson W, Christian S, Kuchinka B, Penaherrera M, Das S, Schuffenhauer S, Malcolm S, Schinzel A, Hassold T, Ledbetter D (2000). Somatic segregation errors predominantly contribute to the gain or loss of a paternal chromosome leading to uniparental disomy for chromosome 15. *Clin Genet* 57: 349–358.

Rougeulle C, Glatt H, Lalande M (1997). The Angelman syndrome candidate gene, UBE3A/E6-AP, is imprinted in brain. *Nat Genet* 17: 14–15.

Rougeulle C, Cardoso C, Fontes M, Colleaux L, Lalande M (1998). An imprinted antisense RNA overlaps UBE3A and a second maternally expressed transcript. *Nat Genet* 19: 15–16.

Ruggieri M, McShane M (1998). Parental view of epilepsy in Angelman syndrome: a questionnaire study. *Arch Dis Child* 79: 423–426.

Runte M, Huttenhofer A, Gross S, Kiefmann M, Horsthemke B, Buiting K (2001). The IC-SNURF-SNRPN transcript serves as a host for multiple small nucleolar RNA species and as an antisense RNA for UBE3A. *Hum Mol Genet* 10: 2687–2700.

Russo S, Cogliati F, Viri M, Cavalleri F, Selicorni A, Turolla L, Belli S, Romeo A, Larizza L (2000). Novel mutations of ubiquitin protein ligase 3A gene in Italian patients with Angelman syndrome. *Hum Mutat* 15: 387.

Stalker H, Williams C (1998). Genetic counseling in Angelman syndrome: the challenges of multiple causes. *Am J Med Genet* 77: 54–59.

Sutcliffe J, Nakao M, Christian S, Orstavik K, Tommerup N, Ledbetter D, Beaudet AL (1994). Deletions of a differentially methylated CpG island at the SNRPN gene define a putative imprinting control region. *Nat Genet* 8: 52–58.

Vu TH, Hoffman AR (1997). Imprinting of the Angelman syndrome gene, UBE3A, is restricted to brain. *Nat Genet* 17: 12–13.

Williams C, Lossie A, Driscoll D (2001). Angelman syndrome: mimicking conditions and phenotypes. *Am J Med Genet* 101: 59–64.

Williams CA, Angelman H, Clayton-Smith J, Driscoll DJ, Hendrickson JE, Knoll JHM, Magenis RE, Schinzel A, Wagstaff J, Whidden EM, et al. (1995a). Angelman syndrome: consensus for diagnostic criteria. *Am J Med Genet* 56: 237–238.

Williams CA, Zori RT, Hendrickson J, Stalker H, Marum T, Whidden E, Driscoll DJ (1995b). Angelman syndrome. *Curr Probl Pediatr* 25: 216–231.

Zackai E, McDonald-McGinn D, Bason L, Bingham P, Pellegrino J, Biegel J, Wolff D, Younkin D, Chance P, Spinner N (1995). Molecular genetics guides clinical geneticist: bedside to bench—now a two way street. *Am J Hum Genet* 57: A106.

Zeschnigk M, Lich C, Buiting K, Doerfler W, Horsthemke B (1997). A single-tube PCR test for the diagnosis of Angelman and Prader-Willi syndrome based on allelic methylation differences at the SNRPN locus. *Eur J Hum Genet* 5: 94–98.

VHL and von Hippel-Lindau Disease

EAMONN R. MAHER

Von Hippel-Lindau (VHL) disease is a dominantly inherited familial cancer syndrome caused by germline mutations in the 3p25 *VHL* tumor-suppressor gene (Latif et al., 1993; Kaelin and Maher, 1998; Clifford and Maher, 2001). VHL is widely expressed in fetal and adult tissues, and the pattern of *VHL* mRNA expression in the fetal kidney was considered to be consistent with a role in normal renal tubular development and differentiation (Richards et al., 1996). A mouse model of VHL disease demonstrated that *VHL* expression is critical for normal extraembryonic vascular development. While mice heterozygous for $VHL^{+/-}$ appeared phenotypically normal, homozygous $VHL^{-/-}$ mice died in utero at 10.5 to 12.5 days of gestation from dysgenesis caused by a failure of embryonic vasculogenesis of the placenta (Gnarra et al., 1997). Later Haase et al. (2001) reported a conditional mouse knockout that developed hepatic hemangiomas. VHL disease tumors such as hemangioblastomas and clear cell renal cell carcinoma (RCC) are highly vascular, also suggesting that pVHL has a role in regulating angiogenesis. While pVHL has not been consistently demonstrated to suppress tumorigenesis in vitro, reintroduction of wild-type pVHL into VHL null RCC cells suppresses tumor formation in vivo in nude mice (Chen et al., 1995a; Iliopoulos et al., 1995).

VHL TUMOR-SUPPRESSOR GENE FUNCTION

Although the *VHL* gene product appears to have multiple functions, the best characterized is the role of pVHL in regulating proteolytic degradation of the HIF (hypoxia inducible factor) transcription factors HIF-1 and HIF-2. The elucidation of the link between pVHL and HIF-1 resulted from concurrent investigations of the potential role of pVHL in angiogenesis regulation and the identification of pVHL-interacting proteins. Thus it was demonstrated that highly vascular VHL tumors overexpressed VEGF and VEGF receptor mRNA (Wizigmann-Voos et al., 1995), and that mRNAs for hypoxia-inducible genes, including vascular endothelial growth factor (VEGF, see Chapter 101), glucose transporter-1 (GLUT-1) and platelet-derived growth factor (PDGF), were constitutively upregulated in VHL null RCC cell lines (Siemester et al., 1996; Maxwell et al., 1999). In addition, normal oxygen-dependent regulation was restored upon reintroduction of wild-type pVHL into VHL null RCC cell lines (Gnarra et al., 1996; Iliopoulos et al., 1996; Levy et al., 1996; Siemeister et al., 1996). Initial experiments suggested that pVHL regulated VEGF mRNA levels by influencing mRNA stability (Gnarra et al., 1996; Knebelmann et al., 1997; Levy et al., 1996), although subsequently the elucidation of the role of pVHL in HIF-1 metabolism demonstrated a major indirect effect of pVHL on VEGF transcription (see later in this chapter).

pVHL-Associated Proteins and Targets

Inspection of the VHL protein sequence did not suggest possible functions, so the identification of elongins B and C and pVHL-interacting proteins provided the first clues to pVHL function (Duan et al., 1995; Kibel et al., 1995). Elongins B and C bind elongin A to generate a transcriptional elongation complex called Elongin or SIII. However, initial suggestions that pVHL might sequester elongins B and C and so down-regulate Elongin activity and transcriptional elongation of target genes, have not been substantiated, and it appears that inhibition of transcriptional elongation is not relevant to pVHL-mediated tumor suppression. Subsequently, Cul-2, a member of the cullin pro-

tein family, was found to associate with pVHL, elongin B, and elongin C to form a tetrameric pVHL/elongin C/elongin B/Cul-2 (VCBC) complex (Pause et al., 1997; Lonergan et al., 1998).

Structural and sequence motif homologies between the VCBC complex and the yeast SCF (Skp1-Cdc53/Cul1-F-box) complex suggested that VCBC might have an SCF-like function and target specific proteins for ubiquitylation and protosomal degradation (Lonergan et al., 1998). In particular, pVHL was predicted to have an "F-box function" and to determine which proteins were targeted. This model was supported by two subsequent reports. First, the Rbx-1 protein was demonstrated to associate with the VCBC complex and to be an essential general component of SCF complexes (Kamura et al., 1999). Second, the elucidation of the crystal structure of the pVHL/elonginB/elonginC complex demonstrated that pVHL has two principal domains: an ~100 residue amino-terminal domain rich in β-sheet (the β-domain) and a smaller carboxy-terminal α-helical domain (the α-domain). A large portion of the α-domain surface interacts with elongin C, and, significantly, a large proportion of disease-causing VHL mutations map to the α-domain and its residues that contact elongin C. A structural analogy was also noted between the F-box protein in SCF complexes and the elongin C binding site in pVHL. Elongin B binds pVHL indirectly through elongin C. Many other *VHL* mutations map to the β-domain, specifically to a patch not implicated in elongin C binding (Stebbins et al., 1999). This suggested that two intact and distinct macromolecular binding sites are required for pVHL function, as well as the possibility that the β-domain may be involved in targeting proteolytic substrates to the general ubiquitylation complex that is bound via the α-domain. Subsequent studies demonstrated that the VCBC complex promoted ubiquitin ligase activity and that promotion of ligase activity was only associated with wild-type pVHL and not disease-causing pVHL mutants (Iwai et al., 1999; Lisztwan et al., 1999).

Maxwell et al. (1999) demonstrated that pVHL plays a critical role in the regulation of the hypoxia-inducible transcription factors HIF-1 and HIF-2. The HIF-1 and HIF-2 transcription factors play a key role in the cellular response to hypoxia (oxygen sensing) and in the regulation of genes involved in energy metabolism, angiogenesis, and apoptosis (e.g., *GLUT-1*, *VEGF*, and other hypoxia-inducible genes previously shown to be regulated by pVHL). HIF-1 and HIF-2 are heterodimers, and their α-subunits are degraded rapidly by the proteasome under normoxic conditions, but are stabilized by hypoxia. pVHL has a critical role in targeting HIF-1α and HIF-2α subunits for oxygen-dependent proteolysis so that pVHL inactivation in RCC results in overexpression of HIF-1 and HIF-2, leading to consequent upregulation of VEGF (and other hypoxia response genes) (Maxwell et al., 1999; Cockman et al., 2000) (see Fig. 82–1). Thus the VHL–HIF-α interaction (via the VHL β-domain surface-binding site) links the SCF-like function of the VCBC complex to the angiogenic phenotype of VHL-associated tumors. While HIF-dysregulation associated with VHL-inactivation provides a plausible explanation for the vascular nature of VHL tumors, the relevance to growth suppression is less clear. However, recent reports suggest that HIF-2 may be oncogenic per se (Kondo et al., 2002; Maranchie et al., 2002).

Further Functional Analysis of pVHL

Several lines of evidence suggest that pVHL is a multifunctional protein. Indirect evidence for this is the complex genotype–phenotype correlations seen in VHL disease (see later in this chapter), which are

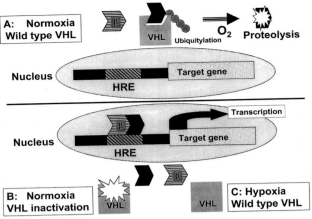

Figure 82–1. Regulation of HIF function. (*A*) In normoxia the HIF-α subunit is captured by the pVHL ubiquitin E3 ligase complex (elongins B and C, Cul2, and Rbx1), ubiquitylated and destroyed in the proteosome. Hence the HIF heterodimer does not form, and there is no transcription of the hypoxia-responsive target gene. (*B*) With VHL inactivation the HIF-α subunit accumulates and dimerizes with the β-subunit, the heterodimer then binds to the hypoxic response element (HRE) of the target genes and activates transcription. (*C*) In the presence of oxygen, specific prolyl residues in HIF-1α are converted to hydroxyproline, thus enabling pVHL to bind to HIF-1α. However, in hypoxia this reaction does not occur, and pVHL is unable to bind to HIF-1α. Hence the HIF-α subunit accumulates and dimerizes with the β-subunit, and the heterodimer then binds to the hypoxic-response element of the target genes and activates transcription.

compatible with multiple and tissue-specific functions. The demonstration that HIF-α-subunits are specifically targeted by the VCBC ubiquitin–ligase complex raised the possibility that pVHL may specify additional protein substrates for VCBC-mediated ubiquitylation. However, although additional targets for pVHL-targeted ubiquitylation have been described (e.g., a novel deubiquitinating enzyme and an atypical protein kinase C [PKCλ] (Okuda et al., 2001; Li et al., 2002), the relevance of these to VHL tumor-suppressor activity has not been established. Additional pVHL functions have been suggested including (*1*) regulation of cell cycle control (Pause et al., 1998), (*2*) reduced mRNA stability of target genes (perhaps through regulating levels of RNA-binding proteins (Pioli and Rigby, 2001), and (*3*) binding of fibronectin and control of extracellular fibronectin matrix (EFM) assembly (Ohh et al., 1998). As yet, the precise relevance of these various functions to pVHL tumor-suppressor activity is unclear. In addition, Feldman et al. (1999) reported that folding and assembly of pVHL into a complex with elongin B and C is directly mediated by the chaperonin TRiC/CCT. However, although it was suggested that exon 2 VHL mutations promote tumorigenesis via loss of pVHL binding to TriC/CCT, a recent analysis suggests that retention of TriC/CCT binding is not of primary importance in VHL tumor-suppressor activity (Hansen et al., 2002).

CLINICAL DESCRIPTION AND INFORMATION FOR GENETIC COUNSELING

VHL disease has an approximate incidence of 1 in 36,000 live births and is dominantly inherited with age-dependent penetrance and variable expression (Maher et al., 1990a; Latif et al., 1993). The three major features of VHL disease are retinal and central nervous system hemangioblastomas and clear cell RCC. The age-dependent penetrance for each of these tumors differs, with mean age at symptomatic diagnosis varying considerably (24.5 years for retinal angioma, 29 years for cerebellar hemangioblastoma, and 44 years for RCC). The earlier onset of retinal angioma and cerebellar hemangioblastoma than for RCC means that the risk of RCC is underestimated in cross-sectional studies and the lifetime probability for each of these three major complications has been estimated as >70% (Maher et al., 1990a), although tumor-specific risks are influenced by allelic heterogeneity (see later). VHL disease may present in childhood or old age, but the usual age of symptomatic presentation is in the second and third decades, and

penetrance is almost complete by age 60 years. Ascertainment of at-risk relatives ensures that many cases are diagnosed presymptomatically following DNA-based predictive testing.

Conventional clinical diagnostic criteria for VHL disease require either (*1*) a typical VHL tumor (hemangioblastoma, pheochromocytoma, or RCC) and a positive family history or (*2*) in isolated cases without a family history, two tumors (e.g., two hemangioblastomas or a hemangioblastoma and a visceral tumor). The necessity for two tumors to have occurred in isolated cases means that diagnosis is often delayed in such cases. The new mutation rate in VHL is $\sim$2–4 $\times$ 10^{-6} (Maher et al., 1991). A diagnosis of VHL disease should be considered in all cases of retinal and central nervous system hemangioblastomas, but also in patients with familial, multicentric, or young-onset pheochromocytoma and RCC. Molecular genetic analysis enables an early diagnosis of VHL disease in patients who do not satisfy conventional clinical diagnostic criteria. Thus $\sim$40% of patients with apparently isolated familial or bilateral pheochromocytoma have germline VHL gene mutations (Woodward et al., 1997, and unpublished observations) and $\sim$4% of patients with an isolated central nervous system hemangioblastoma (and a negative family history and no evidence of subclinical features of VHL disease) have a germline VHL gene mutation (Hes et al., 2000). Estimates of the risk of VHL disease in patients presenting with apparently isolated retinal angioma are available (Webster et al., 2000). For patients with familial RCC and no evidence of VHL disease, a diagnosis of familial papillary RCC and familial clear cell RCC which is not allelic with VHL disease should also be considered (Schmidt et al., 1997; Teh et al., 1997; Woodward et al., 2000b). At-risk children in VHL families with a known VHL mutation are usually considered for predictive testing from age 5 years.

Organ-Specific Features of VHL Disease

Retinal angiomas (histologically hemangioblastomas) are the most common presenting feature of VHL disease and are multiple in many cases. Retinal angiomas (mean 1.85 lesions) are found in almost 70% of cases, and the cumulative risk of visual loss has been estimated as 35% in gene carriers and 55% in patients with retinal angiomas at age 50 years (Webster et al., 1999). However, early detection and treatment of retinal angiomas reduces the risk of visual loss.

Central nervous system hemangioblastomas are a cardinal feature in VHL disease. Cerebellar hemangioblastomas occur in $\sim$70% of cases and symptomatic spinal cord lesions in $\sim$25% (Maher et al., 1990a). The incidence of supratentorial lesions is small. Approximately 30% of all patients with cerebellar hemangioblastoma have VHL disease, and the mean age at diagnosis of those with VHL disease is considerably younger than in sporadic cases (Maher et al., 1990b). Hemangioblastomas are benign tumors, and the results of surgery for single peripherally located cerebellar lesions are often excellent. However, the treatment of multicentric tumors—particularly, brain-stem and spinal tumors—may be hazardous and result in significant morbidity. In the future, anti-angiogenic therapy may offer a medical approach to the treatment of inoperable CNS and retinal hemangioblastomas.

Renal cysts and tumors are major features of VHL disease. The frequency of renal cysts is age-related, and renal cysts are present in most middle-aged patients. Cysts do not usually compromise renal function, but RCC may develop within a cyst, and complex cysts are followed up regularly to detect if solid lesions develop (Choyke et al., 1992). However, most RCC cases do not develop from cysts, and careful examination of the renal parenchyma from patients with clear cell RCC demonstrates numerous microfoci of clear cell RCC (Walther et al., 1995). Early detection and treatment of RCC in VHL disease reduces morbidity and mortality. VHL patients and at-risk relatives are offered annual renal imaging from age 16 years. Solid renal lesions that are detected on routine surveillance are monitored until they reach 3 cm in size, when conservative nephron-sparing surgery is performed. Following surgery there is a high risk of local recurrence (from new primary tumors), but the risk of distant metastasis is low (Steinbach et al., 1995), whereas 25% of VHL patients with a tumor >3 cm develop metastatic disease (Walther et al., 1999).

Pheochromocytoma occurs in $\sim$10% of cases but demonstrates marked interfamilial variability (Richard et al., 1992; Crossey et al.,

1994). Thus in many families pheochromocytoma is absent or rare, but in some families pheochromocytoma is the most frequent feature. Genotype–phenotype correlations are particularly prominent and complex for pheochromocytoma (see later in this chapter). Pheochromocytomas in VHL disease may be extraadrenal, and <5% are malignant. Compared to sporadic cases, onset of pheochromocytoma is earlier in VHL patients, and patients and at-risk relatives are screened from age 10 years.

Pancreas cysts and tumors are both features of VHL disease. Multiple cysts are the most frequent pancreatic manifestation but are rarely of clinical significance, and impairment of pancreatic function is uncommon. Pancreatic tumors occur in 5% to 10% of cases and are usually nonsecretory islet cell tumors. A high frequency of that malignancy has been reported in VHL-associated islet cell tumors, and surgery is indicated in tumors >3 cm while tumors <1 cm may be monitored (Libutti et al., 1998).

Other Organ Involvement in VHL Disease

Endolymphatic sac tumors (ELST) can be detected by MRI in up to 11% of cases (Manski et al., 1997), although only a minority are symptomatic, in which case they present with hearing loss, tinnitus, and vertigo. *Epididymal cysts* are very frequent in males with VHL disease and can, if bilateral, impair fertility. However, because epididymal cysts are not infrequent in the general population, their presence in an at-risk relative does not necessarily indicate carrier status.

GENE STRUCTURE AND MUTATIONS

The *VHL* tumor-suppressor gene (TSG) was isolated by a positional cloning strategy in 1993, five years after it was mapped to chromosome 3p25 by family linkage studies (Seizinger et al., 1988; Latif et al., 1993). The *VHL* gene encodes a 4.7 kb mRNA, which is widely expressed in both fetal and adult tissues, and expression of the VHL transcript and protein is not restricted to those organs involved in VHL disease (Latif et al., 1993; Los et al., 1996; Richards et al., 1996; Corless et al., 1997).

The VHL coding sequence is represented in three exons, and two alternatively spliced VHL transcripts have been detected reflecting the presence (isoform I) or absence (isoform II) of exon 2 (Richards et al., 1994). No endogenous isoform II–associated protein product has been reported to date, and the identification of VHL patients with germline deletions of exon 2 (resulting in the expression of isoform II only from the mutant allele) suggests that isoform II does not encode a functional gene product. A minimal promoter region of 106 bp has been defined, along with the definitions of functional SP1 and AP2 binding sites (Kuzmin et al., 1995; Zatyka et al., 2002a).

The *VHL* gene specifies two translation products: a full-length 213 amino acid protein (pVHL$_{30}$) that migrates with an apparent molecular weight of ~28–30 kDa, and a shorter protein (~18–19 kDa; pVHL$_{19}$), which is translated from an internal translation initiation site at codon 54 and produces a 160 amino acid protein. Evolutionary conservation of VHL sequence is very strong over most of the sequence included in pVHL$_{19}$, but the first 53 amino acids included in pVHL$_{30}$ are much less conserved (Woodward et al., 2000a). Thus the N-terminal sequence of pVHL$_{30}$ contains eight copies of a GXEEX acidic repeat motif in humans and higher primates, but only three copies are present in the marmoset and one copy in rodent *VHL* genes (Woodward et al., 2000a). The primary sequence of pVHL$_{19}$ shows little homology to any known protein.

Germline *VHL* gene mutations have been identified in more than 500 kindreds (Crossey et al., 1994; Chen et al., 1995b; Richards et al., 1995; Maher et al., 1996; Zbar et al., 1996; see also http://www.umd.necker.fr). Although a wide variety of mutations have been described, no mutations have been reported in the first 53 amino acids of pVHL$_{30}$. Germline *VHL* mutations may be divided into three groups: large deletions that account for ~40% of all mutations, intragenic missense mutations (~30%), and protein-truncating mutations (nonsense, frameshift insertions and deletions, splice site mutations) (~30%). Molecular genetic analysis of the complete VHL coding region by direct sequencing and large-deletion detection (e.g.,

quantitative Southern blot and FISH analyses) has been reported to detect mutations in up to 100% of cases (Stolle et al., 1998; Pack et al., 1999). VHL patients without detectable mutations may be mosaic (Sgambati et al., 2000). Recurrent *VHL* gene mutations (e.g., C694T, C712T, G713A, and T505C) mostly represent multiple de novo mutations at hypermutable sequences (e.g., CpG dinucleotides, small repeats) (Richards et al., 1995). However, the T505C (Y98H) mutation common in southwest Germany and in North American kindreds of German origin is a founder mutation in these communities (Brauch et al., 1995).

GENOTYPE–PHENOTYPE CORRELATIONS

Complex genotype-phenotype associations are a notable feature of VHL disease, particularly for pheochromocytoma susceptibility. Thus, VHL disease kindreds have been divided into type 1 (no pheochromocytoma) and type 2 (pheochromocytoma) subsets. Large deletions and truncating mutations typically predispose to hemangioblastomas and RCC but not to pheochromocytomas (type 1 phenotype) (Crossey et al., 1994; Maher et al., 1996; Zbar et al., 1996). Certain missense mutations may produce a type 1 phenotype, but the majority of type 2 kindreds have a missense mutation. Type 2 families are further subdivided according to the presence or absence of RCC and hemangioblastomas. Thus in type 2A kindreds, hemangioblastomas and pheochromocytoma occur but not (or rarely) RCC. The type 2B phenotype is characterized by the development of hemangioblastomas, RCC, and pheochromocytoma, whereas type 2C kindreds develop only pheochromocytoma (Brauch et al., 1995; Neumann et al., 1995; Woodward et al., 1997). These genotype–phenotype correlations may be helpful in clinical management as patients with deletions or truncating mutations have a risk of pheochromocytoma of about 5% at 50 years, but there is a 10-fold higher risk in patients with missense mutations. Missense mutations are heterogeneous, however, and the tumor risks associated with specific mutations may differ markedly so risk estimates should be used with caution. Patients presenting with a familial pheochromocytoma-only history (type 2C) may have a mutation that has been detected in other type 2 subsets (e.g., R167Q, which is seen in type 2B), suggesting that these kindreds are also at risk for hemangioblastomas and RCC. However, some missense mutations are restricted to type 2C kindreds, thus suggesting that they do not predispose to other VHL tumors. These complex correlations are consistent with the hypothesis that the VHL gene product has multiple and tissue-specific functions.

In addition to the phenotypic variability associated with allelic heterogeneity, genetic modifiers may influence the phenotypic expression of VHL disease (Webster et al., 1998). Thus individuals with ocular hemangioblastomas were found to have a significantly increased incidence of cerebellar hemangioblastoma and RCC compared to those without retinal involvement. Relative-pair analysis revealed a significant correlation between numbers of retinal angiomas in close relatives but not in distant relatives (Webster et al., 1998). Recently, allelic variants in the cyclin D1 gene have been reported to influence hemangioblastoma development (Zatyka et al., 2002b).

GENOTYPE, PHENOTYPE, AND pVHL FUNCTION

The definition of the precise relationships between geneotype, phenotype, and specific pVHL functions would provide critical insights into the differing pathways of tumorigenesis in specific VHL tumor types. Structural analysis of the VCBC complex (Stebbins et al., 1999) demonstrated that missense mutations associated with a type 1 phenotype often occur at codons within the hydrophobic core mutations and would be predicted to cause complete disruption to the pVHL structure. In contrast, type 2A/2B mutations show a trend against hydrophobic core mutations, causing mostly local effects, thus suggesting that type 2 mutations have a strong bias against total loss of function (Stebbins et al., 1999). These observations are consistent with the high frequency of loss of function deletion (and truncating mutations) in type 1 families and the rarity of such mutations in type 2 kindreds (Chen et al., 1995; Maher et al., 1996). Furthermore, in vitro analysis of pVHL function demonstrates partial retention of pVHL binding to elongin C or to HIF-1 with pheochromocytoma-associated missense mutations (Clifford et al., 2001). These findings would suggest that complete loss of pVHL function (generally) does not predispose to or is incompatible with pheochromocytoma development. Analysis of HIF-1 regulation by overexpression of mutant VHL proteins demonstrated complete or partial dysregulation with type 1, 2A, and 2B–associated mutations, but type 2C mutants retained the ability to regulate HIF-1 (although fibronectin binding was impaired) (Clifford et al., 2001; Hoffman et al., 2001). These findings suggest that HIF-1 dysregulation is not necessary for pheochromocytoma development in VHL disease.

MANAGEMENT AND PROGNOSIS

Currently the most important aspect of the management of VHL disease is the ascertainment of all at-risk relatives and ensuring annual surveillance of patients and at-risk relatives according to standard protocols (see Hodgson and Maher, 1999). Adherence to screening protocols reduces morbidity and mortality in VHL disease to improve life expectancy. Thus median survival was estimated at 49 years in 1990, but was ~60 years a decade later (Maher et al., 1990a, and unpublished observations). Molecular genetic testing enables surveillance targeted to gene carriers only and so improves the cost effectiveness of screening. The effective management of VHL patients and families requires a multidisciplinary approach. Although specific complications may require expert investigations and treatment from organ-based specialists (e.g., ophthalmologists, neurosurgeons, and urologists), it is essential that responsibility for the overall coordination of family ascertainment and screening is assumed.

It is hoped that in the relatively near future, novel antiangiogenic agents will become widely available and prove to be effective and safe for the medical treatment of hemangioblastomas. Such a development would be a major advance for patients with inoperable CNS tumors.

REFERENCES

Brauch H, Kishida T, Glavac D, Chen F, Pausch F, Hofler H, Latif F, Lerman MI, Zbar B, Neumann HPH (1995). Von Hippel-Lindau (VHL) disease with pheochromocytoma in the Black Forest region of Germany: evidence for a founder effect. *Hum Genet* 95: 551–556.

Chen F, Kishida T, Duh FM, Renbaum P, Orcutt ML, Schmidt L, Zbar B (1995a). Suppression of growth of renal-carcinoma cells by the von Hippel-Lindau tumor-suppressor gene. *Cancer Res* 55: 4804–4807.

Chen F, Kishida T, Yao M, Hustad T, Glavac D, Dean M, Gnarra JR, Orcutt ML, Duh FM, Glenn G, et al. (1995b). Germline mutations in the von Hippel-Lindau disease tumor-suppressor gene: correlations with phenotype. *Hum Mutat* 5: 66–75.

Choyke PL, Glenn GM, Walther MCM, Zbar B, Weiss GH, Alexander RB, Hayes WS, Long JP, Thakore KN, Linehan WM (1992). The natural-history of renal lesions in von Hippel-Lindau disease: a serial CT study in 28 patients. *Am J Roentgenol* 159: 1229–1234.

Clifford SC, Maher ER (2001). Von Hippel-Lindau disease: clinical and molecular perspectives. *Adv Cancer Res* 82: 85–105.

Clifford SC, Cockman ME, Smallwood AC, Mole DR, Woodward ER, Maxwell PH, Ratcliffe PJ, Maher ER (2001). Contrasting effects on HIF-1α regulation by disease-causing pVHL mutations correlate with patterns of tumourigenesis in von Hippel-Lindau disease. *Hum Mol Genet* 10: 1029–1038.

Cockman ME, Masson N, Mole DR, Jaakkola P, Chang GW, Clifford SC, Maher ER, Pugh CW, Ratcliffe PJ, Maxwell PH (2000). Hypoxia inducible factor-α binding and ubiquitylation by the von Hippel-Lindau tumor suppressor protein. *J Biol Chem* 275: 25733–25744.

Corless CL, Kibel AS, Iliopoulos O, Kaelin WG (1997). Immunostaining of the von Hippel-Lindau gene product in normal and neoplastic human tissues. *Hum Pathol* 28: 459–464.

Crossey PA, Richards FM, Foster K, Green JS, Prowse A, Latif F, Lerman MI, Zbar B, Affara NA, Ferguson-Smith MA, Maher ER (1994). Identification of intragenic mutations in the von Hippel-Lindau disease tumor-suppressor gene and correlation with disease phenotype. *Hum Mol Genet* 3: 1303–1308.

Duan DR, Pause A, Burgess WH, Aso T, Chen DYT, Garrett KP, Conaway RC, Conaway JW, Linehan WM, Klausner RD (1995). Inhibition of transcription elongation by the VHL tumor-suppressor protein. *Science* 269: 1402–1406.

Feldman DE, Thulasiraman V, Ferreyra RG, Frydman J (1999). Formation of the VHL-elongin BC tumor suppressor complex is mediated by the chaperonin TRiC. *Mol Cell* 4: 1051–1061.

Gnarra JR, Zhou SB, Merrill MJ, Wagner JR, Krumm A, Papavassiliou E, Oldfield EH, Klausner RD, Linehan WM (1996). Post-transcriptional regulation of vascular endothelial growth factor mRNA by the product of the VHL tumor suppressor gene. *Proc Natl Acad Sci USA* 93: 10589–10594.

Gnarra JR, Ward JM, Porter FD, Wagner JR, Devor DE, Grinberg A, EmmertBuck MR, Westphal H, Klausner RD, Linehan WM (1997). Defective placental vasculogenesis

causes embryonic lethality in VHL-deficient mice. *Proc Natl Acad Sci USA* 94: 9102–9107.

Haase VH, Glickman JN, Socolovsky M, Jaenisch R (2001). Vascular tumors in livers with targeted inactivation of the von Hippel-Lindau tumor suppressor. *Proc Natl Acad Sci USA* 98(4): 1583–1588.

Hes FJ, McKee S, Taphoom MJ, Rehal P, van Der Luijt RB, McMahon R, van Der Smagt JJ, Dow D, Zewald RA, Whittaker J, Lips CJ, MacDonald F, Pearson PL, Maher ER (2000). Cryptic von Hippel-Lindau disease: germline mutations in patients with haemangioblastoma only. *J Med Genet* 37(12): 939–943.

Hodgson SV, Maher ER (1999). *A Practical Guide to Human Cancer Genetics.* Cambridge University Press, Cambridge.

Hoffman MA, Ohh M, Yang H, Klco JM, Ivan M, Kaelin WG Jr. (2001). Von Hippel-Lindau protein mutants linked to type 2C VHL disease preserve the ability to downregulate HIF. *Hum Mol Genet* 10(10): 1019–1027.

Iliopoulos O, Kibel A, Gray S, Kaelin WG (1995). Tumor suppression by the human von Hippel-Lindau gene-product. *Nat Med* 1: 822–826.

Iliopoulos O, Levy AP, Jiang C, Kaelin WG, Goldberg MA (1996). Negative regulation of hypoxia-inducible genes by the von Hippel-Lindau protein. *Proc Natl Acad Sci USA* 93: 10595–10599.

Iwai K, Yamanaka K, Kamura T, Minato N, Conaway RC, Canaway JW, Klausner RD, Pause A (1999). Identification of the von Hippel-Lindau tumor-suppressor protein as part of an active E3 ubiquitin ligase complex. *Proc Natl Acad Sci USA* 96: 12436–12441.

Kaelin WG Jr, Maher ER (1998). The VHL tumour-suppressor gene paradigm. *Trends Genet* 10: 423–426.

Kamura T, Koepp DM, Conrad MN, Skowyra D, Moreland RJ, Iliopoulos O, Lane WS, Kaelin WG, Elledge SJ, Conaway RC, et al. (1999). Rbx1, a component of the VHL tumor suppressor complex and SCF ubiquitin ligase. *Science* 284: 657–661.

Kibel A, Iliopoulos O, Decaprio JA, Kaelin WG (1995). Binding of the von Hippel-Lindau tumor-suppressor protein to elongin-B and elongin-C. *Science* 269: 1444–1446.

Knebelmann B, Ananth S, Cohen HT, Sukhatme VP (1997). The von Hippel-Lindau (VHL) gene product decreases TGF-α mRNA stability in renal carcinoma cells. *J Am Soc Nephrol* 8: A1807.

Kondo K, Klco J, Nakamura E, Lechpammer M, Kaelin WG Jr (2002). Inhibition of HIF is necessary for tumor suppression by the von Hippel-Lindau protein. *Cancer Cell* 1: 237–246

Kuzmin I, Duh FM, Latif F, Geil L, Zbar B, Lerman MI (1995). Identification of the promoter of the human von Hippel-Lindau disease tumor-suppressor gene. *Oncogene* 10: 2185–2194.

Latif F, Tory K, Gnarra J, Yao M, Duh FM, Orcutt ML, Stackhouse T, Kuzmin I, Modi W, Geil L, et al. (1993). Identification of the von Hippel-Lindau disease tumor-suppressor gene. *Science* 260: 1317–1320.

Levy AP, Levy NS, Goldberg MA (1996). Hypoxia-inducible protein binding to vascular endothelial growth factor mRNA and its modulation by the von Hippel-Lindau protein. *J Biol Chem* 271: 25492–25497.

Li Z, Na X, Wang D, Schoen SR, Messing EM, Wu G (2002). Ubiquitination of a novel deubiquitinating enzyme requires direct binding to von Hippel-Lindau tumor suppressor protein. *J Biol Chem* 277: 4656–4662.

Libutti SK, Choyke PL, Bartlett DL, Vargas H, Walther M, Lubensky I, Glenn G, Linehan WM, Alexander HR (1998). Pancreatic neuroendocrine tumors associated with von Hippel-Lindau disease: diagnostic and management recommendations. *Surgery* 124: 1153–1159.

Lisztwan J, Imbert G, Wirbelauer C, Gstaiger M, Krek W (1999). The von Hippel-Lindau tumor suppressor protein is a component of an E3 ubiquitin-protein ligase activity. *Genes Dev* 13: 1822–1833.

Lonergan KM, Iliopoulos O, Ohh M, Kamura T, Conaway RC, Conaway JW, Kaelin WG (1998). Regulation of hypoxia-inducible mRNAs by the von Hippel-Lindau tumor suppressor protein requires binding to complexes containing elongins B/C and Cul2. *Mol Cell Biol* 18: 732–741.

Los M, Jansen GH, Kaelin WG, Lips CJM, Blijham GH, Voest EE (1996). Expression pattern of the von Hippel-Lindau protein in human tissues. *Lab Invest*, 75: 231–238.

Maher ER, Yates JRW, Harries R, Benjamin C, Harris R, Moore AT, Ferguson-Smith MA (1990a). Clinical features and natural history of von Hippel-Lindau disease. *Q J Med* 77: 1151–1163.

Maher ER, Yates JRW, Ferguson-Smith MA (1990b). Statistical analysis of the two stage mutation model in von Hippel-Lindau disease, and in sporadic cerebellar hemangioblastoma and renal cell carcinoma. *J Med Genet* 27: 311–314.

Maher ER, Iselius L, Yates JR, Littler M, Benjamin C, Harris R, Sampson J, Williams A, Ferguson-Smith MA, Morton N (1991). Von Hippel-Lindau disease: a genetic study. *J Med Genet* 28: 443–447.

Maher ER, Webster AR, Richards FM, Green JS, Crossey PA, Payne SJ, Moore AT (1996). Phenotypic expression in von Hippel-Lindau disease: correlations with germline VHL gene mutations. *J Med Genet* 33: 328–332.

Manski TJ, Heffner DK, Glenn GM, Patronas NJ, Pikus AT, Katz D, Lebovics R, Sledjeski K, Choyke PL, Zbar B, et al. (1997). Endolymphatic sac tumors: a source of morbid hearing loss in von Hippel-Lindau disease. *JAMA* 277: 1461–1466.

Maranchie JK, Vasselli JR, Riss J, Bonifacino JS, Linehan WM, Klausner RD (2002). The contribution of VHL substrate binding and HIF1-α to the phenotype of VHL loss in renal cell carcinoma. *Cancer Cell* 1: 247–255

Maxwell PH, Wiesener MS, Chang GW, Clifford SC, Vaux EC, Cockman ME, Wykoff CC, Pugh CW, Maher ER, Ratcliffe PJ (1999). The tumour suppressor protein VHL targets hypoxia-inducible factors for oxygen-dependent proteolysis. *Nature* 399: 271–275.

Neumann HPH, Eng C, Mulligan L, Glavac D, Ponder BAJ, Crossey PA, Maher ER, Brauch H (1995). Consequences of direct genetic testing for germline mutations in the clinical management of families with multiple endocrine neoplasia type 2. *JAMA* 274: 1149–1151.

Ohh M, Yauch RL, Lonergan KM, Whaley JM, Stemmer Rachamimov AO, Louis DN, Gavin BJ, Kley N, Kaelin WG, Iliopoulos O (1998). The von Hippel-Lindau tumor suppressor protein is required for proper assembly of an extracellular fibronectin matrix. *Mol Cell* 1: 959–968.

Okuda H, Saitoh K, Hirai S, Iwai K, Takaki Y, Baba M, Minato N, Ohno S, Shuin T (2001). The von Hippel-Lindau tumor suppressor protein mediates ubiquitination of activated atypical protein kinase C. *J Biol Chem* 276: 43611–43617.

Pack SD, Zbar B, Pak E, Ault DO, Humphrey JS, Pham T, Hurley K, Weil RJ, Park W.S, Kuzmin I, et al. (1999). Constitutional von Hippel-Lindau (VHL) gene deletions detected in VHL families by fluorescence in situ hybridization. *Cancer Res* 59: 5560–5564.

Pause A, Lee S, Worrell RA, Chen DYT, Burgess WH, Linehan WM, Klausner RD (1997). The von Hippel-Lindau tumor-suppressor gene product forms a stable complex with human CUL-2, a member of the Cdc53 family of proteins. *Proc Natl Acad Sci USA* 94: 2156–2161.

Pause A, Lee S, Lonergan KM, Klausner RD (1998). The von Hippel-Lindau tumor suppressor gene is required for cell cycle exit upon serum withdrawal. *Proc Natl Acad Sci USA* 95: 993–998.

Pioli PA, Rigby WF (2001). The von Hippel-Lindau protein interacts with heteronuclear ribonucleoprotein a2 and regulates its expression. *J Biol Chem* 276(43): 40346–40352.

Richard S, Resche F, Vermesse B, Fendler JP, Francillard M, Laroche F, Luton JP, Mery JP, Proye C, Redondo A, Plouin PF (1992). Pheochromocytoma as presenting manifestation of von Hippel-Lindau disease. *Arch Mal Coeur Vaiss* 85: 1153–1156.

Richards FM, Crossey PA, Phipps ME, Foster K, Latif F, Evans G, Sampson J, Lerman MI, Zbar B, Affara NA, et al. (1994). Detailed mapping of germline deletions of the von Hippel-Lindau disease tumor-suppressor gene. *Hum Mol Genet* 3: 595–598.

Richards FM, Payne SJ, Zbar B, Affara NA, Ferguson-Smith MA, Maher ER (1995). Molecular analysis of de-novo germline mutations in the von Hippel-Lindau disease gene. *Hum Mol Genet* 4: 2139–2143.

Richards FM, Schofield PN, Fleming S, Maher ER (1996). Expression of the von Hippel-Lindau disease tumour suppressor gene during human embryogenesis. *Hum Mol Genet* 5: 639–644.

Schmidt L, Duh FM, Chen F, Kishida T, Glenn G, Choyke P, Scherer SW, Zhuang ZP, Lubensky I, Dean M, et al. (1997). Germline and somatic mutations in the tyrosine kinase domain of the MET proto-oncogene in papillary renal carcinomas. *Nat Genet* 16: 68–73.

Seizinger BR, Rouleau GA, Ozelius LJ, Lane AH, Farmer GE, Lamiell JM, Haines J, Yuen JWM, Collins D, Majoorkrakauer D, et al. (1988). Von Hippel-Lindau disease maps to the region of chromosome-3 associated with renal-cell carcinoma. *Nature* 332: 268–269.

Sgambati MT, Stolle C, Choyke PL, Walther MM, Zbar B, Linehan WM, Glenn GM (2000). Mosaicism in von Hippel-Lindau disease: lessons from kindreds with germline mutations identified in offspring with mosaic parents. *Am J Hum Genet* 66: 84–91.

Siemeister G, Weindel K, Mohrs K, Barleon B, Martiny-Baron G, Marme D (1996). Reversion of deregulated expression of vascular endothelial growth factor in human renal carcinoma cells by von Hippel-Lindau tumor suppressor protein. *Cancer Res* 56: 2299–2301.

Stebbins CE, Kaelin WG, Pavletich NP (1999). Structure of the VHL-ElonginC-ElonginB complex: implications for VHL tumor suppressor function. *Science* 284: 455–461.

Steinbach F, Novick AC, Zincke H, Miller DP, Williams RD, Lund G, Skinner DG, Esrig D, Richie JP, Dekernion JB, et al. (1995). Treatment of renal-cell carcinoma in von Hippel-Lindau disease: a multicenter study. *J Urol* 153: 1812–1816.

Stolle C, Glenn G, Zbar B, Humphrey JS, Choyke P, Walther M, Pack S, Hurley K, Andrey C, Klausner R, Linehan WM (1998). Improved detection of germline mutations in the von Hippel-Lindau disease tumor suppressor gene. *Hum Mutat* 12: 417–423.

Teh BT, Giraud S, Sari NF, Hii SI, Bergerat JP, Larsson C, Limacher JM, Nicol D (1997). Familial non-VHL non-papillary clear-cell renal cancer. *Lancet* 349: 848–849.

Walther MM, Lubensky IA, Venzon D, Zbar B, Linehan WM (1995). Prevalence of microscopic lesions in grossly normal renal parenchyma from patients with von Hippel-Lindau disease, sporadic renal cell carcinoma and no renal disease: clinical implications. *J Urol* 154: 2010–2014.

Walther MM, Choyke PL, Glenn G, Lyne JC, Rayford W, Venzon D, Linehan WM (1999). Renal cancer in families with hereditary renal cancer: prospective analysis of a tumor size threshold for renal parenchymal sparing surgery. *J Urol* 161: 1475–1479.

Webster AR, Richards FM, MacRonald FE, Moore AT, Maher ER (1998). An analysis of phenotypic variation in the familial cancer syndrome von Hippel-Lindau disease: Evidence for modifier effects. *Am J Hum Genet* 63: 1025–1035.

Webster AR, Maher ER, Moore AT (1999). Clinical characteristics of ocular angiomatosis in von Hippel-Lindau disease and correlation with germline mutation. *Arch Ophthalmol* 117: 371–378.

Webster AR, Maher ER, Bird AC, Moore AT (2000). Risk of multisystem disease in isolated ocular angioma. *J Med Genet* 37:62–63.

Wizigmann-Voos S, Breier G, Risau W, Plate KH (1995). Up-regulation of vascular endothelial growth factor and its receptors in von Hippel-Lindau disease–associated and sporadic hemangioblastomas. *Cancer Res* 55(6): 1358–1364.

Woodward ER, Eng C, McMahon R, Voutilainen R, Affara NA, Ponder BAJ, Maher ER (1997). Genetic predisposition to phaeochromocytoma: analysis of candidate genes GDNF, RET and VHL. *Hum Mol Genet* 6: 1051–1056.

Woodward ER, Clifford SC, Astuti D, Affara NA, Maher ER (2000b). Familial clear cell renal cell carcinoma (FCRC): clinical features and mutation analysis of the VHL, MET, and CUL2 candidate genes. *J Med Genet* 37: 348–353.

Zatyka M, Morrissey C, Kuzmin I, Lerman MI, Latif F, Richards FM, Maher ER (2002a). Genetic and functional analysis of the von Hippel-Lindau (VHL) tumour suppressor gene promoter. *J Med Genet* 39(7): 463–472.

Zatyka M, da Silva NF, Clifford SC, Morris MR, Wiesener MS, Eckardt K-U, Houlston RS, Richards FM, Latif F, Maher ER (2002b). Identification of cyclin D1 and other novel targets for the von Hippel-Lindau tumour suppressor gene by expression array analysis and investigation of cyclin D1 genotype as a modifier in von Hippel-Lindau disease. *Cancer Res* 62(13): 3803–3811.

Zbar B, Kishida T, Chen F, Schmidt L, Maher ER, Richards FM, Crossey PA, Webster AR, Affara NA, Ferguson-Smith MA, et al. (1996). Germline mutations in the von Hippel-Lindau (VHL) gene in families from North America, Europe, and Japan. *Hum Mutat* 8: 348–357.

83 | *MKKS* and the McKusick-Kaufman and Bardet-Biedl Syndromes

LESLIE G. BIESECKER

McKusick-Kaufman syndrome (MKS) is a rare developmental anomaly syndrome originally described among the Amish that comprises polydactyly, hydrometrocolpos, and congenital heart disease (Kaufman et al., 1972). Bardet-Biedl syndrome (BBS) is more common and more pleiotropic, comprising polydactyly, retinal degeneration, obesity, mental retardation, renal anomalies, and a wide array of other less common malformations (Beales et al., 1999). Both of these developmental anomaly syndromes can be caused by mutations in the *MKKS* gene (Katsanis et al., 2000; Slavotinek et al., 2000; Stone et al., 2000) and are inherited in an autosomal recessive pattern, although the genetics of these disorders may be more complex (Katsanis et al., 2001). Bardet-Biedl syndrome is genetically heterogeneous, and the MKS phenotype may be considered to be a mild form of BBS. The *MKKS* gene encodes a putative group II chaperonin that is most similar to an archebacterial thermosome (Stone et al., 2000). The pathogenetic role of the MKKS chaperonin is unclear.

LOCUS AND DEVELOPMENTAL PATHWAY

The *MKKS* gene has six exons, including a large internal exon of >1400 bp, which encodes a protein of 580 amino acids (Stone et al., 2000). Interestingly, database searches at the time it was identified showed that the most similar protein in the databases was the thermosome from an archebacterium (the so-called third order of life) *Thermoplasma acidophilum*. Subsequently, homologs have been identified in mouse and rat, although homologs in other species have not been described. A second protein that is similar to MKKS is the t-complex-related protein (TCP) family. This large family of proteins includes numerous orthologs in humans and other species. The thermosome, TCP proteins, and, by similarity, MKKS are members of the chaperonin family of proteins. Membership in this family of proteins has interesting implications for the developmental pathogenesis of MKS and is discussed in this chapter. The species distribution of MKKS homologs is interesting because *MKKS* may be an example of a gene that has been transferred from prokaryotes to eukaryotes (Lander et al., 2001). This model would explain the prevalence of the gene in higher animals and archebacteria, while it is apparently absent in *Drosophila*, *C. elegans*, yeast, and other eukaryotes. The alternative hypotheses of the loss of *MKKS* in an early eukaryote evolutionary branch or the existence of functional homologs without similar primary protein structure have not been excluded.

The *MKKS* cDNA open reading frame (ORF) encodes a predicted protein of 580 amino acids. The putative active site of the MKKS protein sequence has been matched to the crystal structure of the *T. acidophilum* active site by threading analysis (Stone et al., 2000). There is evidence of alternative splicing in the 5' UTR of *MKKS*, although the functional significance of this is unknown. The *MKKS* gene appears to be widely expressed throughout development and in adult life in many tissues. This ubiquitous expression begs the question of the specificity of the phenotypes that are attributable to mutations in the gene. Functional studies of the protein and generation of null alleles in mice are under way, but no results are available at the time of this writing.

CLINICAL FEATURES

McKusick-Kaufman Syndrome

This syndrome was originally identified in Amish females as an isolated heritable gynecologic malformation, hydrometrocolpos (McKu-

sick et al., 1964). This term describes a developmental sequence of failure of canalization of the uterovaginal plate at the fusion of the cloaca and the mullerian tubercles (Fig. 83–1). This failure of canalization impedes the outflow of uterine or vaginal secretions that are normal in fetal females. As the fetal uterus is exposed to the maternal hormone milieu, it is highly distensible and can dilate to a large extent. The uterine expansion then leads to displacement or compression of surrounding structures. A common consequence of this is hydronephrosis and pulmonary compression. Soon after the original description of the isolated malformation, it was recognized that many of the affected patients also had polydactyly, and a smaller number had congenital heart disease (CHD), most commonly atrioventricular septal defects (Table 83–1). This led to the identification of the condition as a multiple malformation syndrome (Kaufman et al., 1972). The cardiac defects were not appreciated as many of the patients died soon after birth and the syndrome was not recognized. Some of the siblings of affected individuals had death certificates where the cause of death was simply coded as "blue baby." Since males cannot have hydrometrocolpos, they may only be affected by CHD or polydactyly, or both.

Implicit in these descriptions of MKS is that the disorder has highly variable expressivity. The positional cloning studies used a clinical definition of a female proband as a patient with hydrometrocolpos and polydactyly or congenital heart disease (Stone et al., 1998). Siblings of a proband were diagnosed as affected if they had either polydactyly, hydrometrocolpos, or CHD. In reviewing the more than 20 cases among the Amish, we found that 60% of patients had polydactyly, 70% of affected females had hydrometrocolpos, and 15% of patients had CHD. We noted that these penetrance figures, if they were independent probabilities, predicted that 9% of males and 3% of females who were homozygous for the mutant allele would be expected to be nonpenetrant. Indeed, the linkage studies identified a homozygous female without any of the manifestations of the disorder who was homozygous for the disease haplotype. This woman had five children, four of whom were affected, consistent with pseudodominant inheritance of a nonpenetrant homozygote whose partner was a carrier. To our knowledge, MKS is the first malformation syndrome inherited in an autosomal recessive pattern to be shown to manifest incomplete penetrance. This observation is more than a curiosity and figures prominently in the modeling of gene function and pathogenesis described in this chapter.

The variable expressivity of MKS poses a significant clinical challenge. The diagnostic criteria outlined for research purposes are stringent and may not be appropriate for clinical use. These criteria will not diagnose patients who manifest polydactyly or CHD as a single malformation in a sporadic case, although some children with apparently isolated CHD or limb malformations may harbor *MKKS* mutations. The proportion is expected to be low given the rarity of the syndrome outside the Amish.

In the course of isolating the gene for MKS, there was a critical need for non-Amish patients to confirm that mutations in the *MKKS* gene caused the phenotype. This was necessary because the *MKKS* mutant allele in the Amish had two amino acid substitutions when compared to those in the normal population. We searched assiduously for non-Amish cases with very little success. At that time, there were fewer than 100 known cases of MKS outside of the Amish (Lurie and Wulfsberg, 1994). We and others observed that when these case reports were reanalyzed, one of three observations was made: the patient had died, the family was lost to follow-up, or the child's diag-

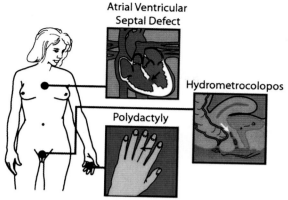

Figure 83–1. Malformations in McKusick-Kaufman syndrome. The triad of hydrometrolcolpos, polydactylyy, and congenital heart disease define this disorder in fully expressing females. Males may have only the limb and cardiac phenotype.

nosis was changed to BBS when they developed retinal degeneration, obesity, and developmental delay, all of which are age-dependant features of BBS (David et al., 1999). In fact, we have identified only one non-Amish case of MKS in a patient who is old enough to be past the age of onset of the BBS-specific features (Slavotinek et al., unpublished observations). From these data we conclude that MKS is exceedingly rare outside the Old Order Amish population. However, the recognition that most infants diagnosed with MKS evolve into a diagnosis of BBS suggested that those disorders might be allelic, as described later in this chapter.

Bardet-Biedl Syndrome

As noted, a number of children who carried a diagnosis of MKS from the neonatal period developed additional symptoms that led their physicians to change their diagnosis to BBS. The Bardet-Biedl syndrome is defined as comprising major and minor manifestations. The major manifestations include pigmentary retinopathy, obesity, learning disability, polydactyly, male hypogonadism, and renal anomalies (Beales et al., 1999). The minor manifestations include speech disorder, eye abnormalities, brachydactyly, developmental delay, nephrogenic diabetes insipidus, ataxia, spasticity, diabetes mellitus, dental anomalies, congenital heart disease, and hepatic fibrosis. Patients are diagnosed with BBS if they have four major criteria or three major and two minor criteria. The average age of a diagnosis for a sporadic patient with BBS is nine years. Although pigmentary retinal degeneration is very common and nearly always leads to complete blindness by the age of 30 years, many of the other manifestations of BBS are highly variable. It is believed that the reported incidence of learning disabilities of 62% is an overestimate due to biased ascertainment (P. Beales, personal communication). It is interesting to note in the context of MKS that genital anomalies in females were not reported among a cohort of 109 patients, and structural CHD is uncommon, affecting only 3% of patients.

Identification of Gene and Mutational Spectrum

The *MKKS* gene was identified by a positional cloning strategy using a large inbred Amish kindred affected with the MKS phenotype from

Table 83–1. Clinical Manifestations of MKS and BBS

	McKusick-Kaufman Syndrome	Bardet-Biedl Syndrome
Hydrometrocolpos	+++	−
Polydactyly	+++	+++
Congenital heart disease	++	+
Renal anomalies	+	++
Pigmentary retinopathy	−	+++
Mental retardation	−	+

+++, common; ++, intermediate frequency; +, uncommon; −, not reported, congenital heart disease.

southeastern Pennsylvania. Because the disorder is prevalent among the Old Order Amish and is inherited in an autosomal recessive pattern, homozygosity mapping was used to map an approximately 400 kb candidate interval (Stone et al., 1998). The linkage mapping of this disorder was the first to use a sophisticated bioinformatics approach to genealogic analysis and pedigree generation in the Old Order Amish (Agarwala et al., 1998, 2001). As the Amish are fastidious record keepers, there are extensive genealogic records that trace many branches of the sect back to a small set of founders in the 18th century. These records were collated and analyzed for errors, and several partially overlapping genealogic data sets were reconciled. This database currently comprises nearly 300,000 individuals. Pedigrees can be generated from this dataset using customized software to query the database for all inheritance paths that connect a given set of nuclear Amish families who have children affected by a given disorder. This pedigree is then optimized by a branch-and-cut algorithm to identify the single pedigree with the simplest structure, representing the most likely true pedigree for that set of families.

Linkage analysis of this pedigree with a full autosomal genome scan identified a candidate region that harbored four genes, one of which harbored mutations in affected persons and was designated *MKKS* (Stone et al., 2000). The *MKKS* allele in the Amish that co-segregated with the disease was found to have two sequence differences, H84Y and A242S, when compared to a set of Caucasian controls. However, this is a situation where homozygosity mapping in closed populations can have limitations. It is formally impossible to prove by genetics that a substitution mutation causes a disease in a closed population. This is because there are no suitable controls who are ethnically matched to the population. In the case of the Amish, the entire North American population was founded by 100 to 200 people who emigrated from Europe. A founder effect could establish a mutation or a polymorphism with very high frequency, and this is impossible to prove 10 to 12 generations later. This problem is compounded by the fact that the phenotype is incompletely penetrant, as it would be expected that one could identify unaffected homozygotes.

The second difficult aspect of the gene identification was that the mutant allele in the Amish had two sequence alterations, as noted here. Because A242S was a relatively conservative change and did not appear to affect secondary protein structure or critical functional sites, we reasoned that it was not significant in the pathogenesis. In contrast, the H84Y change was nonconservative and protruded into the putative ATP hydrolysis domain of the protein, which is necessary for chaperonin substrate refolding. Although this seemed reasonable, it may not be correct.

The confirmation of *MKKS* as the causative gene for MKS was based on a sporadic neonatal case born while the positional cloning efforts were under way. This child had hydrometrocolpos and congenital heart disease and was a *MKKS* compound heterozygote for Y37C and 2111–2112delGG. We concluded that *MKKS* mutations cause the MKS phenotype, although in retrospect this was partially flawed, as will be seen from the following discussion of age-dependant BBS features.

Following the determination that mutations in *MKKS* cause MKS, we turned to the issue of the patients who had a diagnosis change from MKS to BBS. We reasoned that some of these patients might also harbor mutations in *MKKS*, even though we agreed that the most appropriate diagnosis was BBS. At that time it was known that BBS mapped to five loci, although none of those loci were associated with identified genes (Sheffield et al., 2001). In addition to those five loci, it was also recognized that some families (<10%) were not linked to any of the five known loci. To test that hypothesis, we screened 35 sporadic or unlinked BBS patients/families for mutations in *MKKS*. As predicted, about 10% of the cases had mutations in *MKKS* (Slavotinek et al., 2000), a result simultaneously demonstrated by others (Katsanis et al., 2000). This provided the first identification of mutations in patients with BBS and was followed soon after by the identification of BBS2 (Nishimura et al., 2001), BBS4 (Mykytyn et al., 2001), and BBS1 (Mykytyn et al., 2002) (see Chapter 108).

Taking all known cases there are 22 known sequence alterations in the *MKKS* gene (Fig. 83–2), but it has not been established with cer-

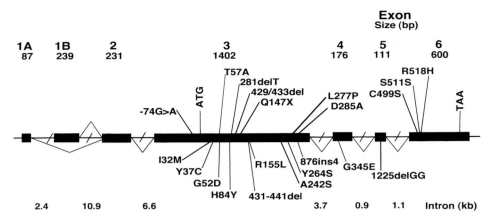

Figure 83–2. The *MKKS* gene, showing six exons with alternative splicing at the 5′ end and 22 mutations that have been described in humans with either the McKusick-Kaufman or the Bardet-Biedl syndrome.

tainty that all of these alterations are pathogenic (Beales et al., 2001; Katsanis et al., 2000, 2001; Slavotinek et al., 2000, 2002; Stone et al., 2000). In addition, there does not appear to be a correlation of the position of these mutations and functional domains of the protein as the mutations are scattered. Only A242S and Y37C have been observed in more than one unrelated family. These mutations include nonsense and missense mutations and small insertions and deletions. Interestingly, we and others noted that there were a large number of patients for whom only one mutation in *MKKS* could be identified. This implied that heterozygous mutations in *MKKS* might contribute to the phenotype when other BBS mutations are identified. This is discussed further in the section on pathogenesis.

COUNSELING AND TREATMENT

Insofar as MKS is concerned, the disorder is inherited as an incompletely penetrant disorder with variable expressivity in an autosomal recessive pattern. Therefore, siblings of an affected child are at a maximum risk of 25% to have a component of the MKS phenotype. However, the real challenge is to determine if the child is affected by MKS or BBS. In many cases this may take several years of careful monitoring including electroretinograms. Readers are referred to the BBS chapter for additional information on this issue (Chapter 108). Mutation analysis of the *MKKS* gene is currently available only on a research basis.

Infants with hydrometrocolpos may require urgent, and in some cases, intensive care. Decompression of the mass and definitive correction of the urogenital anomalies that may accompany the hydrometrocolpos (most commonly fistulae) can be complex. There has been a significant frequency of reproductive limitations in affected Amish women, although those who are currently of reproductive age were operated on two to three decades ago. Current techniques and rapid recognition of the lesion may lead to better reproductive outcome for these children. The CHD can range from simple septal defects to atrioventricular canals that require major cardiac surgery. The polydactyly is most commonly postaxial and straightforward to treat. Duplicated fingers are usually removed in the first year of life. Surgery can be delayed or deferred if the toe duplications do not impede ambulation or shoe fitment. Some patients with MKS have insertional polydactyly, which can be more difficult to repair and should optimally be undertaken by surgeons who have experience with this and other complex hand malformations.

DEVELOPMENTAL PATHOGENESIS

There are few data on which to base a model of the developmental pathogenesis of MKS. What we need to explain are the following attributes of the gene: autosomal recessive inheritance, variable expressivity, incomplete penetrance, ubiquitous gene expression with a limited phenotype, and the possible role of a chaperonin in human development. Furthermore, the anomalies of MKS are not synchronous; polydactyly and septal heart defects most likely occur within 35 to 42

days in utero, whereas perforation of the uterovaginal plate occurs later in development, after the 12th week. That MKS is allelic to one form of BBS must also be explained, with the consequent association of additional malformations and age-dependent features of retinal degeneration, diabetes, and so on. What we know about the gene is limited. It is similar in sequence and predicted secondary structure to a group II chaperonin. Chaperonins function to properly fold nascent proteins as they come off the ribosome or refold them if they become denatured by thermal or other stresses. Chaperonins are one branch of a pathway that folds salvageable proteins, whereas unsalvageable proteins are degraded by the ubiqitination–proteasome system. Other chaperones function to fold nascent protein chains as they extend from the ribosome complex.

Taking these factors into account, a simple model would place the MKKS chaperonin at a point in a developmental cascade where its function may be to salvage or package critical developmental proteins and protect them from environmental stresses. This model allows for the asynchrony of the developmental phenotype and is an attractive candidate for a phenotype that should be highly variable or nonpenetrant. The phenotypic overlap of MKS with BBS, Pallister-Hall syndrome (Chapter 20), and other developmental disorders suggests that some of the gene products associated with those phenotypes may be substrates for the MKKS chaperonin. In this model, MKKS would function as a buffer for environmental stressors such as pH or thermal insults that would typically disrupt the normal control of gene transcription. This model is especially appealing in that it accounts for the extreme phenotypic variation of these disorders, including nonpenetrance (e.g., in fetuses who are not exposed to such stressors). The discovery that MKKS is involved in the BBS phenotype provides another potentially exciting possibility. If MKKS functions as a chaperone, it suggests that some of the age-related features of BBS are related to the accumulated inability of the chaperone to rescue misfolded or unfolded proteins. Age-dependent manifestations of BBS include learning difficulties, obesity, cystic degenerative renal disease, and retinal degeneration. It is possible that these phenotypic manifestations are attributable to chaperone failure, and it suggests that there may be avenues to intervene to delay the onset of these manifestations in BBS. More generally, it suggests that nonsyndromic obesity, retinal degeneration, learning disability, and renal disease may share this pathogenetic mechanism.

Another potential model is that the MKKS protein may function as a transcription factor chaperone analagous to the function of the p23 chaperone in endocrine signaling (Freeman and Yamamoto, 2002). In this model, MKKS would participate in developmental gene regulation by affecting the disruption of transcription factor complexes. It is intriguing to speculate that MKKS may interact with the GLI3 transcription factor in this manner and that this interaction underlies the overlapping phenotypes of MKS, BBS, and Pallister-Hall syndrome. It is also possible that MKKS has structural similarity to chaperones but no functional similarity. If this is the case, it is extremely difficult to predict a model of gene action.

An intriguing hypothesis has been proposed to explain the lack of penetrance in BBS and the finding of many patients who have only a single *MKKS* mutation. It has been proposed that BBS can be considered to be a triallelic disorder where phenotype penetrance requires mutations in three alleles of two of the several BBS genes (Katsanis et al., 2001). This model is attractive in that it explains several observations but does not explain the observation that, at least for Amish MKS and most cases of BBS, a 25% of risk recurrence is observed. However, selection bias may be responsible for this as small families with single cases may be underascertained. The triallelic model also does not explain why five BBS loci were successfully mapped using a parametric recessive model. A related conception of the disorder centers on the variable expressivity to propose that a number of the BBS loci, and perhaps other loci as well, may function as modifiers of mutations in other loci. The *MKKS* gene product is a very attractive candidate for a modifier given its putative biological function as a chaperonin. It is easy to envision that alterations in a chaperonin can modify other mutant alleles, and this has been shown for a number of metabolic disorders (reviewed in Slavotinek and Biesecker, 2001).

REFERENCES

Agarwala R, Biesecker LG, Hopkins KA, Francomano CA, Schäffer AA (1998). Software for constructing and verifying pedigrees within large genealogies and an application to the Old Order Amish of Lancaster County. *Genome Res* 8: 211–221.

Agarwala R, Schäffer AA, Tomlin JF (2001). Towards a complete North American Anabaptist genealogy II: analysis of inbreeding. *Hum Biol* 73: 533–545.

Beales P, Elioglu N, Woolf A, Parker D, Flinter F (1999). New criteria for improved diagnosis of Bardet-Biedl syndrome: results of a population survey. *J Med Genet* 36: 437–446.

Beales P, Katsanis N, Lewis RA, Ansley SJ, Elcioglu N, Raza J, Woods MO, Green JS, Parfrey PS, Davidson WS, Lupski JR (2001). Genetic and mutational analyses of a large multiethnic Bardet-Biedl cohort reveal a minor involvement of BBS6 and delineate the critical intervals of other loci. *Am J Hum Genet* 68: 606–616.

David A, Bitoun P, Lacombe D, Lambert JC, Nivelon A, Vigneron J, Verloes A (1999). Hydrometrocolpos and polydactyly: a common neonatal presentation of Bardet-Biedl and McKusick-Kaufman syndromes. *J Med Genet* 36: 599–603.

Freeman BC, Yamamoto KR (2002). Disassembly of transcriptional regulatory complexes by molecular chaperones. *Science* 296: 2232–2235.

Katsanis N, Beales PL, Woods MO, Lewis RA, Green JS, Parfrey PS, Ansley SJ, David-son WS, Lupski JR (2000). Mutations in MKKS cause obesity, retinal dystrophy and renal malformations associated with Bardet-Biedl syndrome. *Nat Genet* 26: 67–70.

Katsanis N, Ansley SJ, Badano JL, Eichers ER, Lewis RA, Hoskins BE, Scambler PJ, Davidson WS, Beales PL, Lupski JR (2001). Triallelic inheritance in Bardet-Biedl syndrome, a Mendelian recessive disorder. *Science* 293: 2256–2259.

Kaufman RL, Hartmann AF, McAlister WH (1972). Family studies in congenital heart disease, II: a syndrome of hydrometrocolpos, postaxial polydactyly and congenital heart disease. *Birth Defects Orig Artic Ser* 8: 85–87.

Lander ES, Linton LM, Birren B, Nusbaum C, Zody MC, Baldwin J, Devon K, Dewar K, Doyle M, FitzHugh W, et al. (2001). Initial sequencing and analysis of the human genome. *Nature* 409: 860–921.

Lurie IW, Wulfsberg EA (1994). The McKusick-Kaufman syndrome: phenotypic variation observed in familial cases as a clue for the evaluation of sporadic cases. *Genet Couns* 5: 275–281.

McKusick VA, Bauer RL, Koop CE, Scott RB (1964). Hydrometrocolpos as a simply inherited malformation. *JAMA* 189: 813–816.

Mykytyn K, Braun T, Carmi R, Haider NB, Searby CC, Shastri M, Beck G, Wright AF, Iannaccone A, Elbedour K, et al. (2001). Identification of the gene that, when mutated, causes the human obesity syndrome BBS4. *Nat Genet* 28: 188–191.

Mykytyn K, Nishimura DY, Searby CC, Shastri M, Yen HJ, Beck JS, Braun T, Streb LM, Cornier AS, Cox GF, et al. (2002). Identification of the gene (BBS1) most commonly involved in Bardet-Biedl syndrome, a complex human obesity syndrome. *Nat Genet* 31(4): 435–438.

Nishimura DY, Searby CC, Carmi R, Elbedour K, Van Maldergem L, Fulton AB, Lam BL, Powell BR, Swiderski RE, Bugge KE, et al. (2001). Positional cloning of a novel gene on chromosome 16q causing Bardet-Biedl syndrome (BBS2). *Hum Mol Genet* 10: 865–874.

Sheffield VC, Nishimura D, Stone EM (2001). The molecular genetics of Bardet-Biedl syndrome. *Curr Opin Genet Dev* 11: 317–321.

Slavotinek A, Biesecker L (2001). Unfolding the role of chaperones and chaperonins in human disease. *Trends Genet* 17: 528–535.

Slavotinek A, Stone E, Mykytyn K, Heckenlively J, Green J, Heon E, Musarella M, Parfrey P, Sheffield V, Biesecker L (2000). Mutations in *MKKS* cause Bardet-Biedl syndrome. *Nat Genet* 26: 15–16.

Slavotinek A, Mykytyn K, Searby C, Al-Gazali L, Hennekam R, Schrander-Stumpel C, Orcana-Losa M, Pardo-Reoyo S, Kumar D, Cantani A, et al. (2002). Mutation analysis of the MKKS gene in McKusik-Kaufman and Bardet-Biedl syndrome patients. *Hum Genet* 110: 561–567.

Stone D, Agarwala R, Schäffer AA, Weber JL, Vaske D, Oda T, Chandrasekharappa SC, Francomano CA, Biesecker LG (1998). Genetic and physical mapping of the McKusick-Kaufman syndrome. *Hum Mol Genet* 7: 475–481.

Stone D, Slavotinek A, Bouffard G, Banerjee-Basu S, Baxevanis A, Barr M, Biesecker L (2000). Mutations of a gene encoding a putative chaperonin causes McKusick-Kaufman syndrome. *Nat Genet* 25: 79–82.

Part D.
Guanine Nucleotide–Binding Proteins

84 | An Introduction to Guanine Nucleotide–Binding Proteins

SARAH E. NEWEY AND LINDA VAN AELST

Guanine nucleotide–binding proteins (GNBPs) regulate a vast array of physiological processes from cell growth and differentiation to sensory perception. There are two major families. First, the small, monomeric GTPases, whose founder member, Ras, is known to be important in regulating cell growth. Second, the heterotrimeric G proteins that are coupled to G protein–coupled receptors (GPCRs) through which many physiological and developmental processes are regulated. These families of proteins act as molecular switches, cycling between an inactive guanosine diphosphate (GDP) bound state and an active guanosine triphosphate (GTP) bound state, transducing extracellular signals to downstream signaling components. Here we give an introduction to the monomeric and heterotrimeric protein superfamilies and consider how these proteins are regulated, the signaling pathways in which they participate, and, ultimately, how these signals from multiple family members are integrated to generate a biological response.

MONOMERIC AND HETEROTRIMERIC G PROTEINS

Many biological signaling molecules must be transiently activated in order to carry out their function. In the case of guanine nucleotide–binding proteins (GNBPs), activation is achieved by the exchange of guanosine diphosphate (GDP) for guanosine triphosphate (GTP). When GTP is bound, the GNBP assumes an active conformation and can bind to "effector" proteins—proteins that transmit the signal to create a particular biological response. However, when it is hydrolyzed to GDP, the protein undergoes a conformational change and is inactivated. Two structurally distinct families of GNBPs use this approach to execute their function as molecular switches in diverse signaling pathways by cycling between GTP and GDP bound states: the monomeric GTP-binding proteins, also known as the small GTPases, and the heterotrimeric guanine nucleotide–binding proteins, or G proteins. Both families of GNBPs are controlled by positive regulators that promote protein activation by exchanging GDP for GTP and also by negative regulators that lead to protein inactivation by catalyzing the hydrolysis of GTP to GDP (Table 84–1 and Fig. 84–1). These important families of proteins participate in many important developmental and physiological processes which, when perturbed, result in disease.

The basic structural unit that performs nucleotide binding and hydrolysis is called the G-domain and is found, in varying forms, in both small GTPases and in the α-subunits of heterotrimeric G proteins (reviewed in Vetter and Wittinghofer, 2001). The basic G-domain is approximately 20 kDa and consists of six β-strands and five α-helices. Heterotrimeric α-subunits, which have a molecular mass of 39 to 45 kDa, have several extensions and insertions to the basic G-domain.

Table 84–1. Comparison of Some Properties of Small and Heterotrimeric G Proteins

Property	Small GTPases	Heterotrimeric G Proteins
Size	Monomeric 20–40 kDa	Trimeric α subunit: 39–46 kDa β subunit: 35 kDa γ subunit: 7.3–8.5 kDa
GTPase activity	Intrinsic GTPase activity	α subunit has intrinsic GTPase activity
Membrane association	Ras, Rho, and Rab proteins are covalently modified with lipids.	α and γ subunits are covalently modified with lipid moieties
Positive regulators	GEFs	GPCRs
Negative regulators	GAPs; GDIs for Rho and Rab	RGS proteins
Major functions	Ras: Cell proliferation; Rho: Cytoskeletal reorganization; Rab: Vesicle trafficking; Sar1/Arf: Vesicle trafficking; Ran: Nucleocytoplasmic transport	$G\alpha_s$: Activates adenylyl cyclase; $G\alpha_i$: Inhibits adenyly cyclase, modulates ion channel activity; $G\alpha_q$: Activates PLCβ; $G\alpha_{12}$: Activates the Rho signaling pathway

GEFs, GDP/GTP exchange factors; GPCRs, G protein–coupled receptors; GDI, GDP dissociation inhibitors; GAPs, GTPase-activating proteins; PLCβ, phospholipase Cβ; RGS, regulators of G protein signaling.

An important structural element for guanine nucleotide binding is provided by the conserved P-loop (or phosphate-binding loop) that lies near the N terminus of the domain.

In order for G proteins to cycle between "on" (GTP-bound) and "off" (GDP-bound) states, a conformational change, or "switch," occurs within the G-domain. The structures of both GTP-bound and GDP-bound states have been elucidated for a number of G proteins, allowing the details of this molecular switch to be determined. Structural differences between the GTP- and GDP-bound states of small GTPases are mainly restricted to two highly flexible surface loops surrounding the γ-phosphate of GTP, known as switch regions I and II. These switch regions were first identified in the small GTPase Ras and form the effector-binding domains (Milburn et al., 1990). The α-subunits of heterotrimeric G proteins use an additional structural element for this transition, called the switch region III. The switch mechanism, which is thought to be common for all G proteins, is described by Vetter and Wittinghofer (2001) as "a loaded spring mechanism where release of the γ-phosphate after GTP hydrolysis allows the switch regions to relax into the GDP-specific conformation." While these structural studies have shown that the switch apparatus is conserved among GNBPs, albeit with modifications, other studies have revealed that the regulators and effectors adopt a variety of structures and means of interacting with different GNBPs.

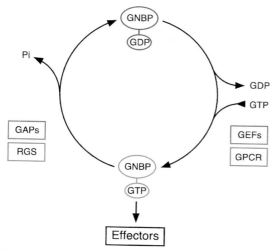

Figure 84–1. Guanine nucleotide–binding proteins (GNBPs) function as molecular switches by cycling between an inactive GDP-bound state (red) and an active GTP-bound state (green). Once in their activated GTP-bound state, GNBPs can stimulate a variety of effector molecules to initiate a biological response. The cycling steps are regulated by positive regulators that promote protein activation—GDP/GTP exchange factors (GEFs) for small GTPases and G protein–coupled receptors (GPCRs) for heterotrimeric G proteins—and also by negative regulators that lead to protein inactivation by catalyzing the hydrolysis of GTP to GDP: GTPase-activating proteins (GAPs) for small GTPases and regulators of G protein signaling (RGS) proteins for heterotrimeric G proteins.

THE SMALL GTPASES

Small GTP-binding proteins are found in all eukaryotes, from yeast to humans, and constitute a protein superfamily that comprises well over 100 members. For the purposes of this chapter we will consider mammalian members of this superfamily, but it should be pointed out that much of the pioneering work on small GTPases was performed in yeast (for reviews see Tamanoi, 1988; Tanaka and Takai, 1998; Arellano et al., 1999; Gotte et al., 2000). Based on structural and functional considerations, the small GTPases can be divided into five subfamilies: Ras, Rho, Rab, Sar1/Arf, and Ran. Ras is the founder member of the small GTPases, and proteins in this subfamily are principally involved in regulating cell growth control (proliferation, senescence, and apoptosis) and differentiation by altering gene expression. Rho family members are best known for their role in remodeling the actin cytoskeleton, but they have many other functions, including regulating gene expression and lipid modification. Members of both the Rab and Sar1/Arf subfamily are involved in regulating intracellular vesicle trafficking, while Ran GTPases shuttle between the nucleus and cytoplasm and regulate nucleo-cytoplasmic transport.

These subfamilies of GTPases utilize an astonishing number of regulator and effector molecules to perform their various functions. Significantly, a number of these regulators and effectors of small GTPases have been implicated in a variety of disease processes, from cancer to mental retardation (Boettner and Van Aelst, 2002). Mutations in several regulatory proteins are also responsible for a number of developmental disorders, such as Aarskog-Scott syndrome, neurofibromatosis type 1, and tuberous sclerosis type 2, which will be discussed in the Chapters 86, 87, and 91. While it is beyond the scope of this section to consider all the small GTPases in detail, we consider some general properties of this protein superfamily, then explore the Ras and Rho subfamilies. In doing this, we use specific examples to illustrate the importance of Ras and Rho proteins as mediators in transducing extracellular signals from the external environment into intracellular responses. For a recent and excellent review of the small GTPases, see Takai et al., (2001).

Distribution of Small GTPases

Small GTPases are widely expressed in mammalian tissues, and most cells express at least some members of the Ras, Rho, Rab, Sar1/Arf, and Ran subfamilies. There are differences however: some small GTPases—such as RhoA, Rac1, and Cdc42—are widely expressed by mammalian cells, whereas others display a more tissue-specific distribution. Rab3A, for example, is expressed in cells that have a regulated secretion pathway, such as neurons, neuroendocrine cells, and exocrine cells (Henry et al., 1996), while Rab17 is detected only in epithelial cells (Lutcke et al., 1993). Within cells, small GTPases are localized throughout, being found in the cytoplasm and being associated with both the plasma membrane and internal membranes. Many small GTPases are also translocated between different intracellular sites. For example, Ran is translocated between the cytoplasm and nucleus via the nuclear pore complex, while Ras and Rho proteins translocate between the cytoplasm and the inner surface of the plasma membrane. These proteins become inserted into the inner surface of the plasma membrane by posttranslational modification with lipid moieties (for review, see Zhang and Casey, 1996; Magee and Marshall, 1999). This is a common feature of small GTPases and is crucial for their activation and biological function.

Regulation of Small GTPases

Small GTPases cycle between two conformational states: an active GTP-bound state and an inactive GDP-bound state. The rate-limiting step of the GDP/GTP exchange is the dissociation of GDP from the inactive state. This step is accelerated by positive regulators called GDP/GTP exchange factors (GEFs), which are activated by upstream signals and facilitate exchange of GDP for GTP. This exchange occurs in a stepwise manner. First, the GEF interacts with the GDP-bound form of the small GTPase, releasing the bound GDP and resulting in a binary complex of nucleotide-free GTPase and GEF. Subsequently, GTP (which is at higher concentration in the cell) replaces the GEF and, in turn, induces a conformational change in the switch regions of the small GTPase. This conformational change enables the small GTPase to interact with one or more downstream effectors. In general, GEFs are specific for a particular subfamily of small GTPases, although there are examples of more promiscuous GEFs that activate multiple family members. For example, Sos is able to activate both Ras and the Rho family member Rac. Each small GTPase subfamily has an associated family of GEFs, which have a characteristic domain responsible for GDP/GTP exchange. GEFs for the Ras proteins contain a Cdc25 domain, while RhoGEFs contain a DH (Dbl homology) domain and ArfGEFs a Sec7 domain (Cherfils and Chardin, 1999). The structures of a number of GEFs have been determined and reveal that the different families of GEFs are not structurally related. However, while the details of the interactions between different subfamilies of small GTPases and their GEFs are all different, the complexes have some similar structural features that suggest underlying mechanistic similarities (Vetter and Wittinghofer, 2001).

The active GTP-bound state of a small GTPase is converted back to its inactive GDP-bound form by the action of negative regulators of GTPase function called GTPase-activating proteins (GAPs). These proteins catalyze the intrinsic ability of a small GTPase to hydrolyze bound GTP to GDP in a reaction that results in the release of bound effectors from the GTPase and halts downstream signaling. As with GEFs, most GAPs are specific for a single GTPase or subfamily of GTPases, and the structures of GAPs for various subfamily GTPases are different (Vetter and Wittinghofer, 2001). Small GTPases of the Rho and Rab subfamilies are also controlled by another class of negative regulators called the GDP-dissociation inhibitors (GDIs) (Olofsson, 1999). GDI proteins bind to and stabilize the GDP-bound form of the GTPase and sequester it in the cytoplasm. These regulators demonstrate a more wide-ranging substrate specificity than either GEFs or GAPs, and both RhoGDIs and RabGDIs are thought to act on most members of their respective subfamilies. A GDI for Ran also has been identified. The nuclear transport factor 2 (NTF2) specifically recognizes the GDP-bound conformation of Ran and recycles it back into the nucleus after a round of import and export involving GTP hydrolysis (Paschal et al., 1996; Yamada et al., 1998).

Thus, small GTPases serve as molecular switches that can be exquisitely controlled by both positive and negative regulators to transduce upstream signals to downstream effectors. In the following sections we use Ras and Rho family members as examples to illustrate the typical structures of small GTPases, their regulation, and their signaling pathways.

Ras Proteins

The viral *H-ras* and *K-ras* oncogenes were the first small GTPases to be identified as the transforming elements of the Harvey and Kirsten strains of rat sarcoma viruses. Interest in these genes was fueled by the discovery that mutations in cellular *ras* genes were present in many human tumors. Indeed, activating mutations in three cellular *ras* genes (*H-ras, K-ras,* and *N-ras*) have been detected in approximately 30% of all human cancers, demonstrating the importance of this gene family in carcinogenesis (reviewed in Bos, 1989). Many other Ras family members have been subsequently identified, such as Ral, Rap, Rit, Rin,

and Rad, but for purposes of this chapter we consider the regulators, effectors, and signaling pathways of the three classic Ras proteins.

K-Ras, N-Ras, and H-Ras are three highly related small GTPases of approximately 189 amino acids. K-Ras exists in two isoforms, A and B, which are generated by alternative splicing (Barbacid, 1987). The N-terminal region of these proteins, consisting of the first 86 amino acids, is 100% identical among the Ras proteins. This region contains the Ras effector-binding domain, which creates the binding site for all known downstream targets of Ras. The following 80 amino acids of the Ras proteins diverge slightly from each other and, together, these two N-terminal regions comprise the critical G-domain important for nucleotide binding and intrinsic GTPase activity. The C-terminal sequence is known as the hypervariable region and shows no sequence similarity between the Ras proteins, with the exception of the CAAX box at the extreme C terminus (CAAX: C, cysteine; A, aliphatic amino acid; X, methionine or serine residue). This sequence is posttranslationally modified to aid the insertion of Ras proteins into the cytoplasmic face of the plasma membrane—an essential step for Ras signaling and function. (Reviewed in Magee and Marshall, 1999; Bar-Sagi, 2001; Prior and Hancock, 2001.)

Activation and Regulation of Ras

Ras proteins are now well known for their role in processing extracellular signals concerned with cell growth, proliferation, survival, and differentiation. Ras is transiently activated by a wide range of extracellular signals that include growth factors, cytokines, hormones, and neurotransmitters that act on receptors that may be either receptor tyrosine kinases (RTKs) (for example the epidermal growth factor receptor [EGFR]), receptors that are associated with non-receptor tyrosine kinases (for example the T-cell antigen receptor), or GPCRs that couple to heterotrimeric G proteins (for example the β-adrenergic receptor). In the best understood case, stimulated RTKs bind adapter proteins and, in turn, recruit a RasGEF from the cytoplasm to create a membrane-associated receptor-adaptor-GEF complex. The GEF is able to activate membrane-associated Ras by converting it from its inactive GDP-bound form to its active GTP-bound form. Activated Ras, like all GTPases, is deactivated to its GDP-bound form by the action of GAPs. A number of GEFs and GAPs for H-Ras, N-Ras, and K-Ras have now been characterized, and we review some examples here.

RasGEFs. The first RasGEF to be identified was the Cdc25 protein in the yeast *S. cerevisiae* (Camonis et al., 1986; Broek et al., 1987; Robinson et al., 1987). The catalytic domains of all other Ras subfamily GEFs are similar in amino acid sequence to Cdc25 and contain the Cdc25 homology domain. Subsequently, this domain has been found in at least a dozen mammalian proteins, and three major classes of RasGEFs have been described: Sos, RasGRFs and RasGRP/CalDAGs. The first of these, Sos (Son of Sevenless), was originally identified in *Drosophila* and was shown in genetic studies to be downstream of Sevenless, a receptor tyrosine kinase that is homologous to the EGF receptor in mammals (Rogge et al., 1991; Simon et al., 1991). Mammalian cells contain two highly related Sos proteins, Sos1 and Sos2 (Bowtell et al., 1992; Chardin et al., 1993). In addition to the Cdc25 domain, both SosGEFs contain proline-rich clusters at their C termini that interact with the Src homology 3 (SH3) domain of the adaptor protein Grb2. The interaction of Sos with the Grb2/(Shc) adaptor complex localizes Sos to the membrane in response to RTK activation where it can efficiently activate Ras (Li et al., 1993; Aronheim et al., 1994; Ravichandran et al., 1995; reviewed in Downward, 1996). Sos1 and Sos2 also contain a DH domain in tandem with a pleckstrin homology (PH) domain, a module that is responsible for GEF activity on Rho GTPases (see section "Activation and Regulation of Rho, Rac, and Cdc 42" following; see also Nimnual et al., 1998). Recent work has shown that Sos1 is a bifunctional GEF and can activate both Ras and Rac (a member of the Rho family). The activation of a specific GTPase appears to depend on the interactions of Sos1: when it is associated with Grb2, Ras is activated, but when it is associated in a tricomplex with two SH3-containing signaling proteins, E3b1 and Eps8, then Rac is stimulated (Scita et al., 2001; Innocenti et al., 2002).

The second major class of RasGEFs includes RasGRF1 (also referred to as Cdc25Mm) (Cen et al., 1992; Shou et al., 1992) and Ras-GRF2 (Fam et al., 1997). Structurally, these are very similar proteins that contain an ilimaquione (IQ) motif that is regulated by Ca^{2+}-bound calmodulin, allowing them to be activated by elevated Ca^{2+} levels (Farnsworth et al., 1995). RasGRF2 is widely expressed (Fam et al., 1997). Meanwhile, RasGRF1 is brain-specific (Shou et al., 1992), is thought to function downstream of heterotrimeric G proteins (Shou et al., 1995; Mattingly and Macara, 1996; Zippel et al., 1996), and can also be activated by phosphorylation (Mattingly and Macara, 1996; Kiyono et al., 2000). RasGRF1 and 2 also contain tandem DH–PH domains that enable them to activate both Rac and Ras (Fan et al., 1998; Kiyono et al., 1999).

The most recent family of RasGEFs to be identified are the Ras-GRP/CalDAG proteins that are regulated by diacylglycerol (DAG) and Ca^{2+}. Three members of this family have been cloned: RasGRP/CalDAG-GEFII (Ebinu et al., 1998; Tognon et al., 1998), CalDAG-GEFI (Kedra et al., 1997; Kawasaki et al., 1998) and an alternatively spliced form called RasGRP2 (Clyde-Smith et al., 2000), and CalDAG-GEFIII (Yamashita et al., 2000). Each posseses EF hands and C1 domains, and are regulated by either Ca^{2+} or DAG, or both. CalDAG-GEFI and II are enriched in the brain, whereas CalDAG-GEFIII is found in glial cells and the kidney.

RasGAPs. Four types of mammalian Ras-specific GAPs have been identified, including p120RasGAP (Trahey and McCormick, 1987), neurofibromin (NF-1) (Xu et al., 1990), SynGAP (Chen et al., 1998; Kim et al., 1998) and the GAP1 family (Cullen et al., 1995). The p120RasGAP and NF1 have received the most attention over the past few years. p120RasGAP acts as a negative regulator of H-Ras, K-ras, and N-Ras (Trahey and McCormick, 1987; Gibbs et al., 1988) and is composed of an N-terminal region that contains two SH2 domains flanking an SH3 domain, a central region that contains a PH domain and a C2 domain, and a C-terminal RasGAP domain. C2 domains are thought to be involved in Ca^{2+}-dependent phospholipid binding, and there is evidence that the C2 domain of p120RasGAP binds to annexin VI, a Ca^{2+}-dependent phospholipid and membrane-binding protein (Davis et al., 1996). It has been suggested that the annexin VI–GAP interaction may play a role in the ability of p120RasGAP to translocate to the membrane in response to increased intracellular Ca^{2+}. p120RasGAP is phosphorylated by a number of tyrosine kinases (Molloy et al., 1989; Ellis et al., 1990) and actually forms a complex with activated platelet-derived growth factor (PDGF) receptors, although the functional relevance of this association is unclear (Kaplan et al., 1990; Kazlauskas et al., 1990). Mutations in the gene that encodes NF1 are responsible for neurofibromatosis type 1, a common familial tumor disposition syndrome that affects 1 in 3500 individuals worldwide (Gutmann, 2001). Our current understanding of the molecular mechanisms that underlie neurofibromatisis type 1 and the regulation and function of NF1 are discussed in Chapter 87.

The more recently discovered GAP1 family comprises GAP1[IP4BP] (Cullen et al., 1995), GAP1m (Maekawa et al., 1994), RASAL (Allen et al., 1998b), and CAPRI (Ca^{2+}-promoted Ras inactivator) (Lockyer et al., 2001), all of which share four conserved structural motifs: Tandem C2 domains, a RasGAP domain, a PH domain, and a Bruton's tyrosine kinase (Btk) motif (reviewed in Cullen, 1998). These molecules associate with the plasma membrane in order to inactivate Ras. Whereas the C2 domains of CAPRI have been shown to mediate Ca^{2+}-dependent-membrane binding and an associated increase in GAP activity (Lockyer et al., 2001), the C2 domains of GAP1[IP4BP] and GAP1m are missing key Ca^{2+}-binding residues and do not regulate Ca^{2+}-mediated membrane association. Instead, membrane targeting is achieved via the PH domains (Nalefski and Falke, 1996; Lockyer et al., 1999), and the GAP activities of GAP1m and GAP1[IP4BP] are stimulated by the heterotrimeric G protein subunit $G\alpha_{12}$ and inositol 1,3,4,5, tetrakisphosphate (IP_4), respectively (Cullen et al., 1995; Jiang et al., 1998).

SynGAP is a brain-specific RasGAP that was identified by its association with the PDZ domains of PSD-95 and SAP102, components of the postsynaptic density (PSD) (Kim et al., 1998) and also during a screen to identify targets of Ca^{2+}/calmodulin-dependent protein ki-

nase II (CAMKII) in rat PSDs (Chen et al., 1998). In addition to the RasGAP domain, SynGAP contains a PH domain and a C2 domain at the N terminus, suggesting that like some of the other RasGAPs, it may respond to changes in Ca^{2+} or phospholipid second messengers. It is highly enriched at excitatory synapses where it is present in a large macromolecular complex with PSD-95 and NMDA receptors and has been suggested to be an important modulator of these proteins (Chen et al., 1998).

Effectors of Ras and Biological Responses to Ras Signaling

Signaling via Ras is now known to control diverse signaling pathways for cell growth, differentiation, and apoptosis. The best characterized Ras effectors and their associated downstream pathways include the kinases Raf and phosphatidylinositol-3 kinase (PI3K) and the family of GEFs for the Ras-related protein Ral (RalGEFs).

One of the primary Ras-dependent pathways in mammalian cells involves the activation of a series of protein kinases: Raf protein kinases (c-raf-1, A-Raf, and B-Raf), MAP kinase kinases 1 and 2 (MAPKK, also known as MEK1 and MEK2) and the p42/p44 MAP kinases (MAPK, also known as ERK1 and ERK2, for extracellular signal–related kinase). This pathway is crucial for Ras's effect on cell proliferation and mediates the transforming effect of oncogenic Ras on many mammalian cells. GTP-bound Ras activates this cascade in response to RTK activation by binding directly to Raf proteins that are recruited from the cytoplasm to the plasma membrane (Moodie et al., 1993; Van Aelst et al., 1993; Vojtek et al., 1993; Warne et al., 1993; Zhang et al., 1993). Raf, a serine/threonine kinase, is activated by a multistep process that involves Ras and other accessory molecules such as 14-3-3, a specific phosphoserine-binding protein (reviewed in Campbell et al., 1998). Once activated, Raf proteins bind to, and phosphorylate, MAPKK 1 and 2 (Dent et al., 1992; Kyriakis et al., 1992), which function as dual-specificity kinases, phosphorylating tandem threonine and tyrosine residues in two MAPKs. Activated MAPKs then translocate to the nucleus, where they phosphorylate and activate a number of transcription factors, including Elk-1, that are required for entry into S phase of the cell cycle (reviewed in Marshall, 1999).

While the Raf/MAPK pathway was the first signaling cascade downstream of Ras to be identified in mammalian cells, it became clear that this was unlikely to be the sole pathway used by Ras to mediate its effects on cell proliferation and differentiation. Direct evidence for the involvement of multiple downstream pathways came from the identification of Ras effector domain mutants that were defective in their associations with Raf, but were able to produce a growth-transformed phenotype (White et al., 1995; Khosravi-Far et al., 1996). These mutants, H-Ras(12V,37G) and H-Ras(12V,40C) no longer activate Raf-1 or MAPKs but are able to activate the RalGEFs or PI3K pathways, respectively.

The phosphoinositide 3-kinases (PI3Ks) are lipid serine/threonine kinases that are important effectors of Ras and are activated by a number of growth factors and cytokines. Multiple isoforms of PI3K can associate with Ras, including members of class 1A and 1B PI3Ks (Rodriguez-Viciana et al., 1997; Wymann and Pirola, 1998). The first PI3K to be isolated and cloned was a heterodimeric complex made up of a p85 regulatory subunit and a p110 catalytic subunit (Kapeller and Cantley, 1994). Ras binds directly to the p110 catalytic subunit to stimulate its lipid kinase activity (Rodriguez-Viciana et al., 1994). The major activity of these kinases is the conversion of phosphatidylinositol (4,5)-bisphosphate (PIP_2) to phophatidylinositol (3,4,5)-triphosphate (PIP_3), which, in turn, activates the serine/threonine kinase Akt/PKB (protein kinase B). There are now a growing number of target proteins for Akt/PKB's kinase activity, many of which contribute to promotion of cell survival and the prevention of apoptosis (reviewed in Downward, 1998; Khwaja, 1999; Brazil and Hemmings, 2001).

PI3K can also activate the Rho GTPase family member Rac, which is an important mediator of actin reorganization and an important downstream effector of Ras function (reviewed in Van Aelst and D'Souza-Schorey, 1997). PI3K-dependent activation of Rac has been shown to mediate growth factor–induced membrane ruffles, as well as Ras-mediated transformation. In mammals, PI3K is thought to activate Rac by regulating at least two RacGEFs—Vav and Sos1 (Han et al., 1998; Nimnual et al., 1998). Activation of these GEFs is thought to occur through binding of PIP₃ (a product of PI3K) to the PH domains of Vav and Sos1.

A third set of effectors for Ras are a family of GEFs for the ras-related GTPases RalA and RalB (Albright et al., 1993). Ral-specific GEFs—including RalGDS, RGL/Rsb2, and RGL2/Rif—are activated by GTP-bound Ras at the plasma membrane, which, in turn, stimulates Ral (reviewed by Wolthuis and Bos, 1999). A number of potential downstream effectors of Ral GTPases have been identified, although their significance in relation to Ras signaling remains to be demonstrated. Activated, GTP-bound Ral proteins can bind to RalBP1 (also known as RLIP1/RIP1), a putative GAP for Cdc42 and Rac GTPases (Cantor et al., 1995; Park and Weinberg, 1995). RalA can also bind to phospholipase D1 (PLD) and enhance its activation by the small GTPase Arf, suggesting that Ral has a scaffolding or targeting role in PLD activation (Jiang et al., 1995; Luo et al., 1998). PLD catalyses the conversion of phosphatidylcholine (PC) to phosphatidic acid (PA) and can also be activated by RhoA. Finally, RalA is thought to influence the actin cytoskeleton by associating with the actin-binding protein filamin, thus contributing to the formation of filopodia (Ohta et al., 1999).

As we have seen, activation of Ras can result in the stimulation of a number of downstream signaling cascades. It has become apparent through the study of Ras in different cell lines that a range of cellular responses can be elicited, depending on the effector pathways activated and the cell type involved. Activated Ras can promote anti-apoptotic or pro-apoptotic responses, it can result in transformation in some and growth inhibition in others, or it can drive differentiation of certain cell types while blocking differentiation in others. In most instances, the specific action of Ras activation in a particular cell type is the result of cooperative actions of multiple effectors or the ratio of activity on the effector pathways. A number of other potential Ras effectors have been reported, including Rin1, an Abl-interacting protein (Han and Colicelli, 1995) that is also a GEF for the Rab family member Rab5 (Tall et al., 2001), the novel protein Nore1 (Vavvas et al., 1998), and a novel Ras-regulated phospholipase C (PLCε) (Cullen, 2001). It appears that the hunt for Ras effectors is not over, but it will be important to determine the physiological relevance of these potential effectors with respect to Ras function and signaling.

The Rho GTPases

There are approximately 20 proteins belonging to the Rho subfamily of small GTPases in mammals, although three members—RhoA (Ras homologous member A), Rac1 (Ras-related C3 botulinum toxin substrate 1), and Cdc42 (cell division cycle 42)—have received by far the most attention. Like Ras family members, these molecules (which will be referred to as Rho, Rac, and Cdc42) regulate signal transduction from cell surface receptors to intracellular effectors and are post-translationally modified by lipid prenylation in order to target these proteins to the plasma membrane (Seabra, 1998). Rho, Rac, and Cdc42 have been shown to function in a diverse array of physiological processes, including cell polarity, cell motility, cytokinesis, cell–cell and cell–matrix adhesion, and cell transformation and invasion. Underlying these effects on cell behavior are the action of Rho GTPases in signaling pathways that regulate actin cytoskeletal reorganization, microtubule dynamics, transcriptional activation, and membrane trafficking. It is now clear that Rho GTPases activate multiple effectors, and it is likely that the coordinated activation of downstream pathways ultimately generates a specific cellular response or behavior (Ridley, 2001a). A large number of regulators (GEFs, GAPs, and GDIs) and effectors for Rho, Rac, and Cdc42 have been identified; although in many cases their mechanism of action has been elucidated, we still have much to learn as to how these molecules are functionally integrated.

Activation and Regulation of Rho, Rac, and Cdc42

Rho GTPases are stimulated in response to the activation of a variety of cell surface receptors, including growth factor receptors, cytokine receptors, GPCRs, and cell-to-cell or extracellular matrix-to-cell adhesion receptors (integrins). In the case of Rho activation, ligands such

as lysophosphatidic acid (LPA), bombesin, and thrombin, which all act through GPCRs, have been most extensively studied (reviewed in Seasholtz et al., 1999). GPCR-independent activation of Rho can also occur, notably through cytokine receptors for TNF-α and IL1. Rac, meanwhile, is activated by tyrosine kinase receptors, including those that are activated by insulin, PDGF, and epidermal growth factor (EGF) (Ridley et al., 1992). No direct link between these receptors and Rac has been documented, but there are several reports implicating PI3K and Src-family kinases in this step. Other activators of Rac include the chemoattractant formyl-methionyl-leucyl-phenylalanine (fMLP) which acts through the heterotrimeric G protein α-subunit Gαᵢ, and bombesin (Ridley et al., 1992; Benard et al., 1999; Kjoller and Hall, 1999). Less is known about how Cdc42 is activated. fMLP working through Gαᵢ has been shown to activate Cdc42, as well as bradykinin, although how this is achieved in unclear (Kozma et al., 1995; Benard et al., 1999). More recent studies have demonstrated that the Rho GTPase activities can be regulated by adhesion receptors, including integrins and cadherins (reviewed in Kjoller and Hall, 1999; Anastasiadis and Reynolds, 2001).

In Swiss 3T3 fibroblasts, a model that has been used extensively to study the effects of Rho GTPases on actin cytoskeletal dynamics, it appears that the activation of the Rho GTPases occurs in a hierarchical cascade in which Cdc42 activates Rac1, which, in turn, activates RhoA (Nobes and Hall, 1995; Hall, 1998). Although the exact molecular links between these small GTPases are poorly understood, they are likely to involve the action of GEFs. In other systems, it appears that crosstalk between the Rho GTPases is more complex. For example, in assays of neurite outgrowth, a mutual antagonism between Cdc42/Rac and Rho has been reported (reviewed in Luo, 2000). Furthermore, in epithelial cells, Rac signaling has been demonstrated to antagonize the activity of Rho, and the reciprocal balance between Rac and Rho activity appears to determine the cell morphology and migratory behavior of these cells (reviewed in Evers et al., 2000).

RhoGEFs. GEFs for the Rho GTPases make up one of the largest families of signaling molecules and outnumber the Rho family proteins (Table 84–2). The reason for so many RhoGEFs is not obvious, but it is consistent with the idea that activation of different combinations of Rho GTPases are designed to produce cell type–specific or signal-specific effects, or both (Ridley, 2001a). All Rho family GEFs contain a DH domain in tandem with a PH domain, which creates the structural module responsible for catalyzing the GDP/GTP exchange reaction. The DH domain was first identified in the Dbl oncogene product (Ron et al., 1991). Subsequently, Dbl was shown to exchange GDP for GTP on human Cdc42, and by deletion analysis it was found that the DH domain was essential for this activity, as well as to induce cellular transformation (Hart et al., 1991; Ron et al., 1991; Hart and Roberts, 1994). The PH domain, which resides at the immediate C terminus of the DH domain, is found in all Dbl family members and appears to be essential for the correct localization of the RhoGEF at the plasma membrane (Zheng et al., 1996). The PH domain can also act as an autoinhibitor of the DH domain in several GEFs such as Vav and Sos. Only when the PH domain binds to phosphoinositides in the plasma membrane is the inhibition on the DH domain relieved (Han et al., 1998; Nimnual et al., 1998).

As their numbers may suggest, members of the RhoGEF family display a wide spectrum of activities and expression profiles (see Table 84–2). Many RhoGEFs have other domains in addition to the DH–PH module that is responsible for GEF activity. Thus, many are likely to be multifunctional proteins that have GEF-independent functions. Identifying these additional functions and establishing how they relate to Rho GTPase signaling pathways will be important in understanding the overall regulation and function of RhoGEFs (Zheng, 2001).

Many RhoGEFs exist in an inactive state in the cell and require stimulation to promote translocation of the GEF to the plasma membrane and stimulation of GEF activity. As alluded to earlier in this chapter, this upstream activating signal may be provided by activation of heterotrimeric G proteins, activation by another upstream Rho GTPase, activation by protein tyrosine or serine/threonine kinases and/or phosphoinositol lipids (reviewed in Zheng, 2001). For instance, the

Table 84–2. GEFs, GAPs, and GDIs for the Rho GTPases Rho, Rac, and Cdc42

Regulator	Rho GTPase Substrates	Disease Involvement and Biological Properties
GEFs		
Abr	Rho, Rac, Cdc42	Widely expressed; highest levels in brain
Alsin	Unknown	Mutations cause amyotrophic lateral sclerosis 2
ARHGEF3 and ARHGEF4	Unknown	ARHGEF4 is restricted to brain
ARHGEF6/Pix/Cool	Rac	Mutations cause nonspecific X-linked mental retardation
Asef	Rac	Binds to and is activated by the tumor supressor APC
Bcr	Rho, Rac, Cdc42	Bcr-abl fusion responsible for chronic myelogenous leukemia
Clg	Cdc42	Implicated in mouse and human cancers
Collybistin	Unknown	Brain specific; interacts with gephyrin
Dbl	Rho, Rac, Cdc42	Transforming potential; implicated in diffuse B-cell lymphoma
Dbs/Ost	Rho, Cdc42	Transforming potential; binds Rac
Ect2	Rho, Rac, Cdc42	Transforming potential; involved in cytokinesis
Ephexin	Rho > Cdc42 > Rac	Involved in axon guidance; transforming potential
FGD1	Cdc42	Mutations result in faciogenital dysplasia, or Aarskog-Scott syndrome
FGD2, FGD3	Unknown	Possible role in embryonic development
Frabin	Cdc42	Involved in cytoskeletal reorganization; binds actin
GEF337	Rho	Promotes stress fiber formation
GEF720	Rho	Brain specific
GEF-H1	Rac, Rho	Associated with microtubules
hPEM-2	Cdc42	Highly expressed in brain
Intersectin-1	Cdc42	Component of endocytic machinery; implicated in Down syndrome
Intersectin-2	Cdc42	Involved in T cell receptor endocytosis; binds WASP
Kalirin	Rac, Rho	Involved in neurite outgrowth and morphology
LARG	Rho	Implicated in acute myeloid leukemia; interacts with $G\alpha_{12}$ and $G\alpha_{13}$
Lbc/Brx/Ht31	Rho	Transforming potential; binds to nuclear hormone receptor and $G\alpha_q$; acts as a protein kinase A anchoring protein
Lfc	Rho	Binds Rac; localizes to microtubules; transforming potential
Net1	Rho	Transforming potential
p114RhoGEF	Rho	Unknown
p115RhoGEF/Lsc	Rho	Transforming potential; GAP for $G\alpha_{12}$ and $G\alpha_{13}$
p190RhoGEF	Rho	Inhibits neurite outgrowth and binds to microtubules
PDZ-RhoGEF/KIAA0380/GTRAP48	Rho	Interacts with $G\alpha_{12}$ and $G\alpha_{13}$
Ras GRF1/RasGRF2	Rac, Ras	Activates both Rac and Ras
Sos1, Sos2	Rac, Ras	Activates both Rac and Ras
Stef	Rac	Required for neurite outgrowth
Tiam-1	Rac	Implicated in T-cell lymphoma and renal cell carcinoma
Tiam-2	Rac	Unknown
Tim	Unknown	Transforming potential
Trio	RhoA, RhoG, Rac1	Two DH-PH domains with distinct specificities for Rac and Rho; important in axon out growth and guidance
Vav1	Rho, Rac, Cdc42	Transforming potential; mainly expressed in hematopoetic cells
Vav2	Rho, Rac, Cdc42	Transforming potential; widely expressed
Vav3	RhoA, RhoG, Rac	Transforming potential; widely expressed
GAPs		
Abr	Rac, Cdc42	Widely expressed; highest levels in brain
ARHGAP4/RhoGAP C1	Rho	Mainly expressed in hematopoetic cells
ARHGAP6	Rho	Implicated in microphthalmia with linear skin defects
ARHGAP7	Unknown	Unknown
ARHGAP9	Cdc42, Rac > Rho	Expressed in hematopoetic cells
Bcr	Rac > Cdc42	Bcr-abl fusion responsible for chronic myelogenous leukemia; cell cycle progression
3BP-1	Rac, Cdc42	Expressed in brain and spleen
CdGAP	Cdc42, Rac	Regulated by the endocytic protein intersectin
$\alpha1$ and $\alpha2$-chimaerin	Rac, Cdc42	Alternatively spliced; expressed in testis and cerebellar granule cells; downregulated in gliomas
N-chimaerin ($\alpha1$ and $\alpha2$-chimaerin)	Rac, Cdc42	Expressed in brain and implicated in neuritogenesis
Graf	Rho, Cdc42	Implicated in myelodysplastic syndrome and acute myeloid leukemia
Graf2	Rho, Cdc42	Highly expressed in muscle
MgcRacGAP	Rac, Cdc42	Implicated in neurogenesis; differentiation of hematopoetic cells and cytokinesis
Myr5, Myr7, Myosin-IXB	Rho	Unconventional myosin IX-RhoGAP
Nadrin	RhoA, Rac1, Cdc42	Expression restricted to neurons; suggested role in exocytosis
Oligophrenin-1	Rho > Cdc42 > Rac	Mutations cause nonspecific X-linked mental retardation
p50RhoGAP/Cdc42GAP	Cdc42 > Rac, Rho in vitro; Rho in vivo	Activated by IGF-binding protein-5; widely expressed
p122RhoGAP	Rho	Stimulates PLC-α1
p190RhoGAP	Rho > Rac, Cdc42	Widely expressed; involved in axon growth and guidance and cell migration and invasion
p190B	Rho, Rac, Cdc42	Widely expressed; linked to integrins
PSGAP	Cdc42, RhoA	Widely expressed; interacts with PYK2 and focal adhesion kinase
RalBP1	Cdc42 > Rac	Binds to Ras-related protein RalA
RICH	Cdc42, Rac1	Widely expressed; binds to CIP4
RIP1	Cdc42 > Rac	Binds to Ras-related protein Ral
RLIP76	Cdc42, Rac	Binds to Ras-related protein Ral1A
GDIs		
RhoGDI-1/RhoGDIα	Rho, Rac, Cdc42	Widely expressed
RhoGDI-2/D4/Ly-GDI/RhoGDIα	Rac, Cdc42 > Rho	Exclusively expressed in hematopoetic cells
RhoGDI-3/RhoGDIα	Rho, Cdc42	Highly expressed in brain and pancreas

References can be found in recent excellent reviews: Zheng, 2001 (RhoGEFs); Jenna and Lamarche-Vane, in press (RhoGAPs); Olofsson, 1999 (RhoGDIs).

p115RhoGEF is stimulated to catalyze nucleotide exchange on Rho on binding the activated heterotrimeric G protein α-subunit Gα_{13} (Hart et al., 1998; Mao et al., 1998). Meanwhile, Vav can be phosphorylated and activated by Src family tyrosine kinases after cytokine or adhesion receptor activation (Bustelo, 2000). Vav can also be activated toward Rac upon binding PIP$_3$ via its PH domain (Han et al., 1998). In general, the pathways that regulate many of the RhoGEFs are not well understood, but it is likely that we will see this shortfall addressed in the coming years as new binding partners and routes for activation are identified.

Of particular interest are the recent observations that a number of RhoGEFs are implicated in a wide range of human disease processes, including certain types of leukemias, mental retardation, and developmental disorders (reviewed in Boettner and Van Aelst, 2002; Table 84–2). Many RhoGEFs are protooncogenes and are highly transforming when overexpressed in cultured cells, highlighting the importance of Rho GTPases in cell growth control. The earliest example was the identification of the Dbl oncogene, which was isolated from a human diffuse B-cell lymphoma (Srivastava et al., 1986). Subsequently, it was discovered that mutations in the FGD1 gene are responsible for faciogenital dysplasia, also known as Aarskog-Scott syndrome, an X-linked developmental disorder in which individuals are of disproportionately short stature and suffer from facial, skeletal, and urogenital abnormalities (Pasteris et al., 1994). The FGD1 gene encodes a Cdc42-specific GEF and is the focus of Chapter 86. A mutation in another X-linked RhoGEF gene encoding ARHGEF6/α-PIX/Cool-2 has been found to be responsible for nonspecific X-linked mental retardation (MRX) in a large Dutch family (Kutsche et al., 2000). Intriguingly, three out of the eight known MRX genes encode regulators or effectors of the Rho GTPases and include oligophrenin-1 (a RhoGAP), and PAK3 (an effector for Rac and Cdc42) (Allen et al., 1998a; Billuart et al., 1998). RhoGEFs are also involved in autosomal disorders, and recently the gene responsible for certain cases of amyotrophic lateral sclerosis (ALS), a progressive neurogenerative disease, was found to encode a putative RhoGEF called alsin (Hadano et al., 2001; Y Yang et al., 2001).

RhoGAPs. Over 50 proteins in the human genome contain a RhoGAP domain (Ridley, 2001a), but only a fraction of these have been characterized in any detail. The RhoGAP domain spans approximately 140 amino acids but does not share any significant sequence identity with the RasGAP motif. Like RhoGEFs, individual RhoGAPs show varying levels of substrate specificity for members of the Rho family, and their tissue expression profiles also vary (see Table 84–2).

Roles for some of the RhoGAPs in cellular processes such as cell cycle progression, adhesion and migration, and neuronal development have been established, although the exact mechanism by which these GAPs exert these effects remains to be defined. However, as with the RhoGEFs, the majority of RhoGAPs contain other protein-binding or lipid-binding modules in addition to the RhoGAP domain, and it has been suggested that these sequences will play a role in recruiting RhoGAPs to specific protein complexes. For example, in the case of p190RhoGAP, there is evidence that Src-induced tyrosine phosphorylation is important for its function (Benard et al., 1999). p190RhoGAP has been shown to play a role in fibroblast migration, melonoma, and breast cancer cell invasion, and a model has now been proposed in which the initial localized suppression of Rho activity by c-Src activation of p190RhoGAP is a critical step to allow cells to migrate (Arthur et al., 2000). Further studies have implicated p190RhoGAP in neuronal development, and p190RhoGAP null mice exhibit several defects in axon guidance and fasciculation (Brouns et al., 2000, 2001). As another example, mouse CdGAP has five SH3-binding motifs within a large C-terminal proline-rich domain, in addition to an N-terminal RhoGAP domain. CdGAP has GAP activity toward Rac1 and Cdc42, but not Rho. This GAP activity appears to be directly regulated through its interaction with the scaffolding protein intersectin, a protein that is implicated in clathrin-dependent endocytosis and mitogenic signaling. Hence, it has been speculated that CdGAP may play a role in these processes (Jenna et al., 2002). For an extensive review of RhoGAPs, see Jenna and Lamarche-Vane (in press).

RhoGDIs. In their inactivated, cytoplasmic located states, Rho and Rac can be purified in a soluble complex with RhoGDIs. In humans, three RhoGDIs have been identified that prevent the activation of many Rho family members. RhoGDI-1, RhoGDI-2/D4/Ly-GDI, and RhoGDI-3 (also known as RhoGDIα, β, and γ) preferentially bind to GDP-bound GTPases and prevent spontaneous and GEF-catalyzed release of nucleotide, thereby maintaining the GTPases in the inactive state (reviewed in Olofsson, 1999). Little is known about how these proteins are regulated, although studies have suggested that association of RhoGDI with the actin-binding ezrin/radixin/moesin (ERM) and/or PKC-mediated phosphorylation of RhoGDI may be important (Takahashi et al., 1997; Mehta et al., 2001). More recently, a novel function for RhoGDI has been identified. It has been shown that RhoGDI, which sequesters Rac in the cytoplasm, also interferes with effector binding and that membrane translocation of Rac displaces RhoGDI, thereby allowing effectors to bind (Del Pozo et al., 2002).

Effectors for the Rho GTPases

Many downstream effectors have been identified for Rho, Rac, and Cdc42 that mediate their effects on actin and microtubule dynamics, membrane trafficking, and transcriptional activation. These are summarized in Table 84–3. The best-understood role for the Rho GTPases involves their regulation of the actin cytoskeleton that underlies many cellular behaviors, including cell motility and migration, changes in cell shape, cell adhesion, and cytokinesis. The actin cytoskeleton is composed of filamenous actin that is organized into three major types of structure, each regulated by a member of the Rho GTPases. Stress fibers are made up of bundles of actin filaments that are linked to the extracellular matrix via focal adhesions. Activation of RhoA is a key step in the formation of stress fibers and focal adhesions (Paterson et al., 1990; Ridley and Hall, 1992). Lamellipodia are thin, protrusive sheets of actin that dominate the edges of cultured fibroblasts. At the leading edge of cells where lamellipodia lift off the substratum and fold backward, they create membrane ruffles. Rac1 activation is responsible for the formation of lamellipodia and membrane ruffles in many cell types (Ridley et al., 1992). Filopodia are long, fingerlike protrusions that each contain a bundle of actin filaments. Neuronal growth cones, for instance, are rich in filopodia, and Cdc42 regulates their formation (Kozma et al., 1995; Nobes and Hall, 1995). Here we discuss a number of the effector molecules that mediate the typical actions of the Rho GTPases on the actin cytoskeleton (Fig. 84–2).

Rho Effectors. The most well characterized effectors for Rho that regulate its effects on the cytoskeleton include the Rho-associated kinase (ROCK) family of protein kinases, members of the diaphanous-related formin (DRF) family and phosphatidylinositol-4-phosphate 5-kinase (PIP5K). The ROCK family comprises p160ROCK (also known as ROKβ) and Rho kinase (also known as ROKα) (Leung et al., 1995, 1996; Ishizaki et al., 1996; Matsui et al., 1996; Nakagawa et al., 1996). These serine/threonine kinases are stimulated by GTP-bound Rho and are involved in the regulation of stress fiber and focal adhesion formation (Leung et al., 1996; Amano et al., 1997; Ishizaki et al., 1997), as well as smooth muscle contraction (reviewed in Fukata et al., 2001), neurite retraction (Amano et al., 1998; Hirose et al., 1998; Katoh et al., 1998), and cytokinesis (Yasui et al., 1998).

ROCK phosphorylates a number of target molecules, including the myosin-binding subunit (MBS) of myosin light chain phosphatase (Kimura et al., 1996), myosin light chain (MLC) (Amano et al., 1996), LIM kinase (LIMK) (Maekawa et al., 1999), and moesin, a member of the ERM family of proteins (Fukata et al., 1998). ROCK, by phosphorylating and inactivating MLC phosphatase as well as by phosphorylating MLC directly, is thought to regulate the level of MLC-phosphorylation and, in turn, control actomyosin assembly and contraction. Phosphorylation of MLC has been shown to induce a conformational change in myosin, which increases its binding to actin filaments and subsequently induces the formation of stress fibers (Chrzanowska-Wodnicka and Burridge, 1996). ROCK also phosphorylates and activates LIMK, a cytosolic serine/threonine kinase that, in turn, phosphorylates cofilin, an actin-depolymerizing factor that mediates the cleavage and disassembly of actin filaments (Arber et al.,

Table 84–3. Effectors for Rho, Rac, and Cdc42

Effector	Selectivity	Protein Type	Function
ROCK/ROK/Rho kinase	Rho	Ser/Thr kinase	Actomyosin assembly and contraction; see text
Citron	Rho	Ser/Thr kinase	Cytokinesis
PKN/PRK1, PRK2	Rho	Ser/Thr kinase	Gene expression
MBS	Rho	Phosphatase subunit	Inactivates MLC
DRFs: Dia1, Dia2	Rho	Scaffold	Actin polymerization and stabilization of microtubules; see text
Rhophilin	Rho	Scaffold	Unknown; expressed in testis
Rhotekin	Rho	Scaffold	Gene transcription
Kinectin	RhoG, RhoA	Scaffold	Binds kinesin
DAG kinase	Rho, Rac	Lipid kinase	Regulates phosphatidic acid
PLD	Rho, Rac, Cdc42	Lipase	Regulates phosphatidic acid
PIP5K	Rho, Rac	Lipid kinase	Regulates PIP_2 levels; actin capping and remodeling; see text
IRSp53	Rac, Cdc42	Scaffold	Actin organization; see text
PI3K	Rac, Cdc42, Rho?	Lipid kinase	PIP_3 levels
P67[phox]	Rac	Part of an enzyme complex	Phagocytosis
p140Sra-1	Rac	Scaffold	Actin organization, membrane ruffling
Por1	Rac	Scaffold	Actin organization, membrane ruffling
POSH	Rac	Scaffold	Gene expression
p70 S6 kinase	Rac, Cdc42	Ser/Thr kinase	Translational regulation
MEK kinase	Rac, Cdc42	Ser/Thr kinase	Gene expression
MLK 2, 3	Rac, Cdc42	Ser/Thr kinase	Gene expression
PAKs	Rac, Cdc42	Ser/Thr kinase	Gene expression and actin reorganization; see text
IQGAP	Rac, Cdc42	Scaffold	Cell–cell adhesion and actin reorganization
PLC-α	Rac, Cdc42	Lipase	DAG/IP_3 levels
MRCK	Cdc42	Ser/Thr kinase	Actin organization, filipodia formation
WASP/N-WASP	Cdc42	Scaffold	Actin nucleation; filipodia formation; see text
Ack	Cdc42	Tyr kinase	Vesicle transport
Par6	Cdc42	Scaffold	Cell polarization
CIP4	Cdc42	Scaffold	Binds to microtubules
MSE55, BORGs	Cdc42	Scaffold	Binds to septin GTPases

References can be found in recent reviews by Kaibuchi et al., 1999; Bishop and Hall, 2000; Ridley, 2001a,b; Takai et al., 2001.
CIP4, Cdc42 interacting protein 4; MRCK, myotonic dystrophy kinase-related Cdc42-binding kinase; MLK, mixed lineage kinase.

1998; Yang et al., 1998; Maekawa et al., 1999). Cofilin's actin-depolymerizing activity is inhibited by phosphorylation by LIMK, resulting in the stabilization of actin filaments and stress fibers.

Another class of Rho effectors that have gained considerable attention over recent years is the DRFs. This family of proteins includes hDia1 in humans, mDia1 (also known as p140mDia) (Watanabe et al., 1997) and mDia2 (Watanabe et al., 1997) in mouse, Diaphanous in *Drosophila* (Castrillon and Wasserman, 1994), and Bni1 in the budding yeast (Kohno et al., 1996). These proteins link the actin filaments with Rho and are required for stress fiber formation, cytokinesis, and establishing and maintaining cell polarity (Wasserman, 1998; Watanabe et al., 1999; Kato et al., 2001). It has recently been shown that

the coordinated action of both mDia and ROCK are required to induce properly aligned stress fibers (Watanabe et al., 1999). In humans, a C-terminally truncated form of hDia1 is associated with an autosomal dominant form of progressive hearing loss (Lynch et al., 1997), and disruption of the gene correlates with premature ovarian failure (Bione et al., 1998).

DRFs contain three formin homology (FH) domains, the first of which binds profilin, an actin-binding protein that is involved in the regulation of actin polymerization (Watanabe et al., 1997). The proline-rich FH1 domain also binds to the SH3 domain of the tyrosine kinase Src, which, in turn, influences stress fiber formation and serum response factor (SRF)–dependent transcription (Tominaga et

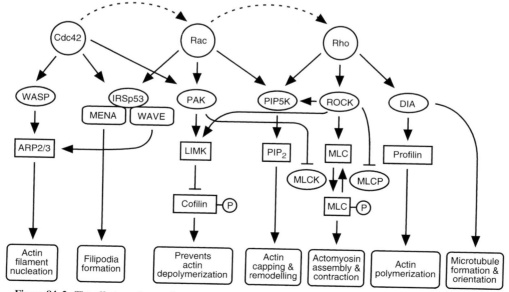

Figure 84–2. The effector pathways downstream of Rho, Rac, and Cdc42 that regulate the dynamic organization of the cytoskeleton. See the section on "Effectors for the Rho GTPases" and Table 84–3 for details and abbreviations.

al., 2000). It is now clear that DRFs not only play a role in regulating the actin cytoskeleton but also function in the formation and maintenance of the microtubules that are essential for cell migration and maintaining cell polarity. Recent evidence has shown that mDia1 is responsible for coordinating microtubules and the actin cytoskeleton during HeLa cell movement (Ishizaki et al., 2001). Furthermore, mDia1 and mDia2 have been shown to mediate Rho-dependent formation and orientation of stable microtubules in 3T3 fibroblasts (Palazzo et al., 2001).

Another way for Rho to affect the actin cytoskeleton is via phosphoinositide kinases. Lipids—in particular, PIP_2—have been shown to have a role in actin cytoskeletal rearrangements. For example, the binding of PIP_2 to actin-capping proteins such as gelsolin can promote their release from actin filaments and thereby increase actin polymerization (Janmey, 1994). Rho and Rac have been shown to stimulate the synthesis of PIP_2 (Chong et al., 1994; Hartwig et al., 1995), which is generated from phosphatidylinositol 4-phosphate (PI4P) by the enzyme phosphatidylinositol-4-phosphate 5-kinase (PIP5K). The mechanism by which Rho induces an increase in PIP_2 is not fully understood. A physical association between Rho and PIP5K has been reported in mouse fibroblasts, although this association does not depend on GTP (Ren et al., 1996) and is not supported by data that demonstrated an association between PIP5K and Rac, but not RhoA (Tolias et al., 1995). More recently, ROCK has been reported to stimulate PIP5K activity (Oude Weernink et al., 2000); it is unknown whether this activation involves the direct phosphorylation of PIP5K. Further investigations have indicated that ROCK may regulate PIP_2 synthesis by controlling PI4P availability (Yamamoto et al., 2001), although, again, exactly how this is achieved is unclear.

Rac and Cdc42 Effectors. The molecular mechanisms by which Rac and Cdc42 regulate the formation of lamellipodia and filopodia, respectively, are beginning to be understood, and several downstream targets have been implicated in these processes. Interestingly, Rac and Cdc42 utilize a number of common effectors, including members of the mammalian p21-activated kinase (Pak) family of serine/threonine kinases that are activated by GTP-bound Rac and Cdc42, but not Rho (Manser et al., 1994; for reviews, see Bagrodia and Cerione, 1999; Daniels and Bokoch, 1999).

Six members of the mammalian Pak family have been identified to date, and these can be separated into two subclasses based on their amino acid sequences. Pak1, Pak2, and Pak3 (Pakα, Pakγ, and Pakβ in rat) belong to class A (Dan et al., 2002) and comprise a carboxyl-terminal kinase domain and an amino-terminal regulatory domain that includes the Cdc42/Rac-interactive-binding (CRIB) domain (also known as the GBD, for GTPase-binding domain) that binds to activated Rac or Cdc42. The CRIB domain is a highly conserved motif that is found in other effectors of Rac and Cdc42 (see later in this section). The regulatory region also contains an autoinhibitory domain that binds to the carboxyl-terminal kinase domain, causing Pak to assume an inactive conformation in the absence of activated Rac or Cdc42. Binding of GTP-Rac or Cdc42 is thought to induce a conformational change in the Pak molecule that relieves this autoinhibitory mechanism and results in the activation of the kinase (Buchwald et al., 2001). Binding sites for the SH3 domain that contains the proteins Nck (an adaptor protein) and Pix/Cool/ARHGEF6 (an exchange factor for the Rho GTPases), together with a motif that binds to the heterotrimeric G protein βγ-subunit, are also found in the regulatory region (reviewed in Daniels and Bokoch, 1999).

Paks 4, 5, and 6 make up subclass B of the Pak family. Pak4 was the first member of this subclass to be identified based on its amino acid sequence (Abo et al., 1998), and although it has a CRIB domain and a carboxyl-terminal kinase domain, it does not appear to have an autoinhibitory domain, a G protein βγ-binding motif, or to bind Nck and Pix/Cool/ARHGEF6. This Pak also differs in that it appears to only bind to activated Cdc42 and not to Rac. Pak5 and Pak6 are recently identified members of this subclass. Pak5 is expressed primarily in brain and has been shown to promote neurite outgrowth in N1E-115 neuroblastoma cells, as well as binding to both the actin and microtubule networks (Cau et al., 2001; Dan et al., 2002). Pak6 is expressed in the testis and prostate and binds to the androgen receptor (F Yang et al., 2001). Both Pak5 and Pak 6 bind to activated Rac and Cdc42, but Pak6 binds only weakly to Rac.

A number of studies have clearly identified roles for Paks in actin cytoskeletal rearrangements. Paks have been reported to induce filopodia and membrane ruffles reminiscent of those induced by Cdc42 and Rac (Sells et al., 1997; Abo et al., 1998); to dissolve stress fibers, down-regulate focal adhesions, and promote cell retraction (Manser et al., 1997; Zeng et al., 2000); and to promote neurite outgrowth (Daniels et al., 1998; Obermeier et al., 1998; Dan et al., 2002). In some cases, these cytoskeletal changes appear to be independent of the kinase activities of the Paks involved, or they are independent of their ability to bind to the Rho GTPases (Sells et al., 1997; Daniels et al., 1998; Obermeier et al., 1998). This suggests that some of the cytoskeletal changes observed may not be mediated by Rac and Cdc42 signaling, and thus it appears that multiple mechanisms exist for Pak to exert its effect on the actin cytoskeleton.

A key discovery linking Cdc42 and Rac to Paks and actin cytoskeletal dynamics was the identification of the Rac/Cdc42-dependent interaction of Pak1 with LIMK (Edwards et al., 1999). Pak1 phosphorylates LIMK and, in turn, promotes LIMK-mediated phosphorylation and inhibition of the actin-depolymerizing protein cofilin. In the kidney cell line used in these experiments, LIMK appears to mediate actin cytoskeletal responses to Rac and to promote membrane ruffling. While Rac and Cdc42 can both activate Pak1, catalytically inactive LIMK was observed to only partially block the morphological changes induced by Cdc42, thus suggesting that Cdc42's effects on the cytoskeleton are likely to involve other pathways. However, it has recently been shown that Pak4—the isoform that is specific for Cdc42 and which regulates filopodia formation—appears to mediate cytoskeletal changes in muscle cells via LIMK and cofilin (Dan et al., 2001). These findings, together with those linking LIMK and cofilin downstream of Rho and ROCK, suggest that LIMK and cofilin can contribute to mediating the cytoskeletal changes that result from the activation of Rho, Rac, and Cdc42, depending on the cellular context and the particular serine/threonine kinase activated.

Another route by which Pak1 can regulate cytoskeletal dynamics is by phosphorylating and down-regulating myosin light chain kinase (MLCK), which, in turn, results in decreased MLC phosphorylation and reduced actomyosin contraction and stress fiber formation (Sanders et al., 1999; see Fig. 84–2). The effects of activated PAK1 on MLC phosphorylation are counter to the effects of ROCK/Rho kinase that result in the formation of stress fibers. This suggests that activated Rho GTPases, through their respective kinases, can act antagonistically to finely regulate the phosphorylation state of MLC and ultimately control the overall levels of actomyosin assembly. Finally, it should be pointed out that Paks also have a role as upstream activators of kinase cascades that result in transcriptional regulation (reviewed in Bagrodia and Cerione, 1999).

Rac and Cdc42 also utilize another family of effectors to regulate their effects on the actin cytoskeleton. The WASP (Wiskott-Aldrich syndrome protein) family includes the founder member WASP together with N-WASP and WAVE/Scar1 (reviewed in Takenawa and Miki, 2001). WASP is exclusively expressed in hematopoietic cells and was originally identified as the product of the X-linked gene that is mutated in patients with the immune-deficiency disorder Wiskott-Aldrich syndrome (Derry et al., 1994). WASP and its ubiquitously expressed homolog N-WASP (neuronally enriched WASP) both contain a CRIB domain and bind to activated Cdc42 (Symons et al., 1996). N-WASP has been shown to be indispensable for the Cdc42-dependent formation of filopodia in fibroblasts (Miki et al., 1998a). Cdc42 in concert with N-WASP has been shown to stimulate the Arp2/3 complex, a multiprotein complex that initiates the nucleation of new actin filaments (Rohatgi et al., 1999; reviewed in Higgs and Pollard, 2001). The Arp2/3 complex is thought to recruit actin monomers to the fast-growing ends of actin filaments. This activity is required for morphological cell shape changes and cell migration, processes that are impaired in WASP-deficient hematopoietic cells.

Actin filament polymerization via the Arp2/3 complex has also been shown to mediate signaling pathways downstream of Rac to induce lamellipodia formation (Miki et al., 1998b, 2000). This cascade incorporates the WASP family member Scar1/WAVE, which, like WASP and N-WASP, binds directly to the Arp2/3 complex (Machesky and Insall, 1998). However, unlike the WASPs, Scar1/WAVE does not contain a CRIB domain and does not bind directly to Rac. This "missing link" between Rac and Scar1/WAVE has been recently identified and occurs via the SH3 domain, which contains scaffold protein IRSp53 (Miki et al., 2000; see Fig. 84–2). IRSp53 is an essential intermediate for Rac-induced membrane ruffling and binds to activated Rac via its amino terminus and to Scar1/WAVE via its carboxy-terminal SH3 domain to form a trimolecular complex.

Interestingly, Cdc42 can also interact with IRSp53 through a partial CRIB motif that, in turn, associates with the Ena/VASP family member Mena to promote filopodia formation (Krugmann et al., 2001). The Ena/VASP family of proteins comprises Mena, VASP, and EVL in mammalian cells (reviewed in Reinhard et al., 2001). These proteins have been implicated in the temporal and spatial control of actin filament dynamics, and Mena has been shown to localize to focal adhesion sites through its N-terminal EVH1 (Ena/VASP homology) domain and to the leading edge of lamellipodia and the tips of filopodia (Gertler et al., 1996; Lanier et al., 1999). It is not clear exactly how IRSp53/Mena complex promotes actin filament assembly and filopodia formation, but Mena is known to contain proline-rich regions that interact with profilin as well as SH3 containing proteins, and also has a C-terminal EVH2 domain that interacts with filamentous actin (Krugmann et al., 2001). The fact that IRSp53 can associate with both Rac and Cdc42 has led to the suggestion that IRSp53 may be a link between Cdc42 and Rac. Such a link may explain the observation that activated Cdc42 can ultimately induce Rac-dependent membrane ruffling (Ridley, 2001a).

As Table 84–3 indicates, many other effectors for Rho, Rac, and Cdc42 have been identified, and it is now understood that the Rho GTPases have important roles in activities beyond regulating the actin cytoskeleton. The reader is referred to a number of excellent reviews for in-depth coverage of the function of Rho GTPases in a range of areas of cell biology, including endocytosis (Ellis and Mellor, 2000), the cell cycle and oncogenesis (Schmitz et al., 2000; Pruitt and Der, 2001; Jaffe and Hall, 2002), cell migration (Ridley, 2001b), neuronal morphogenesis (Luo, 2000), epithelial morphogenesis (Van Aelst and Symons, 2002), and cell adhesion (Fukata and Kaibuchi, 2001).

HETEROTRIMERIC G PROTEINS

The second structurally distinct family of GNBPs to be considered here are the heterotrimeric G proteins. Members of the heterotrimeric G protein superfamily are molecular switches responsible for transducing external signals received by G protein–coupled receptors (GPCRs) to intracellular effectors. GPCRs are activated by a wide range of extracellular ligands and are responsible for initiating signaling cascades that underlie many physiological responses, including cell growth, differentiation, metabolism, neurotransmission, vision, taste, and smell. As their name implies, heterotrimeric G proteins consist of three distinct subunits: α, β, and γ (see Table 84–1).

To date, approximately 20 mammalian α subunits have been cloned; they are divided into four subfamilies based on sequence similarities and function: $G\alpha_s$, $G\alpha_i$, $G\alpha_q$, and $G\alpha_{12}$ (Wilkie et al., 1992). Five β-subunits and 12 γ-subunits have also been identified. Like Rho and Ras family members, the α- and γ-subunits are anchored to the intracellular surface of the plasma membrane via the covalent attachment of lipid moieties (reviewed in Bourne, 1997). The α-subunit ($G\alpha$), which contains a modified G-domain, binds guanine nucleotides and has intrinsic GTPase activity. The inactive GDP-bound form of the $G\alpha$ subunit binds to a dimer consisting of the β- and γ-subunits. Exchange of GDP for GTP on the $G\alpha$ subunit is triggered when the G protein trimer interacts with a ligand-bound GPCR. In this case, the GPCR acts as a GEF analogous to those regulating the small GTPases. Once activated, the $G\alpha$ subunit dissociates from the $G\beta\gamma$ dimer, and both components are free to either generate or activate a variety of second messengers and effector molecules. The deactivation of G protein signaling is also a regulated event, and a family of GAPs termed RGS (regulator of G protein signaling) has been identified. The RGSs promote GTP hydrolysis and allow inactive heterotrimers to reform. These events are summarized in Figure 84–3.

Activation and Regulation of Heterotrimeric G Proteins

GPCRs

GPCRs are targets for many classes of ligand, including most polypeptide hormones, all monoamine neurotransmitters, growth factors, prostaglandins, phospholipids, photons, odorants, and ions, as well as many exogenous therapeutic reagents. This class of receptors makes up the largest superfamily of cell surface molecules involved in signal transduction, and there are more than 700 family members identified in the human genome (Rubin et al., 2000).

Prominent subfamilies of GPCRs include the adrenergic, muscarinic acetylcholine, and chemokine receptors, as well as the photopigments such as rhodopsin. Members of the GPCR superfamily have a common structure consisting of a single polypeptide with seven membrane-spanning α-helical domains that are connected by a series of intracellular and extracellular loops (Dixon et al., 1986; Dohlman et al., 1987). The first high-resolution 3D crystal structure of a GPCR has been elucidated, and the structure of rhodopsin (the light-detecting GPCR found in rod cells of the retina) reveals a highly organized hep-

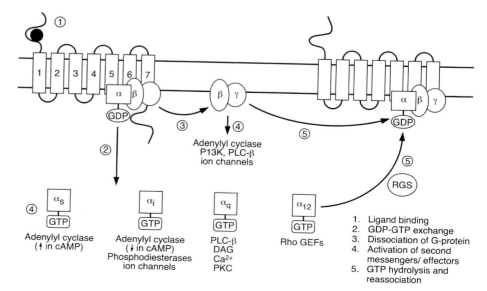

Figure 84–3. Signaling through heterotrimeric G proteins. G protein–coupled receptors (GPCRs) bind to a wide range of ligands such as monoamine neurotransmitters, growth factors, prostaglandins, phospholipids, photons, odorants, and ions. Ligand binding stimulates GDP–GTP exchange on the associated heterotrimeric G protein that dissociates into its constituent $G\alpha$ subunit and $\beta\gamma$-dimer. Four classes of $G\alpha$ subunits have been identified ($G\alpha_s$, $G\alpha_i$, $G\alpha_q$ and $G\alpha_{12}$), and these regulate a variety of downstream effector molecules to initiate key biological responses including cell proliferation, survival, and differentiation. The $\beta\gamma$-dimer also activates a number of effector proteins prior to reassociation with the $G\alpha$ subunit upon GTP hydrolysis. PLC-β, phospholipase C-β; PI3K, phosphoinositide 3-kinase; DAG, diacylglycerol; PKC, protein kinase C; GEFs, GDP/GTP exchange factors; RGS, regulator of G protein signaling.

tahelical transmembrane bundle (Palczewski et al., 2000). These structural findings, together with many prior biochemical, pharmacological, and mutagenesis studies, have led to an understanding of the molecular mechanism of GPCR activation. Many peptide ligands bind to the extracellular loops of GPCRs, whereas biogenic amines and retinal (the covalently bound chromophore of rhodopsin) activate their respective GPCRs via a binding pocket within the bundle of seven α-helices in the plane of the plasma membrane. Ligand binding induces a conformational change in the GPCR which is thought to involve substantial movements of a number of transmembrane helices, resulting in alterations to the receptor's cytoplasmic surface and the exposure of previously masked G protein–binding sites (reviewed in Bourne, 1997; Wess, 1997). Binding of the G protein to the activated receptor promotes the exchange of GDP for GTP on the Gα subunit and finally causes the dissociation of the G protein into its constituent α-subunit and $\beta\gamma$-dimer. The specificity of the interaction between the G protein and the GPCR is largely determined by the carboxy-terminal sequence of the Gα subunit. It has been demonstrated that substituting just three amino acids in this region can alter the specificity of a Gα subunit for particular hormone receptors (Conklin et al., 1993). For a detailed discussion of GPCR structure and activation, see Strader et al., 1995; Bourne, 1997; Wess, 1997; Rohrer and Kobilka, 1998; and Meng and Bourne, 2001.

GAPs for Heterotrimeric G Proteins

The major class of GAPs that regulate heterotrimeric G proteins is the RGS protein family. There are now over 20 mammalian RGS proteins, and most show GAP activity toward G proteins (reviewed in Ross and Wilkie, 2000). The RGS domain encompasses approximately 130 amino acids and is capable of binding to Gα subunits and accelerating GTP hydrolysis. Unlike GAPs for most small GTPases, GAPs for heterotrimeric G proteins do not take part in the chemistry of GTP hydrolysis directly but, rather, change the conformation of the Gα-GTP complex such that the α-subunit becomes a better hydrolase (Tesmer et al., 1997). This mechanism was first described for RGS4, an RGS protein for Gα_i and Gα_q (Berman et al., 1996; Hepler et al., 1997).

RGS proteins have been identified that act as GAPs for all four classes of Gα subunits, including the recently cloned RGS-PX1, which is the first RGS protein specific for Gα_s subunits (Zheng et al., 2001). While some RGS proteins are specific for a particular Gα target (notably RGS-PX1), it has been difficult to show specificity for some RGS proteins that can act as a GAP for both Gα_i and Gα_q subunits when they are transfected into cells. Like GAPs for small GTPases, RGS proteins contain a variety of other protein-binding motifs that link them to other signaling networks where they function as effector-type proteins (reviewed in De Vries and Gist Farquhar, 1999). In addition to the classic RGS proteins, several other molecules can function as GAPs for the heterotrimeric G proteins. These include PLC-β, the principle effector protein regulated by Gα_q, and p115RhoGEF(Berstein et al., 1992; Kozasa et al., 1998). p115RhoGEF contains an RGS-like (RGL) domain (Ross and Wilkie, 2000) that binds to the α-subunits Gα_{12} and Gα_{13} and catalyses GTP hydrolysis. RGL domains have also been identified in two other RhoGEFs—PDZ-RhoGEF and LARG—which also bind to Gα_{12} and Gα_{13}; their GAP activity remains to be demonstrated (Fukuhara et al., 1999, 2000). As discussed next, this class of RGL-containing RhoGEFs provides a direct link between the Gα_{12} subunits and Rho signaling.

Signaling Pathways Downstream of Heterotrimeric G Proteins

The exact signaling pathways that are triggered by dissociation of a G protein into its constituent α-subunit and $\beta\gamma$-dimer depend on the particular combination of α- and $\beta\gamma$-subunits and the availability of effectors and regulatory proteins. Each of the Gα subfamilies signals to a different spectrum of second messengers and effector molecules to initiate a vast array of biological processes. Furthermore, it has become increasingly clear that $\beta\gamma$-dimers are also important for initiating signals downstream of G protein activation. Here we give a brief outline of some of the second-messenger systems and effectors utilized by the various α-subunits and $\beta\gamma$-dimers. There are many ex-

cellent reviews on G protein–linked signaling; see, for example, Hepler and Gilman (1992); Fields and Casey (1997); Hamm (1998); Morris and Malbon (1999); and Marinissen and Gutkind (2001).

Activated α Subunits

The Gα_s class of α-subunits comprises Gα_s and Gα_{olf}. Both these proteins activate adenylyl cyclase (AC), catalyzing the production of the second-messenger cyclic adenosine monophosphate (cAMP). cAMP mediates diverse cellular processes, including cell growth and differentiation, apoptosis, transcriptional regulation, and ion channel conductivity, primarily by activating the cAMP-dependent protein kinase (PKA) (reviewed in Houslay and Milligan, 1997; Simonds, 1999; Skalhegg and Tasken, 2000; Patel et al., 2001; Singh et al., 2001).

Activation of PKA results in the phosphorylation of target proteins, which include other kinases and the transcription factor CREB (cAMP response element–binding) (Mayr and Montminy, 2001). Many hormone-induced cellular responses are mediated by Gα_s. In the heart, stimulation of the prototypical β1-adrenergic receptor activates the Gα_s-AC-cAMP cascade, resulting in the PKA-dependent phosphorylation of a set of regulatory proteins that are involved in cardiac excitation coupling and energy metabolism, including L-type Ca^{2+} channels, the sarcoplasmic reticulum membrane protein phospholamban, myofilament proteins, and glycogen phosphorylase kinase. These events result in increased cardiac contractility, accelerated cardiac relaxation and increased heart rate (reviewed in Xiao, 2001).

The Gα_{olf} subunit transmits signals from activated olfactory receptors expressed on the surface of the olfactory neuronal cilia to AC. In this case, cAMP production results in the depolarization of olfactory neurons via cation influx through cyclic nucleotide-gated channels that are activated by cAMP (Kurahashi and Yau, 1993; reviewed in Pilpel et al., 1998; Zufall and Munger, 2001). Thus, Gα_{olf} processes a chemical signal encoded by an odorant and facilitates its conversion to an electric signal, which is transmitted to the olfactory bulb.

The Gα_i subfamily is the largest and includes the widely expressed subunits Gα_{i1}, Gα_{i2}, and Gα_{i3}; the retinal Gα_t subunits; and the brain-enriched Gα_o subunits, as well as Gα_z. Many receptors for neurotransmitters, hormones, and chemokines utilize Gα_i proteins for transducing extracellular signals. All members of this family, with the exception of Gα_z, are substrates for pertussis toxin ADP-ribosyl transferase, which covalently modifies the subunit and uncouples the G protein from its activating receptor, thus blocking receptor-induced responses (Bokoch and Gilman, 1984). The use of pertussis toxin in many experimental systems has been instrumental in determining the specific cellular signaling pathways utilized by this class of Gα subunits. Activation of Gα_{i1}, Gα_{i2}, and Gα_{i3} results in the inhibition of AC, thereby reducing intracellular levels of cAMP (Wong et al., 1991, 1992). Gα_o also inhibits AC and couples to several receptors in the brain and can regulate both neuronal-type Ca^{2+} channels and some K$^+$ channels (Hescheler et al., 1987; VanDongen et al., 1988).

Gα_t subunits play a central role in phototransduction and couple the GPCR rhodopsin to the second-messenger cyclic guanosine monophosphate (cGMP). Activated Gα_t in rod cells of the retina stimulates cGMP phosphodiesterase (PDE), which hydrolyses cGMP so that cytosolic levels of cGMP drop. As a consequence, cGMP-gated cation channels are closed, resulting in hyperpolarization of the membrane and thus an electrical signal that can be transmitted to the rest of visual system (reviewed in Arshavsky et al., 2002).

Of the members of the Gα_i subfamily, the sequence of Gα_z bears the least similarity to the others and is insensitive to pertussis toxin. Like other members, Gα_z inhibits AC and appears to couple to a wide variety of receptors. Recent studies have indicated that Gα_z may have more complex signaling roles with the identification of functional interactions with some interesting signaling molecules that include PAK (Wang et al., 1999; Section 2.4.2), Rap1GAP (Meng et al., 1999), PKC (Lounsbury et al., 1991) and the RGS protein RGSZ1 (Glick et al., 1998; Wang et al., 1998).

The Gα_q class of α-subunits contains five members—Gα_{11}, Gα_{14}, Gα_{15}, Gα_{16}, and Gα_q. These proteins are key regulators of the β-class of phosphoinositide-specific PLC (PLC-β) and mediate many physiological processes, including smooth muscle contraction and cell growth and differentiation (Sternweis and Smrcka, 1992). Activation of PLC-β hydrolyzes PIP$_2$ to generate two second messengers, inositol 1,4,5-triphosphate (IP$_3$) and DAG (reviewed in Rhee and Bae, 1997; Rebecchi and Pentyala, 2000). IP$_3$ production results in an increase in cytosolic-free Ca^{2+}, released from intracellular stores, while DAG results in the activation of a number of protein kinases, including protein kinase C (PKC) (reviewed in Berridge, 1993; Liu and Heckman, 1998).

Depending on the cell type in question, PKC has a wide range of substrates, including cell surface receptors, ion channels, contractile proteins, transcription factors, and other kinases (reviewed in Keenan and Kelleher, 1998; Kamp and Hell, 2000; Arbuzova et al., 2002). In some cell types, activation of PKC results in the stimulation of the MAPK cascade to induce transcription of the genes involved in cell proliferation. The exact mechanism of activation of MAPK by PKC is unclear; it may require either the direct phosphorylation of Raf by PKC or the activation of Ras, or both (reviewed in Gutkind, 2000). An increase in the intracellular Ca^{2+} concentration can also have a wide range of effects, depending on cell type. In smooth muscle for example, activation of Gα$_q$ initiates the phosphatidylinositol cascade to cause an increase in Ca^{2+} release from the sarcoplasmic reticulum. The increase in intracellular Ca^{2+} enhances binding of Ca^{2+} to calmodulin, which, in turn, activates MLCK to phosphorylate the MLC (reviewed in Fukata et al., 2001). Increased MLC phosphorylation increases smooth muscle contraction, while MLC dephosphorylation, promoted by a reduction in intracellular Ca^{2+}, results in smooth muscle relaxation.

Until recently, little was known about the functions of Gα$_{12}$ and Gα$_{13}$, which make up the final class of Gα subunits. One of the earliest activities associated with this subclass of Gα subunits was their ability to behave as potent transforming genes, thus indicating a role in cell proliferation (Jiang et al., 1993; Xu et al., 1993; Voyno-Yasenetskaya et al., 1994). More recent studies have demonstrated that Gα$_{12}$ and Gα$_{13}$ can stimulate Rho-dependent pathways such as stress fiber formation, and that Rho plays a key role in the transmission of proliferative and transforming signals by the Gα$_{12}$ subfamily of G proteins (Buhl et al., 1995; Fromm et al., 1997; Gohla et al., 1998; reviewed in Fukuhara et al., 2001; Whitehead et al., 2001). The signaling pathway that links Gα$_{13}$ to Rho has been identified and involves p115RhoGEF, a molecule we have met earlier in this chapter as a RhoGEF and a GAP for Gα$_{12}$ and Gα$_{13}$. Following treatment of cells with certain agonists such as LPA, activated Gα$_{13}$ binds to p115RhoGEF, thereby stimulating it to catalyze nucleotide exchange on Rho and activating Rho-dependent signaling (Hart et al., 1998; Kozasa et al., 1998; Mao et al., 1998). The RhoGEFs LARG and PDZ-RhoGEF also associate with Gα$_{12}$ and Gα$_{13}$ (Fukuhara et al., 1999, 2000), thus suggesting further routes by which Gα$_{12}$ proteins can initiate Rho-dependent signaling. This is an excellent illustration of the integration of signaling events by small and heterotrimeric G proteins.

βγ Subunits

There is now a much greater appreciation of the role of Gβγ dimers in the regulation of intracellular effectors including AC (Sunahara et al., 1996), PLC-β (Smrcka and Sternweis, 1993), PI3K (Stephens et al., 1994; Vanhaesebroeck et al., 1997), ion channels (Schneider et al., 1997), and G protein–coupled receptor kinases (GRKs) (Pitcher et al., 1992). One of the most important roles for Gβγ subunits is their involvement in transmitting signals for cell proliferation and survival. There is good evidence that Gβγ dimers stimulate cell proliferation via MAPK pathways and promote cell survival by the activation of PI3K. The pathway or pathways that link Gβγ subunits to MAPKs have yet to be fully defined, but they may involve activation of known Gβγ effectors (e.g., PI3K or PLC-β) or the activation of Src family tyrosine kinases and small G proteins such as Ras (Crespo et al., 1994; reviewed in Gutkind, 2000; Schwindinger and Robishaw, 2001). Gβγ dimers have been shown to directly activate PI3K, which, in turn, initiates many cell survival and antiapoptotic signals through the stimulation of PKB. Although there are no reports of mutations in Gβ or Gγ subunits in tumors, it has been suggested that specific Gβγ dimers may play a role in the pathogenesis of cancer as a result of their effects on the pathways that regulate cell growth and development (reviewed in Schwindinger and Robishaw, 2001).

Signaling through Gβγ dimers can be regulated at different levels. On one level, direct binding of the Gβγ dimer to phosducin (Gaudet et al., 1999) or pleckstrin (Abrams et al., 1996) inhibits Gβγ-mediated signaling. On another level, the Gβγ dimer can indirectly regulate the activation of its GPCR. Ligand-bound GPCRs are downregulated by phosphorylation of the receptor by GRKs, a process that requires Gβγ dimers (Pitcher et al., 1992). The Gβγ dimer mediates the translocation of the GRK from the cytoplasm to the membrane in order that the kinase may phosphorylate activated GPCRs and initiate receptor internalization (Daaka et al., 1997; Stoffel et al., 1997). Thus, the Gβγ dimer, far from being the passive partner of G protein activation, performs important regulatory and effector roles in heterotrimeric G protein signaling.

Heterotrimeric G Proteins and Disease

Malfunctions, or deregulation, of G protein–mediated signaling can give rise to a range of diseases in humans, notably bacterial infections, various cancers, McCune-Albright syndrome, and night blindness. The diarrhea caused by *Vibrio cholera* results from the increased transluminal movement of water and salts into the intestine, a process stimulated by increased concentrations of cAMP in mucosal cells. The increased cAMP is generated by the ADP ribosylation of Gα$_s$ by the bacteria's exotoxin, which results in the α-subunit being locked into its activated GTP-bound form. The activation state of G proteins are altered not only by bacterial toxins but also by heritable or spontaneous mutations. The first oncogenic Gα mutants were identified in the Gα$_s$ gene of pituitary tumors (Landis et al., 1989; Weinstein et al., 1991). The protein encoded by the mutant Gα$_s$ oncogene (termed *gsp* for G stimulatory protein) was found to generate a constitutively active α-subunit, resulting in the persistent production of cAMP. In this case, the activated mutant Gα$_s$ mimicked the intracellular signal induced by growth hormone, which increases cell proliferation (reviewed in Farfel et al., 1999; Lania et al., 2001).

McCune-Albright syndrome is an extreme example of the effects of activating mutations in the Gα$_s$ subunit that reflects the acquisition of a *gsp* mutation early in the developing embryo. This syndrome, together with other endocrine disorders associated with activating or loss of function mutations in Gαs, is the focus of the following chapter. Finally, there are other disorders that are caused by mutations in G protein subunits. Affected members in a family with dominantly inherited night blindness were found to have a point mutation in the gene that encodes Gα$_t$ (Dryja et al., 1996), and, most recently, a mutation in the gene that encodes the Gβ3 subunit has been linked to essential hypertension (Siffert et al., 1998). Thus, there is an expanding list of diseases caused by mutations in G proteins, and it is likely that with further genetic analysis we will see more examples of G protein dysfunction underlying human disease processes.

In conclusion, both small and heterotrimeric G proteins are molecular switches that transduce extracellular signals to downstream effectors. They utilize a vast number of positive and negative regulators and influence many aspects of cell physiology and function. Some components of G protein signaling are implicated in cell dysfunction and human disease. The molecular mechanisms that underlie a number of diseases associated with aberrant G protein signaling are discussed in Chapters 85–87.

ACKNOWLEDGMENTS

We thank Colin Akerman and Benjamin Boettner for their critical reading of the manuscript, and we apologize to our colleagues whose work was not directly cited in this chapter due to space limitations. Sarah Newey is supported by a Wellcome Trust Prize Travelling Research Fellowship, and Linda Van Aelst is supported by grants from the National Institutes of Health, the U.S. Army, and Neurofibromatosis Foundation Inc.

REFERENCES

Abo A, Qu J, Cammarano MS, Dan C, Fritsch A, Baud V, Belisle B, Minden A (1998). PAK4, a novel effector for Cdc42Hs, is implicated in the reorganization of the actin cytoskeleton and in the formation of filopodia. *EMBO J* 17: 6527–6540.

Abrams CS, Zhang J, Downes CP, Tang X, Zhao W, Rittenhouse SE (1996). Phosphopleckstrin inhibits gβγ-activable platelet phosphatidylinositol-4,5-bisphosphate 3-kinase. *J Biol Chem* 271: 25192–25197.

Albright CF, Giddings BW, Liu J, Vito M, Weinberg RA (1993). Characterization of a guanine nucleotide dissociation stimulator for a ras-related GTPase. *EMBO J* 12: 339–347.

Allen KM, Gleeson JG, Bagrodia S, Partington MW, MacMillan JC, Cerione RA, Mulley JC, Walsh CA (1998a). *PAK3* mutation in nonsyndromic X-linked mental retardation. *Nat Genet* 20: 25–30.

Allen M, Chu S, Brill S, Stotler C, Buckler A (1998b). Restricted tissue expression pattern of a novel human rasGAP-related gene and its murine ortholog. *Gene* 218: 17–25.

Amano M, Ito M, Kimura K, Fukata Y, Chihara K, Nakano T, Matsuura Y, Kaibuchi K (1996). Phosphorylation and activation of myosin by Rho-associated kinase (Rho-kinase). *J Biol Chem* 271: 20246–20249.

Amano M, Chihara K, Kimura K, Fukata Y, Nakamura N, Matsuura Y, Kaibuchi K (1997). Formation of actin stress fibers and focal adhesions enhanced by Rho-kinase. *Science* 275: 1308–1311.

Amano M, Chihara K, Nakamura N, Fukata Y, Yano T, Shibata M, Ikebe M, Kaibuchi K (1998). Myosin II activation promotes neurite retraction during the action of Rho and Rho-kinase. *Genes Cells* 3: 177–188.

Anastasiadis PZ, Reynolds AB (2001). Regulation of Rho GTPases by p120-catenin. *Curr Opin Cell Biol* 13: 604–610.

Arber S, Barbayannis FA, Hanser H, Schneider C, Stanyon CA, Bernard O, Caroni P (1998). Regulation of actin dynamics through phosphorylation of cofilin by LIM-kinase. *Nature* 393: 805–809.

Arbuzova A, Schmitz AA, Vergeres G (2002). Cross-talk unfolded: MARCKS proteins. *Biochem J* 362: 1–12.

Arellano M, Coll PM, Perez P (1999). RHO GTPases in the control of cell morphology, cell polarity, and actin localization in fission yeast. *Microsc Res Tech* 47: 51–60.

Aronheim A, Engelberg D, Li N, al-Alawi N, Schlessinger J, Karin M (1994). Membrane targeting of the nucleotide exchange factor Sos is sufficient for activating the Ras signaling pathway. *Cell* 78: 949–961.

Arshavsky VY, Lamb TD, Pugh EN Jr. (2002). G proteins and phototransduction. *Annu Rev Physiol* 64: 153–187.

Arthur WT, Petch LA, Burridge K (2000). Integrin engagement suppresses RhoA activity via a c-Src-dependent mechanism. *Curr Biol* 10: 719–722.

Bagrodia S, Cerione RA (1999). Pak to the future. *Trends Cell Biol* 9: 350–355.

Barbacid M (1987). Ras genes. *Annu Rev Biochem* 56: 779–827.

Bar-Sagi D (2001). A Ras by any other name. *Mol Cell Biol* 21: 1441–1443.

Benard V, Bohl BP, Bokoch GM (1999). Characterization of rac and cdc42 activation in chemoattractant-stimulated human neutrophils using a novel assay for active GTPases. *J Biol Chem* 274: 13198–13204.

Berman DM, Wilkie TM, Gilman AG (1996). GAIP and RGS4 are GTPase-activating proteins for the Gi subfamily of G protein α-subunits. *Cell* 86: 445–452.

Berridge MJ (1993). Inositol trisphosphate and calcium signalling. *Nature* 361: 315–325.

Berstein G, Blank JL, Jhon DY, Exton JH, Rhee SG, Ross EM (1992). Phospholipase C-β 1 is a GTPase-activating protein for Gq/11, its physiologic regulator. *Cell* 70: 411–418.

Billuart P, Bienvenu T, Ronce N, des Portes V, Vinet MC, Zemni R, Roest Crollius H, Carrie A, Fauchereau F, Cherry M, et al. (1998). Oligophrenin-1 encodes a rhoGAP protein involved in X-linked mental retardation. *Nature* 392: 923–926.

Bione S, Sala C, Manzini C, Arrigo G, Zuffardi O, Banfi S, Borsani G, Jonveaux P, Philippe C, Zuccotti M, et al. (1998). A human homologue of the *Drosophila melanogaster* diaphanous gene is disrupted in a patient with premature ovarian failure: evidence for conserved function in oogenesis and implications for human sterility. *Am J Hum Genet* 62: 533–541.

Bishop AL, Hall A (2000). Rho GTPases and their effector proteins. *Biochem J* 348 Pt 2: 241–255.

Boettner B, Van Aelst L (2002). The role of Rho GTPases in disease development. *Gene* 286: 155–174.

Bokoch GM, Gilman AG (1984). Inhibition of receptor-mediated release of arachidonic acid by pertussis toxin. *Cell* 39: 301–308.

Bos JL (1989). *Ras* oncogenes in human cancer: a review. *Cancer Res* 49: 4682–4689.

Bourne HR (1997). How receptors talk to trimeric G proteins. *Curr Opin Cell Biol* 9: 134–142.

Bowtell D, Fu P, Simon M, Senior P (1992). Identification of murine homologues of the *Drosophila son of sevenless* gene: potential activators of ras. *Proc Natl Acad Sci USA* 89: 6511–6515.

Brazil DP, Hemmings BA (2001). Ten years of protein kinase B signalling: a hard Akt to follow. *Trends Biochem Sci* 26: 657–664.

Broek D, Toda T, Michaeli T, Levin L, Birchmeier C, Zoller M, Powers S, Wigler M (1987). The *S. cerevisiae CDC25* gene product regulates the RAS/adenylate cyclase pathway. *Cell* 48: 789–799.

Brouns MR, Matheson SF, Hu KQ, Delalle I, Caviness VS, Silver J, Bronson RT, Settleman J (2000). The adhesion signaling molecule p190 RhoGAP is required for morphogenetic processes in neural development. *Development* 127: 4891–4903.

Brouns MR, Matheson SF, Settleman J (2001). p190 RhoGAP is the principal Src substrate in brain and regulates axon outgrowth, guidance and fasciculation. *Nat Cell Biol* 3: 361–367.

Buchwald G, Hostinova E, Rudolph MG, Kraemer A, Sickmann A, Meyer HE, Scheffzek K, Wittinghofer A (2001). Conformational switch and role of phosphorylation in PAK activation. *Mol Cell Biol* 21: 5179–5189.

Buhl AM, Johnson NL, Dhanasekaran N, Johnson GL (1995). Gα12 and Gα13 stimulate Rho-dependent stress fiber formation and focal adhesion assembly. *J Biol Chem* 270: 24631–24634.

Bustelo XR (2000). Regulatory and signaling properties of the Vav family. *Mol Cell Biol* 20: 1461–1477.

Camonis JH, Kalekine M, Gondre B, Garreau H, Boy-Marcotte E, Jacquet M (1986). Characterization, cloning and sequence analysis of the *CDC25* gene which controls the cyclic AMP level of *Saccharomyces cerevisiae*. *EMBO J* 5: 375–380.

Campbell SL, Khosravi-Far R, Rossman KL, Clark GJ, Der CJ (1998). Increasing complexity of Ras signaling. *Oncogene* 17: 1395–1413.

Cantor SB, Urano T, Feig LA (1995). Identification and characterization of Ral-binding protein 1, a potential downstream target of Ral GTPases. *Mol Cell Biol* 15: 4578–4584.

Castrillon DH, Wasserman SA (1994). *Diaphanous* is required for cytokinesis in *Drosophila* and shares domains of similarity with the products of the *limb deformity* gene. *Development* 120: 3367–3377.

Cau J, Faure S, Comps M, Delsert C, Morin N (2001). A novel p21-activated kinase binds the actin and microtubule networks and induces microtubule stabilization. *J Cell Biol* 155: 1029–1042.

Cen H, Papageorge AG, Zippel R, Lowy DR, Zhang K (1992). Isolation of multiple mouse cDNAs with coding homology to *Saccharomyces cerevisiae* CDC25: identification of a region related to *Bcr, Vav, Dbl* and *CDC24*. *EMBO J* 11: 4007–4015.

Chardin P, Camonis JH, Gale NW, van Aelst L, Schlessinger J, Wigler MH, Bar-Sagi D (1993). Human Sos1: a guanine nucleotide exchange factor for Ras that binds to GRB2. *Science* 260: 1338–1343.

Chen HJ, Rojas-Soto M, Oguni A, Kennedy MB (1998). A synaptic Ras-GTPase activating protein (p135 SynGAP) inhibited by CaM kinase II. *Neuron* 20: 895–904.

Cherfils J, Chardin P (1999). GEFs: structural basis for their activation of small GTP-binding proteins. *Trends Biochem Sci* 24: 306–311.

Chong LD, Traynor-Kaplan A, Bokoch GM, Schwartz MA (1994). The small GTP-binding protein Rho regulates a phosphatidylinositol 4-phosphate 5-kinase in mammalian cells. *Cell* 79: 507–513.

Chrzanowska-Wodnicka M, Burridge K (1996). Rho-stimulated contractility drives the formation of stress fibers and focal adhesions. *J Cell Biol* 133: 1403–1415.

Clyde-Smith J, Silins G, Gartside M, Grimmond S, Etheridge M, Apolloni A, Hayward N, Hancock JF (2000). Characterization of RasGRP2, a plasma membrane-targeted, dual specificity Ras/Rap exchange factor. *J Biol Chem* 275: 32260–32267.

Conklin BR, Farfel Z, Lustig KD, Julius D, Bourne HR (1993). Substitution of three amino acids switches receptor specificity of Gqα to that of Giα. *Nature* 363: 274–276.

Crespo P, Xu N, Simonds WF, Gutkind JS (1994). Ras-dependent activation of MAP kinase pathway mediated by G-protein βγ-subunits. *Nature* 369: 418–420.

Cullen PJ (1998). Bridging the GAP in inositol 1,3,4,5-tetrakisphosphate signalling. *Biochim Biophys Acta* 1436: 35–47.

Cullen PJ (2001). Ras effectors: buying shares in Ras plc. *Curr Biol* 11: R342–344.

Cullen PJ, Hsuan JJ, Truong O, Letcher AJ, Jackson TR, Dawson AP, Irvine RF (1995). Identification of a specific Ins(1,3,4,5)P4-binding protein as a member of the GAP1 family. *Nature* 376: 527–530.

Daaka Y, Pitcher JA, Richardson M, Stoffel RH, Robishaw JD, Lefkowitz RJ (1997). Receptor and Gβγ isoform-specific interactions with G protein-coupled receptor kinases. *Proc Natl Acad Sci USA* 94: 2180–2185.

Dan C, Kelly A, Bernard O, Minden A (2001). Cytoskeletal changes regulated by the PAK4 serine/threonine kinase are mediated by LIM kinase 1 and cofilin. *J Biol Chem* 276: 32115–32121.

Dan C, Nath N, Liberto M, Minden A (2002). PAK5, a new brain-specific kinase, promotes neurite outgrowth in N1E-115 cells. *Mol Cell Biol* 22: 567–577.

Daniels RH, Bokoch GM (1999). p21-activated protein kinase: a crucial component of morphological signaling? *Trends Biochem Sci* 24: 350–355.

Daniels RH, Hall PS, Bokoch GM (1998). Membrane targeting of p21-activated kinase 1 (PAK1) induces neurite outgrowth from PC12 cells. *EMBO J* 17: 754–764.

Davis AJ, Butt JT, Walker JH, Moss SE, Gawler DJ (1996). The Ca2+-dependent lipid binding domain of P120GAP mediates protein–protein interactions with Ca2+-dependent membrane-binding proteins: evidence for a direct interaction between annexin VI and P120GAP. *J Biol Chem* 271: 24333–24336.

Del Pozo MA, Kiosses WB, Alderson NB, Meller N, Hahn KM, Schwartz MA (2002). Integrins regulate GTP-Rac localized effector interactions through dissociation of Rho-GDI. *Nat Cell Biol* 4: 232–239.

Dent P, Haser W, Haystead TA, Vincent LA, Roberts TM, Sturgill TW (1992). Activation of mitogen-activated protein kinase kinase by v-Raf in NIH 3T3 cells and in vitro. *Science* 257: 1404–1407.

Derry JM, Ochs HD, Francke U (1994). Isolation of a novel gene mutated in Wiskott-Aldrich syndrome. *Cell* 78: 635–644.

De Vries L, Gist Farquhar M (1999). RGS proteins: more than just GAPs for heterotrimeric G proteins. *Trends Cell Biol* 9: 138–144.

Dixon RA, Kobilka BK, Strader DJ, Benovic JL, Dohlman HG, Frielle T, Bolanowski MA, Bennett CD, Rands E, Diehl RE, et al. (1986). Cloning of the gene and cDNA for mammalian β-adrenergic receptor and homology with rhodopsin. *Nature* 321: 75–79.

Dohlman HG, Caron MG, Lefkowitz RJ (1987). A family of receptors coupled to guanine nucleotide regulatory proteins. *Biochemistry* 26: 2657–2664.

Downward J (1996). Control of Ras activation. *Cancer Surv* 27: 87–100.

Downward J (1998). Mechanisms and consequences of activation of protein kinase B/Akt. *Curr Opin Cell Biol* 10: 262–267.

Dryja TP, Hahn LB, Reboul T, Arnaud B (1996). Missense mutation in the gene encoding the α-subunit of rod transducin in the Nougaret form of congenital stationary night blindness. *Nat Genet* 13: 358–360.

Ebinu JO, Bottorff DA, Chan EY, Stang SL, Dunn RJ, Stone JC (1998). RasGRP, a Ras guanyl nucleotide-releasing protein with calcium- and diacylglycerol-binding motifs. *Science* 280: 1082–1086.

Edwards DC, Sanders LC, Bokoch GM, Gill GN (1999). Activation of LIM-kinase by Pak1 couples Rac/Cdc42 GTPase signalling to actin cytoskeletal dynamics. *Nat Cell Biol* 1: 253–259.

Ellis C, Moran M, McCormick F, Pawson T (1990). Phosphorylation of GAP and GAP-associated proteins by transforming and mitogenic tyrosine kinases. *Nature* 343: 377–381.

Ellis S, Mellor H (2000). Regulation of endocytic traffic by Rho family GTPases. *Trends Cell Biol* 10: 85–88.

Evers EE, Zondag GC, Malliri A, Price LS, ten Klooster JP, van der Kammen RA, Collard JG (2000). Rho family proteins in cell adhesion and cell migration. *Eur J Cancer* 36: 1269–1274.

Fam NP, Fan WT, Wang Z, Zhang LJ, Chen H, Moran MF (1997). Cloning and charac-

terization of Ras-GRF2, a novel guanine nucleotide exchange factor for Ras. *Mol Cell Biol* 17: 1396–1406.
Fan WT, Koch CA, de Hoog CL, Fam NP, Moran MF (1998). The exchange factor Ras-GRF2 activates Ras-dependent and Rac-dependent mitogen-activated protein kinase pathways. *Curr Biol* 8: 935–938.
Farfel Z, Bourne HR, Iiri T (1999). The expanding spectrum of G protein diseases. *N Engl J Med* 340: 1012–1020.
Farnsworth CL, Freshney NW, Rosen LB, Ghosh A, Greenberg ME, Feig LA (1995). Calcium activation of Ras mediated by neuronal exchange factor Ras-GRF. *Nature* 376: 524–527.
Fields TA, Casey PJ (1997). Signalling functions and biochemical properties of pertussis toxin-resistant G-proteins. *Biochem J* 321(Pt 3): 561–571.
Fromm C, Coso OA, Montaner S, Xu N, Gutkind JS (1997). The small GTP-binding protein Rho links G protein–coupled receptors and $G\alpha_{12}$ to the serum response element and to cellular transformation. *Proc Natl Acad Sci USA* 94: 10098–10103.
Fukata M, Kaibuchi K (2001). Rho-family GTPases in cadherin-mediated cell–cell adhesion. *Nat Rev Mol Cell Biol* 2: 887–897.
Fukata Y, Kimura K, Oshiro N, Saya H, Matsuura Y, Kaibuchi K (1998). Association of the myosin-binding subunit of myosin phosphatase and moesin: dual regulation of moesin phosphorylation by Rho-associated kinase and myosin phosphatase. *J Cell Biol* 141: 409–418.
Fukata Y, Amano M, Kaibuchi K (2001). Rho-Rho-kinase pathway in smooth muscle contraction and cytoskeletal reorganization of non-muscle cells. *Trends Pharmacol Sci* 22: 32–39.
Fukuhara S, Murga C, Zohar M, Igishi T, Gutkind JS (1999). A novel PDZ domain containing guanine nucleotide exchange factor links heterotrimeric G proteins to Rho. *J Biol Chem* 274: 5868–5879.
Fukuhara S, Chikumi H, Gutkind JS (2000). Leukemia-associated Rho guanine nucleotide exchange factor (LARG) links heterotrimeric G proteins of the G_{12} family to Rho. *FEBS Lett* 485: 183–188.
Fukuhara S, Chikumi H, Gutkind JS (2001). RGS-containing RhoGEFs: the missing link between transforming G proteins and Rho? *Oncogene* 20: 1661–1668.
Gaudet R, Savage JR, McLaughlin JN, Willardson BM, Sigler PB (1999). A molecular mechanism for the phosphorylation-dependent regulation of heterotrimeric G proteins by phosducin. *Mol Cell* 3: 649–660.
Gertler FB, Niebuhr K, Reinhard M, Wehland J, Soriano P (1996). Mena, a relative of VASP and *Drosophila* Enabled, is implicated in the control of microfilament dynamics. *Cell* 87: 227–239.
Gibbs JB, Schaber MD, Allard WJ, Sigal IS, Scolnick EM (1988). Purification of ras GTPase activating protein from bovine brain. *Proc Natl Acad Sci USA* 85: 5026–5030.
Glick JL, Meigs TE, Miron A, Casey PJ (1998). RGSZ1, a Gz-selective regulator of G protein signaling whose action is sensitive to the phosphorylation state of $Gz\alpha$. *J Biol Chem* 273: 26008–26013.
Gohla A, Harhammer R, Schultz G (1998). The G-protein G13 but not G12 mediates signaling from lysophosphatidic acid receptor via epidermal growth factor receptor to Rho. *J Biol Chem* 273: 4653–4659.
Gotte M, Lazar T, Yoo JS, Scheglmann D, Gallwitz D (2000). The full complement of yeast Ypt/Rab-GTPases and their involvement in exo- and endocytic trafficking. *Subcell Biochem* 34: 133–173.
Gutkind JS (2000). Regulation of mitogen-activated protein kinase signaling networks by G protein–coupled receptors. *Sci STKE* 2000: RE1.
Gutmann DH (2001). The neurofibromatoses: when less is more. *Hum Mol Genet* 10: 747–755.
Hadano S, Hand CK, Osuga H, Yanagisawa Y, Otomo A, Devon R S, Miyamoto N, Showguchi-Miyata J, Okada Y, Singaraja R, et al. (2001). A gene encoding a putative GTPase regulator is mutated in familial amyotrophic lateral sclerosis 2. *Nat Genet* 29: 166–173.
Hall A (1998). Rho GTPases and the actin cytoskeleton. *Science* 279: 509–514.
Hamm HE (1998). The many faces of G protein signaling. *J Biol Chem* 273: 669–672.
Han J, Luby-Phelps K, Das B, Shu X, Xia Y, Mosteller RD, Krishna UM, Falck JR, White MA, Broek D (1998). Role of substrates and products of PI 3-kinase in regulating activation of Rac-related guanosine triphosphatases by Vav. *Science* 279: 558–560.
Han L, Colicelli J (1995). A human protein selected for interference with Ras function interacts directly with Ras and competes with Raf1. *Mol Cell Biol* 15: 1318–1323.
Hart CM, Roberts JW (1994). Deletion analysis of the λ tR1 termination region. Effect of sequences near the transcript release sites, and the minimum length of rho-dependent transcripts. *J Mol Biol* 237: 255–265.
Hart MJ, Eva A, Evans T, Aaronson SA, Cerione RA (1991). Catalysis of guanine nucleotide exchange on the CDC42Hs protein by the dbl oncogene product. *Nature* 354: 311–314.
Hart MJ, Jiang X, Kozasa T, Roscoe W, Singer WD, Gilman AG, Sternweis PC, Bollag G (1998). Direct stimulation of the guanine nucleotide exchange activity of p115 RhoGEF by $G\alpha_{13}$. *Science* 280: 2112–2114.
Hartwig JH, Bokoch GM, Carpenter CL, Janmey PA, Taylor LA, Toker A, Stossel TP (1995). Thrombin receptor ligation and activated Rac uncap actin filament barbed ends through phosphoinositide synthesis in permeabilized human platelets. *Cell* 82: 643–653.
Henry JP, Johannes L, Dousseau F, Poulain B, Darchen F (1996). Role of Rab3a in neurotransmitter and hormone release: a discussion of recent data. *Biochem Soc Trans* 24: 657–661.
Hepler JR, Gilman AG (1992). G proteins. *Trends Biochem Sci* 17: 383–387.
Hepler JR, Berman DM, Gilman AG, Kozasa T (1997). RGS4 and GAIP are GTPase-activating proteins for $Gq\alpha$ and block activation of phospholipase $C\beta$ by γ-thio-GTP-$Gq\alpha$. *Proc Natl Acad Sci USA* 94: 428–432.
Hescheler J, Rosenthal W, Trautwein W, Schultz G (1987). The GTP-binding protein, Go, regulates neuronal calcium channels. *Nature* 325: 445–447.
Higgs HN, Pollard TD (2001). Regulation of actin filament network formation through ARP2/3 complex: activation by a diverse array of proteins. *Annu Rev Biochem* 70: 649–676.
Hirose M, Ishizaki T, Watanabe N, Uehata M, Kranenburg O, Moolenaar WH, Matsumura F, Maekawa M, Bito H, Narumiya S (1998). Molecular dissection of the Rho-associated protein kinase (p160ROCK)–regulated neurite remodeling in neuroblastoma N1E-115 cells. *J Cell Biol* 141: 1625–1636.
Houslay MD, Milligan G (1997). Tailoring cAMP-signalling responses through isoform multiplicity. *Trends Biochem Sci* 22: 217–224.
Innocenti M, Tenca P, Frittoli E, Faretta M, Tocchetti A, Di Fiore PP, Scita G (2002). Mechanisms through which Sos-1 coordinates the activation of Ras and Rac. *J Cell Biol* 156: 125–136.
Ishizaki T, Maekawa M, Fujisawa K, Okawa K, Iwamatsu A, Fujita A, Watanabe N, Saito Y, Kakizuka A, Morii N, Narumiya S (1996). The small GTP-binding protein Rho binds to and activates a 160 kDa Ser/Thr protein kinase homologous to myotonic dystrophy kinase. *EMBO J* 15: 1885–1893.
Ishizaki T, Naito M, Fujisawa K, Maekawa M, Watanabe N, Saito Y, Narumiya S (1997). p160ROCK, a Rho-associated coiled-coil forming protein kinase, works downstream of Rho and induces focal adhesions. *FEBS Lett* 404: 118–124.
Ishizaki T, Morishima Y, Okamoto M, Furuyashiki T, Kato T, Narumiya S (2001). Coordination of microtubules and the actin cytoskeleton by the Rho effector mDia1. *Nat Cell Biol* 3: 8–14.
Jaffe AB, Hall A (2002). Rho GTPases in transformation and metastasis. *Adv Cancer Res* 84: 57–80.
Janmey PA (1994). Phosphoinositides and calcium as regulators of cellular actin assembly and disassembly. *Annu Rev Physiol* 56: 169–191.
Jenna S, Larmarche-Vane N (In press). The superfamily of Rho GTPase activating proteins. In: *Rho GTPases*. Symons M (ed.) RG Landes, Austin, Tex.
Jenna S, Hussain NK, Danek EI, Triki I, Wasiak S, McPherson PS, Lamarche-Vane N (2002). The activity of the GTPase-activating protein CdGAP is regulated by the endocytic protein intersectin. *J Biol Chem* 277: 6366–6373.
Jiang H, Wu D, Simon MI (1993). The transforming activity of activated $G\alpha_{12}$. *FEBS Lett* 330: 319–322.
Jiang H, Luo JQ, Urano T, Frankel P, Lu Z, Foster DA, Feig LA (1995). Involvement of Ral GTPase in v-Src-induced phospholipase D activation. *Nature* 378: 409–412.
Jiang Y, Ma W, Wan Y, Kozasa T, Hattori S, Huang XY (1998). The G protein $G\alpha_{12}$ stimulates Bruton's tyrosine kinase and a rasGAP through a conserved PH/BM domain. *Nature* 395: 808–813.
Kaibuchi K, Kuroda S, Amano M (1999). Regulation of the cytoskeleton and cell adhesion by the Rho family GTPases in mammalian cells. *Annu Rev Biochem* 68: 459–486.
Kamp TJ, Hell JW (2000). Regulation of cardiac L-type calcium channels by protein kinase A and protein kinase C. *Circ Res* 87: 1095–1102.
Kapeller R, Cantley LC (1994). Phosphatidylinositol 3-kinase. *Bioessays* 16: 565–576.
Kaplan DR, Morrison DK, Wong G, McCormick F, Williams LT (1990). PDGF β-receptor stimulates tyrosine phosphorylation of GAP and association of GAP with a signaling complex. *Cell* 61: 125–133.
Kato T, Watanabe N, Morishima Y, Fujita A, Ishizaki T, Narumiya S (2001). Localization of a mammalian homolog of diaphanous, mDia1, to the mitotic spindle in HeLa cells. *J Cell Sci* 114: 775–784.
Katoh H, Aoki J, Ichikawa A, Negishi M (1998). p160 RhoA-binding kinase $ROK\alpha$ induces neurite retraction. *J Biol Chem* 273: 2489–2492.
Kawasaki H, Springett GM, Toki S, Canales JJ, Harlan P, Blumenstiel JP, Chen EJ, Bany IA, Mochizuki N, Ashbacher A, et al. (1998). A Rap guanine nucleotide exchange factor enriched highly in the basal ganglia. *Proc Natl Acad Sci USA* 95: 13278–13283.
Kazlauskas A, Ellis C, Pawson T, Cooper JA (1990). Binding of GAP to activated PDGF receptors. *Science* 247: 1578–1581.
Kedra D, Seroussi E, Fransson I, Trifunovic J, Clark M, Lagercrantz J, Blennow E, Mehlin H, Dumanski J (1997). The germinal center kinase gene and a novel CDC25-like gene are located in the vicinity of the PYGM gene on 11q13. *Hum Genet* 100: 611–619.
Keenan C, Kelleher D (1998). Protein kinase C and the cytoskeleton. *Cell Signal* 10: 225–232.
Khosravi-Far R, White MA, Westwick JK, Solski PA, Chrzanowska-Wodnicka M, Van Aelst L, Wigler MH, Der CJ (1996). Oncogenic Ras activation of Raf/mitogen-activated protein kinase-independent pathways is sufficient to cause tumorigenic transformation. *Mol Cell Biol* 16: 3923–3933.
Khwaja A (1999). Akt is more than just a Bad kinase. *Nature* 401: 33–34.
Kim JH, Liao D, Lau LF, Huganir RL (1998). SynGAP: a synaptic RasGAP that associates with the PSD-95/SAP90 protein family. *Neuron* 20: 683–691.
Kimura K, Ito M, Amano M, Chihara K, Fukata Y, Nakafuku M, Yamamori B, Feng J, Nakano T, Okawa K, et al. (1996). Regulation of myosin phosphatase by Rho and Rho-associated kinase (Rho-kinase). *Science* 273: 245–248.
Kiyono M, Satoh T, Kaziro Y (1999). G protein $\beta\gamma$-subunit-dependent Rac-guanine nucleotide exchange activity of Ras-GRF1/CDC25(Mm). *Proc Natl Acad Sci USA* 96: 4826–4831.
Kiyono M, Kato J, Kataoka T, Kaziro Y, Satoh T (2000). Stimulation of Ras guanine nucleotide exchange activity of Ras-GRF1/CDC25(Mm) upon tyrosine phosphorylation by the Cdc42-regulated kinase ACK1. *J Biol Chem* 275: 29788–29793.
Kjoller L, Hall A (1999). Signaling to Rho GTPases. *Exp Cell Res* 253: 166–179.
Kohno H, Tanaka K, Mino A, Umikawa M, Imamura H, Fujiwara T, Fujita Y, Hotta K, Qadota H, Watanabe T, et al. (1996). Bni1p implicated in cytoskeletal control is a putative target of Rho1p small GTP binding protein in *Saccharomyces cerevisiae*. *EMBO J* 15: 6060–6068.
Kozasa T, Jiang X, Hart MJ, Sternweis PM, Singer WD, Gilman AG, Bollag G, Sternweis PC (1998). p115 RhoGEF, a GTPase activating protein for $G\alpha_{12}$ and $G\alpha_{13}$. *Science* 280: 2109–2111.
Kozma R, Ahmed S, Best A, Lim L (1995). The Ras-related protein Cdc42Hs and bradykinin promote formation of peripheral actin microspikes and filopodia in Swiss 3T3 fibroblasts. *Mol Cell Biol* 15: 1942–1952.
Krugmann S, Jordens I, Gevaert K, Driessens M, Vandekerckhove J, Hall A (2001). Cdc42 induces filopodia by promoting the formation of an IRSp53 : Mena complex. *Curr Biol* 11: 1645–1655.

Kurahashi T, Yau KW (1993). Co-existence of cationic and chloride components in odorant-induced current of vertebrate olfactory receptor cells. *Nature* 363: 71–74.

Kutsche K, Yntema H, Brandt A, Jantke I, Nothwang HG, Orth U, Boavida MG, David D, Chelly J, Fryns JP, et al. (2000). Mutations in ARHGEF6, encoding a guanine nucleotide exchange factor for Rho GTPases, in patients with X-linked mental retardation. *Nat Genet* 26: 247–250.

Kyriakis JM, App H, Zhang XF, Banerjee P, Brautigan DL, Rapp UR, Avruch J (1992). Raf-1 activates MAP kinase-kinase. *Nature* 358: 417–421.

Landis CA, Masters SB, Spada A, Pace AM, Bourne HR, Vallar L (1989). GTPase inhibiting mutations activate the α-chain of Gs and stimulate adenylyl cyclase in human pituitary tumours. *Nature* 340: 692–696.

Lania A, Mantovani G, Spada A (2001). G protein mutations in endocrine diseases. *Eur J Endocrinol* 145: 543–559.

Lanier LM, Gates MA, Witke W, Menzies AS, Wehman AM, Macklis JD, Kwiatkowski D, Soriano P, Gertler FB (1999). Mena is required for neurulation and commissure formation. *Neuron* 22: 313–325.

Leung T, Manser E, Tan L, Lim L (1995). A novel serine/threonine kinase binding the Ras-related RhoA GTPase which translocates the kinase to peripheral membranes. *J Biol Chem* 270: 29051–29054.

Leung T, Chen XQ, Manser E, Lim L (1996). The p160 RhoA-binding kinase ROKα is a member of a kinase family and is involved in the reorganization of the cytoskeleton. *Mol Cell Biol* 16: 5313–5327.

Li N, Batzer A, Daly R, Yajnik V, Skolnik E, Chardin P, Bar-Sagi D, Margolis B, Schlessinger J (1993). Guanine-nucleotide-releasing factor hSos1 binds to Grb2 and links receptor tyrosine kinases to Ras signalling. *Nature* 363: 85–88.

Liu WS, Heckman CA (1998). The sevenfold way of PKC regulation. *Cell Signal* 10: 529–542.

Lockyer PJ, Wennstrom S, Kupzig S, Venkateswarlu K, Downward J, Cullen PJ (1999). Identification of the ras GTPase-activating protein GAP1(m) as a phosphatidylinositol-3,4,5-trisphosphate-binding protein in vivo. *Curr Biol* 9: 265–268.

Lockyer PJ, Kupzig S, Cullen PJ (2001). CAPRI regulates Ca^{2+}-dependent inactivation of the Ras-MAPK pathway. *Curr Biol* 11: 981–986.

Lounsbury KM, Casey PJ, Brass LF, Manning DR (1991). Phosphorylation of Gz in human platelets: selectivity and site of modification. *J Biol Chem* 266: 22051–22056.

Luo JQ, Liu X, Frankel P, Rotunda T, Ramos M, Flom J, Jiang H, Feig LA, Morris AJ, Kahn RA, Foster DA (1998). Functional association between Arf and RalA in active phospholipase D complex. *Proc Natl Acad Sci USA* 95: 3632–3637.

Luo L (2000). Rho GTPases in neuronal morphogenesis. *Nat Rev Neurosci* 1: 173–180.

Lutcke A, Jansson S, Parton RG, Chavrier P, Valencia A, Huber LA, Lehtonen E, Zerial M (1993). Rab17, a novel small GTPase, is specific for epithelial cells and is induced during cell polarization. *J Cell Biol* 121: 553–564.

Lynch ED, Lee MK, Morrow JE, Welcsh PL, Leon PE, King MC (1997). Nonsyndromic deafness DFNA1 associated with mutation of a human homolog of the *Drosophila* gene diaphanous. *Science* 278: 1315–1318.

Machesky LM, Insall RH (1998). Scar1 and the related Wiskott-Aldrich syndrome protein, WASP, regulate the actin cytoskeleton through the Arp2/3 complex. *Curr Biol* 8: 1347–1356.

Maekawa M, Li S, Iwamatsu A, Morishita T, Yokota K, Imai Y, Kohsaka S, Nakamura S, Hattori S (1994). A novel mammalian Ras GTPase-activating protein which has phospholipid-binding and Btk homology regions. *Mol Cell Biol* 14: 6879–6885.

Maekawa M, Ishizaki T, Boku S, Watanabe N, Fujita A, Iwamatsu A, Obinata T, Ohashi K, Mizuno K, Narumiya S (1999). Signaling from Rho to the actin cytoskeleton through protein kinases ROCK and LIM-kinase. *Science* 285: 895–898.

Magee T, Marshall C (1999). New insights into the interaction of Ras with the plasma membrane. *Cell* 98: 9–12.

Manser E, Leung T, Salihuddin H, Zhao ZS, Lim L (1994). A brain serine/threonine protein kinase activated by Cdc42 and Rac1. *Nature* 367: 40–46.

Manser E, Huang HY, Loo TH, Chen XQ, Dong JM, Leung T, Lim L (1997). Expression of constitutively active α-PAK reveals effects of the kinase on actin and focal complexes. *Mol Cell Biol* 17: 1129–1143.

Mao J, Yuan H, Xie W, Wu D (1998). Guanine nucleotide exchange factor GEF115 specifically mediates activation of Rho and serum response factor by the G protein α-subunit $G\alpha_{13}$. *Proc Natl Acad Sci USA* 95: 12973–12976.

Marinissen MJ, Gutkind JS (2001). G-protein-coupled receptors and signaling networks: emerging paradigms. *Trends Pharmacol Sci* 22: 368–376.

Marshall C (1999). How do small GTPase signal transduction pathways regulate cell cycle entry? *Curr Opin Cell Biol* 11: 732–736.

Matsui T, Amano M, Yamamoto T, Chihara K, Nakafuku M, Ito M, Nakano T, Okawa K, Iwamatsu A, Kaibuchi K (1996). Rho-associated kinase, a novel serine/threonine kinase, as a putative target for small GTP binding protein Rho. *EMBO J* 15: 2208–2216.

Mattingly RR, Macara IG (1996). Phosphorylation-dependent activation of the Ras-GRF/CDC25Mm exchange factor by muscarinic receptors and G-protein $\beta\gamma$-subunits. *Nature* 382: 268–272.

Mayr B, Montminy M (2001). Transcriptional regulation by the phosphorylation-dependent factor CREB. *Nat Rev Mol Cell Biol* 2: 599–609.

Mehta D, Rahman A, Malik AB (2001). Protein kinase C-α signals rho-guanine nucleotide dissociation inhibitor phosphorylation and rho activation and regulates the endothelial cell barrier function. *J Biol Chem* 276: 22614–22620.

Meng EC, Bourne HR (2001). Receptor activation: what does the rhodopsin structure tell us? *Trends Pharmacol Sci* 22: 587–593.

Meng J, Glick JL, Polakis P, Casey PJ (1999). Functional interaction between $G\alpha_z$ and Rap1GAP suggests a novel form of cellular cross-talk. *J Biol Chem* 274: 36663–36669.

Miki H, Sasaki T, Takai Y, Takenawa T (1998a). Induction of filopodium formation by a WASP-related actin-depolymerizing protein N-WASP. *Nature* 391: 93–96.

Miki H, Suetsugu S, Takenawa T (1998b). WAVE, a novel WASP-family protein involved in actin reorganization induced by Rac. *EMBO J* 17: 6932–6941.

Miki H, Yamaguchi H, Suetsugu S, Takenawa T (2000). IRSp53 is an essential intermediate between Rac and WAVE in the regulation of membrane ruffling. *Nature* 408: 732–735.

Milburn MV, Tong L, deVos AM, Brunger A, Yamaizumi Z, Nishimura S, Kim SH (1990). Molecular switch for signal transduction: structural differences between active and inactive forms of protooncogenic ras proteins. *Science* 247: 939–945.

Molloy CJ, Bottaro DP, Fleming TP, Marshall MS, Gibbs JB, Aaronson SA (1989). PDGF induction of tyrosine phosphorylation of GTPase activating protein. *Nature* 342: 711–714.

Moodie SA, Willumsen BM, Weber MJ, Wolfman A (1993). Complexes of Ras.GTP with Raf-1 and mitogen-activated protein kinase kinase. *Science* 260: 1658–1661.

Morris AJ, Malbon CC (1999). Physiological regulation of G protein–linked signaling. *Physiol Rev* 79: 1373–1430.

Nakagawa O, Fujisawa K, Ishizaki T, Saito Y, Nakao K, Narumiya S (1996). ROCK-I and ROCK-II, two isoforms of Rho-associated coiled-coil forming protein serine/threonine kinase in mice. *FEBS Lett* 392: 189–193.

Nalefski EA, Falke JJ (1996). The C2 domain calcium-binding motif: structural and functional diversity. *Protein Sci* 5: 2375–2390.

Nimnual AS, Yatsula BA, Bar-Sagi D (1998). Coupling of Ras and Rac guanosine triphosphatases through the Ras exchanger Sos. *Science* 279: 560–563.

Nobes CD, Hall A (1995). Rho, rac, and cdc42 GTPases regulate the assembly of multimolecular focal complexes associated with actin stress fibers, lamellipodia, and filopodia. *Cell* 81: 53–62.

Obermeier A, Ahmed S, Manser E, Yen SC, Hall C, Lim L (1998). PAK promotes morphological changes by acting upstream of Rac. *EMBO J* 17: 4328–4339.

Ohta Y, Suzuki N, Nakamura S, Hartwig JH, Stossel TP (1999). The small GTPase RalA targets filamin to induce filopodia. *Proc Natl Acad Sci USA* 96: 2122–2128.

Olofsson B (1999). Rho guanine dissociation inhibitors: pivotal molecules in cellular signalling. *Cell Signal* 11: 545–554.

Oude Weernink PA, Schulte P, Guo Y, Wetzel J, Amano M, Kaibuchi K, Haverland S, Voss M, Schmidt M, Mayr GW, Jakobs KH (2000). Stimulation of phosphatidylinositol-4-phosphate 5-kinase by Rho-kinase. *J Biol Chem* 275: 10168–10174.

Palazzo AF, Cook TA, Alberts AS, Gundersen GG (2001). mDia mediates Rho-regulated formation and orientation of stable microtubules. *Nat Cell Biol* 3: 723–729.

Palczewski K, Kumasaka T, Hori T, Behnke CA, Motoshima H, Fox BA, Le Trong I, Teller DC, Okada T, Stenkamp RE, et al. (2000). Crystal structure of rhodopsin: a G protein–coupled receptor. *Science* 289: 739–745.

Park SH, Weinberg RA (1995). A putative effector of Ral has homology to Rho/Rac GTPase activating proteins. *Oncogene* 11: 2349–2355.

Paschal BM, Delphin C, Gerace L (1996). Nucleotide-specific interaction of Ran/TC4 with nuclear transport factor NTF2 and p97. *Proc Natl Acad Sci USA* 93: 7679–7683.

Pasteris NG, Cadle A, Logie LJ, Porteous ME, Schwartz CE, Stevenson RE, Glover TW, Wilroy RS, Gorski JL (1994). Isolation and characterization of the faciogenital dysplasia (Aarskog-Scott syndrome) gene: a putative Rho/Rac guanine nucleotide exchange factor. *Cell* 79: 669–678.

Patel TB, Du Z, Pierre S, Cartin L, Scholich K (2001). Molecular biological approaches to unravel adenylyl cyclase signaling and function. *Gene* 269: 13–25.

Paterson HF, Self AJ, Garrett MD, Just I, Aktories K, Hall A (1990). Microinjection of recombinant p21rho induces rapid changes in cell morphology. *J Cell Biol* 111: 1001–1007.

Pilpel Y, Sosinsky A, Lancet D (1998). Molecular biology of olfactory receptors. *Essays Biochem* 33: 93–104.

Pitcher JA, Inglese J, Higgins JB, Arriza JL, Casey PJ, Kim C, Benovic JL, Kwatra MM, Caron MG, Lefkowitz RJ (1992). Role of $\beta\gamma$-subunits of G proteins in targeting the β-adrenergic receptor kinase to membrane-bound receptors. *Science* 257: 1264–1267.

Prior IA, Hancock JF (2001). Compartmentalization of Ras proteins. *J Cell Sci* 114: 1603–1608.

Pruitt K, Der CJ (2001). Ras and Rho regulation of the cell cycle and oncogenesis. *Cancer Lett* 171: 1–10.

Ravichandran KS, Lorenz U, Shoelson SE, Burakoff SJ (1995). Interaction of Shc with Grb2 regulates association of Grb2 with mSOS. *Mol Cell Biol* 15: 593–600.

Rebecchi MJ, Pentyala SN (2000). Structure, function, and control of phosphoinositide-specific phospholipase C. *Physiol Rev* 80: 1291–1335.

Reinhard M, Jarchau T, Walter U (2001). Actin-based motility: stop and go with Ena/VASP proteins. *Trends Biochem Sci* 26: 243–249.

Ren XD, Bokoch GM, Traynor-Kaplan A, Jenkins GH, Anderson RA, Schwartz MA (1996). Physical association of the small GTPase Rho with a 68-kDa phosphatidylinositol 4-phosphate 5-kinase in Swiss 3T3 cells. *Mol Biol Cell* 7: 435–442.

Rhee SG, Bae YS (1997). Regulation of phosphoinositide-specific phospholipase C isozymes. *J Biol Chem* 272: 15045–15048.

Ridley AJ (2001a). Rho family proteins: coordinating cell responses. *Trends Cell Biol* 11: 471–477.

Ridley AJ (2001b). Rho GTPases and cell migration. *J Cell Sci* 114: 2713–2722.

Ridley AJ, Hall A (1992). The small GTP-binding protein rho regulates the assembly of focal adhesions and actin stress fibers in response to growth factors. *Cell* 70: 389–399.

Ridley AJ, Paterson HF, Johnston CL, Diekmann D, Hall A (1992). The small GTP-binding protein rac regulates growth factor–induced membrane ruffling. *Cell* 70: 401–410.

Robinson LC, Gibbs JB, Marshall MS, Sigal IS, Tatchell K (1987). CDC25: a component of the RAS-adenylate cyclase pathway in *Saccharomyces cerevisiae*. *Science* 235: 1218–1221.

Rodriguez-Viciana P, Warne PH, Dhand R, Vanhaesebroeck B, Gout I, Fry MJ, Waterfield MD, Downward J (1994). Phosphatidylinositol-3-OH kinase as a direct target of Ras. *Nature* 370: 527–532.

Rodriguez-Viciana P, Warne PH, Khwaja A, Marte BM, Pappin D, Das P, Waterfield MD, Ridley A, Downward J (1997). Role of phosphoinositide 3-OH kinase in cell transformation and control of the actin cytoskeleton by Ras. *Cell* 89: 457–467.

Rogge RD, Karlovich CA, Banerjee U (1991). Genetic dissection of a neurodevelopmental pathway: son of sevenless functions downstream of the sevenless and EGF receptor tyrosine kinases. *Cell* 64: 39–48.

Rohatgi R, Ma L, Miki H, Lopez M, Kirchhausen T, Takenawa T, Kirschner MW (1999). The interaction between N-WASP and the Arp2/3 complex links Cdc42-dependent signals to actin assembly. *Cell* 97: 221–231.

Rohrer DK, Kobilka BK (1998). G protein-coupled receptors: functional and mechanistic insights through altered gene expression. *Physiol Rev* 78: 35–52.

Ron D, Zannini M, Lewis M, Wickner RB, Hunt LT, Graziani G, Tronick SR, Aaronson SA, Eva A (1991). A region of proto-dbl essential for its transforming activity shows sequence similarity to a yeast cell cycle gene, CDC24, and the human breakpoint cluster gene, bcr. *New Biol* 3: 372–379.

Ross EM, Wilkie TM (2000). GTPase-activating proteins for heterotrimeric G proteins: regulators of G protein signaling (RGS) and RGS-like proteins. *Annu Rev Biochem* 69: 795–827.

Rubin GM, Yandell MD, Wortman JR, Gabor Miklos GL, Nelson CR, Hariharan IK, Fortini ME, Li PW, Apweiler R, Fleischmann W, et al. (2000). Comparative genomics of the eukaryotes. *Science* 287: 2204–2215.

Sanders LC, Matsumura F, Bokoch GM, de Lanerolle P (1999). Inhibition of myosin light chain kinase by p21-activated kinase. *Science* 283: 2083–2085.

Schmitz AA, Govek EE, Bottner B, Van Aelst L (2000). Rho GTPases: signaling, migration, and invasion. *Exp Cell Res* 261: 1–12.

Schneider T, Igelmund P, Hescheler J (1997). G protein interaction with K^+ and Ca^{2+} channels. *Trends Pharmacol Sci* 18: 8–11.

Schwindinger WF, Robishaw JD (2001). Heterotrimeric G-protein $\beta\gamma$-dimers in growth and differentiation. *Oncogene* 20: 1653–1660.

Scita G, Tenca P, Areces LB, Tocchetti A, Frittoli E, Giardina G, Ponzanelli I, Sini P, Innocenti M, Di Fiore PP (2001). An effector region in Eps8 is responsible for the activation of the Rac-specific GEF activity of Sos-1 and for the proper localization of the Rac-based actin-polymerizing machine. *J Cell Biol* 154: 1031–1044.

Seabra MC (1998). Membrane association and targeting of prenylated Ras-like GTPases. *Cell Signal* 10: 167–172.

Seasholtz TM, Majumdar M, Brown JH (1999). Rho as a mediator of G protein–coupled receptor signaling. *Mol Pharmacol* 55: 949–956.

Sells MA, Knaus UG, Bagrodia S, Ambrose DM, Bokoch GM, Chernoff J (1997). Human p21-activated kinase (Pak1) regulates actin organization in mammalian cells. *Curr Biol* 7: 202–210.

Shou C, Farnsworth CL, Neel BG, Feig LA (1992). Molecular cloning of cDNAs encoding a guanine-nucleotide-releasing factor for Ras p21. *Nature* 358: 351–354.

Shou C, Wurmser A, Suen KL, Barbacid M, Feig LA, Ling K (1995). Differential response of the Ras exchange factor, Ras-GRF, to tyrosine kinase and G protein mediated signals. *Oncogene* 10: 1887–1893.

Siffert W, Rosskopf D, Siffert G, Busch S, Moritz A, Erbel R, Sharma AM, Ritz E, Wichmann HE, Jakobs KH, Horsthemke B (1998). Association of a human G-protein $\beta 3$ subunit variant with hypertension. *Nat Genet* 18: 45–48.

Simon MA, Bowtell DD, Dodson GS, Laverty TR, Rubin GM (1991). Ras1 and a putative guanine nucleotide exchange factor perform crucial steps in signaling by the sevenless protein tyrosine kinase. *Cell* 67: 701–716.

Simonds WF (1999). G protein regulation of adenylate cyclase. *Trends Pharmacol Sci* 20: 66–73.

Singh K, Xiao L, Remondino A, Sawyer DB, Colucci WS (2001). Adrenergic regulation of cardiac myocyte apoptosis. *J Cell Physiol* 189: 257–265.

Skalhegg BS, Tasken K (2000). Specificity in the cAMP/PKA signaling pathway. Differential expression,regulation, and subcellular localization of subunits of PKA. *Front Biosci* 5: D678–693.

Smrcka AV, Sternweis PC (1993). Regulation of purified subtypes of phosphatidylinositol-specific phospholipase Cβ by G protein α- and $\beta\gamma$-subunits. *J Biol Chem* 268: 9667–9674.

Srivastava SK, Wheelock RH, Aaronson SA, Eva A (1986). Identification of the protein encoded by the human diffuse B-cell lymphoma (dbl) oncogene. *Proc Natl Acad Sci USA* 83: 8868–8872.

Stephens L, Smrcka A, Cooke FT, Jackson TR, Sternweis PC, Hawkins PT (1994). A novel phosphoinositide 3 kinase activity in myeloid-derived cells is activated by G protein $\beta\gamma$-subunits. *Cell* 77: 83–93.

Sternweis PC, Smrcka AV (1992). Regulation of phospholipase C by G proteins. *Trends Biochem Sci* 17: 502–506.

Stoffel RH 3rd, Pitcher JA, Lefkowitz RJ (1997). Targeting G protein-coupled receptor kinases to their receptor substrates. *J Membr Biol* 157: 1–8.

Strader CD, Fong TM, Graziano MP, Tota MR (1995). The family of G-protein-coupled receptors. *FASEB J* 9: 745–754.

Sunahara RK, Dessauer CW, Gilman AG (1996). Complexity and diversity of mammalian adenylyl cyclases. *Annu Rev Pharmacol Toxicol* 36: 461–480.

Symons M, Derry JM, Karlak B, Jiang S, Lemahieu V, McCormick F, Francke U, Abo A (1996). Wiskott-Aldrich syndrome protein, a novel effector for the GTPase CDC42Hs, is implicated in actin polymerization. *Cell* 84: 723–734.

Takahashi K, Sasaki T, Mammoto A, Takaishi K, Kameyama T, Tsukita S, Takai Y (1997). Direct interaction of the Rho GDP dissociation inhibitor with ezrin/radixin/moesin initiates the activation of the Rho small G protein. *J Biol Chem* 272: 23371–23375.

Takai Y, Sasaki T, Matozaki T (2001). Small GTP-binding proteins. *Physiol Rev* 81: 153–208.

Takenawa T, Miki H (2001). WASP and WAVE family proteins: key molecules for rapid rearrangement of cortical actin filaments and cell movement. *J Cell Sci* 114: 1801–1809.

Tall GG, Barbieri MA, Stahl PD, Horazdovsky BF (2001). Ras-activated endocytosis is mediated by the Rab5 guanine nucleotide exchange activity of RIN1. *Dev Cell* 1: 73–82.

Tamanoi F (1988). Yeast RAS genes. *Biochim Biophys Acta* 948: 1–15.

Tanaka K, Takai Y (1998). Control of reorganization of the actin cytoskeleton by Rho family small GTP-binding proteins in yeast. *Curr Opin Cell Biol* 10: 112–116.

Tesmer JJ, Berman DM, Gilman AG, Sprang SR (1997). Structure of RGS4 bound to AlF4-activated $G_{i\alpha 1}$: stabilization of the transition state for GTP hydrolysis. *Cell* 89: 251–261.

Tognon CE, Kirk HE, Passmore LA, Whitehead IP, Der CJ, Kay RJ (1998). Regulation of RasGRP via a phorbol ester–responsive C1 domain. *Mol Cell Biol* 18: 6995–7008.

Tolias KF, Cantley LC, Carpenter CL (1995). Rho family GTPases bind to phosphoinositide kinases. *J Biol Chem* 270: 17656–17659.

Tominaga T, Sahai E, Chardin P, McCormick F, Courtneidge SA, Alberts AS (2000). Diaphanous-related formins bridge Rho GTPase and Src tyrosine kinase signaling. *Mol Cell* 5: 13–25.

Trahey M, McCormick F (1987). A cytoplasmic protein stimulates normal N-ras p21 GTPase, but does not affect oncogenic mutants. *Science* 238: 542–545.

Van Aelst L, D'Souza-Schorey C (1997). Rho GTPases and signaling networks. *Genes Dev* 11: 2295–2322.

Van Aelst L, Symons M (2002). Role of Rho family GTPases in epithelial morphogenesis. *Genes Dev* 16: 1032–1054.

Van Aelst L, Barr M, Marcus S, Polverino A, Wigler M (1993). Complex formation between RAS and RAF and other protein kinases. *Proc Natl Acad Sci USA* 90: 6213–6217.

VanDongen AM, Codina J, Olate J, Mattera R, Joho R, Birnbaumer L, Brown AM (1988). Newly identified brain potassium channels gated by the guanine nucleotide binding protein Go. *Science* 242: 1433–1437.

Vanhaesebroeck B, Leevers SJ, Panayotou G, Waterfield MD (1997). Phosphoinositide 3-kinases: a conserved family of signal transducers. *Trends Biochem Sci* 22: 267–272.

Vavvas D, Li X, Avruch J, Zhang XF (1998). Identification of Nore1 as a potential Ras effector. *J Biol Chem* 273: 5439–5442.

Vetter IR, Wittinghofer A (2001). The guanine nucleotide-binding switch in three dimensions. *Science* 294: 1299–1304.

Vojtek AB, Hollenberg SM, Cooper JA (1993). Mammalian Ras interacts directly with the serine/threonine kinase Raf. *Cell* 74: 205–214.

Voyno-Yasenetskaya TA, Pace AM, Bourne HR (1994). Mutant α-subunits of G12 and G13 proteins induce neoplastic transformation of Rat-1 fibroblasts. *Oncogene* 9: 2559–2565.

Wang J, Ducret A, Tu Y, Kozasa T, Aebersold R, Ross EM (1998). RGSZ1, a Gz-selective RGS protein in brain. Structure, membrane association, regulation by Gαz phosphorylation, and relationship to a Gz GTPase-activating protein subfamily. *J Biol Chem* 273: 26014–26025.

Wang J, Frost JA, Cobb MH, Ross EM (1999). Reciprocal signaling between heterotrimeric G proteins and the p21-stimulated protein kinase. *J Biol Chem* 274: 31641–31647.

Warne PH, Viciana PR, Downward J (1993). Direct interaction of Ras and the amino-terminal region of Raf-1 in vitro. *Nature* 364: 352–355.

Wasserman S (1998). FH proteins as cytoskeletal organizers. *Trends Cell Biol* 8: 111–115.

Watanabe N, Madaule P, Reid T, Ishizaki T, Watanabe G, Kakizuka A, Saito Y, Nakao K, Jockusch BM, Narumiya S (1997). p140mDia, a mammalian homolog of *Drosophila diaphanous*, is a target protein for Rho small GTPase and is a ligand for profilin. *EMBO J* 16: 3044–3056.

Watanabe N, Kato T, Fujita A, Ishizaki T, Narumiya S (1999). Cooperation between mDia1 and ROCK in Rho-induced actin reorganization. *Nat Cell Biol* 1: 136–143.

Weinstein LS, Shenker A, Gejman PV, Merino MJ, Friedman E, Spiegel AM (1991). Activating mutations of the stimulatory G protein in the McCune-Albright syndrome. *N Engl J Med* 325: 1688–1695.

Wess J (1997). G-protein-coupled receptors: molecular mechanisms involved in receptor activation and selectivity of G-protein recognition. *FASEB J* 11: 346–354.

White MA, Nicolette C, Minden A, Polverino A, Van Aelst L, Karin M, Wigler MH (1995). Multiple Ras functions can contribute to mammalian cell transformation. *Cell* 80: 533–541.

Whitehead IP, Zohn IE, Der CJ (2001). Rho GTPase-dependent transformation by G protein–coupled receptors. *Oncogene* 20: 1547–1555.

Wilkie TM, Gilbert DJ, Olsen AS, Chen XN, Amatruda TT, Korenberg JR, Trask BJ, de Jong P, Reed RR, Simon MI, et al. (1992). Evolution of the mammalian G protein α-subunit multigene family. *Nat Genet* 1: 85–91.

Wolthuis RM, Bos JL (1999). Ras caught in another affair: the exchange factors for Ral. *Curr Opin Genet Dev* 9: 112–117.

Wong YH, Federman A, Pace AM, Zachary I, Evans T, Pouyssegur J, Bourne HR (1991). Mutant alpha subunits of G_i2 inhibit cyclic AMP accumulation. *Nature* 351: 63–65.

Wong YH, Conklin BR, Bourne HR (1992). Gz-mediated hormonal inhibition of cyclic AMP accumulation. *Science* 255: 339–342.

Wymann MP, Pirola L (1998). Structure and function of phosphoinositide 3-kinases. *Biochim Biophys Acta* 1436: 127–150.

Xiao RP (2001). β-adrenergic signaling in the heart: dual coupling of the $\beta 2$-adrenergic receptor to G_s and G_i proteins. *Sci STKE* 2001: RE15.

Xu GF, O'Connell P, Viskochil D, Cawthon R, Robertson M, Culver M, Dunn D, Stevens J, Gesteland R, White R, et al. (1990). The neurofibromatosis type 1 gene encodes a protein related to GAP. *Cell* 62: 599–608.

Xu N, Bradley L, Ambdukar I, Gutkind JS (1993). A mutant α-subunit of G12 potentiates the eicosanoid pathway and is highly oncogenic in NIH 3T3 cells. *Proc Natl Acad Sci USA* 90: 6741–6745.

Yamada M, Tachibana T, Imamoto N, Yoneda Y (1998). Nuclear transport factor p10/NTF2 functions as a Ran-GDP dissociation inhibitor (Ran-GDI). *Curr Biol* 8: 1339–1342.

Yamamoto M, Hilgemann DH, Feng S, Bito H, Ishihara H, Shibasaki Y, Yin HL (2001). Phosphatidylinositol 4,5-bisphosphate induces actin stress-fiber formation and inhibits membrane ruffling in CV1 cells. *J Cell Biol* 152: 867–876.

Yamashita S, Mochizuki N, Ohba Y, Tobiume M, Okada Y, Sawa H, Nagashima K, Matsuda M (2000). CalDAG-GEFIII activation of Ras, R-ras, and Rap1. *J Biol Chem* 275: 25488–25493.

Yang F, Li X, Sharma M, Zarnegar M, Lim B, Sun Z (2001). Androgen receptor specifically interacts with a novel p21-activated kinase, PAK6. *J Biol Chem* 276: 15345–15353.

Yang N, Higuchi O, Ohashi K, Nagata K, Wada A, Kangawa K, Nishida E, Mizuno K (1998). Cofilin phosphorylation by LIM-kinase 1 and its role in Rac-mediated actin reorganization. *Nature* 393: 809–812.

Yang Y, Hentati A, Deng HX, Dabbagh O, Sasaki T, Hirano M, Hung WY, Ouahchi K, Yan J, Azim AC, et al. (2001). The gene encoding alsin, a protein with three guanine-nucleotide exchange factor domains, is mutated in a form of recessive amyotrophic lateral sclerosis. *Nat Genet* 29: 160–165.

Yasui Y, Amano M, Nagata K, Inagaki N, Nakamura H, Saya H, Kaibuchi K, Inagaki M (1998). Roles of Rho-associated kinase in cytokinesis: mutations in Rho-associated kinase phosphorylation sites impair cytokinetic segregation of glial filaments. *J Cell Biol* 143: 1249–1258.

Zeng Q, Lagunoff D, Masaracchia R, Goeckeler Z, Cote G, Wysolmerski R (2000). Endothelial cell retraction is induced by PAK2 monophosphorylation of myosin II. *J Cell Sci* 113(Pt 3): 471–482.

Zhang FL, Casey PJ (1996). Protein prenylation: molecular mechanisms and functional consequences. *Annu Rev Biochem* 65: 241–269.

Zhang XF, Settleman J, Kyriakis JM, Takeuchi-Suzuki E, Elledge SJ, Marshall MS, Bruder JT, Rapp UR, Avruch J (1993). Normal and oncogenic p21ras proteins bind to the amino-terminal regulatory domain of c-Raf-1. *Nature* 364: 308–313.

Zheng B, Ma YC, Ostrom RS, Lavoie C, Gill GN, Insel PA, Huang XY, Farquhar MG (2001). RGS-PX1, a GAP for GαS and sorting nexin in vesicular trafficking. *Science* 294: 1939–1942.

Zheng Y (2001). Dbl family guanine nucleotide exchange factors. *Trends Biochem Sci* 26: 724–732.

Zheng Y, Zangrilli D, Cerione RA, Eva A (1996). The pleckstrin homology domain mediates transformation by oncogenic dbl through specific intracellular targeting. *J Biol Chem* 271: 19017–19020.

Zippel R, Orecchia S, Sturani E, Martegani E (1996). The brain specific Ras exchange factor CDC25 Mm: modulation of its activity through Gi-protein-mediated signals. *Oncogene* 12: 2697–2703.

Zufall F, Munger SD (2001). From odor and pheromone transduction to the organization of the sense of smell. *Trends Neurosci* 24: 191–193.

GNAS and McCune-Albright Syndrome/Fibrous Dysplasia, Albright Hereditary Osteodystrophy/Pseudohypoparathyroidism Type IA, Progressive Osseous Heteroplasia, and Pseudohypoparathyroidism Type IB

LEE S. WEINSTEIN

The heterotrimeric G protein G_s couples receptors for hormones and other extracellular signals to the stimulation of adenylyl cyclase and intracellular cyclic adenosine monophosphate generation. Ligand-bound receptors activate G_s by promoting the exchange of GTP for GDP on the G_s α-subunit ($G_s\alpha$); an intrinsic GTPase activity of $G_s\alpha$ deactivates the G protein by hydrolyzing bound GTP to GDP. Somatic $G_s\alpha$ mutations that disrupt the GTPase activity result in constitutive signaling and lead to endocrine tumors, fibrous dysplasia of bone, and the McCune-Albright syndrome (OMIM 174800). Conversely, heterozygous inactivating mutations may lead to Albright hereditary osteodystrophy (AHO) (OMIM 13580) or, more rarely, to progressive osseous heteroplasia (OMIM 166350). Within AHO kindreds, paternal transmission of these mutations leads to the AHO phenotype alone (pseudopseudohypoparathyroidism), while maternal transmission leads to AHO plus multihormone resistance (pseudohypoparathyroidism type IA). This is presumably due to the fact that the $G_s\alpha$ gene *GNAS* is imprinted and in certain hormone-sensitive tissues $G_s\alpha$ is primarily expressed from the maternal allele. Patients with isolated renal resistance to parathyroid hormone (pseudohypoparathyroidism type IB) (OMIM 603233) have a *GNAS* imprinting defect that presumably leads to tissue-specific loss of $G_s\alpha$ expression.

$G_s\alpha$ STRUCTURE, FUNCTION, AND EXPRESSION

Heterotrimeric G proteins transmit signals from seven transmembrane-domain cell surface receptors to intracellular effectors, such as ion channels or enzymes, which generate second messengers. Each G protein has a specific α-subunit that binds guanine nucleotide and interacts with specific receptors and effectors. β- and γ-subunits form tightly but noncovalently bound dimers that are targeted to the plasma membrane through lipid modifications. $G\alpha$'s are also targeted to cell membranes by lipid modifications and by association with $\beta\gamma$-dimers.

The G protein G_s couples a wide variety of G protein–coupled receptors to the stimulation of adenylyl cyclase, which catalyzes the synthesis of intracellular cyclic adenosine monophosphate (cAMP) (Weinstein et al., 2001). The G_s α-subunit ($G_s\alpha$) is expressed in virtually all tissues and is required for the cAMP response to a wide variety of extracellular factors, including glycoprotein and peptide hormones, catecholamines and other biogenic amines, and neurotransmitters. $G_s\alpha$ is the only ubiquitously expressed $G\alpha$ shown to be mutated in human diseases (Table 85–1). $G_{olf}\alpha$ also stimulates adenylyl cyclase, but it is only expressed in a small number of tissues (Jones and Reed, 1989).

cAMP mediates many of its downstream effects by activating cAMP-dependent protein kinase (protein kinase A [PKA]) (Fig. 85–1). The physiological consequences of PKA activation vary widely depending on cell type (e.g. hormone secretion in endocrine cells, gluconeogenesis and glycogenolysis in hepatocytes, long-term potentiation in neural cells). PKA is a serine/threonine kinase that mediates many of its metabolic effects by phosphorylating enzymes involved in intermediary metabolism and many of its transcriptional effects by phosphorylating transcription factors such as the cAMP response element–binding protein (CREB) (Montminy, 1997). cAMP can also work through PKA-independent mechanisms (Richards, 2001). For example, cAMP can directly bind to and stimulate both ion channels (Sudlow et al., 1993; Wainger et al., 2001) and guanine nucleotide exchange factors for small Ras-like guanine nucleotide–binding proteins (de Rooij et al., 1998; Kawasaki et al., 1998).

In many cell types (e.g., fibroblasts) cAMP inhibits the mitogenic response to growth factors by disrupting the ability of activated (GTP-bound) Ras to activate its effector Raf-1, a kinase that activates the mitogen-activated protein kinase (MAPK) cascade (Cook and Mc-Cormick, 1993; Wu et al., 1993). cAMP-dependent inhibition of Raf-1 activation is mediated by the PKA-dependent activation of the Ras-like protein Rap1 through a pathway involving Src kinase, the adaptor proteins Cbl and Crk, and the Rap1-specific guanine nucleotide exchange factor C3G (Schmitt and Stork, 2002).

In other cell types, particularly neuroendocrine cells, cAMP is mitogenic. In these cells cAMP directly activates Rap1 by binding to cAMP-regulated guanine nucleotide exchange proteins (cAMP-GEFs) for Rap1; activated Rap1 can stimulate proliferation by activating several downstream pathways, including B-raf (which stimulates MAPK), phosphoinositide-3-kinase (PI3K)/Akt kinase, ralGDS/ralA, and p70S6 kinase (Miller et al., 1997; Vossler et al., 1997; Cass and Meinkoth, 1998; Mei et al., 2002).

$G_s\alpha$ also directly activates other effectors besides adenylyl cyclase (Fig. 85–1), including cardiac Ca^{2+} channels (Yatani et al., 1988; Mattera et al., 1989) and Src tyrosine kinases (Ma et al., 2000). $G_s\alpha$ can also be activated by various tyrosine kinase receptors, including the epidermal growth factor (EGF) (Nair et al., 1990; Sun et al., 1997) and basic fibroblast growth factor receptors (Krieger-Brauer et al., 2000). EGF-dependent activation of $G_s\alpha$ appears to involve phosphorylation of specific $G_s\alpha$ tyrosine residues (Nair and Patel, 1993; Poppleton et al., 1996).

$G_s\alpha$ is targeted to the inner leaflet of cell membranes through palmitoylation at its amino terminus (Degtyarev et al., 1993; Linder et al., 1993; Mumby et al., 1994). $G_s\alpha$ localizes to both plasma membranes, where it functions as a signal transducer, and intracellular membranes, where it may play a role in membrane trafficking (Bomsel and Mostov, 1992). Support for a role of $G_s\alpha$ in membrane trafficking comes from the recent discovery that RGS-PX1, a $G_s\alpha$-specific regulator of G protein signaling (RGS) protein, is also a sorting nexin and is involved in vesicular trafficking (Zheng et al., 2001).

Like all G proteins, G_s is activated and deactivated via a "GTPase" cycle (Fig. 85–1). G_s exists in the inactive state as a $G_s\alpha$-$\beta\gamma$ heterotrimer with GDP bound to $G_s\alpha$. Agonist-bound receptors promote the release of GDP, allowing ambient GTP to bind to $G_s\alpha$. Upon GTP binding, $G_s\alpha$ switches to an active conformation, which leads to release from $\beta\gamma$, depalmitoylation, and probably some release from the plasma membrane (Wedegaertner et al., 1996; Huang et al., 1999; Yu and Rasenick, 2002). GTP-bound $G_s\alpha$ directly activates adenylyl cyclase and other effectors. $G_s\alpha$ is deactivated by an intrinsic GTPase activity that hydrolyzes bound GTP to GDP, which allows $G_s\alpha$ to reassociate with $\beta\gamma$. An RGS protein that stimulates the GTPase activity of $G_s\alpha$ was recently identified (Zheng et al., 2001). Some effectors may also modulate the GTP/GDP cycling of $G_s\alpha$ (Scholich et al., 1999).

Similar to other G protein α-subunits, $G_s\alpha$ contains two structural domains, a Ras-like GTPase domain, which includes the sites for guanine nucleotide binding and effector interaction, and a so-called helical domain (Fig. 85–2) (Sunahara et al., 1997; Tesmer et al., 1997). Alternative splicing leads to two long and two short forms of $G_s\alpha$ with helical domains of slightly differing length (Bray et al., 1986; Kozasa et al., 1988). Although the ratio of long to short $G_s\alpha$ isoforms varies between tissues, there are only subtle biochemical differences between them (Jones et al., 1990; Seifert et al., 1998). Bound guanine nucleotide resides within a cleft between the GTPase and helical do-

Table 85–1. Human Diseases Associated with *GNAS* Defects

Disease	*GNAS* Defect
GH-secreting pituitary tumors	G$_s\alpha$ activating mutations (somatic)
Thyroid adenomas, carcinomas	
Leydig cell tumors	
Pheochromocytoma	
Parathyroid adenoma	
ACTH-secreting pituitary tumor	
McCune-Albright syndrome	
Fibrous dysplasia	
Skeletal muscle myxomas	
Pseudohypoparathyroidism IA	G$_s\alpha$ null mutations (maternal)
Pseudopseudohypoparathyroidism	G$_s\alpha$ null mutations (paternal)
Progressive osseous heteroplasia	G$_s\alpha$ null mutations (?paternal)
Pseudohypoparathyroidism IA with testotoxicosis	G$_s\alpha$ A366S mutation(maternal)
Pseudohypoparathyroidism IB	Exon 1A imprinting defect Paternal UPD G$_s\alpha$ ΔI382 mutation (maternal)

mains. Contacts between the helical domain and the GTPase domain may be important for maintaining guanine nucleotide binding (Mixon et al., 1995; Warner et al., 1998).

GTP binding leads to activation by altering the conformation of three regions (named switch 1, 2 and 3) within the GTPase domain (Noel et al., 1993; Lambright et al., 1994). Upon GTP binding, switches 2 and 3 swing toward each other and stabilize the active state through mutual interactions between acidic and basic residues (Iiri et al., 1997, 1998; Li and Cerione, 1997; Warner et al., 1999). Interactions between switch 3 and helical domain residues may also be important for receptor-mediated activation (Grishina and Berlot, 1998; Marsh et al., 1998; Warner et al., 1998; Warner and Weinstein, 1999). Two highly conserved residues (Arg201 and Gln227 in the long form of G$_s\alpha$) are critical for catalyzing the GTPase reaction (Graziano and Gilman, 1989; Landis et al., 1989; Coleman et al., 1994; Sondek et al., 1994). Both the amino terminus and switch 2 regions interact directly with the β-subunit to form the heterotrimer (Wall et al., 1995; Lambright et al., 1996). The carboxyl terminus is important for receptor interactions and selectivity (Sullivan et al., 1987; Simonds et al., 1989; Schwindinger et al., 1994; Conklin et al., 1996; Grishina and Berlot, 2000; Mazzoni et al., 2000).

STRUCTURE AND IMPRINTING OF THE G$_s\alpha$ GENE

The human G$_s\alpha$ gene *GNAS* is located at 20q13.2–13.3 (Gejman et al., 1991; Levine et al., 1991; Rao et al., 1991) while the mouse ortholog *Gnas* is located within the syntenic region in distal chromosome 2 (Peters et al., 1994). The overall structure and regulation of *GNAS* and *Gnas* are well conserved. The G$_s\alpha$ coding region spans 13 exons (Kozasa et al., 1988) (Fig. 85–3). Alternative splicing of exon 3—an exon that encodes 15 amino acids within the helical domain—results in the generation of long and short forms of G$_s\alpha$ (Bray et al., 1986; Kozasa et al., 1988). Use of an alternative terminal exon located between G$_s\alpha$ exons 3 and 4 generates a neural-specific splice variant of unknown function (Crawford et al., 1993).

Genomic imprinting is an epigenetic phenomenon that affects a small number of genes and results in partial or complete suppression of gene expression from one parental allele (Constancia et al., 1998; Tilghman, 1999; Reik and Walter, 2001). The imprint "mark" that distinguishes the maternal and paternal allele is presumed to be erased in primordial germ cells, reestablished in either male or female gametes, and maintained in all somatic tissues throughout development. DNA methylation is most likely to be the imprint mark, as virtually all imprinted genes have one or more regions that are differentially methylated on the two parental alleles. G$_s\alpha$ is imprinted in a tissue-specific manner in both mice and humans, being expressed primarily from the maternal allele in some tissues (e.g., the pituitary and the renal proximal tubules) but biallelically expressed in the majority of tissues (Davies and Hughes, 1993; Campbell et al., 1994; Yu et al., 1998; Hayward et al., 2001; Weinstein et al., 2001).

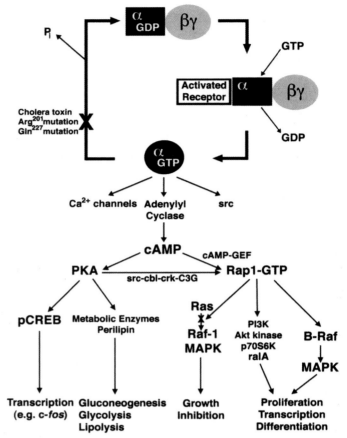

Figure 85–1. The G$_s$ GTPase cycle and downstream signaling pathways. Interaction of activated receptors with G$_s\alpha$-$\beta\gamma$ heterotrimers promotes the exchange of GTP for GDP on G$_s\alpha$, which results in dissociation of G$_s\alpha$ from $\beta\gamma$. GTP binding also changes G$_s\alpha$ into an active conformation that allows it to interact with and activate downstream effectors such as adenylyl cyclase, Ca^{2+} channels, and Src kinase. Adenylyl cyclase catalyzes the formation of cAMP, which activates protein kinase A (PKA), cAMP-regulated guanine nucleotide exchange factors (cAMP-GEF), and ion channels (not shown). PKA phosphorylates many substrates, including the transcription factor CREB, which leads to expression of c-*fos* and other genes; perilipin, which stimulates lipolysis; and metabolic enzymes, which stimulate gluconeogenesis and glycolysis. cAMP-GEFs activate Rap1 by promoting GTP binding. Rap1 activation leads to cell-type specific effects that may include increased proliferation or differentiation (or both) via PI3K, Akt kinase, p70S6 kinase, ralA, and B-Raf activation of MAPK; it may also inhibit growth by inhibiting ras-dependent activation of raf-1/MAPK. In some cells PKA can also activate Rap1 by stimulating the Rap1-GEF C3G via a pathway involving Src kinase and the adapters cbl and crk. G$_s\alpha$ has an intrinsic GTPase activity that hydrolyzes bound GTP to GDP, which deactivates G$_s$ and allows reassociation with $\beta\gamma$. Posttranslational modification of Arg201 by cholera toxin or mutation of Arg201 or Gln227 inhibits the GTPase activity, resulting in constitutive activation. RGS-PX1 (not shown) stimulates the GTPase activity of G$_s\alpha$.

GNAS/Gnas also generates alternative gene products through the use of four alternative promoters and first exons that splice onto a common exon (exon 2; see Fig. 85–3). The most downstream alternative exon is G$_s\alpha$ exon 1, which is located within an unmethylated CpG island, a characteristic of promoter regions of ubiquitously expressed genes (Kozasa et al., 1988; Hayward et al., 1998a; Peters et al., 1999; Liu et al., 2000b). (CpG islands are highly GC-rich regions with a high frequency of CpG dinucleotides.) Therefore G$_s\alpha$ imprinting does not result from methylation of its promoter, as is the case for some other imprinted genes.

The most upstream alternative promoter (~49 kB upstream of G$_s\alpha$ exon 1) generates transcripts that encode the chromogranin-like protein NESP55 (Hayward et al., 1998b; Kelsey et al., 1999; Peters et al., 1999). The entire NESP55 coding sequence is within its specific up-

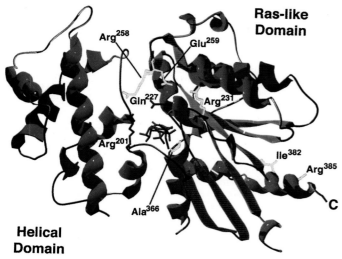

Ras-like Domain

Arg²⁵⁸

Glu²⁵⁹

Gln²²⁷

Arg²³¹

Arg²⁰¹

Ile³⁸²

Arg³⁸⁵

C

Ala³⁶⁶

Helical Domain

Figure 85–2. G$_s\alpha$ protein structure and location of some amino acids that are mutated in human diseases. Tertiary structure of G$_s\alpha$ is shown (α-helices in red, β-sheets in green) with the helical domain on the left and the ras-like domain on the right. Guanine nucleotide (purple) binds within a cleft between the two domains. Mutation of Arg201 and Gln227 (blue) results in constitutive activation as these residues are required for the GTPase "turn-off" reaction. Mutations of Arg231, Arg258, Glu259, and Arg385 (all shown in yellow) inactivate G$_s\alpha$ and result in AHO (see text). Deletion of Ile382 (yellow) uncouples G$_s\alpha$ from PTH1 receptors and leads to PHPIB. Mutation of Ala366 (yellow) increases the basal rate of GDP release and leads to AHO associated with testotoxicosis. (Reproduced from Weinstein et al., 2001.)

stream exon; G$_s\alpha$ exons 2–13 are within the 3' untranslated region of NESP55-specific transcripts (Ischia et al., 1997; Hayward et al., 1998b). NESP55 is only transcribed from the maternal allele, and its promoter region is methylated only on the paternal allele (Hayward et al., 1998b; Peters et al., 1999; Li et al., 2000). In mice, imprinting of NESP55 is not established until after implantation, suggesting that this region is not critical for the establishment of *GNAS/Gnas* imprinting (Liu et al., 2000b).

NESP55 is primarily expressed in neuroendocrine tissues, such as the adrenal medulla, the anterior and posterior pituitary, the hypothalamus, and other midbrain and brainstem regions, and it is present in large, dense core granules (Ischia et al., 1997; Bauer et al., 1999a, 1999b; Lovisetti-Scamiform et al., 1999). In mice, NESP55 transcripts are initially expressed in somites and vasculature during midgestation (Ball et al., 2001). It has been proposed that a proteolytic cleavage

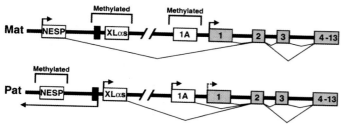

Figure 85–3. Organization and imprinting of *GNAS/Gnas*. The *GNAS* maternal (above) and paternal (below) alleles are shown (not to scale) with G$_s\alpha$ coding exons depicted as gray boxes, three other alternative first exons as white boxes, and the first exon of the antisense transcript as a black box. G$_s\alpha$ exons 4 to 13 are shown as a single box. Transcriptionally active sense and antisense promoters (arrows) are shown above and below the exons, respectively, and the splicing patterns of the sense transcripts are shown below each allele. The striped arrow for the paternal G$_s\alpha$ promoter indicates that the promoter is silenced in some tissues but active in most tissues. Regions that are differentially methylated are bracketed. Long and short forms of G$_s\alpha$ result from alternative splicing of exon 3. An alternative terminal exon between exons 3 and 4, alternative exons downstream of the XLαs exon, and antisense transcript exons are not shown.

product of NESP55 may be an endogenous antagonist of serotonin 1b receptors (Ischia et al., 1997); however, loss of NESP55 expression in humans is not associated with an obvious phenotype (Liu et al., 2000a).

A third alternative promoter (~35 kb upstream of G$_s\alpha$ exon 1) generates transcripts that encode XLαs, an isoform of G$_s\alpha$ with a long amino-terminal extension (Kehlenbach et al., 1994; Hayward et al., 1998a; Kelsey et al., 1999; Peters et al., 1999). The alternative amino-terminal region of XLαs is encoded by its first exon, while the carboxyl-terminal portion of the protein, which is identical to G$_s\alpha$, is encoded by exons 2–13. XLαs is only transcribed from the paternal allele, and its promoter is methylated only on the maternal allele (Hayward et al., 1998a; Peters et al., 1999; Li et al., 2000). Just upstream of the XLαs promoter is a promoter for paternally expressed antisense transcripts that traverse the NESP55 exon from the opposite direction (Hayward and Bonthron, 2000; Li et al., 2000; Wroe et al., 2000). This promoter, like the XLαs promoter, is methylated on the maternal allele. The antisense transcripts do not colocalize with NESP55 transcripts in mouse midgestational embryos, suggesting that they may not be important for NESP55 imprinting (Ball et al., 2001).

In XLαs the first 47 amino acids of G$_s\alpha$ are replaced by a large amino terminal region that is encoded by the XLαs-specific exon (the XL domain) (Kehlenbach et al., 1994; Pasolli et al., 2000). The XL domain contains, in sequential order, Glu-Pro-Ala-Ala (EPAA) repeats, Ala-Ala-Arg-Ala (AARA) repeats, a proline-rich region, and a cysteine-rich region. XLαs is expressed primarily in neural and endocrine tissues (Kehlenbach et al., 1994; Pasolli et al., 2000), and in rats it is first expressed at the onset of neurogenesis (Pasolli and Huttner, 2001). In rats, XLαs is present in the melanotrophs within the pars intermedia of the posterior lobe and, to a lesser extent, in brain, adrenal, heart, and pancreatic islets. The XL domain targets XLαs to the plasma membrane (Pasolli et al., 2000) and possibly also to Golgi membranes (Ugur and Jones, 2000). Small amounts of a basic protein are also translated from an alternative reading frame, and this protein may bind to XLαs (Klemke et al., 2001). Like G$_s\alpha$, XLαs can bind to $\beta\gamma$ and can activate adenylyl cyclase (Klemke et al., 2000).

A fourth alternative promoter and first exon located ~2.5 kb upstream of G$_s\alpha$ exon 1 (exon 1A; see Fig. 85–3) splices onto exon 2 to generate transcripts that are presumed to be untranslated (Ishikawa et al., 1990; Liu et al., 2000b). Exon 1A-specific transcripts are ubiquitously expressed in mice with a tissue-distribution pattern that is similar to that of G$_s\alpha$ (Liu et al., 2000b). The exon 1A promoter region is methylated only on the maternal allele, and exon 1A-specific transcripts are only expressed from the paternal allele (Liu et al., 2000a, 2000b). In mice, maternal-specific methylation of the exon 1A promoter region is established in oocytes and is maintained throughout development, suggesting that this region may be important for the establishment of *GNAS/Gnas* imprinting (Liu et al., 2000b). As discussed in the section on Pseudohypoparathyroidism Type IB, imprinting of exon 1A is lost in patients with pseudohypoparathyroidism type IB (PHPIB), suggesting that this region is important for the tissue-specific imprinting of G$_s\alpha$.

FIBROUS DYSPLASIA, MCCUNE-ALBRIGHT SYNDROME, AND ENDOCRINE TUMORS

Clinical Features

Fibrous dysplasia (FD) is a focal, benign fibrous bone lesion that expands concentrically from the marrow cavity toward the surrounding cortical bone (Weinstein, 2002). Most FD patients have a single bone lesion (monostotic FD) (Nager et al., 1982), and the rest have multiple lesions (polyostotic FD). A small number of polyostotic FD patients also have features of the McCune-Albright syndrome (MAS). With rare exceptions (Hibbs and Rush, 1952; Reitzik and Lownie, 1975; Sarkar et al., 1993), FD or MAS is almost never inherited. FD usually involves the proximal extremities, ribs, and craniofacial bones and can lead to pain, deformity, pathological fractures, or cranial nerve compression (Schlumberger, 1946; Harris et al., 1962; Nager et al., 1982; Danon and Crawford, 1987). Rarely do FD lesions expand beyond the cortical bone (Latham et al., 1992; Dorfman et al., 1994) or undergo malignant degeneration (Yabut et al., 1988; Ruggieri et al., 1994; Blanco et al., 1999; Lopez-Ben et al., 1999). FD is occasionally associated with intramuscular myxomas (Mazabraud syndrome) (Mazabraud and Girard, 1957; Lever and Pettingale, 1983; Prayson and Leeson, 1993; Okamoto et al., 2000).

FD lesions are mainly composed of immature mesenchymal cells with a spindle-shaped fibroblastic appearance (Greco and Steiner, 1986) that express alkaline phosphate and other osteoblast-specific proteins (Riminucci et al., 1997). These lesions usually contain spicules of immature woven bone and occasionally contain islands of hyaline cartilage (Greco and Steiner, 1986; Ishida and Dorfman, 1993). FD lesions have several characteristic features, including flat bone–lining cells with retracted cell bodies and collagen fibrils that are perpendicular to the bone-forming surface (Greco and Steiner, 1986; Riminucci et al., 1997, 1999b; Bianco et al., 2000). Features of osteomalacia are often present (Bianco et al., 2000). Osteoclasts are present at the periphery of the lesions (Yamamoto et al., 1996; Riminucci et al., 1997).

MAS is classically defined by the triad of hyperpigmented (café-au-lait) skin lesions, sexual precocity, and polyostotic FD (McCune, 1936; Albright et al., 1937; Cohen and Howell, 1999; Levine, 1999; Weinstein, 2002). The café-au-lait spots in MAS are hyperpigmented macules with irregular borders that generally follow the developmental lines of Blaschko (Happle, 1986). Many MAS patients also present with other endocrine or nonendocrine abnormalities or with only one or two features of the classic triad (Grant and Martinez, 1983; Rieth et al., 1984; Danon and Crawford, 1987).

Typically, female MAS patients present with premature menses associated with fluctuating estrogen levels and enlarged ovarian follicles (Comite et al., 1984; Rieth et al., 1984; Mauras and Blizzard, 1986; Danon and Crawford, 1987). Sexual development and adult reproductive function are usually otherwise normal. Males present with early onset of puberty and spermatogenesis or with Leydig cell tumors. In one case, premature testicular enlargement without pubertal development was due to selective early maturation of the seminiferous tubules (Giovanelli et al., 1978).

MAS may also be associated with increased growth of and hormone secretion from other endocrine glands (e.g., thyroid, adrenal cortex, and somatotrophs), leading to hyperthyroidism, hypercortisolism, or acromegaly with or without hyperprolactinemia (Benjamin and McRoberts, 1973; Kovacs et al., 1984; Mauras and Blizzard, 1986; Danon and Crawford, 1987; Feuillan et al., 1990; Lair-Milan et al., 1996; Mastorakos et al., 1997; Kirk et al., 1999). In each case the endocrine glands are stimulated even in the presence of low circulating levels of their respective stimulatory pituitary hormones (thyroid stimulating hormone [TSH], adrenocorticotropin [ACTH], and gonadotropins) (Danon et al., 1975; D'Armiento et al., 1983; Foster et al., 1984). Growth hormone (GH) and prolactin are the only pituitary hormones that have been shown to be oversecreted in MAS.

Patients with MAS and polyostotic FD often have hypophosphatemic rickets or osteomalacia associated with increased urinary phosphate excretion (Dent and Gertner, 1976; McArthur et al., 1979; Lever and Pettingale, 1983; Mauras and Blizzard, 1986; Collins et al., 2001). Basal urinary cAMP levels in MAS patients with hypophosphatemia have been reported to be elevated (Zung et al., 1995) or normal (Collins et al., 2001). MAS patients also have a more generalized tubulopathy, with aminoaciduria and mild proteinuria (Collins et al., 2001). Hyperparathyroidism is rarely present in patients with classic MAS (Benedict, 1962; Cavanah and Dons, 1993).

Most MAS patients have only skeletal, skin, and endocrine manifestations with little effect on mortality (Harris et al., 1962; Lee et al., 1986; Danon and Crawford, 1987). However, some patients present with nonendocrine abnormalities that are associated with increased morbidity or mortality (Shenker et al., 1993). These severely affected patients often have extensive polyostotic FD or hypercortisolism. Nonendocrine manifestations of MAS may involve the liver, heart, thymus, spleen, bone marrow, gastrointestinal tract, and the brain (Weinstein et al., 1991; Shenker et al., 1993). Liver abnormalities include severe neonatal jaundice, elevated liver enzymes, and cholestatic and biliary changes on biopsy (Shenker et al., 1993; Silva et al., 2000). Cardiac abnormalities may include cardiomegaly, atypical myocyte hypertrophy, persistent tachycardia, and unexplained sudden death. Other rare clinical manifestations of MAS include thymic hyperplasia, myelofibrosis, gastrointestinal polyps, pancreatitis, breast cancer, and neurological abnormalities (Albright et al., 1937; McCune and Bruch, 1937; MacMahon, 1971; Danon and Crawford, 1987; Tanabeu et al., 1998).

Molecular Genetics

Activating $G_s\alpha$ mutations were first identified in a subset of sporadic GH-secreting pituitary adenomas with elevated basal adenylyl cyclase activity, which account for ~40% of such tumors (Landis et al., 1989; Lyons et al., 1990). These were missense mutations within exons 8 and 9 and encoded substitutions of residues Arg201 (to Cys or His) or Gln227 (to Arg or Lys), respectively. These mutations were heterozygous and presumably dominantly acting; they were also somatic, as the same mutations were not present in peripheral blood samples. An Arg201Ser mutation was subsequently identified in a single tumor (Yang et al., 1996).

Mutation of either Arg201 or Gln227 disrupts the intrinsic GTPase activity of $G_s\alpha$ (Graziano and Gilman, 1989; Landis et al., 1989; Masters et al., 1990) and leads to constitutive activation of $G_s\alpha$ and its downstream effectors. The critical role of these residues in the GTPase reaction is supported by X-ray crystallography (Coleman et al., 1994; Sondek et al., 1994). $G_s\alpha$ alleles with activated mutations have been designated as *gsp* oncogenes due to their role in tumorigenesis (Landis et al., 1989; Lyons et al., 1990).

In 21 of 22 *gsp*-positive GH-secreting tumors, the mutation was in the transcriptionally active maternal allele (Hayward et al., 2001). There may also be some loss of imprinting with variable expression of wild-type $G_s\alpha$ from the paternal allele in some GH-secreting tumors (Hayward et al., 2001). *Gsp* mutations are also present in a small number of nonsecreting and ACTH-secreting pituitary tumors, benign and malignant thyroid tumors (Lyons et al., 1990; O'Sullivan et al., 1991; Suarez et al., 1991; Tordjman et al., 1993; Williamson et al., 1994, 1995a; Esapa et al., 1997), and, more rarely, in parathyroid and adrenal tumors (Yoshimoto et al., 1993; Williamson et al., 1995b).

In MAS patients, a specific Arg201 mutation (either to His or Cys) is present in many tissues in variable abundance (Weinstein et al., 1991; Schwindinger et al., 1992; Shenker et al., 1993, 1994; Kim et al., 1999; Silva et al., 2000). These mutations are present in affected endocrine glands and café-au-lait lesions, as well as in both normal and abnormal nonendocrine tissues. As in sporadic endocrine tumors, the mutations are heterozygous. An Arg201Gly mutation was identified in one MAS patient (Riminucci et al., 1999a) and an Arg201Leu mutation (possibly germline) was identified in a patient with severe skeletal, endocrine, and developmental abnormalities (Mockridge et al., 1999). Gln227 mutations have not been found in MAS, perhaps because these mutations are more activating (Landis et al., 1989) and therefore more lethal.

Somatic *gsp* mutations are also found in FD lesions from patients with MAS, polyostotic FD, and monostotic FD indicating that all forms of FD are caused by a common genetic defect (Malchoff et al., 1994; Shenker et al., 1994, 1995; Alman et al., 1996; Candeliere et al., 1997; Marie et al., 1997; Bianco et al., 2000). The mutations are usually Arg201 to Cys or His, although one polyostotic FD patient had an Arg201Ser mutation (Candeliere et al., 1997). *Gsp* mutations have also been identified in intramuscular myxomas—both those that occur alone and those that present with accompanying FD (Okamoto et al., 2000).

Diagnosis

The diagnosis of MAS is usually obvious, based on its characteristic clinical presentation. Hormonal measurements will confirm hypersecretion of one or more hormones (thyroid hormone, cortisol, GH, or estrogen) in the absence of the respective stimulating hormones. Usually this will be associated with unifocal or multifocal overgrowth of the respective endocrine gland. FD is usually diagnosed by its characteristic ground glass (but occasionally sclerotic) appearance on X-ray (Weinstein, 2002). Some patients with hyperparathyroidism and jaw lesions have been given the diagnosis of MAS (Firat and Stutzman, 1968; Ehrig and Wilson, 1972; Hammami et al., 1997), but these patients more likely have the hyperparathyroidism–jaw tumor syndrome (Szabo et al., 1995).

Management and Counseling

All patients with MAS/FD should be screened for hyperthyroidism, acromegaly, and hypercortisolism. The endocrine manifestations of MAS are managed by surgical removal of abnormal endocrine tissue or by specific medical therapy (e.g., somatostatin analog or bromocryptine for pituitary tumor, radioiodine or thionamides for hyperthyroidism; aromatase inhibitors for precocious puberty). Perioperative sudden death has been reported in a few severely affected MAS patients, possibly resulting from cardiomyopathy and arrythmia (Shenker et al., 1993). There is no specific therapy for the skin manifestations.

Often fibrous dysplasia is minimally symptomatic, and fractures heal well with conservative management (Harris et al., 1962). Both nuclear bone scanning and magnetic resonance imaging are useful for determining the extent of FD (Pfeffer et al., 1990; Inamo et al., 1993). Either surgical excision or curettage and bone grafting is indicated for nonhealing fractures, nerve compression, or severe pain or deformity, particularly on weight-bearing bones (Harris et al., 1962; Grabias and Campbell, 1977; Edgerton et al., 1985). Radiotherapy is ineffective and may increase the risk of sarcomatous degeneration (Yabut et al., 1988; Ruggieri et al., 1994). Pamidronate is effective in many patients, although growth plate widening may occur in children (Liens et al., 1994; Chapurlat et al., 1997; Lala et al., 2000; Zacharin and O'Sullivan, 2000). FD and MAS are virtually never inherited, and therefore no genetic counseling is required.

Animal Models

There are no animal models mimicking the genetic defect of MAS/FD. However, transgenic mice with expression of a cholera toxin gene (which constitutively activates $G_s\alpha$ by covalently modifying Arg201) in GH-secreting pituitary cells (somatotrophs) develop pituitary hyperplasia and excess GH secretion (Burton et al., 1991). Similarly, thyroid-specific expression of the same transgene leads to thyroid hyperplasia and hyperthyroidism (Zeiger et al., 1997).

Pathogenesis

Based on the specific distribution of hyperpigmentation, it was proposed that patients with MAS are mosaics of normal cells and cells bearing a dominant acting mutation, which might arise from an early embryonic somatic mutation or a gametic half-chromatid mutation (Happle, 1986). This was later confirmed by the identification of widespread somatic *gsp* mutations in MAS patients (Weinstein et al., 1991). The specific clinical manifestations in individual patients depend on the relative number and distribution of mutant cells. More limited presentations, such as isolated endocrine tumors or FD, presumably result from somatic *gsp* mutations that occur later in development, leading to mutant cells in only one tissue. *Gsp* mutations are probably germline lethal, as MAS is virtually never inherited.

Since $G_s\alpha$ is preferentially expressed from the maternal allele in some tissues, it might be expected that *gsp* mutations on the maternal allele lead to greater clinical consequences. This possibility is supported by the fact that in GH-secreting pituitary tumors the *gsp* mutation is almost always on the maternal allele (Hayward et al., 2001). As *gsp* mutations also result in constitutive activation of the paternally expressed XLαs protein (Klemke et al., 2000), expression of activated XLαs may contribute to the phenotype in patients with *gsp* mutations on the paternal allele.

By disrupting its intrinsic GTPase activity, *gsp* mutations allow $G_s\alpha$ to remain in the GTP-bound active state for a prolonged time, leading to constitutive activation of $G_s\alpha$ and its downstream effectors, including adenylyl cyclase. cAMP production is increased in affected tissues from MAS/FD patients and from *gsp*-positive GH-secreting tumors (Landis et al., 1989; Zung et al., 1995; Yamamoto et al., 1996; Marie et al., 1997; Kim et al., 1999). It is likely that many, if not all, of the manifestations of MAS result from increased levels of intra-

cellular cAMP in various tissues. cAMP is known to stimulate both growth and hormone secretion in many endocrine glands, and many of the trophic pituitary and hypothalamic hormones stimulate their respective target glands by activating G_s/cAMP pathways. In MAS, the respective endocrine glands are stimulated even in the absence of their respective stimulating hormone because the *gsp* mutation leads to constitutive activation of the G_s/cAMP pathway.

In somatotrophs, G_s/cAMP pathways are normally stimulated by growth hormone–releasing hormone (GHRH) receptors. Constitutive G_s activation stimulates somatotroph proliferation and GH release by inducing the tissue-specific transcription factor GHF1 (Burton et al., 1991; Castrillo et al., 1991). This likely involves PKA-dependent phosphorylation of CREB, as transgenic mice with expression of a nonphosphorylatable form of CREB in somatotrophs develop somatotroph hypoplasia and dwarfism (Struthers et al., 1991). CREB phosphorylation was reported to be higher in GH-secreting tumors than in nonfunctioning pituitary adenomas (Bertherat et al., 1995), but there was no difference between *gsp*-positive and *gsp*-negative tumors (Bertherat et al., 1995; Persani et al., 2001), suggesting that CREB gets phosphorylated by alternative kinase pathways in *gsp*-negative tumors. The effects of chronic G_s activation are mitigated by upregulation of various cAMP-dependent isoforms of phosphodiesterase, which hydrolyzes cAMP to AMP (Persani et al., 2001). Interestingly, *gsp* mutations are rarely present in corticotroph tumors, even though these cells are also hormonally activated via G_s/cAMP pathways.

TSH stimulates thyroid gland growth and hormone secretion through the G_s/cAMP pathway. Constitutively activated $G_s\alpha$ increases thyroid cell proliferation and hormone release in both cultured cells and transgenic mice (Muca and Vallar, 1994; Zeiger et al., 1997). Studies in various cell-culture systems implicate both PKA-dependent and PKA-independent pathways. In thyroid cells, cAMP directly activates Rap1 (and perhaps Ras) through cAMP-regulated guanine nucleotide exchange factors, which leads to activation of PI3K, Akt kinase, p70S6 kinase, and the Ras-related protein RalA, all of which promote mitogenesis (Miller et al., 1997; Cass and Meinkoth, 1998; Tsygankova et al., 2000, 2001; Mei et al., 2002). cAMP fails to activate MAPK in one thyroid cell line (Lamy et al., 1993; Miller et al., 1997), but it is able to activate MAPK in another cell line (Pomerance et al., 2000; Iacovelli et al., 2001), possibly by activating B-Raf through Rap1. PKA is also probably involved in the activation of MAPK (Pomerance et al., 2000), PI3K (Ciullo et al., 2001; Tsygankova et al., 2001), and p70S6 kinase (Tsygankova et al., 2001).

Both ACTH and the gonadotropins stimulate their respective targets, the adrenal cortex and gonads, by activating G_s/cAMP. In MAS these glands appear similar to those observed in patients with excess ACTH and gonadotropins, respectively, even though circulating levels of these hormones are low. In cultured granulosa cells cAMP stimulates various kinases through both PKA-dependent and PKA-independent pathways (Gonzalez-Robayna et al., 2000).

Hyperpigmentation in MAS is the direct consequence of increased cAMP levels in melanocytes. Melanocytes cultured from MAS skin lesions have higher cAMP levels, higher numbers of dendrites and melanosomes, and higher levels of tyrosinase (Kim et al., 1999). Normally the G_s/cAMP pathway in melanocytes is activated by binding of melanocyte-stimulating hormone to melanocortin 1 receptors. cAMP stimulates the expression of tyrosinase, the rate-limiting enzyme for melanin production (Lu et al., 1998), perhaps through inhibition of PI3K and p70S6 kinase (Buscá et al., 1996).

FD results from abnormal proliferation and differentiation of bone marrow stromal cells (Bianco and Robey, 1999). The normal progression of marrow stromal cells to mature osteoblasts consists of a proliferative phase, followed by a postproliferative phase during which the cells differentiate and express osteoblast-specific gene products that support the formation of mineralized bone (Stein and Lian, 1993). Cells isolated from FD lesions have an increased proliferation rate and are poorly differentiated as they express early, but not late, markers of osteoblast differentiation (Marie et al., 1997; Riminucci et al., 1997). Transplantation of these cells into immunocompromised mice produced lesions that are similar to human FD (Bianco et al., 1998, 2000), suggesting that these cells are incapable of forming normal bone. Interestingly, these lesions only formed when both normal and mutant cells were transplanted.

Studies in preosteoblastic cell lines demonstrate that G_s/cAMP inhibits osteoblast differentiation (Bellows et al., 1990; Turksen et al., 1990; Nanes et al., 1995; Tintut et al., 1999) and induces the cellular retraction that is commonly observed in FD lesions (Riminucci et al., 1997). Phosphorylation of CREB by PKA stimulates the transcription of c-*fos* and other genes (Gaiddon et al., 1994; Sassone-Corsi, 1995). Overexpression of the c-*fos* product Fos has been documented in FD lesions (Candeliere et al., 1995), and Fos overexpression in transgenic mice produces fibrous bone lesions similar to FD (Rüther et al., 1987). Fos is one component of the transcriptional factor AP-1 that is present at high levels in proliferating, but not maturing, osteoblasts, and which inhibits the expression of osteoblast-specific genes (Stein and Lian, 1993). High levels of cAMP and Fos in FD also stimulate the expression of the interleukin IL-6, which promotes osteoclast recruitment and bone resorption (Yamamoto et al., 1996; Motomura et al., 1998).

Other mechanisms may also contribute to the generation of FD. PTH-related protein (PTHrP) was highly overexpressed in FD lesions from three patients, suggesting that PTHrP may contribute to the development of FD through an autocrine pathway (Frase et al., 2000). FD lesions also express the β-chain of platelet-derived growth factor (PDGF-B), a factor which stimulates fibroblast proliferation (Alman et al., 1995). Sex steroids stimulate PDGF-B expression (Kaplan et al., 1988; Pensler et al., 1990; Alman et al., 1995), perhaps accounting for why FD lesions sometimes grow during puberty, pregnancy, or the use of oral contraceptives (Stevens-Simon et al., 1991).

It remains to be determined whether hyperphosphaturia in patients with MAS/FD is caused by a phosphaturic factor (phosphatonin) secreted from FD lesions (Dent and Gertner, 1976; McArthur et al., 1979; Collins et al., 2001) or a primary defect in the renal proximal tubule (Tanaka and Suwa, 1977; Lever and Pettingale, 1983). MAS patients have a general tubulopathy similar to that observed in patients with tumor-induced osteomalacia (Collins et al., 2001), suggesting that MAS patients may have increased circulating levels of a phosphatonin, such as fibroblast growth factor 23 (White et al., 2001).

The cardiac hypertrophy and possible sudden death observed in some MAS patients likely reflects constitutive activation of G_s/cAMP pathways in the heart, which are normally activated by sympathetic nerves through β-adrenergic receptors to produce inotropic and chronotropic effects. G_s/cAMP pathway can stimulate MAPK cascades in cardiomyocytes, which may contribute to the observed hypertrophy (Yamazaki et al., 1997a, 1997b; Zheng et al., 2000). While *gsp* mutations are presumably responsible for the other nonendocrine manifestations of MAS, the precise underlying mechanisms are not defined.

ALBRIGHT HEREDITARY OSTEODYSTROPHY

Clinical Features

Albright hereditary osteodystrophy (AHO) (pseudohypoparathyroidism type IA/pseudopseudohypoparathyroidism) is a congenital syndrome that presents with one or more of the following clinical features: short stature, brachydactyly, subcutaneous ossifications, centripetal obesity, facial abnormalities including depressed nasal bridge or hypertelorism, and mental deficits or developmental delay (Fig. 85–4) (Ringel et al., 1996; Weinstein, 1998; Spiegel and Weinstein, 2001; Weinstein et al., 2001). The severity of the phenotype varies greatly, and some patients who carry the genetic trait present with few or no clinical manifestations (Farfel and Friedman, 1986; Weinstein et al., 1990; Miric et al., 1993; Shore et al., 2002).

Ectopic ossifications in AHO (osteoma cutis) can occur in any location and are generally limited to the dermis and subcutaneous tissues. They present as punctate hard nodules or as subcutaneous calcifications on radiographs (Eyre and Reed, 1971; Prendiville et al., 1992; Goeteyn et al., 1999). Occasionally they enlarge to form more platelike lesions but usually do not invade into deeper tissues. These lesions result from intramembranous, as opposed to endochondral, ossification.

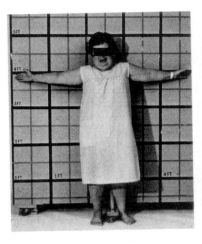
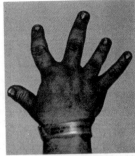
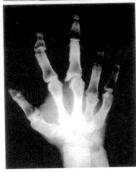

Figure 85–4. Albright hereditary osteodystrophy (AHO). (*Left*) AHO patient showing the cardinal features, including short stature, obesity, and rounded face with depressed nasal bridge. (*Right*) Photograph (above) and radiograph (below) of affected hand with severe brachydactyly affecting the first, fourth, and fifth metacarpals.

Brachydactyly manifests as shortening and widening of long bones in the hands and feet, most often the distal thumb and third, fourth, and fifth metacarpals (Steinbach and Young, 1966; Poznanski et al., 1977; Graudal et al., 1986). This pattern is relatively specific for AHO. Often the pattern of involvement is asymmetric. Brachydactyly is generally not obvious at birth but becomes apparent in early childhood due to premature closure of the growth plate associated with coning of the epiphysis. Spinal cord compression occurs rarely, either from calcifications (Yamamoto et al., 1997) or narrowing of the spinal canal (Goadsby et al., 1991; Okada et al., 1994).

Patients who inherit AHO from their mother also develop multihormone resistance, a condition referred to as pseudohypoparathyroidism type IA (PHPIA) (Davies and Hughes, 1993; Weinstein et al., 2001). In contrast, patients who inherit AHO from their father develop AHO without hormone resistance, a condition also referred to as pseudopseudohypoparathyroidism (PPHP). Both PHPIA and PPHP often occur in the same kindred. Clinically, the multihormone resistance in PHPIA primarily involves three hormones that activate G_s in their target tissues: parathyroid hormone (PTH), TSH, and the gonadotropins. However, there is no clinical resistance to other hormones that also activate G_s, such as glucagon (Levine et al., 1983; Brickman et al., 1986), isoproterenol (Carlson and Brickman, 1983), vasopressin (Moses et al., 1986; Faull et al., 1991), and ACTH (Levine et al., 1983; Faull et al., 1991).

Patients with renal PTH resistance present during childhood or adolescence with acute symptoms of hypocalcemia (seizures, tetany, and numbness), which are associated with hyperphosphatemia and high circulating PTH levels. PTH resistance develops over the first years of life, with hyperphosphatemia and elevated PTH generally preceding hypocalcemia (Werder et al., 1978; Tsang et al., 1984; Barr et al., 1994; Yu et al., 1999). Some PHPIA patients remain eucalcemic with only elevated PTH levels (Balachandar et al., 1975; Drezner and Haussler, 1979; Breslau et al., 1980). Patients often develop chronic features of hypoparathyroidism (e.g., basal ganglia calcification) and rarely develop rickets. Serum 1,25-dihydroxyvitamin D [1,25(OH)$_2$D] levels are low or inappropriately normal for the level of serum PTH and phosphate (Lambert et al., 1980; Braun et al., 1981; Breslau and Weinstock, 1988; Miura et al., 1990). The acute rise in urinary cAMP normally observed in response to administered PTH or PTH analog is almost completely absent in patients with PHPIA, but is maintained in patients with PPHP (Chase et al., 1969; Levine et al., 1986).

Almost all PHPIA patients also have TSH resistance (Werder et al., 1975; Levine et al., 1983) which presents at birth with elevated TSH levels (Levine et al., 1985; Weisman et al., 1985; Yokoro et al., 1990; Yu et al., 1999). TSH levels may normalize for several months before once again becoming elevated (Yu et al., 1999). Typically, TSH levels are mildly elevated, and thyroid hormone levels are normal or slightly low. Goiter is usually absent, and anti-thyroid antibodies are also absent, indicating the absence of autoimmune thyroid disease.

Clinical hypogonadism in female patients with PHPIA presents as delayed or incomplete sexual maturation, oligomenorrhea, or infertility (Wolfsdorf et al., 1978; Shapiro et al., 1980; Levine et al., 1983; Shima et al., 1988; Namnoum et al., 1998). These women are often mildly hypoestrogenic, but studies have not been able to consistently demonstrate increased levels of circulating gonadotropins. Some PHPIA patients also have prolactin deficiency (Carlson et al., 1977; Brickman et al., 1981; Kruse et al., 1981; Levine et al., 1983; Faull et al., 1991; Schuster et al., 1993). Growth hormone deficiency has been reported in some, but not all, PHPIA patients (Urdanivia et al., 1975; Shima et al., 1988; Faull et al., 1991; Scott and Hung, 1995; Germaine-Lee et al., 2001). Olfaction is also impaired in PHPIA, but not in PPHP, patients (Henkin, 1968; Weinstock et al., 1986; Ikeda et al., 1988; Doty et al., 1997). Whether this reflects a true sensory defect or another neurological defect that affects central processing of the signals or olfaction testing is unclear.

Molecular Genetics

A genetic defect of the common signaling component G_s is a plausible explanation for the multihormone resistance in PHPIA. Using an assay that measures G_s signaling in patient membrane samples after reconstitution with membranes lacking $G_s\alpha$ (cyc-negative assay), G_s bioactivity was shown to be reduced by ~50% in various tissues (erythrocytes, fibroblasts, platelets, lymphocytes, and kidney) obtained from PHPIA patients (Farfel and Bourne, 1980; Levine et al., 1980; Bourne et al., 1981; Farfel et al., 1980, 1981; Spiegel et al., 1982; Downs et al., 1983). These initial observations were confirmed by functional studies of patient membrane or cell samples (Mallet et al., 1982; Heinsimer et al., 1984; Ong et al., 1996). G_s bioactivity was later shown to be similarly reduced in PPHP patients, suggesting that PHPIA and PPHP result from a common genetic defect (Levine et al., 1986).

Molecular studies showed that the G_s defect is associated with decreased $G_s\alpha$ mRNA (Carter et al., 1987; Levine et al., 1988) or protein (Patten and Levine, 1990) expression. As would be predicted by $G_s\alpha$ haploinsufficiency, most AHO patients (both PHPIA and PPHP) have a heterozygous inactivating *GNAS* mutation that involves the $G_s\alpha$ coding exons (Patten et al., 1990; Weinstein et al., 1990; Oude Luttikhuis et al., 1994; Shapira et al., 1996; Jan de Beur et al., 1998; Aldred and Trembath, 2000; Aldred et al., 2000; Ahrens et al., 2001; Linglart et al., 2002; Spiegel and Weinstein, 2001). These mutations are spread throughout the $G_s\alpha$ coding exons, with the exception of exon 3, probably due to the fact that splicing out this exon still generates a functional $G_s\alpha$ protein. One specific 4 bp deletion in exon 7 has been identified in at least 22 families (Yu et al., 1995; Aldred and Trembath, 2000; de Sanctis et al., 2000; Mantovani et al., 2000; Ahrens et al., 2001; Linglart et al., 2002; Shore et al., 2002). The frequent de novo occurrence of this mutation is probably due to pausing of DNA polymerase and slipped-strand mispairing (Yu et al., 1995). Nine other mutations have each been reported in two independent kindreds (Iiri et al., 1994; Aldred and Trembath, 2000; Ahrens et al., 2001). In addition, residues Arg231, Ala102, and Pro115 have each been shown to be altered by two different missense mutations (Miric et al., 1993; Farfel et al., 1996; Ahmed et al., 1998; Ahrens et al., 2001). All other mutations have been identified in only one kindred each.

Identical *GNAS* mutations are present in both PHPIA and PPHP patients within the same kindred (Weinstein et al., 1990; Wilson et al., 1994; Fischer et al., 1998; Nakamoto et al., 1998; Walden et al., 1999; Yu et al., 1999; Mantovani et al., 2000; Ahrens et al., 2001), con-

firming that AHO is an autosomal dominant disorder. Whether an individual develops hormone resistance (PHPIA) or not (PPHP) depends on parental inheritance; maternal mutations result in PHPIA, while paternal mutations result in PPHP.

With a few exceptions (see next paragraph) there is no obvious genotype–phenotype correlation, and the vast majority of AHO-associated mutations are complete null mutations, such as frameshift, nonsense, or splice junction mutations that disrupt $G_s\alpha$ mRNA expression. Several missense mutations (listed in Table 85–2 with references) disrupt $G_s\alpha$ protein stability due to either steric effects (e.g., Ser250Arg or Glu259Val) or decreased guanine nucleotide binding (e.g., Arg258Trp or Ala366Ser).

Several other missense mutations have specific effects on $G_s\alpha$ function (Table 85–2). Mutation of the initiator methionine produces a large, inactive form of $G_s\alpha$. Mutation of the basic residue Arg231 within switch 2 results in a receptor-activation defect, probably by disrupting interactions between this residue and acidic residues within switch 3 that stabilize the active conformation. By a similar mechanism, mutation of the acidic residue Glu259 in switch 3 produces the same biochemical phenotype. The Arg258Trp mutation destabilizes GDP binding in the basal state and increases the rate of the GTPase reaction, resulting in a receptor-activation defect. The Ala366Ser mutation results in a syndrome of PHPIA plus gonadotropin-independent precocious puberty in males (testotoxicosis). At core body temperature the mutation leads to thermolability due to increased GDP dissociation, resulting in PHPIA. At the lower temperature of the testis, the mutant protein is stable but constitutively activated as increased basal GDP release allows $G_s\alpha$ to bind GTP independently of receptor stimulation. $G_s\alpha$ activation in the testis leads to testotoxicosis. Several mutations at the carboxyl terminus prevent $G_s\alpha$ from being activated by receptors.

Diagnosis

Many features of AHO are nonspecific, and therefore the diagnosis cannot be made based solely on physical signs and symptoms. Brachydactyly, obesity, and neurological deficits can also be present in other genetic disorders (e.g., Prader-Willi syndrome, brachydactyly syndromes, Turner syndrome, and Rubinstein-Taybi syndrome). An AHO-like syndrome is also associated with deletions at 2q37 (Phelan et al., 1995; Wilson et al., 1995). These alternative syndromes do not present with osteoma cutis or PTH resistance, so the presence of either of these features should increase the suspicion of AHO. Patients with AHO features alone in the absence of family history or hormone resistance should not be diagnosed with AHO unless a $G_s\alpha$ defect is confirmed by biochemical or genetic studies.

All patients with features suggestive of AHO should have serum calcium, phosphorus, PTH, TSH, and thyroid hormone levels measured to look for hormone resistance. In primary hypoparathyroidism, PTH levels are low or normal rather than high. Other forms of secondary hyperparathyroidism (e.g., vitamin D deficiency or resistance and malabsorption) usually present with normal or low serum phosphate levels, but these diagnoses should be considered and ruled out by measurement of 25-hydroxyvitamin D and 1,25(OH)$_2$D levels. Although the PTH analog infusion test is considered the gold standard for diagnosing PTH resistance, the analog is presently not commercially available.

The diagnosis of AHO can be confirmed by evidence of a $G_s\alpha$ defect—either a 50% loss of erythrocyte G_s bioactivity or $G_s\alpha$ expression, or a heterozygous inactivating *GNAS* mutation. Biochemical assays should be performed by stimulating G_s with a receptor ligand such as isoproterenol so that mutant forms of $G_s\alpha$ that are specifically defective in receptor-mediated activation are not missed (Iiri et al., 1997; Linglart et al., 2002). Unfortunately, these biochemical and genetic tests are presently difficult to obtain. There are rare patients who present with both AHO and hormone resistance but do not have a G_s defect, and these patients have been classified as having PHP type IC.

Management and Counseling

There is no specific therapy for the physical and neurocognitive manifestations of the AHO phenotype. The subcutaneous ossifications do

Table 85–2. $G_s\alpha$ Missense Mutations in AHO and PHPIB

Exon	Amino Acid Change*	Functional Consequence†	Reference
1	Met1Val	Abnormal 70 kDa isoform; ↓ cyc assay	Patten et al., 1990; Aldred and Trembath, 2000
1	Arg42Cys	NT	Aldred and Trembath, 2000
4	Val92Glu	NT	Aldred and Trembath, 2000
4	ΔAsn98	NT	Weinstein, unpublished
4	Leu99Pro	↓ $G_s\alpha$ protein expression	Miric et al., 1993
4	Ala102Val	↓ cyc assay	Ahrens et al., 2001
4	Ala102Gln	↓ cyc assay	Ahrens et al., 2001
4	Ile103Thr	NT	Aldred and Trembath, 2000
5	Pro115Ser	NT	Ahmed et al., 1998
5	Pro115Leu	↓ cyc assay	de Sanctis et al., 2000; Ahrens et al., 2001
5	Leu132Pro	NT	Aldred and Trembath, 2000
6	Asp156Asn	↓ cyc assay	Linglart et al., 2002
6	Val159Met	↓ cyc assay	Linglart et al., 2002
6	Arg160Cys	NT	Aldred and Trembath, 2000
6	Arg165Cys	↓ $G_s\alpha$ protein expression	Miric et al., 1993; Ahrens et al., 2001
7	Tyr190Asp	NT	Ringel et al., 1996
9	Arg231His	↓ Activation by receptor	Farfel et al., 1996; Iiri et al., 1997
9	Arg231Cys	↓ cyc assay	Ahrens et al., 2001; Weinstein, unpublished
10	Ser250Arg	↓ $G_s\alpha$ protein expression	Warner et al., 1997
10	Arg258Trp	↑ GDP release; ↑ GTPase activity	Warner et al., 1998; Warner and Weinstein, 1999
10	Glu259Val	↓ $G_s\alpha$ protein stability; ↓ signaling activity	Ahmed et al., 1998; Warner et al., 1999
10	Asn264His	NT	Aldred and Trembath, 2000
10	Arg280Lys	↓ cyc assay	Linglart et al., 2002
11	Leu282Pro	NT	Aldred and Trembath, 2000
11	Ala298Pro	↓ cyc assay	Ahrens et al., 2001
11	Pro313Leu	↓ cyc assay	Ahrens et al., 2001; de Sanctis et al., 2000
12	Arg336Trp	↓ cyc assay	Ahrens et al., 2001
13	His357Leu	↓ cyc assay	Iiri et al., 1994
13	Ala366Ser	PHPIA + Testotoxicosis; ↑ GDP release; ↑ thermolability at 37°C	Aldred et al., 2000
13	366-369dup	NT	Ahrens et al., 2001
13	ΔAsn377	↓ cyc assay	Wu et al., 2001
13	ΔIle382	PHPIB; selectively uncoupled from PTH receptor	Schwindinger et al., 1994
13	Arg385His	Uncoupled from receptors	Linglart et al., 2002
13	Tyr391X	Last 4 residues deleted; Cyc assay normal; uncoupled from receptors	

*Codon numbering based on $G_s\alpha$-1 sequence (GenBank accession no. SEG_HUMGNAS).
†NT, not tested; ↓ cyc assay, decreased G_s bioactivity in patient's erythrocyte membranes after reconstitution with cyc membranes.

not require surgical excision unless they are causing discomfort or disfigurement.

In patients with PHPIA (as well as PHPIB), PTH resistance should be treated aggressively with oral calcium and vitamin D (either ergocalciferol or calcitriol). Unlike patients with primary hypoparathyroidism (who lack PTH), patients with PHP usually do not develop hypercalciuria upon treatment (Mizunashi et al., 1990; Stone et al., 1993). Therefore, the goal of therapy is to normalize both calcium and PTH levels, if possible, while monitoring 24-hour urine specimens for hypercalciuria. Normalizing PTH is important for preventing both the skeletal consequences of high circulating PTH levels and the development of irreversible (so-called tertiary) hyperparathyroidism due to development of autonomous parathyroid tumors. Rarely, patients require surgical excision of these tumors. TSH resistance is treated with levothyroxine to normalize TSH levels. Hypogonadism is treated with oral contraceptives in females and testosterone in males. GH therapy may be beneficial in patients with GH deficiency (Germaine-Lee et al., 2001).

Patients should be counseled that there is a 50% chance of transmission of AHO. Females need to be counseled that their affected offspring will also have multihormone resistance, and males should be counseled that hormone resistance is unlikely to occur in their offspring. Since the AHO phenotype is variable, it is impossible to predict its severity, and even patients with mild disease need to be told that their affected offspring may have severe physical and neurocognitive manifestations. If a GNAS mutation has been identified, then genetic testing will be useful in identifying further affected family members and could be theoretically used for prenatal testing.

Animal Models

Mice with disruption of Gnas exon 2 have been generated by targeted mutagenesis (Yu et al., 1998). Double knockouts (−/−) die in early gestation. Heterozygotes with disruption of the maternal (m−/+) or paternal (+/p−) allele have distinct phenotypes at birth, providing strong evidence that Gnas is imprinted. m−/+ mice are large with broad bodies and transient subcutaneous edema at birth; most develop neurological abnormalities and die within 1 to 3 weeks. In contrast, +/p− mice are small at birth with narrow bodies and fail to suckle; most develop hypoglycemia and die several hours after birth.

Interestingly, mice with paternal uniparental disomy (UPD)/maternal deletion and maternal UPD/paternal deletion of the distal chromosome 2 region including Gnas have almost identical phenotypes to Gnas m−/+ and +/p− mice, respectively (Cattanach and Kirk, 1985; Williamson et al., 1998). A similar mutant mouse was also generated by radiation mutagenesis (Cattanach et al., 2000). The m−/+ and +/p− phenotypes may result from loss of maternal-specific (e.g., $G_s\alpha$) and paternal-specific (e.g., $G_s\alpha$ or XLαs) Gnas gene products, respectively. NESP55 expression is probably not lost in m−/+ mice.

As in humans, disruption of the maternal, but not paternal, Gnas allele results in renal PTH resistance, and molecular studies confirmed that $G_s\alpha$ is preferentially expressed from the maternal allele in renal proximal tubules (Yu et al., 1998). Although $G_s\alpha$ was reported to be preferentially expressed from the paternal allele in glomeruli (Williamson et al., 1996), this was not confirmed in Gnas knockout mice. The imprinting was tissue-specific, as $G_s\alpha$ was equally expressed from both parental alleles in more distal portions of the nephron, as well as in other extrarenal tissues (e.g., lung and skeletal muscle) (Yu et al., 1998; Ecelbarger et al., 1999; Weinstein et al., 2000). Partial $G_s\alpha$ deficiency in the distal nephron leads to diminished urine concentration in response to acute, but not chronic, elevations of circulating vasopressin (Ecelbarger et al., 1999; Yu et al., 1998).

Gnas knockout mice also have unexpected defects in energy metabolism (Yu et al., 2000). M−/+ mice are obese, hypometabolic, and hypoactive, whereas +/p− mice are very lean, hypermetabolic, and hyperactive. Similar weight changes are also observed in mice with a radiation-induced mutation near *Gnas* (Cattanach et al., 2000). These opposite effects possibly result from opposite effects on sympathetic activity (Yu et al., 2000). Both obese m−/+ and lean +/p− mice have increased sensitivity to insulin in vivo and increased insulin-stimulated glucose uptake in skeletal muscle (Yu et al., 2001). This may reflect the fact that $G_s\alpha$ levels in skeletal muscle are similarly reduced in m−/+ and +/p− mice ($G_s\alpha$ is not imprinted in muscle). Although these findings provide in vivo evidence that G_s/cAMP negatively regulates insulin action, there is no evidence that insulin sensitivity is elevated in patients with either PPHP or PHPIA. Differences between the m−/+ and +/p− mouse phenotypes and respective PHPIA and PPHP phenotypes (e.g., lack of ectopic ossifications or TSH resistance, leanness in +/p− mice) might reflect species-specific differences in the importance of *Gnas* gene products or in other physiological or environmental factors.

Pathogenesis

Although $G_s\alpha$ deficiency resulting from heterozygous null mutations would be expected to reduce hormone signaling and lead to clinical hormone resistance, it was initially unclear why some patients developed hormone resistance (PHPIA) while others did not (PPHP). The first clue came from the observation that paternal transmission results in offspring with PPHP, whereas maternal transmission results in PHPIA (Davies and Hughes, 1993; Wilson et al., 1994; Nakamoto et al., 1998), strongly suggesting that *GNAS* is imprinted. $G_s\alpha$ was shown to be imprinted (maternally expressed) in human pituitary glands (Hayward et al., 2001)

If $G_s\alpha$ is primarily expressed from the maternal allele in specific hormone target tissues (e.g., renal proximal tubules [the major site of PTH action in the kidney], thyroid, and gonad), then a null mutation on the active maternal allele would disrupt $G_s\alpha$ expression and hormone signaling (Fig. 85–5). The same mutation on the inactive paternal allele would have little effect on $G_s\alpha$ expression or hormone signaling. This would explain why PTH-stimulated urinary cAMP is markedly reduced in PHPIA but not in PPHP (Chase et al., 1969; Levine et al., 1986). $G_s\alpha$ imprinting would have to be tissue-specific, as $G_s\alpha$ is biallelically expressed in other nonendocrine human tissues (Campbell et al., 1994; Hayward et al., 1998a, 1998b). This would explain why $G_s\alpha$ expression is similarly reduced by ∼50% in both PHPIA and PPHP patients in many tissues (Levine et al., 1986). Tissue-specific imprinting of $G_s\alpha$ has been confirmed in mice (Yu et al., 1998).

PTH activation of G_s/cAMP in renal proximal tubules leads to activation of the 1α-hydroxylase, which converts 25-hydroxyvitamin D to 1,25(OH)₂D, and decreased phosphate reabsorption. $G_s\alpha$ deficiency prevents these downstreams actions, leading to decreased 1,25(OH)₂D synthesis and urinary phosphate excretion. Low 1,25(OH)₂D levels lead to hypocalcemia by decreasing intestinal calcium absorption and skeletal calcium mobilization (Drezner et al., 1976; Drezner and Haussler, 1979; Epstein et al., 1983). Decreased phosphate excretion leads to hyperphosphatemia, which further inhibits the production of 1,25(OH)₂D. Hypocalcemia, hyperphosphatemia, and low 1,25(OH)₂D levels all contribute to secondary hyperparathyroidism.

Hypothyroidism and hypogonadism in PHPIA likely result from decreased TSH and gonadotropin signaling due to partial $G_s\alpha$ deficiency in thyroid and gonads, respectively. TSH-stimulated adenylyl cyclase activity was diminished in thyroid membranes from a PHPIA patient (Mallet et al., 1982). As gonadotropin levels are not clearly elevated in PHPIA, it has been proposed that these patients have a partial resistance that allows for follicular development and estrogen production, but not ovulation (Namnoum et al., 1998). Loss of G_s/cAMP signaling in somatotrophs presumably contributes to the GH deficiency present in some PHPIA patients.

There are several potential explanations for why PHPIA patients lack resistance to other hormones that activate G_s/cAMP in their target tissues (e.g., ACTH or vasopressin). If $G_s\alpha$ is not imprinted in their respective target tissues (e.g., adrenal cortex or renal collecting ducts), then heterozygous mutations will only reduce its expression by 50%. This may fail to produce hormone resistance, either because

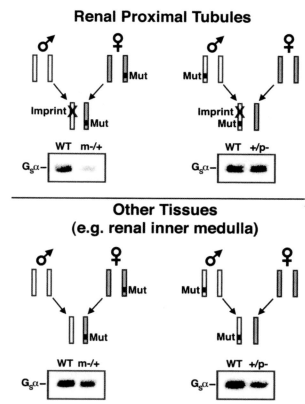

Figure 85–5. Tissue-specific imprinting of $G_s\alpha$ and the effect of heterozygous null mutations. (*Top*) In renal proximal tubules $G_s\alpha$ is paternally imprinted (denoted with an X). Mutation (Mut) of the active allele on the maternally inherited chromosome (gray rectangle) leads to loss of $G_s\alpha$ expression (left) while mutations in the inactive paternal allele have little effect on $G_s\alpha$ expression (right). This is confirmed by immunoblots (shown below) of renal cortical membranes isolated from normal mice (WT) and mice with disruption of the *Gnas* maternal (m−/+) and paternal (+/p−) alleles, respectively (Yu et al., 1998). (*Bottom*) In most other tissues $G_s\alpha$ is not imprinted and is therefore expressed equally from both parental alleles. Mutation of the maternal and paternal alleles should both lead to 50% loss of $G_s\alpha$ expression (haploinsufficiency). Immunoblots of renal inner medulla membranes show that $G_s\alpha$ expression is similarly reduced by 50% in both m−/+ and +/p− mice (Yu et al., 1998). (Figure adapted from Weinstein et al., 2001.)

$G_s\alpha$ is not rate limiting for cAMP generation or because the reduced cAMP levels are still sufficient to elicit the downstream physiological responses (Carlson et al., 1985; Brickman et al., 1986; Weinstein et al., 2000). Lack of $G_s\alpha$ imprinting in the distal nephron may explain why the anticalciuric effect of PTH in the thick ascending limb is unaffected in PHPIA patients (Stone et al., 1993).

While multihormone resistance is almost certainly due to $G_s\alpha$ deficiency, the mechanisms that lead to the AHO phenotype are less clearly defined. It appears unlikely that AHO is due to loss of either the paternal-specific gene product XLαs or the maternal-specific gene product NESP55, because paternal and maternal *GNAS* mutations do not produce different AHO phenotypes. Moreover, loss of NESP55 expression in PHPIB patients does not lead to AHO (Liu et al., 2000a). More likely, AHO results from $G_s\alpha$ haploinsufficiency, which is present in many tissues in both PHPIA and PPHP patients.

Activating *GNAS* mutations inhibit osteoblast differentiation leading to FD, whereas inactivating *GNAS* mutations promote osteoblast differentiation and ectopic ossification, leading to osteoma cutis in AHO patients or occasionally to progressive osseous heteroplasia (POH). The potential mechanisms by which $G_s\alpha$ regulates osteoblast differentiation are discussed in the sections on pathogenesis of MAS/FD and POH.

Brachydactyly most likely results from decreased G_s/cAMP signaling in chondrocytes within the epiphyseal growth plates, which results in premature chondrocyte differentiation and closure of growth plates. Bones normally elongate by endochondral ossification at the growth plates, an orderly process during which proliferating chondrocytes differentiate into hypertrophic chondrocytes, which then become ossified. Locally secreted PTHrP binds to the PTH/PTHrP (PTH1) receptor, which inhibits chondrocyte differentiation via G_s/cAMP pathways (Vortkamp et al., 1996). PTHrP (Karaplis et al., 1994) or PTH1 receptor (Lanske et al., 1996; Jobert et al., 1998) knockout mice develop severe skeletal dysplasia as a result of accelerated chondrocyte differentiation. $G_s\alpha$ deficiency would be expected to result in a similar defect. In fact, a small number of Gnas knockout mice also present with growth plate abnormalities and stunted growth (Yu S, Weinstein LS, unpublished data) and the presence of the same Gnas null allele in growth plate chondrocytes promotes differentiation in vivo (Chung et al., 2000).

Several possible mechanisms may contribute to obesity in AHO patients. Norepinephrine released by innervating sympathetic nerves activate β-adrenergic/G_s/cAMP pathways in adipocytes, which stimulate lipolysis through several mechanisms. One mechanism is PKA-dependent phosphorylation of perilipin, a protein at the surface of lipid droplets. Upon phosphorylation perilipin is released from the lipid surface, allowing access of hormone-sensitive lipase to its substrate. Mice lacking perilipin (Martinez-Botas et al., 2000) or with increased PKA activity in adipocytes (Cummings et al., 1996) are lean. Conversely, mice with an increased ratio of α2- to β-adrenergic receptors in adipocytes (which lowers the catecholamine-stimulated cAMP response) are prone to obesity (Valet et al., 2000). In PHPIA patients, both the cAMP and lipolytic responses to catecholamines are decreased (Kaartinen et al., 1994; Carel et al., 1999), presumably reflecting decreased $G_s\alpha$ levels in adipocytes. However, results in Gnas knockout mice suggest that decreased lipolysis may be secondary to decreased sympathetic nerve activity rather than to resistance of adipocytes to sympathetic stimulation (Yu et al., 2000). This possibility is also supported by the fact that norepinephrine levels are low in PHPIA patients (Carel et al., 1999). $G_s\alpha$ deficiency promotes and $G_s\alpha$ activation prevents adipocyte differentiation, possibly by a cAMP-independent mechanism (Wang et al., 1992; Bianco et al., 1998). The extent to which the metabolic and developmental effects of $G_s\alpha$ deficiency in adipocytes leads to obesity in AHO needs to be better defined.

The mental deficits present in patients with AHO may result from $G_s\alpha$ deficiency in the central nervous system. cAMP and PKA are known to be important for learning and memory (Levin et al., 1992; Wu et al., 1995; Abel et al., 1997; Rotenberg et al., 2000) and studies in neuronal cells show that PKA stimulates Rap1/B-Raf/MAPK pathways and is important for neurite outgrowth and differentiation (Vossler et al., 1997; Jessen et al., 2001). The exact mechanism involved in AHO and why these deficits are only present in a subset of patients are presently not well understood.

PROGRESSIVE OSSEOUS HETEROPLASIA

Clinical Features

POH is characterized by progressive development of dermal and subcutaneous ossifications that grow laterally and coalesce to form large plaques, which eventually grow inwardly to involve deep connective tissues and skeletal muscle (Kaplan and Shore, 2000). These severe ossifications can result in joint stiffness and bone deformity. As in AHO, the ectopic ossifications form by intramembranous ossification. However, in AHO the ossifications are more limited and do not invade into deeper tissues.

POH affects both males and females and can be sporadic or familial. In most cases there are no other features of AHO. While there may be a predilection for POH to be inherited paternally (Shore et al., 2002), there is at least one report of POH being inherited maternally (Eddy et al., 2000). In the latter case the patient also had PHPIA. Another POH patient also had brachydactyly (Eddy et al., 2000). In both of these cases $G_s\alpha$ expression in erythrocyte membranes was reduced by ~50%.

Molecular Genetics

Most POH patients have heterozygous germline GNAS mutations within or surrounding the $G_s\alpha$ coding exons, irrespective of whether they also have other features of AHO (Eddy et al., 2000; Yeh et al., 2000; Shore et al., 2002). There is no obvious difference between the mutations found in AHO versus POH patients, which are mostly frameshift, nonsense, or splice site mutations that fully disrupt $G_s\alpha$ expression. In fact, some of the mutations identified in POH patients (e.g., a 4 bp deletion in exon 7 and a c.348delC mutation in exon 5) are identical to those identified in unrelated AHO kindreds (Yeh et al., 2000; Shore et al., 2002).

In one study, POH was associated with paternal inheritance of GNAS mutations (Shore et al., 2002), although maternal transmission of the disease has been observed in a patient who also had clinical signs of PHPIA (Eddy et al., 2000). In one family, paternal transmission of the common 4 bp exon 7 deletion resulted in five cases of POH, while maternal transmission of the identical mutation resulted in AHO in the next generation (Shore et al., 2002). It was not determined whether these latter cases were in fact PPHP or PHPIA.

Diagnosis

The diagnosis of POH is made based on its characteristic ectopic ossification, which is easily distinguishable from fibrodysplasia ossificans progressiva, a disorder associated with heterotopic endochondral ossification. As POH can be associated with other features of AHO, physical and radiological examination should be performed and baseline calcium, phosphorus, PTH, thyroxine, and TSH should be measured. To confirm the diagnosis, G_s bioactivity in erythrocyte membranes or GNAS mutation analysis can be performed.

Treatment and Counseling

There is no specific therapy for the ossifications. Male patients should be counseled that their offspring each have a 50% chance of developing POH or perhaps other features of AHO, but not hormone resistance. Female patients should be counseled that their offspring have a 50% chance of developing PHPIA and a chance of developing POH. If a specific GNAS mutation has been identified, this could be theoretically used for prenatal diagnosis, although no specific example of such a diagnosis has been reported.

Animal Models

There are no animal models that mimic POH. No ectopic ossification is observed in Gnas knockout mice (Yu et al., 1998).

Pathogenesis

Given that AHO and POH patients have similar null mutations that completely disrupt $G_s\alpha$ expression, it seems likely that the severity of ectopic ossification in an individual patient is determined by genetic background of other "modifying" genes. Such modifiers might influence $G_s\alpha$ expression from the wild-type allele, another component of the signaling pathway, or another pathway involved in bone formation. It is harder to explain why most patients with POH do not also display other features of AHO. The predilection for POH to be paternally transmitted may implicate a paternal-specific GNAS gene product (e.g., XLαs). However, paternal transmission of GNAS mutations more often results in PPHP rather than POH, and maternal transmission can also lead to POH (Eddy et al., 2000).

Activating $G_s\alpha$ mutations lead to FD by inhibiting the differentiation of bone marrow stromal cells to osteoblasts, implicating the G_s/cAMP pathway in the regulation of osteoblast differentiation. Conversely, decreased $G_s\alpha$ expression promotes osteoblast differentiation in cultured cells (Nanes et al., 1995). In AHO and POH, $G_s\alpha$ deficiency (and presumably lower cAMP levels) in mesenchymal precursor cells may promote their differentiation into osteoblasts, resulting in intramembranous ossification in ectopic locations. mRNA for the osteogenic transcription factor Cbfa1/RUNX2 was expressed in dermal fibroblasts derived from a POH patient (Yeh et al., 2000). Recent studies suggest that cAMP may also lower Cbfa1/RUNX2 protein expression by stimulating its degradation (Tintut et al., 1999).

PSEUDOHYPOPARATHYROIDISM TYPE IB

Clinical Features

PHPIB patients have renal PTH resistance in the absence of AHO or resistance to other hormones (except TSH in some cases). In PHPIB, PTH resistance presents in much the same way as in PHPIA. The urinary cAMP response to administered PTH is diminished in PHPIB (Levine et al., 1983), suggesting a proximal signaling defect. Some PHPIB patients present with elevated serum alkaline phosphatase, cortical bone resorption, and/or osteitis fibrosa cystica, presumably due to skeletal effects of chronically elevated PTH levels (Kolb and Steinbach, 1962; Costello and Dent, 1963). PHPIB can be either familial or sporadic. As in patients with AHO, PTH resistance in PHPIB only occurs when it is inherited maternally (Jüppner et al., 1998). Those who inherit the trait paternally are asymptomatic carriers. While most patients with PHPIB are not resistant to TSH (Levine et al., 1983), some of them have slightly elevated TSH levels, which is consistent with borderline TSH resistance (Bastepe et al., 2001a; Weinstein LS, unpublished).

Molecular Genetics

The PTH receptor was first considered as a candidate, but has been ruled out as the PHPIB gene (Schipani et al., 1995; Fukumoto et al., 1996; Jüppner et al., 1998; Jan de Beur et al., 2000). Mapping studies linked PHPIB to 20q13, suggesting that *GNAS* may be the PHPIB locus (Jüppner et al., 1998). However, erythrocyte G$_s$ function is normal in PHPIB patients (Levine et al., 1983; Silve et al., 1986), making it unlikely that these patients have typical G$_s\alpha$ null mutations. Rather, PHPIB is almost always associated with loss of imprinting of the maternal exon 1A promoter region, resulting in a paternal-specific imprinting pattern (unmethylated, transcriptionally active) on both alleles (Liu et al., 2000a; Bastepe et al., 2001b; Jan de Beur et al., 2001). This defect is present in both sporadic and familial cases, and also in patients with severe skeletal changes secondary to excess circulating PTH. In contrast, the NESP55 and XLαs promoters are imprinted normally in most patients, with only a few patients having a paternal-specific imprinting pattern in both alleles. In patients with biallelic NESP55 promoter methylation, NESP55 expression is lost (Liu et al., 2000a). There is no correlation between the phenotype and NESP55 or XLαs imprinting.

Paternal UPD of chromosome 20 is uncommon in PHPIB (Liu et al., 2000a), but it has been reported in one patient with PTH and TSH resistance and other abnormalities (Bastepe et al., 2001a). In the vast majority of patients without UPD, there appears to be a failure to switch to the maternal imprinting pattern in the oocyte. In familial cases, this switching defect is presumed to be caused by genetic mutations that are closely linked to *GNAS* (Jüppner et al., 1998), although no such mutations have been identified. Recent data suggest that such mutations may be located far upstream of the *GNAS* imprinted regions or, in some cases, at other unlinked loci (Bastepe et al., 2001b).

Three siblings with PHPIB were reported to have a 3 bp deletion mutation in exon 13 that deletes G$_s\alpha$ Ile382 within the carboxyl-terminus, which leads to selective uncoupling of G$_s\alpha$ from the PTH1 receptor (Wu et al., 2001). As with other *GNAS* mutations, only maternal transmission of the ΔIle382 mutation resulted in PTH resistance.

Diagnosis

PHPIB is diagnosed by the presence of renal PTH resistance in the absence of AHO or other hormone resistance (except for mild TSH resistance). Renal PTH resistance is diagnosed as discussed above for PHPIA. Measurement of erythrocyte G$_s$ function may be useful, as G$_s$ function is reduced by ~50% in PHPIA but is normal in PHPIB (Levine et al., 1983; Silve et al., 1986). However, this assay is not readily available. The diagnosis can be confirmed by evaluation of *GNAS* exon 1A methylation in blood genomic DNA, which is presently being performed in research laboratories. In rare patients in whom exon 1A methylation is normal, one can perform molecular studies to look for the ΔIle382 mutation.

Treatment and Counseling

In PHPIB, the PTH resistance is treated with oral calcium and vitamin D supplements exactly as in PHPIA. The goal is to try to normalize both serum calcium and PTH if possible while monitoring urine calcium excretion to avoid hypercalciuria. Levothyroxine may be indicated in the few cases with evidence of TSH resistance. Generally no other medical management is required.

In familial cases of PHPIB, PTH resistance only occurs in offspring who inherit the trait maternally. Therefore offspring of affected males will be clinically silent, but may themselves have clinically affected offspring if they are female. There is no way at present to determine which offspring of affected males are silent carriers. Serum calcium, phosphorus, and PTH should be serially measured beginning in childhood in offspring of female patients or potential carriers. Alternatively, these family members could be screened for the *GNAS* methylation defect to determine who is at risk for developing PTH resistance. While prenatal diagnosis could be made by methylation analysis of fetal genomic DNA, this is not indicated, given the limited and easily treatable manifestations of the disorder.

Animal Models

There are presently no animal models that mimic the clinical features or *GNAS* imprinting defect of PHPIB.

Pathogenesis

Expression of an imprinted gene product will be lost if both alleles have the epigenetic characteristics of the silent parental allele (Malcolm et al., 1991; Horsthemke et al., 1997; Reik and Walter, 2001), due to either UPD or so-called imprinting mutations (in which imprinting is abnormal even in the absence of UPD). If both *GNAS* alleles have a paternal-specific imprinting pattern, then renal PTH resistance will result from lack of an "active maternal" G$_s\alpha$ allele in the renal proximal tubules. However, G$_s\alpha$ expression will not be affected in most other tissues where G$_s\alpha$ is expressed equally from both parental alleles. This is precisely the PHPIB phenotype: renal PTH resistance with reduced PTH-stimulated urinary cAMP despite normal G$_s$ expression in other tissues (e.g., erythrocytes). Lack of G$_s\alpha$ haploinsufficiency in most tissues may explain why these patients do not have AHO.

Abnormal imprinting of the exon 1A region in PHPIB strongly suggests that this region is necessary for tissue-specific imprinting of G$_s\alpha$, and perhaps XLαs and NESP55 imprinting as well. In mice, maternal-specific methylation of exon 1A is established in the oocyte and is maintained throughout embryonic development—both characteristics of imprinting control regions critical for the establishment of gene imprinting (Liu et al., 2000b). However, normal NESP55 and XLαs imprinting in most PHPIB patients suggests that imprinting of these regions is not tightly linked to exon 1A imprinting and that PHPIB does not result from NESP55 or XLαs defects.

How tissue-specific imprinting of G$_s\alpha$ may be dependent on exon 1A imprinting is not established. G$_s\alpha$ imprinting does not appear to result from G$_s\alpha$ promoter methylation or promoter competition (Liu et al., 2000b). Tissue-specific G$_s\alpha$ imprinting may involve an interaction between the exon 1A region (which is differentially methylated in all tissues) and a tissue-specific factor (e.g., a tissue-specific DNA-binding factor). One hypothetical model predicts that the exon 1A region contains a silencer element that binds a tissue-specific repressor on the paternal allele but is unable to bind the repressor on the maternal allele because the site is methylated (Ferguson-Smith, 2000) (Fig. 85–6). The repressor leads to paternal-specific suppression of G$_s\alpha$ only in tissues where it is expressed (e.g., renal proximal tubules). In PHPIB, both alleles are unmethylated, allowing the repressor to bind to and suppress G$_s\alpha$ expression from both alleles in the renal proximal tubules. G$_s\alpha$ expression would remain unaffected in other tissues where the repressor is not expressed.

Alternatively, this region could contain a boundary element that insulates the G$_s\alpha$ promoter from an upstream enhancer on the paternal allele through the binding of an insulator protein (Fig. 85–6). The insulator protein cannot bind to the maternal allele due to methylation,

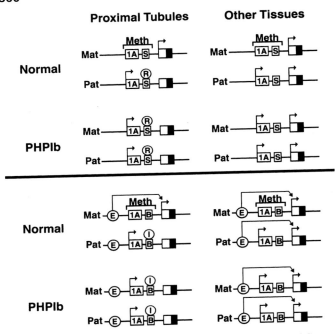

Figure 85–6. Potential mechanisms for tissue-specific imprinting of G$_s\alpha$ and the consequences of the PHPIB imprinting defect. (*Top*) Tissue-specific repressor model. This model predicts that in renal proximal tubules the paternal G$_s\alpha$ promoter (shown as half-filled box) is suppressed because the exon 1A region has a silencer element (S) that binds a tissue-specific repressor (R) on the paternal allele. Methylation of the silencer on the maternal allele prevents repressor binding, allowing the maternal G$_s\alpha$ promoter to remain active. In most other tissues the repressor is not expressed and therefore G$_s\alpha$ is expressed from both alleles even though they are differentially methylated at exon 1A. In PHPIB the silencer on the maternal allele is not methylated, allowing the repressor to bind to and suppress G$_s\alpha$ expression from both alleles in renal proximal tubules. G$_s\alpha$ expression remains unaffected in the majority of tissues where the repressor is not expressed. (*Bottom*) A boundary element model predicts that the exon 1A region has a boundary element (B) that binds an insulator protein (I) on the paternal allele, preventing the paternal G$_s\alpha$ promoter from being activated by an upstream enhancer (E). Methylation prevents binding of the insulator protein on the maternal allele, allowing the enhancer to activate the maternal G$_s\alpha$ promoter. In other tissues, both G$_s\alpha$ alleles are active, either because the insulator protein is expressed in a tissue-specific manner or because G$_s\alpha$ expression does not depend on the upstream enhancer. In either case, loss of maternal-specific methylation of the boundary element would lead to loss of G$_s\alpha$ expression in renal proximal tubules. (Adapted from Weinstein 2001.)

allowing the enhancer to stimulate the maternal G$_s\alpha$ promoter. *Igf2* has been shown to be imprinted by a similar mechanism (Bell and Felsenfeld, 2000; Hark et al., 2000). In the case of G$_s\alpha$, tissue-specific imprinting could result if either insulator protein expression or enhancer activity were limited to specific tissues. In either case, loss of maternal-specific exon 1A methylation in PHPIB would lead to tissue-specific G$_s\alpha$ deficiency.

The ΔIle382 mutation described in one PHPIB kindred selectively uncouples G$_s\alpha$ from the PTH1 receptor (Wu et al., 2001). These patients probably do not develop other manifestations of PHPIA because coupling to other receptors is not affected. As the PTH1 receptor also mediates the effects of PTHrP on bone development, one might expect these patients to also develop skeletal dysplasia, as do patients with other maternal G$_s\alpha$ null mutations. Perhaps this is not observed due to activation of the mutant G$_s\alpha$ by alternative receptors.

REFERENCES

Abel T, Nguyen PV, Barad M, Deuel TA, Kandel ER, Bourtchouladze R (1997). Genetic demonstration of a role for PKA in the late phase of LTP and in hippocampus-based long-term memory. *Cell* 88: 615–626.

Ahmed SF, Dixon PH, Bonthron DT, Stirling HF, Barr DGB, Kelnar CJH, Thakker RV (1998). *GNAS* mutational analysis in pseudohypoparathyroidism. *Clin Endocrinol* 49: 525–531.

Ahrens W, Hiort O, Staedt P, Kirschner T, Marschke C, Kruse K (2001). Analysis of the *GNAS* gene in Albright's hereditary osteodystrophy. *J Clin Endocrinol Metab* 86: 4630–4634.

Albright F, Butler AM, Hampton AO, Smith P (1937). Syndrome characterized by osteitis fibrosa disseminata, areas of pigmentation and endocrine dysfunction, with precocious puberty in females. *N Engl J Med* 216: 727–746.

Aldred MA, Trembath RC (2000). Activating and inactivating mutations in the human *GNAS* gene. *Hum Mutat* 16: 183–189.

Aldred MA, Bagshaw RJ, Macdermot K, Casson D, Murch SH, Walker-Smith JA, Trembath RC (2000). Germline mosaicism for a *GNAS* mutation and Albright hereditary osteodystrophy. *J Med Genet* 37: E35.

Alman BA, Naber SP, Terek RM, Jiranek WA, Goldberg MJ, Wolfe HJ (1995). Platelet derived growth factor in fibrous musculoskeletal disorders: a study of pathologic tissue sections and in vitro primary cell cultures. *J Orthop Res* 13: 67–77.

Alman BA, Wolfe HJ, Greel DA (1996). Activating mutations of Gs protein in monostotic fibrous lesions of bone. *J Orthop Res* 14: 311–315.

Balachandar V, Pahuja J, Maddaiah VT, Collipp PJ (1975). Pseudohypoparathyroidism with normal serum calcium level. *Am J Dis Child* 129: 1092–1095.

Ball ST, Williamson CM, Hayes C, Hacker T, Peters J (2001). The spatial and temporal expression pattern of *Nesp* and its antisense *Nespas*, in mid-gestation mouse embryos. *Mech Develop* 100: 79–81.

Barr DGD, Stirling HF, Darling JAB (1994). Evolution of pseudohypoparathyroidism: an informative family study. *Arch Dis Child* 70: 337–338.

Bastepe M, Lane AH, Jüppner H (2001a). Paternal uniparental disomy of chromosome 20q—and the resulting changes in *GNAS* methylation—as a plausible cause of pseudohypoparathyroidism. *Am J Hum Genet* 68: 1283–1289.

Bastepe M, Pincus JE, Sugimoto T, Tojo K, Kanatani M, Azuma Y, Kruse K, Rosenbloom AL, Koshiyama H, Jüppner H (2001b). Positional dissociation between the genetic mutation responsible for pseudohypoparathyroidism type Ib and the associated methylation defect at exon A/B: evidence for a long-range regulatory element within the imprinted *GNAS* locus. *Hum Mol Genet* 10: 1231–1241.

Bauer R, Ischia R, Marksteiner J, Kapeller I, Fischer-Colbrie R (1999a). Localization of neuroendocrine secretory protein 55 messenger RNA in the rat brain. *Neuroscience* 91: 685–694.

Bauer R, Weiss C, Marksteiner J, Doblinger A, Fischer-Colbrie R, Laslop A (1999b). The new chromogranin-like protein NESP55 is preferentially localized in adrenaline-synthesizing cells of the bovine and rat adrenal medulla. *Neurosci Lett* 263: 13–16.

Bell AC, Felsenfeld G (2000). Methylation of a CTCF-dependent boundary controls imprinted expression of the *Igf2* gene. *Nature* 405: 482–485.

Bellows CG, Ishida H, Aubin JE, Heersche JNM (1990). Parathyroid hormone reversibly suppresses the differentiation of osteoprogenitor cells into functional osteoblasts. *Endocrinology* 127: 3111–3116.

Benedict PH (1962). Endocrine features in Albright's syndrome (fibrous dysplasia of bone). *Metabolism* 11: 30–45.

Benjamin DR, McRoberts JW (1973). Polyostotic fibrous dysplasia associated with Cushing syndrome. *Arch Pathol* 96: 175–178.

Bertherat J, Chanson P, Montminy M (1995). The cyclic adenosine 3′,5′-monophosphate responsive factor CREB is constitutively activated in human somatotroph adenomas. *Mol Endocrinol* 9: 777–783.

Bianco P, Robey PG (1999). Diseases of bone and the stromal cell lineage. *J Bone Miner Res* 14: 336–341.

Bianco P, Kuznetsov SA, Riminucci M, Fisher LW, Spiegel AM, Robey PG (1998). Reproduction of human fibrous dysplasia of bone in immunocompromised mice by transplanted mosaics of normal and Gsα-mutated skeletal progenitor cells. *J Clin Invest* 101: 1737–1744.

Bianco P, Riminucci M, Majolagbe A, Kuznetsov SA, Collins MT, Mankani MH, Corsi A, Bone HG, Wientroub S, Spiegel AM, et al. (2000). Mutations of the *GNAS* gene, stromal cell dysfunction, and osteomalacic changes in non-McCune-Albright fibrous dysplasia of bone. *J Bone Miner Res* 15: 120–128.

Bianco P, Schaeverbeke T, Baillet L, Lequen L, Bannwarth B, Dehais J (1999). Chondrosarcoma in a patient with McCune-Albright syndrome: report of a case. *Rev Rhum Engl Ed* 66: 177–179.

Bomsel M, Mostov K (1992). Role of heterotrimeric G proteins in membrane traffic. *Mol Biol Cell* 3: 1317–1328.

Bourne HR, Kaslow HR, Brickman AS, Farfel Z (1981). Fibroblast defect in pseudohypoparathyroidism, type I: reduced activity of receptor-cyclase coupling protein. *J Clin Endocrinol Metab* 53: 636–640.

Braun JJ, Birkenhäger JC, Visser TJ, Juttmann JR (1981). Lack of response of 1,25-dihydroxycholecalciferol to exogenous parathyroid hormone in a patient with treated pseudohypoparathyroidism. *Clin Endocrinol (Oxf)* 14: 403–407.

Bray P, Carter A, Simons C, Guo V, Puckett C, Kamholz J, Spiegel A, Nirenberg M (1986). Human cDNA clones for four species of G$_{\alpha s}$ signal transduction protein. *Proc Natl Acad Sci USA* 83: 8893–8897.

Breslau NA, Weinstock RS (1988). Regulation of 1,25 (OH)2D synthesis in hypoparathyroidism and pseudohypoparathyroidism. *Am J Physiol* 255: E730–E736.

Breslau NA, Notman DD, Canterbury JM, Moses AM (1980). Studies on the attainment of normocalcemia in patients with pseudohypoparathyroidism. *Am J Med* 68: 856–860.

Brickman AS, Carlson HE, Deftos LJ (1981). Prolactin and calcitonin responses to parathyroid hormone infusion in hypoparathyroid, pseudohypoparathyroid, and normal subjects. *J Clin Endocrinol Metab* 53: 661–664.

Brickman AS, Carlson HE, Levin SR (1986). Responses to glucagon infusion in pseudohypoparathyroidism. *J Clin Endocrinol Metab* 63: 1354–1360.

Burton FH, Hasel KW, Bloom FE, Sutcliffe JG (1991). Pituitary hyperplasia and gigantism in mice caused by a cholera toxin transgene. *Nature* 350: 74–77.

Buscá R, Bertolotto C, Ortonne J-P, Balloti R (1996). Inhibition of the phosphatidylinositol 3-kinase/p70S6-kinase pathway induces B16 melanoma cell differentiation. *J Biol Chem* 271: 31824–31830.

Campbell R, Gosden CM, Bonthron DT (1994). Parental origin of transcription from the human *GNAS* gene. *J Med Genet* 31: 607–614.

Candeliere GA, Glorieux FH, Prud'homme J, St.-Arnaud R (1995). Increased expression of the c-*fos* proto-oncogene in bone from patients with fibrous dysplasia. *N Engl J Med* 332: 1546–1551.

Candeliere GA, Glorieux FH, Roughley PJ (1997). Polymerase chain reaction–based technique for the selective enrichment and analysis of mosaic arg201 mutations in Gαs from patients with fibrous dysplasia of bone. *Bone* 21: 201–206.

Carel JC, Le Stunff C, Condamine L, Mallet E, Chaussain JL, Adnot P, Garabedian M, Bougneres P (1999). Resistance to the lipolytic action of epinephrine: a new feature of protein G_s deficiency. *J Clin Endocrinol Metab* 84: 4127–4131.

Carlson HE, Brickman AS (1983). Blunted plasma cyclic adenosine monophosphate response to isoproterenol in pseudohypoparathyroidism. *J Clin Endocrinol Metab* 56: 1323–1326.

Carlson HE, Brickman AS, Bottazzo GF (1977). Prolactin deficiency in pseudohypoparathyroidism. *N Engl J Med* 296: 140–144.

Carlson HE, Brickman AS, Burns TW, Langley PE (1985). Normal free fatty acid response to isoproterenol in pseudohypoparathyroidism. *J Clin Endocrinol Metab* 61: 382–384.

Carter A, Bardin C, Collins R, Simons C, Bray P, Spiegel A (1987). Reduced expression of multiple forms of the α subunit of the stimulatory GTP-binding protein in pseudohypoparathyroidism type Ia. *Proc Natl Acad Sci USA* 84: 7266–7269.

Cass LA, Meinkoth JL (1998). Differential effects of cyclic adenosine 3′,5′-monophosphate on p70 ribosomal S6 kinase. *Endocrinology* 139: 1991–1998.

Castrillo J -L, Theill LE, Karin M (1991). Function of the homeodomain protein GHF1 in pituitary cell proliferation. *Science* 253: 197–199.

Cattanach BM, Kirk M (1985). Differential activity of maternally and paternally derived chromosome regions in mice. *Nature* 315: 496–498.

Cattanach BM, Peters J, Ball S, Rasberry C (2000). Two imprinted gene mutations: three phenotypes. *Hum Mol Genet* 9: 2263–2273.

Cavanah SFW, Dons RF (1993). McCune-Albright syndrome: how many endocrinopathies can one patient have? *South Med J* 86: 364–367.

Chapurlat RD, Meunier PJ, Liens D, Delmas PD (1997). Long-term effects of intravenous pamidronate in fibrous dysplasia of bone. *J Bone Miner Res* 12: 1746–1752.

Chase LR, Melson GL, Aurbach GD (1969). Pseudohypoparathyroidism: defective excretion of 3′,5′-AMP in response to parathyroid hormone. *J Clin Invest* 48: 1832–1844.

Chung U, Wei W, Schipani E, Humzelman J, Weinstein L, Kronenberg H (2000). In vivo function of stimulatory G protein (Gs) in the growth plate. *J Bone Miner Res* 15(Supp. 1): S175.(Abstract)

Ciullo I, Diez-Roux G, Di Domenico M, Migliaccio A, Avvedimento EV (2001). cAMP signaling selectively influences Ras effectors pathways. *Oncogene* 20: 1186–1192.

Cohen MM Jr, Howell RE (1999). Etiology of fibrous dysplasia and the McCune-Albright syndrome. *Int J Oral Maxillofac Surg* 28: 366–371.

Coleman DE, Berghuis AM, Lee E, Linder ME, Gilman AG, Sprang SR (1994). Structures of active conformations of $G_{i\alpha 1}$ and the mechanism of GTP hydrolysis. *Science* 265: 1405–1412.

Collins MT, Chebli C, Jones J, Kushner H, Consugar M, Rinaldo P, Wientroub S, Bianco P, Robey PG (2001). Renal phosphate wasting in fibrous dysplasia of bone is part of a generalized renal tubular dysfunction similar to that seen in tumor-induced osteomalacia. *J Bone Miner Res* 16: 806–813.

Comite F, Shawker TH, Pescovitz OH, Loriaux DL, Cutler GB Jr. (1984). Cyclical ovarian function resistant to treatment with an analogue of luteinizing hormone releasing hormone in McCune-Albright syndrome. *N Engl J Med* 311: 1032–1036.

Conklin BR, Herzmark P, Ishida S, Voyno-Yasenetskaya TA, Sun Y, Farfel Z, Bourne HR (1996). Carboxyl-terminal mutations of Gqα and Gsα that alter the fidelity of receptor activation. *Mol Pharmacol* 50: 885–890.

Constancia M, Pickard B, Kelsey G, Reik W (1998). Imprinting mechanisms. *Genome Res* 8: 881–900.

Cook SJ, McCormick F (1993). Inhibition by cAMP of Ras-dependent activation of raf. *Science* 262: 1069–1072.

Costello JM, Dent CE (1963). Hypo-hyperparathyroidism. *Arch Dis Child* 38: 397.

Crawford JA, Mutchler KJ, Sullivan BE, Lanigan TM, Clark MS, Russo AF (1993). Neural expression of a novel alternatively spliced and polyadenylated Gsα transcript. *J Biol Chem* 268: 9879–9885.

Cummings DE, Brandon EP, Planas JV, Motamed K, Idzerda RL, McKnight GS (1996). Genetically lean mice result from targeted disruption of the RIIβ subunit of protein kinase A. *Nature* 382: 622–626.

Danon M, Crawford JD (1987). The McCune-Albright syndrome. *Ergeb Inn Med Kinderheilkd* 55: 81–115.

Danon M, Robboy SJ, Kim S, Scully R, Crawford JD (1975). Cushing syndrome, sexual precocity, and polyostotic fibrous dysplasia (Albright syndrome) in infancy. *J Pediatr* 87: 917–921.

D'Armiento M, Reda G, Camagna A, Tardella L (1983). McCune-Albright syndrome: evidence for autonomous multiendocrine hyperfunction. *J Pediatr* 102: 584–586.

Davies SJ, Hughes HE (1993). Imprinting in Albright's hereditary osteodystrophy. *J Med Genet* 30: 101–103.

Degtyarev MY, Spiegel AM, Jones TLZ (1993). The G protein α_s subunit incorporates [^{3}H]palmitic acid and mutation of cysteine-3 prevents this modification. *Biochemistry* 32: 8057–8061.

Dent CE, Gertner JM (1976). Hypophosphataemic osteomalacia in fibrous dysplasia. *Q J Med* 45: 411–420.

de Rooij J, Zwartkruis FJ, Verheijen MH, Cool RH, Nijman SM, Wittinghofer A, Bos JL (1998). Epac is a Rap1 guanine-nucleotide-exchange factor directly activated by cyclic AMP. *Nature* 396: 474–477.

de Sanctis L, Romagnolo D, de Sanctis C, Lala R, Olivero M, Di Renzo F, Dianzani I (2000). Albright hereditary osteodystrophy (AHO) and pseudohypoparathyroidism: three new mutations and a common deletion in *GNAS*. *Am J Hum Genet* 67(Supp 2): 295.(Abstract)

Dorfman HD, Ishida T, Tsuneyoshi M (1994). Exophytic variant of fibrous dysplasia (fibrous dysplasia protuberans). *Hum Pathol* 25: 1234–1237.

Doty RL, Fernandez AD, Levine MA, Moses A, McKeown DA (1997). Olfactory dysfunction in type I pseudohypoparathyroidism: dissociation from $G_s\alpha$ deficiency. *J Clin Endocrinol Metab* 82: 247–250.

Downs RW Jr, Levine MA, Drezner MK, Burch WM Jr, Spiegel AM (1983). Deficient adenylate cyclase regulatory protein in renal membranes from a patient with pseudohypoparathyroidism. *J Clin Invest* 71: 231–235.

Drezner MK, Haussler MR (1979). Normocalcemic pseudohypoparathyroidism: association with normal vitamin D3 metabolism. *Am J Med* 66: 503–508.

Drezner MK, Neelon FA, Haussler M, McPherson HT, Lebovitz HE (1976). 1,25-dihydroxycholecalciferol deficiency: the probable cause of hypocalcemia and metabolic bone disease in pseudohypoparathyroidism. *J Clin Endocrinol Metab* 42: 621–628.

Ecelbarger CA, Yu S, Lee AJ, Weinstein LS, Knepper MA (1999). Decreased Na-K-2Cl cotransporter expression in mice with heterozygous disruption of the gene for heterotrimeric G-protein Gsα. *Am J Physiol* 277: F235–F244.

Eddy MC, Jan de Beur SM, Yandow SM, McAlister WH, Shore EI, Kaplan FS, Whyte MP, Levine MA (2000). Deficiency of the α-subunit of the stimulatory G protein and severe extraskeletal ossification. *J Bone Miner Res* 15: 2074–2083.

Edgerton MT, Persing JA, Jane JA (1985). The surgical treatment of fibrous dysplasia: with emphasis on recent contributions from cranio-maxillo-facial surgery. *Ann Surg* 202: 459–479.

Ehrig U, Wilson DR (1972). Fibrous dysplasia of bone and primary hyperparathyroidism. *Ann Intern Med* 77: 234–238.

Epstein S, Meunier PJ, Lambert PW, Stern PH, Bell NH (1983). 1,25-dihydroxyvitamin D3 corrects osteomalacia in hypoparathyroidism and pseudohypoparathyroidism. *Acta Endocrinol (Copenh)* 103: 241–247.

Esapa C, Foster S, Johnson S, Jameson JL, Kendall-Taylor P, Harris PE (1997). G protein and thyrotropin receptor mutations in thyroid neoplasia. *J Clin Endocrinol Metab* 82: 493–496.

Eyre WG, Reed WB (1971). Albright's hereditary osteodystrophy with cutaneous bone formation. *Arch Dermatol* 104: 634–642.

Farfel Z, Bourne HR (1980). Deficient activity of receptor-cyclase coupling protein in platelets of patients with pseudohypoparathyroidism. *J Clin Endocrinol Metab* 51: 1202–1204.

Farfel Z, Friedman E (1986). Mental deficiency in pseudohypoparathyroidism type I is associated with Ns-protein deficiency. *Ann Intern Med* 105: 197–199.

Farfel Z, Brickman AS, Kaslow HR, Brothers VM, Bourne HR (1980). Defect of receptor-cyclase coupling protein in pseudohypoparathyroidism. *N Engl J Med* 303: 237–242.

Farfel Z, Brothers VM, Brickman AS, Conte F, Neer R, Bourne HR (1981). Pseudohypoparathyroidism: inheritance of deficient receptor-cyclase coupling activity. *Proc Natl Acad Sci USA* 78: 3098–3102.

Farfel Z, Abood ME, Brickman AS, Bourne HR (1982). Deficient activity of receptor-cyclase coupling protein in transformed lymphoblasts of patients with pseudohypoparathyroidism type I. *J Clin Endocrinol Metab* 55: 113–117.

Farfel Z, Iiri T, Shapira H, Roitman A, Mouallem M, Bourne HR (1996). Pseudohypoparathyroidism: a novel mutation in the $\beta\gamma$-contact region of $G_s\alpha$ impairs receptor stimulation. *J Biol Chem* 271: 19653–19655.

Faull CM, Welbury RR, Paul B, Kendall-Taylor P (1991). Pseudohypoparathyroidism: its phenotypic variability and associated disorders in a large family. *Q J Med* 78: 251–264.

Ferguson-Smith AC (2000). Genomic imprinting: silencing elements have their say. *Curr Biol* 10: R872–R875.

Feuillan PP, Shawker T, Rose SR, Jones J, Jeevanram RK, Nisula BC (1990). Thyroid abnormalities in the McCune-Albright syndrome: ultrasonography and hormone studies. *J Clin Endocrinol Metab* 71: 1596–1601.

Firat D, Stutzman L (1968). Fibrous dysplasia of the bone: a review of twenty-four cases. *Am J Med* 44: 421–429.

Fischer JA, Egert F, Werder E, Born W (1998). An inherited mutation associated with functional deficiency of the α-subunit of the guanine nucleotide-binding protein G_s in pseudo- and pseudopseudohypoparathyroidism. *J Clin Endocrinol Metab* 83: 935–938.

Foster CM, Ross JL, Shawker T, Pescovitz OH, Loriaux DL, Cutler GB Jr, Comite F (1984). Absence of pubertal gonadotropin secretion in girls with McCune-Albright syndrome. *J Clin Endocrinol Metab* 58: 1161–1165.

Frase WD, Walsh CA, Birch MA, Durham B, Dillon JP, McGreavy D, Gallagher JA (2000). Parathyroid hormone-related protein in the aetiology of fibrous dysplasia of bone in the McCune-Albright syndrome. *Clin Endocrinol* 53: 621–628.

Fukumoto S, Suzawa M, Takeuchi Y, Kodama Y, Nakayama K, Ogata E, Matsumoto T, Fujita T (1996). Absence of mutations in parathyroid hormone (PTH)/PTH-related protein receptor complementary deoxyribonucleic acid in patients with pseudohypoparathyroidism type Ib. *J Clin Endocrinol Metab* 81: 2554–2558.

Gaiddon C, Boutillier A-L, Monnier D, Mercken L, Loeffler J-P (1994). Genomic effects of the putative oncogene Gαs: chronic transcriptional activation of the c-*fos* proto-oncogene in endocrine cells. *J Biol Chem* 269: 22663–22671.

Gejman PV, Weinstein LS, Martinez M, Spiegel AM, Cao Q, Hsieh W-T, Hoehe MR, Gershon ES (1991). Genetic mapping of the Gs-α subunit gene (*GNAS*) to the distal long arm of chromosome 20 using a polymorphism detected by denaturing gradient gel electrophoresis. *Genomics* 9: 782–783.

Germaine-Lee EL, Willi SM, Key L Jr, Levine MA (2001). Growth hormone secretion is reduced in pseudohypoparathyroidism type IA. *Program and Abstracts of the 83rd Annual Meeting of the Endocrine Society*. Endocrine Society Press, Bethesda, MD, p. 184 (Abstract).

Giovanelli G, Bernasconi S, Banchini G (1978). McCune-Albright syndrome in a male child: a clinical and endocrinologic enigma. *J Pediatr* 92: 220–226.

Goadsby PJ, Lollin Y, Kocen RS (1991). Pseudopseudohypoparathyroidism and spinal cord compression. *J Neurol Neurosurg Psychiatry* 54: 929–931.

Goeteyn V, De Potter CR, Naeyaert JM (1999). Osteoma cutis in pseudohypoparathyroidism. *Dermatology* 198: 209–211.

Gonzalez-Robayna IJ, Falender AE, Ochsner S, Firestone GL, Richards JS (2000). Follicle-stimulating hormone (FSH) stimulates phosphorylation and activation of protein kinase B (PKB/Akt) and serum and glucocorticoid-induced kinase (Sgk): evidence for A kinase–independent signaling by FSH in granulosa cells. *Mol Endocrinol* 14: 1283–1300.

Grabias SL, Campbell CJ (1977). Fibrous dysplasia. *Orthop Clin North Am* 8: 771–783.

Grant DB, Martinez L (1983). The McCune-Albright syndrome without typical skin pigmentation. *Acta Paediatr Scand* 72: 477–478.

Graudal N, Milman N, Nielsen LS, Niebuhr E, Bonde J (1986). Coexistent pseudohypoparathyroidism and D brachydactyly in a family. *Clin Genet* 30: 449–455.

Graziano MP, Gilman AG (1989). Synthesis in *Escherichia coli* of GTPase-deficient mutants of Gsα. *J Biol Chem* 264: 15475–15482.

Greco MA, Steiner GC (1986). Ultrastructure of fibrous dysplasia of bone: a study of its fibrous, osseous, and cartilaginous components. *Ultrastruct Pathol* 10: 55–66.

Grishina G, Berlot CH (1998). Mutations at the interface of $G_{s\alpha}$ impair receptor-mediated activation by altering receptor and guanine nucleotide binding. *J Biol Chem* 273: 15053–15060.

Grishina G, Berlot CH (2000). A surface-exposed region of $G_{s\alpha}$ in which substitutions decrease receptor-mediated activation and increase receptor affinity. *Mol Pharmacol* 57: 1081–1092.

Hammami MM, Hussain SS, Vencer LJ, Butt A, al-Zahrani A (1997). Primary hyperparathyroidism-associated polyostotic fibrous dysplasia: absence of McCune-Albright syndrome mutations. *J Endocrinol Invest* 20: 552–558.

Happle R (1986). The McCune-Albright syndrome: a lethal gene surviving by mosaicism. *Clin Genet* 29: 321–324.

Hark AT, Schoenherr CJ, Katz DJ, Ingram RS, Levorse JM, Tilghman SM (2000). CTCF mediates methylation-sensitive enhancer-blocking activity at the *H19/Igf2* locus. *Nature* 405: 486–489.

Harris WH, Dudley HRJ, Barry RJ (1962). The natural history of fibrous dysplasia. *J Bone Joint Surg* 44-A: 207–233.

Hayward BE, Bonthron DT (2000). An imprinted antisense transcript at the human *GNAS* locus. *Hum Mol Genet* 9: 835–841.

Hayward BE, Kamiya M, Strain L, Moran V, Campbell R, Hayashizaki Y, Bonthron DT (1998a). The human *GNAS* gene is imprinted and encodes distinct paternally and biallelically expressed G proteins. *Proc Natl Acad Sci USA* 95: 10038–10043.

Hayward BE, Moran V, Strain L, Bonthron DT (1998b). Bidirectional imprinting of a single gene: *GNAS* encodes maternally, paternally, and biallelically derived proteins. *Proc Natl Acad Sci USA* 95: 15475–15480.

Hayward BE, Barlier A, Korbonits M, Grossman AB, Jacquet P, Enjalbert A, Bonthron DT (2001). Imprinting of the $G_s\alpha$ gene *GNAS* in the pathogenesis of acromegaly. *J Clin Invest* 107: R31–R36.

Heinsimer JA, Davies AO, Downs RW, Levine MA, Spiegel AM, Drezner MK, De Lean A, Wreggett KA, Caron MG, Lefkowitz RJ (1984). Impaired formation of β-adrenergic receptor-nucleotide regulatory protein complexes in pseudohypoparathyroidism. *J Clin Invest* 73: 1335–1343.

Henkin RI (1968). Impairment of olfaction and of the tastes of sour and bitter in pseudohypoparathyroidism. *J Clin Endocrinol Metab* 28: 624–628.

Hibbs RE, Rush HP (1952). Albright's syndrome. *Ann Intern Med* 37: 587–593.

Horsthemke B, Dittrich B, Buiting K (1997). Imprinting mutations on human chromosome 15. *Hum Mutat* 10: 329–337.

Huang C, Duncan JA, Gilman AG, Mumby SM (1999). Persistent membrane association of activated and depalmitoylated G protein α subunits. *Proc Natl Acad Sci USA* 96: 412–417.

Iacovelli L, Capobianco L, Salvatore L, Sallese M, D'Ancona GM, De Blasi A (2001). Thyrotropin activates mitogen-activated protein kinase pathway in FRTL-5 by a cAMP-dependent protein kinase A–independent mechanism. *Mol Pharmacol* 60: 924–933.

Iiri T, Herzmark P, Nakamoto JM, Van Dop C, Bourne HR (1994). Rapid GDP release from Gs-α in patients with gain and loss of endocrine function. *Nature* 371: 164–167.

Iiri T, Farfel Z, Bourne HR (1997). Conditional activation defect of a human $G_{s\alpha}$ mutant. *Proc Natl Acad Sci USA* 94: 5656–5661.

Iiri T, Farfel Z, Bourne HR (1998). G-protein diseases furnish a model for the turn-on switch. *Nature* 394: 35–38.

Ikeda K, Sakurada T, Sasaki Y, Takasaka T, Furukawa Y (1988). Clinical investigation of olfactory and auditory function in type I pseudohypoparathyroidism: participation of adenylate cyclase system. *J Laryngol Otol* 102: 1111–1114.

Inamo Y, Hanawa Y, Kin H, Okuni M (1993). Findings on magnetic resonance imaging of the spine and femur in a case of McCune-Albright syndrome. *Pediatr Radiol* 23: 15–18.

Ischia R, Lovisetti-Scamihorn P, Hogue-Angeletti R, Wolkersdorfer M, Winkler H, Fischer-Colbrie R (1997). Molecular cloning and characterization of NESP55, a novel chromogranin-like precursor of a peptide with 5-HT_{1B} receptor antagonist activity. *J Biol Chem* 272: 11657–11662.

Ishida T, Dorfman HD (1993). Massive chondroid differentiation in fibrous dysplasia of bone (fibrocartilagenous dysplasia). *Am J Surg Pathol* 17: 924–930.

Ishikawa Y, Bianchi C, Nadal-Ginard B, Homcy CJ (1990). Alternative promoter and 5′ exon generate a novel $G_s\alpha$ mRNA. *J Biol Chem* 265: 8458–8462.

Jan de Beur SM, Deng Z, Ding C, Levine MA (1998). Amplification of the GC-rich exon 1 of *GNAS* and identification of three novel nonsense mutations in Albright's hereditary osteodystrophy. *Program and Abstracts of the 80th Annual Meeting of the Endocrine Society*, Endocrine Society Press, Bethesda, MD, p. 62 (Abstract).

Jan de Beur SM, Ding CL, LaBuda MC, Usdin TB, Levine MA (2000). Pseudohypoparathyroidisim 1b: exclusion of parathyroid hormone and its receptors as candidate disease genes. *J Clin Endocrinol Metab* 85: 2239–2246.

Jan de Beur SM, Deng Z, Cho J, Ding C, Levine MA (2001). Loss of imprinting on the maternal *GNAS* allele in pseudohypoparathyroidism type Ib. *Program and Abstracts of the 83rd Meeting of the Endocrine Society*. Endocrine Society Press, Bethesda, MD, p. 107 (Abstract).

Jessen U, Novitskaya V, Pedersen N, Serup P, Berezin V, Bock E (2001). The transcriptional factors CREB and c-Fos play key roles in NCAM-mediated neuritogenesis in PC12-E2 cells. *J Neurochem* 79: 1149–1160.

Jobert AS, Zhang P, Couvineau A, Bonaventure J, Roume J, LeMerrer M, Silve C (1998). Absence of functional receptors for parathyroid hormone and parathyroid hormone-related peptide in Blomstrand chondrodysplasia. *J Clin Invest* 102: 34–40.

Jones DT, Reed RR (1989). G_{olf}: an olfactory neuron specific–G protein involved in odorant signal transduction. *Science* 244: 790–795.

Jones DT, Masters SB, Bourne HR, Reed RR (1990). Biochemical characterization of three stimulatory GTP-binding proteins: the large and small forms of G_s and the olfactory-specific G-protein, G_{olf}. *J Biol Chem* 265: 2671–2676.

Jüppner H, Schipani E, Bastepe M, Cole DE, Lawson ML, Mannstadt M, Hendy GN, Plotkin H, Koshiyama H, Koh T, et al. (1998). The gene responsible for pseudohypoparathyroidism type Ib is paternally imprinted and maps in four unrelated kindreds to chromosome 20q13.3. *Proc Natl Acad Sci USA* 95: 11798–11803.

Kaartinen JM, Käär M-L, Ohisalo JJ (1994). Defective stimulation of adipocyte adenylate cyclase, blunted lipolysis, and obesity in pseudohypoparathyroidism 1a. *Pediatr Res* 35: 594–597.

Kaplan FS, Shore EI (2000). Progressive osseous heteroplasia. *J Bone Miner Res* 15: 2084–2094.

Kaplan FS, Fallon MD, Boden SD, Schmidt R, Senior M, Haddad JG (1988). Estrogen receptors in bone in a patient with polyostotic fibrous dysplasia (McCune-Albright syndrome). *N Engl J Med* 319: 421–425.

Karaplis AC, Luz A, Glowacki J, Bronson RT, Tybulewicz VLJ, Kronenberg HM, Mulligan RC (1994). Lethal skeletal dysplasia from targeted disruption of the parathyroid hormone-related peptide gene. *Genes Dev* 8: 277–289.

Kawasaki H, Springett GM, Mochizuki N, Toki S, Nakaya M, Matsuda M, Housman DE, Graybiel AM (1998). A family of cAMP-binding proteins that directly activate Rap1. *Science* 282: 2275–2279.

Kehlenbach RH, Matthey J, Huttner WB (1994). XLαs is a new type of G protein. *Nature* 372: 804–809.

Kelsey G, Bodle D, Miller HJ, Beechey CV, Coombes C, Peters J, Williamson CM (1999). Identification of imprinted loci by methylation-sensitive representational difference analysis: application to mouse distal chromosome 2. *Genomics* 62: 129–138.

Kim I, Kim ER, Nam HJ, Chin MO, Moon YH, Oh MR, Yeo UC, Song SM, Kim JS, Uhm MR, et al. (1999). Activating mutation of Gsα in McCune-Albright syndrome causes skin pigmentation by tyrosinase gene activation on affected melanocytes. *Horm Res* 52: 235–240.

Kirk JMW, Brain CE, Carson DJ, Hyde JC, Grant DB (1999). Cushing's syndrome caused by nodular adrenal hyperplasia in children with McCune-Albright syndrome. *J Pediatr* 134: 789–792.

Klemke M, Pasolli HA, Kehlenbach RH, Offermanns S, Schultz G, Huttner WB (2000). Characterization of the extra-large G protein α-subunit XLαs. II. Signal transduction properties. *J Biol Chem* 275: 33633–33640.

Klemke M, Kehlenbach RH, Huttner WB (2001). Two overlapping reading frames in a single exon encode interacting proteins: a novel way of gene usage. *EMBO J* 20: 3849–3860.

Kolb FO, Steinbach HL (1962). Pseudohypoparathyroidism with secondary hyperparathyroidism and osteitis fibrosa. *J Clin Endocrinol Metab* 22: 59–70.

Kovacs K, Horvath E, Thorner MO, Rogol AD (1984). Mammosomatotroph hyperplasia associated with acromegaly and hyperprolactinemia in a patient with the McCune-Albright syndrome. *Virchows Arch* 403: 77–86.

Kozasa T, Itoh H, Tsukamoto T, Kaziro Y (1988). Isolation and characterization of the human Gsα gene. *Proc Natl Acad Sci USA* 85: 2081–2085.

Krieger-Brauer HI, Medda P, Kather H (2000). Basic fibroblast growth factor utilized both types of component subunits of G_s for dual signaling in human adipocytes: stimulation of adenylyl cyclase vis $G\alpha_s$ and inhibition of NADPH oxidase by $G\beta\gamma_s$. *J Biol Chem* 275: 35920–35925.

Kruse K, Gutekunst B, Kracht U, Schwerda K (1981). Deficient prolactin response to parathyroid hormone in hypocalcemic and normocalcemic pseudohypoparathyroidism. *J Clin Endocrinol Metab* 52: 1099–1105.

Lair-Milan F, Le Blevec G, Carel JC, Chaussain JL, Adamsbaum C (1996). Thyroid sonographic abnormalities in McCune-Albright syndrome. *Pediatr Radiol* 26: 424–426.

Lala R, Matarazzo P, Bertelloni S, Buzi F, Rigon F, de Sanctis C (2000). Pamidronate treatment of bone fibrous dysplasia in nine children with McCune-Albright syndrome. *Acta Paediatr* 89: 188–193.

Lambert PW, Hollis BW, Bell NH, Epstein S (1980). Demonstration of a lack of change in serum 1α,25-dihydroxyvitamin D in response to parathyroid extract in pseudohypoparathyroidism. *J Clin Invest* 66: 782–791.

Lambright DG, Noel JP, Hamm HE, Sigler PB (1994). Structural determinants for activation of the α-subunit of a heterotrimeric G protein. *Nature* 369: 621–628.

Lambright DG, Sondek J, Bohm A, Skiba NP, Hamm HE, Sigler PB (1996). The 2.0A crystal structure of a heterotrimeric G protein. *Nature* 379: 297–299.

Lamy F, Wilkin F, Baptist M, Posada M, Roger PP, Dumont JE (1993). Phosphorylation of mitogen-activated protein kinases is involved in the epidermal growth factor and phorbol ester, but not in the thyrotropin/cAMP thyroid mitogenic pathway. *J Biol Chem* 268: 8398–8401.

Landis CA, Masters SB, Spada A, Pace AM, Bourne HR, Vallar L (1989). GTPase inhibiting mutations activate the α chain of G_s and stimulate adenylyl cyclase in human pituitary tumours. *Nature* 340: 692–696.

Lanske B, Karaplis AC, Lee K, Luz A, Vortkamp A, Pirro A, Karperien M, Defize LHK, Ho C, Mulligan RC, et al. (1996). PTH/PTHrP receptor in early development and Indian hedgehog-regulated bone growth. *Science* 273: 663–666.

Latham PD, Athanasou NA, Woods CG (1992). Fibrous dysplasia with locally aggressive malignant change. *Arch Orthop Trauma Surg* 111: 183–186.

Lee PA, Van Dop C, Migeon CJ (1986). McCune-Albright syndrome: long term followup. *JAMA* 256: 2980–2984.

Lever EG, Pettingale KW (1983). Albright's syndrome associated with a soft-tissue myxoma and hypophosphataemic osteomalacia: report of a case and review of the literature. *J Bone Joint Surg [Br]* 65: 621–626.

Levin LR, Han P-L, Hwang PM, Feinstein PG, Davis RL, Reed RR (1992). The *Drosophila* learning and memory gene *rutabaga* encodes a Ca^{2+}/calmodulin-responsive adenylyl cyclase. *Cell* 68: 479–489.

Levine MA (1999). Clinical implications of genetic defects in G proteins: oncogenic mutations in Gαs as the molecular basis for the McCune-Albright syndrome. *Arch Med Res* 30: 522–531.

Levine MA, Downs RW Jr, Singer M, Marx SJ, Aurbach GD, Spiegel AM (1980). Deficient activity of guanine nucleotide regulatory protein in erythrocytes from patients with pseudohypoparathyroidism. *Biochem Biophys Res Commun* 94: 1319–1324.

Levine MA, Downs RW Jr, Moses AM, Breslau NA, Marx SJ, Lasker RD, Rizzoli RE, Aurbach GD, Spiegel AM (1983). Resistance to multiple hormones in patients with pseudohypoparathyroidism: association with deficient activity of guanine nucleotide regulatory protein. *Am J Med* 74: 545–556.

Levine MA, Jap TS, Hung W (1985). Infantile hypothyroidism in two sibs: an unusual presentation of pseudohypoparathyroidism type Ia. *J Pediatr* 107: 919–922.

Levine MA, Jap TS, Mauseth RS, Downs RW, Spiegel AM (1986). Activity of the stimulatory guanine nucleotide-binding protein is reduced in erythrocytes from patients with pseudohypoparathyroidism and pseudopseudohypoparathyroidism: biochemical, endocrine, and genetic analysis of Albright's hereditary osteodystrophy in six kindreds. *J Clin Endocrinol Metab* 62: 497–502.

Levine MA, Ahn TG, Klupt SF, Kaufman KD, Smallwood PM, Bourne HR, Sullivan KA, Van Dop C (1988). Genetic deficiency of the α subunit of the guanine nucleotide-binding protein G_s as the molecular basis for Albright hereditary osteodystrophy. *Proc Natl Acad Sci USA* 85: 617–621.

Levine MA, Modi WS, O'Brien SJ (1991). Mapping of the gene encoding the α subunit of the stimulatory G protein of adenylyl cyclase (*GNAS*) to 20q13.2-q13.3 in human by in situ hybridization. *Genomics* 11: 478–479.

Li QB, Cerione RA (1997). Communication between switch II and switch III of the transducin α subunit is essential for target activation. *J Biol Chem* 272: 21673–21676.

Li T, Vu TH, Zeng ZL, Nguyen BT, Hayward BE, Bonthron DT, Hu JF, Hoffman AR (2000). Tissue-specific expression of antisense and sense transcripts at the imprinted *Gnas* locus. *Genomics* 69: 295–304.

Liens D, Delmas PD, Meunier PJ (1994). Long-term effects of intravenous pamidronate in fibrous dysplasia of bone. *Lancet* 343: 953–954.

Linder ME, Middleton P, Hepler JR, Taussig R, Gilman AG, Mumby SM (1993). Lipid modifications of G proteins: α subunits are palmitoylated. *Proc Natl Acad Sci USA* 90: 3675–3679.

Linglart A, Carel JC, Garabedian M, Le T, Mallet E, Kottler ML (2002). *GNAS* lesions in pseudohypoparathyroidism Ia and Ic: genotype phenotype relationship and evidence of the maternal transmission of the hormonal resistance. *J Clin Endocrinol Metab* 87: 189–197.

Liu J, Litman D, Rosenberg MJ, Yu S, Biesecker LG, Weinstein LS (2000a). A *GNAS* imprinting defect in pseudohypoparathyroidism type IB. *J Clin Invest* 106: 1167–1174.

Liu J, Yu S, Litman D, Chen W, Weinstein LS (2000b). Identification of a methylation imprint mark within the mouse *Gnas* locus. *Mol Cell Biol* 20: 5808–5817.

Lopez-Ben R, Pitt MJ, Jaffe KA, Siegal GP (1999). Osteosarcoma in a patient with McCune-Albright syndrome and Mazabraud's syndrome. *Skeletal Radiol* 28: 522–526.

Lovisetti-Scamiform P, Fischer-Colbrie R, Leitner B, Scherzer G, Winkler H (1999). Relative amounts and molecular forms of NESP55 in various bovine tissues. *Brain Res* 829: 99–106.

Lu D, Haskell-Luevano C, Vage DI, Cone RD (1998). Functional variants of the MSH Receptor (MC1-R), *Agouti*, and their effects in mammalian pigmentation. In: *G Proteins, Receptors, and Disease*. Spiegel AM (ed.). Humana Press, Totowa, N.J., pp. 231–259.

Lyons J, Landis CA, Harsh G, Vallar L, Grünewald K, Feichtinger H, Duh Q-Y, Clark OH, Kawasaki E, Bourne HR, McCormick F (1990). Two G protein oncogenes in human endocrine tumors. *Science* 249: 655–659.

Ma Y, Huang J, Ali S, Lowry W, Huang X (2000). Src tyrosine kinase is a novel direct effector of G proteins. *Cell* 102: 635–646.

MacMahon HE (1971). Albright's syndrome: thirty years later (polyostotic fibrous dysplasia). In: *Pathology Annual*. Sommers SC (ed.) Appleton-Century-Crofts, New York, pp. 81–146.

Malchoff CD, Reardon G, MacGillivray DC, Yamase H, Rogol AD, Malchoff DM (1994). An unusual presentation of McCune-Albright syndrome confirmed by an activating mutation of the G_s α-subunit from a bone lesion. *J Clin Endocrinol Metab* 78: 803–806.

Malcolm S, Clayton-Smith J, Nichols M, Robb S, Webb T, Armour JA, Jeffreys AJ, Pembrey ME (1991). Uniparental paternal disomy in Angelman's syndrome. *Lancet* 337: 694–697.

Mallet E, Carayon P, Amr S, Brunelle P, Ducastelle T, Basuyau JP, de Menibus CH (1982). Coupling defect of thyrotropin receptor and adenylate cyclase in a pseudohypoparathyroid patient. *J Clin Endocrinol Metab* 54: 1028–1032.

Mantovani G, Romoli R, Weber G, Brunelli V, De Menis E, Beccio S, Beck-Peccoz P, Spada A (2000). Mutational analysis of *GNAS* in patients with pseudohypoparathyroidism: identification of two novel mutations. *J Clin Endocrinol Metab* 85: 4243–4248.

Marie PJ, Lomri A, Chanson P, de Pollak C (1997). Increased proliferation of osteoblastic cells expressing the activating Gsα mutation in monostotic and polyostotic fibrous dysplasia. *Am J Pathol* 150: 1059–1069.

Marsh SR, Grishina G, Wilson PT, Berlot CH (1998). Receptor-mediated activation of $G_{s\alpha}$: evidence for intramolecular signal transduction. *Mol Pharmacol* 53: 981–990.

Martinez-Botas J, Anderson JB, Tessler D, Lapillonne A, Chang BH, Quast MJ, Gorenstein D, Chen KH, Chan L (2000). Absence of perilipin results in leanness and reverses obesity in *Lepr* db/db mice. *Nat Genet* 26: 474–479.

Masters SB, Landis CA, Bourne HR (1990). GTPase-inhibiting mutations in the α subunit of Gs. *Adv Second Messenger Phosphoprotein Res* 24: 70–75.

Mastorakos G, Koutras DA, Doufas AG, Mitsiades NS (1997). Hyperthyroidism in McCune-Albright syndrome with a review of thyroid abnormalities sixty years after the first report. *Thyroid* 7: 433–439.

Mattera R, Graziano MP, Yatani A, Zhou Z, Graf R, Codina J, Birnbaumer L, Gilman AG, Brown AM (1989). Splice variants of the α subunit of the G protein Gs activate both adenylyl cyclase and calcium channels. *Science* 243: 804–807.

Mauras N, Blizzard RM (1986). The McCune-Albright syndrome. *Acta Endocrinol Suppl (Copenh)* 279: 207–217.

Mazabraud A, Girard J (1957). Un cas particulier de dysplasia localisations osseus et tendineuses. *Rev Rhum Mal Osteartic* 34: 652–659.

Mazzoni MR, Taddei S, Giusti L, Rovero P, Galoppini C, D'Ursi A, Albrizio S, Triolo A, Novellino E, Greco G, et al. (2000). A $G\alpha_s$ carboxyl-terminal peptide prevents G_s activation by the A_{2A} adenosine receptor. *Mol Pharmacol* 58: 226–236.

McArthur RG, Hayles AB, Lambert PW (1979). Albright's syndrome with rickets. *Mayo Clin Proc* 54: 313–320.

McCune DJ (1936). Osteitis fibrosa cystica: the case of a nine year old girl who also exhibits precocious puberty, multiple pigmentation of the skin and hyperthyroidism. *Am J Dis Child* 52: 743–744.

McCune DJ, Bruch H (1937). Osteodystrophia fibrosa: report of a case in which the condition was combined with precocious puberty, pathologic pigmentation of the skin and hyperthyroidism, with a review of the literature. *Am J Dis Child* 54: 806–848.

Mei FC, Qiao J, Tsygankova OM, Meinkoth JL, Quilliam LA, Cheng X (2002). Differential signaling of cyclic AMP: opposing effects of exchange protein directly activated by cyclic AMP and cAMP-dependent protein kinase on protein kinase B activation. *J Biol Chem* 277: 11497–11504.

Miller MJ, Prigent S, Kupperman E, Rioux L, Park S-H, Feramisco JR, White MA, Rutkowski JL, Meinkoth JL (1997). RalGDS functions in Ras- and cAMP-mediated growth stimulation. *J Biol Chem* 272: 5600–5605.

Miric A, Vechio JD, Levine MA (1993). Heterogeneous mutations in the gene encoding the α subunit of the stimulatory G protein of adenylyl cyclase in Albright hereditary osteodystrophy. *J Clin Endocrinol Metab* 76: 1560–1568.

Miura R, Yumita S, Yoshinaga K, Furukawa Y (1990). Response of plasma 1,25-dihydroxyvitamin D in the human PTH(1-34) infusion test: an improved index for the diagnosis of idiopathic hypoparathyroidism and pseudohypoparathyroidism. *Calcif Tissue Int* 46: 309–313.

Mixon MB, Lee E, Coleman DE, Berghuis AM, Gilman AG, Sprang SR (1995). Tertiary and quaternary structural changes in $G_{i\alpha 1}$. *Science* 270: 954–960.

Mizunashi K, Furukawa Y, Sohn HE, Miura R, Yumita S, Yoshinaga K (1990). Heterogeneity of pseudohypoparathyroidism type I from the aspect of urinary excretion of calcium and serum levels of parathyroid hormone. *Calcif Tissue Int* 46: 227–232.

Mockridge KA, Levine MA, Reed LA, Post E, Kaplan FS, Jan de Beur SM, Deng Z, Ding C, Howard C, Schnur RE (1999). Polyendocrinopathy, skeletal dysplasia, organomegaly, and distinctive facies associated with a novel, widely expressed Gsα mutation. *Am J Hum Genet* 65(Supp): A426. (Abstract)

Montminy M (1997). Transcriptional regulation by cyclic AMP. *Annu Rev Biochem* 66: 807–822.

Moses AM, Weinstock RS, Levine MA, Breslau NA (1986). Evidence for normal antidiuretic responses to endogenous and exogenous arginine vasopressin in patients with guanine nucleotide-binding stimulatory protein-deficient pseudohypoparathyroidism. *J Clin Endocrinol Metab* 62: 221–224.

Motomura T, Kasayama S, Takagi M, Kurebayashi S, Matsui H, Hirose T, Miyashita Y, Yamauchi-Takihara K, Yamamoto T, Okada S, Kishimoto T (1998). Increased interleukin-6 production in mouse osteoblastic MC3T3-E1 cells expressing activating mutant of the stimulatory G protein. *J Bone Miner Res* 13: 1084–1091.

Muca C, Vallar L (1994). Expression of mutationally activated Gαs stimulates growth and differentiation of thyroid FRTL5 cells. *Oncogene* 9: 3647–3653.

Mumby SM, Kleuss C, Gilman AG (1994). Receptor regulation of G-protein palmitoylation. *Proc Natl Acad Sci USA* 91: 2800–2804.

Nager GT, Kennedy DW, Kopstein E (1982). Fibrous dysplasia: a review of the disease and its manifestations in the temporal bone. *Ann Otol Rhinol Laryngol Suppl* 92: 1–52.

Nair BG, Patel TB (1993). Regulation of cardiac adenylyl cyclase by epidermal growth factor (EGF): role of EGF receptor protein tyrosine kinase activity. *Biochem Pharmacol* 46: 1239–1245.

Nair BG, Parikh B, Milligan G, Patel TB (1990). $G_{s\alpha}$ mediates epidermal growth factor–elicited stimulation of rat cardiac adenylate cyclase. *J Biol Chem* 265: 21317–21322.

Nakamoto JM, Sandstrom AT, Brickman AS, Christenson RA, Van Dop C (1998). Pseudohypoparathyroidism type Ia from maternal but not paternal transmission of a $G_s\alpha$ gene mutation. *Am J Med Genet* 77: 61–67.

Namnoum AB, Merriam GR, Moses AM, Levine MA (1998). Reproductive dysfunction in women with Albright's hereditary osteodystrophy. *J Clin Endocrinol Metab* 83: 824–829.

Nanes MS, Boden S, Weinstein LS (1995). Oligonucleotides antisense to Gsα promote osteoblast differentiation. *Program and Abstracts of the 77th Annual Meeting of the Endocrine Society*, Endocrine Society Press, Bethesda, MD, p. 62 (Abstract).

Noel JP, Hamm HE, Sigler PB (1993). The 2.2 Å crystal structure of transducin-α complexed with GTPγS. *Nature* 366: 654–663.

Okada K, Iida K, Sakusabe N, Saitoh H, Abe E, Sato K (1994). Pseudohypoparathyroidism-associated spinal stenosis. *Spine* 19: 1186–1189.

Okamoto S, Hisaoka M, Ushijima M, Nakahara S, Toyoshima S, Hashimoto H (2000). Activating *Gsα* mutation in intramuscular myxomas with and without fibrous dysplasia of bone. *Virchows Arch* 437: 133–137.

Ong OC, Van Dop C, Fung BKK (1996). Real-time monitoring of reduced β-adrenergic response in fibroblasts from patients with pseudohypoparathyroidism. *Anal Biochem* 238: 76–81.

O'Sullivan C, Barton CM, Staddon SL, Brown CL, Lemoine NR (1991). Activating point mutations of the *gsp* oncogene in human thyroid adenomas. *Mol Carcinogenesis* 4: 345–349.

Oude Luttikhuis MEM, Wilson LC, Leonard JV, Trembath RC (1994). Characterization of a de novo 43-bp deletion of the Gsα gene (*GNAS*) in Albright hereditary osteodystrophy. *Genomics* 21: 455–457.

Pasolli HA, Huttner WB (2001). Expression of the extra-large G protein α-subunit XLαs in neuroepithelial cells and young neurons during development of the rat nervous system. *Neurosci Lett* 301: 119–122.

Pasolli HA, Klemke M, Kehlenbach RH, Wang Y, Huttner WB (2000). Characterization of the extra-large G protein α-subunit XLαs: I. Tissue distribution and subcellular localization. *J Biol Chem* 275: 33622–33632.
Patten JL, Levine MA (1990). Immunochemical analysis of the α-subunit of the stimulatory G-protein of adenylyl cyclase in patients with Albright's hereditary osteodystrophy. *J Clin Endocrinol Metab* 71: 1208–1214.
Patten JL, Johns DR, Valle D, Eil C, Gruppuso PA, Steele G, Smallwood PM, Levine MA (1990). Mutation in the gene encoding the stimulatory G protein of adenylate cyclase in Albright's hereditary osteodystrophy. *N Engl J Med* 322: 1412–1419.
Pensler JM, Langman CB, Radosevich JA, Maminta ML, Mangkornkanok M, Higbee R, Molteni A (1990). Sex steroid hormone receptors in normal and dysplastic bone disorders in children. *J Bone Miner Res* 5: 493–498.
Persani L, Borgato S, Lania A, Filopanti M, Mantovani G, Conti M, Spada A (2001). Relevant cAMP-specific phosphodiesterase isoforms in human pituitary: effect of Gs_α mutations. *J Clin Endocrinol Metab* 86: 3795–3800.
Peters J, Beechey CV, Ball ST, Evans EP (1994). Mapping studies of the distal imprinting region of mouse chromosome 2. *Genet Res* 63: 169–174.
Peters J, Wroe SF, Wells CA, Miller HJ, Bodle D, Beechey CV, Williamson CM, Kelsey G (1999). A cluster of oppositely imprinted transcripts at the *Gnas* locus in the distal imprinting region of mouse chromosome 2. *Proc Natl Acad Sci USA* 96: 3830–3835.
Pfeffer S, Molina E, Feullian P, Simon TR (1990). McCune-Albright syndrome: the patterns of scintigraphic abnormalities. *J Nucl Med* 31: 1474–1478.
Phelan MC, Rogers RC, Clarkson KB, Bowyer FP, Levine MA, Estabrooks LL, Severson MC, Dobyns WB (1995). Albright hereditary osteodystrophy and del(2)(q37.3) in four unrelated individuals. *Am J Med Genet* 58: 1–7.
Pomerance M, Abdullah H-B, Kamerji S, Corréze C, Blondeau J-P (2000). Thyroid-stimulating hormone and cyclic AMP activate p38 mitogen-activated protein kinase cascade: involvement of protein kinase A, Rac1, and reactive oxygen species. *J Biol Chem* 275: 40539–40546.
Poppleton H, Sun H, Fulgham D, Bertics P, Patel TB (1996). Activation of $G_s\alpha$ by the epidermal growth factor receptor involves phosphorylation. *J Biol Chem* 271: 6947–6951.
Poznanski AK, Werder EA, Giedion A, Martin A, Shaw H (1977). The pattern of shortening of the bones of the hand in pseudohypoparathyroidism and pseudopseudohypoparathyroidism: a comparison with brachydactyly E, Turner syndrome, and acrodysostosis. *Radiology* 123: 707–718.
Prayson MA, Leeson MC (1993). Soft-tissue myxomas and fibrous dysplasia of bone: a case report and review of the literature. *Clin Orthop Related Res* 291: 222–228.
Prendiville JS, Lucky AW, Mallory SB, Mughal Z, Mimouni F, Langman CB (1992). Osteoma cutis as a presenting sign of pseudohypoparathyroidism. *Pediatr Dermatol* 9: 11–18.
Rao VV, Schnittger S, Hansmann I (1991). G protein Gsα (*GNAS*), the probable candidate gene for Albright hereditary osteodystrophy, is assigned to human chromosome 20q12-q13.2. *Genomics* 10: 257–261.
Reik W, Walter J (2001). Genomic imprinting: parental influence on the genome. *Nat Rev Genet* 2: 21–32.
Reitzik M, Lownie JF (1975). Familial polyostotic fibrous dysplasia. *Oral Surg* 40: 769–774.
Richards JS (2001). New signaling pathways for hormones and cyclic adenosine 3′,5′-monophosphate action in endocrine cells. *Mol Endocrinol* 15: 209–218.
Rieth KG, Comite F, Shawker TH, Cutler GB Jr. (1984). Pituitary and ovarian abnormalities demonstrated by CT and ultrasound in children with features of the McCune-Albright syndrome. *Radiology* 153: 389–393.
Riminucci M, Fisher LW, Shenker A, Spiegel AM, Bianco P, Robey PG (1997). Fibrous dysplasia of bone in the McCune-Albright syndrome: abnormalities in bone formation. *Am J Pathol* 151: 1587–1600.
Riminucci M, Fisher LW, Majolagbe A, Corsi A, Lala R, de Sanctis C, Robey PG, Bianco P (1999a). A novel *GNAS* mutation, R201G, in McCune-Albright syndrome. *J Bone Miner Res* 14: 1987–1989.
Riminucci M, Liu B, Corsi A, Shenker A, Spiegel AM, Robey PG, Bianco P (1999b). The histopathology of fibrous dysplasia of bone in patients with activating mutations of the Gsα gene: site-specific patterns and recurrent histological hallmarks. *J Pathol* 187: 249–258.
Ringel MD, Schwindinger WF, Levine MA (1996). Clinical implications of genetic defects in G proteins: the molecular basis of McCune-Albright syndrome and Albright hereditary osteodystrophy. *Medicine (Baltimore)* 75: 171–184.
Rotenberg A, Abel T, Hawkins RD, Kandel ER, Muller RU (2000). Parallel instabilities of long-term potentiation, place cells, and learning caused by decreased protein kinase A activity. *J Neurosci* 20: 8096–8102.
Ruggieri P, Sim FH, Bond JR, Unni KK (1994). Malignancies in fibrous dysplasia. *Cancer* 73: 1411–1424.
Rüther U, Garber C, Komitowski D, Müller R, Wagner EF (1987). Deregulated c-*fos* expression interferes with normal bone development in transgenic mice. *Nature* 325: 412–416.
Sarkar AK, Ghosh AK, Chowdhury SN, Biswas SK, Bag SK (1993). Fibrous dysplasia in two siblings. *Indian J Pediatr* 60: 301–305.
Sassone-Corsi P (1995). Signaling pathways and c-*fos* transcriptional response-links to inherited diseases. *N Engl J Med* 332: 1576–1577.
Schipani E, Weinstein LS, Bergwitz C, Iida-Klein A, Kong XF, Stuhrmann M, Kruse K, Whyte MP, Murray T, Schmidtke J, et al. (1995). Pseudohypoparathyroidism type Ib is not caused by mutations in the coding exons of the human parathyroid hormone (PTH)/PTH-related peptide receptor gene. *J Clin Endocrinol Metab* 80: 1611–1621.
Schlumberger HG (1946). Fibrous dysplasia of single bones (monostotic fibrous dysplasia). *Mil Surg* 99: 504–527.
Schmitt JM, Stork PJS (2002). PKA phosphorylation of Src mediates cAMP's inhibition of cell growth via Rap1. *Mol Cell* 9: 85–94.
Scholich K, Mullenix JB, Wittpoth C, Poppleton HM, Pierre SC, Lindorfer MA, Garrison JC, Patel TB (1999). Facilitation of signal onset and termination by adenylyl cyclase. *Science* 283: 1328–1331.
Schuster V, Eschenhagen T, Kruse K, Gierschik P, Kreth HW (1993). Endocrine and molecular biological studies in a German family with Albright hereditary osteodystrophy. *Eur J Pediatr* 152: 185–189.
Schwindinger WF, Francomano CA, Levine MA (1992). Identification of a mutation in the gene encoding the α subunit of the stimulatory G protein of adenylyl cyclase in McCune-Albright syndrome. *Proc Natl Acad Sci USA* 89: 5152–5156.
Schwindinger WF, Miric A, Zimmerman D, Levine MA (1994). A novel $G_s\alpha$ mutant in a patient with Albright hereditary osteodystrophy uncouples cell surface receptors from adenylyl cyclase. *J Biol Chem* 269: 25387–25391.
Scott DC, Hung W (1995). Pseudohypoparathyroidism type Ia and growth hormone deficiency in two siblings. *J Pediatr Endocrinol Metab* 8: 205–207.
Seifert R, Wenzel-Seifert K, Lee TW, Gether U, Sanders-Bush E, Kobilka BK (1998). Different effects of $G_s\alpha$ splice variants on β2-adrenoreceptor-mediated signaling: the β2-adrenoreceptor coupled to the long splice variant of $G_s\alpha$ has properties of a constitutively active receptor. *J Biol Chem* 273: 5109–5116.
Shapira H, Mouallem M, Shapiro MS, Weisman Y, Farfel Z (1996). Pseudohypoparathyroidism type Ia: two new heterozygous frameshift mutations in exons 5 and 10 of the Gsα gene. *Hum Genet* 97: 73–75.
Shapiro MS, Bernheim J, Gutman A, Arber I, Spitz IM (1980). Multiple abnormalities of anterior pituitary hormone secretion in association with pseudohypoparathyroidism. *J Clin Endocrinol Metab* 51: 483–487.
Shenker A, Weinstein LS, Moran A, Pescovitz OH, Charest NJ, Boney CM, Van Wyk JJ, Merino MJ, Feuillan PP, Spiegel AM (1993). Severe endocrine and nonendocrine manifestations of the McCune-Albright syndrome associated with activating mutations of stimulatory G protein G_s. *J Pediatr* 123: 509–518.
Shenker A, Weinstein LS, Sweet DE, Spiegel AM (1994). An activating $G_s\alpha$ mutation is present in fibrous dysplasia of bone in the McCune-Albright syndrome. *J Clin Endocrinol Metab* 79: 750–755.
Shenker A, Chanson P, Weinstein LS, Chi P, Spiegel AM, Lomri A, Marie PJ (1995). Osteoblastic cells derived from isolated lesions of fibrous dysplasia contain activating somatic mutations of the $G_s\alpha$ gene. *Hum Mol Genet* 4: 1675–1676.
Shima M, Nose O, Shimizu K, Seino Y, Yabuuchi H, Saito T (1988). Multiple associated endocrine abnormalities in a patient with pseudohypoparathyroidism type 1a. *Eur J Pediatr* 147: 536–538.
Shore EM, Ahn J, Jan de Beur S, Li M, Xu M, Gardner RJM, Zasloff MA, Whyte MP, Levine MA, Kaplan FS (2002). Paternally inherited inactivating mutations of the *GNAS* gene in progressive osseous heteroplasia. *N Engl J Med* 346: 99–106.
Silva ES, Lumbroso S, Medina M, Gillerot Y, Sultan C, Sokal EM (2000). Demonstration of McCune-Albright mutations in the liver of children with high γGT progressive cholestasis. *J Hepatol* 32: 154–158.
Silve C, Santora A, Breslau N, Moses A, Spiegel A (1986). Selective resistance to parathyroid hormone in cultured skin fibroblasts from patients with pseudohypoparathyroidism type Ib. *J Clin Endocrinol Metab* 62: 640–644.
Simonds WF, Goldsmith PK, Woodard CJ, Unson CG, Spiegel AM (1989). Receptor and effector interactions of Gs: functional studies with antibodies to the αs carboxyl-terminal decapeptide. *FEBS Lett* 249: 189–194.
Sondek J, Lambright DG, Noel JP, Hamm HE, Sigler PB (1994). GTPase mechanism of G proteins from the 1.7-Å crystal structure of transducin α-GDP-AlF_4^-. *Nature* 372: 276–279.
Spiegel AM, Weinstein LS (2001). Pseudohypoparathyroidism. In: *The Metabolic and Molecular Bases of Inherited Disease, 8th Edition.* Scriver CR, Beaudet AL, Sly WS, Valle D (eds.) McGraw-Hill, New York, pp. 4205–4221.
Spiegel AM, Levine MA, Aurbach GD, Downs RW Jr, Marx SJ, Lasker RD, Moses AM, Breslau NA (1982). Deficiency of hormone receptor-adenylate cyclase coupling protein: basis for hormone resistance in pseudohypoparathyroidism. *Am J Physiol* 243: E37–E42.
Stein GS, Lian JB (1993). Molecular mechanisms mediating proliferation/differentiation interrelationships during progressive development of the osteoblast phenotype. *Endocr Rev* 14: 424–442.
Steinbach HL, Young DA (1966). The roentgen appearance of pseudohypoparathyroidism (PH) and pseudo-pseudohypoparathyroidism (PPH): differentiation from other syndromes associated with short metacarpals, metatarsals, and phalanges. *Am J Roentgenol Radium Ther Nucl Med* 97: 49–66.
Stevens-Simon C, Stewart J, Nakashima II, White M (1991). Exacerbation of fibrous dysplasia associated with an adolescent pregnancy. *J Adolesc Health* 12: 403–405.
Stone MD, Hosking DJ, Garcia-Himmelstine C, White DA, Rosenblum D, Worth HG (1993). The renal response to exogenous parathyroid hormone in treated pseudohypoparathyroidism. *Bone* 14: 727–735.
Struthers RS, Vale WW, Arias C, Sawehenko PE, Montminy MR (1991). Somatotroph hypoplasia and dwarfism in transgenic mice expressing a non-phosphorylatable CREB mutant. *Nature* 350: 622–624.
Suarez HG, du Villard JA, Caillou B, Schlumberger M, Parmentier C, Monier R (1991). *gsp* mutations in human thyroid tumours. *Oncogene* 6: 677–679.
Sudlow LC, Huang RC, Green DJ, Gillette R (1993). cAMP-activated Na^+ current of molluscum neurons is resistant to kinase inhibitors and is gated by cAMP in the isolated patch. *J Neurosci* 13: 5188–5193.
Sullivan KA, Miller RT, Masters SB, Beiderman B, Heideman W, Bourne HR (1987). Identification of receptor contact site involved in receptor-G protein coupling. *Nature* 330: 758–760.
Sun H, Chen Z, Poppleton H, Scholich K, Mullenix J, Weipz GJ, Fulgham DL, Bertics PJ, Patel TB (1997). The juxtamembrane, cytosolic region of the epidermal growth factor receptor is involved in association with α-subunit of G_s. *J Biol Chem* 272: 5413–5420.
Sunahara RK, Tesmer JJG, Gilman AG, Sprang SR (1997). Crystal structure of the adenylyl cyclase activator $G_{s\alpha}$. *Science* 278: 1943–1947.
Szabo J, Heath B, Hill VM, Jackson CE, Zarbo RJ, Mallette LE, Chew SL, Besser GM, Thakkar RV, Huff V, et al. (1995). Hereditary hyperparathyroidism–jaw tumor syndrome: the endocrine tumor gene HRPT2 maps to chromosome 1q21-q31. *Am J Hum Genet* 56: 944–950.

Tanabeu Y, Nakahara S, Mitsuyama S, Ono M, Toyoshima S (1998). Breast cancer in a patient with McCune-Albright syndrome. *Breast Cancer* 25: 175–178.

Tanaka T, Suwa S (1977). A case of McCune-Albright syndrome with hyperthyroidism and vitamin D–resistant rickets. *Helv Paediatr Acta* 32: 263–273.

Tesmer JJ, Sunahara RK, Gilman AG, Sprang SR (1997). Crystal structure of the catalytic domains of adenylyl cyclase in a complex with $G_s\alpha$·GTPγS. *Science* 278: 1907–1916.

Tilghman SM (1999). The sins of the fathers and mothers: genomic imprinting in mammalian development. *Cell* 96: 185–193.

Tintut Y, Parham F, Le V, Karsenty G, Demer LL (1999). Inhibition of osteoblast-specific transcription factor Cbfa1 by the cAMP pathway in osteoblasts. *J Biol Chem* 274: 28875–28879.

Tordjman K, Stern N, Ouaknine G, Yossiphov Y, Razon N, Nordenskjöld M, Friedman E (1993). Activating mutations of the G_s α-gene in nonfunctioning pituitary tumors. *J Clin Endocrinol Metab* 77: 765–769.

Tsang RC, Venkataraman P, Ho M, Steichen JJ, Whitsett J, Greer F (1984). The development of pseudohypoparathyroidism: involvement of progressively increasing serum parathyroid hormone concentrations, increased 1,25-dihydroxyvitamin D concentrations, and "migratory" subcutaneous calcifications. *Am J Dis Child* 138: 654–658.

Tsygankova OM, Kupperman E, Wen W, Meinkoth JL (2000). Cyclic AMP activates Ras. *Oncogene* 19: 3609–3615.

Tsygankova OM, Saavedra A, Rebhun JF, Quilliam LA, Meinkoth JL (2001). Coordinated regulation of Rap1 and thyroid differentiation by cyclic AMP and protein kinase A. *Mol Cell Biol* 21: 1921–1929.

Turksen K, Grigoriadis AE, Heersche JNM, Aubin JE (1990). Forskolin has biphasic effects on osteoprogenitor cell differentiation in vitro. *J Cell Physiol* 142: 61–69.

Ugur O, Jones TLZ (2000). A proline-rich region and nearby cysteine residues target XLαs to the Golgi complex region. *Mol Biol Cell* 11: 1421–1432.

Urdanivia E, Mataverde A, Cohen MP (1975). Growth hormone secretion and sulfation factor activity in pseudohypoparathyroidism. *J Lab Clin Med* 86: 772–776.

Valet P, Grujic D, Wade J, Ito M, Zingaretti MC, Soloveva V, Ross SR, Graves RA, Cinti S, Lafontan M, Lowell BB (2000). Expression of human α2-adrenergic receptors in adipose tissue of β3-adrenergic receptor deficient mice promotes diet-induced obesity. *J Biol Chem* 275: 34797–34802.

Vortkamp A, Lee K, Lanske B, Segre GV, Kronenberg HM, Tabin CJ (1996). Regulation of rate of cartilage differentiation by Indian hedgehog and PTH-related protein. *Science* 273: 613–622.

Vossler MR, Yao H, York RD, Pan MG, Rim CS, Stork PJ (1997). cAMP activates MAP kinase and Elk-1 through a B-Raf- and Rap1-dependent pathway. *Cell* 89: 73–82.

Wainger BJ, DeGennaro M, Santoro B, Siegelbaum SA, Tibbs GR (2001). Molecular mechanism of cAMP modulation of HCN pacemaker channels. *Nature* 411: 805–810.

Walden U, Weissortel R, Corria Z, Yu D, Weinstein L, Kruse K, Dorr HG (1999). Stimulatory guanine nucleotide binding protein subunit 1 mutation in two siblings with pseudohypoparathyroidism type Ia and mother with pseudopseudohypoparathyroidism. *Eur J Pediatr* 158: 200–203..

Wall MA, Coleman DE, Lee E, Iñiguez-Lluhi JA, Posner BA, Gilman AG, Sprang SR (1995). The structure of the G protein heterotrimer $G_{i\alpha1}\beta_1\gamma_2$. *Cell* 83: 1047–1058.

Wang H, Watkins DC, Malbon CC (1992). Antisense oligodeoxynucleotides to G_s α-subunit sequence accelerate differentiation of fibroblasts to adipocytes. *Nature* 358: 334–337.

Warner DR, Weinstein LS (1999). A mutation in the heterotrimeric stimulatory guanine nucleotide binding protein α-subunit with impaired receptor-mediated activation because of elevated GTPase activity. *Proc Natl Acad Sci USA* 96: 4268–4272.

Warner DR, Gejman PV, Collins RM, Weinstein LS (1997). A novel mutation adjacent to the switch III domain of $G_{s\alpha}$ in a patient with pseudohypoparathyroidism. *Mol Endocrinol* 11: 1718–1727.

Warner DR, Weng G, Yu S, Matalon R, Weinstein LS (1998). A novel mutation in the switch 3 region of $G_s\alpha$ in a patient with Albright hereditary osteodystrophy impairs GDP binding and receptor activation. *J Biol Chem* 273: 23976–23983.

Warner DR, Romanowski R, Yu S, Weinstein LS (1999). Mutagenesis of the conserved residue Glu^{259} of $G_s\alpha$ demonstrates the importance of interactions between switches 2 and 3 for activation. *J Biol Chem* 274: 4977–4984.

Wedegaertner PB, Bourne HR, Von Zastrow M (1996). Activation-induced subcellular redistribution of Gsα. *Mol Biol Cell* 7: 1225–1233.

Weinstein LS (1998). Albright hereditary osteodystrophy, pseudohypoparathyroidism and G_s deficiency. In: *G Proteins, Receptors, and Disease*. Spiegel AM (ed.) Humana Press, Totowa, NJ, pp. 23–56.

Weinstein LS (2001). The stimulatory G protein α-subunit gene: mutations and imprinting lead to complex phenotypes. *J Clin Endocrinol Metab* 86: 4622–4626.

Weinstein LS (2002). Other skeletal diseases resulting from G protein defects: fibrous dysplasia and McCune-Albright syndrome. In: *Principles of Bone Biology, 2nd ed.* Bilezikian JP, Raisz LG, Rodan GA (eds.) Academic Press, San Diego, pp. 1165–1176.

Weinstein LS, Gejman PV, Friedman E, Kadowaki T, Collins RM, Gershon ES, Spiegel AM (1990). Mutations of the G_s α-subunit gene in Albright hereditary osteodystrophy detected by denaturing gradient gel electrophoresis. *Proc Natl Acad Sci USA* 87: 8287–8290.

Weinstein LS, Shenker A, Gejman PV, Merino MJ, Friedman E, Spiegel AM (1991). Activating mutations of the stimulatory G protein in the McCune-Albright syndrome. *N Engl J Med* 325: 1688–1695.

Weinstein LS, Yu S, Ecelbarger CA (2000). Variable imprinting of the heterotrimeric G protein G_s α-subunit within different segments of the nephron. *Am J Physiol* 278: F507–F514.

Weinstein LS, Yu S, Warner DR, Liu J (2001). Endocrine manifestations of stimulatory G protein α-subunit mutations and the role of genomic imprinting. *Endocr Rev* 22: 675–705.

Weinstock RS, Wright HN, Spiegel AM, Levine MA, Moses AM (1986). Olfactory dysfunction in humans with deficient guanine nucleotide-binding protein. *Nature* 322: 635–636.

Weisman Y, Golander A, Spirer Z, Farfel Z (1985). Pseudohypoparathyroidism type Ia presenting as congenital hypothyroidism. *J Pediatr* 107: 413–415.

Werder EA, Illig R, Bernasconi S, Kind H, Prader A (1975). Excessive thyrotropin response to thyrotropin-releasing hormone in pseudohypoparathyroidism. *Pediatr Res* 9: 12–16.

Werder EA, Fischer JA, Illig R, Kind HP, Bernasconi S, Fanconi A, Prader A (1978). Pseudohypoparathyroidism and idiopathic hypoparathyroidism: relationship between serum calcium and parathyroid hormone levels and urinary cyclic adenosine-3′,5′-monophosphate response to parathyroid extract. *J Clin Endocrinol Metab* 46: 872–879.

White KE, Jonsson KB, Carn G, Hampson G, Spector TD, Mannstadt M, Lorenz-Depiereux B, Miyauchi A, Yang IM, Ljunggren O, et al. (2001). The autosomal dominant hypophosphatemic rickets (ADHR) gene is a secreted polypeptide overexpressed by tumors that cause phosphate wasting. *J Clin Endocrinol Metab* 86: 497–500.

Williamson CM, Schofield J, Dutton ER, Seymour A, Beechey CV, Edwards YH, Peters J (1996). Glomerular-specific imprinting of the mouse Gsα gene: how does this relate to hormone resistance in Albright hereditary osteodystrophy? *Genomics* 36: 280–287.

Williamson CM, Beechey CV, Papworth D, Wroe SF, Wells CA, Cobb L, Peters J (1998). Imprinting of distal mouse chromosome 2 is associated with phenotypic anomalies in utero. *Genet Res* 72: 255–265.

Williamson EA, Daniels M, Foster S, Kelly WF, Kendall-Taylor P, Harris PE (1994). Gsα and Gi2α mutations in clinically non-functioning pituitary tumours. *Clin Endocrinol (Oxf)* 41: 815–820.

Williamson EA, Ince PG, Harrison D, Kendall-Taylor P, Harris PE (1995a). G-protein mutations in human pituitary adrenocorticotrophic hormone-secreting adenomas. *Eur J Clin Invest* 25: 128–131.

Williamson EA, Johnson SJ, Foster S, Kendall-Taylor P, Harris PE (1995b). G protein gene mutations in patients with multiple endocrinopathies. *J Clin Endocrinol Metab* 80: 1702–1705.

Wilson LC, Oude Luttikhuis ME, Clayton PT, Fraser WD, Trembath RC (1994). Parental origin of Gsα gene mutations in Albright's hereditary osteodystrophy. *J Med Genet* 31: 835–839.

Wilson LC, Leverton K, Oude Luttikhuis MEM, Oley CA, Flint J, Wolstenholme J, Duckett DP, Barrow MA, Leonard JV, Read AP, Trembath RC (1995). Brachydactyly and mental retardation: an Albright hereditary osteodystrophy-like syndrome localized to 2q37. *Am J Hum Genet* 56: 400–407.

Wolfsdorf JI, Rosenfield RL, Fang VS, Kobayashi R, Razdan AK, Kim MH (1978). Partial gonadotrophin-resistance in pseudohypoparathyroidism. *Acta Endocrinol (Copenh)* 88: 321–328.

Wroe SF, Kelsey G, Skinner JA, Bodle D, Ball ST, Beechey CV, Peters J, Williamson CM (2000). An imprinted transcript, antisense to *Nesp*, adds complexity to the cluster of imprinted genes at the mouse *Gnas* locus. *Proc Natl Acad Sci USA* 97: 3342–3346.

Wu J, Dent P, Jelinek T, Wolfman A, Weber MJ, Sturgill TW (1993). Inhibition of the EGF-activated MAP kinase signaling pathway by adenosine 3′,5′-monophosphate. *Science* 262: 1065–1069.

Wu WI, Schwindinger WF, Aparicio LF, Levine MA (2001). Selective resistance to parathyroid hormone caused by a novel uncoupling mutation in the carboxyl terminus of $G_{\alpha s}$. A cause of pseudohypoparathyroidism type Ib. *J Biol Chem* 276: 165–171.

Wu ZL, Thomas SA, Villacres EC, Xia Z, Simmons ML, Chavkin C, Palmiter RD, Storm DR (1995). Altered behavior and long-term potentiation in type I adenylyl cyclase mutant mice. *Proc Natl Acad Sci USA* 92: 220–224.

Yabut SM, Kenan S, Sissons HA, Lewis MM (1988). Malignant transformation of fibrous dysplasia: a case report and review of the literature. *Clin Orthop* 228: 281–289.

Yamamoto T, Okada S, Kishimoto T, Yamaoka K, Michigami T, Matsumoto S, Takagi M, Hiroshima K, Yoh K, Kasayama S, Ozono K (1996). Increased IL-6-production by cells isolated from the fibrous bone dysplasia tissues in patients with McCune-Albright syndrome. *J Clin Invest* 98: 30–35.

Yamamoto Y, Noto Y, Saito M, Ichizen H, Kida H (1997). Spinal cord compression by heterotopic ossification associated with pseudohypoparathyroidism. *J Int Med Res* 25: 364–368.

Yamazaki T, Komuro I, Zou Y, Kudoh S, Mizuno T, Hiroi Y, Shiojima I, Takano H, Kinugawa K, Kohmoto O, et al. (1997a). Protein kinase A and protein kinase C synergistically activate the Raf-1 kinase/mitogen-activated protein kinase cascade in neonatal rat cardiomyocytes. *J Mol Cell Cardiol* 29: 2491–2501.

Yamazaki T, Komuro I, Zou Y, Kudoh S, Shiojima I, Hiroi Y, Aikawa R, Takano H, Yazaki Y (1997b). Norepinephrine induces the raf-1 kinase/mitogen-activated protein kinase cascade through both α1- and β-adrenoreceptors. *Circulation* 95: 1260–1268.

Yang I, Park S, Ryu M, Woo J, Kim S, Kim J, Kim Y, Choi Y (1996). Characteristics of *gsp*-positive growth hormone-secreting pituitary tumors in Korean acromegalic patients. *Eur J Endocrinol* 134: 720–726.

Yatani A, Imoto Y, Codina J, Hamilton SL, Brown AM, Birnbaumer L (1988). The stimulatory G protein of adenylyl cyclase, Gs, also stimulates dihydropyridine-sensitive Ca^{2+} channels: evidence for direct regulation independent of phosphorylation by cAMP-dependent protein kinase or stimulation by a dihydropyridine agonist. *J Biol Chem* 263: 9887–9895.

Yeh GL, Mathur S, Wivel A, Li M, Gannon FH, Ulied A, Audi L, Olmsted EA, Kaplan FS, Shore EM (2000). *GNAS* mutation and Cbfa1 misexpression in a child with severe congenital platelike osteoma cutis. *J Bone Miner Res* 15: 2063–2073.

Yokoro S, Matsuo M, Ohtsuka T, Ohzeki T (1990). Hyperthyrotropinemia in a neonate with normal thyroid hormone levels: the earliest diagnostic clue for pseudohypoparathyroidism. *Biol Neonate* 58: 69–72.

Yoshimoto K, Iwahana H, Fukuda A, Sano T, Itakura M (1993). Rare mutations of the $G_s\alpha$ subunit gene in human endocrine tumors: mutation detection by polymerase chain reaction-primer-introduced restriction analysis. *Cancer* 72: 1386–1393.

Yu D, Yu S, Schuster V, Kruse K, Clericuzio CL, Weinstein LS (1999). Identification of two novel deletion mutations within the $G_s\alpha$ gene (*GNAS*) in Albright hereditary osteodystrophy. *J Clin Endocrinol Metab* 84: 3254–3259.

Yu JZ, Rasenick MM (2002). Real-time visualization of a fluorescent $G_{\alpha s}$: dissociation of the activated G protein from plasma membrane. *Mol Pharmacol* 61: 352–359.

Yu S, Yu D, Hainline BE, Brener JL, Wilson KA, Wilson LC, Oude-Luttikhuis ME, Trembath RC, Weinstein LS (1995). A deletion hot-spot in exon 7 of the $G_s\alpha$ gene (*GNAS*) in patients with Albright hereditary osteodystrophy. *Hum Mol Genet* 4: 2001–2002.

Yu S, Yu D, Lee E, Eckhaus M, Lee R, Corria Z, Accili D, Westphal H, Weinstein LS (1998). Variable and tissue-specific hormone resistance in heterotrimeric G_s protein α-subunit ($G_s\alpha$) knockout mice is due to tissue-specific imprinting of the $G_s\alpha$ gene. *Proc Natl Acad Sci USA* 95: 8715–8720.

Yu S, Gavrilova O, Chen H, Lee R, Liu J, Pacak K, Parlow AF, Quon MJ, Reitman ML, Weinstein LS (2000). Paternal versus maternal transmission of a stimulatory G protein α-subunit knockout produces opposite effects on energy metabolism. *J Clin Invest* 105: 615–623.

Yu S, Castle A, Chen M, Lee R, Takeda K, Weinstein LS (2001). Increased insulin sensitivity in $G_s\alpha$ knockout mice. *J Biol Chem* 276: 19994–19998.

Zacharin M, O'Sullivan M (2000). Intravenous pamidronate treatment of polyostotic fibrous dysplasia associated with the McCune-Albright syndrome. *J Pediatr* 137: 403–409.

Zeiger MA, Saji M, Gusev Y, Westra WH, Takiyama Y, Dooley WC, Kohn LD, Levine MA (1997). Thyroid-specific expression of cholera toxin A1 subunit causes thyroid hyperplasia and hyperthyroidism in transgenic mice. *Endocrinology* 138: 3133–3140.

Zheng B, Ma Y, Ostrom RS, Lavoie C, Gill GN, Insel PA, Huang X, Farquhar MG (2001). RGS-PX1, a GAP for $G\alpha_s$ and sorting nexin in vesicular trafficking. *Science* 294: 1939–1942.

Zheng M, Zhang S-J, Zhu W-Z, Ziman B, Kobilka BK, Xiao R-P (2000). β_2-adrenergic receptor–induced p38 MAPK activation is mediated by protein kinase A rather than by G_i or $G\beta\gamma$ in adult mouse cardiomyocytes. *J Biol Chem* 275: 40635–40640.

Zung A, Chalew SA, Schwindinger WF, Levine MA, Phillip M, Jara A, Counts DR, Kowarski AA (1995). Urinary cyclic adenosine 3′,5′-monophosphate response in McCune-Albright syndrome: clinical evidence for altered renal adenylate cyclase activity. *J Clin Endocrinol Metab* 80: 3576–3581.

86 | *FGD1* and Faciogenital Dysplasia (Aarskog-Scott Syndrome)

JEROME L. GORSKI

FGD1 mutations result in faciogenital dysplasia (FGDY; Aarskog-Scott syndrome) (OMIM 305400), an X-linked recessive multiple congenital anomaly syndrome. Skeletal anomalies dominate the FGDY phenotype; cardinal clinical features include a distinctive and characteristic set of craniofacial and skeletal anomalies, disproportionate acromelic short stature, delayed skeletal maturation, and urogenital malformations. *FGD1* encodes a guanine nucleotide exchange factor (GEF) that specifically activates Cdc42, a p21 Rho GTPase that is involved in the regulation of the actin cytoskeleton, cell signaling and polarity, vesicular transport, and gene expression. The FGD1 protein is composed of multiple signaling motifs including (in order) a proline-rich N-terminal domain that includes a putative Src homology 3 (SH3)–binding domain, a GEF domain, an immediately adjacent pleckstrin homology (PH) domain, a cysteine-rich zinc-finger FYVE domain, and a second C-terminal PH (PH2) domain. By activating Cdc42, FGD1 stimulates cells to form filopodia, cytoskeletal elements involved in cellular signaling, adhesion, and migration. Through Cdc42, FGD1 also activates the c-Jun N-terminal kinase (JNK) signaling cascade, a pathway that regulates cell growth, apoptosis, and cellular differentiation.

FGD1 is the founding member of an evolutionarily conserved family of *FGD1*-related genes; mammalian genomes contain at least four different *FGD1*-related genes (*FGD1, FGD2, FGD3,* and *Frabin*). All *FGD1*-related genes share a conserved canonical structure of signaling domains (GEF, PH, FYVE, and PH2) that spans about 540 amino acid residues. The observation that, like FGD1, other FGD1-related family members selectively activate Cdc42 strongly suggests that FGD1-related proteins play similar functional roles. Mutations in the *C. elegans FGD1* ortholog, *fgd-1*, result in abnormalities in excretory cell formation. Developmental studies indicate that *fgd-1* plays a critical role in excretory cell morphogenesis and cellular organization. These results suggest that, rather than playing a role in maintaining a specific cellular phenotype, FGD1/fgd-1 signaling is critical in regulating basic cell processes, including Cdc42 signaling.

FGD1 is predominantly expressed in osteoblasts during mammalian development. In osteoblasts, FGD1 is localized at the subcortical actin cytoskeleton and Golgi complex, where it is poised to activate Cdc42 signaling. *FGD1* mutations are heterogeneous; however, to date, all *FGD1* mutations are predicted to result in the loss of GEF activity. The loss of GEF activity is generally equivalent to the loss of the target Rho substrate; thus, these data strongly suggest that faciogenital dysplasia is the result of disrupted FGD1/Cdc42 signaling. Based on an analysis of Cdc42 function, it is reasonable to hypothesize that FGD1/Cdc42 signaling plays a role in the organization of the actin cytoskeleton, osteoblast-extracellular matrix interactions, cell polarity and protein transport, the regulation of gene expression, and osteoblast differentiation.

FGD1, THE GENE RESPONSIBLE FOR FACIOGENITAL DYSPLASIA

FGD1, the gene responsible for faciogenital dysplasia (FGDY), or Aarskog-Scott syndrome, was isolated by using positional cloning techniques. Genetic linkage studies mapped the *FGDY* locus to the pericentric region of the X chromosome (Porteous et al., 1992; Stevenson et al., 1994). A disease-specific chromosome translocation was used as a molecular signpost to clone the *FGD1* gene (Pasteris et al.,

1994). A number of lines of evidence indicate that *FGD1* is the gene responsible for X-linked faciogenital dysplasia. *FGD1* maps to Xp11.21, the region known to contain the FGDY disease locus, and the *FGD1* gene is directly disrupted by an FGDY-specific translocation breakpoint (Pasteris et al., 1994). A variety of different *FGD1* mutations segregate with the FGDY disease phenotype (Pasteris et al., 1994; Orrico et al., 2000; Schwartz et al., 2000). In addition, FGD1 mRNA is predominantly expressed in osteoblasts, a finding consistent with the fact that FGD1 plays a critical role in bone formation during development (Gorski et al., 2000).

Encodes a Cdc42-Specific Guanine Nucleotide Exchange Factor

FGD1 encodes a Rho guanine nucleotide exchange factor (RhoGEF) that specifically activates Cdc42, a member of the Rho family of GT-Pases. Rho (Ras homology) GTPases form a subgroup of the Ras superfamily of 20 to 30 kDa GTP-binding proteins (Van Aelst and D'Souza-Schorey, 1997; see Chapter 84). At least 10 different mammalian Rho GTPases have been identified: Rho (A, B, C isoforms), Rac (1, 2, 3 isoforms), Cdc42, Rnd1/Rho6, Rnd2/Rho7, Rnd3/RhoE, RhoD, RhoG, TC10, and TTF (Bishop and Hall, 2000). Rho GTPases regulate diverse cellular processes, including the organization of the actin cytoskeleton, cellular polarity, vesicular transport, and gene expression. By regulating these processes, Rho proteins regulate a variety of properties that are critical to tissue morphogenesis, including cell shape, adhesion, and differentiation (Van Aelst and D'Souza-Schorey, 1997; Hall 1998).

As shown in Figure 86–1, Rho GTPases function as molecular switches, cycling between an inactive GDP-bound state and an active GTP-bound state. RhoGEFs, including FGD1, activate Rho GTPases by catalyzing the exchange of bound GDP for GTP, thus inducing a conformational change in the GTP-bound GTPase that allows it to interact with downstream effector proteins (Cerione and Zheng, 1996). Through interactions with downstream effectors, activated Rho proteins reorganize the actin cytoskeleton to alter cell shape and morphology, activate different mitogen-activated protein (MAP) kinase cascades to modify patterns of gene expression, and sequentially activate other Rho GTPases (Van Aelst and D'Souza-Schorey, 1997; Bishop and Hall, 2000). GTPase-activating proteins (GAPs) increase the intrinsic rate of GTP hydrolysis by the GTPase and lead to Rho protein inactivation. Although it is formally possible that GTPase activation could occur as the result of GAP inhibition, accumulated data from a variety of systems indicates that GEF stimulation plays a critical role in Rho GTPase activation (Gulli and Peter, 2001).

In vitro and in vivo analyses show that FGD1 is a specific Cdc42 activator (Olson et al., 1996; Zheng et al., 1996). As shown in Figure 86–2, the FGD1 protein is composed of (in order): a proline-rich N-terminal region, a GEF (or Dbl homology, DH) domain and adjacent PH domain, a FYVE domain, and a PH2 domain—structural motifs involved in signaling and subcellular localization (Pasteris et al., 1994). Comparative studies show that all FGD1-related sequences from nematode to humans share this specific structural organization (see below, "The *FGD1*-Related Gene Family"). Studies show that the FGD1 DH domain specifically binds to Cdc42, but not to other Rho GTPases (Zheng et al., 1996). In addition, the FGD1 DH domain stimulates [^{3}H]GDP dissociation from, and [^{35}S]GTP binding to, Cdc42 in vitro. As shown in Figure 86–3, when microinjected into cultured

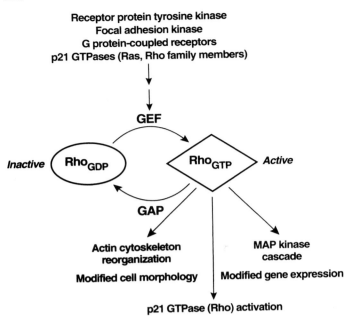

Figure 86–1. Rho GTPases act as molecular switches to regulate a variety of cellular processes. Rho GTPases cycle between an inactive GDP-bound state and an active GTP-bound state. A guanine nucleotide exchange factor (GEF) activates Rho by catalyzing the exchange of bound GDP for GTP. This nucleotide exchange induces a conformational modification in the GTP-bound GTPase that allows it to interact with specific downstream effector proteins. Activated Rho GTPases lead to modified cell morphology by a reorganization of the actin cytoskeleton, changes in gene expression through the activation of mitogen-activated protein (MAP) kinase cascades, and the sequential activation of other Rho family member proteins. A GTPase-activating protein (GAP) increases the intrinsic rate of GTP hydrolysis by the Rho GTPase, leading to a GDP-bound Rho protein and Rho protein inactivation. A variety of stimuli directly, or indirectly, activate different RhoGEFs; these stimuli include activation of receptor protein tyrosine kinases, stimulation of the Ras signaling pathway, and G protein–coupled receptor activation. In principal, GTPase activation can occur by local GEF stimulation or GAP inhibition. However, accumulated data from a variety of systems indicates that GEFs play a critical role in Rho GTPase activation. (From Gorski 1998; used by permission of Humana Press.)

cells, the FGD1 DH domain induces fibroblasts to form filopodia, actin-associated membrane complexes that are generated by activated Cdc42 (Olson et al., 1996). Studies show that the FGD1 DH domain specifically interacts with the Cdc42 protein, and that FGD1-dependent filopodia formation is blocked by competitively binding Cdc42. In FGD1-expressing fibroblasts, JNK activity is stimulated in a manner similar to that obtained with constitutively-activate Cdc42 (Olson et al., 1996; Zheng et al., 1996). In addition, transient coexpression studies indicate that FGD1, in part, regulates the downstream effects of Cdc42 activation (Zhou et al., 1998). Through Cdc42, FGD1 stimulates the passage of fibroblasts through the G_1 phase of the cell cycle (Nagata et al. 1998), and causes tumorigenic transformation (Whitehead et al., 1998). Since FGD1 is a Cdc42 activator, and since *FGD1* mutations result in faciogenital dysplasia, accumulated data strongly suggest that faciogenital dysplasia is a consequence of altered FGD1/Cdc42 signaling.

Composed of Multiple Signaling Domains

Like all RhoGEF proteins, immediately adjacent to the DH (RhoGEF) domain, FGD1 contains a region of sequence homology of approximately 120 residues, termed the pleckstrin homology (PH) domain. As shown in Figure 86–2, FGD1 also contains a second C-terminal PH domain (PH2). PH domains were first identified as duplicated and conserved domains in the protein pleckstrin, the major protein kinase C substrate in platelets (Mayer et al., 1993). PH domains form a diverse family of signaling domains (Lemmon et al., 1996). Some PH domains have been shown to bind to the second-messenger molecule phos-

phatidylinosital-4,5-biphosphate (Harlan et al., 1994); others bind to the $\beta\gamma$-subunits of the G proteins (Touhara et al., 1994), or bind to proteins containing a phosphotyrosine-binding (PTB) domain (Kavanaugh et al., 1995). No specific ligand has yet to be identified for the PH domain(s) associated with the FGD1-related family of proteins.

Based on sequence analyses, FGD1 is predicted to contain at least two additional conserved signaling motifs (Fig. 86–2). The FGD1 amino-terminal proline-rich region is predicted to contain an SH3-binding domain (SH3-BD) that exhibits a strong similarity to the functionally significant regions of several known SH3-BDs, including mouse homolog of *Drosophila* son of sevenless (mSos1), a RasGEF known to bind to the SH3 domain of growth factor receptor-bound protein 2 (Grb2) (Pasteris et al., 1994). SH3 domains have been shown to specifically bind to short (9–10 amino acids) proline-rich structurally conserved motifs (Ren et al., 1993). Grb2, a component of the Ras signaling pathway, was shown to selectively bind to the proline-rich motif of the mSos1 protein to form a link in a signal transduction pathway that functionally ties tyrosine kinase receptors to Ras (Li et al., 1993; Rozakis-Adcock et al., 1993). The identification of a putative SH3-BD in FGD1 infers that, like Sos, proteins that contain an SH3 domain might modify the subcellular distribution or activity of FGD1.

FGD1 also contains a cysteine-rich evolutionarily conserved zinc-finger motif, termed a FYVE domain (Fig. 86–2). At least 30 different proteins of yeast, nematode, plant, insect, and mammalian origin have been found to contain this domain (Gaullier et al., 1998). Most of the proteins containing a FYVE domain are known to be involved in membrane trafficking, including the yeast vacuolar sorting proteins Vac1p and Vps27p (Weisman and Wickner, 1992; Piper et al., 1995), the yeast phophatidylinositol-4-phosphate-5-kinase Fab1 (Yamamoto et al., 1995), and the mammalian ATPase Hrs-2 (Bean et al., 1997). Recent results have illuminated the role the FYVE domain plays in cellular signaling. Stenmark and coworkers have shown that the FYVE domains of both EEA1, a mammalian early endosomal protein, and Hrs-2 selectively bind to phosphatidylinositol-3-phosphate (PtdIns(3)P), and that this binding is necessary for the proteins to localize to the early endosomal membranes (Gaullier et al., 1998; Simonsen et al., 1998). Similar studies show that Vac1p and Vps27 also selectively bind to PtdIns(3)P (Burd and Emr, 1998). The observation that the predicted FGD1 sequence contains an EEA1-like FYVE domain suggests that the FGD1 protein might bind to and interact with phosphatidylinositol second-messenger molecules. Thus, it is likely that the FGD1 protein interacts with, or is regulated by, the components of multiple signal transduction pathways.

Predominantly Expressed in Osteoblasts during Bone Formation

To understand the role that FGD1 plays in development, FGD1 expression was analyzed during mammalian embryogenesis. To facilitate these studies, the FGD1 mouse ortholog, *Fgd1*, was cloned and mapped to a syntenic region of the mouse X chromosome (Pasteris et al., 1995); FGD1 and *Fgd1* have the same structural organization and are 95% identical in nucleotide and amino acid sequence. Studies showed that, during embryogenesis, *Fgd1* was predominantly expressed in bone-forming skeletal tissues (Gorski et al., 2000). For example, *Fgd1* expression was first detected in the base of the skull and cervical vertebrae in E14.5–E15.5 embryos (Fig. 86–4). In these embryos, *Fgd1* transcripts were detected in the cartilage primordia of the neural arches of the cervical vertebrae and the cartilage primordia of the basioccipital bone; these skeletal components are known to contain the earliest centers of ossification that begin to form at about E14–E14.5. *Fgd1* was also expressed in regions of active bone formation in the trabeculae and diaphyseal cortices of developing long bones (Gorski et al., 2000). In ossifying tissue, the onset of *Fgd1* expression correlated with the expression of bone sialoprotein (BSP), a protein specifically expressed in osteoblasts at the onset of matrix mineralization (Fig. 86–4). An analysis of serial sections showed that *Fgd1* was expressed in tissues containing calcified and mineralized extracellular matrix. Immunohistochemical studies showed that FGD1 protein for both mouse and human was specifically expressed in cultured

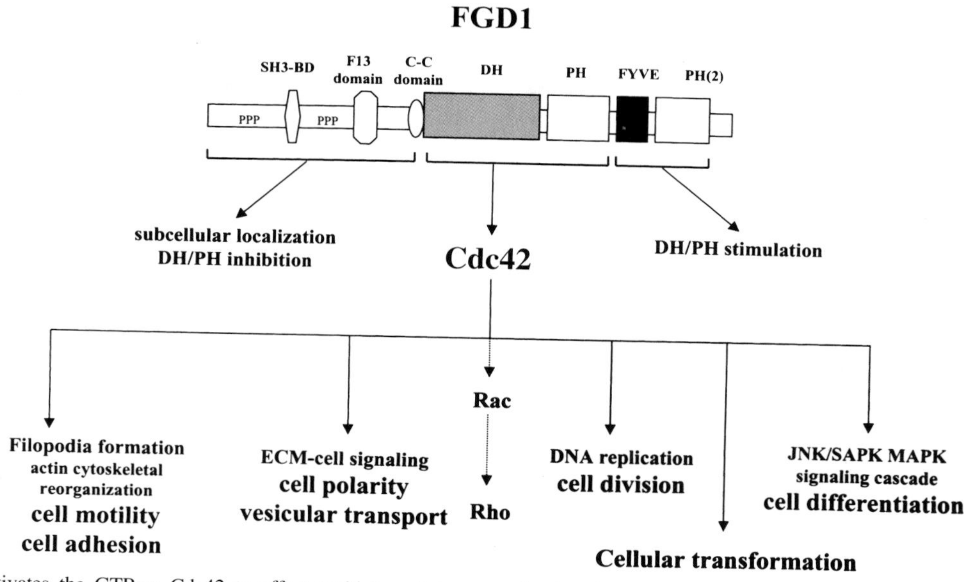

FGD1

subcellular localization
DH/PH inhibition

Cdc42

DH/PH stimulation

Rac

Filopodia formation
actin cytoskeletal
reorganization
**cell motility
cell adhesion**

ECM-cell signaling
**cell polarity
vesicular transport**

Rho

DNA replication
cell division

JNK/SAPK MAPK
signaling cascade
cell differentiation

Cellular transformation

Figure 86–2. FGD1 activates the GTPase Cdc42 to effect multiple cellular changes. This schematic diagram shows that the FGD1 protein contains (in order) a proline-rich N-terminal region, adjacent GEF (or Dbl homology, DH; gray box) and pleckstrin homology (PH; white box) domains, a FYVE domain (black box), and a second C-terminal PH (PH2; white box) domain. As indicated by the arrows, the adjacent DH and PH domains are necessary for activating Cdc42. The N-terminal region is necessary for FGD1 subcellular localization and the intramolecular inhibition of GEF activity (Estrada et al., 2001). This region contains several signaling motifs, including multiple polyproline (PPP) sequence tracts, a putative Src homology 3–binding domain (SH3-BD), a 20-residue sequence tract of unknown function found in other FGD1-related proteins (F13 domain), and a predicted coiled-coil (C-C) domain. The FYVE and PH2 domains stimulate GEF activity (Estrada et al., 2001). Upon activation, Cdc42 interacts with downstream effector proteins to stimulate a variety of cellular processes (Van Aelst and D'Souza-Schorey, 1997; Bishop and Hall, 2000). By stimulating Cdc42, FGD1 stimulates the formation of filopodia, actin-associated membrane complexes, and a reorganization of the actin cytoskeleton to modify cell motility and adhesion. Activated Cdc42 indirectly stimulates the sequential activation of Rac and Rho (Van Aelst and D'Souza-Schorey, 1997; Hall 1998). Cdc42 also mediates signaling from the extracellular matrix (ECM) to the cell to regulate cell polarity and vesicular transport. Through Cdc42, FGD1 stimulates cell division and the passage cells through the cell cycle, and activates the c-Jun N-terminal kinase (JNK) signaling cascade to promote either cell differentiation or cellular transformation, or both.

osteoblasts and osteoblast-like cells, including MC3T3-E1 cells and human osteosarcoma cells, but not in fibroblasts or other mesodermal cells (Gorski et al., 2000). Together, these data showed that *FGD1* was expressed in a variety of regions of incipient and active intramembranous and endochondral ossification, including the craniofacial bones, vertebrae, ribs, long bones, and phalanges. The observed pattern of FGD1 expression correlated with FGDY skeletal manifestations and provided an embryologic basis for skeletal defects observed in faciogenital dysplasia (Gorski et al., 2000). The observation that the initiation of FGD1 expression corresponds to the onset of ossification suggested that FGD1 signaling plays a role in ossification and osteoblast function.

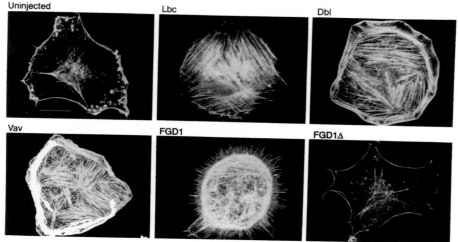

Figure 86–3. FGD1 activates Cdc42 to stimulate the formation of filopodia. Fibroblasts microinjected with RhoGEF expression constructs show the promotion of actin polymerization through the activation of different Rho proteins. Serum-starved Swiss 3T3 cells were microinjected with plasmid DNA encoding epitope-tagged RhoGEF proteins. FGD1, Dbl, Lbc, and Vav promote the polymerization of actin in quiescent cells. Dbl and Vav stimulate the formation of lamellipodia (activation of Rac), and Lbc stimulates the formation of actin stress fibers (activation of Rho). In contrast, by activating Cdc42, FGD1 stimulates the exuberant formation of numerous filopodia, finger-like actin-rich cellular extensions. A construct containing an alternatively spliced form of FGD1 that lacks 36 amino acids near the amino-terminal end of the GEF domain, FGD1Δ, fails to stimulate filopodia formation. Actin cytoskeletal structures in cells expressing the protein constructs were visualized with TRITC-conjugated phalloidin. Scale bar in the uninjected cell represents 20 μm and refers to all panels. (From Olsen et al., 1996; used by permission of *Current Biology.*)

E14.5   E15.5

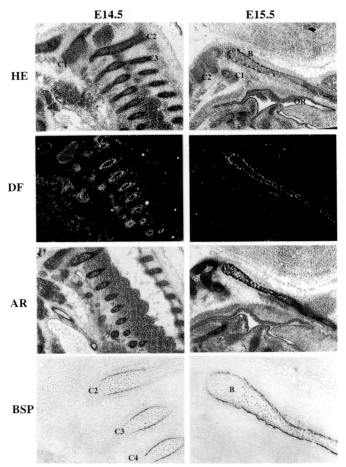

HE

DF

AR

BSP

C2

C3

C4

B

Figure 86–4. *Fgd1* is expressed in the base of the skull and cervical vertebrae during ossification. Serial sagittal sections of the head and neck of E14.5 and E15.5 mouse embryos were used to visualize the spatiotemporal pattern of *Fgd1* expression by in situ hybridization (dark field, DF). The pattern of *Fgd1* expression was compared to the morphology of adjacent tissue sections stained with hematoxylin and eosin (HE), alizarin red (AR), and immunohistochemical staining with bone sialoprotein (BSP) antibody; B, cartilage primordium of the basioccipital bone (clivus); C, cartilage primordium of the body and neural arch of a cervical vertebra (C1, the first vertebra; C2, the second vertebra, etc.); E, epiglottis; OR, oropharynx. White silver grains present in dark field images identify *Fgd1* transcripts (DF). Calcified tissues are stained reddish brown by alizarin red staining. Bound BSP antibody and attached DAB/metal reagent stain black. Photomicrographs showing BSP immunohistochemical staining are at higher magnification. (From Gorski et al., 2000; used by permission of Wiley-Liss, Inc.)

Multiple Signaling Domains and Subcellular Targeting and Activity

Cellular fractionation and immunocytochemical studies show that endogenous FGD1 protein is localized in the cytosol and the Golgi and plasma membranes in osteoblasts. As shown in Figure 86–5, at the plasma membrane, FGD1 protein colocalizes with actin filaments in the subcortical actin cytoskeleton and colocalizes with the Golgi complex (Estrada et al., 2001). The fact that identical distribution patterns were observed for both constitutively and exogenously expressed FGD1 strongly suggested that this localization was accurate and biologically relevant. These results indicated that, by being distributed to the subcortical actin cytoskeleton and the Golgi membranes, FGD1 was poised to activate Cdc42 signaling in either subcellular region (Estrada et al., 2001).

Studies showed that the proline-rich N-terminal region of the FGD1 protein was necessary and sufficient for localization to the plasma membrane and Golgi complex (Estrada et al., 2001). Microinjection studies showed that the N-terminal region was also involved in the in-

tramolecular inhibition of the Fgd1 DH domain and GEF activity. Thus, these data indicated that one or more functional domains within the 350-residue N-terminal region were involved in both the subcellular targeting and the intramolecular regulation of FGD1 GEF activity. Similar studies showed that the Fgd1 C-terminal FYVE and PH2 domains were directly or indirectly involved in relieving the intramolecular inhibition of the N-terminal region and GEF activation (Estrada et al., 2001). Together, these data indicated that the N-terminal region is involved in FGD1 regulation and targeting, and that the C-terminal FYVE and PH2 domains are involved in the regulation of FGD1 GEF activity at the plasma and/or Golgi membranes (Estrada et al., 2001). These data also suggested that FGD1 activation might involve the cooperative interaction of at least two signal types: one that recruits the FGD1 to a particular site, and another that locally modifies FGD1 GEF activity (see Fig. 86–2).

FACIOGENITAL DYSPLASIA: A CLINICAL DESCRIPTION

In 1970, Dagfinn Aarskog observed the association of disproportionate short stature and certain anomalies of the face, hands, feet, and genitalia in seven males from two generations of the same family (Aarskog, 1970). Shortly afterward, three brothers with similar features were reported (Scott, 1971). Since these initial reports, well over 100 cases of Aarskog-Scott syndrome, or faciogenital dysplasia, have been published (Gorlin et al., 1990; Porteous and Goudie, 1991; Gorski et al., 2000). Two reports of similarly affected brothers with osteochondritis dissecans and facial anomalies had been made earlier (Hanley et al., 1967; Ainley 1968). Aarskog observed that the inheritance of this condition was compatible with an X-linked recessive disorder (Aarskog, 1970). Overwhelmingly, most families segregating this disorder have displayed an apparent X-linked recessive pattern of inheritance (Gorlin et al., 1990).

Physical Features

The Aarskog-Scott syndrome phenotype consists of a characteristic set of facial and skeletal anomalies, disproportionate short stature, and urogenital malformations. The cardinal features of this disorder are summarized in Table 86–1 and are illustrated in Figure 86–6. The face is typically round and the forehead broad with ridging of the metopic suture. Facial features typically consist of widely spaced eyes (hypertelorism), ptosis, down-slanting palpebral fissures, and a short up-turned (anteverted) nose. The philtrum is commonly long and the maxilla is typically hypoplastic. A variety of external ear anomalies have been described including low-set ears, posteriorly-rotated auricles, and thickened over-folded helixes (Aarskog, 1970; Gorlin et al., 1990; Porteous and Goudie, 1991; Gorski et al., 2000). Impaired growth is a major manifestation of the disease. Although birth growth parameters are typically normal, growth retardation usually becomes apparent during the first few years of life, and affected males rarely exceed 160 cm in height (Gorlin et al., 1990; Porteous and Goudie, 1991; Gorski et al., 2000). Stature is disproportionate, and the distal extremities are most severely shortened. Isolated growth hormone deficiency has been reported in a significant number of patients (Kodama et al., 1981; Gorlin et al., 1990).

Hands and feet are broad and short (Fig. 86–6). Interphalangeal joints are typically hypermobile, and fifth-digit clinodactyly is common; however, camptodactyly and contractures of the interphalangeal joints have also been observed (Aarskog, 1970; Gorlin et al., 1990; Porteous and Goudie, 1991). The feet are short, broad, and flat with splayed bulbous toes; metatarsus adductus has also been observed. The majority of affected males have a pectus excavatum and inguinal hernias (Gorlin et al., 1990; Porteous and Goudie, 1991). The umbilicus is commonly protuberant and protruding. Affected males commonly have a variety of urogenital anomalies (Aarskog, 1970; Gorlin et al., 1990; Porteous and Goudie, 1991). Typically, the scrotal folds extend ventrally around the base of the penis to form what resembles a shawl; the scrotum commonly appears bifid (Fig. 86–6). Cryptorchidism is common, and penile hypospadius has also been reported. Typically, relative to affected males, the phenotype of obligate female heterozygotes is mild and limited to relative short stature and a subtler form of the characteristic craniofacial anomalies (Gorlin et al.,

Figure 86–5. Endogenous and exogenous Fgd1 protein is distributed to the subcortical actin cytoskeleton and Golgi apparatus in mammalian cells. Osteoblast-like MC3T3-E1 cells (*A–B*) were transfected with either an expression vector encoding a full-length green fluorescent protein (GFP)-Fgd1 fusion construct (panel A), or an expression vector encoding GFP alone (panel B). COS-7 cells were transfected with a myc epitope-tagged expression construct containing a full-length Fgd1 cDNA (*C*). In panels A and C, arrows indicate the localization of epitope-labeled Fgd1 protein at the plasma membrane. COS-7 cells were transfected with the GFP-Fgd1 fusion construct (*D–L*); panels D, G, and J show the localization of the GFP-Fgd1 protein. Panel E shows COS-7 cell stained with TRITC-conjugated phalloidin to show the distribution of filamentous actin. The yellow signal generated in the merged images of panels D and E shows essentially complete colocalization of GFP-Fgd1 and filamentous actin at the subcortical actin cytoskeleton (panel F). (*G–L*) Transfected COS-7 cells were vitally stained with TR-BODIFY ceramide C6, a Texas red-tagged Golgi-specific vital dye, and examined alive. Panel H shows COS-7 cells stained with TR-BODIFY ceramide C6 show the Golgi apparatus. When the images of panels G and H are merged, the generated yellow signal shows significant colocalization of the Golgi apparatus and GFP-Fgd1 (panel I). (*J–L*) Transfected COS-7 cells vitally stained with TR-BODIFY ceramide C6 and treated with brefeldin A (BFA), an agent that disperses the Golgi complex. Panel K shows COS-7 cells stained with TR-BODIFY ceramide C6 and treated with BFA to show a dispersed Golgi apparatus. When the images of panels J and K are merged, the generated yellow signal shows essentially complete colocalization of the dispersed Golgi apparatus and GFP-Fgd1 (panel L). Twelve hours after transfection, cells were fixed and examined by confocal microscopy; magnification at 400×. (From Estrada et al., 2001; used by permission of Oxford University Press.)

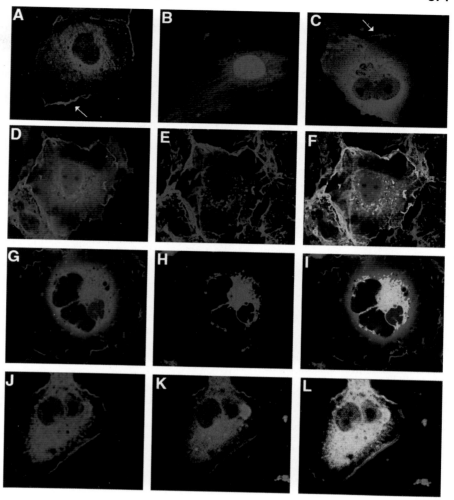

1990; Porteous and Goudie, 1991). Affected males and obligate carrier females both appear to have normal fertility (Porteous and Goudie, 1991). The characteristic facial features are less apparent in affected adult males (Fryns, 1992).

Although mild to moderate mental retardation and attention deficit disorder has been described in some affected males (Fryns, 1992), it does not appear to be a consistent feature (Aarskog, 1970; Gorlin et al., 1990; Porteous and Goudie, 1991). Some affected males have been noted to have ophthalmoplegia and large corneal size (Kirkham et al., 1975). Others have been observed to have enamel hypoplasia and a "col" deformity of the anterior mandible (Melnick and Shields, 1976). Congenitally missing teeth or delays in dental eruption have also been reported (Aarskog, 1970; Gorlin et al., 1990). Affected males occasionally have a cleft lip and palate (Gorlin et al., 1990). Congenital heart defects—including atrial septal defects, ventricular septal defects, aortic valvular stenosis, and pulmonary valvular stenosis—have

been reported (Aarskog, 1970; Fernandez et al., 1994). Affected males with Hirschprung's disease, midgut malrotation, and dolichomegasigmoid have also been reported (Hassinger et al., 1980; Fryns, 1993). Some males have a single palmar crease or distally placed axial tri-radii (Gorlin et al., 1990; Porteous and Goudie, 1991).

Radiographic Features

Radiographic abnormalities are typically limited to those observed in the cervical spine and distal extremities. These abnormalities are summarized in Table 86–1. About half of the affected males have a cervical spine abnormality such as spina bifida occulta, odontoid hypoplasia, fused cervical vertebrae, and ligamentous laxity with subluxation (Gorlin et al., 1990; Porteous and Goudie, 1991; Gorski et al., 2000). Radiographic abnormalities of the hands and feet commonly consist of shortened digits, hypoplasia of the terminal phalanges, clinodactyly, fusion of the middle and distal phalanges, and

Table 86–1. Clinical and Radiographic Features Associated with Faciogenital Dysplasia

Anatomical Region or System	Clinical Features
Craniofacial	Broad forehead, abnormally formed ears, hypertelorism, down-slanted palpebral fissures, ptosis, maxillary hypoplasia, hypodontia and malocclusion; *less common*: cleft lip and palate, enamel hypoplasia
Musculoskeletal	Disproportionate short stature, distally shortened limbs, brachydactyly, pectus excavatum, soft tissue syndactyly of the digits, joint hypermobility, camptodactyly, clinodactyly, broad feet, inguinal hernias; *less common*: single palmar crease, abnormal dermatoglyphics
Urogenital	Shawl and bifid scrotum, cryptorchidism; *less common*: hypospadius
Miscellaneous	Strabismus, growth hormone deficiency; *less common*: mild-to-moderate mental retardation, attention deficit disorder, congenital heart defects
Radiographic	Spina bifida occulta, odontoid hypoplasia, cervical vertebral defects, cervical ligamentous laxity, calcified intervertebral disks, additional ribs, hypoplastic phalanges, retarded bone age; *less common*: osteochondritis

Source: Adapted from Gorski 1998; used by permission of Humana Press.

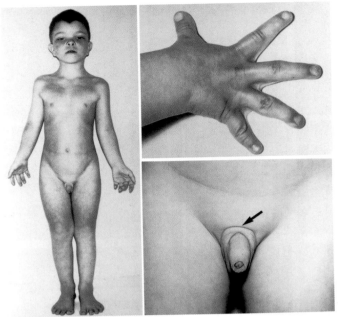

Figure 86–6. A male child with faciogenital dysplasia illustrates the characteristic craniofacial, skeletal, and urogenital features. Facial features are characterized by a broad forehead and a widow's peak, hypertelorism, downsloping palpebral fissures, bilateral ptosis of the upper eyelids, midface hypoplasia with a depressed nasal bridge, an anteverted nose, and low-set ears. Stature is short and disproportionate with shortened distal extremities; hands and feet are short and broad. Hand shows short phalanges, soft-tissue syndactyly between the digits, camptodactyly of the fourth and fifth digits, and fifth-digit clinodactyly. The shawl scrotum is indicated (arrow). Consequential to scrotal folds joining ventrally over the base of the penis, an abnormal penoscrotal configuration is present. Bilateral inguinal herniorrhaphy scars are present. (Courtesy of D. Aarskog, University of Bergen. Adapted from Gorski 1998; used by permission of Humana Press.)

retarded bone maturation. Additional radiographic abnormalities include maxillary hypoplasia, osteochondritis dissecans, additional pairs of ribs and other segmentation anomalies, and calcified intervertebral disks (Taybi, 1983).

MOLECULAR GENETICS OF FACIOGENITAL DYSPLASIA

Analyses of pedigrees segregating faciogenital dysplasia strongly suggested that the disease was inherited in an X-linked recessive fashion (Gorlin et al., 1990; Porteous and Goudie, 1991). In segregating families, X-linked inheritance was strongly supported by the male preponderance of affected individuals and the complete expression in males versus partial expression in females in the same family. Genetic linkage studies mapped the FGDY locus to the pericentric region of the X chromosome (Porteous et al., 1992; Stevenson et al., 1994). An FGDY-specific X,8 translocation breakpoint was used to tentatively map the FGDY disease gene to the Xp11.21 region (Glover et al., 1993). In this family, the observation that an affected female displayed all of the major features of FGDY, and that, in her cells, the rearranged X chromosome was active in the majority of cells examined, suggested that the translocation breakpoint directly interrupted the FGDY disease gene. The FGDY-specific translocation breakpoint region was used to construct a physical map of the translocation breakpoint region and to map the FGDY disease gene to an estimated 350 kb interval within region Xp11.21 (Gorski et al., 1992). Positional cloning techniques were used to isolate and characterize the *FGD1* gene, the gene responsible for faciogenital dysplasia (Pasteris et al., 1994).

In addition to the X-linked form of faciogenital dysplasia, a small number of reports suggest the existence of an autosomal dominant form of the disease (Grier et al., 1983; van de Vooren et al., 1983). To date, there are no genetic mapping data on autosomal dominant

forms of FGDY. However, an individual with a multiple congenital anomaly syndrome similar to Aarskog-Scott syndrome was found to have a partial duplication of the short arm of chromosome 2 (Fryns et al., 1989). This chromosomal rearrangement may be causally associated with a faciogenital dysplasia phenotype and, therefore, may pinpoint a location for an autosomal gene involved in FGDY.

Genomic Organization of the *FGD1* Gene

Structural analyses show that the *FGD1* gene comprises of 18 exons that span an estimated 51 kb of genomic DNA within region Xp11.21 (Pasteris et al., 1997); the structure of the *FGD1* gene is shown schematically in Figure 86–7. RNase protection and primer extension studies show that the *FGD1* gene has multiple transcriptional starts and that the primary start site is located 903 bp upstream of the ATG translation initiation codon (Pasteris et al., 1997). Sequence analyses of the 5′ region of the FGD1 gene indicate that the *FGD1* promoter lacks canonical CAAT and TATA boxes, and this result is consistent with the detection of multiple transcription start sites. Sequence analyses shows that all *FGD1* exon–intron splice sites conform to the AG/GT rule (Pasteris et al., 1997). The first FGD1 exon is the largest, 1210 bp in size; it contains a 903 bp 5′-untranslated region (UTR), the putative ATG start codon, and 307 bp of the open reading frame (ORF). The last exon is 956 bp in size and contains a TAG translation termination site and a 651 bp 3′ UTR. The remaining exons range from 31 to 442 bp in size (Pasteris et al., 1997). Intron sizes were determined directly by sequencing or by exon–exon PCR amplification of genomic DNA. To facilitate an analysis of FGDY patient DNA and the identification of *FGD1* mutations, at least 100 bp of flanking intronic sequence was determined for each FGD1 intron (Pasteris et al., 1997).

Sequence and PCR amplification analyses showed that FGD1 transcripts are alternatively spliced (Pasteris et al., 1997). A comparative analysis of FGD1 cDNAs showed that, relative to clones derived from

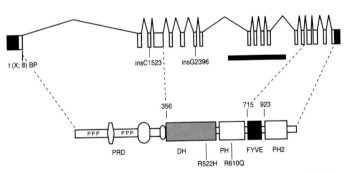

Figure 86–7. A variety of different FGD1 mutations result in faciogenital dysplasia. The top part of the figure illustrates the genomic organization of the FGD1 gene. Exons are depicted as boxes; introns are indicated as lines connecting the boxes. Exons encoding portions of the predicted open reading frame (ORF) are depicted as open boxes; the 5′ and 3′ untranslated regions (UTRs) are depicted as solid black boxes. Identified mutations are indicated below the involved exon. The FGDY-specific X,8 translocation breakpoint [t(X,8)BP] is located in the first exon ORF. Two frameshift mutations—the insertion of a cytosine residue at nucleotide 1523 (insC1523) and the insertion of a guanine residue at nucleotide 2396 (insG2396)—are indicated in exons 3 and 7, respectively. A dark bar indicates the region of the FGD1 gene that is affected by an intragenic deletion (exons 9–12); the exact size of this deletion has not been determined (Schwartz et al., 2000). The bottom part of the figure is a schematic diagram showing the structural organization of the FGD1 protein. FGD1 contains (in order) an N-terminal proline-rich domain (PRD), a DH domain (gray box), a PH domain (white box), a FYVE domain (black box), and a second C-terminal PH (PH2) domain. Dotted lines indicate the exons that encode the different FGD1 structural domains; exons 1–4 encode the PRD, exons 5–14 encode the DH and PH domains, and exons 15–18 encode the FYVE and PH2 domains. The site of the arginine to histidine missense mutation at residue 522 (R522H) and the arginine to glutamine missense mutation at residue 610 (R610Q) are shown at the bottom of the figure.

fetal craniofacial bones, cDNAs derived from fetal brain contained an alternatively spliced sixth exon that effectively removed nucleotides 2095–2202 from the full-length FGD1 transcript. DNA sequence analyses predicted that the alternative FGD1 transcript encoded an abbreviated FGD1 protein that lacked 36 amino acid residues of the amino terminal GEF domain. Microinjection studies showed that, in contrast to the full-length GEF domain, a FGD1 GEF domain containing the alternatively spliced sixth exon failed to activate Cdc42 (Olson et al., 1996; Fig. 86–3). PCR amplification studies showed that the alternatively spliced FGD1 transcript was expressed in a limited number of tissues, including placenta and brain (Pasteris et al., 1997); however, the functional significance of the alternatively spliced transcript remains to be determined.

FGD1 Mutations and Genotype–Phenotype Correlation

Although a limited number of *FGD1* mutations have been identified to date, each of the detected mutations was unique; thus, a high degree of mutation heterogeneity was identified. Characterized *FGD1* mutations are illustrated in Figure 86–7. The FGDY-specific X,8 chromosome translocation was shown to result in a reciprocal translocation that disrupted the first exon of the *FGD1* gene within the ORF; no detectable deletion of the *FGD1* locus was identified (Pasteris et al., 1994). A single intragenic *FGD1* deletion that removed exons 9–12 was recently reported (Schwartz et al., 2000). A previously reported male with faciogenital dysplasia and hematological abnormalities suggestive of sideroblastic anemia might represent another individual with a *FGD1* gene deletion (Escobar and Weaver, 1978). FGD1 and erythroid Δ-aminolevulinate synthase (ALAS2), the gene responsible for X-linked sideroblastic anemia (Cotter et al., 1992), were mapped to a 350 kb interval within Xp11.21 (Gorski et al., 1992). These data suggest that this male might have had FGDY and sideroblastic anemia on the basis of a contiguous gene syndrome as the result of a deletion involving both FGD1 and ALAS2. Unfortunately, the death of this male precludes a confirmation of this hypothesis. A study of over 25 unrelated cases of X-linked FGDY failed to show evidence of an FGD1 deletion (Pasteris et al., 1994). Together, these results suggest that deletions involving the FGD1 locus may occur, but that deletions do not appear to play a common role in the generation of FGD1 mutations.

Two insertional *FGD1* mutations have been identified in families segregating FGDY; both were predicted to result in a prematurely truncated FGD1 protein (Fig. 86–7). The first involved the insertion of an additional guanine residue at nucleotide 2396 within exon 7 (Pasteris et al., 1994). Dagfinn Aarskog has shown that the insertion of a cytosine residue at nucleotide 1523 is the FGD1 mutation segregating in the originally reported Aarskog syndrome family (Boman et al., 2002). Both of these mutations are predicted to result in null *FGD1* alleles and a complete loss of FGD1 function. Two *FGD1* missense mutations have been reported (Fig. 86–7). The first was a guanine to adenosine transition at nucleotide 2296, resulting in the change of amino acid residue 522 from arginine to histidine (Schwartz et al., 2000). The second was a guanine to adenosine transition at nucleotide 2559, resulting in the change of amino acid residue 610 from arginine to glutamine (Orrico et al., 2000). Both mutations were predicted to change strongly conserved residues in the DH and PH FGD1 domains, respectively; thus both missense mutations are predicted to result in a loss of FGD1 GEF function. Together, these data indicate that, to date, all identified *FGD1* mutations are predicted to result in the loss of GEF activity. Since none of the identified mutations have involved the FYVE and PH2 domains and the N-terminal region, it remains to be determined as to whether missense mutations in these domains result in the FGDY phenotype.

ESTABLISHING THE DIAGNOSIS OF FACIOGENITAL DYSPLASIA

Individuals with faciogenital dysplasia typically have a distinctive pattern of characteristic craniofacial abnormalities, disproportionate short stature, acromelic shortening of the distal extremities, and urogenital anomalies that ordinarily provide sufficient diagnostic clues to distinguish them from alternative diagnoses. The cardinal features of this disorder are summarized in Table 86–1. Since many of the cardinal diagnostic features of this condition affect the skeleton, radiological studies are typically performed to detect characteristic abnormalities and to assist in confirming a suspected diagnosis. In families segregating FGDY, clinical analyses show that relatively wide phenotypic variability exists between affected siblings and between affected individuals of different generations (Porteous and Goudie, 1991; Teebi et al., 1993). However, among families segregating the X-linked form of faciogenital dysplasia, an observed X-linked pattern of inheritance provides additional clinical confirmation. Several other inherited conditions, including Noonan syndrome, Robinow syndrome, and Leopard syndrome, share clinical features with faciogenital dysplasia; shared features include short stature, hypertelorism, and cryptorchidism. Pseudohypoparathyroidism and hydantoin embryopathy also share several physical features with FGDY.

Molecular DNA diagnostic studies can now be offered to families with X-linked faciogenital dysplasia in which a specific mutation has been identified. In families in which a mutation has not yet been identified, male individuals can be tested for deletions by Southern blotting, by using *FGD1* cDNA as a probe before proceeding to sequence-based mutation detection. Patients with faciogenital dysplasia who display complex phenotypes should have chromosome analyses performed, and their DNA should be tested with *FGD1* and other Xp11.21 DNA markers in order to detect a contiguous gene syndrome. For X-linked faciogenital dysplasia patients without detectable deletions, direct sequence analyses of the *FGD1* gene should be performed by using primers to directly PCR amplify and sequence *FGD1* exons from male FGDY DNA.

MANAGEMENT AND TREATMENT

Individuals considered to have the potential diagnosis of faciogenital dysplasia should have evaluations directed toward confirming the diagnosis, identifying associated congenital malformations, and treating associated medical problems. Since the cardinal features of this condition affect the skeletal tissues, radiographs are typically obtained to assist in confirming the diagnosis and to identify associated skeletal anomalies such as odontoid hypoplasia, cervical ligamentous laxity, and cervical spine anomalies. Because of the associated problems of cervical spine instability, particular care should be taken to support an affected infant's head and to avoid head and cervical spine trauma. Children with joint contractures, soft tissue syndactyly, and cervical spine anomalies should be referred to the appropriate pediatric subspecialist for surgical correction, and to physical therapy for continued treatment. Affected infants should be evaluated by echocardiography to identify associated congenital heart defects. Common structural malformations such as cryptorchidism, hypospadius, and inguinal hernias should be identified and referred to the appropriate pediatric subspecialist for surgical correction. An ophthalmologic evaluation should be performed to identify associated ocular abnormalities such as strabismus. Children with hypodontia and malocclusion should be referred to a pediatric dentist for care. Endocrinologic evaluations should be performed to identify children with an isolated growth hormone deficiency. At this time, no control studies have been performed to assess the benefits and risks of supplemental growth hormone to individuals with faciogenital dysplasia without isolated growth hormone deficiency.

THE *FGD1*-RELATED GENE FAMILY

FGD1 is the founding member of an evolutionarily conserved gene family. Shortly after *FGD1* was cloned, database searches showed that the *C. elegans* and *Drosophila* genomes contained *FGD1*-related sequences (Bassett et al., 1997). These data indicated that the overall structure of the *FGD1* gene was evolutionarily conserved and implied that the FGD1 signaling pathway was conserved between *C. elegans* and humans. Degenerate PCR and low-stringency hybridization analyses were used to isolate two additional *FGD1*-related gene family members, the mouse (and human ortholog) *Fgd2* (*FGD2*) and *Fgd3* (*FGD3*) genes (Pasteris and Gorski, 1999; Pasteris et al., 2000). Mapping studies showed that the mouse and human *Fgd2* and *FGD2* orthologs mapped to syntenic regions of murine chromosome 17 and human chromosome 6p21.2, respectively (Pasteris and Gorski, 1999). Mapping studies showed that the mouse and human *Fgd3* and *FGD3* orthologs mapped to syntenic regions of murine chromosome 13 and human chromosome 9q22, respectively (Pasteris et al., 2000). No disease genes were mapped to these regions (Pasteris and Gorski, 1999; Pasteris et al., 2000). Biochemical studies were used to isolate a third *FGD1*-related sequence, the rat Frabin gene (Obaishi et al., 1998). More recently, *fgd-1*, the *C. elegans FGD1* gene ortholog, was also isolated and characterized (Gao et al., 2001).

As shown in Figure 86–8, *FGD1*-related gene family members share several distinguishing features. Sequence analyses showed that all *FGD1*-related sequences have a structural organization strikingly similar to human *FGD1*. Like *FGD1*, all of these sequences are predicted to contain (in order) adjacent RhoGEF and PH domains, a FYVE domain, and a second C-terminal PH2 domain. In addition, within each of these domains, each *FGD1*-related sequence was found to be markedly similar to *FGD1* and the other gene family members (Fig. 86–8). By contrast, an examination of the N-terminal regions of the *FGD1*-related gene family members showed that each sequence appeared to contain relatively unique signaling domains (Pasteris and Gorski, 1999; Pasteris et al., 2000). Together, these data indicated that, like *FGD1*, *FGD1*-related genes contained a conserved canonical structure of signaling domains (DH, PH, FYVE, and PH2) that span 540 contiguous amino acid residues. The observation that all *FGD1*-related family members contain identical shared signaling domains suggests that *FGD1*-related gene family members are likely to act as GEFs and interact with a common set of proteins and signaling molecules. The observed N-terminal structural variation suggests that, in addition to acting in a conserved signaling pathway, each protein probably interacts with an additional set of unique signaling molecules to play a unique role in Cdc42 activation. Like *FGD1*, other *FGD1*-related family members selectively activate Cdc42 (Obaishi et al., 1998; Pasteris et al., 2000). This observation supports the hypothesis that FGD1-related proteins have similar functional roles in cell signaling.

Mutations in *fgd-1*, the *C. elegans FGD1* Gene Orthologue

To gain further insight into the function of *FGD1*, we isolated and characterized *fgd-1*, the *C. elegans* ortholog of the human *FGD1* gene (Gao et al., 2001). An analysis of the predicted *fgd-1* sequence showed

that it had a structural organization strikingly similar to *FGD1* and other *FGD1*-related sequences (Fig. 86–8). To determine the biological function of the *fgd-1* gene, RNA interference (RNAi) was used to down-regulate gene expression during development (Gao et al., 2001). As shown in Figure 86–9, these studies showed that disrupted *fgd-1* expression resulted in abnormalities in excretory cell formation and cystic dilation of the excretory cell canal. The single H-shaped excretory cell forms a major component of the nematode renal system (Nelson et al., 1983). From the cell body (located ventral to the pharynx), the excretory cell extends tubular processes, called canals, anteriorly and posteriorly along the basolateral surface of the hypodermis. Each excretory canal is comprised of a fluid-filled channel that is surrounded by a thin continuous wall of cytoplasm. These canals are polarized; the external/basolateral surface of the canal lies against the surface of the surrounding hypodermis and basement membrane, and the internal and apical surface of the excretory cell process faces the extracellular matrix contained in the lumen of the internal channel (Nelson et al., 1983; Buechner et al., 1999).

Molecular genetic analyses showed that Exc-5 worms—nematodes with a specific defect in excretory cell formation—had *fgd-1* mutations (Gao et al., 2001). In addition, transgenic studies showed that *fgd-1* expression rescued the Exc-5 phenotype. Transgenic expression

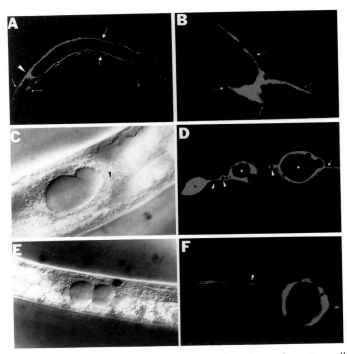

Figure 86–9. Interference of *fgd-1* expression leads to abnormal excretory cell formation in nematodes. (*A and B*) Fluorescent micrographs (A, 20×; B, 100×) showing the pattern of GFP expression in *bgIs310* nematodes; this strain carries a transgenic expression construct insertion that expresses GFP in an excretory cell-specific pattern. The arrowhead indicates the excretory cell body; the small and large arrows indicate the anterior and posterior excretory cell processes, respectively. (*C*) Nomarski micrograph of a typical young adult worm in which RNAi was used to disrupt *fgd-1* expression; the worm has a large excretory canal cyst (100×). The cyst nearly extends across the diameter of the worm. An arrowhead indicates an apparently nonaffected segment of the excretory process and canal; anterior is to the left, ventral is down. (*D*) Fluorescent micrograph of an adult *fgd-1(RNAi); bgIs310* worm showing multiple excretory canal cysts; anterior is to the left, ventral is down (100×). Asterisks (*) and arrowheads indicate large and small cysts, respectively; these cysts communicate with an apparently normal excretory canal (arrow). (*E*) Nomarski micrograph of a typical young adult *exc-5(rh232)* worm showing multiple large excretory canal cysts; anterior is to the left, ventral is down (60×). (*F*) Fluorescent micrograph of an adult *exc-5(rh232) bgIs310* worm showing a large excretory canal cyst; anterior is to the left, ventral is down (100×). An arrowhead indicates an apparently normal excretory canal segment. (From Gao et al., 2001; used by permission of Oxford University Press.)

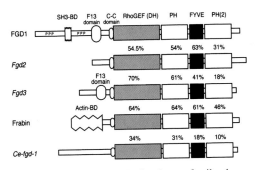

Figure 86–8. Members of the *FGD1*-related gene family share a canonical core structure of signaling domains. Schematic diagrams illustrate the structural organization of human *FGD1*, murine *Fgd2* and *Fgd3*, rat *Frabin*, and *Ce-fgd-1*, the *C. elegans FGD1* ortholog. All FGD1-related proteins contain (in order) an N-terminal region, adjacent RhoGEF (or Dbl homology, DH; gray box) and pleckstrin homology (PH; white box) domains, a FYVE domain (black box), and a second C-terminal PH2 domain (white box). The percentage of residue identity compared to FGD1 is indicated above each of the conserved domains. All FGD1-related sequences are predicted to contain a coiled-coil (C-C) domain immediately upstream of the RhoGEF domain. The FGD1 N-terminal region contains several signaling motifs, including multiple polyproline sequence tracts (PPP) and a putative Src homology 3–binding domain (SH3-BD). The N-terminal domains of *FGD1* and *Fgd3* share a 20-residue sequence tract of unknown function (F13 domain). The *Frabin* N-terminal region contains an actin-binding domain (actin-BD).

studies showed that *fgd-1* has a limited pattern of expression that was confined to the excretory cell during development (Goa et al., 2001). These data suggested that the *C. elegans* FGD-1 protein might function in a cell autonomous manner. Serial observations indicated that *fgd-1* mutations led to developmental excretory cell abnormalities that caused cystic dilation and interfered with canal process extension, a process that is similar to axonal process extension (Hedgecock et al., 1987). Together, these data indicated that *fgd-1* was the *C. elegans* ortholog of the human FGD1 gene, and that *fgd-1* played a critical role in excretory cell morphogenesis and cellular organization.

DEVELOPMENTAL PATHOGENESIS

An analysis of the FGD1 signaling pathway presents a unique opportunity to study RhoGEF signaling in a context relevant to human disease. In marked contrast, most mammalian RhoGEF genes are protooncogenes that were isolated by using transformation assays, and the developmental role of the majority of the isolated RhoGEFs remains to be determined (Cerione and Zheng, 1996; Whitehead et al., 1997). Identified *FGD1* mutations are predicted to result in null *FGD1* alleles and the loss of FGD1 function; thus, a constitutive loss of FGD1 Cdc42GEF activity appears to result in the FGDY phenotype. In *S. cerevisiae*, *S. pombe*, *D. melanogaster*, and *C. elegans*, the loss of a RhoGEF activity is functionally equivalent to the loss of the target Rho protein (Boguski and McCormick, 1993). Although in vitro biochemical studies suggest that FGD1 is but one of at least several Cdc42 activators (Cerione and Zheng, 1996), it is reasonable to expect that, within cells expressing FGD1, loss of FGD1 activity would alter or perturb Cdc42 regulation. Therefore, it is likely that an examination of the molecular biology of Cdc42 and the other Rho proteins will illuminate the biological role of FGD1 signaling during development.

Rho GTPases and Embryonic Development

Several lines of evidence indicate that Rho signaling plays a crucial role during metazoan embryogenesis. Consistent with their role in regulating actin polymerization, Rho GTPases play critical roles in regulating the actin cytoskeleton. For example, in *Drosophila*, Cdc42 and Rac1 dominant-negative mutations result in a variety of developmental defects, including anomalies in axonal and dendritic outgrowth and abnormal myoblast fusion (Luo et al., 1994). Cdc42 and Rac1 mutations result in distinct phenotypes during the development of the fruit fly; these data indicate that different Rho proteins play distinct roles during development. Cdc42 has also been shown to play a critical role in the dorsal closure of the epidermis during fly development (Riesgo-Escovar et al., 1996; Glise and Noselli, 1997). The expression of dominant-negative Cdc42 and Rac1 alleles in a subset of imaginal disc epithelial cells have shown that these mutants have specific and nonoverlapping roles in disc development. Within these cells, Cdc42 controls epithelial cell shape changes by modulating the actin cytoskeleton during pupal and larval development (Eaton et al., 1995). In addition, Cdc42 has been shown to play an important part in wing development by regulating the actin processes that are involved in formation of epithelial wing hairs (Eaton et al., 1996). Cdc42 is also required for multiple processes during fly oogenesis, including the actin-dependent transfer of nurse cell cytoplasm into the oocyte (Luo et al., 1994). Not suprisingly, *Drosophila* RhoGEF mutations have also been associated with the regulation of cell morphology and a variety of different developmental abnormalities during gastrulation (Barrett et al., 1997; Hacker and Perrimon, 1998).

RhoGEFs (or the GTPase they activate) are also known to regulate cell migration. In *C. elegans*, mutations in *unc-73*, the ortholog of the mammalian RhoGEF Trio, exhibit numerous cell migration and axon path-finding defects (Hedgecock et al., 1987). Mutations in *mig-2*, a *C. elegans* Rho GTPase, also result in defects in the migration of a number of different cells and axons (Zipkin et al., 1997). A variety of developmental abnormalities result from mutations in the *C. elegans* ortholog of the mammalian GTPase Rac1, including abnormalities in distal tip cell migration, gonadal morphology, and apoptotic cell phagocytosis (Reddien and Horvitz, 2000). By contrast, other RhoGEFs affect cell morphogenesis; for example, mutations in the *C.*

elegans RhoGEF *unc-89* result in defects in muscle cell organization (Benian et al., 1996). These *unc-89* worms have a disorganized structure of the muscle cells in which thick filaments are not organized into discrete A bands and no M-lines are present. Thus, like *unc-89*, *fgd-1* mutations result in specific defects in cellular organization. Together, these data indicate that RhoGEFs regulate embryonic development and morphogenesis on several scales: from the organization and morphogenesis of single cells, to cell–cell interactions and cellular migration, to tissue morphogenesis.

FGD1/Cdc42 Signaling in Osteoblast Development

FGD1 encodes a Cdc42-specific RhoGEF that is necessary for normal bone formation. Most *FGD1* mutations are predicted null alleles; thus, the FGDY phenotype appears to be the result of a loss of FGD1 GEF activity. Together, these findings imply that the FGDY is a disease of abnormal FGD1/Cdc42 signaling. Data also indicate that the *C. elegans* ortholog of FGD1, *fgd-1*, plays a critical role in nematode excretory cell morphogenesis (Gao et al., 2001). Thus, although these orthologs are expressed in markedly different cell types, data show that both genes play critical roles in development, FGD1 in bone and *fgd-1* in nematode excretory cells. These observations suggest that, rather than playing a role in maintaining a specific cellular phenotype, FGD1/*fgd-1* signaling may be critical in regulating more basic cell processes, such as Cdc42 signaling, the known substrate for FGD1.

Cdc42 coordinately regulates a variety of critical cellular signaling pathways that regulate cell shape, proliferation, differentiation, cellular transformation, and apoptosis (Van Aelst and D'Souza-Schorey, 1997; Bishop and Hall, 2000). Based on an analysis of Cdc42 function, it is reasonable to hypothesize that FGD1/Cdc42 signaling plays a role in osteoblast–extracellular matrix (ECM) interactions, actin cytoskeletal organization, cellular polarity and protein transport, and the regulation of gene expression and osteoblast differentiation. Possible targets for FGD1/Cdc42 signaling are shown in Figure 86–10.

FGD1/Cdc42 Signaling and the Actin Cytoskeleton

Activated Cdc42 induces the formation of filopodia, thin fingerlike actin-containing projections that are probably involved in the recognition of the extracellular environment (Hall, 1998). In contrast, Rac controls the assembly of actin filaments at the cell periphery to produce lamellipodia and membrane ruffles, and Rho regulates the assembly of contractile actin-myosin filaments (stress fibers) and focal adhesions. Cdc42 appears to act through several different effector proteins to regulate filopodia formation (Fig. 86–10). These proteins include neuronal Wiskott-Aldrich syndrome protein (NWASP), an actin-associated protein that directly interacts with the actin-related (Arp2/3) protein complex to nucleate actin filament polymerization (Symons et al., 1996; Machesky et al., 1999; Rohatgi et al., 1999), and the MR-CKα/β (myotonic dystrophy kinase-related Cdc42-binding kinase) proteins, kinases involved in the regulation of myosin light chain phosphorylation (Bishop and Hall, 2000). Data indicate that Cdc42 plays a critical role in integrin-mediated cell signaling in that dominant-negative forms of Cdc42 totally block integrin-dependent cell spreading (Price et al., 1998). Extensive data indicate that Cdc42 signaling regulates the signal transduction pathways that link extracellular stimuli to the organization of the actin cytoskeleton and cell shape (Clark et al., 1998; Giancotti and Rouslahti, 1999; Schoenwaelder and Burridge, 1999; del Pozo et al., 2000). Studies show that osteoblasts are responsive to ECM and that ECM plays a critical role in cell regulation and function (Chen et al., 1997; Gorski and Olsen, 1998; Rodan and Martin, 2000). Specifically, integrin-mediated signaling is necessary for the induction of Cbfa1 expression (Xiao et al., 1998), and osteoblast differentiation (Andrianarivo et al., 1992; Franceschi and Iyer, 1992; Masi et al., 1992; Lynch et al., 1995; Marsh et al., 1995). Based on these data, it is reasonable to hypothesize that FGD1/Cdc42 signaling may play a role in integrin-mediated osteoblast signaling and differentiation.

FGD1/Cdc42 Signaling and Cell Polarity

Numerous studies show that Cdc42 plays a critical role in regulating cell polarity (Van Aelst and D'Souza-Schorey, 1997). Cdc42 was first

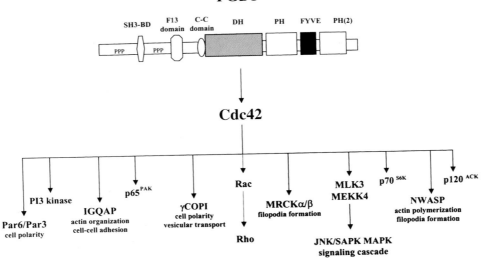

Figure 86–10. FGD1/Cdc42 signaling is likely to play several different but interrelated roles in osteoblast development. FGD1 activates the Cdc42 GTPase to facilitate its interaction with downstream effector proteins. A schematic diagram shows that the FGD1 protein contains a proline-rich N-terminal region, adjacent DH (gray box) and PH (white box) domains, a FYVE domain (black box), and a C-terminal PH2 domain (white box). Cdc42 interacts with a variety of targets in mammalian cells. Cdc42 stimulates the formation of actin-containing filopodial projections by interacting with NWASP and the myotonic dystrophy-related kinase MRCKα/β. Cdc42 regulates cell polarity, in part, by acting through the γ-subunit of the coatomer (γCOPI) complex, as well as through the Par6/Par3 protein complex. Cdc42 regulates cell growth and gene expression by stimulating the MLK3 and MEKK4 kinases to activate the JNK signaling cascade. Activated Cdc42 also stimulates the sequential activation of Rac and Rho. (From van Aelst and D'Souza-Schorey, 1997; Hall, 1998.)

identified in *S. cerevisiae*, where it is required for polarized cell growth and bud formation (Adams et al., 1990). Data show that Cdc42 is important in regulating cell polarity in both mammalian fibroblasts (Nobes and Hall, 1999) and epithelial cells (Korschewski et al., 1999). Cdc42 appears to act through several different effector proteins to regulate cell polarity (Fig. 86–10). Activated Cdc42 binds to the mammalian homolog of Par6 (Joberty et al., 2000; Lin et al., 2000), a *C. elegans* gene that is crucial for determining normal zygotic cell division (Kemphues 2000). Overexpression studies indicate that Cdc42–Par6 interactions play a role in epithelial cell polarity (Joberty et al., 2000; Lin et al., 2000). Activated Cdc42 also binds to the γ-subunit of the coatomer (γCOPI) complex to regulate vesicular membrane transport and epithelial cell polarity (Wu et al., 2000). Together, these studies indicate that, in part, Cdc42 regulates cell polarity in organisms as diverse as yeast and humans. Vesicular transport and cell polarity are also critical to osteoblast function: osteoblasts have an apical-basolateral polarity and secrete ECM in a polarized fashion (Ilvesaro et al., 1999). Based on these data, it is reasonable to hypothesize that the FGD1/Cdc42 pathway has a role in regulating osteoblast vesicular transport and cell polarity.

FGD1/Cdc42 Signaling and the Regulation of Gene Expression

Activated Cdc42 also plays a part in regulating cell growth and gene expression. Like Rac and Rho, Cdc42 has been demonstrated to have transforming and oncogenic potential (Qiu et al., 1997). Cdc42 acts through several different effector proteins to regulate cell growth and modify gene expression (Fig. 86–10). Activated Cdc42 stimulates MLK3 and MEKK4, kinases that activate the JNK signaling cascade (Tibbles et al., 1996; Gerwins et al., 1997). JNK phosphorylates c-Jun and other transcription factors such as ATF-2 and TCF/Elk1. Fos interacts with c-Jun to form the AP-1 transcription factor; c-Jun also interacts with ATF-2 and other members of the ATF family to form additional transcription factors (Treisman, 1996). JNK can stimulate AP-1 through phosphorylation of c-Jun; furthermore, JNK phosphorylation of TCF/Elk1 enhances AP-1 activation. Upsetting the tightly regulated activity of AP-1 may cause a variety of cellular abnormalities such as apoptosis or oncogenic transformation (Treisman, 1996). Considerable evidence shows that c-Fos and c-Jun play critical roles in osteoblast biology. Correlations exist between Fos- and Jun-related

gene expression and osteoblast differentiation (Stein and Lian, 1993); in addition, osteoblast-specific genes, such as osteocalcin, are induced by c-Fos expression (Schule et al., 1990). During embryogenesis, c-Fos is primarily expressed in developing cartilage and bone (Dony and Gruss, 1987). c-Fos is highly expressed in many human and mouse osteosarcomas (Honoki et al., 1992), and *v-fos* expression specifically induces osteosarcomas in rodents (Ward and Young, 1976). In transgenic mice expressing c-Fos and c-Jun, a strong correlation exists between AP-1 activity and osteosarcoma formation (Grigoridadis et al., 1996). These results suggest that AP-1 and related transcription factors have an important role in regulating osteoblast proliferation and differentiation. Since Cdc42 plays an important part in regulating AP-1 activity, it is reasonable to hypothesize that the FGD1/Cdc42 signaling may help regulate osteoblast growth and differentiation.

ACKNOWLEDGMENTS

We thank Dr. D. Aarskog for the patient photographs and Dr. A. Hall for the photomicrograph of the microinjection studies. This work is supported, in part, by the March of Dimes Birth Defects Foundation basic sciences grant 1-93-0326 and National Institutes of Health grant HD34446 to J. L. G.

REFERENCES

Aarskog D (1970). A familial syndrome of short stature associated with facial dysplasia and genital anomalies. *J Pediatr* 77: 856–861.

Adams AE, Johnson DI, Lognecker RM, Sloat BF, Pringle JR (1990). CDC42 and CDC43, two additional genes involved in budding and the establishment of cell polarity in the yeast *Saccharomyces cerevisiae*. *J Cell Biol* 111: 131–142.

Ainley RG (1968). Hypertelorism (Greig's syndrome): a case report. *J Pediatr Ophthalmol* 5: 148–150.

Andrianarivo AG, Robinson JA, Mann KG, Tracy RP (1992). Growth on type I collagen promotes expression of the osteoblastic phenotype in human osteosarcoma MG-63 cells. *J Cell Physiol* 153: 256–265.

Barrett K, Leptin M, Settleman J (1997). The Rho GTPase and a putative RhoGEF mediate a signaling pathway for the cell shape changes in *Drosophila* gastrulation. *Cell* 91: 905–915.

Bassett DE Jr, Boguski MS, Spencer F, Reeves R, Kim S, Weaver T, Hieter P (1997). Genome cross referencing and XREFdb: implications for the identification and analysis of genes mutated in human disease. *Nat Genet* 15: 339–344.

Bean AJ, Seifert R, Chen YA, Sacks R, Scheller RH (1997). Hrs-2 is an ATPase implicated in calcium-regulated secretion. *Nature* 385: 826–829.

Benian GM, Tinley TL, Tang X, Borodovsky M (1996). The *Caenorhabditis elegans* gene *unc-89*, required for muscle M-line assembly, encodes a giant modular protein composed of Ig and signal transduction domains. *J Cell Biol* 32: 835–848.

Bishop AL, Hall A (2000). Rho GTPases and their effector proteins. *Biochem J* 348: 241–255.

Boguski MS, McCormick F (1993). Proteins regulating Ras and its relatives. *Nature* 366: 643–653.

Boman H, Knappskog PM, Aarskog D (2002). FGD1 mutation 1523 ins C in the original Aarskog syndrome family. Unpublished ms.

Buechner M, Hall DH, Bhatt H, Hedgecock EM (1999). Cystic canal mutants in *Caenorhabditis elegans* are defective in the apical membrane domain of the renal (excretory) cell. *Dev Biol* 214: 227–241.

Burd CG, Emr SD (1998). Phosphatidylinositol(3)-phosphate signaling mediated by specific binding to RING FYVE domains. *Mol Cell* 2: 157–162.

Cerione RA, Zheng Y (1996). The Dbl family of oncogenes. *Curr Opin Cell Biol* 8: 216–222.

Chen CS, Mrksich M, Huang S, Whitesides GM, Ingber DE (1997). Geometric control of cell life and death. *Science* 276: 1425–1428.

Clark EA, King WG, Brugge JS, Symons M, Hynes RO (1998). Integrin-mediated signals regulated by members of the Rho family of GTPases. *J Cell Biol* 142: 573–586.

Cotter PD, Willard HF, Gorski JL, Bishop DF (1992). Assignment of human erythroid Δ-aminolevulinate synthase (ALAS2) to a distal subregion of band Xp11.21 by PCR analysis of somatic cell hybrids containing X;autosome translocations. *Genomics* 13: 211–213.

del Pozo MA, Price LS, Alderson NB, Ren X-D, Schwartz MA (2000). Adhesion to the extracellular matrix regulates the coupling of the small GTPase Rac to its effector PAK. *EMBO J* 19: 2008–2014.

Dony C, Gruss P (1987). Proto-oncogene c-*fos* expression in growth regions of fetal bone and mesodermal web tissue. *Nature* 328: 711–714.

Eaton S, Auvinen P, Lou L, Jan YN, Simons K (1995) CDC42 and Rac1 control different actin-dependent processes in the *Drosophila* wing disc epithelium. *J Cell Biol* 131: 151–164.

Eaton S, Wepf R, Simons K (1996). Roles for Rac1 and CDC42 in planar polarization and hair outgrowth in the wing of *Drosophila*. *J Cell Biol* 135: 1277–1289.

Escobar V, Weaver DD (1978). Aarskog syndrome: new findings and genetic analysis. *JAMA* 240: 2638–2641.

Estrada L, Charon E, Gorski JL (2001). *Fgd1*, the Cdc42GEF responsible for faciogenital dysplasia, is localized to the subcortical actin cytoskeleton and Golgi membrane. *Hum Mol Genet* 10: 485–495.

Fernandez I, Tsukahara M, Mito H, Yoshii H, Uchida M, Matsuo K, Kajii T (1994). Congenital heart defects in Aarskog syndrome. *Am J Med Genet* 50: 318–322.

Franceschi RT, Iyer BS (1992). Relationship between collagen synthesis and expression of the osteoblast phenotype in MC3T3-E1 cells. *J Bone Miner Res* 7: 235–246.

Fryns J-P (1992). Aarskog syndrome: the changing phenotype with age. *Am J Med Genet* 43: 420–427.

Fryns J-P (1993). Dolichomegasigmoid in Aarskog syndrome. *Am J Med Genet* 45: 122.

Fryns J-P, Kleczkowska A, Kenis H, Decock P, van den Berghe H (1989). Partial duplication of the short arm of chromosome 2 (dup(2)(p13–p21) associated with mental retardation and an Aarskog-like phenotype. *Ann Genet* 32: 174–176.

Gao J, Estrada L, Cho S, Ellis RE, Gorski JL (2001). The *Caenorhabditis elegans* homolog of FGD1, the human Cdc42GEF gene responsible for faciogenital dysplasia, is critical for excretory cell morphogenesis. *Hum Mol Genet* 10: 3049–3062.

Gaullier J-M, Simonsen A, D'Arrigo A, Bremnes B, Stenmark H (1998). FYVE fingers bind PtdIns(3)P. *Nature* 394: 432–433.

Gerwins P, Blank JL, Johnson GL (1997). Cloning of a novel mitogen-activated protein kinase kinase kinase, MEKK4, that selectively regulates the c-Jun amino terminal kinase pathway. *J Biol Chem* 272: 8288–8295.

Giancotti FG, Rouslahti E (1999). Integrin signaling. *Science* 285: 1028–1032.

Glise B, Noselli S (1997). Coupling of Jun amino-terminal kinase and decapentaplegic signaling pathways in *Drosophila* morphogenesis. *Genes Dev* 11: 1738–1747.

Glover TW, Verga V, Rafael J, Gorski JL, Bawle E, Higgins JV (1993). Translocation breakpoint in Aarskog syndrome maps to Xp11.21 between ALAS2 and DXS323. *Hum Mol Genet* 10: 1717–1718.

Gorlin RJ, Cohen MM, Levin LS (1990). *Syndromes of the Head and Neck, 3rd Edition*. Oxford University Press, New York.

Gorski JL (1998). Aarskog-Scott syndrome. In: *Principles of Molecular Medicine*. Jameson L. (ed.) Humana Press, Totowa, NJ, pp. 1039–1045.

Gorski JP, Olsen BR (1998). Mutations in extracellular matrix molecules. *Curr Opin Cell Biol* 10: 586–593.

Gorski JL, Boehnke M, Reyner EL, Burright EN (1992). A radiation hybrid map of the proximal short arm of the human X chromosome spanning incontinentia pigmenti 1 (IP1) translocation breakpoints. *Genomics* 14: 657–665.

Gorski JL, Estrada L, Hu C, Liu Z (2000). Skeletal-specific expression of *Fgd1* during bone formation and skeletal defects in faciogenital dysplasia (FGDY; Aarskog syndrome). *Dev Dyn* 218: 573–586.

Grier RE, Farrington FH, Kendig R, Mamunes P (1983). Autosomal dominant inheritance of the Aarskog syndrome. *Am J Med Genet* 15: 39–46.

Grigoridadis AE, Wang Z-Q, Wagner EF (1996). Regulation of bone cell differentiation and bone remodelling by the c-Fos/AP-1 transcription factor. In: *Principles of Bone Biology*. Bilezikian JP, Raisz LG, Rodan GA (eds.) Academic Press, San Diego, pp. 1253–1265.

Gulli M-P, Peter M (2001). Temporal and spatial regulation of Rho-type guanine nucleotide exchange factors: the yeast perspective. *Genes Dev* 15: 365–379.

Hacker U, Perrimon N (1998). DRhoGEF2 encodes a member of the Dbl family of oncogenes and controls cell shape changes during gastrulation in *Drosophila*. *Genes Dev* 12: 274–284.

Hall A (1998). Rho GTPases and the actin cytoskeleton. *Science* 279: 509–514.

Hanley WB, McKusick V, Barranci FT (1967). Osteochondritis dissecans and associated malformations in two brothers. *J Bone Jt Surg* 44A: 925.

Harlan JE, Hajduk PJ, Yoon HS, Fesik SW (1994). Pleckstrin homology domains bind to phosphatidylinosital-4,5-biphosphate. *Nature* 371: 168–170.

Hassinger DD, Mulvihill JJ, Chandler JB (1980). Aarskog syndrome with Hirschprung's disease, midgut malrotation, and dental anomalies. *J Med Genet* 17: 235–237.

Hedgecock EM, Culotti JG, Hall DH, Stern BD (1987). Genetics of cell and axon migrations in *Caenorhabditis elegans*. *Development* 100: 365–382.

Honoki K, Tsutsumi M, Tsujiuchi T, Kondoh S, Shiraiwa K, Miyauchi Y, Mii Y, Tamai S, Konishi Y, Bowden GT (1992). Expression of the transin, c-*fos*, and c-*jun* genes in rat transplantable osteosarcomas and malignant fibrous histiocytomas. *Mol Carcinog* 6: 122–128.

Ilvesaro J, Metsikko K, Vaananen K, Tuukkanen J (1999). Polarity of soteoblasts and osteoblast-like UMR-108 cells. *J Bone Miner Res* 14: 1338–1344.

Joberty G, Petersen C, Gao L, Macara I G (2000). The cell-polarity protein Par6 links Par3 and atypical protein kinase C to Cdc42. *Nat Cell Biol* 2: 531–539.

Kavanaugh WM, Turck CW, Williams LT (1995). PTB domain binding to signaling proteins through a sequence motif containing phosphotyrosine. *Science* 268: 1177–1179.

Kemphues K (2000). PARsing embryonic polarity. *Cell* 101: 345–348.

Kirkham TH, Milot J, Berman P (1975). Ophthalmic manifestations of Aarskog (facial-digital-genital) syndrome. *Am J Ophthalmol* 79: 441–445.

Kodama M, Fujimoto S, Namikawa T, Matsuda I (1981). Aarskog syndrome with isolated growth hormone deficiency. *Eur J Pediatr* 135: 273–276.

Korschewski R, Hall A, Mellman I (1999). Cdc42 controls secretory and endocytic transport to the basolateral plasma membrane of MDCK cells. *Nat Cell Biol* 1: 8–13.

Lemmon MA, Ferguson KM, Schlessinger J (1996). PH domains: diverse sequences with a common fold recruit signaling molecules to the cell surface. *Cell* 85: 621–624.

Li N, Batzer A, Daly R, Yajnik V, Skolnik E, Chardin P, Bar-Sagi D, Margolis B, Schlessinger J (1993). Guanine-nucleotide-releasing factor hSos1 binds to Grb2 and links receptor tyrosine kinases to Ras signaling. *Nature* 363: 85–88.

Lin D, Edwards AS, Fawcett JP, Mbamalu G, Scott JD, Pawson T (2000). A mammalian PAR-3–PAR-6 complex implicated in Cdc42/Rac1 and aPKC signaling and cell polarity. *Nat Cell Biol* 2: 540–547.

Lynch MP, Stein JL, Stein GS, Lian JB (1995). The influence of type I collagen on the development and maintenance of the osteoblast phenotype in primary and passaged rat calvarial osteoblasts: modification of expression of genes supporting cell growth, and extracellular matrix mineralization. *Exp Cell Res* 216: 35–45.

Luo L, Liao YJ, Jan LY, Jan YN (1994). Distinct morphogenetic functions of similar small GTPases: *Drosophila* Drac1 is involved in axonal outgrowth and myoblast fusion. *Genes Dev* 8: 1787–1802.

Machesky LM, Mullins RD, Higgs HN, Kaiser DA, Blanchoin L, May RC, Hall ME, Pollard TD (1999). Scar, a WASp-related protein, activates nucleation of actin filaments by the Arp2/3 complex. *Proc Natl Acad Sci USA* 96: 3739–3744.

Marsh ME, Munne AM, Vogel JJ, Cui Y, Franceschi RT (1995). Mineralization of bone-like extracellular matrix in the absence of functional osteoblasts. *J Bone Miner Res* 10: 1635–1643.

Masi L, Franchi A, Santucci M, Danielli D, Arganini L, Giannone V, Formigli L, Benvenuti S, Tanini A, Beghe F, et al. 1992). Adhesion, growth, and matrix production by osteoblasts on collagen substrata. *Calcif Tissue Int* 51: 202–212.

Mayer BJ, Ren R, Clark KL, Baltimore D (1993). A putative modular domain present in diverse signaling proteins. *Cell* 73: 629–630.

Melnick M, Shields ED (1976). Aarskog syndrome: new oral-facial findings. *Clin Genet* 9: 20–24.

Nagata K, Lamarche N, Gorski JL, Hall A (1998). Activation of G_1 progression, JNK MAP kinase and actin filament assembly by the exchange factor FGD1. *J Biol Chem* 273: 15453–15457.

Nelson FK, Albert PS, Riddle DL (1983). Fine structure of the *Caenorhabditis elegans* secretory-excretory system. *J Ultrastruct Res* 82: 156–171.

Nobes CA, Hall A (1999). Rho GTPases control polarity, protrusion, and adhesion during cell movement. *J Cell Biol* 144: 1235–1244.

Obaishi H, Nakanishi H, Mandai K, Satoh K, Satoh A, Takahashi K, Miyahara M, Nishioka H, Takaishi K, Takai Y (1998). Frabin, a novel FGD1-related actin filament-binding protein capable of changing cell shape and activating c-Jun N-terminal kinase. *J Biol Chem* 273: 18697–18700.

Olson MF, Pasteris NG, Gorski JL, Hall A (1996). Faciogenital dysplasia protein (FGD1) and Vav, two related proteins required for normal embryonic development are upstream regulators of Rho GTPases. *Curr Biol* 6: 1628–1633.

Orrico A, Galli L, Falciani M, Bracci M, Cavaliere ML, Rinaldi MM, Musacchio A, Sorrentino V (2000). A mutation in the pleckstrin homology (PH) domain of the FGD1 gene in an Italian family with faciogenital dysplasia (Aarskog-Scott syndrome). *FEBS Lett* 478: 216–220.

Pasteris NG, Gorski JL (1999). Isolation, characterization, and mapping of the mouse and human *Fgd2* genes, faciogenital dysplasia (FGD1; Aarskog syndrome) gene homologues. *Genomics* 60: 57–66.

Pasteris NG, Cadle A, Logie LJ, Porteous MEM, Schwartz CE, Stevenson RE, Glover TW, Wilroy RS, Gorski JL (1994). Isolation and characterization of the faciogenital dysplasia (Aarskog-Scott syndrome) gene: a putative Rho/Rac guanine nucleotide exchange factor. *Cell* 79: 669–678.

Pasteris NG, de Gouyon B, Cadle AB, Campbell K, Herman GE, Gorski JL (1995). Cloning and regional localization of the mouse faciogenital dysplasia (*Fgd1*) gene. *Mamm Genome* 6: 658–661.

Pasteris NG, Buckler JM, Cadle AB, Gorski JL (1997). Genomic organization of the faciogenital dysplasia (FGD1; Aarskog syndrome) gene. *Genomics* 43: 390–394.

Pasteris NG, Nagata K, Hall A, Gorski JL (2000). Isolation, characterization, and mapping of the mouse *Fgd3* gene, a new faciogenital dysplasia (FGD1; Aarskog syndrome) gene homologue. *Gene* 242: 237–247.

Piper RC, Cooper AA, Yang H, Stevens TH (1995). VPS27 controls vacuolar and endocytic traffic through a prevacuolar compartment in *Saccharomyces cerevisiae*. *J Cell Biol* 131: 603–617.

Porteous MEM, Goudie DR (1991). Aarskog syndrome. *J Med Genet* 28: 44–47.

Porteous MEM, Curtis A, Lindsay S, Williams O, Goudie D, Kamakari S, Bhattacharya SS (1992). The gene for Aarskog syndrome is located between DXS255 and DXS566 (Xp11.2–Xq13) *Genomics* 14: 298–301.

Price LS, Leng J, Schwartz MA, Bokoch GM (1998). Activation of Rac and Cdc42 by integrins mediates cell spreading. *Mol Biol Cell* 9: 1863–1871.

Qiu RG, Abo A, McCormick F, Symons M (1997). Cdc42 regulates anchorage-independent growth and is necessary for Ras transformation. *Mol Cell Biol* 17: 3449–3458.

Reddien PW, Horvitz HR (2000). CED-2/CrkII and CED-10/Rac control phagocytosis and cell migration in *Caenorhabditis elegans*. *Nat Cell Biol* 2: 131–136.

Ren R, Mayer BJ, Cicchetti P, Baltimore D (1993). Identification of a ten-amino acid proline-rich SH3 binding site. *Science* 259: 1157–1161.

Riesgo-Escovar JR, Jenni M, Fritz A, Hafen E (1996). The *Drosophila* Jun-N-terminal kinase is required for cell morphogenesis but not for Djun-dependent cell fate specification in the eye. *Genes Dev* 10: 2759–2768.

Rodan GA, Martin TJ (2000). Therapeutic approaches to bone diseases. *Science* 289: 1508–1514.

Rohatgi R, Ma L, Miki H, Lopez M, Kirchhausen T, Takenawa T, Kirschner MW (1999). The interaction between N-WASP and the Arp2/3 complex links Cdc42-dependent signals to actin assembly. *Cell* 97: 221–231.

Rozakis-Adcock M, Fernley R, Wade J, Pawson T, Bowtell D (1993). The SH2 and SH3 domains of mammalian Grb2 couple the EGF receptor to the Ras activator mSos1. *Nature* 363: 83–85.

Schoenwaelder SM, Burridge K (1999). Biderectional signaling between the cytoskeleton and integrins. *Curr Opin Cell Biol* 11: 274–286.

Schule R, Umesono K, Mangelsdorf D, Bolado J, Pike JW, Evans RM (1990). Jun-Fos and receptors for vitamins A and D recognize a common response element in the human osteocalcin gene. *Cell* 61: 497–504.

Schwartz CE, Gillessenkaesbach G, May M, Cappa M, Gorski JL, Steindl K, Neri G (2000). Two novel mutations confirm FGD1 is responsible for the Aarskog syndrome. *Eur J Hum Genet* 8: 869–874.

Scott CI (1971). Unusual facies, joint hypermobility, genital anomaly and short stature: a new dysmorphic syndrome. *Birth Defects* 7(6): 240–246.

Simonsen A, Lippe R, Christoforidis S, Gaullier J-M, Brech A, Callaghan J, Toh B-H, Murphy C, Zerial M, Stenmark H (1998). EEA1 links PI(3)K function to Rab5 regulation of endosome fusion. *Nature* 394: 494–498.

Stein GS, Lian JB (1993). Molecular mechanisms mediating developmental and hormone-regulated expression of genes in osteoblasts. In: *Cellular and Molecular Biology of Bone*. Noda M (ed.) Academic Press, San Diego, pp. 48–95.

Stevenson RE, May M, Arena JF, Millar EA, Scott CI Jr, Schroer RJ, Simensen RJ, Lubs HA, Schwartz CE (1994). Aarskog-Scott syndrome: confirmation of linkage to the pericentric region of the X chromosome. *Am J Med Genet* 52: 339–345.

Symons M, Derry JMJ, Karlak B, Jiang S, Lemahieau V, McCormick F, Francke U, Abo A (1996). Wiskott-Aldrich syndrome protein, a novel effector for the GTPase Cdc42Hs, is implicated in actin polymerization. *Cell* 84: 723–734.

Taybi H (1983). *Radiology of Syndromes and Metabolic Disorders, 2nd Edition*. Year Book Medical Publishers, Chicago.

Teebi AS, Rucquoi JK, Meyn MS (1993). Aarskog syndrome: report of a family with review and discussion of nosology. *Am J Med Genet* 46: 501–509.

Tibbles LA, Ing YL, Kiefer F, Chan J, Iscove N, Woodgett JR, Lassam NJ (1996). MLK-3 activates the SAPK/JNK and p38/RK pathways via SEK1 and MKK3/6. *EMBO J* 15: 7026–7035.

Touhara K, Inglese J, Pitcher JA, Shaw G, Lefkowitz RJ (1994). Binding of G protein $\beta\gamma$-subunits to pleckstrin homology domains. *J Biol Chem* 269: 10217–10220.

Treisman R (1996). Regulation of transcription by MAP kinase cascades. *Curr Opin Cell Biol* 8: 205–215.

Van Aelst L, D'Souza-Schorey C (1997). Rho GTPases and signaling networks. *Genes Dev* 11: 2295–2322.

van de Vooren MJ, Niermeijer MF, Hoogeboom JM (1983). The Aarskog syndrome in a large family, suggestive for autosomal dominant inheritance. *Clin Genet* 24: 439–445.

Ward JM, Young D (1976). Histogenesis and morphology of periosteal sarcomas induced by FBJ virus in NIH Swiss mice. *Cancer Res* 36: 3985–3992.

Weisman LS, Wickner W (1992). Molecular characterization of VAC1, a gene required for vacuole inheritance and vacuole protein sorting. *J Biol Chem* 267: 618–623.

Whitehead IP, Campbell S, Rossman KL, Der CJ (1997). Dbl family proteins. *Biochim et Biophys Acta* 1332: F1–F23.

Whitehead IP, Abe K, Gorski JL, Der CJ (1998). Cdc42 and FGD1 cause distinct signaling and transforming activities. *Mol Cell Biol* 18: 4689–4697.

Wu WJ, Erickson JW, Lin R, Cerione RA (2000). The γ-subunit of the coatomer complex binds Cdc42 to mediate transformation. *Nature* 405: 800–804.

Xiao G, Wang D, Benson MD, Karsenty G, Franceschi RT (1998). Role of the α_2-integrin in osteoblast-specific gene expression and activation of the Osf2 transcription factor. *J Biol Chem* 273: 32988–32994.

Yamamoto A, DeWald DB, Boronenkov IV, Anderson RA, Emr SD, Koshland D (1995). Novel PI(4)P 5-kinase homologue, Fab1p, essential for normal vacuole function and morphology in yeast. *Mol Biol Cell* 6: 525–539.

Zheng Y, Fischer DJ, Tigyi G, Pasteris NG, Gorski JL, Xu Y (1996). The faciogenital dysplasia gene product FGD1 functions as a Cdc42Hs-specific guanine-nucleotide exchange factor. *J Biol Chem* 271: 33169–33172.

Zhou K, Wang Y, Gorski JL, Nomura N, Collard J, Bokoch GM (1998). Guanine nucleotide exchange factors regulate specificity of downstream signaling from Rac and Cdc42. *J Biol Chem* 273: 16782–16786.

Zipkin ID, Kindt RM, Kenyon CJ (1997). Role of a new Rho family member in cell migration and axon guidance in *C. elegans*. *Cell* 90: 883–894.

87 | *NF1* and Neurofibromatosis 1

LAURA A. JANSEN AND DAVID H. GUTMANN

NEUROFIBROMIN

Structure and Function

The neurofibromatosis 1 (NF1) gene product is a 220–250 kDa protein termed neurofibromin (DeClue et al, 1991, Gutmann et al., 1991; Figure 87–1C). It is expressed in a wide variety of tissues, including brain, spinal cord, peripheral nerve, adrenal gland, and Schwann cells, with smaller amounts in liver, spleen, pancreas, and cardiac tissue (DeClue et al., 1991; Gutmann et al. 1991; Daston et al., 1992; Huynh et al., 1994). Within the cell, neurofibromin is localized in the cytoplasm and may be associated with microtubules (Gregory et al., 1993). The protein does not appear to undergo glycosylation or other posttranslational processing events, but it may be phosphorylated (Gutmann and Collins, 1993).

Analysis of the sequence of neurofibromin revealed a region of high similarity to the catalytic domains of the mammalian p120RasGAP and yeast IRA1 and IRA2 (Xu et al., 1990a; Figure 87–1C). These proteins function as GTPase-activating proteins (GAPs) for Ras. Ras is a small GTP-binding protein with diverse functions in the regulation of cell growth and differentiation, as well as oncogenesis (see Chapter 84). Ras activity is tightly regulated (Figure 87–2). Ras is active when bound to GTP and inactive when bound to GDP. GAPs greatly enhance the slow intrinsic GTPase activity of Ras, thereby serving to increase the conversion of active Ras-GTP to inactive Ras-GDP, and thus inhibit Ras activity (Weiss et al., 1999). Ras becomes oncogenic as a result of mutations that impair its inability to hydrolyze GTP, resulting in a constitutively active Ras-GTP, leading to dysregulated cell growth (Wittinghofer, 1998).

Neurofibromin has been shown to function as a GAP for Ras through multiple experimental approaches. Expression of the *NF1* GAP-related domain (GRD) is able to complement mutations in the yeast IRA1 and IRA2 GAP molecules. Peptides containing the *NF1*-GRD as well as full-length neurofibromin, have been demonstrated to directly stimulate the GTPase activity of Ras proteins (Ballester et al., 1990; Martin et al., 1990; Xu et al., 1990b; Bollag et al., 1996). Interestingly, the alternatively spliced type II neurofibromin has reduced GAP activity compared to the type I protein (Andersen et al., 1993). Finally, as will be detailed in this chapter, cell lines and tumors deficient in neurofibromin have absent neurofibromin GAP activity and elevated levels of Ras-GTP.

Neurofibromin likely has functions above and beyond its ability to act as a GAP molecule, since the GAP-related domain comprises just 10% of the protein (Cichowski and Jacks, 2001). In *Drosophila*, the highly conserved NF1 protein has been linked to regulation of the adenylyl cyclase pathway (Guo et al., 1997). Furthermore, neurofibromin binds tubulin and may modulate cellular function through effects on microtubules (Bollag et al., 1993; Xu and Gutmann 1997).

Role of the *NF1* Gene in Development and Differentiation

If the major function of neurofibromin relates to its function as a GAP for Ras, then consideration of its role in differentiation can be addressed by reviewing the Ras signal transduction pathway in development. This has been well studied in *Drosophila*, where expression of an activated Ras1 mutant induces R7 photoreceptor neuron differentiation and also causes nonneuronal cell precursors to form R7 cells (Fortini et al., 1992). Raf-1 acts downstream of Ras, and in *Drosophila*

raf-1 mutants, the development of the posterior three abdominal segments of the fly is affected (Hamilton, 1994).

The actions of many growth factors are at least partially mediated by Ras. DNA synthesis in fibroblasts induced by platelet-derived growth factor, epidermal growth factor, and insulin is blocked by anti-Ras antibodies or dominant inhibitory mutants of Ras (Hamilton, 1994). A dominant *raf*-1 mutant injected into *Xenopus* embryos blocked mesoderm induction by fibroblast growth factor (MacNicol et al., 1993). In PC12 rat pheochromocytoma cells, neurite outgrowth and neuronal differentiation induced by nerve growth factor is mediated by Ras and can be abrogated using Ras antibodies or inhibitory Ras mutant molecules (Hamilton, 1994).

Injection of activated Ras protein into mouse 3T3 fibroblasts stimulated cell growth and induced transformation (Stacey and Kung, 1984). However, other studies have suggested that cell transformation by Ras requires other chemical or genetic factors (Newbold and Overell, 1983; Kinsella et al., 1990). In contrast to fibroblasts, activated *Ras* expression in rat Schwann cells causes growth arrest in the G1 or G1/S phase of the cell cycle. Co-expression of another oncogene together with activated *Ras* in these Schwann cells results in cell division and transformation (Ridley et al., 1988). Similarly, injection of Ras proteins into *Xenopus* oocytes induces maturation (Birchmeier et al., 1985). Collectively, these results suggest a complex role for Ras in oncogenesis, development, and differentiation.

Interestingly, despite its important role in growth and differentiation, there is no evidence for regulation of *Ras* expression during development. In contrast, the expression of neurofibromin is modulated and may function as a method of developmentally regulating Ras activity (Daston and Ratner, 1993; Huynh et al., 1994). In the developing mouse, *Nf1* mRNA is detected as early as embryonic day 8 (E8), predominantly in the primitive central nervous system (CNS), the first branchial arch, and the heart. *Nf1* expression undergoes a marked increase at E11, where it becomes detectable in all embryonic tissues. Type II *Nf1* transcripts predominate between E8 to E10, whereas type I transcripts are most abundantly expressed from E11 through E16 (Huynh et al., 1994). In the developing rat, type I *Nf1* expression is seen in the cerebral cortex, brainstem, and cerebellum throughout embryogenesis. However, in dorsal root ganglia and spinal cord motor neurons, there is an increase in type II mRNA expression as development progresses. In addition, abundant *Nf1* expression is detected into the second postnatal week in the kidney, lung, muscle, and heart, but it is absent in adult tissues (Gutmann et al., 1995).

In human fetal peripheral nerves, neurofibromin is barely detectable during the first trimester of gestation. However, during the second and third trimesters, its expression increases dramatically in Schwann cells, perineurial cells, and axons (Wrabetz et al., 1995; Hirvonen et al., 1998). The CNS-specific isoform of *Nf1* containing the alternatively spliced exon 9a is also regulated during mouse development, as its expression was first detected after postnatal day 2 and increased between P4 and P7 (Geist and Gutmann, 1996; Gutmann et al., 1999b).

CLINICAL DESCRIPTION

NF1 (OMIM 162200) is a common genetic disorder with an estimated prevalence of approximately 1 in 3500, regardless of gender, ethnic background, or race (Friedman, 1999). It is transmitted in an autosomal dominant inheritance pattern with complete penetrance, but variable expressivity.

A. *NF1* genomic DNA-350 kb

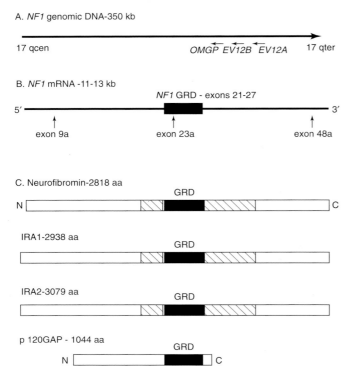

17 qcen   *OMGP EV12B EV12A*   17 qter

B. *NF1* mRNA -11-13 kb

5'   *NF1* GRD - exons 21-27   3'

exon 9a   exon 23a   exon 48a

C. Neurofibromin-2818 aa

GRD

N   C

IRA1-2938 aa

GRD

IRA2-3079 aa

GRD

p 120GAP - 1044 aa

GRD

N   C

Figure 87–1. *NF1* (*A*) gene, (*B*) mRNA, and (*C*) protein structure with areas of homology to other GTPase-activating proteins (GAPs). The presence of the alternatively splicing exons (9a, 23a, and 48a) is shown relative to the GAP-related domain (GRD). Neurofibromin contains regions (shaded areas) with sequence similarity to the yeast IRA proteins.

Fredrick von Recklinghausen first described the clinical features of NF1 in 1882. The most readily recognized features include café-au-lait macules (Fig. 87–3), pigmented iris hamartomas (Lisch nodules), axillary freckling, and dermal and plexiform neurofibromas (Fig. 87–4). Patients with NF1 are predisposed to a variety of benign and malignant tumors, including malignant peripheral nerve sheath tumors (MPNSTs),

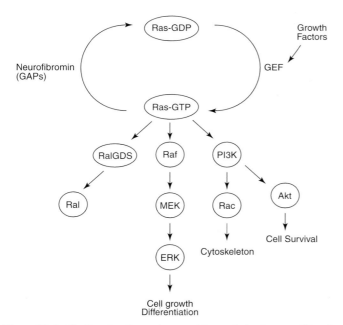

Figure 87–2. The Ras signaling pathway and its regulation by neurofibromin. Neurofibromin as a GAP molecule accelerates the conversion of Ras from its active GTP-bound form to an inactive GDP-bound state. Guanine exchange factors (GEFs) serve to reactivate Ras.

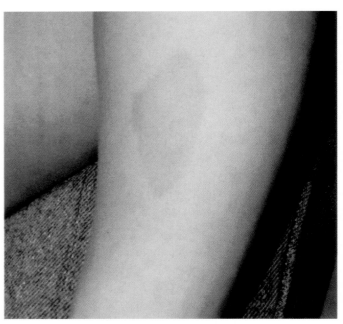

Figure 87–3. Café-au-lait macule on the arm of an individual with neurofibromatosis 1 (NF1).

optic pathway gliomas (Fig. 87–5) and other central nervous system astrocytomas, pheochromocytomas, and juvenile chronic myelogenous leukemia (JCML) (Gutmann et al., 1997; Friedman et al., 1999). There are also many common non-tumor manifestations of NF1, including learning disabilities, macrocephaly, short stature, bony abnormalities, scoliosis, headache, and seizures (North, 2000). Another frequent find-

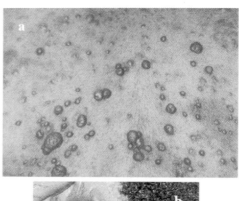

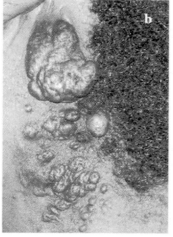

Figure 87–4. (*a*) Dermal neurofibromas in an adult with NF1. (*b*) Facial plexiform neurofibroma in an adult with NF1.

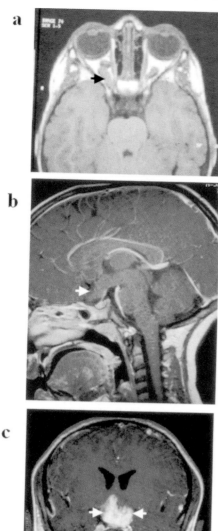

Figure 87–5. Gliomas in NF1. (*a*) Optic nerve glioma in a child with NF1. Arrow denotes swollen and kinked right optic nerve. (*b*) Sagittal section of optic pathway glioma demonstrating both nerve and chiasmal involvement (arrow) in a child with NF1. (*c*) Hypothalamic glioma in a child with NF1 with the tumor extent delineated by the arrows.

ing in individuals with NF1 is T2-weighted hyperintensities on brain MRI imaging (unidentified bright objects, or UBOs), present in 60% to 70% of children with the disease. These are typically located in the basal ganglia, thalamus, brainstem, and cerebellum (North et al., 1997). The pathologic basis of these lesions remains uncertain but does not seem to involve dysplasia or hamartoma development (DiPaolo et al., 1995).

Manifestations of NF1 vary with the developmental age of the patient. Congenitally, the most common features are café-au-lait spots, plexiform neurofibromas, and tibial dysplasia. Axillary freckling and optic pathway gliomas most often make their appearance in the preschool-aged child. Learning disabilities are often diagnosed when the child reaches school age. Dermal neurofibromas tend to appear around the time of puberty and continue to develop during the lifetime of the individual (Gutmann et al., 1997).

NF1 GENE

The *NF1* gene was isolated in 1990 through positional cloning. Linkage was established to the proximal long arm of chromosome 17, and through analysis of individuals with NF1 harboring translocations in-

volving the chromosomal region 17q11.2, cDNA clones of the *NF1* gene were identified (Cawthon et al., 1990; Viskochil et al., 1990; Wallace et al., 1990). The *NF1* gene was found to be quite large, spanning over 350 kb of genomic DNA (Fig. 87–1A). The gene encodes an mRNA of 11 to 13 kb composed of at least 59 exons (Marchuk et al., 1991; Fig. 87–1B). Multiple alternatively spliced *NF1* transcripts have been identified. The most abundant of these are termed type I and type II, which differ in that the type II transcript contains exon 23a, which is excluded in type I (Skuse and Cappione, 1997). *NF1* transcripts have been found to be expressed in a wide variety of tissues, including brain, peripheral nerve, kidney, spleen, stomach, lung, colon, lymphoid cells, skin fibroblasts, and skeletal and cardiac muscle (Huynh et al., 1994; Gutmann et al., 1995). In adult rat tissues, the type I *NF1* transcript predominates in central nervous system neurons and dorsal root ganglia, while the type II transcript predominates in adrenal medullary and Schwann cells (Gutmann et al., 1995). Another *NF1* isoform, containing the alternatively spliced exon 9a, is expressed exclusively in CNS neurons (Geist and Gutmann, 1996; Gutmann et al., 1999b). A final *NF1* mRNA isoform containing the alternatively spliced exon 48a is expressed in high levels in cardiac, skeletal, and smooth muscle (Gutmann et al., 1993).

Approximately one-half of NF1 cases represent new mutations. This proportion of new mutations suggests a high mutational rate for the *NF1* gene, which has been estimated to be about 100-fold higher than the average mutation rate. The exact reason for the high mutational rate is unknown but likely involves a combination of the large size of the *NF1* gene, its genomic position, the presence of GpC dinucleotide "hot spots," and the influence of several pseudogenes (Legius et al., 1992; Cummings et al., 1996; Shen et al., 1996; Lopez-Correa et al., 2001). Interestingly, over 80% of new mutations have been found to be paternal in origin (Friedman, 1999), suggesting that these mutations may occur during male gametogenesis. Although more than 100 different germline *NF1* mutations have been reported, there has been no consistent relationship between mutation size, type, or location and phenotypic expression. It is well known that patients with identical mutations often have different NF1-associated manifestations.

DIAGNOSIS OF NF1

The NIH Consensus Development Conference originally developed criteria for the diagnosis of NF1 in 1988. Individuals can be given the diagnosis of NF1 if two or more of the following features are present: (*1*) six or more café-au-lait macules more than 5 mm in greatest diameter in prepubertal individuals or more than 15 mm in diameter after puberty, (*2*) two or more neurofibromas of any type or one plexiform neurofibroma, (*3*) freckling in the axillary or inguinal regions, (*4*) an optic pathway tumor, (*5*) two or more Lisch nodules, (*6*) sphenoid wing dysplasia or thinning of the cortex of the long bones, and (*7*) a first-degree relative with NF1 by the above criteria (NIH Consensus Development Conference, 1988; Gutmann et al., 1997).

Despite the substanial progress made in the characterization of the *NF1* gene, the diagnosis of NF1 remains a clinical one. Attempts at developing a universal molecular diagnostic approach have been hampered by several factors. As mentioned, approximately 50% of NF1 cases result from new mutations, the *NF1* gene is very large, and over 100 different germline mutations have been identified (Shen et al., 1996). Therefore, undertaking a mutational search in each individual with NF1 would be very laborious. Identification of the specific mutation transmitted in a family affected by NF1 could allow for prenatal diagnosis. However, given the extreme clinical variability in people with the same mutation, no prediction of the manifestations or severity of disease can be made, therefore limiting the usefulness of a prenatal diagnosis (Gutmann et al., 1997).

Proposed Therapies for NF1

Currently, the only therapies available to NF1 patients are conventional treatments that employ surgery or chemotherapeutic agents used for sporadic tumors. However, based on the known functions of the *NF1* gene, targeted therapies have been proposed which address the fundamental pathogenesis of the disease. If the critical function of neurofibromin relates to its ability to inhibit Ras activity, then therapies that result in inhibition of Ras or its downstream effectors may have beneficial effects. One group of compounds—the farnesyl transferase inhibitors, which prevent the addition of a farnesyl group to the CAAX sequence on Ras to allow its translocation to the membrane—have reached early clinical trials (Cox and Der, 1997; Gibbs and Oliff, 1997; Scharovsky et al., 2000; Reed and Gutmann, 2001). These compounds were found to inhibit the growth of NF1-deficient MPNST and myeloid cells in vitro (Yan et al., 1996; Mahgoub et al., 1999b). Compounds that inhibit downstream components of the Ras signaling pathway, such as MEK and phosphoinositol 3-kinase, have also been suggested as possible therapeutic agents in NF1 (Weiss et al., 1999).

Animal Models of NF1

Numerous animal models of NF1 have been developed. In 1994, two groups produced mice with a null mutation at the Nf1 locus (Brannan et al., 1994; Jacks et al., 1994). These mutants demonstrated severe developmental defects. Homozygous Nf1$^{-/-}$ mice die by 14.5 days postcoitum from cardiac failure due to the presence of a double-outlet right ventricle. Further analysis of hearts from these animals revealed overabundant tissue in the endocardial cushions thought to be due to failure of the normal transition from cell proliferation to differentiation and apoptosis (Lakkis and Epstein, 1998). A small percentage (12.5%) of Nf1$^{-/-}$ embryos also show exencephaly in addition to their cardiac defects (Lakkis et al., 1999). Hyperplasia of the sympathetic (Brannan et al., 1994) and dorsal root (Lakkis et al., 1999) ganglia was also reported in Nf1$^{-/-}$ embryos. Schwann cells isolated from Nf1$^{-/-}$ mice exhibited increased Ras-GTP levels, as well as growth inhibition and morphological changes similar to those seen in Schwann cells expressing activated Ras (Kim et al., 1995).

Mice heterozygous for a targeted mutation in the Nf1 gene have been studied in detail. Interestingly, none of these animals develop the neurofibromas, pigmentation defects, or Lisch nodules that are seen in patients with NF1. However, these animals did have an increased rate of tumorigenesis, including adrenal tumors, pheochromocytomas, leukemia, and lymphoma (Jacks et al., 1994). In Nf1$^{+/-}$ mice that developed leukemia, the majority showed loss of heterozygosity (LOH) at the Nf1 locus in hematopoietic tissues (Mahgoub et al., 1999a). Nf1$^{+/-}$ mice have impaired spatial learning and memory (Silva et al., 1997), perhaps paralleling the learning disabilities seen in children with NF1. Astrogliosis, increased astrocyte proliferation, and elevated glial fibrillary acid protein (GFAP) expression have been found in the brains of Nf1$^{+/-}$ mice, which may contribute to the learning deficits in NF1 (Gutmann et al., 1999a; Rizvi et al., 1999; Bajenaru et al., 2001).

To overcome the lethality of the Nf1$^{-/-}$ mutation, alternative strategies have been used, including tissue-specific conditional Nf1 gene disruption, exon-specific ablation, and chimeric mice. Use of a conditional mutation allows induction of Nf1 deficiency in a given cell population, thereby allowing study of the results of Nf1 deficiency in that population while circumventing the embryonic lethality. Using the Cre/loxP system, one group has studied a conditional Nf1 gene mutation that affects neurons (Zhu et al., 2001). A neuronal-specific Cre recombinase transgenic mouse strain was generated by placing Cre recombinase expression under control of the Synapsin I promoter, which drives expression specifically in neurons. These mice were crossed with transgenic mice harboring loxP sites, which flanked exons 31 and 32 in the Nf1 gene. The resultant animals lose Nf1 function in neurons due to NF1 inactivation by Cre-mediated recombination. These neuronal conditional mutants exhibited growth retardation and cerebral astrogliosis, but tumor formation was not seen (Zhu et al., 2001).

Recent studies on Nf1 astrocyte-specific conditional knockout mice have demonstrated that loss of neurofibromin in astrocytes results in increased astrocyte proliferation, supporting the notion that the NF1 gene is a critical growth regulator for astrocytes (Bajenaru et al., unpublished results).

Utilization of exon-specific knockouts has been used to shed light on the functions of the alternatively spliced NF1 variants. A mutant mouse lacking only type II Nf1, generated by deletion of exon 23a, showed impaired spatial learning, abnormal contextual discrimination, and delayed motor skill acquisition, but no tumor formation (Costa et al., 2001). This suggests that type II Nf1 may be important in normal brain development and intellectual function.

The generation of chimeric mice, producing Nf1 loss in some, but not all, cell populations, avoids embryonic lethality while allowing the analysis of the effects of congenital Nf1 deficiency. One group created Nf1$^{-/-}$ chimeric mice through formation of Nf1-deficient embryonic stem cells, which were injected into normal blastocysts. Most of these animals developed multiple plexiform neurofibromas, as well as frequent myelodysplasia, progressive neuromotor defects, and a reduced life span (Cichowski et al., 1999). These findings support the idea that plexiform neurofibromas in humans with NF1 may result from congenital disruption of the NF1 gene.

Additional insights into malignant tumor development were provided by studies of mice harboring both Nf1 and p53 tumor suppressor mutations. Mice who are p53$^{-/-}$ develop lymphomas and hemangiosarcomas by 6 months of age, and p53$^{+/-}$ mice develop osteosarcomas after 9 months of age. When p53$^{+/-}$ and Nf1$^{+/-}$ mice were crossed to produce compound heterozygotes with the genotype Nf1$^{+/-}$; p53$^{+/-}$, accelerated tumor formation was seen (Cichowski et al., 1999; Vogel et al., 1999). Most of these tumors were soft-tissue sarcomas, and a significant portion of these were classified as malignant peripheral nerve sheath tumors. Nf1$^{+/-}$; p53$^{+/-}$ mice generated in a different genetic background developed malignant CNS astrocytomas rather than MPNSTs, suggesting additional genetic contributions to the determination of malignant tumor formation (Reilly et al., 2000). LOH at the Nf1 and p53 alleles was frequently demonstrated in these malignant tumors, supporting the second-hit hypothesis of tumor formation in NF1 (see below in this section) (Cichowski et al., 1999; Vogel et al., 1999; Reilly et al., 2000).

The role of NF1 has also been studied in Drosophila mutants. These results suggest that in Drosophila, NF1 acts as a regulator of both the cyclic AMP (cAMP) and Ras/MAPK (mitogen-activated protein kinase) pathways. NF1 mutant flies showed significant decrements in olfactory learning performance, which was rescued by heat-shock-induced expression of a NF1 transgene (Guo et al., 2000). When NF1 mutant flies were crossed with flies mutant for the rutabaga (rut)-encoded adenylyl cyclase, no further decrement in learning scores was seen, suggesting that NF1 acts through the cAMP pathway. In addition, heat-shock-induced expression of cAMP-dependent protein kinase (PKA) also rescued the learning deficit in NF1 mutant flies (Guo et al., 2000). These results suggest that the mechanism of learning deficits in Drosophila NF1 mutants is through effects on the cAMP pathway.

Studies of Drosophila NF1 mutants also provided evidence for functions of NF1 that are mediated by a pathway involving Ras and MAPK (Williams et al., 2001). Flies with null mutations in NF1 exhibited loss of locomotor circadian rhythms and elevated levels of activated MAPK. The circadian rhythms in these mutants were restored by crosses with flies harboring SOS^{e2H} (guanine nucleotide exchange factor loss-of-function mutation), Ras1^{e1B} (Ras protein mutation), or rl^{x162} (Drosophila MAPK mutation). All of these mutations result in inhibition of the Ras/MAPK pathway, suggesting that the mechanism of loss of circadian rhythms in Drosophila NF1 mutants involves inappropriate activation of Ras (Williams et al., 2001).

MOLECULAR PATHOGENESIS OF NF1-ASSOCIATED FEATURES

The mechanisms by which mutations in the NF1 gene produce the clinical manifestations of NF1 have been widely investigated, especially with respect to tumor formation. The most common tumor in NF1 is the dermal neurofibroma, a benign tumor of the peripheral nerve sheath. These tumors usually begin to appear around adolescence, can number in the hundreds to thousands, and are often disfiguring (Gutmann et al., 1997). Cell types within the dermal neurofibroma include Schwann cells, perineurial cells, fibroblasts, neurons, and mast cells (Peltonen et al., 1988). Plexiform neurofibromas also develop along the peripheral nerve, but they typically involve more than one nerve. These tumors are almost always congenital and can grow to large sizes (Korf 1999). Unlike dermal neurofibromas, plexiform neurofibromas can undergo malignant transformation (King et al., 2000).

There continues to be debate about the precise molecular pathogenesis of neurofibromas. One question involves the cell of origin for tumor formation. Current evidence suggests that the Schwann cell is the initiating cell type, and elevated Ras-GTP levels have been directly demonstrated in Schwann cells from neurofibromas (Sherman et al., 2000). A second question is whether the germline *NF1* mutation is sufficient to trigger neurofibroma development through haploinsufficiency or if a second-hit mutation or LOH is required (Fig. 87–6). This question has been difficult to answer, but studies have demonstrated a low frequency of second-hit mutations or LOH in benign neurofibromas (Colman et al., 1995; Sawada et al., 1996; Serra et al., 1997; Kluwe et al., 1999). Analysis of S100-positive Schwann cells isolated from dermal neurofibromas revealed the absence of *NF1* mRNA, which is consistent with a second genetic hit (Rutkowski et al., 2000). Similar results were obtained by direct analysis of neurofibromas in situ (Perry et al., 2001). One suggestion for the determining event that distinguishes the development of plexiform rather than dermal neurofibromas is the timing of the second-hit mutation: loss of the remaining wild-type *NF1* allele during fetal development may result in plexiform neurofibroma formation, whereas a second-hit mutation later in life could lead to dermal neurofibroma development. Alternatively, dermal neurofibroma formation may result from *NF1* haploinsufficiency combined with other factors, such as local trauma or hormonal changes (Cichowski and Jacks, 2001).

MPNSTs develop in at least 5% of NF1 patients (Ducatman et al., 1986; North, 2000). These tumors have a high rate of local recurrence and metastasis and are associated with poor long-term survival. Most, but not all, of these tumors arise at the site of a pre-existing plexiform neurofibroma (King et al., 2000). Studies have shown *p53* tumor-suppressor gene mutations or chromosome 17p deletions in MPNSTs from NF1 patients (Menon et al, 1990). Mutations in the *INK4* locus, which causes inactivation of the *p16INK4a* and *p14ARF* tumor-suppressor genes, have also been identified in MPNSTs (Legius et al., 1994; Kourea et al., 1999). These findings suggest that a second genetic event is required for the formation of these malignant tumors in NF1 patients.

The most common CNS tumor in NF1 patients is the optic glioma or astrocytoma, which is found in approximately 15% of cases (Listernick et al., 1997, 1999). Optic pathway gliomas are classified as grade I pilocytic astrocytomas, a low-grade tumor, but they can result in visual loss, proptosis, or precocious puberty (Listernick et al., 1997). Gliomas in NF1 can also affect the brainstem, where presenting symptoms include cranial neuropathies and hydrocephalus (Listernick et al., 1999). Astrogliosis has been found in brains from NF1 patients, with a greater number and larger size of GFAP-positive astrocytes (Nordlund et al., 1995). Studies of pilocytic astrocytomas from indi-

viduals affected with NF1 revealed no detectable neurofibromin expression (Gutmann et al., 2000) and increased Ras activity (Lau et al., 2000). These reports suggest that *NF1* haploinsufficiency results in increased astrocyte proliferation, while astrocytoma formation requires a second genetic hit (loss of *NF1* expression).

Children with NF1 harbor a 200-fold to 500-fold risk of developing juvenile chronic myelogenous leukemia over children without NF1. In 8 of 18 children with NF1 and malignant myeloid disorders, LOH at the *NF1* locus was found (Side et al., 1997). Bone marrow cells from individuals with NF1 and leukemia showed reduced neurofibromin GAP activity and elevated Ras-GTP levels (Bollag et al., 1996). These findings support the hypothesis that increased Ras activity results from decreased neurofibromin GAP function, which leads to tumor formation.

Café-au-lait macules in NF1 are composed of melanocytes with a higher content of melanin macroglobules (Kaufmann et al., 1989). Melanocytes and keratinocytes express neurofibromin (Malhotra and Ratner, 1994), and it is thought that the increased melanogenesis is related to a reduction in neurofibromin levels (Kaufmann et al., 1991). However, as opposed to the case in many NF1-associated tumors, LOH was not observed in melanocytes derived from café-au-lait macules (Stark et al., 1992). In addition, alteration of Ras-GTP regulation in melanocytes from NF1 patients was not seen (Griesser et al., 1995). This suggests that reduction in neurofibromin expression results in café-au-lait macule formation through a Ras-independent mechanism.

Learning disabilities are common in NF1, affecting between 30% and 65% of individuals. The mean IQ in patients with NF1 ranges between 89 and 94, with both language-based and nonverbal learning deficits detected (North et al., 1997). The high levels of neurofibromin expression within the CNS and the existence of a CNS-specific isoform of neurofibromin implicate neurofibromin in brain development (Gutmann, 1999). Several studies have found an association between T2 hyperintensities (UBOs) on magnetic resonance imaging (MRI) and cognitive dysfunction in children with NF1 (North et al., 1994; Moore et al., 1996; Samango-Sprouse et al., 1997). In some studies, the number and volume of the hyperintensities were correlated with IQ scores (Hofman et al., 1994). However, other studies have found no such association (Duffner et al., 1989; Dunn and Roos, 1989; Legius et al., 1995). The significance of these MRI lesions to the cognitive phenotype in NF1 remains unclear.

CONCLUSIONS

NF1 is a complex and protean disorder, the study of which has provided valuable insights into the roles of neurofibromin and Ras in development and differentiation. Studies of humans with NF1 and the use of NF1 animal models have demonstrated a critical role for neurofibromin in normal development and have supported the hypothesis that a second genetic event is necessary for tumorigenesis. In addition, loss of neurofibromin-mediated inhibition of Ras activity appears to be critical in NF1 pathogenesis. Further investigation is likely to produce important therapeutic advances, not only for individuals with NF1 but also for those with other disorders.

REFERENCES

Andersen LB, Ballester R, Marchuk DA, Chang E, Gutmann DH, Saulino AM, Camonis J, Wigler M, Collins FS (1993). A conserved alternative splice in the von Recklinghausen neurofibromatosis (NF1) gene produces two neurofibromin isoforms, both of which have GTPase-activating protein activity. *Mol Cell Biol* 13: 487–495.

Ballester R, Marchuk D, Boguski M, Saulino A, Letcher R, Wigler M, Collins F (1990). The NF1 locus encodes a protein functionally related to mammalian GAP and yeast IRA proteins. *Cell* 63: 851–859.

Bajenaru ML, Donahoe J, Corral T, Reilly KM, Brophy S, Pellicer A, Gutmann DH (2001). Neurofibromatosis 1 (NF1) heterozygosity results in a cell-autonomous growth advantage for astrocytes. *Glia* 33: 314–323.

Birchmeier C, Broek D, Wigler M (1985). Ras proteins can induce meiosis in *Xenopus* oocytes. *Cell* 43: 615–621.

Bollag G, McCormick F, Clark R (1993). Characterization of full-length neurofibromin: tubulin inhibits Ras GAP activity. *EMBO J* 12: 1923–1927.

Bollag G, Clapp DW, Shih S, Adler F, Zhang YY, Thompson P, Lange BJ, Freedman MH, McCormick F, Jacks T, Shannon K (1996). Loss of NF1 results in activation of the Ras signaling pathway and leads to aberrant growth in haematopoietic cells. *Nat Genet* 12: 144–148.

Brannan CI, Perkins AS, Vogel KS, Ratner N, Nordlund ML, Reid SW, Buchberg AM,

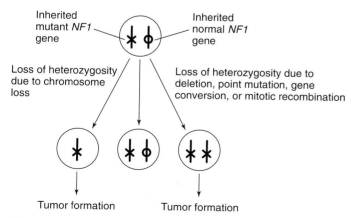

Figure 87–6. Mechanism of loss of heterozygosity and tumor formation in neurofibromatosis 1.

Jenkins NA, Parada LF, Copeland NG (1994). Targeted disruption of the neurofibromatosis type-1 gene leads to developmental abnormalities in heart and various neural crest-derived tissues. *Genes Dev* 8: 1019–1029.

Cawthon RM, Weiss R, Xu GF, Viskochil D, Culver M, Stevens J, Robertson M, Dunn D, Gesteland R, O'Connell P, et al. (1990). A major segment of the neurofibromatosis type 1 gene: cDNA sequence, genomic structure, and point mutations. *Cell* 62: 193–201.

Cichowski K, Jacks T (2001). NF1 tumor suppressor gene function: narrowing the GAP. *Cell* 104: 593–604.

Cichowski K, Shih TS, Schmitt E, Santiago S, Reilly K, McLaughlin ME, Bronson RT, Jacks T (1999). Mouse models of tumor development in neurofibromatosis type 1. *Science* 286: 2172–2176.

Colman SD, Williams CA, Wallace MR (1995). Benign neurofibromas in type 1 neurofibromatosis (NF1) show somatic deletions of the NF1 gene. *Nat Genet* 11: 90–92.

Costa RM, Yang T, Huynh DP, Pulst SM, Viskochil DH, Silva AJ, Brannan CI (2001). Learning deficits, but normal development and tumor predisposition, in mice lacking exon 23a of Nf1. *Nat Genet* 27: 399–405.

Cox AD, Der CJ (1997). Farnesyltransferase inhibitors and cancer tretment: targeting simply Ras? *Biochim Biophys Acta* 1333: F51–F71.

Cummings LM, Trent JM, Marchuk DA (1996). Identification and mapping of type 1 neurofibromatosis (NF1) homologous loci. *Cytogenet Cell Genet* 73: 334–340.

Daston MM, Ratner N (1993). Neurofibromin, a predominantly neuronal GTPase activating protein in the adult, is ubiquitously expressed during development. *Dev Dyn* 195: 216–226.

Daston MM, Crable H, Nordlund M, Sturbaum AK, Nissen LM, Ratner N (1992). The protein product of the neurofibromatosis type 1 gene is expressed at highest abundance in neurons, Schwann cells, and oligodendrocytes. *Neuron* 8: 415–428.

DeClue JE, Cohen BD, Lowy DR (1991). Identification and characterization of the neurofibromatosis type 1 protein product. *Proc Natl Acad Sci USA* 88: 9914–9918.

DiPaolo DP, Zimmerman RA, Rorke LB, Zackai EH, Bilaniuk LT, Yachnis AT (1995). Neurofibromatosis type 1: pathologic substrate of high-signal intensity foci in the brain. *Radiology* 195: 721–724.

Ducatman BS, Scheithauer BW, Peipgras DG, Reiman HM, Ilstrup DM (1986). Malignant peripheral nerve sheath tumors: a clinicopathologic study of 120 cases. *Cancer* 57: 2006–2021.

Duffner PK, Cohen ME, Seidel FG, Shucard DW (1989). The significance of MRI abnormalities in children with neurofibromatosis. *Neurology* 39: 373–378.

Dunn DW, Roos KL (1989). MRI evaluation of learning difficulties and incoordination in neurofibromatosis type 1. *Neurofibromatosis* 2: 1–5.

Fortini ME, Simon MA, Rubin GM (1992) Signaling by the sevenless protein tyrosine kinase is mimicked by Ras1 activation. *Nature* 355: 559–561.

Friedman JM (1999). Epidemiology of neurofibromatosis type 1. *Am J Med Genet (Semin Med Genet)* 89: 1–6.

Friedman JM, Gutmann DH, MacCollin M, Riccardi VM (1999). *Neurofibromatosis: Phenotype, Natural History and Pathogenesis.* Johns Hopkins University Press, Baltimore.

Geist RT, Gutmann DH (1996). Expression of a developmentally-regulated neuron-specific isoform of the neurofibromatosis 1 (NF1) gene. *Neurosci Lett* 211: 85–88.

Gibbs JB, Oliff A (1997). The potential of farnesyltransferse inhibitors as cancer chemotherapeutics. *Annu Rev Pharmacol Toxicol* 37: 143–166.

Gregory PE, Gutmann DH, Mitchell A, Park S, Boguski M, Jacks T, Wood DL, Jove R, Collins FS (1993). Neurofibromatosis type 1 gene product (neurofibromin) associates with microtubules. *Somat Cell Mol Genet* 19: 265–274.

Griesser J, Kaufmann D, Eisenbarth I, Bauerle C, Krone W (1995). Ras-GTP regulation is not altered in cultured melanocytes with reduced levels of neurofibromin derived from patients with neurofibromatosis 1 (NF1). *Biol Chem Hoppe Seyler* 376: 91–101.

Guo HF, The I, Hannan F, Bernards A, Zhong Y (1997) Requirement of *Drosophila* NF1 for activation of adenylyl cyclase by PACAP38-like neuropeptides. *Science* 276: 795–798.

Guo HF, Tong J, Hannan F, Luo L, Zhong Y (2000). A neurofibromatosis-1-regulated pathway is required for learning in *Drosophila*. *Nature* 403: 895–898.

Gutmann DH (1999). Learning disabilities in neurofibromatosis 1: sizing up the brain. *Arch Neurol* 56: 1322–1323.

Gutmann DH, Collins FS (1993). The neurofibromatosis type 1 gene and its protein product, neurofibromin. *Neuron* 10: 335–343.

Gutmann DH, Wood DL, Collins FS (1991). Identification of the neurofibromatosis type 1 gene product. *Proc Natl Acad Sci USA* 88: 9658–9662.

Gutmann DH, Andersen LB, Cole JL, Swaroop M, Collins FS (1993). An alternatively-spliced mRNA in the carboxy terminus of the neurofibromatosis type 1 (NF1) gene is expressed in muscle. *Hum Mol Genet* 2: 989–992.

Gutmann DH, Geist RT, Wright DE, Snider WD (1995). Expression of the neurofibromatosis 1 (NF1) isoforms in developing and adult rat tissues. *Cell Growth Diff* 6: 315–323.

Gutmann DH, Aylsworth A, Carey JC, Korf B, Marks J, Pyeritz RE, Rubenstein A, Viskochil D (1997). The diagnostic evaluation and multidisciplinary management of neurofibromatosis 1 and neurofibromatosis 2. *JAMA* 278: 51–57.

Gutmann DH, Loehr A, Zhang Y, Kim J, Henkemeyer M, Cashen A (1999a). Haploinsufficiency for the neurofibromatosis 1 (NF1) tumor suppressor results in increased astrocyte proliferation. *Oncogene* 18: 4450–4459.

Gutmann DH, Zhang Y, Hirbe A (1999b). Developmental regulation of a neuron-specific neurofibromatosis 1 isoform. *Ann Neurol* 46: 777–782.

Gutmann DH, Donahoe J, Brown T, James CD, Perry A (2000). Loss of neurofibromatosis 1 (NF1) gene expression in NF1-associated pilocytic astrocytomas. *Neuropathol Appl Neurobiol* 26: 361–367.

Hamilton R (1994). The ras signal transduction pathway in development. In: *Growth Factors and Signal Transduction in Development.* Nilsen-Hamilton N (ed). Wiley-Liss, New York, pp. 123–138.

Hirvonen O, Lakkakorpi J, Aaltonen V, Hirvonen H, Rossi M, Karvonen SL, Ylä-Outinen H, Kalima H, Peltonen J (1998). Developmental regulation of NF1 tumor suppressor gene in human peripheral nerve. *J Neurocytol* 27: 939–952.

Hofman KJ, Harris EL, Bryan RN, Denckla MB (1994). Neurofibromatosis 1: the cognitive phenotype. *J Pediatr* 124: S1–S8.

Huynh DP, Nechiporuk T, Pulst SM (1994). Differential expression and tissue distribution of type I and type II neurofibromins during mouse fetal development. *Dev Biol* 161: 538–551.

Jacks T, Shih TS, Schmitt EM, Bronson RT, Bernards A, Weinberg RA (1994). Tumour predisposition in mice heterozygous for a targeted mutation in NF1. *Nat Genet* 7: 353–361.

Kaufmann D, Krone W, Hochsattel R, Martin R (1989). A cell culture study on melanocytes from patients with neurofibromatosis 1. *Arch Dermatol Res* 281: 510–513.

Kaufmann D, Wiandt S, Veser J, Krone W (1991). Increased melanogenesis in melanocytes from patients with neurofibromatosis 1. *Hum Genet* 87: 144–150.

Kim HA, Rosenbaum T, Marchionni MA, Ratner N, DeClue JE (1995). Schwann cells from neurofibromin deficient mice exhibit activation of p21ras, inhibition of cell proliferation and morphological changes. *Oncogene* 11: 325–335.

King AA, DeBaun MR, Riccardi VM, Gutmann DH (2000). Malignant peripheral nerve sheath tumors in neurofibromatosis 1. *Am J Med Genet* 93: 388–392.

Kinsella AR, Fiszer-Maliszewska L, Mitchell EL, Guo YP, Fox M, Scott D (1990). Introduction of activated N-ras oncogene into human fibroblasts by retroviral vector induces morphological transformation and tumorigenicity. *Carcinogenesis* 11: 1803–1809.

Kluwe L, Friedrich RE, Mautner VF (1999). Allelic loss of the NF1 gene in NF1-associated plexiform neurofibromas. *Cancer Genet Cytogenet* 113: 65–69.

Korf BR (1999). Plexiform neurofibromas. *Am J Med Genet* 89: 31–37.

Kourea HP, Cordon-Cardo C, Dudas M, Leung D, Woodruff JM (1999). Expression of p27(kip) and other cell cycle regulators in malignant peripheral nerve sheath tumors and neurofibromas: the emerging role of p27(kip) in malignant transformation of neurofibromas. *Am J Pathol* 155: 1885–1891.

Lakkis MM, Epstein JA (1998). Neurofibromin modulation of ras activity is required for normal endocardial-mesenchymal transformation in the developing heart. *Development* 125: 4359–4367.

Lakkis MM, Golden JA, O'Shea KS, Epstein JA (1999). Neurofibromin deficiency in mice causes exencephaly and is a modifier for Splotch neural tube defects. *Dev Biol* 212: 80–92.

Lau N, Feldkamp MM, Roncari L, Loehr AH, Shannon P, Gutmann DH, Guha A (2000). Loss of neurofibromin is associated with activation of ras/MAPK and PI3-K/Akt signaling in a neurofibromatosis 1 astrocytoma. *J Neuropath Exp Neurol* 59: 759–767.

Legius E, Marchuk DA, Hall BK, Andersen LB, Wallace MR, Collins FS, Glover TW (1992). NF1-related locus on chromosome 15. *Genomics* 13: 1316–1318.

Legius E, Dierick H, Wu R, Hall BK, Marynen P, Cassiman JJ, Glover TW (1994). TP53 mutations are frequent in malignant NF1 tumors. *Genes Chromosomes Cancer* 10: 250–255.

Legius E, Descheemaeker MJ, Steyaert J, Spaepen A, Vlietinck R, Casaer P, Demaeral P, Fryns JP (1995). Neurofibromatosis type 1 in childhood: correlation of MRI findings with intelligence. *J Neurol Neurosurg Psychiatry* 59: 638–640.

Listernick R, Louis DN, Packer RJ, Gutmann DH (1997). Optic pathway gliomas in children with neurofibromatosis 1: consensus statement from the NF1 Optic Pathway Glioma Task Force. *Ann Neurol* 41: 143–149.

Listernick R, Charrow J, Gutmann DH (1999). Intracranial gliomas in neurofibromatosis type 1. *Am J Med Genet (Semin Med Genet)* 89: 38–44.

Lopez-Correa C, Dorschner M, Brems H, Lazaro C, Clementi M, Upadhyaya M, Dooijes D, Moog U, Kehrer-Sawatzki H, Rutkowski JL, et al. (2001). Recombination hotspot in NF1 microdeletion patients. *Hum Mol Genet* 10: 1387–1392.

MacNicol AM, Muslim AJ, Williams LT (1993) Raf-1 kinase is essential for early *Xenopus* development and mediates the induction of mesoderm by FGF. *Cell* 73: 571–583.

Mahgoub N, Taylor BR, Le Beau MM, Gratiot M, Carlson KM, Atwater SK, Jacks T, Shannon KM (1999a). Myeloid malignancies induced by alkylating agents in NF1 mice. *Blood* 93: 3617–3623.

Mahgoub N, Taylor B, Le Beau M, Gratiot M, Carlson K, Jacks T, Shannon KM (1999b). Effects of farnesyl transferase inhibitor (FTI) L744,832 in a Ras-activated murine myeloid leukemia model. *Blood* 90: 497a.

Malhotra R, Ratner N (1994). Localization of neurofibromin to keratinocytes and melanocytes in developing rat and human skin. *J Invest Dermatol* 102: 812–818.

Marchuk DA, Saulino AM, Tavakkol R, Swaroop M, Wallace MR, Andersen LB, Mitchell AL, Gutmann DH, Boguski M, Collins FS (1991). CDNA cloning of the type 1 neurofibromatosis gene: complete sequence of the NF1 gene product. *Genomics* 11: 931–940.

Martin GA, Viskochil D, Bollag G, McCabe PC, Crosier WJ, Haubruck H, Conroy L, Clark R, O'Connell P, Cawthon RM, et al. (1990). The GAP-related domain of the neurofibromatosis type 1 gene product interacts with ras p21. *Cell* 63: 843–849.

Menon AG, Anderson KM, Riccardi VM, Chung RY, Whaley JM, Yandell DW, Farmer GE, Freiman RN, Lee JK, Li FP, et al. (1990) Chromosome 17p deletions and p53 gene mutations associated with the formation of malignant neurofibrosarcomas in von Recklinghausen neurofibromatosis. *Proc Natl Acad Sci USA* 87: 5435–5439.

Moore BD, Slopis JM, Schomer D, Jackson EF, Levy B (1996). Neuropsychological significance of areas of high signal intensity on brain magnetic resonance imaging scans of children with neurofibromatosis. *Neurology* 46: 1660–1668.

National Institutes of Health Consensus Development Conference (1988). Neurofibromatosis: conference statement. *Arch Neurol* 45: 575–578.

Newbold RF, Overell RW (1983). Fibroblast immortality is a prerequisite for transformation by EJ c-Ha-ras oncogene. *Nature* 304: 648–651.

Nordlund ML, Rizvi TA, Brannan CI, Ratner N (1995). Neurofibromin expression and astrogliosis in neurofibromatosis (type 1) brains. *J Neuropathol Exp Neurol* 54: 588–600.

North K (2000). Neurofibromatosis type 1. *Am J Med Genet* 97: 119–127.

North K, Joy P, Yuille D, Cocks N, Hutchins P, McHugh K, de Silva M (1994). Learning difficulties in neurofibromatosis type 1: the significance of MRI abnormalities. *Neurology* 44: 878–883.

North K, Riccardi V, Samango-Sprouse C, Ferner R, Moore B, Legius E, Ratner N, Denckla MB (1997). Cognitive function and academic performance in neurofibromatosis 1: consensus statement from the NF1 cognitive disorders task force. *Neurology* 48: 1121–1127.

Peltonen J, Jaakkola S, Lebwohl M, Renvall S, Risteli L, Virtanen I, Uitto J (1988). Cellular differentiation and expression of matrix genes in type 1 neurofibromatosis. *Lab Invest* 59: 7607–7671.

Perry A, Roth KA, Banerjee R, Fuller CE, Gutmann DH (2001). NF1 deletions in S-100 protein-positive and negative cells of sporadic and neurofibromatosis 1 (NF1)-associated plexiform neurofibromas and malignant peripheral nerve sheath tumors. *Am J Pathol* 159: 57–61.

Reed N, Gutmann DH (2001). Tumorigenesis in neurofibromatosis: new insights and potential therapies. *Trends Mol Med* 7: 157–162.

Reilly KM, Loisel DA, Bronson RT, McLauglin ME, Jacks T (2000). NF1;Trp53 mutant mice develop glioblastoma with evidence of strain-specific effects. *Nat Genet* 26: 109–113.

Ridley AJ, Paterson HG, Noble M, Land H (1988) Ras-mediated cell cycle arrest is altered by nuclear oncogenes to induce Schwann cell transformation. *EMBO J* 7: 1635–1645.

Rizvi TA, Akunuru S, de Courten-Myers G, Switzer RC, Nordlund ML, Ratner N (1999). Region-specific astrogliosis in brains of mice heterozygous for mutations in the neurofibromatosis type 1 (NF1) tumor suppressor. *Brain Res* 816: 111–123.

Rutkowski JL, Wu K, Gutmann DH, Boyer PJ, Legius E (2000). Genetic and cellular defects contributing to benign tumor formation in neurofibromatosis type 1. *Hum Mol Genet* 9: 1059–1066.

Samango-Sprouse C, Vezina LG, Brasseux C, Tifft CJ (1997). Cranial magnetic resonance findings and the neurodevelopmental performance in the young child with neurofibromatosis 1. *Am J Hum Genet* 61: A35.

Sawada S, Florell S, Purandare SM, Ota M, Stephens K, Viskochil D (1996). Identification of NF1 mutations in both alleles of a dermal neurofibroma. *Nat Genet* 14: 110–112.

Scharovsky OG, Rozados VR, Gervasoni SI, Mater P (2000). Inhibition of ras oncogene: a novel approach to antineoplastic therapy. *J Biomed Sci* 7: 292–298.

Serra E, Puig S, Otero D, Gaona A, Kruyer H, Ars E, Estivill X, Lazaro C (1997). Confirmation of a double-hit model for the NF1 gene in benign neurofibromas. *Am J Hum Genet* 61: 512–519.

Shen MH, Harper PS, Upadhyaya M (1996). Molecular genetics of neurofibromatosis type 1 (NF1). *J Med Genet* 33: 2–17.

Sherman LS, Atit R, Rosenbaum T, Cox AD, Ratner N (2000). Single cell Ras-GTP analysis reveals altered Ras activity in a subpopulation of neurofibroma Schwann cells but not fibroblasts. *J Biol Chem* 275: 30740–30745.

Side L, Taylor B, Cayouette M, Conner E, Thompson P, Luce M, Shannon K (1997). Homozygous inactivation of the NF1 gene in bone marrow cells from children with neurofibromatosis type 1 and malignant myeloid disorders. *N Engl J Med* 336: 1713–1720.

Silva AJ, Frankland PW, Marowitz Z, Friedman E, Lazlo G, Cioffi D, Jacks T, Bourtchuladze R (1997). A mouse model for the learning and memory deficits associated with neurofibromatosis type 1. *Nat Genet* 15: 281–284.

Skuse GR, Cappione AJ (1997). RNA processing and clinical variability in neurofibromatosis type 1 (NF1). *Hum Mol Genet* 6: 1707–1712.

Stacey DW, Kung HF (1984). Transformation of NIH 3T3 cells by microinjection of Ha-ras p21 protein. *Nature* 310: 508–511.

Stark M, Assum G, Kaufmann D, Kehrer H, Krone W (1992). Analysis of segregation and expression of an identified mutation at the neurofibromatosis locus. *Hum Genet* 90: 356–359.

Viskochil D, Buchberg AM, Xu G, Cawthon RM, Stevens J, Wolff RK, Culver M, Carey JC, Copeland NG, Jenkins NA, et al. (1990). Deletions and a translocation interrupt a cloned gene at the neurofibromatosis type 1 locus. *Cell* 62: 187–192.

Vogel KS, Klesse LJ, Velasco-Miguel S, Meyers K, Rushing EJ, Parada LF (1999). Mouse tumor model for neurofibromatosis type 1. *Science* 286: 2176–2179.

Wallace MR, Marchuk DA, Andersen LB, Letcher R, Odeh HM, Saulino AM, Fountain JW, Brereton A, Nicholson J, Mitchell AL, et al. (1990). Type 1 neurofibromatosis gene: identification of a large transcript disrupted in three NF1 patients. *Science* 249: 181–186.

Weiss B, Bollag G, Shannon K (1999). Hyperactive Ras as a therapeutic target in neurofibromatosis type 1. *Am J Med Genet* 89: 14–22.

Williams JA, Su HS, Bernards A, Field J, Sehgal A (2001). A circadian output in *Drosophila* mediated by neurofibromatosis-1 and Ras/MAPK. *Science* 293: 2251–2256.

Wittinghofer A (1998). Signal transduction via Ras. *Biol Chem* 379: 933–937.

Wrabetz L, Feltri ML, Kim H, Daston M, Kamholz J, Scherer SS, Ratner N (1995). Regulation of neurofibromin expression in rat sciatic nerve and cultured Schwann cells. *Glia* 15: 22–32.

Xu G, O'Connell P, Viskochil D, Cawthon R, Robertson R, Culver M, Dunn D, Stevens J, Gesteland R, White R, Weiss R (1990a). The neurofibromatosis type 1 gene encodes a protein related to GAP. *Cell* 62: 599–608.

Xu G, Lin B, Tanaka K, Dunn D, Wood D, Gesteland R, White R, Weiss R, Tamanoi F (1990b). The catalytic domain of the neurofibromatosis type 1 gene product stimulates ras GTPase and complements IRA mutants of *S. cerevisiae*. *Cell* 63: 835–841.

Xu H, Gutmann DH (1997). Mutations in the GAP-related domain impair the ability of neurofibromin to associate with microtubules. *Brain Res* 759: 149–152.

Yan N, Ricca C, Fletcher J, Glover T, Seizinger BR, Manne V (1996). Farnesyltransferase inhibitors block the neurofibromatosis type 1 (NF1) malignant phenotype. *Cancer Res* 55: 3569–3575.

Zhu Y, Romero MI, Ghosh P, Ye Z, Charnay P, Rushing EJ, Marth JD, Parada LF (2001). Ablation of NF1 function in neurons induces abnormal development of cerebral cortex and reactive gliosis in the brain. *Genes Dev* 15: 859–876.

Part E.
Kinases and Phosphatases

88 | *ROR2* and Brachydactyly Type B and Recessive Robinow Syndrome

MICHAEL OLDRIDGE AND ANDREW O.M. WILKIE

Mutations of the gene *ROR2*, which maps to 9q22 and encodes an orphan receptor tyrosine kinase, have been identified in two distinct skeletal disorders, dominantly inherited brachydactyly type B (BDB) and recessive Robinow syndrome (RRS). This demonstrates that *ROR2* is required for the development of multiple organs, most prominently bone but also, in the case of RRS, craniofacial structures, the heart, and the urogenital system. A single unlinked paralogue, *Ror1/ROR1*, is present in mice and humans, but mutations of *ROR1* have not yet been identified in any human disorder.

A distinct but confusing pattern of genotype–phenotype correlation is observed for mutations in *ROR2*. The BDB mutations, all of which are predicted to truncate the mutant protein, are localized to two intracellular segments of the polypeptide, whereas the RRS mutations are more widely scattered and diverse in nature. Genetic evidence indicates that BDB mutations act in a dominant positive or dominant negative manner, whereas the recessive RRS mutations lead to loss of protein function; however, a biochemical and developmental explanation of the observed genotype–phenotype correlation is currently lacking.

Analysis of bone development in *Ror2*$^{-/-}$ knockout mice demonstrates abnormalities in cell proliferation and differentiation, both of early mesenchymal condensations and in definitive epiphyseal plates; there is evidence for partial functional redundancy with *Ror1*. ROR orthologues have been identified in *Xenopus laevis*, *Drosophila*

melanogaster, *Aplysia californica*, and *Caenorhabditis elegans*, and recent evidence in *Xenopus* suggests that they interact physically with ont ligands.

ROR FAMILY OF ORPHAN RECEPTOR TYROSINE KINASES

Receptor tyrosine kinases (RTKs) comprise a large and well-studied family of signal transduction molecules; mutations of RTK family members have been described in many developmental and somatic disorders (Robertson et al., 2000; Schlessinger, 2000). A new family of RTKs, the RORs (receptor tyrosine kinase–like, orphan receptors) were first identified in humans through PCR of the conserved tyrosine kinase (TK) region using degenerate oligonucleotides (Masiakowski and Carroll, 1992). The two ROR genes—*ROR1*, located at 1p31-p32 (Reddy et al., 1997), and *ROR2*, located at 9q22 (Deloukas et al., 1998)—encode proteins with 58% amino acid identity. Subsequently, probable orthologues have been described in other species, including mouse (*Ror1* and *Ror2*: Oishi et al., 1999), *Xenopus* (Hikasa et al., 2002), *Drosophila* (*Dror* and *Dnrk*: Wilson et al., 1993; Oishi et al., 1997), *C. elegans* (alternatively termed *cam-1* or *kin-8*: Forrester et al., 1999; Koga et al., 1999), and the marine mollusc *Aplysia* (*Apror*: McKay et al., 2001). The RTKs most closely related to the

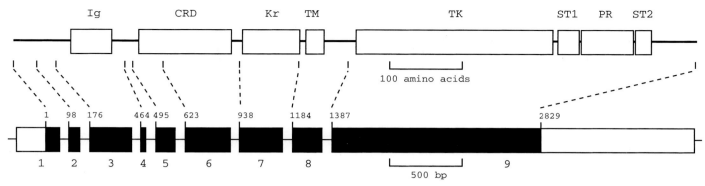

Figure 88–1. Structure of the human *ROR2* gene and its encoded protein. The intron/exon structure of the gene is shown below with rectangular boxes denoting exons, which are drawn to scale; the coding region is shown in black, and nucleotide numbering of the cDNA is indicated. Introns (thin lines) are not drawn to scale. Above, a cartoon of the encoded protein shows major structural motifs as follows: Ig, immunoglobulin-like; CRD, frizzled-like cysteine-rich domain; Kr, kringle; TM, transmembrane region; TK, tyrosine kinase; ST1, ST2, serine-threonine–rich; PR, proline-rich.

RORs are the muscle-specific TK (MuSK: Valenzuela et al., 1995) and the Trk family (Barbacid, 1995).

The RORs are predicted to encode single-pass transmembrane proteins with distinctive features in both extracellular and intracellular regions (Fig. 88–1). The extracellular region includes two motifs—the frizzled-like cysteine-rich domain (CRD) and the kringle (Kr) domain—that characteristically occur together in ROR proteins (MuSK from *Torpedo californica* shares this structure; Jennings et al., 1993). Both domains belong to large and diverse superfamilies, of which other members are involved in protein–protein interactions (Castellino and McCance, 1997; Masiakowski and Yancopoulos, 1998; Xu and Nusse, 1998). The mammalian, *Xenopus*, *C. elegans* and *Aplysia* RORs also feature an Ig-like domain, a frequently used ligand-binding motif for RTKs.

The TK domains of the ROR family share most of the 40 residues that are conserved in most or all TKs, but there are some unusual deviations (Masiakowski and Carroll, 1992). Human ROR2 has five amino acid changes from the consensus residues and therefore is one of the most divergent members of the TK family. Of particular interest is that in mammalian and *Xenopus* RORs (but not in the *Drosophila* or *C. elegans* orthologues), three substitutions occur at positions that are conserved in all other TKs. One of these involves the middle glycine of the glycine-rich loop, which is conserved in all serine/threonine protein kinases as well as other TKs; another involves the phenylalanine in the conserved DFG motif. Both the glycine-rich and DFG motifs are required for Mg-ATP binding, which raises the question of whether the vertebrate ROR proteins actually have associated kinase activity. Although Masiakowski and Carroll (1992) and Oishi et al. (1999) demonstrated phosphorylation of ROR proteins in transfected COS cells (based on radioactive phosphorous incorporation or anti-phosphotyrosine immunoblotting), these experiments do not completely exclude the possibility that RORs are kinase-dead coreceptors for another RTK (Kroiher et al., 2001). Probably the best evidence for the intrinsic activity of the ROR2 TK is provided by an observation in human genetics. The homozygous substitution N620K, which causes RRS (see Mutations of *ROR2* in BDB1 and RRS), locates at a critical residue for Mg-ATP binding and is equivalent to a pathogenic mutation in Bruton's tyrosine kinase (Vorechovsky et al., 1995).

The final distinctive features of RORs are the C-terminal serine/threonine–rich (ST1/ST2) and proline-rich (PR) domains for which the functions have not been determined. The ST1/ST2 domains are found in all family members except *DROR* but the PR domain (which might be a binding target for proteins with SH3 domains) occurs only in the vertebrate orthologues and *Apror*.

The molecular pathways in which mammalian ROR proteins function are currently unknown. The extracellular motifs are likely to be involved in ligand binding but do not indicate with confidence which ligands are involved; similarly, the C-terminal ST1/ST2 and PR regions may be docking sites for intracellular proteins, but no biochemical data on the functions of these motifs are available. Studies of mouse *Ror1* and *Ror2* indicate that both genes are expressed during embryogenesis in a wide variety of tissues, usually in distinct but overlapping patterns.

Expression is especially prominent in the cephalic neural crest, facial primordia, and the developing brain, bone, heart, lungs, gut, urogenital system, limb buds, and dermis (Al-Shawi et al., 2001; DeChiara et al., 2000; Matsuda et al., 2001). *Xenopus Xror2* is expressed initially in the dorsal marginal zone, then in the notochord and neuroectoderm posterior to the midbrain-hindbrain boundary (Hikasa et al., 2002). Both *Drosophila* orthologues and *Aplysia Apror* were reported to be expressed exclusively in the nervous system (Wilson et al., 1993; Oishi et al., 1997; McKay et al., 2001), but in *C. elegans*, *cam-1* is expressed in most cells of the 200-cell–stage embryo, although with a prominent neuronal contribution (Forrester et al., 1999).

At the present, the best clues to the function of the RORs are based on the identification of mutant phenotypes in *C. elegans*, *Xenopus*, mouse (see Mutations in Orthologous Genes), and human. The mapping of two human phenotypes, dominant BDB and RRS, to 9q22 (Gong et al., 1999; Oldridge et al., 1999; van Bokhoven et al., 1999; Afzal et al., 2000a), which coincided with a region of conserved synteny with the location of the mouse *Ror2* gene on chromosome 13 (Oishi et al., 1999), led to the identification of *ROR2* mutations in these disorders (Afzal et al., 2000b; Oldridge et al., 2000; Schwabe et al., 2000; van Bokhoven et al., 2000). Together, these observations implicate mammalian *ROR2* in processes of skeletal, cardiac, and urogenital development.

CLINICAL FEATURES

BDB

The term *brachydactyly* is derived from the Greek word for "short finger." BDB (OMIM 113000) is the most severe of the inherited brachydactylies and clinically is usually very characteristic. Most, but not all, BDB is caused by mutations in *ROR2*; this locus is referred to as *BDB1*. The first recognizable descriptions date back to Kellie (1808) and Mackinder (1857), although the current nomenclature was developed by Bell (1951). The best-documented BDB1 families illustrated in the clinical literature are those of Cragg and Drinkwater (1916), MacArthur and McCullough (1932), Wells and Platt (1947), Degenhardt and Giepel (1954), Malloch (1957), Schott (1978), Battle et al. (1973), Houlston and Temple (1994), Gong et al. (1999) and Schwabe et al. (2000). All exhibited classic autosomal dominant inheritance with complete penetrance. The cases described by Degenhardt and Giepel (1954), Bass (1968), and Cuevas-Sosa and Garcia-Segur (1971) appear to have arisen from fresh mutations; many of the other reports are likely to refer to families inheriting the same English founder mutation (see Mutations of *ROR2* in BDB1 and RRS), falsely giving the impression of greater clinical homogeneity than is necessarily the case.

The most characteristic features of BDB1 (Fig. 88–2A) are symmetrical distal amputations of the fingers, with partially or completely absent fingernails, accompanied by thumbs with a nail that is always present and may be broad or even bifid. The severity of the finger amputations varies considerably, from mild distal hypoplasia with a reduced nail to loss of both the middle and terminal phalanges and hypoplasia of the proximal phalanx with an absent nail. The fourth and fifth digits tend to be more severely affected than the second and third digits. In cases where a single phalanx is missing, Fitch (1979) reviewed the clinical evidence that the missing phalanx is the terminal one, reflecting an old diagnostic term for BDB—*apical dystrophy*.

More occasional features of BDB1 are symphalangism and cutaneous syndactyly, usually between the middle and ring fingers. Occasionally, apparent amputation scars or blebs of tissue are present on the terminal parts of the digits at birth, as described by Battle et al. (1973), Gong et al. (1999), and Oldridge et al. (1999). The feet are also affected but usually more mildly so than the hands. There is a subtle but distinct facial gestalt associated with the common English mutation, with a prominent beaked nose, flared or hypoplastic alae nasae, and a short philtrum (Houlston and Temple, 1994), although not all individuals are considered to share these features (Gong et al., 1999). Congenital phimosis of the penis was described in one case by Wells and Platt (1947), and the authors are aware of another unpublished instance.

The extremes of clinical phenotype currently recognized as heterozygous BDB1 are illustrated by cases reported by Schwabe et al. (2000) and Oldridge et al. (2000). At the mild end of the spectrum, Schwabe et al. (2000) described individuals whose distal phalanges and nails were all present but were variably hypoplastic and frequently associated with distal symphalangism (Fig. 88–2B). At the severe end of the spectrum, Oldridge et al. (2000) described a father and son with severe brachydactyly, syndactyly of digits 2–4 with underlying phalangeal bifurcation or bridging, and duplicated phalanges in the thumbs (Fig. 88–2C). Vari-

ation in the severity of amputations also occurs within families, although symmetry is the rule in the individual; this suggests that genetic background is the major factor modulating severity within a family.

A single case of homozygosity for a *BDB1* mutation, inherited from consanguineous affected parents, was described by Schwabe et al. (2000). This patient had severely hypoplastic hands and feet with the complete absence of the distal and middle phalanges, the absence of some proximal phalanges, and hypoplastic metacarpals and metatarsals. All nails were absent except for rudiments on the great toes. The upper limb long bones were moderately shortened, but the leg bones were of normal length. There were hemivertebrae and fusions of the lower thoracic spine (T8-T12) and malformation of L6/S1, causing thoracolumbar scoliosis. Facial characteristics included borderline hypertelorism and a short narrow nose with a short columella; the alveolar ridges were hyperplastic and the deciduous teeth had severe caries. The anterior fontanelle was still open at the age of 7.5 years. There was a small ventricular septal defect, first-degree atrioventricular heart block, and a small penis. Some (but not all) of these features are reminiscent of Robinow syndrome, as discussed later.

Recessive Robinow Syndrome

Robinow syndrome, or "fetal face" syndrome, was originally described in 1969, and the first cases showed an autosomal dominant mode of inheritance (Robinow et al., 1969). However, Wadlington et al. (1973) described a similar phenotype but with additional multiple vertebral segmentation defects in opposite-sex siblings born to normal parents. Since

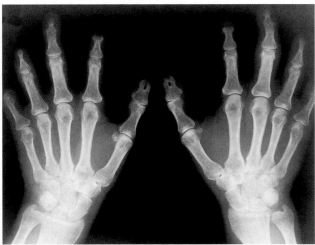
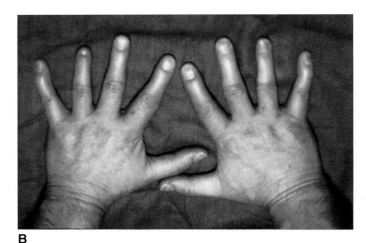
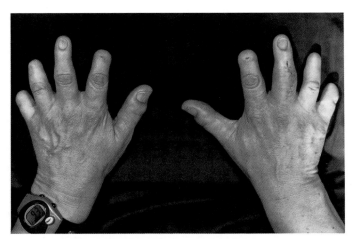

A

B

C

Figure 88–2. Clinical features of BDB1. (*A*) Patient with classic case. Note distal digit amputations with complete loss of some nails but sparing of the thumbnail. Radiological examination reveals that the distal phalanx of the thumb is bifid (Oldridge et al., 2000). (*B*) Patient with mildly affected case. All nails are present, but some are hypoplastic (Schwabe et al., 2000). (*C*) Patient with severely affected case. Note the reduplicated thumb and complex syndactyly involving digits 2–4 (Oldridge et al., 2000). (B courtesy of S. Tinschert, G. Schwabe, and S Mundlos, Berlin.)

then, a number of additional cases have been described in which the disorder is clearly inherited in an autosomal recessive manner (OMIM 268310). The dominant and recessive forms of the syndrome can often be distinguished phenotypically, although there is some overlap (for reviews, see Robinow, 1993, and Patton and Afzal, 2002). From the limited information currently available, RRS appears to be a fairly homogeneous and well-delineated condition, with most cases homozygous for mutations in *ROR2*. The molecular basis of dominant Robinow syndrome has not been reported and is probably heterogeneous.

The largest case studies of definite RRS are those described by Balci et al. (1993) and Soliman et al. (1998), from Turkey and Oman, respectively. Other likely cases of RRS with good illustrations are those reported by Vera-Roman (1973), Wadia et al. (1978), Glaser et al. (1989), Teebi (1990), Schorderet et al. (1992), Türken et al. (1996), Aksit et al. (1997), Balci et al. (1998), and Kantaputra et al. (1999). Features present in virtually all patients include a dysmorphic facies (Fig. 88–3A), with frontal bossing, hypertelorism, prominent eyes, a broad-based nose with anteverted nares, a long philtrum, a wide triangular mouth, micrognathia, gingival hyperplasia with dental crowding, midline cleft of lower lip, and/or ankyloglossia and bilobed tongue. There is short stature (the length at birth may attain the 10th percentile but subsequently declines below the 3rd percentile), caused by a combination of mesomelic limb shortening and costovertebral abnormalities. The mesomelic shortening tends to be more severe in the upper limbs, often with dislocation of the radial head; costovertebral abnormalities include hemivertebrae, butterfly vertebrae, block vertebrae, and costal fusions (Fig. 88–3B). Digital abnormalities are frequent and varied, most commonly consisting of shortening of the terminal phalanges and fifth finger clinodactyly. The genitalia are hypoplastic, with micropenis in males (Fig. 88–3C) and hypoplasia of the clitoris and labia minora in females.

Many other less frequent (<20%) abnormalities have been described in patients with probable RRS. These include broad or bifid thumbs and halluces, cutaneous syndactyly, polydactyly, or ectrodactyly (Balci et al., 1993); inguinal hernia and undescended testes (Türken et al., 1996); vaginal atresia and hydronephrosis (Balci et al., 1993, 1998); and congenital heart disease (Soliman et al., 1998). Death in early infancy and developmental delay have both been described in a few cases (Petit et al., 1980; Percin et al., 2001).

GENETICS

Mutations of *ROR2* in BDB1 and RRS

Linkage of classic BDB to 9q22 was simultaneously reported by two groups (Gong et al., 1999; Oldridge et al., 1999). The four families initially linked to 9q22 all originated from England (in one, the founder had emigrated to Canada), and all had an identical haplotype on the mutant chromosome for multiple microsatellite loci in the 9q22 region. This suggested that the four families shared a common ancestor, enabling a refined localization based on haplotype analysis. Linkage to 9q22 was excluded in a fifth family that exhibited slightly different clinical features (Oldridge et al., 1999; see Diagnosis of BDB).

The discovery that mice homozygous for inactivating mutations of *Ror2* had skeletal anomalies and the mapping of the human orthologue *ROR2* to *9q22* raised the possibility that *ROR2* might be mutated in BDB1 (DeChiara et al., 2000). This was subsequently confirmed (Oldridge et al., 2000). To date, eight distinct mutations in *ROR2*, of which two were shown to have arisen de novo, have been reported in patients with BDB (Oldridge et al., 2000; Schwabe et al., 2000; Bacchelli et al., 2001) (Table 88–1 and Fig. 88–4). The mutations, four nonsense and four frameshift, cluster tightly in two regions

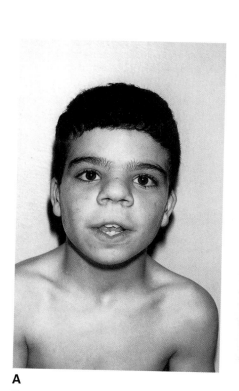

A

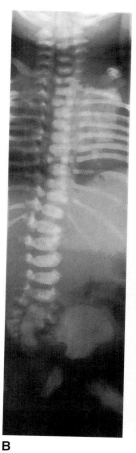

B

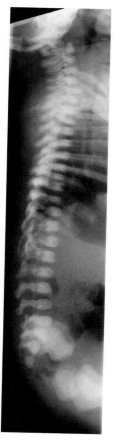

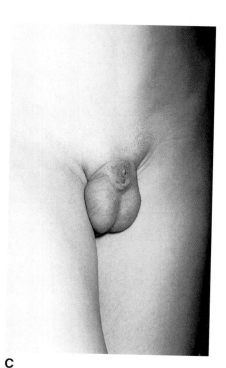

C

Figure 88–3. Clinical features of RRS. (*A*) Facial appearance showing hypertelorism, anteverted nose, long philtrum, and wide mouth. (*B*) Spine radiographs (left, frontal; right, lateral view) showing hemivertebrae, scoliosis, and rib fusions. (*C*) Micropenis with normally developed testes (van Bokhoven et al., 2000). (Courtesy of H. Brunner, Nijmegen, and H. Kayserili, Istanbul.)

Table 88–1. Mutations in *ROR2*

Nucleotide Change	Predicted Amino Acid Change	Protein Domain	Syndrome	Reference
545G>A	C182Y	CRD	RRS	van Bokhoven et al. (2000)
550C>T	R184C	CRD	RRS	Afzal et al. (2000)
565C>T	R189W*	CRD	RRS	Afzal et al. (2000)
613C>T	R205X	CRD	RRS	van Bokhoven et al. (2000)
1096C>T	R366W*	Kr	RRS	Afzal et al. (2000)
1189C>T	R397X	Kr/TM	RRS	van Bokhoven et al. (2000)
1321_1325del	R441fsX456	TM/TK	BDB	Schwabe et al. (2000)
IVS8+3_+5del ins19	A463fsX527†	TM/TK	BDB	Schwabe et al. (2000)
1398_1399insA	E467fsX524	TM/TK	BDB	Schwabe et al. (2000)
1504C>T	Q502X	TK	RRS	Afzal et al. (2000)
1740_1774del	T582fsX704	TK	RRS	van Bokhoven et al. (2000)
1860T>A	N620K	TK	RRS	Afzal et al. (2000)
2160G>A	W720X	TK	RRS	van Bokhoven et al. (2000)
2246G>A	W749X	TK/ST1	BDB	Oldridge et al. (2000)
2247G>A	W749X	TK/ST1	BDB	Bacchelli et al. (2001)
2249delG	G750fsX773	TK/ST1	BDB	Oldridge et al. (2000)
2265C>A	Y755X	ST1	BDB	Oldridge et al. (2000)
2278C>T	Q760X	ST1	BDB	Schwabe et al. (2000)

CRD, cysteine-rich domain; Kr, kringle; TM, transmembrane; TK, tyrosine kinase; ST1, serine/threonine–rich domain.

*These changes are present on the same allele in one affected individual.

†This mutation abolishes the normal intron 8 5′ (donor) splice site, but the inserted sequence contains a new consensus splice site 10 nucleotides downstream, leading to an insertion of three novel amino acids and a frameshift.

of the intracellular part of the ROR2 protein. Three of the mutations (all frameshift) locate in the juxtamembrane region, whereas the other five (four nonsense and one frameshift) locate near the boundary between the end of the TK domain and the start of ST1 region. The severely affected individual born to two affected parents (see Clinical Features section) was shown to be homozygous for the R441fsX456 mutation (Schwabe et al., 2000).

Of population genetic interest, multiple families of English origin harbor an identical mutation (2265C → A/Y755X): in different families, the mutation occurs on the same 9q22 microsatellite haplotype, indicating that these families are related. As well as sharing the mutation, some families share an explanation of its origin (concerning a clergyman, a prized apple tree, and an apple thief who turned out to be the clergyman's wife) that shows remarkable similarities with the legend independently recounted (in delightfully quaint style) in the first two publications of Kellie (1808) and MacKinder (1857). The cultural inheritance of this shared myth directly links the common English mutation to these first two publications.

To interpret the biologic effect of these mutations, it is important to determine whether the mutant mRNA is stably expressed. This was investigated in lymphoblastoid cell lines from four cases (Oldridge et al., 2000; Schwabe et al., 2000), in which gross inequality in the levels of wild-type and mutant transcripts was not observed. This suggests that the mutant mRNA is stable and that the mutations produce truncated proteins: the location of the mutations, within the last two exons of *ROR2* (see Fig. 88–1), presumably means that the mutant mRNA escapes the surveillance mechanism that would lead to nonsense-mediated decay (Frischmeyer and Dietz, 1999; Hentze and Kulozik, 1999).

Shortly after the genetic mapping of BDB1 to 9q22 and the identification of mutations in *ROR2*, linkage of RRS to the same region was reported by homozygosity mapping (van Bokhoven et al., 1999; Afzal et al., 2000a). Because the phenotype of *Ror2⁻/⁻* mice is similar to RRS, mutations in *ROR2* seemed likely to be the cause of RRS; this was subsequently confirmed (Afzal et al., 2000b; van Bokhoven et al., 2000). Nine mutations have been described, all identified in the homozygous state in affected individuals. They are scattered across the

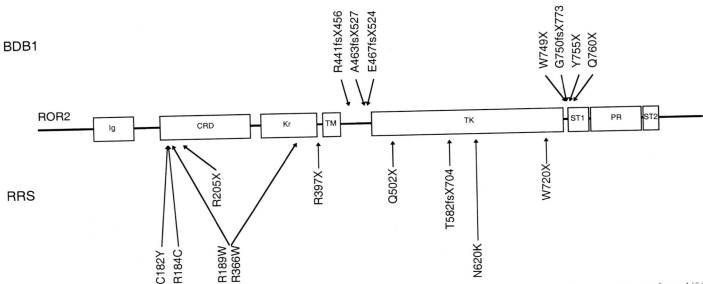

Figure 88–4. Distribution of pathological mutations in BDB1 and RRS. BDB1 mutations are shown above and RRS mutations below a cartoon of the ROR2 protein, which is labeled as in Figure 88–1. The RRS mutations are further divided into two categories: truncating mutations (nonsense or frameshift) (shown in the first row below the protein) and missense mutations (second row).

CRD, Kr, and TK domains and comprise four each of nonsense and missense changes (in one case, two distinct amino acid substitutions are present on the same disease haplotype) and one 35-bp deletion (see Table 88–1 and Fig. 88–4). In contrast to BDB1, these mutations appear to be phenotypically silent in the heterozygous state. Surprisingly, the high frequency of RRS in Turkey (Balci et al., 1993, Aksit et al., 1997) is not explained by a founder effect for a specific mutation; five of the nine distinct *ROR2* mutations described to date have been identified in patients of Turkish origin.

The differences in phenotype and inheritance pattern between cases of BDB1 and RRS with documented *ROR2* mutations indicate that the mutations act via distinct mechanisms. Individuals with 9q22 microdeletions associated with the heterozygous loss of an *ROR2* allele do not have BDB, indicating that the dominantly inherited *ROR2* mutations causing BDB1 must act via a gain-of-function (dominant positive or dominant negative) mechanism (Oldridge et al., 2000). In RRS, by contrast, the scattered mutation distribution in *ROR2*, the uniformity of associated clinical features, and the similarity to the phenotype of *Ror2*$^{-/-}$ mice (DeChiara et al., 2000; Takeuchi et al., 2000) (see later) are more consistent with a loss-of-function mechanism; this provides genetic evidence that the CRD, Kr, and TK domains are all critical for the function of ROR2 (Afzal et al., 2000b; van Bokhoven et al., 2000). In the patient homozygous for the *BDB1* mutation, the blend of features combining severe BDB1 and RRS indicates mixed-gain and loss-of-function effects in the homozygous background.

Genotype–Phenotype Correlations

Analysis of the pattern of *ROR2* mutations shows an intriguing genotype–phenotype correlation (see Fig. 88–4). Although truncating mutations of *ROR2* located either in the extracellular region or in the core of the TK domain are associated with RRS, intracellular truncating mutations that flank either side of the TK domain cause BDB (the more C-terminal cluster of BDB mutations tends to be associated with a more severe phenotype) (Schwabe et al., 2000). No experimental data address this paradoxical pattern; therefore, the mechanism remains a matter of speculation. Although it is expected that truncations in the extracellular part of the protein will completely abrogate function, truncation of RTKs in the TK domain may have a dominant negative effect (Kroiher et al., 2001) or, as in the case of the *C. elegans* orthologue (see Mutations in Orthologous Genes), may not abolish all functions. The BDB mutations are tightly clustered in interdomain regions, suggesting the potential to fold normally, but the partial TK domain truncations predicted by some RRS mutations might lead to misfolding and premature degradation of the protein. However, the apparent loss-of-function (as opposed to dominant negative) effect of the N620K substitution is not readily explained by this model: it will be important to confirm that the heterozygous parents have no associated limb phenotype.

ESTABLISHING THE DIAGNOSIS/MANAGEMENT AND COUNSELING

Diagnosis of BDB

In the diagnosis of classic BDB, particular attention should be given to the appearance of the thumbs: characteristically, the thumbnail is spared in BDB1 and the thumb sometimes appears to be broad and/or flattened. Plain radiographs of the hands may reveal occult bifidity of the thumb, which is pathognomonic of BDB1 in this context. The differential diagnosis includes other forms of nonsyndromic brachydactyly (Temtamy and McKusick, 1978; Fitch, 1979), which are usually easily distinguished by the different pattern of digit involvement. However, at least one other form of BDB exists that is not caused by mutations in *ROR2*; this is sometimes referred to as Cooks syndrome (Cooks et al., 1985, de Ravel et al., 1999). Clinical descriptions of families in which *ROR2* mutations have been excluded (Oldridge et al., 1999; M. Oldridge and A.O.M. Wilkie, unpublished data) have been published by Santos et al. (1981) and Nevin et al. (1995). The fingers may be affected in a pattern very similar to that of classic BDB, but the distal portions of the thumbs are often hypoplastic and tapered,

the thumbnail is reduced or absent, and the nail of the hallux may also be reduced.

Prenatal diagnosis of BDB1 with the careful use of ultrasound scanning was reported to be possible as early as gestational week 14 (Gong et al., 1999). In theory, prenatal diagnosis would also be feasible by molecular genetic analysis, but few at-risk couples are likely to contemplate this option because the condition does not pose any major functional problems in the majority of cases. A minority (10%–20% in the case of the Y755X mutation) do, however, require surgery, usually to correct the duplicated thumb or the syndactyly.

RRS

In sporadic cases of suspected Robinow syndrome, it is important to try to determine whether the clinical features suggest the dominant or recessive form because this will affect the risk of recurrence. Dominantly inherited Robinow syndrome tends to be associated with normal or only mildly reduced stature, less severe mesomelic limb shortening, and abnormal segmentation of no more than one vertebra (Robinow, 1993). The recessive form is generally more severe, with the radius and ulna being very short, thick, and abnormally modeled (often accompanied by dislocation of the radial head), and there are multiple costovertebral segmentation defects. (However, in one of the affected siblings reported by Schorderet et al. [1992], there was only a single bifid rib.) Clinical investigations should include a skeletal survey to document the pattern of bony involvement and the use of cardiac and renal ultrasonography to look for associated congenital malformations. Molecular analysis may in the future provide an objective method to classify sporadic cases with greater confidence, but further work is required to determine what proportion of RRS patients have *ROR2* mutations and whether any dominant Robinow syndrome cases are also caused by mutations in *ROR2*. The prenatal diagnosis of RRS, based on ultrasonographic examination at 13 weeks' gestation, has been described (Percin et al., 2001). Genetic analysis of *ROR2* would be feasible with chorionic villus sampling but has not yet been reported.

Surgical management of malformations associated with RRS (cardiac, renal, limb, and scoliosis) is required in some cases. It has been reported that prepubertal treatment with human chorionic gonadotropin resulted in increased testicular volume and penile length in boys (Soliman et al., 1998).

MUTATIONS IN ORTHOLOGOUS GENES

Loss-of-function mutations of *Ror2* have been engineered in the mouse genome (DeChiara et al., 2000; Takeuchi et al., 2000), as has mutation of the paralogous gene *Ror1* (Nomi et al., 2001). In addition, two natural mutations and an engineered deletion of the *C. elegans* homologue *cam-1/kin-8* have been described (Forrester et al., 1999; Koga et al., 1999), as well as five engineered mutations of *Xenopus Xror2* (Hikasa et al., 2002).

Homozygous *Ror2*$^{-/-}$ mice harboring either a *neo* insertion into the Ig domain (Takeuchi et al., 2000) or an in-phase *LacZ* replacement of the intracellular region (DeChiara et al., 2000) exhibited a similar, predominantly skeletal phenotype. This was unexpected in the light of earlier information suggesting predominantly neuronal expression of both *Ror2* and *Ror1* (Oishi et al., 1999). In both mouse lines, the heterozygotes were reported as normal; homozygous mice died at birth with obvious dwarfism, caused by generalized skeletal deformities that included predominant mesomelic shortening of the limbs, abnormal vertebrae, fusion of adjoining ribs, and a shortened snout and tail (Fig. 88–5) (DeChiara et al., 2000; Takeuchi et al., 2000). Additional features noted in one of the *Ror2*$^{-/-}$ mouse lines were failure of lung alveolae to expand, cardiac septal defects, and cleft palate. Collectively, these features are very similar to those of RRS and indicate a role for *Ror2* in the development of the long bones, axial skeleton, skull, lungs, heart, and reproductive system.

The phenotype of mice homozygous for inactivation of the paralogue *Ror1* was investigated by Nomi et al. (2000). Although the single knockout (*Ror1*$^{-/-}$) mice appear to be normal, the double knockouts (*Ror1*$^{-/-}$; *Ror2*$^{-/-}$) manifest a more severe phenotype than *Ror2*$^{-/-}$ mice. There is greater skeletal deformity (severe hypoplasia

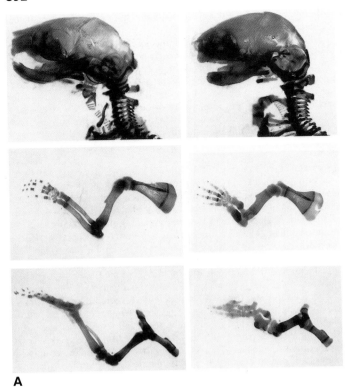

A

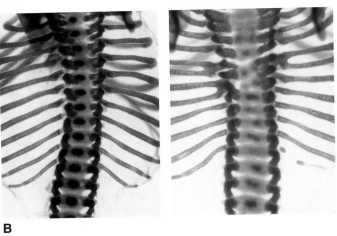

B

Figure 88–5. Skeletal abnormalities in $Ror2^{-/-}$ mice (right) compared with wild type (left), revealed by staining with Alizarin Red (bone) and Alcian Blue (cartilage). (A) Comparison of the skull (top), forelimb (middle), and hindlimb (bottom). Note moderate shortening of the maxilla and mandible, gross mesomelic shortening of the limbs, and reduced number of ossification centers in the digits. (B) The thorax of the $Ror2^{-/-}$, mouse showing multiple costal fusions and abnormal vertebral segmentation (Takeuchi et al., 2000). (Courtesy of I. Oishi and Y. Minami, Kobe.)

of the maxilla, mandible, and proximal long bones; sternal agenesis and dysplasia of the symphysis pubis) and transposition of the great arteries (Nomi et al., 2001). These observations suggest that there is some functional redundancy between *Ror1* and *Ror2*, a possibility compatible with their overlapping expression patterns (Al-Shawi et al., 2001; Matsuda et al., 2001),

In *C. elegans*, two putatively allelic *cam-1* mutants were isolated from a genetic screen for mutations affecting the migration of specific neurons (Forrester and Garriga, 1997). Both are caused by recessive nonsense mutations in the single *C. elegans* homologue of ROR (Forrester et al., 1999). The encoded protein, CAM-1, was shown to act cell autonomously in migrating neurons: overexpression and underexpression resulted in reciprocal cell migration phenotypes (Forrester et al., 1999). Of the two mutations, one (*gm122*) is located in the extracellular CRD domain, and the other (*gm105*) is located just before the start of the intracellular TK domain. The more severe *gm122* mutant showed disrupted migration of several cells along the anteroposterior axis and defects in

asymmetrical cell division and axon outgrowth; interestingly, the *gm105* mutant was normal for a subset of these phenotypes, suggesting that some functions (notably cell migration) did not require the TK activity. Koga et al. (1999) engineered a homozygous deletion mutation of the same gene (*kin*-8), which showed constitutive dauer larva formation.

In *Xenopus*, the effect of mutant *Xror2* mRNA constructs was examined by microinjection (Hisaka et al., 2002). Both wild-type and kinase-dead constructs (engineered either by intracellular truncation, or by point mutation of critical residues) caused head defects, identifying (as for *C. elegans*) a kinase-independent function. All three constructs also interfered with convergent extension during gastrulation and (except for the truncated construct) with neural plate closure. Constructs with part of the extracellular CRD deleted did not show these effects. Co-immunoprecipitation supported a physical interaction between Xror2 and the Wnt ligands Xwnt5a, Xwnt8 and Xwnt11 (Hisaka et al., 2002). This suggests that RORs may be receptors for Wnts, most probably interacting via the frizzled-like CRD.

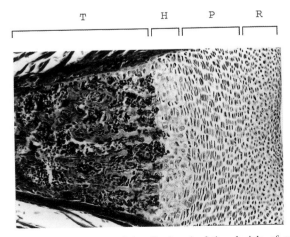

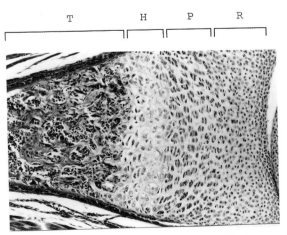

Figure 88–6. Histological section of the distal end of the clavicle of an $Ror2^{-/-}$ neonatal mouse (right) compared with wild type (left). Note reduction in thickness and cellularity of the proliferative (P) zone containing organized columns of flattened cells. The thickness of the hypertrophic (H) zone is increased. Also shown are the resting zone (R) and trabecular bone (T) (Takeuchi et al., 2000). (Courtesy of I. Oishi and Y. Minami, Kobe.)

PATHOGENESIS

Although a detailed understanding of the pathogenesis of the BDB and RRS phenotypes must await studies on the biochemistry of ROR2 mutant proteins and the developmental pathway in which ROR2 acts, the similarity in phenotype between *Ror2*$^{-/-}$ mice and RRS enables the delineation of the major stages of organogenesis at which the abnormal phenotype arises. Preliminary conclusions can be reached on the pathogenesis of the bony abnormalities in RRS. By contrast, the mechanisms for the selective effects of dominant *ROR2* mutations on digit development and the developmental abnormalities in the heart, lungs, and genitalia are not understood.

The *Ror2*$^{-/-}$ mice reported by DeChiara et al. (2000) and Takeuchi et al. (2000) both demonstrated abnormal endochondral bone formation leading to foreshortened and misshapen bones, with the distal portions of the limb being more severely affected. Expression of the Ror2 protein was detectable in the cartilaginous anlage at embryonic day (E) 12.5–E13; within 24 hours (E13–E14), shortening of many of these anlage was evident in the *Ror2*$^{-/-}$ mice, and the anlage of the middle phalanges completely failed to develop (DeChiara et al., 2000). These observations imply that *Ror2* is required during morphogenesis of the cartilaginous anlage. By contrast, the skull bones, which develop directly from membrane, do not express *Ror2* and develop normally.

At later stages, *Ror2* is expressed in articular cartilage, perichondrium, and reserve and proliferative chondrocytes but is not expressed in the hypertrophic chondrocytes. *Ror2*$^{-/-}$ mice had grossly abnormal epiphyseal growth plates, especially in the distal long bones (radius, ulna, tibia, and fibula). Instead of forming a central ossified region flanked by symmetrical growth plates, the *Ror2*$^{-/-}$ growth plates developed eccentrically, leading to bony distortion. Subperiosteal bone formation was relatively spared. Although other growing bones showed fewer gross abnormalities, consistent histological findings were reduction in the height of the proliferative zone and cellular disorganization of the hypertrophic zone, yielding shorter growth plates overall (Fig. 88–6). A very similar defect in endochondral ossification was described in the phalanx of an infant with a clinical diagnosis of RRS, who died in the neonatal period (Petit et al., 1980).

In conclusion, these findings indicate that *Ror2* plays a critical role in controlling the proliferation and differentiation of chondrocytes. Several molecules that control these processes have been identified, such as Indian hedgehog (IHH), parathyroid hormone–related peptide (PTHRP), and fibroblast growth factor receptor 3 (FGFR3) (see Chapter 11). However, expression of the corresponding transcripts was not obviously affected in *Ror2*$^{-/-}$ mice (DeChiara et al., 2000), suggesting that ROR2 may be a component of a novel molecular pathway in bone development.

ACKNOWLEDGMENTS

We thank the Wellcome Trust for personal and laboratory support.

REFERENCES

Afzal AR, Rajab A, Fenske C, Crosby A, Lahiri N, Ternes-Pereira E, Murday VA, Houlston R, Patton MA, Jeffery S (2000a). Linkage of recessive Robinow syndrome to a 4 cM interval on chromosome 9q22. *Hum Genet* 106: 351–354.

Afzal AR, Rajab A, Fenske CD, Oldridge M, Elanko N, Ternes-Pereira E, Tüysüz B, Murday VA, Patton MA, Wilkie AOM, Jeffery S (2000b). Recessive Robinow syndrome, allelic to dominant brachydactyly type B, is caused by mutation of *ROR2*. *Nat Genet* 25: 419–422.

Aksit S, Aydinlioglu H, Dizdarer G, Çaglayan S, Bektaslar D, Cin A (1997). Is the frequency of Robinow syndrome relatively high in Turkey? Four more case reports. *Clin Genet* 52: 226–230.

Al-Shawi R, Ashton SV, Underwood C, Simons JP (2001). Expression of the *Ror1* and *Ror2* receptor tyrosine kinase genes during mouse development. *Dev Genes Evol* 211: 161–171.

Bacchelli C, Goodman FR, Wilson LC, Scambler PJ (2001). A ROR2 mutation in a family with brachydactyly type B in the hands and normal feet. *Eur J Hum Genet* 9: S177–S178.

Balci S, Erçal MD, Say B, Atasü M (1993). Robinow syndrome: with special emphasis on dermatoglyphics and hand malformations (split hand). *Clin Dysmorp* 2: 199–207.

Balci S, Beksaç S, Haliloglu M, Ercis M, Eryilmaz M (1998). Robinow syndrome, vaginal atresia, hematocolpos, and extra middle finger. *Am J Med Genet* 79: 27–29.

Barbacid M (1995). Neurotrophic factors and their receptors. *Curr Opin Cell Biol* 7: 148–155.

Bass HN (1968). Familial absence of middle phalanges with nail dysplasia: a new syndrome. *Pediatrics* 42: 318–323.

Battle HI, Walker NF, Thompson MW (1973). Mackinder's hereditary brachydactyly: phenotypic, radiological, dermatoglyphic and genetic observations in an Ontario family. *Ann Hum Genet (Lond)* 36: 415–424.

Bell J (1951). On brachydactyly and symphalangism. In: *The Treasury of Human Inheritance*. Penrose LS (ed.) Cambridge University Press, Cambridge, pp. 1–31.

Castellino FJ, McCance SG (1997). The kringle domains of human plasminogen. *Ciba Found Symp* 212: 46–65.

Cooks RG, Hertz M, Katznelson MBM, Goodman RM (1985). A new nail dysplasia syndrome with onychonychia and absence and/or hypoplasia of distal phalanges. *Clin Genet* 27: 85–91.

Cragg E, Drinkwater H (1916). Hereditary absence of phalanges through five generations. *J Genet* 6: 81–89.

Cuevas-Sosa A, García-Segur F (1971). Brachydactyly with absence of middle phalanges and hypoplastic nails. *J Bone Joint Surg* 53B: 101–105.

de Ravel TJL, Berkowitz DE, Wagner JM, Jenkins T (1999). Brachydactyly type B with its distinct facies and 'Cooks syndrome' are the same entity. *Clin Dysmorp* 8: 41–45.

DeChiara TM, Kimble RB, Poueymirou WT, Rojas J, Masiakowski P, Valenzuela DM, Yancopoulos GD (2000). *Ror2*, encoding a receptor-like tyrosine kinase, is required for cartilage and growth plate development. *Nat Genet* 24: 271–274.

Degenhardt K-H, Geipel G (1954). Dominant erbliche Perodaktylien in 4 generationen einer sippe. *Z menschl Vererb-u Konstitutionslehre* 32: 227–307.

Deloukas P, Schuler GD, Gyapay G, Beasley EM, Soderlund C, Rodriguez-Tome P, Hui L, Matise TC, McKusick KB, Beckmann JS, et al. (1998). A physical map of 30,000 human genes. *Science* 282: 744–746.

Fitch N (1979). Classification and identification of inherited brachydactylies. *J Med Genet* 16: 36–44.

Forrester WC, Garriga G (1997). Genes necessary for *C. elegans* cell and growth cone migrations. *Development* 124: 1831–1843.

Forrester WC, Dell M, Perens E, Garriga G (1999). A *C. elegans* Ror receptor tyrosine kinase regulates cell motility and asymmetric cell division. *Nature* 400: 881–885.

Frischmeyer PA, Dietz HC (1999). Nonsense-mediated mRNA decay in health and disease. *Hum Mol Genet* 8: 1893–1900.

Glaser D, Herbst J, Roggenkamp K, Tünte W, Lenz W (1989). Robinow syndrome with parental consanguinity. *Eur J Pediatr* 148: 652–653.

Gong Y, Chitayat D, Kerr B, Chen T, Babul-Hirji R, Pal A, Reiss M, Warman ML (1999). Brachydactyly type B: clinical description, genetic mapping to chromosome 9q, and evidence for a shared ancestral mutation. *Am J Hum Genet* 64: 570–577.

Hentze MW, Kulozik AE (1999). A perfect message: RNA surveillance and nonsense-mediated decay. *Cell* 96: 307–310.

Hikasa H, Shibata M, Hiratani I, Taira M (2002). The *Xenopus* receptor tyrosine kinase Xror2 modulates morphogenetic movements of the axial mesoderm and neuroectoderm via Wnt signaling. *Development* 129: 5227–5239.

Houlston RS, Temple IK (1994). Characteristic facies in type B brachydactyly? *Clin Dysmorp* 3: 224–227.

Jennings CGB, Dyer SM, Burden SJ (1993). Muscle-specific *trk*-related receptor with a kringle domain defines a distinct class of receptor tyrosine kinases. *Proc Natl Acad Sci USA* 90: 2895–2899.

Kantaputra PN, Gorlin RJ, Ukarapol N, Unachak K, Sudasna J (1999). Robinow (fetal face) syndrome: report of a boy with dominant type and an infant with recessive type. *Am J Med Genet* 84: 1–7.

Kellie D (1808). Case of defect in the fingers. *Edinb Med J* 4: 252–253.

Koga M, Take-uchi M, Tameishi T, Ohshima Y (1999). Control of DAF-7 TGF-(alpha) expression and neuronal process development by a receptor tyrosine kinase KIN-8 in *Caenorhabditis elegans*. *Development* 126: 5387–5398.

Kroiher M, Miller MA, Steele RE (2001). Deceiving appearances: signaling by "dead" and "fractured" receptor protein-tyrosine kinases. *Bioessays* 23: 69–76.

MacArthur JW, McCullough E (1932). Apical dystrophy. An inherited defect of hands and feet. *Hum Biol* 4: 179–207.

Mackinder D (1857). Deficiency of fingers transmitted through six generations. *Br Med J* 845–846.

Malloch JD (1957). Brachydactyly and symbrachydactyly. *Ann Hum Genet* 22: 36–37.

Masiakowski P, Carroll RD (1992). A novel family of cell surface receptors with tyrosine kinase-like domain. *J Biol Chem* 267: 26181–26190.

Masiakowski P, Yancopoulos GD (1998). The Wnt receptor CRD domain is also found in MuSK and related orphan receptor tyrosine kinases. *Curr Biol* 8: R407.

Matsuda T, Nomi M, Ikeya M, Kani S, Oishi I, Terashima T, Takada S, Minami Y (2001). Expression of the receptor tyrosine kinase genes, *Ror1* and *Ror2*, during mouse development. *Mechan Dev* 105: 153–156.

McKay SE, Hislop J, Scott D, Bulloch AGM, Kaczmarek LK, Carew TJ, Sossin WS (2001). Aplysia Ror forms clusters on the surface of identified neuroendocrine cells. *Mol Cell Neurosci* 17: 821–841.

Nevin NC, Thomas PS, Eedy DJ, Shepherd C (1995). Anonychia and absence/hypoplasia of distal phalanges (Cooks syndrome): report of a second family. *J Med Genet* 32: 638–641.

Nomi M, Oishi I, Kani S, Suzuki H, Matsuda T, Yoda A, Kitamura M, Itoh K, Takeuchi S, Takeda K, et al. (2001). Loss of *mRor1* enhances the heart and skeletal abnormalities in *mRor2* deficient mice: redundant and pleiotropic functions of mRor1 and mRor2 receptor tyrosine kinases. *Mol Cell Biol* 21: 8329–8335.

Oishi I, Sugiyama S, Liu Z-J, Yamamura H, Nishida Y, Minami Y (1997). A novel *Drosophila* receptor tyrosine kinase expressed specifically in the nervous system. *J Biol Chem* 272: 11916–11923.

Oishi I, Takeuchi S, Hashimoto R, Nagabukuro A, Ueda T, Liu Z-J, Hatta T, Akira S, Matsuda Y, Yamamura H, et al. (1999). Spatio-temporally regulated expression of receptor tyrosine kinases, mRor1, mRor2, during mouse development: implications in development and function of the nervous system. *Genes Cells* 4: 41–56.

Oldridge M, Temple IK, Santos HG, Gibbons RJ, Mustafa Z, Chapman KE, Loughlin J, Wilkie AOM (1999). Brachydactyly type B: linkage to chromosome 9q22 and evidence for genetic heterogeneity. *Am J Hum Genet* 64: 578–585.

Oldridge M, Fortuna AM, Maringa M, Propping P, Mansour S, Pollitt C, DeChiara TM, Kimble RB, Valenzuela DM, Yancopoulos GD, et al. (2000). Dominant mutations in *ROR2*, encoding an orphan receptor tyrosine kinase, cause brachydactyly type B. *Nat Genet* 24: 275–278.

Patton MA, Afzal AR (2002). Robinow syndrome. *J Med Genet* 39: 305–310.

Percin EF, Guvenal T, Cetin A, Percin S, Goze F, Arici S (2001). First-trimester diagnosis of Robinow syndrome. *Fetal Diagn Ther* 16: 308–311.

Petit P, Fryns JP, Goddeeris P, Perlmutter-Cremer N (1980). The Robinow syndrome. *Ann Genet* 23: 221–223.

Reddy UR, Phatak S, Allen C, Nycum LM, Sulman EP, White PS, Biegel JA (1997). Localization of the human *Ror1* gene (*NTRKR1*) to chromosome 1p31-p32 by fluorescence *in situ* hybridization and somatic cell hybrid analysis. *Genomics* 41: 283–285.

Robertson SC, Tynan JA, Donoghue DJ (2000). RTK mutations and human syndromes: when good receptors turn bad. *Trends Genet* 16: 265–271.

Robinow M (1993). The Robinow (fetal face) syndrome: a continuing puzzle. *Clin Dysmorp* 2: 189–198.

Robinow M, Silverman FN, Smith HD (1969). A newly recognized dwarfing syndrome. *Am J Dis Child* 117: 645–651.

Santos HG, George FH, Ferreira JR (1981). Braquidactilia hereditária com anoníquia. *Acta Med Port* 3: 147–160.

Schlessinger J (2000). Cell signaling by receptor tyrosine kinases. *Cell* 103: 211–225.

Schorderet DF, Dahoun S, Defrance I, Nusslé D, Morris MA (1992). Robinow syndrome in two siblings from consanguineous parents. *Eur J Pediatr* 151: 586–589.

Schott GD (1978). Hereditary brachydactyly with nail dysplasia. *J Med Genet* 15: 119–122.

Schwabe GC, Tinschert S, Buschow C, Meinecke P, Wolff G, Gillessen-Kaesbach G, Oldridge M, Wilkie AOM, Kömec R, Mundlos S (2000). Distinct mutations in the receptor tyrosine kinase gene *ROR2* cause brachydactyly type B. *Am J Hum Genet* 67: 822–831.

Soliman AT, Rajab A, Alsalmi I, Aziz Bedair SM (1998). Recessive Robinow syndrome: with emphasis on endocrine functions. *Metabolism* 47: 1337–1343.

Takeuchi S, Takeda K, Oishi I, Nomi M, Ikeya M, Itoh K, Tamura S, Ueda T, Hatta T, Otani H, et al. (2000). Mouse Ror2 receptor tyrosine kinase is required for the heart development and limb formation. *Genes Cells* 5: 71–78.

Teebi AS (1990). Autosomal recessive Robinow syndrome. *Am J Med Genet* 35: 64–68.

Temtamy SA, McKusick VA (1978). The genetics of hand malformations. *Birth Defects: Original Article Series* XIV: 215–263.

Türken A, Balci S, Senocak ME, Híçsönmez A (1996). A large inguinal hernia with undescended testes and micropenis in Robinow syndrome. *Clin Dysmorp* 5: 175–178.

Valenzuela DM, Stitt TN, DiStefano PS, Rojas E, Mattsson K, Compton DL, Nunez L, Park JS, Stark JL, Gies DR, et al. (1995). Receptor tyrosine kinase specific for the skeletal muscle lineage: expression in embryonic muscle, at the neuromuscular junction, and after injury. *Neuron* 15: 573–584.

van Bokhoven H, van Beusekom E, Celli J, Kayserili H, Brunner HG (1999). The gene for autosomal recessive Robinow syndrome is located in 9q. *Am J Hum Genet* (suppl) 65: A32.

van Bokhoven H, Celli J, Kayserili H, van Beusekom E, Balci S, Brussel W, Skovby F, Kerr B, Percin EF, Akarsu N, et al. (2000). Mutation of the gene encoding the ROR2 tyrosine kinase causes autosomal recessive Robinow syndrome. *Nat Genet* 25: 423–426.

Vera-Roman JM (1973). Robinow dwarfing syndrome accompanied by penile agenesis and hemivertebrae. *Am J Dis Child* 126: 206–208.

Vorechovsky I, Vihinen M, de Saint Basile G, Honsová S, Hammarström L, Müller S, Nilsson L, Fischer A, Smith CIE (1995). DNA-based mutation analysis of Bruton's tyrosine kinase gene in patients with X-linked agammaglobulinaemia. *Hum Mol Genet* 4: 51–58.

Wadia RS, Shirole DB, Dikshit MS (1978). Recessively inherited costovertebral segmentation defect with mesomelia and peculiar facies (Covesdem syndrome). *J Med Genet* 15: 123–127.

Wadlington WB, Tucker VL, Schimke RN (1973). Mesomelic dwarfism with hemivertebrae and small genitalia (the Robinow syndrome). *Am J Dis Child* 126: 202–205.

Wells NH, Platt M (1947). Hereditary phalangeal agenesis showing dominant mendelian characteristics. *Arch Dis Child* 22: 251–260.

Wilson C, Goberdhan DCI, Steller H (1993). *Dror*, a potential neurotrophic receptor gene, encodes a *Drosophila* homolog of the vertebrate Ror family of Trk-related receptor tyrosine kinases. *Proc Natl Acad Sci USA* 90: 7109–7113.

Xu YK, Nusse R (1998). The Frizzled CRD domain is conserved in diverse proteins including several receptor tyrosine kinases. *Curr Biol* 8: R405–R406.

89 | *PTPN11* and the Noonan Syndrome

MARCO TARTAGLIA AND BRUCE D. GELB

Noonan syndrome (OMIM 163950) is a pleimorphic disorder affecting the cardiovascular, craniofacial, skeletal, hematopoietic, lymphatic, and central nervous systems. It can result from mutations in the *PTPN11* gene, which encodes the protein tyrosine phosphatase (PTP) SHP-2. The disorder is generally transmitted as an autosomal dominant trait, although many cases result from de novo mutations. Defects in the *PTPN11* gene, which resides at chromosomal band 12q24.1, account for approximately 50% of cases. The more than 60 mutations that have been reported are all missense changes, with the vast majority affecting residues clustering at the interface between the N-terminal *src* homology 2 and PTP domains, which plays a role in receptor tyrosine kinase–mediated signal transduction. Mutant SHP-2 proteins have a gain of function, usually through effects on the molecular switching mechanism important for activating/inactivating this enzyme. Clinical manifestations of Noonan syndrome include a typical dysmorphic appearance, congenital heart defects (particularly pulmonic stenosis) or hypertrophic cardiomyopathy, webbing of the neck, short stature, cryptorchidism, eye abnormalities, and skeletal anomalies such as pectus deformities, cubitus valgus, and vertebral anomalies. A minority of affected individuals has bleeding diathesis, hearing loss, and mental retardation. Diagnosis is made by clinical examination. Prenatal diagnosis of Noonan syndrome may be suspected in the presence of ultrasonographic findings such as nuchal edema or cystic hygroma. Therapy in the neonatal period and infancy involves discovering and treating the cardiac disease and managing the feeding problems. Orchidopexy is indicated for undescended testes. Growth hormone therapy has been used to ameliorate the short stature. Preventive pediatric care is appropriate for the hematologic and developmental issues.

THE MOLECULAR GENETICS OF *PTPN11*

Gene Assignment

The locus for human *PTPN11* was assigned to chromosomal band 12q24.1 through the use of fluorescent *in situ* hybridization. Independent analysis with genomic and cDNA probes resulted in similar assignments (Isobe et al., 1994; Dechert et al., 1995).

The *PTPN11* cDNA

Ahmad et al. (1993) cloned the human *PTPN11* cDNA from an umbilical cord library based on its homology to other PTPs in the catalytic domain. The predominant cDNA contained an open reading frame of 1799 nucleotides, resulting in a predicted protein of 593 amino acid residues that is named SHP-2. SHP-2 has a domain arrangement identical to another nonmembranous PTP, SHP-1, with two tandemly arranged *src*-homology 2 (SH2) domains at the N terminus followed by the catalytic, or PTP, domain (Fig. 89–1). There is 60% identity between the PTP domains of SHP-1 and SHP-2 but slightly lower homology across the SH2 domains. Ahmad et al. (1993) also identified a second *PTPN11* transcript that contains an additional 12 bp within the catalytic domain. Little additional information is available about this alternative transcript.

The expression pattern of *PTPN11* has been explored in humans and mice. In humans, a 7.0-kb transcript is detected in several tissues (heart, brain, lung, liver, skeletal muscle, kidney, and pancreas), with the highest steady-state levels in heart and skeletal muscle (Ahmad et

al., 1993). The age of the subjects from whom the RNAs were derived was not specified. The expression pattern of SHP-2 was assessed in adult human brain using immunoblot and immunohistochemistry analyses (Reeves et al., 1996). Although SHP-2 was detected diffusely in the brain, immunohistochemical analysis revealed signal from neurons but not from glial or endothelial cells. In the developing mouse, a 7.0-kb *Ptpn11* transcript was detected at all time points examined (embryonic day [E] 7.5–E18.5) with Northern blot analysis (Feng et al., 1993). *Ptpn11* was detected using in situ hybridization in embryonic and extraembryonic tissues at E7.5. At later time points, signal was present in all tissues, with the highest levels in heart and neural ectoderm.

The *PTPN11* Gene

The *PTPN11* gene spans more than 100 kb and is divided into 16 exons (Tartaglia et al., 2001) (see Fig. 89–1). Exon 1 contains the 5′ untranslated region, the translation initiation ATG, and several additional codons. Exon 15 contains the stop codon, and exon 16 contains a portion of the 3′-untranslated region. This exonic organization is well conserved with *PTPN6*, the gene encoding SHP-1, although the latter has two promoters with alternative first exons (Banville et al., 1995). Other features of the *PTPN11* gene, such as the transcription initiation site and identification of critical enhancer elements, have not been delineated.

CLINICAL DESCRIPTION AND HISTORICAL ASPECTS OF NOONAN SYNDROME

Noonan syndrome is the eponymous name for the disorder described by two pediatric cardiologists, Jacqueline Noonan and Dorothy Ehmke (1963) in an oral presentation and later published by Noonan alone (1968). They based their description of this putatively novel syndrome on observations made in nine patients with valvar pulmonic stenosis; a distinctive dysmorphic facial appearance with hypertelorism, ptosis, and low-set ears; a webbed neck; and chest deformities. Several male patients also had cryptorchidism. John Opitz (1985) suggested that this disorder be called Noonan syndrome, which was subsequently adopted.

As Noonan emphasized (1994), the history of this disorder is long and somewhat complicated. The first known publication of a case of Noonan syndrome was in 1883, in which Kobylinski (1883), then a medical student in Russia, described a 20-year-old man with a webbed neck and several other typical features of Noonan syndrome. In 1930, Ullrich (1930) described several individuals, male and female, with short stature and webbed neck in the German medical literature. Due to possible similarities to a mouse strain that Bonnevie had described, this entity came to be called the Bonnevie-Ullrich phenotype on the European continent (Ullrich, 1949). Independently, Turner (1938) described women with "sexual infantilism" accompanied by webbed neck and short stature in the English literature. With the advent of cytogenetics, it was recognized in 1959 that many women with this disorder either lacked an X chromosome or had an X chromosome rearrangement (Ford et al., 1959). This chromosomal disorder was then named Turner or Ullrich-Turner syndrome. It was apparent, however, that Ullrich had described males with his disorder and that some female patients, who had features resembling the Ullrich-Turner phenotype, had two apparently normal X chromosomes. This led to the

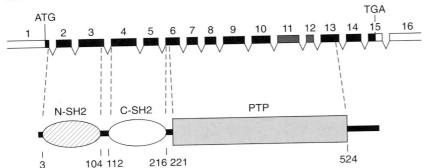

Figure 89–1. *PTPN11* organization and SHP-2 domain structure. The coding exons are shown (*top*) numbered filled boxes, and the positions of the ATG and TGA codons are indicated. The functional domains of the SHP-2 protein, comprising two tandemly arranged SH2 domains at the N terminus (N-SH2 and C-SH2) followed by a protein tyrosine phosphatase (PTP) domain, are shown (*bottom*). Numbers below the domain structure indicate the amino acid boundaries of those domains.

use of confusing terms such as "male Turner syndrome." The work of Noonan, aside from bringing clarity to this semantic muddle, focused on a seminal difference between Turner and Noonan syndromes—the nature and frequency of cardiovascular disease in the latter. The clinical features observed in Noonan syndrome are summarized in Table 89–1.

MOLECULAR PATHOLOGY OF NOONAN SYNDROME

PTPN11 Gene Defects

Tartaglia et al. (2001) identified *PTPN11* as a Noonan syndrome gene. The first genetic mapping studies for Noonan syndrome were performed with small kindreds, with the first report appearing in 1992. Because Noonan syndrome shares some features in common with neurofibromatosis (particularly in certain individuals), markers flanking *NF1* on chromosome 17q and *NF2* on chromosome 22q were used to

Table 89–1. Clinical Features of Noonan Syndrome

Dysmorphia
  Epicanthal folds
  Ptosis
  Downslanting palpebral fissures
  Triangular facies
  Low-set, thickened pinnae
  Light colored irises
  Curly, coarse hair
Cardiovascular
  Congenital heart defects (pulmonic stenosis, atrioventricular septal defects, aortic coarctation, secundum atrial septal defects, mitral valve defects, tetralogy of Fallot, ventricular septal defects, patent ductus arteriosis)
  Hypertrophic cardiomyopathy
Short stature
Webbed neck with low posterior hairline
Skeletal
  Pectus excavatum and/or carinatum
  Cubitus valgus
  Scoliosis
  Vertebral anomalies
Cryptorchidism
Feeding difficulties
Developmental
  Delay
  Attention deficit/hyperactivity disorder
Hematologic
  Bleeding diathesis (von Willebrand disease, factors XI and XII deficiency)
  Thrombocytopenia
  Leukemia
Ophthalmalogic
  Strabismus
  Myopia
Hearing loss
Dental/oral
  Malocclusion
  High arched palate
Lymphatic
  Lymphedema
  Lymphangiectasia

exclude allelism of Noonan syndrome to those traits (Sharland et al., 1992c; Flintoff et al., 1993). Jamieson et al. (1994) used a large Dutch kindred inheriting the disorder to perform a genome-wide scan and observed linkage with several markers at chromosome 12q22-qter, which they named *NS1* (Jamieson et al., 1994). They also documented that Noonan syndrome was genetically heterogeneous, based on linkage exclusion for the *NS1* locus with some other smaller kindreds. The *NS1* locus was refined to a region of approximately 7.5 cM using novel STRs. Legius et al. (1998) studied a four-generation Belgian family in which some affected individuals had findings consistent with Noonan syndrome and others had a phenotype more consistent with cardiofaciocutaneous syndrome. They achieved independent linkage to *NS1* and refined the critical interval further to approximately 5 cM. A positional candidacy approach was taken to identify the Noonan disease gene residing at *NS1*. Ion et al. (2002) mapped the genes encoding epidermal growth factor receptor pathway substrate 8 (*EPS8*) and decorin (*DCN*) out of the *NS1* locus using fluorescent in situ hybridization. They also failed to identify mutations in the genes encoding myosin light chain (*MYL2*) and 60S ribosomal protein L6 (*RPL6*).

Next, Tartaglia et al. (2001) discovered that missense mutations in *PTPN11* cause Noonan syndrome. They studied two medium-sized kindreds inheriting the disorder, documenting probable linkage to *NS1* but failing to further reduce the critical region. *PTPN11* was considered a candidate gene because it mapped to chromosome 12q24.1 between D12S84 and D12S79 and because its protein product, SHP-2, occupied a critical role in several intracellular signal transduction pathways controlling diverse developmental processes, including cardiac semilunar valvulogenesis (Chen et al., 2000). Bidirectional sequencing of the 15 *PTPN11* coding region exons and their intron boundaries for one family revealed a G-to-T transversion at position 214 in exon 3, predicting the substitution of Ala72 by a serine residue (A72S) in the N-SH2 domain. This sequence change was confirmed with a PCR-based RFLP assay that documented its presence in all affected family members and its absence among unaffected ones. This change was not observed in more than 200 control individuals. Sequence comparison of SHP-2 with its orthologues and other closely related PTPs revealed complete conservation of Ala72 (data not shown). Analysis of the second family revealed an A-to-G transition at position 236 in exon 3. This change predicted the substitution of Gln79 by an arginine (Q79R), affecting another highly conserved residue in the N-SH2 domain. This sequence change was confirmed in all affected individuals in this family but was absent in unaffected family members and controls. Taken together, these findings established *PTPN11* as the *NS1* disease gene.

In the original gene discovery article as well as in a subsequent publication, Tartaglia et al. (2001, 2002) investigated the relative importance of *PTPN11* defects in the epidemiology of Noonan syndrome as well as the spectrum of molecular defects observed in the disorder. Mutation screening was performed with 141 apparently unrelated individuals affected with Noonan syndrome, either sporadic (*n* = 81) or familial (*n* = 60) cases. Among the familial cases, the trait was linked to *NS1* in 11 kindreds and excluded in four. For the remaining 45 families, their small size precluded genetic linkage analysis. Missense mutations were identified in 66 cases (47%) (Table 89–2). A total of 22 different molecular defects were observed in this cohort, and one mu-

Table 89–2. *PTPN11* Mutations in Noonan Syndrome

No. of Cases	Nucleotide Substitution	Exon	Amino Acid Substitution	Domain
2	A124 → G	2	T42A	N-SH2
2	G179 → C	3	G60A	N-SH2
1	G181 → A	3	D61N	N-SH2
2	A182 → G	3	D61G	N-SH2
2	T184 → G	3	Y62D	N-SH2
4	A188 → G	3	Y63C	N-SH2
1	G214 → T	3	A72S	N-SH2
2	C215 → G	3	A72G	N-SH2
2	C218 → T	3	T73I	N-SH2
1	G228 → C	3	E76D	N-SH2
6	A236 → G	3	Q79R	N-SH2
3	A317 → C	3	D106A	N-SH2/C-SH2 linker
1	G417 → C	4	E139D	C-SH2
1	G417 → T	4	E139D	C-SH2
1	A836 → G	7	Y279C	PTP
2	A844 → G	7	I282V	PTP
1	T853 → C	7	F285L	PTP
1	T854 → C	8	F285S	PTP
20	A922 → G	8	N308D	PTP
2*	A923 → G	8	N308S	PTP
1	A925 → G	8	I309V	PTP
1	G1502 → A	13	R501K	PTP
4	A1510 → G	13	M504V	PTP

*Affected members of one family exhibited the Noonan-like/multiple giant cell lesion condition.

tation, the 922A-to-G transition that predicted an N308D substitution, constituted nearly one-third of the defects. Several sporadic N308D cases, for whom the parents did not carry that allele, were observed, indicating a mutational hot spot.

It should be noted that there are limitations to the accuracy of the estimate of *PTPN11* mutations in Noonan syndrome. Denaturing HPLC, which has a sensitivity of 96% to 100% under ideal conditions (Xiao and Oefner, 2001), was used for the mutation screening and no attempt was made to look for other types of molecular lesions (large intragenic deletions, promoter defects, and so on). These factors would tend to result in an underestimation of mutation prevalence. On the other hand, the prevalence detected in any Noonan syndrome cohort will be sensitive to the composition of sporadic and familial cases. Because the subjects in the cohort studied were not ascertained in a cross-sectional manner (i.e., there was probably a systematic bias toward familial cases), the prevalence estimate could be too high. With those issues stipulated, the contribution of *PTPN11* mutations to the etiology of Noonan syndrome appears to be approximately 50%.

Two lines of evidence suggest that Noonan syndrome caused by *PTPN11* mutations is almost completely penetrant. First, *PTPN11* mutation analysis with 11 families for which there was significant or suggestive linkage to the *NS1* locus revealed mutations in all affected individuals but none of the unaffected ones. Second, genotyping of a number of unaffected parents for defects discovered in their offspring with apparently sporadic Noonan syndrome provided only a single instance of a genotypically affected, phenotypically normal parent. Although it is possible that similar analysis for "milder" cases of Noonan syndrome might uncover some instances of incomplete penetrance, the strict criteria for Noonan syndrome clinically identifies a cohort with almost 100% penetrance.

The 68 Noonan syndrome mutations identified to date are not randomly distributed in the *PTPN11* gene (Fig. 89–2). Sixty-five of the mutations (96%) affect residues residing at or adjacent to the interface of the N-SH2 and PTP domains. The N-SH2 domain interacts with the PTP domain and binds to phosphotyrosyl-containing targets on activated receptors or docking proteins using two separate sites. These sites show negative cooperativity so that N-SH2 can work as intramolecular switch to control SHP-2 catalytic activity. In the inactive state, the N-SH2 and PTP domains share a broad interaction surface. More precisely, the N-SH2 D'E loop and flanking βD' and βE strands closely interact with the catalytic cleft, blocking the PTP active site. Crystallographic data on SHP-2 in the inactive conformation revealed a complex interdomain hydrogen bonding network involving Asn58, Gly60, Asp61, Cys459, and Gln506, which stabilizes the protein (Hof et al., 1998). Numerous polar interactions between N-SH2 residues located in strands βF and βA, helix αB, and residues of the PTP domain further stabilize the inactive conformation. Significantly, most of the residues mutated in Noonan syndrome either are directly involved in these interdomain interactions (Gly60, Asp61, Ala72, Glu76, and Gln79) or are in close spatial proximity to them (Tyr62, Tyr63, Thr73, Tyr279, Ile282, Phe285, Asn308, Ile309, Arg501, and Met504). This distribution of molecular lesions suggests that the pathogenetic mechanism in Noonan syndrome involves altered N-SH2–PTP interactions that destabilize the inactive conformation without altering the catalytic capability of SHP-2. Consistent with this view, no mutation altered Cys459 (the residue essential for nucleophilic attack), the PTP signature motif (positions 457-467), or the TrpProAsp loop (positions 423-425), which are all essential for phosphatase activity.

Three of the Noonan syndrome mutations affected residues outside of the interacting regions of the N-SH2 and PTP domains (see Fig. 89–2). One recurrent mutation affected Asp106, which is located in the linker stretch connecting the N-SH2 and C-SH2 domains. Although functional studies are required to understand the functional significance of the Asp → Ala substitution, Tartaglia et al. (2002) hypothesized that this mutation might alter the flexibility of the N-SH2 domain, thus inhibiting the N-SH2–PTP interaction. Two mutated residues, Thr42 (N-SH2 domain) and Glu139 (C-SH2 domain), are spatially far from the N-SH2–PTP interaction surfaces. In contrast to

Figure 89–2. Location of mutated residues in SHP-2 in the inactive conformation. Cα trace of N-SH2, C-SH2, and protein tyrosine phosphatase (PTP) domains according to Hof et al. (1998). Mutated residues are indicated with their side chains as thick lines (N-SH2 residues located in or close to the N-SH2–PTP interaction surface, black; linker, C-SH2 and N-SH2-phosphopeptide binding residues, gray; PTP residues located in or close to the N-SH2–PTP interaction surface, gray).

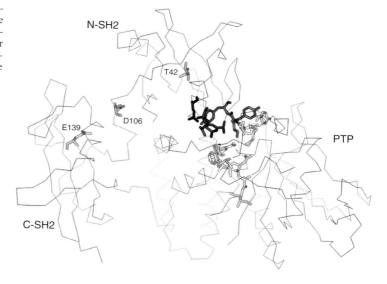

the other mutated residues, Thr42 and Glu139 are implicated in the intermolecular interactions of the SH2 domains with phosphotyrosyl-containing peptides (Lee et al., 1994; Huyer and Ramachandran, 1998). Specifically, Thr42 directly interacts with the tyrosine phosphate and Glu139 is adjacent to Arg138 and Ser140, which form hydrogen bonds to that phosphate. Because the phenotype of the subjects bearing these mutations was typical for Noonan syndrome, molecular characterization is needed to understand how defects in phosphotyrosine binding result in developmental perturbations similar to those affecting SHP-2 inactivation.

The mechanism of action of the mutant SHP-2 proteins appears to be a gain of function. Tartaglia et al. (2001) used thermodynamic analysis to explore the molecular consequences of two Noonan syndrome mutants A72S and A72G. The technique of Monte Carlo (Allen and Tildesley, 1987) with scaled collective variables (Noguti and Go, 1985) was used to determine the energetically accessible conformations of the segment Gly68-Glu76 in the context of N-SH2 in the activated (A) conformation. From this procedure, more than 30 structures were analyzed to relate their structure and energy. For the wild type (Fig. 89–3A), only three low-energy structures had Cα root-mean-square distance (RMSD) of 2 Å or less. The lowest energy structure (RMSD = 0.86 Å) was about 8 kcal/mol below the other two states with small RMSD, supporting the observed stability of the active conformation of isolated N-SH2 (Lee et al., 1994). In addition to the two low-RMSD states around 8 kcal/mol above the lowest energy conformation, several conformations were found at this energy with considerably larger RMSD values. Therefore, shuttling of wild-type SHP-2 between the A and inactivated (I) conformations becomes energetically plausible if, on interaction with the PTP domain, the energy gap between the lowest energy conformation and the nearby states decreases. This would make those conformations accessible and confer the requisite flexibility to this segment of N-SH2. In contrast, both A72G and A72S had large populations with small RMSD and low energies (Figs. 89–3B and 89–C). Even if the energies of these states shifted relative to each other on binding of the PTP domain, there would still be several low-energy conformations available that were close to the A conformation but none that would confer the flexibility required for transition to the I state. Consequently, the ability of these two mutants to shuttle between the A and I states is predicted to be impaired, implying that the equilibrium is shifted toward the A state relative to the wild-type protein.

There are functional data that support the conclusions of the foregoing energetics-based structural analyses. O'Reilly et al. (2000) created and characterized two SHP-2 mutants, D61A and E76A, which they postulated would be gain-of-function changes because both are N-SH2 residues that interact directly with the PTP domain. Both mutants showed increased basal phosphatase activity (E76A > > D61A > wild type) and retained normal phosphopeptide binding properties. When expressed in *Xenopus* ectodermal explants, both mutants induced changes mimicking some aspects of development that are fibroblast growth factor inducible, documenting basal stimulation of some signaling cascades in vivo. D61G, found in a case of Noonan

Table 89–3. Clinical Features in Patients with Noonan Syndrome with and without *PTPN11* Mutations

Clinical Feature	Patients (%) With *PTPN11* Mutation	Patients (%) Without *PTPN11* Mutation	p
Cardiac defects			
Hypertrophic cardiomyopathy	3/51 (5.9)	17/65 (26.1)	0.004
Pulmonic stenosis	36/51 (70.6)	30/65 (46.2)	0.008
Septal defects	6/50 (12.0)	11/63 (17.5)	NS
Short stature	39/51 (76.5)	45/64 (70.3)	NS
Special education class enrollment	11/46 (23.9)	21/59 (35.6)	NS
Pectus deformities	39/50 (78.0)	46/61 (75.4)	NS
Cryptorchidism	26/31 (83.9)	25/35 (71.4)	NS

syndrome, was extremely similar to D61A, providing strong evidence that this mutation has gain-of-function effects. E76D, observed in another case, affected the same residue as the E76A but was a more conservative change. Glu76, however, is invariant among the SHP-2 orthologues and homologues. The similarity in function of Asp61, Ala72, and Glu76 in stabilizing the I state (Hof et al., 1998) provides further evidence that Noonan syndrome is caused by an increased activity of SHP-2.

Genotype–Phenotype Correlation

Because of the clinical heterogeneity observed in Noonan syndrome, Tartaglia et al. (2002) investigated possible associations between genotype and phenotype. The distribution of several major clinical features of Noonan syndrome in subjects with and without mutations in *PTPN11* is shown (Table 89–3). A statistically significant association with pulmonary valve stenosis was found among the group with *PTPN11* mutations (70.6% versus 46.2%, p = 0.008). In contrast, a statistically significant lower incidence of hypertrophic cardiomyopathy was observed in this group (5.9% versus 26.2%, p = 0.004). There was no significant difference in the prevalence of atrial and/or ventricular septal defects or other congenital heart malformations between the *PTPN11* mutation and nonmutation groups. Similarly, there was no difference in the rates of short stature, pectus deformities, cryptorchidism, or enrollment in special education classes (as a marker of developmental delay).

The cohorts with N-SH2 and PTP mutations, respectively, were compared for the same clinical manifestations of NS. Although this analysis had less statistical power due to sample size, no significant differences were identified. The phenotype observed in subjects with the common Asn308Asp substitution (n = 17) was not qualitatively different from that of subjects with other mutations, except none carrying the Asn308Asp change was enrolled in special education classes.

PTPN11 mutations have been identified in two phenotypes related to classic Noonan syndrome. Tartaglia et al. (2002) identified an A-to-G transition at position 923 (Asn308Ser) in a previously described

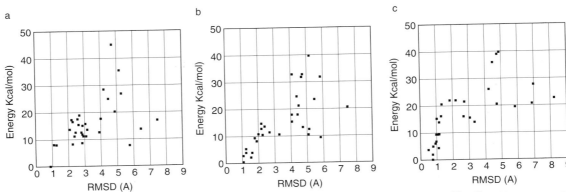

Figure 89–3. Plots of root-mean-square deviation (RMSD) against energy for the wild-type and two mutant N-SH2 segments of SHP-2. For each case, the lowest energy conformation was arbitrarily set to an energy of 0 kcal/mol. (*a*) Wild type. (*b*) Ala72Gly. (*c*) Ala72Ser.

family with Noonan-like syndrome with multiple giant cell lesions in bone (OMIM 163955). In this family, two siblings had lesions in the mandible, whereas their mother only had typical features of Noonan syndrome (Bertola et al., 2001). The same Asn308Ser mutation was observed in another family with Noonan syndrome with no known bony involvement.

Digilio et al. (2002) screened eight independent individuals with LEOPARD syndrome (OMIM 151100) for *PTPN11* defects and identified missense mutations in seven. They also found mutations in two individuals with Noonan syndrome with café-au-lait spots. Among these nine apparently independent mutations, three were A-to-G transitions at position 386 (Tyr279Cys) and six were C-to-T transitions at position 1403 (Thr468Met). The Tyr279Cys mutation had been found previously in an infant diagnosed with Noonan syndrome; reexamination later in life revealed the presence of multiple café-au-lait spots (S. Jeffery, personal communication). These results suggest specificity for these mutations for the development of these dermatological abnormalities.

Ion et al. (2002) searched for *PTPN11* mutations in a cohort of 29 unrelated individuals with cardiofaciocutaneous syndrome. This disorder resembles Noonan syndrome in several respects, and several authors had questioned whether the two were allelic (Fryer et al., 1991; Neri et al., 1991; Ward et al., 1994; Leichtman, 1996; Neri and Zollino, 1996; Wieczorek et al., 1997). No *PTPN11* mutations were found in this cohort.

DIAGNOSIS

Clinical Evaluation

The diagnosis of Noonan syndrome depends on the clinical features (Mendez and Opitz, 1985; Sharland et al., 1992a; Noonan, 1994) (see Table 89–1). Genetic testing is expected to become available and should be capable of detecting approximately 50% of cases. Although a comprehensive scoring system was developed to aid in clinical diagnosis (Duncan et al., 1981), most clinicians continue to use a more subjective assessment. In newborns, the facial features may be less apparent (Allanson et al., 1985) but generalized edema and excess nuchal folds may be present. With time, several features become more obvious, including the facial features (Fig. 89–4), the pectus deformities, and short stature. Hypertrophic cardiomyopathy may also develop during the first few years of life. The webbing of the neck, often subtle in infancy, may become more apparent later in childhood.

As with most clinical genetic assessments, obtaining a careful prenatal and family history is important. Prenatal exposure to certain teratogens such as ethanol must be considered. When evaluating girls, particularly in infancy, a karyotype is usually performed to exclude the diagnosis of Turner syndrome.

Prenatal Diagnosis

The diagnosis of Noonan syndrome can be suspected when a cystic hygroma or nuchal lucency is detected with fetal ultrasonography. Such findings usually prompt further investigation, including a karyotype of chorionic villus samples or amniocytes. Among fetuses with normal chromosomes, the diagnosis of Noonan syndrome will be made in approximately 2% of cases with nuchal edema in the first trimester (Reynders et al., 1997; Adekunle et al., 1999; Nisbet et al., 1999; Hiippala et al., 2001).

TREATMENT

Clinical Management

There are several aspects of the Noonan syndrome phenotype that require medical evaluation and possible treatment. Newborns, infants, and children suspected of having Noonan syndrome need a careful cardiac evaluation, including an echocardiogram. Management of congenital heart defects in these children is dictated by the type and severity of the cardiac disease, which can vary from trivial to life threatening (Burch et al., 1993; Marino et al., 1999; Bertola et al., 2000).

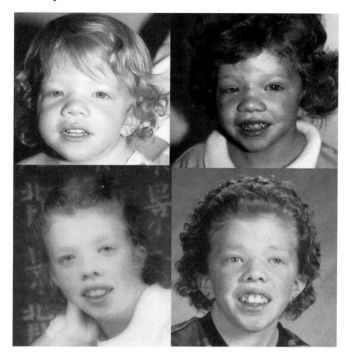

Figure 89–4. Dysmorphic facial features in Noonan syndrome showing the series of one affected girl from age 2 to 17 years, with evolution of the facial features. (Kindly provided by J. Allanson.)

Because patients with Noonan syndrome and pulmonic stenosis tend to have dysplastic valves, outcomes from interventional catheterization are probably less successful than average. Evaluation of the heart in early infancy does not exclude the possibility that an affected child will develop more severe pulmonic stenosis or hypertrophic cardiomyopathy later in childhood. This suggests that serial evaluations during this period are indicated. Data are meager about the time course, including outer limits for presentation, for the development of hypertrophic cardiomyopathy in Noonan syndrome. It is established, however, that Noonan syndrome is a leading cause of hypertrophic cardiomyopathy in young children.

Mothers carrying fetuses at risk for Noonan syndrome (i.e., offspring of affected mothers or fathers) should have fetal echocardiography at about 18 to 20 weeks' gestation to rule out complex congenital heart disease. If disease is present and the pregnancy is continued, such findings might alter the management of the infant at birth as well as suggest a need to change the delivery site to a center able to provide urgent interventions for complex heart defects.

Children with Noonan syndrome need careful pediatric attention during infancy and childhood. Feeding problems are noted in the majority of affected infants and can cause failure to thrive (Shah et al., 1999). For some patients, the inadequacy in oral intake may be severe enough to necessitate placement of gastrostomy tubes, although occupational/feeding therapy is an adequate intervention for most. Visual problems such as strabismus are common, so referral for an ophthalmological assessment is indicated (Lee et al., 1992). Hearing loss has been described in about 40% of patients (Cremers and van der Burgt, 1992; Qiu et al., 1998). Auditory problems have been correlated with the abnormal craniofacial anatomy, particularly of the temporal bone (Naficy et al., 1997). Renal abnormalities are found in a minority of affected children but warrant a screening abdominal ultrasound (George et al., 1993).

Developmental delay and learning problems are quite common in Noonan syndrome, perhaps affecting one-third of patients (Sharland et al., 1992a). Some motor delay can be attributed to the hypotonia often observed in affected infants. Although the learning deficits in Noonan syndrome have not been delineated precisely, increased prevalence of attention deficit/hyperactivity disorder and frank mental retardation is observed. More significant neurological problems, such as epilepsy, are noted in a small minority of patients (Sharland et al., 1992a).

One of the salient features of Noonan syndrome is short stature, with median heights of less than the third centile in children (Witt et al., 1986; Ranke et al., 1988). In an attempt to increase adult stature (averaging 162.5 and 152.7 cm for affected men and women, respectively), efforts have been undertaken to study the effects of growth hormone therapy in cohorts of children with Noonan syndrome (Cotterill et al., 1996; Romano et al., 1996; Kirk et al., 2001; MacFarlane et al., 2001; Noordam et al., 2001b). There appears to be some scientific basis for this because studies of growth hormone secretion in this disorder have documented some quantitative and qualitative abnormalities, although none approach those seen in primary growth hormone deficiency (Ahmed et al., 1991; Tanaka et al., 1992; Noordam et al., 2002). Although initial studies reporting results from a single year of therapy demonstrated significant acceleration in linear growth, more recent reports of longer courses have been less encouraging. Growth in subsequent years of therapy is far less accelerated. For patients reaching later stages of puberty, when linear growth terminates, final heights have been modestly increased compared with predicted ones. A study showed that long-term growth hormone therapy advanced bone age at approximately the same rate as height increased (Noordam et al., 2001b). Because linear growth in Noonan syndrome is often more prolonged due to the later onset of puberty, the advancement of bone age would be expected to result in a decrease in the total years of growth, potentially canceling some of the benefit of more rapid growth early in the treatment course. Efforts are ongoing to determine the extent to which adult height can be augmented with various growth hormone regimens.

One additional concern has been the potential adverse effects of growth hormone on the heart in Noonan syndrome patients with hypertrophic cardiomyopathy. Reports have emphasized the fact that cardiac phenotypes other than hypertrophic cardiomyopathy (considered by some to be a contraindication for growth hormone therapy) were unaffected echocardiographically after growth hormone therapy (Cotterill et al., 1996; MacFarlane et al., 2001; Noordam et al., 2001a; Brown et al., 2002), but revisiting of this issue may be fruitful because there is evidence that the non-*PTPN11* forms of Noonan syndrome are more likely to have the hypertrophic phenotype.

Orthopedic problems are common in Noonan syndrome (Sharland et al., 1992a). For instance, pectus deformities are observed in the vast majority but rarely are severe enough to warrant surgical intervention. Scoliosis occurs in approximately 10% of patients and may become pronounced enough to demand intervention. Other bony defects, such as vertebral anomalies, occur at low frequency.

Patients with Noonan syndrome require evaluation for bleeding diathesis before surgery, dental work, or delivery. The most common abnormalities include von Willebrand disease, deficiencies of factors XI and XII, and thrombocytopenia (Sharland et al., 1992b; Massarano et al., 1996; Singer et al., 1997). Because many affected children will require interventional procedures such as balloon pulmonary valvuloplasty and orchidopexy, this is important to bear in mind to prevent significant hemorrhagic complications.

Malignant hyperthermia is sometimes listed as being associated with Noonan syndrome. There have been rare reports of malignant hyperthermia in patients with Noonan syndrome (Pinsky, 1972; Rissam et al., 1982; Lee et al., 2001). There also is a related disorder, King syndrome, which includes a skeletal myopathy with elevated creatine phosphokinase, malignant hyperthermia, Noonan syndrome–like dysmorphia, short stature, cryptorchidism, and skeletal anomalies, that might be confused with Noonan syndrome (King et al., 1972; Graham et al., 1998). These factors have led to the listing of malignant hyperthermia as associated with Noonan syndrome. Because only about three cases has been reported for isolated Noonan syndrome, which is one of the more common mendelian disorders, it seems unlikely that this is a true association. Careful examination to exclude the diagnosis of King syndrome is appropriate. Practices to avoiding triggering agents during the administration of anesthesia vary among institutions.

The lymphatic system develops abnormally in Noonan syndrome, although the persistence of lymphedema at birth occurs less frequently than observed in Turner syndrome. Lymphangiectasia affecting the gastrointestinal tract and lungs has presented in infants and children with Noonan syndrome (Baltaxe et al., 1975; Herzog et al., 1976; Hernandez et al., 1980; Fisher et al., 1982; Ozturk et al., 2000). The former complication may lead to protein-losing enteropathy and the latter to spontaneous chylothorax; both are difficult to manage. Some older patients with Noonan syndrome have developed peripheral lymphedema, usually most pronounced in the legs, that is treated with compressive bandages (Lanning et al., 1978).

Genetic Counseling

Genetic counseling for Noonan syndrome is complicated because this trait is usually autosomal dominant with nearly complete penetrance and variable expressivity, but there also is genetic heterogeneity and a possible rare autosomal recessive form (van Der Burgt and Brunner, 2000). Emphasis on the variability of the phenotype within families is important, particularly when an affected family member has experienced severe cardiac or neurodevelopmental problems. The recurrence risk for unaffected parents with a prior affected child is quite low because the disorder is almost fully penetrant, mitigated by the theoretical possibility of gonadal mosaicism (Tartaglia et al., 2002). Clinical DNA diagnostics are not available for this disorder but are being developed. Such testing may prove useful to confirm the diagnosis in suspected cases of Noonan syndrome antenatally or postnatally, as well as to diagnose the disorder in families in which a *PTPN11* mutation has already been defined. For the former, DNA testing cannot be exclusionary because of the genetic heterogeneity underlying Noonan syndrome.

MUTATIONS IN ORTHOLOGOUS GENES

A mouse model of Shp-2 deficiency was generated using targeted disruption in embryonic stem cells (Arrandale et al., 1996; Saxton et al., 1997). The allele, which deleted several residues of the N-SH2 domain and obliterated activation of the mitogen-activated protein kinase (MAPK) pathway, was recessive embryonic lethal. Developing embryos nullizygous for Shp-2 had defects in gastrulation and patterning, resulting in severe abnormalities in axial mesoderm development.

Chimeras were generated by associating *Ptpn11*-nullizygous embryonic stem cells with wild-type morulas (Qu et al., 1998; Saxton et al., 2000). Among phenotypically normal chimeric embryos, mutant cells were absent in the heart, somites, limb buds, and nasal placode, all regions that require fibroblast growth factor signaling. There also was an absence of a contribution of *Ptpn11*-mutant cells to hematopoietic progenitors in fetal liver and bone marrow. Extensive characterization of limb development in chimeras demonstrated that the absence of *Ptpn11*-mutant cells in the developing progress zone resulted from abnormal chemokinesis or cell adhesion but not from inadequate proliferation (Saxton et al., 2000). When *Ptpn11*-mutant cells were present in the progress zone, limb development was abnormal, evidence that Shp-2–related signaling is required for limb development.

Of particular relevance to the potential pathogenesis of Noonan syndrome, Shp-2 has a role in semilunar valvulogenesis. Chen et al. (2000) studied the effects of a hypomorphic allele of *Egfr* (called *Egfr*^wa2^), which produces a protein with 10% to 20% residual kinase activity. Mice with combined homozygosity for *Egfr*^wa2^ and heterozygosity for a null *Ptpn11* allele had aortic and pulmonic stenoses due to thickening of the valve leaflets with excessive numbers of mesenchymal cells. Embryos with only *Egfr*^wa2^ homozygosity also had abnormal semilunar valves but to a significantly lesser extent. Although the nature of the *PTPN11* alleles differs between these mice and patients with Noonan syndrome (haploinsufficiency versus gain of function), these data suggest that the pulmonic stenosis associated with Noonan syndrome results from abnormal SHP-2 activity in the epithelial growth factor receptor (EGFR) pathway.

The *Drosophila* orthologue of *PTPN11* is *corkscrew* (*csw*), which was cloned by Perrimon's group (Perkins et al., 1992). This X-linked gene is named for the shape of misshapened fly embryos that result from deficiency of this PTP. Corkscrew is maternally required for de-

Figure 89–5. Torso (TOR) signal transduction pathway from the receptor tyrosine kinase TOR to stimulation of gene transcription by mitogen-activated protein kinase (MAPK) in *Drosophila* embryos. Corkscrew (CSW) binds phosphorylated Y630 residue and dephosphorylates Y918. The latter prevents the binding of GTPase activating protein 1 (GAP1), which negatively regulates the MAPK pathway. Activated TOR also phosphorylates CSW at Y666, potentiating the binding of DRK. This activates the MAPK cascade, resulting in increased expression of TLL and HKB. DRK, Downstream-of-receptor-kinases; SOS, Son-of-sevenless; MEK, MAP kinase kinase; TLL, Tailless; HKB, Huckebein.

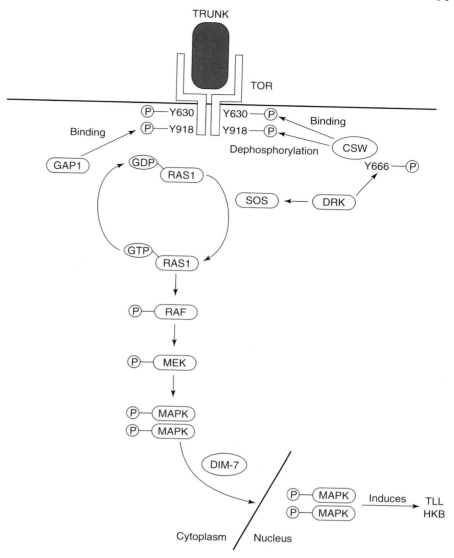

termination of cell fates for terminal structures. Corkscrew acts downstream of torso, which is a receptor tyrosine kinase that is homologous to fibroblast growth factor receptor 3 (Ghiglione et al., 1999; Cleghon et al., 1998; Lu et al., 1993; Perrimon et al., 1995; Perkins et al., 1996). After binding its ligand, torso autophosphorylates and initiates a signal cascade that results in activation of MAPK (Fig. 89–5). Activated MAPK dimerizes and translocates into the nucleus, where it induces expression of two transcription factors, tailless and huckebein, at the anterior and posterior embryonic poles, respectively.

The interactions between torso and corkscrew are complex (see Fig. 89–5). Using an SH2 domain, corkscrew binds to torso at the phosphorylated residue Y630 (Cleghon et al., 1998). This binding activates corkscrew, which then dephosphorylates torso at Y918. This dephosphorylation prevents GAP1, a negative regulator of the MAPK cascade, from binding to torso. Activated torso also phosphorylates corkscrew at Y666, facilitating docking of the protein downstream-of-receptor-kinases (the *Drosophila* homologue of the mammalian adapter protein GRB-2). Downstream-of-receptor-kinases, in turn binds son-of-sevenless, activating it and stimulating the MAPK cascade. Epistatic analyses have also documented that corkscrew interacts with additional members of the MAPK cascade, although its specific targets remain to be determined. It was shown that corkscrew binds with *Drosophila* importin-7, which binds to dimerized MAPK and translocates it across the nuclear membrane (Lorenzen et al., 2001).

In addition to the role of corkscrew in the development of terminal structures through the torso signal cascade, it is also important for sev-

eral other receptor tyrosine kinase pathways that result in MAPK activation (Perkins et al., 1996). Among these, the best characterized is the sevenless pathway in the developing *Drosophila* eye (Raabe, 2000). The *Drosophila* eye is composed of 800 units, called ommatidia, that contain eight photoreceptor cells (R1–R8), as well as lens and accessory cells. Although the development of all photoreceptor cells is dependent on the *Drosophila* epidermal growth factor (EGF) receptor, only R7 development also requires signaling from sevenless. Mutant *corkscrew* alleles perturb R7 development, producing the rough eye phenotype (Allard et al., 1996). Although the sevenless pathway to MAPK is quite similar to that used by torso, the interactions of corkscrew within the cascades are not identical. In particular, corkscrew binds sevenless independent of the phosphorylation state of sevenless (whereas it binds torso only after ligand binding and autophosphorylation). In addition, activated corkscrew binds and dephosphorylates the Gab2 homologue, daughter-of-sevenless, which is phosphorylated by activated sevenless (Herbst et al., 1996, 1999). Daughter-of-sevenless then acts as a multisite adapter in promoting signaling to MAPK in an RAS-dependent or RAS-independent fashion.

Phenotypic characterization of several *corkscrew* alleles has documented that *corkscrew* participates in signal cascades for several other receptor tyrosine kinases (Perkins et al., 1996; Firth et al., 2000). EGF (a.k.a. DER) is important for the development of ventral ectoderm (including the central nervous system), eyes, antennae, legs, and wings. All of these structures develop abnormally when corkscrew is deficient. Similarly, the fibroblast growth factor receptor 1, breathless, is a receptor tyrosine kinase that is critical for tracheal development. When corkscrew is deficient, tracheal cell precursors are produced normally but fail to migrate properly. Finally, another fibroblast growth factor receptor, heartless, is critical for specification of pericardial cells. Deficiency of corkscrew disrupts or deletes their development.

Developmental Pathogenesis of Noonan Syndrome

The phenotype of Noonan syndrome includes developmental defects in several organ systems. Because SHP-2 plays a central role in signaling from a variety of growth factors and hormones and is expressed diffusely, it is not surprising that excessive SHP-2 activity should result in pleiomorphic effects. In previous sections, the relationship between EGFR signaling and semilunar valvulogenesis was discussed, a seminal finding that led to the discovery of *PTPN11* as a Noonan syndrome gene. In addition, the importance of SHP-2 was noted, most likely for FGF signaling, in several developing structures. The heart, limbs, and nasal placode are particularly germane when considering the pathogenesis of Noonan syndrome. All of these observations, however, derive from studies of the loss of SHP-2 function. Future inquiry focusing on the effects of excessive SHP-2 phosphatase activity will provide insights into the pathogenesis of Noonan syndrome per se.

SHP-2 plays a role in the signal transduction resulting from binding of growth hormone to the growth hormone receptor. Because short stature is a cardinal aspect of Noonan syndrome, diminution of growth hormone–induced signaling may be the mechanism through which this feature occurs. As with other aspects of signal transduction and SHP-2 biology, the interactions are complex. In particular, there is evidence that SHP-2 is both a positive and a negative regulator of this pathway. In one study (Kim et al., 1998), SHP-2 was documented to bind to the growth hormone receptor after cell stimulation with growth hormone. Expression of a construct producing a catalytically inactive form of SHP-2 reduced gene activation that results from growth hormone signal transduction, providing evidence of positive regulation. In another study (Stofega et al., 2000), mutation of a critical tyrosine residue on the growth hormone receptor, to which SHP-2 apparently binds after that residue is phosphorylated, resulted in prolonged phosphorylation of STAT5B. Because phosphorylated STAT5B is an activator of transcription, this effect resulted in prolonged signal transduction from growth hormone. In this context, SHP-2 acts as a negative regulator of this pathway. Studies of the cell biologic response to growth hormone in the presence of gain-of-function SHP-2 mutant proteins are necessary to understand with precision the contribution of deranged growth hormone–mediated signal transduction in the pathogenesis of short stature in Noonan syndrome.

SHP-2 has been shown to participate in thrombin-induced platelet aggregation. This effect is mediated in part through the association of SHP-2 with platelet–endothelial cell adhesion molecule-1 (PECAM-1) and other tyrosine-phosphorylated proteins (Jackson et al., 1997; Edmead et al., 1999). PECAM-1 becomes phosphorylated after platelet aggregation, leading to an up-regulation of the integrin system. Because the normal role of SHP-2 in platelet biology appears to favor platelet aggregation, it remains to be determined how an excess of SHP-2 PTP activity can lead to a decreased ability to aggregate. Other contributions to the potential for a bleeding diathesis, such as inadequate levels of coagulations factors, are even more obscure.

ACKNOWLEDGMENTS

We thank Judith Willner for her thoughtful reading. This work was supported in part from grant HBLI38018 from the National Institutes of Health (to B.D.G.).

REFERENCES

Adekunle O, Gopee A, el-Sayed M, Thilaganathan B (1999). Increased first trimester nuchal translucency: pregnancy and infant outcomes after routine screening for Down's syndrome in an unselected antenatal population. *Br J Radiol* 72: 457–460.

Ahmad S, Banville D, Zhao Z, Fischer EH, Shen SH (1993). A widely expressed human protein-tyrosine phosphatase containing src homology 2 domains. *Proc Natl Acad Sci USA* 90: 2197–2201.

Ahmed ML, Foot AB, Edge JA, Lamkin VA, Savage MO, Dunger DB (1991). Noonan's syndrome: abnormalities of the growth hormone/IGF-I axis and the response to treatment with human biosynthetic growth hormone. *Acta Paediatr Scand* 80: 446–450.

Allanson JE, Hall JG, Hughes HE, Preus M, Witt RD (1985). Noonan syndrome: the changing phenotype. *Am J Med Genet* 21: 507–514.

Allard JD, Chang HC, Herbst R, McNeill H, Simon MA (1996). The SH2-containing tyrosine phosphatase corkscrew is required during signaling by sevenless, Ras1 and Raf. *Development* 122: 1137–1146.

Allen M, Tildesley DJ (1987). *Computer Simulation of Liquids.* Clarendon, Oxford.

Arrandale JM, Gore-Willse A, Rocks S, Ren JM, Zhu J, Davis A, Livingston JN, Rabin DU (1996). Insulin signaling in mice expressing reduced levels of Syp. *J Biol Chem* 271: 21353–21358.

Baltaxe HA, Lee JG, Ehlers KH, Engle MA (1975). Pulmonary lymphangiectasia demonstrated by lymphangiography in 2 patients with Noonan's syndrome. *Radiology* 115: 149–153.

Banville D, Stocco R, Shen SH (1995). Human protein tyrosine phosphatase 1C (PTPN6) gene structure: alternate promoter usage and exon skipping generate multiple transcripts. *Genomics* 27: 165–173.

Bertola DR, Kim CA, Pereira AC, Mota GF, Krieger JE, Vieira IC, Valente M, Loreto MR, Magalhaes RP, Gonzalez CH (2001). Are Noonan syndrome and Noonan-like/multiple giant cell lesion syndrome distinct entities? *Am J Med Genet* 98: 230–234.

Bertola DR, Kim CA, Sugayama SM, Albano LM, Wagenfuhr J, Moyses RL, Gonzalez CH (2000). Cardiac findings in 31 patients with Noonan's syndrome. *Arq Bras Cardiol* 75: 409–412.

Brown DC, MacFarlane CE, McKenna WJ, Patton MA, Dunger DB, Savage MO, Kelnar CJ (2002). Growth hormone therapy in Noonan's syndrome: non-cardiomyopathic congenital heart disease does not adversely affect growth improvement. *J Pediatr Endocrinol Metab* 15: 851–852.

Burch M, Sharland M, Shinebourne E, Smith G, Patton M, McKenna W (1993). Cardiologic abnormalities in Noonan syndrome: phenotypic diagnosis and echocardiographic assessment of 118 patients. *J Am Coll Cardiol* 22: 1189–1192.

Chen B, Bronson RT, Klaman LD, Hampton TG, Wang JF, Green PJ, Magnuson T, Douglas PS, Morgan JP, Neel BG (2000). Mice mutant for Egfr and Shp2 have defective cardiac semilunar valvulogenesis. *Nat Genet* 24: 296–299.

Cleghon V, Feldmann P, Ghiglione C, Copeland TD, Perrimon N, Hughes DA, Morrison DK (1998). Opposing actions of CSW and RasGAP modulate the strength of Torso RTK signaling in the Drosophila terminal pathway. *Mol Cell* 2: 719–727.

Cotterill AM, McKenna WJ, Brady AF, Sharland M, Elsawi M, Yamada M, Camacho-Hubner C, Kelnar CJ, Dunger DB, Patton MA, et al. (1996). The short-term effects of growth hormone therapy on height velocity and cardiac ventricular wall thickness in children with Noonan's syndrome. *J Clin Endocrinol Metab* 81: 2291–2297.

Cremers CW, van der Burgt CJ (1992). Hearing loss in Noonan syndrome. *Int J Pediatr Otorhinolaryngol* 23: 81–84.

Dechert U, Duncan AM, Bastien L, Duff C, Adam M, Jirik FR (1995). Protein-tyrosine phosphatase SH-PTP2 (PTPN11) is localized to 12q24.1-24.3. *Hum Genet* 96: 609–615.

Digilio MC, Conti E, Sarkozy A, Mingarelli R, Dottorini T, Marino B, Pizzuti A, Dallapiccola B (2002). Grouping of multiple-lentigines/LEOPARD and Noonan syndromes on the PTPN11 gene. *Am J Hum Genet* 71: 389–394.

Duncan WJ, Fowler RS, Farkas LG, Ross RB, Wright AW, Bloom KR, Huot DJ, Sondheimer HM, Rowe RD (1981). A comprehensive scoring system for evaluating Noonan syndrome. *Am J Med Genet* 10: 37–50.

Edmead CE, Crosby DA, Southcott M, Poole AW (1999). Thrombin-induced association of SHP-2 with multiple tyrosine-phosphorylated proteins in human platelets. *FEBS Lett* 459: 27–32.

Feng GS, Hui CC, Pawson T (1993). SH2-containing phosphotyrosine phosphatase as a target of protein-tyrosine kinases. *Science* 259: 1607–1611.

Firth L, Manchester J, Lorenzen JA, Baron M, Perkins LA (2000). Identification of genomic regions that interact with a viable allele of the Drosophila protein tyrosine phosphatase corkscrew. *Genetics* 156: 733–748.

Fisher E, Weiss EB, Michals K, DuBrow IW, Hastrieter AR, Matalon R (1982). Spontaneous chylothorax in Noonan's syndrome. *Eur J Pediatr* 138: 282–284.

Flintoff WF, Bahuau M, Lyonnet S, Gilgenkrantz S, Lacombe D, Marcon F, Levilliers J, Kachaner J, Munnich A, Le Merrer M (1993). No evidence for linkage to the type 1 or type 2 neurofibromatosis loci in Noonan syndrome families. *Am J Med Genet* 46: 700–705.

Ford CE, Jones KW, Polani PE, de Almeida JC, Bruiggs JH (1959). A sex chromosome anomaly in a case of gonadal dysgenesis (Turner's syndrome). *Lancet* 1: 711–713.

Fryer AE, Holt PJ, Hughes HE (1991). The cardio-facio-cutaneous (CFC) syndrome and Noonan syndrome: are they the same? *Am J Med Genet* 38: 548–551.

George CD, Patton MA, el Sawi M, Sharland M, Adam EJ (1993). Abdominal ultrasound in Noonan syndrome: a study of 44 patients. *Pediatr Radiol* 23: 316–318.

Ghiglione C, Perrimon N, Perkins LA (1999). Quantitative variations in the level of MAPK activity control patterning of the embryonic termini in Drosophila. *Dev Biol* 205: 181–193.

Graham GE, Silver K, Arlet V, Der Kaloustian VM (1998). King syndrome: further clinical variability and review of the literature. *Am J Med Genet* 78: 254–259.

Herbst R, Zhang X, Qin J, Simon MA (1999). Recruitment of the protein tyrosine phosphatase CSW by DOS is an essential step during signaling by the sevenless receptor tyrosine kinase. *EMBO J* 18: 6950–6961.

Herbst R, Carroll PM, Allard JD, Schilling J, Raabe T, Simon MA (1996). Daughter of sevenless is a substrate of the phosphotyrosine phosphatase Corkscrew and functions during sevenless signaling. *Cell* 85: 899–909.

Hernandez RJ, Stern AM, Rosenthal A (1980). Pulmonary lymphangiectasis in Noonan syndrome. *AJR Am J Roentgenol* 134: 75–80.

Herzog DB, Logan R, Kooistra JB (1976). The Noonan syndrome with intestinal lymphangiectasia. *J Pediatr* 88: 270–272.

Hiippala A, Eronen M, Taipale P, Salonen R, Hiilesmaa V (2001). Fetal nuchal translucency and normal chromosomes: a long-term follow-up study. *Ultrasound Obstet Gynecol* 18: 18–22.

Hof P, Pluskey S, Dhe-Paganon S, Eck MJ, Shoelson SE (1998). Crystal structure of the tyrosine phosphatase SHP-2. *Cell* 92: 441–450.

Huyer G, Ramachandran C (1998). The specificity of the N-terminal SH2 domain of SHP-2 is modified by a single point mutation. *Biochemistry* 37: 2741–2747.

Ion A, Tartaglia M, Song X, Kalidas K, van der Burgt I, Crosby AH, Ming JE, Zampino G, Zackai EH, Dean JCS, et al. (2002). Absence of *PTPN11* mutations in 29 cases of Cardiofaciocutaneous (CFC) syndrome. *Hum Genet* 111: 421–427.

Isobe M, Hinoda Y, Imai K, Adachi M (1994). Chromosomal localization of an SH2 containing tyrosine phosphatase (SH-PTP3) gene to chromosome 12q24.1. *Oncogene* 9: 1751–1753.

Jackson DE, Ward CM, Wang R, Newman PJ (1997). The protein-tyrosine phosphatase SHP-2 binds platelet/endothelial cell adhesion molecule-1 (PECAM-1) and forms a distinct signaling complex during platelet aggregation. Evidence for a mechanistic link between PECAM-1- and integrin-mediated cellular signaling. *J Biol Chem* 272: 6986–6993.

Jamieson CR, van der Burgt I, Brady AF, van Reen M, Elsawi MM, Hol F, Jeffery S, Patton MA, Mariman E (1994). Mapping a gene for Noonan syndrome to the long arm of chromosome 12. *Nat Genet* 8: 357–360.

Kim SO, Jiang J, Yi W, Feng GS, Frank SJ (1998). Involvement of the Src homology 2-containing tyrosine phosphatase SHP-2 in growth hormone signaling. *J Biol Chem* 273: 2344–2354.

King JO, Denborough MA, Zapf PW (1972). Inheritance of malignant hyperpyrexia. *Lancet* 1: 365–370.

Kirk JM, Betts PR, Butler GE, Donaldson MD, Dunger DB, Johnston DI, Kelnar CJ, Price DA, Wilton P, Group tU (2001). Short stature in Noonan syndrome: response to growth hormone therapy. *Arch Dis Child* 84: 440–443.

Kobylinski O (1883). Ueber eine flughoutahnbiche ausbreitung. *Am Halse Arch Anthropol* 14: 342–348.

Lanning P, Simila S, Suramo I, Paavilainen T (1978). Lymphatic abnormalities in Noonan's syndrome. *Pediatr Radiol* 7: 106–109.

Lee CH, Kominos D, Jacques S, Margolis B, Schlessinger J, Shoelson SE, Kuriyan J (1994). Crystal structures of peptide complexes of the amino-terminal SH2 domain of the Syp tyrosine phosphatase. *Structure* 2: 423–438.

Lee CK, Chang BS, Hong YM, Yang SW, Lee CS, Seo JB (2001). Spinal deformities in Noonan syndrome: a clinical review of sixty cases. *J Bone Joint Surg Am* 83-A: 1495–1502.

Lee NB, Kelly L, Sharland M (1992). Ocular manifestations of Noonan syndrome. *Eye* 6(pt 3): 328–334.

Legius E, Schollen E, Matthijs G, Fryns JP (1998). Fine mapping of Noonan/cardio-facio cutaneous syndrome in a large family. *Eur J Hum Genet* 6: 32–37.

Leichtman LG (1996). Are cardio-facio-cutaneous syndrome and Noonan syndrome distinct? A case of CFC offspring of a mother with Noonan syndrome. *Clin Dysmorphol* 5: 61–64.

Lorenzen JA, Baker SE, Denhez F, Melnick MB, Brower DL, Perkins LA (2001). Nuclear import of activated D-ERK by DIM-7, an importin family member encoded by the gene moleskin. *Development* 128: 1403–1414.

Lu X, Perkins LA, Perrimon N (1993). The torso pathway in Drosophila: a model system to study receptor tyrosine kinase signal transduction. *Dev Suppl*: 47–56.

MacFarlane CE, Brown DC, Johnston LB, Patton MA, Dunger DB, Savage MO, McKenna WJ, Kelnar CJ (2001). Growth hormone therapy and growth in children with Noonan's syndrome: results of 3 years' follow-up. *J Clin Endocrinol Metab* 86: 1953–1956.

Marino B, Digilio MC, Toscano A, Giannotti A, Dallapiccola B (1999). Congenital heart diseases in children with Noonan syndrome: an expanded cardiac spectrum with high prevalence of atrioventricular canal. *J Pediatr* 135: 703–706.

Massarano AA, Wood A, Tait RC, Stevens R, Super M (1996). Noonan syndrome: coagulation and clinical aspects. *Acta Paediatr* 85: 1181–1185.

Mendez HM, Opitz JM (1985). Noonan syndrome: a review. *Am J Med Genet* 21: 493–506.

Naficy S, Shepard NT, Telian SA (1997). Multiple temporal bone anomalies associated with Noonan syndrome. *Otolaryngol Head Neck Surg* 116: 265–267.

Neri G, Zollino M (1996). More on the Noonan-CFC controversy. *Am J Med Genet* 65: 100.

Neri G, Zollino M, Reynolds JF (1991). The Noonan-CFC controversy. *Am J Med Genet* 39: 367–370.

Nisbet DL, Griffin DR, Chitty LS (1999). Prenatal features of Noonan syndrome. *Prenat Diagn* 19: 642–647.

Noguti T, Go N (1985). Efficient Monte Carlo method for simulation of fluctuating conformations of native proteins. *Biopolymers* 24: 527–546.

Noonan JA (1968). Hypertelorism with Turner phenotype. A new syndrome with associated congenital heart disease. *Am J Dis Child* 116: 373–380.

Noonan JA (1994). Noonan syndrome. An update and review for the primary pediatrician. *Clin Pediatr (Phila)* 33: 548–555.

Noonan J, Ehmke D (1963). Associated non cardiac malformations in children with congenital heart disease. *J Pediatr* 63: 468–470.

Noordam C, Draaisma JM, van den Nieuwenhof J, van der Burgt I, Otten BJ, Daniels O (2001a). Effects of growth hormone treatment on left ventricular dimensions in children with Noonan's syndrome. *Horm Res* 56: 110–113.

Noordam C, Van der Burgt I, Sengers RC, Delemarre-van de Waal HA, Otten BJ (2001b). Growth hormone treatment in children with Noonan's syndrome: four year results of a partly controlled trial. *Acta Paediatr* 90: 889–894.

Noordam K, van der Brunner HG, Otten BJ (2002). The relationship between clinical severity of Noonan's syndrome and growth, growth hormone (GH) secretion and response to GH treatment. *J Pediatr Endocrinol Metab* 15: 175–180.

O'Reilly AM, Pluskey S, Shoelson SE, Neel BG (2000). Activated mutants of SHP-2 preferentially induce elongation of Xenopus animal caps. *Mol Cell Biol* 20: 299–311.

Opitz JM (1985). The Noonan syndrome. *Am J Med Genet* 21: 515–518.

Ozturk S, Cefle K, Palanduz S, Erten NB, Karan MA, Tascioglu C, Umman S, Falay O, Vatansever S, Guler K, et al. (2000). A case of Noonan syndrome with pulmonary and abdominal lymphangiectasia. *Int J Clin Pract* 54: 274–276.

Perkins LA, Larsen I, Perrimon N (1992). corkscrew encodes a putative protein tyrosine phosphatase that functions to transduce the terminal signal from the receptor tyrosine kinase torso. *Cell* 70: 225–236.

Perkins LA, Johnson MR, Melnick MB, Perrimon N (1996). The nonreceptor protein tyrosine phosphatase corkscrew functions in multiple receptor tyrosine kinase pathways in Drosophila. *Dev Biol* 180: 63–81.

Perrimon N, Lu X, Hou XS, Hsu JC, Melnick MB, Chou TB, Perkins LA (1995). Dissection of the Torso signal transduction pathway in Drosophila. *Mol Reprod Dev* 42: 515–522.

Pinsky L (1972). The XX-XY Turner phenotype and malignant hyperthermia. *Lancet* 2: 383.

Qiu WW, Yin SS, Stucker FJ (1998). Audiologic manifestations of Noonan syndrome. *Otolaryngol Head Neck Surg* 118: 319–323.

Qu CK, Yu WM, Azzarelli B, Cooper S, Broxmeyer HE, Feng GS (1998). Biased suppression of hematopoiesis and multiple developmental defects in chimeric mice containing Shp-2 mutant cells. *Mol Cell Biol* 18: 6075–6082.

Raabe T (2000). The sevenless signaling pathway: variations of a common theme. *Biochim Biophys Acta* 1496: 151–163.

Ranke MB, Heidemann P, Knupfer C, Enders H, Schmaltz AA, Bierich JR (1988). Noonan syndrome: growth and clinical manifestations in 144 cases. *Eur J Pediatr* 148: 220–227.

Reeves SA, Ueki K, Sinha B, Difiglia M, Louis DN (1996). Regional expression and subcellular localization of the tyrosine-specific phosphatase SH-PTP2 in the adult human nervous system. *Neuroscience* 71: 1037–1042.

Reynders CS, Pauker SP, Benacerraf BR (1997). First trimester isolated fetal nuchal lucency: significance and outcome. *J Ultrasound Med* 16: 101–105.

Rissam HS, Mittal SR, Wahi PL, Bidwai PS (1982). Postoperative hyperpyrexia in a case of Noonan's syndrome. *Indian Heart J* 34: 180–182.

Romano AA, Blethen SL, Dana K, Noto RA (1996). Growth hormone treatment in Noonan syndrome: the National Cooperative Growth Study experience. *J Pediatr* 128: S18–21.

Saxton TM, Ciruna BG, Holmyard D, Kulkarni S, Harpal K, Rossant J, Pawson T (2000). The SH2 tyrosine phosphatase shp2 is required for mammalian limb development. *Nat Genet* 24: 420–423.

Saxton TM, Henkemeyer M, Gasca S, Shen R, Rossi DJ, Shalaby F, Feng GS, Pawson T (1997). Abnormal mesoderm patterning in mouse embryos mutant for the SH2 tyrosine phosphatase Shp-2. *EMBO J* 16: 2352–2364.

Shah N, Rodriguez M, Louis DS, Lindley K, Milla PJ (1999). Feeding difficulties and foregut dysmotility in Noonan's syndrome. *Arch Dis Child* 81: 28–31.

Sharland M, Burch M, McKenna WM, Paton MA (1992a). A clinical study of Noonan syndrome. *Arch Dis Child* 67: 178–183.

Sharland M, Patton MA, Talbot S, Chitolie A, Bevan DH (1992b). Coagulation-factor deficiencies and abnormal bleeding in Noonan's syndrome. *Lancet* 339: 19–21.

Sharland M, Taylor R, Patton MA, Jeffery S (1992c). Absence of linkage of Noonan syndrome to the neurofibromatosis type 1 locus. *J Med Genet* 29: 188–190.

Singer ST, Hurst D, Addiego JE Jr (1997). Bleeding disorders in Noonan syndrome: three case reports and review of the literature. *J Pediatr Hematol Oncol* 19: 130–134.

Stofega MR, Herrington J, Billestrup N, Carter-Su C (2000). Mutation of the SHP-2 binding site in growth hormone (GH) receptor prolongs GH-promoted tyrosyl phosphorylation of GH receptor, JAK2, and STAT5B. *Mol Endocrinol* 14: 1338–1350.

Tanaka K, Sato A, Naito T, Kuramochi K, Itabashi H, Takemura Y (1992). Noonan syndrome presenting growth hormone neurosecretory dysfunction. *Intern Med* 31: 908–911.

Tartaglia M, Kalidas K, Shaw A, Song X, Musat DL, van der Burgt I, Brunner HG, Bertola DR, Crosby A, Ion A, et al. (2002). PTPN11 mutations in Noonan syndrome: molecular spectrum, genotype-phenotype correlation, and phenotypic heterogeneity. *Am J Hum Genet* 70: 1555–1563.

Tartaglia M, Mehler EL, Goldberg R, Zampino G, Brunner HG, Kremer H, van der Burgt I, Crosby AH, Ion A, Jeffery S, et al. (2001). Mutations in PTPN11, encoding the protein tyrosine phosphatase SHP-2, cause Noonan syndrome. *Nat Genet* 29: 465–468.

Turner H (1938). A syndrome of infantilism, congenital webbed neck, and cubitus valgus. *Endocrinology* 25: 566–574.

Ullrich O (1930). Uber typische kombinationbilder multiper abanturgen. *Z Kinderheilkd* 49: 271–276.

Ullrich O (1949). Turner's syndrome and status Bonnevie-Ullrich; a synthesis of animal phenogenetics and clinical observations on a typical complex of developmental anomalies. *Am J Hum Genet* 1: 179–202.

van Der Burgt I, Brunner H (2000). Genetic heterogeneity in Noonan syndrome: evidence for an autosomal recessive disorder. *Am J Med Genet* 94: 46–51.

Ward KA, Moss C, McKeown C (1994). The cardio-facio-cutaneous syndrome: a manifestation of the Noonan syndrome? *Br J Dermatol* 131: 270–274.

Wieczorek D, Majewski F, Gillessen-Kaesbach G (1997). Cardio-facio-cutaneous (CFC) syndrome—a distinct entity? Report of three patients demonstrating the diagnostic difficulties in delineation of CFC syndrome. *Clin Genet* 52: 37–46.

Witt DR, Keena BA, Hall JG, Allanson JE (1986). Growth curves for height in Noonan syndrome. *Clin Genet* 30: 150–153.

Xiao W, Oefner PJ (2001). Denaturing high-performance liquid chromatography: a review. *Hum Mutat* 17: 439–474.

Part F.
Microtubule Motors and Cytoskeleton

90 | Microtubule Motors: Intracellular Transport, Cell Division, Ciliary Movement, and Nuclear Migration

ANTHONY WYNSHAW-BORIS

Intracellular motility in eukaryotic cells is generated by motor proteins, which drive directional transport along cytoskeletal filaments such as microtubules, the primary intracellular rail system. These cytoplasmic cytoskeletal elements provide not only structure and support to the cell but also an intracellular directional railway that allows components of the cell to be transported outside of organelles (Hirokawa, 1998). This railway system transports molecular complexes and organelles after synthesis in the cell body to their proper peripheral location. Similarly, endocytic vesicles are transported from the cell surface to the center of the cell. In the cell, microtubule plus ends are directed toward the cell membrane and minus ends are anchored at the centrosome, one type of the microtubule organizing center (MTOC) in a cell.

There are two classes of motor proteins that participate in the transport of organelles and molecules along mictrotubules: kinesins and cytoplasmic dyneins. Kinesin is a plus end–directed motor, traveling with cargo along a microtubule from its minus end toward its plus end. Kinesin is thought to mediate transport from the MTOC out toward the plasma membrane in an interphase mitotic cell, while in a postmitotic neuron, transport is mediated from the MTOC in the cell body out toward the synapse (anterograde axonal transport). Cytoplasmic dynein, however, is a minus end–directed motor, mediating transport away from the cell surface and toward the MTOC in mitotic

cells, while also participating in retrograde axonal transport. Finally, cytoplasmic dynein plays a crucial role in an evolutionarily conserved pathway mediating nuclear migration in diverse cells from fungal mycleia to migrating neurons during development.

In addition to their cytoskelatal function, specialized microtubules provide the backbone of flagella and cilia. These extracellular projections extend from the cell surface with connections to the cell membrane and have several functions. They allow cells such as sperm to move independently. They participate in the directional transport of mucus in the respiratory epithelium via the airway cilia. They provide a beating rotor function to direct rotation of structures and/or determine gradients of morphogenes, such as in the node during early development. Movement of cilia and flagella is controlled by axonemal dynein motors, while their assembly is controlled by kinesins.

Finally, the segregation of chromosomes during mitosis and meiosis is choreographed by microtubule motors along the mitotic and meiotic spindles, a structure composed of microtubules organized by MTOCs called *centrosomes* or *basal bodies*. Kinesin motors appear to be most important for these chromosomal movements.

There are many microtubule motors in the cell with specialized functions, and defects in some of these motor proteins that lead to specific human diseases have been identified. For example, mutations in cytoplasmic dynein components result in the severe human neuronal migration defect lissencephaly (see Chapter 92). A signal-transduction pathway that at least in part regulates cytoplasmic dynein activity has been identified, and mutations in a component of this pathway also result in lissencephaly with cerebellar hypoplasia (see Chapter 93). In addition, mutations in axonemal dyneins result in primary ciliary dyskinesia (see Chapter 94). Given the diverse function of microtubule motors, it is likely that other defects may result from mutations in components of these motors and that such defects will be identified in the near future.

The microtubule system and motors will be discussed in this chapter to provide a framework for the following chapters with disorders in members of these pathways. Further details on many of the topics covered in this chapter can be found in several excellent reviews (Hirokawa, 1998; Goldstein and Yang, 2000; Meeks and Bush, 2000; Mountain and Compton, 2000; Sharp et al., 2000; Walczak, 2000; Woehlke and Schliwa, 2000; Brunet and Vernos, 2001).

MICROTUBULES AND MOTOR PROTEINS

Microtubules

Microtubules in the cell have three major functions: as components of the centrosome and mitotic spindle; as cytoskeletal elements that provide substrates for long-distance intracellular transport; and as structural elements for flagella and cilia. Spindle and cytoskeletal microtubules are dynamic 25 nm cylindrical structures composed of two different types of tubulin: α and β. α-Tubulin and β-tubulin assemble into 13 parallel protofilaments for each microtubule. Each of the protofilaments consists of linear tubulin heterodimers. In the axoneme of cilia and flagella, a central pair of microtubules is surrounded by nine pairs of microtubule heterodimers (9 + 2 arrangement). The central pair of the axoneme consists of 13 protofilaments each, while 11 pairs of protofilaments are present in the peripheral doublets of the axoneme. Primary cilia or monocilia are single cilia with nine peripheral pairs of microtubules without a central pair (9 + 0 structure). There are at least seven α-tubulin genes and five β-tubulin genes, although the specific roles of each gene are unknown.

Microtubules have polarity such that each end (plus and minus) of a microtubule is distinct, and this property is considered one of the key elements of cellular polarity (Hirokawa, 1998; Goldstein and Yang, 2000). The position and orientation of microtubules in a cell are highly organized. In a typical animal cell, most microtubules originate near the nucleus and extend in all directions outward toward the periphery, where they are connected to the cell cortex. Microtubules are organized by complexes within a cell known collectively as MTOCs. At the MTOC, microtubules radiate outward with a specified polarity and are shortened or elongated in an organized fashion. There are at least three types of MTOC: the basal body/centriole, the centrosome, and the kinetochore. In a typical animal cell, the centrosome consists of a pair of centrioles surrounded by pericentriolar material, which contains a third type of tubulin, γ-tubulin. γ-Tubulin is involved in nucleating microtubules. A fourth type of tubulin, δ-tubulin, is involved in centriole development and may be a part of centrioles.

Motor Proteins of Cytoplasmic Microtubules

Cytoplasmic microtubules are essential for intracellular trafficking of proteins and organelles as well as for the segregation of chromosomes on the mitotic and meiotic spindle. Trafficking and chromosomal segregation are tightly regulated, and various different types of proteins are known to be involved. Kinesins and dyneins are families of motors that use microtubules as rails for directional movement. Anterograde transport is mainly driven by kinesins, whereas cytoplasmic dynein is responsible for the bulk of retrograde transport. In addition, there are other proteins associated with dyneins and kinesins that are important for transport and function.

Kinesins

Members of the kinesin superfamily of proteins transport organelles, protein complexes, and mRNAs to specific destinations in a microtubule- and ATP-dependent manner (Hirokawa, 1998; Goldstein and Yang, 2000). Kinesins also participate in chromosomal and spindle movements during mitosis and meiosis (Vale and Fletterick, 1997; Hirokawa, 1998). Kinesin superfamily proteins (KIFs) contain a highly conserved motor domain among all eukaryotic phyla studied thus far.

The kinesin superfamily has been completely catalogued since the human genome sequence became available, so comparisons can be made to the fully sequenced genomes of *Drosophila* and *Caenorhabditis elegans* (Miki et al., 2001). *C. elegans* contains 18 different kinesins (kinesin web page: http://www.blocks.fhcrc.org/kinesin/). It was estimated that the *Drosophila* genome contains on the order of 20–30 kinesins, and mammals encode as many as 50–100 different kinesin motor proteins (Goldstein and Yang, 2000). KIFs can be grouped into three classes depending on the location of the motor domain in the molecule. N-kineins and M-kinesins, containing motor domains close to their N terminus or center, have been reported to possess microtubule plus end–directed motility, while KIFs containing a motor domain proximal to the C terminus possess minus end–directed motility. Miki et al. (2001) found 45 KIFs, of which the majority are N-kinesins, with few M- and C-kinesins. There are only three M-kinesins and C-kinesins each, while there are 39 N-kinesins.

Cytoplasmic Dyneins

Cytoplasmic dynein is a member of the dynein superfamily of proteins, which is much less diverse than the kinesin superfamily. *C. elegans* contains two cytoplasmic dynein heavy chains, *Drosophila* encodes one, and mammals appear to have at least three (Goldstein and Yang, 2000). Dyneins are minus end–directed, microtubule-based motor protein complexes that are thought to drive the centrosomal movement of membranous organelles and to propel the beating of cilia and flagella. Cytoplasmic dynein is a high-molecular mass complex ($\sim$1.2 MD) composed of multiple polypeptides, two heavy chains of $\sim$550,000 daltons, three to four 74,000-dalton intermediate chains, four light intermediate chains of $\sim$55,000 daltons, and light chains of 8000–22,000 daltons (Hirokawa, 1998; Goldstein and Yang, 2000). The heavy chain contains the sites for ATP hydrolysis and microtubule binding. The intermediate and light intermediate chains lie at the base of the molecule. The cytoplasmic dynein heavy chain contains phosphate-binding pockets (P-loops) in its central region. The central and COOH-terminal regions are predicted to form a globular domain that interacts with microtubules and has motor activity, and the NH2-terminal region is thought to be the site of the binding of cargoes.

In addition to intermediate and light intermediate chains, cytoplasmic dynein is associated with the protein complex dynactin. Dynactin contains 10 subunits: p150[Glued], p135[Glued] (a brain-specific variant of p150[Glued]), p62, dynamitin (p50), actin-related protein 1 (Arp1), actin, α and β subunits of actin-capping protein, p27, and p24. Cytoplasmic dynein, especially its 74 kDa intermediate chain, is linked to its cargo through the p150[Glued]–Arp1–actin complex, and binding of p150[Glued] to Arp1 is mediated by dynamitin.

Several lines of evidence suggest that cytoplasmic dynein is a motor for the retrograde transport of membranous organelles in axons, the distribution of late endosomes and lysosomes, the centrosomal localization of the Golgi complex, the vesicular transport from early to late endosomes, the apical transport of Golgi-derived membranes in intestinal epithelial cells, and the movement of phagosomes (Hirokawa, 1998; Goldstein and Yang, 2000). For example, microinjection of antibodies to the cytoplasmic dynein heavy chain DHC2 causes dispersion of the Golgi complex (Vaisberg et al., 1996), and cytoplasmic dynein knockout mice display fragmentation of the Golgi complex, while late endosomes are distributed to the periphery of the cells (Harada et al., 1998).

Motor Proteins of Cilia and Flagella: Axonemal Dyneins and Kinesins

As with cytoplasmic microtubule-mediated transport, movement and transport in cilia and flagella are controlled by axonemal dyneins and kinesins (Goldstein and Yang, 2000; Meeks and Bush, 2000). Organized movement of cilia and flagella is controlled by axonemal dyneins, which are distinct genetic loci from the cytoplasmic dyneins.

Recall that in the axoneme, a central pair of microtubules is surrounded by nine pairs of microtubule heterodimers. Axonemal dyneins are present on peripheral microtubule doublets as inner and outer arms. The outer arms consist of two dynein heavy chains (α and β), two or more intermediate chains, and four to eight light chains. The inner arms have a similar organization, but there are distinct inner arm dynein isoforms. These arms mediate displacement of adjacent doublets in an ATP-dependent fashion. The dynein arms disintegrate during movement, allowing the arms to freely slide relative to each other. The axonemal dyneins and primary ciliary dyskinesia will be discussed in more detail in Chapter 94.

As discussed above, axonemal kinesins are motors that regulate transport of proteins in cilia and flagella and, thus, are essential to the assembly of these structures. Unlike dyneins, there are no specific axonemal kinesins.

FUNCTIONS OF MICROTUBULE MOTORS

Microtubule motors are used for several general cellular processes, such as movement of cilia and flagella, intracellular transport along microtubules, and neuronal migration.

Movement of Cilia and Flagella

One of the major functions of microtubule motors is the movement of cilia and flagella. As noted in Chapter 94, cilia are present in the upper and lower airways, middle ear, lacrimal sac, ependyma, vas deferens, endometrium, and certain sensory cells. Flagella are present on sperm. Primary cilia are present on a variety of cells, most notably nodal cells in the gastrulating embryo. The wide distribution of cells with cilia and flagella indicates that these structures play important roles throughout development and in virtually all tissues. One of the important functions appears to be in mucociliary transport of the airways, as will be reviewed in Chapter 94. Other important functions of ciliary transport are in the movement of cerebrospinal fluid, sperm motility, and movement of sperm and eggs in the male and female genital tracts. Additional important functions occur in the node of the gastrulating embryo, where organized ciliary beating results in proper rotation of the embryo to establish left/right asymmetry (Hirokawa, 1998). Thus, there are a variety of functions mediated by ciliary formation and movement, controlled by kinesins and axonemal dyneins, respectively.

Intracellular Transport via Microtubules

Intracellular transport of organelles and some classes of proteins occurs along microtubules using kinesin and dynein motors. The organization of microtubules and how transport occurs differ by cell type (Hirokawa, 1998; Goldstein and Yang, 2000).

Nonneuronal Cells

The mode of transport along the microtubule rails is dependent on the nonneuronal cell type. In nonpolarized cells, microtubules are attached at their minus ends to a centrally located centrosome, with their plus ends directed into the cytoplasm. Plus end–directed kinesin motors move materials such as mitochondria, endoplasmic reticulum, and lysosomes toward the surface of the cell, away from the cell center (reviewed in Goldstein and Philp, 1999). Minus end–directed kinesins and dyneins move materials such as the Golgi apparatus and lysosomes toward the cell center as well (Corthesy-Theulaz et al., 1992; Harada et al., 1998). In polarized epithelial cells, microtubules generally appear to be organized with their minus ends and plus ends pointing toward the apical and basolateral surfaces, respectively (Goldstein and Yang, 2000). Kinesins and dyneins transport cargoes toward the basolateral and apical surfaces, respectively.

Axonal Transport in Neurons

Neurons are polarized cells with multiple processes that can be several orders of magnitude longer than the cell body. Transport in neurons is complex and beyond the scope of this chapter; further details can be found in several recent reviews (Hirokawa, 1998; Baas, 1999; Goldstein and Yang, 2000). Only a few general principles will be dis-

cussed. The neuronal centrosome is not centrally localized in the adult, but after development it is located somewhat randomly in the cell body (Baas, 1999). In axons, microtubules are oriented with the plus and minus ends pointing toward the synapse and cell body, respectively. Anterograde axonal transport moves materials from the cell body out to the synapse, and there are three major classes (Goldstein and Yang, 2000). Fast anterograde transport appears to move most membrane-bound organelles and vesicles and may also be required for the movement of secreted molecules, such as neurotrophins, to the synapse. This component of transport is mostly driven by kinesin superfamily proteins. Several kinesins participate and likely have overlapping functions. Slow component A transport moves microtubule and neurofilament proteins, while slow component B contains microfilaments and other cytoplasmic proteins, such as clathrin, spectrin, and metabolic enzymes. It is unclear which motors drive these forms of transport and whether kinesins and dyneins are even involved since the rate of transport is much slower than the known kinesins or dynein motors. Retrograde axonal transport moves materials such as organelles, vesicles, and perhaps neurotrophic signals from the synapse to the cell body. The majority of retrograde transport is from cytoplasmic dyneins, with some assistance from minus end–directed kinesins such as KIFC2, which are present in neurons. Some of the axonal transport pathways may also be used by viruses to move between neuronal cell bodies and neuronal termini.

Axonemal Transport

Transport in cilia and flagella is necessary to provide structural and membrane components from sites of synthesis in the cell body to sites of utilization or assembly at the flagellar or ciliary tip. It appears that kinesin motors move "rafts" of ciliary components from the cell body to the growing tip (Rosenbaum et al., 1999). Thus, kinesins are necessary for synthetic events and maintenance of cilia and flagella.

Chromosomal Segregation in Mitosis and Meiosis

Chromosomal movement in meiosis and mitosis is also controlled by dyneins and kinesin motors (Mountain and Compton, 2000). Chromosomes are attached at the kinetichore and move to opposite ends of the cell during cell division along the microtubule-based spindle. Kinesin and dynein motors are essential in cell division. They organize various aspects of spindle assembly and function, including the establishment of spindle polarity, spindle pole organization, chromosomal alignment and segregation, regulation of microtubule dynamics, and cytokinesis. Some of these kinesins were noted above. For example, N- and C-kinesins are required for the movement of centrosomes to opposite ends of the cell. In addition, dynein is required for attachment of microtubules to the centrosomes, cross-linking microtubules, and driving convergence of microtubule minus ends at spindle poles (Gaglio et al., 1997). Although the details of kinesin and dynein motor function in mitosis and meiosis remain to be fully worked out, it is clear that both superfamilies of proteins have essential roles in cell division.

Nuclear Movement, Neuronal Migration, and Cytoplasmic Dynein Function

In the filamentous fungus *Aspergillus nidulans*, nuclei migrate toward the growing tip of hyphae to establish regular spacing, a process termed *nucleokinesis* (Oakley and Morris, 1980). Nuclear movement is a microtubule-dependent process (Oakley and Morris, 1980, 1981). Several nuclear distribution mutants (*nud* mutants) have been generated to study nucleokinesis in this organism (Morris, 1976; Xiang et al., 1999). The identification of *nud* mutants directly implicated cytoplasmic dynein and dynactin in this process. For example, the *nudA* and *nudG* genes code for the heavy chain and the 8 kDa light chain of cytoplasmic dynein, respectively (Xiang et al., 1994; Beckwith et al., 1998). From a large series of *nud* mutants, at least 10 new loci involved in nucleokinesis, *nudI* through *nudR*, were identified (Xiang et al., 1999). The *nudK* gene codes for the actin-related protein Arp1, part of the dynactin complex.

Thus, a surprising finding from the study of nuclear movement in several fungi was that this process was controlled by dyneins. Even more surprising, however, was that the discovery of this pathway was instrumental in illuminating the function of human LIS1, the protein product of the first gene identified that was responsible for the neuronal migration defect lissencephaly when mutated. The value of model organisms is truly underscored by this linkage since a slime mold provided key insight into mammalian brain development.

Lissencephaly (smooth brain) is a term used to describe the smooth surface of the cortex seen in human brain malformations caused by certain types of neuronal migration defect. Classical, or type I, lissencephaly defines a subgroup of human neuronal migration disorders characterized by generalized agyria (absence of gyri) and pachygyria (reduced numbers of broadened gyri), four abnormal cortical layers, enlarged ventricles, and generalized neuronal heterotopias (Barkovich et al., 1991; Dobyns and Truwit, 1995). As discussed in detail in Chapter 92, many patients with lissencephaly have visible or submicroscopic deletions of human chromosome 17p13.3 (Dobyns et al., 1993; Chong et al., 1997). The *LIS1* gene was cloned from 17p13.3 and was the first gene responsible for neuronal migration defects to be identified (Reiner et al., 1993). *LIS1* was disrupted in an isolated lissencephaly sequence (ILS) patient with a translocation and several other key Miller-Dieker syndrome (MDS) patients (Chong et al., 1997). Point mutations and an intragenic deletion in *LIS1* were identified in ILS patients who showed no gross structural chromosomal rearrangements (Lo Nigro et al., 1997; Pilz et al., 1998).

One of these *nud* mutants, *nudF*, is the fungal homologue of *LIS1* (Xiang et al., 1995). Like the mammalian protein, NudF contains WD-40 repeats and remarkably is 42% identical and 64% similar to the human LIS1 protein. A mutant allele of *nudF*, *nudF6*, can be suppressed by mutations in *nudA*, the cytoplasmic dynein heavy chain, providing genetic evidence that NUDA and NUDF are in the same genetic pathway (Willins et al., 1997) and suggesting that LIS1 might directly interact with cytoplasmic dynein.

Another protein important for LIS1 function was found in a screen for multicopy suppressors of the *nudF* phenotype and was termed *nudE* (Efimov and Morris, 2000). The double mutants *nudF;nudE* and *nudE;nudA* were similar to the *nudF* and *nudA* (cytoplasmic dynein heavy chain) single mutants, indicating that NudF, NudE, and NudA are part of the same genetic pathway. NudE is a homologue of the nuclear distribution protein RO11 in *Neurospora crassa,* the mitotic protein MP43 in *Xenopus laevis,* and two murine homologues of nudE, NUDEL (for NudE-like) and NudE (Feng et al., 2000; Niethammer

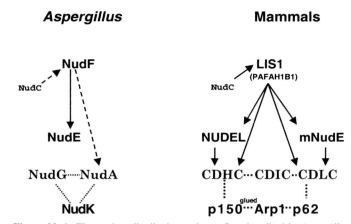

Figure 90–1. The nuclear distribution pathway first described in *Aspergillus nidulans* (*left*) is conserved in mammals (*right*). Direct interactions of NudF or LIS1 with other proteins are indicated by a solid arrow. Genetic interactions are represented by a dashed arrow. The directions of arrows represent the presumed directions of information transfer. Dotted lines connect proteins in a complex with no attempt to represent the molecular interactions.

et al., 2000; Sasaki et al., 2000). The nud pathway is remarkably conserved in eukaryotes (Fig. 90–1). *NudF* is the *LIS1* homologue in *A. nidulans.* Cytoplasmic dynein and dynactin are conserved throughout eukaryotic evolution. Homologues have been cloned in *Drosophila* and several mammalian species.

The process of nuclear migration in fungi is strikingly similar to neuronal migration in mammals. Migrating neurons initially extend a leading process along radial glial fibers. After completion of this process, the nuclei of migrating neurons must relocate from their birth place to their final destination in the nervous system. Nuclear distribution in *A. nidulans* is also similar to nuclear movement and cellular transport in *Drosophila.* Therefore, it is not surprising that the same molecular mechanism utilizing NUDEL, NudE, LIS1, and cytoplasmic dynein motors may underlie these processes in all eukaryotes.

The regulation of dynein motor function by LIS1 (Fig. 90–2) and microtubule organization are conserved in mammalian cells (Smith et al., 2000). LIS1 interaction with cytoplasmic dynein and dynactin ap-

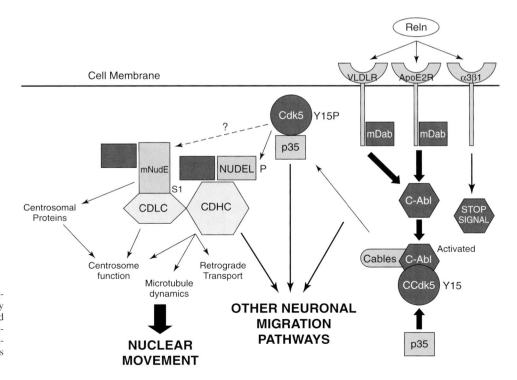

Figure 90–2. Integration of pathways that regulate neuronal migration. The RELN pathway is to the *right*, Cdk5/p35 in the *middle*, and LIS1 on the *left*. Although it is possible to connect all pathways, the situation is more complex, and each component pathway likely has additional effects on neuronal migration.

pears to be important for mitotic cell division and cytokinesis, based on overexpression and antisense or antibody inhibition experiments (Faulkner et al., 2000). These results suggest that LIS1 plays a critical role in cell division and chromosomal segregation. They imply that defects seen in human lissencephaly due to haploinsufficiency of LIS1 may be the result of altered neurogenesis in the proliferative ventricular zone as well as defective migration of neurons into the cortical plate. In support of this, LIS1 dosage reduction in mice is associated with progressive thinning of the cortex, implying that LIS1 may be important for neuronal proliferation (Hirotsune et al., 1998). In addition, proliferation of cells in the ventricular zone of murine *Lis1* mutants is disrupted, and embryonic fibroblasts from *Lis1* mutants have slow doubling times (Gambello et al., 2002).

Potential Regulation of LIS1/Dynein Activity by Other Neuronal Migration Pathways

Several other human and mouse proteins that participate in neuronal migration have been identified either by cloning the human and murine genes responsible for migration defects or based on phenotypes displayed in gene-targeted mice. These proteins can be placed into three functional groups based on integrated functioning of the components. These groups have independent functions, but there is clearly crosstalk among them (for reviews, see Wynshaw-Boris and Gambello, 2001; Gupta et al., 2002).

RELN

RELN is a large extracellular matrix-like secreted protein produced by the Cajal-Retzius cells lining the outer layer of the preplate (for reviews, see (Wynshaw-Boris and Gambello, 2001; Gupta et al., 2002). RELN binds at least two types of cell surface receptor: the lipoprotein receptors, such as VLDLR and ApoER2, and $\alpha_3\beta_1$-integrin (Fig. 90–2). The relative importance and interactions of these RELN receptors are currently unknown, although RELN binding to $\alpha_3\beta_1$ integrin is an apparent stop signal for migration. *mDab1 (mouse disabled-1)*, the vertebrate homologue of the *Drosophila disabled (dab)* gene, codes for a phosphoprotein that transduces the downstream signal of the lipoprotein RELN receptors. *mDab1*-deficient mice display a *reeler* phenotype. MDab1 is a target of Cdk5 kinase.

RELN is mutated in the human disorder lissencephaly with cerebellar hypoplasia, as will be discussed in Chapter 93.

Cdk5 and Its Activators

Homozygous mice with targeted disruption of the serine-threonine kinase *Cdk5* or its regulatory subunit *p35* also demonstrate severe defects in cortical lamination (for reviews, see Wynshaw-Boris and Gambello, 2001; Gupta et al., 2002). Though these mice display a reeler-like phenotype, further analysis of *Cdk5$^{-/-}$* mutants has demonstrated a distinct difference from *reeler*. However, the similar phenotype of Cdk5 and RELN pathway mutants suggests that many of these proteins participate in a common signal-transduction pathway that is crucial for cortical lamination (Fig. 90–2). Cables is an activator of Cdk5 that binds to Cdk5 in the brain along with the c-abl tyrosine kinase. Active c-abl phosphorylates and activates Cdk5, and Cdk5 phosphorylation is enhanced by Cables. mDab1 also binds to c-abl and is activated by RELN pathway signals. Thus, these two pathways are potentitally linked.

NUDEL Is Phosphorylated by Cdk5/p35

NUDEL is a substrate for Cdk5/p35 in vitro (Niethammer et al., 2000; Sasaki et al., 2000) and *in vivo* (Niethammer et al., 2000). The latter studies were particularly convincing and suggest that Cdk5 phosphorylation of NUDEL on three serine/threonine residues controls its cellular localization and probably influences dynein motor function. These same serine residues are conserved in mNudE, suggesting that mNudE may also be a target of Cdk5 (Fig. 90–2).

In summary (Fig. 90–2), LIS1 regulates dynein motor function and localization of dynein-associated proteins. LIS1 binds two different NudE homologues to regulate dynein motor function and centrosomal localization. At least one of these homologues, NUDEL, is directly phosphorylated by Cdk5 and its coactivators p35 and p39. It appears that each of these proteins regulates dynein motor function in a positive fashion since decreasing the activity, decreasing the amount, or eliminating the protein completely results in decreased dynein motor function and mislocalization of dynein components and centrosomal proteins. Thus, the apparent function of the LIS1 pathway is to activate dynein motors and place them in the proper cellular location for function. The RELN pathway may somehow regulate Cdk5/p35 activity, thus integrating at some level all of these pathways important for neuronal migration.

SUMMARY

As will be discussed in the next few chapters, several distinct disorders have been described with defects in microtubule motors or related proteins. Primary ciliary dyskinesia and laterality defects are caused by defects in axonemal dyneins (Chapter 94). These may also be associated with infertility. Neuronal migration defects, such as lissencephaly, can be caused by mutations in proteins that bind to dynein motors and regulate dynein function, such as *LIS1* (Chapter 92). Related disorders are caused by mutations in *Doublecortin (DCX)*, a gene that codes for a microtubule-binding protein of unknown function (Chapter 92), or *RELN* (Chapter 93), a component of a pathway that may regulate dynein function via Cdk5/p35.

Given the broad distribution and function of microtubule motors, as well as the diversity of motor proteins and regulatory molecules, it is likely that these known disorders are just the beginning of our understanding of genetic disorders of microtubule motor proteins. For example, several types of cell have cilia, including specialized sensory cells, germ cells (sperm), and cells lining the reproductive tract. Mutations in ciliary dyneins or kinesins important for the assembly of cilia could result in deafness, visual defects, other sensory defects, or isolated infertility. Since kinesins and cytoplasmic dyneins are used in intracellular transport in neuronal and nonneuronal cells, the cellular function of virtually any can be compromised. This is particularly true for the CNS, since neuronal transport must occur over very long distances. It has been suggested that neural degeneration disorders such as Alzheimers disease could result from transport defects. Finally, abnormalities in the segregation of chromosomes at mitosis and meiosis, a process choreographed by microtubule motors, can result in aneuploidy during development or in the adult cell, leading to characteristic dysmorphic syndromes or cancer. Thus, microtubule motor proteins can be considered candidates for virtually any disorder, from those of early development to those of aging.

REFERENCES

Baas P (1999). Microtubules and neuronal polarity: lessons from mitosis. *Neuron* 22: 23–31.

Barkovich AJ, Koch TK, Carrol CL (1991). The spectrum of lissencephaly: report of ten patients analyzed by magnetic resonance imaging. *Ann Neurol* 30: 139–146.

Beckwith SM, Roghi CH, Liu B, Ronald Morris N (1998). The "8-kD" cytoplasmic dynein light chain is required for nuclear migration and for dynein heavy chain localization in *Aspergillus nidulans. J Cell Biol* 143: 1239–1247.

Brunet S, Vernos I (2001). Chromosome motors on the move. From motion to spindle checkpoint activity. *EMBO Rep* 2: 669–673.

Chong SS, Pack SD, Roschke AV, Tanigami A, Carrozzo R, Smith AC, Dobyns WB, Ledbetter DH (1997). A revision of the lissencephaly and Miller-Dieker syndrome critical regions in chromosome 17p13.3. *Hum Mol Genet* 6: 147–155.

Corthesy-Theulaz I, Pauloin A, Rfeffer SR (1992). Cytoplasmic dynein participates in the centrosomal localization of the Golgi complex. *J Cell Biol* 118: 1333–1345.

Dobyns WB, Truwit CL (1995). Lissencephaly and other malformations of cortical development: 1995 update. *Neuropediatrics* 26: 132–147.

Dobyns WB, Reiner O, Carrozzo R, Ledbetter DH (1993). Lissencephaly. A human brain malformation associated with deletion of the LIS1 gene located at chromosome 17p13. *JAMA* 270: 2838–2842.

Efimov VP, Morris NR (2000). The LIS1-related NUDF protein of *Aspergillus nidulans* interacts with the coiled-coil domain of the NUDE/RO11 protein. *J Cell Biol* 150: 681–688.

Faulkner NE, Dujardin DL, Tai CY, Vaughan KT, O'Connell CB, Wang Y, Vallee RB (2000). A role for the lissencephaly gene *LIS1* in mitosis and cytoplasmic dynein function. *Nat Cell Biol* 2: 784–791.

Feng Y, Olson EC, Stukenberg PT, Flanagan LA, Kirschner MW, Walsh CA (2000). LIS1 regulates CNS lamination by interacting with mNudE, a central component of the centrosome. *Neuron* 28: 665–679.

Gaglio T, Dionne MA, Compton DA (1997). Mitotic spindle poles are organized by structural and motor proteins in addition to centrosomes. *J Cell Biol* 138: 1055–1066.

Gambello MJ, Darling DL, Yingling J, Tanaka T, Gleeson JG, Wynshaw-Boris A (2003).

Multiple dose dependent effects of *Lis1* on cerebral cortical development. *J Neurosci* 23: 1719–1729.

Goldstein LS, Philp AV (1999). The road less traveled: emerging principles of kinesin motor utilization. *Annu Rev Cell Dev Biol* 15: 141–183.

Goldstein LS, Yang Z (2000). Microtubule-based transport systems in neurons: the roles of kinesins and dyneins. *Annu Rev Neurosci* 23: 39–71.

Gupta A, Tsai LH, Wynshaw-Boris A (2002). Life is a journey: a genetic look at neo-cortical development. *Nat Rev Genet* 3: 342–355.

Harada A, Takei Y, Kanai Y, Tanaka Y, Nonaka S, Hirokawa N (1998). Golgi vesiculation and lysosome dispersion in cells lacking cytoplasmic dynein. *J Cell Biol* 141: 51–59.

Hirokawa N (1998). Kinesin and dynein superfamily proteins and the mechanism of organelle transport. *Science* 279: 519–526.

Hirotsune S, Fleck MW, Gambello MJ, Bix GJ, Chen A, Clark GD, Ledbetter DH, McBain CJ, Wynshaw-Boris A (1998). Graded reduction of Pafah1b1 (Lis1) activity results in neuronal migration defects and early embryonic lethality. *Nat Genet* 19: 333–339.

Lo Nigro C, Chong CS, Smith AC, Dobyns WB, Carrozzo R, Ledbetter DH (1997). Point mutations and an intragenic deletion in LIS1, the lissencephaly causative gene in isolated lissencephaly sequence and Miller-Dieker syndrome. *Hum Mol Genet* 6: 157–164.

Meeks M, Bush A (2000). Primary ciliary dyskinesia (PCD). *Pediatr Pulmonol* 29: 307–316.

Miki H, Setou M, Kaneshiro K, Hirokawa N (2001). All kinesin superfamily protein, KIF, genes in mouse and human. *Proc Natl Acad Sci USA* 98: 7004–7011.

Morris NR (1976). A temperature-sensitive mutant of *Aspergillus nidulans* reversibly blocked in nuclear division. *Exp Cell Res* 98: 204–210.

Mountain V, Compton DA (2000). Dissecting the role of molecular motors in the mitotic spindle. *Anat Rec* 261: 14–24.

Niethammer M, Smith DS, Ayala R, Peng J, Ko J, Lee MS, Morabito M, Tsai LH (2000). NUDEL is a novel Cdk5 substrate that associates with LIS1 and cytoplasmic dynein. *Neuron* 28: 697–711.

Oakley BR, Morris NR (1980). Nuclear movement is beta-tubulin-dependent in *Aspergillus nidulans*. *Cell* 19: 255–262.

Oakley BR, Morris NR (1981). A beta-tubulin mutation in *Aspergillus nidulans* that blocks microtubule function without blocking assembly. *Cell* 24: 837–845.

Pilz DT, Matsumoto N, Minnerath S, Mills P, Gleeson JG, Allen KM, Walsh CA, Barkovich AJ, Dobyns WB, Ledbetter DH, et al. (1998). LIS1 and XLIS (DCX) muta-tions cause most classical lissencephaly, but different patterns of malformation. *Hum Mol Genet* 7: 2029–2037.

Reiner O, Carrozzo R, Shen Y, Wehnert M, Faustinella F, Dobyns WB, Caskey CT, Ledbetter DH (1993). Isolation of a Miller-Dieker lissencephaly gene containing G protein beta-subunit-like repeats. *Nature* 364: 717–721.

Rosenbaum J, Cole D, Diener D (1999). Intraflagellar transport: the eyes have it. *J Cell Biol* 144: 385–388.

Sasaki S, Shionoya A, Ishida M, Gambello MJ, Yingling J, Wynshaw-Boris A, Hirotsune S (2000). A LIS1/NUDEL/cytoplasmic dynein heavy chain complex in the developing and adult nervous system. *Neuron* 28: 681–696.

Sharp DJ, Rogers GC, Scholey JM (2000). Roles of motor proteins in building microtubule-based structures: a basic principle of cellular design. *Biochim Biophys Acta* 1496: 128–141.

Smith DS, Niethammer M, Ayala R, Zhou Y, Gambello MJ, Wynshaw-Boris A, Tsai LH. (2000). Regulation of cytoplasmic dynein behaviour and microtubule organization by mammalian Lis1. *Nat Cell Biol* 2: 767–775.

Vaisberg EA, Grissom PM, McIntosh JR (1996). Mammalian cells express three distinct dynein heavy chains that are localized to different cytoplasmic organelles. *J Cell Biol* 133: 831–842.

Vale RD, Fletterick RJ (1997). The design plan of kinesin motors. *Annu Rev Cell Dev Biol* 13: 745–777.

Walczak CE (2000). Molecular mechanisms of spindle function. *Genome Biol* 1: reviews 101.1–101.4.

Willins DA, Liu B, Xiang X, Morris NR (1997). Mutations in the heavy chain of cytoplasmic dynein suppress the nudF nuclear migration mutation of *Aspergillus nidulans*. *Mol Gen Genet* 255: 194–200.

Woehlke G, Schliwa M (2000). Walking on two heads: the many talents of kinesin. *Nat Rev Mol Cell Biol* 1: 50–58.

Wynshaw-Boris A, Gambello MJ (2001). LIS1 and dynein motor function in neuronal migration and development. *Genes Dev* 15: 639–651.

Xiang X, Beckwith SM, Morris NR (1994). Cytoplasmic dynein is involved in nuclear migration in *Aspergillus nidulans*. *Proc Natl Acad Sci USA* 91: 2100–2104.

Xiang X, Osmani AH, Osmani SA, Roghi CH, Willins DA, Beckwith S, Goldman G, Chiu Y, Xin M, Liu B, et al. (1995). Analysis of nuclear migration in *Aspergillus nidulans*. *Cold Spring Harb Symp Quant Biol* 60: 813–819.

Xiang X, Zuo W, Efimov VP, Morris NR (1999). Isolation of a new set of *Aspergillus nidulans* mutants defective in nuclear migration. *Curr Genet* 35: 626–630.

91 | *TSC1* and *TSC2* and Tuberous Sclerosis

DAVID J. KWIATKOWSKI

Tuberous sclerosis complex (TSC) is an autosomal dominant disease characterized by the development of hamartomas and hamartias in several organ systems. It is caused by inactivating mutations in either the *TSC1* gene, which encodes the protein hamartin, or the *TSC2* gene, which encodes the protein tuberin. Some, but not all, TSC lesions have been shown to follow the first germline hit–second somatic hit tumor suppressor gene paradigm. The biochemical functions of tuberin and hamartin have been elusive. It is known that the proteins form a strong, stoichiometric complex and that both can be phosphorylated. The strongest hypothesis for a function to date relates to their involvement in a conserved pathway regulating cell size, discovered through work on the *Drosophila* homologues, and extended to mammalian cells. Clinically, TSC is characterized by involvement of brain with the hallmark tubers, several types of cutaneous lesions, renal angiomyolipomas, cardiac rhabdomyomas, and pulmonary lymphangioleiomyomatosis. There is a high sporadic case rate, and both genes have a wide spectrum of mutations, although mutations in *TSC2* are seen five times more commonly than in *TSC1*. *TSC2* disease is significantly more severe than *TSC1* disease. Clinical management focuses on seizure control, neurodevelopmental assessment and educational assistance, and monitoring of brain and kidney for lesion growth.

SPECIFIC LOCI AND DEVELOPMENTAL PATHWAY

Expression and Subcellular Localization of Tuberin and Hamartin

Expression analyses, including Northern blot, in situ hybridization, immunoblotting, and immunohistochemical studies, have indicated that tuberin and hamartin are widely expressed at low levels (Johnson et al., 2001; Murthy et al., 2001). Both proteins show a higher level of expression during fetal development, in both humans and rodents, than in adults (Murthy et al., 2001). Most, but not all, cell lines of diverse origin also express both proteins. Certain brain cells, including cortical neurons, and vascular smooth muscle cells express tuberin and hamartin at high levels (Gutmann et al., 2000). In general, there is a parallel level of expression of the two proteins, although some renal and brain cells appear to express hamartin at levels higher than those of tuberin (Gutmann et al., 2000; Johnson et al., 2001; Murthy et al., 2001). The intracellular distribution of tuberin and hamartin has been analyzed in cultured cells, but antibody limitations have been problematic. Tuberin has been reported to occur in a perinuclear distribution in association with the *cis*-medial Golgi (Wienecke et al., 1996), whereas hamartin is reported to occur in a punctate distribution (Plank et al., 1998) or more diffusely in cortical cytoplasm (Lamb et al., 2000).

Biochemical Functions of Tuberin and Hamartin

Much effort has been directed at determining the biochemical functions of tuberin and hamartin. This research has not been conclusive to date, and there are several candidate biochemical activities for these proteins. Clarification of which of these activities is physiologically relevant, particularly for the tumor supressor function of these proteins, is very much needed.

Tuberin contains a region of homology to a large family of proteins that have GTPase activating protein (GAP) activity for small GTPases such as ras. Tuberin has been shown to have modest GAP activity on rap1a, but not rap2, ras, rho, or rac (Wienecke et al., 1995). Tuberin

has also been shown to have GAP activity toward rab5 (Xiao et al., 1997). Loss of these functions in cells could lead to persistent stimulation through the signaling pathways that these two GTPases engage, which could contribute to hamartoma formation. However, hypotheses that these are critical functions of tuberin await confirmation.

Increased fluid phase endocytosis has been noted in a single Eker rat cell line, potentially consistent with hyperactivation of rab5 signaling, because rab5 is thought to regulate endosome fusion (Xiao et al., 1997). In addition, in an Eker rat kidney-derived cell line in which there is homozygous loss of tuberin, there is aberrant retention of polycystin-1 (product of the *PKD1* gene) in the Golgi apparatus, consistent with an endosomal pathway defect (Kleymenova et al., 2001).

Transcriptional activity of tuberin has been suggested, based on autoactivation results seen in the yeast two-hybrid system assays and related observations on transcriptional effects in HeLa and NIH3T3 cells. Although these results could be artifactual, tuberin has been shown to migrate to the nucleus in some cells under some conditions (Lou et al., 2001).

Hamartin was shown to bind to ezrin in endothelial cells under some conditions after its discovery as a prominent binding partner for ezrin, radixin, and moesin in a yeast two-hybrid assay (Lamb et al., 2000). Transient loss of hamartin was also noted to cause endothelial cell retraction with loss of focal adhesions and substrate detachment. Overexpression of hamartin or certain fragments induces the fomation of actin stress fibers in Swiss 3T3 cells through activation of the rho GTPase (Lamb et al., 2000). Changes in the actin cytoskeleton are seen in Tsc1-null NIH3T3 cells but are relatively mild (Kwiatkowski et al., 2002).

High-level overexpression of tuberin or hamartin in many types of cells leads to growth arrest, with accumulation of cells in G_0/G_1 phases of the cell cycle (Soucek et al., 1998; Benvenuto et al., 2000; Miloloza et al., 2000). Associated with this cell cycle arrest is an increase in the level of expression of the *cdk* inhibitor p27KIP (Soucek et al., 1998; Miloloza et al., 2000). Analysis of a single tuberin-null Eker rat cell line indicated that *p27* expression was reduced compared with a control line, consistent with some type of interaction between tuberin and p27KIP (Soucek et al., 1998). However, expression of mutant forms of tuberin at high levels also induces cell cycle arrest and increased p27KIP expression, suggesting that this set of observations may be nonspecific or artifacts of high-level expression.

We observed that *Tsc1*-null embryo fibroblast lines have persistent phosphorylation of S6K and its substrate S6 (Kwiatkowski et al., 2002). The activation of S6K in these hamartin-null cells is sensitive to treatment with rapamycin, consistent with constitutive activation of the mTOR-S6K pathway due to loss of hamartin (Fig. 91–1). Similar findings have been made in *Tsc2*-null fibroblast and neuroepithelial lines (H. Onda, M. Zhang, and D.J. Kwiatkowski, unpublished observations). Hyperphosphorylation of S6 is also seen in kidney tumors in the *Tsc1* and *Tsc2* heterozygote mice. Thus, these data overall are consistent with genetic studies in *Drosophila* (see later), suggesting this is an important activity of tuberin and hamartin. The mechanism of this effect is uncertain at the present. Nonetheless, inhibition of this pathway may have benefit in the control of TSC hamartomas (Kwiatkowski et al., 2002).

Binding Partners and Phosphorylation of Tuberin and Hamartin

Although missed in early yeast two-hybrid experiments, tuberin and hamartin form a complex that appears to be highly stable, with ap-

Figure 91–1. Model of interactions in the phosphatidylinositol-3 kinase (PI3K)/Akt/S6K signaling cascade. This figure portrays a portion of a more complex pathway. Receptors illustrated by the parallel lines at left undergo tyrosine phosphorylation (Y-P), which leads to activation of PI3K, which phosphorylates phosphoinositides at the 3 position to yield phosphatidylinositol-3,4-biphosphate [PI(3,4)P2] and phosphatidylinositol-3,4,5-triphosphate [PI(3,4,5)P3]. These molecules lead to recruitment of *PDK1* and Akt to the membrane and activation of Akt. Activated Akt then phosphorylates and inactivates tuberin, leading to activation of mTOR, which then phosphorylates S6K and 4E-BP1. These events lead to activation of translation. The results in *Drosophila* and murine systems suggest that tuberin–hamartin normally act to turn off activation of this pathway.

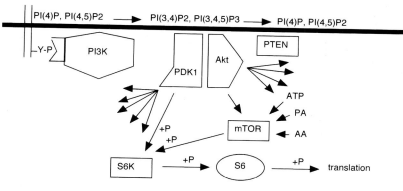

proximate 1:1 stoichiometry (Plank et al., 1998; van Slegtenhorst et al., 1998). It also appears that the majority, although not all, of each protein present in the cell occurs in a complex with the other member (Nellist et al., 1999; H. Zhang and D.J. Kwiatkowski, unpublished observations). These observations are consistent with *Drosophila* experiments in which overexpression of either dTsc1 or dTsc2 alone has no effect on development, whereas the expression of both had marked effects (see later). Overexpression of tuberin in COS cells leads to degradation via ubiquitination in a proteasome-dependent pathway (Benvenuto et al., 2000), whereas overexpression of hamartin leads to its mislocalization and apparent precipitation in complexes (Nellist et al., 1999). These observations further suggest that it is the tuberin–hamartin complex that is the functional unit in the cell.

The effects of about 10 different tuberin missense mutations and a single *Tsc1* in-frame insertion–deletion mutation on the interaction between tuberin and hamartin have been studied (Hodges et al., 2001; Nellist et al., 2001). Most of these mutations abrogate the binding between tuberin and hamartin, although three *Tsc2* missense mutations do not appear to affect the interaction (Nellist et al., 2001). The pathogenicity of these latter mutations, however, has not been clearly established.

Both tuberin and hamartin are substrates for phosphorylation (Aicher et al., 2001; Lou et al., 2001; Nellist et al., 2001). Tuberin contains both phospho-serine and phospho-tyrosine (Aicher et al., 2001), whereas hamartin contains at least phospho-tyrosine (Nellist et al., 2001). Serum stimulation of transfected COS cells leads to tuberin phosphorylation (Aicher et al., 2001). Tuberin within the tuberin–hamartin complex does not appear to be tyrosine-phosphorylated, whereas hamartin is tyrosine-phosphorylated (Nellist et al., 2001). In addition, mutant forms of tuberin are not phosphorylated (Nellist et al., 2001).

Two other binding partners have been described for tuberin–rabaptin (Xiao et al., 1997) and CDK1 (Catania et al., 2001). The physiologic significance of these observations is uncertain.

Involvement of the TSC Genes in Other Disorders

The wide variety of tumors and lesions associated with TSC has suggested the possibility that many different forms of cancer might be associated with inactivation of either *TSC1* or *TSC2*. There is strong evidence that both sporadic angiomyolipomas (AMLs) and sporadic lymphangiomyomatosis (LAM) are due to two-hit inactivation of either *TSC1* or *TSC2* (Henske et al., 1995; Carsillo et al., 2000). *TSC1* and *TSC2* may also be involved in atypical adenomatous hyperplasia of the lung and some lung adenocarcinomas (Takamochi et al., 2001), and *TSC1* may be involved in bladder carcinoma (Hornigold et al., 1999). However, the TSC genes do not appear to be involved in the pathogenesis of usual renal cell carcinoma, glial and glioneuronal cancers, or medulloblastoma.

CLINICAL FEATURES OF TSC

Overview and Diagnostic Criteria

TSC is a relatively variable clinical syndrome, in which several pathologic manifestations are highly specific for the disease (Gomez et al.,

1999). The cardinal feature is the cortical tuber, which is a distinctive form of brain hamartia. Hamartias and hamartomas usually involve several different organ systems in TSC patients, in addition to the brain. Involvement of the skin, heart, and kidney are particularly frequent, occurring at some point during the lifetime of most patients. For clarity, a *hamartia* is a focal developmental defect within an organ without unusual growth. A *hamartoma* is a benign tumor-like nodule composed of an overgrowth of mature cells and tissues that normally occur in the affected organ.

Brain Involvement

Cortical tubers, the hallmark finding in TSC, are found grossly as firm, smooth, somewhat raised, pale lesions of the cerebral cortex (Gomez et al., 1999). Up to 40 such lesions have been seen in one brain, and they range in size from a few millimeters to several centimeters. The second most common brain lesion seen in TSC is the subependymal nodule (SEN), which is typically found in the thalamostriate sulcus of the lateral ventricle. SENs occur grossly as smooth, round to ovoid elevations projecting into the ventricle. They typically calcify in patients past the age of 10 years. Both lesions can be visualized on MRI and CT, although tubers are best seen with MRI, using the T2-weighted technique (Fig. 91–2A).

Histologically, cortical tubers are characterized by architectural disarray with particular disruption of cortical lamination (Crino and Henske, 1999; Gomez et al., 1999). Tubers contain a mixture of cells, including normal and dysplastic neurons, astrocytes, and the hallmark giant cell. Giant cells extend short aberrant processes; staining studies suggest they are of mixed glioneuronal lineage. Dysplastic neurons in tubers show disrupted radial orientation and abnormal dendritic arbors and express both typical neuronal markers and markers indicative of an undifferentiated state, such as nestin. Neuroglial heterotopias are also present in the subcortical white matter in most TSC patients but are much less frequent than either tubers or SENs. SENs consist of large cells in a vascular stroma, with occasional cells that attain giant cell proportions with aberrant and/or multiple nuclei.

Subependymal giant cell astrocytomas (SEGAs) develop in 5% to 10% of TSC patients. These lesions represent a form of SEN with progressive growth and enlargement to a size of more than 1 cm. Histologically, they are nearly identical to SENs, with expression of both astrocytic and neuronal markers.

The major presenting symptoms and signs of cerebral TSC are a variety of epileptic seizures (Crino and Henske, 1999; Gomez et al., 1999). These seizures have their origin in the cortical tubers or in nearby transitional cortex. Nearly all types of seizures can be seen in TSC, but the most common types are infantile spasms and partial motor, complex partial, and partial secondarily generalized seizures. Approximately two-thirds of TSC patients first present with infantile spasms, usually between the ages of 3 and 9 months. The great majority of TSC patients will have experienced some form of epileptic seizure by the age of 1 year. There is a general correlation between the number of cortical tubers in a TSC patient and both a younger age at onset of seizures and severity of seizures.

The molecular basis for epileptogenesis in cortical tubers is uncertain, beyond the general lack of organization of the cortex in these lesions. There is increased transcription of genes encoding glutamater-

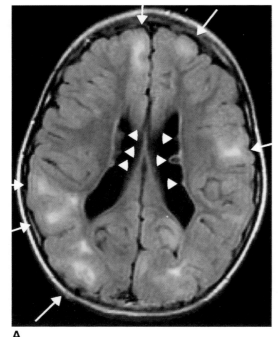

A

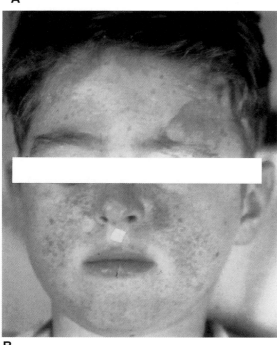

B

Figure 91–2. Manifestations of tuberous sclerosis complex. (*A*) Brain MRI of an 8-year-old boy using the FLAIR technique demonstrates several cortical tubers (white, cortical lesions, indicated by *arrows*) and subependymal nodules lining the ventricles (*arrowheads*). (Courtesy of J. Egelhoff.) (*B*) Facial angiofibroma and forehead fibrous plaque in a 10-year-old boy.

gic receptors in dysplastic neurons and giant cells, with reduced expression of γ-aminobutyric acid (GABA)-ergic receptors. These expression changes may contribute to epileptogenesis in TSC (White et al., 2001).

Mental retardation and developmental problems are serious consequences of brain involvement by cortical tubers. Mental retardation is variable but can be profound and rarely occurs in the absence of a generalized seizure disorder. Developmental problems are very common in TSC and include autistic behavior, hyperactivity, sleep disorders, and aggressive behavior. Autism, hyperactivity, and aggressive

behavior are all seen nearly exclusively in mentally retarded TSC patients. The association between TSC and autism is quite striking in that autism is rarely seen in other neurogenetic disorders and TSC is the most common genetic cause of autism as a whole, accounting for about 3% of all cases. Based on MRI and PET scans, generalized epilepsy in early life and functional imbalance in subcortical circuits appear to be associated with autistic features in children with TSC (Asano et al., 2001).

Growing SEGAs will cause significant intracranial hypertension due to obstruction of ventricular cerebrospinal fluid flow, with symptoms of headache and vomiting. Surgical resection is required for symptomatic SEGAs and is typically quite effective, although occasional cases require repeat procedures.

Kidney Involvement

AMLs are the most common lesion to occur in the kidney of a TSC patient, being seen in about 75% of children by adolescence using ultrasound imaging (Ewalt et al., 1998). These lesions consist of a variable mixture of aberrant vessels, smooth muscle, and fat, being more muscle like early in life and becoming more adipose with age (Gomez et al., 1999). Some smooth muscle and other more epithelioid cells seen in AMLs stain with the HMB-45 antibody, which recognizes an antigen normally expressed exclusively in the melanosome. Lesions frequently appear during the ages of 5 to 10 years and often grow in the adolescent interval (Ewalt et al., 1998). In TSC patients, AMLs are typically bilateral and of varying sizes. Lesions of more than 5 cm in diameter are not rare, and larger lesions are associated with a significant risk of bleeding as well as loss of nephrons due to compression.

Renal cysts are seen in about 10% to 20% of young adults with TSC (Ewalt et al., 1998). The cysts have a distinctive lining epithelium (Gomez et al., 1999). About 3% of TSC patients have severe progressive polycystic kidney disease, which is due to combined mutation of the *TSC2* and *PKD1* genes, as described later.

Renal malignancy appears to occur at an elevated rate and at an unusually young age in TSC patients (Gomez et al., 1999), with a lifetime risk of about 2% to 3%. A proportion of these tumors are typical renal cell carcinoma, whereas others appear to be malignant AMLs, based on spindle cell architecture and other histologic features, as well as positive staining with HMB-45.

Skin Involvement

Cutaneous findings are present in the great majority of TSC patients and are the most easily identified sign of the disease. Most lesions are of minor clinical significance, but facial angiofibromas can be a significant cosmetic issue (Gomez et al., 1999).

Hypomelanotic macules or white spots typically have a lance-ovate shape ("ash leaf") and are most common over the trunk and buttocks. Three or more of these lesions are very unusual in the general population and thus are considered a major diagnostic criterion (Table 91–1). Histopathologic examination shows reduced number, pigment content, and size of melanosomes within the melanocytes in a hypomelanotic macule. The lesions are present at birth and do not change, although they are more easily observed after a suntan is obtained.

Facial angiofibromas (formerly known as adenoma sebaceum) are red to pink papules or nodules with a smooth surface that are found in a malar distribution and extend to the chin (Fig. 91–2B). They typically first appear between the ages of 2 and 6 years and progress to a variable extent during puberty. Histologic findings are dermal fibrosis and vasodilatation, with occasional large glial-appearing cells. They are found in about 85% of all TSC patients. Forehead fibrous plaque (Fig. 91–2B) is a larger lesion related to facial angiofibroma; Shagreen patch is also a related lesion found typically on the upper buttock.

Ungual fibromas are another common cutaneous manifestation of TSC, being seen in up to 90% of adults over the age of 30 years (Gomez et al., 1999). These lesions are red or flesh-colored papules or nodules occurring in the finger or toe nail beds and along the proximal or distal nail fold or under the nail plate. Their histopathology is similar to that of facial angiofibromas.

Table 91–1. Diagnostic Criteria for Tuberous Sclerosis Complex*

Major Features	Minor Features
Facial angiofibromas or forehead plaque	Multiple, randomly distributed pits in dental enamel
Nontraumatic ungual or periungual fibroma	Hamartomatous rectal polyps
Hypomelanotic macules (three or more)	Bone cysts
Shagreen patch (connective tissue nevus)	Cerebral white matter radial migration lines†
Multiple retinal nodular hamartomas	Gingival fibromas
Cortical tuber†	Nonrenal hamartoma
Subependymal nodule	Retinal achromic patch
Subependymal giant cell astrocytoma	"Confetti" skin lesions
Cardiac rhabdomyoma, single or multiple	Multiple renal cysts
Lymphangiomyomatosis‡	
Renal angiomyolipoma‡	

*Definite tuberous sclerosis complex, either two major features or one major feature plus two minor features; probable tuberous sclerosis complex, one major feature plus one minor feature; possible tuberous sclerosis complex, either one major feature or two or more minor features.

†When cerebral cortical dysplasia and cerebral white matter migration tracts occur together, they should be counted as one feature rather than as two features of tuberous sclerosis.

‡When both lymphangiomyomatosis and renal angiomyolipomas are present, other features of tuberous sclerosis should be present before a definite diagnosis is assigned.

Source: Modified from Roach et al. (1998).

Other Sites of Involvement

LAM is a disorder seen almost exclusively in females that is characterized pathologically by smooth muscle and other cellular proliferation and cystic changes in the lung parenchyma. Some LAM cells stain positive with HMB-45 like AML cells, and these tend to be cells of an epithelioid nature (Matsumoto et al., 1999). Most LAM patients also have AMLs in the kidney or elsewhere in the abdomen. LAM presents clinically as progressive dyspnea or as acute dyspnea due to pneumothorax. The natural history of LAM is poorly defined. There are women in whom it is progressive and fatal. Recent studies have documented that about 40% of women with TSC have CT evidence of LAM. It is likely that most of those in whom it is asymptomatic and detected with CT will not have significant symptoms from this condition.

The retina is involved in about 50% of TSC patients with hamartomas. Rhabdomyomas are also common in infants and children with TSC (Gomez et al., 1999). These lesions can be up to several centimeters in diameter and consist of glycogen-filled myocytes. With echocardiographic screening, more than 50% of TSC infants are found to have rhabdomyomas. In most cases, there are no symptoms and the lesions spontaneously decrease in size or disappear over time. Less often, rhabdomyomas cause heart failure due to obstruction, affect myocardial function by replacement, or cause rhythm disturbances, and surgical resection is considered.

CLINICAL AND MOLECULAR GENETICS OF TSC

Clinical Genetics of TSC

TSC occurs as an autosomal dominant disorder. Large families with the condition are rare due to reduced reproduction rates among those affected. About two-thirds of cases of TSC are sporadic, representing new mutations. TSC occurs in up to 1:6000 live births without apparent ethnic clustering. Linkage of TSC to chromosome 9q34 was first reported in 1987, and the corresponding *TSC1* gene was identified in 1997 (van Slegtenhorst et al., 1997). Linkage of TSC to chromosome 16p13 was discovered in 1992, and the corresponding *TSC2* gene identified in 1993 (European Tuberous Sclerosis Consortium, 1993). Among families large enough to permit linkage analysis, approximately half show linkage to 9q34 and half show linkage to 16p13 (Cheadle et al., 2000). There is no evidence of a third locus.

Gene Structure

The *TSC1* gene consists of 23 exons, of which 21 encode hamartin, with an 8.6-kb mRNA that includes a 4.5-kb 3′-untranslated region. There is variable splicing of the second, untranslated exon. The gene is found in a genomic region of 55 kb on 9q34. The *TSC2* gene consists of 42 exons, of which 41 encode tuberin, with a 5.4-kb mRNA and relatively short 5′- and 3′-untranslated regions. There is alterna-

tive splicing of exon 25, the first 3 bp of exon 26, and exon 31, although the significance of these alternative forms of tuberin with respect to function is not known (Cheadle et al., 2000).

Mutations in *TSC1* and *TSC2*

More than 600 mutations in the *TSC1* and *TSC2* genes have been identified (http://expmed.bwh.harvard.edu/ts/review/). Here we discuss a set of 594 patients with TSC mutations (172 in *TSC1* and 422 in *TSC2*, Table 91–2) published before January 2001 (Cheadle et al., 2000; Dabora et al., 2001). There are a total of 427 different reported mutations, 115 of *TSC1* and 312 of *TSC2*. Fifty-four mutations have been reported recurrently (21 in *TSC1* and 33 in *TSC2*), accounting for 176 of the 591 (30%) mutations.

In *TSC1*, 82 (48%) of the mutations are single-base substitutions, of which 82% are nonsense mutations (Table 91–2, Fig. 91–3). Just over half of the nonsense mutations are recurrent C-to-T transitions at six of the seven CGA codons within the *TSC1* coding region. Splicing mutations account for 16% of all single-base changes in *TSC1*. Two missense mutations have been reported in *TSC1*, but neither have been conclusively shown to be disease causing as opposed to polymorphisms.

In *TSC2*, 222 (53%) of the mutations are single-base substitutions (see Table 91–2, Fig. 91–3). Nonsense mutations in *TSC2* make up only 39% (86 of 222) of this class, but again they commonly (36%) occur at five of the seven CpG sites that can transition to nonsense codons in *TSC2*. In contrast to *TSC1*, missense mutations account for 38% of the single-base substitutions (84 of 222) in *TSC2*. *TSC2* has two CpG sites that are mutational hot spots that lead to missense mutations: 1831-2 (611R → W and 611R → Q) and 5024-5 (1675P → L). These two CpG sites account for 35 (42%) of the 84 missense mutations in *TSC2*. Splice mutations make up the remaining 23% of point mutations in *TSC2*.

About one-third of *TSC1* mutations are small deletions (less than 29 bp), whereas 17% are small insertions (less than 34 bp), and nearly all of these cause frameshifts in the *TSC1* mRNA. Nearly all small insertions arise as duplication of an adjacent single or multiple bases.

Table 91–2. Types and Numbers of *TSC1* and *TSC2* Mutations

Type of Mutation	*TSC1* Number (%)	*TSC2* Number (%)
Large deletions/rearrangements	3 (2)	69 (16)
Insertions	29 (17)	34 (8)
Deletions	58 (34)	97 (23)
Nonsense	67 (39)	86 (20)
Point splicing	13 (7)	52 (12)
Missense	2 (1)	84 (20)
Total	172	422

TSC1

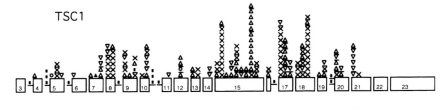

Figure 91–3. Map of the sites of several hundred small mutations in *TSC1* and *TSC2*. Proportional drawings (boxes) of all of the exons of *TSC1* and *TSC2* are shown. Intron regions are not drawn to scale and are expanded only when a mutation is present. Mutation symbols are x, nonsense; ■, splice site; △, deletion; ▽, insertion; ○, missense; ▲, in-frame deletion. A line separates mutations occurring at nearby, but not identical, nucleotide positions.

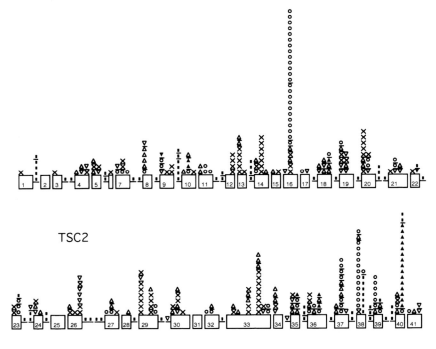

TSC2

Similarly, most deletions (62%) are the deletion of an element of a tandem repeat. Similar observations apply to small deletions and insertions found in *TSC2*.

Large deletions and rearrangements are strikingly more common in *TSC2* than in *TSC1* (69 versus 3). They show no consistency in either the size or junction fragments involved, ranging in size from 1 kb to more than 100 kb (Sampson et al., 1997; Dabora et al., 2000).

Large sets of TSC patients (150 and 224) have undergone comprehensive screens for mutations in *TSC1* and *TSC2*, with an overall rate of mutation detection of 80% to 90% (Jones et al., 1999; Dabora et al., 2001). *TSC1* mutations have been identified in 10% to 15% of sporadic TSC patients, whereas *TSC2* mutations have been found in about 70%. Several differences between the genes and their mutations appear to explain these differences in mutation rate. First, missense mutations do not (or perhaps rarely) occur in *TSC1*. Second, a much higher rate of large rearrangements and deletions occurs in *TSC2*, probably reflecting differences in chromosomal location, genomic structural features, or the specific sequences present at the two loci. Third, the TSC2 coding region is about 1.5 times longer than TSC1 and has approximately twice the number of splice sites, providing increased opportunity for all types of small mutations (Cheadle et al., 2000).

TSC Patients without Mutations in *TSC1* or *TSC2*

Even with comprehensive effort, there remains 10% to 20% of TSC patients for whom no mutation can be identified (Jones et al., 1999; Dabora et al., 2001). There are several possible explanations for this, including incomplete sensitivity of mutation detection and unidentified intronic and promoter region mutations. Through protein truncation test screening, four intronic mutations in *TSC2* (15, 15, 18, and 281 bp from the exon border) have been identified to date (Mayer et al., 2000). Thus, these mutations may contribute to the 10% to 20% of patients in whom mutation detection by exon amplification and screening fails. Another explanation for mutation detection failure is

low-level mosaicism for a mutation in *TSC1* or *TSC2*, which could cause a full TSC phenotype but be very difficult to detect. Another possibility is that there are additional genes, of which a mutation causes a TSC syndrome. However, all reported large TSC families show linkage to either *TSC1* or *TSC2*, arguing against this last possibility.

We have observed that patients without identified mutations in *TSC1* or *TSC2* in our set of 224 intensively screened patients have clinical features that are milder than those of patients with defined *TSC2* mutations but similar to those of patients with defined *TSC1* mutations (Dabora et al., 2001). This observation seems most consistent with the occurrence of mosaicism for a *TSC2* mutation in these patients, to explain both the lack of mutation identification and the milder clinical features.

No verified pathogenic missense mutations in *TSC1* have yet been discovered. Because there is no reason why such mutations would not occur, this observation suggests that missense mutations might either have no effect or cause a unique clinical phenotype distinct from that of TSC. It seems possible that some *TSC1* missense mutations may have a dominant negative effect on hamartin produced by the normal *TSC1* allele, leading to an embryonic lethal or other severe phenotype.

Mosaicism in TSC

Mosaicism for a TSC gene mutation occurs when the mutation occurs early during embryogenesis but after the fertilized egg undergoes one or more divisions. Both somatic (generalized) and germline (confined gonadal) mosaicism for *TSC1* and *TSC2* mutations have been described. Mosaicism has been observed in 10% to 26% of TSC families (Sampson et al., 1997; Verhoef et al., 1999). Some of the founder individuals with somatic mosaicism had relatively mild signs of TSC, not meeting diagnostic criteria, but other patients with somatic mosaicism have classic TSC features.

Ten sets of siblings affected by TSC but with apparently normal parents have been reported (Rose et al., 1999). In some of these cases, identical *TSC2* mutations have been found in DNA from affected siblings but not in blood-derived DNA from their parents. These observations strongly implicate gonadal mosaicism in a parent. The frequency of germline mosaicism is low in TSC, probably less than 5% of all parents of sporadic TSC children.

GENOTYPE–PHENOTYPE CORRELATIONS

TSC1 versus *TSC2* Disease

The discordance between the frequency of *TSC1* and *TSC2* mutations in sporadic TSC patients (10% to 15% *TSC1*, 70% *TSC2*) and their frequencies in large TSC families (50% *TSC1*, 50% *TSC2*) has suggested for several years that TSC due to *TSC1* mutations might be less severe than TSC due to *TSC2* mutations. However, the equal frequency observation in large families was based on analysis of a relatively small number of large TSC families. Moreover, in some series, the mutation distribution in small to moderate-sized TSC families is also very much skewed toward *TSC2* (Dabora et al., 2001).

We performed a detailed analysis of this hypothesis using a comprehensive TSC clinical data instrument (Dabora et al., 2001). Twenty-two sporadic TSC patients with *TSC1* mutations and 129 sporadic cases with *TSC2* mutations were compared. Eight of 16 clinical features occurred at a significantly higher frequency and/or with greater severity in *TSC2* than in *TSC1* sporadic cases (Table 91–3). These features included seizures, moderate to severe mental retardation, mean number of subependymal nodules, tuber count, kidney AMLs, mean grade of facial angiofibromas, forehead plaque, and retinal hamartomas. Thus, this study provides strong evidence that *TSC1* disease is less severe than *TSC2* disease in multiple respects, consistent with the original discordance between sporadic case and large family frequency of *TSC1* versus *TSC2* mutations.

The observations that there is a lower frequency of sporadic TSC patients with *TSC1* compared with *TSC2* mutations and that there is a smaller number of cortical tubers and subependymal nodules in *TSC1* patients (4.9 and 1.7) than in *TSC2* patients (12.9 and 6.7) are consistent with the model that both germline and somatic mutations occur less frequently in *TSC1* than in *TSC2*. Although this is a straightforward explanation of these data, it is certain that brain MRI does not detect all cortical tubers or SENs. Thus, an alternative explanation could be that *TSC1* gene loss (presumed to occur in the cortical tubers and SENs of a *TSC1* patient) leads to the development of smaller tubers, which are less often detected on brain MRI, compared with *TSC2* patients.

A Contiguous Gene Deletion Syndrome Involving *TSC2* and PKD1

Renal cysts are common in TSC patients, but in most patients they are small in number and pose no significant health risk. About 3% of TSC patients develop severe renal cystic disease similar to that seen in polycystic kidney disease (PKD). Large genomic deletions involving both *TSC2* and *PKD1*, which are directly adjacent in the genome, are present in most of these patients (Sampson et al., 1997). Interestingly, the PKD that develops in these patients is more severe than the usual PKD associated with mutation in *PKD1* alone, with cystic changes in the kidney in early childhood and progression to renal failure by age 20 (Sampson et al., 1997). It appears likely that this accelerated pathogenesis is due to the genetic mechanism of genomic deletion of the second allele of both genes occurring as a single somatic event. In such cells, there would be loss of expression of both tuberin and polycystin (the product of the *PKD1* gene) to produce a synergistic effect in cystogenesis.

A Mild TSC Phenotype?

Two exceptional families from the same region have been reported with the same *TSC2* missense mutation (1503Q → P) (Khare et al., 2001). In these families, relatively mild TSC features are seen, and some family members carrying the mutation do not appear to have any clinical signs of TSC. However, a detailed clinical evaluation of these families has not been performed, limiting the clinical implications. Nonetheless, it is possible that there are families in which a milder variant form of TSC is seen with a unique mutational spectrum in either *TSC1* or *TSC2*.

ESTABLISHING THE DIAGNOSIS

The diversity of hamartias and hamartomas that occur in TSC has led to the development of formal diagnostic criteria (Roach et al., 1998; see Table 91–1). Many features of TSC appear as the patient ages (Jozwiak et al., 2000; see Table 91–4).

MANAGEMENT

Eventually, gene therapy may be a potential form of treatment for TSC. However, neurologic morbidity in the form of seizures, mental retardation, and developmental disorders is the most serious aspect of TSC. Cortical tubers are the main cause of these neurologic morbidi-

Table 91–3. Comparison of Clinical Features in Sporadic Tuberous Sclerosis Complex (TSC) Patients with *TSC1* versus *TSC2* Mutations

	TSC1 Sporadic Cases	*TSC2* Sporadic Cases	p Value *TSC1* versus *TSC2*
No. of patients	22	129	
Age range (average) (yr)	2–51 (13.4)	1–44 (11.2)	NS
Median age (yr)	9	10	
Neurologic			
Seizures	19/22 (86%)	127/128 (99%)	0.02
Mental handicap (age >6 yr)			
Moderate plus severe	2/14 (14%)	41/90 (46%)	0.04
Mean MR gr (scale 0–3)	0.67	1.4	0.007
Subependymal nodules	15/20 (75%)	127/136 (93%)	0.02
Mean No. of nodules	1.7	6.7	0.0002
Tubers (any)	13/15 (87%)	55/60 (92%)	NS
>10 Tubers	1/9 (11%)	29/42 (69%)	0.002
Mean No. of tubers	4.4	12.9	0.002
Renal			
Kidney angiomyolipomas	6/19 (31%)	72/121 (60%)	0.03
Mean grade (scale 0–3)	0.32	0.97	0.006
Skin			
Facial angiofibromas (age >2 yr)	13/22 (59%)	95/121 (78%)	NS
Mean grade (scale 0–3)	0.9	1.5	0.02
Forhead plaque	2/20 (10%)	51/128 (40%)	0.01
Other			
Retinal hamartomas	0/16	32/117 (27%)	0.01

Source: Dabora et al. (2001).

Table 91–4. Frequency of Diagnostic Features of Tuberous Sclerosis Complex in Children, According to Age

Diagnostic Feature	Age (yr)				
	0–2	2–5	5–9	9–14	14–18
Hypomelanotic macules (%)	90	95	97	97	97
Cardia rhabdomyoma (%)	83	21	21	41	75
Epilepsy, usually infantile spasms (%)	83	91	94	96	96
Subependymal nodules on CT/MRI (%)	83	97	97	100	100
Renal angiomyolipomas (%)	17	42	64	65	92
Facial angiofibromas (%)	10	63	74	77	77
Retinal hamartoma (%)	8	17	21	17	31
Shagreen patch (%)	0	21	35	47	48
Forehead plaque (%)	0	9	16	19	19
Liver angiomyolipomas (%)	0	0	11	24	46
Periungual fibromas (%)	0	0	0	11	15

n = 13–40 for each age/diagnostic feature comparison.
Source: Modified from Jozwiak et al. (2000).

ties, and the development of both the brain and cortical tubers is essentially complete by birth. Therefore, any approach directed at elimination or modification of tuber development is particularly challenging as therapy in utero would be required.

Effective management of TSC patients can improve the quality of life of the affected individual to a dramatic extent. There are at least four areas where intervention is recommended: clinical monitoring, seizure control, renal AML management, and care of facial angiofibromas.

Regular clinical evaluation is recommended (Table 91–5) to identify potential clinical problems at an early stage and permit effective intervention (Roach et al., 1999). Neurodevelopmental testing is recommended at the time of diagnosis and at school entry because neurodevelopment problems are so common in TSC children and children can benefit from early intervention. Renal ultrasonography is recommended every 1 to 3 years from the age of diagnosis until age 20 to permit monitoring of renal AMLs. In 10% to 20% of children, these lesions grow to a significant extent, and early intervention, as described later, may lead to preservation of renal function and avoidance of morbidity. Repeated brain MRI or brain CT scans are also recommended every 1 to 3 years from age of diagnosis until age 20 to permit serial follow-up of subependymal nodules, and early intervention for growing lesions.

Aggressive seizure control is recommended for all TSC patients with seizures due to the connection between poor seizure control and poor intellectual outcome. An expanding armamentarium of drugs are available for seizure control, with two relatively new drugs that are effective in TSC: vigabatrin and lamotrogine (Curatolo et al., 2001; Franz et al., 2001). Vigabatrin appears to be the best drug for control of infantile spasms in TSC; more than 50% of patients have complete cessation of spasms while on vigabatrin (Curatolo et al., 2001). Unfortunately, use of vigabatrin is associated with the late appearance of visual-field defects in up to 50% of patients, so monitoring is required. Steroid treatment, usually in the form of corticotropin injections, is an alternative treatment method for infantile spasms in TSC and is also effective in some infants. Lamotrigine also appears to be particularly effective in the treatment of a variety of seizure types occurring in TSC (Franz et al., 2001). Surgical resection of seizure foci is another

approach that can be effective in TSC patients who have proved to be refractory to a number of antiepileptic drugs. Innovative approaches using neurotransmitter precursors to specifically label epileptogenic foci by PET scanning are also being explored (Asano et al., 2000) and may assist in targetting surgery.

Surgical approaches are available for the treatment of AMLs that grow or are symptomatic and for the facial angiofibromas of TSC. Nephron-sparing approaches, including selective arterial embolization, are recommended for AML management because bilateral disease is common and the natural history is unpredictable. Facial angiofibromas are a significant cosmetic issue in many patients with TSC, and a variety of approaches have been used.

GENETIC COUNSELING

Genetic counseling is appropriate for every TSC patient (Gomez et al., 1999). TSC patients should have a thorough investigation of their family history. Although nonpenetrance of TSC is uncommon, manifestations of TSC can go unrecognized. Specific inquiry should be made as to all of the clinical features described in Table 91–1, as well as seizures, mental retardation or developmental delay, autism, cardiac arrhythmias, stillbirths, lung disease, renal failure or cancer, pneuomothorax, and skin disease of any kind. If additional children are contemplated, the parents of sporadic cases of TSC should have a thorough evaluation, including general physical examination with Wood's light evaluation of the skin, ophthalmologic examination, renal ultrasonography or CT, and brain MRI or CT. These studies should be interpreted by physicians familiar with TSC findings.

A parent who has one or two findings consistent with TSC but who does not meet formal diagnostic criteria should be considered cautiously. Such individuals may be full carriers of a TSC gene mutation with low expression, may be mosaic for a mutation, or may not carry a mutation at all. Such a parent's risk of having a second TSC child should be considered to be elevated over that of the general population but is uncertain.

Even with a completely normal clinical and radiographic evaluation, there remains the possibility that one of the parents has confined

Table 91–5. Summary of Testing Recommendations for Children with Tuberous Sclerosis Complex

Assessment	Initial Testing	Repeat Testing
Neurodevelopmental testing	At diagnosis and at school entry	As indicated
Ophthalmic examination	At diagnosis	As indicated
Electroencephalography	If seizures occur	As indicated for seizure management
Electrocardiography	At diagnosis	As indicated
Echocardiography	If cardiac symptoms occur	If cardiac dysfunction occurs
Renal ultrasonography	At diagnosis	Every 1–3 years
Chest CT	At adulthood (women only)	If pulmonary dysfunction occurs
Cranial CT or MRI*	At diagnosis	Children/adolescents: every 1–3 years

CT, computed tomography; MRI, magnetic resonance imaging.
Source: Roach et al. (1999).

gonadal mosaicism for a TSC mutation (Rose et al., 1999). Recurrent sporadic cases born to entirely normal parents are quite uncommon; therefore, the recurrence risk in this situation should be estimated as about 2% and definitely no greater than 5%.

Mutational testing with identification of a specific *TSC1* or *TSC2* mutation in a sporadic patient enables direct testing of parental DNA samples for the mutation. However, low-level somatic mosaicism as well as gonadal mosaicism present in a parent can be missed by such testing. An alternative approach that parents may wish to consider is prenatal fetal sampling (e.g., by amniocentesis) to directly examine whether the fetus is carrying the mutation present in the sporadic child.

When one parent is affected with TSC, the risk of transmission of the mutant allele is 50%. However, prospective parents in this situation should be aware that the severity of tuberous sclerosis is not predictable and an affected child may have relatively few medical problems. There are several professionals with advanced degrees who have TSC. Although many mothers with TSC have had uneventful pregnancies, there appears to be some additional risk due to AML hemorrhage and worsening of pulmonary LAM.

Prenatal diagnosis of TSC can be made on the basis of the identification of cardiac rhabdomyomas with ultrasonography and/or cortical tubers with ultrasonography or rapid-sequence MRI. However, the frequency of positive findings in fetuses with TSC using these modalities is uncertain. In addition, the earliest time at which definite findings have been identified is 22 weeks' gestation. Nonetheless, such findings may be helpful in the management of delivery and in the care of the neonate.

ANIMAL MODELS

Drosophila

Studies have used the power of genetic analysis in *Drosophila* to discover a connection between *Drosophila dTsc1* and *dTsc2* and the regulation of cell and organ size (Gao and Pan, 2001; Potter et al., 2001; Tapon et al., 2001). In parallel studies from three laboratories, fly mutagenesis was followed by a screen using FRT/FLP recombination to search for mutations affecting cell and organ size in the eye. *dTsc1* turned up as a positive hit in this screen and was shown to have similar effects on organ development as disruption of the *Tsc2* gene, which had earlier been shown to be the gene termed *gigas* responsible for a classic large cell mutant in *Drosophila* (Ito and Rubin, 1999).

Homozygous inactivation of either *dTsd1* or *dTsc2* leads to an identical phenotype. When restricted to the eye or wing, organogenesis and differentiation proceed fairly normally, but there is an increase in the size of the overall organ that is nearly entirely due to an increase in cell size. *dTsd1-* or *dTsc2*-null cells in these organs continue to enter S phase at an elevated rate compared with wild-type cells; there is a slight (~1%) increase in the number of cells per organ, and some mild developmental abnormalities are seen. Null cells isolated from these organs show a normal DNA content but are shifted from G_1 to the S and G_2 phases of the cell cycle, and there is increased expression of cyclins E, A, and B (Tapon et al., 2001). Increased expression of *dTsd1* alone or *dTsc2* alone has no effect, but their combined expression in the *Drosophila* eye leads to an opposite phenotype in which there are small eyes with fewer individual subunits, with parallel findings with wing expression (Gao and Pan, 2001; Potter et al., 2001; Tapon et al., 2001).

Epistasis studies, examining the interaction of null or overexpression mutations in *dTsd1* and *dTsc2*, focused on genes previously identified as important in the regulation of cell size in *Drosophila*, the PI3K–Akt–p70S6K pathway (see Fig. 91–1), and cell cycle components (Tapon et al., 2001) . Ablation of *dTsd1* or *dTsc2*, or overexpression of both, had effects that were dominant in effect over mutations in the insulin receptor, PI3K, and dAkT. A synergistic effect was seen with dPTEN, suggesting that *dTsd1/dTsc2* may act in parallel to the kinase cascade of this pathway, for which dPTEN is a critical regulator. In contrast, dS6K inactivation or overexpression was dominant in effect to mutations in *dTsd1* and/or *dTsc2*. Overexpression of cyclin D with *cdk4* or cyclin E or *myc* also suppressed the effects of in-

creased expression of *dTsd1* and *dTsc2*, suggesting that *dTsd1* and *dTsc2* act through a cyclin-dependent mitotic pathway to achieve their effects on cell size and growth. Thus, the observations suggest that *dTsd1* and *dTsc2* participate in this conserved pathway that regulates cell growth in *Drosophila*, but the precise level of interaction is uncertain, and the mechanism involved is unknown.

Mice and Rats

Null mutations in each of *Tsc1* and *Tsc2* have been engineered in mice (Kobayashi et al., 1999, 2001; Onda et al., 1999; Kwiatkowski et al., 2002), and there is a spontaneously occurring null allele of *Tsc2* in the Eker rat (Eker et al., 1981; Yeung et al., 1994; Kobayashi et al., 1995). The pathology in all of these animal models is similar and is discussed in aggregate.

Tsc1- or *Tsc2*-null embryos do not survive past embryonic day 13. The survival is about 1 day longer in the *Tsc1*-null embryos than in the *Tsc2*-null embryos (Kobayashi et al., 2001; Kwiatkowski et al., 2002). In both cases, the null embryos tend to be smaller than wild-type embryos from the same litter, whereas the pathology is a little more severe in *Tsc2*-null embryos than in *Tsc1*-null embryos. Null embryos show abnormalities in the form of liver and gut hypoplasia and of hyperplasia with abnormal development in the heart. The cause of death appears to be liver hypoplasia resulting in cardiac failure, but primary cardiac pathology may also contribute. Exencephaly with abnormal skull and brain development has been seen in a proportion of null embryos, particularly in the Eker rat, *Tsc2*-null mice, and one of the *Tsc1*-null alleles. However, the finding is not consistent among all null pups and appears to correlate with strain in the rat.

Mice heterozygous for mutations in either *Tsc1* or *Tsc2*, as well as the Eker rat, develop several tumors that are very unusual in the rodent. Renal cystadenomas develop by 6 months of age and grow progressively and slowly throughout the life of the animal. Histologically, these lesions appear as a continuous spectrum from pure cysts to cysts with papillary projections to solid adenomas. In both rodents, progression of these lesions to carcinoma is a rare event given the number of cystadenomas per animal and has been estimated at less than 1:1000 cystadenomas (Onda et al., 1999). Such carcinomas are characterized by nuclear atypia (common), massive growth (less common), and metastasis (very rare). The cell of origin of these tumors is tubular epithelial cells. In the mouse the cystadenomas uniformly express gelsolin, consistent with an origin in the intercalated cell of the cortical collecting duct (Onda et al., 1999). Cystadenomas appear to be unrelated to any human TSC pathology.

Liver hemangiomas, characterized by endothelial and smooth muscle cell proliferation with large vascular spaces, are also commonly seen in both *Tsc1* and *Tsc2* heterozygote mice. These lesions thus are similar to the kidney AMLs and pulmonary lesions seen in TSC patients. Interestingly, they are also more common and more extensive and cause greater mortality rates in female than in male *Tsc1* heterozygote mice (Kwiatkowski et al., 2002).

Tsc1 and *Tsc2* heterozygote mice also develop angiosarcomas on their tails, legs, and mouths at a low frequency (about 1:20 by age 18 months). Eker rats do not develop liver hemangiomas but rather develop pituitary adenomas, uterine leiomyomas and leiomyosarcomas, and splenic hemangiomas, each at a frequency of about 50% at 2 years of age.

Brain hamartomas resembling TSC subependymal nodules have been identified in 63% of Eker rats at age 1.5 to 2 years (Yeung et al., 1997). The lesions consist of a mixture of large and elongated cells that express glial markers, are often calcified, and are found in both subcortical and subependymal regions. No brain lesions have been seen in the *Tsc1* and *Tsc2* heterozygote mice.

Variation in the severity of expression of the heterozygote phenotype according to genetic background has been shown for both the mouse and rat models of TSC and influence kidney, liver, and brain (Rennebeck et al., 1998; Onda et al., 1999; Kwiatkowski et al., 2002). A locus *Mot1* has been mapped genetically that accounts for 35% of the variation in the severity of renal tumor development in the Fisher 344 and Brown Norway rat strains (Yeung et al., 2001).

MOLECULAR PATHOGENESIS

Tumor Suppressor Gene Mechanism

The focal nature of the lesions that occur in tuberous sclerosis has suggested for many years that a fundamental pathogenetic mechanism in this disease was the classic Knudson model of a first germline hit and a second somatic hit, ablating both alleles of either *TSC1* or *TSC2* in lesions. Large somatic deletions of the wild-type *TSC1* or *TSC2* allele have been identified in the form of loss of heterozygosity (LOH) using nearby microsatellite or other polymorphic markers in numerous TSC lesions (Green et al., 1994; Carbonara et al., 1996; Henske et al., 1996; Au et al., 1999; Niida et al., 2001). However, the rate of LOH varies considerably according to the site of the lesion and is highest (~75%) in renal AMLs. LOH has been difficult to demonstrate in TSC cutaneous lesions, primarily due to a lack of access to pathologic material.

LOH has been seen very rarely in brain lesions from TSC patients, in fewer than 1:30 lesions examined (Henske et al., 1996; Niida et al., 2001). Because cortical tubers always contain apparently normal cells, this could mask LOH. However, SENs are typically relatively free of normal cells and do not show LOH. It is possible that brain lesions undergo loss of the second allele via a different mechanism of inactivation than that detectable by LOH analysis. Immunohistochemical analyses of tuberin and hamartin expression in cortical tubers have yielded conflicting results in different laboratories, with some indicating robust expression of both proteins in cortical tuber giant cells and others indicating reduced expression of both (Henske et al., 1997; Johnson et al., 1999; Mizuguchi et al., 2000). Thus, the pathogenic mechanism of cortical tuber development remains unproved.

ACKNOWLEDGMENTS

The author wishes to apologize for not citing all relevant references due to space limitations. He also thanks his colleagues, fellows, students, technicians, and TSC family members who have stimulated his thinking on this subject for many years and Mary Pat Reeve for maintenance of the TSC mutation database. He acknowledges the support of the National Institutes of Health, Tuberous Sclerosis Association, March of Dimes, and William Watts.

NOTE ADDED IN PROOF

Advances in our understanding of the biochemical function of tuberin and hamartin which suggest potential therapies have recently been made. Additional genetic interaction studies in *Drosophila* have positioned *Tsc1/Tsc2* in the PI3Kinase-Akt-S6Kinase pathway at about the level of Tor. Furthermore, the *Drosophila* Tsc2 protein was recognized to contain two to four Akt1 phosphorylation sites, and Akt1 phosphorylation of Tsc2 was shown to cause disruption of the Tsc1-Tsc2 complex (Gao et al., 2002; Potter et al., 2002). Evidence for activation of the pathway downstream of mTOR has now also been seen in TSC patient lesions (Goncharova et al., 2002; El-Hashemite et al., 2003). Furthermore, in mammalian cells, activated Akt also phosphorylates TSC2 at two to four different sites (Dan et al., 2002; Inoki et al., 2002; Manning et al., 2002), which appears to reduce its activity in inhibiting mTOR. High-level expression of TSC1/TSC2 by transfection leads to inhibition of signaling pathways downstream of mTOR (Inoki et al., 2002).

Thus, in normal cells the TSC1-TSC2 complex acts as an inhibitor of mTOR. When stimulated by growth factors or other agents, activation of Akt leads to phosphorylation of TSC2, which leads to inactivation of the inhibitory activity of the TSC1/TSC2 complex. In cells that are lacking either TSC1 or TSC2, mTOR/S6Kinase activity is increased severalfold and is no longer dependent upon several signals that normally regulate their activity, including signals acting through the PI3Kinase pathway. This appears to be a fundamental biochemical defect that contributes to the growth of TSC hamartomas in cells lacking TSC1 or TSC2. It is a remarkably fortuitous circumstances that rapamycin, a clinically approved compound, has selective activity in the inhibition of mTOR and appears to be effetive in short-term trials in mouse models of TSC (Kenerson et al., 2002; Kwiatkowski et al., unpublished observations). Therefore, there is currently guarded enthusiasm for the possibility that rapamycin will provide benefit for some of the clinical manifestations of TSC, and clinical trials are just beginning.

REFERENCES

Aicher LD, Campbell JS, Yeung RS (2001). Tuberin phosphorylation regulates its interaction with hamartin. Two proteins involved in tuberous sclerosis. *J Biol Chem* 276: 21017–21021.

Asano E, Chugani DC, Muzik O, Behen M, Janisse J, Rothermel R, Mangner TJ, Chakraborty PK, Chugani HT (2001). Autism in tuberous sclerosis complex is related to both cortical and subcortical dysfunction. *Neurology* 57: 1269–1277.

Asano E, Chugani DC, Shen C, Juhasz C, Janisse J, Ager J, Canady A, Shah JR, Shah AK, et al. (2000). Multimodality imaging for improved detection of epileptogenic foci in tuberous sclerosis complex. *Neurology* 54: 1976–1984.

Au KS, Hebert AA, Roach ES, Northrup H (1999). Complete inactivation of the TSC2 gene leads to formation of hamartomas. *Am J Hum Genet* 65: 1790–1795.

Benvenuto G, Li S, Brown SJ, Braverman R, Vass WC, Cheadle JP, Halley DJ, Sampson JR, Wienecke R, DeClue JE (2000). The tuberous sclerosis-1 (TSC1) gene product hamartin suppresses cell growth and augments the expression of the TSC2 product tuberin by inhibiting its ubiquitination. *Oncogene* 19: 6306–6316.

Carbonara C, Longa L, Grosso E, Mazzucco G, Borrone C, Garre ML, Brisigotti M, Filippi G, Scabar A, Giannotti A, et al. (1996). Apparent preferential loss of heterozygosity at TSC2 over TSC1 chromosomal region in tuberous sclerosis hamartomas. *Genes Chromosomes Cancer* 15: 18–25.

Carsillo T, Astrinidis A, Henske EP (2000). Mutations in the tuberous sclerosis complex gene TSC2 are a cause of sporadic pulmonary lymphangioleiomyomatosis. *Proc Natl Acad Sci USA* 97: 6085–6090.

Catania MG, Mischel PS, Vinters HV (2001). Hamartin and tuberin interaction with the G2/M cyclin-dependent kinase CDK1 and its regulatory cyclins A and B. *J Neuropathol Exp Neurol* 60: 711–723.

Cheadle JP, Reeve MP, Sampson JR, Kwiatkowski DJ (2000). Molecular genetic advances in tuberous sclerosis. *Hum Genet* 107: 97–114.

Crino PB, Henske EP (1999). New developments in the neurobiology of the tuberous sclerosis complex. *Neurology* 53: 1384–1390.

Curatolo P, Verdecchia M, Bombardieri R (2001). Vigabatrin for tuberous sclerosis complex. *Brain Dev* 23: 649–653.

Dabora SL, Nieto AA, Franz D, Jozwiak S, Van Den Ouweland A, Kwiatkowski DJ (2000). Characterisation of six large deletions in TSC2 identified using long range PCR suggests diverse mechanisms including Alu mediated recombination. *J Med Genet* 37: 877–883.

Dabora SL, Jozwiak S, Franz DN, Roberts PS, Nieto A, Chung J, Choy YS, Reeve MP, Thiele E, Egelhoff JC, et al. (2001). Mutational analysis in a cohort of 224 tuberous sclerosis patients indicates increased severity of TSC2, compared with TSC1, disease in multiple organs. *Am J Hum Genet* 68: 64–80.

Dan HC, Sun M, Yang L, Feldman RI, Sui XM, Yeung RS, Halley DJ, Nicosia SV, Pledger WJ, Cheng JQ (2002). PI3K/AKT pathway regulates TSC tumor suppressor complex by phosphorylation of tuberin. *J Biol Chem* 277: 35364–35370.

Eker R, Mossige J, Johannessen JV, Aars H (1981). Hereditary renal adenomas and adenocarcinomas in rats. *Diagn Histopathol* 4: 99–110.

El-Hashemite N, Zhang H, Henske EP, Kwiatkowski DJ (2003). Mutation in TSC2 and activation of mammalian target of rapamycin signaling pathway in renal angiomyolipoma. *Lancet* 361: 1348–1349.

European Tuberous Sclerosis Consortium (1993). Identification and characterization of the tuberous sclerosis gene on chromosome 16. *Cell* 75: 1305–1315.

Ewalt DH, Sheffield E, Sparagana SP, Delgado MR, Roach ES (1998). Renal lesion growth in children with tuberous sclerosis complex. *J Urol* 160: 141–145.

Franz DN, Tudor C, Leonard J, Egelhoff JC, Byars A, Valerius K, Sethuraman G (2001). Lamotrigine therapy of epilepsy in tuberous sclerosis. *Epilepsia* 42: 935–940.

Gao X, Pan D (2001). TSC1 and TSC2 tumor suppressors antagonize insulin signaling in cell growth. *Genes Dev* 15: 1383–1392.

Gao X, Zhang Y, Arrazola P, Hino O, Kobayashi T, Yeung RS, Ru B, Pan D (2002). Tsc tumour suppressor proteins antagonize amino-acid TOR signalling. *Nat Cell Biol* 4: 699–704.

Gomez MR, Sampson JR, Whittemore VH (eds) (1999) *The tuberous sclerosis complex*, 3rd edit. (Oxford, New York).

Goncharova EA, Goncharov DA, Eszterhas A, Hunter DS, Glassberg MK, Yeung RS, Walker CL, Noonan D, Kwiatkowski DJ, Chou MM, Panettieri RA Jr, Krymskaya VP (2002). Tuberin regulates p70 S6 kinase activation and ribosomal protein S6 phosphorylation: a role for the TSC2 tumor suppressor gewne in pulmonary lymphangioleiomyomatosis (LAM). *J Biol Chem* 277: 30958–30967.

Green AJ, Smith M, Yates JR (1994). Loss of heterozygosity on chromosome 16p13.3 in hamartomas from tuberous sclerosis patients. *Nat Genet* 6: 193–196.

Gutmann DH, Zhang Y, Hasbani MJ, Goldberg MP, Plank TL, Petri Henske E (2000). Expression of the tuberous sclerosis complex gene products, hamartin and tuberin, in central nervous system tissues. *Acta Neuropathol (Berl)* 99: 223–230.

Henske EP, Neumann HP, Scheithauer BW, Herbst EW, Short MP, Kwiatkowski DJ (1995). Loss of heterozygosity in the tuberous sclerosis (TSC2) region of chromosome band 16p13 occurs in sporadic as well as TSC-associated renal angiomyolipomas. *Genes Chromosomes Cancer* 13: 295–298.

Henske EP, Scheithauer BW, Short MP, Wollmann R, Nahmias J, Hornigold N, van Slegtenhorst M, Welsh CT, Kwiatkowski DJ (1996). Allelic loss is frequent in tuberous sclerosis kidney lesions but rare in brain lesions. *Am J Hum Genet* 59: 400–406.

Henske EP, Wessner LL, Golden J, Scheithauer BW, Vortmeyer AO, Zhang Z, Klein-Szanto AJP, Kwiatkowski DJ, Yeung RS (1997). Loss of tuberin in both subependymal giant cell astrocytomas and angiomyolipomas supports a two-hit model for the pathogenesis of tuberous sclerosis tumors. *Am J Pathol* 151: 1639–1647.

Hodges AK, Li S, Maynard J, Parry L, Braverman R, Cheadle JP, DeClue JE, Sampson

JR (2001). Pathological mutations in TSC1 and TSC2 disrupt the interaction between hamartin and tuberin. *Hum Mol Genet* 10: 2899–2905.

Hornigold N, Devlin J, Davies AM, Aveyard JS, Habuchi T, Knowles MA (1999). Mutation of the 9q34 gene TSC1 in sporadic bladder cancer. *Oncogene* 18: 2657–2661.

Inoki K, Li Y, Zhu T, Wu J, Guan KL (2002). TSC2 is phosphorylated and inhibited by Akt and suppresses mTOR signalling. *Nat Cell Biol* 4: 648–657.

Ito N, Rubin GM (1999). gigas, a Drosophila homolog of tuberous sclerosis gene product-2, regulates the cell cycle. *Cell* 96: 529–539.

Johnson MW, Emelin JK, Park SH, Vinters HV (1999). Co-localization of TSC1 and TSC2 gene products in tubers of patients with tuberous sclerosis. *Brain Pathol* 9: 45–54.

Johnson MW, Kerfoot C, Bushnell T, Li M, Vinters HV (2001). Hamartin and tuberin expression in human tissues. *Mod Pathol* 14: 202–210.

Jones AC, Shyamsundar MM, Thomas MW, Maynard J, Idziaszczyk S, Tomkins S, Sampson JR, Cheadle JP (1999). Comprehensive mutation analysis of TSC1 and TSC2 and phenotypic correlations in 150 families with tuberous sclerosis. *Am J Hum Genet* 64: 1305–1315.

Jozwiak S, Schwartz RA, Janniger CK, Bielicka-Cymerman J (2000). Usefulness of diagnostic criteria of tuberous sclerosis complex in pediatric patients. *J Child Neurol* 15: 652–659.

Kenerson HL, Aicher LD, True LD, Yeung RS (2002). Activated mammalian target of rapamycin pathway in the pathogenesis of tuberous sclerosis complex renal tumors. *Cancer Res* 62: 5645–5650.

Khare L, Strizheva GD, Bailey JN, Au KS, Northrup H, Smith M, Smalley SL, Henske EP (2001). A novel missense mutation in the GTPase activating protein homology region of TSC2 in two large families with tuberous sclerosis complex. *J Med Genet* 38: 347–349.

Kleymenova E, Ibraghimov-Beskrovnaya O, Kugoh H, Everitt J, Xu H, Kiguchi K, Landes G, Harris P, Walker C (2001). Tuberin-dependent membrane localization of polycystin-1: a functional link between polycystic kidney disease and the TSC2 tumor suppressor gene. *Mol Cell* 7: 823–832.

Kobayashi T, Hirayama Y, Kobayashi E, Kubo Y, Hino O (1995). A germline insertion in the tuberous sclerosis (Tsc2) gene gives rise to the Eker rat model of dominantly inherited cancer. *Nat Genet* 9: 70–74.

Kobayashi T, Minowa O, Kuno J, Mitani H, Hino O, Noda T (1999). Renal carcinogenesis, hepatic hemangiomatosis, and embryonic lethality caused by a germ-line Tsc2 mutation in mice. *Cancer Res* 59: 1206–1211.

Kobayashi T, Minowa O, Sugitani Y, Takai S, Mitani H, Kobayashi E, Noda T, Hino O (2001). A germ-line Tsc1 mutation causes tumor development and embryonic lethality that are similar, but not identical, to those caused by Tsc2 mutation in mice. *Proc Natl Acad Sci USA* 98: 8762–8767.

Kwiatkowski DJ, Zhang H, Bandura JL, Heiberger KM, Glogauer M, el-Hashemite N, Onda H (2002). A mouse model of TSC1 reveals sex-dependent lethality from liver hemangiomas, and up-regulation of p70S6K kinase activity in Tsc1 null cells. *Hum Mol Genet* 11: 525–534.

Lamb RF, Roy C, Diefenbach TJ, Vinters HV, Johnson MW, Jay DG, Hall A (2000). The TSC1 tumour suppressor hamartin regulates cell adhesion through ERM proteins and the GTPase Rho. *Nat Cell Biol* 2: 281–287.

Lou D, Griffith N, Noonan DJ (2001). The tuberous sclerosis 2 gene product can localize to nuclei in a phosphorylation-dependent manner. *Mol Cell Biol Res Commun* 4: 374–380.

Manning BD, Tee AR, Logsdon MN, Blenis J, Cantley LC (2002). Identification of the tuberous sclerosis complex-2 tumor suppressor gene product tuberin as a target of the phosphoinositide 3-kinase/akt pathway. *Mol Cell* 10: 151–162.

Matsumoto Y, Horiba K, Usuki J, Chu SC, Ferrans VJ, Moss J (1999). Markers of cell proliferation and expression of melanosomal antigen in lymphangioleiomyomatosis. *Am J Respir Cell Mol Biol* 21: 327–336.

Mayer K, Ballhausen W, Leistner W, Rott H (2000). Three novel types of splicing aberrations in the tuberous sclerosis TSC2 gene caused by mutations apart from splice consensus sequences. *Biochim Biophys Acta* 1502: 495–507.

Miloloza A, Rosner M, Nellist M, Halley D, Bernaschek G, Hengstschlager M (2000). The TSC1 gene product, hamartin, negatively regulates cell proliferation. *Hum Mol Genet* 9: 1721–1727.

Mizuguchi M, Ikeda K, Takashima S (2000). Simultaneous loss of hamartin and tuberin from the cerebrum, kidney and heart with tuberous sclerosis. *Acta Neuropathol (Berl)* 99: 503–510.

Murthy V, Stemmer-Rachamimov AO, Haddad LA, Roy JE, Cutone AN, Beauchamp RL, Smith N, Louis DN, Ramesh V (2001). Developmental expression of the tuberous sclerosis proteins tuberin and hamartin. *Acta Neuropathol (Berl)* 101: 202–210.

Nellist M, van Slegtenhorst MA, Goedbloed M, van den Ouweland AM, Halley DJ, van der Sluijs P (1999). Characterization of the cytosolic tuberin-hamartin complex. Tuberin is a cytosolic chaperone for hamartin. *J Biol Chem* 274: 35647–35652.

Nellist M, Verhaaf B, Goedbloed MA, Reuser AJ, van Den Ouweland AM, Halley DJ (2001). TSC2 missense mutations inhibit tuberin phosphorylation and prevent formation of the tuberin-hamartin complex. *Hum Mol Genet* 10: 2889–2898.

Niida Y, Stemmer-Rachamimov AO, Logrip M, Tapon D, Perez R, Kwiatkowski DJ, Sims K, MacCollin M, Louis DN, Ramesh V (2001). Survey of somatic mutations in tuberous sclerosis complex (TSC) hamartomas suggests different genetic mechanisms for pathogenesis of TSC lesions. *Am J Hum Genet* 69: 493–503.

Onda H, Lueck A, Marks PW, Warren HB, Kwiatkowski DJ (1999). Tsc2(+/−) mice develop tumors in multiple sites that express gelsolin and are influenced by genetic background. *J Clin Invest* 104: 687–695.

Plank TL, Yeung RS, Henske EP (1998). Hamartin, the product of the tuberous sclerosis 1 (TSC1) gene, interacts with tuberin and appears to be localized to cytoplasmic vesicles. *Cancer Res* 58: 4766–4770.

Potter CJ, Huang H, Xu T (2001). Drosophila tsc1 functions with tsc2 to antagonize insulin signaling in regulating cell growth, cell proliferation, and organ size. *Cell* 105: 357–368.

Potter CJ, Pedraza LG, Xu T (2002). Akt regulates growth by directly phosphorylating Tsc2. *Nat Cell Biol* 4: 658–665.

Rennebeck G, Kleymenova EV, Anderson R, Yeung RS, Artzt K, Walker CL (1998). Loss of function of the tuberous sclerosis 2 tumor suppressor gene results in embryonic lethality characterized by disrupted neuroepithelial growth and development. *Proc Natl Acad Sci USA* 95: 15629–15634.

Roach ES, Gomez MR, Northrup H (1998). Tuberous Sclerosis Complex Consensus Conference: revised clinical diagnostic criteria. *J Child Neurol* 13: 624–628.

Roach ES, DiMario FJ, Kandt RS, Northrup H (1999). Tuberous Sclerosis Consensus Conference: recommendations for diagnostic evaluation. National Tuberous Sclerosis Association. *J Child Neurol* 14: 401–407.

Rose VM, Au KS, Pollom G, Roach ES, Prashner HR, Northrup H (1999). Germ-line mosaicism in tuberous sclerosis: how common? *Am J Hum Genet* 64: 986–992.

Sampson JR, Maheshwar MM, Aspinwall R, Thompson P, Cheadle JP, Ravine D, Roy S, Haan E, Bernstein J, Harris PC (1997). Renal cystic disease in tuberous sclerosis: role of the polycystic kidney disease 1 gene. *Am J Hum Genet* 61: 843–851.

Soucek T, Yeung RS, Hengstschlager M (1998). Inactivation of the cyclin-dependent kinase inhibitor p27 upon loss of the tuberous sclerosis complex gene-2. *Proc Natl Acad Sci USA* 95: 15653–15658.

Takamochi K, Ogura T, Suzuki K, Kawasaki H, Kurashima Y, Yokose T, Ochiai A, Nagai K, Nishiwaki Y, Esumi H (2001). Loss of heterozygosity on chromosomes 9q and 16p in atypical adenomatous hyperplasia concomitant with adenocarcinoma of the lung. *Am J Pathol* 159: 1941–1948.

Tapon N, Ito N, Dickson BJ, Treisman JE, Hariharan IK (2001). The drosophila tuberous sclerosis complex gene homologs restrict cell growth and cell proliferation. *Cell* 105: 345–355.

van Slegtenhorst M, de Hoogt R, Hermans C, Nellist M, Janssen B, Verhoef S, Lindhout D, van den Ouweland A, Halley D, Young J, et al. (1997). Identification of the tuberous sclerosis gene TSC1 on chromosome 9q34. *Science* 277: 805–808.

van Slegtenhorst M, Nellist M, Nagelkerken B, Cheadle J, Snell R, van den Ouweland A, Reuser A, Sampson J, Halley D, van der Sluijs P (1998). Interaction between hamartin and tuberin, the TSC1 and TSC2 gene products. *Hum Mol Genet* 7: 1053–1058.

Verhoef S, Bakker L, Tempelaars AM, Hesseling-Janssen AL, Mazurczak T, Jozwiak S, Fois A, Bartalini G, Zonnenberg BA, van Essen AJ, et al. (1999). High rate of mosaicism in tuberous sclerosis complex. *Am J Hum Genet* 64: 1632–1637.

White R, Hua Y, Scheithauer B, Lynch DR, Henske EP, Crino PB (2001). Selective alterations in glutamate and GABA receptor subunit mRNA expression in dysplastic neurons and giant cells of cortical tubers. *Ann Neurol* 49: 67–78.

Wienecke R, Konig A, DeClue JE (1995). Identification of tuberin, the tuberous sclerosis-2 product. Tuberin possesses specific Rap1GAP activity. *J Biol Chem* 270: 16409–16414.

Wienecke R, Maize JC, Shoarinejad F, Vass WC, Reed J, Bonifacino JS, Resau JH, de Gunzberg J, Yeung RS, DeClue JE (1996). Co-localization of the TSC2 product tuberin with its target rap1 in the Golgi apparatus. *Oncogene* 13: 913–923.

Xiao GH, Shoarinejad F, Jin F, Golemis EA, Yeung RS (1997). The tuberous sclerosis 2 gene product, tuberin, functions as a Rab5 GTPase activating protein (GAP) in modulating endocytosis. *J Biol Chem* 272: 6097–6100.

Yeung RS, Katsetos CD, Klein-Szanto A (1997). Subependymal astrocytic hamartomas in the Eker rat model of tuberous sclerosis. *Am J Pathol* 151: 1477–1486.

Yeung RS, Gu H, Lee M, Dundon TA (2001). Genetic Identification of a locus, Mot1, that affects renal tumor size in the rat. *Genomics* 78: 108–112.

Yeung RS, Xiao GH, Jin F, Lee WC, Testa JR, Knudson AG (1994). Predisposition to renal carcinoma in the Eker rat is determined by germ-line mutation of the tuberous sclerosis 2 (TSC2) gene. *Proc Natl Acad Sci USA* 91: 11413–11416.

92 | *LIS1* and *DCX* and Classical Lissencephaly

JOSEPH G. GLEESON

Classical lissencephaly (LIS) is either a sporadic autosomal disorder or an X-linked dominant disorder that affects approximately 1 in 40,000 individuals. It is characterized by the presence of a severely thickened cerebral cortical gray matter with widely spaced gyri and sulci. Diagnosis of LIS is made by the characteristic MRI appearance of the brain. Associated clinical features include significant mental retardation, intractable epilepsy, and shortened life expectancy. Syndromes related to classical lissencephaly include the double cortex syndrome, a less-severe genocopy syndrome, lissencephaly with cerebellar hypoplasia, polymicrogyria, and cobblestone (or type II lissencephaly) with associated congenital muscular dystrophy and eye disease. Positional cloning identified the *LIS1* gene on chromosome 17p13.3 and the *DCX* gene on chromosome Xq22.3–23 as independently responsible for cases of classical lissencephaly. The two genes encode for microtubule-associated proteins and are critical for neuronal migration. While their exact role in migration remains unclear, they appear to function with dynein, the main minus-end-directed microtubule motor, to mediate movement of the neuronal soma. Most *LIS1* mutations are germline submicroscopic deletions. With larger deletions, additional features constitute the contiguous gene deletion Miller-Dieker syndrome. Most *DCX* mutations are single-base mutations that lead to amino acid substitutions or frameshift mutations. Genetic counseling largely depends on the results of mutation analysis and whether prenatal diagnosis is available. Treatment consists of supportive measures and seizure prevention, with a focus on maintaining quality of life.

CLINICAL ASPECTS

Lissencephaly (agyria) is a developmental malformation characterized by an absence of cerebral convolutions. Pachygyria is a related malformation with relatively few broad gyri and shallow sulci. Subcortical band heterotopia (SBH, or double cortex) is also a related malformation with a second layer of gray matter situated within the subcortical white matter.

Historical Perspectives

In the late 1800s and early 1900s, lissencephaly (Erhardt, 1914; De Lange, 1939), pachygyria (Bielschowsky, 1923; Jacob, 1940), and SBH (Matell, 1893) were described pathologically and hypothesized to result from arrested migration of neuroblasts from the proliferative zone (along the lining of the lateral ventricle) to the cerebral cortex. These hypotheses were based on the association of these disorders with extensive subcortical heterotopic neurons that appeared to have arrested in migration.

Two major genetic forms of lissencephaly have been differentiated: type I and type II, now known as classical lissencephaly (herein referred to as LIS) and cobblestone lissencephaly, respectively. However, with more careful delineation of syndromes, it is clear that there are over 10 forms of lissencephaly (OMIM, 2000) and therefore the numbering system has been dropped in favor of more descriptive terminology based on radiographic or pathological hallmark. A review of the pathological and genetic forms of lissencephaly is presented in Table 92–1.

Miller and Dieker independently identified children with LIS, together with additional systemic features that now constitute the Miller-Dieker syndrome (MDS). Miller (1963) described lissencephaly in a brother and sister who were the fifth and sixth children of unrelated parents. The features were microcephaly, small mandible, bizarre facies, failure to thrive, retarded motor development, dysphagia, decorticate and decerebrate posturing, and death at 3 and 4 months of life. Autopsy showed anomalies of the brain, kidney, heart, and gastrointestinal tract. The brains were smooth with large ventricles and a histological architecture similar to a fetal brain of 3 to 4 months gestation. Dieker et al. (1969) described two affected brothers and an affected female maternal first cousin. They emphasized the features associated with LIS, including malformations of the heart, kidneys, and other organs, as well as polydactyly and unusual facial appearance. MDS is now defined as the combination of LIS with additional systemic features and facial dysmorphisms. Of historical note, although MDS is nearly always a sporadic condition, the original families had several affected members, each of whom was later found to harbor a translocation (Stratton et al., 1984), thus explaining this apparent discrepancy.

Since 1991, a biannual conference held in the United States has brought together families, physicians, and researchers who are interested in the disease with the goal of improving diagnosis and treatment. This organization, known as the Lissencephaly Network, has helped diagnose and treat thousands of children and provided support for families.

Incidence

Few studies exist on the incidence of LIS. In addition, lissencephaly is a rare disease, and because of the subtle differences in brain MRI, many cases may be incorrectly classified. In the Netherlands (de Rijk-van Andel et al., 1991) 22 patients with lissencephaly were identified from 11.7 million births between 1980 and 1988, for an incidence of 1 in 500,000 without a clear sex difference. The actual incidence is estimated to be perhaps 10 times higher. Because most patients present with new or relatively recent mutations, there is not thought to be any racial or ethnic predilection. Because mutations in *LIS1* lead to lissencephaly in both sexes and mutations in *DCX* lead to LIS predominantly in males, the incidence of LIS may be somewhat higher in males whereas SBH is higher in females.

Radiographic and Pathological Hallmarks

The agyria-pachygyria-band spectrum is the most common type of lissencephaly, and hence has been described as LIS. Characteristic findings of LIS on MRI are the lack of cerebral gyri (agyria) or abnormally broad cerebral gyri (pachygyria) and an abnormally thick cerebral cortex (1–2 cm, compared to the normal 0.5 cm) (Barkovich et al., 1991; Dobyns and Truwit, 1995) (Fig. 92–1). Associated findings are enlarged ventricles, dysmorphic or hypoplastic but not absent corpus callosum, and cavum septum pellucidum. The brain stem and cerebellum are usually normal except for mild vermis upward rotation and hypoplasia in some patients. Characteristic histological findings consist of an abnormally thick and poorly organized cortex, with four layers consisting of (*1*) a relatively well-preserved marginal zone, (*2*) a superficial cortical gray zone with diffusely scattered neurons, (*3*) a relatively neuron-sparse zone, and (*4*) a thick cortical zone with neurons often oriented in random columns (Kuchelmeister et al., 1993; Norman et al., 1995).

A less severe variant of LIS is known as subcortical band heterotopia (SBH) (Barkovich et al., 1989, 1994). Characteristic findings of SBH

Table 92–1. Phenotypic and Genetic Characterization of Syndromes with Lissencephaly

	Classical Lissencephaly	Pachygyria	Subcortical Band Heterotopia	Cobblestone Lissencephaly	Polymicrogyria	Microlissencephaly	Lissencephaly with Cerebellar Hypoplasia	Lissencephaly with Absent Corpus Callosum (XLAG)	Norman-Roberts Syndrome	Miller-Dieker Syndrome
Cortex surface	Completely to partially smooth	Widely spaced gyri	Normal to partially smooth	Rough	Excessive gyri packed too tightly	Simplified gyral pattern	Completely to partially smooth	Completely to partially smooth	Completely to partially smooth	Completely smooth
Cortex lamination	Four-layered	Four-layered	Six-layered	Unlayered	Variable	Unknown	Unknown	Three-layered	Four-layered	Four-layered
Subcortex	Scattered heterotopic neurons	Scattered heterotopic neurons	Band of neurons	Scattered heterotopic neurons		Unknown	Unknown	Scattered heterotopic neurons	Unknown	Scattered heterotopic neurons
Hydrocephalus	—	—	—	Frequent	—	—	—	—	—	—
Ventriculomegaly	Variable	Variable	Variable	Variable	—	—	Variable	Variable	Variable	Variable
Cerebellum	Scattered heterotopic neurons	Scattered heterotopic neurons	Scattered heterotopic neurons	Severely dysplastic	Normal	Variable	Severely hypoplastic and dysplastic	Scattered heterotopic neurons	Scattered heterotopic neurons	Scattered heterotopic neurons
Corpus callosum	Thinned	Thinned	Slightly thinned	Dysplastic	Normal	Normal	Thinned	Absent	Thinned	Thinned
Head circumference	Acquired microcephaly	Acquired microcephaly	Normal	Acquired microcephaly	Acquired microcephaly	<3 SD below mean	Acquired microcephaly	<3 SD below mean	Acquired microcephaly	Acquired microcephaly
Inheritance pattern	Sporadic or X-linked	Sporadic or X-linked	Sporadic or X-linked	AR	AD, AR, X-linked, sporadic	AR or sporadic	AR or sporadic	X-linked	AR	Sporadic
Associated dysmorphic features	—	—	—	Congenital muscular dystrophy, severe eye abnormalities	Spastic quadriparesis	Abnormal myelination, arthrogryposis, cardiac, spinal and urogenital defects	Ataxia, lymphedema	Ambiguous genitalia	Sloping forehead, prominent nasal bridge	Prominent forehead, short nose with anteverted nares, etc.

AD, autosomal dominant; AR, autosomal recessive.

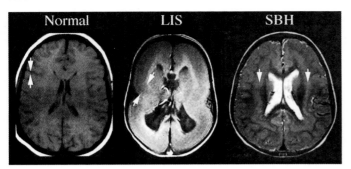

Figure 92–1. Radiographic hallmarks of classical lissencephaly (LIS) and subcortical band heterotopia (SBH). Normal brain MRI shows typical appearance of cortical gyri and sulci. Gray matter thickness is approximately 0.5 cm (area between arrowheads), and white matter is several cm in thickness. In LIS, there are no cortical gyri or sulci; in addition, gray matter thickness is 2 to 3 cm, and there is relative loss of white matter volume. In SBH there is a bilaterally symmetrical band of subcortical gray matter located within the white matter (arrows).

on MRI are a normal or mildly simplified gyral pattern, a normal cortical thickness, and a striking subcortical band of heterotopic gray matter that is located just beneath the cortex and separated from it by a thin zone of normal white matter (Fig. 92–1). The bands are most often symmetric and diffuse, extending from frontal to occipital regions, although asymmetric and partial frontal or partial posterior bands have been observed. Characteristic histological findings consist of relatively preserved architecture of the outer cortex, readily distinguishable white matter including U-fibers, scattered neurons in the outer portion of the band, a somewhat columnar arrangement of neurons in the inner part of the bands accentuated by radially oriented bundles of myelinated fibers, and scattered inverted neurons (Harding, 1996).

A grading system characterizing the brain malformations ranges from grade 1 (the most severe) to grade 6 (the least severe) (Table 92–2) (Dobyns et al., 1999). Grades 1–4 are considered "classical lissencephaly." Grade 5 consists of pachygyria and subcortical band heterotopia in different regions of the same brain, while grade 6 refers to SBH alone. Lissencephaly and SBH are further classified based on the gradient of the malformation (Dobyns and Truwit, 1995; Pilz et al., 1998): in some patients, the LIS or SBH is more severe posteriorly and is referred to as a posterior to anterior (P-A) gradient; others display a reverse anterior to posterior (A-P) gradient. When the malformation is severe, it may be difficult to appreciate a gradient on cranial MRI examination. The grading system shown in Table 92–2 (grades 1a–6a for a P-A gradient, and grades 1b–6b for an A-P gradient) may be helpful in identifying the underlying genetic causes of LIS and SBH.

MOLECULAR GENETICS OF LISSENCEPHALY

Chromosome 17 Locus

A ring chromosome 17 in a patient with MDS prompted the study of two other cases; Dobyns et al. (1983) found partial monosomy of 17p13 in one of these. To confirm the importance of chromosome 17 in MDS, the original families reported by Miller and Dieker were

tested, and unsuspected chromosome 17 abnormalities were identified (Stratton et al., 1984). The father of Miller's sibs had a 15q;17p translocation; the father of Dieker's patients 1 and 3 had a 12q;17p translocation. In all of the seven patients studied, Ledbetter et al. (1989) found that three overlapping cosmids (spanning more than 100 kb) were completely deleted, thus providing a minimum estimate of the size of the MDS critical region. A hypomethylated island and some evolutionarily conserved sequences were identified within this 100 kb region—indications of the presence of one or more expressed sequences that are potentially involved in the pathophysiology of this disorder. Nonoverlapping deletions involving either the 5' or the 3' end of a novel gene named *LIS1* (*lissencephaly-1*) were found in two patients, identifying it as a possible candidate gene (Reiner et al., 1993). Subsequent identification of intragenic gene mutations confirmed that mutations in *LIS1* are causative (Lo Nigro et al., 1997). Because most mutations resulted in complete or partial deletions, haploinsufficiency is thought to be the genetic mechanism.

The *LIS1* Gene

The *LIS1* gene spans 92 kb at the genomic level (Chong et al., 1997) and consists of 11 exons and a coding region of 1233 bp from exons 2 to 11. There are two alternative transcripts (5.5 and 7.5 kb) that differ in the length of their respective 3' UTR regions (Lo Nigro et al., 1997), but their functional significance is unknown. *LIS1* is ubiquitously expressed, although there is some enrichment of expression in the brain during the period of neuronal migration (Reiner et al., 1995).

The LIS1 Protein Product

Both *LIS1* transcripts encode a protein of 410 amino acids known at LIS1, or PAFAH1B1. The protein has no close neighbors in terms of primary amino acid sequence, but low homology is shared with the β-subunits of heterotrimeric G proteins, including transducin (Reiner et al., 1993). The WD40 repeats are predicted to take the structure of a propeller, with each of the repeats forming one of the blades (Garcia-Higuera et al., 1996). The N-terminal portion contains a predicted coiled-coil domain (Cardoso et al., 2000) (Fig. 92–2). The WD40 repeat is most similar to those found in several other disease-related proteins, including the encoded proteins from the Treacher Collins syndrome gene and the oral-facial-digital type 1 syndrome gene (Emes and Ponting, 2001). It was proposed that this repeat, called the *Lis1* homology motif (LisH) motif, may contribute to an unknown shared function.

The highly similar LIS1 bovine homolog was also found to function as a component of the brain platelet-activating factor acetylhydrolase Ib (PAF-AH Ib) (Hattori et al., 1994), which is involved in a variety of biologic and pathologic processes (Arai et al., 2002). PAF-AH inactivates PAF by removing the acetyl group at the sn-2 position; it consists of three subunits of molecular weight 45, 30, and 29 kDa. LIS1 corresponds to the 45 kDa fragment, and therefore the *LIS1* gene is also known as *PAFAH1B1*. These results raised the possibility that PAF and PAF-AH are important in the formation of the cortex during differentiation and development. Which enzyme (PAF or PAF-AH) has a role in brain development is unclear, but altering PAF signaling does affect some neuronal functions (Clark et al., 1995). Recent data suggest that the function of LIS1 in neuronal migration may not relate to its role as a subunit of PAF-AH, as the complex does not appear to form in *Drosophila* (Sheffield et al., 2000), yet *Lis1* still plays a critical role in migration (Lei and Warrior, 2000).

Table 92–2. Grading System Used for LIS and SBH

Grade	Description
1a or 1b	Complete agyria
2a or 2b	Diffuse agyria with a few undulations at the frontal or occipital poles
3a or 3b	Mixed agyria and pachygyria
4a or 4b	Diffuse pachygyria, or mixed pachygyria and normal or simplified gyri
5a or 5b	Mixed pachygyria and subcortical band heterotopia
6a or 6b	Subcortical band heterotopia only

The "a" classification denotes cases with a P-A gradient (more severe posteriorly), whereas the "b" classification denotes cases with an A-P gradient. The "a" gradient is more frequently associated with *LIS1* mutations and the "b" gradient with *DCX* mutations.

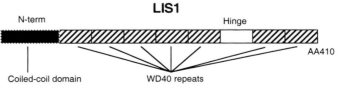

Figure 92–2. LIS1 encodes for a 410 amino acid protein with a predicted coiled-coil domain followed by seven WD40 repeats with an internal hinge. The seven WD40 repeats are predicted to form a β-propeller structure and may have a role in its interaction with other proteins including dynein. AA, amino acid.

LIS1 was also found to bind to microtubules and to contain a microtubule-binding domain (Sapir et al., 1997, 1999). Purified LIS1 decreases the catastrophe rate of native microtubules—that is, the rate at which spontaneous depolymerization occurs. LIS1 was shown to be phosphorylated on serine and threonine in the brain by unknown kinases (Sapir et al., 1999).

MDS is likely to be a contiguous gene-deletion syndrome, in which deletion of both the *LIS1* gene and unknown contiguous genes is required to produce the full phenotype. This supposition is based on the finding that patients with isolated LIS display either intragenic mutations or small deletions that encompass only a small number of genes, whereas MDS mutations are uniformly larger and encompass additional genes. The critical genes that contribute to the full MDS syndrome are yet to be identified.

Chromosome X Locus

An X-linked locus for LIS was suspected because of two observations: (*1*) a female with LIS and an X;2 balanced reciprocal translocation and classical lissencephaly (Dobyns et al., 1992), and (*2*) families displaying an X-linked inheritance pattern for LIS, with only males displaying LIS (Pinard et al., 1994). These X-linked families also displayed SBH in obligate carrier females (Berg et al., 1998), thus suggesting that mutations in an X-linked gene might produce LIS in males and SBH in females.

The X-linked locus was identified by linkage analysis to lie within a 20 cM candidate interval in Xq22.3–q24 (des Portes et al., 1997) with a peak two-point LOD score of 3.3 (Ross et al., 1997). Cloning of the breakpoint from the X;2 translocation demonstrated a novel 9.5 kB mRNA encoding a 40 kDa novel predicted protein named *doublecortin* (*DCX*) (des Portes et al., 1998; Gleeson et al., 1998). Independent missense and nonsense mutations were also identified in families and sporadic patients.

Mutations in *DCX* are found in 60% to 80% of female patients with SBH and in 5% to 20% of males with LIS. No patients with MDS have been reported with a *DCX* mutation.

The *DCX* Gene

The *DCX* gene spans 100 kb at the genomic level (Gleeson et al., 1998) and consists of nine exons and a coding region of 1083 bases between exons 4 and 9. Several alternative splice variants predominate in the 5′ UTR of the gene, but they do not significantly alter the size of the message (des Portes et al., 1998). In addition, two splice variants affect the coding region, with a 6 amino acid insert between coding exons 4 and 5 and a 1 amino acid insert between coding exons 5 and 6. The function of these alternative transcripts is not known.

The *DCX* transcript is expressed predominantly during periods of neuronal migration in both humans and mouse. Expression initiates at low levels in neurons in the ventricular zone and increases in the intermediate zone and in the cortical plate. At the completion of migration, there is down-regulation of expression. The message is expressed throughout adulthood by populations of neuroblasts that are generated during periods of migration, including those in the rostral migratory stream (Gleeson et al., 1999a) and in neurons that are generated after neurons in the cortex have been damaged (Magavi et al., 2000).

The DCX Protein Product

The 361 amino acid protein encoded by the *DCX* gene, known as DCX, encodes a novel protein with a C-terminal serine/proline-rich tail found in many signaling molecules. The N-terminal portion of the protein has similarity to two other proteins (Fig. 92–3A). The DCAMKL1 protein is encoded on chromosome 13 and displays 90% homology at the amino acid level over the length of the DCX region, but DCAMKL1 extends an additional 300 amino acids and encodes for a CaM kinase domain (des Portes et al., 1998; Gleeson et al., 1998). The role of this gene is unknown. The RP1 protein is encoded on chromosome 8q11–12 and displays 80% homology at the amino acid level over the length of the DCX region (Bowne et al., 1999), but RP1 encodes for an additional 1900 amino acids with poor sequence similarity to other proteins (Liu et al., 2002). Interestingly, mutations in the RP1 protein were found in families and in sporadic patients with retinitis pigmentosa (Pierce et al., 1999).

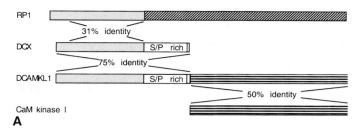

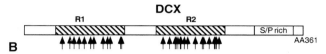

Figure 92–3. *DCX* encodes a 361 amino acid protein containing an internal repeated domain. (*A*) DCX has sequence similarity with RP1 and DCAMKL1 over their N-terminal regions, but both proteins encode for additional domains. DCAMKL1 encodes a CaM kinase I domain in its C terminus. (*B*) DCX encodes an internal duplication and a serine/proline (S/P)–rich region. The R1 and R2 regions have a 60% amino acid similarity, and each region binds tubulin. In addition, all of the reported patient missense mutations cluster in one of the two repeated domains (arrows) and interfere with normal microtubule interactions.

DCX was found to colocalize and copurify with microtubules in newly generated neurons. Furthermore, the addition of purified DCX to purified tubulin led to polymerization of tubulin into microtubules in a fashion similar to known microtubule-associated proteins. Misexpression of DCX in neural cells led to a dramatic effect on the microtubule cytoskeleton, with bundling and polymerization of the microtubule cytoskeleton. These effects indicated that DCX in neuronal migration may affect microtubule stability or organization during neuronal migration (Francis et al., 1999; Gleeson et al., 1999a).

The patient missense amino acid mutations in DCX were found to cluster tightly in two regions of the protein, suggesting functional domains (Gleeson et al., 1999b; Sapir et al., 2000) (Fig. 92–3B). These domains were found to display low amino acid sequence similarity, indicating that DCX contains a tandem duplication (Sapir et al., 2000). Each repeat was found to bind to tubulin, and the two tandem repeats are sufficient for tubulin polymerization. In addition, intact tandem repeats are necessary for tubulin polymerization, as patient missense mutations in either repeat significantly impair the tubulin-polymerizing ability of DCX (Taylor et al., 2000).

GENOTYPE–PHENOTYPE CORRELATIONS

MDS vs. LIS

Typically, patients with MDS display additional non-brain phenotypes, as well as more severe grades of lissencephaly. As some patients with isolated lissencephaly displayed complete deletions of the *LIS1* gene but lacked features of MDS, deletions of the *LIS1* gene do not appear to be sufficient to produce MDS. Moreover, patients with MDS typically display larger deletions than do patients with isolated lissencephaly, always extending in excess of 250 kb in the telomeric direction. Further physical mapping found that the *LIS1* locus was smaller than the 400 kb originally proposed, instead encompassing approximately 80 kb, and that immediately telomeric to the *LIS1* gene were additional genes, including the 14-3-3e gene. These data raise the questions of whether additional genes telomeric to the *LIS1* gene modify the phenotype and whether deletions of *LIS1* in addition to these genes are necessary to express the full MDS phenotype (Chong et al., 1997). As patients with the facial features of MDS in absence of lissencephaly have not been described, this issue remains unclear.

Modifiers of *LIS1* Phenotypes

While most of the mutations in *LIS1* are heterozygous, whole-gene deletions (suggesting haploinsufficiency as a disease mechanism), recent work suggests that patients with missense mutations are less severely affected and that some mutations may represent hypomorphic alleles (Cardoso et al., 2000). In 29 nondeletion patients with a LIS1 mutation, 15 novel mutations were identified. Patients with missense mutations had a milder LIS grade than did those with mutations that led to a shortened or truncated protein. Additionally, early truncation mutations in the putative microtubule-binding domain resulted in a more severe LIS grade than did later mutations. Patients with mutations that were predicted to result in a shortened protein did not show evidence of a truncated protein based on Western analysis of lysates from lymphoblastoid cell lines, thus suggesting that either mutated mRNA or truncated proteins may be unstable. This last result brings into question the mechanism by which late-truncating mutations may ameliorate the phenotype.

Because even complete deletions of the *LIS1* gene produces a less severe grade of LIS than is seen in association with the MDS with deletions encompassing neighboring genes, it has been hypothesized that mutations or deletions in these neighboring genes may worsen or modify the grade of LIS (Cardoso et al., 2000).

Modifiers of *DCX* Phenotypes

The *DCX* phenotype is significantly affected by the sex of the patient, as males inherit a single X chromosome from their mother, whereas females inherit two X chromosomes. In males with a *DCX* mutation, all cells will express the same mutant allele, whereas in females due to random X-inactivation, half of the cells, including neurons, will express the wild-type allele. It is thought that the heterotopic band of neurons arises from the mutant neurons, whereas the normal outer cortex arises from the wild-type neurons. Skewed X-inactivation could either worsen or ameliorate the phenotype, depending on the direction of skewing. While this mechanism seems likely, it has not been demonstrated to affect the severity in SBH.

Several different types of mutations have been identified in the *DCX* gene, including nonsense, missense, frameshift, and splice site mutations, as well as deletions that encompass one to several base pairs and larger deletions. Protein truncation and single amino acid substitutions were found with equal frequency, but pedigrees with transmission of the mutation exclusively displayed substitution mutations, suggesting that these mutations may have less of a reproductive disadvantage than truncation mutations have. This reproductive disadvantage could have arisen from an effect of the mutation on reproductive capabilities, but *DCX* is not expressed outside of the brain. Therefore, the truncation mutations might be associated with a more severe phenotype, and thus these females might be less likely to conceive and bear children (Gleeson et al., 1999b). Consistent with this hypothesis, the thickness of the band in SBH is greater with truncation mutations (Matsumoto et al., 2001). Additionally, our unpublished data suggest greater deficits on IQ testing in female SBH patients with truncation mutations. Together, these data suggest that the missense mutations are likely to represent partial loss of gene function, whereas the truncation mutations may represent near complete or complete loss-of-function. Consistent with this hypothesis, missense mutations displayed impaired but not absent microtubule-polymerizing ability, compared to wild-type protein (Taylor et al., 2000).

Mosaicism has been shown to modify the phenotype in males with a *DCX* mutation. Males with mosaic mutations display the female phenotype (SBH) (Gleeson et al., 2000b; Kato et al., 2001). This is not unexpected, as *DCX* somatic mosaic mutations should produce a population of both wild-type and mutant neurons and thus mimic the mosaicism normally seen in females following X-inactivation. While somatic mosaicism has been demonstrated in females, the phenotype that was reported in the two females was indistinguishable from SBH females with germline mutations, suggesting that these patients are at risk for the full clinical severity of the disease (Gleeson et al., 2000b).

LIS1 Associated with a P-A Gradient, *DCX* Associated with an A-P Gradient

Patients with *LIS1* and *DCX* mutations can display the same severity of LIS, but the gradient of severity on brain MRI is opposite. Many but not all patients with LIS display a clear gradient in severity of the lissencephaly that may be helpful in predicting gene mutations. Patients

with a *LIS1* mutation display more severe pachygyria/agyria posteriorly (P-A gradient), whereas patients with a *DCX* mutation display more severe pachygyria/agyria anteriorly (A-P) (Pilz et al., 1998; Dobyns et al., 1999). Presumably, these effects reflect selective requirements for the causative genes during brain development, but the pathophysiological basis for the different gradients has not been elucidated.

SBH can been seen with either a P-A gradient or an A-P gradient, and like LIS, *LIS1* mutations tend to produce SBH with a P-A gradient, whereas *DCX* mutations tend to produce an A-P gradient. *DCX* mutations were found exclusively in SBH females with an A-P gradient or no discernable gradient, whereas no *DCX* mutations were found in SBH females with a P-A gradient (Gleeson et al., 2000a). Likewise, a *LIS1* mutation was found in an SBH male with a P-A gradient, and *DCX* mutations were found in two SBH males with an A-P gradient (Pilz et al., 1999). Therefore, the general observation that *LIS1* mutations are associated with a P-A gradient and *DCX* mutations are associated with an A-P gradient appears to be valid irrespective of the phenotype. Whether *LIS1* mutations account for female SBH with a P-A gradient has not yet been determined.

ESTABLISHING THE DIAGNOSIS

Diagnostic criteria for lissencephaly rest primarily with the brain MRI scan, because the clinical presentations for the related syndromes are often indistinguishable. The typical features seen on brain MRI are listed in Table 92–1 and are contrasted with those for related syndromes.

Establishing the correct diagnosis for a given patient involves obtaining a family history and a medical history; performing physical and neurological examinations and reviewing brain MRI, biopsy, and autopsy material; obtaining chromosomal evaluation; and obtaining results of molecular studies, including FISH and DNA-based mutation analysis.

Family History

Special emphasis should be placed on discerning a possible family history of similar neurological abnormalities, as well as mental retardation and epilepsy. The presence of miscarriages, stillbirths, or live-born children with birth defects or with short survival times should be identified. As several different inheritance patterns have been identified, the presence of a positive family history, even remote, can affect the diagnosis. History of consanguinity should be noted. Whenever possible, potentially affected relatives should be evaluated by brain MRI or chromosomal karyotype (or both), together with molecular studies.

Clinical Examination

Careful examination and documentation of several aspects of the physical examinations are important. The different forms of lissencephaly are associated with different syndromic features. Classical lissencephaly is associated with mild dysmorphic facial features and acquired microcephaly, but the characteristic facial features of MDS are absent. MDS is associated with facial features including bitemporal hollowing, widely spaced eyes, prominent forehead, short nose with upturned nares, prominent upper lip, thin vermilion border of the upper lip, and small jaw. MDS is associated with systemic dysmorphic features including abnormal palmar creases, clinodactyly, polydactyly, cryptorchidism, sacral dimples, congenital heart defects, and other visceral abnormalities (Dobyns et al., 1984). Systemic features seen in Walker-Waarburg, Fukuyama, and HARD syndromes, including developmental eye abnormalities (micropthalmia, retinal dysplasia, and coloboma) and congenital muscular dystrophy, as well as systemic features in XLAG, including micropenis and small adrenal glands, are absent in MDS and LIS.

Neurological Examination

While it is important to document the degree of developmental delay and neuromotor impairment, clinical findings overlap among all of the lissencephaly syndromes. However, several features can be helpful in making a specific diagnosis. Patients with classical lissencephaly typically display severe to profound mental retardation, with seizures beginning at several months of age. Infantile spasms are not infrequent, and atypical absence seizures are common. Seizures are often intractable. Patients with SBH typically display mild to moderate mental retardation, with seizures beginning in childhood. Atypical absence or tonic-clonic seizures predominate. The motor exam shows poor coordination and mild global hypotonia. Spasticity is not a component. This clinical picture can be contrasted with other lissencephaly syndromes. Polymicrogyria has the least similar presentation, characterized by severe spasticity, with often very mild cognitive impairments. Patients with cobblestone lissencephaly display a mixed motor examination with hypotonia, spasticity, and exaggerated reflexes (Dobyns et al., 1985).

Brain Imaging

The study of choice is cranial MRI examination, preferably obtained with adequate sedation at a center experienced in evaluating children for developmental brain abnormalities. Review of the study by a radiologist or clinician familiar with the different types of LIS, SBH and related malformations is essential. Table 92–1 lists the key features seen on brain MRI with classical lissencephaly versus other forms of lissencephaly.

Chromosome Analysis and FISH

Chromosome analysis and FISH for chromosome 17 submicroscopic deletions are indicated in most patients with LIS or SBH, unless a specific syndrome with a known pattern of inheritance is recognized. High-resolution karyotype should be performed routinely. FISH analysis of the LIS1 locus at chromosome 17p13.3 using the PAC95H6 probe detects submicroscopic deletions at a much higher percentage than older probes.

Testing Strategy for LIS

The strategy for testing children with LIS depends on the clinical diagnosis, the type and gradient, the sex of the child, and the family history (Table 92–3). However, most patients with a P-A gradient (LIS grades 2a or 3a) and no other major congenital anomalies have isolated lissencephaly sequence (ILS). In these patients and most other patients with LIS, the testing pathway should begin with high-resolution chromosome analysis and continue sequentially with FISH using a *LIS1*-specific probe, mutation analysis of *LIS1*, and finally mutation analysis of *DCX*. This strategy detects the underlying genetic mechanism in all children with MDS and in 76% of children with ILS. In boys with an A-P gradient or a family history that is consistent with X-linked inheritance, it is more effective to begin with mutation analysis of *DCX* (Pilz et al., 1998; Dobyns et al., 1999). Many clinical laboratories will perform FISH using the PAC95H6 probe or the Vysis LIS1 probe. In the United States, sequencing of the *LIS1* and *DCX* gene can be arranged through the University of Chicago Genetics Services Laboratory, at 888-UC-GENES or http://www.genetics.uchicago.edu. In Europe, mutation analysis can be arranged through the Institute for Medical Genetics at the University Hospital of Wales at telephone number 44 (0)29-207-43922.

In children with other types of LIS, chromosome analysis should be obtained. More detailed studies of the *LIS1* and *DCX* genes may still be indicated if the diagnosis is not clear. This is most relevant for children with LIS with cerebellar hypoplasia (LCH) (Ross et al., 2001). These patients may be difficult to distinguish from children with LIS, many of whom have mild cerebellar hypoplasia, and from children with MDS, approximately 10% of whom have mild cerebellar hypoplasia. Children with atypical phenotypes, negative results with the above testing strategy, or chromosomal abnormalities should be referred for further evaluation. Please contact the author (Dr. Joseph Gleeson) directly for more information.

Testing Strategy for SBH

The most useful diagnostic test in patients with SBH is direct sequencing of the *DCX* gene, which will detect deletions in about 40% to 80% of female patients (Gleeson et al., 1999b, 2000a), especially those with an A-P gradient or a family history consistent with X-linked inheritance. In patients with atypical, especially P-A gradient SBH, sequencing of *DCX* will be negative, and thus sequencing of *LIS1* may be considered. These patients should also be referred for research testing.

Prenatal Diagnosis

While prenatal diagnosis is possible, it is hindered by the fact that until midgestation, the human cerebral cortex lacks gyri and suchi and therefore appears smooth. Moreover, no other characteristic feature—such as severe cerebellar hypoplasia or hydrocephalus—has helped in the prenatal diagnosis of other forms of lissencephaly (Kojima et al., 2002). For this reason, imaging with level 2 sonography or MRI has not been particularly helpful in the prenatal diagnosis of unsuspected LIS. Some nonspecific findings before midgestation may suggest the possibility of an underlying developmental brain abnormality (Holzgreve et al., 1993; Pilu et al., 1999), but the imaging findings are not specific for LIS. Once an index case has been diagnosed within a family and a molecular diagnosis is made, it is possible to use the same molecular test to evaluate the genotype, and thus the likely affection status of a fetus at any time during the pregnancy, as has been performed for mutations in *LIS1* (Saltzman et al., 1991) and *DCX* (Gleeson et al., 2000b).

MANAGEMENT

Extreme care should be taken in counseling families regarding prognosis and life expectancy, as these can vary widely. The clinical course of the disease varies, but most children will display profound mental retardation and intractable epilepsy. Death between 5 and 10 years of age is not uncommon, due to medical complications of the severe grades of lissencephaly, although some children have survived into their 30s. The less severe grades of lissencephaly and all forms of SBH are not associated with a shortened life span.

There are no specific treatments once the diagnosis of lissencephaly has been made. Generally, medical care is aimed at treating the complications of the disease, including intractable epilepsy, feeding intolerance, compromised respiratory status, and severe motor impairment.

Although mild ventriculomegaly is seen with both LIS and SBH, it is not associated with hydrocephalus and does not require a ventricular shunt. This is to be contrasted with cobblestone lissencephaly, which is often associated with acqueductal stenosis and obstructive hydrocephalus that requires a ventricular shunt (Martinez-Lage et al., 1995).

GENETIC COUNSELING

Lissencephaly can result from several different gene mutations and with several different modes of inheritance. Therefore, the risks of recurrence in subsequent pregnancies can be calculated once the type of lissencephaly and genetic diagnosis is known.

LIS1 Mutations

For MDS and LIS due to a *LIS1* mutation, approximately 80% of patients display de novo deletions at the *LIS1* locus, and approximately

Table 92–3. Frequency of Identifying a *LIS1* or a *DCX* Mutation

Mutation Identified	Miller-Dieker Syndrome	Lissencephaly in Males	Lissencephaly in Females	SBH in Males	SBH in Females
LIS1	Common	Common	Common	Rare	NR
DCX	NR	Common	Rare	Rare	Common

NR, not reported; SBH, subcortical band heterotopia.

20% have inherited a deletion from a parent who carries a balanced chromosome rearrangement (unpublished data, Lissencephaly Network, http://www.lissencephaly.org). Parental karyotypes and FISH using a *LIS1* probe should be obtained from both parents to evaluate for a possible cryptic chromosomal translocation involving 17p13.3. No recurrences for MDS have been reported in cases in which a submicroscopic deletion has been detected in a child, but there is up to a 50% chance of recurrence in the setting of a balanced translocation (in practice, the risk of an adverse outcome in this setting was found to be approximately 33% [Pollin et al., 1999]). It is possible to identify subsequent pregnancies carrying the chromosomal abnormality for prenatal diagnosis.

DCX Mutations

For LIS and SBH with intragenic *DCX* mutations, the inheritance is X-linked dominant with full penetrance if the mutation is transmitted from the parental germline. When a *DCX* mutation is identified in a proband, mutation analysis can be performed on the mother to determine if the *DCX* mutation was de novo in the proband or was inherited from the mother, who would then be a carrier. This may be combined with brain MRI analysis in the mother to determine affection status. Because in males, a *DCX* mutation should not be phenotypically silent, generally the father is not tested. If it can be determined that a parent transmitted the *DCX* mutation, then the risk of recurrence of SBH in females and LIS in males is 50%.

There appears to be a high rate of somatic mosaicism in patients and their parents (with *DCX* mutations), and even if neither parent carries the *DCX* mutation based on lymphocyte DNA mutation analysis, there is still a 10% chance of recurrence. We found that of children with a *DCX* mutation, approximately 10% of the parents carry a somatic mutation, some of which may be identifiable by mutation analysis (Gleeson et al., 2000b). An example included a mutation detected in lymphocyte DNA from the unaffected mother of an SBH female. Additionally, there were two families in which there were two affected children (one male, one female), each displaying an identical *DCX* mutation that must be present in the mother's germ cells; however, neither mother carried the mutation in lymphocyte DNA, suggesting germ cell mosaicism. Because approximately 10% of parents carry a somatic or germline mosaic mutation, the risk of recurrence for a DCX mutation if the parent does not carry the mutation is roughly 10%. In this situation, prenatal mutation analysis on subsequent fetuses can be diagnostic (Gleeson et al., 2000b).

MUTATIONS IN ORTHOLOGOUS GENES

Mutations in *LIS1* Orthologs

Even though the phenotype produced by *LIS1* mutations in humans appears to be restricted to brain cells, *Lis1* orthologs are found throughout evolution, even in single-cell organisms, which appear to share function. This finding has greatly aided the delineation of evolutionarily conserved biochemical and genetic pathways. The human *LIS1* gene is highly conserved through evolution, displaying 99% amino acid identity with mouse, 96% identity with *Xenopus laevis*, 70% identity and 87% similarity with *Drosophila melanogaster*, 42% identity and 62% similarity with *Aspergillus nidulans* (named NudF), and 29% identity and 47% similarity with *Saccharomyces cerevisiae* (named PAC1). A single copy is present in each organism, which suggests that the *LIS1* gene may have retained an ancient and conserved function that is essential for development or survival.

Lis1 Mutations in *Aspergillus*

Perhaps the most important finding about the potential role for LIS1 in neuronal migration has come from work in the slime mold *A. nidulans*. Formation of spores consists of four basic steps: (*1*) nuclear replication in the mother cell to produce daughter nuclei, (*2*) extension of a stalk or hyphae of cell membrane extending from the mother cell, (*3*) migration of the daughter nuclei into the stalk, and (*4*) septation of the stalk into individual spores (Fig. 92–4). The mutants, named Nuclear Distribution (NUD), included a mutation in an ortholog

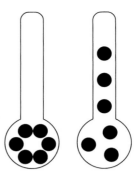

Figure 92–4. During spore formation in *A. nidulans*, a stalk of cell membrane extends from the mother cell followed by migration of the daughter nuclei (black circles) into the stalk. The *LIS1* ortholog *nudF* is required for the latter function, suggesting that nuclear migration in *A. nidulans* may relate to neuronal migration in the brain.

of *LIS1* named *nudF*. Other mutations included *nudA*, *nudG*, and *nudK*, which encoded cytoplasmic dynein heavy chain, the 8 kDa dynein light chain, and the dynactin component Actin-related protein-1 (Arp-1), respectively (Xiang et al., 1994, 1999). Arp-1, with 50% homology to actin, was later found to encode a component of dynactin (Waterman-Storer et al., 1995). The *nudC* and *nudE* genes are novel but have orthologs in higher organisms. Additional evidence to support the importance of this pathway came from epistasis experiments, showing that NUDF overexpression rescued the *nudC* phenotype, NUDE overexpression rescued the *nudF* phenotype, and *nudA* mutations suppressed the *nudF* phenotype in an allele-specific fashion. The finding that NUDF has homology to LIS1 and that it functions with several dynein components to regulate nuclear migration suggests that nuclear migration in *A. nidulans* may relate to neuronal migration in the brain. Similar pathways have been constructed in several other organisms, including *S. cervesiae* (Geiser et al., 1997; Fujiwara et al., 1999) and *C. elegans* (Dawe et al., 2001).

Lis1 Mutations in *Drosophila*

Lis1 is required in *Drosophila* for embryonic development, as homozygous mutants die between the L2 and L3 stages, and their development up to this point is likely rescued by maternal Lis1 protein. *Lis1* was also found to be required for germline cell division and oocyte differentiation (Liu et al., 1999). During germline cell division, Lis1 is required for transport from nurse cell to oocyte and for proper positioning of the nucleus (Swan et al., 1999; Lei and Warrior, 2000).

Lis1 was found to act together with the Bicaudal-D (Bic-D) and Egalitarian (Egl) complex, which is required for axis determination in *Drosophila* (Mach and Lehmann, 1997). A *Lis1* mutation was identified as a dominant enhancer of the Bic-D phenotype (Swan et al., 1999) and was further shown to be required in nuclear positioning within the oocyte and the developing eye. *Lis1* was found to function with dynein, an additional regulator of these events in *Drosophila*. Together, these results suggested that Lis1 interacts genetically with several factors and appears to be required for several stages during development, all of which require proper nuclear movement within cells (Swan et al., 1999).

Lis1 is strongly expressed in the *Drosophila* nervous system and is required in a cell-autonomous fashion for neuroblast proliferation, axonal transport, and dendritic morphology (Liu et al., 2000). Because homozygous *Lis1* mutations are embryonic lethal in *Drosophila* as in mice, the MARCM technique was used. This technique created uniquely marked homozygous *Lis1*-deleted cells in otherwise heterozygous animals, essentially producing low-level chimeras. When deleted from a subset of cells in the developing CNS, there was a marked reduction in proliferation of neuroblasts; in dendritic growth, branching, and maturation; and in axonal transport. There was also formation of large swellings along axons in marked cells. Similar defects were observed with a nonlethal dynein-heavy-chain mutation, suggesting similar mechanisms of action. These results demonstrate that Lis1 is required for diverse physiological functions in the nervous system.

Lis1 Mutations in Mice

In mouse, heterozygous null mutations created by introducing a premature stop codon produced a defect in brain development, and this is consistent with the hypothesis of haploinsufficiency as a mutation mechanism in human (Hirotsune et al., 1998). Homozygous mutants are lethal soon after implantation indicating that the gene is essential for survival of the embryo. Several additional mutations have been engineered in mouse, including a hypomorphic allele (through introduction of a neomycin resistance gene between exons 2 and 3) that partially silences gene transcription by approximately 50%. This is called the CKO *Lis1* allele; when combined with the null allele, this allele reduces LIS1 expression to approximately 30% of that in the wild-type allele and is associated with a more severe brain phenotype (Hirotsune et al., 1998). These compelling data indicate that *Lis1* dosage is a major determinant of phenotype and supports the haploinsufficiency mechanism of disease.

The brain phenotype in these mice demonstrated impaired and delayed neuronal migration, with improper targeting of neurons to the correct cortical layer. Cortical layering was severely disrupted, although the neurons were roughly positioned in an "inside-out" gradient, suggesting that events prior to neuronal migration are likely intact. There was also a striking hippocampal and cerebellar phenotype, which was particularly evident in compound heterozygous mice (Hirotsune et al., 1998). Neuronal migration appeared to be impaired in a cell-autonomous fashion, as cultures of mixed mutant and wild-type neurons displayed impaired migration of only the mutant neurons.

In the brains of *Lis1* mutant mice, normally positioned neurons displayed normal morphology and electrophysiological properties, whereas heterotopically positioned neurons displayed bizarre dendritic branching and hyperexcitable electrophysiological properties. These findings may relate to the seizures observed in patients with LIS (Fleck et al., 2000). Furthermore, mice with heterozygous mutations in *Lis1* displayed impaired learning and motor behavior, which may relate to the mental retardation seen in patients with LIS (Paylor et al., 1999).

An additional *Lis1* mutant allele was created in mouse by removing the first coding exon, and this resulted in a shorter protein that initiates from the second methionine. In heterozygous mice, neuronal migration was delayed, and radial glia and neuronal morphology were abnormal (Cahana et al., 2001).

Two mammalian counterparts for NudE were identified, mNudE and NUDEL, and found to form a complex with dynein heavy chain and LIS1. Also, misexpression of the LIS1-binding domain of mNudE in *Xenopus* embryos disrupted the architecture and lamination of the CNS. Furthermore, the NUDEL protein was shown to be a substrate for serine/threonine phosphorylation by cdk5, a known regulator of neuronal migration. Therefore, these studies showed that the LIS1-dynein-NUDEL pathway is evolutionarily conserved and likely functions to mediate neuronal migration (Feng et al., 2000; Niethammer et al., 2000; Sasaki et al., 2000).

Mutations in *DCX* Orthologs

In contrast to LIS1, nonmammalian isofoms of DCX do not appear to exist, although there is clear evidence for proteins with sequence similarity to DCX in lower organisms. The human *DCX* gene is highly conserved among mammals, displaying 99% amino acid identity with mouse and rat. Although DCX orthologs have not been identified from other mammals to date, the *DCAMKL1* gene appears to be represented evolutionarily in *D. melanogaster, X. laevis, C. elegans,* and *Dictyostelium discoideum,* with sequence similarity of approximately 50% over both the DCX domain and the kinase domain. In *C. elegans,* loss-of-function mutations in the *zyg-8* gene, an ortholog of *DCAMKL1,* produces a defect in stabilization of microtubules during cell division at the one-cell stage that is phenocopied by administration of colchicine, a microtubule-depolymerizing drug (Gönczy et al., 2001). Mutations were identified in both the DCX domain and the kinase domain, suggesting that both domains

are necessary for proper function. These zyg-8 mutations that result in poorly stabilized microtubules are consistent with the hypothesis that DCX-based stabilization of microtubules is required for proper neuronal migration.

DEVELOPMENTAL PATHOGENESIS OF THE CONDITION

The pathogenesis of lissencephaly and how mutations in *LIS1* or *DCX* lead to the disease is still unclear, but several findings suggest that the proteins function to stabilize microtubules, interact with other migration genes, and mediate movement of the cell body as the neuron migrates.

LIS1 and a Cell-Autonomous Role in Migration

The main effect of LIS1 insufficiency is likely due to a cell-autonomous defect in neuronal migration of cortical and subcortical neurons during brain development (Gleeson and Walsh, 2000). During weeks 8–20 of human gestation, neurons generated in proliferative zones migrate hundreds of cell-body distances to achieve final positioning within the developing cortical plate (Fig. 92–5). Long-distance neuronal migration occurs at all levels of the neural axis, and humans and mice with dosage reduction in LIS1 display defects in this migration at several locations. The phenotype is most striking in the cerebral cortex, but it is also seen in the cerebellum, where it results in cerebellar hypoplasia (Ross et al., 2001), and at the inferior olive, where it results in disrupted development (Sarnat, 1992). It appears that LIS1 has an essential role in neuronal migration for most, if not all, populations of postmitotic migrating neurons.

Neuronal migration is characterized by a repeating of three main events: neurite outgrowth in the direction of migration, translocation of the soma or nucleus, and retraction of the trailing process (Edmondson and Hatten, 1987) (Fig. 92–6). It has been hypothesized that a defect in movement of the nucleus during neuronal migration accounts for the pathogenesis of the condition, based on the finding of

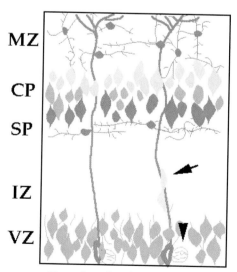

Cortical Plate Stage

Figure 92–5. Neurons migrate hundreds of cell body distances to reach final position within the developing cerebral cortex. Neuroblasts undergo cell division (indicated by mitotic spindles, arrowhead) within the ventricular zone (VZ), followed by migration toward the developing cortical plate (CP). This migration can occur along radial glial fibers (long fibers extending from VZ to MZ) or may be independent of these fibers. (Arrow indicates radially migrating neuron.) Neurons penetrate the subplate layer, part of the protomap of the cortex, and deposit at the outer margin of the cortical plate (indicated by progressively lighter shading of CP neurons). VZ, ventricular zone; IZ, intermediate zone; SP, subplate; CP, cortical plate; MZ, marginal zone.

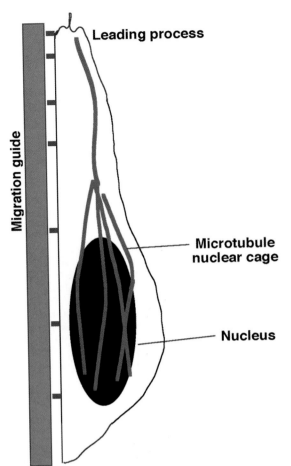

Leading process

Microtubule nuclear cage

Nucleus

Migration guide

Figure 92–6. Neuron migrating along a glial fiber. Neuron migration consists of three basic events: extension of the leading process, translocation of the cell soma and other cellular components, retraction of the trailing process. A distinct "cage" of microtubules has been described as surrounding the nucleus during migration.

defective nuclear migration in lower organisms with mutations in *LIS1* orthologs (Gupta et al., 2002). Because dynein functions with LIS1, this suggests that the LIS1–dynein interaction is critical for this phase of migration.

One central question is whether the LIS phenotype is purely a disorder of migration of cortical neurons or whether additional defects contribute to the phenotype. These additional defects may be of two types. First, in addition to enabling migration of neurons, LIS1 may play a part either in establishment of the protomap of the cortex or in neuronal proliferation. Prior to migration of the majority of cortical neurons, the protomap consists of a population of neurons known as the "preplate," and the correct formation of this structure is essential for subsequent formation of the cortical plate (Meyer et al., 2000). There is a suggestion that the preplate is not properly formed in mice deficient for LIS1, suggesting that part of the phenotype in LIS may relate to impaired protomap formation. There is also the suggestion that LIS1 may have a role in cell division (Faulkner et al., 2000), and therefore some of the LIS phenotype may relate to impaired neuron generation during fetal development.

LIS1 and Roles in Cell Division and Dynein-Mediated Transport

While LIS1 haploinsufficiency leads to a defect in neuronal migration, the findings that homozygous null embryos die prior to implantation, that it is ubiquitously expressed, and that orthologs are present in species without a nervous system suggest that LIS1 plays a part in nonneuronal functioning. The finding that LIS1 functions with dynein in cell division (Faulkner et al., 2000) and is required for dynein-based

intracellular trafficking in nonneuronal cells clearly suggest extraneuronal functions for the protein. However, it is unclear whether heterozygous LIS1 mutations lead to extranervous system disorders that contribute to the phenotype. For instance, many patients with a LIS1 mutation display multiple organ dysfunction, but it is unclear whether these are primary defects or secondary to overall poor health and multiple medications.

DCX and a Cell-Autonomous Role in Neuronal Migration

The main effect of a mutation of DCX is likely due to a cell-autonomous defect in neuronal migration of cortical and subcortical neurons during brain development. This hypothesis is based on the observation that DCX mutations produce the mosaic phenotypes of SBH in females and LIS in males. It is thought likely that the neurons in the heterotopic band have inactivated the normal X chromosome, and thus females with SBH essentially display a mosaic genotype due to random X-inactivation.

It is more difficult to speculate on the molecular mechanism that underlies the LIS caused by *DCX* mutations because no animal model has been described and because molecular pathways of DCX have yet to be defined. However, given the similarity in phenotype, the mechanism of the migration defect may be the same for both genetic forms of LIS.

Data indicate that DCX and LIS1 may directly bind to one another and function to cooperatively polymerize microtubules (Caspi et al., 2000). These data suggest that DCX and LIS1 may function on the same pathway to mediate their effect on migration. However, the relation of these findings to migration is still unclear.

ACKNOWLEDGMENTS

Thanks to the support group, the Lissencephaly Network. See http://www. lissencephaly.org.

REFERENCES

Arai H, Koizumi H, Aoki J, Inoue K (2002). Platelet-activating factor acetylhydrolase (PAF-AH). *J Biochem (Tokyo)* 131: 635–640.
Barkovich AJ, Jackson DE Jr, Boyer RS (1989). Band heterotopias: a newly recognized neuronal migration anomaly. *Radiology* 171: 455–458.
Barkovich AJ, Koch TK, Carrol CL (1991). The spectrum of lissencephaly: report of ten patients analyzed by magnetic resonance imaging. *Ann Neurol* 30: 139–146.
Barkovich AJ, Guerrini R, Battaglia G, Kalifa G, N'Guyen T, Parmeggiani A, Santucci M, Giovanardi-Rossi P, Granata T, D'Incerti L (1994). Band heterotopia: correlation of outcome with magnetic resonance imaging parameters. *Ann Neurol* 36: 609–617.
Berg MJ, Schifitto G, Powers JM, Martinez-Capolino C, Fong CT, Myers GJ, Epstein LG, Walsh CA (1998). X-linked female band heterotopia-male lissencephaly syndrome. *Neurology* 50: 1143–1146.
Bielschowsky M (1923). Über die Oberflächengestaltung des Grosshirnmantels bei Pachygyrie, Microgyrie und bei normaler Entwicklung. *J Psychol Neurol* 30: 29–76.
Bowne SJ, Daiger SP, Hims MM, Sohocki MM, Malone KA, McKie AB, Heckenlively JR, Birch DG, Inglehearn CF, Bhattacharya SS, et al. (1999). Mutations in the RP1 gene causing autosomal dominant retinitis pigmentosa. *Hum Mol Genet* 8: 2121–2128.
Cahana A, Escamez T, Nowakowski RS, Hayes NL, Giacobini M, von Holst A, Shmueli O, Sapir T, McConnell SK, Wurst W, et al. (2001). Targeted mutagenesis of Lis1 disrupts cortical development and LIS1 homodimerization. *Proc Natl Acad Sci USA* 98: 6429–6434.
Cardoso C, Leventer RJ, Matsumoto N, Kuc JA, Ramocki MB, Mewborn SK, Dudlicek LL, May LF, Mills PL, Das S, et al. (2000). The location and type of mutation predict malformation severity in isolated lissencephaly caused by abnormalities within the *LIS1* gene. *Hum Mol Genet* 9: 3019–3028.
Caspi M, Atlas R, Kantor A, Sapir T, Reiner O (2000). Interaction between LIS1 and doublecortin, two lissencephaly gene products. *Hum Mol Genet* 9: 2205–2213.
Chong SS, Pack SD, Roschke AV, Tanigami A, Carrozzo R, Smith AC, Dobyns WB, Ledbetter DH (1997). A revision of the lissencephaly and Miller-Dieker syndrome critical regions in chromosome 17p13.3. *Hum Mol Genet* 6: 147–155.
Clark GD, McNeil RS, Bix GJ, Swann JW (1995). Platelet-activating factor produces neuronal growth cone collapse. *Neuroreport* 6: 2569–2575.
Dawe AL, Caldwell KA, Harris PM, Morris NR, Caldwell GA (2001). Evolutionarily conserved nuclear migration genes required for early embryonic development in *Caenorhabditis elegans*. *Dev Genes Evol* 211: 434–441.
De Lange C (1939). Lissenzephalie beim Meinschem. *Msch Psychiat Neurol* 101: 350.
de Rijk-van Andel JF, Arts WF, Hofman A, Staal A, Niermeijer MF (1991). Epidemiology of lissencephaly type I. *Neuroepidemiology* 10: 200–204.
des Portes V, Pinard JM, Smadja D, Motte J, Boespfüg-Tanguy O, Moutard ML, Desguerre I, Billuart P, Carrie A, Bienvenu T, et al. (1997). Dominant X linked subcortical laminar heterotopia and lissencephaly syndrome (XSCLH/LIS): evidence for the occurence of mutations in males and mapping of a potential locus in Xq22. *J Med Genet* 34: 177–183.

des Portes V, Pinard JM, Billuart P, Vinet MC, Koulakoff A, Carrie A, Gelot A, Dupuis E, Motte J, Berwald-Netter Y, et al. (1998). A novel CNS gene required for neuronal migration and involved in X-linked subcortical laminar heterotopia and lissencephaly syndrome. *Cell* 92: 51–61.

Dieker H, Edwards RH, Zurhein G, Chou SM, Hartman HA, Opitz JM (1969). The lissencephaly syndrome. *Birth Defects* 5: 53–64.

Dobyns WB, Truwit CL (1995). Lissencephaly and other malformations of cortical development: 1995 update. *Neuropediatrics* 26: 132–147.

Dobyns WB, Stratton RF, Parke JT, Greenberg F, Nussbaum RL, Ledbetter DH (1983). Miller-Dieker syndrome: lissencephaly and monosomy 17p. *J Pediatr* 102: 552–558.

Dobyns WB, Stratton RF, Greenburg F (1984). Syndromes with lissencephaly. I: Miller-Dieker and Norman-Roberts syndromes and isolated lissencephaly. *Am J Med Genet* 18: 509–526.

Dobyns WB, Kirkpatrick JB, Hittner HM, Roberts RM, Kretzer FL (1985). Syndromes with lissencephaly. II: Walker-Warburg and cerebro-oculo-muscular syndromes and a new syndrome with type II lissencephaly. *Am J Med Genet* 22: 157–195.

Dobyns WB, Elias ER, Newlin AC, Pagon RA, Ledbetter DH (1992). Causal heterogeneity in isolated lissencephaly. *Neurology* 42: 1375–1388.

Dobyns WB, Truwit CL, Ross ME, Matsumoto N, Pilz DT, Ledbetter DH, Gleeson JG, Walsh CA, Barkovich AJ (1999). Differences in the gyral pattern distinguish chromosome 17-linked and X-linked lissencephaly. *Neurology* 53: 270–277.

Edmondson JC, Hatten ME (1987). Glial-guided granule neuron migration in vitro: a high-resolution time-lapse video microscopic study. *J Neurosci* 7: 1928–1934.

Emes RD, Ponting CP (2001). A new sequence motif linking lissencephaly, Treacher Collins and oral-facial-digital type 1 syndromes, microtubule dynamics and cell migration. *Hum Mol Genet* 10: 2813–2820.

Erhardt A (1914). Über Agyrie und Heterotopie im Grosshirn. *Allg Z Psychiat* 71: 656.

Faulkner NE, Dujardin DL, Tai CY, Vaughan KT, O'Connell CB, Wang Y, Vallee RB (2000). A role for the lissencephaly gene LIS1 in mitosis and cytoplasmic dynein function. *Nat Cell Bio* 2: 784–791.

Feng Y, Olson EC, Stukenberg PT, Flanagan LA, Kirschner MW, Walsh CA (2000). LIS1 regulates CNS lamination by interacting with mNudE, a central component of the centrosome. *Neuron* 28: 665–679.

Fleck MW, Hirotsune S, Gambello MJ, Phillips-Tansey E, Suares G, Mervis RF, Wynshaw-Boris A, McBain CJ (2000). Hippocampal abnormalities and enhanced excitability in a murine model of human lissencephaly. *J Neurosci* 20: 2439–2450.

Francis F, Koulakoff A, Boucher D, Chafey P, Schaar B, Vinet MC, Friocourt G, McDonnell N, Reiner O, Kahn A, et al. (1999). Doublecortin is a developmentally regulated, microtubule-associated protein expressed in migrating and differentiating neurons. *Neuron* 23: 247–256.

Fujiwara T, Tanaka K, Inoue E, Kikyo M, Takai Y (1999). Bni1p regulates microtubule-dependent nuclear migration through the actin cytoskeleton in *Saccharomyces cerevisiae*. *Mol Cell Biol* 19: 8016–8027.

Garcia-Higuera I, Fenoglio J, Li Y, Lewis C, Panchenko MP, Reiner O, Smith TF, Neer EJ (1996). Folding of proteins with WD-repeats: comparison of six members of the WD-repeat superfamily to the G protein β subunit. *Biochemistry* 35: 13985–13994.

Geiser JR, Schott EJ, Kingsbury TJ, Cole NB, Totis LJ, Bhattacharyya G, He L, Hoyt MA (1997). *Saccharomyces cerevisiae* genes required in the absence of the CIN8-encoded spindle motor act in functionally diverse mitotic pathways. *Mol Biol Cell* 8: 1035–1050.

Gleeson JG, Walsh CA (2000). Neuronal migration disorders: from genetic diseases to developmental mechanisms. *Trends Neurosci* 23: 352–359.

Gleeson JG, Allen KM, Fox JW, Lamperti ED, Berkovic S, Scheffer I, Cooper EC, Dobyns WB, Minnerath SR, Ross ME, Walsh CA (1998). *Doublecortin*, a brain-specific gene mutated in human X-linked lissencephaly and double cortex syndrome, encodes a putative signaling protein. *Cell* 92: 63–72.

Gleeson JG, Lin PT, Flanagan LA, Walsh CA (1999a). Doublecortin is a microtubule-associated protein and is expressed widely by migrating neurons. *Neuron* 23: 257–271.

Gleeson JG, Minnerath SR, Fox JW, Allen KM, Luo RF, Hong SE, Berg MJ, Kuzniecky R, Reitnauer PJ, Borgatti R, et al. (1999b). Characterization of mutations in the gene doublecortin in patients with double cortex syndrome. *Ann Neurol* 45: 146–153.

Gleeson JG, Luo RF, Grant PE, Guerrini R, Huttenlocher PR, Berg MJ, Ricci S, Cusmai R, Wheless JW, Berkovic S, et al. (2000a). Genetic and neuroradiological heterogeneity of double cortex syndrome. *Ann Neurol* 47: 265–269.

Gleeson JG, Minnerath S, Kuzniecky RI, Dobyns WB, Young ID, Ross ME, Walsh CA (2000b). Somatic and germline mosaic mutations in the doublecortin gene are associated with variable phenotypes. *Am J Hum Genet* 67: 574–581.

Gönczy P, Bellanger J-M, Kirkham M, Pozniakowski A, Baumer K, Phillips JB, Hyman AA (2001). zyg-8: a gene required for spindle positioning in C. elegans: encodes a doublecortin-related kinase that promotes microtubule assembly. *Dev Cell* 1: 363–375.

Gupta A, Tsai LH, Wynshaw-Boris A (2002). Life is a journey: a genetic look at neocortical development. *Nat Rev Genet* 3: 342–355.

Harding B (1996). Grey matter heterotopia. In: *Dysplasias of Cerebral Cortex and Epilepsy*. Guerrini R, Andermann F, Canapicchi R, Roger J, Zifkin BG, Pfanner P (eds.) Lippincott-Raven, Philadelphia, pp. 81–88.

Hattori M, Adachi H, Tsujimoto M, Arai H, Inoue K (1994). Miller-Dieker lissencephaly gene encodes a subunit of brain platelet-activating factor acetylhydrolase. *Nature* 370: 216–218.

Hirotsune S, Fleck MW, Gambello MJ, Bix GJ, Chen A, Clark GD, Ledbetter DH, McBain CJ, Wynshaw-Boris A (1998). Graded reduction of Pafah1b1 (Lis1) activity results in neuronal migration defects and early embryonic lethality. *Nat Genet* 19: 333–339.

Holzgreve W, Feil R, Louwen F, Miny P (1993). Prenatal diagnosis and management of fetal hydrocephaly and lissencephaly. *Childs Nerv Syst* 9: 408–412.

Jacob J. (1940). Die feinere Oberflachengestaltung der Hirnwindungen, die Hirnwarzenbildung und die Mikroplygyrie. *Neurol Psychiat* 170: 64–84.

Kato M, Kanai M, Soma O, Takusa Y, Kimura T, Numakura C, Matsuki T, Nakamura S, Hayasaka K (2001). Mutation of the doublecortin gene in male patients with double cortex syndrome: somatic mosaicism detected by hair root analysis. *Ann Neurol* 50: 547–551.

Kojima K, Suzuki Y, Seki K, Yamamoto T, Sato T, Tanaka T, Suzumori K (2002). Prenatal diagnosis of lissencephaly (type II) by ultrasound and fast magnetic resonance imaging. *Fetal Diagn Ther* 17: 34–36.

Ledbetter DH, Ledbetter SA, vanTuinen P, Summers KM, Robinson TJ, Nakamura Y, Wolff R, White R, Barker DF, Wallace MR, et al. (1989). Molecular dissection of a contiguous gene syndrome: frequent submicroscopic deletions, evolutionarily conserved sequences, and a hypomethylated "island" in the Miller-Dieker chromosome region. *Proc Natl Acad Sci USA* 86: 5136–5140.

Lei Y, Warrior R (2000). The *Drosophila* Lissencephaly1 (DLis1) gene is required for nuclear migration. *Dev Biol* 226: 57–72.

Liu Z, Xie T, Steward R (1999). Lis1, the *Drosophila* homolog of a human lissencephaly disease gene, is required for germline cell division and oocyte differentiation. *Development* 126: 4477–4488.

Liu Z, Steward R, Luo L (2000). *Drosophila* Lis1 is required for neuroblast proliferation, dendritic elaboration and axonal transport. *Nat Cell Biol* 2: 776–783.

Liu Q, Zhou J, Daiger SP, Farber DB, Heckenlively JR, Smith JE, Sullivan LS, Zuo J, Milam AH, Pierce EA (2002). Identification and subcellular localization of the RP1 protein in human and mouse photoreceptors. *Invest Ophthalmol Vis Sci* 43: 22–32.

Lo Nigro C, Chong CS, Smith AC, Dobyns WB, Carrozzo R, Ledbetter DH (1997). Point mutations and an intragenic deletion in LIS1, the lissencephaly causative gene in isolated lissencephaly sequence and Miller-Dieker syndrome. *Hum Mol Genet* 6: 157–164.

Mach JM, Lehmann R (1997). An Egalitarian–BicaudalD complex is essential for oocyte specification and axis determination in *Drosophila*. *Genes Dev* 11: 423–435.

Magavi SS, Leavitt BR, Macklis JD (2000). Induction of neurogenesis in the neocortex of adult mice. *Nature* 405: 951–955.

Martinez-Lage JF, Garcia Santos JM, Poza M, Puche A, Casas C, Rodriguez Costa T (1995). Neurosurgical management of Walker-Warburg syndrome. *Childs Nerv Syst* 11: 145–153.

Matell M (1893). Heterotopie der grauen Substanz in den beiden Hemisphären des Grosshirns. *Arch Psychiat Nervenkr* 25: 124–136.

Matsumoto N, Leventer RJ, Kuc JA, Mewborn SK, Dudlicek LL, Ramocki MB, Pilz DT, Mills PL, Das S, Ross ME, et al. (2001). Mutation analysis of the DCX gene and genotype/phenotype correlation in subcortical band heterotopia. *Eur J Hum Genet* 9: 5–12.

Meyer G, Schaaps JP, Moreau L, Goffinet AM (2000). Embryonic and early fetal development of the human neocortex. *J Neurosci* 20: 1858–1868.

Miller JQ (1963). Lissencephaly in two siblings. *Neurology* 13: 841–850.

Niethammer M, Smith DS, Ayala R, Peng J, Ko J, Lee MS, Morabito M, Tsai LH (2000). NUDEL is a novel Cdk5 substrate that associates with LIS1 and cytoplasmic dynein. *Neuron* 28: 697–711.

OMIM (2000). Online Mendelian Inheritance in Man, OMIM (TM). Available at http://www.ncbi.nlm.nih.gov/omim/, J. H. U. B. McKusick-Nathans Institute for Genetic Medicine, MD) and National Center for Biotechnology Information, National Library of Medicine (Bethesda, MD), eds.

Paylor R, Hirotsune S, Gambello MJ, Yuva-Paylor L, Crawley JN, Wynshaw-Boris A (1999). Impaired learning and motor behavior in heterozygous Pafah1b1 (Lis1) mutant mice. *Learn Mem* 6: 521–537.

Pierce EA, Quinn T, Meehan T, McGee TL, Berson EL, Dryja TP (1999). Mutations in a gene encoding a new oxygen-regulated photoreceptor protein cause dominant retinitis pigmentosa. *Nat Genet* 22: 248–254.

Pilu G, Falco P, Gabrielli S, Perolo A, Sandri F, Bovicelli L (1999). The clinical significance of fetal isolated cerebral borderline ventriculomegaly: report of 31 cases and review of the literature. *Ultrasound Obstet Gynecol* 14: 320–326.

Pilz DT, Matsumoto N, Minnerath S, Mills P, Gleeson JG, Allen KM, Walsh CA, Barkovich AJ, Dobyns WB, Ledbetter DH, Ross ME (1998). LIS1 and XLIS (DCX) mutations cause most classical lissencephaly, but different patterns of malformation. *Hum Mol Genet* 7: 2029–2037.

Pilz DT, Kuc J, Matsumoto N, Bodurtha J, Bernadi B, Tassinari CA, Dobyns WB, Ledbetter DH (1999). Subcortical band heterotopia in rare affected males can be caused by missense mutations in DCX (XLIS) or LIS1. *Hum Mol Genet* 8: 1757–1760.

Pinard JM, Motte J, Chiron C, Brian R, Andermann E, Dulac O (1994). Subcortical laminar heterotopia and lissencephaly in two families: a single X linked dominant gene. *J Neurol Neurosurg Psychiatry* 57: 914–920.

Pollin TI, Dobyns WB, Crowe CA, Ledbetter DH, Bailey-Wilson JE, Smith AC (1999). Risk of abnormal pregnancy outcome in carriers of balanced reciprocal translocations involving the Miller-Dieker syndrome (MDS) critical region in chromosome 17p13.3. *Am J Med Genet* 85: 369–375.

Reiner O, Carrozzo R, Shen Y, Wehnert M, Faustinella F, Dobyns WB, Caskey CT, Ledbetter DH (1993). Isolation of a Miller-Dieker lissencephaly gene containing G protein β-subunit-like repeats. *Nature* 364: 717–721.

Reiner O, Albrecht U, Gordon M, Chianese KA, Wong C, Gal-Gerber O, Sapir T, Siracusa LD, Buchberg AM, Caskey CT, et al. (1995). Lissencephaly gene (LIS1) expression in the CNS suggests a role in neuronal migration. *J Neurosci* 15: 3730–3738.

Ross ME, Allen KM, Srivastava AK, Featherstone T, Gleeson JG, Hirsch B, Harding BN, Andermann E, Abdullah R, Berg M, et al. (1997). Linkage and physical mapping of X-linked lissencephaly/SBH (XLIS): a gene causing neuronal migration defects in human brain. *Hum Mol Genet* 6: 555–562.

Ross ME, Swanson K, Dobyns WB (2001). Lissencephaly with cerebellar hypoplasia (LCH): a heterogeneous group of cortical malformations. *Neuropediatrics* 32: 256–263.

Saltzman DH, Krauss CM, Goldman JM, Benacerraf BR (1991). Prenatal diagnosis of lissencephaly. *Prenat Diagn* 11: 139–143.

Sapir T, Elbaum M, Reiner O (1997). Reduction of microtubule catastrophe events by LIS1, platelet-activating factor acetylhydrolase subunit. *EMBO J* 16: 6977–6984.

Sapir T, Cahana A, Seger R, Nekhai S, Reiner O (1999). LIS1 is a microtubule-associated phosphoprotein. *Eur J Biochem* 265: 181–188.

Sapir T, Horesh D, Caspi M, Atlas R, Burgess HA, Wolf SG, Francis F, Chelly J, Elbaum M, Pietrokovski S, Reiner O (2000). Doublecortin mutations cluster in evolutionarily conserved functional domains. *Hum Mol Genet* 9: 703–712.

Sarnat HB (1992). *Cerebral Dysgenesis: Embryology and Clinical Expression*. Oxford University Press, New York.

Sasaki S, Shionoya A, Ishida M, Gambello MJ, Yingling J, Wynshaw-Boris A, Hirotsue S (2000). A LIS1/NUDEL/cytoplasmic dynein heavy chain complex in the developing and adult nervous system. *Neuron* 28: 681–696.

Sheffield PJ, Garrard S, Caspi M, Aoki J, Arai H, Derewenda U, Inoue K, Suter B, Reiner O, Derewenda ZS (2000). Homologs of the α- and β-subunits of mammalian brain platelet-activating factor acetylhydrolase Ib in the *Drosophila melanogaster* genome. *Proteins* 39: 1–8.

Stratton RF, Dobyns WB, Airhart SD, Ledbetter DH (1984). New chromosomal syndrome: Miller-Dieker syndrome and monosomy 17p13. *Hum Genet* 67: 193–200.

Swan A, Nguyen T, Suter B (1999). *Drosophila* Lissencephaly-1 functions with Bic-D and dynein in oocyte determination and nuclear positioning. *Nat Cell Biol* 1: 444–449.

Taylor KR, Holzer AK, Bazan JF, Walsh CA, Gleeson JG (2000). Patient mutations in doublecortin define a repeated tubulin-binding domain. *J Biol Chem* 275: 34442–34450.

Waterman-Storer CM, Karki S, Holzbaur EL (1995). The p150Glued component of the dynactin complex binds to both microtubules and the actin-related protein centractin (Arp-1). *Proc Natl Acad Sci USA* 92: 1634–1638.

Xiang X, Beckwith SM, Morris NR (1994). Cytoplasmic dynein is involved in nuclear migration in *Aspergillus nidulans*. *Proc Natl Acad Sci USA* 91: 2100–2104.

Xiang X, Zuo W, Efimov VP, Morris NR (1999). Isolation of a new set of *Aspergillus nidulans* mutants defective in nuclear migration. *Curr Genet* 35: 626–630.

93 | *RELN* and Lissencephaly with Cerebellar Hypoplasia

CHRISTOPHER A. WALSH

Lissencephaly, meaning literally "smooth cortex," refers to a global malformation of the cerebral cortex resulting from widespread abnormal migration of neurons. Whereas "classical lissencephaly" (Chapter 92) typically spares the cerebellum, a more recently described syndrome causes abnormal development in both the cerebral cortex and the cerebellum, resulting in lissencephaly with cerebellar hypoplasia (LCH). This condition is inherited in autosomal recessive fashion and is associated with profound neurological disability—with ataxia, hypotonia, mental retardation, and seizures. One form of LCH is associated with mutations in the human *Reelin* gene (*RELN*), which encodes a very large (>400 kDa) secreted glycoprotein that associates with the extracellular matrix and regulates the migration and organization of neurons in a noncell-autonomous fashion. *RELN* represents the human ortholog of the murine *Reelin* gene, which was originally discovered as mutated in the mutant mouse called *reeler*. A great deal of progress has recently been made in understanding the signaling mechanisms triggered by Reelin, and many members of the Reelin signaling pathway are candidate genes for other forms of human LCH.

The *reeler* mouse, characterized by its ataxic "reeling" gait, is one of the oldest and most familiar of the neurological mutant mice (Rice and Curran, 2001), but only recently has a corresponding human disease been described (Hong et al., 2000). In *reeler* mutants, the distinct "reeling" gait is caused by profound hypoplasia of the cerebellum, in which the normal cerebellar folia are missing due to a failure of migration of both Purkinje cells and granule cells (Lambert de Rouvroit and Goffinet, 1998). The cerebral cortex shows a severe abnormality of neuronal migration as well; here the normal layering pattern of the neocortex is severely effaced and difficult to appreciate (Caviness, 1982; Lambert de Rouvroit and Goffinet, 1998). Studies of the sequence of neuronal "birthdates," as determined by exposure of embryos to pulses of DNA analogs such as ^{3}H-labeled thymidine or Bromo-deoxyuridine, indicate that the cortical neurons are produced over the normal time frame of development and in the normal numbers (Caviness, 1982). However, the sequence of migration of these neurons is severely disrupted: neurons that belong in the upper layers of the cortex tend instead to be arrested at lower layers of the cortex (though without forming the tight layer that they would normally form), whereas neurons that are normally destined for deeper cortical layers are instead positioned more superficially. Because neurons destined for the neocortex normally migrate past earlier formed neurons (an "inside-out" sequence of neurogenesis), this prominent disruption and partial inversion of the normal layering is generally explained as a failure of newly generated neurons to migrate past their older counterparts (Pinto-Lord et al., 1982).

Although it had previously been suggested that the *reeler* mutation acted noncell-autonomously (Mikoshiba et al., 1985), it was nonetheless surprising when the identification of the *reeler* gene demonstrated it to encode a large secreted extracellular matrix glycoprotein that is synthesized by only a small minority of cerebral cortical neurons (D'Arcangelo et al., 1995; Hirotsune et al., 1995). The gene, referred to as *Reelin*, encodes a 400 kDa protein that encodes an amino-terminal region homologous to F-spondin, and eight consecutive repeats that are fairly unique (D'Arcangelo et al., 1997). The mRNA and protein are synthesized and secreted mainly by neurons at the outermost surface of the developing cortex, called Cajal-Retzius neurons (Ogawa et al., 1995). Ironically, these are essentially the only neurons in the *reeler* mutant that are normally positioned, while Reelin appears to regulate the migration of all other cortical neurons during development.

Although disorders of human neuronal migration have been well characterized neuropathologically for over a century (Walsh, 1999; Ross and Walsh, 2001), their genetic basis has only come to be appreciated more recently. Moreover, the syndrome that ultimately corresponded to the *reeler* mouse was just described in the clinical literature in the last decade, and its genetic basis revealed in the last few years. Like *reeler*, human mutations at the *Reelin* locus cause prominent disruptions of neuronal migration and architecture in the cerebellum and cerebral cortex (Hong et al., 2000), producing a syndrome referred to as lissencephaly with cerebellar hypoplasia (LCH).

CLINICAL FEATURES

The earliest known clinical report of a family that ultimately showed mutations in the *Reelin* gene was published in 1993. Three children, two of them identical twins, had a phenotype that was characterized by severe ataxia, hypotonia, developmental delay, mental retardation, and seizures (Hourihane et al., 1993). The children achieved few developmental milestones, with little or no ability to walk or talk. All of the children were described as having congenital lymphedema, and in one case there was frank chylous ascites, with an accumulation of lipid-containing fluid in the abdominal cavity, suggesting a defect in lymphatic drainage. MRI of the brain of these children showed reduction of the cerebral cortical gyri, with unfolding of the hippocampus (Fig. 93–1). The cortex was thickened, especially in the frontal regions, while the occipital cortex appeared almost normal in thickness. The cerebellum was profoundly hypoplastic, with a complete absence of detectable cerebellar folia in all children, and the brain stem also showed severe hypoplasia. Autosomal recessive inheritance was suggested by the fact that the parents were half-first cousins (Hourihane et al., 1993). A similar patient was presented as a case report a few years later by al-Shahwan et al. (1996), who also described a second, more extensive pedigree with three affected offspring of a marriage between first cousins (Hong et al., 2000). The clinical features and radiographic features were both quite similar to those of the Hourihane cases, though congenital lymphedema was not noted in these patients.

IDENTIFICATION OF THE GENE AND MUTATIONAL SPECTRUM

Given the similarity of LCH to the *reeler* mouse, the possibility that they were orthologous conditions was tested first by analyzing markers near the human *Reelin* locus for linkage to LCH (Hong et al., 2000). Markers in and around the *Reelin* locus showed strong evidence of linkage to LCH (LOD score > 4.5 at O), and both families subsequently showed mutations in the *Reelin* gene (Fig. 93-2). The Saudi family showed a mutation (CAG to CAA) at the splice acceptor for exon 37, causing predicted skipping of this exon and early termination of the predicted protein. Interestingly, a naturally occurring mouse reeler allele, Albany2, skips this same exon, albeit by another mechanism (Royaux et al., 1997). The British family showed a distinct allele with two different potentially deleterious mutations. In RT-PCR experiments, there was apparent skipping of exon 43, though the DNA mutation that causes this abnormal splicing has not been

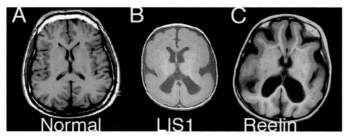

Figure 93–1. Axial MRI images. (*A*) The normal cortex represents a thin lining of gray matter atop the white matter, and is characterized by innumerable gyri (folds) and sulci (grooves). (*B*) In classical lissencephaly, the gray matter is smoother, lacking almost all gyri, while the gray matter is also considerably increased in thickness. The amount of white matter is reduced, the ventricles are enlarged, and the overall volume of the brain is generally reduced as well. (*C*) In lissencephaly due to *Reelin* mutations, the cortex is roughly normal in thickness and has more gyri than in classical lissencephaly, though far fewer than normal. The white matter is less severely reduced, though it is still abnormal, and the overall size of the brain is generally normal.

identified. Moreover, downstream of this splicing abnormality, a T to G point mutation changes isoleucine at position 3222 to serine at a highly conserved position that is likely to affect the secretion of the protein (Hong et al., 2000).

Reelin is expressed in many tissues, including peripheral serum, and thus allows a simple assay for protein expression (Smalheiser et al., 2000). Affected individuals homozygous for the Saudi allele showed absolutely no detectable Reelin protein in serum, with intermediate levels in obligatory heterozygotes. Similarly, the British allele resulted in only very small amounts of detectable Reelin protein in the peripheral serum of affected individuals, though some could be seen. The clinical features of the two families are indistinguishable, suggesting that both alleles are probably null alleles (Hong et al., 2000).

COUNSELING AND TREATMENT

LCH is a very rare autosomal recessive condition, and so recurrence rate counseling should be for an autosomal recessive condition. However, there are other forms of LCH that resemble *Reelin* mutations but have other potential diagnoses (Ross et al., 2001) and patterns of inheritance. In our experience, only patients with a complete absence of

cerebellar folia on MRI have *Reelin* mutations (Walsh et al., unpublished observations), and other patients with similar, but distinct MRI patterns have other syndromes. Thus, careful interpretation of the MRI governs the genetic counseling advice.

While there is no known definitive treatment for the profound developmental delay and hypotonia caused by *Reelin* mutations, the ataxia has been treated with splints and supports. The seizures have responded well to a variety of agents, including carbamezipine (Hong et al., 2000), and are not as catastrophic as seizures typically can be in the setting of other severe neuronal migration disorders in humans. The relatively mild seizure pattern in humans with LCH again recalls the *reeler* mutant mouse, which, despite the profound neuronal architectural disturbance, has never been reported to suffer from seizures (Lambert de Rouvroit and Goffinet, 1998).

MUTATIONS IN ORTHOLOGOUS GENES

Reelin encodes one of the largest of all mRNA (>12,000 bp of coding sequence) and hence proteins (>400 kDa), and so it is hardly surprising to see spontaneous mutations in this gene in several different species. Indeed, the "creeping" rat has histological and behavioral features that resemble *reeler* mice, and there is evidence that the creeping mutation maps to the rat *Reelin* locus and that creeping rats are deficient in *Reelin* mRNA (Yokoi et al., 2000). Another mutant rat, Kawasaki shaking (Aikawa et al., 1988; Ikeda and Terashima, 1997), is also similar histologically to *reeler* and may represent a second *Reelin* allele. Although a *reeler* gene has been identified in all other vertebrates studied (e.g., Fugu, zebrafish, turtle, lizard, chicken, cow), the effects of mutations in nonmammalian species are not known. A highly homologous gene has not been identified in invertebrates to date.

MOLECULAR PATHOGENESIS

Several key elements of the Reelin signaling pathway have been identified over the past few years, largely by the study of a number of mutant mice that precisely copy the *reeler* phenotype. The *scrambler* (Sweet et al., 1996) and *yotari* (Yoneshima et al., 1997) mutants are phenotypically indistinguishable from *reeler* (Goldowitz et al., 1997; Gonzalez et al., 1997), but these two mutants reflect mutations in an unlinked gene called *Dab1* (Howell et al., 1997b; Sheldon et al., 1997; Ware et al., 1997). Dab1 was originally identified as a cytoplasmic adaptor protein that is expressed in migrating cortical neurons (How-

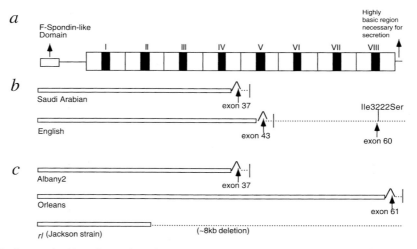

Figure 93–2. Domains of the Reelin protein (*a*), and mutations that cause lissencephaly with cerebellar hypoplasia in humans (*b*) or the reeler phenotype in mice (*c*). The N terminus off Reelin includes a domain homologous to F-spondin, an extracellular matrix protein. Most of the protein is composed of eight "Reelin" repeats whose exact function is unknown. The carboxy terminus of the protein is highly basic and is required for proper secretion of the protein. The Saudi Arabian allele is caused by a mutation at the splice acceptor for exon 37, which is consequently skipped, causing a frameshift mutation and a truncated protein that is undetectable by Western blot. The English al-

lele shows some evidence of skipping of exon 43 by RT-PCR, but the genomic mutation causing this has not been identified. In addition, a point mutation in exon 60 changes isoleucine 3222 to serine, which may interfere with secretion of any residual full length protein. In (*c*), the Albany 2 mouse allele skips exon 37 as well, due to a retrotransposon insertion. The Orleans allele skips exon 61 due to an insertion, and this blocks secretion by truncating the carboxy terminus. The original Jackons rl mutations represent a deletion of much of the locus. This figure is modified from Hong et al. (2000) in order to make exon numbering in human and mouse correspond.

ell et al., 1997a). Moreover, engineered mutations in the mouse VLDL (very low density lipoprotein) receptor and ApoE (apolipoprotein E) receptors, when present in combination, also cause the *reeler* phenotype (Trommsdorff et al., 1999). Biochemical analysis suggests that the Reelin protein binds to the functionally redundant VLDL and ApoER2 proteins, and that Dab1 binds to the NPXY motif present in the cytoplasmic tails of these receptors (Trommsdorff et al., 1998; D'Arcangelo et al., 1999; Hiesberger et al., 1999). Dab1 becomes phosphorylated in response to Reelin application, though the kinase that mediates this phosphorylation event is still not identified for certain (Howell et al., 1999; Keshvara et al., 2002). Additional potential binding partners of Reelin that may serve as coreceptors or targets include members of the protocadherin superfamily (Senzaki et al., 1999) and $\alpha 3\beta 1$ integrin (Dulabon et al., 2000). No naturally occurring mutations in Dab1, VLDLR, ApoER2, or other components of the Reelin pathway have been observed in humans or other nonrodent mammals, but mutations in these genes may also ultimately prove to be a significant cause of human neurological disease.

OTHER HUMAN SYNDROMES DUE TO MUTATIONS AT THE *Reelin* LOCUS

Other neurological and psychiatric disorders have recently been associated with abnormalities of Reelin expression. There have been reports of decreased levels of *Reelin* mRNA in the brain of schizophrenics (Impagnatiello et al., 1998; Guidotti et al., 2000) and of decreased Reelin protein in the serum of schizophrenics (Fatemi et al., 2001). Moreover, there was a recent report of apparent linkage of a polymorphic trinucleotide marker in the *Reelin* gene to autism spectrum disorders (Persico et al., 2001), though a second report has not reproduced the original finding (Krebs et al., 2002). Not only does Reelin have critical roles in the developing cortex and hippocampus and throughout the CNS, but also it is persistently expressed in the adult, with likely roles there as well (Pappas et al., 2001; Weeber et al., 2002). However, it seems unlikely that schizophrenia or autism spectrum disorders represent simple mendelian disorders linked to the *Reelin* locus. In LCH pedigrees neither severely affected individuals with homozygous *Reelin* mutations nor related individuals with heterozygous *Reelin* mutations showed evidence of schizophrenia or autism (Hong et al., 2000). Nevertheless, the presence of congenital lymphedema and chylous ascites in patients with homozygous *Reelin* mutations suggest potential roles for Reelin in vascular or lymphatic development that were not apparent in the mouse model. Thus, the investigation of additional roles for Reelin inside and outside of the brain will continue.

ACKNOWLEDGMENTS

Work in the author's lab is supported by grants from the March of Dimes, the McKnight Endowment, and the National Institutes of Neurological Disease and Stroke.

REFERENCES

Aikawa H, Nonaka I, Woo M, Tsugane T, Esaki K (1988). Shaking rat Kawasaki (SRK): a new neurological mutant rat in the Wistar strain. *Acta Neuropathol* 76: 366–372.

Caviness VS Jr. (1982). Neocortical histogenesis and reeler mice: a developmental study based upon [³H]thymidine autoradiography. *Dev Brain Res* 4: 293–302.

D'Arcangelo G, Miao G, Chen S, Soares H, Morgan J, Curran T (1995). A protein related to extracellular matrix proteins deleted in the mouse mutant reeler. *Nature* 734: 719–723.

D'Arcangelo G, Nakajima K, Miyata T, Ogawa M, Mikoshiba K, Curran T (1997). Reelin is a secreted glycoprotein recognized by the CR-50 monoclonal antibody. *J Neurosci* 17: 23–31.

D'Arcangelo G, Homayouni R, Keshvara L, Rice DS, Sheldon M, Curran T (1999). Reelin is a ligand for lipoprotein receptors. *Neuron* 24: 471–479.

Dulabon L, Olson EC, Taglienti MG, Eisenhuth S, McGrath B, Walsh CA, Kreidberg JA, Anton ES (2000). Reelin binds α3β1 integrin and inhibits neuronal migration. *Neuron* 27: 33–44.

Fatemi SH, Kroll JL, Stary JM (2001). Altered levels of Reelin and its isoforms in schizophrenia and mood disorders. *Neuroreport* 12: 3209–3215.

Goldowitz D, Cushing RC, Laywell E, D'Arcangelo G, Sheldon M, Sweet HO, Davisson M, Steindler D, Curran T (1997). Cerebellar disorganization characteristic of reeler in scrambler mutant mice despite presence of reelin. *J Neurosci* 17: 8767–8777.

Gonzalez JL, Russo CJ, Goldowitz D, Sweet HO, Davisson MT, Walsh CA (1997). Birthdate and cell marker analysis of scrambler: a novel mutation affecting cortical development with a reeler-like phenotype. *J Neurosci* 17: 9204–9211.

Guidotti A, Auta J, Davis JM, Di-Giorgi-Gerevini V, Dwivedi Y, Grayson DR, Impagnatiello F, Pandey G, Pesold C, Sharma R, et al. (2000). Decrease in reelin and glutamic acid decarboxylase67 (GAD67) expression in schizophrenia and bipolar disorder: a postmortem brain study. *Arch Gen Psychiatry* 57: 1061–1069.

Hiesberger T, Trommsdorff M, Howell BW, Goffinet A, Mumby MC, Cooper JA, Herz J (1999). Direct binding of Reelin to VLDL receptor and ApoE receptor 2 induces tyrosine phosphorylation of disabled-1 and modulates tau phosphorylation. *Neuron* 24: 481–489.

Hirotsune S, Takahara T, Sasaki N, Hirose K, Yoshiki A, Ohashi T, Kusakabe M, Murakami Y, Muramatsu M, Watanabe S, et al. (1995). The reeler gene encodes a protein with an EGF-like motif expressed by pioneer neurons. *Nat Genet* 10: 77–83.

Hong SE, Shugart YY, Huang DT, Shahwan SA, Grant PE, Hourihane JO, Martin ND, Walsh CA (2000). Autosomal recessive lissencephaly with cerebellar hypoplasia is associated with human RELN mutations. *Nat Genet* 26: 93–96.

Hourihane JO, Bennett CP, Chaudhuri R, Robb SA, Martin ND (1993). A sibship with a neuronal migration defect, cerebellar hypoplasia and congenital lymphedema. *Neuropediatrics* 24: 43–46.

Howell BW, Gertler FB, Cooper JA (1997a). Mouse disabled (mDab1): a Src binding protein implicated in neuronal development. *EMBO J* 16: 121–132.

Howell BW, Hawkes R, Soriano P, Cooper JA (1997b). Neuronal position in the developing brain is regulated by mouse disabled-1. *Nature* 389: 733–737.

Howell BW, Herrick TM, Cooper JA (1999). Reelin-induced tryosine phosphorylation of disabled 1 during neuronal positioning. *Genes Dev* 13: 643–648.

Ikeda Y, Terashima T (1997). Corticospinal tract neurons are radially malpositioned in the sensory-motor cortex of the Shaking rat Kawasaki. *J Comp Neurol* 383: 370–380.

Impagnatiello F, Guidotti AR, Pesold C, Dwivedi Y, Caruncho H, Pisu MG, Uzunov DP, Smalheiser NR, Davis JM, Pandey GN, et al. (1998). A decrease of reelin expression as a putative vulnerability factor in schizophrenia. *Proc Natl Acad Sci USA* 95: 15718–15723.

Keshvara L, Magdaleno S, Benhayon D, Curran T (2002). Cyclin-dependent kinase 5 phosphorylates disabled 1 independently of Reelin signaling. *J Neurosci* 22: 4869–4877.

Krebs MO, Betancur C, Leroy S, Bourdel MC, Gillberg C, Leboyer M (2002). Absence of association between a polymorphic GGC repeat in the 5′ untranslated region of the reelin gene and autism. *Mol Psychiatry* 7: 801–804.

Lambert de Rouvroit C, Goffinet AM (1998). The reeler mouse as a model of brain development. *Adv Anat Embryol Cell Biol* 150: 1–106.

Mikoshiba K, Yokoyama M, Nishimura Y, Katsuki M, Nomura T, Tsukada Y (1985). Mosaic expression of the Reeler and normal phenotypes in the cerebral cortex in Reeler-normal chimeras at a late embryonic stage. *Dev Growth Differ* 27: 737–744.

Ogawa M, Miyata T, Nakajima K, Yagyu K, Seike M, Ikenaka K, Yamamoto H, Mikoshiba K (1995). The reeler gene-associated antigen on Cajal-Retzius neurons is a crucial molecule for laminar organization of cortical neurons. *Neuron* 14: 899–912.

Pappas GD, Kriho V, Pesold C (2001). Reelin in the extracellular matrix and dendritic spines of the cortex and hippocampus: a comparison between wild type and heterozygous reeler mice by immunoelectron microscopy. *J Neurocytol* 30: 413–425.

Persico AM, D'Agruma L, Maiorano N, Totaro A, Militerni R, Bravaccio C, Wassink TH, Schneider C, Melmed R, Trillo S, et al. (2001). Reelin gene alleles and haplotypes as a factor predisposing to autistic disorder. *Mol Psychiatry* 6: 150–159.

Pinto-Lord MC, Evrard P, Caviness VS Jr. (1982). Obstructed neuronal migration along radial glial fibers in the neocortex of the reeler mouse: a Golgi-EM analysis. *Brain Res* 256: 379–393.

Rice DS, Curran T (2001). Role of the reelin signaling pathway in central nervous system development. *Annu Rev Neurosci* 24: 1005–1039.

Ross ME, Walsh CA (2001). Human brain malformations and their lessons for neuronal migration. *Annu Rev Neurosci* 24: 1041–1070.

Ross ME, Swanson K, Dobyns WB (2001). Lissencephaly with cerebellar hypoplasia (LCH): a heterogeneous group of cortical malformations. *Neuropediatrics* 32: 256–263.

Royaux I, Bernier B, Montgomery JC, Flaherty L, Goffinet AM (1997). Reln^{rlAlb2}, an allele of Reeler isolated from a chlorambucil screen, is due to an IAP insertion with exon skipping. *Genomics* 42: 479–482.

Senzaki K, Ogawa M, Yagi T (1999). Proteins of the CNR family are multiple receptors for reelin. *Cell* 99: 635–647.

al-Shahwan SA, Bruyn GW, al Deeb SM (1996). Lissencephaly with pontocerebellar hypoplasia. *J Child Neurol* 11: 241–244.

Sheldon M, Rice DS, D'Arcangelo G, Yoneshima H, Nakajima K, Mikoshiba K, Howell BW, Cooper JA, Goldowitz D, Curran T (1997). Scrambler and yotari disrupt the disabled gene and produce a reeler-like phenotype in mice. *Nature* 389: 730–733.

Smalheiser NR, Costa E, Guidotti A, Impagnatiello F, Auta J, Lacor P, Kriho V, Pappas GD (2000). Expression of reelin in adult mammalian blood, liver, pituitary pars intermedia, and adrenal chromaffin cells. *Proc Natl Acad Sci USA* 97: 1281–1286.

Sweet HO, Bronson RT, Johnson KR, Cook SA, Davisson MT (1996). *Scrambler*, a new neurological mutation of the mouse with abnormalities of neuronal migration. *Mamm Genome* 7: 798–802.

Trommsdorff M, Borg JP, Margolis B, Herz J (1998). Interaction of cytosolic adaptor proteins with neuronal apolipoprotein E receptors and the amyloid precursor protein. *J Biol Chem* 273: 33556–33560.

Trommsdorff M, Gotthardt M, Hiesberger T, Shelton J, Stockinger W, Nimpf J, Hammer RE, Richardson JA, Herz J (1999). Reeler/Disabled-like disruption of neuronal migration in knockout mice lacking the VLDL receptor and ApoE receptor 2. *Cell* 97: 689–701.

Walsh CA (1999). Genetic malformations of the human cerebral cortex. *Neuron* 23: 19–29.

Ware ML, Fox JW, Gonzalez JL, Davis NM, Lambert de Rouvroit C, Russo CJ, Chua SC Jr, Goffinet AM, Walsh CA (1997). Aberrant splicing of a mouse disabled homolog, mdab1, in the scrambler mouse. *Neuron* 19: 239–249.

Weeber EJ, Beffert U, Jones C, Christian JM, Forster E, Sweatt JD, Herz J (2002). Reelin and ApoE receptors cooperate to enhance hippocampal synaptic plasticity and learning. *J Biol Chem* 277: 39944–39952.

Yokoi N, Shimizu S, Ishibashi K, Kitada K, Iwama H, Namae M, Sugawara M, Serikawa T, Komeda K (2000). Genetic mapping of the rat mutation creeping and evaluation of its positional candidate gene twitchh. *Mamm Genome* 11: 111–114.

Yoneshima H, Nagata E, Matsumoto M, Yamada M, Nakajima K, Miyata T, Ogawa M, Mikoshiba K (1997). A novel neurological mutant mouse, yotari, which exhibits reeler-like phenotype but expresses CR-50 antigen/reelin. *Neurosci Res* 29: 217–223.

94 | *DNAI1* and *DNAH5* and Primary Ciliary Dyskinesia or Kartagener Syndrome

MICHAL WITT

Primary ciliary dyskinesia (PCD), formerly known as immotile cilia syndrome (ICS), belongs to a relatively small group of human genetic disorders caused by dysfunctions of particular organelles and analogous to mitochondrial, lysosomal, or peroxisomal disease. PCD is the only known human disorder caused by a primary dysfunction of the ciliary apparatus. In 1933 the Swiss physician Manes Kartagener described four cases of coexisting *situs inversus*, bronchiectasis, and chronic sinusitis (Kartagener, 1933). Later this set of symptoms was named the Kartagener triad, or Kartagener syndrome. In fact, a Russian author, Siewert, was first to describe a case of the disease in 1904, but it was Kartagener who suggested the common pathomechanism of all three symptoms described. In the 1970s it was found that the sperm and respiratory cilia of males with Kartagener syndrome are immobile due to the impairment of ciliary ultrastructure observed under the electron microscope and that this causes both chronic bronchopulmonary diseases and male infertility (Afzelius, 1976; Elliason et al., 1977). Afzelius (1976) coined the term "immotile cilia syndrome," which has been gradually replaced by "dysmotile cilia syndrome" and finally by "primary ciliary dyskinesia."

Kartagener syndrome (KS) is considered a subtype of primary ciliary dyskinesia (McKusick, 2002). It is "situs inversus," a mirror reversal of the usual left–right asymmetry of the abdominal and thoracic internal organ locations, which distinguishes KS from other forms of PCD. All forms of PCD are characterized by dysmotility or immotility of cilia/flagella in airway epithelial cells, spermatozoa, and other ciliated cells of the body (Schidlow, 1994; Afzelius and Mossberg, 1995; Afzelius, 1998; McKusick, 2002). To differentiate this inherited syndrome from the ultrastructural abnormalities observed during or after injuries (e.g., respiratory infections), the term "secondary ciliary dyskinesia" (SCD) is used for the acquired forms of the disorder (Sleigh, 1981; Jorissen et al., 2000a).

CILIA

Structure and Occurrence

Cilia and flagella are organelles present on protozoan, animal, and some plant cells; they extend from the cell surface with which they share the cell membrane. The main body of the organelle—the axoneme—consists of nine peripheral microtubular doublets surrounding a central pair of microtubules (Fig. 94–1). Microtubular doublets are composed of heterodimers of α and β tubulin assembled into 13 or 11 protofilaments (in tubules A and B, respectively). The 13 protofilaments of the central microtubular pair are spatially oriented with respect to the central pair of the adjacent cilia. Tubulins are accompanied by microtubule-associated proteins (MAPs). The most extensively studied MAPs are dyneins, forming inner (IDA) and outer (ODA) dynein arms that extend from the microtubular doublets. All these structures are composed of various kinds of MAPs. The dynein molecule shows ATPase activity that depends on Ca^{2+} and Mg^{2+} and is composed of several peptide subunits. Dynein molecules of the outer dynein arms are constructed of two heavy chains (α and β), two or more intermediate chains, and four to eight light chains. The inner dynein arms have a basic structure similar to the outer ones, but there are three structurally distinct types of inner arms that contain different dynein isoforms: I1, I2, and I3. Dynein arms undergo disintegration during ATP hydrolysis, causing reciprocal displacement of mi-

crotubules A and B. This forms the physical basis of the mechanism of ciliary movement. Dynein arms of one doublet slide along the adjacent microtubular doublet. The tubulin–dynein complex, typical for ciliary and flagellar inner structure, constitutes a functional equivalent of the myofibrillar actin–myosin complex. Radial spokes connect peripheral and central microtubules, while peripheral doublets are connected with each other by nexin links. The axoneme at its basis is connected with the kinetosome (basal body).

Cilia present on human cells are 0.2 μm wide and 5 to 7 μm long, while sperm flagella are 40 μm long (Schidlow, 1994). The organelles with the typical 9 + 2 internal structure are present in:

- upper airways (nasal cavity, paranasal sinuses, eustachian tubes, pharynx)
- lower airways (from the trachea, through the primary and secondary bronchi, to bronchioles)
- middle ear
- lacrimal sac
- ependymal lining of the brain and spinal cord
- vas deferens
- endometrium of uterus and oviducts
- sperm (ca. 45 μm long flagella, regarded as modified cilia, in distal parts having the typical 9 + 2 structure)
- sensory cells (olfactory cells, vestibular organ, spiral organ in the fetal and perinatal period)

Single cilia that lack the central pair of microtubules (9 + 0 structure), called primary cilia or monocilia, are present on the surface of ganglion cells, as well as on the pineal gland, adrenal gland, pancreas, liver, kidney, heart, cartilage, connective tissue, dermis, epidermis, and some fetal cells.

The total number of cilia on all ciliated cells of the human body is approximately 3×10^{12}. The estimated density of cilia in the respiratory tract is 10^9 per cm^2, and each ciliated epithelial cell has about 200 cilia. The largest number of cilia per cell is in the trachea, where the ciliary transport is the most intensive. Ciliated epithelium occupies approximately 150 cm^2 in the nasal cavity, 300 cm^2 in sinuses, and over 500 cm^2 in lower airways (Afzelius and Mossberg, 1995).

Ciliary Function

The major role of ciliary movement (beat) is to mobilize naturally occurring mucus, which is composed of two layers, each 5 μm thick: the low-density sol forms a periciliary environment, and the higher density and higher viscosity upper gel serves as a sticky trap for inhaled particles of dust, bacteria, and so on. Mucus is produced by submucosal glands and goblet cells, in the smaller parts of the airways probably also by serous cells and Clara cells. Mucus consists of water (95%), inorganic salts (1%), and macromolecules, like glycoproteins and lipids (4%).

The cilia beat in a coordinated and controlled manner. The maximum velocity of the tip of the cilium reaches 30 mm per minute. Ciliary beat frequency (CBF) varies between 6 and 8 per second in bronchioli and 22 per second in the trachea. This translates into a velocity of the ciliary transport of 0.5 to 2 mm per minute in bronchioli and up to 10 to 24 mm per minute in the trachea. The intensity of mucus secretion in a bronchial tree is approximately 0.5 ml/kg body weight per day. The respiratory mucus-propelling cilia display a rhythmical beating pattern. Every beating cycle consists of two active components: a recovery stroke when cilia bend in a direction opposite to the

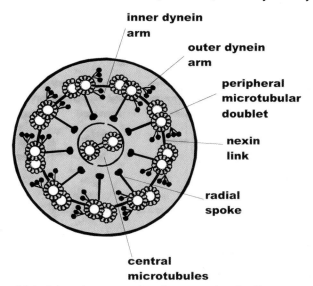

Figure 94–1. Schematic representation of a cross section of a ciliary axoneme. See text for discussion.

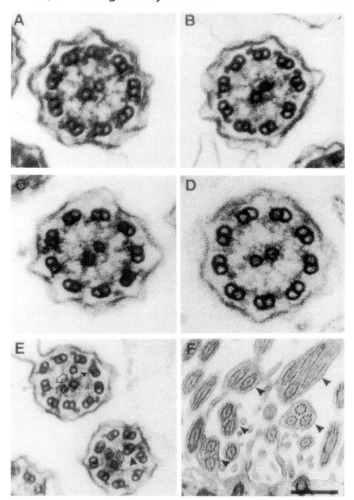

Figure 94–2. Cross sections of ciliary axonemes: (*A*) healthy subject, all ultrastructural elements present; (*B*) PCD patient, absence of inner dynein arms; (*C*) PCD patient, reduced numbers of outer dynein arms (remnants of outer dynein arms are seen on some microtubules); (*D*) PCD patient, reduction of both inner and outer dynein arms; (*E*) PCD patient, absent inner dynein arms, eccentrically located central microtubules (open arrows), displaced peripheral doublet (larger arrowhead), and an extra single microtubule (smaller arrowheads) inside the peripheral ring of doublets; (*F*) compound cilia (arrowheads) from a patient with bronchiectasis not due to PCD. Scale bars: *A* through *D*, 0.1 μm; *E*, 0.13 μm; *F*, 0.6 μm. (From de Iongh and Rutland, 1995, Ciliary Defects in Healthy Subjects, Bronchiectasis, and Primary Ciliary Dyskinesia, *American Journal of Respiratory and Critical Care Medicine*, 151, 1559–1567).

vector of ciliary transport, and an effective stroke when the cilium dives into the gel layer, moving it actively. The duration of the recovery stroke is 2 to 3 times that of the effective stroke. After the effective stroke there is a short resting phase before the next recovery stroke. The upper layer is moved toward the oropharynx, where it is automatically swallowed, clearing small particles and bacteria from the peripheral airways. This coordinated activity of ciliary lining is called "mucociliary clearance" (MC). Mucociliary clearance is directed downward and backward in the upper airways, and upward in the lower airways. The permanent clearance of the mucus toward the pharynx is the most important defense mechanism in the upper and lower airways. Ciliary motility also enables a constant flow of cerebrospinal fluid in the central nervous system, flow of sperm from the testis toward the epidydimis, and movement of the ovary cell along the oviduct (in addition to the natural oviductal peristalsis).

Ultrastructural Defects of Cilia

In typical cases, clinical symptoms of primary ciliary dyskinesia are caused by an impaired motility of the ciliary lining. Usually, ultrastructural lesions of the internal ciliary anatomy constitute a physical basis for immotility and dysmotility, although certain structural defects lead to specific variations of ciliary dysmotility. In any case, inefficient ciliary beating results in the incorrect movement of the upper layer of bronchial mucus, which triggers specific clinical consequences.

Most of the cases of ciliary dysmotility or immotility reported to date are associated with visible ultrastructural defects of cilia, predominantly with a total or partial absence of dynein arms (70%–80% of all defects detected under the electron microscope) (Fig. 94–2). Other defects involve changes in microtubular structure or organization (e.g., absence of the central pair with transposition of a peripheral doublet to the center; extraperipheral microtubules), absence of radial spokes (usually coinciding with the absence of inner dynein arms), or presence of compound cilia. Ciliary beat discoordination can also occur as a result of random ciliary orientation; in Rutland ciliary disorientation syndrome, the mean standard deviation of angles between the central doublets in adjacent central cilia in nose and bronchi exceeds 20° and does not change with treatment (Rutland and de Iongh, 1990) (Fig. 94–3). Cases of abnormally elongated cilia (Afzelius et al., 1985), total loss of cilia (complete ciliary aplasia) (Lungarella et al., 1982), and abnormal structure of the basal body (Lungarella et al., 1985) have also been described. In our cohort of 45 PCD patients, 73% of the analyzed cilia displayed total absence of dynein arms, 27% showed absence of outer dynein arms, and 21% had absence of inner dynein arms (Witt et al., 1999a).

Similar abnormalities of the ciliary ultrastructure can occur as effects of infection (bacterial or viral), inflammation, smoking, environmental pollutants, and so on. However, in contrast to the primary, inborn abnormalities, such secondary defects can change with time and treatment (ultrastructural normalization in the biopsy samples). These secondary ciliary abnormalities consist mainly of microtubular defects and can occur in up to 10% of the cilia in normal individuals (Afzelius, 1981). Chronic inflammation of upper airways, in particular, can lead to destruction of cilia and even to a total denudation of ciliary tapestry.

Certain defects of ultrastructural ciliary architecture lead to various abnormalities of ciliary movement (Afzelius, 1979; Schidlow, 1994):
1. Absence of dynein arms causes eggbeater-like rotation or movement of a distal part of the axoneme.
   - With the absence of both arms or of outer arms only, cilia are usually completely immotile.
   - The absence of inner dynein arms is usually less devastating, but the resulting rigid beating of cilia is ineffective for mucociliary clearance.

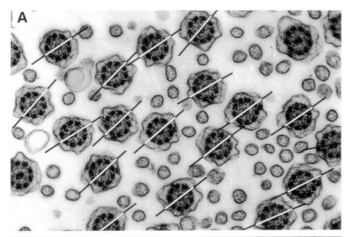

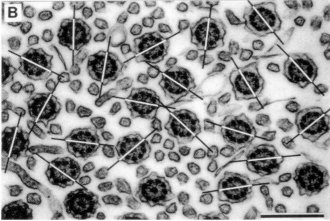

Figure 94–3. Aligned ciliary orientation in a healthy nonsmoking subject (*A*), and a random orientation of the ciliary axes and eccentrically located central tubules (arrowheads) in a PCD patient (*B*). The ciliary axes are shown for five cilia in each field. Scale bar: 0.3 μm. (From de Iongh and Rutland, 1995, Ciliary Defects in Healthy Subjects, Bronchiectasis, and Primary Ciliary Dyskinesia, *American Journal of Respiratory and Critical Care Medicine*, 151, 1559–1567.)

2. Defects of radial spokes result in increased axonemal flexibility, leading to a corkscrew rotational beat; some residual movement of cilia can be noted, but again it is completely ineffective for mucociliary clearance.
3. Translocational defects cause increased rigidity of proximal parts of cilia, with grabbing-type motion of distal parts; cilia beat, but in a very disorganized circular manner, again ineffective for mucociliary clearance.
4. In some patients, cilia with a normal internal architecture quiver only, which results in functionally ineffective movement.

CLINICAL PICTURE

Clearance of mucus and other debris from the airways is achieved by two main mechanisms: mucociliary clearance and coughing. Disorders of ciliary structure or function result in impaired mucociliary clearance, which leads to a chronic sinopulmonary disease manifested as chronic sinusitis, otitis media, nasal polyposis, and, ultimately, bronchiectasis. In addition, situs inversus, dextrocardia, and infertility may be associated with dysfunctional ciliary activity (Fig. 94–4). The prognosis in PCD is good, but morbidity can be high if patients are not correctly managed (Bush et al., 1998).

Airway Disease Phenotype

This condition is one of very few in which symptoms appear in the early neonatal period. Symptoms of respiratory tract involvement are detectable in at least 50% of newborns with PCD (Bush, 2000). The earliest symptoms are tachypnea or neonatal pneumonia (or both), particularly in term babies with no risk factor for congenital infection. Neonatal respiratory distress syndrome of unknown cause should be added to the list of early clinical presentations of PCD (Whitelaw et al., 1981; Holzmann and Felix, 2000). Other symptoms in the neonatal period may include rhinitis, dextrocardia, complex congenital heart disease (with laterality anomalies), esophageal or biliary atresia, and hydrocephalus (Greenstone et al., 1984; Baruch et al., 1989; Gemou Engesaeth et al., 1993).

In infants, older children, and adults, the major symptom of lower airway involvement is recurrent cough, which tends to be rather diurnal than nocturnal and is typically productive. In this light, any case of "atypical asthma-like" symptoms (not responding to regular treatment) with chronic productive cough and excessive sputum production should be considered as possible PCD. Sputum flora in PCD is similar to that observed in adult chronic bronchitis, with predominance of *Haemophilus influenzae* (Sannuti et al., 2001), but *Staphylococcus aureus* and *Streptococcus pneumoniae* are also common (Perraudeau, 1994). In adults, *Pseudomonas aeruginosa* colonization is not rare (Pedersen and Mygind, 1983). Diffuse bronchiolitis might be one of the characteristic features of the lungs in some patients with Kartagener syndrome (Homma et al., 1999).

Malfunction of the mucociliary clearance apparatus causes chronic stasis, impaction, and infection, leading to erosion and distention of the bronchial wall. Chest radiograph abnormalities are observed in all patients. The changes cover a wide spectrum, and the most typical include bronchial wall thickening and hyperinflation, segmental atelectasis or consolidation, and bronchiectasis (visible on chest radiographs) in older children and adults. No radiographic pattern related to particular ultrastructural abnormalities of cilia has been established (Nadel et al., 1985).

Use of imaging techniques (bronchography, computer tomography) confirms tubular or saccular ectasia. The irreversible bronchial abnormalities (bronchiectases) are usually found in at least half of the patients. The incidence of bronchiectases changes with age and reaches 23% in persons younger than 10 years, 56% in persons 10 to 18 years old, and 88% in adulthood. This suggests the acquired origin and the progressive nature of pulmonary damage. Bronchographic abnormalities are mainly located in the right middle lobe, thus confirming the role of the right middle lobe bronchus as a *locus minoris resistentiae*

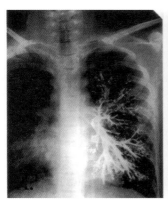
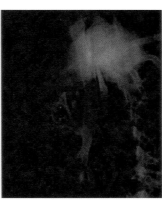
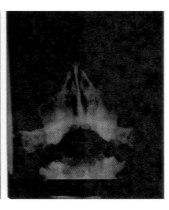

Figure 94–4. Kartagener triad: situs inversus (and bronchiectases) (*left*), bronchiectases (*middle*), and chronic sinusitis (maxillar) (*right*).

in diseases with impaired mucociliary clearance (Pawlik et al., 1998). Digital clubbing may coincide with bronchiectasis (Turner et al., 1991) but is never as severe as that seen in cystic fibrosis.

Results of lung function tests indicate mainly obstructive airway disease, air trapping (ratio of increased residual volume and residual volume to total lung capacity), and unequal ventilation caused by mucus impaction, inflammation, and segmental pulmonary fibrosis (Reyes de la Rocha, 1987).

Chronic rhinosinusitis is one of the most frequent clinical findings in PCD patients, combining nasal congestion and discharge of a mostly thin nasal secretion with chronic or recurrent involvement of mainly maxillary and ethmoidal paranasal sinuses; frontal sinuses frequently fail to develop, and the mastoid cells display poor aeration (Mygind et al., 1983). The radiological signs of sinusitis can be recognized as early as at 6 months of age. Hyponasal speech is very common, but anosmia is an occasional feature. Chronic and severe secretory otitis media, frequently with continuous, long-lasting and offensive discharge from the ears after tympanostomy tube (grommet) insertion, is almost always present in childhood, with occasional eruptions of the acute form of the disease. Sclerosis of the mastoid or middle ear region is often present on radiological examination. A moderate conductive hearing loss between 10 and 40 dB is not infrequent (Pedersen and Mygind, 1983). The sense of balance is normally unaffected (Eliasson et al., 1977). PCD patients usually grow out of most of these symptoms at puberty.

Corneal abnormalities are another side symptom (Svedbergh et al., 1981). Dull, chronic headaches and increased risk of hydrocephalus are most probably caused by impaired circulation of the cerebro-spinal fluid (Afzelius and Mossberg, 1995).

Reproductive Tract Phenotype

Since both sperm flagella and respiratory cilia have an identical internal ultrastructure, affected males are usually characterized by absent or decreased sperm motility (azoospermia, asthenozoospermia). It is worth remembering that the disease was first fully characterized in fertility clinics where the association of male infertility due to abnormal sperm motility and chronic sinopulmonary symptoms was noted (Afzelius, 1976; Elliason et al., 1977). Sterility is almost a rule, although exceptions exist, so fertility does not exclude the diagnosis of PCD in males (Bush et al., 1998). There are many incongruities concerning male infertility in PCD: Kartagener's syndrome has been diagnosed in men with normal ciliary and flagellar ultrastructure (Greenstone et al., 1985), in patients having cilia without dynein arms and normal flagella (Jonsson et al., 1982), and in individuals with flagella without dynein arms and with normal cilia (Wilton et al., 1986). Usually semen analysis shows normal ejaculate volume and sperm concentration, viscosity, liquefaction, and pH also within normal range, but it also shows markedly reduced mean motility: spermatozoa display straight nonprogressive motility with minimal amplitude of lateral head displacement and no potential for hyperactivation (Kay and Irvine, 2000). Patients with hydrocoele or oligospermia are also known. Spermatozoa from men with PCD have a normal ability to capacitate, but, due to a poor motility and absence of hyperactivation, they are unlikely to achieve fertilization in vivo.

The fallopian tubes are lined with ciliated epithelium. As the kinetic activity of ciliated endosalpinx is an important factor in normal ovum transport, ciliary dyskinesia may cause female infertility. Nevertheless, women affected with PCD may be fertile (McComb et al., 1986). The existence of some ciliary activity, although abnormal, may account for fertility in some women with PCD (Halbert et al., 1997). Theoretically, ectopic pregnancy should be more common in affected women because of malfunction of oviduct cilia, but displacement of the egg cell along the oviduct also depends on other mechanisms, such as muscular propulsion (Schidlow, 1994). The problem of female fertility and PCD still lacks reliable analysis.

EPIDEMIOLOGY AND GENETICS

Prevalence and Inheritance

Estimates of prevalence of PCD range from 1 in 15,000 to 1 in 60,000 live births (Afzelius and Mossberg, 1995). Since about half of PCD

cases display situs inversus, incidence of KS is estimated to range between 1 in 30,000 and 1 in 120,000 live births, but the possibly frequent occurrence of PCD without respiratory complaints in situs inversus cases and other circumstances, as noted in this chapter, suggest an incidence of PCD as high as 1 in 12,500 (Kroon et al., 1991; Teknos et al., 1997). It is certain that the frequency of PCD is markedly underestimated. Late diagnosis is common (Gomez de Terreros Caro et al., 1999), even at the age of 60 to 75 years as an extreme, and mild cases are often picked up by screening the nuclear family of the proband. Particularly the group of PCD patients with usual visceral arrangement (theoretically 50% of patients) is often diagnosed later than those with mirror image arrangement: in the absence of malposition of organs, the diagnosis becomes much more difficult.

Inheritance in most cases appears to be via a single major locus with an autosomal recessive mode of transmission (Afzelius and Mossberg, 1995; Afzelius, 1998; McKusick, 2002), although pedigrees showing autosomal dominant or X-linked modes of inheritance have also been reported (Narayan et al., 1994b). The genetic basis of a variety of defects affecting ciliary structure and function in PCD is not clear. Nearly 200 different polypeptides have been identified within the ciliary axoneme of lower organisms, and at least the same number of proteins can be expected in axonemes of humans (Luck et al., 1982). It is rather unlikely that mutations of as many as 200 different genes coding for various ciliary proteins cause the same or similar pathologic consequences of ciliary dysfunction. If this were true, one might expect the incidence of PCD to be much higher than actually reported (McKusick, 2002). It is possible that many ciliary protein gene mutations may be lethal even if heterozygous, while mutations in other genes may not affect ciliary function at all, perhaps due to redundancy of functions of gene families such as dyneins. In any case, the low incidence of KS and PCD suggests that perhaps mutations in a small number of genes may underlie these diseases. This potentially reduced level of locus heterogeneity provides cautious optimism for success of gene mapping efforts.

Candidate Genes and Chromosomal Regions

A number of animal models of PCD have been identified, including examples in the mouse (*iv/iv, inv/inv, hop*) (Handel, 1985; Brueckner et al., 1989; Yokoyama et al., 1993), rat (WIC-Hyd rat) (Torikata et al., 1991), dog (Edwards et al., 1983; Watson et al., 1998), and pig (Roperto et al., 1993). Both dogs (springer spaniels, English setters, Newfoundlands) and pigs have a relatively high incidence of respiratory disease, with the phenotype almost identical to the primary ciliary dyskinesia of humans, but in both species hydrocephalus is an additional prominent component of the syndrome. *Chlamydomonas reinhardtii,* a unicellular alga with two flagella, has an axonemal structure similar to that of human respiratory cilia and sperm tails and thus became a good model for studies of mutational events related to ciliary ultrastructural abnormalities (Blair and Dutcher, 1992). Studies on some of these models helped to focus attention on particular regions of the human genome that contain homologs of genes involved in animal models of PCD, thus creating a list of candidate genes and possible chromosomal locations to be taken into account in genetic mapping of humans (Table 94–1). So far, two human genes have been identified in which mutations underlying the ultrastructural phenotype were found in PCD patients.

DNAI1 (Chromosome 9p13–21)

DNAI1, a human homolog of the *C. reinhardtii* gene *IC78,* was the very first human gene in which mutations causing the ultrastructural phenotype were described in PCD patients (Pennarun et al., 1999). The *DNAI1* gene is highly expressed in the trachea and testes and is composed of 20 exons located at 9p13–21. This gene encodes a dynein intermediate chain found in the outer dynein arms. Originally, two loss-of-function mutations of this gene were identified in a patient with PCD characterized by immotile cilia lacking outer dynein arms: (*1*) maternal insertion of four nucleotides in exon 5, causing a frameshift, and (*2*) paternal T insertion at +3 position of the intron 1 donor site, resulting in absence of splicing. Both mutations generate severely truncated polypeptides lacking 85% and 95%, respectively,

Table 94–1. PCD Candidate Genes and Chromosomal Regions

Chromosomal Region	Gene	Mutations Detected†	Reference
1p35.1	HP28	—	Pennarun et al., 2001
2p14–q14.3	CFC1	In heterotaxy	Bamford et al., 2000
3p21.3	DNAH1		Neesen et al., 2001
4q*			Blouin et al., 2000
5p15–p14	DNAH5		Omran et al., 2000
5q31	KIF3A		Takeda et al., 1999
6p21.3	TUBB	—	Bianchi et al., 1992; Janitz et al., 1999
	MLN	—	
	KNSL2	—	
	HSET	—	
7p15	DNAH11	In PCD	Witt et al., 1999a; Bartoloni et al., 2000
7q33–q34			Handel, 1985
8q*			Blouin et al., 2000
9p13–21	DNAI1	In PCD/KS	Pennarun et al., 1999; Guichard et al., 2001; Zariwala et al., 2001
9q31	Encoding inversin		Morgan et al., 1998
10p*			Blouin et al., 2000
11q*			Blouin et al., 2000
13q*			Blouin et al., 2000
14q32	EMAPL	In Usher syndrome type A1	Bonneau et al., 1993; Narayan et al., 1994a; Eudy et al., 1997
	DNCH1		
15q24			Witt et al., 1999b
16pter*			Blouin et al., 2000
17p12 (17q25)	DNAH9		Bartoloni et al., 2001
17q*			Blouin et al., 2000
19q13.3	RSHL1	In X-linked and sporadic heterotaxy	Gebbia et al., 1997; Blouin et al., 2000; Meeks et al., 2000; Eriksson et al., 2001
	ZIC3		
20	KIF3B		Nonaka et al., 1998

PCD, primary ciliary dyskinesia; KS, Kartagener syndrome.
*Results of a genome-wide low-density linkage analysis.
†Human disorders are shown.

of the DNAI1 protein. However, linkage between this gene and PCD has been excluded in five other families, demonstrating locus heterogeneity of the disease. Further studies of a series of 34 KS families (Guichard et al., 2001) and 7 PCD families with outer dynein arm (ODA) defects (Zariwala et al., 2001) revealed four other mutations of the DNAI1 gene: (3) transition G → A (position 1714or5) in exon 16, resulting in a Gly (highly conserved, potential N-myristoylation site) to Ser transposition at position 515; (4) 12 bp deletion in exon 17, resulting in protein truncation, removing a highly conserved Phe at position 556; (5) G1874C transversion leading to a missense mutation (W568S); and (6) G1875A transition leading to a nonsense mutation (W568X). The last two mutations were present at the conserved Trp residue in the WD-repeat region, which is predicted to lead to an abnormal folding of the DNAI1 protein. The splice defect caused by T insertion of intron 1 is the most common mutation: it is present on one allele in all cases analyzed so far. Mutations of the DNAI1 gene cause either situs solitus (normal) or situs inversus.

The other human dynein intermediate chain 2 gene (DNAI2), located at 17q25, with a similar pattern of tissue specificity of expression, showed no mutations of the coding sequence in 12 PCD patients investigated (Pennarun et al., 2000).

DNAH11 (Chromosome 7p15)

The gene for a β heavy chain of the outer dynein arm maps to the 7p15 region (Kastury et al., 1997), and clones containing sequences homologous to the dynein gene family map to 7q21–q22 and to 7p21. The second gene documented in literature as causative for PCD is the human dynein heavy chain 11 gene (DNAH11) also mapped to chromosome 7. Its homolog is mutated in the mouse iv/iv model of situs inversus (Bartoloni et al., 2000). The mutation analysis of all 40 exons of the human DNAH11 gene was performed, and a nonsense mutation (R to X) was identified in homozygosity in one of the exons coding for the motor domain of DNAH11. The mutation was detected in a patient previously reported as having uniparental disomy of chromosome 7 (UPD7) (Pan et al., 1998). The patient expressed complete situs inversus, motionless respiratory cilia, and cystic fibrosis (due to the homozygous ΔF508 mutation of the CFTR gene located on human chromosome 7). His mother was not a carrier of the CF mutation, and both chromosomes 7 were inherited from his father—a doc-

umented CF carrier—as false maternity was excluded. Electron microscopy analysis in this patient revealed normal cilia and dynein arms, which is compatible with the nonsense mutation in the middle of the motor domain of a heavy chain dynein. The mutant DNAH11 truncated protein could theoretically be incorporated in dynein arms but is inactive due to the lack of microtubule-binding domain.

Before this report, linkage data were obtained from 30 PCD families recruited in Poland, with a multipoint LOD score of < −2.0, which strongly excluded a putative KS gene (at least for a high proportion of families studied) for all or most of chromosome 7 (Witt et al., 1999a, 1998). In this study, PCD families were subclassified either as Kartagener's syndrome (KS) families (if at least one PCD-affected member was diagnosed as having KS—i.e., exhibiting situs inversus) or as ciliary dysfunction only (CDO) families (if none of the members affected with PCD exhibited situs inversus). The KS and CDO families were analyzed separately because of the possibility that different molecular pathologies could underlie these subtypes of PCD. Such a hypothesis is consistent with the fact that mice carrying the hop mutation that maps to a region syntenic to human 7q33–q34 exhibit CDO but not situs inversus. The results of pairwise and multipoint LOD scoring provided a weak suggestion of linkage in only the CDO subset of PCD families. The highest multipoint LOD score of 1.41 for these families occurred precisely at the position where the gene for the β-heavy chain of the outer dynein arm is located. These linkage data remain in perfect agreement with existence of the mutation in the DNAH11 gene in a PCD patient with normal situs.

Chromosome 7q33–q34 is syntenic to a fragment of mouse chromosome 6 containing the hop mutation (previously named hpy). In homozygous form, this mutation causes a dynein defect in cilia and flagella, similar to that seen in PCD and resulting in, for example, male infertility; in contrast to all other mouse models of PCD, these mutants do not show laterality defects (Johnson and Hunt, 1971; Handel, 1985).

Other Genes and Regions Coding for Axonemal Proteins

In other studies, mutations were not detected in six unspecified axonemal dynein heavy chain genes (Poller et al., 1999) or in the DNAH9 gene (Bartoloni et al., 2001). The latter was mapped by FISH and radiation hybrid analysis to 17p12 (Bartoloni et al., 1999; Maiti et al.,

2000b); the alternative map position of this locus is 17q25 (Milisav et al., 1996).

Disruption by homologous recombination of the mouse dynein heavy chain 7 (*Mdhc7*) gene, a homolog of the human *DNAH1* gene, results in male infertility due to dramatically reduced sperm motility and in a ciliary beat frequency reduction, but not in defects in the axonemal structure of tracheal cilia or sperm flagella (Neesen et al., 2001). The *DNAH1* gene was mapped to 3p21.3, which is syntenic to mouse chromosome 14 region B–C that contains the *Mdhc7* gene (Neesen et al., 1997).

Another human candidate gene studied is *HP28* located at 1p35.1 (Pennarun et al., 2001). It is a human ortholog of the *Chlamydomonas p28* gene that encodes a dynein light chain, whose mutations lead to an absence of inner dynein arms in flagellar axonemes of this model organism. The *HP28* gene did not show any mutations in PCD patients analyzed by Pennarun et al. (2001).

Several other human genes or chromosomal regions can be considered candidates for PCD gene locations. A total genome scan performed in a large consanguineous family of Arabic origin (ciliary akinesia, absence of ODA) resulted in localization of a new gene locus for PCD in a region of homozygosity by descent on chromosome 5p15–p14 with a multipoint LOD score of 3.51 (Omran et al., 2000). The gene encoding for a *Chlamydomonas*-related axonemal heavy dynein chain DNAH5 was localized within the critical disease interval.

Another genome scan in five PCD (defect of ODA) families of Arabic origin (four with reported consanguinity) revealed a maximum multipoint LOD score of 4.4 on chromosome 19q13.3, defining a 15 cM critical region of a possible PCD locus location (Meeks et al., 2000). Linkage was not found for this region in two of these families, again confirming locus heterogeneity. Chromosome 19q13.3–qter is a gene-rich region that contains at least two candidates for a PCD locus: (*1*) radial spokehead-like 1 gene (*RSHL1*) residing at the myotonic dystrophy-1 locus—*RSHL1*, expressed in adult testis, codes for radial spokehead-like protein characterized by high homology to proteins of sea urchins and *Chlamydomonas*, important in normal ciliary or flagellar action, including that of sea urchin spermatozoa (Eriksson et al., 2001); (*2*) ZIC3 locus coding for zinc finger transcription factor that is mutated in subjects with X-linked and sporadic laterality defects (Gebbia et al., 1997).

The echinoderm microtubule-associate protein-like gene (*EMAPL*) is located on chromosome 14q32. Mutations in this gene have been shown to cause Usher's syndrome type 1A, and these patients sometimes exhibit ultrastructural defects in the axonemes of their respiratory cilia similar to PCD (Bonneau et al., 1993; Eudy et al., 1997). Human chromosome 14qter contains an axonemal dynein heavy chain gene *DNCH1* (Narayan et al., 1994a).

Genes and Regions Involved in L-R Asymmetry

Candidates for primary ciliary dyskinesia include a whole group of genes that are involved in determination of a left/right asymmetry of internal organs. Left–right (L–R) axis abnormalities or laterality defects are relatively common in humans (1 in 8500 live births). Only a few genes associated with a small percentage of human situs defects have been identified. These include *ZIC3* (Gebbia et al., 1997), *CFC1* (encoding the CRYPTIC protein) (Bamford et al., 2000), *LEFTB* (formerly *LEFTY2*) (Meno et al., 1999), and *ACVR2B* (encoding activin receptor IIB) (Kosaki et al., 1999). Mutations in *ZIC3* (chromosome 19q13.3–qter) and *CFC1* (chromosome 2p14–q14.3) were found in individuals who exhibited heterotaxic phenotypes (randomized organ positioning) (Gebbia et al., 1997; Bamford et al., 2000).

A link between ciliary motility and lateralization has already been provided by mouse mutants defective in the genes that are required for ciliary growth or beating. Randomization of L–R asymmetry due to complete absence of cilia was observed in mice homozygous for mutation of the hepatocyte nuclear factor 3/forkhead homolog-4 (*Hfh)-4* (alias *Foxj1*) gene. Homozygous *Foxj1*$^{-/-}$ mutant mice revealed heterotaxy, or situs inversus totalis, in 50% of the animals and a complete absence of respiratory cilia and spermatic flagella. In addition, left–right dynein (lrd) expression was not observed in the embryonic lungs, suggesting that *Foxj1* may act by regulating expression of

dyneins (Chen et al., 1998). The human homolog *HFH-4*, also called *FKHL13* and recently renamed *FOXJ1*, has been mapped to chromosome 17q22–q25, but mutations of this candidate gene have not been detected in a number of PCD patients studied (Maiti et al., 2000a; Pennarun et al., 2001).

It has been shown that proteins KIF3A and KIF3B of the kinesin superfamily determine L–R asymmetry by participating in the assembly of motile cilia that produce the leftward nodal flow of the extraembryonic fluid in mouse embryo (Nonaka et al., 1998; Takeda et al., 1999; Supp et al., 2000). These genes are located on human chromosomes 5q31 (*KIF3A*) and 20 (*KIF3B*).

Another mouse mutant, *inv* (inversion of embryonic turning), is the only mutation that causes almost 100% of homozygous embryos to develop situs inversus (Yokoyama et al., 1993). These embryos do not survive, and they have cardiovascular, renal, and pancreatic defects. However, cilia show no structural or activity abnormalities. The gene that causes the *inv* mutation has been cloned, and the protein, called "inversin," has ankyrin-like repeats and potential nuclear localization signals (Morgan et al., 1998). This gene reverses the left–right pattern of expression of the *nodal*, *lefty-1*, and *lefty-2* genes, suggesting that inversin acts upstream of these TGF-β-like genes, which are also involved in left–right asymmetry (Supp et al., 2000). The human inversin gene is located on chromosome 9q31.

The mouse mutants *iv/iv* have laterality defects in 50% of offspring, but ciliary abnormalities have not been described (Brueckner et al., 1989). It has been shown that mutations of the *lrd* gene (encoding left/right dynein) are the cause of the *iv* and *legless* (*lgl*) mutants, which exhibit randomization of L–R asymmetry (Supp et al., 1997) through effects on cilia of the embryonic ventral node (Supp et al., 2000). The region to which it is likely to map in humans is on chromosome 7q. This finding definitely confirms the role of the dynein protein family in both ciliary structure/function and lateralization.

Other Genes and Regions

A high-density genomic scan of chromosome 15 using 66 microsatellite markers specific for this chromosomal region was performed separately on 51 families with Kartagener's syndrome and on 19 families of Polish origin with ciliary dysfunction only (Witt et al., 1999b). A maximum pairwise LOD score of 4.23 was obtained for the KS families. This, together with results of nonparametric analyses, localized a *KS* gene to a 10 cM region of 15q24. In CDO families, linkage to this chromosomal location was negative, demonstrating locus heterogeneity dependent on the presence or absence of situs inversus among PCD individuals.

A genome-wide linkage search performed in 31 multiplex PCD families failed to identify the major disease locus, confirming the common conviction on extensive locus heterogeneity (Blouin et al., 2000). Potential genomic regions harboring PCD loci were localized on chromosomes 3p, 4q, 5p, 7p, 8q, 10p, 11q, 13q, 15q, 16p, 17q, and 19q. Linkage analyses in PCD families with a documented dynein arm deficiency provided suggestive evidence for linkage to chromosomal regions 8q and 16pter, while analyses carried out exclusively in Kartagener's syndrome families resulted in pointing toward 8q and 19q as possible locations of the *KS* locus.

The *HLA* region of chromosome 6p contains the β-tubulin gene (*TUBB*) (Volz et al., 1994) and was suggested to be linked to PCD in one study (Bianchi et al., 1992). However, the motilin gene (*MLN*), which also resides in this region, was not supported as a candidate for involvement in PCD etiology in another study (Gasparini et al., 1994b), and recombination was also observed in another family (Gasparini et al., 1994a). Another candidate gene located in the HLA region is the kinesin-like 2 gene (*KNSL2*) (Janitz et al., 1999). Kinesins are involved in ciliary beating (Supp et al., 2000), and this gene is located at the centromeric end of the major histocompatibility complex. Four single-base substitutions were detected in the *HSET* gene (kinesin-related protein), mapped also to 6p21.3, in two PCD families studied (Janitz et al., 1999).

It is clear that PCD is genetically heterogeneous, with different genes involved in different families, depending, in part, on whether situs inversus is present (i.e., KS versus CDO subtypes of PCD). The successes obtained thus far already confirm that PCD is not commonly caused by hundreds of different genes, even though the cilia themselves have many structural and assembly and regulatory proteins. Future priorities are to identify the genes that reside in the mapped regions and to identify new genes by combinations of linkage and linkage disequilibrium gene-mapping strategies and by mutation screening of appropriate candidate genes. With the imminent final completion of the human genome sequences, and with mouse and *Chlamydomonas* sequences coming in the near future, information on many genes that affect cilia and left–right asymmetry—such as dyneins, nexins, kinesins, myosins, and others (Hirokawa, 1998; Mermall et al., 1998; Izraeli et al., 1999; Tamura et al., 1999; Rankin et al., 2000)—rapidly accumulates in genomic databases, making new promises toward identification of the genes that cause primary ciliary dyskinesia.

DIAGNOSTIC STANDARDS AND PROBLEMS

Certain criteria for diagnosis of primary ciliary dyskinesia have been established, but in reality most, if not all, create significant problems in reliable interpretation.

Clinical Diagnosis

Patients with the complete or partial syndrome may present to a wide variety of practitioners and specialists: family doctors, neonatologists, pediatricians, pulmonologists, laryngologists, ophthalmologists, allergologists, urologists, andrologists, and gynecologists. All these specialists should be aware of the existence of PCD and be able to diagnose the syndrome in cases of high index of clinical suspicion. In practice, PCD often remains unrecognized, hence underdiagnosed and poorly treated.

The following groups of patients require in-depth screening for PCD:
- Newborns with sital congenital anomalies
- Children with atypical or refractory "asthma"
- Allergic children and adults
- Children and adults with rhinosinusitis or chronic severe otitis media, particularly when discharge persists after grommet insertion
- Children and adults with a chronic respiratory infection, with or without bronchiectases, and particularly children producing purulent sputum
- Sub- or infertile males and females, particularly when respiratory infection coexists

In differential diagnosis, PCD should be distinguished from cystic fibrosis, allergy, immune deficiency, Young syndrome, and asplenia or polysplenia (Shidlow, 1994).

Diagnostic Laboratory Tests

Nasal Nitric Oxide Level

Nasal nitric oxide (NO) level is a relatively recent measurement that has recently been proved to be of utmost importance in diagnosing PCD (Karadag et al., 1999). Nitric oxide influences various aspects of airway homeostasis, the regulation of ciliary motility, and host defense. NO is generated by the paranasal sinus epithelium and then diffuses into the nasal cavities. It is present in measurable quantities in the exhaled air of normal subjects. Higher concentrations are recorded in patients with asthma and bronchiectasis (not treated with glucocorticoids), and lower concentrations are found in patients with cystic fibrosis, diffused panbronchiolitis, and systemic sclerosis with pulmonary hypertension; the lowest are definitely in patients with primary ciliary dyskinesia (Lundberg, 1996). Similarly, nasal concentrations of NO are markedly reduced in children with PCD and CF: normal level >250 ppb, in CF about 180 ppb, in PCD 25 ppb or less. A simple, noninvasive chemiluminescent test can be applied for measurements (Larj et al., 2001). Interestingly, NO levels in PCD carriers (e.g., parents of affected children) are intermediate between normal concentrations and levels found in CF patients. The phenomenon of reduced NO level in PCD is caused by the lack of inducible nitric oxide synthetase in the nasal epithelium of patients with primary ciliary dyskinesia (Wodehouse et al., 2001). Assessment of nasal NO level is the best way to distinguish between primary and secondary ciliary dyskinesia, which is a diagnostic dilemma of particular clinical importance.

Saccharin Test

This test requires cooperation of the patient; thus it is suitable for older children and adults rather than for young children. This is the most widely used screening test for PCD. A small particle of saccharin is placed on the nasal inferior turbinate about 10 mm from the anterior end. The time to a sweet taste of saccharin in the mouth is a measure of nasal mucociliary clearance (NMCC): extension of the time beyond 60 minutes indicates an impairment of NMCC (Greenstone and Cole, 1985). Currently, a modified version of this test with the use of albumin labeled with radioactive technetium (instead of saccharin) is being applied.

Light Microscopy

The most frequently used way to obtain ciliated cells for microscopic analysis is by brushing the inferior meatus at the lateral aspect of the inferior turbinate with a special cytology brush (Rutland et al., 1982). Alternatively, ciliated mucosa may be obtained from the middle turbinate or from the bronchus through bronchoscopy. Epithelial chunks are then dislodged to a cell culture medium, or saline and ciliary motility can be evaluated under the light microscope, with a subsequent oscillometric assessment of a ciliary beat frequency, or waveform. The approximate normal range of ciliary beat frequency in vivo in nasal biopsies is 11 to 16 per second. The interpretation of results may be difficult because of inadequate quality of nasal specimens due to nasal infections: ideally the patient should be free from upper respiratory tract infections for 4 to 6 weeks before the examination (Bush et al., 1998).

Electron Microscopy

For ultrastructural studies, biopsied nasal or bronchial epithelium or sperm specimens should be fixed immediately and processed for transmission electron microscopy. The specimen should be examined by an experienced pathologist. At least five ciliary cross-sections of good quality from each of 10 different nonadjacent cells should be studied as a minimum at magnifications of about × 100,000 to 150,000; ideally, the ciliated cells should be derived from at least two different sites in the respiratory tract (Bush et al., 1998). Abnormalities in up to 10% of cilia should be considered not indicative of pathology (de Iongh and Rutland, 1995). No clearly defined clinical differences have been attributed so far to the different ultrastructural defects.

In vitro Ciliogenesis

Another frequent problem in PCD diagnostics is a distinction between primary and secondary defects in ciliary structure and function. Primary (PCD) and secondary (SCD) ciliary dyskinesia are frequently associated (Jorissen et al., 2000a, 2000b). Respiratory infections and inflammations triggered by PCD may easily cause SCD. The secondary abnormalities may be superimposed on primary ones, altering the complete picture and interpretation. The primary abnormality may be missed, or the secondary abnormality may be taken as primary, and so on. Evaluation of cilia without secondary abnormalities being present would facilitate the diagnosis or exclusion of PCD. This can be achieved by structural and functional analysis of cilia resulting from in vitro ciliogenesis in the sequential monolayer-suspension culture instead of biopsied cilia: respiratory epithelial cells cultured in monolayer lose their cilia; these deciliated cells brought in suspension regain respiratory-type morphology and coordinated ciliary activity (Jorissen et al., 1989). Cilia obtained through such in vitro ciliogenesis express only primary, inherited structural and functional abnormalities not influenced by secondary phenomena.

PCD-like Syndrome

The problem faced by a pathologist or clinician team is a PCD-like syndrome with all the clinical manifestations of the classical PCD but with normal ciliary beat frequency and normal ultrastructural architecture. Measurement of nasal NO level defines the diagnosis but does not present any morphological basis for the syndrome. Ciliary disorientation was described as a possible variant of PCD (Rutland and de Iongh, 1990), in which ultrastructural anatomical deficiency is replaced by a random ciliary orientation. Similarly to ultrastructural deficiency, this can also be either primary or secondary, but the latter does not necessarily revert to normal along with proper treatment. It turns out that ciliary disorientation in PCD-like syndrome does not exceed disorientation in, for example, idiopathic bronchiectasis, which raises the question whether the primary ciliary disorientation really exists.

Diagnostic Algorithm

The rational, widely accepted, general diagnostic algorithm in standard cases (Bush et al., 1998) encompasses the following steps:
1. Physical examination
   if the index of clinical suspicion for PCD is high
   ↓
2. Saccharin test (to be skipped in young children) and/or NO level measurement
   if pathological
   ↓
3. Examination of ciliary beat frequency on nasal brushings
   if pathological
   ↓
4. Ultrastructural anatomy analysis and/or orientation studies
   ↓
5. To be repeated after treatment and in clinically atypical cases.

PRINCIPLES OF TREATMENT

The treatment of PCD is essentially symptomatic. The aim of treatment of respiratory problems should be prevention of chronic lung damage and bronchiectasis. Suppression of cough, which is the sole clearance mechanism in the affected lungs, should be avoided. Two main treatment modalities applicable to PCD are antibiotic treatment and chest physiotherapy with postural drainage. In contrast to cystic fibrosis, a prophylactic regimen of antibiotic therapy does not appear to be significantly helpful in PCD. Prolonged, high-dose oral antibiotics should be prescribed at any sign of increase of respiratory symptoms or deterioration of lung function. Intravenous treatment should be applied when the patient's improvement on regular treatment is not satisfactory. Daily physiotherapy is essential for augmenting airway clearance in order to delay the onset and progression of obstructive airway disease; it is also extremely important when bronchiectasis is present. After encouraging experiences in cystic fibrosis, nebulized recombinant human DNase (rhDNase) is currently recommended for some PCD patients: the drug reduces sputum viscosity and volume, improves pulmonary function, and results in a small reduction in the acute respiratory exacerbations that require intravenous antibiotics (Desai et al., 1995; ten Berge et al., 1999). Surgical resection of affected lung lobes may be considered if saccular bronchiectasis is precisely localized. Physical exercise may enhance sputum clearance in PCD more effectively than bronchodilator (β-2 agonist) treatment (Bush et al., 1998). Abandonment of smoking seems to be one of the most important preventive measures.

If secretory recurrent otitis media affects hearing, speech, and educational ability, insertion of bilateral myringotomy tubes (grommets) is being applied almost universally. Alternatively, unilateral grommet insertion and use of hearing aids may be considered (Ernesson et al.,1984; Hadfield et al., 1997). However, grommet insertion does not earn unequivocal support due to the common complication of prolonged and severe chronic otorrhea in these patients (Meeks and Bush, 2000). Maxillary sinusitis can be treated through endoscopic surgery, especially in older patients refractory to pharmacological treatment (Schidlow, 1994).

Until recently there was no treatment available for male infertility due to PCD. The development of assisted reproductive techniques has allowed rational treatment for these patients, and there are some reports on pregnancies resulting from subzonal insemination (SUZI) (Nijs et al., 1996) and intracytoplasmic sperm injection (ICSI)

(Chemes et al., 1998). Moreover, a successful treatment by in vitro fertilization (IVF) recently has been described; the male partner of the couple had Kartagener's syndrome characterized by deficient dynein arms and disordered microtubular configuration in flagellar ultrastructure (Kay and Irvine, 2000).

GENETIC COUNSELING

For technical purposes of genetic counseling, a general scheme of counseling of cystic fibrosis families can be followed. The risk of PCD in children of an affected parent is either 50% or zero, depending on the carrier status of the spouse. Assuming theoretically an incidence of PCD of about 1 in 15,000, the frequency of heterozygotes (according to the Hardy-Weinberg equilibrium for low incidence) is about 1:61, and the occurrence risk of PCD in a child is about 0.8%. Assuming the genetic heterogeneity of PCD, this risk is somewhat overestimated (Rott, 1998). A 25% recurrence risk should be thoroughly discussed with the family at risk, according to usual rules. At present, neither diagnostic identification of mutations for index cases nor heterozygosity testing can be routinely applied to PCD due to the still unsolved problem of the gene or genes that cause the disorder. On the basis of the author's experience in counseling these families, a presentation of differences between PCD and cystic fibrosis is frequently expected and appreciated by patients.

A micromanipulative-assisted reproduction (ICSI, SUZI) becomes a preferentially applied treatment modality for male sterility in PCD. Since application of these procedures may cause an increase in the overall genetic risk of the resulting pregnancies—for example, with sex chromosome abnormalities (Levron et al., 2001)—a full spectrum of routine prenatal genetic testing should be offered in such cases (Meschede et al., 1995). However, there is no specific prenatal diagnosis for PCD available. Cardiac dextroposition in fetuses affected with Kartagener's syndrome may be recognized by ultrasound analysis (Abdullah et al., 2000). Since PCD seems to be evenly distributed among different ethnic groups, there is no apparent racial predilection in prevalence of the disorder.

MOUSE MODELS

The anomalous phenotypes caused by defects of the left–right thoracoabdominal asymmetry development are strikingly similar in mice and humans. Over 20 different mouse genes involved in this process have already been identified (Schneider and Brueckner, 2000). Among them four categories can be distinguished.

Genes Involved in Formation of the Embryonic Node

The node (organizer) is a separate structure at the distal tip of the murine gastrulating embryo, the mammalian equivalent of Hensen's node in chicken and Spemann's organizer in *Xenopus*, displaying a direct contact between the ectoderm and endoderm and being a major organizing center in early-stage embryos that regulates pattern formation. The "organizing" function is restricted to endodermal, ventral cells of the node. Each ventral node cell carries a single cilium (monocilium) that points away from the embryo into the extracellular fluid (Bellomo et al., 1996). The node is essential for both gastrulation and body axes formation. Defects of genes directly affecting its formation, such as mutant *nodal* (−/−), are lethal early in development (Conlon et al., 1994). Mutations of other genes of this group have less severe effects: mutations of the transcription factor *Hnf3* gene result in a failure to develop a node (Collignon et al. 1996), and situs inversus has been detected in 50% of mouse mutants *brachyury*, having mutations in the *T* gene (a transcription factor) and lacking the mature notochord (King et al., 1998).

Genes Required to Assemble and Move Nodal Monocilia

Ciliary structure and function are defective in several mouse mutants and affect L–R axis development. These mutations occur in various genes and their only commonality, besides abnormal development of LR asymmetry, is the effect on cilia. This fact lends strong support to the argument that L–R asymmetry is established by specific functions of cilia during embryogenesis (Brueckner, 2001). Out of a group of genes that affect either the assembly of cilia or ciliary kinetic activity (or both), targeted mutagenesis of kinesins KIF3A and KIF3B results in failure to assemble motile ciliary axonemes (Morris and Scholey, 1997). KIF3A and KIF3B proteins form a heterotrimeric complex with an associated protein KAP3 (Yamazaki et al., 1995). Heterotrimeric kinesin homologs are found in many species, including mice, *C. elegans, Chlamydomonas,* and sea urchins. Kif3A/kif3B homozygous mutants have no node monocilia and display abnormal L–R expression of markers of embryonal asymmetry (Nonaka et al., 1998; Takeda et al., 1999). A similar phenotype is displayed by mice that lack the tetratricorepeat protein *polaris,* with absent node monocilia and defective L–R development (Murcia et al., 2000); in fact, phenotypes of both mutants are indistinguishable from each other. Like heterotrimeric kinesin, the *Chlamydomonas* homolog of *polaris* functions in intraflagellar transport (IFT) (Pazour et al., 2000). Therefore, both kinesin and *polaris* are likely to be required to assemble functional node cilia. The recessive mutation *iv (inversus viscerum)* results in random asymmetry, with 50% of liveborn homozygous mutants displaying situs inversus in the absence of any other defects (Supp et al., 1999). The *iv* phenotype is caused by a missense mutation in the motor domain of an axonemal dynein heavy-chain gene *LR dynein* (*lrd*) (Supp et al., 1997): the node cilia in mice with mutated *lrd* are present, being normal in size and distribution but immotile, frozen in a rigorlike state (Supp et al., 1999). The *inv/inv* insertional mouse mutants (*inversion of embryonal turning*) display situs inversus in 100% (Yokoyama et al., 1993), and the mutant results from disruption of the gene coding for inversin (Morgan et al., 1998). In addition to the aberrant shape of the *inv/inv* node itself, the defective monocilia rotate more rapidly than they usually do (Okada et al., 1999).

A further link between ciliary morphogenesis and L–R asymmetry has been provided by targeted mutants of the transcription factor Hfh4 (hepatocyte nuclear factorB3/forkhead homolog 4), a member of the forkhead/winged-helix family of transcription factors. Hfh4 is expressed in ciliated cells, both embryonal and epithelial. Hfh4$^{-/-}$ mice are devoid of all 9 + 2 cilia, but their 9 + 0 cilia at the embryonic node are present. These mutants show random development of L–R asymmetry, accompanied by heart defects and hydrocephalus (Chen et al., 1998; Brody et al., 2000). Positioning of the basal bodies in Hfh4$^{-/-}$ ciliated epithelia is abnormal, and the ultrastructure of their node monocilia is unknown (Brueckner, 2001). It is possible that Hfh4 is necessary for assembly of the more complex 9 + 2 cilia or for transport of ciliary components required for normal motility into 9 + 0 node cilia (Schneider and Brueckner, 2000). It has been shown as a surprise by videomicroscopy (Nonaka et al., 1998) that, in fact, node monocilia are motile and move in a directional, vortical manner, distinct from the bending movement of 9 + 2 cilia. The motility of node monocilia drives directional, leftward movement of the extracellular fluid surrounding the node (Brueckner, 2001). All the mutants described here show that disturbance of motility of the node monocilia results for the embryo in wrongly distinguishing its left side from the right.

Genes Responsible for Conveying the Nodal Asymmetry

This group of genes and their protein products form a complex signaling pathway that is required to expand L–R asymmetry information generated at the embryonic node to the immediately adjacent developing embryo (Schneider and Brueckner, 2000). *Nodal* plays a direct and pivotal role in L–R patterning, initially being expressed symmetrically around the node and further in the development getting restricted exclusively to the left side, functioning downstream of the node monocilia and LR dynein (in the *iv/iv* mice all the asymmetric *nodal* expression becomes random [Lowe et al., 1996]). *Nodal*$^{-/-}$ mutants do not gastrulate, but compound double heterozygous mutants *nodal/HNF-3β* or *nodal/Smad2* display obvious laterality defects. This effect is due to haploinsufficiency for *nodal,* since both *Smad2* and *HNF-3β* single heterozygotes are perfectly normal (Schneider and Brueckner, 2000). The *nodal* signaling of L–R asymmetry informa-

tion, requires the EGF-CFC protein *cryptic* as a cofactor to expand L–R asymmetric gene expression from the area immediately surrounding the node to the periphery: *cryptic*$^{-/-}$ mice express *nodal* at the node early in development but never come to the stage of normal left-side peripheral *nodal* expression (Yashiro et al., 2000). *Lefty-2,* another member of the TGF-β family, undergoing asymmetric peripheral expression during mouse embryo development, most probably acts as an inhibitor of the *nodal* signaling pathway (Meno et al., 1999). Factors downstream of *nodal,* conveying L–R information to individual organ primordia, are activin receptor type II and a bicoid-related homeobox gene *Pitx2*: both *ActRIIB*$^{-/-}$ and *Pitx2*$^{-/-}$ mice display certain abnormalities of laterality (Kosaki et al., 1999; Lu et al., 1999).

Genes Involved in Forming and Maintaining the Midline

Mouse and zebrafish mutants that display defects in axial midline structures frequently also have defects in L–R patterning and expression of left-side specific genes (Schneider and Brueckner, 2000). Such a midline barrier could have either a biochemical or a physical nature (or both) (Meno et al., 1998). *Sonic hedgehog (Shh)* is required for development of the midline and of L–R asymmetry, at least partly through the induction of *lefty-1* expression (Chiang et al., 1996; Meyers and Martin, 1999): *lefty-1* is a candidate for the "midline barrier" molecule required to maintain L–R asymmetry (Meno et al., 1998). *Shh*$^{-/-}$ mice display randomized developmental laterality, while *lefty-1*$^{-/-}$ show left pulmonary isomerism and heterotaxia. It seems that absence of *lefty-1* results in bilateral (or ectopic right-hand-side) expression of downstream signaling molecules, like *lefty-2* and *Pitx2,* which are thought to determine "leftness" (Schneider and Brueckner, 2000). Other mouse mutations that affect the midline include defects of FGF-8 and hGDF-1, both resulting in right pulmonary isomerism and in situs inversus displayed by some of the mutants (Meyers and Martin, 1999; Rankin et al., 2000).

DEVELOPMENTAL PATHOGENESIS OF PCD

Our understanding of human heterotaxy syndromes comes mainly from striking analogies between humans and mice with regard to a highly conserved fundamental mechanism governing left–right axis development. All of the described mouse genes, mutants, and phenotypes point to the role of node monocilia in signaling L–R asymmetry to the developing embryo. At first, asymmetry requires properly assembled and motile node monocilia. The major mechanism linking ciliary activity with development of the L–R axis seems to be based on the fact that directional vortical, anticlockwise movement of node monocilia generates a net leftward flow of the extracellular fluid that surrounds the node. The detailed cascade of events breaking the embryonic internal bilateral symmetry still remains elusive, however. Most probably, the nodal flow results in an uneven distribution of a putative soluble morphogen: higher concentration on the left, and lower concentration on the right side of the node. The concentrated morphogenic substance interacts with its receptor molecule with a far higher ratio on the left than on the right. The candidates for a putative soluble asymmetry factor actually include any protein secreted into the perinodal fluid (Schneider and Brueckner, 2000), especially those involved in midline maintenance, like sonic hedgehog (Chiang et al., 1996), fgf8 (Meyers and Martin, 1999), or GDF1 (growth and differentiation factor 1) (Rankin et al., 2000). This initially obtained, subtle asymmetry of the node and of the perinodal area is then amplified and communicated to the neighboring region or regions by a complex feedback loop that involves *nodal,* the TGF-β growth factor, as a pivotal factor. Then, this embryonal "left identity" (marked by a left-sided expression of *nodal*) triggers the cascade of asymmetric expression of various genes to signal this early stable asymmetry to the developing organ primordia.

The resulting asymmetric pattern of localization of various proteins is prevented from diffusing back across the midline (Schneider and Brueckner, 2000). The extent of the asymmetric nature of the soluble morphogen influence is conditioned by the velocity of nodal flow and by the kinetics of the ligand–receptor interaction (both coupling and breakdown of the complex). In this model, the absence of a functional morphogen or its receptor (or both) will result in maintenance of bilateral symmetry instead of asymmetry. If the nodal flow were inhibited by the absence or dysfunction-causing defect of node monocilia, but both the soluble morphogen and its receptor remain intact, the nondirectional nodal flow generated most probably by the physical movement of the embryo within the uterus would disperse the asymmetry chemical factor evenly in the vicinity of the node, resulting in random activation of its receptor. The effect of such an action would be randomization of asymmetry of the developing embryo. Such a random distribution between situs solitus and situs inversus (50% : 50%) is precisely the phenotype observed in humans with Kartagener's syndrome and in mice with mutation in *lrd* (Brueckner, 2001). Several human homologs of genes required for L–R development in mice have already been identified, including *LR dynein*, *fgf-8*, *nodal*, *lefty-1* and *lefty-2*, *Pitx2*, and *ActR2B*. As in mice, human phenotypes resulting from mutations in the genes that control L–R development correlate with the specific defective developmental steps. Most frequently, human mutations causing various L–R defects (heterotaxy syndromes) in heterozygous form cause similar effects as the corresponding homozygous mouse mutations (Schneider and Brueckner, 2000).

One explanation for the relationship between axonemal ultrastructural defects and situs inversus in PCD may be that normal ciliary function plays a part in organ orientation, whereas organ orientation in PCD is a random event because of dysfunctional cilia in early embryonic development. An alternative hypothesis for the association between PCD and situs inversus is that the same gene mutation in PCD-affected subjects causes both defective cilia and organ laterality through independent molecular pathways, rather than the cilia defect itself directly causing the loss of left right asymmetry. This mechanism could involve either pleiotropic effects of a single KS gene or action of a relatively common variation at a situs inversus modifier gene or genes linked or unlinked to the KS gene, but expressed only when the KS gene mutation is present (i.e., gene interaction). A pair of monozygotic PCD twins was reported to be discordant in their organ laterality, with one diagnosed as KS, the other as PCD without situs inversus (Noone et al., 1999). This observation is most consistent with the view that the KS gene mutation itself causes a randomization of the direction of left–right asymmetry and argues against the influence of genetic variation at "modifier" genes affecting the outcome. Caution should be exercised, however, against generalizing too broadly to all cases of KS and PCD from this one observation.

NOTE ADDED IN PROOF

Recently an important candidate gene for PCD pathogenesis, *DNAH5* has been characterized (Olbrich et al., 2002). It is expressed mainly in lung and kidney, but also in brain, heart, and testis. Eight various mutations were found in PCD families, both with and without situs inversus, all with outer dynein arms defect. Murine homolog *Dnahc5* is expressed in the embryonal node. Mutations in *DNAH5* cause PCD with randomiation of LR asymmetry. DNAH5 is the first recognized axonemal dynein heavy chain that is essential for nodal and respiratory cilia function.

ACKNOWLEDGMENTS

This chapter was written in part within the grant 3PO5E 019 23 of the State Committee for Scientific Research (KBN). X-ray pictures were generously supplied by Dr. Jacek Pawlik (Rabka, Poland) and EM-grams by Dr. Robbert de Iongh and Dr. Jonathan Rutland (Sydney, Australia). The manuscript was critically read by Dr. Ewa Zietkiewicz (who also contributed the computer drawing of ciliary cross section) and Dr. Lucyna Majka (both Poznan, Poland).

REFERENCES

Abdullah MM, Lacro RV, Smallhorn J, Chitayat D, van der Velde ME, Yoo SJ, Oman-Ganes L, Hornberg LK (2000). Fetal cardiac dextroposition in the absence of an intrathoracic mass: sign of significant right lung hypoplasia. *J Ultrasound Med* 19: 669–676.

Afzelius BA (1976). A human syndrome caused by immotile cilia. *Science* 193: 317–319.

Afzelius BA (1979). The immotile cilia syndrome and other ciliary diseases. *Int Rev Exp Pathol* 19: 1–43.

Afzelius BA (1981). "Immotile cilia" syndrome and ciliary abnormalities induced by infection and injury. *Am Rev Respir Dis* 124: 107–109.

Afzelius BA (1998). Immotile cilia syndrome: past, present, and prospects for the future. *Thorax* 53: 894–897.

Afzelius BA, Mossberg B (1995). Immotile-cilia syndrome (primary ciliary dyskinesia), including Kartagener syndrome. In: *The Metabolic and Molecular Bases of Inherited Diseases, 7th edition*. Scriver C, Beaudet AL, Sly W, Valle D (eds.) McGraw-Hill, New York, pp. 3943–3954.

Afzelius BA, Gargani G, Romano C (1985). Abnormal length of cilia as a possible cause of defective mucociliary clearance. *Eur J Respir Dis* 66:173–180.

Bamford RN, Roessler E, Burdine RD, Saplakoglu U, dela Cruz J, Splitt M, Towbin J, Bowers P, Marino B, Schier AF, et al. (2000). Loss-of-function mutations in the EGF-CFC gene *CFC1* are associated with human left–right laterality defects. *Nat Genet* 26: 365–369.

Bartoloni L, Blouin J-L, Sainsbury AJ, Gos A, Morris MA, Affara NA, DeLozier-Blanchet CD, Antonarakis SE (1999). Assignment of the human dynein heavy chain gene DNAH17L to human chromosome 17p12 by in situ hybridization and radiation hybrid mapping. *Cytogenet Cell Genet* 84: 188–189.

Bartoloni L, Pan Y, Rossier C, Blouin J-L, Craigen WJ, Antonarakis SE (2000). The DNAH11 (axonemal heavy chainb dynein type 11) gene is mutated in one form of primary ciliary dyskinesia. *Am J Hum Genet* 67 (Suppl): 27.

Bartoloni L, Blouin J-L, Maiti AK, Sainsbury A, Rossier C, Gehrig C, She J-X, Marron MP, Lander ES, Meeks M, et al. (2001). Axonemal β heavy chain dynein DNAH9: cDNA sequence, genomic structure, and investigation of its role in primary ciliary dyskinesia. *Genomics* 72: 21–33.

Baruch GR, Gottfried E, Pery M, Sahin A, Etzioni A (1989). Immotile cilia syndrome including polysplenia, situs inversus and extrahepatic biliary atresia. *Am J Med Genet* 33: 390–393.

Bellomo D, Lander A, Harragan I, Brown NA (1996). Cell proliferation in mammalian gastrulation: the ventral node and notochord are relatively quiescent. *Dev Dyn* 205: 471–485.

Bianchi E, Savasta S, Calligaro A, Beluffi G, Poggi P, Tinelli M, Mevio E, Martinetti M (1992). HPA haplotype segregation and ultrastructural study in familial immotile-cilia syndrome. *Hum Genet* 89: 270–274.

Blair DF, Dutcher SK (1992). Flagella in prokaryotes and lower eukaryotes. *Curr Opin Genet Dev* 2: 756–767.

Blouin JL, Meeks M, Radhakrishna U, Sainsbury A, Gehring C, Sail GD, Bartolini L, Dombi V, O'Rawe A, Walne A, et al. (2000). Primary ciliary dyskinesia: a genome-wide linkage analysis reveals extensive locus heterogeneity. *Eur J Hum Genet* 8: 109–118.

Bonneau D, Raymond F, Kremer C, Klossek J-M, Kaplan J, Patte F (1993). Usher syndrome type I associated with bronchiectasis and immotile nasal cilia in two brothers. *J Med Genet* 30: 253–254.

Brody SL, Yan XH, Wuerffel MK, Song SK, Shapiro SD (2000). Ciliogenesis and left-right axis defects in forkhead factor HFH-4-null mice. *Am J Respir Cell Mol Biol* 23: 45–51.

Brueckner M (2001). Cilia propel the embryo in the right direction. *Am J Med Genet* 101: 339–344.

Brueckner M, D'Eustachio P, Horwich AL (1989). Linkage mapping of a mouse gene, "*iv*," that controls left–right asymmetry of the heart and viscera. *Proc Natl Acad Sci USA* 86: 5035–5038.

Bush A (2000). Primary ciliary dyskinesia. *Acta Otorhinolaryngol Belg* 54: 317–324.

Bush A, Cole P, Hariri M, Mackay I, Phillips G, O'Callaghan C, Wilson R, Warner JO (1998). Primary ciliary dyskinesia: diagnosis and standards of care. *Eur Respir J* 12: 982–988.

Chemes HE, Brugo Olmedo S, Carrere C, Oses R, Carizza C, Leisner M, Blaquier J (1998). Ultrastructural pathology of the sperm flagellum: association between flagellar pathology and fertility prognosis in severely asthenozoospermic men. *Hum Reprod* 13: 2521–2526.

Chen J, Knowles HJ, Hebert JL, Hackett BP (1998). Mutation of the mouse hepatocyte nuclear factor/forkhead homologue 4 gene results in an absence of cilia and random left–right asymmetry. *J Clin Invest* 102: 1077–1082.

Chiang C, Litingtung Y, Lee E, Young KE, Corden JL, Westphal H, Beachy PA (1996). Cyclopia and defective axial patterning in mice lacking sonic hedgehog gene function. *Nature* 383: 407–413.

Collignon J, Varlet I, Robertson EJ (1996). Relationship between asymmetric nodal expression and the direction of embryonic turning. *Nature* 381: 155–158.

Conlon FL, Lyons KM, Takaesu N, Barth KS, Kispert A, Herrmann B, Robertson EJ (1994). A primary requirement for nodal in the formation and maintenance of the primitive streak in the mouse. *Development* 120: 1919–1928.

de Iongh RU, Rutland J (1995). Ciliary defects in healthy subjects, bronchiectasis, and primary ciliary dyskinesia. *Am J Respir Crit Care Med* 151: 1559–1567.

Desai M, Weller PH, Spencer DA (1995). Clinical benefit from nebulized human recombinant DNase in Kartagener's syndrome. *Pediatr Pulmonol* 20: 307–308.

Edwards DF, Patton CS, Bemis DA (1983). Immotile cilia syndrome in three dogs from a litter. *J Am Vet Med Assoc* 183: 667–672.

Eliasson R, Mossberg B, Camner P, Afzelius BA (1977). The immotile-cilia syndrome: a congenital ciliary abnormality as an etiologic factor in chronic airway infections and male sterility. *N Engl J Med* 297: 1–5.

Eriksson M, Ansved T, Anvret M, Carey N (2001). A mammalian radial spokehead-like gene, RSHL1, at the myotonic dystrophy-1 locus. *Biochem Biophys Res Commun* 281: 835–841.

Ernesson S, Afzelius BA, Mossberg B (1984). Otologic manifestation of the immotile-cilia syndrome. *Acta Otolaryngol (Stockholm)* 97: 83–85.

Eudy JD, Edmonds M, Yao SF, Talmadge CB, Kelley PM, Weston MD, Kimberling WJ, Sumegi J (1997). Isolation of a novel human homologue of the gene coding for echinoderm microtubule-associated protein (EMAP) from the Usher syndrome type 1a locus at 14q32. *Genomics* 43: 104–106.

Gasparini P, Griffa A, Oggiano N, Fabrizzi E, Giorgi PL (1994a). Immotile cilia syndrome: a recombinant family at HLA-linked gene locus. *Am J Med Genet* 49: 450–451.

Gasparini P, Grifa A, Savasta S, Merlo I, Bisceglia L, Totaro A, Zelante L (1994b). The motilin gene: subregional localisation, tissue expression, DNA polymorphisms and exclusion as a candidate gene for the HLA-associated immotile cilia syndrome. *Hum Genet* 94: 671–674.

Gebbia M, Ferrero GB, Pilia G, Bassi MT, Aylsworth A, Penman-Split M, Bird LM, Bamforth JS, Burn J, et al. (1997). X-linked situs abormalities result from mutations in ZIC3. *Nat Genet* 17: 305–308.

Gemou Engesaeth V, Warner JO, Bush A (1993). New associations of primary ciliary dyskinesia syndrome. *Pediatr Pulmonol* 16: 9–12.

Gomez de Terreros Caro FJ, Gomez-Stern Aguilar C, Alvarez-Sala R, Prados Sanchez C, Garcia Rio F, Villamor Leon J (1999). Kartagener's syndrome: diagnosis in a 75-year-old woman. *Arch Bronconeumol* 35: 242–244.

Greenstone M, Cole PJ (1985). Ciliary function in health and disease. *Br J Dis Chest* 79: 9–26.

Greenstone M, Rutman A, Pavia D (1985). Normal axonemal structure and function in Kartagener's syndrome: an explicable paradox. *Thorax* 40: 956–957.

Greenstone MA, Jones RWA, Dewar A, Neville BGR, Cole PJ (1984). Hydrocephalus and primary ciliary dyskinesia. *Arch Dis Child* 59: 481–482.

Guichard C, Harricane M-C, Lafitte J-J, Godard P, Zaegel M, Tack V, Lalau G, Bouvagnet P (2001). Axonemal dynein intermediate-chain gene (*DNAI1*) mutations result in situs inversus and primary ciliary dyskinesia (Kartagener syndrome). *Am J Hum Genet* 68: 1030–1035.

Hadfield PJ, Rowe-Jones JM, Bush A, Mackay IS (1997). Treatment of otitis media with effusion in children with primary ciliary dyskinesia. *Clin Otolaryngol* 22: 302–306.

Halbert SA, Patton DL, Zarutskie PW, Soules MR (1997). Function and structure of cilia in the fallopian tube of an infertile woman with Kartagener's syndrome. *Hum Reprod* 12: 55–58.

Handel MA (1985). Allelism of *hop* and *hpy*. *Mouse News Lett* 72: 124.

Hirokawa N (1998). Kinesin and dynein superfamily proteins and the mechanism of organelle transport. *Science* 279: 519–526.

Holzmann D, Felix H (2000). Neonatal respiratory distress syndrome: a sign of primary ciliary dyskinesia? *Eur J Pediatr* 159: 857–860.

Homma S, Kawabata M, Kishi K, Tsuboi E, Narui K, Nakatani T, Saiki S, Nakata K (1999). Bronchiolitis in Kartagener's syndrome. *Eur Respir J* 14: 1332–1339.

Izraeli S, Lowe LA, Bertness VL, Good DJ, Dorward DW, Kirsch IR, Kuehn MR (1999). The SIL gene is required for mouse embryonic axial development and left–right specification. *Nature* 399: 691–694.

Janitz K, Wild A, Beck S, Savasta S, Beluffi G, Ziegler A, Volz A (1999). Genomic organization of the HSET locus and the possible association of HLA-linked genes with immotile cilia syndrome (ICS). *Immunogenetics* 49: 644–652.

Johnson DR, Hunt DM (1971). Hop-sterile, a mutant gene affecting sperm tail development in the mouse. *J Embryol Exp Morphol* 25: 223–236.

Jonsson MS, McCormick JR, Gillies CG (1982). Kartagener's syndrome with motile spermatozoa. *N Engl J Med* 18: 1131–1133.

Jorissen M, van der Schueren B, van den Berghe H, Cassiman JJ (1989). The preservation and regeneration of cilia on human nasal epithelial cells cultured in vitro. *Arch Otorhinolaryngol* 246: 308–314.

Jorissen M, Willems T, van der Schueren B, Verbeken E (2000a). Secondary ciliary dyskinesia is absent after ciliogenesis in culture. *Acta Otorhinolaryngol Belg* 54: 333–342.

Jorissen M, Willems T, van der Schueren B, Verbeken E, de Boeck K (2000b). Ultrastructural expression of primary ciliary dyskinesia after ciliogenesis in culture. *Acta Otorhinolaryngol Belg* 54: 343–356.

Karadag B, James AJ, Gultekin E, Wilson NM, Bush A (1999). Nasal and lower airway level of nitric oxide in children with primary ciliary dyskinesia. *Eur Respir J* 13: 1402–1405.

Kartagener M (1933). Zur Pathogenese der Bronchiektasien bei Situs viscerum inversus. *Beitr Klin Tuberk* 83: 489–501.

Kastury K, Taylor WE, Gutierrez M, Ramirez L, Coucke PJ, Van Hauwe P, Van Camp G, Bhasin S (1997). Chromosomal mapping of two members of the human dynein gene family to chromosome regions 7p15 and 11q13 near the deafness loci DFNA 5 and DFNA 11. *Genomics* 44: 362–364.

Kay VJ, Irvine DS (2000). Succesful in-vitro fertilization pregnancy with spermatozoa from a patient with Kartagener's syndrome: case report. *Hum Reprod* 15: 135–138.

King T, Beddington RS, Brown NA (1998). The role of the brachyury gene in heart development and left–right specification in the mouse. *Mech Dev* 79: 29–37.

Kosaki R, Gebbia M, Kosaki K, Lewin M, Bowers P, Towbin JA, Casey B (1999). Left–right axis malformations associated with mutations in ACVR2B, the gene for human activin receptor type IIB. *Am J Med Genet* 82: 70–76.

Kroon AA, Heij JM, Kuijper WA, Veerman AJ, van der Baan S (1991). Function and morphology of respiratory cilia in situs inversus. *Clin Otolaryngol* 16: 294–297.

Larj MJ, Hazucha M, Sannuti A, Zariwala M, Minnix SL, Carson JL, Knowles MR, Noone PG (2001). Levels of nasal nitric oxide are reduced in conjunction with genetic mutations associated with pulmonary ciliary dyskinesia. Presented at the American Thoracic Society 97th International Conference. San Francisco, May 19–21, 2001.

Levron J, Aviram-Goldring A, Madgar I, Raviv G, Barkai G, Dor J (2001). Sperm chromosome abnormalities in men with severe male factor infertility who are undergoing in vitro fertilization with intracytoplasmic sperm injection. *Fertil Steril* 76: 479–484.

Lowe LA, Supp DM, Sampath K, Yokoyama T, Wright CV, Potter SS, Overbeek P, Kuehn MR (1996). Conserved left–right asymmetry of nodal expression and alterations in murine situs inversus. *Nature* 381: 158–161.

Lu ME, Pressman C, Dyer R, Johnson RL, Marin JF (1999). Function of Rieger syndrome gene in left–right asymmetry and craniofacial development. *Nature* 401: 276–278.

Luck DJL, Huang B, Piperno G (1982). Genetic and biochemical analysis of the eukaryotic flagellum. *Soc Exp Biol Symp* 35: 399–407.

Lundberg JO (1996). Airborne nitric oxide: inflammatory marker and aerocrine messenger in man. *Acta Physiol Scand Suppl* 633: 1–27.

Lungarella G, de Santi MM, Palatresi R (1982). Lack of kinocilia in the immotile cilia syndrome. *Eur J Respir Dis* 63: 558–563.

Lungarella G, de Santi MM, Palatresi R, Tosi P (1985). Ultrastructural observations on basal apparatus of respiratory cilia in immotile cilia syndrome. *Eur J Respir Dis* 66: 165–172.

Maiti AK, Bartoloni L, Mitchison HM, Meeks M, Chung E, Spiden S, Gehrig C, Rossier C, DeLozier-Blanchet CD, Blouin J-L, et al. (2000a). No deletorious mutations in the *FOXJ1* (alias *HFH-4*) gene in patients with primary ciliary dyskinesia (PCD). *Cytogenet Cell Genet* 90: 119–122.

Maiti AK, Mattei M-G, Jorissen M, Volz A, Ziegler A, Bouvagnet P (2000b). Identification, tissue specific expression, and chromosomal localization of several human dynein heavy chain genes. *Eur J Hum Genet* 8: 923–932.

McComb P, Langley L, Villalon M, Verdugo P (1986). The oviductal cilia and Kartagener's syndrome. *Fertil Steril* 46: 412–416.

McKusick V (ed.) (2002). Kartagener syndrome (244400) and immotile cilia syndrome (242650). Available at: http://www.ncbi.nlm.nih.gov/omim/ *Online Mendelian Inheritance of Man.*

Meeks M, Bush A (2000). Primary ciliary dyskinesia (PCD). *Pediatr Pulmonol* 29: 307–316.

Meeks M, Walne A, Spiden S, Simpson H, Mussafi-Georgy H, Hamam HD, Fehaid EL, Cheehab M, Al-Dabbagh M, Polak-Charcon S, et al. (2000). A locus for primary ciliary dyskinesia maps to chromosome 19q. *J Med Genet* 37: 241–244.

Meno C, Shimono A, Saijoh Y, Yashiro K, Mochida K, Ohishi S, Noji S, Kondoh H, Hamada H (1998). Lefty-1 is required for left-right determination as a regulator of lefty-2 and nodal. *Cell* 94: 287–297.

Meno C, Gritsman K, Ohishi S, Ohfuji Y, Hecksher E, Mochida K, Shimono A, Kondoh H, Talbot WS, Robertson EJ, et al. (1999). Mouse Lefty-2 and zebrafish antivin are feedback inhibitors of nodal signaling during vertebrate gastrulation. *Mol Cell* 4: 287–298.

Mermall V, Post PL, Moosaker MS (1998). Unconventional myosins in cell movement, membrane traffic, and signal transduction. *Science* 279: 527–533.

Meschede D, De Geyter C, Nieschlag E, Horst J (1995). Genetic risk in micomanipulative assisted reproduction. *Hum Reprod* 11: 2880–2886.

Meyers EN, Martin GR (1999). Differences in left–right axis pathways in mouse and chick: functions of FGF8 and SHH. *Science* 285: 403–406.

Milisav I, Jones MH, Affara NA (1996). Characterization of a novel human dynein-related gene that is specifically expressed in testis. *Mamm Genome* 7: 667–672.

Morgan D, Turnpenny L, Goodship J, Dai W, Majumder K, Matthews L, Gardner A, Schuster G, Vien L, Harrison W, et al. (1998). Inversin, a novel gene in the vertebrate left–right axis pathway, is partially deleted in the inv mouse. *Nat Genet* 20: 149–156.

Morris RL, Scholey JM (1997). Heterotrimeric kinesin-II is required for the assembly of motile 9 + 2 ciliary axonemes in sea-urchin embryos. *J Cell Biol* 138: 1009–1022.

Murcia NS, Richards WG, Yoder BK, Mucenski ML, Dunlap JR, Woychik RP (2000). The Oak Ridge polycystic kidney disease (orpk) disease gene is required for left–right axis determination. *Development* 127: 2347–2355.

Mygind NG, Pedersen M, Toremalm NG (1983). Lay cilia make the otologist busy. *Clin Otolaryngol* 8: 148–151.

Nadel HR, Stringer DA, Levison H, Turner JAP, Sturgess JM (1985). The immotile cilia syndrome: radiological manifestations. *Radiology* 154: 651–655.

Narayan D, Desai T, Banks A, Patanjali SR, Ravikumar TS, Ward DC (1994a). Localization of the human cytoplasmic dynein heavy chain (DNECL) to 14qter by fluorescence in situ hybridization. *Genomics* 22: 660–661.

Narayan D, Krishnan SN, Upender M, Ravikumar TS, Mahoney MJ, Dolan TF Jr, Teebi AS, Haddad GG (1994b). Unusual inheritance of primary ciliary dyskinesia (Kartagener syndrome). *J Med Genet* 31: 493–496.

Neesen J, Koehler MR, Kirschner R, Steinlein C, Kreutzberger J, Engel W, Schmid M (1997). Identification of dynein heavy chain genes expressed in human and mouse testis: chromosomal localization of an axonemal dynein gene. *Gene* 200: 193–202.

Neesen J, Kirschner R, Ochs M, Schmiedl A, Habermann B, Mueller C, Holstein AF, Nuesslein T, Adham I, Engel W (2001). Disruption of an inner arm dynein heavy chain gene results in asthenozoospermia and reduced ciliary beat frequency. *Hum Mol Genet* 10: 1117–1128.

Nijs M, Vanderzwalmen P, Vandamme B, Segal-Bertin G, Lejeune B, Segal L, van Rosendaal, Schoysman R (1996). Fertilizing ability of immotile spermatozoa after intracytoplasmic sperm injection. *Hum Reprod* 11: 2180–2185.

Nonaka S, Tanaka Y, Okada Y, Takeda S, Harada A, Kanai Y, Kido M, Hirokawa N (1998). Randomizaton of left–right asymmetry due to loss of nodal cilia generating leftward flow of extraembryonic fluid in mice lacking KIF3B motor protein. *Cell* 95: 829–837.

Noone PG, Bali D, Carson JL, Sannuti A, Gipson CL, Ostrowski LE, Bromberg PA, Boucher RC, Knowles MR (1999). Discordant organ laterality in monozygotic twins with primary ciliary dyskinesia. *Am J Med Genet* 15: 155–160.

Okada Y, Nonaka S, Tanaka Y, Saijoh Y, Hamada H, Hirokawa N (1999). Abnormal nodal flow precedes situs inversus in iv and inv mice. *Mol Cell* 4: 459–468.

Olbrich H, Haffner K, Kispert A, Volkel A, Volz A, Sasmaz G, Reinhardt R, Hennig S, Lehrach H, Konietzko N, Zariwala M, Noone PG, Knowles M, Mitchison HM, Meeks M, Chung EM, Hildebrandt F, Sudbrak R, Omran H (2002). Mutations in DNAH5 cause primary ciliary dyskinesia and randomization of left-right asymmetry. *Nat Genet* 30: 143–144.

Omran H, Haffner K, Volkel A, Kuehr J, Ketelsen UP, Ross UH, Konietzko N, Wienker T, Brandis M, Hildebrandt F (2000). Homozygosity mapping of a gene locus for primary ciliary dyskinesia on chromosome 5p and identification of the heavy dynein chain DNAH5 as a candidate gene. *Am J Respir Cell Mol Biol* 23: 696–702.

Pan Y, McCaskill CD, Thompson KH, Hicks J, Casey B, Shaffer LG, Craigen WJ (1998). Paternal isodisomy of chromosome 7 associated with complete situs inversus and immotile cilia. *Am J Hum Genet* 62: 1551–1555.

Pawlik J, Zebrak J, Pogorzelski A, Witt M (1998). Character of bronchopulmonary changes in patients with primary ciliary dyskinesia. In: *Cilia, Mucus and Mucociliary Interactions*, Baum GL, Priel Z, Roth Y, Liron N, Ostfeld E (eds., Marcel Dekker, New York, pp. 543–550.

Pazour GJDB, Vucica Y, Seeley ES, Rosenbaum JL, Witman GB, Cole DG (2000). Chlamydomonas IFT88 and its mouse homologue, polycystic kidney disease gene tg 737, are required for assembly of cilia and flagella. *J Cell Biol* 151: 709–718.

Pedersen M, Mygind N (1983). Rhinitis, sinusitis and otitis media in Kartagener's syndrome. *Clin Otolaryngol* 7: 373–377.

Pennarun G, Escudier E, Chapelin C, Bridoux AM, Cacheux V, Roger G, Clement A, Goossens M, Amselem S, Duriez B (1999). Loss-of-function mutations in a human gene related to *Chlamydomonas reinhardti* dynein IC78 result in primary ciliary dyskinesia. *Am J Hum Genet* 65: 1508–1519.

Pennarun G, Chapelin C, Escudier E, Bridoux A-M, Dastot F, Cacheux V, Goossens M, Amselem S, Duriez B (2000). The human dynein intermediate chain 2 gene (*DNAI2*): cloning, mapping, expression pattern, and evaluation as a candidate for primary ciliary dyskinesia. *Hum Genet* 107: 642–649.

Pennarun G, Bridoux AM, Escudier E. Amselem S, Duriez B (2001) The human *HP28* and *HFH4* genes: evaluation as candidate genes for primary ciliary dyskinesia. Presented at the American Thoracic Society 97th International Conference. San Francisco, May 19–21, 2001.

Perraudeau M (1994). Grand rounds Hammersmith Hospital: late presentation of Kartagener's syndrome. *Br Med J* 308: 519–521.

Poller WC, Knoll R, Fechner H, Gaub R, Serbest Y, Wang H (1999). Molecular genetic analysis of the axonemal dynein heavy chain gene family in patients with Kartagener syndrome. Presented at the American Thoracic Society 95th International Conference. San Francisco, May 19–21, 2001.

Rankin CT, Bunton T, Lawler AM, Lee SJ (2000). Regulation of left–right patterning in mice by growth/differentiation factor-1. *Nat Genet* 24: 262–265.

Reyes de la Rocha S, Pysher T, Leonard J (1987). Dyskinetic cilia syndrome: clinical, radiographic and scintigraphic findings. *Pediatr Radiol* 17: 97–103.

Roperto F, Galati O, Rossacco P (1993). Immotile cilia syndrome in pigs: a model for human disease. *Am J Pathol* 143: 634–647.

Rott HD (1998). Genetic counseling of adults with primary ciliary dyskinesia or cystic fibrosis. In: *Cilia, Mucus and Mucociliary Interactions*, Baum GL, Priel Z, Roth Y, Liron N, Ostfeld E (eds.) Marcel Dekker, New York, pp. 551–555.

Rutland J, de Iongh RU (1990). Random ciliary orientation: a cause of respiratory tract disease. *N Engl J Med* 323: 1681–1684.

Rutland J, Dewar A, Cox T, Cole PJ (1982). Nasal brushing for the study of ciliary utrastructure. *J Clin Pathol* 35: 356–359.

Sannuti A, Minnix SL, Carson JL, Hazucha M, Daines CL, Burns KA, Zariwala MA, Leigh MW, Knowles MR. Noone PG (2001). Primary ciliary dyskinesia: an analysis of the clinical and cell biologic phenotype. Presented at the American Thoracic Society 97th International Conference. San Francisco, May 19–21, 2001.

Schidlow DV (1994). Primary ciliary dyskinesia (the immotile cilia syndrome). *Ann Allergy* 73: 457–470.

Schneider H, Brueckner M (2000). Of mice and men: dissecting the genetic pathway that controls left–right assymetry in mice and humans. *Am J Med Genet* 97: 258–270.

Sleigh MA (1981). Primary ciliary dyskinesia (letter). *Lancet* ii, 476.

Supp DM, Witte DP, Potter SS, Brueckner M (1997). Mutation of an axonemal dynein affects left–right asymmetry in inversus viscerum mice. *Nature* 389: 963–966.

Supp DM, Brueckner M, Kuehn MR, Witte DP, Lowe LA, McGrath J, Corrales J, Potter SS (1999). Targeted deletion of the ATP binding domain of left–right dynein confirms its role in specifying development of left–right asymmetries. *Development* 126: 5495–5504.

Supp DM, Potter S, Brueckner M (2000). Molecular motors: the driving force behind mammalian left–right development. *Trends Cell Biol* 10: 41–45.

Svedbergh B, Johnsson V, Afzelius BA (1981). Immotile-cilia syndrome and the cilia of the eye. *Graefes Arch Klin Exp Ophthalmol* 215: 265–272.

Takeda S, Yonekawa Y, Tanaka Y, Okada Y, Nonaka S, Hirokawa N (1999). Left-right asymmetry and kinesin superfamily protein KIF3 new insights in determination of laterality and mesoderm induction by kif3A$^{-/-}$ mice analysis. *J Cell Biol* 145: 825–836.

Tamura K, Yonei-Tamura S, Belmonte JC (1999). Molecular basis of left–right asymmetry. *Dev Growth Differ* 41: 645–656.

Teknos TN, Metson R, Chasse T, Balercia G, Dickersin GR (1997). New developments in the diagnosis of Kartagener's syndrome. *Otolaryngol Head Neck Surg* 116: 68–74.

ten Berge M, Brinkhorst G, Kroon AA, de Jongste JC (1999). DNase treatment in primary ciliary dyskinesia: assessment by nocturnal pulse oximetry. *Pediatr Pulmonol* 27: 59–61.

Torikata C, Kijimoto C, Koto M (1991). Ultrastructure of respiratory cilia of WIV-Hyd male rats: an animal model for human immotile cilia syndrome. *Am J Pathol* 138: 341–347.

Turner P, Corkey C, Lee J, Levison H, Sturgess J (1991). Clinical expression of immotile cilia syndrome. *Pediatrics* 67: 805–809.

Volz A, Weiss E, Trowsdale J, Ziegler A (1994). Presence of an expressed β-tubulin gene (TUBB) in the HLA class I region may provide the genetic basis for HLA-linked microtubule dysfunction. *Hum Genet* 93: 42–46.

Watson PJ, Herrtege ME, Sargan D (1998). Primary ciliary dyskinesia in Newfoundland dogs. *Vet Rec* 143: 484.

Whitelaw A, Evans A, Corrin B (1981). Immotile cilia syndrome: a new cause of neonatal respiratory distress. *Arch Dis Child* 56: 432–435.

Wilton LJ, Teichtahl H, Templesmith PD (1986). Kartagener's syndrome with motile cilia and immotile spermatozoa: axonemal ultrastructure and function. *Am Rev Respir Dis* 134: 1233–1236.

Witt M, Gillanders E, Wan S, Freas-Lutz D, Sun C, Zebrak J, Pawlik J, Rutkiewicz E, Diehl S (1998). Preliminary exclusion of chromosome 7 as a potential location of a gene for primary ciliary dyskinesia. In: *Cilia, Mucus and Mucociliary Interactions*, Baum GL, Priel Z, Roth Y, Liron N, Ostfeld E (eds.) Marcel Dekker, New York, pp. 557–562.

Witt M, Wang Y-F, Wang S, Sun C, Pawlik J, Rutkiewicz E, Zebrak J, Diehl SR (1999a). Exclusion of chromosome 7 for Kartagener syndrome but suggestion of linkage in families with other forms of primary ciliary dyskinesia. *Am J Hum Genet* 64: 313–318.

Witt MP, Wyszynski DF, Wang Y-F, Miller-Chisholm A, Pawlik J, Khoshnevisan MH, Sun C, Wang S, Zhang Y-J, Rutkiewicz E, Zebrak J, Kapelerova A, Diehl SR (1999b). Linkage of a gene for Kartagener syndrome to chromosome 15q. *Am J Hum Genet* 65: A31.

Wodehouse T, Nicholson AG, Mackay IS, Bishop AE, Wilson R, Polak JM, Cole PJ (2001). Lack of inducible nitric oxide synthetase in the nasal epithelium of patients with primary ciliary dyskinesia. Presented at the American Thoracic Society 97th International Conference. San Francisco, May 19–21, 2001.

Yamazaki H, Nakata T, Okada Y, Hirokawa N (1995). KIF3A/B: a heterodimeric kinesin superfamily protein that works as a microtubule plus end-directed motor for membrane organelle transport. *J Cell Biol* 130: 1387–1399.

Yashiro K, Saijoh Y, Sakuma R, Tada M, Tomita N, Amano K, Matsuda Y, Monden M, Okada S, Hamada H (2000). Distinct transcriptional regulation and phylogenetic divergance of human LEFTY genes. *Genes Cells* 5: 343–357.

Yokoyama T, Copeland N, Jenkins N, Montgomery C, Elder F, Overbeek P (1993). Reversal of left–right asymmetry: a situs inversus mutation. *Science* 260: 679–682.

Zariwala MA, Noone PG, Sannuti A, Minnix SL, Leigh MW, Carson JL, Knowles MR (2001) Mutation analyses of *DNAI1* (IC78) gene in patients with pulmonary ciliary dyskinesia (PCD). Presented at the American Thoracic Society 97th International Conference. San Francisco, May 19–21, 2001.

Part G.
Extracellular Matrix

95 | Extracellular Matrix and Signaling during Development

SCOTT B. SELLECK AND SALLY E. STRINGER

There was a time when the biology of the extracellular matrix was considered quite separately from study of signaling or morphogenesis. This was even reflected in the terminology of the field, where "ground substance" was used to refer to the extracellular matrix. "Ground substance" certainly does not evoke images of dynamic processes that involve interactions between cells and their environment. We now know that it is impossible to understand the biology of multicellular organisms without appreciating that cells create the extracellular matrix that surrounds them and that the matrix reciprocally affects virtually all aspects of cellular behavior.

The matrix regulates the availability of growth factors and the migration of cells through it. It influences cell shape and cell division. In addition, different assemblies of extracellular matrix molecules provide for a stunning array of material designs, from the transparent matrix of the cornea to the durability and hardness of enamel. Diseases involving the matrix are not limited to those that affect the structure of bone, cartilage, or connective tissue but include those where the fundamental defect is in signaling. Proteoglycans, components of both cell surfaces and the extracellular matrix, have been found to have profound influences on signaling mediated by the principal growth factors that govern development, including the Wnts, transforming growth factor-β (TGF-β)/bone morphogenetic proteins (BMP), and Hedgehog families of secreted signaling molecules (Selleck, 2000,

2001). They consist of a protein core with covalently attached polysaccharide chains (glycosaminoglycans) that have the ability to bind to a range of growth factors, cytokines, matrix proteins, and enzymes. Matrix molecules have also been shown to regulate tumor neovascularization and apoptosis during the development of malignancy (see, for example, Lawler et al. [2001]). In short, there are few, if any, biological processes that do not involve the interactions between cells and the matrix that surrounds them. Furthermore, cell biology and "matrix biology" are operationally inseparable, and an understanding of the complexity of human disease requires a thorough appreciation of the interplay between cells and matrix.

Like many areas of biology, understanding of the molecular basis of inborn errors in development that affect the extracellular matrix increasingly comes from an analysis of a number of model systems combined with the genetics and pathophysiology of human disease. These systems include invertebrate organisms where powerful genetic tools have been assembled, namely, the fruitfly *Drosophila melanogaster*, the nematode worm *Caenorhabditis elegans,* the zebrafish *Danio rerio*, and the mouse *Mus domesticus*. The completion of the genome projects for the human, worm, fruitflies, and, in the near future, the mouse have revealed the stunning degree of functional homology among all of these organisms. For example, more than 70% of the human genes known to play a role in cancer development have functional orthologs in the fruitfly (Fortini et al., 2000; Rubin et al., 2000). And the complexity of the human genome is not as daunting as predicted. The complement of approximately 32,000 open reading frames found in the human genome is not far from the nearly 14,000 documented for fruitflies. These are both humbling and powerful statistics. First, it is clear that understanding the molecular basis of human diseases can in some measure be derived from molecular genetic studies of relatively simple organisms. Nonetheless, understanding the interplay of many genes together with the environmental influences on the expressivity of disease states remains a challenge. Even with a very detailed understanding of a disease, effective medical treatments often remain in the far future. However, there is good reason to be optimistic that studies of the molecular basis of developmental anomalies will provide the foundation to treat a number of devastating diseases, including cancer.

The chapters that follow provide a few examples of how defects in extracellular matrix components contribute to inborn errors of development. A comprehensive treatment would require a volume on its own, but the cases described here illustrate the diverse biological processes affected by extracellular matrix components and how mutations affecting these molecules can alter human development.

A FEW DEFINITIONS: WHAT IS THE EXTRACELLULAR MATRIX?

The *extracellular matrix* is in simplest terms the network of proteins, polysaccharides, and glycoproteins that are secreted by cells. The complex interactions between these matrix components are illustrated by the genetic disorder pseudoachondroplasia, in which misfolding of cartilage oligomeric protein (COMP)/thrombospondin-5 results in the retention of a number of matrix molecules in the rough endoplasmic reticulum. The giant rough endoplasmic reticulum cisternae disrupt chondrocyte function and eventually lead to cell death (see Chapter 99). The interactions among matrix components create the molecular network that surrounds all cells, an intimate element affecting virtually all aspects of cellular behavior (Fig. 95–1). Although this general definition includes all matrix types, there are some specialized assemblies of extracellular matrix that are worth mentioning.

Basement membranes, or *basal laminae*, are specialized sheets of matrix associated with the basal surface of all epithelia (Fig. 95–2). Endothelial cells that form blood vessels are also surrounded by basement membranes, providing a critical determinant of cellular extravasation into tissues by either normal cells such as lymphocytes, or abnormal cells, such as metastatic tumor cells. Basal laminae additionally surround a number of other cell types, including muscle, fat and Schwann cells. Specializations of the basement membrane at the neuromuscular junction provide important cues that organize the molecular architecture of the muscle, such as the clustering of neurotransmitter receptors mediated by the release of agrin from the axon

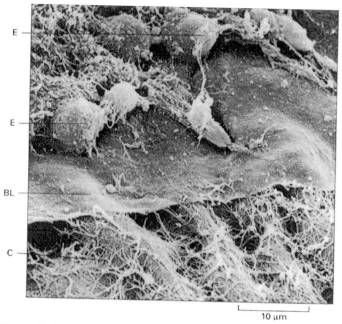

Figure 95–2. Scanning electron micrograph of basal lamina in chick cornea. Epithelial cells (E) have been removed to expose the surface of the basal lamina (BL). Collagen fibrils (C) in the underlying connective tissue make contact with the lower face of the basal lamina. (From Alberts et al., 2002.)

terminal. Another basement membrane specialization is found in the kidney, providing a filter between blood and urine. Defects in collagen IV, a nonfibrillar collagen component of the basement membrane, are the cause of Alport's syndrome, a disease characterized by proteinuria and glomerular nephritis.

Connective tissue, a term frequently encountered in discussions of the extracellular matrix, refers to the matrix and associated cells that form the physical support system for tissues (see Fig. 95–1) or to the elements below the epidermis (cartilage and bone) (see Fig. 95–1). Connective tissue is a mixture of cells and extracellular matrix molecules; principal among these is collagen. *Collagens* are a family of proteins that comprise approximately 25% of the total protein mass of mammals. Defects in collagens are responsible for a variety of human syndromes, such as osteogenesis imperfecta and Ehlers-Danlös syndrome, disorders that affect the assembly and structure of bone and skin, respectively.

Extracellular material is also of importance in more fluid environments, such as the vitreous humour of the eye and the synovial fluid that nourishes and lubricates the joints and tendons. These gel-like

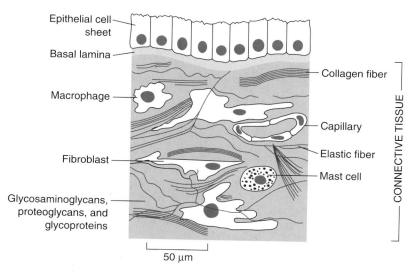

Figure 95–1. Organization of the extracellular matrix, including basal lamina and connective tissue. Illustrated is the overall organization of an epithelial sheet and associated connective tissue. A columnar epithelium is bounded by the basal lamina, or basement membrane, a specialized form of extracellular matrix. Below the basal lamina is connective tissue, a mixture of cells and matrix material that provides physical support for the tissue. (From Alberts et al., 2002.)

fluids are enriched in proteoglycans. Mutations in the gene encoding camptodactyly-arthropathy-coxa vara-pericarditis (CACP)/lubricin/megakaryocyte stimulating factor precursor/superficial zone protein, a novel proteoglycan found in synovial fluid, result in the recessive disorder CACP syndrome (Marcelino et al., 1999). This proteoglycan is secreted by both synoviocytes, the cells that line the joint cavities and tendon sheaths, and the chondrocytes and is thought to be glycosylated with two types of glycosaminoglycans: keratan sulfate and chondroitin sulfate. The principal pathological feature of this syndrome is synoviocyte hyperplasia, and the phenotype includes noninflammatory large joint arthropy.

COMPOSITION OF THE EXTRACELLULAR MATRIX

The extracellular matrix was once considered simply as an inert scaffold for surrounding cells, providing a structural framework. It has now been realized that the matrix also plays a role in orchestrating cellular responses in both normal and pathological situations. The extracellular matrix consists of fibrous proteins, which can be mainly structural or adhesive; glycosaminoglycans; and the molecules that are transiently bound to them, such as growth factors and matrix metalloproteinases (MMP) (Houck et al., 1992; Yu and Woessner, 2000). The glycosaminoglycans such as hyaluronan form a highly hydrated gel-like substance in which the fibrous proteins are embedded. Many extracellular proteins are large multifunctional proteins with multiple protein domains to allow interaction with each other and cell surfaces, and link domains for binding to hyaluronan. Collagens form rod-like structures or fibers to strengthen and organize the matrix, whereas elastic fibers, composed of elastin and fibrillin, provide resilience. In arteries where elasticity is critical, elastin is the major extracellular protein, constituting 50% of the dry weight of the aorta. For example, elastin deficiency in people with Williams syndrome is associated with supravalvular aortic stenosis and other vascular stenosis. Adhesive proteins such as fibronectin and laminin anchor the cells to the collagen via cell surface integrin receptors. Studies (Thelen et al., 2002) suggest that the neuronal cell adhesion molecule L1CAM can potentiate the interaction between $\beta 1$ integrins and extracellular matrix molecules such as fibronectin and laminin, which may be important for its role in neuronal growth and guidance (see Chapter 98).

The plethora of glycosaminoglycans that reside in the matrix appear to be key to its biological significance. The most abundant glycosaminoglycan, hyaluronan, is a huge 10^3 to 10^4-kDa polymer of the repeating disaccharide glucuronic acid with N-acetyl glucosamine. Hyaluronan is believed to be crucial in many cellular processes, including tissue remodeling, inflammation, and tumorigenesis (Sherman et al., 1994). Hyaluronan is unique among glycosaminoglycans in that it is synthesized as a carbohydrate polymer at the cell surface by a transmembrane protein, hyaluronan synthase, as opposed to in the endoplasmic reticulum. Besides several well-characterized proteins within the matrix that associate with hyaluronan, it is clear that hyaluronan also interacts directly with the cell surface hyaluronan binding proteins CD44 and RHAMM, which have been implicated in cell migration, lymphocyte activation, and tumor progression.

In contrast to hyaluronan, the other glycosaminoglycans in the matrix are attached to protein cores. These proteoglycans can be subdivided into three groups: the hyalectans, which are proteoglycans that interact with hyaluronan and lectin, the small leucine-rich proteoglycans (SLRPs), and the basement membrane proteoglycans. (For a more extensive review of proteoglycans in the matrix, see Iozzo [1998]). The hyalectans include versican, aggrecan, neurocan, and brevican. A common feature is their tridomain structure. Their N-terminal domain binds hyaluronan, the central domain carries the glycosaminoglycan side chains, and the C-terminal binds lectins, proteins with specific carbohydrate binding properties. They may be substituted with as few as 2 or as many as 100 chondroitin/dermatan sulfate chains, a linear sulfated glycosaminoglycan polymer of uronic acid and galactosamine. Chondroitin sulfate proteoglycans have been implicated in the regulation of cell migration and pattern formation in the developing peripheral nervous system, and their expression is increased in response to central nervous system injury, limiting the capacity for axonal regeneration (Asher et al., 2002). The functional properties of aggrecan lie in its high con-

centration of chondroitin sulfate side chains and formation of large supramolecular aggregates with hyaluronan (Roughley and Lee, 1994). Each aggrecan monomer occupies a large hydrodynamic volume, which can be displaced by compressive forces. The functional roles of the two brain proteoglycans neurocan and brevican are less well understood.

The family of SLRPs contains at least nine distinct proteins, including decorin, biglycan, fibromodulin, and lumican, and appears to be modulators of collagen fibrillogenesis. Phenotypic effects of biglycan deficiency in mice were linked to collagen fibril abnormalities and mimic Ehlers-Danlös syndrome–like changes in bone and other connective tissues (Corsi et al., 2002). The sugar chains that the SLRPs carry can be chondroitin/dermatan sulfate or keratan sulfate, a complex branching polymer mainly composed of galactose and glucosamine-6-sulfate.

Three proteoglycans are characteristically found in vascular and epithelial mammalian basement membranes—perlecan, agrin, and the relatively recently cloned bamacan, all of which are complex pentadomain proteins. Perlecan and agrin primarily carry heparan sulfate side chains, whereas bamacan primarily is a chondroitin sulfate proteoglycan. Perlecan has regions homologous to the ligand binding portion of the low-density lipoprotein receptor, laminin, and immunoglobulins and has been implicated in lipid uptake and metabolism, cell adhesion, and cell growth (Iozzo, 1998). Agrin is the major heparan sulfate proteoglycan of neuromuscular junctions and renal tubular basement membranes. One of its functions is the aggregation of acetylcholine receptors (Liyanage et al., 2002).

An increasing number of growth factors and enzymes have been found to associate with extracellular matrix, including the insulin growth factors, fibroblast growth factors (FGFs), TGFs, vascular endothelial growth factors, and hepatocyte growth factors. For example, MMPs, which are capable of specifically degrading the matrix, are bound tightly to it, and at least in the case of MMP-7, this is mediated by heparan sulfate proteoglycans (Yu and Woessner, 2000). These enzymes are critical for the processes of growth, repair, and development. For example, a deficiency in MMP-2 results in a rare group of disorders characterized by destruction and reabsorption of the bone (see Chapter 100). Rapid and localized changes in the activity of these growth factors and enzymes can be induced by release from matrix storage or by activation of latent forms, resulting in control of their activities. The regulation of many of these factors has been attributed to the presence of heparan sulfate in the matrix. For instance, the bioavailability of vascular endothelial growth factor splice variant 165 appears to be regulated by matrix heparan sulfate proteoglycans (Houck et al., 1992), and basic fibroblast growth factor-2 could be released from perlecan by either protease or heparanase (heparan sulfate–degrading) enzymes (Whitelock et al., 1996).

The heparan sulfate polysaccharide is composed of alternating hexuronic acid and D-glucosamine residues (Fig. 95–3). (For a review on heparan sulfate, see Esko and Selleck [2002].) The uronic acid can be D-glucuronic acid or L-iduronic acid, and N-sulfation of the glucosamine residues, which are otherwise mostly N-acetylated, occurs mainly in blocks along the chain, commonly referred to as sulfated domains. O-Sulfation occurs predominantly in the sulfated domains, at the C2 position of the iduronate and the C3 and C6 positions of the N-sulfated glucosamine. More rarely, N-acetylated glucosamine may be 6-O-sulfated, and glucuronic acid may be 2-O-sulfated. This produces a hypervariable tissue/cell type–specific structure that is capable of specifically binding to a wide variety of growth factors and their receptors, cytokines, enzymes, and matrix proteins.

EXTRACELLULAR MATRIX AND SIGNALING

Cellular responses to Wnts, TGF-βs, hepatocyte growth factor, FGF, and Hedgehogs, to name a few, are all influenced by heparan sulfate–modified proteoglycans. The appreciation of how proteoglycans can affect signaling began with the demonstration that normal cellular responses to FGF require cell surface heparan sulfate (Rapraeger et al., 1991; Olwin and Rapraeger, 1992). The most current models invoke heparan sulfate proteoglycans as a means of dimerizing FGF, as well as promoting the interaction of FGF receptors at the cell surface (Plotnikov et al., 1999). This co-receptor model may also explain the ability of heparan sulfate proteoglycans to promote signaling of

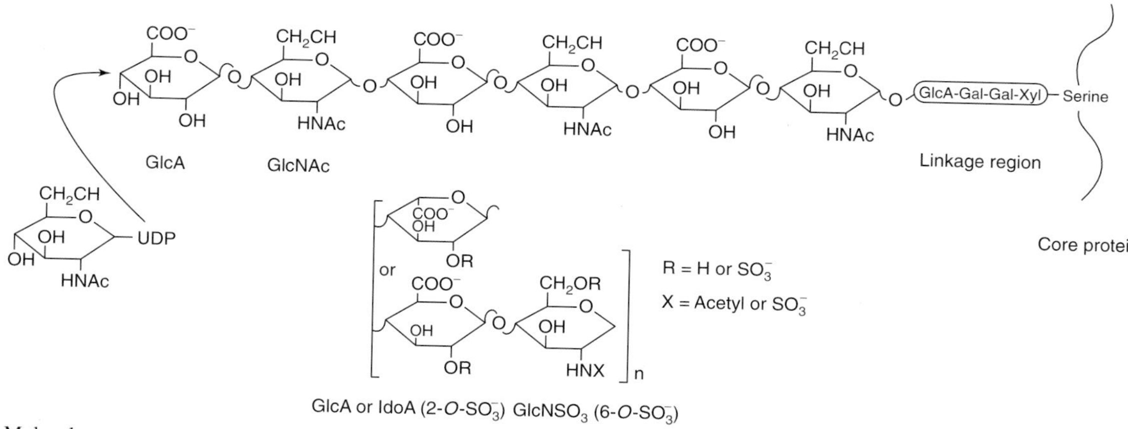

Figure 95–3. Molecular structure of heparan sulfate, a glycosaminoglycan. The heparan sulfate polymer, comprised of a repeat of the disaccharide *N*-acetylglucosamine (GlcNAc) and glucuronic acid (GluA), is attached to the polypeptide via a tetrasaccharide linker. The linker is generated at specific serine residues of the protein core, providing for distinct attachment sites for the glycosaminoglycan. The polymer is elongated by the sequential addition of GlcNAc and GluA residues from UDP-sugar donors. A number of structural modifications to the polymer provide for a great deal of structural diversity along the length of the chain, and in heparan sulfate chains found in different tissues. The disaccharide illustrated in brackets shows some of the structural modifications known, including epimerization of glucuronic acid to iduronic acid, *N*-deacetylation and sulfation of GlcNAc, and three different *O*-linked sulfations: 2-*O*-sulfation of iduronic acid, 6-*O*-sulfation of GlcNSO$_4$, and 3-*O*-sulfation of GlcNSO$_4$.

other growth factors, but there is little direct evidence in those other cases that the proteoglycans are true co-receptors.

There is, however, considerable genetic data showing that heparan sulfate proteoglycans are critical for normal signaling during development. Some of those findings come from the analysis of human syndromes, such as Simpson-Golabi-Behmel syndrome (see Chapter 96). This overgrowth and tumor susceptibility syndrome is caused by mutations in glypican-3, a glycosylphosphatidylinositol-linked proteoglycan. Mutation of the basement membrane heparan sulfate proteoglycan perlecan can result in Schwartz-Jampel syndrome, a recessive inherited condition. This syndrome is characterized by abnormal endochondral ossification and permanent myotonia due to severe muscle hyperexcitability (see Chapter 97). Control of FGF signaling by perlecan during development may have a role in the skeletal abnormalities found in this disorder. Perlecan has also been proposed to be the major receptor of acetylcholine esterase at the neuromuscular junction, so its absence in these tissues may prevent hydrolysis of the neurotransmitter acetylcholine, resulting in continued muscle stimulation.

A great deal of the genetic analysis of proteoglycan and glycosaminoglycan function comes from studies in model organisms: the fruitfly *D. melanogaster,* the nematode *C. elegans,* the zebrafish, and the mouse. These studies have collectively shown that proteoglycans are required for patterning events directed by Wnts, TGF-β/BMPs, FGF, and Hedgehogs in vivo.

The analysis of mutants with defects in enzymes required for heparan sulfate biosynthesis or modification have also been instrumental in documenting that specific structural features of the heparan sulfate chain are essential for normal patterning. Heparan sulfate biosynthesis (Sasisekharan and Venkataraman, 2000) is initiated in the Golgi apparatus by formation of a tetrasaccharide linkage sequence consisting of glucuronic acid-β1,3-galactose-β1,3-galactose-β1-4-xylose-β-*O*-serine at serine-glycine sites on the proteoglycan core. After addition of the first *N*-acetylated glucosamine to the chain, committing it to heparan sulfate rather than chondroitin sulfate, elongation of the polysaccharide occurs by the addition of alternating glucuronic acid and *N*-acetylated glucosamine residues. The growing polymer is partially *N*-deacetylated and *N*-sulfated by a combination of up to four mammalian *N*-deacetylase-*N*-sulfotransferase enzymes. C5 epimerase of the glucuronic acid and the various *O*-sulfations take place near the *N*-sulfated groups and result in the formation of the sulfated domains. At most stages of this biosynthesis, there are a number of possible isoforms of each enzyme type, which are expressed in a specific temporal and spacial manner. Abrogation of the activity of any one of these enzymes will change the structure of the heparan sulfate and its abil-

ity to regulate key ligands, such as the growth factors. For example, mutations affecting a heparan sulfate 2-*O*-sulfotransferase produce renal agenesis by disrupting mesenchymal condensation and branching morphogenesis of the ureteric bud (Bullock et al., 1998). The *Drosophila* gene *pipe,* which bears considerable homology to the mammalian heparan sulfate 2-*O*-sulfotransferases, was found to play a role in the proteolytic activation of Spatzle, the proposed ligand for the Toll receptor, which is required to specify the ventral fate of early embryonic cells (Sen et al., 1998). This suggests that a proteoglycan may control the activation of a protease in this developmental context. Mutations compromising a heparan sulfate co-polymerase in *Drososphila* (the gene is called *tout velu [ttv],* a French term for "all hairy," which describes the appearance of the *ttv* mutant embyros) rather selectively disrupt Hedgehog signaling, whereas mutants with defective *N*-deacetylase *N*-sulfotransferase (*sulfateless* in *Drosophila*) show abnormalities in Hedgehog, Wg, and FGF signaling.

Another hereditary tumor syndrome, multiple hereditary exostoses (MHE) (see Chapter 96), is the result of mutations in genes encoding heparan sulfate copolymerases related to *ttv* in *Drosophila*. MHE is a genetically dominant disorder associated with mutations at *EXT1* (exostosin) or *EXT2* that produce benign tumors at the growth plates of endochondral bone. Loss of heterozygosity at either *EXT1* or *EXT2,* however, is associated with a malignant osteosarcoma. The molecular basis of how heparan sulfate proteoglycans affect tumor development in MHE patients remains a mystery, but the sensitivity of Hedgehog signaling to changes in EXT function in *Drosophila* suggest this is a good place to begin looking for a molecular mechanism.

The sugar donor for all glucuronate-containing glycosaminoglycans, including heparan sulfate and chondroitin sulfate, is UDP-glucuronic acid. Consequently, the enzyme responsible for the biosynthesis of this building block, UDP glucose dehydrogenase, is critical for biosynthesis of these glycosaminoglycans. Analysis of mutants affecting Wg, decapentaplegic (Dpp, a BMP-related factor), FGF receptor, and Hedgehog signaling in *Drosophila,* uncovered the gene for this enzyme, now referred to as *sugarless* (*sgl*). Patterning events in the embryo that are known to be directed by Wg are compromised in *sgl* mutants, indicating that this gene affects Wg signaling (Hacker, 1997). *sgl* is also required for Dpp and FGF receptor signaling (mediated by *branchless,* an FGF-like molecule, and *breathless,* the FGF receptor), further demonstrating the importance of glycosaminoglycans in all of these signaling pathways (Haerry et al., 1997, Lin et al., 1999).

Genetic studies in *Drosophila* have implicated matrix components in the assembly and maintenance of morphogen gradients. Morphogens are secreted protein growth factors that provide distinct instructions to cells at different extracellular concentrations. Morphogens are critical for patterning during development, directing a variety of cell fates based on a graded distribution of the protein across epithelial fields. Wnts, TGF-βs/activins, and Hedgehogs have all been shown to possess morphogen activity, and studies indicate that heparan sulfate proteoglycans are required for the normal formation of these activity gradients. For example, loss of *ttv* prevents the normal distribution of Hedgehog across a 10-cell-wide dimension of the developing wing epithelium (Bellaiche et al., 1998; The et al., 1999). Cells defective for *sulfateless* produce reductions in the levels of extracellular Wingless (a *Drosophila wnt* family member) surrounding the mutant cells (Baeg et al., 2001; see Chapter 22). The molecular basis for the effects of heparan sulfate proteoglycans on morphogen gradient formation and maintenance are not known. However, the clear role of proteoglycans in the control of morphogen distributions illustrates that these molecules serve to not only affect how cells respond to growth factors but also govern the levels of growth factors that reach cell surfaces.

Two different classes of secreted proteins have been shown to affect Wnt Wingless signaling. Both enzymes show sequence homology to enzymes that could potentially modify the structure of glycosaminoglycans on cell surfaces and in the matrix. One of these, Qsulf1 is proposed to remove a specific sulfate group on heparan sulfate and hence affect Wnt signaling by modifying a proteoglycan co-receptor (Dhoot et al., 2001). The other, named *wingful* and *Notum* by two different groups (Gerlitz and Basler, 2002; Giraldez et al., 2002), encodes a gene with homology to plant pectin acetyl esterases and is proposed to modify heparan sulfate by removing the *N*-linked acetyl group of *N*-acetyl glucosamine, one of the two sugars that comprise the disaccharide repeat of heparan sulfate (see Fig. 95–3). This modification is postulated to affect the interaction of Wingless with its proteoglycan co-receptor, potentially affecting both cellular responses to Wingless and its distributions in tissues. These discoveries suggest that signaling mediated by proteoglycans is sculpted by the secretion of enzymes that modify their associated glycosaminoglycan chains.

The dynamic nature of matrix composition is illustrated by the ability of cell surface proteoglycans to be shed in a controlled fashion. Syndecan-1 and -4, two related transmembrane proteoglycans, are released from cell surfaces in response to a number of stimuli, including mechanical stress, heat shock, and secreted products of bacterial pathogens (Subramanian et al., 1997; Fitzgerald et al., 2000; Park et al., 2001). Syndecan shedding occurs at wound sites and may serve to regulate the activity of growth factors involved in wound repair, including heparin-binding endothelial growth factor and FGF-2. These behaviors and activities of syndecans illustrate that matrix composition is tightly regulated and can serve to alter the signaling activities of growth factors released into the extracellular space.

Although the molecular details of how matrix components impinge on signaling events remain largely unknown, some working models can be plausibly suggested. First, matrix molecules can affect the assembly of ligands and their receptors, promoting or inhibiting the formation of signaling complexes. Proteoglycans serving as co-receptors for growth factors such as FGF provide an example of this type of mechanism. Second, matrix molecules can serve as allosteric regulators of enzymes in extracellular spaces. The ability of heparin to produce a conformation of antithrombin III that is able to inhibit the factor X protease (Rosenberg et al., 1997) illustrates that carbohydrates can be allosteric effectors of important extracellular enzymes. Third, extracellular matrix molecules could alter the stability and distributions of protein growth factors in extracellular spaces. Given that certain growth factors serve as morphogens, where the level of signaling dictates the biological outcome, extracellular determinants of growth factor distributions are critical to the normal assembly of tissues during development.

REFERENCES

Alberts B, Johnson A, Lewis J, Raff M, Roberts K, Walter P (2002). Cell junctions, cell adhesion and the extracellular matrix. In: *Molecular Biology of the Cell, 4th Edition.* Garland Science, New York, pp. 1066–1125.

Asher RA, Morgenstern DA, Shearer MC, Adcock KH, Pesheva P, Fawcett JW (2002). Versican is upregulated in CNS injury and is a product of oligodendrocyte lineage cells. *J Neurosci* 22: 2225–2236.

Baeg GH, Lin X, Khare N, Baumgartner S, Perrimon N (2001). Heparan sulfate proteoglycans are critical for the organization of the extracellular distribution of Wingless. *Development* 128: 87–94.

Bellaiche Y, The I, Perrimon N (1998). Tout-velu is a *Drosophila* homologue of the putative tumour suppressor EXT-1 and is needed for Hh diffusion. *Nature* 394: 85–88.

Bullock SL, Fletcher JM, Beddington RS, Wilson VA (1998). Renal agenesis in mice homozygous for a gene trap mutation in the gene encoding heparan sulfate 2-sulfotransferase. *Genes Dev* 12: 1894–1906.

Corsi A, Xu T, Chen XD, Boyde A, Liang J, Mankani M, Sommer B, Iozzo RV, Eichstetter I, Robey PG, et al. (2002). Phenotypic effects of biglycan deficiency are linked to collagen fibril abnormalities, are synergized by decorin deficiency, and mimic Ehlers-Danlos-like changes in bone and other connective tissues. *J Bone Miner Res* 17: 1180–1189.

Dhoot GK, Gustafsson MK, Ai X, Sun W, Standiford DM, Emerson CP Jr (2001). Regulation of Wnt signaling and embryo patterning by an extracellular sulfatase. *Science* 293: 1663–1666.

Esko JD, Selleck SB (2002). Order out of chaos: assembly of ligand binding sites in heparan sulfate. *Annu Rev Biochem* 71:435–471.

Fitzgerald ML, Wang Z, Park PW, Murphy G, Bernfield M (2000). Shedding of syndecan-1 and -4 ectodomains is regulated by multiple signaling pathways and mediated by a TIMP-3-sensitive metalloproteinase. *J Cell Biol* 148: 811–824.

Fortini ME, Skupski MP, Boguski MS, Hariharan IK (2000). A survey of human disease gene counterparts in the *Drosophila* genome. *J Cell Biol* 150: F23–F29.

Gerlitz O, Basler K (2002). Wingful, an extracellular feedback inhibitor of Wingless. *Genes Dev* 16: 1055–1059.

Giraldez AJ, Copley RR, Cohen SM (2002). HSPG modification by the secreted enzyme notum shapes the Wingless morphogen gradient. *Dev Cell* 2: 667–676.

Haerry TE, Heslip TR, Marsh JL, O'Connor MB (1997). Defects in glucuronate biosynthesis disrupt Wingless signaling in *Drosophila*. *Development* 124: 3055–3064.

Houck KA, Leung DW, Rowland AM, Winer J, Ferrara N (1992). Dual regulation of vascular endothelial growth factor bioavailability by genetic and proteolytic mechanisms. *J Biol Chem* 267: 26031–26037.

Iozzo RV (1998). Matrix proteoglycans: from molecular design to cellular function. *Annu Rev Biochem* 67: 609–652.

Lawler J, Miao WM, Duquette M, Bouck N, Bronson RT, Hynes RO (2001). Thrombospondin-1 gene expression affects survival and tumor spectrum of p53-deficient mice. *Am J Pathol* 159: 1949–1956.

Lin X, Buff EM, Perrimon N, Michelson AM (1999). Heparan sulfate proteoglycans are essential for FGF receptor signaling during Drosophila embryonic development. *Development* 126: 3715–3723.

Liyanage Y, Hoch W, Beeson D, Vincent A (2002). The agrin/muscle-specific kinase pathway: new targets for autoimmune and genetic disorders at the neuromuscular junction. *Muscle Nerve* 25: 4–16.

Marcelino J, Carpten JD, Suwairi WS, Gutierrez OM, Schwartz S, Robbins C, Sood R, Makalowska I, Baxevanis A, Johnstone B, et al. (1999). CACP, encoding a secreted proteoglycan, is mutated in camptodactyl-arthropathy-coxa vara-pericarditis syndrome. *Nat Genet* 23: 319–322.

Olwin BB, Rapraeger A (1992). Repression of myogenic differentiation by aFGF, bFGF, and K-FGF is dependent on cellular heparan sulfate. *J Cell Biol* 118: 631–639.

Park PW, Pier GB, Hinkes MT, Bernfield M (2001). Exploitation of syndecan-1 shedding by Pseudomonas aeruginosa enhances virulence. *Nature* 411: 98–102.

Plotnikov AN, Schlessinger J, Hubbard SR, Mohammadi M (1999). Structural basis for FGF receptor dimerization and activation. *Cell* 98: 641–650.

Rapraeger AC, Krufka A, Olwin BB (1991). Requirement of heparan sulfate for bFGF-mediated fibroblast growth and myoblast differentiation. *Science* 252: 1705–1708.

Rosenberg RD, Shworak NW, Liu J, Schwartz JJ, Zhang L (1997). Heparan sulfate proteoglycans of the cardiovascular system. Specific structures emerge but how is synthesis regulated? *J Clin Invest* 100: S67–S75.

Roughley PJ, Lee ER (1994). Cartilage proteoglycans: structure and potential functions. *Microsc Res Tech* 28: 385–397.

Rubin GM, Yandell MD, Wortman JR, Gabor Miklos GL, Nelson CR, Hariharan IK, Fortini ME, Li PW, Apweiler R, Fleischmann W, et al. (2000). Comparative genomics of the eukaryotes. *Science* 287: 2204–2215.

Sasisekharan R, Venkataraman G (2000). Heparin and heparan sulfate: biosynthesis, structure and function. *Curr Opin Chem Biol* 4: 626–631.

Selleck SB (2000). Proteoglycans and pattern formation: sugar biochemistry meets developmental genetics. *Trends Genet* 16: 206–212.

Selleck SB (2001). Genetic dissection of proteoglycan function. *Semin Cell Dev Biol* 12: 127–134.

Sen J, Goltz JS, Stevens L, Stein D (1998). Spatially restricted expression of pipe in the *Drosophila* egg chamber defines embryonic dorsal-ventral polarity. *Cell* 95: 471–481.

Sherman L, Sleeman J, Herrlich P, Ponta H (1994). Hyaluronate receptors: key players in growth, differentiation, migration and tumor progression. *Curr Opin Cell Biol* 6: 726–733.

Subramanian SV, Fitzgerald ML, Bernfield M (1997). Regulated shedding of syndecan-1 and -4 ectodomains from growth and extracellular factor activation. *J Biol Chem* 272: 14713–14720.

The I, Bellaiche Y, Perrimon N (1999). Hedgehog movement is regulated through tout velu-dependent synthesis of a heparan sulfate proteoglycan. *Mol Cell* 4: 633–639.

Thelen K, Kedar V, Panicker AK, Schmid RS, Midkiff BR, Maness PF (2002). The neural cell adhesion molecule L1 potentiates integrin-dependent cell migration to extracellular matrix proteins. *J Neurosci* 22: 4918–4931.

Whitelock JM, Murdoch AD, Iozzo RV, Underwood PA (1996). The degradation of human endothelial cell-derived perlecan and release of bound basic fibroblast growth factor by stromelysin, collagenase, plasmin, and heparanases. *J Biol Chem* 271: 10079–10086.

Yu WH, Woessner JF Jr (2000). Heparan sulfate proteoglycans as extracellular docking molecules for matrilysin (matrix metalloproteinase 7). *J Biol Chem* 275: 4183–4191.

96 | *GPC3* and the Simpson-Golabi-Behmel Syndrome

SCOTT SAUNDERS, RICK A. MARTIN, AND MICHAEL R. DEBAUN

LOCUS AND DEVELOPMENTAL PATHWAY

Most genetically characterized cases of Simpson-Golabi-Behmel syndrome (SGBS) in humans have been linked with mutations in the *GPC3* gene located at Xq26 (Pilia et al., 1996), a gene encoding for glypican-3, a glycosylphosphatidylinositol-linked cell surface heparan sulfate proteoglycan (Fig. 96–1). However, a severe form of SGBS has also been reported that maps to Xp22 (Brzustowicz et al., 1999), and many patients with the clinical diagnosis of SGBS have as yet no detectable mutations identified within their *GPC3* gene. These data suggest that not all cases of SGBS result solely from *GPC3* mutations. Six distinct glypican genes have been identified in vertebrates, all encoding heparan sulfate proteoglycans with structural features similar to those shown in Figure 96–1 (Paine-Saunders et al., 1999; Veugelers et al., 1999). Interestingly, the *GPC4* gene is located immediately centromeric to *GPC3* in both humans (Huber et al., 1998; Veugelers et al., 1998) and mice (Matsuki et al., 1998), and at least one patient with SGBS has been identified with a deletion involving both *GPC3* and *GPC4* (Veugelers et al., 1998). However, isolated *GPC4* mutations have not been identified in any patients with SGBS, and there is no evidence to suggest that patients with mutations involving both *GPC3* and *GPC4* have any distinct alteration or enhancement of their phenotype. Furthermore, none of the remaining glypican genes have been mapped to loci linked either specifically with SGBS or, more generally, with overgrowth phenotypes in humans, and mutant alleles of other glypican genes in mice do not seem to phenocopy SGBS (Scott Saunders, unpublished data). Therefore, cases of SGBS not arising from *GPC3* mutations are unlikely to be due to mutations in genes encoding other members of the glypican gene family. On the other hand, salient and undoubtedly essential structural features of glypican-3 are its heparan sulfate chains. More than a half dozen distinct gene products are required for the posttranslational modification of glypican-3 with heparan sulfate, and alterations in the activities of any one or more of these gene products could hypothetically alter the functions of glypican-3 in vivo, resulting in the SGBS phenotype. Supporting this speculation is the fact that loss-of-function mutations for some of these enzymes have been reported in a number of organisms, all resulting in highly complex phenotypes (Perrimon and Bernfield, 2000).

Heparan sulfate is an O-linked posttranslational modification consisting of large, highly acidic, and unbranched carbohydrate chains that occur on select serine residues of only certain core proteins. Indeed, although heparan sulfate is found abundantly in the tissues of all metazoan species, posttranslational modification of proteins with heparan sulfate chains has been predominantly reserved for a highly restricted subset of proteins. In the case of cell surface proteins, heparan sulfate is found predominantly on members of just two gene families: syndecans (Saunders et al., 1989) and glypicans (David et al., 1990). Orthologs of these gene families evolved apparently in concert with gastrulation, appearing first in *Cnidaria*, suggesting a function for heparan sulfate proteoglycans in the control of extracellular signaling events in complex tissues (Park et al., 2000). Consistent with this, heparan sulfate proteoglycans bind and regulate the activities of a wide variety of extracellular ligands essential to multiple cellular functions. These activities of heparan sulfate proteoglycans appear themselves to be developmentally regulated through modifications in the structure of the heparan sulfate chains; there is mounting evidence

that structural sequence variation of individual heparan sulfate chains provides tissue selectivity to the functional binding of ligands. Heparan sulfate chains in vivo are typically hundreds of saccharides in length, and given the 32 potential disaccharides that can occur in varying order along the length of individual chains, there are more than 1 million potential unique structural sequence combinations within any single eight-saccharide-long region of sequence (Sasisekharan and Venkataraman, 2000; Gallagher, 2001). Specific heparan sulfate structures have been found to have differential binding selectivity for individual ligands in vitro, and several studies have strongly suggested that heparan sulfate sequences with distinct ligand binding and functional specificity are developmentally expressed in vivo (Allen et al., 2001; Rubin et al., 2002).

CLINICAL DESCRIPTION

SGBS is a well-described but frequently unrecognized overgrowth syndrome whose incidence is currently unknown. The syndrome was independently described by Simpson et al. (1975), by Golabi and Rosen (1984), and by Behmel et al. (1984), and is now known as SGBS. In 1996, the molecular basis for this syndrome was reported by Pilia et al. (1996) when they identified mutations in *GPC3* at Xq26 in an SGBS patient with a translocation. Subsequently, three research groups have independently generated and characterized mice with targeted disruption of the *glypican-3* gene, all of which display phenotypic features consistent with SGBS and thus confirms the relationship between mutations in *GPC3* and SGBS (Cano-Gauci et al., 1999; Paine-Saunders et al., 2000; Chiao et al., 2002). However, subsequent human studies have demonstrated that only 40% of SGBS patients have an identifiable mutation or deletion in the *GPC3* gene (Li et al., 2001) which suggests that in some cases mutations in additional genes are responsible. A common pattern of malformation can be easily identified in SGBS patients with documented *GPC3* mutations (Table 96–1). Other less frequently described and reported features are listed in Table 96–2, although these features have not been similarly confirmed in children or adults with *GPC3* mutations. Because this is an X-linked disorder, obligate carrier females have been described with various minor manifestations of SGBS, however, systematic documentation of anomalies in the mothers of affected patients has not been reported.

Overgrowth

Prenatal and postnatal overgrowth (length, weight and occipitofrontal circumference OFC of >95%) is a virtual sine-qua-non for SGBS. However, macrosomia is not a specific finding and may be a feature in several other conditions that should be considered in the differential diagnosis of SGBS, such as Beckwith-Wiedemann syndrome (BWS), Perlman syndrome, Sotos syndrome, and Weaver syndrome.

Craniofacial

The SGBS facies is distinctive. In the newborn period hypertelorism, epicanthal folds, macrostomia, macroglossia, and anteverted nares are evident. These features persist, and with age the child's face takes on a coarse appearance due in part to growth of the mandible and nasal tip (Fig. 96–2). The lower lip is often full with a midline groove, and the midline of the tongue may reveal a deep furrow (Fig. 96–3). The

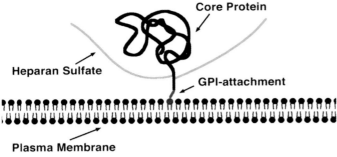

Figure 96–1. Schematic representation of the fully processed glypican-3 glycoprotein. The N terminus is believed to be stabilized in a highly folded conformation through disulfide bonds, whereas the C terminus, which bears two heparan sulfate chains, is anchored to the plasma membrane via a glycosylphosphatidylinositol (GPI) linkage.

palate, if not cleft, is often narrow. Cleft lip can often occur along with various minor ear malformations, including posterior creases.

Extremities

Anomalies of the hands are frequent and include brachydactyly, broad thumbs, cutaneous syndactyly, and, occasionally, polydactyly. These malformations may also be seen in the feet, but hallux valgus is more common. Nail hypoplasia or flat nails are often noted. Broad distal femoral metaphyses are notable in a number of children with SGBS whom we follow.

Chest Wall

One of the most consistent minor malformations seen in SGBS is a supernumerary nipple (Fig. 96–4). Extra nipples can be unilateral or bilateral, and there may be several present in the axillary line, sometimes to the level of the axilla. Areolar skin tags, pectus excavatum, and rib defects can also be present.

Abdominal Wall

Minor abdominal wall anomalies such as diastasis recti and umbilical hernia are often present. The abdominal wall musculature may be underdeveloped but, unlike in BWS, true omphalocele is rare.

Internal Organs

Renal dysplasia and cardiac malformations are the most commonly reported organ anomalies. Renal dysplasia is often associated with nephromegaly; ureteral anomalies may also be present. Structural cardiopulmonary anomalies are varied, but most are flow-related defects such as ventricular and atrial septal defects. A significant number of conduction defects have also been noted. Diaphragmatic hernia occurs occasionally, as do gastrointestinal malformations. Defects of the genitalia include hypospadius and cryptorchidism.

Table 96–1. Features Associated with Documented Deletions of *GPC3* in 26 Simpson-Golabi-Behmel Syndrome Patients (All Patients Had at Least Three of These Features in Addition to Overgrowth)

Always present	Common
Prenatal overgrowth	Congenital heart defect
Postnatal overgrowth	Occasional
Very common	Cleft lip/palate
Coarse facial appearance	Embryonal tumor
Macroglossia	
Urinary tract anomalies	
Skeletal defects of thorax	
Hand/nail malformations	
Supernumerary nipples	
Umbilical/inguinal hernia	
Developmental delay	

Source: Pilia et al. (1996), Hughes-Benzie et al. (1996), Lindsay et al. (1997), Veugelers et al. (2000), and Li et al. (2001).

Table 96–2. Other Features Described in Simpson-Golabi-Behmel Syndrome

Macrostomia	Diastasis recti
Hypertelorism	Coccygeal skin tag
Midline groove in tongue and/or upper lip	Diaphragmatic defect
	Organomegaly
Down slanting palpebral fissures	Cryptorchidism/hypospadius

Neurologic

A spectrum of neurologic problems have been described in SGBS, but any cause-and-effect relationship is unclear. Neurologic findings may include hypotonia, seizures, absent primitive reflexes, abnormal electroencephalogram, and central nervous system malformations. Reports of developmental delay and subnormal IQs are inconsistent; therefore, the frequency of developmental delay and other neurologic characteristics associated with SGBS requires further study.

Cancer

Despite being recognized as an embryonal cancer predisposition syndrome, relatively little information is known about the incidence, age group risks, and full spectrum of cancers in this overgrowth syndrome. Similar to BWS, patients with SGBS have an increased risk of developing Wilms' tumor and neuroblastoma. Patients with SGBS may also have a greater frequency of hepatic cancer and testicular gonadoblastoma.

Differential Diagnosis

Newborns and infants presenting with macrosomia and congenital malformations require a differential diagnosis that should include BWS, Perlman syndrome, and Weaver syndrome. Of these diagnoses, BWS is the one syndrome with the greatest clinical overlap with SGBS (see Chapter 73). Features commonly ascribed to both syndromes include macrosomia, macroglossia, abdominal wall defects, minor ear anomalies, and an increased frequency of genitourinary malformations, including hypospadius, nephromegaly, and elevated risk of Wilms' tumor and neuroblastoma. Careful evaluation for the physical features outlined in the previous section should be helpful in clinically distinguishing these syndromes. In particular, the facial features of these two syndromes are distinctly different. The face of an SGBS patient is typically more coarse than that of a patient with BWS, with hypertelorism, broad nose, prominent jaw, and midline groove in the lower lip and/or tongue. By contrast, the characteristic BWS facies is manifest by midface hypoplasia with a flat nasal bridge, facial nevus flammeus, and characteristic ear creases and/or pits. Other features that help distinguish these two syndromes are supernumerary nipples and the increased frequency of skeletal malformations such as polydactyly, syndactyly, and rib malformations found in association with SGBS. Clinical centers have begun to provide CLIA-certified genetic tests for SGBS and BWS, but the SGBS test is limited to the identi-

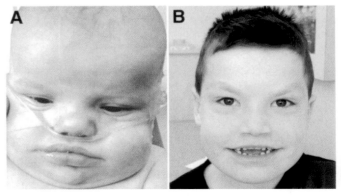

Figure 96–2. Typical facies of Simpson-Golabi-Behmel syndrome demonstrating coarse appearance, hypertelorism, epicanthal folds, macrostomia, and full lower lip. (*A*) A 5-month-old child. (*B*) A 6-year-old child.

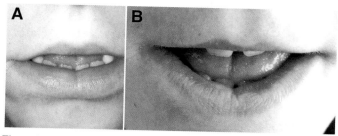

Figure 96–3. (*A*) Midline groove in lower lip of a boy with Simpson-Golabi-Behmel syndrome (SGBS). (*B*) A different SGBS patient revealing a midline groove in both the lower lip and tongue.

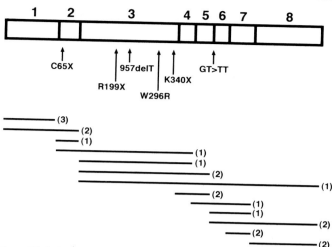

Figure 96–5. Schematic representation of the eight exons composing the glypican-3 cDNA, and the known mutations resulting in Simpson-Golabi-Behmel syndrome (SGBS) as reported in the literature. *Arrows*, Relative positions of the six known point mutations causing SGBS. (From Veugelers et al., 2000.) Below are shown the reported deletions of the *GPC3* gene involving all or a portion of the exons indicated schematically. In parentheses are the total number of reported patients bearing similar deletions. (From Hughes-Benzie et al., 1996; Lindsay et al., 1997; Okamoto et al., 1999; Veugelers et al., 2000; Li et al., 2001.) Not shown are the two described SGBS patients with translocations involving the regions of exons 2 and exon 7-8, respectively, of *GPC3* (Pilia et al., 1996).

fication of deletion mutations within the *GPC3* gene and is unable to detect a wider variety of potential mutations involving the *GPC3* gene. Therefore, although a positive test result is confirmatory for the diagnosis of SGBS, a good history and physical examination by a pediatric dysmorphologist/geneticist remain the cornerstone of making the diagnosis of SGBS until more extensive forms of genetic testing become commercially available.

IDENTIFICATION OF GENE AND MUTATIONAL SPECTRUM

Although no useful structure–function relationships have been identified, significant progress is being made to define specific *GPC3* mutations in patients with SGBS. *GPC3* is a large gene that includes eight exons that span more than 500 kb (Fig. 96–5). Deletions within this gene have been found in 40% of the SGBS patients who have been evaluated and reported in the literature (Li et al., 2001). All exons within the *GPC3* gene have been equally represented in the deletions reported, and there is no obvious phenotypic correlation with any specific deletion. This most likely reflects the fact that these larger deletions of the *GPC3* gene result in null alleles. Although no functional relationships have been associated, several SGBS patients have been identified who have more discrete mutations within the coding region of their *GPC3* gene. For example, one family has been reported with a deletion within *GPC3* (345-357del; base numbering according to GenBank accession No. L47125) resulting in a frameshift that causes premature termination of the coding region (Xuan et al., 1999), and a sporadic case of SGBS has been reported due to deletion of a single nucleotide (1666delC; GenBank accession No. L47125) in exon 7 (Okamoto et al., 1999). In addition, six SGBS patients have been reported who bear point mutations in *GPC3*, including a splice site mutation (IVS5 + 1G → T), a frameshift mutation (957delT; GenBank accession No. L47125), three nonsense mutations (C65X, R199X, and K340X), and a missense mutation (W269R) in a residue found thus far to be conserved in all glypicans (Veugelers et al., 2000). Further evaluation of the biology of this specific mutation is warranted, but preliminary studies have suggested that this single missense mutation results in a failure to undergo normal processing when expressed in vitro (Veugelers et al., 2000). As might be anticipated, most of the point mutations identified in this study were found within the largest exon of the *GPC3* gene, exon 3. Although there appears to be no ev-

idence of a mutational hot spot, addressing this issue with certainty can only come after the analysis of larger samples from patients with SGBS. In a study by Li et al. (2001) that reported some newly identified patients, several patients with deletions were described. Sequencing of the *GPC3* gene coding region was performed on the SGBS patients without deletions, but no additional mutations were identified.

COUNSELING AND TREATMENT

Due to the rarity of SGBS, most of the clinical descriptions of SGBS have been case reports. Few centers, including our own, which established an SGBS registry in 1999, have systematically followed the clinical course of more than a few patients with this disorder. As such, recommendations for clinical management of these patients have primarily been extrapolated from the recommendations of centers that follow large numbers of patients with the clinically related syndrome BWS.

In the perinatal period, it has been suggested that SGBS can be categorized into two presentations—a severe neonatal form and a less severe form; the two forms occur with relatively similar frequencies (Neri et al., 1988; Konig et al., 1991). In the severe form, infants frequently die in utero or during early infancy. Although the immediate cause has not been established in all cases of neonatal death in suspected SGBS patients, death has been attributed in several cases to cor pulmonale, heart failure from congenital heart disease, conduction defects, diaphragmatic hernia, overwhelming sepsis, and hypoglycemia (Neri et al., 1988; Terespolsky et al., 1995). Given the potential, as discussed earlier, for cases of SGBS arising from mutations in genes other than *GPC3*, it is tempting to speculate that these two presentations arise from distinct gene mutations. However, it should be noted that several research groups have independently observed neonatal death in mice bearing null alleles for *Gpc3* (Cano-Gauci et al., 1999; Paine-Saunders et al., 2000; Chiao et al., 2002). The frequency of death in these studies was found to vary widely depending on the genetic background of the mice, suggesting that unknown genes that modify the *glypican-3*–deficient phenotype are equally important in determining the risk for neonatal death. As such, families with known inherited mutations in *GPC3* should be counseled with respect to the potential risks for neonatal death in future offspring, and con-

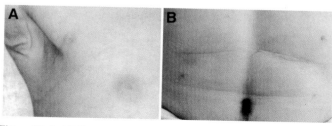

Figure 96–4. (*A*) Supernumerary nipple in the anterior axillae of a boy with Simpson-Golabi-Behmel syndrome (SGBS). (*B*) An adult male with SGBS displaying multiple supernumerary nipples.

siderations should be given for higher-level surveillance during pregnancy with possible delivery at a tertiary care center offering neonatal intensive care if warranted.

In the newborn period, management of de novo cases of suspected SGBS should include prompt assessment for hypoglycemia as in the case of other overgrowth syndromes. Although the prevalence and severity of this problem are unknown, newborn hypoglycemia has been reported in SGBS patients. The etiology of this hypoglycemia is also unknown but is believed to be related to hyperinsulinemia resulting from increased numbers of islet of Langerhans cells (Neri et al., 1988). Most patients are likely to be asymptomatic and have transient hypoglycemia; however, if the pathophysiology is analogous to hypoglycemia in BWS, it is reasonable to anticipate that some children may be at risk for persistent hypoglycemia requiring long-term management. Also, in the newborn period, a cardiac evaluation that includes chest radiography, electrocardiography, and echocardiography is indicated, as is a detailed genitalia examination coupled with a renal and abdominal ultrasound examination to assess for genitourinary abnormalities as well as occult tumors of the adrenal glands and liver. Thorough evaluation should also obviously be done for less life-threatening congenital malformations associated with SGBS that may nonetheless require referral to surgical subspecialists. Possible referrals include a craniofacial specialist for management of cleft lip or palate and macroglossia and an orthopedist for management of syndactyly or polydactyly.

Beyond infancy, the clinical consequences of SGBS have been even less systematically described and require further clarification. A wide spectrum of neurological findings have been inconsistently reported in patients with SGBS, but the cause-and-effect relationship of these findings is uncertain. Prudent advice for the clinician following a patient with SGBS would be increased vigilance for signs and symptoms consistent with any of these findings, along with normal attention to any specific signs of developmental delay. In our experience, most of the patients we have followed appeared to benefit from speech therapy. Although the average age of long-term survival for patients surviving infancy is unknown, it is likely similar to adults without the condition. Therefore, in the absence of severe cardiac conduction defects (Konig et al., 1991), the single major cause of long-term morbidity and mortality in these patients is likely to be cancer.

Because the incidence of cancer in children with SGBS is increased, a major consideration for clinicians is whether their patients should undergo long-term cancer surveillance. Before the implementation of any screening program, certain features must be considered. The minimum criteria required for a successful cancer screening program should include but are not limited to (1) early identification of the specific cancer leads to a decrease in morbidity and/or mortality rates; (2) a screening method that is easy to use, accessible, and acceptable to the parent/patient; (3) a population to be served that is easily identified; and (4) a specific incidence of cancer that is high enough to justify screening if the other conditions are met (DeBaun et al., 1996).

Despite the paucity of data regarding specific cancer risks in children with SGBS, cancer surveillance in these children is prudent for several reasons. First, identification of either Wilms' tumor or hepatic cancer at an early tumor stage results in increased survival and decreased morbidity. Choyke et al. (1999) demonstrated that no child (0 of 12) with either BWS or idiopathic hemihypertrophy and a Wilms' tumor who was screened with sonography at an interval of at least every 4 months had late-stage Wilms' tumor, whereas 42% of children (24 of 59) who were screened at intervals of greater than 4 months or not screened at all had late-stage Wilms' tumor when diagnosed.

We recommend screening of SGBS patients at least every 4 months with abdominal sonography (Table 96–3). Second, hepatic cancer can theoretically be identified early in its course by detection of an elevated alpha–fetal protein (AFP). Because of the increased risk of hepatic cancer in SGBS patients, we believe that obtaining an AFP level every 6 to 12 weeks to detect any pattern of increasing AFP until age 3 years is reasonable (Table 96–3). The decision to stop screening should be based on the age-specific incidence of Wilms' tumor and hepatic cancer, the costs, and consultation with the parents. In general, Wilms' tumor screening could stop at about 8 years of age, when 92% of these tumors have occurred in other overgrowth syndromes such as BWS and isolated hemihypertrophy (Beckwith, 1998). The age-specific incidence of hepatic cancer is highest in children younger than 3 years (Ross and Gurney, 1998); consequently, we recommend screening until that age. In contrast, no data are available suggesting that early identification of neuroblastoma is beneficial (Schilling et al., 2002). The lack of data to support cancer screening for neuroblastoma and other cancers requires a balanced discussion with parents to ensure that they are informed of the benefits and risks.

MUTANTS IN ORTHOLOGOUS GENES AND DEVELOPMENTAL PATHOGENESIS

Although loss-of-function mutations in *GPC3* are known to cause SGBS, the molecular basis of that function is only beginning to be unraveled, primarily through studies of mouse models of SGBS. Based on the phenotypic overlap between SGBS and BWS, as well as the similarity in phenotypes between SGBS and transgenic mice with functional overexpression of insulin-like growth factor II (IGF-II) (Eggenschwiler et al., 1997), a role for glypican-3 in the control of IGF-II levels was initially proposed (Pilia et al., 1996; Pellegrini et al., 1998). Specifically, one model proposed that glypican-3, much like IGF-2R, binds IGF-II directly and normally mediates its uptake and degradation (Pilia et al., 1996; Pellegrini et al., 1998). Because IGF-II is not a heparan sulfate binding protein, this binding was suggested to occur through the glypican-3 core protein. However, subsequent studies have been unable to confirm any direct physical interaction between IGF-II and glypican-3 (Song et al., 1997), and glypican-3–deficient mice do not appear to have altered levels of IGF-II (Cano-Gauci et al., 1999). Furthermore, recent studies have more directly tested the relationship between glypican-3 and IGF-II function through genetic experiments involving the breeding of glypican-3–deficient animals to mice with various mutations involving the IGF signaling pathway (Chiao et al., 2002). These studies concluded that it was unlikely that glypican-3 functions as a growth suppressor by primarily inhibiting or down-regulating an IGF ligand. However, certain phenotypic features of glypican-3–deficient animals were enhanced in the setting of increased levels of IGF-II (Chiao et al., 2002), suggesting there might be some intersection of these signaling pathways, which certainly deserves further investigation.

In contrast, given that glypican-3 is a heparan sulfate proteoglycan, it is reasonable to expect that functions of glypican-3 could be in large part dependent on its interactions with heparan sulfate binding proteins. In this regard, cell surface heparan sulfate proteoglycans regulate in vitro the function of a number of proteins directly related to the control of cell growth, including fibroblast growth factors (FGFs) (Rapraeger et al., 1991; Yayon et al., 1991), heparin binding epidermal growth factor (Aviezer and Yayon, 1994), hepatocyte growth factor (Zioncheck et al., 1995), Wnts (Reichsman et al., 1996), bone mor-

Table 96–3. Cancer Screening Guidelines

Recommendation	Strength of Evidence	Reference
Abdominal sonography to detect Wilms' tumor, from birth until at least 7 or 8 years of age, every 4 months	Moderate	Choyke et al. (1999)
Abdominal sonography to detect hepatoblastoma and/or adrenocortical carcinoma until 3 years of age	Weak	M. R. DeBaun, unpublished data
Alpha-fetal protein level to detect hepatocellular carcinoma every 6 to 12 weeks until 3 years of age	Weak	M. R. DeBaun, unpublished data
Urine vanillylmandelic acid/homovanillic acid level to detect neuroblastoma	None	Schilling et al. (2002)

phogenetic proteins (BMPs) (Ruppert et al., 1996; Ohkawara et al., 2002), endostatin (Karihaloo et al., 2001), and members of the hedgehog gene family products (The et al., 1999; Rubin et al., 2002). Furthermore, genetic studies in model organisms have in particular implicated glypicans in the control of cellular responsiveness to both Wnts (Lin and Perrimon, 1999; Tsuda et al., 1999; Baeg et al., 2001) and bone morphogenetic proteins (BMPs) (Jackson et al., 1997; Paine-Saunders et al., 2000) in vivo. Specifically, skeletal growth and patterning defects seen in *GPC3*-deficient mice are significantly enhanced when bred onto a background of *BMP4* haploinsufficiency (Paine-Saunders et al., 2000). Although some of the resulting phenotypes from this cross are synthetic, others, such as postaxial polydactyly, are frequently seen in patients with SGBS, thus suggesting that a reduction in BMP signaling in SGBS is in part responsible for these phenotypes. Subsequently, other investigators have demonstrated an apparently similar requirement for glypican-3 in BMP, FGF (Grisaru et al., 2001), and endostatin (Karihaloo et al., 2001) signaling during kidney morphogenesis, using cultured cell lines derived from glypican-3–deficient animals. In the case of FGF and endostatin signaling, heparan sulfate participates as a co-receptor in the formation of an activated signaling complex. Although BMPs also bind directly to heparan sulfate (Sampath et al., 1987; Wang et al., 1988; Ruppert et al., 1996), the role for heparan sulfate proteoglycans in BMP signaling is less well defined and does not appear to be as an essential co-receptor. However, cell surface heparan sulfate has also been found to bind and localize BMP antagonists such as noggin to the cell surface and offers another mechanism by which these proteins could modulate BMP signaling in vivo (Paine-Saunders et al., 2002). Interestingly, *Drosophila* glypicans have been found to participate in distinctly different signaling pathways in a highly tissue- and developmental context–dependent manner. Thus, it seems likely that various phenotypes associated with SGBS will be found to occur as a result of heparan sulfate–dependent functions other than just the regulation of BMP and FGF signaling.

ACKNOWLEDGMENTS

The work from the laboratory of Scott Saunders cited here was supported in part by National Institutes of Health grants DK56063 and HD39952, as well as by funding from the March of Dimes Birth Defects Foundation.

REFERENCES

Allen BL, Filla MS, Rapraeger AC (2001). Role of heparan sulfate as a tissue-specific regulator of FGF-4 and FGF receptor recognition. *J Cell Biol* 155(5): 845–858.

Aviezer D, Yayon A (1994). Heparin-dependent binding and autophosphorylation of epidermal growth factor (EGF) receptor by heparin-binding EGF-like growth factor but not by EGF. *Proc Natl Acad Sci USA* 91(25): 12173–12177.

Baeg GH, Lin X, Khare N, Baumgartner S, Perrimon N (2001). Heparan sulfate proteoglycans are critical for the organization of the extracellular distribution of Wingless. *Development* 128(1): 87–94.

Beckwith JB (1998). Nephrogenic rests and the pathogenesis of Wilms tumor: developmental and clinical considerations. *Am J Med Genet* 79(4): 268–273.

Behmel A, Plochl E, Rosenkranz W (1984). A new X-linked dysplasia gigantism syndrome: identical with the Simpson dysplasia syndrome? *Hum Genet* 67(4): 409–413.

Brzustowicz LM, Farrell S, Khan MB, Weksberg R (1999). Mapping of a new SGBS locus to chromosome Xp22 in a family with a severe form of Simpson-Golabi-Behmel syndrome. *Am J Hum Genet* 65(3): 779–783.

Cano-Gauci DF, Song HH, Yang H, McKerlie C, Choo B, Shi W, Pullano R, Piscione TD, Grisaru S, Soon S, et al. (1999). Glypican-3-deficient mice exhibit developmental overgrowth and some of the abnormalities typical of Simpson-Golabi-Behmel Syndrome. *J Cell Biol* 146: 255–264.

Chiao E, Fisher P, Crisponi L, Deiana M, Dragatsis I, Schlessinger D, Pilia G, Efstratiadis A (2002). Overgrowth of a mouse model of the Simpson-Golabi-Behmel syndrome is independent of IGF signaling. *Dev Biol* 243(1): 185–206.

Choyke PL, Siegel MJ, Craft AW, Green DM, DeBaun MR (1999). Screening for Wilms tumor in children with Beckwith-Wiedemann syndrome or idiopathic hemihypertrophy. *Med Pediatr Oncol* 32(3): 196–200.

David G, Lories V, Decock B, Marynen P, Cassiman J-J, van der Berghe H (1990). Molecular cloning of a phosphatidylinositol-anchored membrane heparan sulfate proteoglycan from human lung fibroblasts. *J Cell Biol* 111: 3165–3176.

DeBaun MR, Brown M, Kessler L (1996). Screening for Wilms' tumor in children with high-risk congenital syndromes: considerations for an intervention trial. *Med Pediatr Oncol* 27(5): 415–421.

Eggenschwiler J, Ludwig T, Fisher P, Leighton PA, Tilghman SM, Efstratiadis A (1997). Mouse mutant embryos overexpressing IGF-II exhibit phenotypic features of the Beckwith-Wiedemann and Simpson-Golabi-Behmel syndromes. *Genes Dev* 11: 3128–3142.

Gallagher JT (2001). Heparan sulfate: growth control with a restricted sequence menu. *J Clin Invest* 108(3): 357–361.

Golabi M, Rosen L (1984). A new X-linked mental retardation-overgrowth syndrome. *Am J Med Genet* 17(1): 345–358.

Grisaru S, Cano-Gauci D, Tee J, Filmus J, Rosenblum ND (2001). Glypican-3 modulates BMP- and FGF-mediated effects during renal branching morphogenesis. *Dev Biol* 231(1): 31–46.

Huber R, Mazzarella R, Chen CN, Chen E, Ireland M, Lindsay S, Pilia G, Crisponi L (1998). Glypican 3 and glypican 4 are juxtaposed in Xq26.1. *Gene* 225(1–2): 9–16.

Hughes-Benzie R, Pilia G, Xuan J, Hunter AG, Chen E, Golabi M, Hurst JA, Kobori J, Marymee K, Pagon RA, et al. (1996). Simpson-Golabi-Behmel syndrome: genotype/phenotype analysis of 18 affected males from 7 unrelated families. *Am J Med Genet* 66: 227–234.

Jackson SM, Nakato H, Sugiura M, Jannuzi A, Oakes R, Kaluza V, Golden C, Selleck SB (1997). Division abnormally delayed, a *Drosophila* glypican, controls cellular responses to the TGF-β related morphogen, Dpp. *Development* 124: 4113–4120.

Karihaloo A, Karumanchi SA, Barasch J, Jha V, Nickel CH, Yang J, Grisaru S, Bush KT, Nigam S, Rosenblum ND, et al. (2001). Endostatin regulates branching morphogenesis of renal epithelial cells and ureteric bud. *Proc Natl Acad Sci USA* 98(22): 12509–12514.

Konig R, Fuchs S, Kern C, Langenbeck U (1991). Simpson-Golabi-Behmel syndrome with severe cardiac arrhythmias. *Am J Med Genet* 38(2–3): 244–247.

Li M, Shuman C, Fei YL, Cutiongco E, Bender HA, Stevens C, Wilkins-Haug L, Day-Salvatore D, Yong SL, Geraghty MT, et al. (2001). GPC3 mutation analysis in a spectrum of patients with overgrowth expands the phenotype of Simpson-Golabi-Behmel syndrome. *Am J Med Genet* 102(2): 161–168.

Lin X, Perrimon N (1999). Dally cooperates with Drosophila Frizzled 2 to transduce Wingless signalling. *Nature* 400: 281–284.

Lindsay S, Ireland M, O'Brien O, Clayton-Smith J, Hurst JA, Mann J, Cole T, Sampson J, Slaney S, Schlessinger D, et al. (1997). Large scale deletions in the GPC3 gene may account for a minority of cases of Simpson-Golabi-Behmel syndrome. *J Med Genet* 34(6): 480–483.

Matsui Y, Kaname T, Suematsu S, Yamaguchi Y, Abe K, Yamamura K (1998). Mouse K-glypican gene, gpc4, maps to chromosome X. *Genomics* 54(2): 358–359.

Neri G, Marini R, Cappa M, Borrelli P, Opitz JM (1988). Simpson-Golabi-Behmel syndrome: an X-linked encephalo-tropho-schisis syndrome. *Am J Med Genet* 30(1–2): 287–299.

Ohkawara B, Iemura S, ten Dijke P, Ueno N (2002). Action range of BMP is defined by its N-terminal basic amino acid core. *Curr Biol* 12(3): 205–209.

Okamoto N, Yagi M, Imura K, Wada Y (1999). A clinical and molecular study of a patient with Simpson-Golabi-Behmel syndrome. *J Hum Genet* 44(5): 327–329.

Paine-Saunders S, Viviano BL, Economides AN, Saunders S (2002). Heparan sulfate proteoglycans retain Noggin at the cell surface: a potential mechanism for shaping bone morphogenetic protein gradients. *J Biol Chem* 277(3): 2089–2096.

Paine-Saunders S, Viviano BL, Saunders S (1999). GPC6, a novel member of the glypican gene family, encodes a product structurally related to GPC4 and is colocalized with GPC5 on human chromosome 13. *Genomics* 57: 455–458.

Paine-Saunders S, Viviano BL, Zupicich J, Skarnes WC, Saunders S (2000). glypican-3 controls cellular responses to Bmp4 in limb patterning and skeletal development. *Dev Biol* 225(1): 179–187.

Park PW, Reizes O, Bernfield M (2000). Cell surface heparan sulfate proteoglycans: selective regulators of ligand-receptor encounters. *J Biol Chem* 275(39): 29923–29926.

Pellegrini M, Pilia G, Pantano S, Lucchini F, Uda M, Fumi M, Cao A, Schessinger D, Forabosco A (1998). Gpc3 expression correlates with the phenotype of the Simpson-Golabi-Behmel syndrome. *Dev Dyn* 213: 431–439.

Perrimon N, Bernfield M (2000). Specificities of heparan sulphate proteoglycans in developmental processes. *Nature* 404(6779): 725–728.

Pilia G, Hughes-Benzie RM, MacKenzie A, Baybayan P, Chen EY, Huber R, Neri G, Cao A, Foarabosco A, Schlessinger D. (1996). Mutations in GPC3, a glypican gene, cause the Simpson-Golabi-Behmel overgrowth syndrome. *Nat Genet* 12: 241–247.

Rapraeger A, Krufka A, Olwin BB (1991). Requirement of heparan sulfate for bFGF-mediated fibroblast growth and myoblast differentiation. *Science* 252: 1705–1708.

Reichsman F, Smith L, Cumberledge S (1996). Glycosaminoglycans can modulate extracellular localization of the wingless protein and promote signal transduction. *J Cell Biol* 135: 819–827.

Ross JA, Gurney JG (1998). Hepatoblastoma incidence in the United States from 1973 to 1992. *Med Pediatr Oncol* 30(3): 141–142.

Rubin JB, Choi Y, Segal RA (2002). Cerebellar proteoglycans regulate sonic hedgehog responses during development. *Development* 129(9): 2223–2232.

Ruppert R, Hoffmann E, Sebald W (1996). Human bone morphogenetic protein 2 contains a heparin-binding site which modifies its biological activity. *Eur J Biochem* 237: 295–302.

Sampath TK, Muthukumaran N, Reddi AH (1987). Isolation of osteogenin, an extracellular matrix-associated, bone-inductive protein, by heparin affinity chromatography. *Proc Natl Acad Sci USA* 84: 7109–7113.

Sasisekharan R, Venkataraman G (2000). Heparin and heparan sulfate: biosynthesis, structure and function. *Curr Opin Chem Biol* 4(6): 626–631.

Saunders S, Jalkanen M, O'Farrell S, Bernfield M (1989). Molecular cloning of syndecan, an integral membrane proteoglycan. *J Cell Biol* 108: 1547–1556.

Schilling FH, Spix C, Berthold F, Erttmann R, Fehse N, Hero B, Klein G, Sander J, Schwarz K, Treuner J, et al. (2002). Neuroblastoma screening at one year of age. *N Engl J Med* 346(14): 1047–1053.

Simpson JL, Landey S, New M, German J (1975). A previously unrecognized X-linked syndrome of dysmorphia. *Birth Defects Orig Artic Ser* 11(2): 18–24.

Song HH, Shi W, Filmus J (1997). OCI-5/rat glypican-3 binds to fibroblast growth factor-2 but not to insulin-like growth factor-2. *J Biol Chem* 272: 7574–7577.

Terespolsky D, Farrell SA, Siegel-Bartelt J, Weksberg R (1995). Infantile lethal variant of Simpson-Golabi-Behmel syndrome associated with hydrops fetalis. *Am J Med Genet* 59(3): 329–333.

The I, Bellaiche Y, Perrimon N (1999). Hedgehog movement is regulated through tout velu-dependent synthesis of a heparan sulfate proteoglycan. *Mol Cell* 4: 633–639.

Topczewski J, Sepich DS, Myers DC, Walker C, Amores A, Lele Z, Hammerschmidt M, Postlethwait J, Solnica-Krezel L (2001). The zebrafish glypican knypek controls cell polarity during gastrulation movements of convergent extension. *Dev Cell* 1(2): 251–264.

Tsuda M, Kamimura K, Nakato H, Archer M, Staatz W, Fox B, Humphrey M, Olson S, Futch T, Kaluza V, et al. (1999). The cell-surface proteoglycan Dally regulates Wingless signalling in Drosophila. *Nature* 400: 276–280.

Veugelers M, De Cat B, Ceulemans H, Bruystens AM, Coomans C, Durr J, Vermeesch J, Marynen P, David G (1999). Glypican-6, a new member of the glypican family of cell surface heparan sulfate proteoglycans. *J Biol Chem* 274(38): 26968–26977.

Veugelers M, De Cat B, Muyldermans SY, Reekmans G, Delande N, Frints S, Legius E, Fryns JP, Schrander-Stumpel C, Weidle B, et al. (2000). Mutational analysis of the GPC3/GPC4 glypican gene cluster on Xq26 in patients with Simpson-Golabi-Behmel syndrome: identification of loss-of-function mutations in the GPC3 gene. *Hum Mol Genet* 9(9): 1321–1328.

Veugelers M, Vermeesch J, Watanabe K, Yamaguchi Y, Marynen P, David G (1998).

GPC4, the gene for human K-glypican, flanks GPC3 on xq26: deletion of the GPC3-GPC4 gene cluster in one family with Simpson-Golabi-Behmel syndrome. *Genomics* 53(1): 1–11.

Wang EA, Rosen V, Cordes P, Hewick RM, Kriz MJ, Luxenberg DP, Sibley BS, Wozney JM (1988). Purification and characterization of other distinct bone-inducing factors. *Proc Natl Acad Sci USA* 85: 9484–9488.

Xuan JY, Hughes-Benzie RM, MacKenzie AE (1999). A small interstitial deletion in the GPC3 gene causes Simpson-Golabi-Behmel syndrome in a Dutch-Canadian family. *J Med Genet* 36(1): 57–58.

Yayon A, Klagsbrun M, Esko JD, Leder P, Ornitz DM (1991). Cell surface, heparin-like molecules are required for binding of basic fibroblast growth factor to its high affinity receptor. *Cell* 64: 841–848.

Zioncheck TF, Richardson L, Liu J, Chang L, King KL, Bennett GL, Fugedi P, Chamow SM, Schwall RH, Stack RJ (1995). Sulfated oligosaccharides promote hepatocyte growth factor association and govern its mitogenic activity. *J Biol Chem* 270: 16871–16878.

97 | *HSPG2* (Perlecan) and the Schwartz-Jampel Syndrome and Dyssegmental Dysplasia, Silverman-Handmaker Type

SOPHIE NICOLE AND BERTRAND FONTAINE

Schwartz-Jampel syndrome (SJS) (OMIM 255800) and dyssegmental dysplasia, Silverman-Handmaker type (DDSH) (OMIM 224410) are two infrequent human disorders transmitted with an autosomal recessive mode of inheritance. Both are characterized by abnormal endochondral ossification resulting in skeletal malformations. However, they differ on their degree of severity; DDSH is lethal and unlike SJS is not. In addition, SJS is characterized by a permanent myotonia due to a severe muscle hyperexcitability, which has not been reported in DDSH. Both disorders have been linked to loss of function mutations in the gene encoding perlecan, the major heparan sulfate (HS) proteoglycan (HSPG) of basement membranes (BMs). The functions of perlecan have been, at least in part, elucidated, and animal models with perlecan deficiency are available. These advances led us to propose SJS and DDSH physiopathological models.

PERLECAN

Perlecan is a mammoth protein found in BMs. BMs are thin sheets of extracellular matrix associated with many different cell types (see Chapter 95). Major components of BM include collagen type IV, laminin, glycoproteins such as nidogen (entactin) and fibronectin, and proteoglycans. Proteoglycans are macromolecules composed of a core protein covalently bound to polyanionic glycosaminoglycans (GAGs), which confer charge-dependent functions to the core element. One of the major BM proteoglycans is perlecan. Its name comes from its appearance on rotary-shadowing electron micrographs, looking like pearls on a string (*perle*), and its posttranslational GAG modifications (*can*) (Yurchenco et al., 1987; Noonan et al., 1991).

Structure of Perlecan

The perlecan gene has been cloned in humans, mice, and *Caenorhabditis elegans* and displays a high degree of conservation through evolution (72.4% and 24.9% of identity between human and mouse and between human and nematode proteins, respectively). The human perlecan gene (*HSPG2*, for HSPG 2) is localized on 1p35-p36.1 and is composed of 97 exons (Cohen et al., 1993; Nicole et al., 2000). It is one of the largest human genes described so far; it codes for an open reading frame of 13.2 kb (Kallunki and Tryggvason, 1992; Murdoch et al., 1992). The mature core protein, without the N-terminal signal peptide of 21 amino acids, is composed of 4370 residues in human (compared with 3686 and 3357 residues in mouse and *C. elegans*, respectively) with a predicted molecular weight of 467 kDa. This gigantic protein is subdivided into five domains on the basis of sequence homology to other proteins (Fig. 97–1). These domains are referred to as I to V from the N to the C terminus (Iozzo, 1998).

Domain I contains three SGD consensus sequences whose serine residues serve as attachment sites for HS chains and an SEA (named after the three proteins, sperm protein, enterokinase, and agrin, in which it was identified) module, which enhances the HS attachment (Costell et al., 1997; Dolan et al., 1997). Domain II is arranged in four cysteine-rich modular units (low-density lipoprotein [LDL] receptor class A or LA module) that exhibit structural homology to the ligand-binding domain of the LDL receptor. Domain III displays striking homology to the α chains of laminins. This domain consists of an alternating arrangement of three cysteine-free globular modules inserted within a laminin epidermal growth factor–like (LE) motif (L4 module) and eight connecting LE modules (Schulze et al., 1996). Each LE module contains six to eight cysteine residues that form three or four disulfide bonds. Domain IV is the largest and the most repetitive domain; it consists of a tandem array of 21 immunoglobulin (Ig)-like repeats (14 and 15 in mice and *C. elegans*, respectively), similar to those observed in the extracellular region of neural cell adhesion molecules (NCAMs). Alternate splicing of domain IV has been suggested to generate multiple perlecan isoforms in mice and humans, but no clear data have confirmed these observations (Noonan and Hassell, 1993). Domain V consists in a tandem arrangement of three laminin-type G (LG) and four epidermal growth factor–like (EG) modules and displays structural homology to agrin, another HSPG. It may be partially substituted with GAG chains (Brown et al., 1997a).

Posttranslational modifications add to the complexity of the protein core. Although primarily substituted with HS chains, perlecan may carry chondroitin/dermatan sulfate side chains, even in a hybrid configuration (Brown et al., 1997a; Dolan et al., 1997). Whether this variety in GAG chain attachment is tissue, cell, or time specific remains to be elucidated.

Expression Pattern of Perlecan

Perlecan has been found in all surveyed BMs (Couchman and Ljubimov, 1989; Murdoch et al., 1994). Extensive analyses of perlecan expression during mouse development were performed by in situ hybridization or immunostaining analyses (Handler et al., 1997; Smith et al., 1997). Perlecan is first detected in two-cell embryos before the formation of BMs. Later, perlecan expression occurs in tissue during vasculogenesis that coincides with the formation of the cardiovascular system. Its expression is also correlated with the differentiation of various organs such as skeletal muscle, kidney, lung, liver and spleen. Although lacking a true BM, developing cartilage undergoing endochondral ossification is the tissue that displays the greatest perlecan accumulation. Perlecan is observed in the cartilage primordia and is still observed in adult cartilage, where it is mostly accumulated within the pericellular (the cartilage matrix nearest the chondrocytes) and the territorial matrices throughout the growth plate (SundarRaj et al., 1995).

In vitro Investigations of Perlecan Function

Various functions have been attributed to BMs, such as cell–cell and cell–matrix interactions, growth factor storage and signaling, and passive molecular filtration. Because perlecan is the most abundant HSPG of BMs, a key role of this proteoglycan, either in assembly or in function of BMs, has been suggested and extensively explored.

BM Assembly and Cell Adhesion Properties

The BM architecture results from specific interactions between its components. Type IV collagen chains and laminin isoforms self-assemble to form frameworks. These two distinct networks are connected to each other by nidogen and to the cells by cell surface receptors (Timpl and Brown, 1996). To determine whether mammalian perlecan has an essential role in BM architecture, its interactions with other BM components have been investigated, and various perlecan partners have been identified. Perlecan may self-assemble into dimers or oligomers, probably through domain V (Yurchenco et al., 1987). The HS chains of perlecan mediate interactions with laminin-1, collagen IV, and fibronectin (Battaglia et al., 1992; Sasaki et al., 1998). Domain IV displays a particularly rich binding repertoire, because it interacts with nidogen-1 and -2, fibulin-2, fibronectin, collagen IV, and heparin (Hopf et al., 1999,

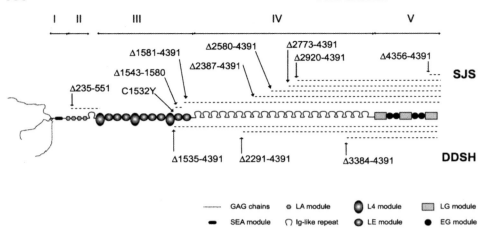

Figure 97–1. Structure of the perlecan core element and perlecan mutations in Schwartz-Jampel syndrome (SJS) and dyssegmental dysplasia, Silverman-Handmaker type (DDSH). The core protein of perlecan consists of five domains (I–V) containing structural motifs found in other proteins. The location and the expected consequences of the mutations are indicated. *Dotted lines*, truncated regions resulting from the mutations.

2001). Domain V binds to heparin, fibulin-2, nidogen-1, and laminin-1 (Brown et al., 1997a; Friedrich et al., 1999).

The major cell surface receptors involved in cell–matrix interactions are integrins, which are transmembrane α/β heterodimers. Collagen IV and laminins are the primary BM integrin ligands, but perlecan also seems to be a BM cell-adhesive component. Perlecan promotes integrin-mediated adherence of a variety of cells, including chondrocytes (Hayashi et al., 1992; SundarRaj et al., 1995). Domain III has been proposed to mediate this cell-adhesion property, but divergent results have been reported, and additional domains seem to be involved in the cell-attachment properties of perlecan (Chakravarti et al., 1995; Schulze et al., 1996). One of these domains could be domain V because it mediates the $\beta1$ integrin cell adhesion of several cell lines (Brown et al., 1997a). In addition, domain V of perlecan is one of the strongest BM partners for the α chain of dystroglycan, another cell surface receptor (Friedrich et al., 1999; Talts et al., 1999). Perlecan may therefore have a crucial role not only in BM architecture, but also in BM–cell interactions.

Growth Factor Signaling

BMs are scaffolds for the cells and also control their phenotypes notably through their ability to modulate the turnover and to control the release and activation status of some growth factors. Because perlecan displays a wide range of expression and is substituted with HS chains, it has been proposed as a candidate for these properties. Perlecan effectively binds several growth factors through both its HS chains, and its core protein. The HS-substituted domain I mediates interactions with fibroblast growth factor (FGF)-2 and platelet-derived growth factor (PDGF)-BB (Whitelock et al., 1996; Gohring et al., 1998). Domain III interacts with PDGF-AA and -BB, FGF-7, and FGF-binding protein (FGF-BP), a secreted protein that binds to FGFs and modulates their activity (Gohring et al., 1998; Mongiat et al., 2000, 2001). Domain V also binds FGF-7 but displays a lower affinity than domain III (Brown et al., 1997a).

Cell assays have demonstrated that perlecan promotes the biological activity of growth factors. Perlecan acts as a low-affinity receptor that assists the binding of FGF-2 and -7 to their receptors and modulates their mitogenic activity (Aviezer et al., 1997; Sharma et al., 1998). However, the apparant FGF mitogenic activity promoted by perlecan depends on the cells. For instance, perlecan is a potent inhibitor of FGF-2 mitogenic stimulation on vascular smooth muscle cells, whereas it promotes FGF-2 signaling on mouse fibroblasts and human melanoma cells (Forsten et al., 1997). The GAG chains that substitute perlecan, or a balance between active and inactive FGF-signaling HSPGs, could contribute to the modulation of perlecan activity on growth factor signaling.

ASSOCIATED DISEASES

Mutations in the human perlecan gene have been identified in two infrequent human diseases: SJS (Nicole et al., 2000) and DDSH (Arikawa-Hirasawa et al., 2001). These two conditions share osteoarticular deformities but diverge in their degree of severity and involvement of skeletal muscle.

Schwartz-Jampel Syndrome

SJS was first reported by Schwartz and Jampel (1962). These two ophthalmologists described two sibs with a blepharophimosis associated with generalized myopathy and skeletal malformations. The same sibs were later characterized in greater detail by Aberfeld et al. (1965), who also noted myotonia (i.e., slowed muscle relaxation caused by an increased muscle excitability). An additional 100 cases have been published in the medical literature.

Giedion et al. (1997) proposed an SJS classification that is based on genetic data, age of manifestation, and radiological features of the disease. Two types are distinguished. Type 1 (SJS1) is the more frequent form and is recognized in childhood. Type 2 is a neonatal form with a more severe course; it generally leads to death of the patient during infancy.

Clinical Features of SJS1

SJS1 is a slowly progressive disorder of abnormal bone and cartilage growth, associated with myotonia. The symptoms and signs become obvious within the first 3 years of life and may begin with either myotonia (type 1A, or SJS1A) or bone deformities (type 1B, or SJS1B). Although few adult patients have been reported, the disease course seems to be slowly progressive until mid-adolescence. The condition then remains stable, and does not alter the life span (Brown et al., 1975; Edwards and Root, 1982).

One of the most recognizable sign of SJS1 is a peculiar facies for which the term "mask-like face" is often used. It is characterized by narrow palpebral fissures with a blepharospasm, a ptosis, pursed lips, and reduced mobility of the facial muscles (Fig. 97–2). This facial expression results from the generalized myotonia that occurs in SJS. It manifests clinically by slowed muscle relaxation and may be elicited by percussion. It is not influenced by exercise, body temperature, or blood potassium levels, unlike other human myotonic disorders (Fontaine et al., 1997). Muscle trophicity may be changed: either hypertrophy or atrophy has been reported. Resistance to passive motion at joints, and fixed flexion contractures are present. The tendon reflexes are generally diminished. Patients complain of pain and fatigue after exercise.

Osteoarticular deformities help to distinguish SJS from other myotonic syndromes. Dwarfism, which may reach −4 to −5 standard deviation, is a constant feature. Bilateral dislocation of the hips frequently occurs, requiring abduction casts. Pectus carinatum (pigeon breast-deformity of the chest) with deformity of the sternum and ribs, kyphoscoliosis, lumbar lordosis, bowing of the long bone, and equinovarus deformity of the feet are other usual findings (see Fig. 97–2).

Additional clinical features may include a high-pitched voice due to an hypoplastic larynx, low-set ears, short neck, paucity of subcutaneous tissue, high arched palate, inguinal hernias, and general hirsutism. Mental development is unaffected. Complications include mechanical difficulties during intubation (Viljoen and Beighton, 1992), malignant hyperthermia during anesthesia (Seay and Ziter, 1978),

A

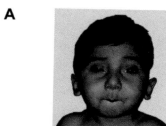

B

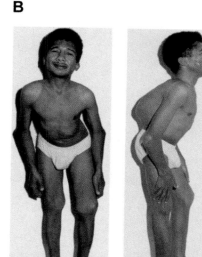

Figure 97–2. Schwartz-Jampel syndrome (SJS). (*A*) SJS1A in a 5-year-old boy. Note the narrow palpebral fissure, low-set ears, and pursed lips. (Photograph kindly provided by J. A. Urtizberea, University of Paris V, Raymond Poincaré Hospital, Garches, France). (*B*) SJS1B in a 20-year-old boy. Osteoarticular deformities include cyphosis, bowing of the long bones, and equinovarus deformity of the feet. (Adapted from Viljoen D, Beighton P [1992]. *J Med Genet,* 20: 58–62, with BMJ Publishing Group permission.)

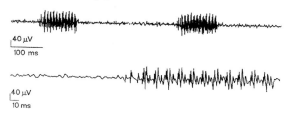

Figure 97–3. Electromyographic recordings from quadriceps of a boy with Schwartz-Jampel syndrome (SJS) with typical SJS spontaneous repetitive discharges observed at rest. (Kindly provided by F. Lehmann-Horn, University of Ulm, Ulm, Germany.)

carpal tunnel syndrome (Cruz Martinez and Arpa, 1998), and compressive myelopathy (Smith et al., 1981).

Laboratory Findings
The results of routine examinations of blood and urine are in normal ranges, except for mild to moderate elevation of serum aldolase or creatine kinase in some cases. Electrocardiograms, electroencephalograms, and motor nerve conduction velocity tests are normal. Decreased conduction of somatosensory evoked potentials through the cervical spinal cord has been reported, but it remains to be determined whether this observation is due to SJS or results from spinal cord compression (Singh et al., 1997).

Electromyographic (EMG) findings in SJS are peculiar, and puzzling contradictions remain. In some investigations, typical myotonic discharges that wax and wane with characteristic musical frequency have been observed in response to muscle stimuli (Mereu et al., 1969; Aberfeld et al., 1970; Desbois et al., 1977). According to the myogenic origin of these discharges, they were still observed during local inhibition of neuromuscular transmission (Cadilhac et al., 1975; Greze et al., 1975). However, spontaneous sustained discharges that persist for long periods are the most frequent and characteristic electromyographic findings of SJS. These high-frequency discharges, also described as pseudomyotonic or complex repetitive discharges, do not wax and wane in amplitude, are present at rest without any stimulating mechanism, and display a relatively constant frequency, thus differing from classic myotonic discharges (Fig. 97–3). They have been observed even in apparent relaxation or after general anesthesia (Huttenlocher et al., 1969; Greze et al., 1975). These discharges have been

suggested to be neurogenic in origin because they are strongly sensitive to neuromuscular block (Taylor et al., 1972). An association of both typical myotonic discharges and spontaneous activities has been observed (Cadilhac et al., 1975; Cruz Martinez et al., 1984; Arimura et al., 1996; Ishpekova et al., 1996).

Muscle biopsy findings are nonspecific and are not required to establish the SJS diagnosis. Findings include mild dystrophic changes with variation in the size of muscle fibers, few central nuclei, increase in endomysial connective tissue, and light fibrosis (Huttenlocher et al., 1969; Desbois et al., 1977; Ben Hamida et al., 1991). The most specific modifications are vacuolation of some muscle fibers. These vacuoles contain granular material and might result from a focal dilatation of the sarcotubular system.

Distinguishing radiographic features are decreased bone age, platyspondyly with frequent coronal cleft vertebrae, epimetaphyseal dysplasia, and paralytic chest (Kozlowski and Wise, 1974; Horan and Beighton, 1975). Severe bilateral coxa vara and iliac base shortening with acetabular dysplasia are noted. Anterior bowing of the diaphyses, metaphyseal widening, and flattening of the epiphyses of the long bones are observed. One biopsy of epiphyseal cartilage revealed relatively inactive resting cartilage with poor columnar organization of chondrocytes (Aberfeld et al., 1965).

Genetic Basis of SJS1
SJS1 is transmitted with an autosomal recessive mode of inheritance. Despite its low frequency, it has been reported in all populations, although it is more frequent in regions of northern Africa, the Middle East, and India where consanguineous marriages are observed. The karyotype was normal in all cases that were studied. SJS1 was mapped to chromosome 1p34-p36.1, and genetic homogeneity of the condition was demonstrated by linkage analyses (Nicole et al., 1995; Fontaine et al., 1996). Types 1A and 1B are allelic disorders, as demonstrated by both genetic linkage and perlecan mutation analyses (Nicole et al., 2000). These molecular studies prove that characteristic facies, continuous muscle hyperexcitability, and osteoarticular deformities, confirmed on electromyography and radiography, respectively, are adequate criteria for the SJS1 diagnosis (Nicole et al., 2003) (Table 97–1).

An autosomal dominant inheritance has been proposed in two families (Ferrannini et al., 1982; Pascuzzi et al., 1990). However, no major bone deformities were observed in these families, suggesting that they may have another myotonic disease.

Table 97–1. Diagnostic Criteria for Schwartz-Jampel Syndrome

Positive Criteria	Exclusion Criteria
Age at onset delayed after birth	Neonatal onset or onset after the first decade
Blepharospasm and mask-like face	
Myotonia confirmed at electromyography	Absence of osteochondrodysplasia at X-rays
Short stature	
Osteochondrodysplasia at X-rays	
Autosomal recessive mode of inheritance	

Patients with a severe form of *myotonia congenita* (mutations in the muscle voltage-gated chloride channel gene) or *myotonia permanens* (mutations in the muscle voltage-gated sodium channel gene) can present with a mask-like face.
Source: The 102nd ENMC meeting, "Advances on Schwartz-Jampel Syndrome," December 2001, Naarden, the Netherlands.

SJS2

Both myotonia and bone dysplasia are manifest at birth in patients with the proposed SJS2 type. Only 30 cases have been reported since its first description by Cao et al. (1978). Clinical findings include an expressionless, flat face with short palpebral fissures, severe dwarfism, marked muscle hypertrophy with stiffness, myotonia, and multiple skeletal deformities (Al Gazali, 1993). These features are apparent at birth or even during pregnancy, when low fetal movements may be noted by the pregnant woman and osteoarticular deformities such as shortening and bowing of the long bones may be seen on ultrasonographic examination (Hunziker et al., 1989). Respiratory difficulties with hypoventilation and life-threatening episodes of hyperthermia are observed in SJS2 that generally lead to early death of the patient due to respiratory complications (Al Gazali et al., 1996).

SJS2 is transmitted with an autosomal recessive mode. SJS2 is not genetically linked to the SJS1 locus, indicating that SJS1 and SJS2 are not allelic disorders (Brown et al., 1997b; Giedion et al., 1997). The reminiscence of clinical signs and the similarity of radiological findings have suggested that SJS2 and Stüve-Wiedemann syndrome (SWS) (OMIM 601559), another infrequent human disorder, are a single entity (Cormier-Daire et al., 1998; Superti-Furga et al., 1998). Identification of SJS2 and SWS on a molecular basis will help to determine whether they are effectively a single entity. Because the clinical picture of SJS2 is differs from that initially described by Schwartz and Jampel and is a distinct genetic entity from SJS1, we propose that the designation of Schwartz-Jampel syndrome type 2 be abandoned (Nicole et al., 2003).

DDSH

DDSH is a rare lethal form of neonatal short-limbed dwarfism. This syndrome was first described by Silverman, who used the term *dysostotic dwarfism*. In 1977, the term *dyssegmental dysplasia* was coined by Handmaker et al. (1977) because of the pronounced malformations in size and shape of the vertebral bodies, which are the primary radiographic features of this condition. Another dyssegmental dysplasia type is the Rolland-Desbuquois syndrome, which displays similar but much less severe dysplastic changes (Aleck et al., 1987). Fewer than 30 cases of DDSH have been reported, that makes this syndrome more rare than SJS.

Clinical Features

DDSH is a fatal condition that manifests at birth, with the affected infants being stillborn or dying within 48 hours after birth. Newborns display an unusual facial appearance with a flat face, short neck, small mouth, low-set ears, frequent prominence of eyes with hypoplastic supraorbital bridges, and narrow palpebral fissures (Handmaker et al., 1977; Fasanelli et al., 1985). Occipital encephalocele and cleft palate may be present. Bone deformities are very severe and include marked dwarfism, narrow and short thorax, bowing of the bones, and micromelia. Reduced joint mobility with flexion contractures is observed. Equinovarus deformity of the feet and general hirsutism are other findings.

Accurate prenatal diagnosis is possible on ultrasonography as early as 16 to 18 weeks' gestation by measurement of the relative femoral length (Andersen et al., 1988; Izquierdo et al., 1990; Stoll et al., 1998; Hsieh et al., 1999). Spine malsegmentation and occipital encephalocele may also be detected.

Radiological and Laboratory Findings

The radiographic findings in DDSH are unique. Severe midface hypoplasia with micrognathia is observed. The skull is small but appears normal except for an opening if there is encephalocele, and thinning of the vault. The most striking feature on skeletal radiographs is a severe segmentation defect of the spine characterized by an extreme anisospondyly due to delayed ossification of the vertebral bodies (Fig. 97–4). These spinal features range from a complete lack of primary and secondary ossification centers to oversized or cleft vertebral bodies. Varying degrees of platyspondyly may also be present. The ilia of patients with DDSH are small and rounded with narrow sacrosciatic notches. The tubular bones are extremely short and bowed and

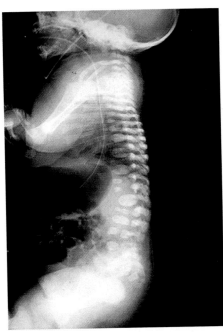

Figure 97–4. Lateral radiograph of the spine from a newborn patient with dyssegmental dysplasia, Silverman-Handmaker type showing severe anisospondyly. (X-ray kindly provided by P. Maroteaux and V. Cormier-Daire, INSERM U393, Hôpital Necker, Paris, France.)

often display midshaft angulation. Flaring and cupping of metaphyses are observed, and epiphyseal ossification at major joints may be absent.

Chondroosseous morphology shows severe abnormalities. Disorganization of the growth plate is observed with no columnar organization of chondrocytes (Handmaker et al., 1977; Fasanelli et al., 1985; Aleck et al., 1987). Calcospherites in the hypertrophic zone are readily visible because they are abnormally large and fail to aggregate. Mucoid degeneration and paucity in collagen fiber patches are noted in the resting cartilage. All of these features indicate a severe defect of endochondral ossification in patients with DDSH.

Autopsies of patients have revealed urinary tract malformations with bilateral hydroureters and early hydronephrosis, and dextrocardia as well as patent ductus arteriosus in some cases. In other cases, the genitourinary tract and the cardiovascular system were intact, indicating that these changes are nonspecific (Handmaker et al., 1977). The skeletal muscular system has never been explored in DDSH.

Inheritance

Affected sibs of both sexes have been observed in DDSH, which indicates an autosomal recessive mode of inheritance. Although DDSH has been proved to result from loss-of-function mutations in the perlecan gene (Arikawa-Hirasawa et al., 2001), it remains to be determined whether this condition is genetically homogeneous. The molecular basis of the milder Rolland-Desbuquois form of dyssegmental dysplasia is still unknown, and whether this form is due to perlecan mutations remains to be documented.

MOLECULAR GENETICS OF THE DISEASES

Two distinct approaches have been used to demonstrate that SJS and DDSH result from mutations in the perlecan gene. A positional cloning strategy was performed to identify perlecan as the SJS gene. The SJS1 locus was located on human chromosome 1p35-p36.1 by genetic linkage analyses (Nicole et al., 1995). Cloning the candidate locus led to the demonstration that the perlecan gene was contained within the SJS1 critical region. Therefore, the perlecan gene was considered as a candidate, and loss-of-function mutations were found (Nicole et al., 2000). A candidate gene approach was used to identify perlecan as the DDSH causative gene. Knockout of the perlecan gene was performed in mice (Arikawa-Hirasawa et al., 1999; Costell et al., 1999), and human diseases with skeletal abnormalities similar to those observed in perlecan-deficient mice were studied for perlecan mutations. Using this approach, DDSH was considered to be a candidate disease, and search for mutations led to the identification of perlecan as responsible for DDSH (Arikawa-Hirasawa et al., 2001).

Review of Human Perlecan Mutations

To date, 13 mutations have been described in the perlecan gene (Table 97–2). Ten of them are associated with SJS, and three are associated with DDSH (Nicole et al., 2000; Arikawa-Hirasawa et al., 2001, 2002a; Nicole et al., 2001). Most of the mutations identified so far are predicted to result in a truncated protein (see Fig. 97–1). Both SJS and DDSH mutations include unusual splicing mutations that do not involve the invariant AG-GT sequences at the splice acceptor and donor sites, respectively. Other mutations include genomic deletions, one genomic duplication, and one missense mutation that affects a highly conserved cysteine residue located within domain III. Nonsense mutations have not been reported. The mutations are located along the entire gene; exons encoding parts of domain II, III, IV or V are altered. Neither hot spot nor founder effect has been observed; each family studied displayed a peculiar mutation.

Phenotype–Genotype Correlation

No phenotype–genotype correlation has been established at the perlecan locus. Both SJS and DDSH are associated with either splicing mutations or genomic rearrangements that are predicted to result in a truncated core element. In addition, the perlecan domains altered by SJS mutations overlap those affected in DDSH. Thus, the molecular genetic analysis of the perlecan gene defect cannot help to establish the resulting phenotype.

If genetic analyses fail to establish a genotype–phenotype correlation, biochemical studies appear to be more efficient. Immunostaining analyses have established that perlecan was secreted by neither cultured fibroblast cells nor chondrocytes in the cartilage matrix from patients with DDSH (Arikawa-Hirasawa et al., 2001). On the contrary, a small amount of perlecan is secreted by cells from SJS patients (Arikawa-Hirasawa et al., 2002a). These observations strongly suggest the concept of a dosage effect for perlecan mutations. Mutations leading to a nearly complete deficiency of perlecan would result in DDSH, whereas hypomorph mutations resulting in a partial perlecan deficiency would be responsible for the milder SJS phenotype.

ESTABLISHING THE SJS AND DDSH DIAGNOSES AND CURRENT THERAPIES

Clinical differential diagnosis for SJS includes severe myotonic and osteochondrodysplasic disorders. Severe *myotonia congenita* and *myotonia permanens* may be confused with SJS (Rüdel et al., 1993) (see

Table 97–1). Although myotonia permanens results from a dominant missense mutation (G1306E) in the muscular voltage-gated sodium channel, only sporadic cases have been described that may be confused with an autosomal recessive transmission. Identification of mutations into the *CLCN1* (responsible for myotonia congenita) or *SCN4A* (responsible for myotonia permanens) genes may help to definitely exclude the diagnosis of SJS (Fontaine et al, 1997). SJS1B, in which myotonia appears later than bone deformities, may be first diagnosed as another chondrodysplasia disease such as micromelic chondrodysplasia, kyphomelic dysplasia, or Burton skeletal dysplasia (Spranger et al., 2000; Arikawa-Hirasawa et al., 2002a).

No efficient therapies have been proposed for SJS and DDSH. Antiepileptic or antiarrhythmic drugs such as carbamazepine, phenytoin, and procainamide have been shown to slightly improve muscle stiffness in SJS (Topaloglu et al., 1993; Ishpekova et al., 1996). Osteoarticular deformities require orthopedic management and often surgery. Due to the severity of the disease and the lack of therapy, a prenatal diagnosis may be desired for DDSH. However, the unusual length of the perlecan gene and the absence of recurrent mutations will render a molecular diagnosis difficult. One way to circumvent these difficulties is to look for perlecan mutations either by genetic linkage, when a first family case has been reported, or by biochemical analyses, when DDSH is suspected on ultrasonography.

ANIMAL MODELS WITH PERLECAN MUTATIONS

C. elegans: Perlecan and Myofilament Attachment

The first animal model resulting from perlecan mutations was described in the nematode *C. elegans*. Perlecan has been designated UNC-52 in this species because it was first identified as responsible for the uncoordinated (unc)-52 phenotype (Rogalski et al., 1993). Five domains are also distinguishable in UNC-52. Interestingly, three major UNC-52 isoforms are produced through alternative splicing: a short isoform composed of domains I to III, a medium isoform extending from domain I to domain IV, and a long form, that contains all five domains (Mullen et al., 1999). Alternative splicing of complete exons generates additional diversity within domains III and IV. These isoforms exhibit differences in expression, as demonstrated by immunostaining analyses using domain-specific antibodies. The short isoform was observed in the pharynx and anal muscles, whereas expression of the medium isoform was restricted to the body-wall musculature.

Two major classes of *unc-52* mutants have been described. Both mutants display a paralytic phenotype due to the disorganization of the myofilament lattice of the body-wall musculature used for locomotion. The first class (class 1) is viable, whereas the second (class 2) is lethal (Kramer, 1997). The class 1 mutants move normally in early larval stages but become progressively less motile. Electron microscopic views of paralyzed adult muscles showed little sarcomere

Table 97–2. Perlecan Mutations in Schwartz-Jampel Syndrome and Dyssegmental Dysplasia, Silverman-Handmaker Type

Mutation	Gene Location	Effect on the Protein	Disease
Genomic deletion	del 720-1654 (exons 8–13)	Δaa235-551? (DII-III)	SJS1A
Missense mutation	G4595A (exon 36)	C1532Y (DIII)	SJS1A
Genomic duplication	4603-4604 ins 89 bp (exon 36)	Δaa1535-4391 (DIII-V)	DDSH
Splicing mutation	G4740A (SD, intron 37)	Δaa1543-1580? (DIII)	SJS1A
Splicing mutation	IVS37-10t → g (SA, intron 37)	Δaa1581-4391? (DIII-V)	SJS1A
Splicing mutation	IVS54+5g → a (SD, intron 54)	Δaa2291-4391 (DIV-V)	DDSH
Splicing mutation	IVS56+4a → g (SD, intron 56)	Δaa2387-4391 (DIV-V)	SJS1A
Genomic deletion	del intron 60	Δaa2580-4391 (DIV-V)	SJS1A
Splicing mutation	G8464A (SD, intron 64)	Δaa2773-4391 (DIV-V)	SJS1B
Splicing mutation	IVS64+4a → g (SD, intron 64)	Δaa2773-4391 (DIV-V)	SJS1A
Genomic deletion	del 8759-8764 (SA, intron 66–exon 67)	Δaa2920-4391 (DIV-V)	SJS1B
Splicing mutation	C10248T (exon 75)	Δaa3384-4391 (DIV-V)	DDSH
Genomic deletion	del 12920 (exons 96–97)	Δaa4356-4391 (DV)	SJS1B

All nucleotide positions refer to the coding sequence (GenBank accession No. M85289) with nucleotide +1 corresponding to the "A" of the first methionine codon. Bases in exon are denoted by uppercase letters and in introns by lowercase letters. ?, Consequence of the mutation is putative; Δ and del, deletion; ins, insertion; SD, splice donor site; SA, splice acceptor site.

organization and fractured dense bodies (the worm analog of Z line), so that the myofilament lattice was no longer associated with the cell membrane. The class 2 mutants result in an elongation arrest at the twofold stage of embryogenesis, when normal embryos begin to move. A severe retarded assembly of myofilament lattice was observed in this class. Both classes result from loss-of-function mutations in the *unc-52* gene, including transposon insertion, genomic deletion, splice donor and nonsense mutations (Rogalski et al., 1995). Interestingly, all of the class 1 mutant alleles are located in alternatively spliced exons, suggesting the presence of a protein with reduced or altered function. The detection of domain IV–containing isoforms in class 1 mutant embryos is consistent with an hypomorphic effect of the class 1 mutations (Rogalski et al., 1995). The class 2 alleles lead to the loss of domain IV, because the medium isoform is not immunodetectable, whereas the short isoform is still observed in the class 2 mutants (Mullen et al., 1999).

The phenotype resulting from perlecan-null mutations indicates that domain IV–containing isoforms are required to initiate and to stabilize the organization of sarcomere units of the body wall musculature. Dense bodies, which are finger-shaped structures that project from the sarcolemma into the cytoplasm, are responsible for anchoring the actin-containing thin filaments to the cell membrane (Moerman and Fire, 1997). They are anchored to the BM, which lies between the muscle cells and the hypodermis, through transmembrane attachments. Perlecan resides in the BM adjacent to the body-wall muscle cells, with an increased concentration at the bases of dense bodies and M-lines (Francis and Waterston, 1991). Its expression overlaps that of integrins at the plasma membrane, and the integrin staining pattern, normally localized at dense bodies and M-lines, is disrupted in *unc-52* class 2 mutants (Hresko et al., 1994). Interestingly, deficiency in integrins also results in a failure to organize sarcomeres in *C. elegans* (Moerman and Fire, 1997). These data strongly support the view that perlecan is necessary for the assembly and the maintenance of the cell muscle attachment structures in *C. elegans*, probably through its interaction with integrin.

Mouse: Perlecan, Basal Lamina Maintenance, Endochondral Ossification, and Muscle Excitability

No spontaneous murine perlecan mutant has been identified so far. To gain insight into the function of mammalian perlecan in vivo, mice lacking perlecan gene expression have been generated through homologous recombination (Arikawa-Hirasawa et al., 1999; Costell et al., 1999). Heterozygous mice were phenotypically normal. From 40% to 80% of homozygous mice for the perlecan-null mutation died between embryonic day (E) 10 and E13 from intrapericardial hemorrhages that result from a local deterioration of BMs submitted to mechanical stress, such as the contracting myocardium (Costell et al., 1999). However, BMs in perlecan-deficient mice appeared normal until E10–E13. The progressive disorganization of BMs when perlecan is lacking supports a critical perlecan function in the structural maintenance of BMs when subjected to mechanical stress, whereas it rejects a key role of perlecan in BM formation.

The mutants surviving to the E10–E13 critical period developed a severe osteochondrodysplasia with frequent exencephaly and died just after birth. The bone deformities included dwarfism, anisospondyly, bowing of limbs, and craniofacial abnormalities resembling those observed in DDSH. Examination of growth plates showed highly disorganized growth zones with a reduced columnar organization of hypertrophic chondrocytes and a poorly organized collagen network with reduced density and shorter collagen fibrils. These data indicate that perlecan is a key element of endochondral ossification, as already suggested by its expression pattern.

Expression of major muscle components appeared normal at E18.5 in perlecan-null mice, suggesting that perlecan is dispensable for the structural organization of skeletal muscle in mammals (Arikawa-Hirasawa et al., 2002b). However, data strongly suggest that perlecan plays a crucial role in the anchoring of acetylcholinesterase (AChE), the primary terminator of neuromuscular transmission, to the synaptic BM. AChE exists in an asymmetric form at the neuromuscular junction (NMJ), which results from the disulfide linkage of AChE catalytic subunits to a collagen-like tail ColQ. Although predominantly present within the BM in a fibrillar network, perlecan was observed at the surface of *Xenopus laevis* muscle cells in a punctuate pattern that was co-localized with AChE (Peng et al., 1998, 1999). In addition, perlecan was found to bind asymmetric AChE in vitro (Peng et al., 1999). The absence of AChE at the NMJ in perlecan-null mice strongly supports the view that perlecan is necessary to the AChE localization to the NMJ (Arikawa-Hirasawa et al., 2002b). Perlecan could therefore take part in the regulation of the muscle excitability through its ability to bind AChE.

TOWARD UNDERSTANDING THE PATHOPHYSIOLOGICAL MECHANISMS THAT LEAD TO DDSH AND SJS

Both in vitro and in vivo data indicate that perlecan acts on the maintenance of BM integrity, endochondral ossification, and organization of NMJ. The biochemical observations performed on patients strongly suggest that DDSH is due to a complete lack of functional perlecan, whereas SJS results from a partial deficiency of this HSPG. The developmental pathways altered in DDSH and SJS are therefore suspected to be the same, with a range of severity that depends on the dosage of perlecan. Although further investigations are required to definitively define the DDSH and SJS pathophysiological mechanisms, the following models emerge from the current knowledge.

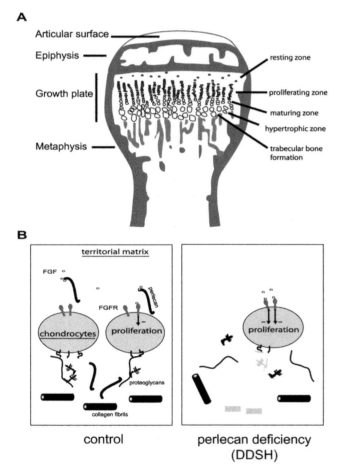

Figure 97–5. Endochondral ossification and perlecan deficiency. (*A*) Longitudinal growth of the long bones occurs in the growth plate located between epiphysis and metaphysis. Chondrocytes located within the growth plate proliferate, mature, and become hypertrophic. The cartilage matrix within the hypertrophic zone will serve as a scaffold for new trabecular bone formation. (*B*) Perlecan is mainly localized within the territorial zone of cartilage matrix. It may act as a reservoir for fibroblast growth factors (FGFs) or help to maintain the integrity of the cartilage matrix. Lack of perlecan would lead to either an increase FGF signaling that inhibits the chondrocyte proliferation or a disassembly of cartilage matrix. FGFR, FGF receptor.

Perlecan and Endochondral Ossification

Endochondral ossification is the bone development process by which an initial cartilage matrix serves as a template for bone formation. *Cartilage* is a specialized form of supportive connective tissue composed of cells, the chondrocytes, that synthesize the cartilage matrix. Chondrocytes develop from resting to hypertrophic states within the growth plate. In the hypertrophic zone, calcification of the matrix provides a scaffold for the formation of new trabecular bone (Fig. 97–5). Chondrogenesis and skeleton pattern formation are triggered by both expression of homeobox genes, which confers information to precursor cells, and cell condensation, allowing autocrine/paracrine signals (Erlebacher et al., 1995; Olsen et al., 2000). Perlecan promotes chondrogenic differentiation in vitro (French et al., 1999, 2002). However, perlecan accumulation follows that of collagen II, a hallmark of chondrocyte differentiation, indicating that perlecan is dispensable for the initial aspects of chondrogenesis (French et al., 1999). In accord with this hypothesis is the finding of normal early events of chondrocyte differentiation in perlecan-null mice.

Perlecan is predominantly observed in the maturing and hypertrophic zones of growth plate where FGF receptor (FGFR3) is also expressed (SundarRaj et al., 1995; Arikawa-Hirasawa et al., 1999). FGF signaling has a critical role in skeletal development, as revealed by the identification of activating FGFR3 mutations in hypochondroplasia, achondroplasia, and thanatophoric dysplasia (Horton, 1997). FGFR3 activation inhibits proliferation and terminal differentiation of chondrocytes in vitro (Kato and Iwamoto, 1990; Sahni et al., 1999). Perlecan, which binds growth factors such as FGF2 and FGF7, could play a critical role in this process. If perlecan acts as a FGF sequestration factor in cartilage matrix, its loss could lead to an increased FGFR3 activation and a subsequent inhibition of chondrocyte proliferation and/or differentiation. However, the DDSH phenotype is quite different from the human diseases associated with activating FGFR3 mutations.

Another possible reason for abnormal endochondral ossification in DDSH and SJS is a role of perlecan in cartilage matrix structure and cell–matrix connections. The collagen fibrils of cartilage matrix are reduced in quantity and size in perlecan-null mice (Costell et al., 1999). The mechanical properties of the cartilage matrix have been suggested to be necessary for proper endochondral ossification (Talts et al., 1998). Because perlecan has been found to protect BMs from mechanical degradation, a perlecan protective effect against cartilage matrix degradation may also be suggested. An excessive degradation of cartilage matrix when perlecan is lacking, resulting in abnormal organization of growth plate and subsequent altered endochondral ossification, might account for the osteoarticular deformities in DDSH and SJS. Studies of perlecan-deficient mice, which represent a good model for DDSH, would help to test this hypothesis.

Perlecan and Skeletal Muscle Excitability

The skeletal NMJ is a chemical synapse that transmits the signal from a motor nerve terminal (the presynaptic membrane) to the muscle fiber (the postsynaptic membrane). The synaptic space between the presynaptic and postsynaptic membranes is lined with a specialized BM, where AChE is located (Sanes and Lichtman, 1999). Arrival of the action potential at the motor neuron terminal leads to neurotransmitter release into the synaptic space. The released neurotransmitter, acetylcholine (ACh), crosses the synaptic space and binds to nicotinic acetylcholine receptors (nAChRs) that are concentrated at the crests of the postsynaptic folds. These ligand-gated cation channels are thus activated, and the subsequent local membrane depolarization, or end-plate potential, activates the voltage-gated sodium channels that generate the muscle action potential (Fig. 97–6).

AChE located at synaptic BMs restricts both the temporal and spatial extents of the action of a nerve impulse on muscle by hydrolyzing ACh. It is selectively localized to the synaptic BM by two events: (1) its gene expression is restricted to subsynaptic muscle nuclei and (2) its collagen-like tail fastly links synaptic BM components (Legay, 2000). Perlecan is suggested to be one of the BM components involved in the selective location of AChE at the NMJ. A lack of perlecan may lead to a reduced synaptic AChE level, as observed in perlecan-null mice. Without hydrolysis, ACh disappearance at the NMJ can occur only via passive diffusion. AChE deficiency may therefore result in a sustained ACh level that will act both on presynaptic and postsynaptic membranes. Hydrolyzing activity of AChE modulates the neurotransmitter release at the NMJ by involving presynaptic muscarinic AChRs (Minic et al., 2002). At the postsynaptic membrane, sustained ACh could rebind to nAChRs, which would lead to multiple activation of nAChRs, and repetitive end-plate potentials after a single nerve impulse. A fine balance between the presynaptic and postsynaptic

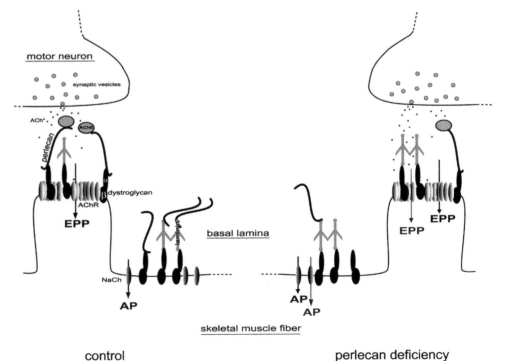

Figure 97–6. The neuromuscular junction and the synaptic transmission. The synaptic space between the motor nerve terminal and the muscle fiber is filled with a specialized basement membrane. When the action potential (AP) raises the motor nerve terminal, it provokes a release of acetylcholine (ACh) into the synaptic cleft. ACh goes through the synapse and binds to ACh receptor (AChR), causing an end-plate potential (EPP). This slight depolarization activates the voltage-gated sodium channels (NaCh), that generates the muscle AP. Perlecan interacts with both the α chain of dystroglycan and AChE to concentrate this enzyme at the neuromuscular junction. When perlecan is missing, a deficiency in AChE occurs. The remaining ACh generates repetitive EPPs and APs that might account for the Schwartz-Jampel syndrome (SJS) muscle hyperexcitability. Another mechanism would be an interaction of extrajunctional perlecan with voltage-gated ion channels to modulate the functional properties of these channels.

effects of perlecan deficiency could result in multiple action potentials in response to each nerve impulse and in a subsequent muscle hyperexcitability.

If a deficiency in AChE can account for a neurogenic myotonia, it does not explain the intrinsic muscle hyperexcitability observed in patients with SJS. Although predominantly present at the NMJ, perlecan is observed within the muscle extrasynaptic BM. Data have demonstrated that the extracellular matrix protein tenascin-R binds to voltage-gated sodium channels and modulates their electrophysiological properties (Xiao et al., 1999). The observation of reduced motor axon conduction velocities observed in tenascin-R–null mice is in agreement with an effect of this extracellular matrix protein on voltage-gated ion channel properties (Weber et al., 1999). Whether extrasynaptic perlecan can act on the regulation of muscle voltage-gated ion channel properties remains to be investigated. Another role for extrasynaptic perlecan would be to maintain BM architecture, as observed in *C. elegans* and mice. Although the major muscle dysfunction in SJS is myotonia, patients also have mild dystrophy. An animal model that circumvents the lethality of complete perlecan deficiency is required to definitively assess the function of perlecan in mammal skeletal muscles and its relationship to skeletal muscle excitability.

ACKNOWLEDGMENTS

Our work was financially supported by Institut National de la Santé et de la Recherche Médicale (INSERM), RESOCANAUX, and Association Française contre les Myopathies (AFM).

REFERENCES

Aberfeld DC, Hinterbuchner LP, Schneider M (1965). Myotonia, dwarfism, diffuse bone disease and unusual ocular and facial abnormalities (a new syndrome). *Brain* 88: 313–322.

Aberfeld DC, Namba T, Vye MV, Grob D (1970). Chondrodystrophic myotonia: report of two cases. Myotonia, dwarfism, diffuse bone disease, and unusual ocular and facial abnormalities. *Arch Neurol* 22: 455–462.

Al Gazali LI (1993). The Schwartz-Jampel syndrome. *Clin Dysmorphol* 2: 47–54.

Al Gazali LI, Varghese M, Varady E, Al Talabani J, Scorer J, Bakalinova D (1996). Neonatal Schwartz-Jampel syndrome: a common autosomal recessive syndrome in the United Arab Emirates. *J Med Genet* 33: 203–211.

Aleck K, Grix A, Clericuzio C, Kaplan P, Adomian G, Lachman R, Rimoin D (1987). Dyssegmental dysplasias: clinical, radiographic, and morphologic evidence of heterogeneity. *Am J Med Genet* 27: 295–312.

Andersen P, Hauge M, Bang J (1988). Dyssegmental dysplasia in siblings: prenatal ultrasonic diagnosis. *Skeletal Radiol* 17: 29–31.

Arikawa-Hirasawa E, Watanabe H, Takami H, Hassell JR, Yamada Y (1999). Perlecan is essential for cartilage and cephalic development. *Nat Genet* 23: 354–358.

Arikawa-Hirasawa E, Wilcox WR, Le A, Silverman N, Govindraj P, Hassell J, Yamada Y (2001). Dyssegmental dysplasia, Silverman-Handmaker type, is caused by functional null mutations of the perlecan gene. *Nat Genet* 27: 431–434.

Arikawa-Hirasawa E, Le AH, Nishino I, Nonaka I, Ho NC, Francomano CA, Govindraj P, Hassell JR, Devaney JM, Spranger J, et al. (2002a). Structural and functional mutations of the perlecan gene cause Schwartz-Jampel syndrome, with myotonic myopathy and chondrodysplasia. *Am J Hum Genet* 70: 1368–1375.

Arikawa-Hirasawa E, Rossi SG, Rotundo RL, Yamada Y (2002b). Absence of acetylcholinesterase at the neuromuscular junctions of perlecan-null mice. *Nat Neurosci* 5: 119–123.

Arimura K, Takenaga S, Nakagawa M, Osame M, Stalberg E (1996). Stimulation single fibre EMG study in a patient with Schwartz-Jampel syndrome. *J Neurol Neurosurg Psychiatry* 61: 425–426.

Aviezer D, Iozzo RV, Noonan DM, Yayon A (1997). Suppression of autocrine and paracrine functions of basic fibroblast growth factor by stable expression of perlecan antisense cDNA. *Mol Cell Biol* 17: 1938–1946.

Battaglia C, Mayer U, Aumailley M, Timpl R (1992). Basement-membrane heparan sulfate proteoglycan binds to laminin by its heparan sulfate chains and to nidogen by sites in the protein core. *Eur J Biochem* 208: 359–366.

Ben Hamida M, Miladi N, Ben Hamida C (1991). Schwartz-Jampel syndrome. Clinical and histopathological study of 4 cases. *Rev Neurol (Paris)* 147: 279–284.

Brown JC, Sasaki T, Gohring W, Yamada Y, Timpl R (1997a). The C-terminal domain V of perlecan promotes beta1 integrin-mediated cell adhesion, binds heparin, nidogen and fibulin-2 and can be modified by glycosaminoglycans. *Eur J Biochem* 250: 39–46.

Brown KA, al-Gazali LI, Moynihan LM, Lench NJ, Markham AF, Mueller RF (1997b). Genetic heterogeneity in Schwartz-Jampel syndrome: two families with neonatal Schwartz-Jampel syndrome do not map to human chromosome 1p34-p36.1. *J Med Genet* 34: 685–687.

Brown SB, Garcia-Mullin R, Murai Y (1975). The Schwartz-Jampel syndrome (myotonic chondrodystrophy) in the adult. *Neurology* 25: 365–366.

Cadilhac J, Baldet P, Greze J, Duday H (1975). E.M.G. studies of two family cases of the Schwartz and Jampel syndrome (osteo-chondro-muscular dystrophy with myotonia). *Electromyogr Clin Neurophysiol* 15: 5–12.

Cao A, Cianchetti C, Calisti L, de Virgiliis S, Ferreli A, Tangheroni W (1978). Schwartz-Jampel syndrome. Clinical, electrophysiological and histopathological study of a severe variant. *J Neurol Sci* 35: 175–187.

Chakravarti S, Horchar T, Jefferson B, Laurie GW, Hassell JR (1995). Recombinant domain III of perlecan promotes cell attachment through its RGDS sequence. *J Biol Chem* 270: 404–409.

Cohen IR, Grassel S, Murdoch AD, Iozzo RV (1993). Structural characterization of the complete human perlecan gene and its promoter. *Proc Natl Acad Sci USA* 90: 10404–10408.

Cormier-Daire V, Superti-Furga A, Munnich A, Lyonnet S, Rustin P, Delezoide AL, De Lonlay P, Giedion A, Maroteaux P, Le Merrer M (1998). Clinical homogeneity of the Stuve-Wiedemann syndrome and overlap with the Schwartz-Jampel syndrome type 2. *Am J Med Genet* 78: 146–149.

Costell M, Mann K, Yamada Y, Timpl R (1997). Characterization of recombinant perlecan domain I and its substitution by glycosaminoglycans and oligosaccharides. *Eur J Biochem* 243: 115–121.

Costell M, Gustafsson E, Aszodi A, Morgelin M, Bloch W, Hunziker E, Addicks K, Timpl R, Fassler R (1999). Perlecan maintains the integrity of cartilage and some basement membranes. *J Cell Biol* 147: 1109–1122.

Couchman JR, Ljubimov AV (1989). Mammalian tissue distribution of a large heparan sulfate proteoglycan detected by monoclonal antibodies. *Matrix* 9: 311–321.

Cruz Martinez A, Arpa J (1998). Carpal tunnel syndrome in childhood: study of 6 cases. *Electroencephalogr Clin Neurophysiol* 109: 304–308.

Cruz Martinez A, Arpa J, Perez Conde MC, Ferrer MT (1984). Bilateral carpal tunnel in childhood associated with Schwartz-Jampel syndrome. *Muscle Nerve* 7: 66–72.

Desbois J, Guyou J, Grenet P, Herrault A (1977). Chondrodystrophie myotonique (ou syndrome de Schwartz-Jampel). Etude d'une fratrie et revue de la littérature. *Ann Pediatr* 24: 563–574.

Dolan J, Horchar T, Rigatti B, Hassell JR (1997). Identification of sites in domain I of perlecan that regulate heparan sulfate synthesis. *J Biol Chem* 272: 4316–4322.

Edwards WC, Root AW (1982). Chondrodystrophic myotonia (Schwartz-Jampel syndrome): report of a new case and follow-up of patients initially reported in 1969. *Am J Med Genet* 13: 51–56.

Erlebacher A, Filvaroff E, Gitelman S, Derynck R (1995). Toward a molecular understanding of skeletal development. *Cell* 80: 371–378.

Fasanelli S, Kozlowski K, Reiter S, Sillence D (1985). Dyssegmental dysplasia (Report of two cases with a review of the literature). *Skeletal Radiol* 14: 173–177.

Ferrannini E, Perniola T, Krajewska G, Serlenga L, Trizio M (1982). Schwartz-Jampel syndrome with autosomal-dominant inheritance. *Eur Neurol* 21: 137–146.

Fontaine B, Plassart-Schiess E, Nicole S (1997). Diseases caused by voltage-gated ion channels. *Mol Aspects Med* 18: 415–463.

Fontaine B, Nicole S, Topaloglu H, Ben Hamida C, Beighton P, Spaans F, Cantu JM, Bakouri S, Romero N, Ricker K, et al. (1996). Recessive Schwartz-Jampel syndrome (SJS): confirmation of linkage to chromosome 1p, evidence of genetic homogeneity and reduction of the SJS locus to a 3-cM interval. *Hum Genet* 98: 380–385.

Forsten KE, Courant NA, Nugent MA (1997). Endothelial proteoglycans inhibit bFGF binding and mitogenesis. *J Cell Physiol* 172: 209–220.

Francis R, Waterston R (1991). Muscle cell attachment in *Caenorhabditis elegans*. *J Cell Biol* 114: 465–479.

French MM, Gomes RR Jr, Timpl R, Hook M, Czymmek K, Farach-Carson MC, Carson DD (2002). Chondrogenic activity of the heparan sulfate proteoglycan perlecan maps to the N-terminal domain I. *J Bone Miner Res* 17: 48–55.

French MM, Smith SE, Akanbi K, Sanford T, Hecht J, Farach-Carson MC, Carson DD (1999). Expression of the heparan sulfate proteoglycan, perlecan, during mouse embryogenesis and perlecan chondrogenic activity in vitro. *J Cell Biol* 145: 1103–1115.

Friedrich MV, Gohring W, Morgelin M, Brancaccio A, David G, Timpl R (1999). Structural basis of glycosaminoglycan modification and of heterotypic interactions of perlecan domain V. *J Mol Biol* 294: 259–270.

Giedion A, Boltshauser E, Briner J, Eich G, Exner G, Fendel H, Kaufmann L, Steinmann B, Spranger J, Superti-Furga A (1997). Heterogeneity in Schwartz-Jampel chondrodystrophic myotonia. *Eur J Pediatr* 156: 214–223.

Gohring W, Sasaki T, Heldin CH, Timpl R (1998). Mapping of the binding of platelet-derived growth factor to distinct domains of the basement membrane proteins BM-40 and perlecan and distinction from the BM-40 collagen-binding epitope. *Eur J Biochem* 255: 60–66.

Greze J, Baldet P, Dumas R, Cadilhac J, Pages A, Jean J (1975). Schwartz-Jampel osteo-chondro-muscular dystrophy. 2 familial cases. *Arch Fr Pediatr* 21: 59–75.

Handler M, Yurchenco PD, Iozzo RV (1997). Developmental expression of perlecan during murine embryogenesis. *Dev Dyn* 210: 130–145.

Handmaker S, Robinson L, Campbell J, Chinwah O, Gorlin R (1977). Dyssegmental dwarfism: a new syndrome of lethal dwarfism. *Birth Defects Orig Art Ser* XIII (3D): 79–90.

Hayashi K, Madri JA, Yurchenco PD (1992). Endothelial cells interact with the core protein of basement membrane perlecan through beta 1 and beta 3 integrins: an adhesion modulated by glycosaminoglycan. *J Cell Biol* 119: 945–959.

Hopf M, Gohring W, Mann K, Timpl R (2001). Mapping of binding sites for nidogens, fibulin-2, fibronectin and heparin to different IG modules of perlecan. *Mol Biol* 311: 529–541.

Hopf M, Gohring W, Kohfeldt E, Yamada Y, Timpl R (1999). Recombinant domain IV of perlecan binds to nidogens, laminin-nidogen complex, fibronectin, fibulin-2 and heparin. *Eur J Biochem* 259: 917–925.

Horan F, Beighton P (1975). Orthopaedic aspects of the Schwartz-Jampel syndrome. *J Bone Joint Surg (Am)* 57: 542–544.

Horton WA (1997). Fibroblast growth factor receptor 3 and the human chondrodysplasias. *Curr Opin Pediatr* 9: 437–442.

Hresko M, Williams B, Waterston R (1994). Assembly of body wall muscle and muscle cell attachment structures in *Caenorhabditis elegans*. *J Cell Biol* 124: 491–506.

Hsieh Y, Chang C, Tsai H, Lee C, Tsai F, Tsai C (1999). Prenatal diagnosis of dyssegmental dysplasia. A case report. *J Reprod Med* 44: 303–305.

Hunziker UA, Savoldelli G, Boltshauser E, Giedion A, Schinzel A (1989). Prenatal diagnosis of Schwartz-Jampel syndrome with early manifestation. *Prenat Diagn* 9: 127–131.

Huttenlocher PR, Landwirth J, Hanson V, Gallagher BB, Bensch K (1969). Osteo-chondro-muscular dystrophy. A disorder manifested by multiple skeletal deformities, myotonia, and dystrophic changes in muscle. *Pediatrics* 44: 945–958.

Iozzo RV (1998). Matrix proteoglycans: from molecular design to cellular function. *Annu Rev Biochem* 67: 609–652.

Ishpekova B, Rasheva M, Moskov M (1996). Schwartz-Jampel syndrome: clinical, electromyographic and genetic studies. *Electromyogr Clin Neurophysiol* 36: 151–155.

Izquierdo L, Kushnir O, Aase J, Lantz P, Castellano T, Curet L (1990). Antenatal ultrasonic diagnosis of dyssegmental dysplasia: a case report. *Prenat Diagn* 10: 587–592.

Kallunki P, Tryggvason K (1992). Human basement membrane heparan sulfate proteoglycan core protein: a 467-kD protein containing multiple domains resembling elements of the low density lipoprotein receptor, laminin, neural cell adhesion molecules, and epidermal growth factor. *J Cell Biol* 116: 559–571.

Kato Y, Iwamoto M (1990). Fibroblast growth factor is an inhibitor of chondrocyte terminal differentiation. *J Biol Chem* 265: 5903–5909.

Kozlowski K, Wise G (1974). Spondylo-epi-metaphyseal dysplasia with myotonia. A radiographic study (Catel-Hempel syndrome, Schwarz-Jampel syndrome, Aberfeld syndrome, chondrodystrophic myotonia). *Radiol Diagn (Berl)* 15: 817–824.

Kramer J (1997). Extracellular matrix. In: *C. elegans* II. Riddle D, Blumenthal T, Meyer B, Priess J (eds). Cold Spring Harbor Laboratory Press, Cold Spring Harbor, NY, pp. 471–500.

Legay C (2000). Why so many forms of acetylcholinesterase? *Microsc Res Tech* 49: 56–72.

Mereu TR, Porter IH, Hug G (1969). Myotonia, shortness of stature, and hip dysplasia. Schwartz-Jampel syndrome. *Am J Dis Child* 117: 470–478.

Minic J, Molgo J, Karlsson E, Krejci E (2002). Regulation of acetylcholine release by muscarinic receptors at the mouse neuromuscular junction depends on the activity of acetylcholinesterase. *Eur J Neurosci* 15: 439–448.

Moerman D, Fire A (1997). Muscle: structure, function and development. In: *C. elegans* II. Riddle D Blumenthal T, Meyer B, Priess J (eds). Cold Spring Harbor Laboratory Press, Cold Spring Harbor, NY, pp. 417–470.

Mongiat M, Otto J, Oldershaw R, Ferrer F, Sato JD, Iozzo RV (2001). Fibroblast growth factor-binding protein is a novel partner for perlecan core protein. *J Biol Chem* 276: 10263–10271.

Mongiat M, Taylor K, Otto J, Aho S, Uitto J, Whitelock JM, Iozzo RV (2000). The protein core of the proteoglycan perlecan binds specifically to fibroblast growth factor-7. *J Biol Chem* 275: 7095–7100.

Mullen GP, Rogalski TM, Bush JA, Gorji PR, Moerman DG (1999). Complex patterns of alternative splicing mediated the spatial and temporal distribution of perlecan/UNC-52 in *Caenorhabditis elegans*. *Mol Biol Cell* 10: 3205–3221.

Murdoch AD, Dodge GR, Cohen I, Tuan RS, Iozzo RV (1992). Primary structure of the human heparan sulfate proteoglycan from basement membrane (HSPG2/perlecan). A chimeric molecule with multiple domains homologous to the low density lipoprotein receptor, laminin, neural cell adhesion molecules, and epidermal growth factor. *J Biol Chem* 267: 8544–8557.

Murdoch AD, Liu B, Schwarting R, Tuan RS, Iozzo RV (1994). Widespread expression of perlecan proteoglycan in basement membranes and extracellular matrices of human tissues as detected by a novel monoclonal antibody against domain III and by in situ hybridization. *J Histochem Cytochem* 42: 239–249.

Nicole S, Topaloglu H, Fontaine B (2003). 102nd ENMC international workshop: Advances in Schwartz-Jampel syndrome. *Neuromusc Disord* 13:347–351.

Nicole S, Vicart S, Davoine C, Fontaine B (2001). Mutations of perlecan, the major proteoglycan of basement membranes, cause Schwartz-Jampel syndrome: a new mechanism for myotonia? *Acta Myol* XX: 130–133.

Nicole S, Ben Hamida C, Beighton P, Bakouri S, Belal S, Romero N, Viljoen D, Ponsot G, Sammoud A, Weissenbach J, et al. (1995). Localization of the Schwartz-Jampel syndrome (SJS) locus to chromosome 1p34-p36.1 by homozygosity mapping. *Hum Mol Genet* 4: 1633–1636.

Nicole S, Davoine C-S, Topaloglu H, Cattolico L, Barral D, Beighton P, Ben Hamida C, Hammouda H, Cruaud C, White P, et al. (2000). Perlecan, the major proteoglycan of basement membranes, is altered in patients with Schwartz-Jampel syndrome (chondrodystrophic myotonia). *Nature Genet* 26: 480–483.

Noonan DM, Hassell JR (1993). Perlecan, the large low-density proteoglycan of basement membranes: structure and variant forms. *Kidney Int* 43: 53–60.

Noonan DM, Fulle A, Valente P, Cai S, Horigan E, Sasaki M, Yamada Y, Hassell JR (1991). The complete sequence of perlecan, a basement membrane heparan sulfate proteoglycan, reveals extensive similarity with laminin A chain, low density lipoprotein-receptor, and the neural cell adhesion molecule. *J Biol Chem* 266: 22939–22947.

Olsen BR, Reginato AM, Wang W (2000). Bone development. *Annu Rev Cell Dev Biol* 16: 191–220.

Pascuzzi RM, Gratianne R, Azzarelli B, Kincaid JC (1990). Schwartz-Jampel syndrome with dominant inheritance. *Muscle Nerve* 13: 1152–1163.

Peng HB, Ali AA, Daggett DF, Rauvala H, Hassell JR, Smalheiser NR (1998). The relationship between perlecan and dystroglycan and its implication in the formation of the neuromuscular junction. *Cell Adhes Commun* 5: 475–489.

Peng HB, Xie H, Rossi SG, Rotundo RL (1999). Acetylcholinesterase clustering at the neuromuscular junction involves perlecan and dystroglycan. *J Cell Biol* 145: 911–921.

Rogalski TM, Gilchrist EJ, Mullen GP, Moerman DG (1995). Mutations in the unc-52 gene responsible for body wall muscle defects in adult Caenorhabditis elegans are located in alternatively spliced exons. *Genetics* 139: 159–169.

Rogalski TM, Williams BD, Mullen GP, Moerman DG (1993). Products of the unc-52 gene in Caenorhabditis elegans are homologous to the core protein of the mammalian basement membrane heparan sulfate proteoglycan. *Genes Dev* 7: 1471–1484.

Rüdel R, Ricker K, Lehmann-Horn F (1993). Genotype-phenotype correlations in human skeletal muscle sodium channel diseases. *Arch Neurol* 50: 1241–1248.

Sahni M, Ambrosetti DC, Mansukhani A, Gertner R, Levy D, Basilico C (1999). FGF signaling inhibits chondrocyte proliferation and regulates bone development through the STAT-1 pathway. *Genes Dev* 13: 1361–1366.

Sanes JR, Lichtman JW (1999). Development of the neuromuscular junction. *Annu Rev Neurosci* 22: 389–442.

Sasaki T, Costell M, Mann K, Timpl R (1998). Inhibition of glycosaminoglycan modification of perlecan domain I by site-directed mutagenesis changes protease sensitivity and laminin-1 binding activity. *FEBS Lett* 435: 169–172.

Schulze B, Sasaki T, Costell M, Mann K, Timpl R (1996). Structural and cell-adhesive properties of three recombinant fragments derived from perlecan domain III. *Matrix Biol* 15: 349–357.

Schwartz O, Jampel R (1962). Congenital blepharophimosis associated with a unique generalized myopathy. *Arch Ophthalmol* 68: 82–87.

Seay A, Ziter F (1978). Malignant hyperpyrexia in a patient with Schwartz-Jampel syndrome. *J Pediatr* 93: 83–84.

Sharma B, Handler M, Eichstetter I, Whitelock JM, Nugent MA, Iozzo RV (1998). Antisense targeting of perlecan blocks tumor growth and angiogenesis in vivo. *J Clin Invest* 102: 1599–1608.

Silverman F (1969). Forms of dysostotic dwarfism of uncertain classification. *Ann Radiol (Paris)* 19: 139.

Singh B, Biary N, Jamil AA, al-Shahwan SA (1997). Schwartz-Jampel syndrome: evidence of central nervous system dysfunction. *J Child Neurol* 12: 214–217.

Smith D, Schoumaker R, Shuman R (1981). Compressive myelopathy in the Schwartz-Jampel syndrome. *Ann Neurol* 10: 497.

Smith SE, French MM, Julian J, Paria BC, Dey SK, Carson DD (1997). Expression of heparan sulfate proteoglycan (perlecan) in the mouse blastocyst is regulated during normal and delayed implantation. *Dev Biol* 184: 38–47.

Spranger J, Hall BD, Hane B, Srivastava A, Stevenson RE (2000). Spectrum of Schwartz-Jampel syndrome includes micromelic chondrodysplasia, kyphomelic dysplasia, and Burton disease. *Am J Med Genet* 94: 287–295.

Stoll C, Langer B, Gasser B, Alembik Y (1998). Sporadic case of dyssegmental dysplasia with antenatal presentation. *Genet Couns* 9: 125–130.

SundarRaj N, Fite D, Ledbetter S, Chakravarti S, Hassell JR (1995). Perlecan is a component of cartilage matrix and promotes chondrocyte attachment. *J Cell Sci* 108: 2663–2672.

Superti-Furga A, Tenconi R, Clementi M, Eich G, Steinmann B, Boltshauser E, Giedion A (1998). Schwartz-Jampel syndrome type 2 and Stuve-Wiedemann syndrome: a case for "lumping." *Am J Med Genet* 78: 150–154.

Talts JF, Andac Z, Gohring W, Brancaccio A, Timpl R (1999). Binding of the G domains of laminin alpha1 and alpha2 chains and perlecan to heparin, sulfatides, alpha-dystroglycan and several extracellular matrix proteins. *EMBO J* 18: 863–870.

Talts JF, Pfeifer A, Hofmann F, Hunziker EB, Zhou XH, Aszodi A, Fassler R (1998). Endochondral ossification is dependent on the mechanical properties of cartilage tissue and on intracellular signals in chondrocytes. *Ann N Y Acad Sci* 857: 74–85.

Taylor RG, Layzer RB, Davis HS, Fowler WM, Jr. (1972). Continuous muscle fiber activity in the Schwartz-Jampel syndrome. *Electroencephalogr Clin Neurophysiol* 33: 497–509.

Timpl R, Brown JC (1996). Supramolecular assembly of basement membranes. *Bioessays* 18: 123–132.

Topaloglu H, Serdaroglu A, Okan M, Gucuyener K, Topcu M (1993). Improvement of myotonia with carbamazepine in three cases with the Schwartz-Jampel syndrome. *Neuropediatrics* 24: 232–234.

Viljoen D, Beighton P (1992). Schwartz-Jampel syndrome (chondrodystrophic myotonia). *J Med Genet* 29: 58–62.

Weber P, Bartsch U, Rasband M, Czaniera R, Lang Y, Bluethmann H, Margolis R, Levinson S, Shrager P, Montag D, et al. (1999). Mice deficient for tenascin-R display alterations of the extracellular matrix and decreased axonal conduction velocities in the CNS. *J Neurosci* 19: 4245–4262.

Whitelock JM, Murdoch AD, Iozzo RV, Underwood PA (1996). The degradation of human endothelial cell-derived perlecan and release of bound basic fibroblast growth factor by stromelysin, collagenase, plasmin, and heparanases. *J Biol Chem* 271: 10079–10086.

Xiao ZC, Ragsdale DS, Malhotra JD, Mattei LN, Braun PE, Schachner M, Isom LL (1999). Tenascin-R is a functional modulator of sodium channel beta subunits. *J Biol Chem* 274: 26511–26517.

Yurchenco PD, Chang YS, Ruben GC (1987). Self-assembly of a high molecular weight basement membrane heparan sulfate proteoglycan into dimers and oligomers. *J Biol Chem* 262: 17668–17676.

CONNIE SCHRANDER-STUMPEL AND JEAN-PIERRE FRYNS

Mutations in the *L1CAM* gene encoding for the neural (L1) cell adhesion molecule L1CAM, located at Xq28, result in a varying clinical spectrum. Manifestations range from lethal congenital hydrocephalus in males (X-linked hydrocephalus or hereditary stenosis of the aquaductus of Sylvius [HSAS], OMIM 307000) to mild to moderate mental retardation combined with spastic paraplegia (with or without hydrocephalus on brain imaging): MASA syndrome (mental retardation, aphasia or slow speech development, shuffling gait or spastic paraplegia, and adducted thumbs; OMIM 303350). X-linked spastic paraplegia (SPG1, OMIM 312900) is included in the spectrum, as is "L1 syndrome" (OMIM 308840), which includes the X-linked agenesis of the corpus callosum and mental retardation with clasped thumb.

L1CAM belongs to the immunoglobulin superfamily of cell adhesion molecules and is involved in neuronal cell migration, fasciculation, outgrowth, and regeneration in the brain and in the peripheral nervous system. L1CAM has a prominent role in the formation of the pyramids and the corticospinal tract (see Chapter 95). There are specific neuropathological findings on MRI and brain autopsy.

The great majority of *L1CAM* mutations in well-documented families are private. With a proved linkage to Xq28 or (preferably) proved *L1* gene mutation, carrier detection and prenatal diagnosis can be offered. Prenatal diagnosis based on an early ultrasonography scan is not reliable because ventriculomegaly usually starts after 20 weeks' of gestation. We stress the importance of mutation analysis, even in sporadic cases, after careful neuropathological workup based on a standardized protocol.

Congenital hydrocephalus is a serious condition that can arise from multiple causes. It comprises a diverse group of conditions that result in impaired circulation and absorption of cerebrospinal fluid. Congenital malformations of the central nervous system, infections, hemorrhage, trauma, teratogens, and, occasionally, tumors can all give rise to hydrocephalus. In this chapter, we focus on the X-linked type of hydrocephalus that comprises approximately 5% of all cases of congenital hydrocephalus (Schrander-Stumpel, 1995).

In this condition caused by mutations in the *L1* gene at Xq28 coding for L1CAM, a neural cell adhesion molecule, clinical variability is great and extends from massive, (sub)lethal hydrocephalus to complicated spastic paraplegia to mental retardation with clasped thumbs as the mildest manifestation (Fryns et al., 1991; Schrander-Stumpel, 1995).

CLINICAL DESCRIPTION

HSAS (Bickers and Adams, 1949) is the most common genetic form of congenital hydrocephalus, with an incidence of approximately 1:30,000. This accounts for approximately 2% of newborns with nonsyndromal hydrocephalus (Editorial, 1962) to a maximum of 25% in male newborns (Burton, 1979). A general estimate of approximately 5% of children with nonsyndromal congenital hydrocephalus seems appropriate (Schrander-Stumpel and Fryns, 1998). Clinical variability ranges from lethality in utero or early infancy to survival with mental retardation, spastic paraplegia and adducted thumbs (Edwards, 1961; Schrander-Stumpel, 1995). The clinical diagnosis is based on the finding of a boy with hydrocephalus and clasped thumbs, which are present in more than 50% of reported cases (Schrander-Stumpel and Fryns, 1998) (Figs. 98–1 through 98–3). Family history is gener-

ally positive for similarly affected boys or for affected males with complicated spastic paraplegia. De novo occurences, however, have been reported and encountered (M. Jouet and S. Kenwrick, 1995, personal observations). If family history is negative and a deceased boy had no clasped thumbs but had a severe hydrocephalus, neuropathological examination provides an important diagnostic contribution. Bilateral absence of the pyramids is an important and almost pathognomonic finding in autopsies and MRI studies (Chow et al., 1985; Schander-Stumpel et al., 2000). Aqueductal stenosis is not a constant feature in the condition (Landrieu et al., 1979; Varadi et al., 1987; Yamasaki et al., 1995). Many concomitant nervous system anomalies have been reported, such as corpus callosal a/dysgenesis, small brain stem, and absence of the pyramidal tract (Willems et al., 1987; Yamasaki et al., 1995). A protocol for the neuropathological workup in male children with hydrocephalus of unknown cause and without family history was proposed by Schrander-Stumpel et al. (2000) and it was hypothesized that the L1 syndrome can be recognized with a high specificity by a standardized workup (Table 98–1).

Clinical features in surviving patients with HSAS show great overlap with the patients affected with MASA syndrome (Bianchine and Lewis, 1974; Schrander-Stumpel et al., 1990). Corpus callosal agenesis (CCA) is commonly reported in surviving patients with the syndrome (Willems et al., 1987; Boyd et al., 1993; Yamasaki et al., 1995). In the literature, there are a number of reports of X-linked complicated CCA (Schrander-Stumpel, 1995). Although no DNA linkage analysis with distal Xq probes is available in these families, we suggest that at least some X-linked CCA families may fit into the spectrum. Hirschsprung disease accompanies the clinical features in some patients (Parisi et al., 2002).

The clinical spectrum of X-linked hydrocephalus thus is variable, with diagnostic problems occurring in about 10% of the surviving patients. X-linked mental retardation can be regarded as the minimal clinical criterion, but in general there are additional neurological features. Because clinical overlap with the second X-linked locus for complicated spastic paraplegia exists (*PLP* locus at Xq22), there may be pitfalls in making the diagnosis of the *L1* syndrome on clinical grounds only, especially when hydrocephalus is absent in the affected males.

Preferential X chromosome inactivation in lymphocytes has been shown in manifesting carriers of one family, suggesting that nonrandom X inactivation is responsible for a phenotype in females (Kaepernick et al., 1994). In females, minor clinical features of the spectrum can be found, such as adducted thumbs, subnormal intelligence, and sometimes the full-blown clinical picture that includes hydrocephalus (Fryns et al., 1991; Macias et al., 1992; Kaepernick et al., 1994).

MOLECULAR GENETICS, MUTATIONS, AND GENOTYPE–PHENOTYPE CORRELATIONS

The *L1* gene is located at Xq28 and consists of 28 exons, distributed across 16 kb of genomic DNA. The 1256–amino acid human L1CAM protein is encoded by a open reading frame of 3825 bp contained within a 4.5-kb messenger RNA (mRNA) (Hlavin and Lemmon, 1991; Reid and Hemperley, 1992). L1CAM is a cell surface glycoprotein. It belongs to the large immunoglobulin superfamily of neural cell adhesion molecules that mediate cell–cell adhesion. It is an important component of the ligand–receptor network of guidance forces that in-

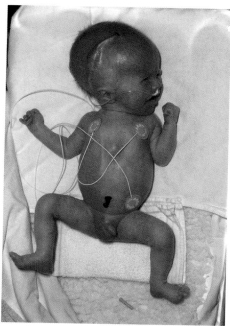

Figure 98–1. Male neonate with enlarged skull. (The parents give their full support and permission for publication.)

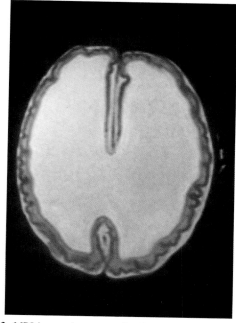

Figure 98–3. MRI in a male neonate showing massive hydrocephalus. (The parents give their full support and permission for publication.)

fluence axonal growth and guidance (Lemmon et al., 1989). For this reason, L1 is more of a neural recognition molecule than an adhesion molecule. It consists of six inmunoglobulin and five fibronectin type III–like domains in its extracellular domains, a single-pass transmembrane domain, and a short cytoplasmic domain (Hlavin and Lemmon, 1991).

There is a wide mutational spectrum in the of *L1* gene, and so far at least 134 different mutations have been reported in 154 families with L1 syndrome (Weller and Gärtner, 2001). The actual situation can be seen at the *L1CAM* mutation Web page (http://dnalab-www.uia.ac.be/dnalab/l1/; Van Camp et al., 1996). Most mutations are private, occurring in single families.

The *L1* mutations are subdivided into four classes, according to the effect they are expected to have on the L1 protein (Fransen et al., 1998). Class I includes mutations in the extracellular part of L1 expected to lead to a truncation or an absence of the protein. These mutations include frameshift mutations or point mutations leading to a stop codon. They were found to cause a severe phenotype in all families. Class II includes missense mutations resulting in an amino acid substitution in the extracellular part of L1. If it affects "key amino

acid residues," it is crucial for the structural buildup of one of the L1 domains, or even of the entire L1 protein, and also leads to a severe clinical picture. If it affects "surface residues," it has a varied effect on the whole protein and produces a variable phenotype. Class III includes any mutation in the cytoplasmic domain, which may cause only partial loss of the function of L1, leading to a significantly milder phenotype. Class IV consists of extracellular mutations resulting in aberrant splicing of pre-mRNA, with an unpredictable effect on the protein and no genotype–phenotype correlation found. In their review, Weller and Gärtner (2001) confirmed that missense mutations in extracellular domains or mutations in cytoplasmic regions cause milder phenotypes than those leading to truncation in extracellular domains or to nondetectable L1 protein.

ESTABLISHING A DIAGNOSIS

Prenatally

Fetal hydrocephalus occurs in 1:2000 pregnancies (Vintzileos et al., 1983), with the X-linked type of hydrocephalus being present in a mi-

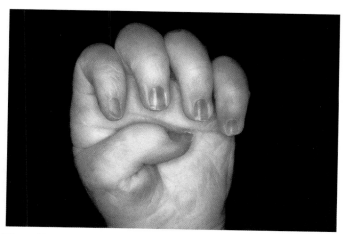

Figure 98–2. Adducted thumb in a deceased male neonate. (The parents give their full support and permission for publication.)

Table 98–1. Protocol for Neuropathology Studies

When there is a clinical suspicion, brain CT or MRI is preferred.
A. Morphometry and photodocument
    Brain weight
    Head size
    Brain components (photographs)
    Cerebral cortex thickness
    Cerebellar hemisphere (weight)
B. Dissection and tissue harvest; emphasize
    a. Cerebral cortex (surface)
    b. Ventricular size (plus hydrocephalus)
    c. Neuronal migration pattern
    d. Aqueduct histology
    e. Corpus callosum: thickness, morphology, length
    f. Cerebellum
        Cerebellar weight
        Vermis morphology
        Pyramids
    g. Brain stem (crytical)
        Pyramidal tracts and size
        Corticospinal tracts and size

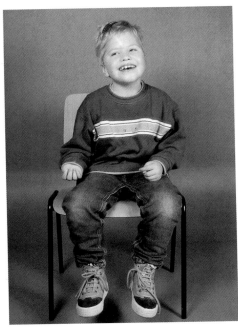

Figure 98–4. The same patient as shown in Figures 98–1 and 98–3 at the age of 7 years. He is a boy with a pleasant personality with mental retardation and spasticity. (The parents give their full support and permission for publication.)

nority of cases. With a positive family history and/or a proved carrier mother, prenatal monitoring is based on the recurrence risk (see Genetic Counseling), and DNA analysis after chorionic villus sampling at 10 to 11 weeks will provide a prenatal diagnosis. In the absence of DNA testing, fetal ultrasonography is offered at intervals of a few weeks starting at 18 to 20 weeks. However, without DNA analysis, a reliable prenatal diagnosis is not available. Because of the intrafamilial variation, it is not possible to guarantee an ultrasonographic diagnosis before 20 to 24 weeks' gestation or even during the third trimester of pregnancy.

In Affected Individuals

The clinical diagnosis of X-linked hydrocephalus in a male child with massive hydrocephalus and adducted thumbs is not difficult. Without adducted thumbs however, the L1 syndrome cannot be excluded. Finckh at al. (2000) summarized data on the prevalence of *L1* mutations in cases of hydrocephalus. They found a mutation detection rate of 22.4% in isolated male cases. The chance of finding a mutation obviously is related to clinical features but also to the number of patients in a family.

Diagnosis in male children and adults with developmental delay and mental retardation with neurological features of early hypotonia changing to spastic paraplegia during childhood, with or without adducted thumbs, is not straightforward. Differential diagnosis in this group of X-linked mental retardation includes many conditions along with the L1 syndrome. In the case of a positive family history, early diagnosis is usually possible. In nonfamilial cases, brain imaging with a positive finding of hydrocephalus and careful neuropathological studies are helpful. *L1* mutation analysis should be performed in familial and nonfamilial cases with a suggested clinical diagnosis.

GENETIC COUNSELING AND PRENATAL DIAGNOSIS

In families with the spectrum of conditions that includes L1 or X-linked hydrocephalus/MASA, the recurrence risk is high when the mother is a carrier: for a boy, 50% and for a girl, 50% chance of being a carrier with a low (<5%) risk of manifesting clinical features. Female relatives at risk of being a carrier cannot be informed about their status without DNA linkage analysis or mutation analysis. For

these reasons, all efforts should be made to perform DNA studies, preferably *L1* mutation analysis. Of importance for genetic counselling is that there is no indication of genetic heterogeneity in X-linked hydrocephalus. The finding of an *L1* mutation in the family enables the possibility of a reliable prenatal diagnosis.

If mutation analysis is not possible, genetic counseling is given with a recurrence risk according to the X-linked mode of inheritance. As stated earlier, no reliable prenatal diagnosis can be offered without *L1* mutation analysis: the results of prenatal ultrasonography are nonreliable, and the diagnosis of even severe hydrocephalus cannot be guaranteed before 20 to 24 weeks' gestation or even the third trimester of pregnancy.

Girls may have minor symptoms of the clinical spectrum, with severe hydrocephalus being an exception; ultrasonographic examination in case of a carrier (or at-risk) female fetus should be considered.

DATA IN KNOCKOUT MICE

L1CAM is expressed both in the brain and in the peripheral nervous system (primarily on the axons of postmitotic neurons) and functions as a membrane-bound protein with an extracellular and intracellular cytoplasmatic domain linked by a transmembrane domain. The high degree of conservation between the cytoplasmic portion of human *L1CAM* and its homologues in mouse, rat, and chick suggests an important role for this region (Hlavin and Lemmon, 1991; Jouet et al., 1993b). The *L1* knockout mice show dilated ventricles, vermis hypoplasia, and impaired exploration patterns (Fransen et al., 1998). Knockout mice also show hypoplasia of the corticospinal tract, failure of corticospinal axonal decussation, and projection beyond the cervical spinal cord (Dobson et al., 2001). L1 function seems not to be necessary for the establishment or maintenance of long-term potentiation in the hippocampus (Bliss et al., 2000). In another mouse model, it was suggested that stenosis of the aqueduct is a secondary event due to massively enlarged ventricles (Rolf et al., 2001).

DEVELOPMENTAL PATHOGENESIS

Although it is not yet clear how mutations in *L1CAM* lead to specific patterns of defective development of the central nervous system, there is hope of learning more about the pathogenesis of this clinical spectrum. The mouse models are very helpfull in this respect.

Similarities between patients with fetal alcohol syndrome and *L1* mutations suggested that the mechanism of developmental neurotoxicity of ethanol is in part due to effects on L1 cell adhesion molecule (Bearer, 2001). At this stage, the following hypothesis can be made: Different mutations in *L1CAM* may give rise to different abnormal or even absent protein products, resulting in various types of central nervous system maldevelopment, with clinical variability as a result. This hypothesis, however, does not explain the variability seen in the different patients in one family who were all affected with the same *L1CAM* mutation (e.g., Schrander-Stumpel et al., 1990). Thus, additional further insight into environmental factors or modifying factors (genes) in the individual patient are needed to understand and explain this intrafamilial variability.

REFERENCES

Bearer CF (2001). Mechanisms of brain injury: L1 cell adhesion molecule as a target for ethanol-induced prenatal brain injury. *Semin Pediatr Neurol* 8: 100.

Bianchine JW, Lewis RC Jr (1974).The MASA syndrome: a new heritable mental retardation syndrome. *Clin Genet* 5: 298–306.

Bickers DA, Adams RD (1949). Hereditary stenosis of the aqueduct of Sylvius as a cause of congenital hydrocephalus. *Brain* 72: 246–262.

Bliss T, Errington M, Fransen E, Godfraind JM, Kauer JA, Kooy R, Maness PF, Furley AJ (2000). Long-term potentiation in mice lacking the neural cell adhesion molecule L1. *Curr Biol* 14: 1607.

Boyd E, Schwartz CE, Schroer RJ, May MM, Shapiro SD, Arena JF, Lubs HA, Stevenson RE (1993). Agenesis of the corpus callosum associated with MASA syndrome. *Clin Dysmorphol* 2: 332–341.

Burton BK (1979). Recurrence risks for congenital hydrocephalus. *Clin Genet* 16: 47–53.

Chow CW, Halliday JL, Anderson RM, Danks DM, Fortune DW (1985). Congenital absence of pyramids and its significance in genetic diseases. *Acta Neuropathol (Berl)* 65: 313–317.

Dobson CB, Villagra F, Clowry GJ, Smith M, Kenwrick S, Donnai D, Miller S, Eyre JA (2001). Abnormal corticospinal function but normal axonal guidance in human L1CAM mutations. *Brain* 124: 2393–2406.

Editorial (1962). Sex linked hydrocephalus with severe mental retardation. *Br Med J* I: 168.

Edwards JH (1961). The syndrome of sex-linked hydrocephalus. *Arch Dis Child* 36: 486–493.

Finckh U, Schröder J, Ressler B, Veske A, Gal A (2000). Spectrum and detection rate of L1CAM mutations in isolated and familial cases with clinically susptected L1-disease. *Am J Med Genet* 92: 40–46.

Fransen E, Van Camp G, D'Hooge R, Vits L, Willems P (1998). Genotype-phenotype correlation in L1 associated disease. *J Med Genet* 35: 399–404.

Fransen E, D'Hooge R, Van Camp G, Verhoye M, Sijbers J, Reyniers E, Soriano P, Kamiguchi H, Willemsen R, Koekkoek SK, et al. (1998). L1 knockout mice show dilated ventricles, vermis hypoplasia and impaired exploration patterns. *Hum Mol Genet* 7: 999–1009.

Fryns JP, Spaepen A, Cassiman JJ, van den Berghe H (1991). X-linked complicated spastic paraplegia, MASA syndrome and X-linked hydrocephaly due to congenital stenosis of the aqueduct of Sylvius: a variable expression of the same mutation at Xq28 (letter). *J Med Genet* 28: 429–432.

Hlavin ML, Lemmon V (1991). Molecular structure and functional testing of human L1. *Genomics* 11: 416–423.

Jouet M, Rosenthal A, Macfarlane J, Donnai D, Kenwrick S (1993). A missense mutation confirms the L1 defect in X-linked hydrocephalus (HSAS). *Nat Genet* 4: 331.

Jouet N, Kenwrick S (1995). Gene analysis of L1 neural cell adhesion molecule in prenatal diagnosis of hydrocephalus. *Lancet* 345: 161–162.

Kaepernick LA, Legius E, Higgins J, Kapur S (1994). Clinical aspects of MASA syndrome in a large family including expressing females. *Clin Genet* 45: 181–185.

Landrieu P, Ninane J, Ferriäre, Lyon G (1979). Aqueductal stenosis in X-linked hydrocephalus: a secondary phenomenon? *Dev Med Child Neurol* 21: 637–652.

Lemmon V, Farr KL, Lagenaur C (1989). L1-mediated axon outgrowth occurs via a homophilic binding mechanism. *Neuron* 2: 1597–1603.

Macias VR, Day DW, King TE, Wilson G (1992). Clasped-thumb mental retardation (MASA) syndrome: confirmation of linkage to Xq28. *Am J Med Genet* 43: 408–414.

Parisi MA, Kapur RP, Neilson I, Hofstra RMW, Holloway LW, Michaelis RC, Leppig KA (2002). Hydrocephalus and intestinal aganglionosis: is L1CAM a modifier gene in Hirschsprung disease? *Am J Med Genet* 108: 51–56.

Reid RA, Hemperley JJ (1992). Variants of human L1 cell adhesion molecule arise through alternate splicing of RNA. *J Mol Neurosci* 3: 127–135.

Rolf B, Kutsche M, Bartsch U (2001). Severe hydrocephalus in L1-deficient mice. *Brain Res* 891: 247–252.

Schrander-Stumpel CTRM, Legius E, Fryns JP, Cassiman JJ (1990). MASA syndrome: new clinical features and linkage analysis using DNA probes. *J Med Genet* 27: 688–692.

Schrander-Stumpel CTRM (1995). Clinical and genetic aspects of the X-linked hydrocephalus/MASA spectrum. Thesis, Maastricht Datawyse/University Press.

Schrander-Stumpel CTRM, Fryns JP (1998). Congenital hydrocephalus: nosology and guidelines for clinical approach and genetic counselling. *Eur J Pediatr* 157: 355–362.

Schrander-Stumpel CTRM, Krijne-Kubat B, Vandevijver N, Offermans J, Blanco C, Blackburn W, den Hartog J, Cooley NR (2000). Studies of congenital hydrocephalus with special emphasis on the X-linked type: the need for a protocol. *Proc Greenwood Genet Center* 19: 74.

Van Camp G, Fransen E, Vits L, Raes G, Willems PJ (1996). A locus-specific mutation database for the neural cell adhesion molecule L1CAM (Xq28). *Hum Mutat* 8: 391.

Varadi V, Csécsei K, Szeifert GT, Tóth Z, Papp Z (1987). Prenatal diagnosis of X linked hydrocephalus without aquaductal stenosis. *J Med Genet* 24: 207–209.

Vintzileos AM, Ingardia CJ, Nochimson DJ (1983). Congenital hydrocephalus: a review and protocol for perinatal management. *Obstet Gynecol* 62: 539–549.

Weller S, Gärtner J (2001). Genetic and clinical aspects of X-linked hydrocephalus (L1 disease): mutations in the L1CAM gene. *Hum Mutat* 18: 1–12.

Willems PJ, Brouwer OF, Dijkstra I, Wilmink J (1987). X-Linked hydrocephalus. *Am J Med Genet* 27: 921–928.

Yamasaki M, Arita N, Hiraga S, Izumoto S, Morimoto K, Nakatani S, Fujitani K, Sato N, Hayakawa T (1995). A clinical and neuroradiological study of X-linked hydrocephalus in Japan. *J Neurosurg* 83: 50–55.

99 | *COMP* and Pseudoachondroplasia

DANIEL H. COHN

Pseudoachondroplasia (PSACH) is a dominantly inherited form of short-limb short stature. Both mild and typical forms are recognized, comprising a spectrum of clinical severity. A definitive diagnosis can be made on the basis of radiographs showing delayed epiphyseal ossification, epiphyseal and metaphyseal irregularities, and a characteristic anterior beaking of the vertebral bodies apparent on lateral projection. In addition to short stature, loose joints due to ligamentous laxity, joint pain, varus and/or valgus deformities at the knees, and scoliosis characterize the phenotype. The major complication is degenerative joint disease, particularly in the hips, which can lead to joint replacement in the third or fourth decade of life. Patients with PSACH have defects in cartilage oligomeric matrix protein (COMP), a pentameric glycoprotein of the extracellular matrix. All patients with PSACH studied to date have been shown to be heterozygous for structural mutations in the *COMP* gene, either missense mutations or small deletions. The phenotype appears to primarily result from reduced secretion of COMP, the presence of abnormal COMP in the extracellular matrix, and disrupted interactions between COMP and other matrix molecules.

LOCUS and DEVELOPMENTAL PATHWAY

COMP is a 524-kDa pentameric extracellular matrix glycoprotein originally isolated from cartilage (Hedbom et al., 1992). It is a member of the thrombospondin family of proteins (Oldberg et al., 1992) and is also known as thrombospondin 5 (TSP5). Among the TSPs, COMP is most closely related to TSP3 and TSP4, both of which arose through duplication of an ancestral gene (Newton et al., 1994). Human COMP is a 757-residue modular protein containing an amino-terminal cysteine-rich domain, four epidermal growth factor (EGF)–like repeats, eight calmodulin-like or calcium-binding repeats, and a large carboxyl-terminal globular domain (Fig. 99–1A). After translation, the primary posttranslational glycosylation steps, folding of the monomers, and pentamer formation occur in the lumen of the rough endoplasmic reticulum (RER). Pentamerization results from the formation of disulfide bonds among the α-helical amino-terminal domains of the five chains (Efimov et al., 1994), forming a coiled coil structure (Malashkevich et al., 1996). The functions of the EGF-like and calcium-binding domains are not known, but both appear to be structural elements for which calcium binding is an essential component. The carboxyl-terminal domain may be involved in interactions between COMP and other extracellular matrix molecules as well as chondrocytes (Dicesare et al., 1994a; Holden et al., 2001). Bovine COMP has two amino-linked glycosylation sites: one within the EGF-like repeat domain and a second in the carboxyl-terminal globular region (Zaia et al., 1997). Maturation of the sugars takes place during secretion through the Golgi apparatus. The secreted COMP molecule forms a five-armed structure (Figs. 99–1B and 99–C), which can be visualized with rotary shadowing electron microscopy (Morgelin et al., 1992).

Although the function of the COMP protein in cartilage remains largely undiscovered, it is beginning to appear that COMP carries out a bridging function in the extracellular matrix. The carboxyl-terminal globular domain of COMP has been shown to interact with noncollagenous regions of type IX collagen (Holden et al., 2001; Thur et al., 2001), which is itself a component of the major collagenous fibril of cartilage. A direct, zinc-dependent interaction between COMP and type II collagen has also been demonstrated (Rosenberg et al., 1998), providing a type IX collagen–independent link with the collagen fibril network. Similar binding of COMP with type I collagen suggests

interactions that may be important to its function in extraskeletal tissues. Chondrocyte binding has been demonstrated for bovine COMP (Dicesare et al., 1994a), suggesting that the molecule may mediate communication between the extracellular environment and the chondrocyte. Based on comparisons with the thrombospondins, which bind cells via the integrin-associated CD47 molecule (Gao and Frazier, 1994; Gao et al., 1996), it has been hypothesized that COMP may have a chondrocyte-binding site in the carboxyl-terminal domain of the molecule (Briggs et al., 1998). Thus, there is the possibility that COMP has a role in matrix–chondrocyte signaling.

The *COMP* gene, which has been localized to chromosome 19p13.1 (Newton et al., 1994), consists of 19 exons with canonical splice junction consensus sequences at their margins (Briggs et al., 1995). There is only limited information regarding the regulation of *COMP* gene expression, and the regulatory steps that confer the complex developmental expression pattern observed for *COMP* are unknown. The promoter lacks TATA or CAAT box consensus sequences, and four closely spaced transcription start sites are used in chondrocytes (Deere et al., 2001). The promoter contains at least one functional SP-1 binding site, and consensus sequences for many additional transcription factor binding sites are present immediately upstream of the translation start site. Additional functional regulatory elements have also been detected in the promoter of the mouse *Comp* gene in a region in which there are conserved sequence elements with the orthologous human *COMP* gene (Issack et al., 2000).

Expression of COMP during development and within the growth plate has been studied in the mouse, rat, and porcine systems. COMP is expressed early in fetal development and has been detected in the undifferentiated mesenchymal cells that give rise to the cartilaginous anlagen of the developing skeleton (Fang et al., 2000). Within the cartilage rudiments, COMP expression is initially seen in the proliferating and hypertrophic chondrocytes of the growth plate (Murphy et al., 1999). Although present in all areas of the cartilage matrix, the highest level of COMP is detected in the territorial matrix surrounding the proliferating and hypertrophic cells, with lower concentrations in the pericellular and interterritorial matrix (Shen et al., 1995; Ekman et al., 1997). Subsequently, COMP expression increases in the developing articular chondrocytes, the major site of COMP expression in adults. In articular cartilage, COMP has a primarily interterritorial distribution. Thus, COMP plays a role in skeletal pattern formation, in endochondral ossification, and in articular cartilage.

Albeit at lower levels than in cartilage, COMP is also expressed in extraskeletal tissues, most notably in tendon and ligament cells (Dicesare et al., 1994b; Smith et al., 1997; Muller et al., 1998). This pattern of expression is compatible with abnormalities in these tissues in PSACH. COMP expression has also been identified in synovial cells, dermal fibroblasts, osteoblasts, and vascular smooth muscle cells (Dicesare et al., 1997, 2000; Dodge et al., 1998; Recklies et al., 1998; Riessen et al., 2001), and is represented among many tissues in the UniGene expressed sequence *tag* database, suggesting possible functional roles beyond tissues known to be affected in PSACH.

CLINICAL FEATURES

The term *pseudoachondroplasia* is somewhat of a misnomer, reflecting that the disease was recognized and distinguished from achondroplasia early in the development of the nosology of the osteochon-

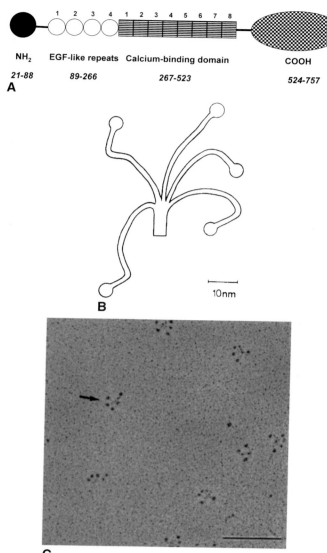

Figure 99–1. (A) Domain structure of the cartilage oligomeric matrix protein (COMP) monomer. The amino acid residue numbers corresponding to each domain are listed below. EGF, endothelial growth factor. (B) Model of the COMP pentamer showing chain association among the amino-terminal domains of the monomers. The scale bar represents 10 nm. (C) Image of COMP, isolated from rat chondrosarcoma, visualized by rotary shadowing electron microscopy. The scale bar represents 200 nm. (B and C are reprinted with permission from Morgelin et al., 1992.)

drodysplasias (Maroteaux and Lamy, 1959; McKusick and Scott, 1971). At one time, as the classification evolved, four subtypes, including dominant and recessive forms, were recognized (Hall and Dorst, 1969; Young and Moore, 1985; Wynne-Davies et al., 1986; Hall et al., 1987). However, the current classification (Hall, 2002) recognizes a single entity with exclusively dominant inheritance. Both mild (Maroteaux et al., 1980; Rimoin et al., 1994) and typical forms can be distinguished, constituting a spectrum of clinical severity. At the mild end of severity, there is overlap with some forms of multiple epiphyseal dysplasia (MED), which can result from defects in COMP or other matrix molecules.

The diagnosis of PSACH is best made on the basis of childhood radiographs that reveal small, irregular epiphyses and metaphyseal abnormalities of the long bones, hands, and spine (Fig. 99–2). The hands are characterized by small, irregular carpal bones and short metacarpals and phalanges, with delayed epiphyseal ossification. The

hips show short femoral necks with small, dysplastic capital femoral epiphyses. The acetabulae are hypoplastic with irregular margins. The ends of the long bones show small irregular epiphyses and flared metaphyses with irregularities at the metaphyseal–epiphyseal junction. The spine has a distinctive and diagnostic appearance, with anterior beaking of the vertebral bodies. The anterior vertebral abnormalities normalize over time, so it is most helpful to obtain prepubertal radiographs to firmly establish the diagnosis.

The major extraskeletal feature observed in patients with PSACH is loose joints due to ligamentous laxity. This finding reflects the expression of COMP in the tendons and ligaments and is particularly evident in the hands, knees, and ankles during childhood. By contrast, at the elbows and hips there can be limitation in extension.

The PSACH phenotype is not usually apparent at birth but can be recognized at the onset of walking due to a waddling gait. At about the same time, the growth of affected individuals begins to fall below the standard growth curve (Horton et al., 1982). In addition to moderately severe short stature, deformity of the lower extremities is common. There may be bilateral valgus or varus deformity at the knees, or a combination of a varus deformity of one knee and a valgus deformity of the other knee, leading to a windswept appearance. Beginning with joint pain in childhood, there is progressive, early-onset osteoarthropathy that leads to total hip replacement in early adulthood in about half of patients (McKeand et al., 1996). There is pain in other large joints, but surgical intervention is much less common. Abnormalities of the spine, lumbar lordosis, and a mild degree of scoliosis are common. Odontoid hypoplasia leading to atlantoaxial instability has been reported (Svensson and Aaro, 1988), but the frequency of this complication has not been well documented.

IDENTIFICATION OF THE GENE AND MUTATIONAL SPECTRUM

The PSACH disease gene was localized to chromosome 19 through a genome-wide screen in a single large family with a mild form of the disease (Briggs et al., 1993). The identified locus was also defined in a large family with MED (Oehlmann et al., 1993), and the two phenotypes were subsequently shown to be allelic in some cases. Based on the linkage in the mild form of PSACH, linkage to the same region was then demonstrated for the more severe typical form of PSACH (Hecht et al., 1993). There was no evidence of locus heterogeneity, an observation since borne out by mutation analysis.

Within the genetic interval defined by linkage, the gene encoding COMP, a candidate gene of unknown function, had been localized (Newton et al., 1994). Through mutation analysis in families with typical PSACH and MED, it was determined that COMP was the disease gene for these osteochondrodysplasia phenotypes (Briggs et al., 1995; Hecht et al., 1995).

Sufficient mutations have been defined in PSACH to accurately define the molecular basis of the phenotype (Briggs et al., 1995, 1998; Hecht et al., 1995; Maddox et al., 1997; Susic et al., 1997; Deere et al., 1998, 1999; Ikegawa et al., 1998; Loughlin et al., 1998; Susic et al., 1998; Delot et al., 1999; Mabuchi et al., 2001; Shotelersuk and Punyashthiti, 2002). Only COMP mutations have been identified in patients with PSACH, providing confirmation of the lack of apparent locus heterogeneity in this phenotype initially apparent from linkage studies (Hecht et al., 1993). The majority of mutations are in the region of the gene encoding the calcium-binding repeats. A common mutation, deletion of a single aspartic acid codon within a run of five consecutive GAC codons, is found in about one third of all genetically independent patients (Hecht et al., 1995; Briggs et al., 1998). Slipped mispairing at DNA replication is the likely mutational mechanism (Briggs et al., 1998), explaining the high frequency of this molecular defect. Duplication of two of the GAC codons also produces typical PSACH (Delot et al., 1999). Most of the remaining mutations are unique to each patient and are either missense mutations or deletions of one or a few codons. Most of these mutations either alter a negatively charged residue involved in calcium binding or change one of the cysteine residues essential for disulfide binding within the calcium-binding domain. Therefore, most PSACH mutations affect the structure of COMP either di-

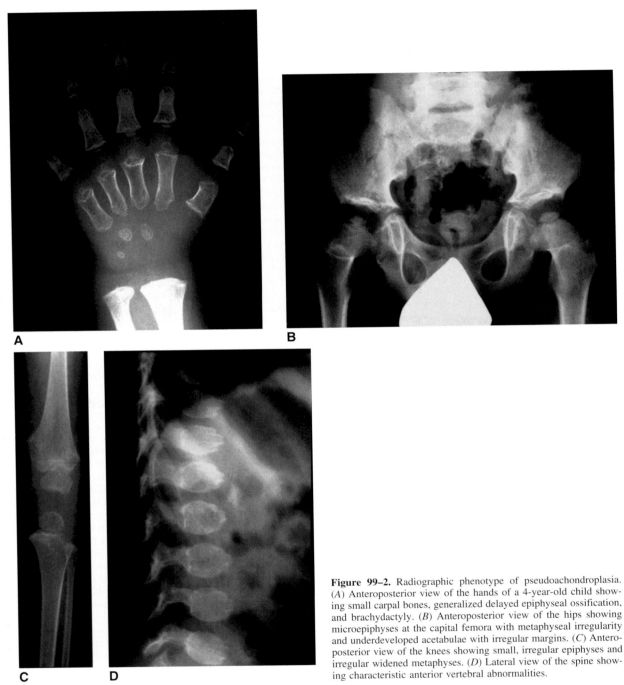

Figure 99–2. Radiographic phenotype of pseudoachondroplasia. (*A*) Anteroposterior view of the hands of a 4-year-old child showing small carpal bones, generalized delayed epiphyseal ossification, and brachydactyly. (*B*) Anteroposterior view of the hips showing microepiphyses at the capital femora with metaphyseal irregularity and underdeveloped acetabulae with irregular margins. (*C*) Anteroposterior view of the knees showing small, irregular epiphyses and irregular widened metaphyses. (*D*) Lateral view of the spine showing characteristic anterior vertebral abnormalities.

rectly by altering a cysteine residue or deleting one or more codons or indirectly via an effect on calcium binding.

A small proportion of patients have mutations that alter an amino acid residue in the carboxyl-terminal globular region of the protein (Briggs et al., 1998; Deere et al., 1998, 1999; Mabuchi et al., 2001). It is not yet clear whether the mechanism leading to the phenotype is different than that for mutations in the calcium-binding region, but these mutations identify unique functional domains within the COMP protein. Mutations have not been identified in the region of the gene that encodes either the amino-terminal domain or the EGF-like repeats. It remains to be determined whether sequence changes in these regions produce osteochondrodysplasia phenotypes that are not yet recognized. Similarly, null mutations in the *COMP* gene have not been observed among PSACH and MED patients.

About 20% to 25% of patients with MED have dominant mutations

in the *COMP* gene. The mutations are similar to those identified in patients with PSACH, with most resulting in amino acid substitutions in the calcium-binding repeats. A few mutations cluster in the carboxyl-terminal domain (Briggs et al., 1998; Deere et al., 1999; Czarny-Ratajczak et al., 2001). These mutations presumably have a milder effect on the structure of COMP than do the mutations that produce PSACH. It has been subsequently shown that MED can also result from mutations in at least five additional genes, those encoding the three chains of type IX collagen and the matrilin 3 gene in dominantly inherited forms (Muragaki et al., 1996; Paassilta et al., 1999; Chapman et al., 2001; Czarny-Ratajczak et al., 2001), and the *DTDST* (*SLC26A2*) gene in a recessively inherited MED phenotype (Superti-Furga et al., 1999). All of the identified loci appear to account for only about half of cases of MED, making MED the most genetically heterogeneous of the osteochondrodysplasias.

COUNSELING AND TREATMENT

PSACH is an autosomal dominant disorder with complete penetrance. As with many dominantly inherited disorders, there is some variability in phenotypic expression, but the range of intrafamilial variability is relatively narrow. The wider spectrum of clinical severity is seen across PSACH families, likely reflecting mutation-specific determinants of phenotype.

Based on the autosomal dominant inheritance pattern, the risk to offspring of an affected individual with an average stature partner is 50%. When the affected parent is female, the rate of delivery by cesarean section is extremely high (Allanson and Hall, 1986). For sporadic PSACH cases, risk to siblings of the affected individual is based on the frequency of germline mosaicism for the mutation in one of the parents. Recurrence due to germline mosaicism has been observed in PSACH (Hall et al., 1987; Ferguson et al., 1997; Deere et al., 1999), but the frequency has not been calculated. However, the risk is likely to be on the order of a few percent.

Assortative mating among individuals with short stature leads to the risk of double heterozygosity for both dominant disorders among their offspring. PSACH in combination with achondroplasia, osteogenesis imperfecta type III, and spondyloepiphyseal dysplasia congenita has been described (Langer et al., 1993; Kitoh et al., 1994; Unger et al., 2001). In most cases, the resulting double dominant phenotype is quite severe and may have features and complications not common to either disorder alone.

Because prenatal ultrasonographic features of PSACH have not been defined, ultrasonographic prenatal diagnosis is not possible. With the advent of more sophisticated imaging techniques, such as three-dimensional ultrasonography (Garjian et al., 2000; Krakow et al., 2003), it might be possible to define subtle skeletal features that could prenatally identify the phenotype. DNA level prenatal diagnosis has been facilitated by the definition of the molecular defect in PSACH and should be applicable to at-risk families in which the mutation has been defined. Any accessible fetal tissue, chorionic villus or amniocytes, could be used for this purpose. Given the difficulty of recognizing PSACH at birth, presymptomatic diagnosis in early childhood, again for at-risk children, could also be accomplished through molecular analysis. This may have benefits in anticipatory counseling for families as well as to aid in guiding affected individuals toward activities that will preserve joint function.

Treatment options for patients with PSACH primarily involve management of the complications of the disorder. During childhood, the need for orthopedic approaches for treatment of the skeletal deformities in PSACH is common. Genu varum, genu valgum, or windswept deformity of the lower limbs results from proximal relative fibular overgrowth and is compounded by ligamentous laxity at the knees and ankles (Rimoin et al., 2002). Correction of the limb deformity by osteotomy is the treatment of choice, but correction may be temporary and require revision in subsequent years (Hunter, 1999), likely due to the ongoing effects of lax ligaments. Although thoracolumbar scoliosis is common, it is generally mild and usually does not require surgical intervention. Atlantoaxial instability due to odontoid hypoplasia is a rare complication but can require cervical vertebral fusion when present. Progressive osteoarthropathy leads to joint pain, beginning in childhood. Pharmacologic management of joint pain is common, but no systematic study of the treatments of choice and efficacy has been reported. The major joints that most commonly fail are the hips, and hip replacement surgery during the third or fourth decade of life can be of great benefit to patients. There is only a single report of a PSACH patient who has undergone extended limb lengthening (Aldegheri, 1999); therefore, it is difficult to make conclusions about the effectiveness of the procedure for the phenotype.

(MUTATIONS IN) PARALOGOUS AND ORTHOLOGOUS GENES

A *Comp* knockout mouse strain has been reported, and it has normal growth and development, with neither an overt osteochondrodysplasia phenotype nor abnormalities in the histology or ultrastructure of cartilage (Svensson et al., 2002). There were no apparent radiographic abnormalities of the skeleton, the structure of the growth plate was comparable to that of control animals, and the extracellular matrix collagen fibril network was normal. Although it might be expected that, over the longer term, the absence of the protein might lead to cartilage instability and subsequent degenerative joint disease, there was no evidence of osteoarthritis in 14-month-old knockout animals.

Mouse knockout strains lacking either of the paralogous TSP 1 (*Tsp1*) or TSP 2 (*Tsp2*) gene have been described (Kyriakides et al., 1998a; Lawler et al., 1998; reviewed in Adams, 2001). The *Tsp1* knockout strain had defective lung homeostasis, with alveolar hemorrhage and pneumonia. The *Tsp2* knockout strain had a pleiotropic phenotype that included increased bone density and an increased bleeding time. There were irregularities in type I collagen fibrils, consistent with a structural role for some members of the TSP family in the extracellular matrix. Although the knockout strains reveal greater importance for these molecules in tissues other than cartilage, the combination of a defect in *Comp* with a defect in one of the other TSPs might produce an abnormality in cartilage, potentially revealing overlap among the functions of TSP family members in the tissue. Although their level of expression is not altered in the *Comp*-null mice, *Tsp1*, *Tsp2*, and *Tsp3* are all expressed in chondrocytes (Kyriakides et al., 1998b; Svensson et al., 2002); therefore, complementation of the *Comp* deficiency by one or more of the other TSP family members might not be entirely unexpected.

DEVELOPMENTAL PATHOGENESIS

Patients with PSACH have been found to be heterozygous for missense mutations in the *COMP* gene. Transcripts derived from the mutant allele appear to be stable and the abnormal protein is expressed in chondrocytes and other tissues. At least for cells in culture, there is little intracellular accumulation of monomeric COMP and there are approximately normal levels of COMP pentamer biosynthesis, leading to the conclusion that the abnormal monomers are efficiently incorporated into pentamers within the RER (Delot et al., 1998). Thus, it is likely that PSACH results from the presence of abnormal COMP. Because COMP is a pentameric molecule, random association of monomers in an individual heterozygous for a COMP mutation predicts that 97% of assembled pentamers should have one or more abnormal chains. Provided that pentamers with at least one abnormal chain will have altered function, this implies a dominant negative effect acting at the level of the pentamer.

Alterations in the sequence of the calcium-binding repeats of the COMP protein have a marked effect on the structure of the molecule. The mutations appear to act by decreasing the ability of the molecule to bind calcium, leading to a less compact molecular structure (Chen et al., 2000). The magnitude of the decrease in calcium binding is greater than would be expected by disruption of a single calcium-binding module (Hou et al., 2000; Maddox et al., 2000; Kleerekoper et al., 2002), compatible with the cooperative nature of calcium binding in this domain by members of the TSP protein family (Misenheimer and Mosher, 1995).

PSACH chondrocytes have inclusions in the RER (Maynard et al., 1972; Stanescu et al., 1982). The inclusions have a characteristic and diagnostic lamellar appearance (Fig. 99–3) and stain with antibodies to COMP (Maddox et al., 1997; Delot et al., 1998). Thus, abnormal COMP molecules are secreted less efficiently than normal molecules, although the extent of the implied quantitative deficiency in the matrix has not been examined in sufficient detail. The presence of inclusions implies a quality control mechanism in the RER tied to monitoring of the folded state of the COMP protein (acting at the level of the pentamer) to prevent the secretion of abnormal molecules. In this context, the levels of chaperones heat shock protein 47 and protein disulfide isomerase (PDI) increase in PSACH chondrocytes compared with normal tissue (Vranka et al., 2001), supporting the hypothesis that both of these molecules participate in COMP folding and are derepressed when COMP accumulates in the RER.

In addition to COMP, the material retained in the RER of PSACH chondrocytes stains with antibodies to type IX collagen (Maddox et

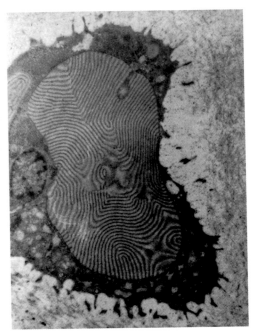

Figure 99–3. Lamellar inclusions in the rough endoplastic reticulum of a pseudoachondroplasia chondrocyte as viewed by transmission electron microscopy.

al., 1997; Delot et al., 1999). Because an interaction between COMP and type IX collagen has been demonstrated (Holden et al., 2001; Thur et al., 2001), retention of type IX collagen may reflect binding of type IX collagen by the retained COMP protein. Paradoxically, mutant COMP has reduced affinity for type IX collagen in vitro (Thur et al., 2001), suggesting that decreased binding efficiency may not be significant enough to prevent retention of type IX collagen in the RER. For molecules that are secreted into the cartilage matrix, reduced interactions between mutant COMP and type IX collagen suggest a mechanism for the cartilage matrix destabilization seen in PSACH. There are contradictory reports that aggrecan, the major proteoglycan in the cartilage extracellular matrix, accumulates in the RER of PSACH chondrocytes. Aggrecan has been localized in the inclusions in some studies (Stanescu et al., 1993; Hecht et al., 2001) but not in others (Delot et al., 1999; Vranka et al., 2001). Whether *COMP* mutations lead to decreased aggrecan secretion, whether the two proteins interact, and the possible contribution of decreased aggrecan in the cartilage matrix to phenotypic expression in PSACH are unresolved. To some extent, PSACH chondrocytes also accumulate type XI collagen, type XII collagen, decorin, and fibromodulin (Vranka et al., 2001). The overall implication that decreased secretion of several components of the cartilage matrix contributes to the PSACH phenotype is intriguing but merits further quantitative and functional analysis before firm conclusions can be reached.

Extraskeletal tissues from patients with PSACH have been examined to only a limited extent, but retention of abnormal COMP in the RER also has been observed in tendon from patients with *COMP* mutations (Delot et al., 1999). These data suggest that a reduced amount of COMP in extraskeletal tissues, similar to that observed in cartilage, is a component of phenotypic expression in all tissues that express COMP.

An additional element of phenotypic expression may be related to the effect of RER accumulation of COMP and other proteins on chondrocyte physiology and metabolism. At least in cultured cells, increased apoptosis in PSACH cells compared with normal cells has been observed (Hecht et al., 1998). The significance of these data *in vivo* is unclear but worth a more in-depth investigation.

Finally, there is evidence that COMP can bind chondrocytes (Dicesare et al., 1994a) and speculation that COMP may consequently have a signaling function (Briggs et al., 1998). An axis of communication between the matrix and chondrocyte, mediated by COMP, represents

an additional component of possible pathophysiological significance that merits further exploration.

At the tissue level, the PSACH cartilage matrix is disorganized with short columns of growth plate chondrocytes that appear more like clusters than like columns (Pedrini-Mille, 1984). Thus, the net effect of the presence of abnormal COMP in the growth plate is alteration of the orderly progression from resting to proliferating to hypertrophic chondrocytes, leading to a disordered and foreshortened axis of linear growth. In the articular cartilage, the cartilage matrix is destabilized, reducing the ability to sustain compressive loads and increasing the rate of degeneration.

PERSPECTIVE

PSACH results from structural mutations in the gene encoding cartilage oligomeric matrix protein. Identification of the disease gene has clarified the genetics of the disorder, a fully penetrant autosomal dominant condition with no apparent locus heterogeneity. The genetic data have facilitated counseling for families and provided opportunities for diagnostic testing in the prenatal and presymptomatic setting. From the viewpoint of disease pathogenesis, the phenotype appears to be primarily produced by a dominant negative mechanism, with decreased COMP secretion, presence of abnormal COMP in the extracellular matrix, and disruption of specific intermolecular interactions between COMP and other extracellular matrix molecules—all contributing to phenotypic expression. However, there is much remaining to be uncovered about the range and relative importance of each possible element in defining the disease phenotype.

From a therapeutic viewpoint, management of the skeletal complications of the disorder is the primary capability, and this should continue to improve with experience. However, longer-term therapies aimed at ameliorating the severity of the disorder are the ultimate goal of uncovering the molecular basis and pathogenetic mechanism of PSACH. Under the hypothesis that the presence of abnormal COMP in the extracellular matrix underlies the phenotype, strategies aimed at reducing or eliminating the abundance of COMP in the matrix could be useful. This might be accomplished by gene therapy with the goal of delivering a therapeutic reagent capable of reducing the level of expression of the mutant allele. As an initial step, stabilizing the articular cartilage of the large joints, which may be the most relevant and accessible therapeutic sites, could delay the onset and/or severity of degenerative joint disease and osteoarthrosis. Given the normal phenotype of the *Comp* knockout mouse, it might be possible to eliminate COMP expression from both alleles and improve chondrocyte function. Perhaps pharmacological reagents that specifically affect COMP biosynthesis would be relevant from this viewpoint. A deeper understanding of *COMP* gene regulation could provide further suggestions of profitable avenues for controlling COMP biosynthesis. An alternative to gene therapy would be to integrate a therapeutic chondrocyte population into articular cartilage, creating a state of tissue mosaicism that could improve cartilage stability and function.

The approaches outlined here do not address the short stature that characterizes the PSACH phenotype. To effect therapy, the much more difficult task of targeting growth plate chondrocytes, or their resting chondrocyte precursors, would be required. For all such approaches, creating relevant animal models for testing therapeutic modalities is an essential first step.

REFERENCES

Adams JC (2001). Thrombospondins: multifunctional regulators of cell interactions. *Annu Rev Cell Dev Biol* 17: 25–51.

Aldegheri R (1999). Distraction osteogenesis for lengthening of the tibia in patients who have limb-length discrepancy or short stature. *J Bone Joint Surg Am* 81: 624–634.

Allanson JE, Hall JG (1986). Obstetric and gynecologic problems in women with chondrodystrophies. *Obstet Gynecol* 67: 74–78.

Briggs MD, Rasmussen IM, Weber JL, Yuen J, Reinker K, Garber AP, Rimoin DL, Cohn DH (1993). Genetic linkage of pseudoachondroplasia to markers in the pericentromeric region of chromosome 19. *Genomics* 18: 656–660.

Briggs MD, Hoffman SMG, King LM, Olsen AS, Mohrenweiser H, Leroy JG, Mortier GR, Rimoin DL, Lachman RS, Gaines ES, et al. (1995). Pseudoachondroplasia and multiple epiphyseal dysplasia due to mutations in the cartilage oligomeric matrix protein gene. *Nat Genet* 10: 330–336.

Briggs MD, Mortier GR, Cole WG, King LM, Golik SS, Bonaventure J, Nuytinck L, De-paepe A, Leroy JG, Biesecker L, et al. (1998). Diverse mutations in the gene for cartilage oligomeric matrix protein in the pseudoachondroplasia-multiple epiphyseal dysplasia disease spectrum. *Am J Hum Genet* 62: 311–319.

Chapman KL, Mortier GR, Chapman K, Loughlin J, Grant ME, Briggs MD (2001). Mutations in the region encoding the von Willebrand factor A domain of matrilin-3 are associated with multiple epiphyseal dysplasia. *Nat Genet* 28: 393–396.

Chen H, Deere M, Hecht JT, Lawler J (2000). Cartilage oligomeric matrix protein is a calcium-binding protein, and a mutation in its type 3 repeats causes conformational changes. *J Biol Chem* 275: 26538–26544.

Czarny-Ratajczak M, Lohiniva J, Rogala P, Kozlowski K, Perala M, Carter L, Spector TD, Kolodziej L, Seppanen U, Glazar R, et al. (2001). A mutation in COL9A1 causes multiple epiphyseal dysplasia: further evidence for locus heterogeneity. *Am J Hum Genet* 69: 969–980.

Deere M, Sanford T, Ferguson HL, Daniels K, Hecht JT (1998). Identification of twelve mutations in cartilage oligomeric matrix protein (COMP) in patients with pseudoachondroplasia. *Am J Med Genet* 80: 510–513.

Deere M, Sanford T, Francomano CA, Daniels K, Hecht JT (1999). Identification of nine novel mutations in cartilage oligomeric matrix protein in patients with pseudoachondroplasia and multiple epiphyseal dysplasia. *Am J Med Genet* 85: 486–490.

Deere M, Hall CR, Gunning KB, Lefebvre V, Ridall AL, Hecht JT (2001). Analysis of the promoter region of human cartilage oligomeric matrix protein (*COMP*). *Matrix Biol* 19: 783–792.

Delot E, Brodie S, King LM, Wilcox WR, Cohn DH (1998). Physiological and pathological secretion of cartilage oligomeric matrix protein by cells in culture. *J Biol Chem* 26692–26697.

Delot E, King LM, Briggs MD, Wilcox WR, Cohn DH (1999). Trinucleotide expansion mutations in the cartilage oligomeric matrix protein (COMP) gene. *Hum Mol Genet* 8: 123–128.

Dicesare PE, Morgelin M, Mann K, Paulsson M (1994a). Cartilage oligomeric matrix protein and thrombospondin: 1. Purification from articular cartilage, electron microscopic structure and chondrocyte binding. *Eur J Biochem* 223: 927–937.

Dicesare PE, Carlson CS, Stollerman ES, Chen FS, Leslie M, Perris R (1997). Expression of cartilage oligomeric matrix protein by human synovium. *FEBS Lett* 412: 249–252.

Dicesare P, Hauser N, Lehman D, Pasumarti S, Paulsson M (1994b). Cartilage oligomeric matrix protein (COMP) is an abundant component of tendon. *FEBS Lett* 354: 237–240.

Dicesare PE, Fang C, Leslie MP, Tulli H, Perris R Carlson CS (2000). Expression of cartilage oligomeric matrix protein (COMP) by embryonic and adult osteoblasts. *J Orthop Res* 18: 713–720.

Dodge GR, Hawkins D, Boesler E, Sakai L, Jiminez SA (1998). Production of cartilage oligomeric matrix protein (COMP) by cultured human dermal and synovial fibroblasts. *Osteoarthritis Cartilage* 6: 435–440.

Efimov VP, Lustig A, Engel J (1994). The thrombospondin-like chains of cartilage oligomeric matrix protein are assembled by a five-stranded [alpha]-helical bundle between residues 20 and 83. *FEBS Lett* 341: 54–58.

Ekman S, Reinholt FP, Hultenby K, Heinegard D (1997). Ultrastructural immunolocalization of cartilage oligomeric matrix protein (COMP) in porcine growth cartilage. *Calcif Tiss Int* 60: 547–553.

Fang C, Carlson CS, Leslie MP, Tulli H, Stolerman E, Perris R, Ni L, Dicesare PE (2000). Molecular cloning, sequencing, and tissue and developmental expression of mouse cartilage oligomeric matrix protein (COMP). *J Orthop Res* 18: 593–603.

Ferguson HL, Deere M, Evans R, Rotta J, Hall JG, Hecht JT (1997). Mosaicism in pseudoachondroplasia. *Am J Med Genet* 70: 287–291.

Gargian KV, Pretorius DH, Budorick NE, Cantrell CJ, Johnson DD, Nelson TR (2000). Fetal skeletal dysplasia: three-dimensional US—initial experience. *Radiology* 214: 717–723.

Gao A, Frazier WA (1994). Identification of a receptor candidate for the carboxyl-terminal cell binding domain of thrombospondins. *J Biol Chem* 269: 29650–29657.

Gao A, Lindberg FP, Finn MB, Blystone SD, Brown EJ, Frazier WA (1996). Integrin-associated protein is a receptor for the C-terminal domain of thrombospondin. *J Biol Chem* 271: 21–24.

Hall CM (2002). International nosology and classification of constitutional disorders of bone (2001). *Am J Med Genet* 113: 65–77.

Hall JG, Dorst JP (1969). Pseudoachondroplastic SED, recessive Maroteaux-Lamy type. The Clinical Delineation Of Birth Defects. *Birth Defects Orig Artic Ser* 5: 242–257.

Hall JG, Dorst JP, Rotta J, McKusick VA (1987). Gonadal mosaicism in pseudoachondroplasia. *Am J Med Genet* 28: 143–151.

Hecht JT, Montufar-Solis D, Decker G, Lawler J, Daniels K, Duke J (1998). Retention of cartilage oligomeric matrix protein (COMP) and cell death in redifferentiated pseudoachondroplasia chondrocytes. *Matrix Biol* 17: 625–633.

Hecht JT, Francomano CA, Briggs MD, Williams M, Conner B, Horton WA, Warman ML, Cohn DH, Blanton SH (1993). Linkage of typical pseudoachondroplasia to chromosome 19. *Genomics* 18: 661–666.

Hecht JT, Hayes E, Snuggs M, Decker G, Montufar-Solis D, Doege K, Mwalle F, Poole R, Stevens J, Duke PJ (2001). Calreticulin, PDI, Grp94, and BiP chaperone proteins are associated with retained COMP in pseudoachondroplasia chondrocytes. *Matrix Biol* 20: 251–262.

Hecht JT, Nelson LD, Crowder E, Wang Y, Elder FFB, Harrison WR, Francomano CA, Prange CK, Lennon GG, Deere M, et al. (1995). Mutations in exon 17B of cartilage oligomeric matrix protein (COMP) cause pseudoachondroplasia. *Nat Genet* 10: 325–329.

Hedbom E, Antonsson P, Hjerpe A, Aeschlimann D, Paulsson M, Rosa-Pimental E, Sommarin Y, Wendel M, Oldberg A, Heinegard D (1992). Cartilage matrix proteins: an acidic oligomeric protein (COMP) detected only in cartilage. *J Biol Chem* 267: 6132–6136.

Holden P, Meadows RS, Chapman KL, Grant ME, Kadler KE, Briggs MD (2001). Cartilage oligomeric matrix protein interacts with type IX collagen, and disruptions to these interactions identify a pathogenetic mechanism in a bone dysplasia family. *J Biol Chem* 276: 6046–6055.

Horton WA, Hall JG, Scott CI, Pyeritz RE, Rimoin DL (1982). Growth curves for height

for diastrophic dysplasia, spondyloepiphyseal dysplasia congenita, and pseudoachondroplasia. *Am J Dis Child* 136: 316–319.

Hou J, Putkey JA, Hecht JT (2000). Delta 469 mutation in the type 3 repeat calcium binding domain of cartilage oligomeric matrix protein disrupts calcium binding. *Cell Calcium* 27: 309–314.

Hunter AG (1999). Perceptions of the outcome of orthopedic surgery in patients with chondrodysplasias. *Clin Genet* 56: 434–440.

Ikegawa S, Ohashi H, Nishimura G, Kim KC, Sannohe A, Kimizuka M, Fukushima Y, Nagai T, Nakamura Y (1998). Novel and recurrent COMP (cartilage oligomeric matrix protein) mutations in pseudoachondroplasia and multiple epiphyseal dysplasia. *Hum Genet* 103: 633–638.

International Working Group On Constitutional Diseases Of Bone (1998). International nomenclature and classification of the osteochondrodysplasias. *Am J Med Genet* 79: 376–382.

Issack PS, Fang C, Leslie MP, Dicesare PE (2000). Chondrocyte-specific enhancer regions in the *COMP* gene. *J Orthop Res* 18: 345–350.

Kitoh H, Oki T, Arao K, Nogami H (1994). Bone dysplasia in a child born to parents with osteogenesis imperfecta and pseudoachondroplasia. *Am J Med Genet* 51: 187–190.

Kleerekoper Q, Hecht JT, Putkey JA (2002). Disease-causing mutations in cartilage oligomeric matrix protein cause an unstructured Ca^{2+} binding domain. *J Biol Chem* 277: 10581–10589.

Krakow D, Williams J, Poehl M, Rimoin D, Platt L (2003). Use of 3D ultrasound imaging in the diagnosis of prenatal-onset skeletal dysplasias. *Ultrasound Obstet Gynecol*. in press.

Kyriakides TR, Zhu YH, Yang Z, Bornstein P (1998b). The distribution of the matricellular protein TSP–2 in tissues of embryonic and adult mice. *J Histochem Cytochem* 46: 1007–1015.

Kyriakides TR, Zhu Y-H, Smith LT, Bain ST, Yang Z, Lin MT, Danielsson KG, Iozzo RV, Lamarca M, McKinney CE, et al. (1998a). Mice that lack TSP-2 display connective tissue abnormalities that are associated with disordered collagen fibrillogenesis, an increased vascular density and a bleeding diathesis. *J Cell Biol* 140: 419–430.

Langer LO, Schaefer GB, Wadsworth DT (1993). Patient with double heterozygosity for achondroplasia and pseudoachondroplasia, with comments on these conditions and the relationship between pseudoachondroplasia and multiple epiphyseal dysplasia, Fairbank type. *Am J Med Genet* 47: 772–781.

Lawler J, Sunday M, Thibert V, Duquette M, George EL, Rayburn H, Hynes RO (1998). Thrombospondin-1 is required for normal murine pulmonary homeostasis and its absence causes pneumonia. *J Clin Invest* 101: 982–992.

Loughlin J, Irven C, Mustafa Z, Briggs MD, Carr A, Lynch SA, Knowlton RG, Cohn DH, Sykes B (1998). Identification of five novel mutations in cartilage oligomeric matrix protein gene in pseudoachondroplasia and multiple epiphyseal dysplasia. *Hum Mutat* (suppl 1): S10–S17.

Mabuchi A, Haga N, Ikeda T, Manabe N, Ohashi H, Takatori Y, Nakamura K, Ikegawa S (2001). Novel mutation in exon 18 of the cartilage oligomeric matrix protein gene causes a severe pseudoachondroplasia. *Am J Med Genet* 104: 135–139.

Maddox BK, Mokashi A, Keene DR, Bachinger HP (2000). A cartilage oligomeric matrix protein mutation associated with pseudoachondroplasia changes the structural and functional properties of the type 3 domain. *J Biol Chem* 275: 11412–11427.

Maddox BK, Keene DR, Sakai LY, Charbonneau NL, Morris NP, Ridgway CC, Boswell BA, Sussman MD, Horton WA, Bachinger HP, et al. (1997). The fate of cartilage oligomeric matrix protein is determined by the cell type in the case of a novel mutation in pseudoachondroplasia. *J Biol Chem* 272: 30993–30997.

Malashkevich VN, Kammerer RA, Efimov VP, Schulthess T, Engel J (1996). The crystal structure of a five-stranded coiled coil in COMP: a prototype ion channel? *Science* 274: 761–765.

Maroteaux P, Lamy M (1959). Les formes pseudoachondroplasiques des dysplasies spondyloepiphysaires. *Press Med* 67: 383–386.

Maroteaux P, Stanescu R, Stanescu V, Fontaine G (1980). The mild form of pseudoachondroplasia. *Eur J Pediatr* 133: 227–231.

Maynard JA, Cooper RR, Ponseti IV (1972). A unique rough surfaced endoplasmic reticulum inclusion in pseudoachondroplasia. *Lab Invest* 26: 40–44.

McKeand J, Rotta J, Hecht JT (1996). Natural history study of pseudoachondroplasia. *Am J Med Genet* 63: 406–410.

McKusick VA, Scott CI (1971). A nomenclature for constitutional disorders of bone. *J Bone Joint Surg Am* 53: 978–986.

Misenheimer T, Mosher DF (1995). Calcium ion binding to thrombospondin-1. *J Biol Chem* 270: 1729–1733.

Mörgelin M, Heinegård D, Engel J, Paulsson M (1992). Electron microscopy of native cartilage oligomeric matrix protein purified from the Swarm rat chondrosarcoma reveals a five-armed structure. *J Biol Chem* 267: 6137–6141.

Muller G, Michel A, Altenburg E (1998). COMP (cartilage oligomeric matrix protein) is synthesized in ligament, tendon, meniscus, and articular cartilage. *Connect Tiss Res* 39: 233–244.

Muragaki Y, Mariman ECM, Van Beersum SEC, Perala M, Van Mourik JBA, Warman ML, Olsen BR, Hamel BCJ (1996). A mutation in the gene encoding the $\alpha 2$ chain of the fibril-associated collagen IX, COL9A2, causes multiple epiphyseal dysplasia (EDM2). *Nat Genet* 12: 103–105.

Murphy JM, Heinegard D, McIntosh A, Sterchi D, Barry FP (1999). Distribution of cartilage molecules in the developing mouse joint. *Matrix Biol* 18: 487–497.

Newton G, Weremowicz S, Morton CC, Copeland NG, Gilbert DJ, Jenkins NA, Lawler J (1994). Characterization of human and mouse cartilage oligomeric matrix protein. *Genomics* 24: 435–439.

Oehlmann R, Summerville GP, Yeh G, Weaver EJ, Jiminez SA, Knowlton RG (1994). Genetic linkage mapping of multiple epiphyseal dysplasia to the pericentromeric region of chromosome 19. *Am J Hum Genet* 54: 3–10.

Oldberg A, Antonsson P, Lindblom K, Heinegard D (1992). COMP (cartilage oligomeric matrix protein) is structurally related to the thrombospondins. *J Biol Chem* 267: 22346–22350.

Paassilta P, Lohinva J, Annunen S, Bonaventure J, Le Merrer M, Pai L, Ala-Kokko L (1999). COL9A3: a third locus for multiple epiphyseal dysplasia. *Am J Hum Genet* 64:1036–1044.

Pedrini-Mille A, Maynard JA, Pedrini VA (1984). Pseudoachondroplasia: biochemical and histochemical studies of cartilage. *J Bone Joint Surg* 66-A: 1408–1414.

Recklies AD, Baillargeon L, White C (1998). Regulation of cartilage oligomeric matrix protein synthesis in human synovial cells and articular chondrocytes. *Arthritis Rheum* 41: 997–1006.

Riessen R, Fenchel M, Chen H, Axel D, Karch K, Lawler J (2000). Cartilage oligomeric matrix protein (thrombospondin-5) is expressed by vascular smooth muscle cells. *Arterioscler Thromb Vasc Biol* 21: 47–54.

Rimoin DL, Lachman RS, Unger S (2002). Chondrodysplasias. In: Emery and Rimoin's *Principles and Practices of Medical Genetics, 4th edition.* Connor JM, Pyeritz R, Korf B, et al. (eds.) Churchill Livingstone, London. p. 4076.

Rimoin DL, Rasmussen IM, Briggs MD, Roughley PJ, Gruber HE, Warman ML, Olsen BR, Hsia YE, Yuen J, Reinker K, et al. (1994). A large family with features of pseudoachondroplasia and multiple epiphyseal dysplasia: exclusion of seven candidate loci that encode proteins of the cartilage extracellular matrix. *Hum Genet* 93: 236–242.

Rosenberg K, Olsson H, Morgelin M, Heinegard D (1998). Cartilage oligomeric matrix protein shows high affinity zinc–dependent interaction with triple helical collagen. *J Biol Chem* 273: 20397–20403.

Shen Z, Heinegard D, Sommarin Y (1995). Distribution and expression of cartilage oligomeric matrix protein and bone sialoprotein show marked changes during rat femoral head development. *Matrix Biol* 14: 773–781.

Shotelersuk V, Punyashthiti R (2002). A novel mutation of the COMP gene in a Thai family with pseudoachondroplasia. *Int J Mol Med* 9: 81–84.

Smith RKW, Zunino L, Webbon RM, Heinegard D (1997). The distribution of cartilage oligomeric matrix protein (COMP) in tendon and its variation with tendon site, age, and load. *Matrix Biol* 16: 255–271.

Stanescu V, Maroteaux P, Stanescu R (1982). The biochemical defect of pseudoachondroplasia. *Eur J Pediatr* 138: 221–225.

Stanescu R, Stanescu V, Muriel M-P, Maroteaux P (1993). Multiple epiphyseal dysplasia, Fairbank type: morphologic and biochemical study of cartilage. *Am J Med Genet* 45: 501–507.

Superti-Furga A, Neumann L, Riebel T, Eich G, Steinmann B, Spranger J, Kunze J (1999). Recessively inherited multiple epiphyseal dysplasia with normal stature, club foot, and double layered patella caused by a DTDST mutation. *J Med Genet* 36: 621–624.

Susic S, Ahier J, Cole WG (1998). Pseudoachondroplasia due to the substitution of the highly conserved Asp482 by Gly in the seventh calmodulin-like repeat of cartilage oligomeric matrix protein. *Hum Mutat* (suppl 1): S125–S127.

Susic S, McGrory J, Ahier J, Cole WG (1997). Multiple epiphyseal dysplasia and pseudoachondroplasia due to novel mutations in the calmodulin-like repeats of cartilage oligomeric matrix protein. *Clin Genet* 51: 219–224.

Svensson O, Aaro S (1988). Cervical instability in skeletal dysplasia. Report of 6 surgicall fused cases. *Acta Orthop Scand* 59: 66–70.

Svensson L, Aszodi A, Heinegard D, Hunziker EB, Reinholt FP, Fassler R, Oldberg A (2002). Cartilage oligomeric matrix protein-deficient mice have normal skeletal development. *Mol Cell Biol* 22: 4366–4371.

Thur J, Rosenberg K, Nitsche DP, Pihlajamaa T, Ala-Kokko L, Heinegard D, Paulsson M, Maurer P (2001). Mutations in cartilage oligomeric matrix protein causing pseudoachondroplasia and multiple epiphyseal dysplasia affect binding of calcium and collagen I, II, and IX. *J Biol Chem* 276: 6083–6092.

Unger S, Korkko J, Krakow D, Lachman RS, Rimoin DL, Cohn DH (2001) Double heterozygosity for pseudoachondroplasia and spondyloepiphyseal dysplasia congenita. *Am J Med Genet* 104: 140–146.

Vranka J, Mokashi A, Keene DR, Tufa S, Corson G, Sussman M, Horton WA, Maddox K, Sakai L, Bächinger HP (2001). Selective intracellular retention of extracellular matrix proteins and chaperones associated with pseudoachondroplasia. *Matrix Biol* 20: 439–450.

Wynne-Davies R, Hall CM, Young ID (1986). Pseudoachondroplasia: clinical diagnosis at different ages and comparison of autosomal dominant and recessive types. A review of 32 patients (26 kindreds). *J Med Genet* 23: 425–434.

Young ID, Moore JR (1985). Severe pseudoachondroplasia with parental consanguinity. *J Med Genet* 22: 150–153.

Zaia J, Boynton RE, Mcintosh A, Marshak DR, Olsson H, Heinegard D, Barry FP (1997). Post-translational modifications in cartilage oligomeric matrix protein. Characterization of the N-linked oligosaccharides by matrix-assisted laser desorption ionization time-of-flight mass spectrometry. *J Biol Chem* 272: 14120–14126.

MMP2 and Multicentric Osteolysis with Nodulosis and Arthritis Syndrome

OONAGH DOWLING AND JOHN A. MARTIGNETTI

The inherited osteolyses, or "vanishing bone" syndromes, are a group of rare skeletal disorders of previously unknown etiology (Torg and Steel, 1968; Torg et al., 1969; Whyte et al., 1978; Fryns et al., 1980; Hemingway et al., 1983; Hardegger et al., 1985; Petit and Fryns, 1986; Raat et al., 1994; Brennan and Pauli, 2001). They are distinguished by their differing anatomic distribution, degrees of severity, inheritance pattern, and associated syndromic features, including mental retardation and nephropathy (Hardegger et al., 1985; Petit and Fryns, 1986). Multicentric osteolysis with nodulosis and arthritis (MONA, NAO, or Al Aqeel-Sewairi, syndrome [OMIM 605156]) is an autosomal recessive member of this group notable for the extent of carpal and tarsal osteolysis and interphalangeal joint erosions, facial dysmorphia, and the presence of fibrocollagenous nodules (Al Aqeel et al., 2000). The availability of three large and unrelated Saudi Arabian families with this syndrome permitted a positional cloning approach to identify the causative gene. A genome-wide search was performed for regions that were homozygous by descent using polymerase chain reaction–(PCR)-based microsatellite markers, and the disease gene was localized to 16q12-21. Molecular analysis of the candidate genes within this locus identified that all MONA affecteds of Saudi Arabian origin completely lacked matrix metalloproteinase (MMP)-2 gelatinolytic activity and that this deficiency was the result of inactivating mutations in the *MMP2* gene (Martignetti et al., 2001).

The MMPs are important mediators of extracellular matrix turnover, and cell signaling and disruption of their activity have been implicated in many disease processes (Birkedal-Hansen 1993; Cockett et al., 1998; Akagi et al., 1999; Clegg and Carter 1999). MMP2, a gelatinase and type IV collagenase, has broad substrate specificity and is expressed constitutively by many cell types. Previously, the majority of disease studies have implicated increased MMP2 activity in processes such as arthritis (Brinckerhoff, 1991; Konttinen et al., 1999), angiogenesis (Sang, 1998), and tumor invasion and metastasis (Kleiner and Stetler-Stevenson, 1999; Duffy et al., 2000; Stetler-Stevenson, 2001). The mechanism of development of the osteolytic, arthritic, and osteopenic phenotype in MMP2–deficient patients appears counterintuitive to the *in vitro* disease association theories of MMP2 function. In addition, the MMP2–deficient mouse model phenotype has not been particularly informative because these animals, apart from being slightly smaller at birth, appear physiologically normal (Itoh et al., 1997). This subtle growth phenotype, although not thoroughly investigated, is suggestive of a functional redundancy in the mouse and makes understanding the disease mechanism and the development of specific treatments challenging.

Therefore, the unexpected discovery that MONA is the result of MMP2 inactivation not only defines the first hereditary disease caused by mutations in an MMP but, more important, provides valuable insight into the *in vivo* role of MMP2 in skeletal and joint development and pathophysiology. Although there is no specific MONA therapy, identification of the genetic defect immediately suggests a role for targeted enzyme replacement.

LOCUS AND DEVELOPMENTAL PATHWAY: THE MATRIX METALLOPROTEINASES

The MMP family, a group of structurally related, secreted, and membrane-associated proteinases, are involved in degrading the structural components of the extracellular matrix (ECM) as well as other extracellular and nonmatrix proteins (McQuibban et al., 2000; Yu and Stamenkovic, 2000; Agnihotri et al., 2001; McCawley and Matrisian, 2001). ECM turnover is a crucial and highly regulated part of normal physiological processes, development, and tissue remodeling. Disruption of tightly orchestrated ECM turnover processes can lead to pathological states associated with excessive or inadequate matrix removal, such as arthritis (Brinckerhoff, 1991; Konttinen et al., 1999), cancer invasion, metastasis (Kleiner and Stetler-Stevenson, 1999; Duffy et al., 2000; Stetler-Stevenson, 2001), and fibrosis (Preaux et al., 1999; Corbel et al., 2002). These zinc- and calcium-dependent neutral endopeptidases have traditionally been divided into subgroups based on substrate preference and the presence of particular structural domains (Fig. 100–1). Twenty-two MMPs have been identified in humans. Members include gelatinases, collagenases, stromelysins, matrilysins, and membrane-type MMPs (Woessner, 2000).

All of the MMPs share a high degree of sequence and structural homology, and the proteins are organized into three distinctive and conserved domains: an amino propeptide, a catalytic domain, and a carboxy-terminal hemopexin domain (Fridman et al., 1992; Massova et al., 1998). In addition to these three basic domains, subgroups of this family have evolved by incorporating and/or deleting certain unique structural and functional domains. For example, the gelatinases (MMP2 and MMP9) comprise a subfamily that possesses three repeat structures homologous to type II fibronectin in their primary sequence. This MMP-novel functional motif allows MMP2 and MMP9 to bind to denatured collagen or gelatin, and its presence suggests a shared evolution and potential functional overlap between these two MMPs (Murphy et al., 1994). Membrane-type MMPs contain a transmembrane domain of approximately 25 hydrophobic amino acids, which allows localization to the cell surface (Woessner, 2000) (Fig. 100–1).

The MMPs are thought to act as mediators of ECM turnover, and although their in vivo substrate preferences have not yet been fully characterized, in vitro substrates include collagens, fibronectin, vitronectin, aggrecan, and laminin (Murphy et al., 1981; Fosang et al., 1992; Imai et al., 1995). This substrate specificity ensures their role in many normal developmental and tissue repair processes, including morphogenesis (Schnaper et al., 1993; Werb and Chin, 1998), angiogenesis (Fisher et al., 1994; Itoh et al., 1998; Vu et al., 1998; Sang, 1998; Stetler-Stevenson, 2001), skeletogenesis (Bord et al., 1998; Holmbeck et al., 1999), and wound healing (Madlener et al., 1998; Pilcher et al., 1999) as well as some pathological tissue-reshaping processes such as the arthritic erosion of joints (Brinckerhoff, 1991; Konttinen et al., 1999). MMPs may also participate in ECM-dependent cellular processes by mobilizing a number of pathways including cellular signals such as ECM-associated growth factors and altering cellular behavior in response to ECM environment changes (see Chapter 95). These cellular signals can in turn modulate activities such as cell migration, proliferation, and apoptosis (Sternlicht and Werb, 2001). Disregulation of ECM-related activity has been implicated in a number of pathological conditions with usually an increased activity associated with processes such as arthritic erosion of joints (Brinckerhoff, 1991; Konttinen et al., 1999), tumor metastasis (Kleiner and Stetler-Stevenson, 1999; Duffy et al., 2000; Stetler-Stevenson, 2001), emphysema (Ohnishi et al., 1998), and atherosclerosis (Prescott et al., 1999). The MMPs are also thought to process a number of nonmatrix proteins, including growth factors, cytokines, and other proteinases (McCawley and Matrisian, 2001). For example, MMP2 and MMP9

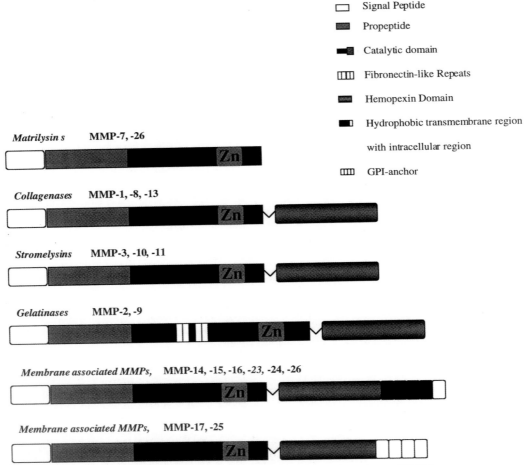

Figure 100–1. Basic domain structure of the matrix metalloproteinases (MMPs).

process transforming growth factor (TGF)-β into an active ligand that has a major role in the promotion of matrix synthesis and homeostasis (Yu and Stamenkovic, 2000).

To ensure ECM homeostasis, MMP activities have to be very tightly regulated at many different levels. One level of regulation is achieved because MMPs are synthesized as inactive precursors or zymogens that contain a prodomain. Structurally, this domain resides within the catalytic site and blocks substrate access. Dislocation of the prodomain via proteolysis renders the enzyme active (Morgunova et al., 1999). This mechanism of activation, the existence of specific endogenous tissue inhibitors of metalloproteinases (TIMPs), and other transcriptional, posttranscriptional regulatory mechanisms, as well as differential tissue-specific and developmentally regulated patterns of expression and cell surface localization, all ensure an exquisite coordination of MMP-mediated processes (Van Wart and Birkedal-Hansen, 1990; Overall et al., 1991; Whitelock et al., 1993; Brassart et al., 1998; Kusano et al., 1998). Another level of control is provided by the TIMPs. Four TIMPs (TIMP1, 2, 3, and 4) have been identified in vertebrates. These molecules not only can inhibit active MMPs but also can regulate MMP function at the level of activation (Shofuda et al., 1998; Brew et al., 2000). The activation of pro-MMP2 by MT1-MMP is greatly enhanced in the presence of small amounts of TIMP2 with the formation of a ternary pro-MMP2/TIMP2/MT1-MMP complex at the cell surface. In this model, the MT1-MMP catalytic domain binds to the amino-terminal portion of TIMP-2. The MT1-MMP–bound TIMP-2 then acts as a molecular link providing its negatively charged terminus to bind to the hemopexin-like domain of pro-MMP2. Cleavage at Asn66-Leu77 in the MMP2 prodomain by a free MT1-MMP molecule generates an intermediate that is autocatalyzed to produce fully active MMP2 (Strongin et al., 1995; Butler et al., 1997; Lehti et al., 1998; Shofuda et al., 1998).

The multiplicity of MMPs, overlapping substrate specificity, and wide tissue distribution, although suggestive of involvement in many diverse biological processes, may also imply a redundancy of function. This possible redundancy has made the deduction of natural enzyme-substrate relationships and the in vivo role of these enzymes in pathological conditions a very difficult task (Parks, 1999). Many studies have suggested an in vitro disregulation of MMP enzymatic activity with a particular disease process. For example, the MMPs have been implicated in the process of tumor growth and invasion with an overexpression of activity in malignant tumors. Overexpression of MMPs has also been found in many inflammatory and degenerative processes, including rheumatoid arthritis (Brinckerhoff, 1991; Konttinen et al., 1999), osteoarthritis (Clark et al., 1993), and periodontitis (Birkedal-Hansen, 1993).

With the exception of Sorsby fundal dystrophy, a disease caused by mutations in the *TIMP3* gene (Weber et al., 1994), there has been difficulty in understanding the in vivo significance of a specific MMP's contribution to particular disease states. This difficulty has arisen from the genetic complexity of the diseases wherein MMPs are most likely involved. Traditional approaches for the mapping of causative genes in simple mendelian traits becomes exceedingly cumbersome and difficult to interpret for complex diseases like arthritis or artherosclerosis. There has, however, been some success in molecular studies involving genetic variations in the form of single-nucleotide polymorphisms (SNPs) in MMP genes and disease susceptibility (Table 100–1). Epidemiological studies have suggested that a functional polymorphism in the MMP-1 gene promoter that increases the binding of the Ets-1 transcription factor is associated with ovarian cancer predisposition (Kanamori et al., 1999). Studies in atherosclerosis have identified MMP-3 promoter allele differences with increased risk for acute myocardial infarction (Ye et al., 1996).

As well as these genetic studies, a number of mouse MMP-deficient models have been generated with the aim of defining the role of specific MMPs in normal development and disease-specific pathophysiol-

Table 100–1. Disease Association of Matrix Metalloproteinase (MMP) Promoter Polymorphisms

Gene	Position/Polymorphism	Disease Association	Proposed Mechanism
MMP1	−1607, 1G/1G → 1G/2G 2G/2G	Increased lung cancer susceptibility (Zhu et al., 2001) Colorectal cancer invasiveness (Ghilardi et al., 2001) Ovarian cancer invasiveness (Kanamori et al., 1999) Endometrial carcinoma development (Nishioka et al., 2000) Susceptibility to preterm premature rupture of the fetal membrane (Fujimoto et al., 2002)	Creation of an Ets transcription factor binding site resulting in increased expression
MMP2	−735 C → T	Increased allele frequency in patients with psoriasis (Vasku et al., 2002)	Increased promoter activity
MMP3	−1612/5A/5AG → 5A/6A	Age-related stiffening of arteries (Kingwell et al., 2001) Risk factor for acute myocardial infarction (Terashima et al., 1999)	Decreased expression due to increased binding of transcription repressor
MMP9	−1562 C → T −90 (CA)n	Severity of coronary atherosclerosis (Wang et al., 2001) (CA)23 allele associated with risk of intracranial aneurysm (Zhang et al., 2001)	Increased transcriptional activity Increased promoter activity
MMP12	−82 G → A	Influence on luminal diameter in diabetic patients with coronary artery disease (Jormsjo et al., 2000)	Increased binding affinity to AP-1 transcription factor resulting in higher transcriptional activities

ogy (Table 100–2). Disease targets have included tumorigenesis, aneurysmal degeneration, wound healing, and Alzheimer's disease. The gelatinase B/MMP9–deficient mouse has probably been the most extensively studied MMP-deficient model and has provided valuable information on the significance of this gelatinase in experimental models of traumatic brain injury, tumorigenesis, lung injury, multiple sclerosis, wound healing, and normal biological processes such as osteoclast recruitment and reproductive capacity. It was only the discovery that an MMP2 deficiency in humans resulted in a severe osteolytic phenotype that provided definitive evidence of an *in vivo* role for one of these enzymes in normal human skeletal development (Martignetti et al., 2001).

CLINICAL DESCRIPTION OF MONA AFFECTEDS

The multicentric osteolyses, or "vanishing bone," syndromes are a group of hereditary autosomal dominant and recessive skeletal disorders generally characterized by marked and progressive bone and joint destruction resulting in skeletal deformities and significant functional impairment (Torg et al., 1969; Tyler and Rosenbaum, 1976; Fuchs,

1991; Rizzo et al., 1993; Al Aqeel et al., 2000; Al-Mayouf et al., 2000; Teebi et al., 2001). The first case of "disappearing bone" disease was described by Jackson in 1838. Since then, a number of clinically distinguishable forms have been described under many different designations as originally catalogued by Tyler and Rosenbaum (1976). These designations have included idiopathic osteolysis, essential osteolysis, progressive essential osteolysis, essential acroosteolysis, hereditary osteolysis, familial osteolysis, hereditary multicentric osteolysis, carpal and tarsal agenesis, bone agenesis, familial dysostosis, and carpal and bilateral carpal necroses. These rare syndromes, although sharing many phenotypic characteristics, can differ from each other in mode of transmission and in clinical features, including the presence or absence of mental retardation and nephropathy and the extent and anatomic distribution of osteolysis (Table 100–3). Based on clinical, radiographic, and hereditary criteria, the International Skeletal Dysplasia Registry has provided a useful comparative classification of the multicentric disorders into four groups (Table 100–4). The group with carpal, tarsal, and interphalangeal joint destruction previously included only Torg (OMIM 259600), Winchester (OMIM

Table 100–2. Some MMP- and TIMP-Deficient Mouse Models

MMP/TIMP	Phenotype
MMP2/Gelatinase A	Reduced corneal and tumor-induced angiogenesis (Itoh et al., 1998; Kato et al., 2001)
MMP3/Stromelysin1	Absence of cartilage erosions, MMP-induced and collagen cleavage-site neoepitopes in an experimental model of immune-mediated arthritis (van Meurs et al., 1999) Prevention of contact hypersensitivity response (Pilcher et al., 1999) Reduced lung injury in experimental acute lung injury (Warner et al., 2001)
MMP7/Matrilysin	Suppressed intestinal tumorigenesis (Wilson et al., 1997)
MMP9/Gelatinase B	Delayed osteoclast recruitment in developing long bones (Engsig et al., 2000) Defect in endochondral bone formation, delayed vascular invasion, and apoptosis of hypertrophic cartilage chrondrocytes (Vu et al., 1998) Improved morphological and motor outcome after traumatic brain injury (Wang et al., 2000) Reduced lung injury in experimental acute lung injury (Warner et al., 2001) Increased severity of nephritis in antiglomerular basement membrane nephritis model (Lelongt et al., 2001) Suppressed development of experimental abdominal aortic aneurysms (Pyo et al., 2000) Increased resistance to experimental bullous pemphigoid (Liu et al., 1998) Suppressed experimental metastasis (Itoh et al., 1999) Resistance to experimental autoimmune encephalomyelitis (Dubois et al., 1999) Decreased alveolar bronchiolization in a fibrosing alveolitis model (Betsuyaku et al., 2000)
MMP11/Stromelysin3	Defective remodeling of ECM at epithelial basement membrane zone (Mohan et al., 2002) Suppression of intestinal tumorigenesis and increased cancer cell apoptosis and necrosis (Boulay et al., 2001) Accelerated neointima formation after vascular injury (Lijnen et al., 1999) Adipocyte hypertrophy in nutritionally induced obesity model (Lijnen et al., 2002)
MMP14/MT1-MMP	Impaired skeletal development, craniofacial dysmorphism, dwarfism, arthritis, osteopenia, fibrotic periskeletal soft tissue, defective cartilage and corneal angiogenesis, increased mortality (Holmbeck et al., 1999; Zhou et al., 2000)
TIMP1	Reduced atherosclerotic plaque formation and enhanced aneurysm formation (Silence et al., 2002) Altered cardiac left ventricular structure (Roten et al., 2000) Accelerated neointima formation after vascular injury (Lijnen et al., 1999)
TIMP3	Spontaneous lung air space enlargement, impaired lung function, and increased mortality (Leco et al., 2001)

MMP, matrix metalloproteinase; TIMP, tissue inhibitor of matrix metalloproteinase; ECM, extracellular matrix.

Table 100–3. Comparison of Features of Some of the Autosomal Recessive Multicentric Osteolysis

Feature	MONA Syndrome	Torg Syndrome	Winchester Syndrome	Francois Syndrome	Juvenile Hyaline Fibromatosis	Farber Lipogranulomatosis
Face						
Corneal opacities	−	−/+	+	+	−	+
Proptosis	+	+	−	−		
Bulbous nose	+	−/+	+	−		
Maxillary hypoplasia	+	+	−			
Micrognathia	+	+	−			
Gum hypertrophy	−	−	+		+	−
Skin						
Subcutaneous nodules	+	+	+	+	+	+
Nodule biopsy	Fibrofatty	Fibrofatty			Tumor-like	Erythematous
Nodule location	Palmar/plantar	Palmar/plantar			Scalp/neck/face	Widespread
Wound healing	Abnormal					
Hyperpigmented lesions	−	+	−			
Swelling of digits	+	+	+			
Deformity of hands/feet	+	+	+	+		+
Joint contractures	+	+	+		+	+
Radiological features						
Osteolysis	Severe	Moderate	Severe		Mild/moderate	Mild
Carpal/tarsal	+	+	+			
Metacarpal/metatarsal	+	+	+			
Interphalangeal/phalangeal	+	+	+			
Other joints	+	+	+		+	+
Spine	−	−/+	+			
Osteopenia	Severe	Mild	Severe		Severe	Mild
Other features						
Nephropathy	−	−/+	−	−	−	−/+
Hirsutism	+	−	−	−	−	−
Miscellaneous				Abnormal EEG and seizures		Hoarse cry and respiratory insufficiency
Diagnostic markers	MMP2 deficiency					Acid ceramidase deficiency

Source: Information on multicentric osteolysis with nodulosis and arthritis (MONA) syndrome from Al Aqeel et al. (2000); Torg syndrome, Torg and Steel, 1968, and Eisenstein et al., 1998; Winchester syndrome, Prapanpoch et al., 1992, and Matthiesen et al., 2001; Francois sydnrome, Bierly et al., 1992; juvenile hyaline fibromatosis, Breier et al., 1997; and Farber lipogranulomatosis, Kim et al., 1998.

277950), Francois (OMIM 221800), and Whyte Hemingway syndromes (Lachman, 1998). MONA (or NAO) is an autosomal recessive member of this group that was recently identified by two independent groups in 12 affected offspring of six consanguineous Saudi Arabian families (Al Aqeel et al., 2000; Al-Mayouf et al., 2000).

The features of MONA overlap with many phenotypic attributes of the other autosomal recessive multicentric osteolyses, most notably Torg and Winchester syndromes (see Table 100–3). Torg syndrome may in fact be genetically identical to MONA; however, biological samples from the originally diagnosed Torg affecteds are not available for biochemical and genetic testing (J. S. Torg, personal communication). In addition, the bone loss and joint destruction seen in MONA patients are comparable to the complications experienced by patients with severe juvenile rheumatoid arthritis (Davidson, 2000; Wihlborg et al., 2001). MONA affecteds tend to develop symptoms

in the first 2 to 3 years of life with the development and progression of painful swellings of the proximal interphalangeal joints of hands, feet, and wrists. Children may also present with decreased range of motion or a deformity of the hands and/or wrists. Of particular note, on physical examination, the presence of firm subcutaneous nodules has been universal. These nodules are composed of fibrocollagenous tissue that extends throughout the entire thickness of the reticular dermis and into the subcutaneous tissue. Magnetic resonance imaging studies are consistent with this presence of dense fibrous tissue and may suggest areas of inflammation near margins (Fig. 100–2) (Al Aqeel et al., 2000; Al-Mayouf et al., 2000).

Interestingly, nodules have been described in a number of children with osteolysis, and their presence and distribution may be a marker for MONA syndrome. These nodules should be distinguished from the xanthomatous nodules present on the pinnae of those affected with Fran-

Table 100–4. International Skeletal Dysplasia Registry Classification of the Multicentric Osteolyses

	Mode of Inheritance	OMIM	Chromosomal Locus
Multicentric predominantly carpal and tarsal in the hand			
Multicentric carpal-tarsal osteolysis with and without nephropathy	AD	166300	
Nodulosis arthropathy and osteolysis syndrome			
Shinohara carpal-tarsal osteolysis			
Multicentric predominantly carpal, tarsal, and interphalangeal			
Francois syndrome	AR	221800	
Winchester syndrome	AR	277950	
Torg syndrome	AR	259600	
Whyte-Hemingway carpal-tarsal phalangeal osteolysis	AD		
Predominantly distal phalanges			
Hadju-Cheney syndrome	AD	102500	
Giacci familial neurogenic acroosteolysis	AR	201300	
Mandibulo acral syndrome	AR		
Predominantly involving diaphyses and metaphyses			
Familial expansile osteolysis	AD	174810	18q21.1-22
Juvenile hyaline fibromatosis	AR	228600	

AD, autosomal dominant; AR, autosomal recessive.
Source: Lachman, 1998.

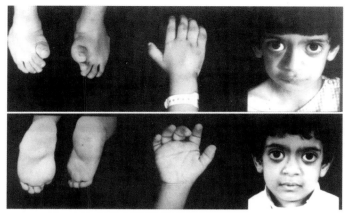

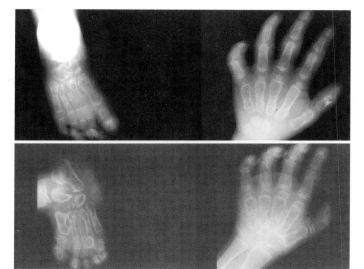

Figure 100–2. The multicentric osteolysis with nodulosis and arthritis (MONA) syndrome affected at 2 (*top*) and 4 (*bottom*) years of age. The feet display planovarus deformity and fixed hyperextension of the halluces and a subcutaneous plantar nodule over the sole of the foot. Fusiform swelling of fingers with hyperextension of metacarpophalangeal joints and flexion of interphalangeal joints is evident. Subcutaneous painful nodules are seen covering the whole palm of the hand, and a scar on the dorsum of the hand indicates the site of a nodule biopsy. The facial features are notable for bilateral proptosis, bulbous nose, narrow nasal bridge, and small chin. (From Al Aqeel et al., 2000 with permission.)

cois syndrome (Bierly et al., 1992) and juvenile hyaline fibromatosis. Physical examination of patients may also reveal significant muscle wastage and restricted growth. Facial features are also quite distinctive and help distinguish MONA from other osteolysis syndromes. These minor facial anomalies include proptosis, frontal bossing, hypertelorism, and a bulbous nose with a flat nasal ridge (see Fig. 100–2). Unlike Winchester syndrome, no affecteds have shown signs of corneal clouding, gum hypertrophy, or renal dysfunction (see Table 100–3). Two affecteds of the group reported by Al Mayouf et al. (2000), showed signs of mental retardation. Affecteds from the family reported by Al Aqeel et al. (2000), displayed generalized hirsutism. With age, hands and feet become progressively deformed with short fingers and thick skin (see Fig. 100–2). Large, painful subcutaneous fibrocollagenous pads can present on hands and feet, and wound healing after biopsy of these nodules resulted in abnormal scarring and keloid formation (see Fig. 100–3). Flexion deformities are also detected in elbows, knees, wrists, and hips, and flexion contractures in interphalangeal joints are very apparent. All fingers have painful fusiform swellings with hyperextension over the metacarpophalangeal joints. Radiological analysis of these children have revealed generalized osteopenia, contractures of the phalanges, osteolysis of carpal and tarsal bones (Figs. 100–4, 100–5 and 100–6), and brachycephaly with frontal bone and maxillary hypoplasia. As affecteds get older, the osteolysis progresses and results in chaotic destruction of carpals and tarsals and destruction of the metatarsal, phalangeal, and interphalangeal joints. Hands and feet in the few older patients assessed tend to become markedly distorted with even the loss of digits

Figure 100–4. Plain radiographs of the hands and feet of multicentric osteolysis with nodulosis and arthritis (MONA) syndrome affected. *Top right,* Hands at 2 years of age with osteopenia, fusiform swelling of fingers, and osteolysis of interphalangeal joints. *Bottom right,* Hands at 4 years of age showing further destruction of the carpal bones, progressive involvement of the metacarpal bones with proximal tapering, and bilateral distal notching and shadowing by the subcutaneous palmar nodule. *Left,* Feet at 2 (*top*) and 4 (*right*) years of age. The progression of an obvious and marked tarsal osteolysis is evident. (From Al Aqeel et al., 2000 with permission.)

and telescoping of the overlying tissue (Figs. 100–5 and 100–6). Ankylosis of remaining bones becomes apparent with elbows, knees, and hips eventually becoming completely fixed with radiological analysis of knees revealing cortical thinning, epiphyseal enlargement, and reduced joint spaces. Radiological analysis also demonstrates severe and universal osteopenia, destruction of the femoral heads, and pelvic distortions. Laboratory evaluations, including complete blood cell counts, liver and kidney functions, bone and rheumatology panels, erythrocyte

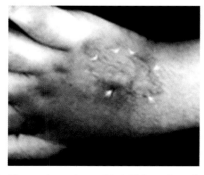

Figure 100–3. Abnormal scarring and keloid formation after skin biopsy of the multicentric osteolysis with nodulosis and arthritis (MONA) syndrome affected. Arrows indicate margins of keloid.

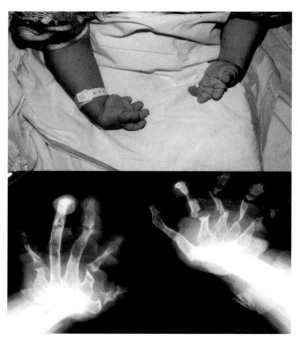

Figure 100–5. Hands and radiological features of a 20-year-old multicentric osteolysis with nodulosis and arthritis (MONA) syndrome affected. Hands show complete destruction and loss of all carpal bones, marked destruction of metacarpals, and phalanges with ankylosis of the remaining bones. (From Al Aqeel et al., 2000 with permission.)

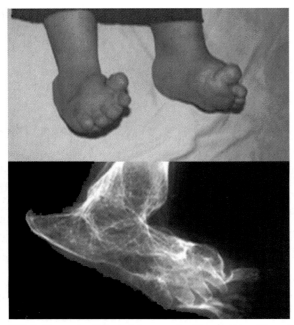

Figure 100–6. Feet and radiological features of a 20-year-old multicentric osteolysis with nodulosis and arthritis (MONA) syndrome affected. (From Al Aqeel et al., 2000 with permission.)

sedimentation rate and metabolic screening of serum and urine, are all within normal limits (Al Aqeel et al., 2000; Al-Mayouf et al., 2000).

IDENTIFICATION OF GENE AND MUTATIONAL SPECTRUM: MMP2 DEFICIENCY RESULTS IN MONA SYNDROME

The identification of MONA affected individuals in three large and unrelated Saudi Arabian consanguineous families, where the parents were first cousins suggested an autosomal recessive mode of inheritance and allowed gene identification by linkage analysis. A genome-wide search was performed for regions homozygous-by-descent using PCR-based microsatellite markers. Based on an initial genetic screen using two families, linkage was established for marker D16S3253 on chromosome 16q12 with a maximal LOD score of 4.59 at $\theta = 0$. Additional markers in this region, as defined by the 1999 Marshfield Map (Broman et al., 1998), were selected, and haplotype analysis defined the 13-cM interval between markers D16S3396 and GATA67G11 as the critical region. Mapping of a third Saudi family established a maximum multipoint LOD score of 1.61 at $\theta = 0$ for marker D16S3140, which was present within this region. Haplotype analysis of this family allowed refined localization of the disease locus to a 1.2-cM region, flanked telomerically by marker D16S3140 and centromerically by marker D16S3032.

Inspection of this mapped region revealed several candidate genes, including the *MMP2* gene. Accordingly affecteds and their families were screened for MMP2 biochemical activity. Affecteds completely lacked serum and fibroblast MMP2 gelatinolytic activity, whereas parents of affected children, all obligate heterozygotes, had half-normal levels of MMP2 activity (Martignetti et al., 2001).

Efforts were then directed to determine whether these three MMP2–deficient families had the same or different mutations, with the latter being predicted by their different haplotypes. The *MMP2* gene had been previously cloned and its sequence analyzed. It contains 13 exons, of which exons 1 through 4 and 8 through 12 show extensive homology to the interstitial collagenase and stromelysin genes, whereas exons 5 through 7 each encode one complete internal repeat, resembling the collagen-binding fibronectin type II domains (Collier et al., 1991). In one family, all affected individuals were homoallelic for a nonsense mutation (TCA → TAA) in codon 244 of exon 5, predicting replacement of a tyrosine residue by a stop codon in the first fibronectin type II domain (Y244X) and premature trun-

cation. Comparison of the mutant Y224X protein with the wild type, along with previous biochemical studies exploring domain properties, resulted in the predicted loss of all three MMP2 functional domains: the Zn^{2+} binding site catalytic domain (which is present in all prokaryotic and eukaryotic metalloproteinases), the three fibronectin type II–like domains, and the hemopexin domain (Martignetti et al., 2001).

The second familial mutation is a missense variation in exon 2, predicting the replacement of an arginine with a histidine in the highly conserved prodomain region. Although these amino acids are structurally very different and the change could significantly disrupt the prodomain, it is not immediately apparent why this mutation in the prodomain could result in complete loss of gelatinolytic activity (Martignetti et al., 2001). One explanation might lie in the effect of this mutation on the structural characteristics of the folded native enzyme. Structurally, the native arginine residue is adjacent to the cysteine residue integral to the cysteine switch mechanism. In the inactive proform of this enzyme, this cysteine interacts with the catalytic zinc ion (Morgunova et al., 1999). Replacement of this arginine with a histidine may disrupt two adjacent salt bridges with an adjacent asparagine thus destabilizing the structure necessary for the cysteine switch mechanism to function. Alternatively the proximity of this mutation to the active site coupled with the bulkiness of the mutant histidine residue could simply disrupt the tertiary structure, destabilizing all essential domain structures and rendering the peptidase inactive and/or unstable. Although linkage and haplotype analyses demonstrate that the disease locus in the third family maps to the same finite region as the other two families and no gelatinolytic activity was found in patient serum samples, no inactivating mutations were found in the exonic sequences of the gene. Perhaps an undetected homoallelic mutation is present in the promoter or intronic regions. A nonpathogenic homoallelic polymorphism was nonetheless present in affected individuals in codon 210 of exon 4. This GT transversion is predicted to result in the substitution of an aspartate with a tyrosine residue (D210Y). Analysis of 50 unrelated and unaffected members of this particular Saudi tribe shows that the polymorphism is a relatively common allele and suggest the possibility of future MMP2 association studies (Martignetti et al., 2001).

MMP2, a 72-kDa gelatinase and type IV collagenase, was originally isolated from rheumatoid arthritis synovial tissue culture media (Harris and Krane, 1972) and is thought to be involved in normal collagen turnover (Creemers et al., 1998). Although very little is known about the *in vivo* substrates of MMP2, many studies have implicated it in the degradation of a wide array of ECM and nonmatrix substrates, including gelatin (Murphy and Crabbe, 1995), elastin (Okada et al., 1993), fibronectin, collagen, laminin (Murphy et al., 1981), aggrecan (Fosang et al., 1992), vitronectin (Imai et al., 1995), MCP-3 (McQuibban et al., 2000), pro–tumor necrosis factor (TNF)-α (Shubayev and Myers, 2002), pro–interleukin 1β (Schonbeck et al., 1998), and pro-TGF-β2 (Yu and Stamenkovic, 2000). This wide substrate specificity and ubiquitous expression pattern of this enzyme confound simple explanations of the disease mechanism. Moreover, the discovery that MONA arises from an MMP2 deficiency raises questions about the previously implied role of MMP2 in normal and pathological bone processes. Paradoxical to the finding that MMP2 defiency leads to a severe osteolytic and arthritic phenotype is the multitude of studies suggesting that MMPs, and specifically MMP2 overexpression and increased activity, result in bone, cartilage, and joint destruction and abnormal wound repair (Brinckerhoff, 1991; Agren 1994; Konttinen et al., 1999; Yoshihara et al., 2000). MMP2 has been implicated in concert with MT1-MMP and TIMP-2 in contributing to the loosening and osteolysis of periprosthetic joints, and augmented levels of activated MMP2 have been observed in the synovia of patients with early erosive rheumatoid arthritis (Goldbach-Mansky et al., 2000; Takei et al., 2000).

DIAGNOSIS AND MANAGEMENT OF MONA AFFECTEDS

The many shared and overlapping features of the osteolysis syndromes make an accurate diagnosis between them a clinical challenge. In addition, some of the features of these syndromes during early childhood can also mimic findings of severe juvenile rheumatoid arthritis, juvenile hyaline fibromatosis, and Farber disease (OMIM 228000), (see Table 100–3). However, establishing an accurate diagnosis will be crucial for understanding and establishing the natural history of these diseases, management, treatment, genetic counseling, and future gene discovery projects. Because the etiology of these disorders, with the exception of MONA, remains unknown, definitive diagnosis is a future goal. Clinicians must therefore rely on a combination of long-term radiological and physical characteristics with the extent and locus of tissue damage to establish disease categorization. In this regard, the outline provided by the International Skeletal Dysplasia Registry is quite useful (see Table 100–4) (Lachman, 1998). However, as demonstrated by the identification and description of MONA syndrome, new syndromes will undoubtedly be discovered. The discovery of MMP2–inactivating gene mutations as the causative factor of MONA has made molecular diagnosis a reality. A small aliquot of blood allows definitive assessment of MMP2 gelatinolytic activity by gel zymography (Johansson and Smedsrod, 1986). The zymographic assay for detecting serum MMP2 activity represents the gold standard for diagnosis, while DNA sequence analysis allows confirmation and understanding of the mechanism of gene inactivation. In the future, DNA sequence information may provide genotype/phenotype correlations. However, it must be stressed that lack of demonstrable *MMP2* DNA mutations, in the face of absent biochemical activity, should suggest the presence of functional changes within promoter or intronic sequences. In fact, the possibility of genotype/phenotype correlations further stresses the importance of a thorough clinical and radiological evaluation for defining disease progression and establishng the full clinical spectrum of the disorder. Before biochemical and genetic testing, establishment of a family history, which may include parental consanguinity and/or affected sibs in only one generation, should suggest the autosomal recessive nature of the disease. Including MONA, the autosomal recessive multicentric osteolyses comprise a group of about four syndromes with similar clinical and radiological findings (see Table 100–3). Although a number of clinical features are useful in distinguishing MONA from Francois syndrome, a significant amount of overlap is seen among MONA, Torg, and Winchester syndromes. Indeed, based on molecular analysis, we have reclassified a number of affected individuals previously diagnosed with Torg and Winchester syndromes, as true MONA affecteds (unpublished data).

Unfortunately, no specific treatments are yet available for MONA or any of the multicentric osteolysis disorders. Utimately, enzyme or gene replacement therapy with MMP2 would represent the most specific therapeutic approach. Enzyme replacement therapy has already become a reality for some lysosomal storage diseases such as Gaucher and Fabry disease, but its efficacy in treating defects in ECM metabolism still has not been tested (Desnick, 2001). In addition, because of the biochemical activation of MMP2 by MT1-MMP and inhibition by TIMP2, one could imagine that regulation of these MMPs could also represent a potential future therapeutic research strategy.

Methotrexate and D-penicillamine have previously been used in this disorder with apparently encouraging results. Although osteolysis in these patients was not halted, deterioration in both joint contracture and nodule formation was suggested to be prevented (Al-Mayouf et al., 2000). Short-term improvement in skin and joint mobility was also reported in a Winchester patient treated with methotrexate (Matthiesen et al., 2001). In addition, agents traditionally used to treat juvenile rheumatoid arthritis, osteoporosis, and other childhood skeletal dysplasias may provide additional therapeutic strategies; however, no long-term or well-controlled studies are available.

We believe that with respect to the osteopenic phenotype of MONA, biphosphonates have the potential to be a useful treatment. Bisphosphonates have been shown to inhibit osteoclast-mediated bone resorption and are used in the treatment of a number of disorders characterized by increased bone resorption, including osteoporosis, Paget's disease, osteolytic bone disease of malignancy, and the very rare congenital disease fibrous dysplasia of bone (Chapurlat and Meunier, 2000; Devogelaer, 2000). However, although bisphosphonates such as pamidronate used in combination with antirheumatic drugs such as

TNF blockers and methotrexate present a very promising treatment strategy, care will have to be taken in determining the optimal regimen with respect to efficacy and long-term patient safety.

MUTANTS IN ORTHOLOGOUS GENES

Before the report demonstrating mutations in the human *MMP2* gene, *MMP2* knockout mice had been generated to examine the role of MMP2 in amyloid precursor protein (APP) processing and secretion *in vivo*. In these mice, a knockout mutation was introduced by replacing its promoter and first exon with the *pgk-neo* cassette by gene targeting. Although no significant phenotypic differences were found between wild-type and mutant animals in their APP processing ability, MMP2–deficient animals were smaller at birth and exhibited a slower growth rate (Itoh et al., 1997). This growth-restricted phenotype most likely parallels the skeletal defects seen in MONA affecteds and would suggest that a directed analysis of bone and joint development in these knockouts is required. Despite size differences, these MMP2 knockout mice were reported to develop normally with no obvious skeletal or joint problems and no functional impairment (Itoh et al., 1997). More recent studies on these mice have revealed MMP2–dependent effects on corneal and tumor-induced angiogenesis (Itoh et al., 1998, 1999). The potential skeletal or metabolic mechanisms underlying their growth delay has not yet been fully explored. The apparent lack of a suitable mouse knockout model for MONA has restricted progress in helping to determine the pathogenic mechanisms in the human disease, but there have been intriguing developments in the description of other MMP-deficient mouse models.

Of the MMP mouse models generated, only MT1-MMP– and MMP9–deficient animals have shown skeletal developmental anomalies (Vu et al., 1998; Holmbeck et al., 1999; Zhou et al., 2000). The most relevant of these in relation to MONA syndrome appears to be the previously unstated finding that MT1-MMP–deficient mice share human MONA clinical characteristics. This is especially interesting given that activation of MMP2 is mediated by MT1-MMP on the cell membrane (Strongin et al., 1995). MT1-MMP knockouts are dwarfed and have dysmorphic craniofacial features, osteopenia, arthritis, and skeletal dysplasia. The mechanisms behind these developmental abnormalities appear to be in part due to a disruption of matrix homeostasis or, more specifically, a loss of a collagenolytic activity essential for the development, growth, and maintenance of skeletal structures (Holmbeck et al., 1999). Craniofacial structures should under normal conditions be formed by membranous ossification, an event dependent on the removal of the cartilage primordia. Failure to remove this matrix probably results in disruption of the membranous ossification process and incomplete suture closure. Epiphyseal ossification in the long bones is also disrupted in these animals. Vascularization, a process dependent on uncalcified cartilage removal, appears to be completely obstructed. Failure of this angiogenic process then results in diminished longitudinal bone growth as a function of impaired growth plate function. Increased osteoclastic bone resorption was found at the bone surface of soft tissue insertion sites. Remodeling of these periskeletal soft tissues was severely impaired to the extent that a compensatory mechanism of osteoclastic resorption was activated, perhaps in response to the build up of this collagen-rich fibrotic tissue, to accommodate growth. Osteoblast function was also impaired in response to this failure to remodel their surrounding collagenous matrix for the ensuing ossification process. Although these animals do not develop lytic bone lesions to the same extent as the human MONA affecteds, they do show an increased mortality. The majority of animals die before 3 months of age (Holmbeck et al., 1999; Zhou et al., 2000). This increased mortality could possibly be attributed to malnutrition, secondary to craniofacial anomalies resulting in inefficient feeding (Zhou et al., 2000). It is very tempting to credit the MT1-MMP mouse phenotype to impaired MMP2 activation, but this theory is completely at odds with the lack of any comparable MMP2–deficient mouse phenotype. Although MT1-MMP in conjunction with TIMP2 is thought to be the major physiological activator of pro-MMP2 with minimal conversion to its active form in tissue extracts from MT1-MMP–deficient mice, it is clear it has a very important role in collagen I degradation and angiogenesis in mice (Holmbeck et al., 1999). It is also worth noting that mice deficient in TIMP-2, although lacking efficient pro-MMP2 conversion, have no overt phenotype, skeletal or otherwise (Caterina et al., 1999, 2000). Perhaps in mice there is a redundancy in MMP2 function, not found in humans, with some other matrix-degrading enzyme, perhaps MT1-MMP, compensating for the loss in collagenolytic activity.

DEVELOPMENTAL PATHOGENESIS: HOW DOES MMP2 DEFICIENCY RESULT IN THE MONA PHENOTYPE IN HUMANS?

The discovery that MMP2 deficiency results in a disorder characterized by tissue destruction in the form of osteolysis and arthritis has raised questions about the complex role of this gelatinase in normal bone development and joint maintenance processes. Studies had previously associated an increased presence of certain MMP family members, including MMP2, with bone and joint destruction, as the end point of the arthritic disease process and osteolytic metastasis (Yoneda et al., 1997; Konttinen et al., 1998; Yoshihara et al., 2000). Traditionally, therefore, one might have associated an osteopetrotic or bone "overgrowth" phenotype with MMP2 deficiency. An interesting overgrowth parallel is seen in the inherited form of cathepsin K deficiency, which in humans results in pycnodysostosis (Gelb et al., 1996; Hou et al., 1999) and in mice results in an osteopetrotic phenotype (Lazner et al., 1999). The ambiguity about the *in vivo* function of MMP2 and the lack of a skeletal phenotype in the MMP2–deficient mouse mean that the cellular mechanism behind the MONA phenotype remains unknown. Also, the differences in functional redundancy of MMPs between humans and mice are still unappreciated. Therefore, the genetics of a rare human disorder suggests a reevaluation of our understanding of MMP2 function in the context of in vivo physiology. For instance, are MMP2 deficiency and its direct effect on structural components of the ECM responsible for tissue damage? Is MMP2 an essential activator of some other molecule(s) critical to the bone remodeling process? Ultimately, MMP2 effects will be translated by one of three mechanisms: a decrease in osteoblastic function, an increase in osteoclastic resorption, or a combination of these events. An understanding of the cellular events responsible for the progression of bone lesions, joint destruction, and osteopenia not only could be central in establishing effective treatment regimens for MONA but also could provide greater understanding of the pathogenesis of arthritis and osteoporosis.

MONA may result from MMP2–deficient remodeling of the skeletal and periskeletal matrix. Structural components and regulators of the extracellular matrix play a crucial role in skeletal development and homeostasis (Rice et al., 1997; Bord et al., 1998; Aszodi et al., 2000, 2001; Wu et al., 2001; see Chapter 95). Mutations in bone and cartilage matrix molecules have been associated with a large number of skeletal dysplasias and fibromatosis, some of which share the overlapping features of fibrotic skin nodules, osteolysis, joint destruction, and contractures (Lewkonia and Pope, 1985; Tsipouras et al., 1986; Thur et al., 2001). Juvenile hyaline fibromatosis is a disease characterized by osteolytic bone lesions and multiple subcutaneous tumors, joint contractures, short stature, and skull deformities. Juvenile hyaline-fibromatosis affected-derived fibroblasts demonstrated decreased collagen III metabolism and increased collagen I synthesis and degradation (Breier et al., 1997). These features suggest a defect in ECM metabolism. Another potential insight into understanding the pathogenesis is provided by analysis of the MT1-MMP–deficient mouse model. This animal model, which to date has no recognized human counterpart, is another excellent example of how an MMP deficiency can lead to tissue destruction. As discussed earlier, the MT1-MMP–deficient phenotype has been attributed to disruption of several processes critical to bone homeostasis and joint maintenance. Inadequate collagen turnover was found to be responsible, with the accumulation of collagen-rich fibrotic periskeletal soft tissue linked to increased osteoclastic resorption and decreased bone formation. This animal model also illustrates the importance of remodeling of soft connective tissue matrix in the development and maintenance of the skeleton (Holmbeck et al., 1999; Zhou et al., 2000).

Finally another possibility is that MMP2 loss could disrupt some critical cellular process by the loss of activation of some essential cell signal such as TGF-β (Vu, 2001). This potent osteotropic peptide has an important role in the coupling process between bone formation and bone resorption. Active TGF-β not only promotes osteoblast recruitment and proliferation but also has both an inhibitory effect on osteoclast formation and a stimulatory effect on differentiation and survival of osteoclasts (Bonewald and Dallas, 1994; Centrella et al., 1994; Erlebacher et al., 1998; Chambers, 2000). This important regulator of bone remodeling already has an established role in human skeletal irregularities with polymorphisms and mutations in the TGF-β gene associated with susceptibility to osteoporosis and a hereditary sclerotic bone disease respectively (Janssens et al., 2000; Hinke et al., 2001). MMP2, by virtue of its ability to activate TGF-β *in vitro*, could play a role in complementary bone remodeling processes (Yu and Stamenkovic, 2000). However, there is no *in vivo* evidence for participation of MMP2 in the activation of TGF-β, and given its very broad in vitro substrate specificity, the disruption of any number of MMP2–related signaling processes could be responsible and should be investigated.

REFERENCES

Agnihotri R, Crawford HC, Haro H, Matrisian LM, Havrda MC, Liaw L (2001). Osteopontin, a novel substrate for matrix metalloproteinase-3 (stromelysin-1) and matrix metalloproteinase-7 (matrilysin). *J Biol Chem* 276: 28261–28267.

Agren MS (1994). Gelatinase activity during wound healing. *Br J Dermatol* 131: 634–640.

Akagi A, Tajima S, Ishibashi A, Yamaguchi N, Nagai Y (1999). Expression of type XVI collagen in human skin fibroblasts: enhanced expression in fibrotic skin diseases. *J Invest Dermatol* 113: 246–250.

Al Aqeel A, Al Sewairi W, Edress B, Gorlin RJ, Desnick RJ, Martignetti JA (2000). Inherited multicentric osteolysis with arthritis: a variant resembling Torg syndrome in a Saudi family. *Am J Med Genet* 93: 11–18.

Al-Mayouf SM, Majeed M, Hugosson C, Bahabri S (2000). New form of idiopathic osteolysis: nodulosis, arthropathy and osteolysis (NAO) syndrome. *Am J Med Genet* 93: 5–10.

Aszodi A, Hunziker EB, Olsen BR, Fassler R (2001). The role of collagen II and cartilage fibril-associated molecules in skeletal development. *Osteoarthritis Cartilage* 9: S150–159.

Aszodi A, Bateman JF, Gustafsson E, Boot-Handford R, Fassler R (2000). Mammalian skeletogenesis and extracellular matrix: what can we learn from knockout mice? *Cell Struct Funct* 25: 73–84.

Betsuyaku T, Fukuda Y, Parks WC, Shipley JM, Senior RM (2000). Gelatinase B is required for alveolar bronchiolization after intratracheal bleomycin. *Am J Pathol* 157: 525–535.

Bierly JR, George SP, Volpicelli M (1992). Dermochondral corneal dystrophy (of Francois). *Br J Ophthalmol* 76: 760–761.

Birkedal-Hansen H (1993). Role of matrix metalloproteinases in human periodontal diseases. *J Periodontol* 64: 474–484.

Bonewald LF, Dallas SL (1994). Role of active and latent transforming growth factor beta in bone formation. *J Cell Biochem* 55: 350–357.

Bord S, Horner A, Hembry RM, Compston JE (1998). Stromelysin-1 (MMP-3) and stromelysin-2 (MMP-10) expression in developing human bone: potential roles in skeletal development. *Bone* 23: 7–12.

Boulay A, Masson R, Chenard MP, El Fahime M, Cassard L, Bellocq JP, Sautes-Fridman C, et al. (2001). High cancer cell death in syngeneic tumors developed in host mice deficient for the stromelysin-3 matrix metalloproteinase. *Cancer Res* 61: 2189–2193.

Brassart B, Randoux A, Hornebeck W, Emonard H (1998). Regulation of matrix metalloproteinase-2 (gelatinase A, MMP2), membrane-type matrix metalloproteinase-1 (MT1-MMP) and tissue inhibitor of metalloproteinases-2 (TIMP-2) expression by elastin-derived peptides in human HT-1080 fibrosarcoma cell line. *Clin Exp Metast* 16: 489–500.

Breier F, Fang-Kircher S, Wolff K, Jurecka W (1997). Juvenile hyaline fibromatosis: impaired collagen metabolism in human skin fibroblasts. *Arch Dis Child* 77: 436–440.

Brennan AM, Pauli RM (2001). Hajdu-Cheney syndrome: evolution of phenotype and clinical problems. *Am J Med Genet* 100: 292–310.

Brew K, Dinakarpandian D, Nagase H (2000). Tissue inhibitors of metalloproteinases: evolution, structure and function. *Biochim Biophys Acta* 1477: 267–283.

Brinckerhoff CE (1991). Joint destruction in arthritis: metalloproteinases in the spotlight. *Arthritis Rheum* 34: 1073–1075.

Broman KW, Murray JC, Sheffield VC, White RL, Weber JL (1998). Comprehensive human genetic maps: individual and sex-specific variation in recombination. *Am J Hum Genet* 63: 861–869.

Butler GS, Will H, Atkinson SJ, Murphy G (1997). Membrane-type-2 matrix metalloproteinase can initiate the processing of progelatinase A and is regulated by the tissue inhibitors of metalloproteinases. *Eur J Biochem* 244: 653–657.

Caterina J, Caterina N, Yamada S, Holmback K, Longenecker G, Shi J, Netzel-Arnett S, et al. (1999). Murine TIMP-2 gene-targeted mutation. *Ann N Y Acad Sci* 878: 528–530.

Caterina JJ, Yamada S, Caterina NC, Longenecker G, Holmback K, Shi J, Yermovsky AE, et al (2000). Inactivating mutation of the mouse tissue inhibitor of metalloproteinases-2 (Timp-2) gene alters proMMP2 activation. *J Biol Chem* 275: 26416–26422.

Centrella M, Horowitz MC, Wozney JM, McCarthy TL (1994). Transforming growth factor-beta gene family members and bone. *Endocr Rev* 15: 27–39.

Chambers TJ (2000). Regulation of the differentiation and function of osteoclasts. *J Pathol* 192: 4–13.

Chapurlat RD, Meunier PJ (2000). Fibrous dysplasia of bone. *Baillieres Best Pract Res Clin Rheumatol* 14: 385–398.

Clark IM, Powell LK, Ramsey S, Hazleman BL, Cawston TE (1993). The measurement of collagenase, tissue inhibitor of metalloproteinases (TIMP), and collagenase-TIMP complex in synovial fluids from patients with osteoarthritis and rheumatoid arthritis. *Arthritis Rheum* 36: 372–379.

Clegg PD, Carter SD (1999). Matrix metalloproteinase-2 and -9 are activated in joint diseases. *Equine Vet J* 31: 324–330.

Cockett MI, Murphy G, Birch ML, O'Connell JP, Crabbe T, Millican AT, Hart IR, et al. (1998). Matrix metalloproteinases and metastatic cancer. *Biochem Soc Symp* 63: 295–313.

Collier IE, Bruns GA, Goldberg GI, Gerhard DS (1991). On the structure and chromosome location of the 72- and 92-kDa human type IV collagenase genes. *Genomics* 9: 429–434.

Corbel M, Belleguic C, Boichot E, Lagente V (2002). Involvement of gelatinases (MMP2 and MMP-9) in the development of airway inflammation and pulmonary fibrosis. *Cell Biol Toxicol* 18: 51–61.

Creemers LB, Jansen ID, Docherty AJ, Reynolds JJ, Beertsen W, Everts V (1998). Gelatinase A (MMP2) and cysteine proteinases are essential for the degradation of collagen in soft connective tissue. *Matrix Biol* 17: 35–46.

Davidson J (2000). Juvenile idiopathic arthritis: a clinical overview. *Eur J Radiol* 33: 128–134.

Desnick RJ (2001). Enzyme replacement and beyond. *J Inherit Metab Dis* 24: 251–265.

Devogelaer JP (2000). Treatment of bone diseases with bisphosphonates, excluding osteoporosis. *Curr Opin Rheumatol* 12: 331–335.

Dubois B, Masure S, Hurtenbach U, Paemen L, Heremans H, van den Oord J, Sciot R, et al. (1999). Resistance of young gelatinase B-deficient mice to experimental autoimmune encephalomyelitis and necrotizing tail lesions. *J Clin Invest* 104: 1507–1515.

Duffy MJ, Maguire TM, Hill A, McDermott E, O'Higgins N (2000). Metalloproteinases: role in breast carcinogenesis, invasion and metastasis. *Breast Cancer Res* 2: 252–257.

Eisenstein DM, Poznanski AK, Pachman LM (1998). Torg osteolysis syndrome. *Am J Med Genet* 80: 207–212.

Engsig MT, Chen QJ, Vu TH, Pedersen AC, Therkidsen B, Lund LR, Henriksen K, et al. (2000). Matrix metalloproteinase 9 and vascular endothelial growth factor are essential for osteoclast recruitment into developing long bones. *J Cell Biol* 151: 879–890.

Erlebacher A, Filvaroff EH, Ye JQ, Derynck R (1998). Osteoblastic responses to TGF-beta during bone remodeling. *Mol Biol Cell* 9: 1903–1918.

Fisher C, Gilbertson-Beadling S, Powers EA, Petzold G, Poorman R, Mitchell MA (1994). Interstitial collagenase is required for angiogenesis in vitro. *Dev Biol* 162: 499–510.

Fosang AJ, Neame PJ, Last K, Hardingham TE, Murphy G, Hamilton JA (1992). The interglobular domain of cartilage aggrecan is cleaved by PUMP, gelatinases, and cathepsin B. *J Biol Chem* 267: 19470–19474.

Fridman R, Fuerst TR, Bird RE, Hoyhtya M, Oelkuct M, Kraus S, Komarek D, et al. (1992). Domain structure of human 72-kDa gelatinase/type IV collagenase. Characterization of proteolytic activity and identification of the tissue inhibitor of metalloproteinase-2 (TIMP-2) binding regions. *J Biol Chem* 267: 15398–15405.

Fryns JP, Pedersen JC, Hauglustaine D, Michielsen P, Van den Berghe H (1980). Carpal and tarsal osteolysis. *Ann Genet* 23: 123–125.

Fuchs GA (1991). [Idiopathic multicentric osteolysis and the delimitation of the cranio-carpal-tarsal-osteolysis syndrome]. *Z Orthop Ihre Grenzgeb* 129: 542–548.

Fujimoto T, Parry S, Urbanek M, Sammel M, Macones G, Kuivaniemi H, Romero R, et al. (2002). A single nucleotide polymorphism in the matrix metalloproteinase-1 (MMP-1) promoter influences amnion cell MMP-1 expression and risk for preterm premature rupture of the fetal membranes. *J Biol Chem* 277: 6296–6302.

Gelb BD, Shi GP, Chapman HA, Desnick RJ (1996). Pycnodysostosis, a lysosomal disease caused by cathepsin K deficiency. *Science* 273: 1236–1238.

Ghilardi G, Biondi ML, Mangoni J, Leviti S, DeMonti M, Guagnellini E, Scorza R (2001). Matrix metalloproteinase-1 promoter polymorphism 1G/2G is correlated with colorectal cancer invasiveness. *Clin Cancer Res* 7: 2344–2346.

Goldbach-Mansky R, Lee JM, Hoxworth JM, Smith D, 2nd, Duray P, Schumacher RH Jr, Yarboro CH, et al. (2000). Active synovial matrix metalloproteinase-2 is associated with radiographic erosions in patients with early synovitis. *Arthritis Res* 2: 145–153.

Hardegger F, Simpson LA, Segmueller G (1985). The syndrome of idiopathic osteolysis. Classification, review, and case report. *J Bone Joint Surg Br* 67: 88–93.

Harris ED Jr, Krane SM (1972). An endopeptidase from rheumatoid synovial tissue culture. *Biochim Biophys Acta* 258: 566–576.

Hemingway AP, Leung A, Lavender JP (1983). Familial vanishing limbs: four generations of idiopathic multicentric osteolysis. *Clin Radiol* 34: 585–588.

Hinke V, Seck T, Clanget C, Scheidt-Nave C, Ziegler R, Pfeilschifter J (2001). Association of transforming growth factor-beta1 (TGFbeta1) T29 → C gene polymorphism with bone mineral density (BMD), changes in BMD, and serum concentrations of TGF-beta1 in a population-based sample of postmenopausal german women. *Calcif Tissue Int* 69: 315–320.

Holmbeck K, Bianco P, Caterina J, Yamada S, Kromer M, Kuznetsov SA, Mankani M, et al. (1999). MT1-MMP-deficient mice develop dwarfism, osteopenia, arthritis, and connective tissue disease due to inadequate collagen turnover. *Cell* 99: 81–92.

Hou WS, Bromme D, Zhao Y, Mehler E, Dushey C, Weinstein H, Miranda CS, et al. (1999). Characterization of novel cathepsin K mutations in the pro and mature polypeptide regions causing pycnodysostosis. *J Clin Invest* 103: 731–738.

Imai K, Shikata H, Okada Y (1995). Degradation of vitronectin by matrix metalloproteinases-1, -2, -3, -7 and -9. *FEBS Lett* 369: 249–251.

Itoh T, Ikeda T, Gomi H, Nakao S, Suzuki T, Itohara S (1997). Unaltered secretion of beta-amyloid precursor protein in gelatinase A (matrix metalloproteinase 2)-deficient mice. *J Biol Chem* 272: 22389–22392.

Itoh T, Tanioka M, Yoshida H, Yoshioka T, Nishimoto H, Itohara S (1998). Reduced angiogenesis and tumor progression in gelatinase A-deficient mice. *Cancer Res* 58: 1048–1051.

Itoh T, Tanioka M, Matsuda H, Nishimoto H, Yoshioka T, Suzuki R, Uehira M (1999). Experimental metastasis is suppressed in MMP-9-deficient mice. *Clin Exp Metast* 17: 177–181.

Jackson JBS (1838). A boneless arm. *Boston Med Surg J* 18:368–369.

Janssens K, Gershoni-Baruch R, Guanabens N, Migone N, Ralston S, Bonduelle M, Lissens W, et al. (2000). Mutations in the gene encoding the latency-associated peptide of TGF-beta 1 cause Camurati-Engelmann disease. *Nat Genet* 26: 273–275.

Johansson S, Smedsrod B (1986). Identification of a plasma gelatinase in preparations of fibronectin. *J Biol Chem* 261: 4363–4366.

Jormsjo S, Ye S, Moritz J, Walter DH, Dimmeler S, Zeiher AM, Henney A, et al. (2000). Allele-specific regulation of matrix metalloproteinase-12 gene activity is associated with coronary artery luminal dimensions in diabetic patients with manifest coronary artery disease. *Circ Res* 86: 998–1003.

Kanamori Y, Matsushima M, Minaguchi T, Kobayashi K, Sagae S, Kudo R, Terakawa N, et al. (1999). Correlation between expression of the matrix metalloproteinase-1 gene in ovarian cancers and an insertion/deletion polymorphism in its promoter region. *Cancer Res* 59: 4225–4227.

Kato T, Kure T, Chang JH, Gabison EE, Itoh T, Itohara S, Azar DT (2001). Diminished corneal angiogenesis in gelatinase A-deficient mice. *FEBS Lett* 508: 187–190.

Kim YJ, Park SJ, Park CK, Kim SH, Lee CW (1998). A case of Farber lipogranulomatosis. *J Korean Med Sci* 13: 95–98.

Kingwell BA, Medley TL, Waddell TK, Cole TJ, Dart AM, Jennings GL (2001). Large artery stiffness: structural and genetic aspects. *Clin Exp Pharmacol Physiol* 28:1040–1043.

Kleiner DE, Stetler-Stevenson WG (1999). Matrix metalloproteinases and metastasis. *Cancer Chemother Pharmacol* 43: S42–S51.

Konttinen YT, Ainola M, Valleala H, Ma J, Ida H, Mandelin J, Kinne RW, et al. (1999). Analysis of 16 different matrix metalloproteinases (MMP-1 to MMP20) in the synovial membrane: different profiles in trauma and rheumatoid arthritis. *Ann Rheum Dis* 58: 691–697.

Konttinen YT, Ceponis A, Takagi M, Ainola M, Sorsa T, Sutinen M, Salo T, et al. (1998). New collagenolytic enzymes/cascade identified at the pannus-hard tissue junction in rheumatoid arthritis: destruction from above. *Matrix Biol* 17: 585–601.

Kusano K, Miyaura C, Inada M, Tamura T, Ito A, Nagase H, Kamoi K, et al. (1998). Regulation of matrix metalloproteinases (MMP2, -3, -9, and -13) by interleukin-1 and interleukin-6 in mouse calvaria: association of MMP induction with bone resorption. *Endocrinology* 139: 1338–1345.

Lachman RS (1998). International nomenclature and classification of the osteochondrodysplasias. *Pediatr Radiol* 28: 737–744.

Lazner F, Gowen M, Kola I (1999). An animal model for pycnodysostosis: the role of cathepsin K in bone remodelling. *Mol Med Today* 5: 413–414.

Leco KJ, Waterhouse P, Sanchez OH, Gowing KL, Poole AR, Wakeham A, Mak TW, et al. (2001). Spontaneous air space enlargement in the lungs of mice lacking tissue inhibitor of metalloproteinases-3 (TIMP-3). *J Clin Invest* 108: 817–829.

Lehti K, Lohi J, Valtanen H, Keski-Oja J (1998). Proteolytic processing of membrane-type-1 matrix metalloproteinase is associated with gelatinase A activation at the cell surface. *Biochem J* 334: 345–353.

Lelongt B, Bengatta S, Delauche M, Lund LR, Werb Z, Ronco PM (2001). Matrix metalloproteinase 9 protects mice from anti-glomerular basement membrane nephritis through its fibrinolytic activity. *J Exp Med* 193: 793–802.

Lewkonia RM, Pope FM (1985). Joint contractures and acroosteolysis in Ehlers-Danlos syndrome type IV. *J Rheumatol* 12: 140–144.

Lijnen HR, Soloway P, Collen D (1999). Tissue inhibitor of matrix metalloproteinases-1 impairs arterial neointima formation after vascular injury in mice. *Circ Res* 85: 1186–1191.

Lijnen HR, Van HB, Frederix L, Rio MC, Collen D (2002). Adipocyte hypertrophy in stromelysin-3 deficient mice with nutritionally induced obesity. *Thromb Haemost* 87: 530–535.

Liu Z, Shipley JM, Vu TH, Zhou X, Diaz LA, Werb Z, Senior RM (1998). Gelatinase B-deficient mice are resistant to experimental bullous pemphigoid. *J Exp Med* 188: 475–482.

Madlener M, Parks WC, Werner S (1998). Matrix metalloproteinases (MMPs) and their physiological inhibitors (TIMPs) are differentially expressed during excisional skin wound repair. *Exp Cell Res* 242: 201–210.

Martignetti JA, Aqeel AA, Sewairi WA, Boumah CE, Kambouris M, Mayouf SA, Sheth KV, et al. (2001). Mutation of the matrix metalloproteinase 2 gene (MMP2) causes a multicentric osteolysis and arthritis syndrome. *Nat Genet* 28: 261–265.

Massova I, Kotra LP, Fridman R, Mobashery S (1998). Matrix metalloproteinases: structures, evolution, and diversification. *FASEB J* 12: 1075–1095.

Matthiesen G, Pedersen VF, Helin P, Jacobsen GK, Nielsen NS (2001). Winchester syndrome. *Int Orthop* 25: 331–333.

McCawley LJ, Matrisian LM (2001). Matrix metalloproteinases: they're not just for matrix anymore! *Curr Opin Cell Biol* 13: 534–540.

McQuibban GA, Gong JH, Tam EM, McCulloch CA, Clark-Lewis I, Overall CM (2000). Inflammation dampened by gelatinase A cleavage of monocyte chemoattractant protein-3. *Science* 289: 1202–1206.

Mohan R, Chintala SK, Jung JC, Villar WV, McCabe F, Russo LA, Lee Y, et al. (2002). Matrix metalloproteinase gelatinase B (MMP-9) coordinates and effects epithelial regeneration. *J Biol Chem* 277: 2065–2072.

Morgunova E, Tuuttila A, Bergmann U, Isupov M, Lindqvist Y, Schneider G, Tryggvason K (1999). Structure of human pro-matrix metalloproteinase-2: activation mechanism revealed. *Science* 284: 1667–1670.

Murphy G, Crabbe T (1995). Gelatinases A and B. *Methods Enzymol* 248: 470–484.

Murphy G, Cawston TE, Galloway WA, Barnes MJ, Bunning RA, Mercer E, Reynolds JJ, et al. (1981). Metalloproteinases from rabbit bone culture medium degrade types IV and V collagens, laminin and fibronectin. *Biochem J* 199: 807–811.

Murphy G, Nguyen Q, Cockett MI, Atkinson SJ, Allan JA, Knight CG, Willenbrock F, et al. (1994). Assessment of the role of the fibronectin-like domain of gelatinase A by analysis of a deletion mutant. *J Biol Chem* 269: 6632–6636.

Nishioka Y, Kobayashi K, Sagae S, Ishioka S, Nishikawa A, Matsushima M, Kanamori Y, et al. (2000). A single nucleotide polymorphism in the matrix metalloproteinase-1 promoter in endometrial carcinomas. *Jpn J Cancer Res* 91: 612–615.

Ohnishi K, Takagi M, Kurokawa Y, Satomi S, Konttinen YT (1998). Matrix metalloproteinase-mediated extracellular matrix protein degradation in human pulmonary emphysema. *Lab Invest* 78: 1077–1087.

Okada Y, Katsuda S, Nakanishi I (1993). An elastinolytic enzyme detected in the culture medium of human arterial smooth muscle cells. *Cell Biol Int* 17: 863–869.

Overall CM, Wrana JL, Sodek J (1991). Transcriptional and post-transcriptional regulation of 72-kDa gelatinase/type IV collagenase by transforming growth factor-beta 1 in human fibroblasts. Comparisons with collagenase and tissue inhibitor of matrix metalloproteinase gene expression. *J Biol Chem* 266: 14064–14071.

Parks WC (1999). Matrix metalloproteinases in repair. *Wound Repair Regen* 7: 423–432.

Petit P, Fryns JP (1986). Distal osteolysis, short stature, mental retardation, and characteristic facial appearance: delineation of an autosomal recessive subtype of essential osteolysis. *Am J Med Genet* 25: 537–541.

Pilcher BK, Wang M, Qin XJ, Parks WC, Senior RM, Welgus HG (1999). Role of matrix metalloproteinases and their inhibition in cutaneous wound healing and allergic contact hypersensitivity. *Ann N Y Acad Sci* 878: 12–24.

Prapanpoch S, Jorgenson RJ, Langlais RP, Nummikoski PV (1992). Winchester syndrome. A case report and literature review. *Oral Surg Oral Med Oral Pathol* 74: 671–677.

Preaux AM, Mallat A, Nhieu JT, D'Ortho MP, Hembry RM, Mavier P (1999). Matrix metalloproteinase-2 activation in human hepatic fibrosis regulation by cell-matrix interactions. *Hepatology* 30: 944–950.

Prescott MF, Sawyer WK, Von Linden-Reed J, Jeune M, Chou M, Caplan SL, Jeng AY (1999). Effect of matrix metalloproteinase inhibition on progression of atherosclerosis and aneurysm in LDL receptor-deficient mice overexpressing MMP-3, MMP-12, and MMP-13 and on restenosis in rats after balloon injury. *Ann N Y Acad Sci* 878: 179–190.

Pyo R, Lee JK, Shipley JM, Curci JA, Mao D, Ziporin SJ, Ennis TL, et al. (2000). Targeted gene disruption of matrix metalloproteinase-9 (gelatinase B) suppresses development of experimental abdominal aortic aneurysms. *J Clin Invest* 105: 1641–1649.

Raat H, De Witte B, Lateur L (1994). Idiopathic multicentric osteolysis. *J Belge Radiol* 77: 220.

Rice DP, Kim HJ, Thesleff I (1997). Detection of gelatinase B expression reveals osteoclastic bone resorption as a feature of early calvarial bone development. *Bone* 21: 479–486.

Rizzo R, Sorge G, Denaro V, Carpinato C, Tine A (1993). Idiopathic multicentric osteolysis: family report and review of the literature. *Clin Dysmorphol* 2: 251–256.

Roten L, Nemoto S, Simsic J, Coker ML, Rao V, Baicu S, Defreyte G, et al. (2000). Effects of gene deletion of the tissue inhibitor of the matrix metalloproteinase-type1 (TIMP-1) on left ventricular geometry and function in mice. *J Mol Cell Cardiol* 32: 109–120.

Sang QX (1998). Complex role of matrix metalloproteinases in angiogenesis. *Cell Res* 8: 171–177.

Schnaper HW, Grant DS, Stetler-Stevenson WG, Fridman R, D'Orazi G, Murphy AN, Bird RE, et al. (1993). Type IV collagenase(s) and TIMPs modulate endothelial cell morphogenesis in vitro. *J Cell Physiol* 156: 235–246.

Schonbeck U, Mach F, Libby P (1998). Generation of biologically active IL-1 beta by matrix metalloproteinases: a novel caspase-1-independent pathway of IL-1 beta processing. *J Immunol* 161: 3340–3346.

Shofuda K, Moriyama K, Nishihashi A, Higashi S, Mizushima H, Yasumitsu H, Miki K, et al. (1998). Role of tissue inhibitor of metalloproteinases-2 (TIMP-2) in regulation of pro-gelatinase A activation catalyzed by membrane-type matrix metalloproteinase-1 (MT1-MMP) in human cancer cells. *J Biochem (Tokyo)* 124: 462–470.

Shubayev VI, Myers RR (2002). Endoneurial remodeling by TNFalph- and TNFalpha-releasing proteases. A spatial and temporal co-localization study in painful neuropathy. *J Peripher Nerv Syst* 7: 28–36.

Silence J, Collen D, Lijnen HR (2002). Reduced atherosclerotic plaque but enhanced aneurysm formation in mice with inactivation of the tissue inhibitor of metalloproteinase-1 (TIMP-1) gene. *Circ Res* 90: 897–903.

Sternlicht MD, Werb Z (2001). How matrix metalloproteinases regulate cell behavior. *Annu Rev Cell Dev Biol* 17: 463–516.

Stetler-Stevenson WG (2001). The role of matrix metalloproteinases in tumor invasion, metastasis, and angiogenesis. *Surg Oncol Clin N Am* 10: 383–392, x.

Strongin AY, Collier I, Bannikov G, Marmer BL, Grant GA, Goldberg GI (1995). Mechanism of cell surface activation of 72-kDa type IV collagenase. Isolation of the activated form of the membrane metalloprotease. *J Biol Chem* 270: 5331–5338.

Takei I, Takagi M, Santavirta S, Ida H, Ishii M, Ogino T, Ainola M, et al. (2000). Messenger ribonucleic acid expression of 16 matrix metalloproteinases in bone-implant interface tissues of loose artificial hip joints. *J Biomed Mater Res* 52: 613–620.

Teebi AS, Elliott AM, Azouz EM, Lachman RS (2001). Progressive erosive arthropathy with contractures, multicentric osteolysis-like changes, characteristic craniofacial appearance, and dermatological abnormalities: A new syndrome? *Am J Med Genet* 100: 198–203.

Terashima M, Akita H, Kanazawa K, Inoue N, Yamada S, Ito K, Matsuda Y, et al. (1999). Stromelysin promoter 5A/6A polymorphism is associated with acute myocardial infarction. *Circulation* 99: 2717–2719.

Thur J, Rosenberg K, Nitsche DP, Pihlajamaa T, Ala-Kokko L, Heinegard D, Paulsson M, et al. (2001). Mutations in cartilage oligomeric matrix protein causing pseudoachondroplasia and multiple epiphyseal dysplasia affect binding of calcium and collagen I, II, and IX. *J Biol Chem* 276: 6083–6092.

Torg JS, Steel HH (1968). Essential osteolysis with nephropathy. A review of the literature and case report of an unusual syndrome. *J Bone Joint Surg Am* 50: 1629–1638.

Torg JS, DiGeorge AM, Kirkpatrick JA Jr, Trujillo MM (1969). Hereditary multicentric osteolysis with recessive transmission: a new syndrome. *J Pediatr* 75: 243–252.

Tsipouras P, Byers PH, Schwartz RC, Chu ML, Weil D, Pepe G, Cassidy SB, et al. (1986). Ehlers-Danlos syndrome type IV: cosegregation of the phenotype to a COL3A1 allele of type III procollagen. *Hum Genet* 74: 41–46.

Tyler T, Rosenbaum HD (1976). Idiopathic multicentric osteolysis. *AJR Am J Roentgenol* 126: 23–31.

van Meurs J, van Lent P, Stoop R, Holthuysen A, Singer I, Bayne E, Mudgett J, et al. (1999). Cleavage of aggrecan at the Asn341-Phe342 site coincides with the initiation of collagen damage in murine antigen-induced arthritis: a pivotal role for stromelysin 1 in matrix metalloproteinase activity. *Arthritis Rheum* 42: 2074–2084.

Van Wart HE, Birkedal-Hansen H (1990). The cysteine switch: a principle of regulation of metalloproteinase activity with potential applicability to the entire matrix metalloproteinase gene family. *Proc Natl Acad Sci U S A* 87: 5578–5582.

Vasku V, Vasku A, Tschoplova S, Izakovicova Holla L, Semradova V, Vacha J (2002). Genotype association of C(-735)T polymorphism in matrix metalloproteinase 2 gene with G(8002)A endothelin 1 gene with plaque psoriasis. *Dermatology* 204: 262–265.

Vu TH (2001). Don't mess with the matrix. *Nat Genet* 28: 202–203.

Vu TH, Shipley JM, Bergers G, Berger JE, Helms JA, Hanahan D, Shapiro SD, et al. (1998). MMP-9/gelatinase B is a key regulator of growth plate angiogenesis and apoptosis of hypertrophic chondrocytes. *Cell* 93: 411–422.

Wang J, Warzecha D, Wilcken D, Wang XL (2001). Polymorphism in the gelatinase B gene and the severity of coronary arterial stenosis. *Clin Sci (Lond)* 101: 87–92.

Wang X, Jung J, Asahi M, Chwang W, Russo L, Moskowitz MA, Dixon CE, et al. (2000). Effects of matrix metalloproteinase-9 gene knock-out on morphological and motor outcomes after traumatic brain injury. *J Neurosci* 20: 7037–7042.

Warner RL, Beltran L, Younkin EM, Lewis CS, Weiss SJ, Varani J, Johnson KJ (2001). Role of stromelysin 1 and gelatinase B in experimental acute lung injury. *Am J Respir Cell Mol Biol* 24: 537–544.

Weber BH, Vogt G, Pruett RC, Stohr H, Felbor U (1994). Mutations in the tissue inhibitor of metalloproteinases-3 (TIMP3) in patients with Sorsby's fundus dystrophy. *Nat Genet* 8: 235–236.

Werb Z, Chin JR (1998). Extracellular matrix remodeling during morphogenesis. *Ann N Y Acad Sci* 857: 110–118.

Whitelock JM, Paine ML, Gibbins JR, Kefford RF, O'Grady RL (1993). Multiple levels of post-transcriptional regulation of collagenase (matrix metalloproteinase 1) in an epithelial cell line. *Immunol Cell Biol* 71: 39–47.

Whyte MP, Murphy WA, Kleerekoper M, Teitelbaum SL, Avioli LV (1978). Idiopathic multicentric osteolysis. Report of an affected father and son. *Arthritis Rheum* 21: 367–376.

Wihlborg C, Babyn P, Ranson M, Laxer R (2001). Radiologic mimics of juvenile rheumatoid arthritis. *Pediatr Radiol* 31: 315–326.

Wilson CL, Heppner KJ, Labosky PA, Hogan BL, Matrisian LM (1997). Intestinal tumorigenesis is suppressed in mice lacking the metalloproteinase matrilysin. *Proc Natl Acad Sci U S A* 94: 1402–1407.

Woessner JF (2000). *Matrix Metalloproteinases and TIMPs*. Oxford University Press, New York.

Wu W, Mwale F, Tchetina E, Kojima T, Yasuda T, Poole AR (2001). Cartilage matrix resorption in skeletogenesis. *Novartis Found Symp* 232: 158–166.

Ye S, Eriksson P, Hamsten A, Kurkinen M, Humphries SE, Henney AM (1996). Progression of coronary atherosclerosis is associated with a common genetic variant of the human stromelysin-1 promoter which results in reduced gene expression. *J Biol Chem* 271: 13055–13060.

Yoneda T, Sasaki A, Dunstan C, Williams PJ, Bauss F, De Clerck YA, Mundy GR (1997). Inhibition of osteolytic bone metastasis of breast cancer by combined treatment with the bisphosphonate ibandronate and tissue inhibitor of the matrix metalloproteinase-2. *J Clin Invest* 99: 2509–2517.

Yoshihara Y, Nakamura H, Obata K, Yamada H, Hayakawa T, Fujikawa K, Okada Y (2000). Matrix metalloproteinases and tissue inhibitors of metalloproteinases in synovial fluids from patients with rheumatoid arthritis or osteoarthritis. *Ann Rheum Dis* 59: 455–461.

Yu Q, Stamenkovic I (2000). Cell surface-localized matrix metalloproteinase-9 proteolytically activates TGF-beta and promotes tumor invasion and angiogenesis. *Genes Dev* 14: 163–176.

Zhang B, Dhillon S, Geary I, Howell WM, Iannotti F, Day IN, Ye S (2001). Polymorphisms in matrix metalloproteinase-1, -3, -9, and -12 genes in relation to subarachnoid hemorrhage. *Stroke* 32: 2198–2202.

Zhou Z, Apte SS, Soininen R, Cao R, Baaklini GY, Rauser RW, Wang J, et al. (2000). Impaired endochondral ossification and angiogenesis in mice deficient in membrane-type matrix metalloproteinase I. *Proc Natl Acad Sci U S A* 97: 4052–4057.

Zhu Y, Spitz MR, Lei L, Mills GB, Wu X (2001). A single nucleotide polymorphism in the matrix metalloproteinase-1 promoter enhances lung cancer susceptibility. *Cancer Res* 61: 7825–7829.

Part H.
Angiogenesis

101 | Angiopoietins, TIEs, Ephrins, Vascular Endothelial Growth Factors, and Vascular Endothelial Growth Factor Receptors

MIIKKA VIKKULA, MARIKA J. KARKKAINEN, AND KARI ALITALO

Development of the vascular and lymphatic networks is pivotal already early in embryogenesis. Angiogenesis is also implicated in wound healing and tumor growth. As vessels develop, they acquire tissue-specific phenotypes. This complex morphogenetic differentiation process is regulated by a plethora of molecules, among which receptors expressed in differentiating and mature vascular endothelial cells (ECs) and their ligands, often expressed by adjacent cells, are especially important. In this chapter, we summarize the three most important signaling pathways for vascular morphogenesis: vascular endothelial growth factors (VEGFs) and their receptors (VEGFRs), angiopoietins (Angpts) and their receptors, *T*yrosine kinases with *I*g and *EGF* homology domains (TIEs), and ephrins and their Eph receptors. The roles of VEGFR-3 and TIE2 in vascular phenotypes caused by inherited mutations in humans are also discussed. We start with a short review on vasculogenesis, angiogenesis, and development of the lymphatic vessels.

FORMATION OF THE VASCULAR AND LYMPHATIC NETWORKS

The blood vasculature forms in a coordinated manner through a combination of vasculogenesis and angiogenesis, and supports the growth of the developing embryo. In the yolk sac, the mesoderm-derived pre-

cursors, hemangioblasts, form blood islands and give rise to both endothelial and hematopoietic lineages (Fig. 101–1). The ECs proliferate, differentiate, and assemble to form the early vascular plexus, in a process termed *vasculogenesis* (Flamme et al., 1997). In addition to the extraembryonic formation of the vasculature, hematopoiesis and vasculogenesis take place intraembryonically, and the blood vessels differentiating in the embryo are connected to the yolk sac by vitelline vessels. After the development of the primary vascular plexus, the mature vasculature forms by sprouting and remodeling from preexisting vessels, in a process called *angiogenesis* (Risau, 1997).

Angiogenic sprouting requires programmed proteolytic activity to selectively dissolve the extracellular matrix (ECM). The basement membrane and ECM are degraded by cooperation between adhesive and proteolytic mechanisms (reviewed in Werb, 1997). For example, the plasminogen–plasmin system and matrix metalloproteinases are involved in the breakdown of many ECM and basement membrane proteins. Migration of ECs is also facilitated by integrins, which are ECM receptors with distinct cellular and adhesive specificities. Sprouting EC tubes fuse and coalesce into loops, allowing blood circulation in the newly vascularized region.

In addition to sprouting angiogenesis, the mature vascular network develops via nonsprouting angiogenesis. New vessels can split into individual daughter vessels through the formation of transendothelial

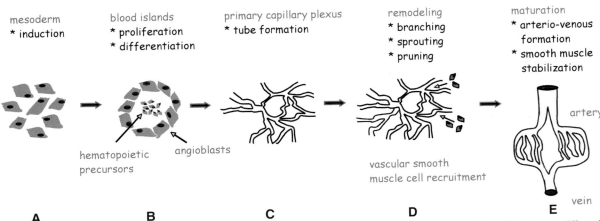

Figure 101–1. Vasculogenesis and angiogenesis. Endothelial and hematopoietic cells are derived from a common precursor, the hemangioblast (*A*). The hemangioblasts aggregate and the cells in the interior of the cell clusters become hematopoietic cells, whereas the cells in the periphery differentiate into primi-tive endothelial cells, angioblasts (*B*). Via proliferation and differentiation, a primary capillary plexus is formed (*C*). Modification leads to vessels with variable size and structure (*D*), which, with the concomitant recruitment of vascular smooth muscular cells leads to development of the mature vasculature (*E*).

cell bridges or through intussusception, whereby the daughter vessels form via insertion of interstitial tissue columns into the lumen of pre-existing vessels (Risau, 1997; Djonov et al., 2000; Conway et al., 2001). In the course of maturation, the newly formed vessels are supported by a basement membrane and a pericyte layer, and thus become less vulnerable to vessel regression (Benjamin et al., 1998). The ECs themselves also secrete growth factors, such as platelet-derived growth factor-B, which are important in the recruitment of the supporting pericytes. The mature vasculature consists of a complex organized network assembled into arteries, capillaries, and veins with variation in mural structure and other properties, such as EC phenotype.

It has also been suggested that circulating endothelial precursor cells participate in angiogenesis in adults (Shi et al., 1998). These cells are immobilized after vascular trauma, possibly due to the elevated circulating levels of VEGF, further supporting the idea that the endothelial precursors are also involved in neo-angiogenesis (Takahashi et al., 1999; Gill et al., 2001). Findings also suggest that a population of VEGFR-2–positive cells may give rise to cells of both EC and smooth muscle cell lineages (Yamashita et al., 2000).

The pivotal molecules in the formation of the vascular system are the VEGFs, Angpts, ephrins, and their receptors. Studies using transgenic technology have shown that the early steps of vascular morphogenesis, comprising EC differentiation, blood island formation and organization, formation of the primitive vascular plexus, and developmental angiogenesis, are all dependent on VEGF signaling often in collaboration with the Angpt/TIE signaling pathway. In addition, ephrin signaling has been shown to be crucial for the formation of vascular identity (Wang et al., 1998).

The circulatory system, formed by the heart and blood vessels, requires the adjacent lymphatic system to collect extravasated protein-rich fluid and lymphocytes from the tissues, and to transport them back to the blood circulation. These two systems communicate with each other and are intimately associated during development. The development of the cardiovascular system precedes the development of the lymphatic system. One theory postulates that the fetal lymphatic sacs are formed from the large central veins in the jugular and perimesonephric regions (Sabin, 1902, 1912). The lymphatic vessels then arise from these sacs by sprouting toward the peripheral regions. All lymphatic vessel links to the venous system are disconnected, except for the region of the left thoracic duct that drains the lymph into the subclavian vein.

In contrast to sprouting from pre-existing veins, another theory suggests that the lymphatic vessels develop via in situ differentiation from mesenchymal cells in different tissues (Huntington and McClure, 1908; Kampmeier, 1912) or by a combination of sprouting and in situ formation (van der Jagt, 1932). It has been shown that mesodermal lymphangioblasts participate in the development of the avian lymphatic system, supporting the theory that the peripheral lymphatic vessels develop via multiple mechanisms (Schneider et al., 1999; Wilting et al., 2000a, 2000b). Whether these lymphangioblasts also participate in lymphangiogenesis in adults is unknown.

RECEPTOR TYROSINE KINASES

Targeted EC signaling is achieved by specific receptor tyrosine kinases (RTKs), which mediate growth factor signals from the extracellular space to the cytosol and finally to the nucleus of the target cell. RTKs are classified into subclasses based on sequence similarities and distinct structural characteristics (van der Geer et al., 1994). X-ray crystallographic studies of the unphosphorylated RTKs have revealed molecular mechanisms by which RTKs are kept in an unphosphorylated state (review in Hubbard et al., 1998). The activation loop of the kinase seems to be autoinhibitory in a monomeric receptor, preventing ligand-independent phosphorylation. The juxtamembrane domain also seems to have an important role in inhibition of RTK autophosphorylation (Huse et al., 2001; Wybenga-Groot et al., 2001).

Most known ligands for RTKs are secreted soluble proteins. In the case of VEGFs, the dimeric ligand binds to the extracellular part of the receptor, resulting in a symmetric receptor dimer (Wiesmann et al., 1997). Dimerization is followed by transphosphorylation of the tyrosine residues in the activation loop, which stabilizes an active state of the kinase via a conformation favorable for catalysis (Hubbard et al., 1998; Schlessinger, 2000). Receptor phosphorylation generates docking sites for downstream signaling proteins. The phosphorylated tyrosine residues and their adjacent sequences act as specific activation sites for downstream signaling proteins containing the Src homology 2 (SH2) or phosphotyrosine-binding domains. Further activation of multiple signal transduction cascades eventually leads to biochemical changes in the cell, such as readjustment of gene expression.

VEGFs

VEGF family contains five mammalian members, VEGF, VEGF-B, VEGF-C, VEGF-D and placental growth factor (PlGF). VEGFs and their receptors are critical regulators of both angiogenesis and lymphangiogenesis (Table 101–1) (review in Veikkola et al., 2000). VEGFs share a common VEGF homology domain with eight conserved cysteine residues and they all are secreted glycoproteins that form either disulfide-linked or noncovalently bound dimers, whose subunits are arranged in an antiparallel manner (Muller et al., 1997). Although VEGFs structurally form a unified family, they differ in their expres-

Table 101–1. Summary of the Biological Roles of VEGFs, VEGFRs, TIEs, and Angiopoietins

Gene	Phenotype in Gene-Deficient Mice and in Human (*) Disorder	Lethal	Biological Role
VEGF	Defective blood vessel and blood island development (Carmeliet et al., 1996; Ferrara et al., 1996)	−/− E8–9 +/− E11–12	Vasculogenesis, developmental and pathological angiogenesis
VEGF-B	Normal heart development (Aase et al., 2001) or Defective heart development (Bellomo et al., 2000)	Viable	Modulates biological activity of VEGF (?)
PlGF	Normal vascular development (Carmeliet et al., 2001)	Viable	Pathological angiogenesis, amplifies responsiveness to VEGF
VEGF-C	Failure in lymphatic vascular development (Karkkainen et al., submitted)	During the fetal period	Lymphangiogenesis
VEGF-D	?	?	Lymphangiogenesis (?)
VEGFR-1	Disorganization of vascular system, increased number of endothelial precursors (Fong et al., 1995, 1999)	E8.5	Negative regulator of VEGF-mediated angiogenesis (?) Monocyte recruitment
VEGFR-2	No mature endothelial or hematopoietic cells (Shalaby et al., 1995)	E8.5–9.5	Hemangioblast differentiation, proliferation, and migration, vascular permeability
VEGFR-3 (*)	Pericardial effusion, defective large blood vessels, congenital lymphedema (Dumont et al., 1998; Irrthum et al., 2000; Karkkainen et al., 2000)	E9.5–10.5	Vascular remodeling, migration and survival of lymphatic ECs
NRP-1	Anomalies in cardiovascular system and efferent nerve fibers (Kitsukawa et al., 1995; Kawasaki et al., 1999)	E12.5	Axon guidance in PNS, cardiovascular development, enhances effect of $VEGF_{165}$
NRP-2	Defects in the development of central and peripheral nerves (Chen et al., 2000; Giger et al., 2000)	Viable	Axon guidance
ANGPT-1	Fewer branches, homogeneously sized vessels, defects in endocardium and myocardium (Suri et al., 1996)	E12.5	Recruitment of perivascular cells, vessel stabilization
TIE-1	Defective angiogenic expansion and integrity of blood vessels (Puri et al., 1995; Sato et al., 1995)	E10.5	Vascular network formation, survival of ECs
TIE-2 (*)	Defects in maturation and organization of blood vessels, mucocutaneous venous malformation (Sato et al., 1995; Vikkula et al., 1996)	E10.5	Recruitment of perivascular cells, vessel stabilization

sion patterns, receptor specificities, and biological activities (Table 101–1, Fig. 101–2).

VEGF

The parent molecule VEGF has been shown to be a potent mitogen of ECs and to induce migration *in vitro* (Ferrara et al., 1992). The crusial function of VEGF during embryogenesis has also been implicated, as inactivation of even a single *Vegf* allele resulted in lethality of murine embryos between embryonic days (E) 11 and 12. The *Vegf*+/− embryos were growth retarded and exhibited a number of developmental anomalies due to impaired formation of blood islands and decreased sprouting (Carmeliet et al., 1996; Ferrara et al., 1996). This was the first case in which the loss of a single allele is lethal.

VEGF gene is differentially spliced to produce several mRNA species, encoding putative proteins of 121, 145, 165, 189, and 206 amino acids (Leung et al., 1989; Houck et al., 1992; Poltorak et al., 1997). VEGF165 and VEGF121 appear to be the most abundant forms *in vivo*. The bioavailability of VEGFs is regulated by the differential affinities of the isoforms to the heparan sulfate proteoglycans. VEGF121 is non-heparin-binding protein that is freely secreted into the interstitial space, whereas VEGF165 is both found in the interstitial space and associated with the extracellular matrix. The longer forms, VEGF189 and VEGF206, have highly basic, heparin-binding C-terminal tails and are sequestered on the extracellular matrix (Park et al., 1993).

The biological functions of the various VEGF isoforms have been studied by using genetically engineered mice. Interestingly, mice with targeted deletion of two murine Vegf isoforms, Vegf164 and Vegf188, have impaired myocardial angiogenesis rather than vascular deregulation, resulting in ischemic cardiomyopathy (Carmeliet et al., 1999). This suggests that specific isoforms are required for an optimal angiogenic response *in vivo* and that this is likely to depend on the tissue type. The biological functions of different VEGF isoforms were also underscored by observations of retinal angiogenesis in mice expressing only specific Vegf isoforms. Vegf (164/164) mice had normal retinal angiogenesis, whereas the Vegf(120/120) mice exhibited severe defects in vascular outgrowth and patterning. Moreover, Vegf(188/188) mice displayed normal

venular outgrowth but impaired arterial development (Stalmans et al., 2002).

In addition to physiological angiogenesis, VEGF has a crucial role in the pathogenesis of several disorders, including cancer and diabetic retinopathy. VEGF levels are highly upregulated by hypoxia, leading to increased angiogenesis (Shweiki, et al., 1992). In addition, VEGF induces vascular permeability via its VEGFR-2 receptor, which may also contribute to tumor induced angiogenesis and growth. Increased number of blood vessels have been implicated in increased metastasis rate and poor prognosis of the patients in several cancer types. Thus, several studies are now focusing on the mechanisms by which VEGF function could be blocked in various disease conditions (Review in Ferrara et al., 2002).

VEGF-B

VEGF-B resembles PlGF in several aspects: both have two currently known splice isoforms and both bind selectively VEGFR-1 (Olofsson et al., 1996) (Fig. 101–2). Of the splice isoforms, VEGF-B167 remains cell associated via C-terminal basic sequences. On the other hand, VEGF-B186 lacking the highly basic region is *O*-glycosylated and freely secreted from cells. Both forms of VEGF-B are produced as disulfide-linked homodimers, but they can also form heterodimers with VEGF (Olofsson et al., 1996). The VEGF-B167 isoform is predominantly expressed in tissues, accounting for more than 80% of the total VEGF-B transcripts, whereas the VEGF-B186 isoform is expressed at lower levels and only in a limited number of tissues (Li et al., 2001). The VEGF-B186 isoform is also involved in tumor-induced angiogenesis, because it is up-regulated in murine and human tumor cell lines and primary tumors.

VEGF-B is a mitogen for ECs. VEGF-B–containing conditioned medium was able to stimulate thymidine incorporation into DNA in human umbilical vein ECs and bovine capillary ECs (Olofsson et al., 1996). However, so far this has not been reproduced using recombinant VEGF-B, suggesting that the activity could be due to VEGF-B/VEGF heterodimers in transfected cells (Olofsson et al., 1996). In addition to binding to VEGFR1, VEGF-B binds to NRP-1 (Makinen et al., 1999). VEGF-B is particularly abundant in the heart and skeletal muscle. In contrast to Vegf-deficient mice, *Vegfb*−/− mice are vi-

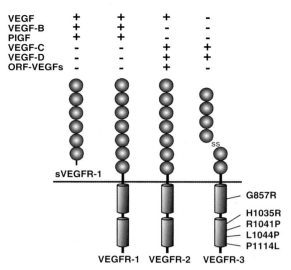

Figure 101–2. Binding specificity of vascular endothelial growth factor (VEGF) family members to the VEGF receptors (VEGFRs). Five amino acid substitutions causing congenital hereditary lymphedema are marked next to the kinase domain of VEGFR-3. PlGF, placental growth factor; ORF, open reading frame. (From Terman et al., 1992; De Vries et al., 1992; Park et al., 1994; Joukov et al., 1996; Achen et al., 1998; Ogawa et al., 1998; Olofsson et al., 1998; Meyer et al., 1999; Wise et al., 1999). Ball = Ig homology domain; box = kinase domain.

able and fertile, but their hearts are smaller and their recovery from induced myocardial ischemia is impaired (Bellomo et al., 2000; Aase et al., 2001).

VEGF-C and VEGF-D

VEGF-C and VEGF-D are the two VEGF family members that are thought to mainly stimulate lymphangiogenesis *in vivo*. The biological functions of VEGF-C and -D are mediated through VEGFR-2 and VEGFR-3. Unlike other VEGFs, VEGF-C and VEGF-D have N- and C-terminal extensions, and they are proteolytically cleaved on secretion (Joukov et al., 1997; Stacker et al., 1999). The cleavage is an important regulator of receptor binding and biological activity because only the fully processed forms of these growth factors can bind to VEGFR-2. This binding may explain the conditional angiogenic potential of VEGF-C and VEGF-D (Cao et al., 1998; Marconcini et al., 1999). The VEGF-C–induced blood vessel permeability is also mediated via VEGFR-2 (Joukov et al., 1998). Interestingly, mouse VEGF-D does not bind mouse VEGFR-2, suggesting that the biological functions of VEGF-D differ in mouse and humans and that VEGF-D interaction with VEGFR-2 is not crucial for normal development (Baldwin et al., 2001).

VEGF-C and -D signaling through VEGFR-3 is a key regulator of lymphangiogenesis (Joukov et al., 1996; Lee et al., 1996; Orlandini et al., 1996; Yamada et al., 1997; Achen et al., 1998). During development, the distribution of the *VEGFR-3* mRNA follows a somewhat similar spatiotemporal pattern to VEGF-C expression, suggesting paracrine ligand–receptor signaling (Kukk et al., 1996). Although VEGF-C and VEGF-D show different expression patterns during embryogenesis, it is possible that they compensate for each other at sites of overlapping expression, such as in the lung and in the kidney mesenchyme (Kukk et al., 1996; Avantaggiato et al., 1998). Both VEGF-C and VEGF-D are lymphangiogenic. VEGF-C is mitogenic toward lymphatic ECs and shows a selective lymphangiogenic response in differentiated avian chorioallantoic membrane (Oh et al., 1997). Accordingly, overexpression of VEGF-C in transgenic mice induces the development of a hyperplastic lymphatic vessel network (Jeltsch et al., 1997; Mandriota et al., 2001). Data also show that VEGF-D and a VEGF-3–specific mutant of VEGF-C (VEGF-C156S) are lymphangiogenic when overexpressed in the skin of transgenic mice (Joukov et al., 1998; Veikkola et al., 2001). Conversely, inhibition of lymphatic growth is obtained when a soluble form of VEGFR-3 is expressed in a similar transgenic mouse model (Makinen et al., 2001).

These results and the expression patterns of VEGF-C and VEGFR-3 suggest that lymphatic growth is induced by VEGF-C and VEGF-D and mediated via VEGFR-3.

VEGF-E

A VEGF121 homologue has been found to be encoded by the Orf virus. The parapox orf virus induces skin lesions characterized by massive capillary proliferation and dilation (Groves et al., 1991; Lyttle et al., 1994). Viral ORF-VEGF (VEGF-E) is a dimer that is able to bind and activate only VEGFR-2, and similar to VEGF121, it does not contain the heparin-binding domain (Ogawa et al., 1998; Meyer et al., 1999). VEGF and ORF-VEGFs have remarkably similar bioactivities because they both can induce EC proliferation, migration and sprouting in vitro, and angiogenesis in vivo (Meyer et al., 1999).

VEGF RECEPTORS

VEGFR-1 and VEGFR-2 in Vasculogenesis and Angiogenesis

Two receptor families, VEGFRs and neuropilins (NRPs), have been found to bind VEGFs. VEGFRs are expressed predominantly on the surface of ECs. The three known members of this family (VEGF-1 through -3) all contain seven extracellular Ig-homology domains, except for VEGFR3 for which one is cleaved, but bridged by a disulphide bond (Shibuya et al., 1990; Matthews et al., 1991; Terman et al., 1991; Pajusola et al., 1992; Galland et al., 1993; Fig. 101–2). The second and third Ig-homology domains are necessary for ligand binding and specificity (Davis-Smyth et al., 1996; Wiesmann et al., 1997; Fuh et al., 1998; Makinen et al., 2001). The intracellular catalytic kinase domain of VEGFRs is split by a kinase insert.

VEGFR-2 (KDR/Flk1) is a key marker of hemangioblasts and angioblasts, but its expression is down-regulated in hematopoietic cells. The crucial role of VEGFR-2 for normal vasculogenesis has been shown, as $Vegfr2^{-/-}$ embryos fail to develop blood islands and embryonic vasculature and die in utero between E8.5 to E9.5 (Shalaby et al., 1995). Furthermore, analysis of chimeric mice showed that *Vegfr2* is required cell autonomously for both extraembryonic and intraembryonic EC development and hematopoiesis (Shalaby et al., 1995). The interaction of VEGF with VEGFR-2 seems to be a critical requirement for the full spectrum of VEGF-induced biological responses. Receptor-selective VEGF mutants, which bind only to VEGFR-2, are fully active EC mitogens, whereas the mutants binding only to the VEGFR-1 have a substantially reduced ability to promote EC growth (Keyt et al., 1996). In addition, the virus-encoded ORF-VEGFs bind to VEGFR-2 but not to VEGFR-1 and are capable of inducing EC proliferation, migration, and permeability (Ogawa et al., 1998; Meyer et al., 1999; Wise et al., 1999). EC survival is also mediated via VEGFR-2 (Gerber et al., 1998).

VEGFR-1 (Flt1) is a weak signaling receptor that seems to act in concert with VEGFR-2 to regulate physiological angiogenesis. In murine embryos, Vegfr1 deficiency results in increased proliferation of endothelial precursors, whereas EC differentiation is normal (Fong et al., 1995, 1999). Surprisingly, mice lacking the Vegfr-1 tyrosine kinase domain appeared normal, as did *Vegfr1* and *Vegfr2* heterozygous mice (Hiratsuka et al., 1998). Only VEGF-induced macrophage migration was suppressed in these mice, suggesting that VEGFR-1 signaling is not required for vasculogenesis and that VEGFR-1 may play a role in inhibition of EC proliferation. However, VEGFR-1 may have an important role in pathological angiogenesis and hematopoietic cell/monocyte function. VEGFR-1 is up-regulated by hypoxia at the transcriptional level (Gerber et al., 1997). In addition, it has been shown that PlGF, which binds only to VEGFR-1, is required for pathological angiogenesis (Carmeliet et al., 2001).

VEGFR-1 ligands also act as chemoattractants for cells of the monocyte/macrophage lineage, which express VEGFR-1 (Barleon et al., 1996). VEGFR-1 signaling is required for migration of these cells, and inflammatory cells play an important role in pathological angiogenesis and collateral vessel growth (Hiratsuka et al., 1998). It was shown that VEGF administration enhances the formation of atherosclerotic plaques in an experimental setting (Celletti et al., 2001). This effect may occur via monocyte/macrophage recruitment from the bone marrow.

VEGFR-3 in Lymphangiogenesis and Primary Lymphedema

The first characterized marker for the lymphatic endothelium was VEGFR-3 (FLT4) (Pajusola et al., 1992; Galland et al., 1993). During embryogenesis, VEGFR-3 is first expressed in a subset of blood vascular ECs (Kaipainen et al., 1995). Accordingly, mice deficient in the *Vegfr3* gene show abnormal remodeling of the primary vascular plexus and die at E9.5 (Dumont et al., 1998). However, during further development, *Vegfr3* expression becomes mainly restricted to the lymphatic vessels (Kaipainen et al., 1995; Dumont et al., 1998), and several studies have indicated the importance of VEGF-C/VEGF-D signaling via VEGFR-3 as a mediator of lymphangiogenesis (Jeltsch et al., 1997; Irrthum et al., 2000; Karkkainen et al., 2000; Veikkola et al., 2001).

The essential role of VEGFR-3 in the lymphatic development was confirmed as inactivating *VEGFR-3* missense mutations were identified as causative for congenital primary lymphedema (Ferrell et al., 1998; Witte et al., 1998; Evans et al., 1999; Irrthum et al., 2000; Karkkainen et al., 2000) (see Chapter 102). Lymphatic vessels play a key role in maintaining fluid homeostasis in tissues. Accordingly, hypoplasia or abnormal development of the superficial lymphatic vessels leads to disfiguring swelling of the extremities in lymphedema patients. The heterozygous *VEGFR-3* mutations in lymphedema patients result in inactivation of the RTK, insufficient downstream signaling, and accumulation of the mutant receptors on the lymphatic EC surface. Thus, the mutant VEGFR-3s function in a dominant negative manner and interfere with normal lymphangiogenesis. Interestingly, VEGF-C overexpression resulted in formation of a functional lymphatic vessel network in the skin of the *Chy* lymphedema mice, which normally lack the cutaneous lymphatic vessels. This suggests that VEGFR-3 ligand therapy could be used in treatment of human lymphedema (Karkkainen et al., 2001; Saaristo et al., 2002).

NRPs

NRPs were characterized as receptors for semaphorins, which have a key role in mediating axonal guidance during neural development (Chen et al., 1997; He and Tessier-Lavigne, 1997; Kolodkin et al., 1997). However, it was demonstrated that in addition to normal neural development, NRP-1 is crucial for the formation of the embryonic vasculature (Kitsukawa et al., 1995; Kawasaki et al., 1999). NRPs have the ability to bind various VEGFs in an isoform-specific manner (Fig. 101–3) (Migdal et al., 1998; Soker et al., 1998; Makinen et al., 1999; Gluzman-Poltorak et al., 2000).

It has been demonstrated that NRP-1 has a functional role in VEGF/VEGFR signaling, as it enhances VEGF165 binding to VEGFR-2 and the VEGFR-2–mediated chemotactic response of ECs

(Soker et al., 1998). The extracellular domain of NRP-1 also binds with high affinity to immunoglobulin homology domains 3 and 4 of VEGFR-1 (Fuh et al., 1998). In addition, a naturally occurring soluble form of NRP-1 binds VEGF165 and shows antitumor activity in an experimental rat prostate carcinoma model, possibly by antagonizing VEGF165 binding to its cell surface receptors (Gagnon et al., 2000). *Nrp 1*$^{-/-}$ mice exhibit severe cardiac defects, such as agenesis and transposition of great vessels (Kawasaki et al., 1999). In contrast, mice with a targeted *Nrp2* deletion are viable until adulthood (Chen et al., 2000; Giger et al., 2000) and have normal vasculature yet have several problems in the peripheral and central nervous systems.

It seems that the cytoplasmic tails of NRPs do not possess signaling capabilities, but instead, NRPs use other receptors in signal transduction. For example, plexins, which themselves do not bind secreted semaphorins, form complexes with NRPs (Takahashi et al., 1999; Tamagnone et al., 1999). The plexin-1/NRP-1 complex has a higher affinity to Sema3A than NRP-1 alone, and the intracellular signaling is transmitted via this complex and activation of a plexin-associated tyrosine kinase. Thus, also in ECs, NRPs may signal by forming complexes with VEGFRs.

In addition to the cell surface receptors for VEGFs, naturally occurring soluble forms of VEGFR-1, NRP-1, and NRP-2 have been found (Kendall and Thomas, 1993; Gagnon et al., 2000; Rossignol et al., 2000). By inhibiting ligand binding to the membrane receptors, these soluble molecules may act as naturally occurring regulators of the angiogenic processes. They seem to be able to bind at least VEGF, VEGF-B, and PlGF. Whether additional regulation is achieved by VEGFR heterodimer formation remains to be seen.

ANGIOPOIETINS AND TIE RECEPTORS

Tie receptors (tyrosine kinase with Ig and EGF homology domains) are another family of EC-specific RTKs (Fig. 101–4). In gene targeting studies, Tie1 and Tie2/Tek (tunica interna endothelial cell kinase) have been shown to have distinct roles in vascular development (Jones et al., 2001). The orphan receptor Tie1 is needed for the structural integrity of blood vascular ECs, and its deficiency results in edema and localized hemorrhaging in embryos (Puri et al., 1995; Sato et al., 1995). Signaling via the Tie2 receptor is particularly important in angiogenic sprouting, vessel remodeling, and maturation (Dumont et al., 1994; Sato et al., 1995; Vikkula et al., 1995).

Three distinct Tie2 ligands, Angpt1, Angpt2, and Angpt3 (or Angpt4 for the human gene), have been cloned (Davis et al., 1996; Maisonpierre et al., 1997; Valenzuela et al., 1999) (Fig. 101–4). Agpt1 induces Tie2 autophosphorylation, whereas Angpt2 inhibits this activation (Davis et al., 1996; Maisonpierre et al., 1997; Teichert-

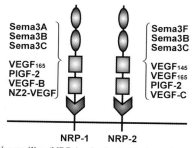

Figure 101–3. Neuropilins (NRPs) selectively bind members of the semaphorin and vascular endothelial growth factor (VEGF) families. NRPs are transmembrane proteins containing two CUB (complement-binding) domains (ovals), two coagulation factor (V/VIII) domains (boxes), and a MAM (meprin, A5, μ) domain (arrowhead) in the extracellular part, a single transmembrane domain, and a short cytoplasmic tail. PlGF, placental growth factor.

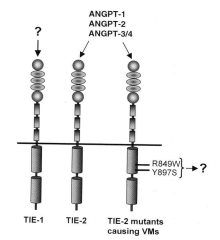

Figure 101–4. TIE receptors and angiopoietins (ANGPTs). The altered signaling causing mucocutaneous venous malformations (VMCMs) due to two identified inherited mutations in the kinase domain of TIE2 remains unclear.

Kuliszewska et al., 2001). A similar inhibitory effect is seen with Angpt3 in mice, whereas its human homologue, ANGPT4, has an agonistic effect similar to that of Angpt1 (Valenzuela et al., 1999). Accessory receptor proteins might also exist, because Angpt2 induces TIE2 phosphorylation in TIE2-transfected NIH3T3 fibroblasts, although it acts as an inhibitory ligand in ECs (Maisonpierre et al., 1997; Witzenbichler et al., 1998). In hematopoietic cells that express TIE2, Angpt2 also acts as an inducer of TIE2 phosphorylation (Sato et al., 1998). Thus, Angpt2 action is cell type specific, and due to counteracting ligands, TIE2 phosphorylation is under tight control.

A severe defect in vascular remodeling results in mice, when the activity of this signaling pathway is reduced due to deficiency of the Tie2 receptor or its agonistic ligand Angpt1 (Dumont et al., 1994; Sato et al., 1995; Suri et al., 1996). Both $Tie2^{-/-}$ and $Angpt1^{-/-}$ embryos die due to generalized defective angiogenesis. Although vasculogenesis is normal, the primary capillary plexus does not undergo remodeling and sprouting, resulting in a lack of formation of small and large vessels. Moreover, in $Angpt1^{-/-}$ embryos, this deregulated angiogenesis is marked by deficiency in pericyte recruitment (Suri et al., 1996). This could involve interactions with the surrounding matrix and mesenchyme, as suggested by Suri et al. (1996). This concept is further supported by the notion that Angpt1-induced, but not uninduced, cellular adhesion of cultured TIE2-expressing hematopoietic cells could be diminished by an antibody against β_1 integrin (Takakura et al., 1998). Thus, TIE2 activation is linked to β_1 integrin expression, and because complete block of adhesion was not achieved by β_1 integrin antibody, other integrins (such as $\alpha_v\beta_3$) might be involved (Takakura et al., 1998). The anti-apoptotic effect that Angpt1 has on cultured ECs could thus be mediated by integrin-mediated cell adhesion (Holash et al., 1999; Kwak et al., 1999; Papapetropoulos et al., 1999). Interestingly, overexpression of the inhibitory ligand Angpt2 using the Tie2 promoter causes similar, but more pronounced, effects than Tie2 and Angpt1 in knockout mice (Maisonpierre et al., 1997).

VEGF and Angpts act in a cooperative and coordinated manner in the formation and maintenance of vessels. VEGF is thought to promote EC proliferation, differentiation, and migration, whereas Angpt signaling via Tie2 mediates vessel maturation and EC interaction with the supporting cells. Data suggest that Angpt1 can inhibit vascular permeability and stabilize existing vessels. Transgenic overexpression of Angpt1 in mouse skin results in enlarged vessels at normal density due to circumferential growth, whereas the dermal microvessels induced by VEGF in the same model were numerous, tortuous, and leaky (Detmar et al., 1998; Suri et al., 1998). Surprisingly, mice coexpressing both Angpt1 and VEGF in the skin showed enlarged and more numerous, but leakage-resistant, vessels, suggesting that Angpt1 is capable of inhibiting the VEGF-induced permeability (Thurston et al., 1999). Similar results were obtained when adenoviral VEGF and/or Angpt1 were intravenously administered to mice (Thurston et al., 2000).

In vessels undergoing active remodeling, the stabilizing function of Angpt1 is overcome by an excess of Angpt2 expression. It has been speculated that Angpt2 is able to trigger detachment of pericytes from the ECs, which would then be more vulnerable to an angiogenic stimulus, such as VEGF (Gerber et al., 1999). Indeed, Angpt2 expression precedes that of VEGF at sites of active vessel growth in adults, such as during the vascular remodeling in the ovary and in tumors (Maisonpierre et al., 1997; Stratmann et al., 1998; Holash et al., 1999a, 1999b). Surprising data suggest that Angpt2 also has a role in lymphatic development. The Angpt2 knockout mice exhibit chylous ascites with defects in the patterning and function of the lymphatic vasculature (Gale et al., 2002).

VENOUS MALFORMATIONS IN HUMANS

An R849W mutation in the kinase domain of the TIE2 receptor, which confers constitutive, ligand-independent autophosporylation, has been identified in four families with inherited mucocutaneous venous malformations (Boon et al., 1994; Gallione et al., 1995; Vikkula et al., 1996; Calvert et al., 1999; A. Irrthum, L. M. Boon, and M. Vikkula, unpublished results) (Fig. 101–4). In addition, a Y8975 mutation was identified in an additional family (Calvert et al., 1999). The affected individuals have defective veins, not capillaries or arteries. Moreover, only mucocutaneous veins are affected (for a review, see Vikkula et al., 1998, 2001; Brouillard and Vikkula, 2003). This suggests that TIE2 signaling is different in venous channels and that this function may be nonexistent or redundant in other vessels. In fact, vascular type specificity of TIE2 signaling was suggested on the basis of the notion that TIE2 interacts with a vascular endothelial protein tyrosine phosphatase (VE-PTP) that shows vessel-type–specific expression (Fachinger et al., 1999). This murine receptor-type protein tyrosine phosphatase is more strongly expressed in vessels invested with smooth muscle than in capillaries and small veins. VE-PTP could protect arteries and large veins from increased autophosphorylation activity, whereas small cutaneous venules, not expressing VE-PTP, become malformed.

An interesting phenotypic difference exists between venous malformations in humans and the $Tie2^{-/-}$, $Angpt1^{-/-}$, and Angpt2-overexpressing mice. Detachment between endocardium and myocardium is evidenced in the mouse phenotypes (Dumont et al., 1994; Suri et al., 1996; Maisonpierre et al., 1997), whereas no such separation is observed underlying the endothelium of venous malformations. Moreover, ECs in these mouse models are rounded, whereas they are flat and elongated in venous malformations (Vikkula et al., 1996). It could be that the cardiac phenotype in mice is a secondary phenomenon due to the severe angiogenic problems in the embryo. The difference may also be due to the altered intracellular signaling of TIE2 caused by the human mutation (Korpelainen et al., 1999).

Interestingly, a novel molecule with unknown function, *glomulin*, was identified as being mutated in individuals with another type of cutaneous venous malformation, glomuvenous malformation ("glomangioma") (Boon et al., 1999; Brouillard et al., 2002). These lesions are clinically similar to the TIE2-caused lesions; however, histologically they contain a varying number of "glomus cells" in the walls of the distended vein–like channels (Boon et al., 1999). The glomus cells are thought to be non–well-differentiated vascular smooth muscle cells (Brouillard et al., 2002). In the mucocutaneous venous malformations caused by the activating TIE2 mutations, glomus cells are not present, but rather a relative lack of morphologically normal vascular smooth muscle cells is observed (Vikkula et al., 1996, 2001; Boon et al., 1999; Brouillard and Vikkula, 2003). Thus, it is not clear whether glomulin function is linked to TIE2 signaling in vascular morphogenesis.

EPHRINS AND Eph RECEPTORS

During vascular network formation, blood vessels assemble to form a hierarchic pattern of arteries and veins, connected by a capillary network. Ephrins and their Eph receptors form an interesting ligand–receptor system that is likely to play an important role in creating vascular identity. The Eph family contains at least 14 receptors and 8 ligands (for a review, see Cheng et al., 2002) (Fig. 101–5). The Eph receptors are divided into EphA and EphB receptors according to sequence homologies, and the ligands are grouped into ephrin As and ephrin Bs, which mainly bind to EphA and EphB receptors, respectively. However, in both classes, ligand–receptor binding is promiscuous, and specificity is created by microenvironment and cell-specific localization of the molecules. Moreover, the RTKs bind multimeric, membrane-bound ligands, resulting in a bidirectional signaling in the interacting cells (for a review, see Schmucker, 2001).

Ephrin and Eph receptors were first identified as being important for neuronal development, including axon guidance. Reciprocal expression of ligands and receptors in axons and surrounding mesenchyme led to the hypothesis that the molecules may signal repulsive forces that are important for directional growth of the axon. Additional data have implicated ephrins and their receptors in cell morphology, survival, and cell–cell and cell–matrix attachment, especially via the integrins and cadherins (for a review, see Cheng et al., 2002). Some ephrins and Eph RTKs have also been implicated in defining the arterial/venous patterning of vessels and in EC–matrix interactions. From the beginning of angiogenesis, arterial ECs express ephrinB2, a transmembrane ligand, whereas venous ECs express its receptor, EphB4 (Wang et al., 1998). Other ephrins or their receptors are also expressed in the developing vasculature, notably ephrinB1

Figure 101–5. Ephrins and Eph receptors. Eph receptors are transmembrane molecules with a large ligand-binding domain in the N-terminal end of the extracellular domain. Phosphotyrosines are marked with P. Signaling molecules with PDZ domains bind both Eph receptors and Ephrin-B ligands at their C-terminal intracellular domains. Ephrin A molecules bind to membranes via GPI anchor. (Adopted from Cheng et al., 2002).

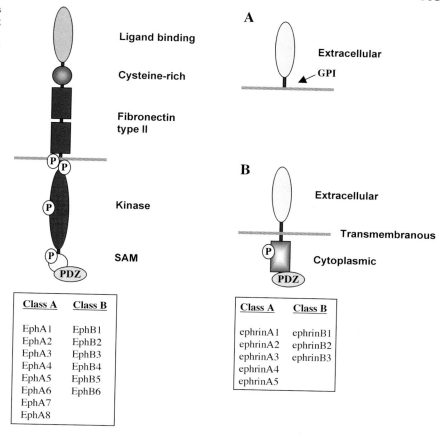

and EphB3 in veins and some arteries (for a review, see Gale and Yancopoulos, 1999). Thus, ephrins and the Eph receptors serve to distinguish between the two vessel types. In fact, ephrin-B2 and EphB4 are the best markers for differentiating between arterial and venous endothelia. It has been speculated that mixing of the two developing vessel types is prevented via the repulsive effect of ephrin-B2/EphB4 signaling (Wang et al., 1998). Interestingly, it was noted that the expression of ephrin-B2 on the arterial side seems to extend midway in capillaries, suggesting that these vessels also have arterial/venous identity (Gale et al., 2001). Because aortic smooth muscle cells also express ephrin-B2, its role is not limited to ECs but may extent to mural cells (Gale et al., 2001; Othman-Hassan et al., 2001).

Ephrin As, more specifically ephrin-A1 and its receptor EphA2, have also been implicated in angiogenesis, especially in tumor-induced angiogenesis. Both molecules were expressed in ECs and in tumor cells of various human tumors, including breast, lung, and kidney cancer (Ogawa et al., 2000). Because ephrin-A1 is not strongly expressed in adult vasculature, but rather in embryonic vessels, its presence in tumor vessels suggests a role in neovascularization. Because expression is not limited to ECs, ephrin-A1 and EphA2 probably also influence EC–tumor cell interactions, which might be important for sprouting angiogenesis. Interestingly, ephrin-A1 expression is upregulated by VEGF, and blocking class A Eph receptor signaling results in inhibition of VEGF-induced EC survival, migration, and sprouting angiogenesis (Cheng et al., 2002). Thus, concerted action occurs between ephrin/Eph signaling and VEGF-related angiogenesis.

Surprisingly, mice lacking ephrin-B2 or EphB4 resemble mice lacking either Angpt1 or Tie2, with aberrant vessel remodeling, sprouting, and cardiac trabeculation (Wang et al., 1998; Adams et al., 1999; Gerety et al., 1999). Thus, reciprocal interactions between venous and arterial ECs via the bidirectional signaling ligands and receptors is crucial for proper vascular morphogenesis. Moreover, mice lacking the intracellular part of ephrin-B2 show similar defects (Adams et al., 2001), underscoring the importance of signaling downstream of ephrin-B2. EphB2 and EphB3 knockouts have normal vascular de-

velopment, yet 30% of *EphB2/B3* double-knockout mice have defects in vascular morphogenesis similar to ephrin-B2 and EphB4 knockouts (Adams et al., 1999). Therefore, redundancy most likely exists between Eph receptor function. These results also suggest that the Angpt1/Tie2 and ephrin-B2/EphB4 signaling pathways interact.

CONCLUDING REMARKS

Vasculogenesis and angiogenesis are multistep processes involving a concerted action of a number of molecules. Differentiation, proliferation, aggregation, migration, and cell–cell and cell–matrix adhesion are needed for the vascular and lymphatic networks to be developed. Among the growth factors and the RTKs that are crucial in these processes, VEGFs, Angpt, and ephrins play a central role. Without them, both vasculogenesis and angiogenesis are severely deranged or halted. This is especially due to the pivotal function of VEGFs and VEGFRs in vascular EC proliferation and migration and the role of angiopoietins and TIE2 in EC survival and migration. In addition, ephrins and Eph receptors are needed for morphology and adhesion. These signaling pathways are intertwined and act together. Altered angiogenesis occurs if any of the pathways are dysregulated. Thus, in therapeutic approaches, one molecule alone most likely will not lead to the desired effect, but balanced intervention is needed. Alterations in these pathways and interacting molecules are also likely to be responsible for the various kinds of vascular anomalies seen in humans, as underscored by the VEGF-3 and TIE2 mutations identified as being responsible for congenital primary lymphedema and venous malformations in the skin and mucosa.

ACKNOWLEDGMENTS

The studies in the authors' laboratories have been supported by the Fonds Spéciaux de Recherche-Université catholique de Louvain, the Belgian Federal Service for Scientific, Technical and Cultural Affairs, the Fonds National de la Recherche Scientifique (F.N.R.S.) (to M.V., a "chercheur qualifié du F.N.R.S) and the Finnish Cancer Organization, Finnish Cultural Foundation, Ida Montini Foundation, Emil Aaltonen Foundation, Paulo Foundation, Research and Science Foundation of Farmos, Ella and Georg Ehrnrooth's Foundation, Academy of Finland (grant 204312), Novo Nordisk Foundation, National Institutes of Health grant HD37243, and the European Union (Biomed grant PL963380). The authors thank Liliana Niculescu for expert secretarial help.

REFERENCES

Aase K, von Euler G, Li X, Ponten A, Thoren P, Cao R, Cao Y, Olofsson B, Gebre-Medhin S, Pekny M (2001). Vascular endothelial growth factor-B-deficient mice display an atrial conduction defect. *Circulation* 104: 358–64.

Achen MG, Jeltsch M, Kukk E, Makinen T, Vitali A, Wilks AF, Alitalo K, Stacker S. A (1998). Vascular endothelial growth factor D (VEGF-D) is a ligand for the tyrosine kinases VEGF receptor 2 (Flk1) and VEGF receptor 3 (Flt4). *Proc Natl Acad Sci USA* 95: 548–553.

Adams RH, Diella F, Hennig S, Helmbacher F, Deutsch U, Klein R (2001). The cytoplasmic domain of the ligand ephrinB2 is required for vascular morphogenesis but not cranial neural crest migration. *Cell* 104: 57–69.

Adams RH, Wilkinson GA, Weiss C, Diella F, Gale NW, Deutsch U, Risau W, Klein R (1999). Roles of ephrinB ligands and EphB receptors in cardiovascular development: demarcation of arterial/venous domains, vascular morphogenesis, and sprouting angiogenesis. *Genes Dev* 13: 295–306.

Avantaggiato V, Orlandini M, Acampora D, Oliviero S, Simeone A (1998). Embryonic expression pattern of the murine fegf gene, a growth factor belonging to platelet-derived growth factor/vascular endothelial growth factor family. *Mech Dev* 73: 221–224.

Baldwin ME, Catimel B, Nice EC, Roufail S, Hall NE, Stenvers KL, Karkkainen MJ, Alitalo K, Stacker SA, Achen MG (2001). The specificity of receptor binding by vascular endothelial growth factor-D is different in mouse and man. *J Biol Chem* 276: 19166–19171.

Barleon B, Sozzani S, Zhou D, Weich HA, Mantovani A, Marme D (1996). Migration of human monocytes in response to vascular endothelial growth factor (VEGF) is mediated via the VEGF receptor flt-1. *Blood* 87: 3336–3343.

Bellomo D, Headrick JP, Silins GU, Paterson CA, Thomas PS, Gartside M, Mould A, Cahill MM, Tonks ID, Grimmond SM, et al. (2000). Mice lacking the vascular endothelial growth factor-B gene (Vegfb) have smaller hearts, dysfunctional coronary vasculature, and impaired recovery from cardiac ischemia. *Circ Res* 86: E29–E35.

Benjamin LE, Hemo I, Keshet E (1998). A plasticity window for blood vessel remodelling is defined by pericyte coverage of the preformed endothelial network and is regulated by PDGF-B and VEGF. *Development* 125: 1591–1598.

Boon LM, Mulliken JB, Vikkula M, Watkins H, Seidman J, Olsen BR, Warman ML (1994). Assignment of a locus for dominantly inherited venous malformations to chromosome 9p. *Hum Mol Genet* 3: 1583–1587.

Boon LM, Brouillard P, Irrthum A, Karttunen L, Warman ML, Rudolph R, Mulliken JB, Olsen BR, Vikkula M (1999). A gene for inherited cutaneous venous anomalies ("glomangiomas") localizes to chromosome 1p21-22. *Am J Hum Genet* 65: 125–133.

Brouillard P, Boon LM, Mulliken JB, Enjolras O, Ghassibe M, Warman ML, Tan OT, Olsen BR, Vikkula M (2002). Mutations in a novel factor, glomulin, are responsible for glomuvenous malformations ("glomangiomas"). *Am J Hum Genet* 70: 866–874.

Brouillard P, Vikkula M (2003). Vascular malformation: localized defects in vascular morphogenesis. *Clinical Genetics* 63: 340–351.

Calvert JT, Riney TJ, Kontos CD, Cha EH, Prieto VG, Shea CR, Berg JN, Nevin NC, Simpson SA, Pasyk KA, et al. (1999). Allelic and locus heterogeneity in inherited venous malformations. *Hum Mol Genet* 8: 1279–1289.

Cao Y, Linden P, Farnebo J, Cao R, Eriksson A, Kumar V, Qi JH, Claesson-Welsh L, Alitalo K (1998). Vascular endothelial growth factor C induces angiogenesis in vivo. *Proc Natl Acad Sci U S A* 95: 14389–14394.

Carmeliet P, Ferreira V, Breier G, Pollefeyt S, Kieckens L, Gertsenstein M, Fahrig M, Vandenhoeck A, Harpal K, Eberhardt C, et al. (1996). Abnormal blood vessel development and lethality in embryos lacking a single VEGF allele. *Nature* 380: 435–439.

Carmeliet P, Moons L, Luttun A, Vincenti V, Compernolle V, De Mol M, Wu Y, Bono F, Devy L, Beck H, et al. (2001). Synergism between vascular endothelial growth factor and placental growth factor contributes to angiogenesis and plasma extravasation in pathological conditions. *Nat Med* 7: 575–583.

Carmeliet P, Ng YS, Nuyens D, Theilmeier G, Brusselmans K, Cornelissen I, Ehler E, Kakkar VV, et al. (1999). Impaired myocardial angiogenesis and ischemic cardiomyopathy in mice lacking the vascular endothelial growth factor isoforms VEGF164 and VEGF188. *Nat Med* 5: 495–502.

Celletti FL, Waugh JM, Amabile PG, Brendolan A, Hilfiker PR, Dake MD (2001). Vascular endothelial growth factor enhances atherosclerotic plaque progression. *Nat Med* 7: 425–429.

Chen H, Chedotal A, He Z, Goodman CS, Tessier-Lavigne M (1997). Neuropilin-2, a novel member of the neuropilin family, is a high affinity receptor for the semaphorins Sema E and Sema IV but not Sema III. *Neuron* 19: 547–559.

Chen H, Bagri A, Zupicich JA, Zou Y, Stoeckli E, Pleasure SJ, Lowenstein DH, Skarnes WC, Chedotal A, Tessier-Lavigne M (2000). Neuropilin-2 regulates the development of selective cranial and sensory nerves and hippocampal mossy fiber projections. *Neuron* 25: 43–56.

Cheng N, Brantley DM, Chen J (2002). The ephrins and Eph receptors in angiogenesis. *Cytokine Growth Factor Rev* 13: 75–85.

Conway EM, Collen D, Carmeliet P (2001). Molecular mechanisms of blood vessel growth. *Cardiovasc Res* 49: 507–521.

Davis S, Aldrich TH, Jones PF, Acheson A, Compton DL, Jain V, Ryan TE, Bruno J, Radziejewski C, Maisonpierre PC, et al. (1996). Isolation of angiopoietin-1, a ligand for the TIE2 receptor, by secretion-trap expression cloning. *Cell* 87: 1161–1169.

Davis-Smyth T, Chen H, Park J, Presta LG, Ferrara N (1996). The second immunoglobulin-like domain of the VEGF tyrosine kinase receptor Flt-1 determines ligand binding and may initiate a signal transduction cascade. *EMBO J* 15: 4919–4927.

Detmar M, Brown LF, Schon MP, Elicker BM, Velasco P, Richard L, Fukumura D, Monsky W, Claffey KP, Jain RK (1998). Increased microvascular density and enhanced leuko-

cyte rolling and adhesion in the skin of VEGF transgenic mice. *J Invest Dermatol* 111: 1–6.

Djonov V, Schmid M, Tschanz SA, Burri PH (2000). Intussusceptive angiogenesis: Its role in embryonic vascular network formation. *Circ Res* 86: 286–292.

Dumont DJ, Gradwohl G, Fong GH, Puri MC, Gertsenstein M, Auerbach A, Breitman ML (1994). Dominant-negative and targeted null mutations in the endothelial receptor tyrosine kinase, tek, reveal a critical role in vasculogenesis of the embryo. *Genes Dev* 8: 1897–1909.

Dumont DJ, Jussila L, Taipale J, Lymboussaki A, Mustonen T, Pajusola K, Breitman M, Alitalo K (1998). Cardiovascular failure in mouse embryos deficient in VEGF receptor-3. *Science* 282: 946–949.

Evans AL, Brice G, Sotirova V, Mortimer P, Beninson J, Burnand K, Rosbotham J, Child A, Sarfarazi M (1999). Mapping of primary congenital lymphedema to the 5q35.3 region. *Am J Hum Genet* 64: 547–555.

Fachinger G, Deutsch U, Risau W (1999). Functional interaction of vascular endothelial-protein-tyrosine phosphatase with the angiopoietin receptor Tie-2. *Oncogene* 18: 5948–5953.

Ferrara N, Houck K, Jakeman L, Leung DW (1992). Molecular and biological properties of the vascular endothelial growth factor family of proteins. *Endocr Rev* 13: 18–32.

Ferrara N, Carver-Moore K, Chen H, Dowd M, Lu L, O'Shea KS, Powell-Braxton L, Hillan KJ, Moore MW (1996). Heterozygous embryonic lethality induced by targeted inactivation of the VEGF gene. *Nature* 380: 439–442.

Ferrara N (2002). Role of vascular endothelial growth factor in physiologic and pathologic angiogenesis: therapeutic implications. *Semin Oncol* 29(6 Suppl 16): 10–14.

Ferrell RE, Levinson KL, Esman JH, Kimak MA, Lawrence EC, Barmada MM, Finegold DN (1998). Hereditary lymphedema: evidence for linkage and genetic heterogeneity. *Hum Mol Genet* 7: 2073–2078.

Flamme I, Frolich T, Risau W (1997). Molecular mechanisms of vasculogenesis and embryonic angiogenesis. *J Cell Physiol* 173: 206–210.

Fong GH, Zhang L, Bryce DM, Peng J (1999). Increased hemangioblast commitment, not vascular disorganization, is the primary defect in flt-1 knock-out mice. *Development* 126: 3015–3025.

Fong GH, Rossant J, Gertsenstein M, Breitman ML (1995). Role of the Flt-1 receptor tyrosine kinase in regulating the assembly of vascular endothelium. *Nature* 376: 66–70.

Fuh G, Li B, Crowley C, Cunningham B, Wells JA (1998). Requirements for binding and signaling of the kinase domain receptor for vascular endothelial growth factor. *J Biol Chem* 273: 11197–11204.

Gagnon ML, Bielenberg DR, Gechtman Z, Miao HQ, Takashima S, Soker S, Klagsbrun M (2000). Identification of a natural soluble neuropilin-1 that binds vascular endothelial growth factor: in vivo expression and antitumor activity. *Proc Natl Acad Sci U S A* 97: 2573–2578.

Gale NW, Yancopoulos GD (1999). Growth factors acting via endothelial cell-specific receptor tyrosine kinases: VEGFs, angiopoietins, and ephrins in vascular development. *Genes Dev* 13: 1055–1066.

Gale NW, Baluk P, Pan L, Kwan M, Holash J, DeChiara TM, McDonald DM, Yancopoulos GD (2001). Ephrin-B2 selectively marks arterial vessels and neovascularization sites in the adult, with expression in both endothelial and smooth-muscle cells. *Dev Biol* 230: 151–160.

Gale NW, Thurston G, Hackett SF, Renard R, Wang Q, McClain J, Martin C, Witte C, Witte MH, Jackson D, Suri C, Campochiaro PA, Wiegand SJ, Yancopoulos GD (2002). Angiopoietin-2 is required for postnatal angiogenesis and lymphatic patterning, and only the latter role is rescued by Angiopoietin-1. *Dev Cell* 3: 411–423.

Galland F, Karamysheva A, Pebusque MJ, Borg JP, Rottapel R, Dubreuil P, Rosnet O, Birnbaum D (1993). The FLT4 gene encodes a transmembrane tyrosine kinase related to the vascular endothelial growth factor receptor. *Oncogene* 8: 1233–1240.

Gallione CJ, Pasyk KA, Boon LM, Lennon F, Johnson DW, Helmbold EA, Markel DS, Vikkula M, Mulliken JB, Warman ML, et al. (1995). A gene for familial venous malformations maps to chromosome 9p in a second large kindred. *J Med Genet* 32: 197–199.

Gerber HP, Condorelli F, Park J, Ferrara N (1997). Differential transcriptional regulation of the two vascular endothelial growth factor receptor genes. Flt-1, but not Flk-1/KDR, is up-regulated by hypoxia. *J Biol Chem* 272: 23659–23667.

Gerber HP, McMurtrey A, Kowalski J, Yan M, Keyt BA, Dixit V, Ferrara N (1998). Vascular endothelial growth factor regulates endothelial cell survival through the phosphatidylinositol 3'-kinase/Akt signal transduction pathway. Requirement for Flk-1/KDR activation. *J Biol Chem* 273: 30336–30343.

Gerber HP, Hillan KJ, Ryan AM, Kowalski J, Keller GA, Rangell L, Wright BD, Radtke F, Aguet M, Ferrara N (1999). VEGF is required for growth and survival in neonatal mice. *Development* 126: 1149–1159.

Gerety SS, Wang HU, Chen ZF, Anderson DJ (1999). Symmetrical mutant phenotypes of the receptor EphB4 and its specific transmembrane ligand ephrin-B2 in cardiovascular development. *Mol Cell* 4: 403–414.

Giger RJ, Cloutier JF, Sahay A, Prinjha RK, Levengood DV, Moore SE, Pickering S, Simmons D, Rastan S, Walsh FS, et al. (2000). Neuropilin-2 is required in vivo for selective axon guidance responses to secreted semaphorins. *Neuron* 25: 29–41.

Gill M, Dias S, Hattori K, Rivera ML, Hicklin D, Witte L, Girardi L, Yurt R, Himel H, Rafii S (2001). Vascular trauma induces rapid but transient mobilization of VEGFR2(+)AC133(+) endothelial precursor cells. *Circ Res* 88: 167–174.

Gluzman-Poltorak Z, Cohen T, Herzog Y, Neufeld G (2000). Neuropilin-2 and neuropilin-1 are receptors for the 165-amino acid form of vascular endothelial growth factor (VEGF) and of placenta growth factor-2, but only neuropilin-2 functions as a receptor for the 145-amino acid form of VEGF. *J Biol Chem* 275: 18040–18045.

Groves RW, Wilson-Jones E, MacDonald DM (1991). Human orf and milkers' nodule: a clinicopathologic study. *J Am Acad Dermatol* 25: 706–711.

He Z, Tessier-Lavigne M (1997). Neuropilin is a receptor for the axonal chemorepellent semaphorin III. *Cell* 90: 739–751.

Hiratsuka S, Minowa O, Kuno J, Noda T, Shibuya M (1998). Flt-1 lacking the tyrosine kinase domain is sufficient for normal development and angiogenesis in mice. *Proc Natl Acad Sci U S A* 95: 9349–9354.

Holash J, Maisonpierre PC, Compton D, Boland P, Alexander CR, Zagzag D, Yancopoulos GD, Wiegand SJ (1999a). Vessel cooption, regression, and growth in tumors mediated by angiopoietins and VEGF. *Science* 284: 1994–1998.
Holash J, Wiegand SJ, Yancopoulos GD (1999b). New model of tumor angiogenesis: dynamic balance between vessel regression and growth mediated by angiopoietins and VEGF. *Oncogene* 18: 5356–5362.
Houck KA, Leung DW, Rowland AM, Winer J, Ferrara N (1992). Dual regulation of vascular endothelial growth factor bioavailability by genetic and proteolytic mechanisms. *J Biol Chem* 267: 26031–26037.
Hubbard SR, Mohammadi M, Schlessinger J (1998). Autoregulatory mechanisms in protein-tyrosine kinases. *J Biol Chem* 273: 11987–11990.
Huntington G, McClure C (1908). The anatomy and development of the jugular lymph sac in the domestic cat (*Felis domestica*). *Anat Rec* 2: 1–19.
Huse M, Muir TW, Xu L, Chen YG, Kuriyan J, Massague J (2001). The TGF beta receptor activation process: an inhibitor- to substrate-binding switch. *Mol Cell* 8: 671–682.
Irrthum A, Karkkainen MJ, Devriendt K, Alitalo K, Vikkula M (2000). Congenital hereditary lymphedema caused by a mutation that inactivates VEGFR3 tyrosine kinase. *Am J Hum Genet* 67: 295–301.
Jeltsch M, Kaipainen A, Joukov V, Meng X, Lakso M, Rauvala H, Swartz M, Fukumura D, Jain RK, Alitalo K (1997). Hyperplasia of lymphatic vessels in VEGF-C transgenic mice. *Science* 276: 1423–1425.
Jones N, Iljin K, Dumont DJ, Alitalo K (2001). Tie receptors: new modulators of angiogenic and lymphangiogenic responses. *Nat Rev Mol Cell Biol* 2: 257–267.
Joukov V, Kumar V, Sorsa T, Arighi E, Weich H, Saksela O, Alitalo K (1998). A recombinant mutant vascular endothelial growth factor-C that has lost vascular endothelial growth factor receptor-2 binding, activation, and vascular permeability activities. *J Biol Chem* 273: 6599–6602.
Joukov V, Kaipainen A, Jeltsch M, Pajusola K, Olofsson B, Kumar V, Eriksson U, Alitalo K (1997). Vascular endothelial growth factors VEGF-B and VEGF-C. *J Cell Physiol* 173: 211–215.
Joukov V, Pajusola K, Kaipainen A, Chilov D, Lahtinen I, Kukk E, Saksela O, Kalkkinen N, Alitalo K (1996). A novel vascular endothelial growth factor, VEGF-C, is a ligand for the Flt4 (VEGFR-3) and KDR (VEGFR-2) receptor tyrosine kinases (published erratum appears in *EMBO J* 19961;15:1751). *EMBO J* 15: 290–298.
Joukov V, Sorsa T, Kumar V, Jeltsch M, Claesson Welsh L, Cao Y, Saksela O, Kalkkinen N, Alitalo K (1997). Proteolytic processing regulates receptor specificity and activity of VEGF-C. *EMBO-J* 16: 3898–3911.
Kaipainen A, Korhonen J, Mustonen T, van Hinsbergh VW, Fang GH, Dumont D, Breitman M, Alitalo K (1995). Expression of the fms-like tyrosine kinase 4 gene becomes restricted to lymphatic endothelium during development. *Proc Natl Acad Sci USA* 92: 3566–3570.
Kampmeier O (1912). The value of the injection method in the study of lymphatic development. *Anat Rec* 6: 223–232.
Karkkainen MJ, Ferrell RE, Lawrence EC, Kimak MA, Levinson KL, McTigue MA, Alitalo K, Finegold DN (2000). Missense mutations interfere with VEGFR-3 signalling in primary lymphoedema. *Nat Genet* 25: 153–159.
Karkkainen MJ, Saaristo A, Jussila L, Karila KA, Lawrence EC, Pajusola K, Bueler H, Eichmann A, Kauppinen R, Kettunen MI, et al. (2001). A model for gene therapy of human hereditary lymphedema. *Proc Natl Acad Sci U S A* 98: 12677–12682.
Kawasaki T, Kitsukawa T, Bekku Y, Matsuda Y, Sanbo M, Yagi T, Fujisawa H (1999). A requirement for neuropilin-1 in embryonic vessel formation. *Development* 126: 4895–902.
Kendall RL, Thomas KA (1993). Inhibition of vascular endothelial cell growth factor activity by an endogenously encoded soluble receptor. *Proc Natl Acad Sci U S A* 90: 10705–10709.
Kitsukawa T, Shimono A, Kawakami A, Kondoh H, Fujisawa H (1995). Overexpression of a membrane protein, neuropilin, in chimeric mice causes anomalies in the cardiovascular system, nervous system and limbs. *Development* 121: 4309–4318.
Kolodkin AL, Levengood DV, Rowe EG, Tai YT, Giger RJ, Ginty DD (1997). Neuropilin is a semaphorin III receptor. *Cell* 90: 753–762.
Korpelainen EI, Kärkkäinen M, Gunji Y, Vikkula M, Alitalo K (1999). Endothelial receptor tyrosine kinases activate the STAT signaling pathway: mutant TIE-2 causing venous malformations signals a distinct STAT activation response. *Oncogene* 18: 1–8.
Kukk E, Lymboussaki A, Taira S, Kaipainen A, Jeltsch M, Joukov V, Alitalo K (1996). VEGF-C receptor binding and pattern of expression with VEGFR-3 suggests a role in lymphatic vascular development. *Development* 122: 3829–3837.
Kwak HJ, So JN, Lee SJ, Kim I, Koh GY (1999). Angiopoietin-1 is an apoptosis survival factor for endothelial cells. *FEBS Lett* 448: 249–253.
Lee J, Gray A, Yuan J, Luoh SM, Avraham H, Wood WI (1996). Vascular endothelial growth factor-related protein: a ligand and specific activator of the tyrosine kinase receptor Flt4. *Proc Natl Acad Sci U S A* 93: 1988–1992.
Leung DW, Cachianes G, Kuang WJ, Goeddel DV, Ferrara N (1989). Vascular endothelial growth factor is a secreted angiogenic mitogen. *Science* 246: 1306–1309.
Li X, Aase K, Li H, von Euler G, Eriksson U (2001). Isoform-specific expression of VEGF-B in normal tissues and tumors. *Growth Factors* 19: 49–59.
Lyttle DJ, Fraser KM, Fleming SB, Mercer AA, Robinson AJ (1994). Homologs of vascular endothelial growth factor are encoded by the poxvirus orf virus. *J Virol* 68: 84–92.
Maisonpierre PC, Suri C, Jones PF, Bartunkova S, Wiegand S, Radziejewski C, Compton D, McClain J, Aldrich TH, Papadopoulos N, et al. (1997). Angiopoietin 2, a natural antagonist for Tie2 that disrupts in vivo angiogenesis. *Science* 277 (5322): 55–60.
Makinen T, Olofsson B, Karpanen T, Hellman U, Soker S, Klagsbrun M, Eriksson U, Alitalo K (1999). Differential binding of vascular endothelial growth factor B splice and proteolytic isoforms to neuropilin-1. *J Biol Chem* 274: 21217–21222.
Makinen T, Jussila L, Veikkola T, Karpanen T, Kettunen MI, Pulkkanen KJ, Kauppinen R, Jackson DG, Kubo H, Nishikawa S, et al. (2001). Inhibition of lymphangiogenesis with resulting lymphedema in transgenic mice expressing soluble VEGF receptor-3. *Nat Med* 7: 199–205.
Mandriota SJ, Jussila L, Jeltsch M, Compagni A, Baetens D, Prevo R, Banerji S, Huarte J, Montesano R, Jackson DG, et al. (2001). Vascular endothelial growth factor-C-mediated lymphangiogenesis promotes tumour metastasis. *EMBO J* 20: 672–682.
Marconcini L, Marchio S, Morbidelli L, Cartocci E, Albini A, Ziche M, Bussolino F, Oliviero S (1999). c-fos-induced growth factor/vascular endothelial growth factor D induces angiogenesis in vivo and in vitro. *Proc Natl Acad Sci U S A* 96: 9671–9676.
Matthews W, Jordan CT, Gavin M, Jenkins NA, Copeland NG, Lemischka IR (1991). A receptor tyrosine kinase cDNA isolated from a population of enriched primitive hematopoietic cells and exhibiting close genetic linkage to c-kit. *Proc Natl Acad Sci U S A* 88: 9026–9030.
Meyer M, Clauss M, Lepple-Wienhues A, Waltenberger J, Augustin HG, Ziche M, Lanz C, Buttner M, Rziha HJ, Dehio C (1999). A novel vascular endothelial growth factor encoded by Orf virus, VEGF-E, mediates angiogenesis via signalling through VEGFR-2 (KDR) but not VEGFR-1 (Flt-1) receptor tyrosine kinases. *EMBO J* 18: 363–374.
Migdal M, Huppertz B, Tessler S, Comforti A, Shibuya M, Reich R, Baumann H, Neufeld G (1998). Neuropilin-1 is a placenta growth factor-2 receptor. *J Biol Chem* 273: 22272–22278.
Muller YA, Li B, Christinger HW, Wells JA, Cunningham BC, de Vos AM (1997). Vascular endothelial growth factor: crystal structure and functional mapping of the kinase domain receptor binding site. *Proc Natl Acad Sci U S A* 94: 7192–7197.
Ogawa K, Pasqualini R, Lindberg RA, Kain R, Freeman AL, Pasquale EB (2000). The ephrin-A1 ligand and its receptor, EphA2, are expressed during tumor neovascularization. *Oncogene* 19: 6043–6052.
Ogawa S, Oku A, Sawano A, Yamaguchi S, Yazaki Y, Shibuya M (1998). A novel type of vascular endothelial growth factor, VEGF-E (NZ-7 VEGF), preferentially utilizes KDR/Flk-1 receptor and carries a potent mitotic activity without heparin-binding domain. *J Biol Chem* 273: 31273–31282.
Oh SJ, Jeltsch MM, Birkenhager R, McCarthy JE, Weich HA, Christ B, Alitalo K, Wilting J (1997). VEGF and VEGF-C: specific induction of angiogenesis and lymphangiogenesis in the differentiated avian chorioallantoic membrane. *Dev Biol* 188: 96–109.
Olofsson B, Pajusola K, Kaipainen A, von Euler G, Joukov V, Saksela O, Orpana A, Pettersson RF, Alitalo K, Eriksson U (1996). Vascular endothelial growth factor B, a novel growth factor for endothelial cells. *Proc Natl Acad Sci USA* 93: 2576–2581.
Orlandini M, Marconcini L, Ferruzzi R, Oliviero S (1996). Identification of a c-fos-induced gene that is related to the platelet-derived growth factor/vascular endothelial growth factor family. *Proc Natl Acad Sci U S A* 93: 11675–11680.
Othman-Hassan K, Patel K, Papoutsi M, Rodriguez-Niedenfuhr M, Christ B, Wilting J (2001). Arterial identity of endothelial cells is controlled by local cues. *Dev Biol* 237: 398–409.
Pajusola K, Aprelikova O, Korhonen J, Kaipainen A, Pertovaara L, Alitalo R, Alitalo K (1992). FLT4 receptor tyrosine kinase contains seven immunoglobulin-like loops and is expressed in multiple human tissues and cell lines. *Cancer Res* 52: 5738–5743.
Papapetropoulos A, Garcia-Cardena G, Dengler TJ, Maisonpierre PC, Yancopoulos GD, Sessa WC (1999). Direct actions of angiopoietin-1 on human endothelium: evidence for network stabilization, cell survival, and interaction with other angiogenic growth factors. *Lab Invest* 79: 213–223.
Park JE, Keller GA, Ferrara N (1993). The vascular endothelial growth factor (VEGF) isoforms: differential deposition into the subepithelial extracellular matrix and bioactivity of extracellular matrix-bound VEGF. *Mol Biol Cell* 4: 1317–1326.
Poltorak Z, Cohen T, Sivan R, Kandelis Y, Spira G, Vlodavsky I, Keshet E, Neufeld G (1997). VEGF145, a secreted vascular endothelial growth factor isoform that binds to extracellular matrix. *J Biol Chem* 272: 7151–7158.
Puri MC, Rossant J, Alitalo K, Bernstein A, Partanen J (1995). The receptor tyrosine kinase TIE is required for integrity and survival of vascular endothelial cells. *EMBO J* 14: 5884–5891.
Risau W (1997). Mechanisms of angiogenesis. *Nature* 386: 671–674.
Rossignol M, Gagnon ML, Klagsbrun M (2000). Genomic organization of human neuropilin-1 and neuropilin-2 genes: identification and distribution of splice variants and soluble isoforms. *Genomics* 70: 211–222.
Saaristo A, Veikkola T, Tammela T, Enholm B, Karkkainen MJ, Pajusola K, Bueler H, Ylä-Herttuala S, Alitalo K (2002). Lymphangiogenic gene therapy with minimal blood vascular side effects. *J Exp Med* 196: 719–730.
Sabin F (1902). On the origin of the lymphatic system from the veins and the development of the lymph hearts and toracic duct in the pig. *Am J Anat* 1: 367–391.
Sabin F (1912). On the origin of the abdominal lymphatics in mammals from the vena cava and renal veins. *Anat Rec* 6: 335–343.
Sato A, Iwama A, Takakura N, Nishio H, Yancopoulos GD, Suda T (1998). Characterization of TEK receptor tyrosine kinase and its ligands, Angiopoietins, in human hematopoietic progenitor cells. *Int Immunol* 10: 1217–1227.
Sato TN, Tozawa Y, Deutsch U, Wolburg-Buchholz K, Fujiwara Y, Gendron-Maguire M, Gridley T, Wolburg H, Risau W, Qin Y (1995). Distinct roles of the receptor tyrosine kinases Tie-1 and Tie-2 in blood vessel formation. *Nature* 376: 70–74.
Schlessinger J (2000). Cell signaling by receptor tyrosine kinases. *Cell* 103: 211–225.
Schmucker D, Zipursky SL (2001). Signaling downstream of Eph receptors and ephrin ligands. *Cell* 105: 701–704.
Schneider M, Othman-Hassan K, Christ B, Wilting J (1999). Lymphangioblasts in the avian wing bud. *Dev Dyn* 216: 311–319.
Shalaby F, Rossant J, Yamaguchi TP, Gertsenstein M, Wu XF, Breitman ML, Schuh AC (1995). Failure of blood-island formation and vasculogenesis in Flk-1-deficient mice. *Nature* 376: 62–66.
Shi Q, Rafii S, Wu MH, Wijelath ES, Yu C, Ishida A, Fujita Y, Kothari S, Mohle R, Sauvage LR, et al. (1998). Evidence for circulating bone marrow-derived endothelial cells. *Blood* 92: 362–367.
Shibuya M, Yamaguchi S, Yamane A, Ikeda T, Tojo A, Matsushime H, Sato M (1990). Nucleotide sequence and expression of a novel human receptor-type tyrosine kinase gene (flt) closely related to the fms family. *Oncogene* 5: 519–524.
Shweiki D, Itin A, Soffer D, Keshet E (1992). Vascular endothelial growth factor induced by hypoxia may mediate hypoxia-initiated angiogenesis. *Nature* 359: 843–845.

Soker S, Takashima S, Miao HQ, Neufeld G, Klagsbrun M (1998). Neuropilin-1 is expressed by endothelial and tumor cells as an isoform-specific receptor for vascular endothelial growth factor. *Cell* 92: 735–745.

Stacker SA, Stenvers K, Caesar C, Vitali A, Domagala T, Nice E, Roufail S, Simpson RJ, Moritz R, Karpanen T, et al. (1999). Biosynthesis of vascular endothelial growth factor-D involves proteolytic processing which generates non-covalent homodimers. *J Biol Chem* 274: 32127–32136.

Stalmans I, Ng YS, Rohan R, Fruttiger M, Bouche A, Yuce A, Fujisawa H, Hermans B, Shani M, Jansen S, et al. (2002). Arteriolar and venular patterning in retinas of mice selectively expressing VEGF isoforms. *J Clin Invest* 109: 327–336.

Stratmann A, Risau W, Plate KH (1998). Cell type-specific expression of angiopoietin-1 and angiopoietin-2 suggests a role in glioblastoma angiogenesis. *Am J Pathol* 153: 1459–1466.

Suri C, Jones PF, Patan S, Bartunkova S, Maisonpierre PC, Davis S, Sato TN, Yancopoulos GD (1996). Requisite role of angiopoietin-1, a ligand for the TIE2 receptor, during embryonic angiogenesis. *Cell* 87: 1171–1180.

Suri C, McClain J, Thurston G, McDonald DM, Zhou H, Oldmixon EH, Sato TN, Yancopoulos GD (1998). Increased vascularization in mice overexpressing angiopoietin-1. *Science* 282: 468–471.

Takakura N, Huang XL, Naruse T, Hamaguchi I, Dumont DJ, Yancopoulos GD, Suda T (1998). Critical role of the TIE2 endothelial cell receptor in the development of definitive hematopoiesis. *Immunity* 9: 677–686.

Takahashi T, Fournier A, Nakamura F, Wang LH, Murakami Y, Kalb RG, Fujisawa H, Strittmatter SM (1999). Plexin-neuropilin-1 complexes form functional semaphorin-3A receptors. *Cell* 99: 59–69.

Takahashi T, Kalka C, Masuda H, Chen D, Silver M, Kearney M, Magner M, Isner JM, Asahara T (1999). Ischemia- and cytokine-induced mobilization of bone marrow-derived endothelial progenitor cells for neovascularization. *Nat Med* 5: 434–438.

Tamagnone L, Artigiani S, Chen H, He Z, Ming GI, Song H, Chedotal A, Winberg ML, Goodman CS, Poo M, et al. (1999). Plexins are a large family of receptors for transmembrane, secreted, and GPI-anchored semaphorins in vertebrates. *Cell* 99: 71–80.

Teichert-Kuliszewska K, Maisonpierre PC, Jones N, Campbell AI, Master Z, Bendeck MP, Alitalo K, Dumont DJ, Yancopoulos GD, Stewart DJ (2001). Biological action of angiopoietin-2 in a fibrin matrix model of angiogenesis is associated with activation of Tie2. *Cardiovasc Res* 49: 659–670.

Terman BI, Carrion ME, Kovacs E, Rasmussen BA, Eddy RL, Shows TB (1991). Identification of a new endothelial cell growth factor receptor tyrosine kinase. *Oncogene* 6: 1677–1683.

Thurston G, Suri C, Smith K, McClain J, Sato TN, Yancopoulos GD, McDonald DM (1999). Leakage-resistant blood vessels in mice transgenically overexpressing angiopoietin-1. *Science* 286: 2511–2514.

Thurston G, Rudge JS, Ioffe E, Zhou H, Ross L, Croll SD, Glazer N, Holash J, McDonald DM, Yancopoulos GD (2000). Angiopoietin-1 protects the adult vasculature against plasma leakage. *Nat Med* 6: 460–463.

Valenzuela DM, Griffiths JA, Rojas J, Aldrich TH, Jones PF, Zhou H, McClain J, Copeland NG, Gilbert DJ, Jenkins NA, et al. (1999). Angiopoietins 3 and 4: diverging gene counterparts in mice and humans. *Proc Natl Acad Sci USA* 96: 1904–1909.

van der Geer P, Hunter T, Lindberg R (1994). Receptor protein-tyrosine kinases and their signal transduction pathways. *Annu Rev Cell Biol* 10: 251–337.

van der Jagt E (1932). The origin and development of the anterior lymph sacs in the sea turtle (*Thalassochelys caretta*). *Q J Microbiol Sci* 75: 151–165.

Veikkola T, Karkkainen M, Claesson-Welsh L, Alitalo K (2000). Regulation of angiogenesis via vascular endothelial growth factor receptors. *Cancer Res* 60: 203–212.

Veikkola T, Jussila L, Makinen T, Karpanen T, Jeltsch M, Petrova TV, Kubo H, Thurston G, McDonald DM, Achen MG, et al. (2001). Signalling via vascular endothelial growth factor receptor-3 is sufficient for lymphangiogenesis in transgenic mice. *EMBO J* 20: 1223–1231.

Vikkula M, Boon LM, Mulliken JB (2001). Molecular genetics of vascular malformations. *Matrix Biol* 20: 327–335.

Vikkula M, Boon LM, Mulliken JB, Olsen BR (1998). Molecular basis of vascular anomalies. *Trends Cardiovasc Med* 8: 281–292.

Vikkula M, Boon LM, Carraway KLI, Calvert JT, Diamonti AJ, Goumnerov B, Pasyk KA, Marchuk DA, Warman ML, Cantley LC, et al. (1996). Vascular dysmorphogenesis caused by an activating mutation in the receptor tyrosine kinase TIE2. *Cell* 87:1181–1190.

Wang HU, Chen Z-F, Anderson DJ (1998). Molecular distinction and angiogenic interaction between embryonic arteries and veins revealed by ephrin-B2 and its receptor Eph-B4. *Cell* 93: 741–753.

Werb Z (1997). ECM and cell surface proteolysis: regulating cellular ecology. *Cell* 91: 439–442.

Wiesmann C, Fuh G, Christinger HW, Eigenbrot C, Wells JA, de Vos AM (1997). Crystal structure at 1.7 A resolution of VEGF in complex with domain 2 of the Flt-1 receptor. *Cell* 91: 695–704.

Wilting J, Papoutsi M, Schneider M, Christ B (2000a). The lymphatic endothelium of the avian wing is of somitic origin. *Dev Dyn* 217: 271–278.

Wilting J, Schneider M, Papoutski M, Alitalo K, Christ B (2000b). An avian model for studies of embryonic lymphangiogenesis. *Lymphology* 33: 81–94.

Wise LM, Veikkola T, Mercer AA, Savory LJ, Fleming SB, Caesar C, Vitali A, Makinen T, Alitalo K, Stacker SA (1999). Vascular endothelial growth factor (VEGF)-like protein from orf virus NZ2 binds to VEGFR2 and neuropilin-1. *Proc Natl Acad Sci U S A* 96: 3071–3076.

Witte MH, Erickson R, Bernas M, Andrade M, Reiser F, Conlon W, Hoyme HE, Witte CL (1998). Phenotypic and genotypic heterogeneity in familial Milroy lymphedema. *Lymphology* 31: 145–155.

Witzenbichler B, Maisonpierre PC, Jones P, Yancopoulos GD, Isner JM (1998). Chemotactic properties of angiopoietin-1 and -2, ligands for the endothelial-specific receptor tyrosine kinase Tie2. *J Biol Chem* 273: 18514–18521.

Wybenga-Groot LE, Baskin B, Ong SH, Tong J, Pawson T, Sicheri F (2001). Structural basis for autoinhibition of the Ephb2 receptor tyrosine kinase by the unphosphorylated juxtamembrane region. *Cell* 106: 745–757.

Yamada Y, Nezu J, Shimane M, Hirata Y (1997). Molecular cloning of a novel vascular endothelial growth factor, VEGF-D. *Genomics* 42: 483–488.

Yamashita J, Itoh H, Hirashima M, Ogawa M, Nishikawa S, Yurugi T, Naito M, Nakao K (2000). Flk1-positive cells derived from embryonic stem cells serve as vascular progenitors. *Nature* 408: 92–96.

102 | *VEGFR3* and Milroy Disease

ROBERT E. FERRELL AND DAVID N. FINEGOLD

The vascular endothelial growth factor receptor-3 (VEGFR3) is a member of the VEGFR family that binds both VEGFs C and D. VEGFR3 is expressed on lymphatic endothelia and appears to be required for normal development of the lymphatic system, a process that is still poorly understood. Mutations in the gene *VEGFR3* have been found to cause Milroy disease, an inherited abnormality of the lymphatic system. This autosomal dominant disorder is characterized by swelling of the extremities, with the lower usually affected to a greater degree than the upper. Imaging studies reveal hypoplasia or aplasia of the lymphatics. The management is symptomatic, limited to manual massage and compression. Multiple, independent, nonconservative mutations in the tyrosine kinase domains of *VEGFR3* have been identified that segregate with the lymphedema phenotype in families and show defective protein kinase activity and altered stability in *in vitro* expression studies. The *Chy* mouse, a chemically mutagenized model, demonstrates a comparable mutation in the kinase domain of the mouse homolog of *VEGFR3*, and the dermal lymphatic phenotype is corrected by *VEGFC* gene therapy. This developmental abnormality appears to be an attractive model for future gene therapy trials in humans.

VEGFR3 AND LYMPHATIC DEVELOPMENT

VEGFR3 is a member of the platelet-derived growth factor receptor subfamily of class III receptor tyrosine kinases (van der Geer et al., 1994; Klagsbrun and D'Amore, 1996). VEGFR3 and the related family members VEGFR1 and VEGFR2 are expressed almost exclusively on endothelial cells and mediate the actions of the VEGF members VEGFA, VEGFB, VEGFC, and VEGFD. VEGFC and VEGFD bind to VEGFR3 and activate downstream signaling (Joukov et al., 1996; Achen et al., 1998). The VEGFRs participate in several processes essential in angiogenesis and lymphangiogenesis, including endothelial cell migration, proliferation, and survival. VEGFR3 appears to be the most critical of these receptors in the context of normal lymphatic development and the pathological development characteristic of Milroy congenital lymphedema. VEGFR3 is essential in the formation of the cardiovascular network, and *VEGFR3* knockout mouse embryos die around embryonic day (E) 9.5 due to cardiovascular failure (Dumont et al., 1998) before emergence of the lymphatic vessels. Normally, by E13 and in subsequent development, VEGFR3 expression is largely restricted to the lymphatic endothelium (Kaipainen et al., 1995; Kukk et al., 1996), and ablation of VEGFR3 signaling at this stage of development leads to aplasia of the lymphatics (Makinen et al., 2001), indicating that VEGFR3 is essential for both lymphatic development and maintenance.

MILROY DISEASE: CONGENITAL LYMPHEDEMA

In 1892 in a report to the *New York Medical Journal*, Dr. W. F. Milroy described a remarkable kindred that came to his attention when he was asked to perform an insurance physical examination on a 31-year-old man (Milroy, 1892). This individual, who was otherwise healthy, had prominent edema of one leg that extended to the knee and demonstrated a reddish discoloration with pea-sized white spots over the legs. He reported to Milroy that the swelling had been present since birth. It had grown with the limb, was never painful, did not tend to ulcerate, and had never interfered with his activities. Most re-

markable was the fact that he described this condition as a characteristic inherited from his mother. His mother, who was living in New England, had a relative who had compiled a volume of the family's history in the Americas for a period of 250 years that showed this phenotype seemed to have entered the family pedigree through marriage in 1768. Milroy summarized the occurrence of the phenotype over the subsequent six generations. Affected individuals were all similar to his proband in having one or both lower extremities demonstrating varying degrees of swelling from the feet to the entire leg. None of the family members had swelling in the upper extremities. Unique in the pedigree, one male developed "testicular swelling" to a degree that he sought removal of the testes. Milroy was at a loss to explain these observations, and when he sought advice from Dr. William Welch and Professor William Osler in Baltimore, angioneurotic edema was the only possible explanation offered. We now recognize that insufficient information was available to resolve Milroy's conundrum. He revisited this family in a 1928 report in the *Journal of the American Medical Association*, where he was able to identify 30 additional family members in the fifth, sixth, and seventh generations (Milroy, 1928). Only two additional affected individuals were identified from this group, and Milroy concluded that the trait was disappearing from the family "by attenuation of the taint through marriage with normal persons."

Sufficient evidence had accumulated by this time to suggest that the condition resulted from a defect in development of the lymphatic system. Since the original report by Milroy, many descriptions clearly documented congenital inherited lymphedema. They are monotonously similar, with lower extremity swelling consistently being the prominent feature with only rare upper extremity involvement. Dominant inheritance with varying penetrance and expressivity and congenital onset are hallmarks of the disease.

Large families continued to be identified after Milroy's account. In 1949, Schroeder and Helweg-Larsen (1950) reviewed about 100 reports of what appeared to be various forms of inherited lymphedema reported since the original descriptions of Milroy (1892, 1928), Nonne (1891), and Letessier (1865) in the 1800s. Esterly (1965) described a large seven-generation family with Milroy disease and reported the first linkage studies using traditional blood group markers and phenylthiocarbamide tasting. He meticulously addressed the inheritance patterns in his family, and others, and showed that there was no linkage between lymphedema and the genetic markers available at that time.

The true incidence of Milroy disease is unknown. Dale (1985) estimated an incidence of about 1:6000. Although this figure is frequently cited, it is likely that this is an overestimate of the incidence of Milroy disease because Dale's estimate included individuals with an age at diagnosis of up to 35 years. Smeltzer et al. (1985) estimated an annual incidence of 1.15:100,000, which may be too low; the true incidence probably is somewhere between these estimates. Because there is no reliable, inexpensive, noninvasive technique for identifying clinically indolent lymphedema, there are no true population-based estimates of the incidence. Estimating the incidence of Milroy disease is further complicated by the overlapping phenotypic manifestations of several clinically defined lymphedema syndromes. Phenotypic heterogeneity is observed, even within lymphedema families defined by the presence of a specific mutation in *VEGFR3* or *FOXC2*, the two molecularly defined forms of lymphedema.

DIAGNOSIS OF MILROY DISEASE

The diagnosis of lymphedema is a consideration in the differential diagnosis of the swollen limb (Young, 1991; Rockson, 2001). In advanced stages of the disease, a typical clinical history and physical examination often make lymphedema the logical consideration with minimal testing. However, in the early stages of swelling, a broad range of conditions must be considered. General medical conditions such as congestive heart failure, hepatic cirrhosis with concomitant increased intraabdominal pressure, and hypoalbuminemia secondary to conditions such as nephrotic syndrome are usually obvious causes of swelling of the lower extremities. Peripheral venous insufficiency is common in older patients and is the most common cause of lower extremity edema. Myxedema in older individuals will sometimes result in a brawny texture and swelling, which may be confused with lymphedema. Determination of a serum thyroid-stimulating hormone level quickly differentiates these two entities. Deep venous thrombosis may result in a swollen limb on an acute basis, but the circumstance under which it appears and the pain and rubor associated with deep venous thrombosis make lymphedema an unlikely consideration. Pelvic and abdominal malignancy may obstruct both venous and lymphatic flow, resulting in limb edema. Situations in which lymphedema develops associated with a malignancy may be entirely mechanical, but no studies have evaluated whether genetic variation exists in such patients that may predispose them to lymphatic insufficiency. Medications, especially antihypertensive drugs, and male and female hormones may cause fluid retention with resultant swelling. Lipedema is a poorly understood condition that is most typically seen in females and is associated with an unusual collection of fat commonly between the ankles and pelvis (Beninson and Edelglass, 1984; Rudkin and Miller, 1994). Sparing of the feet differentiates this condition from lymphedema.

The current standard for the diagnosis of lymphedema is lymphoscintigraphy (Mortimer, 1997). Radiolabeled macromolecular tracers such as isotopic sulfur colloid are injected infradermally into the distal affected limb. The passage of the dye through the limb is followed with use of a gamma camera. The test may be performed in a static fashion, or multiple timed images may provide a more dynamic assessment. Other noninvasive techniques such as magnetic resonance imaging, ultrasonography, and computerized axial tomography have been proposed with varying success (Rockson, 2001). At some centers, techniques such as tissue tonometry and bioelectrical impedance are used to assess small changes in tissue turgor, and the changes are used to monitor the efficacy of therapy. These procedures remain largely experimental. Direct visualization with lymphangiography is only rarely performed because of the risk of further damage to compromised lymphatics.

TREATMENT OF MILROY DISEASE

The treatment of Milroy disease has in large part been based on a multidisciplinary approach that is focused on the avoidance of traumatic and infectious complications, which might further damage a limb compromised with lymphedematous swelling. In all instances, meticulous skin hygiene is emphasized. Regular cleansing of the affected areas with a mild antiseptic soap assists in the prevention of local infection (Kinmonth, 1972). Hardened or cracked skin may be softened with creams. Avoidance of trauma is always a prudent recommendation. Blood pressure measurements should be taken in an unaffected limb, if possible, and blood should also be drawn from an unaffected limb. If suprainfections occur, they should be aggressively and promptly treated with antibiotics. Limbs with lymphedema should be treated as at risk, like the limbs of a patient with long-standing diabetes mellitus. Tinea pedis may cause cracking of the skin on the feet and should be aggressively treated. Skin complications such as hyperkeratosis, verrucae, and allergic eczema should be treated symptomatically. Early phases of swelling are treated with elevation and a fitted pressure garment.

Patient education and cooperation are key elements in preventing progressive, more recalcitrant swelling that results in chronic changes to the limb. Exercise and muscular activity augment physiological lymphatic drainage. Physical therapy and regular exercise are important to augmentation of lymphatic flow. Various techniques of gentle massage, referred to as *manual lymphatic drainage*, have become the treatment of choice for many patients despite the labor-intensive nature of this therapy. Pneumatic pumps are used in selected situations.

The critical evaluation of treatment strategies was difficult without a molecular or genetic classification scheme. This has resulted in patients being grouped on the basis of physical description of the sizes of their extremities or, rarely, on the lymphoscintographic characterization of the pattern of or absence of dermal lymphatics. Size classification is often normalized to the contralateral (normal) extremity. It is recognized that, in families with defined *VEGFR3* or *FOXC2* mutations, mutation carriers may have asymmetrical swelling. This may preclude the use of the contralateral limb as a control for treatment studies. More extensive lymphedema is usually approached more aggressively with a complex regimen of massage by the patient, family members, and therapists and coordinated bandaging followed by the application of a compressive garment to sustain the reduction in limb volume. Hafez (1996) reviewed multiple series of lymphedema treatments, including groups managed with physical therapy, drugs, and varying surgical approaches. Physical therapy, in skilled hands, is usually effective in producing some reduction in limb volume. The factors that determine the interpatient variability within a series have been speculative, again limited by lack of a classification other than anatomical.

Benzopyrones have been used mostly in filarial lymphedema, with fewer reports in hereditary and post mastectomy lymphedema (Casley-Smith, 1985, 1988). The mechanism of response for this drug appears to be through a process of macrophage activation of and reduction in the protein content of the lymphatic fluid. Other drugs have been used with varied and limited success.

Surgery appears to be indicated only in very severe cases of swelling where conservative methods have failed. No surgical procedure has been consistently effective. The results vary widely with the experience of the surgeon and the procedure chosen to create lymphatic drainage. The emerging molecular understanding of lymphedema holds the best hope for rational therapy.

MOLECULAR GENETICS OF MILROY DISEASE

The molecular basis of Milroy disease was established by linkage and candidate gene analysis in families characterized by lymphedema with a congenital or childhood diagnosis and the absence of clinical features characteristic of other described lymphedema syndromes. Linkage to chromosome 5q35 was independently established by three groups (Ferrell et al., 1998; Witte et al., 1998; Evans et al., 1999). Ferrell et al. (1998) identified a missense mutation in the positional candidate gene *VEGFR3* in one linked family and subsequently identified mutations in three additional families (Karkkainen et al., 2000). These mutations, and a subsequent mutation reported by Irrthum et al. (2000), occur exclusively in the tyrosine kinase domains of VEGFR3 and lead to an inactivation of tyrosine kinase activity (Karkkainen et al., 2000). The nature and location of the reported mutations are shown in Figure 102–1. All are nonconservative mutations in kinase domain I or II of the mature receptor. Transient overexpression of the wild-type VEGFR3 in human embryonic kidney cells, which do not normally express VEGFR3, leads to ligand-independent receptor dimerization, activation of the tyrosine kinase, and autophosphorylation. Tyrosine phosphorylation is not observed when these mutant receptors are overexpressed in the same system. When stably transfected into NIH 3T3 cells, the wild-type allele undergoes autophosphorylation in response to VEGFC stimulation, whereas none of the mutant alleles are phosphorylated after VEGFC stimulation (Irrthum et al., 2000; Karkkainen et al., 2000). Cotransfection of embryonic human kidney cells with wild-type or mutant *VEGFR3* and luciferase reporter constructs containing activating protein-1– and nuclear-factor-κB *cis*-acting transcription factor–binding sequences verified defective downstream signaling function of the mutant receptors. Receptor expression and function have not been characterized in lymphatic endothelial cells derived from mutation carriers.

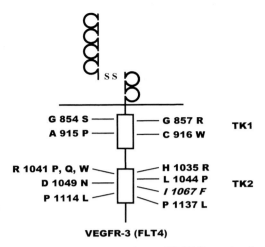

Figure 102–1. Missense mutations in human VEGFR3 tyrosine domains −1 (TK1) and −2 (TK2) in primary lymphedema (Milroy disease) and in the *Chy* Mouse. Schematic of the genomic structure of human vascular endothelial growth factor receptor-3 (*VEGFR3*) showing the location of the tyrosine kinase domains. The expanded view of the tyrosine kinase domains shows the location of six mutations identified in families with primary lymphedema and shown to be kinase negative in vitro. The kinase domain II I1067F mutation is responsible for the *Chy* phenotype in the mouse. The extracellular P641S variation is a common single-nucleotide polymorphism.

Families with mutations in *VEGFR3* are characterized by an early onset age, with 96% of cases being congenital. Lymphedema is the predominant phenotypic manifestation in families with documented *VEGFR3* mutations. The overall penetrance in these families is 0.62, with sex-specific penetrance of 0.53 and 0.71 in males and females, respectively. The female/male ratio of 1.5 estimated from families with *VEGFR3* mutations is similar to that reported by Smeltzer et al. (1985) but not as skewed as that estimated from earlier phenotype-based studies (Kinmonth et al., 1957; Schirger et al., 1962; Feins et al., 1977). Neither the reduced penetrance nor the skewed sex ratio among affecteds in families with molecularly defined mutations is understood.

It is unclear whether there are yet-to-be-detected mutations in *VEGFR3*, occurring outside the kinase domains, that cause lymphedema. Small families compatible with linkage to chromosome 5q, but with no detected mutation in *VEGFR3*, have been reported by several groups (Ferrell et al., 1998; Witte et al., 1998). Holberg et al. (2001) described several families with a clinical presentation indistinguishable from the phenotype of Milroy's families with *VEGFR3* mutations in which there was evidence of linkage to other chromosomal locations. These results suggest the possibility that Milroy disease is genetically heterogeneous.

MODELS OF MILROY DISEASE

In the mouse, disruption of members of the *VEGFR* family leads to early embryonic death due to failure of blood vessel development. Vegfr3-deficient embryos appear grossly normal through E9.0 with normal appearing myocardium, endocardium, and small blood vessels. However, defects are observed in sites of Vegfr3 expression, with irregularly formed large vessels with defective lumens. By E10, embryos are severely growth retarded with underdeveloped yolk sac vasculature. Vegfr3 appears to be necessary for normal remodeling of the yolk sac capillary network into complex vitelline vessels (Dumont et al., 1998). Heterozygous embryos and newborns are phenotypically normal, with normal appearing lymphatics. Because deficiency of Vegfr3 is developmentally lethal before the emergence of the lymphatic vessels, a more informative model for altered lymphangiogenesis is the targeted dermal expression of soluble Vegfr3. Expression of a chimeric protein consisting of the extracellular, ligand-binding domain of VEGFR3 and the Fc domain of the Ig-γ chain under control of the keratin 14 promoter leads to high-level expression around E14.5 and neutralizes the activities of VegfC and VegfD. This disruption of Vegfr3 signaling inhibits the formation of dermal lymphatics. Expression of the *VEGFR3-Ig* transgene also leads to the regression of previously formed lymphatics, indicating that intact signaling through Vegfr3 is vital to both the formation and maintenance of the normal lymphatic vasculature (Makinen et al., 2001). The gross phenotype of the *VEGFR3-Ig* mouse resembles that of Milroy disease with hypoplasia or aplasia of the dermal lymphatics with impaired macromolecular transport and increased fluid accumulation with visible swelling of the extremities. Older mice show thickening of the skin and dermal fibrosis.

Congenital lymphedema characterized by aplasia or hyperplasia of the lymphatics has been described in the dog (Luginbuhl et al., 1967; Patterson et al., 1967), the pig (van der Putte, 1978), and cattle (Morris et al., 1954), but none of these animal models have been characterized at the molecular level. The *Chy* mouse was first described by Lyon and Glenister (1984, 1986) as an ethyl nitrosourea–induced mutation characterized by a gross phenotype of chylous ascites and swollen, edematous hind feet. The *Chy* phenotype maps to mouse chromosome 11 in a region homologous to human chromosome 5q. Like humans with Milroy disease, the *Chy* mouse has an inactivating mutation in the tyrosine kinase II domain of VEGFR3 and hypoplastic cutaneous lymphatic vessels (Karkkainen et al., 2001). When the *Chy* mouse was mated with the heterozygous *VEGFR3*-null mouse, no viable *Chy*⁻ offspring were born. At E105, *Chy*⁻ embryos were growth retarded similar to *Vegfr3*-null embryos.

Local delivery of VEGFC, a ligand for Vegfr3, via adeno-associated virus–mediated delivery of recombinant human VEGFC stimulated the production of functional lymphatic vessels in the ears of *Chy* mice. In addition, crosses between the *Chy* mouse and the K14-VEGF-C156S mouse, which overexpresses the VEGFR3-specific ligand VEGF-C1565 in skin keratinocytes (Veikkola et al., 2001) led to restored lymphatic function in the *Chy* × K14-VEGF-C156S offspring. These experiments demonstrate that normal lymphatic function can be restored in the *Vegfr3* mutant *Chy* mouse via delivery of an excess of receptor ligand.

MOLECULAR PATHOGENESIS OF MILROY DISEASE

Milroy congenital lymphedema due to *VEGFR3* mutation is inherited as an autosomal dominant phenotype. Mice heterozygous for a null allele at the *Vegfr3* locus display no overt phenotype, and humans with chromosomal abnormalities leading to deletion of the chromosome region containing the *VEGFR3* gene do not display lymphedema as a phenotype (Barber et al., 1996; Groen et al., 1998). This suggests that lymphedema is not due to haploinsufficiency for *VEGFR3*.

Endocytosis of activated tyrosine kinase receptors through clathrin-coated pits is a well-established mechanism for regulating the duration of receptor-mediated signaling (DiFiore and deCamilli, 2001). When coexpressed with the wild-type receptor in stably transfected cells, the mutant VEGFR3 is weakly transphosphorylated in response to VEGFC stimulation, indicating that dimers between mutant and wild-type receptors are formed. However, the rate of decay of wild-type receptors was faster than that of mutant receptors and the mutant receptor is highly stable on the cell surface. In cells coexpressing the receptors, the half-life of the mutant receptor was 40% longer than that of the wild-type. Altered processing of mutant receptors suggests a mechanism by which mutant receptors accumulating on the cell surface may interfere with normal VEGFC signaling in individuals heterozygous for a kinase-defective allele. This is consistent with the observation that the expression of a kinase-negative mutant of *VEGFR1* in glioblastoma cells abrogates their response to the mitogenic actions of VEGFA (Millauer et al., 1994). The dominant mode of inheritance of Milroy disease reflects the dominant-negative action of tyrosine kinase domain mutations.

There are no biologically based therapies for lymphedema, and therapies offer only symptomatic relief. Although primary lymphedema is a rare condition, the demonstration by Karkkainen et al. (2001) that local delivery of VEGFC can ameliorate the cutaneous lymphatic hypoplasia of primary lymphedema in the mouse model of Milroy disease suggests a possible route to rational therapeutic intervention. Secondary lymphedema arising after surgical disruption of the lymphatic network may be an even more promising target for local VEGFC therapy. In this case, the site of the lymphatic damage is localized, and the underlying lymphatic endothelium has functional VEGFC receptors. However, native VEGFC also binds VEGFR2 expressed on vascular endothelium and has the potential to increase vascular permeability and perhaps stimulate abnormal angiogenesis. The findings that, at least in the mouse, the mutant *VEGFC, VEGF-C156S*, is specific for Vegfr3, has a very short biological half-life, and stimulates lymphaniogenesis but not angiogenesis (Veikkola et al., 2001) suggest that the potential risks of VEGFC therapy can be reduced through targeted mutagenesis. The potential therapeutic usefulness of VEGFC is supported by the report that human VEGFC delivered locally via injection stimulated lymphatic regeneration in a rabbit model of postsurgical lymphatic insufficiency (Szuba et al., 2002). The potential for growth factor therapy in lymphedema syndromes such as lymphedemadistichiasis syndrome or in secondary lymphedema associated with filariasis awaits a more thorough understanding of the molecular pathology of these conditions.

REFERENCES

Achen MG, Jeltsch M, Kukk E, Makinen T, Vitali A, Wilks AF, Alitalo K, Stacker SA (1998). Vascular endothelial growth factor D (VEGFD) is a ligand for the tyrosine kinases VEGF receptor 2 (Flk1) and VEGF receptor 3 (Flt4). *Proc Nat Acad Sci USA* 95: 548–553.

Barber JCK, Temple IK, Campbell PL, Collinson MN, Campbell CM, Renshaw RM, Dennis NR (1996). Unbalanced translocation in a mother and her son in one of two 5;10 translocation families. *Am J Med Genet* 62: 84–90.

Beninson J, Edelglass JW (1984). Lipedema—the non-lymphatic masquerader. *Angiology* 35: 506–510.

Casley-Smith JR (1985). The effects of diosmin (a benzo-pyrone) upon some high-protein oedemas: lung contusion, and burn and lymphoedema of rat legs. *Agents Actions* 17: 14–20.

Casley-Smith JR (1988). The pathophysiology of lymphedema and the action of benzopyrones in reducing it. *Lymphology* 21: 190–194.

Dale RF (1985). The inheritance of primary lymphoedema. *J Med Genet* 22: 274–278.

DiFiore PP, DeCamilli P (2001). Endocytosis and signaling: An inseparable partnership. *Cell* 106: 1–4.

Dumont DJ, Jussila L, Taipale J, Lymboussaki A, Mustonen T, Pajusola K, Breitman M, Alitalo K (1998). Cardiovascular failure in mouse embryos deficient in VEGF receptor-3. *Science* 282: 946–949.

Esterly JR (1965). Congenital hereditary lymphoedema. *J Med Genet* 2: 93–98.

Evans AL, Brice G, Sotirova V, Mortimer P, Beninson J, Burnand K, Rosbotham J, Child A, Sarfarazi M (1999). Mapping of primary congenital lymphedema to the 5q35.3 region. *Am J Hum Genet* 64: 547–555.

Feins NR, Rubin R, Crais T, O'Connor JF (1977). Surgical management of thirty-nine children with lymphedema. *J Pediatr Surg* 12: 471–476.

Ferrell RE, Levinson KL, Esman JH, Kimak MA, Lawrence EC, Barmada MM, Finegold DN (1998). Hereditary lymphedema: evidence for linkage and genetic heterogeneity. *Hum Mol Genet* 7: 2073–2078.

Groen SE, Drewes JG, deBoer EG, Hoovers JMN, Hennekam RCM (1998). Repeated unbalanced offspring due to a familial translocation involving chromosomes 5 and 6. *Am J Med Genet* 80: 448–453.

Hafez HM, Wolfe JH (1996). Lymphedema: basic data underlying clinical decision making. *Ann Vasc Surg* 10: 88–95.

Holberg CJ, Erickson RP, Bernas MJ, Witte MH, Fultz KE, Andrade M, Witte CL (2001). Segregation analysis and a genome-wide linkage search confirm genetic heterogeneity and suggest oligogenic inheritance in some Milroy congenital primary lymphedema families. *Am J Med Genet* 98: 303–312.

Irrthum A, Karkkainen MJ, Devriendt K, Alitalo K, Vikkula M (2000). Congenital hereditary lymphedema caused by a mutation that inactivates VEGFR3 tyrosine kinase. *Am J Hum Genet* 67: 295–301.

Joukov V, Pajusola K, Kaipainen A, Chilov D, Lahtinen I, Kukk E, Saksela O, Kalkkinen N, Alitalo K (1996). A novel vascular endothelial growth factor, VEGFC, is a lig-

and for the Flt4 (VEGFR3) and KDR (VEGFR2) receptor tyrosine kinases. *EMBO J* 15: 290–298.

Kaipainen A, Korhonen J, Mustonen T, van Hinsbergh VWM, Fang GH, Dumont D, Breitman M, Alitalo K (1995). Expression of the fms-like tyrosine kinase-4 gene becomes restricted to lymphatic endothelium during development. *Proc Natl Acad Sci USA* 92: 3566–3570.

Karkkainen MJ, Ferrell RE, Lawrence EC, Kimak MA, Levinson KL, McTigue MA, Alitalo K, Finegold DN (2000). Missense mutations interfere with VEGFR3 signalling in primary lymphedema. *Nat Genet* 25: 153–159.

Karkkainen MJ, Saaristo A, Jussila L, Karila KA, Lawrence EC, Pajusola K, Bueler H, Eichmann A, Kauppinen R, Kettunen MI, et al. (2001). A model for gene therapy of human hereditary lymphedema. *Proc Natl Acad Sci USA* 98: 12677–12682.

Kinmonth JB (1972). 17-Conservative treatment of lymphoedema. In: *The Lymphatics: Diseases, Lymphography and Surgery.* Kinmonth JB (ed.) Edward Arnold Ltd, Edinburgh.

Kinmonth JB, Taylor GW, Tracy GD, Marsh JD (1957). Primary lymphedema: clinical and lymphangiographic studies of a series of 107 patients in which the lower limbs were affected. *Br J Surg* 45: 1–10.

Klagsbrun M, D'Amore PA (1996). Vascular endothelial growth factor and its receptor. *Cytokine Growth Factor Rev* 7: 259–270.

Kukk E, Lymboussaki A, Taira S, Kaipainen A, Jeltsch M, Joukov V, Alitalo K (1996). VEGF-C receptor binding and pattern of expression with VEGFR-3 suggests a role in lymphatic vascular development. *Development* 122: 3829–3837.

Letessier EE (1865). De l'elephhantiasis des arabes et de son heredite. Thesis, Strassbourg.

Luginbuhl H, Chacko SK, Patterson DF, Medway W (1967). Congenital hereditary lymphedema in the dog. Pathological studies. *J Med Genet* 4: 153–165.

Lyon MF, Glenister PH (1984) Chylous ascites (*Chy*). *Mouse News Lett* 71: 26.

Lyon MF, Glenister PH (1986). Gene order of *chy-vt-re* on mouse chromosome 11. *Mouse News Lett* 74: 96.

Makinen T, Jussila L, Veikkola T, Karpanen T, Kettunen MI, Pulkkanen KJ, Kauppinen R, Jackson DG, Kubo H, Nishikawa SI, et al. (2001). Inhibition of lymphangiogenesis with resulting lymphedema in transgenic mice expressing soluble VEGF-receptor-3. *Nat Med* 7: 199–205.

Millauer B, Shawver LK, Plate KH, Risau W, Ulrich A (1994). Glioblastoma growth inhibited *in vivo* by a dominant-negative Flk-1 mutant. *Nature* 367: 576–579.

Milroy WF (1892). An undescribed variety of hereditary oedema. *N Y Med J* 56: 505–508.

Milroy WF (1928). Chronic hereditary edema: Milroy disease. *JAMA* 91: 1172–1175.

Morris B, Blood DC, Sidman WR, Steel JD, Whittem JH (1954). Congenital lymphatic oedema in Ayrshire calves. *Austral J Exp Biol* 32: 265–274.

Mortimer PS (1997). Therapy approaches for lymphedema. *Angiology* 48: 87–91.

Nonne M (1891). Vier falle von elephantiasis congenita heredituria. *Arch Pathol Anat Physiol* 125: 189–190.

Patterson DF, Medway W, Luginbuhl H, Chacko S (1967). Congenital hereditary lymphedema in the dog. Clinical and genetic studies. *J Med Genet* 4: 145–152.

Rockson SG (2001). Lymphedema. *Am J Med* 110: 288–295.

Rudkin GH, Miller TA (1994). Lipedema: a clinical entity distinct from lymphedema. *Plast Reconstr Surg* 94: 841–847.

Schirger A, Harrison EG Jr, James JM (1962). Idiopathic lymphedema: review of 131 cases. *JAMA* 182: 14–22.

Schroeder E, Helweg-Larsen HF (1950). Chronic hereditary lymphedema (Nonne-Milroy-Meige's disease). *Acta Med Scand* 87: 198–216.

Smeltzer DM, Stickler GB, Schirger A (1985). Primary lymphedema in children and adolescents: a follow-up study and review. *Pediatrics* 76: 206–218.

Szuba A, Skoke M, Shin W, Beynet DP, Rockson NB, Dakhil N, Goris ML, Strauss HW, Quertermous T, Alitalo K (2002). Therapeutic lymphangiogenesis in a rabbit ear model of chronic post-surgical lymphatic insufficiency. *FASEB J* 16: A516.

van der Geer P, Hunter T, Lindberg RA (1994). Receptor protein-tyrosine kinases and their signal transduction pathways. *Annu Rev Cell Biol* 10: 251–337.

van der Putte (1978). Congenital hereditary lymphedema in the pig. *Lymphology* 11: 1–9.

Veikkola T, Jussila L, Makinen T, Karpanen T, Jeltsch M, Petrova TV, Kubo H, Thurston G, McDonald DM, Achen MG, et al. (2001). Signaling via vascular endothelial growth factor receptor-3 is sufficient for lymphangiogenesis in transgenic mice. *EMBO J* 20: 1223–1231.

Witte MH, Erickson R, Bernas M, Andrade M, Reiser F, Conlon W, Hoyme HE, Witte CL (1998). Phenotypic and genotypic heterogeneity in familial Milroy lymphedema. *Lymphology* 31: 145–155.

Young JR (1991). The swollen leg: clinical significance and differential diagnosis. *Cardiol Clin Peripheral Vasc Dis Elderly* 9: 443–456.

Part I.
Transporters

103 | ## *KCNJ2* (Kir2.1) and Andersen Syndrome

DAVID R. RENNER, RABI TAWIL, MARTIN TRISTANI-FIROUZI,
AND LOUIS J. PTÁČEK

Andersen syndrome (AS) (OMIM 170390) is a rare autosomal dominant disorder characterized by the triad of dysmorphic features, prolonged QT intervals with ventricular dysrhythmias, and episodic paralysis (Tawil et al., 1994; Sansone et al., 1997; Canún et al., 1999). Prior studies excluded linkage to the hyperkalemic periodic paralysis *SCN4A* locus on chromosome 17, the long QT syndrome (LQTS) locus on chromosome 11 (*KCNQ1*), and the *CACNA1S* locus on chromosome 1. An AS gene was linked to markers on chromosome 17q23 near the inward rectifying potassium channel gene *KCNJ2*, encoding Kir2.1. Sequencing *KCNJ2* in the linked family identified a mutation D71V in the N terminus of the protein. Twelve additional mutations were identified in highly conserved regions of the channel. This disorder is the first to illustrate a direct link between skeletal and cardiac muscle excitability, as well as a link between paroxysmal cell hyper-excitability and developmental phenotypes. One of the authors (L.P.) has proposed renaming the syndrome the Andersen/Tawil syndrome (ATS) (Donaldson et al., 2003).

ION CHANNELS ARE REQUISITE FOR THE PROPER FUNCTIONING OF ELECTRICALLY EXCITABLE TISSUE

The periodic paralyses and nondystrophic myotonias compose a group of disorders in which patients experience myotonia (delayed relaxation of muscle after voluntary contraction or mechanical stimulation) and/or paroxysmal weakness of their extremities. Although classification of these periodic paralyses and nondystrophic myotonias has previously been based on the presence or absence of myotonia with weakness, effect of administered potassium, and temperature sensitivity, we now understand that these entities result from mutations in specific genes encoding ion channels. (McClatchey et al., 1992; Ptáček et al., 1993). The result of these specific ion channel abnormalities, or channelopathies, affects excitable tissues such as nerve, skeletal muscle, and cardiac muscle, as well as nonexcitable tissues, such as the kidney.

The first mutations in an ion channel to account for a human paroxysmal disorder was characterized one decade ago when mutations in *SCN4A*, the gene that encodes a voltage-gated sodium channel, was shown to cause hyperkalemic periodic paralysis (Ptáček et al., 1991; Rojas et al., 1991). The understanding that channelopathies could account for paroxysmal symptoms led to predictions that cardiac dysrhythmias could be accounted for by mutations in homologous genes (Ptáček et al., 1991). Since that time, periodic paralysis has been associated with mutations in voltage-gated K^+, Na^+, Ca^{2+}, and Cl^- channels (Jen and Ptáček, 2001) (Table 103–1). In addition, LQTS has been associated with mutations in the voltage-gated K^+ and Na^+ channels (Sanguinetti, 2001).

An understanding of basic membrane physiology has implicated ion channels as candidates for heritable diseases of muscle and cardiac excitability. Muscle membrane excitability is dependent on intracellular versus extracellular concentrations of numerous ions. In the rest-

Table 103–1. Ion Channel Mutations and Their Respective Neuromuscular Disorders

Sodium channel disorders: chromosome 17q locus (*SCN4A*)
  Hyperkalemic periodic paralysis
  Paramyotonia congenita
  Potassium aggravated myotonia
  Hyperkalemic periodic paralysis with paramyotonia congenita
  Hypokalemic periodic paralysis
Calcium channel disorders: chromosome 1q locus (*CACNA1S*)
  Hypokalemic periodic paralysis
Chloride channel disorders: chromosome 7q locus (*CLCN1*)
  Myotonia congenita
    Becker's disease
    Thomsen's disease
Potassium channel disorders: chromosome 21q locus (*KCNE2*)
  Andersen syndrome
  Hyperkalemic periodic paralysis
  Hypokalemic periodic paralysis
Unknown potential channel disorders
  Thyrotoxic periodic paralysis
  Chondrodystrophic myotonia

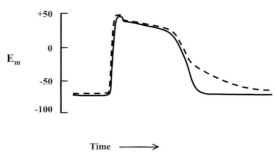

Figure 103–2. Delayed repolarization in the heart could lead to hyperexcitability. Kir2.1 assists in generating the cardiac inward rectifier current (I_{K1}). I_{K1} contributes repolarizing current during the terminal phase of the cardiac action potential. The normal cardiac action potential is depicted by the solid line. Reduction of Kir2.1 function is believed to prolong the cardiac action potential (dotted line) and QT intervals by reducing the amount of repolarizing current during the terminal phase. Prolongation of the action potential is a prerequisite for early afterdepolarizations and a possible trigger for ventricular tachycardia.

ing state, Na^+ and Ca^{2+} ions are at higher concentrations extracellularly than intracellularly. In contrast, K^+ and Cl^- ions are held in higher concentrations intracellularly. This balance between high intracellular potassium and low intracellular sodium is maintained by active transport through specific ion transporters. When the muscle membrane is depolarized, threshold potentials are reached, and voltage-gated Na^+ channels become activated, leading to an increase in Na^+ conductance, and fast Na^+ influx into a cell. As the negative interior of the cell becomes positive (depolarization), Na^+ channels inactivate and Cl^- and K^+ conductances rise, allowing K^+ ions to diffuse out of the cell through K^+-selective channels, and Cl^- to move inside. This reestablishes the negative membrane potential (E_m), after which active transporters reestablish the ionic gradients. When this balance of ion flux is disrupted, as with mutations in Kir2.1, K^+ conductance becomes reduced, shifting toward the depolarized direction and thus inactivating Na^+ channels, making them unavailable for the initiation and propagation of action potentials (Fig. 103–1).

Cardiac membrane excitability is similar to that of muscle. With the depolarization of myocardium, the transmemembrane potential reverses, resulting in positive overshoot. Immediately after this upstroke, there is a brief period of partial repolarization (phase 1) followed by a plateau (phase 2) that persists for about 0.1 to 0.2 second. The potential becomes progressively more negative (phase 3) until the resting state of repolarization is again achieved (Fig. 103–2). Inward rectifying K^+ (Kir) channels contribute to cell excitability and resting membrane potential during the final repolarization phase by passing small amounts of K^+ out of the myocyte and bringing the membrane potential back to resting membrane potential (Plaster et al., 2001). Reduction in the function of the inward rectifying current (as can be seen

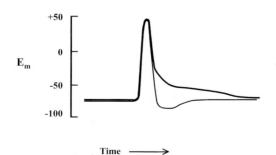

Figure 103–1. Delayed repolarization in muscle could lead to inexcitability. Kir2.1 modulates skeletal muscle excitability. Wild-type Kir2.1 function normally (thin line). Mutations in Kir2.1 reduce the resting K^+ conductance such that E_m is shifted in the depolarized direction (thick line), toward the equilibrium potential of Cl^-. Depolarization of cell membrane inactivates Na^+ channels, making them unavailable for initiation and propagation of action potentials.

with mutations in Kir2.1) is believed to prolong the cardiac action potential and QT intervals by reducing the amount of repolarizing current during the terminal phase. Prolonged action potentials are believed to be prerequisites for early afterdepolarizations, a possible trigger for ventricular tachycardia.

Proper ion channel functioning is requisite for the normal functioning of skeletal and cardiac muscle. With specific ion channel abnormalities, defects in membrane excitability of nerve, skeletal muscle, and cardiac myocytes may manifest.

POTASSIUM ION CHANNELS

The potassium channels are ion-specific macromolecular proteins that span the lipid bilayer of cells, including nerves, skeletal muscle, and cardiac myocytes. Voltage-gated skeletal muscle potassium channels are composed in part of an α subunit with a single domain with six putative membrane-spanning segments (S1 to S6) (Fig. 103–3A). Four α subunits associate to form a tetramer, which is requisite for a functional channel. Often, this tetramer associates with β subunits. The N-terminal portion of the a subunit protein serves as an inactivation gate of the Shaker-like class of voltage-gated K^+ channels (Hoshi et al., 1990). Inactivation of potassium channels can be eliminated via removal of this N terminus, as demonstrated by site-directed mutagenesis. This inactivation can be restored with coexpression of the N-terminal peptide along with truncated α subunits (Hoshi et al., 1990).

Kir channels are similar in structure to voltage-gated K^+ channels, although they are missing the four N-terminal transmembrane domains, including the S4 voltage sensor. Kir channels consist of an intracellular N-terminal domain, two transmembrane segments (M1 and M2) flanking a pore region, and an intracellular C-terminal segment. M1 and M2 correspond to S5 and S6 of the voltage-gated K^+ channel (Plaster et al., 2001) (see Fig. 103–3B). Kir subunits organize to form either homotetramers or heterotetramers (Yang et al., 1995) (Fig. 103–4).

There are multiple families of potassium channels. One subfamily of these potassium channels is encoded by *KCNE* genes, which encode MinK-related peptides, single transmembrane subunits that function as regulatory β subunits. Of the five members of this subfamily already identified (*KCNE1* through *KCNE5*), one (*KCNE3*) has been shown through two hybrid screening techniques, co-immunoprecipitation, and co-localization to associate with a pore-forming Kv3.4 potassium channel a subunit (Abbott et al., 2001).

KCNE3 is located on chromosome 11q and codes for a 103-residue peptide (MiRP2) that is expressed in skeletal muscle. MiRP2 is a β subunit that associates with the Kv3.4 pore-forming potassium channel α subunit to form stable complexes. Together, these MiRP2-Kv3.4 heteromultimers co-localize to plasma membranes and are most abundantly expressed in skeletal muscle. Four α subunits are requisite for a functional unit; however, Kv3.4 attains functionally distinct properties when it associates with MiRP2.

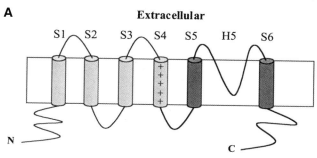

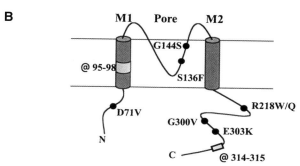

Figure 103–3. (*A*) Voltage-gated potassium channel. The potassium channel α subunit is depicted containing six membrane-spanning segments (S1 to S6). An auxiliary protein, MiRP2, associates with pore-forming Kv3.4 potassium channel α subunits (comprised of S1 to S6). S4 contains positively charged residues every third position and acts as a voltage sensor. Together, the MiRP2-Kv3.4 heteromultimers localize to skeletal muscle membranes to form a rapidly recovering potassium channel. A functional voltage-gated potassium channel is formed by four α subunits clustered around a central ion pore. (*B*) Inward rectifying potassium channel (Kir2.1). Kir channels are similar to voltage-gated potassium channels, although they are missing four of the N-terminal transmembrane domains, including the S4 voltage sensor. The channel consists of an intracellular N-terminal domain, two transmembrane segments (M1 and M2) flanking a central pore, and an intracellular C-terminal segment. M1 and M2 correspond to S5 and S6 of the voltage gated K$^+$ channel. Kir2.1 mutations are depicted.

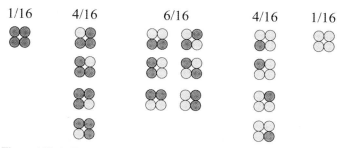

Figure 103–4. Homotetramers and heterotetramers of the Kir subunits. Kir subunits organize to form either homomultimers or heteromultimers. Because Andersen syndrome is inherited in an autosomal dominant manner, with affected individuals possessing one normal (dark) and one mutant (light) *KCNJ2* allele, 15 of 16 channels will contain one or more mutant subunits.

mandibular hypoplasia, soft and hard palate defects, scaphocephaly, clinodactyly, short stature, ventricular extrasystoles, and paroxysmal weakness was made by Andersen et al. (1971). The disorder was subsequently characterized in detail years later by Tawil, who named the triad *Andersen syndrome* (Tawil et al., 1994; Sansone et al., 1997).

Dysmorphisms are often mild, can vary between affected family members, and are occasionally absent. When present, significant examination findings include short stature, low-set ears, broad nose, hyperteleorism, micrognathia, high arched palate, scaphocephaly, and scoliosis (Renner and Ptáček, 2001) (Fig. 103–5). The severity of dysmorphisms does not correlate with the involvement of heart or skeletal muscle, illustrating the variability of expressivity in AS (Canún et al., 1999, Tristani-Firouzi et al., 2002).

Patients with AS usually experience their first episode of paralysis between ages 4 to 18 years. The attacks often present during rest after exercise and follow stressful or emotional events. The attacks usually last hours to several days and are followed by a return of strength to baseline. In individuals with AS and hypokalemic attacks of weakness, potassium ingestion can result in a more rapid recovery of strength. Weakness can be incapacitating, at worst leading to tetraparesis and a nonambulatory state. Most often, the degree of ictal weakness is mild to moderate. As with other forms of periodic paralyses, continued gentle exercise can ameliorate the weakness (Canún et al., 1999). Temperature and intakes of sodium and carbohydrate usually have no effect on these paroxysms of weakness.

Objective examination during an attack usually demonstrates proximal more than distal weakness with minimal (if any) weakness of swallowing and respiratory muscles. Between attacks, strength is initially normal. However, approximately 50% of patients with AS will develop varying degrees of interattack weakness. Myotonia is not gen-

CLINICAL DESCRIPTION

AS is a rare syndrome that is characterized by the triad of (1) hyperkalemic, normokalemic, or hypokalemic periodic paralysis, (2) prolonged QT interval with ventricular arrhythmias, and (3) dysmorphic features. The first clinical description of a male with hyperteleorism,

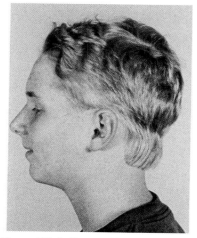

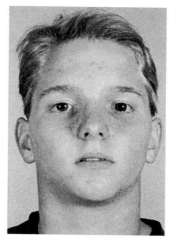

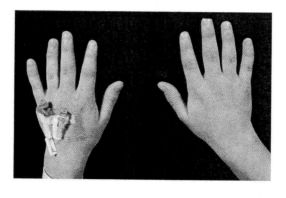

Figure 103–5. Dysmorphisms. This profile of an individual with Andersen syndrome reveals prominent micrognathia and low-set ears. Hyperteleorism is evident in the frontal view. His fingers curve medially at the distal interpha-langeal joints of the fifth fingers bilaterally (clinodactyly). (Reproduced with modifications from Plaster et al., 2001.)

erally elicited on examination. Sensory examination is normal. Deep tendon reflexes are usually preserved.

The onset of cardiac arrhythmias does not correlate with the onset of muscle weakness. However, like the weakness, cardiac symptoms tend to start within the first two decades of life. Syncope and palpitations are the most common cardiac presenting symptoms. Patients rarely present with cardiac arrest (Canún et al., 1999). Characteristic rhythm disturbances range from asymptomatic polymorphic ventricular ectopy to runs of ventricular tachycardia (typically polymorphic, but occasionally bidirectional), to potentially fatal sustained ventricular tachycardia and torsades des pointes (Levitt et al., 1972; Canún et al., 1999). The underlying cause for these rhythm disturbances is abnormality of cardiac repolarization that results in a prolonged QT interval.

MOLECULAR GENETICS

Because long QT intervals are associated with this syndrome, linkage to the LQTS (*LQT1*, *LQT2*, and *LQT3*) on chromosome 11 was tested and excluded (Tawil et al., 1994). In addition, prior reports of AS patients manifesting hyperkalemia during episodes of weakness raised suspicion that the a subunit of the skeletal muscle sodium channel may be involved. This also was tested and excluded (Sansone et al., 1997). Mutational analysis did not implicate the dihydropyridine receptor (*DHPR*) gene.

An AS allele was identified and localized on chromosome 17q23, an area that contains three ion channel genes: *KCNJ2* (encoding the Kir channel), *CACNG1* (encoding the calcium channel), and *SCN4A* (encoding the sodium channel) (Fig. 103–6). Prior studies demonstrated that *SCN4A* was responsible for periodic paralysis without cardiac or developmental abnormalities (Ptácek et al., 1991); *CACNG1* mRNA was not detectable in the heart. Given the known function and expression pattern of the gene product of *KCNJ2* (Kir2.1), *KCNJ2* was considered the best candidate gene for AS.

Kir2.1 is a member of the Kir2.x family of inward rectifying K^+ channels and is encoded by the gene *KCNJ2* (Fig. 103–7). It is expressed in the heart, brain, and skeletal muscle, although its function has been studied primarily in the heart (Kubo et al., 1993). (Inward rectification refers to the inward flux of K^+ ions at potentials negative to the K^+ equilibrium potential [E_k] more readily than outward flux at potentials positive to E_k.) Kir2.1 is one component of the inward rectifier K^+ current, I_{k1}. As a strong inward rectifier, it prevents the excess loss of K^+ during the plateau phase (phase 2) of the cardiac action potential. In addition, it allows outward K^+ flux during terminal repolarization and diastolic phases of the action potential (Sanguinetti and Tristani-Firouzi, 2000). Although it has been studied extensively in the heart, much less is known about its role in skeletal muscle and neurons; however, its function is likely similar in these tissues, that is, controlling the resting membrane potential and the terminal repolarization phase of the action potential.

DNA from 15 members of a kindred with a clinical diagnosis of

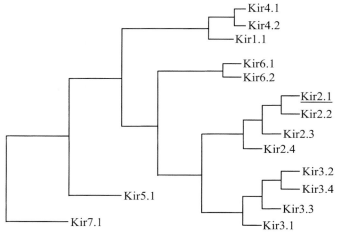

Figure 103–7. Kirs are composed of seven subfamilies.

AS was amplified and sequenced. An A-to-T transversion corresponding to the D71V mutation was identified in all affected members but not in any unaffected members. Subsequently, 29 additional unrelated probands with a clinical diagnosis of AS were examined for mutations in the *KCNJ2*. Thirteen mutations were identified in 20 of these probands. Eleven of 13 mutations were missense mutations. All mutations occurred at highly conserved residues (see Fig. 103–3B).

The mutations in D71V and R218W cause varying degrees of dominant-negative suppression of channel function. Co-expression of wild-type and D71V or R218W Kir2.1 has been found experimentally to induce an inwardly rectifying K^+ current that was markedly reduced. AS is inherited in an autosomal dominant manner. Based on the assumptions that affected individuals possess one normal and one mutant *KCNJ2* allele, that wild-type and mutant alleles are expressed equally, and that co-assembly between wild-type and mutant subunits is random, then one-sixteenth of channels would be predicted to be composed entirely of wild-type homomultimers (containing no mutant subunits), with fifteen-sixteenths of channels containing at least one mutant subunit. Therefore, if a single mutant subunit (or possibly two) is sufficient to disrupt the function of these tetramers, then a large majority of the tetramers (approximately fifteen-sixteenths) would be expected to be dysfunctional, resulting in a strong dominant negative effect. As expected, the reduction in current induced by co-expressed wild type and D71V subunits approximates fifteen-sixteenths of the wild-type current, suggesting that one mutant subunit is sufficient to markedly reduce channel function (Plaster et al., 2001).

ESTABLISHING THE DIAGNOSIS

Little has been published regarding criteria needed to diagnose AS. Previous studies, which have taken into account the variable penetrance of AS, have classified individuals as affected if two of the following three criteria were met: paroxysmal weakness, prolonged corrected QT interval (QTc) with or without ventricular dysrhythmias, and characteristic dysmorphic features. AS should be included in the differential diagnosis of any individual with documented LQTS, even in the absence of periodic paralysis or dysmorphism, because some family members of patients with the full triad demonstrate only prolonged QT intervals. Similarly, electrocardiograms should be performed on all patients with suspected periodic paralysis for careful measurement of the QTc interval.

The diagnosis of AS is often rendered when an individual with a history of paroxysmal weakness is noted to have electrocardiographic abnormalities. The diagnosis is often overlooked, however, because the cardiac abnormalities, as with periodic muscle weakness, can be transient and thus may be missed on routine electrocardiography. Thus, when AS is suspected and the electrocardiogram is unremarkable, a Holter monitor can capture episodic dysrhythmias and provide longer tracings for QT-interval analysis. Cardiac monitoring under provocative

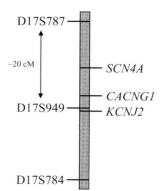

Figure 103–6. Andersen syndrome allele location with surrounding ion channel genes. An Andersen syndrome allele was identified and located on chromosome 17q23. This area contained three ion channel genes: Kir channel *KCNJ2*, calcium channel *CACNG1*, and sodium channel *SCN4A*.

maneuvers such as tilt-table testing or graded exercise protocols may allow dysrhythmias to surface and should be used when the diagnosis of AS is highly suspected but prior cardiac evaluation is unremarkable.

Laboratory testing during episodes of weakness often reveals normal creatine kinase levels, although occasionally these levels may be elevated to 2 times normal. Ictal K^+ levels are inconsistent; they usually are abnormally low but can be high or normal. Profound hypokalemia of less than 2.0 mmol/L in individuals over the age of 20 years should alert the physician to an alternate diagnosis of thyrotoxic periodic paralysis. In the diagnosis of common forms of periodic paralysis, hypokalemic and hyperkalemic challenges were frequently done when it was not possible to check potassium levels during spontaneous attacks of weakness. Hypokalemic challenges should be especially avoided because hypokalemia in patients with AS may exacerbate preexisting QT prolongation and could cause life-threatening ventricular arrhythmias.

Skeletal muscle biopsy may be performed to substantiate the diagnosis of AS. The histology of proximal muscle may demonstrate tubular aggregates; their presence signifies damage to the sarcoplasmic reticulum (Fig. 103–8). Tubular aggregates are not specific for AS; they may be seen in other types of periodic paralyses and toxic myopathies.

The results of nerve conduction studies are normal. Electromyography results are usually normal or may show myopathic motor units but without evidence of myotonia even after cooling. An exercise nerve conduction study may be helpful in documenting the presence of abnormalities of muscle membrane excitability.

The differential diagnosis of AS is limited and often be can narrowed by taking a thorough history, with special attention to age of onset of weakness, the presence of dysmorphisms, and the presence of palpitations and syncope. Attacks of weakness in AS are less stereotyped than are those of other forms of periodic paralysis. Although vigorous exercise, as in other periodic paralyses, is a common precipitating factor, patients with AS rarely relate the onset of attack to their diet. Careful examination of the patient for dysmorphic features is crucial, as is obtaining a history and examining other family members. Other secondary and primary forms of periodic paralysis have to be ruled out. Thyrotoxic periodic paralysis usually presents later in life and often is associated with ictal K^+ levels of 2.5 mmol/L or less. Hyperkalemic periodic paralysis usually presents in infancy with weakness or hypotonia, usually after vigorous activity. Serum potassium levels may be elevated at onset but often fall to normokalemic levels. Many patients have clinical or subclinical (detected on electromyography) myotonia. Hypokalemic periodic paralysis, by contrast, usually begins in puberty and is often precipitated by meals high in sodium and carbohydrates. Chondrodystrophic myotonia, which is also known as Schwartz-Jampel syndrome (SJS), should be included in the differential diagnosis of any patient with dysmorphisms who does not possess the complete triad of AS. Patients with SJS may resemble the dysmorphic AS patients but do not manifest cardiac dysrhythmias or weakness as a part of their syndrome. Patients with SJS also have facial dysmorphology and chondrodystrophy, in addition to myotonia. SJS is caused by mutations in the gene encoding perlecan (HSPG2) (Nicole et al., 2000).

At this time, no method is available for prenatal testing.

MANAGEMENT AND TREATMENT

The treatment of AS patients is directed at controlling underlying cardiac arrhythmias, in addition to decreasing the frequency, severity, and duration of attacks of weakness. This may be difficult because some treatments for arrhythmias can produce weakness, and treatments for weakness have been shown to exacerbate cardiac dysrhythmias (Gould et al., 1985). It therefore is imperative, in treating patients with AS, that there be close coordination between the treating neurologist and the treating cardiologist.

There are no approved treatments for the periodic paralyses, although a recent randomized controlled study has demonstrated the efficacy of dichlorphenamide (a carbonic anhydrase inhibitor) in both hypokalemic and hyperkalemic periodic paralysis (Tawil et al., 2000). The periodic paralysis of AS usually responds to carbonic anhydrase inhibitors. Although thiazide diuretics may also be used in patients with associated hyperkalemia, carbonic anhydrase inhibitors are preferred because they cause only mild, if any, hypokalemia and are less likely to exacerbate cardiac dysrhythmias (Renner and Ptáček, 2001). In a patient with AS with hypokalemic weakness, oral potassium ingestion can be used to treat acute attacks. Prophylaxis with daily sustained-release potassium tablets may prevent attacks of weakness. Maintaining a high serum potassium level (>4.5 mEq/L) has the additional advantage of narrowing the QT interval, thus reducing the likelihood of the development of ventricular arrhythmias.

Treating the arrhythmias of AS may be difficult because of the lack of response to antiarrhythmic agents, some of which may exacerbate muscle weakness (Andersen et al., 1971; Lisak et al., 1972; Yoshimura et al., 1983; Gould et al., 1985). Imipramine, a mild antiarrhythmic agent, has been reported to be of benefit in one patient (Gould et al., 1985). The primary aim of therapy for the cardiac manifestations of AS is to treat the underlying prolonged QT interval. Such intervention depends on the severity of the underlying arrhythmias. β-Blockers are one of the mainstays of treatment in syndromes with a long QT, and clinical experience has shown that these agents are well tolerated by patients with AS. In the presence of syncope due to sustained ventricular tachycardia, it is becoming clear that such patients benefit from aggressive treatment with the placement of an implantable defibrillator. Other antiarrhythmic agents should be used judiciously in AS. With the discovery of one AS gene, a gene-specific treatment approach may be feasible.

COUNSELING

There is a high rate of de novo mutations in AS. AS occurs either sporadically or is inherited in an autosomal dominant manner. However, given the prominent phenotypic variability of this syndrome, in addition to the often asymptomatic nature of the arrhythmias, individuals and their physicians may not realize the affected status. Sporadic mutations (some of which may be de novo), recessive inheritance with incomplete penetrance, multiple gene influences, or nongenetic factors may contribute to this striking phenotypic variability. At this time, 10 of 30 probands with AS have not demonstrated mutations in KCNJ2, and their disease may, in theory, be explained by locus heterogeneity. Spontaneous mutations in Kir2.1 may be transmitted to future generations. Genetic counseling may be offered to affected individuals who are contemplating pregnancy.

Affected family members should be screened for cardiac dysrhyth-

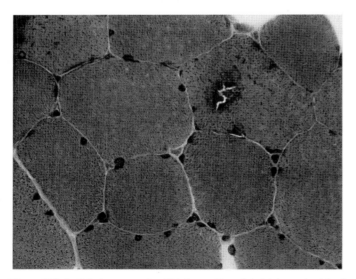

Figure 103–8. Tubular aggregates. This is a section of skeletal muscle stained with Gomori's trichrome. Tubular aggregates can be seen accumulating in the subsarcolemmal regions in the interior of muscle fibers. They appear red on the modified trichrome stain (as seen here), dark on the NADH-tetrazolium reductase stain, and blue on the hematoxylin and eosin stain.

mias starting at age 10, even if they are asymptomatic. Pregnancy and anesthesia have no known effects on AS patients.

MUTATIONS IN ORTHOLOGOUS GENES

The role of Kir2.1 and Kir2.2 has been studied in genetically engineered mice lacking these channels (Zaritsky et al., 2001). Knockout mice lacking Kir2.1 have a cleft palate and die shortly after birth; thus they can only be studied as newborns. Electrophysiologic recordings of Kir2.1$^{-/-}$ ventricular myocytes confirm that Kir2.1 is the major component of I_{k1} in mouse. The electrocardiograms of Kir2.1 knockout mice revealed neither ectopic beats nor reentrant arrhythmias, although the mice had consistently slower heart rates and their myocytes had broader action potentials and more frequent spontaneous action potentials than wild-type myocytes.

A homologous gene mutation is illustrated by the *weaver* mouse, which possesses a missense mutation in a gene encoding a G protein–coupled inward rectifier potassium channel (Kir3.2). Homozygous animals have ataxia, tremor, and hyperactivity due to depletion of the major cell type (granule cell). Heterozygous animals are not ataxic, but they have an intermediate number of surviving granule cells (Rakic and Sidman, 1973). The phenotype is produced by a G-to-A substitution replacing a glycine with serine at a highly conserved residue (156) in the GIRK2 protein (Patil et al., 1995). Gly156 is the first residue that is highly conserved in the H5 domain of the voltage-gated, Ca^{2+}-dependent, and inward rectifying families of potassium channels (Hoshi et al., 1993).

DEVELOPMENTAL PATHOGENESIS OF AS

Kir2.1 is encoded by the gene *KCNJ2*. It is expressed in the heart, skeletal muscle, brain, and placenta in various cell types, such as neurons, glia, Schwann cells, osteoclasts, macrophages, and myocytes. Functioning as a homotetramer, Kir2.1 plays an important role in controlling membrane excitability of skeletal and cardiac muscle. It is a major contributor to terminal repolarization and the resting membrane potential in the heart. It is not necessary for normal heart development in mice because Kir2.1 knockout mice have no observed heart defects, although murine arteries do not dilate normally in response to elevated extracellular K^+ concentrations. The fact that Kir2.1 knockout mice have a complete cleft of the secondary palate and narrowing of the maxilla supports laboratory evidence of Kir2.1 mRNA and its association with bone structures in the head, limbs, and body (Karschin and Karschin, 1997). The role that Kir2.1 plays in the morphogenesis of facial and skeletal structure is not understood at this time.

AS is a rare and highly variable disorder caused by mutations in the gene encoding Kir2.1 (*KCNJ2)* and is characterized by the triad of dysmorphic features, prolonged QT intervals with ventricular dysrhythmias, and episodic paralysis. Given the variable penetrance and prominent phenotypic variability of AS, it is underrecognized and often misdiagnosed. The recognition and treatment of AS are important given its associated cardiac conduction defects and risk for interattack weakness. New mutations continue to be discovered within ion channel genes, allowing researchers to implement animal models to study the pathogenesis of AS in vivo. Whether genotype influences treatment remains to be seen and may best be assessed in future clinical trials with molecular genetic characterization before patient entry.

REFERENCES

Abbott GW, Butler MH, Bendahhou S, Dalakas MC, Ptácek LJ, Goldenstein SAN (2001). MiRP2 forms potassium channels in skeletal muscle with Kv3.4 and is associated with periodic paralysis. *Cell* 104: 217–231.

Andersen ED, Krasilnikoff PA, Overvad H (1971). Intermittent muscular weakness, extrasystoles, and multiple developmental anomalies. *Acta Paediatr Scand* 60: 559–564.

Canún S, Pérez N, Beirana LG (1999). Andersen syndrome autosomal dominant in three generations. *Am J Med Genet* 85: 147–156.

Donaldson MR, Jensen JL, Tristani Firouzi M, Tawil R, Bendahhou S, Suarez WA, Cobo AM, et al., PIP$_2$ binding residues of KIR2.1 are common targets of mutations causing Andersen syyndrome. *Neurology* 60: in press.

Gould RJ, Streeg CN, Eastwood AB, et al. (1985). Potentially fatal cardiac dysrhythmia and hyperkalemic periodic paralysis. *Neurology* 35: 1208–1212.

Hoshi T, Zagotta WN (1993). Recent advances in the understanding of potassium channel function. *Curr Opin Neurobiol* 3: 283–290.

Hoshi T, Zagotta WN, Aldrich RW (1990). Biophysical and molecular mechanisms of Shaker potassium channel inactivation. *Science* 250: 533–538.

Jen J, Ptáček LJ (2001). Channelopathies: episodic disorders of the nervous system. In: *Metabolic and Molecular Bases of Inherited Disease, 8th edition.* Schriver CR, Beaudet AL, Sly WS, et al. (eds.) McGraw-Hill, New York. pp. 5223–5238.

Karschin C, Karschin A (1997). Ontogeny of gene expression of Kir channel subunits in the rat. *Mol Cell Neurosci* 10: 131–148.

Kubo Y, Baldwin TJ, Jan YN, Jan LY (1993). Primary structure and functional expression of a mouse inward rectifier potassium channel. *Nature* 362: 127–133.

Levitt LP, Rose LI, Dawson D (1972). Hypokalemic periodic paralysis with arrhythmia. *N Engl J Med* 286: 253–254.

Lisak RP, Lebeau J, Tucker SH, Rowland LP (1972). Hyperkalemic periodic paralysis and cardiac arrhythmia. *Neurology* 22: 810–815.

McClatchey AI, Van den Bergh P, Pericak Vance MA, et al. (1992). Temperature-sensitive mutations in the III-IV cytoplasmic loop region of the skeletal muscle sodium channel gene in paramyotonia congenita. *Cell* 68: 769–774.

Nicole S, Davoine CS, Topaloglu H, Cattolico L, Barral D, Beighton P, Ben Hamida C, Hammouda H, Cruaud C, White PS, et al. (2000). Perlecan, the major proteoglycan of basement membranes, is altered in patients with Schwartz-Jampel syndrome (chondrodystrophic myotonia). *Nat Genet* 26: 480–483.

Patil N, et al. (1995). A potassium channel mutation in weaver mice implicates membrane excitability in granule cell differentiation. *Nat Genet* 11(2): 126–129.

Plaster NM, et al. (2001). Mutations in kir2.1 cause the developmental and episodic electrical phenotypes of andersen's syndrome. *Cell* 105: 511–519.

Ptáček LJ (1997). Channelopathies: ion channel disorders of muscle as a paradigm for paroxysmal disorders of the nervous system. *Neuromusc Disord* 7: 250–255.

Ptáček LJ (1998). Channelopathies: ion channels and paroxysmal disorders of the nervous system. In: *Genetics of Focal Epilepsies.* Genton P (ed.) John Libbey. London, pp. 204–213.

Ptáček LJ (1999). Ion channel diseases: episodic disorders of the nervous system. *Semin Neurol* 19: 363–369.

Ptáček LJ, Griggs RC (1996). Familial periodic paralyses. In: *The Molecular Biology of Membrane Transport Disorders, 3rd edition.* Andreoli T (ed.) Plenum, New York.

Ptáček LJ, Johnson KJ, Griggs RC (1993). Genetics and physiology of the myotonic muscle disorders. *N Engl J Med* 328: 482–489.

Ptáček LJ, George AL, Griggs RC, et al. (1991). Identification of a mutation in the gene causing hyperkalemic periodic paralysis. *Cell* 67: 1021–1027.

Ptáček LJ, Tawil R, Griggs RC, et al. (1992). Linkage of atypical myotonia congenita to a sodium channel locus. *Neurology* 42: 431–433.

Rakic P, Sidman RL (1973). Organization of cerebellar cortex secondary to deficit of granule cells in weaver mutant mice. *J Comp Neurol* 152: 133–161.

Renner DR, Ptáček LJ (2001). Periodic paralyses and nondystrophic myotonias. *Adv Neurol* 88: 235–252.

Rojas CV, Wang JZ, Schwartz LS, Hoffman EP, Powell BR, and Brown RH (1991). A Met-to-Val mutation in the skeletal muscle Na+ channel alpha-subunit in hyperkalaemic periodic paralysis. *Nature* 354: 387–389.

Sanguinetti MT (2001). Molecular and cellular mechanisms of cardiac arrhythmias. *Cell* 104: 569–580.

Sanguinetti MC, Tristani-Firouzi M (2000). Delayed and inward rectifier potassium channels. In: *Cardiac Electrophysiology: From Cell to Bedside.* Zipes DP, Jalife J (eds.) WB Saunders, Philadelphia. pp. 79–86.

Sansone V, Griggs RC, Meola G, et al. (1997). Andersen's syndrome: a distinct periodic paralysis. *Ann Neurol* 42: 305–312.

Tawil R, Ptáček LJ, Pavlakis SG, et al. (1994). Andersen's syndrome: potassium-sensitive periodic paralysis, ventricular ectopy, and dysmorphic features. *Ann Neurol* 35: 326–330.

Tawil R, McDermott MP, Brown R Jr, Shapiro BC, Ptáček LJ, McManis PG, Dalakas MC, Spector SA, Mendell JR, Hahn AF, et al. (2000). Randomized trials of dichlorphenamide in the periodic paralyses. Working Group on Periodic Paralysis. *Ann Neurol* 47: 46–53.

Tristani-Firouzi M, Jensen J, Donaldson M, Sansone V, Meola G, Hahn A, Bendahhou S, Kwiecinski H, Fidzianska A, Plaster N, et al. (2002). Functional and clinical characterization of KCNJ2 mutations associated with LQT7 (Andersen syndrome). *J Clin Invest* 110: 381–388.

Yang J, Jan YN, Jan LY (1995). Determination of the subunit stoichiometry of an inwardly rectifying potassium channel. *Neuron* 15: 1441–1447.

Yoshimura T, Kaneuji M, Okuno T, et al. (1983). Periodic paralysis with cardiac arrhythmia. *Eur J Pediatr* 140: 338–343.

Zaritsky JJ, Eckman DM, Wellman GC, Nelson MT, Schwartz TL (2000). Targeted disruption of Kir2.1 and Kir2.2 genes reveals the essential role of the inwardly rectifying K(+) current in the K(+)-mediated vasodilation. *Circ Res* 87: 160–166.

Zaritsky JJ, Redell JB, Tempel BL, Schwarz TL (2001). The consequences of disrupting cardiac inwardly rectifying K$^+$ current (I_{K1}) as revealed by the targeted deletion of the murine Kir2.1 and Kir2.2 genes. *J Phys* 533.3: 697–710.

PETER NÜRNBERG AND SIGRID TINSCHERT

Craniometaphyseal dysplasia (CMD) is a bone dysplasia characterized by overgrowth and sclerosis of the craniofacial bones and abnormal modeling of the metaphyses of the tubular bones. Affected individuals display highly variable features ranging from barely discernible anomalies to severe nasal obstruction, compression and functional impairment of cranial nerves, and increased intracranial pressure. An autosomal dominant form of the disorder (CMDD; OMIM 123000) was linked to chromosome 5p15.2-p14.1 within a region harboring the human ortholog of the mouse *progressive ankylosis (Ank)* gene. The gene codes for a protein with a putative role in the transport of inorganic pyrophosphate (PP$_i$), a major inhibitor of physiologic and pathologic calcification, bone mineralization, and bone resorption. Sequencing of the 12 exons of *ANKH* revealed six different heterozygous mutations in several unrelated CMD patients, including sporadic cases with supposed autosomal recessive CMD (CMDR; OMIM 218400). The mutations occurred at highly conserved amino acid residues presumed to be located in the cytosolic portion of the multipass transmembrane ANK protein. The dominant effect of the *ANKH* mutations in CMD patients contrasts with the recessive character of the truncating mutation in the *ank* mouse and suggests a gain of function as the molecular basis of the CMD pathology. So far, no phenotype–genotype correlation is evident. Pronounced intrafamiliar variability suggests that additional modifying factors may be involved.

THE *ANKH* LOCUS AND ITS ROLE IN CMD AND OTHER DISEASES

The *ANKH* locus is the human ortholog of the gene mutated in the *ank* mouse (see later), a spontaneous mouse mutant that has progressive ankylosis (Sweet and Green, 1981). The *ank* locus was originally mapped to proximal mouse chromosome 15 (Sweet and Green, 1981). Fine mapping with microsatellite markers in a total of 923 affected F$_2$ progeny from a cross with *Mus musculus castaneus* placed the *ank* mutation next to markers D15Mit20 and D15Mit164 at map position 14.4 cM (Ho et al., 2000). This region is homologous to a region around D5S1954 on human chromosome 5p. Using several BAC clones from a contig spanning the critical region to generate transgenic *ank/ank* mice, Ho et al. (2000) were able to rescue the *ank* mutant phenotype with a particular clone of about 190 kb. Shotgun sequencing of the BAC clone identified 11 candidate genes. None of them showed any obvious relation to arthritis. However, a nonsense mutation in the open reading frame (ORF) of the gene later called *Ank* revealed this one to be the culprit. The sequence was predicted to encode a 492-amino-acid integral transmembrane protein of unknown function.

Interestingly, the first idea about the possible function of the ANK protein came from patients with familiar articular chondrocalcinosis. Some families with chondrocalcinosis (CCAL2; OMIM 118600) showed linkage to a region on chromosome 5p (Hughes et al., 1995; Andrew et al., 1999) where the human ortholog of *Ank (ANKH)* was mapped using radiation hybrid panels (Ho et al., 2000). In one of these families, twofold increased levels of intracellular PP$_i$ had previously been reported in cultured skin fibroblasts and lymphoblasts of the affected family members compared with the unaffected members or normal unrelated control subjects (Lust et al., 1981). This prompted Ho et al. (2000) to test *ank* mutants for a similar defect in PP$_i$ metabolism. Indeed, fibroblasts from *ank* mutants displayed a similar twofold

increase in intracellular PP$_i$ levels over wild-type cells, and transfection of *ank* mutant fibroblasts with a construct driving expression of wild-type ANK restored the normal PP$_i$ levels. Furthermore, overexpression of ANK in COS-7 cells led to a dramatic drop in intracellular PP$_i$ and rise in extracellular PP$_i$ levels, an effect that was blocked by the anion transport inhibitor probenecid. These data together with the verification of its subcellular localization at the plasma membrane through immunofluorescence staining and confocal microscopy led to the hypothesis that ANK might be a transmembrane transporter that shuttles PP$_i$ between intracellular and extracellular compartments (Ho et al., 2000).

Similar changes in PP$_i$ levels reported for patients who were members of a French CCAL2 family (Lust et al., 1981) and for *ank* mice (Ho et al., 2000), as well as the coincidence of the map position on 5p, strongly suggested that *ANKH* was involved in CCAL2. However, fine mapping of the CCAL2 disease interval in an Argentinean family (Andrew et al., 1999) and precise determination of the *ANKH* locus (Nürnberg et al., 2001) placed the latter about 2 cM apart from the disease interval (Fig. 104–1). Commensurate with the recent mapping data, mutation screening of *ANKH* in patients of 12 CCAL2 kindreds that included two large pedigrees (the pedigree from Argentina and another one from North America) failed to identify disease-causing mutations in *ANKH* (Peariso et al., 2001). A substitution of threonine for proline 5 (P5T) in one family did not occur on the disease haplotype and also was seen in control subjects. However, in the large French family mentioned earlier, a heterozygous missense mutation in exon 2 changing a methionine into a threonine at position 48 (M48T) has been reported to completely cosegregate with the disease phenotype (Johnson et al., 2001). Strikingly, the phenotype of the affected recombinant VII:19 (Andrew et al., 1999), originally excluding *ANKH* from the disease interval, was deemed "unaffected" (Maldonado et al., 2001). In a large British pedigree (Hughes et al., 1995) with obligate recombinants defining the CCAL2 disease interval between markers D5S810 and D5S416, and thus including the *ANKH* locus, a heterozygous transition from C to T in the 5′ untranslated region (UTR) was found in all affected individuals within the kindred. This base substitution is supposed to create a new translational initiation codon ATG four codons upstream from the original start codon. The mutation was absent from all unaffected family members and from 100 unrelated controls (Pendleton et al., 2001).

The only clear link of a disease phenotype to *ANKH* mutations has been found in two studies on CMD patients (Nürnberg et al., 2001; Reichenberger et al., 2001). The positional cloning approach started with a large German pedigree, in which a locus for CMD was mapped to 5p15.2-p14.1 (Nürnberg et al., 1997). Linkage mapping of the CMDD locus to this region of the short arm of chromosome 5 was confirmed in a large Australian pedigree and a second German family (Chandler et al., 2001). Using obligate recombinants of all three families, the critical region could be narrowed down to a 4-cM interval between markers D5S1987 and D5S1991 (Chandler et al., 2001). Sequence comparisons between the human *ANKH* mRNA and the draft version of the human genome allowed us to locate the *ANKH* gene next to *D5S1991*, positioning *ANKH* within the refined CMD interval (see Fig. 104–1). We tested *ANKH* as a positional candidate in nine unrelated families. Genomic sequencing of all 12 *ANKH* exons, including their flanking splice sites, revealed six different mutations in eight of these families (Nürnberg et al., 2001). All mutations affected

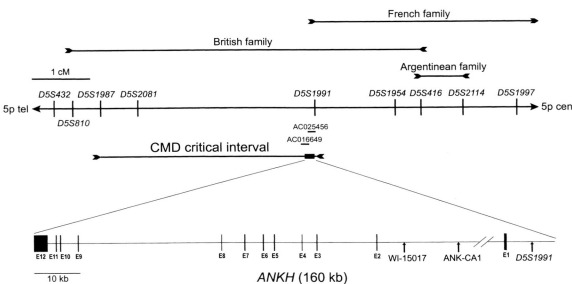

Figure 104–1. Mapping of disease intervals for craniometaphyseal dysplasia (CMD) and familial articular chondrocalcinosis type 2 (CCAL2) on chromosome 5p15.1. Part of the Généthon map is shown. The CMD interval is defined distally by *D5S1987* and proximally by *D5S1991*. The smallest interval for CCAL2 (Argentinean family) maps between markers *D5S416* and *D5S2114*. Two overlapping BAC clones spanning *D5S1991* and *ANKH* are de-noted by bars. The accession numbers of the corresponding clone sequences are given above the bars. Position of *ANKH* (shaded box) is within the CMD critical interval distal from *D5S1991*. The genomic exon/intron structure of *ANKH* is delineated approximately to scale. A new (CA)$_n$ repeat marker, ANK-CA1, and STS marker WI-15017 were identified in the sequence. (Adapted from Nürnberg et al., 2001.)

single amino acid positions. The spectrum included four missense mutations, three single amino acid deletions, and one presumed single amino acid insertion due to the formation of a new splice acceptor in intron 9. Demonstration of complete cosegregation of the CMD phenotype with the *ANKH* mutations in the families and the absence of the mutant variants from DNA of at least 100 control individuals suggested the mutations to be disease causing. The observed allelic heterogeneity together with the two verified de novo mutations provided even stronger evidence for a causal relationship between mutations in *ANKH* and CMD. Further evidence came from evolutionary, structural, and functional considerations of the ANK protein sequence and

the predicted amino acid changes (see later). *ANKH* was subsequently tested as a positional candidate in 10 unrelated CMD families by another group (Reichenberger et al., 2001). They detected three different mutations in five families. Interestingly, they found the same splice acceptor mutation and 3-bp deletions as we did in our patients. Then we identified three additional cases of sporadic CMD with a deletion of Ser375 (unpublished data). A summary of *ANKH* mutation screening in CMD patients is shown in Table 104–1. Notably, a high proportion of the sporadic CMD patients are carriers of heterozygous *ANKH* mutations and hence do not belong to the group of recessive CMD cases. No phenotype–genotype correlation is evident from the

Table 104–1. *ANKH* Mutations in Patients with Craniometaphyseal Dysplasia

Family	Origin	No. of Patients	Sporadic (S)/ Familial (F)	Location	DNA Change*	Amino Acid Change	Reference
1	Russia	1	S	Exon 7	942T → C	W292R	Nürnberg et al., 2001
2	Germany	13	F	Exon 8	1059T → C	C331R	Nürnberg et al., 2001
3	USA	2	F	Exon 9	1192delCCT	S375del	Nürnberg et al., 2001
10	Switzerland	1	S	Exon 9	1192delCCT	S375del	Unpublished
11	USA	1	S	Exon 9	1192delCCT	S375del	Unpublished
12	Australia	1	S	Exon 9	1192delCCT	S375del	Unpublished
D		1	S	Exon 9	1192delCCT	S375del	Reichenberger et al., 2001
S		1	S	Exon 9	1192delCCT	S375del	Reichenberger et al., 2001
4	Germany	2	F	Exon 9	1196delCTT	F377del	Nürnberg et al., 2001
C		9	F	Exon 9	1196delCTT	F377del	Reichenberger et al., 2001
F		?	F	Exon 9	1196delCTT	F377del	Reichenberger et al., 2001
5	Germany	2	F	Exon 9	1196delCTT	F377del	Nürnberg et al., 2001
6	Israel	1	S	Intron 9	1210-4A → G†	P380insA	Nürnberg et al., 2001
G		≥4	F	Intron 9	1210-4A → G†	P380insA	Reichenberger et al., 2001
7	Australia	11	F	Exon 10	1233G → A	G389R	Nürnberg et al., 2001
8	Switzerland	2	F	Exon 10	1233G → A	G389R	Nürnberg et al., 2001
9	Israel	1	S	—	—	—	Nürnberg et al., 2001
13	Brazil	1	S	—	—	—	Unpublished
A		3	F	—	—	—	Reichenberger et al., 2001
B		?	F	—	—	—	Reichenberger et al., 2001
E		1	S	—	—	—	Reichenberger et al., 2001
X1		1	S	—	—	—	Reichenberger et al., 2001
X2		1	S	—	—	—	Reichenberger et al., 2001

*Sequence numbering follows the published sequence for human *ANKH* mRNA (AF274753).
†New splice acceptor.

data available. This and the pronounced intrafamiliar variability both point to modifying factors that may be of major importance for the highly variable expressivity of the disease phenotype.

CLINICAL DESCRIPTION

CMD is characterized by hyperostosis and sclerosis of the craniofacial bones combined with abnormal modeling of the tubular bones, resulting in metaphyseal widening that resembles metaphyseal dysplasia (MD) type Pyle (OMIM 265900). Even after the delineation of CMD by Jackson et al. (1954), both conditions, CMD and MD, often were lumped together and referred to as "Pyle's disease." CMD may be genetically heterogeneous. An autosomal dominant form (OMIM 123000) and a more severe autosomal recessive form (OMIM 218400) were delineated (Gorlin et al., 1969). However, the considerable overlap between the two forms does not allow them to be distinguished clinically in sporadic cases.

Reports on CMDD include more than 100 patients, with nearly half coming from a few large kindreds from the United States (Rimoin et al., 1969), South Africa/England (Beighton et al., 1979), Mexico (Carnevale et al., 1983), Australia (Colavita et al., 1988; Taylor and Sprague, 1989), and Germany (Tinschert and Braun, 1998). In contrast, the autosomal recessive form is suggested only in about 15 unrelated patients, mostly on the basis of a severe manifestation (Halliday, 1949; Jackson et al., 1954; Lélek, 1961; Wemmer and Böttger, 1978; Boltshauser et al., 1996; Elcioglu and Hall, 1998) with only one sibship born to consanguineous parents reported twice (Millard et al., 1967; Ross and Altman, 1967). On the other hand, Penchaszadeh et al. (1980) reported two families, each with two affected sibs clinically not distinguishable from CMDD, as it is the case in the two sibs reported by Komins (1954) and in the three sibs reported by Lehmann (1957). Iughetti et al. (2000) reported an inbred kindred with 10 affected individuals and suggested a more severe involvement of diaphyses than in the autosomal dominant form. Parental consanguinity was reported in some instances of sporadic patients (Sommer, 1954; Lièvre and Fischgold, 1956).

Persons with CMD have no serious complaints in most cases, as has been reported for the affected members of some large kindreds (Beighton et al., 1979; Taylor and Sprangue, 1989; Beighton, 1995; Tinschert and Braun, 1998). However, there is great variability in the phenotypical expression of CMD even within individual families (Beighton et al., 1979; Carnevale et al., 1983; Taylor and Sprangue, 1989; Tinschert and Braun, 1998). The major and earliest clinical finding of CMD, usually apparent within the first year of life, is a typical facial appearance (Figs. 104–2A and 104–2B). This is caused by a bony prominence of the nasal root and the paranasal regions extending bilaterally to the zygomatic arch (inverse Y shape) in combination with hypertelorism and a relatively small nose (Spranger et al., 1965; Gorlin et al., 1969). These facial features, which are striking in infancy, change with time and are often less marked in adults (Beighton et al., 1979; Taylor and Sprangue, 1989; Tinschert and Braun, 1998). Usually, the skull is enlarged and the frontal and parietal bones are prominent, as is the mandibular bone. Changes in the long bones do not seem to cause any obvious clinical manifestations with the exception of genu valgum, which is sometimes severe (Ross and Altman, 1967; Tinschert and Braun, 1998).

If present, complaints are related to the extent of hyperostotic changes of calvarial and facial bones. Massive hyperostosis has been observed mostly in sporadic cases, contributing to the idea of an autosomal recessive gene mutation underlying the rare severe cases. Mouth breathing, nasorespiratory infections, and chronic otitis media are due to a stenosis of the nasal cavity and underpneumatization of the paranasal sinuses and mastoids. Respiratory distress at birth, caused by bilateral choanal narrowing, is reported (Cheung et al., 1997). Increasing expansion and thickening of the mandible are associated with mandibular prognathism and dental malocclusion. Delayed eruption of permanent teeth occurs (Hayashibara et al., 2000). Deafness is common and mostly mixed in type. Conductive hearing loss is caused primarily by alteration of middle ear structures, including fixation of the ossicles or obliteration of the fenestrae as due to fre-

quent episodes of otitis and upper respiratory tract infections. Sensorineural hearing loss is attributed to auditory nerve compression by stenosis of the internal auditory meatus (Millard, 1967; Shea et al 1981; Franz et al., 1996; Richards et al., 1996). Bony overgrowth of the nerve canals or encroachment on cranial foramina may also compress other cranial nerves. Facial and optic nerves are primarily affected, resulting in facial palsy and blindness. Facial palsy is much more frequent than is visual loss, which is very rare. Narrowing of the foramen magnum with medullary compression may lead to headache, syncope, reflex changes, pareses, hydrocephalus, or sudden death (Boltshauser et al., 1996; Day et al., 1997).

DIAGNOSIS OF CMD

To establish the diagnosis in an affected individual, radiographic manifestations are most important. Hyperostosis and sclerosis involve the calvarium (especially in the frontal and occipital parts), the base of the skull and the facial bones (with underpneumatization of the paranasal sinuses and mastoid cells), and the mandible (Fig. 104–2C). The metaphyses of the long bones show a club-shaped widening (Erlenmeyer flask deformity) with thinned cortex most evident in the distal femora. In early infancy, the metaphyses are flared. Diaphyseal sclerosis is also present but disappears with age (Fig. 104–2D). Sequencing of the *ANKH* gene is used to confirm the clinical diagnosis. However, several sporadic cases do not seem to have a mutated *ANKH* (Nürnberg et al., 2001; Reichenberger et al., 2001). Intriguingly, two CMD families have been reported to have no mutation in *ANKH* although they show linkage to the CMDD locus on 5p (Reichenberger et al., 2001). This finding gave rise to speculations about the existence of mutations in *cis*-acting regulatory elements, such as in the promotor or enhancer/silencer regions of *ANKH*, in these families.

MANAGEMENT AND SPECIFIC TREATMENT

Therapeutic trials to reduce hyperostosis have included the application of calcitonin (Fanconi at al., 1988) or calcitriol (Key et al., 1988; Richards et al., 1996). Although metabolic responses in the patients indicated some effects on osteoblasts or osteoclasts, none of these patients showed convincingly beneficial results.

Decompressive surgical treatment of patients with CMD have been reported with varying results. It is complicated because of the hardness of the sclerotic bone, especially in massive craniofacial hyperostosis. Successful results on facial palsy with facial canal decompression (Gorlin et al., 1969; Stool and Caruso, 1973) and on conductive hearing loss with ossicular replacement (Shea et al., 1981; Franz et al., 1996) were shown. Decompression of the optic canal bears an increased risk of blindness (Satoh et al., 1994), but in an other report, visual impairment was also avoided (Boltshauser et al., 1996). In dangerous foramen magnum stenosis, neurosurgery was helpful (Bolts-hauser et al., 1996; Day et al., 1997).

GENETIC COUNSELING GUIDELINES AND PROGNOSTIC INFORMATION

Both autosomal dominant and autosomal recessive patterns of inheritance have been reported in CMD. Based on the early reports of CMD patients, it was stated that the recessive form is more severe with massive involvement of craniofacial bones (Boltshauser et al., 1996; Elcioglu and Hall, 1998). However, recent reports do not confirm this concept (Iughetti et al., 2000), and further studies are needed to elucidate the difference between the autosomal recessive and autosomal dominant forms of CMD. Thus, a decision between dominant and recessive forms is not possible in a sporadic case unless sequencing of *ANKH* reveals a mutation. This may make genetic counseling difficult, especially when no *ANKH* mutation is found. Furthermore, as shown in families with vertical transmission, expressivity can be highly variable, and therefore gene carriers without any clinical signs must be taken into account. Their status may be confirmed by molecular diagnosis. A DNA test also makes a first-trimester prenatal diagnosis an option in some families. However, because molecular di-

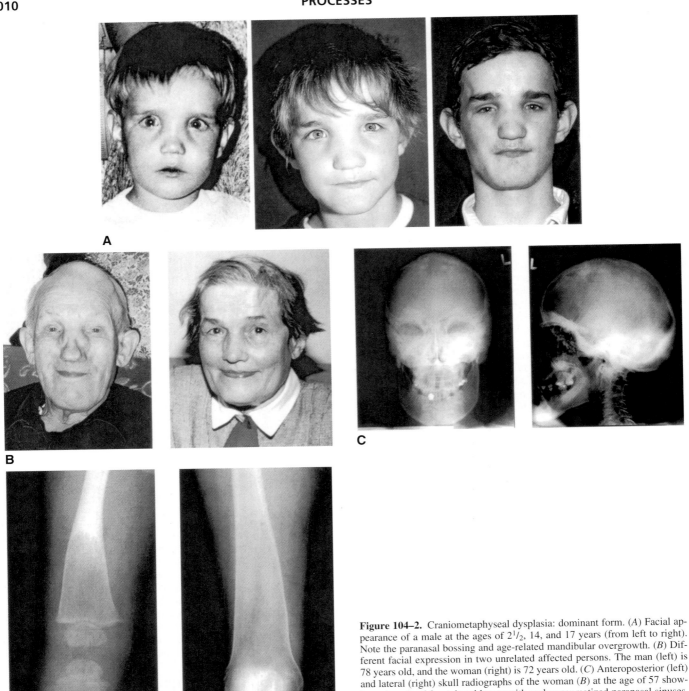

Figure 104–2. Craniometaphyseal dysplasia: dominant form. (*A*) Facial appearance of a male at the ages of $2^{1}/_{2}$, 14, and 17 years (from left to right). Note the paranasal bossing and age-related mandibular overgrowth. (*B*) Different facial expression in two unrelated affected persons. The man (left) is 78 years old, and the woman (right) is 72 years old. (*C*) Anteroposterior (left) and lateral (right) skull radiographs of the woman (*B*) at the age of 57 showing sclerosis of frontobasal bones with underpneumatized paranasal sinuses, frontooccipital hyperostosis, and prominent mandible. (*D*) Anteroposterior knee radiographs of an affected girl at age 1 year (left) and of the woman (*B*) at the age of 56 (right) showing the age-related metaphyseal modeling defect.

agnosis cannot predict clinical severity, a decision about reproductive options is very difficult.

MUTATIONS IN ORTHOLOGOUS GENES IN ANIMAL MODELS

The *progressive ankylosis* (*ank*) mutation arose spontaneously at the Jackson Laboratory Mouse Mutant Stocks Center. Homozygotes have a severe joint disease. The phenotype is characterized by a flat-footed gait in young mice due to decreased mobility of ankle and toe joints. Affected mice are first recognizable at about 5 weeks of age on the basis of stiffness of the toes of the forefeet. Loss of joint mobility be-

comes more severe with age and spreads to most joints throughout the limbs and vertebral column, leading to complete rigidity and death around 6 month of age (Sweet and Green, 1981). Mice carrying the *ank* mutation have been studied as a model of arthritis during the past 20 years (Sweet and Green, 1981; Hakim et al., 1984; Hakim and Brown, 1986; Sampson and Davis, 1988; Mahowald et al., 1989; Krug et al., 1997). It was demonstrated that hydroxyapatite crystals develop in articular surfaces and synovial fluid, accompanied by joint space narrowing, cartilage erosion, and formation of bony outgrowths or osteophytes that cause fusion (ankylosis) and joint immobility. Although the distribution and severity of pathological features do not precisely mimic any single form of human arthritis, many of the features ob-

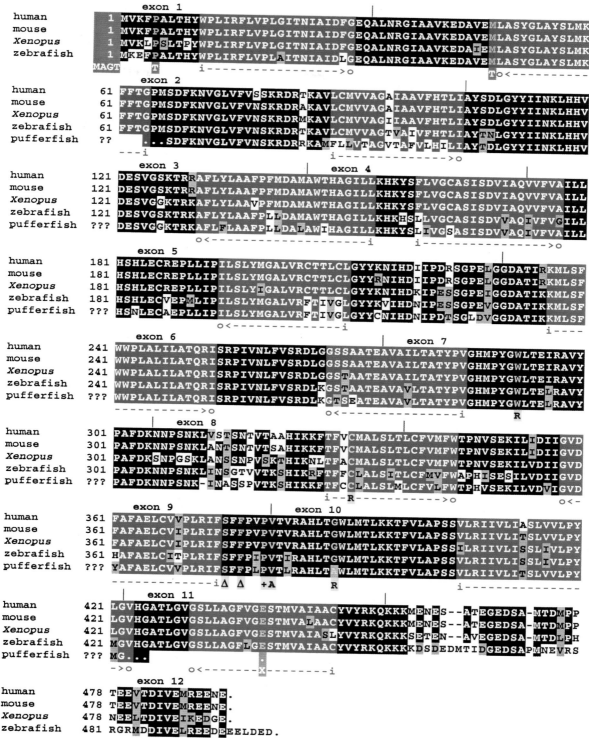

Figure 104–3. Sequence alignment of ANK proteins from different vertebrate species. White letters represent identical amino acids. Black letters on a gray background represent conserved amino acids. The whole sequence is highly conserved. Amino acid sequence identity between human and zebrafish (*Danio rerio*) is above 82%. Predicted membrane-spanning helices are highlighted in red. Their inside/out (i → o) orientation, as well as mutations are given in the bottom line. Mutations were found in CCAL2 families (exons 1 and 2, high- lighted in green; note that mutation P5T did not occur on the disease haplo- type [Peariso et al., 2001]), in craniometaphyseal dysplasia (CMD) patients (exons 7 to 10, highlighted in blue), and in the *ank* mouse (exon 11, high- lighted in blue). The kind of change is given in the top line; triangles indicate deletions. Mutations of CMD patients are highlighted in gray. The vertical bars in the top line indicate exon boundaries. (Adapted from Nürnberg et al., 2001.)

served in *ank* mice are reminiscent of cardinal features in important arthritic diseases, such as ectopic calcification in mineral deposition disease, cartilage erosion and osteophyte formation in osteoarthritis, and vertebral fusion in ankylosing spondylitis (Sweet and Green, 1981; Hakim et al., 1984; Sampson and Davis, 1988; Mahowald et al., 1989).

The genetic defect in *ank* mice has been identified by positional

cloning (Ho et al., 2000). Among 11 candidate genes, the authors iden- tified one with a nonsense mutation in the ORF. This is called the *Ank* gene; it consists of 12 exons, and its ORF codes for 492 amino acids. The *ank* mutation (E440X) is situated in the middle of exon 11 (Fig. 104–3) and is predicted to result in a truncated protein of only 439 amino acids. However, the truncated protein has not yet been detected, and it remains to be seen whether the mutation results in a nonfunctional protein or rather in a complete loss of the gene product by nonsense-mediated decay of its mRNA (Hentze and Kulozik, 1999) and/or by instability of the truncated protein. As a matter of fact, the mutation E440X causes a loss of function that has been described as a block of PP$_i$ transport from the intracellular to the extracellular compartment (see earlier). The reduced extracelluar PP$_i$ level observed in *ank* mutant mouse fibroblasts may account for the ectopical mineralization of the joints because PP$_i$ is known to be a potent inhibitor of calcification and bone mineralization in vitro and in vivo (Fleisch, 1981). This scenario is in line with the situation found in another mouse mutant where ectopic mineralization of the joints and ligaments is observed. This mouse mutant, called *tiptoe walking*, carries a genetic defect in a cell surface ectoenzyme (PC-1) that normally generates extracellular PP$_i$ from nucleotide triphosphate (Okawa et al., 1998).

DEVELOPMENTAL PATHOGENESIS

The few reports on bone biopsy findings are inconsistent. Increased osteoblastic activity suggesting enhanced bone matrix synthesis (Halliday, 1949; Jackson, 1954; Fanconi et al., 1982), lack of osteoclastic activity suggesting failure of endostal resorption (Millard et al., 1967; Shea et al., 1981), and normal osteoblastic or osteoclastic activity (Jackson, 1954; Kaitila and Rimoin, 1976) have been reported. Experiments with bone marrow–derived osteoclast-like cells from a patient with CMD suggested an osteoclast dysfunction due to impaired expression of the osteoclast-reactive vacuolar proton pump (Yamamoto et al., 1993). However, ANK is expressed in osteoblasts but not in osteoclasts (Reichenberger et al., 2001). Thus, if osteoclasts are involved in the pathological process, it would be an indirect effect, such as osteoclast recruitment by the osteoblasts. Interestingly, mouse and human ANK is expressed in a wide variety of tissues, with highest expression found in brain, heart, and skeletal muscle (Ho et al., 2000; Guo et al., 2002). Moreover, it has been characterized as a growth factor–regulated delayed-early response gene in mammalian cells (Guo et al., 2002). The authors suggest that the observed increase in ANK expression during mitogen-stimulated cell cycle progression may be necessary for the efficient removal of the excess intracellular PP$_i$ generated in the proliferating cells.

It is well established that CMD is caused by heterozygous mutations of *ANKH*. However, the mechanism is still far from being understood, and all models presented so far are highly speculative. Protein alignment shows a high degree of conservation among a wide variety of species, suggesting that the function of ANK is of major importance for vertebrate species (see Fig. 104–3). All mutations occurred at conserved amino acid residues, which further underlines their functional relevance. It is indeed tempting to speculate about a dysregulation of PP$_i$ levels as a direct result of the *ANKH* mutations occurring in patients with CMD. Ho et al. (2000) described ANK as a transmembrane transporter for PP$_i$. Using a hydrophobicity plot together with experimental results from cell membrane staining by antibodies against three extrahelical epitopes, they proposed a 10–helical transmembrane topology as one of several possible models for the ANK molecule. We have reevaluated the transmembrane topology and propose an alternative and somewhat more detailed model strongly suggesting that ANK serves as a conduit for PP$_i$ with proper structural prerequisites for selectivity (Nürnberg et al., 2001). Our analyses of the sequence data predict 12 membrane–spanning helices with an alternate inside/out orientation (see Fig. 104–3). A plot of the overall hydrophobicity of the 12 consecutive helices against helix number revealed an alternating hydrophobicity behavior suggesting that only every second helix contributes directly to the channel by forming a six-member parallel assembly. The other six helices probably stabilize the interaction of these channel helices by interacting with the membrane lipid bilayer. If the inner helices are oriented in such a way that the more polar sides (as derived from a helical wheel presentation) point toward the channel, there is a preference of basic residues at the pore-oriented sides, resulting in a positive potential of the channel inner surface. This may be significant for the transport of

the negatively charged pyrophosphate ion through this channel. A schematic presentation of the proposed topology is given in Figure 104–4. In our model, all except one of the observed mutations associated with CMD occurred at the cytosolic side of the channel, with the only exception being the substitution of Cys331 in helix 9. Furthermore, all missense mutations are changes to arginine that introduce an additional positive charge next to the pore entry. This might influence the passage of the channel by PP$_i$. The amino acid deletions and the putative insertion in the loop between helices 10 and 11 suggest that this interhelical region is involved in the regulation of the PP$_i$ transport through the channel. This domain may also be involved in complex formation with other proteins.

It can be speculated that the mutations result in a gain of function, that is, "leaky" PP$_i$ channels in CMD. However, as long as experimental evidence is lacking, we do not know if PP$_i$ levels are really changed in CMD patients or in which direction they are changed. Changes in extracellular PP$_i$ levels in both directions are conceivable in hyperostotic and sclerotic patients because PP$_i$ is an inhibitor of both bone mineralization and bone resorption (Fleisch, 1981). Knowing that increased extracellular PP$_i$ concentrations, such as in hypophosphatasia (OMIM 146300), have a negative effect on bone density, Reichenberger et al. (2001) suggested a dominant negative effect of the CMD mutations on the ANK protein function, resulting in decreased extracellular PP$_i$ levels. This raises the question of why mice heterozygous for the nonfunctional *ank* mutation do not show any phenotypic abnormality (Sweet and Green, 1981). Obviously, haploinsufficiency is not a valid concept for CMD. The dominant negative effect suggests an interaction between

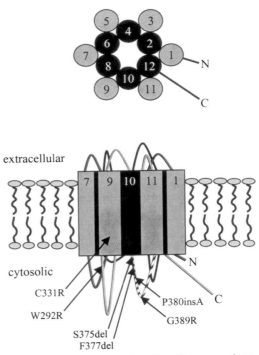

Figure 104–4. Schematic representation of ANK transmembrane helix assembly with sites of mutation indicated by arrows. Views from above and from the side are shown. Only even-numbered helices (in black) are predicted to contribute directly to the channel. The six-membered helical assembly results in a central channel wide enough to permit the passage of a pyrophosphate molecule, whereas the channel of a five-membered ring would be too narrow (e.g., the five-helix channel of phospholamban [PDB code 1PLN] has an inner diameter of about 4 Å, but the lowest diameter for inorganic pyrophosphate is 5.3 Å, even without Mg^{2+} or water ligands), and that of a circular 12- (or 10-) membered helix assembly would be far too wide to be selective for pyrophosphate. Note that nearly all mutations identified in craniometaphyseal dysplasia patients occurred at the cytosolic side. Loops in black are in the background connecting helices not visible in the side view. The fact that the majority of *ANKH* mutations found in this study affect only one of the five intracellular loops (hatched) suggests that this loop may play a critical role in control of ANK function. (Published with permission, Nürnberg et al., 2001.)

mutant and wild-type ANK protein with an impairment of the function of the latter. This might occur if at least two molecules form a complex. However, our model does not provide any hint to dimer formation. We are favoring the gain-of-function concept for the CMD mutations. This is supported by the lack of a CMD-like phenotype in patients with cri-du-chat syndrome, many of whom have deletions of chromosome 5p that include the *ANKH* locus (Overhauser et al., 1994). A gain of function could also explain the dominant nature of the mutations and the profound difference between the human and the mouse phenotype and provide a rationale for the increased bone formation, sclerosis, and abnormal bone remodeling seen in human CMD.

REFERENCES

Andrew LJ, Brancolini V, de la Pena LS, Devoto M, Caeiro F, Marchegiani R, Reginato A, Gaucher A, Netter P, Gillet P, et al. (1999). Refinement of the chromosome 5p locus for familial calcium pyrophosphate dihydrate deposition disease. *Am J Hum Genet* 64: 136–145.

Beighton P (1995). Craniometaphyseal dysplasia (CMD), autosomal dominant form. *J Med Genet* 32: 370–374.

Beighton P, Hamersma H, Horan F (1979). Craniometaphyseal dysplasia—variability of expression within a large family. *Clin Genet* 15: 252–258.

Boltshauser E, Schmitt B, Wichmann W, Valavanis A, Sailer H, Yonekawa Y (1996). Cerebellomedullary compression in recessive craniometaphyseal dysplasia. *Neuroradiology* 38(suppl 1): S193–S195.

Carnevale A, Grether P, del Castillo V, Takenaga R, Orzechowski A (1983). Autosomal dominant craniometaphyseal dysplasia. Clinical variability. *Clin Genet* 23: 17–22.

Colavita N, Kozlowski K, Sprague P (1988). Cranio-metaphyseal dysplasia. (Report of 3 cases—two infants and one adult). *Australas Radiol* 32: 257–262.

Chandler D, Tinschert S, Lohan K, Harrop K, Goldblatt J, Nagy M, Hummel S, Braun HS, Laing N, Nürnberg P (2001). Refinement of the chromosome 5p locus for craniometaphyseal dysplasia. *Hum Genet* 108: 394–397.

Cheung VG, Boechat MI, Barrett CT (1997). Bilateral choanal narrowing as a presentation of craniometaphyseal dysplasia. *J Perinatol* 17: 241–243

Day RA, Park TS, Ojemann JG, Kaufman BA (1997). Foramen magnum decompression for cervicomedullary encroachment in craniometaphyseal dysplasia: case report. *Neurosurgery* 41: 960–964.

Elcioglu N, Hall CM (1998). Temporal aspects in craniometaphyseal dysplasia: autosomal recessive type. *Am J Med Genet* 76: 245–251.

Fanconi S, Fischer JA, Wieland P, Giedion A, Boltshauser E, Olah AJ, Landolt AM, Prader A (1988). Craniometaphyseal dysplasia with increased bone turnover and secondary hyperparathyroidism: therapeutic effect of calcitonin. *J Pediatr* 112: 587–591.

Fleisch H (1981). Diphosphonates: history and mechanisms of action. *Metab Bone Dis Relat Res* 3: 279–288.

Franz DC, Horn KL, Aase J (1996). Craniometaphyseal dysplasia: operative findings and treatment. *Am J Otol* 17: 283–287.

Gorlin RJ, Spranger J, Koszalka MF (1969): Genetic craniotubular bone dysplasias and hyperostoses: a critical analysis. *Birth Defects Orig Art Ser V* 4: 79–95.

Guo Y, Hsu DK, Feng SL, Richards CM, Winkles JA (2002). Polypeptide growth factors and phorbol ester induce progressive ankylosis (ank) gene expression in murine and human fibroblasts. *J Cell Biochem* 84: 27–38.

Hakim FT, Brown KS, Oppenheim JJ (1986). Hereditary joint disorder in progressive ankylosis (ank/ank) mice. II. Effect of high-dose hydrocortisone treatment on inflammation and intraarticular calcium hydroxyapatite deposits. *Arthritis Rheum* 29: 114–123.

Hakim FT, Cranley R, Brown KS, Eanes ED, Harne L, Oppenheim JJ (1984). Hereditary joint disorder in progressive ankylosis (*ank/ank*) mice. I. Association of calcium hydroxyapatite deposition with inflammatory arthropathy. *Arthritis Rheum* 27: 1411–1420.

Halliday J (1949). A rare case of bone dystrophy. *Br J Surg* 37: 52–63.

Hayashibara T, Komura T, Sobue S, Ooshima T (2000). Tooth eruption in a patient with craniometaphyseal dysplasia: case report. *J Oral Pathol Med* 29: 460–462.

Hentze MW, Kulozik AE (1999). A perfect message: RNA surveillance and nonsense-mediated decay. *Cell* 96: 307–310.

Ho AM, Johnson MD, Kingsley DM (2000). Role of the mouse ank gene in control of tissue calcification and arthritis. *Science* 289: 265–270.

Hughes AE, McGibbon D, Woodward E, Dixey J, Doherty M (1995). Localisation of a gene for chondrocalcinosis to chromosome 5p. *Hum Mol Genet* 4: 1225–1228.

Iughetti P, Alonso LG, Wilcox W, Alonso N, Passos-Bueno MR (2000). Mapping of the autosomal recessive (AR) craniometaphyseal dysplasia locus to chromosome region 6q21-22 and confirmation of genetic heterogeneity for mild AR spondylocostal dysplasia. *Am J Med Genet* 95: 482–491.

Jackson WPU, Albright F, Drewery G, Hanelin J, Rubin ML (1954). Metaphyseal dysplasia, epiphyseal dysplasia, diaphyseal dysplasia and related conditions. *Arch Intern Med* 94: 871–885.

Johnson M, Ho A, McGrath R, Netter P, Loeuille D, Gillet P, Jonveaux P, Gaucher A, Reginato A, Gurley K, et al. (2001). Analysis of the ank gene reveals a heterozygous missense mutation in a French family with calcium pyrophosphate deposition disease (CPPDD). *Arthritis Rheum* 44: S161.

Kaitila I, Rimoin DL (1976). Histologic heterogeneity in the hyperostotic bone dysplasias. *Birth Defects Orig Artic Ser* 12: 71–79.

Key LL Jr, Volberg F, Baron R, Anast CS (1988). Treatment of craniometaphyseal dysplasia with calcitriol. *J Pediatr* 112: 583–587.

Komins C (1954). Familial metaphyseal dysplasia (Pyle's disease). *Br J Radiol* 27: 670–675.

Krug HE, Wietgrefe MM, Ytterberg SR, Taurog JD, Mahowald ML (1997). Murine progressive ankylosis is not immunologically mediated. *J Rheumatol* 24: 115–122.

Lehmann ECH (1957). Familial osteodystrophy of the skull and face. *J Bone Joint Surg* 39B: 313–315.

Lélek I (1961). Camurati-Engelmannsche Erkrankung. *Fortschr Röntgenstr* 94: 702–713.

Lièvre JA, Fischgold H (1956). Leontiasis ossea chez l'enfant (ostéopetrose partielle probable). *Presse Med* 64: 763–765.

Lust G, Faure G, Netter P, Seegmiller JE (1981). Increased pyrophosphate in fibroblasts and lymphoblasts from patients with hereditary diffuse articular chondrocalcinosis. *Science* 214: 809–810.

Mahowald ML, Krug H, Halverson P (1989). Progressive ankylosis (ank/ank) in mice: an animal model of spondyloarthropathy. II. Light and electron microscopic findings. *J Rheumatol* 16: 60–66.

Maldonado I, Reginato AM, Reginato AJ (2001). Familial calcium crystal diseases: what have we learned? *Curr Opin Rheumatol* 13: 225–233.

Millard DR, Maisels DO, Batstone JHF, Yates BW (1967): Craniofacial surgery in craniometaphyseal dysplasia. *Am J Surg* 113: 615–621.

Nürnberg P, Tinschert S, Mrug M, Hampe J, Müller CR, Fuhrmann E, Braun HS, Reis A (1997). The gene for autosomal dominant craniometaphyseal dysplasia maps to chromosome 5p and is distinct from the growth hormone-receptor gene. *Am J Hum Genet* 61: 918–923.

Nürnberg P, Thiele H, Chandler D, Höhne W, Cunningham ML, Ritter H, Leschik G, Uhlmann K, Mischung C, Harrop K, et al. (2001). Heterozygous mutations in *ANKH*, the human ortholog of the mouse progressive ankylosis gene, result in craniometaphyseal dysplasia. *Nat Genet* 28: 37–41.

Okawa A, Nakamura I, Goto S, Moriya H, Nakamura Y, Ikegawa S (1998). Mutation in *Npps* in a mouse model of ossification of the posterior longitudinal ligament of the spine. *Nat Genet* 19: 271–273.

Overhauser J, Huang X, Gersh M, Wilson W, McMahon J, Bengtsson U, Rojas K, Meyer M, Wasmuth JJ (1994). Molecular and phenotypic mapping of the short arm of chromosome 5: sublocalization of the critical region for the cri-du-chat syndrome. *Hum Mol Genet* 3: 247–252.

Peariso S, McGrath R, Bonavita G, Reginato A, Caeiro F, Marchegiani R, Iglesias A (2001). Characterization of sequence variants in *ank* in familial calcium pyrophosphate deposition disease (CPPD). *Arthritis Rheum* 44: S162.

Penchaszadeh VB, Gutierriz ER, Figueeroa EP (1980). Autosomal recessive craniometaphyseal dysplasia. *Am J Med Genet* 5: 43–55.

Pendleton A, Johnston M, Ho A, Gurley K, Kingsley D, Wright GD, Dixey J, Doherty M, Hughes AE (2001). A heterozygous mutation in the human *ank* gene in a British family with adult onset chondrocalcinosis due to calcium pyrophosphate crystal deposition. *Arthritis Rheum* 44: S101.

Reichenberger E, Tiziani V, Watanabe S, Park L, Ueki Y, Santanna C, Baur ST, Shiang R, Grange DK, Beighton P, et al. (2001). Autosomal dominant craniometaphyseal dysplasia is caused by mutations in the transmembrane protein ANK. *Am J Hum Genet* 68: 1321–1326.

Richards A, Brain C, Dillon MJ, Bailey CM (1996). Craniometaphyseal and craniodiaphyseal dysplasia, head and neck manifestations and management. *J Laryngol Otol* 110: 328–338.

Rimoin DL, Woodruff SL, Holman BL (1969). Craniometaphyseal dysplasia (Pyle's disease): autosomal dominant inheritance in a large kindred. *Birth Defects Orig Art Ser* 5: 96–104.

Ross MW, Altman DH (1967). Familial metaphyseal dysplasia. Review of the clinical and radiologic feature of Pyle's disease. *Clin Pediatr (Phila)* 6: 143–149.

Sampson HW, Davis JS (1988). Histopathology of the intervertebral disc of progressive ankylosis mice. *Spine* 13: 650–654.

Satoh K, Iwata T, Ikeda H (1994). Unsuccessful consequence of optic canal decompression for a case of craniometaphyseal dysplasia. *Plast Reconstr Surg* 94: 705–708.

Shea J, Gerbe R, Ayani N (1981). Craniometaphyseal dysplasia: the first successful surgical treatment for associated hearing loss. *Laryngoscope* 91: 1369–1374.

Sommer F (1954). Eine besondere Form einer generalisierten Hyperostose mit Leontiasis ossea faciei et cranii. *Radiol Clin (Basel)* 23: 65–75.

Spranger J, Paulsen K, Lehmann W (1965). Die kraniometaphysäre Dysplasie (Pyle). *Z Kinderheilkd* 93: 64–79.

Stool SE, Caruso VG (1973). Cranial metaphyseal dysplasia. *Arch Otolaryngol* 97: 410–412.

Sweet HO, Green MC (1981). Progressive ankylosis, a new skeletal mutation in the mouse. *J Hered* 72: 87–93.

Taylor DB, Sprague P (1989). Dominant craniometaphyseal dysplasia—a family study over five generations. *Australas Radiol* 33: 84–89.

Tinschert S, Braun H-S (1998). Craniometaphyseal dysplasia in six generations of a German kindred. *Am J Med Genet* 77: 175–181.

Wemmer U, Böttger E (1978). Die kraniometaphysäre Dysplasie (Jackson). *Fortschr Röntgenstr* 128: 66–69.

Yamamoto T, Kurihara N, Yamaoka K, Ozono K, Okada M, Yamamoto K, Matsumoto S, Michigami T, Ono J, Okada S (1993). Bone marrow-derived osteoclast-like cells from a patient with craniometaphyseal dysplasia lack expression of osteoclast-reactive vacuolar proton pump. *J Clin Invest* 91: 362–367.

VI

DYSMORPHIC DISEASE GENES OF UNKNOWN FUNCTION

105 | *p63* and the Ectodermal Dysplasia, Ectrodactyly, and Cleft Lip and/or Palate (EEC), Limb-Mammary (LMS), Ankyloblepharon, Ectrodactyly, and Cleft Lip/Palate (AEC, Hay-Wells), and Acro-Dermato-Ungual-Lacrimal-Digit (ADULT) Syndromes and Ectrodactyly (Split Hand/Foot Malformation)

MICHAEL J. BAMSHAD

*T*P63 encodes a homologue of the prototypic tumor suppressor gene, *TP53*. Mutations in *TP63* are found in 90% of individuals who have one of four different multiple malformation syndromes: (1) ectodermal dysplasia, ectrodactyly, and cleft lip and/or palate (EEC) syndrome (OMIM 604292); (2) limb-mammary syndrome (LMS) (OMIM 603543); (3) ankyloblepharon, ectrodactyly, and cleft lip/palate (AEC) syndrome (or Hay-Wells syndrome) (OMIM 106260); and (4) acro-dermato-ungual-lacrimal-digit (ADULT) syndrome (OMIM 103285). All of these syndromes are characterized by ectodermal defects accompanied by limb malformations that range from subtle to severe. A small percentage of patients with isolated ectrodactyly (split hand/foot malformation) syndrome (OMIM 605289) also have mutations in *TP63*. All of these conditions can usually be distinguished from each other and from rarer disorders through the use of clinical criteria, although mutation analysis can be helpful, particularly in sporadic cases. The long-term care of patients with syndromes caused by mutations in *TP63* can be challenging, but in general, most patients do well. None of these conditions are associated with an increased predisposition to cancer, underscoring the divergent role of p63 compared with that of p53. *TP63* is widely expressed in the progenitor epithelial cells of many different tissues and organs; this includes the region of specialized ectoderm covering the developing limb that in part controls outgrowth of the limb bud. *TP63*-deficient mice have malformations of the epidermis and its appendages, severe truncation defects of the limbs, and craniofacial abnormalities, fully recapitulating EEC syndrome. Individuals heterozygous for deletions of *TP63* do not have EEC syndrome. This is consistent with in vitro studies of mutant p63 proteins that suggest development is disrupted by either gain-of-function or dominant-negative effect. As a consequence, the proliferative capacities of progenitor cells may be limited because of early terminal differentiation or increased cell death.

One of the striking revelations about the human genome is that it contains only 30,000 to 40,000 genes (Lander et al., 2001; Venter et al., 2001), far fewer than many predictions. Equally surprising is the observation that this is only about twice as many genes as found in the roundworm (*C. elegans*) and only slightly more than the approximately 26,000 genes of the mustard plant (*A. thaliana*). This leads to the somewhat puzzling inference that organisms with approximately the same number of genes, many of which are homologous, can look strikingly different from one another.

One difference contributing to this wide assortment of morphologies is the diversity of proteins and interactions among the proteins produced by homologous genes in different species. In the human genome, it is clear that many genes encode multiple products that have myriad roles in metabolism, growth, and development. It is not surprising, therefore, that mutations in different parts of the same gene might perturb different functions, resulting in dramatically different phenotypes. Examples of genes in which different mutations cause similar but distinct syndromes include *FGFR2*, *FGFR3*, *GLI3*, and *GNAS1*.

It has been discovered that at least five different syndromes are caused by mutations in the gene *TP53*. Characterization of these mutations coupled with structural and functional studies of p63 has revealed an explicit genotype–phenotype correlation among these different syndromes. This is providing valuable new insights into the role of p63 in molecular, cellular, and developmental processes. Moreover, it is facilitating the diagnosis and clinical management of individuals with an assortment of malformation syndromes.

TP63 is located on chromosome 3q27 and is composed of 16 exons (Figure 105–1) that encode at least six different alternatively spliced transcripts from four different transcription initiation sites (Schmale and Bamberger, 1997; Yang et al., 1998; Haigwara et al., 1999). Each of these transcripts encodes a protein that shares substantial amino acid identity with the DNA-binding (DBD), transactivation (TA), and tetramerization (ISO) domains of *p53*, the prototypic tumor suppressor in mammals (Levine, 1997). In general, the use of two of the initiation sites yields two different classes of proteins: those with a TA domain (TA-p63) and those with a truncated amino terminus (ΔN-p63) lacking this region. Further complexity is added by alternatively splicing one of three different carboxyl-terminal domains (α, β, and γ) onto the TA and ΔN isoforms. The DBD and ISO are found in all of these isoforms of p63. The α isoforms of p63 encode a motif that is similar to the sterile-α-motif (SAM) domain. SAM domains are involved in protein–protein interactions via homodimerization or heterodimerization with other SAM domains, although p63 SAM domains do not oligomerize with each other (Chi et al., 1999).

Although the presence of a TA domain is necessary for transactivation activity, not all TA isoforms of p63 can activate TA. TA-p63γ and TA-p63β can transactivate reporter genes containing consensus *p53*-binding sites, whereas TA-p63α lacks this ability. Originally, the SAM domain was thought to be a key regulatory element of TA-p63α. However, it is apparent that the post-SAM region of the carboxyl terminus is necessary for the lack of TA properties of TA-p63α. This domain is now called the transactivation inhibitory domain (TID).

None of the ΔN-p63 proteins, which lack a TA domain, can transactivate p53-responsive genes. Moreover, the ΔN-p63 isoforms effectively block the function of p53 as well as the function of TA-p63 isoforms. Thus, they not only function as dominant-negative repressors of transcription but also have opposing properties compared with the TA isoforms of p63. RNA and protein expression studies in mice have demonstrated that the ΔN-p63 isoforms are the major products found in the epithelial tissues of embryos and appear to play a role in the modulation of p53 activity.

MALFORMATION SYNDROMES CAUSED BY MUTATIONS IN *TP63*

Mutations in *TP63* are sufficient to cause at least five distinct malformation syndromes, each of which is characterized by defects of organs, structures, and/or body areas whose normal development is dependent on the integrity of the ectoderm (Table 105–1). These syndromes include EEC syndrome, LMS syndrome, AEC or Hay-Wells syndrome, ADULT syndrome, and isolated ectrodactyly or split hand/foot malformation (SHFM) syndrome. All of these disorders are transmitted in an autosomal dominant pattern.

The most consistent abnormality observed in individuals with EEC, LMS, AEC, or ADULT syndrome is an overlapping combination of varying defects of ectoderm-derived structures such as the skin, hair, teeth, nails, and apocrine glands, including the breasts. The frequency of each of these defects varies widely among these disorders, and no specific defect is found in all individuals with any one of these conditions. Limb defects can be found in individuals affected with any of these five disorders. They are typically least severe in AEC syndrome and most severe in EEC or isolated SHFM syndrome. As its name

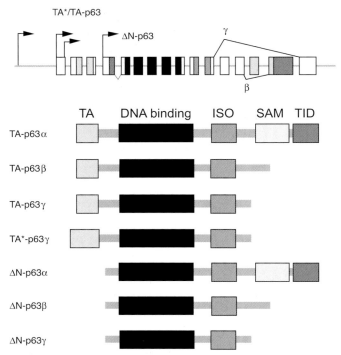

Figure 105–1. Schematic representation of the genomic structure of *TP63* and its major isoforms. There are at least four sites (*arrows*) where the transcription of *TP63* is initiated. Alternative splicing is used to generate a wide variety of different mRNAs. All of these transcripts contain DNA-binding and tetramerization (ISO) domains that are highly homologous to the corresponding domains of p53. Only TA-p63β and TA-p63γ are capable of transactivating gene expression. SAM, sterile-α-motif domain; TA, transactivation; TID, transactivation inhibitory domain.

suggests, isolated SHFM syndrome is the only one of these conditions in which the skin and ectoderm-derived appendages are normal, although normal limb development is dependent on signals emanating from a specialized region of ectoderm. Thus, all five disorders are caused by primary abnormalities of ectoderm. The best characterized of these disorders is EEC syndrome. Investigation of the molecular etiology of EEC syndrome led to the identification of *TP63* as a major cause of human malformations.

EEC Syndrome

EEC syndrome is an uncommon syndrome characterized by SHFM; anomalies of hair, teeth, nails, nasolacrimal ducts, and sweat glands; and cleft lip with or without cleft palate (Buss et al., 1995; Roelfsema and Cobbens, 1996; Gorlin et al., 2001). Although there are earlier reports of patients with EEC syndrome (Eckholdt and Martens, 1804), a comprehensive description of this disorder was first provided by Cockayne in 1936. The acronym *EEC syndrome* was coined by Rudiger et al., (1970).

The most common and consistent feature of individuals with EEC syndrome is the presence of ectodermal defects (Buss et al., 1995; Roelfsema and Cobbens, 1996). The scalp hair, eyebrows, and eyelashes are affected in nearly all cases, with the scalp hair generally being coarse and dry and growing slowly (Figure 105–2). In some individuals, it is also sparse. Individuals of European ancestry typically have light-colored hair, whereas in individuals of African descent, pigmentation of the hair is usually normal. Axillary hair in males and females and facial hair in males are usually normal.

The teeth are nearly always affected. The primary dentition may be complete although morphologically abnormal. Malformations of the secondary dentition are common and most often include microdontia and oligodontia. Dental caries is common and often severe. This may be a consequence of xerostomia coupled with hypoplasia of the dental enamel.

Abnormalities of the skin are common although usually relatively minor. The most common manifestation is excessively dry, scaly skin. Erosions and cutis aplasia are not observed in individuals with EEC syndrome. Multiple pigmented nevi have been reported in about 10% of cases. Hypohydrosis and abnormalities of the sweat glands have been reported but are not common features of EEC (Temtamy and McKusick, 1978; Freire-Maia and Pinheiro, 1984; Roelfsema and Cobbens, 1996). The nails are affected in more than 75% of cases. They are typically slow growing, and the presence of transverse ridges, pitting, or splitting is common (Figure 105–3). In the absence of ectodermal defects, the diagnosis of EEC syndrome is virtually excluded. However, the expression of ectodermal defects is highly variable both within and among families, and some individuals have only subtle abnormalities.

Orofacial clefts are found in approximately 60% to 70% of affected individuals (Buss et al., 1995; Roelfsema and Cobbens, 1996). These include unilateral or bilateral cleft lip and palate or cleft palate without cleft lip (Figure 105–4). In EEC syndrome, cleft lip/palate and isolated cleft palate sometimes occur in the same pedigree, whereas for most malformation syndromes, families manifest one or the other. This phenomenon is called *mixed clefting*. It is a feature of only several malformation syndromes, of which the best known is van der Woude

Table 105–1. Body Areas Affected in Syndromes Caused by Mutation in *TP63*

Body Area	Syndrome				
	EEC	AEC	LMS	SHFM	ADULT
Limb					
Split hand/foot	++	−	++	+++	++
Syndactyly	+++	+/−	++	++	++
Ectodermal	+++	+++	+	−	++
Hair	++	+++	−	−	+
Skin	+	+++	−	−	++
Nail	++	++	+/−	−	+
Teeth	++	++	+/−	−	++
Lacrimal ducts	++	+	+	−	+
Sweat glands	+	++	+	−	−
Fused eyelid	−	+++	−	−	−
Breast/nipple hypoplasia	+	−	+++	−	+
Supernumerary nipples	+/−	+	−	−	−
Facial					
Cleft lip/palate	+++	+	−	−	−
Cleft palate	+	+	+	−	−
Other					
Genitourinary defects	++	+	−	−	−
Urethra/bladder	+	−	−	−	−
Hearing loss	+	+	−	−	−
freckling	+	−	−	−	+++

ADULT, acro-dermato-ungual-lacrimal-digit syndrome; AEC, ankyloblepharon, ectrodactyly, and cleft lip/palate syndrome; EEC, ectodermal dysplasia, ectrodactyly, and cleft lip and/or palate syndrome; LMS, limb-mammary syndrome; SHFM, split hand/foot malformation; −, not observed; +/−, rare; +, uncommon; ++, common; +++, very common.

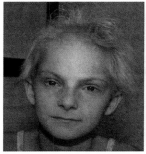
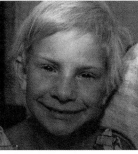

Figure 105–2. Two sisters with ectodermal dyslasia, ectrodactyly, and cleft lip and/or palate (EEC) syndrome. Note the sparse, bright blonde scalp hair accompanied by blonde eyebrows and eyelashes. The nasal root, bridge, and tip are broad, and the malar surfaces are flattened. The periorbital regions are somewhat darkened as a consequence of chronic blepharitis caused by dysfunction of the meibomian and lacrimal glands coupled with obstruction/stenosis of the lacrimal ducts.

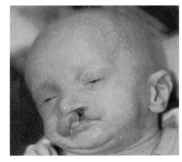

Figure 105–4. A newborn with ectodermal dysplasia, ectrodactyly, and cleft lip and/or palate (EEC) syndrome and a left-sided cleft lip. Note the sparse scalp hair and the prominence of the scalp vessels. (Courtesy of Dr. Steve Braddock, University of Missouri.)

syndrome (Neilson et al., 2002). Two other conditions, Rapp-Hodgkin and Hay-Wells (AEC) syndromes, also exhibit mixed clefting, with the latter also caused by mutations in *TP63*.

Lacrimal duct anomalies are observed in nearly 90% of affected individuals (Buss et al., 1995). These anomalies include lacrimal duct stenosis, obstruction, and atresia that may be unilateral or bilateral. Dacrocystitis secondary to a lacrimal duct defect is common. Lacrimal duct obstruction occurs in 1% to 2% of the general pediatric population and is even more common in children with cleft palate. Isolated lacrimal duct atresia can also be transmitted in an autosomal dominant pattern (McNab et al., 1989). However, when accompanied by split hand/foot malformations, the combination is nearly pathognomonic for EEC syndrome.

Other ophthamologic abnormalities that have been reported in patients with EEC syndrome include blepharitis, chronic conjunctivitis, corneal scarring, pannus formation with photophobia, and corneal perforation (McNab et al., 1989). Although, the orofacial clefts and limb defects produce considerable disabilities, the secondary consequences of the ophthamologic abnormalities are responsible for the bulk of adult morbidity associated with EEC syndrome. Visual impairment is caused by recurrent infections caused by lacrimal duct obstructions, defective tearing due to aplasia of the meibomian glands, and primary epithelial defects of the cornea (Kasmann and Ruprecht, 1997). All of these anomalies are quite variable and not unique to EEC syndrome. SHFM has been reported in association with a retinal macular dystrophy that has been called the EEM syndrome (Albrecsten and Svendsen, 1956; Ohdo et al., 1983), although the etiology of this condition is unknown.

Individuals with EEC syndrome may exhibit a variety of breast malformations, including inverted nipples, hypoplastic areolae, absence of the areolae, and unilateral or bilateral hypoplasia of the breasts (Maas et al., 1996; O'Quinn et al., 1998). Unilateral or bilateral ab-

sence of the breast is uncommon. Supernumerary nipples have also been reported (van Bokhoven et al., 2001). Although the range of breast defects is well understood, the incidence of these defects is poorly documented.

Malformations of the limb are found in more than 80% to 90% of individuals with EEC syndrome (Buss et al., 1995; Roelfsema et al., 1996). The defect most commonly associated with EEC syndrome is called *ectrodactyly*, a term derived from the Greek words *ektroma* ("abortion") and *daktylos* ("finger"). Thus, *ectrodactyly* means a partial or total absence of the hand with the proximal segments that are more or less normal. However, the term has been widely and variably interpreted, with some authors using it to describe the absence of one or more digits. Originally, Geoffrey Saint-Hilaire used the term to describe an abnormality characterized by having only two digits, the thumb, and the fifth digit (Temtamy and McKusick, 1978). This defect was designated first by Meller in 1893 as a split-hand (*spalthand*). Today, this malformation is more appropriately referred to as a split-hand/foot malformation (SHFM). SHFMs are commonly divided into typical and atypical forms.

In typical SHFM, the hand/foot is divided into two parts separated by a cleft with or without syndactyly of the digits on either side of the cleft (Figure 105–5). In the mildest form, only the third digit is absent, and the corresponding metacarpal or metatarsal is normal. Increasingly severe defects are characterized by additional hypoplastic or missing digits and metacarpals. The most severe SHFM is characterized by the complete absence of all digits, metcarpals/metatarsals, and carpals/tarsals. SHFM characterized by hypoplasia or the absence of digits 1 and/or 5 is called *atypical SHFM*.

EEC syndrome is characterized by a remarkably broad range of limb defects. Asymmetry between the right and left sides is common. One to four limbs may be affected, including only both upper limbs or only both lower limbs. The observation that SHFM is the most common limb defect observed in EEC syndrome may be biased because it is the identification of an SHFM that often leads to ascertainment of a case. However, there are numerous reports of families in which only one or a few of multiple individuals affected with EEC syndrome have an SHFM (Kuster et al., 1985; Anneren et al., 1991; Bamshad et al.,

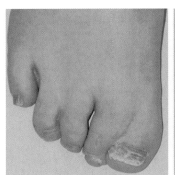
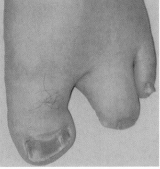

Figure 105–3. Dysplasia of the nails in an individual with ectodermal dysplasia, ectrodactyly, and cleft lip and/or palate (EEC) syndrome. Note that the nails are thickened, splitting, and chipped. (Courtesy of Dr. Louanne Hudgins and Dr. Anita Beck, Stanford University.)

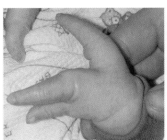
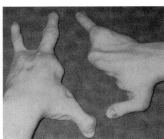

Figure 105–5. Typical split hand malformations. *Left*, metacarpals and phalanges of digits 3 and 4 are absent, producing a deep cleft of the hand. *Right*, abnormalities of the hand are similar, although digit 2 is also missing.

2000). The most common defect in familial cases appears to be syndactyly, usually of digits 3 and 4. Moreover, some individuals with EEC syndrome have only nonspecific limb abnormalities (e.g., camptodactyly, anterior or posterior polydactyly) or normal limbs (Wallis et al., 1988; Maas et al., 1996; Bamshad et al., 2000).

Abnormalities of the genitourinary tract are observed in about 50% of individuals with EEC syndrome (Rollnick and Hoo, 1988; Nardi et al., 1992). This estimate is probably low because individuals with EEC syndrome often are not evaluated for genitourinary anomalies unless they are symptomatic. Any portion of the genitourinary tract, including the kidneys, ureters, bladder, and urethra, may be abnormal. Defects of the kidneys range from mild, unilateral hydronephrosis to unilateral renal agenesis (Kaiser-Kupfer, 1973). Duplication of the kidney, collecting system, and ureter has also been reported (Preus and Fraser, 1973; Rodini and Richieri-Costa, 1990). Cystic/dysplastic kidneys are uncommon, although they may occur coincidentally. Any segment of the ureter may be stenotic and present as an obstruction. Stricture of the distal urethra has been reported in both males and females (Maas et al., 1996). The gonads and external genitalia are usually normal, although males with cryptorchidism and/or glandular hypospadias have been observed (da Silva et al., 1984; Rodini and Richieri-Costa, 1990; Maas et al., 1996).

A genitourinary abnormality that appears relatively unique to EEC among disorders caused by mutations in *TP63* is an atrophic/dysplastic bladder epithelium (Maas et al., 1996). Although the pathogenic mechanism is unknown, thinning of the epithelium results in dysuria, an urgency to void, and an increased voiding frequency. These symptoms resemble those observed in individuals with urinary tract infection. However, the urine is sterile and the symptoms do not respond to antibiotic treatment.

The facial phenotype of individuals with EEC syndrome is characteristic but nonspecific (see Figures 105–2 and 105–3). The extent of deviation from the facial characteristics representative of the family background is dependent on the presence and severity of malformations of the lacrimal ducts, lip, and palate. However, even individuals with EEC syndrome who do not have severe ectodermal defects or cleft lip and/or palate often have facial features like those of other individuals with EEC syndrome. These features include a broad nasal root, bridge, and tip and flared ala nasi. This suggests that there may be subtle midface/palatal abnormalities even in individuals with EEC syndrome without cleft lip and/or palate.

A myriad of abnormalities that occur at low frequency have been reported in individuals with EEC syndrome (Buss et al., 1995; Roelfsema et al., 1996; van Bokhoven et al., 2001). One of the most notable abnormalities is hearing loss, which in some series (Buss et al., 1995) has been found in more than 40% of affected individuals. In most cases of hearing loss, a conductive deficit was observed. Some patients have reported a frequently dry mouth, probably secondary to dysfunction of the salivary glands.

Early reports suggested that developmental delay and mental retardation were common features of children with EEC syndrome (Bixler et al., 1971). However, it has become clear that most individuals with EEC syndrome experience normal development, are enrolled in regular classrooms, and are cognitively normal. As a secondary consequence of cleft lip and/or palate or hearing impairment, language development is delayed in some children with EEC syndrome.

LMS

LMS is a condition that differs from EEC syndrome in at least three ways (van Bokhoven et al., 1999). First, abnormalities of the breasts, such as hypoplasia of the areola, athelia, or hypoplasia of the breast, are consistent features of individuals affected with LMS. Second, the hair and skin of individuals with LMS are usually normal, although dry skin has been reported (van Bokhoven et al., 2001). Third, although cleft lip and/or palate is observed in individuals with EEC syndrome, only clefting of the palate has been reported in individuals with LMS.

Additional features of LMS are hypodontia, anodontia, lacrimal duct atresia, and dystrophic nails. Malformations of the limb include cutaneous syndactyly, hypoplasia of the fifth digit, and typical SHFMs. Some individuals have normal limbs.

LMS has been reported in a single large, extended kindred exhibiting wide variation in phenotypic expression among the 29 affected individuals (van Bokhoven et al., 1999). The most subtly affected individual had only athelia. There was no evidence of nonpenetrance. A few sporadic cases of LMS have also been reported (van Bokhoven et al., 2001).

AEC Syndrome

AEC syndrome is a condition first fully described by Hay and Wells (1976) in which the hallmark feature is the presence of an *ankyloblepharon*, the partial or complete fusion of the eyelids. The ankyloblepharon found in individuals with AEC syndrome is usually not complete (Vanderhooft et al., 1993). Typically, it consists of strands of vascularized connective tissue that bridge the eyelids at the medial or lateral margins of the lid; this is called *ankyloblepharon filiforme adnatum* (Figure 105–6). These strands are sometimes so friable at birth that they are easily disrupted by unintended, gentle manipulation of the lids. Thus, it is sometimes difficult to ascertain whether ankyloblepharon filiforme adenatum was present in a newborn. Other abnormalities of the skin include severe erosions, dry skin, palmer or plantar hyperkeratosis, and dermatitis.

Additional characteristics of AEC syndrome include cleft lip and palate or cleft palate, lacrimal duct atresia, hypodontia, dystrophic nails, sparse scalp hair, hypoplastic or supernumerary nipples, and hypohidrosis. Genital anomalies, including micropenis, hypospadias, and filamentous bands of tissue spanning the lateral walls of the vagina, have been reported (Hay and Wells, 1976). Limb malformations observed in AEC syndrome are in general less severe than those in individuals with EEC syndrome. The most common malformation reported is cutaneous syndactyly of digits 3 and 4 and/or toes 2 and 3.

ADULT Syndrome

ADULT syndrome is a rare condition characterized by SHFMs, hypodontia and/or early loss of permanent teeth, nail dysplasia, lacrimal duct obstruction, and breast abnormalities. Individuals with ADULT syndrome commonly develop an exfoliative dermatitis of the digits and exhibit excessive freckling. It is differentiated from EEC syndrome by the absence of facial clefting.

Expression of the hand and foot malformations ranges from cutaneous syndactyly to the absence of a single digit to typical SHFMs, although affected individuals may have normal limbs. Some patients have primary hypodontia of their permanent teeth, whereas others have a normal number of permanent teeth but begin to loose them in their teens.

ADULT syndrome has been described in only a few sporadic cases and families (Propping and Zerres, 1993; Amiel et al., 2001; van Bokhoven et al., 2001). The few families with ADULT syndrome display extensive intrafamilial variation. This appears to be a general characteristic of disorders caused by mutations in *TP63*. In addition, many of the features of ADULT syndrome are also features of EEC syndrome and LMS. However, ADULT syndrome differentiated from EEC syndrome by the absence of facial clefting. Distinguishing ADULT syndrome from LMS in the absence of excessive freckling may prove to be challenging.

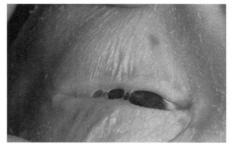

Figure 105–6. Ankyloblepharon filiforme adnatum in a newborn with ankyloblepharon, ectrodactyly, and cleft lip/palate (AEC) syndrome. (Courtesy of Dr. Virginia Sybert, University of Washington.)

Isolated SHFMs

Approximately 60% of SHFMs occur without accompanying defects of additional organs or body areas. These malformations are referred to as *isolated SHFMs* and have a prevalence of approximately 1:15,000 to 20,000 (Czeizel et al., 1993; Evans et al., 1994). The phrase *split hand/foot* is somewhat of a misnomer because many affected individuals do not have a typical split hand or foot. In individuals ascertained by having at least one family member with a typical SHFM, limb involvement ranges from cutaneous syndactyly of the proximal portion of digits 3 and 4 to absence of the hands and feet accompanied by the absence of or reduction in the long bones of the upper and lower limbs. One or more limbs may be involved, and the pattern of malformations between the upper and lower limbs and/or the left and right sides is usually asymmetric. Amelia of one or more limbs is not a common feature of isolated SHFMs. The penetrance of isolated SHFMs appears to be high in families in which no affected individual has tibial hemimelia. The presence of tibial hemimelia may distinguish a subset of families with isolated SHFMs in whom the penetrance is substantially lower (Majewski et al., 1985; Zlotogora, 1994).

Isolated SHFMs can be transmitted in autosomal dominant, autosomal recessive, and X-linked recessive patterns. Also, isolated SHFM has been associated with a variety of karyotypic abnormalities, such as deletions or rearrangements of chromosome 2q31-34 (Boles et al., 1993) or 6q21 (Braverman et al., 1993; Viljoen et al., 1993; Gurrieri et al., 1995). The most commonly reported karyotypic abnormalities are rearrangements involving chromosome 7q11-7q22 (Klep-de Pater et al., 1979; Del Porto et al., 1983; Pfeiffer 1984; Tajara et al., 1989; Morey and Higgins, 1990; Roberts et al., 1991; Sharland et al., 1991; Scherer et al., 1994). Abnormalities of this region have also been reported to cause a condition resembling EEC syndrome (Hasegawa et al., 1991; Fukushima et al., 1993). The latter conclusion is based in large part on the analysis of a few sporadic cases and a single family in which a balanced translocation involving chromosome 7q11 was segregating. None of the affected individuals with these chromosome abnormalities were reported to have lacrimal duct, genitourinary, or nail anomalies, and two individuals had uncommon features of EEC syndrome (i.e., bilateral accessory nipples and mental retardation). A locus causing dominantly inherited isolated SHFM has been mapped to chromosome 10q24-q25 (Nunes et al., 1995; Raas-Rothschild et al., 1996), and the critical interval has been narrowed to just a few centimorgans (Ozën et al., 1999). However, the gene responsible for isolated SHFM has not yet been identified.

DIAGNOSIS

Diagnostic Criteria

The varying expressivity and overlapping characteristics of the different syndromes caused by mutations in *TP63* can make the assignment of a specific diagnosis challenging. As a consequence, specific criteria have been proposed to facilitate the diagnostic process. These criteria were originally developed for EEC syndrome, but with the exception of isolated SHFM, they can be applied to other conditions caused by mutations in *TP63* with only minor modification.

For a sporadic case of EEC, an individual must have at least three of the following findings: (1) ectodermal defects involving the hair, teeth, and/or nails, (2) limb defects including typical or atypical SHFMs, oligodactyly, and simple or complex syndactyly, (3) cleft lip with or without cleft palate—not cleft palate alone, (4) lacrimal duct or lacrimal gland defects, (5) an atrophic bladder epithelium, (6) breast abnormalities, and (7) genitourinary defects. If at least one individual in a family meets the diagnostic criteria for a sporadic case, the criteria are relaxed, and additional family members are required to have only two or more findings of the criteria for EEC syndrome.

For LMS, the criteria are modified to make breast abnormalities mandatory while hair and skin defects or a cleft lip virtually excludes the diagnosis. The presence of ankyloblepharon filiforme adnatum is required in a sporadic case of AEC syndrome, and the limbs of individuals with AEC syndrome are in general normal. Individuals with ADULT syndrome have extensive freckling but do not exhibit cleft lip and/or cleft palate.

These criteria only facilitate diagnosis; they cannot be used to exclude all alternatives, including other syndromes with similar phenotypes caused by mutations in genes other than *TP63*. For example, some individuals with mutations in *TBX3*, causing ulnar-mammary syndrome (see Chapter 69), meet the diagnostic criteria for EEC syndrome.

Differential Diagnosis

All five syndromes caused by mutations in *TP63* are characterized by abnormalities of tissues and structures that develop in part from epithelial tissues. These abnormalities include defects of skin, hair, teeth, nails, apocrine glands including the breasts, palate, and limbs. As a consequence, many of the phenotypic characteristics of these different syndromes are shared (see Table 105–1). It is usually possible to distinguish which of these syndromes affects an individual, although a specific diagnosis can be difficult to make if individuals within a family have uncommon findings or lack common findings and in sporadic cases. There are numerous reports of multiplex families in which none, one, or only a few individuals affected with EEC syndrome have an SHFM (Küster et al., 1985; Rodini and Richieri-Costa, 1990; Anneren et al., 1991) or cleft lip/palate (Wallis et al., 1988). Each of the features found in these five syndromes has been observed in individuals with an alternative diagnosis. Thus, none of these features is pathognomonic of any of one of these disorders.

Depending on how one chooses to distinguish between syndromes, approximately one-half to a dozen additional syndromes have been reported that share many of the characteristics of the five syndromes caused by mutations in *TP63* (Table 105–2). Although each of these should be considered in the differential diagnosis, in many cases it is easy to distinguish between these conditions and those caused by mutations in *TP63*.

Many of the individual phenotypic characteristics of syndromes caused by mutations in *TP63* can be transmitted as isolated finding in an autosomal dominant pattern; these include cleft palate, lacrimal duct atresia, hypodontia, and hypoplasia of the breasts. SHFM accompanied by aplasia cutis of the scalp has also been reported (Bonafede and Beighton, 1979).

There is a plethora of reports describing individuals with SHFMs and one or two characteristics of EEC syndrome such as lacrimal duct obstruction or hearing impairment. Few, if any, of these cases would meet the diagnostic criteria for EEC syndrome. Nevertheless, it is possible that some of these conditions are caused by mutations in *TP63*; this hypothesis remains to be tested. There also are a handful of case reports in which an individual or members of a family manifest the cardinal features of EEC syndrome yet have been labeled with a different, sometimes provisionally unique syndrome. For example, Reed et al., (1971) described a mother and daughter with SHFM, lacrimal duct obstruction, alopecia, and atrophic, pigmented macules and called it REEDS syndrome.

Table 105–2. Syndromes Sharing Features with Syndrome Caused by *TP63* Mutations

Syndrome	Characteristics
REEDS	SHFM; lacrimal duct obstruction; alopecia; atrophic, pigmented macules
Rapp-Hodgkin	Cleft palate; hypohydrosis; sparse hair; dry skin; abnormal nails and teeth
Zanier-Roubicek	Hypohydrosis; hypodontia; breast hypoplasia; hypotrichosis; normal limbs
Roselli-Gulienetti	Thumb hypoplasia; cleft lip/palate; skin, hair, dental, nail defects; genital hypoplasia
Bowen-Armstrong	Limb defects; cleft lip/palate; skin, hair, dental, nail defects; genital hypoplasia
Lacrimo-auriculo-dento-digital (LADD)	Clinodactyly/triphalangeal thumbs; lacrimal duct obstruction; cupped ears; dental defects
Ectrodactyly/cleft palate (ECP)	SHFM; cleft palate but no cleft lip
Adams-Oliver	Aplasia cutis congenita, oligodactyly, brachydactyly, limb deficiency

SHFM, split hand/foot malformation.

Other syndromes that resemble those caused by mutations in *TP63* are clearly distinct conditions. Rapp-Hodgkin (RH) syndrome is a disorder characterized by hypohydrosis, cleft lip and palate, and defects of the hair, nails, and teeth (Rapp and Hodgkin, 1968). The limbs of most individuals with RH syndrome are normal. RH syndrome is virtually indistinguishable from a condition described by Zanier and Roubicek (1976) in a single kindred of more than 20 affected individuals. These individuals had hypohydrosis, hypodontia, hypotrichosis, breast hypoplasia, and normal limbs. It is likely that RH syndrome and Zanier-Roubicek syndrome are the same entity. RH syndrome has also been reported in the mother of a child with EEC syndrome (Moerman and Fryns, 1996). This suggests that some cases of RH, EEC, and Zanier-Roubicek syndromes may have a common etiology. To date, no mutations in *TP63* have been reported in classic cases of RH or Zanier-Roubicek syndrome.

AEC syndrome overlaps with at least two other conditions: Rosselli-Gulienetti and Bowen-Armstrong syndromes. Rosselli-Gulienetti syndrome was originally described in four individuals with hair, dental, nail, limb, palate, breast, and sweating abnormalities (Rosselli and Gulienetti, 1971). Genital hypoplasia, hyperpigmented macules, and popliteal pterygia were observed in two of the cases, a pair of affected sibs. In 1976, Bowen and Armstrong reported a family of three girls with hair, dental, nail, skin, and limb defects, cleft lip and palate, genital hypoplasia, breast hypoplasia, hyperpigmented macules, and ankyloblepharon. This overlap suggests that Bowen-Armstrong and Roselli-Gulienetti syndromes are the same entity (Hall, 1982). Zenteno et al. (1999) described a 2-year-old girl with AEC syndrome accompanied by hyperpigmented macules and hypoplastic external genitalia. They proposed that AEC and Bowen-Armstrong syndromes are the same entity. The similarity of the phenotypes of affected individuals in these reports suggests that both of these conditions may be variants of AEC syndrome.

An individual with SHFMs in a family with lacrimo-auriculo-dento-digital (LADD) syndrome has been reported (Lacombe et al., 1993). LADD syndrome is characterized by clinodactyly, triphalangeal thumbs, lacrimal duct obstruction, misshapen ears, and small, peg-shaped teeth with enamel hypoplasia (Bamforth and Kaurah, 1992). Some individuals with LADD syndrome also have renal anomalies. Cleft lip/palate is not a feature of LADD syndrome. *TP63* has been screened in a few families with LADD syndrome, but no mutations have been reported.

SPECTRUM OF MUTATIONS IN *TP63*

More than 95% of unrelated individuals diagnosed with EEC syndrome have been found to have mutations in *TP63* (Celli et al., 1999; Ianakiev et al., 2000; Wessagowit et al., 2000; Kosaki et al 2001; van Bokhoven et al., 2001; van Bokhoven and Brunner, 2002). Thus, mutations in *TP63* cause EEC syndrome in most cases. More than 20 different mutations in *TP63* have been identified (Figure 105–7); most of these mutations are missense mutations predicted to cause substitution of amino acid residues in the DBD of p63 common to all isoforms of p63. These amino acids are important for direct and indirect interaction of p63 with target DNA sequences. Substitutions at any one of five different different amino acid residues (i.e., 204, 227, 279, 280, and 304) account for about 75% of mutations found in individuals with EEC syndrome. Interestingly, these sites correspond to the same sites that are frequently mutated in p53 in tumors. Half of the mutations were de novo, whereas the other half were found in familial cases. Several mutations have been found in multiple unrelated individuals, suggesting the presence of mutational hotspots.

There are several explanations for the specific distribution of mutations found in individuals with EEC syndrome (van Bokhoven et al., 1999). First, the mutation rate of these sites may be higher than that of other sites in *TP63*. This is supported by the high frequency of transitions, the large number of de novo mutations, and the observation that many of the same sites are mutated in *TP53*. Second, missense mutations disrupting the DBD may initiate a specific pathogenetic mechanism that results in the spectrum of phenotypic findings that characterize EEC syndrome. Third, it is possible, if not likely, that

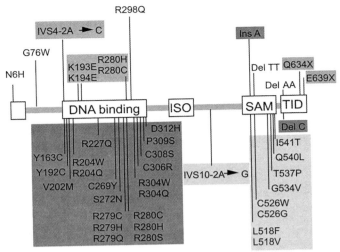

Figure 105–7. Distribution of mutations in *TP63*. The approximate position of truncating mutations and the amino acid changes are indicated. Ectodermal dysplasia, ectrodactyly, and cleft lip and/or palate (EEC) syndrome is caused by amino acid substitutions in the DNA-binding domain (dark gray box). Most mutations in the sterile-α-motif (SAM) domain cause ankyloblepharon, ectrodactyly, and cleft lip/palate (AEC) syndrome (light gray boxes). Note that some mutations in the DNA-binding domain (e.g., R280H, C) can cause either ectodermal dysplasia, ectrodactyly, and cleft lip and/or palate (EEC) syndrome or isolated split hand/foot malformations (medium gray boxes). ISO, tetramerization; TID, transactivation inhibitory domain.

this pattern is a consequence of the ascertainment procedure used to identify cases of EEC. None of these explanations are mutually exclusive, and the evidence suggests that all of them may be correct.

Mutations in *TP63* also cause LMS, ADULT syndrome, AEC syndrome, and some cases of isolated SHFM. Most of the mutations that cause each of these conditions are different than those that cause EEC syndrome. Nine different mutations that cause AEC syndrome have been found in *TP63*, the best characterized of these syndromes. Eight of these mutations are unique missense mutations that cause amino acid substitutions in the SAM domain (McGrath et al., 2001). All of these mutations are predicted to disrupt protein–protein interactions mediated by the SAM domain. The SAM domain is included only in α isoforms which in contrast to β and γ isoforms, have no TA. Indeed, the ΔN-p63α isoform exhibits dominant-negative activity toward TA by TA-p63γ. This is thought to be caused in part by competing with TA-p63γ for a shared DNA-binding site. Missense mutations in the SAM domain cause a loss of this inhibitory activity, suggesting that isoforms with mutations in the SAM domain have lost their capacity to compete for the DNA-binding site of transactivating isoforms.

A single family with AEC syndrome has a mutation in intron 10 that causes a splicing defect that deletes exon 11 (van Bokhoven and McKeon, 2002). This is predicted to disrupt the carboxyl terminus of α and β isoforms of *p63*, while keeping the SAM domain intact. The mechanism by which deletion of this exon causes a phenotype similar to that caused by substitutions in the SAM domain is unknown.

Three mutations have been found in families with LMS. One is a deletion of two thymines at nucleotide positions 1693–1694 in exon 13, and the other is a deletion of two adenines at nucleotide positions 1860–1861 in exon 14. Both are predicted to cause frameshifts that produce truncated products that lack the TID and part of the SAM domain in α isoforms while leaving β and γ isoforms intact. The multiplex kindred that was used to demonstrate that LMS mapped to chromosome 3q27 was reported to have a missense mutation in exon 4 that results in a substitution of tryptophan for glycine at amino acid residue 76 (van Bokhoven and Brunner 2002).

Mutations in *TP63* have been found in two families with ADULT syndrome. Similar to the mutations that cause EEC syndrome, one of these is a missense mutation that causes the substitution of glutamine for arginine at amino acid residue 298 of the DBD of p63. This amino acid does not appear to be critical for DNA binding but perturbs p63-mediated TA (van Bokhoven and McKeon, 2002). The other mutation was reported in a sporadic case of ADULT syndrome. It is a missense mutation in exon 3 that results in an asparagine-to-histidine substitution at amino acid residue 6 that is part of only the ΔN-p63 isoforms. The mechanism by which this mutation causes the unique constellation of abnormalities found in ADULT syndrome is unknown.

Six mutations have been found in *TP63* that cause isolated SHFM. However, this represents fewer than 10% of cases of isolated SHFM that have been screened. Four of these mutations are found only in individuals with isolated SHFM; these include substitutions of lysine for glutamic acid at amino acid residues 193 and 194, a splice site mutation (IVS4-2A → C), and nonsense mutation resulting in a change of glutamine to stop at position 634. The latter mutation is predicted to truncate eight amino acid residues from the carboxyl terminus of α isoforms. Missense mutations causing an arginine-to-cytosine or an arginine-to-histidine substitution at amino acid residue 280 have been reported in individuals with isolated SHFM and EEC syndrome.

TP63 has been screened in a handful of cases of sporadic and familial cases of RH syndrome and LADD syndrome, but no mutations have been reported. For other syndromes with phenotypes that overlap EEC syndrome, no analysis of *TP63* has been performed.

MANAGEMENT

The management of an individual with a multiple malformation syndrome caused by a mutation in *TP63* often requires a multidisciplinary approach. Specialties that should participate include orthopedics, plastic and craniofacial surgery, dentistry, and ophthalmology. Early diagnosis affords important information about natural history. This allows an opportunity to implement preventive measures and to institute screening to facilitate early diagnosis and intervention. The management of individuals with EEC syndrome provides a general model that can be adapted to care for patients with limb-mammary, ADULT, and AEC syndromes.

Initial Evaluation

The initial assessment of an individual suspected to have EEC syndrome or a related disorder should be focused on the broad collection of phenotypic data. Data to be collected include detailed obstetric, medical, developmental, and family histories and a comprehensive physical examination. Documentation of at least a three-generation pedigree is also recommended. It is also often helpful to examine photographs of the parents that were taken when they were children, of siblings, and of extended family members. This is especially useful when attempting to determine whether a particular physical characteristic is a diagnostic clue or part of the phenotypic background of the family or both (i.e., when a parent or relative is unknowingly affected as well).

In addition to general inquiries about medical history, more detailed questions should be asked about the organ systems and body areas typically affected. For example, it is important to inquire about the rate of growth of hair, whether the hair is unusually brittle, and hair color (some adults who dyes to color their hair darker). Children and adults are often symptomatic with excessive tearing caused by lacrimal duct stenosis, obstruction, or absence. Other symptoms of ocular abnormalities about which direct inquires should be made include excessive dryness, chronic irritation, photophobia, blurred vision, and pain. Some individuals may not consider some subtle skin findings abnormal, particularly if there are multiple affected family members. Thus, each individual should be asked about excessively dry and/or flaky skin, slow growth of nails, and reduced sweating. However, it should be noted that diminished sweating and heat intolerance are not common characteristics of these syndromes, although they may be present in some individuals and in cases of AEC or EEC syndrome. In individuals with EEC syndrome who experience hypohydrosis, sweating of the scalp, axillary region, groin, and palmer/plantar surfaces are retained.

One of the more unusual findings in EEC syndrome is pain with voiding, often accompanied by increased urgency and frequency.

These symptoms mimic those of a urinary tract infection, and frequently these patients have been erroneously diagnosed with recurrent or chronic UTIs despite having repeatedly been shown to have sterile urine.

The physical examination should include a detailed survey of the individual and overall morphologic characteristics of the head and face. The facial gestalt of an individual with the classic features of EEC syndrome is often characteristic (see Figure 105–2). The puncta of the lacrimal ducts should be identified, and the palate should be inspected and palpated. The general relationships among the parts of the hands and feet (e.g., length of digits, spacing between digits) should be observed, and subsequently each part should be examined individually. The thumb is a particularly complex body part that requires skill in differentiating between normal variations and abnormal findings.

All individuals provisionally diagnosed with EEC syndrome should (1) be referred for specialized ocular, dental, orthopedic, and craniofacial examinations; (2) have a baseline hearing evaluation; and (3) undergo imaging of the kidneys and collecting system, typically via ultrasonography. Imaging of the limbs to better define the underlying skeletal structure is of interest but usually not necessary for diagnostic purposes. However, before surgical palliation or correction of a limb malformation, the skeletal structures of the affected limb(s) should be imaged with standard radiography or MRI.

Repair of Malformations

Many of the abnormalities found in individuals with syndromes caused by mutations in *TP63* require only symptomatic treatment. However, some of the major malformations always require surgical palliation or correction.

The first surgical procedure that many individuals undergo is repair of cleft lip and/or palate. This is typically completed within the first 6 months of life. If the lacrimal ducts are obstructed or stenotic, this is often treated during the same surgical procedure. The ankyloblepharon filiforme adnatum of neonates with AEC syndrome can often be disrupted with gentle traction, circumventing the need for surgical intervention.

The need for surgical intervention to treat the limb defects found in individuals with mutations in *TP63* is highly variable. The overwhelming principle to keep in mind is that the function of the limbs should be optimized, and sometimes this means that no surgical procedure is indicated. It is common to separate fingers that are fused together, particularly when a separated finger is needed to facilitate opposition with the thumb. Isolated defects of the thumb are uncommon, although the thumb can be severely hypoplastic or absent. In these cases, it is necessary to reconstruct the thumb or to create an equivalent digit from another finger. Limb defects that result in truncations of the arm or leg may necessitate amputation if it is likely to improve the fit of a prosthesis.

Long-term Care and Prognosis

The long-term care of individuals with syndromes caused by mutations in *TP63* can be challenging. Although the physical impairments caused by limb malformations may present the most salient problem, the most difficult symptoms to manage are usually the consequence of ectodermal defects. Simple emollients can be used to treat dry skin, whereas cosmetics, dyes, and wigs can be used to alter hair color or to conceal very sparse scalp hair. Ongoing dental care is often necessary to preserve the permanent teeth. Most individuals do not have full dentures, although caps are common and partial dentures are occasionally recommended.

Ocular abnormalities can be difficult to treat and sometimes require lifelong therapy. Excessive tearing due to lacrimal duct abnormalities or excessive dryness caused by lacrimal gland dysfunction is common. The latter can lead to chronic conjunctivitis, corneal scarring, and perforation.

A relatively small number of individuals with EEC syndrome have been reported to have intermittent pelvic pain, dysuria, urgency, and increased voiding frequency in the absence of a urinary tract infection. These symptoms are thought to result from a defect of the transitional epithelium of the bladder. Biopsies in a few individuals have demonstrated thinning of the bladder epithelium with an inflammatory cell infiltrate in the underlying connective tissue (Maas et al., 1996). Some patients have responded positively to treatment with synthetic glycosaminoglycans with virtually complete resolution of symptoms. However, this treatment appears, in some cases, to lose its effectiveness over time. Others have stopped the treatment intentionally with no recurrence of symptoms.

Despite the need for specialized medical care throughout life, the overall prognosis for individuals with syndromes caused by mutations in *TP63* is quite good. As awareness has increased among health professionals, the practical management of cases has improved. Likewise, among the general public, there is growing acceptance of individuals with medical disabilities. It is not clear that this has diminished the psychologic impact of these disorders on affected individuals, although the perception of isolation felt by some patients may have been lessened.

A variety of different advocacy groups with people with *TP63*-related disorders exist. These groups concentrate of disseminating accurate information to health care providers and families of affected individuals, promoting the exchange of information among patients and their families, advocating for issues directly pertinent to the perceived needs of their community, and, to a limited extent, supporting clinical research.

Recurrence Risk

All disorders caused by mutations in *TP63* are transmitted in an autosomal dominant pattern. Accordingly, once a diagnosis is established, the recurrence risk for each disorder is 50%. Case reports of multiple affected children within the same sibship born to unaffected parents suggest that EEC syndrome and EEC-like disorders may segregate in an autosomal recessive pattern or exhibit germline mosaicism. However, to date, neither of these possibilities has been demonstrated in individuals confirmed to have mutations in *TP63*.

MODELS OF DISEASE

TP53 is the prototypic tumor suppressor gene in mammals (Levine, 1997). Since its discovery in 1979, there has been broad interest in elucidating its role in inducing cell-cycle arrest and promoting cellular senescence or death. In the late 1990s, two homologues of *TP53* were discovered, *TP73* and *TP63*, and it was initially suspected that they might also be important tumor suppressors (Kaghad et al., 1998; Yang et al., 1998). Thus, the role of *p63* in normal cellular and developmental processes has been an intense area of investigation. One strategy used to clarify the function of *TP63* was to create loss-of-function murine mutants (i.e., knockout mice). In 1999, two groups independently reported the phenotypic characteristics of mice lacking functional *TP63* (i.e., *TP63*$^{-/-}$ mutants). One group replaced exons 6, 7, and 8 with a neomycin-resistance cassette, thereby disrupting the DBD of p63 (Yang et al., 1999). The other group created two different mutant alleles; the first was predicted to truncate the transcript in exon 6, eliminating the DBD of p63 (Mills et al., 1999). The second allele was predicted to truncate the transcript in exon 10. Thus, if translated, this isoform of p63 would retain the DBD but lack the wild-type amino-terminal region. However, animals homozygous for either mutant allele did not express p63 transcripts, indicating that both are likely null alleles.

Mice bearing one nonfunctional allele of *TP63* could not be distinguished from wild-type mice (i.e., mice without targeted mutations of their genome). In contrast, mice with two nonfunctional alleles of *TP63* (i.e., *TP63*$^{-/-}$ mice) were born with multiple malformations, including absence of the epidermis and its appendages (e.g., hair follicles; tooth primordia; mammary, sebaceous, lacrimal, and salivary glands), severe truncation defects of the limbs, and craniofacial abnormalities. This closely recapitulated the spectrum of malformations observed in individuals with EEC syndrome. Despite the breeding of these null mutants on a highly inbred strain of mice, the phenotypes observed among null mutants were varied, particularly the defects of the forelimbs. This parallels the marked intrafamilial variation observed in EEC syndrome, although variation in humans extends to the asymmetric involvement of the left and right sides of the body and the upper and lower limbs of the same individual.

Abnormal morphogenesis of the limbs was evident as early as embryonic day 9.5 (E9.5) and progressed throughout gestation. All newborn *TP63*$^{-/-}$ mice had truncated forelimbs and absent hindlimbs. In the forelimbs, the phalanges, carpals, and radius were always absent, whereas the ulna was present in about 40% of mice. The humerus was present in each mutant, although it was always hypoplastic and misshapen. Electron micrography and histologic analyses of the limb bud revealed that the apical ectodermal ridge (AER) of each bud was absent. The AER is a layer of stratified ectoderm that forms along the anteroposterior boundary of the bud at the junction of the dorsal and ventral surfaces. The AER is responsible in part for signals that maintain proximodistal outgrowth of the limb. In *TP63*$^{-/-}$ mice, the AER is absent, with the ectoderm of the tip of the limb bud indistinguishable from the surrounding ectoderm.

In classic experiments performed in chick, extirpation of the AER results in truncation or absence of the limb depending on when the AER is removed. The presence of some skeletal structures in the forelimb of *TP63*$^{-/-}$ mice suggests that the AER must function weakly and/or transiently and that this activity is absent in the hindlimbs. One signaling molecule produced in the AER that is in part responsible for the maintenance of limb outgrowth is fibroblast growth factor 8 (FGF8). *FGF8* expression in the AER of forelimbs of *TP63*$^{-/-}$ mice is present, but very weak compared with that in the AER of wild-type mice and is absent in the hindlimbs of *TP63* null mutants. FGF8 promotes outgrowth by maintaining cells in the underlying mesenchyme (the progress zone) in a highly proliferative state, reflected by the expression of genes such as *Msx1*. Thus, reduced expression of *Msx1* is an indirect indicator of the activity of the AER. *Msx1* expression was diminished in the AER of *TP63*$^{-/-}$ mice, indicating that AER activity was also reduced.

TP63-deficient embryos are notable for the absence of skin and related appendages. Histologic analysis revealed the absence of a stratified epidermis, with the surface of *TP63*$^{-/-}$ mice being covered with a single layer of flattened cells, without spongiosum, granulosum, or corneum strata. Similarly, the stratified epithelium of the tongue was replaced with one or two layers of cubodial cells. The single layer of the epidermis in *TP63*$^{-/-}$ mice expressed low levels of keratin-14, a protein normally expressed in proliferating keratinocytes. Keratin-1, an early marker of epithelial differentiation found throughout the suprabasal layers of the epidermis, was not detected in *TP63*-deficient mice. Loricrin, a marker for mature, terminally differentiated cells in the cornified layer of the epidermis, was expressed in the tufts of cells on the otherwise denuded surface of *TP63*$^{-/-}$ mice. Together, these results suggested that *TP63*-deficient mice lacked an adequate supply of progenitor cells to form the epidermis and its appendages.

TP63 is expressed in the basal or progenitor epithelial cells of the esophagus, the anterior portion of the stomach, urogenital tract, bladder, prostate, cervix, and breast. In each of these organs in *TP63*$^{-/-}$ mice, the normal stratified epithelium was replaced with a simpler epithelium, often with a cell type different than that found in wild-type animals. For example, the esophageal epithelium contained ciliated and goblet cells, neither of which is found in wild-type mice. In the bladder, the transitional epithelium was thinner than normal or absent.

DEVELOPMENTAL PATHOGENESIS

Before mutations in *TP63* were found to cause EEC syndrome or related disorders, it was suggested that the common theme among the disparate malformations observed in individuals with EEC syndrome was a defect in epithelium–mesenchyme signaling that disrupted the integrity of the ectoderm. As it turned out, the complex malformation phenotypes observed in mice, and, by inference, the human phenotypes as well, have a common, although slightly different, basis. All of the epithelial tissues affected in *TP63*-deficient mice are normally stratified, with immature progenitor cells located in the basal layer and more differentiated cells located above. This is most obvious in the stratified layers of the epidermis. In the *TP63*$^{-/-}$ mice, the population of basal cells is markedly reduced. This indicates that *p63* is required to maintain the regenerative capacity of basal stem cells. Mice deficient in *p63* can produce some basal stem cells that are capable of terminal differentiation; however, insufficient stem cells are available to sustain normal growth and development.

The development of the limb and of all of the appendages of the epidermis, including hair follicles and glands such as the breast, is dependent on signaling between the mesenchyme and overlying ectoderm. Failure to create an adequate population of ectodermal cells in these signaling centers (e.g., the AER) disrupts the growth and patterning of the underlying mesenchyme. Thus, an intrinsic defect of growth and patterning is caused by abnormal histogenesis, an observation that may be a generalized phenomenon of all primary ectodermal dysplasia disorders accompanied by malformations.

It has been suggested that the signaling pathways used to build the morphologically diverse structures affected by mutations in *TP63* are similar, although data on the identity of these effector molecules are very limited. In any case, the role of p63 appears to be similar in all of these developmental processes. This makes it more challenging to explain the mechanism by which disruption of different domains of p63 can produce overlapping but distinct phenotypes.

Although *TP63*$^{-/-}$ mice recapitulate the EEC syndrome phenotype, mice heterozygous for a null allele of *TP63* are normal. Moreover, individuals with deletions of chromosome 3q27 including *TP63* do not manifest any characteristics of EEC syndrome or related disorders. These observations suggest that functional haploinsufficiency is not the mechanism by which mutations in *TP63* cause disease. Virtually all of the mutations in *TP63* that cause EEC have a direct or an indirect disruptive effect on the DNA-binding characteristics of all isoforms of p63. However, the effects of these mutations on the activities of p53-responsive genes and wild-type p63 isoforms is varied. Some mutants exhibit gain-of-function, whereas others demonstrate dominant-negative activities. The varied phenotypes of individuals with mutations in *TP63* may be the consequence of the complex interaction of different aberrant p63 isoforms with their normal targets, including the modification of other isoforms of p63. Therefore, understanding the consequences of mutations in *TP63* will be challenging.

Examination of the activities of p53 and expression patterns of p63 isoforms in developing epidermis may provide some insights that can be generalized to explain the pathogenesis of developmental defects observed in individuals with mutations in *TP63*. In immature keratinocytes, the level of p53 protein is high although p53-TA activities are low, whereas in differentiating keratinocytes the level of p53 is low, and p53-TA activities are high. In contrast, levels of ΔN-p63 are high in the immature keratinocytes and diminished in differentiating keratinocytes. A similar reciprocal relationship between levels of p53 and ΔN-p63 isoforms is induced as a consequence of ultraviolet B–induced DNA damage. Thus, down-regulation of ΔN-p63 isoforms and up-regulation of TA-p63 isoforms may be required for p-53–mediated apoptosis (Liefer et al., 2000). It is possible that ΔN-p63 isoforms inhibit p53-TA activities in immature keratinocytes and that this inhibition is released as keratinocytes differentiate. This is supported by the observation that the application of retinoic acid, which prevents degradation of ΔN-p63α, blocks the differentiation of cultured keratinocytes (Bamberger et al., 2002). Loss of normal ΔN-p63 inhibitory activity in *TP63*$^{-/-}$ mice and patients with mutations in *TP63* may lead to reduced inhibition of p53-TA activities in ectoderm. As a consequence, the proliferative capacities of basal progenitor cells may be diminished because of early terminal differentiation or increased cell death.

Little is known about the upstream regulators that control *TP63* expression and the downstream targets of p63. The expression of ΔN-p63α is up-regulated by two common mediators of bone morphogenetic protein (BMP) signaling, Smad4 and Smad5. Binding sites for both of these proteins are found in the ΔN-p63 promoter. Thus, some of the actions of BMPs appear to be mediated, at least in part, by ΔN-p63α (Bakkers et al., 2002).

Two genes that are up-regulated by p63 are *Jagged1* (*JAG1*) and *Jagged2* (*JAG2*), of which both encode ligands for the Notch family of transmembrane receptors (Sasaki et al., 2002). p63 appears to interact directly with a binding site in the second intron of *JAG1* lead-

ing to activation of the Notch signaling pathway. Activation of the Notch signaling pathway induces the proteolytic release of the intracellular domain of the receptor and TA of its target genes that modulate cell proliferation and differentiation. Mutations in *JAG1* that disrupt Notch signaling cause Alagille syndrome, an autosomal dominant disorder characterized by malformations of the heart, liver, skeleton, and eye (see Chapter 40). These defects are dissimilar from those caused by mutations in *TP63*. In contrast, mice homozygous for null alleles of *JAG2* have cleft palate and syndactyly of the forelimbs and hindlimbs (Jiang et al., 1998), a phenotype that overlaps with those caused by mutations in *TP63*.

It is tempting to speculate that the upstream regulators and downstream targets of p63 may act as modifiers of the phenotypes caused by mutations in *TP63*. In particular, the action modifiers may explain the broad within-family variability that characterizes EEC syndrome. At least one large family with EEC syndrome and a mutation in *TP63* exhibits a marginally significant linkage result on chromosome 19 (O'Quinn et al., 1998). Whether this is a spurious result or the location of a modifier remains to be explored. Regardless, the characterization of modifiers will not only be an important step toward better understanding the pathophysiology of the various disorders caused by mutations in *TP63* but also facilitate clinical management. However, although there is a clear genotype–phenotype correlation among the different syndromes caused by mutations in *TP63*, no significant associations have been found between mutations in *TP63* and specific phenotypic characteristics. This is underscored by the observation that not only is there wide intrafamilial phenotypic variation, also limb defects can also vary substantially between the left and right sides or the upper and lower limbs of an affected individual. Thus, stochastic factors are certain to play an important role in influencing the phenotypic consequences of mutations in *TP63*.

REFERENCES

Albrectsen B, Svendsen IB (1956). Hypotrichosis, syndactyly, and retinal degeneration in two siblings. *Acta Derm Venerol* 1: 96–101.

Amiel J, Bougeard G, Francannet C, Raclin V, Munnich A, Lyonnet S, Frebourg T (2001). TP63 gene mutation in ADULT syndrome. *Eur J Hum Genet* 9: 642–645.

Anneren G, Andersson T, Lindgren PG, Kjartansson S (1991). Ectrodactyly-ectodermal dysplasia-clefting syndrome (EEC): the clinical variation and prenatal diagnosis. *Clin Genet* 40: 257–262.

Bakkers J, Hild M, Kramer C, Furutani-Seiki M, Hammerschmidt M (2002). Zebrafish DeltaNp63 is a direct target of Bmp signaling and encodes a transcriptional repressor blocking neural specification in the ventral ectoderm. *Dev Cell* 2: 617–627.

Bamberger C, Pollet D, Schmale H (2002). Retinoic acid inhibits downregulation of DeltaNp63alpha expression during terminal differentiation of human primary keratinocytes. *J Invest Dermatol* 118: 133–138.

Bamforth JS, Kaurah P (1992). Lacrimo-auriculo-dento-digital syndrome: evidence for lower limb involvement and severe congenital renal abnormalities. *Am J Med Genet* 43: 932–937.

Bamshad M, Jorde LB, Carey JC (2000). Getting a LEAD on EEC. *Am J Med Genet* 90: 179–182.

Bixler D, Fogh-Andersen P, Conneally PM (1971). Incidence of cleft lip and palate in the offspring of cleft parents. *Clin Genet* 2: 155–159.

Boles RG, Pober BR, Gibson LH, Willis CR, McGrath J, Roberts DJ, Yang-Feng TL (1995). Deletion of chromosome 2q24-q31 causes characteristic digital anomalies: case report and review. *Am J Med Genet* 55: 155–160.

Bonafede RP, Beighton P. (1979). Autosomal dominant inheritance of scalp defects with ectrodactyly. *Am J Med Genet* 3: 35–41.

Braverman A, Kline A, Pyeritz RE (1993). Interstitial deletion of 6q associated with ectrodactyly. *Am J Hum Genet* 53(suppl): 410.

Buss PW, Hughes HE, Clarke A (1995). Twenty-four cases of the EEC syndrome: clinical presentation and management. *J Med Genet* 32: 716–723.

Celli J, Duijf P, Hamel BCJ, Bamshad M, Kramer B, Newbury-Ecob R, Hennekam RC, Van Buggenhout G, van Haeringen A, Woods CG, et al. (1999). Heterozygous mutations in the p53 homologue p63 cause limb malformations and ectodermal dysplasia in humans. *Cell* 99: 143–153.

Chi SW, Ayed A, Arrowsmith CH (1999). Solution structure of a conserved C-terminal domain of p73 with structural homology to the SAM domain. *EMBO J* 18: 4438–4445.

Cockayne EA. 1936. Cleft palate, hare lip, dacryocystitis, and cleft hand and feet. *Biometrika* XXVIII (pt I and II): 58–63.

Czeizel AE, Vitez M, Kodaj I, Lenz W. 1993. An epidemiological study of isolated split hand/foot in Hungary, 1975–1984. *J Med Genet* 30: 593–596.

da-Silva EO, Alves JG, Almeida E. 1984. Is the EEC syndrome genetically heterogeneous? *Rev Bras Genet* 7: 735–742.

Del Porto G, D'Alessandro E, De Matteis C, Lo Re ML, Ivaldi M, Di Fusco C. 1983. Interstitial deletion of the long arm of chromosome 7 and its clinical correlations. *Pathologica* 75(suppl): 268–271.

Eckoldt JG, Martens FH (1804). *Uber eine sehr Komplicierte Hasenscharte*. Steinacker, Leipzig.

Evans JA, Vitez M, Czeizel A (1994). Congenital abnormalities associated with limb deficiency defects: a population study based on cases from the Hungarian Congenital Malformation Registry (1975–1984). *Am J Med Genet* 49: 52–66.

Freire-Maia N, Pinheiro M (1984). *Ectodermal Dysplasias: A Clinical and Genetic Study.* Alan R. Liss, Inc, New York.

Fukushima Y, Ohashi H, Hasegawa T (1993). The breakpoints of the EEC syndrome (ectrodactyly, ectodermal dysplasia and cleft lip/palate) confirmed to 7q11.21 and 9p12 by fluorescence in situ hybridization. *Clin Genet* 44: 50.

Gorlin RJ, Cohen MM, Hennekam RCM (2001). *Syndromes of the Head and Neck.* Oxford University Press, New York.

Gurrieri F, Cammarata M, Avarello RM, Genuardi M, Pomponi MG, Neri G, Giuffre L (1995). Ulnar ray defect in an infant with a 6q21;7q31.2 translocation: further evidence for the existence of a limb defect gene in 6q21. *Am J Med Genet* 55: 315–318.

Hay RJ, Wells RS (1975). The syndrome of ankyloblepharon, ectodermal defects and cleft lip and palate: an autosomal dominant condition. *Br J Dermatol* 94: 277–289.

Hagiwara K, McMenamin MG, Miura K, Harris CC (1999). Mutational analysis of the p63/p73L/p51/p40/CUSP/KET gene in human cancer cell lines using intronic primers. *Cancer Res* 59: 4165–4169.

Hall JG, Reed SD, Greene G (1982). The distal arthrogryposis: delineation of new entities—review and nosologic discussion. *Am J Med Genet* 11: 185–129.

Hasegawa T, Hasegawa Y, Asamura S, Nagai T, Tsuchiya Y, Ninomiya M, Fukushima Y (1991). EEC syndrome (ectrodactyly, ectodermal dysplasia and cleft lip/palate) with a balanced reciprocal translocation between 7q11.21 and 9p12 (or 7p11.2 and 9q12) in three generations. *Clin Genet* 40: 202–206.

Ianakiev P, Kilpatrick MW, Toudjarska I, Basel D, Beighton P, Tsipouras P (2000). Split-hand/split-foot malformation is caused by mutations in the p63 gene on 3q27. *Am J Hum Genet* 67: 59–66.

Jiang R, Lan Y, Chapman HD, Shawber C, Norton CR, Serreze DV, Weinmaster G, Gridley T (1998). Defects in limb, craniofacial, and thymic development in Jagged2 mutant mice. *Genes Dev* 12: 1046–1057.

Kaghad M, Bonnet H, Yang A, Creancier L, Biscan JC, Valent A, Minty A, Chalon P, Lelias JM, Dumont X, et al. (1997). Monoallelically expressed gene related to p53 at 1p36, a region frequently deleted in neuroblastoma and other human cancers. *Cell.* 90: 809–819.

Kaiser-Kupfer M (1973). Ectrodactyly, ectodermal dysplasia, and clefting syndrome. *Am J Ophthalmol* 76: 992–998.

Kasmann B, Ruprecht KW (1997). Ocular manifestations in a father and son with EEC syndrome. *Graefes Arch Clin Exp Ophthalmol* 235: 512–516.

Klep-de Pater JM, Bijlsma JB, Bleeker-Wagemakers EM, de France HF, de Vries-Ekkers CM (1979). Two cases with different deletions of the long arm of chromosome 7. *J Med Genet* 16: 151–154.

Kosaki R, Ohashi H, Yoshihashi H, Suzuki T, Kosaki K (2001). A de novo mutation (R279C) in the P63 gene in a patient with EEC syndrome. *Clin Genet* 60: 314–315.

Kuster W, Majewski F, Meinecke P (1985). EEC syndrome without ectrodactyly? Report of 8 cases. *Clin Genet* 28: 130–135.

Lacombe D, Serville F, Marchand D, Battin J (1993). Split hand/split foot deformity and LADD syndrome in a family: overlap between EEC and LADD syndromes. *J Med Genet* 30: 700–703.

Lander ES, Linton LM, Birren B, Nusbaum C, Zody MC, Baldwin J, Devon K, Dewar K, Doyle M, FitzHugh W, et al. (2001). Initial sequencing and analysis of the human genome. *Nature* 409: 860–921.

Levine AJ (1997). p53, the cellular gatekeeper for growth and division. *Cell* 88: 323–331.

Liefer KM, Koster MI, Wang XJ, Yang A, McKeon F, Roop DR (2000). Down-regulation of p63 is required for epidermal UV-B-induced apoptosis. *Cancer Res* 60: 4016–4020.

Maas SM, de Jong TP, Buss P, Hennekam RC (1996). EEC syndrome and genitourinary anomalies: an update. *Am J Med Genet* 63: 472–478.

Majewski F, Kuster W, ter Haar B, Goecke T (1985). Aplasia of tibia with split-hand/split-foot deformity. Report of six families with 35 cases and considerations about variability and penetrance. *Hum Genet* 70: 136–147.

McGrath JA, Duijf PH, Doetsch V, Irvine AD, de Waal R, Vanmolkot KR, Wessagowit V, Kelly A, Atherton DJ, Griffiths WA, et al. (2001). Hay-Wells syndrome is caused by heterozygous missense mutations in the SAM domain of p63. *Hum Mol Genet* 10: 221–229.

McNab AA, Potts, MJ, Welham RA. 1989. The EEC syndrome and its ocular manifestations. *Br J Ophthalmol* 73: 261–264.

Meller J (1893). Ein Fall von angeborener Spaltbildung der HÑnde und Füsse. *Berl Klin Wschr* 30: 232.

Mills AA, Zheng B, Wang XJ, Vogel H, Roop DR, Bradley A (1999). p63 is a p53 homologue required for limb and epidermal morphogenesis. *Nature* 398: 708–713.

Moerman P, Fryns JP (1996). Ectodermal dysplasia, Rapp-Hodgkin type in a mother and severe ectrodactyly-ectodermal dysplasia-clefting syndrome (EEC) in her child. *Am J Med Genet* 63: 479–481.

Morey MA, Higgins RR (1990). Ectro-amelia syndrome associated with an interstitial deletion of 7q. *Am J Med Genet* 35: 95–99.

Nardi AC, Ferreira U, Netto Junior NR, Magna LA, Rodini ES, Richieri-Costa A (1992). Urinary tract involvement in EEC syndrome: a clinical study in 25 Brazilian patients. *Am J Med Genet* 44: 803–806.

Neilson DE, Brunger JW, Heeger S, Bamshad M, Robin NH (2002). Mixed clefting type in Rapp-Hodgkin syndrome. *Am J Med Genet* 108: 281–284.

Nunes ME, Schutt G, Kapur RP, Luthardt F, Kukolich M, Byers P, Evans JP (1995). A second autosomal split hand/split foot locus maps to chromosome 10q24-q25. *Hum Mol Genet* 4: 2165–2170.

O'Quinn JR, Hennekam RC, Jorde LB, Bamshad M (1998). Syndromic ectrodactyly with severe limb, ectodermal, urogenital, and palatal defects maps to chromosome 19. *Am J Hum Genet* 62: 130–135.

Ohdo S, Hirayama K, Terawaki T (1983). Association of ectodermal dysplasia, ectrodactyly, and macular dystrophy: the EEM syndrome. *J Med Genet* 20: 52–57.

Ozen RS, Baysal BE, Devlin B, Farr JE, Gorry M, Ehrlich GD, Richard CW (1999). Fine mapping of the split-hand/split-foot locus (SHFM3) at 10q24: evidence for anticipation and segregation distortion. *Am J Hum Genet* 64: 1646–1654.

Pfeiffer RA (1984). Interstitial deletion of a chromosome 7 (q11.2q22.1) in a child with splithand/splitfoot malformation. *Ann Genet* 27: 45–48.

Preus M, Fraser FC (1973). The lobster claw defect with ectodermal defects, cleft lip-palate, tear duct anomaly and renal anomalies. *Clin Genet* 4: 369–375.

Propping P, Zerres K (1993). ADULT-syndrome: an autosomal-dominant disorder with pigment anomalies, ectrodactyly, nail dysplasia, and hypodontia. *Am J Med Genet* 45: 642–648.

Raas-Rothschild A, Manouvrier S, Gonzales M, Farriaux JP, Lyonnet S, Munnich A (1996). Refined mapping of a gene for split hand-split foot malformation (SHFM3) on chromosome 10q25. *J Med Genet* 33: 996–1001.

Rapp RS, Hodgkin WE (1968). Anhidrotic ectodermal dysplasia: autosomal dominant inheritance with palate and lip anomalies. *J Med Genet* 5: 269–272.

Reed WB, Brown AC, Sugarman GI, Schlesinger L (1974). The REEDS syndrome. *Birth Defects Orig Artic Ser* 10: 61–73.

Roberts SH, Hughes HE, Davies SJ, Meredith AL (1991). Bilateral split hand and split foot malformation in a boy with a de novo interstitial deletion of 7q21.3. *J Med Genet* 28: 479–481.

Rodini ESO, Richieri-Costa A (1990). EEC syndrome: report on 20 new patients, clinical and genetic considerations. *Am J Med Genet* 37: 42–53.

Roelfsema NM, Cobben JM (1996). The EEC syndrome: a literature study. *Clin Dysmorphol* 5: 115–127.

Rollnick BR, Hoo JJ (1988). Genitourinary anomalies are a component manifestation in the ectodermal dysplasia, ectrodactyly, cleft lip/palate (EEC) syndrome. *Am J Med Genet* 29: 131–136.

Roselli D, Gulienetti R (1961). Ectodermal dysplasia. *Br J Plast Surg* 14: 190–204.

Rudiger RA, Haase W, Passarge E (1970). Association of ectrodactyly ectodermal dysplasia, and cleft lip-palate. *Am J Dis Child* 120: 160–163.

Sasaki Y, Ishida S, Morimoto I, Yamashita T, Kojima T, Kihara C, Tanaka T, Imai K, Nakamura Y, Tokino T (2002). The p53 family member genes are involved in the Notch signal pathway. *J Biol Chem* 277: 719–724.

Scherer SW, Poorkaj P, Massa H, Soder S, Allen T, Nunes M, Geshuri D, Wong E, Belloni E, Little S, et al. (1994). Physical mapping of the split hand/split foot locus on chromosome 7 and implication in syndromic ectrodactyly. *Hum Mol Genet* 3: 1345–1354.

Schmale H, Bamberger C (1997). A novel protein with strong homology to the tumor suppressor p53. *Oncogene* 15: 1363–1367.

Senecky Y, Halpern GJ, Inbar D, Attias J, Shohat M (2001). Ectodermal dysplasia, ectrodactyly and macular dystrophy (EEM syndrome) in siblings. *Am J Med Genet* 101: 195–197.

Sharland M, Patton MA, Hill L. 1991. Ectrodactyly of hands and feet in a child with a complex translocation including 7q21.2. *Am J Med Genet* 39: 413–414.

Tajara EH, Varella-Garcia M, Gusson AC (1989). Interstitial long-arm deletion of chromosome 7 and ectrodactyly. *Am J Med Genet* 32: 192–194.

Temtamy SA, McKusick VA (1978). The genetics of hand malformations. *Birth Defects Orig Artic Ser* 14: i–xviii, 1–619.

Van Bokhoven H, Brunner HG. 2002. Splitting p63. *Am J Hum Genet* 71: 1–13.

Van Bokhoven H, McKeon F. 2002. Mutations in the p53 homolog p63: allele-specific developmental syndromes in humans. *Trends Mol Med* 8: 133–139.

Van Bokhoven H, Hamel BCJ, Bamshad M, Sangiorgi E, Gurrieri F, Duijf PPHG, Vanmolkot KRJ, Beusekom EV, Van Berrsum SEC, Celli J, et al. (2001). p63 gene mutations in ECC syndrome, limb-mammary syndrome, and isolated split hand-foot malformation suggest a genotype-phenotype correlation. *Am J Hum Genet* 69: 481–492.

Van Bokhoven H, Jung M, Smits APT, van Beersum S, Ruschendorf F, van Steensel M, Veenstra M, Tuerlings JH, Mariman EC, Brunner HG, et al. (1999). Limb mammary syndrome: a new genetic disorder with mammary hypoplasia, ectrodactyly, and other hand/foot anomalies maps to human chromosome 3q27. *Am J Hum Genet* 64: 538–546.

Vanderhooft SL, Stephan MJ, Sybert VP (1993). Severe skin erosions and scalp infections in AEC syndrome. *Pediatr Dermatol* 10: 334–340.

Venter JC, Adams MD, Myers EW, Li PW, Mural RJ, Sutton GG, Smith HO, Yandell M, Evans CA, Holt RA, et al. 2001. The sequence of the human genome. *Science* 291: 1304–1351.

Viljoen DL, Smart R (1993). Split-foot anomaly, microphthalmia, cleft-lip and cleft-palate, and mental retardation associated with a chromosome 6;13 translocation. *Clin Dysmorphol* 2: 274–277.

Wallis CE (1988). Ectrodactyly (split-hand/split-foot) and ectodermal dysplasia with normal lip and palate in a four-generation kindred. *Clin Genet* 34: 252–257.

Wessagowit V, Mellerio JE, Pembroke AC, McGrath JA (2000). Heterozygous germline missense mutation in the p63 gene underlying EEC syndrome. *Clin Exp Dermatol* 25: 441–443.

Yang A, Kaghad M, Wang Y, Gillett E, Fleming MD, Dotsch V, Andrews NC, Caput D (1998). p63, a p53 homolog at 3q27-29, encodes multiple products with transactivating, death-inducing, and dominant-negative activities. *Mol Cell* 2: 305–316.

Yang A, Schweitzer R, Sun D, Kaghad M, Walker N, Bronson RT, Tabin C, Sharpe A, Caput D, Crum C, et al (1999). p63 is essential for regenerative proliferation in limb, craniofacial and epithelial development. *Nature* 398: 714–718.

Zanier JM, Roubicek MM (1976). Hypohidrotic ectodermal dysplasia with autosomal dominant transmission. Presented at the Fifth International Congress of Human Genetics, Mexico, Comunication 273.

Zenteno JC, Venegas C, Kofman-Alfaro S (1999). Evidence that AEC syndrome and Bowen-Armstrong syndrome are variable expressions of the same disease. *Pediatr Dermatol* 16: 103–107.

Zlotogora J (1994). On the inheritance of the split hand/split foot malformation. *Am J Med Genet* 53: 29–32.

JILL DIXON AND MICHAEL J. DIXON

Treacher Collins syndrome (TCS) (OMIM 154500) is an autosomal dominant disorder of facial development that occurs with an incidence of 1:50,000 live births. Because the tissues that are affected in TCS arise during early embryonic development from the first and second branchial arches, it has long been considered that TCS may result from abnormal neural crest cell development, migration, or differentiation. Positional cloning strategies were used to isolate the gene mutated in TCS, designated *TCOF1,* which was found to encode a low-complexity, serine/alanine-rich, nucleolar phosphoprotein, which was named Treacle. A series of predominantly family-specific mutations that result in the introduction of a premature termination codon are spread throughout *TCOF1,* suggesting that the mechanism underlying TCS is haploinsufficiency. To date, the human, murine, and canine genes have been characterized, and much information about the locus has been determined. Data generated from ablating one copy of the murine gene, using gene-targeting strategies, have indicated that elevated levels of cell death in the neuroepithelium of the neural folds result in the depletion of neural crest cells. However, the precise mechanism underlying TCS remains unknown. Determination of the pathway in which Treacle functions and with what the protein interacts should help to elucidate why mutations affecting the function of a widely expressed nucleolar protein result in a craniofacial disorder.

TCS (OMIM 154500) (also known as mandibulofacial dysostosis or Franceschetti-Zwahlen-Klein syndrome) is a craniofacial disorder that is inherited in an autosomal dominant fashion. TCS occurs with an estimated incidence of 1:50,000 live births (Rovin et al., 1964; Fazen et al., 1967). More than 60% of patients do not appear to have a previous family history, and these cases are thought to arise as the result of a de novo mutation (Jones et al., 1975). On the basis that the tissues affected in TCS are derived from the first and second branchial arches, which are populated extensively by cranial neural crest cells, several theories have been suggested to explain the cellular basis of this disorder. These include abnormal neural crest cell migration (Poswillo, 1975), improper cellular differentiation during development (Wiley et al., 1983), or an abnormality of the extracellular matrix (Herring et al., 1979). In the absence of any naturally occurring mouse models or compelling candidate genes, positional cloning strategies were used to determine the molecular basis of TCS. These studies demonstrated that the disorder results from mutations in the gene *TCOF1,* which encodes Treacle (The Treacher Collins Syndrome Collaborative Group, 1996).

CLINICAL FEATURES OF THE DISORDER

TCS is characterized by numerous developmental anomalies, which are restricted to the head and neck. These abnormalities include alterations in the shape, size, and position of the external ears, which are frequently associated with atresia of the external auditory canals and anomalies of the middle ear ossicles. Radiographic analysis of the middle ears of patients with TCS has revealed irregular or absent auditory ossicles with fusion between rudiments of the malleus and incus, partial absence of the stapes and oval window, and even complete absence of the middle ear and epitympanic space (Stovin et al., 1960). As a result, bilateral conductive hearing loss is common, whereas mixed or sensorineural hearing loss is rare (Phelps et al., 1981). Audiologic examination of patients with TCS is therefore very important because at least 50% of patients may have significant hearing loss. Hypoplasia of the facial bones, particularly the mandible and zygomatic complex, are also extremely common features of TCS (Figure 106–1A). In severe cases, the zygomatic arches may be absent (Poswillo, 1975). The hypoplasia of the facial bones may result in dental malocclusion, with anterior open bite a common finding. The teeth may be widely spaced, malpositioned, or reduced in number. In a large proportion of cases, the palate is high, arched, and occasionally cleft. Ophthalmic abnormalities include downward slanting of the palpebral fissures with colobomas of the lower eyelids and a paucity of lid lashes medial to the defect (Figure 106–1B).

A high degree of both interfamilial and intrafamilial variability has been observed in TCS (Dixon et al., 1994; Marres et al., 1995), but there usually is a reasonable degree of bilateral symmetry in the affected features (Kay and Kay, 1989). Some individuals are so mildly affected that it can be extremely difficult to establish an unequivocal diagnosis and to provide accurate genetic counseling. Indeed, some mildly affected patients with TCS may be diagnosed only after the birth of a more severely affected child. At the other end of the spectrum, severe cases may result in perinatal death due to a compromised airway. The variation in the severity of the affected features and how this may affect the advice offered by genetic counselors are illustrated in Figures 106–2 and 106–3, which depict a number of affected individuals from a large multigenerational TCS family. The members of this family were initially analyzed through clinical examination, which was complemented by haplotype analysis (Dixon et al., 1994). Within this family, the clinical features vary from extremely mild to severe. Individuals III-1 (Figure 106–3, G and H) and IV-1 (Figure 106–3, I and J) could not be diagnosed on clinical grounds alone, but individual III-1 was determined to be affected because he had an affected daughter, individual IV-2 (Figure 106–3, K and L). Haplotype analysis using short tandem repeat polymorphisms (STRPs) was used to determine that a particular haplotype was inherited by the remaining affected family members; therefore, individual IV-1 was considered to be "at risk" of inheriting the mutated allele from his affected father. Subsequently, the mutation nucleotide 2386 del(G) was identified as causing TCS in this family, and individual IV-1 was confirmed to have inherited the mutation, giving him a 50% risk of passing on the mutation to any future children.

In a review of the literature, Jones et al. (1975) documented that the most common clinical abnormalities (with their percentage occurrence where available), include down-slanting palpebral fissures (89%), zygomatic hypoplasia (81%), mandibular hypoplasia (78%), abnormalities of the external ear (77%) frequently associated with atresia of the external auditory canals (36%) and leading to conductive deafness (50% of cases), coloboma of the lower eyelids (69%), paucity of eyelashes medial to the coloboma (69%), and cleft palate (28%). In most patients with TCS, a spectrum of affected features is observed; in fact, rarely is any single abnormality alone sufficient to lead to a diagnosis of TCS. More often, the entire facial profile and structure are considered when trying to arrive at a diagnosis, particularly in mildly affected patients.

MOLECULAR ANALYSIS OF THE *TCOF1* LOCUS

To date, the underlying developmental basis of TCS remains unknown, despite the fact that several groups have directed their efforts toward characterizing the *TCOF1* locus and toward determining the nature

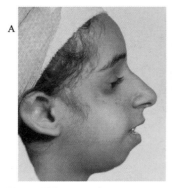
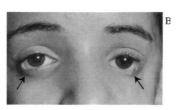

Figure 106–1. A patient with Treacher Collins syndrome. (*A*) A lateral view of the patient illustrates the mandibular hypoplasia and the abnormal external ear. (*B*) A frontal view of the same individual illustrates the colobomas (*arrows*) and paucity of eyelid lashes on the medial side of the abnormality. Immediately beneath the eyes, some flattening of the zygomatic complex is apparent.

and function of the encoded protein. The gene has an open reading frame of 4233 bp and is composed of 25 coding exons that predict a protein of 1411 amino acids with a theoretical molecular weight of 144 kDa (Dixon et al., 1997a). In addition, a 5′ untranslated region of 93 nucleotides and a 3′ untranslated region of 507 nucleotides containing a noncoding exon have been identified. Analysis of Treacle has indicated that the protein is of low complexity and is particularly rich in serine, alanine, lysine, proline, and glutamic acid residues, which together account for more than 60% of the total protein. Bioinformatic analyses identified that the protein contains three distinct domains, unique amino and carboxyl termini and a characteristic central repeat domain (Dixon et al., 1997b; Wise et al., 1997). The repeated domain consists of 10 acidic serine clusters containing numerous sites for potential casein kinase II (CKII) phosphorylation, alternating with alanine-, lysine-, and proline-rich stretches. The repeat units are highly homologous and are encoded by individual exons, extending from exon 6 to exon 16. A multiple alignment of the units indicated that exons 7, 8, 9, 10, 13, and 16 are particularly homologous, with the most closely related being exons 8 and 16, which share 77.41% identity and 87.10% similarity. Even the least closely related, which are exons 7 and 13, still share a surprising degree of homology and are 50% identical and 59.09% similar to each other (Dixon et al., 1997b).

Database searches revealed that Treacle did not exhibit strong homologies to any previously identified genes or gene families. These searches did indicate, however, that Treacle exhibited weak homology to rat nucleolar phosphoprotein Nopp140, with the greatest homology arising in the region of the repeated domain, suggesting that Treacle may be structurally related to Nopp140 and may be a nucle-

olar protein (Dixon et al., 1997b; Wise et al., 1997). Further analysis of Treacle identified a number of potential monopartite nuclear localisation signals (NLSs) of the consensus sequence K-K/R-x-R/K (Chelsky et al., 1989), embedded in the lysine-rich carboxyl terminus of the protein. Subsequently, several groups have used fusion proteins tagged to green fluorescent protein (GFP) reporters and anti-Treacle antibodies to investigate the subcellular localization of Treacle. These combined experiments demonstrated that the NLSs at the carboxyl terminus of Treacle are functional, as full-length fusion proteins localized to the nucleolus, whereas constructs in which the carboxyl terminus was deleted were excluded from the nucleus and remained in the cytoplasm (Marsh et al., 1998; Winokur and Shiang, 1998). In addition, anti-Treacle antibodies generated bright punctate nucleolar staining patterns in a range of mammalian cell types (Marsh et al., 1998). The subnucleolar localization of Treacle has been refined and the expression domain found to lie within that of nucleolin, precisely mirroring that of fibrillarin, suggesting localization to the dense fibrillar component of the nucleolus (Isaac et al., 2000). However, unlike Nopp140, Treacle is absent from the coiled (Cajal) bodies.

Biochemical analyses have also been performed to further characterize the protein. Western blotting indicated that anti-Treacle antibodies recognized a single protein band of approximately 220 kDa in cell lysates (Isaac et al., 2000). However, because the predicted molecular weight of Treacle is 144 kDa, in vitro transcription and translation studies were used to confirm that this is the correct molecular weight of Treacle as determined by sodium dodecyl sulfate–polyacrylamide gel electrophoresis analyses. The authors of this study noted that the discrepancy between the theoretical molecular weight of Treacle and its mobility on SDS-PAGE was reminiscent of that of Nopp140, as first demonstrated by Meier and Blobel (1992) (Isaac et al., 2000). Because most of the aberrant mobility of Nopp140 is due to phosphorylation in its central repeat domain, which shares homology with that of Treacle, the in vitro translated Treacle protein was treated with alkaline phosphatase in the presence or absence of phosphatase inhibitors. Treacle, like Nopp140, showed an approximate 40-kDa mobility shift on phosphatase treatment and migrated at about 180 kDa, indicating a high degree of phosphorylation (Isaac et al., 2000). Subsequently, it has also been determined that CKII and Treacle co-immunoprecipitate from HeLa cell lysates and that CKII is likely to be the kinase responsible for the posttranslational modification of Treacle (Isaac et al., 2000). This is consistent with the results of Jones et al. (1999), who showed that avian branchial arches contain a kinase activity that can phosphorylate Treacle peptides consistent with CKII site recognition.

Analogous to the signal-mediated import of large proteins into the nucleus, protein export is also thought to be regulated by such signals. To date, regions that confer nuclear export have been defined in many proteins, including the HIV-1 Rev protein (Fischer et al., 1995), the protein kinase A inhibitor (Wen et al., 1995), the T-cell leukaemia virus type 1 Rex protein (Bogerd et al., 1996), and Smad 1 and 4 (Pierreux et al., 2000; Xiao et al., 2001). The nuclear export signal (NES) consensus sequence was initially defined as a set of critically spaced hydrophobic residues, usually leucines in the form LxxLxxLxL, where x indicates any residue (Wen et al., 1995). Later, this consensus sequence was revised to the format L-x$_{(2-3)}$-(L/I/V/M/F)-x$_{(2-3)}$-L-x-(L/I) (Bogerd et al., 1996). In this regard, it is important to note that the amino terminus of the Treacle protein contains a leucine-rich sequence motif, L̲AQPV̲TLL̲DI̲, between amino acid positions 40 and 49, which conforms to the consensus NES. Currently, the functional significance of this putative export signal is unclear as no biochemical evidence to date suggests that the protein is exported from the nucleus. This motif is, however, highly conserved among the human, mouse, and dog Treacle proteins, suggesting that the region of the protein surrounding this motif is essential to the correct function of Treacle. It is also interesting to note that three of the four disease-associated missense mutations that have been documented reside in this region of the protein, indeed, one of the missense mutations, A41V, is located within the NES signal itself (see later and Table 106–1), raising the possibility that these sequence changes interfere with the correct function

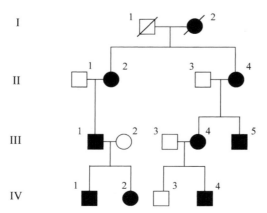

Figure 106–2. A partial pedigree of the family illustrated in Figure 106–3, plates *A* to *L*.

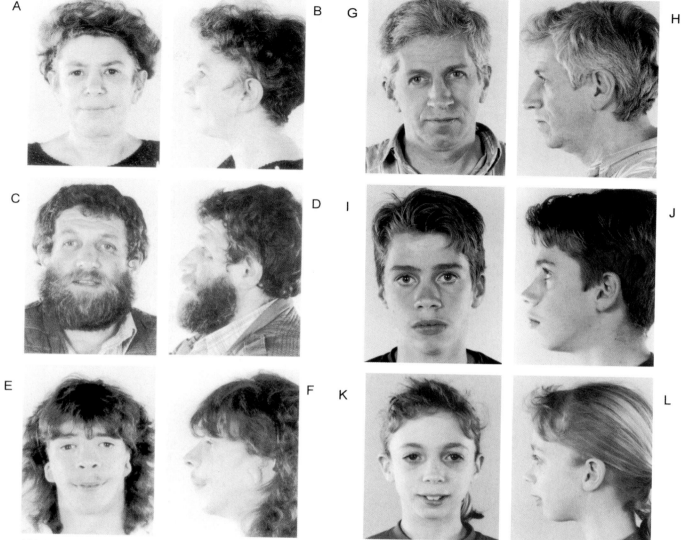

Figure 106–3. A series of affected individuals from the same Treacher Collins syndrome family whose differences in clinical severity serve to illustrate the diagnostic problems presented to clinicians. Individuals from this family were initially evaluated by clinical examination, followed by genetic linkage analysis (Dixon et al., 1994). Subsequently, the underlying mutation within this family has been identified. (*A* through *F*) These individuals are moderately to severely affected. Individual III-4 (*A* and *B*) exhibits mandibular hypoplasia and low-set ears, with slight downslanting of the palpebral fissures. Her brother III-5 (*C* and *D*) is more severely affected and displays downslating palpebral fissures and coloboma of the lower eyelids. This individual also has significant hearing loss. Individual IV-4 (*E* and *F*) is very severely affected and displays micrognathia, abnormal external ears, and complete hearing loss. (*G* through *L*) These closely related individuals, in contrast, are mildly affected. Individuals III-1 (*G* and *H*) and IV-1 (*I* and *J*) could not be diagnosed on clinical grounds alone; however, in the case of individual III-1, he was diagnosed as having TCS because his daughter, individual IV-2 (*K* and *L*), has Treacher Collins syndrome and exhibits hypoplasia of the mandible and zygomatic complex and downslanting palpebral fissures. His son, individual IV-1, has no visible signs of Treacher Collins syndrome, even after radiologic examination.

of Treacle by impeding nuclear export of the protein, possibly by altering protein conformation.

Another motif has been documented within the protein sequence of Treacle, an LIS1 homology (LisH) motif at amino acid positions 5 to 38 (Emes and Ponting, 2001). The *LIS1* gene is mutated in patients with lissencepahly, a brain malformation that results in severe retardation, epilepsy, and premature death (Lo Nigro et al., 1997) (see Chapter 92). In this bioinformatics-based study, more than 100 eukaryotic intracellular proteins were found to contain an LisH motif, and from their diverse functions the authors suggested that these motifs might contribute to the regulation of microtubule dynamics, either by mediating dimerization or by directly binding cytoplasmic dynein heavy chain or microtubules. There have been no laboratory-based studies that support this hypothesis, however, it is interesting to note that Nopp140 also contains a LisH motif, reinforcing previous obser-

vations that Treacle and Nopp140 share structural and functional similarities.

THE MUTATIONAL SPECTRUM OBSERVED IN TCS

Several studies have been performed on the human *TCOF1* gene, resulting in the identification of more than 120 mutations. In a subset of cases, the identification of the mutation that causes TCS in a particular family has facilitated both prenatal and postnatal diagnostic predictions (Gladwin et al., 1996; The Treacher Collins Syndrome Collaborative Group, 1996; Edwards et al., 1997; Wise et al., 1997, Dawson, 1999; Ellis et al., 2002; Splendore et al., 2000; Dixon et al., unpublished observations). Table 106–1 details all of the mutations that have been published to date, together with unpublished data from our laboratory. The combined results of these studies indicate that mu-

Table 106–1. A List of All *TCOF1* Mutations that Have Been Reported, Including Unpublished Data from Our Laboratory

Location	Mutation	Familial (F) or Sporadic (S)	Reference
Exon 1	nt 28 del(C)	F	Ellis et al., 2000
Exon 1	nt 38 del(T)	S	Ellis et al., 2000
Exon 1	nt 59 del(G)	F	Present study
Exon 1	Q36X	F	Edwards et al., 1997
Exon 1	I14F	F	Present study
Intron 1	nt 109-1 del(G)	F	Edwards et al., 1997
Exon 2	A41V	F	Ellis et al., 2000
Exon 2	W53C	S	Ellis et al., 2000
Exon 2	W53R	S	Edwards et al., 1997
Exon 2	Q55X	S	Ellis et al., 2000
Exon 3	nt 274 del(G)	F	Edwards et al., 1997
Exon 3	E93X	S	Edwards et al., 1997
Intron 3	nt 304 + 5 G → C	F	Edwards et al., 1997
Intron 3	nt 304 + 5 G → C	F	Edwards et al., 1997
Intron 3	nt 304 + 5 G → C	S	Present study
Exon 5	nt 389 ins(A)	F	Present study
Exon 5	nt 405 del(TG)	F	Gladwin et al., 1996
Exon 5	nt 422 ins(A)	F	Wise et al., 1997
Exon 5	nt 497 del(ATAC)	ND	Wise et al., 1997
Exon 5	nt 513 del(AG)	S	Ellis et al., 2000
Exon 6	nt 630 del(AG)	S	Gladwin et al., 1996
Exon 7	Q252X	F	The TCSCG, 1996
Exon 7	Q252X	S	Ellis et al., 2000
Exon 7	nt 658 del(A)	S	Ellis et al., 2000
Exon 7	nt 698 del(C)	S	Present study
Exon 7	nt 724 ins(C)	F	The TCSCG, 1996
Exon 7	nt 786 del(AG)	S	Ellis et al., 2000
Exon 7	nt 786 del(AG)	S	Ellis et al., 2000
Exon 7	nt 689 (CCAAGGGGACCC) → (GGAGGCCT)	S	Ellis et al., 2000
Exon 8	nt 864 del(AG)	F	Present study
Exon 9	nt 1106 ins(C)	S	Present study
Exon 9	nt 1120 del(G)	F	Gladwin et al., 1996
Exon 9	nt 1164 ins(T)	S	Splendore et al., 2000
Exon 9	nt 1216 ins(A)	S	Gladwin et al., 1996
Exon 10	nt 1287 ins(G)	S	Splendore et al., 2000
Exon 10	nt 1327 ins(A)	F	The TCSCG, 1996
Exon 10	nt 1334 del 29bp	S	Ellis et al., 2000
Exon 10	nt 1406 del(AGAG)	S	Splendore et al., 2000
Exon 10	nt 1408 del(AG)	F	Wise et al., 1997
Exon 10	nt 1408 del(AG)	S	Splendore et al., 2000
Exon 10	nt 1441 ins(GG)	F	The TCSCG, 1996
Exon 12	nt 1866 del(AGATAGTG)	F	Splendore et al., 2000
Exon 12	nt 1867 del(GA)	F	Splendore et al., 2000
Exon 12	nt 1879 del(GAGAA)	S	Ellis et al., 2000
Exon 12	nt 1879 del(GAGAA)	S	Edwards et al., 1997
Exon 12	S617X	S	Ellis et al., 2000
Exon 13	nt 1915 del(AA)	S	Present study
Exon 13	nt 2014 ins(G)	F	The TCSCG, 1996
Exon 13	nt 2018 del(CAGTCACC)	S	Splendore et al., 2000
Exon 13	nt 2019 del (AGTCACC)	S	Present study
Exon 13	nt 2054 del(CT)	F	Present study
Exon 13	nt 2082 del(TGAG)	S	Present study
Exon 13	Q676X	S	Present study
Exon 14	nt 2247 G → A transition (K749K)	F	Gladwin et al., 1996
Exon 14	K749K	S	Splendore et al., 2000
Exon 14	nt 2110 del(G)	F	Present study
Exon 15	nt 2259 del(A)	F	Ellis et al., 2000
Exon 15	nt 2297 del(G)	S	Edwards et al., 1997
Exon 15	nt 2354 del(CAGGGCCAGA)	F	Splendore et al., 2000
Exon 15	nt 2354 del(CAGGGCCAGA)	F	Splendore et al., 2000
Exon 15	nt 2355 del(AG)	S	Ellis et al., 2000
Exon 15	nt 2355 del(AG)	F	Splendore et al., 2000
Exon 15	nt 2386 del(G)	F	Edwards et al., 1997
Exon 15	nt 2399 del(GTGA)	F	Present study
Exon 15	nt 2399 del(GTGA)	F	Edwards et al., 1997
Exon 15	Q758X	F	Present study
Exon 15	E796X	F	Splendore et al., 2000
Intron 15	nt 2428-2 A → C	S	Ellis et al., 2000
Exon 16	nt 2442 del(G)	F	Edwards et al., 1997
Exon 16	nt 2490 del(C)	F	Wise et al., 1997
Exon 16	nt 2497 del(G)	S	Ellis et al., 2000

(continued)

Table 106–1. *Continued*

Location	Mutation	Familial (F) or Sporadic (S)	Reference
Exon 16	nt 2526 del(AG)	F	Wise et al., 1997
Exon 16	nt 2527 ins(A)	S	Splendore et al., 2000
Exon 16	nt 2552 del(A)	S	Wise et al., 1997
Exon 16	nt 2561 del(A)	F	Wise et al., 1997
Exon 16	nt 2565 del(AG)	S	Wise et al., 1997
Exon 16	nt 2622 ins(T)	F	Present study
Exon 17	S913X	S	Present study
Exon 18	nt 2822 del(GA)	F	Splendore et al., 2000
Exon 19	nt 2998 del(C)	F	Edwards et al., 1997
Exon 20	Q1041X	F	Edwards et al., 1997
Exon 20	Q1087X	S	Ellis et al., 2000
Exon 20	nt3086 del(CACTCCC)	F	Splendore et al., 2000
Exon 20	nt 3100 del(A)	S	Splendore et al., 2000
Exon 20	nt 3101 del 40bp	S	Ellis et al., 2000
Exon 21	nt 3311 del(C)	S	Splendore et al., 2000
Intron 22	nt 3550 + 1 G → A	S	Edwards et al., 1997
Exon 22	nt 3376 del(CTCTC)	S	Present study
Exon 23	nt 3606 del(AG)	S	Edwards et al., 1997
Exon 23	nt 3700 del(G)	F	Present study
Exon 23	nt 3711 del(AG)	S	Splendore et al., 2000
Exon 23	nt 3792 del(C)	S	Ellis et al., 2000
Exon 23	nt 3941 del(AG)	F	Ellis et al., 2000
Exon 23	nt 3987 ins(G)	F	Splendore et al., 2000
Exon 23	nt 3987 ins(G)	F	Splendore et al., 2000
Exon 23	nt 4108 del(AA)	F	Edwards et al., 1997
Exon 23	nt 4108 del(AA)	S	Ellis et al., 2000
Intron 23	nt4111 + 1 G → T	F	Ellis et al., 2000
Exon 24	nt 4127-4134 del(A)	S	Ellis et al., 2000
Exon 24	nt 4130 del(AAAAA)	F	Edwards et al., 1997
Exon 24	nt 4135 del(GAAAA)	S	Splendore et al., 2000
Exon 24	nt 4135 del(GAAAA)	S	Splendore et al., 2000
Exon 24	nt 4135 del(GAAAA)	S	Splendore et al., 2000
Exon 24	nt 4135 del(GAAAA)	S	Splendore et al., 2000
Exon 24	nt 4135 del(GAAAA)	ND	Splendore et al., 2000
Exon 24	nt 4135 del(GAAAA)	S	Splendore et al., 2000
Exon 24	nt 4135 del(GAAAA)	F	Edwards et al., 1997
Exon 24	nt 4135 del(GAAAA)	F	Edwards et al., 1997
Exon 24	nt 4135 del(GAAAA)	F	Edwards et al., 1997
Exon 24	nt 4135 del(GAAAA)	F	Edwards et al., 1997
Exon 24	nt 4135 del(GAAAA)	F	Edwards et al., 1997
Exon 24	nt 4135 del(GAAAA)	F	Edwards et al., 1997
Exon 24	nt 4135 del(GAAAA)	F	Ellis et al., 2000
Exon 24	nt 4135 del(GAAAA)	F	Ellis et al., 2000
Exon 24	nt 4135 del(GAAAA)	F	Ellis et al., 2000
Exon 24	nt 4135 del(GAAAA)	F	Ellis et al., 2000
Exon 24	nt 4135 del(GAAAA)	F	Ellis et al., 2000
Exon 24	nt 4135 del(GAAAA)	F	Present study
Exon 24	nt 4135 del(GAAAA)	S	Ellis et al., 2000
Exon 24	nt 4135 del(GAAAA)	S	Ellis et al., 2000
Exon 24	nt 4135 del(GAAAA)	S	Ellis et al., 2000
Exon 24	nt 4135 del(GAAAA)	S	Present study

ND, not determined; nt, nucleotide; TCSCG, Treacher Collins Syndrome Collaborative Group.

tations occur in almost all of the 25 exons of the gene (Figure 106–4), and the vast majority result in the introduction of a premature termination codon, suggesting that the mechanism underlying TCS is haploinsufficiency. The mutations are predominantly family specific, but the most notable exception to this rule is the mutation nucleotide (nt) 4135 del(GAAAA), which occurs in exon 24 of *TCOF1*. This mutation has been documented in 23 of 123 cases, for a frequency of 18.6%. Several authors have proposed that this mutation represents a "mutation hotspot" within the gene, which may be due to the fact that the nucleotide sequence in this region contains a homopolymeric stretch of adenine residues, which may result in replication slippage (Splendore et al., 2000; Ellis et al., 2002). Because nt 4135 del(GAAAA) occurs with a relatively high frequency, it represents a very useful starting point in the search for mutations. The mutations that have been documented include splicing mutations, insertions, and nonsense mutations, by far the majority of the mutations are deletions, and these range in size from 1 to 40 nucleotides. Deletions have been observed in 68% of cases, in contrast to insertions, which have been documented in only 10% of cases.

A number of missense mutations have been identified in *TCOF1* (Gladwin et al., 1996; Dawson, 1999; Splendore et al., 2000; Ellis et al., 2002), one of which has been documented in two independent studies (Gladwin et al., 1996; Splendore et al., 2000). This mutation, K749K, is interesting in that the last nucleotide of codon 749 was the subject of a G-to-A transition in a child with no previous family history of TCS. Although apparently silent, this transition occurred in the last nucleotide of exon 14. In this particular exon, the 5' splice donor site immediately following the G-to-A transition is gc rather than the more usual gt, a variation that is present in the human, mouse, and dog *TCOF1* genes (Dixon et al., 1997a, 1997b; Haworth et al., 2001). In vitro studies have shown that gc is the only substitution that will allow the 5' splice site to be accurately cleaved, although in such cases the surrounding sequence is usually very closely matched to the consensus AG/gcaagt (Aebi et al., 1987; Jackson, 1991). In the affected

Mutations in *TCOF1*

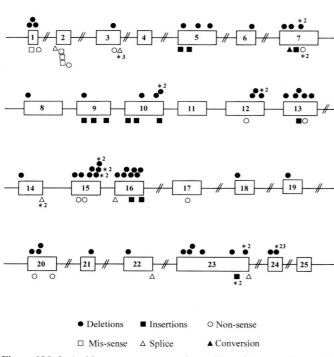

- ● Deletions   ■ Insertions   ○ Non-sense
- □ Mis-sense   △ Splice   ▲ Conversion

Figure 106–4. An ideogram to represent the position of the mutations within *TCOF1*. Exons are represented as open boxes, and introns are represented with a line. Introns indicated with a double-hatched line were not sized. A numbered star indicates any mutations documented more than once; the number indicates how many times the mutation has been documented. The drawing is not to scale.

TCS individual, the silent transition, when coupled with the gc splice site, provided two separate mismatches that resulted in aberrant splicing (Gladwin et al., 1996). RT-PCR assays indicated that the intron immediately following exon 14 was not correctly spliced out and a portion of intron 14 was present in the *TCOF1* transcript in this affected individual. A termination codon was encountered after 14 amino acids of intron 14, followed by a cryptic splice site, whereupon the remainder of intron 14 was spliced out (Gladwin et al., 1996).

The remaining missense mutations I14F, A41V, W53C, and W53R (see Table 106–1) arise in the first two exons of *TCOF1* and were detected in DNA samples from classically affected TCS patients. The amino terminus of Treacle is the most highly conserved region of the protein between humans and mice with the region encoded by exons 1 and 2 displaying 92.6% identity, as opposed to 54.8% identity for the entire protein (Dixon et al., 1997a). Although I14F and A41V are semiconservative changes, both W53C and W53R are nonconservative changes. The occurrence of these missense changes strongly suggests that alterations to this region of the protein are not tolerated as they could affect the function of Treacle, possibly by altering protein folding. This theory is supported by two findings. First, although a number of studies have demonstrated that a high frequency of single nucleotide polymorphisms (SNPs) arise within the coding exons of *TCOF1*, suggesting that this gene accumulates a high level of genetic variation (Splendore et al., 2000), no SNPs have been documented in either exon 1 or exon 2 in more than 100 normal individuals (Gladwin et al., 1996; The Treacher Collins Syndrome Collaborative Group, 1996; Wise et al., 1997). Although a number of these polymorphisms have been detected in noncoding sequence, the majority are located in the central repeated region of the gene (Splendore et al., 2000). In addition, where such sequence variants result in an amino acid change in affected individuals, they have also been detected in control individuals, confirming that they were not disease causing (The Treacher

Collins Syndrome Collaborative Group, 1996; Wise et al., 1997; Splendore et al., 2000). Second, Haworth et al. (2001) identified nine genetic variants between human and canine *TCOF1*, three of which lead to amino acid substitutions. In this study, however, no polymorphic variants were detected in exons 1 to 3, suggesting that the amino terminus may be under strong selective pressure. Nevertheless, until the exact function of Treacle is determined and, in particular, the role that the unique amino and carboxyl termini play in contributing to that function, these missense changes should only be considered as "putative" mutations.

DO THE MUTATIONS RESULT IN MISLOCALIZATION OF THE PROTEIN?

As discussed earlier, TCS has been shown to result from a wide variety of mutations. The effect of the majority of these mutations is the introduction of a premature termination codon into the protein. It seems possible, therefore, that the region that encodes the majority of the nuclear localization signals would be deleted from a "mutant" protein and may result in mislocalization of such a protein. Marsh et al. (1998) investigated this hypothesis by using site-directed mutagenesis to recreate mutations that have been observed in TCS patients into GFP reporter constructs. Three mutations were examined in these experiments: Q36X, E93X, and nt 405 del(TG). Although the GFP-fusion protein produced by the construct containing the mutation Q36X was of an insufficient length to visualize via direct fluorescence microscopy, both of the constructs containing the mutations E93X and nt405 del(TG) exhibited abnormal localization of the protein. This was characterized by nuclear staining with sparing of the nucleolus and cytoplasm. Examination of the sequence within these two constructs subsequently identified an additional NLS signal at position 74 of the amino terminus, which was sufficient to drive these truncated proteins into the nucleus. However, when interpreting these results, it must be remembered that this assay was an overexpression assay, as the GFP-Treacle fusion proteins were under the control of a ubiquitous and highly expressed promoter, and that the endogenous protein would still be present in the transfected cells.

Although regions sufficient to target nucleolar localization have been reported within several genes (Hatanaka, 1990; Moroianu and Riordan, 1994), a comprehensive analysis of the human nucleolus has indicated that nucleolar proteins do not share any simple targeting motifs and that their localization in the nucleolus probably involves a diverse range of mechanisms (Andersen et al., 2002). The major function of the nucleolus is the transcription and processing of ribosomal RNAs and their subsequent assembly into ribosomal subunits. Because Treacle is a nucleolar protein, it has previously been proposed that Treacle may function in some aspect of ribosome biogenesis (Marsh et al., 1998; Winokur and Shiang, 1998; Dixon et al., 2000). However, data have shown that nucleoli have a surprisingly high protein complexity, which in turn provides evidence that the nucleolus may perform functions in addition to its role as a ribosome factory (Andersen et al., 2002). As such, the localization of Treacle does not shed any light on the function of the protein.

Interestingly, no alterations to the localization of Treacle could be determined in fibroblasts from either healthy individuals or patients with TCS via indirect immunofluorescence with two different anti-Treacle antibodies (Isaac et al., 2000). This observation suggests that no truncated forms of Treacle are expressed in the cells of TCS patients. It is likely, therefore, that any protein produced from the mutant allele is degraded by nonsense-mediated mRNA degradation (Frischmeyer and Dietz, 1999). This pathway is essentially a proofreading mechanism to ensure accurate production of proteins within the cell by removing transcripts that encode truncated, nonfunctional or potentially harmful proteins by monitoring for premature termination of translation. However, quantification of the cellular amounts of Treacle, through antibody reactivity on Western blots, was unable to demonstrate any differences in the amount of Treacle in cell lines established by Epstein-Barr virus transformation of primary fibroblasts and peripheral lymphoblasts from either healthy individuals or patients with TCS (Isaac et al., 2000). This finding suggests that mature fibroblast cells of TCS patients possess a mechanism to compensate for the lower levels of Treacle produced by the mutant allele. This may regulate levels of Treacle within the cell and bring them to a level indistinguishable from that of unaffected individuals, indicating that certain levels of this protein are essential for normal development. This hypothesis is supported by the observation that high levels of the murine gene are expressed during the period of facial development (Dixon et al., 1997a). If embryonic fibroblast cells carrying a mutation in the *TCOF1* gene were unable to maintain an appropriately high level of Treacle, it is possible that the normal function of the protein would be restricted and that correct cellular development, migration, or differentiation could be impeded.

PHENOTYPE–GENOTYPE CORRELATIONS

As several groups have documented, there do not appear to be any genotype–phenotype correlations emerging in TCS (Gladwin et al., 1996; Edwards et al., 1997; Splendore et al., 2000). To evaluate the interfamilial and intrafamilial variability observed in TCS, Splendore et al. (2000) scored for the presence or absence of seven readily identifiable clinical abnormalities, including downslanting palpebral fissures, maxillary and mandibular hypoplasia, ear abnormalities, coloboma and the paucity of eyelashes, and cleft palate. They found no significant difference in the number or severity of the affected features between sporadic and familial cases or between male and female patients. This work supports earlier studies that indicated that marked interfamilial and intrafamilial variability in the affected features is observed regardless of the position of the mutation within the gene (Dixon, 1996; Edwards et al., 1997).

ESTABLISHING THE DIAGNOSIS

Before identification of the *TCOF1* gene, diagnosis of TCS was possible only by clinical evaluation or by using linked STRPs (Dixon et al., 1994). Penetrance of the genetic mutation is very high, indeed, there is only a single case in the literature where nonpenetrance has been established unequivocally (Dixon et al., 1994). There is, however, extreme variation in the clinical features. A number of attempts have been made to classify the condition based on the severity of the affected features, but these classifications are arbitrary and of little use because they cannot be used to make predictions about future pregnancies. Although concordance of severity in affected siblings has been reported (Nicolaides et al., 1984), anticipation, in which the severity of the disease increases with successive generations, is not thought to be a feature of TCS. Analysis of large cohorts of affected individuals suggests that a degree of ascertainment bias, where affected individuals are readily diagnosed due to the presence of another affected family member, may often be encountered (Marres et al., 1995; Gladwin et al., 1996; Edwards et al., 1997). The extreme variability in the degree to which individuals can be affected, together with the high rate of de novo mutations, has previously complicated the provision of genetic counseling, particularly where the diagnosis of either of an affected child's parents was equivocal. Because TCS is inherited in an autosomal dominant fashion, the risk to future pregnancies if either parent is affected is 50%. If, however, genuinely unaffected parents produce an affected child, they have a negligible recurrence risk of producing another affected child, even though their first affected child will themselves possess a 50% chance of passing on the mutated allele. In the case of apparently unaffected individuals who were clinically evaluated, it was extremely important to ensure that even minimal features of TCS were not present. In this regard, the use of craniofacial radiographs, particularly the occipitomental view, which enables visualization of the zygomatic complex, have been extremely useful in detecting zygomatic hypoplasia (Dixon et al., 1991; Marres et al., 1995). Since the identification of the gene in 1996, both prenatal and postnatal molecular diagnoses have been possible. Nevertheless, the wide spectrum of mutations observed in TCS complicates the provision of such diagnosis because it is necessary to identify the mutation in each individual case, before undertaking diagnostic predictions. Although the identification of the recurrent mutation nt 4135 del(GAAAA) provides a starting point in the search for a mutation in an affected individual, more than 120 mutations have been documented throughout 23 of the 25 coding exons (see Table 106–1). Such a wide spread of possible mutations renders a "quick" diagnosis impossible, in the event of an unexpected pregnancy in a family in which the mutation has not previously been identified. In addition, although molecular diagnosis has proved extremely valuable in establishing the affected status of individuals within a family, when using these techniques it must be remembered that it is not possible to predict how severe the clinical abnormalities may be when a prenatal case of TCS is diagnosed. In such cases, the use of ultrasonography to monitor the pregnancy can be an invaluable aid to prenatal diagnosis, because severely affected babies may be detected by such means and enhanced levels of clinical care provided in the perinatal period (Edwards et al., 1996).

DIFFERENTIAL DIAGNOSIS

A number of conditions have a similar facial profile to TCS, including Nager and Miller syndromes and the oculoauriculovertebral (OAV) spectrum. It is usually a straightforward matter to differentiate these conditions from TCS on the basis of the facial gestalt, but caution should be exercised where individuals are only mildly affected so that the minimal diagnostic criteria that constitute TCS are not overlooked. Nager syndrome has facial features similar to those of TCS, particularly in the region of the eyes, which are downslanting with a deficiency of eyelashes (Chemke et al., 1988). However, the mandible is usually more hypoplastic than in TCS. Lower lid colobomas are rare, but preaxial limb abnormalities are a consistent feature of Nager syndrome, unlike TCS. Thumbs may be hypoplastic, aplastic, or duplicated, and the radius and ulna may be fused. Cases of Nager syndrome are generally sporadic, although affected siblings have been reported in rare cases (Chemke et al., 1988).

Miller syndrome also has features in common with TCS, with the additional diagnostic feature of ectropion or out-turning of the lower lids (Gorlin et al., 1990). Cleft lip, with or without cleft palate, is more common than in TCS. The limb anomalies are postaxial, most commonly with absence or incomplete development of the fifth digital ray of all four limbs. In addition, there may be shortening of the radius and ulna. Some patients may exhibit congenital heart defects. The inheritance of Miller syndrome is somewhat unclear, because both autosomal dominant with variable expression (Allanson and McGillivray, 1985) and autosomal recessive forms (Ogilvy-Stuart and Parsons, 1991) have been reported.

The OAV spectrum is a complex and heterogeneous set of conditions that includes hemifacial microsomia and Goldenhar syndrome, which primarily affect the development of the ear, mouth, and mandible. These conditions vary from mild to severe and usually affect only one side of the face. Bilateral involvement has occasionally been documented, but, in such cases, expression is usually more severe on one side of the face (Kay and Kay, 1989). Goldenhar syndrome has vertebral anomalies and epibulbar dermoids in addition to the facial involvement. In most instances, OAV spectrum occurs sporadically, although 1% to 2% of cases have a previous family history.

To investigate whether these conditions are allelic with TCS, mutation studies have been undertaken in a limited number of patients with Nager or Goldenhar syndrome (Edwards et al., 1997; Dawson, 1999; Ellis et al., 2002). The combined results of these studies have detected three unusual sequence variants. These sequence changes occurred in exon 23 in two Goldenhar syndrome patients [Q1235E and nt3853 del(AAG)] and a Nager syndrome patient [nt 4095 del(GAA)]. The net result of the deletions is that although the reading frame of the protein is not altered, a single amino acid is deleted from Treacle at position 1285–1289 and at position 1365–1366, respectively. The importance of these sequence changes is unknown, however, it is possible that they represent polymorphisms that must be extremely rare, because none of these changes have been detected in more than 100 control individuals.

MUTATION DETECTION RATES AND GENETIC HETEROGENEITY

The mutation studies that have been performed have reported widely varying mutation detection rates. Initially, Edwards et al. (1997) documented a rate of 60% using single-strand conformation polymorphism (SSCP) analysis, followed by sequence analysis of mobility shifts. In contrast, Splendore et al. (2000) published a mutation detection rate of 89% using SSCP analysis and sequence analysis. There may be several reasons for the lower rates documented by Edwards et al. (1997). First, the patient cohort examined in this study was examined and referred to our laboratory by a number of different clinicians, resulting in the possibility that some individuals were atypical and exhibited only some of the features of TCS. In addition, ^{35}S-dATP was used to label the PCR products, which is likely to result in loss of sensitivity (Hayashi and Yandell, 1993). Indeed, in the study by Splendore et al. (2000), the mutation underlying TCS in three individuals could not be identified with SSCP analysis alone. To investigate this further, the entire *TCOF1* coding sequence in these individuals was examined by direct sequence analysis and one further mutation was identified, raising the mutation detection rate to 93%. Because the mutations in two individuals remained unidentified after this analysis, and after ruling out the possibility that "atypical" cases of TCS had been included in the study, Splendore et al. (2000) suggested that it is possible that mutations affecting the function of Treacle occur in the 5' and 3' untranslated regions of the gene or in the promoter, which has not yet been identified. It is also possible that mutations may reside in alternatively spliced exons. Several lines of evidence suggest that *TCOF1* exhibits alternative splicing, including unpublished data from our laboratory. Genomic and cDNA sequencing studies have identified two alternative exons: exon 6a, which is 228 nucleotides in length and is present in the human gene only, and exon 16a, which is 108 nucleotides in length and is present in both the human and mouse genes. RT-PCR assays have determined that both of the alternatively spliced exons do not show any tissue type or developmental age specificity and were present in all of the samples tested. In addition, Haworth et al. (2001) reported that the dog equivalent of exon 10 is absent and that exon 19 also appears to be alternatively spliced, with the splice variant that does not contain exon 19 being the major mRNA form.

Because the mutations underlying TCS remain unidentified in some patients, this also raises the possibility that mutations in another gene may result in the same disorder. Although genetic heterogeneity is not thought to be a feature of TCS, because all of the multigenerational families exhibit linkage to the region of chromosome 5 in which the *TCOF1* gene resides (Dixon et al., 1991; 1993), the majority of TCS families are small with few affected individuals, rendering linkage studies impossible in every case. To exclude the possibility that TCS is heterogeneous may not be trivial, because it would require the remaining individuals in whom the mutations remain undetected to be examined by the minimal number of different clinicians and would require detailed examination of case notes and radiographs. Also, because SSCP analysis alone may not detect all of the mutations, sequence analysis of the entire coding region, the promoter, and the untranslated regions of *TCOF1* may be necessary. As such, the question of whether TCS exhibits heterogeneity is likely to remain unresolved.

TREATMENT

The care of individuals affected by TCS often requires a multidisciplinary approach. In addition to intricate surgery to correct underdeveloped or abnormal facial structures, patients may exhibit a range of symptoms such as hearing loss, speech problems, and sleeping and breathing difficulties. All of these symptoms may have a significant impact on learning ability, self-esteem, and social interaction, and many of these require the care of a number of health care professionals at different times, both preoperatively and postoperatively (Arndt et al., 1987). Surgical procedures may be required in the immediate postnatal period, because children presenting with severe micrognathia may require an emergency tracheotomy to enable them to maintain their airway. In general, the tracheotomy will be maintained until reconstructive surgery can be performed. Such surgery may include maxillomandibular osteotomies, in which the chin is moved farther forward through a simultaneous vertical movement of the maxilla, sagittal split osteotomy, and body osteotomy of the mandible or through mandibular distraction osteogenesis. In a review of this relatively new surgical advance, 10 patients with craniofacial disorders who presented with micrognathia were evaluated with cephalometric analysis both before and after distraction (Denny et al., 2001). The disorders included Pierre Robin sequence, TCS, and Nager syndrome, and the age of the patients ranged from 3 months to 8 years. All patients had obstructive airway symptoms. Measurable airway increase occurred in all patients, independent of the syndrome considered, as did clinical improvement in their airway symptoms. This study indicates that mandibular distraction osteogenesis appears to generate a good surgical outcome in terms of airway management, at least in a subset of well-selected cases of micrognathia. In a number of children affected by TCS, particularly those with severe mandibular hypoplasia, general anaesthesia may prove more complicated, mainly due to the restricted airway. In such situations, the use of a laryngeal mask to induce anesthesia, rather than intubation, may prove effective (Jones et al., 2001). Postoperative complications such as nausea and vomiting may also require specialized care in patients with micrognathia.

In terms of the audiologic problems, in the vast majority of cases, the hearing loss may be alleviated by the use of bone-anchored hearing aids. Historically, surgical middle ear reconstruction has been attempted in some patients; however, this technique infrequently produces adequate hearing (Granstrom and Tjellstrom, 1997).

In addition, the provision of percutaneous titanium screws allows prosthetic ears to be fitted for those patients with severe anomalies of the external ears, and for appropriate cases, the aesthetic result achieved in this way is superior to that which can be achieved by surgery.

MOUSE MODELS OF TCS

Induced by Teratogens

On the basis that the tissues affected in *TCOF1* arise during early embryonic development from the first and second branchial arches, two main theories have been advanced to explain the underlying developmental basis of the disorder, both of which result from teratologic experiments in animals. These theories are (1) interference with neural crest cell migration and (2) excessive cell death in the ectodermal placodes. The first of these hypotheses was reported by Poswillo (1975), who produced a phenocopy of TCS in the rat by the administration of teratogenic doses of vitamin A palmitate during early development. This appeared to cause localized cell death in the neural crest cell population before, or during, their migration from the neural folds, resulting in severe disruption of the preotic neural crest. It was therefore proposed that selective destruction of the neural crest cells destined for migration into the first and second branchial arches had occurred. Because morphogenesis appeared to continue normally, it was proposed that the anomalies resulted from a lack of available tissue. A later study by Sulik et al. (1987) suggested that TCS resulted from excessive cell death in the ectodermal placodes. In this study, phenocopies of TCS and Nager or Miller syndrome were produced in mice by acute maternal exposure to 13-*cis*-retinoic acid, a vitamin A analogue that is not stored in the maternal liver, at 9.0 to 9.5 days postfertilization. These studies demonstrated that the facial and limb anomalies resulted from excessive cell death in the proximal aspect of the maxillary and mandibular processes of the first branchial arch and the apical ectodermal ridge of the limb bud. From these studies, Sulik et al. (1987) hypothesized that the cell death observed was a direct result of damage to the ectodermal placodes, with the resulting local tissue damage causing altered or abnormal migration of the neural crest cells, rather than a defect of the neural crest cells themselves.

Although both of these studies initially provided insights into the cellular mechanisms that may affect facial development, it has been established that TCS results from mutations in the *TCOF1* gene. To investigate the contribution of this gene to facial development and to determine why mutations in a gene encoding a widely expressed nucleolar phosphoprotein result in a purely craniofacial disorder, genetic targeting studies were undertaken.

Targeting of the *Tcof1* Locus

To investigate the molecular basis of TCS by targeting the *Tcof1* locus, the murine gene was isolated and the locus was characterized (Dixon et al., 1997a; Paznekas et al., 1997). The mouse and human genes display 65.9% identity at the nucleotide level and 54.8% identity and 71.6% similarity at the protein level. The 3′ untranslated regions also display 62.8% identity, which is relatively high and might indicate an important role in maintaining the function of the protein or stabilizing the transcript. Northern blot analysis, RT-PCR, and whole-mount in situ hybridization assays determined that the gene is expressed in a wide variety of both embryonic and adult tissues. Peak expression levels were detected with whole-mount in situ hybridization in the developing branchial arches during embryonic days 8, 9, and 10, which decreased as development progressed and reduced to background levels by day 11 of gestation (Dixon et al., 1997a). These data suggest that high expression levels of the gene are required during times of critical morphogenetic events. To ensure complete functional inactivation of *Tcof1*, Dixon et al. (2000) replaced the first coding exon of *Tcof1* with a neomycin-resistance cassette and generated chimeric animals. Chimeric males were then crossed with C57BL/6 female mice to produce heterozygous offspring. Surprisingly, however, the phenotypic effect of ablation of a single *Tcof1* allele is more severe in mice than in humans, and a lethal phenotype was observed, precluding any further breeding strategies. Profound craniofacial anomalies, including agenesis of the nasal passages, abnormal development of the maxilla, acrania, exencephaly, and a complete absence of eye development, were observed in *Tcof1* heterozygous mice, resulting in their death shortly after birth due to asphyxia (Dixon et al., 2000). These abnormalities were first detected in *Tcof1* heterozyygous mice at embryonic day 8, after which they exhibited a generalized developmental delay and showed no signs of optic development (Figure 106–5). Wild-type mouse embryos normally undergo an axial turning

sequence and have closed their rostral neuropore by embryonic day 9. Their heterozygous littermates, however, remained unturned with an open rostral neuropore. This delay in closure of the neural tube was never recovered, and heterozygous embryos went on to develop exencephaly, with developing brain tissue protruding through the open rostral neuropore (Figure 106–5, C and D). By birth, the *Tcof1* heterozygous mice displayed mandibular hypoplasia and severe retrognathia of the middle third of the face and had no discernible skull vault. Histologic and skeletal analyses revealed an absence of the frontal, parietal, and interparietal bones. The nasal capsule and the maxilla were extremely malformed, and the zygomatic arch, tympanic ring, and middle ear ossicles were hypoplastic and misshapen. Whole-mount TUNEL analysis, a technique that identifies cells undergoing apoptosis, revealed that the number of apoptotic cells was markedly elevated in the *Tcof1* heterozygous embryos—in particular, the neuroepithelium of the cranial neural folds and the neural tube displayed a profusion of apoptotic cells. These abnormally high levels of apoptosis were observed in *Tcof1* heterozygous mice throughout embryonic days 8 and 9, but thereafter they declined. The high levels of cell death in the neuroepithelium, together with the gross morphologic phenotype, strongly suggested that a proportion of the premigratory neural crest cells were depleted. In addition, immunohistochemistry of embryonic day 10.5 mice with an antineurofilament antibody indicated that the neural crest cell–derived cranial ganglia were severely hypoplastic, the ophthalmic branch of the trigeminal nerve and the glossopharyngeal ganglia/nerves were absent, and the dorsal root ganglia were markedly disorganized. These results suggest that the TCS phenotype results, at least in part, from a massive increase in apoptosis in the prefusion neural folds. Although exencephaly and anophthalmia have not been reported in patients with TCS, the exencephaly observed in *Tcof1* heterozygous mice is most likely to be a secondary defect caused by the failure of neural tube fusion, rather than an intrinsic defect in the bones that comprise the vault of the skull. A large number of both transgenic and naturally occurring mouse mutants exhibit neural tube fusion defects, of which exencephaly is a nonspecific feature (Harris and Juriloff, 1999). In addition, these phenotypic differences may reflect species-specific variation in craniofacial development between humans and mice.

Subsequent studies in our laboratory have investigated the contribution of different genetic backgrounds to the phenotype of the heterozygous mice. To date, the *Tcof1* chimeras have been bred with females from different three inbred strains, including C3H, CBA/Ca, and DBA/1. These studies indicate that the heterozygous mice exhibit strain-dependent phenotypes ranging from moderately abnormal to extremely severe (J. Dixon, unpublished observations). CBA/Ca *Tcof1* heterozygous mice are even more severely affected than C57BL/6 mice, with exencephaly present in all of the embryos examined, a severe developmental delay, and major craniofacial abnormalities, including excessive cartilage development in the nasal complex, micrognathia, and microphthalmia. C3H *Tcof1* heterozygous mice are less severely affected but still exhibit exencephaly and abnormalities of the facial complex. DBA/1 *Tcof1* heterozygous mice are moderately affected, but a large proportion of embryos exhibit abnormal brain development, micrognathia, and microphthalmia. Studies to further characterize these developmental abnormalities are ongoing, but these preliminary studies indicate that different genetic backgrounds have a significant contribution to the phenotypic outcome in *Tcof1* heterozygous mice.

PATHOGENESIS OF THE DISORDER

The underlying pathogenesis of TCS and the function of Treacle remain undetermined. It has been demonstrated, however, that the correct dosage of this protein is crucial to the development of the facial complex (Dixon et al., 2000). Although there is some evidence to suggest that adult fibroblasts are able to maintain the levels of Treacle in the event of haploinsufficiency (Isaac et al., 2000), no studies have been performed on embryonic, immature, or untransformed fibroblasts. It is not known, therefore, whether the cells of the neural crest are normally able to regulate their levels of this protein during devel-

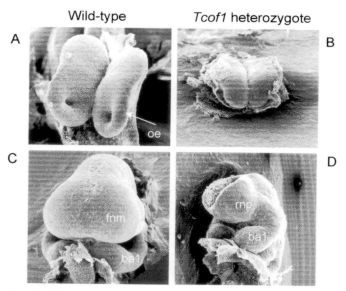

Figure 106–5. Scanning electron microscope (SEM) analysis of wild-type and *Tcof1* heterozygous embryos. (*A* and *B*) Embryonic day 8.5. The forebrain region of the wild-type embryo (*A*) exhibits a distinct optic evagination (oe), whereas no optic development is evident in the *Tcof1* heterozygous embryo (*B*). The neural folds of the *Tcof1* heterozygote are smaller and more rounded than the wild-type embryo. (*C* and *D*) Embryonic day 9.5. Comparison of wild-type (*C*) and *Tcof1* heterozygous (*D*) embryos reveals that the rostral neuropore of the *Tcof1* heterozygous embryos has not fused by this point in development and neural tissue appears to be spilling from the defect. fnm, frontonasal mass; ba1, first branchial arch; rnp, rostral neuropore.

opment and migration and, if so, whether being heterozygous for the *Tcof1* gene renders them unable to do so. Data from the mouse model indicate that the phenotype results from massively elevated levels of cell death in the developing neural folds, although it is unclear what proportion of the neural crest cells survive, what proportion undergo cell death, and what induces them to enter this inappropriate program of cell death. Studies to investigate this are ongoing.

Perhaps one of the most interesting features of TCS is that affected individuals from within the same family, who all have the same genetic mutation, exhibit wide variation in the clinical severity of their symptoms. The reason for this is unknown, but hypotheses to explain this variability include the effect of either stochastic processes or environmental influences and the contribution of different genetic backgrounds. Indeed, evidence from the mouse studies indicate that different genetic backgrounds can have a major effect on the phenotype of *Tcof1* heterozygous mice and that interactions with other, as-yet-undefined genes, contribute to the overall phenotype. It is also possible that variation in other genes in the same or a related pathway affects the function of the protein in different individuals.

In conclusion, although much work has been completed on the *TCOF1* gene, elucidation of the function of the protein and the identification of the pathway of Treacle and of what interacts with this protein will be central to determining how mutations in this locus result in TCS.

ACKNOWLEDGMENTS

We thank the numerous TCS patients and their families who have provided blood samples and an endless source of inspiration during the past 14 years and the clinicians who have collected samples on our behalf. We would also like to thank the people that have worked on the TCS project during that time and our many collaborators during the project, including the late Professor J. Wasmuth, Dr. S. Loftus, Dr. T. Meier, Dr. D. Newgreen, Professor R. Fassler, Dr. C. Brakebusch, Professor R. Williamson, and Professor M.W.J. Ferguson. The financial support for this project has arisen from many different sources, and the Medical Research Council, the Wellcome Trust, and the Birth Defects Foundation are gratefully acknowledged. J.D. is an MRC Research Training Fellow.

REFERENCES

Aebi M, Hornig H, Weissmann C (1987). 5' Cleavage site in eukaryotic pre-mRNA splicing is determined by the overall 5' splice region, not by the conserved GU. *Cell* 50: 237–246.

Allanson JE, McGillivray BC (1985). Familial clefting syndrome with ectropion and dental anomaly without limb anomalies. *Clin Genet* 27: 426–429.

Andersen JS, Lyon CE, Fox AH, Leung AK, Lam YW, Steen H, Mann M, Lamond AI (2002). Directed proteomic analysis of the human nucleolus. *Curr Biol* 8: 1–11.

Arndt EM, Travis F, Lefebvre A, Munro IR (1987). Psychosocial adjustment of 20 patients with Treacher Collins syndrome before and after reconstructive surgery. *Br J Plast Surg* 40: 605–609.

Bogerd HP, Fridell RA, Benson RE, Hua J, Cullen BR (1996). Protein sequence requirements for function of the human T-cell leukemia virus type 1 Rex nuclear export signal delineated by a novel in vivo randomization-selection assay. *Mol Cell Biol* 16: 4207–4214.

Chelsky D, Ralph R, Jonak G (1989). Sequence requirement for synthetic peptide mediated translocation to the nucleus. *Mol Cell Biol* 9: 2487–2492.

Chemke J, Mogliner BM, Ben-Itzahak I, Zurkowski L, Ophir D (1988). Autosomal recessive inheritance pattern of Nager acrofacial dysostosis. *J Med Genet* 25: 230–232.

Dawson M (1999). *Mutational Analysis of Treacher Collins Syndrome*. Masters Thesis, University of Manchester.

Denny AD, Talisman R, Hanson PR, Recinos RF (2001). Mandibular distraction osteogenesis in very young patients to correct airway obstruction. *Plast Reconstr Surg* 108: 302–311.

Dixon MJ (1996). Treacher Collins syndrome. *Hum Mol Genet* 5: 1391–1396.

Dixon J, Brakebusch C, Fässler R, Dixon MJ (2000). Increased levels of apoptosis in the prefusion neural folds underlie the craniofacial disorder, Treacher Collins syndrome. *Hum Mol Genet* 10: 1473–1480.

Dixon J, Hovanes K, Shiang R, Dixon MJ (1997a). Sequence analysis, identification of evolutionary conserved motifs and expression analysis of murine *TCOF1* provide further evidence for a potential function for the gene and its human homologue, *TCOF1*. *Hum Mol Genet* 6: 727–737.

Dixon J, Edwards SJ, Anderson I, Brass A, Scambler PJ, Dixon MJ (1997b). Identification of the complete coding sequence and genomic organisation of the Treacher Collins syndrome gene. *Genome Res* 7: 223–234.

Dixon MJ, Marres HAM, Edwards SJ, Dixon J, Cremers CWRJ (1994). Treacher Collins syndrome: Correlation between clinical and genetic linkage studies. *Clin Dysmorphol* 3: 96–103.

Dixon MJ, Dixon J, Houseal T, Bhatt M, Ward DC, Klinger K, Landes GM (1993). Narrowing the position of the Treacher Collins syndrome locus to a small interval between three new microsatellite markers at 5q32-33.1. *Am J Hum Genet* 52: 907–914.

Dixon MJ, Haan E, Baker E, David D, McKenzie N, Williamson R, Mulley J, Farrall M, Callen D (1991). Association of Treacher Collins syndrome and translocation 6p21.31/16p13.11: Exclusion of the locus from these candidate regions. *Am J Hum Genet* 48: 274–280.

Edwards SJ, Gladwin AJ, Dixon MJ (1997). The mutational spectrum in Treacher Collins syndrome reveals a predominance of mutations that create a premature termination codon. *Am J Hum Genet* 60: 515–524.

Edwards SJ, Fowlie A, Cust MP, Liu DTY, Young ID, Dixon MJ (1996). Prenatal diagnosis in Treacher Collins syndrome using combined linkage analysis and ultrasound imaging. *J Med Genet* 33: 603–606.

Ellis PE, Dawson M, Dixon MJ (2002). Mutation testing in Treacher Collins syndrome. *J Orthod* 29: 293–298.

Emes RD, Ponting CP (2001). A new sequence motif linking lissencephaly, Treacher Collins and oral-facial-digital type 1 syndromes, microtubule dynamics and cell migration. *Hum Mol Genet* 10: 2813–2820.

Fazen LE, Elmore J, Nadler HL (1967). Mandibulo-facial dysostosis (Treacher Collins syndrome). *Am J Dis Child* 113: 406–410.

Fischer U, Huber J, Boelens WC, Mattaj IW, Luhrmann R (1995). The HIV-1 Rev activation domain is a nuclear export signal that accesses an export pathway used by specific cellular RNAs. *Cell* 82: 475–483.

Frischmeyer PA, Dietz HC (1999). Nonsense-mediated mRNA decay in health and disease. *Hum Mol Genet* 8: 1893–1900.

Gladwin AJ, Dixon J, Loftus SK, Edwards SJ, Wasmuth JJ, Hennekam RCM, Dixon MJ (1996). Treacher Collins syndrome may result from insertions, deletions or splicing mutations, which introduce a termination codon into the gene. *Hum Mol Genet* 5: 1533–1538.

Gorlin RJ, Cohen MM, Levin LS (1990). *Syndromes of the Head and Neck*. Oxford University Press, Oxford.

Granstrom G, Tjellstrom A (1997). The bone-anchored hearing aid (BAHA) in children with auricular malformations. *Ear Nose Throat J* 76: 238–240.

Harris MJ, Juriloff DM (1999). Mini-review: towards understanding mechanisms of genetic neural tube defects in mice. *Teratology* 60: 292–305.

Hatanaka M (1990). Discovery of the nucleolar targeting signal. *BioEssays* 12: 143–148.

Haworth KE, Islam I, Breen M, Putt W, Makrinou E, Binns M, Hopkinson D, Edwards Y (2001). Canine TCOF1; cloning, chromosome assignment and genetic analysis in dogs with different head types. *Mamm Genome* 12: 622–629.

Hayashi K, Yandell DW (1993). How sensitive is PCR-SSCP? *Hum Mutat* 2: 338–346.

Herring SW, Rowlatt UF, Pruzansky S (1979). Anatomical abnormalities in mandibulofacial dysostosis. *Am J Med Genet* 3: 225–259.

Isaac C, Marsh KL, Dixon J, Paznekas W, Dixon MJ, Jabs EW, Meier UT (2000). Characterization of the nucleolar gene product of Treacher Collins syndrome in patient and control cells. *Mol Biol Cell* 11: 3061–3071.

Jackson I (1991). A reappraisal of non-consensus mRNA splice sites. *Nucl Acids Res* 19: 3795–3798.

Jones KL, Smith DW, Harvey MA, Hall BD, Quan L (1975). Older paternal age and fresh gene mutation: data on additional disorders. *J Pediatr* 86: 84–88.

Jones NC, Farlie PG, Minichiello J, Newgreen DF (1999). Detection of an appropriate kinase activity in branchial arches I and II that coincide with peak expression of the Treacher Collins sydrome gene product, treacle. *Hum Mol Genet* 8: 2239–2245.

Jones SE, Dickson U, Moriarty A (2001). Anaesthesia for insertion of bone-anchored hearing aids in children: a 7-year audit. *Anaesthesia* 56: 777–780.

Kay ED, Kay CN (1989). Dysmorphogenesis of the mandible, zygoma, and middle ear ossicles in hemifacial microsomia and mandibulofacial dysostosis. *Am Med Genet* 32: 27–31.

Lo Nigro C, Chong CS, Smith AC, Dobyns WB, Carrozzo R, Ledbetter DH (1997). Point mutations and an intragenic deletion in LIS1, the lissencephaly causative gene in isolated lissencephaly sequence and Miller-Dieker syndrome. *Hum Mol Genet* 6: 157–164.

Marres HAM, Cremers CWRJ, Dixon MJ, Huygen PLM, Joosten BM (1995). The Treacher Collins syndrome: A clinical, radiological and genetic linkage study on two pedigrees. *Arch Otolaryngol Head Neck Surg* 121: 509–514.

Marsh KL, Dixon J, Dixon MJ (1998). Mutations in the Treacher Collins syndrome gene lead to mislocalisation of the nucleolar protein treacle. *Hum Mol Genet* 7: 1795–1800.

Meier UT, Blobel G (1992). Nopp140 shuttles on tracks between nucleolus and cytoplasm. *Cell* 70: 127–138.

Moroianu J, Riordan JF (1994). Identification of the nucleolar targeting signal of human angiogenin. *Biochem Biophys Res Commun* 203: 1765–1772.

Nicolaides KH, Johansson D, Donnai D, Rodeck CH (1984). Prenatal diagnosis of mandibulofacial dysostosis. *Prenatal Diagn* 4: 201–205.

Ogilvy-Stuart AL, Parsons AC (1991). Miller syndrome (postaxial acrofacial dysostosis): Further evidence for autosomal recessive inheritance and expansion of the phenotype. *J Med Genet* 28: 695–700.

Paznekas WA, Zhang N, Gridley T, Jabs EW (1997). Mouse TCOF1 is expressed widely, has motifs conserved in nucleolar phosphoproteins, and maps to chromosome 18. *Biochem Biophys Res Commun* 238: 1–6.

Phelps PD, Poswillo D, Lloyd GAS (1981). The ear deformities in mandibulofacial dysostosis (Treacher Collins syndrome). *Clin Otolaryngol* 6: 15–28.

Pierreux CE, Nicolas FJ, Hill CS (2000). Transforming growth factor beta-independent shuttling of Smad4 between the cytoplasm and nucleus. *Mol Cell Biol* 20: 9041–54.

Poswillo D (1975). The pathogenesis of Treacher Collins syndrome (mandibulofacial dysostosis). *Br J Oral Surg* 13: 1–26.

Rovin S, Dachi SF, Borenstein DB, Cotter WB (1964). Mandibulofacial dysostosis, a familial study of five generations. *J Pediatr* 65: 215–221.

Splendore A, Silva EO, Alonso LG, Richieri-Costa A, Alonso N, Rosa A, Carakushanky G, Cavalcanti DP, Brunoni D, Passos-Bueno MR (2000). High mutation detection rate in *TCOF1* among Treacher Collins syndrome patients reveals clustering of mutations and 16 novel pathogenic changes. *Hum Mutat* 16: 315–322.

Stovin JJ, Lyon JA, and Clemens RL (1960). Mandibulofacial dysostosis. *Radiology* 74: 225–231.

Sulik KK, Johnston MC, Smiley SJ, Speight HS, Jarvis BE (1987). Mandibulofacial dyostosis (Treacher Collins syndrome): A new proposal for its pathogenesis. *Am J Med Genet* 27: 359–372.

The Treacher Collins Syndrome Collaborative Group (1996). Positional cloning of a gene involved in the pathogenesis of Treacher Collins syndrome. *Nat Genet* 12: 130–136.

Wen W, Meinkoth JL, Tsien RY, Taylor SS (1995). Identification of a signal for rapid export of proteins from the nucleus. *Cell* 82: 463–473.

Wiley MJ, Cauwenbergs P, Taylor IM (1983). Effects of retinoic acid on the development of the facial skeleton in hamsters: Early changes involving cranial neural crest cells. *Acta Anat* 116: 180–192.

Winokur ST, Shiang R (1998). The Treacher Collins syndrome (*TCOF1*) gene product, treacle, is targeted to the nucleolus by signals in its C-terminus. *Hum Mol Genet* 7: 1947–1952.

Wise CA, Chiang LC, Paznekas WA, Sharma M, Musy MM, Ashley JA, Lovett M, Jabs EW (1997). *TCOF1* gene encodes a putative nucleolar phosphoprotein that exhibits mutations in Treacher Collins syndrome throughout its coding region. *Proc Natl Acad Sci USA* 94: 3110–3115.

Xiao Z, Watson N, Rodriguez C, Lodish HF (2001). Nucleocytoplasmic shuttling of Smad1 conferred by its nuclear localization and nuclear export signals. *J Biol Chem* 276: 39404–39410.

LMBR1 and Acheiropodia and Preaxial Polydactyly

PETROS TSIPOURAS AND MICHAEL W. KILPATRICK

Acheiropodia (OMIM 200500) is a genetically inherited limb malformation that is detected at birth. The condition was initially described in 1929 by Peacock; since then, several reports have delineated its clinical and radiographic phenotype (Toledo and Saldanha, 1969, 1972; Marcallo et al., 1979; Grimaldi et al., 1983; Fett-Conte and Richieri-Costa, 1990; Lemos Silveira and Freire-Maia, 1998). Acheiropodia was mapped to 7q36 (Escamilla et al., 2000; Ianakiev et al., 2001) in a region overlapping that of preaxial polydactyly (PPD) (OMIM 174500) (Heutink et al., 1994; Tsukurov et al., 1994). The two conditions, albeit phenotypically distinct, appear to originate from structural disruptions of the *C7orf2* gene locus (Ianakiev et al., 2001), which encodes the orthologue of the murine *Lmbr1* gene (Clark et al., 2000). Although a null mutation of the *C7orf2* gene transcript results in acheiropodia, PPD probably results from the inability of the same locus to function as a *cis*-acting regulator for the *Sonic hedgehog* gene (Lettice et al., 2002).

CLINICAL PHENOTYPE

Acheiropodia is a rare limb reduction malformation. Affected individuals typically lack hands and feet their limbs terminate to a conical stump (Toledo and Saldanha, 1969, 1972). In the upper extremity, the limb terminates at the distal third of the humerus, and in the lower extremity, there is a knee joint and the proximal third of the tibia (Marcallo et al., 1979) (Figure 107–1). On radiograph, the fibula is missing. In addition, an accessory bone is found either parallel or in tandem to the humerus (Bohomoletz bone). Occasionally, a skeletal appendage that resembles a finger composed of two or three digits and is attached to the upper extremity stump has been detected (Fett-Conte and Richieri-Costa 1990; Lemos Silveira and Freire-Maia, 1998) (Figure 107–1). There are no other skeletal or organ malformations reported in this condition.

PPD describes the duplication of the thumb and/or the index finger and corresponding toes; it is one of several manifestations in a phenotypic continuum that includes triphalangeal thumb, syndactyly, and associated thenar hypoplasia, tibial hypoplasia, and sternal deformity (Zguricas et al.,1994, 1999; Dundar et al., 2001) (Figure 107–2).

Combinations of these phenotypic manifestations segregate in families as autosomal dominant traits with almost complete penetrance. This has led to a phenotypic classification scheme of PPD in four types (I through IV) (Temtamy and McKusick, 1978). In contrast to acheiropodia, polydactyly is one of the most commonly observed malformations of the extremities, and it has been detected in several populations (Temtamy and McKusick, 1978).

CHROMOSOMAL LOCALIZATION AND FINE MAPPING OF THE ACHEIROPODIA/PPD LOCUS

All reported cases of acheiropodia, with the exception of one family, have originated from Brazil (Kruger and Kumar, 1994). Furthermore, a high degree of consanguinity is present in a significant proportion of families with affected individuals (Freire-Maia et al., 1975a, 1975b). This feature of acheiropodia-affected families has been used for chromosomal localization and fine mapping (Kruglyak et al., 1995; Escamilla et al., 2000; Ianakiev et al., 2001).

The mapping of the acheiropodia locus to 7q36 was initially achieved by undertaking a complete genome screen of an extended pedigree that included three affected siblings. Homozygosity mapping was used to identify regions most likely to harbor the gene for acheiropodia in this pedigree. Multipoint linkage analysis generated a Z_{max} of 4.2 for markers D7S2546 and D7S550. These studies localized acheiropodia to 7q36 and defined a critical region for the disease gene of 8.6 cM (Escamilla et al., 2000) (Figure 107–3).

Further refinement of the critical region was achieved by haplotype analysis of five families segregating acheiropodia (Ianakiev et al., 2001). Genotyping of these families for a series of 15 highly polymorphic 7q36 markers defined a long region of homozygosity in affected individuals from all five families. These regions overlapped in identical alleles at the D7S3037–D7S3036 interval, suggesting that the most likely region for the acheiropodia locus could be reduced to the region between D7S550 and D7S2465. Thus, analysis of this family panel reduced the acheiropodia critical region from 8.4 cM (Escamilla et al., 2000) to 1.3 cM, on the basis of identity by descent (Ianakiev et al., 2000) (see Figure 107–3).

The physical map of the region (Integrated Chromosome 7 Database [The Chromosome 7 Project; see http://www.genet.sickkids.on.ca/chromosome7]) suggested that it comprised less than 1 Mb (see Figure 107–3).

In each of the five affected individuals, homozygosity was observed in no fewer than eight consecutive microsatellite markers. Within these overlapping regions of homozygosity, a two-marker haplotype was observed that was shared identically among all these affected individuals and that was not seen in homozygous form in any unaffected individuals in these families. Because these alleles are normally found in low frequency in the general population, their concordant segregation in all five families strongly indicated that this segment, which spans 1.3 cM, was inherited by descent from a single ancestor (Ianakiev et al., 2001). The length of the shared 7q36 region suggested a relatively recent age (31 generations) for this common mutation (Ianakiev et al., 2001).

Interestingly, this 1.3-cM region was completely contained within the 8.4-cM region implicated by Escamilla et al., (2000), and the shared alleles near this region matched the shared haplotype in that study (see Figure 107–3). This observation strongly suggested that all affected individuals in the two reports shared homozygosity for a common haplotype and confirmed the expectation that a single common ancestral mutation (Freire-Maia et al., 1975b) is the cause of nearly all cases of acheiropodia in Brazil.

In 1994, two independent studies reported linkage of two different types of PPD to 7q36 (Heutink et al., 1994; Tsukurov et al., 1994). Subsequently, haplotype analysis in 12 PPD families enabled the localization of PPD to a region of 1.9 cM between D7S550 and D7S2423 (Zguricas et al., 1999) (see Figure 107–3). Saturation mapping allowed the critical region to be further refined to the 1-cM interval between CGR17 and D7S3037 (Heus et al., 1999). This defined an approximate 450 kb region (see Figure 107–3). Thus, analysis of the genetic data for the acheiropodia and PPD demonstrated a shared minimum critical region on 7q36 (see Figure 107–3).

MUTATION ANALYSIS OF *C7orf2*

Physical and transcriptional mapping of the acheiropodia/PPD region on 7q36 identified a previously undescribed transcript, which was designated C7orf2 (Heus et al., 1999). The gene encoding the C7orf2 tran-

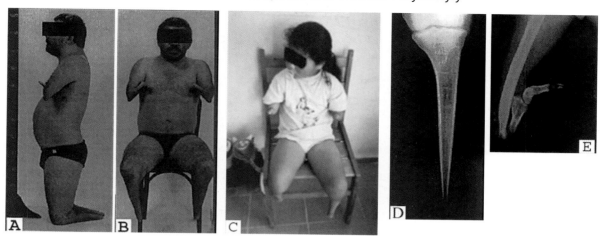

Figure 107–1. Affected individuals with acheiropodia. Note the small finger-like appendages at the end of the arm, which are present bilaterally (*A–C*). (*D* and *E*) Radiographs of individuals in *A* and *B* showing tapered amputation of the distal tibia with well-preserved proximal epiphysis and dysplastic distal humerus articulating with a rudimentary forearm composed of three dysplastic long bones, respectively. (Modified from Ianakiev et al., 2001.)

script is the human orthologue of the mouse *Limb region 1 gene* (*Lmbr1*) that was identified in the course of positional cloning of genes disrupted by the mouse *Hemimelic extra-toes (Hx)* and *Hammertoe (Hm)* mutations (Clark et al., 2000). The mouse *Lmbr1* gene shows striking alterations of expression in the limbs of *Hx* mice (see later). The *Hx* mutation causes hemimelia of the radius and tibia and preaxial polydactyly on both forelimbs and hindlimbs. The involvement of the mouse *Lmbr1* gene in a limb phenotype, combined with its genomic location on 7q36, suggested *C7orf2* as a candidate gene for Acheiropodia/PPD.

The C7orf2 transcript sequence encoded a 492-amino-acid open reading frame (ORF) that starts with a methionine residue. The C7orf2 ORF predicts a protein that contains nine transmembrane domains and a coiled-coil domain and is likely to be located in the plasma membrane, suggesting that this protein might be a receptor. The *C7orf2* gene comprises 17 exons that encompass 200 kb of genomic DNA (Ianakiev et al., 2001).

Genomic DNA from affected individuals from each of five families with acheiropodia was amplified by sets of primers for the entire gene. All exons amplified successfully, with the exception of exon 4, which consistently failed to amplify in affected individuals, in contrast to its reproducible amplification in both obligate carriers and normal controls. Analysis of the C7orf2 transcript obtained from affected individuals, obligate carriers, and normal controls demonstrated both by size and sequence the presence of a deletion of the coding sequence corresponding to exon 4 in the homozygous affected. This mutation is predicted to introduce a frameshift leading to a premature stop codon in exon 6. It therefore appears to be a true null mutation, consistent with the lack of any phenotypic effect in heterozygotes (Ianakiev et al., 2001) (see Figure 107–3).

PCR-based analysis of genomic DNA from affected individuals indicated a deletion of 4 to 6 kb. Analysis of the *C7orf2* gene identified a common acheiropodia mutation in all unrelated affected individuals studied. However, no coding-sequence alterations of *C7orf2* were detected in affected individuals in any PPD families studied. A PPD patient presenting with bilateral duplication of the triphalangeal thumb and triplication of the big toe was shown to carry a de novo reciprocal translocation t(5,7);(q11,q36) (Lettice et al., 2002). FISH analysis of a cell line derived from this patient identified a BAC clone that spanned the translocation breakpoint. Analysis of this clone and of genomic DNA from the patient-derived cell line showed that the translocation breakpoint is located in intron 5 of the *c7orf2/LMBR1* gene (see Figure 107–3).

CLINICAL DIAGNOSIS

Acheiropodia is present at birth. The clinical evaluation should include a radiographic survey of the extremities. Acheiropodia should not be confused with terminal transverse limb defects, which also present with the absence of hands and feet but with the ulna/radius and tibia/fibula present (Horn and Kolb, 1994). Genetic counseling and molecular diagnostic analysis of the *C7orf2* gene should be offered to the parents after the birth of an affected child. Based on the findings of Ianakiev et al. (2001), a single mutation could be the underlying cause of all cases in Brazil. Prenatally, acheiropodia could be diagnosed by molecular testing or by ultrasonographic examination. The management of the condition involves the use of orthopedic prostheses to confer a certain level of function.

PPD is apparent at birth. Clinical evaluation and radiographic assessment are necessary to establish whether the phenotype segregates independently or as a constituent part of a syndromic entity. PPD is inherited as an autosomal dominant trait with very high penetrance; thus, it is likely to segregate in either the maternal or paternal side of the family. Molecular studies should be offered only as an investigational test at present. Ultrasonographic examination should be offered for pregnancies at risk; however, its sensitivity has not been fully assessed. The management could include amputation of supernumerary digits and surgical repositioning of the triphalangeal thumb for improved function.

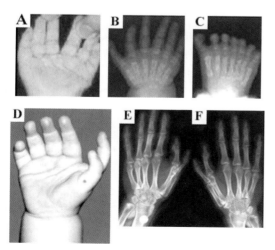

Figure 107–2. Affected individuals with preaxial polydactyly. Note duplication of the triphalangeal thumb (*A*), bilateral duplications in the radiogram of the right hand (*B*), and triplication of the great toe (*C*). (*D*) Hexadactyly with a fully developed thumb placed in a normal "thumb" plane at an angle of 90 degrees to the digital rays. (*E* and *F*) Radiograms showing the complete duplication of both thumbs. (Modified from Lettice et al., 2002 [*A–C*] and Zguricas et al., 1999 [*D–F*]).

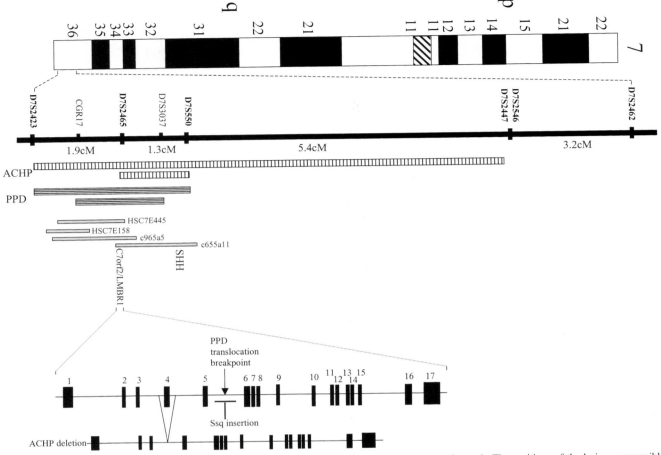

Figure 107–3. Integrated schematic map of the 7q36 region. The genetic map of the region is shown at the top, with the initial and subsequently refined acheiropodia and preaxial polydactyly (PPD) critical regions shown as vertically or horizontally striped bars, respectively. Solid gray bars depict some of the YACs that define the physical map of the region with the structure of the *C7orf2/LMBR1* gene underneath. The positions of the lesions responsible for acheiropodia, PPD, and *Ssq* are shown along with the position of the neighboring *SHH* gene suggested to be involved in the mechanism of these mutations.

ANIMAL MODELS

Hx and *Hm* Mice

In mice, the dominant limb deformity mutations *Hx* and *Hm* map to chromosome 5, to a region syntenic to the human 7q36 (Green, 1964; Knudsen and Kochhar, 1981; Clark et al., 2000). These mouse mutations cause related limb abnormalities. The *Hx* mutation causes hemimelia of the tibia and radius and PPD on both the forelimbs and hindlimbs (Knudsen and Kochhar, 1981), and the anterior digits in *Hx* mice are typically triphalangeal (Masuya et al., 1995), which is seen in many patients from human PPD families (Heutinck et al., 1994; Hing et al., 1995; Zguricas et al., 1999) (Figure 107–4; see Figures 107–2). *Hm* mice have correct numbers of digits but extensive webbing between the digits (Green, 1964), and it has been suggested that the syndactyly in *Hm* mice may be analogous to that observed in humans with complex polysyndactyly (Tsukurov et al., 1994; Clark et al., 2000).

Although the mouse *Hx* and *Hm* mutations are closely linked, they are distinct (one recombinant in 3664 meioses) (Sweet, 1982), which suggests that they might disrupt the same or closely linked genes that control limb development. The mouse and the human mutations are also linked to the *Sonic hedgehog (Shh)* locus (Chang et al., 1994; Marigo et al., 1995), and alteration of Shh signaling has been proposed to underlie both mouse and human limb abnormalities (see later).

Lmbr1 is ubiquitously expressed, including the developing limbs, but in the *Hx* mutant, the level of expression is significantly reduced during a specific period of limb development (embryonic days 10.5–12.5) (Clark et al., 2000). This aberrant expression coincides with the ectopic expression of *Shh* at the anterior aspect of the apical ectodermal ridge, as opposed to its normal expression, which is restricted to the posterior aspect (Riddle et al., 1993; Masuya et al., 1995).

Clark et al. (2000) defined a 450-kb interval for the mouse *Hm* and *Hx* mutations and identified several genes within this critical region. However, extensive mutational analysis in mouse failed to identify le-

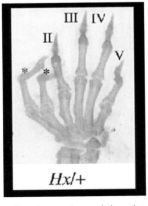

Figure 107–4. Limb phenotypes observed in mice heterozygous for the *Hemimelic extra-toes* (*Hx*). Dorsal view of an Hx/+ forelimb stained with alizarin red is shown. In the preaxial polydactyly, digit I is replaced by extra triphalangeal digits (asterisks). (Modified from Clark et al., 2001.)

sions in the coding sequences of any candidate genes. The absence of coding region mutations raised the possibility that the dominant mouse and human mutations are regulatory alleles that disrupt the expression of a gene or genes in the interval.

An *Lmbr1* Loss-of-Function Mouse Mutant

One of the genes within the mouse *Hx* and *Hm* critical region *Lmbr1* is normally expressed in developing limbs at the times that both the *Hx* and *Hm* phenotypes arise. More important, *Lmbr1* was found to be dynamically misexpressed in *Hx* limbs at the exact time that abnormal limb morphology first appears (Clark et al., 2000). Expression changes included a possible overexpression of the gene followed by a dramatic decrease in *Lmbr1* transcript levels at later stages. The human *Lmbr1* orthologue (C7orf2) is contained entirely within the human critical region for acheiropodia/PPD, and the striking correlation between the appearance of defects in *Hx* mice and *Lmbr1* misregulation suggested that the mouse and human limb mutations might be alleles of the *Lmbr1* gene. In addition, the creation of a loss-of-function allele of the *Lmbr1* gene was undertaken to test whether this gene is required for normal limb development (Clark et al., 2001). Mice with reduced *Lmbr1* function showed distal limb reductions, including oligodactyly (Figure 107–5). These phenotypes are reciprocal to those caused by the classic *Hx* and *Ssq* dominant mutations (Sharpe et al., 1999; Clark et al., 2001). The complementary defects suggested that levels of expression of the *Lmbr1* gene play a key role in controlling the development of skeletal structures in the vertebrate limb.

The *Sasquatch* (*Ssq*) Mouse

The semidominant *Ssq* mouse mutation results in supernumerary-preaxial digits on the hindfeet in heterozygotes and additional preaxial digits on both forelimbs and hindlimbs, with occasional shortening and apparent twisting of the limbs, in homozygotes (Sharpe et al., 1999) (Figure 107–6). The limb abnormalities consistently correlated with the presence of the transgene in more than six generations of backcrosses to wild-type mice, suggesting that the phenotype resulted from an insertional mutation. The insertion site was found to be close to the *Shh* locus on mouse chromosome 5 (see later) (see Figure

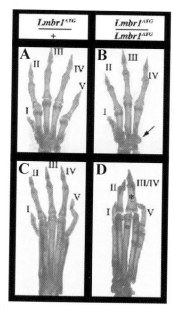

Figure 107–5. Limb phenotypes observed in mice with reduced *Lmbr1* function. Heteroygous (*A* and *C*) and homozygous (*B* and *D*) *Lmbr1* mutant mice. (*A* and *B*) Dorsal views of alizarin red–stained forefeet showing normal digit number and morphology in the heterozygote (*A*) and reduced digit number in the homozygote (*B*). *Arrow*, Apparent rudimentary fifth metacarpal. (*C* and *D*) Dorsal views of hindfeet showing normal morphology in the heterozygote (*C*) and reduced digit number resulting from syndactyly of digits III and IV to produce a single digit (asterisked) in the homozygote (*D*). (Modified from Clark et al., 2001.)

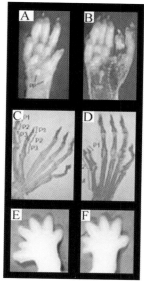

Figure 107–6. Limb phenotypes observed in mice expressing the *Sasquatch* mutation. The ventral surface of the adult hindfoot shows preaxial polydactyly in *Ssq/+* mouse (*B*) compared with wild-type (*A*). (*C* and *D*) Skeletal morphology of strong and weak, respectively, *Ssq/+* hindlimb digit phenotype. (*E* and *F*) Varying severity of polydactyly in 14.5-day *Ssq/+* embryos. (Modified from Sharpe et al. 1999.)

107–3). In adult heterozygous *Ssq* mutants, the forelimbs were normal; however, the anterior region of the hindlimbs displayed preaxial polydactyly and syndactyly. Occasionally, on a supernumerary digit, a second claw inverted along the dorsoventral axis was observed. The ventral metatarsal pads of the affected digit were replaced with fur typical of the dorsal skin. These changes to the foot demonstrated that the *Ssq* mutation disrupts both anteroposterior and dorsoventral patterning in the ectopic digits. More extensive abnormalities were observed in homozygous animals in the form of more severe hindlimb polydactyly and hemimelia (Sharpe et al., 1999).

Examination of molecular alterations in the limb bud demonstrated that the *Shh*, *Fgf4*, *Fgf8*, *Hoxd12*, and *Hoxd13* genes were all ectopically expressed in the anterior region. Analysis of expression patterns also demonstrated that expression of the transgene reporter had come under the control of a regulatory element that directs a pattern mirroring the endogenous expression of *Shh* in the limb. In abnormal limbs, expression of both *Shh* and the reporter was ectopically induced in the anterior region in contrast to the situation in normal limbs, where expression of *Shh* and the reporter was restricted to the zone of polarizing activity. This suggests that the Sasquatch phenotype is caused by interference with the *cis*-regulation of the *Shh* gene (see later).

Analysis of clones isolated from a genomic library made from *Ssq/Ssq* mice identified one that contained the junction of the transgene and the insertion site. Analysis of the insertion site showed that multiple copies of the transgene had incorporated into a predominantly repeat containing a region that lies within intron 5 of the *Lmbr1* gene (Lettice et al., 2002) (see Figure 107–3).

The *Shh* Knockout Mouse

Mice lacking *Shh* gene function, generated by targeted disruption of the *Shh* gene, demonstrated the critical role played by this gene in the patterning of vertebrate embryonic tissues, including the brain and spinal cord, the axial skeleton, and the limbs (Chiang et al., 1996, 2001). Detailed analysis of *Shh*$^{-/-}$ mutant limbs showed that each mutant embryo has four limbs with a recognizable humerus/femur displaying anteroposterior polarity, but that distal to the elbow/knee joints, zeugopod skeletal elements form but lack identifiable anteroposterior polarity (Figure 107–7). *Shh* appears, therefore, to specifically become necessary for normal limb development at or just distal to the stylopod/zeugopod junction (elbow/knee joints) during mouse limb development. The apical ectodermal ridge is induced in the *Shh*

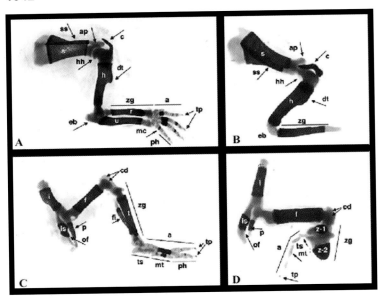

Figure 107–7. Limb phenotypes observed in mice lacking *Sonic hedgehog* gene function. Alizarin red/alcian blue–stained forelimbs (*A* and *B*) and hindlimbs (*C* and *D*) from wild-type (*A* and *C*) and *Shh*[−/−] (*B* and *D*) mice are shown at 17.5 days post coitum. Note that at the mutant elbow joint (eb), the humerus (h) is connected by solid cartilage to a single zeugopod element (zg) that is ossified along its length and ends in a cartilaginous extension. (Modified from Chiang et al., 2001.)

mutant buds with relatively normal morphology but is gradually disrupted over developmental time in parallel with a reduction in *Fgf8* expression in the ridge (Chiang et al., 1996, 2001).

MUTATIONAL MECHANISM

The elucidation of the molecular basis of acheiropodia led to a better understanding of the role of *Lmbr1* in the genetic regulation of development of the distal part of the limb. It appears that *Lmbr1* plays a pivotal role as displayed by the limb abnormalities resulting from its abnormal expression. Two categories of malformations have been identified in human and mouse: limb reduction defects as in acheiropodia and duplications, fusions, and aplasias of skeletal elements as in PPD, *Hx*, and *Ssq*. The acheiropodia phenotype appears to result from a loss-of-function mutation, whereas PPD, *Hx*, and *Ssq* appear to be the consequence of gain-of-function mutations of the same gene (Figure 107–8).

The loss-of-function nature of the common acheiropodia mutation is supported by the autosomal recessive mode of inheritance and the absence of discernible phenotypic effects in the heterozygotes. This

is further supported by the prediction of a stop codon in exon 6 of the human orthologue of *Lmbr1* leading to a null mutant. In contrast, all three antithetical phenotypes, PPD, Hx, and Ssq, are expressed in the heterozygous state and more severely as homozygotes. The latter supports a gain-of-function mechanism rather than haploinsufficiency. Interestingly, both the acheiropodia and the *Sasquatch* mutations point to the possible role of mutant *Lmbr1* in the misregulation of *sonic hedgehog*.

Shh is involved in the specification of the anteroposterior and proximodistal axes of the limb. The observed ectopic expression of *Shh* in the *Hx* mutant could be explained by *C7orf2/Lmbr1* acting as a regulator of *Shh*, either through direct interaction or mediated through other factors. The similarity of the limb phenotype in acheiropodia and the *Shh*[−/−] mouse offers additional evidence as to the role *Lmbr1* may be playing in regulating *Shh* expression.

Genetic analysis of *Sasquatch* shows that the mutation interrupts a long-range *cis*-acting regulatory element that acts on *Shh* 1 Mb away. Consequently, disruption of *Shh* regulation is a likely mechanism for PPD in humans. In addition, the acheiropodia mutation removes 4 to 6 kb of genomic DNA adjacent to the PPD translocation breakpoint and *Ssq* integration site. Thus, long-range disruption of the regulation of *Shh* expression may also be involved in the Acheiropodia phenotype.

REFERENCES

Chang DT, Lopez A, von Kessler DP, Chiang C, Simandl BK, Zhao R, Seldin MF, Fallon JF, Beachy PA (1994). Products, genetic linkage and limb patterning activity of a murine hedgehog gene. *Development* 120: 3339–53.

Chiang C, Litingtung Y, Harris MP, Simandl BK, Li Y, Beachy PA, Fallon JF (2001). Manifestation of the limb prepattern: limb development in the absence of sonic hedgehog function. *Dev Biol* 236: 421–435.

Chiang C, Litingtung Y, Lee E, Young KE, Corden JL, Westphal H, Beachy PA (1996). Cyclopia and defective axial patterning in mice lacking Sonic hedgehog gene function. *Nature* 383: 407–413.

Clark RM, Marker PC, Kingsley DM (2000). A novel candidate gene for mouse and human preaxial polydactyly with altered expression in limbs of hemimelic extra-toes mutant mice. *Genomics* 67: 19–27.

Clark RM, Marker PC, Roessler E, Dutra A, Schimenti JC, Muenke M, Kingsley DM (2001). Reciprocal mouse and human limb phenotypes caused by gain- and loss-of-function mutations affecting Lmbr1. *Genetics* 159: 715–726.

Dundar M, Gordon TM, Ozyazgan I, Oguzkaya F, Ozkul Y, Cooke A, Wilkinson AG, Holloway S, Goodman FR, Tolmie JL (2001). A novel acropectoral syndrome maps to chromosome 7q36. *J Med Genet* 38: 304–309.

Escamilla MA, DeMille MC, Benavides E, Roche E, Almasy L, Pittman S, Hauser J, Lew DF, Freimer B, Whittle MR (2000). A minimalist approach to gene mapping: locating the gene for a acheiropodia by homozygosity analysis. *Am J Hum Genet* 66: 1995–2000.

Fett-Conte AC, Richieri-Costa A (1990). Acheiropodia: report on four new Brazilian patients. *Am J Med Genet* 36: 341–344.

Freire-Maia A, Li WH, Maruyama T (1975a). Genetics of acheiropodia (the handless and footless families of Brazil) VII. Population dynamics. *Am J Hum Genet* 27: 665–675.

Freire-Maia A, Freire-Maia N, Morton NE, Azevedo ES, Quelce-Salgado A (1975b). Genetics of acheiropodia (the handless and footless families of Brazil). VI. Formal genetic analysis. *Am J Hum Genet* 27: 521–527.

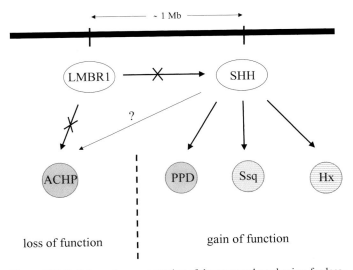

Figure 107–8. Schematic representation of the proposed mechanism for loss-of-function or gain-of-function *Lmbr1* mutations. The *Lmbr1* and *Shh* loci lie within 1 Mb of each other in both humans and mice, and no other genes have been identified in the region between them. Mouse and human mutations are depicted as solid or striped gray circles, respectively.

Green MC (1964). New mutation. *Mouse News Lett* 31: 27.

Grimaldi A, Masiero D, Richieri-Costa A, Freire-Maia A (1983). Variable expressivity of the acheiropodia gene. *Am J Med Genet* 16: 631–634.

Heus CH, Hing A, van Baren MJ, Joosse M, Breedveld GJ, Wang JC, Burgess A, et al. (1999). A physical and transcriptional map of the preaxial polydactyly locus on chromosome 7q36. *Genomics* 57: 342–351.

Heutink P, Zguricas J, van Oosterhout L, Breedveld GJ, Testers L, Sandkuijl LA, Snijders PJ, Weissenbach J, Lindhout D, Hovius SER, et al. (1994). The gene for triphalangeal thumb maps to the subtelomeric region of chromosome 7q. *Nat Genet* 6: 287–292.

Hing AV, Helms C, Slaugh R, Burgess A, Wang JC, Herman T, Dowton SB, Donis-Keller H (1995). Linkage of preaxial polydactyly type 2 to 7q36. *Am J Med Genet* 58: 128–135.

Horn D, Kolb GP (1994). Two isolated cases with symmetrically absent hands and feet. *Clin Dysmorphol* 3: 228–233.

Ianakiev P, Kilpatrick MW, Daly MJ, Zolindaki A, Bagley D, Beighton G, Beighton P, Tsipouras P (2000). Localization of an acromesomelic dysplasia on chromosome 9 by homozygosity mapping. *Clin Genet* 57: 278–283.

Ianakiev P, van Baren MJ, Daly MJ, Toledo SPA, Cavalcanti MG, Correa Neto J, Lemos Silveira E, Freire-Maia A, Heutink P, Kilpatrick MW, Tsipouras P (2001). Acheiropodia is caused by mutations in C7orf2 the human orthologue of the Lmbr1 gene. *Am J Hum Genet* 68: 38–45.

Knudsen TB, Kochhar DM (1981). The role of morphogenetic cell death during abnormal limb-bud outgrowth in mice heterozygous for the dominant mutation hemimelia-extra toe (Hmx). *J Embryol Exp Morphol Suppl* 65: 289–307.

Kruger LM, Kumar A (1994). Acheiropody: a report of two cases. *J Bone Joint Surg* 76A: 1557–1560.

Kruglyak L, Daly MJ, Lander ES (1995). Rapid multipoint linkage analysis of recessive traits in nuclear families including homozygosity mapping. *Am J Hum Genet* 56: 519–517.

Lemos Silveira E, Freire-Maia A (1998). Acheiropodia: new cases from Brazil. *Clin Genet* 54: 256–257.

Lettice LA, Horikoshi T, Heaney SJH, van Baren MJ, van der Linde HC, Breedveld GJ, Joosse M, Akarsu N, Oostra BA, Endo N, et al. (2002). Disruption of a long-range cis-acting regulator for Shh causes preaxial polydactyly. *Proc Natl Acad Sci USA* 99: 7548–7553.

Marcallo FA, Pilotto RF, Freire-Maia A (1979). Genetics of acheiropodia ('the handless and footless families of Brazil'): XI. pathologic aspects. *Am J Med Genet* 4: 287–291.

Marigo V, Roberts DJ, Lee SM, Tsukurov O, Levi T, Gastier JM, Epstein DJ, Gilbert DJ, Copeland NG, Seidman CE, et al. (1995). Cloning, expression, and chromosomal location of SHH and IHH: two human homologues of the *Drosophila* segment polarity gene hedgehog. *Genomics* 28: 44–51.

Masuya H, Sagai T, Wakana S, Moriwaki K, Shiroishi T (1995). A duplicated zone of polarizing activity in polydactylous mouse mutants. *Genes Dev* 9: 1645–1653.

Peacock W (1929). Hereditary absence of hands and feet. *Eugenical News* 14: 46–47.

Riddle RD, Johnson RL, Laufer E, Tabin C (1993). Sonic hedgehog mediates the polarizing activity of the ZPA. *Cell* 75: 1401–1416.

Sharpe J, Lettice L, Hecksher-Sorensen J, Fox M, Hill R, Krumlauf R (1999). Identification of sonic hedgehog as a candidate gene responsible for the polydactylous mouse mutant Sasquatch. *Curr Biol* 9: 97–100.

Sweet HO (1982). Hm and Hx are not alleles. *Mouse News Lett* 66: 66.

Temtamy S, McKusick V (1978). The genetics of hand malformations. *Birth Defects* 14: 3–128.

Toledo SP, Saldanha PH (1969). A radiological and genetical investigation of acheiropody in a kindred including six cases. *J Genet Hum* 17: 81–94.

Toledo SP, Saldanha PH (1972). Further data on acheiropody. *J Genet Hum* 20: 253–258.

Tsukurov O, Boehmer A, Flynn J, Nicolai JP, Hamel BC, Traill S, Zaleske D, Mankin HJ, Yeon H, Ho C, et al. (1994). A complex bilateral polysyndactyly disease locus maps to chromosome 7q36. *Nat Genet* 6: 282–286.

Zguricas J, Snijders PJLM, Hovius SER, Heutink P, Oostra BA, Lindhout D (1994). Phenotypic analysis of triphalangeal thumb and associated hand malformations. *J Med Genet* 31: 462–467.

Zguricas J, Heus H, Morales-Peralta E, Breedveld G, Kuyt B, Mumcu EF, Bakker W, Akarsu N, Kay SP, Hovius SE, et al. (1999). Clinical and genetic studies on 12 preaxial polydactyly families and refinement of the localisation of the gene responsible to a 1.9 cM region on chromosome 7q36. *J Med Genet* 36: 32–40.

VAL C. SHEFFIELD, ELISE HEON, EDWIN M. STONE, AND RIVKA CARMI

Bardet-Biedl syndrome (BBS) (OMIM 209900) is a genetically heterogeneous autosomal recessive disorder involving genes that map to six known loci. The disorder is characterized by a combination of clinical findings that include obesity, photoreceptor degeneration, polydactyly, hypogenitalism, renal abnormalities and developmental delay (Ammann, 1970; Alton and McDonald, 1973; Harnett et al., 1988; Green et al., 1989). Clinical characterization and the nomenclature describing this syndrome have evolved over time. In 1866, Laurence and Moon reported a syndrome consisting of mental retardation, retinal degeneration, hypogonadism, ataxia, and spastic paraplegia. Nearly six decades later, Bardet (1920) and Biedl (1922) independently described patients with the additional clinical features of polydactyly and obesity. Subsequently, Solis-Cohen and Weiss (1924) reported a single family that had features that overlapped those described by Laurence and Moon (1866), Bardet (1920), and Biedl (1922), suggesting the name *Laurence-Moon-Biedl syndrome*. The disorder was later referred to in the scientific and medical literature as *Laurence-Moon-Bardet-Biedl syndrome* (McLoughlin and Shanklin, 1967; Klein and Ammann, 1969). The Laurence-Moon-Bardet-Biedl syndrome has in general been viewed as two distinct clinical disorders. *Bardet-Biedl syndrome* is used to refer to patients and families that have the minimum findings of retinopathy, obesity, and polydactyly without spastic paraplegia. Patients affected with Laurence-Moon syndrome do not have polydactyly (Ammann, 1970). Although BBS is considered to be rare, it is the more common of the two syndromes. The incidence in the general population is often cited as being less than 1:100,000 (Klein and Ammann, 1969; Lofterod, et al., 1990; Croft et al., 1995; Beales et al., 1997). However, in some isolated populations, BBS has been reported to have a 10-fold higher incidence (Farag, 1989; Green, 1989). There has been considerable interest in the identification of genes that cause BBS due to the pleiotropic nature of the disorder, as well as the fact that components of the phenotype are common (i.e., obesity, diabetes, and hypertension). It is hypothesized that genes involved in BBS may provide clues to the identification of biochemical and developmental pathways involved in these more common disorders, as well as to provide additional understanding of normal developmental processes.

BBS is genetically heterogeneous with six known disease-causing loci. The genes at four of these loci have been identified (Kwitek-Black et al., 1993; Leppert et al., 1994; Sheffield et al., 1994; Carmi et al., 1995; Young et al., 1999; Katsanis et al., 2000; Slavotinek et al., 2000b; Woods et al., 2000; Mykytyn et al., 2001, 2002; Nishimura et al., 2001). One of these genes, *MKKS* (also referred to as *BBS6*), was identified based on the fact that abnormal variants of this gene cause McKusick-Kaufman syndrome (MKS), a disorder characterized by hydrometrocolpos, polydactyly, and congenital heart defects (Robinow and Shaw, 1979; Stone et al., 1998, 2000). The MKKS protein has sequence similarity to the chaperonin family of proteins (see Chapter 83). Clearly, the identification of MKKS as a putative chaperonin was the first molecular clue to the understanding of the pathophysiology of BBS. It was hypothesized that the identification of the first BBS gene would facilitate the identification of other BBS genes, as well as genes involved in BBS-associated phenotypes and developmental anomalies. Based on the observation that MKKS has chaperonin homology, other BBS genes might be expected to code for proteins that collaborate with MKKS in the formation of a multimeric chaperonin complex or code for proteins that are substrates of the MKKS protein.

Three other BBS genes—*BBS1*, *BBS2*, and *BBS4*—have been identified using positional cloning methods (Mykytyn et al., 2001, 2002; Nishimura et al., 2001). The predicted BBS1 and BBS2 proteins have no sequence homology to other known proteins that provide clues to their function, although they do show limited homology to each other (Nishimura et al., 2000; Mykytyn et al., 2002). The predicted BBS4 protein shows weak homology to *O*-linked *N*-acetylglucosamine (O-GlcNAc) transferase (OGT) from several species (Mykytyn et al., 2001). However, the sequence similarity between BBS4 and OGT is of unclear significance and biochemical data supporting this role for BBS4 has not yet been generated. Therefore, BBS1, BBS2 and BBS4 are classified as proteins with unknown functions.

CLINICAL OVERVIEW OF BBS

BBS is recognized to have the primary or cardinal features of obesity, photoreceptor degeneration, polydactyly, hypogenitalism, renal abnormalities, and developmental delay (Figure 108–1). Secondary features of BBS include diabetes, hypertension, and congenital heart defects (Green et al., 1989; Elbedour et al., 1994). The detailed clinical features of the BBS phenotype are discussed here.

Ophthalmologic Findings

BBS is associated with a severe form of retinitis pigmentosa in which a decrease in visual function is observed early in childhood and relentlessly progresses to legal blindness because of severe central and peripheral visual loss (Figure 108–2). Retinal disease is reported to occur in 100% of patients with BBS. Legal blindness has been reported to affect 73% of affected individuals by the second and third decade of life (Riise et al., 1987; Leys et al., 1988; Green et al., 1989; Jacobson et al., 1990; Fulton et al., 1993). Loss of light perception in adulthood had been observed on several occasions. Although the retinal degeneration varies both among families and within families, there are few patients who retain useful vision until later in life. Nystagmus is usually not seen, and the pupillary response is usually normal until later in the disease, when it can become sluggish.

Electroretinographic responses are abnormal in all affected individuals (Jacobson et al., 1990) and often become nonrecordable in the first decade of life. The rod-cone dystrophy, detected with electroretinography, is a major feature of the disease (Jacobson et al., 1990). However, the ratio of rod-cone involvement to severity of electroretinographic changes varies, and cases with recordable rod-cone responses can occur even later in life (personal communication, Dr. Carol Westall). The photoreceptor abnormality first manifests as night-blindness in early childhood and progresses in parallel to the central and peripheral vision loss occurs in the first decade of life.

The fundus changes observed are variable (see Figure 108–2). Often, especially early in life, the retinopathy is *sine pigmento*. The fundus changes observed can include surface retinal wrinkling or mild bone spicule-like pigmentation later in life. Retinopathy can be detected as early as age 5 years, when mild peripapillary atrophy, equatorial mottling of the retinal pigment epithelium, and mild patchy changes at the level of the internal limiting membrane can be observed. The retinal atrophy progresses slowly with age, with macular atrophic changes that are often seen in the adults. The retinal dystrophy is often associated with surface retinal wrinkling, which can be detected quite early. In some cases, choroidosclerosis-type changes are ob-

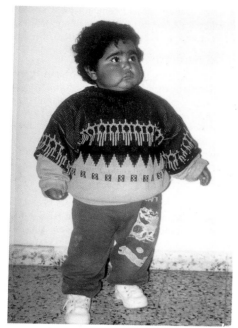

Figure 108–1. A young girl with Bardet-Biedl syndrome.

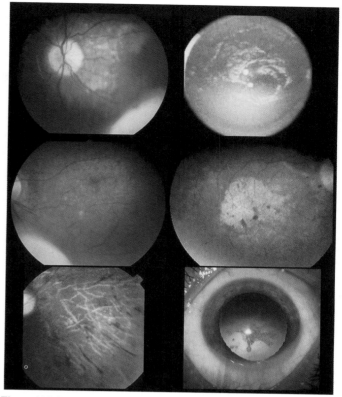

Figure 108–2. (*Top left*) Fundus photograph of a 5-year-old boy with early peripapillary atrophy and optic nerve pallor. (*Top right*) Fundus photograph of a 5-year-old boy with early surface retinal wrinkling. Second row, left, fundus photograph showing more prominent surface retinal wrinkling in the region of the macula in a 14-year-old patient. Second row, right, fundus photograph of a 30-year-old man with atrophic macular changes. (*Bottom left*) Fundus photograph showing bone spiculing and mottling of the retinal pigmented epithelium in a 55-year-old patient. (*Bottom right*) Photograph of the anterior segment showing a typical posterior subcapsular cataract in a 37-year-old patient.

served. The narrowing of vessels can be appreciated as early as the first decade and is progressive. The optic nerve inevitably becomes pale as the disease progresses.

Significant refractive errors (range −17 to +4.0 diopters) have been observed and should be looked for to optimize visual development. As seen in other forms of retinitis pigmentosa, cataracts can manifest early and typically involve the posterior subcapsular area. This central opacity can lead to significant visual impairment when the visual fields are constricted.

Obesity

Birth weight in patients with BBS has been reported to be within normal limits. The obesity in BBS patients begins in infancy and is often severe but can be quite variable. The incidence of obesity is generally reported to be high and to increase with age (Green et al., 1989; Beales et al., 1997). However, the incidence of obesity in BBS patients may be somewhat overestimated, especially in studies using singleton cases due to ascertainment bias. Nevertheless, obesity is common in BBS patients. For example, in a study of three large Bedouin BBS kindreds, 16 of 28 (57%) patients had a weight greater or equal to the 97th percentile. Seven of 10 (70%) patients older than 15 years in these kindreds had a body mass index (BMI) of 30 kg/m^2 or greater (Carmi et al., 1995a). Some patients are extremely obese, with BMIs in the morbid obesity range (>40 kg/m^2) (Klein et al., 1969; Carmi et al., 1995a).

The cause of the obesity has not been determined. Hyperphagia is not present to the degree that it is seen in patients with Prader-Willi syndrome, although parents report hyperphagia to be a problem in childhood (Beales et al., 1997). Obesity in BBS patients is likely to result from a combination of increased caloric intake and decreased use of calories. Dietary control of caloric intake can be beneficial in weight control.

Linear growth has been reported to be normal in childhood, but adult height generally is diminished (Green et al., 1989).

Skeletal Findings

The most common skeletal abnormality found in BBS patients is postaxial polydactyly (Figure 108–3). In addition, patients may have other digit anomalies such as brachydactyly, clinodactyly, and/or syndactyly. Polydactyly may be found on all four extremities, or it may be limited to a single limb (Carmi et al., 1995a). Extra digits may be well developed or rudimentary. Although polydactyly is not a uni-

versal finding in all patients with BBS, the incidence is extremely high, ranging from 93% to 98% (Green et al., 1989). In a study of three large Bedouin kindreds, 27 of 28 (96%) patients had polydactyly of at least one extremity (Carmi et al., 1995a). Affected members of the Bedouin kindred mapping to chromosome 3 (BBS3) generally had polydactyly on all four extremities, whereas patients with BBS2 or BBS4 often had polydactyly limited to a single extremity. The variability in the digit anomalies observed is likely to be genetically determined. Ten patients of the Bedouin BBS4 kindred were found to have dysgenesis of various epiphyses, including vertebrae, proximal

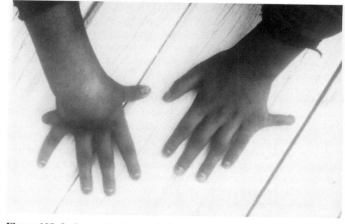

Figure 108–3. Postaxial polydactyly in a patient with Bardet-Biedl syndrome.

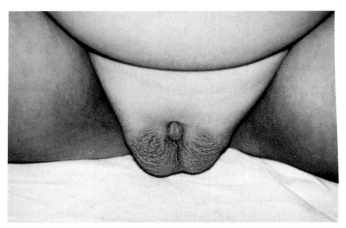

Figure 108–4. The genitalia of a male patient with Bardet-Biedl syndrome, showing a micropenis.

femur, proximal tibia, capitellum, tarsal navicular, and distal epiphysis of the first metatarsal (Moses et al., 1998).

Urogenital and Renal Anomalies

Hypogenitalism was first reported to be part of the syndrome by Biedl in 1922, and renal abnormalities are recognized to be a major component of the syndrome. Harnett et al. (1988) and Green et al. (1989) reported a wide variation in renal involvement including structural abnormalies in 95% of patients. Eighteen percent of patients who were evaluated had a partial defect in the ability to concentrate urine. A small percentage of patients develop chronic renal failure and end-stage renal disease, which contribute to the observed shorten life expectancy in 50% of patients with BBS (O'dea et al., 1996; Riise, 1996).

Most male patients have small testes and micropenises (Green et al., 1989) (Figure 108–4). Genital abnormalities in females include vaginal atresia, ovarian cysts, hypoplastic ovaries, hypoplastic uterus, and hydrometrocolpos (Klein and Ammann, 1969; Stoler et al., 1995). Hypogonadism has been documented based on endocrine studies in some patients. Fertility has been reported in both male and female patients, although fertility is decreased, particularly in males (Klein and Ammann, 1969; Green et al., 1989, O'dea et al., 1996).

Molecular studies have shown that the phenotypic overlap between BBS and MKS is due to some cases of BBS being caused by mutations in the *MKKS* gene, the gene that causes MKS. Typically, MKS is diagnosed in infancy based on the presence of polydactyly and, in females, vaginal abnormalities. The diagnosis of BBS is usually delayed until the appearance of the pigmented retinopathy or the abnormal weight gain. Clinicians have begun to recognize the association of vaginal atresia with BBS (Mehrota et al., 1997; David et al., 1999; Oguzkurt et al., 1999; Slavotinek et al., 2000b). David et al. (1999) reported nine patients who were initially diagnosed with MKS because of vaginal atresia and postaxial polydactyly. These patients later developed obesity and retinal dystrophy, resulting in the diagnosis of BBS. Oguzkurt et al. (1999) reported two cases of teenage girls with vaginal atresia and the classic features of BBS. These authors concluded that BBS should be considered in the differential diagnosis of any girl with vaginal atresia.

Central Nervous System Findings

Historically, mental retardation is reported to be a major component of BBS syndrome (Bell, 1958; Klein and Ammann, 1969). However, the degree of mental retardation may have been overestimated due to the difficulty in assessing mental function in some patients with visual impairment. It is now recognized that severe mental retardation is rare in this disorder. Green et al. (1989) reported that 41% of patients were considered to be mentally retarded. However, learning disabilities and developmental delay are common in patients with BBS (Beales et al., 1997). Many patients are able to remain in mainstream education when appropriate support for visual impairment is provided. Speech delay in early development is common, and behavior problems and emotional instability in children also occur. Structural abnormalities of the brain and seizures do not appear to be components of BBS.

Other Clinical Findings

Up to 45% of patients have been reported to have diabetes mellitus of the insulin-resistant form (type II diabetes) (Escallon et al., 1989; Green et al., 1989; O'dea et al., 1996). Hypertension is reported to occur in up to 60% of adult patients (O'dea et al., 1996). The hypertension can be associated with chronic renal failure, although in other cases the hypertension is unexplained by the renal disease. Croft and Swift (1990) have observed obesity, hypertension, diabetes mellitus, and renal disease in first-degree and other relatives of patients with BBS, raising the possibility that BBS heterozygotes are predisposed to these disorders.

A wide variety of cardiac abnormalities have been reported to occur in BBS patients. In a study of 22 Bedouin BBS patients who underwent echocardiographic testing, 50% had a cardiac abnormality. A wide range of defects, including congenital and acquired abnormalities, were reported. No specific consistent malformations were observed (Elbedour et al., 1994). In addition, myocardial infarction was a prominent cause of death (Riise, 1996). In a study of the cause of death in patients with BBS, it was reported that death occurred at a significantly younger age than in the general population.

DIAGNOSIS

Because variable expressivity is common in patients with BBS (Warkany et al., 1937), establishment of the diagnosis generally requires the presence of four of the cardinal symptoms (obesity, photoreceptor degeneration, polydactyly, hypogenitalism, renal abnormalities and developmental delay) (Churchill et al., 1981; Schachat and Maumenee, 1982; Green et al., 1989). Most authors consider retinopathy a requirement for diagnosis, although this may not be present in a young patient. An abnormal electroretinogram precedes visible retinal anomalies and can be helpful in establishing the diagnosis in early childhood (Marmor, 1979; Jacobson et al., 1990). Renal ultrasonography may also aid in the establishment of the diagnosis. Diagnosis in the presence of a family history can be established with fewer than four cardinal symptoms. In the absence of a family history, one must be cautious in making the diagnosis based on retinopathy and obesity alone. In some familial cases, linkage studies may be helpful. Mutation screening of the *BBS1*, *BBS2*, *BBS4*, and *MKKS* genes is useful in some cases for establishing the diagnosis. The identification of the *BBS1* gene and a common *BBS1* mutation will facilitate molecular diagnosis (Mykytyn et al., 2002).

Prenatal diagnosis has been accomplished using fetal ultrasonography to look for limb and renal anomalies (Farag and Teebi, 1988; Riise, 1996). In addition, prenatal diagnosis has been performed using linkage analyis (R. Carmi and V. C. Sheffield, unpublished observations).

GENETIC HETEROGENEITY OF BBS

It is important to recognize the extent of the genetic heterogeneity of BBS. What was once thought to be a single locus autosomal recessive disorder has turned out to be a genetically heterogeneous disease caused by multiple individual loci (Kwitek-Black et al., 1993; Leppert et al., 1994; Sheffield et al., 1994; Carmi et al., 1995; Young et al., 1999; Woods et al., 2000). Furthermore, there has been the suggestion that some cases of BBS result from the interaction of two or more loci (Beales et al., 2001; Katsanis et al., 2001, 2002). Genetic heterogeneity of BBS was first shown by studying isolated Bedouin populations in the Negev region of Israel. The high rate of consanguinity in these populations results in an increase in the frequency of recessive genetic disorders (Carmi et al., 1998). Three tribes with BBS were identified among the Bedouin Arabs of Israel. In each tribe, the disorder was shown to be linked to a different region of the human genome: *BBS2*, *BBS3*, and *BBS4* (Kwitek-Black et al., 1993; Sheffield et al., 1994; Carmi et al., 1995).

Six BBS loci have been identified on chromosomes 11q13 (*BBS1*) (Leppert et al., 1994), 16q21 (*BBS2*) (Kwitek-Black et al., 1993), 3p (*BBS3*) (Sheffield et al., 1994), 15q22.3-q23 (*BBS4*) (Carmi et al., 1995), 2q31 (*BBS5*) (Young et al., 1999), and 20p12 (*BBS6; MKKS*) (Katsanis et al., 2000; Slavotanik et al., 2000b; Woods et al., 2000). A seventh locus is hypothesized to exist based on the existence of a small proportion of families that do not map to any of the known loci (Beales et al., 2001). In addition, a pericentric inversion of chromosome 1 (p36.3;q23) has been reported to be associated with the BBS phenotype in multiple members of a single extended family (Tayel et al., 1999).

Several linkage studies indicate that *BBS1* is the most common causative locus (Leppert et al., 1994: Bruford et al., 1997; Katsanis et al., 1999; Beales et al., 1999, 2001), and this finding was confirmed through mutation analysis of the *BBS1* gene (Mykytyn et al., 2002; 2003). The majority of BBS1 cases are caused by a single missense mutation (M390R). *BBS2* is the next most common locus (Bruford et al., 1997; Beales et al., 1999). Mutations in the *BBS4* and *MKKS (BBS6)* genes are each thought to cause fewer than 5% of cases (Beales et al., 2001; Katsanis et al., 2002). *BBS3* and *BBS5* appear to be the rarest known loci associated with the disorder. *BBS3* and *BBS5* were each initially mapped by using individual large inbred kindreds (Sheffield et al., 1994; Young et al., 1999). Two additional families have been shown to map to the BBS3 locus, confirming the existence of this locus (Beales et al., 1999; Ghadami et al., 2000).

The extensive locus heterogeneity and the fact that not all families map to the known loci raise the possibility that some cases of BBS may be associated with mutations at two or more loci. Katsanis et al. (2001, 2002) suggested triallelic inheritance of BBS. This hypothesis is based on the identification of two BBS mutations at one locus and one BBS variant at a second locus. The hypothesis that one BBS locus might act in conjunction with or modify a second BBS locus is intriguing but needs further investigation. Mykytyn et al. (2002) found no evidence of involvement of the most common BBS mutation (*BBS1* M390R) in triallelic inheritance.

MOLECULAR CHARACTERIZATION OF BBS

BBS is characterized by allelic and nonallelic genetic heterogeneity. The mutations identified in the four known *BBS* genes are summarized in Table 108–1. No clear genotype–phenotype correlations have been established, with the exception of the compound His84Tyr and Ala242Ser *MKKS* allele that is found in the homozygous state in the Amish population. This compound allele causes MKS without obesity and retinal degeneration, rather than BBS. The His84Tyr/Ala242Ser allele has been reported to show incomplete penetrance (Stone et al., 2000). Intrafamilial variation in BBS has been established and is thought to be as great as interfamilial variation, which would suggest that factors other than the primary mutation influence the phenotype in patients with BBS. It should be noted that studies have not yet focused on defining locus-specific phenotypic features of BBS.

The *BBS1* gene was identified based on the finding of a common missense mutation in BBS probands, as well as termination, splice site, and frameshift mutations in BBS1 families. The M390R mutation was found in the homozygous state in 15 of 60 BBS probands and in the heterozygous state in 7 of the same 60 probands (Mykytyn et al., 2002).

Ten homozygous mutations have been identified in *BBS2* with some variability in the associated phenotype. One homozygous missense mutation (Val75Gly) found in the *BBS2* gene may result in a leaner phenotype based on data from a large Bedouin family (Nishimura et al., 2001). Several heterozygous sequence variants have been identified, including two variants that have been suggested to contribute to disease when found in combination with mutations in the *MKKS* gene (Katsanis et al., 2001).

Six homozygous *BBS4* mutations have been identified in BBS families. The Arg259Pro *BBS4* mutation found in the Bedouin population may result in early-onset profound obesity (Mykytyn et al., 2001).

Table 108–1. Reported Disease-Associated Variants in Known BBS Genes

MKKS
Y37C homozygote
Y37C/2111delGG (reported to cause McKussick-Kaufman syndrome)
H84Y;A242S homozygote (reported to cause McKussick-Kaufman syndrome)
A242S heterozygote**
Y26rter/G52D
1167delT homozygote
1167delT/L277P
1316delC;1324-1326delGTA homozygote
1316delC;1324-1326delGTA/1167delT
T57A heterozygote
Q147ter heterozygote†
C499S heterozygote†
T57A
I32M
S235P
D285A
R518H
S511A
BBS1
M390R homozygote
E549X homozygote
M390R/E549X compound heterozygote
C,432+1G → A heterozygote
Y284fsX288 homozygote
BBS2
940delA homozygote
V75G homozygote
R272ter homozygote
R275ter homozygote
D170fsX171 homozygote
1206insA homozygote
Y24ter homozygote*
Y24ter/Q59ter*
R315W homozygote
R315Q homozygote
C210fsX246 homozygote
D104A/R634P
V158fsX200 heterozygote
N70S heterozygote†
L168FS/R216ter*
T560I homozygote‡
IVS1-1G → C heterozygote
IVS4+1G → C heterozygote
BBS4
R294P homozygote
EX3-4 DEL homozygote
c.220+1G → C homozygote
c.406-2A → C homozygote
c.585-586insTG heterozygote
IVS3-2A → G homozygote
A364E homozygote‡
L327P heterozygote
N165H heterozygote
S457I heterozygote

BBS, Bardet-Biedl syndrome; MKKS, McKussick-Kaufman syndrome.
Note: 1316delC;1324-1226delGTA is also known as 429delCT;433delAG, and 1167delT is also known as 280delT.
*Found in the presence of a third mutant allele
†Reported to be the third mutant allele found in an individual with two mutations in another BBS gene.
‡Reported to be involved in tetra-allelic inheritance.

MANAGEMENT AND GENETIC COUNSELING

There is no specific treatment for patients with BBS, although evaluation and management of the individual symptoms are important. It is important to manage the obesity through dietary methods because successful dietary management of BBS has been documented. Patients should receive an initial renal ultrasound to look for congenital renal anomalies and an echocardiogram to evaluate the patient for congenital heart defects. Evaluation of female BBS patients for vaginal atresia and other genital anomalies is important due to life-threatening complications that result from this anomaly if left untreated. Refraction of children with BBS is warranted because refractive errors are frequently observed and can range from hyperopia to high myopia. These patients should be assessed early and continuously to prevent ametropic amblyopia and unnecessary visual sensory deprivation. An audiologic examination should also be performed to evaluate patients for hearing loss.

Specifically, we recommend a yearly evaluation of patients with BBS that should include at a minimum blood pressure measurement, renal function studies, serum electrolytes, serum glucose, serum cholesterol, ophthalmologic examination, and dietary counseling.

Unaffected parents with a child with BBS are at 25% risk of having another BBS child in subsequent pregnancies. Despite reports suggesting triallelic inheritance of BBS (Katsanis et al., 2001, 2002), the data do not warrant anything other than autosomal recessive genetic counseling (Mykytyn et al., 2002). Due to the genetic heterogeneity of the disorder, prenatal diagnosis can be offered only in cases of well-established linkage within larger families or for specific known mutations within smaller families.

ANIMAL MODELS

No animal models of BBS, either naturally occurring or generated using transgenetic or homologous recombination technologies, have been reported. However, Cox et al. (2000) used positional cloning to identify the gene responsible for the mouse mutant, fidget. Fidget mice have a characteristic head shaking and circling behavior due to reduced or absent semicircular canals. They also have features partially overlapping the BBS phenotype consisting of small eyes, due to insufficient growth of the retina, and polydactyly. The fidgetin gene (*Fign*) encodes a member of the subfamily-7 (SF7) group of ATPases associated with diverse cellular activities (AAA proteins) (Patel and Latterich, 1998). Of interest, the human *FIGN* gene maps within or near the *BBS5* locus on chromosome 2. Mutations within this gene causing BBS have not been reported.

DEVELOPMENTAL PATHOGENESIS

Little is known about the developmental pathogenesis of BBS despite the fact that four genes have been identified. The four known genes show very similar spatial and temporal pattern of expression. All are expressed early in development and continue to be widely expressed in adult tissues (Stone et al., 2000; Nishimura et al., 2001; Mykytyn et al., 2001, 2002). As previously mentioned, one of these genes, *MKKS*, is predicted to code for a protein that has sequence similarity to the chaperonin family of proteins. Molecular chaperones are proteins that participate in the folding or assembly of nascent proteins into a higher order structure. MKKS has the highest sequence homology to the α subunit of the *Thermoplasma acidophilum* thermosome (Stone et al., 2000), a prokaryotic chaperonin complex with structural similarity to an eukaryotic chaperonin called tailess complex polypeptide ring complex, a hetero-oligomeric chaperonin involved in the folding of many proteins, including tubulin and actin (Frydman et al., 1992). Based on sequence homology, BBS1, BBS2, and BBS4 do not appear to play a chaperonin role, suggesting that these proteins may require MKKS for proper folding and function. Other clues to the function of BBS1, BBS2, and BBS4 are limited. The predicted BBS1 and BBS2 proteins have no sequence homology to other known proteins that provide clues to their function (Nishimura et al., 2001). The BBS4 protein sequence shows strongest homology to OGT from several species, including archaebacteria and plants (Mykytyn et al., 2001). The plant OGT, known as SPINDLY, has been shown to be a signal transduction protein that is involved in a variety of developmental processes in *Arabidopsis*. It remains to be seen whether the multiple BBS genes will prove to code for proteins that are a part of a multisubunit complex or whether BBS proteins do not directly interact with each other but are part of a common biochemical and developmental pathway.

REFERENCES

Alton DJ, McDonald P (1973). Urographic findings in Laurence-Moon-Biedl syndrome. *Radiology* 109: 659–663.

Ammann F. Investigations cliniques et genetiques sur le syndrome de Bardet-Biedl en Suisse. *J Genet Hum* 18(suppl): 1–310.

Bardet G (1920). *Sur un Syndrome d'Obesite Infantile avec Polydactylie et Retinite Pigmentaire (Contribution a l'Etude des Formes Cliniques de l'Obesite Hypophysaire).* Thesis, Paris, Note, no. 479.

Beales PL, Warner AM, Hitman GA, Thakker R, Flinter FA (1997). Bardet-Biedl syndrome: a molecular and phenotypic study of 18 families. *J Med Genet* 34: 92–98.

Beales PL, Elcioglu, N, Woolf, AS, Parker, D, Flinter, FA (1999). New criteria for improved diagnosis of Bardet-Biedl syndrome: results of a population survey. *J Med Genet* 36: 437–446.

Beales PL, Katsanis N, Lewis RA, Ansley SJ, Elcioglu N, Raza J, Woods MO, Green JS, Parfrey PS, Davidson WS, et al. (2001). Genetic and mutational analyses of a large multiethnic Bardet-Biedl cohort reveal a minor involvement of BBS6 and delineate the critical intervals of other loci. *Am J Hum Genet* 68: 606–616.

Biedl A (1922). Ein Geschwisterpaar mit adiposo-genitaler Dystrophie. *Dtsch Med Wschr* 48: 1630.

Bell J (1958). The Laurence-Moon syndrome. In: *Treasury of Human Inheritance.* Cambridge University Press London, 5: 51–96.

Bruford EA, Riise R, Teague PW, Porter K, Thomson KL, Moore AT, Jay M, Warburg M, Schinzel A, Tommerup N, et al. (1997). Linkage mapping in 29 Bardet-Biedl syndrome families confirms loci in chromosomal regions 11q13, 15q22.3-q23, and 16q21. *Genomics* 41: 93–99.

Carmi R, Rokhlina T, Kwitek-Black AE, Elbedour K, Nishimura D, Stone EM, Sheffield VC (1995). Use of a DNA pooling strategy to identify a human obesity syndrome locus on chromosome 15. *Mol Genet* 4: 9–13.

Carmi R, Elbedour K, Stone EM, Sheffield VC (1995a). Phenotypic differences among patients with Bardet-Biedl syndrome linked to three different chromosome loci. *Am J Med Genet* 59: 199–203.

Carmi R, Elbedour K, Wietzman D, Sheffield V, Shoham-Vardi I (1998). Lowering the burden of hereditary diseases in a traditional, inbred community: Ethical aspects of genetic research and its application. *Sci Context* 11: 391–394.

Churchill DN, McMannamon P, Hurley RM (1981). Renal disease: a sixth cardinal feature of the Laurence-Moon-Biedl syndrome. *Clin Nephrol* 16: 151–154.

Cox GA, Mahaffey CL, Nystuen A, Letts VA, Frankel WN (2000). The mouse fidgetin gene defines a new role for AAA family proteins in mammalian development. *Nat Genet* 26: 198–202.

Croft JB, Swift M (1990). Obesity, hypertension, and renal disease in relatives of Bardet-Biedl syndrome sibs. *Am J Med Genet* 36: 37–42.

Croft JB, Morrell D, Chase CL, Swift M (1995). Obesity in heterozygous carriers of the gene for the Bardet-Biedl syndrome. *Am J Med Genet* 55: 12–15.

David A, Bitoun P, Lacombe D, Lambert J-C, Nivelson A, Nigneron J, Verloes A (1999). Hydrometrocolpos and polydactyly: a common neonatal presenation of Bardet-Biedl and McKusick-Kaufman syndromes. *J Med Genet* 36: 599–603.

Elbedour K, Kucker N, Zalstein E, Barki Y, Carmi R (1994). Cardiac abnormalities in the Bardet-Biedl syndrome: echocardiographic studies of 22 patients. *Am J Med Genet* 52: 164–169.

Escallon F, Traboulsi EI Infante R (1989). A family with the Bardet-Biedl syndrome and diabetes mellitus. *Arch Ophthalmol* 107: 855–857.

Farag TI, Teebi AS (1988). Bardet-Biedl and Laurence-Moon syndromes in a mixed Arab population. *Clin Genet* 33: 78–82.

Farag TI, Teebi AS (1989). High incidence of Bardet-Biedl syndrome among the Bedouin (Letter) *Clin Genet* 36: 463–465.

Frydman J, Nimmesgern E, Erdjument-Bromage H, Wall JS, Tempst P, Hartl FU (1992). Function in protein folding of TriC, a cytosolic ring complex containing TCP-1 and structurally related subunits. *EMBO J* 11(13): 4767–78.

Fulton AB, Hansen RM, Glynn RJ (1993). Natural course of visual functions in the Bardet-Biedl syndrome. *Arch Opthalmol* 111: 1500–1506.

Green JS, Parfrey PS, Harnett JD, Faried NR, Cramer BC, Johnson G, Health O, McManamon PJ, O'Leary E, Pryse-Phillips W (1989). The cardinal manifestations at Bardet-Biedl syndrome, a form of Laurence-Moon-Biedl syndrome. *New Eng J Med* 321: 1002–1009.

Ghadami M, Tomita H-A, Najafi M-T, Damavandi E, Farahvash M-S, Yamada K, Majidzadeh-AK, Niikawa N (2000). Bardet-Biedl syndrome type 3 in an Iranian family: clinical study and confirmation of disease localization. *Amer J Med Genet* 94: 433–437.

Harnett JD, Green JS, Cramer BC, Johnson G, Chafe L, McManamon P, Farid NR, Pryse-Phillips W, Parfrey PS (1988). The spectrum of renal disease in Laurence-Moon-Biedl syndrome. *N Engl J Med* 319: 615–618.

Jacobson SG, Borruat FX, Apathy PP (1990). Patterns of rod and cone dysfunction in Bardet-Biedl syndrome. *Am J Ophthalmol* 109: 676–88.

Katsanis N, Lewis RA, Stockton DW, Mai PMT, Baird L, Beales PL, Leppert M, Lupski JR (1999). Delineation of the critical interval of Bardet-Biedl syndrome 1 (BBS1) to a small region of 11q13, through linkage and haplotype analysis of 91 pedigrees. *Am J Hum Genet* 65: 1672–1679.

Katsanis N, Beales PL, Woods MO, Lewis RA, Green JS, Parfrey PS, Ansley SJ, Davidson WS, Lupski JR (2000). Mutations in *MKKS* cause obesity, retinal dystrophy and renal malformations associated with Bardet-Biedl syndrome. *Nat Genet* 26: 67–70.

Katsanis N, Ansley SJ, Badano JL, Eichers ER, Lewis RA, Hoskins BE, Scambler PJ, Davidson WS, Beales PL, Lupski JR (2001). Triallelic inheritance in Bardet-Biedl syndrome, a mendelian recessive disorder. *Science* 293: 2256–2261.

Katsanis N, Eichers ER, Ansley SJ, Lewis RA, Kayserili H, Hoskins BE, Scambler PJ, Beales PL, and Lupski JR (2002). *BBS4* is a minor contributor to Bardet-Biedl syndrome and may also participate in triallelic inheritance. *Am J Hum Genet* 71: 22–29.

Klein D, Amman F (1969). The syndrome of Laurence-Moon-Bardet-Biedl and allied disease in Switzerland. Clinical, Genetic and epidemiological studies. *J Neurol Sci* 9: 479–513.

Kwitek-Black AE, Carmi R, Duyk GM, Buetow KH, Elbedour K, Parvari R, Yandava CN, Stone EM, Sheffield VC (1993). Linkage of Bardet-Biedl syndrome to chromosome 16q and evidence for non-allelic genetic heterogeneity. *Nat Genet* 5: 392–396.

Laurence JZ, Moon RC (1866). Four cases of retinitis pigmentosa occurring in the same family and accompanied by general imperfection of development. *Ophthal Rev* 2: 32–41.

Leppert M, Baird L, Anderson KL, Otterud B, Lupski JR, Lewis RA (1994). Bardet-Biedl syndrome is linked to DNA markers on chromosome 11q and is genetically heterogeneous. *Nat Genet* 7: 108–112.

Leys MJ, Schreiner LA, Hansen RM, Mayer DL, Fulton AB (1988). Visual acuities and dark-adapted thresholds of children with Bardet-Biedl syndrome. *Am J Ophthalmol* 106: 561–569.

Lofterod B, Riise R, Skuseth T, Storhaug K (1990). Laurence-Moon-Bardet-Biedl syndrome. *Nord Med* 105: 146–148.

Marmor MF (1979). The electroretinogram in retinitis pigmentosa. *Arch Ophthalmol* 97: 1300–1304.

McLoughlin TG, Shanklin DR (1967). Pathology of Laurence-Moon-Bardet-Biedl syndrome. *J Pathol Bacteriol* 93: 65–79.

Mehrota N, Taub S, Covert RF (1997). Hydrometrocolpos as a neonatal manifestation of the Bardet-Beidl syndrome. (Letter) *Am J Med Genet* 69: 220.

Moses G, Howard C, Bar-Ziv J, Dekel S, Nyska M (1998). Epiphyseal dysgenesis in Laurence-Monn-Biedl-Bardet syndrome. *J Pediatr Orthop B* 7: 193–198.

Mykytyn K, Braun T, Carmi R, Haider NB, Searby CC, Shastri M, Beck G, Wright AF, Iannaccone A, Elbedour K, et al. (2001). Identification of a gene that, when mutated, causes the human obesity syndrome BBS4. *Nat Genet* 28: 188–191.

Mykytyn K, Nishimura DY, Searby CC, Shastri M, Yen H-J, Beck JS, Braun T, Streb LM, Cornier AS, Cox GF, et al. (2002). Identification of the gene most commonly involved in Bardet-Biedl syndrome (BBS1), a complex human obesity syndrome. *Nat Genet* 31: 435–438.

Nishimura DY, Searby CC, Carmi R, Elbedour K, Van Maldergem L, Fulton AB, Lam BL, Powell BR, Swiderski RE, Bugge KE, et al. (2001). Positional cloning of a novel gene on chromosome 16q causing Bardet Biedl syndrome (BBS2). *Hum Mol Genet* 10: 864–874.

O'dea D, Parfrey PS, Harnett JD, Heffeton D, Cramer BC, Green J (1996). The importance of renal impairment in the natural history of Bardet-Biedl syndrome. *Am J Kidney Dis* 27: 776–783.

Oguzkurt P, Tanyel FC, Hicsonmez A (1999). Vaginal atresia and Bardet-Biedl syndrome association: A component or a distinct entity? *J Pediatr Surg* 34(3): 504–506.

Patel S, Latterich M (1998). The AAA team: related ATPases with diverse functions. *Trends Cell Biol* 8: 65–71.

Riise R (1987). Visual function in Laurence-Moon-Bardet-Biedl syndrome. A survey of 26 cases. *Acta Ophthalmol Scand* 182(suppl): 128–131.

Riise R (1996). The cause of death in Laurence-Moon-Bardet-Biedl syndrome. *Acta Ophthalmol Scand* 74(suppl): 45–47.

Robinow M, Shaw A (1979). The McKusick-Kaufman syndrome: recessively inherited vaginal atresia, hydrometrocolpos, uterovaginal duplications, anorectal anomalies, postaxial polydactyly, and congenital heart disease. *J Pediatr* 94: 776–778.

Schachat AP, Maumenee IH (1982). The Bardet-Biedl syndrome and related disorders. *Arch Ophthalmol* 100: 285–288.

Sheffield VC, Carmi R, Kwitek-Black A, Rokhlina T, Nishimura D, Duyk GM, Elbedour K, Sunden SL, Stone EM (1994). Identification of a Bardet-Biedl syndrome locus on chromosome 3 and evaluation of an efficient approach to homozygosity mapping. *Hum Mol Genet* 3: 1331–1335.

Slavotinek AM, Stone EM, Mykytyn K, Heckenlively JR, Green JS, Heon E, Musarella MA, Parfrey PS, Sheffield VC, Biesecker LG (2000a). Mutations in *MKKS* cause Bardet-Biedl syndrome. *Nat Genet* 26: 15–16.

Slavotinek AM, Biesecker LG (2000b). Phenotypic overlap of McKusick-Kaufman syndrome with Bardet-Biedl syndrome: a literature review. *Am J Med Genet* 95: 208–215.

Solis-Cohen S, Weiss E (1924). Dystrophia adiposogenitalis, with atypical retinitis pigmentosa and mental deficiency, possibly of cerebral origin: a report of four cases in one family. *Trans Assoc Am Phys* 39: 356–358.

Stoler JM, Herrin JT, Holmes LB (1995). Genital abnormalities in females with Bardet-Biedl syndrome. *Am J Med Genet* 55: 276–278.

Stone DL, Slavotinek A, Bouffard GG, Banerjee-Basu S, Baxevanis AD, Barr M, Biesecker LG (2000). Mutation of a gene encoding a putative chaperonin causes McKusick-Kaufman syndrome. *Nat Genet* 25: 79–82.

Stone DL, Agarwala R, Schaffer AA, Weber JL, Vaske D, Oda T, Chandrasekharappa SC, Francomanono CA, Biesecker LG (1998). Genetic and physical mapping of the McKusick-Kaufman syndrome. *Hum Mol Genet* 7: 475–481.

Tayel SM, Al-Naggar RL, Krishna Murthy DS, Naguib KK, Al-Awadi SA (1999). Familial pericentric inversion of chromosome 1 (p36.3q23) and Bardet-Biedl syndrome. *J Med Genet* 36: 418–419.

Warkany J, Frauenberger GS, Mitchell AG (1937). Heredofamilial deviations. I. The Laurence-Moon-Biedl syndrome. *Am J Dis Child* 53: 455–470.

Woods MO, Parfrey PS, Green JS, Davidson WS (2000). Evidence for yet another novel Bardet-Biedl syndrome (BBS) locus in the Newfoundland population (abstract). *Am J Hum Genet* 67(suppl): 1730.

Young T-L, Penney L, Woods MO, Parfrey PS, Green JS, Hefferton D, Davidson WS (1999). A fifth locus for Bardet-Biedl syndrome maps to chromosome 2q31 (letter). *Am J Hum Genet* 64: 901–904.

Index

Page numbers followed by f and t indicate figures and tables, respectively.